P9-CAT-077

Goodman & Gilman's

The Pharmacological Basis of THERAPEUTICS

Notice

Goodman & Gilman's

The Pharmacological Basis of THERAPEUTICS

twelfth edition

editor

Laurence L. Brunton, PhD
Professor of Pharmacology and Medicine
School of Medicine, University of California, San Diego
La Jolla, California

associate editors

Bruce A. Chabner, MD
Professor of Medicine
Harvard Medical School
Director of Clinical Research
Massachusetts General Hospital Cancer Center
Boston, Massachusetts

Björn C. Knollmann, MD, PhD
Professor of Medicine and Pharmacology
Oates Institute for Experimental Therapeutics
Division of Clinical Pharmacology
Vanderbilt University School of Medicine
Nashville, Tennessee

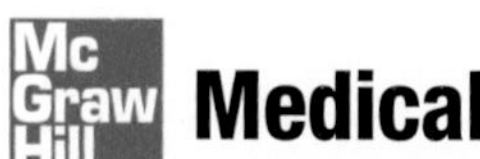

New York Chicago San Francisco Lisbon London Madrid Mexico City Milan
New Delhi San Juan Seoul Singapore Sydney Toronto

Goodman and Gilman's
The Pharmacological Basis of Therapeutics, Twelfth Edition

1 2 3 4 5 6 7 8 9 0 CTP/CTP 14 13 12 11 10

ISBN 978-0-07-162442-8
MHID 0-07-162442-2
Book ISBN 978-0-07-175352-4 Book MHID 0-07-175352-4
DVD ISBN 978-0-07-175306-7 DVD MHID 0-07-175306-0
Set ISBN 978-0-07-162442-8 Set MHID 0-07-162442-2

This book was set in Times by Glyph International.
The editors were James F. Shanahan and Christie Naglieri.
The production manager was Sherri Souffrance.
Project management was provided by Rajni Pisharody, Glyph International.
The illustration manager was Armen Ovsepyan.
The designer was Janice Bielawa.
The cover art director was Anthony Landi; the cover designer was Thomas De Pierro.
The indexer was Coughlin Indexing Services.
China Translation & Printing Services, Ltd., was printer and binder.

This book is printed on acid-free paper.

Library of Congress Cataloging-in-Publication Data

Goodman & Gilman's pharmacological basis of therapeutics.—12th ed. / editor, Laurence L. Brunton ; associate editors, Bruce A. Chabner, Björn C. Knollmann.
p. ; cm.
Other title: Goodman and Gilman's pharmacological basis of therapeutics
Other title: Pharmacological basis of therapeutics
Rev. ed. of: Goodman & Gilman's the pharmacological basis of therapeutics. 11th ed. / editor, Laurence L. Brunton. c2006.
Includes bibliographical references and index.
ISBN-13: 978-0-07-162442-8 (hardcover : alk. paper)
ISBN-10: 0-07-162442-2
1. Pharmacology. 2. Therapeutics. I. Goodman, Louis Sanford, 1906- II. Brunton, Laurence L. III. Chabner, Bruce. IV. Knollmann, Björn C. V. Goodman & Gilman's the pharmacological basis of therapeutics. VI. Title: Goodman and Gilman's pharmacological basis of therapeutics. VII. Title: Pharmacological basis of therapeutics.
[DNLM: 1. Pharmacological Phenomena. 2. Drug Therapy. QV 4 G6532 2011]
RM300.G644 2011
615'.7–dc22

2010000236

McGraw-Hill books are available at special quantity discounts to use as premiums or sales promotions, or for use in corporate training programs. To contact a representative, please email us at bulksales@mcgraw-hill.com.

In Memoriam
Keith L. Parker
(1954-2008)

Contents

SECTION III
Modulation of Cardiovascular Function 669

SECTION IV
Inflammation, Immunomodulation, and Hematopoiesis 909

SECTION V
Hormones and Hormone Antagonists 1101

SECTION VI
Drugs Affecting Gastrointestinal Function 1307

SECTION VII
Chemotherapy of Microbial Diseases 1363

Contributors

Edward P. Acosta, PharmD
Professor of Clinical Pharmacology
University of Alabama, Birmingham

Peter J. Barnes, DM, DSc, FRCP, FMedSci, FRS
Professor and Head of Respiratory Medicine
National Heart & Lung Institute
Imperial College, London

Jeffrey A. Barnes, MD, PhD
Fellow in Hematology-Oncology
Dana-Farber Cancer Institute
Boston, Massachusetts

Leslie Z. Benet, PhD
Professor of Bioengineering and Therapeutic Sciences
Schools of Pharmacy and Medicine
University of California, San Francisco

John E. Bennett, MD
Chief of Clinical Mycology
National Institute of Allergy and Infectious Diseases
Bethesda, Maryland

William Bennett, MD
Professor (Emeritus) of Medicine and Pharmacology
Oregon Health & Science University, Portland

Thomas P. Bersot, MD, PhD
Professor of Medicine; Associate Investigator
Gladstone Institute of Cardiovascular Disease
University of California, San Francisco

Joseph R. Bertino, MD
Professor of Medicine and Pharmacology
Robert Wood Johnson Medical School
University of Medicine & Dentistry of New Jersey
New Brunswick

Donald K. Blumenthal, PhD
Associate Professor of Pharmacology & Toxicology
College of Pharmacy
University of Utah, Salt Lake City

Viengngeun Bounkeua, PhD
Medical Scientist Training Program, School of Medicine
University of California, San Diego

Gregory A. Brent, MD
Professor of Medicine and Physiology
Geffen School of Medicine
University of California, Los Angeles

Joan Heller Brown, PhD
Professor and Chair of Pharmacology
University of California, San Diego

Craig N. Burkhart, MD
Assistant Professor of Dermatology, School of Medicine
University of North Carolina, Chapel Hill

Iain L. O. Buxton, PharmD
Professor of Pharmacology
University of Nevada School of Medicine, Reno

Michael C. Byrns, PhD
Fellow in Pharmacology
University of Pennsylvania School of Medicine, Philadelphia

William A. Catterall, PhD
Professor and Chair of Pharmacology
University of Washington School of Medicine, Seattle

Bruce A. Chabner, MD
Professor of Medicine, Harvard Medical School
Director of Clinical Research, Massachusetts General Hospital Cancer Center
Boston, Massachusetts

Henry F. Chambers, MD
Professor of Medicine and Chief of Infectious Diseases
San Francisco General Hospital
University of California, San Francisco

Jérôme Clain, PharmD, PhD
Research Fellow in Microbiology and Immunology
College of Physicians and Surgeons
Columbia University, New York

James M. Cleary MD, PhD
Attending Physician
Dana-Farber Cancer Institute
Boston, Massachusetts

Michael W.H. Coughtrie, PhD
Professor of Biochemical Pharmacology
Division of Medical Sciences
University of Dundee, Scotland

David D'Alessio, MD
Professor of Endocrinology and Medicine
University of Cinncinnati, Ohio

Richard T. Eastman, PhD
Fellow in Microbiology
Columbia University, New York

Ervin G. Erdös, MD
Professor (Emeritus) of Pharmacology
University of Illinois-Chicago

David A. Fidock, PhD
Associate Professor of Microbiology and Medicine
College of Physicians and Surgeons
Columbia University, New York

Garret A. FitzGerald, MD
Professor of Medicine, Pharmacology and Translational Medicine and Therapeutics;
Chair of Pharmacology
University of Pennsylvania School of Medicine, Philadelphia

Charles W. Flexner, MD
Professor of Medicine, Pharmacology and Molecular Sciences, and International Health
The Johns Hopkins University School of Medicine and Bloomberg School of Public Health
Baltimore, Maryland

Peter A. Friedman, PhD
Professor of Pharmacology and Chemical Biology School of Medicine
University of Pittsburgh, Pennsylvania

John W. Funder, AO, MD, BS, PhD, FRACP
Professor of Medicine, Prince Henry's Institute
Monash Medical Centre
ClaytonVictoria, Australia

James C. Garrison, PhD
Professor of Pharmacology, School of Medicine
University of Virginia, Charlottesville

Kathleen M. Giacomini, PhD
Professor and Chair of Biopharmaceutical Sciences School of Pharmacy
University of California, San Francisco

Alfred G. Gilman, MD, PhD
Professor (Emeritus) of Pharmacology
University of Texas Southwestern Medical School
Chief Scientific Officer, Cancer Prevention and Research Institute of Texas, Dallas

Lowell A. Goldsmith, MD, MPH
Professor of Dermatology, School of Medicine
University of North Carolina, Chapel Hill, North Carolina

Frank J. Gonzalez, PhD
Chief, Laboratory of Metabolism
Center for Cancer Research, National Cancer Institute
Bethesda, Maryland

Tilo Grosser, MD
Assistant Professor of Pharmacology
Institute for Translational Medicine and Therapeutics
University of Pennsylvania, Philadelphia

Tawanda Gumbo, MD
Associate Professor of Internal Medicine
University of Texas Southwestern Medical School, Dallas

Stephen R. Hammes, MD, PhD
Professor of Medicine, Chief of Endocrinology and Metabolism
School of Medicine and Dentistry
University of Rochester, New York

R. Adron Harris, PhD
Professor of Molecular Biology; Director, Waggoner Center for Alcohol and Addiction Research
University of Texas, Austin

Lisa A. Hazelwood, PhD
Research Fellow, Molecular Neuropharmacology Section
National Institute of Neurological Disorders and Stroke
Bethesda, Maryland

Jeffrey D. Henderer, MD
Professor and Chair of Ophthalmology
Temple University School of Medicine
Philadelphia, Pennsylvania

Ryan E. Hibbs, PhD
Research Fellow, Vollum Institute
Oregon Health & Science University, Portland

Randa Hilal-Dandan, PhD
Lecturer in Pharmacology
University of California, San Diego

Brian B. Hoffman, MD
Professor of Medicine, Harvard Medical School
Physician, VA-Boston Health Care System
Boston, Massachusetts

Peter J. Hotez, MD, PhD
Professor and Chair of Microbiology, Immunology, and Tropical Medicine
George Washington University Washington, DC

Nina Isoherranen, PhD
Assistant Professor of Pharmaceutics, School of Pharmacy
University of Washington, Seattle

Edwin K. Jackson, PhD
Professor of Pharmacology and Chemical Biology School of Medicine
University of Pittsburgh, Pennsylvania

Allen P. Kaplan, MD
Clinical Professor of Medicine
Medical University of South Carolina, Charleston

Robert S. Kass, PhD
Professor and Chair of Pharmacology Vice Dean for Research
College of Physicians and Surgeons Columbia University, New York

Kenneth Kaushansky, MD
Dean, School of Medicine and Senior Vice President of Health Sciences
SUNY Stony Brook, New York

Thomas J. Kipps, MD, PhD
Professor of Medicine, Moores Cancer Center
University of California, San Diego

Ronald J. Koenig, MD, PhD
Professor of Metabolism, Endocrinology and Diabetes
Department of Internal Medicine
University of Michigan Health System, Ann Arbor

Alan M. Krensky, MD
Senior Investigator, National Cancer Institute, Bethesda, Maryland

Nora Laiken, PhD
Lecturer in Pharmacology and Medicine
University of California, San Diego

Andrew A. Lane, MD, PhD
Fellow, Dana-Farber Cancer Institute
Massachusetts General Hospital Cancer Center, Boston

Richard J. Lee, MD, PhD
Professor of Medicine, Harvard Medical School
Physician, Massachusetts General Hospital
Boston, Massachusetts

Ellis R. Levin, MD
Professor of Medicine; Chief of Endocrinology
Diabetes and Metabolism
University of California, Irvine, and Long Beach
VA Medical Center, Long Beach

Dan L. Longo, MD
Scientific Director, National Institute on Aging
National Institutes of Health, Bethesda, Maryland

Alex Loukas, PhD
Professor of Public Health, Tropical Medicine and Rehabilitation Sciences
James Cook University, Cairns, Australia

Conan MacDougall, PharmD, MAS
Associate Professor of Clinical Pharmacy School of Pharmacy
University of California, San Francisco

Kenneth P. Mackie, MD
Professor of Neuroscience
Indiana University, Bloomington

Bradley A. Maron, MD
Fellow in Cardiovascular Medicine
Harvard Medical School and Brigham and Women's Hospital
Boston, Massachusetts

James McCarthy, MD
Associate Professor of Clinical Tropical Medicine
University of Queensland
Brisbane, Australia

James O. McNamara, MD
Professor and Chair of Neurobiology
Director of Center for Translational Neuroscience
Duke University Medical Center
Durham, North Carolina

Jonathan M. Meyer, MD
Assistant Adjunct Professor of Psychiatry
University of California, San Diego

Thomas Michel, MD, PhD
Professor of Medicine and Biochemistry
Harvard Medical School
Senior Physician in Cardiovascular Medicine
Brigham and Women's Hospital
Boston, Massachusetts

S. John Mihic, PhD
Professor of Neurobiology
Waggoner Center for Alcohol & Addiction Research
Institute for Neuroscience and Cell & Molecular Biology
University of Texas, Austin

Constantine S. Mitsiades, MD, PhD
Professor of Medical Oncology
Dana-Farber Cancer Institute, Harvard Medical School
Boston, Massachusetts

Perry Molinoff, MD
Professor of Pharmacology, School of Medicine
University of Pennsylvania, Philadelphia

Dean S. Morrell, MD
Associate Professor of Dermatology
University of North Carolina, Chapel Hill

Beverly Moy, MD, MPH
Assistant Professor of Medicine
Harvard Medical School
Massachusetts General Hospital, Needham

Hamza Mujagic, MD, MR. SCI, DR. SCI
Visiting Professor of Hematology and Oncology
Harvard Medical School
Massachusetts General Hospital, Needham

Joel W. Neal, MD, PhD
Assistant Professor of Medicine-Oncology,
Stanford University School of Medicine,
Palo Alto, California

Charles P. O'Brien, MD, PhD
Professor of Psychiatry, School of Medicine
University of Pennsylvania, Philadelphia

James O'Donnell, PhD
Professor of Behavioral Medicine and Psychiatry
School of Medicine
West Virginia University, Morgantown

Erin M. Olson, MD
Fellow in Medical Oncology
Dana-Farber Cancer Institute
Boston, Massachusetts

Taylor M. Ortiz, MD
Clinical Fellow in Medical Oncology
Dana-Farber Cancer Institute
General Hospital Cancer Center
Boston, Massachusetts

Kevin Osterhoudt, MD, MSCE, FAAP, FACMT
Associate Professor of Pediatrics
School of Medicine, University of Pennsylvania;
Medical Director, Poison Control Center, Children's Hospital
of Philadelphia, Pennsylvania

Keith L. Parker, MD, PhD (deceased)
Professor of Internal Medicine and Pharmacology
Chief of Endocrinology and Metabolism
University of Texas Southwestern Medical School, Dallas

Hemal H. Patel, PhD
Associate Professor of Anesthesiology
University of California, San Diego Dean, School of Medicine
and Senior Vice President of Health Sciences
SUNY Stony Brook, New York

Piyush M. Patel, MD, FRCPC
Professor of Anesthesiology
University of California, San Diego

Trevor M. Penning, PhD
Professor of Pharmacology
Director, Center of Excellence in Environmental Toxicology
School of Medicine
University of Pennsylvania, Philadelphia

William A. Petri, Jr, MD, PhD
Professor of Medicine; Chief, Division of Infectious Diseases
University of Virginia, Charlottesville

Margaret A. Phillips, PhD
Professor of Pharmacology
University of Texas Southwestern Medical School, Dallas

Alvin C. Powers, MD
Professor of Medicine, Molecular Physiology and Biophysics
Vanderbilt University Medical Center
Nashville, Tennessee

Christopher Rapuano, MD
Director, Cornea Service and Refractive Surgery
Department, Wills Eye Institute
Philadelphia, Pennsylvania

Robert F. Reilly, Jr, MD
Professor of Internal Medicine
University of Texas Southwestern Medical School, Dallas
Chief of Nephrology
VA-North Texas Health Care System, Dallas

Mary V. Relling, PharmD
Chair of Pharmaceutical Sciences
St. Jude Childrens' Research Hospital
Memphis, Tennessee

Paul G. Richardson, MD
Associate Professor of Medicine, Harvard Medical School
Clinical Director, Lipper Center for Multiple Myeloma
Dana-Farber Cancer Institute
Boston, Massachusetts

Suzanne M. Rivera, PhD, MSW
Assistant Professor of Clinical Sciences
University of Texas Southwestern Medical Center, Dallas

Erik Roberson, MD, PhD
Assistant Professor of Neurology and Neurobiology
University of Alabama, Birmingham

Thomas P. Rocco, MD
Associate Professor of Medicine
Harvard Medical School
VA-Boston Healthcare System
Boston, Massachusetts

David M. Roth, MD, PhD
Professor of Anesthesiology
University of California, San Diego
VA-San Diego Healthcare System

David P. Ryan, MD
Associate Professor of Medicine
Harvard Medical School
Massachusetts General Hospital Cancer Center, Boston

Kevin J. Sampson, PhD
Postdoctoral Research Scientist in Pharmacology
Columbia University, New York

Elaine Sanders-Bush, PhD
Professor (Emerita) of Pharmacology
School of Medicine, Vanderbilt University
Nashville, Tennessee

Bernard P. Schimmer, PhD
Professor (Emeritus) of Medical Research and Pharmacology
University of Toronto, Ontario

Marc A. Schuckit, MD
Distinguished Professor of Psychiatry
University of California, San Diego
Director, Alcohol Research Center
VA-San Diego Healthcare System

Lecia Sequist, MD, MPH
Assistant Professor of Medicine
Harvard Medical School, Massachusetts General Hospital Cancer Center, Boston

Keith A. Sharkey, PhD
Professor of Physiology & Pharmacology and Medicine
University of Calgary, Alberta

Richard C. Shelton, MD
Professor of Psychiatry and Pharmacology
School of Medicine, Vanderbilt University
Nashville, Tennessee

Danny Shen, PhD
Professor and Chair of Pharmacy
Professor of Pharmaceutics, School of Pharmacy
University of Washington, Seattle

Randal A. Skidgel, PhD
Professor of Pharmacology and Anesthesiology
College of Medicine, University of Illinois-Chicago

Matthew R. Smith, MD, PhD
Associate Professor of Medicine, Harvard Medical School
Physician, Massachusetts General Hospital, Boston

Emer M. Smyth, PhD
Research Assistant, Professor of Pharmacology
University of Pennsylvania, Philadelphia

Peter J. Snyder, MD
Professor of Medicine
University of Pennsylvania, Philadelphia

David Standaert, MD, PhD
Professor of Neurology
Director, Center for Neurodegeneration and Experimental Therapeutics
University of Alabama, Birmingham

Samuel L. Stanley, Jr, MD
Professor of Medicine and President
SUNY Stony Brook, New York

Yuichi Sugiyama, PhD
Professor and Chair of Molecular Pharmacokinetics
University of Tokyo, Japan

Jeffrey G. Supko, PhD
Associate Professor of Medicine, Harvard Medical School
Massachusetts General Hospital, Boston

Palmer W. Taylor, PhD
Professor of Pharmacology, School of Medicine
Dean, Skaggs School of Pharmacy and Pharmaceutical Sciences
University of California, San Diego

Kenneth E. Thummel, PhD
Professor and Chair, Department of Pharmaceutics
University of Washington, Seattle

Robert H. Tukey, PhD
Professor of Pharmacology and Chemistry/Biochemistry
University of California, San Diego

Flavio Vincenti, MD
Professor of Clinical Medicine
Medical Director, Pancreas Transplant Program
University of California, San Francisco

Joseph M. Vinetz, MD
Professor of Medicine, Division of Infectious Diseases
University of California, San Diego

Mark S. Wallace, MD
Professor of Clinical Anesthesiology
University of California, San Diego

John L. Wallace, PhD, MBA, FRSC
Professor and Director, Farncombe Family Digestive Health Research Institute
McMaster University, Hamilton, Ontario

Jeffrey I. Weitz, MD, FRCP(C), FACP
Professor of Medicine, Biochemistry and Biomedical Sciences McMaster University
Executive Director, Thrombosis & Atherosclerosis
Research Institute, Hamilton, Ontario

David P. Westfall, PhD
Professor (Emeritus) of Pharmacology
University of Nevada School of Medicine, Reno

Thomas C. Westfall, PhD
Professor and Chair of Pharmacological and Physiological Science
St. Louis University School of Medicine, Missouri

Wyndham Wilson, MD, PhD
Senior Investigator and Chief of Lymphoid Therapeutics Section,
Center for Cancer Research, National Cancer Institute
Bethesda Maryland

Tony L. Yaksh, PhD
Professor of Anesthesiology and Pharmacology
University of California, San Diego

Alexander C. Zambon, PhD
Assistant Professor of Pharmacology
University of California, San Diego

Preface

The publication of the twelfth edition of this book is a testament to the vision and ideals of the original authors, Alfred Gilman and Louis Goodman, who, in 1941 set forth the principles that have guided the book through eleven editions: to correlate pharmacology with related medical sciences, to reinterpret the actions and uses of drugs in light of advances in medicine and the basic biomedical sciences, to emphasize the applications of pharmacodynamics to therapeutics, and to create a book that will be useful to students of pharmacology and to physicians. These precepts continue to guide the current edition.

As with editions since the second, expert scholars have contributed individual chapters. A multiauthored book of this sort grows by accretion, posing challenges to editors but also offering memorable pearls to the reader. Thus, portions of prior editions persist in the current edition, and I hasten to acknowledge the contributions of previous editors and authors, many of whom will see text that looks familiar. However, this edition differs noticeably from its immediate predecessors. Fifty new scientists, including a number from outside the U.S., have joined as contributors, and all chapters have been extensively updated. The focus on basic principles continues, with new chapters on drug invention, molecular mechanisms of drug action, drug toxicity and poisoning, principles of antimicrobial therapy, and pharmacotherapy of obstetrical and gynecological disorders. Figures are in full color. The editors have continued to standardize the organization of chapters; thus, students should easily find the basic physiology, biochemistry, and pharmacology set forth in regular type; bullet points highlight important lists within the text; the clinician and expert will find details in extract type under clear headings.

Online features now supplement the printed edition. The entire text, updates, reviews of newly approved drugs, animations of drug action, and hyperlinks to relevant text in the prior edition are available on the Goodman & Gilman section of McGraw-Hill's websites, *AccessMedicine.com* and *AccessPharmacy.com*. An Image Bank CD accompanies the book and makes all tables and figures available for use in presentations.

The process of editing brings into view many remarkable facts, theories, and realizations. Three stand out: the invention of new classes of drugs has slowed to a trickle; therapeutics has barely begun to capitalize on the information from the human genome project; and, the development of resistance to antimicrobial agents, mainly through their overuse in medicine and agriculture, threatens to return us to the pre-antibiotic era. We have the capacity and ingenuity to correct these shortcomings.

Many, in addition to the contributors, deserve thanks for their work on this edition; they are acknowledged on an accompanying page. In addition, I am grateful to Professors Bruce Chabner (Harvard Medical School/Massachusetts General Hospital) and Björn Knollmann (Vanderbilt University Medical School) for agreeing to be associate editors of this edition at a late date, necessitated by the death of my colleague and friend Keith Parker in late 2008. Keith and I worked together on the eleventh edition and on planning this edition. In anticipation of the editorial work ahead, Keith submitted his chapters before anyone else and just a few weeks before his death; thus, he is well represented in this volume, which we dedicate to his memory.

Laurence L. Brunton
San Diego, California
December 1, 2010

Preface to the First Edition

Three objectives have guided the writing of this book—the correlation of pharmacology with related medical sciences, the reinterpretation of the actions and uses of drugs from the viewpoint of important advances in medicine, and the placing of emphasis on the applications of pharmacodynamics to therapeutics.

Although pharmacology is a basic medical science in its own right, it borrows freely from and contributes generously to the subject matter and technics of many medical disciplines, clinical as well as preclinical. Therefore, the correlation of strictly pharmacological information with medicine as a whole is essential for a proper presentation of pharmacology to students and physicians. Further more, the reinterpretation of the actions and uses of well-established therapeutic agents in the light of recent advances in the medical sciences is as important a function of a modern text book of pharmacology as is the description of new drugs. In many instances these new interpretations necessitate radical departures from accepted but outworn concepts of the actions of drugs. Lastly, the emphasis throughout the book, as indicated in its title, has been clinical. This is mandatory because medical students must be taught pharmacology from the standpoint of the actions and uses of drugs in the prevention and treatment of disease. To the student, pharmacological data per se are value less unless he/she is able to apply this information in the practice of medicine. This book has also been written for the practicing physician, to whom it offers an opportunity to keep abreast of recent advances in therapeutics and to acquire the basic principles necessary for the rational use of drugs in his/her daily practice.

The criteria for the selection of bibliographic references require comment. It is obviously unwise, if not impossible, to document every fact included in the text. Preference has therefore been given to articles of a review nature, to the literature on new drugs, and to original contributions in controversial fields. In most instances, only the more recent investigations have been cited. In order to encourage free use of the bibliography, references are chiefly to the available literature in the English language.

The authors are greatly indebted to their many colleagues at the Yale University School of Medicine for their generous help and criticism. In particular they are deeply grateful to Professor Henry Gray Barbour, whose constant encouragement and advice have been invaluable.

Louis S. Goodman
Alfred Gilman
New Haven, Connecticut
November 20, 1940

Acknowledgments

The editors appreciate the assistance of:

John E. Bennett, MD
Chief of Clinical Mycology
National Institute of Allergy and Infectious Diseases

Nancy J. Brown, MD
Professor and Chair of Medicine
Professor of Pharmacology
Vanderbilt University School of Medicine

Laura Collins
Editorial Assistant
Massachusetts General Hospital

Randa Hilal-Dandan, PhD
Lecturer in Pharmacology
University of California, San Diego

Renée Johnson
Executive Assistant
Massachusetts General Hospital

Laura Libretti
Administrative Assistant
McGraw-Hill

Nelda Murri, PharmD, MBA
Consulting Pharmacist

Christie Naglieri
Senior Project Development Editor
McGraw-Hill

Rajni Pisharody
Senior Project Manager
Glyph International

L. Jackson Roberts II, MD
Professor of Pharmacology and Medicine
Vanderbilt University School of Medicine

Sherri Souffrance
Senior Production Supervisor
McGraw-Hill

Cynthia E. Stalmaster, MS, MPH
Editorial Assistant
University of California, San Diego

James F. Shanahan
Editor-in-Chief, Internal Medicine
McGraw-Hill

Russell A. Wilke, MD, PhD
Associate Professor of Medicine
Director, Genomics and Cardiovascular Risk Reduction
Vanderbilt University School of Medicine

Bobbi Sherg, Mike Vonderkret
FedEx Office RBLCE, San Diego, CA

Section I

General Principles

Drug Invention and the Pharmaceutical Industry

Suzanne M. Rivera and
Alfred Goodman Gilman*

The first edition of this textbook, published in 1941, is often credited with organizing the field of pharmacology, giving it intellectual validity and an academic identity. That first edition began: "The subject of pharmacology is a broad one and embraces the knowledge of the source, physical and chemical properties, compounding, physiological actions, absorption, fate, and excretion, and therapeutic uses of drugs. A *drug* may be broadly defined as any chemical agent that affects living protoplasm, and few substances would escape inclusion by this definition." These two sentences still serve us well. This first section of the 12th edition of this textbook provides the underpinnings for these definitions by exploring the processes of drug invention and development into a therapeutic entity, followed by the basic properties of the interactions between the drug and biological systems: *pharmacodynamics*, *pharmacokinetics* (including drug transport and metabolism), and *pharmacogenomics*. Subsequent sections deal with the use of drugs as therapeutic agents in human subjects.

We intentionally use the term *invention* to describe the process by which a new drug is identified and brought to medical practice, rather than the more conventional term *discovery*. This significant semantic change was suggested to us by our colleague Michael S. Brown, MD, and it is appropriate. In the past, drugs were discovered as natural products and used as such. Today, useful drugs are rarely discovered hiding somewhere waiting to be found; rather, they are sculpted and brought into being based on experimentation and optimization of many independent properties. The term *invention* emphasizes this process; there is little serendipity.

*Alfred G. Gilman serves on the Board of Directors of Eli Lilly & Co. and Regeneron Pharmaceuticals, and acknowledges potential conflicts of interests.

FROM EARLY EXPERIENCES WITH PLANTS TO MODERN CHEMISTRY

Man's fascination—and sometimes infatuation—with chemicals (i.e., drugs) that alter biological function is ancient and arose as a result of experience with and dependence on plants. Most plants are root-bound, and many have become capable of elaborate chemical syntheses, producing harmful compounds for defense that animals learned to avoid and man learned to exploit. Many examples are described in earlier editions of this text: the appreciation of coffee (caffeine) by the prior of an Arabian convent who noted the behavior of goats that gamboled and frisked through the night after eating the berries of the coffee plant, the use of mushrooms or the deadly nightshade plant (containing the belladonna alkaloids atropine and scopolamine) by professional poisoners, and a rather different use of belladonna ("beautiful lady") to dilate pupils. Other examples include the uses of the Chinese herb ma huang (containing ephedrine) for over 5000 years as a circulatory stimulant, curare-containing arrow poisons used for centuries by South American Indians to paralyze and kill animals hunted for food, and poppy juice (opium) containing morphine (from the Greek Morpheus, the god of dreams) for pain relief and control of dysenteries. Morphine, of course, has well-known addicting properties, mimicked in some ways by other problematic ("recreational") natural products—nicotine, cocaine, and ethanol.

While many terrestrial and marine organisms remain valuable sources of naturally occurring compounds with various pharmacological activities, especially including lethal effects on both microorganisms and eukaryotic cells, drug invention became more allied with synthetic organic chemistry as that discipline flourished over the past 150 years. This revolution began in the dye industry. Dyes, by definition, are colored compounds with selective affinity for biological tissues. Study of these interactions stimulated Paul Ehrlich to postulate the existence of chemical receptors in tissues that interacted with and "fixed" the dyes. Similarly, Ehrlich thought that unique receptors on microorganisms or parasites might react specifically with certain dyes and that such selectivity could spare normal tissue. Ehrlich's work culminated in the invention of arsphenamine in 1907, which was patented as "salvarsan," suggestive of the hope that the chemical would be the salvation of humankind. This arsenic-containing compound and other organic arsenicals were invaluable for the chemotherapy of syphilis until the discovery of penicillin. During that period and thanks to the work of Gerhard Domagk, another dye, prontosil (the first clinically useful sulfonamide) was shown to be dramatically effective in treating streptococcal infections. The era of antimicrobial chemotherapy was born, and the fascination with dyes soon spread to the entire and nearly infinite spectrum of organic chemicals. The resulting collaboration of pharmacology with chemistry on the one hand, and with clinical medicine on the other, has been a major contributor to the effective treatment of disease, especially since the middle of the 20th century.

SOURCES OF DRUGS

Small Molecules Are the Tradition

With the exception of a few naturally occurring hormones such as insulin, most drugs were small organic molecules (typically <500 Da) until recombinant DNA technology permitted synthesis of proteins by various organisms (bacteria, yeast) and mammalian cells, starting in the 1980s. The usual approach to invention of a small-molecule drug is to screen a collection of chemicals ("library") for compounds with the desired features. An alternative is to synthesize and focus on close chemical relatives of a substance known to participate in a biological reaction of interest (e.g., congeners of a specific enzyme substrate chosen to be possible inhibitors of the enzymatic reaction), a particularly important strategy in the discovery of anticancer drugs.

While drug discovery in the past often resulted from serendipitous observations of the effects of plant extracts or individual chemicals administered to animals or ingested by man, the approach today relies on high-throughput screening of libraries containing hundreds of thousands or even millions of compounds for their ability to interact with a specific molecular target or elicit a specific biological response (see "Targets of Drug Action" later in the chapter). Chemical libraries are synthesized using modern organic chemical synthetic approaches such as combinatorial chemistry to create large collections of related chemicals, which can then be screened for activity in high-throughput systems. Diversity-oriented synthetic approaches also are of obvious value, while natural products (plant or marine animal collections) are sources of novel and sometimes exceedingly complex chemical structures.

Automated screening procedures employing robotic systems can process hundreds of thousands of samples in just a few days. Reactions are carried out in small trays containing a matrix of tiny wells (typically 384 or 1536). Assay reagents and samples to be tested are coated onto plates or distributed by robots, using ink-jet technology. Tiny volumes are used and chemical samples are thus conserved. The assay must be sensitive, specific, and designed to yield a readily detectable signal, usually a change in absorption or emission of light (fluorescence, luminescence, phosphorescence) or alteration of a radioactive substrate. The signal may result from the interaction of a candidate chemical with a specific protein target, such as an enzyme or a biological receptor protein that one hopes to inhibit or activate with a drug. Alternatively, cell-based high-throughput screens may be performed. For example, a cell may be engineered to emit a fluorescent signal when Ca^{2+} fluxes into the cell as a result of a ligand-receptor interaction. Cellular engineering is accomplished by transfecting the necessary genes into the cell, enabling it to perform the functions of interest. It is of enormous value that the specific protein target in an assay or the molecules used to engineer a cell for a high-throughput screen are of human origin, obtained by transcription and translation of the cloned human gene. The potential drugs that are identified in the screen ("hits") are thus known to react with the human protein and not just with its relative (ortholog) obtained from mouse or another species.

Several variables affect the frequency of hits obtained in a screen. Among the most important are the "drugability" of the target and the stringency of the screen in terms of the concentrations of compounds that are tested. The slang term "drugability" refers to the ease with which the function of a target can be altered in the desired fashion by a small organic molecule. If the protein target has a well-defined binding site for a small molecule (e.g., a catalytic or allosteric site), chances are excellent that hits will be obtained. If the goal is to employ a small molecule to mimic or disrupt the interaction between two proteins, the challenge is much greater.

From Hits to Leads

Only rarely do any of the initial hits in a screen turn out to be marketable drugs. Initial hits often have modest affinity for the target, and lack the desired specificity and pharmacological properties of a successful pharmaceutical. Skilled medicinal chemists synthesize derivatives of the hits, making substitutions at accessible positions, and begin in this way to define the relationship between chemical structure and biological activity. Many parameters may require optimization, including affinity for the target, agonist/antagonist activity, permeability across cell membranes, absorption and distribution in the body, metabolism of the drug, and unwanted effects. While this approach was driven largely by instinct and trial and error in the past, modern drug development frequently takes advantage of determination of a high-resolution structure of the putative drug bound to its target. X-ray crystallography offers the most detailed structural information if the target protein can be crystallized with the lead drug bound to it. Using techniques of molecular modeling and computational chemistry, the structure provides the chemist with information about substitutions likely to improve the "fit" of the drug with the target and thus enhance the affinity of the drug for its target (and, hopefully, optimize selectivity of the drug simultaneously). Nuclear magnetic resonance (NMR) spectroscopy is another valuable technique for learning the structure of a drug-receptor complex. NMR studies are done in solution, with the advantage that the complex need not be crystallized. However, the structures obtained by NMR spectroscopy usually are not as precise as those from X-ray crystallography, and the protein target must not be larger than roughly 35–40 kDa.

The holy grail of this approach to drug invention will be to achieve success entirely through computation. Imagine a database containing detailed chemical information about millions of chemicals and a second database containing detailed structural information about all human proteins. The computational approach is to "roll" all the chemicals over the protein of interest to find those with high-affinity interactions. The dream gets bolder if we acquire the ability to roll the chemicals that bind to the target of interest over all other human proteins to discard compounds that have unwanted interactions. Finally, we also will want to predict the structural and functional consequences of a drug binding to its target (a huge challenge), as well as all relevant pharmacokinetic properties of the molecules of interest. We are a long way from realization of this fabulous dream; however, we are sufficiently advanced to imagine it and realize that it could someday be a reality. Indeed, computational approaches have suggested new uses for old drugs and offered explanations for recent failures of drugs in the later stages of clinical development (e.g., torcetrapib; see below) (Kim et al., 2010; Kinnings et al., 2009; Xie et al., 2007, 2009).

Large Molecules Are Increasingly Important

Protein therapeutics were uncommon before the advent of recombinant DNA technology. Insulin was introduced into clinical medicine for the treatment of diabetes following the experiments of Banting and Best in 1921. Insulin could be produced in great quantities by purification from porcine or bovine pancreas obtained from slaughter houses. These insulins are active in man, although antibodies to the foreign proteins are occasionally problematic.

Growth hormone, used to treat pituitary dwarfism, is a case of more stringent species specificity: only the human hormone could be used after purification from pituitary glands harvested during autopsy. The danger of this approach was highlighted when patients who had received the human hormone developed Creutzfeldt-Jakob disease (the human equivalent of mad cow disease), a fatal degenerative neurological disease caused by prion proteins that contaminated the drug preparation. Thanks to gene cloning and the ability to produce large quantities of proteins by expressing the cloned gene in bacteria or eukaryotic cells grown in enormous (30,000-liter) bioreactors, protein therapeutics now utilize highly purified preparations of human (or humanized) proteins. Rare proteins can now be produced in quantity, and immunological reactions are minimized. Proteins can be designed, customized, and optimized using genetic engineering techniques. Other types of macromolecules may also be used therapeutically. For example, antisense oligonucleotides are used to block gene transcription or translation, as are small interfering RNAs (siRNAs).

Proteins utilized therapeutically include various hormones, growth factors (e.g., erythropoietin, granulocyte-colony stimulating factor), and cytokines, as well as a rapidly increasing number of monoclonal antibodies now widely used in the treatment of cancer and autoimmune diseases. Murine monoclonal antibodies can be "humanized" (by substituting human for mouse amino acid sequences). Alternatively, mice have now been "engineered" by replacement of critical mouse genes with their human equivalents, such that they make completely human antibodies. Protein therapeutics are administered parenterally, and their receptors or targets must be accessible extracellularly.

The earliest drugs came from observation of the effects of plants after their ingestion by animals. One could observe at least some of the effects of the chemical(s) in the plant and, as a side benefit, know that the plant extract was active when taken orally. Valuable drugs were discovered with no knowledge of their mechanism or site of action. While this approach is still useful (e.g., in screening for the ability of natural products to kill microorganisms or malignant cells), modern drug invention usually takes the opposite approach—starting with a statement (or hypothesis) that a certain protein or pathway plays a critical role in the pathogenesis of a certain disease, and that altering the protein's activity would therefore be effective against that disease. Crucial questions arise:

- can one find a drug that will have the desired effect against its target?
- does modulation of the target protein affect the course of disease?
- does this project make sense economically?

The effort that may be expended to find the desired drug will be determined by the degree of confidence in the answers to the latter two questions.

Is the Target "Drugable"?

The drugability of a target with a low-molecular-weight organic molecule relies on the presence of a binding site for the drug that can be approached with considerable affinity and selectivity. If the target is an enzyme or a receptor for a small ligand, one is encouraged. If the target is related to another protein that is known to have, for example, a binding site for a regulatory ligand, one is hopeful. However, if the known ligands are large peptides or proteins with an extensive set of contacts with their receptor, the challenge is much greater. If the goal is to disrupt interactions between two proteins, it may be necessary to find a "hot spot" that is crucial for the protein-protein interaction, and such a region may not be detected. Accessibility of the drug to its target also is critical. Extracellular targets are intrinsically easier to approach and, in general, only extracellular targets are accessible to macromolecular drugs.

Has the Target Been Validated?

This question is obviously a critical one. A negative answer, frequently obtained only retrospectively, is a common cause of failure in drug invention. Based on extensive study of a given biological process, one may believe that protein X plays a critical role in pathological alterations of that process. However, biological systems frequently contain redundant elements, and they are adaptable. When the activity of protein X is, e.g., inhibited by a drug, redundancy in the system may permit compensation. The system also may adapt to the presence of the drug, perhaps by regulating the expression of the target or of functionally related gene products. In general, the more important the function, the greater the complexity of the system. For example, many mechanisms control feeding and appetite, and drugs to control obesity have been notoriously difficult to find. The discovery of the hormone leptin, which suppresses appetite, was based on mutations in mice that cause loss of either leptin or its receptor; either kind of mutation results in enormous obesity in both mice and people. Leptin thus appeared to be a marvelous opportunity to treat obesity. However, obese individuals have high circulating concentrations of leptin and appear quite insensitive to its action.

Modern techniques of molecular biology offer new and powerful tools for validation of potential drug targets, to the extent that the biology of model systems resembles human biology. Genes can be inserted, disrupted, and altered in mice. One can thereby create models of disease in animals or mimic the effects of long-term disruption or activation of a given biological process. If, for example, disruption of the gene encoding a specific enzyme or receptor has a beneficial effect in a valid murine model of a human disease, one may believe that the potential drug target has been validated. Mutations in humans also can provide extraordinarily valuable information. For example, loss-of-function mutations in the PCSK9 gene (encoding proprotein convertase subtilisin/kexin type 9) greatly lower concentrations of LDL cholesterol in plasma and reduce the risk of myocardial infarction (Horton et al., 2009). This single powerful observation speaks to a well-validated drug target. Based on these findings, many drug companies are actively seeking inhibitors of PCSK9 function.

Is This Drug Invention Effort Economically Viable?

Drug invention and development is extraordinarily expensive, as discussed later in the chapter. Economic realities influence the direction of science. For example, investor-owned companies generally cannot afford to develop products for rare diseases or for diseases that are common only in economically underdeveloped parts of the world. Funds to invent drugs targeting rare diseases or diseases primarily affecting developing countries (especially parasitic diseases) can come from taxpayers or very wealthy philanthropists; such funds generally will not come from private investors involved in running for-profit companies.

ADDITIONAL PRECLINICAL RESEARCH

Following the path just described can yield a potential drug molecule that interacts with a validated target and alters its function in the desired fashion (either enhancing or inhibiting the functions of the target). Now one must consider all aspects of the molecule in question—its affinity and selectivity for interaction with the target, its pharmacokinetic properties (absorption, distribution, excretion, metabolism), issues with regard to its large-scale synthesis or purification from a natural source, its pharmaceutical properties (stability, solubility, questions of formulation), and its safety. One hopes to correct, to the extent possible, any obvious deficiencies by modification of the molecule itself or by changes in the way the molecule is presented for use.

Before being administered to people, potential drugs are tested for general toxicity by monitoring the activity of various systems in two species of animals for extended periods of time. Compounds also are evaluated for carcinogenicity, genotoxicity, and reproductive toxicity. Animals are used for much of this testing, although the predictive value of results obtained in non-human species is certainly not perfect. Usually one rodent (usually mouse) and one non-rodent (often rabbit) species are used. *In vitro* and *ex vivo* assays are utilized when possible, both to spare animals and to minimize cost. If an unwanted effect is observed, an obvious question is whether it is mechanism-based (i.e., caused by interaction of the drug with its intended target) or due to an off-target effect of the drug. If the latter, there is hope of minimizing the effect by further optimization of the molecule.

Before clinical trials of a potential new drug may proceed in the U.S. (that is, before the drug candidate can be administered to a human subject), the sponsor must file an IND (Investigational New Drug) application, which is a request to the U.S. Food and Drug Administration (FDA; see the next section) for permission to administer the drug to human test subjects. The IND describes the rationale and preliminary evidence for efficacy in experimental systems, as well as pharmacology, toxicology, chemistry, manufacturing, and so forth. It also describes the plan for investigating the drug in human subjects. The FDA has 30 days to review the application, by which time the agency may disapprove the application, ask for more data, or allow initial clinical testing to proceed. In the absence of an objection or request for more information within 30 days by the FDA, a clinical trial may begin.

CLINICAL TRIALS AND THE ROLE OF THE FDA

The FDA is a regulatory agency within the U.S. Department of Health and Human Services. As its mission statement indicates, the FDA:

> is responsible for protecting the public health by assuring the safety, efficacy, and security of human and veterinary drugs, biological products, medical devices, our nation's food supply, cosmetics, and products that emit radiation. The FDA is also responsible for advancing the public health by helping to speed innovations that make medicines and foods more effective, safer, and more affordable; and helping the public get the accurate, science-based information they need to use medicines and foods to improve their health (FDA, 2009).

The first drug-related legislation in the U.S., the Federal Food and Drug Act of 1906, was concerned only with the interstate transport of adulterated or misbranded foods and drugs. There were no obligations to establish drug efficacy or safety. This act was amended in 1938, after the deaths of 105 children from "elixir sulfanilamide," a solution of sulfanilamide in diethylene glycol, an excellent but highly toxic solvent and an ingredient in antifreeze. The enforcement of the amended act was entrusted to the FDA. Toxicity studies as well as approval of a New Drug Application (NDA; see the next section) were required before a drug could be promoted and distributed. Although a new drug's safety had to be demonstrated, no proof of efficacy was required. In the 1960s, thalidomide, a hypnotic drug with no obvious advantages over others, was introduced in Europe. Epidemiological research eventually established that this drug, taken early in pregnancy, was responsible for an epidemic of a relatively rare and severe birth defect, phocomelia. In reaction to this catastrophe, the U.S. Congress passed the Harris-Kefauver amendments to the Food, Drug, and Cosmetic Act in 1962. These amendments established the requirement for proof of efficacy as well of documentation of relative safety in terms of the risk-to-benefit ratio for the disease entity to be treated (the more serious the disease, the greater the acceptable risk).

One of the agency's primary responsibilities is to protect the public from harmful medications. However, the FDA clearly faces an enormous challenge, especially in view of the widely held belief that its mission cannot possibly be accomplished with the available resources. Moreover, harm from drugs that cause unanticipated adverse effects is not the only risk of an imperfect system; harm also occurs when the approval process delays the marketing of a new drug with important beneficial effects. Determining safety and efficacy prior to mass marketing requires careful consideration.

The Conduct of Clinical Trials

Clinical trials (as applied to drugs) are investigations in human subjects intended to acquire information about the pharmacokinetic and pharmacodynamic properties of a potential drug. Depending on the nature and phase of the trial, it may be designed to evaluate a drug's safety, its efficacy for treatment or prevention of specific conditions in patients, and its tolerability and side effects. Efficacy must be proven and an adequate margin of safety established for a drug to be approved for sale in the U.S. The U.S. National Institutes of Health notes seven ethical requirements that must be met before a clinical trial can begin. These include social value, scientific validity, fair and objective selection of subjects, informed consent, favorable ratio of risks to benefits, approval and oversight by an independent review board (IRB), and respect for human subjects.

FDA-regulated clinical trials typically are conducted in four phases. The first three are designed to establish safety and efficacy, while Phase IV post-marketing trials delineate additional information regarding new indications, risks, and optimal doses and schedules. Table 1–1 and Figure 1–1 summarize the important features of each phase of clinical trials, especially the attrition at each successive stage over a relatively long and costly process.

When initial Phase III trials are complete, the sponsor (usually a pharmaceutical company) applies to the FDA for approval to market the drug; this application is called either a New Drug Application (NDA) or a Biologics License Application (BLA). These applications contain comprehensive information, including individual case-report forms from the hundreds or thousands of individuals who have received the drug during its Phase III testing. Applications are reviewed by teams of specialists, and the FDA may call on the help of panels of external experts in complex cases. The use of such external advisory committees greatly expands the

Table 1–1

Typical Characteristics of the Various Phases of the Clinical Trials Required for Marketing of New Drugs.

PHASE I First in Human	PHASE II First in Patient	PHASE III Multi-Site Trial	PHASE IV Post-Marketing Surveillance
10-100 participants	50-500 participants	A few hundred to a few thousand participants	Many thousands of participants
Usually healthy volunteers; occasionally patients with advanced or rare disease	Patient-subjects receiving experimental drug	Patient-subjects receiving experimental drug	Patients in treatment with approved drug
Open label	Randomized and controlled (can be placebo-controlled); may be blinded	Randomized and controlled (can be placebo-controlled) or uncontrolled; may be blinded	Open label
Safety and tolerability	Efficacy and dose ranging	Confirm efficacy in larger population	Adverse events, compliance, drug-drug interactions
Months to 1 year	1-2 years	3-5 years	No fixed duration
U.S. $10 million	US $20 million	US $50-100 million	—
Success rate: 50%	Success rate: 30%	Success rate: 25-50%	—

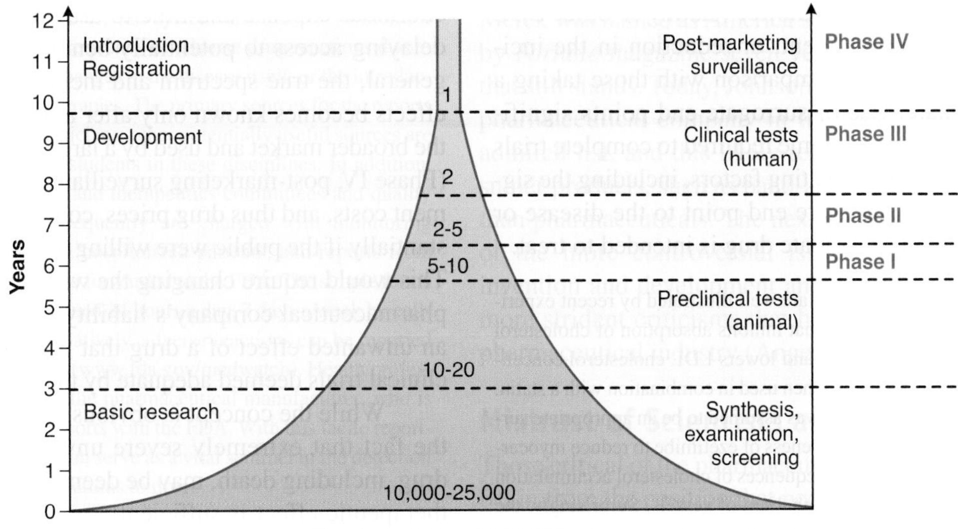

Figure 1–1. *The phases, time lines, and attrition that characterize the invention of new drugs.* See also Table 1–1.

talent pool available to assist in making important and difficult decisions.

Under the provisions of the Prescription Drug User Fee Act (PDUFA, enacted initially in 1992 and renewed in 2007), pharmaceutical companies now provide a significant portion of the FDA budget via user fees, a legislative effort to expedite the drug approval review process. PDUFA also broadened the FDA's drug safety program and increased resources for review of television drug advertising. The larger FDA staffing now in place has shortened the time required for review; nevertheless, the process is a lengthy one. A 1-year review time is considered standard, and 6 months is the target if the drug candidate is granted priority status because of its importance in filling an unmet need. Unfortunately, these targets are not always met.

Before a drug is approved for marketing, the company and the FDA must agree on the content of the "label" (package insert)—the official prescribing information. This label describes the approved indications for use of the drug and clinical pharmacological information including dosage, adverse reactions, and special warnings and precautions (sometimes posted in a "black box"). Promotional materials used by pharmaceutical companies cannot deviate from information contained in the package insert. Importantly, the physician is not bound by the package insert; a physician in the U.S. *may* legally prescribe a drug for any purpose that she or he deems reasonable. However, third-party payers (insurance companies, Medicare, and so on) generally will not reimburse a patient for the cost of a drug used for an "off-label" indication unless the new use is supported by one of several compendia such as the U.S. Pharmacopeia. Furthermore, a physician may be vulnerable to litigation if untoward effects result from an unapproved use of a drug.

Determining "Safe" and "Effective"

To demonstrate efficacy to the FDA requires performing "adequate and well-controlled investigations," generally interpreted to mean two replicate clinical trials that are usually, but not always, randomized, double-blind, and placebo-controlled. Is a placebo the proper control? The World Medical Association's *Declaration of Helsinki* (2000) discourages use of placebo controls when an alternative treatment is available for comparison. What must be measured in the trials? In a straightforward trial, a readily quantifiable parameter (a secondary or surrogate end point), thought to be predictive of relevant clinical outcomes, is measured in matched drug- and placebo-treated groups. Examples of surrogate end points include LDL cholesterol as a predictor of myocardial infarction, bone mineral density as a predictor of fractures, or hemoglobin A_{1c} as a predictor of the complications of diabetes mellitus. More stringent trials would require demonstration of reduction of the incidence of myocardial infarction in patients taking a candidate drug in comparison with those taking an

it to market as therapeutic agents. Consequently, drugs must be priced to recover the substantial costs of invention and development, and to fund the marketing efforts needed to introduce new products to physicians and patients. Nevertheless, as U.S. healthcare spending continues to rise at an alarming pace, prescription drugs account for only ~10% of total healthcare expenditures (Kaiser Family Foundation, 2009), and a significant fraction of this drug cost is for low-priced nonproprietary medicines. Although the increase in prices is significant in certain classes of drugs (e.g., anticancer agents), the total price of prescription drugs is growing at a slower rate than other healthcare costs. Even drastic reductions in drug prices that would severely limit new drug invention would not lower the overall healthcare budget by more than a few percent.

Are profit margins excessive among the major pharmaceutical companies? There is no objective answer to this question. Pragmatic answers come from the markets and from company survival statistics. A free-market system says that rewards should be greater for particularly risky fields of endeavor, and the rewards should be greater for those willing to take the risk. The pharmaceutical industry is clearly one of the more risky. The costs to bring products to market are enormous; the success rate is low (accounting for much of the cost); effective patent protection is only about a decade (see "Intellectual Property and Patents" later in the chapter), requiring every company to completely reinvent itself on a roughly 10-year cycle (about equal to the lifespan of a CEO or an executive vice president for research and development); regulation is stringent; product liability is great even after an approved product has reached the market; competition is fierce.

The ratio of the price of a company's stock to its annual earnings per share of stock is called the price-to-earnings ratio (P/E) and is a measure of the stock market's predictions about a company's prospects. A decade ago, pharmaceutical companies' stocks on average were priced at a 20% premium to the market; today they sell at a 34% discount; this is a dramatic change. A decade or two ago, the pharmaceutical industry was incredibly fragmented, with the biggest players commanding only very modest shares of the total market. Mergers and acquisitions continue to narrow the field. For example, Hoechst AG, Roussel Uclaf, and Marion Merrell Dow plus Rhone-Poulenc became Aventis, which then merged with Sanofi-Synthélabo to become Sanofi-Aventis. The giant Pfizer represents the consolidation of Warner Lambert, Park Davis, Searle, Monsanto, Pharmacia, Upjohn, and Agouron, among others. Pfizer's acquisition of Wyeth is currently pending; Wyeth is the result of the consolidation of American Home Products, American Cyanamid, Ayerst, A. H. Robbins, Ives Laboratories, and Genetics Institute. The pharmaceutical world is shrinking.

Who Pays?

Healthcare in the U.S. is funded by a mix of private payers and government programs. Correspondingly, the cost of prescription drugs is borne by consumers ("out-of-pocket"), private insurers, and public insurance programs like Medicare, Medicaid, and the State Children's Health Insurance Program (SCHIP). Recent initiatives by major retailers and mail-order pharmacies run by private insurers to offer consumer incentives for purchase of generic drugs have helped to contain the portion of household expenses spent on pharmaceuticals; however, more than one-third of total retail drug costs in the U.S. are paid with public funds—tax dollars.

Healthcare in the U.S. is more expensive than everywhere else, but it is not, on average, demonstrably better than everywhere else. However, the U.S. is considerably more socio-economically diverse than many of the countries with which comparisons are made. Forty-five million Americans are uninsured and seek routine medical care in emergency rooms. Remedies are the current subjects of complex medical, public health, economic, and political debates. Solutions to these real problems must recognize both the need for effective ways to incentivize innovation and to permit, recognize, and reward compassionate medical care.

Intellectual Property and Patents

Drug invention, like any other, produces intellectual property eligible for patent protection. Without patent protection, no company could think of making the investments necessary for drug invention and development. With the passage of the Bayh-Dole Act (35 USC 200) in 1980, the federal government created strong incentives for scientists at academic medical centers to approach drug invention with an entrepreneurial spirit. The Act transferred intellectual property rights to the researchers themselves and in some instances to their respective institutions in order to encourage the kinds of partnerships with industry that would bring new products to market, where they could benefit the public. This resulted in the development of "technology transfer" offices at virtually every major university, which help scientists to apply for patents and to negotiate licensing arrangements with industry (Geiger and Sá, 2008). While the need to protect intellectual property is generally accepted, the encouragement of public-private research collaborations has given rise to concerns about conflicts of interest by scientists and universities (Kaiser, 2009).

Despite the complications that come with university-industry relations, patent protection is enormously important for innovation. As noted in 1859 by Abraham Lincoln (the only U.S. president to ever hold a patent [# 6469, for a device to lift boats over shoals]), by giving the inventor exclusive use of his or her invention for limited time, the patent system "added the fuel of interest to the fire of genius, in the discovery and production of new and useful things." The U.S. patent protection system mandates that when a new drug is invented, the patent covering the property lasts only 20 years from the time the patent is filed. During this period, the patent owner may bring suit to prevent others from marketing the product, giving the manufacturer of the brand-name version exclusive rights to market and sell the drug. When the patent expires, equivalent products can come on the market, where they are sold much more cheaply than the original drug, and without the huge development costs borne by the original patent holder. The marketer of the so-called generic product must demonstrate "therapeutic equivalence" of the new product: it must contain equal amounts of the same active chemical ingredient and achieve equal concentrations in blood when administered by the same routes.

Note, however, that the long time course of drug development, usually more than 10 years (Figure 1–1), dramatically reduces the time during which patent protection functions as intended. Although The Drug Price Competition and Patent Term Restoration Act of 1984 (the "Hatch-Waxman Act") permits a patent holder to apply for extension of a patent term to compensate for delays in marketing due to FDA approval processes, patents can be extended only for half the time period consumed by the regulatory approval process, for a maximum of 14 years. The average new drug brought to market now enjoys only ~10-12 years of patent protection. Some argue that patent protection for drugs should be shortened, based on the hope that earlier generic competition will lower healthcare costs. The counter-argument is that new drugs would have to bear higher prices to provide adequate compensation to companies during a shorter period of protected time. If that is true, lengthening patent protection would actually permit lower prices. Recall that patent protection is worth little if a superior competitive product is invented and brought to market at any time in the patent cycle.

Drug Promotion

In an ideal world, physicians would learn all they need to know about drugs from the medical literature, and good drugs would thereby sell themselves; we are a long way from the ideal. Instead we have print advertising and visits from salespeople directed at physicians, and extensive so-called "direct-to-consumer" advertising aimed at the public (in print, on the radio, and especially on television). There are roughly 100,000 pharmaceutical sales representatives in the U.S. who target ~10 times that number of physicians. It has been noted that college cheerleading squads are attractive sources for recruitment of this sales force. The amount spent on promotion of drugs approximates or perhaps even exceeds that spent on research and development. Pharmaceutical companies have been especially vulnerable to criticism for some of their marketing practices.

Promotional materials used by pharmaceutical companies cannot deviate from information contained in the package insert. In addition, there must be an acceptable balance between presentation of therapeutic claims for a product and discussion of unwanted effects. Nevertheless, direct-to-consumer advertising of drugs remains controversial and is permitted only in the U.S. and New Zealand. Physicians frequently succumb with misgivings to patients' advertising-driven requests for specific medications. The counter-argument is that patients are educated by such marketing efforts and in many cases will then seek medical care, especially for conditions that they may have been denying (e.g., depression) (Donohue et al., 2007).

The major criticism of drug marketing involves some of the unsavory approaches used to influence physician behavior. Gifts of value (e.g., sports tickets) are now forbidden, but dinners where drug-prescribing information is presented are widespread. Large numbers of physicians are paid as "consultants" to make presentations in such settings. It has been noted that the pharmaceutical companies' sales representatives frequently deliver more pizza and free drug samples than information to a doctor's office. These practices have now been brought squarely into the public view, and acceptance of any gift, no matter how small, from a drug company by a physician, is now forbidden at many academic medical centers and by law in several states (e.g., Vermont and Minnesota).

The board of directors of the Pharmaceutical Research and Manufacturers of America (PhRMA) has recently adopted an enhanced code on relationships with U.S. healthcare professionals. This code prohibits the distribution of non-educational items, prohibits company sales representatives from providing restaurant meals to healthcare professionals, and requires companies to ensure that their representatives are trained about laws and regulations that govern interactions with healthcare professionals.

Exploitation or "Medical Imperialism"

There is concern about the degree to which U.S. and European patent protection laws have restricted access to potentially life-saving drugs in developing countries. Because development of new drugs is so expensive, private-sector investment in pharmaceutical innovation naturally has focused on products that will have lucrative markets in wealthy countries such as the U.S., which combines patent protection with a free-market economy. However, to lower costs, companies increasingly test their experimental drugs outside the U.S. and the E.U., in countries such as China, India, Russia, and Mexico, where there is less regulation and easier access to large numbers of patients. If the drug is successful in obtaining marketing approval, consumers in these countries often cannot afford the drugs they helped to develop. Some ethicists have argued that this practice violates the justice principle articulated in The Belmont Report (1979), which states that "research should not unduly involve persons from groups unlikely to be among the beneficiaries of subsequent applications of the research." On the other hand, the conduct of trials in developing nations also frequently brings needed medical attention to underserved populations. Some concerns about the inequitable access to new pharmaceuticals in the very countries where they have been tested have been alleviated by exemptions made to the World Trade Organization's Agreement on Trade Related Aspects of Intellectual Property Rights (TRIPS) agreement. The TRIPS agreement originally made pharmaceutical product patent protection mandatory for all developing countries beginning in 2005. However, recent amendments have exempted the least developed countries from pharmaceutical patent obligations at least through 2016. Consequently, those developing countries that do not currently provide patent protection for pharmaceutical products can legally import less expensive versions of the same drugs from countries such as India where they are manufactured.

Product Liability

Product liability laws are intended to protect consumers from defective products. Pharmaceutical companies can be sued for faulty design or manufacturing, deceptive promotional practices, violation of regulatory requirements, or failure to warn consumers of known risks. So-called "failure to warn" claims can be made against drug makers even when the product is approved by the FDA. Although the traditional defense offered by manufacturers in such cases is that a "learned intermediary" (the patient's physician) wrote the prescription for the drug in question, the rise of direct-to-consumer advertising by drug companies has undermined this argument. With greater frequency, courts are finding companies that market prescription drugs directly to consumers responsible when these advertisements fail to provide an adequate warning of potential adverse effects.

Although injured patients are entitled to pursue legal remedies when they are harmed, the negative effects of product liability lawsuits against pharmaceutical companies may be considerable. First, fear of liability that causes pharmaceutical companies to be overly cautious about testing also delays access to the drug. Second, the cost of drugs increases for consumers when pharmaceutical companies increase the length and number of trials they perform to identify even the smallest risks, and when regulatory agencies increase the number or intensity of regulatory reviews. To the extent that these price increases may actually reduce the number of people who can afford to buy the drugs, there can be a negative effect on public health. Third, excessive liability costs create disincentives for development of so-called "orphan drugs," pharmaceuticals that would be of benefit to a very small number of patients. Should pharmaceutical companies be liable for failure to warn when all of the rules were followed and the product was approved by the FDA but the unwanted effect was not detected because of its rarity or another confounding factor? The only way to find "all" of the unwanted effects that a drug may have is to market it—to conduct a Phase IV "clinical trial" or observational study. Enlightened self-interest works both ways, and this basic friction between risk to patients and the financial risk of drug development does not seem likely to be resolved except on a case-by-case basis.

The Supreme Court of the U.S. added further fuel to these fiery issues in 2009 in the case *Wyeth v. Levine*. A patient (Levine) suffered gangrene of an arm following inadvertent arterial administration of the drug promethazine. The health-care provider had intended to administer the drug by so-called intravenous push. The FDA-approved label for the drug *warned against* but did not prohibit administration by intravenous push. The state courts and then the U.S. Supreme Court held both the health-care provider *and the company* liable for damages. FDA approval of the label apparently neither protects a company from liability nor prevents individual states from imposing regulations more stringent than those required by the federal government. Perhaps this decision rested more on the intricacies of the law than on consideration of proper medical practice.

"Me Too" Versus True Innovation: The Pace of New Drug Development

"Me-too drug" is a term used to describe a pharmaceutical that is usually structurally similar to one or more drugs that already are on the market. The other names for this phenomenon are "derivative medications, "molecular modifications," and "follow-up drugs." In some cases, a me-too drug is a different molecule developed deliberately by a competitor company to take market share from the company with existing drugs on the market. When the market for a class of drugs is especially large, several companies can share the market and make a profit. Other me-too drugs result coincidentally from numerous companies developing products simultaneously without knowing which drugs will be approved for sale.

Some me-too's are simply slightly altered formulations of a company's own drug, packaged and promoted as if it really offers something new. An example of this type of me-too is the heartburn medication esomeprazole, which is marketed by the same company that makes omeprazole. Omeprazole is a mixture of two stereoisomers; esomeprazole contains only one of the isomers and is eliminated less rapidly. Development of esomeprazole created a new period of market exclusivity, although generic versions of omeprazole are marketed, as are branded congeners of omeprazole/esomeprazole.

There are valid criticisms of me-too drugs. First, it is argued that an excessive emphasis on profit will stifle true innovation. Of the 487 drugs approved by the FDA between 1998 and 2003,

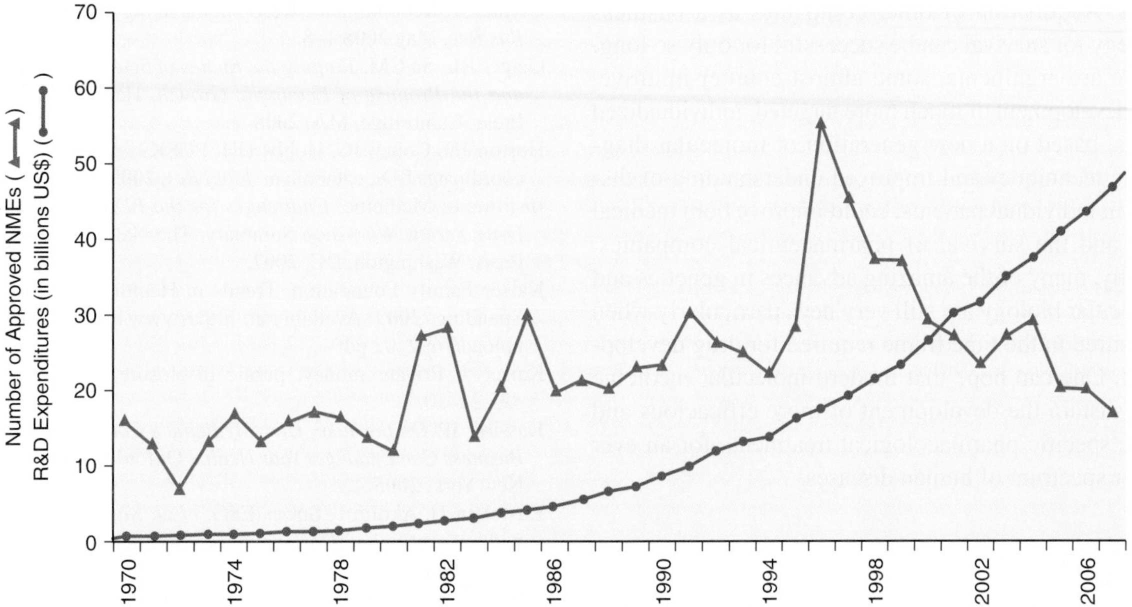

Figure 1–2. *The cost of drug invention is rising dramatically while productivity is declining.* The past several decades have seen enormous increases in spending for research and development by the pharmaceutical industry. While this was associated with increasing numbers of new molecular entities (NMEs) approved for clinical use during the latter years of the 20th century, this trend has been reversed over the past decade, leading to unsustainable costs per new molecular entity approved by the FDA. The peak in the mid-1990s was caused by the advent of PDUFA (see text), which facilitated elimination of a backlog.

only 67 (14%) were considered by the FDA to be new molecular entities. Second, to the extent that some me-too drugs are more expensive than the older versions they seek to replace, the costs of healthcare are increased without corresponding benefit to patients. Nevertheless, for some patients, me-too drugs may have better efficacy or fewer side effects or promote compliance with the treatment regimen. For example, the me-too that can be taken but once a day and not more frequently is convenient and promotes compliance. Some "me-toos" add great value from a business and medical point of view. Atorvastatin was the seventh statin to be introduced to market; it subsequently became the best-selling drug in the world.

Introduction of similar products in other industries is viewed as healthy competition. Such competition becomes most evident in the pharmaceutical business when one or more members of a group loses patent protection. Now that non-proprietary versions of simvastatin are available, sales of atorvastatin are declining. Billions of dollars might be saved, likely with little loss of benefit, if nonproprietary simvastatin were substituted for proprietary atorvastatin, with appropriate adjustment of dosages.

Critics of the pharmaceutical companies argue that they are not innovative and do not take risks and, further, that medical progress is actually slowed by their excessive concentration on me-too products. Figure 1–2 summarizes a few of the facts behind this and some of the other arguments just discussed. Clearly, smaller numbers of new molecular entities have been approved by the FDA over the past decade, despite the industry's enormous investment in research and development. This disconnect has occurred at a time when combinatorial chemistry was blooming, the human genome was being sequenced, highly automated techniques of screening were being developed, and new techniques of molecular biology and genetics were offering novel insights into the pathophysiology of human disease. Some blame mismanagement of the companies. Some say that industry science is not of high quality, an argument readily refuted. Some believe that the low-hanging fruit has been plucked, that drugs for complex diseases, such as neural degeneration or psychiatric and behavioral disorders, will be harder to develop. The biotechnology industry has had its successes, especially in exploiting relatively obvious opportunities that the new recombinant DNA technologies made available (e.g., insulin, growth hormone, erythropoietin, and more recently, monoclonal antibodies to approachable extracellular targets). Despite their innovations, the biotechnology companies have not, on balance, been more efficient at drug invention or discovery than the traditional major pharmaceutical companies.

Whatever the answers, the trends evident in Figure 1–2 must be reversed (Garnier, 2008). The current path will not sustain today's companies as they face a major wave of patent expirations over the next several years. Acquisition of other companies as a business strategy for survival can be successful for only so long. There are arguments, some almost counter-intuitive, that development of much more targeted, individualized drugs, based on a new generation of molecular diagnostic techniques and improved understanding of disease in individual patients, could improve both medical care and the survival of pharmaceutical companies. Finally, many of the amazing advances in genetics and molecular biology are still very new, particularly when measured in the time frame required for drug development. One can hope that modern molecular medicine will sustain the development of more efficacious and more specific pharmacological treatments for an ever wider spectrum of human diseases.

BIBLIOGRAPHY

Aagard L, Hansen EH. Information about ADRs explored by pharmacovigilance approaches: A qualitative review of studies on antibiotics, SSRIs and NSAIDs. *BMC Clin Pharmacol*, **2009,** *9*:4.

Angell M. *The Truth about the Drug Companies*. Random House, New York, **2004**.

The Belmont Report. Ethical Principles and Guidelines for the Protection of Human Subjects of Research. The National Commission for the Protection of Human Subjects of Biomedical and Behavioral Research, **1979**.

Brewer T, Colditz GA. Postmarketing surveillance and adverse drug reactions: current perspectives and future needs. *JAMA*, **1999**, *281*:824–829.

Brody B. *Ethical Issues in Drug Testing, Approval, and Pricing*. Oxford University Press, New York, **1995.**

Cutler DM. The demise of a blockbuster? *N Engl J Med,* **2007,** *356*:1292–1293.

Donohue JM, Cevasco M, Rosenthal MB. A decade of direct-to-consumer advertising of prescription drugs. *N Engl J Med,* **2007,** *357*:673–681.

FDA (U.S. Food and Drug Administration). *What We Do*. **2009**. Available at: http://www.fda.gov/AboutFDA/WhatWeDo/default.htm. Accessed 9/28/09.

Fontarosa PB, Rennie D, DeAngelis CD. Postmarketing surveillance—lack of vigilance, lack of trust. *JAMA*, **2004**, *292*:2647–2650.

Garnier JP. Rebuilding the R&D engine in big pharma. *Harvard Bus Rev*, May **2008**:1–8.

Geiger RL, Sá CM. *Tapping the Riches of Science. Universities and the Promise of Economic Growth.* Harvard University Press, Cambridge, MA, **2008**.

Horton JD, Cohen JC, Hobbs HH. PCSK9: A convertase that coordinates LDL catabolism. *Lipid Res*, **2009**, *50*:S172–S177.

Institute of Medicine. *Challenges for the FDA. The Future of Drug Safety.* Workshop Summary. The National Academies Press, Washington, DC, **2007.**

Kaiser Family Foundation. Trends in Health Care Costs and Spending. **2009.** Available at: http://www.kff.org/insurance/upload/7692_02.pdf

Kaiser J. Private money, public disclosure. *Science*, **2009**, *325*:28–30.

Kassirer JP. *On the Take. How Medicine's Complicity with Big Business Can Endanger Your Health.* Oxford University Press, New York, **2005.**

Kastelein JJ, Akdim F, Stroes ESG, *et al*. Simvastatin with or without ezetimibe in familial hypercholesterolemia. *N Engl J Med*, **2008**, *358*:1421–1443.

Kessler DA and "the Working Group." Introducing MEDWatch: A new approach to reporting medication and device adverse effects and product problems. *JAMA*, **1993**, *269*:2765–2768.

Kim J, Tang JY, Gong R, et al. Itraconazole, a commonly used antifungal that inhibits hedgehog pathway activity and cancer growth. *Cancer Cell*, **2010**, *17*:388–399.

Kinnings SL, Liu N, Buchmeier N, et al. Drug discovery using chemical systems biology: Repositioning the safe medicine Comtan to treat multi-drug and extensively drug resistant tuberculosis. *PLoS Comput Biol*, **2009**, *5*:e1000423.

Ng R. *Drugs: From Discovery to Approval*. Wily-Liss, Hoboken, NJ, **2004**.

Trontell A. Expecting the unexpected—drug safety, pharmacovigilance, and the prepared mind. *N Eng J Med*, **2004**, *351*:1385–1387.

World Medical Association. World Medical Association declaration of Helsinki: Ethical principles for medical research involving human subjects. *JAMA*, **2000**, *284*:3043–3045.

Xie L, Li J, Xie L, Bourne PE. Drug discovery using chemical systems biology: identification of the protein-ligand binding network to explain the side effects of CETP inhibitors. *PLoS Comput Biol*, **2009**, *5*:e1000387.

Xie L, Wang J, Bourne PE. In silico elucidation of the molecular mechanism defining the adverse effect of selective estrogen receptor modulators. *PLoS Comput Biol*, **2007**, *3*:e217.

Pharmacokinetics: The Dynamics of Drug Absorption, Distribution, Metabolism, and Elimination

Iain L. O. Buxton and
Leslie Z. Benet

In order to understand and control the therapeutic action of drugs in the human body, one must know how much drug will reach the site(s) of drug action and when this will occur. The absorption, distribution, metabolism (biotransformation), and elimination of drugs are the processes of *pharmacokinetics* (Figure 2–1). Understanding and employing pharmacokinetic principles can increase the probability of therapeutic success and reduce the occurrence of adverse drug effects in the body.

PHYSICOCHEMICAL FACTORS IN TRANSFER OF DRUGS ACROSS MEMBRANES

The absorption, distribution, metabolism, excretion, and action of a drug all involve its passage across cell membranes. Mechanisms by which drugs cross membranes and the physicochemical properties of molecules and membranes that influence this transfer are critical to understanding the disposition of drugs in the human body. The characteristics of a drug that predict its movement and availability at sites of action are its molecular size and structural features, degree of ionization, relative lipid solubility of its ionized and non-ionized forms, and its binding to serum and tissue proteins. In most cases, a drug must traverse the plasma membranes of many cells to reach its site of action. Although barriers to drug movement may be a single layer of cells (intestinal epithelium) or several layers of cells and associated extracellular protein (skin), the plasma membrane represents the common barrier to drug distribution.

Cell Membranes. The plasma membrane consists of a bilayer of amphipathic lipids with their hydrocarbon chains oriented inward to the center of the bilayer to form a continuous hydrophobic phase and their hydrophilic heads oriented outward. Individual lipid molecules in the bilayer vary according to the particular membrane and can move laterally and organize themselves with cholesterol (e.g., sphingolipids), endowing the membrane with fluidity, flexibility, organization, high electrical resistance, and relative impermeability to highly polar molecules. Membrane proteins embedded in the bilayer serve as structural anchors, receptors, ion channels, or transporters to transduce electrical or chemical signaling pathways and provide selective targets for drug actions. In contrast to earlier proposals that cell membranes are fluid and thus proteins collide in an unordered fashion, we now understand that membranes are highly ordered and compartmented (Pinaud et al., 2009; Singer, 2004). These proteins may be associated with caveolin and sequestered within caveolae; they may be excluded from caveolae; or they may be organized in signaling domains rich in cholesterol and sphingolipid not containing caveolin or other scaffolding proteins (i.e., lipid rafts).

Cell membranes are relatively permeable to water either by diffusion or by flow resulting from hydrostatic or osmotic differences across the membrane, and bulk flow of water can carry with it drug molecules. However, proteins with drug molecules bound to them are too large and polar for this type of membrane passage to occur. Transmembrane movement of drug generally is limited to unbound drug; thus drug-protein complexes constitute an inactive reservoir of drug that can influence both therapeutic as well as unwanted drug effects. Paracellular passage through intercellular gaps is sufficiently large that transfer across capillary endothelium is generally limited by blood flow and not by other factors. As described later, such membrane passage is an important factor in filtration across the glomerulus in the kidney. Important exceptions exist in such capillary diffusion; "tight" intercellular junctions are present in specific tissues, and paracellular passage in them is limited. Capillaries of the central nervous system (CNS) and a variety of epithelial tissues have tight junctions. Bulk flow of water can carry with it small water-soluble substances, but bulk-flow transfer is limited when the molecular mass of the solute exceeds 100–200 Da. Accordingly, most large lipophilic drugs must pass through the cell membrane itself (Figure 2–2).

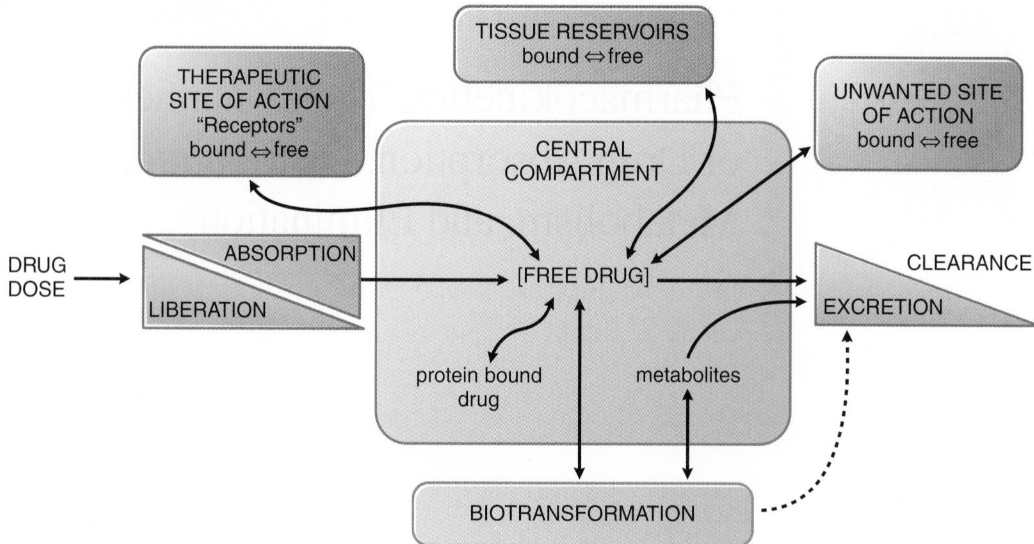

Figure 2–1 *The interrelationship of the absorption, distribution, binding, metabolism, and excretion of a drug and its concentration at its sites of action.* Possible distribution and binding of metabolites in relation to their potential actions at receptors are not depicted.

Passive Flux Across Membranes. Drugs cross membranes either by passive processes or by mechanisms involving the active participation of components of the membrane. In passive transfer, the drug molecule usually penetrates by diffusion along a concentration gradient by virtue of its solubility in the lipid bilayer. Such transfer is directly proportional to the magnitude of the concentration gradient across the membrane, to the lipid-water partition coefficient of the drug, and to the membrane surface area exposed to the drug. The greater the partition coefficient, the higher is the concentration of drug in the membrane and the faster is its diffusion. After a steady state is attained, the concentration of the unbound drug is the same on both sides of the membrane if the drug is a non-electrolyte. For ionic compounds, the steady-state concentrations depend on the electrochemical gradient for the ion and on differences in pH across the membrane, which will influence the state of ionization of the molecule disparately on either side of the membrane and can effectively trap drug on one side of the membrane.

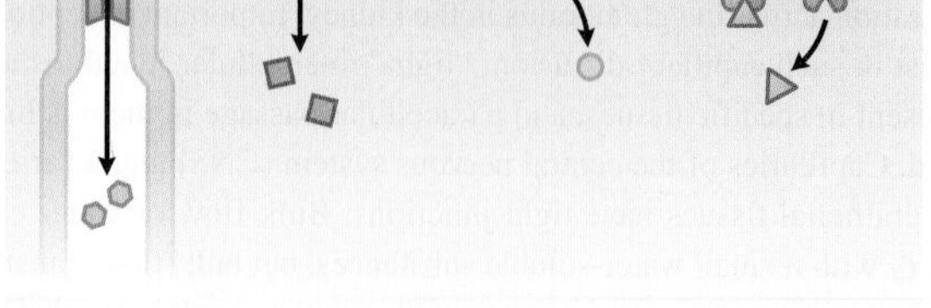

PASSIVE TRANSPORT — Paracellular transport, Diffusion; ACTIVE TRANSPORT — Facilitated diffusion, Drug transporters

Figure 2–2. *The variety of ways drugs move across cellular barriers in their passage throughout the body.*

Weak Electrolytes and the Influence of pH. Many drugs are weak acids or bases that are present in solution as both the non-ionized and ionized species. The non-ionized molecules usually are more lipid soluble and can diffuse readily across the cell membrane. In contrast, the ionized molecules usually are less able to penetrate the lipid membrane because of their low lipid solubility, and passage will depend on the leakiness of the membrane related to the membrane's electrical resistance. Therefore, the transmembrane distribution of a weak electrolyte is influenced by its pK_a and the pH gradient across the membrane. The pK_a is the pH at which half the drug (weak acid or base electrolyte) is in its ionized form.

To illustrate the effect of pH on distribution of drugs, the partitioning of a weak acid ($pK_a = 4.4$) between plasma (pH = 7.4) and gastric juice (pH = 1.4) is depicted in Figure 2–3. Assume that the gastric mucosal membrane behaves as a simple lipid barrier with a high electrical resistance that is permeable only to the lipid-soluble, non-ionized form of the acid. The ratio of non-ionized to ionized drug at each pH is readily calculated from the Henderson-Hasselbalch equation:

$$\log \frac{[\text{protonated form}]}{[\text{unprotonated form}]} = pK_a - pH \quad \text{(Equation 2–1)}$$

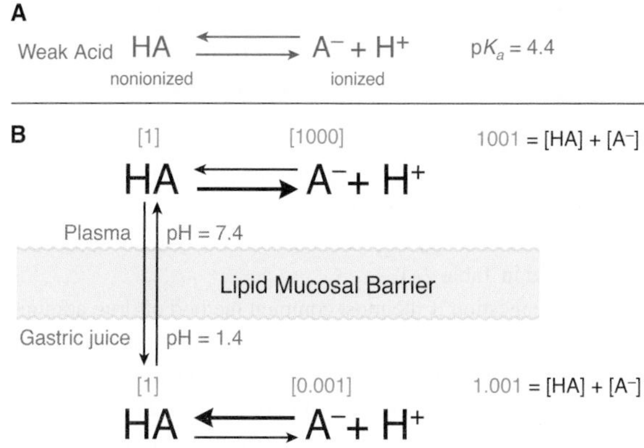

Figure 2–3 *Influence of pH on the distribution of a weak acid between plasma and gastric juice separated by a lipid barrier.* **A.** The dissociation of a weak acid, $pK_a = 4.4$. **B**. Dissociation of the weak acid in plasma (pH 7.4) and gastric acid (pH 1.4). The uncharged from, HA, equibrates across the membrane. Blue numbers in brackets show relative concentrations of HA and A^-.

This equation relates the pH of the medium around the drug and the drug's acid dissociation constant (pK_a) to the ratio of the protonated (HA or BH^+) and unprotonated (A^- or B) forms, where $HA \leftrightarrow A^- + H^+$ ($K_a = [A^-][H^+]/[HA]$) describes the dissociation of an acid, and $BH^+ \leftrightarrow B + H^+$ ($K_a = [B][H^+]/[BH^+]$) describes the dissociation of the protonated form of a base.

In the example of Figure 2–3, the ratio of non-ionized to ionized drug in plasma is 1:1000; in gastric juice, the ratio is 1:0.001, as given in brackets in Figure 2–3. The total concentration ratio between the plasma and the gastric juice therefore would be 1000:1 if such a system came to a steady state. For a weak base with a pK_a of 4.4 (e.g., chlordiazepoxide), the ratio would be reversed, as would the thick horizontal arrows in Figure 2–3, which indicate the predominant species at each pH. Accordingly, at steady state, an acidic drug will accumulate on the more basic side of the membrane and a basic drug on the more acidic side.

Common ionizable groups on drug molecules are carboxylic acids (pK_a~4.5) and primary amino groups (pK_a~9.5), but myriad others are possible. Resonance structures and electron withdrawing groups can change the pK_a, and many compounds have multiple ionizable groups; thus, pK_a values vary over a broad range. Furthermore, some drugs contain quaternary amines with a permanent positive change. One consequence of a drug being ionized at physiological pH is illustrated by the relative lack of sedative effects of second generation histamine H_1 antagonists: second generation antihistamines are ionized molecules (less lipophilic) that cross the blood-brain barrier poorly compared to first generation agents (uncharged at pH 7.4). The effects of net charge are observable elsewhere in the body, in the kidney tubules, for instance. Urine pH can vary over a ride range, from 4.5 to 8. As urine pH drops (as $[H^+]$ increases), weak acids (A^-) and weak bases (B) will exist to a greater extend in their protonated forms (HA and BH^+); the reverse is true as pH rises, where A^- and B will be favored. In the kidney tubules where a lipid soluble (uncharged) drug can be reabsorbed by passive diffusion, excretion of the drug can be promoted by altering the pH of the urine to favor the ionized state (A^- or BH^+). Thus, alkaline urine favors excretion of weak acids; acid urine favors excretion of weak bases. Elevation of urine pH (by giving sodium bicarbonate) will promote urinary excretion of weak acids such as aspirin (pK_a~3.5) and urate (pK_a~5.8). This principle of *in trapping* is an important process in drug distribution.

These considerations have obvious implications for the absorption and excretion of many drugs, as will be discussed more specifically. The establishment of concentration gradients of weak electrolytes across membranes with a pH gradient is a physical process and does not require an active electrolyte transport system. All that is necessary is a membrane preferentially permeable to one form of the weak electrolyte and a pH gradient across the membrane. The establishment of the pH gradient, however, is an active process.

Carrier-Mediated Membrane Transport. While passive diffusion through the bilayer is dominant in the disposition of most drugs, carrier-mediated mechanisms also play an important role. *Active transport* is characterized by a direct requirement for energy, movement against an electrochemical gradient, saturability, selectivity, and competitive inhibition by co-transported compounds. Na^+,K^+-ATPase is an important example of an active transport mechanism that is a therapeutic target of digoxin in the treatment of heart failure (Chapter 28). Secondary active transport uses the electrochemical energy stored in a gradient to move another molecule against a concentration gradient; e.g., the Na^+–Ca^{2+} exchange protein uses the energy stored in the Na^+ gradient established by the Na^+, K^+-ATPase mechanism to export cytosolic Ca^{2+} and maintain it at a low basal level, ~100 nM in most cells (Chapter 3); similarly, the Na^+-dependent glucose transporters SGLT1 and SGLT2 move glucose across membranes of gastrointestinal (GI) epithelium and renal tubules by coupling glucose transport to downhill Na^+ flux.

Facilitated diffusion describes a carrier-mediated transport process in which there is no input of energy, and therefore enhanced movement of the involved substance is down a chemical gradient as in the permeation of glucose across a muscle cell membrane mediated by the insulin-sensitive glucose transporter GLUT4. Such mechanisms, which may be highly selective for a specific conformational structure of a drug, are involved in the transport of endogenous compounds whose rate of transport by passive diffusion otherwise would be too slow (Figure 5–4). In other cases, they function as exporters, creating a barrier to prevent the intracellular accumulation of potentially toxic substances. Pharmacologically important transporters may mediate either drug uptake or efflux and often facilitate vectorial transport across polarized cells. An important efflux transporter is the P-glycoprotein encoded by the multidrug resistance-1 (*MDR1*) gene (Table 5–4). P-glycoprotein localized in the enterocyte limits the oral absorption of transported drugs because it exports compounds back into the lumen of the GI tract subsequent to their absorption by passive diffusion. The P-glycoprotein also can confer resistance to some cancer chemotherapeutic agents (Chapters 60-63). Transporters and their roles in drug action are presented in detail in Chapter 5.

DRUG ABSORPTION, BIOAVAILABILITY, AND ROUTES OF ADMINISTRATION

Absorption is the movement of a drug from its site of administration into the central compartment (Figure 2–1) and the extent to which this occurs. For solid dosage forms, absorption first requires dissolution of the tablet or capsule, thus liberating the drug. The clinician is concerned primarily with bioavailability rather than absorption. *Bioavailability* is a term used to indicate the fractional extent to which a dose of drug reaches its site of action or a biological fluid from which the drug has access to its site of action. For example, a drug given orally must be absorbed first from the GI tract, but net absorption may be limited by the characteristics of the dosage form, the drug's physicochemical properties, by intestinal metabolism, and by transporter export back into the intestinal lumen. The absorbed drug then passes through the liver, where metabolism and biliary excretion may occur before the drug enters the systemic circulation. Accordingly, a fraction of the administered and absorbed dose of drug will be inactivated or diverted in the intestine and liver before it can reach the general circulation and be distributed to its sites of action. If the metabolic or excretory capacity of the liver and the intestine for the drug is large, bioavailability will be reduced substantially (*first-pass effect*). This decrease in availability is a function of the anatomical site from which absorption takes place; other anatomical, physiological, and pathological factors can influence bioavailability (described later), and the choice of the route of drug administration must be based on an understanding of these conditions. Moreover, knowledge of drugs that undergo significant metabolism or require active transport across the intestinal and hepatic membranes instructs our understanding of adverse events in therapeutics, since some drugs are substrates for the same drug metabolizing enzymes or drug transporters and thus compete for metabolism and transport.

Oral (Enteral) Versus Parenteral Administration. Often there is a choice of the route by which a therapeutic agent may be administered, and knowledge of the advantages and disadvantages of the different routes of administration is then of primary importance. Some characteristics of the major routes employed for systemic drug effect are compared in Table 2–1.

Oral ingestion is the most common method of drug administration. It also is the safest, most convenient, and most economical. Disadvantages to the oral route include limited absorption of some drugs because of their physical characteristics (e.g., low water solubility or poor membrane permeability), emesis as a result of irritation to the GI mucosa, destruction of some drugs by digestive enzymes or low gastric pH, irregularities in absorption or propulsion in the presence of food or other drugs, and the need for cooperation on the part of the patient. Such cooperation is frequently not forthcoming, since tolerating certain oral medications means accepting unwanted effects, such as GI pain, which may require use of an alternate route of administration (Cosman, 2009). In addition, drugs in the GI tract may be metabolized by the enzymes of the intestinal flora, mucosa, or liver before they gain access to the general circulation.

Parenteral injection of drugs has certain distinct advantages over oral administration. In some instances, parenteral administration is essential for the drug to be delivered in its active form, as in the case of monoclonal antibodies such as infliximab, an antibody directed against tumor necrosis factor α (TNF α) used in the treatment of rheumatoid arthritis. Availability usually is more rapid, extensive, and predictable when a drug is given by injection. The effective dose can therefore be delivered more accurately. In emergency therapy and when a patient is unconscious, uncooperative, or unable to retain anything given by mouth, parenteral therapy may be a necessity. The injection of drugs, however, has its disadvantages: asepsis must be maintained, and this is of particular concern when drugs are given over time, such as in intravenous or intrathecal administration; pain may accompany the injection; and it is sometimes difficult for patients to perform the injections themselves if self-medication is necessary.

Oral Administration. Absorption from the GI tract is governed by factors such as surface area for absorption, blood flow to the site of absorption, the physical state of the drug (solution, suspension, or solid dosage form), its water solubility, and the drug's concentration at the site of absorption. For drugs given in solid form, the rate of dissolution may limit their absorption, especially drugs of low aqueous solubility. Since most drug absorption from the GI tract occurs by passive diffusion, absorption is favored when the drug is in the non-ionized and more lipophilic form. Based on the pH-partition concept (Figure 2–3), one would predict that drugs that are weak acids would be better absorbed from the stomach (pH 1-2) than from the upper intestine (pH 3-6), and vice versa for weak bases. However, the epithelium of the stomach is lined with a thick mucus layer, and its surface area is small; by contrast, the villi of the upper intestine provide an extremely large surface area (~200 m^2). Accordingly, the rate of absorption of a drug from the intestine will be greater than that from the stomach even if the drug is predominantly ionized in the intestine and largely non-ionized in the stomach. Thus, any factor that accelerates gastric emptying (recumbent position, right side)

Table 2–1

Some Characteristics of Common Routes of Drug Administration[a]

ROUTE	ABSORPTION PATTERN	SPECIAL UTILITY	LIMITATIONS AND PRECAUTIONS
Intravenous	Absorption circumvented Potentially immediate effects Suitable for large volumes and for irritating substances, or complex mixtures, when diluted	Valuable for emergency use Permits titration of dosage Usually required for high-molecular-weight protein and peptide drugs	Increased risk of adverse effects Must inject solutions *slowly* as a rule Not suitable for oily solutions or poorly soluble substances
Subcutaneous	Prompt from aqueous solution Slow and sustained from repository preparations	Suitable for some poorly soluble suspensions and for instillation of slow-release implants	Not suitable for large volumes Possible pain or necrosis from irritating substances
Intramuscular	Prompt from aqueous solution Slow and sustained from repository preparations	Suitable for moderate volumes, oily vehicles, and some irritating substances Appropriate for self-administration (e.g., insulin)	Precluded during anticoagulant therapy May interfere with interpretation of certain diagnostic tests (e.g., creatine kinase)
Oral ingestion	Variable, depends on many factors (*see* text)	Most convenient and economical; usually more safe	Requires patient compliance Bioavailability potentially erratic and incomplete

[a]*See* text for more complete discussion and for other routes.

will be likely to increase the rate of drug absorption (Queckenberg and Fuhr, 2009), whereas any factor that delays gastric emptying is expected to have the opposite effect, regardless of the characteristics of the drug. Gastric motor activity and gastric emptying rate are governed by neural and humoral feedback provided by receptors found in the gastric musculature and proximal small intestine. In healthy individuals, gastric emptying rate is influenced by a variety of factors including the caloric content of food; volume, osmolality, temperature, and pH of ingested fluid; diurnal and inter-individual variation; metabolic state (rest/exercise); and the ambient temperature. Such factors will influence ingested drug absorption. Gastric emptying is influenced in women by the effects of estrogen (i.e., slower than in men for premenopausal women and those taking estrogen replacement therapy).

Drugs that are destroyed by gastric secretions and low pH or that cause gastric irritation sometimes are administered in dosage forms with an enteric coating that prevents dissolution in the acidic gastric contents. These pharmacologically inactive coatings, often of cellulose polymers, have a threshold of dissolution between pH 5 and 6. Enteric coatings are useful for drugs such as aspirin, which can cause significant gastric irritation in many patients, and for presenting a drug such as mesalamine to sites of action in the ileum and colon (Figure 47–4).

Controlled-Release Preparations. The rate of absorption of a drug administered as a tablet or other solid oral dosage form is partly dependent on its rate of dissolution in GI fluids. This is the basis for *controlled-release, extended-release, sustained-release,* and *prolonged-action* pharmaceutical preparations that are designed to produce slow, uniform absorption of the drug for 8 hours or longer. Such preparations are offered for medications in all major drug categories. Potential advantages of such preparations are reduction in the frequency of administration of the drug as compared with conventional dosage forms (often with improved compliance by the patient), maintenance of a therapeutic effect overnight, and decreased incidence and/or intensity of both undesired effects (by dampening of the peaks in drug concentration) and nontherapeutic blood levels of the drug (by elimination of troughs in concentration) that often occur after administration of immediate-release dosage forms.

Many controlled-release preparations fulfill these expectations and may be preferred in some therapeutic situations (e.g., therapy for depression [Nemeroff, 2003] and ADHD [Manos et al., 2007]) or treatment with dihydropyridine Ca^{2+} entry blockers (Chapters 26-28). However, such products do have drawbacks: variability of the systemic concentration achieved may be greater for controlled-release than for immediate-release dosage forms; the dosage form may fail, and "dose dumping" with resulting toxicity can occur because the total dose of drug in a controlled-release preparation may be several times the amount contained in the conventional preparation, although current regulatory approval requirements generally preclude such occurrences. Controlled-release dosage forms are most appropriate for drugs with short half-lives ($t_{1/2}$ <4 hours) or in selected patient groups such as those receiving anti-epileptics (Bialer, 2007; Pellock et al., 2004). So-called controlled-release dosage forms are sometimes developed for drugs with long $t_{1/2}$ values (>12 hours). These usually more expensive products should not be prescribed unless specific advantages have been demonstrated. The availability of controlled-release dosage forms of some drugs can lead to abuse, as in the case of controlled-release oxycodone marketed as OXYCONTIN. Crushing and snorting the delayed-release tablets results in a rapid release of the drug, increased absorption, and high peak serum concentrations (Aquina et al., 2009).

Sublingual Administration. Absorption from the oral mucosa has special significance for certain drugs despite the fact that the surface area available is small. Venous drainage from the mouth is to the superior vena cava, bypassing the portal circulation and thereby protecting the drug from rapid intestinal and hepatic first-pass metabolism. For example, nitroglycerin is effective when retained sublingually because it is non-ionic and has very high lipid solubility. Thus, the drug is absorbed very rapidly. Nitroglycerin also is very potent; absorption of a relatively small amount produces the therapeutic effect ("unloading" of the heart; Chapter 27).

Transdermal Absorption. Not all drugs readily penetrate the intact skin. Absorption of those that do is dependent on the surface area over which they are applied and their lipid solubility because the epidermis behaves as a lipid barrier (Chapter 65). The dermis, however, is freely permeable to many solutes; consequently, systemic absorption of drugs occurs much more readily through abraded, burned, or denuded skin. Inflammation and other conditions that increase cutaneous blood flow also enhance absorption. Toxic effects sometimes are produced by absorption through the skin of highly lipid-soluble substances (e.g., a lipid-soluble insecticide in an organic solvent). Absorption through the skin can be enhanced by suspending the drug in an oily vehicle and rubbing the resulting preparation into the skin. Because hydrated skin is more permeable than dry skin, the dosage form may be modified or an occlusive dressing may be used to facilitate absorption. Controlled-release topical patches have become increasingly available, including nicotine for tobacco-smoking withdrawal, scopolamine for motion sickness, nitroglycerin for angina pectoris, testosterone and estrogen for replacement therapy, various estrogens and progestins for birth control, and fentanyl for pain relief.

Rectal Administration. Approximately 50% of the drug that is absorbed from the rectum will bypass the liver; the potential for hepatic first-pass metabolism thus is less than that for an oral dose; furthermore, a major drug metabolism enzyme, CYP3A4, is present in the upper intestine but not in the lower intestine. However, rectal absorption can be irregular and incomplete, and certain drugs can cause irritation of the rectal mucosa. The use of special mucoadhesive microspheres may increase the number of medications that can be given by the rectal route (Patil and Sawant, 2008).

Parenteral Injection. The major routes of parenteral administration are intravenous, subcutaneous, and intramuscular. Absorption from subcutaneous and intramuscular sites occurs by simple diffusion along the gradient from drug depot to plasma. The rate is limited by the area of the absorbing capillary membranes and by the solubility of the substance in the interstitial fluid. Relatively large aqueous channels in the endothelial membrane account for the indiscriminate diffusion of molecules regardless of their lipid solubility. Larger molecules, such as proteins, slowly gain access to the circulation by way of lymphatic channels.

Drugs administered into the systemic circulation by any route, excluding the intra-arterial route, are subject to possible first-pass elimination in the lung prior to distribution to the rest of the body. The lungs serve as a temporary storage site for a number of agents, especially drugs that are weak bases and are predominantly non-ionized at the blood pH, apparently by their partition into lipid. The lungs also serve as a filter for particulate matter that may be given intravenously, and they provide a route of elimination for volatile substances.

Intravenous. Factors limiting absorption are circumvented by intravenous injection of drugs in aqueous solution because bioavailability is complete and rapid. Also, drug delivery is controlled and achieved with an accuracy and immediacy not possible by any other procedure. In some instances, as in the induction of surgical anesthesia, the dose of a drug is not predetermined but is adjusted to the response of the patient. Also, certain irritating solutions can be given only in this manner because the drug, if injected slowly, is greatly diluted by the blood. There are both advantages and disadvantages to the use of this route of administration. Unfavorable reactions can occur because high concentrations of drug may be attained rapidly in both plasma and tissues. There are therapeutic circumstances where it is advisable to administer a drug by bolus injection (small volume given rapidly, e.g., tissue plasminogen activator immediately following an acute myocardial infarction) and other circumstances where slower administration of drug is advisable, such as the delivery of drugs by intravenous "piggyback" (e.g., antibiotics). Intravenous administration of drugs warrants close monitoring of the patient's response. Furthermore, once the drug is injected, there is often no retreat. Repeated intravenous injections depend on the ability to maintain a patent vein. Drugs in an oily vehicle, those that precipitate blood constituents or hemolyze erythrocytes, and drug combinations that cause precipitates to form must not be given by this route.

Subcutaneous. Injection into a subcutaneous site can be done only with drugs that are not irritating to tissue; otherwise, severe pain, necrosis, and tissue sloughing may occur. The rate of absorption following subcutaneous injection of a drug often is sufficiently constant and slow to provide a sustained effect. Moreover, altering the period over which a drug is absorbed may be varied intentionally, as is accomplished with insulin for injection using particle size, protein complexation, and pH to provide short-acting (3-6 hours), intermediate-acting (10-18 hours), and long-acting (18-24 hours) preparations. The incorporation of a vasoconstrictor agent in a solution of a drug to be injected subcutaneously also retards absorption. Thus, the injectable local anesthetic lidocaine incorporates epinephrine into the dosage form. Absorption of drugs implanted under the skin in a solid pellet form occurs slowly over a period of weeks or months; some hormones (e.g., contraceptives) are administered effectively in this manner, and implantable devices (e.g., a plastic rod delivering etonogestrel) can provide effective contraception for 3 years (Blumenthal et al., 2008).

Intramuscular. Drugs in aqueous solution are absorbed quite rapidly after intramuscular injection depending on the rate of blood flow to the injection site. This may be modulated to some extent by local heating, massage, or exercise. For example, while absorption of insulin generally is more rapid from injection in the arm and abdominal wall than the thigh, jogging may cause a precipitous drop in blood sugar when insulin is injected into the thigh rather than into the arm or abdominal wall because running markedly increases blood flow to the leg. A hot bath accelerates absorption from all these sites owing to vasodilation. Generally, the rate of absorption following injection of an aqueous preparation into the deltoid or vastus lateralis is faster than when the injection is made into the gluteus maximus. The rate is particularly slower for females after injection into the gluteus maximus. This has been attributed to the different distribution of subcutaneous fat in males and females and because fat is relatively poorly perfused. Very obese or emaciated patients may exhibit unusual patterns of absorption following intramuscular or subcutaneous injection. Slow, constant absorption from the intramuscular site results if the drug is injected in solution in oil or suspended in various other repository (depot) vehicles. Antibiotics often are administered in this manner. Substances too irritating to be injected subcutaneously sometimes may be given intramuscularly.

Intra-arterial. Occasionally, a drug is injected directly into an artery to localize its effect in a particular tissue or organ, such as in the treatment of liver tumors and head/neck cancers. Diagnostic agents sometimes are administered by this route (e.g., technetium-labeled human serum albumin). Intra-arterial injection requires great care and should be reserved for experts. The dampening, first-pass, and cleansing effects of the lung are not available when drugs are given by this route.

Intrathecal. The blood-brain barrier and the blood-cerebrospinal fluid (CSF) barrier often preclude or slow the entrance of drugs into the CNS. Therefore, when local and rapid effects of drugs on the meninges or cerebrospinal axis are desired, as in spinal anesthesia or treatment of acute CNS infections, drugs sometimes are injected directly into the spinal subarachnoid space. Brain tumors also may be treated by direct intraventricular drug administration. More recent developments include special targeting of substances to the brain via receptor-mediated transcytosis (Jones and Shusta, 2007) and modulation of tight junctions (Matsuhisa et al., 2009).

Pulmonary Absorption. Provided that they do not cause irritation, gaseous and volatile drugs may be inhaled and absorbed through the pulmonary epithelium and mucous membranes of the respiratory tract. Access to the circulation is rapid by this route because the lung's surface area is large. The principles governing absorption and excretion of anesthetic and other therapeutic gases are discussed in Chapter 19. In addition, solutions of drugs can be atomized and the fine droplets in air (aerosol) inhaled. Advantages are the almost instantaneous absorption of a drug into the blood, avoidance of hepatic first-pass loss, and in the case of pulmonary disease, local application of the drug at the desired site of action. For example, owing to the ability to meter doses and create fine aerosols, drugs can be given in this manner for the treatment of allergic rhinitis or bronchial asthma (Chapter 36). Pulmonary absorption is an important route of entry of certain drugs of abuse and of toxic environmental substances of varied composition and physical states. Both local and systemic reactions to allergens may occur subsequent to inhalation.

Topical Application

Mucous Membranes. Drugs are applied to the mucous membranes of the conjunctiva, nasopharynx, oropharynx, vagina, colon, urethra, and urinary bladder primarily for their local effects. Occasionally, as in the application of synthetic anti-diuretic hormone to the nasal mucosa, systemic absorption is the goal. Absorption through mucous membranes occurs readily. In fact, local anesthetics applied for local effect sometimes may be absorbed so rapidly that they produce systemic toxicity.

Eye. Topically applied ophthalmic drugs are used primarily for their local effects (Chapter 64). Systemic absorption that results from drainage through the nasolacrimal canal is usually undesirable. Because drug that is absorbed via drainage is not subject to first-pass intestinal and hepatic metabolism, unwanted systemic pharmacological effects may occur when β adrenergic receptor antagonists or corticosteroids are administered as ophthalmic drops. Local effects usually require absorption of the drug through the cornea; corneal infection or trauma thus may result in more rapid absorption. Ophthalmic delivery systems that provide prolonged duration of action (e.g., suspensions and ointments) are useful additions to ophthalmic therapy. Ocular inserts, such as the use of pilocarpine-containing inserts for the treatment of glaucoma, provide continuous delivery of small amounts of drug. Very little is lost through drainage; hence systemic side effects are minimized.

Novel Methods of Drug Delivery

Drug-eluting stents and other devices are being used to target drugs locally and minimize systemic exposure. The systemic toxicity of potentially important compounds can be decreased significantly by combination with a variety of drug carrier vehicles that modify distribution. For example, linkage of the cytotoxic agent calicheamicin to an antibody directed to an antigen found on the surface of certain leukemic cells can target the drug to its intended site of action, improving the therapeutic index of calicheamicin.

Recent advances in drug delivery include the use of biocompatible polymers with functional monomers attached in such a way as to permit linkage of drug molecules to the polymer. A drug-polymer conjugate can be designed to be a stable, long-circulating prodrug by varying the molecular weight of the polymer and the cleavable linkage between the drug and the polymer. The linkage is designed to keep the drug inactive until it released from the backbone polymer by a disease-specific trigger, typically enzyme activity in the targeted tissue that delivers the active drug at or near the site of pathology. Nanoparticles are offering new opportunities for diagnosis, targeted drug delivery, and imaging of clinical effect (Prestidge et al., 2010; Sajja et al., 2009).

Bioequivalence

Drug products are considered to be pharmaceutical equivalents if they contain the same active ingredients and are identical in strength or concentration, dosage form, and route of administration. Two pharmaceutically equivalent drug products are considered to be *bioequivalent* when the rates and extents of bioavailability of the active ingredient in the two products are not significantly different under suitable test conditions. In the past, dosage forms of a drug from different manufacturers and even different lots of preparations from a single manufacturer sometimes differed in their bioavailability. Such differences were seen primarily among oral dosage forms of poorly soluble, slowly absorbed drugs such as the urinary anti-infective, metronidazole (FLAGYL). When first introduced, the generic form was not bioequivalent because the generic manufacturer was not able to mimic the proprietary process used to microsize the drug for absorption initially. Differences in crystal form, particle size, or other physical characteristics of the drug that are not rigidly controlled in formulation and manufacture affect disintegration of the dosage form and dissolution of the drug and hence the rate and extent of drug absorption.

The potential non-equivalence of different drug preparations has been a matter of concern (Meredith, 2009). However, no prospective clinical study has shown an FDA-approved generic drug product to yield significantly different therapeutic effects, even when testing published anecdotal reports of non-equivalence. Because of the legitimate concern of clinicians and the financial consequences of generic prescribing, this topic will continue to be actively addressed. Generic versus brand name prescribing is further discussed in connection with drug nomenclature and the choice of drug name in writing prescription orders (Appendix I).

DISTRIBUTION OF DRUGS

Following absorption or systemic administration into the bloodstream, a drug distributes into interstitial and intracellular fluids. This process reflects a number of physiological factors and the particular physicochemical properties of the individual drug. Cardiac output, regional blood flow, capillary permeability, and tissue volume determine the rate of delivery and potential amount of drug distributed into tissues. Initially, liver, kidney, brain, and other well-perfused organs receive most of the drug; delivery to muscle, most viscera, skin, and fat is slower, and this second distribution phase may require minutes to several hours before the concentration of drug in tissue is in equilibrium with that in blood. The second phase also involves a far larger fraction of body mass (e.g., muscle) than does the initial phase and generally accounts for most of the extravascularly distributed drug. With exceptions such as the brain, diffusion of drug into the interstitial fluid occurs rapidly because of the highly permeable nature of the capillary endothelial membrane. Thus, tissue distribution is determined by the partitioning of drug between blood and the particular tissue. Lipid solubility and transmembrane pH gradients are important determinants of such uptake for drugs that are either weak acids or bases. However, in general, ion trapping associated with transmembrane pH gradients is not large because the pH difference between tissue and blood (~7.0 versus 7.4) is small. The more important determinant of blood-tissue partitioning is the relative binding of drug to plasma proteins and tissue macromolecules that limits the concentration of free drug.

Plasma Proteins. Many drugs circulate in the bloodstream bound to plasma proteins. Albumin is a major carrier for acidic drugs; α_1-acid glycoprotein binds basic drugs. Nonspecific binding to other plasma proteins generally occurs to a much smaller extent. The binding is usually reversible; covalent binding of reactive drugs such as alkylating agents occurs occasionally. In addition to the binding of drugs to carrier proteins such as albumin, certain drugs may bind to proteins that function as specific hormone carrier proteins, such as the binding of estrogen or testosterone to sex hormone–binding globulin or the binding of thyroid hormone to thyroxin-binding globulin.

The fraction of total drug in plasma that is bound is determined by the drug concentration, the affinity of binding sites for the drug, and the number of binding sites. Mass-action relationships determine the unbound and bound concentrations (described later). At low concentrations of drug (less than the plasma protein binding dissociation constant), the fraction bound is a function of the concentration of binding sites and the dissociation constant. At high drug concentrations (greater than the dissociation constant), the fraction bound is a function of the number of binding sites and the drug concentration. Therefore, plasma binding is a nonlinear, saturable process. For most drugs, the therapeutic range of plasma concentrations is limited; thus, the extent of binding and the unbound fraction are relatively constant. The percentage values listed for protein binding in Appendix II refer to binding in the therapeutic range unless otherwise indicated. The extent of plasma protein binding also may be affected by disease-related factors. For example, hypoalbuminemia secondary to severe liver disease or nephrotic syndrome results in reduced binding and an increase in the unbound fraction. Also, conditions resulting in the acute-phase reaction response (e.g., cancer, arthritis, myocardial infarction, Crohn's disease) lead to elevated levels of α_1-acid glycoprotein and enhanced binding of basic drugs. Changes in protein binding due to disease states and drug-drug interactions are clinically relevant mainly for a small subset of so-called high-clearance drugs of narrow therapeutic index (described later) that are administered intravenously, such as lidocaine (Benet and Hoener, 2002). When changes in plasma protein binding occur in patients, unbound drug rapidly equilibrates throughout the body and only a transient significant change in unbound plasma concentration will occur. Only drugs that show an almost instantaneous relationship between free plasma concentration and effect (e.g., anti-arrhythmics) will show a measureable effect. Thus, unbound plasma drug concentrations will really exhibit significant changes only when either drug input or clearance of unbound drug occurs, as a consequence of metabolism or active transport. A more common problem resulting from competition of drugs for plasma protein-binding sites is misinterpretation of measured concentrations of drugs in plasma because most assays do not distinguish free drug from bound drug.

Importantly, binding of a drug to plasma proteins limits its concentration in tissues and at its site of action because only unbound drug is in equilibrium across membranes. Accordingly, after distribution equilibrium is achieved, the concentration of active, unbound drug in intracellular water is the same as that in plasma except when carrier-mediated transport is involved. Binding of a drug to plasma protein also limits the drug's glomerular filtration because this process does not immediately change the concentration of free drug in the plasma (water is also filtered). However, plasma protein binding generally does not limit renal tubular secretion or biotransformation because these processes lower the free drug concentration, and this is followed rapidly by dissociation of drug from the drug-protein complex, thereby reestablishing equilibrium between bound and free drug. Drug transport and metabolism also are limited by binding to plasma proteins, except when these are especially efficient, and drug clearance, calculated on the basis of unbound drug, exceeds organ plasma flow.

Tissue Binding. Many drugs accumulate in tissues at higher concentrations than those in the extracellular fluids and blood. For example, during long-term administration of the anti-malarial agent quinacrine, the concentration of drug in the liver may be several thousand times that in the blood. Such accumulation may be a result of active transport or, more commonly, binding. Tissue binding of drugs usually occurs with cellular constituents such as proteins, phospholipids, or nuclear proteins and generally is reversible. A large fraction of drug in the body may be bound in this fashion and serve as a reservoir that prolongs drug action in that same tissue or at a distant site reached through the circulation. Such tissue binding and accumulation also can produce local toxicity, as in the case of the accumulation of the aminoglycoside antibiotic gentamicin in the kidney and vestibular system.

Fat as a Reservoir. Many lipid-soluble drugs are stored by physical solution in the neutral fat. In obese persons, the fat content of the body may be as high as 50%, and even in lean individuals fat constitutes 10% of body weight; hence fat may serve as a reservoir for lipid-soluble drugs. For example, as much as 70% of the highly lipid-soluble barbiturate thiopental may be present in body fat 3 hours after administration, when plasma concentrations are negligible and no anesthetic effects are measurable. Fat is a rather stable reservoir because it has a relatively low blood flow. However, among highly lipophilic drugs (e.g., remifentanil and some β blockers), the degree of lipophilicity does not predict their distribution in obese individuals.

Bone. The tetracycline antibiotics (and other divalent metal-ion chelating agents) and heavy metals may accumulate in bone by adsorption onto the bone crystal surface and eventual incorporation into the crystal lattice. Bone can become a reservoir for the slow release of toxic agents such as lead or radium into the blood; their effects thus can persist long after exposure has ceased. Local destruction of the bone medulla also may lead to reduced blood flow and prolongation of the reservoir effect because the toxic agent becomes sealed off from the circulation; this may further enhance the direct local damage to the bone. A vicious cycle results, whereby the greater the exposure to the toxic agent, the slower is its rate of elimination. The adsorption of drug onto the bone crystal surface and incorporation into the crystal lattice have therapeutic advantages for the treatment of osteoporosis. Phosphonates such as sodium etidronate bind tightly to hydroxyapatite crystals in mineralized bone matrix. However, unlike naturally occurring pyrophosphates, etidronate is resistant to degradation by pyrophosphatases and thus stabilizes the bone matrix.

Redistribution. Termination of drug effect after withdrawal of a drug usually is by metabolism and excretion but also may result from redistribution of the drug from its site of action into other tissues or sites. Redistribution is a factor in terminating drug effect primarily when a highly lipid-soluble drug that acts on the brain or cardiovascular system is administered rapidly by intravenous injection or by inhalation. A good example of this is the use of the intravenous anesthetic thiopental, a highly lipid-soluble drug. Because blood flow to the brain is so high, the drug reaches its maximal concentration in brain within a minute of its intravenous injection. After injection is concluded, the plasma concentration falls as thiopental diffuses into other tissues, such as muscle. The concentration of the drug in brain follows that of the plasma because there is little binding of the drug to brain constituents. Thus, in this example, the onset of anesthesia is rapid, but so is its termination. Both are related directly to the concentration of drug in the brain.

CNS and Cerebrospinal Fluid. The distribution of drugs into the CNS from the blood is unique. One reason for this is that the brain capillary endothelial cells have continuous tight junctions; therefore, drug penetration into the brain depends on transcellular rather than paracellular transport. The unique characteristics of brain capillary endothelial cells and pericapillary glial cells constitute the blood-brain barrier. At the choroid plexus, a similar blood-CSF barrier is present, except that it is epithelial cells that are joined by tight junctions rather than endothelial cells. The lipid solubility of the nonionized and unbound species of a drug is therefore an important determinant of its uptake by the brain; the more lipophilic a drug, the more likely it is to cross the blood-brain barrier. This situation often is used in drug design to alter drug distribution to the brain; e.g., the so-called second-generation antihistamines, such as loratadine, achieve far lower brain concentrations than do agents such as diphenhydramine and thus are nonsedating. Drugs may penetrate into the CNS by specific uptake transporters normally involved in the transport of nutrients and endogenous compounds from blood into the brain and CSF.

Another important factor in the functional blood-brain barrier involves membrane transporters that are efflux carriers present in the brain capillary endothelial cell and capable of removing a large number of chemically diverse drugs from the cell. MDR1 (P-gp) and the organic anion–transporting polypeptide (OATP) are two of the more notable of these. The effects of these exporters are to dramatically limit access of the drug to the tissue expressing the efflux transporter. Together, P-gp and the OATP family export a large array of structurally diverse drugs (see Chapter 5 and Maeda et al., 2008). Expression of OATP isoforms and their polymorphic forms in the GI tract, liver, and kidney, as well as the blood-brain barrier, has important implications for drug absorption and elimination, as well as tissue penetration. Expression of these efflux transporters accounts for the relatively restricted pharmacological access to the brain and other tissues such as the testes, where drug concentrations may be below those necessary to achieve a desired effect despite adequate blood flow. This situation occurs with HIV protease inhibitors and with loperamide, a potent, systemically active opioid that lacks the central effects characteristic of other opioids (Chapter 19). Efflux transporters that actively secrete drug from the CSF into the blood also are present in the choroid plexus (see Chapter 5 for details of the contribution of drug transporters to barrier function). Drugs also may exit the CNS along with the bulk flow of CSF through the arachnoid villi. In general, the blood-brain barrier's function is well maintained; however, meningeal and encephalic inflammation increase local permeability. Recently, blood-brain barrier disruption has emerged as a strategy in the treatment of certain brain tumors such as primary CNS lymphomas (Angelov et al., 2009).The goal of this treatment is to enhance delivery of chemotherapy to the brain tumor while maintaining cognitive function that is often damaged by conventional radiotherapy.

Placental Transfer of Drugs. The transfer of drugs across the placenta is of critical importance because drugs may cause anomalies in the developing fetus. Administered immediately before delivery, as is often the case with the use of tocolytics in the treatment of preterm labor, they also may have adverse effects on the neonate. Lipid solubility, extent of plasma binding, and degree of ionization of weak acids and bases are important general determinants in drug transfer across the placenta. The fetal plasma is slightly more acidic than that of the mother (pH 7.0-7.2 versus 7.4), so that ion trapping of basic drugs occurs. As in the brain, P-gp and other export transporters are present in the placenta and function to limit fetal exposure to potentially toxic agents. The view that the placenta is an absolute barrier to drugs is, however, inaccurate, in part because a number of influx transporters are also present (Weier et al., 2008). The fetus is to some extent exposed to all drugs taken by the mother.

EXCRETION OF DRUGS

Drugs are eliminated from the body either unchanged by the process of excretion or converted to metabolites. Excretory organs, the lung excluded, eliminate polar compounds more efficiently than substances with high lipid solubility. Lipid-soluble drugs thus are not readily eliminated until they are metabolized to more polar compounds.

The kidney is the most important organ for excreting drugs and their metabolites. Substances excreted in the feces are principally unabsorbed orally ingested drugs or drug metabolites excreted either in the bile or secreted directly into the intestinal tract and not reabsorbed. Excretion of drugs in breast milk is important not because of the amounts eliminated, but because the excreted drugs are potential sources of unwanted pharmacological effects in the nursing infant (Buhimschi and Weiner, 2009). Excretion from the lung is important mainly for the elimination of anesthetic gases (Chapter 19).

Renal Excretion. Excretion of drugs and metabolites in the urine involves three distinct processes: glomerular filtration, active tubular secretion, and passive tubular reabsorption. Changes in overall renal function generally affect all three processes to a similar extent. Even in healthy persons, renal function is not constant. In neonates, renal function is low compared with body mass but matures rapidly within the first few months after birth. During adulthood, there is a slow decline in renal function, ~1% per year, so that in elderly patients a substantial degree of functional impairment may be present.

The amount of drug entering the tubular lumen by filtration depends on the glomerular filtration rate and the extent of plasma binding of the drug; only unbound drug is filtered. In the proximal renal tubule, active, carrier-mediated tubular secretion also may add drug to the tubular fluid. Transporters such as P-gp and the multidrug-resistance–associated protein type 2 (MRP2), localized in the apical brush-border membrane, are responsible for the secretion of amphipathic anions and conjugated metabolites (such as glucuronides, sulfates, and glutathione adducts), respectively (Chapters 5 and 6). Solute carrier transporters that are more selective for organic cationic drugs are involved in the secretion of organic bases. Membrane transporters, mainly located in the distal renal tubule, also are responsible for any active reabsorption of drug from the tubular lumen back into the systemic circulation; however, most such reabsorption occurs by non-ionic diffusion.

In the proximal and distal tubules, the non-ionized forms of weak acids and bases undergo net passive reabsorption. The concentration gradient for back-diffusion is created by the reabsorption of water with Na^+ and other inorganic ions. Since the tubular cells are less permeable to the ionized forms of weak electrolytes, passive reabsorption of these substances depends on the pH. When the tubular urine is made more alkaline, weak acids are largely ionized and thus are excreted more rapidly and to a greater extent. When the tubular urine is made more acidic, the fraction of drug ionized is reduced, and excretion is likewise reduced. Alkalinization and acidification of the urine have the opposite effects on the excretion of weak bases. In the treatment of drug poisoning, the excretion of some drugs can be hastened by appropriate alkalinization or acidification of the urine. Whether alteration of urine pH results in a significant change in drug elimination depends on the extent and persistence of the pH change and the contribution of pH-dependent passive reabsorption to total drug elimination. The effect is greatest for weak acids and bases with pK_a values in the range of urinary pH (5-8). However, alkalinization of urine can produce a 4-6-fold increase in excretion of a relatively strong acid such as salicylate when urinary pH is changed from 6.4 to 8.0 and the fraction of non-ionized drug is reduced from 1% to 0.04%.

Biliary and Fecal Excretion. Transporters are also present in the canalicular membrane of the hepatocyte, and these actively secrete drugs and metabolites into bile. P-gp and BCRP (breast cancer resistance protein, or ABCG2) transport a plethora of amphipathic lipid-soluble drugs, whereas MRP2 is mainly involved in the secretion of conjugated metabolites of drugs (e.g., glutathione conjugates, glucuronides, and some sulfates). Ultimately, drugs and metabolites present in bile are released into the GI tract during the digestive process. Because secretory transporters also are expressed on the apical membrane of enterocytes, direct secretion of drugs and metabolites may occur from the systemic circulation into the intestinal lumen. Subsequently, drugs and metabolites can be reabsorbed back into the body from the intestine, which, in the case of conjugated metabolites such as glucuronides, may require their enzymatic hydrolysis by the intestinal microflora. Such enterohepatic recycling, if extensive, may prolong significantly the presence of a drug (or toxin) and its effects within the body prior to elimination by other pathways. For this reason, drugs may be given orally to bind substances excreted in the bile. In the case of mercury poisoning, for example, a resin can be administered orally that binds with dimethyl mercury excreted in the bile, thus preventing reabsorption and further toxicity.

Enterohepatic recycling also can be an advantage in the design of drugs. Ezetimibe is the first of a class of drugs that specifically reduces the intestinal absorption of cholesterol (Lipka, 2003). The drug is absorbed into the intestinal epithelial cell, where it is believed to interfere with the sterol transporter system, preventing both free cholesterol and plant sterols (phytosterols) from being transported into the cell from the intestinal lumen. The drug is absorbed rapidly and glucuronidated to an active metabolite in the intestinal cell before secretion into the blood. Absorbed ezetimibe is avidly taken up by the liver from the portal blood and excreted into the bile, resulting in low peripheral blood concentrations. The glucuronide conjugate is hydrolyzed and absorbed, and is equally effective in inhibiting sterol absorption. This enterohepatic recycling is responsible for a $t_{1/2}$ in the body of >20 hours. The principal benefit is a reduction in low-density lipoprotein cholesterol (see Chapter 31 and Dembowki and Davidson, 2009).

Excretion by Other Routes. Excretion of drugs into sweat, saliva, and tears is quantitatively unimportant. Elimination by these routes depends mainly on diffusion of the non-ionized lipid-soluble form of drugs through the epithelial cells of the glands and depends on the pH. Drugs excreted in the saliva enter the mouth, where they are usually swallowed. The concentration of some drugs in saliva parallels that in plasma. Saliva therefore may be a useful biological fluid in which to determine drug concentrations when it is difficult or inconvenient to obtain blood. The same principles apply to excretion of drugs in breast milk. Since milk is more acidic than plasma, basic compounds may be slightly concentrated in this fluid; conversely, the concentration of acidic compounds in the milk is lower than in plasma. Non-electrolytes, such as ethanol and urea, readily enter breast milk and reach the same concentration as in plasma, independent of the pH of the milk. Thus, the administration of drugs to breast-feeding women carries the general caution that the suckling infant will be exposed to some extent to the medication and/or its metabolites. In certain cases, such as treatment with the β blocker atenolol, the infant may be exposed to significant amounts of drug (Ito and Lee, 2003). Although excretion into hair and skin is quantitatively unimportant, sensitive methods of detection of drugs in these tissues have forensic significance.

METABOLISM OF DRUGS

The lipophilic characteristics of drugs that promote their passage through biological membranes and subsequent access to their sites of action hinder their excretion from the body. Renal excretion of unchanged drug is a major route of elimination for 25–30% of drugs administered to humans. The majority of therapeutic agents are lipophilic compounds filtered through the glomerulus and reabsorbed into the systemic circulation during passage through the renal tubules. The metabolism of drugs and other xenobiotics into more hydrophilic metabolites is essential for their elimination from the body, as well as for termination of their biological and pharmacological activity. In general, biotransformation reactions generate more polar, inactive metabolites that are readily excreted from the body. However, in some cases, metabolites with potent biological activity or toxic properties are generated. Many of the enzyme systems that transform drugs to inactive metabolites also generate biologically active metabolites of endogenous compounds, as in steroid biosynthesis. Understanding drug metabolism has spawned the new disciplinary focus of pharmacogenetics, which offers the promise that understanding the expression and activities of specific metabolizing enzyme isoforms in a given individual will permit the clinician to tailor treatments, particularly in chemotherapy (Dawood and Leyland-Jones, 2009), to maximize therapeutic outcomes and minimize risks of toxicity or drug-drug interactions.

Drug metabolism or biotransformation reactions are classified as either phase I functionalization reactions or phase II biosynthetic (conjugation) reactions. Phase I reactions introduce or expose a functional group on the parent compound such as occurs in hydrolysis reactions. Phase I reactions generally result in the loss of pharmacological activity, although there are examples of retention or enhancement of activity. In rare instances, metabolism is associated with an altered pharmacological activity. *Prodrugs* are pharmacologically inactive compounds designed to maximize the amount of the active species that reaches its site of action. Inactive prodrugs are converted rapidly to biologically active metabolites often by the hydrolysis of an ester or amide linkage. Such is the case with a number of angiotensin-converting enzyme (ACE) inhibitors employed in the management of high blood pressure. Enalapril, for instance, is relatively inactive until converted by esterase activity to the diacid enalaprilat. If not excreted rapidly into the urine, the products of phase I biotransformation reactions then can react with endogenous compounds to form a highly water-soluble conjugate.

Phase II conjugation reactions lead to the formation of a covalent linkage between a functional group on the parent compound or phase I metabolite and endogenously derived glucuronic acid, sulfate, glutathione, amino acids, or acetate. These highly polar conjugates generally are inactive and are excreted rapidly in the urine and feces. An example of an active conjugate is the 6-glucuronide metabolite of morphine, which is a more potent analgesic than its parent.

The enzyme systems involved in the biotransformation of drugs are localized primarily in the liver, although every tissue examined has some metabolic activity. Other organs with significant metabolic capacity include the GI tract, kidneys, and lungs. Following oral administration of a drug, a significant portion of the dose may be metabolically inactivated in either the intestinal epithelium or the liver before the drug reaches the systemic circulation. This so-called first-pass metabolism significantly limits the oral availability of highly metabolized drugs. Within a given cell, most drug-metabolizing activity is found in the smooth endoplasmic reticulum and the cytosol, although drug biotransformations also can occur in the mitochondria, nuclear envelope, and plasma membrane. The enzyme systems involved in phase I reactions are located primarily in the endoplasmic reticulum, whereas the phase II conjugation enzyme systems are mainly cytosolic. Often, drugs biotransformed through a phase I reaction in the endoplasmic reticulum are conjugated at this same site or in the cytosolic fraction of the same cell in a sequential fashion. These biotransforming reactions are carried out by CYPs (cytochrome P450 isoforms) and by a variety of transferases. These enzyme families, the major reactions they catalyze, and their roles in drug metabolism and adverse drug responses are presented in detail in Chapter 6.

CLINICAL PHARMACOKINETICS

The fundamental tenet of clinical pharmacokinetics is that a relationship exists between the pharmacological effects of a drug and an accessible concentration of the drug (e.g., in blood or plasma). This relationship has been documented for many drugs and is of benefit in the therapeutic management of patients. For some drugs, no clear or simple relationship has been found between pharmacological effect and concentration in plasma, whereas for other drugs, routine measurement of drug concentration is impractical as part of therapeutic monitoring. In most cases, as depicted in Figure 2–1, the concentration of drug at its sites of action will be related to the concentration of drug in the systemic circulation. The pharmacological effect that results may be the clinical effect desired, a toxic effect, or in some cases an effect unrelated to the known therapeutic efficacy or toxicity. Clinical pharmacokinetics attempts to provide both a quantitative relationship between dose and effect and a framework within which to interpret measurements of concentrations of drugs in biological fluids and their adjustment through changes in dosing for the benefit of the patient. The importance of pharmacokinetics in patient care is based on the improvement in therapeutic efficacy and the avoidance of unwanted effects that can be attained by application of its principles when dosage regimens are chosen and modified.

The four most important parameters governing drug disposition are *bioavailability*, the fraction of drug absorbed as such into the systemic circulation; *volume of distribution,* a measure of the apparent space in the body available to contain the drug based on how much is given versus what is found in the systemic circulation; *clearance,* a measure of the body's efficiency in eliminating drug from the systemic circulation; and *elimination* $t_{1/2}$, a measure of the rate of removal of drug from the systemic circulation. We will deal with each of these parameters in turn, and will explore mathematical relationships that use them to describe the time course of plasma drug accumulation and to design dosage regimens based on physiologic and pathophysiologic variables of individual patients.

Clearance

Clearance is the most important concept to consider when designing a rational regimen for long-term drug administration. The clinician usually wants to maintain steady-state concentrations of a drug within a *therapeutic window* or range associated with therapeutic efficacy and a minimum of toxicity for a given agent. Assuming complete bioavailability, the steady-state concentration of drug in the body will be achieved when the rate of drug elimination equals the rate of drug administration. Thus:

$$\text{Dosing rate} = CL \cdot C_{ss} \qquad \text{(Equation 2–2)}$$

where CL is clearance of drug from the systemic circulation and C_{ss} is the steady-state concentration of drug. If the desired steady-state concentration of drug in plasma or blood is known, the rate of clearance of drug by the patient will dictate the rate at which the drug should be administered.

The concept of clearance is extremely useful in clinical pharmacokinetics because its value for a particular drug usually is constant over the range of concentrations encountered clinically. This is true because systems for elimination of drugs such as metabolizing enzymes and transporters usually are not saturated, and thus the absolute rate of elimination of the drug is essentially a linear function of its concentration in plasma. That is, the elimination of most drugs follows first-order kinetics, where a constant fraction of drug in the body is eliminated per unit of time. If mechanisms for elimination of a given drug become saturated, the kinetics approach zero order, in which a constant amount of drug is eliminated per unit of time.

Under such a circumstance, clearance (CL) will vary with the concentration of drug, often according to the equation

$$CL = v_m/(K_m + C) \quad \text{(Equation 2–3)}$$

where K_m represents the concentration at which half the maximal rate of elimination is reached (in units of mass/volume) and v_m is equal to the maximal rate of elimination (in units of mass/time). Thus, clearance is derived in units of volume/time. This equation is analogous to the Michaelis-Menten equation for enzyme kinetics. Design of dosage regimens for drugs with zero-order elimination kinetics is more complex than when elimination is first-order (described later).

Principles of drug clearance are similar to those of renal physiology, where, e.g., creatinine clearance is defined as the rate of elimination of creatinine in the urine relative to its concentration in plasma. At the simplest level, clearance of a drug is its rate of elimination by all routes normalized to the concentration of drug C in some biological fluid where measurement can be made:

$$CL = \text{rate of elimination}/C \quad \text{(Equation 2–4)}$$

Thus, when clearance is constant, the rate of drug elimination is directly proportional to drug concentration. Note that clearance does not indicate how much drug is being removed, but rather the volume of biological fluid such as blood or plasma from which drug would have to be completely removed to account for the clearance per unit of body weight (e.g., mL/min per kg). Clearance can be defined further as blood clearance (CL_b), plasma clearance (CL_p), or clearance based on the concentration of unbound drug (CL_u), depending on the measurement made (C_b, C_p, or C_u).

Clearance of drug by several organs is additive. Elimination of drug from the systemic circulation may occur as a result of processes that occur in the kidney, liver, and other organs. Division of the rate of elimination by each organ by a concentration of drug (e.g., plasma concentration) will yield the respective clearance by that organ. Added together, these separate clearances will equal systemic clearance:

$$CL_{renal} + CL_{hepatic} + CL_{other} = CL \quad \text{(Equation 2–5)}$$

Other routes of elimination could include loss of drug in saliva or sweat, secretion into the GI tract, volatile elimination from the lung, and metabolism at other sites such as skin. Note that changes in clearance in one organ will change the overall calculation; thus, renal failure alters CL for drugs excreted unchanged from the plasma.

Systemic clearance may be determined at steady state by using Equation 2–2. For a single dose of a drug with complete bioavailability and first-order kinetics of elimination, systemic clearance may be determined from mass balance and the integration of Equation 2–4 over time:

$$CL = \text{Dose}/AUC \quad \text{(Equation 2–6)}$$

where AUC is the total area under the curve that describes the measured concentration of drug in the systemic circulation as a function of time (from zero to infinity), as in Figure 2–6.

Examples. The plasma clearance for the antibiotic cephalexin is 4.3 mL/min/kg, with 90% of the drug excreted unchanged in the urine. For a 70-kg man, the clearance from plasma would be 301 mL/min, with renal clearance accounting for 90% of this elimination. In other words, the kidney is able to excrete cephalexin at a rate such that the drug is completely removed (cleared) from ~270 mL of plasma every minute (renal clearance = 90% of total clearance). Because clearance usually is assumed to remain constant in a medically stable patient (e.g., no acute decline in kidney function), the rate of elimination of cephalexin will depend on the concentration of drug in the plasma (Equation 2–4).

The β adrenergic receptor antagonist propranolol is cleared from the blood at a rate of 16 mL/min/ kg (or 1120 mL/min in a 70-kg man), almost exclusively by the liver. Thus, the liver is able to remove the amount of propranolol contained in 1120 mL of blood in 1 minute. Even though the liver is the dominant organ for elimination, the plasma clearance of some drugs exceeds the rate of blood flow to this organ. Often this is so because the drug partitions readily into red blood cells (RBCs) and the rate of drug delivered to the eliminating organ is considerably higher than expected from measurement of its concentration in plasma. The relationship between plasma (subscript p; acellular) and blood (subscript b; all components) clearance at steady state is given by

$$\frac{CL_p}{CL_b} = \frac{C_b}{C_p} = 1 + H\left[\frac{C_{rbc}}{C_p} - 1\right] \quad \text{(Equation 2–7)}$$

Clearance from the blood therefore may be estimated by dividing the plasma clearance by the drug's blood-to-plasma concentration ratio, obtained from knowledge of the hematocrit ($H = 0.45$) and the red cell to plasma concentration ratio. In most instances, the blood clearance will be less than liver blood flow (1.5 L/min) or, if renal excretion also is involved, the sum of the blood flows to each eliminating organ. For example, the plasma clearance of the immunomodulator, tacrolimus, ~2 L/min, is more than twice the hepatic plasma flow rate and even exceeds the organ's blood flow despite the fact that the liver is the predominant site of this drug's extensive metabolism. However, after taking into account the extensive distribution of tacrolimus into red cells, its clearance from the blood is only ~63 mL/min, and it is actually a low- rather than high-clearance drug, as might be interpreted from the plasma clearance value alone. Sometimes, however, clearance from the blood by metabolism exceeds liver blood flow, and this indicates extrahepatic metabolism. In the case of the β_1 receptor antagonist, esmolol, the blood clearance value (11.9 L/min) is greater than cardiac output (~5.3 L/min) because the drug is metabolized efficiently by esterases present in red blood cells.

A further definition of clearance is useful for understanding the effects of pathological and physiological variables on drug elimination, particularly with respect to an individual organ. The rate of presentation of drug to the organ is the product of blood flow (Q) and the arterial drug concentration (C_A), and the rate of exit of drug from the organ is the product of blood flow and the venous drug concentration (C_V). The difference between these rates at steady state is the rate of drug elimination by that organ:

$$\begin{aligned}\text{Rate of elimination} &= Q \cdot C_A - Q \cdot C_V \\ &= Q(C_A - C_V) \quad \text{(Equation 2–8)}\end{aligned}$$

Division of Equation 2–8 by the concentration of drug entering the organ of elimination C_A yields an expression for clearance of the drug by the organ in question:

$$CL_{organ} = Q\left[\frac{C_A - C_V}{C_A}\right] = Q \cdot E \qquad \text{(Equation 2–9)}$$

The expression $(C_A - C_V)/C_A$ in Equation 2–9 can be referred to as the *extraction ratio (E)* of the drug. While not employed in general medical practice, calculations of a drug's extraction ratio(s) are useful for modeling the effects of disease of a given metabolizing organ on clearance and in the design of ideal therapeutic properties of drugs in development.

Hepatic Clearance. The concepts developed in Equation 2–9 have important implications for drugs that are eliminated by the liver. Consider a drug that is removed efficiently from the blood by hepatic processes—metabolism and/or excretion of drug into the bile. In this instance, the concentration of drug in the blood leaving the liver will be low, the extraction ratio will approach unity, and the clearance of the drug from blood will become limited by hepatic blood flow. Drugs that are cleared efficiently by the liver (e.g., drugs in Appendix II with systemic clearances >6 mL/min/kg, such as diltiazem, imipramine, lidocaine, morphine, and propranolol) are restricted in their rate of elimination not by intra-hepatic processes but by the rate at which they can be transported in the blood to the liver.

Additional complexities also may be considered. For example, the equations presented earlier do not account for drug binding to components of blood and tissues, nor do they permit an estimation of the intrinsic capacity of the liver to eliminate a drug in the absence of limitations imposed by blood flow, termed *intrinsic clearance*. In biochemical terms and under first-order conditions, intrinsic clearance is a measure of the ratio of the Michaelis-Menten kinetic parameters for the eliminating process (i.e., v_m/K_m) and thus reflects the maximum metabolic or transport capability of the clearing organ. Extensions of the relationships of Equation 2–9 to include expressions for protein binding and intrinsic clearance have been proposed for a number of models of hepatic elimination (Hallifax and Houston, 2009). Models indicate that when the capacity of the eliminating organ to metabolize the drug is large in comparison with the rate of presentation of drug to the organ, clearance will approximate the organ's blood flow. By contrast, when the drug-metabolizing capacity is small in comparison with the rate of drug presentation, clearance will be proportional to the unbound fraction of drug in blood and the drug's intrinsic clearance. Appreciation of these concepts allows understanding of a number of possibly puzzling experimental results. For example, enzyme induction or hepatic disease may change the rate of drug metabolism in an isolated hepatic microsomal enzyme system but not change clearance in the whole animal. For a drug with a high extraction ratio, clearance is limited by blood flow, and changes in intrinsic clearance owing to enzyme induction or hepatic disease should have little effect. Similarly, for drugs with high extraction ratios, changes in protein binding owing to disease or competitive binding interactions by other drugs should have little effect on clearance. Conversely, changes in intrinsic clearance and protein binding will affect the clearance of drugs with low intrinsic clearances such as warfarin, and thus extraction ratios, but changes in blood flow will have little effect.

Renal Clearance. Renal clearance of a drug results in its appearance in the urine. In considering the impact of renal disease on the clearance of a drug, complications that relate to filtration, active secretion by the kidney tubule, and reabsorption from it must be considered along with blood flow. The rate of filtration of a drug depends on the volume of fluid that is filtered in the glomerulus and the unbound concentration of drug in plasma, because drug bound to protein is not filtered. The rate of secretion of drug by the kidney will depend on the drug's intrinsic clearance by the transporters involved in active secretion as affected by the drug's binding to plasma proteins, the degree of saturation of these transporters, and the rate of delivery of the drug to the secretory site. In addition, processes involved in drug reabsorption from the tubular fluid must be considered. The influences of changes in protein binding and blood flow and in the number of functional nephrons are analogous to the examples given earlier for hepatic elimination.

DISTRIBUTION

Volume of Distribution. Volume is a second fundamental parameter that is useful in considering processes of drug disposition. The volume of distribution (*V*) relates the amount of drug in the body to the concentration of drug (*C*) in the blood or plasma depending on the fluid measured. This volume does not necessarily refer to an identifiable physiological volume but rather to the fluid volume that would be required to contain all of the drug in the body at the same concentration measured in the blood or plasma:

$$\text{Amount of drug in body}/V = C \quad \text{or} \qquad \text{(Equation 2–10)}$$
$$V = \text{amount of drug in body}/C$$

A drug's volume of distribution therefore reflects the extent to which it is present in extravascular tissues and not in the plasma. It is reasonable to view V as an imaginary volume, since for many drugs the volume of distribution exceeds the known volume of any and all body compartments. For example, the value of V for the highly lipophilic anti-malarial chloroquine is some 15,000 L, yet the plasma volume of a typical 70-kg man is 3 L, blood volume is ~5.5 L, extracellular fluid volume outside the plasma is 12 L, and the volume of total-body water is ~42 L.

Many drugs exhibit volumes of distribution far in excess of these values. For example, if 500 μg of the cardiac glycoside digoxin were in the body of a 70-kg subject, a plasma concentration of ~0.75 ng/mL would be observed. Dividing the amount of drug in the body by the plasma concentration yields a volume of distribution for digoxin of ~667 L, or a value ~15 times greater than the total-body volume of a 70-kg man. In fact, digoxin distributes preferentially to muscle and adipose tissue and to its specific receptors (Na^+,K^+-ATPase), leaving a very small amount of drug in the plasma to be measured. For drugs that are bound extensively to plasma proteins but that are not bound to tissue components, the volume of distribution will approach that of the plasma volume because drug bound to plasma protein is measurable in the assay of most drugs. In contrast, certain drugs have high volumes of distribution even though most of the drug in the circulation is bound to albumin because these drugs are also sequestered elsewhere.

The volume of distribution may vary widely depending on the relative degrees of binding to high-affinity receptor sites, plasma and tissue proteins, the partition coefficient of the drug in fat, and accumulation in poorly perfused tissues. As might be expected, the volume of distribution for a given drug can differ according to patient's age, gender, body composition, and presence of disease. Total-body water of infants younger than 1 year of age, for example, is 75–80% of body weight, whereas that of adult males is 60% and that of females is 55%.

Several volume terms are used commonly to describe drug distribution, and they have been derived in a number of ways. The volume of distribution defined in Equation 2–10 considers the body as a single homogeneous compartment. In this one-compartment model, all drug administration occurs directly into the central compartment, and distribution of drug is instantaneous throughout the volume (V). Clearance of drug from this compartment occurs in a first-order fashion, as defined in Equation 2–4; that is, the amount of drug eliminated per unit of time depends on the amount (concentration) of drug in the body compartment. Figure 2–4A and Equation 2–11 describe the decline of plasma concentration with time for a drug introduced into this central compartment:

$$C = [\text{dose}/V][e^{-kt}] \qquad \text{(Equation 2–11)}$$

where k is the rate constant for elimination that reflects the fraction of drug removed from the compartment per unit of time. This rate constant is inversely related to the $t_{1/2}$ of the drug [$kt_{1/2} = 0.693 = \ln 2$].

The idealized one-compartment model discussed earlier does not describe the entire time course of the plasma concentration. That is, certain tissue reservoirs can be distinguished from the central compartment, and the drug concentration appears to decay in a manner that can be described by multiple exponential terms (Figure 2–4B).

Rate of Distribution. The multiple exponential decay observed for a drug that is eliminated from the body with first-order kinetics results from differences in the rates at which the drug equilibrates to and within tissues. The rate of equilibration will depend on the ratio of the perfusion of the tissue to the partition of drug into the tissue. In many cases, groups of tissues with similar perfusion-partition ratios all equilibrate at essentially the same rate such that only one apparent phase of distribution is seen (rapid initial fall of concentration of intravenously injected drug, as in Figure 2–4B). It is as though the drug starts in a "central" volume (Figure 2–1), which

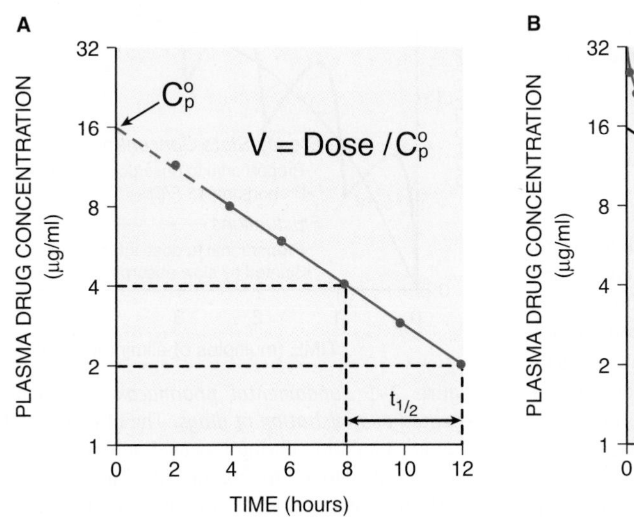

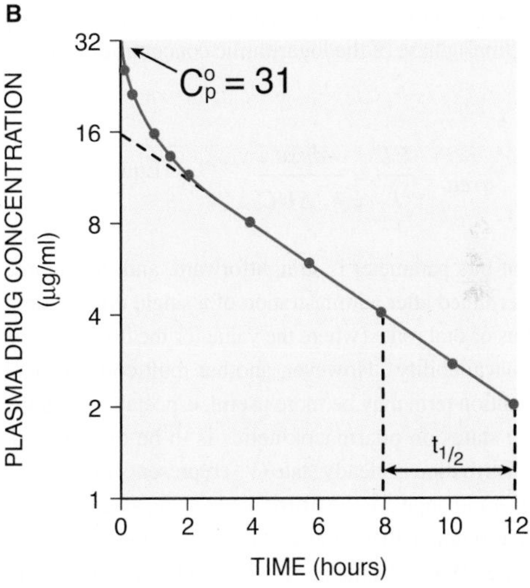

Figure 2–4 *Plasma concentration-time curves following intravenous administration of a drug (500 mg) to a 70-kg patient.*
A. Drug concentrations are measured in plasma at 2-hour intervals following drug administration. The semi-logarithmic plot of plasma concentration (C_p) versus time appears to indicate that the drug is eliminated from a single compartment by a first-order process (Equation 2–11) with a $t_{1/2}$ of 4 hours ($k = 0.693/t_{1/2} = 0.173\ hr^{-1}$). The volume of distribution (V) may be determined from the value of C_p obtained by extrapolation to $t = 0$ ($C_p^o = 16\ \mu g/mL$). Volume of distribution (Equation 2–10) for the one-compartment model is 31.3 L, or 0.45 L/kg ($V = \text{dose}/C_p^o$). The clearance for this drug is 90 mL/min; for a one-compartment model, $CL = kV$.
B. Sampling before 2 hours indicates that in fact the drug follows multi-exponential kinetics. The terminal disposition $t_{1/2}$ is 4 hours, clearance is 84 mL/min (Equation 2–6), V_{area} is 29 L (Equation 2–11), and V_{ss} is 26.8 L. The initial or "central" distribution volume for the drug ($V_1 = \text{dose}/C_p^o$) is 16.1 L. The example chosen indicates that multicompartment kinetics may be overlooked when sampling at early times is neglected. In this particular case, there is only a 10% error in the estimate of clearance when the multicompartment characteristics are ignored. For many drugs, multicompartment kinetics may be observed for significant periods of time, and failure to consider the distribution phase can lead to significant errors in estimates of clearance and in predictions of the appropriate dosage. Also, the difference between the "central" distribution volume and other terms reflecting wider distribution is important in deciding a loading dose strategy.

consists of plasma and tissue reservoirs that are in rapid equilibrium with it, and distributes to a "final" volume, at which point concentrations in plasma decrease in a log-linear fashion with a rate constant of k (Figure 2–4B). The multicompartment model of drug disposition can be viewed as though the blood and highly perfused lean organs such as heart, brain, liver, lung, and kidneys cluster as a single central compartment, whereas more slowly perfused tissues such as muscle, skin, fat, and bone behave as the final compartment (the tissue compartment).

If the pattern or ratio of blood flow to various tissues changes within an individual or differs among individuals, rates of drug distribution to tissues also will change. However, changes in blood flow also may cause some tissues that were originally in the "central" volume to equilibrate sufficiently more slowly so as to appear only in the "final" volume. This means that central volumes will appear to vary with disease states that cause altered regional blood flow (such as would be seen in cirrhosis of the liver). After an intravenous bolus dose, drug concentrations in plasma may be higher in individuals with poor perfusion (e.g., shock) than they would be if perfusion were better. These higher systemic concentrations may in turn cause higher concentrations (and greater effects) in tissues such as brain and heart, whose usually high perfusion has not been reduced by the altered hemodynamic state. Thus, the effect of a drug at various sites of action can vary depending on perfusion of these sites.

Multicompartment Volume Terms. Two different terms have been used to describe the volume of distribution for drugs that follow multiple exponential decay. The first, designated V_{area}, is calculated as the ratio of clearance to the rate of decline in concentration during the elimination (final) phase of the logarithmic concentration versus time curve:

$$V_{area} = \frac{CL}{k} = \frac{dose}{k \cdot AUC} \qquad \text{(Equation 2–12)}$$

The estimation of this parameter is straightforward, and the volume term may be determined after administration of a single dose of drug by the intravenous or oral route (where the value for the dose must be corrected for bioavailability). However, another multicompartment volume of distribution term may be more useful, especially when the effect of disease states on pharmacokinetics is to be determined. The volume of distribution at steady state (V_{ss}) represents the volume in which a drug would appear to be distributed during steady state if the drug existed throughout that volume at the same concentration as that in the measured fluid (plasma or blood). V_{ss} also may be appreciated as shown in Equation 2–13, where V_c is the volume of distribution of drug in the central compartment and V_T is the volume term for drug in the tissue compartment:

$$V_{ss} = V_C + V_T \qquad \text{(Equation 2–13)}$$

Although V_{area} is a convenient and easily calculated parameter, it varies when the rate constant for drug elimination changes, even when there has been no change in the distribution space. This is so because the terminal rate of decline of the concentration of drug in blood or plasma depends not only on clearance but also on the rates of distribution of drug between the "central" and "final" volumes. V_{ss} does not suffer from this disadvantage. The value of V_{area} will always be greater than V_{ss}. As will be described, the extent of this difference will depend on the difference in $t_{1/2}$ observed during a dosing interval at steady state versus the value found for the terminal $t_{1/2}$. V_{ss} can only be determined accurately if the drug is given intravenously.

Steady State. Equation 2–2 (dosing rate = CL · C_{ss}) indicates that a steady-state concentration eventually will be achieved when a drug is administered at a constant rate. At this point, drug elimination (the product of clearance and concentration; Equation 2–4) will equal the rate of drug availability. This concept also extends to regular intermittent dosage (e.g., 250 mg of drug every 8 hours). During each interdose interval, the concentration of drug rises with absorption and falls by elimination. At steady state, the entire cycle is repeated identically in each interval (Figure 2–5). Equation 2–2

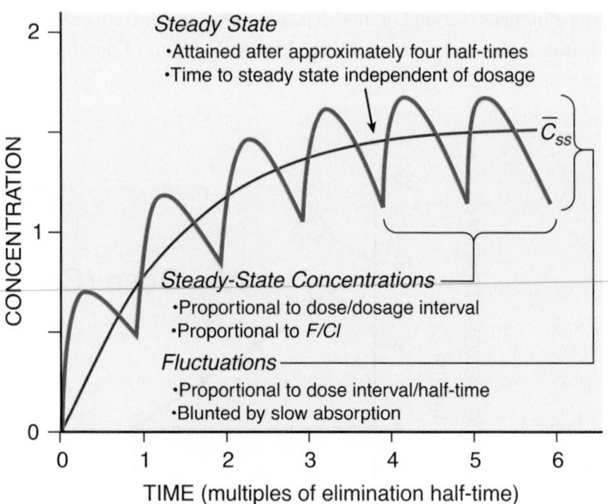

Figure 2–5 ***Fundamental pharmacokinetic relationships for repeated administration of drugs.*** The blue line is the pattern of drug accumulation during repeated administration of a drug at intervals equal to its elimination half-time when drug absorption is 10 times as rapid as elimination. As the rate of absorption increases, the concentration maxima approach 2 and the minima approach 1 during the steady state. The black line depicts the pattern during administration of equivalent dosage by continuous intravenous infusion. Curves are based on the one-compartment model. Average concentration ($\bar{C}_{ss}$) when the steady state is attained during intermittent drug administration is

where F is fractional bioavailability of the dose and T is dosage interval (time). By substitution of infusion rate for $F \cdot$ dose/T, the formula is equivalent to Equation 2–2 and provides the concentration maintained at steady state during continuous intravenous infusion.

still applies for intermittent dosing, but it now describes the average steady-state drug concentration ($\bar{C}_{ss}$) during an interdose interval.

Half-Life. The $t_{1/2}$ is the time it takes for the plasma concentration to be reduced by 50%. For a one-compartment model (Figure 2–4A), $t_{1/2}$ may be determined readily by inspection and used to make decisions about drug dosage. However, as indicated in Figure 2–4B, drug concentrations in plasma often follow a multi-exponential pattern of decline, reflecting the changing amount of drug in the body. When using pharmacokinetics to calculate drug dosing in disease, note in Equation 2-14 that $t_{1/2}$ changes as a function of both clearance and volume of distribution.

$$t_{1/2} \cong 0.693 \cdot V_{ss}/CL \qquad \text{(Equation 2–14)}$$

This $t_{1/2}$ reflects the decline of systemic drug concentrations during a dosing interval at steady-state as depicted in Figure 2–5.

Examples of the marked differences in terminal versus steady-state $t_{1/2}$ (which reflect the difference between V_{area} and V_{ss}) are gentamicin and indomethacin. A terminal $t_{1/2}$ of 53 hours is observed for gentamicin (versus the steady-state value of 2-3 hours); biliary cycling probably is responsible for the 120-hour terminal value for indomethacin (compared to the steady-state value of 2.4 hours). The appreciation of longer terminal $t_{1/2}$ values for some medications may relate to their accumulation in tissues during chronic dosing or shorter periods of high-dose treatment. Such is the case for gentamicin, where the terminal $t_{1/2}$ is associated with renal and ototoxicities. The relevance of a particular $t_{1/2}$ may be defined in terms of the fraction of the clearance and volume of distribution that is related to each $t_{1/2}$ and whether plasma concentrations or amounts of drug in the body are best related to measures of response.

Clearance is the measure of the body's ability to eliminate a drug; thus, as clearance decreases, owing to a disease process, e.g., $t_{1/2}$ would be expected to increase. However, this reciprocal relationship is valid only when the disease does not change the volume of distribution. For example, the $t_{1/2}$ of diazepam increases with increasing age; however, it is not clearance that changes as a function of age but rather the volume of distribution. Similarly, changes in protein binding of a drug may affect its clearance as well as its volume of distribution, leading to unpredictable changes in $t_{1/2}$ as a function of disease. The $t_{1/2}$ of tolbutamide, e.g., decreases in patients with acute viral hepatitis in a fashion opposite from what one might expect. The disease alters the drug's protein binding in both plasma and tissues, causing no change in volume of distribution but an increase in clearance because higher concentrations of unbound drug are present in the bloodstream.

Although it can be a poor index of drug elimination from the body *per se* (disappearance of drug may be the result of formation of undetected metabolites that have therapeutic or unwanted effects), the $t_{1/2}$ defined in Equation 2–14 provides an approximation of the time required to reach steady state after a dosage regimen is initiated or changed (e.g., four half-lives to reach ~94% of a new steady state) and a means to estimate the appropriate dosing interval (see the later discussion and Sahin and Benet, 2008).

Extent and Rate of Bioavailability

Bioavailability. It is important to distinguish between the rate and extent of drug absorption and the amount of drug that ultimately reaches the systemic circulation. The amount of the drug that reaches the systemic circulation depends not only on the administered dose but also on the fraction of the dose (F) that is absorbed and escapes any first-pass elimination. This fraction is the drug's *bioavailability*. Reasons for incomplete absorption were discussed earlier. Also, as noted previously, if the drug is metabolized in the intestinal epithelium or the liver, or excreted in bile, some of the active drug absorbed from the GI tract will be eliminated before it can reach the general circulation and be distributed to its sites of action.

Knowing the extraction ratio (E_H) for a drug across the liver (Equation 2–9), it is possible to predict the maximum oral availability (F_{max}), assuming that hepatic elimination follows first-order processes:

$$F_{max} = 1 - E_H = 1 - (CL_{hepatic}/Q_{hepatic}) \qquad \text{(Equation 2–15)}$$

Thus, if the hepatic blood clearance for the drug is large relative to hepatic blood flow, the extent of availability will be low when the drug is given orally (e.g., lidocaine or propranolol). This reduction in availability is a function of the physiological site from which absorption takes place, and no modification of dosage form will improve the availability under conditions of linear kinetics. Incomplete absorption and/or intestinal metabolism following oral dosing will, in practice, reduce this predicted maximal value of F.

When drugs are administered by a route that is subject to first-pass loss, the equations presented previously that contain the terms *dose* or *dosing rate* (Equations 2–2, 2–6, 2–11, and 2–12) also must include the bioavailability term F such that the available dose or dosing rate is used. For example, Equation 2–2 is modified to

$$F \cdot \text{dosing rate} = CL \cdot C_{ss} \qquad \text{(Equation 2–16)}$$

where the value of F is between 0 and 1. The value of F varies widely for drugs administered by mouth. Etidronate, a bisphosphonate used to stabilize bone matrix in the treatment of Paget's disease and osteoporosis, has an F of 0.03, meaning that only 3% of the drug appears in the bloodstream following oral dosing. In the case of etidronate, therapy using oral administration is still useful, and the dose of the drug administered per kilogram is larger than would be given by injection.

Rate of Absorption. Although the rate of drug absorption does not, in general, influence the average steady-state concentration of the drug in plasma, it may still influence drug therapy. If a drug is absorbed rapidly (e.g., a dose given as an intravenous bolus) and has a small "central" volume, the concentration of drug initially will be high. It will then fall as the drug is distributed to its "final" (larger) volume (Figure 2–4B). If the same drug is absorbed more slowly (e.g., by slow infusion), a significant amount of the drug will be distributed while it is being administered, and peak concentrations will be lower and will occur later. Controlled-release oral preparations are designed to provide a slow and sustained rate of absorption in order to produce smaller fluctuations in the plasma concentration-time profile during the dosage interval compared with more immediate-release formulations. A given drug may act to produce both desirable and undesirable effects at several sites in the body, and the rates of distribution of drug to these sites may not be the same. The relative intensities of these different effects of a drug thus may vary transiently when its rate of administration is changed. Since the beneficial, nontoxic effects of drugs are based on knowledge of an ideal or desired plasma concentration range, maintaining that range while avoiding large swings between peak and trough concentrations can improve therapeutic outcome.

Nonlinear Pharmacokinetics

Nonlinearity in pharmacokinetics (i.e., changes in such parameters as clearance, volume of distribution, and $t_{1/2}$ as a function of dose or concentration of drug) usually is due to saturation of either protein binding, hepatic metabolism, or active renal transport of the drug.

Saturable Protein Binding. As the molar concentration of drug increases, the unbound fraction eventually also must increase (as all binding sites become saturated). This usually occurs only when drug concentrations in plasma are in the range of tens to hundreds of micrograms per milliliter. For a drug that is metabolized by the liver with a low intrinsic clearance-extraction ratio, saturation of plasma-protein binding will cause both V and CL to increase as drug concentrations increase; $t_{1/2}$ thus may remain constant (Equation 2–14). For such a drug, C_{ss} will not increase linearly as the rate of drug administration is increased. For drugs that are cleared with high intrinsic clearance-extraction ratios, C_{ss} can remain linearly proportional to the rate of drug administration. In this case, hepatic clearance will not change, and the increase in V will increase the half-time of disappearance by reducing the fraction of the total drug in the body that is delivered to the liver per unit of time. Most drugs fall between these two extremes, and the effects of nonlinear protein binding may be difficult to predict.

Saturable Elimination. In this situation, the Michaelis-Menten equation (Equation 2–3) usually describes the nonlinearity. All active processes are undoubtedly saturable, but they will appear to be linear if values of drug concentrations encountered in practice are much less than K_m. When drug concentrations exceed K_m, nonlinear kinetics are observed. The major consequences of saturation of metabolism or transport are the opposite of those for saturation of protein binding. Saturation of protein binding will lead to increased CL because CL increases as drug concentration increases, whereas saturation of metabolism or transport may decrease CL. When both conditions are present simultaneously, they may virtually cancel each others' effects, and surprisingly linear kinetics may result; this occurs over a certain range of concentrations for salicylic acid, for example.

Saturable metabolism causes oral first-pass metabolism to be less than expected (higher F), and there is a greater fractional increase in C_{ss} than the corresponding fractional increase in the rate of drug administration. The latter can be seen most easily by substituting Equation 2–3 into Equation 2–2 and solving for the steady-state concentration:

$$C_{ss} = \frac{\text{dosing rate} \cdot K_m}{v_m - \text{dosing rate}} \qquad \text{(Equation 2–17)}$$

As the dosing rate approaches the maximal elimination rate (v_m), the denominator of Equation 2–17 approaches zero, and C_{ss} increases disproportionately. Because saturation of metabolism should have no effect on the volume of distribution, clearance and the relative rate of drug elimination decrease as the concentration increases; therefore, the log C_p time curve is concave-decreasing until metabolism becomes sufficiently desaturated and first-order elimination is present. Thus, the concept of a constant $t_{1/2}$ is not applicable to nonlinear metabolism occurring in the usual range of clinical concentrations. Consequently, changing the dosing rate for a drug with nonlinear metabolism is difficult and unpredictable because the resulting steady state is reached more slowly, and importantly, the effect is disproportionate to the alteration in the dosing rate.

The anti-seizure medication phenytoin provides an example of a drug for which metabolism becomes saturated in the therapeutic range of concentrations. Its $t_{1/2}$ is 6-24 hours. For clearance, K_m (5-10 mg/L) is typically near the lower end of the therapeutic range (10-20 mg/L). For some individuals, especially young children and newborns being treated for emergent seizures, K_m may be as low as 1 mg/L. If, for an adult, the target concentration is 15 mg/L and this is attained at a dosing rate of 300 mg/day, then from Equation (2–17), v_m equals 320 mg/day. For such a patient, a dose that is 10% less than optimal (i.e., 270 mg/day) will produce a C_{ss} of 5 mg/L, well below the desired value. In contrast, a dose that is 10% greater than optimal (330 mg/day) will exceed metabolic capacity (by 10 mg/day) and cause a long, slow and unending climb in concentration during which toxicity will occur. Dosage cannot be controlled so precisely (<10% error). Therefore, for patients in whom the target concentration for phenytoin is more than ten times greater than the K_m, alternating between inefficacious therapy and toxicity is almost unavoidable. For a drug such as phenytoin that has a narrow therapeutic index and exhibits nonlinear metabolism, therapeutic drug monitoring (described later) is most important. When the patient is a neonate, appreciation of this concept is of particular concern because signs and symptoms of toxicity are particularly difficult to monitor. In such cases, a pharmacokinetic consult is appropriate.

Design and Optimization of Dosage Regimens

Following administration of a dose of drug, its effects usually show a characteristic temporal pattern (Figure 2–6).

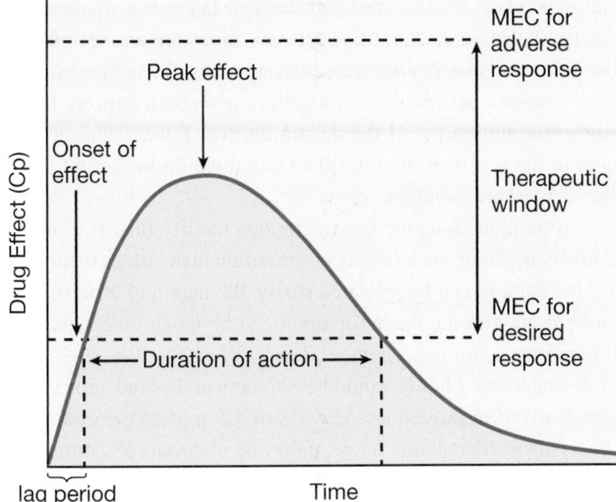

Figure 2–6 *Temporal characteristics of drug effect and relationship to the therapeutic window (e.g., single dose, oral administration).* A lag period is present before the plasma drug concentration (Cp) exceeds the minimum effective concentration (MEC) for the desired effect. Following onset of the response, the intensity of the effect increases as the drug continues to be absorbed and distributed. This reaches a peak, after which drug elimination results in a decline in Cp and in the effect's intensity. Effect disappears when the drug concentration falls below the MEC. Accordingly, the duration of a drug's action is determined by the time period over which concentrations exceed the MEC. An MEC exists for each adverse response, and if drug concentration exceeds this, toxicity will result. The therapeutic goal is to obtain and maintain concentrations within the therapeutic window for the desired response with a minimum of toxicity. Drug response below the MEC for the desired effect will be subtherapeutic; above the MEC for an adverse effect, the probability of toxicity will increase. Increasing or decreasing drug dosage shifts the response curve up or down the intensity scale and is used to modulate the drug's effect. Increasing the dose also prolongs a drug's duration of action but at the risk of increasing the likelihood of adverse effects. Unless the drug is nontoxic (e.g., penicillins), increasing the dose is not a useful strategy for extending the duration of action. Instead, another dose of drug should be given, timed to maintain concentrations within the therapeutic window. The area under the blood concentration-time curve (area under the curve, or AUC, shaded in gray) can be used to calculate the clearance (Equation 2–6) for first-order elimination. The AUC is also used as a measure of bioavailability (defined as 100% for an intravenously administered drug). Bioavailability will be <100% for orally administered drugs, due mainly to incomplete absorption and first-pass metabolism and elimination.

Onset of the effect is preceded by a lag period, after which the magnitude of the effect increases to a maximum and then declines; if a further dose is not administered, the effect eventually disappears as the drug is eliminated. This time course reflects changes in the drug's concentration as determined by the pharmacokinetics of its absorption, distribution, and elimination. Accordingly, the intensity of a drug's effect is related to its concentration above a minimum effective concentration, whereas the duration of the drug's effect reflects the length of time the drug level is above this value. These considerations, in general, apply to both desired and undesired (adverse) drug effects, and as a result, a *therapeutic window* exists that reflects a concentration range that provides efficacy without unacceptable toxicity.

Similar considerations apply after multiple dosing associated with long-term therapy, and they determine the amount and frequency of drug administration to achieve an optimal therapeutic effect. In general, the lower limit of a drug's therapeutic range is approximately equal to the drug concentration that produces about half the greatest possible therapeutic effect, and the upper limit of the therapeutic range is such that no more than 5-10% of patients will experience a toxic effect. For some drugs, this may mean that the upper limit of the range is no more than twice the lower limit. Of course, these figures can be highly variable, and some patients may benefit greatly from drug concentrations that exceed the therapeutic range, whereas others may suffer significant toxicity at much lower values (e.g., with digoxin).

For a limited number of drugs, some effect of the drug is easily measured (e.g., blood pressure, blood glucose) and can be used to optimize dosage using a trial-and-error approach. Even in an ideal case, certain quantitative issues arise, such as how often to change dosage and by how much. These usually can be settled with simple rules of thumb based on the principles discussed (e.g., change dosage by no more than 50% and no more often than every 3-4 half-lives). Alternatively, some drugs have very little dose-related toxicity, and maximum efficacy usually is desired. In such cases, doses well in excess of the average required will ensure efficacy (if this is possible) and prolong drug action. Such a "maximal dose" strategy typically is used for penicillins.

For many drugs, however, the effects are difficult to measure (or the drug is given for prophylaxis), toxicity and lack of efficacy are both potential dangers, or the therapeutic index is narrow. In these circumstances, doses must be titrated carefully, and drug dosage is limited by toxicity rather than efficacy. Thus, the therapeutic goal is to maintain steady-state drug levels within the therapeutic window. For most drugs, the actual concentrations associated with this desired range are not known and need not be known. It is sufficient to understand that efficacy and toxicity generally depend on concentration and how drug dosage and frequency of administration affect the drug level. However, for a small number of drugs for which there is a small (2-3 fold) difference between concentrations resulting in efficacy and toxicity (e.g., digoxin, theophylline, lidocaine, aminoglycosides, cyclosporine, tacrolimus, sirolimus, warfarin, and anticonvulsants), a plasma concentration range associated with effective therapy has been defined. In these cases, a target-level strategy is reasonable, wherein a desired (target) steady-state concentration of the drug (usually in plasma) associated with efficacy and minimal toxicity is chosen, and a dosage is computed that is expected to achieve this value. Drug concentrations are subsequently measured, and dosage is adjusted if necessary to approximate the target more closely (described later).

Maintenance Dose

In most clinical situations, drugs are administered in a series of repetitive doses or as a continuous infusion to maintain a steady-state concentration of drug associated with the therapeutic window. Calculation of the appropriate maintenance dosage is a primary goal. To maintain the chosen steady-state or target concentration, the rate of drug administration is adjusted such that the rate of input equals the rate of loss. This relationship was defined previously in Equations 2–2 and 2–16 and is expressed here in terms of the desired target concentration:

$$\text{Dosing rate} = \text{target } C_p \cdot CL/F \qquad \text{(Equation 2–18)}$$

If the clinician chooses the desired concentration of drug in plasma and knows the clearance and bioavailability for that drug in a particular patient, the appropriate dose and dosing interval can be calculated.

Example. Oral digoxin is to be used as a maintenance dose to gradually "digitalize" a 63 year old, 84-kg patient with congestive heart failure. A steady-state plasma concentration of 0.7-0.9 ng/mL is selected as an appropriate conservative target based on prior knowledge of the action of the drug in patients with heart failure to maintain levels at or belowin the 0.5-1.0 ng/mL range (Bauman et al., 2006). Based on the fact that the patient's creatinine clearance (CL_{Cr}) is 56 mL/min, digoxin's clearance may be estimated from data in Appendix II.

$$\begin{aligned} CL &= 0.88\ CL_{CR} + 0.33\ \text{mL} \cdot \text{min}^{-1} \cdot \text{kg}^{-1} \\ &= 0.88 \times 56/84 + 0.33\ \text{mL} \cdot \text{min}^{-1} \cdot \text{kg}^{-1} \\ &= 0.92\ \text{mL} \cdot \text{min}^{-1} \cdot \text{kg}^{-1} \\ &= 77\ \text{mL} \cdot \text{min}^{-1} = 4.6\ \text{L} \cdot \text{hour}^{-1} \end{aligned}$$

Equation (2–18) then is used to calculate an appropriate dosing rate knowing that the oral bioavailability of digoxin is 70% ($F = 0.7$).

$$\begin{aligned} \text{Dosing rate} &= \text{Target } C_p \cdot CL/F \\ &= 0.75\ \text{ng} \cdot \text{mL}^{-1} \times (0.92/0.7)\ \text{mL} \cdot \text{min}^{-1} \cdot \text{kg}^{-1} \\ &= 0.99\ \text{ng} \cdot \text{min}^{-1} \cdot \text{kg}^{-1} \\ &\quad \text{or } 83\ \text{ng} \cdot \text{min}^{-1} \text{ for an 84-kg patient} \\ &\quad \text{or } 83\ \text{ng} \cdot \text{min}^{-1} \times 60\ \text{min} \times 24/24\ \text{hr} \\ &= 0.12\ \text{mg}/24\ \text{hr} \end{aligned}$$

In practice, the dosing rate would be rounded to the closest dosage size, 0.125 mg/24 hr, which would result in a steady-state plasma concentration of 0.78 ng/mL (0.75 × 125/120). Digoxin is a well characterized example of a drug that is difficult to dose and must be monitored regularly. While guidelines based on calculations of the sort suggested here are useful (Bauman et al., 2006), it is clear that tablet sizes are limiting and tablet sizes intermediate to those available are needed. Since the coefficient of variation for the clearance equation when used for digoxin treatment in this patient group is large (52%), it is common for patients who are not monitored regularly to require hospital admission to adjust medication. Monitoring the clinical status of patients (new or increased ankle edema, inability to sleep in a recumbent position, decreased exercise tolerance) whether accomplished by home health follow up or regular visits to the clinician, is essential to avoid untoward results.

Dosing Interval for Intermittent Dosage. In general, marked fluctuations in drug concentrations between doses are not desirable. If absorption and distribution were instantaneous, fluctuations in drug concentrations between doses would be governed entirely by the drug's elimination $t_{1/2}$. If the dosing interval T were chosen to be equal to the $t_{1/2}$, then the total fluctuation would be 2-fold; this is often a tolerable variation.

Pharmacodynamic considerations modify this. If a drug is relatively nontoxic such that a concentration many times that necessary for therapy can be tolerated easily, the maximal-dose strategy can be used, and the dosing interval can be much longer than the elimination $t_{1/2}$ (for convenience). The $t_{1/2}$ of amoxicillin is ~2 hours, but dosing every 2 hours would be impractical. Instead, amoxicillin often is given in large doses every 8 or 12 hours. For some drugs with a narrow therapeutic range, it may be important to estimate the maximal and minimal concentrations that will occur for a particular dosing interval. The minimal steady-state concentration $C_{ss,min}$ may be reasonably determined by the use of Equation 1–19:

$$C_{ss,\,min} = \frac{F \cdot \text{dose}/V_{SS}}{1 - \exp(-kT)} \cdot \exp(-kT) \qquad \text{(Equation 2–19)}$$

where k equals 0.693 divided by the clinically relevant plasma $t_{1/2}$, and T is the dosing interval. The term $\exp(-kT)$ is, in fact, the fraction of the last dose (corrected for bioavailability) that remains in the body at the end of a dosing interval.

For drugs that follow multi-exponential kinetics and are administered orally, estimation of the maximal steady-state concentration $C_{ss,max}$ involves a complicated set of exponential constants for distribution and absorption. If these terms are ignored for multiple oral dosing, one easily may predict a maximal steady-state concentration by omitting the $\exp(-kT)$ term in the numerator of Equation 2–19 (see Equation 2–20). Because of the approximation, the predicted maximal concentration from Equation 2–20 will be greater than that actually observed.

Example. In the patient with congestive heart failure discussed earlier, an oral maintenance dose of 0.125 mg digoxin per 24 hours was calculated to achieve an average plasma concentration of 0.78 ng/mL during the dosage interval. Digoxin has a narrow therapeutic index, and plasma levels ≤1.0 ng/mL usually are associated with efficacy and minimal toxicity. What are the maximum and minimum plasma concentrations associated with the preceding regimen? This first requires estimation of digoxin's volume of distribution based on available pharmacokinetic data (Appendix II).

$$\begin{aligned} V_{ss} &= 3.1\ CL_{CR} + 3.8\ \text{L} \cdot \text{kg}^{-1} \\ &= 3.1 \times (56/84) + 3.8\ \text{L} \cdot \text{kg}^{-1} \end{aligned}$$

Combining this value with that of digoxin's clearance provides an estimate of digoxin's elimination $t_{1/2}$ in the patient (Equation 2–14).

$$\begin{aligned} t_{1/2} &= 0.693\ V_{SS}/CL \\ &= \frac{0.693 \times 496\ \text{L}}{4.4\ \text{L} \cdot \text{hour}^{-1}} = 75\ \text{hr} = 3.1\ \text{days} \end{aligned}$$

Accordingly, the fractional rate constant of elimination is equal to 0.22 day^{-1} (0.693/3.1 days). Maximum and minimum digoxin plasma concentrations then may be predicted depending on the dosage interval. With T = 1 day (i.e., 0.125 mg given every day):

$$C_{SS,\ max} = \frac{F \cdot \text{dose} / V_{SS}}{1 - \exp(-kT)} = \frac{0.7 \times 0.125\ \text{mg} / 496\ \text{L}}{0.2} = 0.88\ \text{ng/mL} \quad \text{(Equation 2–20)}$$

$$C_{SS,\ min} = C_{SS,\ max} \cdot \exp(-kT) = (0.88\ \text{ng/mL})(0.8) = 0.7\ \text{ng/mL} \quad \text{(Equation 2–21)}$$

Thus, the plasma concentrations would fluctuate minimally about the steady-state concentration of 0.78 ng/mL, well within the recommended therapeutic range of 0.5-1.0 ng/mL. In this patient example, twice the daily dose (2 × 0.125 mg) could be given every other day. The average steady-state concentration would remain at 0.78 ng/mL, while the predicted maximum concentration would be 0.98 ng/mL (in Equation 2–20; dose = 0.25 mg and T = 2 days) and the minimum concentration would be 0.62 ng/mL (in Equation 2–21; 0.98 × 0.64). While this result would maintain a therapeutic concentration and avoid large excursions from it between doses, it does not favor patient compliance. Dosing must be compatible with the patient's routine and every other day dosing is problematic in this patient population.

Loading Dose

The *loading dose* is one or a series of doses that may be given at the onset of therapy with the aim of achieving the target concentration rapidly. The appropriate magnitude for the loading dose is

$$\text{Loading dose} = \text{target } C_p \cdot V_{ss}/F \quad \text{(Equation 2–22)}$$

A loading dose may be desirable if the time required to attain steady state by the administration of drug at a constant rate (4 elimination $t_{1/2}$ values) is long relative to the temporal demands of the condition being treated. For example, the $t_{1/2}$ of lidocaine is usually 1-2 hours. Arrhythmias encountered after myocardial infarction obviously may be life-threatening, and one cannot wait 4-8 hours to achieve a therapeutic concentration of lidocaine by infusion of the drug at the rate required to attain this concentration. Hence, use of a loading dose of lidocaine in the coronary care unit is standard.

The use of a loading dose also has significant disadvantages. First, the particularly sensitive individual may be exposed abruptly to a toxic concentration of a drug. Moreover, if the drug involved has a long $t_{1/2}$, it will take a long time for the concentration to fall if the level achieved is excessive. Loading doses tend to be large, and they are often given parenterally and rapidly; this can be particularly dangerous if toxic effects occur as a result of actions of the drug at sites that are in rapid equilibrium with plasma. This occurs because the loading dose calculated on the basis of V_{ss} subsequent to drug distribution is at first constrained within the initial and smaller "central" volume of distribution. It is therefore usually advisable to divide the loading dose into a number of smaller fractional doses that are administered over a period of time. Alternatively, the loading dose should be administered as a continuous intravenous infusion over a period of time. Ideally, this should be given in an exponentially decreasing fashion to mirror the concomitant accumulation of the maintenance dose of the drug, and this is accomplished using computerized infusion pumps.

Example. Accumulation of digitalis ("digitalization") in the patient described earlier is gradual if only a maintenance dose is administered (for at least 12 days, based on $t_{1/2}$ = 3.1 days). A more rapid response could be obtained (if deemed necessary) by using a loading-dose strategy and Equation 2–22. Here a target C_p of 0.9 ng/mL is chosen as a target below the recommended maximum of 1.0 ng/mL.

$$\text{Loading dose} = 0.9\ \text{ng} \cdot \text{mL}^{-1} \times 496\ \text{L}/0.7 = 638\ \mu\text{g, or} \sim 0.625\ \text{mg}$$

To avoid toxicity, this oral loading dose, would be given as an initial 0.25-mg dose followed by a 0.25-mg dose 6 -8 hours later, with careful monitoring of the patient and the final 0.125-mg dose given 12-14 hours later.

Individualizing Dosage

A rational dosage regimen is based on knowledge of *F, CL,* V_{ss}, and $t_{1/2}$ and some information about rates of absorption and distribution of the drug together with potential effects of the disease on these parameters. Recommended dosage regimens generally are designed for an "average" patient; usual values for the important determining parameters and appropriate adjustments that may be necessitated by disease or other factors are presented in Appendix II. This "one size fits all" approach, however, overlooks the considerable and unpredictable inter-patient variability that usually is present in these pharmacokinetic parameters. For many drugs, one standard deviation in the values observed for *F, CL,* and V_{ss} is ~20%, 50%, and 30%, respectively. This means that 95% of the time the C_{ss} that is achieved will be between 35% and 270% of the target; this is an unacceptably wide range for a drug with a low therapeutic index. Individualization of the dosage regimen to a particular patient therefore is critical for optimal therapy. The pharmacokinetic principles described earlier provide a basis for modifying the dosage regimen to obtain a desired degree of efficacy with a minimum of unacceptable adverse effects. In situations where the drug's plasma concentration can be measured and related to the therapeutic window, additional guidance for dosage modification is obtained from blood levels taken during therapy and evaluated in a pharmacokinetic consult available in many institutional settings. Such measurement and adjustment are appropriate for many drugs with low therapeutic indices (e.g., cardiac glycosides, anti-arrhythmic agents, anticonvulsants, immunosuppressants, theophylline, and warfarin).

Therapeutic Drug Monitoring

The major use of measured concentrations of drugs (at steady state) is to refine the estimate of *CL*/*F* for the patient being treated, using Equation 2–16 as rearranged below:

$$CL/F\ (\text{patient}) = \text{dosing rate}/C_{ss}(\text{measured}) \quad \text{(Equation 2–23)}$$

The new estimate of *CL/F* can be used in Equation 2–18 to adjust the maintenance dose to achieve the desired target concentration.

Certain practical details and pitfalls associated with therapeutic drug monitoring should be kept in mind. The first of these relates to the time of sampling for measurement of the drug concentration. If intermittent dosing is used, when during a dosing interval should samples be taken? It is necessary to distinguish between two possible uses of measured drug concentrations to understand the possible answers. A concentration of drug measured in a sample taken at virtually any time during the dosing interval will provide information that may aid in the assessment of drug toxicity. This is one type of therapeutic drug monitoring. It should be stressed, however, that such use of a measured concentration of drug is fraught with difficulties because of inter-individual variability in sensitivity to the drug. When there is a question of toxicity, the drug concentration is just one of many items used to interpret the clinical situation.

Changes in the effects of drugs may be delayed relative to changes in plasma concentration because of a slow rate of distribution or pharmacodynamic factors. Concentrations of digoxin, e.g., regularly exceed 2 ng/mL (a potentially toxic value) shortly after an oral dose, yet these peak concentrations do not cause toxicity; indeed, they occur well before peak effects. Thus, concentrations of drugs in samples obtained shortly after administration can be uninformative or even misleading.

The purpose of sampling during supposed steady state is to modify the estimate of *CL/F* and thus the choice of dosage. Early post-absorptive concentrations do not reflect clearance; they are determined primarily by the rate of absorption, the "central" (rather than the steady-state) volume of distribution, and the rate of distribution, all of which are pharmacokinetic features of virtually no relevance in choosing the long-term maintenance dosage. When the goal of measurement is adjustment of dosage, the sample should be taken well after the previous dose, as a rule of thumb, just before the next planned dose, when the concentration is at its minimum. The exceptions to this approach are drugs that are eliminated nearly completely between doses and act only during the initial portion of each dosing interval. If it is questionable whether efficacious concentrations of such drugs are being achieved, a sample taken shortly after a dose may be helpful. On the other hand, if a concern is whether low clearance (as in renal failure) may cause accumulation of drug, concentrations measured just before the next dose will reveal such accumulation and are considerably more useful for this purpose than is knowledge of the maximal concentration. For such drugs, determination of both maximal and minimal concentrations is recommended. These two values can offer a more complete picture of the behavior of the drug in a specific patient (particularly if obtained over more that one dosing period) can better support pharmacokinetic modeling.

A second important aspect of the timing of sampling is its relationship to the beginning of the maintenance-dosage regimen. When constant dosage is given, steady state is reached only after four $t_{1/2}$ have passed. If a sample is obtained too soon after dosage is begun, it will not reflect this state and the drug's clearance accurately. Yet, for toxic drugs, if sampling is delayed until steady state is ensured, the damage may have been done. Some simple guidelines can be offered. When it is important to maintain careful control of concentrations, the first sample should be taken after two $t_{1/2}$ (as calculated and expected for the patient), assuming that no loading dose has been given. If the concentration already exceeds 90% of the eventual expected mean steady-state concentration, the dosage rate should be halved, another sample obtained in another two (supposed) $t_{1/2}$, and the dosage halved again if this sample exceeds the target. If the first concentration is not too high, the initial rate of dosage is continued; even if the concentration is lower than expected, it is usually reasonable to await the attainment of steady state in another two estimated $t_{1/2}$ and then to proceed to adjust dosage as described earlier.

If dosage is intermittent, there is a third concern with the time at which samples are obtained for determination of drug concentrations. If the sample has been obtained just prior to the next dose, as recommended, concentration will be a minimal value, not the mean. However, as discussed earlier, the estimated mean concentration may be calculated by using Equation 2–16.

If a drug follows first-order kinetics, the average, minimum, and maximum concentrations at steady state are linearly related to dose and dosing rate (see Equations 2–16, 2–19, and 2–20). Therefore, the ratio between the measured and desired concentrations can be used to adjust the dose, consistent with available dosage sizes:

$$\frac{C_{ss}\,(\text{measured})}{C_{ss}\,(\text{predicted})} = \frac{\text{Dose (previous)}}{\text{Dose (new)}} \qquad \text{(Equation 2–24)}$$

In the previously described patient given 0.125 mg digoxin every 24 hours, for example, if the measured minimum (trough) steady-state concentration were found to be 0.35 ng/mL rather than the predicted level of 0.7 ng/mL, an appropriate, practical change in the dosage regimen would be to *increase* the daily dose by 0.125 mg to 0.25-mg digoxin daily.

$$\text{Dose (new)} = \frac{C_{SS}\text{(predicted)}}{C_{SS}\text{(measured)}} \times \text{Dose (previous)}$$

$$= \frac{0.7}{0.35} \times 0.125 = 0.25/24 \text{ hour}$$

In practice, one would change the dose from the 0.125-mg tablet to the 0.25-mg tablet by providing a new prescription.

Compliance. Ultimately, therapeutic success depends on the patient actually taking the drug according to the prescribed dosage regimen—"Drugs don't work if you don't take them." Noncompliance with the prescribed dosing schedule is a major reason for therapeutic failure, especially in the long-term treatment of heart failure as in our example patient being administered digoxin where the absence of intermediate tablet sizes influences the regimens that can be practically constructed (our patient ultimately required an alternate day or alternate dose schedule). Moreover, treatment of chronic disease using antihypertensive, anti-retroviral, and anticonvulsant agents also represents a compliance problem. When no special efforts are made to address this issue, only about 50% of patients follow the prescribed dosage regimen in a reasonably satisfactory fashion, approximately one-third comply only partly, and about one in six patients is essentially noncompliant (Devabhaktuni and Bangalore 2009). Missed doses are more common than too many doses. The number of drugs does not appear to be as important as the number of times a day doses must be remembered (Ho et al., 2009). Reducing the number of required dosing occasions can improve adherence to a prescribed dosage regimen. Equally important is the need to involve patients in the responsibility for their own health using a variety of strategies based on improved communication regarding the nature of the disease and the overall therapeutic plan (Appendix I).

BIBLIOGRAPHY

Angelov L, Doolittle ND, Kraemer DF, et al. Blood-brain barrier disruption and intra-arterial methotrexate-based therapy for newly diagnosed primary CNS lymphoma: A multi-institutional experience. *J Clin Oncol,* **2009**, *27*:3503–3509.

Aquina CT, Marques-Baptista A, Bridgeman P, Merlin MA. OxyContin abuse and overdose. *Postgrad Med,* **2009**, *121*:163–167.

Bauman JL, DiDomenico RJ, Viana M, Fitch M. A method of determining the dose of digoxin for heart failure in the modern era. *Arch Intern Med,* **2006**, *166*:2539–2545.

Benet LZ, Hoener BA. Changes in plasma protein binding have little clinical relevance. *Clin Pharmacol Ther,* **2002**, *71*:115–121.

Bialer M. Extended-release formulations for the treatment of epilepsy. *CNS Drugs,* **2007**, *21*:765–774.

Blumenthal PD, Gemzell-Danielsson K, Marintcheva-Petrova M. Tolerability and clinical safety of Implanon. *Eur J Contracept Reprod Health Care*, **2008**, *13*(suppl 1):29–36.

Buhimschi CS, Weiner CP. Medications in pregnancy and lactation. *Obstet Gynecol*, **2009**, *114*:167–168.

Cosman F. Treatment of osteoporosis and prevention of new fractures: Role of intravenously administered bisphosphonates. *Endocr Pract*, **2009**, *15*:483–493.

Dawood S, Leyland-Jones B. Pharmacology and pharmacogenetics of chemotherapeutic agents. *Cancer Invest,* **2009**, *27*:482–488.

Dembowski E, Davidson MH. Statin and ezetimibe combination therapy in cardiovascular disease. *Curr Opin Endocrinol Diabetes Obes,* **2009**, *16*:183–188.

Devabhaktuni M, Bangalore S. Fixed combination of amlodipine and atorvastatin in cardiovascular risk management: Patient perspectives. *Vasc Health Risk Manag,* **2009**, *5*:377–387.

Hallifax D, Houston JB. Methodological uncertainty in quantitative prediction of human hepatic clearance from in vitro experimental systems. *Curr Drug Metab,* **2009**, *10*:307–321.

Ho PM, Bryson CL, Rumsfeld JS. Medication adherence: Its importance in cardiovascular outcomes. *Circulation,* **2009**, *119*:3028–3035.

Ito S, Lee A. Drug excretion into beast milk: Overview. *Adv Drug Deliv Rev*, **2003**, *55*:617–627.

Jones AR, Shusta EV. Blood-brain barrier transport of therapeutics via receptor-mediation. *Pharm Res*, **2007**, *24*:1759–1771.

Lipka LJ. Ezetimibe: a first-in-class, novel cholesterol absorption inhibitor. *Cardiovasc Drug Rev*, **2003**, *21*:293–312.

Maeda K, Sugiyama Y. Impact of genetic polymorphisms of transporters on the pharmacokinetic, pharmacodynamic and toxicological properties of anionic drugs. *Drug Metab Pharmacokinet,* **2008**, *23*:223–235.

Manos MJ, Tom-Revzon C, Bukstein OG, Crismon ML. Changes and challenges: Managing ADHD in a fast-paced world. *J Manag Care Pharm*, **2007**, *13*:S2–S13.

Matsuhisa K, Kondoh M, Takahashi A, Yagi K. Tight junction modulator and drug delivery. *Expert Opin Drug Deliv*, **2009**, *6*:509–515.

Meredith PA. Potential concerns about generic substitution: Bioequivalence versus therapeutic equivalence of different amlodipine salt forms. *Curr Med Res Opin,* **2009**, *25*:2179–2189.

Nemeroff CB. Improving antidepressant adherence. *J Clin Psychiatry*, **2003**, *64 Suppl 18*:25–30.

Patil SB, Sawant KK. Mucoadhesive microspheres: A promising tool in drug delivery. *Curr Drug Deliv,* **2008**, *5*:312–318.

Pellock JM, Smith MC, Cloyd JC, et al. Extended-release formulations: simplifying strategies in the management of antiepileptic drug therapy. *Epilepsy Behav*, **2004**, *5*:301–307.

Pinaud F, Michalet X, Iyer G, et al. Dynamic partitioning of a glycosyl-phosphatidylinositol-anchored protein in glycosphingolipid-rich microdomains imaged by single-quantum dot tracking. *Traffic*, **2009**, *10*:691–712.

Prestidge CA, Tan A, Simovic S, et al. Silica nanoparticles to control the lipase-mediated digestion of lipid-based oral delivery systems. *Mol Pharm*, **2010**, DOI: 10.1021/mp9002442.

Queckenberg C, Fuhr U. Influence of posture on pharmacokinetics. *Eur J Clin Pharmacol,* **2009**, *65*:109–119.

Sahin S, Benet LZ. The operational multiple dosing half-life: A key to defining drug accumulation in patients and to designing extended release dosage forms. *Pharm Res,* **2008**, *25*:2869–2877.

Sajja HK, East MP, Mao H, et al. Development of multifunctional nanoparticles for targeted drug delivery and noninvasive imaging of therapeutic effect. *Curr Drug Discov Technol,* **2009**, *6*:43–51.

Singer SJ. (2004). Some early history of membrane molecular biology. *Annu Rev Physiol*, **2004**, *66*:1–27.

Weier N, He SM, Li XT, et al. Placental drug disposition and its clinical implications. *Curr Drug Metab*, **2008**, *9*:106–121.

Pharmacodynamics: Molecular Mechanisms of Drug Action

Donald K. Blumenthal and
James C. Garrison

Pharmacodynamics is the study of the biochemical and physiological effects of drugs and their mechanisms of action. Understanding pharmacodynamics can provide the basis for the rational therapeutic use of a drug and the design of new and superior therapeutic agents. Simply stated, pharmacodynamics refers to the effects of a drug on the body. In contrast, the effects of the body on the actions of a drug are *pharmacokinetic* processes (Chapter 2), and include absorption, distribution, metabolism, and excretion of drugs (often referred to collectively as ADME). Many adverse effects of drugs and drug toxicities can be anticipated by understanding a drug's mechanism(s) of action, its pharmacokinetics, and its interactions with other drugs. Thus, both the pharmacodynamic properties of a drug and its pharmacokinetics contribute to safe and successful therapy. The effects of many drugs, both salutory and deleterious, may differ widely from patient to patient due to genetic differences that alter the pharmacokinetics and the pharmacodynamics of a given drug. This aspect of pharmacology is termed *pharmacogenetics* and is covered in Chapter 7.

PHARMACODYNAMIC CONCEPTS

The effects of most drugs result from their interaction with macromolecular components of the organism. These interactions alter the function of the pertinent component and initiate the biochemical and physiological changes that are characteristic of the response to the drug. The term drug *receptor* or drug *target* denotes the cellular macromolecule or macromolecular complex with which the drug interacts to elicit a cellular response, i.e., a change in cell function. Drugs commonly alter the rate or magnitude of an intrinsic cellular response rather than create new responses. Drug receptors are often located on the surface of cells, but may also be located in specific intracellular compartments such as the nucleus. Many drugs also interact with *acceptors* (e.g., serum albumin) within the body. Acceptors are entities that do not directly cause any change in biochemical or physiological response. However, interactions of drugs with acceptors such as serum albumin can alter the pharmacokinetics of a drug's actions.

From a numerical standpoint, proteins form the most important class of drug receptors. Examples include the receptors for hormones, growth factors, transcription factors, and neurotransmitters; the enzymes of crucial metabolic or regulatory pathways (e.g., dihydrofolate reductase, acetylcholinesterase, and cyclic nucleotide phosphodiesterases); proteins involved in transport processes (e.g., Na^+,K^+-ATPase); secreted glycoproteins (e.g., Wnts); and structural proteins (e.g., tubulin). Specific binding of drugs to other cellular constituents such as DNA is also exploited for therapeutic purposes. For example, nucleic acids are particularly important drug receptors for certain cancer chemotherapeutic agents and antiviral drugs.

Physiological Receptors

A major group of drug receptors consists of proteins that normally serve as receptors for endogenous regulatory ligands. These drug targets are termed *physiological receptors*. Many drugs act on physiological receptors and are particularly selective because physiological receptors have evolved to recognize and respond to individual signaling molecules with great selectivity. Drugs that bind to physiological receptors and mimic the regulatory effects of the endogenous signaling compounds are termed *agonists*. If the drug binds to the same *recognition site* as the endogenous agonist (the primary or orthosteric site on the receptor) the drug is said to be a *primary agonist*. *Allosteric (allotopic)* agonists bind to a different region on the receptor referred to as an allosteric or allotopic site. Drugs that block or reduce the action of an agonist are termed *antagonists*. Antagonism most commonly results from competition with an agonist for the same or overlapping site on the receptor (a *syntopic* interaction), but can also occur by interacting with other sites on the receptor (allosteric antagonism), by combining with the agonist (chemical antagonism), or by functional antagonism by indirectly inhibiting the cellular or physiological effects of the agonist. Agents that are only partly as effective as agonists regardless of the concentration employed are termed *partial agonists*. Many receptors exhibit some constitutive activity in the absence of a regulatory ligand; drugs that stabilize such receptors in an inactive conformation are termed *inverse agonists* (Figure 3–1) (Kenakin, 2004; Milligan, 2003). Note that partial agonists and inverse agonists that interact syntopically with a full agonist will behave as competitive antagonists.

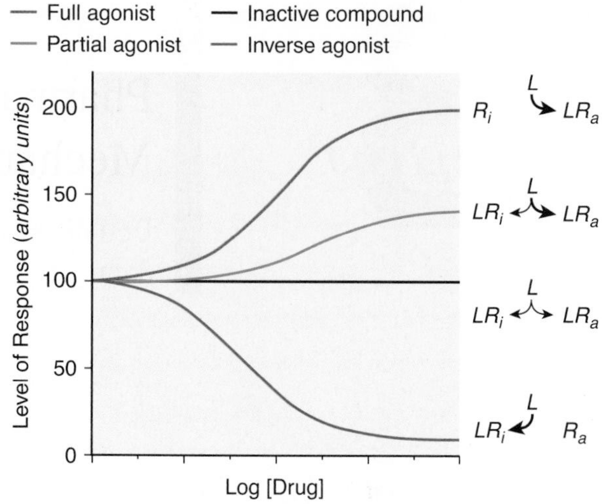

Figure 3–1. *Regulation of the activity of a receptor with conformation-selective drugs.* The ordinate is the activity of the receptor produced by R_a, the active receptor conformation (e.g., stimulation of adenylyl cyclase by a β adrenergic receptor). If a drug *L* selectively binds to R_a, it will produce a maximal response. If *L* has equal affinity for R_i and R_a, it will not perturb the equilibrium between them and will have no effect on net activity; *L* would appear as an inactive compound. If the drug selectively binds to R_i, then the net amount of R_a will be diminished. If *L* can bind to receptor in an active conformation R_a but also bind to inactive receptor R_i with lower affinity, the drug will produce a partial response; *L* will be a partial agonist. If there is sufficient R_a to produce an elevated basal response in the absence of ligand (agonist-independent constitutive activity), then activity will be inhibited; *L* will then be an inverse agonist. Inverse agonists selectively bind to the inactive form of the receptor and shift the conformational equilibrium toward the inactive state. In systems that are not constitutively active, inverse agonists will behave like competitive antagonists, which helps explain why the properties of inverse agonists and the number of such agents previously described as competitive antagonists were only recently appreciated. Receptors that have constitutive activity and are sensitive to inverse agonists include benzodiazepine, histamine, opioid, cannabinoid, dopamine, bradykinin, and adenosine receptors.

Drug Specificity

The strength of the reversible interaction between a drug and its receptor, as measured by the *dissociation constant*, is defined as the affinity of one for the other. Both the affinity of a drug for its receptor and its *intrinsic activity* are determined by its chemical structure. The chemical structure of a drug also contributes to the drug's *specificity*. A drug that interacts with a single type of receptor that is expressed on only a limited number of differentiated cells will exhibit high specificity. An example of such a drug is ranitidine, an H_2 receptor antagonist used to treat ulcers (Chapter 45). If, however, a receptor is expressed ubiquitously on a variety of cells throughout the body, drugs acting on such a widely expressed receptor will exhibit widespread effects, and could produce serious side effects or toxicities if the receptor serves important functions in multiple tissues.

There are numerous examples of drugs that work through a discrete action, but have effects throughout the body. These include the inotropic drug digoxin, which inhibits the ubiquitously expressed enzyme Na^+,K^+-ATPase (Chapter 28), and the antifolate anticancer drugs such as methotrexate that inhibit dihydrofolate reductase, an enzyme required by all cells for the synthesis of purines and thymidylate (Chapters 60 and 61). The Na^+ channel blocker lidocaine has effects in peripheral nerves, the heart, and the central nervous system (CNS) because Na^+ channels are highly expressed in all these tissues (Chapters 20 and 29). Lidocaine has local anesthetic effects when administered locally to prevent or relieve pain, but can also have cardiac and CNS effects if it reaches the systemic circulation. Even if the primary action of a drug is localized, as might be the case with injected lidocaine, the subsequent physiological effects of the drug may be widespread. One example would be immunosuppressant drugs (Chapter 35) that specifically inhibit cells of the immune system; their use is limited by the risk of opportunistic systemic infections. Other examples of drugs that act locally but have global effects are diuretics (Chapter 25) that act on cells in the kidney to alter serum electrolytes such as K^+. However, the hypokalemia that a diuretic such as furosemide can cause can significantly increase the risk of skeletal muscle cramps and cardiac arrhythmias.

Many clinically important drugs exhibit a broad (low) specificity because the drug is able to interact with multiple receptors in different tissues. Such broad specificity might enhance the clinical utility of a drug, but also contribute to a spectrum of adverse side effects due to off-target interactions. One example of a drug that interacts with multiple receptors is amiodarone, an agent used to treat cardiac arrhythmias. In cardiac muscle, amiodarone inhibits Na^+, Ca^{2+}, and K^+ channels, and noncompetitively inhibits β adrenergic receptors (Table 29–3). All of these drug-receptor interactions may contribute to its therapeutic efficacy and widespread use to treat many forms of arrhythmia. However, amiodarone also has a number of serious toxicities, some of which are due to the drug's structural similarity to thyroid hormone and its ability to interact with nuclear thyroid receptors. Amiodarone's salutary effects and toxicities may also be mediated through interactions with receptors that are poorly characterized or unknown.

Some drugs are administered as racemic mixtures of stereoisomers. The stereoisomers can exhibit different pharmacodynamic as well as pharmacokinetic properties. For example, the antiarrhythmic drug sotalol is prescribed as a racemic mixture; the d- and l-enantiomers are equipotent as K^+ channel blockers, but the l-enantiomer is a much more potent β adrenergic antagonist (Chapter 29). Labetolol (Chapter 12) is another drug that has complex pharmacodynamic properties because it is used clinically as a racemic mixture containing equal amounts of four diastereomers. The *R,R* isomer is a potent β_1 adrenergic antagonist and partial β_2 receptor agonist; the *S,R* and *S,S* isomers have little or no β antagonist activity but do possess significant α_1 adrenergic antagonist activity, and the *R,S* isomer is essentially devoid of adrenergic blocking activity. It should always be considered that a given drug has multiple mechanisms of action that depend upon many factors, including receptor specificity, the tissue-specific expression of the receptor(s), drug access to target tissues, drug concentration in different tissues, pharmacogenetics, and interactions with other drugs.

The pharmacological properties of many drugs differ depending upon whether the drug is used acutely or chronically. In some cases, chronic administration of a drug causes a *down-regulation* or *desensitization* of receptors that can require dose adjustments to maintain adequate therapy. Chronic administration of nitrovasodilators to treat angina results in the rapid development of complete tolerance, a process known as *tachyphylaxis*. To avoid tachyphylaxis, it is necessary to interrupt nitrovasodilator therapy every night for at least 18 hours (Chapter 27). Differential development of tolerance to different effects of a drug can also occur. Tolerance to the analgesic effects of opioids can develop with chronic administration, whereas little tolerance to the effects of these agents on respiratory depression occurs under the same dosing conditions (Chapter 18). Drug resistance may also develop due to pharmacokinetic mechanisms (i.e., the drug is metabolized more rapidly with chronic exposure), the development of mechanisms that prevent the drug from reaching its receptor (i.e., increased expression of the multidrug resistance transporter in drug-resistant cancer cells; see Chapter 5), or the clonal expansion of cancer cells containing drug-resistant mutations in the drug receptor (e.g., imatinib-resistant mutations in BCR-ABL; Chapter 62).

Some drug effects do not occur by means of macromolecular receptors, such as the therapeutic neutralization of gastric acid by the antacid bases aluminum and magnesium hydroxides [$Al(OH)_3$ and $Mg(OH)_2$]. Drugs such as mannitol act according to colligative properties to increase the osmolarity of various body fluids and cause changes in the distribution of water to promote diuresis, catharsis, expansion of circulating volume in the vascular compartment, or reduction of cerebral edema (Chapter 25). The oral administration of cholesterol-binding agents (e.g., cholestyramine resin) is used to decrease serum cholesterol by limiting absorption of dietary cholesterol from the intestine (Chapter 31).

Anti-infective drugs such as antibiotics, antivirals, and drugs used to treat parasitic infections target receptors or cell processes that are critical for the growth or survival of the infective agent but are nonessential or lacking in the host organism. Thus, the therapeutic goal of anti-infective drugs involves delivering drugs to the pathogenic organism in sufficient concentrations to kill or suppress the growth of the pathogen without causing untoward effects on the patient. For instance, antibiotics such as penicillin inhibit a key enzyme required for synthesis of bacterial cell walls, an enzyme not present in humans or animals. A major challenge with many anti-infectives is the rapid development of drug resistance. Resistance to antibiotics, antivirals, and other drugs can result through a variety of mechanisms including mutation of the target receptor, increased expression of enzymes that degrade or increase efflux of the drug from the infective agent, and development of alternative biochemical pathways that circumvent the drug's effects on the infective agent (Chapter 48).

Structure-Activity Relationships and Drug Design

A significant number of clinically useful drugs were developed in an era when drug discovery primarily involved screening compounds for their capacity to elicit salutary effects in patients or an animal disease model such as the spontaneously hypertensive rat or seizure-prone mouse. The receptors responsible for the clinical effects of many of these drugs have yet to be identified, although significant efforts are devoted toward identifying their mechanisms of action. Conversely, sequencing of the entire human genome has identified novel genes related by sequence to known receptors, but because the endogenous and exogenous ligands for these putative receptors are still unknown, these are referred to as *orphan receptors*. Orphan receptors are still found in the G–protein coupled receptor and nuclear hormone receptor families. Detailed knowledge of a drug's molecular target(s) can inform the development of new drugs with greater efficacy and lower toxicities. With the advent of transgenic animal models, it is now feasible to develop animal models that can test hypotheses regarding the possible physiological effects of altering a specific receptor's function and to predict the effects of receptor antagonists and agonists by genetically altering the receptor's expression and function. The methods and rationale currently used by the pharmaceutical industry to design and invent new drugs is covered fully in Chapter 1 and outlined briefly below.

Both the affinity of a drug for its receptor and its intrinsic activity are determined by its chemical structure. This relationship frequently is quite stringent. Relatively minor modifications in the drug molecule may result in major changes in its pharmacological properties based on altered affinity for one or more receptors. The stringent nature of chemical structure to specificity of binding of a drug to its receptor is illustrated by the capacity of receptors to interact selectively with optical isomers, as described for the antimuscarinic actions of dl-hyoscyamine (atropine, effects of which are due to the l-isomer) versus d-hyoscyamine.

Exploitation of structure-activity relationships on many occasions has led to the synthesis of valuable therapeutic agents. Because changes in molecular configuration need not alter all actions and effects of a drug equally, it is sometimes possible to develop a congener with a more favorable ratio of therapeutic to adverse effects, enhanced selectivity among different cells or tissues, or more acceptable secondary characteristics than those of the parent drug. Therapeutically useful antagonists of hormones or neurotransmitters have been developed by chemical modification of the structure of the physiological agonist. Minor modifications of structure also can have profound effects on the pharmacokinetic properties of drugs. For example, addition of a phosphate ester at the N3 position in the antiseizure drug phenytoin (5,5-diphenyl-2,4-imidazolidinedione) produces a prodrug (FOSPHENYTOIN) that is more soluble in intravenous solutions than its parent. This modification results in far more reliable distribution in the body and a drug that must be cleaved by esterase to become active.

Given adequate information about both the molecular structures and the pharmacological activities of a relatively large group of congeners, it is possible to use computer analysis to identify the chemical properties (i.e., the pharmacophore) required for optimal action at the receptor: size, shape, position, and orientation of charged groups or hydrogen bond donors, and so on. Advances in molecular modeling of organic compounds and the methods for drug target (receptor) discovery and biochemical measurement of the primary actions of drugs at their receptors have enriched the quantitation of structure-activity relationships and its use in drug design (Carlson and McCammon, 2000). The importance of specific drug-receptor interactions can be evaluated further by analyzing the responsiveness of receptors that have been selectively mutated at individual amino acid residues. Such information increasingly is allowing the optimization or design of chemicals that can bind to a receptor with improved affinity, selectivity, or regulatory effect. Similar structure-based approaches also are used to improve pharmacokinetic properties of drugs, particularly if knowledge of their metabolism is known. Knowledge of the structures of receptors and of drug-receptor complexes, determined at atomic resolution by x-ray crystallography, is even more helpful in the design of ligands and in understanding the molecular basis of drug resistance and circumventing it (i.e., x-ray crystal structures of BCR-ABL and BCR-ABL mutants in complex with imatinib and other small molecule inhibitors). Emerging technology in the field of pharmacogenetics (Chapter 7) is improving our understanding of the nature of and variation in receptors, and is positioned to permit molecular diagnostics in individual patients to predict those who will most benefit from a particular drug (Jain, 2004).

QUANTITATIVE ASPECTS OF DRUG INTERACTIONS WITH RECEPTORS

Receptor occupancy theory assumes that response emanates from a receptor occupied by a drug, a concept that has its basis in the law of mass action. The basic currency of receptor pharmacology is the *dose-response* (or concentration-response) *curve*, a depiction of the observed effect of a drug as a function of its concentration in the receptor compartment. Figure 3–2 shows a typical dose-response curve; it reaches a maximal asymptotic value when the drug occupies all the receptor sites.

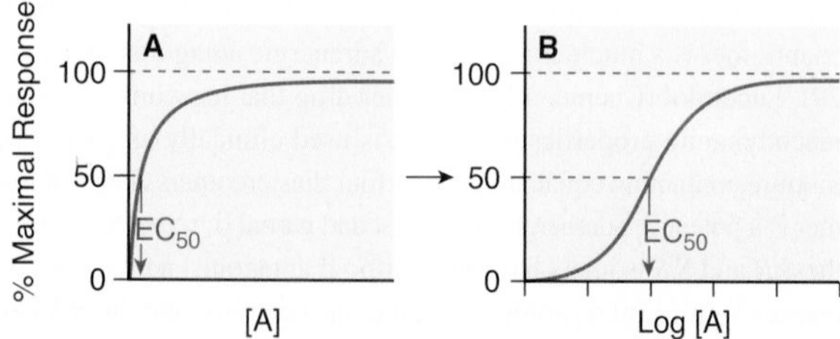

Figure 3–2. *Graded responses (y axis as a percentage of maximal response) expressed as a function of the concentration of drug A present at the receptor.* The hyperbolic shape of the curve in panel **A** becomes sigmoid when plotted semi-logarithmically, as in panel **B**. The concentration of drug that produces 50% of the maximal response quantifies drug activity and is referred to as the EC_{50} (effective concentration for 50% response). The range of concentrations needed to fully depict the dose-response relationship (~3 $\log_{10}$ [10] units) is too wide to be useful in the linear format of Figure 3–2A; thus, most dose-response curves use log [Drug] on the x axis, as in Figure 3–2B. Dose-response curves presented in this way are sigmoidal in shape and have three properties: threshold, slope, and maximal asymptote. These three parameters quantitate the activity of the drug.

Some drugs cause low-dose stimulation and high-dose inhibition of response. These U-shaped relationships for some receptor systems are said to display *hormesis*. Several drug-receptor systems can display this property (e.g., prostaglandins, endothelin, and purinergic and serotonergic agonists, among others), which is likely to be at the root of some drug toxicities (Calabrese and Baldwin, 2003).

Affinity, Efficacy, and Potency. In general, the drug-receptor interaction is characterized by (1) binding of drug to receptor and (2) generation of a response in a biological system, as illustrated in Equation 3-1 where the drug or ligand is denoted as *L* and the inactive receptor as *R*. The first reaction, the reversible formation of the ligand-receptor complex LR, is governed by the chemical property of *affinity*.

$$L + R \underset{k_{-1}}{\overset{k_{+1}}{\rightleftharpoons}} LR \underset{k_{-2}}{\overset{k_{+2}}{\rightleftharpoons}} LR^* \qquad \text{(Equation 3-1)}$$

where LR* is produced in proportion to [LR] and leads to a response. This simple relationship illustrates the reliance of the affinity of the ligand (*L*) with receptor (*R*) on both the forward or *association rate* (k_{+1}) and the reverse or *dissociation rate* (k_{-1}). At any given time, the concentration of ligand-receptor complex [LR] is equal to the product of $k_{+1}[L][R]$, the rate of formation of the bi-molecular complex LR, minus the product k_{-1}[LR], the rate dissociation of LR into L and R. At equilibrium (i.e., when $\delta[LR]/\delta t = 0$), $k_{+1}[L][R] = k_{-1}[LR]$. The *equilibrium dissociation constant* (K_D) is then described by ratio of the *off* and *on* rate constants (k_{-1}/k_{+1}).

Thus, at equilibrium,

$$K_D = \frac{[L][R]}{[LR]} = \frac{k_{-1}}{k_{+1}} \qquad \text{(Equation 3-2)}$$

The *affinity constant* or *equilibrium association constant* (K_A) is the reciprocal of the equilibrium dissociation constant (i.e., $K_A = 1/K_D$); thus a high-affinity drug has a low K_D and will bind a greater number of a particular receptor at a low concentration than a low-affinity drug. As a practical matter, the affinity of a drug is influenced most often by changes in its off-rate (k_{-1}) rather than its on-rate (k_{+1}).

Equation 3-2 permits us to write an expression of the fractional occupancy (*f*) of receptors by agonist:

$$f = \frac{\text{[ligand-receptor complexes]}}{\text{[total receptors]}} = \frac{[LR]}{[R] + [LR]} \qquad \text{(Equation 3-3)}$$

This can be expressed in terms of K_A (or K_D) and [L]:

$$f = \frac{K_A[L]}{1 + K_A[L]} = \frac{[L]}{[L] + K_D} \qquad \text{(Equation 3-4)}$$

This relationship illustrates that when the concentration of drug equals the K_D (or $1/K_A$), f = 0.5, that is, the drug will occupy 50% of the receptors. Note that this relationship describes only receptor occupancy, not the eventual response that is often amplified by the cell. Many signaling systems reach a full biological response with only a fraction of receptors occupied (described later). Potency is defined by example in Figure 3–3. Basically, when two drugs produce equivalent responses, the drug whose dose-response curve (plotted as in Figure 3-3A) lies to the left of the other (i.e., the concentration producing a half-maximal effect [EC_{50}] is smallest) is said to be the more potent.

Response to Drugs. The second reaction shown in Equation 3-1 is the reversible formation of the active

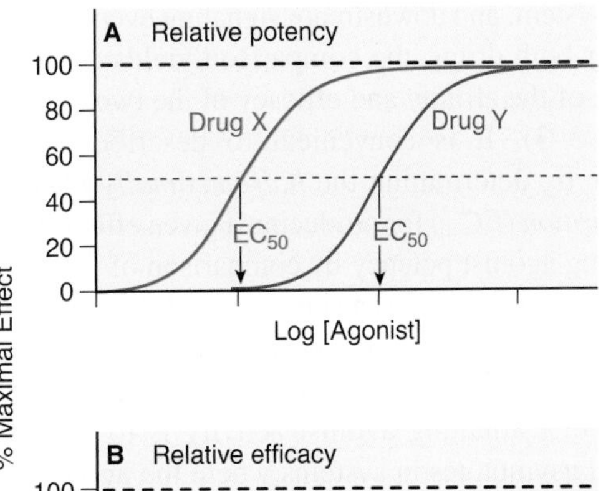

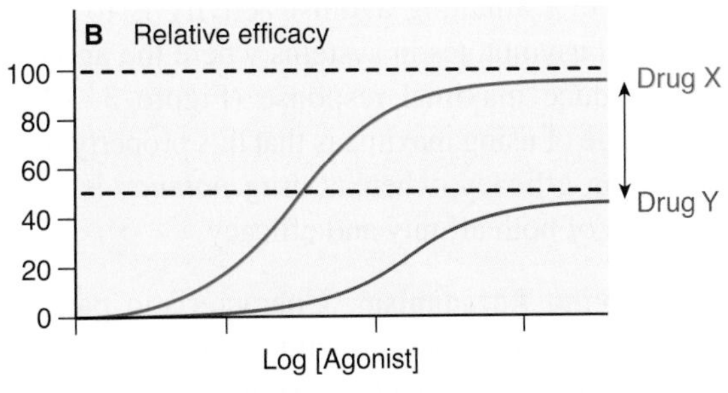

Figure 3–3. *Two ways of quantifying agonism.* **A.** The relative potency of two agonists (Drug X, *red line;* Drug Y, *purple line*) obtained in the same tissue is a function of their relative affinities and intrinsic efficacies. The EC_{50} of Drug X occurs at a concentration that is one-tenth the EC_{50} of Drug Y. Thus, Drug X is more potent than Drug Y. **B.** In systems where the two drugs do not both produce the maximal response characteristic of the tissue, the observed maximal response is a nonlinear function of their relative intrinsic efficacies. Drug X is more efficacious than Drug Y; their asymptotic fractional responses are 100% (Drug X) and 50% (Drug Y).

ligand-receptor complex, LR*. The ability of a drug to activate a receptor and generate a cellular response is a reflection of its *efficacy*. Historically, efficacy has been treated as a proportionality constant that quantifies the extent of functional change imparted to a receptor-mediated response system on binding a drug. Thus, a drug with high efficacy may be a full agonist, eliciting, at some concentration, a full response. A drug with a lower efficacy at the same receptor may not elicit a full response at any dose (Figure 3–1). When it is possible to describe the relative efficacy of drugs at a particular receptor, a drug with a low intrinsic efficacy will be a partial agonist. A drug that binds to a receptor and exhibits zero efficacy is an antagonist. When the response of an agonist is measured in a simple biological system, the *apparent dissociation constant*, K_{app}, is a macroscopic equilibrium constant that reflects both the ligand binding equilibrium and the subsequent equilibrium that results in the formation of the active receptor LR*.

Quantifying Agonism. When the relative potency of two agonists of equal efficacy is measured in the same biological system, and downstream signaling events are the same for both drugs, the comparison yields a relative measure of the affinity and efficacy of the two agonists (Figure 3–3). It is convenient to describe agonist response by determining the *half-maximally effective concentration* (EC_{50}) for producing a given effect. Thus, measuring agonist potency by comparison of EC_{50} values is one method of measuring the capability of different agonists to induce a response in a test system and for predicting comparable activity in another. Another method of estimating agonist activity is to compare maximal asymptotes in systems where the agonists do not produce maximal response (Figure 3–3B). The advantage of using maxima is that this property depends solely on efficacy, whereas drug *potency* is a mixed function of both affinity and efficacy.

Quantifying Antagonism. Characteristic patterns of antagonism are associated with certain mechanisms of blockade of receptors. One is straightforward *competitive antagonism*, whereby a drug with affinity for a receptor but lacking intrinsic efficacy competes with the agonist for the primary binding site on the receptor (Ariens, 1954; Gaddum, 1957). The characteristic pattern of such antagonism is the concentration-dependent production of a parallel shift to the right of the agonist dose-response curve with no change in the maximal response (Figure 3–4A). The magnitude of the rightward shift of the curve depends on the concentration of the antagonist and its affinity for the receptor (Schild, 1957).

A partial agonist similarly can compete with a "full" agonist for binding to the receptor. However, increasing concentrations of a partial agonist will inhibit response to a finite level characteristic of the drug's intrinsic efficacy; a competitive antagonist will reduce the response to zero. Partial agonists thus can be used therapeutically to buffer a response by inhibiting excessive receptor stimulation without totally abolishing receptor stimulation (for instance, pindolol, a β antagonist with slight intrinsic agonist activity, will prevent overstimulation of the heart by blocking effects of endogenous catecholamines but will assure slight receptor stimulation in patients overly sensitive to the negative inotropic and negative chronotropic effects of β blockade).

An antagonist may dissociate so slowly from the receptor that its action is exceedingly prolonged, as with the opiate partial agonist buprenorphine and the Ca^{2+} channel blocker amlodipine. In the presence of a slowly dissociating antagonist, the maximal response to the agonist will be depressed at some antagonist concentrations (Figure 3–4B). Operationally, this is referred to as *noncompetitive antagonism,* although the molecular mechanism of action really cannot be inferred unequivocally from the effect. An antagonist may also interact irreversibly (covalently) with a receptor, as do the α adrenergic antagonist phenoxybenzamine and the acetylcholinesterase inhibitor DFP (diisopropylfluorophosphate), to produce relatively irreversible effects. An *irreversible antagonist* competing for the same binding site as the agonist can produce the pattern of antagonism shown in Figure 3–4B. Noncompetitive antagonism can also be produced by another type of drug, referred to as an *allosteric* or *allotopic antagonist.* This type of drug produces its effect by binding to a site on the receptor distinct from that of the primary agonist, thereby changing the affinity of the receptor for the agonist. In the case of an allosteric antagonist, the affinity of the receptor for the agonist is decreased by the antagonist (Figure 3–4C). In contrast, a drug binding at an allosteric site could potentiate the effects of primary agonists (Figure 3–4D); such a drug would be referred to as an *allosteric agonist* or *co-agonist* (May et al., 2007).

The affinity of a competitive antagonist (K_i) for its receptor can be determined in radioligand binding assays or by measuring the functional response of a system to a drug in the presence of the antagonist (Cheng, 2004; Cheng and Prusoff, 1973; Limbird, 2005). Concentration curves are run with the agonist alone and with the

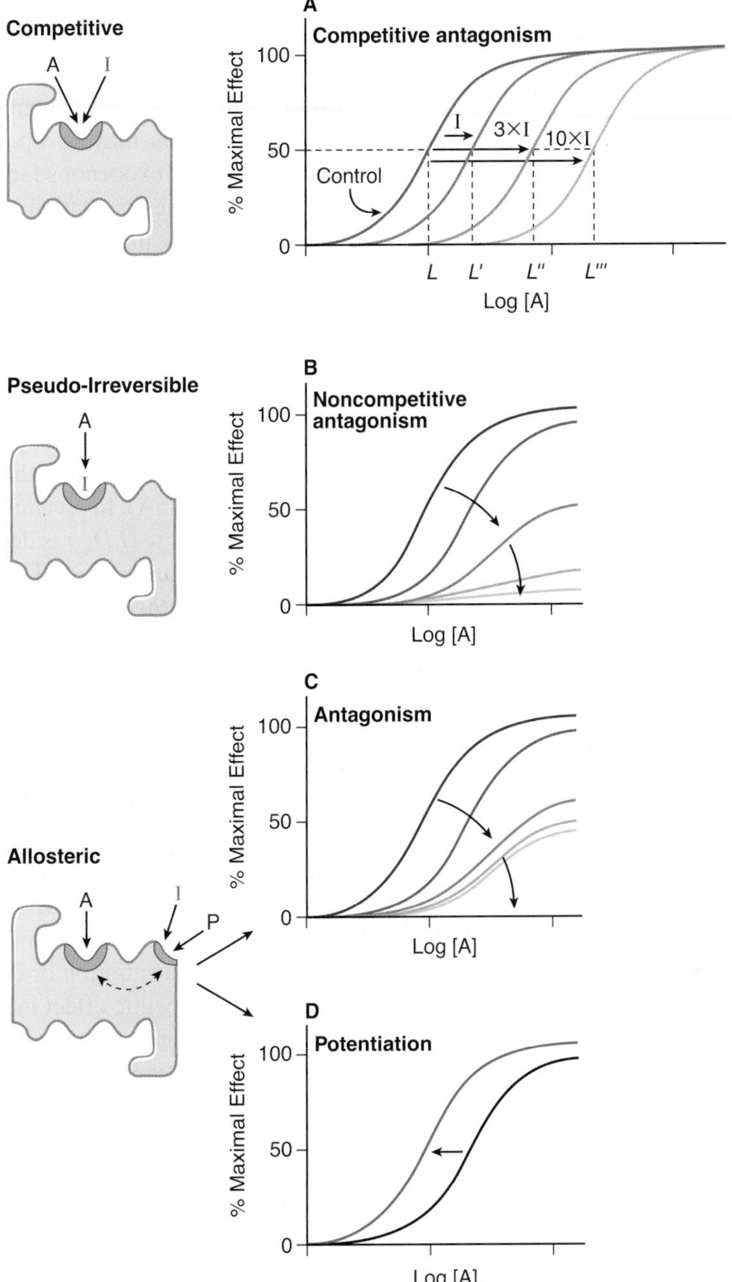

Figure 3–4. *Mechanisms of receptor antagonism.* **A**. Competitive antagonism occurs when the agonist A and antagonist I compete for the same binding site on the receptor. Response curves for the agonist are shifted to the right in a concentration-related manner by the antagonist such that the EC_{50} for the agonist increases (e.g., L versus L', L'', and L''') with the concentration of the antagonist. **B**. If the antagonist binds to the same site as the agonist but does so irreversibly or pseudo-irreversibly (slow dissociation but no covalent bond), it causes a shift of the dose-response curve to the right, with further depression of the maximal response. Allosteric effects occur when an allosteric ligand I or P binds to a different site on the receptor to either inhibit (I) the response (see panel **C**) or potentiate (P) the response (see panel **D**). This effect is saturable; inhibition or potentiation reaches a limiting value when the allosteric site is fully occupied.

agonist plus an effective concentration of the antagonist (Figure 3–4A). As as more antagonist (I) is added, a higher concentration of the agonist (A) is needed to produce an equivalent response (the half-maximal or 50%, response is a convenient and accurately determined level of response).

The extent of the rightward shift of the concentration-dependence curve is a measure of the affinity of the inhibitor, and a higher-affinity inhibitor will cause a greater rightward shift than a lower-affinity inhibitor at the same inhibitor concentration. Using Equations 3–3 and 3–4, one may write mathematical expressions of *fractional occupancy* (f) of the receptor by agonist for the agonist alone (control) and agonist in the presence of inhibitor.

For the agonist drug (L) alone,

$$f_{\text{control}} = \frac{[L]}{[L] + K_D} \quad \text{(Equation 3-5)}$$

For the case of agonist plus antagonist (I),

$$f_{+I} = \frac{[L]}{[L] + K_D\left(1 + \frac{[I]}{K_i}\right)} \quad \text{(Equation 3-6)}$$

Assuming that equal responses result from equal fractional receptor occupancies in both the absence and presence of antagonist, one can set the fractional occupancies equal at agonist concentrations (L and L') that generate equivalent responses in Figure 3–4A. Thus,

$$\frac{L}{L + K_D} = \frac{L'}{L' + K_D\left(1 + \frac{[I]}{K_i}\right)} \quad \text{(Equation 3-7)}$$

Simplifying, one gets:

$$\frac{L'}{L} - 1 = \frac{[I]}{K_i} \quad \text{(Equation 3-8)}$$

where all values are known except K_i. Thus, one can determine the K_i for a reversible, competitive antagonist without knowing the K_D for the agonist and without needing to define the precise relationship between receptor and response.

PHARMACODYNAMIC VARIABILITY: INDIVIDUAL AND POPULATION PHARMACODYNAMICS

Individuals vary in the magnitude of their response to the same concentration of a single drug or to similar drugs, and a given individual may not always respond in the same way to the same drug concentration. Attempts have been made to define and measure individual "sensitivity" (or "resistance") to drugs in the clinical setting, and progress has been made in understanding some of the determinants of sensitivity to drugs that act at specific receptors. Drug responsiveness may change because of disease or because of previous drug administration. Receptors are dynamic, and their concentration and function may be up- or down-regulated by endogenous and exogenous factors.

Data on the correlation of drug levels with efficacy and toxicity must be interpreted in the context of the pharmacodynamic variability in the population (e.g., genetics, age, disease, and the presence of co-administered drugs). The variability in pharmacodynamic response in the population may be analyzed by constructing a quantal concentration-effect curve (Figure 3–5A). The dose of a drug required to produce a specified effect in 50% of the population is the *median effective dose* (*ED_{50}*, Figure 3–5A). In preclinical studies of drugs, the *median lethal dose* (*LD_{50}*) is determined in experimental animals (Figure 3-5B). The LD_{50}/ED_{50} ratio is an indication of the *therapeutic index*, which is a statement of how selective the drug is in producing its desired effects versus its adverse effects. A similar term, the *therapeutic window,* is the range of steady-state concentrations of drug that provides therapeutic efficacy with minimal toxicity (Figure 3–6). In clinical studies, the dose, or preferably the concentration, of a drug required to produce toxic effects can be compared with the concentration required for therapeutic effects in the population to evaluate the *clinical therapeutic index*. Since pharmacodynamic variation in the population may be marked, the concentration or dose of drug required to produce a therapeutic effect in most of the population usually will overlap the concentration required to produce toxicity in some of the population, even though the drug's therapeutic index in an individual patient may be large. Also, the concentration-percent curves for efficacy and toxicity need not be parallel, adding yet another complexity to determination of the therapeutic index in patients. Finally, no drug produces a single effect, and the therapeutic index for a drug will vary depending on the effect being measured.

A clear demonstration of the relation of plasma drug concentration to efficacy or toxicity is not achievable for many drugs; even when such a relationship can be determined, it usually predicts only a probability of efficacy or toxicity. In trials of antidepressant drugs, such a high proportion of patients respond to placebo that it is difficult to determine the plasma drug level associated with efficacy. There is a quantal concentration-response curve for efficacy and adverse effects (Figure 3–5B); for many drugs, the concentration that achieves efficacy in all the population may produce adverse effects in some individuals. Thus, a *population therapeutic window* expresses a range of concentrations at which the likelihood of

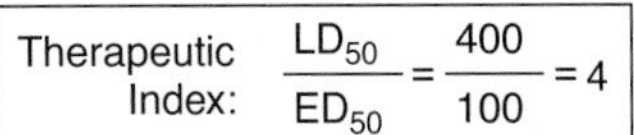

Therapeutic Index: $\frac{LD_{50}}{ED_{50}} = \frac{400}{100} = 4$

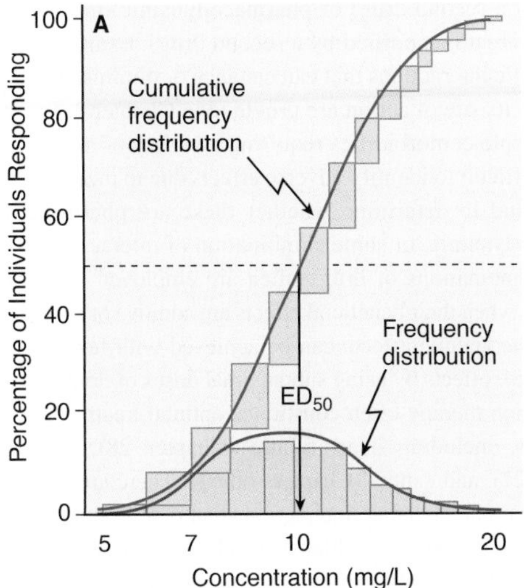

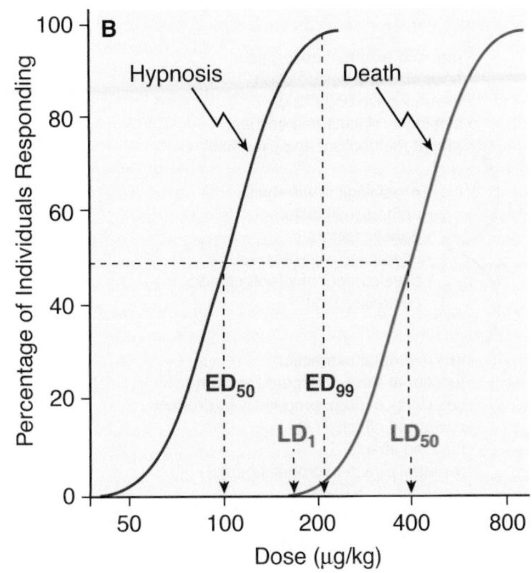

Figure 3–5. *Frequency distribution curves and quantal concentration-effect and dose-effect curves.* **A.** *Frequency distribution curves.* An experiment was performed on 100 subjects, and the effective plasma concentration that produced a quantal response was determined for each individual. The number of subjects who required each dose is plotted, giving a log-normal frequency distribution (*purple bars*). The red bars demonstrate that the normal frequency distribution, when summated, yields the cumulative frequency distribution—a sigmoidal curve that is a quantal concentration-effect curve. **B.** *Quantal dose-effect curves.* Animals were injected with varying doses of a drug and the responses were determined and plotted. The calculation of the therapeutic index, the ratio of the LD_{50} to the ED_{50}, is an indication of how selective a drug is in producing its desired effects relative to its toxicity. See text for additional explanation.

efficacy is high and the probability of adverse effects is low (Figure 3–6). It does not guarantee either efficacy or safety. *Therefore, use of the population therapeutic window to adjust dosage of a drug should be complemented by monitoring appropriate clinical and surrogate markers for drug effect(s).*

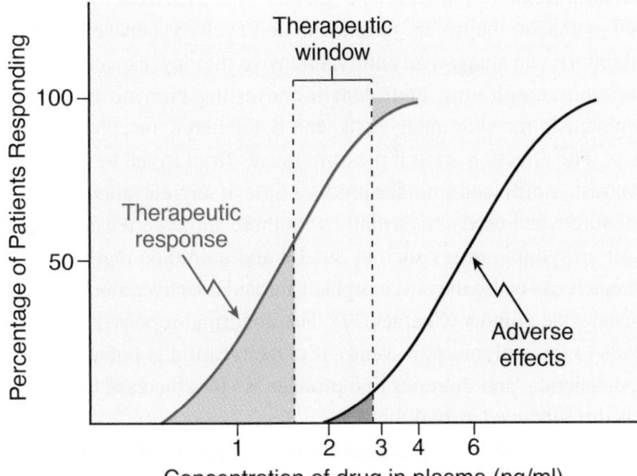

Figure 3–6. *The relation of the therapeutic window of drug concentrations to the therapeutic and adverse effects in the population.* The ordinate is linear; the abcissa is logarithmic.

Factors Modifying Drug Action. Many factors can influence the therapeutic efficacy and safety of a drug in an individual patient. These same factors give rise to inter-individual variability in the dose required to obtain optimal therapeutic effect with minimal adverse effects. Some of the factors that contribute to the wide patient-to-patient variability in the dose required for optimal therapy observed with many drugs are shown in Figure 3–7. Therapeutic success and safety result from integrating evidence of efficacy and safety with knowledge of the individual factors that determine response in a given patient. Determinants of inter-individual variation in response to drugs that are due to pharmacokinetics include disease-related alterations such as impaired renal and liver clearance due to renal and hepatic disease, circulatory failure, altered drug binding to plasma proteins, impaired GI absorption, and pharmacokinetic drug interactions. The effects of these factors on variability of drug pharmacokinetics are described more thoroughly in Chapters 2 and 5-7.

Pharmacogenetics. Pharmacogenetics refers to the genetic and genomic variations that give rise to variability in both pharmacokinetic and pharmacodynamic aspects of drug therapy. These factors

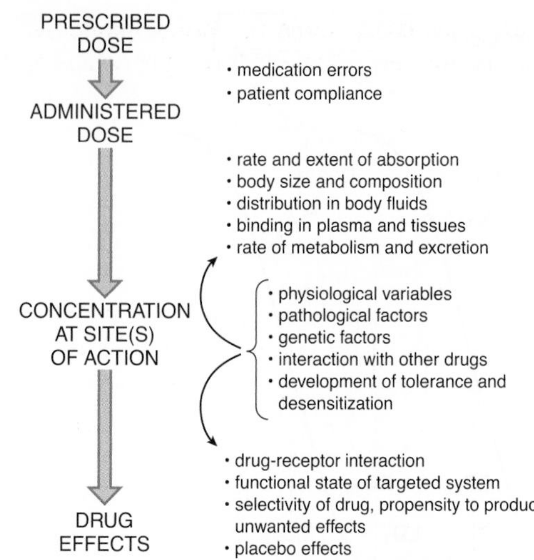

Figure 3–7. *Factors that influence the relationship between prescribed dosage and drug effects.* (Modified with permission from Koch-Weser J. Serum drug concentrations as therapeutic guides. *N Engl J Med*, **1972**, *287*:227–231. Copyright © Massachusetts Medical Society. All rights reserved.)

contribute significantly to the inter-individual variability of responsiveness to many drugs (Chapter 7). Among the best examples of a drug with significant inter-individual sensitivity due to genetic factors affecting both pharmacokinetics and pharmacodynamics is the anticoagulant drug warfarin (Chapter 30). In order to achieve optimal anticoagulant therapy with minimal adverse effects (i.e., excessive clotting due to under dosing, or excessive bleeding due to overdosing), it is necessary to stay within a very narrow dose range (i.e., warfarin's therapeutic index is very low). There is considerable inter-individual variation in this optimal dose range, on the order of 10-fold or more, and nearly 60% of the variability is due to genetic variation in the primary metabolizing enzyme (CYP2C9) and in the drug's receptor, vitamin K epoxide reductase complex, subunit 1 (VKORC1). Polymorphisms in CYP2C9 (especially homozygosity in the *3/*3 allele) increase sensitivity towards warfarin, whereas coding region polymorphisms in VKORC1 result in a warfarin-resistant phenotype. In 2007, the FDA recommended that pharmacogenetics be used to optimize warfarin dosing, but did not provide specific protocols to be used. Subsequently, an algorithm that incorporates clinical and pharmacogenetic data was shown to be significantly better than algorithms that lack genetic data in predicting the initial appropriate dose of warfarin that is close to the required stable dose. The patients who benefited most by the pharmacogenetic algorithm were the 46% who required either low or high dosing to achieve optimal anticoagulation (Klein et al., 2009).

Combination Therapy. Marked alterations in the effects of some drugs can result from co-administration with other agents, including prescription and non-prescription drugs, as well as supplements and nutraceuticals. Such interactions can cause toxicity, or inhibit the drug effect and the therapeutic benefit. Drug interactions always should be considered when unexpected responses to drugs occur. Understanding the mechanisms of drug interactions provides a framework for preventing them. Drug interactions may be pharmacokinetic (the delivery of a drug to its site of action is altered by a second drug) or pharmacodynamic (the response of the drug target is modified by a second drug). Examples of pharmacokinetic interactions that can enhance or diminish the delivery of drug to its site of action are provided in Chapter 2. In a patient with multiple comorbidities requiring a variety of medications, it may be difficult to identify adverse effects due to medication interactions, and to determine whether these are pharmacokinetic, pharmacodynamic, or some combination of interactions.

Combinations of drugs often are employed to therapeutic advantage when their beneficial effects are additive or synergistic, or because therapeutic effects can be achieved with fewer drug-specific adverse effects by using submaximal doses of drugs in concert. Combination therapy often constitutes optimal treatment for many conditions, including heart failure (Chapter 28), hypertension (Chapter 27), and cancer (Chapters 60-63). There are many examples of pharmacodynamic interactions that can produce significant adverse effects. Nitrovasodilators produce relaxation of vascular smooth muscle (vasodilation) via NO-dependent elevation of cyclic GMP in vascular smooth muscle. The pharmacologic effects of sildenafil, tadalafil, and vardenafil result from inhibition of the type 5 cyclic nucleotide phosphodiesterase (PDE5) that hydrolyzes cyclic GMP to 5′GMP in the vasculature. Thus, co-administration of an NO donor (e.g., nitroglycerin) with a PDE5 inhibitor can cause potentially catastrophic hypotension. The oral anticoagulant warfarin has a narrow margin between therapeutic inhibition of clot formation and bleeding complications and is subject to numerous important pharmacokinetic and pharmacodynamic drug interactions. Alterations in dietary vitamin K intake may also significantly affect the pharmacodynamics of warfarin and dosing changes may be required if a patient's diet is inconsistent. Similarly, antibiotics that alter the intestinal flora reduce the bacterial synthesis of vitamin K, thereby enhancing the effect of warfarin. Nonsteroidal anti-inflammatory drugs (NSAIDs) cause gastric and duodenal ulcers (Chapter 34), and their concurrent administration with warfarin increases the risk of GI bleeding almost 4-fold compared with warfarin alone. By inhibiting platelet aggregation, aspirin increases the incidence of bleeding in warfarin-treated patients. A subset of NSAIDs, including indomethacin, ibuprofen, piroxicam, and cyclooxygenase (COX)-2 inhibitors, can antagonize antihypertensive therapy, especially with regimens employing angiotensin-converting enzyme inhibitors, angiotensin receptor antagonists, and β adrenergic receptor antagonists. The effect on arterial pressure ranges from trivial to severe. In contrast, aspirin and sulindac produce little, if any, elevation of blood pressure when used concurrently with these antihypertensive drugs. Anti-arrhythmic drugs such as sotalol and quinidine that block K^+ channels can cause the polymorphic ventricular tachycardia known as torsades de pointes (Chapter 29). The abnormal repolarization that leads to this polymorphic ventricular tachycardia is potentiated by hypokalemia, and diuretics that produce K^+ loss increase the risk of this drug-induced arrhythmia.

Most drugs are evaluated in young and middle-aged adults, and data on their use in children and the elderly are sparse. At the extremes of age, drug pharmacokinetics and pharmacodynamics can be altered, possibly requiring substantial alteration in the dose or dosing regimen to safely produce the desired clinical effect.

MECHANISMS OF DRUG ACTION

Receptors That Affect Concentrations of Endogenous Ligands

A large number of drugs act by altering the synthesis, storage, release, transport, or metabolism of endogenous ligands such as neurotransmitters, hormones, and other intercellular mediators. For instance, there are many examples of drugs that act on neuroeffector junctions by altering neurotransmitter synthesis, storage of neurotransmitter in vesicles, release of neurotransmitters into the synaptic cleft, and subsequent removal of the neurotransmitter from the synaptic cleft by hydrolysis or transport into the pre-synaptic or post-synaptic neuron. The effects of these drugs can either enhance or diminish the effects of the neurotransmitter in order to achieve the desired therapeutic effect. For instance, some of the drugs acting on adrenergic neurotransmission (Chapters 8 and 12) include α-methyltyrosine (inhibits synthesis of norepinephrine (NE)), cocaine (blocks NE reuptake), amphetamine (promotes NE release), and selegeline (inhibits NE breakdown). There are similar examples for other neurotransmitter systems including acetylcholine (ACh; Chapters 8 and 10), dopamine (DA), and serotonin (5HT; Chapters 13-15). Drugs that affect the synthesis of circulating mediators such as vasoactive peptides (e.g., angiotensin-converting enzyme inhibitors; Chapter 26) and lipid-derived autocoids (e.g., cyclooxygenase inhibitors; Chapter 33) are also widely used in the treatment of hypertension, inflammation, myocardial ischemia, and other disease states.

Receptors That Regulate the Ionic Milieu

A relatively small number of drugs act by affecting the ionic millieu of blood, urine, and the GI tract. The receptors for these drugs are ion pumps and transporters, many of which are expressed only in specialized cells of the kidney and GI system. Drug effects on many of these receptors can have effects throughout the body due to changes in blood electrolytes and pH. For instance, most of the diuretics (e.g., furosemide, chlorothiazide, amiloride) act by directly affecting ion pumps and transporters in epithelial cells of the nephron that increase the movement of Na^+ into the urine, or by altering the expression of ion pumps in these cells (e.g., aldosterone). Chapter 25 provides a detailed description of the mechanisms of action of diuretic drugs. Another therapeutically important target is the H^+,K^+-ATPase (proton pump) of gastric parietal cells. Irreversible inhibition of this proton pump by drugs such as esomeprazole reduces gastric acid secretion by 80-95% (Chapter 45) and is a mainstay of therepy for peptic ulcer.

Cellular Pathways Activated by Physiological Receptors

Signal Transduction Pathways. Physiological receptors have at least two major functions, ligand binding and message propagation (i.e., signaling). These functions imply the existence of at least two functional domains within the receptor: a *ligand-binding domain* and an *effector domain*. The structure and function of these domains in many families of receptors have been deduced from high-resolution crystal structures of the receptor proteins and/or by analysis of the behavior of intentionally mutated receptors. Many drugs target the extracelluar ligand-binding domain of physiological receptors. Examples include the widely used β adrenergic antagonists. However, drugs can affect the receptor by targeting either domain, as in the case of anticancer drugs used to target the epidermal growth factor receptor (EGFR; Chapters 60-62). Cetuximab is a monoclonal antibody that targets the extracellular ligand-binding domain of the EGFR and inhibits epidermal growth factor (EGF) signaling, whereas the small molecule drugs gefitinib and erlotinib bind the intracellular effector domain and block the protein tyrosine kinase activity of the activated EGFR.

The regulatory actions of a receptor may be exerted directly on its cellular target(s), on *effector protein(s)*, or may be conveyed by intermediary cellular signaling molecules called *transducers*. The receptor, its cellular target, and any intermediary molecules are referred to as a *receptor-effector system* or *signal transduction pathway*. Frequently, the proximal cellular effector protein is not the ultimate physiological target but rather is an enzyme, ion channel, or transport protein that creates, moves, or degrades a small molecule (e.g., a cyclic nucleotide, inositol trisphosphate, or NO) or ion (e.g., Ca^{2+}) termed a *second messenger*. If the effector is an ion channel or ion pump, the effect of ligand binding can be a change in membrane potential that alters the excitability of the cell. Second messengers can diffuse in the proximity of their synthesis or release and convey information to a variety of targets, which may integrate multiple signals. Even though these second messengers originally were thought of as freely diffusible molecules within the cell, imaging studies show that their diffusion and intracellular actions are constrained by compartmentation—selective localization of receptor-transducer-effector-signal termination complexes—established by protein-lipid and protein-protein interactions (Baillie, 2009). All cells express multiple forms of proteins designed to localize signaling pathways by protein-protein interactions; these proteins are termed scaffolds or anchoring proteins. Examples of scaffold molecules include the AKAPs (A-kinase anchoring proteins) that bind the regulatory subunit of the cyclic AMP dependent protein kinase (PKA) near its substrate(s) in various subcellular compartments (Carnegie et al., 2009).

Signal Integration and Amplification. Receptors and their associated effector and transducer proteins also act as integrators of information as they coordinate signals from multiple ligands with each other and with the differentiated activity of the target cell. For example, signal transduction systems regulated by changes in cyclic AMP (cAMP) and intracellular Ca^{2+} are integrated in many excitable tissues. In cardiac myocytes, an increase in cellular cAMP caused by activation of β adrenergic receptors enhances cardiac contractility by augmenting the rate and amount of Ca^{2+} delivered to the contractile apparatus; thus, cAMP and Ca^{2+} are positive contractile signals in cardiac myocytes. By contrast, cAMP and Ca^{2+} produce opposing effects on the contractility of smooth muscle cells: as usual, Ca^{2+} is a contractile signal, however, activation of β adrenergic receptors on these cells activates the cAMP-PKA pathway, which leads to relaxation through the phosphorylation of proteins that mediate Ca^{2+} signaling, such as myosin light chain kinase and ion channels that hyperpolarize the cell membrane. Thus, the distinct patterns of integration of signal transduction systems within target cells can lead to a variety of pharmacodynamic effects that result from functional interactions downstream from the receptors. These functional interactions can be synergistic, additive, or antagonistic.

Another important property of physiological receptors is their capacity to significantly amplify a physiological signal. Neurotransmitters, hormones, and other extracellular ligands are often present at the ligand-binding domain of a receptor in very low concentrations (nM to μM levels). However, the effector domain or the signal transduction pathway often contains enzymes and enzyme cascades to catalytically amplify the intended signal. In this regard, the description of receptor occupancy-cellular response in Equation 3-1 is an oversimplification. The ability of virtually all receptors to amplify physiological signals makes them excellent targets for natural ligands and drugs. When, e.g., a single agonist molecule binds to a receptor that is an ion channel, hundreds of thousands to millions of ions flow through the channel every second. Similarly, the binding of a single photon to *cis*-retinal in the photoreceptor rhodpsin is eventually amplified ~1×10^6-fold. In the case of nuclear receptors, a single steroid hormone molecule binding to its receptor initiates the transcription of many copies of specific mRNAs, which in turn can give rise to multiple copies of a single protein.

Structural and Functional Families of Physiological Receptors

Receptors for physiological regulatory molecules can be assigned to functional families whose members share similar molecular structures and biochemical mechanisms with common features. Table 3–1 outlines six major families of receptors with examples of their physiological ligands, signal transduction systems, and drugs that affect these systems. The basic structure of their ligand-binding domains, effector domains, and how agonist binding influences the regulatory activity of the receptor is well understood for each of these signal transduction systems. The relatively small number of biochemical mechanisms and structural formats used for cellular signaling is fundamental to the ways in which target cells integrate signals from multiple receptors to produce additive, sequential, synergistic, or mutually inhibitory responses.

G Protein–Coupled Receptors (GCPRs)

Receptors and G Proteins. GPCRs span the plasma membrane as a bundle of seven α-helices (Palczewski et al., 2000) (Figure 3–8). Humans express over 800 GPCRs that make up the third largest family of genes in humans, with roughly half of these GPCRs dedicated to sensory perception (smell, taste, and vision). The remaining receptors regulate an impressive number of physiological functions including nerve activity, tension of smooth muscle, metabolism, rate and force of cardiac contraction, and the secretion of most glands in the body. Included among the ligands for GPCRs are neurotransmitters such as ACh, biogenic amines such as NE, all eicosanoids and other lipid signaling molecules, peptide hormones, opioids, amino acids such as GABA, and many other peptide and protein ligands. GPCRs are important regulators of nerve activity in the CNS and are the receptors for the neurotransmitters of the peripheral autonomic nervous system. For example, ACh released by the parasympathetic nervous system regulates the functions of glands and smooth muscle through

Table 3–1

Physiological Receptors

STRUCTURAL FAMILY	FUNCTIONAL FAMILY	PHYSIOLOGICAL LIGANDS	EFFECTORS AND TRANSDUCERS	EXAMPLE DRUGS
GPCR	β Adrenergic receptors	NE, Epi, DA	G_s; AC	Dobutamine, propranolol
	Muscarinic cholinergic receptors	ACh	G_i and G_q; AC, ion channels, PLC	Atropine
	Eicosanoid receptors	Prostaglandins, leukotrienes, thromboxanes	G_s, G_i and G_q proteins	Misoprostol, montelukast
	Thrombin receptors (PAR)	Receptor peptide	$G_{12/13}$, GEFs	(in development)
Ion channels	Ligand-gated	ACh (M_2), GABA, 5-HT	Na^+, Ca^{2+}, K^+, Cl^-	Nicotine, gabapentin
	Voltage-gated	None (activated by membrane depolarization)	Na^+, Ca^{2+}, K^+, other ions	Lidocaine, verapamil
Transmembrane enzymes	Receptor tyrosine kinases	Insulin, PDGF, EGF, VEGF, growth factors	SH2 domain and PTB-containing proteins	Herceptin, imatinib
	Membrane-bound GC Tyrosine phosphatases	Natriuretic peptides	Cyclic GMP	Neseritide
Transmembrane, non-enzymes	Cytokine receptors	Interleukins and other cytokines	Jak/STAT, soluble tyrosine kinases	
	Toll-like receptors	LPS, bacterial products	MyD88, IARKs, NF-κB	
Nuclear receptors	Steroid receptors	Estrogen, testosterone	Co-activators	Estrogens, androgens, cortisol
	Thyroid hormone receptors	Thyroid hormone		Thyroid hormone
	PPARγ	PPARγ		Thiazolidinediones
Intracellular enzymes	Soluble GC	NO, Ca^{2+}	Cyclic GMP	Nitrovasodilators

AC, adenylyl cyclase; GC, guanylyl cyclase; PAR, protease-activated receptor; PLC, phospholipase C; PPAR, peroxisome proliferator-activated receptor.

its action on muscarinic receptors. NE released by the sympathetic nervous system interacts with α and β adrenergic receptors to regulate cardiac function and the tone of vascular smooth muscle (Chapters 8-12). Because of their number and physiological importance, GPCRs are the targets for many drugs; perhaps half of all non-antibiotic prescription drugs act at these receptors.

Receptor Subtypes. There are multiple receptor subtypes within families of receptors. Ligand-binding studies with multiple chemical entities initially identified receptor subtypes; molecular cloning has greatly accelerated the discovery and definition of additional receptor subtypes; their expression as recombinant proteins has facilitated the discovery of subtype-selective drugs. Distinct but related receptors may display distinctive

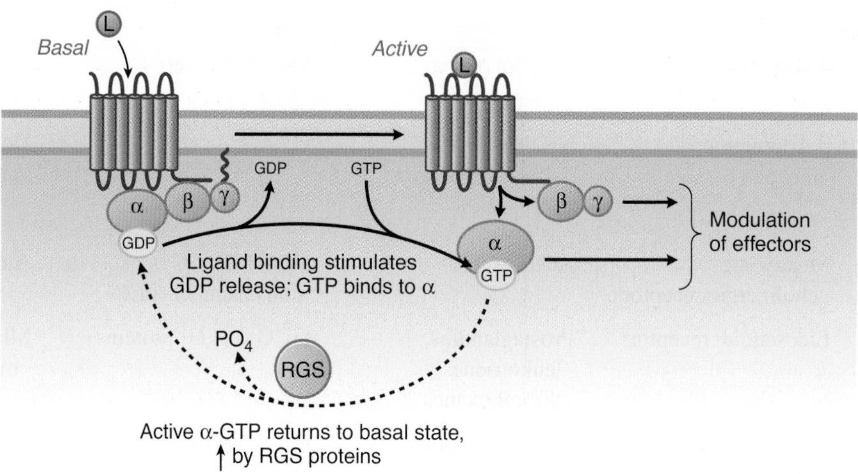

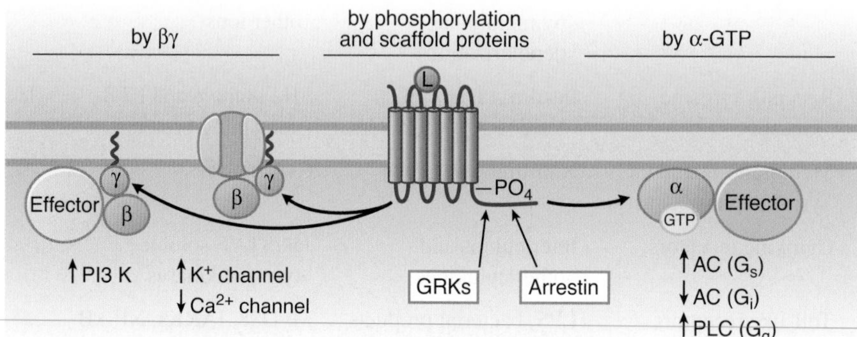

Figure 3–8. *Diagram showing the stimulation of a G–protein coupled receptor by ligand, the activation of the G protein, and stimulation of selected effectors.* Schematic diagram of the mechanisms involved in the control of cell function by G–protein coupled receptors, G proteins, and effectors. In the absence of ligand, the receptor and G protein heterotrimer form a complex in the membrane with the Gα subunit bound to GDP. Following binding of ligand, the receptor and G protein α subunit undergo a conformational change leading to release of GDP, binding of GTP, and dissociation of the complex. The activated GTP-bound Gα subunit and the freed βγ dimer bind to and regulate effectors. The system is returned to the basal state by hydrolysis of the GTP on the α subunit; a reaction that is markedly enhanced by the RGS proteins. Prolonged stimulation of the receptor can lead to down-regulation of the receptor. This event is initiated by G protein receptor kinases (GRKs) that phosphorylate the C terminal tail of the receptor, leading to recruitment of proteins termed arrestins; arrestins bind to the receptor on the internal surface, displacing G proteins and inhibiting signaling. Detailed descriptions of these signaling pathways are given throughout the text in relation to the therapeutic actions of drugs affecting these pathways.

patterns of selectivity among agonist or antagonist ligands. When selective ligands are not known, the receptors are more commonly referred to as isoforms rather than as subtypes. The distinction between classes and subtypes of receptors, however, is often arbitrary or historical. The α_1, α_2, and β adrenergic receptors differ from each other both in ligand selectivity and in coupling to G proteins (G_q, G_i, and G_s, respectively), yet α and β are considered receptor classes and α_1 and α_2 are considered subtypes. The α_{1A}, α_{1B}, and α_{1C} receptor isoforms differ little in their biochemical properties, although their tissue distributions are distinct. The β_1, β_2, and β_3 adrenergic receptor subtypes exhibit differences in both tissue distribution and regulation by phosphorylation by G–protein receptor kinases (GRKs) and PKA.

Pharmacological differences among receptor subtypes are exploited therapeutically through the development and use of receptor-selective drugs. Such drugs may be used to elicit different responses from a single tissue when receptor subtypes initiate different intracellular signals, or they may serve to differentially modulate different cells or tissues that express one or another receptor subtype. For example, β_2 adrenergic agonists such as terbutaline are used for bronchodilation in the treatment of asthma in the hope of minimizing cardiac side effects caused by stimulation of the β_1 adrenergic receptor (Chapter 12). Conversely, the use of β_1-selective antagonists minimizes the chance of bronchoconstriction in patients being treated for hypertension or angina (Chapters 12 and 27). Increasing the selectivity of a drug among tissues or among responses elicited from a single tissue may determine whether the drug's therapeutic benefits outweigh its unwanted effects.

Receptor Dimerization. Receptor-ligand interactions alone do not regulate all GPCR signaling. GPCRs undergo both homo- and heterodimerization and possibly oligomerization. Heterodimerization can result in receptor units with altered pharmacology compared with either individual receptor. As an example, opioid receptors can exist as homodimers of μ or δ receptors, or as μδ heterodimers with distinctly different pharmacodynamic properties than either homodimer (Chapter 18). Evidence is emerging that dimerization of receptors may regulate the affinity and specificity of the complex for G proteins, and regulate the sensitivity of the receptor to phosphorylation by receptor kinases and the binding of arrestin, events important in termination of the action of agonists and removal of receptors from the cell surface. Dimerization also may permit binding of receptors to other regulatory proteins such as transcription factors. Thus, the receptor-G protein-effector systems are complex networks of convergent and divergent interactions involving both receptor-receptor and receptor-G protein coupling that permit extraordinarily versatile regulation of cell function. Dimerization of single membrane spanning receptors is central to their activation (described later in the chapter).

G Proteins. GPCRs couple to a family of heterotrimeric GTP-binding regulatory proteins termed G proteins. G proteins are signal transducers that convey the information that agonist is bound to the receptor from the receptor to one or more effector proteins (Gilman, 1987). G–protein-regulated effectors include enzymes such as adenylyl cyclase, phospholipase C, cyclic GMP phosphodiesterase (PDE6), and membrane ion channels selective for Ca^{2+} and K^+ (Table 3–1, Figure 3–8). The G protein heterotrimer is composed of a guanine nucleotide-binding α subunit, which confers specific recognition to both receptors and effectors, and an associated dimer of β and γ subunits that helps confer membrane localization of the G protein heterorimer by prenylation of the γ subunit. In the basal state of the receptor-heterotrimer complex, the α subunit contains bound GDP and the α-GDP:βγ complex is bound to the unliganded receptor (Figure 3-8). The G protein family is comprised of 23 α subunits (which are the products of 17 genes), 7 β subunits, and 12 γ subunits. The α subunits fall into four families (G_s, G_i, G_q, and $G_{12/13}$) which are responsible for coupling GPCRs to relatively distinct effectors. The G_s α subunit uniformly activates adenylyl cyclase; the G_i α subunit can inhibit certain isoforms of adenylyl cyclase; the G_q α subunit activates all forms of phospholipase Cβ; and the $G_{12/13}$ α subunits couple to guanine nucleotide exchange factors (GEFs), such as p115RhoGEF for the small GTP-binding proteins Rho and Rac. The signaling specificity of the large number of possible βγ combinations is not yet clear; nonetheless, it is known that K^+ channels, Ca^{2+} channels, and PI-3 kinase (PI3K) are some of the effectors of free βγ dimer (Figure 3–8).

G Protein Activation. When an agonist binds to a GPCR, there is a conformational change in the receptor that is transmitted from the ligand-binding pocket to the second and third intracellular loops of the receptor which couple to the G protein heterotrimer. This conformational change causes the α subunit to exchange its bound GDP for GTP (Figure 3-8). Binding of GTP activates the α subunit and causes it to release both the βγ dimer and the receptor, and both the GTP-bound α subunit and the βγ heterodimer become active signaling molecules (Gilman, 1987). The interaction of the agonist-bound GPCR with the G protein is transient; following activation of one G protein, the receptor is freed to interact with other G proteins. Depending on the nature of the α subunit, the active, GTP-bound form binds to and regulates effectors such as adenylyl cyclase (via G_s α) or phospholipase Cβ (via G_q α). The βγ subunit can regulate many effectors including ion channels and enzymes such as PI3-K (Figure 3–8). The G protein remains active until the GTP bound to the α subunit is hydrolyzed to GDP. The α subunit has a slow intrinsic rate of GTP hydrolysis that is modulated by a family of proteins termed *regulators of G protein signaling* (RGSs). The RGS proteins greatly accelerate the hydrolysis of GTP and are potentially attractive drug targets (Ross and Wilkie, 2000). Once the GDP bound to the α subunit is hydrolyzed to GDP, the βγ subunit and receptor recombine to form the inactive receptor-G protein heterotrimer basal complex that can be reactivated by another ligand-binding event (Figure 3–8).

Cyclic AMP. Cyclic AMP is synthesized by adenylyl cyclase under the control of many GPCRs; stimulation is mediated by the G_s α subunit, inhibition by the G_i α subunit. The cyclic AMP pathway provides a good basis for understanding the architecture and regulation of many second messenger signaling systems (for an overview of cyclic nucleotide action, *see* Beavo and Brunton, 2002).

There are nine membrane-bound isoforms of adenylyl cyclase (AC) and one soluble isoform found in mammals (Hanoune and Defer, 2001). The membrane-bound ACs are glycoproteins of ~120 kDa with considerable sequence homology: a small cytoplasmic domain; two hydrophobic transmembrane domains, each with six membrane-spanning helices; and two large cytoplasmic domains. Membrane-bound ACs exhibit basal enzymatic activity that is modulated by binding of GTP-liganded α subunits of the stimulatory and inhibitory G proteins (G_s and G_i). Numerous other regulatory interactions are possible, and these enzymes are catalogued based on their structural homology and their distinct regulation by G protein α and βγ subunits, Ca^{2+}, protein kinases, and the actions of the diterpene forskolin. Cyclic AMP generated by adenylyl cyclases has three major targets in most cells, the cyclic AMP dependent protein kinase (PKA), cAMP-regulated guanine nucleotide exchange factors termed EPACs (exchange factors directly activated by cAMP), and via PKA phosphorylation, a transcription factor termed CREB (cAMP response element binding protein). In cells with specialized functions, cAMP can have additional targets such as cyclic nucleotide-gated ion channels (Wahl-Schott and Biel, 2009), cyclic nucleotide-regulated phosphodiesterases (PDEs), and several ABC transporters (MRP4 and MRP5) for which it is a substrate (see Chapter 7).

PKA. The best understood target of cyclic AMP is the PKA holoenzyme consisting of two catalytic (C) subunits reversibly bound to a regulatory (R) subunit dimer to form a heterotetramer complex (R_2C_2). At low concentrations of cAMP, the R subunits inhibit the C subunits; thus the holoenzyme is inactive. When AC is activated and cAMP concentrations are increased, four cyclic AMP molecules bind to the R_2C_2 complex, two to each R subunit, causing a conformational change in the R subunits that lowers their affinity for the C subunits, causing their activation. The active C subunits phosphorylate serine and threonine residues on specific protein substrates.

There are multiple isoforms of PKA; molecular cloning has revealed α and β isoforms of both the regulatory subunits (RI and RII), as well as three C subunit isoforms Cα, Cβ, and Cγ. The R subunits exhibit different subcellular localization and binding affinities for cAMP, giving rise to PKA holoenzymes with different thresholds for activation (Taylor et al., 2008). Both the R and C subunits interact with other proteins within the cell, particularly the R subunits, and these interactions can be isoform-specific. For instance, the RII isoforms are highly localized near their substrates in cells through interactions with a variety of A kinase anchoring proteins (AKAPs) (Carnegie et al., 2009; Wong and Scott, 2004).

PKA can phosphorylate a diverse array of physiological targets such as metabolic enzymes and transport proteins, and numerous regulatory proteins including other protein kinases, ion channels, and transcription factors. For instance, phosphorylation of the cAMP response element–binding protein, CREB, on serine 133 recruits CREB-binding protein (CBP), a histone acetyltransferase that interacts with RNA polymerase II (POLII) and leads to enhanced transcription of ~105 genes containing the cAMP response element motif (CRE) in their promoter regions (e.g., tyrosine hydroxylase, iNOS, AhR, angiotensinogen, insulin, the glucocorticoid receptor, BC12, and CFTR) (Mayr and Montminy, 2001; Sands and Palmer, 2008).

Cyclic AMP–Regulated Guanine Nucleotide Exchange Factors (GEFs). The small GTP-binding proteins are monomeric GTPases and key regulators of cell function. The small GTPases operate as binary switches that exist in GTP- or GDP-liganded conformations. They integrate extracellular signals from membrane receptors with cytoskeletal changes and activation of diverse signaling pathways, regulating such processes as phagocytosis, progression through the cell cycle, cell adhesion, gene expression, and apoptosis (Etienne-Manneville and Hall, 2002). A number of extracellular stimuli signal to the small GTPases directly or through second messengers such as cyclic AMP.

For example, many small GTPases are regulated by GEFs. GEFs act by binding to the GDP-liganded GTPase and catalyzing the exchange of GDP for GTP. The two GEFs regulated by cAMP are able to activate members of the Ras small GTPase family, Rap1 and Rap2; these GEFs are termed *exchange proteins activated by cyclic AMP* (EPAC-1 and EPAC-2). The EPAC pathway provides an additional effector system for cAMP signaling and drug action that can act independently or cooperatively with PKA (Cheng et al., 2008; Roscioni et al., 2008).

PKG. Stimulation of receptors that raise intracellular cyclic GMP concentrations (Figure 3-11) leads to the activation of the cyclic GMP-dependent protein kinase (PKG) that phosphorylates some of the same substrates as PKA and some that are PKG-specific. In some tissues, PKG can also be activated by cAMP. Unlike the heterotetramer (R_2C_2) structure of the PKA holoenzyme, the catalytic domain and cyclic nucleotide-binding domains of PKG are expressed as a single polypeptide, which dimerizes to form the PKG holoenzyme.

PKG exists in two homologous forms, PKG-I and PKG-II. PKG-I has an acetylated N terminus, is associated with the cytoplasm and has two isoforms (Iα and Iβ) that arise from alternate splicing. PKG-II has a myristylated N terminus, is membrane-associated and can be localized by PKG-anchoring proteins in a manner analogous to that known for PKA, although the docking domains of PKA and PKG are very different structurally. Pharmacologically important effects of elevated cyclic GMP include modulation of platelet activation and relaxation of smooth muscle (Rybalkin et al., 2003).

PDEs. Cyclic nucleotide phosphodiesterases form another family of important signaling proteins whose activities are regulated via the rate of gene transcription as well as by second messengers (cyclic nucleotides or Ca^{2+}) and interactions with other signaling proteins such as β arrestin and protein kinases. PDEs hydrolyze the cyclic 3′,5′-phosphodiester bond in cAMP and cGMP, thereby terminating their action.

The enzymes comprise a superfamily with >50 different PDE proteins divided into 11 subfamilies on the basis of amino acid sequence, substrate specificity, pharmacological properties, and allosteric regulation (Conti and Beavo, 2007). PDEs share a conserved catalytic domain at the carboxyl terminus, as well as regulatory domains and targeting domains that localize a given enzyme to a specific cellular compartment. The substrate specificities of the different PDEs include those specific for cAMP hydrolysis, cGMP hydrolysis, and some that hydrolyze both cyclic nucleotides. PDEs (mainly PDE3 forms) are drug targets for treatment of diseases such as asthma, cardiovascular diseases such as heart failure, atherosclerotic coronary and peripheral arterial disease, and neurological disorders. PDE5 inhibitors (e.g., sildenafil) are used in treating chronic obstructive pulmonary disease and erectile dysfunction. By inhibiting PDE5, these drugs increase accumulation of cellular cGMP in the smooth muscle of the corpus caverosum, thereby enhancing its relaxation and improving its capacity for engorgement (Mehats et al., 2002).

Other Second Messengers

Ca^{2+}. Calcium is an important messenger in all cells and can regulate diverse responses including gene expression, contraction, secretion, metabolism, and electrical activity. Ca^{2+} can enter the cell through Ca^{2+} channels in the plasma membrane (See "Ion Channels", below) or be released by hormones or growth factors from intracellular stores. In keeping with its role as a signal, the basal Ca^{2+} level in cells is maintained in the 100 n range by membrane Ca^{2+} pumps that extrude Ca^{2+} to the extracellular space and a sarcoplasmic reticulum (SR) Ca^{2+}-ATPase (SERCA) in the membrane of the endoplasmic reticulum (ER) that accumulates Ca^{2+} into its storage site in the ER/SR.

Hormones and growth factors release Ca^{2+} from its intracellular storage site, the ER, via a signaling pathway that begins with activation of phospholipase C at the plasma membrane, of which there are two primary forms, PLCβ and PLCγ. GPCRs that couple to G_q or G_i activate PLCβ by activating the G protein α subunit (Figure 3–8) and releasing the $\beta\gamma$ dimer. Both the active, G_q-GTP bound α subunit and the $\beta\gamma$ dimer can activate certain isoforms of PLCβ. PLCγ isoforms are activated by tyrosine phosphorylation, including phosphorylation by receptor and non-receptor tyrosine kinases. For example, growth factor receptors such as the epidermal growth factor receptor (EGFR) are receptor tyrosine kinases (RTKs) that autophosphorylate on tyrosine residues upon binding their cognate growth factor. The phosphotyrosine formed on the cytoplasmic domain of the RTK is a binding site for signaling proteins that contain SH2 domains, such as PLCγ. Once recruited to the RTK's SH2 domain, PLCγ is phosphorylated/activated by the RTK.

PLCs are cytosolic enzymes that translocate to the plasma membrane upon receptor stimulation. When activated, they hydrolyze a minor membrane phospholipid, phosphatidylinositol-4, 5-bisphosphate, to generate two intracellular signals, inositol-1,4,5-trisphosphate (IP_3) and the lipid, diacylglycerol (DAG). Both of these molecules lead to signaling events by activating families of protein kinases. DAG directly activates members of the protein kinase C (PKC) family. IP_3 diffuses to the ER where it activates the IP_3 receptor in the ER membrane causing release of stored Ca^{2+} from the ER. Release of Ca^{2+} from these intracellular stores raises Ca^{2+} levels in the cytoplasm many fold within seconds and activates calmodulin-sensitive enzymes such as cyclic AMP PDE and a family of Ca^{2+}/calmodulin-sensitive protein kinases (e.g., phosphorylase kinase, myosin light chain kinase, and CaM kinases II and IV) (Hudmon and Schulman, 2002). Depending on the cell's differentiated function, the Ca^{2+}/calmodulin kinases and PKC may regulate the bulk of the downstream events in the activated cells. For example, release of the sympathetic transmitter norepinephrine onto vascular smooth muscle cells stimulates α adrenergic receptors, activates the G_q-PLC-IP_3 pathway, triggers the release of Ca^{2+}, and leads to contraction by stimulating the Ca^{2+}/calmodulin-sensitive myosin light chain kinase to phosphorylate the regulatory subunit of the contractile protein, myosin.

The IP_3-stimulated release of Ca^{2+} from the ER, its reuptake, and the refilling of the ER pool of Ca^{2+} are regulated by a novel set of Ca^{2+} channels. The IP_3 receptor is a ligand-gated Ca^{2+} channel found in high concentrations in the membrane of the ER (Patterson et al., 2004). It is a large protein of ~2700 amino acids with three major domains. The N-terminal region contains the IP3-binding site, and the middle region contains a regulatory domain that can be phosphorylated by a number of protein kinases including PKA and PKG. The C-terminal region contains six membrane-spanning helices that form the Ca^{2+} pore. The functional channel is formed by four subunits arranged as a tetramer. In addition to IP_3, which markedly stimulates Ca^{2+} flux, the IP_3 channel is regulated by Ca^{2+} and by the activities of PKA and PKG. Ca^{2+} concentrations in the 100-300 nM range enhance Ca^{2+} release, but concentrations near 1 μM inhibit release, which can create the oscillatory patterns of Ca^{2+} release seen in certain cells. Phosphorylation of the IP_3 receptor by PKA enhances Ca^{2+} release, but phosphorylation of an accessory protein, IRAG, by PKG inhibits Ca^{2+} release. In smooth muscle, this effect of PKG represents part of the mechanism by which cyclic GMP relaxes vessel tone. In skeletal and cardiac muscle, Ca^{2+} release from intracellular stores (the sarcoplasmic reticulum) occurs through a process termed Ca^{2+}-induced Ca^{2+} release, and is primarily mediated by the ryanodine receptor (RyR). Ca^{2+} entry into a skeletal or cardiac myocyte through L-type Ca^{2+} channels causes conformational changes in the ryanodine receptor that induce the release of large quantities of Ca^{2+} into the sarcoplasm. Drugs that activate the RyR include caffeine; drugs that inhibit the RyR include dantrolene.

Calcium released into the cytoplasm from the ER is rapidly removed by plasma membrane Ca^{2+} pumps, and the ER pool of Ca^{2+} is refilled with extracellular Ca^{2+} flowing through store-operated Ca^{2+} channels (SOC) in the plasma membrane. These currents are termed Ca^{2+} release-activated currents, or I_{CRAC}. The mechanism by which ER store depletion opens the store-operated channels requires two proteins, the channel itself, termed Orai1, and an ER sensor termed STIM1. The Orai1 channel is a 33-kDa protein with four membrane-spanning helices and no homology with other Ca^{2+} channels (Prakriya, 2009). Orai1 is highly selective for Ca^{2+}. The C terminal end of the channel contains coiled-coil domains thought to interact with the STIM1 sensor. STIM1 is a 77-kDa protein containing a Ca^{2+} sensor domain termed an EF hand. This domain is located at the N-terminus of the protein on the inside of the ER membrane before the single membrane-spanning domain. There are multiple protein-protein interaction motifs in the middle and C-terminal end of the molecule. Specifically, there are two coiled-coil domains on the C-terminal side of the transmembrane domain in STIM1 that may interact with coiled-coil domains in the Orai1 channel. Under resting conditions, the STIM1 protein is uniformly distributed on the ER membrane. Release of Ca^{2+} from the ER stores results in dimerization of STIM1 and movement to the plasma membrane where STIM1 and Orai1 form clusters, opening the Ca^{2+} pore of Orai1 and refilling of the ER Ca^{2+} pool (Fahrner et al., 2009).

Ion Channels

The lipid bilayer of the plasma membrane is impermeable to anions and cations, yet changes in the flux of ions across the plasma membrane are critical regulatory events in both excitable and non-excitable cells. To establish and maintain the electrochemical gradients required to maintain a membrane potential, all cells express ion transporters for Na^+, K^+, Ca^{2+}, and Cl^-. For example, the Na^+,K^+-ATPase pump expends cellular ATP to pump Na^+ out of the cell and K^+ into the cell. The electrochemical gradients thus established are used by excitable tissues such as nerve and muscle to generate and transmit electrical impulses, by non-excitable cells to trigger biochemical and secretory events, and by all cells to support a variety of secondary symport and antiport processes (Chapter 5).

Passive ion fluxes down cellular electrochemical gradients are regulated by a large family of ion channels located in the membrane. Humans express ~232 distinct ion channels to precisely regulate the flow of Na^+, K^+, Ca^{2+}, and Cl^- across the cell membrane (Jegla et al., 2009). Because of their roles as regulators of cell function, these proteins are important drug targets. The diverse ion channel family can be divided into subfamilies based on the mechanisms that open the channels, their architecture, and the ions they conduct. They can also be classified as voltage-activated, ligand-activated, store-activated, stretch-activated, and temperature-activated channels. Examples of channels that are major drug targets are detailed next.

Voltage-Gated Channels. Humans express multiple isoforms of voltage-gated channels for Na^+, K^+, Ca^{2+}, and Cl^- ions. In nerve and muscle cells, voltage-gated Na^+ channels are responsible for the generation of robust action potentials that depolarize the membrane from its resting potential of –70 mV up to a potential of +20 mV within a few milliseconds. These Na^+ channels are composed of three subunits, a pore-forming α subunit and two regulatory β subunits. The α subunit is a 260 kDa protein containing four domains that form a Na^+ ion-selective pore by arranging into a pseudo-tetramer shape. The β subunits are ~36 kDa proteins that span the membrane once (Figure 3–9A). Each domain of the α subunit contains six membrane-spanning helices (S1-S6) with an extracellular loop between S5 and S6, termed the pore-forming or P loop; the P loop dips back into the pore and, combined with residues from the corresponding P loops from the other domains, provides a selectivity filter for the Na^+ ion. Four other helices surrounding the pore (one S4 helix from each of the domains) contain a set of charged amino acids that form the voltage sensor and cause a conformational change in the pore at more positive voltages leading to opening of the pore and depolarization of the membrane (Purves and McNamara, 2008). The voltage-activated Na^+ channels in pain neurons are targets for local anesthetics such as lidocaine and tetracaine, which block the pore, inhibit depolarization, and thus block the sensation of pain. They are also the targets of the naturally occurring marine toxins, tetrodotoxin and saxitoxin (Chapter 20). Voltage-activated Na^+ channels are also important targets of many drugs used to treat cardiac arrhythmias (Chapter 29).

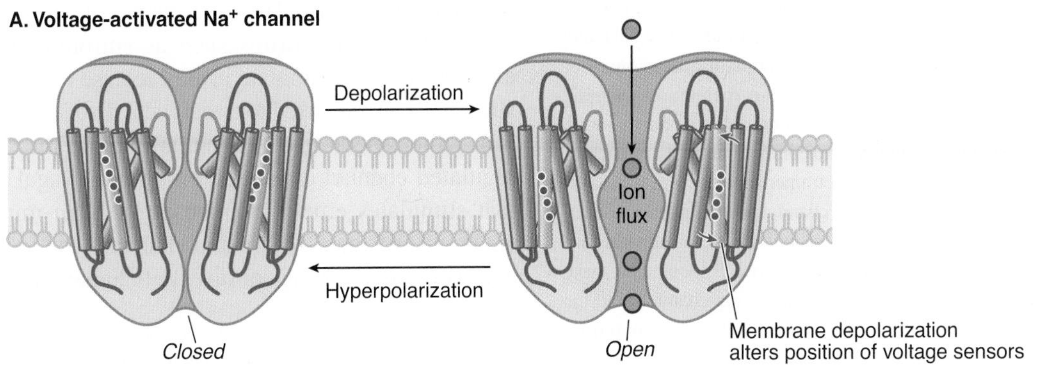

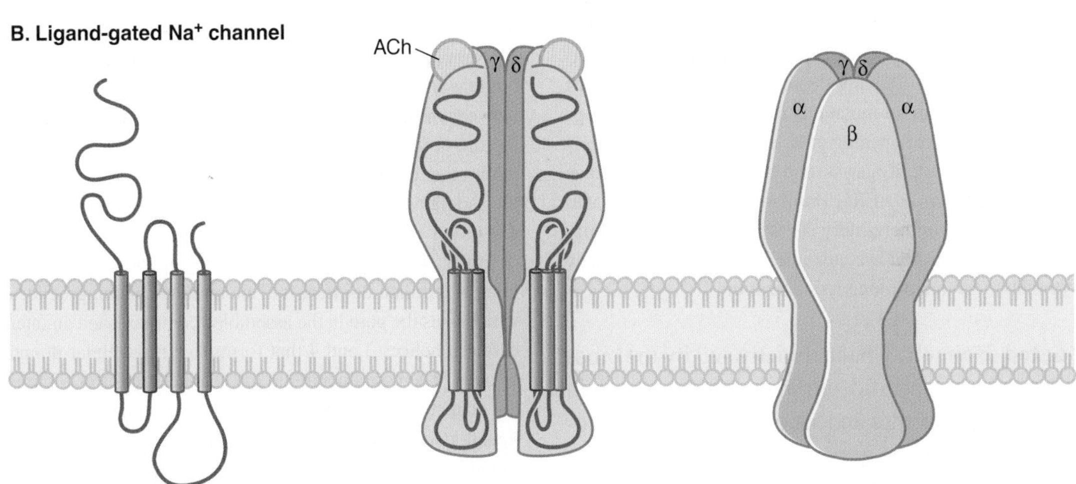

Figure 3–9. *Schematic diagram of two types of ion channels regulated by receptors and drugs.* **A.** Diagram of a voltage-activated Na^+ channel with the pore in the open and closed state. The P loops are shown in blue, angled into the pore to form the selectivity filter. The S4 helices forming the voltage sensor are shown in orange, with the positively charged amino acids displayed as red dots. **B.** Ligand-gated nicotinic acetylcholine receptor expressed in the skeletal muscle neuromuscular junction. The pore is made up of five subunits, each with a large extracellular domain and four transmembrane helices (one of these subunits is shown at the left of panel **B**). The helix that lines the pore is shown in blue. The receptor is composed of 2 α subunits, and β, γ, and δ subunits. See text for discussion of other ligand-gated ion channels. Detailed descriptions of specific channels are given throughout the text in relation to the therapeutic actions of drugs affecting these channels (see especially Chapters 11, 14 and 20). (Adapted with permission from Purves, D, Augustine, GJ, Fitzpatrick, D, Hall, WC, LaMantia, AS, McNamara, JO, and White, LE (eds). *Neuroscience*, 4ed. Sinauer Associates, Inc., 2008.)

Voltage-gated Ca^{2+} channels have a similar architecture to voltage-gated Na^+ channels with a large α subunit (four domains of six membrane-spanning helices) and three regulatory subunits (the β, δ and γ subunits). There are multiple isoforms of these channels that are widely expressed in nerve, cardiac and smooth muscle cells. Ca^{2+} channels can be responsible for initiating an action potential (as in the pacemaker cells of the heart), but are more commonly responsible for modifying the shape and duration of an action potential initiated by fast voltage-gated Na^+ channels (Purves and McNamara, 2008). These channels initiate the influx of Ca^{2+} that stimulates the release of neurotransmitters in the central, enteric, and autonomic nervous systems, and that control heart rate and impulse conduction in cardiac tissue (Chapters 8, 14, and 27). The L-type voltage-gated Ca^{2+} channels are subject to additional regulation via phosphorylation by PKA. Thus, when the sympathetic nervous system releases norepinephrine onto β adrenergic receptors in cardiac tissue, raising cAMP and activating PKA, the phosphorylated L-type channels allow more Ca^{2+} to flow into the cytoplasm, increasing the force of contraction. Voltage-gated Ca^{2+} channels expressed in smooth muscle regulate vascular tone; the intracelluar concentration of Ca^{2+} is critical to regulating the phosphorylation state of the contractile apparatus via the activity of the Ca^{2+}/calmodulin-sensitive myosin light chain kinase. Accordingly, the Ca^{2+} channel antagonists such as nifedipine, diltiazem, and verapamil are effective vasodilators and are widely used to treat angina, cardiac arrhythmias, and hypertension.

Voltage-gated K^+ channels are the most numerous and structurally diverse members of the voltage-gated channel family. Humans express ~78 distinct K^+ channels and nearly all of them are voltage-gated (Jegla et al., 2009). The voltage-gated K_v channels form channels as tetramers with topology similar to the Na+ and Ca^{2+} channels, but rather than having four domains, they consist of four separate subunits that each incorporate six membrane-spanning domains. The inwardly rectifying K^+ channel subunits only contain two membrane-spanning domains surrounding the pore. In each of these cases, the native channel is a tetramer formed from four individual subunits. A final group of K^+ channels is the tandem or two-pore domain "leak" K^+ channels; each subunit in this group has four membrane-spanning domains surrounding two P loops, and these form channels as dimers. The inwardly rectifying channels and the two-pore channels are voltage insensitive and are regulated by G proteins and H^+ ions and are greatly stimulated by general anesthetics. All these channels are expressed in nerve, cardiac tissue, skeletal and smooth muscle, as well as non-excitable tissues. Increasing K^+ conductance through these channels drives the membrane potential more negative; thus, these channels are important in regulating resting membrane potential and resetting the resting membrane at –70 to –90 mV following depolarizaion. Some forms of epilepsy are caused by natural mutations in K_v channels, and drugs such as retigabine that favor opening of K_v channels are under study for the treatment of epilepsy (Rogawski and Bazil, 2008). The cardiac KCNH2 channel, known as hERG (human ether-a-go-go-related gene), is responsible for hereditary as well as acquired (drug-induced) long QT syndrome. It is also the primary target of many anti-arrhythmic drugs that prolong repolarization.

Ligand-Gated Channels. Channels activated by the binding of a ligand to a specific site in the channel protein have a diverse architecture and set of ligands. Major ligand-gated channels in the nervous system are those that respond to excitatory neurotransmitters such as acetylcholine or glutamate (or agonists such as AMPA and NMDA) and inhibitory neurotransmitters such as glycine or γ-aminobutyric acid (GABA) (Purves and McNamara, 2008). Activation of these channels is responsible for the majority of synaptic transmission by neurons both in the CNS and in the periphery (Chapters 8, 11, and 14). In addition, there are a variety of more specialized ion channels that are activated by intracellular small molecules, and are structurally distinct from conventional ligand-gated ion channels. These include ion channels that are formally members of the K_v family, such as the hyperpolarization and cAMP-gated (HCN) channel expressed in the heart (Wahl-Schott and Biel, 2009) that is responsible for the slow depolarization seen in phase 4 of AV and SA nodal cell action potentials (Chapter 29), and the cyclic nucleotide-gated (CNG) channels important for vision (Chapter 64). The intracellular small molecule category of ion channels also includes the IP_3-sensitive Ca^{2+} channel responsible for release of Ca^{2+} from the ER and the sulfonylurea "receptor" (SUR1) that associates with the $K_{ir}6.2$ channel to regulate the ATP-dependent K^+ channel (K_{ATP}) in pancreatic beta cells. The K_{ATP} channel is the target of oral hypoglycemic drugs such as sulfonylureas and meglitinides that stimulate insulin release from pancreatic β cells and are used to treat type 2 diabetes (Chapter 43). Other specialized channels include the 5-HT_3-regulated channel expressed on afferent vagal nerves that stimulates emesis. Ondansetron is an important antagonist of the 5-HT_3-gated channel used to inhibit emesis caused by drugs or disease (Chapter 46).

The nicotinic acetylcholine receptor provides an instructive example of a ligand-gated ion channel. Isoforms of this channel are expressed in the CNS, autonomic ganglia and at the neuromuscular junction (Figure 3–9B). The pentameric channel consists of four different subunits (2α, β, δ, γ) in the neuromuscular junction or two different subunits (2α, 3β) in autonomic ganglia (Purves and McNamara, 2008). Each α subunit has an identical acetylcholine binding site; the different compositions of the other three subunits between the neuronal and neuromuscular junction receptors accounts for the ability of competitive antagonists such as rocuronium to inhibit the receptor in the neuromuscular junction without effect on the ganglionic receptor. This property is exploited to provide muscle relaxation during surgery with minimal autonomic side effects (Chapter 11). Each subunit of the receptor contains a large, extracellular N-terminal domain, four membrane-spanning helices (one of which lines the pore in the assembled complex), and an internal loop between helices 3 and 4 that forms the intracellular domain of the channel. The pore opening in the channel measures ~3 nm whereas the diameter of a Na^+ or K^+ ion is only 0.3 nm or less. Accordingly, ligand-gated ion channels do not possess the exquisite ion selectivity found in most voltage-activated channels and activation of the nicotinic acetylcholine receptor allows passage of both Na^+ and K^+ ions.

The major excitatory transmitter at CNS synapses is glutamate. There are three types of ionotropic glutamate receptors (AMPA, NMDA, and kainate), named after the ligands that selectively activate them. They have a topology similar to that of the nicotinic acetylcholine receptor: the channel is made up of five subunits organized with a large extracellular region, a pore, and a small intracellular face. Activation of these channels with glutamate markedly increases Na^+ and K^+ conductance leading to depolarization. NMDA receptors are less ion-selective; activation increases Na^+, K^+, and Ca^{2+} conductance, with the Ca^{2+} signal being used for additional signaling events.

Over one-third of synapses in the brain are inhibitory; the major inhibitory transmitters are glycine and γ-aminobutyric acid (GABA). Glycine and ionotropic $GABA_A$ receptors have a topology like that of the glutamate and nicotinic acetylcholine receptors, with five subunits (α, β, γ, δ and ρ), a ligand-binding domain, and pore-forming helices. Activation of these channels increases Cl^- conductance, which hyperpolarizes the cell membrane and inhibits excitability (Purves and McNamara, 2008). $GABA_A$ receptors are targets of important sedative-hypnotic drugs such as the benzodiazepines and barbituates, and are also important in the mechanisms of ethanol and general anesthetics (Chapters 17, 19, and 23).

TRP Channels. The transient receptor potential (TRP) channels comprise a superfamily of ubiquitously expressed ion channels that is remarkable in its diversity and domain strucutre (Clapham 2003; Venkatachalam and Montell, 2007). Although the TRP channels are not presently targets of approved drugs, there is significant interest in developing drugs that can alter the function of these ion channels because of their roles in various sensory phenomena such as pain, temperature, osmolarity, touch, olfaction, vision, and hearing. Because these channels contain multiple domains, they can act as signal integrators and most can be activated by multiple mechanisms. There are 27 TRP channel genes in humans, representing six different TRP channel families. TRP channels contain six membrane-spanning segments and the functional ion channels consist of tetrameric complexes. Closely related TRP channels can form heterotetramers. The TRP channels are cation channels, but as with other heteromultimeric ion channels, the subunit composition of the multimeric channels can prescribe a number of important channel characteristics, including ion selectivity and activation properties. The intracellular domains of TRP channels can include ankyrin domains, protein kinase domains, and ADP-ribose pyrophosphatase domains. Mutations in TRP channels are known to cause several disease including hypomagnesemia and hypocalcemia, and various renal disorders and neurodegenerative diseases.

Transmembrane Receptors Linked to Intracellular Enzymes

Mammalian cells express a diverse group of physiological membrane receptors with extracellular ligand-binding domains and an intrinsic enzymatic activity on the cytoplasmic surface of the cell. These molecules include the receptor tyrosine kinases (RTKs) such as the epidermal growth factor (EGF) and insulin receptors, which contain intrinsic tyrosine kinases in the cytoplasmic domain of the receptor; tyrosine kinase-associated receptors without enzymatic activity, such as the receptors for γ-interferon, which recruit the cytoplasmic Janus tyrosine kinases (JAKs); receptor serine-threonine kinases such as the TGF-β receptor; and receptors linked to other enzyme activities such as the receptors for natriuretic pepides, which have a cytoplasmic guanylate cyclase activity that produces a soluble second messenger, cyclic GMP (see the next section). Receptors responsible for innate immunity, the Toll-like receptors and those for tumor necrosis factors (TNF-α), have many features in common with the JAK-STAT receptors.

Receptor Tyrosine Kinases. The receptor tyrosine kinases include receptors for hormones such as insulin, for multiple growth factors such EGF, platelet-derived growth factor (PDGF), nerve growth factor (NGF), fibroblast growth factor (FGF), vascular endothelial growth factor (VEGF), and ephrins. With the exception of the insulin receptor, which has α and β chains (Chapter 43), these molecules consist of single polypeptide chains with large, cysteine-rich extracellular domains, short transmembrane domains, and an intracellular region containing one (or in some cases two) protein tyrosine kinase domains. Activation of growth factor receptors leads to cell survival, cell proliferation, and differentiation. Activation of the ephrin receptors leads to neuronal angiogenesis, axonal migration, and guidance (Ferguson, 2008; Hubbard and Till, 2000).

The inactive state of growth factor receptors is monomeric; binding of ligand induces dimerization of the receptor and cross-phosphorylation of the kinase domains on multiple tyrosine residues. Some of these tyrosine residues are in the activation loop of the kinase and their phosphorylation serves to further activate the receptor kinase (Figure 3–10A). The phosphorylation of other tyrosine residues forms docking sites for the SH2 domains contained in a large number of signaling proteins (Ferguson, 2008). There are over 100 proteins encoded in the human genome containing SH2 domains, and following receptor activation, large signaling complexes are formed on the receptor that eventually lead to cell proliferation. Molecules recruited to phosphotyrosine-containing proteins by their SH2 domains include PLCγ which raises intracellular levels of Ca^{2+} and activates PKC, as described earlier. The α and β isoforms of phosphatidylinositiol 3-kinase (PI3-K) contain SH2 domains, dock at the phosphorylated receptor, are activated, and increase the level of phosphatidylinositol 3,4,5 trisphosphate (PIP_3), a molecule that forms other kinds of docking sites at the plasma membrane for signaling molecules such as protein kinase B (PKB, also known as Akt). PKB can regulate the mammalian target of rapamycin (mTOR) in the various signaling pathways and the Bad protein that is important in apoptosis.

In addition to recruiting enzymes, phosphotyrosine-presenting proteins can attract SH2 domain-containing adaptor molecules without activity such as Grb2, which in turn attract guanine nucleotide exchange factors (GEFs) such as Sos that can activate the small GTP-binding protein, Ras. The small GTP binding proteins Ras and Rho belong to a large family of small monomeric GTPases; only members of the Ras and Rho subfamilies are activated by extracelluar receptors. The Ras family includes four isoforms H-ras, K-ras, n-Ras, and Rheb (activated by the insulin receptor). Spontaneous activating mutations in Ras are responsible for a large fraction of human cancers; thus, molecules that inhibit Ras are of great interest in cancer chemotherapy. The Rho family includes Rho, Rac, and Cdc42, which are responsible for relaying signals from the membrane to the cytoskeleton. All of the small GTPases are activated by GEFs that are regulated by a variety of mechanisms and inhibited by GTPase activating proteins (GAPs) (Etienne-Manneville and Hall, 2002).

upon binding ligand. Other members of the family such as the LXR and FXR receptors reside in the nucleus and are activated by changes in the concentration of hydrophobic lipid molecules.

Nuclear hormone receptors contain four major domains in a single polypeptide chain. The N-terminal domain can contain an activation region (AF-1) essential for transcriptional regulation followed by a very conserved region with two zinc fingers that bind to DNA (the *DNA-binding domain*). The N-terminal activation region (AF-1) is subject to regulation by phosphorylation and other mechanisms that stimulate or inhibit the overall ability of the nuclear receptor to activate transcription. The C terminal half of the molecule contains a *hinge region* (which can be involved in binding DNA), the domain responsible for binding the hormone or ligand (the *ligand-binding domain* or LBD), and specific sets of amino acid residues for binding co-activators and co-repressors in a second activation region (AF-2). The x-ray structures of nuclear hormone receptors show that the LBD is formed from a bundle of 12 helices and that ligand binding induces a major conformational change in helix 12 (Privalsky, 2004; Tontonoz and Spiegelman, 2008). This conformational change also affects the binding of the co-regulatory proteins essential for activation of the receptor-DNA complex (Figure 3–12).

When bound to DNA, most of the nuclear hormone receptors act as dimers—some as homodimers, others as heterodimers. Steroid hormone receptors such as the glucocorticoid receptor are commonly homodimers, whereas those for lipids are heterodimers with the RXR receptor. The receptor dimers bind to repetitive DNA sequences, either direct repeat sequences or an inverted repeat termed hormone response elements (HRE) that are specific for each type of receptor (e.g., AGGTCA half-sites oriented as an inverted repeat with a three-base spacer for the estrogen receptor). The hormone response elements in DNA are found upstream of the regulated genes or in some cases within the regulated genes. An agonist-bound nuclear hormone receptor often activates a large number of genes to carry out a program of cellular differentiation or metabolic regulation. For example, stimulation of the LXR receptor in hepatocytes activates 29 genes and inhibits 14 others (Kalaany and Mangelsdorf, 2006).

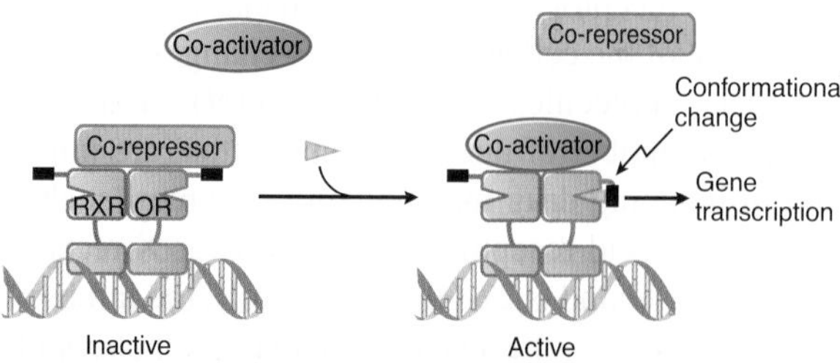

Figure 3–12. *Diagram of nuclear hormone receptor activation.* A nuclear hormone receptor (OR) is shown in complex with the retinoic acid receptor (RXR). When an agonist (yellow triangle) and co-activator bind, a conformational change occurs in helix 12 (black bar) and gene transcription is stimulated. If co-repressors are bound, activation does not occur. See text for details; see also Figure 6–13.

An important property of these receptors is that they must bind their ligand, the appropriate HRE, and a co-regulator (from a family of over 100 proteins co-regulators) to regulate their target genes. There are co-activators such as the steroid receptor co-activator (SRC) family, the p160 family proteins, CARM and CBP/p300 or PCG-1α, and co-repressors such as the silencing mediator of retinoid hormone receptor (SMRT) and nuclear hormone receptor co-repressor (NCor) (Privalsky, 2004). The activity of the nuclear hormone receptors in a given cell depends not only on the ligand, but the ratio of co-activators and co-repressors recruited to the complex. Co-activators recruit enzymes to the transcription complex that modify chromatin, such as histone acetylase, which serves to unravel DNA for transcription. Co-repressors recruit proteins such as histone deacetylase, which keeps DNA tightly packed and inhibits transcription.

Depending on the chemical nature of the bound ligand and the combination of co-activatiors and co-repressors recruited to the complex, nuclear hormone receptors may differentially regulate their target genes. This property explains the ability of certain drugs to act as selective modulators of the receptor and gene expression. For example, compounds such as 17β-estradiol are estrogen receptor agonists in all tissues, whereas tamoxifen and raloxifene are termed selective estrogen receptor modulators (SERMs). Tamoxifen and raloxifene are partial agonists at the estrogen receptor; upon binding, these agents elicit unique confomations of the ligand-binding domain. Thus, depending on the specific tissue, different combinations of co-activators and co-repressors are bound to the receptor-DNA complex, yielding gene-selective functions. For example, tamoxifen is an antagonist in breast tissue by virtue of recruiting co-repressors to the transcription factor complex but is an agonist in the endometrium because it recruits co-activators (Riggs and Hartmann, 2003) (Chapter 40).

APOPTOSIS

The maintenance of many organs requires the continuous renewal of cells. Examples include mucosal cells lining the intestine and a variety of cells in the immune system including T-cells and neutrophils. Cell renewal requires a balance between survival and expansion of the cell population, or cell death and removal. The process by which cells are genetically programmed for death is termed *apoptosis*. Apoptosis is a highly regulated program of biochemical reactions that leads to cell rounding, shrinking of the cytoplasm, condensation of the nucleus and nuclear material, and changes in the cell membrane that eventually lead to presentation of phosphatidylserine on the outer surface of the cell. Phosphatidylserine is recognized as a sign of apoptosis by macrophages, which engulf and phagocytize the dying cell. Notably, during this process the membrane of the apoptotic cell remains intact and the cell does not release its cytoplasm or nuclear material. Thus, unlike necrotic cell death, the apoptotic process does not initiate an inflammatory response. Understanding the pathways regulating apoptosis is important because apoptosis plays an important role in normal cells and because alterations in apoptotic pathways are implicated in a variety of diseases such as cancer, and neurodegenerative and autoimmune diseases (Bremer et al., 2006; Ghavami et al., 2009). Thus, maintaining or restoring normal apoptotic pathways is the goal of major drug development efforts to treat diseases that involve dysregulated apoptotic pathways (Fesik, 2005) and selectively stimulating apoptotic pathways could be useful in removing unwanted cells.

Two major signaling pathways induce apoptosis. Apoptosis can be initiated by external signals that have features in common with those used by ligands such as TNF-α or by an internal pathway activated by DNA damage, improperly folded proteins, or withdrawal of cell survival factors (Figure 3-13). Regardless of the mode of initiation, the apoptotic program is carried out by a large family of cysteine proteases termed caspases. The caspases are highly specific cytoplasmic proteases that are inactive in normal cells but become activated by apoptotic signals (Danial and Korsmeyer, 2004; Ghobrial et al., 2005; Strasser et al., 2000).

The external apoptosis signaling pathway can be activated by ligands such as TNF, FAS (another member of the TNF family, also called Apo-1), or the TNF-related apoptosis-inducing ligand (TRAIL). The receptors for FAS and TRAIL are transmembrane receptors with no enzymatic activity, similar to the organization of the TNF receptor described above. They have large external ligand-binding domains, short transmembrane domains, and a cytoplasmic death domain capable of binding intracelllular adaptor proteins. Upon binding TNF, FAS ligand, or TRAIL, these receptors form a receptor dimer, undergo a conformational change, and recruit adapter proteins to the death domain. The adaptor proteins are TNF-associated death domain binding protein (TRADD), FADD, or TRAF2. These adaptor proteins then recruit the receptor-interacting protein kinase (RIP1) and caspase 8 to form a complex of RIP1, TRADD/

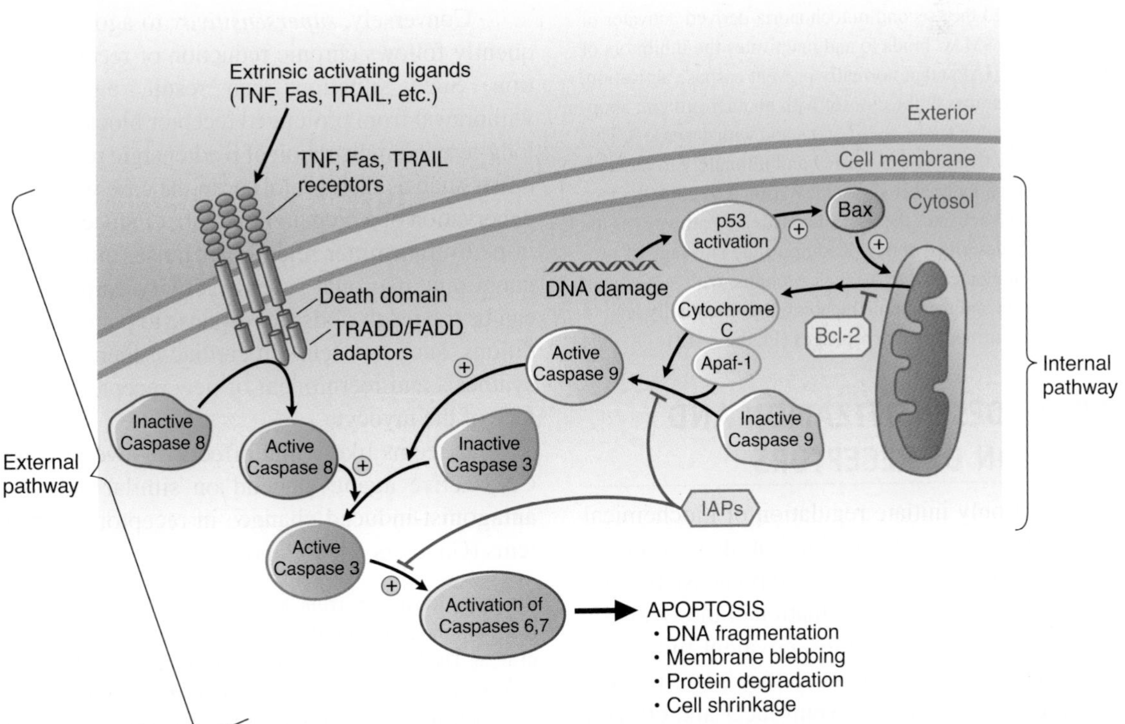

Figure 3–13. *Two pathways leading to apoptosis.* Apoptosis can be initiated by external ligands such as TNF, FAS, or TRAIL at specific transmembrane receptors (left half of figure). Activation leads to trimerization of the receptor, and binding of adaptor molecules such as TRADD, to the intracellular death domain. The adaptors recruit caspase 8, activate it leading to cleavage and activation of the effector caspase, caspase 3, which activates the caspase pathway, leading to apoptosis. Apoptosis can also be initiated by an intrinsic pathway regulated by Bcl-2 family members suc as BAX and Bcl-2. BAX is activated by DNA damage or malformed proteins via p53 (right half of figure). Activation of this pathway leads to release of cytochrome c form the mitochondria, formation of a complex with Apaf-1 and caspase 9. Caspase 9 is activated in the complex and initiates apoptosis thru activation of caspase 3. Either the extrinsic or the intrinsic pathway can overwhelm the inhibitors of apoptosis proteins (IAPs) that otherwise keep apoptosis in check. See text for details.

FADD/TRAF2, and caspase 8, which results in the activation of caspase 8. The FAS and TRAIL receptors recruit different adaptors, termed FADD/MORT, which are capable of attracting and then activating caspase 8 by autoproteoyltic cleavage. Regardless of the upstream complexes that activate caspase 8, stimulation of its proteolytic activity leads to the activation of caspase 3, which initiates the apoptotic program. The final steps of apoptosis are carried out by caspase 6 and 7, leading to degradation of enzymes, structural proteins, and DNA fragmentation characteristic of cell death (Danial and Korsmeyer, 2004; Wilson et al., 2009) (Figure 3–13).

The internal apoptosis pathway can be activated by signals such as DNA damage leading to increased transcription of the p53 gene and involves damage to the mitochondria by pro-apoptotic members of the Bcl-2 family of proteins. This family includes pro-apoptotic members such as BAX, Bak, and Bad, which induce damage at the mitochondrial membrane. There are also anti-apoptotic Bcl-2 members, such as Bcl-2, Bcl-X, and Bcl-W, which serve to inhibit mitochondrial damage and are negative regulators of the system (Rong and Distelhorst, 2008). When DNA damage occurs, p53 transcription is activated and holds the cell at a cell cycle check point until the damage is repaired. If the damage cannot be repaired, apoptosis is initiated through the pro-apoptotic Bcl-2 members such as BAX. BAX is activated, translocates to the mitochondria, overcomes the anti-apoptotic proteins, and induces the release of cytochrome c and a protein termed the "second mitochondria-derived activator of caspase" (SMAC). SMAC binds to and inactivates the inhibitors of apoptosis proteins (IAPs) that normally prevent caspase activation. Cytochrome C combines in the cytosol with another protein, apoptotic activating protease factor -1 (Apaf-1), and with caspase 9. This complex leads to activation of caspase 9 and ultimately to the activation of caspase 3 (Ghobrial et al., 2005; Wilson et al., 2009). Once activated, caspase 3 activates the same downstream pathways as the external pathway described above, leading to the cleavage of proteins, cytoskeletal elements, DNA repair proteins, with subsequent DNA condensation and membrane blebbing that eventually lead to cell death and engulfment by macrophages (Figure 3–13)

RECEPTOR DESENSITIZATION AND REGULATION OF RECEPTORS

Receptors not only initiate regulation of biochemical events and physiological function but also are themselves subject to many regulatory and homeostatic controls. These controls include regulation of the synthesis and degradation of the receptor, covalent modification, association with other regulatory proteins, and relocalization within the cell. Transducer and effector proteins are regulated similarly. Modulatory inputs may come from other receptors, directly or indirectly, and receptors are almost always subject to feedback regulation by their own signaling outputs.

Continued stimulation of cells with agonists generally results in a state of *desensitization* (also referred to as *adaptation, refractoriness,* or *down-regulation*) such that the effect that follows continued or subsequent exposure to the same concentration of drug is diminished. This phenomenon, called *tachyphylaxis,* occurs rapidly and is important therapeutically; an example is attenuated response to the repeated use of β adrenergic receptor agonists as bronchodilators for the treatment of asthma (Chapters 12 and 36).

Desensitization can result from temporary inaccessibility of the receptor to agonist or from fewer receptors being synthesized and available at the cell surface (e.g., down-regulation of receptor number). Phosphorylation of GPCR receptors by specific GPCR kinases (GRKs) plays a key role in triggering rapid desensitization. Phosphorylation of agonist-occupied GPCRs by GRKs facilitates the binding of cytosolic proteins termed *arrestins* to the receptor, resulting in the uncoupling of G protein from the receptor (Moore et al., 2007). The β-arrestins recruit proteins, such as PDE4, that limit cyclic AMP signaling, and clathrin and β2-adaptin, that promote sequestration of receptor from the membrane (*internalization*), thereby providing a scaffold that permits additional signaling steps.

Conversely, *supersensitivity* to agonists also frequently follows chronic reduction of receptor stimulation. Such situations can result, e.g., following withdrawal from prolonged receptor blockade (e.g., the long-term administration of β adrenergic receptor antagonists such as metoprolol) or in the case where chronic denervation of a preganglionic fiber induces an increase in neurotransmitter release per pulse, indicating postganglionic neuronal supersensitivity. Supersensitivity can be the result of tissue response to pathological conditions, such as occurs in cardiac ischemia due to the synthesis and recruitment of new receptors to the surface of the myocyte.

It seems likely that effects of several classes of CNS-active agents depend on similar agonist- and antagonist-induced changes in receptor-effector systems (Chapters 14, 15, and 18).

Diseases Resulting from Receptor Malfunction. Alteration in receptors and their immediate signaling effectors can be the cause of disease. The loss of a receptor in a highly specialized signaling system may cause a relatively limited, if dramatic, phenotypic disorder (e.g., deficiency of the androgen receptor and testicular feminization syndrome; Chapter 41). Deficiencies in widely employed signaling pathways have broad effects, as are seen in myasthenia gravis and some forms of insulin-resistant diabetes mellitus, which result from autoimmune depletion of nicotinic cholinergic receptors (Chapter 11) or insulin receptors (Chapter 43), respectively. The expression of constitutively active, aberrant, or ectopic receptors, effectors, and coupling proteins potentially can lead to supersensitivity, subsensitivity, or other untoward responses (Smit et al., 2007). Among the most significant events is the appearance of aberrant receptors as products of oncogenes that transform otherwise normal cells into malignant cells. Virtually any type of signaling system may have oncogenic potential.

PHARMACODYNAMIC INTERACTIONS IN A MULTICELLULAR CONTEXT

It is instructive to examine the pharmacodynamic interactions of physiological ligands and drugs that can occur in the context of a pathophysiological setting. Consider the vascular wall of an arteriole (Figure 3–14). Several cell types interact at this site, including vascular smooth muscle cells (SMCs), endothelial cells (ECs), platelets, and post-ganglionic sympathetic neurons. A variety of physiological receptors and ligands are represented, including ligands that cause SMCs to contract (angiotensin II [AngII], norepinephrine [NE]) and relax (nitric oxide [NO], B-type natriuretic peptide [BNP], and epinephrine), as well as ligands that alter SMC gene expression (platelet-derived growth factor [PDGF], AngII, NE, and eicosanoids). The intracellular second messengers Ca^{2+}, cAMP, and cGMP are also shown.

AngII has both acute and chronic effects on SMC. Interaction of AngII with AT_1 receptors (AT_1-R) causes the formation of the second messenger IP_3 through the action of the AT_1-R with the G_q-PLC-IP_3 pathway. IP_3 causes the release of Ca^{2+} from the endoplasmic reticulum; the Ca^{2+} binds and activates calmodulin and its target protein, myosin light chain kinase (MLCK). The activation of MLCK results in the phosphorylation of myosin, leading to smooth muscle cell contraction. Activation of the sympathetic nervous system also regulates SMC tone through release of NE from post-ganglionic sympathetic neurons impinging on SMCs. NE binds α_1 adrenergic receptors that couple to the G_q-PLC-IP_3 pathway, causing an increase in intracellular Ca^{2+} and, as a result, contraction, an effect that is additive to that of AngII. The contraction of SMCs is opposed by several physiological mediators that promote relaxation, including NO, BNP, and epinephrine. NO is formed in ECs by the action of two NO synthase enzymes, eNOS and iNOS. The NO formed in ECs diffuses into SMCs, and activates the soluble form of guanylate cyclase (sGC), which catalyzes the formation of cyclic GMP from GTP. The increase in cyclic GMP activates PKG, which phosphorylates protein substrates in SMCs that reduce intracellular concentrations of Ca^{2+} by several different mechanisms including reducing entry of extracellular Ca^{2+} through L-type voltage-gated Ca^{2+} channels. Intracellular concentrations

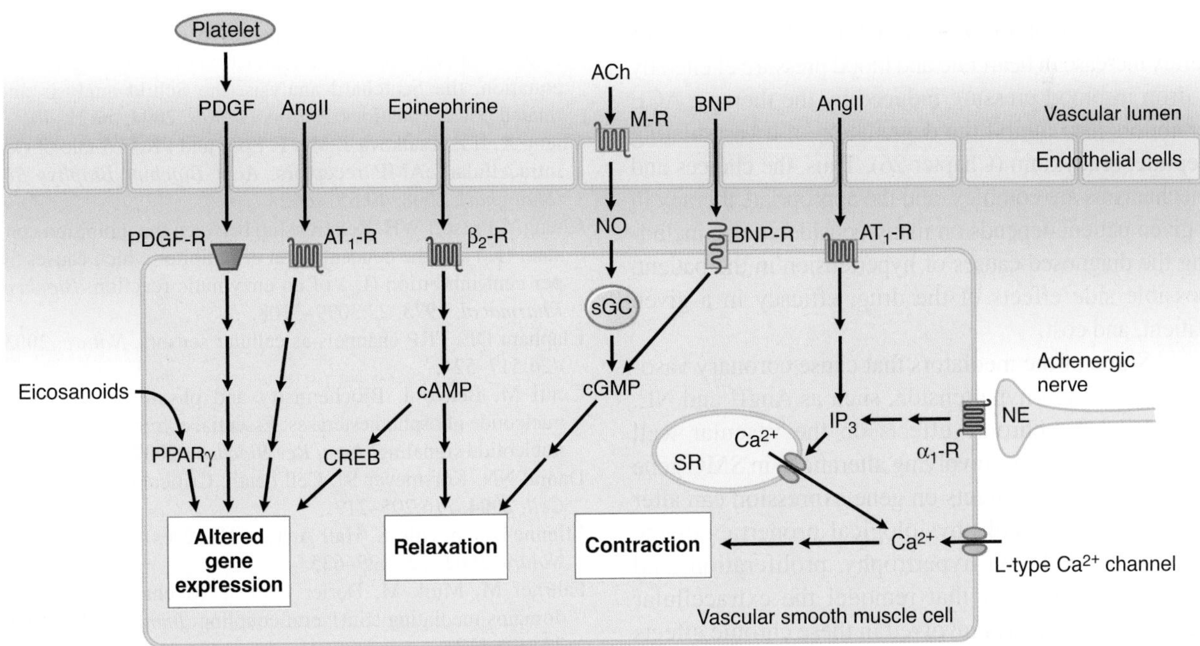

Figure 3–14. *Interaction of multiple signaling systems regulating vascular smooth muscle cells.* The membrane receptors and channels are sensitive to pharmacological antagonists. See text for explanation of signaling and contractile pathways and abbreviations.

of cyclic GMP are also increased by activation of the transmembrane BNP receptor (BNP-R), whose guanylate cyclase activity is increased when BNP binds. BNP is released from cardiac muscle in response to increased filling pressures. The contractile state of the arteriole is thus regulated acutely by a variety of physiological mediators working through a number of signal transduction pathways. In a patient with hypertension, SMC tone in an arteriole may be elevated above normal due to one or more changes in endogenous ligands or signaling pathways. These include elevated circulating concentrations of AngII, increased activity of the sympathetic nervous system, and decreased NO production by endothelial cells. Pharmacotherapy might include the use of one or more drugs to block or counteract the acute pathological changes in blood pressure as well as to prevent long-term changes in vessel wall structure due to stimulation of SMC proliferation and alterations in SMC gene expression.

Drugs commonly used to treat hypertension include β_1 antagonists to reduce secretion of renin (the rate-limiting first step in AngII synthesis), a direct renin inhibitor (aliskiren) to block the rate-limiting step in AngII production, angiotensin-converting enzyme (ACE) inhibitors (e.g., enalapril) to reduce the concentrations of circulating AngII, AT_1 receptor blockers (e.g., losartan) to block AngII binding to AT_1 receptors on SMCs, α_1 adrenergic blockers to block NE binding to SMCs, sodium nitroprusside to increase the quantities of NO produced, or a Ca^{2+} channel blocker (e.g., nifedipine) to block Ca^{2+} entry into SMCs. β_1 antagonists would also block the baroreceptor reflex increase in heart rate and blood pressure elicited by a drop in blood pressure induced by the therapy. ACE inhibitors also inhibit the degradation of a vasodilating peptide, bradykinin (Chapter 26). Thus, the choices and mechanisms are complex, and the appropriate therapy in a given patient depends on many considerations, including the diagnosed causes of hypertension in the patient, possible side effects of the drug, efficacy in a given patient, and cost.

Some of the mediators that cause coronary vasoconstriction and hypertension, such as AngII and NE, can also have chronic effects on the vascular wall through mechanisms involving alterations in SMC gene expression. These effects on gene expression can alter the biochemical and physiological properties of the SMC by stimulating hypertrophy, proliferation, and synthesis of proteins that remodel the extracellular matrix. The pathways involved in these chronic effects include many of the same pathways used by growth factor receptors, such as PDGF which can also be involved in the vascular wall remodeling that occurs in neointimal hyperplasia associated with coronary artery restenosis. One of the beneficial effects of using ACE inhibitors and AT_1 receptor blockers in the treatment of hypertension is their ability to prevent the long-term pathological remodeling of the vascular wall that results from chronic activation of AT_1 receptors by AngII.

BIBLIOGRAPHY

Alexander WS, Hilton DJ. The role of suppressors of cytokine signaling (socs) proteins in regulation of the immune response. *Annu Rev Immunol,* **2004**, *22*:503–529.

Ariens EJ. Affinity and intrinsic activity in the theory of competitive inhibition. I. Problems and theory. *Arch Int Pharmacodyn Ther,* **1954**, *99*:32–49.

Baillie GS. Compartmentalized signalling: Spatial regulation of cAMP by the action of compartmentalized phosphodiesterases. *FEBS J,* **2009**, *276*:1790–1799.

Beavo JA, Brunton LL. Cyclic nucleotide research—still expanding after half a century. *Nat Rev Mol Cell Biol,* **2002**, *3*:710–718.

Bremer E, van Dam G, Kroesen BJ, et al. Targeted induction of apoptosis for cancer therapy: Current progress and prospects. *Trends Mol Med,* **2006**, *12*:382–393.

Calabrese EJ, Baldwin LA. Hormesis: The dose-response revolution. *Annu Rev Pharmacol Toxicol,* **2003**, *43*:175–197.

Carlson HA, McCammon JA. Accommodating protein flexibility in computational drug design. *Mol Pharmacol,* **2000**, *57*:213–218.

Carnegie GK, Means CK, Scott JD. A-kinase anchoring proteins: From protein complexes to physiology and disease. *IUBMB Life,* **2009**, *61*:394–406.

Cheng HC. The influence of cooperativity on the determination of dissociation constants: Examination of the Cheng-Prusoff equation, the Scatchard analysis, the Schild analysis and related power equations. *Pharmacol Res,* **2004**, *50*:21–40.

Cheng X, Ji Z, Tsalkova T, Mei F. Epac and PKA: A tale of two intracellular cAMP receptors. *Acta Biochim Biophys Sin (Shanghai),* **2008**, *40*:651–662.

Cheng Y, Prusoff WH. Relationship between the inhibition constant (K_i) and the concentration of inhibitor which causes 50 per cent inhibition (I_{50}) of an enzymatic reaction. *Biochem Pharmacol,* **1973**, *22*:3099–3108.

Clapham DE. TRP channels as cellular sensors. *Nature,* **2003**, *426*:517–524.

Conti M, Beavo J. Biochemistry and physiology of cyclic nucleotide phosphodiesterases: Essential components in cyclic nucleotide signaling. *Annu Rev Biochem,* **2007**, *76*:481–511.

Danial NN, Korsmeyer SJ. Cell death: Critical control points. *Cell,* **2004**, *116*:205–219.

Etienne-Manneville S, Hall A. Rho GTPases in cell biology. *Nature,* **2002**, *420*:629–635.

Fahrner M, Muik M, Derler I, et al. Mechanistic view on domains mediating stim1-orai coupling. *Immunol Rev,* **2009**, *231*:99–112.

Ferguson KM. Structure-based view of epidermal growth factor receptor regulation. *Annu Rev Biophys,* **2008**, *37*:353–373.

Fesik SW. Promoting apoptosis as a strategy for cancer drug discovery. *Nat Rev Cancer,* **2005**, 5:876–885.

Gaddum JH. Theories of drug antagonism. *Pharmacol Rev,* **1957**, *9*:211–218.

Gay NJ, Gangloff M. Structure and function of toll receptors and their ligands. *Annu Rev Biochem,* **2007**, 76:141–165.

Ghavami S, Hashemi M, Ande SR, et al. Apoptosis and cancer: Mutations within caspase genes. *J Med Genet,* **2009**, *46*:497–510.

Ghobrial IM, Witzig TE, Adjei AA. Targeting apoptosis pathways in cancer therapy. *CA Cancer J Clin,* **2005**, *55*:178–194.

Ghosh S, Hayden MS. New regulators of NFκB in inflammation. *Nat Rev Immunol,* **2008**, *8*:837–848.

Gilman AG. G proteins: Transducers of receptor-generated signals. *Annu Rev Biochem,* **1987**, *56*:615–649.

Gough DJ, Levy DE, Johnstone RW, Clarke CJ. IFN-γ signaling-does it mean JAK-STAT? *Cytokine Growth Factor Rev,* **2008**, *19*:383–394.

Hanoune J, Defer N. Regulation and role of adenylyl cyclase isoforms. *Annu Rev Pharmacol Toxicol,* **2001**, *41*:145–174.

Hayden MS, Ghosh S. Shared principles in NFκB signaling. *Cell,* **2008**, *132*:344–362.

Hubbard SR, Till JH. Protein tyrosine kinase structure and function. *Annu Rev Biochem,* **2000**, *69*:373–398.

Hudmon A, Schulman H. Structure-function of the multifunctional Ca^{2+}/calmodulin-dependent protein kinase II. *Biochem J,* **2002**, *364*:593–611.

Jain KK. Role of pharmacoproteomics in the development of personalized medicine. *Pharmacogenomics,* **2004**, *5*:331–336.

Jegla TJ, Zmasek CM, Batalov S, Nayak SK. Evolution of the human ion channel set. *Comb Chem High Throughput Screen,* **2009**, *12*:2–23.

Kalaany NY, Mangelsdorf DJ. LXRs and FXR: The yin and yang of cholesterol and fat metabolism. *Annu Rev Physiol,* **2006**, *68*:159–191.

Kataoka T. Chemical biology of inflammatory cytokine signaling. *J Antibiot (Tokyo),* **2009**.

Kenakin T. Efficacy as a vector: The relative prevalence and paucity of inverse agonism. *Mol Pharmacol,* **2004**, *65*:2–11.

Klein TE, Altman RB, Eriksson N, et al. Estimation of the warfarin dose with clinical and pharmacogenetic data. *N Engl J Med,* **2009**, *360*:753–764.

Limbird LE. *Cell Surface Receptors: A Short Course on Theory and Methods*. Springer-Verlag, **2005**.

Manning AM, Davis RJ. Targeting JNK for therapeutic benefit: From junk to gold? *Nat Rev Drug Discov,* **2003**, *2*:554–565.

May LT, Leach K, Sexton PM, Christopoulos A. Allosteric modulation of G protein-coupled receptors. *Annu Rev Pharmacol Toxicol,* **2007**, *47*:1–51.

Mayr B, Montminy M. Transcriptional regulation by the phosphorylation-dependent factor creb. *Nat Rev Mol Cell Biol,* **2001**, *2*:599–609.

McEwan IJ. Nuclear receptors: One big family. *Methods Mol Biol,* **2009**, *505*:3–18.

Mehats C, Andersen CB, Filopanti M, et al. Cyclic nucleotide phosphodiesterases and their role in endocrine cell signaling. *Trends Endocrinol Metab,* **2002**, *13*:29–35.

Milligan G. Constitutive activity and inverse agonists of G protein-coupled receptors: A current perspective. *Mol Pharmacol,* **2003**, *64*:1271–1276.

Moore CA, Milano SK, Benovic JL. Regulation of receptor trafficking by GRKs and arrestins. *Annu Rev Physiol,* **2007**, *69*:451–482.

Palczewski K, Kumasaka T, Hori T, et al. Crystal structure of rhodopsin: A G protein-coupled receptor. *Science,* **2000**, *289*:739–745.

Patterson RL, Boehning D, Snyder SH. Inositol 1,4,5-trisphosphate receptors as signal integrators. *Annu Rev Biochem,* **2004**, *73*:437–465.

Potter LR, Yoder AR, Flora DR, et al. Natriuretic peptides: Their structures, receptors, physiologic functions and therapeutic applications. *Handb Exp Pharmacol,* **2009**, 341–366.

Prakriya M. The molecular physiology of CRAC channels. *Immunol Rev,* **2009**, *231*:88–98.

Privalsky ML. The role of corepressors in transcriptional regulation by nuclear hormone receptors. *Annu Rev Physiol,* **2004**, *66*:315–360.

Purves D, Augustine GJ, Fitzpatrick D, et al. Channels and transporters. In, *Neuroscience.* Sinauer, Sunderland, MA, **2008**, pp. 61–84.

Riggs BL, Hartmann LC. Selective estrogen-receptor modulators—mechanisms of action and application to clinical practice. *N Engl J Med,* **2003**, *348*:618–629.

Rogawski MA, Bazil CW. New molecular targets for antiepileptic drugs: $\alpha_2\delta$, SV2a, and K_v7/KCNQ Potassium Channels. *Curr Neurol Neurosci Rep,* **2008**, *8*:345–352.

Rong Y, Distelhorst CW. Bcl-2 protein family members: Versatile regulators of calcium signaling in cell survival and apoptosis. *Annu Rev Physiol,* **2008**, *70*:73–91.

Roscioni SS, Elzinga CR, Schmidt M. Epac: Effectors and biological functions. *Naunyn Schmiedebergs Arch Pharmacol,* **2008**, *377*:345–357.

Ross EM, Wilkie TM. GTPase-activating proteins for heterotrimeric G proteins: Regulators of G protein signaling (RGS) and RGS-like proteins. *Annu Rev Biochem,* **2000**, *69*:795–827.

Rybalkin SD, Yan C, Bornfeldt KE, Beavo JA. Cyclic GMP phosphodiesterases and regulation of smooth muscle function. *Circ Res,* **2003**, *93*:280–291.

Sands WA, Palmer TM. Regulating gene transcription in response to cyclic AMP elevation. *Cell Signal,* **2008**, *20*:460–466.

Schild HO. Drug antagonism and pA_2. *Pharmacol Rev,* **1957**, *9*:242–246.

Skaug B, Jiang X, Chen ZJ. The role of ubiquitin in NFκB regulatory pathways. *Annu Rev Biochem,* **2009**, *78*: 769–796.

Smit MJ, Vischer HF, Bakker RA, et al. Pharmacogenomic and structural analysis of constitutive G protein-coupled receptor activity. *Annu Rev Pharmacol Toxicol,* **2007**, *47*:53–87.

Strasser A, O'Connor L, Dixit VM. Apoptosis signaling. *Annu Rev Biochem,* **2000**, *69*:217–245.

Taylor SS, Kim C, Cheng CY, et al. Signaling through cAMP and cAMP-dependent protein kinase: Diverse strategies for drug design. *Biochim Biophys Acta,* **2008**, *1784*:16–26.

Tontonoz P, Spiegelman BM. Fat and beyond: The diverse biology of PPARγ. *Annu Rev Biochem,* **2008**, *77*: 289–312.

Tsai EJ, Kass DA. Cyclic GMP signaling in cardiovascular pathophysiology and therapeutics. *Pharmacol Ther,* **2009**, *122*:216–238.

Venkatachalam K, Montell C. TRP Channels. *Annu Rev Biochem,* **2007**, *76*:387–417.

Vo NK, Gettemy JM, Coghlan VM. Identification of cGMP-dependent protein kinase anchoring proteins (GKAPs). *Biochem Biophys Res Comm*, **1998**, *246*:831–835.

Wahl-Schott C, Biel M. HCN channels: Structure, cellular regulation and physiological function. *Cell Mol Life Sci*, **2009**, *66*:470–494.

Wang X, Lupardus P, Laporte SL, Garcia KC. Structural biology of shared cytokine receptors. *Annu Rev Immunol*, **2009**, *27*:29–60.

Wilson NS, Dixit V, Ashkenazi A. Death receptor signal transducers: Nodes of coordination in immune signaling networks. *Nat Immunol*, **2009**, *10*:348–355.

Wong W, Scott JD. AKAP signalling complexes: Focal points in space and time. *Nat Rev Mol Cell Biol*, **2004**, *5*:959–970.

Drug Toxicity and Poisoning

Kevin C. Osterhoudt
and Trevor M. Penning

Pharmacology deals with drugs and their chemical properties or characteristics, their mode of action, the physiological response to drugs, and the clinical uses of drugs. Pharmacology intersects with *toxicology* when the physiological response to a drug is an *adverse effect*. Toxicology is often regarded as the science of poisons or poisoning, but developing a strict definition for poison is problematic. A *poison* is any substance, including any drug, that has the capacity to harm a living organism. The Renaissance physician Paracelsus (1493-1541) is famously credited with offering the philosophical definition of poisons: "What is there that is not poison? All things are poison and nothing is without poison. Solely the dose determines that a thing is not a poison." However, *poisoning* inherently implies that damaging physiological effects result from exposure to pharmaceuticals, illicit drugs, or chemicals. So each drug in the pharmacopeia is a potential poison, and individual dose-, situation-, environment-, and gene-related factors contribute to a drug's ability to achieve its adverse potential.

Some chemicals may inherently be poisons, such as lead, which has no known necessary physiological role in the human body, and which is known to cause neuronal injury even at very low exposure levels. Most pharmaceuticals are threshold poisons; at therapeutic dosing the drug is used to confer a health advantage, but at higher doses the drug may produce a toxic effect. For instance, iron is a nutrient essential for heme synthesis and numerous physiological enzyme functions, but overdose of ferrous sulfate can lead to life-threatening multi-organ dysfunction.

DOSE-RESPONSE

Evaluation of the dose-response or the dose-effect relationship is crucially important to toxicologists. There is a graded dose-response relationship in an *individual* and a quantal dose-response relationship in the *population* (see Chapters 2 and 3). Graded doses of a drug given to an individual usually result in a greater magnitude of response as the dose is increased. In a quantal dose-response relationship, the percentage of the population affected increases as the dose is raised; the relationship is quantal in that the effect is specified to be either present or absent in a given individual (Figure 4–1). This quantal dose-response phenomenon is extremely important in toxicology and is used to determine the *median lethal dose* (LD_{50}) of drugs and other chemicals.

The LD_{50} of a compound is determined experimentally, usually by administration of the chemical to mice or rats (orally or intraperitoneally) at several doses in the lethal range (Figure 4–1A).

To linearize such data, the response (death) can be converted to units of *deviation from the mean,* or *probits* (*probability units*). The probit designates the deviation from the median; a probit of 5 corresponds to a 50% response, and because each probit equals one standard deviation, a probit of 4 equals 16% and a probit of 6 equals 84%. A plot of the percentage of the population responding, in probit units, against log dose yields a straight line (Figure 4–1B). The LD_{50} is determined by drawing a vertical line from the point on the line where the probit unit equals 5 (50% mortality). The slope of the dose-effect curve also is important. The LD_{50} for both compounds depicted in Figure 4–1 is the same (~10 mg/kg); however, the slopes of the dose-response curves are quite different. At a dose equal to one-half the LD_{50} (5 mg/kg), less than 5% of the animals exposed to compound **B** would die, but 30% of the animals given compound **A** would die.

Figure 4–2 illustrates the relationship between a quantal dose-response curve for the therapeutic effect of a drug to generate a median effective dose (ED_{50}), the concentration of drug at which 50% of the population will have the desired response, and a quantal dose-response curve for lethality by the same agent. These two curves can be used to generate a therapeutic index (TI), which quantifies the relative safety of a drug. Clearly, the higher the ratio, the safer the drug.

$$TI = LD_{50}/ED_{50}$$

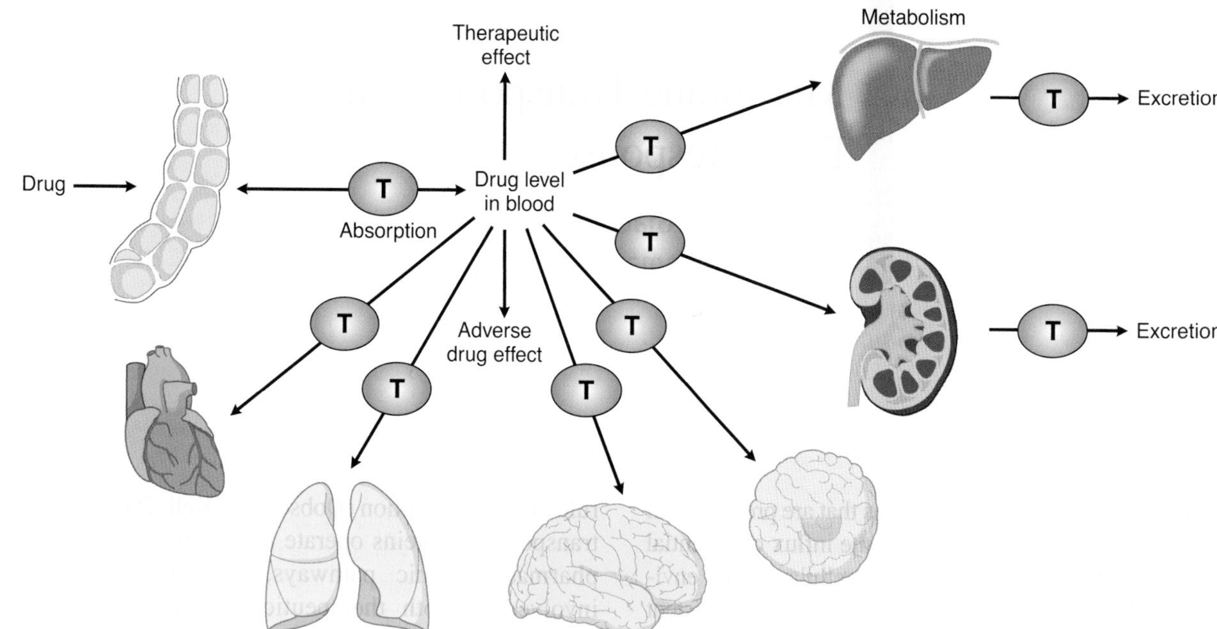

Figure 5–1. *Roles of membrane transporters in pharmacokinetic pathways.* Membrane transporters (T) play roles in pharmacokinetic pathways (drug absorption, distribution, metabolism, and excretion), thereby setting systemic drug levels. Drug levels often drive therapeutic and adverse drug effects.

transporters are the targets for drugs used in the treatment of neuropsychiatric disorders (Murphy et al., 2004; Torres and Amara, 2007). SERT (*SLC6A4*) is a target for a major class of antidepressant drugs, the selective serotonin reuptake inhibitors (SSRIs). Other neurotransmitter reuptake transporters serve as drug targets for the tricyclic antidepressants, various amphetamines (including amphetamine-like drugs used in the treatment of attention deficit disorder in children), and anticonvulsants (Elliott and Beveridge,

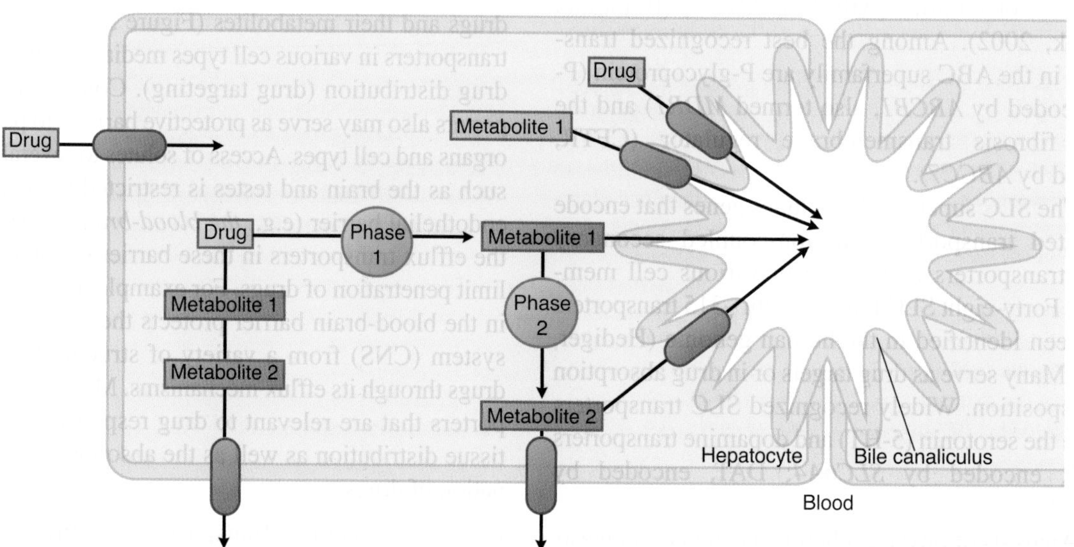

Figure 5–2. *Hepatic drug transporters.* Membrane transporters, shown as red ovals with arrows, work in concert with phase 1 and phase 2 drug-metabolizing enzymes in the hepatocyte to mediate the uptake and efflux of drugs and their metabolites.

2005; Torres and Amara, 2007). These transporters also may be involved in the pathogenesis of neuropsychiatric disorders, including Alzheimer's and Parkinson's diseases (Shigeri et al., 2004; Sotnikova et al., 2006). Transporters that are non-neuronal also may be potential drug targets, e.g., cholesterol transporters in cardiovascular disease, nucleoside transporters in cancers, glucose transporters in metabolic syndromes, and Na^+-H^+ antiporters in hypertension (Bobulescu et al., 2005; Kidambi and Patel, 2008; Pascual et al., 2004; Rader, 2006; Zhang et al., 2007).

Drug Resistance. Membrane transporters play critical roles in the development of resistance to anticancer drugs, antiviral agents, and anticonvulsants. Drug resistance, particularly to cytotoxic drugs, generally occurs by multiple mechanisms, two of which involve membrane transporters. *Decreased uptake of drugs* such as folate antagonists, nucleoside analogs, and platinum complexes, is mediated by reduced expression of influx transporters required for these drugs to access the tumor. *Enhanced efflux of hydrophobic drugs* is one of the most frequently encountered mechanisms of antitumor resistance in cellular assays of resistance. For example, P-glycoprotein is overexpressed in tumor cells after exposure to cytotoxic anticancer agents (Lin and Yamazaki, 2003; Leslie et al., 2005; Szakacs et al., 2006). P-glycoprotein pumps out the anticancer drugs, rendering cells resistant to their cytotoxic effects. Other efflux transporters, including breast cancer resistance protein (BCRP), and multidrug resistance-associated proteins (MRPs), also have been implicated in resistance to anticancer drugs (Clarke et al., 2002; Toyoda et al., 2008). The over-expression of multidrug resistance protein 4 (MRP4) is associated with resistance to antiviral nucleoside analogs (Imaoka et al., 2006; Schuetz et al., 1999).

MEMBRANE TRANSPORTERS AND ADVERSE DRUG RESPONSES

Through import and export mechanisms, transporters ultimately control the exposure of cells to chemical carcinogens, environmental toxins, and drugs. Thus, transporters play crucial roles in the cellular toxicities of these agents. Transporter-mediated adverse drug responses generally can be classified into three categories (Figure 5–3).

Transporters expressed in the liver and kidney, as well as metabolic enzymes, are key determinants of drug exposure in the circulating blood, thereby affecting exposure, and hence toxicity, in all organs (Figure 5–3, top panel) (Mizuno et al., 2003). For example, after oral administration of an HMG-CoA reductase inhibitor (e.g., pravastatin), the efficient first-pass hepatic uptake of the drug by the organic anion-transporting polypeptide OATP1B1 maximizes the effects of such drugs on hepatic HMG-CoA reductase. Uptake by OATP1B1 also minimizes the escape of these drugs into the systemic circulation, where they can cause adverse responses such as skeletal muscle myopathy.

Transporters in toxicological target organs or at barriers to such organs affect exposure of the target organs to drugs. Transporters expressed in tissues that may be targets for drug toxicity (e.g., brain) or in barriers to such tissues (e.g., the blood-brain barrier [BBB]) can tightly control local drug concentrations and thus control the exposure of these tissues to the drug (Figure 5–3, middle panel). For example, to restrict the penetration of compounds into the brain, endothelial cells in the BBB are closely linked by tight junctions, and some efflux transporters are expressed on the blood-facing (luminal) side. The importance of the ABC transporter multidrug resistance protein (*ABCB1*, MDR1; P-glycoprotein, P-gp) in the BBB has been demonstrated in *mdr1a* knockout mice (Schinkel et al., 1994). The brain concentrations of many P-glycoprotein substrates, such as digoxin, used in the treatment of heart failure (Chapter 28), and cyclosporin A (Chapter 35), an immunosuppressant, are increased dramatically in *mdr1a*(–/–) mice, whereas their plasma concentrations are not changed significantly.

Another example of transporter control of drug exposure can be seen in the interactions of loperamide and quinidine. Loperamide is a peripheral opioid used in the treatment of diarrhea and is a substrate of P-glycoprotein. Co-administration of loperamide and the potent P-glycoprotein inhibitor quinidine results in significant respiratory depression, an adverse response to the loperamide (Sadeque et al., 2000). Because plasma concentrations of loperamide are not changed in the presence of quinidine, it has been suggested that quinidine inhibits P-glycoprotein in the BBB, resulting in an increased exposure of the CNS to loperamide and bringing about the respiratory depression. Inhibition of P-glycoprotein-mediated efflux in the BBB thus would cause an increase in the concentration of substrates in the CNS and potentiate adverse effects.

The case of oseltamivir (the antiviral drug TAMIFLU) provides an example that dysfunction of an active barrier may cause a CNS effect. Abnormal behavior appears to be a rare adverse reaction of oseltamivir. Oseltamivir and its active form, Ro64-0802, undergo active efflux across the BBB by P-glycoprotein, organic anion transporter 3 (OAT3), and multidrug resistance-associated protein 4 (MRP4) (Ose et al., 2009). Decreased activities of these transporters at the BBB caused by concomitant drugs, ontogenetic and genetic factors, or disease may enhance the CNS exposure to oseltamivir and Ro64-0802, contributing to an adverse effect on the CNS.

Drug-induced toxicity sometimes is caused by the concentrative tissue distribution mediated by influx transporters. For example, biguanides (e.g., metformin and phenformin), widely used as oral

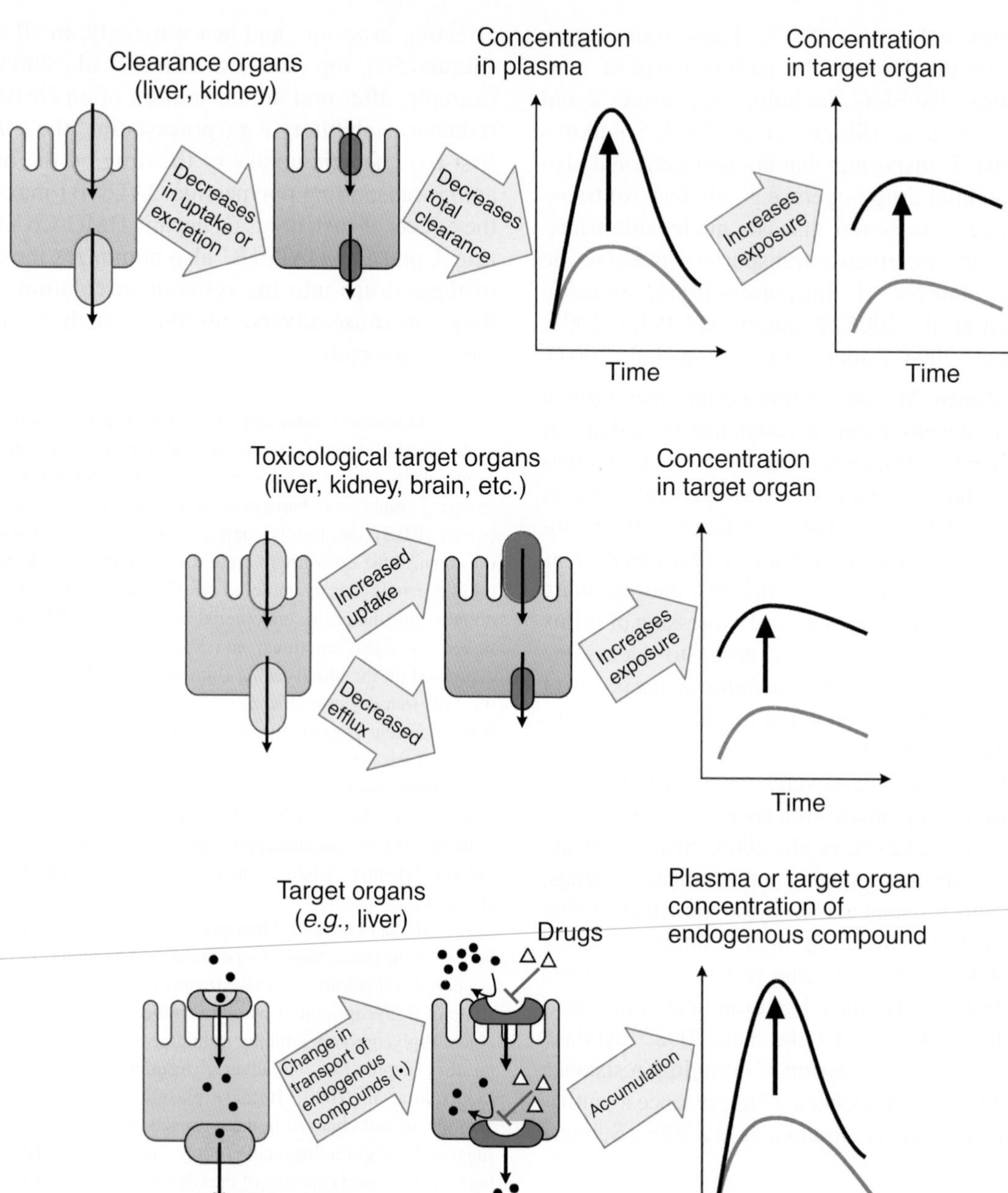

Figure 5–3. *Major mechanisms by which transporters mediate adverse drug responses.* Three cases are given. The *left panel* of each case provides a cartoon representation of the mechanism; the *right panel* shows the resulting effect on drug levels. (*Top panel*) Increase in the plasma concentrations of drug due to a decrease in the uptake and/or secretion in clearance organs such as the liver and kidney. (*Middle panel*) Increase in the concentration of drug in toxicological target organs due either to the enhanced uptake or to reduced efflux of the drug. (*Bottom panel*) Increase in the plasma concentration of an endogenous compound (e.g., a bile acid) due to a drug's inhibiting the influx of the endogenous compound in its eliminating or target organ. The diagram also may represent an increase in the concentration of the endogenous compound in the target organ owing to drug-inhibited efflux of the endogenous compound.

hypoglycemic agents for the treatment of type II diabetes mellitus, can produce lactic acidosis, a lethal side effect. Phenformin was withdrawn from the market for this reason. Biguanides are substrates of the organic cation transporter OCT1, which is highly expressed in the liver. After oral administration of metformin, the distribution of the drug to the liver in *oct1*(–/–) mice is markedly reduced compared with the distribution in wild-type mice. Moreover, plasma lactic acid concentrations induced by metformin are reduced in *oct1*(–/–) mice compared with wild-type mice, although the plasma concentrations of metformin are similar in the wild-type and knockout mice. These results indicate that the OCT1-mediated hepatic uptake of biguanides plays an important role in lactic acidosis (Wang et al., 2003).

The organic anion transporter 1 (OAT1) and organic cation transporters (OCT1 and OCT2) provide other examples of transporter-related toxicity. OAT1 is expressed mainly in the kidney and is responsible for the renal tubular secretion of anionic compounds. Substrates of OAT1, such as cephaloridine (a β-lactam antibiotic), and adefovir and cidofovir (antiviral drugs), reportedly cause nephrotoxicity. *In vitro* experiments suggest that cephaloridine, adefovir, and cidofovir are substrates of OAT1 and that OAT1-expressing cells are more susceptible to the toxicity of these drugs than control cells (Ho et al., 2000; Takeda et al., 1999). Exogenous expression of OCT1 and OCT2 enhances the sensitivities of tumor cells to the cytotoxic effect of oxaliplatin for OCT1, and cisplatin and oxaliplatin for OCT2 (Zhang et al., 2006b).

Drugs may modulate transporters for endogenous ligands and thereby exert adverse effects (Figure 5–3, bottom panel). For example, bile acids are taken up mainly by *Na*$^+$-*t*aurocholate *c*otransporting *p*olypeptide (NTCP) (Hagenbuch et al., 1991) and excreted into the bile by the *b*ile *s*alt *e*xport *p*ump (BSEP, *ABCB11*) (Gerloff et al., 1998). Bilirubin is taken up by OATP1B1 and conjugated with glucuronic acid, and bilirubin glucuronide is excreted by the *m*ultidrug-*r*esistance-associated *p*rotein (MRP2, *ABCC2*). Inhibition of these transporters by drugs may cause cholestasis or hyperbilirubinemia. Troglitazone, a thiazolidinedione insulin-sensitizing drug used for the treatment of type II diabetes mellitus, was withdrawn from the market because it caused hepatotoxicity. The mechanism for this troglitazone-induced hepatotoxicity remains unclear. One hypothesis is that troglitazone and its sulfate conjugate induced cholestasis. Troglitazone sulfate potently inhibits the efflux of taurocholate (K_i = 0.2 μM) mediated by the ABC transporter BSEP. These findings suggest that troglitazone sulfate induces cholestasis by inhibition of BSEP function. BSEP-mediated transport is also inhibited by other drugs, including cyclosporin A and the antibiotics rifamycin and rifampicin (Stieger et al., 2000).

Thus, uptake and efflux transporters determine the plasma and tissue concentrations of endogenous compounds and xenobiotics, and thereby can influence the systemic or site-specific toxicity of drugs.

BASIC MECHANISMS OF MEMBRANE TRANSPORT

Transporters Versus Channels. Both channels and transporters facilitate the membrane permeation of inorganic ions and organic compounds (Reuss, 2000). In general, channels have two primary states, open and closed, that are totally stochastic phenomena. Only in the open state do channels appear to act as pores for the selected ions, allowing their permeation across the plasma membrane. After opening, channels return to the closed state as a function of time. In contrast, a transporter forms an intermediate complex with the substrate (solute), and subsequently a conformational change in the transporter induces translocation of the substrates to the other side of the membrane. Therefore, there is a marked difference in turnover rates between channels and transporters. The turnover rate constants of typical channels are 10^6 to 10^8 s^{-1}, whereas those of transporters are, at most, 10^1 to 10^3 s^{-1}. Because a particular transporter forms intermediate complexes with specific compounds (referred to as *substrates*), transporter-mediated membrane transport is characterized by saturability and inhibition by substrate analogs, as described in "Kinetics of Transport."

The basic mechanisms involved in solute transport across biological membranes include passive diffusion, facilitated diffusion, and active transport. Active transport can be further subdivided into primary and secondary active transport. These mechanisms are depicted in Figure 5–4 and described in the next sections.

Passive Diffusion. Simple diffusion of a solute across the plasma membrane consists of three processes: partition from the aqueous to the lipid phase, diffusion across the lipid bilayer, and repartition into the aqueous phase on the opposite side. Diffusion of any solute (including drugs) occurs down an electrochemical potential gradient of the solute.

Such diffusion may be described by the equation:

$$\Delta\mu = zE_m F + RT \ \text{In}\left(\frac{C_i}{C_o}\right) \qquad \text{(Equation 5–1)}$$

where $\Delta\mu$ is the potential gradient, z is the charge valence of the solute, E_m is the membrane voltage, F is the Faraday constant, R is the gas constant, T is the absolute temperature, C is the concentration of the solute inside (i) and outside (o) of the plasma membrane. The first term on the right side in Equation (5–1) represents the electrical potential, and the second represents the chemical potential.

For non-ionized compounds, the flux J owing to simple diffusion is given by Fick's first law (permeability multiplied by the concentration difference). For ionized compounds, the difference in electrical potential across the plasma membrane needs to be taken into consideration. Assuming that the electrical field is constant, the flux is given by the Goldman-Hodgkin-Katz equation:

$$J = -P\frac{zE_m F}{RT}\left[\frac{C_i - C_o \exp\left(E_m F / RT\right)}{1 - \exp\left(E_m F / RT\right)}\right] \qquad \text{(Equation5–2)}$$

where P represents the permeability. The lipid and water solubility and the molecular weight and shape of the solute are determinants of

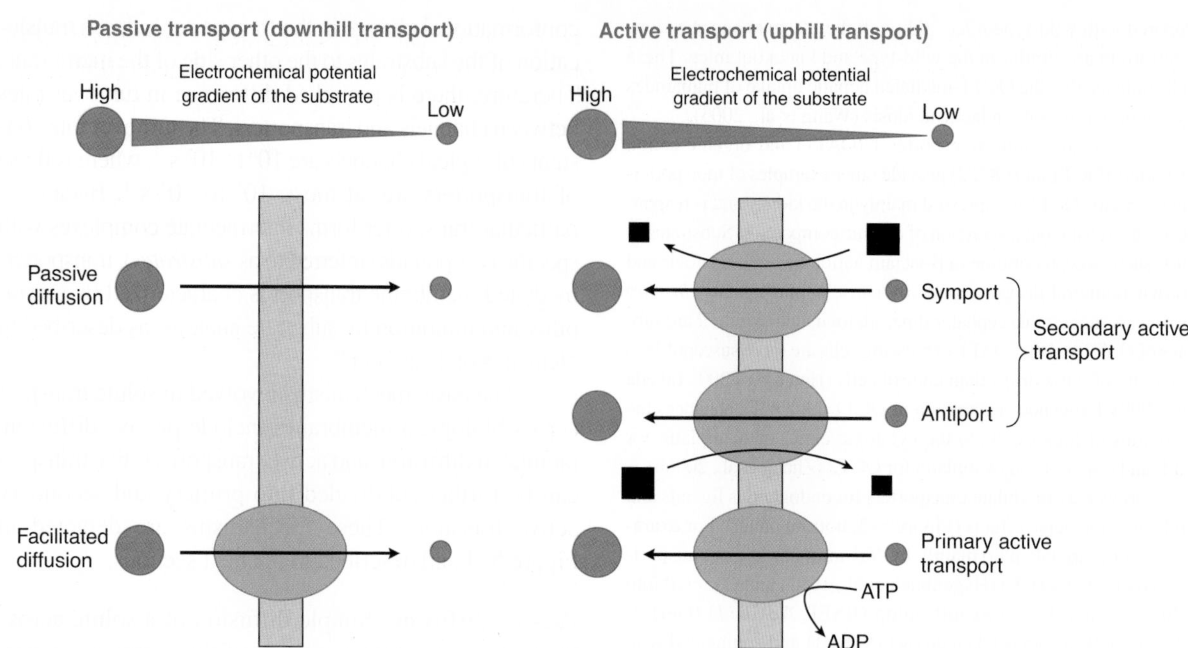

Figure 5–4. *Classification of membrane transport mechanisms. Red circles* depict the substrate. Size of the circles is proportional to the concentration of the substrate. *Arrows* show the direction of flux. *Black squares* represent the ion that supplies the driving force for transport (size is proportional to the concentration of the ion). *Blue ovals* depict transport proteins.

the flux in passive diffusion; they are incorporated in the permeability constant P. The permeability constant positively correlates with the lipophilicity, determined by the partition between water and organic solvents, such as octanol, and is also related to the inverse of the square root of the molecular weight of the solute. At steady state, the electrochemical potentials of all compounds become equal across the plasma membrane. In the case of non-ionized compounds, the steady-state concentrations are equal across the plasma membrane. For ionized compounds, however, the steady-state concentration ratio across the plasma membrane is affected by the membrane voltage and given by the Nernst equation:

$$\frac{C_i}{C_o} = \exp\left(\frac{-zE_m F}{RT}\right) \quad \text{(Equation 5–3)}$$

The membrane voltage is maintained by the ion gradients across the membrane.

Facilitated Diffusion. Diffusion of ions and organic compounds across the plasma membrane may be facilitated by a membrane transporter. Facilitated diffusion is a form of transporter-mediated membrane transport that does not require energy input. Just as in passive diffusion, the transport of ionized and non-ionized compounds across the plasma membrane occurs down their electrochemical potential gradient. Therefore, steady state will be achieved when the electrochemical potentials of the compound on both sides of the membrane become equal.

Active Transport. Active transport is the form of membrane transport that requires the input of energy. It is the transport of solutes against their electrochemical gradients, leading to the concentration of solutes on one side of the plasma membrane and the creation of potential energy in the electrochemical gradient formed. Active transport plays an important role in the uptake and efflux of drugs and other solutes. Depending on the driving force, active transport can be subdivided into primary and secondary active transport (Figure 5–4).

Primary Active Transport. Membrane transport that directly couples with ATP hydrolysis is called *primary active transport*. ABC transporters are examples of primary active transporters. They contain one or two ATP-binding cassettes that are highly conserved domains in the intracellular loop region and exhibit ATPase activity. In mammalian cells, ABC transporters mediate the unidirectional efflux of solutes across biological membranes. The molecular mechanism by which ATP hydrolysis is coupled to the active transport of substrates by ABC transporters is a subject of current investigation.

Secondary Active Transport. In secondary active transport, the transport across a biological membrane of one solute S_1 against its concentration gradient is energetically driven by the transport of another solute S_2 in accordance with its concentration gradient. The driving force for this type of transport therefore is stored in the electrochemical potential created by the concentration difference of S_2 across the plasma membrane. For example, an inwardly directed Na^+ concentration gradient across the plasma membrane is created by Na^+, K^+-ATPase. Under these conditions, inward movement of Na^+ produces the energy to drive the movement of a substrate S_1 against its concentration gradient by a secondary active transporter as in Na^+/Ca^{2+} exchange.

Depending on the transport direction of the solute, secondary active transporters are classified as either symporters or antiporters. *Symporters*, also termed *co-transporters*, transport S_2 and S_1 in the same direction, whereas *antiporters*, also termed *exchangers*, move their substrates in opposite directions (Figure 5–4). The free energy produced by one extracellular sodium ion (Na^+) is given by the difference in the electrochemical potential across the plasma membrane:

$$\Delta\mu_{Na} = E_m F + RT \ln\left(\frac{C_{Na,i}}{C_{Na,o}}\right) \quad \text{(Equation 5–4)}$$

The electrochemical potential of a non-ionized compound $\Delta\mu_s$ acquired from one extracellular Na^+ is less than this value:

$$\Delta\mu_s + \Delta\mu_{Na} \leq 0 \quad \text{(Equation 5–5)}$$

Therefore, the concentration ratio of the compound is given by the following equation:

$$\frac{S_i}{S_o} \leq \left(\frac{C_{Na,o}}{C_{Na,i}}\right)\exp\left(\frac{-E_m F}{RT}\right) \quad \text{(Equation 5–6)}$$

Assuming that the concentration ratio of Na^+ is 10 and that E_m is –60 mV, ideally, symport of one non-ionized organic compound with one Na^+ ion can achieve a 100-fold difference in the intracellular substrate concentration compared with the extracellular concentration. When more than one Na^+ ion is coupled to the movement of the solute, a synergistic driving force results. For the case in which two Na^+ ions are involved,

$$\frac{S_i}{S_o} \leq \left(\frac{C_{Na,o}}{C_{Na,i}}\right)^2\exp\left(\frac{-2E_m F}{RT}\right) \quad \text{(Equation 5–7)}$$

In this case, the substrate ideally is concentrated intracellularly 1000-fold relative to the extracellular space under the same conditions. The Na^+/Ca^{2+} antiporter shows the effect of this dependence in the square of the concentration ratio of Na^+; Ca^{2+} is transported from the cytosol (0.1 μM < $[Ca^{2+}]$ < 1 μM) to the plasma $[Ca^{2+}]_{free}$ ~1.25 mM.

KINETICS OF TRANSPORT

The flux of a substrate (rate of transport) across a biological membrane *via* transporter-mediated processes is characterized by saturability. The relationship between the flux v and substrate concentration C in a transporter-mediated process is given by the Michaelis-Menten equation:

$$v = \frac{V_{max} C}{K_m + C} \quad \text{(Equation 5–8)}$$

where V_{max} is the maximum transport rate and is proportional to the density of transporters on the plasma membrane, and K_m is the Michaelis constant, which represents the substrate concentration at which the flux is half the V_{max} value. K_m is an approximation of the dissociation constant of the substrate from the intermediate complex. When C is small compared with the K_m value, the flux is increased in proportion to the substrate concentration (roughly linear with substrate concentration). However, if C is large compared with the K_m value, the flux approaches a constant value (V_{max}). The K_m and V_{max} values can be determined by examining the flux at different substrate concentrations. The Eadie-Hofstee plot often is used for graphical interpretation of saturation kinetics. Plotting clearance v/C on the y axis and flux v on the x axis gives a straight line. The y intercept represents the ratio V_{max}/K_m, and the slope of the line is the inverse of the K_m value:

$$\frac{v}{C} = \frac{V_{max}}{K_m} - \frac{C}{K_m} \quad \text{(Equation 5–9)}$$

Involvement of multiple transporters with different K_m values gives an Eadie-Hofstee plot that is curved. In algebraic terms, the Eadie-Hofstee plot of kinetic data is equivalent to the Scatchard plot of equilibrium binding data.

Transporter-mediated membrane transport of a substrate is also characterized by inhibition by other compounds. The manner of inhibition can be categorized as one of three types: competitive, noncompetitive, and uncompetitive.

Competitive inhibition occurs when substrates and inhibitors share a common binding site on the transporter, resulting in an increase in the apparent K_m value in the presence of inhibitor. The flux of a substrate in the presence of a competitive inhibitor is

$$v = \frac{V_{max} C}{K_m(1 + I/K_i) + C} \quad \text{(Equation 5–10)}$$

where I is the concentration of inhibitor, and K_i is the inhibition constant.

Noncompetitive inhibition assumes that the inhibitor has an allosteric effect on the transporter, does not inhibit the formation of an intermediate complex of substrate and transporter, but does inhibit the subsequent translocation process.

$$v = \frac{V_{max} / (1 + I / K_i) \cdot C}{K_m + C} \quad \text{(Equation 5–11)}$$

Uncompetitive inhibition assumes that inhibitors can form a complex only with an intermediate complex of the substrate and transporter and inhibit subsequent translocation.

$$v = \frac{V_{max} / \left(1 + I / K_i\right) \cdot C}{K_m / \left(1 + I / K_i\right) + C} \quad \text{(Equation 5–12)}$$

VECTORIAL TRANSPORT

Asymmetrical transport across a monolayer of polarized cells, such as the epithelial and endothelial cells of brain capillaries, is called *vectorial transport* (Figure 5–5). Vectorial transport is important in the efficient transfer of solutes across epithelial or endothelial barriers. For example, vectorial transport is important for the absorption of nutrients and bile acids in the intestine. From the viewpoint of drug absorption and disposition, vectorial transport plays a major role in hepatobiliary and urinary excretion of drugs from the blood to the lumen and in the intestinal absorption of drugs. In addition, efflux of drugs from the brain via brain endothelial cells and brain choroid plexus epithelial cells involves vectorial transport. The ABC transporters mediate only unidirectional efflux, whereas SLC transporters mediate either drug uptake or efflux.

For lipophilic compounds that have sufficient membrane permeability, ABC transporters alone are able to achieve vectorial transport without the help of influx transporters (Horio et al., 1990). For relatively hydrophilic organic anions and cations, coordinated uptake and efflux transporters in the polarized plasma membranes are necessary to achieve the vectorial movement of solutes across an epithelium. Common substrates of coordinated transporters are transferred efficiently across the epithelial barrier (Cui et al., 2001; Sasaki et al., 2002).

In the liver, a number of transporters with different substrate specificities are localized on the sinusoidal membrane (facing blood). These transporters are involved in the uptake of bile acids, amphipathic organic anions, and hydrophilic organic cations into the hepatocytes. Similarly, ABC transporters on the canalicular membrane (facing bile) export such compounds into the bile. Multiple combinations of uptake (OATP1B1, OATP1B3, OATP2B1) and efflux transporters (MDR1, MRP2, and BCRP) are involved in the efficient transcellular transport of a wide variety of compounds in the liver by using a model cell system called "doubly transfected cells," which express both uptake and efflux transporter on each side (Ishiguro et al., 2008; Kopplow et al., 2005; Matsushima et al., 2005). In many cases, overlapping substrate specificities between the uptake transporters (OATP family) and efflux transporters (MRP family) make the vectorial transport of organic anions highly efficient. Similar transport systems also are present in the intestine, renal tubules, and endothelial cells of the brain capillaries (Figure 5–5).

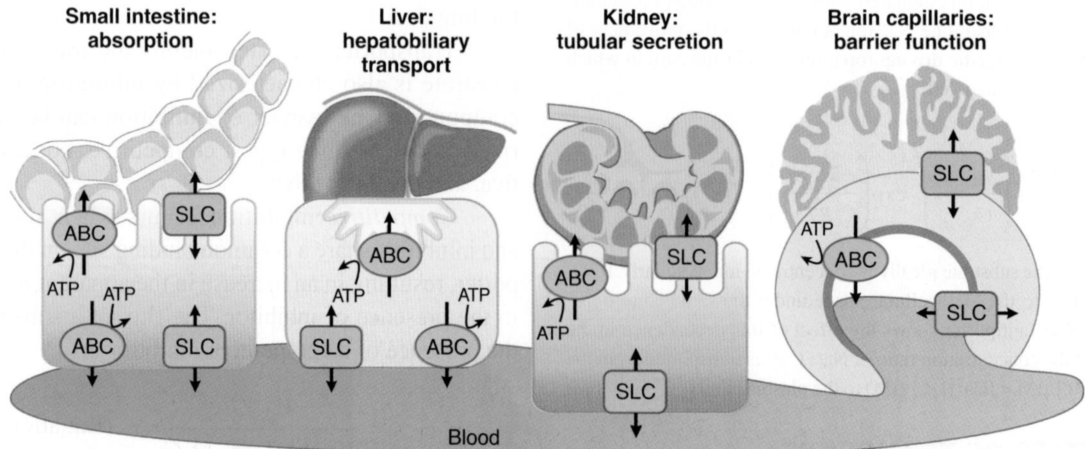

Figure 5–5. *Transepithelial or transendothelial flux.* Transepithelial or transendothelial flux of drugs requires distinct transporters at the two surfaces of the epithelial or endothelial barriers. These are depicted diagrammatically for transport across the small intestine (absorption), the kidney and liver (elimination), and the brain capillaries that comprise the blood-brain barrier.

Regulation of Transporter Expression. Transporter expression can be regulated transcriptionally in response to drug treatment and pathophysiological conditions, resulting in induction or down-regulation of transporter mRNAs. Recent studies have described important roles of type II nuclear receptors, which form heterodimers with the 9-cis-retinoic acid receptor (RXR), in regulating drug-metabolizing enzymes and transporters (see Table 6–4 and Figure 6–12) (Kullak-Ublick et al., 2004; Wang and LeCluyse, 2003). Such receptors include pregnane X receptor (PXR/NR1I2), constitutive androstane receptor (CAR/NR1I3), farnesoid X receptor (FXR/ NR1H4), PPARα (peroxisome proliferator-activated receptor α), and retinoic acid receptor (RAR). Except for CAR, these are ligand-activated nuclear receptors that, as heterodimers with RXR, bind specific elements in the enhancer regions of target genes. CAR has constitutive transcriptional activity that is antagonized by inverse agonists such as androstenol and androstanol and induced by barbiturates. PXR, also referred to as *steroid X receptor* (SXR) in humans, is activated by synthetic and endogenous steroids, bile acids, and drugs such as clotrimazole, phenobarbital, rifampicin, sulfinpyrazone, ritonavir, carbamazepine, phenytoin, sulfadimidine, paclitaxel, and hyperforin (a constituent of St. John's wort). Table 5–1 summarizes the effects of drug activation of type II nuclear receptors on expression of transporters. The potency of activators of PXR varies among species such that rodents are not necessarily a model for effects in humans. There is an overlap of substrates between CYP3A4 and P-glycoprotein, and PXR mediates coinduction of CYP3A4 and P-glycoprotein, supporting their synergy in efficient detoxification.

DNA methylation is one of the mechanisms underlying the epigenetic control of gene expression. Reportedly, the tissue-selective expression of transporters is achieved by DNA methylation (silencing in the transporter-negative tissues) as well as by transactivation in the transporter-positive tissues. Transporters subjected to epigenetic control include OAT3, URAT1, OCT2, Oatp1b2, Ntcp, and PEPT2 in the SLC families; and MDR1, BCRP, BSEP, and ABCG5/ABCG8 (Aoki et al., 2008; Imai et al., 2009; Kikuchi et al., 2006; Turner et al., 2006; Uchiumi et al., 1993).

MOLECULAR STRUCTURES OF TRANSPORTERS

Predictions of secondary structure of membrane transport proteins based on hydropathy analysis indicate that membrane transporters in the SLC and ABC superfamilies are multi-membrane-spanning proteins. A typical predicted secondary structure of the ABC transporter MRP2 (*ABCC2*) is shown in Figure 5–6. However, understanding the secondary structure of a membrane transporter provides little information on how the transporter functions to translocate its substrates. For this, information on the tertiary structure of the transporter is needed, along with complementary molecular information about the residues in the transporter that are involved in the recognition, association, and dissociation of its substrates. X-ray diffraction data on representative membrane transporters illustrate some basic structural properties of membrane transporters.

ABC Transporter Crystal Structures. To date, four full ABCs have been crystallized; three are importers and one is an exporter reminiscent of human ABC transporters (Figure 5–7). The importers are the vitamin B_{12} transporter BtuCD from *E. coli* (Locher et al., 2002), the metal-chelate-type transporter HI1470/1 from *H. influenzae* (Pinkett et al., 2007), and the molybdate/tungstate transporter ModBC from *A. fulgidus* (Hollenstein et al., 2007). The exporter is *Sav1866*, a multidrug resistance transporter from *S. aureus* (Dawson et al., 2006, 2007). The nucleotide-binding domains (NBDs), which are present in the cytoplasm, are considered the motor domains of ABC transporters and contain conserved motifs (e.g., Walker-A motif, ABC signature motif) that participate in binding and hydrolysis of ATP. Crystal structures of all four full ABC transporters show two NBDs, which are in contact with each other, and a conserved fold. The transmembrane domains of Sav1866 serve as a good model for the basic architecture of human ABC transporters. Note how the transmembrane domains of Sav1866 extend into the cytoplasm and how in the observed crystal structure, the two major bundles are visible at the extracelluar surface. The mechanism, shared by these ABC transporters, appears to involve binding of ATP to the NBDs, which subsequently triggers an outward-facing conformation of the transporters. Dissociation of the hydrolysis products of ATP appears to result in an inward-facing conformation. In the case of drug extrusion, when ATP binds, the transporters open to the outside, releasing their substrates to the extracellular media. Upon dissociation of the hydrolysis products, the transporters return to the inward-facing conformation, permitting the binding of ATP and substrate.

Lactose Permease Symporter (LacY). Lactose permease is a bacterial transporter that belongs to the *m*ajor *f*acilitator *s*uperfamily (MFS). This transporter is a proton-coupled symporter. A high-resolution X-ray crystal structure has been obtained for the protonated form of a mutant of LacY (C154G) (Abramson et al., 2003) (Figure 5–8). LacY consists of two units of six membrane-spanning α-helices. The crystal structure locates substrate at the interface of the two units and in the middle of the membrane. This location is consistent with an alternating-access transport mechanism in which the substrate recognition site is accessible to the cytosolic and then the extracellular surface but not to both simultaneously (Figure 5–9). Eight helices form the surface of the hydrophilic cavity, and each contains proline and glycine residues that result in kinks in the cavity. From LacY, we now know that, as in the case of MsbA, six membrane-spanning α-helices are critical structural units for transport by LacY.

Table 5–1

Regulation of Transporter Expression by Nuclear Receptors

TRANSPORTER	SPECIES	TRANSCRIPTION FACTOR	LIGAND (DOSE)	EFFECT
MDR1 (P-gp)	human	PXR	Rifampin (rifampicin)	↑ Transcription activity (promoter assay)
			Rifampin (600mg/day, 10 days)	↑ Expression in duodenum in healthy subjects
			Rifampin (600mg/day, 10 days)	↓ Oral bioavailability of digoxin in healthy subjects
			Rifampin (600mg/day, 9 days)	↓ AUC of talinolol after in and oral administration in healthy subjects
			St John's wort (300mg t.i.d., 14 days)	↑ Expression in duodenum in healthy subjects
			St John's wort (300mg t.i.d., 14 days)	↓ Oral bioavailability of digoxin in healthy subject
		PXR	Rifampin	↑ Expression in human primary hepatocye
		CAR	Phenobarbital	↑ Expression in human primary hepatocye
Mdr1a	mouse	PPARα	Clofibrate (500mg/kg, 10 days)	↑ Expression in liver
MRP2	human	PXR	Rifampin (600mg/day, 9 days)	↑ Expression in duodenum in healthy subjects
			Rifampin/hyperforin	↑ Expression in human primary hepatocye
		FXR	GW4064/ chenodeoxycholate	↑ Expression in HepG2-FXR
		CAR	Phenobarbital	↑ Expression in human hepatocye
	rat	PXR/FXR/CAR	PCN/GW4064/ phenobarbital	↑ Expression in rat hepatocyte
		PXR/FXR/CAR	PCN/GW4064/ phenobarbital	↑ Transcription activity (promoter assay)
	mouse	PXR	Pregnenolone 16α-carbonitrile/ dexamethasone	↑ Expression in mouse hepatocyte
		CAR	Phenobarbital	↑ Expression in hepatocyte from PXR(–/–) mice
			Phenobarbital	↑ Transcription activity (promoter assay)
			TCPOBOP (3mg/kg, 3 or 4 days)	↑ Expression in liver
BCRP	human	PXR	Rifampin	↑ Expression in human primary hepatocye
		CAR	Phenobarbital	↑ Expression in human primary hepatocye
	mouse	PPARα	Clofibrate (500mg/kg, 10 days)	↑ Expression in liver
MRP3	human	PXR	Rifampin	↑ Expression in human hepatocye
	rat	CAR	Phenobarbital (75 mg/kg, 4 days)	↑ Expression in liver
	mouse	PXR	Pregnenolone 16α-carbonitrile (200mg/kg, 4 days)	↑ Expression in liver
		CAR	Phenobarbital (100mg/kg, 3 days)	↑ Expression in liver
			TCPOBOP (3mg/kg, 3 or 4 days)	↑ Expression in liver
		PPARα	Clofibrate (500mg/kg, 4 or 10 days)	↑ Expression in liver

Table 5–1

Regulation of Transporter Expression by Nuclear Receptors (*Continued*)

TRANSPORTER	SPECIES	TRANSCRIPTION FACTOR	LIGAND (DOSE)	EFFECT
MRP4	mouse	CAR	Phenobarbital (100mg/kg, 3 days) TCPOBOP (3mg/kg, 4 days)	↑ Expression in liver and kidney
		PPARα	Clofibrate (500mg/kg, 10 days)	↑ Expression in liver
OATP1B1	human	SHP1	Cholic acid	indirect effect on HNF1α expression
		PXR	Rifampin	↑ Expression in human hepatocye
OATP1B3	human	FXR	Chenodeoxycholate	↑ Expression in Hepatoma cells
Oatp1a4	rat	PXR	Pregnenolone 16α-carbonitrile (75 mg/kg, 4 days)	↑ Expression in liver
		CAR	Phenobarbital (80 mg/kg, 5 days)	↑ Expression in liver, ↑ hepatic uptake of digoxin
	mouse	PXR	Pregnenolone 16α-carbonitrile (75 mg/kg, 3 days)	↑ Expression in liver
		CAR	Phenobarbital (100mg/kg, 3 days) TCPOBOP (3mg/kg, 3 days)	↑ Expression in liver
BSEP	human	FXR	Chenodeoxycholate	↑ Transcription activity (promoter assay)
Ntcp	rat	SHP1	Cholic acid	↓ RAR mediated transcription
OSTα/β	human	FXR	Chenodeoxycholate/ GW4064	↑ Transcription activity (promoter assay)
		FXR	Chenodeoxycholate	↑ Expression in ileal biopsies
	mouse	FXR	GW4064 (30 mg/kg, twice daily, 4 days)	↑ Expression in intestine and kidney
MDR2	mouse	PPARα	Ciprofibrate (0.05% w/w in diet)	↑ Expression in the liver

See Geick et al., 2001; Greiner et al., 1999; Kok et al., 2003.

Sodium Galactose Transporter (vSGLT). vSGLT is a sodium galactose transporter of *Vibrio parahaemolyticus.* vSGLT is a member of the solute sodium symporters (SSS). This bacterial transporter is ~30% homologous to the human SGLT1, an important transporter for the intestinal absorption of sugars. Crystal structure at ~3 Å resolution suggests that like LacY, vSGLT operates as an alternating-access transport mechanism (Faham et al., 2008). However, vSGLT operates as a gated pore rather than a rocker switch mechanism (Figure 5–9) (Kanner, 2008; Karpowich and Wang, 2008). The 12 transmembrane domains consist of two symmetrical halves (six domains each). Galactose and sodium are bound at the center of the membrane at two broken helices, one from each of the symmetrical halves. These broken helices appear to rotate to achieve alternating access of extracellular and intracellular sides. This mechanism, though similar to LacY, involves less molecular dynamic changes than LacY, which operates as a rocker switch. Figure 5–9 shows an alternating access model for SGLT (Karpowich and Wang, 2008). In this model, a binding pocket faces the extracellular side. The substrate, glucose, is bound to this binding pocket. Movement of a bundle of helices, triggered by binding of glucose and sodium, simultaneously closes the access of the binding pocket to the extracellular face and opens the exit pathway to the intracellular spaces. The model is based on symmetrical arrangement of helices.

TRANSPORTER SUPERFAMILIES IN THE HUMAN GENOME

Two major gene superfamilies play critical roles in the transport of drugs across plasma and other biological membranes: the SLC and ABC superfamilies. Web sites that have information on these families include *http://nutrigene.4t.com/humanabc.htm* (ABC superfamily),

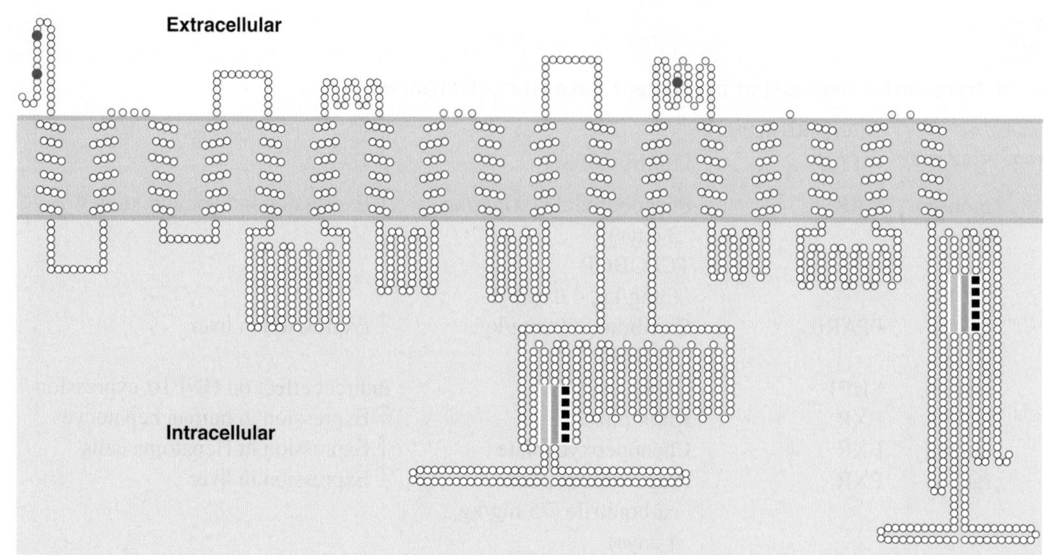

Figure 5–6. *Predicted secondary structure of MRP2 based on hydropathy analysis.* The *dark blue circles* depict glycosylation sites; Walker A motif is colored *light blue; black* boxes represent the Walker B motif. *Light gray* is the middle region between the two motifs. The Walker A motifs interact with α and β phosphates of di- and tri-nucleotides; the Walker B motifs help to coordinate Mg^2.

http://www.bioparadigms.org/slc/intro.asp (SLC superfamily), *http://www.pharmaconference.org/slctable.asp* (SLC superfamily), and *http://www.TP_Search.jp/* (drug transporters). Information on pharmacogenetics of these transporters can be found in Chapter 7 and at *http://www.pharmgkb.org* and *http://www.pharmacogenetics.ucsf.edu*.

SLC Transporters. The solute carrier (SLC) superfamily includes 48 families and represents ~315 genes in the human genome. The nomenclature of the transporters within each family is listed at *http://www.genenames.org/aboutHGNC.html.* Table 5–2 lists the families in the human SLC superfamily and some of the genetic diseases that are associated with members of selected

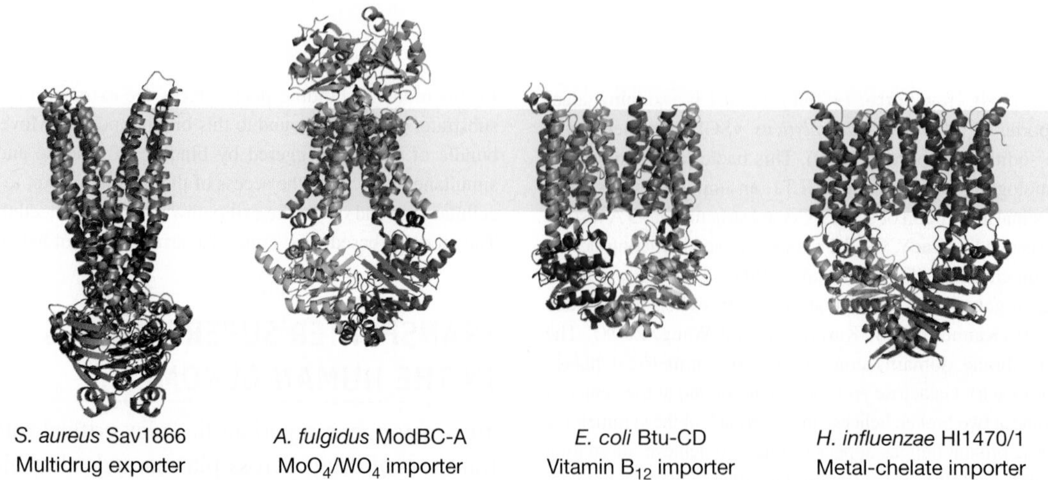

Figure 5–7. *Structure of four crystallized ABC transporters from microorganisms.* The structures show the intracellular nucleotide binding domains (NBDs) along with the transmembrane alpha helices. Structure was reconstructed by Libusha Kelly using the coordinates deposited in the Protein Data Bank (PDB; *http://www.rcsb.org/pdb/*).

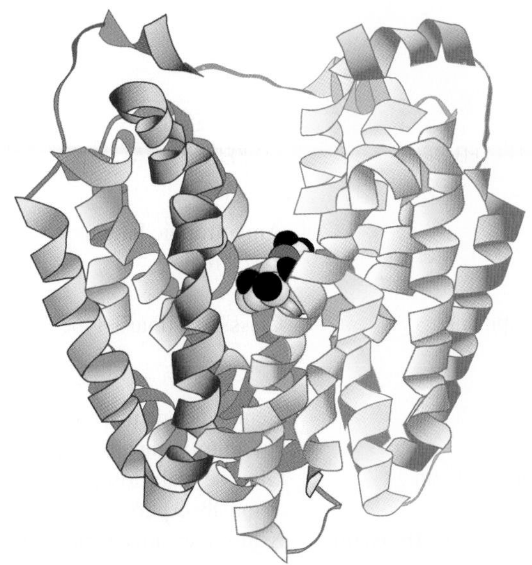

Figure 5–8. *Structure of the protonated form of a mutant of LacY.* Two units of six-membrane-spanning α-helices (shown as *ribbons*) are present. Substrate (depicted as *green and black balls*) is bound to the interface of the two units and in the middle of the membrane. Structure has been redrawn from coordinates in Protein Data Bank (http://www.rcsb.org/pdb/).

families. The family name provides a description of the function(s) of each family. However, some caution should be exercised in interpretation of family names because individual family members may have vastly different specificities or functional roles (Hediger, 2004).

Transporters in the SLC superfamily transport diverse ionic and non-ionic endogenous compounds and xenobiotics. SLC superfamily transporters may be facilitated transporters or secondary active symporters or antiporters. The first SLC family transporter was cloned in 1987 by expression cloning in *Xenopus laevis* oocytes (Hediger et al., 1987). Since then, many transporters in the SLC superfamily have been cloned and characterized functionally. Predictive models defining important characteristics of substrate binding and knockout mouse models defining the *in vivo* role of specific transporters have been constructed for many SLC transporters (Chang et al., 2004; Ocheltree et al., 2004).

ABC Superfamily. ABC transporters can be divided into seven groups based on their sequence homology: ABCA (12 members), ABCB (11 members), ABCC (13 members), ABCD (4 members), ABCE (1 member), ABCF (3 members), and ABCG (5 members). ABC genes are essential for many cellular processes, and mutations in at least 13 of these genes cause or contribute to human genetic disorders (Table 5–3). In addition to conferring multidrug resistance (Sadee et al., 1995), an important pharmacological aspect of these transporters is xenobiotic export from healthy tissues. In particular, MDR1/ABCB1, MRP2/ABCC2, and BCRP/ABCG2 have been shown to be involved in overall drug disposition (Leslie et al., 2005). ABC transporters including MDR1, BCRP, and MRP4 play pivotal roles in the blood-tissue barriers in the brain, placenta, testis, and retina. Active efflux against concentration gradient in the blood-to-tissue direction on the blood-facing plasma membranes limits the tissue penetration from the blood.

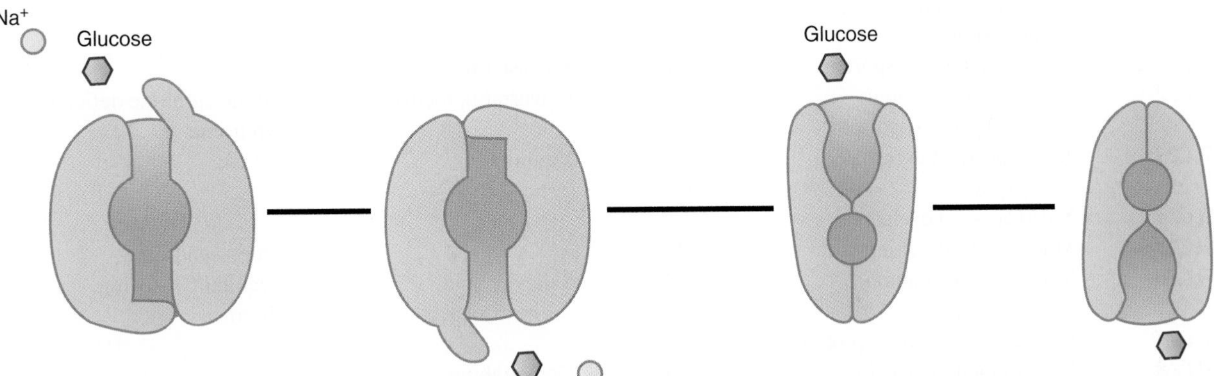

Figure 5–9. *Alternating access models of the transport function of two transporters.* The gated pore represents the model for SGLT in which the rotation of two broken helices facilitates alternating access of substrates to the intracellular and extracellular sides of the plasma membrane. The rocker switch represents the model by which MFS proteins, such as LacY, work. This example models a facilitated glucose transporter, GLUT2.

Table 5–2

Families in the Human Solute Carrier Superfamily

GENE NAME	FAMILY NAME	NUMBER OF FAMILY MEMBERS	SELECTED DRUG SUBSTRATES	EXAMPLES OF LINKED HUMAN DISEASES
SLC1	High-affinity glutamate and neutral amino acid transporter	7		Amyotrophic lateral sclerosis
SLC2	Facilitative GLUT transporter	14		
SLC3	Heavy subunits of the heteromeric amino acid transporters	2	Melphalan	Classic cystinuria type I
SLC4	Bicarbonate transporter	10		Hemolytic anemia, blindness–auditory impairment
SLC5	Na^+ glucose cotransporter	8	Dapagliflozin	Glucose–galactose malabsorption syndrome
SLC6	Na^+- and Cl^--dependent neurotransmitter transporter	16	Paraoxetine, fluoxetine	X-linked creatine deficiency syndrome
SLC7	Cationic amino acid transporter	14	Melphalan	Lysinuric protein intolerance
SLC8	Na^+/Ca^{2+} exchanger	3	N, N-Dimethylarginine	
SLC9	Na^+/H^+ exchanger	8	Thiazide diuretics	Congenital secretory diarrhea
SLC10	Na^+ bile salt cotransporter	6	Benzothiazepines	Primary bile salt malabsorption
SLC11	H^+ coupled metal ion transporter	2		Hereditary hemochromatosis
SLC12	Electroneutral cation–Cl^- cotransporter family	9		Gitelman's syndrome
SLC13	Na^+–sulfate/carboxylate cotransporter	5	Sulfate conjugates, cysteine conjugates	
SLC14	Urea transporter	2		Kidd antigen blood group
SLC15	H^+–oligopeptide cotransporter	4	Valacyclovir	
SLC16	Monocarboxylate transporter	14	Salicylic acid, atorvastatin	Muscle weakness
SLC17	Vesicular glutamate transporter	8		Sialic acid storage disease
SLC18	Vesicular amine transporter	3	Reserpine	Myasthenic syndromes
SLC19	Folate/thiamine transporter	3	Methotrexate	Thiamine-responsive megaloblastic anemia
SLC20	Type III Na^+–phosphate cotransporter	2		
SLC21/SLCO	Organic anion transporter	11	Pravastatin	
SLC22	Organic cation/anion/ zwitterion transporter	18	Pravastatin, metformin	Systemic carnitine deficiency syndrome
SLC23	Na^+-dependent ascorbate transporter	4	Vitamin C	
SLC24	$Na^+/(Ca^{2+}\text{-}K^+)$ exchanger	5		
SLC25	Mitochondrial carrier	27		Senger's syndrome
SLC26	Multifunctional anion exchanger	10	Salicylic acid, ciprofloxacin	Congenital Cl^--losing diarrhea
SLC27	Fatty acid transporter protein	6		
SLC28	Na^+-coupled nucleoside transport	3	Gemcitabine, cladribine	

Table 5–2

Families in the Human Solute Carrier Superfamily (*Continued*)

GENE NAME	FAMILY NAME	NUMBER OF FAMILY MEMBERS	SELECTED DRUG SUBSTRATES	EXAMPLES OF LINKED HUMAN DISEASES
SLC29	Facilitative nucleoside transporter	4	Dipyridamole, gemcitabine	
SLC30	Zinc efflux	9		
SLC31	Copper transporter	2	Cisplatin	
SLC32	Vesicular inhibitory amino acid transporter	1	Vigabatrin	
SLC33	Acetyl-CoA transporter	1		
SLC34	Type II Na^+–phosphate cotransporter	3		Autosomal-dominant hypophosphatemic rickets
SLC35	Nucleoside-sugar transporter	17		Leukocyte adhesion deficiency type II
SLC36	H^+-coupled amino acid transporter	4	D-Serine, cycloserine	
SLC37	Sugar-phosphate/phosphate exchanger	4		Glycogen storage disease (non-la)
SLC38	System A and N, Na^+-coupled neutral amino acid transporter	6		
SLC39	Metal ion transporter	14		Acrodermatitis enteropathica
SLC40	Basolateral iron transporter	1		Type IV hemochromatosis
SLC41	MgtE-like magnesium transporter	3		
SLC42	Rh ammonium transporter	3		Rh-null regulator
SLC43	Na^+-independent system-L-like amino acid transporter	2		

In 1976, Juliano and Ling reported that overexpression of a membrane protein in colchicine-resistant Chinese hamster ovary cells also resulted in acquired resistance to many structurally unrelated drugs (i.e., multidrug resistance) (Juliano and Ling, 1976). Since the cDNA cloning of this first mammalian ABC protein (P-glycoprotein/MDR1/ABCB1), knowledge of the ABC superfamily has grown to include 49 genes, each containing one or two conserved ABC regions (Borst and Elferink, 2002). The ABC region is a core catalytic domain of ATP hydrolysis and contains Walker A and B sequences and an ABC transporter-specific signature C sequence (Figure 5–6). The ABC regions of these proteins bind and hydrolyze ATP, and the proteins use the energy for uphill transport of their substrates across the membrane. Although some ABC superfamily transporters contain only a single ABC motif, they form homodimers (BCRP/ABCG2) or heterodimers (ABCG5 and ABCG8) that exhibit a transport function. ABC transporters (e.g., MsbA) (Figure 5–7) also are found in prokaryotes, where they are involved predominantly in the import of essential compounds that cannot be obtained by passive diffusion (sugars, vitamins, metals, etc.). By contrast, most ABC genes in eukaryotes transport compounds from the cytoplasm to the outside or into an intracellular compartment (endoplasmic reticulum, mitochondria, peroxisomes).

Properties of ABC Transporters Related to Drug Action

The tissue distribution of drug-related ABC transporters in the body is summarized in Table 5–4 together with information about typical substrates.

Tissue Distribution of Drug-Related ABC Transporters. MDR1 (*ABCB1*), MRP2 (*ABCC2*), and BCRP (*ABCG2*) are all expressed in the apical side of the intestinal epithelia, where they serve to pump out xenobiotics, including many orally administered drugs. MRP3 (ABCC3) is expressed in the basal side of the epithelial cells.

The kidney and liver are major organs for overall systemic drug elimination from the body. The liver also plays a role in presystemic drug elimination. Key to the vectorial excretion of drugs into

Table 5–3

The ATP Binding Cassette (ABC) Superfamily in the Human Genome and Linked Genetic Diseases

GENE NAME	FAMILY NAME	NUMBER OF FAMILY MEMBERS	EXAMPLES OF LINKED HUMAN DISEASES
ABCA	ABC A	12	Tangier disease (defect in cholesterol transport; ABCA1), Stargardt syndrome (defect in retinal metabolism; ABCA4)
ABCB	ABC B	11	Bare lymphocyte syndrome type I (defect in antigen-presenting; ABCB3 and ABCB4), progressive familial intrahepatic cholestasis type 3 (defect in biliary lipid secretion; MDR3/ABCB4), X-linked sideroblastic anemia with ataxia (a possible defect in iron homeostasis in mitochondria; ABCB7), progressive familial intrahepatic cholestasis type 2 (defect in biliary bile acid excretion; BSEP/ABCB11)
ABCC	ABC C	13	Dubin-Johnson syndrome (defect in biliary bilirubin glucuronide excretion; MRP2/ABCC2), pseudoxanthoma (unknown mechanism; ABCC6), cystic fibrosis (defect in Cl^- channel regulation; ABCC7), persistent hyperinsulinemic hypoglycemia of infancy (defect in inwardly rectifying K^+ conductance regulation in pancreatic B cells; SUR1)
ABCD	ABC D	4	Adrenoleukodystrophy (a possible defect in peroxisomal transport or catabolism of very long-chain fatty acids; ABCD1)
ABCE	ABC E	1	
ABCF	ABC F	3	
ABCG	ABC G	5	Sitosterolemia (defect in biliary and intestinal excretion of plant sterols; ABCG5 and ABCG8)

urine or bile, ABC transporters are expressed in the polarized tissues of kidney and liver: MDR1, MRP2, and MRP4 (*ABCC4*) on the brush-border membrane of renal epithelia; MDR1, MRP2, and BCRP on the bile canalicular membrane of hepatocytes; and MRP3 and MRP4 on the sinusoidal membrane of hepatocytes. Some ABC transporters are expressed specifically on the blood side of the endothelial or epithelial cells that form barriers to the free entrance of toxic compounds into tissues: the BBB (MDR1 and MRP4 on the luminal side of brain capillary endothelial cells), the blood-cerebrospinal fluid (CSF) barrier (MRP1 and MRP4 on the basolateral blood side of choroid plexus epithelia), the blood-testis barrier (MRP1 on the basolateral membrane of mouse Sertoli cells and MDR1 in several types of human testicular cells), and the blood-placenta barrier (MDR1, MRP2, and BCRP on the luminal maternal side and MRP1 on the anti-luminal fetal side of placental trophoblasts).

Substrate Specificity of ABC Transporters. MDR1/ABCB1 substrates tend to share a hydrophobic planar structure with positively charged or neutral moieties (see Table 5–4 and Ambudkar et al., 1998). These include structurally and pharmacologically unrelated compounds, many of which are also substrates of CYP3A4, a major drug-metabolizing enzyme in the human liver and GI tract. Such overlapping substrate specificity implies a synergistic role for MDR1 and CYP3A4 in protecting the body by reducing the intestinal absorption of xenobiotics (Zhang and Benet, 2001). After being taken up by enterocytes, some drug molecules are metabolized by CYP3A4. Drug molecules that escape metabolic conversion are eliminated from the cells by MDR1 and then reenter the enterocytes. The intestinal residence time of the drug is prolonged with the aid of MDR1, thereby increasing the chance of local metabolic conversion by the CYP3A4 (see Chapter 6).

MRP/ABCC Family. The substrates of transporters in the MRP/ABCC family are mostly organic anions. The substrate specificities of MRP1 and MRP2 are similar: both accept glutathione and glucuronide conjugates, sulfated conjugates of bile salts, and non-conjugated organic anions of an amphipathic nature (at least one negative charge and some degree of hydrophobicity). They also transport neutral or cationic anticancer drugs, such as vinca alkaloids and anthracyclines, possibly by means of a cotransport or symport mechanism with reduced glutathione (GSH).

MRP3 also has a substrate specificity that is similar to that of MRP2 but with a lower transport affinity for glutathione conjugates compared with MRP1 and MRP2. Most characteristic MRP3 substrates are monovalent bile salts, which are never transported by MRP1 and MRP2. Because MRP3 is expressed on the sinusoidal side of hepatocytes and is induced under cholestatic conditions, backflux of toxic bile salts and bilirubin glucuronides into the blood circulation is considered to be its physiological function.

Table 5–4

ABC Transporters Involved in Drug Absorption, Distribution, and Excretion Processes

TRANSPORTER NAME	TISSUE DISTRIBUTION	PHYSIOLOGICAL FUNCTION	SUBSTRATES
MDR1 (ABCB1)	Liver Kidney Intestine BBB BTB BPB	Natural detoxification system against xenobiotics	**Characteristics:** Neutral or cationic compounds with bulky structure **Anticancer drugs:** etoposide, doxorubicin, vincristine **Ca^{2+} channel blockers:** diltiazem, verapamil **HIV protease inhibitors:** indinavir, ritonavir **Antibiotics/Antifungals:** erythromycin, ketoconazole **Hormones:** testosterone, progesterone **Immunosuppressants:** cyclosporine, tacrolimus **Others:** digoxin, quinidine, fexofenadine, loperamide
MRP1 (ABCC1)	Ubiquitous (Kidney, BCSFB, BTB)	Leukotriene C_4 secretion from leukocyte	**Characteristics:** Amphiphilic with at least one negative net charge **Anticancer drugs:** vincristine (with GSH), methotrexate **Glutathione conjugates:** leukotriene C_4, glutathione conjugate of ethacrynic acid **Glucuronide conjugates:** estradiol-17-D-glucuronide, bilirubin mono(or bis)glucuronide **Sulfated conjugates:** estrone-3-sulfate (with GSH) **HIV protease inhibitors:** saquinavir **Antibiotics:** grepafloxacin **Others:** folate, GSH, oxidized glutathione
MRP2 (ABCC2)	Liver Kidney Intestine BPB	Excretion of bilirubin glucuronide and GSH into bile	**Characteristics:** Amphiphilic with at least one negative net charge (similar to MRP1) **Anticancer drugs:** methotrexate, vincristine **Glutathione conjugates:** leukotriene C4, glutathione conjugate of ethacrynic acid **Glucuronide conjugates:** estradiol-17-D-glucuronide, bilirubin mono(or bis)glucuronide **Sulfate conjugate of bile salts:** taurolithocholate sulfate **Amphipathic organic anions**: statins, angiotensin II receptor antagonists, temocaprilat **HIV protease inhibitors:** indinavir, ritonavir **Others:** GSH, oxidized glutathione
MRP3 (ABCC3)	Liver Kidney Intestine	?	**Characteristics:** Amphiphilic with at least one negative net charge (Glucuronide conjugates are better substrates than glutathione conjugates.) **Anticancer drugs**: etoposide, methotrexate **Glutathione conjugates:** leukotriene C_4, glutathione conjugate of 15-deoxy-delta prostaglandin J2 **Glucuronide conjugates:** estradiol-17-D-glucuronide, etoposide glucuronide, morphine-3-glucuronide, morphine-6-glucuronide, acetaminophen glucuronide, hymecromone glucuronide, and harmol glucuronide **Sulfate conjugates of bile salts:** taurolithocholate sulfate **Bile salts:** glycocholate, taurocholate **Others:** folate, leucovorin

(*Continued*)

Table 5–4

ABC Transporters Involved in Drug Absorption, Distribution, and Excretion Processes (*Continued*)

TRANSPORTER NAME	TISSUE DISTRIBUTION	PHYSIOLOGICAL FUNCTION	SUBSTRATES
MRP4 (ABCC4)	Ubiquitous (Kidney, Prostate, Lung, Muscle, Pancreas, Testis, Ovary, Bladder, Gallbladder, BBB, BCSFB)	?	**Characteristics:** Nucleotide analogs **Anticancer drugs:** 6-mercaptopurine, methotrexate **Glucuronide conjugates:** estradiol-17-D-glucuronide **Sulfate conjugates:** dehydroepiandrosterone sulfate **Cyclic nucleotides**: cAMP, cGMP **Diuretics:** furosemide, trichlormethiazide **Antiviral drugs**: adefovir, tenofovir **Antibiotics:** cefazolin, ceftizoxime **Others**: folate, leucovorin, taurocholate (with GSH)
MRP5 (ABCC5)	Ubiquitous	?	**Characteristics:** Nucleotide analogs **Anticancer drugs:** 6-mercaptopurine **Cyclic nucleotides:** cAMP, cGMP **HIV protease inhibitors:** adefovir
MRP6 (ABCC6)	Liver Kidney	?	**Anticancer drugs:** doxorubicin*, etoposide* **Glutathione conjugates:** leukotriene C_4 **Other:** BQ-123 (cyclic peptide)
BCRP (MXR) (ABCG2)	Liver Intestine BBB	Normal heme metabolism/ transport during maturation of erythrocytes?	**Anticancer drugs:** methotrexate, mitoxantrone, camptothecins SN-38, topotecan, imatinib **Glucuronide conjugates:** 4-methylumbelliferone glucuronide, estradiol-17-D-glucuronide **Sulfate conjugates:** dehydroepiandrosterone sulfate, estrone-3-sulfate **Antibiotics:** nitrofurantoin, fluoroquinolones **Statins:** pitavastatin, rosuvastatin **Others:** cholesterol, estradiol, dantrolene, prazosin, sulfasalazine, phytoestrogens, PhIP, pheophorbide A
MDR3 (ABCB4)	Liver	Excretion of phospholipids into bile	**Characteristics:** Phospholipids
BSEP (ABCB11)	Liver	Excretion of bile salts into bile	**Characteristics:** Bile salts
ABCG5 and ABCG8	Liver Intestine	Excretion of plant sterols into bile and intestinal lumen	**Characteristics:** Plant sterols

Representative substrates and cytotoxic drugs with increased resistance (*) are included in this table (cytotoxicity with increased resistance is usually caused by the decreased accumulation of the drugs). Although MDR3 (ABCB4), BSEP (ABCB11), ABCG5 and ABCG8 are not directly involved in drug disposition, inhibition of these physiologically important ABC transporters will lead to unfavorable side effects.
BBB, blood-brain barrier; BTB, blood-testis barrier; BPB, blood-placental barrier; BCSFB, blood-cerebrospinal fluid barrier.

MRP4 accepts negatively charged molecules, including cytotoxic compounds (e.g., 6-mercaptopurine and methotrexate), cyclic nucleotides, antiviral drugs (e.g., adefovir and tenofovir), diuretics (e.g., furosemide and trichlorothiazide), and cephalosporins (e.g., ceftizoxime and cefazolin). Glutathione enables MRP4 to accept taurocholate and leukotriene B_4.

MRP5 has a narrower substrate specificity and accepts nucleotide analog and clinically important anti–human immunodeficiency virus (HIV) drugs. Although some transport substrates have been identified for MRP6, no physiologically important endogenous substrates have been identified that explain the mechanism of the MRP6-associated disease, pseudoxanthoma.

BCRP/ABCG2. BCRP accepts both neutral and negatively charged molecules, including cytotoxic compounds (e.g., topotecan, flavopiridol, and methotrexate), sulfated conjugates of therapeutic drugs and hormones (e.g., estrogen sulfate), antibiotics (e.g., nitrofurantoin and fluoroquinolones), statins (e.g., pitavastatin and rosuvastatin), and toxic compounds found in normal food [phytoestrogens, 2-amino-1-methyl-6-phenylimidazo[4,5-*b*]pyridine (PhIP) and pheophorbide A, a chlorophyll catabolite].

Physiological Roles of ABC Transporters. The physiological significance of the ABC transporters is illustrated by studies involving knockout animals or patients with genetic defects in these transporters.

Mice deficient in MDR1 function are viable and fertile and do not display obvious phenotypic abnormalities other than hypersensitivity to toxic drugs, including the neurotoxic pesticide ivermectin (100-fold) and the cytotoxic drug vinblastine (3-fold) (Schinkel et al., 1994). *Mrp1* (–/–) mice are also viable and fertile without any obvious difference in litter size. However, these mice are hypersensitive to the anticancer drug etoposide. Damage is especially severe in the testis, kidney, and oropharyngeal mucosa, where MRP1 is expressed on the basolateral membrane. Moreover, these mice have an impaired response to an arachidonic acid–induced inflammatory stimulus, which is likely due to a reduced secretion of leukotriene C_4 from mast cells, macrophages, and granulocytes. MRP2-deficient rats (TR– and EHBR) and Dubin-Johnson syndrome patients are normal in appearance except for mild jaundice owing to impaired biliary excretion of bilirubin glucuronide (Büchler M et al., 1996; Ito et al., 1997; Paulusma et al., 1996). *Mrp4* (–/–) mice are hypersensitive to adefovir and thiopurine. Damage induced by adefovir is especially severe in the bone marrow, thymus, spleen, and intestine, and that by thiopurine is in the myeloid progenitor cells (Belinsky et al., 2007; Krishnamurthy et al., 2008; Takenaka et al., 2007). MRP4 modulates the signal transduction by active efflux of cAMP and cGMP across the plasma membrane. *Mrp4* (–/–) mice are sensitive to CFTR-mediated secretory diarrhea (Li et al., 2007), and exhibit an increase in inflammatory pain threshold. In addition, MRP4 is associated with proliferation of smooth muscle through modulation of cAMP/cGMP signaling (Sassi et al., 2008).

BCRP (–/–) mice are viable but highly sensitive to the dietary chlorophyll catabolite phenophorbide, which induces phototoxicity (Jonker et al., 2002). These mice also exhibit protoporphyria, with a 10-fold increase in protoporphyrin IX accumulation in erythrocytes, resulting in photosensitivity. This protoporphyria is caused by the impaired function of BCRP in bone marrow: knockout mice transplanted with bone marrow from wild-type mice become normal with respect to protoporphyrin IX level in the erythrocytes and photosensitivity.

BSEP has a narrower substrate specificity. It accepts bile acids (Gerloff et al., 1998) and its physiological role is to provide the osmotic driving force for bile flow by biliary excretion of bile acids in an ATP-dependent manner. Hereditary functional defect of this transporter results in the acquisition of progressive familial intrahepatic cholestasis (PFIC2), a fatal liver disease (Strautnieks et al., 1998). In addition, several drugs such as cyclosporin A inhibit the transport function of BSEP at clinically relevant concentrations, thereby causing the disruption of bile formation usually called drug-induced cholestasis (Stieger et al., 2000).

As described earlier, complete absence of these drug-related ABC transporters is not lethal and can remain unrecognized in the absence of exogenous perturbations due to food, drugs, or toxins. Thus, inhibition of physiologically important ABC transporters (especially those related directly to the genetic diseases described in Table 5–3) by drugs should be avoided to reduce the incidence of drug-induced side effects.

ABC Transporters in Drug Absorption and Elimination. With respect to clinical medicine, MDR1 is the most important ABC transporter yet identified, and digoxin is one of the most widely studied of its substrates. The systemic exposure to orally administered digoxin (as assessed by the area under the plasma digoxin concentration–time curve) is decreased by coadministration of rifampin (an MDR1 inducer) and is negatively correlated with the MDR1 protein expression in the human intestine. MDR1 is also expressed on the brush-border membrane of renal epithelia, and its function can be monitored using digoxin as a probe. Digoxin undergoes very little degradation in the liver, and renal excretion is the major elimination pathway (>70%) in humans. Several studies in healthy subjects have been performed with MDR1 inhibitors (e.g., quinidine, verapamil, vaspodar, spironolactone, clarythromycin, and ritonavir) with digoxin as a probe drug, and all resulted in a marked reduction in the renal excretion of digoxin.

The intestinal absorption of cyclosporine is also related mainly to the MDR1 level rather than to the CYP3A4 level, although cyclosporine is a substrate of both CYP3A4 and MDR1. Alteration of MDR1 activity by inhibitors (drug-drug interactions) affects oral absorption and renal clearance. Drugs with narrow therapeutic windows (such as the cardiac glycoside digoxin and the immunosuppressants cyclosporine and tacrolimus) should be used with great care if MDR1-based drug-drug interactions are likely.

Despite the broad substrate specificity and distinct localization of MRP2 and BCRP in drug-handling tissues (both are expressed on the canalicular membrane of hepatocytes and the brush-border membrane of enterocytes), there has been little integration of clinically relevant information. Part of the problem lies in distinguishing the biliary transport activities of MRP2 and BCRP from the contribution of the hepatic uptake transporters of the OATP family. Most MRP2 or BCRP substrates also can be transported by the OATP family transporters on the sinusoidal membrane. The rate-limiting process for systemic elimination is uptake in most cases. Under such conditions, the effect of drug-drug interactions (or genetic variants) in these biliary transporters may be difficult to identify. Despite such practical difficulties, there is a steady increase in the information about genetic variants and their effects on transporter expression and activity *in vitro*. Variants of BCRP with high allele frequencies (0.184 for V12M and 0.239 for Q141K) have been found to alter the protein expression in cellular assays. One variant is associated with greater oral availability of rosuvastatin and sulfasalazine following oral administration although the impact of the variant on the intestinal absorption and biliary excretion has not been separately evaluated (Yamasaki et al., 2008; Zhang et al., 2006c).

MRP3 is characterized by its localization in the plasma membrane of epithelial cells facing blood (basolateral membrane in the intestine epithelial cells, and sinusoidal membrane in the liver).

In the intestine, MRP3 can mediate the intestinal absorption in conjunction with uptake transporters. MRP3 mediates sinusoidal efflux in the liver, decreasing the efficacy of the biliary excretion from the blood, and excretion of intracellularly formed metabolites, particularly, glucuronide conjugates. Thus, dysfunction of MRP3 results in a shortening of the elimination half-life (Kitamura et al., 2008; Zelcer et al., 2005).

MRP4 substrates also can be transported by the OAT family transporters (OAT1 and OAT3) on the basolateral membrane of the epithelial cells in the kidney. MRP4 is involved in the directional transport in conjunction with OAT1 and/or OAT3 in the kidney (Hasegawa et al., 2007). The rate-limiting process in renal tubular secretion is likely the uptake process at the basolateral surface. Dysfunction of MRP4 enhances the renal concentration, but has limited impact on the blood concentration.

GENETIC VARIATION IN MEMBRANE TRANSPORTERS: IMPLICATIONS FOR CLINICAL DRUG RESPONSE

Inherited defects in membrane transport have been known for many years, and the genes associated with several inherited disorders of membrane transport have been identified [Tables 5–2 (SLC) and 5–3 (ABC)]. Reports of polymorphisms in membrane transporters that play a role in drug response have appeared only recently, but the field is growing rapidly. Cellular studies have focused on genetic variation in only a few drug transporters, but progress has been made in characterizing the functional impact of variants in these transporters, including characterization of the effects of single-nucleotide polymorphisms (SNPs) (Burman et al., 2004; Gray et al., 2004; Leabman et al., 2003; Osato et al., 2003; Shu et al., 2003; see also Chapter 7).

The clinical impact of membrane transporter variants on drug response has been studied only recently. Clinical studies have focused on a limited number of transporters, relating genetic variation in membrane transporters to drug disposition and response. For example, two common SNPs in *SLCO1B1* (OATP1B1) have been associated with elevated plasma levels of pravastatin, a widely used drug for the treatment of hypercholesterolemia (Mwinyi et al., 2004; Niemi et al., 2004) (see Chapter 31). Recent studies using genome-wide association methods have determined that genetic variants in SLCO1B1 (OATP1B1) predispose patients to risk for muscle toxicity associated with use of simvastatin (Search Collaborative Group, 2008). Other studies indicate that genetic variants in transporters in the SLC22A family associate with variation in renal clearance and response to various drugs including the anti-diabetic drug, metformin (Shu et al., 2007; Song et al., 2008; Wang et al., 2008). Further genetic variants in MRP2 and MRP4 have been associated with various drug related phenotypes (Han et al., 2007; Kiser et al., 2008; Naesens et al., 2006). Chapter 7 presents a more thorough discussion of the effects of genetic variation in membrane transporters on drug disposition and response.

TRANSPORTERS INVOLVED IN PHARMACOKINETICS

Drug transporters play a prominent role in pharmacokinetics (Figure 5–1). Transporters in the liver and kidney have important roles in removal of drugs from the blood and hence in metabolism and excretion.

Hepatic Transporters

Hepatic uptake of organic anions (e.g., drugs, leukotrienes, and bilirubin), cations, and bile salts is mediated by SLC-type transporters in the basolateral (sinusoidal) membrane of hepatocytes: OATPs (SLCO) (Abe et al., 1999; Konig et al., 2000) and OATs (SLC22) (Sekine et al., 1998), OCTs (SLC22) (Koepsell, 1998), and NTCP (SLC10A1) (Hagenbuch et al., 1991), respectively. These transporters mediate uptake by either facilitated or secondary active mechanisms.

ABC transporters such as MRP2, MDR1, BCRP, BSEP, and MDR2 in the bile canalicular membrane of hepatocytes mediate the efflux (excretion) of drugs and their metabolites, bile salts, and phospholipids against a steep concentration gradient from liver to bile. This primary active transport is driven by ATP hydrolysis. Moreover, SLC type transporter, MATE1 (SLC47A1), is also located on the canalicular membrane of hepatocytes. As a cation-proton antiporter, it works as an efflux transporter of organic cations, though its role in the biliary excretion of drugs has not been clearly demonstrated so far.

Some ABC transporters are also present in the basolateral membrane of hepatocytes and may play a role in the efflux of drugs back into the blood, although their physiological role remains to be elucidated. Drug uptake followed by metabolism and excretion in the liver is a major determinant of the systemic clearance of many drugs. Since clearance ultimately determines systemic blood levels, transporters in the liver play key roles in setting drug levels.

Vectorial transport of drugs from the circulating blood to the bile using an uptake transporter (OATP family) and an efflux transporter (MRP2) is important

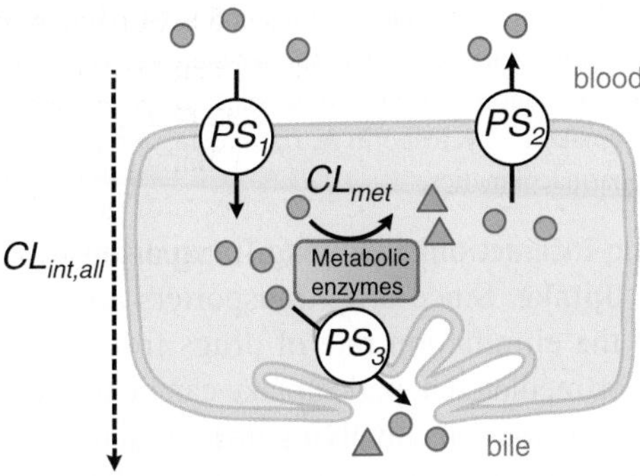

Figure 5–10. *Diagram showing hepatic uptake, backflux into blood, metabolism, and efflux into bile.* The red circles represent parent drugs; the green triangles represent drug metabolites. PS, permeability surface product; CL_{met}, metabolic clearance; CL_{int}, intrinsic clearance.

for determining drug exposure in the circulating blood and liver. Moreover, there are many other uptake and efflux transporters in the liver (Figures 5–10 and 5–11). The following examples illustrate the importance of vectorial transport in determining drug exposure in the circulating blood and liver.

HMG-CoA Reductase Inhibitors. Statins are cholesterol-lowering agents that reversibly inhibit HMG-CoA reductase, which catalyzes a rate-limiting step in cholesterol biosynthesis (see Chapter 31). Statins affect serum cholesterol by inhibiting cholesterol biosynthesis in the liver, and this organ is their main target. On the other hand, exposure of extrahepatic cells in smooth muscle to these drugs may cause adverse effects. Among the statins, pravastatin, fluvastatin, cerivastatin, atorvastatin, rosuvastatin, and pitavastatin are given in a biologically active open-acid form, whereas simvastatin and lovastatin are administered as inactive prodrugs with lactone rings. The open-acid statins are relatively hydrophilic and have low membrane permeabilities. However, most of the statins in the acid form are substrates of uptake transporters, so they are taken up efficiently by the liver and undergo enterohepatic circulation (Figures 5–5 and 5–11). In this process, hepatic uptake transporters such as OATP1B1 and efflux transporters such as MRP2 act cooperatively to produce vectorial trans-cellular transport of bisubstrates in the liver. The efficient first-pass hepatic uptake of these statins by OATP1B1 after their oral administration helps to exert the pharmacological effect and also minimizes the escape of drug molecules into the circulating blood, thereby minimizing the exposure in a target of adverse response, smooth muscle. Recent studies indicate that the genetic polymorphism of OATP1B1 also affects the function of this transporter (Tirona et al., 2001).

Temocapril. Temocapril is an ACE inhibitor (see Chapter 26). Its active metabolite, temocaprilat, is excreted both in the bile and in

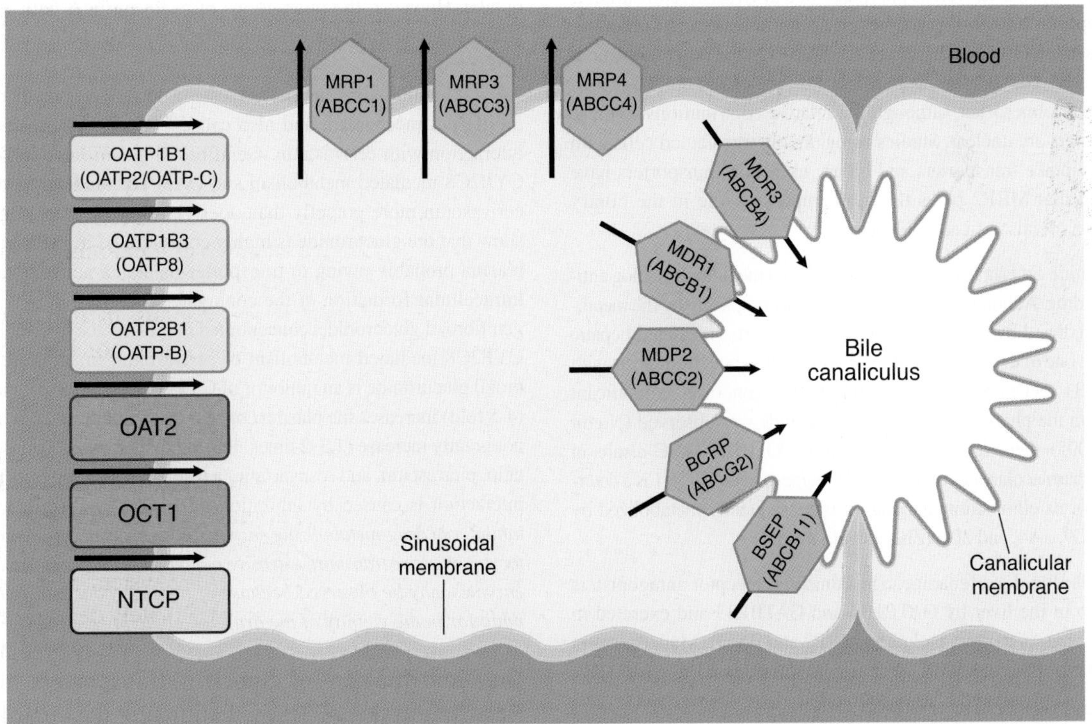

Figure 5–11. *Transporters in the hepatocyte that function in the uptake and efflux of drugs across the sinusoidal membrane and efflux of drugs into the bile across the canalicular membrane.* See text for details of the transporters pictured.

the urine by the liver and kidney, respectively, whereas other ACE inhibitors are excreted mainly by the kidney. The special feature of temocapril among ACE inhibitors is that the plasma concentration of temocaprilat remains relatively unchanged even in patients with renal failure. However, the plasma area under the curve (*AUC*) of enalaprilat and other ACE inhibitors is markedly increased in patients with renal disorders. Temocaprilat is a bisubstrate of the OATP family and MRP2, whereas other ACE inhibitors are not good substrates of MRP2 (although they are taken up into the liver by the OATP family). Taking these findings into consideration, the affinity for MRP2 may dominate in determining the biliary excretion of any series of ACE inhibitors. Drugs that are excreted into both the bile and urine to the same degree thus are expected to exhibit minimum inter-individual differences in their pharmacokinetics.

Irinotecan (CPT-11). Irinotecan hydrochloride (CPT-11) is a potent anticancer drug, but late-onset gastrointestinal toxic effects, such as severe diarrhea, make it difficult to use CPT-11 safely. After intravenous administration, CPT-11 is converted to SN-38, an active metabolite, by carboxylesterase. SN-38 is subsequently conjugated with glucuronic acid in the liver. SN-38 and SN-38 glucuronide are then excreted into the bile by MRP2. The inhibition of MRP2-mediated biliary excretion of SN-38 and its glucuronide by co-administration of probenecid reduces the drug-induced diarrhea, at least in rats. For additional details, see Figures 6–5 and 6–7.

Angiotensin II Receptor Antagonists. Angiotensin II receptor antagonists are used for the treatment of hypertension, acting on AT_1 receptors expressed in vascular smooth muscle, proximal tubule, and adrenal medullary cells, and elsewhere. For most of these drugs, hepatic uptake and biliary excretion are important factors for their pharmacokinetics as well as pharmacological effects. Telmisartan is taken up into human hepatocytes in a saturable manner, predominantly via OATP1B3 (Ishiguro et al., 2006). On the other hand, both OATPs 1B1 and 1B3 are responsible for the hepatic uptake of valsartan and olmesartan, although the relative contributions of these transporters are unclear. Studies using doubly transfected cells with hepatic uptake transporters and biliary excretion transporters have clarified that MRP2 plays the most important role in the biliary excretion of valsartan and olmesartan.

Repaglinide and Nateglinide. Repaglinide is a meglitinide analog antidiabetic drug. Although it is eliminated almost completely by the metabolism mediated by CYPs 2C8 and 3A4, transporter-mediated hepatic uptake is one of the determinants of its elimination rate. In subjects with SLCO1B1 (gene code for OATP1B1) 521CC genotype, a significant change in the pharmacokinetics of repaglinide was observed (Niemi et al., 2005). Genetic polymorphism in SLCO1B1 521T>C results in altered pharmacokinetics of nateglinide, suggesting OATP1B1 is a determinant of its elimination, although it is subsequently metabolized by CYPs 2C9, 3A4, and 2D6 (Zhang et al., 2006a).

Fexofenadine. Fexofenadine, a histamine H_1 receptor antagonist, is taken up in the liver by OATP1B1 and OATP1B3 and excreted in the bile via transporters including MRP2 and BSEP (Matsushima et al., 2008). Patients with genetic polymorphism in SLCO1B1 521T>C, show altered pharmacokinetics.

Bosentan. Bosentan is an endothelin antagonist used to treat pulmonary arterial hypertension. It is taken up in the liver by OATP1B1 and OATP1B3, and subsequently metabolized by CYP2C9 and CYP3A4 (Treiber et al., 2007). Transporter-mediated hepatic uptake can be a determinant of elimination of bosentan, and the inhibition of hepatic uptake by cyclosporin A, rifampicin, and sildenafil can affect its pharmacokinetics.

Drug-Drug Interactions Involving Transporter-Mediated Hepatic Uptake. Since drug transporters are determinants of the elimination rate of drugs from the body, transporter-mediated hepatic uptake can be the cause of drug-drug interactions involving drugs that are actively taken up into the liver and metabolized and/or excreted in the bile.

Cerivastatin (currently withdrawn), an HMG-CoA reductase inhibitor, is taken up into the liver via transporters (especially OATP1B1) and subsequently metabolized by CYPs 2C8 and 3A4. Its plasma concentration is increased 1-5 fold when co-administered with cyclosporin A. Transport studies using cryopreserved human hepatocytes and OATP1B1-expressing cells suggest that this drug-drug interaction is caused by inhibition of OATP1B1-mediated hepatic uptake (Shitara et al., 2003). However, cyclosporin A inhibits the metabolism of cerivastatin only to a limited extent, suggesting a low possibility of serious drug-drug interactions involving the inhibition of metabolism. Cyclosporin A also increases the plasma concentrations of other HMG-CoA reductase inhibitors. It markedly increases the plasma *AUC* of pravastatin, pitavastatin, and rosuvastatin, which are minimally metabolized and eliminated from the body by transporter-mediated mechanisms. Therefore, these pharmacokinetic interactions also may be due to transporter-mediated hepatic uptake. However, the interactions of cyclosporin A with pro-drug statins (lactone form) such as simvastatin and lovastatin are mediated by CYP3A4.

Gemfibrozil is another cholesterol-lowering agent that acts by a different mechanism and also causes a severe pharmacokinetic interaction with cerivastatin. Gemfibrozil glucuronide inhibits the CYP2C8-mediated metabolism and OATP1B1-mediated uptake of cerivastatin more potently than does gemfibrozil. Laboratory data show that the glucuronide is highly concentrated in the liver versus plasma probably owing to transporter-mediated active uptake and intracellular formation of the conjugate. Therefore, it may be that gemfibrozil glucuronide, concentrated in the hepatocytes, inhibits the CYP2C8-mediated metabolism of cerivastatin. In addition, gemfibrozil glucuronide is an inhibitor of CYP2C8. Gemfibrozil markedly (4-5 fold) increases the plasma concentration of cerivastatin but does not greatly increase (1.3-2 times) that of unmetabolized statins pravastatin, pitavastatin, and rosuvastatin, a result that also suggests that this interaction is caused by inhibition of metabolism. *Thus, when an inhibitor of drug-metabolizing enzymes is highly concentrated in hepatocytes by active transport, extensive inhibition of the drug-metabolizing enzymes may be observed because of the high concentration of the inhibitor in the vicinity of the drug-metabolizing enzymes.*

The Contribution of Specific Transporters to the Hepatic Uptake of Drugs. Estimating the contribution of transporters to the total hepatic uptake is necessary for understanding their importance in drug disposition.

This estimate can help to predict the extent to which a drug-drug interaction or a genetic polymorphism of a transporter may affect drug concentrations in plasma and liver. The contribution to hepatic uptake has been estimated successfully for CYP-mediated metabolism by using neutralizing antibody and specific chemical inhibitors. Unfortunately, specific inhibitors or antibodies for important transporters have not been identified yet, although some *relatively specific* inhibitors have been discovered.

The contribution of transporters to hepatic uptake can be estimated from *in vitro* studies. Injection of cRNA results in transporter expression on the plasma membrane of *Xenopus laevis* oocytes (Hagenbuch et al., 1996). Subsequent hybridization of the cRNA with its antisense oligonucleotide specifically reduces its expression. Comparison of the drug uptake into cRNA-injected oocytes in the presence and absence of antisense oligonucleotides clarifies the contribution of a specific transporter. Second, a method using reference compounds for specific transporters has been proposed. The reference compounds should be specific substrates for a particular transporter. The contribution of a specific transporter can be calculated from the uptake of test compounds and reference compounds into hepatocytes and transporter-expressing systems (Hirano et al., 2004):

$$\text{Contribution} = \frac{CL_{\text{hep,ref}} \,/\, CL_{\text{exp,ref}}}{CL_{\text{hep,test}} \,/\, CL_{\text{exp,test}}} \qquad \text{(Equation 5–13)}$$

where $CL_{\text{hep,ref}}$ and $CL_{\text{exp,ref}}$ represent the uptake of reference compounds into hepatocytes and transporter-expressing cells, respectively, and $CL_{\text{hep,test}}$ and $CL_{\text{exp,test}}$ represent the uptake of test compounds into the corresponding systems. For example, the contributions of OATP1B1 and OATP1B3 to the hepatic uptake of pitavastatin have been estimated using estrone-3-sulfate and cholecystokinine octapeptide (CCK8) as reference compounds for OATP1B1 and OATP1B3, respectively. However, for many transporters, reference compounds specific to the transporter are not available. Another approach to estimate the relative contribution of OATP1B1 and OATP1B3 is to use estrone-3-sulfate as a selective inhibitor for OATP1B1 (Ishiguro et al., 2006). The difference in uptake clearance of test compound in human hepatocytes in the absence and presence of estrone-3-sulfate represents OATP1B1-mediated hepatic uptake.

Renal Transporters

Secretion in the kidney of structurally diverse molecules including many drugs, environmental toxins, and carcinogens is critical in the body's defense against foreign substances. The specificity of secretory pathways in the nephron for two distinct classes of substrates, organic anions and cations, was first described decades ago, and these pathways were well characterized using a variety of physiological techniques including isolated perfused nephrons and kidneys, micro-puncture techniques, cell culture methods, and isolated renal plasma membrane vesicles. More recently, molecular studies have identified and characterized the renal transporters that play a role in drug elimination, toxicity, and response.

Although the pharmacological focus is often on the kidney, there is useful information on the tissue distribution of these transporters. Molecular studies using site-directed mutagenesis have identified substrate-recognition and other functional domains of the transporters, and genetic studies of knockout mouse models have been used to characterize the physiological roles of individual transporters. Recently, studies have identified and functionally analyzed genetic polymorphisms and haplotypes of the relevant transporters in humans. In some cases, transporters that are considered organic anion or organic cation transporters have dual specificity for anions and cations. The following section summarizes recent work on transporters in humans and other mammals. For more detail, refer to recent reviews of renal organic cation and anion transport (Ciarimboli, 2008; El-Sheikh et al., 2008; Koepsell et al., 2007; Srimaroeng et al., 2008; Wright and Dantzler, 2004).

Organic Cation Transport. Structurally diverse organic cations are secreted in the proximal tubule (Ciarimboli, 2008; Koepsell et al., 2007; Wright and Dantzler, 2004). Many secreted organic cations are endogenous compounds (e.g., choline, *N*-methylnicotinamide, and dopamine), and renal secretion appears to be important in eliminating excess concentrations of these substances. However, a primary function of organic cation secretion is ridding the body of xenobiotics, including many positively charged drugs and their metabolites (e.g., cimetidine, ranitidine, metformin, procainamide, and *N*-acetylprocainamide) and toxins from the environment (e.g., nicotine). Organic cations that are secreted by the kidney may be either hydrophobic or hydrophilic. Hydrophilic organic drug cations generally have molecular weights < 400 daltons; a current model for their secretion in the proximal tubule of the nephron is shown in Figure 5–12.

For the transepithelial flux of a compound (e.g., secretion), the compound must traverse two membranes sequentially, the basolateral membrane facing the blood side and the apical membrane facing the tubular lumen. Distinct transporters on each membrane mediate each step of transport. Organic cations appear to cross the basolateral membrane in human proximal tubule by two distinct transporters in the SLC family 22 (SCL22):

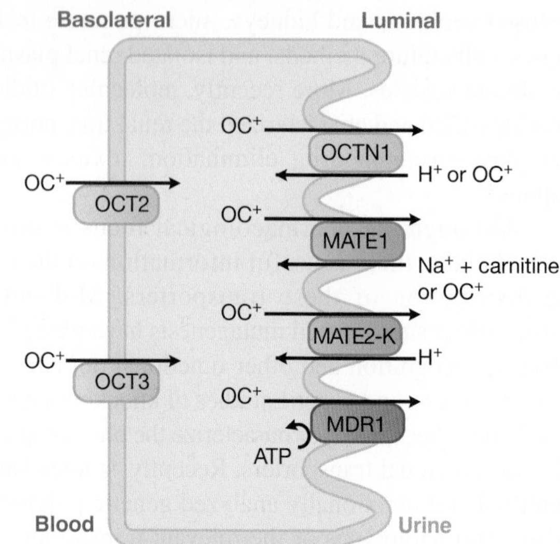

Figure 5–12. *Model of organic cation secretory transporters in the proximal tubule.* OC^+, organic cation.

OCT2 (*SLC22A2*) and OCT3 (*SLC22A3*). Organic cations are transported across this membrane down an electrochemical gradient. Previous studies in isolated basolateral membrane vesicles demonstrate the presence of a potential-sensitive mechanism for organic cations. The cloned transporters OCT2 and OCT3 are potential sensitive and mechanistically coincide with previous studies of isolated basolateral membrane vesicles.

Transport of organic cations from cell to tubular lumen across the apical membrane occurs *via* an electroneutral proton–organic cation exchange mechanism in a variety of species, including human, dog, rabbit, and cat. The recent discovery of a new transporter family, SLC47A, *m*ultidrug *a*nd *t*oxin *e*xtrusion family (MATEs), has provided the molecular identities of the previously characterized electroneutral proton–organic cation antiport mechanism (Otsuka et al., 2005; Tanihara et al., 2007). Transporters in the MATE family, assigned to the apical membrane of the proximal tubule, appear to play a key role in moving hydrophilic organic cations from tubule cell to lumen. In addition, *novel organic cation transporters* (OCTNs), located on the apical membrane, appear to contribute to organic cation flux across the proximal tubule. In humans, these include OCTN1 (*SLC22A4*) and OCTN2 (*SLC22A5*). These bifunctional transporters are involved not only in organic cation secretion but also in carnitine reabsorption. In the reuptake mode, the transporters function as Na^+ co-transporters, relying on the inwardly driven Na^+ gradient created by Na^+,K^+-ATPase to move carnitine from tubular lumen to cell. In the secretory mode, the transporters appear to function as proton–organic cation exchangers. That is, protons move from tubular lumen to cell interior in exchange for organic cations, which move from cytosol to tubular lumen. The inwardly directed proton gradient (from tubular lumen to cytosol) is maintained by transporters in the SLC9 family, which are Na^+/H^+ exchangers (NHEs, antiporters). Of the two steps involved in secretory transport, transport across the luminal membrane appears to be rate-limiting.

OCT2 (*SLC22A2*). OCT2 (SLC22A2) was first cloned from a rat kidney cDNA library in 1996 (Okuda et al., 1996). Human, rabbit, mouse, and pig orthologs all have been cloned. Mammalian orthologs range in length from 553 through 555 amino acids. OCT2 is predicted to have 12 transmembrane domains, including one *N*-linked glycosylation site. OCT2 is located adjacent to OCT1 on chromosome 6 (6q26). A single splice variant of human OCT2, termed *OCT2-A*, has been identified in human kidney. OCT2-A, which is a truncated form of OCT2, appears to have a lower K_m (or greater affinity) for substrates than OCT2, although a lower affinity has been observed for some inhibitors (Urakami et al., 2002). Human, mouse, and rat orthologs of OCT2 are expressed in abundance in human kidney and to some extent in neuronal tissue such as choroid plexus. In the kidney, OCT2 is localized to the proximal tubule and to distal tubules and collecting ducts. In the proximal tubule, OCT2 is restricted to the basolateral membrane. OCT2 mammalian species orthologs are > 80% identical, whereas the OCT2 paralog found primarily in the liver, OCT1, is ~70% identical to OCT2. OCT2-mediated transport of model organic cations MPP^+ and TEA is electrogenic, and both OCT2 and OCT1 can support organic cation–organic cation exchange (Koepsell et al., 2007). OCT2 generally accepts a wide array of monovalent organic cations with molecular weights < 400 daltons (Ciarimboli, 2008; Koepsell et al., 2007). The apparent affinities of the human paralogs, OCT1 and OCT2, for some organic cation substrates and inhibitors are different in side-by-side comparison studies. Isoform-specific inhibitors of the OCTs are needed to determine the relative importance of OCT2 and OCT1 in the renal clearance of compounds in rodents, in which both isoforms are present in kidney. OCT2 is also present in neuronal tissues; however, monoamine neurotransmitters have low affinities for OCT2. OCT2 may play a housekeeping role in neurons, taking up only excess concentrations of neurotransmitters. OCT2 also may be involved in recycling of neurotransmitters by taking up breakdown products, which in turn enter monoamine synthetic pathways.

OCT3 (*SLC22A3*). OCT3 (SLC22A3) was cloned initially from rat placenta (Kekuda et al., 1998). Human and mouse orthologs have also been cloned. OCT3 consists of 551 amino acids and is predicted to have 12 transmembrane domains, including three *N*-linked glycosylation sites. hOCT3 is located in tandem with OCT1 and OCT2 on chromosome 6. Tissue distribution studies suggest that human OCT3 is expressed in liver, kidney, intestine, and placenta, although it appears to be expressed in considerably less abundance than OCT2 in the kidney. Like OCT1 and OCT2, OCT3 appears to support electrogenic potential-sensitive organic cation transport. Although the specificity of OCT3 is similar to that of OCT1 and OCT2, it appears to have quantitative differences in its affinities for many organic cations. Some studies have suggested that OCT3 is the extraneuronal monoamine transporter based on its substrate specificity and potency of interaction with monoamine neurotransmitters. Because of its relatively low abundance in the kidney (in the basolateral membrane of the proximal tubule (Koepsell et al., 2007)), OCT3 may play only a limited role in renal drug elimination.

OCTN1 (*SLC22A4*). OCTN1, cloned originally from human fetal liver, is expressed in the adult kidney, trachea, and bone marrow (Tamai et al., 1997). The functional characteristics of OCTN1 suggest that it operates as an organic cation–proton exchanger. OCTN1-mediated influx of model organic cations is enhanced at alkaline pH, whereas efflux is increased by an inwardly directed proton gradient. OCTN1 contains a nucleotide-binding sequence motif, and transport of its substrates appears to be stimulated by cellular ATP. OCTN1 also can function as an organic cation–organic cation exchanger. Although the subcellular localization of OCTN1 has not been demonstrated clearly, available data collectively suggest that OCTN1 functions as a bidirectional pH- and ATP-dependent transporter at the apical membrane in renal tubular epithelial cells. OCTN1 appears to transport the anti-epileptic agent, gabapentin, in the kidney (Urban et al., 2007).

OCTN2 (*SLC22A5*). OCTN2 was first cloned from human kidney and determined to be the transporter responsible for systemic carnitine deficiency (Tamai et al., 1998). Rat OCTN2 mRNA is expressed predominantly in the cortex, with very little expression in the medulla, and is localized to the apical membrane of the proximal tubule.

OCTN2 is a bifunctional transporter, i.e., it transports *L*-carnitine with high affinity in an Na^+-dependent manner, whereas, Na^+ does not influence OCTN2-mediated transport of organic cations such as TEA. Thus, OCTN2 is thought to function as both an Na^+-dependent carnitine transporter and an Na^+-independent organic cation transporter. Similar to OCTN1, OCTN2 transport of organic cations is sensitive to pH, suggesting that OCTN2 may function as an organic cation exchanger. The transport of *L*-carnitine by OCTN2 is a Na^+-dependent electrogenic process, and mutations in OCTN2 appear to be the cause of primary systemic carnitine deficiency (Nezu et al., 1999).

MATE1 and MATE2-K (*SLC47A1* and *SLC47A2*). Database searches for human orthologs of bacterial multidrug resistance transporters have identified two genes in the human genome that code for membrane transporters (Otsuka et al., 2005). Multidrug and toxin extrusion family members MATE1 (*SLC47A1*) and MATE2-K (*SLC47A2*) interact with structurally diverse hydrophilic organic cations including the anti-diabetic drug metformin, the H_2 antagonist cimetidine, and the anticancer drug, topotecan (Tanihara et al., 2007). In addition to cationic compounds, the transporters also recognize some anions, including the antiviral agents acyclovir and ganciclovir. The zwitterions cephalexin and cephradine are specific substrates of MATE1, but not MATE2-K. The herbicide paraquat, a bisquaternary ammonium compound, which is nephrotoxic in humans, is a potent substrate of MATE1 (Chen et al., 2007). Both MATE1 and MATE2-K have been localized to the apical membrane of the proximal tubule (Tanihara et al., 2007). MATE1, but not MATE2-K, is also expressed on the canalicular membrane of the hepatocyte. These transporters appear to be the long-searched-for organic cation proton antiporters on the apical membrane of the proximal tubule, i.e., an oppositely directed proton gradient can drive the movement of organic cations via MATE1 or MATE2-K. The antibiotics, levofloxacin and ciprofloxacin, though potent inhibitors, are not translocated by either MATE1 or MATE2-K.

Polymorphisms of OCTs. Polymorphisms of OCTs have been identified in large post–human genome SNP discovery projects (Kerb et al., 2002; Leabman et al., 2003; Shu et al., 2003). OCT1 exhibits the greatest number of amino acid polymorphisms, followed by OCT2 and then OCT3. Furthermore, allele frequencies of OCT1 amino acid variants in human populations generally are greater than those of OCT2 and OCT3 amino acid variants. Functional studies of OCT1 and OCT2 polymorphisms have been performed. OCT1 exhibits five variants with reduced function. These variants may have important implications clinically in terms of hepatic drug disposition and targeting of OCT1 substrates. In particular, individuals with OCT1 variants may have reduced liver uptake of OCT1 substrates and therefore reduced metabolism. Recent studies suggest that genetic variants of OCT1 and OCT2 are associated with alterations in the renal elimination and response to the anti-diabetic drug, metformin (Shu et al., 2007; Song et al., 2008; Wang et al., 2008).

Organic Anion Transport. Myriad structurally diverse organic anions are secreted in the proximal tubule (Burckhardt and Burckhardt, 2003; El-Sheikh et al, 2008; Srimaroeng et al., 2008; Wright and Dantzler, 2004). As with organic cation transport, the primary function of organic anion secretion appears to be the removal from the body of xenobiotics, including many weakly acidic drugs [e.g., pravastatin, captopril, *p*-aminohippurate (PAH), and penicillins] and toxins (e.g., ochratoxin). Organic anion transporters move both hydrophobic and hydrophilic anions but also may interact with cations and neutral compounds.

A current model for the transepithelial flux of organic anions in the proximal tubule is shown in Figure 5–13. Two primary transporters on the basolateral membrane mediate the flux of organic anions from interstitial fluid to tubule cell: OAT1 (*SLC22A6*) and OAT3 (*SLC22A8*). Energetically, hydrophilic organic anions are

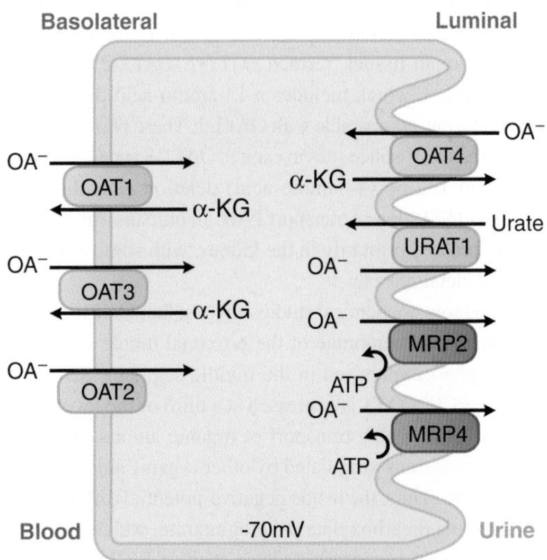

Figure 5–13. *Model of organic anion secretory transporters in the proximal tubule.* OA, organic anion; α-KG, α-ketoglutarate.

transported across the basolateral membrane against an electrochemical gradient in exchange with intracellular α-ketoglutarate, which moves down its concentration gradient from cytosol to blood. The outwardly directed gradient of α-ketoglutarate is maintained at least in part by a basolateral Na^+-dicarboxylate transporter (NaDC3). The Na^+ gradient that drives NaDC3 is maintained by Na^+,K^+-ATPase. Transport of small-molecular-weight organic anions by the cloned transporters OAT1 and OAT3 can be driven by α-ketoglutarate; coupled transport of α-ketoglutarate and small-molecular-weight organic anions (e.g., *p*-aminohippurate) occurs in isolated basolateral membrane vesicles. The molecular pharmacology and molecular biology of OATs have recently been reviewed (El-Sheikh et al., 2008; Srimaroeng et al., 2008).

The mechanism responsible for the apical membrane transport of organic anions from tubule cell cytosol to tubular lumen remains controversial. Some studies suggest that OAT4 may serve as the luminal membrane transporter for organic anions. However, recent studies show that the movement of substrates *via* this transporter can be driven by exchange with α-ketoglutarate, suggesting that OAT4 may function in the reabsorptive, rather than secretory, flux of organic anions. Other studies have suggested that in the pig kidney, OATV1 serves as an electrogenic facilitated transporter on the apical membrane (Jutabha et al., 2003). The human ortholog of OATV1 is NPT1, or NaPi-1, originally cloned as a phosphate transporter. NPT1 can support the low-affinity transport of hydrophilic organic anions such as PAH. Other transporters that may play a role in transport across the apical membrane include MRP2 and MRP4, multidrug-resistance transporters in the ATP binding cassette family C (ABCC). Both transporters interact with some organic anions and may actively pump their substrates from tubule cell cytosol to tubular lumen.

OAT1 (*SLC22A6*). OAT1 was cloned from rat kidney (Sekine et al., 1997; Sweet et al., 1997). This transporter is > 30% identical to OCTs in the SLC22 family. Mouse, human, pig, and rabbit orthologs have been cloned and are ~80% identical to human OAT1. Mammalian isoforms of OAT1 vary in length from 545-551 amino acids. The gene for the human OAT1 is mapped to chromosome 11 and is found in an SLC22 cluster that includes OAT3 and OAT4. There are four splice variants in human tissues, termed *OAT1-1, OAT1-2, OAT1-3*, and *OAT1-4*. OAT1-2, which includes a 13-amino-acid deletion, transports PAH at a rate comparable with OAT1-1. These two splice variants use the alternative 5′-splice sites in exon 9. OAT1-3 and OAT1-4, which result from a 132-bp (44-amino-acid) deletion near the carboxyl terminus of OAT1, do not transport PAH. In humans, rat, and mouse, OAT1 is expressed primarily in the kidney, with some expression in brain and skeletal muscle.

Immunohistochemical studies suggest that OAT1 is expressed on the basolateral membrane of the proximal tubule in human and rat, with highest expression in the middle segment, S2. Based on quantitative PCR, OAT1 is expressed at a third of the level of OAT3. OAT1 exhibits saturable transport of organic anions such as PAH. This transport is trans-stimulated by other organic anions, including α-ketoglutarate. Thus, the inside negative-potential difference drives the efflux of the dicarboxylate α-ketoglutarate, which, in turn, supports the influx of monocarboxylates such as PAH. Regulation of expression levels of OAT1 in the kidney appears to be controlled by sex steroids.

OAT1 generally transports small-molecular-weight organic anions that may be endogenous (e.g., PGE_2 and urate) or ingested drugs and toxins. Some neutral compounds are also transported by OAT1 at a lower affinity (e.g., cimetidine). Key residues that contribute to transport by OAT1 include the conserved K394 and R478, which are involved in the PAH–glutarate exchange mechanism.

OAT2 (*SLC22A7*). OAT2 was cloned first from rat liver (and named NLT at the time) (Sekine et al., 1998; Simonson et al., 1994). OAT2 is present in both kidney and liver. In the kidney, the transporter is localized to the basolateral membrane of the proximal tubule, and appears to function as a transporter for nucleotides, particularly guanine nucleotides such as cyclic GMP (Cropp et al., 2008). Cellular studies suggest that OAT2 functions in both the influx and efflux of guanine nucleotides. Organic anions such as PAH and methotrexate are also transported with low affinity by OAT2, which transports PGE_2 with a high affinity.

OAT3 (*SLC22A8*). OAT3 (*SLC22A8*) was cloned originally from rat kidney (Kusuhara et al., 1999). Human OAT3 consists of two variants, one of which transports a wide variety of organic anions, including model compounds, PAH and estrone sulfate, as well as many drug products (e.g., pravastatin, cimetidine, 6-mercaptopurine, and methotrexate) (Srimaroeng et al., 2008). The longer OAT3 in humans, a 568-amino-acid protein, does not support transport. It is likely that the two OAT3 variants are splice variants. Human OAT3 is confined to the basolateral membrane of the proximal tubule.

OAT3 clearly has overlapping specificities with OAT1, although kinetic parameters differ. For example, estrone sulfate is transported by both OAT1 and OAT3, but OAT3 has a much higher affinity in comparison with OAT1. The weak base cimetidine (an H_2 receptor antagonist) is transported with high affinity by OAT1, whereas the cation TEA is not transported.

OAT4 (*SLC22A9*). OAT4 (SLC22A9) was cloned from a human kidney cDNA library (Cha et al., 2000). OAT4 is expressed in human kidney and placenta; in human kidney, OAT4 is present on the luminal membrane of the proximal tubule. At first, OAT4 was thought to be involved in the second step of secretion of organic anions, i.e., transport across the apical membrane from cell to tubular lumen. However, studies demonstrate that organic anion transport by OAT4 can be stimulated by transgradients of α-ketoglutarate (Ekaratanawong et al., 2004), suggesting that OAT4 may be involved in the reabsorption of organic anions from tubular lumen into cell. The specificity of OAT4 includes the model compounds estrone sulfate and PAH, as well as zidovudine, tetracycline, and methotrexate (El-Sheikh et al., 2008; Srimaroeng et al., 2008). Interestingly, the affinity for PAH is low (>1 mM). Collectively, emerging studies suggest that OAT4 may be involved not in secretory flux of organic anions but in reabsorption instead.

Other Anion Transporters. URAT1 (*SLC22A12*), first cloned from human kidney, is a kidney-specific transporter confined to the apical membrane of the proximal tubule (Enomoto et al., 2002). Data suggest that URAT1 is primarily responsible for urate reabsorption, mediating electroneutral urate transport that can be trans-stimulated by Cl^- gradients. The mouse ortholog of URAT1 is involved in the renal secretory flux of organic anions including benzylpenicillin and urate.

NPT1 (*SLC17A1*), cloned originally as a phosphate transporter in humans, is expressed in abundance on the luminal membrane of the proximal tubule as well as in the brain (Werner et al., 1991). NPT1 transports PAH, probenecid, and penicillin G. It appears to be part of the system involved in organic anion efflux from tubule cell to lumen.

MRP2 (*ABCC2*), an ABC transporter, initially called the *GS-X pump* (El-Sheikh et al., 2008; Ishikawa et al., 1990; Toyoda et al., 2008), has been considered to be the primary transporter involved in efflux of many drug conjugates such as glutathione conjugates across the canalicular membrane of the hepatocyte. However, MRP2 is also found on the apical membrane of the proximal tubule, where it is thought to play a role in the efflux of organic anions into the tubular lumen. Its role in the kidney may be to secrete glutathione conjugates of drugs, but it also may support the translocation (with glutathione) of various non-conjugated substrates. In general, MRP2 transports larger, bulkier compounds than do most of the organic anion transporters in the SLC22 family.

MRP4 (*ABCC4*) is found on the apical membrane of the proximal tubule and transports a wide array of conjugated anions, including glucuronide and glutathione conjugates (El-Sheikh et al., 2008; Toyoda et al., 2008). However, unlike MRP2, MRP4 appears to interact with various drugs, including methotrexate, cyclic nucleotide analogs, and antiviral nucleoside analogs. Recent studies in *Mrp4* knockout mice suggest that the transporter is involved in the renal elimination of the antiviral drugs adefovir and tenofovir (Imaoka et al., 2006). Other MRP efflux transporters also have been identified in human kidney, including MRP3 and MRP6, both on the basolateral membrane. Their roles in the kidney are not yet known.

Polymorphisms of OATs. Polymorphisms in OAT1 and OAT3 have been identified in ethnically diverse human populations (Leabman et al., 2003; Srimaroeng et al., 2008). Two amino acid polymorphisms (allele frequencies >1%) in OAT1 have been identified in African-American populations. Three amino acid polymorphisms and seven rare amino acid variants in OAT3 have been identified in ethnically diverse U.S. populations (see www.pharmgkb.org).

TRANSPORTERS INVOLVED IN PHARMACODYNAMICS: DRUG ACTION IN THE BRAIN

Neurotransmitters are packaged in vesicles in presynpatic neurons, released in the synapse by fusion of the vesicles with the plasma membrane, and, excepting acetylcholine, are then taken back into the presynaptic neurons or postsynaptic cells (see Chapter 8). Transporters involved in the neuronal reuptake of the neurotransmitters and the regulation of their levels in the synaptic cleft belong to two major superfamilies, SLC1 and SLC6. Transporters in both families play roles in reuptake of γ-aminobutyric acid (GABA), glutamate, and the monoamine neurotransmitters norepinephrine, serotonin, and dopamine. These transporters may serve as pharmacologic targets for neuropsychiatric drugs (Gether et al., 2006; Hog et al., 2006; Schousboe et al., 2004).

SLC6 family members localized in the brain and involved in the reuptake of neurotransmitters into presynaptic neurons include the norepinephrine transporters (NET, *SLC6A2*), the dopamine transporter (DAT, *SLC6A3*), the serotonin transporter (SERT, *SLC6A4*), and several GABA reuptake transporters (GAT1, GAT2, and GAT3) (Chen et al., 2004; Elliott and Beveridge, 2005; Hediger, 2004). Each of these transporters appears to have 12 transmembrane secondary structures and a large extracellular loop with glycosylation sites between transmembrane domains 3 and 4. These proteins are typically ~ 600 amino acids in length. SLC6 family members depend on the Na^+ gradient to actively transport their substrates into cells. Cl^- is also required, although to a variable extent depending on the family member. Residues and domains that form the substrate recognition and permeation pathways are currently being identified.

Through reuptake mechanisms, the neurotransmitter transporters in the SLC6A family regulate the concentrations and dwell times of neurotransmitters in the synaptic cleft; the extent of transmitter uptake also influences subsequent vesicular storage of transmitters. Many of these transporters are present in other tissues (e.g., kidney and platelets) and may serve other roles. Further, the transporters can function in the reverse direction. That is, the transporters can export neurotransmitters in an Na^+-independent fashion. The characteristics of each member of the SLC6A family of transporters that play a role in reuptake of monoamine neurotransmitters and GABA merit a brief description.

SLC6A1 **(GAT1),** ***SLC6A11*** **(GAT3), and** ***SLC6A13*** **(GAT2).** GAT1 (599 amino acids) is the most important GABA transporter in the brain, expressed in GABAergic neurons and found largely on presynaptic neurons (Høg et al., 2006; Schousboe et al., 2004). GAT1 is found in abundance in the neocortex, cerebellum, basal ganglia, brainstem, spinal cord, retina, and olfactory bulb. GAT3 is found only in the brain, largely in glial cells. GAT2 is found in peripheral tissues, including the kidney and liver, and within the CNS in the choroid plexus and meninges.

GAT1, GAT2, and GAT3 are ~50% identical in amino acid sequence. Functional analysis indicates that GAT1 transports GABA with a 2:1 Na^+:$GABA^-$ stoichiometry. Cl^- is required. Residues and domains responsible for the recognition of GABA and subsequent translocation have been identified. Physiologically, GAT1 appears to be responsible for regulating the interaction of GABA at receptors. The presence of GAT2 in the choroid plexus and its absence in presynaptic neurons suggest that this transporter may play a primary role in maintaining the homeostasis of GABA in the CSF. GAT1 and GAT3 are drug targets (Schousboe et al., 2004). GAT1 is the target of the anti-epileptic drug tiagabine, which presumably acts to

Hasegawa M, Kusuhara H, Adachi M, et al. Multidrug resistance-associated protein 4 is involved in the urinary excretion of hydrochlorothiazide and furosemide. *J Am Soc Nephrol*, **2007,** *18*:37–45.

Hediger MA (ed.). In, Special Issue: The ABCs of solute carriers: Physiological, pathological and therapeutic implications of human membrane transport proteins. *Pflügers Arch*, **2004**, *447*:465–468.

Hediger MA, Coady MJ, Ikeda TS, Wright EM. Expression cloning and cDNA sequencing of the Na^+/glucose co-transporter. *Nature*, **1987,** *330*:379–381.

Hirano M, Maeda K, Shitara Y, Sugiyama Y. Contribution of OATP2 (OATP1B1) and OATP8 (OATP1B3) to the hepatic uptake of pitavastatin in humans. *J Pharmacol Exp Ther*, **2004,** *311*:139–146.

Ho ES, Lin DC, Mendel DB, Cihlar T. Cytotoxicity of antiviral nucleotides adefovir and cidofovir is induced by the expression of human renal organic anion transporter 1. *J Am Soc Nephrol*, **2000**, *11*:383–393.

Hog S, Greenwood JR, Madsen KB, et al. Structure-activity relationships of selective GABA uptake inhibitors. *Curr Top Med Chem,* **2006**, *6*:1861–1882.

Hollenstein K, Dawson R, Locher K. Strucutre and mechanism of ABC transporter proteins. *Curr Opin Structural Biol*, **2007**, *17*:412–418.

Horio M, Pastan I, Gottesman MM, Handler JS. Transepithelial transport of vinblastine by kidney-derived cell lines: Application of a new kinetic model to estimate in situ K_m of the pump. *Biochem Biophys Acta*, **1990,** *1027*:116–122.

Imai S, Kikuchi R, Kusuhara H, et al. Analysis of DNA methylation and histone modification profiles of liver-specific transporters. *Mol Pharmacol*, **2009**, *75*:568–576.

Imaoka T, Kusuhara H, Adachi M, et al. Functional involvement of multidrug resistance-associated protein 4 (MRP4/ABCC4) in the renal elimination of the antiviral drugs adefovir and tenofovir. *Mol Pharmacol*, **2006**, *71*:619–627.

Ishiguro N, Maeda K, Kishimoto W, et al. Predominant contribution of OATP1B3 to the hepatic uptake of telmisartan, an angiotensin II receptor antagonist, in humans. *Drug Metab Dispos*, **2006,** *34*:1109–1115.

Ishiguro, N, Maeda, K, Saito, A, et al., Establishment of a set of double transfectants coexpressing organic anion transporting polypeptide 1B3 and hepatic efflux transporters for the characterization of the hepatobiliary transport of telmisartan acylglucuronide. *Drug Metab Dispos*, **2008,** *36*:796–805.

Ishikawa T, Muller M, Klunemann C, et al. ATP-dependent primary active transport of cysteinyl leukotrienes across liver canalicular membrane: Role of the ATP-dependent transport system for glutathione *S*-conjugates. *J Biol Chem*, **1990,** *265*:19279–19286.

Ito K, Suzuki H. Hirohashi T, et al. Molecular cloning of canalicular multispecific organic anion transporter defective in EHBR. *Am J Physiol*, **1997,** *272*:G16–G22.

Jonker JW, Buitelaar M, Wagenaar E, et al. The breast cancer resistance protein protects against a major chlorophyll-derived dietary phototoxin and protoporphyria. *Proc Natl Acad Sci USA*, **2002,** *99*:15649–15654.

Juliano RL, Ling V. A surface glycoprotein modulating drug permeability in Chinese hamster ovary cell mutants. *Biochem Biophys Acta*, **1976,** *455*:152–162.

Jutabha P, Kanai Y, Hosoyamada M, et al. Identification of a novel voltage-driven organic anion transporter present at apical membrane of renal proximal tubule. *J Biol Chem*, **2003,** *278*:27930–27938.

Kanner B. It's not all in the family. *Nature*, **2008**, *454*:593–594.

Karpowich N, Wang D. Symmetric transporters for asymmetric transport. *Science*, **2008**, *321*:781–782.

Kekuda R, Prasad PD, Wu X, et al. Cloning and functional characterization of a potential-sensitive polyspecific organic cation transporter (OCT3) most abundantly expressed in placenta. *J Biol Chem*, **1998,** *273*:15971–15979.

Kerb R, Brinkmann U, Chatskaia N, et al. Identification of genetic variations of the human organic cation transporter hOCT1 and their functional consequences. *Pharmacogenetics*, **2002,** *12*:591–595.

Kidambi S, Patel S. Cholesterol and non-cholesterol sterol transporters: ABCG5, ABCG8 and NPC1L1: A review. *Xenobiotica*, **2008**, *38*:1119–1139.

Kikuchi R, Kusuhara H, Abe T, et al. Involvement of multiple transporters in the efflux of 3-hydroxy-3-methylglutaryl-CoA reductase inhibitors across the blood–brain barrier. *J Pharmacol Exp Ther*, **2004,** *311*:1147–1153.

Kikuchi R, Kusuhara H, Hattori N, et al. Regulation of the expression of human organic anion transporter 3 by hepatocyte nuclear factor 1α/beta and DNA methylation. *Mol Pharmacol*, **2006,** *70*:887–896.

Kiser J, Aquilante C, Anderson P, et al. Clinical and genetic determinants of intracellular tenofovir diphosphate concentrations in HIV-infected patients. *J Acquir Immune Defic Syndr*, **2008**, *47*:298–303.

Kitamura Y, Hirouchi M, Kusuhara H, et al. Increasing systemic exposure of methotrexate by active efflux mediated by multidrug resistance-associated protein 3 (MRP3/ABCC3). *J Pharmacol Exp Ther*, **2008,** *327*:465–473.

Koepsell H. Organic cation transporters in intestine, kidney, liver, and brain. *Annu Rev Physiol*, **1998,** *60*:243–266.

Koepsell H, Lips K, Volk C. Polyspecific organic cation transporters: Structure, function, physiological roles, and biopharmaceutical implications. *Pharm Res*, **2007**, *24*:1227–1251.

Konig J, Cui Y, Nies AT, Keppler D. Localization and genomic organization of a new hepatocellular organic anion transporting polypeptide. *J Biol Chem*, **2000,** *275*:23161–23168.

Kopplow K, Letschert K, Konig J, et al. Human hepatobiliary transport of organic anions analyzed by quadruple-transfected cells. *Mol Pharmacol*, **2005,** *68*:1031–1038.

Krishnamurthy P, Schwab M, Takenaka K, et al. Transporter-mediated protection against thiopurine-induced hematopoietic toxicity. *Cancer Res*, **2008,** *68*:4983–4989.

Kullak-Ublick GA, Stieger B, Meier PJ. Enterohepatic bile salt transporters in normal physiology and liver disease. *Gastroenterology*, **2004,** *126*:322–342.

Kusuhara H, Sekine T, Utsunomiya-Tate N, et al. Molecular cloning and characterization of a new multispecific organic anion transporter from rat brain. *J Biol Chem*, **1999,** *274*:13675–13680.

Leabman MK, Huang CC, DeYoung J, et al. Natural variation in human membrane transporter genes reveals evolutionary and functional constraints. *Proc Natl Acad Sci USA*, **2003,** *100*:5896–5901.

Leggas M, Adachi M, Scheffer GL, et al. MRP4 confers resistance to topotecan and protects the brain from chemotherapy. *Mol Cell Biol*, **2004,** *24*:7612–7621.

Lesch KP, Bengel D, Heils A, et al. Association of anxiety-related traits with a polymorphism in the serotonin transporter gene regulatory region. *Science*, **1996,** *274*:1527–1531.

Leslie E, Deeley R, Cole S. Multidrug resistance proteins: role of P-glycoprotein, MRP1, MRP2 and BCRP (ABCG2) in tissue defense. *Toxicol Appl Pharmacol*, **2005,** *204*:216–237.

Li C, Krishnamurthy PC, Penmatsa H, et al. Spatiotemporal coupling of cAMP transporter to CFTR chloride channel function in the gut epithelia. *Cell*, **2007**, *131*:940–951.

Lin JH, Yamazaki M. Clinical relevance of P-glycoprotein in drug therapy. *Drug Metab Rev*, **2003,** *35*:417–454.

Locher KP, Lee AT, Rees DC. The E.coli BtuCD structure: A framework for ABC transporter architecture and mechanism. *Science*, **2002**, *296*:1091–1098.

Matsushima S, Maeda K, Ishiguro N, et al. Investigation of the inhibitory effects of various drugs on the hepatic uptake of fexofenadine in humans. *Drug Metab Dispos*, **2008**, *36*:663–669.

Matsushima S, Maeda K, Kondo C, et al. Identification of the hepatic efflux transporters of organic anions using double-transfected Madin-Darby canine kidney II cells expressing human organic anion-transporting polypeptide 1B1 (OATP1B1)/ multidrug resistance-associated protein 2, OATP1B1/multidrug resistance 1, and OATP1B1/breast cancer resistance protein. *J Pharmacol Exp Ther*, **2005,** *314*:1059–1067.

Mizuno N, Niwa T, Yotsumoto Y, Sugiyama Y. Impact of drug transporter studies on drug discovery and development. *Pharmacol Rev*, **2003,** *55*:425–461.

Mori S, Takanaga H, Ohtsuki S, et al. Rat organic anion transporter 3 (rOAT3) is responsible for brain-to-blood efflux of homovanillic acid at the abluminal membrane of brain capillary endothelial cells. *J Cereb Blood Flow Metab*, **2003,** *23*:432–440.

Murphy DL, Lerner A, Rudnick G, Lesch KP. Serotonin transporter: Gene, genetic disorders, and pharmacogenetics. *Mol Interven*, **2004,** *4*:109–123.

Mwinyi J, Johne A, Bauer S, et al. Evidence for inverse effects of OATP-C (SLC21A6) 5 and 1b haplotypes on pravastatin kinetics. *Clin Pharmacol Ther*, **2004,** *75*:415–421.

Naesens M, Kuypers DRJ, Verbeke K, Vanrenterghem Y. Multidrug resistance protein 2 genetic polymorphisms influence mycophenolic acid exposure in renal allograft recipients. *Transplantation*, **2006**, *82*:1074–1084.

Nezu J, Tamai I, Oku A, et al. Primary systemic carnitine deficiency is caused by mutations in a gene encoding sodium ion–dependent carnitine transporter. *Nature Genet*, **1999,** *21*:91–94.

Niemi M, Backman JT, Kajosaari LI, et al. Polymorphic organic anion transporting polypeptide 1B1 is a major determinant of repaglinide pharmacokinetics. *Clin Pharmacol Ther*, **2005,** *77*:468–478.

Niemi M, Schaeffeler E, Lang T, et al. High plasma pravastatin concentrations are associated with single nucleotide polymorphisms and haplotypes of organic anion transporting polypeptide-C (OATP-C, SLCO1B1). *Pharmacogenetics*, **2004,** *14*:429–440.

Ocheltree SM, Shen H, Hu Y, et al. Mechanisms of cefadroxil uptake in the choroid plexus: Studies in wild-type and PEPT2 knockout mice. *J Pharmacol Exp Ther*, **2004,** *308*:462–467.

Okuda M, Saito H, Urakami Y, et al. cDNA cloning and functional expression of a novel rat kidney organic cation transporter, OCT2. *Biochem Biophys Res Commun*, **1996,** *224*:500–507.

Olivier B, Soudijn W, van Wijngaarden I. Serotonin, dopamine and norepinephrine transporters in the central nervous system and their inhibitors. *Prog Drug Res*, **2000,** *54*:59–119.

Oostendorp RL, Buckle T, Beijnen JH, et al. The effect of P-gp, BCRP and P-gp/BCRP inhibitors on the in vivo absorption, distribution, metabolism and excretion of imatinib. *Invest New Drugs*, **2008,** *27*:31–40.

Osato DH, Huang CC, Kawamoto M, et al. Functional characterization in yeast of genetic variants in the human equilibrative nucleo-side transporter, ENT1. *Pharmacogenetics*, **2003,** *13*:297–301.

Ose A, Ito M, Kusuhara H, et al. Limited brain distribution of [3R,4R,5S]-4-acetamido-5-amino-3-(1-ethylpropoxy)-1-cyclohexene-1-carboxylate phosphate (Ro 64-0802), a pharmacologically active form of oseltamivir, by active efflux across the blood-brain barrier mediated by organic anion transporter 3 (OAT3/SLC22A8) and multidrug resistance-associated protein 4 (MRP4/ABCC4). *Drug Metab Dispos*, **2009**, *37*:315–321.

Otsuka M, Matsumoto T, Morimoto R, et al. A human transporter protein that mediates the final excretion step for toxic organic cations. *Proc Natl Acad Sci USA*, **2005**, *102*:17923–17928.

Pascual JM, Wang D, Lecumberri B, et al. GLUT1 deficiency and other glucose transporter diseases. *Eur J Endocrinol*, **2004,** *150*:627–633.

Paulusma CC, Bosma PJ, Zaman GJ, et al. Congenital jaundice in rats with a mutation in a multidrug resistance-associated protein gene. *Science*, **1996,** *271*:1126–1128.

Pinkett HW, Lee AT, Lum P, et al. An inward-facing conformation of a putative metal-chelate-type ABC transporter. *Science*, **2006**, *315*:373–377.

Polli JW, Olson KL, Chism JP, et al. An unexpected synergist role of P-glycoprotein and breast cancer resistance protein on the CNS penetration of the tyrosine kinase inhibitor lapatinib (GW572016). *Drug Metab Dispos*, **2009,** *37*:439–442.

Rader, D.J. Regulation of reverse cholesterol transport and clinical implications. *Am J Cardiol*, **2003,** *92*:42J–49J.

Rader DJ. Molecular regulation of HDL metabolism and function: Implications for novel therapies. *J Clin Invest*, **2006**, *116*:3090–3100.

Reuss L. Basic mechanisms of ion transport. In, *The Kidney: Physiology and Pathophysiology* (Seldin D, Giebisch G, eds.), Lippincott Williams & Wilkins, Baltimore, **2000,** pp. 85–106.

Sadee W, Drubbisch V, Amidon GL. Biology of membrane transport proteins. *Pharm Res*, **1995,** *12*:1823–1837.

Sadeque AJ, Wandel C, He H. Increased drug delivery to the brain by P-glycoprotein inhibition. *Clin Pharmacol Ther*, **2000,** *68*:231–237.

Sasaki M, Suzuki H, Ito K. Transcellular transport of organic anions across a double-transfected Madin-Darby canine kidney II cell monolayer expressing both human organic anion-transporting polypeptide (OATP2/SLC21A6) and multidrug resistance-associated protein 2 (MRP2/ABCC2). *J Biol Chem*, **2002,** *277*:6497–6503.

Sassi Y, Lipskaia L, Vandecasteele G, et al. Multidrug resistance-associated protein 4 regulates cAMP-dependent signaling pathways and controls human and rat SMC proliferation. *J Clin Invest*, **2008,** *118*:2747–2757.

Schinkel AH, Smit JJ, van Tellingen O. Disruption of the mouse mdrla P-glycoprotein gene leads to a deficiency in the blood–brain barrier and to increased sensitivity to drugs. *Cell*, **1994,** *77*:491–502.

Schuetz JD, Connelly MC, Sun D. MRP4: A previously unidentified factor in resistance to nucleoside-based antiviral drugs. *Nature Med*, **1999,** *5*:1048–1051.

Search Collaborative Group. SLC01B1 variants and statin-induced myopathy—a genomewide study. *N Engl J Med*, **2008**, *359*:789–799.

Sekine T, Cha SH, Tsuda M, et al. Identification of multispecific organic anion transporter 2 expressed predominantly in the liver. *FEBS Lett*, **1998,** *429*:179–182.

Sekine T, Watanabe N, Hosoyamada M, et al. Expression cloning and characterization of a novel multispecific organic anion transporter. *J Biol Chem*, **1997,** *272*:18526–18529.

Schousboe A, Sarup A, Larsson OM, White HS. GABA transporters as drug targets for modulation of GABAergic activity. *Biochem Pharmacol*, **2004**, *68*:1557–1563.

Shigeri Y, Seal RP, Shimamoto K. Molecular pharmacology of glutamate transporters, EAATs and VGLUTs. *Brain Res Rev*, **2004,** *45*:250–265.

Shitara Y, Horie T, Sugiyama Y. Transporters as a determinant of drug clearance and tissue distribution. *Eur J Pharm Sci*, **2006**, *27*:425-446.

Shitara Y, Itoh T, Sato H, et al. Inhibition of transporter-mediated hepatic uptake as a mechanism for drug–drug interaction between cerivastatin and cyclosporin A. *J Pharmacol Exp Ther*, **2003,** *304*:610–616.

Shitara Y, Sato H, Sugiyama Y. Evaluation of drug-drug interaction in the hepatobiliary and renal transport of drugs. *Annu Rev Pharmacol Toxicol*, **2005**, *45*:689–723.

Shu Y, Leabman MK, Feng B, et al. Evolutionary conservation predicts function of variants of the human organic cation transporter, OCT1. *Proc Natl Acad Sci USA*, **2003,** *100*: 5902–5907.

Shu Y, Sheardown SA, Brown C, et al. Effect of genetic variation in the organic cation transporter 1 (OCT1) on metformin action. *J Clin Invest*, **2007**, *117*:1422–1431.

Simonson GD, Vincent AC, Roberg KJ, et al. Molecular cloning and characterization of a novel liver-specific transport protein. *J Cell Sci*, **1994,** *107*:1065–1072.

Song IS, Shin HJ, Shim EJ, et al. Genetic variants of the organic cation transporter 2 influence the disposition of metformin. *Nature Pub Group*, **2008**, *84*:559–562.

Sotnikova TD, Beaulieu JM, Gainetdinov RR, Caron MG. Molecular biology, pharmacology and functional role of the plasma membrane dopamine transporter. *CNS Neurol Disord Drug Targets*, **2006**, *5*:45–56.

Srimaroeng C, Perry JL, Pritchard JB. Physiology, structure, and regulation of the cloned organic anion transporters. *Xenobiotica*, **2008**, *38*:889–935.

Stieger B, Fattinger K, Madon J, et al. Drug- and estrogen-induced cholestasis through inhibition of the hepatocellular bile salt export pump (BSEP) of rat liver. *Gastroenterology*, **2000,** *118*:422–430.

Strautnieks SS, Bull LN, Knisely AS, et al. A gene encoding a liver-specific ABC transporter is mutated in progressive familial intrahepatic cholestasis. *Nat Genet,* **1998**, *20*:233–238.

Sun H, Dai H, Shaik N, Elmquist WF. Drug efflux transporters in the CNS. *Adv Drug Deliv Rev*, **2003,** *55*:83–105.

Sweet DH, Wolff NA, Pritchard JB. Expression cloning and characterization of ROAT1: The basolateral organic anion transporter in rat kidney. *J Biol Chem*, **1997,** *272*:30088–30095.

Szakacs G, Paterson J, Ludwig J, et al. Targeting multidrug resistance in cancer. *Nature Rev*, **2006**, *5*:219–234.

Takeda M, Tojo A, Sekine T, et al. Role of organic anion transporter 1 (OAT1) in cephaloridine (CER)-induced nephrotoxicity. *Kidney Int,* **1999**, 56:2128–2136.

Takenaka K, Morgan JA, Scheffer GL, et al. Substrate overlap between MRP4 and ABCG2/BCRP affects purine analogue drug cytotoxicity and tissue distribution. *Cancer Res*, **2007,** *67*:6965–6972.

Tamai I, Ohashi R, Nezu J, et al. Molecular and functional identification of sodium ion–dependent, high affinity human carnitine transporter OCTN2. *J Biol Chem*, **1998,** *273*:20378–20382.

Tamai I, Yabuuchi H, Nezu J, et al. Cloning and characterization of a novel human pH-dependent organic cation transporter, OCTN1. *FEBS Lett*, **1997,** *419*:107–111.

Tanihara Y, Masuda S, Sato T, et al. Substrate specificity of MATE1 and MATE2-K, human multidrug and toxin extrusions/H$^+$-organic cation antiporters. *Biochem Pharmacol*, **2007**, *74*:359–371.

Tirona RG, Leake BF, Merino G, Kim RB. Polymorphisms in OATP-C: Identification of multiple allelic variants associated with altered transport activity among European- and African-Americans. *J Biol Chem*, **2001,** *276*: 35669–35675.

Torres G, Amara S. Glutamate and monoamine transporters: New visions of form and function. *Curr Opin Neurobiol*, **2007**, *17*:304–312.

Toyoda Y, Hagiya Y, Adachi T, et al. MRP class of human ATP binding cassette (ABC) transporters: Historical background and new research directions. *Xenobiotica,* **2008**, *38*:833–862.

Treiber A, Schneiter R, Häusler S, et al. Bosentan is a substrate of human OATP1B1 and OATP1B3: inhibition of hepatic uptake as the common mechanism of its interactions with cyclosporin A, rifampicin, and sildenafil. *Drug Metab Dispos,* **2007**, *35*:1400–1407.

Turner JG, Gump JL, Zhang C, et al. ABCG2 expression, function, and promoter methylation in human multiple myeloma. *Blood*, **2006,** *108*:3881–3889.

Uchiumi T, Kohno K, Tanimura H, et al. Enhanced expression of the human multidrug resistance 1 gene in response to UV light irradiation. *Cell Growth Differ*, **1993,** *4*:147–157.

Uhl GR. Dopamine transporter: basic science and human variation of a key molecule for dopaminergic function, locomotion, and parkinsonism. *Mov Disord*, **2003,** *18*:S71–S80.

Urakami Y, Akazawa M, Saito H, et al. cDNA cloning, functional characterization, and tissue distribution of an alternatively spliced variant of organic cation transporter hOCT2 predominantly expressed in the human kidney. *J Am Soc Nephrol*, **2002,** *13*:1703–1710.

Urban TJ, Sebro R, Hurowitz EH, et al. Functional genomics of membrane transporters in human populations. *Genome Res,* **2006**, *16*:223–230.

Wang DS, Kusuhara H, Kato Y, et al. Involvement of organic cation transporter 1 in the lactic acidosis caused by metformin. *Mol Pharmacol*, **2003,** *63*:844–848.

Wang H, LeCluyse EL. Role of orphan nuclear receptors in the regulation of drug-metabolising enzymes. *Clin Pharmacokinet*, **2003,** *42*:1331–1357.

Wang ZJ, Yin OQP, Tomlinson B, Chow MSS. OCT2 polymorphisms and in-vivo renal functional consequence: studies with metformin and cimetidine. *Pharmacogenet Genom*, **2008**, *18*:637–645.

Werner A, Moore ML, Mantei N, et al. Cloning and expression of cDNA for a Na/P_i cotransport system of kidney cortex. *Proc Natl Acad Sci USA*, **1991,** *88*:9608–9612.

Wright SH, Dantzler WH. Molecular and cellular physiology of renal organic cation and anion transport. *Physiol Rev*, **2004,** *84*:987–1049.

Xu F, Gainetdinov RR, Wetsel WC, et al. Mice lacking the norepinephrine transporter are supersensitive to psychostimulants. *Nature Neurosci*, **2000,** *3*:465–471.

Yamasaki Y, Ieiri I, Kusuhara H, et al. Pharmacogenetic characterization of sulfasalazine disposition based on NAT2 and ABCG2 (BCRP) gene polymorphisms in humans. *Clin Pharmacol Ther*, **2008,** *84*:95–103.

Zelcer N, van de Wetering K, Hillebrand M, et al. Mice lacking multidrug resistance protein 3 show altered morphine pharmacokinetics and morphine-6-glucuronide antinociception. *Proc Natl Acad Sci USA*, **2005,** *102*:7274–7279.

Zhang Y, Benet LZ. The gut as a barrier to drug absorption: Combined role of cytochrome P450 3A and P-glycoprotein. *Clin Pharmacokinet*, **2001,** *40*:159–168.

Zhang W, He YJ, Han CT, et al. Effect of SLCO1B1 genetic polymorphism on the pharmacokinetics of nateglinide. *Br J Clin Pharmacol,* **2006a,** *62*:567–572.

Zhang S, Lovejoy KS, Shima JE, et al. Organic cation transporters are determinants of oxaliplatin cytotoxicity. *Cancer Res*, **2006b,** *66*:8847–8857.

Zhang J, Visser F, King KM, et al. The role of nucleoside transporters in cancer chemotherapy with nucleoside drugs. *Cancer Metastasis Rev*, **2007**, *26*:85–110.

Zhang W, Yu BN, He YJ, et al. Role of BCRP 421C>A polymorphism on rosuvastatin pharmacokinetics in healthy Chinese males. *Clin Chim Acta*, **2006c,** *373*:99–103.

Drug Metabolism

Frank J. Gonzalez, Michael Coughtrie, and Robert H. Tukey

COPING WITH EXPOSURE TO XENOBIOTICS

Humans come into contact with thousands of foreign chemicals, medicines, or xenobiotics (substances foreign to the body) through intentional exposure, accidental exposure to environmental contaminants, as well as through diet. Fortunately, humans have developed a means to rapidly eliminate xenobiotics so that they do not accumulate in the tissues and cause harm. The ability of humans to metabolize and clear drugs is a natural process that involves the same enzymatic pathways and transport systems that are used for normal metabolism of dietary constituents. In fact, plants are a common source of xenobiotics in the diet, contributing many structurally diverse chemicals, some of which are associated with pigment production and others of which are toxins (called phytoallexins) that protect plants against predators. For example, poisonous mushrooms produce toxins that are lethal to mammals, including amanitin, gyromitrin, orellanine, muscarine, ibotenic acid, muscimol, psilocybin, and coprine. Animals must be able to metabolize and eliminate such chemicals in order to consume vegetation.

Drugs are considered xenobiotics and most are extensively metabolized in humans. Many drugs are derived from chemicals found in plants, some of which have been used in Chinese herbal medicines for thousands of years. Thus, it is not surprising that humans also metabolize synthetic drugs by pathways that mimic the disposition of chemicals found in the diet. This capacity to metabolize xenobiotics, while mostly beneficial, has made development of drugs very time consuming and costly due in large part to:

- Inter-individual variations in the capacity of humans to metabolize drugs
- Drug-drug interactions
- Metabolic activation of chemicals to toxic and carcinogenic derivatives
- Species differences in expression of enzymes that metabolize drugs, thereby limiting the use of animal models for drug testing to predict effects in humans

A large number of diverse enzymes have evolved in animals that apparently function only to metabolize foreign chemicals. As will be discussed later, there are such large differences among species in the ability to metabolize xenobiotics, that animal models cannot be solely relied upon to predict how humans will metabolize a drug. Enzymes that metabolize xenobiotics have historically been called drug-metabolizing enzymes, although they are involved in the metabolism of many foreign chemicals to which humans are exposed. Thus, a more appropriate name would be *xenobiotic-metabolizing enzymes.* Dietary differences among species during the course of evolution could account for the marked species variation in the complexity of the drug-metabolizing enzymes. Additional diversity within these enzyme systems has also derived from the necessity to detoxify a host of endogenous chemicals that would otherwise prove harmful to the organism, such as bilirubin, steroid hormones, and catecholamines. Many of these compounds are detoxified by the same or closely related xenobiotic-metabolizing enzymes.

Xenobiotics to which humans are exposed come from sources that include environmental pollution, food additives, cosmetic products, agrochemicals, processed foods, and drugs. In general, most xenobiotics are lipophilic chemicals that, in the absence of metabolism, would not be efficiently eliminated, and thus would accumulate in the body, potentially resulting in toxicity. With very few exceptions, xenobiotics are subjected to one or multiple enzymatic pathways that constitute *phase 1 oxidation* and *phase 2 conjugation*. As a general paradigm, metabolism serves to convert these hydrophobic chemicals into more hydrophilic derivatives that can easily be eliminated from the body through the urine or the bile.

In order to be accessible to cells and reach their sites of action, drugs generally must possess physical properties that allow them to move down a concentration gradient into the cell. Many drugs are hydrophobic, a property that allows entry through the lipid bilayers into cells where the agents can interact with their target receptors or proteins. With some compounds, entry into cells is facilitated by a large number of transporters on the plasma membrane (see Chapter 5). This property of hydrophobicity renders drugs difficult to eliminate, since in the absence of metabolism, they accumulate in fat and cellular phospholipid bilayers in cells. The xenobiotic-metabolizing enzymes serve to convert drugs and other xenobiotics into derivatives that are more hydrophilic and thus easily eliminated through excretion into the aqueous compartments of the tissues.

The process of drug metabolism that leads to elimination also plays a major role in diminishing the biological activity of a drug. For example, (S)-phenytoin, an anticonvulsant used in the treatment of epilepsy, is virtually insoluble in water. Metabolism by the phase 1 cytochromes P450 (CYPs) followed by phase 2 uridine diphosphate-glucuronosyltransferases (UGTs) produces a metabolite that is highly water soluble and readily eliminated from the body (Figure 6–1). Metabolism also terminates the biological activity of the drug. Since conjugates are generally hydrophobic, elimination via the bile and/or urine is dependent on the actions of many efflux transporters (see Chapter 5).

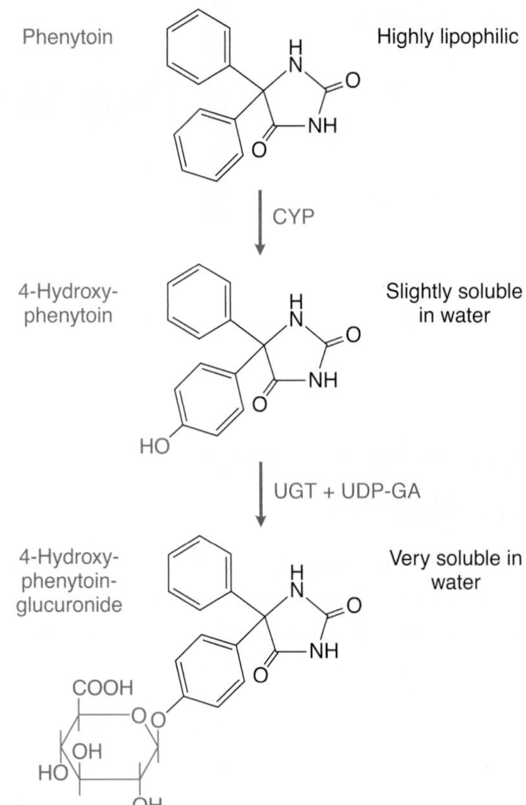

Figure 6–1. *Metabolism of phenytoin by phase 1 cytochrome P450 (CYP) and phase 2 uridine diphosphate-glucuronosyltransferase (UGT).* CYP facilitates 4-hydroxylation of phenytoin. The hydroxy group serves as a substrate for UGT that conjugates a molecule of glucuronic acid (in green) using UDP-glucuronic acid (UDP-GA) as a cofactor. This converts a very hydrophobic molecule to a larger hydrophilic derivative that is eliminated *via* the bile.

While xenobiotic-metabolizing enzymes are responsible for facilitating the elimination of chemicals from the body, paradoxically these same enzymes can also convert certain chemicals to highly reactive, toxic, and carcinogenic metabolites. This occurs when an unstable intermediate is formed that has reactivity toward other cellular constituents. Chemicals that can be converted by xenobiotic metabolism to cancer-causing derivatives are called *carcinogens*. Depending on the structure of the chemical substrate, xenobiotic-metabolizing enzymes can produce electrophilic metabolites that react with nucleophilic cellular macromolecules such as DNA, RNA, and protein. This can cause cell death and organ toxicity. Reaction of these electrophiles with DNA can sometimes result in cancer through the mutation of genes, such as oncogenes or tumor suppressor genes. It is generally believed that most human cancers are due to exposure to chemical carcinogens. This potential for carcinogenic activity makes testing the safety of drug candidates of vital importance. Testing for potential cancer-causing activity is particularly critical for drugs that will be used for the treatment of chronic diseases. Since each species has evolved a unique combination of xenobiotic-metabolizing enzymes, non-primate rodent models cannot be the only animal models used for testing the safety of new drug candidates targeted for human diseases. Nevertheless, testing in rodent models, such as mice and rats, can usually identify potential carcinogens. If a drug tests negative for carcinogenicity in rodents, it is unlikely to cause cancer in humans, albeit some rodent carcinogens are not associated with human cancer. However, many cytotoxic cancer drugs have the potential to cause cancer; this risk potential is minimized by their time-limited use in cancer therapy.

THE PHASES OF DRUG METABOLISM

Xenobiotic metabolizing enzymes have historically been grouped into those that carry out *phase 1 reactions*, which include oxidation, reduction, or hydrolytic reactions, and the *phase 2 reactions*, in which enzymes catalyze the conjugation of the substrate (the phase 1 product) with a second molecule (Table 6–1). The phase 1

Table 6–1

Xenobiotic Metabolizing Enzymes

ENZYMES	REACTIONS
Phase 1 "oxygenases"	
Cytochrome P450s (P450 or CYP)	C and O oxidation, dealkylation, others
Flavin-containing monooxygenases (FMO)	N, S, and P oxidation
Epoxide hydrolases (mEH, sEH)	Hydrolysis of epoxides
Phase 2 "transferases"	
Sulfotransferases (SULT)	Addition of sulfate
UDP-glucuronosyltransferases (UGT)	Addition of glucuronic acid
Glutathione-S-transferases (GST)	Addition of glutathione
N-acetyltransferases (NAT)	Addition of acetyl group
Methyltransferases (MT)	Addition of methyl group
Other enzymes	
Alcohol dehydrogenases	Reduction of alcohols
Aldehyde dehydrogenases	Reduction of aldehydes
NADPH-quinone oxidoreductase (NQO)	Reduction of quinones

mEH and sEH are microsomal and soluble epoxide hydrolase. UDP, uridine diphosphate; NADPH, reduced nicotinamide adenine dinucleotide phosphate.

enzymes lead to the introduction of functional groups such as –OH, –COOH, –SH, –O–, or NH_2. The addition of functional groups does little to increase the water solubility of the drug, but can dramatically alter the biological properties of the drug. Reactions carried out by phase 1 enzymes usually lead to the inactivation of a drug. However, in certain instances, metabolism, usually the hydrolysis of an ester or amide linkage, results in bioactivation of a drug. Inactive drugs that undergo metabolism to an active drug are called *prodrugs*. Examples are the anti-tumor drug cyclophosphamide, which is bioactivated to a cell-killing electrophilic derivative (see Chapter 61); and clofibrate, which is converted in the cell from an ester to an active acidic metabolite. Phase 2 enzymes facilitate the elimination of drugs and the inactivation of electrophilic and potentially toxic metabolites produced by oxidation. While many phase 1 reactions result in the biological inactivation of the drug, phase 2 reactions produce a metabolite with improved water solubility, a change that facilitates the elimination of the drug from the tissue, normally via efflux transporters.

Superfamilies of evolutionarily related enzymes and receptors are common in the mammalian genome; the enzyme systems responsible for drug metabolism are good examples. The phase 1 oxidation reactions are carried out by CYPs, flavin-containing monooxygenases (FMO), and epoxide hydrolases (EH). The CYPs and FMOs are composed of superfamilies of enzymes. Each superfamily contains multiple genes. The phase 2 enzymes include several superfamilies of conjugating enzymes. Among the more important are the glutathione-S-transferases (GST), UDP-glucuronosyltransferases (UGT), sulfotransferases (SULT), *N*-acetyltransferases (NAT), and methyltransferases (MT). These conjugation reactions usually require the substrate to have oxygen (hydroxyl or epoxide groups), nitrogen, or sulfur atoms that serve as acceptor sites for a hydrophilic moiety, such as glutathione, glucuronic acid, sulfate, or an acetyl group. The example of phase 1 and phase 2 metabolism of phenytoin is shown in Figure 6–1. The oxidation by phase 1 enzymes either adds or exposes a functional group, permitting the products of phase 1 metabolism to serve as substrates for the phase 2 conjugating or synthetic enzymes. In the case of the UGTs, glucuronic acid is delivered to the functional group, forming a glucuronide metabolite that is more water soluble and is targeted for excretion either in the urine or bile. When the substrate is a drug, these reactions usually convert the original drug to a form that is not able to bind to its target receptor, thus attenuating the biological response to the drug.

SITES OF DRUG METABOLISM

Xenobiotic metabolizing enzymes are found in most tissues in the body with the highest levels located in the GI tract (liver, small and large intestines). Drugs that are orally administered, absorbed by the gut, and taken to the liver, can be extensively metabolized. The liver is considered the major "metabolic clearing house" for both endogenous chemicals (e.g., cholesterol, steroid hormones, fatty acids, and proteins) and xenobiotics. The small intestine plays a crucial role in drug metabolism since drugs that are orally administered are absorbed by the gut and taken to the liver through the portal vein. The xenobiotic-metabolizing enzymes located in the epithelial cells of the GI tract are responsible for the initial metabolic processing of most oral medications. This should be considered the initial site of drug metabolism. The absorbed drug then enters the portal circulation for its first pass through the liver, where it can undergo significant metabolism. While a portion of active drug escapes metabolism in the GI tract and liver, subsequent passes through the liver result in more metabolism of the parent drug until the agent is eliminated. Thus, drugs that are poorly metabolized remain in the body for longer periods of time and their pharmacokinetic profiles show much longer elimination half-lives than drugs that are rapidly metabolized. Other organs that contain significant xenobiotic-metabolizing enzymes include tissues of the nasal mucosa and lung, which play important roles in the metabolism of drugs that are administered through aerosol sprays. These tissues are also the first line of contact with hazardous chemicals that are airborne.

Within the cell, xenobiotic-metabolizing enzymes are found in the intracellular membranes and in the cytosol. The phase 1 CYPs, FMOs, and EHs, and some phase 2 conjugating enzymes, notably the UGTs, are all located in the endoplasmic reticulum of the cell (Figure 6–2). The endoplasmic reticulum consists of phospholipid bilayers, organized as tubes and sheets throughout the cytoplasm, forming a network that has an inner lumen that is physically distinct from the rest of the cytosolic components of the cell and has connections to the plasma membrane and nuclear envelope. This membrane localization is ideally suited for the metabolic function of these enzymes: hydrophobic molecules enter the cell and become embedded in the lipid bilayer, where they come into direct contact with the

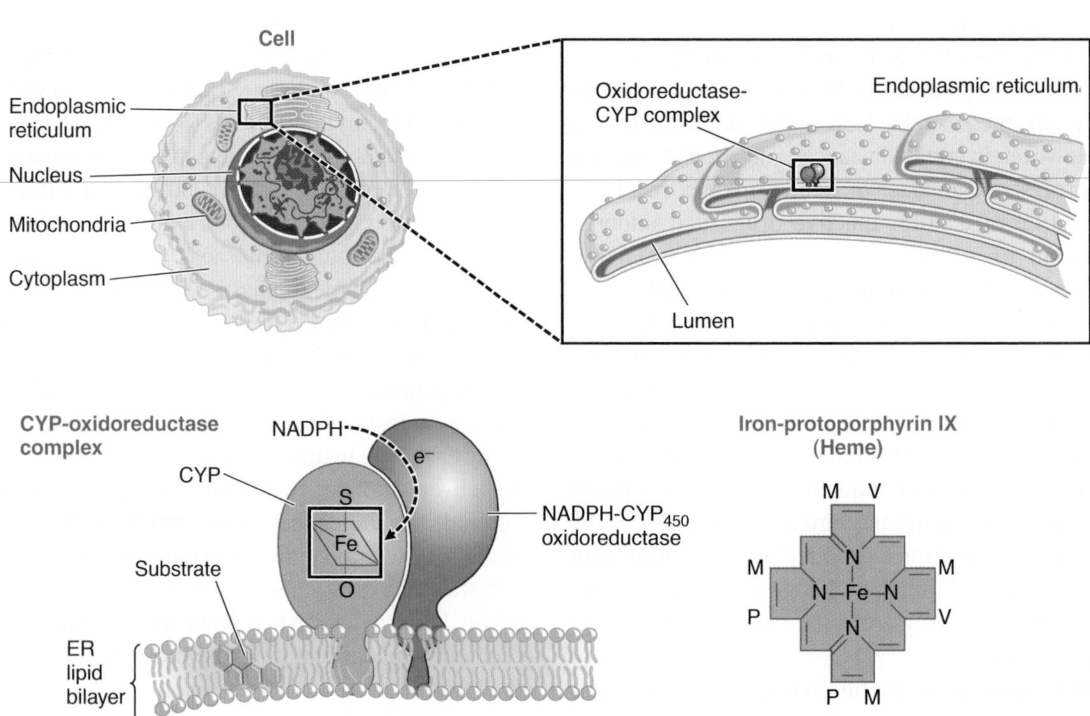

Figure 6–2. *Location of CYPs in the cell.* The figure shows increasingly microscopic levels of detail, sequentially expanding the areas within the black boxes. CYPs are embedded in the phospholipid bilayer of the endoplasmic reticulum (ER). Most of the enzyme is located on the cytosolic surface of the ER. A second enzyme, NADPH-cytochrome P_{450} oxidoreductase, transfers electrons to the CYP where it can, in the presence of O_2, oxidize xenobiotic substrates, many of which are hydrophobic and dissolved in the ER. A single NADPH-CYP oxidoreductase species transfers electrons to all CYP isoforms in the ER. Each CYP contains a molecule of iron-protoporphyrin IX that functions to bind and activate O_2. Substituents on the porphyrin ring are methyl (M), propionyl (P), and vinyl (V) groups.

phase 1 enzymes. Once subjected to oxidation, drugs can be directly conjugated by the UGTs (in the lumen of the endoplasmic reticulum) or by the cytosolic transferases such as GST and SULT. The metabolites can then be transported out of the cell through the plasma membrane where they are deposited into the bloodstream. Hepatocytes, which constitute >90% of the cells in the liver, carry out most drug metabolism and can produce conjugated substrates that can also be transported though the bile canalicular membrane into the bile, from which they are eliminated into the gut (see Chapter 5).

PHASE 1 REACTIONS

The Cytochrome P-450 Superfamily: the CYPs

The CYPs are a superfamily of enzymes, all of which contain a molecule of heme that is non-covalently bound to the polypeptide chain (Figure 6–2). Many other enzymes that use O_2 as a substrate for their reactions also contain heme. Heme is the oxygen-binding moiety found in hemoglobin, where it functions in the binding and transport of molecular oxygen from the lung to other tissues. Heme contains one atom of iron in a hydrocarbon cage that functions to bind oxygen in the CYP active site as part of the catalytic cycle of these enzymes. CYPs use O_2, plus H^+ derived from the cofactor-reduced nicotinamide adenine dinucleotide phosphate (NADPH), to carry out the oxidation of substrates. The H^+ is supplied through the enzyme NADPH-cytochrome P450 oxidoreductase. Metabolism of a substrate by a CYP consumes one molecule of molecular oxygen and produces an oxidized substrate and a molecule of water as a by-product. However, for most CYPs, depending on the nature of the substrate, the reaction is "uncoupled," consuming more O_2 than substrate metabolized and producing what is called activated oxygen or O_2^-. The O_2^- is usually converted to water by the enzyme superoxide dismutase. Elevated O_2^-, a *reactive oxygen species* (ROS), can give rise to oxidative stress that is detrimental to cellular physiology and associated with diseases including hepatic cirrhosis.

Among the diverse reactions carried out by mammalian CYPs are *N*-dealkylation, *O*-dealkylation, aromatic hydroxylation, *N*-oxidation, *S*-oxidation, deamination, and dehalogenation (Table 6–2). More than 50 individual CYPs have been identified in humans. As a family of enzymes, CYPs are involved in the metabolism of dietary and xenobiotic chemicals, as well as the synthesis of endogenous compounds (e.g., steroids; fatty acid-derived signaling molecules, such as epoxyeicosatrienoic acids). CYPs also participate in the production of bile acids from cholesterol.

In contrast to the drug-metabolizing CYPs, the CYPs that catalyze steroid and bile acid synthesis have very specific substrate preferences. For example, the CYP that produces estrogen from testosterone, CYP19 or aromatase, can metabolize only testosterone or androstenedione and does not metabolize xenobiotics. Specific inhibitors for aromatase, such as *anastrozole*, have been developed for use in the treatment of estrogen-dependent tumors (see Chapters 40 and 60-63). The synthesis of bile acids from cholesterol occurs in the liver, where, subsequent to CYP-catalyzed oxidation, the bile acids are conjugated with amino acids and transported through the bile duct and gallbladder into the small intestine. Bile acids are emulsifiers that facilitate the elimination of conjugated drugs from the liver and the absorption of fatty acids and vitamins from the diet. In this capacity, > 90% of bile acids are reabsorbed by the gut and transported back to the hepatocytes. Similar to the steroid biosynthetic CYPs, CYPs involved in bile acid production have strict substrate requirements and do not participate in xenobiotic or drug metabolism.

The CYPs that carry out xenobiotic metabolism have the capacity to metabolize diverse chemicals. This is due both to multiple forms of CYPs and to the capacity of a single CYP to metabolize many structurally distinct chemicals. There is also significant overlapping substrate specificity amongst CYPs; a single compound can also be metabolized, albeit at different rates, by different CYPs. Additionally, CYPs can metabolize a single compound at different positions on the molecule. In contrast to most enzymes in the body that carry out highly specific reactions involved in the biosynthesis and degradation of important cellular constituents in which there is a single substrate and one or more products, or two simultaneous substrates, the CYPs are promiscuous in their capacity to bind and metabolize multiple substrates (Table 6–2). This property, which is due to large and fluid substrate binding sites in the CYP, sacrifices metabolic turnover rates; CYPs metabolize substrates at a fraction of the rate of more typical enzymes involved in intermediary metabolism and mitochondrial electron transfer. As a result, drugs have, in general, half-lives in the range of 3-30 hours, while endogenous compounds have half-lives of the order of seconds or minutes (e.g., dopamine and insulin). Even though CYPs have slow catalytic rates, their activities are sufficient to metabolize drugs that are administered at high concentrations in the body. This unusual feature of extensive overlapping substrate specificities by the CYPs is one of the underlying reasons for the predominance of drug-drug interactions. When two co-administered drugs are both metabolized by a single CYP, they compete for binding to the enzyme's active site. This can result in the inhibition of metabolism of one or both of the drugs, leading to elevated plasma levels. If there is a narrow therapeutic index for the drugs, the elevated serum levels may elicit unwanted toxicities. Drug-drug interactions are among the leading causes of adverse drug reactions (ADRs).

The Naming of CYPS. The CYPs are the most actively studied of the xenobiotic metabolizing enzymes since they are responsible for metabolizing the vast majority of therapeutic drugs. Genome sequencing has revealed the existence of 102 putatively functional

Table 6–2

Major Reactions Involved in Drug Metabolism

	REACTION	EXAMPLES
I. Oxidative reactions		
N-Dealkylation	$RNHCH_3 \rightarrow RNH_2 + CH_2O$	Imipramine, diazepam, codeine, erythromycin, morphine, tamoxifen, theophylline, caffeine
O-Dealkylation	$ROCH_3 \rightarrow ROH + CH_2O$	Codeine, indomethacin, dextromethorphan
Aliphatic hydroxylation	$RCH_2CH_3 \rightarrow RCHOHCH_3$	Tolbutamide, ibuprofen, phenobarbital, meprobamate, cyclosporine, midazolam
Aromatic hydroxylation	$R\text{-}C_6H_5 \rightarrow$ arene epoxide $\rightarrow R\text{-}C_6H_4\text{-}OH$	Phenytoin, phenobarbital, propanolol, ethinyl estradiol, amphetamine, warfarin
N-Oxidation	$RNH_2 \rightarrow RNHOH$ $R_1R_2NH \rightarrow R_1R_2N{-}OH$	Chlorpheniramine, dapsone, meperidine
S-Oxidation	$R_1R_2S \rightarrow R_1R_2S{=}O$	Cimetidine, chlorpromazine, thioridazine, omeprazole
Deamination	$RCH(NH_2)CH_3 \rightarrow R{-}C(OH)(NH_2){-}CH_3 \rightarrow R{-}C(=O){-}CH_3 + NH_3$	Diazepam, amphetamine
II. Hydrolysis reactions	epoxide $\rightarrow$ trans-dihydrodiol (H, OH / H, OH)	Carbamazepine (see Figure 6-4)
	$R_1C(=O)OR_2 \rightarrow R_1COOH + R_2OH$	Procaine, aspirin, clofibrate, meperidine, enalapril, cocaine
	$R_1C(=O)NHR_2 \rightarrow R_1COOH + R_2NH_2$	Lidocaine, procainamide, indomethacin
III. Conjugation reactions		
Glucuronidation	R + UDP-glucuronic acid (COOH, OH, OH, OH, O–UDP) $\rightarrow$ R–O-glucuronide (COOH, OH, OH, OH) + UDP	Acetaminophen, morphine, oxazepam, lorazepam
Sulfation	$PAPS + ROH \rightarrow R{-}O{-}SO_2{-}OH + PAP$	Acetaminophen, steroids, methyldopa
Acetylation	$CoAS{-}CO{-}CH_3 + RNH_2 \rightarrow RNH{-}CO{-}CH_3 + CoA\text{-}SH$	Sulfonamides, isoniazid, dapsone, clonazepam
Methylation	RO-, RS-, RN- + AdoMet $\rightarrow$ RO-CH_3 + AdoHomCys	L-Dopa, methyldopa, mercaptopurine, captopril
Glutathionylation	GSH + R $\rightarrow$ R-GSH	Adriamycin, fosfomycin, busulfan

PAPS, 3′-phosphoadenosine-5′ phosphosulfate; PAP 3′-phosphoadenosine-5′-phosphate.

genes and 88 pseudogenes in the mouse, and 57 putatively functional genes and 58 pseudogenes in humans. These genes are grouped, based on amino acid sequence similarity, into a superfamily composed of families and subfamilies with increasing sequence similarity. CYPs are named with the root CYP followed by a number designating the family, a letter denoting the sub-family, and another number designating the CYP form. Thus, *CYP3A4* is family 3, subfamily A, and gene number 4.

A Dozen CYPs Suffice for Metabolism of Most Drugs. While several CYP families are involved in the synthesis of steroid hormones and bile acids, and the metabolism of retinoic acid and fatty acids (including prostaglandins and eicosanoids), a limited number of CYPs that fall into families 1 to 3 are primarily involved in xenobiotic metabolism. Since a single CYP can metabolize myriad structurally diverse compounds, these enzymes can collectively metabolize scores of chemicals found in the diet and environment, and administered as drugs. In humans, 12 CYPs (CYP1A1, 1A2, 1B1, 2A6, 2B6, 2C8, 2C9, 2C19, 2D6, 2E1, 3A4, and 3A5) are known to be important for metabolism of xenobiotics. The liver contains the greatest abundance of xenobiotic-metabolizing CYPs, thus ensuring efficient first-pass metabolism of drugs. CYPs are also expressed throughout the GI tract, and in lower amounts in lung, kidney, and even in the CNS. The expression of the different CYPs can differ markedly as a result of dietary and environmental exposure to inducers, or through inter-individual changes resulting from heritable polymorphic differences in gene structure; tissue-specific expression patterns can affect overall drug metabolism and clearance. The most active CYPs for drug metabolism are those in the CYP2C, CYP2D, and CYP3A sub-families. CYP3A4, the most abundantly expressed in liver, is involved in the metabolism of over 50% of clinically used drugs (Figure 6–3A). The CYP1A, CYP1B, CYP2A, CYP2B, and CYP2E subfamilies are not significantly involved in the metabolism of therapeutic drugs, but they do catalyze the metabolic activation of many protoxins and procarcinogens to their ultimate reactive metabolites.

There are large differences in levels of expression of each CYP amongst individuals as assessed both by clinical pharmacological studies and by analysis of expression in human liver samples. This large inter-individual variability in CYP expression is due to the presence of genetic polymorphisms and differences in gene regulation (see following discussion). Several human CYP genes exhibit polymorphisms, including *CYP2A6*, *CYP2C9*, *CYP2C19*, and *CYP2D6*. Allelic variants have been found in the *CYP1B1* and *CYP3A4* genes, but they are present at low frequencies in humans and appear not to have a major role in inter-individual levels of expression of these enzymes. However, homozygous mutations in the *CYP1B1* gene are associated with primary congenital glaucoma.

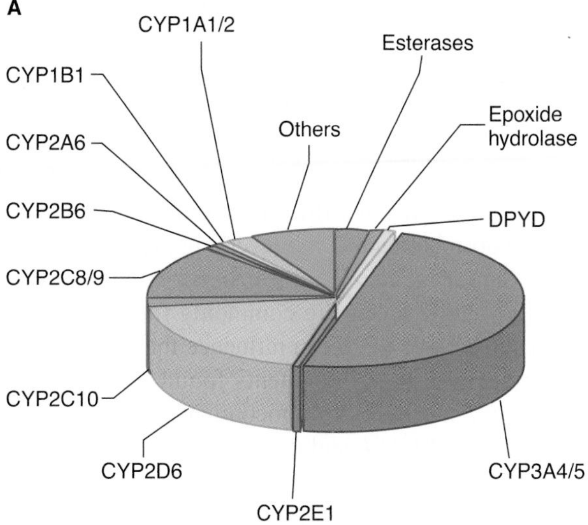

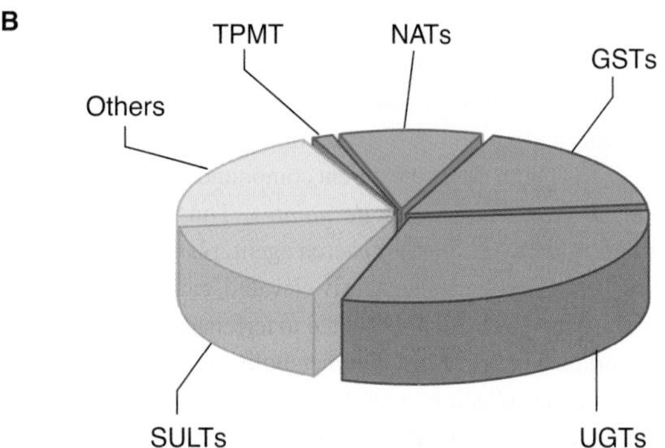

Figure 6–3. *The fraction of clinically used drugs metabolized by the major phase 1 and phase 2 enzymes.* The relative size of each pie section represents the estimated percentage of drugs metabolized by the major phase 1 (panel ***A***) and phase 2 (panel ***B***) enzymes, based on studies in the literature. In some cases, more than a single enzyme is responsible for metabolism of a single drug. CYP, cytochrome P450; DPYD, dihydropyrimidine dehydrogenase; GST, glutathione-S-transferase; NAT, N-acetyltransferase; SULT, sulfotransferase, TPMT, thiopurine methyltransferase; UGT, UDP-glucuronosyltransferase.

CYPs and Drug-Drug Interactions. Differences in the rate of metabolism of a drug can be due to drug interactions. Most commonly, this occurs when two drugs (e.g., a statin and a macrolide antibiotic or antifungal agent) are co-administered and subjected to metabolism by the same enzyme. Thus, it is important to determine the identity of the CYP that metabolizes a particular drug and to avoid co-administering drugs that are metabolized by the same enzyme. Some drugs can also inhibit CYPs independently of being substrates for a CYP. For example, the common antifungal agent, ketoconazole (NIZORAL), is a potent inhibitor of *CYP3A4* and other CYPs, and co-administration of ketoconazole with an anti-HIV viral protease inhibitor reduces the clearance of the protease inhibitor and increases its plasma concentration and the risk of toxicity. For most drugs, information found on the package insert lists the CYP that metabolizes the drug and determines the potential for drug interactions. Some drugs are CYP inducers that can increase not only their own rates of metabolism, but also induce metabolism of other co-administered drugs (see later discussion and Figure 6–12). For example, steroid hormones and herbal products such as St. John's wort can increase hepatic levels of *CYP3A4*, thereby increasing the metabolism of many orally administered drugs. Indeed, St, John's wort can induce hepatic metabolism of the steroid components of birth control pills, rendering the standard dose ineffective in preventing pregancy. Drug metabolism can also be influenced by diet. CYP inhibitors and inducers are commonly found in foods and in some cases these can influence the toxicity and efficacy of a drug. Components found in grapefruit juice (e.g., naringin, furanocoumarins) are potent inhibitors of *CYP3A4*, and thus some drug inserts recommend not taking medication with grapefruit juice because it could increase the bioavailability of the drug.

Terfenadine, a once popular antihistamine, was removed from the market because its metabolism was inhibited *by CYP3A4* substrates such as erythromycin and grapefruit juice. Terfenadine was actually a prodrug that required oxidation by *CYP3A4* to its active metabolite, and at high doses the parent compound caused the potentially fatal arrhythmia *torsades de pointes*. Thus, as a result of *CYP3A4* inhibition by a co-administered agent, plasma levels of the parent drug could become dangerously elevated, causing ventricular tachycardia in some individuals; this led to terfenadine's withdrawal from the market. Subsequently, the metabolite was developed as a drug, fexofenadine, which retains the therapeutic properties of the parent compound but avoids the step involving *CYP3A4*.

In addition, inter-individual differences in drug metabolism are significantly influenced by polymorphisms in CYPs. The *CYP2D6* polymorphism has led to the withdrawal of several clinically used drugs (e.g., debrisoquine and perhexiline) and the cautious use of others that are known *CYP2D6* substrates (e.g., encainide and flecainide [anti-arrhythmics], desipramine and nortriptyline [antidepressants], and codeine).

FLAVIN-CONTAINING MONOOXYGENASES (FMOs)

The FMOs are another superfamily of phase 1 enzymes involved in drug metabolism. Similar to CYPs, the FMOs are expressed at high levels in the liver and are bound to the endoplasmic reticulum, a site that favors interaction with and metabolism of hydrophobic drug substrates. There are six families of FMOs, with FMO3 being the most abundant in liver. FMO3 is able to metabolize nicotine, as well as H_2 receptor antagonists (cimetidine and ranitidine), antipsychotics (clozapine), and anti-emetics (itopride). A genetic deficiency in this enzyme causes the *fish-odor syndrome* due to a lack of metabolism of trimethylamine *N*-oxide (TMAO) to trimethylamine (TMA); in the absence of this enzyme, TMAO accumulates in the body and causes a socially offensive fish odor. TMAO is found at high concentrations, up to 15% by weight, in marine animals, where it acts as an osmotic regulator. FMOs are considered minor contributors to drug metabolism and they almost always produce benign metabolites. In addition, FMOs are not induced by any of the xenobiotic receptors (see below) or easily inhibited; thus, in contrast to CYPs, FMOs would not be expected to be involved in drug-drug interactions. In fact, this has been demonstrated by comparing the pathways of metabolism of two drugs used in the control of gastric motility, itopride, and cisapride. Itopride is metabolized by FMO3 while cisapride is metabolized by *CYP3A4*; thus, itopride is less likely to be involved in drug-drug interactions than is cisapride. *CYP3A4* participates in drug-drug interactions through induction and inhibition of metabolism, whereas FMO3 is not induced or inhibited by any clinically used drugs. FMOs could be of importance in the development of new drugs. A candidate drug could be designed by introducing a site for FMO oxidation with the knowledge that favorable metabolism and pharmacokinetic properties could be accurately predicted.

HYDROLYTIC ENZYMES

Two forms of epoxide hydrolase carry out hydrolysis of epoxides, most of which are produced by CYPs. The soluble epoxide hydrolase (sEH) is expressed in the cytosol while the microsomal epoxide hydrolase (mEH) is localized to the membrane of the endoplasmic reticulum. Epoxides are highly reactive electrophiles that can bind to cellular nucleophiles found in protein, RNA, and DNA, resulting in cell toxicity and transformation. Thus, epoxide hydrolases participate in the deactivation of potentially toxic metabolites generated by CYPs. There are a few examples of the influence of mEH on drug metabolism. The anti-epileptic drug carbamazepine is a prodrug that is converted to its pharmacologically active derivative, carbamazepine-10, 11-epoxide by a CYP. This metabolite is efficiently hydrolyzed to a dihydrodiol by mEH, resulting in inactivation of the drug (Figure 6–4). Inhibition of mEH can cause an elevation in plasma concentrations of the active metabolite, causing side effects. The tranquilizer valnoctamide and anticonvulsant valproic acid inhibit mEH, resulting in clinically significant drug interactions with carbamazepine. This has led to efforts to develop new anti-epileptic drugs such as gabapentin and levetiracetam that are metabolized by CYPs and not by EHs.

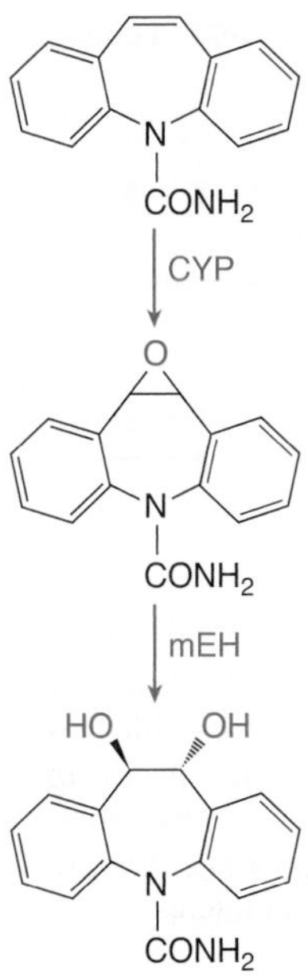

Figure 6–4. Metabolism of carbamazepine by CYP and microsomal epoxide hydrolase (mEH). Carbamazepine is oxidized to the pharmacologically-active metabolite carbamazepine-10, 11-epoxide by CYP. The epoxide is converted to a trans-dihydrodiol by mEH. This metabolite is biologically inactive and can be conjugated by phase 2 enzymes.

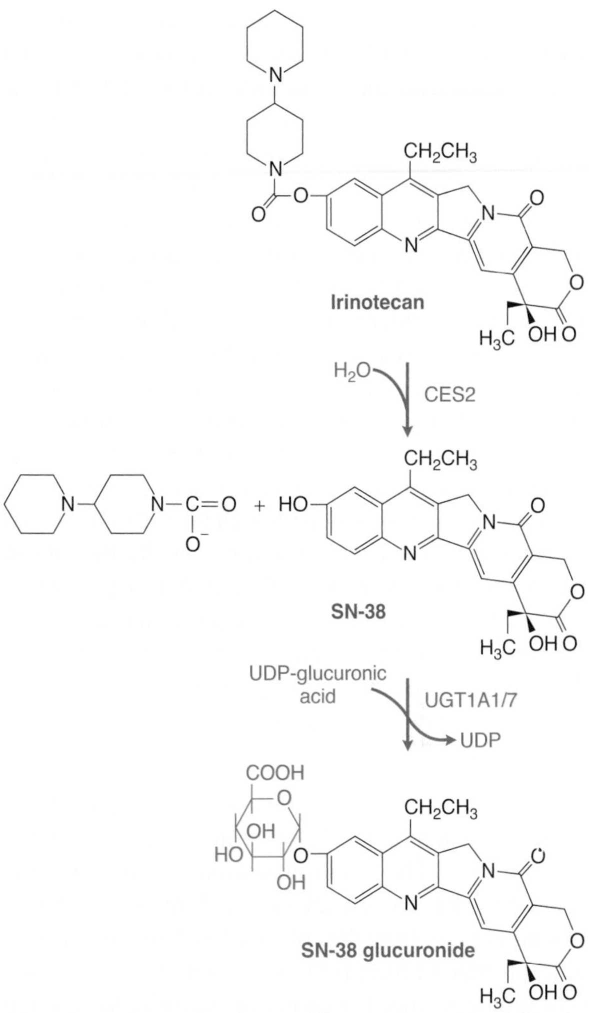

The carboxylesterases comprise a superfamily of enzymes that catalyze the hydrolysis of ester- and amide-containing chemicals. These enzymes are found in both the endoplasmic reticulum and the cytosol of many cell types and are involved in detoxification or metabolic activation of various drugs, environmental toxicants, and carcinogens. Carboxylesterases also catalyze the activation of prodrugs to their respective free acids. For example, the prodrug and cancer chemotherapeutic agent irinotecan is a camptothecin analog that is bioactivated by plasma and intracellular carboxylesterases to SN-38 (Figure 6–5), a potent inhibitor of topoisomerase 1.

Figure 6–5. Metabolism of irinotecan (CPT-11). The pro-drug CPT-11 is initially metabolized by a serum esterase (CES2) to the topoisomerase inhibitor SN-38, which is the active camptothecin analog that slows tumor growth. SN-38 is then subject to glucuronidation, which results in loss of biological activity and facilitates elimination of the SN-38 in the bile.

CONJUGATING ENZYMES (PHASE 2 REACTIONS)

There are a large number of phase 2 conjugating enzymes, all of which are considered to be synthetic in nature since they result in the formation of a metabolite with an increased molecular mass. Phase 2 reactions also normally terminate the biological activity of the drug, although for drugs like morphine and minoxidil, glucuronide and sulfate conjugates, respectively, are more pharmacologically active than the parent. The contributions of different phase 2 reactions to drug metabolism are shown in Figure 6–3B. Two of the phase 2 reactions, glucuronidation and sulfation, result in the formation of metabolites with a significantly increased water-to-lipid partition coefficient, resulting in hydrophilicity and facilitating metabolite accumulation in the aqueous compartments of the cell and the body. While sulfation and acetylation terminate the biological activity of drugs, the solubility properties of these metabolites are altered through minor changes in the overall charge of the molecule. Characteristic of the phase 2 reactions is the dependency on the catalytic reactions for cofactors, (or more correctly, co-substrates) such as UDP-glucuronic acid (UDP-GA) and 3′-phosphoadenosine-5′-phosphosulfate (PAPS), for UDP-glucuronosyltransferases (UGT) and sulfotransferases (SULT), respectively, which react with available functional groups on the substrates. The reactive functional groups are often generated by the phase 1 CYPs, although there are many drugs (e.g., acetaminophen) where glucuronidation and/or sulfation occur directly without prior oxidative metabolism. All of the phase 2 reactions are carried out in the cytosol of the cell, with the exception of glucuronidation, which is localized to the luminal side of the endoplasmic reticulum. *The catalytic rates of phase 2 reactions are significantly faster than the rates of the CYPs.* Thus, if a drug is targeted for phase 1 oxidation through the CYPs, followed by a phase 2 conjugation reaction, usually the rate of elimination will depend upon the initial (phase 1) oxidation reaction. Since the rate of conjugation is faster and the process leads to an increase in hydrophilicity of the drug, phase 2 reactions are generally considered to assure the efficient elimination and detoxification of most drugs.

Glucuronidation. Among the more important of the phase 2 reactions in the metabolism of drugs is that catalyzed by UDP-glucuronosyltransferases (UGTs) (Figure 6–3B). These enzymes catalyze the transfer of glucuronic acid from the cofactor UDP-glucuronic acid to a substrate to form β-D-glucopyranosiduronic acids (glucuronides), metabolites that are sensitive to cleavage by β-glucuronidase. The generation of glucuronides can be formed through alcoholic and phenolic hydroxyl groups, carboxyl, sulfuryl, and carbonyl moieties, as well as through primary, secondary, and tertiary amine linkages. Examples of glucuronidation reactions are shown in Table 6–2 and Figure 6–5. The structural diversity in the many different types of drugs and xenobiotics that are processed through glucuronidation assures that most clinically efficacious therapeutic agents will be excreted as glucuronides.

There are 19 human genes that encode the UGT proteins. Nine are encoded by the *UGT1* locus and 10 are encoded by the *UGT2* family of genes. Both families of proteins are involved in the metabolism of drugs and xenobiotics, while the UGT2 family of proteins appears to have greater specificity for the glucuronidation of endogenous substances such as steroids. The UGT2 proteins are encoded by unique genes on chromosome 4 and the structure of each gene includes six exons. The clustering of the *UGT2* genes on the same chromosome, with a comparable organization of the regions encoding the open reading frames, is evidence that gene duplication has occurred, a process of natural selection that has resulted in the multiplication and eventual diversification of the potential to detoxify the plethora of compounds that are targeted for glucuronidation.

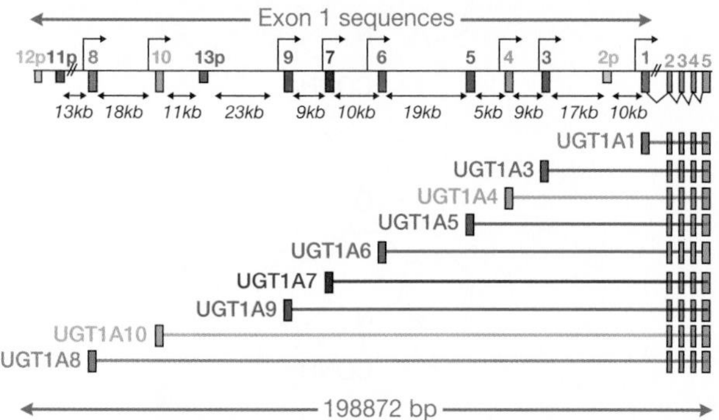

Figure 6–6. *Organization of the UGT1A Locus.* Transcription of the *UGT1A* genes commences with the activation of PolII, which is controlled through tissue-specific events. Conserved exons 2-5 are spliced to each respective exon 1 sequence, resulting in the production of unique *UGT1A* sequences. The *UGT1A* locus encodes nine functional proteins.

The nine functional UGT1 proteins are all encoded by the *UGT1* locus (Figure 6–6), which is located on chromosome 2. The *UGT1* locus spans nearly 200 kb, with over 150 kb of a tandem array of cassette exonic regions that encode ~280 amino acids of the amino terminal portion of the UGT1A proteins. Four exons are located at the 3′ end of the locus that encode the carboxyl 245 amino acids that combine with one of the consecutively numbered array of first exons to form the individual *UGT1* gene products. Since exons 2-5 encode the same sequence for each UGT1A protein, the variability in substrate specificity for each of the UGT1A proteins results from the significant divergence in sequence encoded by the exon 1 regions. The 5′ flanking region of each first-exon cassette contains a fully functional promoter capable of initiating transcription in an inducible and tissue-specific manner.

From a clinical perspective, the expression of UGT1A1 assumes an important role in drug metabolism, since the glucuronidation of bilirubin by UGT1A1 is the rate-limiting step in assuring efficient bilirubin clearance, and this rate can be affected by both genetic variation and competing substrates (drugs). Bilirubin is the breakdown product of heme, 80% of which originates from circulating hemoglobin and 20% from other heme-containing proteins such as the CYPs. Bilirubin is hydrophobic, associates with serum albumin, and must be metabolized further by glucuronidation to assure its elimination. The failure to efficiently metabolize bilirubin by glucuronidation leads to elevated serum levels and a clinical symptom called hyperbilirubinemia or jaundice. There are >50 genetic lesions in the *UGT1A1* gene that can lead to inheritable unconjugated hyperbilirubinemia. Crigler-Najjar syndrome type I is diagnosed as a complete lack of bilirubin glucuronidation; Crigler-Najjar syndrome type II is differentiated by the detection of low amounts of bilirubin glucuronides in duodenal secretions. Types I and II Crigler-Najjar syndrome are rare, and result from genetic polymorphisms in the open reading frames of the *UGT1A1* gene, resulting in abolished or highly diminished levels of functional protein.

Gilbert's syndrome is a generally benign condition that is present in up to 10% of the population; it is diagnosed clinically because circulating bilirubin levels are 60-70% higher than those seen in normal subjects. The most common genetic polymorphism associated with Gilbert's syndrome is a mutation in the *UGT1A1* gene promoter, identified as the UGT1A1*28 allele, which leads to reduced expression levels of UGT1A1. Subjects diagnosed with Gilbert's syndrome may be predisposed to ADRs (Table 6-3) that result from a reduced capacity of UGT1A1 to metabolize drugs. If a drug undergoes selective metabolism by UGT1A1, competition for drug metabolism with bilirubin glucuronidation will exist, resulting in pronounced hyperbilirubinemia as well as reduced clearance of the metabolized drug. Tranilast [N-(3′4′-demethoxycinnamoyl)-anthranilic acid] is an investigational drug used for the prevention of restenosis in patients who have undergone transluminal coronary revascularization (intracoronary stents). Tranilast therapy in patients with Gilbert's syndrome can to lead to hyperbilirubinemia, as well as hepatic complications resulting from elevated levels of tranilast.

Gilbert's syndrome also alters patient responses to irinotecan. Irinotecan, a prodrug used in chemotherapy of solid tumors (see Chapter 61), is metabolized to its active form, SN-38, by serum carboxylesterases (Figure 6–5). SN-38, a potent topoisomerase inhibitor, is inactivated by UGT1A1 and excreted in the bile (Figures 6–7 and 6–8). Once in the lumen of the intestine, the SN-38 glucuronide undergoes cleavage by bacterial β-glucuronidase and reenters the circulation through intestinal absorption. Elevated levels of SN-38 in the blood lead to bone marrow toxicities characterized by leukopenia and neutropenia, as well as damage to the intestinal epithelial cells (Figure 6–8), resulting in acute and life-threatening diarrhea. Patients with Gilbert's syndrome who are receiving irinotecan therapy are predisposed to the hematological and GI toxicities resulting from elevated serum levels of SN-38.

While most of the drugs that are metabolized by UGT1A1 compete for glucuronidation with bilirubin, Gilbert's patients who are HIV-positive and on protease inhibitor therapy with atazanavir (REYATAZ) develop hyperbilirubinemia because the drug inhibits UGT1A1 function. Although atazanavir is not a substrate for glucuronidation, severe hyperbilirubinemia can develop in Gilbert's patients who have inactivating mutations in their *UGT1A3* and *UGT1A7* genes. Clearly, drug-induced side effects attributed to the inhibition of the UGT enzymes can be a significant concern and can be complicated in the presence of gene inactivating polymorphisms.

The UGTs are expressed in a tissue-specific and often inducible fashion in most human tissues, with the highest concentration of enzymes found in the GI tract and liver. Based upon their physicochemical properties, glucuronides are excreted by the kidneys into the urine or through active transport processes through the apical surface of the liver hepatocytes into the bile ducts where they are transported to the duodenum for excretion with components of the bile. Most of the bile acids that are conjugated are reabsorbed from the gut back to the liver via *enterohepatic recirculation*; many drugs that are glucuronidated and excreted in the bile can re-enter the circulation by this same process. The β-D-glucopyranosiduronic acids are targets for β-glucuronidase activity found in resident strains of bacteria that are common in the lower GI tract, thus liberating the free drug into the intestinal lumen. As water is reabsorbed into the large intestine, the free drug can then be transported by passive diffusion or through apical transporters back into the intestinal epithelial cells, from which the drug can then re-enter the circulation. Through portal venous return from the large intestine to the liver, the reabsorption process allows for the reentry of drug into the systemic circulation (Figures 3–7 and 3–8).

Table 6–3

Drug Toxicity and Gilbert's Syndrome

PROBLEM	FEATURE
Gilbert's syndrome	UGT1A1*28 (main variant in Caucasians)
Established toxicity reactions	Irinotecan
	Atazanavir
UGT1A1 substrates (potential risk?)	Gemfibrozil†
	Ezetimibe
	Simvastatin, atorvastatin, cerivastatin†
	Ethinylestradoil
	Buprenorphine
	Fulvestrant
	Ibuprofen, ketoprofen

†A severe drug reaction owing to the inhibition of glucuronidation (UGT1A1) and CYP2C8 and CYP2C9 when both drugs were combined led to the withdrawal of cerivastatin. Reproduced with permission from Strassburg CP. Pharmacogenetics of Gilbert's syndrome. *Pharmacogenomics*, **2008**, 9: 703–715.

Sulfation. The sulfotransferases (SULTs) are cytosolic and conjugate sulfate derived from 3′-phosphoadenosine-5′-phosphosulfate (PAPS) to the hydroxyl and, less frequently, amine groups of aromatic and aliphatic compounds. Like all of the xenobiotic metabolizing enzymes, the SULTs metabolize a wide variety of endogenous and exogenous substrates.

In humans, 13 SULT isoforms have been identified, and based on sequence comparisons, have been classified into the SULT1 (SULT1A1, SULT1A2, SULT1A3/4, SULT1B1, SULT1C1, SULT1C2, SULT1C4, SULT1E1), SULT2 (SULT2A1, SULT2B1a, SULT2B1b), SULT4 (SULT4A1), and SULT6 (SULT6A1) families. SULTs play an important role in normal human homeostasis. For example, SULT2B1b non-covalent and sometimes covalent interactions with compounds that are not substrates for glutathione conjugation. The cytosolic pool of GSTs, once identified as *ligandin*, has been shown to bind steroids, bile acids, bilirubin, cellular hormones, and environmental toxicants, in addition to complexing with other cellular proteins.

Over 20 human GSTs have been identified and divided into two subfamilies: the cytosolic and the microsomal forms. The major differences in function between the microsomal and cytosolic GSTs reside in the selection of substrates for conjugation; the cytosolic forms have more importance in the metabolism of drugs and xenobiotics, whereas the microsomal GSTs are important in the endogenous metabolism of leukotrienes and prostaglandins. The cytosolic GSTs are divided into seven classes termed alpha (GSTA1 and 2), mu (GSTM1 through 5), omega (GSTO1), pi (GSTP1), sigma (GSTS1), theta (GSTT1 and 2), and zeta (GSTZ1). Those in the alpha and mu classes can form heterodimers, allowing for a large number of active transferases to form. The cytosolic forms of GST catalyze conjugation, reduction, and isomerization reactions.

The high concentrations of GSH in the cell and the plenitude of GSTs mean that few reactive molecules escape detoxification. However, while there appears to be an overcapacity of enzyme and reducing equivalents, there is always concern that some reactive intermediates will escape detoxification, and by nature of their electrophilicity, will bind to cellular components, and cause toxicity. The potential for such an occurrence is heightened if GSH is depleted or if a specific form of GST is polymorphic. While it is difficult to deplete cellular GSH levels, reactive therapeutic agents that require large doses for clinical efficacy have the greatest potential to lower cellular GSH levels. Acetaminophen, which is normally metabolized by glucuronidation and sulfation, is also a substrate for oxidative metabolism by CYP2E1 and CYP3A4, which generate the toxic metabolite *N*-acetyl-*p*-benzoquinone imine (NAPQI) that, under normal dosing, is readily neutralized through conjugation with GSH. However, an overdose of acetaminophen can lead to depletion of cellular GSH levels, thereby increasing the potential for NAPQI to interact with other cellular components resulting in toxicity and cell death (see Figure 4-5). Acetaminophen toxicity is associated with increased levels of NAPQI and hepatic necrosis.

Like many of the enzymes involved in drug and xenobiotic metabolism, all of the GSTs have been shown to be polymorphic. The mu (GSTM1*0) and theta (GSTT1*0) genotypes express a null phenotype; thus, individuals that are polymorphic at these loci are predisposed to toxicities by agents that are selective substrates for these GSTs. For example, the mutant GSTM1*0 allele is observed in 50% of the Caucasian population and has been linked genetically to human malignancies of the lung, colon, and bladder. Null activity in the GSTT1 gene has been associated with adverse side effects and toxicity in cancer chemotherapy with cytostatic drugs; the toxicities result from insufficient clearance of the drugs by GSH conjugation. Expression of the null genotype can be as high as 60% in Chinese and Korean populations. GST polymorphisms may influence efficacies and severity of adverse side effects of drugs.

While the GSTs play an important role in cellular detoxification, their activities in cancerous tissues have been linked to the development of drug resistance toward chemotherapeutic agents that are both substrates and nonsubstrates for the GSTs. Many anticancer drugs are effective because they initiate cell death or apoptosis, which is linked to the activation of mitogen-activated protein (MAP) kinases such as JNK and p38. Investigational studies have demonstrated that overexpression of GSTs is associated with resistance to apoptosis and the inhibition of MAP kinase activity. In a variety of tumors, GSTs are overexpressed, leading to a reduction in MAP kinase activity and reduced efficacy of chemotherapy. Taking advantage of the relatively high levels of GST in tumor cells, inhibition of GST activity has been exploited as a therapeutic strategy to modulate drug resistance by sensitizing tumors to anticancer drugs. TLK199, a glutathione analog, serves as a prodrug that undergoes activation by plasma esterases to a GST inhibitor, TLK117, which potentiates the toxicity of different anticancer agents (Figure 6–10). Alternatively, the elevated GST activity in cancer cells has been utilized to develop pro-drugs that can be activated by the GSTs to form electrophilic intermediates. For example, TLK286 is a substrate for GST that undergoes a β-elimination reaction, forming a glutathione conjugate and a nitrogen mustard (Figure 6–11) capable of alkylating cellular nucleophiles, resulting in anti-tumor activity.

N-Acetylation. The cytosolic N-acetyltransferases (NATs) are responsible for the metabolism of drugs and environmental agents that contain an aromatic amine or hydrazine group. The addition of the acetyl group from the cofactor acetyl-coenzyme A often leads to a metabolite that is less water soluble because the potential

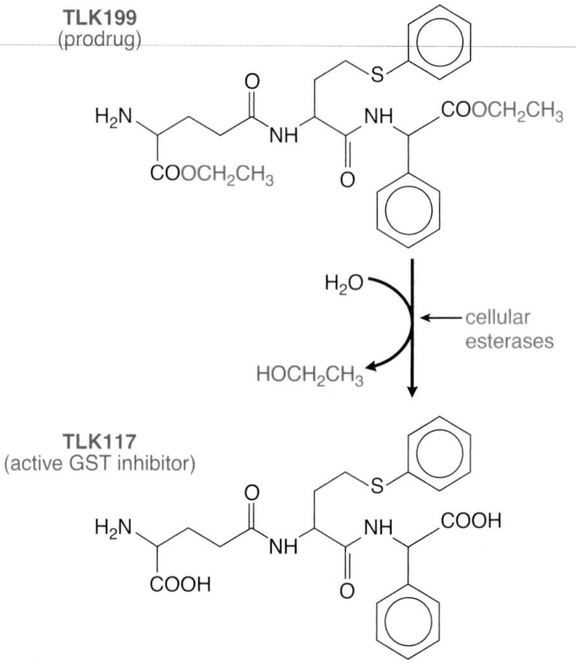

TLK199
(prodrug)

H_2N … NH … S … NH … $COOCH_2CH_3$
$COOCH_2CH_3$

H_2O → cellular esterases → $HOCH_2CH_3$

TLK117
(active GST inhibitor)

H_2N … NH … S … NH … COOH
COOH

Figure 6-10. *Activation of TLK199 by cellular esterases to the glutathione-S-transferase (GST) inhibitor TLK117.* (For additional information, see Townsend and Tew, 2003.)

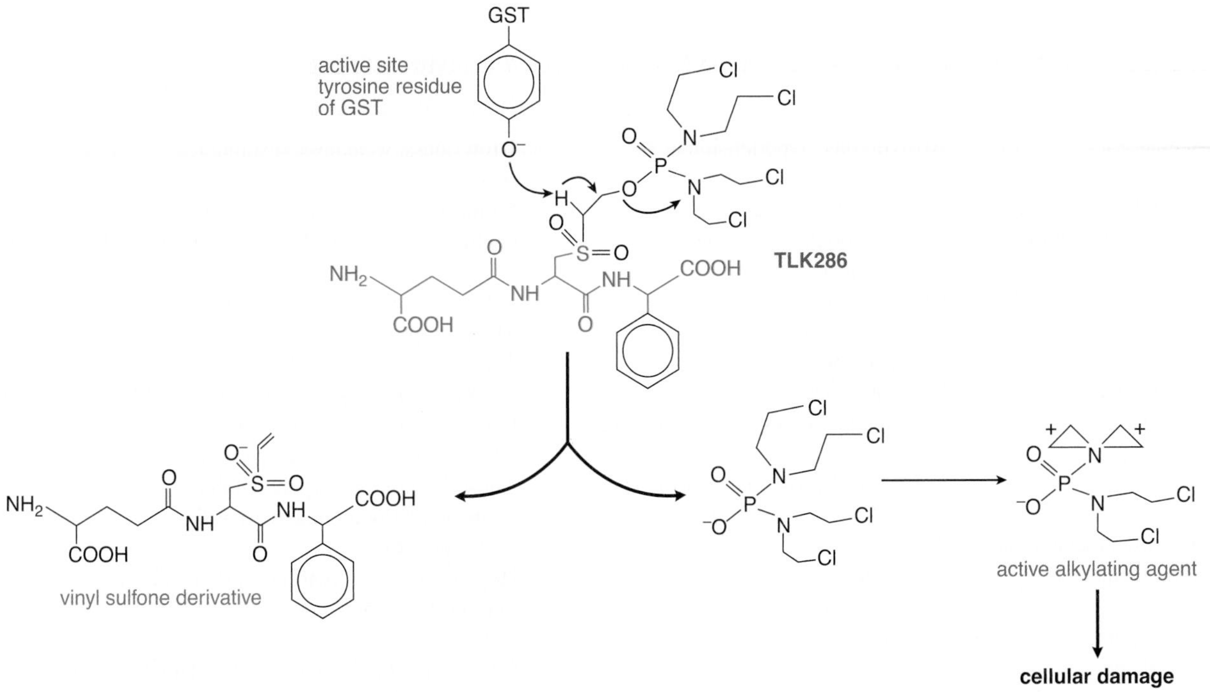

Figure 6-11. *Generation of the reactive alkylating agent following the conjugation of glutathione to TLK286.* GST interacts with the prodrug and GSH analog, TLK286, *via* a tyrosine in the active site of GST. GSH portion is shown in red. The interaction promotes β-elimination and cleavage of the prodrug to a vinyl sulfone and an active alkylating fragment. (*See* Townsend and Tew, 2003.)

ionizable amine is neutralized by the covalent addition of the acetyl group. NATs are among the most polymorphic of all the human xenobiotic drug-metabolizing enzymes.

The characterization of an acetylator phenotype in humans was one of the first hereditary traits identified, and was responsible for the development of the field of pharmacogenetics (see Chapter 7). Following the discovery that isonicotinic acid hydrazide (isoniazid, INH) could be used in the cure of tuberculosis, a significant proportion of the patients (5-15%) experienced toxicities that ranged from numbness and tingling in their fingers to CNS damage. After finding that isoniazid was metabolized by acetylation and excreted in the urine, researchers noted that individuals suffering from the toxic effects of the drug excreted the largest amount of unchanged drug and the least amount of acetylated isoniazid. Pharmacogenetic studies led to the classification of "rapid" and "slow" acetylators, with the "slow" phenotype being predisposed to toxicity. Purification and characterization of N-acetyltransferase and the eventual cloning of its RNA provided sequence characterization of the gene, revealing polymorphisms that correspond to the "slow" acetylator phenotype. There are two functional NAT genes in humans, *NAT1* and *NAT2*. Over 25 allelic variants of *NAT1* and *NAT2* have been characterized, and in individuals in whom acetylation of drugs is compromised, homozygous genotypes for at least two variant alleles are required to predispose a patient to lowered drug metabolism. Polymorphism in the *NAT2* gene, and its association with the slow acetylation of isoniazid, was one of the first completely characterized genotypes shown to affect drug metabolism, thereby linking pharmacogenetic phenotype to a genetic polymorphism. Although nearly as many mutations have been identified in the *NAT1* gene as the *NAT2* gene, the frequency of the slow acetylation patterns are attributed mostly to the polymorphism in the *NAT2* gene.

Drugs that are subject to acetylation and their known toxicities are listed in Table 6–4. The therapeutic relevance of NAT polymorphisms is in avoiding drug-induced toxicities. The adverse drug response in a slow acetylator resembles a drug overdose; thus, reducing the dose or increasing the dosing interval is recommended. Aromatic amine or a hydrazine groups exist in many classes of clinically used drugs, and if a drug is

Table 6–4

Indications and Unwanted Side Effects of Drug Metabolized by *N*-Acetyltransferases

DRUG	INDICATION	MAJOR SIDE EFFECTS
Acebutolol	Arrhythmias, hypertension	Drowsiness, weakness, insomnia
Amantadine	Influenza A, parkinsonism	Appetite loss, dizziness, headache, nightmares
Aminobenzoic acid	Skin disorders, sunscreens	Stomach upset, contact sensitization
Aminoglutethimide	Adrenal cortex carcinoma, breast cancer	Clumsiness, nausea, dizziness, agranulocytosis
Aminosalicylic acid	Ulcerative colitis	Allergic fever, itching, leukopenia
Amonafide	Prostate cancer	Myelosuppression
Amrinone	Advanced heart failure	Thrombocytopenia, arrhythmias
Benzocaine	Local anesthesia	Dermatitis, itching, rash, methemoglobinemia
Caffeine	Neonatal respiratory distress syndrome	Dizziness, insomnia, tachycardia
Clonazepam	Epilepsy	Ataxia, dizziness, slurred speech
Dapsone	Dermatitis, leprosy, AIDS-related complex	Nausea, vomiting, hyperexcitability, methemoglobinemia, dermatitis
Dipyrone, metamizole	Analgesic	Agranulocytosis
Hydralazine	Hypertension	Hypotension, tachycardia, flush, headache
Isoniazid	Tuberculosis	Peripheral neuritis, hepatotoxicity
Nitrazepam	Insomnia	Dizziness, somnolence
Phenelzine	Depression	CNS excitation, insomnia, orthostatic hypotension, hepatotoxicity
Procainamide	Ventricular tachyarrhythmia	Hypotension, systemic lupus erythematosus
Sulfonamides	Antibacterial agents	Hypersensitivity, hemolytic anemia, fever, lupus-like syndromes

For details, *see* Meisel, 2002.

known to be metabolized through acetylation, determining an individual's phenotype can be important in maximizing outcome in subsequent therapy. For example, hydralazine, a once popular orally active antihypertensive (vasodilator) drug, is metabolized by NAT2; the administration of therapeutic doses of hydralazine to a slow acetylator can result in extreme hypotension and tachycardia. Several drugs, such as the sulfonamides, that are known targets for acetylation have been implicated in idiosyncratic hypersensitivity reactions; in such instances, an appreciation of a patient's acetylating phenotype is particularly important. Sulfonamides are transformed into hydroxylamines that interact with cellular proteins, generating haptens that can elicit autoimmune responses. Individuals who are slow acetylators are predisposed to drug-induced autoimmune disorders.

Tissue-specific expression patterns of NAT1 and NAT2 have a significant impact on the fate of drug metabolism and the potential for eliciting a toxic episode. NAT1 is ubiquitously expressed among most human tissues, whereas NAT2 is found predominantly in liver and the GI tract. Both NAT1 and NAT2 can form *N*-hydroxy–acetylated metabolites from bicyclic aromatic hydrocarbons, a reaction that leads to the non-enzymatic release of the acetyl group and the generation of highly reactive nitrenium ions. Thus, *N*-hydroxy acetylation is thought to activate certain environmental toxicants. In contrast, direct *N*-acetylation of bicyclic aromatic amines is stable and leads to detoxification. Individuals who are NAT2 fast acetylators are able to efficiently metabolize and detoxify bicyclic aromatic amines through liver-dependent acetylation. Slow acetylators (NAT2 deficient), however, accumulate bicyclic aromatic amines, which then become substrates for CYP-dependent *N*-oxidation. These N-OH metabolites are eliminated in the urine. In tissues such as bladder epithelium, NAT1 is highly expressed and can efficiently catalyze the *N*-hydroxy acetylation of bicyclic aromatic amines, a process that leads to de-acetylation and the formation of the mutagenic nitrenium ion, especially in NAT2-deficient subjects. Epidemiological studies have shown that slow acetylators are predisposed to bladder cancer if exposed environmentally to bicyclic aromatic amines.

Methylation. In humans, drugs and xenobiotics can undergo O-, N-, and S-methylation. The identification of the individual methyltransferase (MT) is based on the substrate and methyl conjugate. Humans express three *N*-methyltransferases, one catechol-*O*-methyltransferase (COMT), a phenol-*O*-methyltransferase (POMT), a thiopurine *S*-methyltransferase (TPMT), and a thiol methyltransferase (TMT). These MTs exist as monomers and use *S*-adenosyl-methionine (SAM;

AdoMet) as the methyl donor. With the exception of a signature sequence that is conserved among the MTs, there is limited conservation in sequence, indicating that each MT has evolved to display a unique catalytic function. Although the common theme among the MTs is the generation of a methylated product, substrate specificity is high and distinguishes the individual enzymes.

Nicotinamide *N*-methyltransferase (NNMT) methylates serotonin and tryptophan as well as pyridine-containing compounds such as nicotinamide and nicotine. Phenylethanolamine *N*-methyltransferase (PNMT) is responsible for the methylation of the neurotransmitter norepinephrine, forming epinephrine; the histamine *N*-methyltransferase (HNMT) metabolizes drugs containing an imidazole ring such as that found in histamine. COMT methylates the ring hydroxyl groups of neurotransmitters containing a catechol moiety, such as dopamine and norepinephrine, in addition to drugs such as methyldopa and drugs of abuse such as ecstasy (MDMA; 3, 4-methylenedioxymethamphetamine).

From a clinical perspective, the most important MT may be thiopurine *S*-methyltransferase (TPMT), which catalyzes the S-methylation of aromatic and heterocyclic sulfhydryl compounds, including the thiopurine drugs azathioprine (AZA), 6-mercaptopurine (6-MP); and thioguanine. AZA and 6-MP are used for the management of inflammatory bowel disease (see Chapter 47), as well as autoimmune disorders such as systemic lupus erythematosus and rheumatoid arthritis. Thioguanine is used in the treatment of acute myeloid leukemia, and 6-MP is used worldwide for the treatment of childhood acute lymphoblastic leukemia (see Chapters 61-63). Because TPMT is responsible for the detoxification of 6-MP, a genetic deficiency in TPMT can result in severe toxicities in patients taking these drugs. When given orally at clinically established doses, 6-MP serves as a prodrug that is metabolized by hypoxanthine guanine phosphoribosyl transferase (HGPRT) to 6-thioguanine nucleotides (6-TGNs), which become incorporated into DNA and RNA, resulting in arrest of DNA replication and cytotoxicity. The toxic side effects arise when a lack of 6-MP methylation by TPMT causes a buildup of 6-MP, resulting in the generation of toxic levels of 6-TGNs. The identification of the inactive TPMT alleles and the development of a genotyping test to identify homozygous carriers of the defective allele have now made it possible to identify individuals who may be predisposed to the toxic side effects of 6-MP therapy. Simple adjustments in the patient's dosage regiment have been shown to be a life-saving intervention for those with TPMT deficiencies.

ROLE OF XENOBIOTIC METABOLISM IN THE SAFE AND EFFECTIVE USE OF DRUGS

Any xenobiotics entering the body must be eliminated through metabolism and excretion in the urine or bile/feces. This mechanism keeps foreign compounds from accumulating in the body and possibly causing toxicity. In the case of drugs, metabolism normally results in the inactivation of their therapeutic effectiveness and facilitates their elimination. The extent of metabolism can determine the efficacy and toxicity of a drug by controlling its biological $t_{1/2}$. Among the most serious considerations in the clinical use of drugs are ADRs. If a drug is metabolized too quickly, it rapidly loses its therapeutic efficacy. This can occur if specific enzymes involved in metabolism are naturally overly active or are induced by dietary or environmental factors. If a drug is metabolized too slowly, the drug can accumulate in the bloodstream; as a consequence, the pharmacokinetic parameter AUC (area under the plasma concentration-time curve) is elevated and the plasma clearance of the drug is decreased. This increase in AUC can lead to overstimulation or excessive inhibition of some target receptors or undesired binding to other cellular macromolecules. An increase in AUC often results when specific xenobiotic-metabolizing enzymes are inhibited, which can occur when an individual is taking a combination of different therapeutic agents and one of those drugs targets the enzyme involved in drug metabolism. For example, the consumption of grapefruit juice with drugs taken orally can inhibit intestinal CYP3A4, blocking the metabolism of many of these drugs. The inhibition of specific CYPs in the gut by dietary consumption of grapefruit juice alters the oral bioavailability of many classes of drugs, such as certain antihypertensives, immunosuppressants, antidepressants, antihistamines, and statins, to name a few. Among the components of grapefruit juice that inhibit CYP3A4 are naringin and furanocoumarins.

While environmental factors can alter the steady-state levels of specific enzymes or inhibit their catalytic potential, these phenotypic changes in drug metabolism are also observed clinically in groups of individuals that are genetically predisposed to adverse drug reactions because of pharmacogenetic differences in the expression of xenobiotic-metabolizing enzymes (see Chapter 7). Most of the xenobiotic-metabolizing enzymes display polymorphic differences in their expression, resulting from heritable changes in the structure of the genes. For example, as discussed earlier, a significant population was found to be hyperbilirubinemic, resulting from a reduction in the ability to glucuronidate circulating bilirubin due to a lowered expression of the *UGT1A1* gene (Gilbert's syndrome). Drugs that are subject to glucuronidation by UGT1A1, such as the topoisomerase inhibitor SN-38 (Figures 6–5, 6–7, and 6–8), will display an increased AUC because individuals with Gilbert's syndrome are unable to detoxify these drugs. Since most cancer chemotherapeutic agents have a very narrow therapeutic index, increases in the circulating levels of the active form can result in significant toxicities. There are a number of genetic differences in CYPs that can have a major impact on drug therapy.

Nearly every class of therapeutic agent has been reported to initiate an adverse drug response (ADR). In the U.S., the annual costs of ADRs have been estimated at over 100,000 deaths and $100 billion. It has been estimated that 56% of drugs that are associated with adverse responses are subjected to metabolism by the xenobiotic-metabolizing enzymes, notably the CYPs and UGTs. Since many of the CYPs and UGTs are subject to induction as well as inhibition by drugs, dietary factors, and other environmental agents, these enzymes play an important role in most ADRs. Thus, before a new drug application (NDA) is filed with the Food and Drug Administration, the route of metabolism and the enzymes involved in the metabolism must be known. As a result, it is now routine practice in the pharmaceutical industry to establish which enzymes are involved in metabolism of a drug candidate and to identify the metabolites and determine their potential toxicity.

Induction of Drug Metabolism

Xenobiotics can influence the extent of drug metabolism by activating transcription and inducing the expression of genes encoding drug-metabolizing enzymes. Thus, a foreign compound may induce its own metabolism, as may certain drugs. One potential consequence of this is a decrease in plasma drug concentration over the course of treatment, resulting in loss of efficacy, as the auto-induced metabolism of the drug exceeds the rate at which new drug enters the body. Many ligands and receptors participate in this way to induce drug metabolism (Table 6–5). A particular receptor, when activated by a ligand, can induce the transcription of a battery of target genes. Among these target genes are certain CYPs and drug transporters. Thus, any drug that is a ligand for a receptor that induces CYPs and transporters could lead to drug interactions. Figure 6–12 shows the scheme by which a drug may interact with nuclear receptors to induce its own metabolism.

The aryl hydrocarbon receptor (AHR) is a member of a superfamily of transcription factors with diverse roles in mammals, such as a regulatory role in the development of the mammalian CNS and modulating the response to chemical and oxidative stress. This superfamily of transcription factors includes Period (Per) and Simpleminded (Sim), two transcription factors involved in development of the CNS, and the HIF (hypoxia-inducible factor) family of transcription factors that activate genes in response to low cellular O_2 levels. The AHR induces expression of genes encoding CYP1A1, CYP1A2, and CYP1B1, three CYPs that are able to metabolically activate chemical carcinogens, including environmental contaminants and carcinogens derived from food. Many of these substances are inert unless metabolized by CYPs. Thus, induction of these CYPs by a drug could potentially result in an increase in the toxicity and carcinogenicity of procarcinogens. For example, omeprazole, a proton pump inhibitor used to treat gastric and duodenal ulcers (see Chapter 45), is a ligand for the AHR and can induce CYP1A1 and CYP1A2, with the possible consequences of toxin/carcinogen activation as well as drug-drug interactions in patients receiving agents that are substrates for either of these CYPs.

Another important induction mechanism is due to type 2 nuclear receptors that are in the same superfamily as the steroid hormone receptors. Many of these receptors, identified on the basis of their structural similarity to steroid hormone receptors, were originally termed "orphan receptors," because no endogenous ligands were known to interact with them. Subsequent studies revealed that some of these receptors are activated by xenobiotics, including drugs. The type 2 nuclear receptors of most importance to drug metabolism and drug therapy include the pregnane X receptor (PXR), constitutive androstane receptor (CAR), and the peroxisome proliferator activated receptors (PPARs). PXR, discovered because it is activated by the synthetic steroid pregnenolone-16α-carbonitrile, is also activated by a number of other drugs including, antibiotics (rifampicin and troleandomycin), Ca^{2+} channel blockers (nifedipine), statins (mevastatin), anti-diabetic drugs

Table 6–5

Nuclear Receptors That Induce Drug Metabolism

RECEPTOR	LIGANDS
Aryl hydrocarbon receptor (AHR)	Omeprazole
Constitutive androstane receptor (CAR)	Phenobarbital
Pregnane X receptor (PXR)	Rifampin
Farnesoid X receptor (FXR)	Bile acids
Vitamin D receptor	Vitamin D
Peroxisome proliferator activated receptor (PPAR)	Fibrates
Retinoic acid receptor (RAR)	*all-trans*-Retinoic acid
Retinoid X receptor (RXR)	9-*cis*-Retinoic acid

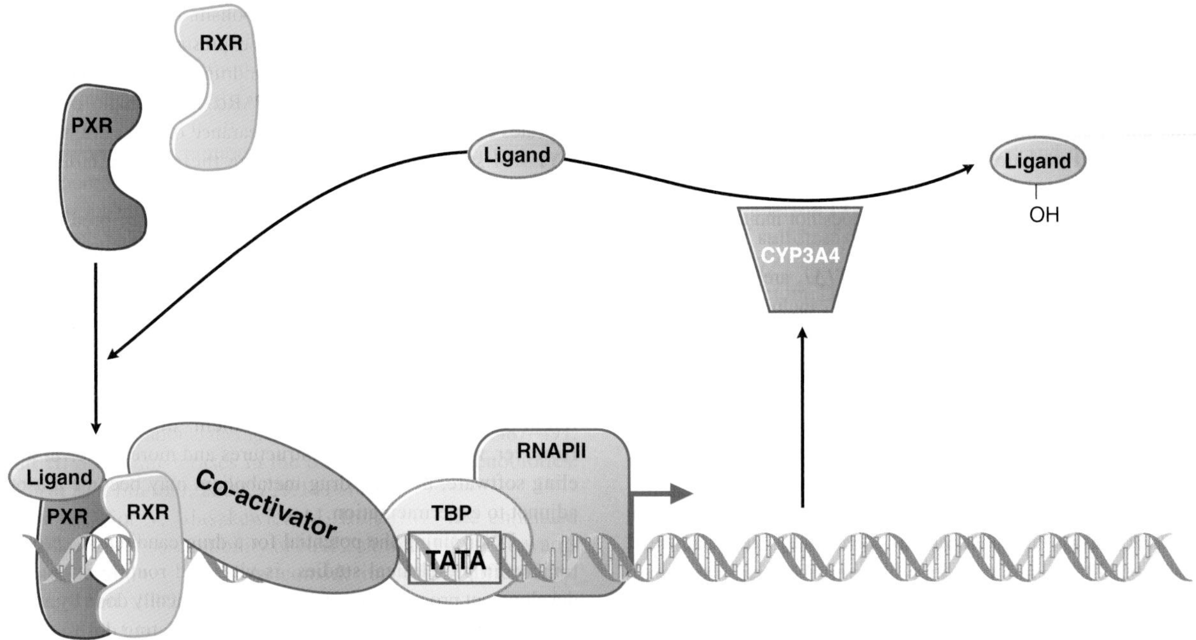

Figure 6–12. *Induction of drug metabolism by nuclear receptor–mediated signal transduction.* When a drug such as atorvastatin (Ligand) enters the cell, it can bind to a nuclear receptor such as the pregnane X receptor (PXR). PXR then forms a complex with the retinoid X receptor (RXR), binds to DNA upstream of target genes, recruits coactivator (which binds to the TATA box binding protein, TBP), and activates transcription by RNA polymerase II (RNAP II). Among PXR target genes are CYP3A4, which can metabolize the atorvastatin and decrease its cellular concentration. Thus, atorvastatin induces its own metabolism. Atorvastatin undergoes both *ortho* and *para* hydroxylation. (*See* Handschin and Meyer, 2003.)

(troglitazone), HIV protease inhibitors (ritonavir), and anticancer drugs (paclitaxel). Hyperforin, a component of St. John's wort, an over-the-counter herbal remedy used for depression, also activates PXR. This activation is thought to be the basis for the increase in failure of oral contraceptives in individuals taking St. John's wort: Activated PXR is an inducer of CYP3A4, which can metabolize steroids found in oral contraceptives. PXR also induces the expression of genes encoding certain drug transporters and phase 2 enzymes including SULTs and UGTs. Thus, PXR facilitates the metabolism and elimination of xenobiotics, including drugs, with notable consequences (Figure 6–12).

The nuclear receptor CAR was discovered based on its ability to activate genes in the absence of ligand. Steroids such as androstanol, the antifungal agent clotrimazole, and the anti-emetic meclizine are inverse agonists that inhibit gene activation by CAR, while the pesticide 1,4-bis[2-(3,5-dichloropyridyloxy)]benzene, the steroid 5-β-pregnane-3,20-dione, and probably other endogenous compounds, are agonists that activate gene expression when bound to CAR. Genes induced by CAR include those encoding several CYPs (*CYP2B6*, *CYP2C9*, and *CYP3A4*), various phase 2 enzymes (including GSTs, UGTs, and SULTs), and drug and endobiotic transporters. CYP3A4 is induced by both PXR and CAR and thus its level is highly influenced by a number of drugs and other xenobiotics. In addition to a potential role in inducing the degradation of drugs including the over-the-counter analgesic acetaminophen, this receptor may function in the control of bilirubin degradation, the process by which the liver decomposes heme.

Clearly, PXR and CAR have a capacity for binding a great variety of ligands. As with the xenobiotic-metabolizing enzymes, species differences also exist in the ligand specificities of these receptors. For example, rifampin activates human PXR, but not mouse or rat PXR, while pregnenolone-16α-carbonitrile preferentially activates the mouse and rat PXR. Paradoxically, meclizine activates mouse CAR, but inhibits gene induction by human CAR. These findings further underscore that data from rodent model systems do not always reflect the response of humans to drugs.

Members of a receptor family do not always show similar activities toward xenobiotics. The peroxisome proliferator activated receptor (PPAR) family has three members, α, β, and γ. PPARα is

Pharmacogenetics

Mary V. Relling and
Kathleen M. Giacomini

Pharmacogenetics is the study of the genetic basis for variation in drug response. In this broadest sense, pharmacogenetics encompasses pharmacogenomics, which employs tools for surveying the entire genome to assess multigenic determinants of drug response. Prior to the technical advances in genomics of the last decade, pharmacogenetics proceeded using a forward genetic, phenotype-to-genotype approach. Drug response outliers were compared to individuals with "normal" drug response to identify the pharmacologic basis of altered response. An inherited component to response was demonstrated using family studies or imputed through intra- *vs.* intersubject reproducibility studies. With the explosion of technology in genomics, a reverse genetic, genotype-to-phenotype approach is feasible whereby genomic polymorphisms can serve as the starting point to assess whether genomic variability translates into phenotypic variability.

Individuals differ from each other approximately every 300-1000 nucleotides, with an estimated total of 10 million single nucleotide polymorphisms (SNPs; single base pair substitutions found at frequencies ≥1% in a population) and thousands of copy number variations in the genome (International HapMap et al., 2007; Redon et al., 2006; Stranger et al., 2007). Identifying which of these variants or combinations of variants have functional consequence for drug effects is the task of modern pharmacogenetics.

Historical Context. In the pre-genomics era, the frequency of genetic variation was hypothesized to be relatively uncommon, and the demonstration of inherited drug-response traits applied to a relatively small number of drugs and pathways (Eichelbaum and Gross, 1990; Evans and Relling, 2004; Johnson and Lima, 2003). Historically, uncommon severe drug-induced phenotypes served as the triggers to investigate and document pharmacogenetic phenotypes. Prolonged neuromuscular blockade following normal doses of succinylcholine, neurotoxicity following isoniazid therapy (Hughes et al., 1954), and methemoglobinemia in glucose-6-phosphate dehydrogenase (G6PD) deficiency (Alving et al., 1956) were discovered to have a genetic basis in the first half of the 20th century. In the 1970s and 1980s, debrisoquine hydroxylation and exaggerated hypotensive effects from that drug were related to an autosomal recessive inherited deficiency in the cytochrome P450 isoenzyme 2D6 (CYP2D6) (Evans and Relling, 2004). Since the elucidation of the molecular basis of the phenotypic polymorphism in CYP2D6 (Gonzalez et al., 1988), the molecular bases of many other monogenic pharmacogenetic traits have been identified (Meyer and Zanger, 1997).

Importance of Pharmacogenetics to Variability in Drug Response

Drug response is considered to be a gene-by-environment phenotype. That is, an individual's response to a drug depends on the complex interplay between environmental factors and genetic factors (Figure 7–1). Variation in drug response therefore may be explained by variation in environmental and genetic factors, alone or in combination. What proportion of drug-response variability is likely to be genetically determined? Classical family studies provide some information (Weinshilboum and Wang, 2004).

Because estimating the fraction of phenotypic variability that is attributable to genetic factors in pharmacogenetics usually requires administration of a drug to twins or trios of family members, data are somewhat limited. Twin studies have shown that drug metabolism is highly heritable, with genetic factors accounting for most of the variation in metabolic rates for many drugs (Vesell, 2000). Results from a twin study in which the $t_{1/2}$ of antipyrine was measured are typical (Figure 7–2). Antipyrine, a pyrazolone analgesic, is eliminated exclusively by metabolism and is a substrate for multiple CYPs. There is considerably greater concordance in the $t_{1/2}$ of antipyrine between the monozygotic (identical) twin pairs in comparison to the dizygotic (fraternal) twin pairs. Comparison of intra-twin *vs.* inter-pair variability suggests that ~75-85% of the variability in pharmacokinetic half-lives for drugs that are eliminated by metabolism is heritable (Penno et al., 1981). It has also been proposed that heritability can be estimated by comparing intra-subject *vs.* inter-subject variability in drug response or disposition in unrelated individuals (Kalow et al., 1998), with the assumption that high intra-subject reproducibility translates into high heritability; the validity of this method across pharmacologic phenotypes remains to be established. In any case, such studies provide only an estimate of

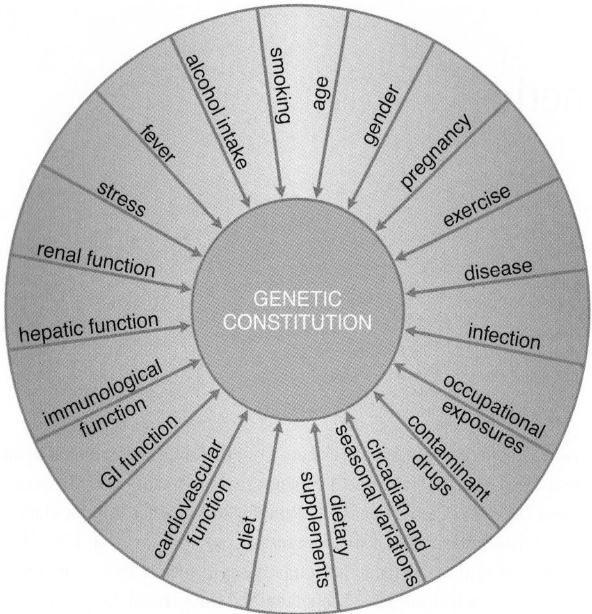

Figure 7–1. *Exogenous and endogenous factors contribute to variation in drug response.* (Reproduced with permission from Vesell, 1991. Copyright © Elsevier.)

the overall contribution of inheritance to the phenotype; because multiple gene products contribute to antipyrine disposition, most of which have unelucidated mechanisms of genetic variability, the predictability of antipyrine disposition based on known genetic variability is poor.

Extended kindreds may be used to estimate heritability. This approach to estimating the degree of heritability of a pharmacogenetic phenotype uses *ex vivo* experiments with cell lines derived from related individuals from extended multigenerational families. Inter- *vs.* intrafamily variability and relationships among members of a kindred are used to estimate heritability. Using this approach with lymphoblastoid cells, cytotoxicity from chemotherapeutic agents was shown to be heritable, with ~20-70% of the variability in sensitivity to 5-fluorouracil, cisplatin, docetaxel and other anticancer agents estimated as inherited (Hartford and Dolan, 2007; Watters et al., 2004).

For the "monogenic" phenotypic traits of G6PD deficiency, CYP2D6, or thiopurine methyltransferase (TPMT) metabolism, it is often possible to predict phenotype based on genotype. Several genetic polymorphisms of drug metabolizing enzymes result in monogenic traits. Based on a retrospective study, 49% of adverse drug reactions were associated with drugs that are substrates for polymorphic drug metabolizing enzymes, a proportion larger than estimated for all drugs (22%) or for top-selling drugs (7%) (Phillips et al., 2001). Prospective genotype determinations may result in the ability to prevent adverse drug reactions.

Defining multigenic contributors to drug response will be much more challenging. For some multigenic phenotypes, such as response to antihypertensives, the large numbers of candidate genes will necessitate a large patient sample size to produce the statistical power required to solve the "multigene" problem.

GENOMIC BASIS OF PHARMACOGENETICS

Phenotype-Driven Terminology

Because initial discoveries in pharmacogenetics were driven by variable phenotypes and defined by family and twin studies, the classic genetic terms for monogenic traits apply to some pharmacogenetic polymorphisms. A trait (e.g., CYP2D6 "poor metabolism") is deemed autosomal recessive if the responsible gene is located on an autosome (i.e., it is not sex-linked) and a distinct

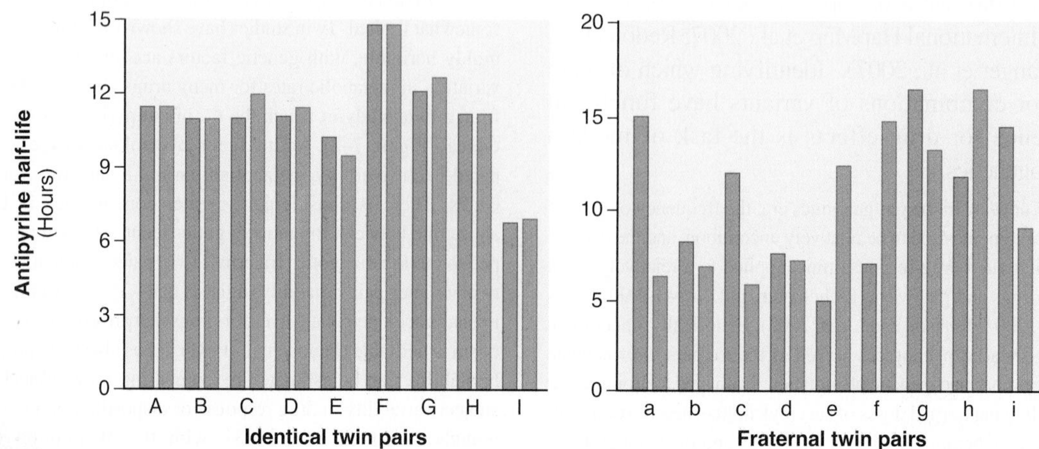

Figure 7–2. *Pharmacogenetic contribution to pharmacokinetic parameters.* $t_{1/2}$ of antipyrine is more concordant in identical in comparison to fraternal twin pairs. Bars show the $t_{1/2}$ of antipyrine in identical (monozygotic) and fraternal (dizygotic) twin pairs. (Redrawn from data in Vesell and Page, 1968.)

phenotype is evident only with nonfunctional alleles on both the maternal and paternal chromosomes. An autosomal recessive trait does not appear in heterozygotes. A trait is deemed codominant if heterozygotes exhibit a phenotype that is intermediate to that of homozygotes for the common allele and homozygotes for the variant allele. For example, TPMT catabolism of thiopurines exhibits three relatively distinct phenotypes, and thus was deemed codominant even in the pre-molecular era. With the advances in molecular characterization of polymorphisms and a genotype-to-phenotype approach, many polymorphic traits (e.g., CYP2C19 metabolism of drugs such as mephenytoin and omeprazole) are now recognized to exhibit some degree of codominance. Some pharmacogenetic traits, such as the long QT syndrome, segregate as dominant traits; the long QT syndrome is associated with heterozygous loss-of-function mutations of ion channels. A prolonged QT interval is seen on the electrocardiogram, either basally or in the presence of certain drugs, and individuals with prolonged QT intervals are predisposed to cardiac arrhythmias (see Chapter 29).

In an era of detailed molecular characterization, two major factors complicate the historical designation of recessive, co-dominant, and dominant traits. *First*, even within a single gene, a vast array of polymorphisms (promoter, coding, noncoding, completely inactivating, or modestly modifying) are possible. Each polymorphism may produce a different effect on gene function and therefore differentially affect a measured trait. For example, the effect of a polymorphism with only a modest effect on the function of an enzyme will only be observed in individuals who are homozygous for the polymorphism. Heterozygotes will not exhibit any measureable changes in enzyme activity. In contrast, the effect of a polymorphism that exhibits complete loss of function of the enzyme will be large and may be observed phenotypically in heterozygotes. *Secondly*, most traits (pharmacogenetic and otherwise) are multigenic, not monogenic. Thus, even if the designations of recessive, co-dominant, and dominant are informative for a given gene, their utility in describing the genetic variability that underlies variability in drug response phenotype is diminished, because most phenotypic variability is likely to be multigenic.

Types of Genetic Variants

A *polymorphism* is a variation in the DNA sequence that is present at an allele frequency of 1% or greater in a population. Two major types of sequence variation have been associated with variation in human phenotype: *single nucleotide polymorphisms* (SNPs) and *insertions/deletions* (indels) (Figure 7–3). In comparison to base pair

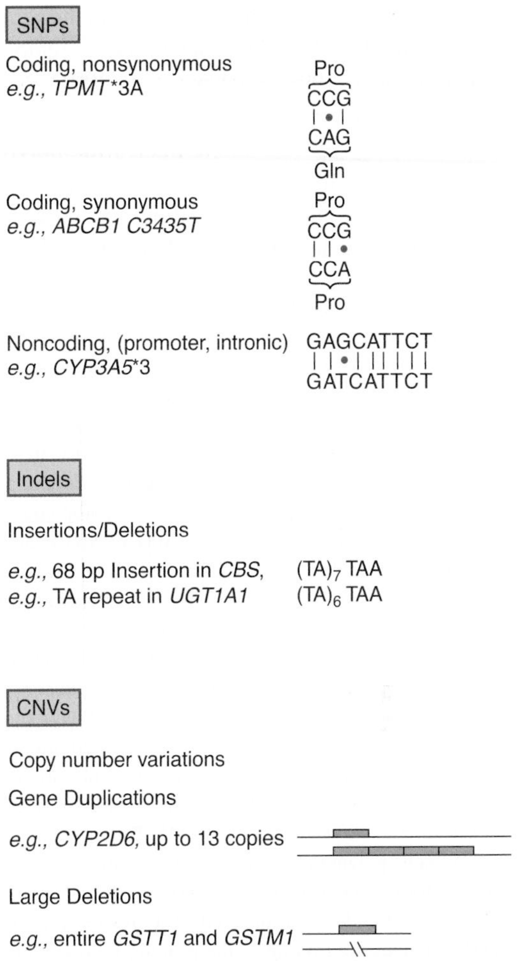

SNPs

Coding, nonsynonymous
*e.g., TPMT**3A
Pro CCG / CAG Gln

Coding, synonymous
e.g., ABCB1 C3435T
Pro CCG / CCA Pro

Noncoding, (promoter, intronic)
*e.g., CYP3A5**3
GAGCATTCT / GATCATTCT

Indels

Insertions/Deletions

e.g., 68 bp Insertion in *CBS*, (TA)$_7$ TAA
e.g., TA repeat in *UGT1A1* (TA)$_6$ TAA

CNVs

Copy number variations

Gene Duplications

e.g., CYP2D6, up to 13 copies

Large Deletions

e.g., entire *GSTT1* and *GSTM1*

Figure 7–3. *Molecular mechanisms of genetic polymorphisms.* The most common genetic variants are single nucleotide polymorphism substitutions (SNPs). Coding non-synonymous SNPs result in a nucleotide substitution that changes the amino acid codon (here proline to glutamine), which could change protein structure, stability, substrate affinities, or introduce a stop codon. Coding synonymous SNPs do not change the amino acid codon, but may have functional consequences (transcript stability, splicing). Noncoding SNPs may be in promoters, introns, or other regulatory regions that may affect transcription factor binding, enhancers, transcript stability, or splicing. The second major type of polymorphism is indels (insertion/deletions). SNP indels can have any of the same effects as SNP substitutions: short repeats in the promoter (which can affect transcript amount), or insertions/deletions that add or subtract amino acids. Copy number variations (CNVs) involve large segments of genomic DNA that may involve gene duplications (stably transmitted inherited germline gene replication that causes increased protein expression and activity), gene deletions that result in the complete lack of protein production, or inversions of genes that may disrupt gene function. All of these mechanisms have been implicated in common germline pharmacogenetic polymorphisms. TPMT, thiopurine methyltransferase; ABCB1, the multidrug resistance transporter (P-glycoprotein); CYP, cytochrome P450; CBS, cystathionine β-synthase; UGT, UDP-glucuronyl transferase; GST, glutathione-S-transferase.

substitutions, indels are much less frequent in the genome and are of particularly low frequency in coding regions of genes (Cargill et al., 1999; Stephens et al., 2001). Single base pair substitutions that are present at frequencies ≥1% in a population are termed single nucleotide polymorphisms (SNPs) and are present in the human genome at ~1 SNP every few hundred to a thousand base pairs, depending on the gene region (Stephens et al., 2001).

SNPs in the coding region are termed cSNPs, and are further classified as non-synonymous (or *missense*) if the base pair change results in an amino acid substitution, or synonymous (or *sense*) if the base pair substitution within a codon does not alter the encoded amino acid. Typically, substitutions of the third base pair, termed the *wobble position*, in a three base pair codon, such as the G to A substitution in proline shown in Figure 7–3, do not alter the encoded amino acid. Base pair substitutions that lead to a stop codon are termed *nonsense* mutations. In addition, ~10% of SNPs can have more than two possible alleles (e.g., a C can be replaced by either an A or G), so that the same polymorphic site can be associated with amino acid substitutions in some alleles but not others.

Synonymous polymorphisms have sometimes been found to contribute directly to a phenotypic trait. One of the most notable examples is a polymorphism in ABCB1, which encodes P-glycoprotein, an efflux pump that interacts with many clinically used drugs. The synonymous polymorphism, C3435T, is associated with various phenotypes and has been the subject of numerous studies (Hoffmeyer et al., 2000; Kim et al., 2006; Sills et al., 2005; Turgut et al., 2007). This synonymous polymorphism results in a change from a preferred codon for isoleucine to a less preferred codon. Presumably, the less preferred codon is translated at a slower rate, which apparently changes the folding of the protein, its insertion into the membrane, and its interaction with drugs (Kimchi-Sarfaty et al., 2007).

Polymorphisms in noncoding regions of genes may occur in the 3′ and 5′ untranslated regions, in promoter or enhancer regions, in intronic regions, or in large regions between genes, intergenic regions (Figure 7–4). Polymorphisms in introns found near exon-intron boundaries are often treated as a separate category from other intronic polymorphisms since these may affect splicing, and thereby affect function. Noncoding SNPs in promoters or enhancers may alter *cis*- or *trans*-acting elements that regulate gene transcription or transcript stability. Noncoding SNPs in introns or exons may create alternative exon splicing sites, and the altered transcript may have fewer or more exons, or shorter or larger exons, than the wild-type transcript. Introduction or deletion of exonic sequence can cause a frame shift in the translated protein and thereby change protein structure or function, or result in an early stop codon, which makes an unstable or nonfunctional protein. Because 95% of the genome is intergenic, most polymorphisms are unlikely to directly affect the encoded transcript or protein. However, intergenic polymorphisms may have biological consequences by affecting DNA tertiary structure, interaction with chromatin and topoisomerases, or DNA replication. Thus, intergenic polymorphisms cannot be assumed to be without pharmacogenetic importance.

A remarkable degree of diversity in the types of insertions/deletions that are tolerated as germline polymorphisms is evident. A common glutathione-S-transferase M1 (*GSTM1*) polymorphism is caused by a 50-kilobase (kb) germline deletion, and the null allele has a population frequency of 0.3-0.5, depending on race/ethnicity. Biochemical studies indicate that livers from homozygous null individuals have only ~50% of the glutathione conjugating capacity of those with at least one copy of the *GSTM1* gene (Townsend and Kew, 2003). The number of TA repeats in the *UGT1A1* promoter affects the quantitative expression of this crucial glucuronosyl transferase in liver; although 4-9 TA repeats exist in germline-inherited alleles, 6 or 7 repeats constitute the most common alleles (Monaghan et al., 1996). Cystathionine β-synthase has a common 68 base pair insertion/deletion polymorphism that has been linked to folate levels (Kraus et al., 1998). Some deletion and duplication polymorphisms can be seen as a special case of copy number variations (CNVs) (Beckmann et al., 2007; Redon et al., 2006; Stranger et al., 2007). A CNV is a segment of DNA in which a variable number of that segment has been found in one or more populations. CNVs, which range in size from 1 kb to many megabases, are caused by genomic rearrangements including duplications, deletions, and inversions. CNVs appear to occur in ~10% of the human genome and in one study accounted for ~18% of the detected genetic variation in expression of around 15,000 genes in lymphoblastoid cell lines (Stranger et al., 2007). Because of their size, CNVs are likely to affect phenotype. There are notable examples of CNVs in pharmacogenetics; gene duplications of CYP2D6 are associated with an ultra-rapid metabolizer phenotype.

A *haplotype*, which is defined as a series of alleles found at a linked locus on a chromosome, specifies the DNA sequence variation

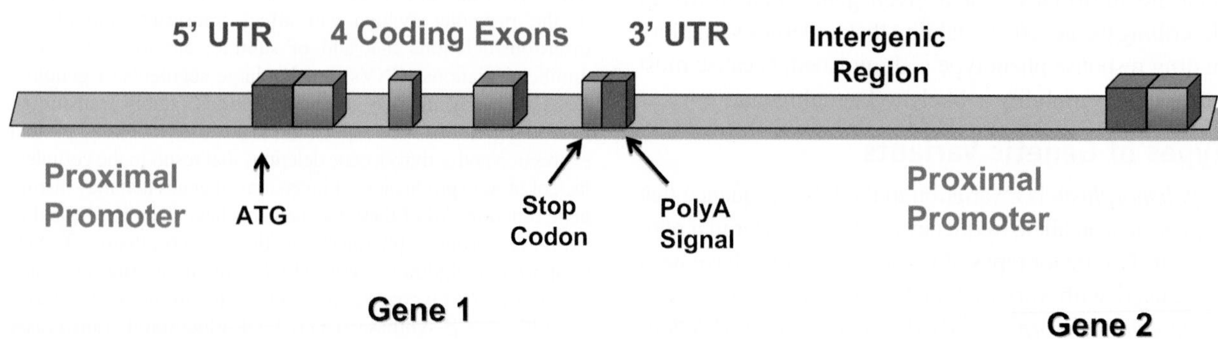

Figure 7–4. *Nomenclature of genomic regions.*

in a gene or a gene region on one chromosome. For example, consider two SNPs in *ABCB1*, which encodes for the multidrug resistance protein, P-glycoprotein. One SNP is a T to A base pair substitution at position 3421 and the other is a C to T change at position 3435. Possible haplotypes would be $T_{3421}C_{3435}$, $T_{3421}T_{3435}$, $A_{3421}C_{3435}$, and $A_{3421}T_{3435}$. For any gene, individuals will have two haplotypes, one maternal and one paternal in origin, which may or may not be identical. Haplotypes are important because they are the functional unit of the gene. That is, a haplotype represents the constellation of variants that occur together for the gene on each chromosome. In some cases, this constellation of variants, rather than the individual variant or allele, may be functionally important. In others, however, a single mutation may be functionally important regardless of other linked variants within the haplotype(s).

Two terms are useful in describing the relationship of genotypes at two loci: linkage equilibrium and linkage disequilibrium. Linkage equilibrium occurs when the genotype present at one locus is independent of the genotype at the second locus. Linkage disequilibrium occurs when the genotypes at the two loci are not independent of one another. In complete linkage disequilibrium, genotypes at two loci always occur together. As recombination occurs then linkage disequilibrium between two alleles will decay and linkage equilibrium will result. Over many generations, with many recombination events, linkage disequilibrium will be eliminated. Patterns of linkage disequilibrium are population specific. For any gene region, linkage disequilibrium among individuals between SNPs in that region may be viewed using a software tool such as Haploview (Barrett et al., 2005) (Figure 7–5).

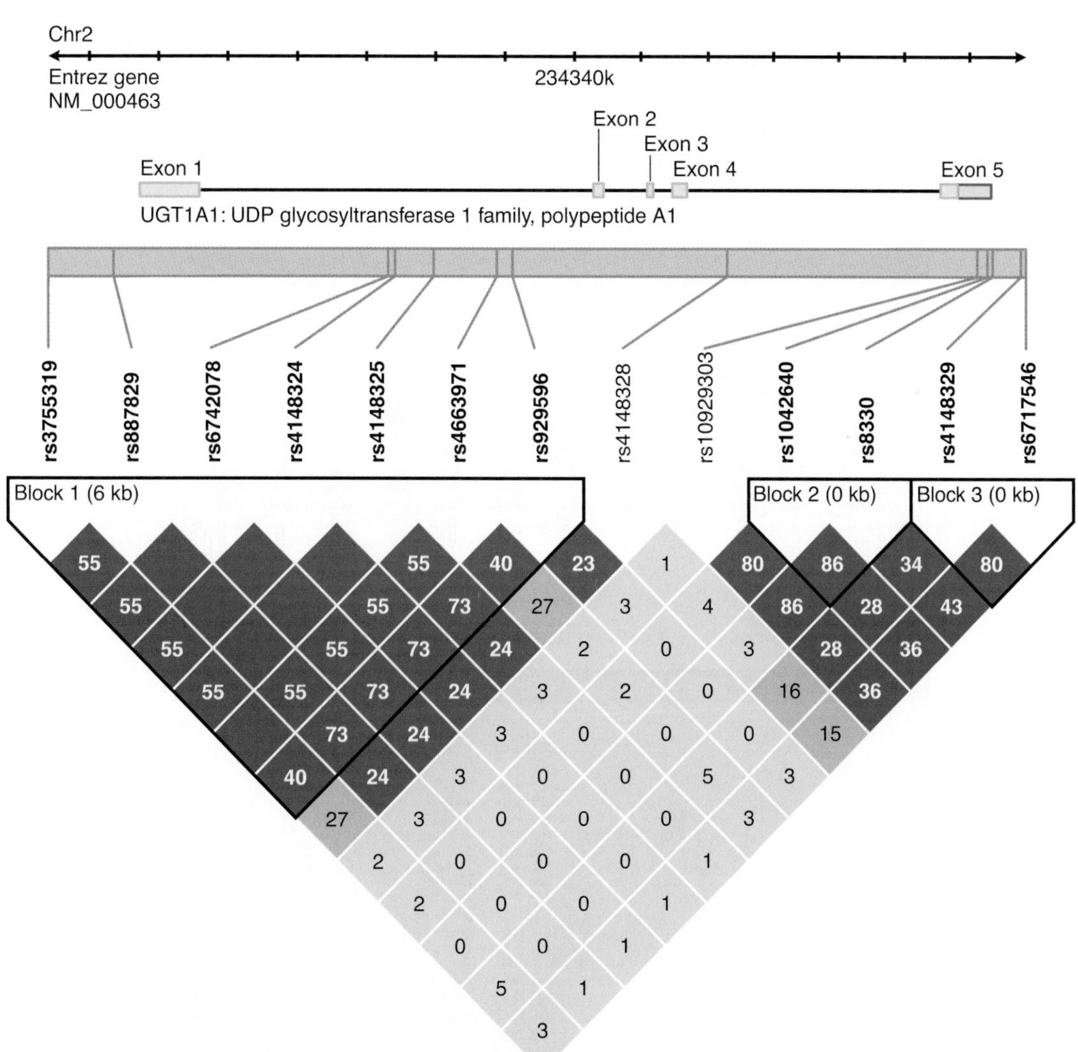

Figure 7–5. *Haplotype blocks in UGT1A1 generated by Haploview version 4.1.* Linkage disequilibrium between SNPs in *UGT1A1* in Europeans is shown. SNPs present at allele frequencies of 20% or greater are included and identified by rs numbers. The r^2 values indicating linkage disequilibrium values between any two SNPs are shown in the blocks below as whole numbers (e.g., 86 = r^2 of 0.86 between SNPs at rs4148238 and rs8330. Those that are dark blue without numbers have an r^2 = 1.0. The relationships among the SNP genotypes in this population for this gene indicate that there are three primary linkage disequilibrium blocks (Block 1, Block 2, and Block 3), which in this case, were generated by the Haploview program. (Source: Broad Institute, http://www.broad.mit.edu/haploview/haploview.)

Ethnic Diversity

Polymorphisms differ in their frequencies within human populations (Burchard et al., 2003; Rosenberg et al., 2002, 2003). Frequencies of polymorphisms in ethnically or racially diverse human populations have been examined in whole genome scanning studies (Cargill et al., 1999; Stephens et al., 2001). In these studies, polymorphisms have been classified as either cosmopolitan or population (or race and ethnic) specific. Cosmopolitan polymorphisms are those polymorphisms present in all ethnic groups, although frequencies may differ among ethnic groups. Cosmopolitan polymorphisms are usually found at higher allele frequencies in comparison to population-specific polymorphisms. Likely to have arisen before migrations of humans from Africa, cosmopolitan polymorphisms are generally older than population-specific polymorphisms.

The presence of ethnic and race-specific polymorphisms is consistent with geographical isolation of human populations (Xie et al., 2001). These polymorphisms probably arose in isolated populations and then reached a certain frequency because they are advantageous (positive selection) or more likely, neutral, conferring no advantage or disadvantage to a population. Large-scale sequence studies in ethnically diverse populations in the U.S. demonstrate that African Americans have the highest number of population-specific polymorphisms in comparison to European Americans, Mexican Americans, and Asian Americans (Leabman et al., 2003; Stephens et al., 2001). Africans are believed to be the oldest population and therefore have both recently derived, population-specific polymorphisms, and a large number of older polymorphisms that occurred before migrations out of Africa.

Consider the coding region variants of two membrane transporters identified in 247 ethnically diverse DNA samples (Figure 7–6).

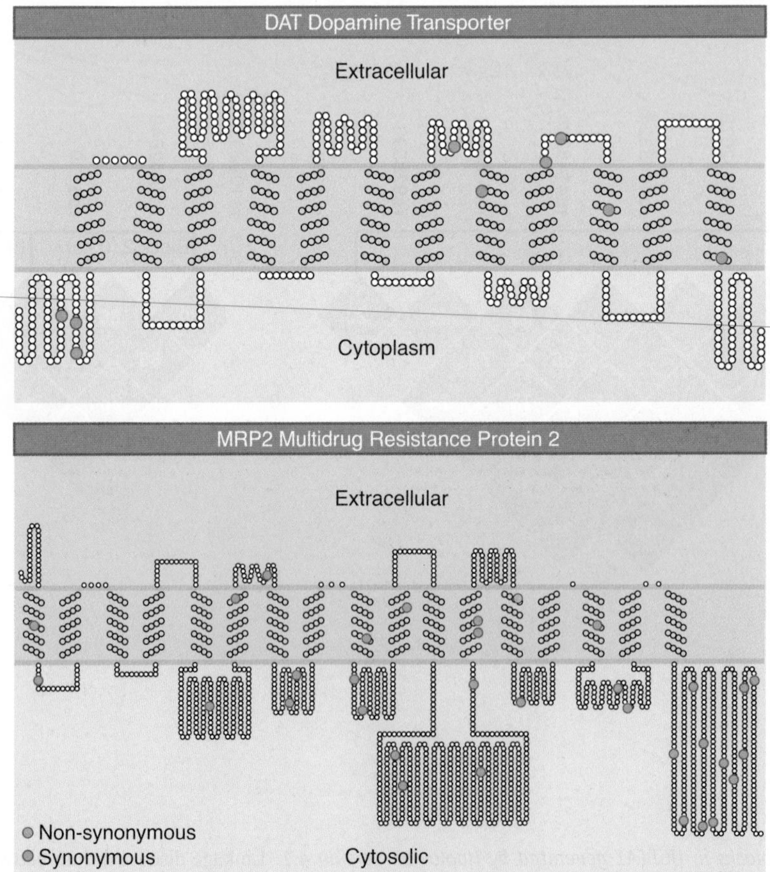

Figure 7–6. *Coding region polymorphisms in two membrane transporters.* Shown are the dopamine transporter, DAT (encoded by *SLC6A3*) and multidrug resistance associated protein, MRP2 (encoded by *ABCC2*). Coding region variants were identified in 247 ethnically diverse DNA samples (100 African Americans, 100 European Americans, 30 Asians, 10 Mexicans, and 7 Pacific islanders). Shown in blue circles are synonymous variants, and in red circles, non-synonymous variants.

Shown are non-synonymous and synonymous SNPs; population-specific non-synonymous cSNPs are indicated in the figure. The multidrug resistance associated protein, MRP2, has a large number of non-synonymous cSNPs. There are fewer synonymous variants than non-synonymous variants, but the allele frequencies of the synonymous variants are greater than those of the non-synonymous variants (Leabman et al., 2003). By comparison, DAT, the dopamine transporter, has a number of synonymous variants but no non-synonymous variants, suggesting that selective pressures have acted against substitutions that led to changes in amino acids.

In a survey of coding region haplotypes in 313 different genes in 80 ethnically diverse DNA samples, most genes were found to have between 2 and 53 haplotypes, with the average number of haplotypes in a gene being 14 (Stephens et al., 2001). Like SNPs, haplotypes may be cosmopolitan or population specific and ~ 20% of the over 4000 identified haplotypes were cosmopolitan (Stephens et al., 2001). Considering the frequencies of the haplotypes, cosmopolitan haplotypes actually accounted for over 80% of all haplotypes, whereas population-specific haplotypes accounted for only 8%. Similarly, recent studies suggest that population-specific CNVs and cosmopolitan CNVs also exist (Redon et al., 2006). As with SNPs and haplotypes, African populations have the greatest numbers of CNVs.

Polymorphism Selection

Genetic variation that results in penetrant and constitutively evident biological variation sometimes causes a "disease" phenotype. Cystic fibrosis, sickle-cell anemia, and Crigler-Najjar syndrome are examples of inherited diseases caused by single gene defects (Pani et al., 2000). In the case of Crigler-Najjar syndrome, the same gene (*UGT1A1*) that is targeted by rare inactivating mutations (and associated with a serious disease) is also targeted by modest polymorphisms (and associated with modest hyperbilirubinemia and altered drug clearance) (Monaghan et al., 1996). Due to the disease, some evolutionary selection against these single-gene polymorphisms is present. Polymorphisms in other genes have highly penetrant effects in the drug-challenged but not in the constitutive state, which are the causes of monogenic pharmacogenetic traits. There is unlikely to be any selective pressure for or against these polymorphisms (Evans and Relling, 2004; Meyer, 2000; Weinshilboum, 2003). The vast majority of genetic polymorphisms have a modest impact on the affected genes, are part of a large array of multigenic factors that impact on drug effect, or affect genes whose products play a minor role in drug action relative to a large nongenetic effect. For example, phenobarbital induction of metabolism may be such an overwhelming "environmental" effect that polymorphisms in the affected transcription factors and drug-metabolizing genes have modest effects by comparison.

PHARMACOGENETIC STUDY DESIGN CONSIDERATIONS

Pharmacogenetic Measures

What are pharmacogenetic traits and how are they measured? A *pharmacogenetic trait* is any measurable or discernible trait associated with a drug. Thus, enzyme activity, drug or metabolite levels in plasma or urine, blood pressure or lipid lowering produced by a drug, and drug-induced gene expression patterns are examples of pharmacogenetic traits. Directly measuring a trait (e.g., enzyme activity) has the advantage that the net effect of the contributions of all genes that influence the trait is reflected in the phenotypic measure. However, it has the disadvantage that it is also reflective of nongenetic influences (e.g., diet, drug interactions, diurnal or hormonal fluctuation) and thus, may be "unstable."

For CYP2D6, if a patient is given an oral dose of dextromethorphan, and the urinary ratio of parent drug to metabolite is assessed, the phenotype is reflective of the genotype for CYP2D6 (Meyer and Zanger, 1997). However, if dextromethorphan is given with quinidine, a potent inhibitor of CYP2D6, the phenotype may be consistent with a poor metabolizer genotype, even though the subject carries wild-type CYP2D6 alleles. In this case, quinidine administration results in a drug-induced haploinsufficiency, and the assignment of a CYP2D6 poor metabolizer phenotype would not be accurate for that subject in the absence of quinidine. If a phenotypic measure, such as the erythromycin breath test (for CYP3A), is not stable within a subject, this is an indication that the phenotype is highly influenced by nongenetic factors, and may indicate a multigenic or weakly penetrant effect of a monogenic trait.

Because most pharmacogenetic traits are multigenic rather than monogenic (Figure 7–7), considerable effort is being made to identify the important genes and their polymorphisms that influence variability in drug response.

Genetic Testing. Most genotyping methods use constitutional or germline DNA, i.e., DNA extracted from any somatic, diploid cells, usually white blood cells or buccal cells (due to their ready accessibility). DNA is extremely stable if appropriately extracted and stored, and unlike many laboratory tests, genotyping need to be performed only once, because DNA sequence is generally invariant throughout an individual's lifetime. Progress continues in moving genotyping tests from research laboratories into patient care. Because genotyping tests are directed at specific known polymorphic sites using a variety of strategies, and not all known functional polymorphisms are likely to be known for any particular gene, it is critical that the methodology for interrogating the polymorphic sites be understood, so that the probability of a negative genotyping test being falsely negative can be estimated.

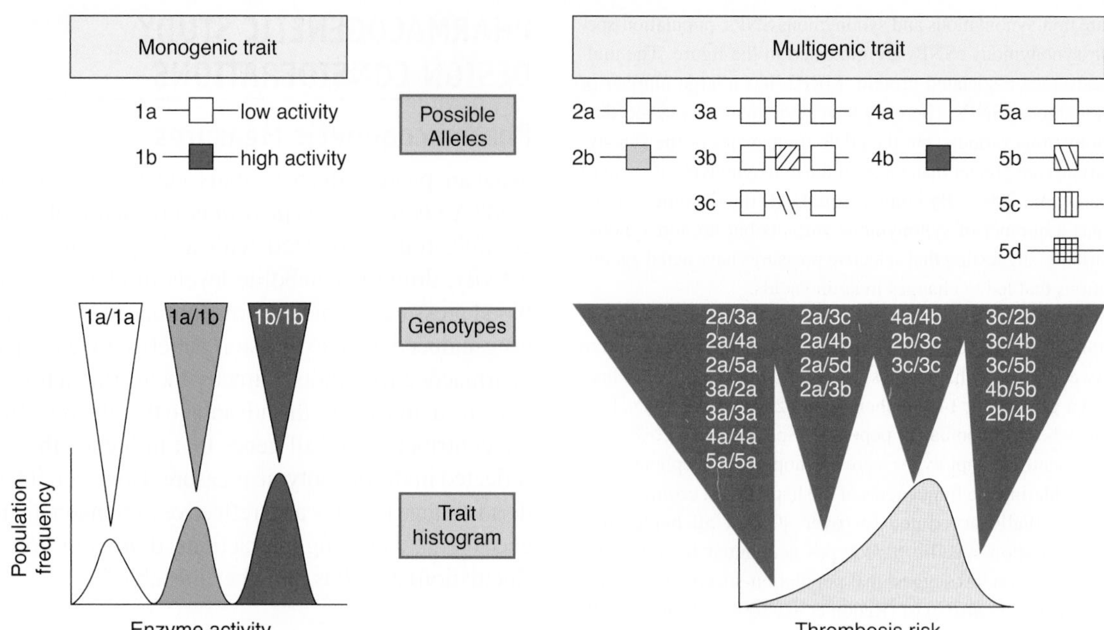

Figure 7–7. *Monogenic versus multigenic pharmacogenetic traits.* Possible alleles for a monogenic trait (*upper left*), in which a single gene has a low-activity (1a) and a high-activity (1b) allele. The population frequency distribution of a monogenic trait (*bottom left*), here depicted as enzyme activity, may exhibit a trimodal frequency distribution with relatively distinct separation among low activity (homozygosity for 1a), intermediate activity (heterozygote for 1a and 1b), and high activity (homozygosity for 1b). This is contrasted with multigenic traits (e.g., an activity influenced by up to four different genes, genes 2 through 5), each of which has 2, 3, or 4 alleles (a through d). The population histogram for activity is unimodal-skewed, with no distinct differences among the genotypic groups. Multiple combinations of alleles coding for low activity and high activity at several of the genes can translate into low-, medium-, and high-activity phenotypes.

One method to assess the reliability of any specific genotype determination in a group of individuals is to assess whether the relative number of homozygotes to heterozygotes is consistent with the overall allele frequency at each polymorphic site. *Hardy-Weinberg equilibrium* is maintained when mating within a population is random and there is no natural selection effect on the variant. Such assumptions are described mathematically when the proportions of the population that are observed to be homozygous for the variant genotype (q^2), homozygous for the wild-type genotype (p^2), and heterozygous ($2*p*q$) are not significantly different from that predicted from the overall allele frequencies (p = frequency of wild-type allele; q = frequency of variant allele) in the population. Proportions of the observed three genotypes must add up to one; significant differences from those predicted may indicate a genotyping error.

Candidate Gene Versus Genome-Wide Approaches

Because pathways involved in drug response are often known or at least partially known, pharmacogenetic studies are highly amenable to candidate gene association studies. After genes in drug response pathways are identified, the next step in the design of a candidate gene association pharmacogenetic study is to identify the genetic polymorphisms that are likely to contribute to the therapeutic and/or adverse responses to the drug. There are several databases that contain information on polymorphisms and mutations in human genes (Table 7–1); these databases allow the investigator to search by gene for reported polymorphisms. Some of the databases, such as the Pharmacogenetics and Pharmacogenomics Knowledge Base (PharmGKB), include phenotypic as well as genotypic data.

In candidate gene association studies, specific genes are prioritized as playing a role in response or adverse response to a drug, it is important to select polymorphisms in those genes for association studies. For this purpose, there are two categories of polymorphisms. The first are polymorphisms that do not, in and of themselves, cause altered function or expression level of the encoded protein (e.g., an enzyme that metabolizes the drug or the drug receptor). Rather, these polymorphisms are linked to the variant allele(s) that produces the altered function. These polymorphisms serve as biomarkers for drug-response phenotype. One way to select SNPs in each gene is to use a tag SNP approach. That is, all SNPs in a gene including SNPs in and around the gene (e.g., 25 kb upstream and downstream of the

Table 7–1

Databases Containing Information on Human Genetic Variation

DATABASE NAME	URL (AGENCY)	DESCRIPTION OF CONTENTS
Pharmacogenetics and Pharmacogenomics Knowledge Base (PharmGKB)	www.pharmgkb.org (NIH Sponsored Research Network and Knowledge Database)	Genotype and phenotype data related to drug response
EntrezSNP (Single Nucleotide Polymorphism) (dbSNP)	www.ncbi.nlm.nih.gov/SNP (National Center for Biotechnology Information [NCBI])	SNPs and frequencies
Human Genome Variation Database (HGVbase)	www.hgvbaseg2p.org	Genotype/phenotype associations
HuGE Navigator	www.hugenavigator.net	Literature annotations for genotype/ phenotype associations
Online Mendelian Inheritance in Man	www.ncbi.nlm.nih.gov/sites/entrez/?db=OMIM (NCBI)	Human genes and genetic disorders
International HapMap Project	www.hapmap.org	Genotypes, frequency and linkage data for variants in ethnic and racial populations
UCSC Genome Browser	http://genome.ucsc.edu	Sequence of the human genome; variant alleles
Genomics Institute of Novartis Research Foundation	http://symatlas.gnf.org/SymAtlas/	Gene expression data for human genes in multiple tissues and cell lines
The Broad Institute Software	http://www.broad.mit.edu/science/software/software	Software tools for the analysis of genetic studies

gene) are identified from SNP databases (e.g., HapMap Database: http://www.hapmap.org/). SNPs with allele frequencies equal to or greater than a target allele frequency are selected. From this set of SNPs, tag SNPs are selected to serve as representatives of multiple SNPs that tend to be in linkage disequilibrium. These tag SNPs are then genotyped in the candidate gene studies.

The second type of polymorphism is the causative polymorphism, which directly precipitates the phenotype. For example, a causative SNP may change an amino acid residue at a site that is highly conserved throughout evolution. This substitution may result in a protein that is nonfunctional or has reduced function. If biological information indicates that a particular polymorphism alters function, e.g., in cellular assays of non-synonymous variants, this polymorphism is an excellent candidate to use in an association study. When causative SNPs are unknown, tag SNPs can be typed to represent important, relatively common blocks of variation within a gene. Once a tag SNP is found to associate with a drug response phenotype, the causative variant or variants, which may be in linkage with the tag SNP, should be identified. Because the causative variant may be an unknown variant, sequencing the gene may be necessary to identify potential causative variants. These additional causative variants may be uncovered by further deep resequencing of the gene.

Genome-Wide and Alternative Large-Scale Approaches. A potential drawback of the candidate gene approach is that the wrong genes may be studied. Genome-wide approaches, using gene expression arrays, genome-wide scans, or proteomics, can complement and feed into the candidate gene approach by providing a relatively unbiased survey of the genome to identify previously unrecognized candidate genes. For example, RNA, DNA, or protein from patients who have unacceptable toxicity from a drug can be compared with identical material from identically treated patients who did not have such toxicity. Differences in gene expression, DNA polymorphisms, or relative amounts of proteins can be ascertained using computational tools, to identify genes, genomic regions, or proteins that can be further assessed for germline polymorphisms differentiating the phenotype. Gene expression and proteomic approaches have the advantage that the abundance of signal may itself directly reflect some of the relevant genetic variation; however, both types of expression are highly influenced by choice of tissue type, which may not be available from the relevant tissue; e.g., it may not be feasible to obtain biopsies of brain tissue for studies on CNS toxicity. DNA has the advantage that it is readily available and independent of tissue type, but the vast majority of genomic variation is not in genes, and the large number of polymorphisms presents the danger of *type I error* (finding differences in genome-wide surveys that are false positives). Current research challenges include prioritizing among the many possible differentiating variations in genome-wide surveys of RNA, DNA, and protein to focus on those that hold the most promise for future pharmacogenomic utility.

Functional Studies of Polymorphisms

For most polymorphisms, functional information is not available. Therefore, to select polymorphisms that are likely to be causative, it is important to predict whether a polymorphism may result in a change in expression level of a protein or a change in protein function, stability, or subcellular localization. One way to gain an understanding of the functional effects of various types of genomic variations is to survey the mutations that have been associated with human Mendelian disease. The greatest numbers of DNA variations associated with Mendelian diseases or traits are missense and nonsense mutations, followed by deletions. Further studies suggest that among amino acid replacements associated with human disease, there is a high representation at residues that are most evolutionarily conserved (Miller and Kumar, 2001; Ng and Henikoff, 2003).

These data have been supplemented by a large survey of genetic variation in membrane transporters important in drug response (Leabman et al., 2003). That survey shows that non-synonymous SNPs that alter evolutionarily conserved amino acids are present at lower allele frequencies on average than those that alter residues that are not conserved across species. A functional genomics study of almost 90 variants in membrane transporters demonstrated that the variants that altered function were likely to change an evolutionarily conserved amino acid residue and to be at low allele frequencies (Urban et al., 2006; SEARCH Group et al., 2008). These data indicate that SNPs that alter evolutionarily conserved residues are most deleterious. The nature of chemical change of an amino acid substitution determines the functional effect of an amino acid variant. More radical changes in amino acids are more likely to be associated with disease than more conservative changes. For example, substitution of a charged amino acid (Arg) for a nonpolar, uncharged amino acid (Cys) is more likely to affect function than substitution of residues that are more chemically similar (e.g., Arg to Lys). The data also suggest that rare SNPs, at least in the coding region, are likely to alter function. New sequencing methods to identify SNPs in pharmacogenetic studies will likely uncover many new rare SNPs which cause variation in drug response.

Among the first pharmacogenetic examples to be discovered was glucose-6-phosphate dehydrogenase (G6PD) deficiency, an X-linked monogenic trait that results in severe hemolytic anemia in individuals after ingestion of fava beans or various drugs, including many antimalarial agents (Alving et al., 1956). G6PD is normally present in red blood cells and helps to regulate levels of glutathione (GSH), an antioxidant. Antimalarials such as primaquine increase red blood cell fragility in individuals with G6PD deficiency, leading to profound hemolytic anemia. Interestingly, the severity of the deficiency syndrome varies among individuals and is related to the amino acid variant in G6PD. The severe form of G6PD deficiency is associated with changes at residues that are highly conserved across evolutionary history. Chemical change is also more radical on average in mutations associated with severe G6PD deficiency in comparison to mutations associated with milder forms of the syndrome. Collectively, studies of Mendelian traits and polymorphisms suggest that non-synonymous SNPs that alter residues that are highly conserved among species and those that result in more radical changes in the nature of the amino acid are likely to be the best candidates for causing functional changes. The information in Table 7–2 (categories of polymorphisms and the likelihood of each polymorphism to alter function) can be used as a guide for prioritizing polymorphisms in candidate gene association studies.

With the increasing number of SNPs that have been identified in large-scale SNP discovery projects, it is clear that computational methods are needed to predict the functional consequences of SNPs. To this end, predictive algorithms have been developed to identify potentially deleterious amino acid substitutions. These methods can be classified into two groups. The first group relies on sequence comparisons alone to identify and score substitutions according to their degree of conservation across multiple species; different scoring matrices have been used (e.g., BLOSUM62, SIFT and PolyPhen) (Henikoff and Henikoff, 1992; Ng and Henikoff, 2003; Ramensky, 2002). The second group of methods relies on mapping of SNPs onto protein structures, in addition to sequence comparisons (Mirkovic et al., 2004). For example, rules have been developed that classify SNPs in terms of their impact on folding and stability of the native protein structure as well as shapes of its binding sites. Such rules depend on the structural context in which SNPs occur (e.g., buried in the core of the fold or exposed to the solvent, in the binding site or not), and are inferred by machine learning methods from many functionally annotated SNPs in test proteins.

Functional activity of amino acid variants for many proteins can be studied in cellular assays. An initial step in characterizing the function of a non-synonymous variant would be to isolate the variant gene or construct the variant by site-directed mutagenesis, express it in cells, and compare its functional activity to that of the reference or most common form of the protein. Large-scale functional analyses have been performed on genetic variants in membrane transporters and phase II enzymes. Figure 7–8 shows the function of all non-synonymous variants and coding region insertions and deletions of two membrane transporters, the organic cation transporter, OCT1 (encoded by *SLC22A1*) and the nucleoside transporter, CNT3 (encoded by *SLC28A3*). Most of the naturally occurring variants have functional activity similar to that of the reference transporters. However, several variants exhibit reduced function; in the case of OCT1, a gain-of-function variant is also present. Results such as these indicate heterogeneity exists in the functionality of natural amino acid variants in normal healthy human populations.

For many proteins, including enzymes, transporters, and receptors, the mechanisms by which amino acid substitutions alter function have been characterized in kinetic studies. Figure 7–9 shows simulated curves depicting the rate of metabolism of a substrate by two amino acid variants of an enzyme and the most common genetic form of the enzyme. The kinetics of metabolism of substrate by one variant enzyme, Variant A, are characterized by an

Table 7–2

Predicted Functional Effect and Relative Risk That a Variant Will Alter Function of SNP Types in the Human Genome

TYPE OF VARIANT	LOCATION	FREQUENCY IN GENOME	PREDICTED RELATIVE RISK OF PHENOTYPE	FUNCTIONAL EFFECT
Nonsense	Coding region	Very low	Very high	Stop codon
Nonsynonymous Evolutionarily conserved	Coding region	Low	High	Amino acid substitution of a residue conserved across evolution
Nonsynonymous Evolutionarily unconserved	Coding region	Low	Low to moderate	Amino acid substitution of a residue not conserved across evolution
Nonsynonymous Radical chemical change	Coding region	Low	Moderate to high	Amino acid substitution of a residue that is chemically dissimilar to the original residue
Nonsynonymous Low to moderate chemical change	Coding region	Low	Low to high	Amino acid substitution of a residue that is chemically similar to the original residue
Insertion/deletion	Coding/noncoding region	Low	Low to high	Coding region: can cause frameshift
Synonymous	Coding region	Medium	Low	Can affect mRNA stability or splicing
Regulatory region	Promoter, 5′ UTR, 3′ UTR	Medium	Low to High	Can affect the level of mRNA transcript by changing rate of transcription or stability of transcript
Intron/exon boundary	Within 8 bp of intron	Low	High	May affect splicing
Intronic	Deep within intron	Medium	Unknown	May affect mRNA transcript levels through enhancer mechanism
Intergenic	Noncoding region between genes	High	Unknown	May affect mRNA transcript levels through enhancer mechanisms

Data adapted from Tabor et al., 2002.

increased K_m. Such an effect can occur if the amino acid substitution alters the binding site of the enzyme leading to a decrease in its affinity for the substrate. An amino acid variant may also alter the maximum rate of metabolism (V_{max}) of substrate by the enzyme, as exemplified by Variant B. The mechanisms for a reduced V_{max} are generally related to a reduced expression level of the enzyme, which may occur because of decreased stability of the protein or changes in protein trafficking or recycling (Shu et al., 2003; Tirona et al., 2001; Xu et al., 2002).

In contrast to the studies with SNPs in coding regions, we know much less about noncoding region SNPs. The principles of evolutionary conservation that have been shown to be important in predicting the function of non-synonymous variants in the coding region need to be refined and tested as predictors of function of SNPs in noncoding regions. New methods in comparative genomics are being refined to identify conserved elements in noncoding regions of genes that may be functionally important (Bejerano et al., 2004; Boffelli et al., 2004; Brudno et al., 2003). SNPs identified in genome-wide association studies as being associated with clinical phenotypes including drug response phenotypes have largely been in noncoding regions, either intergenic or intronic regions, of the genome (Figure 7–10). It is a challenge in human genetics and pharmacogenetics to understand the functional effects of noncoding region variants. Such variants may be in potential enhancer regions of the genome and may enhance (or repress) gene transcription.

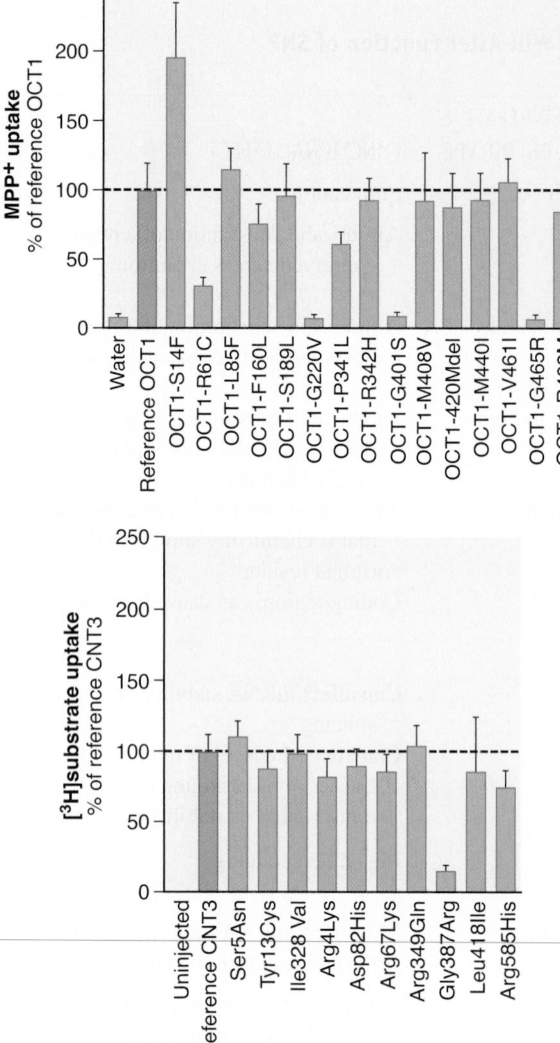

Figure 7–8. *Functional activity of natural variants of two membrane transporters.* Data for the organic cation transporter (OCT1, *top panel*) and the nucleoside transporter (CNT3, *bottom panel*). Variants, identified in ethnically diverse populations, were constructed by site-directed mutagenesis and expressed in *Xenopus laevis* oocytes. Blue bars represent uptake of the model compounds by variant transporters. Red bars represent uptake of the model compounds by reference transporters. MPP+, 1-methyl-4-phenylpyridium. (Reproduced with permission from Shu et al., 2003. Copyright © National Academy of Sciences, USA.)

An example of profound functional effect of a noncoding SNP is provided by CYP3A5; a common noncoding intronic SNP in CYP3A5 accounts for its polymorphic expression in humans. It was well known that only ~10% of whites but a higher percentage of blacks expressed CYP3A5. The SNP accounting for variation in CYP3A5 protein lies in intron 3, 1618 nucleotides 3′ from exon 3 and 377 nucleotides 5′ of exon 4. This SNP creates an alternative splice site, resulting in a transcript with a larger exon 3 but also the introduction of an early stop codon in this 13 exon transcript (Figure 7–11). The resultant protein, in the majority of whites who are homozygous for the *3 nonfunctional allele, is thus truncated so early that the protein is completely non-detectable. Thus, even SNPs quite distant from intron/exon borders can profoundly affect splicing and thus affect protein function (Kuehl et al., 2001).

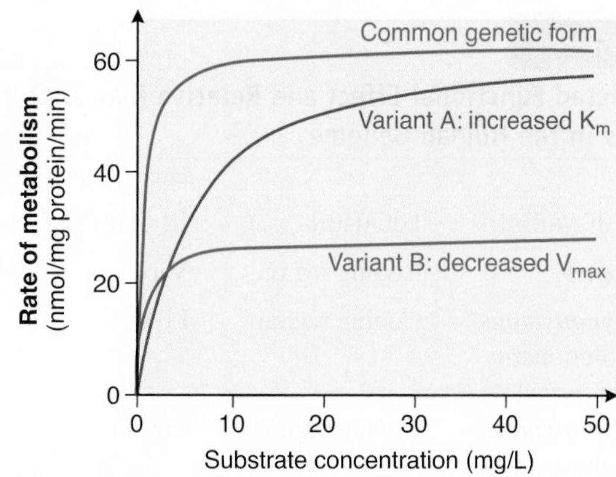

Figure 7–9. *Simulated concentration-dependence curves showing the rate of metabolism of a hypothetical substrate by the common genetic form of an enzyme and two non-synonymous variants.* Variant A exhibits an increased K_m and likely reflects a change in the substrate binding site of the protein by the substituted amino acid. Variant B exhibits a change in the maximum rate of metabolism (V_{max}) of the substrate. This may be due to reduced expression level of the enzyme.

Pharmacogenetic Phenotypes

Candidate genes for therapeutic and adverse response can be divided into three categories: *pharmacokinetic*, *receptor/target*, and *disease modifying*.

Pharmacokinetics. Germline variability in genes that encode determinants of the pharmacokinetics of a drug, in particular metabolizing enzymes and transporters, affect drug concentrations, and are therefore major determinants of therapeutic and adverse drug response (Table 7–3; Nebert et al., 1996). Multiple enzymes and transporters may be involved in the pharmacokinetics of a single drug. Several polymorphisms in drug metabolizing enzymes were discovered as monogenic phenotypic trait variations, and thus may be referenced using their phenotypic designations (e.g., slow *vs.* fast acetylation, extensive *vs.* poor metabolizers of debrisoquine or sparteine) rather than their genotypic designations that reference the polymorphic gene (NAT2 and CYP2D6, respectively) (Grant et al., 1990). CYP2D6 is now known to catabolize the two initial probe drugs (sparteine and debrisoquine), each of which was associated with exaggerated responses in 5-10% of treated

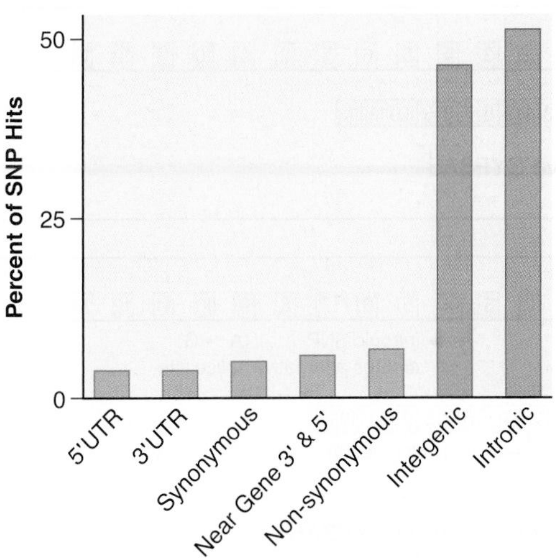

	Percent of SNP Hits
5' UTR	3
3' UTR	3
Synonymous	4
Near Gene	5
Non-synonymous	6
Intergenic	45
Intronic	50

Figure 7–10. *Types of genetic variants that have been significantly associated with complex human traits and disease in 208 genome-wide association studies.* Approximately 500 SNPs were associated with human disease and complex traits. Intergenic and intronic SNPs comprise the largest fraction of associated variants. See www.genome.gov/gwastudies/.

individuals. The exaggerated responses are an inherited trait (Eichelbaum et al., 1975; Mahgoub et al., 1977). At present, a very large number of medications (estimated at 15-25% of all medicines in use) have been shown to be substrates for CYP2D6 (Table 7–3 and Figure 6–3A). The molecular and phenotypic characterization of multiple racial and ethnic groups has shown that seven variant alleles account for well over 90% of the "poor metabolizer" low-activity alleles for this gene in most racial groups; that the frequency of variant alleles varies with geographic origin; and that a small percentage of individuals carry stable duplications of CYP2D6, with "ultra-rapid" metabolizers having up to 13 copies of the active gene (Ingelman-Sundberg and Evans, 2001). Phenotypic consequences of the deficient CYP2D6 phenotype (Table 7–3) include increased risk of toxicity of antidepressants or antipsychotics (catabolized by the enzyme), lack of analgesic effects of codeine (anabolized by the enzyme), and lack of activation of tamoxifen, leading to a greater risk of relapse or recurrence in breast cancer (Borges et al., 2006; Goetz et al., 2008; Ingle, 2008). Conversely, the ultra-rapid phenotype is associated with extremely rapid clearance and thus inefficacy of antidepressants (Kirchheiner et al., 2001).

A promoter region variant in the enzyme UGT1A1, UGT1A1*28, which has an additional TA in comparison to the more common form of the gene, has been associated with a reduced transcription rate of *UGT1A1* and lower glucuronidation activity of the enzyme. This reduced activity has been associated with higher levels of the active metabolite of the cancer chemotherapeutic agent *irinotecan* (see Chapters 6). The metabolite, SN38, which is eliminated by glucuronidation, is associated with the risk of toxicity (Iyer et al., 2002; Rosner and Panetta, 2008), which will be more severe in individuals with genetically lower *UGT1A1* activity (see Figures 6–5, 6–7, and 6–8).

CYP2C19, historically termed mephenytoin hydroxylase, displays penetrant pharmacogenetic variability, with just a few SNPs accounting for the majority of the deficient, poor metabolizer phenotype (Mallal et al., 2002). The deficient phenotype is much more common in Chinese and Japanese populations. Several proton pump inhibitors, including omeprazole and lansoprazole, are inactivated by CYP2C19. Thus, the deficient patients have higher exposure to active parent drug, a greater pharmacodynamic effect (higher gastric pH), and a higher probability of ulcer cure than heterozygotes or homozygous wild-type individuals (Figure 7–12).

Both pharmacokinetic and pharmacodynamic polymorphisms affect warfarin dosing. The anticoagulant warfarin is catabolized by CYP2C9, and its action is partly dependent upon the baseline level of reduced vitamin K (catalyzed by vitamin K epoxide reductase; Figures 7–13 and 30–7). Inactivating polymorphisms in *CYP2C9* are common (Goldstein, 2001), with 2-10% of most populations being homozygous for low-activity variants, and are associated with lower warfarin clearance, a higher risk of bleeding complications, and lower dose requirements (see Table 30–2 and Aithal et al., 1999). Combined with

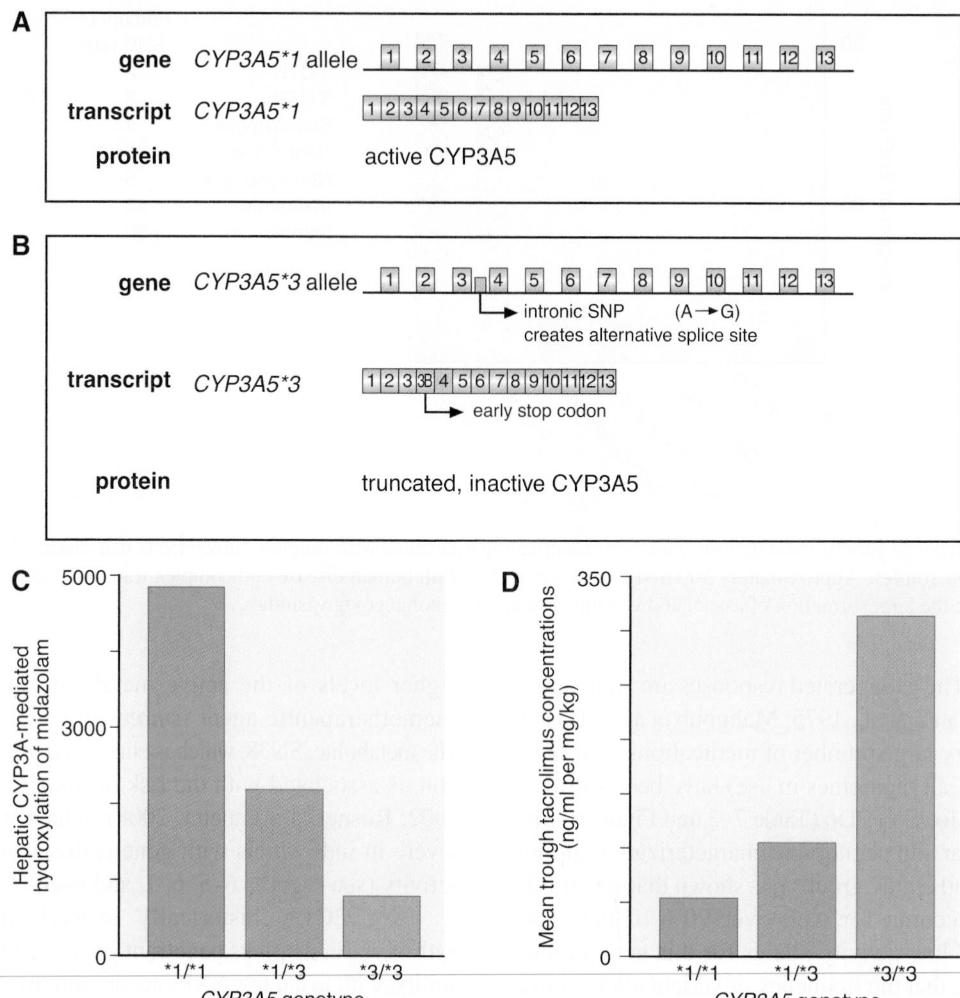

Figure 7–11. *An intronic SNP can affect splicing and account for polymorphic expression of CYP3A5.* A common polymorphism (A>G) in intron 3 of CYP3A5 defines the genotypes associated with the wild-type CYP3A5*1 allele, or the variant nonfunctional CYP3A5*3 allele. This intronic SNP creates an alternative splice site that results in the production of an alternative CYP3A5 transcript carrying an additional intron 3B (panel B), with an accompanying early stop codon and truncated CYP3A5 protein. Whereas the wild-type gene (more common in African than Caucasian or Asian populations) results in production of active CYP3A5 protein (panel A), the *3 variant results in a truncated and inactive CYP3A5 protein. Thus, metabolism of CYP3A5 substrates is diminished *in vitro* (panel C, shown for midazolam) and blood concentrations of such medications are higher *in vivo* (panel D, shown for tacrolimus) for these with the *3 than the *1 allele. (Based on data from Haufroid et al., 2004; Kuehl et al., 2001; Lin et al., 2002.)

genotyping for a common polymorphism in *VKORC1*, inherited variation in these two genes account for 20-60% of the variability in warfarin doses needed to achieve the desired INR, and use of these tests in the clinic can result in fewer bleeding complications and shorter time of trial-and-error to achieve the desired steady state level of anticoagulation. (Caraco et al., 2008; Lesko, 2008; Schwarz et al., 2008).

Thiopurine methyltransferase (TPMT) methylates thiopurines such as mercaptopurine (an anti-leukemic drug that is also the product of azathioprine metabolism; Figure 47–5). One in 300 individuals is homozygous deficient, 10% are heterozygotes, and ~90% are homozygous for the wild-type alleles for *TPMT* (Weinshilboum and Sladek, 1980). Three SNPs account for over 90% of the inactivating alleles (Yates et al., 1997). Because methylation of mercaptopurine competes with activation of the drug to thioguanine nucleotides, the concentration of the active (but also toxic) thioguanine metabolites is inversely related to

Table 7–3

Examples of Genetic Polymorphisms Influencing Drug Response

GENE PRODUCT (*GENE*)	DRUGS*	RESPONSES AFFECTED
Drug Metabolism and Transport		
CYP2C9	Tolbutamide, warfarin,* phenytoin, nonsteroidal anti-inflammatory	Anticoagulant effect of warfarin
CYP2C19	Mephenytoin, omeprazole, voriconazole*, hexobarbital, mephobarbital, propranolol, proguanil, phenytoin, clopidogrel	Peptic ulcer response to omeprazole; cardiovascular events after clopidogrel
CYP2D6	β blockers, antidepressants, anti-psychotics, codeine, debrisoquine, atomoxetine*, dextromethorphan, encainide, flecainide, fluoxetine, guanoxan, *N*-propylajmaline, perhexiline, phenacetin, phenformin, propafenone, sparteine, tamoxifen	Tardive dyskinesia from antipsychotics, narcotic side effects, codeine efficacy, imipramine dose requirement, β blocker effect; breast cancer recurrence after tamoxifen
CYP3A4/3A5/3A7	Macrolides, cyclosporine, tacrolimus, Ca^{2+} channel blockers, midazolam, terfenadine, lidocaine, dapsone, quinidine, triazolam, etoposide, teniposide, lovastatin, alfentanil, tamoxifen, steroids	Efficacy of immunosuppressive effects of tacrolimus
Dihydropyrimidine dehydrogenase	Fluorouracil, capecitabine*	5-Fluorouracil toxicity
N-acetyltransferase (*NAT2*)	Isoniazid, hydralazine, sulfonamides, amonafide, procainamide, dapsone, caffeine	Hypersensitivity to sulfonamides, amonafide toxicity, hydralazine-induced lupus, isoniazid neurotoxicity
Glutathione transferases (*GSTM1, GSTT1,GSTP1*)	Several anticancer agents	Decreased response in breast cancer, more toxicity and worse response in acute myelogenous leukemia
Thiopurine methyltransferase (*TPMT*)	Mercaptopurine*, thioguanine*, azathioprine*	Thiopurine toxicity and efficacy, risk of second cancers
UDP-glucuronosyl-transferase (*UGT1A1*)	Irinotecan*, bilirubin	Irinotecan toxicity
P-glycoprotein (*ABCB1*)	Natural product anticancer drugs, HIV protease inhibitors, digoxin	Decreased CD4 response in HIV-infected patients, decreased digoxin AUC, drug resistance in epilepsy
UGT2B7	Morphine	Morphine plasma levels
Organic anion transporter (*SLC01B1*)	Statins, methotrexate, ACE inhibitors	Statin plasma levels, myopathy; methotrexate plasma levels, mucositis
COMT	Levodopa	Enhanced drug effect
Organic cation transporter (*SLC22A1, OCT1*)	Metformin	Pharmacologic effect and pharmacokinetics
Organic cation transporter (*SLC22A2, OCT2*)	Metformin	Renal clearance
Novel organic cation transporter (*SLC22A4, OCTN1*)	Gabapentin	Renal clearance
CYP2B6	Cyclophosphamide	Ovarian failure

(*Continued*)

Table 7–3

Examples of Genetic Polymorphisms Influencing Drug Response (*Continued*)

GENE PRODUCT (*GENE*)	DRUGS*	RESPONSES AFFECTED
Targets and Receptors		
Angiotensin-converting enzyme (ACE)	ACE inhibitors (e.g., enalapril)	Renoprotective effects, hypotension, left ventricular mass reduction, cough
Thymidylate synthase	5-Fluorouracil	Colorectal cancer response
Chemokine receptor 5 (CCR5)	Antiretrovirals, interferon	Antiviral response
β_2 Adrenergic receptor (*ADBR2*)	β_2 Antagonists (e.g., albuterol, terbutaline)	Bronchodilation, susceptibility to agonist-induced desensitization, cardiovascular effects (e.g., increased heart rate, cardiac index, peripheral vasodilation)
β_1 Adrenergic receptor (*ADBR1*)	β_1 Antagonists	Blood pressure and heart rate after β_1 antagonists
5-Lipoxygenase (ALOX5)	Leukotriene receptor antagonists	Asthma response
Dopamine receptors (D_2, D_3, D_4)	Antipsychotics (e.g., haloperidol, clozapine, thioridazine, nemonapride)	Antipsychotic response (D_2, D_3, D_4), antipsychotic-induced tardive dyskinesia (D_3) and acute akathisia (D_3), hyperprolactinemia in females (D_2)
Estrogen receptor α	Estrogen hormone replacement therapy	High-density lipoprotein cholesterol
Serotonin transporter (5-HTT)	Antidepressants (e.g., clomipramine, fluoxetine, paroxetine, fluvoxamine)	Clozapine effects, 5-HT neurotransmission, antidepressant response
Serotonin receptor (5-HT_{2A})	Antipsychotics	Clozapine antipsychotic response, tardive dyskinesia, paroxetine antidepression response, drug discrimination
HMG-CoA reductase	Pravastatin	Reduction in serum cholesterol
Vitamin K oxidoreductase (VKORC1)	Warfarin*	Anticoagulant effect, bleeding risk
Corticotropin releasing hormone receptor (CRHR1)	Glucocorticoids	Bronchodilation, osteopenia
Ryanodine receptor (RYR1)	General anesthetics	Malignant hyperthermia
Modifiers		
Adducin	Diuretics	Myocardial infarction or strokes, blood pressure
Apolipoprotein E	Statins (e.g., simvastatin), tacrine	Lipid-lowering; clinical improvement in Alzheimer's disease
Human leukocyte antigen	Abacavir, carbamazepine, phenytoin	Hypersensitivity reactions

(*Continued*)

Table 7–3

Examples of Genetic Polymorphisms Influencing Drug Response (*Continued*)

GENE PRODUCT (*GENE*)	DRUGS*	RESPONSES AFFECTED
G6PD deficiency	Rasburicase*, dapsone*	Methemoglobinemia
Cholesteryl ester transfer protein	Statins (e.g., pravastatin)	Slowing atherosclerosis progression
Ion channels (*HERG, KvLQT1, Mink, MiRP1*)	Erythromycin, cisapride, clarithromycin, quinidine	Increased risk of drug-induced *torsades de pointes*, increased QT interval (Roden, 2003; Roden, 2004)
Methylguanine-methyltransferase	DNA methylating agents	Response of glioma to chemotherapy
Parkin	Levodopa	Parkinson disease response
MTHFR	Methotrexate	GI toxicity (Ulrich et al., 2001)
Prothrombin, factor V	Oral contraceptives	Venous thrombosis risk
Stromelysin-1	Statins (e.g., pravastatin)	Reduction in cardiovascular events and in repeat angioplasty
Inosine triphosphatase (ITPA)	Azathioprine, mercaptopurine	Myelosuppression
Vitamin D receptor	Estrogen	Bone mineral density

* Information on genetics-based dosing, adverse events, or testing added to FDA-approved drug label (Grossman, 2007).

TPMT activity and directly related to the probability of pharmacologic effects. Dose reductions (from the "average" population dose) may be required to avoid myelosuppression in 100% of homozygous deficient patients, 35% of heterozygotes, and only 7-8% of those with homozygous wild-type activity (Relling et al., 1999). The rare homozygous deficient patients can tolerate 10% or less of the mercaptopurine doses tolerated by the homozygous wild-type patients, with heterozygotes often requiring an intermediate dose. Conversely, homozygous wild-type patients show less anti-leukemic response to a short course of mercaptopurine than

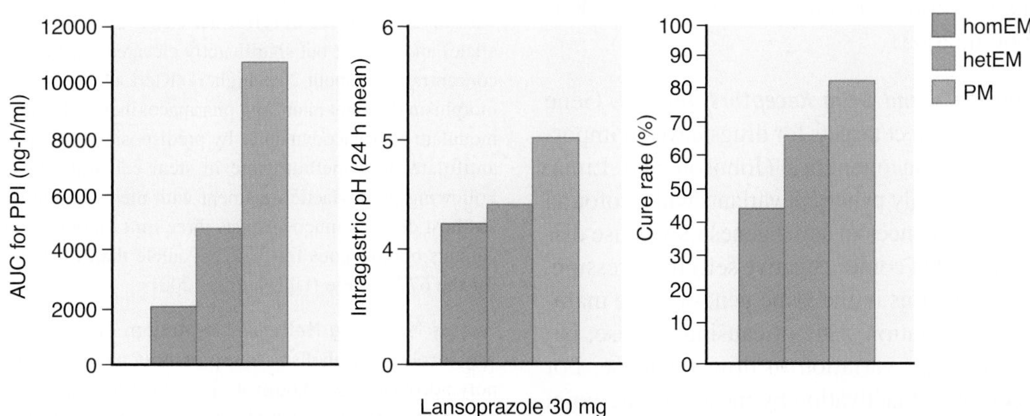

Figure 7–12. *Effect of CYP2C19 genotype on proton pump inhibitor (PPI) pharmacokinetics (AUC), gastric pH, and ulcer cure rates.* Depicted are the average variables for *CYP2C19* homozygous extensive metabolizers (homEM), heterozygotes (hetEM), and poor metabolizers (PM). (Reproduced with permission from Furuta T et al. Pharmcogenomics of proton pump inhibitors. *Pharmacogenomics*, **2004**, 5: 181–202. Copyright © 2004 Future Medicine Ltd. All rights reserved.)

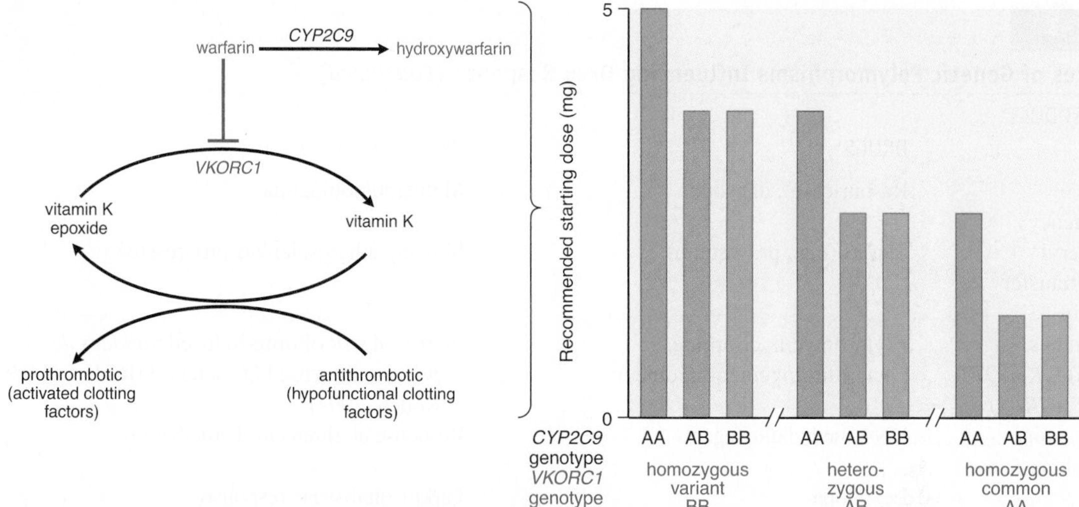

Figure 7–13. *Pharmacogenetics of warfarin dosing.* Warfarin is metabolized by *CYP2C9* to inactive metabolites, and exerts its anticoagulant effect partly via inhibition of *VKORC1* (vitamin K epoxide hydrolase), an enzyme necessary for reduction of inactive to active vitamin K. Common polymorphisms in both genes, *CYP2C9* and *VKORC1*, impact on warfarin pharmacokinetics and pharmacodynamics, respectively, to affect the population mean therapeutic doses of warfarin necessary to maintain the desired degree of anticoagulation (often measured by the international normalized ratio [INR] blood test) and minimize the risk of too little anticoagulation (thrombosis) or too much anticoagulation (bleeding). (Based on data from Caraco et al., 2008; Schwarz et al., 2008; Wen et al., 2008.)

those with at least one inactive *TPMT* allele (Stanulla et al., 2005). Mercaptopurine has a narrow therapeutic range, and dosing by trial and error can place patients at higher risk of toxicity; thus, prospective adjustment of *thiopurine* doses based on *TPMT* genotype has been suggested (Lesko and Woodcock, 2004). Life-threatening toxicity has also been reported when thiopurines have been given to patients with nonmalignant conditions (such as Crohn's disease, arthritis, or for prevention of solid organ transplant rejection) (Evans and Johnson, 2001; Evans and Relling, 2004; Weinshilboum, 2003).

Pharmacogenetics and Drug Receptors/Targets. Gene products that are direct targets for drugs have an important role in pharmacogenetics (Johnson and Lima, 2003). Whereas highly penetrant variants with profound functional consequences in some genes may cause disease phenotypes that confer negative selective pressure, more subtle variations in the same genes can be maintained in the population without causing disease, but nonetheless causing variation in drug response. For example, complete inactivation by means of rare point mutations in methylenetetrahydrofolate reductase (MTHFR) causes severe mental retardation, cardiovascular disease, and a shortened lifespan (Goyette et al., 1994). MTHFR reduces 5,10-CH_2- to 5-CH_3-tetrahydrofolate, and thereby interacts with folate-dependent one-carbon synthesis reactions, including homocysteine/methionine metabolism and pyrimidine/purine synthesis (see Chapter 61). This pathway is the target of several antifolate drugs. For details, see the methotrexate pathway at www.pharm GKB.org.

Whereas rare inactivating variants in *MTHFR* may result in early death, the 677C→T SNP causes an amino acid substitution that is maintained in the population at a high frequency (variant allele, q, frequency in most white populations = 0.4). This variant is associated with modestly lower MTHFR activity (~30% less than the 677C allele) and modest but significantly elevated plasma homocysteine concentrations (about 25% higher) (Klerk et al., 2002). This polymorphism does not alter drug pharmacokinetics, but does appear to modulate pharmacodynamics by predisposing to GI toxicity to the antifolate drug methotrexate in stem cell transplant recipients. Following prophylactic treatment with methotrexate for graft-versus-host disease, mucositis was three times more common among patients homozygous for the 677T allele than those homozygous for the 677C allele (Ulrich et al., 2001).

Factors Modifying Methotrexate Action. The methotrexate pathway involves metabolism, transport, drug modifier, and drug target polymorphisms. Methotrexate is a substrate for transporters and anabolizing enzymes that affect its intracellular pharmacokinetics and that are subject to common polymorphisms (see methotrexate pathway at www.pharm GKB.org). Several of the direct targets (dihydrofolate reductase, purine transformylases, and thymidylate synthase [TYMS]) are also subject to common polymorphisms.

A polymorphic indel in *TYMS* (two vs. three repeats of a 28-base pair repeat in the enhancer) affects the amount of enzyme expression in both normal and tumor cells. The polymorphism is quite common, with alleles equally split between the lower-expression two-repeat and the higher-expression three-repeat alleles. The *TYMS* polymorphism can affect both toxicity and efficacy of anticancer agents (e.g., fluorouracil and methotrexate) that target TYMS (Krajinovic et al., 2002). Thus, the genetic contribution to variability in the pharmacokinetics and pharmacodynamics of methotrexate cannot be understood without assessing genotypes at a number of different loci.

Other Examples of Drug Target Polymorphisms. Many drug target polymorphisms have been shown to predict responsiveness to drugs (Table 7–3). Serotonin receptor polymorphisms predict not only the responsiveness to antidepressants, but also the overall risk of depression (Murphy et al., 2003). β Adrenergic receptor polymorphisms have been linked to asthma responsiveness (degree of change in 1-second forced expiratory volume after use of a β agonist) (Tan et al., 1997), renal function following angiotensin-converting enzyme (ACE) inhibitors (Essen et al., 1996), and heart rate following β blockers (Taylor and Kennedy, 2001). Polymorphisms in 3-hydroxy-3-methylglutaryl coenzyme A (HMG-CoA) reductase have been linked to the degree of lipid lowering following statins, which are HMG-CoA reductase inhibitors (see Chapter 31), and to the degree of positive effects on high-density lipoproteins among women on estrogen replacement therapy (Herrington et al., 2002). Ion channel polymorphisms have been linked to a risk of cardiac arrhythmias in the presence and absence of drug triggers (Roden, 2004).

Polymorphism-Modifying Diseases and Drug Responses. Some genes may be involved in an underlying disease being treated, but do not directly interact with the drug. Modifier polymorphisms are important for the *de novo* risk of some events and for the risk of drug-induced events. The *MTHFR* polymorphism, e.g., is linked to homocysteinemia, which in turn affects thrombosis risk (den Heijer, 2003). The risk of a drug-induced thrombosis is dependent not only on the use of prothrombotic drugs, but on environmental and genetic predisposition to thrombosis, which may be affected by germline polymorphisms in *MTHFR*, factor V, and prothrombin (Chanock, 2003). These polymorphisms do not directly act on the pharmacokinetics or pharmacodynamics of prothrombotic drugs, such as glucocorticoids, estrogens, and asparaginase, but may modify the risk of the phenotypic event (thrombosis) in the presence of the drug.

Likewise, polymorphisms in ion channels (e.g., *HERG*, KvLQT1, Mink, and *MiRP1*) may affect the overall risk of cardiac dysrhythmias, which may be accentuated in the presence of a drug that can prolong the QT interval in some circumstances (e.g., macrolide antibiotics, antihistamines) (Roden, 2003). These modifier polymorphisms may impact on the risk of "disease" phenotypes even in the absence of drug challenges; in the presence of drug, the "disease" phenotype may be elicited.

Cancer As a Special Case. Cancer pharmacogenetics have an unusual aspect in that tumors exhibit somatically acquired mutations in addition to the underlying germline variation of the host. Thus, the efficacy of some anticancer drugs depends on the genetics of both the host and the tumor. For example, non-small-cell lung cancer is treated with an inhibitor of epidermal growth factor receptor (EGFR), gefitinib. Patients whose tumors have activating mutations in the tyrosine kinase domain of *EGFR* appear to respond better to gefitinib than those without the mutations (Lynch et al., 2004). Thus, the receptor is altered, and at the same time, individuals with the activating mutations may be considered to have a distinct category of non-small-cell lung cancer. Breast cancer patients with expression of the Her2 antigen (as an acquired genetic changes) are more likely to benefit from the antibody trastuzumab than are those who are negative for Her2 expression, and this results in a common tailoring of anticancer therapy in patients with breast cancer based on tumor genetics. As an example of a gene that affects both tumor and host, the presence of two instead of three copies of a *TYMS* enhancer repeat polymorphism increases the risk of host toxicity but also increases the chance of tumor susceptibility to thymidylate synthase inhibitors (Evans, and McLeod, 2003; Relling and Dervieux, 2001; Villafranca et al., 2001).

Pharmacogenetics and Drug Development

Pharmacogenetics will likely impact drug regulatory considerations in several ways (Evans and Relling, 2004; Lesko and Woodcock, 2004; Weinshilboum and Wang, 2004). Genome-wide approaches hold promise for identification of new drug targets and therefore new drugs. In addition, accounting for genetic/genomic inter-individual variability may lead to genotype-specific development of new drugs, and to genotype-specific dosing regimens. Recently, the U.S. Food and Drug Administration (FDA) altered the labels of several drugs in clinical use to indicate a pharmacogenetic issue (Table 7–3). With time and study, other drug labels will likely be changed as well.

Pharmacogenomics can identify new targets. For example, genome-wide assessments using microarray technology could identify genes whose expression differentiates inflammatory processes; a compound could be identified that changes expression of that gene; and then that compound could serve as a starting point for anti-inflammatory drug development. Proof of principle has been demonstrated for identification of anti-leukemic agents (Stegmaier et al., 2004) and antifungal drugs (Parsons et al., 2004), among others.

Pharmacogenetics may identify subsets of patients who will have a very high or a very low likelihood of responding to an agent. This will permit testing of the drug in a selected population that is more likely to respond, minimizing the possibility of adverse events in patients who derive no benefit, and more tightly defining the parameters of response in the subset more likely to benefit. Somatic mutations in the *EGFR* gene strongly identify patients with lung cancer who are likely to respond to the tyrosine kinase inhibitor gefitinib (Lynch et al., 2004); germline variations in 5-lipoxygenase (*ALOX5*) determine which asthma patients are likely to respond to ALOX inhibitors (Drazen et al., 1999); and vasodilation in response to β_2 agonists has been linked to β_2 adrenergic receptor polymorphisms (Johnson and Lima, 2003).

A related role for pharmacogenomics in drug development is to identify which genetic subset of patients is at highest risk for a serious adverse drug effect, and to avoid testing the drug in that subset of patients (Lesko and Woodcock, 2004). For example, the identification of HLA subtypes associated with hypersensitivity to the HIV-1 reverse transcriptase inhibitor abacavir (Mallal et al., 2002, 2008) identifies a subset of patients who should receive alternative antiretroviral therapy, and this has been shown to decrease the frequency of hypersensitivity as an adverse effect of this agent. Children with acute myeloid leukemia who are homozygous for germline deletions in GSH transferase (*GSTT1*) are almost three times as likely to die of toxicity as those patients who have at least one wild-type copy of *GSTT1* following intensively timed antileukemic therapy but not after "usual" doses of antileukemic therapy (Davies et al., 2001). These latter results suggest an important principle: pharmacogenetic testing may help to identify patients who require altered dosages of medications, but will not necessarily preclude the use of the agents completely.

Pharmacogenetics in Clinical Practice

Despite considerable research activity, pharmacogenetics are not yet widely utilized in clinical practice. There are three major types of evidence that should accumulate in order to implicate a polymorphism in clinical care (Figure 7–14):

- screens of tissues from multiple humans linking the polymorphism to a trait
- complementary preclinical functional studies indicating that the polymorphism is plausibly linked with the phenotype
- multiple supportive clinical phenotype/genotype association studies

Because of the high probability of type I error in genotype/phenotype association studies, replication of clinical findings will generally be necessary. Although the impact of the polymorphism in TPMT on mercaptopurine dosing in childhood leukemia is a good example of a polymorphism for which all three types of evidence are available, proactive individualized dosing of thiopurines based on genotype has not been widely incorporated into clinical practice (Lesko et al., 2004).

Most drug dosing relies on a population "average" dose of drug. Adjusting dosages for variables such as renal or liver dysfunction is often accepted in drug dosing, even in cases in which the clinical outcome of such adjustments has not been studied. Even though there are many examples of significant effects of polymorphisms on drug disposition (e.g., Table 7–3), there is much more hesitation from clinicians to adjust doses based on genetic testing than on indirect clinical measures of renal and liver function. Whether this hesitation reflects resistance to abandon the "trial-and-error" approach that has defined most drug dosing, concern about genetic discrimination, or unfamiliarity with the principles of genetics is not clear. Nonetheless, broad public initiatives, such as the NIH-funded Pharmacogenetics and Pharmacogenomics Knowledge Base (www.pharmGKB.org), provide useful resources to permit clinicians to access information on pharmacogenetics (see Table 7–1). The passage of laws to prevent genetic discrimination (Erwin, 2008) may also assuage concerns that genetic data placed in medical records could penalize those with "unfavorable" genotypes.

The fact that functionally important polymorphisms are so common means that complexity of dosing will be likely to increase substantially in the postgenomic era. Even if every drug has only one important polymorphism to consider when dosing, the scale of complexity could be large. Many individuals take multiple drugs simultaneously for different diseases, and many therapeutic regimens for a single disease consist of multiple agents. This situation translates into a large number of possible drug-dose combinations. Much of the excitement regarding the promise of human genomics has emphasized the hope of discovering individualized "magic bullets," and ignored the reality of the added complexity of additional testing and need for interpretation of results to capitalize on individualized dosing. This is illustrated in a potential pharmacogenetic example in Figure 7–14. In this case, a traditional anticancer treatment approach is replaced with one that incorporates pharmacogenetic information with the stage of the cancer determined by a variety of standardized pathological criteria. Assuming just one important genetic polymorphism for each of the

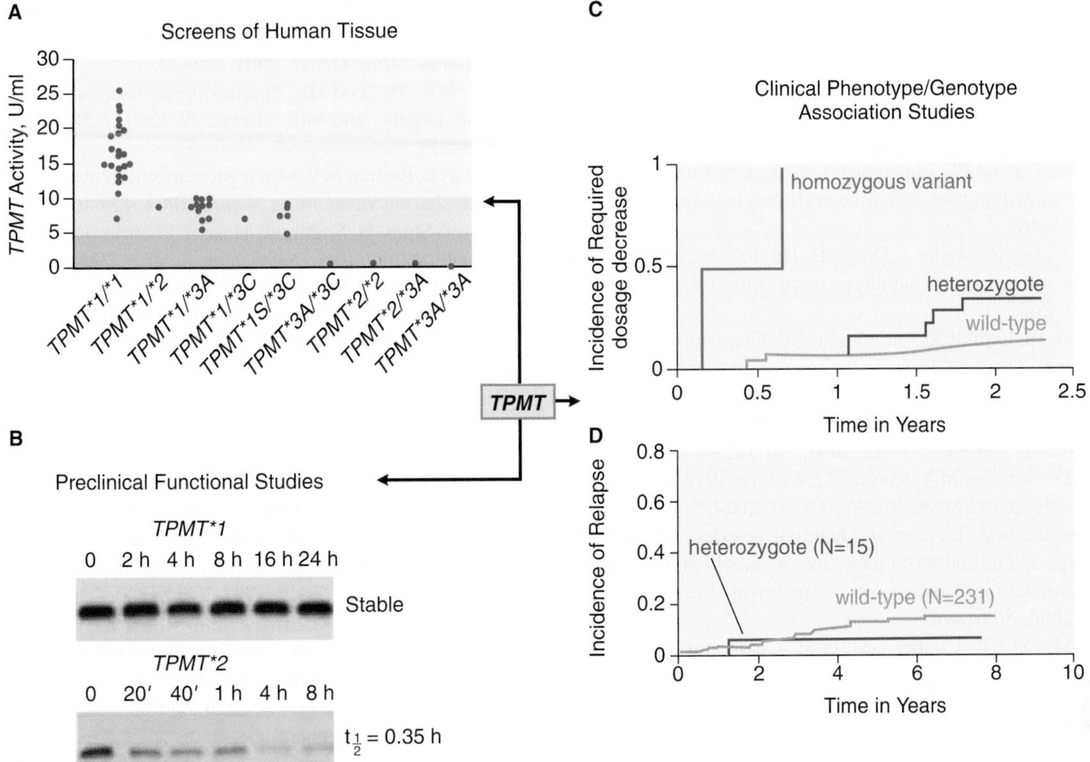

Figure 7–14. *Three primary types of evidence in pharmacogenetics.* Screens of human tissue (***A***) link phenotype (thiopurine methyltransferase activity in erythrocytes) with genotype (germline *TPMT* genotype). The two alleles are separated by a slash (/); the ∗1 and ∗1S alleles are wild-type, and the ∗2, ∗3A, and ∗3C are nonfunctional alleles. Shaded areas indicate low and intermediate levels of enzyme activity: those with the homozygous wild-type genotype have the highest activity, those heterozygous for at least one ∗1 allele have intermediate activity, and those homozygous for two inactive alleles have low or undetectable TPMT activity (Yates et al., 1997). Directed preclinical functional studies (***B***) can provide biochemical data consistent with the *in vitro* screens of human tissue, and may offer further confirmatory evidence. Here, the heterologous expression of the *TPMT∗1* wild-type and the *TPMT∗2* variant alleles indicate that the former produces a more stable protein, as assessed by Western blot (Tai et al., 1997). The third type of evidence comes from clinical phenotype/genotype association studies (***C*** and ***D***). The incidence of required dosage decrease for thiopurine in children with leukemia (***C***) differs by *TPMT* genotype: 100%, 35%, and 7% of patients with homozygous variant, heterozygous, or homozygous wild-type, respectively, require a dosage decrease (Relling et al., 1999). When dosages of thiopurine are adjusted based on *TPMT* genotype in the successor study (***D***), leukemic relapse is not compromised, as indicated by comparable relapse rates in children who were wild-type *vs.* heterozygous for *TPMT*. Taken together, these three data sets indicate that the polymorphism should be accounted for in dosing of thiopurines. (Reproduced with permission from Relling et al., 1999. Copyright © Oxford University Press.)

three different anticancer drugs, 11 individual drug regimens can easily be generated.

Nonetheless, the potential utility of pharmacogenetics to optimize drug therapy is great. After adequate genotype/phenotype studies have been conducted, molecular diagnostic tests will be developed, and genetic tests have the advantage that they need only be conducted once during an individual's lifetime. With continued incorporation of pharmacogenetics into clinical trials, the important genes and polymorphisms will be identified, and data will demonstrate whether dosage individualization can improve outcomes and decrease short- and long-term adverse effects. Significant covariates will be identified to allow refinement of dosing in the context of drug interactions and disease influences. Although the challenges are substantial, accounting for the genetic basis of variability in response to medications is already being used in specific pharmacotherapeutics decisions, and is likely to become a fundamental component of diagnosing any illness and guiding the choice and dosage of medications.

Aithal GP, Day CP, Kesteven PJ, Daly AK. Association of polymorphisms in the cytochrome p450 cyp2c9 with warfarin dose requirement and risk of bleeding complications. *Lancet*, **1999**, *353*:717–719.

Alving AS, Carson PE, Flanagan CL, Ickes CE. Enzymatic deficiency in primaquine-sensitive erythrocytes. *Science*, **1956**, *124*:484–485.

Barrett JC, Fry B, Maller J, Daly MJ. Haploview: Analysis and visualization of ld and haplotype maps. *Bioinformatics*, **2005**, *21*:263–265.

Beckmann JS, Estivill X, Antonarakis SE. Copy number variants and genetic traits: Closer to the resolution of phenotypic to genotypic variability. *Nat Rev Genet*, **2007**, *8*:639–646.

Bejerano G, Pheasant M, Makunin I, et al. Ultraconserved elements in the human genome. *Science*, **2004**, *304*:1321–1325.

Boffelli D, Nobrega MA, Rubin EM. Comparative genomics at the vertebrate extremes. *Nat Rev Genet*, **2004**, *5*:456–465.

Borges S, Desta Z, Li L, et al. Quantitative effect of CYP2D6 genotype and inhibitors on tamoxifen metabolism: Implication for optimization of breast cancer treatment. *Clin Pharmacol Ther*, **2006**, *80*:61–74.

Brudno M, Do CB, Cooper GM, et al. Lagan and multi-lagan: Efficient tools for large-scale multiple alignment of genomic DNA. *Genome Res*, **2003**, *13*:721–731.

Burchard EG, Ziv E, Coyle N, et al. The importance of race and ethnic background in biomedical research and clinical practice. *N Engl J Med*, **2003**, *348*:1170–1175.

Caraco Y, Blotnick S, Muszkat M. CYP2C9 genotype-guided warfarin prescribing enhances the efficacy and safety of anticoagulation: A prospective randomized controlled study. *Clin Pharmacol Ther*, **2008**, *83*:460–470.

Cargill M, Altshuler D, Ireland J, et al. Characterization of single-nucleotide polymorphisms in coding regions of human genes. *Nat Genet*, **1999**, *22*:231–238.

Chanock S. Genetic variation and hematology: Single-nucleotide polymorphisms, haplotypes, and complex disease. *Semin Hematol*, **2003**, *40*:321–328.

Davies SM, Robison LL, Buckley JD, et al. Glutathione S-transferase polymorphisms and outcome of chemotherapy in childhood acute myeloid leukemia. *J Clin Oncol*, **2001**, *19*: 1279–1287.

den Heijer HM. Hyperhomocysteinaemia as a risk factor for venous thrombosis: An update of the current evidence. *Clin Chem Lab Med*, **2003**, *41*:1404–1407.

Drazen JM, Yandava CN, Dube L, et al. Pharmacogenetic association between alox5 promoter genotype and the response to anti-asthma treatment. *Nat Genet*, **1999**, *22*:168–170.

Eichelbaum M, Gross AS. The genetic polymorphism of debrisoquine/sparteine metabolism-clinical aspects. *Pharmacol Ther*, **1990**, *46*:377–394.

Eichelbaum M, Spannbrucker N, Dengler HJ. Proceedings: N-oxidation of sparteine in man and its interindividual differences. *Naunyn Schmiedebergs Arch Pharmacol*, **1975**, *287 (Suppl)*: R94.

Erwin C. Legal update: Living with the genetic information nondiscrimination act. *Genet Med*, **2008**, *10*:869–873.

Essen GGV, Rensma PL, Zeeuw DD, et al. Association between angiotensin-conferting-enzyme gene polymorphism and failure of renoprotective therapy. *Lancet*, **1996**, *347*:94–95.

Evans WE, Johnson JA. Pharmacogenomics: The inherited basis for interindividual differences in drug response. *Annu Rev Genomics Hum Genet*, **2001**, *2*:9–39.

Evans WE, McLeod HL. Pharmacogenomics—drug disposition, drug targets, and side effects. *N Engl J Med*, **2003**, *348*: 538–549.

Evans WE, Relling MV. Moving towards individualized medicine with pharmacogenomics. *Nature*, **2004**, *429*:464–468.

Furuta T, Shirai N, Sugimoto M, et al. Pharmacogenomics of proton pump inhibitors. *Pharmacogenomics*, **2004**, *5*:181–202.

Goetz MP, Kamal A, Ames MM. Tamoxifen pharmacogenomics: The role of CYP2D6 as a predictor of drug response. *Clin Pharmacol Ther*, **2008**, *83*:160–166.

Goldstein JA. Clinical relevance of genetic polymorphisms in the human CYP2C subfamily. *Br J Clin Pharmacol*, **2001**, *52*:349–355.

Gonzalez FJ, Skoda RC, Kimura S, et al. Characterization of the common genetic defect in humans deficient in debrisoquine metabolism. *Nature*, **1988**, *331*:442–446.

Goyette P, Sumner JS, Milos R, et al. Human methylenetetrahydrofolate reductase: Isolation of cDNA, mapping and mutation identification. *Nat Genet*, **1994**, *7*:195–200.

Grant DM, Morike K, Eichelbaum M, Meyer UA. Acetylation pharmacogenetics. The slow acetylator phenotype is caused by decreased or absent arylamine N-acetyltransferase in human liver. *J Clin Invest*, **1990**, *85*:968–972.

Grossman I. Routine pharmacogenetic testing in clinical practice: Dream or reality? *Pharmacogenomics*, **2007**, *8*:1449–1459.

Hartford CM, Dolan ME. Identifying genetic variants that contribute to chemotherapy-induced cytotoxicity. *Pharmacogenomics*, **2007**, *8*:1159–1168.

Haufroid V, Mourad M, Van Kerckhove V, et al. The effect of CYP3A5 and MDR1 (ABCB1) polymorphisms on cyclosporine and tacrolimus dose requirements and trough blood levels in stable renal transplant patients. *Pharmacogenetics*, **2004**, *14*:147–154.

Henikoff S, Henikoff JG. Amino acid substitution matrices from protein blocks. *Proc Natl Acad Sci USA*, **1992**, *89*:10915–10919.

Herrington DM, Howard TD, Hawkins GA, et al. Estrogen-receptor polymorphisms and effects of estrogen replacement on high-density lipoprotein cholesterol in women with coronary disease. *N Engl J Med*, **2002**, *346*:967–974.

Hoffmeyer S, Burk O, von Richter O, et al. Functional polymorphisms of the human multidrug-resistance gene: Multiple sequence variations and correlation of one allele with P-glycoprotein expression and activity in vivo. *Proc Natl Acad Sci USA*, **2000**, *97*:3473–3478.

Hughes HB, Biehl JP, Jones AP, Schmidt LH. Metabolism of isoniazid in man as related to occurrence of peripheral neuritis. *Am Rev Tuberc*, **1954**, *70*:266–273.

Ingelman-Sundberg M, Evans WE. Unravelling the functional genomics of the human CYP2D6 gene locus. *Pharmacogenetics*, **2001**, *11*:553–554.

Ingle JN. Pharmacogenomics of tamoxifen and aromatase inhibitors. *Cancer*, **2008**, *112*:695–699.

International HapMap C, Frazer KA, Ballinger DG, et al. A second generation human haplotype map of over 3.1 million snps. *Nature*, **2007**, *449*:851–861.

Iyer L, Das S, Janisch L, et al. UGT1A1*28 polymorphism as a determinant of irinotecan disposition and toxicity. *Pharmacogenomics J*, **2002**, *2*:43–47.

Johnson JA, Lima JJ. Drug receptor/effector polymorphisms and pharmacogenetics: Current status and challenges. *Pharmacogenetics*, **2003**, *13*:525–534.

Kalow W, Tang BK, Endrenyi L. Hypothesis: Comparisons of inter- and intra-individual variations can substitute for twin studies in drug research. *Pharmacogenetics*, **1998**, *8*: 283–289.

Kim DW, Kim M, Lee SK, et al. Lack of association between C3435T nucleotide MDR1 genetic polymorphism and multidrug-resistant epilepsy. *Seizure*, **2006**, *15*:344–347.

Kimchi-Sarfaty C, Oh JM, Kim IW, et al. A "silent" polymorphism in the MDR1 gene changes substrate specificity1. *Science*, **2007**, *315*:525–528.

Kirchheiner J, Brosen K, Dahl ML, et al. CYP2D6 and CYP2C19 genotype-based dose recommendations for antidepressants: A first step towards subpopulation-specific dosages. *Acta Psychiatr Scand*, **2001**, *104*:173–192.

Klerk M, Verhoef P, Clarke R, et al. MTHFR 677C—>T polymorphism and risk of coronary heart disease: A meta-analysis. *JAMA*, **2002**, *288*:2023–2031.

Krajinovic M, Costea I, Chiasson S. Polymorphism of the thymidylate synthase gene and outcome of acute lymphoblastic leukaemia. *Lancet*, **2002**, *359*:1033–1034.

Kraus JP, Oliveriusova J, Sokolova J, et al. The human cystathionine beta-synthase (CBS) gene: Complete sequence, alternative splicing, and polymorphisms. *Genomics*, **1998**, *52*: 312–324.

Kuehl P, Zhang J, Lin Y, et al. Sequence diversity in CYP3A promoters and characterization of the genetic basis of polymorphic CYP3A5 expression. *Nat Genet*, **2001**, *27*:383–391.

Leabman MK, Huang CC, DeYoung J, et al. Natural variation in human membrane transporter genes reveals evolutionary and functional constraints. *Proc Natl Acad Sci USA*, **2003**, *100*:5896–5901.

Lesko LJ. The critical path of warfarin dosing: Finding an optimal dosing strategy using pharmacogenetics. *Clin Pharmacol Ther*, **2008**, *84*:301–303.

Lesko LJ, Woodcock J. Opinion: Translation of pharmacogenomics and pharmacogenetics: A regulatory perspective. *Nat Rev Drug Discov*, **2004**, *3*:763–769.

Lin YS, Dowling AL, Quigley SD, et al. Co-regulation of CYP3A4 and CYP3A5 and contribution to hepatic and intestinal midazolam metabolism. *Mol Pharmacol*, **2002**, *62*:162–172.

Lynch TJ, Bell DW, Sordella R, et al. Activating mutations in the epidermal growth factor receptor underlying responsiveness of non-small-cell lung cancer to gefitinib. *N Engl J Med*, **2004**, *350*:2129–2139.

Mahgoub A, Idle JR, Dring LG, et al. Polymorphic hydroxylation of debrisoquine in man. *Lancet*, **1977**, *2*:584–586.

Mallal S, Nolan D, Witt C, et al. Association between presence of HLA-B*5701, HLA-DR7, and HLA-DQ3 and hypersensitivity to HIV-1 reverse-transcriptase inhibitor abacavir. *Lancet*, **2002**, *359*:727–732.

Mallal S, Phillips E, Carosi G, et al. Hla-b*5701 screening for hypersensitivity to abacavir. *N Engl J Med*, **2008**, *358*: 568–579.

McDonald OG, Krynetski EY, Evans WE. Molecular haplotyping of genomic DNA for multiple single nucleotide polymorphisms located kilobases apart using long range polymerase chain reaction and intramolecular ligation. *Pharmacogenetics*, **2002**, *12*:93–99.

Meyer UA. Pharmacogenetics and adverse drug reactions. *Lancet*, **2000**, *356*:1667–1671.

Meyer UA, Zanger UM. Molecular mechanisms of genetic polymorphisms of drug metabolism. *Annu Rev Pharmacol Toxicol*, **1997**, *37*:269–296.

Miller MP, Kumar S. Understanding human disease mutations through the use of interspecific genetic variation. *Hum Mol Genet*, **2001**, *10*:2319–2328.

Mirkovic N, Marti-Renom MA, Weber BL, et al. Structure-based assessment of missense mutations in human BRCA1: Implications for breast and ovarian cancer predisposition. *Cancer Res*, **2004**, *64*:3790–3797.

Monaghan G, Ryan M, Seddon R, et al. Genetic variation in bilirubin upd-glucuronosyltransferase gene promoter and gilbert's syndrome. *Lancet*, **1996**, *347*:578–581.

Murphy GM Jr, Kremer C, Rodrigues HE, Schatzberg AF. Pharmacogenetics of antidepressant medication intolerance. *Am J Psychiatry*, **2003**, *160*:1830–1835.

Nebert DW, McKinnon RA, Puga A. Human drug-metabolizing enzyme polymorphisms: Effects on risk of toxicity and cancer. *DNA Cell Biol*, **1996**, *15*:273–280.

Ng LC, Forslund O, Koh S, et al. The response of murine macrophages to infection with *Yersinia pestis* as revealed by DNA microarray analysis. *Adv Exp Med Biol*, **2003**, *529*: 155–160.

Pani MA, Knapp M, Donner H, et al. Vitamin D receptor allele combinations influence genetic susceptibility to type 1 diabetes in germans. *Diabetes*, **2000**, *49*:504–507.

Parsons AB, Brost RL, Ding H, et al. Integration of chemical-genetic and genetic interaction data links bioactive compounds to cellular target pathways. *Nat Biotechnol*, **2004**, *22*:62–69.

Penno MB, Dvorchik BH, Vesell ES. Genetic variation in rates of antipyrine metabolite formation: A study in uninduced twins. *Proc Natl Acad Sci USA*, **1981**, *78*:5193–5196.

Phillips KA, Veenstra DL, Oren E, et al. Potential role of pharmacogenomics in reducing adverse drug reactions: A systematic review. *JAMA*, **2001**, *286*:2270–2279.

Ramensky V, Bork P, Sunyaev S. Human non-synonymous SNPs: Server and survey. *Nucleic Acids Res*, **2002**, *30*: 3894–3900.

Redon R, Ishikawa S, Fitch KR., et al. Global variation in copy number in the human genome. *Nature*, **2006**, *444*:444–454.

Relling MV, Dervieux T. Pharmacogenetics and cancer therapy. *Nature Rev Cancer*, **2001**, *1*:99–108.

Relling MV, Hancock ML, Rivera GK, et al. Mercaptopurine therapy intolerance and heterozygosity at the thiopurine S-methyltransferase gene locus. *J Natl Cancer Inst*, **1999**, *91*:2001–2008.

Roden DM. Cardiovascular pharmacogenomics. *Circulation*, **2003**, *108*:3071–3074.

Roden DM. Drug-induced prolongation of the QT interval. *N Engl J Med*, **2004**, *350*:1013–1022.

Rosenberg NA, Li LM, Ward R, Pritchard JK. Informativeness of genetic markers for inference of ancestry. *Am J Hum Genet*, **2003**, *73*:1402–1422.

Rosenberg NA, Pritchard JK, Weber JL, et al. Genetic structure of human populations. *Science*, **2002**, *298*:2381–2385.

Rosner GL, Panetta JC, Innocenti F, Ratain MJ. Pharmacogenetic pathway analysis of irinotecan. *Clin Pharmacol Ther*, **2008**, *84*:393–402.

Schwarz UI, Ritchie MD, Bradford Y, et al. Genetic determinants of response to warfarin during initial anticoagulation. *N Engl J Med*, **2008**, *358*:999–1008.

SEARCH Collaborative Group, Link E, Parish S, et al. SLCO1B1 Variants and Statin-Induced Myopathy—A Genomewide Study. *N Engl J Med*, **2008**, *359*:789–799.

Shu Y, Leabman MK, Feng B, et al. Evolutionary conservation predicts function of variants of the human organic cation transporter, OCT1. *Proc Natl Acad Sci USA*, **2003**, *100*: 5902–5907.

Sills GJ, Mohanraj R, Butler E, et al. Lack of association between the C3435T polymorphism in the human multidrug resistance (MDR1) gene and response to antiepileptic drug treatment. *Epilepsia*, **2005**, *46*:643–647.

Stanulla M, Schaeffeler E, Flohr T, et al. Thiopurine methyltransferase (tpmt) genotype and early treatment response to mercaptopurine in childhood acute lymphoblastic leukemia. *JAMA*, **2005**, *293*:1485–1489.

Stegmaier K, Ross KN, Colavito SA, et al. Gene expression-based high-throughput screening(GE-HTS) and application to leukemia differentiation. *Na.Genet*, **2004**, *36*:257–263.

Stephens JC, Schneider JA, Tanguay DA., et al. Haplotype variation and linkage disequilibrium in 313 human genes. *Science*, **2001**, *293*:489–493.

Stranger BE, Forrest MS, Dunning M, et al. Relative impact of nucleotide and copy number variation on gene expression phenotypes. *Science*, **2007**, *315*:848–853.

Tabor HK, Risch NJ, Myers RM. Candidate-gene approaches for studying complex genetic traits: Practical considerations. *Nat Rev Genet*, **2002**, *3*:391–397.

Tai HL, Krynetski EY, Schuetz EG, et al. W.E. Enhanced proteolysis of thiopurine S-methyltransferase (TPMT) encoded by mutant alleles in humans (TPMT*3a, TPMT*2): Mechanisms for the genetic polymorphism of tpmt activity. *Proc Natl Acad Sci USA*, **1997**, *94*:6444–6449.

Tan S, Hall IP, Dewar J, et al. Association between beta 2-adrenoceptor polymorphism and susceptibility to bronchodilator desensitisation in moderately severe stable asthmatics. *Lancet*, **1997**, *350*:995–999.

Taylor DR, Kennedy MA. Genetic variation of the beta(2)-adrenoceptor: Its functional and clinical importance in bronchial asthma. *Am J Pharmacogenom*, **2001**, *1*:165–174.

Tirona RG, Leake BF, Merino G, Kim RB. Polymorphisms in OATP-C: Identification of multiple allelic variants associated with altered transport activity among European- and African-americans. *J Biol Chem*, **2001**, *276*:35669–35675.

Townsend DM, Tew KD. The role of glutathione-S-transferase in anti-cancer drug resistance. *Oncogene*, **2003**, *22*:7369–7375.

Turgut S, Yaren A, Kursunluoglu R, Turgut G. MDR1 C3435T polymorphism in patients with breast cancer. *Arch Med Res*, **2007**, *38*:539–544.

Ulrich CM, Yasui Y, Storb R, et al. Pharmacogenetics of methotrexate: Toxicity among marrow transplantation patients varies with the methylenetetrahydrofolate reductase C677T polymorphism. *Blood*, **2001**, *98*:231–234.

Urban TJ, Gallagher RC, Brown C, et al. Functional genetic diversity in the high-affinity carnitine transporter OCTN2 (SLC22A5). *Mol Pharmacol*, **2006**, *70*:1602–1611.

Vesell ES. Genetic and environmental factors causing variation in drug response. *Mutat Res*, **1991**, *247*:241–257.

Vesell ES. Advances in pharmacogenetics and pharmacogenomics. *J Clin Pharmacol*, **2000**, *40*:930–938.

Vesell ES, Page JG. Genetic control of drug levels in man: Antipyrine. *Science*, **1968**, *161*:72–73.

Villafranca E, Okruzhnov Y, Dominguez MA, et al. Polymorphisms of the repeated sequences in the enhancer region of the thymidylate synthase gene promoter may predict downstaging after preoperative chemoradiation in rectal cancer. *J Clin Oncol*, **2001**, *19*:1779–1786.

Watters JW, Kraja A, Meucci MA, et al. Genome-wide discovery of loci influencing chemotherapy cytotoxicity. *Proc Natl Acad Sci USA*, **2004**, *101*:11809–11814.

Weinshilboum R. Inheritance and drug response. *N Engl J Med*, **2003**, *348*:529–537.

Weinshilboum R, Wang, L. Pharmacogenomics: Bench to bedside. *Nat Rev Drug Discov*, **2004**, *3*:739–748.

Weinshilboum RM, Sladek SL. Mercaptopurine pharmacogenetics: Monogenic inheritance of erythrocyte thiopurine methyltransferase activity. *Am J Hum Genet*, **1980**, *32*:651–662.

Wen MS, Lee M, Chen JJ, et al. Prospective study of warfarin dosage requirements based on CYP2C9 and VKORC1 genotypes. *Clin Pharmacol Ther*, **2008**, *84*:83–89.

Xie HG, Kim RB, Wood AJ, Stein CM. Molecular basis of ethnic differences in drug disposition and response. *Annu Rev Pharmacol Toxicol*, **2001**, *41*:815–850.

Xu ZH, Freimuth RR, Eckloff B, et al. Human 3′-phosphoadenosine 5′-phosphosulfate synthetase 2 (PAPSS2) pharmacogenetics: Gene resequencing, genetic polymorphisms and functional characterization of variant allozymes. *Pharmacogenetics*, **2002**, *12*:11–21.

Yates CR, Krynetski EY, Loennechen T, et al. Molecular diagnosis of thiopurine S-methyltransferase deficiency: Genetic basis for azathioprine and mercaptopurine intolerance. *Ann Intern Med*, **1997**, *126*:608–614.

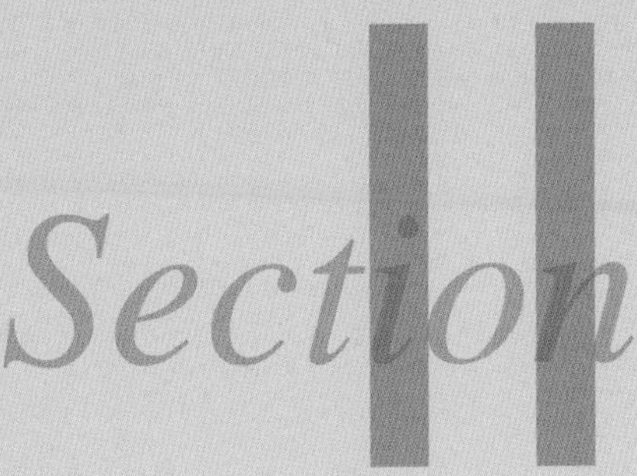

Neuropharmacology

Neurotransmission: The Autonomic and Somatic Motor Nervous Systems

Thomas C. Westfall and
David P. Westfall

ANATOMY AND GENERAL FUNCTIONS

The autonomic nervous system, also called the *visceral, vegetative,* or *involuntary nervous system,* is distributed widely throughout the body and regulates autonomic functions that occur without conscious control. In the periphery, it consists of nerves, ganglia, and plexuses that innervate the heart, blood vessels, glands, other visceral organs, and smooth muscle in various tissues.

Differences Between Autonomic and Somatic Nerves. The efferent nerves of the involuntary system supply all innervated structures of the body except skeletal muscle, which is served by somatic nerves. The most distal synaptic junctions in the autonomic reflex arc occur in ganglia that are entirely outside the cerebrospinal axis. These ganglia are small but complex structures that contain axodendritic synapses between preganglionic and postganglionic neurons. Somatic nerves contain no peripheral ganglia, and the synapses are located entirely within the cerebrospinal axis. Many autonomic nerves form extensive peripheral plexuses, but such networks are absent from the somatic system. Whereas motor nerves to skeletal muscles are myelinated, postganglionic autonomic nerves generally are nonmyelinated. When the spinal efferent nerves are interrupted, the denervated skeletal muscles lack myogenic tone, are paralyzed, and atrophy, whereas smooth muscles and glands generally retain some level of spontaneous activity independent of intact innervation.

Visceral Afferent Fibers. The afferent fibers from visceral structures are the first link in the reflex arcs of the autonomic system. With certain exceptions, such as local axon reflexes, most visceral reflexes are mediated through the central nervous system (CNS).

Information on the status of the visceral organs is transmitted to the CNS through two main sensory systems: the cranial nerve (parasympathetic) visceral sensory system and the spinal (sympathetic) visceral afferent system (Saper, 2002). The cranial visceral sensory system carries mainly mechanoreceptor and chemosensory information, whereas the afferents of the spinal visceral system principally convey sensations related to temperature and tissue injury of mechanical, chemical, or thermal origin. Cranial visceral sensory information enters the CNS by four cranial nerves: the trigeminal (V), facial (VII), glossopharyngeal (IX), and vagus (X) nerves. These four cranial nerves transmit visceral sensory information from the internal face and head (V); tongue (taste, VII); hard palate and upper part of the oropharynx (IX); and carotid body, lower part of the oropharynx, larynx, trachea, esophagus, and thoracic and abdominal organs (X), with the exception of the pelvic viscera. The pelvic viscera are innervated by nerves from the second through fourth sacral spinal segments.

The visceral afferents from these four cranial nerves terminate topographically in the solitary tract nucleus (STN) (Altschuler et al., 1989). The most massive site for termination of the fibers from the STN is the parabrachial nucleus, which is thus the major relay station. The parabrachial nucleus consists of at least 13 separate subnuclei, which in turn project extensively to a wide range of sites in the brainstem, hypothalamus, basal forebrain, thalamus, and cerebral cortex. Other direct projections from the STN also innervate these brain structures.

Sensory afferents from visceral organs also enter the CNS from the spinal nerves. Those concerned with muscle chemosensation may arise at all spinal levels, whereas sympathetic visceral sensory afferents generally arise at the thoracic levels where sympathetic preganglionic neurons are found. Pelvic sensory afferents from spinal segments S2–S4 enter at that level and are important for the regulation of sacral parasympathetic outflow. In general, visceral afferents that enter the spinal nerves convey information concerned with temperature as well as nociceptive visceral inputs related to mechanical, chemical, and thermal stimulation. The primary pathways taken by ascending spinal visceral afferents are complex and controversial (Saper, 2002). Most probably converge with musculoskeletal and cutaneous afferents and ascend by the spinothalamic and spinoreticular tracts. Others ascend by the dorsal column. An important feature of the ascending pathways is that they provide collaterals that converge with the cranial visceral sensory pathway at virtually every level (Saper, 2000). At the brainstem level, collaterals from the spinal system converge with the cranial nerve sensory system in the STN, the ventrolateral medulla, and the parabrachial nucleus. At the level of the forebrain, the spinal system appears to form a posterolateral continuation of the cranial nerve visceral sensory thalamus and cortex (Saper, 2000).

The neurotransmitters that mediate transmission from sensory fibers have not been characterized unequivocally. Substance P and calcitonin gene–related peptide (CGRP), which are present in afferent sensory fibers, in the dorsal root ganglia, and in the dorsal horn of the spinal cord, are leading candidates for neurotransmitters that communicate nociceptive stimuli from the periphery to the spinal cord and higher structures. Other neuroactive peptides, including somatostatin, vasoactive intestinal polypeptide (VIP), and cholecystokinin, also have been found in sensory neurons (Hökfelt et al., 2000), and one or more such peptides may play a role in the transmission of afferent impulses from autonomic structures. ATP appears to be a neurotransmitter in certain sensory neurons, including those that innervate the urinary bladder. Enkephalins, present in interneurons in the dorsal spinal cord (within an area termed the *substantia gelatinosa*), have antinociceptive effects that appear to arise from presynaptic and postsynaptic actions to inhibit the release of substance P and diminish the activity of cells that project from the spinal cord to higher centers in the CNS. The excitatory amino acids glutamate and aspartate also play major roles in transmission of sensory responses to the spinal cord.

Central Autonomic Connections. There probably are no purely autonomic or somatic centers of integration, and extensive overlap occurs. Somatic responses always are accompanied by visceral responses, and vice versa. Autonomic reflexes can be elicited at the level of the spinal cord. They clearly are demonstrable in experimental animals or humans with spinal cord transection and are manifested by sweating, blood pressure alterations, vasomotor responses to temperature changes, and reflex emptying of the urinary bladder, rectum, and seminal vesicles. Extensive central ramifications of the autonomic nervous system exist above the level of the spinal cord. For example, integration of the control of respiration in the medulla oblongata is well known. The hypothalamus and the STN generally are regarded as principal loci of integration of autonomic nervous system functions, which include regulation of body temperature, water balance, carbohydrate and fat metabolism, blood pressure, emotions, sleep, respiration, and reproduction. Signals are received through ascending spinobulbar pathways, the limbic system, neostriatum, cortex, and to a lesser extent other higher brain centers. Stimulation of the STN and the hypothalamus activates bulbospinal pathways and hormonal output to mediate autonomic and motor responses (Andresen and Kunze, 1994; (see Chapter 14). The hypothalamic nuclei that lie posteriorly and laterally are sympathetic in their main connections, whereas parasympathetic functions evidently are integrated by the midline nuclei in the region of the tuber cinereum and by nuclei lying anteriorly.

The CNS can produce a wide range of patterned autonomic and somatic responses from discrete activation of sympathetic or parasympathetic neurons to more generalized activation of these nerves with highly integrated patterns of response. There are highly differentiated patterns of activity during a wide range of physiological conditions consistent with the need for modulation of different organ functions. There is evidence for organotropical organization of neuronal pools at multiple levels of the CNS that generate these various patterns of sympathetic and parasympathetic responses. The pattern generators at these different levels of the neuroaxis are often organized in a hierarchical manner that allows individual response or larger responses made up of multiple individual units.

Highly integrated patterns of response generally are organized at a hypothalamic level and involve autonomic, endocrine, and behavioral components. On the other hand, more limited patterned responses are organized at other levels of basal forebrain, brainstem, and spinal cord.

Divisions of the Peripheral Autonomic System. On the efferent side, the autonomic nervous system consists of two large divisions: (1) the sympathetic or thoracolumbar outflow and (2) the parasympathetic or craniosacral outflow. A brief outline of those anatomical features is necessary for an understanding of the actions of autonomic drugs.

The arrangement of the principal parts of the peripheral autonomic nervous system is presented schematically in Figure 8–1. The neurotransmitter of all preganglionic autonomic fibers, most postganglionic parasympathetic fibers, and a few postganglionic sympathetic fibers is acetylcholine (ACh). Some postganglionic parasympathetic nerves use nitric oxide (NO) as a neurotransmitter; nerves that release NO are referred to as *nitrergic* (Toda and Okamura, 2003). The adrenergic fibers comprise the majority of the postganglionic sympathetic fibers; here the primary transmitter is norepinephrine (NE, noradrenaline, levarterenol). The terms *cholinergic* and *adrenergic* were proposed originally by Dale to describe neurons that liberate ACh or norepinephrine, respectively. Not all the transmitter(s) of the primary afferent fibers, such as those from the mechano- and chemoreceptors of the carotid body and aortic arch, have been identified conclusively. Substance P and glutamate are thought to mediate many afferent impulses; both are present in high concentrations in the dorsal spinal cord.

Sympathetic Nervous System. The cells that give rise to the preganglionic fibers of this division lie mainly in the intermediolateral columns of the spinal cord and extend from the first thoracic to the second or

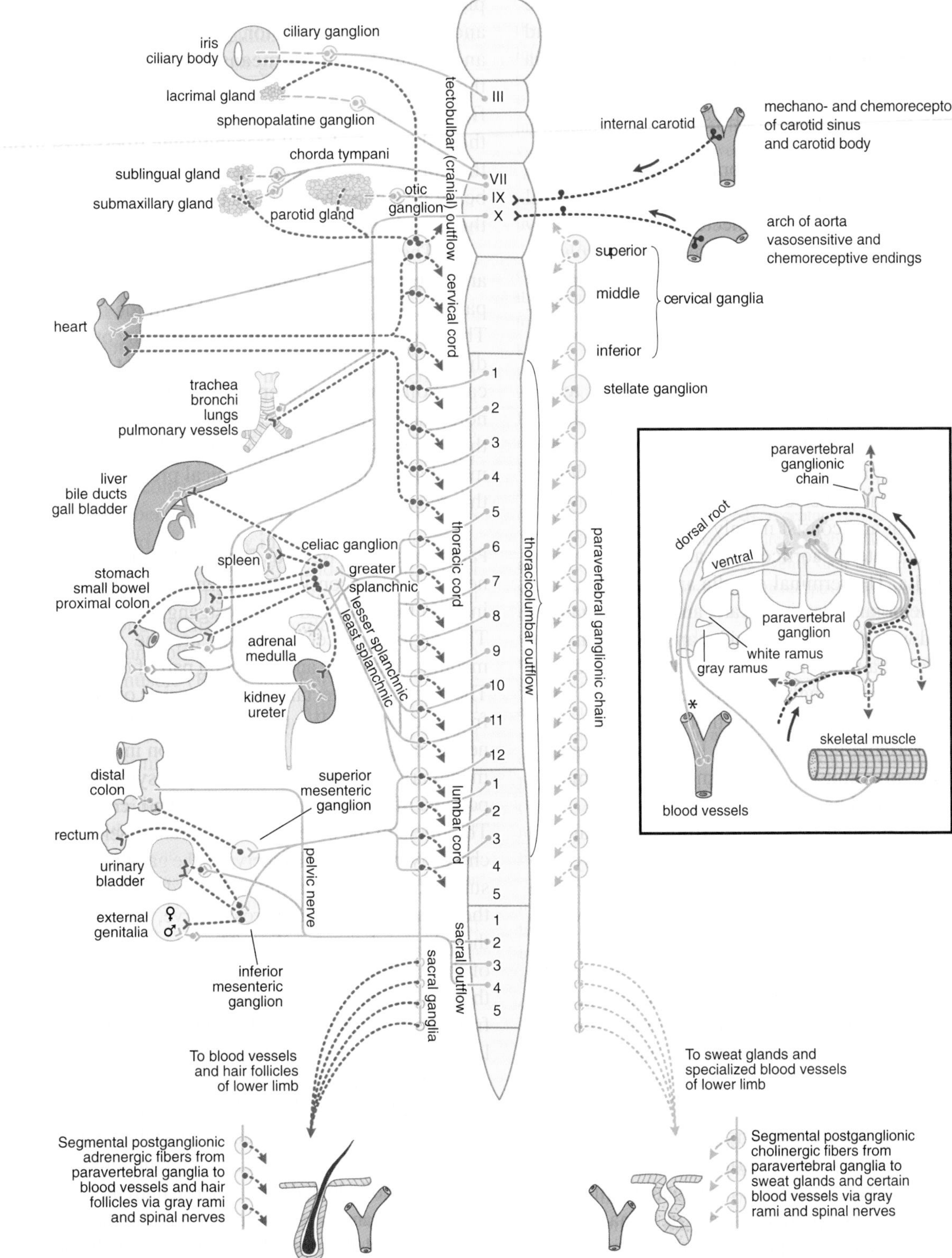

Figure 8–1. *The autonomic nervous system.* Schematic representation of the autonomic nerves and effector organs based on chemical mediation of nerve impulses. Yellow, cholinergic; red, adrenergic; dotted blue, visceral afferent; solid lines, preganglionic; broken lines, postganglionic. In the upper rectangle at the right are shown the finer details of the ramifications of adrenergic fibers at any one segment of the spinal cord, the path of the visceral afferent nerves, the cholinergic nature of somatic motor nerves to skeletal muscle, and the presumed cholinergic nature of the vasodilator fibers in the dorsal roots of the spinal nerves. The asterisk (*) indicates that it is not known whether these vasodilator fibers are motor or sensory or where their cell bodies are situated.

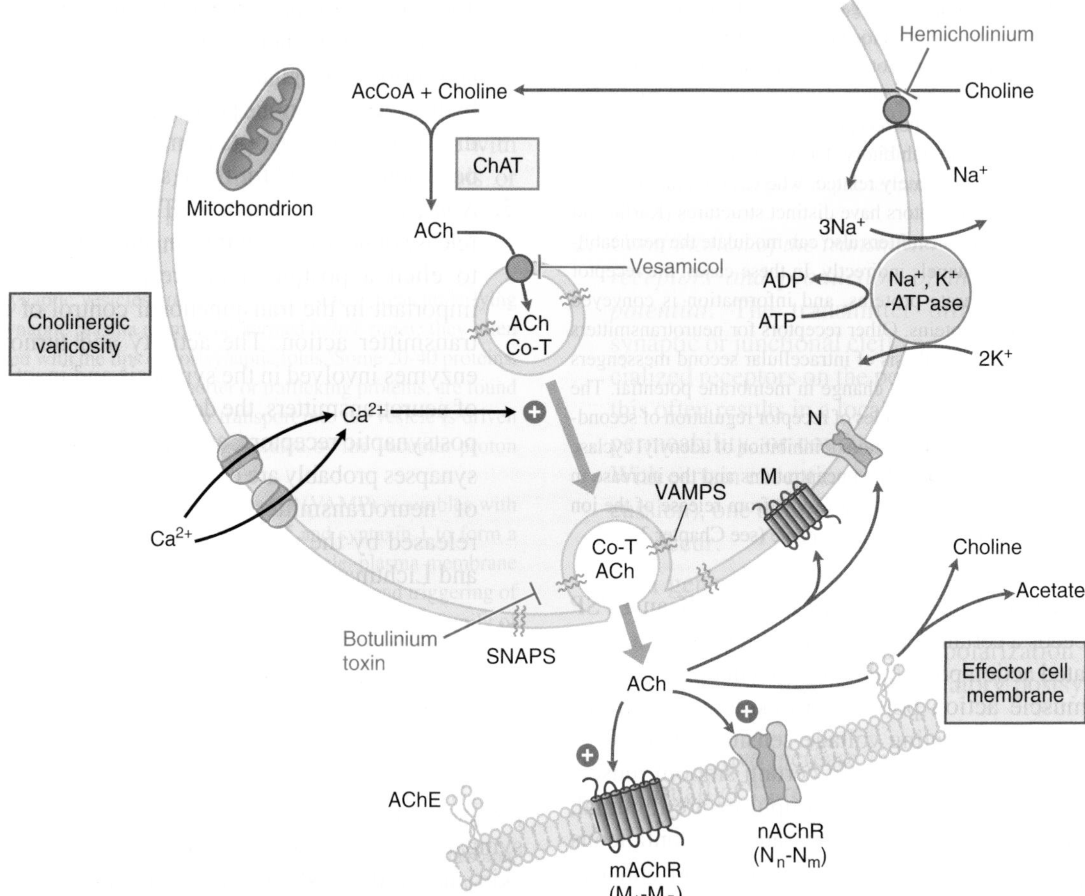

Figure 8–4. *A cholinergic neuroeffector junction showing features of the synthesis, storage, and release of acetylcholine (ACh) and receptors on which ACh acts.* The synthesis of ACh in the varicosity depends on the uptake of choline *via* a sodium-dependent carrier. This uptake can be blocked by hemicholinium. Choline and the acetyl moiety of acetyl coenzyme A, derived from mitochondria, form ACh, a process catalyzed by the enzyme choline acetyl transferase (ChAT). ACh is transported into the storage vesicle by another carrier that can be inhibited by vesamicol. ACh is stored in vesicles along with other potential cotransmitters (Co-T) such as ATP and VIP at certain neuroeffector junctions. Release of ACh and the Co-T occurs on depolarization of the varicosity, which allows the entry of Ca^{2+} through voltage-dependent Ca^{2+} channels. Elevated $[Ca^{2+}]_{in}$ promotes fusion of the vesicular membrane with the cell membrane, and exocytosis of the transmitters occurs. This fusion process involves the interaction of specialized proteins associated with the vesicular membrane (VAMPs, vesicle-associated membrane proteins) and the membrane of the varicosity (SNAPs, synaptosome-associated proteins). The exocytotic release of ACh can be blocked by botulinum toxin. Once released, ACh can interact with the muscarinic receptors (M), which are GPCRs, or nicotinic receptors (N), which are ligand-gated ion channels, to produce the characteristic response of the effector. ACh also can act on presynaptic mAChRs or nAChRs to modify its own release. The action of ACh is terminated by metabolism to choline and acetate by acetylcholinesterase (AChE), which is associated with synaptic membranes.

sequestered within synaptic vesicles. Although moderately potent inhibitors of choline acetyltransferase exist, they have no therapeutic utility, in part because the uptake of choline is the rate-limiting step in ACh biosynthesis.

Choline and Choline Transport. The availability of choline is critical to the synthesis of acetylcholine and is provided from the diet as there is little *de novo* synthesis of choline in cholinergic neurons. Choline is also an essential component for the normal function of all cells, necessary for the structural integrity and signaling functions for cell membranes. Choline is taken up from the extracellular space by two transport systems: a ubiquitous low affinity, Na^+-independent transport system that is inhibited by hemicholinium-3 with a K_i of ~50 μM, and high affinity Na^+- and Cl^--dependent choline transport system that is also sensitive to inhibition by hemicholinium-3 (K_i = 10-100 nM). This second transport system is found predominantly in cholinergic neurons and is responsible for providing choline for ACh synthesis. Once ACh is released from cholinergic neurons following the arrival of action potentials, ACh is hydrolyzed by acetylcholine esterase (AChE) to acetate and choline. Choline is recycled after reuptake into the nerve terminal of cholinergic cells and reused for ACh synthesis. Under many circumstances this reuptake and availability of choline appear to serve as the rate limiting step in acetylcholine synthesis.

The gene for the high-affinity choline transporter (CHT1) has been cloned from a variety of species including human and it is homologous to the Na^+-dependent glucose transport family. The location of CHT1 is in intracellular vesicular structures rather than the nerve terminal plasma membrane and co-localizes with synaptic vesicle markers such as vesicle-associated membrane protein 2 (VAMP2) and vesicular ACh transporter (VAChT). Although the details are incomplete there is evidence that in response to the cascade of events that culminate in transmitter release, there is also increased trafficking of CHT1 to the plasma membrane, where it functions to take up choline after hydrolysis of acetylcholine. Since choline transport is rate limiting for acetylcholine synthesis, increased availability of choline via its transport by CHT1 would favor an increase in ACh stores to maintain high levels of transmitter release during neuronal stimulation. This also suggests that the availability of CHT1 at the cell surface is dynamically regulated in a manner very similar to the regulation of the exocytosis of synaptic vesicles. The precise mechanisms involved in maintaining the distribution of CHT1 predominantly in intracellular vesicles rather than at the terminal surface like other neurotransmitter transporters are unclear (Ferguson and Blakely, 2004; Chaudhry et al. 2008).

Storage of Acetylcholine. Following the synthesis of acetylcholine, which takes place in the cytoplasm of the nerve terminal, ACh is transported into synaptic vesicles by VAChT using a proton electrochemical gradient to move ACh to the inside of the organelle. VAChT is thought to be a protein comprising 12 transmembrane domains with hydrophilic N- and C-termini in the cytoplasm. By sequence homology, VAChT appears to be a member of a family of transport proteins that includes two vesicular monoamine transporters. Transport of protons out of the vesicle is coupled to uptake of ACh into the vesicle and against a concentration gradient via the acetylcholine antiporter.

There appear to be two types of vesicles in cholinergic terminals: electron-lucent vesicles (40-50 nm in diameter) and dense-cored vesicles (80-150 nm). The core of the vesicles contains both ACh and ATP, at an estimated ratio of 10:1, which are dissolved in the fluid phase with metal ions (Ca^{2+} and Mg^{2+}) and a proteoglycan called vesiculin. Vesiculin is negatively charged and is thought to sequester the Ca^{2+} or ACh. It is bound within the vesicle, with the protein moiety anchoring it to the vesicular membrane. In some cholinergic terminals there are peptides, such as VIP, that act as co-transmitters at some junctions. The peptides usually are located in the dense-cored vesicles. Vesicular membranes are rich in lipids, primarily cholesterol and phospholipids, as well as protein. The proteins include ATPase, which is ouabain-sensitive and thought to be involved in proton pumping and in vesicular inward transport of Ca^{2+}. Other proteins include protein kinases (involved in phosphorylation mechanisms of Ca^{2+} uptake), calmodulin, atractyloside-binding protein (which acts as an ATP carrier), and synapsin (which is thought to be involved with exocytosis).

The vesicular transporter allows for the uptake of ACh into the vesicle, has considerable concentrating power, is saturable, and is ATPase-dependent. The process is inhibited by vesamicol (Figure 8–4). Inhibition by vesamicol is noncompetitive and reversible and does not affect the vesicular ATPase. The gene for choline acetyltransferase and the vesicular transporter are found at the same locus, with the transporter gene positioned in the first intron of the transferase gene. Hence a common promoter regulates the expression of both genes (Eiden, 1998).

Estimates of the ACh content of synaptic vesicles range from 1000 to over 50,000 molecules per vesicle, and it has been calculated that a single motor nerve terminal contains 300,000 or more vesicles. In addition, an uncertain but possibly significant amount of ACh is present in the extravesicular cytoplasm. Recording the electrical events associated with the opening of single channels at the motor end plate during continuous application of ACh has permitted estimation of the potential change induced by a single molecule of ACh (3×10^{-7} V); from such calculations it is evident that even the lower estimate of the ACh content per vesicle (1000 molecules) is sufficient to account for the magnitude of the mepps.

Release of Acetylcholine. Release of acetylcholine and co-transmitters (e.g., ATP and VIP or in some neurons, NO) occurs on depolarization of the nerve terminals and takes place by exocytosis. Depolarization of the terminals allows the entry of Ca^{2+} through voltage-gated Ca^{2+} channels. Elevated Ca^{2+} concentration promotes fusion of the vesicular membrane with the plasma membrane, allowing exocytosis to occur.

The molecular mechanisms involved in the release and regulation of release are not completely understood (Südhof, 2004). ACh, like other neurotransmitters, is stored in vesicles located at special release sites, close to presynaptic membranes and ready for release following the appropriate stimulus. The vesicles initially dock and are primed for release. A multiprotein complex appears to form and attach the vesicle to the plasma membrane close to other signaling elements. The complex involves proteins from the vesicular membrane and the presynaptic neuronal membrane, as well as other components that help link them together. Various synaptic proteins, including the plasma membrane protein syntaxin and synaptosomal protein 25 kDa (SNAP-25), and the vesicular membrane protein, synaptobrevin, form a complex. This complex interacts in an ATP-dependent manner with soluble N-ethylmalemide-sensitive fusion protein and soluble SNAPs. The ability of synaptobrevin, sytaxin, and SNAP-25 to bind SNAPs has led to their designation as SNAP regulators (SNARES). It has been hypothesized that most, if not all, intracellular fusion events are mediated by SNARE interactions. Important evidence supporting the involvement of SNARE proteins in transmitter release comes from the fact that botulinum neurotoxins and tetanus toxin, which block neurotransmitter release, proteolyze these three proteins (Südhof, 2004).

Two pools of acetylcholine appear to exist. One pool, the "depot" or "readily releasable" pool, consists of vesicles located near the plasma membrane of the nerve terminals; these vesicles contain newly synthesized transmitter. Depolarization of the terminals causes these vesicles to release ACh rapidly or readily. The other pool, the "reserve pool," seems to replenish the readily releasable pool and may be required to sustain ACh release during periods of prolonged or intense nerve stimulation.

Acetylcholinesterase (AChE). For ACh to serve as a neurotransmitter in the motor system and at other neuronal synapses, it must be removed or inactivated within the time limits imposed by the response characteristics of the synapse. At the neuromuscular junction, immediate removal is required to prevent lateral diffusion and sequential activation of adjacent receptors. Modern biophysical methods have revealed that the time required for hydrolysis of ACh at the neuromuscular junction is less than a millisecond. The K_m of AChE for ACh is ~50-100 μM. Choline has only 10^{-3} to 10^{-5} the potency of ACh at the neuromuscular junction.

While AChE is found in cholinergic neurons (dendrites, perikarya, and axons), it is distributed more widely than cholinergic synapses. It is highly concentrated at the postsynaptic end plate of the neuromuscular junction. Butyrylcholinesterase (BuChE; also known as pseudocholinesterase) is present in low abundance in glial or satellite cells but is virtually absent in neuronal elements of the central and peripheral nervous systems. BuChE is synthesized primarily in the liver and is found in liver and plasma; its likely physiological function is the hydrolysis of ingested esters from plant sources. AChE and BuChE typically are distinguished by the relative rates of ACh and butyrylcholine hydrolysis and by effects of selective inhibitors (Chapter 10). Almost all pharmacological effects of the anti-ChE agents are due to the inhibition of AChE, with the consequent accumulation of endogenous ACh in the vicinity of the nerve terminal. Distinct but single genes encode AChE and BuChE in mammals; the diversity of molecular structure of AChE arises from alternative mRNA processing (Taylor et al., 2000).

Numerous reports suggest that AChE plays other roles in addition to its classical function in terminating impulse transmission at cholinergic synapses. Non-classical functions of AChE might include hydrolysis of ACh in a non-synaptic context, action as an adhesion protein involved in synaptic development and maintenance, as a bone matrix protein, involvement in neurite outgrowth, and acceleration of the assembly of Aβ peptide into amyloid fibrils (Silman and Sussman, 2005).

Characteristics of Cholinergic Transmission at Various Sites. There are marked differences among various sites of cholinergic transmission with respect to architecture and fine structure, the distributions of AChE and receptors, and the temporal factors involved in normal function. In skeletal muscle, e.g., the junctional sites occupy a small, discrete portion of the surface of the individual fibers and are relatively isolated from those of adjacent fibers; in the superior cervical ganglion, ~100,000 ganglion cells are packed within a volume of a few cubic millimeters, and both the presynaptic and postsynaptic neuronal processes form complex networks.

Skeletal Muscle. Stimulation of a motor nerve results in the release of ACh from perfused muscle; close intra-arterial injection of ACh produces muscular contraction similar to that elicited by stimulation of the motor nerve. The amount of ACh (10^{-17}mol) required to elicit an end-plate potential (EPP) following its microiontophoretic application to the motor end plate of a rat diaphragm muscle fiber is equivalent to that recovered from each fiber following stimulation of the phrenic nerve.

The combination of ACh with nicotinic ACh receptors at the external surface of the postjunctional membrane induces an immediate, marked increase in cation permeability. On receptor activation by ACh, its intrinsic channel opens for ~1 ms; during this interval, ~50,000 Na^+ ions traverse the channel. The channel-opening process is the basis for the localized depolarizing EPP within the end plate, which triggers the muscle AP. The latter, in turn, leads to contraction.

Following section and degeneration of the motor nerve to skeletal muscle or of the postganglionic fibers to autonomic effectors, there is a marked reduction in the threshold doses of the transmitters and of certain other drugs required to elicit a response; that is, denervation supersensitivity occurs. In skeletal muscle, this change is accompanied by a spread of the receptor molecules from the end-plate region to the adjacent portions of the sarcoplasmic membrane, which eventually involves the entire muscle surface. Embryonic muscle also exhibits this uniform sensitivity to ACh prior to innervation. Hence, innervation represses the expression of the receptor gene by the nuclei that lie in extrajunctional regions of the muscle fiber and directs the subsynaptic nuclei to express the structural and functional proteins of the synapse (Sanes and Lichtman, 1999).

Autonomic Effector Cells. Stimulation or inhibition of autonomic effector cells occurs on activation of muscarinic acetylcholine receptors (discussed later in the chapter). In this case, the effector is coupled to the receptor by a G protein (Chapter 3). In contrast to skeletal muscle and neurons, smooth muscle and the cardiac conduction system [sinoatrial (SA) node, atrium, atrioventricular (AV) node, and the His-Purkinje system] normally exhibit intrinsic activity, both electrical and mechanical, that is modulated but not initiated by nerve impulses.

In the basal condition, unitary smooth muscle exhibits waves of depolarization and/or spikes that are propagated from cell to cell at rates considerably slower than the AP of axons or skeletal muscle. The spikes apparently are initiated by rhythmic fluctuations in the membrane resting potential. Application of ACh (0.1 to 1 μM) to isolated intestinal muscle causes a decrease in the resting potential (i.e., the membrane potential becomes less negative) and an increase in the frequency of spike production, accompanied by a rise in tension. A primary action of ACh in initiating these effects through muscarinic receptors is probably partial depolarization of the cell membrane brought about by an increase in Na^+ and, in some instances, Ca^{2+} conductance. ACh also can produce contraction of some smooth muscles when the membrane has been depolarized completely by high concentrations of K^+, provided that Ca^{2+} is present. Hence, ACh stimulates ion fluxes across membranes and/or mobilizes intracellular Ca^{2+} to cause contraction.

In the heart, spontaneous depolarizations normally arise from the SA node. In the cardiac conduction system, particularly in the SA and AV nodes, stimulation of the cholinergic innervation or the direct application of ACh causes inhibition, associated with hyperpolarization of the membrane and a marked decrease in the rate of depolarization. These effects are due, at least in part, to a selective increase in permeability to K^+ (Hille, 1992).

Autonomic Ganglia. The primary pathway of cholinergic transmission in autonomic ganglia is similar to that at the neuromuscular junction of skeletal muscle. Ganglion cells can be discharged by injecting very small amounts of ACh into the ganglion. The initial depolarization is the result of activation of nicotinic ACh receptors, which are ligand-gated cation channels with properties similar to those found at the neuromuscular junction. Several secondary transmitters or modulators either enhance or diminish the sensitivity of the postganglionic cell to ACh. This sensitivity appears to be related to the membrane potential of the postsynaptic nerve cell body or its dendritic branches. Ganglionic transmission is discussed in more detail in Chapter 11.

Prejunctional Sites. As described earlier, both cholinergic and adrenergic nerve terminal varicosities contain autoreceptors and heteroreceptors. ACh release therefore is subject to complex regulation by mediators, including ACh itself acting on M_2 and M_4 autoreceptors, and other transmitters (e.g., NE acting on α_{2A} and α_{2C} adrenergic receptors) (Philipp and Hein, 2004; Wess, 2004) or substances produced locally in tissues (e.g., NO). ACh-mediated inhibition of ACh release following activation of M_2 and M_4 autoreceptors is thought to represent a physiological negative-feedback control mechanism. At some neuroeffector junctions such as the myenteric plexus in the GI tract or the SA node in the heart, sympathetic and parasympathetic nerve terminals often lie juxtaposed to each other. The opposing effects of norepinephrine and ACh, therefore, result not only from the opposite effects of the two transmitters on the smooth muscle or cardiac cells but also from the inhibition of ACh release by NE or inhibition of NE release by ACh acting on heteroreceptors on parasympathetic or sympathetic terminals. The muscarinic autoreceptors and heteroreceptors also represent drug targets for both agonists and antagonists. Muscarinic agonists can inhibit the electrically induced release of ACh, whereas antagonists will enhance the evoked release of transmitter. The parasympathetic nerve terminal varicosities also may contain additional heteroreceptors that could respond by inhibition or enhancement of ACh release by locally formed autacoids, hormones, or administered drugs. In addition to α_{2A} and α_{2C} adrenergic receptors, other inhibitory heteroreceptors on parasympathetic terminals include adenosine A_1 receptors, histamine H_3 receptors, and opioid receptors. Evidence also exists for β_2-adrenergic facilitatory receptors.

Extraneuronal Sites. A large body of evidence now indicates that all elements of the cholinergic system including the enzyme ChAT, ACh synthesis, ACh release mechanisms, and both mAChRs and nAChRs, are functionally expressed independently of cholinergic innervation in numerous non-neuronal cells including those of humans. These non-neuronal cholinergic systems can both modify and control phenotypic cell functions such as proliferation, differentiation, formation of physical barriers, migration, and ion and water movements. The widespread synthesis of ACh in non-neuronal cells has changed the thinking that ACh acts only as a neurotransmitter. Each component of the cholinergic system in non-neuronal cells can be affected by pathophysiological conditions or secondary to disease states. For instance, blockade of mAChRs and nAChRs on non-neuronal cells can cause cellular dysfunction and cell death. Moreover, dysfunctions of non-neuronal cholinergic systems may be involved in the pathogenesis of diseases (e.g., inflammatory processes) (Kalamida et al., 2007; Wessler and Kirkpatrick, 2008).

Cholinergic Receptors and Signal Transduction

Sir Henry Dale noted that the various esters of choline elicited responses that were similar to those of either nicotine or muscarine depending on the pharmacological preparation. A similarity in response also was noted between muscarine and nerve stimulation in those organs innervated by the craniosacral divisions of the autonomic nervous system. Thus, Dale suggested that ACh or another ester of choline was a neurotransmitter in the autonomic nervous system; he also stated that the compound had dual actions, which he termed a "nicotine action" (*nicotinic*) and a "muscarine action" (*muscarinic*).

The capacities of tubocurarine and atropine to block nicotinic and muscarinic effects of ACh, respectively, provided further support for the proposal of two distinct types of cholinergic receptors. Although Dale had access only to crude plant alkaloids of then unknown structure from *Amanita muscaria* and *Nicotiana tabacum,* this classification remains as the primary subdivision of cholinergic receptors. Its utility has survived the discovery of several distinct subtypes of nicotinic and muscarinic receptors.

Although ACh and certain other compounds stimulate both muscarinic and nicotinic cholinergic receptors, several other agonists and antagonists are selective for one of the two major types of receptors. ACh is a flexible molecule, and indirect evidence suggests that the conformations of the neurotransmitter are distinct when it is bound to nicotinic or muscarinic cholinergic receptors.

Nicotinic receptors are ligand-gated ion channels whose activation always causes a rapid (millisecond) increase in cellular permeability to Na^+ and Ca^{2+}, depolarization, and excitation. By contrast, muscarinic receptors are G protein–coupled receptors (GPCRs). Responses to muscarinic agonists are slower; they may be either excitatory or inhibitory, and they are not necessarily linked to changes in ion permeability.

The primary structures of various species of nicotinic receptors (Changeux and Edelstein, 1998; Numa et al., 1983) and muscarinic receptors (Bonner, 1989; Caulfield and Birdsall, 1998) have been deduced from the sequences of their respective genes. That these two types of receptors belong to distinct families of proteins is not surprising, retrospectively, in view of their distinct differences in chemical specificity and function.

Subtypes of Nicotinic Acetylcholine Receptors. The nicotinic ACh receptors (nAChRs) are members of a superfamily of ligand-gated ion channels. The receptors exist at the skeletal neuromuscular junction, autonomic ganglia, adrenal medulla, the CNS and in non-neuronal tissues. The nAChRs are composed of five homologous subunits organized around a central pore (see Chaper 11). In general the nAChRs are further divided into two groups:

- muscle type, found in vertebrate skeletal muscle, where they mediate transmission at the neuromuscular junction (NMJ)
- neuronal type, found mainly throughout the peripheral nervous system, central nervous system, and also non-neuronal tissues

Both the mAChRs and nAChRs are the natural targets of ACh, synthesized, stored, and released from cholinergic neurons as well as numerous pharmacologically administered drugs (agonists and antagonists), including the alkaloids muscarine and nicotine.

cDNAs for 17 types of nAChRs subunits have been cloned from several species. These consist of α subunits (α1-α10) that compose the main ligand binding sites, β (β1-4), γ, δ, and ε subunits. The nAChRs have been further divided into two main types based on different binding properties to the toxin α-bungarotoxin (αβgtx): 1) the αβgtx binding nAChRs, which can be either homopentamers of α7, α8, or α9 subunits or heteropentamers (e.g., $\alpha_2\beta\varepsilon[\gamma]\delta$); and 2) nAChRs that do not bind αβgtx. These contain the α2-α6 and β2-β4 subunits, exist only as heteropentamers, and bind agonists with high affinity (Albuquerque et al., 2009).

Muscle-Type nAChRs. In fetal muscle prior to innervation, in adult muscle after denervation, and in fish electric organs, the nAChR subunit stoichiometry is $(\alpha 1)_2\beta 1\gamma\delta$, whereas in adult muscle the γ subunit is replaced by ε to give the $(\alpha 1)_2\beta 1\varepsilon\delta$ stoichiometry (Table 8–2). The γ/ε and δ subunits are involved together with the α1 subunits in forming the ligand-binding sites and in the maintenance of cooperative interactions between the α1 subunit. Different affinities to the two binding sites are conferred by the presence of different non α-subunits. Binding of ACh to the αγ and αδ sites is thought to induce a conformational change predominantly in the α1 subunits which interacts with the transmembrane region to cause channel opening.

Neuronal-Type nAChRs. Neuronal nAChRs are widely expressed in peripheral ganglia, the adrenal medulla, numerous areas of the brain, and non-neuronal cells such as epithelial cells and cells of the immune system. To date, nine α (α_2-α_{10}) and three β (β_2-β_4) subunit genes have been cloned. The α_7-α_{10} subunits are found either as homopentamers (of five α_7, α_8, and α_9 subunits) or as heteropentamers of α7, α8, and α_9/α_{10}. By contrast, the α_2-α_6 and β_2-β_4 subunits form heteropentamers usually with $(\alpha x)_2(\beta y)_3$ stoichiometry. The α_5 and β_3 subunits do not appear to be able to form functional receptors when expressed alone or in paired combinations with α or β subunits, respectively (Kalamida et al., 2007).

The precise function of many of the neuronal nAChRs in the brain is not known; presumably, the considerable molecular diversity of the subunits can result in numerous nAChRs being formed with different physiological properties. There are few examples of neuronal nAChRs in the CNS mediating fast signaling propogation in a manner similar to that at the NMJ, and it is thought that they act more as synaptic modulators. Neuronal nAChRs are widely distributed in the CNS and are found at presynaptic, perisynaptic, and postsynaptic sites. At pre- and perisynaptic sites, nAChRs appear to act as autoreceptors or heteoreceptors to regulate the release of several neurotransmitters (ACh, DA, NE, glutamate, and 5-HT) at several diverse sites throughout the brain (Exley and Cragg, 2008). The synaptic release of a particular neurotransmitter can be regulated by different neuronal type nAChR subtypes in different CNS regions. For instance, DA release from striatal and thalamic dopamine neurons can be controlled by the $\alpha_4\beta_2$ subtype or both $\alpha_4\beta_2$ and $\alpha_6\beta_2\beta_3$ subtypes, respectively. In contrast, glutametergic neurotransmission is regulated everywhere by α7 nAChRs (Kalamida et al., 2007).

Subtypes of Muscarinic Receptors. In mammals, five distinct subtypes of muscarinic ACh receptors (mAChRs) have been identified, each produced by a different gene. Like the different forms of nicotinic receptors, these variants have distinct anatomic locations in the periphery and CNS and differing chemical specificities. The mAChRs are GPCRs (see Table 8–3 for characteristics of the mAChRs and Chapter 9 for further details).

Different experimental approaches including immunohistochemical and mRNA hybridization studies have shown that mAChRs are present in virtually all organs, tissues, and cell types (Table 8–3). Although most cell types have multiple mAChR subtypes, certain subtypes often predominate in specific sites. For example, the M_2 receptor is the predominant subtype in the heart and in CNS neurons is mostly located presynaptically, whereas the M_3 receptor is the predominant subtype in the detrusor muscle of the bladder (Dhein et al., 2001; Fetscher et al., 2002) (see Table 8–3). M_1, M_4, and M_5 receptors are richly expressed in the CNS, whereas the M_2 and M_4 receptor subtypes are widely distributed both in the CNS and peripheral tissue (Wess et al., 2007). M_3 receptors are widely distributed in the periphery, and although they are also widely distributed in the CNS, they are at lower levels than other subtypes.

In the periphery, mAChRs mediate the classical muscarinic actions of ACh in organs and tissues innervated by parasympathetic nerves, although receptors may be present at sites that lack parasympathetic innervation (e.g., most blood vessels). In the CNS, mAChRs are involved in regulating a large number of cognitive, behavioral, sensory, motor, and autonomic functions. Owing to the lack of specific muscarinic agonists and antagonists that demonstrate selectivity for individual mAChRs and the fact that most organs and tissues express multiple mAChRs, it has been a challenge to assign specific pharmacological functions to distinct mAChRs. The development of gene-targeting techniques in mice has been very helpful in defining specific functions (Table 8–3) (Wess, 2004).

The basic functions of muscarinic cholinergic receptors are mediated by interactions with G proteins

Table 8–2

Characteristics of Subtypes of Nicotinic Acetylcholine Receptors (nAChRs)

RECEPTOR (Primary Receptor Subtype)[a]	MAIN SYNAPTIC LOCATION	MEMBRANE RESPONSE	MOLECULAR MECHANISM	AGONISTS	ANTAGONISTS
Skeletal Muscle (N_m) $(\alpha_1)_2\beta_1\varepsilon\delta$ adult $(\alpha_1)_2\ \beta_1\gamma\delta$ fetal	Skeletal neuromuscular junction (postjunctional)	Excitatory; end-plate depolarization; skeletal muscle contraction	Increased cation permeability (Na^+; K^+)	ACh Nicotine Succinylcholine	Atracurium Vecuronium *d*-Tubocurarine Pancuronium α-Conotoxin α-Bungarotoxin
Peripheral Neuronal (N_n) $(\alpha_3)_2(\beta_4)_3$	Autonomic ganglia; adrenal medulla	Excitatory; depolarization; firing of postganglion neuron; depolarization and secretion of catecholamines	Increased cation permeability (Na^+; K^+)	ACh Nicotine Epibatidine Dimethylphenyl-piperazinium	Trimethaphan Mecamylamine
Central Neuronal (CNS) $(\alpha_4)_2(\beta_4)_3$ (α-btox-insensitive)	CNS; pre- and postjunctional	Pre- and post-synaptic excitation Prejunctional control of transmitter release	Increased cation permeability (Na^+; K^+)	Cytosine, epibatidine Anatoxin A	Mecamylamine Dihydro-β-erythrodine Erysodine Lophotoxin
$(\alpha_7)_5$ (α-btox-sensitive)	CNS; Pre- and post-synaptic	Pre- and post-synaptic excitation Prejunctional control of transmitter release	Increased permeability (Ca^{2+})	Anatoxin A	Methyllycaconitine α-Bungarotoxin α-Conotoxin ImI

[a]Nine α (α_2-α_{10}) and three β (β_2-β_4) subunits have been identified and cloned in human brain, which combine in various conformations to form individual receptor subtypes. The structure of individual receptors and the subtype composition are incompletely understood. Only a finite number of naturally occurring functional nAChR constructs have been identified. α-btox, β-bungarotoxin.

and by G protein–induced changes in the function of distinct member-bound effector molecules. The M_1, M_3, and M_5 subtypes couple through the pertussis toxin–insensitive $G_{q/11}$ responsible for stimulation of phospholipase C (PLC) activity. The immediate result is hydrolysis of membrane phosphatidylinositol 4,5 diphosphate to form inositol polyphosphates. Inositol trisphosphate (IP_3) causes release of intracellular Ca^{2+} from the endoplasmic reticulum, with activation of Ca^{2+}-dependent phenomena such as contraction of smooth muscle and secretion (Chapter 3). The second product of the PLC reaction, diacylglycerol, activates PKC (in conjunction with Ca^{2+} and phosphatidylserine). This arm of the pathway plays a role in the phosphorylation of numerous proteins, leading to various physiological responses. Activation of M_1, M_3, and M_5 receptors can also cause the activation of phospholipase A_2, leading to the release of arachidonic acid and consequent eicosanoid synthesis, resulting in autocrine/paracrine stimulation of adenylyl cyclase and

Table 8–3

Characteristics of Muscarinic Acetylcholine Receptor Subtypes (mAChRs) (continued)

RECEPTOR	SIZE; CHROMOSOME	CELLULAR AND TISSUE LOCATION[a]	CELLULAR RESPONSE[b]	FUNCTIONAL RESPONSE[c]	DISEASE RELEVANCE
M_1	460 aa llq 12-13	CNS; Most abundant in cerebral cortex, hippocampus, striatum and thalamus Autonomic ganglia Glands (gastric and salivary) Enteric nerves	Couples by $G_{q/11}$ Activation of PLC; ↑ IP_3 and ↑ DAG → ↑ Ca^{2+} and PKC Depolarization and excitation (↑ sEPSP) Activation of PLD_2, PLA_2; ↑ AA	Increased cognitive function (learning and memory) Increased seizure activity Decrease in dopamine release and locomotion Increase in depolarization of autonomic ganglia Increase in secretions	Alzheimer's disease Cognitive dysfunction Schizophrenia
M_2	466 aa 7q 35-36	Widely expressed in CNS, hind brain, thalamus, cerebral cortex, hippocampus, striatum, heart, smooth muscle, autonomic nerve terminals	Couples by G_i/G_o (PTX-sensitive) Inhibition of AC, ↓ cAMP Activation of inwardly rectifying K^+ channels Inhibition of voltage-gated Ca^{2+} channels Hyperpolarization and inhibition	***Heart:*** SA node: slowed spontaneous depolarization; hyperpolarization, ↓ HR AV node: decrease in conduction velocity Atrium: ↓ refractory period, ↓ contraction Ventricle: slight ↓ contraction ***Smooth muscle:*** ↑ Contraction ***Peripheral nerves:*** Neural inhibition *via* autoreceptors and heteroreceptor ↓ Ganglionic transmission. ***CNS:*** Neural inhibition ↑ Tremors; hypothermia; analgesia	Alzheimer's disease Cognitive dysfunction Pain

(*Continued*)

an increase in cyclic AMP. These effects of M_1, M_3, and M_5 mAChRs are generally secondary to elevations of intracellular Ca^{++} (Eglen, 2005).

Stimulation of M_2 and M_4 cholinergic receptors leads to interaction with other G proteins, (e.g., G_i and G_o) with a resulting inhibition of adenylyl cyclase, leading to a decrease in cyclic AMP, activation of inwardly rectifying K^+ channels, and inhibition of voltage-gated Ca^{2+} channels (van Koppen and Kaiser, 2003). The functional consequences of these effects are hyperpolarization

Table 8–3

Characteristics of Muscarinic Acetylcholine Receptor Subtypes (mAChRs) (*Continued*)

RECEPTOR	SIZE; CHROMOSOME	CELLULAR AND TISSUE LOCATION[a]	CELLULAR RESPONSE[b]	FUNCTIONAL RESPONSE[c]	DISEASE RELEVANCE
M_3	590 aa 1q 43-44	Widely expressed in CNS (< than other mAChRs), cerebral cortex, hippocampus Abundant in smooth muscle and glands Heart	Couples by $G_{q/11}$ Activation of PLC; ↑ IP_3 and ↑ DAG → ↑ Ca^{2+} and PKC Depolarization and excitation (↑ sEPSP) Activation of PLD_2, PLA_2; ↑ AA	*Smooth muscle* ↑ contraction (predominant in some, *e.g.* bladder) *Glands:* ↑ secretion (predominant in salivary gland) Increases food intake, body weight fat deposits Inhibition of DA release Synthesis of NO	Chronic obstructive pulmonary disease (COPD) Urinary incontinence Irritable bowel disease
M_4	479 aa 11p 12-11.2	Preferentially expressed in CNS, particularly forebrain, also striatum, cerebral cortex, hippocampus	Couples by G_i/G_0 (PTX-sensitive) Inhibition of AC, ↓ cAMP Activation of inwardly rectifying K^+ channels Inhibition of voltage-gated Ca^{2+} channels Hyperpolarization and inhibition	Autoreceptor- and heteroreceptor-mediated inhibition of transmitter release in CNS and periphery. Analgesia; cataleptic activity Facilitation of DA release	Parkinson disease Schizophrenia Neuropathic pain
M_5	532 aa 15q 26	Substantia nigra Expressed in low levels in CNS and periphery Predominant mAchR in neurons in VTA and substantia nigra	Couples by $G_{q/11}$ Activation of PLC; ↑ IP_3 and ↑ DAG → ↑ Ca^{2+} and PKC Depolarization and excitation (↑ sEPSP) Activation of PLD_2, PLA_2; ↑ AA	Mediator of dilation in cerebral arteries and arterioles (?) Facilitates DA release Augmentation of drug-seeking behavior and reward (e.g., opiates, cocaine)	Drug dependence Parkinson disease Schizophrenia

[a]Most organs, tissues, and cells express multiple mAChRs.

[b]M_1, M_3, and M_5 mAChRs appear to couple to the same G proteins and signal through similar pathways. Likewise, M_2 and M_4 mAChRs couple through similar G proteins and signal through similar pathways.

[c]Despite the fact that in many tissues, organs, and cells multiple subtypes of mAChRs coexist, one subtype may predominate in producing a particular function; in others, there may be equal predominance.

PLC, phospholipase C; IP_3, inositol-l,4,5-triphosphate; DAG, diacylglycerol; PLD_2, phospholipase D; AA, arachidonic acid; PLA, phospholipase A; AC, adenylyl cyclase; DA, dopamine; cAMP, cyclic AMP; SA node, sinoatrial node; AV node, atrioventricular node; HR, heart rate; PTX, pertussis toxin; VTA, ventral tegmentum area.

and inhibition of excitable membranes. These are most clear in myocardium, where inhibition of adenylyl cyclase and activation of K^+ conductances account for the negative inotropic and chronotropic effects of ACh. The specificity is not absolute, however, and depends on proper trafficking of the G protein subunits within the cell; consequently, heterologous systems may exhibit alternative interactions between mAChRs and G–protein coupled pathways (Nathanson, 2008). In addition, there are numerous reports suggesting the differential subcellular location of specific mAChR subtypes in a variety of cell types in the nervous system and in a variety of non-neuronal polarized cells.

Following activation by classical or allosteric agonists, mAChRs can be phosphorylated by a variety of receptor kinases and second-messenger regulated kinases; the phosphorylated mAChR subtypes then can interact with *β*-arrestin and possibly other adaptor proteins. As a result, mAChR signaling pathways may be differentially altered. Agonist activation of mAChRs also may induce receptor internalization and down-regulation (van Koppen and Kaiser, 2003). Muscarinic AChRs can also regulate other signal transduction pathways that have diverse effects on cell growth, survival, and physiology, such as the MAP kinase, phosphoinositide-3-kinase, RhoA, and Rac1 (Nathanson, 2008).

Changes in mAChR levels and activity have been implicated in the pathophysiology of numerous major diseases in the CNS and in the autonomic nervous system (Table 8–3). Phenotypic analysis of mAChR-mutant mice as well as the development of selective agonists and antagonists has led to a wealth of new information regarding the physiological and potential pathophysiological roles of the individual mAChR subtype (Langmead et al., 2008; Wess et al., 2007).

Adrenergic Transmission

Under this general heading are norepinephrine (NE), the principal transmitter of most sympathetic postganglionic fibers and of certain tracts in the CNS; dopamine (DA), the predominant transmitter of the mammalian extrapyramidal system and of several mesocortical and mesolimbic neuronal pathways; and epinephrine, the major hormone of the adrenal medulla. Collectively, these three amines are called *catecholamines.*

A tremendous amount of information about catecholamines and related compounds has accumulated in recent years partly because of the importance of interactions between the endogenous catecholamines and many of the drugs used in the treatment of hypertension, mental disorders, and a variety of other conditions. The details of these interactions and of the pharmacology of the sympathomimetic amines themselves will be found in subsequent chapters. The basic physiological, biochemical, and pharmacological features are presented here.

Synthesis of Catecholamines. The steps in the synthesis of DA, NE (noradrenaline), and epinephrine (adrenaline) are shown in Figure 8–5. Tyrosine is sequentially 3-hydroxylated and decarboxylated to form dopamine. Dopamine is *β*-hydroxylated to yield norepinephrine, which is *N*-methylated in chromaffin tissue to give epinephrine. The enzymes involved have been identified,

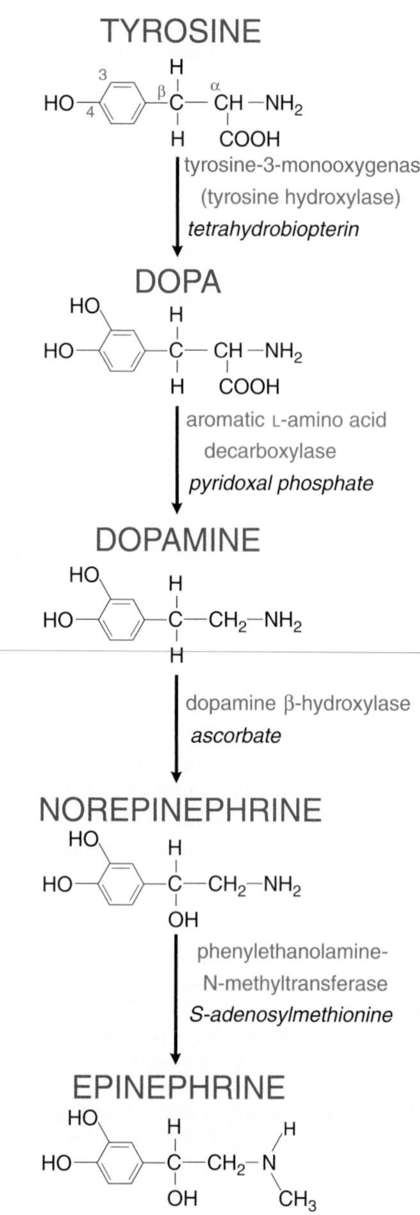

Figure 8–5. *Steps in the enzymatic synthesis of dopamine, norepinephrine and epinephrine.* The enzymes involved are shown in red; essential cofactors in italics. The final step occurs only in the adrenal medulla and in a few epinephrine-containing neuronal pathways in the brainstem.

Table 8–4

Enzymes for Synthesis of Catecholamines

ENZYME	OCCURRENCE	SUBCELLULAR DISTRIBUTION	COFACTOR REQUIREMENT	SUBSTRATE SPECIFICITY	COMMENTS
Tyrosine hydroxylase	Widespread; sympathetic nerves	Cytoplasmic	Tetrahydrobiopterin, O_2, Fe^{2+}	Specific for L-tyrosine	Rate limiting step. Inhibition can deplete NE
Aromatic L-amino acid decarboxylase	Widespread; sympathetic nerves	Cytoplasmic	Pyridoxal phosphate	Nonspecific	Inhibition does not alter tissue NE and Epi appreciably
Dopamine *β*-hydroxylase	Widespread; sympathetic nerves	Synaptic vesicles	Ascorbic acid, O_2 (contains copper)	Nonspecific	Inhibition can decrease NE and Epi levels
Phenylethanolamine *N*-methyltransferase	Largely in adrenal gland	Cytoplasmic	*S*-Adenosyl methionine (CH_3 donor)	Nonspecific	Inhibition can decrease adrenal E_{pi}/NE; regulated by glucocorticoids

cloned, and characterized (Nagatsu, 1991). Table 8–4 summarizes some of the important characteristics of the four enzymes. These enzymes are not completely specific; consequently, other endogenous substances, as well as certain drugs, are also substrates. For example, 5-hydroxytryptamine (5-HT, serotonin) can be produced from 5-hydroxy-*L*-tryptophan by aromatic *L*-amino acid decarboxylase (or dopa decarboxylase). Dopa decarboxylase also converts dopa into DA (Chapter 13) and methyldopa to *α*-methyldopamine, which in turn is converted by dopamine *β*-hydroxylase (D*β*H) to methylnorepinephrine.

The hydroxylation of tyrosine by tyrosine hydroxylase (TH) generally is regarded as the rate-limiting step in the biosynthesis of catecholamines (Zigmond et al., 1989); this enzyme is activated following stimulation of sympathetic nerves or the adrenal medulla. The enzyme is a substrate for PKA, PKC, and CaM kinase; phosphorylation is associated with increased hydroxylase activity. This is an important acute mechanism for increasing catecholamine synthesis in response to elevated nerve stimulation. In addition, there is a delayed increase in TH gene expression after nerve stimulation. This increased expression can occur at multiple levels of regulation, including transcription, RNA processing, regulation of RNA stability, translation, and enzyme stability (Kumer and Vrana, 1996). These mechanisms serve to maintain the content of catecholamines in response to increased transmitter release. In addition, TH is subject to feedback inhibition by catechol compounds, which allosterically modulate enzyme activity.

TH deficiency has been reported in humans and is characterized by generalized rigidity, hypokinesia, and low cerebrospinal fluid (CSF) levels of NE and DA metabolites homovanillic acid and 3-methoxy-4-hydroxyphenylethylene glycol (Wevers et al., 1999). TH knockout is embryonically lethal in mice, presumably because the loss of catecholamines results in altered cardiac function. Interestingly, residual levels of DA are present in these mice. It has been suggested that tyrosinase may be an alternate source for catecholamines, although tyrosinase-derived catecholamines are clearly not sufficient for survival (Carson and Robertson, 2002).

D*β*H deficiency in humans is characterized by orthostatic hypotension, ptosis of the eyelids, retrograde ejaculation, and elevated plasma levels of dopamine. In the case of DβH-deficient mice, there is ~90% embryonic mortality (Carson and Robertson, 2002).

Our understanding of the cellular sites and mechanisms of synthesis, storage, and release of catecholamines derives from studies of sympathetically innervated organs and the adrenal medulla. Nearly all the NE content of innervated organs is confined to the postganglionic sympathetic fibers; it disappears within a few days after section of the nerves. In the adrenal medulla, catecholamines are stored in chromaffin granules (Aunis, 1998). These vesicles contain extremely high concentrations of catecholamines (~21% dry weight), ascorbic acid, and ATP, as well as specific proteins such as chromogranins, D*β*H, and peptides including enkephalin and neuropeptide Y. Vasostatin-1, the *N*-terminal fragment of chromogranin A, has been found to have antibacterial and antifungal activity (Lugardon et al., 2000), as have other chromogranin A fragments such as chromofungin, vasostatin II, prochromacin, and chromacins I and II (Taupenot et al., 2003). Two types of storage vesicles are found in sympathetic nerve terminals: large dense-core vesicles corresponding to chromaffin granules; and small dense-core vesicles containing NE, ATP, and membrane-bound DβH.

The main features of the mechanisms of synthesis, storage, and release of catecholamines and their modifications by drugs are summarized in Figure 8–6. In the case of adrenergic neurons, the enzymes that participate in the formation of NE are synthesized in the cell bodies of the neurons and then are transported along the axons to their terminals. In the course of synthesis (Figure 8–6), the hydroxylation of tyrosine to dopa and the decarboxylation of dopa to dopamine take place in the cytoplasm. DA formed in the cytoplasm then is actively transported into the DβH-containing storage vesicles, where it is converted to NE. About 90% of the dopamine is converted to NE by DβH in sympathetic nerves; the remainder is metabolized. DA is converted by MAO to a aldehyde intermediate DOPAL, and then mainly converted to 3,4-dihydroxyphenyl acetic acid (DOPAC) by aldehyde dehydrogenase and to a minor extent 3,4-dihydroxyphenylethanol (DOPET) by aldehyde reductase. DOPAC is further converted to homovanillic acid (HVA) by o-methylation in non-neuronal sites.

The adrenal medulla has two distinct catecholamine-containing cell types: those with NE and those with primarily epinephrine. The latter cell population contains the enzyme phenylethanolamine-*N*-methyltransferase (PNMT). In these cells, the NE formed in the granules leaves these structures, presumably by diffusion, and is methylated in the cytoplasm to epinephrine. Epinephrine then reenters the chromaffin granules, where it is stored until released. In adults, epinephrine accounts for ~80% of the catecholamines of the adrenal medulla, with NE making up most of the remainder.

A major factor that controls the rate of synthesis of epinephrine, and hence the size of the store available for release from the adrenal medulla, is the level of glucocorticoids secreted by the adrenal cortex. The intra-adrenal portal vascular system carries the corticosteroids directly to the adrenal medullary chromaffin cells, where they induce the synthesis of PNMT (Figure 8–5). The activities of both TH and DβH also are increased in the adrenal medulla when the secretion of glucocorticoids is stimulated (Viskupic et al., 1994). Thus, any stress that persists sufficiently to evoke an enhanced secretion of corticotropin mobilizes the appropriate hormones of both the adrenal cortex (predominantly cortisol in humans) and medulla (epinephrine). This remarkable relationship is present only in certain mammals, including humans, in which the adrenal chromaffin cells are enveloped entirely by steroid-secreting cortical cells. In the dogfish, e.g., where the chromaffin cells and steroid-secreting cells are located in independent, noncontiguous glands, epinephrine is not formed. Nonetheless, there is evidence indicating that PMNT is expressed in mammalian tissues such as brain, heart, and lung, leading to extra-adrenal epinephrine synthesis (Kennedy et al., 1993).

In addition to *de novo* synthesis, NE stores in the terminal portions of the adrenergic fibers are also replenished by reuptake and restorage of NE following its release. At least two distinct carrier-mediated transport systems are involved: one across the axoplasmic membrane from the extracellular fluid to the cytoplasm (NET, the norepinephrine transporter, previously called *uptake 1*); and the other from the cytoplasm into the storage vesicles (VMAT2, the vesicular monoamine transporter) (Chandhry et al., 2008). A third transporter, ENT (the extraneuronal transporter, also called *uptake 2*), is responsible for the facilitated entry of catecholamines into non-neuronal cells.

For norepinephrine released by neurons, uptake by NET is more important than extraneuronal uptake and metabolism of norepinephrine. Sympathetic nerves as a whole remove ~87% of released norepinephrine by NET, compared with 5% by extraneuronal uptake (ENT) and 8% by diffusion to the circulation. In contrast, clearance of circulating catecholamines is primarily by non-neuronal mechanisms, with liver and kidney accounting for over 60% of the clearance of circulating catecholamines. Because the VMAT2 has a much higher affinity for norepinephrine than does monoamine oxidase (MAO), over 70% of recaptured norepinephrine is sequestered into storage vesicles (Eisenhofer, 2001).

Storage of Catecholamines. Catecholamines are stored in vesicles, ensuring their regulated release; this storage decreases intraneuronal metabolism of these transmitters and their leakage outside the cell. The vesicular amine transporter (VMAT2) appears to be driven by pH and potential gradients that are established by an ATP-dependent proton translocase. For every molecule of amine taken up, two H^+ ions are extruded (Brownstein and Hoffman, 1994). Monoamine transporters are relatively promiscuous and transport DA, NE, epinephrine, and 5-HT, e.g., as well as meta-iodobenzylguanidine, which can be used to image chromaffin cell tumors (Schuldiner, 1994). Reserpine inhibits monoamine transport into storage vesicles and ultimately leads to depletion of catecholamine from sympathetic nerve endings and in the brain. Several vesicular transport cDNAs have been cloned; these cDNAs reveal open reading frames predictive of proteins with 12 transmembrane domains (Chapter 5). Regulation of the expression of these various transporters may be important in the regulation of synaptic transmission (Varoqui and Erickson, 1997).

NET is Na^+-dependent and is blocked selectively by a number of drugs, including cocaine and tricyclic antidepressants such as imipramine. This transporter has a high affinity for NE and a somewhat lower affinity for epinephrine (Table 8–5); the synthetic β adrenergic

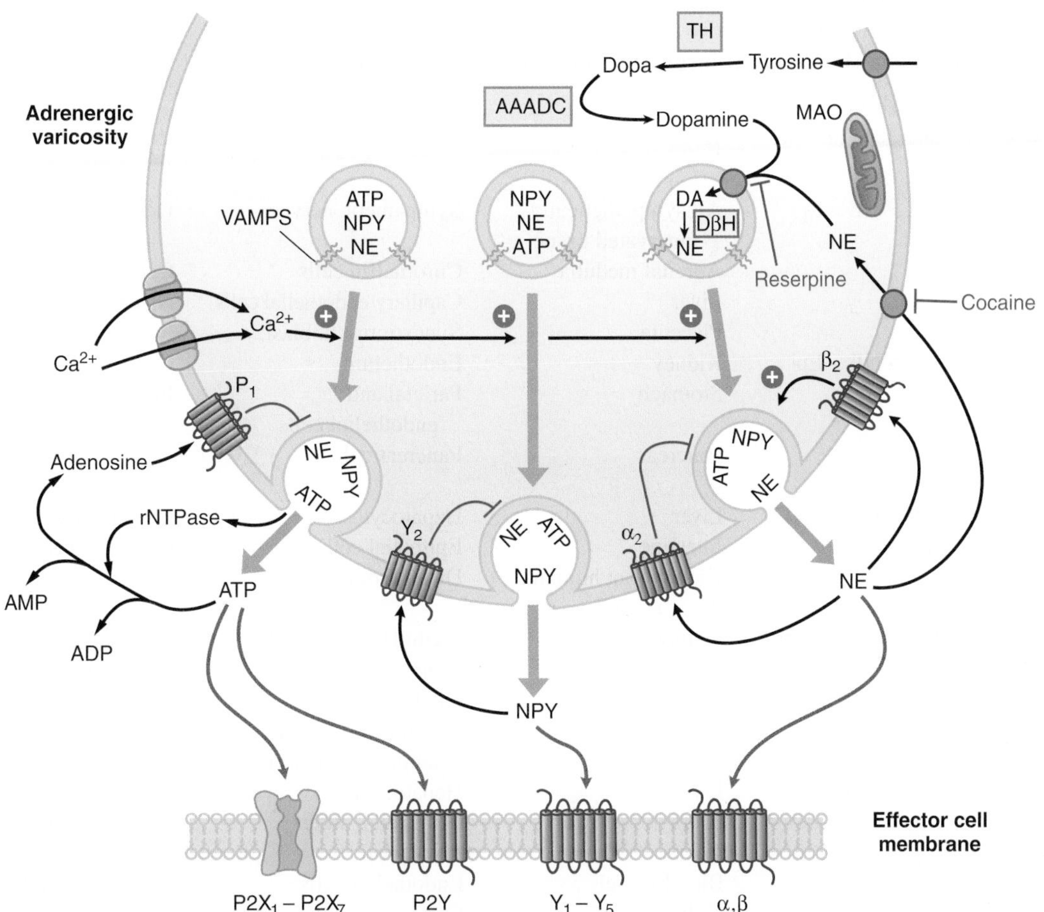

Figure 8–6. *An adrenergic neuroeffector junction showing features of the synthesis, storage, release, and receptors for norepinephrine (NE), the cotransmitters neuropeptide Y (NPY), and ATP.* Tyrosine is transported into the varicosity and is converted to DOPA by tyrosine hydroxylase (TH) and DOPA to dopamine (DA) by the action of aromatic L-amino acid decarboxylase (AAADC). Dopamine is taken up into the vesicles of the varicosity by a transporter, VMAT2, that can be blocked by reserpine. Cytoplasmic NE also can be taken up by this transporter. Dopamine is converted to NE within the vesicle *via* the action of dopamine-β-hydroxylase (DβH). NE is stored in vesicles along with other cotransmitters, NPY and ATP, depending on the particular neuroeffector junction. Release of the transmitters occurs upon depolarization of the varicosity, which allows entry of Ca^{2+} through voltage-dependent Ca^{2+} channels. Elevated levels of Ca^{2+} promote the fusion of the vesicular membrane with the membrane of the varicosity, with subsequent exocytosis of transmitters. This fusion process involves the interaction of specialized proteins associated with the vesicular membrane (VAMPs, vesicle-associated membrane proteins) and the membrane of the varicosity (SNAPs, synaptosome-associated proteins). In this schematic representation, NE, NPY, and ATP are stored in the same vesicles. Different populations of vesicles, however, may preferentially store different proportions of the cotransmitters. Once in the synapse, NE can interact with α and β adrenergic receptors to produce the characteristic response of the effector. The adrenergic receptors are GPCRs. α and β *R*eceptors also can be located presynaptically where NE can either diminish (α_2), or facilitate (β) its own release and that of the cotransmitters. The principal mechanism by which NE is cleared from the synapse is *via* a cocaine-sensitive neuronal uptake transporter, NET. Once transported into the cytosol, NE can be re-stored in the vesicle or metabolized by monoamine oxidase (MAO). NPY produces its effects by activating NPY receptors, of which there are at least five types (Y_1 through Y_2). NPY receptors are GPCRs. NPY can modify its own release and that of the other transmitters *via* presynaptic receptors of the Y_2 type. NPY is removed from the synapse by metabolic breakdown by peptidases. ATP produces its effects by activating P2X receptors or P2Y receptors. P2X receptors are ligand-gated ion channels; P2Y receptors are GPCRs. There are multiple subtypes of both P2X and P2Y receptors. As with the other cotransmitters, ATP can act prejunctionally to modify its own release *via* receptors for ATP or *via* its metabolic breakdown to adenosine that acts on P1 (adenosine) receptors. ATP is cleared from the synapse primarily by releasable nucleotidases (rNTPase) and by cell-fixed ectonucleotidases.

Table 8–5

Characteristics of Plasma Membrane Transporters for Endogenous Catecholamines

TYPE OF TRANSPORTER	SUBSTRATE SPECIFICITY	TISSUE	REGION/CELL TYPE	INHIBITORS
Neuronal				
NET	DA > NE > Epi	All sympathetically innervated tissue	Sympathetic nerves	Desipramine
		Adrenal medulla	Chromaffin cells	Cocaine
		Liver	Capillary endothelial cells	Nisoxetine
		Placenta	Syncytiotrophoblast	
DAT	DA > NE > Epi	Kidney	Endothelium	Cocaine
		Stomach	Parietal and endothelial cells	Imazindol
		Pancreas	Pancreatic duct	
Non-neuronal				
OCT1	DA > Epi >> NE	Liver	Hepatocytes	Isocyanines
		Intestine	Epithelial cells	Corticosterone
		Kidney (not human)	Distal tubule	
OCT2	DA >> NE > Epi	Kidney	Medullary proximal and distal tubules	Isocyanines Corticosterone
		Brain	Glial cells of DA-rich regions, some non-adrenergic neurons	
ENT (OCT 3)	Epi >> NE > DA	Liver	Hepatocytes	Isocyanines
		Brain	Glial cells, others	Corticosterone
		Heart	Myocytes	*O*-methyl-isoproterenol
		Blood vessels	Endothelial cells	
		Kidney	Cortex, proximal and distal tubules	
		Placenta	Syncytiotrophoblasts (basal membrane)	
		Retina	Photoreceptors, ganglion amacrine cells	

NET, norepinephrine transporter, originally known as uptake 1; DAT, dopamine transporter; ENT (OCT3), extraneuronal transporter, originally known as uptake 2; OCT 1, OCT 2, organic cation transporters; Epi, epinephrine; NE, norepinephrine; DA, dopamine.

receptor agonist isoproterenol is not a substrate for this system.

There are actually two neuronal membrane transporters for catecholamines, the NE transporter (NET) mentioned above and the DA transporter (DAT); their characteristics are depicted in Table 8–5.

The NET is also present in the adrenal medulla, the liver, and the placenta, whereas the DAT is present in the stomach, pancreas, and kidney (Eisenhofer, 2001). NET and DAT are members of an extended family of biogenic amine and amino acid neurotransmitter transporters. Members share common structural motifs, particularly the putative 12-transmembrane helices. These plasma membrane transporters appear to have greater substrate specificity than do vesicular transporters and are targets for specific drugs such as cocaine (catecholamine transporters) and fluoxetine (serotonin transporter).

Certain sympathomimetic drugs (e.g., ephedrine and tyramine) produce some of their effects indirectly by displacing NE from the nerve terminals to the extracellular fluid, where it then acts at receptor sites of the effector cells. The mechanisms by which these drugs release NE from nerve endings are complex. All such agents are substrates for NET. As a result of their transport across the neuronal membrane and release into the axoplasm, they make carrier available at the inner surface of the membrane for the outward transport of NE ("facilitated exchange diffusion"). In addition, these amines are able to mobilize NE stored in the vesicles by competing for the vesicular uptake process. Reserpine, which depletes vesicular stores of NE, also inhibits this uptake mechanism, but in contrast with the indirect-acting sympathomimetic amines, it enters the adrenergic nerve ending by passive diffusion across the axonal membrane.

The actions of indirect-acting sympathomimetic amines are subject to *tachyphylaxis*. For example, repeated administration of tyramine results in rapidly decreasing effectiveness, whereas repeated administration of NE does not reduce effectiveness and, in fact, reverses the tachyphylaxis to tyramine. Although these phenomena have not been explained fully, several hypotheses have been proposed. One possible explanation is that the pool of neurotransmitter available for displacement by these drugs is small relative to the total amount stored in the sympathetic nerve ending. This pool is presumed to reside in close proximity to the plasma membrane, and the NE of such vesicles may be replaced by the less potent amine following repeated administration of the latter substance. In any case, neurotransmitter release by displacement is not associated with the release of DβH and does not require extracellular Ca^{2+}; thus, it is presumed not to involve exocytosis.

There are also three extraneuronal transporters that handle a wide range of endogenous and exogenous substrates. The extraneuronal amine transporter (ENT), originally named uptake-2 and also designated OCT3, is an organic cation transporter. Relative to NET, ENT exhibits lower affinity for catecholamines, favors epinephrine over NE and DA, and shows a higher maximum rate of catecholamine uptake. The ENT is not Na^+- dependent and displays a different profile of pharmacological inhibition. Other members of this family are the organic cation transporters OCT1 and OCT2 (Chapter 5). All three can transport catecholamines in addition to a wide variety of other organic acids, including 5-HT, histamine, choline, spermine, guanidine, and creatinine. The characteristics and location of the non-neuronal transporters are summarized in Table 8–5.

Release of Catecholamines. The full sequence of steps by which the nerve impulse effects the release of NE from sympathetic neurons is not known. In the adrenal medulla, the triggering event is the liberation of ACh by the preganglionic fibers and its interaction with nicotinic receptors on chromaffin cells to produce a localized depolarization; a subsequent step is the entrance of Ca^{2+} into these cells, which results in the extrusion by exocytosis of the granular contents, including epinephrine, ATP, some neuroactive peptides or their precursors, chromogranins, and DβH. Influx of Ca^{2+} likewise plays an essential role in coupling the nerve impulse, membrane depolarization, and opening of voltage-gated Ca^{2+} channels with the release of norepinephrine at sympathetic nerve terminals. Blockade of N-type Ca^{2+} channels leads to hypotension likely owing to inhibition of NE release. Ca^{2+}-triggered secretion involves interaction of highly conserved molecular scaffolding proteins leading to docking of granules at the plasma membrane and ultimately leading to secretion (Aunis, 1998).

Reminiscent of the release of ACh at cholinergic terminals, various synaptic proteins, including the plasma membrane proteins syntaxin and SNAP-25, and the vesicle membrane protein synaptobrevin form a complex that interacts in an ATP-dependent manner with the soluble proteins *N*-ethylmaleimide-sensitive fusion protein (NSF) and soluble NSF attachment proteins (SNAPs). The ability of synaptobrevin, syntaxin, and SNAP-25 to bind SNAPs has led to their designation as *SNAP receptors* (SNAREs). It has been hypothesized that most, if not all, intracellular fusion events are mediated by SNARE interactions (Boehm and Kubista, 2002). As with cholinergic neurotransmission, important evidence supporting the involvement of SNARE proteins (e.g., SNAP-25, syntaxin, and synaptobrevin) in transmitter release comes from the fact that botulinum neurotoxins and tetanus toxin, which potently block neurotransmitter release, proteolyse these proteins.

Enhanced activity of the sympathetic nervous system is accompanied by an increased concentration of both DβH and chromogranins in the circulation, supporting the argument that the process of release following adrenergic nerve stimulation also involves exocytosis.

Adrenergic fibers can sustain the output of norepinephrine during prolonged periods of stimulation without exhausting their reserve supply, provided that synthesis and uptake of the transmitter are unimpaired. To meet increased needs for NE acute regulatory mechanisms are evoked involving activation of tyrosine hydroxylase and DβH (described earlier in the chapter).

Prejunctional Regulation of Norepinephrine Release. The release of the three sympathetic co-transmitters can be modulated by prejunctional autoreceptors and heteroreceptors. Following their release from sympathetic terminals, all three co-transmitters—NE, neuropeptide Y (NPY), and ATP—can feed back on prejunctional receptors to inhibit the release of each other (Westfall, 2004; Westfall et al., 2002). The most thoroughly studied have been prejunctional α_2 adrenergic receptors. The α_{2A} and α_{2C} adrenergic receptors are the principal prejunctional receptors that inhibit sympathetic neurotransmitter release, whereas the α_{2B} adrenergic receptors also may inhibit transmitter release at selected sites. Antagonists of this receptor, in turn, can enhance the electrically evoked release of sympathetic neurotransmitter. NPY, acting on Y_2 receptors, and ATP-derived adenosine, acting on P1 receptors, also can inhibit sympathetic neurotransmitter release. Numerous heteroreceptors on sympathetic nerve varicosities also inhibit the release of sympathetic neurotransmitters; these include: M_2 and M_4 muscarinic, 5-HT, PGE_2, histamine, enkephalin, and DA receptors. Enhancement of sympathetic neurotransmitter release can be produced by activation of β_2 adrenergic receptors, angiotensin AT_2 receptors, and nACh receptors. All of these receptors can be targets for agonists and antagonists (Kubista and Boehm, 2006).

Termination of the Actions of Catecholamines. The actions of NE and epinephrine are terminated by:

- reuptake into nerve terminals by NET
- dilution by diffusion out of the junctional cleft and uptake at extraneuronal sites by ENT, OCT 1, and OCT 2

Following uptake, catecholamines can be metabolized (in neuronal and non-neuronal cells) or re-stored in vesicles (in neurons). Two enzymes are important in the initial steps of metabolic transformation of catecholamines—monoamine oxidase (MAO) and catechol-*O*-methyltransferase (COMT). In addition, catecholamines are metabolized by sulfotransferases (Dooley, 1998) (Chapter 6). However, termination of action by a powerful degradative enzymatic pathway, such as that provided by AChE at sites of cholinergic transmission, is absent from the adrenergic nervous system. The importance of neuronal reuptake of catecholamines is shown by observations that inhibitors of this process (e.g., cocaine and imipramine) potentiate the effects of the neurotransmitter; inhibitors of MAO and COMT have relatively little effect. However, MAO metabolizes transmitter that is released within the nerve terminal. COMT, particularly in the liver, plays a major role in the metabolism of endogenous circulating and administered catecholamines.

Both MAO and COMT are distributed widely throughout the body, including the brain; the highest concentrations of each are in the liver and the kidney. However, little or no COMT is found in sympathetic neurons. In the brain, there is also no significant COMT in presynaptic terminals, but it is found in some postsynaptic neurons and glial cells. In the kidney, COMT is localized in proximal tubular epithelial cells, where DA is synthesized, and is thought to exert local diuretic and natriuretic effects. The physiological substrates for COMT include L-dopa, all three endogenous catecholamines (DA, NE, and epinephrine), their hydroxylated metabolites, catecholestrogens, ascorbic acid, and dihydroxyindolic intermediates of melanin (Männistö and Kaakkola, 1999). There are distinct differences in the cytological locations of the two enzymes; MAO is associated chiefly with the outer surface of mitochondria, including those within the terminals of sympathetic or central noradrenergic neuronal fibers, whereas COMT is largely cytoplasmic except in the chromaffin cells of the adrenal medulla, where COMT is present as a membrane-bound form. These factors are of importance both in determining the primary metabolic pathways followed by catecholamines in various circumstances and in explaining the effects of certain drugs. Two different isozymes of MAO (MAO-A and MAO-B) are found in widely varying proportions in different cells in the CNS and in peripheral tissues. In the periphery, MAO-A is located in the syncytiotrophoblast layer of term placenta and liver, whereas MAO-B is located in platelets, lymphocytes, and liver. In the brain, MAO-A is located in all regions containing catecholamines, with the highest abundance in the locus ceruleus. MAO-B, on the other hand, is found primarily in regions that are known to synthesize and store 5-HT. MAO-B is most prominent in the nucleus raphe dorsalis but also in the posterior hypothalamus and in glial cells in regions known to contain nerve terminals. MAO-B is also present in osteocytes around blood vessels (Abell and Kwan, 2001). Selective inhibitors of these two isozymes are available (Chapter 15). Irreversible antagonists of MAO-A (e.g., phenelzine, tranylcypromine, and isocarboxazid) enhance the bioavailability of tyramine contained in many foods; tyramine-induced NE release from sympathetic neurons may lead to markedly increased blood pressure (hypertensive crisis). Selective MAO-B inhibitors (e.g., selegiline) or reversible MAO-A–selective inhibitors (e.g., moclobemide) are less likely to cause this potential interaction (Volz and Geiter, 1998; Wouters, 1998). MAO inhibitors are useful in the treatment of Parkinson's disease and mental depression (Chapters 15 and 22).

Inhibitors of MAO (e.g., pargyline and nialamide) can cause an increase in the concentration of NE, DA, and 5-HT in the brain and other tissues accompanied by a variety of pharmacological effects. No striking pharmacological action in the periphery can be attributed to the inhibition of COMT. However, the COMT inhibitors entacapone and tocapone have been found to be efficacious in the therapy of Parkinson's disease (Chong and Mersfelder, 2000) (Chapter 22).

There is ongoing passive leakage of catecholamines from vesicular storage granules of sympathetric neurons and adrenal medullary chromaffin cells. As a consequence, most metabolism of catecholamines takes place in the same cells where the amines are synthesized and stored. VMAT2 effectively sequesters ~90% of the amines leaking into the cytoplasm back into storage vesicles; ~10% escapes sequestration and is metabolized (Eisenhofer et al., 2004).

Sympathetic nerves contain MAO but not COMT, and this MAO catalyzes only the first step of a two-step reaction. MAO converts NE or epinephrine into a short-lived intermediate, DOPGAL, which undergoes further metabolism in a second step catalyzed by another group of enzymes forming more stable alcohol- or acid-deaminated metabolites. Aldehyde dehydrogenase metabolizes DOPGAL to 3,4-dihydroxymandelic acid (DOMA), while aldehyde reductase metabolized DOPGAL to 3,4-dihydroxyphenyl glycol (DOPEG). In addition to aldehyde reductase, a related enzyme, aldose reductase, can also reduce a catecholamine to its corresponding alcohol. This latter enzyme is present in sympathetic neurons and adrenal chromaffin cells. Under normal circumstances, DOMA is an insignificant metabolite of NE and epinephrine, with DOPEG being the main metabolite produced by deamination in sympathetic neurons and adrenal medullary chromaffin cells.

Once it leaves the sites of formation (sympathetic neurons, adrenal medulla), DOPEG is converted to 3-methyl, 4-hydroxy phenylglycol (MOPEG) by COMT. Therefore most MOPEG comes from the extraneuronal *O*-methylation of DOPEG produced in and diffusing rapidly from sympathetic neurons into the extracellular fluid. MOPEG is then converted to vanillylmandelic acid (VMA) by the sequential action of alcohol and aldehyde dehydrogenase. MOPEG is first converted to the unstable aldehyde metabolite

MOPGAL and then to VMA, with VMA being the major end product of NE and epinephrine metabolism. Another route for the formation of VMA is conversion of NE and epinephrine into normetanephrine and metaneprhine, respectively, by COMT followed by deamination to MOPGAL and ultimately VMA. This is now thought to be only a minor pathway, as indicated by the size of the arrows on Figure 8–7.

In contrast to sympathetic neurons, adrenal medullary chromaffin cells contain both MAO and COMT. In chromaffin cells, the COMT is mainly present as the membrane-bound form of the enzyme in contrast to the form found in the cytoplasm of extra-neuronal tissue. This isoform of COMT has a higher affinity for catecholamines than does the soluble form found in most other tissues (e.g., liver and kidney). In adrenal medullary chromaffin cells, leakage of NE and epinephrine from storage vesicles leads to substantial intracellular production of the *O*-methylated metabolites normetanephrine and metanephrine. It is estimated that in humans, over 90% of circulating metanephrine and 25-40% of circulating normetanephrine are derived from catecholamines metabolized within adrenal chromaffin cells.

The sequence of cellular uptake and metabolism of catecholamines in extraneuronal tissues contributes very little (~25%) to the total metabolism of endogenously produced NE in sympathetic neurons or the adrenal medulla. However, extraneuronal metabolism is an important mechanism for the clearance of circulating and exogenously administered catecholamines.

Classification of Adrenergic Receptors. Crucial to understanding the remarkably diverse effects of the catecholamines and related sympathomimetic agents is an understanding of the classification and properties of the different types of adrenergic receptors (or adrenoceptors). Elucidation of the characteristics of these receptors and the biochemical and physiological pathways they regulate has increased our understanding of the seemingly contradictory and variable effects of catecholamines on various organ systems. Although structurally related (discussed later), different receptors regulate distinct physiological processes by controlling the synthesis or release of a variety of second messengers (Table 8–6).

Based on studies of the abilities of epinephrine, norepinephrine, and other related agonists to regulate various physiological processes, Ahlquist first proposed the existence of more than one adrenergic receptor. It was known that these drugs could cause either contraction or relaxation of smooth muscle depending on the site, the dose, and the agent chosen. For example, NE was known to have potent excitatory effects on smooth muscle and correspondingly low activity as an inhibitor; isoproterenol displayed the opposite pattern of activity. Epinephrine could both excite and inhibit smooth muscle. Thus, Ahlquist proposed the designations α and β for receptors on smooth muscle where catecholamines produce excitatory and inhibitory responses, respectively. An exception is the gut, which generally is relaxed by activation of either α or β receptors. The rank order of potency of agonists is isoproterenol > epinephrine ≥ norepinephrine for β adrenergic receptors and epinephrine ≥ norepinephrine >> isoproterenol for α adrenergic receptors (Table 8–3). This initial classification was corroborated by the finding that certain antagonists produce selective blockade of the effects of adrenergic nerve impulses and sympathomimetic agents at α receptors (e.g., phenoxybenzamine), whereas others produce selective β receptor blockade (e.g., propranolol).

β Receptors later were subdivided into β_1 (e.g., those in the myocardium) and β_2 (smooth muscle and most other sites) because epinephrine and norepinephrine essentially are equipotent at the former sites, whereas epinephrine is 10-50 times more potent than norepinephrine at the latter. Antagonists that discriminate between β_1 and β_2 receptors were subsequently developed (Chapter 12). A human gene that encodes a third β receptor (designated β_3) has been isolated (Emorine et al., 1989). Since the β_3 receptor is about tenfold more sensitive to norepinephrine than to epinephrine and is relatively resistant to blockade by antagonists such as propranolol, it may mediate responses to catecholamine at sites with "atypical" pharmacological characteristics (e.g., adipose tissue). Although the adipocytes are a major site of β_3 adrenergic receptors, all three β adrenergic receptors are present in both white adipose tissue and brown adipose tissue. Animals treated with β_3 receptor agonists exhibit a vigorous thermogenic response as well as lipolysis (Robidoux et al., 2004). Polymorphisms in the β_3 receptor gene may be related to risk of obesity or type 2 diabetes in some populations (Arner and Hoffstedt, 1999). Also, there has been interest in the possibility that β_3 receptor–selective agonists may be beneficial in treating these disorders (Weyer et al., 1999). The existence of a fourth type of βAR, β_4AR, has been proposed. Despite intense efforts, β_4AR, like α_{1L}AR, has not been cloned. Current thinking is that the β_4AR represents an affinity state of β_1AR rather than a descrete receptor (Hieble, 2007).

There is also heterogeneity among α adrenergic receptors. The initial distinction was based on functional and anatomic considerations when it was realized that NE and other α-adrenergic receptors could profoundly inhibit the release of norepinephrine from neurons (Westfall, 1977) (Figure 8–6). Indeed, when sympathetic nerves are stimulated in the presence of certain α receptor antagonists, the amount of NE liberated by each nerve impulse increases markedly. This

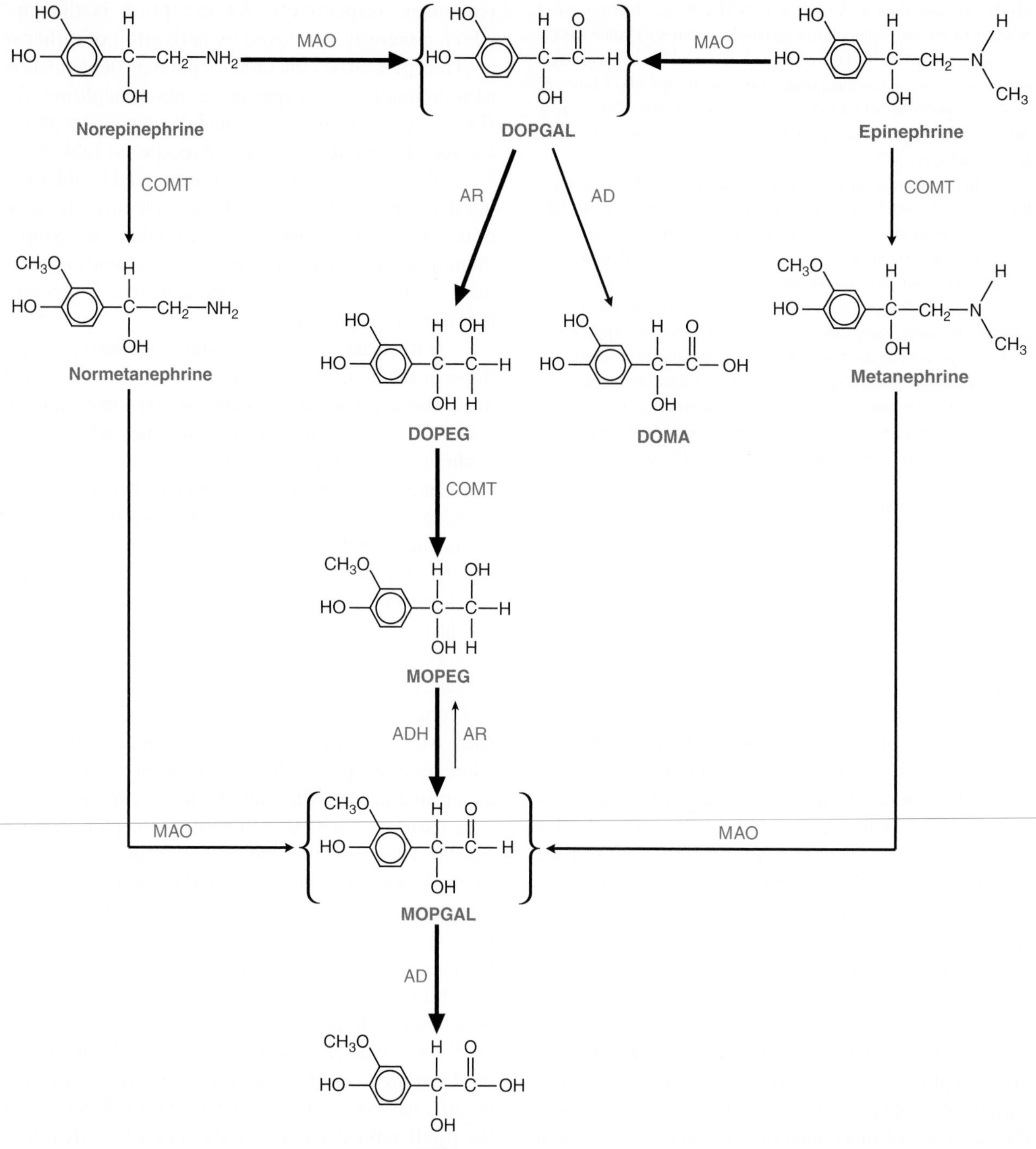

Norepinephrine
MAO
DOPGAL
MAO
Epinephrine
COMT
AR
AD
COMT
Normetanephrine
DOPEG
DOMA
Metanephrine
COMT
MOPEG
ADH
AR
MAO
MOPGAL
MAO
AD
VMA

Figure 8-7. *Steps in the metabolic disposition of catecholamines.* Norepinephrine and epinephrine are first oxidatively deaminated to a short lived intermediate (DOPGAL) by monoamine oxidase (MAO). DOPGAL then undergoes further metabolism to more stable alcohol or acid deaminated metabolites. Aldehyde dehydrogenase (AD) metabolizes DOPGAL to 3,4-dihydroxymandelic acid (DOMA) while aldehyde reductase (AR) metabolizes DOPGAL to 3,4-dihydroxyphenyl glycol (DOPEG). Under normal circumstances DOMA is a minor metabolite with DOPEG being the major metabolite produced from norepinephrine and epinephrine. Once DOPEG leaves the major sites of its formation (sympathetic nerves; adrenal medulla), it is converted to 3-methoxy, 4-hydroxyphenylglycol (MOPEG) by catechol-*0*-methyl transferase (COMT). MOPEG is then converted to the unstable aldehyde (MOPGAL) by alcohol dehydrogenase (ADH) and finally to vanillyl mandelic acid (VMA) by aldehyde dehydrogenase. VMA is the major end product of norepinephrine and epinephrine metabolism. Another route for the formation of VMA is conversion of norepinephrine or epinephrine into normetanephrine or metanephrine by COMT either in the adreneal medulla or extraneuronal sites,with subsequent metabolism to MOPGAL and thence to VMA.

Table 8–6

Characteristics for Adrenergic Receptor Subtypes

SUBTYPE[a]	GENE LOCATION IN HUMAN CHROMOSOME	G-PROTEIN COUPLING	PRINCIPLE EFFECTORS	TISSUE LOCALIZATION	SUBTYPE DOMINANT EFFECTS[b]
α_{1A}	8p21-p11.2	$G\alpha_q$ ($\alpha_{11}/\alpha_{14}/\alpha_{16}$)	↑ PLC, ↑ PLA_2 ↑ Ca^{2+} channels ↑ Na^+/H^+ exchanger Modulation of K^+ channels ↑ MAPK Signaling	Heart Liver Smooth muscle Blood vessels Lung Vas deferens Prostate Cerebellum Cortex Hippocampus	• Predominant receptor causing contraction of vascular smooth muscle • Promotes cardiac growth and structure • Vasoconstriction of large resistant arterioles in skeletal muscle
α_{1B}	5q23-q32	$G\alpha_q$ ($\alpha_{11}/\alpha_{14}/\alpha_{16}$)	↑ PLC, ↑ PLA_2 ↑ Ca^{2+} channels ↑ Na^+/H^+ exchanger Modulation of K^+ channels ↑ MAPK Signaling	Kidney Spleen Lung Blood vessels Cortex Brainstem	• Most abundant subtype in heart • Promotes cardiac growth and structure
α_{1D}	20p13	$G\alpha_q$ ($\alpha_{11}/\alpha_{14}/\alpha_{16}$)	↑ PLC, ↑ PLA_2 ↑ Ca^{2+} channels ↑ Na^+/H^+ exchanger Modulation of K^+ channels ↑ MAPK Signaling	Platelets Prostate Aorta Coronary artery Cortex Hippocampus	• Predominant receptor causing vasoconstriction in aorta and coronary artery
α_{2A}	10q24-q26	$G\alpha_i$ Family $G\alpha_o$ Family (α_{o1}/α_{o2})	Inhibition of AC ↓ cAMP ↓ PKA activity	Platelets Sympathetic neurons Autonomic ganglia Pancreas Coronary/CNS vessels Locus ceruleus Brainstem Spinal cord	• Predominant inhibitory receptor on sympathetic neurons • Vasoconstriction of small procapillary vessels in skeletal muscle
α_{2B}	2q12-q13	$G\alpha_i$ Family $G\alpha_o$ Family (α_{o1}/α_{o2})	Inhibition of AC ↓ cAMP ↓ PKA activity	Liver Kidney Blood vessels Coronary/CNS vessels Diencephalon Pancreas Platelets	• Predominant receptor mediating α_2 vasoconstriction
α_{2C}	4p16	$G\alpha_i$ Family ($\alpha_{11}/\alpha_{12}/\alpha_{13}$) $G\alpha_o$ Family (α_{o1}/α_{o2})	Inhibition of AC ↓ cAMP ↓ PKA activity	Basal ganglia Cortex Cerebellum Hippocampus	• Predominant receptor modulating dopamine neurotransmission • Predominant receptor inhibiting hormone release from adrenal medulla

(Continued)

Table 8–6

Characteristics for Adrenergic Receptor Subtypes (*Continued*)

SUBTYPE[a]	GENE LOCATION IN HUMAN CHROMOSOME	G-PROTEIN COUPLING	PRINCIPLE EFFECTORS	TISSUE LOCALIZATION	SUBTYPE DOMINANT EFFECTS[b]
β_1	10q240q26	$G\alpha_s$	Activation of AC ↑ cAMP ↑ PKA activation Activation of L type Ca^{2+} channels	Heart Kidney Adipocytes Skeletal muscle Olfactory nucleus Cortex Cerebellar nuclei Brain stem Spinal cord	• Predominant receptor in heart producing positive inotropic and chronotropic effects
β_2[c]	531-q32	$G\alpha_s$	Activation of AC ↑ cAMP ↑ PKA activation Activation of Ca^{2+} channels	Heart, Lung Blood vessels Bronchial and GI smooth muscle Kidney Skeletal muscle Olfactory bulb Piriform cortex Cortex Hippocampus	• Predominant receptor in smooth muscle relaxation • Skeletal muscle hypertrophy
β_3[c,d]	8p12-p11.2	$G\alpha_s$	Activation of AC ↑ cAMP ↑ PKA activation Activation of Ca^{2+} channels	Adipose tissue GI tract Heart	• Predominant receptor producing metabolic effects

[a]At least three subtypes each of α_1 and α_2 adrenergic receptors are known, but distinctions in their mechanisms of action have not been clearly defined.
[b]In some species (e.g., rat), metabolic responses in the liver are mediated by α_1 adrenergic receptors, whereas in others (e.g., dog) β_2 adrenergic receptors are predominantly involved. Both types of receptors appear to contribute to responses in human beings.
[c]β Receptor coupling to cell signaling can be more complex. In addition to coupling to G_s to stimulate AC, β_2 receptors can activate signaling via a GRK/β-arrestin pathway (Violin and Lefkowitz, 2007). β_2 and β_3 receptors can couple to both G_s and G_i in a manner that may reflect agonist stereochemistry (Woo et al., 2009). See also Chapter 12.
[d]Metabolic responses in adipocytes and certain other tissues with atypical pharmacological characteristics may be mediated by this subtype of receptor. Most β adrenergic receptor antagonists (including propranolol) do not block these responses.
AC, adenylyl cyclase; Epi, epinephrine; NE, norepinephrine; Iso, isoproterenol; GI, gastrointestinal; GU, genitourinary.

feedback-inhibitory effect of NE on its release from nerve terminals is mediated by α receptors that are pharmacologically distinct from the classical postsynaptic α receptors. Accordingly, these presynaptic α adrenergic receptors were designated α_2, whereas the postsynaptic "excitatory" α receptors were designated α_1 (Langer, 1997). Compounds such as clonidine are more potent agonists at α_2 than at α_1 receptors; by contrast, phenylephrine and methoxamine selectively activate postsynaptic α_1 receptors. Although there is little evidence to suggest that α_1 adrenergic receptors function presynaptically in the autonomic nervous system, it is now clear that α_2 receptors also are present at postjunctional or nonjunctional sites in several tissues. For example, stimulation of postjunctional α_2 receptors in the brain is associated with reduced sympathetic outflow from the CNS and appears to be responsible for a significant component of the antihypertensive effect of drugs such as clonidine (Chapter 12). Thus, the anatomic concept of prejunctional

α_2 and postjunctional α_1 adrenergic receptors has been abandoned in favor of a pharmacological and functional classification (Tables 8–6 and 8–7).

Cloning revealed additional heterogeneity of both α_1 and α_2 adrenergic receptors (Bylund, 1992). There are three pharmacologically defined α_1 receptors (α_{1A}, α_{1B}, and α_{1D}) with distinct sequences and tissue distributions, and three cloned subtypes of α_2 receptors (α_{2A}, α_{2B}, and α_{2C}) (Table 8–6). A fourth type of α_1 receptor, α_{1L}AR, has been defined on the basis of a low affinity for a number of selective antagonists including prazosin (Hieble, 2007). This phenotype could be of physiological significance since the α_{1L} profile has been identified in a variety of tissues across a number of different species, where it appears to regulate smooth muscle contractility in the vasculature and lower urinary tract. It also appears (at least in the mouse prostate smooth muscle) to be dependent upon expression of the α_{1A}AR gene product. Moreover, an intact cellular environment is important for the manifestation of the α_{1L}AR phenotype *in vivo*. Despite intense efforts, α_{12}AR has not been cloned and it is doubtful that α_{1L} is a discrete AR (Hieble, 2007).

Owing to the lack of sufficiently subtype-selective ligands, the precise physiological function and therapeutic potential of the subtypes of adrenergic receptors have not been elucidated fully. Great advances in our understanding have been made through the use of genetic approaches using transgenic and receptor knockout experiments in mice (discussed later). These mouse models have been used to identify the particular receptor subtypes and pathophysiological relevance of individual adrenergic receptors subtypes (Philipp and Hein, 2004; Tanoue et al., 2002a, 2002b; Xiao et al., 2006).

Molecular Basis of Adrenergic Receptor Function. All of the adrenergic receptors are GPCRs that link to heterotrimeric G proteins. Each major type shows preference for a particular class of G proteins, i.e., α_1 to G_q, α_2 to G_i, and β to G_s (Table 8–6). The responses that follow activation of all types of adrenergic receptors result from G protein–mediated effects on the generation of second messengers and on the activity of ion channels, as discussed in Chapter 3. The pathways overlap broadly with those discussed for muscarinic acetylcholine receptors and are summarized in Table 8–6 (Drake et al., 2006; Park et al., 2008).

Structure of Adrenergic Receptors. Adrenergic receptors constitute a family of closely related proteins that are related both structurally and functionally to GPCRs for a wide variety of other hormones and neurotransmitters (see Chapter 3). Ligand binding, site-directed labeling, and mutagenesis have revealed that the conserved membrane-spanning regions are crucially involved in ligand binding (Hutchins, 1994; Strader et al.,1994). These regions appear to create a ligand-binding pocket analogous to that formed by the membrane-spanning regions of rhodopsin to accommodate the covalently attached chromophore, retinal, with molecular models placing catecholamines either horizontally (Strader et al., 1994) or perpendicularly (Hutchins, 1994) in the bilayer. The crystal structure of mammalian rhodopsin confirms a number of predictions about the structure of GPCRs (Palczewski et al., 2000).

β Adrenergic Receptors. The three β receptors share ~60% amino acid sequence identity within the presumed membrane-spanning domains where the ligand-binding pocket for epinephrine and norepinephrine is found. Based on results of site-directed mutagenesis, individual amino acids in the β_2 receptor that interact with each of the functional groups on the catecholamine agonist molecule have been identified.

β Receptors regulate numerous functional responses, including heart rate and contractility, smooth muscle relaxation, and multiple metabolic events in numerous tissues including adipose and hepatic cells and skeletal muscle (Lynch and Ryall, 2008) (Table 8–1). All three of the β receptor subtypes (β_1, β_2, and β_3) couple to G_s and activate adenylyl cyclase (Table 8–7). However, recent data suggest differences in downstream signals and events activated by the three β receptors (Lefkowitz, 2000; Ma and Huang, 2002). Catecholamines promote β receptor feedback regulation, that is, desensitization and receptor down-regulation (Kohout and Lefkowitz, 2003). β Receptors differ in the extent to which they undergo such regulation, with the β_2 receptor being the most susceptible. Stimulation of β adrenergic receptors leads to the accumulation of cyclic AMP, activation of the PKA, and altered function of numerous cellular proteins as a result of their phosphorylation (Chapter 3). In addition, G_s can enhance directly the activation of voltage-sensitive Ca^{2+} channels in the plasma membrane of skeletal and cardiac muscle.

Several reports demonstrate that β_1, β_2, and β_3 receptors can differ in their intracellular signaling pathways and subcellular location (Brodde et al., 2006; Violin and Lefkowitz, 2007; Woo, et al., 2009). While the positive chronotropic effects of β_1 receptor activation are clearly mediated by G_s in myocytes, dual coupling of β_2 receptors to G_s and G_i occurs in myocytes from newborn mice. Stimulation of β_2 receptors caused a transient increase in heart rate that is followed by a prolonged decrease. Following pretreatment with pertussis toxin, which prevents activation of G_i, the negative chronotropic effect of β_2 activation is abolished. It is thought that these specific signaling properties of β receptor subtypes are linked to subtype-selective association with intracellular scaffolding and signaling proteins (Baillie and Houslay, 2005). β_2 Receptors normally are confined to caveolae in cardiac myocyte membranes. The activation

Table 8–7

Representative Agents Acting at Peripheral Cholinergic and Adrenergic Neuroeffector Junctions

MECHANISM OF ACTION	SYSTEM	AGENTS	EFFECT
1. Interference with synthesis of transmitter	Cholinergic	Choline acetyl transferase inhibitors	Minimal depletion of ACh
	Adrenergic	α-Methyltyrosine (inhibition of tyrosine hydroxylase)	Depletion of NE
2. Metabolic transformation by same pathway as precursor of transmitter	Adrenergic	Methyldopa	Displacement of NE by α-methyl-NE, which is an α_2 agonist, similar to clonidine, that reduces sympathetic outflow from CNS.
3. Blockade of transport system at nerve terminal membrane	Cholinergic	Hemicholinium	Block of choline uptake with consequent depletion of ACh
	Adrenergic	Cocaine, imipramine	Accumulation of NE at receptors
4. Blockade of transport system of storage vesicle	Cholinergic	Vesamicol	Block of ACh storage
	Adrenergic	Reserpine	Destruction of NE by mitochondrial MAO, and depletion from adrenergic terminals
5. Promotion of exocytosis or displacement of transmitter from storage sites	Cholinergic	Latrotoxins	Cholinomimetic followed by anticholinergic
	Adrenergic	Amphetamine, tyramine	Sympathomimetic
6. Prevention of release of transmitter	Cholinergic	Botulinum toxin	Anti-cholinergic
	Adrenergic	Bretylium, guanadrel	Anti-adrenergic
7. Mimicry of transmitter at postjunctional sites	Cholinergic		
	Muscarinic[a]	Methacholine, bethanachol	Cholinomimetic
	Nicotinic[b]	Nicotine, epibatidine, cytisine	Cholinomimetic
	Adrenergic		
	α_1	Phenylephrine	Selective α_1 agonist
	α_2	Clonidine	Sympathomimetic (periphery); reduced sympathetic outflow (CNS)
	α_1,α_2	Oxymetazoline	Non-selective α adrenomimetic
	β_1	Dobutamine	Selective cardiac stimulation (also activates α_1 receptors)
	β_2	Terbutaline, albuterol metaproterenol	Selective β_2 receptor agonist (selective inhibition of smooth muscle contraction)
	β_1,β_2	Isoproterenol	Nonselective β agonist
8. Blockade of postsynaptic receptor	Cholinergic		
	Muscarinic[a]	Atropine	Muscarinic blockade
	Nicotinic (N_m)[b]	*d*-tubucurarine, atracurium	Neuromuscular blockade
	Nicotinic (N_n)[b]	Trimethaphan	Ganglionic blockade
	Adrenergic		
	α_1,α_2	Phenoxybenzamine	Nonselective α receptor blockade (irreversible)
	α_1,α_2	Phentolamine	Nonselective α receptor blockade (reversible)
	α_1	Prazosin, terazosin, doxasozin	Selective α_1 receptor blockade (reversible)

(*Continued*)

Table 8–7

Representative Agents Acting at Peripheral Cholinergic and Adrenergic Neuroeffector Junctions (*Continued*)

MECHANISM OF ACTION	SYSTEM	AGENTS	EFFECT
	α_2	Yohimbine	Selective α_2 receptor blockade
	β_1, β_2	Propranolol	Nonselective β receptor blockade
	β_1	Metoprolol, atenolol	Selective β_1 receptor blockade (cardiomyocytes; renal j-g cells)
	β_2	—	Selective β_2 receptor blockade (smooth muscle)
9. Inhibition of enzymatic breakdown of transmitter	Cholinergic	AChE inhibitors Edrophonium, neostigmine, pyridostigmine	Cholinomimetic (muscarinic sites) Depolarization blockade (nicotinic sites)
	Adrenergic	Nonselective MAO inhibitors Pargyline, nialamide	Little direct effect on NE or sympathetic response; potentiation of tyramine
		Selective MAO-B inhibitor Selegeline	Adjunct in Parkinson disease
		Peripheral COMT inhibitor Entacapone	Adjunct in Parkinson disease
		COMT inhibitor Tolcapone	

[a]At least five subtypes of muscarinic receptors exist. Agonists show little selectivity for subtypes whereas several antagonists show partial subtype selectivity (see Table 8–3).
[b]Two subtypes of muscle acetylcholine nicotinic receptors and several subtypes of neuronal receptors have been identified (seeTable 8–2).
ACh, acetylcholine; AChE, acetylcholine esterase; COMT, catechol-*O*-methyl transferase; MAO, monoamine oxidase; NE, norepinephrine; j-g cells, renin-secreting cells in the juxta-glomerular complex of the kidney.

of PKA by cyclic AMP and the importance of compartmentation of components of the cyclic AMP pathway are discussed in Chapter 3. A representation of the general structure of adrenergic receptors is shown in Figure 8–8.

α Adrenergic Receptors. The deduced amino acid sequences from the three α_1 receptor genes (α_{1A}, α_{1B}, and α_{1D}) and three α_2 receptor genes (α_{2A}, α_{2B}, and α_{2C}) conform to the well-established GPCR paradigm (Bylund, 1992; Zhong and Minneman, 1999). The general structural features of α receptors and their relation to the functions of ligand binding and G protein activation appear to agree with those set forth in Chapter 3 and earlier in this chapter for the β receptors. Within the membrane-spanning domains, the three α_1 adrenergic receptors share ~75% identity in amino acid residues, as do the three α_2 receptors, but the α_1 and α_2 subtypes are no more similar than are the α and β subtypes (~30-40%).

α_2 Adrenergic Receptors. As shown in Table 8–6, α_2 receptors couple to a variety of effectors (Aantaa et al., 1995; Bylund, 1992; Tan and Limbird, 2005). Inhibition of adenylyl cyclase activity was the first effect observed, but in some systems the enzyme actually is stimulated by α_2 adrenergic receptors, either by G_i $\beta\gamma$ subunits or by weak direct stimulation of G_s. The physiological significance of these latter processes is not currently clear. α_2 Receptors activate G protein–gated K^+ channels, resulting in membrane hyperpolarization. In some cases (e.g., cholinergic neurons in the myenteric plexus) this may be Ca^{2+}-dependent, whereas in others (e.g., muscarinic ACh receptors in atrial myocytes) it results from direct interaction of $\beta\gamma$ subunits with K^+ channels. α_2 Receptors also can inhibit voltage-gated Ca^{2+} channels; this is mediated by G_o. Other second-messenger systems linked to α_2 receptor activation include acceleration of Na^+/H^+ exchange, stimulation of $PLC_{\beta 2}$ activity and arachidonic acid mobilization, increased phosphoinositide hydrolysis, and increased intracellular availability of Ca^{2+}. The latter is involved in the smooth muscle–contracting effect of

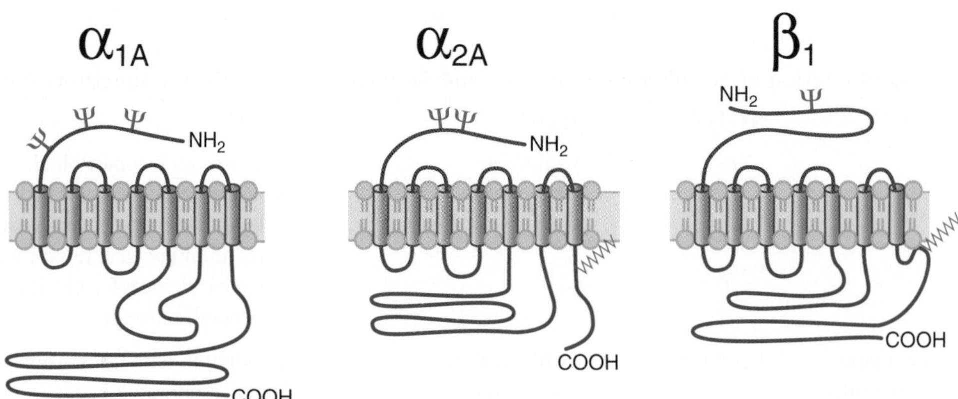

Figure 8-8. *Subtypes of adrenergic receptors.* All of the adrenergic receptors are heptaspanning GPCRs. A representative of each type is shown; each type has three subtypes: α_{1A}, α_{1B}, and α_{1D}; α_{2A}, α_{2B}, and α_{2C}; and β_1, β_2, and β_3. The principle effector systems affected by α_1, α_2 and β receptors are depicted in Table 8–6. (Ψ) indicates a site for *N*-glycosylation. ww indicates a site for thio-acetylation.

α_2 adrenergic receptor agonists. In addition, the α_2 receptors activate mitogen-activated protein kinases (MAPKs) likely by means of $\beta\gamma$ subunits released from pertussis toxin–sensitive G proteins (Della Rocca et al., 1997; Richman and Regan, 1998). This and related pathways lead to activation of a variety of tyrosine kinase–mediated downstream events. These pathways are reminiscent of pathways activated by tyrosine kinase activities of growth factor receptors. Although α_2 receptors may activate several different signaling pathways, the exact contribution of each to many physiological processes is not clear. The α_{2A} receptor plays a major role in inhibiting NE release from sympathetic nerve endings and suppressing sympathetic outflow from the brain, leading to hypotension (Kable et al., 2000).

In the CNS, α_{2A} receptors, which appear to be the most dominant adrenergic receptor, probably produce the antinociceptive effects, sedation, hypothermia, hypotension, and behavioral actions of α_2 agonists (Lakhlani et al., 1997). The α_{2C} receptor occurs in the ventral and dorsal striatum and hippocampus. It appears to modulate dopamine neurotransmission and various behavioral responses. The α_{2B} receptor is the main receptor mediating α_2-induced vasoconstriction, whereas the α_{2C} receptor is the predominant receptor inhibiting the release of catecholamines from the adrenal medulla and modulating dopamine neurotransmission in the brain.

α_1 Adrenergic Receptors. Stimulation of α_1 receptors results in the regulation of multiple effector systems. A primary mode of signal transduction involves activation of the G_q-PLC_β-IP_3-Ca^{2+} pathway and the activation of other Ca^{2+} and calmodulin sensitive pathways such as CaM kinases (Chapter 3). For example, α_1 receptors regulate hepatic glycogenolysis in some animal species; this effect results from the activation of phosphorylase kinase by the mobilized Ca^{2+}, aided by the inhibition of glycogen synthase caused by PKC-mediated phosphorylation. PKC phosphorylates many substrates, including membrane proteins such as channels, pumps, and ion-exchange proteins (e.g., Ca^{2+}-transport ATPase). These effects presumably lead to regulation of various ion conductances.

α_1 Receptor stimulation of PLA_2 leads to the release of free arachidonate, which is then metabolized by the cyclooxygenase and lipoxygenase pathways to the bioactive prostaglandins and leukotrienes, respectively (Chapter 33). Stimulation of PLA_2 activity by various agonists (including epinephrine acting at α_1 receptors) is found in many tissues and cell lines, suggesting that this effector is physiologically important. PLD hydrolyzes phosphatidylcholine to yield phosphatidic acid (PA). Although PA itself may act as a second messenger by releasing Ca^{2+} from intracellular stores, it also is metabolized to the second messenger DAG. PLD is an effector for ADP-ribosylating factor (ARF), suggesting that PLD may play a role in membrane trafficking. Finally, some evidence in vascular smooth muscle suggests that α_1 receptors are capable of regulating a Ca^{2+} channel by means of a G protein.

In most smooth muscles, the increased concentration of intracellular Ca^{2+} ultimately causes contraction as a result of activation of Ca^{2+}-sensitive protein kinases such as the calmodulin-dependent myosin light-chain kinase; phosphorylation of the light chain of myosin is associated with the development of tension (see Chapter 3). In contrast, the increased concentration of intracellular Ca^{2+} that result from stimulation of α_1 receptors in GI smooth muscle causes hyperpolarization and relaxation by activation of Ca^{2+}-dependent K^+ channels (McDonald et al., 1994).

As with α_2 receptors, there is considerable evidence demonstrating that α_1 receptors activate MAPKs and other kinases such as PI3 kinase leading to important effects on cell growth and proliferation (Dorn and Brown, 1999; Gutkind, 1998). For example, prolonged stimulation of α_1 receptors promotes growth of cardiac myocytes and vascular smooth muscle cells. The α_{1A} receptor is the predominant receptor causing vasoconstriction in many vascular beds, including the following arteries: mammary, mesenteric, splenic, hepatic, omental, renal, pulmonary, and epicardial coronary. It is also the predominant subtype in the vena cava and the saphenous and pulmonary veins (Michelotti et al., 2001). Together with the α_{1B} receptor subtype, it promotes cardiac growth and structure. The α_{1B} receptor subtype is the most abundant subtype in the heart, whereas the α_{1D} receptor subtype is the predominant receptor causing vasoconstriction in the aorta. There is evidence to support the idea that α_{1B} receptors mediate behaviors such as reaction to novelty and exploration and are involved in behavioral sensitizations and in the vulnerability to addiction (see Chapter 24).

Adrenergic Receptor Polymorphism. Numerous polymorphisms and slice variants of adrenergic receptors continue to be identified. Receptors α_{1A}, α_{1B} and β_{1D}, β_1, and β_2 are polymorphic. Such polymorphisms in these adrenergic receptors could result in altered physiological responses to activation of the sympathetic nervous system, contribute to disease states and alter the responses to adrenergic agonists and/or antagonists (Brodde, 2008). Knowledge of the functional consequences of specific polymorphisms could theoretically result in the individualization of drug therapy based on a patient's genetic makeup and could explain marked inter-individual variability within the human population.

Localization of Adrenergic Receptors. Presynaptically located α_2 and β_2 receptors fulfill important roles in the regulation of neurotransmitter release from sympathetic nerve endings. Presynaptic α_2 receptors also may mediate inhibition of release of neurotransmitters other than norepinephrine in the central and peripheral nervous systems. Both α_2 and β_2 receptors are located at postsynaptic sites (Table 8–6), such as on many types of neurons in the brain. In peripheral tissues, postsynaptic α_2 receptors are found in vascular and other smooth muscle cells (where they mediate contraction), adipocytes, and many types of secretory epithelial cells (intestinal, renal, endocrine). Postsynaptic β_2 receptors can be found in the myocardium (where they mediate contraction) as well as on vascular and other smooth muscle cells (where they mediate relaxation) and skeletal muscle (where they can mediate hypertrophy). Indeed, most normal human cell types express β_2 receptors. Both α_2 and β_2 receptors may be situated at sites that are relatively remote from nerve terminals releasing NE. Such extrajunctional receptors typically are found on vascular smooth muscle cells and blood elements (platelets and leukocytes) and may be activated preferentially by circulating catecholamines, particularly epinephrine.

In contrast, α_1 and β_1 receptors appear to be located mainly in the immediate vicinity of sympathetic adrenergic nerve terminals in peripheral target organs, strategically placed to be activated during stimulation of these nerves. These receptors also are distributed widely in the mammalian brain (Table 8–6).

The cellular distributions of the three α_1 and three α_2 receptor subtypes still are incompletely understood. *In situ* hybridization of receptor mRNA and receptor subtype-specific antibodies indicates that α_{2A} receptors in the brain may be both pre- and postsynaptic. These findings and other studies indicate that this receptor subtype functions as a presynaptic autoreceptor in central noradrenergic neurons (Aantaa et al., 1995; Lakhlani et al., 1997). Using similar approaches, α_{1A} mRNA was found to be the dominant subtype message expressed in prostatic smooth muscle (Walden et al., 1997).

Refractoriness to Catecholamines. Exposure of catecholamine-sensitive cells and tissues to adrenergic agonists causes a progressive diminution in their capacity to respond to such agents. This phenomenon, variously termed *refractoriness, desensitization,* or *tachyphylaxis,* can limit the therapeutic efficacy and duration of action of catecholamines and other agents (Chapter 3). The mechanisms are incompletely understood. They have been studied most extensively in cells that synthesize cyclic AMP in response to β_2 receptor agonists.

Multiple mechanisms are involved in desensitization, including rapid events such as receptor phosphorylation by both G-protein receptor kinases (GRKs) and by signaling kinases such as PKA and PKC, receptor sequestration, uncoupling from G proteins, and activation of specific cyclic nucleotide phosphodiesterases. More slowly occurring events also are seen, such as receptor endocytosis, which decreases receptor number. An understanding of the mechanisms involved in regulation of GPCR desensitization has developed over the last few years (Kohout and Lefkowitz, 2003; Violin and Lefkowitz, 2007). Such regulation is very complex and exceeds the simplistic model of GPCR phosphorylation by GRKs followed by arrestin binding and uncoupling of G-protein signaling. It is known that GRK activities are extensively regulated by numerous interactions with and modifications by other proteins. β-Arrestin, now recognized as a scaffolding protein, can physically interrupt signaling to the G proteins as well as to further enhance GPCR desensitization by causing translocation of cytosolic proteins to the receptor (e.g., phosphodiesterase and cSrc). These, in turn, can turn off signaling at its source by degrading cyclic AMP or phosphorylating GRK2 to enhance its activity toward the receptor (DeFea, 2008; DeWire et al., 2007; Hanyaloglu and VonZastrow, 2008).

RELATIONSHIP BETWEEN THE NERVOUS AND ENDOCRINE SYSTEMS

The theory of neurohumoral transmission by its very designation implies at least a superficial resemblance between the nervous and endocrine systems. It is now clear that the similarities extend considerably deeper, particularly with respect to the autonomic nervous system. In the regulation of homeostasis, the autonomic nervous system is responsible for rapid adjustments to changes in the environment, which it effects at both its ganglionic synapses and its postganglionic terminals by the liberation of chemical agents that act transiently at their immediate sites of release. The endocrine system, in contrast, regulates slower, more generalized adaptations by releasing hormones into the systemic circulation to act at distant, widespread sites over periods of minutes to hours or days. Both systems have major central representations in the hypothalamus, where they are integrated with each other and with subcortical, cortical, and spinal influences. The neurohumoral theory provides a unitary concept of the functioning of the nervous and endocrine systems in which the differences largely relate to the distances over which the released mediators travel.

PHARMACOLOGICAL CONSIDERATIONS

The foregoing sections contain numerous references to the actions of drugs considered primarily as tools for the dissection and elucidation of physiological mechanisms. This section presents a classification of drugs that act on the peripheral nervous system and its effector organs at some stage of neurotransmission. In the subsequent four chapters, the systematic pharmacology of the important members of each of these classes is described.

Each step involved in neurotransmission (Figures 8–3, 8–4, and 8–6) represents a potential point of therapeutic intervention. This is depicted in the diagrams of the cholinergic and adrenergic terminals and their postjunctional sites (Figure 8–4 and 8–6). Drugs that affect processes involved in each step of transmission at both cholinergic and adrenergic junctions are summarized in Table 8–7, which lists representative agents that act through the mechanisms described next.

Interference with the Synthesis or Release of the Transmitter

Cholinergic. Hemicholinium (HC-3), a synthetic compound, blocks the transport system by which choline accumulates in the terminals of cholinergic fibers, thus limiting the synthesis of the ACh store available for release. Vesamicol blocks the transport of ACh into its storage vesicles, preventing its release. The site on the presynaptic nerve terminal for block of ACh release by botulinum toxin was discussed previously; death usually results from respiratory paralysis unless patients with respiratory failure receive artificial ventilation. Injected locally, botulinum toxin type A is used in the treatment of certain ophthalmological conditions associated with spasms of ocular muscles (e.g., strabismus and blepharospasm) (Chapter 64) and for a wide variety of unlabeled uses ranging from treatment of muscle dystonias and palsy (Chapter 11) to cosmetic erasure of facial lines and wrinkles (Chapter 65).

Adrenergic. α-Methyltyrosine (metyrosine) blocks the synthesis of NE by inhibiting TH, the enzyme that catalyzes the rate-limiting step in catecholamine synthesis. This drug occasionally may be useful in treating selected patients with pheochromocytoma. On the other hand, methyldopa, an inhibitor of aromatic *L*-amino acid decarboxylase, is—like dopa itself—successively decarboxylated and hydroxylated in its side chain to form the putative "false neurotransmitter" α-methylnorepinephrine. The use of methyldopa in the treatment of hypertension is discussed in Chapter 27. Bretylium, guanadrel, and guanethidine act by preventing the release of NE by the nerve impulse. However, such agents can transiently stimulate the release of NE because of their capacity to displace the amine from storage sites.

Promotion of Release of the Transmitter

Cholinergic. The ability of cholinergic agents to promote the release of ACh is limited presumably because ACh and other cholinomimetic agents are quaternary amines and do not readily cross the axonal membrane into the nerve ending. The latrotoxins from black widow spider venom and stonefish are known to promote neuroexocytosis by binding to receptors on the neuronal membrane.

Adrenergic. Several drugs that promote the release of the adrenergic mediator already have been discussed. On the basis of the rate and duration of the drug-induced release of norepinephrine from adrenergic terminals, one of two opposing effects can predominate. Thus tyramine, ephedrine, amphetamine, and related drugs cause a relatively rapid, brief liberation of the transmitter and produce a sympathomimetic effect. On the other hand, reserpine, by blocking the vesicular amine transporter (VAMT2) uptake of amines, produces a slow, prolonged depletion of the adrenergic transmitter from adrenergic storage vesicles, where it is largely metabolized by intraneuronal MAO. The resulting depletion of transmitter produces the equivalent of adrenergic blockade. Reserpine also causes the depletion of 5-HT, DA, and possibly other, unidentified amines from central and peripheral sites, and many of its major effects may be a consequence of the depletion of transmitters other than NE.

As discussed earlier, deficiencies of tyrosine hydroxylase in humans cause a neurologic disorder (Carson and Robertson, 2002) that can be treated by supplementation with the dopamine precursor levodopa.

A syndrome caused by congenital DβH deficiency has been described; this syndrome is characterized by the absence of NE and epinephrine, elevated concentrations of DA, intact baroreflex afferent fibers and cholinergic innervation, and undetectable concentrations of plasma DβH activity (Carson and Robertson, 2002). Patients have severe orthostatic hypotension, ptosis of the eyelids, and retrograde ejaculations. Dihydroxyphenylserine (L-DOPS) has been shown to improve postural hypotension in this rare disorder. This therapeutic approach cleverly takes advantage of the nonspecificity of aromatic *L*-amino acid decarboxylase, which synthesizes NE directly from this drug in the absence of DβH (Man in't Veld et al., 1988; Robertson et al., 1991). Despite the restoration of plasma NE in humans with L-DOPS, epinephrine levels are not restored, leading to speculations that PNMT may require DβH for appropriate functioning (Carson and Robertson, 2002).

Agonist and Antagonist Actions at Receptors

Cholinergic. The nicotinic receptors of autonomic ganglia and skeletal muscle are not identical; they respond differently to certain stimulating and blocking agents, and their pentameric structures contain different combinations of homologous subunits (Table 8–2). *Dimethylphenylpiperazinium* (DMPP) and phenyltrimethylammonium (PTMA) show some selectivity for stimulation of autonomic ganglion cells and end plates of skeletal muscle, respectively. Trimethaphan and hexamethonium are relatively selective competitive and noncompetitive ganglionic blocking agents. Although tubocurarine effectively blocks transmission at both motor end plates and autonomic ganglia, its action at the former site predominates. Succinylcholine, a depolarizing agent, produces selective neuromuscular blockade. Transmission at autonomic ganglia and the adrenal medulla is complicated further by the presence of muscarinic receptors in addition to the principal nicotinic receptors (see Chapter 11).

Various toxins in snake venoms exhibit a high degree of specificity toward cholinergic receptors. The α-neurotoxins from the Elapidae family interact with the agonist-binding site on the nicotinic receptor. α-Bungarotoxin is selective for the muscle receptor and interacts with only certain neuronal receptors, such as those containing α_7 through α_9 subunits. Neuronal bungarotoxin shows a wider range of inhibition of neuronal receptors. A second group of toxins, called the *fasciculins,* inhibits AChE. A third group of toxins, termed the *muscarinic toxins* (MT_1 through MT_4), includes partial agonists and antagonists for the muscarinic receptors. Venoms from the Viperidae family of snakes and the fish-hunting cone snails also have relatively selective toxins for nicotinic receptors.

Muscarinic ACh receptors, which mediate the effects of ACh at autonomic effector cells, now can be divided into five subclasses. Atropine blocks all the muscarinic responses to injected ACh and related cholinomimetic drugs whether they are excitatory, as in the intestine, or inhibitory, as in the heart. Newer muscarinic agonists, pirenzepine for M_1, tripitramine for M_2, and darifenacin for M_3, show selectivity as muscarinic blocking agents. Several muscarinic antagonists show sufficient selectivity in the clinical setting to minimize the bothersome side effects seen with the nonselective agents at therapeutic doses (see Chapter 9).

Adrenergic. A vast number of synthetic compounds that bear structural resemblance to the naturally occurring catecholamines can interact with α and β adrenergic receptors to produce sympathomimetic effects (see Chapter 12). Phenylephrine acts selectively at α_1 receptors, whereas clonidine is a selective α_2 adrenergic agonist. Isoproterenol exhibits agonist activity at both β_1 and β_2 receptors. Preferential stimulation of cardiac β_1 receptors follows the administration of dobutamine. Terbutaline is an example of a drug with relatively selective action on β_2 receptors; it produces effective bronchodilation with minimal effects on the heart. The main features of adrenergic blockade, including the selectivity of various blocking agents for α and β adrenergic receptors, are considered in detail in Chapter 12. Partial dissociation of effects at β_1 and β_2 receptors has been achieved by subtype-selective antagonists, as exemplified by the β_1 receptor antagonists metoprolol and atenolol, which antagonize the cardiac actions of catecholamines while causing somewhat less antagonism at bronchioles. Prazosin and yohimbine are representative of α_1 and α_2 receptor antagonists, respectively, although prazosin has a relatively high affinity at α_{2B} and α_{2C} subtypes compared with α_{2A} receptors. Several important drugs that promote the release of norepinephrine or deplete the transmitter resemble, in their effects, activators or blockers of postjunctional receptors (e.g., tyramine and reserpine, respectively).

Interference with the Destruction of the Transmitter

Cholinergic. The anti-ChE agents (see Chapter 10) constitute a chemically diverse group of compounds, the primary action of which is inhibition of AChE, with the consequent accumulation of endogenous ACh. At the neuromuscular junction, accumulation of ACh produces depolarization of end plates and flaccid paralysis. At postganglionic muscarinic effector sites, the response is either excessive stimulation resulting in contraction and secretion or an inhibitory response mediated by hyperpolarization. At ganglia, depolarization and enhanced transmission are observed.

Adrenergic. The reuptake of NE by the adrenergic nerve terminals by means of NET is the major mechanism for terminating its transmitter action. Interference with this process is the basis of the potentiating effect of cocaine on responses to adrenergic impulses and injected catecholamines. It also has been suggested that the antidepressant actions and some of the adverse effects of imipramine and related drugs are due to a similar action at adrenergic synapses in the CNS (Chapter 15).

Entacapone and tolcapone are nitro catechol-type COMT inhibitors. Entacapone is a peripherally acting COMT inhibitor, whereas tolcapone also inhibits COMT activity in the brain. COMT inhibition has been shown to attenuate levodopa toxicity on dopamine neurons and enhance dopamine action in the brain of patients with Parkinson disease (Chapter 22). On the other hand, nonselective MAO inhibitors, such as tranylcypromine, potentiate the effects of tyramine and may potentiate effects of neurotransmitters. While most MAO inhibitors used as antidepressants inhibit both MAO-A and MAO-B, selective MAO-A and MAO-B inhibitors are available. Selegiline is a selective and irreversible MAO-B inhibitor that also has been used as an adjunct in the treatment of Parkinson disease.

OTHER AUTONOMIC NEUROTRANSMITTERS

The vast majority of neurons in both the central and peripheral nervous systems contain more than one substance with potential or demonstrated activity at relevant postjunctional sites (see Chapter 14). In some cases, especially in peripheral structures, it has been possible to demonstrate that two or more such substances are contained within individual nerve terminals and are released simultaneously on nerve stimulation. Although the anatomic separation of the parasympathetic and sympathetic components of the autonomic nervous system and the actions of ACh and NE (their primary neurotransmitters) still provides the essential framework for studying autonomic function, a host of other chemical messengers such as purines, eicosanoids, NO, and peptides modulate or mediate responses that follow stimulation of the autonomic nervous system. An expanded view of autonomic neurotransmission has evolved to include instances where substances other than ACh or NE are released and may function as co-transmitters, neuromodulators, or even primary transmitters. For example, it appears that some postganglionic parasympathetic nerves utilize NO as a neurotransmitter (Toda and Okamura, 2003).

The evidence for co-transmission in the autonomic nervous system usually encompasses the following considerations:

- A portion of responses to stimulation of preganglionic or postganglionic nerves or to field stimulation of target structures persists in the presence of concentrations of muscarinic or adrenergic antagonists that completely block their respective agonists.
- The candidate substance can be detected within nerve fibers that course through target tissues.
- The substance can be recovered on microdialysis or in the venous or perfusion effluent following electrical stimulation; such release often can be blocked by tetrodotoxin.
- Effects of electrical stimulation are mimicked by the application of the substance and are inhibited in the presence of specific antagonists, neutralizing antibodies, or selective desensitization produced by prior exposure to the substance.

A more recent approach to this challenging problem is the use of knockout mice that do not express the putative co-transmitter.

A number of problems confound interpretation of such evidence. It is particularly difficult to establish that substances that fulfill all the listed criteria originate within the autonomic nervous system. In some instances, their origin can be traced to sensory fibers, to intrinsic neurons, or to nerves innervating blood vessels. Also, there may be marked synergism between the candidate substance and known or unknown transmitters. In knockout mice, compensatory mechanisms or transmitter redundancy may disguise even well-defined actions (Hökfelt et al., 2000). Finally, it should be recognized that the putative co-transmitter may have primarily a trophic function in maintaining synaptic connectivity or in expressing a particular receptor.

ATP and ACh coexist in cholinergic vesicles (Dowdall et al., 1974) and ATP, NPY, and catecholamine are found within storage granules in nerves and the adrenal medulla (*see* above). ATP is released along with the transmitters, and either it or its metabolites have a significant function in synaptic transmission in some circumstances (see below). Recently, attention has focused on the growing list of peptides that are found in the adrenal medulla, nerve fibers, or ganglia of the autonomic nervous system or in the structures that are innervated by the autonomic nervous system. This list includes the encephalin, substance P and other tachykinins, somatostatin, gonadotropin-releasing hormone, cholecystokinin, calcitonin gene–related peptide, galanin, pituitary adenylyl cyclase–activating peptide, VIP, chromogranins, and NPY (Hökfelt et al., 2000). Some of the orphan GPCRs discovered in the course of genome-sequencing projects may represent receptors for undiscovered peptides or other co-transmitters. The evidence for widespread transmitter function in the autonomic nervous system is substantial for VIP and NPY, and further discussion is confined to these peptides. The possibility that abnormalities in function of neuropeptide co-transmitters, in type 2 diabetes, e.g., contribute to disease pathogenesis remains of interest (Ahren, 2000).

Co-transmission in the Autonomic Nervous System. The evidence is substantial that ATP plays a role in sympathetic nerves as a co-transmitter with norepinephrine (Silinsky et al., 1998; Westfall et al., 1991, 2002). For example, the rodent vas deferens is supplied with a dense sympathetic innervation, and stimulation of the nerves results in a biphasic mechanical response that consists of an initial rapid twitch followed by a sustained contraction. The first phase of the response is mediated by ATP acting on postjunctional P2X receptors, whereas the second phase is mediated mainly by norepinephrine acting on α_1 receptors (Sneddon and Westfall, 1984). The co-transmitters apparently are released from the same types of nerves because pretreatment with 6-hydroxydopamine, an agent that specifically destroys adrenergic nerves, abolishes both phases of the neurogenically induced biphasic contraction. It has been assumed that the sympathetic nerves store ATP and NE in the same synaptic vesicles, and therefore, on release, the two co-transmitters are released together (Stjärne, 1989). This may not always be the case, and ATP and NE may be released from separate subsets of vesicles and subject to differential regulation (Todorov et al., 1996).

While part of the metabolism of ATP, once released into the neuroeffector junction, is by extracellularly directed membrane-bound nucleotidases to ADP, AMP, and adenosine (Gordon, 1986), the majority of the metabolism occurs by the action of releasable nucleotidases. There is also evidence that ATP and its metabolites exert presynaptic modulatory effects on transmitter release by P2 receptors and receptors for adenosine. In addition to evidence showing that ATP is a co-transmitter with norepinephrine, there is also evidence that ATP may be a co-transmitter with ACh in certain postganglionic parasympathetic nerves, such as in the urinary bladder.

The NPY family of peptides is distributed widely in the central and peripheral nervous systems and consists of three members: NPY, pancreatic polypeptide, and peptide YY. NPY has been shown to be colocalized and core-leased with NE and ATP in most sympathetic nerves in the peripheral nervous system, especially those innervating blood vessels (Westfall, 2004). There is also convincing evidence that NPY exerts prejunctional modulatory effects on transmitter release and synthesis. Moreover, there are numerous examples of postjunctional interactions that are consistent with a co-transmitter role for NPY at various sympathetic neuroeffector junctions. Thus, it seems that NPY, together with NE and ATP, is the third sympathetic co-transmitter. The functions of NPY include 1) direct postjunctional contractile effects; 2) potentiation of the contractile effects of the other sympathetic co-transmitters; and 3) inhibitory modulation of the nerve stimulation–induced release of all three sympathetic co-transmitters.

Studies with selective NPY-Y_1 antagonists provide evidence that the principal postjunctional receptor is of the Y_1 subtype, although other receptors are also present at some sites and may exert physiological actions. Studies with selective NPY-Y_2 antagonists suggest that the principal prejunctional receptor is of the Y_2 subtype both in the periphery and in the CNS. Again, there is evidence for a role for other NPY receptors, and clarification awaits the further development of selective antagonists. NPY also can act prejunctionally to inhibit the release of ACh, CGRP, and substance P. In the CNS, NPY exists as a co-transmitter with catecholamine in some neurons and with peptides and mediators in others. A prominent action of NPY is the presynaptic inhibition of the release of various neurotransmitters, including NE, DA, GABA, glutamate, and 5-HT, as well as inhibition or stimulation of various neurohormones such as gonadotropin-releasing hormone, vasopressin, and oxytocin. Evidence also exists for stimulation of NE and DA release. NPY also acts on autoreceptors to inhibit its own release. NPY may use several mechanisms to produce its presynaptic effects, including: inhibition of Ca^{2+} channels, activation of K^+ channels, and perhaps regulation of the vesicle release complex at some point distal to Ca^{2+} entry. NPY also may play a role in several pathophysiological conditions. The further development of selective NPY agonists and antagonists should enhance understanding about the physiological and pathophysiological roles of NPY.

The pioneering studies of Hökfelt and coworkers, which demonstrated the existence of VIP and ACh in peripheral autonomic neurons, initiated interest in the possibility of peptidergic co-transmission in the autonomic nervous system. Subsequent work has confirmed the frequent association of these two substances in autonomic fibers, including parasympathetic fibers that innervate smooth muscle and exocrine glands and cholinergic sympathetic neurons that innervate sweat glands (Hökfelt et al., 2000).

The role of VIP in parasympathetic transmission has been studied most extensively in the regulation of salivary secretion. The evidence for co-transmission includes the release of VIP following stimulation of the chorda lingual nerve and the incomplete blockade by atropine of vasodilation when the frequency of stimulation is raised; the latter observation may indicate independent release of the two substances, which is consistent with histochemical evidence for storage of ACh and VIP in separate populations of vesicles. Synergism between ACh and VIP in stimulating vasodilation and secretion also has been described. VIP may be involved in parasympathetic responses in the GI tract, where it may facilitate sphincter relaxation, and the trachea.

Nonadrenergic, Noncholinergic Transmission by Purines. The smooth muscle of many tissues that are innervated by the autonomic nervous system shows inhibitory junction potentials following stimulation by field electrodes. Since such responses frequently are undiminished in the presence of adrenergic and muscarinic cholinergic antagonists, these observations have been taken as evidence for the existence of nonadrenergic, noncholinergic (NANC) transmission in the autonomic nervous system.

Burnstock (1996) and colleagues have compiled compelling evidence for the existence of purinergic neurotransmission in the GI tract, genitourinary tract, and certain blood vessels; ATP has fulfilled all the criteria for a neurotransmitter listed earlier. However, in at least some circumstances, primary sensory axons may be an important source of ATP (Burnstock, 2000). Although adenosine is generated from the released ATP by ectoenzymes and releasable nucleotidases, its primary function appears to be modulatory by causing feedback inhibition of release of the transmitter.

Adenosine can be transported from the cell cytoplasm to activate extracellular receptors on adjacent cells. The efficient uptake of adenosine by cellular transporters and its rapid rate of metabolism to inosine or to adenine nucleotides contribute to its rapid turnover. Several inhibitors of adenosine transport and metabolism are known to influence extracellular adenosine and ATP concentrations (Sneddon et al., 1999).

The purinergic receptors found on the cell surface may be divided into the adenosine (P1) receptors and the receptors for ATP (P2X and P2Y receptors) (Fredholm et al., 2000). Both of the P1 and P2 receptors have various subtypes. Methylxanthines such as caffeine and theophylline preferentially block adenosine receptors (Chapter 36). There are four adenosine receptors (A_1, A_{2A}, A_{2B}, and A_3) and multiple sub-types of P2X and P2Y receptors throughout the body. The adenosine receptors and the P2Y receptors mediate their responses *via* G proteins, whereas the P2X receptors are a subfamily of ligand-gated ion channels (Burnstock, 2000).

Modulation of Vascular Responses by Endothelium-Derived Factors; NO and Eendothelin. Furchgott and colleagues demonstrated that an intact endothelium is necessary to achieve vascular relaxation in response to ACh (Furchgott, 1999). This inner cellular layer of the blood vessel now is known to modulate autonomic and hormonal effects on the contractility of blood vessels. In response to a variety of vasoactive agents and even physical stimuli, the endothelial cells release a short-lived vasodilator called endothelium-derived relaxing factor (EDRF), now known to be NO. Less commonly, an endothelium-derived hyperpolarizing factor (EDHF) and endothelium-derived contracting factor (EDCF) of as yet undefined compositions are released (Vanhoutte, 1996). EDCF formation depends on cyclooxygenase activity.

Products of inflammation and platelet aggregation (e.g., 5-HT, histamine, bradykinin, purines, and thrombin) exert all or part of their action by stimulating the production of NO. Endothelial cell–dependent mechanisms of relaxation are important in a variety of vascular beds, including the coronary circulation (Hobbs et al., 1999). Activation of specific GPCRs on endothelial cells promotes NO production. NO diffuses readily to the underlying smooth muscle and induces relaxation of vascular smooth muscle by activating the soluble form of guanylyl cyclase, which increases cyclic GMP concentrations. Nitrovasodilating drugs used to lower blood pressure or to treat ischemic heart disease probably act through conversion to or release of NO (Chapters 3 and 27). NO also has been shown to be released from certain nerves (*nitrergic*) innervating blood vessels and smooth muscles of the GI tract. NO has a negative inotropic action on the heart.

Alterations in the release or action of NO may affect a number of major clinical situations such as atherosclerosis (Hobbs et al., 1999; Ignarro et al., 1999). Furthermore, there is evidence suggesting that the hypotension of endotoxemia or that induced by cytokines is mediated by induction of enhanced production and release of NO; consequently, increased NO production may have pathological significance in septic shock.

Full contractile responses of cerebral arteries also require an intact endothelium. A family of peptides, termed *endothelins,* is stored in vascular endothelial cells. Their release onto smooth muscle promotes contraction by stimulation of endothelin receptors. Endothelins contribute to the maintenance of vascular homostasis by acting *via* multiple endothelin receptors (Sokolovsky, 1995) to reverse the response to NO (Rubanyi and Polokoff, 1994). In isolated cell systems, several G-protein-linked responses to endothelins are quasi-irreversible (Hilal-Dandan et al., 1997).

BIBLIOGRAPHY

Aantaa R, Marjamaki A, Scheinin M. Molecular pharmacology of α_2-adrenoceptor subtypes. *Ann Med,* **1995,** *27*:439–449.

Abell CW, Kwan SW. Molecular characterization of monoamine oxidases A and B. *Prog Nucleic Acid Res Mol Biol,* **2001,** *65*:129–156.

Ahren B. Autonomic regulation of islet hormone secretion: Implications for health and disease. *Diabetologia,* **2000,** *43*:393–410.

Albuquerque EX, Pereira EFR, Alkondon M, Rogers SW. Mammalian nicotinic acetylcholine receptors: From structure to function. *Physiol Rev,* **2009,** *89*:73–120.

Altschuler SM, Bao XM, Bieger D, et al. Viscerotopic representation of the upper alimentary tract in the rat: Sensory ganglia and nuclei of the solitary and spinal trigeminal tracts. *J Comp Neurol,* **1989,** *283*:248–268.

Andresen MC, Kunze DL. Nucleus tractus solitarius: Gateway to neural circulatory control. *Annu Rev Physiol,* **1994,** *56*:93–116.

Arner P, Hoffstedt J. Adrenoceptor genes in human obesity. *J Intern Med,* **1999,** *245*:667–672.

Aunis D. Exocytosis in chromaffin cells of the adrenal medulla. *Int Rev Cytol,* **1998,** *181*:213–320.

Baillie G, Houslay M. Arrestin times for compartmentalized cAMP signalling and phosphodiesterase-4 enzymes. *Curr Opin Cell Biol,* **2005,** *17*:129–134.

Boehm S, Kubista H. Fine tuning of sympathetic transmitter release via ionotropic and metabotropic presynaptic receptors. *Pharmacol Rev,* **2002,** *54*:43–99.

Bonner TI. The molecular basis of muscarinic receptor diversity. *Trends Neurosci,* **1989,** *12*:148–151.

Bowman WC, Prior C, Marshall IG. Presynaptic receptors in the neuromuscular junction. *Ann NY Acad Sci,* **1990,** *604*: 69–81.

Brodde OE. β_1 and β_2 adrenoceptor polymorphisms: Functional importance, impact on cardiovascular disease and drug responses. *Pharmacol Ther,* **2008,** *117*:1–29.

Brodde OE, Bruck H, Leineweber K. Cardiac adrenoceptors: physiological and pathophysiological relevance. *J Pharmacol Sci,* **2006,** *100*:323–337.

Burnstock G. Purinergic neurotransmission. *Semin Neurosci,* **1996,** *8*:171–257.

Burnstock G. P_{2X} receptors in sensory neurons. *Br J Anaesth,* **2000,** *84*:476–488.

Bylund DB. Subtypes of α_1- and α_2-adrenergic receptors. *FASEB J,* **1992,** *6*:832–839.

Carson RP, Robertson D. Genetic manipulation of noradrenergic neurons. *J Pharmacol Exp Ther,* **2002,** *301*:407–410.

Catterall WA. From ionic currents to molecular mechanisms: The structure and function of voltage-gated sodium channels. *Neuron,* **2000,** *26*:13–25.

Caulfield MP, Birdsall NJ. International Union of Pharmacology: XVII. Classification of muscarinic acetylcholine receptors. *Pharmacol Rev,* **1998,** *50*:279–290.

Changeux JP, Edelstein SJ. Allosteric receptors after 30 years. *Neuron,* **1998,** *21*:959–980.

Chaudhry FA, Edwards RH, Fonnum F. Vesicular neurotransmitter transporters as targets for endogenous and exogenous toxic substances. *Annu Rev Pharmacol Toxicol,* **2008,** *48*: 277–301.

Chen H, Ordög T, Chen J, et al. Differential gene expression in functional classes of interstitial cells of Cajal in murine small intestine. *Physiol Genomics,* **2007,** *31*:492–509.

Chong BS, Mersfelder TL. Entacapone. *Ann Pharmacother,* **2000,** *34*:1056–1065.

Cooke HJ. "Enteric tears": Chloride secretion and its neural regulation. *News Physiol Sci,* **1998,** *13*:269–274.

Costa M, Brookes SJ, Hennig GW. Anatomy and physiology of the enteric nervous system. *Gut,* **2000,** *47*:15–19.

Costa M, Brookes SJ, Steele PA, *et al.* Neurochemical classification of myenteric neurons in the guinea-pig ileum. *Neuroscience,* **1996,** *75*:949–967.

DeFea K. β-arrestins and heterotrimeric G proteins: Collaborators and competitors in signal transduction. *Br J Pharmacol,* **2008,** *153*:5298–5309.

Della Rocca GJ, van Biesen T, Daaka Y, *et al.* Ras-dependent mitogen-activated protein kinase activation by G protein–coupled receptors: Convergence of G_i- and G_q-mediated pathways on calcium/ calmodulin, Pyk2, and Src kinase. *J Biol Chem,* **1997,** *272*:19125–19132.

DeWire SM, Ahn S, Lefkowitz RT, Shenoy SK. β arrestins and cell signaling. *Annu Rev Physiol,* **2007**, *69*:483–510.

Dhein S, van Koppen CJ, Brodde OE. Muscarinic receptors in the mammalian heart. *Pharmacol Res,* **2001,** *44*: 161–182.

Dooley TP. Cloning of the human phenol sulfotransferase gene family: Three genes implicated in the metabolism of catecholamine, thyroid hormones and drugs. *Chem Biol Interact,* **1998,** *109*:29–41.

Dorn GW, Brown JH. G_q signaling in cardiac adaptation and maladaptation. *Trends Cardiovasc Med,* **1999,** *9*:26–34.

Dowdall MJ, Boyne AF, Whittaker VP. Adenosine triphosphate, a constituent of cholinergic synaptic vesicles. *Biochem J,* **1974,** *140*:1–12.

Drake MT, Shenoy SK, Lefkowitz RJ. Trafficking of G-proteins coupled receptors. *Circ Res,* **2006,** *99*:570–582.

Eglen RM. Muscarinic receptor subtype. *Pharmacol Physiol Prog Med Chem,* **2005,** *43*:105–136.

Eiden LE. The cholinergic gene locus. *J Neurochem,* **1998,** *70*:2227–2240.

Eisenhofer G. The role of neuronal and extraneuronal plasma membrane transporters in the inactivation of peripheral catecholamine. *Pharmacol Ther,* **2001,** *91*:35–62.

Eisenhofer G, Kopin IJ, Goldstein DS. Catecholamine metabolism: A contemporary view with implications for physiology and medicine. *Pharmacol Rev,* **2004,** *56*:331–349.

Emorine LJ, Marullo S, Briend-Sutren MM, *et al.* Molecular characterization of the human β_3-adrenergic receptor. *Science,* **1989,** *245*:1118–1121.

Exley R, Cragg SJ. Presynaptic nicotinic receptors: A dynamic and diverse cholinergic filter of striatal dopamine neurotransmission. *Br J Pharmacol,* **2008,** *153*:5283–5297.

Ferguson S, Blakely R. The choline transporter resurfaces: New roles for synaptic vesicles? *Mol Interv,* **2004,** *4*:22–37.

Fetscher C, Fleichman M, Schmidt M, et al. M_3 muscarinic receptors mediate contraction of human urinary bladder. *Br J Pharmacol,* **2002,** *136*:641–643.

Fredholm BB, Ijzerman AP, Jacobson KA, Linden J. Adenosine receptors. In, *The IUPHAR Compendium of Receptor Characterization and Classification.* **2000,** pp. 78–87.

Furchgott RF. Endothelium-derived relaxing factor: Discovery, early studies, and identification as nitric oxide. *Biosci Rep,* **1999,** *19*:235–251.

Gordon JL. Extracellular ATP: Effects, sources and fate. *Biochem J,* **1986,** *233*:309–319.

Gutkind JS. The pathways connecting G protein–coupled receptors to the nucleus through divergent mitogen-activated protein kinase cascades. *J Biol Chem,* **1998,** *273*: 1839–1842.

Hanyaloglu A, von Zastrow M. Regulation of GPCRs by endocytic membrane trafficking and its potential implications. *Annu Rev Pharmacol Toxicol,* **2008,** *48*:537–568.

Hein L, Schmitt JP. α_1-Adrenoceptors in the heart: Friend or foe? *J Mol Cell Cardiol,* **2003,** *35*:1183–1185.

Hieble J P. Subclassification and nomenclature of α- and β-adrenoceptors. *Curr Top Med Chem,* **2007,** *7*:129–134.

Hilal-Dandan R, Villegas S, Gonzalez A, Brunton L. The quasi-irreversible nature of endothelin binding and G protein-linked signaling in cardiac myocytes. *J Pharmacol Exp Ther*, **1997,** *281*:267–273.

Hille B. *Ionic Channels of Excitable Membranes,* 2d ed. Sinauer Associates, Sunderland, MA, **1992.**

Hobbs AJ, Higgs A, Moncada S. Inhibition of nitric oxide synthase as a potential therapeutic target. *Annu Rev Pharmacol Toxicol,* **1999,** *39*:191–220.

Hökfelt T, Broberger C, Xu ZQ, et al. Neuropeptides: An overview. *Neuropharmacology,* **2000,** *39*:1337–1356.

Hutchins C. Three-dimensional models of the D_1 and D_2 dopamine receptors. *Endocr J,* **1994,** *2*:7–23.

Ignarro LJ, Cirino G, Casini A, Napoli C. Nitric oxide as a signaling molecule in the vascular system: An overview. *J Cardiovasc Pharmacol,* **1999,** *34*:879–886.

Jahn R, Lang T, Südhof T. Membrane fusion. *Cell,* **2003,** *112*:519–533.

Kable JW, Murrin LC, Bylund DB. In Vivo Gene Modification Elucidates Subtype-Specific Functions of α_2-Adrenergic Receptors. *J Pharmacol Exp Ther,* **2000,** *293*:1–7.

Kalamida D, Poulas K, Avramopoulou V, et al. Muscle and neuronal nicotinic acetylcholine receptors structure function and pathogenicity. *FEBS J,* **2007,** *274*:3799–3845.

Karlin A, Akabas MH. Toward a structural basis for the function of nicotinic acetylcholine receptors and their cousins. *Neuron,* **1995,** *15*:1231–1244.

Kennedy B, Elayan H, Ziegler MG. Glucocorticoid elevation of mRNA encoding epinephrine-forming enzyme in lung. *Am J Physiol,* **1993,** *265*:L117–L120.

Kohout TA, Lefkowitz RJ. Regulation of G protein–coupled receptor kinases and arrestins during receptor desensitization. *Mol Pharmacol,* **2003,** *63*:9–18.

Kubista H, Boehm S. Molecular mechanisms underlying the modulation of exocytoxic noradrenaline release via presynaptic receptors. *Pharmacol Ther,* **2006,** *112*:213–242.

Kumer SC, Vrana KE. Intricate regulation of tyrosine hydroxylase activity and gene expression. *J Neurochem,* **1996,** *67*: 443–462.

Kunze WAA, Furness JB. The enteric nervous system and regulation of intestinal motility. *Annu Rev Physiol,* **1999,** *61*:117–142.

Lakhlani PP, MacMillan LB, Guo TZ, *et al.* Substitution of a mutant α_{2A}-adrenergic receptor via "hit and run" gene targeting reveals the role of this subtype in sedative, analgesic, and anesthetic-sparing responses in vivo. *Proc Natl Acad Sci USA,* **1997,** *94*:9950–9955.

Langmead CJ, Watson J, Reavill C. Muscarinic acetylcholine receptors as CNS drug targets. *Pharmacol Ther,* **2008,** *117*:232–243.

Lefkowitz RJ. G protein–coupled receptors: III. New roles for receptor kinases and β-arrestins in receptor signaling and desensitization. *J Biol Chem,* **1998,** *273*:18677–18680.

Lefkowitz RJ. The superfamily of heptahelical receptors. *Nature Cell Biol,* **2000,** *2*:E133–E136.

Lugardon K, Raffner R, Goumon Y, et al. Antibacterial and antifungal activities of vasostatin-1, the N-terminal fragment of chromogranin A. *J Biol Chem,* **2000,** *275*:10745–10753.

Lynch GS, Ryall JG. Role of β-adrenoceptor signaling in skeletal muscle: Implications for muscle wasting and disease. *Physiol Rev,* **2008,** *88*:729-767.

Ma YC, Huang XY. Novel signaling pathways through the β-adrenergic receptors. *Trends Cardiovasc Med,* **2002,** *12*: 46–49.

MacDermott AB, Role LW, Siegelbaum SA. Presynaptic ionotropic receptors and the control of transmitter release. *Annu Rev Neurosci,* **1999,** *22*:443–485.

Man in't Veld A, Boomsma F, Lenders J, et al. Patients with congenital dopamine β-hydroxylase deficiency: A lesson in catecholamine physiology. *Am J Hypertens,* **1988,** *1*: 231–238.

Männistö PT, Kaakkola S. Catechol-*O*-methyltransferase (COMT): Biochemistry, molecular biology, pharmacology, and clinical efficacy of the new selective COMT inhibitors. *Pharmacol Rev,* **1999,** *51*:593–628.

Masson J, Sagne C, Hamon M, Mestikawy SE. Neurotransmitter transporters in the central nervous system. *Pharmacol Rev,* **1999,** *51*:439–464.

McDonald TF, Pelzer S, Trautwein W, Pelzer DJ. Regulation and modulation of calcium channels in cardiac, skeletal, and smooth muscle cells. *Physiol Rev,* **1994,** *74*:365–507.

Meir A, Ginsburg S, Butkevich A, et al. Ion channels in presynaptic nerve terminals and control of transmitter release. *Physiol Rev,* **1999,** *79*:1019–1088.

Michelotti GA, Price DT, Schwinn DA. α_1-Adrenergic receptor regulation: Basic science and clinical implications. *Pharmacol Ther,* **2000,** *88*:281–309.

Miller RJ. Presynaptic receptors. *Annu Rev Pharmacol Toxicol,* **1998,** *38*:201–227.

Moncada S, Higgs A, Furchgott R. International Union of Pharmacology nomenclature in nitric oxide research. *Pharmacol Rev,* **1997,** *49*:137–142.

Murthy VN, Stevens CF. Synaptic vesicles retain their identity through the endocytic cycle. *Nature,* **1998,** *392*:497–501.

Mutafova-Yambolieva VN, Hwang SF, Hao X, et al. β-nicotinamide adenine dinucleotide is an inhibitory neurotransmitter in visceral smooth muscle. *Proc Natl Acad Sci USA,* **2007**.

Nagatsu T. Genes for human catecholamine-synthesizing enzymes. *Neurosci Res,* **1991,** *12*:315–345.

Nathanson NM. Synthesis, trafficking and localization of muscarinic acetylcholine receptors. *Pharmacol Ther,* **2008,** *119*:33–43.

Numa S, Noda M, Takahashi H, et al. Molecular structure of the nicotinic acetylcholine receptor. *Cold Spring Harbor Symp Quant Biol,* **1983,** *48*:57–69.

Palczewski K, Kumasaka T, Hori T, *et al.* Crystal structure of rhodopsin: A G protein–coupled receptor. *Science,* **2000,** *289*:739–745.

Park PS-H, Lodowski DT, Palczewski K. Activation of G-protein-coupled receptors: Beyond two state models and tertiary conformational changes. *Annu Rev Pharmacol Toxicol* **2008,** *48*:107–141.

Philipp M, Hein L. Adrenergic receptor knockout mice: Distinct functions of 9 receptor subtypes. *Pharmacol Ther,* **2004,** *101*:65–74.

Richman JG, Regan JW. α_2-Adrenergic receptors increase cell migration and decrease F-actin labeling in rat aortic smooth muscle cells. *Am J Physiol,* **1998,** *274*:C654–C662.

Robertson D, Haile V, Perry SE, *et al.* Dopamine β-hydroxylase deficiency: A genetic disorder of cardiovascular regulation. *Hypertension,* **1991,** *18*:1–8.

Robidoux J, Martin TL, Collins S. β-Adrenergic receptors and regulation of energy expenditure: A family affair. *Annu Rev Pharmacol Toxicol,* **2004,** *44*:297–323.

Rubanyi GM, Polokoff MA. Endothelins: Molecular biology, biochemistry, pharmacology, physiology, and pathophysiology. *Pharmacol Rev,* **1994,** *46*:325–415.

Sanes JR, Lichtman JW. Development of the vertebrate neuromuscular junction. *Annu Rev Neurosci,* **1999,** *22*:389–442.

Saper CB. Pain as a visceral sensation. *Prog Brain Res,* **2000,** *122*:237–243.

Saper CB. The central autonomic nervous system: Conscious visceral perception and autonomic pattern generation. *Annu Rev Neurosci,* **2002,** *25*:433–469.

Schuldiner S. A molecular glimpse of vesicular monoamine transporters. *J Neurochem,* **1994,** *62*:2067–2078.

Silinsky EM, von Kügelgen I, Smith A, Westfall DP. Functions of extracellular nucleotides in peripheral and central neuronal tissues. In, *The P_2 Nucleotide Receptors.* (Turner JT, Weisman GA, Fedan JS, eds.) Humana Press, Totowa, NJ, **1998,** pp. 259–290.

Silman I, Sussman JL. Acetylcholinesterase: "classical and non-classical" functions and pharmacology. *Curr Opin Pharmacol,* **2005**, *5*:293–302.

Sneddon P, Westfall DP. Pharmacological evidence that adenosine trisphosphate and noradrenaline are co-transmitters in the guinea-pig vas deferens. *J Physiol,* **1984,** *347*:561–580.

Sneddon P, Westfall TD, Todorov LD, *et al.* Modulation of purinergic neurotransmission. *Prog Brain Res,* **1999,** *120*:11–20.

Sokolovsky M. Endothelin receptor subtypes and their role in transmembrane signaling mechanisms. *Pharmacol Ther,* **1995,** *68*:435–471.

Strader CD, Fong TM, Tota MR, *et al.* Structure and function of G protein–coupled receptors. *Annu Rev Biochem,* **1994,** *63*:101–132.

Südhof TC. The synaptic vesicle cycle. *Annu Rev Neurosci,* **2004,** *27*:509–547.

Tan CM, Limbird LE. The α_2-adrenergic receptors: Lessons from knockouts. Clifton, NJ *Humana*, **2005**, pp. 241–266.

Tanoue A, Koshimizu TA, Tsujimoto G. Transgenic studies of α_1-adrenergic receptor subtype function. *Life Sci,* **2002a,** *71*:2207–2215.

Tanoue A, Nasa Y, Koshimizu T, *et al.* The α_{1D}-adrenergic receptor directly regulates arterial blood pressure via vasoconstriction. *J Clin Invest,* **2002b,** *109*:765–775.

Taupenot L, Harper KL, O'Connor DT. The chromogranin–secretogranin family. *N Engl J Med,* **2003,** *348*:1134–1149.

Taylor P, Luo ZD, Camp S. The genes encoding the cholinesterases: Structure, evolutionary relationships and regulation of their expression. In, *Cholinesterase and Cholinesterase Inhibitors.* (Giacobini E, ed.) London, Martin Dunitz, **2000,** pp. 63–80.

Toda N, Okamura J. The pharmacology of nitric oxide in the peripheral nervous system of blood vessels. *Pharmacol Rev,* **2003,** *55*:271–324.

Todorov LD, Mihaylova-Todorova S, Craviso GL, *et al.* Evidence for the differential release of the cotransmitters ATP and noradrenaline from sympathetic nerves of the guinea-pig vas deferens. *J Physiol,* **1996,** *496*:731–748.

Tsien RW, Lipscombe D, Madison DV, *et al.* Multiple types of neuronal calcium channels and their selective modulation. *Trends Neurosci,* **1988,** *11*:431–438.

Vanhoutte PM. Endothelium-dependent responses in congestive heart failure. *J Mol Cell Cardiol,* **1996,** *28*:2233–2240.

van Koppen CJ, Kaiser B. Regulation of muscarinic acetylcholine signaling. *Pharmacol Ther,* **2003,** *98*:197–220.

Varoqui H, Erickson JD. Vesicular neurotransmitter transporters: Potential sites for the regulation of synaptic function. *Mol Neurobiol,* **1997,** *15*:165–191.

Violin JD, Lefkowitz RJ, β-arrestin-biased ligands at seven-transmembrane receptors. *Trends Pharmacol Sci*, **2007**, *28*:416–422.

Viskupic E, Kvetnansky R, Sabban EL, *et al.* Increase in rat adrenal phenylethanolamine *N*-methyltransferase mRNA level caused by immobilization stress depends on intact pituitary-adrenocortical axis. *J Neurochem,* **1994,** *63*: 808–814.

Volz HP, Gleiter CH. Monoamine oxidase inhibitors: A perspective on their use in the elderly. *Drugs Aging,* **1998,** *13*:341–355.

von Euler. U.S. Synthesis, uptake and storage of catecholamine in adrenergic nerves: The effects of drugs. In, *Catecholamine: Handbuch der Experimentellen Pharmakologie,* vol. 33. (Blaschko H, Muscholl E, eds.) Springer-Verlag, Berlin, **1972,** pp. 186–230.

Walden PD, Durkin MM, Lepor H, *et al.* Localization of mRNA and receptor binding sites for the α_{1A}-adrenoceptor subtype in the rat, monkey and human urinary bladder and prostate. *J Urol,* **1997,** *157*:1032–1038.

Wang Z, Shi H, Wang H. Functional M_3 muscarinic acetylcholine receptors in mammalian hearts. *Br J Pharmacol,* **2004,** *142*:395–408.

Ward SE, Beckett EAH, Wang XY, et al. Interstitial cells of cajal mediate cholinergic neurotransmission from enteric motor neurons *J Neurosci*, **2000**, *20*:1393–1403.

Wess J. Muscarinic acetylcholine receptor knockout mice: Novel phenotypes and clinical implication. *Annu Rev Pharmacol Toxicol,* **2004,** *44*:423–450.

Wess J, Eglen RM, Gantam D. Muscarinic acetylcholine receptors: mutant mice provide new insights for drug development. *Nature Rev/Drug Discov*, **2007,** *6*:721–733.

Wessler I, Kirkpatrick CJ. Acetylcholine beyond neurons: the non-neuronal cholinergic system in humans. *Br J Pharmacol* **2008,** *154*:1558–1571.

Westfall DP, Dalziel HH, Forsyth KM. ATP as neurotransmitter, cotransmitter and neuromodulator. In, *Adenosine and Adenine*

Nucleotides as Regulators of Cellular Function. (Phillis T, ed.) CRC Press, Boca Raton, FL, **1991,** pp. 295–305.

Westfall DP, Todorov LD, Mihaylova-Todorova ST. ATP as a cotransmitter in sympathetic nerves and its inactivation by releasable enzymes. *J Pharmacol Exp Ther,* **2002,** *303*: 439–444.

Westfall TC. Local regulation of adrenergic neurotransmission. *Physiol Rev,* **1977,** *57*:659–728.

Westfall TC. Prejunctional effects of neuropeptide Y and its role as a cotransmitter. *Exp Pharmacol,* **2004,** *162*:138–183.

Wevers RA, de Rijk-van Andel JF, Brautigam C, *et al.* A review of biochemical and molecular genetic aspects of tyrosine hydroxylase deficiency including a novel mutation (291delC). *J Inherit Metab Dis,* **1999,** *22*:364–373.

Weyer C, Gautier JF, Danforth E. Development of β_3-adrenoceptor agonists for the treatment of obesity and diabetes: An update. *Diabetes Metab,* **1999,** *25*:11–21.

Woo AY-H, Wang T-B, Zeng X, et al. Stereochemistry of an agonist determines coupling preference of β_2-adrenoceptor to different G proteins in cardiomyocytes. *Mol Pharmacol,* **2000,** *75*:158–165.

Wouters J. Structural aspects of monoamine oxidase and its reversible inhibition. *Curr Med Chem,* **1998,** *5*:137–162.

Wu D, Hersh LB. Choline acetyltransferase: Celebrating its fiftieth year. *J Neurochem,* **1994,** *62*:1653–1663.

Xiao RP, Zhu W, Zheng M, *et al.* Sutype-specific α_1- and β-adrenoceptor signaling in the heart. *Trends Pharm Sci,* **2006,** *27*:330–337.

Zhong H, Minneman KP. α_1-Adrenoceptor subtypes. *Eur J Pharmacol,* **1999,** *375*:261–276.

Zigmond RE, Schwarzschild MA, Rittenhouse AR. Acute regulation of tyrosine hydroxylase by nerve activity and by neurotransmitters via phosphorylation. *Annu Rev Neurosci,* **1989,** *12*:415–461.

Muscarinic Receptor Agonists and Antagonists

Joan Heller Brown and
Nora Laiken

ACETYLCHOLINE AND ITS MUSCARINIC RECEPTOR TARGET

Muscarinic acetylcholine receptors in the peripheral nervous system occur primarily on autonomic effector cells innervated by postganglionic parasympathetic nerves. Muscarinic receptors are also present in autonomic ganglia and on some cells (e.g., vascular endothelial cells) that, paradoxically, receive little or no cholinergic innervation. Within the central nervous system (CNS), the hippocampus, cortex, and thalamus have high densities of muscarinic receptors.

Acetylcholine (ACh), the naturally occurring neurotransmitter for these receptors, has virtually no systemic therapeutic applications because its actions are diffuse, and its hydrolysis, catalyzed by both acetylcholinesterase (AChE) and plasma butyrylcholinesterase, is rapid. Muscarinic agonists mimic the effects of ACh at these sites. These agonists typically are longer-acting congeners of ACh or natural alkaloids, some of which stimulate nicotinic as well as muscarinic receptors.

The mechanisms of action of endogenous ACh at the postjunctional membranes of the effector cells and neurons that represent different types of cholinergic synapses are discussed in Chapter 8. To recapitulate, these synapses are found at: 1) autonomic effector sites innervated by postganglionic parasympathetic nerves (or, in the sweat glands, by postganglionic sympathetic nerves); 2) sympathetic and parasympathetic ganglia and the adrenal medulla, innervated by preganglionic autonomic nerves; 3) motor end plates on skeletal muscle, innervated by somatic motor nerves; and 4) certain synapses in the CNS (Krnjevic, 2004), where ACh can have either pre- or postsynaptic actions. When ACh is administered systemically, it can potentially act at all of these sites; however, as a quaternary ammonium compound, its penetration to the CNS is limited, and the amount of ACh that reaches peripheral areas with low blood flow is limited due to hydrolysis by plasma butyrylcholinesterase.

The actions of ACh and related drugs at autonomic effector sites are referred to as *muscarinic*, based on the observation that the alkaloid muscarine acts selectively at those sites and produces the same qualitative effects as ACh. The muscarinic, or parasympathomimetic, actions of the drugs considered in this chapter are practically equivalent to the parasympathetic effects of ACh listed in Table 8–1. Muscarinic receptors are present in autonomic ganglia and the adrenal medulla but primarily function to modulate the nicotinic actions of ACh at these sites (Chapter 11). In the CNS, muscarinic receptors are widely distributed and have a role in mediating many important responses. The differences between the actions of ACh and other muscarinic agonists are largely quantitative, with limited selectivity for one organ system or another. All of the actions of ACh and its congeners at muscarinic receptors can be blocked by atropine.

Properties and Subtypes of Muscarinic Receptors

Muscarinic receptors were characterized initially by analysis of the responses of cells and organ systems in the periphery and the CNS. For example, differential effects of two muscarinic agonists, bethanechol and McN-A-343, on the tone of the lower esophageal sphincter led to the initial designation of muscarinic receptors as M_1 (ganglionic) and M_2 (effector cell) (Goyal and Rattan, 1978). The cloning of the cDNAs that encode muscarinic receptors identified five distinct gene products (Bonner et al., 1987), now designated as

M_1 through M_5 muscarinic receptors (Chapter 8). All of the known muscarinic receptors are G protein-coupled receptors that in turn couple to various cellular effectors (Chapter 3). Although selectivity is not absolute, stimulation of M_1, M_3, and M_5 receptors causes hydrolysis of polyphosphoinositides and mobilization of intracellular Ca^{2+} as a consequence of activation of the G_q-PLC pathway (Chapter 8), resulting in a variety of Ca^{2+}-mediated responses. In contrast, M_2 and M_4 muscarinic receptors inhibit adenylyl cyclase and regulate specific ion channels via their coupling to the pertussis toxin–sensitive G proteins, G_i and G_o (Chapter 3).

The binding site for the endogenous agonist ACh, the *orthosteric site* (Neubig et al., 2003), is highly conserved among muscarinic receptor subtypes (Hulme et al., 2003). By analogy with the position of retinal in the orthosteric site of the mammalian rhodopsin receptor structure (Palczewski et al., 2000), the ACh orthosteric binding site is putatively located toward the extracellular regions of a cleft formed by several of the receptor's seven transmembrane helices. An aspartic acid present in the *N*-terminal portion of the third transmembrane helix of all five muscarinic receptor subtypes is believed to form an ionic bond with the cationic quaternary nitrogen in ACh and the tertiary or quaternary nitrogen of antagonists (Caulfield and Birdsall, 1998; Wess, 1996).

The five muscarinic receptor subtypes are widely distributed in both the CNS and peripheral tissues; most cells express at least two subtypes (Abrams et al., 2006; Wess, 1996; Wess et al., 2007). Identifying the role of a specific subtype in mediating a particular muscarinic response to ACh has been difficult due to the lack of subtype-specific agonists and antagonists. More recently, gene-targeting techniques have been used to elucidate the functions of each subtype (Wess et al., 2007). These techniques have allowed the creation of mutant mice with null alleles for the genes of each of the muscarinic receptor subtypes (Gomeza et al., 1999; Hamilton et al., 1997; Matsui et al., 2000; Wess, 2004; Yamada et al., 2001a, 2001b). All of these muscarinic receptor knockout mice are viable and fertile. The minimal phenotypic alteration that accompanies deletion of a single receptor subtype suggests functional redundancy between receptor subtypes in various tissues. For example, abolition of cholinergic bronchoconstriction, salivation, pupillary constriction, and bladder contraction generally requires deletion of more than a single receptor subtype. Such knockout mice studies have resulted in an increased understanding of the physiological roles of the individual muscarinic receptor subtypes (Wess et al., 2007; Table 8–3); many of the findings are consistent with the results obtained from examining the localization of muscarinic receptor subtypes in human tissues (Abrams et al., 2006). Although there is functional redundancy, the M_2 receptor is the predominant subtype in the cholinergic control of the heart, while the M_3 receptor is the predominant subtype in the cholinergic control of smooth muscle, secretory glands, and the eye. The M_1 receptor has an important role in the modulation of nicotinic cholinergic transmission in ganglia.

Although antagonists that can discriminate between various muscarinic receptor subtypes have been identified, the development of selective agonists and antagonists has generally been difficult because of the high conservation of the orthosteric site across subtypes (Conn et al., 2009b). Muscarinic receptors seem to possess topographically distinct *allosteric binding sites*, with at least one being located in the extracellular loops and outermost segments of different transmembrane helices; these sites are less conserved across receptor subtypes than the orthosteric binding site and thus offer the potential for greater subtype-selective targeting (Birdsall and Lazareno, 2005; May et al., 2007). Ligands that bind to allosteric sites are called allosteric modulators, because they can change the conformation of the receptor to modulate the affinity or efficacy of the orthosteric ligand. Progress has been made in developing selective positive allosteric modulators (PAMs) as important candidates for drugs with muscarinic receptor subtype selectivity, especially in the CNS (Conn et al., 2009a, 2009b). Selective negative allosteric modulators (NAMs), which act at an allosteric site to reduce the responsiveness of specific muscarinic receptor subtype(s) to ACh, also may become important therapeutic agents in the future. In both instances, the modulators do not activate the receptor by themselves, but can potentiate (in the case of PAMs) or inhibit (in the case of NAMs) receptor activation by ACh at specific muscarinic receptor subtype(s). Allosteric agonists have also been identified that appear to mediate receptor activation through a distinct allosteric site even in the absence of an orthosteric agonist (Nawaratne et al., 2008). Another potential mechanism for achieving selectivity is though the development of hybrid, bitopic orthosteric/allosteric ligands, which interact with both the orthosteric site and an allosteric site, a mechanism recently demonstrated to explain the unique effects of the M_1 selective agonist McN-A-343 (Valant et al., 2008).

Pharmacological Effects of Acetylcholine

The influence of ACh and parasympathetic innervation on various organs and tissues was introduced in Chapter 8; a more detailed description of the effects of ACh is presented here as background for understanding the physiological basis for the therapeutic uses of the muscarinic receptor agonists and antagonists.

Cardiovascular System. ACh has four primary effects on the cardiovascular system:

- vasodilation
- decrease in heart rate (negative chronotropic effect)
- decrease in the conduction velocity in the atrioventricular (AV) node (negative dromotropic effect)
- decrease in the force of cardiac contraction (negative inotropic effect)

The last effect is of lesser significance in the ventricles than in the atria. Some of the above responses can be obscured by baroreceptor and other reflexes that dampen the direct responses to ACh.

Although ACh rarely is given systemically, its cardiac actions are important because the cardiac effects of cardiac glycosides, anti-arrhythmic agents, and many other drugs are at least partly due to changes in parasympathetic (vagal) stimulation of the heart; in addition, afferent stimulation of the viscera during surgical interventions can reflexly increase the vagal stimulation of the heart.

The intravenous injection of a small dose of ACh produces a transient fall in blood pressure owing to generalized vasodilation (mediated by vascular endothelial NO), which is usually accompanied by reflex tachycardia. A considerably larger dose is required to see direct effects of ACh on the heart, such as eliciting bradycardia or AV nodal conduction block. The generalized vasodilation produced by exogenously administered ACh is due to the stimulation of muscarinic receptors, primarily of the M_3 subtype (Khurana et al., 2004; Lamping et al., 2004), located on vascular endothelial cells despite the apparent lack of cholinergic innervation. Occupation of the receptors by agonist activates the G_q–PLC–IP_3 pathway, leading to Ca^{2+}-calmodulin–dependent activation of endothelial NO synthase and production of NO (endothelium-derived relaxing factor) (Moncada and Higgs, 1995), which diffuses to adjacent vascular smooth muscle cells and causes them to relax (Furchgott, 1999; Ignarro et al., 1999) (Chapters 3 and 8). If the endothelium is damaged, as occurs under various pathophysiological conditions, ACh acts predominantly on M_3 receptors located on vascular smooth muscle cells, causing vasoconstriction.

Although endogenous ACh does not have a significant role in the physiological regulation of peripheral vascular tone, there is evidence that baroreceptor or chemoreceptor reflexes or direct stimulation of the vagus can elicit parasympathetic coronary vasodilation mediated by ACh and the consequent production of NO by the endothelium (Feigl, 1998). However, neither parasympathetic vasodilator nor sympathetic vasoconstrictor tone plays a major role in the regulation of coronary blood flow relative to the effects of local oxygen tension, activation of K_{ATP} channels, and autoregulatory metabolic factors such as adenosine (Berne and Levy, 2001).

ACh affects cardiac function directly and also indirectly through inhibition of the adrenergic stimulation of the heart. Cardiac effects of ACh are mediated primarily by M_2 muscarinic receptors (Stengel et al., 2000), which couple to G_i/G_o. The direct effects include an increase in the ACh-activated K^+ current ($I_{K\text{-}ACh}$) due to activation of K-ACh channels, a decrease in the L-type Ca^{2+} current ($I_{Ca\text{-}L}$) due to inhibition of L-type Ca^{2+} channels, and a decrease in the cardiac pacemaker current (I_f) due to inhibition of HCN (pacemaker) channels (DiFrancesco and Tromba, 1987). The indirect effects include a G_i-mediated decrease in cyclic AMP, which opposes and counteracts the β_1 adrenergic/G_s–mediated increase in cyclic AMP, and an inhibition of the release of norepinephrine from sympathetic nerve terminals. The inhibition of norepinephrine release is mediated by presynaptic M_2 and M_3 receptors, which are stimulated by ACh released from adjacent parasympathetic postganglionic nerve terminals (Trendelenburg et al., 2005). There are also presynaptic M_2 receptors that inhibit ACh release from parasympathetic postganglionic nerve terminals in the human heart (Oberhauser et al., 2001).

In the SA node, each normal cardiac impulse is initiated by the spontaneous depolarization of the pacemaker cells (Chapter 29). At a critical level (the threshold potential), this depolarization initiates an action potential. ACh slows the heart rate primarily by decreasing the rate of spontaneous depolarization; attainment of the threshold potential and the succeeding events in the cardiac cycle are therefore delayed. Until recently it was widely accepted that β adrenergic and muscarinic cholinergic effects on heart rate resulted from regulation of the cardiac pacemaker current (I_f). Unexpected findings made through genetic deletion of HCN4 and pharmacological inhibition of I_f have generated an alternative, albeit controversial, theory involving a pacemaking function for an intracellular Ca^{2+} "clock" (Lakatta and DiFrancesco, 2009) that might mediate effects of ACh on heart rate (Lyashkov et al., 2009).

In the atria, ACh causes hyperpolarization and a decreased action potential duration by increasing $I_{K\text{-}ACh}$. ACh also inhibits cyclic AMP formation and norepinephrine release, decreasing atrial contractility. The rate of impulse conduction is either unaffected or may increase in response to ACh; the increase probably is due to the activation of additional Na^+ channels in response to ACh-induced hyperpolarization. In contrast, in the AV node (which has Ca^{2+} channel-dependent action potentials; see Chapter 29), ACh slows conduction and increases the refractory period by inhibiting $I_{Ca\text{-}L}$; the decrement in AV conduction is responsible for the complete heart block that may be observed when large quantities of cholinergic agonists are administered systemically. With an increase in parasympathetic (vagal) tone, such as is produced by the digitalis glycosides, the increased refractory period of the AV node can contribute to the reduction in the frequency with which aberrant atrial impulses are transmitted to the ventricles and thereby decrease the ventricular rate during atrial flutter or fibrillation.

Cholinergic (vagal) innervation of the His-Purkinje system and ventricular myocardium is sparse (Kent et al., 1974; Levy and Schwartz, 1994) and the effects of ACh are smaller than those observed in the atria and nodal tissues. In the ventricles, ACh, whether released by vagal stimulation or applied directly, has a small negative inotropic effect; this inhibition is most apparent when there is concomitant adrenergic stimulation or underlying sympathetic tone (Brodde and Michel, 1999; Levy and Schwartz, 1994; Lewis et al., 2001). Automaticity of Purkinje fibers is suppressed, and the threshold for ventricular fibrillation is increased (Kent and Epstein, 1976).

Respiratory Tract. The parasympathetic nervous system plays a major role in regulating bronchomotor tone. A diverse set of stimuli cause reflex increases in parasympathetic activity that contributes to bronchoconstriction. The effects of ACh on the respiratory system include not only bronchoconstriction but also increased tracheobronchial secretion and stimulation of the chemoreceptors of the carotid and aortic bodies. These effects are mediated primarily by M_3 muscarinic receptors (Fisher et al., 2004).

Urinary Tract. Parasympathetic sacral innervation causes detrusor muscle contraction, increased voiding pressure, and ureteral peristalsis. These responses are difficult to observe with administered ACh because poor perfusion of visceral organs and rapid hydrolysis by plasma butyrylcholinesterase limit access of systemically administered ACh to visceral muscarinic receptors. Control of bladder contraction apparently is mediated by multiple muscarinic receptor subtypes. Receptors of the M_2 subtype appear most prevalent in the bladder, yet studies with selective antagonists and M_3 knockout mice suggest that the M_3 receptor mediates detrusor muscle contraction (Matsui et al., 2000). The M_2 receptor may act to inhibit β adrenergic receptor–mediated relaxation of the bladder and may be involved primarily in the filling stages to diminish urge incontinence (Chapple, 2000; Hegde and Eglen, 1999).

GI Tract. Although stimulation of vagal input to the GI tract increases tone, amplitude of contractions, and secretory activity of the stomach and intestine, such responses are inconsistently seen with administered ACh for the same reasons that urinary tract responses are difficult to observe. As in the urinary tract, muscarinic receptors of the M_2 subtype are most prevalent, but M_3 muscarinic receptors appear to be primarily responsible for mediating the cholinergic control of GI motility (Matsui et al., 2002).

Miscellaneous Peripheral Effects. In addition to its above-mentioned stimulatory effects on the tracheobronchial and GI secretions, ACh stimulates secretion from other glands that receive parasympathetic or sympathetic cholinergic innervation, including the lacrimal, nasopharyngeal, salivary, and sweat glands. All of these effects are mediated primarily by M_3 muscarinic receptors (Caulfield and Birdsall, 1998); M_1 receptors also contribute significantly to the cholinergic stimulation of salivary secretion (Gautam et al., 2004). When instilled into the eye, ACh produces miosis by contracting the pupillary sphincter muscle and accommodation for near vision by contracting the ciliary muscle (Chapter 64); both of these effects are mediated primarily by M_3 muscarinic receptors, but other subtypes may contribute to the ocular effects of cholinergic stimulation.

CNS Effects. While systemically administered ACh has limited CNS penetration, muscarinic agonists that can cross the blood-brain barrier evoke a characteristic cortical arousal or activation response, similar to that produced by injection of anticholinesterase agents or by electrical stimulation of the brainstem reticular formation. All five muscarinic receptor subtypes are found in the brain (Volpicelli and Levey, 2004), and recent studies suggest that muscarinic receptor-regulated pathways may have an important role in cognitive function, motor control, appetite regulation, nociception, and other processes (Wess et al., 2007).

MUSCARINIC RECEPTOR AGONISTS

Muscarinic cholinergic receptor agonists can be divided into two groups: 1) choline esters, including ACh and several synthetic esters; and 2) the naturally occurring cholinomimetic alkaloids (particularly pilocarpine, muscarine, and arecoline) and their synthetic congeners.

Of several hundred synthetic choline derivatives investigated, only methacholine, carbachol, and bethanechol (Figure 9–1) have had clinical applications. Methacholine (acetyl-β-methylcholine), the β-methyl analog of ACh, is a synthetic choline ester that differs from ACh chiefly in its greater duration and selectivity of action. Its action is more prolonged because the added methyl group increases its resistance to hydrolysis by cholinesterases. Its selectivity is reflected in a predominance of muscarinic with only minor nicotinic actions, the former manifest most clearly in the cardiovascular system (Table 9–1).

Carbachol, and its β-methyl analog, bethanechol, are unsubstituted carbamoyl esters that are almost completely resistant to hydrolysis by cholinesterases; their $t_{1/2}$ are thus sufficiently long that they become distributed to areas of low blood flow. Carbachol retains substantial nicotinic activity, particularly on autonomic ganglia. Bethanechol has mainly muscarinic actions, with prominent effects on motility of the GI tract and urinary bladder.

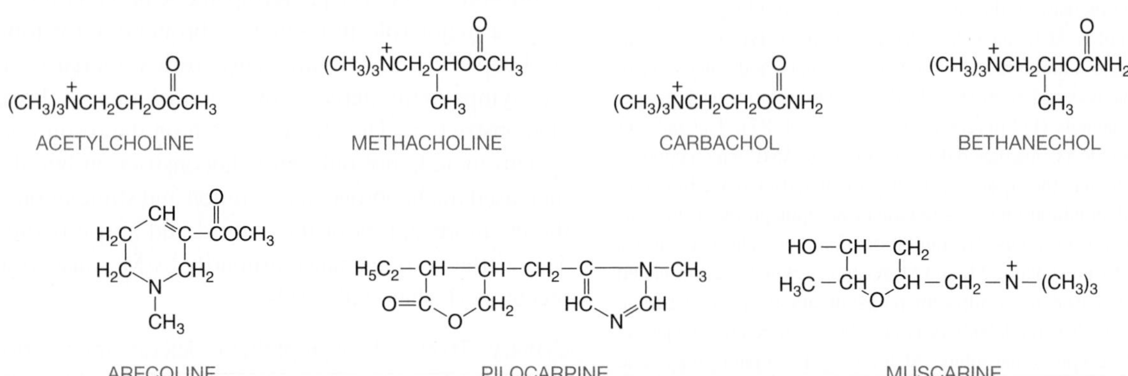

Figure 9–1. *Structural formulas of acetylcholine, choline esters, and natural alkaloids that stimulate muscarinic receptors.*

Table 9–1

Some Pharmacological Properties of Choline Esters and Natural Alkaloids

MUSCARINIC AGONIST	SUSCEPTIBILITY TO CHOLINESTERASES	MUSCARINIC ACTIVITY: *Cardio-vascular*	*Gastro-intestinal*	*Urinary Bladder*	*Eye (Topical)*	*Antagonism by Atropine*	NICOTINIC ACTIVITY
Acetylcholine	+++	++	++	++	+	+++	++
Methacholine	+	+++	++	++	+	+++	+
Carbachol	–	+	+++	+++	++	+	+++
Bethanechol	–	±	+++	+++	++	+++	–
Muscarine[a]	–	++	+++	+++	++	+++	–
Pilocarpine	–	+	+++	+++	++	+++	–

[a]Not used therapeutically

The major natural alkaloid muscarinic agonists—muscarine, pilocarpine, and arecoline—have the same principal sites of action as the choline esters. Muscarine acts almost exclusively at muscarinic receptor sites, and the classification of these receptors derives from the actions of this alkaloid. Pilocarpine has a dominant muscarinic action but is a partial rather than a full agonist; the sweat glands are particularly sensitive to pilocarpine. Arecoline also acts at nicotinic receptors. Although these naturally occurring alkaloids are of great value as pharmacological tools and muscarine has toxicological significance (discussed later), present clinical use is restricted largely to the employment of pilocarpine as a sialagogue and miotic agent (Chapter 64).

History and Sources. The alkaloid muscarine was isolated from the mushroom *Amanita muscaria* by Schmiedeberg in 1869; its toxicology is discussed later. Pilocarpine is the chief alkaloid obtained from the leaflets of South American shrubs of the genus *Pilocarpus*. Although it was long known by the natives that the chewing of leaves of *Pilocarpus* plants caused salivation, the first experiments were apparently performed in 1874 by the Brazilian physician Coutinhou. The alkaloid was isolated in 1875, and shortly thereafter the actions of pilocarpine on the pupil and on the sweat and salivary glands were described by Weber. Arecoline is the chief alkaloid of areca or betel nuts, the seeds of *Areca catechu*. The red-staining betel nut is consumed as a euphoretic by the natives of the Indian subcontinent and East Indies in a masticatory mixture known as betel and composed of the nut, shell lime, and leaves of *Piper betle*, a climbing species of pepper. Methacholine was synthesized and studied by Hunt and Taveau as early as 1911. Carbachol and bethanechol were synthesized and investigated in the 1930s.

Absorption, Distribution, and Elimination

The absorption and distribution of these compounds may be predicted from their structures: muscarine and the choline esters are quaternary amines; pilocarpine and arecoline are tertiary amines (Figure 9–1).

Because they are quaternary amines, the choline esters are poorly absorbed following oral administration and have a limited ability to cross the blood-brain barrier. Even though these drugs resist hydrolysis, the choline esters are short-acting agents due to rapid elimination by the kidneys.

Pilocarpine and arecoline, being tertiary amines, are readily absorbed and can cross the blood-brain barrier. In contrast, muscarine, a quaternary amine, is poorly absorbed. Muscarine can still, however, be toxic when ingested and can even have CNS effects. Although the specific metabolic pathways have not been elucidated, pilocarpine clearance is decreased in patients with hepatic impairment, in whom doses may need to be reduced. The natural alkaloids are primarily eliminated by the kidneys; excretion of the tertiary amines can be accelerated by acidification of the urine.

Therapeutic Uses of Muscarinic Receptor Agonists

Muscarinic agonists are currently used in the treatment of urinary bladder disorders and xerostomia and in the diagnosis of bronchial hyperreactivity. They are also used in ophthalmology as miotic agents and for the treatment of glaucoma.

There is growing interest in the role of muscarinic receptors in cognition. The potential utility of M_1 agonists in treating the cognitive impairment associated with Alzheimer's disease has long been considered. Other receptor subtypes including M_2 and M_5 also appear to be involved in the regulation of cognitive function, at least in animal models (Wess et al., 2007).

The difficulty in developing subtype selective muscarinic receptor agonists, coupled with the lack of efficacy and the significant peripheral side effects of available muscarinic agonists, have prompted a search for other strategies for selectively activating specific muscarinic receptor subtypes, such as allosteric agonists and positive allosteric modulators (PAMs) (Conn et al., 2009b). Selective muscarinic subtype activators may be useful in the treatment of additional CNS disorders, including schizophrenia and drug addiction, and as analgesic agents (Conn et al., 2009b). For example, xanomeline, a muscarinic agonist with some selectivity for the M_1 and M_4 subtypes that was in clinical development for Alzheimer's disease, has an antipsychotic profile in animal models and therapeutic efficacy in patients with schizophrenia (Mirza et al., 2003; Shekhar et al., 2008).

Acetylcholine. Although rarely given systemically, ACh (MIOCHOL-E) is used topically for the induction of miosis during ophthalmologic surgery; it is instilled into the eye as a 1% solution (Chapter 64).

Methacholine. Methacholine (PROVOCHOLINE) is administered by inhalation for the diagnosis of bronchial airway hyperreactivity in patients who do not have clinically apparent asthma (Crapo et al., 2000). While muscarinic agonists can cause bronchoconstriction and increased tracheobronchial secretions in all individuals, asthmatic patients respond with intense bronchoconstriction and a reduction in vital capacity. Accordingly, contraindications to methacholine testing include severe airflow limitation, recent myocardial infarction or stroke, uncontrolled hypertension, or pregnancy. The response to methacholine also may be exaggerated or prolonged in patients taking β adrenergic receptor antagonists. Emergency resuscitation equipment, oxygen, and medications to treat severe bronchospasm (e.g., $β_2$ adrenergic receptor agonists for inhalation) should be available during testing. Methacholine is available as a powder that is diluted with 0.9% sodium chloride and administered via a nebulizer.

Bethanechol. Bethanechol (URECHOLINE, others) primarily affects the urinary and GI tracts. In the urinary tract, bethanechol has utility in treating urinary retention and inadequate emptying of the bladder when organic obstruction is absent, as in postoperative urinary retention, diabetic autonomic neuropathy, and certain cases of chronic hypotonic, myogenic, or neurogenic bladder (Wein, 1991); catheterization can thus be avoided. When used chronically, 10-50 mg of the drug is given orally three to four times daily; the drug should be administered on an empty stomach (i.e., 1 hour before or 2 hours after a meal) to minimize nausea and vomiting.

In the GI tract, bethanechol stimulates peristalsis, increases motility, and increases resting lower esophageal sphincter pressure. Bethanechol formerly was used to treat postoperative abdominal distention, gastric atony, gastroparesis, adynamic ileus, and gastroesophageal reflux; more efficacious therapies for these disorders are now available (Chapters 45 and 46).

Carbachol. Carbachol (MIOSTAT, ISOPTO CARBACHOL, others) is used topically in ophthalmology for the treatment of glaucoma and the induction of miosis during surgery; it is instilled into the eye as a 0.01-3% solution (Chapter 64).

Pilocarpine. Pilocarpine hydrochloride (SALAGEN, others) is used for the treatment of xerostomia that follows head and neck radiation treatments or that is associated with Sjögren's syndrome (Porter et al., 2004;Wiseman and Faulds, 1995), an autoimmune disorder occurring primarily in women in whom secretions, particularly salivary and lacrimal, are compromised (Anaya and Talal, 1999). Provided salivary parenchyma maintains residual function, enhanced salivary secretion, ease of swallowing, and subjective improvement in hydration of the oral cavity are achieved. Side effects typify cholinergic stimulation, with sweating being the most common complaint. The usual dose is 5-10 mg three times daily; the dose should be lowered in patients with hepatic impairment.

Pilocarpine (ISOPTO CARPINE, others) is used topically in ophthalmology for the treatment of glaucoma and as a miotic agent; it is instilled in the eye as a 0.5-6% solution and also can be delivered via an ocular insert (Chapter 64).

Cevimeline. Cevimeline (EVOXAC), a quinuclidine derivative of ACh, is a muscarinic agonist with a high affinity for M_3 muscarinic receptors on lacrimal and salivary gland epithelia. Cevimeline has a long-lasting sialogogic action and may have fewer side effects than pilocarpine (Anaya and Talal, 1999). Cevimeline also enhances lacrimal secretions in Sjögren's syndrome (Ono et al., 2004). The usual dose is 30 mg three times daily.

Contraindications, Precautions, and Adverse Effects

Most contraindications, precautions, and adverse effects are predictable consequences of muscarinic receptor stimulation. Thus, important contraindications to the use of muscarinic agonists include asthma, chronic obstructive pulmonary disease, urinary or GI tract obstruction, acid-peptic disease, cardiovascular disease accompanied by bradycardia, hypotension, and hyperthyroidism (muscarinic agonists may precipitate atrial fibrillation in hyperthyroid patients). Common adverse effects include diaphoresis; diarrhea, abdominal cramps, nausea/vomiting, and other GI side effects; a sensation of tightness in the urinary bladder; difficulty in visual accommodation;

and hypotension, which can severely reduce coronary blood flow, especially if it is already compromised. These contraindications and adverse effects are generally of limited concern with topical administration for ophthalmic use.

Toxicology

Poisoning from the ingestion of plants containing pilocarpine, muscarine, or arecoline is characterized chiefly by exaggeration of their various parasympathomimetic effects and resembles that produced by consumption of mushrooms of the genus *Inocybe* (described in the next section). Treatment consists of the parenteral administration of atropine in doses sufficient to cross the blood-brain barrier and measures to support the respiratory and cardiovascular systems and to counteract pulmonary edema.

Mushroom Poisoning (Mycetism). Mushroom poisoning has been known for centuries. The Greek poet Euripides (fifth century B.C.E.) is said to have lost his wife and three children from this cause. In recent years, the number of cases of mushroom poisoning has been increasing as the result of the current popularity of the consumption of wild mushrooms. Various species of mushrooms contain many toxins, and species within the same genus may contain distinct toxins.

Although *Amanita muscaria* is the source from which muscarine was isolated, its content of the alkaloid is so low (~ 0.003%) that muscarine cannot be responsible for the major toxic effects. Much higher concentrations of muscarine are present in various species of *Inocybe* and *Clitocybe*. The symptoms of intoxication attributable to muscarine develop within 30-60 minutes of ingestion; they include salivation, lacrimation, nausea, vomiting, headache, visual disturbances, abdominal colic, diarrhea, bronchospasm, bradycardia, hypotension, and shock. Treatment with atropine (1-2 mg intramuscularly every 30 minutes) effectively blocks these effects (Goldfrank, 2006; Köppel, 1993).

Intoxication produced by *A. muscaria* and related *Amanita* species arises from the neurologic and hallucinogenic properties of muscimol, ibotenic acid, and other isoxazole derivatives. These agents stimulate excitatory and inhibitory amino acid receptors. Symptoms range from irritability, restlessness, ataxia, hallucinations, and delirium to drowsiness and sedation. Treatment is mainly supportive; benzodiazepines are indicated when excitation predominates; atropine often exacerbates the delirium.

Mushrooms from *Psilocybe* and *Panaeolus* species contain psilocybin and related derivatives of tryptamine. They also cause short-lasting hallucinations. *Gyromitra* species (false morels) produce GI disorders and a delayed hepatotoxicity. The toxic substance, acetaldehyde methylformylhydrazone, is converted in the body to reactive hydrazines. Although fatalities from liver and kidney failure have been reported, they are far less frequent than with amatoxin-containing mushrooms.

The most serious form of mycetism is produced by *Amanita phalloides*, other *Amanita* species, *Lepiota*, and *Galerina* species (Goldfrank, 2006). These species account for > 90% of all fatal cases. Ingestion of as little as 50 g of *A. phalloides* (deadly nightcap) can be fatal. The principal toxins are the amatoxins (α- and β-amanitin), a group of cyclic octapeptides that inhibit RNA polymerase II and thereby block mRNA synthesis. This causes cell death, manifested particularly in the GI mucosa, liver, and kidneys. Initial symptoms, which often are unnoticed or when present are due to other toxins, include diarrhea and abdominal cramps. A symptom-free period lasting up to 24 hours is followed by hepatic and renal malfunction. Death occurs in 4-7 days from renal and hepatic failure (Goldfrank, 2006). Treatment is largely supportive; penicillin, thioctic acid, and silibinin may be effective antidotes, but the evidence is based largely on anecdotal studies (Köppel, 1993).

Because the severity of toxicity and treatment strategies for mushroom poisoning depend on the species ingested, their identification should be sought. Often symptomatology is delayed, limiting the value of gastric lavage and administration of activated charcoal. Regional poison control centers in the U.S. maintain up-to-date information on the incidence of poisoning in the region and treatment procedures.

MUSCARINIC RECEPTOR ANTAGONISTS

The muscarinic receptor antagonists include: 1) the naturally occurring alkaloids, atropine and scopolamine; 2) semisynthetic derivatives of these alkaloids, which primarily differ from the parent compounds in their disposition in the body or their duration of action; and 3) synthetic derivatives, some of which show selectivity for subtypes of muscarinic receptors. Noteworthy agents among the latter two categories are homatropine and tropicamide, which have a shorter duration of action than atropine, and methscopolamine, ipratropium, and tiotropium, which are quaternized and do not cross the blood-brain barrier or readily cross membranes. The synthetic derivatives possessing some degree of receptor selectivity include pirenzepine, which shows selectivity for M_1 receptors; and darifenacin and solifenacin, which show selectivity for M_3 receptors.

Muscarinic antagonists prevent the effects of ACh by blocking its binding to muscarinic receptors on effector cells at parasympathetic (and sympathetic cholinergic) neuroeffector junctions, in peripheral ganglia, and in the CNS. In general, muscarinic antagonists cause little blockade of nicotinic receptors. However, the quaternary ammonium antagonists generally exhibit a greater degree of nicotinic blocking activity and therefore are more likely to interfere with ganglionic or neuromuscular transmission.

While many effects of muscarinic antagonists can be predicted from an understanding of the physiological responses mediated by muscarinic receptors at parasympathetic (and sympathetic cholinergic) neuroeffector junctions, paradoxical responses are sometimes seen. For example, presynaptic muscarinic receptors of variable subtype are present on postganglionic parasympathetic nerve terminals. Since blockade of presynaptic receptors generally augments neurotransmitter release, the presynaptic effects of muscarinic antagonists may counteract their postsynaptic receptor blockade. Blockade of the modulatory muscarinic receptors in peripheral ganglia represents an additional mechanism for paradoxical responses.

An important consideration in the therapeutic use of muscarinic antagonists is the fact that physiological functions in different organs vary in their sensitivity to muscarinic receptor blockade (Table 9–2). Small doses of atropine depress salivary and bronchial secretion and sweating. With larger doses, the pupil dilates, accommodation of the lens to near vision is inhibited, and vagal effects on the heart are blocked so that the heart rate increases. Larger doses antagonize parasympathetic control of the urinary bladder and GI tract, thereby inhibiting micturition and decreasing intestinal tone and motility. Still larger doses are required to inhibit gastric motility and particularly secretion. Thus, doses of atropine and most related muscarinic antagonists that depress gastric secretion also almost invariably affect salivary secretion, ocular accommodation, micturition, and GI motility. This hierarchy of relative sensitivities is not a consequence of differences in the affinity of atropine for the muscarinic receptors at these sites because atropine lacks selectivity toward different muscarinic receptor subtypes. More likely determinants include the degree to which the functions of various end organs are regulated by parasympathetic tone, the "spareness" of receptors and signaling mechanisms, the involvement of intramural neurons and reflexes, and the presence of other regulatory mechanisms.

Most clinically available muscarinic antagonists are nonselective and their actions differ little from those of atropine, the prototype of the group. No subtype-selective antagonist, including pirenzepine, is completely selective (i.e., can be used to define a single receptor subtype relative to all other receptor subtypes). In fact, the clinical efficacy of some agents may arise from a balance of antagonistic actions on two or more receptor subtypes.

Table 9–2

Effects of Atropine in Relation to Dose

DOSE (mg)	EFFECTS
0.5	Slight cardiac slowing; some dryness of mouth; inhibition of sweating
1	Definite dryness of mouth; thirst; acceleration of heart, sometimes preceded by slowing; mild dilation of pupils
2	Rapid heart rate; palpitation; marked dryness of mouth; dilated pupils; some blurring of near vision
5	Above symptoms marked; difficulty in speaking and swallowing; restlessness and fatigue; headache; dry, hot skin; difficulty in micturition; reduced intestinal peristalsis
≥10	Above symptoms more marked; pulse rapid and weak; iris practically obliterated; vision very blurred; skin flushed, hot, dry, and scarlet; ataxia, restlessness, and excitement; hallucinations and delirium; coma

The clinical picture of a high (toxic) dose of atropine may be remembered by an old mnemonic device that summarizes the symptoms: *Red as a beet, Dry as a bone, Blind as a bat, Hot as firestone, and Mad as a hatter.*

History. The naturally occurring muscarinic receptor antagonists atropine and scopolamine are alkaloids of the belladonna (Solanaceae) plants. Preparations of belladonna were known to the ancient Hindus and have long been used by physicians. During the time of the Roman Empire and in the Middle Ages, the deadly nightshade shrub was frequently used to produce an obscure and often prolonged poisoning, prompting Linnaeus to name the shrub *Atropa belladonna*, after Atropos, the oldest of the three Fates, who cuts the thread of life. The name *belladonna* derives from the alleged use of this preparation by Italian women to dilate their pupils; modern-day fashion models are known to use this same device for visual appeal. Atropine (d,l-hyoscyamine) also is found in *Datura stramonium* (Jamestown or jimson weed). Scopolamine (l-hyoscine) is found chiefly in *Hyoscyamus niger* (henbane). In India, the root and leaves of jimson weed were burned and the smoke inhaled to treat asthma. British colonists observed this ritual and introduced the belladonna alkaloids into western medicine in the early 1800s.

Accurate study of the actions of belladonna dates from the isolation of atropine in pure form by Mein in 1831. Bezold and Bloebaum (1867) showed that atropine blocked the cardiac effects of vagal stimulation, and Heidenhain (1872) found that it prevented salivary secretion produced by stimulation of the chorda tympani. Many semisynthetic congeners of the belladonna alkaloids and a large number of synthetic muscarinic receptor antagonists have been prepared, primarily with the objective of altering GI or bladder activity without causing dry mouth or pupillary dilation.

Chemistry. Atropine and scopolamine are esters formed by combination of an aromatic acid, tropic acid, and complex organic bases, either tropine (tropanol) or scopine. Scopine differs from tropine only in having an oxygen bridge between the carbon atoms designated as 6 and 7 (Figure 9–2). Homatropine is a semisynthetic compound produced by combining the base tropine with mandelic acid. The corresponding quaternary ammonium derivatives, modified by the addition of a second methyl group to the nitrogen, are methylatropine nitrate, methscopolamine bromide, and homatropine methylbromide. Ipratropium and tiotropium also are quaternary tropine

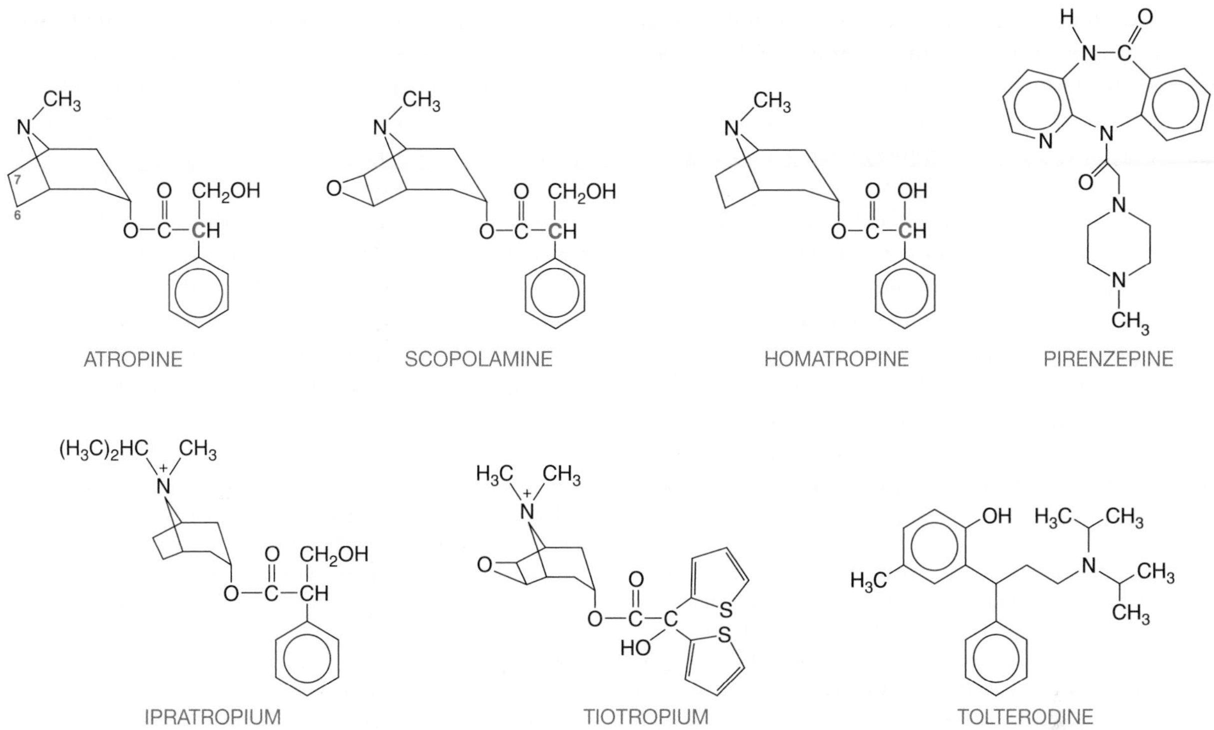

Figure 9–2. *Structural formulas of the belladonna alkaloids and semisynthetic and synthetic analogs.* The red C identifies an asymmetric carbon atom.

analogs esterified with synthetic aromatic acids. A similar agent, *oxitropium bromide*, an *N*-ethyl-substituted, quaternary derivative of scopolamine, is available in Europe.

Structure-Activity Relationships. An intact ester of tropine and tropic acid is essential for antimuscarinic action, since neither the free acid nor the basic alcohol exhibits significant antimuscarinic activity. The presence of a free OH group in the acyl portion of the ester also is important for activity. When given parenterally, quaternary ammonium derivatives of atropine and scopolamine are generally more potent than their parent compounds in both muscarinic and ganglionic (nicotinic) blocking activities. The quaternary derivatives, when given orally, are poorly and unreliably absorbed.

Both tropic and mandelic acids have an enantiomeric center (boldface red **C** in the formulas in Figure 9–2). Scopolamine is *l*-hyoscine and is much more active than *d*-hyoscine. Atropine is racemized during extraction and consists of *d,l*-hyoscyamine, but antimuscarinic activity is almost wholly due to the naturally occurring *l* isomer. Synthetic derivatives show a wide range of structures that spatially replicate the aromatic acid and the bridged nitrogen of the tropine.

Mechanism of Action. Atropine and related compounds compete with ACh and other muscarinic agonists for a common binding site on the muscarinic receptor. Since antagonism by atropine is competitive, it can be overcome if the concentration of ACh at muscarinic receptors of the effector organ is increased sufficiently. Muscarinic receptor antagonists inhibit responses to postganglionic cholinergic nerve stimulation less effectively than they inhibit responses to injected choline esters. The difference may be explained by the fact that release of ACh by cholinergic nerve terminals occurs in close proximity to the receptors, resulting in very high concentrations of the transmitter at the receptors.

Pharmacological Effects of Muscarinic Antagonists

The pharmacological effects of atropine, the prototypical muscarinic antagonist, provide a good background for understanding the therapeutic uses of the various muscarinic antagonists. The effects of other muscarinic antagonists will be mentioned only when they differ significantly from those of atropine. The major pharmacological effects of increasing doses of atropine, summarized in Table 9–2, offer a general guide to the problems associated with administration of this class of agents.

Cardiovascular System

Heart. The main effect of atropine on the heart is to alter the rate. Although the dominant response is tachycardia, the heart rate often decreases transiently with average clinical doses (0.4-0.6 mg; Table 9–2). The slowing is modest (4-8 beats per minute) and is usually absent after rapid intravenous injection. There are no accompanying changes in blood pressure or cardiac output. This unexpected effect has been attributed to the block of presynaptic M_1 muscarinic receptors on parasympathetic postganglionic nerve terminals in the SA node, which normally inhibit ACh release (Wellstein and Pitschner, 1988).

Larger doses of atropine cause progressive tachycardia by blocking M_2 receptors on the SA nodal pacemaker cells, thereby antagonizing parasympathetic (vagal) tone to the heart. The resting heart rate is increased by ~35-40 beats per minute in young men given 2 mg of atropine intramuscularly. The maximal heart rate (e.g., in response to exercise) is not altered by atropine. The influence of atropine is most noticeable in healthy young adults, in whom vagal tone is considerable. In infancy and old age, even large doses of atropine may fail to accelerate the heart. Atropine often produces cardiac arrhythmias, but without significant cardiovascular symptoms.

Atropine can abolish many types of reflex vagal cardiac slowing or asystole, such as from inhalation of irritant vapors, stimulation of the carotid sinus, pressure on the eyeballs, peritoneal stimulation, or injection of contrast dye during cardiac catheterization. Atropine also prevents or abruptly abolishes bradycardia or asystole caused by choline esters, acetylcholinesterase inhibitors, or other parasympathomimetic drugs, as well as cardiac arrest from electrical stimulation of the vagus.

The removal of vagal tone to the heart by atropine also may facilitate AV conduction. Atropine shortens the functional refractory period of the AV node and can increase ventricular rate in patients who have atrial fibrillation or flutter. In certain cases of second-degree AV block (e.g., Wenckebach AV block), in which vagal activity is an etiological factor (as with digitalis toxicity), atropine may lessen the degree of block. In some patients with complete AV block, the idioventricular rate may be accelerated by atropine; in others it is stabilized. Atropine may improve the clinical condition of patients with inferior or posterior wall myocardial infarction by relieving severe sinus or nodal bradycardia or AV block.

Circulation. Atropine, in clinical doses, completely counteracts the peripheral vasodilation and sharp fall in blood pressure caused by choline esters. In contrast, when given alone, its effect on blood vessels and blood pressure is neither striking nor constant. This result is expected because most vascular beds lack significant cholinergic innervation. In toxic and occasionally in therapeutic doses, atropine can dilate cutaneous blood vessels, especially those in the blush area (atropine flush). This may be a compensatory reaction permitting the radiation of heat to offset the atropine-induced rise in temperature that can accompany inhibition of sweating.

Respiratory System. Although atropine can cause some bronchodilation and decrease in tracheobronchial secretion in normal individuals by blocking parasympathetic (vagal) tone to the lungs, its effects on the respiratory system are most significant in patients with respiratory disease. Atropine can inhibit the bronchoconstriction caused by histamine, bradykinin, and the eicosanoids, which presumably reflects the participation of reflex parasympathetic (vagal) activity in the bronchoconstriction elicited by these agents. The ability to block the indirect bronchoconstrictive effects of these mediators forms the basis for the use of muscarinic receptor antagonists, along with β adrenergic receptor agonists, in the treatment of asthma (Chapter 36). Muscarinic antagonists also have an important role in the treatment of chronic obstructive pulmonary disease (Chapter 36).

Atropine inhibits the secretions of the nose, mouth, pharynx, and bronchi, and thus dries the mucous membranes of the respiratory tract. This action is especially marked if secretion is excessive and formed the basis for the use of atropine and other muscarinic antagonists to prevent irritating inhalational anesthetics such as diethyl ether from increasing bronchial secretion. While the newer inhalational anesthetics are less irritating, muscarinic antagonists are similarly used to decrease the rhinorrhea associated with the common cold or with allergic and nonallergic rhinitis. Reduction of mucous secretion and mucociliary clearance can, however, result in mucus plugs, a potentially undesirable side effect of muscarinic antagonists in patients with airway disease.

Eye. Muscarinic receptor antagonists block the cholinergic responses of the pupillary sphincter muscle of the iris and the ciliary muscle controlling lens curvature (Chapter 64). Thus, they dilate the pupil (mydriasis) and paralyze accommodation (cycloplegia). The wide pupillary dilation results in photophobia; the lens is fixed for far vision, near objects are blurred, and objects may appear smaller than they are. The normal pupillary reflex constriction to light or upon convergence of the eyes is abolished. These effects can occur after either local or systemic administration of the alkaloids.

However, conventional systemic doses of atropine (0.6 mg) have little ocular effect, in contrast to equal doses of scopolamine, which cause evident mydriasis and loss of accommodation. Locally applied atropine produces ocular effects of considerable duration; accommodation and pupillary reflexes may not fully recover for 7-12 days. Other muscarinic receptor antagonists with shorter durations of action are therefore preferred as mydriatics in ophthalmologic practice (Chapter 64). Pilocarpine and choline esters (e.g., carbachol) in sufficient concentrations can reverse the ocular effects of atropine.

Muscarinic receptor antagonists administered systemically have little effect on intraocular pressure except in patients predisposed to angle-closure glaucoma, in whom the pressure may occasionally rise dangerously. The rise in pressure occurs when the anterior chamber is narrow and the iris obstructs outflow of aqueous humor into the trabeculae. Muscarinic antagonists may precipitate a first attack in unrecognized cases of this relatively rare condition. In patients with open-angle glaucoma, an acute rise in pressure is unusual. Atropine-like drugs generally can be used safely in this latter condition, particularly if the glaucoma is being treated appropriately.

GI Tract. Knowledge of the actions of muscarinic receptor agonists on the stomach and intestine led to the use of muscarinic receptor antagonists as antispasmodic agents for GI disorders and in the treatment of peptic ulcer disease. Although atropine can completely abolish the effects of ACh (and other parasympathomimetic drugs) on GI motility and secretion, it inhibits only incompletely the gastrointestinal responses to vagal stimulation. This difference, which is particularly striking in the effects of atropine on gut motility, can be attributed to the fact that preganglionic vagal fibers innervating the GI tract synapse not only with postganglionic cholinergic fibers, but also with a network of noncholinergic intramural neurons. These neurons, which form the plexuses of the enteric nervous system, utilize numerous neurotransmitters or neuromodulators including serotonin (5-HT), dopamine, and peptides, the effects of which are not blocked by atropine. Another reason that atropine only incompletely inhibits the GI responses to vagal activity is that vagal stimulation of gastrin secretion is mediated by gastrin-releasing peptide (GRP), not ACh. The parietal cell secretes acid in response to at least three agonists: gastrin, histamine, and acetylcholine; furthermore, stimulation of muscarinic receptors on enterochromaffin-like cells will cause histamine release. Atropine will inhibit the component of acid secretion that results from muscarinic stimulation of enterochromafin cells (histamine secretors) and parietal cells (acid secretors).

Secretions. Salivary secretion is particularly sensitive to inhibition by muscarinic receptor antagonists, which can completely abolish the copious, watery secretion induced by parasympathetic stimulation. The mouth becomes dry, and swallowing and talking may become difficult. *Gastric secretion* during the cephalic and fasting phases is also reduced markedly by muscarinic receptor antagonists. In contrast, the intestinal phase of gastric secretion is only partially inhibited. The concentration of acid is not necessarily lowered because secretion of HCO_3^- as well as that of H^+ is blocked. The gastric cells that secrete mucin and proteolytic enzymes are more directly under vagal influence than are the acid-secreting cells, and atropine decreases their secretory function. Although muscarinic antagonists can reduce gastric secretion, the doses required also affect salivary secretion, ocular accommodation, micturition, and GI motility (Table 9–2). Thus, histamine H_2 receptor antagonists and, more recently, proton pump inhibitors have replaced muscarinic antagonists as inhibitors of acid secretion (Chapter 45).

In contrast to most muscarinic receptor antagonists, pirenzepine, which shows some selectivity for M_1 receptors, inhibits gastric acid secretion at doses that have little effect on salivation or heart rate. Since the muscarinic receptors on the parietal cells are primarily M_3 receptors and do not appear to have a high affinity for pirenzepine, the M_1 receptor responsible for alterations in gastric acid secretion is postulated to be localized in intramural ganglia (Eglen et al., 1996). Blockade of ganglionic muscarinic receptors (rather than those at the neuroeffector junction) may underlie the ability of pirenzepine to inhibit the relaxation of the lower esophageal sphincter. The physiology and pharmacology here are complex: Pirenzepine reportedly inhibits carbachol-stimulated acid secretion in KO mice lacking M_1 receptors (Aihara et al., 2005).

Motility. The parasympathetic nerves enhance both tone and motility and relax sphincters, thereby favoring the passage of gastrointestinal contents. Both in normal subjects and in patients with gastrointestinal disease, muscarinic antagonists produce prolonged inhibitory effects on the motor activity of the stomach, duodenum, jejunum, ileum, and colon, characterized by a reduction in tone and in amplitude and frequency of peristaltic contractions. Relatively large doses are needed to produce such inhibition. This probably can be explained by the ability of the enteric nervous system to regulate motility independently of parasympathetic control; parasympathetic nerves serve only to modulate the effects of the enteric nervous system (Chapter 8).

Other Smooth Muscle

Urinary Tract. Muscarinic antagonists decrease the normal tone and amplitude of contractions of the ureter and bladder, and often eliminate drug-induced enhancement of ureteral tone. However, this inhibition cannot be achieved in the absence of inhibition of salivation and lacrimation and blurring of vision (Table 9–2).

Biliary Tract. Atropine exerts a mild antispasmodic action on the gallbladder and bile ducts in humans. However, this effect usually is not sufficient to overcome or prevent the marked spasm and increase in biliary duct pressure induced by opioids. The nitrates (Chapter 27) are more effective than atropine in this respect.

Sweat Glands and Temperature. Small doses of atropine inhibit the activity of sweat glands innervated by sympathetic cholinergic fibers, and the skin becomes hot and dry. Sweating may be depressed enough to raise the body temperature, but only notably so after large doses or at high environmental temperatures.

Central Nervous System. Atropine has minimal effects on the CNS at therapeutic doses, although mild stimulation of the parasympathetic medullary centers may occur. With toxic doses of atropine, central excitation becomes more prominent, leading to restlessness, irritability, disorientation, hallucinations, or delirium (see the discussion of atropine poisoning later in the chapter). With still larger doses, stimulation is followed by depression, leading to circulatory collapse and respiratory failure after a period of paralysis and coma.

In contrast to atropine, scopolamine has prominent central effects at low therapeutic doses; atropine therefore is preferred over scopolamine for many purposes. The basis for this difference is probably the greater permeation of scopolamine across the blood-brain barrier. Specifically, scopolamine in therapeutic doses normally causes CNS depression manifest as drowsiness, amnesia, fatigue, and dreamless sleep, with a reduction in rapid eye movement (REM) sleep. It also causes euphoria and can therefore be subject to abuse. The depressant and amnesic effects formerly were sought when scopolamine was used as an adjunct to anesthetic agents or for preanesthetic medication. However, in the presence of severe pain, the same doses of scopolamine can occasionally cause excitement, restlessness, hallucinations, or delirium. These excitatory effects resemble those of toxic doses of atropine. Scopolamine also is effective in preventing motion sickness, probably by blocking neural pathways from the vestibular apparatus in the inner ear to the emetic center in the brainstem.

Muscarinic receptor antagonists have long been used in the treatment of Parkinson disease. These agents can be effective adjuncts to treatment with levodopa (Chapter 22). Muscarinic receptor antagonists also are used to treat the extrapyramidal symptoms that commonly occur as side effects of conventional antipsychotic drug therapy (Chapter 16). Certain antipsychotic drugs are relatively potent muscarinic receptor antagonists (Richelson, 1999; Roth et al., 2004) and, perhaps for this reason, cause fewer extrapyramidal side effects.

Ipratropium and Tiotropium

The quaternary ammonium compounds ipratropium and tiotropium are used exclusively for their effects on the respiratory tract. When inhaled, their action is confined almost completely to the mouth and airways. Dry mouth is the only frequently reported side effect, as the absorption of these drugs from the lungs or the GI tract is very inefficient. The degree of bronchodilation achieved by these agents is thought to reflect the level of basal parasympathetic tone, supplemented by reflex activation of cholinergic pathways brought about by various stimuli. In normal individuals, inhalation of the drugs can provide virtually complete protection against the bronchoconstriction produced by the subsequent inhalation of such irritants as sulfur dioxide, ozone, or cigarette smoke. However, patients with atopic asthma or patients with demonstrable bronchial hyperresponsiveness are less well protected. Although these drugs cause a marked reduction in sensitivity to methacholine in asthmatic subjects, more modest inhibition of responses to challenge with histamine, bradykinin, or $PGF_{2\alpha}$ is achieved, and little protection is afforded against the bronchoconstriction induced by 5-HT or leukotrienes. A therapeutically important property of ipratropium and tiotropium is their minimal inhibitory effect on mucociliary clearance relative to atropine. Hence, the choice of these agents for use in patients with airway disease minimizes the increased accumulation of lower airway secretions encountered with atropine.

Ipratropium appears to block all subtypes of muscarinic receptors and accordingly also antagonizes the inhibition of ACh release by presynaptic M_2 receptors on parasympathetic postganglionic nerve terminals in the lung; the resulting increase in ACh release may counteract its blockade of M_3 receptor-mediated bronchoconstriction. In contrast, tiotropium shows some selectivity for M_1 and M_3 receptors; its lower affinity for M_2 receptors minimizes its presynaptic effect to enhance ACh release (Barnes, 2004; Disse et al., 1999)

Absorption, Distribution, and Elimination. The belladonna alkaloids and the *tertiary* synthetic and semisynthetic derivatives are absorbed rapidly from the GI tract. They also enter the circulation when applied locally to the mucosal surfaces of the body. Absorption from intact skin is limited, although efficient absorption does occur in the postauricular region for some agents (e.g., scopolamine, allowing delivery by transdermal patch). Systemic absorption of inhaled or orally ingested *quaternary* muscarinic receptor antagonists is limited. The quaternary ammonium derivatives of the belladonna alkaloids also penetrate the conjunctiva of the eye less readily, and central effects are lacking because the quaternary agents do not cross the blood-brain barrier. Atropine has a $t_{1/2}$ of ~4 hours; hepatic metabolism accounts for the elimination of about half of a dose; the remainder is excreted unchanged in the urine.

Ipratropium is administered as an aerosol or solution for inhalation whereas tiotropium is administered as a dry powder. As with most drugs administered by inhalation, ~90% of the dose is swallowed. Most of the swallowed drug appears in the feces. After inhalation, maximal responses usually develop over 30-90 minutes, with tiotropium having the slower onset. The effects of ipratropium last for 4-6 hours, while tiotropium's effects persist for 24 hours so that the drug is amenable to once-daily dosing (Barnes and Hansel, 2004).

Therapeutic Uses of Muscarinic Receptor Antagonists

Muscarinic receptor antagonists have been used in the treatment of a wide variety of clinical conditions, predominantly to inhibit effects of parasympathetic activity in the respiratory tract, urinary tract, GI tract, eye, and heart. Their CNS effects have resulted in their use in the treatment of Parkinson disease, the management of extrapyramidal side effects of antipsychotic drugs, and the prevention of motion sickness. The major limitation in the use of the nonselective drugs is often failure to obtain desired therapeutic responses without concomitant side effects. While the latter usually are not serious, they can be sufficiently disturbing to decrease patient compliance, particularly during long-term administration. To date, selectivity has mainly been achieved by local administration, e.g., by pulmonary inhalation or instillation in the eye, since few available muscarinic antagonists show absolute selectivity. The development of allosteric modulators that recognize sites unique to particular receptor subtypes is currently considered an important approach to the development of selective drugs for the treatment of specific clinical conditions (Conn et al., 2009b).

Respiratory Tract. Ipratropium (ATROVENT, others) and tiotropium (SPIRIVA) are important agents in the treatment of chronic obstructive pulmonary disease; they are less effective in most asthmatic patients (Barnes, 2004; Barnes and Hansel, 2004; Gross, 2004). These agents often are used with inhaled long-acting β_2 adrenergic receptor agonists, although there is little evidence of true synergism. Ipratropium is administered four times daily via a metered-dose inhaler or nebulizer; tiotropium is administered once daily via a dry powder inhaler. The therapeutic uses of ipratropium and tiotropium are discussed further in Chapter 36.

Ipratropium also is FDA-approved for use in nasal inhalers for the treatment of the rhinorrhea associated with the common cold or with allergic or nonallergic perennial rhinitis. Although the ability of muscarinic antagonists to reduce nasopharyngeal secretions may provide some symptomatic relief, such therapy does not affect the natural course of the condition. It is probable that the contribution of first-generation antihistamines employed in nonprescription cold medications is due primarily to their antimuscarinic properties, except in conditions with an allergic basis (Chapter 32). *The uncomplicated common cold will generally last 2 weeks if treated and 14 days if untreated; cold medications may, however, ameliorate some of the symptoms.*

Genitourinary Tract. Overactive urinary bladder can be successfully treated with muscarinic receptor antagonists. These agents can lower intravesicular pressure, increase capacity, and reduce the frequency of contractions by antagonizing parasympathetic control of the bladder; they also may alter bladder sensation during filling (Chapple et al., 2005). Muscarinic antagonists can be used to treat enuresis in children, particularly when a progressive increase in bladder capacity is the objective, and to reduce urinary frequency and increase bladder capacity in spastic paraplegia (Chapple, 2000; Goessl et al., 2000).

The muscarinic receptor antagonists indicated for overactive bladder are oxybutynin (DITROPAN, others), tolterodine (DETROL), trospium chloride (SANCTURA), darifenacin (ENABLEX), solifenacin (VESICARE), and fesoterodine (TOVIAZ); available preparations and dosages are summarized in Table 9–3. Although some comparison trials have demonstrated small but statistically significant differences in efficacy between agents (Chapple et al., 2005), whether these efficacy differences are clinically significant is uncertain. The most important adverse reactions are consequences of muscarinic receptor blockade and include xerostomia, blurred vision, and GI side effects such as constipation and dyspepsia. CNS-related antimuscarinic effects, including drowsiness, dizziness, and confusion, can occur and are particularly problematic in elderly patients. CNS effects appear to be less likely with trospium, a quaternary amine, and with darifenacin and solifenacin; the latter agents are relatively selective for M_3 receptors and therefore have minimal effects on M_1 receptors in the CNS, which appear to play an important role in memory and cognition (Kay et al., 2006). Adverse effects can limit the tolerability of these drugs with continued use, and patient acceptance declines. Xerostomia is the most common reason for discontinuation.

Oxybutynin, the oldest of the antimuscarinics currently used to treat overactive bladder disorders, is associated with a high incidence of antimuscarinic side effects, particularly xerostomia. In an attempt to increase patient acceptance, oxybutynin is marketed as a transdermal system (OXYTROL) that is associated with a lower incidence of side effects than the oral immediate- or extended-release formulations; a topical gel formulation of oxybutynin (GELNIQUE) also appears to offer a more favorable side effect profile. Because of the extensive metabolism of oral oxybutynin by enteric and hepatic CYP3A4, higher doses are used in oral than transdermal administration; the dose may need to be reduced in patients taking drugs that inhibit CYP3A4.

Tolterodine shows selectivity for the urinary bladder in animal models and in clinical studies, resulting in greater patient acceptance; however, studies on isolated receptors do not reveal a unique subtype selectivity (Abrams et al., 1998, 1999; Chapple, 2000).

Table 9–3

Muscarinic Receptor Antagonists Used in the Treatment of Overactive Urinary Bladder

NONPROPRIETARY NAME	TRADE NAME	$t_{1/2}$ (HOURS)	PREPARATIONS[a]	DAILY DOSE (ADULT)
Oxybutynin	DITROPAN, others	2-5	IR	10-20 mg[b]
	OXYTROL		ER	5-30 mg[b]
	GELNIQUE		Transdermal patch	3.9 mg
			Topical gel	100 mg
Tolterodine	DETROL	2-9.6[c]	IR	2-4 mg[b,d]
		6.9-18[c]	ER	4 mg[b,d]
Trospium chloride	SANCTURA	20	IR	20-40 mg[e]
		35	ER	60 mg[e]
Solifenacin	VESICARE	55	IR	5-10 mg[b]
Darifenacin	ENABLEX	13-19	ER	7.5-15 mg[f]
Fesoterodine	TOVIAZ	7	ER	4-8 mg

[a]Preparations are designated as follows: IR, immediate-release tablet; ER, extended-release tablet or capsule.
[b]Doses may need to be reduced in patients taking drugs that inhibit CYP3A4.
[c]Longer times in indicated ranges are seen in poor metabolizers.
[d]Doses should be reduced in patients with significant renal or hepatic impairment.
[e]Doses should be reduced in patients with significant renal impairment; dosage adjustments also may be needed in patients with hepatic impairment.
[f]Doses may need to be reduced in patients taking drugs that inhibit CYPs 3A4 or 2D6.

Inhibition of a particular complement of receptors in the bladder may give rise to synergism and clinical efficacy. Tolterodine is metabolized by CYP2D6 to 5-hydroxymethyltolterodine. Since this metabolite possesses similar activity to the parent drug, variations in CYP2D6 levels do not affect the net antimuscarinic activity or duration of action of the drug. However, in patients who poorly metabolize tolterodine via CYP2D6, the CYP3A4 pathway becomes important in tolterodine elimination. Because it is often difficult to assess which patients will be poor metabolizers, tolterodine doses may need to be reduced in patients taking drugs that inhibit CYP3A4 (dosage adjustments generally are not necessary in patients taking drugs that inhibit CYP2D6). Patients with significant renal or hepatic impairment also should receive lower doses of the drug. Fesoterodine, a new agent, is a prodrug that is rapidly hydrolyzed to the active metabolite of tolterodine.

Trospium, a quaternary amine, is as effective as oxybutynin with better tolerability. Trospium is the only antimuscarinic used for overactive bladder that is eliminated primarily by the kidneys; 60% of the absorbed trospium dose is excreted unchanged in the urine, and dosage adjustment is necessary for patients with impaired renal function.

Solifenacin is relatively selective for muscarinic receptors of the M_3 subtype, giving it a favorable efficacy:side effect ratio (Chapple et al., 2004). Solifenacin is significantly metabolized by CYP3A4; thus, patients taking drugs that inhibit CYP3A4 should receive lower doses.

Like solifenacin, darifenacin is relatively selective for M_3 receptors. It is metabolized by CYP2D6 and CYP3A4; as with tolterodine, the latter pathway becomes more important in patients who poorly metabolize the drug by CYP2D6. Darifenacin doses may need to be reduced in patients taking drugs that inhibit either of these CYPs.

Flavoxate hydrochloride, a drug with direct spasmolytic actions on smooth muscle, especially of the urinary tract, is used for the relief of dysuria, urgency, nocturia, and other urinary symptoms associated with genitourinary disorders (e.g., cystitis, prostatitis, urethritis). Flavoxate also has weak antihistaminic, local anesthetic, analgesic, and, at high doses, antimuscarinic effects.

GI Tract. Muscarinic receptor antagonists were once widely used for the management of peptic ulcer. Although they can reduce gastric motility and the secretion of gastric acid, antisecretory doses produce pronounced side effects, such as xerostomia, loss of visual accommodation, photophobia, and difficulty in urination (Table 9–2). As a consequence, patient compliance in the long-term management of symptoms of acid-peptic disease with these drugs is poor.

Pirenzepine, a tricyclic drug similar in structure to imipramine, has selectivity for M_1 over M_2 and M_3 receptors (Caulfield, 1993; Caulfield and Birdsall, 1998). However, pirenzepine's affinities for M_1 and M_4 receptors are comparable, so it does not possess total M_1 selectivity. Telenzepine, an analog of pirenzepine, has higher potency and similar selectivity for M_1 muscarinic receptors. Both drugs are used in the treatment of acid-peptic disease in Europe, Japan, and Canada, but not currently in the U.S. At therapeutic doses of pirenzepine, the incidence of xerostomia, blurred vision, and central muscarinic disturbances is relatively low. Central effects are not seen because of the drug's limited penetration into the CNS.

Most studies indicate that pirenzepine (100-150 mg per day) produces about the same rate of healing of duodenal and gastric ulcers as the H_2 receptor antagonists cimetidine or ranitidine; it also may be effective in preventing the recurrence of ulcers (Carmine and Brogden, 1985; Tryba and Cook, 1997). Side effects necessitate drug withdrawal in <1% of patients. Studies in human subjects have shown pirenzepine to be more potent in inhibiting gastric acid secretion produced by neural stimuli than by muscarinic agonists, supporting the postulated localization of M_1 receptors at ganglionic sites. Nevertheless, H_2 receptor antagonists and proton pump inhibitors generally are considered to be the current drugs of choice to reduce gastric acid secretion (Chapter 45).

Myriad conditions known or supposed to involve increased tone (spasticity) or motility of the GI tract are treated with belladonna alkaloids (e.g., atropine, hyoscyamine sulfate [ANASPAZ, others], and scopolamine) alone or in combination with sedatives (e.g., phenobarbital [DONNATAL, others]) or antianxiety agents (e.g., chlordiazepoxide [LIBRAX]). The belladonna alkaloids and their synthetic substitutes can reduce tone and motility when administered in maximally tolerated doses, and they might be expected to be efficacious in conditions simply involving excessive smooth muscle contraction, a point that is often in doubt. M_3-selective antagonists might achieve more selectivity but are unlikely to be better tolerated, as M_3 receptors also have an important role in the control of salivation, bronchial secretion and contraction, and bladder motility. Glycopyrrolate (ROBINUL, others), a muscarinic antagonist that is structurally unrelated to the belladonna alkaloids, also is used to reduce GI tone and motility; being a quaternary amine, it is less likely to cause adverse CNS effects than atropine, scopolamine, and other tertiary amines. Alternative agents for treatment of increased GI motility and its associated symptoms are discussed in Chapter 46.

Diarrhea associated with irritation of the lower bowel, such as mild dysenteries and diverticulitis, may respond to atropine-like drugs, an effect that likely involves actions on ion transport as well as motility. However, more severe conditions such as *Salmonella* dysentery, ulcerative colitis, and Crohn's disease respond little if at all to muscarinic antagonists. The belladonna alkaloids and synthetic substitutes are very effective in reducing excessive salivation, such as drug-induced salivation and that associated with heavy-metal poisoning and Parkinson disease.

Dicyclomine hydrochloride (BENTYL, others) is a weak muscarinic receptor antagonist that also has nonspecific direct spasmolytic effects on smooth muscle of the GI tract. It is occasionally used in the treatment of diarrhea-predominant irritable bowel syndrome.

Eye. Effects limited to the eye are obtained by topical administration of muscarinic receptor antagonists to produce mydriasis and cycloplegia. Cycloplegia is not attainable without mydriasis and requires higher concentrations or more prolonged application of a given agent. Mydriasis often is necessary for thorough examination of the retina and optic disc and in the therapy of iridocyclitis and keratitis. The belladonna mydriatics may be alternated with miotics for breaking or preventing the development of adhesions between the iris and the lens. Complete cycloplegia may be necessary in the treatment of iridocyclitis and choroiditis and for accurate measurement of refractive errors.

Homatropine hydrobromide (ISOPTO HOMATROPINE, others), a semisynthetic derivative of atropine (Figure 9–2), cyclopentolate hydrochloride (CYCLOGYL, others), and tropicamide (MYDRIACYL, others) are agents used in ophthalmological practice. These agents are preferred to topical atropine or scopolamine because of their shorter duration of action. Additional information on the ophthalmological properties and preparations of these and other drugs is provided in Chapter 64.

Cardiovascular System. The cardiovascular effects of muscarinic receptor antagonists are of limited clinical utility. Generally, these agents are used only in coronary care units for short-term interventions or in surgical settings.

Atropine may be considered in the initial treatment of patients with acute myocardial infarction in whom excessive vagal tone causes sinus bradycardia or AV nodal block. Sinus bradycardia is the most common arrhythmia seen during acute myocardial infarction of the inferior or posterior wall. Atropine may prevent further clinical deterioration in cases of high vagal tone or AV block by restoring heart rate to a level sufficient to maintain adequate hemodynamic status and to eliminate AV nodal block. Dosing must be judicious; doses that are too low can cause a paradoxical bradycardia (described earlier), while excessive doses will cause tachycardia that may extend the infarct by increasing the demand for oxygen.

Atropine occasionally is useful in reducing the severe bradycardia and syncope associated with a hyperactive carotid sinus reflex. It has little effect on most ventricular rhythms. In some patients, atropine may eliminate premature ventricular contractions associated with a very slow atrial rate. It also may reduce the degree of AV block when increased vagal tone is a major factor in the conduction defect, such as the second-degree AV block that can be produced by digitalis. Selective M_2 receptor antagonists would be of potential utility in blocking ACh-mediated bradycardia or AV block; however, none is currently available for clinical use.

Central Nervous System. The belladonna alkaloids were among the first drugs to be used in the prevention of motion sickness. Scopolamine is the most effective prophylactic agent for short (4-6 hour) exposures to severe motion, and probably for exposures of up to several days. All agents used to combat motion sickness should be given prophylactically; they are much less effective after severe nausea or vomiting has developed. A transdermal preparation of scopolamine (TRANSDERM SCOP) has been shown to be highly effective when used prophylactically for the prevention of motion sickness. The drug, incorporated into a multilayered adhesive unit, is applied to the postauricular mastoid region, an area where transdermal absorption of the drug is especially efficient, resulting in the delivery of ~ 0.5 mg of scopolamine over 72 hours.

Xerostomia is common, drowsiness is not infrequent, and blurred vision occurs in some individuals. Mydriasis and cycloplegia can occur by inadvertent transfer of the drug to the eye from the fingers after handling the patch. Rare but severe psychotic episodes have been reported. As noted earlier, the preoperative use of scopolamine to produce tranquilization and amnesia is no longer recommended. Given alone in the presence of pain or severe anxiety, scopolamine may induce outbursts of uncontrolled behavior.

For many years, the belladonna alkaloids and subsequently synthetic substitutes were the only agents helpful in the treatment of Parkinson disease. Levodopa combined with carbidopa (SINEMET) and dopamine receptor agonists are currently the most important treatments for Parkinson disease, but alternative or concurrent therapy with muscarinic receptor antagonists may be required in some patients (Chapter 22). Centrally acting muscarinic antagonists are efficacious in preventing extrapyramidal side effects such as dystonias or parkinsonian symptoms in patients treated with antipsychotic drugs (Chapter 16). The muscarinic antagonists used for Parkinson disease and drug-induced extrapyramidal symptoms include benztropine mesylate (COGENTIN, others), trihexyphenidyl hydrochloride (ARTANE, others), and biperiden; all are tertiary amines that readily gain access to the CNS.

Current evidence based on studies using muscarinic receptor knockout mice, subtype-selective drugs, and early-stage clinical trials suggest that selective blockade of specific muscarinic receptor subtypes in the CNS may have important therapeutic applications. For example, selective M_1 and M_4 muscarinic antagonists may be efficacious for the treatment of Parkinson disease with fewer side effects than nonselective muscarinic antagonists, while selective M_3 antagonists may be useful in the treatment of obesity and associated metabolic abnormalities (Wess et al., 2007).

Uses in Anesthesia. The use of anesthetics that are relatively nonirritating to the bronchi has virtually eliminated the need for prophylactic use of muscarinic receptor antagonists. Atropine commonly is given to block responses to vagal reflexes induced by surgical manipulation of visceral organs. Atropine or glycopyrrolate is used with neostigmine to block its parasympathomimetic effects when the latter agent is used to reverse skeletal muscle relaxation after surgery (Chapter 11). Serious cardiac arrhythmias have occasionally occurred, perhaps because of the initial bradycardia produced by atropine combined with the cholinomimetic effects of neostigmine.

Anticholinesterase Poisoning. The use of atropine in large doses for the treatment of poisoning by anticholinesterase organophosphorus insecticides is discussed in Chapter 10. Atropine also may be used to antagonize the parasympathomimetic effects of pyridostigmine or other anticholinesterases administered in the treatment of myasthenia gravis. It does not interfere with the salutary effects at the skeletal neuromuscular junction. It is most useful early in therapy, before tolerance to muscarinic side effects of anticholinesterases have developed.

Other Therapeutic Uses of Muscarinic Antagonists. Methscopolamine bromide (PAMINE) is a quaternary ammonium derivative of scopolamine and therefore lacks the central actions of scopolamine. Although formerly used to treat peptic ulcer disease, at present it is primarily used in certain combination products for the temporary relief of symptoms of allergic rhinitis, sinusitis, and the common cold.

Homatropine methylbromide, the methyl derivative of homatropine, is less potent than atropine in antimuscarinic activity but four times more potent as a ganglionic blocking agent. Formerly used for the treatment of irritable bowel syndrome and peptic ulcer disease, at present it is primarily used with hydrocodone as an antitussive combination (HYCODAN, others).

Contraindications and Adverse Effects

Most contraindications, precautions, and adverse effects are predictable consequences of muscarinic receptor blockade: xerostomia, constipation, blurred vision, dyspepsia, and cognitive impairment. Important contraindications to the use of muscarinic antagonists include urinary tract obstruction, GI obstruction, and uncontrolled (or susceptibility to attacks of) angle-closure glaucoma. Muscarinic receptor antagonists also are contraindicated (or should be used with extreme caution) in patients with benign prostatic hyperplasia. These adverse effects and contraindications generally are of more limited concern with muscarinic antagonists that are administered by inhalation or used topically in ophthalmology.

Toxicology of Drugs with Antimuscarinic Properties

The deliberate or accidental ingestion of natural belladonna alkaloids is a major cause of poisonings. Many histamine H_1 receptor antagonists, phenothiazines, and tricyclic antidepressants also block muscarinic receptors, and in sufficient dosage, produce syndromes that include features of atropine intoxication.

Among the tricyclic antidepressants, protriptyline and amitriptyline are the most potent muscarinic receptor antagonists, with an affinity for the receptor that is ~ one-tenth of that reported for atropine. Since these drugs are administered in therapeutic doses considerably higher than the effective dose of atropine, antimuscarinic effects are often observed clinically (Chapter 15). In addition, overdose with suicidal intent is a danger in the population using antidepressants. Fortunately, most of the newer antidepressants and selective serotonin reuptake inhibitors have more limited anticholinergic properties (Cusack et al., 1994).

Like the tricyclic antidepressants, many of the older antipsychotic drugs have antimuscarinic effects. These effects are most likely to be observed with the less potent drugs, e.g., chlorpromazine and thioridazine, which must be given in higher doses. The newer antipsychotic drugs, classified as "atypical" and characterized by their low propensity for inducing extrapyramidal side effects, also include agents that are potent muscarinic receptor antagonists. In particular, clozapine binds to human brain muscarinic receptors with high affinity (10 nM, compared to 1-2 nM for atropine); olanzapine also is a potent muscarinic receptor antagonist (Richelson, 1999; Roth et al., 2004). Accordingly, xerostomia is a prominent side effect of these drugs. A paradoxical side effect of clozapine is increased salivation and drooling, possibly the result of partial agonist properties of this drug (Richelson, 1999).

Infants and young children are especially susceptible to the toxic effects of muscarinic antagonists. Indeed, cases of intoxication in children have resulted from conjunctival instillation for ophthalmic refraction and other ocular effects. Systemic absorption occurs either from the nasal mucosa after the drug has traversed the nasolacrimal duct or from the GI tract if the drug is swallowed. Poisoning with diphenoxylate-atropine (LOMOTIL, others), used to treat diarrhea, has been extensively reported in the pediatric literature. Transdermal preparations of scopolamine used for motion sickness have been noted to cause toxic psychoses, especially in children and in the elderly. Serious intoxication may occur in children who ingest berries or seeds containing belladonna alkaloids. Poisoning from ingestion and smoking of jimson weed is seen with some frequency today.

Table 9–2 shows the oral doses of atropine causing undesirable responses or symptoms of overdosage. These symptoms are predictable results of blockade of parasympathetic innervation. In cases of full-blown atropine poisoning, the syndrome may last 48 hours or longer. Intravenous injection of the anticholinesterase agent physostigmine may be used for confirmation. If physostigmine does not elicit the expected salivation, sweating, bradycardia, and intestinal hyperactivity, intoxication with atropine or a related agent is almost certain. Depression and circulatory collapse are evident only in cases of severe intoxication; the blood pressure declines, convulsions may ensue, respiration becomes inadequate, and death due to respiratory failure may follow after a period of paralysis and coma.

Measures to limit intestinal absorption should be initiated without delay if the poison has been taken orally. For symptomatic treatment, slow intravenous injection of physostigmine rapidly abolishes the delirium and coma caused by large doses of atropine, but carries some risk of overdose in mild atropine intoxication. Since physostigmine is metabolized rapidly, the patient may again lapse into coma within 1-2 hours, and repeated doses may be needed (Chapter 10). If marked excitement is present and more specific treatment is not available, a benzodiazepine is the most suitable agent for sedation and for control of convulsions. Phenothiazines or agents with antimuscarinic activity should not be used, because their antimuscarinic action is likely to intensify toxicity. Support of respiration and control of hyperthermia may be necessary. Ice bags and alcohol sponges help to reduce fever, especially in children.

CLINICAL SUMMARY

Drugs that target muscarinic receptors have a wide variety of therapeutic uses. For example, muscarinic agonists are used in the treatment of urinary retention and xerostomia; muscarinic antagonists are used in the treatment of overactive bladder, chronic obstructive pulmonary disease, and increased GI motility; and both groups of agents have important uses in ophthalmology. The cloning of five distinct muscarinic receptor subtypes and their subsequent genetic deletion in mice has raised the expectation that one might greatly improve the therapeutic utility of drugs that interact with muscarinic receptors by the development of subtype-selective agonists and antagonists. By targeting unique subsets of receptors that control muscarinic responses within a particular organ, unwanted side effects that typify the use of these drugs could be avoided. Subtype-selective muscarinic receptor agonists and antagonists show particular promise in the treatment of CNS disorders such as Alzheimer's disease and Parkinson disease. Although complete selectivity has been difficult to achieve, the development of allosteric modulators may allow enhanced selectivity and new therapeutic uses in the future.

BIBLIOGRAPHY

Abrams P, Andersson K-E, Buccafusco JJ, et al. Muscarinic receptors: their distribution and function in body systems, and the implications for treating overactive bladder. *Br J Pharmacol*, **2006**, *148*:565–578.

Abrams P, Freeman R, Anderstrom C, Mattiasson A. Tolterodine, a new antimuscarinic agent: as effective but better tolerated than oxybutynin in patients with an overactive bladder. *Br J Urol*, **1998,** *81*:801–810.

Abrams P, Larsson G, Chapple C, Wein AJ. Factors involved in the success of antimuscarinic treatment. *BJU Int*, **1999**, *83*(suppl 2):42–47.

Aihara T, Nakamura Y, Taketo MM, et al. Cholinergically stimulated gastric acid secretion is mediated by M_3 and M_5 but not M_1 muscarinic acetylcholine receptors in mice. *Am J Physiol*, **2005,** *288*:G1199–G1207.

Anaya JM, Talal N. Sjögren's syndrome comes of age. *Semin Arthritis Rheum*, **1999**, *28*:355–359.

Barnes PJ. The role of anticholinergics in chronic obstructive pulmonary disease. *Am J Med*, **2004**, *117*(suppl 12A):24S–32S.

Barnes PJ, Hansel TT. Prospects for new drugs for chronic obstructive pulmonary disease. *Lancet*, **2004**, *364*:985–996.

Berne RM, Levy MN. In, *Cardiovascular Physiology*, 8th ed. Mosby, St. Louis, **2001**.

Birdsall NJM, Larenzo S. Allosterism at muscarinic receptors: ligands and mechanisms. *Mini Rev Med Chem*, **2005**, *5*:523–543.

Bonner TI, Buckley NJ, Young AC, Brann MR. Identification of a family of muscarinic acetylcholine receptor genes. *Science*, **1987**, *237*:527–532.

Brodde OE, Michel MC. Adrenergic and muscarinic receptors in the human heart. *Pharmacol Rev*, **1999**, *51*:651–690.

Carmine AA, Brogden RN. Pirenzepine. A review of its pharmacodynamic and pharmacokinetic properties and therapeutic efficacy in peptic ulcer disease and other allied diseases. *Drugs*, **1985**, *30*:85–126.

Caulfield MP. Muscarinic receptors—characterization, coupling and function. *Pharmacol Ther*, **1993**, *58*:319–379.

Caulfield MP, Birdsall NJ. International Union of Pharmacology, XVII. Classification of muscarinic acetylcholine receptors. *Pharmacol Rev*, **1998**, *50*:279–290.

Chapple CR. Muscarinic receptor antagonists in the treatment of overactive bladder. *Urology*, **2000**, *55*(suppl. 5A):33–46.

Chapple C, Khullar V, Gabriel Z, Dooley JA. The effects of antimuscarinic treatments in overactive bladder: a systematic review and meta-analysis. *Eur Urol*, **2005**, *48*:5–26.

Chapple RR, Rechberger T, Al-Shukri S, et al. Randomized, double-blind placebo- and tolterodine-controlled trial of the once-daily antimuscarinic agent solifenacin in patients with symptomatic overactive bladder. *BJU Int*, **2004**, *93*:303–310.

Conn PJ, Christopoulos A, Lindsley CW. Allosteric modulators of GPCRs: A novel approach for the treatment of CNS disorders. *Nature Rev Drug Discov*, **2009a**, *8*:41–54.

Conn PJ, Jones CK, Lindsley CW. Subtype-selective allosteric modulators of muscarinic receptors for the treatment of CNS disorders. *Trends Pharmacol Sci*, **2009b**, *30*:148–155.

Crapo RO, Casaburi R, Coates AL, et al. Guidelines for methacholine and exercise challenge testing–1999. *Am J Respir Crit Care Med*, **2000**, *161*:309–329.

Cusack B, Nelson A, Richelson E. Binding of antidepressants to human brain receptors: focus on newer generation compounds. *Psychopharmacology (Berl)*, **1994**, *114*:559–565.

DiFrancesco D, Tromba C. Acetylcholine inhibits activation of the cardiac hyperpolarizing-activated current, i_f. *Pflugers Arch*, **1987**, *410*:139–142.

Disse B, Speck GA, Rominger KL, et al. Tiotropium (Spiriva): mechanistical considerations and clinical profile in obstructive lung disease. *Life Sci*, **1999**, *64*:457–464.

Eglen RM, Hegde SS, Watson, N. Muscarinic receptor subtypes and smooth muscle function. *Pharmacol Rev*, **1996**, *48*:531–565.

Feigl EO. Neural control of coronary blood flow. *J Vasc Res*, **1998,** *35*:85–92.

Fisher JT, Vincent SG, Gomeza, J, et al. Loss of vagally mediated bradycardia and bronchoconstriction in mice lacking M_2 or M_3 muscarinic acetylcholine receptors. *FASEB J*, **2004**, *18*:711–713.

Furchgott RF. Endothelium-derived relaxing factor: Discovery, early studies, and identification as nitric oxide. *Biosci Rep*, **1999**, *19*:235–251.

Gautam D, Heard TS, Cui Y, et al. Cholinergic stimulation of salivary secretion studied with M_1 and M_3 muscarinic receptor single- and double-knockout mice. *Mol Pharmacol*, **2004**, *66*:260–267.

Goessl C, Sauter T, Michael T, et al. Efficacy and tolerability of tolterodine in children with detrusor hyperreflexia. *Urology*, **2000**, *55*:414–418.

Goldfrank LR. Mushrooms. In, *Goldfrank's Toxicologic Emergencies*, 8th ed. (Flomenbaum NE, Goldfrank LR, Hoffman RS, et al., eds.) McGraw-Hill, New York, **2006**, pp. 1564–1576.

Gomeza J, Shannon H, Kostenis E, et al. Pronounced pharmacologic deficits in M_2 muscarinic acetylcholine receptor knockout mice. *Proc Natl Acad Sci USA*, **1999**, *96*:1692–1697.

Goyal RK, Rattan S. Neurohumoral, hormonal, and drug receptors for the lower esophageal sphincter. *Gastroenterology*, **1978**, *74*:598–619.

Gross NJ. Tiotropium bromide. *Chest*, **2004**, *126*:1946–1953.

Hamilton SE, Loose MD, Qi M, et al. Disruption of the M_1 receptor gene ablates muscarinic receptor-dependent M current regulation and seizure activity in mice. *Proc Natl Acad Sci USA*, **1997**, *94*:13311–13316.

Hegde SS, Eglen RM. Muscarinic receptor subtypes modulating smooth muscle contractility in the urinary bladder. *Life Sci*, **1999**, *64*:419–428.

Hulme EC, Lu ZL, Bee MS. Scanning mutagenesis studies of the M_1 muscarinic acetylcholine receptor. *Recept Chann*, **2003**, *9*:215–228.

Ignarro LJ, Cirino G, Casini A, Napoli C. Nitric oxide as a signaling molecule in the vascular system: An overview. *J Cardiovasc Pharmacol*, **1999**, *34*:879–886.

Kay G, Crook, T, Rekeda L, et al. Differential effects of the antimuscarinic agents darifenacin and oxybutynin ER on memory in older subjects. *Eur Urol*, **2006**, *50*:317–326.

Kent KM, Epstein SE. Neural basis for the genesis and control of arrhythmias associated with myocardial infarction. *Cardiology*, **1976**, *61*:61–74.

Kent KM, Epstein SE, Cooper T, Jacobowitz DM. Cholinergic innervation of the canine and human ventricular conducting system. Anatomic and electrophysiologic correlations. *Circulation*, **1974**, *50*:948–955.

Khurana S, Chacon I, Xie G, et al. Vasodilatory effects of cholinergic agonists are greatly dimished in aorta from $M_3R^{-/-}$ mice. *Eur J Pharmacol*, **2004**, *493*:127–132.

Köppel C. Clinical sympatomatology and management of mushroom poisoning. *Toxicon*, **1993**, *31*:1513–1540.

Krnjevíc K. Synaptic mechanisms modulated by acetylcholine in cerebral cortex. *Prog Brain Res*, **2004**, *145*:81–93.

Lakatta EG, DiFrancesco D. What keeps us ticking: a funny current, a calcium clock, or both? *J Mol Cell Cardiol*, **2009**, *47*:157–170.

Lamping KG, Wess J, Cui Y, et al. Muscarinic (M) receptors in coronary circulation. *Arterioscler Thromb Vasc Biol*, **2004**, *24*:1253–1258.

Levy MN, Schwartz PJ, eds. *Vagal Control of the Heart: Experimental Basis and Clinical Implications*. Futura, Armonk, NY, **1994.**

Lewis ME, Al-Khalidi AH, Bonser RS, et al. Vagus nerve stimulation decreases left ventricular contractility in vivo in the human and pig heart. *J Physiol*, **2001**, *534*:547–552.

Lyashkov AE, Vinogradova TM, Zahanich I, et al. Cholinergic receptor signaling modulates spotaneous firing of sinoatrial nodal cells via integrated effects on PKAH-dependent Ca^{2+} cycling and I_{KACh}. *Am J Physiol,* **2009**, *297*:949-959.

Matsui M, Motomura D, Fujikawa T, et al. Mice lacking M_2 and M_3 muscarinic acetylcholine receptors are devoid of cholinergic smooth muscle contractions but still viable. *J Neurosci*, **2002**, *22*:10627–10632.

Matsui M, Motomura D, Karasawa H, et al. Multiple functional defects in peripheral autonomic organs in mice lacking muscarinic acetylcholine receptor gene for the M_3 subtype. *Proc Natl Acad Sci USA*, **2000**, *97*:9579–9584.

May LT, Leach K, Sexton PM, Christopoulos A. Allosteric modulation of G protein-coupled receptors. *Annu Rev Pharmacol Toxicol*, **2007**, *47*:1–51.

Mirza NR, Peters D, Sparks RG. Xanomeline and the antipsychotic potential of muscarinic receptor subtype selective agonists. *CNS Drug Rev*, **2003**, *9*:159–186.

Moncada S, Higgs EA. Molecular mechanisms and therapeutic strategies related to nitric oxide. *FASEB J*, **1995**, *9*: 1319–1330.

Nawaratne V, Leach K, Suratman N, et al. New insights into the function of M_4 muscarinic acetylcholine receptors gained using a novel allosteric modulator and a DREADD (Designer Receptor Exclusively Activated by a Designer Drug). *Mol Pharmacol,* **2008**, *74*:1119–1131.

Neubig RR, Spedding M, Kenakin T, Christopoulos A. International Union of Pharmacology Committee on Receptor Nomenclature and Drug Classification. XXXVIII. Update on terms and symbols in quantitative pharmacology. *Pharmacol Rev*, **2003**, *55*:597–606.

Oberhauser V, Schwertfeger E, Rutz T, et al. Acetylcholine release in human heart atrium: influence of muscarinic autoreceptors, diabetes, and age. *Circulation*, **2001**, *103*: 1638–1643.

Ono M, Takamura E, Shinozaki K, et al. Therapeutic effect of cevimeline on dry eye in patients with Sjögren's syndrome: a randomized, double-blind clinical study. *Am J Ophthalmol*, **2004**, *138*:6–17.

Palczewski K, Kumasaka T, Hori T, et al. Crystal structure of rhodopsin: A G protein–coupled receptor. *Science*, **2000**, *289*:739–745.

Porter SR, Scully C, Hegarty AM. An update of the etiology and management of xerostomia. *Oral Surg Oral Med Oral Pathol Oral Radiol Endod*, **2004**, *97*:28–46.

Richelson E. Receptor pharmacology of neuroleptics: Relation to clinical effects. *J Clin Psychiatry*, **1999**, *10* (suppl 10):5–14.

Roth B, Sheffler DJ, Kroeze WK. Magic shotguns versus magic bullets: selectively non-selective drugs for mood disorders and schizophrenia. *Nature Rev Drug Discov*, **2004**, *3*:353–359.

Shekhar A, Potter WZ, Lightfoot J, et al. Selective muscarinic receptor agonist xanomeline as a novel treatment approach for schizophrenia. *Am J Psychiatry*, **2008**, *165*:1033–1039.

Stengel PW, Gomeza J, Wess J, Cohen ML. M_2 and M_4 receptor knockout mice: muscarinic receptor function in cardiac and smooth muscle *in vitro*. *J Pharmacol Exp Ther*, **2000**, *292*:877–885.

Trendelenburg AU, Meyer A, Wess J, Starke K. Distinct mixtures of muscarinic receptor subtypes mediate inhibition of noradrenaline release in different mouse peripheral tissues, as studied with receptor knockout mice. *Br J Pharmacol*, **2005**, *145*:1153–1159.

Tryba M, Cook D. Current guidelines on stress ulcer prophylaxis. *Drugs*, **1997**, *54*:581–596.

Valant C, Gregory, KJ, Hall NE, et al. A novel mechanism of G protein-coupled receptor functional selectivity. *J Biol Chem*, **2008**, *283*:29312–29321.

Volpicelli LA, Levey AI. Muscarinic acetylcholine receptor subtypes in cerebral cortex and hippocampus. *Progr Brain Res*, **2004**, *145*:59–66.

Wein AJ. Practical uropharmacology. *Urol Clin North Am*, **1991**, *18*:269–281.

Wellstein A, Pitschner HF. Complex dose-response curves of atropine in man explained by different functions of M_1- and M_2-cholinoceptors. *Naunyn Schmiedebergs Arch Pharmacol*, **1988**, *338*:19–27.

Wess J. Molecular biology of muscarinic acetylcholine receptors. *Crit Rev Neurobiol*, **1996**, *10*:69–99.

Wess J. Muscarinic acetylcholine receptor knockout mice: novel phenotypes and clinical implications. *Annu. Rev. Pharmacol. Toxicol.*, **2004**, *44*: 423–450.

Wess J, Eglen RM, Gautam D. Muscarinic acetylcholine receptors: mutant mice provide new insights for drug development. *Nature Rev Drug Discov*, **2007**, *6*:721–733.

Wiseman LR, Faulds D. Oral pilocarpine: A review of its pharmacological properties and clinical potential in xerostomia. *Drugs*, **1995**, *49*:143–155.

Yamada M, Lamping KG, Duttaroy A, et al. Cholinergic dilation of cerebral blood vessels is abolished in M_5 muscarinic acetylcholine receptor knockout mice. *Proc Natl Acad Sci USA*, **2001a**, *98*:14096–14101.

Yamada M, Miyakawa T, Duttaroy A, et al. Mice lacking the M_3 muscarinic acetylcholine receptor are hypophagic and lean. *Nature*, **2001b**, *410*:207–212.

Anticholinesterase Agents

Palmer Taylor

The function of acetylcholinesterase (AChE) in terminating the action of acetylcholine (ACh) at the junctions of the various cholinergic nerve endings with their effector organs or postsynaptic sites is considered in Chapter 8. Drugs that inhibit AChE are called anti-cholinesterase (anti-ChE) agents. They cause ACh to accumulate in the vicinity of cholinergic nerve terminals and thus are potentially capable of producing effects equivalent to excessive stimulation of cholinergic receptors throughout the central and peripheral nervous systems. In view of the widespread distribution of cholinergic neurons across animal species, it is not surprising that the anti-ChE agents have received extensive application as toxic agents, in the form of agricultural insecticides, pesticides, and potential chemical warfare "nerve gases." Nevertheless, several compounds of this class are widely used therapeutically; others that cross the blood-brain barrier have been approved or are in clinical trials for the treatment of Alzheimer's disease.

Prior to World War II, only the "reversible" anti-ChE agents were generally known, of which physostigmine is the prototype. Shortly before and during World War II, a new class of highly toxic chemicals, the organophosphates, was developed first as agricultural insecticides and later as potential chemical warfare agents. The extreme toxicity of these compounds was found to be due to their "irreversible" inactivation of AChE, which resulted in prolonged enzyme inhibition. Since the pharmacological actions of both the reversible and irreversible anti-ChE agents are qualitatively similar, they are discussed here as a group. Interactions of anti-ChE agents with other drugs acting at peripheral autonomic synapses and the neuromuscular junction are described in Chapters 9 and 11.

History. Physostigmine, also called *eserine,* is an alkaloid obtained from the Calabar or ordeal bean, the dried, ripe seed of *Physostigma venenosum,* a perennial plant found in tropical West Africa. The Calabar bean once was used by native tribes of West Africa as an "ordeal poison" in trials for witchcraft, in which guilt was judged by death from the poison, innocence by survival after ingestion of a bean. A pure alkaloid was isolated by Jobst and Hesse in 1864 and named physostigmine. The first therapeutic use of the drug was in 1877 by Laqueur, in the treatment of glaucoma, one of its clinical uses today. Accounts of the history of physostigmine have been presented by Karczmar (1970) and Holmstedt (2000).

After basic research elucidated the chemical basis of the activity of physostigmine, scientists began systematic investigations of a series of substituted aromatic esters of alkyl carbamic acids. Neostigmine was introduced into therapeutics in 1931 for its stimulant action on the GI tract and subsequently was reported to be effective in the symptomatic treatment of myasthenia gravis.

Remarkably, the first account of the synthesis of a highly potent organophosphorus anti-ChE, tetraethyl pyrophosphate (TEPP), was published by Clermont in 1854. It is even more remarkable that the investigator survived to report on the compound's taste; a few drops should have been lethal. Modern investigations of the organophosphorus compounds date from the 1932 publication of Lange and Krueger on the synthesis of dimethyl and diethyl phosphorofluoridates.

Upon synthesizing ~2000 compounds, Schrader defined the structural requirements for insecticidal activity [(and, as learned subsequently, for anti-ChE) (discussed later) (Gallo and Lawryk, 1991)]. One compound in this early series, parathion (a phosphorothioate), later became the most widely used insecticide of this class. Malathion, which currently is used extensively, also contains the thionophosphorus bond found in parathion. Prior to and during World War II, the efforts of Schrader's group were directed toward the development of chemical warfare agents. The synthesis of several compounds of much greater toxicity than parathion, such as sarin, soman, and tabun, was kept secret by the German government. Investigators in the Allied countries also followed Lange and Krueger's lead in the search for potentially toxic compounds; diisopropyl phosphorofluoridate (diisopropyl fluorophosphate; DFP), synthesized by McCombie and Saunders, was studied most extensively by British and American scientists.

In the 1950s, a series of aromatic carbamates was synthesized and found to have substantial selective toxicity against insects and to be potent anti-ChE agents (Ecobichon, 2000).

Structure of Acetylcholinesterase. AChE exists in two general classes of molecular forms: simple homomeric oligomers of catalytic subunits (monomers, dimers, and tetramers) and heteromeric associations of catalytic subunits with structural subunits (Massoulié, 2000; Taylor et al., 2000). The homomeric forms are found as soluble species in the cell, presumably destined for export or for association with the outer membrane of the cell, typically through an attached glycophospholipid. One heteromeric form, largely found in neuronal synapses, is a tetramer of catalytic subunits disulfide-linked to a 20,000-Da lipid-linked subunit and localized to the outer surface of the cell membrane. The other heteromeric form consists of tetramers of catalytic subunits, disulfide linked to each of three strands of a collagen-like structural subunit. This molecular species, whose molecular mass approaches 10^6 Da, is associated with the basal lamina of junctional areas of skeletal muscle.

Molecular cloning revealed that a single gene encodes vertebrate AChEs (Schumacher et al., 1986; Taylor et al., 2000). However, multiple gene products arise from alternative processing of the mRNA that differ only in their carboxyl-termini; the portion of the gene encoding the catalytic core of the enzyme is invariant. Hence, the individual AChE species can be expected to show identical substrate and inhibitor specificities.

A separate, structurally related gene encodes butyrylcholinesterase, which is synthesized in the liver and is primarily found in plasma (Lockridge et al., 1987). The cholinesterases define a superfamily of proteins whose structural motif is the α, β hydrolase-fold (Cygler et al., 1993). The family includes several esterases, other hydrolases not found in the nervous system, and surprisingly, proteins without hydrolase activity such as thyroglobulin and members of the tactin and neuroligin families of proteins (Taylor et al., 2000).

The three-dimensional structures of AChEs show the active center to be nearly centrosymmetric to each subunit, residing at the base of a narrow gorge ~20 Å in depth (Bourne et al., 1995; Sussman et al., 1991). At the base of the gorge lie the residues of the catalytic triad: Ser203, His447, and Glu334 in mammals (Figure 10–1). The catalytic mechanism resembles that of other hydrolases; the serine hydroxyl group is rendered highly nucleophilic through a charge-relay system involving the carboxylate anion from glutamate, the imidazole of histidine, and the hydroxyl of serine (Figure 10–2A).

During enzymatic attack of ACh, an ester with trigonal geometry, a tetrahedral intermediate between enzyme and substrate is formed (Figure 10–2A) that collapses to an acetyl enzyme conjugate with the concomitant release of choline. The acetyl enzyme is

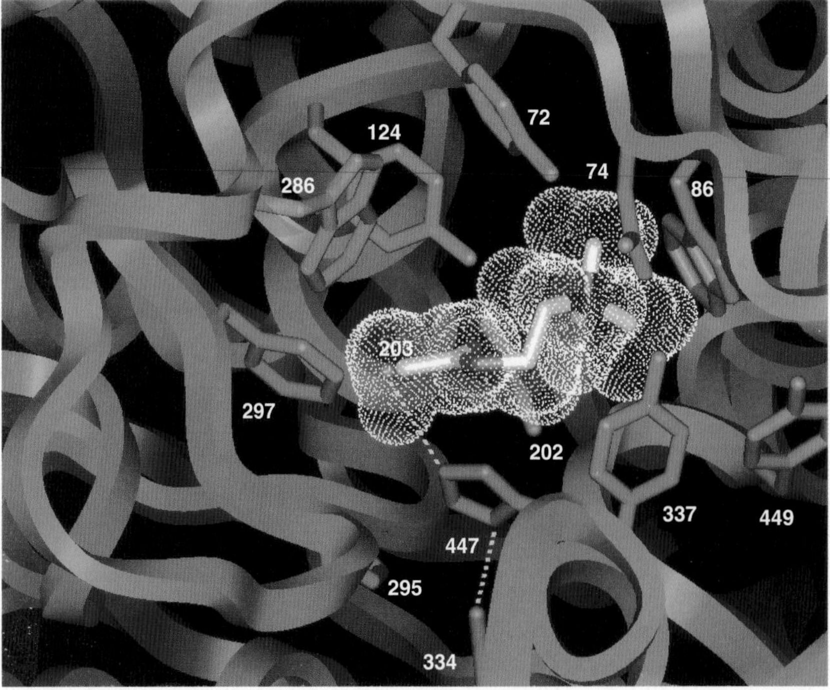

Figure 10–1. *The active center gorge of mammalian acetylcholinesterase.* Bound acetylcholine is shown by the dotted structure depicting its van der Waals radii. The crystal structure of mouse cholinesterase active center, which is virtually identical to human AChE, is shown (Bourne et al., 1995). Included are the side chains of (a) the catalytic triad, Glu334, His447, Ser203 (hydrogen bonds are denoted by the dotted lines); (b) acyl pocket, Phe295 and Phe297; (c) choline subsite, Trp86, Glu202, and Tyr337; and (d) the peripheral site: Trp286, Tyr72, Tyr124, and Asp74. Tyrosines 337 and 449 are further removed from the active center but likely contribute to stabilization of certain ligands. The catalytic triad, choline subsite, and acyl pocket are located at the base of the gorge, while the peripheral site is at the lip of the gorge. The gorge is 18-20 Å deep, with its base centrosymmetric to the subunit.

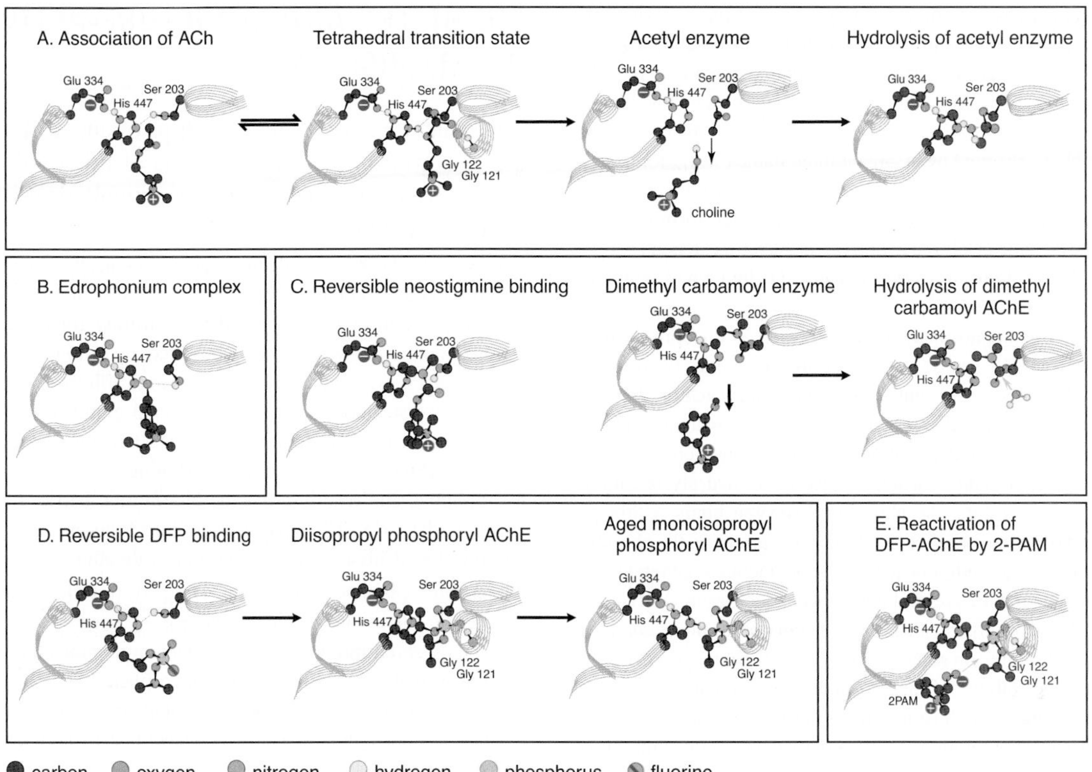

Figure 10–2. *Steps involved in the hydrolysis of acetylcholine by acetylcholinesterase and in the inhibition and reactivation of the enzyme.* Only the three residues of the catalytic triad shown in Figure 10–1 are depicted. The associations and reactions shown are: ***A.*** Acetylcholine (ACh) catalysis: binding of ACh, formation of a tetrahedral transition state, formation of the acetyl enzyme with liberation of choline, rapid hydrolysis of the acetyl enzyme with return to the original state. ***B.*** Reversible binding and inhibition by edrophonium. ***C.*** Neostigmine reaction with and inhibition of AChE: reversible binding of neostigmine, formation of the dimethyl carbamoyl enzyme, slow hydrolysis of the dimethyl carbamoyl enzyme. ***D.*** Diisopropyl fluorophosphate (DFP) reaction and inhibition of AChE: reversible binding of DFP, formation of the diisopropyl phosphoryl enzyme, formation of the aged monoisopropyl phosphoryl enzyme. Hydrolysis of the diisopropyl enzyme is very slow and is not shown. The aged monoisopropyl phosphoryl enzyme is virtually resistant to hydrolysis and reactivation. The tetrahedral transition state of ACh hydrolysis resembles the conjugates formed by the tetrahedral phosphate inhibitors and accounts for their potency. Amide bond hydrogens from Gly121 and Gly122 stabilize the carbonyl and phorphoryl oxygens. ***E.*** Reactivation of the diisopropyl phosphoryl enzyme by pralidoxime (2-PAM). 2-PAM attack of the phosphorus on the phosphorylated enzyme will form a phospho-oxime with regeneration of active enzyme. The individual steps of phosphorylation reaction and oxime reaction have been characterized by mass spectrometry (Jennings et al., 2003).

very labile to hydrolysis, which results in the formation of acetate and active enzyme (Froede and Wilson, 1971; Rosenberry, 1975). AChE is one of the most efficient enzymes known: one molecule of AChE can hydrolyze 6×10^5 ACh molecules per minute; this yields a turnover time of 100 microseconds.

Mechanism of Action of AChE Inhibitors. The mechanisms of the action of compounds that typify the three classes of anti-ChE agents are also shown in Figure 10–2.

Three distinct domains on AChE constitute binding sites for inhibitory ligands and form the basis for specificity differences between AChE and butyrylcholinesterase: the acyl pocket of the active center, the choline subsite of the active center, and the peripheral anionic site (Reiner and Radić, 2000; Taylor and Radić, 1994). Reversible inhibitors, such as edrophonium and tacrine, bind to the choline subsite in the vicinity of Trp86 and Glu202 (Silman and Sussman, 2000) (Figure 10–2B). Edrophonium has a brief duration of action because its quaternary structure facilitates renal elimination and it binds reversibly to the AChE active center. Additional reversible inhibitors, such as donepezil, bind with higher affinity to the active center.

Other reversible inhibitors, such as propidium and the snake peptidic toxin fasciculin, bind to the peripheral anionic site on AChE. This site resides at the rim of the gorge and is defined by Try286 and Tyr72 and Tyr124 (Figure 10–1).

Drugs that have a carbamoyl ester linkage, such as physostigmine and neostigmine, are hydrolyzed by AChE, but much more slowly than is ACh. The quaternary amine neostigmine and the tertiary amine physostigmine exist as cations at physiological pH. By serving as alternate substrates to ACh (Figure 10–2C), attack by the active center serine generates the carbamoylated enzyme. The carbamoyl moiety resides in the acyl pocket outlined by Phe295 and Phe297. In contrast to the acetyl enzyme, methylcarbamoyl AChE and dimethylcarbamoyl AChE are far more stable (the $t_{1/2}$ for hydrolysis of the dimethylcarbamoyl enzyme is 15-30 minutes). Sequestration of the enzyme in its carbamoylated form thus precludes the enzyme-catalyzed hydrolysis of ACh for extended periods of time. When administered systemically, the duration of inhibition by the carbamoylating agents is 3-4 hours.

The organophosphate inhibitors, such as diisopropyl fluorophosphate (DFP), serve as true hemisubstrates, since the resultant conjugate with the active center serine phosphorylated or phosphonylated is extremely stable (Figure 10–2D). The organophosphorus inhibitors are tetrahedral in configuration, a configuration that resembles the transition state formed in carboxyl ester hydrolysis. Similar to the carboxyl esters, the phosphoryl oxygen binds within the oxyanion hole of the active center. If the alkyl groups in the phosphorylated enzyme are ethyl or methyl, spontaneous regeneration of active enzyme requires several hours. Secondary (as in DFP) or tertiary alkyl groups further enhance the stability of the phosphorylated enzyme, and significant regeneration of active enzyme usually is not observed. The stability of the phosphorylated enzyme is enhanced through "aging," which results from the loss of one of the alkyl groups. Hence, the return of AChE activity depends on synthesis of a new enzyme.

Thus, the terms *reversible* and *irreversible* as applied to the carbamoyl ester and organophosphate anti-ChE agents, respectively, reflect only quantitative differences in rates of decarbamoylation or dephosphorylation of the conjugated enzyme. Both chemical classes react covalently with the active center serine in essentially the same manner as does ACh.

Action at Effector Organs. The characteristic pharmacological effects of the anti-ChE agents are due primarily to the prevention of hydrolysis of ACh by AChE at sites of cholinergic transmission. Transmitter thus accumulates, enhancing the response to ACh that is liberated by cholinergic impulses or that is spontaneously released from the nerve ending. Virtually all acute effects of moderate doses of organophosphates are attributable to this action. For example, characteristic miosis that follows local application of DFP to the eye is not observed after chronic postganglionic denervation of the eye because there is no source from which to release endogenous ACh. The consequences of enhanced concentrations of ACh at motor end-plates are unique to these sites and are discussed later.

The tertiary amine and particularly the quaternary ammonium anti-ChE compounds may have additional direct actions at certain cholinergic receptor sites. For example, the effects of neostigmine on the spinal cord and neuromuscular junction are based on a combination of its anti-ChE activity and direct cholinergic stimulation.

CHEMISTRY AND STRUCTURE-ACTIVITY RELATIONSHIPS

The structure-activity relationships of anti-ChE agents are reviewed in previous editions of this book. Only agents of general therapeutic or toxicological interest are considered here.

Noncovalent Inhibitors. While these agents interact by reversible and noncovalent association with the active site in AChE, they differ in their disposition in the body and their affinity for the enzyme. Edrophonium, a quaternary drug whose activity is limited to peripheral nervous system synapses, has a moderate affinity for AChE. Its volume of distribution is limited and renal elimination is rapid, accounting for its short duration of action. By contrast, tacrine and donepezil (Figure 10–3) have higher affinities for AChE, are more hydrophobic, and readily cross the blood-brain barrier to inhibit AChE in the CNS. Their partitioning into lipid and their higher affinities for AChE account for their longer durations of action.

"Reversible" Carbamate Inhibitors. Drugs of this class that are of therapeutic interest are shown in Figure 10–3. Early studies showed that the essential moiety of the physostigmine molecule was the methylcarbmate of an amine-substituted phenol. The quaternary ammonium derivative neostigmine is a compound of equal or greater potency. Pyridostigmine is a close congener that also is used to treat myasthenia gravis.

An increase in anti-ChE potency and duration of action can result from the linking of two quaternary ammonium moieties. One such example is the miotic agent demecarium, which consists of two neostigmine molecules connected by a series of ten methylene groups. The second quaternary group confers additional stability to the interaction by associating with a negatively charged amino side chain, Asn74, near the rim of the gorge. Carbamoylating inhibitors with high lipid solubilities (e.g., rivastigmine), which readily cross the blood-brain barrier and have longer durations of action, are approved or in clinical trial for the treatment of Alzheimer's disease (Cummings, 2004; Giacobini, 2000) (Chapter 22).

The carbamate insecticides carbaryl (SEVIN), propoxur (BAYGON), and aldicarb (TEMIK), which are used extensively as garden insecticides, inhibit ChE in a fashion identical with other carbamoylating inhibitors. The symptoms of poisoning closely resemble those of the organophosphates (Baron, 1991; Ecobichon, 2000). Carbaryl has a particularly low toxicity from dermal absorption. It is used topically for control of head lice in some countries. Not all carbamates in garden formulations are ChE inhibitors; the dithiocarbamates are fungicidal.

Organophosphorus Compounds. The general formula for this class of ChE inhibitors is presented in Table 10–1. A great variety of substituents is possible: R_1 and R_2 may be alkyl, alkoxy, aryloxy, amido, mercaptan, or other groups; and X, the leaving group, typically a conjugate base of a weak acid, is a halide, cyanide, thiocyanate, phenoxy, thiophenoxy, phosphate, thiocholine, or carboxylate group. For a compilation of the organophosphorus compounds and their toxicity, see Gallo and Lawryk (1991).

DFP produces virtually irreversible inactivation of AChE and other esterases by alkylphosphorylation. Its high lipid solubility, low molecular weight, and volatility facilitate inhalation, transdermal

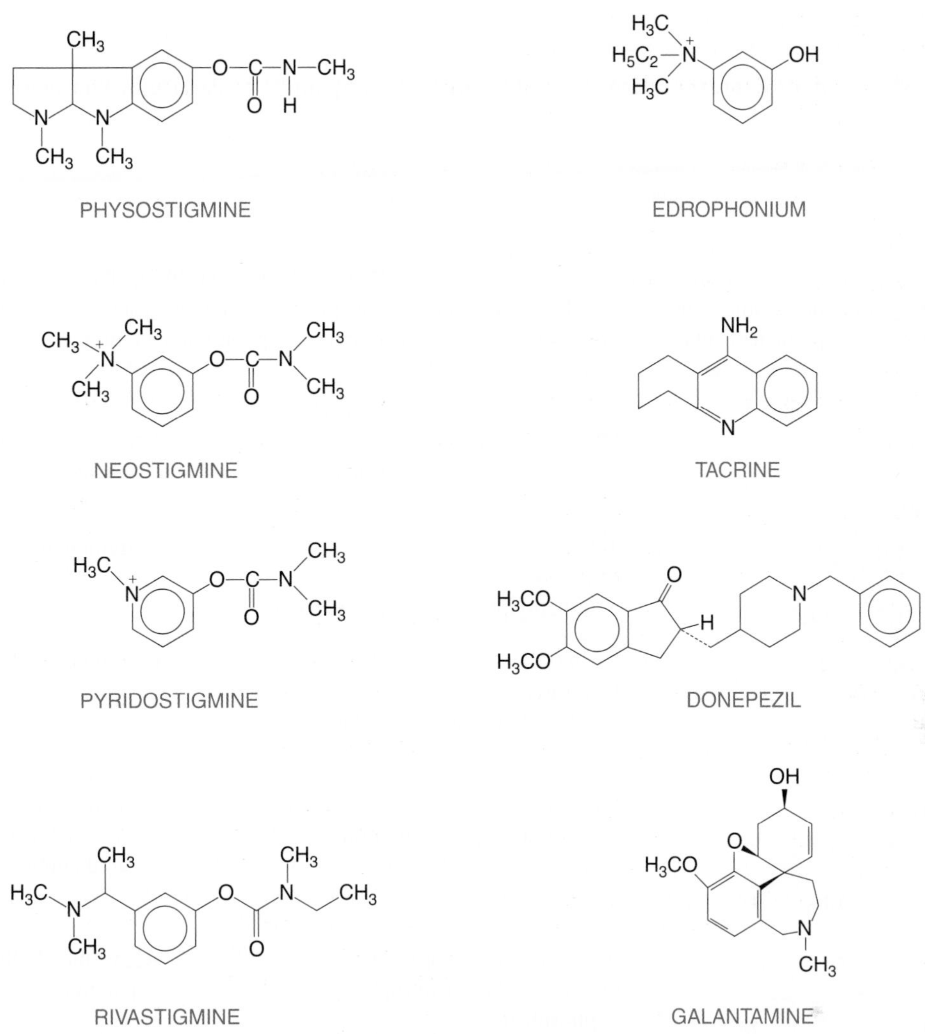

PHYSOSTIGMINE

EDROPHONIUM

NEOSTIGMINE

TACRINE

PYRIDOSTIGMINE

DONEPEZIL

RIVASTIGMINE

GALANTAMINE

Figure 10–3. *Representative "reversible" anticholinesterase agents employed clinically.*

absorption, and penetration into the CNS. After desulfuration, the insecticides in current use form the dimethoxy or diethoxyphosphoryl enzyme.

The "nerve gases"—tabun, sarin, and soman—are among the most potent synthetic toxins known; they are lethal to laboratory animals in nanogram doses. Insidious employment of these agents has occurred in warfare and terrorism attacks (Nozaki and Aikawa, 1995).

Because of their low volatility and stability in aqueous solution, parathion and methylparathion were widely used as insecticides. Acute and chronic toxicity has limited their use, and potentially less hazardous compounds have replaced them for home and garden use, now largely throughout the world. These compounds are inactive in inhibiting AChE *in vitro*; paraoxon is the active metabolite. The phosphoryl oxygen for sulfur substitution is carried out predominantly by hepatic CYPs. This reaction also occurs in the insect, typically with more efficiency. Other insecticides possessing the phosphorothioate structure have been widely employed for home, garden, and agricultural use. These include *diazinon* (SPECTRACIDE, others) and *chlorpyrifos* (DURSBAN, LORSBAN). Both of these agents have been placed under restricted use because of evidence of chronic toxicity in the newborn animal. They have been banned from indoor and outdoor residential use since 2005.

Malathion (CHEMATHION, MALA-SPRAY) also requires replacement of a sulfur atom with oxygen *in vivo,* conferring resistance to mammalian species. Also, this insecticide can be detoxified by hydrolysis of the carboxyl ester linkage by plasma carboxylesterases, and plasma carboxylesterase activity dictates species resistance to malathion. The detoxification reaction is much more rapid in mammals and birds than in insects (Costa et al., 2003). In recent years, malathion has been employed in aerial spraying of relatively populous areas for control of citrus orchard-destructive Mediterranean fruit flies and mosquitoes that harbor and transmit viruses harmful to human beings, such as the West Nile encephalitis virus.

Evidence of acute toxicity from malathion arises only with suicide attempts or deliberate poisoning. The lethal dose in mammals is ~1 g/kg. Exposure to the skin results in a small fraction (<10%) of systemic absorption. Malathion is used topically in the treatment of pediculosis (lice) infestations.

Table 10–1

Chemical Classification of Representative Organophosphorus Compounds of Particular Pharmacological or Toxicological Interest

General formula

Group **A**, X = halogen, cyanide, or thiocyanate leaving group; group **B**, X = alkylthio, arylthio, alkoxy, or aryloxy leaving group; group **C**, thionophosphorus or thio-thionophosphorus compounds; group **D**, quaternary ammonium leaving group. R_1 can be an alkyl (phosphonates), alkoxy (phosphorates) or an alkylamino (phosphoramidates) group.

GROUP	STRUCTURAL FORMULA	COMMON, CHEMICAL, AND OTHER NAMES	COMMENTS
A	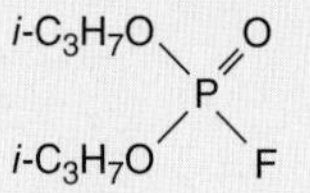 $i\text{-}C_3H_7O$, O, P, $i\text{-}C_3H_7O$, F	DFP; Isoflurophate; diisopropyl fluorophosphate	Potent, irreversible inactivator
	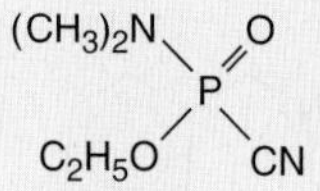 $(CH_3)_2N$, O, P, C_2H_5O, CN	Tabun Ethyl N-dimethylphosphoramidocyanidate	Extremely toxic "nerve gas"
	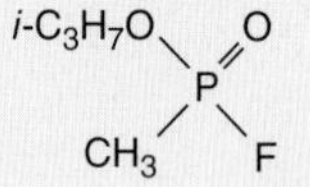 $i\text{-}C_3H_7O$, O, P, CH_3, F	Sarin (GB) Isopropyl methylphosphonofluoridate	Extremely toxic "nerve gas"
	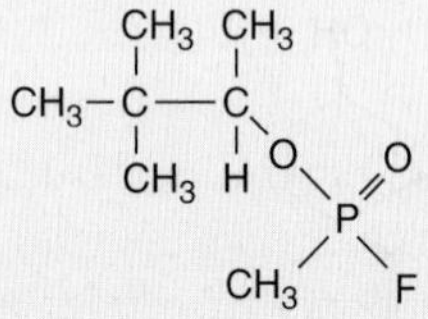 CH_3 CH_3, CH_3-C-C, CH_3 H, O, O, P, CH_3, F	Soman (GD) Pinacolyl methylphosphonofluoridate	Extremely toxic "nerve gas"; greatest potential for irreversible action/rapid aging
B	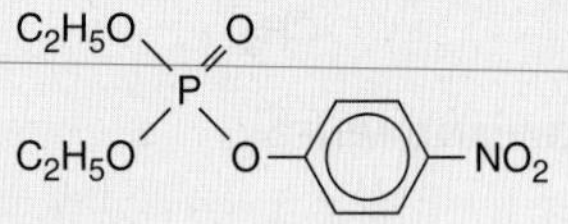 C_2H_5O, O, P, C_2H_5O, O–(phenyl)–NO_2	Paraoxon (MINTACOL), E 600 *O,O*-Diethyl *O*-(4-nitrophenyl)-phosphate	Active metabolite of parathion
	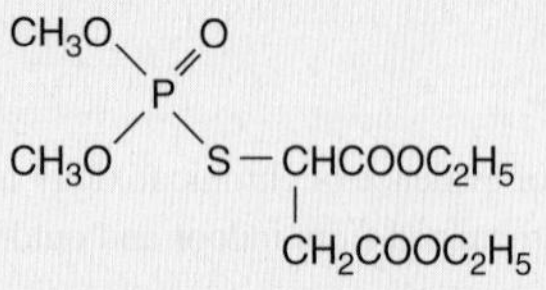 CH_3O, O, P, CH_3O, $S-CHCOOC_2H_5$, $CH_2COOC_2H_5$	Malaoxon *O,O*-Dimethyl S-(1,2-dicarboxyethyl)-phosphorothioate	Active metabolite of malathion
C	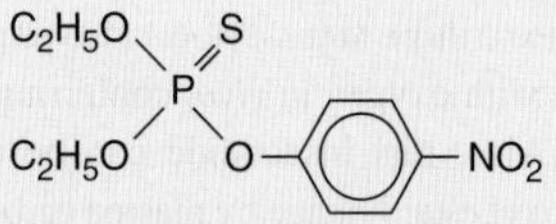 C_2H_5O, S, P, C_2H_5O, O–(phenyl)–NO_2	Parathion *O,O*-Diethyl *O*-(4-nitrophenyl)-phosphorothioate	Agricultural insecticide, resulting in numerous cases of accidental poisoning; phased out in 2003.
	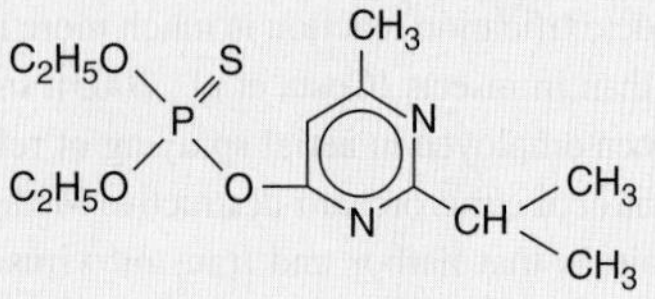 C_2H_5O, S, P, C_2H_5O, O–(pyrimidinyl: CH_3, N, N)–$CH(CH_3)_2$	Diazinon, Dimpylate *O,O*-Diethyl *O*-(2-isopropyl-6-methyl-4-pyrimidinyl) phosphorothioate	Insecticide; use limited to non-residential agricultural settings

(Continued)

Table 10–1

Chemical Classification of Representative Organophosphorus Compounds of Particular Pharmacological or Toxicological Interest (Continued)

GROUP	STRUCTURAL FORMULA	COMMON, CHEMICAL, AND OTHER NAMES	COMMENTS
C	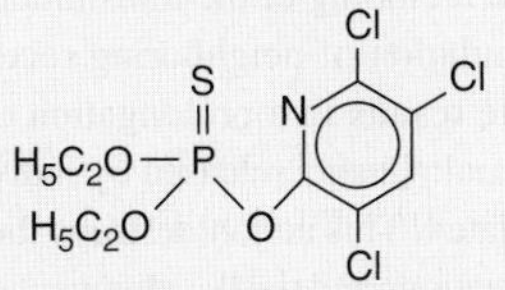 $(H_5C_2O)_2P(=S)O$–(3,5,6-trichloro-2-pyridyl)	Chlorpyrifos *O,O*-Diethyl *O*-(3,5,6-trichloro-2-pyridyl) phosphorothioate	Insecticide; use limited to non-residential agricultural settings
	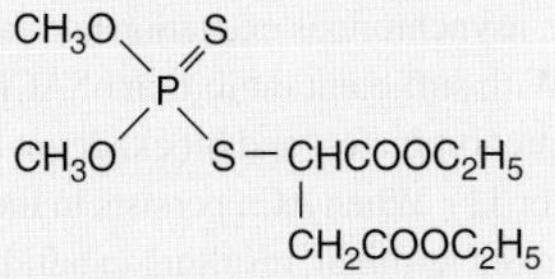 $(CH_3O)_2P(=S)S-CHCOOC_2H_5$ $\quad\quad\quad\quad\quad\quad\;\; CH_2COOC_2H_5$	Malathion *O,O*-Dimethyl S-(1,2-dicarbethoxyethyl) phosphorodithioate	Widely employed insecticide of greater safety than parathion or other agents because of rapid detoxification by higher organisms
D	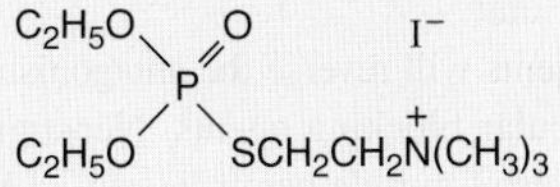 $(C_2H_5O)_2P(=O)SCH_2CH_2\overset{+}{N}(CH_3)_3\ I^-$	Echothiophate (PHOSPHOLINE IODIDE), MI-217 Diethoxyphosphinylthiocholine iodide	Extremely potent choline derivative; administered locally in treatment of glaucoma; relatively stable in aqueous solution

Among the quaternary ammonium organophosphorus compounds (group D in Table 10–1), only echothiophate is useful clinically and is limited to ophthalmic administration. Being positively charged, it is not volatile and does not readily penetrate the skin.

Metrifonate is a low-molecular-weight organophosphate that is spontaneously converted to the active phosphoryl ester, dimethyl 2,2-dichlorovinyl phosphate (DDVP, dichlorvos). Both metrifonate and DDVP readily cross the blood-brain barrier to inhibit AChE in the CNS. Metrifonate originally was developed for the treatment of schistosomiasis (Chapter 51). Its capacity to inhibit AChE in the CNS and its reported low toxicity led to its clinical trial in treatment of Alzheimer's disease (Cummings, 2004); a low incidence of skeletal muscle paralysis has limited its acceptance.

PHARMACOLOGICAL PROPERTIES

Generally, the pharmacological properties of anti-ChE agents can be predicted by knowing those loci where ACh is released physiologically by nerve impulses, the degree of nerve impulse activity, and the responses of the corresponding effector organs to ACh (see Chapter 8). The anti-ChE agents potentially can produce all the following effects:

- stimulation of muscarinic receptor responses at autonomic effector organs
- stimulation, followed by depression or paralysis, of all autonomic ganglia and skeletal muscle (nicotinic actions)
- stimulation, with occasional subsequent depression, of cholinergic receptor sites in the CNS.

Following toxic or lethal doses of anti-ChE agents, most of these effects are evident (discussed later). However, with smaller doses, particularly those used therapeutically, several modifying factors are significant. In general, compounds containing a quaternary ammonium group do not penetrate cell membranes readily; hence, anti-ChE agents in this category are absorbed poorly from the GI tract or across the skin and are excluded from the CNS by the blood-brain barrier after moderate doses. On the other hand, such compounds act preferentially at the neuromuscular junctions of skeletal muscle, exerting their action both as anti-ChE agents and as direct agonists. They have comparatively less effect at autonomic effector sites and ganglia. In contrast, the more lipid-soluble agents are well absorbed after oral administration, have ubiquitous effects at both peripheral and central cholinergic sites, and may be sequestered in lipids for long periods of time. Lipid-soluble organophosphorus agents also are well absorbed through the skin, and the volatile agents are transferred readily across the alveolar membrane (Storm et al., 2000).

The actions of anti-ChE agents on autonomic effector cells and on cortical and subcortical sites in the CNS, where the receptors are largely of the muscarinic type, are blocked by atropine. Likewise, atropine blocks some of the excitatory actions of anti-ChE agents on autonomic ganglia, since both nicotinic and muscarinic receptors are involved in ganglionic neurotransmission (Chapter 11).

The sites of action of anti-ChE agents of therapeutic importance are the CNS, eye, intestine, and the neuromuscular junction of skeletal muscle; other actions are of toxicological consequence.

Eye. When applied locally to the conjunctiva, anti-ChE agents cause conjunctival hyperemia and constriction of the pupillary sphincter muscle around the pupillary margin of the iris (miosis) and the ciliary muscle (block of accommodation reflex with resultant focusing to near vision). Miosis is apparent in a few minutes and can last several hours to days. Although the pupil may be "pinpoint" in size, it generally contracts further when exposed to light. The block of accommodation is more transient and generally disappears before termination of miosis. Intraocular pressure, when elevated, usually falls as the result of facilitation of outflow of the aqueous humor (Chapter 64).

GI Tract. In humans, neostigmine enhances gastric contractions and increases the secretion of gastric acid. After bilateral vagotomy, the effects of neostigmine on gastric motility are greatly reduced. The lower portion of the esophagus is stimulated by neostigmine; in patients with marked achalasia and dilation of the esophagus, the drug can cause a salutary increase in tone and peristalsis.

Neostigmine also augments motor activity of the small and large bowel; the colon is particularly stimulated. Atony produced by muscarinic receptor antagonists or prior surgical intervention may be overcome, propulsive waves are increased in amplitude and frequency, and movement of intestinal contents is thus promoted. The total effect of anti-ChE agents on intestinal motility probably represents a combination of actions at the ganglion cells of Auerbach's plexus and at the smooth muscle fibers, as a result of the preservation of ACh released by the cholinergic preganglionic and postganglionic fibers, respectively (Chapter 46).

Neuromuscular Junction. Most of the effects of potent anti-ChE drugs on skeletal muscle can be explained adequately on the basis of their inhibition of AChE at neuromuscular junctions. However, there is good evidence for an accessory direct action of neostigmine and other quaternary ammonium anti-ChE agents on skeletal muscle. For example, the intra-arterial injection of neostigmine into chronically denervated muscle, or muscle in which AChE has been inactivated by prior administration of DFP, evokes an immediate contraction, whereas physostigmine does not.

Normally, a single nerve impulse in a terminal motor-axon branch liberates enough ACh to produce a localized depolarization (end-plate potential) of sufficient magnitude to initiate a propagated muscle action potential. The ACh released is rapidly hydrolyzed by AChE, such that the lifetime of free ACh within the nerve-muscle synapse (~200 μsec) is shorter than the decay of the end-plate potential or the refractory period of the muscle. Therefore, each nerve impulse gives rise to a single wave of depolarization. After inhibition of AChE, the residence time of ACh in the synapse increases, allowing for lateral diffusion and rebinding of the transmitter to multiple receptors. Successive stimulation of neighboring receptors to the release site in the end plate results in a prolongation of the decay time of the end-plate potential. Quanta released by individual nerve impulses are no longer isolated. This action destroys the synchrony between end-plate depolarizations and the development of the action potentials. Consequently, asynchronous excitation and fasciculations of muscle fibers occur. With sufficient inhibition of AChE, depolarization of the end plate predominates, and blockade owing to depolarization ensues (Chapter 11). When ACh persists in the synapse, it also may depolarize the axon terminal, resulting in antidromic firing of the motoneuron; this effect contributes to fasciculations that involve the entire motor unit.

The anti-ChE agents will reverse the antagonism caused by competitive neuromuscular blocking agents. Neostigmine is not effective against the skeletal muscle paralysis caused by succinylcholine; this agent also produces neuromuscular blockade by depolarization, and depolarization will be enhanced by neostigmine.

Actions at Other Sites. Secretory glands that are innervated by postganglionic cholinergic fibers include the bronchial, lacrimal, sweat, salivary, gastric (antral G cells and parietal cells), intestinal, and pancreatic acinar glands. Low doses of anti-ChE agents augment secretory responses to nerve stimulation, and higher doses actually produce an increase in the resting rate of secretion.

Anti-ChE agents increase contraction of smooth muscle fibers of the bronchioles and ureters, and the ureters may show increased peristaltic activity.

The cardiovascular actions of anti-ChE agents are complex, since they reflect both ganglionic and postganglionic effects of accumulated ACh on the heart and blood vessels and actions in the CNS. The predominant effect on the heart from the peripheral action of accumulated ACh is bradycardia, resulting in a fall in cardiac output. Higher doses usually cause a fall in blood pressure, often as a consequence of effects of anti-ChE agents on the medullary vasomotor centers of the CNS.

Anti-ChE agents augment vagal influences on the heart. This shortens the effective refractory period of atrial muscle fibers and increases the refractory period and conduction time at the SA and AV nodes. At the ganglionic level, accumulating ACh initially is excitatory on nicotinic receptors, but at higher concentrations, ganglionic blockade ensues as a result of persistent depolarization of the cell membrane. The excitatory action on the parasympathetic ganglion cells would tend to reinforce the diminished cardiac output, whereas the opposite sequence would result from the action of ACh on sympathetic ganglion cells. Excitation followed by inhibition also is elicited by ACh at the central medullary vasomotor and cardiac centers. All of these effects are complicated further by the hypoxemia resulting from the bronchoconstrictor and secretory actions of increased ACh on the respiratory system; hypoxemia, in turn, can reinforce both sympathetic tone and ACh-induced discharge of epinephrine from the adrenal medulla. Hence, it is not surprising that an increase in heart rate is seen with severe ChE inhibitor poisoning. Hypoxemia probably is a major factor in the CNS depression that appears after large doses of anti-ChE agents. The CNS-stimulant effects are antagonized by larger doses of atropine, although not as completely as are the muscarinic effects at peripheral autonomic effector sites.

Absorption, Fate, and Excretion. Physostigmine is absorbed readily from the GI tract, subcutaneous tissues, and mucous membranes. The conjunctival instillation of solutions of the drug may result in systemic effects if measures (e.g., pressure on the inner canthus) are not taken to prevent absorption from the nasal mucosa. Parenterally administered physostigmine is largely destroyed within 2-3 hours, mainly by hydrolytic cleavage by plasma esterases; renal excretion plays only a minor role in its elimination.

Neostigmine and pyridostigmine are absorbed poorly after oral administration, such that much larger doses are needed than by the parenteral route. Whereas the effective parenteral dose of neostigmine is 0.5-2 mg, the equivalent oral dose may be 15-30 mg or more. Neostigmine and pyridostigmine are destroyed by plasma esterases, and the quaternary aromatic alcohols and parent compounds are excreted in the urine; the half-lives of these drugs are only 1-2 hours (Cohan et al., 1976).

Organophosphate anti-ChE agents with the highest risk of toxicity are highly lipid-soluble liquids; many have high vapor pressures. The less volatile agents that are commonly used as agricultural insecticides (e.g., diazinon, malathion) generally are dispersed as aerosols or as dusts adsorbed to an inert, finely particulate material. Consequently, the compounds are absorbed rapidly through the skin and mucous membranes following contact with moisture, by the lungs after inhalation, and by the GI tract after ingestion (Storm et al., 2000).

Following their absorption, most organophosphates are excreted almost entirely as hydrolysis products in the urine. Plasma and liver esterases are responsible for hydrolysis to the corresponding phosphoric and phosphonic acids. However, the CYPs are responsible for converting the inactive phosphorothioates containing a phosphorus-sulfur (thiono) bond to phosphorates with a phosphorus-oxygen bond, resulting in their activation. These enzymes also play a role in the inactivation of certain organophosphorus agents, and allelic differences are known to affect rates of metabolism (Furlong, 2007).

The organophosphate anti-ChE agents are hydrolyzed by two families of enzymes: the carboxylesterases and the paraoxonases (A-esterases). These enzymes are found in the plasma and liver and scavenge or hydrolyze a large number of organophosphates by cleaving the phosphoester, anhydride, PF, or PCN bonds. The paraoxonases are low-molecular-weight enzymes, requiring Ca^{2+} for catalysis, whose natural substrate may be lactones. Some of the isozymes are associated with high density lipoproteins, and in addition to their capacity to hydrolyze organophosphates, they may control low density lipoprotein oxidation, thereby exerting a protective effect in atherosclerosis (Harel et al., 2004; Mackness et al., 2004). Genetic polymorphisms that govern organophosphate substrate specificity and possible susceptibility to atherosclerosis have been found (Costa et al., 2003; Mackness et al., 2004). Wide variations in paraoxonase activity exist among animal species. Young animals are deficient in carboxylesterases and paraoxonases, which may account for age-related toxicities seen in newborn animals and suspected to be a basis for toxicity in human beings (Padilla et al., 2004).

Plasma and hepatic carboxylesterases (aliesterases) and plasma butyrylcholinesterase are inhibited irreversibly by organophosphates (Lockridge and Masson, 2000); their scavenging capacity for organophosphates can afford partial protection against inhibition of AChE in the nervous system. The carboxylesterases also catalyze hydrolysis of malathion and other organophosphates that contain carboxyl-ester linkages, rendering them less active or inactive. Since carboxylesterases are inhibited by organophosphates, toxicity from simultaneous exposure to two organophosphorus insecticides can be synergistic.

TOXICOLOGY

The toxicological aspects of the anti-ChE agents are of practical importance to clinicians. In addition to cases of accidental intoxication from the use and manufacture of organophosphorus compounds as agricultural insecticides, these agents have been used frequently for homicidal and suicidal purposes. Organophosphates account for as many as 80% of pesticide-related hospital admissions. The World Health Organization documents pesticide toxicity as a widespread global problem associated with over 200,000 deaths a year; most poisonings occur in Southeast Asia (Eddleston et al., 2008). Occupational exposure occurs most commonly by the dermal and pulmonary routes, while oral ingestion is most common in cases of non-occupational poisoning.

In the U.S., the Environmental Protection Agency (EPA), by virtue of revised risk assessments and the Food Quality Protection Act of 1996, has placed several organophosphate insecticides, including diazinon and chlorpyrifos, on restricted use and phase-out status in consumer products for home and garden use. A primary concern relates to children, since the developing nervous system may be particularly susceptible to certain of these agents (Eaton et al., 2008). The Office of Pesticide Programs of the EPA provides continuous reviews of the status of organophosphate pesticides, their tolerance reassessments, and revisions of risk assessments through their Web site (www.epa.gov/pesticides/op/).

Acute Intoxication. The effects of acute intoxication by anti-ChE agents are manifested by muscarinic and nicotinic signs and symptoms, and, except for compounds of extremely low lipid solubility, by signs referable to the CNS (Costa, 2006). Systemic effects appear within minutes after inhalation of vapors or aerosols. The onset of symptoms is delayed after GI and percutaneous absorption. The duration of toxic symptoms is determined largely by the properties of the compound: its lipid solubility, whether it must be activated to form the oxon, the stability of the organophosphate-AChE bond, and whether "aging" of the phosphorylated enzyme has occurred.

After local exposure to vapors or aerosols or after their inhalation, ocular and respiratory effects generally appear first. Ocular manifestations include marked miosis, ocular pain, conjunctival congestion, diminished vision, ciliary spasm, and brow ache. With acute systemic absorption, miosis may not be evident due to sympathetic discharge in response to hypotension. In addition to rhinorrhea and hyperemia of the upper respiratory tract, respiratory responses consist of tightness in the chest and wheezing respiration, caused by the combination of bronchoconstriction and increased bronchial secretion. GI symptoms occur earliest after ingestion and include anorexia, nausea and vomiting, abdominal cramps, and diarrhea. With percutaneous absorption of liquid, localized sweating and muscle fasciculations in the immediate vicinity are generally the earliest symptoms. Severe intoxication is manifested by extreme salivation, involuntary defecation and urination, sweating, lacrimation, penile erection, bradycardia, and hypotension.

Nicotinic actions at the neuromuscular junctions of skeletal muscle usually consist of fatigability and generalized weakness, involuntary twitchings, scattered fasciculations, and eventually severe weakness and paralysis. The most serious consequence is paralysis of the respiratory muscles. Knockout mice lacking the gene encoding AChE can survive under highly supportive conditions and with a special diet, but they exhibit continuous tremors and are stunted in growth (Xie et al., 2000). Mice that selectively lack AChE expression in skeletal muscle but have normal or near normal expression in brain and organs innervated by the autonomic nervous system can reproduce, but have continuous tremors and severe compromise of skeletal muscle strength. By contrast, mice with selective reductions of CNS AChE by elimination of the exons encoding alternative splices or expression of the structural subunits influencing expression in brain yield no obvious phenotype. This arises from large compensatory reductions of acetylcholine synthesis and storage and receptor responses (Camp et al., 2008; Dobbertin et al., 2009). These studies show that cholinergic systems in the CNS adapt in development to chronically diminished hydrolytic capacity for AChE.

The broad spectrum of effects of acute AChE inhibition on the CNS includes confusion, ataxia, slurred speech, loss of reflexes, Cheyne-Stokes respiration, generalized convulsions, coma, and central respiratory paralysis. Actions on the vasomotor and other cardiovascular centers in the medulla oblongata lead to hypotension.

The time of death after a single acute exposure may range from < 5 minutes to nearly 24 hours, depending on the dose, route, agent, and other factors. The cause of death primarily is respiratory failure, usually accompanied by a secondary cardiovascular component. Peripheral muscarinic and nicotinic as well as central actions all contribute to respiratory compromise; effects include laryngospasm, bronchoconstriction, increased tracheobronchial and salivary secretions, compromised voluntary control of the diaphragm and intercostal muscles, and central respiratory depression. Blood pressure may fall to alarmingly low levels and cardiac arrhythmias intervene. These effects usually result from hypoxemia and often are reversed by assisted pulmonary ventilation.

Delayed symptoms appearing after 1-4 days and marked by persistent low blood ChE and severe muscle weakness are termed the *intermediate syndrome* (Lotti, 2002). Delayed neurotoxicity also may be evident after severe intoxication (discussed later).

Diagnosis and Treatment. The diagnosis of severe, acute anti-ChE intoxication is made readily from the history of exposure and the characteristic signs and symptoms. In suspected cases of milder acute or chronic intoxication, determination of the ChE activities in erythrocytes and plasma generally will establish the diagnosis (Storm et al., 2000). Although these values vary considerably in the normal population, they usually are depressed well below the normal range before symptoms are evident.

Atropine in sufficient dosage (described later in the chapter) effectively antagonizes the actions at muscarinic receptor sites, including increased tracheobronchial and salivary secretion, bronchoconstriction, bradycardia, and to a moderate extent, peripheral ganglionic and central actions. Larger doses are required to get appreciable concentrations of atropine into the CNS. Atropine is virtually without effect against the peripheral neuromuscular compromise, which can be reversed by pralidoxime (2-PAM), a cholinesterase reactivator.

In moderate or severe intoxication with an organophosphorus anti-ChE agent, the recommended adult dose of pralidoxime is 1-2 g, infused intravenously over not < 5 minutes. If weakness is not relieved or if it recurs after 20-60 minutes, the dose should be repeated. Early treatment is very important to assure that the oxime reaches the phosphorylated AChE while the latter still can be reactivated. Many of the alkylphosphates are extremely lipid soluble, and if extensive partitioning into body fat has occurred and desulfuration is required for inhibition of AChE, toxicity will persist and symptoms may recur after initial treatment. With severe toxicities from the lipid-soluble agents, it is necessary to continue treatment with atropine and pralidoxime for a week or longer.

General supportive measures also are important, including:

- termination of exposure, by removal of the patient or application of a gas mask if the atmosphere remains contaminated, removal and destruction of contaminated clothing, copious washing of contaminated skin or mucous membranes with water, or gastric lavage

- maintenance of a patent airway, including endobronchial aspiration
- artificial respiration, if required administration of oxygen
- alleviation of persistent convulsions with diazepam (5-10 mg, intravenously)
- treatment of shock

Atropine should be given in doses sufficient to cross the blood-brain barrier. Following an initial injection of 2-4 mg, given intravenously if possible, otherwise intramuscularly, 2 mg should be given every 5-10 minutes until muscarinic symptoms disappear, if they reappear, or until signs of atropine toxicity appear. More than 200 mg may be required on the first day. A mild degree of atropine block then should be maintained for as long as symptoms are evident. The AChE reactivators can be of great benefit in the therapy of anti-ChE intoxication (described below), but their use is supplemental to the administration of atropine.

Cholinesterase Reactivators. Although the phosphorylated esteratic site of AChE undergoes hydrolytic regeneration at a slow or negligible rate, nucleophilic agents, such as hydroxylamine (NH_2OH), hydroxamic acids (RCONH—OH), and oximes (RCH=NOH), reactivate the enzyme more rapidly than does spontaneous hydrolysis. Researchers reasoned that selective reactivation could be achieved by a site-directed nucleophile, wherein interaction of a quaternary nitrogen with the negative subsite of the active center would place the nucleophile in close apposition to the phosphorus. This goal was achieved to a remarkable degree with pyridine-2-aldoxime methyl chloride (pralidoxime); reactivation with this compound occurs at a million times the rate of that with hydroxylamine. The oxime is oriented proximally to exert a nucleophilic attack on the phosphorus; a phosphoryloxime is formed, leaving the regenerated enzyme (Figure 10–2E).

Several *bis*-quaternary oximes are even more potent as reactivators for insecticide and nerve gas poisoning (described later); an example is HI-6, which is used in Europe as an antidote.

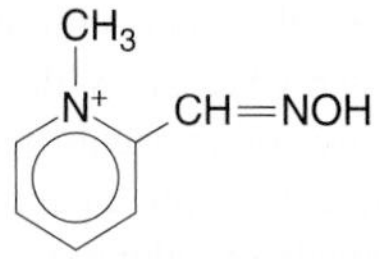

PRALIDOXIME (2-PAM)

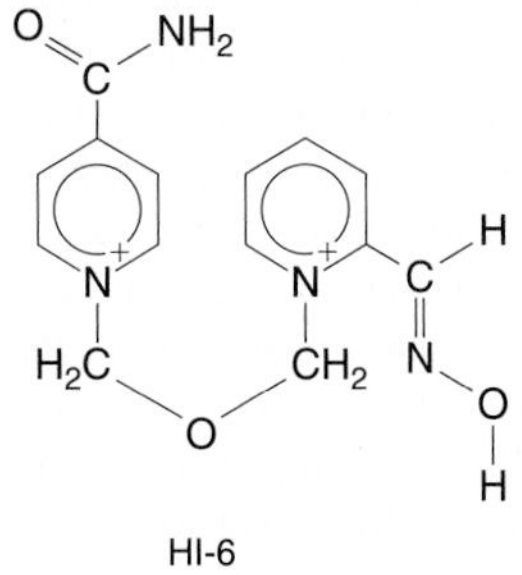

HI-6

The velocity of reactivation of phosphorylated AChE by oximes depends on their accessibility to the impacted active center serine (Wong et al., 2000). Furthermore, certain phosphorylated AChEs can undergo a fairly rapid process of "aging," so that within the course of minutes or hours they become completely resistant to the reactivators. "Aging" is due to the loss of one alkoxy group, leaving a much more stable monoalkyl- or monoalkoxy-phosphoryl-AChE (Figure 10–2D and E). Organophosphorus compounds containing tertiary alkoxy groups are more prone to "aging" than are congeners containing the secondary or primary alkoxy groups. The oximes are not effective in antagonizing the toxicity of the more rapidly hydrolyzing carbamoyl ester inhibitors; since pralidoxime itself has weak anti-ChE activity, it is not recommended for the treatment of overdosage with neostigmine or physostigmine or poisoning with carbamoylating insecticides such as carbaryl.

Pharmacology, Toxicology, and Disposition. The reactivating action of oximes *in vivo* is most marked at the skeletal neuromuscular junction. Following a dose of an organophosphorus compound that produces total blockade of transmission, the intravenous injection of an oxime can restore the response to stimulation of the motor nerve within a few minutes. Antidotal effects are less striking at autonomic effector sites, and the quaternary ammonium group restricts entry into the CNS (Eddleston et al., 2009)

Although high doses or accumulation of oximes can inhibit AChE and cause neuromuscular blockade, they should be given until one can be assured of clearance of the offending organophosphate. Many organophosphates partition into lipid and are released slowly as the active entity. Current antidotal therapy for organophosphate exposure resulting from warfare or terrorism includes parenteral atropine, an oxime (2-PAM or HI-6), and a benzodiazepine as an anticonvulsant. The oximes and their metabolites are readily eliminated by the kidney.

Parenterally administered human butyrylcholinesterase is under development as an antidote, to scavenge the AChE inhibitor in the plasma before it reaches peripheral and central tissue sites (Cerasoli et al., 2005). Because this effect of butyrylcholinesterase is stoichiometric rather than catalytic, large quantities are required.

Delayed Neurotoxicity of Organophosphorus Compounds. Certain fluorine-containing organophosphorus anti-ChE agents (e.g., DFP, mipafox) have the property of inducing delayed neurotoxicity, a property they share with the triarylphosphates, of which triorthocresyl phosphate (TOCP) is the classical example. This syndrome first received wide-spread attention following the demonstration that TOCP, an adulterant of Jamaica ginger, was responsible for an outbreak of thousands of cases of paralysis that occurred in the U.S. during Prohibition.

The clinical picture is that of a severe polyneuropathy manifested initially by mild sensory disturbances, ataxia, weakness, muscle fatigue and twitching, reduced tendon reflexes, and tenderness to palpation. In severe cases, the weakness may progress to flaccid paralysis and muscle wasting. Recovery may require several years and may be incomplete.

Toxicity from this organophosphate-induced delayed polyneuropathy is not dependent upon inhibition of cholinesterases; instead a distinct esterase, termed *neurotoxic esterase,* is linked to the lesions (Johnson, 1993). This enzyme has a specificity for hydrophobic esters, but its natural substrate and function remain unknown (Glynn, 2000). Myopathies that result in generalized necrotic lesions and changes in end-plate cytostructure also are found in experimental animals after long-term exposure to organophosphates (De Bleecker et al., 1992).

THERAPEUTIC USES

Current use of anti-AChE agents is limited to four conditions in the periphery:

- atony of the smooth muscle of the intestinal tract and urinary bladder
- glaucoma
- myasthenia gravis
- reversal of the paralysis of competitive neuromuscular blocking drugs (Chapter 11)

Long-acting and hydrophobic ChE inhibitors are the only inhibitors with well-documented efficacy, albeit limited, in the treatment of dementia symptoms of Alzheimer's disease. Physostigmine, with its shorter duration of action, is useful in the treatment of intoxication by atropine and several drugs with anticholinergic side effects (discussed later); it also is indicated for the treatment of Friedreich's or other inherited ataxias. Edrophonium has been used for terminating attacks of paroxysmal supraventricular tachycardia.

Available Therapeutic Agents. The compounds described here are those commonly used as anti-ChE drugs and ChE reactivators in the U.S. Preparations used solely for ophthalmic purposes are described in Chapter 64. Conventional dosages and routes of administration are given in the later discussion of therapeutic applications.

Physostigmine salicylate (ANTILIRIUM) is available for injection. Physostigmine sulfate ophthalmic ointment and physostigmine salicylate ophthalmic solution also are available. Pyridostigmine bromide is available for oral (MESTINON) or parenteral (REGONOL, MESTINON) use. Neostigmine bromide (PROSTIGMIN) is available for oral use. Neostigmine methylsulfate (PROSTIGMIN) is marketed for parenteral injection. Ambenonium chloride (MYTELASE) is available for oral use. *Tacrine* (COGNEX), donepezil (ARICEPT), rivastigmine (EXELON), and galantamine (REMINYL) have been approved for the treatment of Alzheimer's disease.

Pralidoxime chloride (PROTOPAM CHLORIDE) is the only AChE reactivator currently available in the U.S. and can be obtained in a parenteral formulation. HI-6 is available in several European and Near Eastern countries.

Paralytic Ileus and Atony of the Urinary Bladder. In the treatment of both these conditions, neostigmine generally is preferred among the anti-ChE agents. Directly acting muscarinic agonists (Chapter 9) are employed for the same purposes.

Neostigmine is used for the relief of abdominal distension and acute colonic pseudo-obstruction from a variety of medical and surgical causes (Ponec et al., 1999). The usual subcutaneous dose of neostigmine methylsulfate for postoperative paralytic ileus is 0.5 mg, given as needed. Peristaltic activity commences 10-30 minutes after parenteral administration, whereas 2-4 hours are required after oral administration of neostigmine bromide (15-30 mg). It may be necessary to assist evacuation with a small low enema or gas with a rectal tube.

When neostigmine is used for the treatment of atony of the detrusor muscle of the urinary bladder, postoperative dysuria is relieved, and the time interval between operation and spontaneous urination is shortened. The drug is used in a similar dose and manner as in the management of paralytic ileus. Neostigmine should not be used when the intestine or urinary bladder is obstructed, when peritonitis is present, when the viability of the bowel is doubtful, or when bowel dysfunction results from inflammatory bowel disease.

Glaucoma and Other Ophthalmologic Indications. Glaucoma is a complex disease characterized by an increase in intraocular pressure that, if sufficiently high and persistent, leads to damage to the optic disc at the juncture of the optic nerve and the retina; irreversible blindness can result. Of the three types of glaucoma—primary, secondary, and congenital—anti-AChE agents are of value in the management of the primary as well as of certain categories of the secondary type (e.g., aphakic glaucoma, following cataract extraction); congenital glaucoma rarely responds to any therapy other than surgery. Primary glaucoma is subdivided into narrow-angle (acute congestive) and wide-angle (chronic simple) types, based on the configuration of the angle of the anterior chamber where the aqueous humor is reabsorbed.

Narrow-angle glaucoma is nearly always a medical emergency in which drugs are essential in controlling the acute attack, but the long-range management is often surgical (e.g., peripheral or complete iridectomy). Wide-angle glaucoma, on the other hand, has a gradual, insidious onset and is not generally amenable to surgical improvement; in this type, control of intraocular pressure usually is dependent upon continuous drug therapy.

Since the cholinergic agonists and ChE inhibitors also block accommodation and induce myopia, these agents produce transient blurring of far vision, limited visual acuity in low light, and loss of vision at the margin when instilled in the eye. With long-term administration of the cholinergic agonists and anti-ChE agents, the compromise of vision diminishes. Nevertheless, other agents without these side effects, such as β adrenergic receptor antagonists, prostaglandin analogs, or carbonic anhydrase inhibitors, have become the primary topical therapies for open-angle glaucoma (Alward, 1998), with AChE inhibitors held in reserve for the chronic conditions when patients become refractory to the above agents. Topical treatment with long-acting ChE inhibitors such as echothiophate gives rise to symptoms characteristic of systemic ChE inhibition. Echothiophate treatment in advanced glaucoma may be associated with the production of cataracts (Alward, 1998).

Anti-ChE agents have been employed locally in the treatment of a variety of other less common ophthalmologic conditions, including accommodative esotropia and myasthenia gravis confined to the extraocular and eyelid muscles. Adie (or tonic pupil) syndrome results from dysfunction of the ciliary body, perhaps because of local nerve degeneration. Low concentrations of physostigmine are reported to decrease the blurred vision and pain associated with this condition. In alternation with a mydriatic drug such as atropine, short-acting anti-ChE agents have proven useful for breaking adhesions between the iris and the lens or cornea. (For a complete account of the use of anti-ChE agents in ocular therapy, see Chapter 64).

Myasthenia Gravis. Myasthenia gravis is a neuromuscular disease characterized by weakness and marked fatigability of skeletal muscle (Drachman, 1994); exacerbations and partial remissions occur frequently. The similarity between the symptoms of myasthenia gravis and curare poisoning in animals suggested to Jolly that physostigmine, an agent known to antagonize curare, might be of therapeutic value. Forty years elapsed before his suggestion was given systematic trial.

The defect in myasthenia gravis is in synaptic transmission at the neuromuscular junction. When a motor nerve of a normal subject is stimulated at 25 Hz, electrical and mechanical responses are well sustained. A suitable margin of safety exists for maintenance of neuromuscular transmission. Initial responses in the myasthenic patient may be normal, but they diminish rapidly, consistent with the rapid muscle fatigue seen in patients.

The relative importance of prejunctional and postjunctional defects in myasthenia gravis was a matter of considerable debate until Patrick and Lindstrom found that rabbits immunized with the nicotinic receptor purified from electric eels slowly developed muscular weakness and respiratory difficulties that resembled the symptoms of myasthenia gravis. The rabbits also exhibited decremental responses following repetitive nerve stimulation, enhanced sensitivity to curare, and following the administration of anti-AChE agents, symptomatic and electrophysiological improvement of neuromuscular transmission. This animal model prompted intense investigation into whether the natural disease represented an autoimmune response directed toward the ACh receptor. Antireceptor antibodies are detectable in sera of 90% of patients with the disease, although the clinical status of the patient does not correlate precisely with antibody titers (Drachman, 1994; Lindstrom, 2000). Sequences and the structural location in the $\alpha 1$ subunit constituting the main immunogenic region are well defined (Lindstrom 2008).

The picture that emerges is that myasthenia gravis is caused by an autoimmune response primarily to the ACh receptor at the post-junctional end plate. These antibodies reduce the number of receptors detectable either by snake α-neurotoxin-binding assays (Fambrough et al., 1973) or by electrophysiological measurements of ACh sensitivity (Drachman, 1994). Immune complexes along with marked ultrastructural abnormalities appear in the synaptic cleft and enhance receptor degradation through complement-mediated lysis in the end plate. A related disease that also compromises neuromuscular transmission is Lambert-Eaton syndrome. Here, antibodies are directed against Ca^{2+} channels that are necessary for presynaptic release of ACh (Lang et al., 1998).

In a subset of ~10% of patients presenting with a myasthenic syndrome, muscle weakness has a congenital rather than an autoimmune basis. Characterization of biochemical and genetic bases of the congenital condition has shown mutations to occur in the acetylcholine receptor which affect ligand-binding and channel-opening kinetics and durations (Engel et al., 2008; Sine and Engel, 2006). Other mutations occur as a deficiency in the form of AChE that contains the collagen-like tail unit. As expected, following administration of anti-ChE agents (see following discussion), subjective improvement is not seen in most congenital myasthenic patients, although some of the above channel syndromes can be ameliorated pharmacologically.

Diagnosis. Although the diagnosis of autoimmune myasthenia gravis usually can be made from the history, signs, and symptoms, its differentiation from certain neurasthenic, infectious, endocrine, congenital, neoplastic, and degenerative neuromuscular diseases can be challenging. However, myasthenia gravis is the only condition in which the aforementioned deficiencies can be improved dramatically by anti-ChE medication. The edrophonium test for evaluation of possible myasthenia gravis is performed by rapid intravenous injection of 2 mg of edrophonium chloride, followed 45 seconds later by an additional 8 mg if the first dose is without effect; a positive response consists of brief improvement in strength, unaccompanied by lingual fasciculation (which generally occurs in nonmyasthenic patients).

An excessive dose of an anti-ChE drug results in a *cholinergic crisis*. The condition is characterized by weakness resulting from generalized depolarization of the motor end plate; other features result from overstimulation of muscarinic receptors. The weakness resulting from depolarization blockade may resemble myasthenic weakness, which is manifest when anti-ChE medication is insufficient. The distinction is of obvious practical importance, since the former is treated by withholding, and the latter by administering, the anti-ChE agent. When the edrophonium test is performed cautiously, limiting the dose to 2 mg and with facilities for respiratory resuscitation available, a further decrease in strength indicates cholinergic crisis, while improvement signifies myasthenic weakness. Atropine sulfate, 0.4-0.6 mg or more intravenously, should be given immediately if a severe muscarinic reaction ensues (for complete details, see Drachman, 1994; Osserman et al., 1972). Detection of antireceptor antibodies in muscle biopsies or plasma is now widely employed to establish the diagnosis.

Treatment. Pyridostigmine, neostigmine, and ambenonium are the standard anti-ChE drugs used in the symptomatic treatment of myasthenia gravis. All can increase the response of myasthenic muscle to repetitive nerve impulses, primarily by the preservation of endogenous ACh. Following AChE inhibition, receptors over a greater cross-sectional area of the end plate presumably are exposed to concentrations of ACh that are sufficient for channel opening and production of a postsynaptic end-plate potential.

When the diagnosis of myasthenia gravis has been established, the optimal single oral dose of an anti-ChE agent can be determined empirically. Baseline recordings are made for grip strength, vital capacity, and a number of signs and symptoms that reflect the strength of various muscle groups. The patient then is given an oral dose of pyridostigmine (30-60 mg), neostigmine (7.5-15 mg), or ambenonium (2.5-5 mg). The improvement in muscle strength and changes in other signs and symptoms are noted at frequent intervals until there is a return to the basal state. After an hour or longer in the basal state, the drug is given again, with the dose increased to one and one-half times the initial amount, and the same observations are repeated. This sequence is continued, with increasing increments of one-half the initial dose, until an optimal response is obtained.

The duration of action of these drugs is such that the interval between oral doses required to maintain muscle strength usually is 2-4 hours for neostigmine, 3-6 hours for pyridostigmine, or 3-8 hours for ambenonium. However, the dose required may vary from day to day; physical or emotional stress, intercurrent infections, and menstruation usually necessitate an increase in the frequency or size of the dose. Unpredictable exacerbations and remissions of the myasthenic state may require adjustment of dosage. Pyridostigmine is available in sustained-release tablets containing a total of 180 mg, of which 60 mg is released immediately and 120 mg over several hours; this preparation is of value in maintaining patients for 6–8-hour periods, but should be limited to use at bedtime. Muscarinic cardiovascular and GI side effects of anti-ChE agents generally can be controlled by atropine or other anticholinergic drugs (Chapter 9). However, these anticholinergic drugs mask many side effects of an excessive dose of an anti-ChE agent. In most patients, tolerance develops eventually to the muscarinic effects. Several drugs, including curariform agents and certain antibiotics and general anesthetics, interfere with neuromuscular transmission (Chapter 11); their administration to patients with myasthenia gravis requires proper adjustment of anti-ChE dosage and other precautions.

Other therapeutic measures are essential elements in the management of this disease. Glucocorticoids promote clinical improvement in a high percentage of patients. However, when treatment with steroids is continued over prolonged periods, a high incidence of side effects may result (Chapter 42). Gradual lowering of maintenance doses and alternate-day regimens of short-acting steroids are used to minimize side effects. Initiation of steroid treatment augments muscle weakness; however, as the patient improves with continued administration of steroids, doses of anti-ChE drugs can be reduced (Drachman, 1994). Other immunosuppressive agents such as azathioprine and cyclosporine also have been beneficial in more advanced cases (Chapter 35).

Thymectomy should be considered in myasthenia associated with a thymoma or when the disease is not controlled adequately by anti-ChE agents and steroids. The relative risks and benefits of the surgical procedure *versus* anti-ChE and glucocorticoid treatment require careful assessment. Since the thymus contains myoid cells with nicotinic receptors (Schluep et al., 1987), and a predominance of patients have thymic abnormalities, the thymus may be responsible for the initial pathogenesis. It also is the source of autoreactive T-helper cells.

In keeping with the presumed autoimmune etiology of myasthenia gravis, plasmapheresis and immune therapy have proven beneficial in patients who have remained disabled in the face of other treatments (Drachman, 1994, 1996). Improvement in muscle strength correlates with the reduction of the titer of antibody directed against the nicotinic ACh receptor.

Prophylaxis in Cholinesterase Inhibitor Poisoning. Studies in experimental animals have shown that pretreatment with pyridostigmine reduces the incapacitation and mortality associated with nerve agent poisoning, particularly for agents such as soman that show rapid aging. The first large-scale administration of pyridostigmine to humans occurred in 1990 in anticipation of nerve-agent attack in the first Persian Gulf War. At an oral dose of 30 mg every 8 hours, the incidence of side effects was around 1%, but fewer than 0.1% of the subjects had responses sufficient to warrant discontinuing the drug in the setting of military action (Keeler et al., 1991). Long-term follow-up indicates that veterans of the Persian Gulf War who received pyridostigmine showed a low incidence of a neurologic syndrome, now termed the *Persian Gulf War syndrome.* It is characterized by impaired cognition, ataxia, confusion, myoneuropathy, adenopathy, weakness, and incontinence (Haley et al., 1997; Institute of Medicine, 2003). While pyridostigmine has been implicated by some as the causative agent, the absence of similar neuropathies in pyridostigmine-treated myasthenic patients makes it far more likely that a combination of agents, including combusted organophosphates and insect repellents in addition to pyridostigmine, contributed to this persisting syndrome. It also is difficult to distinguish residual chemical toxicity from post-traumatic stress experienced after combat action. Pyridostigmine is FDA-approved for prophylaxis against soman, an organophosphate that rapidly "ages" following inhibition of cholinesterases.

Intoxication by Anticholinergic Drugs. In addition to atropine and other muscarinic agents, many other drugs, such as the phenothiazines, antihistamines, and tricyclic antidepressants, have central and peripheral anticholinergic activity. Physostigmine is potentially useful in reversing the central anticholinergic syndrome produced by overdosage or an unusual reaction to these drugs (Nilsson, 1982). The effectiveness of physostigmine in reversing the anticholinergic effects of these agents has been clearly documented. However, other toxic effects of the tricyclic antidepressants and phenothiazines (Chapters 15 and 16), such as intraventricular conduction deficits and ventricular arrhythmias, are not reversed by physostigmine. In addition, physostigmine may precipitate seizures; hence, its usually small potential benefit must be weighed against this risk. The initial intravenous or intramuscular dose of physostigmine is 2 mg, with additional doses given as necessary. Physostigmine, a tertiary amine, crosses the blood-brain barrier, in contrast to the quaternary anti-AChE drugs. The use of anti-ChE agents to reverse the effects of competitive neuromuscular blocking agents is discussed in Chapter 11.

Alzheimer's Disease. A deficiency of intact cholinergic neurons, particularly those extending from subcortical areas such as the nucleus basalis of Meynert, has been observed in patients with progressive dementia of the Alzheimer type (Chapter 22). Using a rationale similar to that in other CNS degenerative diseases, therapy for enhancing concentrations of cholinergic neurotransmitters in the CNS was investigated.

In 1993, the FDA approved tacrine (tetrahydroaminoacridine) for use in mild to moderate Alzheimer's disease, but a high incidence of enhanced alanine aminotransferase and hepatotoxicity limited the utility of this drug. Other side effects were typical of AChE inhibitors.

Subsequently, donepezil was approved for clinical use. Improved cognition and global clinical function were seen in the 21–81-week intervals studied (Dooley and Lamb, 2000). In long-term studies, the drug delayed symptomatic progression of the disease for periods up to 55 weeks. Side effects are largely attributable to excessive cholinergic stimulation, with nausea, diarrhea, and vomiting being most frequently reported. The drug is well tolerated in single daily doses. Usually, 5-mg doses are administered at night; if this dose is well tolerated, the dose can be increased to 10 mg daily.

Rivastigmine, a long-acting carbamoylating inhibitor, is approved for use in the U.S. and Europe. Although fewer studies have been conducted, its efficacy, tolerability, and side effects are similar to those of donepezil (Corey-Bloom et al., 1998; Giacobini, 2000). Galantamine is another AChE inhibitor recently approved by the FDA. It has a side-effect profile similar to those of donepezil and rivastigmine.

These three cholinesterase inhibitors, which have the requisite affinity and hydrophobicity to cross the blood-brain barrier and exhibit a prolonged duration of action, along with an excitatory amino acid transmitter mimic, memantine, constitute current modes of therapy. These agents are not disease modifying and have no well-documented actions on the pathology of Alzheimer's disease. However, the bulk of the evidence indicates that they slow the decline in cognitive function and behavioral manifestation for limited intervals of time (Chapter 22). Associated symptoms, such as depression, may be preferentially delayed (Lu et al., 2009). Current clinical research efforts are directed to synergistic actions of arresting inflammatory processes or neurodegeneration and combining cholinesterase inhibition with selective cholinergic receptor modulation.

BIBLIOGRAPHY

Alward WLM. Medical management of glaucoma. *N Engl J Med,* **1998,** *339:*1298–1307.

Baron RL. Carbamate insecticides. In, *Handbook of Pesticide Toxicology,* vol. 3. (Hayes WJ Jr., Laws ER Jr., eds.) Academic Press, San Diego, **1991,** pp. 1125–1190.

Bourne Y, Marchot P, Taylor P. Acetylcholinesterase inhibition by fasciculin: crystal structure of the complex. *Cell,* **1995,** *83:*493–506.

Burkhart CG. Relationship of treatment resistant head lice to the safety and efficacy of pediculicides. *Mayo Clin Proc,* **2004,** *79:*661–666.

Camp S, DeJaco A, Zhang L, *et al.* Acetylcholinesterase expression in muscle is specifically controlled by a promoter selective enhancesome in the first intron. *J Neurosci,* **2008,** *28:*2459–2470.

Cerasoli DM, Griffiths EM, Doctor BP, et al. In vitro and in vivo characterization of recombinant human butyrylcholinesterase (Protexia) as a potential nerve agent scavenger. *Chem Biol Interactions,* **2005**, 157-158:363–365.

Cohan SL, Pohlmann JLW, Mikszewski J, O'Doherty DS. The pharmacokinetics of pyridostigmine. *Neurology,* **1976,** *26:*536–539.

Corey-Bloom J, Anand R, Veach J. A randomized trial evaluating the efficacy and safety of ENA 713 (rivastigmine tartrate), a new acetylcholinesterase inhibitor, in patients with mild to moderately severe Alzheimer's disease. *Int J Psychopharmacol,* **1998,** *1:*55–65.

Costa LG. Current issues in organophosphate toxicology. *Clin Chim Acta,* **2006**, *366:*1–13.

Costa LG, Cole TB, Furlong CE. Polymorphisms of paroxonase and their significance in clinical toxicology of organophosphates. *J Toxicol Clin Toxicol,* **2003,** *41:*37–45.

Cummings JL. Alzheimer's disease. *N Engl J Med,* **2004,** *351:*56–67.

Cygler M, Schrag J, Sussman JL, *et al.* Relationship between sequence conservation and three dimensional structure in a large family of esterases, lipases and related proteins. *Protein Sci,* **1993,** *2:*366–382.

De Bleecker J, Willems J, De Reuck J, Santens P, Lison D. Histological and histochemical study of paraoxon myopathy in the rat. *Acta Neurol Belg,* **1991,** *91:*255–70.

Dobbertin A, Hrabouska A, Dembele K, *et al.* Targeting acetylcholinesterase in neurons: A dual processing function for the praline rich membrane anchor and the attachment domain of the catalytic subunit. *J Neurosci,* **2009**, *29:*4519–4530.

Dooley M, Lamb HM Donepezil: A review of its use in Alzheimer's disease. *Drugs Aging,* **2000,** *16:*199–226.

Drachman DB. Myasthenia gravis. *N Engl J Med,* **1994,** *330:*1797–1810.

Drachman DB. Immunotherapy in neuromuscular disorders: Current and future strategies. *Muscle Nerve,* **1996,** *19:*1239–1251.

Eaton DL, Daroff RB, Autrup H, *et al.* Review of the toxicology of chlorpyrifos with an emphasis on human exposure and neurodevelopment. *Clin Rev Toxicol,* **2008,** *38:*1–125.

Ecobichon DJ. Carbamates. In, *Experimental and Clinical Neurotoxicology,* 2nd ed. (Spencer, PS, Schauburg HH, eds.) Oxford University Press, New York, **2000.**

Eddleston M, Buckley NA, Eyer P, Dawson AR. Management of acute organophosphorous pesticide poisoning. *Lancet,* **2008**, *371:*597–607.

Eddleston M, Eyer P, Worek F, Juszczak E, et al. Pralidoxime in acute organophosphorus insecticide poisoning—a randomized controlled trial. *PLoS Med,* **2009**, 6: e1000104.

Engel AG, Shen X-M, Selcen D, Sine SM. Further observations in congenital myasthenic syndromes. *Ann NY Acad Sci,* **2008,** *1132:*104–113.

Fambrough DM, Drachman DB, Satyamurti S. Neuromuscular junction in myasthenia gravis: decreased acetylcholine receptors. *Science,* **1973,** *182:*293–295.

Froede HC, Wilson IB. Acetylcholinesterase. In, *The Enzymes,* vol. 5. (Boyer PD, ed.) Academic Press, New York, **1971,** pp. 87–114.

Furlong CE. Genetic variability in the cytochrome P450–paraoxonase 1 pathway for detoxication of organophosphorus compounds. *J Biochem Molec Toxicol,* **2007**, *21:197*–205.

Gallo MA, Lawryk NJ. Organic phosphorus pesticides. In, *Handbook of Pesticide Toxicology,* vol. 2. (Hayes WJ Jr., Laws ER Jr., eds.) Academic Press, San Diego, CA, **1991,** pp. 917–1123.

Giacobini E. Cholinesterase inhibitors: From the Calabar bean to Alzheimer's therapy. In, *Cholinesterases and Cholinesterase Inhibitors.* (Giacobini E, ed.) Martin Dunitz, London, **2000,** pp. 181–227.

Glynn P. Neural development and neurodegeneration: Two faces of neuropathy target esterase. *Prog Neurobiol,* **2000,** *61:*61–74.

Haley RW, Kurt TL, Hom J. Is there a Gulf War syndrome? *JAMA,* **1997,** *277:*215–222.

Harel M, Aharoni A, Gaidukov L, *et al.* Structure and evolution of the serum paraoxonase family of detoxifying and anti-atherosclerotic enzymes. *Nat Struct Mol Biol,* **2004,** *11:*412–419.

Holmstedt B. Cholinesterase inhibitors: an introduction. In, *Cholinest-erases and Cholinesterase Inhibitors.* (Giacobini E, ed.) Martin Dunitz, London, **2000,** pp. 1–8.

Institute of Medicine (National Academy of Science–USA). *Gulf War and Health Volume 2,* National Academies Press, Washington, DC, **2003.**

Jennings LL, Malecki M, Komives EA, Taylor P. Direct analysis of the kinetic profiles of organophosphate-acetylcholinesterase adducts by MALDI-TOF mass spectrometry. *Biochemistry,* **2003,** *42:*11083–11091.

Johnson MK. Symposium introduction: retrospect and prospects for neuropathy target esterase (NTE) and the delayed polyneuropathy (OPIDP) induced by some organophosphorus esters. *Chem Biol Interact,* **1993,** *87:*339–346.

Karczmar AG. History of the research with anticholinesterase agents. In, *Anticholinesterase Agents,* vol. 1, *International Encyclopedia of Pharmacology and Therapeutics,* section 13. (Karczmar AG, ed.) Pergamon Press, Oxford, **1970,** pp. 1–44.

Keeler JR, Hurst CG, Dunn MA. Pyridostigmine used as a nerve agent pretreatment under wartime conditions. *JAMA,* **1991,** *266:*693–695.

Lang B, Waterman S, Pinto A, *et al.* The role of autoantibodies in Lambert-Eaton myasthenic syndrome. *Ann NY Acad Sci,* **1998,** *841:*596–605.

Lindstrom JM. Acetylcholine receptors and myasthenia. *Muscle Nerve,* **2000,** *23:*453–477.

Lindstrom JM. Myasthenia gravis and the tops and bottoms of AChRs-antigenic structure of the MIR and specific immunosuppression of EAMG using AChR cytoplasmic domains. *Ann NY Acad Sci,* **2008,** *1132*:29–41.

Lockridge O, Bartels CF, Vaughan TA, *et al.* Complete amino acid sequence of human serum cholinesterase. *J Biol Chem,* **1987,** *262:*549–557.

Lockridge O, Masson P. Pesticides and susceptible populations: People with butyrylcholinesterase genetic variants may be at risk. *Neurotoxicology,* **2000,** *21:*113–126.

Lotti M. Low-level exposures to organophosphorus esters and peripheral nerve function. *Muscle Nerve,* **2002,** *25:*492–504.

Lu PH, Edland SD, Teng E, *et al.* Donepezil delays progression of A.D. in MCI subjects with depressive symptoms. *Neurology* **2009**, *72:*2115–2212.

Mackness M, Durrington P, Mackness B. Paraoxonase 1 activity, concentration and genotype in cardiovascular disease. *Curr Opin Lipidol,* **2004,** *15:*399–404.

Markesbery WR (ed.). *Neuropathology of Dementing Disorders.* Arnold, London, **1998.**

Massoulié J. Molecular forms and anchoring of acetylcholinesterase. In, *Cholinesterases and Cholinesterase Inhibitors.* (Giacobini E, ed.) Martin Dunitz, London, **2000,** pp. 81–103.

Nilsson E. Physostigmine treatment in various drug-induced intoxications. *Ann Clin Res,* **1982,** *14:*165–172.

Nozaki H, Aikawa N. Sarin poisoning in Tokyo subway. *Lancet,* **1995,** *346:*1446–1447.

Osserman KE, Foldes FF, Genkins G. Myasthenia gravis. In, *Neuromuscular Blocking and Stimulating Agents,* vol. 11, *International Encyclopedia of Pharmacology and Therapeutics,* section 14. (Cheymol J, ed.) Pergamon Press, Oxford, **1972,** pp. 561–618.

Padilla S, Sung HJ, Moser VC. Further assessment of an in vitro screen that may help identify organophosphate insecticides that are more acutely toxic to the young. *J Toxicol Environ Health,* **2004,** *67:*1477–1489.

Patrick J, Lindstrom J. Autoimmune response to acetylcholine receptor. *Science,* **1973,** *180:*871–872.

Ponec RJ, Saunders MD, Kimmey MB. Neostigmine for the treatment of acute colonic pseudo-obstruction. *N Engl J Med,* **1999,** *341:*137–141.

Reiner E, Radić Z. Mechanism of action of cholinesterase inhibitors. In, *Cholinesterases and Cholinesterase Inhibitors.* (Giacobini E, ed.) Martin Dunitz, London, **2000,** pp. 103–120.

Rosenberry TL. Acetylcholinesterase. *Adv Enzymol Relat Areas Mol Biol,* **1975,** *43:*103–218.

Schluep M, Wilcox N, Vincent A, *et al.* Acetylcholine receptors in human thymic myoid cells in situ: An immunohistological study. *Ann Neurol,* **1987,** *22:*212–222.

Schumacher M, Camp S, Maulet Y, *et al.* Primary structure of *Torpedo californica* acetylcholinesterase deduced from its cDNA sequence. *Nature,* **1986,** *319:*407–409.

Silman I, Sussman JL. Structural studies on acetylcholinesterase. In, *Cholinesterases and Cholinesterase Inhibitors.* (Giacobini E, ed.) Martin Dunitz, London, **2000,** pp. 9–26.

Sine SM, Engel AG. Recent advances in Cys-loop receptor structure and function. *Nature (London)* **2006**, *440*:448–455.

Storm JE, Rozman KK, Doull J. Occupational exposure limits for 30 organophosphate pesticides based on inhibition of red blood cell acetylcholinesterase. *Toxicology,* **2000,** *150:*1–29.

Sussman JL, Harel M, Frolow F, *et al.* Atomic structure of acetylcholinesterase from *Torpedo californica:* A prototypic acetylcholine-binding protein. *Science,* **1991,** *253:*872–879.

Taylor P, Luo ZD, Camp S. The genes encoding the cholinesterases: structure, evolutionary relationships and regulation of their expression. In, *Cholinesterases and Cholinesterase Inhibitors.* (Giacobini E, ed.) Martin Dunitz, London, **2000,** pp. 63–80.

Taylor P, Radić Z. The cholinesterases: from genes to proteins. *Annu Rev Pharmacol Toxicol,* **1994,** *34:*281–320.

Wong L, Radić Z, Bruggemann RJ, *et al.* Mechanism of oxime reactivation of acetylcholinesterase analyzed by chirality and mutagenesis. *Biochemistry,* **2000,** *39:*5750–5757.

Xie W, Stribley JA, Chatonnet A, *et al.* Postnatal development delay and supersensitivity to organophosphate in gene-targeted mice lacking acetylcholinesterase. *J Pharmacol Exp Ther,* **2000,** *293:*892–902.

Agents Acting at the Neuromuscular Junction and Autonomic Ganglia

Ryan E. Hibbs and
Alexander C. Zambon

The nicotinic acetylcholine (ACh) receptor mediates neurotransmission postsynaptically at the neuromuscular junction and peripheral autonomic ganglia; in the CNS, it largely controls release of neurotransmitters from presynaptic sites. The receptor is called the *nicotinic acetylcholine receptor* because both the alkaloid nicotine and the neurotransmitter ACh can stimulate the receptor. Distinct subtypes of nicotinic receptors exist at the neuromuscular junction and the ganglia, and several pharmacological agents discriminate between the receptor subtypes.

THE NICOTINIC ACETYLCHOLINE RECEPTOR

The binding of ACh to the nicotinic ACh receptor initiates the end-plate potential (EPP) in muscle or an excitatory postsynaptic potential (EPSP) in peripheral ganglia, as was introduced in Chapter 8. Classical studies of the actions of curare and nicotine defined the concept of the nicotinic ACh receptor over a century ago and made this the prototypical pharmacological receptor. By taking advantage of specialized structures that have evolved to mediate cholinergic neurotransmission and of natural toxins that block motor activity, peripheral and then central nicotinic receptors were isolated and characterized. These accomplishments represent landmarks in the development of molecular pharmacology.

History. The electrical organs from the aquatic species of *Electrophorus* and *Torpedo* provide rich sources of nicotinic receptor. The electrical organ is derived embryologically from myoid tissue; however, in contrast to vertebrate skeletal muscle, in which motor end plates occupy 0.1% or less of the cell surface, up to 40% of the surface of the electric organ's membrane is excitable and contains cholinergic receptors. The discovery of seemingly irreversible antagonism of neuromuscular transmission by α-toxins from venoms of the krait, *Bungarus multicinctus*, or varieties of the cobra, *Naja naja,* offered suitable markers for identification of the receptor. The α-toxins are peptides of ~7 kDa. Radioisotope-labeled toxins were used in 1970 to assay the isolated cholinergic receptor *in vitro* (Changeux and Edelstein, 1998). The α-toxins have extremely high affinities and slow rates of dissociation from the receptor, yet the interaction is noncovalent. *In situ* and *in vitro,* their behavior resembles that expected for a high-affinity antagonist. Since cholinergic neurotransmission mediates motor activity in marine vertebrates and mammals, a large number of peptide, terpinoid, and alkaloid toxins that block the nicotinic receptors have evolved to enhance predation or protect plant and animal species from predation (Taylor *et al.*, 2007).

Purification of the receptor from *Torpedo* ultimately led to isolation of complementary DNAs for each of the subunits. These cDNAs, in turn, permitted the cloning of genes encoding the multiple receptor subunits from mammalian neurons and muscle (Numa et al., 1983). By simultaneously expressing various permutations of the genes that encode the individual subunits in cellular systems and then measuring binding and the electrophysiological events that result from activation by agonists, researchers have been able to correlate functional properties with details of primary structures of the receptor subtypes (Changeux and Edelstein, 2005; Karlin, 2002; Sine et al., 2008).

Nicotinic Receptor Structure. The nicotinic receptor of the electrical organ and vertebrate skeletal muscle is a pentamer composed of four distinct subunits (α, β, γ, and δ) in the stoichiometric ratio of 2:1:1:1, respectively. In mature, innervated muscle end plates, the γ subunit is replaced by ε, a closely related subunit. The individual subunits arose from a common primordial gene and are ~ 40% identical in their amino acid sequences.

The nicotinic receptor became the prototype for other pentameric ligand-gated ion channels, which include the receptors for the inhibitory amino acids (γ-aminobutyric acid and glycine; Chapter 14) and certain serotonin (5-HT_3) receptors (Chapter 13). Each of the subunits in the pentameric receptor has a molecular mass of 40-60 kDa. In each subunit, the amino-terminal ~210 residues constitute a large extracellular domain. This is followed by four transmembrane-spanning (TM) domains; the region between TM3 and TM4 forms most of the cytoplasmic component (Figure 11–1).

The five subunits are arranged around a pseudo-axis of symmetry to circumscribe a channel (Changeux and Edelstein, 1998; Karlin, 2002; Unwin, 2005). The resulting receptor is an asymmetrical molecule (16 × 8 nm) of 290 kDa, with the bulk of the non-membrane-spanning domain on the extracellular surface. The receptor is present at high densities (10,000/μm^2) in junctional areas (i.e., the motor end plate in skeletal muscle and the ventral surface of the electrical organ). The regular packing of receptors in these membranes has facilitated electron microscopic image reconstruction of the molecular structure (Figure 11–2). Agonist-binding sites are found at the subunit interfaces; in muscle, only two of the five subunit interfaces, $\alpha\gamma$ and $\alpha\delta$, have evolved to bind ligands (Figure 11-2D). Both of the subunits forming the subunit interface contribute to ligand specificity. The binding of agonists and reversible competitive antagonists involves overlapping surfaces on the receptor and is mutually exclusive.

Measurements of membrane conductance demonstrate that rates of ion translocation are sufficiently rapid (5×10^7 ions per second) to require ion translocation through an open channel rather than by a rotating carrier. Moreover, agonist-mediated changes in ion permeability (typically an inward movement of Na^+, and secondarily, of Ca^{2+}) occur through a cation channel intrinsic to the receptor structure. The TM2 regions of the five subunits form the internal perimeter of the channel. The agonist-binding site is intimately coupled with an ion channel; in the muscle receptor, simultaneous binding of two agonist molecules results in a rapid conformational change that opens the channel. Both the binding and gating response show positive cooperativity. Details on the kinetics of channel opening have emerged from electrophysiological patch-clamp techniques that distinguish the individual opening and closing events of a single receptor (Sakmann, 1992).

An ACh-binding protein homologous to only the extracellular domain of the nicotinic receptor has been identified in fresh- and saltwater snails and characterized structurally and pharmacologically (Brejc et al., 2001). This protein assembles as a homomeric pentamer and binds nicotinic receptor ligands with selectivity similar to neuronal nicotinic ACh receptors; its crystal structure reveals an atomic organization expected of the nicotinic receptor. Moreover, fusion of the ACh-binding protein and the transmembrane spans of the receptor yields a functional protein that exhibits the channel gating and changes in state expected of the receptor (Bouzat et al., 2004). This binding protein serves as both a structural and functional surrogate of the receptor and has provided a detailed understanding of the determinants governing ligand specificity of the nicotinic receptor.

Neuronal Nicotinic Receptor Composition. Cloning by sequence homology identified the genes encoding the vertebrate nicotinic receptor. Neuronal nicotinic receptors found in ganglia and the CNS also exist as pentamers of one, two, or more types of subunits. A single subunit of the α-type sequence (denoted as $\alpha 1$) is found in

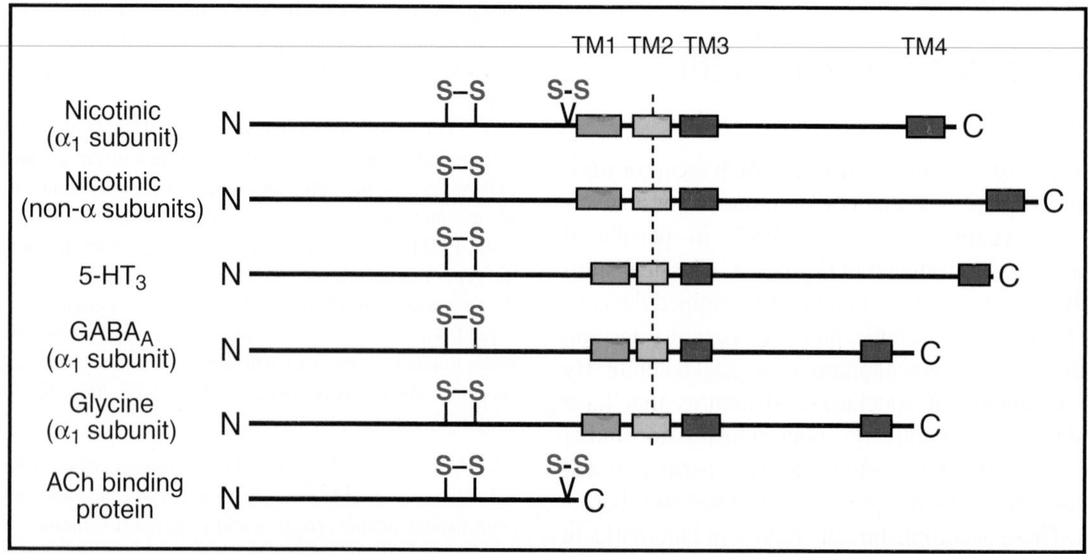

Figure 11–1. *Subunit organization of pentameric ligand-gated ion channels and the ACh binding protein.* For each receptor, the amino terminal region of ~ 210 amino acids is found at the extracellular surface. It is then followed by four hydrophobic regions that span the membrane (TM1-TM4), leaving the small carboxyl terminus on the extracellular surface. The TM2 region is α-helical, and TM2 regions from each subunit of the pentameric receptor line the internal pore of the receptor. Two disulfide loops at positions 128–142 and 192–193 are found in the α-subunit of the nicotinic receptor. The 128–142 motif is conserved in the family of receptors, whereas the vicinal cysteines at 192 and 193 distinguish α- subunits and the acetylcholine binding protein from β, γ, δ, and ε in the nicotinic receptor.

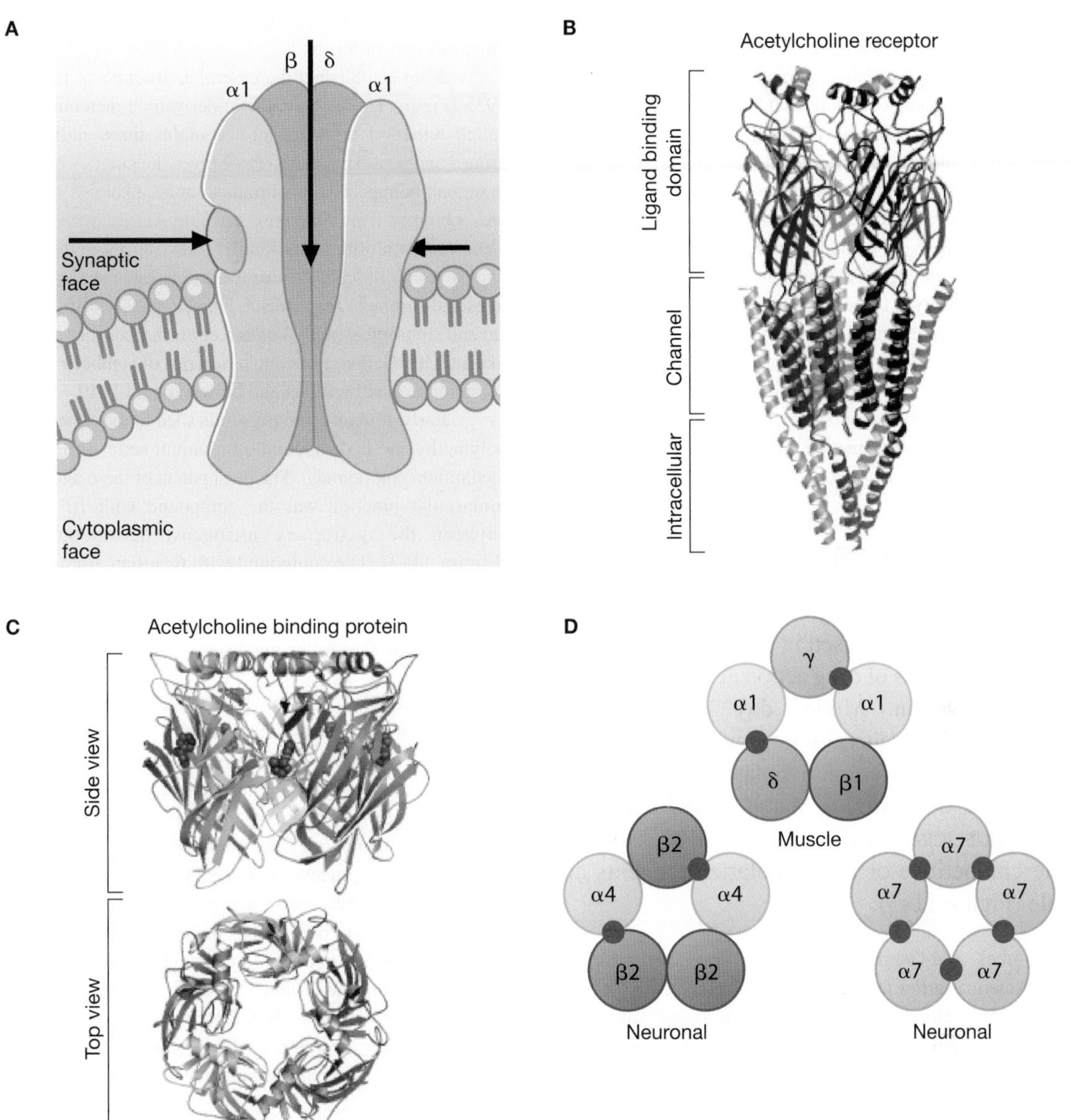

Figure 11–2. *Subunit arrangement and molecular structure of the nicotinic acetylcholine receptor.* **A.** Longitudinal view of receptor schematic with the γ subunit removed. The remaining subunits, two copies of α, one of β, and one of δ, are shown to surround an internal channel with an outer vestibule and its constriction located deep in the membrane bilayer region. Spans of α-helices with slightly bowed structures form the perimeter of the channel and come from the TM2 region of the linear sequence (Figure 11–1). Acetylcholine (ACh) binding sites, indicated by arrows, are found at the $\alpha\gamma$ and $\alpha\delta$ (not visible) interfaces. **B.** Longitudinal view of the receptor from *Torpedo* showing secondary structure and membrane topology from 4 Å electron micrograph data (Unwin, 2005). The ACh binding protein (panel ***C***) is homologous to the extracellular domain of the nicotinic receptor (Figure 11–1). The protein is a homopentamer that binds nicotinic receptor ligands with the expected selectivity and, when fused to the TM portions of the receptor, yields a functional ligand-gated channel. The subunit structure of the ACh binding protein is clear from the top view (panel ***C***, *upper orientation*) and side view (panel ***C***, *lower orientation*). The agonist nicotine is shown bound to the ACh binding protein with its atoms modeled as spheres in ***C***. Nicotinic receptor subunit arrangement is shown in ***D***, with examples of subunit assembly and location of agonist binding sites (small red circles) at α subunit-containing interfaces in nicotinic receptors. A total of 17 functional receptor isoforms have been observed *in vivo*, with different ligand specificity, relative Ca^{2+}/Na^{+} permeability, and physiological function as determined by their subunit composition. The only isoform found at the neuromuscular junction (and in the electric organ of *Torpedo*) is that shown here. The 16 neuronal receptor isoforms, found at autonomic ganglia and in the central nervous system, form homo- and heteropentameric nicotinic receptors composed of α2-α10 and β2-β4 subunits.

abundance in muscle, along with β, δ, and γ or ε. At least eight subtypes of α ($\alpha 2$ through $\alpha 9$) and three of the non-α type (designated as $\beta 2$ through $\beta 4$) are found in neuronal tissues (Figure 11–2). Studies of neuronal receptor subunit abundance and associations in brain and the periphery have enabled investigators to identify subunit combinations that confer function. Although not all permutations of α and β subunits lead to functional receptors, the diversity in subunit composition is large and exceeds the capacity of ligands to distinguish subtypes on the basis of their selectivity. For example, the $\alpha 3/\beta 4$ and $\alpha 3/\beta 2$ subtypes are prevalent in peripheral ganglia, whereas the $\alpha 4/\beta 2$ subtype is most prevalent in brain. The subtypes $\alpha 2$ through $\alpha 6$ and $\beta 2$ through $\beta 4$ associate as heteromeric pentamers composed of two or three distinct subtypes, whereas $\alpha 7$ through $\alpha 9$ often are seen as homomeric associations. Distinctive selectivities of the receptor subtypes for Na^+ and Ca^{2+} suggest that certain subtypes may possess functions other than rapid trans-synaptic signaling.

NEUROMUSCULAR BLOCKING AGENTS

The classical neuromuscular blocker, curare, was the tool that Claude Bernard used in the mid-19th century to demonstrate a locus of drug action at or near the neuromuscular junction. Modern-day neuromuscular blocking agents fall generally into two classes, depolarizing and competitive/non-depolarizing. At present, only a single depolarizing agent, succinylcholine (ANECTINE, QUELICIN), is in general clinical use, whereas multiple competitive or non-depolarizing agents are available (Figure 11–3).

History, Sources, and Chemistry. Curare is a generic term for various South American arrow poisons. The drug has been used for centuries by Indians along the Amazon and Orinoco Rivers for immobilizing and paralyzing wild animals used for food; death results from paralysis of skeletal muscles. The preparation of curare was long shrouded in mystery and was entrusted only to tribal witch doctors. Soon after the discovery of the American continent, European explorers and botanists became interested in curare, and late in the 16th century, samples of the native preparations were brought to Europe. Following the pioneering work of the scientist/explorer von Humboldt in 1805, the botanical sources of curare became the object of much field research. The curares from eastern Amazonia come from *Strychnos* species; these and other South American species of *Strychnos* contain chiefly quaternary neuromuscular-blocking alkaloids. The Asiatic, African, and Australian species nearly all contain tertiary strychnine-like alkaloids.

The modern clinical use of curare apparently dates from 1932, when West employed highly purified fractions in patients with tetanus and spastic disorders. Research on curare was accelerated greatly by the work of Gill, who, after prolonged and intimate study of the native methods of preparing curare, brought to the U.S. a sufficient amount of the authentic drug to permit chemical and pharmacological investigations. Griffith and Johnson reported the first trial of curare for promoting muscular relaxation in general anesthesia in 1942. Details of the fascinating history of curare and the chemical identification of the curare alkaloids are presented in previous editions of this book.

King established the essential structure of tubocurarine in 1935 (Figure 11–3). A synthetic derivative, metocurine (formerly called dimethyl tubocurarine), contains three additional methyl groups and possesses two to three times the potency of tubocurarine in human beings. The most potent curare alkaloids are the toxiferines, obtained from *Strychnos toxifera*. A semisynthetic derivative, alcuronium chloride (*N,N*′-diallylnortoxiferinium dichloride), was widely used clinically in Europe and elsewhere. The seeds of the trees and shrubs of the genus *Erythrina,* widely distributed in tropical and subtropical areas, contain erythroidines that possess curare-like activity. Gallamine is one of a series of synthetic substitutes for curare described by Bovet and co-workers in 1949.

Early structure-activity studies led to the development of the polymethylene *bis*-trimethyl-ammonium series (referred to as the methonium compounds). The most potent of these agents at the neuromuscular junction was the compound with 10 carbon atoms between the quaternary nitrogens: decamethonium (C10) (Figure 11–3). The compound with 6 carbon atoms in the chain, hexamethonium (C6), was found to be essentially devoid of neuromuscular blocking activity but particularly effective as a ganglionic blocking agent (see following discussion).

Structure-Activity Relationships. Several structural features distinguish competitive and depolarizing neuromuscular blocking agents. The competitive agents (e.g., tubocurarine, the benzylisoquinolines, the ammonio steroids, and the asymmetric mixed-onium chlorofumarates) are relatively bulky, rigid molecules, whereas the depolarizing agents (e.g., decamethonium [no longer marketed in the U.S. and succinylcholine) generally have more flexible structures that enable free bond rotations (Figure 11–3). While the distance between quaternary groups in the flexible depolarizing agents can vary up to the limit of the maximal bond distance (1.45 nm for decamethonium), the distance for the rigid competitive blockers is typically 1.0 ± 0.1 nm. L-Tubocurarine is considerably less potent than D-tubocurarine, perhaps because the D-isomer has all the hydrophilic groups localized uniquely to one surface.

Pharmacological Properties

Actions on Organ Systems

Skeletal Muscle. Claude Bernard first described a localized paralytic action of curare in the 1850s. The site of action of D-tubocurarine and other competitive blocking agents was identified as the motor end plate (a thickened region of postjunctional membrane) by fluorescence and electron microscopy, micro-iontophoretic application of drugs, patch-clamp analysis of single channels, and intracellular recording. Competitive antagonists combine with the nicotinic ACh receptor at the end plate and thereby competitively block the binding of ACh. When the drug is applied directly to the end plate of a single isolated muscle fiber, the muscle cell becomes insensitive to motor-nerve impulses and to directly applied ACh; however, the end-plate region

Depolarizing Neuromuscular Blockers

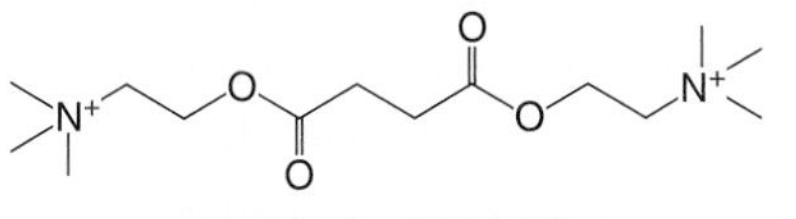

SUCCINYLCHOLINE

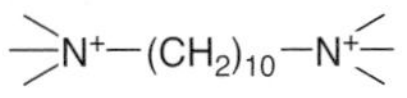

DECAMETHONIUM

Benzylisoquinoline Competitive Neuromuscular Blockers

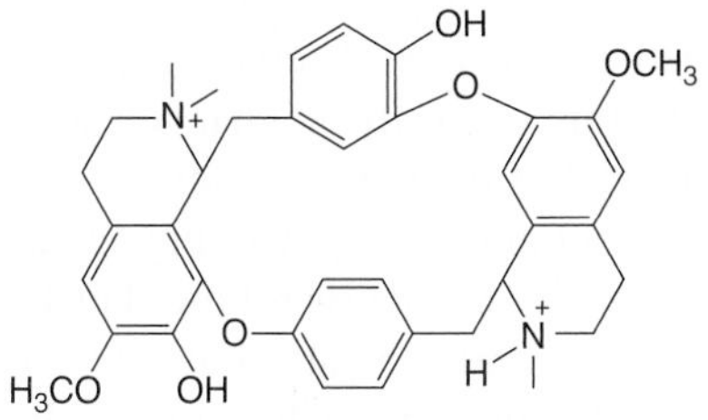

TUBOCURARINE

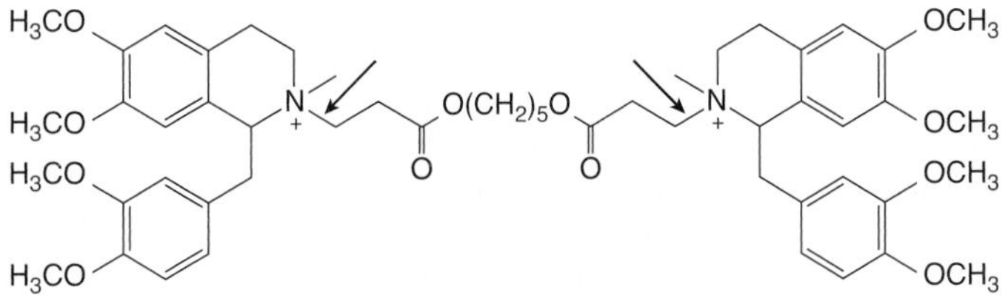

ATRACURIUM/CISTRACURIUM
arrows: cleavage sites for Hofmann elimination

Ammino Steroid Competitive Neuromuscular Blockers

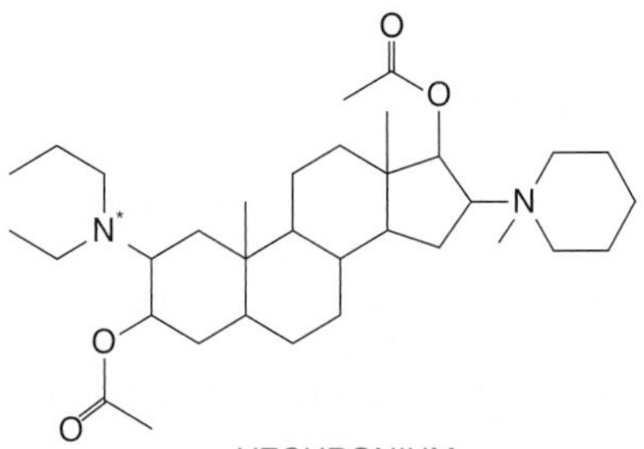

VECURONIUM
PANCURONIUM: addition of CH_3 at N*

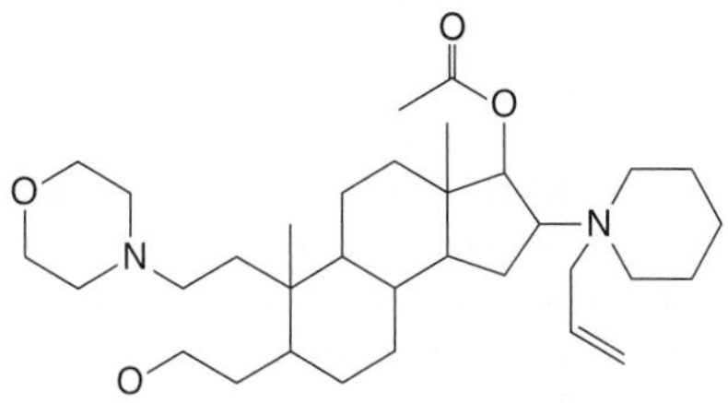

ROCURONIUM

Mixed-onium Chlorofumarate Competitive Neuromuscular Blockers

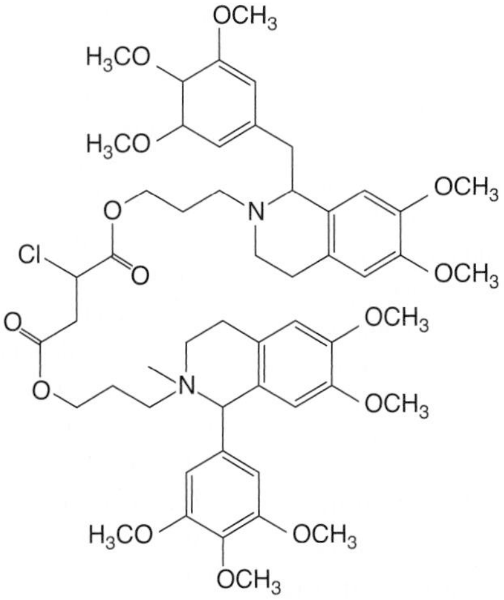

GANTACURIUM

Figure 11–3. *Structural formulas of major neuromuscular blocking agents.*

and the remainder of the muscle fiber membrane retain their normal sensitivities to K^+ depolarization and direct electrical stimulation.

The steps involved in ACh release by the nerve action potential, the development of miniature end-plate potentials (MEPPs), their summation to form a postjunctional end-plate potential (EPP), the triggering of the muscle action potential, and contraction are described in Chapter 8. Biophysical studies with patch electrodes reveal that the fundamental event elicited by ACh or other agonists is an "all or none" opening of the individual receptor channels, which gives rise to a square wave pulse with an average open-channel conductance of 20-30 picosiemens (pS) and a duration that is exponentially distributed around a time of ~1 ms. The *duration* of channel opening is far more dependent on the nature of the agonist than is the magnitude of the open-channel conductance (Sakmann, 1992).

Increasing concentrations of the competitive antagonist tubocurarine progressively diminish the amplitude of the excitatory postjunctional EPP. The amplitude of this potential may fall to below 70% of its initial value before it is insufficient to initiate the propagated muscle action potential; this provides a safety factor in neuromuscular transmission. Analysis of the antagonism of tubocurarine on single-channel events shows that, as expected for a competitive antagonist, tubocurarine reduces the frequency of channel-opening events but does not affect the conductance or duration of opening for a single channel (Katz and Miledi, 1978). At higher concentrations, curare and other competitive antagonists block the channel directly in a fashion that is noncompetitive with agonists and dependent on membrane potential (Colquhoun et al., 1979).

The decay time of the MEPP is similar to the average lifetime of channel opening (1-2 ms). MEPPs are a consequence of the spontaneous release of one or more quanta of ACh (~10^5 molecules); individual molecules of ACh in the synapse have only a transient opportunity to activate the receptor and do not rebind successively to receptors to activate multiple channels before being hydrolyzed by acetylcholinesterase (AChE). The concentration of unbound ACh in the synapse from nerve-released ACh diminishes more rapidly than does the decay of the EPP (or current). In the presence of anticholinesterase drugs, the EPP is prolonged up to 25-30 ms, which is indicative of the rebinding of transmitter to neighboring receptors before hydrolysis by AChE or diffusion from the synapse.

Simultaneous binding by two agonist molecules at the respective $\alpha\gamma$ and $\alpha\delta$ subunit interfaces of the receptor is required for activation. Activation shows positive cooperativity and thus occurs over a narrow range of concentrations (Changeux and Edelstein, 1998; Sine and Claudio, 1991). Although two molecules of competitive antagonist or snake α-toxin can bind to each receptor molecule at the agonist sites, the binding of one molecule of antagonist to each receptor is sufficient to render it nonfunctional (Taylor et al., 1983).

The depolarizing agents, such as succinylcholine, act by a different mechanism. Their initial action is to depolarize the membrane by opening channels in the same manner as ACh. However, they persist for longer durations at the neuromuscular junction primarily because of their resistance to AChE. The depolarization is thus longer-lasting, resulting in a brief period of repetitive excitation that may elicit transient and repetitive muscle excitation (fasciculations). This initial depolarization is followed by block of neuromuscular transmission and flaccid paralysis (called *phase I block*). The block arises because, after an initial opening, perijunctional sodium channels close and will not reopen until the end plate is repolarized. At this point, neural release of ACh results in the binding of ACh to receptors on an already depolarized end plate. These closed perijunctional channels keep the depolarization signal from affecting downstream channels and effectively shield the rest of the muscle from activity at the motor end plate. In humans, depolarizing agents elicit a sequence of repetitive excitation followed by block of transmission and neuromuscular paralysis; however, this sequence is influenced by such factors as the anesthetic agent used concurrently, the type of muscle, and the rate of drug administration. The characteristics of depolarization and competitive blockade are contrasted in Table 11–3.

In other animal species and occasionally in humans, depolarizing agents produce a blockade that has unique features, some of which combine those of the depolarizing and the competitive agents; this type of action is termed a *dual mechanism*. In such cases, the depolarizing agent initially produces characteristic fasciculations and potentiation of the maximal twitch, followed by the rapid onset of neuromuscular block. This phase I block is potentiated by anticholinesterase agents (e.g., ambenonium, edrophonium, neostigmine, pyridostigmine, donepezil, galantamine, rivastigmine, and tacrine): Inhibition of ACh degradation results in additional depolarizing agent, in this case endogenous ACh, at the neuromuscular junction. Following the onset of blockade, there is a poorly sustained response to tetanic stimulation of the motor nerve, intensification of the block by tubocurarine, and lack of potentiation by anti-cholinesterase agents. The dual action of the depolarizing blocking agents is also seen in intracellular recordings of membrane potential; when agonist is applied continuously, the initial depolarization is followed by a gradual repolarization, which in many respects resembles receptor desensitization.

Under clinical conditions, with increasing concentrations of succinylcholine and over time, the block may convert slowly from a depolarizing phase I block to a non-depolarizing, *phase II block* (Durant and Katz, 1982). The pattern of neuromuscular blockade produced by depolarizing drugs in anesthetized patients appears to depend, in part, on the anesthetic; fluorinated hydrocarbons may be more apt to predispose the motor end plate to non-depolarization blockade after prolonged use of succinylcholine (Fogdall and Miller, 1975). While the response to peripheral stimulation during phase II block resembles that of the competitive agents, reversal of phase II block by administration of anti-cholinesterase agents (e.g., with neostigmine) is difficult to predict and should be undertaken with much caution. The characteristics of phase I and phase II blocks are shown in Table 11–1.

Although the observed fasciculations also may be a consequence of stimulation of the prejunctional nerve terminal by the

Table 11–1

Clinical Responses and Monitoring of Phase I and Phase II Neuromuscular Blockade by Succinylcholine Infusion

RESPONSE	PHASE I	PHASE II
End-plate membrane potential	Depolarized to –55 mV	Repolarization toward –80 mV
Onset	Immediate	Slow transition
Dose-dependence	Lower	Usually higher or follows prolonged infusion
Recovery	Rapid	More prolonged
Train of four and tetanic stimulation	No fade	Fade [a]
Acetylcholinesterase inhibition	Augments	Reverses or antagonizes
Muscle response	Fasciculations → flaccid paralysis	Flaccid paralysis

[a]Post-tetanic potentiation follows fade.

depolarizing agent, giving rise to stimulation of the motor unit in an antidromic fashion, the primary site of action of both competitive and depolarizing blocking agents is the post-junctional membrane. Presynaptic actions of the competitive agents may become significant on repetitive high-frequency stimulation because pre-junctional nicotinic receptors may be involved in the mobilization of ACh for release from the nerve terminal (Bowman et al., 1990; Van der Kloot and Molgo, 1994).

Many drugs and toxins block neuromuscular transmission by other mechanisms, such as interference with the synthesis or release of ACh (Chapter 8), but most of these agents are not employed clinically for this purpose. One exception is botulinum toxin, which has been administered locally into muscles of the orbit in the management of ocular blepharospasm and strabismus and has been used to control other muscle spasms and to facilitate facial muscle relaxation (Chapters 8 and 64). This toxin also has been injected into the lower esophageal sphincter to treat achalasia (Chapter 47). The sites of action and interrelationship of several agents that serve as pharmacological tools are shown in Figure 11–4.

Sequence and Characteristics of Paralysis. When an appropriate dose of a competitive blocking agent is injected intravenously in human beings, motor weakness progresses to a total flaccid paralysis. Small, rapidly moving muscles such as those of the eyes, jaw, and larynx relax before those of the limbs and trunk. Ultimately, the intercostal muscles and finally the diaphragm are paralyzed, and respiration then ceases. Recovery of muscles usually occurs in the reverse order to that of their paralysis, and thus the diaphragm ordinarily is the first muscle to regain function (Feldman and Fauvel, 1994; Viby-Mogensen, 2005).

After a single intravenous dose of 10-30 mg of succinylcholine, muscle fasciculations, particularly over the chest and abdomen, occur briefly; then relaxation occurs within 1 minute, becomes maximal within 2 minutes, and generally disappears within 5 minutes. Transient apnea usually occurs at the time of maximal effect. Muscle relaxation of longer duration is achieved by continuous intravenous infusion. After infusion is discontinued, the effects of the drug usually disappear rapidly because of its efficient hydrolysis by plasma and hepatic butyrylcholinesterase. Muscle soreness may follow the administration of succinylcholine. Small prior doses of competitive blocking agents have been employed to minimize fasciculations and muscle pain caused by succinylcholine, but this procedure is controversial because it increases the requirement for the depolarizing drug.

During prolonged depolarization, muscle cells may lose significant quantities of K^+ and gain Na^+, Cl^-, and Ca^{2+}. In patients with extensive injury to soft tissues, the efflux of K^+ following continued administration of succinylcholine can be life-threatening. The life-threatening complications of succinylcholine-induced hyperkalemia are discussed later, but it is important to stress that there are many conditions for which succinylcholine administration is contraindicated or should be undertaken with great caution. The change in the nature of the blockade produced by succinylcholine (from phase I to phase II) presents an additional complication with long-term infusions.

Central Nervous System. Tubocurarine and other quaternary neuromuscular blocking agents are virtually devoid of central effects following ordinary clinical doses because of their inability to penetrate the blood-brain barrier. The most decisive experiment performed to resolve whether curare significantly affects central functions in the dose range used clinically was that of Smith and associates (1947). Smith (an anesthesiologist) daringly permitted himself to receive, intravenously, two and one-half times the amount of tubocurarine necessary for paralysis of all skeletal muscles. Adequate respiratory exchange was maintained by artificial respiration. At no time was there any evidence of lapse of consciousness, clouding of sensorium, analgesia, or disturbance of special senses. Despite adequate artificially controlled respiration, Smith experienced "shortness of breath" and the sensation of choking due to the accumulation of unswallowed saliva in the pharynx. The experience was decidedly unpleasant,

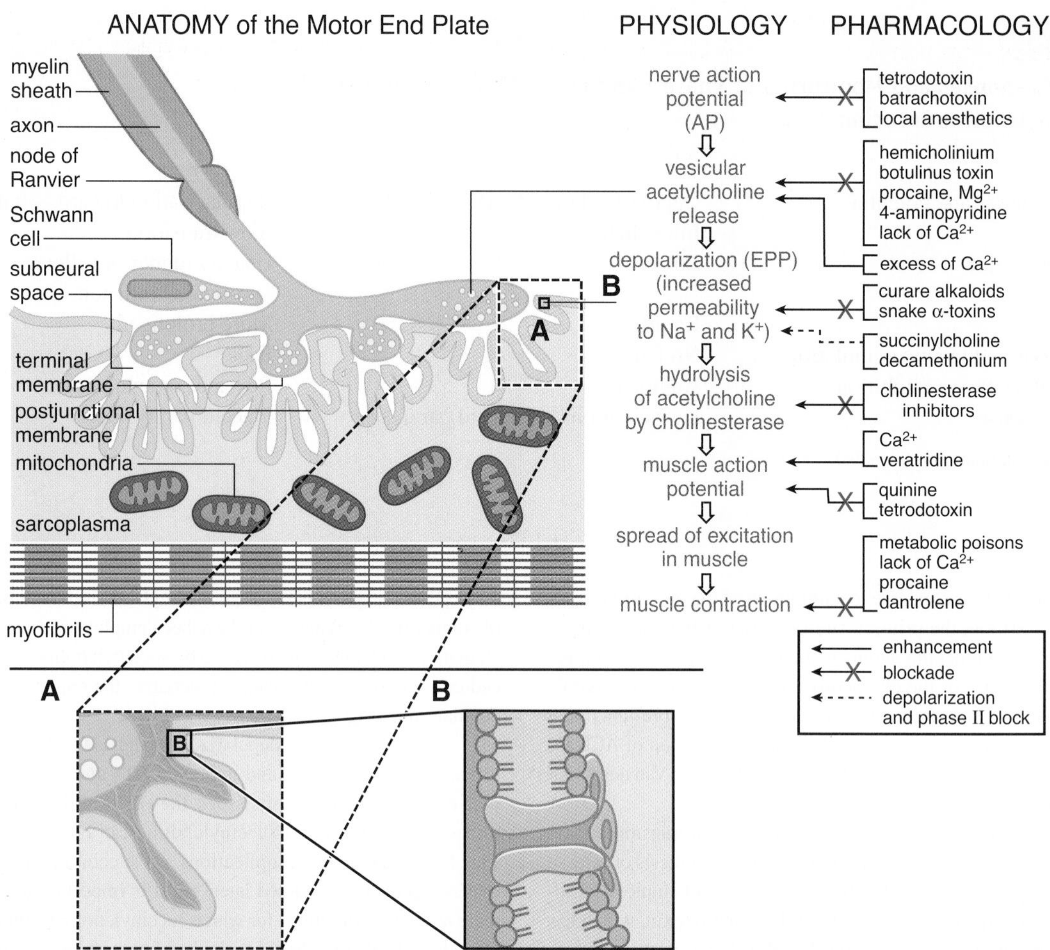

Figure 11–4. *Sites of action of agents at the neuromuscular junction and adjacent structures.* The anatomy of the motor end plate, shown at the left, and the sequence of events from liberation of acetylcholine (ACh) by the nerve action potential (AP) to contraction of the muscle fiber, indicated by the middle column, are described in Chapter 8. The modification of these processes by various agents is shown on the right; an arrow marked with an X indicates inhibition or block; an unmarked arrow indicates enhancement or activation. The insets are enlargements of the indicated structures. The highest magnification depicts the receptor in the bilayer of the postsynaptic membrane. A more detailed view of the receptor is shown in Figure 11–2.

but the results were clear: Tubocurarine given intravenously, even in large doses, has no significant central stimulant, depressant, or analgesic effects.

Autonomic Ganglia and Muscarinic Sites. Neuromuscular blocking agents show variable potencies in producing ganglionic blockade. Just as at the motor end plate, ganglionic blockade by tubocurarine and other stabilizing drugs is reversed or antagonized by anti-ChE agents.

At the doses of tubocurarine once used clinically, partial blockade probably is produced both at autonomic ganglia and at the adrenal medulla, which results in a fall in blood pressure and tachycardia. Pancuronium shows less ganglionic blockade at common clinical doses. Atracurium, vecuronium, doxacurium, pipecuronium, mivacurium, and rocuronium are even more selective (Naguib and Lien, 2005; Pollard, 1994)). The maintenance of cardiovascular reflex responses usually is desired during anesthesia. Pancuronium has a vagolytic action, presumably from blockade of muscarinic receptors, which leads to tachycardia.

Of the depolarizing agents, succinylcholine at doses producing neuromuscular relaxation rarely causes effects attributable to ganglionic blockade. However, cardiovascular effects are sometimes observed, probably owing to the successive stimulation of vagal ganglia (manifested by bradycardia) and sympathetic ganglia (resulting in hypertension and tachycardia).

Mast Cells and Histamine Release. Tubocurarine produces typical histamine-like wheals when injected intracutaneously or intra-arterially in humans, and some clinical responses to neuromuscular blocking agents (e.g., bronchospasm, hypotension, excessive bronchial and salivary secretion) appear to be caused by the release of histamine. Succinylcholine, mivacurium, and atracurium also cause histamine release, but to a lesser extent unless administered rapidly. The ammonio steroids, pancuronium, vecuronium, pipecuronium, and rocuronium, have even less tendency to release histamine after intradermal or systemic injection (Basta, 1992; Watkins, 1994). Histamine release typically is a direct action of the muscle relaxant on the mast cell rather than IgE-mediated anaphylaxis (Watkins, 1994).

Release of Cellular K^+. Depolarizing agents can release K^+ rapidly from intracellular sites; this may be a factor in several of the clinical toxicities of these drugs (see "Toxicology" later in the chapter).

Absorption, Distribution, and Elimination

Quaternary ammonium neuromuscular blocking agents are very poorly absorbed from the GI tract, a fact well known to the South American Indians, who ate with impunity the flesh of game killed with curare-poisoned arrows. Absorption is quite adequate from intramuscular sites. Rapid onset is achieved with intravenous administration. The more potent agents, of course, must be given in lower concentrations, and diffusional requirements slow their rate of onset.

When long-acting competitive blocking agents such as D-tubocurarine and pancuronium are administered, blockade may diminish after 30 minutes owing to redistribution of the drug, yet residual blockade and plasma levels of the drug persist. Subsequent doses show diminished redistribution. Long-acting agents may accumulate with multiple doses.

The ammonio steroids contain ester groups that are hydrolyzed in the liver. Typically, the metabolites have about one-half the activity of the parent compound and contribute to the total relaxation profile. Ammonio steroids of intermediate duration of action, such as vecuronium and rocuronium (Table 11–2), are cleared more rapidly by the liver than is pancuronium. The more rapid decay of neuromuscular blockade with compounds of intermediate duration argues for sequential dosing of these agents rather than administering a single dose of a long-duration neuromuscular blocking agent. There is a modified γ-cyclodextrin available as an investigational chelating agent specific for rocuronium and vecuronium (see "Reversal of Effects by Chelation Therapy" later in the chapter).

Atracurium is converted to less active metabolites by plasma esterases and spontaneous Hofmann elimination (Figure 11–3). Cisatracurium is also subject to this spontaneous degradation. Because of these alternative routes of metabolism, atracurium and cisatracurium do not exhibit an increased $t_{1/2}$ in patients with impaired renal function and therefore are good choices in this setting (Hunter, 1994; Naguib and Lien, 2005).

The extremely brief duration of action of succinylcholine is due largely to its rapid hydrolysis by the butyrylcholinesterase synthesized by the liver and found in the plasma. Among the occasional patients who exhibit prolonged apnea following the administration of succinylcholine or mivacurium, most have an atypical plasma cholinesterase or a deficiency of the enzyme owing to allelic variations (Pantuck, 1993; Primo-Parmo et al., 1996), hepatic or renal disease, or a nutritional disturbance; however, in some, the enzymatic activity in plasma is normal (Whittaker, 1986).

Gantacurium is degraded by two chemical mechanisms, a rapid cysteine adduction and a slower hydrolysis of the ester bond adjacent to the chlorine. Both processes are purely chemical and hence not dependent on enzymatic activities. The adduction process has a $t_{1/2}$ of 1-2 minutes and is likely the basis for the ultrashort duration of action of gantacurium. Administration of exogenous cysteine, which may have excitotoxic side effects, can accelerate the antagonism of gantacurium-induced neuromuscular blockade (Naguib and Brull, 2009).

Clinical Pharmacology

Choice of Agent

Therapeutic selection of a neuromuscular blocking agent should be based on achieving a pharmacokinetic profile consistent with the duration of the interventional procedure and minimizing cardiovascular compromise or other side effects, with attention to drug-specific modes of elimination in patients with renal or hepatic failure (Table 11–2).

Two characteristics are useful in distinguishing side effects and pharmacokinetic behavior of neuromuscular blocking agents. The first relates to the duration of drug action: These agents are categorized as long-, intermediate-, or short-acting. The persistent blockade and difficulty in complete reversal after surgery with D-tubocurarine, metocurine, doxacurium, and pancuronium led to the development of vecuronium (NORCURON, others) and atracurium (TRACRIUM, others), agents of intermediate duration; cisatracurium (NIMBEX) is one of ten isomers of atracurium with three times its potency. This was followed by the development of a short-acting agent, mivacurium (not available in the U.S.). Often, the long-acting agents are the more potent, requiring the use of low concentrations (Table 11–3). The necessity of administering potent agents in low concentrations delays their onset. Rocuronium (ZEMURON, others) is an agent of intermediate duration but of rapid onset and lower potency. Its rapid onset allows its use as an alternative to succinylcholine in rapid-induction anesthesia and in relaxing the laryngeal and jaw muscles to facilitate tracheal intubation (Bevan, 1994; Naguib and Lien, 2005). Gantacurium, a mixed-onium chlorofumarate, recently completed phase 2 clinical trials and is the first in a new class of ultra-short acting, competitive neuromuscular blocking agents designed to replace succinylcholine in rapid-induction anesthesia (Naguib and Brull, 2009; Savarese, 2006).

The second useful classification is derived from the chemical nature of the agents and includes the natural alkaloids or their congeners, the ammonio steroids, the benzylisoquinolines, and the asymmetric mixed-onium chlorofumarates (Table 11–2, Figure 11–3). The natural alkaloid D-tubocurarine and the semisynthetic alkaloid alcuronium are not approved for use in the U.S. Apart from a shorter duration of action, newer agents exhibit greatly diminished frequency of side effects, chief of which are ganglionic blockade, block

Table 11–2

Classification of Neuromuscular Blocking Agents

AGENT	CHEMICAL CLASS	PHARMACOLOGICAL PROPERTIES	TIME OF ONSET (MIN)[a]	CLINICAL DURATION (MIN)[a]	MODE OF ELIMINATION
Succinyl choline (ANECTINE, others)	Dicholine ester	Ultrashort duration; depolarizing	0.8-1.4	6-11	Hydrolysis by plasma cholinesterases
D-Tubocurarine[b]	Natural alkaloid (cyclic benzyl-isoquinoline)	Long duration; competitive	6	80	Renal and hepatic elimination
Metocurine[b]	Benzylisoquinoline	Long duration; competitive	4	110	Renal elimination
Atracurium (TRACRIUM, others)	Benzylisoquinoline	Intermediate duration; competitive	3	45	Hofmann elimination; hydrolysis by plasma esterases
Cisatracurium (NIMBEX)	Benzylisoquinoline	Intermediate duration; competitive	2-8	45-90	Hofmann and renal elimination
Doxacurium[b]	Benzylisoquinoline	Long duration; competitive	4-8	120	Renal elimination
Mivacurium	Benzylisoquinoline	Short duration; competitive	2-3	15-21	Hydrolysis by plasma cholinesterases
Pancuronium (generic)	Ammonio steroid	Long duration; competitive	3-4	85-100	Renal and hepatic elimination
Pipecuronium[b]	Ammonio steroid	Long duration; competitive	3-6	30-90	Renal elimination; hepatic metabolism and clearance
Rocuronium (ZEMURON, others)	Ammonio steroid	Intermediate duration; competitive	0.9-1.7	36-73	Hepatic elimination
Vecuronium (NORCURON, others)	Ammonio steroid	Intermediate duration; competitive	2-3	40-45	Hepatic and renal elimination
Gantacurium[c]	Asymmetric mixed-onium chlorofumarate	Ultra-short duration, competitive	1-2	5-10	Cysteine adduction and ester hydrolysis

[a]Time of onset and clinical duration achieved from dose ranges in Table 11–3.
[b]D-Tubocurarine, doxacurium, metocurine, and pipecuronium are no longer available in the U.S.
[c]Gantacurium is in investigational status.

of vagal responses, and histamine release. The prototypical ammonio steroid, pancuronium, induces virtually no histamine release; however, it blocks muscarinic receptors, and this antagonism is manifested primarily in vagal blockade and tachycardia. Tachycardia is eliminated in the newer ammonio steroids, vecuronium and rocuronium.

The benzylisoquinolines appear to be devoid of vagolytic and ganglionic blocking actions but show a slight propensity to cause histamine release. The unusual metabolism of the prototype compound atracurium and its congener mivacurium confers special indications for use of these compounds. For example, atracurium's disappearance from the body depends on hydrolysis of the ester

Table 11–3

Dosing Ranges for Neuromuscular Blocking Agents

AGENT	INITIATION DOSE (mg/kg)	MAINTENANCE DOSE: INTERMITTENT INJECTION (mg/kg)	MAINTENANCE DOSE: CONTINUOUS INFUSION (μg/kg/min)
Succinylcholine	0.5-1	0.04-0.07	N/A
D-Tubocurarine[a]	0.6	0.25-0.5	2-3
Metocurine[a]	0.4	0.5-1	N/A
Atracurium	0.5	0.08-0.1	5-10
Cisatracurium	0.1-0.4	0.03	1-3
Mivacurium	0.15-0.25	0.1	9-10
Doxacurium[a]	0.03-0.06	0.005-0.01	N/A
Pancuronium	0.08-0.1	0.01-0.015	1
Rocuronium	0.6-1.2	0.1-0.2	10-12
Vecuronium	0.1	0.01-0.015	0.8-1
Gantacurium[a]	0.2-0.5	N/A	N/A

[a]Not commercially available in the U.S.

moiety by plasma esterases and by a spontaneous or Hofmann degradation (cleavage of the *N*-alkyl portion in the benzylisoquinoline). Hence two routes for degradation are available, both of which remain functional in renal failure. Mivacurium is extremely sensitive to catalysis by cholinesterase or other plasma hydrolases, accounting for its short duration of action.

Side effects are not yet fully characterized for gantacurium, but transient adverse cardiovascular effects suggestive of histamine release have been observed at doses over three times the ED_{95}.

Clinical Uses

Muscle Relaxation. The main clinical use of the neuromuscular blocking agents is as an adjuvant in surgical anesthesia to obtain relaxation of skeletal muscle, particularly of the abdominal wall, to facilitate operative manipulations. With muscle relaxation no longer dependent on the depth of general anesthesia, a much lighter level of anesthesia suffices. Thus, the risk of respiratory and cardiovascular depression is minimized, and post-anesthetic recovery is shortened. These considerations notwithstanding, neuromuscular blocking agents cannot be used to substitute for inadequate depth of anesthesia. Otherwise, a risk of reflex responses to painful stimuli and conscious recall may occur.

Muscle relaxation is also of value in various orthopedic procedures, such as the correction of dislocations and the alignment of fractures. Neuromuscular blocking agents of short duration often are used to facilitate endotracheal intubation and have been used to facilitate laryngoscopy, bronchoscopy, and esophagoscopy in combination with a general anesthetic agent.

Neuromuscular blocking agents are administered parenterally, nearly always intravenously. As potentially hazardous drugs, they should be administered to patients only by anesthesiologists and other clinicians who have had extensive training in their use and in a setting where facilities for respiratory and cardiovascular resuscitation are immediately at hand. Detailed information on dosage and monitoring the extent of muscle relaxation can be found in anesthesiology textbooks (Naguib and Lien, 2005; Pollard, 1994).

Measurement of Neuromuscular Blockade in Humans. Assessment of neuromuscular block usually is performed by stimulation of the ulnar nerve. Responses are monitored from compound action potentials or muscle tension developed in the adductor pollicis (thumb) muscle. Responses to repetitive or tetanic stimuli are most useful for evaluation of blockade of transmission because individual measurements of twitch tension must be related to control values obtained prior to the administration of drugs. Thus, stimulus schedules such as the "train of four" and the "double burst" or responses to tetanic stimulation are preferred procedures (Drenck et al., 1989; Waud and Waud, 1972). Rates of onset of blockade and recovery are more rapid in the airway musculature (jaw, larynx, and diaphragm) than in the thumb. Hence, tracheal intubation can be performed before onset of complete block at the adductor pollicis, whereas partial recovery of function of this muscle allows sufficient recovery of respiration for extubation (Naguib and Lien, 2005). Differences in rates of onset of blockade, recovery from blockade, and intrinsic sensitivity between the stimulated muscle and those of the larynx, abdomen, and diaphragm should be considered.

Preventing Trauma During Electroshock Therapy. Electroconvulsive therapy (ECT) of psychiatric disorders occasionally is complicated by trauma to the patient; the seizures induced may cause dislocations or fractures. Inasmuch as the muscular component of the convulsion is not essential for benefit from the procedure, neuromuscular blocking agents, usually succinylcholine, and a short-acting barbiturate, usually methohexital or thiopental, are employed. The combination of the blocking drug, the anesthetic agent, and postictal depression usually results in respiratory depression or temporary apnea. An endotracheal tube and oxygen always should be available. An oropharyngeal airway should be inserted as soon as the jaw muscles relax (after the seizure) and provision made to prevent aspiration of mucus and saliva. A cuff may be applied to one extremity to prevent the effects of the drug in that limb; evidence of an effective electroshock is provided by contraction of the group of protected muscles. After the procedure, ventilation with oxygen by mask should be continued until adequate breathing resumes (Stensrud, 2005). These agents are also used in capital punishment by electrocution. Although a convulsive response is blocked, ethical concerns have been raised because all motor function is blocked.

Control of Muscle Spasms and Rigidity. Botulinum toxins and dantrolene act peripherally to reduce muscle contraction; a variety of other agents act centrally to reduce skeletal muscle tone and spasm.

The anaerobic bacterium *Clostridium botulinum* produces a family of toxins targeted to presynaptic proteins that block the release of ACh (Chapter 8). Onabotulinum toxin A (BOTOX), abobotulinum toxin A (DYSPORT), and rimabotulinum toxin B (MYOBLOC), by blocking ACh release, produce flaccid paralysis of skeletal muscle and diminished activity of parasympathetic and sympathetic cholinergic synapses. Inhibition lasts from several weeks to 3 to 4 months, and restoration of function requires nerve sprouting. Immunoresistance is uncommon but may develop with continued use (Davis and Barnes, 2000). Originally approved for the treatment of the ocular conditions of strabismus and blepharospasm and for hemifacial spasms, botulinum toxin has been used to treat spasms and dystonias such as adductor spasmodic dysphonia, oromandibular dystonia, cervical dystonia, and spasms associated with the lower esophageal sphincter and anal fissures. Its dermatological uses include treatment of hyperhidrosis of the palms and axillae that is resistant to topical and iontophoretic remedies and removal of facial lines associated with excessive nerve stimulation and muscle activity. Treatment involves local intramuscular or intradermal injections (Boni et al., 2000; Flynn, 2006). Botox treatments also have become a popular cosmetic procedure for those seeking a wrinkle-free face. Like the bloom of youth, the reduction of wrinkles is temporary; unlike the bloom of youth, the effect of Botox can be renewed by re-administration. The FDA has issued a safety alert, warning of respiratory paralysis from unexpected spread of the toxin from the site of injection (Chapter 65).

Dantrolene (DANTRIUM, others) inhibits Ca^{2+} release from the sarcoplasmic reticulum of skeletal muscle by limiting the capacity of Ca^{2+} and calmodulin to activate RYR-1 (Fruen et al., 1997). RYR-1 and the L-type Ca^{2+} channel are juxtaposed to associate at a triadic junction formed between the T-tubule and the sarcoplasmic reticulum. The L-type channel with its T-tubular location serves as the voltage sensor receiving the depolarizing activation signal. The intimate coupling of the two proteins at the triad, along with a host of modulatory proteins in the two organelles and the surrounding cytoplasm, regulates the release of and response to Ca^{2+} (Lehmann-Horn and Jurkat-Rott, 1999). Because of its efficacy in managing an acute attack of malignant hyperthermia (described under "Toxicology"), dantrolene has been used experimentally in the treatment of muscle rigidity and hyperthermia in neuroleptic malignant syndrome (NMS). NMS is a life-threatening complication of treatment with both typical and atypical antipsychotic drugs (Chapter 16) characterized by fever, severe muscle rigidity, mental status change, and dysautonomia. Administration of 1-2.5 mg/kg dantrolene in severe NMS cases, concurrent with immediate discontinuation of antipsychotic therapy, usually results in rapid reversal of hyperthermia and rigidity (Strawn et al., 2007). Dantrolene is also used in treatment of spasticity and hyperreflexia. With its peripheral action, it causes a generalized weakness. Thus, its use should be reserved to non-ambulatory patients with severe spasticity. Hepatotoxicity has been reported with continued use, requiring liver function tests (Kita and Goodkin, 2000).

Several agents, many of limited efficacy, have been used to treat spasticity involving the α-motor neuron with the objective of increasing functional capacity and relieving discomfort. Agents that act in the CNS at either higher centers or the spinal cord to block spasms are considered in Chapter 22. These include baclofen (LIORESAL, others), the benzodiazepines, tizanidine (ZANAFLEX, others), and cyclobenzaprine (FLEXARIL, others). A number of other agents used as muscle relaxants seem to rely on sedative properties and blockade of nociceptive pathways; this group includes carisoprodol (which is metabolized to meprobamate; SOMA, others); metaxalone (SKELAXIN); methocarbamol (ROBAXIN, others); and orphenadrine (NORFLEX, others). Tetrabenazine (XENAZINE) is available for treatment of the chorea associated with Huntington's disease; the drug is a VMAT2 inhibitor that depletes vesicular stores of dopamine in the CNS (Chapters 8 and 22).

Synergisms and Antagonisms. Interactions between competitive and depolarizing neuromuscular blocking agents already have been considered (Table 11–4). From a clinical viewpoint, important pharmacological interactions of these drugs are with certain general anesthetics, certain antibiotics, Ca^{2+} channel blockers, and anti-cholinesterase (anti-ChE) compounds.

Since the anti-ChE agents neostigmine, pyridostigmine, and edrophonium preserve endogenous ACh and also act directly on the neuromuscular junction, they have been used in the treatment of overdosage with competitive blocking agents. Similarly, on completion of the surgical procedure, many anesthesiologists employ neostigmine or edrophonium to reverse and decrease the duration of competitive neuromuscular blockade. A muscarinic antagonist (atropine or glycopyrrolate) is used concomitantly to prevent stimulation of muscarinic receptors and thereby to avoid slowing of the heart rate. Since

Table 11–4

Comparison of Competitive (D-Tubocurarine) and Depolarizing (Decamethonium) Blocking Agents

	D-TUBOCURARINE	DECAMETHONIUM
Effect of D-tubocurarine administered previously	Additive	Antagonistic
Effect of decamethonium administered previously	No effect, or antagonistic	Some tachyphylaxis; but may be additive
Effect of anticholinesterase agents on block	Reversal of block	No reversal
Effect on motor end plate	Elevated threshold to acetylcholine; no depolarization	Partial, persisting depolarization
Initial excitatory effect on striated muscle	None	Transient fasciculations
Character of muscle response to indirect tetanic stimulation during *partial* block	Poorly sustained contraction	Well-sustained contraction

anti-cholinesterase agents will not reverse depolarizing neuromuscular blockade and, in fact, can enhance it, the distinction between competitive and depolarizing types of neuromuscular blocking agent must be clearly communicated in healthcare settings to avoid potential adverse clinical outcomes.

Many inhalational anesthetics exert a stabilizing effect on the postjunctional membrane and therefore potentiate the activity of competitive blocking agents. Consequently, when such blocking drugs are used for muscle relaxation as adjuncts to these anesthetics, their doses should be reduced. The rank of order of potentiation is desflurane > sevoflurane > isoflurane > halothane > nitrous oxide-barbiturate-opioid or propofol anesthesia (Naguib and Lien, 2005).

Aminoglycoside antibiotics produce neuromuscular blockade by inhibiting ACh release from the preganglionic terminal (through competition with Ca^{2+}) and to a lesser extent by noncompetitively blocking the receptor. The blockade is antagonized by Ca^{2+} salts but only inconsistently by anti-ChE agents (Chapter 54). The tetracyclines also can produce neuromuscular blockade, possibly by chelation of Ca^{2+}. Additional antibiotics that have neuromuscular blocking action, through both presynaptic and postsynaptic actions, include polymyxin B, colistin, clindamycin, and lincomycin (Pollard, 1994). Ca^{2+} channel blockers enhance neuromuscular blockade produced by both competitive and depolarizing antagonists. It is not clear whether this is a result of a diminution of Ca^{2+}-dependent release of transmitter from the nerve ending or is a postsynaptic action. When neuromuscular blocking agents are administered to patients receiving these agents, dose adjustments should be considered; if recovery of spontaneous respiration is delayed, Ca^{2+} salts may facilitate recovery.

Miscellaneous drugs that may have significant interactions with either competitive or depolarizing neuromuscular blocking agents include trimethaphan (no longer marketed in the U.S.), lithium, opioid analgesics, procaine, lidocaine, quinidine, phenelzine, carbamazemine, phenytoin, propranolol, dantrolene, azathioprine, tamoxifen, magnesium salts, corticosteroids, digitalis glycosides, chloroquine, catecholamines, and diuretics (Naguib and Lien, 2005; Pollard, 1994).

Toxicology

The important untoward responses of the neuromuscular blocking agents include prolonged apnea, cardiovascular collapse, those resulting from histamine release, and rarely, anaphylaxis. Failure of respiration to become adequate in the postoperative period may not always be due directly to excessive muscle paralysis from the drug. An obstruction of the airway, decreased arterial PCO_2 secondary to hyperventilation during the operative procedure, or the neuromuscular depressant effect of excessive amounts of neostigmine used to reverse the action of the competitive blocking drugs, may also be implicated. Directly related factors may include alterations in body temperature; electrolyte imbalance, particularly of K^+ (see the next paragraph); low plasma butyrylcholinesterase levels, resulting in a reduction in the rate of destruction of succinylcholine; the presence of latent myasthenia gravis or of malignant disease such as small cell carcinoma of the lung with Eaton-Lambert myasthenic syndrome; reduced blood flow to skeletal muscles, causing delayed removal of the blocking drugs; and decreased elimination of the muscle relaxants secondary to hepatic dysfunction (cisatricurium, rocuronium, vecuronium) or reduced renal function (pancuronium). Great care should be taken when administering neuromuscular blockers to dehydrated or severely ill patients.

The depolarizing agents can release K^+ rapidly from intracellular sites; this may be a factor in production of the prolonged apnea in patients who receive these drugs while in electrolyte imbalance. Succinylcholine-induced hyperkalemia is a life-threatening complication of that drug (Yentis, 1990). For example, such alterations in the distribution of K^+ are of particular concern in patients with congestive heart failure who are receiving digoxin or diuretics. For the same reason, caution should be used or depolarizing blocking agents should be avoided in patients with extensive soft-tissue trauma or burns. A higher dose of a competitive blocking agent often is indicated in these patients. In addition, succinylcholine administration is contraindicated or should be given with great caution in patients with nontraumatic rhabdomyolysis, ocular lacerations, spinal cord injuries with paraplegia or quadriplegia, or muscular dystrophies. Succinylcholine no longer is indicated for children ≤8 years of age unless emergency intubation or securing an airway is necessary. Hyperkalemia, rhabdomyolysis, and cardiac arrest have been reported. A subclinical dystrophy is frequently associated with these adverse responses. Neonates may also have an enhanced sensitivity to competitive neuromuscular blocking agents.

Malignant Hyperthermia. Malignant hyperthermia is a potentially life-threatening event triggered by the administration of certain anesthetics and neuromuscular blocking agents. The clinical features include contracture, rigidity, and heat production from skeletal muscle resulting in severe hyperthermia (increases of up to 1°C/5 min), accelerated muscle metabolism, metabolic acidosis, and tachycardia. Uncontrolled release of Ca^{2+} from the sarcoplasmic reticulum of skeletal muscle is the initiating event. Although the halogenated hydrocarbon anesthetics (e.g., halothane, isoflurane, and sevoflurane) and succinylcholine alone have been reported to precipitate the response, most of the incidents arise from the combination of depolarizing blocking agent and anesthetic. Susceptibility to malignant hyperthermia, an autosomal dominant trait, is associated with certain congenital myopathies such as *central core disease*. In the majority of cases, however, no clinical signs are visible in the absence of anesthetic intervention.

Determination of susceptibility is made with an *in vitro* contracture test on a fresh biopsy of skeletal muscle, where contractures in the presence of halothane and caffeine are measured. In over 50% of affected families, a linkage is found between the phenotype as measured by the contracture test and a mutation in the gene encoding the skeletal muscle ryanodine receptor (RYR-1). Over 30 mutations in a region of the gene that encodes the cytoplasmic face of the receptor have been described. Other loci have been identified on the L-type Ca^{2+} channel (voltage-gated dihydropyridine receptor) and on other associated proteins or channel subunits. The large number of mutations in the *RYR-1* gene, combined with genetic and metabolic heterogeneity of the condition, have precluded reliable genotypic determination of susceptibility to malignant hyperthermia (Rosenberg et al., 2007).

Treatment entails intravenous administration of dantrolene (DANTRIUM, others), which blocks Ca^{2+} release from the sarcoplasmic reticulum of skeletal muscle (see "Control of Muscle Spasms and Rigidity" earlier in the chapter). Rapid cooling, inhalation of 100% oxygen, and control of acidosis should be considered adjunct therapy in malignant hyperthermia. Declining fatality rates for malignant hyperthermia relate to anesthesiologists' awareness of the condition and the efficacy of dantrolene.

Patients with central core disease, so named because of the presence of myofibrillar cores seen on biopsy of slow-twitch muscle fibers, show muscle weakness in infancy and delayed motor development. These individuals are highly susceptible to malignant hyperthermia with the combination of an anesthetic and a depolarizing neuromuscular blocker. Central core disease has five allelic variants of *RYR-1* in common with malignant hyperthermia. Patients with other muscle syndromes or dystonias also have an increased frequency of contracture and hyperthermia in the anesthesia setting. Succinylcholine in susceptible individuals also induces *trismus-masseter spasm,* an increase in jaw muscle tone, which may complicate endotracheal tube insertion and airway management (van der Spek et al., 1990). This condition has been correlated with a mutation in the gene encoding the α subunit of the voltage-sensitive Na^+ channel (Vita et al., 1995). This increase in jaw muscle tone can be an early sign of the onset of malignant hyperthermia, and when observed along with rigidity in other muscles, is a signal that anesthesia should be halted and treatment of malignant hyperthermia begun (Gronert et al., 2005).

Respiratory Paralysis. Treatment of respiratory paralysis arising from an adverse reaction or overdose of a neuromuscular blocking agent should be by positive-pressure artificial respiration with oxygen and maintenance of a patent airway until recovery of normal respiration is ensured. With the competitive blocking agents, this may be hastened by the administration of neostigmine methylsulfate (0.5-2 mg IV) or edrophonium (10 mg IV, repeated as required up to a total of 40 mg) (Watkins, 1994).

Interventional Strategies for Other Toxic Effects. Neostigmine effectively antagonizes only the skeletal muscular blocking action of the competitive blocking agents and may aggravate such side effects as hypotension or induce bronchospasm. In such circumstances, sympathomimetic amines may be given to support the blood pressure. Atropine or glycopyrrolate is administered to counteract muscarinic stimulation. Antihistamines are definitely beneficial to counteract the responses that follow the release of histamine, particularly when administered before the neuromuscular blocking agent.

Reversal of Effects by Chelation Therapy. There is now an investigational chelating agent specific for rocuronium and vecuronium, sugammadex (BRIDION), a modified γ-cyclodextrin. Administration of sugammadex at doses >2 mg/kg is able to reverse neuromuscular blockade from rocuronium within 3 minutes. The majority of sugammadex and its complex with rocuronium is eliminated in the urine. In patients with impaired renal function, sugammadex clearance is markedly reduced and this agent should be avoided. Theoretically, neuromuscular blockade can reoccur if rocuronium or vecuronium become displaced from the sugammadex complex, necessitating careful monitoring and repeat dosing if necessary. Sugammadex is approved for clinical use in Europe but not yet in the U.S. (Naguib and Brull, 2009). Side effects include dysgeusia and rare self-limiting hypersensitivity.

GANGLIONIC NEUROTRANSMISSION

Neurotransmission in autonomic ganglia is a complex process involving multiple neurotransmitter-receptor systems. The primary event involves release of ACh and the rapid depolarization of postsynaptic membranes via the activation of neuronal nicotinic (N_n) receptors by ACh. Intracellular recordings from postganglionic neurons indicate that at least four different changes in postsynaptic membrane potential can be elicited by stimulation of the preganglionic nerve (Figure 11–5):

1. An initial excitatory postsynaptic potential (EPSP, via nicotinic receptors) that may result in an action potential
2. An inhibitory postsynaptic potential (IPSP) mediated by M_2 muscarinic receptors
3. A secondary slow EPSP mediated by M_1 muscarinic receptors
4. A late, slow EPSP mediated by myriad peptides

There are multiple nicotinic receptor subunits (e.g., $\alpha 3$, $\alpha 5$, $\alpha 7$, $\beta 2$, and $\beta 4$) in ganglia, with $\alpha 3$ and $\beta 2$ being most abundant. The ganglionic nicotinic ACh receptors are sensitive to classical blocking agents such as hexamethonium and trimethaphan.

An action potential is generated in the postganglionic neuron when the initial EPSP attains a critical amplitude. In mammalian sympathetic ganglia *in vivo,* it is common for multiple synapses to be activated before transmission is effective. Unlike the neuromuscular junction, discrete end plates with focal localization of receptors do not exist in ganglia; rather, the dendrites and nerve cell bodies contain the receptors. Iontophoretic application of ACh to the ganglion results in a depolarization with a latency < 1 ms; this decays over a period of 10-50 ms (Ascher et al., 1979). Measurements of single-channel conductances indicate that the characteristics of nicotinic-receptor channels of the ganglia and the neuromuscular junction are quite similar.

The secondary events that follow the initial depolarization (IPSP; slow EPSP; late, slow EPSP) are insensitive to hexamethonium or other N_n antagonists. The IPSP is unaffected by the classical nicotinic-receptor blocking agents. Electrophysiological and neurochemical evidence suggests that catecholamines participate in the generation of the IPSP. Dopamine and norepinephrine cause hyperpolarization of ganglia; however, in some ganglia IPSPs are mediated by M_2 muscarinic receptors (Chapter 9). Since the IPSP is sensitive in most systems to blockade by both atropine and α adrenergic receptor antagonists, ACh that is released at the preganglionic terminal may act on catecholamine-containing interneurons to stimulate the release of dopamine or norepinephrine; the catecholamine in turn produces hyperpolarization (an IPSP) of ganglion cells. Histochemical studies indicate that dopamine- or norepinephrine-containing small, intensely fluorescent (SIF) cells and adrenergic nerve terminals are present in ganglia. Details of the functional linkage between the SIF cells and the electrogenic mechanism of the IPSP remain to be resolved (Prud'homme et al., 1999; Slavikova et al., 2003).

The slow EPSP is generated by ACh activation of M_1 (G_q-coupled) muscarinic receptors and is blocked by atropine or antagonists

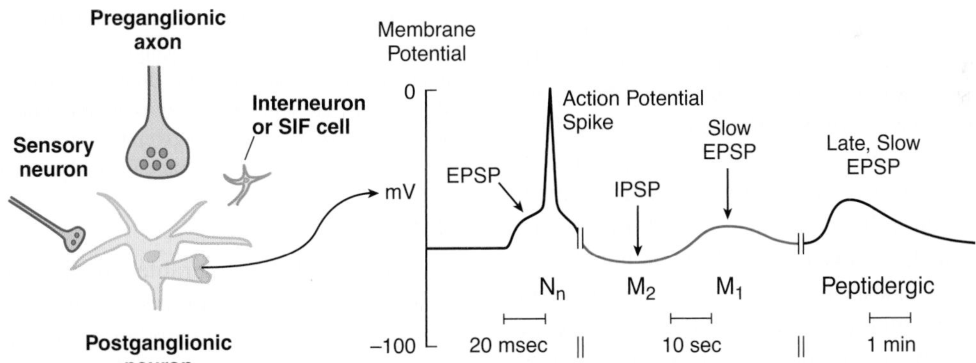

Figure 11–5. *Postsynaptic potentials recorded from an autonomic postganglionic nerve cell body after stimulation of the preganglionic nerve fiber.* The preganglionic nerve releases ACh onto postganglionic cells. The initial EPSP results from the inward Na^+ current (and perhaps Ca^{2+} current) through the nicotinic receptor channel. If the EPSP is of sufficient magnitude, it triggers an action potential spike, which is followed by a slow IPSP, a slow EPSP, and a late, slow EPSP. The slow IPSP and slow EPSP are not seen in all ganglia. The electrical events subsequent to the initial EPSP are thought to modulate the probability that a subsequent EPSP will reach the threshold for triggering a spike. Other interneurons, such as catecholamine-containing, small, intensely fluorescent (SIF) cells, and axon terminals from sensory, afferent neurons also release transmitters and that may influence the slow potentials of the postganglionic neuron. A number of cholinergic, peptidergic, adrenergic, and amino acid receptors are found on the dendrites and soma of the postganglionic neuron and the interneurons. The preganglionic fiber releases ACh and peptides; the interneurons store and release catecholamines, amino acids, and peptides; the sensory afferent nerve terminals release peptides. The initial EPSP is mediated through nicotinic (N_n) receptors, the slow IPSP and EPSP through M_2 and M_1 muscarinic receptors, and the late, slow EPSP through several types of peptidergic receptors.

that are selective for M_1 muscarinic receptors (Chapter 9). The slow EPSP has a longer latency and greater duration (10-30 seconds) than the initial EPSP. Slow EPSPs result from decreased K^+ conductance, the *M current* that regulates the sensitivity of the cell to repetitive fast-depolarizing events (Adams et al., 1982). In contrast, the late slow EPSP lasts for several minutes and is mediated by peptides released from presynaptic nerve endings or interneurons in specific ganglia, as discussed in the next section. The peptides and ACh may be co-released at the presynaptic nerve terminals; the relative stability of the peptides in the ganglion extends its sphere of influence to postsynaptic sites beyond those in the immediate proximity of the nerve ending.

The secondary synaptic events modulate the initial EPSP. The importance of the secondary pathways and the nature of the modulating transmitters appear to differ among individual ganglia and between parasympathetic and sympathetic ganglia. A variety of peptides, including gonadotropin-releasing hormone, substance P, angiotensin, calcitonin gene–related peptide, vasoactive intestinal polypeptide, neuropeptide Y, and enkephalins, have been identified in ganglia by immunofluorescence. They appear localized to particular cell bodies, nerve fibers, or SIF cells, are released on nerve stimulation, and are presumed to mediate the late slow EPSP (Elfvin et al., 1993). Other neurotransmitter substances, such as 5-hydroxytryptamine and γ-aminobutyric acid, are known to modify ganglionic transmission. Precise details of their modulatory actions are not understood, but they appear to be most closely associated with the late slow EPSP and inhibition of the M current in various ganglia. Conventional ganglionic blocking agents can inhibit ganglionic transmission completely; the same cannot be said for muscarinic antagonists or α adrenergic receptor agonists (Volle, 1980).

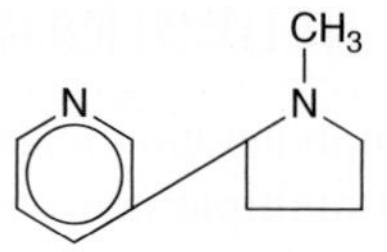

NICOTINE

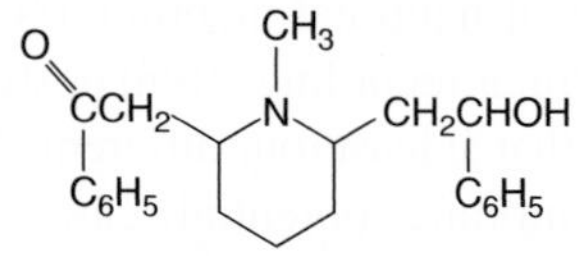

LOBELINE

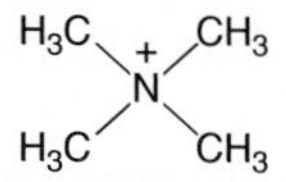

TETRAMETHYLAMMONIUM (TMA)

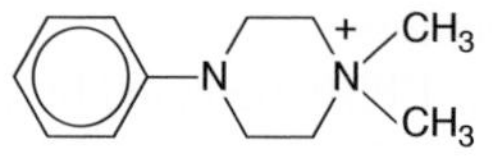

1,1-DIMETHYL-4-PHENYLPIPERAZINIUM (DMPP)

Figure 11–6. *Ganglionic stimulants.*

GANGLIONIC STIMULATING DRUGS

Drugs that stimulate cholinergic receptor sites on autonomic ganglia have been essential for analyzing the mechanism of ganglionic function; however, these ganglionic agonists have very limited therapeutic use. They can be grouped into two categories. The first group consists of drugs with nicotinic specificity, including nicotine, itself, which millions of tobacco users ingest on a daily basis. Nicotine's excitatory effects on ganglia are rapid in onset, are blocked by ganglionic nicotinic-receptor antagonists, and mimic the initial EPSP. The second group consists of muscarinic receptor agonists such as muscarine, McN-A-343, and methacholine (Chapter 9); their excitatory effects on ganglia are delayed in onset, blocked by atropine-like drugs, and mimic the slow EPSP.

History. Two natural alkaloids, nicotine and lobeline, exhibit peripheral actions by stimulating autonomic ganglia. Nicotine (Figure 11–6) was first isolated from leaves of tobacco, *Nicotiana tabacum,* by Posselt and Reiman in 1828; Orfila initiated the first pharmacological studies of the alkaloid in 1843. Langley and Dickinson painted the superior cervical ganglion of rabbits with nicotine and demonstrated that its site of action was the ganglion rather than the preganglionic or postganglionic nerve fiber. Lobeline, from *Lobelia inflata,* has many of the same actions as nicotine but is less potent.

Other ganglionic stimulants include tetramethylammonium (TMA) and 1,1-dimethyl-4-phenylpiperazinium iodide (DMPP) (Figure 11–6). Stimulation of ganglia by TMA or DMPP differs from that produced by nicotine in that the initial stimulation is not followed by a dominant blocking action. DMPP is about three times more potent and slightly more ganglion-selective than nicotine. Although parasympathomimetic drugs stimulate ganglia, their effects usually are obscured by stimulation of other neuroeffector sites. McN-A-343 represents an exception: in certain tissues its primary action appears to occur at muscarinic M_1 receptors in ganglia.

Nicotine

Nicotine is of considerable medical significance because of its toxicity, presence in tobacco, and propensity for conferring a dependence on its users. The chronic effects of nicotine and the untoward effects of the chronic use of tobacco are considered in Chapter 24. Nicotine is one of the few natural liquid alkaloids. It is a colorless, volatile base ($pK_a = 8.5$) that turns brown and acquires the odor of tobacco on exposure to air.

Pharmacological Actions. The complex and often unpredictable changes that occur in the body after administration of nicotine are due not only to its actions on a variety of neuroeffector and chemosensitive sites but also to the fact that the alkaloid can both stimulate and desensitize receptors. The ultimate response of any one system represents the summation of stimulatory and inhibitory effects of nicotine. For example, the drug can increase heart rate by excitation of sympathetic ganglia or by paralysis of parasympathetic cardiac ganglia, and it can slow heart rate by paralysis of sympathetic or stimulation of parasympathetic cardiac ganglia. In addition, the effects of the drug on the chemoreceptors of the carotid and aortic bodies and on regions of the CNS can influence heart rate, as can the compensatory baroreceptor reflexes resulting from changes in blood pressure caused by nicotine. Finally, nicotine elicits a discharge of epinephrine from the adrenal medulla, which accelerates heart rate and raises blood pressure.

Peripheral Nervous System. The major action of nicotine consists initially of transient stimulation and subsequently of a more persistent depression of all autonomic ganglia. Small doses of nicotine stimulate the ganglion cells directly and may facilitate impulse transmission. Following larger doses, the initial stimulation is followed very quickly by a blockade of transmission. Whereas stimulation of the ganglion cells coincides with their depolarization, depression of transmission by adequate doses of nicotine occurs both during the depolarization and after it has subsided. Nicotine also possesses a biphasic action on the adrenal medulla: small doses evoke the discharge of catecholamines; larger doses prevent their release in response to splanchnic nerve stimulation.

The effects of high doses of nicotine on the neuromuscular junction are similar to those on ganglia. However, with the exception of avian and denervated mammalian muscle, the stimulant phase is obscured largely by the rapidly developing paralysis. In the latter stage, nicotine also produces neuromuscular blockade by receptor desensitization. At lower concentrations, such as those typically achieved by recreational tobacco use (~200 nM), nicotine's effects reflect its higher affinity for a neuronal nicotinic receptor ($\alpha 4\beta 2$) than for the neuromuscular junction receptor ($\alpha 1\beta 1\gamma\delta$), as explained in molecular detail by Xiu and associates (2009). This high affinity, coupled with the ability of nicotine to cross the blood-brain barrier, allows nicotine to selectively activate neuronal receptors without causing intolerable contractions or paralysis of skeletal muscle.

Nicotine, like ACh, stimulates a number of sensory receptors. These include mechanoreceptors that respond to stretch or pressure of the skin, mesentery, tongue, lung, and stomach; chemoreceptors of the carotid body; thermal receptors of the skin and tongue; and pain receptors. Prior administration of hexamethonium prevents stimulation of the sensory receptors by nicotine but has little, if any, effect on the activation of sensory receptors by physiological stimuli.

Central Nervous System. Nicotine markedly stimulates the CNS. Low doses produce weak analgesia; with higher doses, tremors leading to convulsions at toxic doses are evident. The excitation of respiration is a prominent action of nicotine; although large doses act directly on the medulla oblongata, smaller doses augment respiration reflexly by excitation of the chemoreceptors of the carotid and aortic bodies. Stimulation of the CNS with large doses is followed by depression, and death results from failure of respiration owing to both central paralysis and peripheral blockade of the diaphragm and intercostal muscles that facilitate respiration.

Nicotine induces vomiting by both central and peripheral actions. The central component of the vomiting response is due to stimulation of the emetic chemoreceptor trigger zone in the area postrema of the medulla oblongata. In addition, nicotine activates vagal and spinal afferent nerves that form the sensory input of the reflex pathways involved in the act of vomiting. Studies in isolated higher centers of the brain and spinal cord reveal that the primary sites of action of nicotine in the CNS are prejunctional, causing the release of other transmitters. Accordingly, the stimulatory and pleasure–reward actions of nicotine appear to result from release of excitatory amino acids, dopamine, and other biogenic amines from various CNS centers (MacDermott et al., 1999). Release of excitatory amino acids may account for much of nicotine's stimulatory action.

Chronic exposure to nicotine in several systems causes a marked increase in the density or number of nicotinic receptors, possibly contributing to tolerance and dependence. Nicotine acts as an intracellular molecular chaperone to promote the assembly of receptor subunits by inducing an active conformation in the nascent subunits that assemble more efficiently. Chronic low dose exposure to nicotine also significantly increases the $t_{1/2}$ of receptors on the cell surface (Kuryatov et al., 2005; Lester et al., 2009).

Cardiovascular System. When administered intravenously to dogs, nicotine characteristically produces an increase in heart rate and blood pressure. The latter is usually more sustained. In general, the cardiovascular responses to nicotine are due to stimulation of sympathetic ganglia and the adrenal medulla, together with the discharge of catecholamines from sympathetic nerve endings. Contributing to the sympathomimetic response to nicotine is the activation of chemoreceptors of the aortic and carotid bodies, which reflexly results in vasoconstriction, tachycardia, and elevated blood pressure.

GI Tract. The combined activation of parasympathetic ganglia and cholinergic nerve endings by nicotine results in increased tone and motor activity of the bowel. Nausea, vomiting, and occasionally diarrhea are observed following systemic absorption of nicotine in an individual who has not been exposed to nicotine previously.

Exocrine Glands. Nicotine causes an initial stimulation of salivary and bronchial secretions that is followed by inhibition.

Absorption, Distribution, and Elimination. Nicotine is readily absorbed from the respiratory tract, buccal membranes, and skin. Severe poisoning has resulted from percutaneous absorption. As a relatively strong base, nicotine has limited absorption from the stomach. Intestinal absorption is far more efficient. Nicotine in chewing tobacco, because it is absorbed more slowly than inhaled nicotine, has a longer duration of effect. The average cigarette contains 6-11 mg nicotine and delivers ~1-3 mg nicotine systemically to the smoker; bioavailability can increase as much as 3-fold with the intensity of puffing and technique of the smoker (Benowitz, 1998).

Approximately 80-90% of nicotine is altered in the body, mainly in the liver but also in the kidney and lung. Cotinine is the major metabolite, with nicotine-1′-*N*-oxide and 3-hydroxycotinine and conjugated metabolites found in lesser quantities (Benowitz, 1998). The profile of metabolites and the rate of metabolism appear to be similar in smokers and nonsmokers. The $t_{1/2}$ of nicotine following inhalation or parenteral administration is ~2 hours. Nicotine

gastric emptying. Although the absorption of mecamylamine is less erratic, a danger exists of reduced bowel activity leading to frank paralytic ileus.

After absorption, the quaternary ammonium- and sulfonium-blocking agents are confined primarily to the extracellular space and are excreted mostly unchanged by the kidney. Mecamylamine concentrates in the liver and kidney and is excreted slowly in an unchanged form.

Untoward Responses and Severe Reactions. Among the milder untoward responses observed are visual disturbances, dry mouth, conjunctival suffusion, urinary hesitancy, decreased potency, subjective chilliness, moderate constipation, occasional diarrhea, abdominal discomfort, anorexia, heartburn, nausea, eructation, and bitter taste and the signs and symptoms of syncope caused by postural hypotension. More severe reactions include marked hypotension, constipation, syncope, paralytic ileus, urinary retention, and cycloplegia.

Clinical Summary

Neuromuscular blocking agents paralyze skeletal muscle by blocking neurotransmission through nicotinic ACh receptors at the neuromuscular junction. They have no sedative, amnestic, or analgesic properties, and are mainly used in combination with narcotic or volatile anesthetics to relax skeletal muscle and facilitate surgical procedures. Depolarizing neuromuscular blocking agents cause an initial depolarization of the motor end plate that renders it refractory to further stimulation. Competitive or non-depolarizing blocking agents compete directly with ACh at its receptor in the motor end plate. Neuromuscular blocking agents are preferably administered as a single or as intermittent intravenous injections. Depth of blockade is monitored by peripheral nerve stimulation. Competitive agents can be reversed by administration of anti-cholinesterase agents.

Succinylcholine, the most common depolarizing neuromuscular blocking agent, is used to facilitate endotracheal intubation during rapid-sequence induction of anesthesia due to its rapid onset and short duration of action. The numerous non-depolarizing neuromuscular blocking agents provide a spectrum of pharmacokinetic and pharmacodynamic profiles; vecuronium and pancuronium are used frequently. Due to differences in metabolism/elimination, certain non-depolarizing agents are appropriate for patients with compromised renal, hepatic, or cardiovascular function. Vecuronium or rocuronium are appropriate for patients with cardiovascular disease, atracurium for patients with hepatic or renal insufficiency, and pancuronium for patients with normal hepatic and renal function. Gantacurium, currently in clinical trial, represents a new class of competitive agents with ultrashort duration of action comparable to succinylcholine but reportedly with fewer side effects.

Ganglionic blocking agents have been supplanted by superior agents for the treatment of chronic hypertension (Chapter 28). Alternative agents also are available for management of acute hypertensive crises and for the production of controlled hypotension (e.g., reduction in blood pressure during surgery to minimize hemorrhage in the operative field, to reduce blood loss in various orthopedic procedures, and to facilitate surgery on blood vessels).

BIBLIOGRAPHY

Adams PR, Brown DA, Constanti A. Pharmacological inhibition of the M-current. *J Physiol,* **1982,** *332*:223–262.

Ascher P, Large WA, Rang HP. Studies on the mechanism of action of acetylcholine antagonists on rat parasympathetic ganglion cells. *J Physiol,* **1979,** *295*:139–170.

Basta SJ. Modulation of histamine release by neuromolecular blocking drugs. *Curr Opin Anaesthesiol,* **1992,** *5*:512–566.

Benowitz NL. In, *Nicotine Safety and Toxicity.* (Benowitz NL, ed.) Oxford University Press, New York, **1998,** pp. 3–28.

Benowitz NL. Nicotine addiction. *Primary Care,* **1999,** *26*:611–653.

Bevan DR. Newer neuromuscular blocking agents. *Pharmacol Toxicol,* **1994,** *74*:3–9.

Boni R, Kryden OP, Burg G. Revival of the use of botulinum toxin: Application in dermatology. *Dermatology,* **2000,** *200*:287–291.

Bouzat C, Gumilar F, Spitzmaul G, et al. Coupling of agonist binding to channel gating in an ACh-binding protein linked to an ion channel. *Nature,* **2004,** *430*:896–900.

Bowman WC, Prior C, Marshall IG. Presynaptic receptors in the neuromuscular junction. *Ann NY Acad Sci,* **1990,** *604*:69–81.

Brejc K, van Dijk WJ, Klaassen RV, et al. Crystal structure of an ACh-binding protein reveals the ligand-binding domain of nicotinc receptors. *Nature*, **2001,** *411*:269–276.

Changeux JP, Edelstein SJ. Allosteric receptors after 30 years. *Neuron,* **1998,** *21*:959–980.

Changeux JP, Edelstein SJ. *Nicotinic Acetylcholine Receptors*, Odile Jacob, New York, **2005**.

Colquhoun D, Dreyer F, Sheridan RE. The actions of tubocurarine at the frog neuromuscular junction. *J Physiol,* **1979,** *293*:247–284.

Davis E, Barnes MP. Botulinum toxin and spasticity. *J Neurol Neurosurg Psychiatry,* **2000,** *68*:141–147.

Drenck NE, Ueda N, Olsen NV, et al. Manual evaluation of residual curarization using double-burst stimulation: A comparison with train-of-four. *Anesthesiology,* **1989,** *70*: 578–581.

Durant NN, Katz RL. Suxamethonium. *Br J Anaesth,* **1982,** *54*:195–208.

Elfvin LG, Lindh B, Hokfelt T. The chemical neuroanatomy of sympathetic ganglia. *Annu Rev Neurosci,* **1993,** *16*:471–507.

Fant RV, Owen LL, Henningfield JE. Nicotine replacement therapy. *Primary Care,* **1999,** *26*:633–652.

Feldman SA, Fauvel N. Onset of neuromuscular block. In, *Applied Neuromuscular Pharmacology.* (Pollard BJ, ed.) Oxford University Press, Oxford, England, **1994**, pp. 69–84.

Flynn TC. Update on botulinum toxin. *Semin Cutan Med Surg*, **2006**, *25*:115–121.

Fogdall RP, Miller RD. Neuromuscular effects of enflurane, alone and combined with D-tubocurarine, pancuronium, and succinylcholine, in man. *Anesthesiology,* **1975**, *42*:173–178.

Frishman WH. Smoking cessation pharmacotherapy. *Ther Adv Cardiovasc Dis*, **2009**, *3*:287–308.

Fruen BR, Mickelson JR, Louis CF. Dantrolene inhibition of sarcoplasmic reticulum Ca^{2+} release by direct and specific action at skeletal muscle ryanodine receptors. *J Biol Chem,* **1997,** *272*:26965–26971.

Fukusaki M, Miyako M, Hara T, et al. Effects of controlled hypotension with sevoflurane anesthesia on hepatic function of surgical patients. *Eur J Anaesthesiol,* **1999,** *16*:111–116.

Gronert GA, Pessah IN, Muldoon SM, et al. Malignant Hyperthermia. In, *Miller's Anesthesia*, 6th ed. (Miller RD, ed.) Churchill-Livingstone, Philadelphia, **2005,** pp. 1169–1190.

Gurney AM, Rang HP. The channel-blocking action of methonium compounds on rat submandibular ganglion cells. *Br J Pharmacol,* **1984,** *82*:623–642.

Hunter JM. Muscle relaxants in renal disease. *Acta Anaesthesiol Scand Suppl,* **1994,** *102*:2–5.

Karlin A. Emerging structures of nicotinic acetylcholine receptors. *Nature Rev Neurosci,* **2002,** *3*:102–114.

Katz B, Miledi R. A re-examination of curare action at the motor end plate. *Proc R Soc Lond [Biol],* **1978,** *203*:119–133.

Kita M, Goodkin DE. Drugs used to treat spasticity. *Drugs,* **2000,** *59*:487–495.

Kuryatov A, Luo J, Cooper J, et al. Nicotine acts as a pharmacological chaperone to up-regulate human a4b2 acetylcholine receptors. *Mol Pharm,* **2005**, *68*: 1839–1851.

Lehmann-Horn F, Jurkat-Rott K. Voltage-gated ion channels and hereditary disease. *Physiol Rev,* **1999,** *79*:1317–1372.

Lester HA, Xiao C, Srinivasan R, et al. Nicotine is a selective pharmacological chaperone of acetylcholine receptor number and stoichiometry. Implications for drug discovery. *AAPS J,* **2009**, *11*:167–177.

MacDermott AB, Role LW, Siegelbaum SA. Presynaptic ionotropic receptors and the control of transmitter release. *Annu Rev Neurosci,* **1999,** *22*:443–485.

Mihalak KB, Carroll FI, Luetje CW. Varenicline is a partial agonist at α4β2 and a full agonist at α7 neuronal nicotinic receptors. *Mol Pharmacol,* **2006**, *70*: 801–805.

Naguib M, Brull SJ. Update on neuromuscular pharmacology. *Curr Opin Anaesthesiol*, **2009**, *22*:483–490.

Naguib M, Lien CA. Pharmacology of Muscle Relaxants and Their Antagonists. In, *Miller's Anesthesia*, 6th ed. (Miller RD, ed.) Churchill-Livingstone, Philadelphia, **2005**, pp. 481–572.

Numa S, Noda M, Takahashi H, et al. Molecular structure of the nicotinic acetylcholine receptor. *Cold Spring Harbor Symp Quant Biol,* **1983,** *48*:57–69.

Pantuck EJ. Plasma cholinesterase: gene and variations. *Anesth Analg,* **1993,** *77*:380–386.

Pollard BJ. Interactions involving relaxants. In, *Applied Neuromuscular Pharmacology.* (Pollard BJ, ed.) Oxford University Press, Oxford, England, **1994,** pp. 202–248.

Primo-Parmo SL, Bartels CF, Wiersema B, et al. Characterization of 12 silent alleles of the human butyrylcholinesterase (*BCHE*) gene. *Am J Hum Genet,* **1996,** *58*:52–64.

Prud'homme M, Houdeau E, Serghini R, et al. Small intensely fluorescent cells of the rat paracervical ganglion. *Brain Res,* **1999,** *821*:141–149.

Rollema H, Coe JW, Chambers LK, et al. Rationale, pharmacology and clinical efficacy of partial agonists of α4β2 nACh receptors for smoking cessation. *Trends Pharmacol Sci*, **2007**, *28*:316–325.

Rosenberg H, Davis M, James D, et al. Malignant Hyperthermia. *Orphanet J Rare Dis,* **2007**, *2*:21–35

Sakmann B. Elementary steps in synaptic transmission revealed by currents through single ion channels. *Science,* **1992,** *256*:503–512.

Savarese JJ. Upcoming Improvements in Relaxation & Reversal. In, *Clinical Anesthesiology,* 4th ed. (Morgan GE Jr., Mikhail MS, Murray MJ, eds.) McGraw-Hill, New York, **2006**, pp. 216–217.

Sine SM, Claudio T. γ- and δ-subunits regulate the affinity and cooperativity of ligand binding to the acetylcholine receptor. *J Biol Chem*, **1991,** *266*:19369–19377.

Sine SM, Gao F, Lee WY, et al. Recent structural and mechanistic insights into endplate acetylcholine receptors. *Ann NY Acad Sci,* **2008,** *1132*:53-60.

Slavikova J, Kuncova J, Reischig J, et al. Catecholaminergic neurons in the rat intrinsic cardiac nervous system. *Neurochem Res*, **2003,** *28*:593–598.

Smith S, Brown H, Toman J, Goodman L. The lack of cerebral effects of D-tubocurarine. *Anesthesiology*, **1947**, *8*:1–14.

Stensrud PE. Anesthesia at Remote Locations. In, *Miller's Anesthesia*, 6th ed. (Miller RD, ed.) Churchill-Livingstone, Philadelphia, **2005,** pp. 2637–2664.

Strawn JR, Keck PE Jr, Caroff SN. Neuroleptic Malignant Syndrome. *Am J Psychiatry*, **2007**, *164*:870–876.

Taylor P, Brown RD, Johnson DA. The linkage between ligand occupation and response of the nicotinic acetylcholine receptor. In, *Current Topics in Membranes and Transport,* vol. 18. (Kleinzeller A, Martin BR, eds.) Academic Press, New York, **1983,** pp. 407–444.

Taylor P, Talley TT, Radic Z, et al. Structure-guided drug design: Conferring selectivity among neuronal nicotinic receptor and acetylcholine-binding protein subtypes. *Biochem Pharmacol,* **2007**, *74*:1164–1171.

Unwin N. Nicotinic acetylcholine receptor at 9 Å resolution. *J Mol Biol,* **1993,** *229*:1101–1124.

Unwin N. Refined structure of the nicotinic acetylcholine receptor at 4 Å resolution. *J Mol Biol*, **2005,** *346*:967–989.

Van der Kloot W, Molgo J. Quantal acetylcholine release at the vertebrate neuromuscular junction. *Physiol Rev,* **1994,** *74*:899–991.

van der Spek AF, Reynolds PI, Fang WB, et al. Changes in resistance to mouth opening induced by depolarizing and nondepolarizing neuromuscular relaxants. *Br J Anaesth,* **1990,** *64*:21–27.

Viby-Mogensen J. Neuromuscular Monitoring. In, *Miller's Anesthesia*, 6th ed. (Miller RD, ed.) Churchill-Livingstone, Philadelphia, **2005,** pp. 1551–1569.

Vita GM, Olckers A, Jedlicka AE, et al. Masseter muscle rigidity associated with glycine 1306-to-alanine mutation in the adult muscle sodium channel α-subunit gene. *Anesthesiology,* **1995,** *82*:1097–1103.

Volle RL. Nicotinic ganglion-stimulating agents. In, *Pharmacology of Ganglionic Transmission.* (Kharkevich DA, ed.) Springer-Verlag, Berlin, **1980,** pp. 281–312.

Watkins J. Adverse reaction to neuromuscular blockers: Frequency, investigation, and epidemiology. *Acta Anaesthesiol Scand Suppl,* **1994,** *102*:6–10.

Waud BE, Waud DR. The relation between the response to "train-of-four" stimulation and receptor occlusion during competitive neuromuscular block. *Anesthesiology,* **1972,** *37*:413–416.

Whittaker M. Cholinesterase. In, *Monographs in Human Genetics,* vol. 11. (Beckman L, ed.) S. Karger, Basel, **1986,** p. 231.

Xiu X, Paskar NL, Shanata JAP, et al. Nicotine binding to brain receptors requires a strong cation-π interaction. *Nature*, **2009**, *458*:534-537.

Yentis SM. Suxamethonium and hyperkalaemia. *Anaesth Intensive Care*, **1990**, *18*:92–101.

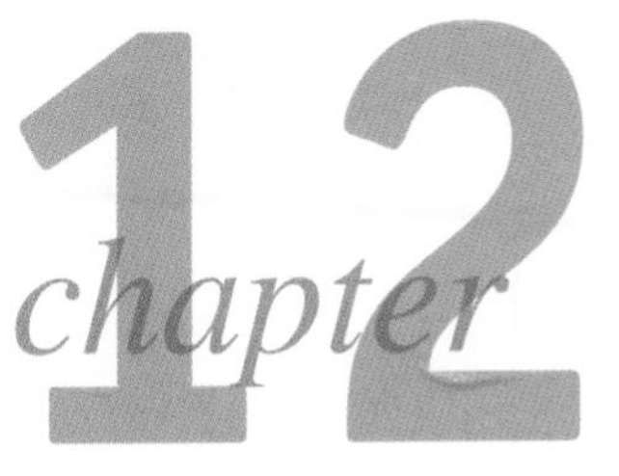

Adrenergic Agonists and Antagonists

Thomas C. Westfall
and David P. Westfall

Catecholamines and Sympathomimetic Drugs

Most of the actions of catecholamines and sympathomimetic agents can be classified into seven broad types:

1. A peripheral excitatory action on certain types of smooth muscle, such as those in blood vessels supplying skin, kidney, and mucous membranes; and on gland cells, such as those in salivary and sweat glands.
2. A peripheral inhibitory action on certain other types of smooth muscle, such as those in the wall of the gut, in the bronchial tree, and in blood vessels supplying skeletal muscle.
3. A cardiac excitatory action that increases heart rate and force of contraction.
4. Metabolic actions, such as an increase in the rate of glycogenolysis in liver and muscle and liberation of free fatty acids from adipose tissue.
5. Endocrine actions, such as modulation (increasing or decreasing) of the secretion of insulin, renin, and pituitary hormones.
6. Actions in the central nervous system (CNS), such as respiratory stimulation, an increase in wakefulness and psychomotor activity, and a reduction in appetite.
7. Prejunctional actions that either inhibit or facilitate the release of neurotransmitters, the inhibitory action being physiologically more important.

Many of these actions and the receptors that mediate them are summarized in Tables 8–1 and 8–8. Not all sympathomimetic drugs show each of the above types of action to the same degree; however, many of the differences in their effects are only quantitative. The pharmacological properties of these drugs as a class are described in detail for the prototypical agent, epinephrine.

Appreciation of the pharmacological properties of the drugs described in this chapter depends on an understanding of the classification, distribution, and mechanism of action of α and β adrenergic receptors (Chapter 8).

CLASSIFICATION OF SYMPATHOMIMETIC DRUGS

Catecholamines and sympathomimetic drugs are classified as direct-acting, indirect-acting, or mixed-acting sympathomimetics (Figure 12–1). Direct-acting sympathomimetic drugs act directly on one or more of the adrenergic receptors. These agents may exhibit considerable selectivity for a specific receptor subtype (e.g., phenylephrine for α_1, terbutaline for β_2) or may have no or minimal selectivity and act on several receptor types (e.g., epinephrine for α_1, α_2, β_1, β_2, and β_3 receptors; norepinephrine for α_1, α_2, and β_1 receptors). Indirect-acting drugs increase the availability of norepinephrine (NE) or epinephrine to stimulate adrenergic receptors. This can be accomplished in several ways:

- by releasing or displacing NE from sympathetic nerve varicosities
- by blocking the transport of NE into sympathetic neurons (e.g., cocaine)
- by blocking the metabolizing enzymes, monoamine oxidase (MAO) (e.g., pargyline) or catechol-*O*-methyltransferase (COMT) (e.g., entacapone)

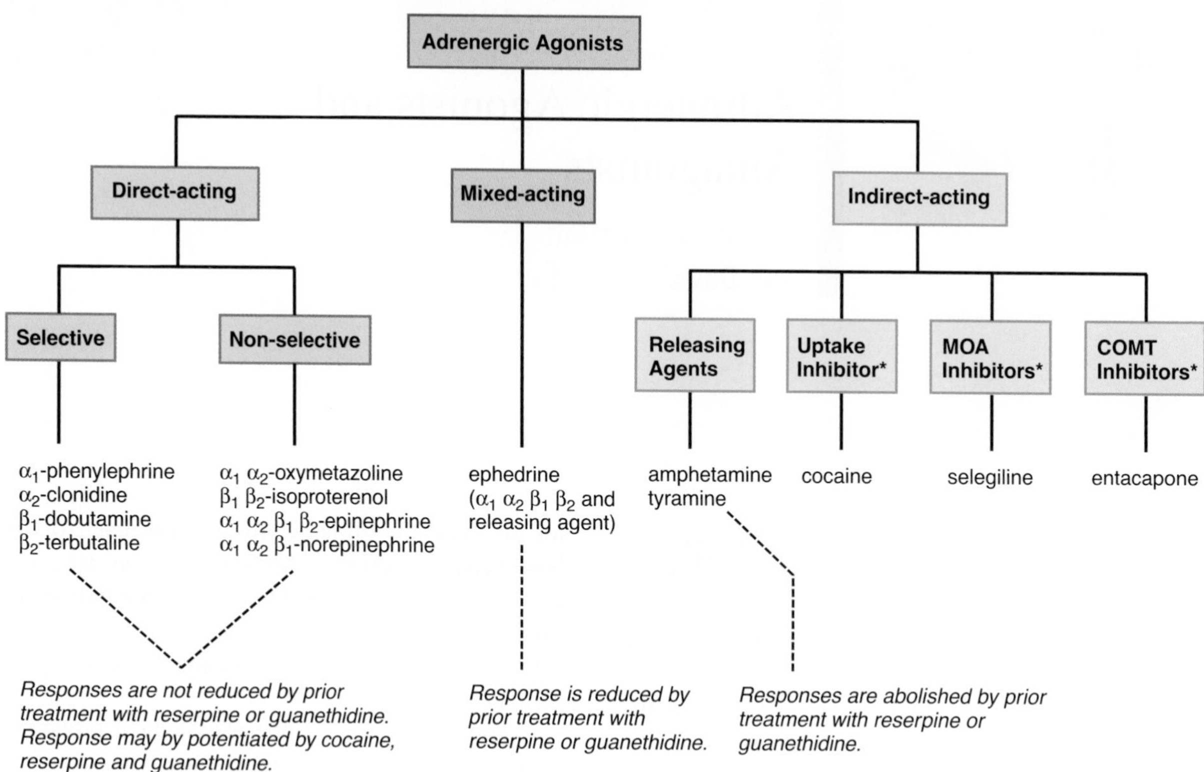

Figure 12–1. *Classification of adrenergic receptor agonists (sympathomimetic amines) or drugs that produce sympathomimetic-like effects. For each category, a prototypical drug is shown. (*Not actually sympathetic drugs but produce sympathomimetic-like effects.)*

Drugs that indirectly release NE and also directly activate receptors are referred to as mixed-acting sympathomimetic drugs (e.g., ephedrine, DA).

Prototypical drugs for these various mechanisms are listed in Figure 12–1. Although this classification is convenient, there probably is a continuum of activity from predominantly direct-acting to predominantly indirect-acting drugs. Thus, this classification is relative rather than absolute.

A feature of direct-acting sympathomimetic drugs is that their responses are not reduced by prior treatment with reserpine or guanethidine, which deplete NE from sympathetic neurons. After transmitter depletion, the actions of direct-acting sympathomimetic drugs actually may increase because the loss of the neurotransmitter induces compensatory changes that up-regulate receptors or enhance the signaling pathway. In contrast, the responses of indirect-acting sympathomimetic drugs (e.g., amphetamine, tyramine) are abolished by prior treatment with reserpine or guanethidine. The cardinal feature of mixed-acting sympathomimetic drugs is that their effects are blunted, but not abolished, by prior treatment with reserpine or guanethidine.

Since the actions of NE are more pronounced on α and β_1 receptors than on β_2 receptors, many non-catecholamines that release NE have predominantly α receptor–mediated and cardiac effects. However, certain non-catecholamines with both direct and indirect effects on adrenergic receptors show significant β_2 activity and are used clinically for these effects. Thus, ephedrine, although dependent on release of NE for some of its effects, relieves bronchospasm by its action on β_2 receptors in bronchial smooth muscle, an effect not seen with NE. Moreover, some non-catecholamines (e.g., phenylephrine) act primarily and directly on target cells. It therefore is impossible to predict precisely the effects of non-catecholamines solely on their ability to provoke NE release.

Chemistry and Structure-Activity Relationship of Sympathomimetic Amines. β-Phenylethylamine (Table 12–1) can be viewed as the parent compound of the sympathomimetic amines, consisting of a benzene ring and an ethylamine side chain. The structure permits substitutions to be made on the aromatic ring, the α- and β-carbon atoms, and the terminal amino group to yield a variety of compounds with sympathomimetic activity. NE, epinephrine, DA, isoproterenol, and a few other agents have hydroxyl groups substituted at positions 3 and 4 of the benzene ring. Since *o*-dihydroxybenzene is also known as catechol, sympathomimetic amines with these hydroxyl substitutions in the aromatic ring are termed catecholamines.

Table 12–1

Chemical Structures and Main Clinical Uses of Important Sympathomimetic Drugs[b]

	Ring (positions 1–6)	β CH	α CH	NH	MAIN CLINICAL USES: α RECEPTOR A	N	P	V	β RECEPTOR B	C	U	CNS, O
Phenylethylamine		H	H	H								
Epinephrine	3-OH, 4-OH	OH	H	CH_3	A		P	V	B	C		
Norepinephrine (NE)	3-OH, 4-OH	OH	H	H			P					
Dopamine (DA)	3-OH, 4-OH	H	H	H			P					
Dobutamine	3-OH, 4-OH	H	H	1[a]						C		
Colterol	3-OH, 4-OH	OH	H	$C(CH_3)_3$					B			
Ethylnorepinephrine	3-OH, 4-OH	OH	CH_2CH_3	H					B			
Isoproterenol	3-OH, 4-OH	OH	H	$CH(CH_3)_2$					B	C		
Isoetharine	3-OH, 4-OH	OH	CH_2CH_3	$CH(CH_3)_2$					B			
Metaproterenol	3-OH, 5-OH	OH	H	$CH(CH_3)_2$					B			
Terbutaline	3-OH, 5-OH	OH	H	$C(CH_3)_3$					B		U	
Metaraminol	3-OH	OH	CH_3	H			P					
Phenylephrine	3-OH	OH	H	CH_3		N	P					
Tyramine	4-OH	H	H	H								
Hydroxyamphetamine	4-OH	H	CH_3	H								
Ritodrine	4-OH	OH	CH_3	2[a]							U	
Prenalterol	4-OH	OH‡	H	$-CH(CH_3)_2$						C		
Methoxamine	2-OCH_3, 5-OCH_3	OH	CH_3	H			P					
Albuterol	3-CH_2OH, 4-OH	OH	H	$C(CH_3)_3$					B		U	
Amphetamine		H	CH_3	H								CNS, O
Methamphetamine		H	CH_3	CH3								CNS, O
Benzphetamine		H	CH_3	3[a]								O
Ephedrine		OH	CH_3	CH_3		N	P		B	C		
Phenylpropanolamine		OH	CH_3	H		N						O
Mephentermine		H	4[a]	CH_3		N	P					
Phentermine		H	4[a]	H								O
Propylhexedrine	5[a]	H	CH_3	CH_3		N						
Diethylpropion			6[a]									O
Phenmetrazine			7[a]									O
Phendimetrazine			8[a]									O

(Continued)

Table 12–1

Chemical Structures and Main Clinical Uses of Important Sympathomimetic Drugs[b] (Continued)

				MAIN CLINICAL USES							
				α RECEPTOR				β RECEPTOR			
				A	N	P	V	B	C	U	CNS, 0
1: $-CH(CH_3)-(CH_2)_2-C_6H_4-OH$		2: $-CH_2-CH_2-C_6H_4-OH$		3: $-N(CH_3)-CH_2-C_6H_5$				4: $-C(CH_3)_2-$			
5: (cyclohexyl ring)	6: $-C(=O)-CH(CH_3)-N(C_2H_5)-C_2H_5$		7: $-CH$ (ring: O—CH_2—CH_2—NH—CH(CH_3)—)					8: $-CH$ (ring: O—CH_2—CH_2—N(CH_3)—CH(CH_3)—)			

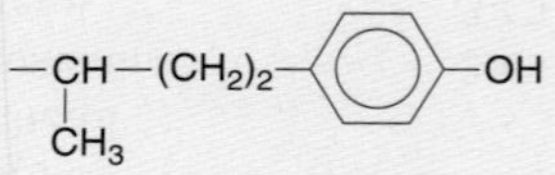

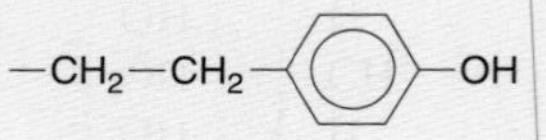

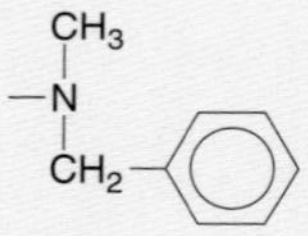

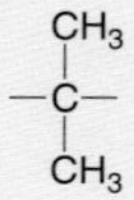

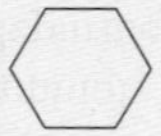

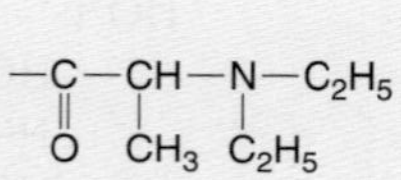

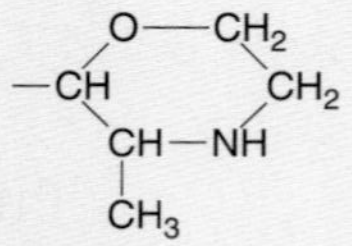

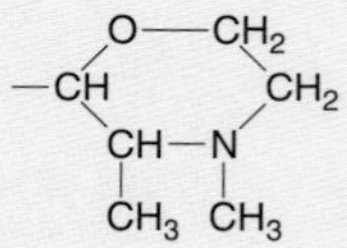

α Activity
A = Allergic reactions (includes action)
N = Nasal decongestion
P = Pressor (may include action)
V = Other local vasoconstriction
(e.g., in local anesthesia)

β Activity
B = Bronchodilator
C = Cardiac
U = Uterus

CNS = Central nervous system
0 = Anorectic

[a]Numbers bearing an asterisk refers to substituents numbered in the bottom rows of the table; substituent 3 replaces the N atom, substituent 5 replaces the phenyl ring and 6,7 and 8 are attached directly to the phenyl ring, replacing the ethylamine side chain.

[b]The α and β in the prototypical formula refer to positions of the C atoms in the ethylamine side chain. Prenalterol has $-OCH_2$-between the aromatic ring and the carbon atom designated as β in the prototypical formula.

Many directly acting sympathomimetic drugs influence both α and β receptors, but the ratio of activities varies among drugs in a continuous spectrum from predominantly α activity (phenylephrine) to predominantly β activity (isoproterenol). Despite the multiplicity of the sites of action of sympathomimetic amines, several generalizations can be made (Table 12–1).

Separation of Aromatic Ring and Amino Group. By far the greatest sympathomimetic activity occurs when two carbon atoms separate the ring from the amino group. This rule applies with few exceptions to all types of action.

Substitution on the Amino Group. The effects of amino substitution are most readily seen in the actions of catecholamines on α and β receptors. Increase in the size of the alkyl substituent increases β receptor activity (e.g., isoproterenol). NE has, in general, rather feeble β_2 activity; this activity is greatly increased in epinephrine by the addition of a methyl group. A notable exception is phenylephrine, which has an *N*-methyl substituent but is an α-selective agonist. β_2-Selective compounds require a large amino substituent, but depend on other substitutions to define selectivity for β_2 rather than for β_1 receptors. In general, the smaller the substitution on the amino group, the greater the selectivity for α activity, although *N*-methylation increases the potency of primary amines. Thus, α activity is maximal in epinephrine, less in NE and almost absent in isoproterenol.

Substitution on the Aromatic Nucleus. Maximal α and β activity depends on the presence of hydroxyl groups on positions 3 and 4. When one or both of these groups are absent, with no other aromatic substitution, the overall potency is reduced. Phenylephrine is thus less potent than epinephrine at both α and β receptors, with β_2 activity almost completely absent. Studies of the β adrenergic receptor suggest that the hydroxyl groups on serine residues 204 and 207 probably form hydrogen bonds with the catechol hydroxyl groups at positions 3 and 4, respectively. It also appears that aspartate 113 is a point of electrostatic interaction with the amine group on the ligand. Since the serines are in the fifth membrane-spanning region and the aspartate is in the third (Chapter 8), it is likely that catecholamines bind parallel to the plane of the membrane, forming a bridge between the two membrane spans. However, models involving DA receptors suggest alternative possibilities.

Hydroxyl groups in positions 3 and 5 confer β_2 receptor selectivity on compounds with large amino substituents. Thus, metaproterenol, terbutaline, and other similar compounds relax the bronchial musculature in patients with asthma, but cause less direct cardiac stimulation than do the non-selective drugs. The response to non-catecholamines is partly determined by their capacity to release NE from storage sites. These agents thus cause effects that are mostly mediated by α and β_1 receptors, since NE is a weak β_2 agonist. Phenylethylamines that lack hydroxyl groups on the ring and the β-hydroxyl group on the side chain act almost exclusively by causing the release of NE from sympathetic nerve terminals.

Since substitution of polar groups on the phenylethylamine structure makes the resultant compounds less lipophilic, unsubstituted or alkyl-substituted compounds cross the blood-brain barrier more readily and have more central activity. Thus, ephedrine, amphetamine, and methamphetamine exhibit considerable CNS activity. In addition, as noted, the absence of polar hydroxyl groups results in a loss of direct sympathomimetic activity.

Catecholamines have only a brief duration of action and are ineffective when administered orally, because they are rapidly inactivated in the intestinal mucosa and in the liver before reaching the systemic circulation (Chapter 8). Compounds without one or both hydroxyl substituents are not acted upon by COMT, and their oral effectiveness and duration of action are enhanced.

Groups other than hydroxyls have been substituted on the aromatic ring. In general, potency at α receptors is reduced and β receptor activity is minimal; the compounds may even block β receptors. For example, methoxamine, with methoxy substituents at positions 2 and 5, has highly selective α-stimulating activity, and in large doses blocks β receptors. Albuterol, a β_2-selective agonist, has a substituent at position 3 and is an important exception to the general rule of low β receptor activity.

Substitution on the α-Carbon Atom. This substitution blocks oxidation by MAO, greatly prolonging the duration of action of non-catecholamines because their degradation depends largely on the action of this enzyme. The duration of action of drugs such as ephedrine or amphetamine is thus measured in hours rather than in minutes. Similarly, compounds with an α-methyl substituent persist in the nerve terminals and are more likely to release NE from storage sites. Agents such as metaraminol exhibit a greater degree of indirect sympathomimetic activity.

Substitution on the β-Carbon Atom. Substitution of a hydroxyl group on the β carbon generally decreases actions within the CNS, largely because it lowers lipid solubility. However, such substitution greatly enhances agonist activity at both α and β adrenergic receptors. Although ephedrine is less potent than methamphetamine as a central stimulant, it is more powerful in dilating bronchioles and increasing blood pressure and heart rate.

Optical Isomerism. Substitution on either α- or β-carbon yields optical isomers. Levorotatory substitution on the β-carbon confers the greater peripheral activity, so that the naturally occurring *l*-epinephrine and *l*-NE are at least 10 times as potent as their unnatural *d*-isomers. Dextrorotatory substitution on the α-carbon generally results in a more potent compound. *d*-Amphetamine is more potent than *l*-amphetamine in central but not peripheral activity.

Physiological Basis of Adrenergic Receptor Function. An important factor in the response of any cell or organ to sympathomimetic amines is the density and proportion of α and β adrenergic receptors. For example, NE has relatively little capacity to increase bronchial airflow, since the receptors in bronchial smooth muscle are largely of the β_2 subtype. In contrast, isoproterenol and epinephrine are potent bronchodilators. Cutaneous blood vessels physiologically express almost exclusively α receptors; thus, NE and epinephrine cause constriction of such vessels, whereas isoproterenol has little effect. The smooth muscle of blood vessels that supply skeletal muscles has both β_2 and α receptors; activation of β_2 receptors causes vasodilation, and stimulation of α receptors constricts these vessels. In such vessels, the threshold concentration for activation of β_2 receptors by epinephrine is lower than that for α receptors, but when both types of receptors are activated at high concentrations of epinephrine, the response to α receptors predominates. Physiological concentrations of epinephrine primarily cause vasodilation.

The ultimate response of a target organ to sympathomimetic amines is dictated not only by the direct effects of the agents but also by the reflex homeostatic adjustments of the organism. One of the most striking effects of many sympathomimetic amines is a rise in arterial blood pressure caused by stimulation of vascular α adrenergic receptors. This stimulation elicits compensatory reflexes that are mediated by the carotid–aortic baroreceptor system. As a result, sympathetic tone is diminished and vagal tone is enhanced; each of these responses leads to slowing of the heart rate. Conversely, when a drug (e.g., a β_2 agonist) lowers mean blood pressure at the mechanoreceptors of the carotid sinus and aortic arch, the baroreceptor reflex works to restore pressure by reducing parasympathetic (vagal) outflow from the CNS to the heart, and increasing sympathetic outflow to the heart and vessels. The baroreceptor reflex effect is of special importance for drugs that have little capacity to activate β receptors directly. With diseases such as atherosclerosis, which may impair baroreceptor mechanisms, the effects of sympathomimetic drugs may be magnified.

False-Transmitter Concept. Indirectly acting amines are taken up into sympathetic nerve terminals and storage vesicles, where they replace NE in the storage complex. Phenylethylamines that lack a β-hydroxyl group are retained there poorly, but β-hydroxylated phenylethylamines and compounds that subsequently become hydroxylated in the synaptic vesicle by dopamine β-hydroxylase are retained in the synaptic vesicle for relatively long periods of time. Such substances can produce a persistent diminution in the content of NE at functionally critical sites. When the nerve is stimulated, the contents of a relatively constant number of synaptic vesicles are apparently released by exocytosis. If these vesicles contain phenylethylamines that are much less potent than NE, activation of postsynaptic α and β receptors will be diminished.

This hypothesis, known as the false-transmitter concept, is a possible explanation for some of the effects of MAO inhibitors. Phenylethylamines normally are synthesized in the GI tract as a result of the action of bacterial tyrosine decarboxylase. The tyramine formed in this fashion usually is oxidatively deaminated in the GI tract and the liver, and the amine does not reach the systemic circulation in significant concentrations. However, when an MAO inhibitor is administered, tyramine may be absorbed systemically and transported into sympathetic nerve terminals, where its catabolism again is prevented because of the inhibition of MAO at this site; the tyramine then is β-hydroxylated to octopamine and stored in the vesicles in this form. As a consequence, NE gradually is displaced, and stimulation of the nerve terminal results in the release of a relatively small amount of NE along with a fraction of octopamine. The latter amine has relatively little ability to activate either α or β receptors. Thus, a functional impairment of sympathetic transmission parallels long-term administration of MAO inhibitors.

Despite such functional impairment, patients who have received MAO inhibitors may experience severe hypertensive crises if they ingest cheese, beer, or red wine. These and related foods, which are produced by fermentation, contain a large quantity of tyramine, and to a lesser degree, other phenylethylamines. When GI and hepatic MAO are inhibited, the large quantity of tyramine that is ingested is absorbed rapidly and reaches the systemic circulation in high concentration. A massive and precipitous release of NE can result, with consequent hypertension that can be severe enough to cause myocardial infarction or a stroke. The properties of various MAO inhibitors (reversible or irreversible; selective or non-selective at MAO-A and MAO-B) are discussed in Chapter 15.

ENDOGENOUS CATECHOLAMINES

Epinephrine

Epinephrine (adrenaline) is a potent stimulant of both α and β adrenergic receptors, and its effects on target organs are thus complex. Most of the responses listed in Table 8–1 are seen after injection of epinephrine, although the occurrence of sweating, piloerection, and mydriasis depends on the physiological state of the subject. Particularly prominent are the actions on the heart and on vascular and other smooth muscle.

Blood Pressure. Epinephrine is one of the most potent vasopressor drugs known. If a pharmacological dose is given rapidly by an intravenous route, it evokes a characteristic effect on blood pressure, which rises rapidly to a peak that is proportional to the dose. The increase in systolic pressure is greater than the increase in diastolic pressure, so that the pulse pressure increases. As the response wanes, the mean pressure may fall below normal before returning to control levels.

The mechanism of the rise in blood pressure due to epinephrine is 3-fold:

- a direct myocardial stimulation that increases the strength of ventricular contraction (positive inotropic action)
- an increased heart rate (positive chronotropic action)
- vasoconstriction in many vascular beds—especially in the precapillary resistance vessels of skin, mucosa, and kidney—along with marked constriction of the veins

The pulse rate, at first accelerated, may be slowed markedly at the height of the rise of blood pressure by compensatory vagal discharge. Small doses of epinephrine (0.1 μg/kg) may cause the blood pressure to fall.

The depressor effect of small doses and the biphasic response to larger doses are due to greater sensitivity to epinephrine of vasodilator β_2 receptors than of constrictor α receptors.

The effects are somewhat different when the drug is given by slow intravenous infusion or by subcutaneous injection. Absorption of epinephrine after subcutaneous injection is slow due to local vasoconstrictor action; the effects of doses as large as 0.5-1.5 mg can be duplicated by intravenous infusion at a rate of 10-30 μg/min. There is a moderate increase in systolic pressure due to increased cardiac contractile force and a rise in cardiac output (Figure 12–2). Peripheral resistance decreases, owing to a dominant action on β_2 receptors of vessels in skeletal muscle, where blood flow is enhanced; as a consequence, diastolic pressure usually falls. Since the mean blood pressure is not, as a rule, greatly elevated, compensatory baroreceptor reflexes do not appreciably antagonize the direct cardiac actions. Heart rate, cardiac output, stroke volume, and left ventricular work per beat are increased as a result of direct cardiac stimulation and increased venous return to the heart, which is reflected by an increase in right atrial pressure. At slightly higher rates of infusion, there may be no change or a slight rise in peripheral resistance and diastolic pressure, depending on the dose and the resultant ratio of α to β responses in the various vascular beds; compensatory reflexes also may come into play. The details of the effects of intravenous infusion of epinephrine, NE, and isoproterenol in humans are compared in Table 12–2 and Figure 12–2.

Vascular Effects. The chief vascular action of epinephrine is exerted on the smaller arterioles and precapillary sphincters, although veins and large arteries also respond to the drug. Various vascular beds react differently, which results in a substantial redistribution of blood flow.

Injected epinephrine markedly decreases cutaneous blood flow, constricting precapillary vessels and small venules. Cutaneous vasoconstriction accounts for a marked decrease in blood flow in the hands and feet. The "after congestion" of mucosa following the vasoconstriction from locally applied epinephrine probably is due to changes in vascular reactivity as a result of tissue hypoxia rather than to β-agonist activity of the drug on mucosal vessels.

Blood flow to skeletal muscles is increased by therapeutic doses in humans. This is due in part to a powerful β_2-mediated vasodilator action that is only partially counterbalanced by a vasoconstrictor action on the α receptors that also are present in the vascular bed. If an α receptor antagonist is given, the vasodilation in muscle is more pronounced, the total peripheral resistance is decreased, and the mean blood pressure

Table 12–2

Comparison of the Effects of Infusion of Epinephrine and Norepinephrine in Human Beings[a]

EFFECT	EPI	NE
Cardiac		
Heart rate	+	–[b]
Stroke volume	++	++
Cardiac output	+++	0,–
Arrhythmias	++++	++++
Coronary blood flow	++	++
Blood Pressure		
Systolic arterial	+++	+++
Mean arterial	+	++
Diastolic arterial	+,0,–	++
Mean pulmonary	++	++
Peripheral Circulation		
Total peripheral resistance	–	++
Cerebral blood flow	+	0,–
Muscle blood flow	+++	0,–
Cutaneous blood flow	–	–
Renal blood flow	–	–
Splanchnic blood flow	+++	0,+
Metabolic Effects		
Oxygen consumption	++	0,+
Blood glucose	+++	0,+
Blood lactic acid	+++	0,+
Eosinopenic response	+	0
Central Nervous System		
Respiration	+	+
Subjective sensations	+	+

[a]0.1-0.4 μg/kg per minute. [b]Abbreviations: Epi, epinephrine; NE norepinephrine; +, increase; 0, no change; –, decrease; [b], after atropine, + After Goldenberg et al, 1950.

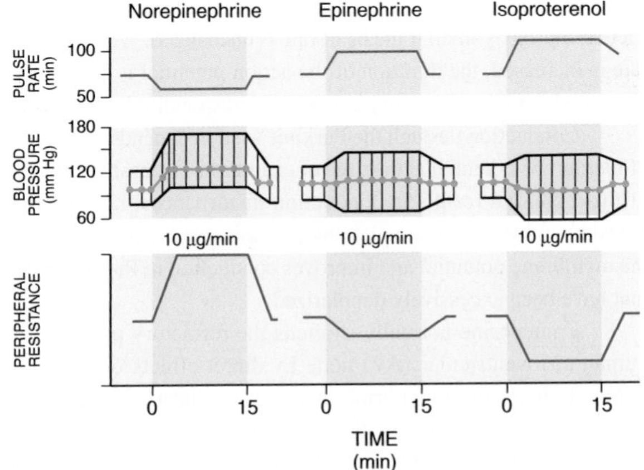

Figure 12–2. *Effects of intravenous infusion of norepinephrine, epinephrine or isoproterenol in humans.* (Modified from Allwood et al., 1963, with permission from Oxford University Press.)

falls (epinephrine reversal). After the administration of a non-selective β receptor antagonist, only vasoconstriction occurs, and the administration of epinephrine is associated with a considerable pressor effect.

The effect of epinephrine on cerebral circulation is related to systemic blood pressure. In usual therapeutic doses, the drug has relatively little constrictor action on cerebral arterioles. It is physiologically advantageous that the cerebral circulation does not constrict in response to activation of the sympathetic nervous system by stressful stimuli. Indeed, autoregulatory mechanisms tend to limit the increase in cerebral blood flow caused by increased blood pressure.

Doses of epinephrine that have little effect on mean arterial pressure consistently increase renal vascular resistance and reduce renal blood flow by as much as 40%. All segments of the renal vascular bed contribute to the increased resistance. Since the glomerular filtration rate is only slightly and variably altered, the filtration fraction is consistently increased. Excretion of Na^+, K^+, and Cl^- is decreased; urine volume may be increased, decreased, or unchanged. Maximal tubular reabsorptive and excretory capacities are unchanged. The secretion of renin is increased as a consequence of a direct action of epinephrine on β_1 receptors in the juxtaglomerular apparatus.

Arterial and venous pulmonary pressures are raised. Although direct pulmonary vasoconstriction occurs, redistribution of blood from the systemic to the pulmonary circulation, due to constriction of the more powerful musculature in the systemic great veins, doubtless plays an important part in the increase in pulmonary pressure. Very high concentrations of epinephrine may cause pulmonary edema precipitated by elevated pulmonary capillary filtration pressure and possibly by "leaky" capillaries.

Coronary blood flow is enhanced by epinephrine or by cardiac sympathetic stimulation under physiological conditions. The increased flow, which occurs even with doses that do not increase the aortic blood pressure, is the result of two factors. The first is the increased relative duration of diastole at higher heart rates (described later); this is partially offset by decreased blood flow during systole because of more forceful contraction of the surrounding myocardium and an increase in mechanical compression of the coronary vessels. The increased flow during diastole is further enhanced if aortic blood pressure is elevated by epinephrine; as a consequence, total coronary flow may be increased. The second factor is a metabolic dilator effect that results from the increased strength of contraction and myocardial O_2 consumption due to the direct effects of epinephrine on cardiac myocytes. This vasodilation is mediated in part by adenosine released from cardiac myocytes, which tends to override a direct vasoconstrictor effect of epinephrine that results from activation of α receptors in coronary vessels.

Cardiac Effects. Epinephrine is a powerful cardiac stimulant. It acts directly on the predominant β_1 receptors of the myocardium and of the cells of the pacemaker and conducting tissues; β_2, β_3, and α receptors also are present in the heart, although there are considerable species differences. Substantial recent interest has focused on the role of β_1 and β_2 receptors in the human heart, especially in heart failure. The heart rate increases, and the rhythm often is altered. Cardiac systole is shorter and more powerful, cardiac output is enhanced, and the work of the heart and its oxygen consumption are markedly increased. Cardiac efficiency (work done relative to oxygen consumption) is lessened. Direct responses to epinephrine include increases in contractile force, accelerated rate of rise of isometric tension, enhanced rate of relaxation, decreased time to peak tension, increased excitability, acceleration of the rate of spontaneous beating, and induction of automaticity in specialized regions of the heart.

In accelerating the heart, epinephrine preferentially shortens systole so that the duration of diastole usually is not reduced. Indeed, activation of β receptors increases the rate of relaxation of ventricular muscle. Epinephrine speeds the heart by accelerating the slow depolarization of sinoatrial (SA) nodal cells that takes place during diastole, that is, during phase 4 of the action potential (Chapter 29). Consequently, the transmembrane potential of the pacemaker cells rises more rapidly to the threshold level of action potential initiation. The amplitude of the action potential and the maximal rate of depolarization (phase 0) also are increased. A shift in the location of the pacemaker within the SA node often occurs, owing to activation of latent pacemaker cells. In Purkinje fibers, epinephrine also accelerates diastolic depolarization and may activate latent pacemaker cells. These changes do not occur in atrial and ventricular muscle fibers, where epinephrine has little effect on the stable, phase 4 membrane potential after repolarization. If large doses of epinephrine are given, premature ventricular contractions occur and may herald more serious ventricular arrhythmias. This rarely is seen with conventional doses in humans, but ventricular extrasystoles, tachycardia, or even fibrillation may be precipitated by release of endogenous epinephrine when the heart has been sensitized to this action of epinephrine by certain anesthetics or by myocardial ischemia. The mechanism of induction of these cardiac arrhythmias is not clear.

Some effects of epinephrine on cardiac tissues are largely secondary to the increase in heart rate and are small or inconsistent when the heart rate is kept constant. For example, the effect of epinephrine on repolarization of atrial muscle, Purkinje fibers, or ventricular muscle is small if the heart rate is unchanged. When the heart rate is increased, the duration of the action potential is consistently shortened, and the refractory period is correspondingly decreased.

Conduction through the Purkinje system depends on the level of membrane potential at the time of excitation. Excessive reduction of this potential results in conduction disturbances, ranging from slowed conduction to complete block. Epinephrine often increases the membrane potential and improves conduction in Purkinje fibers that have been excessively depolarized.

Epinephrine normally shortens the refractory period of the human atrioventricular (AV) node by direct effects on the heart, although doses of epinephrine that slow the heart through reflex vagal discharge may indirectly tend to prolong it. Epinephrine also decreases the grade of AV block that occurs as a result of disease, drugs, or vagal stimulation. Supraventricular arrhythmias are apt to occur from the combination of epinephrine and cholinergic stimulation. Depression of sinus rate and AV conduction by vagal discharge probably plays a part in epinephrine-induced ventricular arrhythmias, since various drugs that block the vagal effect confer some protection. The actions of epinephrine in enhancing cardiac automaticity and in causing arrhythmias are effectively antagonized by β receptor antagonists such as propranolol. However, α_1 receptors exist in most regions of the heart, and their activation prolongs the refractory period and strengthens myocardial contractions.

Cardiac arrhythmias have been seen in patients after inadvertent intravenous administration of conventional subcutaneous doses of epinephrine. Premature ventricular contractions can appear, which may be followed by multifocal ventricular tachycardia or ventricular fibrillation. Pulmonary edema also may occur.

Epinephrine decreases the amplitude of the T wave of the electrocardiogram (ECG) in normal persons. In animals given relatively larger doses, additional effects are seen on the T wave and the ST segment. After decreasing in amplitude, the T wave may become biphasic, and the ST segment can deviate either above or below the isoelectric line. Such ST-segment changes are similar to those seen in patients with angina pectoris during spontaneous or epinephrine-induced attacks of pain. These electrical changes therefore have been attributed to myocardial ischemia. Also, epinephrine as well as other catecholamines may cause myocardial cell death, particularly after intravenous infusions. Acute toxicity is associated with contraction band necrosis and other pathological changes. Recent interest has focused on the possibility that prolonged sympathetic stimulation of the heart, such as in congestive cardiomyopathy, may promote apoptosis of cardiomyocytes.

Effects on Smooth Muscles. The effects of epinephrine on the smooth muscles of different organs and systems depend on the type of adrenergic receptor in the muscle (Table 8–1). The effects on vascular smooth muscle noted above are of major physiological importance, whereas those on smooth muscle of the GI tract are relatively minor. GI smooth muscle is, in general, relaxed by epinephrine. This effect is due to activation of both α and β receptors. Intestinal tone and the frequency and amplitude of spontaneous contractions are reduced. The stomach usually is relaxed and the pyloric and ileocecal sphincters are contracted, but these effects depend on the pre-existing tone of the muscle. If tone already is high, epinephrine causes relaxation; if low, contraction.

The responses of uterine muscle to epinephrine vary with species, phase of the sexual cycle, state of gestation, and dose given. Epinephrine contracts strips of pregnant or nonpregnant human uterus *in vitro* by interaction with α receptors. The effects of epinephrine on the human uterus *in situ*, however, differ. During the last month of pregnancy and at parturition, epinephrine inhibits uterine tone and contractions. Effects of adrenergic agents and other drugs on the uterus are discussed later in this chapter and in Chapter 66.

Epinephrine relaxes the detrusor muscle of the bladder as a result of activation of β receptors and contracts the trigone and sphincter muscles owing to its α-agonist activity. This can result in hesitancy in urination and may contribute to retention of urine in the bladder. Activation of smooth muscle contraction in the prostate promotes urinary retention.

Respiratory Effects. Epinephrine affects respiration primarily by relaxing bronchial muscle. It has a powerful bronchodilator action, most evident when bronchial muscle is contracted because of disease, as in bronchial asthma, or in response to drugs or various autacoids. In such situations, epinephrine has a striking therapeutic effect as a physiological antagonist to substances that cause bronchoconstriction.

The beneficial effects of epinephrine in asthma also may arise from inhibition of antigen-induced release of inflammatory mediators from mast cells, and to a lesser extent from diminution of bronchial secretions and congestion within the mucosa. Inhibition of mast cell secretion is mediated by β_2 receptors, while the effects on the mucosa are mediated by α receptors; however, other drugs, such as glucocorticoids and leukotriene receptor antagonists, have much more profound anti-inflammatory effects in asthma (Chapters 33 and 34).

Effects on the CNS. Because of the inability of this rather polar compound to enter the CNS, epinephrine in conventional therapeutic doses is not a powerful CNS stimulant. While the drug may cause restlessness, apprehension, headache, and tremor in many persons, these effects in part may be secondary to the effects of epinephrine on the cardiovascular system, skeletal muscles, and intermediary metabolism; that is, they may be the result of somatic manifestations of anxiety. Some other sympathomimetic drugs more readily cross the blood-brain barrier.

Metabolic Effects. Epinephrine has a number of important influences on metabolic processes. It elevates the concentrations of glucose and lactate in blood by mechanisms described in Chapter 8. Insulin secretion is inhibited through an interaction with α_2 receptors and is enhanced by activation of β_2 receptors; the predominant effect seen with epinephrine is inhibition. Glucagon secretion is enhanced by an action on the β receptors of the α cells of pancreatic islets. Epinephrine also decreases the uptake of glucose by peripheral tissues, at least in part because of its effects on the secretion of insulin, but also possibly due to direct effects on skeletal muscle. Glycosuria rarely occurs. The effect of epinephrine to stimulate glycogenolysis in most tissues and in most species involves β receptors.

Epinephrine raises the concentration of free fatty acids in blood by stimulating β receptors in adipocytes. The result is activation of triglyceride lipase, which accelerates the triglyceride breakdown to free fatty acids and glycerol. The calorigenic action of epinephrine (increase in metabolism) is reflected in humans by an increase of 20-30% in oxygen consumption after conventional doses. This effect mainly is due to enhanced breakdown of triglycerides in brown adipose tissue, providing an increase in oxidizable substrate (Chapter 8).

Miscellaneous Effects. Epinephrine reduces circulating plasma volume by loss of protein-free fluid to the extracellular space, thereby increasing hematocrit and plasma protein concentration. However, conventional doses of epinephrine do not significantly alter plasma volume or packed red cell volume under normal conditions, although such doses are reported to have variable effects in the presence of shock, hemorrhage, hypotension, or anesthesia. Epinephrine rapidly increases the number of circulating polymorphonuclear leukocytes, likely due to β receptor–mediated demargination of these cells. Epinephrine accelerates blood coagulation in laboratory animals and humans and promotes fibrinolysis.

The effects of epinephrine on secretory glands are not marked; in most glands secretion usually is inhibited, partly owing to the reduced blood flow caused by vasoconstriction. Epinephrine stimulates lacrimation and a scanty mucus secretion from salivary glands. Sweating and pilomotor activity are minimal after systemic administration of epinephrine, but occur after intradermal injection of very dilute solutions of either epinephrine or NE. Such effects are inhibited by α receptor antagonists.

Mydriasis is readily seen during physiological sympathetic stimulation but not when epinephrine is instilled into the conjunctival sac of normal eyes. However, epinephrine usually lowers intraocular pressure; the mechanism of this effect is not clear but probably reflects reduced production of aqueous humor due to vasoconstriction and enhanced outflow (Chapter 64).

Although epinephrine does not directly excite skeletal muscle, it facilitates neuromuscular transmission, particularly that following prolonged rapid stimulation of motor nerves. In apparent contrast to the effects of α receptor activation at presynaptic nerve terminals in the autonomic nervous system (α_2 receptors), stimulation of α receptors causes a more rapid increase in transmitter release from the somatic motor neuron, perhaps as a result of enhanced influx of Ca^{2+}. These responses likely are mediated by α_1 receptors. These actions may explain in part the ability of epinephrine (given intra-arterially) to briefly increase strength of the injected limb of patients with myasthenia gravis. Epinephrine also acts directly on white, fast-twitch muscle fibers to prolong the active state, thereby increasing peak tension. Of greater physiological and clinical importance is the capacity of epinephrine and selective β_2 agonists to increase physiological tremor, at least in part due to β receptor–mediated enhancement of discharge of muscle spindles.

Epinephrine promotes a fall in plasma K^+, largely due to stimulation of K^+ uptake into cells, particularly skeletal muscle, due to activation of β_2 receptors. This is associated with decreased renal K^+ excretion. These receptors have been exploited in the management of hyperkalemic familial periodic paralysis, which is characterized by episodic flaccid paralysis, hyperkalemia, and depolarization of skeletal muscle. The β_2-selective agonist albuterol apparently is able to ameliorate the impairment in the ability of the muscle to accumulate and retain K^+.

The administration of large or repeated doses of epinephrine or other sympathomimetic amines to experimental animals damages arterial walls and myocardium, even inducing necrosis in the heart indistinguishable from myocardial infarction. The mechanism of this injury is not yet clear, but α and β receptor antagonists and Ca^{2+} channel blockers may afford substantial protection against the damage. Similar lesions occur in many patients with pheochromocytoma or after prolonged infusions of NE.

Absorption, Fate, and Excretion. Epinephrine is not effective after oral administration because it is rapidly conjugated and oxidized in the GI mucosa and liver. Absorption from subcutaneous tissues occurs relatively slowly because of local vasoconstriction and the rate may be further decreased by systemic hypotension, for example in a patient with shock. Absorption is more rapid after intramuscular injection. In emergencies, it may be necessary to administer epinephrine intravenously. When relatively concentrated solutions are nebulized and inhaled, the actions of the drug largely are restricted to the respiratory tract; however, systemic reactions such as arrhythmias may occur, particularly if larger amounts are used.

Epinephrine is rapidly inactivated in the body. The liver, which is rich in both of the enzymes responsible for destroying circulating epinephrine (COMT and MAO), is particularly important in this regard (see Figure 8–7 and Table 8–4). Although only small amounts appear in the urine of normal persons, the urine of patients with pheochromocytoma may contain relatively large amounts of epinephrine, NE and their metabolites.

Epinephrine is available in a variety of formulations geared for different clinical indications and routes of administration, including self-administration for anaphylactic reactions (EpiPen). Several practical points are worth noting. First, epinephrine is unstable in alkaline solution; when exposed to air or light, it turns pink from oxidation to adrenochrome and then brown from formation of polymers. Epinephrine injection is available in 1 mg/mL (1:1000), 0.1 mg/mL (1:10,000), and 0.5 mg/mL (1:2,000) solutions. The usual adult dose given subcutaneously ranges from 0.3-0.5 mg. Fatal medication errors have occurred as a consequence of confusing these dilutions. The intravenous route is used cautiously if an immediate and reliable effect is mandatory. If the solution is given by vein, it must be adequately diluted and injected very slowly. The dose is seldom as much as 0.25 mg, except for cardiac arrest, when larger doses may be required.

Toxicity, Adverse Effects, and Contraindications. Epinephrine may cause disturbing reactions, such as restlessness, throbbing headache, tremor, and palpitations. The effects rapidly subside with rest, quiet, recumbency, and reassurance. More serious reactions include cerebral hemorrhage and cardiac arrhythmias. The use of large doses or the accidental, rapid intravenous injection of epinephrine may result in cerebral hemorrhage from the sharp rise in blood pressure. Ventricular arrhythmias may follow the administration of epinephrine. Angina may be induced by epinephrine in patients with coronary artery disease. The use of epinephrine generally is contraindicated in patients who are receiving non-selective β receptor antagonists, since its unopposed actions on vascular α_1 receptors may lead to severe hypertension and cerebral hemorrhage.

Therapeutic Uses. The clinical uses of epinephrine are based on its actions on blood vessels, heart, and bronchial muscle. In the past, the most common use of epinephrine was to relieve respiratory distress due to bronchospasm; however, β_2-selective agonists now are preferred. A major use is to provide rapid, emergency relief of hypersensitivity reactions, including anaphylaxis, to drugs and other allergens. Epinephrine also is used to prolong the action of local anesthetics, presumably by decreasing local blood flow (Chapter 20). Its cardiac effects may be of use in restoring cardiac rhythm in patients with cardiac arrest due to various causes. It also is used as a topical hemostatic agent on bleeding surfaces such as in the mouth or in bleeding peptic ulcers during endoscopy of the stomach and duodenum. Systemic absorption of the drug can occur with dental application. In addition, inhalation of epinephrine may be useful in the treatment of post-intubation and infectious croup. The therapeutic uses of epinephrine, in relation to other sympathomimetic drugs, are discussed later in this chapter.

Norepinephrine

Norepinephrine (levarterenol, *l*-noradrenaline, *l*-β-[3,4-dihydroxyphenyl]-α-aminoethanol, NE) is a major chemical mediator liberated by mammalian postganglionic sympathetic nerves. It differs from epinephrine only by lacking the methyl substitution in the amino group (Table 12–1). NE constitutes 10-20% of the catecholamine content of human adrenal medulla and as much as 97% in some pheochromocytomas, which may not express the enzyme phenylethanolamine-*N*-methyltransferase. The history of its discovery and its role as a neurohumoral mediator are discussed in Chapter 8.

Pharmacological Properties. The pharmacological actions of NE and epinephrine have been extensively compared *in vivo* and *in vitro* (Table 12–2). Both drugs are direct agonists on effector cells, and their actions differ mainly in the ratio of their effectiveness in stimulating α and β_2 receptors. They are approximately equipotent in stimulating β_1 receptors. NE is a potent α agonist and has relatively little action on β_2 receptors; however, it is somewhat less potent than epinephrine on the α receptors of most organs.

Cardiovascular Effects. The cardiovascular effects of an intravenous infusion of 10 μg/min of NE in humans are shown in Figure 12–2. Systolic and diastolic pressures, and usually pulse pressure, are increased. Cardiac output is unchanged or decreased, and total peripheral resistance is raised. Compensatory vagal reflex activity slows the heart, overcoming a direct cardioaccelerator action, and stroke volume is increased. The peripheral vascular resistance increases in most vascular beds, and renal blood flow is reduced. NE constricts mesenteric vessels and reduces splanchnic and hepatic blood flow. Coronary flow usually is increased, probably owing both to indirectly induced coronary dilation, as with epinephrine, and to elevated blood pressure. Although generally a poor β_2 receptor agonist, NE may increase coronary blood flow directly by stimulating β_2 receptors on coronary vessels The physiological significance of this is not yet established. Patients with Prinzmetal's variant angina may be supersensitive to the α adrenergic vasoconstrictor effects of NE.

Unlike epinephrine, small doses of NE do not cause vasodilation or lower blood pressure, since the blood vessels of skeletal muscle constrict rather than dilate; α adrenergic receptor antagonists therefore abolish the pressor effects but do not cause significant reversal (i.e., hypotension).

Other Effects. Other responses to NE are not prominent in humans. The drug causes hyperglycemia and other metabolic effects similar to those produced by epinephrine, but these are observed only when large doses are given because NE is not as effective a "hormone" as epinephrine. Intradermal injection of suitable doses causes sweating that is not blocked by atropine.

Absorption, Fate, and Excretion. NE, like epinephrine, is ineffective when given orally and is absorbed poorly from sites of subcutaneous injection. It is rapidly inactivated in the body by the same enzymes that methylate and oxidatively deaminate epinephrine (discussed earlier). Small amounts normally are found in the urine. The excretion rate may be greatly increased in patients with pheochromocytoma.

Toxicity, Adverse Effects, and Precautions. The untoward effects of NE are similar to those of epinephrine, although there typically is greater elevation of blood pressure with NE. Excessive doses can cause severe hypertension, so careful blood pressure monitoring generally is indicated during systemic administration of this agent.

Care must be taken that necrosis and sloughing do not occur at the site of intravenous injection owing to extravasation of the drug. The infusion should be made high in the limb, preferably through a long plastic cannula extending centrally. Impaired circulation at injection sites, with or without extravasation of NE, may be relieved by infiltrating the area with phentolamine, an α receptor antagonist. Blood pressure must be determined frequently during the infusion and particularly during adjustment of the rate of the infusion. Reduced blood flow to organs such as kidney and intestines is a constant danger with the use of NE.

Therapeutic Uses and Status. NE (LEVOPHED, others) is used as a vasoconstrictor to raise or support blood pressure under certain intensive care conditions. The use of it and other sympathomimetic amines in shock is discussed later in this chapter. In the treatment of low blood pressure, the dose is titrated to the desired pressor response.

Dopamine

Dopamine (3,4-dihydroxyphenylethylamine, DA) (Table 12–1) is the immediate metabolic precursor of NE and epinephrine; it is a central neurotransmitter particularly important in the regulation of movement (Chapters 14, 16, and 22) and possesses important intrinsic pharmacological properties. In the periphery, it is synthesized in epithelial cells of the proximal tubule and is thought to exert local diuretic and natriuretic effects. DA is a substrate for both MAO and COMT and thus is ineffective when administered orally. Classification of DA receptors is described in Chapter 13.

Pharmacological Properties.

Cardiovascular Effects. The cardiovascular effects of DA are mediated by several distinct types of receptors that vary in their affinity for DA (Chapter 13). At low concentrations, the primary interaction of DA is with vascular D_1 receptors, especially in the renal, mesenteric, and coronary beds. By activating adenylyl cyclase and raising intra-cellular concentrations of cyclic AMP, D_1 receptor stimulation leads to vasodilation. Infusion of low doses of DA causes an increase in glomerular filtration rate, renal blood flow, and Na^+ excretion. Activation of D_1 receptors on renal tubular cells decreases Na^+ transport by cAMP-dependent and cAMP-independent mechanisms. Increasing cAMP production in the proximal tubular cells and the medullary part of the thick ascending limb of the loop of Henle inhibits the Na^+-H^+ exchanger and the Na^+,K^+-ATPase pump. The renal tubular actions of DA that cause natriuresis may be augmented by the increase in renal blood flow and the small increase in the glomerular filtration rate that follow its administration. The resulting increase in hydrostatic pressure in the peritubular capillaries and reduction in oncotic pressure may contribute to diminished reabsorption of Na^+ by the proximal tubular cells. As a consequence, DA has pharmacologically appropriate effects in the management of states of low cardiac output associated with compromised renal function, such as severe congestive heart failure.

At somewhat higher concentrations, DA exerts a positive inotropic effect on the myocardium, acting on β_1 adrenergic receptors. DA also causes the release of NE from nerve terminals, which contributes to its effects on the heart. Tachycardia is less prominent during infusion of DA than of isoproterenol (discussed later). DA usually increases systolic blood pressure and pulse pressure and either has no effect on diastolic blood pressure or increases it slightly. Total peripheral resistance usually is unchanged when low or intermediate doses of DA are given, probably because of the ability of DA to reduce regional arterial resistance in some vascular beds, such as mesenteric and renal, while causing only minor increases in others. At high concentrations, DA activates vascular α_1 receptors, leading to more general vasoconstriction.

Other Effects. Although there are specific DA receptors in the CNS, injected DA usually has no central effects because it does not readily cross the blood-brain barrier.

Precautions, Adverse Reactions, and Contraindications. Before DA is administered to patients in shock, hypovolemia should be corrected by transfusion of whole blood, plasma, or other appropriate fluid. Untoward effects due to overdosage generally are attributable to excessive sympathomimetic activity (although this also may be the response to worsening shock). Nausea, vomiting, tachycardia, anginal pain, arrhythmias, headache, hypertension, and peripheral vasoconstriction may be encountered during dopamine infusion. Extravasation of large amounts of DA during infusion may cause ischemic necrosis and sloughing. Rarely, gangrene of the fingers or toes has followed prolonged infusion of the drug.

DA should be avoided or used at a much reduced dosage (one-tenth or less) if the patient has received a MAO inhibitor. Careful adjustment of dosage also is necessary in patients who are taking tricyclic antidepressants.

Therapeutic Uses. DA is used in the treatment of severe congestive heart failure, particularly in patients with oliguria and low or normal peripheral vascular resistance. The drug also may improve physiological parameters in the treatment of cardiogenic and septic shock. While DA may acutely improve cardiac and renal function in severely ill patients with chronic heart disease or renal failure, there is relatively little evidence supporting long-term benefit in clinical outcome (Marik and Iglesias, 1999). The management of shock is discussed later.

Dopamine hydrochloride is used only intravenously, preferably into a large vein to prevent perivasular infiltration; extravasation may cause necrosis and sloughing of the surrounding tissue. The use of a calibrated infusion pump or other device capable of controlling the rate of flow is necessary. The drug initially is administered at a rate of 2-5 μg/kg per minute; this rate may be increased gradually up to 20-50 μg/kg per minute or more as the clinical situation dictates. During the infusion, patients require clinical assessment of myocardial function, perfusion of vital organs such as the brain, and the production of urine. Most patients should receive intensive care, with monitoring of arterial and venous pressures and the ECG. Reduction in urine flow, tachycardia, or the development of arrhythmias may be indications to slow or terminate the infusion. The duration of action of DA is brief, and hence the rate of administration can be used to control the intensity of effect.

Related drugs include fenoldopam and dopexamine. Fenoldopam (CORLOPAM, others), a benzazepine derivative, is a rapidly acting vasodilator used for control of severe hypertension (e.g., malignant hypertension with end-organ damage) in hospitalized patients for not more than 48 hours. Fenoldopam is an agonist for peripheral D_1 receptors and binds with moderate affinity to α_2 adrenergic receptors; it has no significant affinity for D_2 receptors or α_1 or β adrenergic receptors. Fenoldopam is a racemic mixture; the R-isomer is the active component. It dilates a variety of blood vessels, including coronary arteries, afferent and efferent arterioles in the kidney, and mesenteric arteries (Murphy et al., 2001). Fenoldopam must be administered using a calibrated infusion pump; the usual dose rate ranges from 0.01-1.6 μg/kg per minute.

Less than 6% of an orally administered dose is absorbed because of extensive first-pass formation of sulfate, methyl, and glucuronide conjugates. The elimination $t_{1/2}$ of intravenously infused fenoldopam, estimated from the decline in plasma concentration in hypertensive patients after the cessation of a 2-hour infusion, is 10 minutes. Adverse effects are related to the vasodilation and include headache, flushing, dizziness, and tachycardia or bradycardia.

Dopexamine (DOPACARD) is a synthetic analog related to DA with intrinsic activity at dopamine D_1 and D_2 receptors as well as at β_2 receptors; it may have other effects such as inhibition of catecholamine uptake (Fitton and Benfield, 1990). It appears to have favorable hemodynamic actions in patients with severe congestive heart failure, sepsis, and shock. In patients with low cardiac output, dopexamine infusion significantly increases stroke volume with a decrease in systemic vascular resistance. Tachycardia and hypotension can occur, but usually only at high infusion rates. Dopexamine is not currently available in the U.S.

β ADRENERGIC RECEPTOR AGONISTS

β adrenergic receptor agonists have been utilized in many clinical settings but now play a major role only in the treatment of bronchoconstriction in patients with asthma (reversible airway obstruction) or chronic obstructive pulmonary disease (COPD). Minor uses include management of preterm labor, treatment of complete heart block in shock, and short-term treatment of cardiac decompensation after surgery or in patients with congestive heart failure or myocardial infarction.

Epinephrine first was used as a bronchodilator at the beginning of the past century, and ephedrine was introduced into western medicine in 1924, although it had been used in China for thousands of years. The next major advance was the development in the 1940s of isoproterenol, a β receptor–selective agonist; this provided a drug for asthma that lacked α receptor activity. The recent development of β_2-selective agonists has resulted in drugs with even more valuable characteristics, including adequate oral bioavailability, lack of α adrenergic activity, and diminished likelihood of some adverse cardiovascular effects.

β Receptor agonists may be used to stimulate the rate and force of cardiac contraction. The chronotropic effect is useful in the emergency treatment of arrhythmias such as torsades de pointes, bradycardia, or heart block (Chapter 29), whereas the inotropic effect is useful when it is desirable to augment myocardial contractility. The therapeutic uses of β agonists are discussed later in the chapter.

Isoproterenol

Isoproterenol (isopropylarterenol, isopropyl norepinephrine, isoprenaline, isopropyl noradrenaline, *d,l*-β-[3,4-dihydroxyphenyl]-α-isopropylaminoethanol) (Table 12–1) is a potent, non-selective β receptor agonist with very low affinity for α receptors. Consequently, isoproterenol has powerful effects on all β receptors and almost no action at α receptors.

Pharmacological Actions. The major cardiovascular effects of isoproterenol (compared with epinephrine and NE) are illustrated in Figure 12–2. Intravenous infusion of isoproterenol lowers peripheral vascular resistance, primarily in skeletal muscle but also in renal and mesenteric vascular beds. Diastolic pressure falls. Systolic blood pressure may remain unchanged or rise, although mean arterial pressure typically falls. Cardiac output is increased because of the positive inotropic and chronotropic effects of the drug in the face of diminished peripheral vascular resistance. The cardiac effects of isoproterenol may lead to palpitations, sinus tachycardia, and more serious arrhythmias; large doses of isoproterenol may cause myocardial necrosis in animals.

Isoproterenol relaxes almost all varieties of smooth muscle when the tone is high, but this action is most pronounced on bronchial and GI smooth muscle. It prevents or relieves bronchoconstriction. Its effect in asthma may be due in part to an additional action to inhibit antigen-induced release of histamine and other mediators of inflammation; this action is shared by β_2-selective stimulants.

Absorption, Fate, and Excretion. Isoproterenol is readily absorbed when given parenterally or as an aerosol. It is metabolized primarily in the liver and other tissues by COMT. Isoproterenol is a relatively poor substrate for MAO and is not taken up by sympathetic neurons to the same extent as are epinephrine and NE. The duration of action of isoproterenol therefore may be longer than that of epinephrine, but it still is brief.

Toxicity and Adverse Effects. Palpitations, tachycardia, headache, and flushing are common. Cardiac ischemia and arrhythmias may occur, particularly in patients with underlying coronary artery disease.

Therapeutic Uses. Isoproterenol (ISUPREL, others) may be used in emergencies to stimulate heart rate in patients with bradycardia or heart block, particularly in anticipation of inserting an artificial cardiac pacemaker or in patients with the ventricular arrhythmia torsades de pointes. In disorders such as asthma and shock, isoproterenol largely has been replaced by other sympathomimetic drugs (discussed later in this chapter and in Chapter 36).

Dobutamine

Dobutamine resembles DA structurally but possesses a bulky aromatic substituent on the amino group (Table 12–1). The pharmacological effects of dobutamine are due to direct interactions with α and β receptors; its actions do not appear to result from release of NE from sympathetic nerve endings, nor are they exerted by dopaminergic receptors.

Although dobutamine originally was thought to be a relatively selective β_1 receptor agonist, it now is clear that its pharmacological effects are complex. Dobutamine possesses a center of asymmetry; both enantiomeric forms are present in the racemic mixture used clinically. The (–) isomer of dobutamine is a potent agonist at α_1 receptors and is capable of causing marked pressor responses. In contrast, (+)-dobutamine is a potent α_1 receptor antagonist, which can block the effects of (–)-dobutamine. The effects of these two isomers are mediated by β receptors. The (+) isomer is a more potent β receptor agonist than the (–) isomer (~10-fold). Both isomers appear to be full agonists.

Cardiovascular Effects. The cardiovascular effects of racemic dobutamine represent a composite of the distinct pharmacological properties of the (–) and (+) stereoisomers. Dobutamine has relatively more prominent inotropic than chronotropic effects on the heart compared to isoproterenol. Although not completely understood, this useful selectivity may arise because peripheral resistance is relatively unchanged. Alternatively, cardiac α_1 receptors may contribute to the inotropic effect. At equivalent inotropic doses, dobutamine enhances automaticity of the sinus node to a lesser extent than does isoproterenol; however, enhancement of atrioventricular and intraventricular conduction is similar for both drugs.

In animals, administration of dobutamine at a rate of 2.5-15 μg/kg per minute increases cardiac contractility and cardiac output. Total peripheral resistance is not greatly affected. The relatively constant peripheral resistance presumably reflects counterbalancing of α_1 receptor–mediated vasoconstriction and β_2 receptor–mediated vasodilation (Ruffolo, 1987). Heart rate increases only modestly when the rate of administration of dobutamine is maintained at < 20 μg/kg per minute. After administration of β receptor antagonists, infusion of dobutamine fails to increase cardiac output, but total peripheral resistance increases, confirming that dobutamine has modest direct effects on α adrenergic receptors in the vasculature.

Adverse Effects. In some patients, blood pressure and heart rate increase significantly during dobutamine administration; this may require reduction of the rate of infusion. Patients with a history of hypertension may exhibit such an exaggerated pressor response more frequently. Since dobutamine facilitates atrioventricular conduction, patients with atrial fibrillation are at risk of marked increases in ventricular response rates; digoxin or other measures may be required to prevent this from occurring. Some patients may develop ventricular ectopic activity. As with any inotropic agent, dobutamine potentially may increase the size of a myocardial infarct by increasing myocardial O_2 demand. This risk must be balanced against the patient's overall clinical status. The efficacy of dobutamine over a period of more than a few days is uncertain; there is evidence for the development of tolerance.

Therapeutic Uses. Dobutamine (DOBUTREX) is indicated for the short-term treatment of cardiac decompensation that may occur after cardiac surgery or in patients with congestive heart failure or acute myocardial infarction. Dobutamine increases cardiac output and stroke volume in such patients, usually without a marked increase in heart rate. Alterations in blood pressure or peripheral resistance usually are minor, although some patients may have marked increases in blood pressure or heart rate. Clinical evidence of longer-term efficacy remains uncertain. An infusion of dobutamine in combination with echocardiography is useful in the noninvasive assessment of patients with coronary artery disease. Stressing of the heart with dobutamine may reveal cardiac abnormalities in carefully selected patients.

Dobutamine has a $t_{1/2}$ ≈2 minutes; the major metabolites are conjugates of dobutamine and 3-*O*-methyldobutamine. The onset of effect is rapid. Consequently, a loading dose is not required, and steady-state concentrations generally are achieved within 10 minutes of initiation of the infusion by calibrated infusion pump. The rate of infusion required to increase cardiac output typically is between 2.5 and 10 μg/kg per minute, although higher infusion rates occasionally are required. The rate and duration of the infusion are determined by the clinical and hemodynamic responses of the patient.

β_2-Selective Adrenergic Receptor Agonists

Some of the major adverse effects of β receptor agonists in the treatment of asthma or chronic obstructive pulmonary disease (COPD) are caused by stimulation of β_1 receptors in the heart. Accordingly, drugs with preferential affinity for β_2 receptors compared with β_1 receptors have been developed. However, this selectivity is relative, not absolute, and is lost at high concentrations of these drugs. Moreover up to 40% of the β receptors in the human heart are β_2 receptors, activation of which can cause cardiac stimulation (Brodde and Michel, 1999).

A second strategy that has increased the usefulness of several β_2-selective agonists in the treatment of asthma and COPD has been structural modification that results in lower rates of metabolism and enhanced oral bioavailability (compared with catecholamines).

Modifications have included placing the hydroxyl groups at positions 3 and 5 of the phenyl ring or substituting another moiety for the hydroxyl group at position 3. This has yielded drugs such as metaproterenol, terbutaline, and albuterol, which are not substrates for COMT. Bulky substituents on the amino group of catecholamines contribute to potency at β receptors with decreased activity at α receptors and decreased metabolism by MAO. A final strategy to enhance preferential activation of pulmonary β_2 receptors is the administration by inhalation of small doses of the drug in aerosol form. This approach typically leads to effective activation of β_2 receptors in the bronchi but very low systemic drug concentrations. Consequently, there is less potential to activate cardiac β_1 or β_2 receptors or to stimulate β_2 receptors in skeletal muscle, which can cause tremor and thereby limit oral therapy.

Administration of β receptor agonists by aerosol (Chapter 36) typically leads to a very rapid therapeutic response, generally within minutes, although some agonists such as salmeterol have a delayed onset of action (discussed later). While subcutaneous injection also causes prompt bronchodilation, the peak effect of a drug given orally may be delayed for several hours. Aerosol therapy depends on the delivery of drug to the distal airways. This, in turn, depends on the size of the particles in the aerosol and respiratory parameters such as inspiratory flow rate, tidal volume, breath-holding time, and airway diameter. Only ~10% of an inhaled dose actually enters the lungs; much of the remainder is swallowed and ultimately may be absorbed. Successful aerosol therapy requires that each patient master the technique of drug administration. Many patients, particularly children and the elderly, do not use optimal techniques, often because of inadequate instructions or incoordination. In these patients, spacer devices may enhance the efficacy of inhalation therapy.

In the treatment of asthma and COPD, β receptor agonists are used to activate pulmonary receptors that relax bronchial smooth muscle and decrease airway resistance. Although this action appears to be a major therapeutic effect of these drugs in patients with asthma, evidence suggests that β receptor agonists also may suppress the release of leukotrienes and histamine from mast cells in lung tissue, enhance mucociliary function, decrease microvascular permeability, and possibly inhibit phospholipase A_2 (Seale, 1988). These additional actions seem to contribute to the beneficial effects of β agonists in the treatment of human asthma It is becoming increasingly clear that airway inflammation is also directly involved in airway hyper-responsiveness; consequently, the use of anti-inflammatory drugs such as inhaled steroids has primary importance. Most authorities recommend that long-acting β agonists should not be used without concomitant anti-inflammatory therapy in the treatment of asthma (Drazen and O'Byrne, 2009; Fanta, 2009). The use of β agonists for the treatment of asthma and COPD is discussed in Chapter 36.

Short Acting β_2 Adrenergic Agonists

Metaproterenol. Metaproterenol (called orciprenaline in Europe), along with terbutaline and fenoterol, belongs to the structural class of resorcinol bronchodilators that have hydroxyl groups at positions 3 and 5 of the phenyl ring (rather than at positions 3 and 4 as in catechols) (Table 12–1). Consequently, metaproterenol is resistant to methylation by COMT, and a substantial fraction (40%) is absorbed in active form after oral administration. It is excreted primarily as glucuronic acid conjugates. Metaproterenol is considered to be β_2-selective, although it probably is less selective than albuterol or terbutaline and hence is more prone to cause cardiac stimulation; as noted earlier, up to 40% of the β receptors in the human heart are of the β_2 subtype, thus even β_2-selective agents have the potential to cause cardiac stimulation.

Effects occur within minutes of inhalation and persist for several hours. After oral administration, onset of action is slower, but effects last 3-4 hours. Metaproterenol is used for the long-term treatment of obstructive airway diseases, asthma, and for treatment of acute bronchospasm (Chapter 36). Side effects are similar to the short- and intermediate-acting sympathomimetic bronchodilators.

Albuterol. Albuterol (VENTOLIN-HFA, PROVENTIL-HFA, others; Table 12-1) is a selective β_2 receptor agonist with pharmacological properties and therapeutic indications similar to those of terbutaline. It is administered either by inhalation or orally for the symptomatic relief of bronchospasm.

When administered by inhalation, it produces significant bronchodilation within 15 minutes, and effects persist for 3-4 hours. The cardiovascular effects of albuterol are considerably weaker than those of isoproterenol when doses that produce comparable bronchodilation are administered by inhalation. Oral albuterol has the potential to delay preterm labor. Although rare, CNS and respiratory side effects are sometimes observed.

Albuterol has been made available in a metered dose inhaler free of chlorofluorcarbons (CFC); CFC-containing albuterol inhalers have been taken off the market. Like CFCs, the alternate propellant, hydrofluoroalkane (HFA) is inert in the human airway, but unlike CFCs, it does not contribute to depletion of the stratospheric ozone layer.

Levalbuterol. Levalbuterol (XOPENEX) is the R-enantiomer of albuterol which is a racemic drug used to treat asthma and COPD. Although originally available only as a solution for nebulizer, it is now available as a CFC-free metered dose inhaler. Levalbuterol is β_2-selective and acts like other β_2 adrenergic agonists. In general, levalbuterol has similar pharmacokinetic and pharmacodynamics properties to albuterol. Although it has been claimed to have fewer side effects than albuterol, these claims have not been supported by clinical trials.

Pirbuterol. Pirbuterol is a relatively selective β_2 agonist. Its structure is identical to albuterol except for the substitution of a pyridine ring for the benzene ring. Pirbuterol acetate (MAXAIR) is available for inhalation therapy; dosing is typically every 4-6 hours. Pirbuterol is

agonist that has twice the potency of racemic formoterol. It is FDA-approved for the long-term treatment of bronchoconstriction in patients with COPD, including chronic bronchitis and emphysema (Matera and Cazzola, 2007). It is the first long-acting β_2 agonist developed as inhalational therapy to use with a nebulizer (Abdelghany, 2007). Like other β_2 agonists, arformoterol activates the cyclic AMP pathway, thereby relaxing bronchial smooth muscle and inhibiting release of mast cell mediators (e.g., histamine and leukotrienes).

A substantial portion of systemic exposure to arformoterol is due to pulmonary absorption with plasma levels reaching peak levels in 0.25-1 hour. Plasma protein binding is 52-65%. It is primarily metabolized by direct conjugation to glucuronide or sulfate conjugates and secondarily by O-demethylation by CYP2D6 and CYP2C19. It does not inhibit any of the common CYPs. The drug is well tolerated and the most common side effects are skeletal muscle tremor and cramps, insomnia, tachycardia, decreases in plasma potassium, and increases in plasma glucose. As mentioned previously, a black-box warning has been instituted in response to findings of the SMART trials (Fanta, 2009; Lipworth, 2007).

Carmoterol. Carmoterol is a pure (R,R)-isomer and a non-catechol with a *p*-methoxyphenyl group on the carbostyril aromatic ring. It is a potent and selective β_2 adrenergic agonist with a selectivity for β_2 over β_1 receptors of 53. It is claimed to be 5 times more selective for the β_2 adrenergic receptor in tracheal preparations than those in the right atrium. Carmoterol has a rapid onset and long duration of action and shows a bronchodilator effect over 24 hours with once a day dosing. Indications for carmoterol include asthma and COPD (Cazzola and Matera, 2008; Matera and Cazzola, 2007).

Indacaterol. Indacaterol is a once-daily long-acting β adrenergic agonist in development for asthma and COPD. It has a fast onset of action, appears well tolerated, and has been shown to be effective in both asthma and COPD with little tachyphalaxis upon continued use. Indacaterol behaves as a potent β_2 agonist with high intrinsic efficacy, which, in contrast to salmeterol, does not antagonize the bronchorelaxant effect of short-acting β_2 adrenergic agonists. Evidence indicates that indacaterol has a longer duration of action than salmeterol and formoterol.

Both indacaterol and carmoterol are currently in Phase III clinical trials in the U.S. (Cazzola and Matera, 2008; Matera and Cazzola, 2007).

Ritodrine. Ritodrine is a β_2-selective agonist that was developed specifically for use as a uterine relaxant. Nevertheless, its pharmacological properties closely resemble those of the other agents in this group.

Ritodrine is rapidly but incompletely (30%) absorbed following oral administration, and 90% of the drug is excreted in the urine as inactive conjugates; ~50% of ritodrine is excreted unchanged after intravenous administration. The pharmacokinetic properties of ritodrine are complex and incompletely defined, especially in pregnant women.

Ritodrine may be administered intravenously to selected patients to arrest premature labor. Ritodrine and related drugs can prolong pregnancy. However, β_2-selective agonists may not have clinically significant benefits on perinatal mortality and may actually increase maternal morbidity. Ritodrine is not available in the U.S. See Chapter 66 for the pharmacology of tocolytic agents.

Adverse Effects of β_2-Selective Agonists. The major adverse effects of β receptor agonists occur as a result of excessive activation of β receptors. Patients with underlying cardiovascular disease are particularly at risk for significant reactions. However, the likelihood of adverse effects can be greatly decreased in patients with lung disease by administering the drug by inhalation rather than orally or parenterally.

Tremor is a relatively common adverse effect of the β_2-selective receptor agonists. Tolerance generally develops to this effect; it is not clear whether tolerance reflects desensitization of the β_2 receptors of skeletal muscle or adaptation within the CNS. This adverse effect can be minimized by starting oral therapy with a low dose of drug and progressively increasing the dose as tolerance to the tremor develops. Feelings of restlessness, apprehension, and anxiety may limit therapy with these drugs, particularly oral or parenteral administration.

Tachycardia is a common adverse effect of systemically administered β receptor agonists. Stimulation of heart rate occurs primarily by means of β_1 receptors. It is uncertain to what extent the increase in heart rate also is due to activation of cardiac β_2 receptors or to reflex effects that stem from β_2 receptor–mediated peripheral vasodilation. However, β_2 receptors are also present in the human myocardium and all β_2 adrenergic agonists have the potential to produce cardiac stimulation. During a severe asthma attack, heart rate actually may decrease during therapy with a β agonist, presumably because of improvement in pulmonary function with consequent reduction in endogenous cardiac sympathetic stimulation. In patients without cardiac disease, β agonists rarely cause significant arrhythmias or myocardial ischemia; however, patients with underlying coronary artery disease or preexisting arrhythmias are at greater risk. The risk of adverse cardiovascular effects also is increased in patients who are receiving MAO inhibitors. In general, at least 2 weeks should elapse between the use of MAO inhibitors and administration of β_2 agonists or other sympathomimetics.

Large doses of β receptor agonists cause myocardial necrosis in laboratory animals. When given parenterally, these drugs also may increase the concentrations of glucose, lactate, and free fatty acids in plasma and decrease the concentration of K^+. The decrease in K^+ concentration may be especially important in patients with cardiac disease, particularly those taking digoxin and diuretics. In some diabetic patients, hyperglycemia may be worsened by these drugs, and higher doses of insulin may be required. All these adverse effects are far less likely with inhalation therapy than with parenteral or oral therapy.

α_1-SELECTIVE ADRENERGIC RECEPTOR AGONISTS

The major clinical effects of a number of sympathomimetic drugs are due to activation of α adrenergic receptors in vascular smooth muscle. As a result, peripheral vascular resistance is increased and blood pressure is maintained or elevated. Although the clinical utility of these drugs is limited, they may be useful in the treatment of some patients with hypotension, including orthostatic hypotension, or shock. Phenylephrine and methoxamine (discontinued in the U.S.) are direct-acting vasoconstrictors and are selective activators of α_1 receptors. Mephentermine and metaraminol act both directly and indirectly. Midodrine is a prodrug that is converted, after oral administration, to desglymidodrine, a direct-acting α_1 agonist.

Phenylephrine

Phenylephrine (NEO-SYNEPHRINE, others) is a α_1-selective agonist; it activates β receptors only at much higher concentrations. Chemically, phenylephrine differs from epinephrine only in lacking a hydroxyl group at position 4 on the benzene ring (Table 12–1). The pharmacological effects of phenylephrine are similar to those of methoxamine. The drug causes marked arterial vasoconstriction during intravenous infusion. Phenylephrine (NEO-SYNEPHRINE, others) also is used as a nasal decongestant and as a mydriatic in various nasal and ophthalmic formulations (see Chapter 64 for ophthalmic uses).

Mephentermine. Mephentermine is a sympathomimetic drug that acts both directly and indirectly; it has many similarities to ephedrine (discussed later). After an intramuscular injection, the onset of action is prompt (within 5-15 minutes), and effects may last for several hours. Since the drug releases NE, cardiac contraction is enhanced, and cardiac output and systolic and diastolic pressures usually are increased. The change in heart rate is variable, depending on the degree of vagal tone. Adverse effects are related to CNS stimulation, excessive rises in blood pressure, and arrhythmias. Mephentermine is used to prevent hypotension, which frequently accompanies spinal anesthesia. The drug has been discontinued in the U.S.

Metaraminol. Metaraminol is a sympathomimetic drug with prominent direct effects on vascular α adrenergic receptors. Metaraminol also is an indirectly acting agent that stimulates the release of NE. The drug has been used in the treatment of hypotensive states or off-label to relieve attacks of paroxysmal atrial tachycardia, particularly those associated with hypotension (see Chapter 29 for preferable treatments of this arrhythmia).

Midodrine. Midodrine (PROAMATINE, others) is an orally effective α_1 receptor agonist. It is a prodrug; its activity is due to its conversion to an active metabolite, desglymidodrine, which achieves peak concentrations ~1 hour after a dose of midodrine. The $t_{1/2}$ of desglymidodrine is ~3 hours. Consequently, the duration of action is ~4-6 hours. Midodrine-induced rises in blood pressure are associated with both arterial and venous smooth muscle contraction. This is advantageous in the treatment of patients with autonomic insufficiency and postural hypotension (McClellan et al., 1998). A frequent complication in these patients is supine hypertension. This can be minimized by administering the drug during periods when the patient will remain upright, avoiding dosing within 4 hours of bedtime, and elevating the head of the bed. Very cautious use of a short-acting antihypertensive drug at bedtime may be useful in some patients. Typical dosing, achieved by careful titration of blood pressure responses, varies between 2.5 and 10 mg three times daily.

α_2-SELECTIVE ADRENERGIC RECEPTOR AGONISTS

α_2-Selective adrenergic agonists are used primarily for the treatment of systemic hypertension. Their efficacy as antihypertensive agents is somewhat surprising, since many blood vessels contain postsynaptic α_2 adrenergic receptors that promote vasoconstriction (Chapter 8). Indeed, clonidine, the prototypic α_2 agonist, was initially developed as a vasoconstricting nasal decongestant. Its capacity to lower blood pressure results from activation of α_2 receptors in the cardiovascular control centers of the CNS; such activation suppresses the outflow of sympathetic nervous system activity from the brain.

In addition, α_2 agonists reduce intraocular pressure by decreasing the production of aqueous humor. This action first was reported for clonidine and suggested a potential role for α_2 receptor agonists in the management of ocular hypertension and glaucoma. Unfortunately, clonidine lowered systemic blood pressure even if applied topically to the eye (Alward, 1998). Two derivatives of clonidine, apraclonidine and brimonidine, have been developed that retain the ability to decrease intraocular pressure with little or no effect on systemic blood pressure.

Clonidine

Clonidine, an imidazoline, was originally tested as a vasoconstrictor acting at peripheral α_2 receptors. During clinical trials as a topical nasal decongestant, clonidine was found to cause hypotension, sedation, and bradycardia.

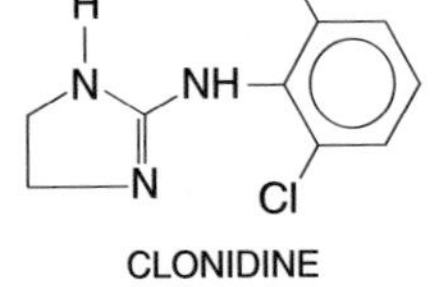

Cl
H
N NH
N Cl

CLONIDINE

Pharmacological Effects. The major pharmacological effects of clonidine involve changes in blood pressure and heart rate, although the drug has a variety of other important actions. Intravenous infusion of clonidine causes an acute rise in blood pressure, apparently because of activation of postsynaptic α_2 receptors in vascular smooth muscle. The affinity of clonidine for these receptors is high, although the drug is a partial agonist with relatively low efficacy at these sites. The hypertensive response that follows parenteral administration of clonidine generally is not seen when the drug is given orally. However, even after intravenous administration, the transient vasoconstriction is followed by a more prolonged hypotensive response that results from decreased sympathetic outflow from the CNS. The exact mechanism by which clonidine lowers blood pressure is not completely understood. The effect appears to result, at least in part, from activation of α_2 receptors in the lower brainstem region. This central action has been demonstrated by infusing small amounts of the drug into the vertebral arteries or by injecting it directly into the cisterna magna.

Questions remain about whether the sympatho-inhibitory action of clonidine results solely from its α_2 receptor agonism or whether part or all of its actions are mediated by imidazoline receptors. Imidazoline receptors include three subtypes (I_1, I_2, and I_3) and are widely distributed in the body, including the CNS. Clonidine, as an imidazoline, binds to these imidazoline receptors, in addition to its well-described binding to α_2 receptors. Two newer antihypertensive imidazolines, rilmenidine and moxonidine, have profiles of action similar to clonidine's, suggesting a role for I_1 receptors. However, the lack of an antihypertensive effect of clonidine in knockout mice lacking α_{2A} receptors supports a key role for these receptors in blood pressure regulation (Zhu et al., 1999). Others argue that, while the action of clonidine may be mediated by α_2 receptors, the I_1 receptor mediates the effects of moxonidine and rilmenidine. Finally, α_2 and imidazoline receptors may cooperatively regulate vasomotor tone and may jointly mediate the hypotensive actions of centrally acting drugs with affinity for both receptor types.

Clonidine decreases discharges in sympathetic preganglionic fibers in the splanchnic nerve and in postganglionic fibers of cardiac nerves. These effects are blocked by α_2-selective antagonists such as yohimbine. Clonidine also stimulates parasympathetic outflow, which may contribute to the slowing of heart rate as a consequence of increased vagal tone and diminished sympathetic drive. In addition, some of the antihypertensive effects of clonidine may be mediated by activation of presynaptic α_2 receptors that suppress the release of NE, ATP, and NPY from postganglionic sympathetic nerves. Clonidine decreases the plasma concentration of NE and reduces its excretion in the urine.

Absorption, Fate, and Excretion. Clonidine is well absorbed after oral administration, and its bioavailability is nearly 100%. The peak concentration in plasma and the maximal hypotensive effect are observed 1-3 hours after an oral dose. The elimination $t_{1/2}$ of the drug ranges from 6-24 hours, with a mean of ~12 hours. About half of an administered dose can be recovered unchanged in the urine, and the $t_{1/2}$ of the drug may increase with renal failure. There is good correlation between plasma concentrations of clonidine and its pharmacological effects. A transdermal delivery patch permits continuous administration of clonidine as an alternative to oral therapy. The drug is released at an approximately constant rate for a week; 3-4 days are required to reach steady-state concentrations in plasma. When the patch is removed, plasma concentrations remain stable for ~8 hours and then decline gradually over a period of several days; this decrease is associated with a rise in blood pressure.

Adverse Effects. The major adverse effects of clonidine are dry mouth and sedation. These responses occur in at least 50% of patients and may require drug discontinuation. However, they may diminish in intensity after several weeks of therapy. Sexual dysfunction also may occur. Marked bradycardia is observed in some patients. These and some of the other adverse effects of clonidine frequently are related to dose, and their incidence may be lower with transdermal administration of clonidine, since antihypertensive efficacy may be achieved while avoiding the relatively high peak concentrations that occur after oral administration of the drug. About 15-20% of patients develop contact dermatitis when using clonidine in the transdermal system. Withdrawal reactions follow abrupt discontinuation of long-term therapy with clonidine in some hypertensive patients (Chapter 27).

Therapeutic Uses. The major therapeutic use of clonidine (CATAPRES, others) is in the treatment of hypertension (Chapter 27). Clonidine also has apparent efficacy in the off-label treatment of a range of other disorders. Stimulation of α_2 receptors in the GI tract may increase absorption of sodium chloride and fluid and inhibit secretion of bicarbonate. This may explain why clonidine has been found to be useful in reducing diarrhea in some diabetic patients with autonomic neuropathy. Clonidine also is useful in treating and preparing addicted subjects for withdrawal from narcotics, alcohol, and tobacco (Chapter 24). Clonidine may help ameliorate some of the adverse sympathetic nervous activity associated with withdrawal from these agents, as well as decrease craving for the drug. The long-term benefits of clonidine in these settings and in neuropsychiatric disorders remain to be determined. Clonidine may be useful in selected patients receiving anesthesia because it may decrease the requirement for anesthetic and increase hemodynamic stability (Hayashi and Maze, 1993; Chapter 19). Other potential benefits of clonidine and related drugs such as dexmedetomidine (PRECEDEX; a relatively selective α_2 receptor agonist with sedative properties) in anesthesia include preoperative sedation and anxiolysis, drying of secretions, and analgesia. Transdermal administration of clonidine (CATAPRESTTS) may be useful in reducing the incidence of menopausal hot flashes.

Acute administration of clonidine has been used in the differential diagnosis of patients with hypertension and suspected pheochromocytoma. In patients with primary hypertension, plasma concentrations of NE are markedly suppressed after a single dose of clonidine; this response is not observed in many patients with pheochromocytoma. The capacity of clonidine to activate postsynaptic α_2 receptors in vascular smooth muscle has been exploited in a limited number of patients whose autonomic failure is so severe that reflex sympathetic responses on standing are absent; postural hypotension is thus marked. Since the central effect of clonidine on blood pressure is unimportant in these patients, the drug can elevate blood pressure and improve the symptoms of postural hypotension. Among the other off-label uses of clonidine are atrial fibrillation, attention-deficit/hyperactivity disorder, constitutional growth delay in children, cyclosporine-associated nephrotoxicity, Tourette's syndrome, hyperhidrosis, mania, posthepatic neuralgia, psychosis, restless leg syndrome, ulcerative colitis, and allergy-induced inflammatory reactions in patients with extrinsic asthma.

Apraclonidine. Apraclonidine (IOPIDINE) is a relatively selective α_2 receptor agonist that is used topically to reduce intraocular pressure. It can reduce elevated as well as normal intraocular pressure whether accompanied by glaucoma or not. The reduction in intraocular pressure occurs with minimal or no effects on systemic cardiovascular parameters; thus apraclonidine is more useful than clonidine for ophthalmic therapy. Apparently apraclonidine does not cross the blood-brain barrier. The mechanism of action of apraclonidine is related to α_2 receptor–mediated reduction in the formation of aqueous humor.

The clinical utility of apraclonidine is most apparent as short-term adjunctive therapy in glaucoma patients whose intraocular pressure is not well controlled by other pharmacological agents such as β receptor antagonists, parasympathomimetics, or carbonic anhydrase inhibitors. The drug also is used to control or prevent elevations in intraocular pressure that occur in patients after laser trabeculoplasty or iridotomy (Chapter 64).

Brimonidine. Brimonidine (ALPHAGAN, others), is another clonidine derivative that is administered ocularly to lower intraocular pressure in patients with ocular hypertension or open-angle glaucoma. Brimonidine is a α_2-selective agonist that reduces intraocular pressure both by decreasing aqueous humor production and by increasing outflow (Chapter 64). The efficacy of brimonidine in reducing intraocular pressure is similar to that of the β receptor antagonist timolol. Unlike apraclonidine, brimonidine can cross the blood-brain barrier and can produce hypotension and sedation, although these CNS effects are slight compared to those of clonidine. As with all α_2 agonists, this drug should be used with caution in patients with cardiovascular disease.

Guanfacine. Guanfacine (TENEX, others) is an α_2 receptor agonist that is more selective for α_2 receptors than is clonidine. Like clonidine, guanfacine lowers blood pressure by activation of brainstem receptors with resultant suppression of sympathetic activity. A sustained-release form (INTUNIV) has recently been FDA-approved for treatment of ADHD in children aged 6-17 years.

The drug is well absorbed after oral administration and has a large volume of distribution (4-6 L/kg). About 50% of guanfacine appears unchanged in the urine; the rest is metabolized. The $t_{1/2}$ for elimination ranges from 12-24 hours. Guanfacine and clonidine appear to have similar efficacy for the treatment of hypertension. The pattern of adverse effects also is similar for the two drugs, although it has been suggested that some of these effects may be milder and occur less frequently with guanfacine. A withdrawal syndrome may occur after the abrupt discontinuation of guanfacine, but it appears to be less frequent and milder than the syndrome that follows clonidine withdrawal. Part of this difference may relate to the longer $t_{1/2}$ of guanfacine.

Guanabenz. Guanabenz (WYTENSIN, others) is a centrally acting α_2 agonist that decreases blood pressure by a mechanism similar to those of clonidine and guanfacine. Guanabenz has a $t_{1/2}$ of 4-6 hours and is extensively metabolized by the liver. Dosage adjustment may be necessary in patients with hepatic cirrhosis. The adverse effects caused by guanabenz (e.g., dry mouth and sedation) are similar to those seen with clonidine.

Methyldopa. Methyldopa (α-methyl-3,4-dihydroxyphenylalanine) is a centrally acting antihypertensive agent. It is metabolized to α-methylnorepinephrine in the brain, and this compound is thought to activate central α_2 receptors and lower blood pressure in a manner similar to that of clonidine (Chapter 27).

Tizanidine. Tizanidine (ZANAFLEX, others) is a muscle relaxant used for the treatment of spasticity associated with cerebral and spinal disorders. It is also an α_2 agonist with some properties similar to those of clonidine (Wagstaff and Bryson, 1997).

MISCELLANEOUS SYMPATHOMIMETIC AGONISTS

Amphetamine

Amphetamine, racemic β phenylisopropylamine (Table 12–1), has powerful CNS stimulant actions in addition to the peripheral α and β actions common to indirect-acting sympathomimetic drugs. Unlike epinephrine, it is effective after oral administration and its effects last for several hours.

Cardiovascular System. Amphetamine given orally raises both systolic and diastolic blood pressure. Heart rate often is reflexly slowed; with large doses, cardiac arrhythmias may occur. Cardiac output is not enhanced by therapeutic doses, and cerebral blood flow does not change much. The *l*-isomer is slightly more potent than the *d*-isomer in its cardiovascular actions.

Other Smooth Muscles. In general, smooth muscles respond to amphetamine as they do to other sympathomimetic amines. The contractile effect on the sphincter of the urinary bladder is particularly marked, and for this reason amphetamine has been used in treating enuresis and incontinence. Pain and difficulty in micturition occasionally occur. The GI effects of amphetamine are unpredictable. If enteric activity is pronounced, amphetamine may cause relaxation and delay the movement of intestinal contents; if the gut already is relaxed, the opposite effect may occur. The response of the human uterus varies, but there usually is an increase in tone.

CNS. Amphetamine is one of the most potent sympathomimetic amines in stimulating the CNS. It stimulates the medullary respiratory center, lessens the degree of central depression caused by various drugs, and produces other signs of CNS stimulation. These effects are thought to be due to cortical stimulation and possibly to stimulation of the reticular activating system. In contrast, the drug can obtund the maximal electroshock seizure discharge and prolong the ensuing period of depression. In eliciting of CNS excitatory effects, the *d*-isomer (dextroamphetamine) is 3-4 times more potent than the *l*-isomer.

The psychic effects depend on the dose and the mental state and personality of the individual. The main results of an oral dose of 10-30 mg include wakefulness, alertness, and a decreased sense of fatigue; elevation of mood, with increased initiative, self-confidence, and ability to concentrate; often, elation and euphoria; and increase in motor and speech activities. Performance of simple mental tasks is improved, but, although more work may be accomplished, the number of errors may increase. Physical performance—in athletes, e.g.—is improved, and the drug often is abused for this purpose. These effects are not invariable and may be reversed by overdosage or repeated usage. Prolonged use or large doses are nearly always followed by depression and fatigue. Many individuals given amphetamine experience headache, palpitation, dizziness, vasomotor disturbances, agitation, confusion, dysphoria, apprehension, delirium, or fatigue (Chapter 24).

Fatigue and Sleep. Prevention and reversal of fatigue by amphetamine have been studied extensively in the laboratory, in military field studies, and in athletics. In general, the duration of adequate performance is prolonged before fatigue appears, and the effects of fatigue are at least partly reversed. The most striking improvement appears to occur when performance has been reduced by fatigue and lack of sleep. Such improvement may be partly due to alteration of unfavorable attitudes toward the task. However, amphetamine reduces the frequency of attention lapses that impair performance after prolonged sleep deprivation and thus improves execution of tasks requiring sustained attention. The need for sleep may be postponed, but it cannot be avoided indefinitely. When the drug is discontinued after long use, the pattern of sleep may take as long as 2 months to return to normal.

Analgesia. Amphetamine and some other sympathomimetic amines have a small analgesic effect, but it is not sufficiently pronounced to be therapeutically useful. However, amphetamine can enhance the analgesia produced by opiates.

Respiration. Amphetamine stimulates the respiratory center, increasing the rate and depth of respiration. In normal individuals, usual doses of the drug do not appreciably increase respiratory rate or minute volume. Nevertheless, when respiration is depressed by centrally acting drugs, amphetamine may stimulate respiration.

Depression of Appetite. Amphetamine and similar drugs have been used for the treatment of obesity, although the wisdom of this use is at best questionable. Weight loss in obese humans treated with amphetamine is almost entirely due to reduced food intake and only in small measure to increased metabolism. The site of action probably is in the lateral hypothalamic feeding center; injection of amphetamine into this area, but not into the ventromedial region, suppresses food intake. Neurochemical mechanisms of action are unclear but may involve increased release of NE and/or DA. In humans, tolerance to the appetite suppression develops rapidly. Hence, continuous weight reduction usually is not observed in obese individuals without dietary restriction.

Mechanisms of Action in the CNS. Amphetamine appears to exert most or all of its effects in the CNS by releasing biogenic amines from their storage sites in nerve terminals. In addition, the neuronal dopamine transporter (DAT) and the vesicular monoamine transporter 2 (VMAT2) appear to be two of the principal targets of amphetamine's action (Fleckenstein, 2007). These mechanisms include amphetamine-induced exchange diffusion, reverse transport, channel-like transport phenomena, and effects resulting from the weakly basic properties of amphetamine. Amphetamine analogs affect monamine transporters through phosphorylation, transporter trafficking, and the production of reactive oxygen and nitrogen species. These mechanisms may have potential implications for neurotoxicity as well as dopaminergic neurodegenerative diseases (discussed later) (Fleckenstein, 2007).

The alerting effect of amphetamine, its anorectic effect, and at least a component of its locomotor-stimulating action presumably are mediated by release of NE from central noradrenergic neurons. These effects can be prevented in experimental animals by treatment with metyrosine (α-methyltyrosine), an inhibitor of tyrosine hydroxylase, and therefore of catecholamine synthesis. Some aspects of locomotor activity and the stereotyped behavior induced by amphetamine probably are a consequence of the release of DA from dopaminergic nerve terminals, particularly in the neostriatum. Higher doses are required to produce these behavioral effects, and this correlates with the higher concentrations of amphetamine required to release DA from brain slices or synaptosomes *in vitro*. With still higher doses of amphetamine, disturbances of perception and overt psychotic behavior occur. These effects may be due to release of 5-hydroxytryptamine (serotonin, 5-HT) from serotonergic neurons and of DA in the mesolimbic system. In addition, amphetamine may exert direct effects on CNS receptors for 5-HT (Chapter 13).

Toxicity and Adverse Effects. The acute toxic effects of amphetamine usually are extensions of its therapeutic actions, and as a rule result from overdosage. CNS effects commonly include restlessness, dizziness, tremor, hyperactive reflexes, talkativeness, tenseness, irritability, weakness, insomnia, fever, and sometimes euphoria. Confusion, aggressiveness, changes in libido, anxiety, delirium, paranoid hallucinations, panic states, and suicidal or homicidal tendencies occur, especially in mentally ill patients. However, these psychotic effects can be elicited in any individual if sufficient quantities of amphetamine are ingested for a prolonged period. Fatigue and depression usually follow central stimulation. Cardiovascular effects are common and include headache, chilliness, pallor or flushing, palpitation, cardiac arrhythmias, anginal pain, hypertension or hypotension, and circulatory collapse. Excessive sweating occurs. GI symptoms include dry mouth, metallic taste, anorexia, nausea, vomiting, diarrhea, and abdominal cramps. Fatal poisoning usually terminates in convulsions and coma, and cerebral hemorrhages are the main pathological findings.

The toxic dose of amphetamine varies widely. Toxic manifestations occasionally occur as an idiosyncratic reaction after as little as 2 mg, but are rare with doses of < 15 mg. Severe reactions have occurred with 30 mg, yet doses of 400-500 mg are not uniformly fatal. Larger doses can be tolerated after chronic use of the drug.

Treatment of acute amphetamine intoxication may include acidification of the urine by administration of ammonium chloride; this enhances the rate of elimination. Sedatives may be required for the CNS symptoms. Severe hypertension may require administration of sodium nitroprusside or an α adrenergic receptor antagonist.

Chronic intoxication with amphetamine causes symptoms similar to those of acute overdosage, but abnormal mental conditions are more common. Weight loss may be marked. A psychotic reaction with vivid hallucinations and paranoid delusions, often mistaken for schizophrenia, is the most common serious effect. Recovery usually is rapid after withdrawal of the drug, but occasionally the condition becomes chronic. In these persons, amphetamine may act as a precipitating factor hastening the onset of incipient schizophrenia.

The abuse of amphetamine as a means of overcoming sleepiness and of increasing energy and alertness should be discouraged. The drug should be used only under medical supervision. The amphetamines are schedule II drugs under federal regulations. The additional contraindications and precautions for the use of amphetamine generally are similar to those described above for epinephrine. Its use is inadvisable in patients with anorexia, insomnia, asthenia, psychopathic personality, or a history of homicidal or suicidal tendencies.

Dependence and Tolerance. Psychological dependence often occurs when amphetamine or dextroamphetamine is used chronically, as discussed in Chapter 24. Tolerance almost invariably develops to the anorexigenic effect of amphetamines, and often is seen also in the need for increasing doses to maintain improvement of mood in psychiatric patients. Tolerance is striking in individuals who are dependent on the drug; a daily intake of 1.7 g without apparent ill effects has been reported. Development of tolerance is not invariable, and cases of narcolepsy have been treated for years without requiring an increase in the initially effective dose.

Therapeutic Uses. Amphetamine is used chiefly for its CNS effects. Dextroamphetamine (DEXEDRINE, others), with greater CNS action and less peripheral action, was used off-label for obesity (but no longer is approved for this purpose because of the risk of abuse) and is FDA-approved for the treatment of narcolepsy and attention-deficit/hyperactivity disorder (see below, "Therapeutic Uses of Sympathomimetic Drugs").

Methamphetamine

Methamphetamine (DESOXYN) is closely related chemically to amphetamine and ephedrine (Table 12–1). In the brain, methamphetamine releases DA and other biogenic amines, and inhibits neuronal and vesicular monoamine transporters as well as MAO.

Small doses have prominent central stimulant effects without significant peripheral actions; somewhat larger doses produce a sustained rise in systolic and diastolic blood pressures, due mainly to cardiac stimulation. Cardiac output is increased, although the heart rate may be reflexly slowed. Venous constriction causes peripheral venous pressure to increase. These factors tend to increase the venous return, and thus cardiac output. Pulmonary arterial pressure is raised, probably owing to increased cardiac output. Methamphetamine is a schedule II drug under federal regulations and has high potential for abuse (Chapter 24). It is widely used as a cheap, accessible recreational drug and its abuse is a widespread phenomenon. Illegal production of methamphetamine in clandestine laboratories throughout the U.S. is common. It is used principally for its central effects, which are more pronounced than those of amphetamine and are accompanied by less prominent peripheral actions (see below, Therapeutic Uses of Sympathomimetic Drugs).

Methylphenidate

Methylphenidate is a piperidine derivative that is structurally related to amphetamine. Methylphenidate (RITALIN, others) is a mild CNS stimulant with more prominent effects on mental than on motor activities. However, large doses produce signs of generalized CNS stimulation that may lead to convulsions.

METHYLPHENIDATE

Its pharmacological properties are essentially the same as those of the amphetamines. Methylphenidate also shares the abuse potential of the amphetamines and is listed as a schedule II controlled substance in the U.S. Methylphenidate is effective in the treatment of narcolepsy and attention-deficit/hyperactivity disorder, as described in the subsequent paragraphs.

Methylphenidate is readily absorbed after oral administration and reaches peak concentrations in plasma in ~2 hours. The drug is a racemate; its more potent (+) enantiomer has a $t_{1/2}$ of ~6 hours, and the less potent (–) enantiomer has a $t_{1/2}$ of ~4 hours. Concentrations in the brain exceed those in plasma. The main urinary metabolite is a de-esterified product, ritalinic acid, which accounts for 80% of the dose. The use of methylphenidate is contraindicated in patients with glaucoma.

Dexmethylphenidate. Dexmethylphenidate (FOCALIN) is the *d*-threo enantiomer of racemic methylphenidate. It is FDA-approved for the treatment of attention-deficit/hyperactivity disorder and is listed as a schedule II controlled substance in the U.S.

Pemoline. Pemoline (CYLERT, others) is structurally dissimilar to methylphenidate but elicits similar changes in CNS function with minimal effects on the cardiovascular system. It is employed in treating attention-deficit/hyperactivity disorder. It can be given once daily because of its long $t_{1/2}$. Clinical improvement may require treatment for 3-4 weeks. Use of pemoline has been associated with severe hepatic failure. The drug was discontinued in the U.S. in 2006.

Ephedrine

Ephedrine is an agonist at both α and β receptors; in addition, it enhances release of NE from sympathetic neurons and therefore is a mixed-acting sympathomimetic drug. Ephedrine contains two asymmetrical carbon atoms (Table 12–1); only *l*-ephedrine and racemic ephedrine are used clinically.

Pharmacological Actions. Ephedrine does not contain a catechol moiety and is effective after oral administration. The drug stimulates heart rate and cardiac output and variably increases peripheral resistance; as a result, ephedrine usually increases blood pressure. Stimulation of the α receptors of smooth muscle cells in the bladder base may increase the resistance to the outflow of urine. Activation of β receptors in the lungs promotes bronchodilation. Ephedrine is a potent CNS stimulant. After oral administration, effects of the drug may persist for several hours. Ephedrine is eliminated in the urine largely as unchanged drug, with a $t_{1/2}$ of 3-6 hours.

Therapeutic Uses and Toxicity. In the past, ephedrine was used to treat Stokes-Adams attacks with complete heart block and as a CNS stimulant in narcolepsy and depressive states. It has been replaced by alternate treatments in each of these disorders. In addition, its use as a bronchodilator in patients with asthma has become much less extensive with the development of β_2-selective agonists. Ephedrine has been used to promote urinary continence, although its efficacy is not clear. Indeed, the drug may cause urinary retention, particularly in men with benign prostatic hyperplasia. Ephedrine also has been used to treat the hypotension that may occur with spinal anesthesia.

Untoward effects of ephedrine include hypertension, particularly after parenteral administration or with higher-than-recommended oral dosing. Insomnia is a common CNS adverse effect. Tachyphylaxis may occur with repetitive dosing. Concerns have been raised about the safety of ephedrine. Usual or higher-than-recommended doses may cause important adverse effects in susceptible individuals and are especially of concern in patients with underlying cardiovascular disease that might be unrecognized. Of potentially greater cause for concern, large amounts of herbal preparations containing ephedrine (ma huang, ephedra) are utilized around the world. There can be considerable variability in the content of ephedrine in these preparations, which may lead to inadvertent consumption of higher-than-usual doses of ephedrine and its isomers. Because of this, the FDA has banned the sale of dietary supplements containing ephedra. In addition, the Combat Methamphetamine Epidemic Act of 2005 regulates the sale of ephedrine, phenylpropanolamine, and pseudoephedrine, which can be used as precursors in the illicit manufacture of amphetamine and methamphetamine.

Other Sympathomimetic Agents

Several sympathomimetic drugs are used primarily as vasoconstrictors for local application to the nasal mucous membrane or the eye. The structures of propylhexedrine (BENZEDREX, others), naphazoline (PRIVINE, NAPHCON, others), oxymetazoline (AFRIN, OCU-CLEAR, others), and xylometazoline (OTRIVIN, others) are depicted in Table 12–1 and Figure 12–4.

Phenylephrine (described earlier), pseudoephedrine (SUDAFED, others) (a stereoisomer of ephedrine), and phenylpropanolamine are the sympathomimetic drugs that have been used most commonly in oral preparations for the relief of nasal congestion. Pseudoephedrine is available without a prescription in a variety of solid and liquid dosage forms. Phenylpropanolamine shares the pharmacological properties of ephedrine and is approximately equal in potency except that it causes less CNS stimulation. Due to concern about the possibility that phenylpropanolamine increases the risk of hemorrhagic stroke, the drug is no longer licensed for marketing in the U.S.

THERAPEUTIC USES OF SYMPATHOMIMETIC DRUGS

The variety of vital functions that are regulated by the sympathetic nervous system and the success that has attended efforts to develop therapeutic agents that can

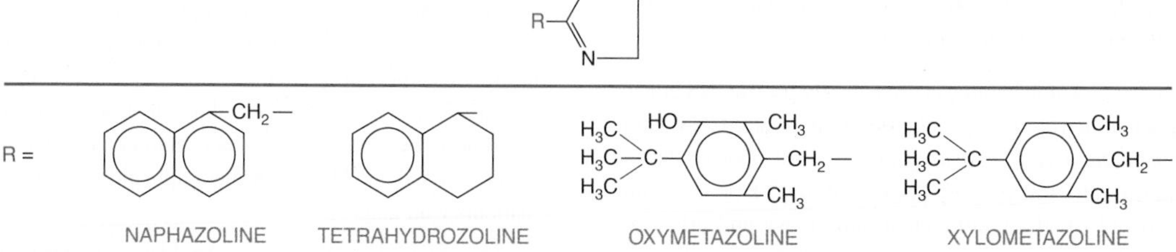

R =

NAPHAZOLINE TETRAHYDROZOLINE OXYMETAZOLINE XYLOMETAZOLINE

Figure 12–4. *Chemical structures of imidazoline derivatives.*

influence adrenergic receptors selectively have resulted in a class of drugs with a large number of important therapeutic uses.

Shock. Shock is a clinical syndrome characterized by inadequate perfusion of tissues; it usually is associated with hypotension and ultimately with the failure of organ systems (Hollenberg et al., 1999). Shock is an immediately life-threatening impairment of delivery of oxygen and nutrients to the organs of the body. Causes of shock include hypovolemia (due to dehydration or blood loss), cardiac failure (extensive myocardial infarction, severe arrhythmia, or cardiac mechanical defects such as ventricular septal defect), obstruction to cardiac output (due to pulmonary embolism, pericardial tamponade, or aortic dissection), and peripheral circulatory dysfunction (sepsis or anaphylaxis). Recent research on shock has focused on the accompanying increased permeability of the GI mucosa to pancreatic proteases, and on the role of these degradative enzymes on microvascular inflammation and multi-organ failure (Schmid-Schoenbein and Hugli, 2005). The treatment of shock consists of specific efforts to reverse the underlying pathogenesis as well as nonspecific measures aimed at correcting hemodynamic abnormalities. Regardless of etiology, the accompanying fall in blood pressure generally leads to marked activation of the sympathetic nervous system. This, in turn, causes peripheral vasoconstriction and an increase in the rate and force of cardiac contraction. In the initial stages of shock these mechanisms may maintain blood pressure and cerebral blood flow, although blood flow to the kidneys, skin, and other organs may be decreased, leading to impaired production of urine and metabolic acidosis.

The initial therapy of shock involves basic life-support measures. It is essential to maintain blood volume, which often requires monitoring of hemodynamic parameters. Specific therapy (e.g., antibiotics for patients in septic shock) should be initiated immediately. If these measures do not lead to an adequate therapeutic response, it may be necessary to use vasoactive drugs in an effort to improve abnormalities in blood pressure and flow. This therapy generally is empirically based on response to hemodynamic measurements. Many of these pharmacological approaches, while apparently clinically reasonable, are of uncertain efficacy. Adrenergic receptor agonists may be used in an attempt to increase myocardial contractility or to modify peripheral vascular resistance. In general terms, β receptor agonists increase heart rate and force of contraction, α receptor agonists increase peripheral vascular resistance, and DA promotes dilation of renal and splanchnic vascular beds, in addition to activating β and α receptors (Breslow and Ligier, 1991).

Cardiogenic shock due to myocardial infarction has a poor prognosis; therapy is aimed at improving peripheral blood flow. Definitive therapy, such as emergency cardiac catheterization followed by surgical revascularization or angioplasty, may be very important. Mechanical left ventricular assist devices also may help to maintain cardiac output and coronary perfusion in critically ill patients. In the setting of severely impaired cardiac output, falling blood pressure leads to intense sympathetic outflow and vasoconstriction. This may further decrease cardiac output as the damaged heart pumps against a higher peripheral resistance. Medical intervention is designed to optimize cardiac filling pressure (preload), myocardial contractility, and peripheral resistance (afterload). Preload may be increased by administration of intravenous fluids or reduced with drugs such as diuretics and nitrates. A number of sympathomimetic amines have been used to increase the force of contraction of the heart. Some of these drugs have disadvantages: isoproterenol is a powerful chronotropic agent and can greatly increase myocardial O_2 demand; NE intensifies peripheral vasoconstriction; and epinephrine increases heart rate and may predispose the heart to dangerous arrhythmias. DA is an effective inotropic agent that causes less increase in heart rate than does isoproterenol. DA also promotes renal arterial dilation; this may be useful in preserving renal function. When given in high doses ($>$ 10-20 μg/kg per minute), DA activates α receptors, causing peripheral and renal vasoconstriction. Dobutamine has complex pharmacological actions that are mediated by its stereoisomers; the clinical effects of the drug are to increase myocardial contractility with little increase in heart rate or peripheral resistance.

In some patients in shock, hypotension is so severe that vasoconstricting drugs are required to maintain a blood pressure that is adequate for CNS perfusion. Alpha agonists such as NE, phenylephrine, metaraminol, mephentermine, midodrine, ephedrine, epinephrine, DA, and methoxamine all have been used for this purpose. This approach may be advantageous in patients with hypotension due to failure of the sympathetic nervous system (e.g., after spinal anesthesia or injury). However, in patients with other forms of shock, such as cardiogenic shock, reflex vasoconstriction generally is intense, and α receptor agonists may further compromise blood flow to organs such as the kidneys and gut and adversely increase the work of the heart. Indeed, vasodilating drugs such as nitroprusside are more likely to improve blood flow and decrease cardiac work in such patients by decreasing afterload if a minimally adequate blood pressure can be maintained.

The hemodynamic abnormalities in septic shock are complex and poorly understood. Most patients with septic shock initially have low or barely normal peripheral vascular resistance, possibly owing to excessive effects of endogenously produced NO as well as normal or increased cardiac output. If the syndrome progresses, myocardial depression, increased peripheral resistance, and impaired tissue oxygenation occur. The primary treatment of septic shock is antibiotics. Data on the comparative value of various adrenergic agents in the treatment of septic shock are limited. Therapy with drugs such as DA or dobutamine is guided by hemodynamic monitoring, with individualization of therapy depending on the patient's overall clinical condition.

Hypotension. Drugs with predominantly α agonist activity can be used to raise blood pressure in patients with decreased peripheral resistance in conditions such as spinal anesthesia or intoxication with antihypertensive medications. However, hypotension *per se* is not an indication for treatment with these agents unless there is inadequate perfusion of organs such as the brain, heart, or kidneys. Furthermore, adequate replacement of fluid or blood may be more appropriate than drug therapy for many patients with hypotension. In patients with spinal anesthesia that interrupts sympathetic activation of the heart, injections of ephedrine increase heart rate as well as peripheral vascular resistance; tachyphylaxis may occur with repetitive injections, necessitating the use of a directly acting drug.

Patients with orthostatic hypotension (excessive fall in blood pressure with standing) often represent a pharmacological challenge. There are diverse causes for this disorder, including the Shy-Drager syndrome and idiopathic autonomic failure. Therapeutic approaches include physical maneuvers and a variety of drugs (fludrocortisone, prostaglandin synthesis inhibitors, somatostatin analogs, caffeine, vasopressin analogs, and DA antagonists). A number of sympathomimetic drugs also have been used in treating this disorder. The ideal agent would enhance venous constriction prominently and produce relatively little arterial constriction so as to avoid supine hypertension. No such agent currently is available. Drugs used in this disorder to activate α_1 receptors include both direct- and indirect-acting agents. Midodrine shows promise in treating this challenging disorder.

Hypertension. Centrally acting α_2 receptor agonists such as clonidine are useful in the treatment of hypertension. Drug therapy of hypertension is discussed in Chapter 27.

Cardiac Arrhythmias. Cardiopulmonary resuscitation in patients with cardiac arrest due to ventricular fibrillation, electromechanical dissociation, or asystole may be facilitated by drug treatment. Epinephrine is an important therapeutic agent in patients with cardiac arrest; epinephrine and other α agonists increase diastolic pressure and improve coronary blood flow. Alpha agonists also help to preserve cerebral blood flow during resuscitation. Cerebral blood vessels are relatively insensitive to the vasoconstricting effects of catecholamines, and perfusion pressure is increased. Consequently, during external cardiac massage, epinephrine facilitates distribution of the limited cardiac output to the cerebral and coronary circulations. Although it had been thought that the β adrenergic effects of epinephrine on the heart made ventricular fibrillation more susceptible to conversion with electrical countershock, tests in animal models have not confirmed this hypothesis. The optimal dose of epinephrine in patients with cardiac arrest is unclear. Once a cardiac rhythm has been restored, it may be necessary to treat arrhythmias, hypotension, or shock.

In patients with paroxysmal supraventricular tachycardias, particularly those associated with mild hypotension, careful infusion of an α agonist (e.g., phenylephrine) to raise blood pressure to ~160 mm Hg may end the arrhythmia by increasing vagal tone. However, this method of treatment has been replaced largely by Ca^{2+} channel blockers with clinically significant effects on the AV node, β antagonists, adenosine, and electrical cardioversion (Chapter 29). Beta agonists such as isoproterenol may be used as adjunctive or temporizing therapy with atropine in patients with marked bradycardia who are compromised hemodynamically; if long-term therapy is required, a cardiac pacemaker usually is the treatment of choice.

Congestive Heart Failure. Sympathetic stimulation of β receptors in the heart is an important compensatory mechanism for maintenance of cardiac function in patients with congestive heart failure. Responses mediated by β receptors are blunted in the failing human heart. While β agonists may increase cardiac output in acute emergency settings such as shock, long-term therapy with β agonists as inotropic agents is not efficacious. Indeed, interest has grown in the use of β receptor antagonists in the treatment of patients with congestive heart failure (Chapter 28).

Local Vascular Effects of α Adrenergic Receptor Agonists. Epinephrine is used in many surgical procedures in the nose, throat, and larynx to shrink the mucosa and improve visualization by limiting hemorrhage. Simultaneous injection of epinephrine with local anesthetics retards the absorption of the anesthetic and increases the duration of anesthesia (Chapter 20). Injection of α agonists into the penis may be useful in reversing priapism, a complication of the use of α receptor antagonists or PDE5 inhibitors (e.g., sildenafil) in the treatment of erectile dysfunction. Both phenylephrine and oxymetazoline are efficacious vasoconstrictors when applied locally during sinus surgery.

Nasal Decongestion. α Receptor agonists are used extensively as nasal decongestants in patients with allergic or vasomotor rhinitis and in acute rhinitis in patients with upper respiratory infections. These drugs probably decrease resistance to airflow by decreasing the volume of the nasal mucosa; this may occur by activation of α receptors in venous capacitance vessels in nasal tissues that have erectile characteristics. The receptors that mediate this effect appear to be α_1 receptors. Interestingly, α_2 receptors may mediate contraction of arterioles that supply nutrition to the nasal mucosa. Intense constriction of these vessels may cause structural damage to the mucosa. A major limitation of therapy with nasal decongestants is loss of efficacy, "rebound" hyperemia, and worsening of symptoms with chronic use or when the drug is stopped. Although mechanisms are uncertain, possibilities include receptor desensitization and damage to the mucosa. Agonists that are selective for α_1 receptors may be less likely to induce mucosal damage.

For decongestion, α agonists may be administered either orally or topically. Oral ephedrine often causes CNS adverse effects. Pseudoephedrine is a stereoisomer of ephedrine that is less potent than ephedrine in producing tachycardia, increased blood pressure, and CNS stimulation. Sympathomimetic decongestants should be used with great caution in patients with hypertension and in men with prostatic enlargement, and they are contraindicated in patients who are taking MAO inhibitors. A variety of compounds (see under Ephedrine, earlier) are available for topical use in patients with rhinitis. Topical decongestants are particularly useful in acute rhinitis because of their more selective site of action, but they are apt to be used excessively by patients, leading to rebound congestion. Oral decongestants are much less likely to cause rebound congestion but carry a greater risk of inducing adverse systemic effects. Indeed, patients with uncontrolled hypertension or ischemic heart disease generally should carefully avoid the oral consumption of over-the-counter products or herbal preparations containing sympathomimetic drugs.

Asthma. Use of β adrenergic agonists in the treatment of asthma and chronic obstructive pulmonary disease (COPD) is discussed in Chapter 36.

Allergic Reactions. Epinephrine is the drug of choice to reverse the manifestations of serious acute hypersensitivity reactions (e.g., from food, bee sting, or drug allergy). A subcutaneous injection of epinephrine rapidly relieves itching, hives, and swelling of lips, eyelids, and tongue. In some patients, careful intravenous infusion of epinephrine may be required to ensure prompt pharmacological effects. This treatment may be life-saving when edema of the glottis threatens airway patency or when there is hypotension or shock in patients with anaphylaxis. In addition to its cardiovascular effects, epinephrine is thought to activate β receptors that suppress the release from mast cells of mediators such as histamine and leukotrienes. Although glucocorticoids and antihistamines frequently are administered to patients with severe hypersensitivity reactions, epinephrine remains the mainstay. Epinephrine auto-injectors (EPIPEN, others) are employed widely for the emergency self-treatment of anaphylaxis.

Ophthalmic Uses. Application of various sympathomimetic amines for diagnostic and therapeutic ophthalmic use is discussed in Chapter 64.

Narcolepsy and Related Syndromes. Narcolepsy is characterized by hypersomnia, including attacks of sleep that may occur suddenly under conditions that are not normally conducive to sleep. Some patients respond to treatment with tricyclic antidepressants or MAO inhibitors. Alternatively, CNS stimulants such as amphetamine, dextroamphetamine, or methamphetamine may be useful. Modafinil (PROVIGIL), a CNS stimulant, may have benefit in narcolepsy. In the U.S., it is a schedule IV controlled substance. Its mechanism of action in narcolepsy is unclear and may not involve adrenergic receptors. Therapy with amphetamines is complicated by the risk of abuse and the likelihood of the development of tolerance. Depression, irritability, and paranoia also may occur. Amphetamines may disturb nocturnal sleep, which increases the difficulty of avoiding daytime attacks of sleep in these patients. Armodafinil (NUVIGIL), the R-enantiomer of modafinil (a mixture of R- and S-enantiomers) is also indicated for narcolepsy, to improve wakefulness in shift workers, and to combat excessive sleepiness in patients with obstructive sleep apnea-hypopnea syndrome.

Narcolepsy in rare individuals is caused by mutations in the related orexin neuropeptides (also called hypocretins), which are expressed in the lateral hypothalamus, or in their G protein–coupled receptors (Mignot, 2004). Although such mutations are not present in most subjects with narcolepsy, the levels of orexins in the CSF are markedly diminished, suggesting that deficient orexin signaling may play a pathogenic role. The association of these neuropeptides and their cognate GPCRs with narcolepsy provides an attractive target for the development of novel pharmacotherapies for this disorder.

Weight Reduction. Obesity arises as a consequence of positive caloric balance. Optimally, weight loss is achieved by a gradual increase in energy expenditure from exercise combined with dieting to decrease the caloric intake. However, this obvious approach has a relatively low success rate. Consequently, alternative forms of treatment, including surgery or medications, have been developed in an effort to increase the likelihood of achieving and maintaining weight loss. Amphetamine was found to produce weight loss in early studies of patients with narcolepsy and was subsequently used in the treatment of obesity. The drug promotes weight loss by suppressing appetite rather than by increasing energy expenditure. Other anorexic drugs include methamphetamine, dextroamphetamine (and a prodrug form, lisdexamfetamine), phentermine, benzphetamine, phendimetrazine, phenmetrazine, diethylpropion, mazindol, phenylpropanolamine, and sibutramine (a mixed adrenergic/serotonergic drug). Phenmetrazine, mazindol, and phenylpropanolamine have been discontinued in the U.S. In short-term (up to 20 weeks), double-blind controlled studies, amphetamine-like drugs have been shown to be more effective than placebo in promoting weight loss; the rate of weight loss typically is increased by ~ 0.5 pound per week with these drugs. There is little to choose among these drugs in terms of efficacy. However, long-term weight loss has not been demonstrated unless these drugs are taken continuously. In addition, other important issues have not yet been resolved, including the selection of patients who might benefit from these drugs, whether the drugs should be administered continuously or intermittently, and the duration of treatment. Adverse effects of treatment include the potential for drug abuse and habituation, serious worsening of hypertension (although in some patients blood pressure actually may fall, presumably as a consequence of weight loss), sleep disturbances, palpitations, and dry mouth. These agents may be effective adjuncts in the treatment of obesity. However, available evidence does not support the isolated use of these drugs in the absence of a more comprehensive program that stresses exercise and modification of diet. β_3 Receptor agonists have remarkable anti-obesity and anti-diabetic effects in rodents. However, pharmaceutical companies have not yet succeeded in developing β_3 receptor agonists for the treatment of these conditions in humans, perhaps because of important differences in β_3 receptors between humans and rodents. With the cloning of the human β_3 receptor, compounds with favorable metabolic effects have been developed. The use of β_3 agonists in the treatment of obesity remains a possibility for the future (Fernandez-Lopez et al., 2002; Robidoux et al., 2004).

Attention-Deficit/Hyperactivity Disorder (ADHD). This syndrome, usually first evident in childhood, is characterized by excessive motor activity, difficulty in sustaining attention, and impulsiveness. Children with this disorder frequently are troubled by difficulties in school, impaired interpersonal relationships, and excitability. Academic underachievement is an important characteristic. A substantial number of children with this syndrome have characteristics that persist into adulthood, although in modified form. Behavioral therapy may be helpful in some patients. Catecholamines may be involved in the control of attention at the level of the cerebral cortex. A variety of stimulant drugs have been utilized in the treatment of ADHD, and they are particularly indicated in moderate-to-severe cases. Dextroamphetamine has been demonstrated to be more effective than placebo. Methylphenidate is effective in children with ADHD and is the most common intervention (Swanson and Volkow, 2003). Treatment may start with a dose of 5 mg of methylphenidate in the morning and at lunch; the dose is increased gradually over a period of weeks depending on the response as judged by parents, teachers, and the clinician. The total daily dose generally should not exceed 60 mg; because of its short duration of action, most children require two or three doses of methylphenidate each day. The timing of doses is adjusted individually in accordance with rapidity of onset of effect and duration of action. Methylphenidate, dextroamphetamine, and amphetamine probably have similar efficacy in ADHD and are the preferred drugs in this disorder. Sustained-release preparations of dextroamphaetamine, methylphenidate (RITALIN SR, CONCERTA, META-DATE), dexmethylphenidate (FOCALIN XR), and amphetamine (ADDERAL XR) may be used once daily in children and adults. Lisdexamfetamine (VYVANSE) can be administered once daily and a transdermal formulation of methylphenidate (DAYTRANA) is marketed for daytime use. Potential adverse effects of these medications include insomnia, abdominal pain, anorexia, and weight loss that may be associated with suppression of growth in children. Minor symptoms may be transient or may respond to adjustment of dosage or administration of the drug with meals. Other drugs that have been utilized include tricyclic antidepressants, antipsychotic agents, and clonidine. A sustained release formulation of guanfacine (INTUNIV), an α_{2A} receptor agonist, has recently been approved for use in children (ages 6-17 years) in treating ADHD.

Adrenergic Receptor Antagonists

Many types of drugs interfere with the function of the sympathetic nervous system and thus have profound effects on the physiology of sympathetically innervated organs. Several of these drugs are important in clinical medicine, particularly for the treatment of cardiovascular diseases.

The remainder of this chapter focuses on the pharmacology of adrenergic receptor *antagonists*, drugs that inhibit the interaction of NE, epinephrine, and other sympathomimetic drugs with α and β receptors (Figure 12–5). Almost all of these agents are competitive antagonists; an important exception is phenoxybenzamine, an irreversible antagonist that binds covalently to α receptors. There are important structural differences among the various types of adrenergic receptors (Chapter 8). Since compounds have been developed that have different affinities for the various receptors, it is possible to interfere selectively with responses that result from stimulation of the sympathetic nervous system. For example, selective antagonists of β_1 receptors block most actions of epinephrine and NE on the heart, while having less effect on β_2 receptors in bronchial smooth muscle and no effect on responses mediated by α_1 or α_2 receptors. Detailed knowledge of the autonomic nervous system and the sites of action of drugs that act on adrenergic receptors is essential for understanding the pharmacological properties and therapeutic uses of this important class of drugs. Additional background material is presented in Chapter 8. Agents that block DA receptors are considered in Chapter 13.

α ADRENERGIC RECEPTOR ANTAGONISTS

The α adrenergic receptors mediate many of the important actions of endogenous catecholamines. Responses of particular clinical relevance include α_1 receptor–mediated contraction of arterial, venous and visceral smooth muscle. The α_2 receptors are involved in suppressing sympathetic output, increasing vagal tone, facilitating platelet aggregation, inhibiting the release of NE and ACh from nerve endings, and regulating metabolic effects. These effects include suppression of insulin secretion and inhibition of lipolysis. The α_2 receptors also mediate contraction of some arteries and veins.

α receptor antagonists have a wide spectrum of pharmacological specificities and are chemically

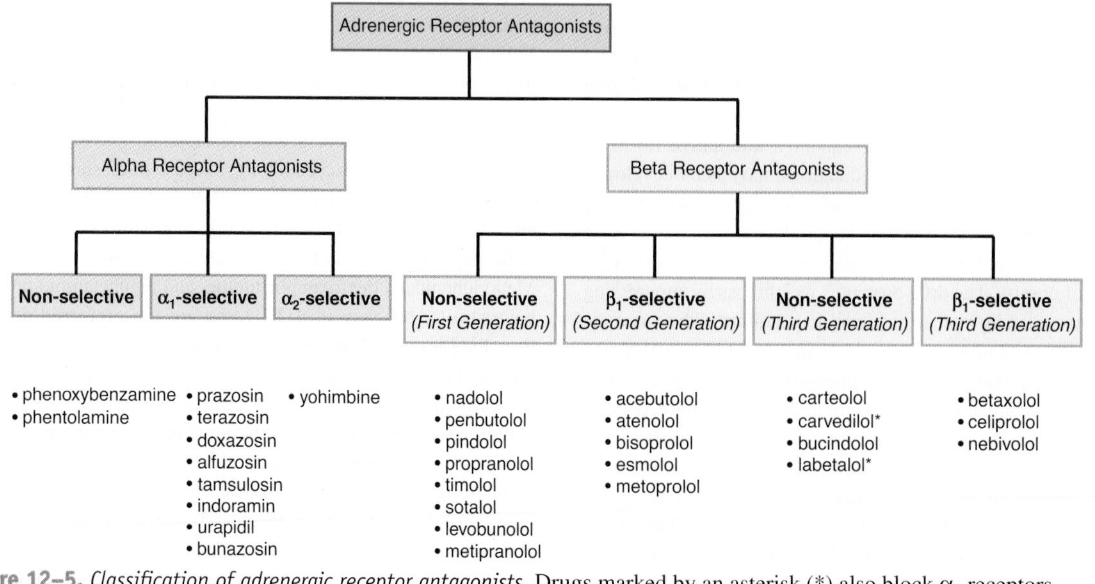

Figure 12–5. *Classification of adrenergic receptor antagonists.* Drugs marked by an asterisk (*) also block α_1 receptors.

heterogeneous. Some of these drugs have markedly different affinities for α_1 and α_2 receptors. For example, prazosin is much more potent in blocking α_1 than α_2 receptors (i.e., α_1 selective), whereas yohimbine is α_2 selective; phentolamine has similar affinities for both of these receptor subtypes. More recently, agents that discriminate among the various subtypes of a particular receptor have become available; e.g., tamsulosin has higher potency at α_{1A} than at α_{1B} receptors. Figure 12–6 shows the structural formulas of many of these agents. Prior editions of this textbook contain information about the chemistry of α receptor antagonists.

Some of the most important effects of α receptor antagonists observed clinically are on the cardiovascular system. Actions in both the CNS and the periphery are involved; the outcome depends on the cardiovascular status of the patient at the time of drug administration and the relative selectivity of the agent for α_1 and α_2 receptors.

Catecholamines increase the output of glucose from the liver; in humans this effect is mediated predominantly by β receptors, although α receptors may contribute. α Receptor antagonists therefore may reduce glucose release. Receptors of the α_{2A} subtype facilitate platelet aggregation; the effect of blockade of platelet α_2 receptors *in vivo* is not clear. Activation of α_2 receptors in the pancreatic islets suppresses insulin secretion; conversely, blockade of pancreatic α_2 receptors may facilitate insulin release (Chapter 43).

α_1 Receptor Antagonists

General Pharmacological Properties. Blockade of α_1 adrenergic receptors inhibits vasoconstriction induced by endogenous catecholamines; vasodilation may occur in both arteriolar resistance vessels and veins. The result is a fall in blood pressure due to decreased peripheral resistance. The magnitude of such effects depends on the activity of the sympathetic nervous system at the time the antagonist is administered, and thus is less in supine than in upright subjects and is particularly marked if there is hypovolemia. For most α receptor antagonists, the fall in blood pressure is opposed by baroreceptor reflexes that cause increases in heart rate and cardiac output, as well as fluid retention. These reflexes are exaggerated if the antagonist also blocks α_2 receptors on peripheral sympathetic nerve endings, leading to enhanced release of NE and increased stimulation of postsynaptic β_1 receptors in the heart and on juxtaglomerular cells (Chapter 8) (Starke et al., 1989). Although stimulation of α_1 receptors in the heart may cause an increased force of contraction, the importance of blockade at this site in humans is uncertain.

Blockade of α_1 receptors also inhibits vasoconstriction and the increase in blood pressure produced by the administration of a sympathomimetic amine. The pattern of effects depends on the adrenergic agonist that is administered: pressor responses to phenylephrine can be completely suppressed; those to NE are only incompletely blocked because of residual stimulation of cardiac β_1 receptors; and pressor responses to epinephrine may be transformed to vasodepressor effects because of residual stimulation of β_2 receptors in the vasculature with resultant vasodilation.

Blockade of α_1 receptors can alleviate some of the symptoms of benign prostatic hyperplasia (BPH). The symptoms of BPH include a resistance to urine outflow. This results from mechanical pressure on the urethra due to an increase in smooth muscle mass and an α adrenergic receptor mediated increase in smooth muscle tone in the prostate and neck of the bladder. Antagonism of α_1 receptors permits relaxation of the smooth muscle and decreases the resistance to the outflow of urine. The prostate and lower urinary tract tissues exhibit a high proportion of α_{1A} receptors (Michel and Vrydag, 2006).

Available Agents

Prazosin and Related Drugs. Due in part to its greater α_1 receptor selectivity, this class of α receptor antagonists exhibits greater clinical utility and has largely replaced the non-selective haloalkylamine (e.g., phenoxybenzamine) and imidazoline (e.g., phentolamine) α receptor antagonists.

Prazosin is the prototypical α_1-selective antagonist. The affinity of prazosin for α_1 adrenergic receptors is ~1000-fold greater than that for α_2 adrenergic receptors. Prazosin has similar potencies at α_{1A}, α_{1B}, and α_{1D} subtypes. Interestingly, the drug also is a relatively potent inhibitor of cyclic nucleotide phosphodiesterases, and it originally was synthesized for this purpose. The pharmacological properties of prazosin have been characterized extensively. Prazosin and the related α receptor antagonists, doxazosin and tamsulosin, frequently are used for the treatment of hypertension (Chapter 27).

Pharmacological Properties. The major effects of prazosin result from its blockade of α_1 receptors in arterioles and veins. This leads to a fall in peripheral vascular resistance and in venous return to the heart. Unlike other vasodilating drugs, administration of prazosin usually does not increase heart rate. Since prazosin has little or no α_2 receptor–blocking effect at concentrations achieved clinically, it probably does

Alkylating agent

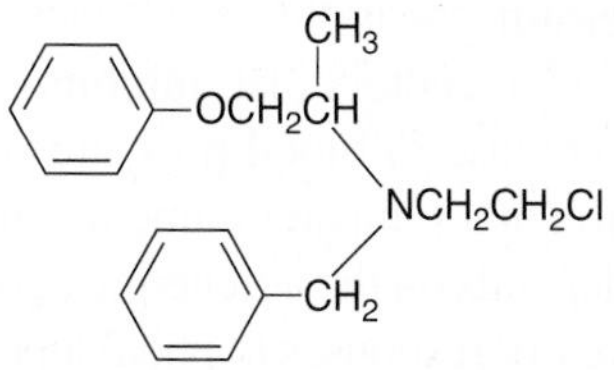

PHENOXYBENZAMINE

Benzenesulfonamide

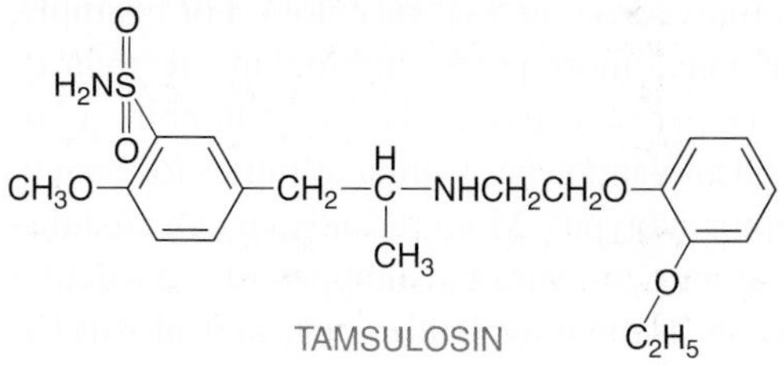

TAMSULOSIN

Imidazolines

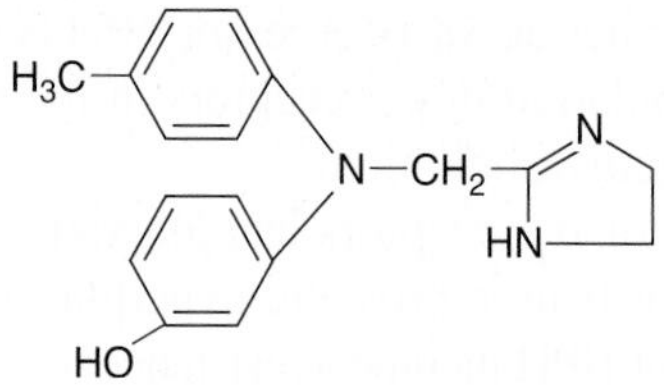

PHENTOLAMINE

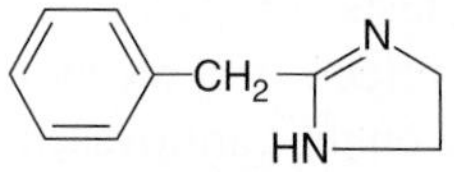

TOLAZOLINE

Piperazinyl quinazolines

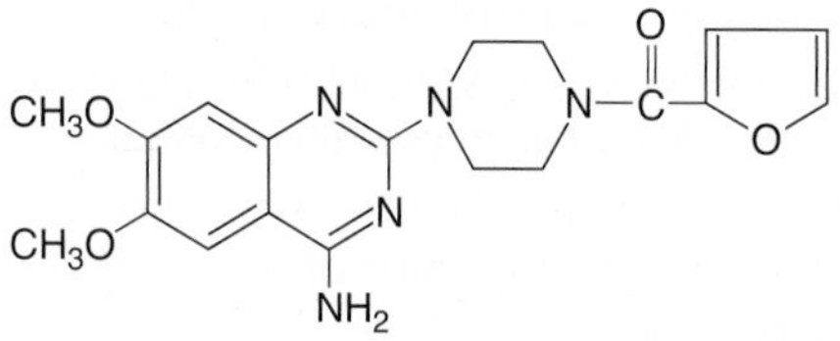

PRAZOSIN

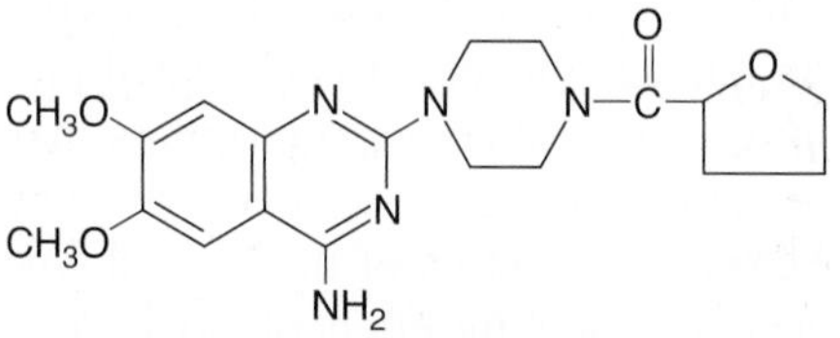

TERAZOSIN

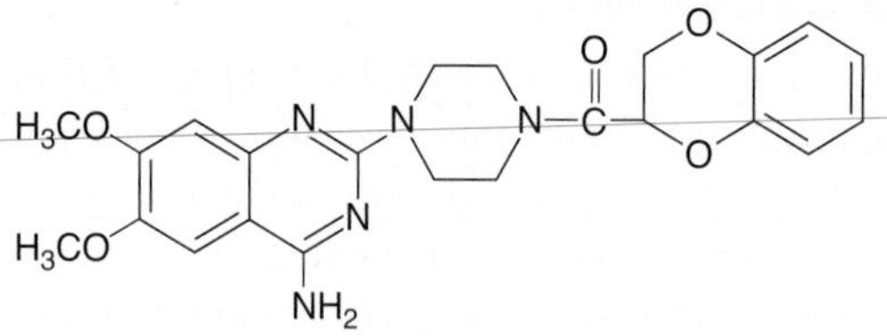

DOXAZOSIN

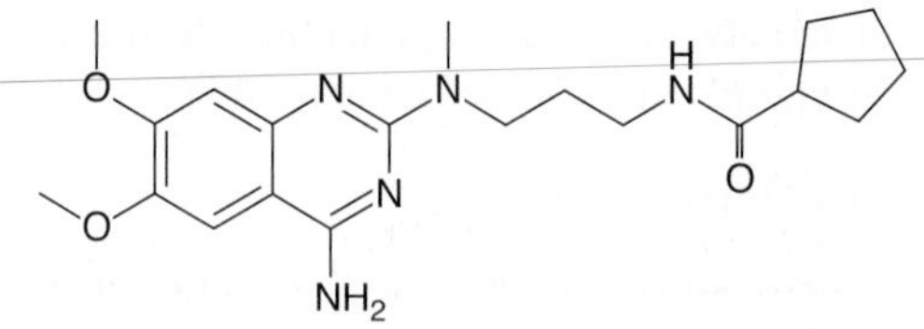

ALFUZOSIN

Indoles

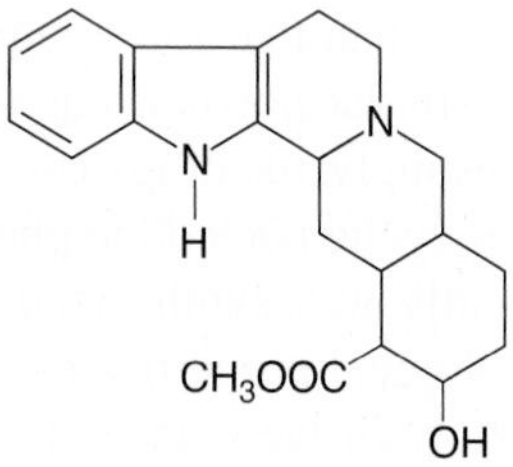

YOHIMBINE

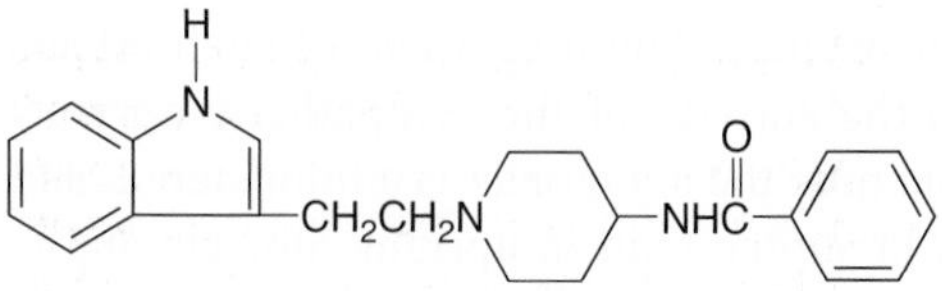

INDORAMIN

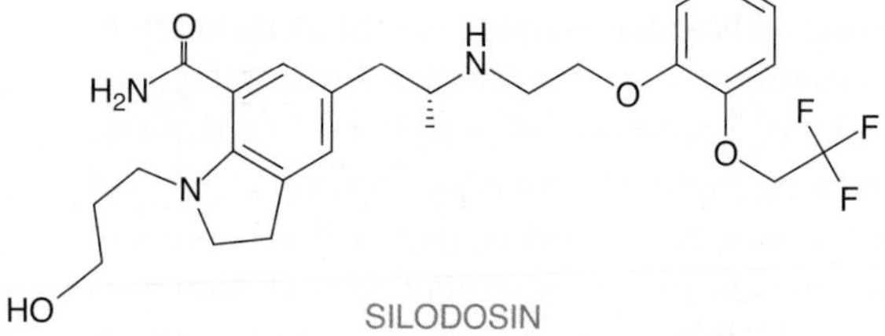

SILODOSIN

Figure 12–6. *Structural formulas of some α adrenergic receptor antagonists.*

not promote the release of NE from sympathetic nerve endings in the heart. In addition, prazosin decreases cardiac preload and thus has little tendency to increase cardiac output and rate, in contrast to vasodilators such as hydralazine that have minimal dilatory effects on veins. Although the combination of reduced preload and selective α_1 receptor blockade might be sufficient to account for the relative absence of reflex tachycardia, prazosin also may act in the CNS to suppress sympathetic outflow. Prazosin appears to depress baroreflex function in hypertensive patients. Prazosin and related drugs in this class tend to have favorable effects on serum lipids in humans, decreasing low-density lipoproteins (LDL) and triglycerides while increasing concentrations of high-density lipoproteins (HDL). Prazosin and related drugs may have effects on cell growth unrelated to antagonism of α_1 receptors (Hu et al., 1998).

Prazosin (MINIPRESS, others) is well absorbed after oral administration, and bioavailability is ~ 50-70%. Peak concentrations of prazosin in plasma generally are reached 1-3 hours after an oral dose. The drug is tightly bound to plasma proteins (primarily α_1-acid glycoprotein), and only 5% of the drug is free in the circulation; diseases that modify the concentration of this protein (e.g., inflammatory processes) may change the free fraction. Prazosin is extensively metabolized in the liver, and little unchanged drug is excreted by the kidneys. The plasma $t_{1/2}$ is ~3 hours (may be prolonged to 6-8 hours in congestive heart failure). The duration of action of the drug typically is 7-10 hours in the treatment of hypertension.

The initial dose should be 1 mg, usually given at bedtime so that the patient will remain recumbent for at least several hours to reduce the risk of syncopal reactions that may follow the first dose of prazosin. Therapy is begun with 1 mg given two or three times daily, and the dose is titrated upward depending on the blood pressure. A maximal effect generally is observed with a total daily dose of 20 mg in patients with hypertension. In the off-label treatment of benign prostatic hyperplasia (BPH), doses from 1-5 mg twice daily typically are used.

Terazosin. Terazosin (HYTRIN, others) is a close structural analog of prazosin. It is less potent than prazosin but retains high specificity for α_1 receptors; terazosin does not discriminate among α_{1A}, α_{1B}, and α_{1D} receptors. The major distinction between the two drugs is in their pharmacokinetic properties.

Terazosin is more soluble in water than is prazosin, and its bioavailability is high (>90%). The $t_{1/2}$ of elimination of terazosin is ~12 hours, and its duration of action usually extends beyond 18 hours. Consequently, the drug may be taken once daily to treat hypertension and BPH in most patients. Terazosin has been found more effective than finasteride in treatment of BPH (Lepor et al., 1996). An interesting aspect of the action of terazosin and doxazosin in the treatment of lower urinary tract problems in men with BPH is the induction of apoptosis in prostate smooth muscle cells. This apoptosis may lessen the symptoms associated with chronic BPH by limiting cell proliferation. The apoptotic effect of terazosin and doxazosin appears to be related to the quinazoline moiety rather than α_1 receptor antagonism; tamsulosin, a non-quinazoline α_1 receptor antagonist, does not produce apoptosis (Kyprianou, 2003). Only ~10% of terazosin is excreted unchanged in the urine. An initial first dose of 1 mg is recommended. Doses are slowly titrated upward depending on the therapeutic response. Doses of 10 mg/day may be required for maximal effect in BPH.

Doxazosin. Doxazosin (CARDURA, others) is another structural analog of prazosin and a highly selective antagonist at α_1 receptors. It is non-selective among α_1 receptor subtypes, and differs from prazosin in its pharmacokinetic profile.

The $t_{1/2}$ of doxazosin is ~20 hours, and its duration of action may extend to 36 hours. The bioavailability and extent of metabolism of doxazosin and prazosin are similar. Most doxazosin metabolites are eliminated in the feces. The hemodynamic effects of doxazosin appear to be similar to those of prazosin. As in the cases of prazosin and terazosin, doxazosin should be given initially as a 1-mg dose in the treatment of hypertension or BPH. Doxazosin also may have beneficial actions in the long-term management of BPH related to apoptosis that are independent of α_1 receptor antagonism. Doxazosin is typically administered once daily. An extended-release formulation marketed for BPH is not recommended for the treatment of hypertension.

Alfuzosin. Alfuzosin (UROXATRAL) is a quinazoline-based α_1 receptor antagonist with similar affinity at all of the α_1 receptor subtypes. It has been used extensively in treating BPH; it is not approved for treatment of hypertension. Its bioavailability is ~64%; it has a $t_{1/2}$ of 3-5 hours. Alfuzosin is a substrate of CYP3A4 and the concomitant administration of CPY3A4 inhibitors (e.g., ketoconazole, clarithromycin, itraconazole, ritonavir) is contraindicated. Alfuzosin should be avoided in patients at risk for prolonged QT syndrome. The recommended dosage is one 10-mg extended-release tablet daily to be taken after the same meal each day.

Tamsulosin. Tamsulosin (FLOMAX), a benzenesulfonamide, is an α_1 receptor antagonist with some selectivity for α_{1A} (and α_{1D}) subtypes compared to the α_{1B} subtype (Kenny et al., 1996). This selectivity may favor blockade of α_{1A} receptors in prostate. Tamsulosin is efficacious in the treatment of BPH with little effect on blood pressure (Beduschi et al., 1998); tamsulosin is not approved for the treatment of hypertension. Tamsulosin is well absorbed and has a $t_{1/2}$ of 5-10 hours. It is extensively metabolized by CYPs. Tamsulosin may be administered at a 0.4-mg starting dose; a dose of 0.8 mg ultimately will be more efficacious in some patients. Abnormal ejaculation is an adverse effect of tamsulosin, experienced by ~18% of patients receiving the higher dose.

Silodosin. Silidosin (RAPAFLO) also exhibits selectivity for the α_{1A}, over the α_{1B} adrenergic receptor. The drug is metabolized by several pathways; the main metabolite is a glucuronide formed by UGT2B7; co-administration with inhibitors of this enzyme (e.g., probenecid, valproic acid, fluconazole) increases systemic exposure to silodosin. The drug is approved for the treatment of BPH and is reported, as is tamsulosin, to have lesser effects on blood pressure than the non-α_1 subtype selective antagonists. Nevertheless, dizziness and orthostatic hypotension can occur. The chief side effect of silodosin is retrograde ejaculation (in 28% of those treated). Silodosin is available as 4-mg and 8-mg capsules.

Adverse Effects. A major potential adverse effect of prazosin and its congeners is the first-dose effect; marked postural hypotension and syncope sometimes are seen 30-90 minutes after an initial dose of prazosin and 2-6 hours after an initial dose of doxazosin.

Syncopal episodes also have occurred with a rapid increase in dosage or with the addition of a second antihypertensive drug to the regimen of a patient who already is taking a large dose of prazosin. The mechanisms responsible for such exaggerated hypotensive responses or for the development of tolerance to these effects are not clear. An action in the CNS to reduce sympathetic outflow may contribute (described earlier). The risk of the first-dose phenomenon is minimized by limiting the initial dose (e.g., 1 mg at bedtime), by increasing the dosage slowly, and by introducing additional antihypertensive drugs cautiously.

Since orthostatic hypotension may be a problem during long-term treatment with prazosin or its congeners, it is essential to check standing as well as recumbent blood pressure. Nonspecific adverse effects such as headache, dizziness, and asthenia rarely limit treatment with prazosin. The nonspecific complaint of dizziness generally is not due to orthostatic hypotension. Although not extensively documented, the adverse effects of the structural analogs of prazosin appear to be similar to those of the parent compound. For tamsulosin, at a dose of 0.4 mg daily, effects on blood pressure are not expected, although impaired ejaculation may occur.

Therapeutic Uses

Hypertension. Prazosin and its congeners have been used successfully in the treatment of essential hypertension (Chapter 28). Considerable interest has also focused on the tendency of these drugs to improve rather than worsen lipid profiles and glucose-insulin metabolism in patients with hypertension who are at risk for atherosclerotic disease (Grimm, 1991). Catecholamines are also powerful stimulators of vascular smooth muscle hypertrophy, acting by α_1 receptors. To what extent these effects of α_1 antagonists have clinical significance in diminishing the risk of atherosclerosis is not known.

Congestive Heart Failure. α receptor antagonists have been used in the treatment of congestive heart failure, as have other vasodilating drugs. The short-term effects of prazosin in these patients are due to dilation of both arteries and veins, resulting in a reduction of preload and afterload, which increases cardiac output and reduces pulmonary congestion. In contrast to results obtained with inhibitors of angiotensin-converting enzyme or a combination of hydralazine and an organic nitrate, prazosin has not been found to prolong life in patients with congestive heart failure.

Benign Prostatic Hyperplasia (BPH). In a significant percentage of older men, BPH produces symptomatic urethral obstruction that leads to weak stream, urinary frequency, and nocturia. These symptoms are due to a combination of mechanical pressure on the urethra due to the increase in smooth muscle mass and the α_1 receptor–mediated increase in smooth muscle tone in the prostate and neck of the bladder (Kyprianou, 2003).

α_1 receptors in the trigone muscle of the bladder and urethra contribute to the resistance to outflow of urine. Prazosin reduces this resistance in some patients with impaired bladder emptying caused by prostatic obstruction or parasympathetic decentralization from spinal injury. The efficacy and importance of α receptor antagonists in the medical treatment of benign prostatic hyperplasia have been demonstrated in multiple controlled clinical trials. Transurethral resection of the prostate is the accepted surgical treatment for symptoms of urinary obstruction in men with BPH; however, there are some serious potential complications (e.g., risk of impotence), and improvement may not be permanent. Other, less invasive procedures also are available.

Medical therapy has utilized α receptor antagonists for many years. Finasteride (PROPECIA, PROSCAR, others) and dutasteride (AVODART), two drugs that inhibit conversion of testosterone to dihydrotestosterone (Chapter 41) and can reduce prostate volume in some patients, are approved as monotherapy and in combination with α receptor antagonists. α_1-Selective antagonists have efficacy in BPH owing to relaxation of smooth muscle in the bladder neck, prostate capsule, and prostatic urethra. These drugs rapidly improve urinary flow, whereas the actions of finasteride are typically delayed for months. Combination therapy with doxazosin and finasteride reduces the risk of overall clinical progression of BPH significantly more than treatment with either drug alone (McConnell et al., 2003). Tamsulosin at the recommended dose of 0.4 mg daily and silodosin at 0.8 mg are less likely to cause orthostatic hypotension than are the other drugs. There is growing evidence that the predominant α_1 receptor subtype expressed in the human prostate is the α_{1A} receptor (Michel and Vrydag, 2006). Developments in this area will provide the basis for the selection of α receptor antagonists with specificity for the relevant subtype of α_1 receptor. However, the possibility remains that some of the symptoms of BPH are due to α_1 receptors in other sites, such as bladder, spinal cord, or brain.

Other Disorders. Though anecdotal evidence suggested that prazosin might be useful in the treatment of patients with variant angina (Prinzmetal's angina) due to coronary vasospasm, several small controlled trials have failed to demonstrate a clear benefit. Some studies have indicated that prazosin can decrease the incidence of digital vasospasm in patients with Raynaud's disease; however, its relative efficacy as compared with other vasodilators (e.g., Ca^{2+} channel blockers) is not known. Prazosin may have some benefit in patients with other vasospastic disorders. Prazosin decreases ventricular arrhythmias induced by coronary artery ligation or reperfusion in laboratory animals; the therapeutic potential for this use in humans is not known. Prazosin also may be useful for the treatment of patients with mitral or aortic valvular insufficiency, presumably because of reduction of afterload.

α_2 ADRENERGIC RECEPTOR ANTAGONISTS

The α_2 receptors have an important role in regulation of the activity of the sympathetic nervous system, both peripherally and centrally. As mentioned earlier, activation of presynaptic α_2 receptors inhibits the release of NE and other co-transmitters from peripheral sympathetic nerve endings. Activation of α_2 receptors in the pontomedullary region of the CNS inhibits sympathetic nervous system activity and leads to a fall in blood pressure; these receptors are a site of action for drugs such as clonidine. Blockade of α_2 receptors with selective antagonists such as yohimbine thus can increase sympathetic outflow and potentiate the release of NE from nerve endings, leading to activation of α_1 and β_1 receptors in the heart and peripheral vasculature with a consequent rise in blood pressure. Antagonists that also block α_1 receptors give rise to similar effects on sympathetic outflow and release of NE, but the net increase in blood pressure is prevented by inhibition of vasoconstriction.

Although certain vascular beds contain α_2 receptors that promote contraction of smooth muscle, it is thought that these receptors are preferentially stimulated by circulating catecholamines, whereas α_1 receptors are activated by NE released from sympathetic nerve fibers. In other vascular beds, α_2 receptors reportedly promote vasodilation by stimulating the release of NO from endothelial cells. The physiological role of vascular α_2 receptors in the regulation of blood flow within various vascular beds is uncertain. The α_2 receptors contribute to smooth muscle contraction in the human saphenous vein, whereas α_1 receptors are more prominent in dorsal hand veins. The effects of α_2 receptor antagonists on the cardiovascular system are dominated by actions in the CNS and on sympathetic nerve endings.

Yohimbine. Yohimbine (YOCON, APHRODYNE) is a competitive antagonist that is selective for α_2 receptors. The compound is an indolealkylamine alkaloid and is found in the bark of the tree *Pausinystalia yohimbe* and in *Rauwolfia* root; its structure resembles that of reserpine. Yohimbine readily enters the CNS, where it acts to increase blood pressure and heart rate; it also enhances motor activity and produces tremors. These actions are opposite to those of clonidine, an α_2 agonist. Yohimbine also antagonizes effects of 5-HT. In the past, it was used extensively to treat male sexual dysfunction (Tam et al., 2001). Although efficacy never was clearly demonstrated, there is renewed interest in the use of yohimbine in the treatment of male sexual dysfunction. The drug enhances sexual activity in male rats and may benefit some patients with psychogenic erectile dysfunction. However, the efficacies of PDE5 inhibitors (e.g., sildenafil, vardenafil, and tadalafil) and apomorphine (off-label) have been much more conclusively demonstrated in oral treatment of erectile dysfunction. Several small studies suggest that yohimbine also may be useful for diabetic neuropathy and in the treatment of postural hypotension. In the U.S., yohimbine can be legally sold as a dietary supplement; however, labeling claims that it will arouse or increase sexual desire or improve sexual performance are prohibited. Yohimbine (ANTAGONIL, YOBINE) is approved in veterinary medicine for the reversal of xylazine anesthesia.

Non-selective α Adrenergic Antagonists: Phenoxybenzamine and Phentolamine. Phenoxybenzamine and phentolamine are non-selective α receptors antagonists. Phenoxybenzamine, a haloalkylamine compound, produces an irreversible antagonism; while phentolamine, an imidazaline, produces a competitive antagonism. Phenoxybenzamine and phentolamine have played an important role in the establishment of the importance of α receptors in the regulation of the cardiovascular and other systems. They are sometimes referred to as "classical" α blockers to distinguish them from more recently developed compounds such as prazosin.

The actions of phenoxybenzamine and phentolamine on the cardiovascular system are similar. These "classical" α blockers cause a progressive decrease in peripheral resistance, due to antagonism of α receptors in the vasculature, and an increase in cardiac output that is due in part to reflex sympathetic nerve stimulation. The cardiac stimulation is accentuated by enhanced release of NE from cardiac sympathetic nerve due to antagonism of presynaptic α_2 receptors by these non-selective α blockers. Postural hypotension is a prominent feature with these drugs and this, accompanied by reflex tachycardia that can precipitate cardiac arrhythmias, severely limits the use of these drugs to treat essential hypertension. The more recently developed α_1-selective antagonists, such as prazosin, have replaced the "classical" α blockers in the management of essential hypertension. Phenoxybenzamine and phentolamine are still marketed for several specialized uses.

Therapeutic Uses. A use of phenoxybenzamine (DIBENZYLINE) is in the treatment of pheochromocytoma. Pheochromocytomas are tumors of the adrenal medulla and sympathetic neurons that secrete enormous quantities of catecholamines into the circulation. The usual result is hypertension, which may be episodic and severe. The vast majority of pheochromocytomas are treated surgically; however, phenoxybenzamine is often used in preparing the patient for surgery. The drug controls episodes of severe hypertension and minimizes other adverse effects of catecholamines, such as contraction of plasma volume and injury of the myocardium. A conservative approach is to initiate treatment with phenoxybenzamine (at a dosage of 10 mg twice daily) 1-3 weeks before the operation. The dose is increased every other day until the desired effect on blood pressure is achieved. Therapy may be limited by postural hypotension; nasal stuffiness is another frequent adverse effect. The usual daily dose of phenoxybenzamine in patients with pheochromocytoma is 40-120 mg given in two or three divided portions. Prolonged treatment with phenoxybenzamine may be necessary in patients with inoperable or malignant pheochromocytoma. In some patients, particularly those with malignant disease, administration of metyrosine may be a useful adjuvant. Metyrosine (DEMSER) is a competitive inhibitor of tyrosine hydroxylase, the rate-limiting enzyme in the synthesis of catecholamines (Chapter 8). β Receptor antagonists also are used to treat pheochromocytoma, but only after the administration of an α receptor antagonist (described later).

Phentolamine can also be used in short-term control of hypertension in patients with pheochromocytoma. Rapid infusions of phentolamine may cause severe hypotension, so the drug should be administered cautiously. Phentolamine also may be useful to relieve pseudo-obstruction of the bowel in patients with pheochromocytoma; this condition may result from the inhibitory effects of catecholamines on intestinal smooth muscle.

Phentolamine has been used locally to prevent dermal necrosis after the inadvertent extravasation of an α receptor agonist. The drug also may be useful for the treatment of hypertensive crises that follow the abrupt withdrawal of clonidine or that may result from the ingestion of tyramine-containing foods during the use of non-selective MAO inhibitors. Although excessive activation of α receptors is important in the development of severe hypertension in these settings, there is little information about the safety and efficacy of phentolamine compared with those of other antihypertensive agents in the treatment of such patients. Direct intracavernous injection of phentolamine (in combination with papaverine) has been proposed as a treatment for male sexual dysfunction. The long-term efficacy of this treatment is not known. Intracavernous injection of phentolamine may cause orthostatic hypotension and priapism; pharmacological reversal of drug-induced erections can be achieved with an α receptor agonist such as phenylephrine. Repetitive intrapenile injections may cause fibrotic reactions. Buccally or orally administered phentolamine may have efficacy in some men with sexual dysfunction.

In 2008, the FDA approved the use of phentolamine (ORAVERSE) to reverse or shorten the duration of soft-tissue anesthesia. Sympathomimetics are frequently administered with local anesthetics to slow the removal of the anesthetic by causing vasoconstriction. When the need for anesthesia is over, phentolamine can help reverse it by antagonizing the α-receptor induced vasoconstriction.

Phenoxybenzamine has been used off-label to control the manifestations of autonomic hyperreflexia in patients with spinal cord transection.

Toxicity and Adverse Effects. Hypotension is the major adverse effect of phenoxybenzamine and phentolamine. In addition, reflex cardiac stimulation may cause alarming tachycardia, cardiac arrhythmias, and ischemic cardiac events, including myocardial infarction. Reversible inhibition of ejaculation may occur due to impaired smooth muscle contraction in the vas deferens and ejaculatory ducts. Phenoxybenzamine is mutagenic in the Ames test, and repeated administration of this drug to experimental animals causes peritoneal sarcomas and lung tumors. The clinical significance of these findings is not known. Phentolamine stimulates GI smooth muscle, an effect antagonized by atropine, and also enhances gastric acid secretion due in part to histamine release. Thus, phentolamine should be used with caution in patients with a history of peptic ulcer.

Additional α Adrenergic Receptor Antagonists

Ergot Alkaloids. The ergot alkaloids were the first adrenergic receptor antagonists to be discovered, and most aspects of their general pharmacology were disclosed in the classic studies of Dale. Ergot alkaloids exhibit a complex variety of pharmacological properties. To varying degrees, these agents act as partial agonists or antagonists at α receptors, DA receptors, and serotonin receptors. Additional information about the ergot alkaloids can be found in Chapter 13 and in previous editions of this book.

Indoramin. Indoramin is a selective, competitive α_1 receptor antagonist that is used outside the U.S. for the treatment of hypertension, BPH, and in the prophylaxis of migraine. Competitive antagonism of histamine H_1 and 5-HT receptors also is evident. As an α_1-selective antagonist, indoramin lowers blood pressure with minimal tachycardia. The drug also decreases the incidence of attacks of Raynaud's phenomenon.

The bioavailability of indoramin generally is < 30% (with considerable variability), and it undergoes extensive first-pass metabolism. Little unchanged drug is excreted in the urine, and some of the metabolites may be biologically active. The elimination $t_{1/2}$ is ~5 hours. Some of the adverse effects of indoramin include sedation, dry mouth, and failure of ejaculation. Although indoramin is an effective antihypertensive agent, it has complex pharmacokinetics and lacks a well-defined place in current therapy.

Ketanserin. Although developed as a 5-HT-receptor antagonist, ketanserin also blocks α_1 receptors. Ketanserin (not available in the U.S.) is discussed in Chapter 13.

Urapidil. Urapidil is a novel, selective α_1 receptor antagonist that has a chemical structure distinct from those of prazosin and related compounds; the drug is not commercially available in the U.S. Blockade of peripheral α_1 receptors appears to be primarily responsible for the hypotension produced by urapidil, although it has actions in the CNS as well. The drug is extensively metabolized and has a $t_{1/2}$ of 3 hours. The role of urapidil in the treatment of hypertension remains to be determined.

Bunazosin. Bunazosin is an α_1-selective antagonist of the quinazoline class that has been shown to lower blood pressure in patients with hypertension. Bunazosin is available in Germany, Japan, Thailand, and Indonesia.

Neuroleptic Agents. Natural and synthetic compounds of several other chemical classes developed primarily because they are antagonists of D_2 dopamine receptors also exhibit α receptor blocking activity. Chlorpromazine, haloperidol, and other neuroleptic drugs of the phenothiazine and butyrophenone types produce significant α receptor blockade in both laboratory animals and humans.

β ADRENERGIC RECEPTOR ANTAGONISTS

Competitive antagonists of β adrenergic receptors, or β blockers, have received enormous clinical attention because of their efficacy in the treatment of hypertension, ischemic heart disease, congestive heart failure, and certain arrhythmias.

History. Ahlquist's hypothesis that the effects of catecholamines were mediated by activation of distinct α and β receptors provided the initial impetus for the synthesis and pharmacological evaluation of β receptor antagonists (Chapter 8). The first such selective agent was dichloroisoproterenol, a partial agonist. Sir James Black and his colleagues initiated a program in the late 1950s to develop additional β blockers, with the resulting synthesis and characterization of propranolol.

Chemistry. The structural formulas of some β receptor antagonists in general use are shown in Figures 12–7 and 12–8. The structural similarities between agonists and antagonists that act on β receptors are closer than those between α receptor agonists and antagonists. Substitution of an isopropyl group or other bulky substituent on the amino nitrogen favors interaction with β receptors. There is a rather wide tolerance for the nature of the aromatic moiety in the non-selective β receptor antagonists; however, the structural tolerance for β_1-selective antagonists is far more constrained.

Overview. Propranolol is a competitive β receptor antagonist and remains the prototype to which other β antagonists are compared. β antagonists can be distinguished

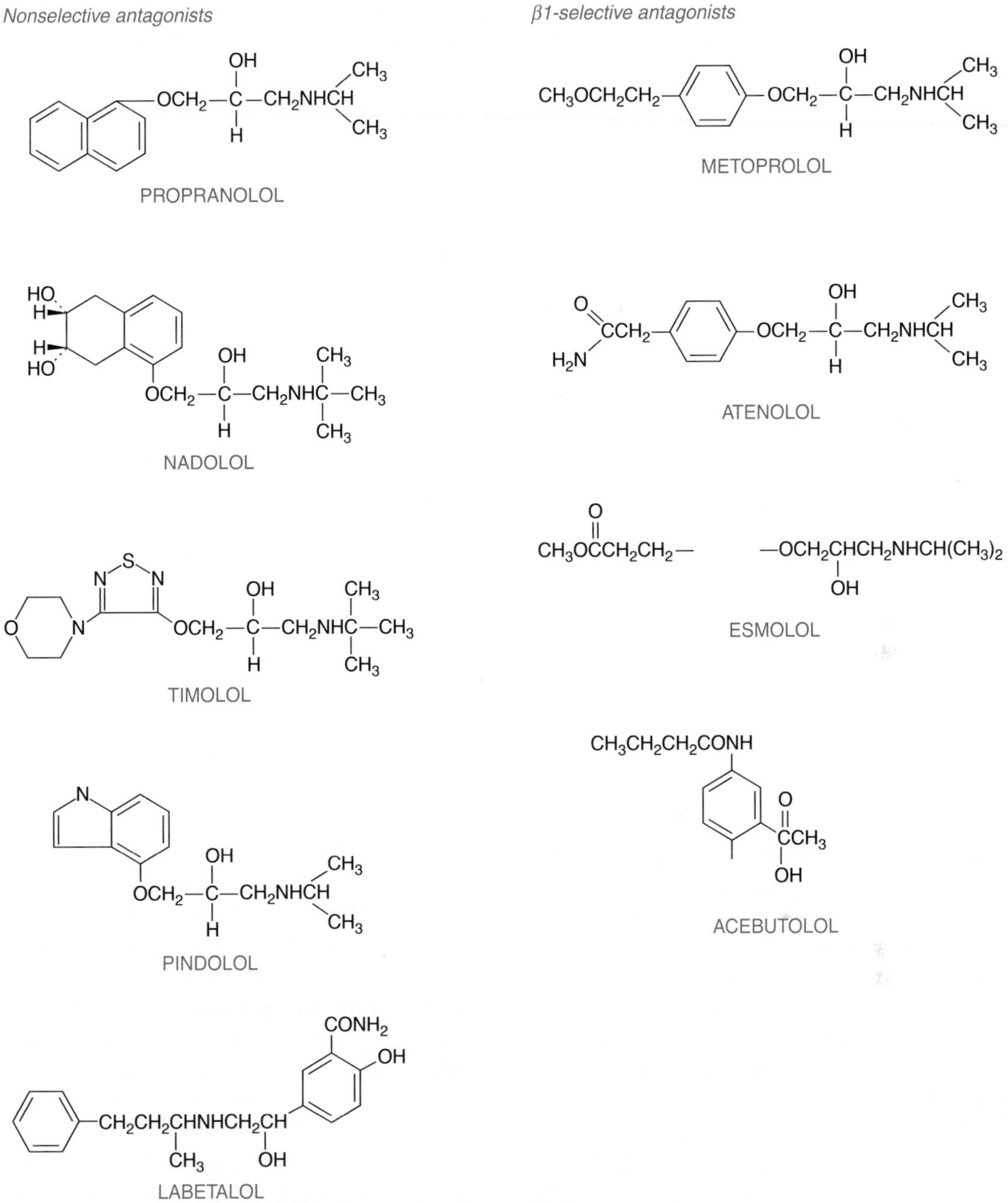

Nonselective antagonists

PROPRANOLOL

NADOLOL

TIMOLOL

PINDOLOL

LABETALOL

β1-selective antagonists

METOPROLOL

ATENOLOL

ESMOLOL

ACEBUTOLOL

Figure 12–7. *Structural formulas of some β adrenergic receptor antagonists.*

by the following properties: relative affinity for β_1 and β_2 receptors, intrinsic sympathomimetic activity, blockade of α receptors, differences in lipid solubility, capacity to induce vasodilation, and pharmacokinetic parameters. Some of these distinguishing characteristics have clinical significance and help guide the appropriate choice of a β receptor antagonist for an individual patient.

Propranolol has equal affinity for β_1 and β_2 adrenergic receptors; thus, it is a non-selective β adrenergic receptor antagonist. Agents such as metoprolol, atenolol, acebutolol, bisoprolol, and esmolol have somewhat greater affinity for β_1 than for β_2 receptors; these are examples of β_1-selective antagonists, even though the selectivity is not absolute. Propranolol is a pure antagonist, and it has no capacity to activate β receptors.

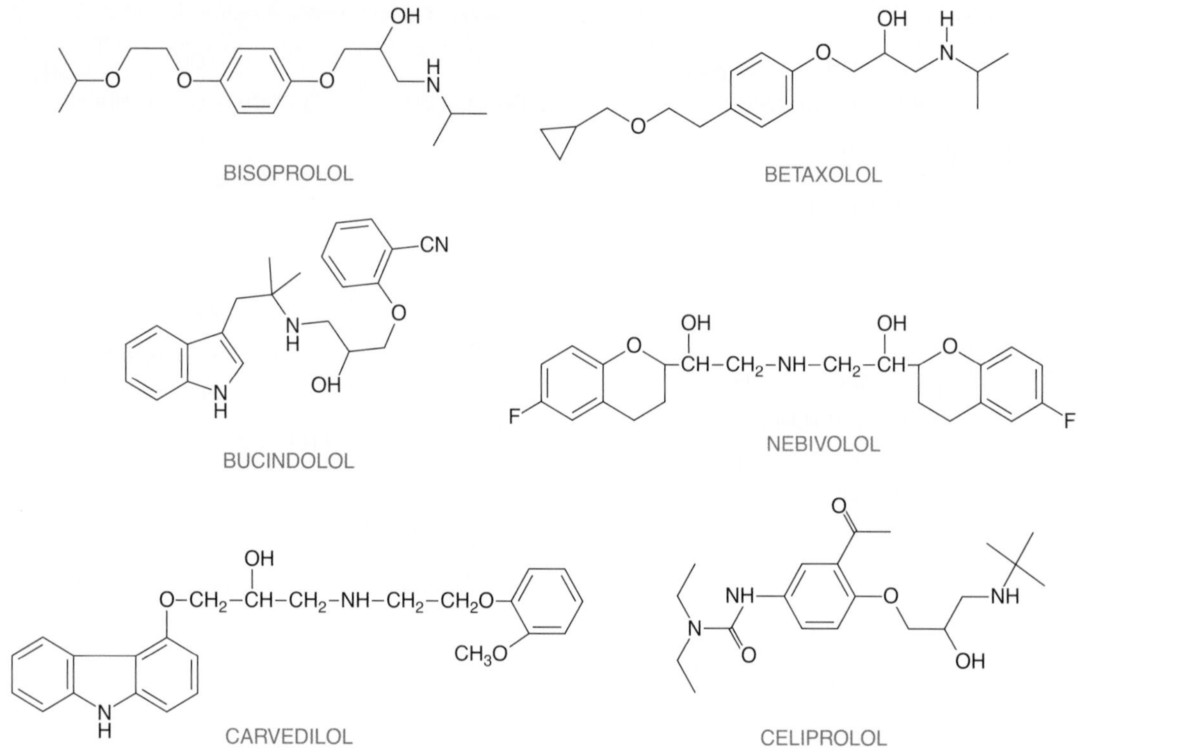

BISOPROLOL

BETAXOLOL

BUCINDOLOL

NEBIVOLOL

CARVEDILOL

CELIPROLOL

Figure 12–8. *Structural formulas of some "third-generation" β adrenergic receptor antagonists with additional cardiovascular effects.*

Several β blockers (e.g., pindolol and acebutolol) activate β receptors partially in the absence of catecholamines; however, the intrinsic activities of these drugs are less than that of a full agonist such as isoproterenol. These partial agonists are said to have intrinsic sympathomimetic activity. Substantial sympathomimetic activity would be counterproductive to the response desired from a β antagonist; however, slight residual activity may, e.g., prevent profound bradycardia or negative inotropy in a resting heart. The potential clinical advantage of this property, however, is unclear and may be disadvantageous in the context of secondary prevention of myocardial infarction (described under Therapeutic Uses). In addition, other β receptor antagonists have been found to have the property of inverse agonism (Chapter 3). These drugs can decrease basal activity of β receptor signaling by shifting the equilibrium of spontaneously active receptors toward the inactive state (Chidiac et al., 1994). Several β receptor antagonists also have local anesthetic or membrane-stabilizing activity, similar to lidocaine, that is independent of β blockade. Such drugs include propranolol, acebutolol, and carvedilol. Pindolol, metoprolol, betaxolol, and labetalol have slight membrane-stabilizing effects. Although most β receptor antagonists do not block α adrenergic receptors, labetalol, carvedilol, and bucindolol are examples of agents that block both α_1 and β adrenergic receptors. In addition to carvedilol, labetalol, and bucindolol, many other β receptor antagonists have vasodilating properties due to various mechanisms discussed below. These include celiprolol, nebivolol, nipradilol, carteolol, betaxolol, bopindolol, and bevantolol (Toda, 2003).

Pharmacological Properties

As in the case of α receptor blocking agents, the pharmacological properties of α receptor antagonists can be explained largely from knowledge of the responses elicited by the receptors in the various tissues and the activity of the sympathetic nerves that innervate these tissues (Table 8–1). For example, β receptor blockade has relatively little effect on the normal heart of an individual at rest, but has profound effects when sympathetic control of the heart is dominant, as during exercise or stress.

In this chapter, β adrenergic receptor antagonists are classified as non–subtype-selective ("first generation"), β_1-selective ("second generation"), and non–subtype or subtype-selective *with additional cardiovascular actions* ("third generation"). These latter drugs have additional cardiovascular properties (especially vasodilation) that seem unrelated to β blockade. Table 12–3 summarizes important pharmacological and pharmacokinetic properties of β receptor antagonists.

Cardiovascular System. The major therapeutic effects of β receptor antagonists are on the cardiovascular system. It is important to distinguish these effects in normal subjects from those in subjects with cardiovascular disease such as hypertension or myocardial ischemia.

Since catecholamines have positive chronotropic and inotropic actions, β receptor antagonists slow the heart rate and decrease myocardial contractility. When tonic stimulation of β receptors is low, this effect is correspondingly modest. However, when the sympathetic nervous system is activated, as during exercise or stress, β receptor antagonists attenuate the expected rise in heart rate. Short-term administration of β receptor antagonists such as propranolol decreases cardiac output; peripheral resistance increases in proportion to maintain blood pressure as a result of blockade of vascular β_2 receptors and compensatory reflexes, such as increased sympathetic nervous system activity, leading to activation of vascular α receptors. However, with long-term use of β antagonists, total peripheral resistance returns to initial values (Mimran and Ducailar, 1988) or decreases in patients with hypertension (Man in't Veld et al., 1988). With β antagonists that also are α_1 receptor antagonists, such as labetalol, carvedilol, and bucindolol, cardiac output is maintained with a greater fall in peripheral resistance. This also is seen with β receptor antagonists that are direct vasodilators.

β Receptor antagonists have significant effects on cardiac rhythm and automaticity. Although it had been thought that these effects were due exclusively to blockade of β_1 receptors, β_2 receptors likely also regulate heart rate in humans (Altschuld and

Table 12–3

Pharmacological/Pharmacokinetic Properties of β Adrenergic Receptor Blocking Agents

DRUG	MEMBRANE STABILIZING ACTIVITY	INTRINSIC AGONIST ACTIVITY	LIPID SOLUBILITY	EXTENT OF ABSORPTION (%)	ORAL AVAI-LABILITY (%)	PLASMA $t_{1/2}$(HOURS)	PROTEIN BINDING (%)
Classical non-selective β blockers: First generation							
Nadolol	0	0	Low	30	30-50	20-24	30
Penbutolol	0	+	High	~100	~100	~5	80-98
Pindolol	+	+++	Low	>95	~100	3-4	40
Propranolol	++	0	High	<90	30	3-5	90
Timolol	0	0	Low to moderate	90	75	4	<10
β_1-Selective β blockers: Second generation							
Acebutolol	+	+	Low	90	20-60	3-4	26
Atenolol	0	0	Low	90	50-60	6-7	6-16
Bisoprolol	0	0	Low	≤90	80	9-12	~30
Esmolol	0	0	Low	NA	NA	0.15	55
Metoprolol	+*	0	Moderate	~100	40-50	3-7	12
Non-selective β blockers with additional actions: Third generation							
Carteolol	0	++	Low	85	85	6	23-30
Carvedilol	++	0	Moderate	>90	~30	7-10	98
Labetalol	+	+	Low	>90	~33	3-4	~50
β_1-selective β blockers with additional actions: Third generation							
Betaxolol	+	0	Moderate	>90	~80	15	50
Celiprolol	0	+	Low	~74	30-70	5	4-5
Nebivolol	0	0	Low	NA	NA	11-30	

*Detectable only at doses much greater than required for β blockade.

Billman, 2000; Brodde and Michel, 1999). β_3 Receptors also have been identified in normal myocardial tissue in several species, including humans (Moniotte et al., 2001). Signal transduction for β_3 receptors is complex and includes G_s but also G_i/G_o; stimulation of cardiac β_3 receptors inhibits cardiac contraction and relaxation. The physiological role of β_3 receptors in the heart remains to be established (Morimoto et al., 2004). β Receptor antagonists reduce sinus rate, decrease the spontaneous rate of depolarization of ectopic pacemakers, slow conduction in the atria and in the AV node, and increase the functional refractory period of the AV node.

Although high concentrations of many β blockers produce quinidine-like effects (membrane-stabilizing activity), it is doubtful that this is significant at usual doses of these agents. However, this effect may be important when there is overdosage. Interestingly, *d*-propranolol may suppress ventricular arrhythmias independently of β receptor blockade.

The cardiovascular effects of β receptor antagonists are most evident during dynamic exercise. In the presence of β receptor blockade, exercise-induced increases in heart rate and myocardial contractility are attenuated. However, the exercise-induced increase in cardiac output is less affected because of an increase in stroke volume. The effects of β receptor antagonists on exercise are somewhat analogous to the changes that occur with normal aging. In healthy elderly persons, catecholamine-induced increases in heart rate are smaller than in younger individuals; however, the increase in cardiac output in older people may be preserved because of an increase in stroke volume during exercise. β Blockers tend to decrease work capacity, as assessed by their effects on intense short-term or more prolonged steady-state exertion. Exercise performance may be impaired to a lesser extent by β_1-selective agents than by non-selective antagonists. Blockade of β_2 receptors tends to blunt the increase in blood flow to active skeletal muscle during submaximal exercise. Blockade of β receptors also may attenuate catecholamine-induced activation of glucose metabolism and lipolysis.

Coronary artery blood flow increases during exercise or stress to meet the metabolic demands of the heart. By increasing heart rate, contractility, and systolic pressure, catecholamines increase myocardial oxygen demand. However, in patients with coronary artery disease, fixed narrowing of these vessels attenuates the expected increase in flow, leading to myocardial ischemia. β Receptor antagonists decrease the effects of catecholamines on the determinants of myocardial O_2 consumption. However, these agents may tend to increase the requirement for oxygen by increasing end-diastolic pressure and systolic ejection period. Usually, the net effect is to improve the relationship between cardiac O_2 supply and demand; exercise tolerance generally is improved in patients with angina, whose capacity to exercise is limited by the development of chest pain (Chapter 28).

Activity as Antihypertensive Agents. β Receptor antagonists generally do not reduce blood pressure in patients with normal blood pressure. However, these drugs lower blood pressure in patients with hypertension. Despite their widespread use, the mechanisms responsible for this important clinical effect are not well understood. The release of renin from the juxtaglomerular apparatus is stimulated by the sympathetic nervous system by means of β_1 receptors, and this effect is blocked by β receptor antagonists (Chapter 25). However, the relationship between this phenomenon and the fall in blood pressure is not clear. Some investigators have found that the antihypertensive effect of propranolol is most marked in patients with elevated concentrations of plasma renin, as compared with patients with low or normal concentrations of renin. However, β receptor antagonists are effective even in patients with low plasma renin, and pindolol is an effective antihypertensive agent that has little or no effect on plasma renin activity.

Presynaptic β receptors enhance the release of NE from sympathetic neurons, but the importance of diminished release of NE to the antihypertensive effects of β antagonists is unclear. Although β blockers would not be expected to decrease the contractility of vascular smooth muscle, long-term administration of these drugs to hypertensive patients ultimately leads to a fall in peripheral vascular resistance (Man in't Veld *et al.*, 1988). The mechanism for this important effect is not known, but this delayed fall in peripheral vascular resistance in the face of a persistent reduction of cardiac output appears to account for much of the antihypertensive effect of these drugs. Although it has been hypothesized that central actions of β blockers also may contribute to their antihypertensive effects, there is relatively little evidence to support this possibility, and drugs that poorly penetrate the blood-brain barrier are effective antihypertensive agents.

As indicated, some β receptor antagonists have additional effects that may contribute to their capacity to lower blood pressure. These drugs all produce peripheral vasodilation; at least six properties have been proposed to contribute to this effect, including production of nitric oxide, activation of β_2 receptors, blockade of α_1 receptors, blockade of Ca^{2+} entry, opening of K^+ channels, and antioxidant activity. The ability of vasodilating β receptor antagonists to act through one or more of these mechanisms is depicted in Table 12–4 and Figure 12–9. These mechanisms appear to contribute to the antihypertensive effects by enhancing hypotension, increasing peripheral blood flow, and decreasing afterload. Two of these agents (e.g., celiprolol and nebivolol) also have been observed to produce vasodilation and thereby reduce preload.

Although further clinical trials are needed, these agents may be associated with a lower incidence of bronchospasm, impaired lipid metabolism, impotence, reduced regional blood flow, increased vascular resistance, and withdrawal symptoms. A lower incidence of these adverse effects would be particularly beneficial in patients who have insulin resistance and diabetes mellitus in addition to hypertension (Toda, 2003). The clinical significance in humans of some of these relatively subtle differences in pharmacological properties still is unclear. Particular interest has focused on patients with congestive heart failure or peripheral arterial occlusive disease.

Propranolol and other non-selective β receptor antagonists inhibit the vasodilation caused by isoproterenol and augment the pressor response to epinephrine. This is particularly significant in patients with pheochromocytoma, in whom β receptor antagonists should be used only after adequate α receptor blockade has been

Table 12–4

Third Generation β Receptor Antagonists with Putative Additional Mechanisms of Vasodilation

NITRIC OXIDE PRODUCTION	β_2 RECEPTOR AGONISM	α_1 RECEPTOR ANTAGONISM	Ca^{2+} ENTRY BLOCKADE	K^+ CHANNEL OPENING	ANTIOXIDANT ACTIVITY
Celiprolol[a]	Celiprolol[a]	Carvedilol	Carvedilol	Tilisolol[a]	Carvedilol
Nebivolol	Carteolol	Bucindolol[a]	Betaxolol		
Carteolol	Bopindolol[a]	Bevantolol[a]	Bevantolol[a]		
Bopindolol[a]		Nipradilol[a]			
Nipradilol[a]		Labetalol			

[a]Not currently available in the U.S., where most are under investigation for use.

established. This avoids uncompensated α receptor–mediated vasoconstriction caused by epinephrine secreted from the tumor.

Pulmonary System. Non-selective β receptor antagonists such as propranolol block β_2 receptors in bronchial smooth muscle. This usually has little effect on pulmonary function in normal individuals. However, in patients with COPD, such blockade can lead to life-threatening bronchoconstriction. Although β_1-selective antagonists or antagonists with intrinsic sympathomimetic activity are less likely than propranolol to increase airway resistance in patients with asthma, these drugs should be used only with great caution, if at all, in patients with bronchospastic diseases. Drugs such as celiprolol, with β_1 receptor selectivity and β_2 receptor partial agonism, are of potential promise, although clinical experience is limited.

Metabolic Effects. β Receptor antagonists modify the metabolism of carbohydrates and lipids. Catecholamines promote glycogenolysis and mobilize glucose in response to hypoglycemia. Non-selective β blockers may delay recovery from hypoglycemia in type 1 (insulin-dependent) diabetes mellitus, but infrequently in type 2 diabetes mellitus. In addition to blocking glycogenolysis, β receptor antagonists can interfere with the counter-regulatory effects of catecholamines secreted during hypoglycemia by blunting the perception of symptoms such as tremor, tachycardia, and nervousness. Thus, β adrenergic receptor antagonists should be used with great caution in patients with labile diabetes and frequent hypoglycemic reactions. If such a drug is indicated, a β_1-selective antagonist is preferred, since these drugs are less likely to delay recovery from hypoglycemia (DiBari et al., 2003).

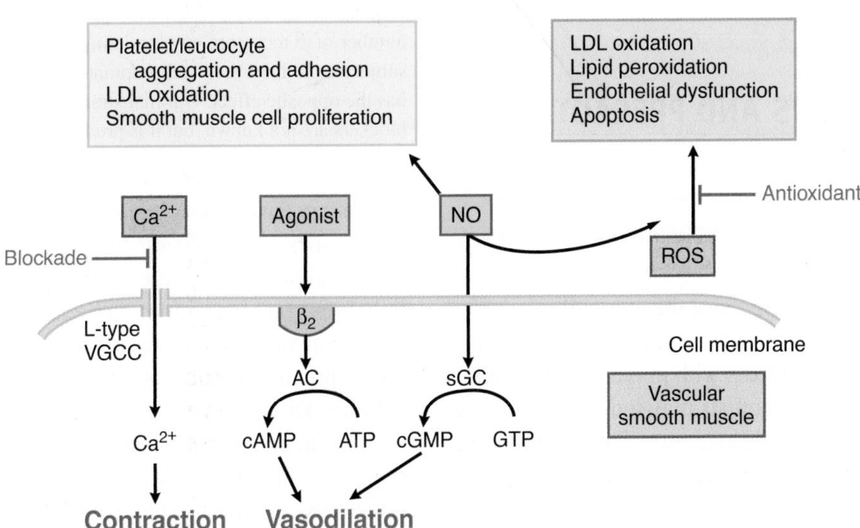

Figure 12–9. *Mechanisms underlying actions of vasodilating β blockers in blood vessels.* ROS, reactive oxygen species; sGC, soluble guanylyl cyclase; AC adenylyl cyclase; L-type VGCC, L-type voltage gated Ca^{2+} channel.) (Modified with permission from Toda, 2003. Copyright © Elsevier.)

The β receptors mediate activation of hormone-sensitive lipase in fat cells, leading to release of free fatty acids into the circulation (Chapter 8). This increased flux of fatty acids is an important source of energy for exercising muscle. β Receptor antagonists can attenuate the release of free fatty acids from adipose tissue. Non-selective β receptor antagonists consistently reduce HDL cholesterol, increase LDL cholesterol, and increase triglycerides. In contrast, β_1-selective antagonists, including celiprolol, carteolol, nebivolol, carvedilol, and bevantolol, reportedly improve the serum lipid profile of dyslipidemic patients. While drugs such as propranolol and atenolol increase triglycerides, plasma triglycerides are reduced with chronic celiprolol, carvedilol, and carteolol (Toda, 2003).

In contrast to classical β blockers, which decrease insulin sensitivity, the vasodilating β receptor antagonists (e.g., celiprolol, nipradilol, carteolol, carvedilol, and dilevalol) increase insulin sensitivity in patients with insulin resistance. Together with their cardioprotective effects, improvement in insulin sensitivity from vasodilating β receptor antagonists may partially counterbalance the hazard from worsened lipid abnormalities associated with diabetes. If β blockers are to be used, β_1-selective or vasodilating β receptor antagonists are preferred. In addition, it may be necessary to use β receptor antagonists in conjunction with other drugs, (e.g., HMGCoA reductase inhibitors) to ameliorate adverse metabolic effects (Dunne et al., 2001).

β Receptor agonists decrease the plasma concentration of K^+ by promoting the uptake of the ion, predominantly into skeletal muscle. At rest, an infusion of epinephrine causes a decrease in the plasma concentration of K^+. The marked increase in the concentration of epinephrine that occurs with stress (such as myocardial infarction) may cause hypokalemia, which could predispose to cardiac arrhythmias. The hypokalemic effect of epinephrine is blocked by an experimental antagonist, ICI 118551, which has a high affinity for β_2 and β_3 receptors. Exercise causes an increase in the efflux of K^+ from skeletal muscle. Catecholamines tend to buffer the rise in K^+ by increasing its influx into muscle. β Blockers negate this buffering effect.

Other Effects. β Receptor antagonists block catecholamine-induced tremor. They also block inhibition of mast-cell degranulation by catecholamines.

ADVERSE EFFECTS AND PRECAUTIONS

The most common adverse effects of β receptor antagonists arise as pharmacological consequences of blockade of β receptors; serious adverse effects unrelated to β receptor blockade are rare.

Cardiovascular System. Because the sympathetic nervous system provides critical support for cardiac performance in many individuals with impaired myocardial function, β receptor antagonists may induce congestive heart failure in susceptible patients. Thus, β receptor blockade may cause or exacerbate heart failure in patients with compensated heart failure, acute myocardial infarction, or cardiomegaly. It is not known whether β receptor antagonists that possess intrinsic sympathomimetic activity or peripheral vasodilating properties are safer in these settings. Nonetheless, there is convincing evidence that chronic administration of β receptor antagonists is efficacious in prolonging life in the therapy of heart failure in selected patients (discussed later in this chapter and in Chapter 28).

Bradycardia is a normal response to β receptor blockade; however, in patients with partial or complete AV conduction defects, β antagonists may cause life-threatening bradyarrhythmias. Particular caution is indicated in patients who are taking other drugs, such as verapamil or various anti-arrhythmic agents, which may impair sinus-node function or AV conduction.

Some patients complain of cold extremities while taking β receptor antagonists. Symptoms of peripheral vascular disease may worsen, although this is uncommon, or Raynaud's phenomenon may develop. The risk of worsening intermittent claudication probably is very small with this class of drugs, and the clinical benefits of β antagonists in patients with peripheral vascular disease and coexisting coronary artery disease may be very important.

Abrupt discontinuation of β receptor antagonists after long-term treatment can exacerbate angina and may increase the risk of sudden death. The underlying mechanism is unclear, but it is well established that there is enhanced sensitivity to β receptor agonists in patients who have undergone long-term treatment with certain β receptor antagonists after the blocker is withdrawn abruptly. For example, chronotropic responses to isoproterenol are blunted in patients who are receiving β receptor antagonists; however, abrupt discontinuation of propranolol leads to greater-than-normal sensitivity to isoproterenol. This increased sensitivity is evident several days after stopping propranolol and may persist for at least 1 week. Such enhanced sensitivity can be attenuated by tapering the dose of the β blocker for several weeks before discontinuation. Supersensitivity to isoproterenol also has been observed after abrupt discontinuation of metoprolol, but not of pindolol. This enhanced β responsiveness may result from up-regulation of β receptors. The number of β receptors on circulating lymphocytes is increased in subjects who have received propranolol for long periods; pindolol has the opposite effect. Optimal strategies for discontinuation of β blockers are not known, but it is prudent to decrease the dose gradually and to restrict exercise during this period.

Pulmonary Function. A major adverse effect of β receptor antagonists is caused by blockade of β_2 receptors in bronchial smooth muscle. These receptors are particularly important for promoting bronchodilation in patients with bronchospastic disease, and β blockers may cause a life-threatening increase in airway resistance in such patients. Drugs with selectivity for β_1 receptors or those with intrinsic sympathomimetic activity at β_2 receptors seem less likely to induce bronchospasm. Since the selectivity of current β blockers for β_1 receptors is modest, these drugs should be avoided if at all possible in patients with asthma. However, in selected patients with chronic obstructive pulmonary disease and cardiovascular disease (hypertension, heart failure, coronary artery disease), the advantages of using β_1 receptor antagonists may outweigh the risk of worsening pulmonary function (Salpeter et al., 2005).

CNS. The adverse effects of β receptor antagonists that are referable to the CNS may include fatigue, sleep disturbances (including insomnia and nightmares), and depression. The previously ascribed association between these drugs and depression is unclear (Gerstman et al., 1996; Ried et al., 1998). Interest has focused on the relationship between the incidence of the adverse effects of β receptor antagonists and their lipophilicity; however, no clear correlation has emerged.

Metabolism. As already described, β adrenergic blockade may blunt recognition of hypoglycemia by patients; it also may delay recovery from insulin-induced hypoglycemia. β Receptor antagonists should be used with great caution in patients with diabetes who are prone to hypoglycemic reactions; β_1-selective agents may be preferable for these patients. The benefits of β receptor antagonists in type 1 diabetes with myocardial infarction may outweigh the risk in selected patients (Gottlieb et al., 1998).

Miscellaneous. The incidence of sexual dysfunction in men with hypertension who are treated with β receptor antagonists is not clearly defined. Although experience with the use of β adrenergic receptor antagonists in pregnancy is increasing, information about the safety of these drugs during pregnancy still is limited.

Overdosage. The manifestations of poisoning with β receptor antagonists depend on the pharmacological properties of the ingested drug, particularly its β_1 selectivity, intrinsic sympathomimetic activity, and membrane-stabilizing properties. Hypotension, bradycardia, prolonged AV conduction times, and widened QRS complexes are common manifestations of overdosage. Seizures and depression may occur. Hypoglycemia and bronchospasm can occur. Significant bradycardia should be treated initially with atropine, but a cardiac pacemaker often is required. Large doses of isoproterenol or an α receptor agonist may be necessary to treat hypotension. Glucagon, acting through its own GPCR and independently of the β adrenergic receptor, has positive chronotropic and inotropic effects on the heart, and the drug has been useful in some patients suffering from an overdose of a β receptor antagoinst.

Drug Interactions. Both pharmacokinetic and pharmacodynamic interactions have been noted between β receptor antagonists and other drugs. Interactions with sympathomimetics, α blockers, and β agonists are predictable from the pharmacology. Aluminum salts, cholestyramine, and colestipol may decrease the absorption of β blockers. Drugs such as phenytoin, rifampin, and phenobarbital, as well as smoking, induce hepatic biotransformation enzymes and may decrease plasma concentrations of β receptor antagonists that are metabolized extensively (e.g., propranolol). Cimetidine and hydralazine may increase the bioavailability of agents such as propranolol and metoprolol by affecting hepatic blood flow. β Receptor antagonists can impair the clearance of lidocaine.

Other drug interactions have pharmacodynamic explanations. For example, β antagonists and Ca^{2+} channel blockers have additive effects on the cardiac conducting system. Additive effects on blood pressure between β blockers and other antihypertensive agents often are employed to clinical advantage. However, the antihypertensive effects of β receptor antagonists can be opposed by indomethacin and other nonsteroidal anti-inflammatory drugs (Chapter 34).

THERAPEUTIC USES

Cardiovascular Diseases

β Receptor antagonists are used extensively in the treatment of hypertension, angina and acute coronary syndromes, and congestive heart failure (Chapters 27 and 28). These drugs also are used frequently in the treatment of supraventricular and ventricular arrhythmias (Chapter 29).

Myocardial Infarction. A great deal of interest has focused on the use of β receptor antagonists in the treatment of acute myocardial infarction and in the prevention of recurrences for those who have survived an initial attack. Numerous trials have shown that β receptor antagonists administered during the early phases of acute myocardial infarction and continued long-term may decrease mortality by ~25% (Freemantle et al., 1999). The precise mechanism is not known, but the favorable effects of β receptor antagonists may stem from decreased myocardial oxygen demand, redistribution of myocardial blood flow, and anti-arrhythmic actions. There is likely much less benefit if β adrenergic receptor antagonists are administered for only a short time. In studies of secondary prevention, the most extensive, favorable clinical trial data are available for propranolol, metoprolol, and timolol. In spite of these proven benefits, many patients with myocardial infarction do not receive a β adrenergic receptor antagonist.

Congestive Heart Failure. It is a common clinical observation that acute administration of β receptor antagonists can worsen markedly or even precipitate congestive heart failure in compensated patients with multiple forms of heart disease, such as ischemic or congestive cardiomyopathy. Consequently, the hypothesis that β receptor antagonists might be efficacious in the long-term treatment of heart failure originally seemed counterintuitive to many physicians. However, the reflex sympathetic responses to heart failure may stress the failing heart and exacerbate the progression of the disease, and blocking those responses could be beneficial. A number of well-designed randomized clinical trials involving numerous patients have demonstrated that certain β receptor antagonists are highly effective

Table 12–5

Summary of Adrenergic Agonists and Antagonists (continued)

CLASS	DRUGS	PROMINENT PHARMACOLOGICAL ACTIONS	PRINCIPAL THERAPEUTIC APPLICATIONS	UNTOWARD EFFECTS	COMMENTS
β_2-selective (intermediate acting)	Albuterol Bitolterol Fenoterol Isoetharine Levalbuterol Metaproterenol Pirbuterol Procaterol Terbutaline	Relaxation of bronchial smooth muscle Relaxation of uterine smooth muscle Activation of other β_2 receptors after systemic administration	Bronchodilators for treatment of asthma and COPD Short/intermediate-acting drugs for acute bronchospasm	Skeletal muscle tremor Tachycardia and other cardiac effects seen after systemic administration (much less with inhalational use)	Use with caution in patients with CV disease (reduced by inhalational administration) Minimal side effects
(Long acting)	Formoterol Salmeterol Arformoterol Carniterol Indacaterol Ritodrine		Best choice for prophylaxis due to long action Ritodrine, to stop premature labor		Long action favored for prophylaxis
α Receptor agonists					
α_1-selective	Methoxamine Phenylephrine Mephentermine Metaraminol Midodrine	Vasoconstriction	Nasal congestion (used topically) Postural hypotension	Hypertension Reflex bradycardia Dry mouth, sedation, rebound hypertension upon abrupt withdrawal	Mephentermine and metaraminol also act indirectly to release NE Midodrine, a prodrug activated *in vivo*
α_2-selective	Clonidine Apraclonidine Guanfacine Guanabenz Brimonidine α-methyldopa	↓ sympathetic outflow from brain to periphery resulting in ↓ PVR and blood pressure ↓ nerve-evoked release of sympathetic transmitters ↓ production of aqueous humor	Adjunctive therapy in shock Hypertension To reduce sympathetic response to withdrawal from narcotics, alcohol, and tobacco Glaucoma		Apraclonidine and brimonidine used topically for glaucoma and ocular hypertension Methyldopa is converted in CNS to α-methyl NE, an effective α_2 agonist

Indirect-acting	Amphetamine Methamphetamine Methyphenidate (releases NE peripherally; NE, DA, 5-HT centrally)	CNS stimulation ↑ blood pressure Myocardial stimulation	Treatment of ADHD Narcolepsy Obesity (rarely)	Restlessness Tremor Insomnia Anxiety Tachycardia Hypertension Cardiac arrhythmias	Schedule II drugs Marked tolerance occurs Chronic use leads to dependence Can result in hemorrhagic stroke in patients with underlying disease Long-term use can cause paranoid schizophrenia
Mixed-acting	Dopamine (α_1; α_2, β_1, D_1; releases NE)	Vasodilation (coronary, renal mesenteric beds) ↑ GFR and natriuresis ↑ heart rate and contractility ↑ systolic blood pressure	Cardiogenic shock Congestive heart failure Treatment of acute renal failure	High doses lead to vasoconstriction	Important for its ability to maintain renal blood flow Administered IV
	Ephedrine (α_1, α_2, β_1, β_2; releases NE)	Similar to epinephrine but longer lasting CNS stimulation	Bronchodilator for treatment of asthma Nasal congestion Treatment of hypotension and shock	Restlessness Tremor Insomnia Anxiety Tachycardia Hypertension	Administered by all routes Not commonly used
α Blockers					
Non-selective (classical α blockers)	PBZ Phentolamine Tolazoline	↓ PVR and blood pressure Venodilation	Treatment of catecholamine excess (e.g., pheochromocytoma)	Postural hypotension Failure of ejaculation	Cardiac stimulation due to initiation of reflexes and to enhanced release of NE via α_2 receptor blockade.

(Continued)

Table 12–5

Summary of Adrenergic Agonists and Antagonists (continued)

CLASS	DRUGS	PROMINENT PHARMACOLOGICAL ACTIONS	PRINCIPAL THERAPEUTIC APPLICATIONS	UNTOWARD EFFECTS	COMMENTS
α-selective	Prazosin Terazosin Doxazosin Trimazosin Alfuzosin Tamsulosin Silodosin	↓ PVR and blood pressure Relax smooth muscles in neck of urinary bladder and in prostate	Primary hypertension Increase urine flow in BPH	Postural hypotension when therapy instituted	PBZ produces long-lasting α receptor blockade, can block neuronal and extraneuronal uptake of amines Prazosin and related quinazolines are selective for α_1 receptors Tamsulosin exhibits some selectivity for α_{1A} receptors
β Blockers					
Non-selective (first generation)	Nadolol Penbutolol Pindolol Propranolol Timolol	↓ heart rate ↓ contractility ↓ cardiac output Slow conduction in atria and AV node ↑ refractory period, AV node Bronchoconstriction Prolonged hypoglycemia ↓ plasma FFA ↓ HDL cholesterol ↑ LDL cholesterol and triglycerides Hypokalemia	Angina pectoris Hypertension Cardiac arrhythmias CHF Pheochromocytoma Glaucoma Hypertropic obstructive cardiomyopathy Hyperthyroidism Migraine prophylaxis Acute panic symptoms Substance abuse withdrawal Variceal bleeding in portal hypertension	Bradycardia Negative inotropy ↓ in cardiac output Bradyarrhythmias ↓ AV conduction Bronchoconstriction Fatigue Sleep disturbances (insomnia, nightmares) Prolongation of hypoglycemia Sexual dysfunction in men Drug interactions	Effects depend on sympatho-adrenal tone Bronchoconstriction (of concern in asthmatics and COPD) Hypoglycemia (of concern in hypoglycemics and diabetics) Membrane stabilizing effect (propranolol, and betaxolol) ISA (strong for pindolol; weak for penbutolol, carteolol, labetalol, and betaxolol)

β_1-selective (second generation)	Acebutolol Atenolol Bisoprolol Betaxolol Esmolol Metoprolol		
Non-selective (third generation) vasodilators	Carteolol Carvedilol Bucindolol Labetalol	(Membrane stabilizing effect) (ISA) (Vasodilation)	Vasodilation seen in 3rd generation drugs; multiple mechanisms (see Figure 12–9)
β_1-selective (third generation) vasodilators	Celiprolol Nebivolol		

ADHD, attention-deficit/hyperactivity disorder; AV, atrioventricular; BPH, benign prostatic hypertrophy; CAD, coronary artery disease; CHF, congestive heart failure; COPD, chronic obstructive pulmonary disease; CV, cardiovascular; DA, dopamine; D_1, subtype 1 dopamine receptor; Epi, epinephrine; FFA, free fatty acids; 5-HT, serotonin; GFR, glomerular filtration rate; ISA, intrinsic sympathomimetic activity; MI, myocardial infarction; NE, norepinephrine; NO, nitric oxide; PBZ, phenoxybenzamine; PVR, peripheral vascular resistance.

nadolol is its relatively long $t_{1/2}$. It can be used to treat hypertension and angina pectoris. Unlabeled uses have included migraine prophylaxis, parkinsonian tremors, and variceal bleeding in portal hypertension.

Absorption, Fate, and Excretion. Nadolol is very soluble in water and is incompletely absorbed from the gut; its bioavailability is ~35%. Interindividual variability is less than with propranolol. The low lipid solubility of nadolol may result in lower concentrations of the drug in the brain as compared with more lipid-soluble β receptor antagonists. Although it frequently has been suggested that the incidence of CNS adverse effects is lower with hydrophilic β receptor antagonists, data from controlled trials to support this contention are limited. Nadolol is not extensively metabolized and is largely excreted intact in the urine. The $t_{1/2}$ of the drug in plasma is ~20 hours; consequently, it generally is administered once daily. Nadolol may accumulate in patients with renal failure, and dosage should be reduced in such individuals.

Timolol

Timolol (BLOCADREN, others) is a potent, non-selective β receptor antagonist. It has no intrinsic sympathomimetic or membrane-stabilizing activity. It is used for hypertension, congestive heart failure, acute MI, andmigraine prophylaxis. In ophthalmology, timolol has been used in the treatment of open-angle glaucoma and intraocular hypertension. Its mechanism of action in treating open angle glaucoma is not precisely known; but the drug appears to reduce aqueous humour production through blockade of β receptors on the ciliary epithelium.

Absorption, Fate, and Excretion. Timolol is well absorbed from the GI tract. It is metabolized extensively by CYP2D6 in the liver and undergoes first-pass metabolism. Only a small amount of unchanged drug appears in the urine. The $t_{1/2}$ in plasma is ~4 hours. Interestingly, the ocular formulation of timolol (TIMOPTIC, others), used for the treatment of glaucoma, may be extensively absorbed systemically (Chapter 64); adverse effects can occur in susceptible patients, such as those with asthma or congestive heart failure. The systemic administration of cimetidine with topical ocular timolol increases the degree of β blockade, resulting in a reduction of resting heart rate, intraocular pressure, and exercise tolerance (Ishii et al., 2000). For ophthalmic use timolol is available combined with other medications (e.g., with dorzolamide or travoprost). Timolol also provide benefits to patients with coronary heart disease: in the acute post MI period, timolol produced a 39% reduction in mortality in the Norwegian Multicenter Study.

Pindolol

Pindolol (VISKEN, others) is a non-selective β receptor antagonist with intrinsic sympathomimetic activity. It has low membrane-stabilizing activity and low lipid solubility. It is used to treat angina pectoris and hypertension.

Although only limited data are available, β blockers with slight partial agonist activity may produce smaller reductions in resting heart rate and blood pressure. Hence, such drugs may be preferred as antihypertensive agents in individuals with diminished cardiac reserve or a propensity for bradycardia. Nonetheless, the clinical significance of partial agonism has not been substantially demonstrated in controlled trials but may be of importance in individual patients. Agents such as pindolol block exercise-induced increases in heart rate and cardiac output.

Absorption, Fate, and Excretion. Pindolol is almost completely absorbed after oral administration and has moderately high bioavailability. These properties tend to minimize interindividual variation in the plasma concentrations of the drug that are achieved after its oral administration. Approximately 50% of pindolol ultimately is metabolized in the liver. The principal metabolites are hydroxylated derivatives that subsequently are conjugated with either glucuronide or sulfate before renal excretion. The remainder of the drug is excreted unchanged in the urine. The plasma $t_{1/2}$ of pindolol is ~4 hours; clearance is reduced in patients with renal failure.

β_1 SELECTIVE ADRENERGIC RECEPTOR ANTAGONISTS

Metoprolol

Metoprolol (LOPRESSOR, others) is a β_1-selective receptor antagonist that is devoid of intrinsic sympathomimetic activity and membrane-stabilizing activity.

Absorption, Fate, and Excretion. Metoprolol is almost completely absorbed after oral administration, but bioavailability is relatively low (~40%) because of first-pass metabolism. Plasma concentrations of the drug vary widely (up to 17-fold), perhaps because of genetically determined differences in the rate of metabolism. Metoprolol is extensively metabolized in the liver, with CYP2D6 the major enzyme involved, and only 10% of the administered drug is recovered unchanged in the urine. The $t_{1/2}$ of metoprolol is 3-4 hours, but can increase to 7-8 hours in CYP2D6 poor metabolizers. It recently has been reported that CYP2D6 poor metabolizers have a 5-fold higher risk for developing adverse effects during metoprolol treatment than patients who are not poor metabolizers (Wuttke et al., 2002). An extended-release formulation (TOPROL XL) is available for once-daily administration.

Therapeutic Uses. Metoprolol has been used to treat essential hypertension, angina pectoris, tachycardia, heart failure, vasovagal syncope, and as secondary prevention after myocardial infarction, an adjunct in treatment of hyperthyroidism, and for migraine prophylaxis. For the treatment of hypertension, the usual initial dose is 100 mg/day. The drug sometimes is effective when given once daily, although it frequently is used in two divided doses. Dosage may be increased at weekly intervals until optimal reduction of blood pressure is achieved. If the drug is taken only once daily, it is important to confirm that blood pressure is controlled for the entire 24-hour period. Metoprolol generally is used in two divided doses for the treatment of stable angina. For the initial treatment of patients with acute myocardial infarction, an intravenous formulation of metoprolol tartrate is available. Oral dosing is initiated as soon as the clinical situation permits. Metoprolol generally is contraindicated for the treatment of acute myocardial infarction in patients with heart rates of < 45 beats per minute, heart block greater than first-degree (PR interval ≥ 0.24 second), systolic blood pressure <100 mm Hg, or moderate to severe heart failure. Metoprolol also has been proven to be effective in chronic heart failure. Its use is associated with a striking reduction in all-cause mortality and hospitalization for worsening heart failure and a modest reduction in all-cause hospitalization (MERIT-HF Study Group, 1999; Prakash and Markham, 2000).

Atenolol

Atenolol (TENORMIN, others) is a β_1-selective antagonist that is devoid of intrinsic sympathomimetic and membrane stabilizing activity. Atenolol is very hydrophilic and appears to penetrate the CNS only to a limited extent. Its $t_{1/2}$ is somewhat longer than that of metoprolol.

Absorption, Fate, and Excretion. Atenolol is incompletely absorbed (~50%), but most of the absorbed dose reaches the systemic circulation. There is relatively little interindividual variation in the plasma concentrations of atenolol; peak concentrations in different patients vary over only a 4-fold range. The drug is excreted largely unchanged in the urine, and the elimination $t_{1/2}$ is 5-8 hours. The drug accumulates in patients with renal failure, and dosage should be adjusted for patients whose creatinine clearance is < 35 mL/min.

Therapeutic Uses. Atenol can be used to treat hypertension, coronary heart disease, arrhythmias, and angina pectoris, and to treat or reduce the risk of heart complications following myocardial infarction. It is also used to treat Graves disease until anti-thyroid medication can take effect. The initial dose of atenolol for the treatment of hypertension usually is 50 mg/day, given once daily. If an adequate therapeutic response is not evident within several weeks, the daily dose may be increased to 100 mg; higher doses are unlikely to provide any greater antihypertensive effect. Atenolol has been shown to be efficacious, in combination with a diuretic, in elderly patients with isolated systolic hypertension. Atenolol causes fewer CNS side effects (depression, nightmares) than most β blockers and few bronchospatic reactions due to its pharmacological and pharmacokinetic profile (Varon, 2008).

Esmolol

Esmolol (BREVIBLOC, others) is a β_1-selective antagonist with a rapid onset and a very short duration of action. It has little if any intrinsic sympathomimetic activity and lacks membrane-stabilizing actions. Esmolol is administered intravenously and is used when β blockade of short duration is desired or in critically ill patients in whom adverse effects of bradycardia, heart failure, or hypotension may necessitate rapid withdrawal of the drug. It is a class II anti-arrhythmic agent (Chapter 29).

Absorption, Fate, and Excretion. Esmolol is given by slow IV injection and has a $t_{1/2}$ of ~8 minutes and an apparent volume of distribution of ~2 L/kg. The drug contains an ester linkage, and it is hydrolyzed rapidly by esterases in erythrocytes. The $t_{1/2}$ of the carboxylic acid metabolite of esmolol is far longer (4 hours), and it accumulates during prolonged infusion of esmolol. However, this metabolite has very low potency as a β receptor antagonist (1/500 of the potency of esmolol); it is excreted in the urine.

Esmolol is commonly used in patients during surgery to prevent or treat tachycardia and in the treatment of supraventricular tachycardia. The onset and cessation of β receptor blockade with esmolol are rapid; peak hemodynamic effects occur within 6-10 minutes of administration of a loading dose, and there is substantial attenuation of β blockade within 20 minutes of stopping an infusion. Esmolol may have striking hypotensive effects in normal subjects, although the mechanism of this effect is unclear.

Because esmolol is used in urgent settings where immediate onset of β blockade is warranted, a partial loading dose typically is administered, followed by a continuous infusion of the drug. If an adequate therapeutic effect is not observed within 5 minutes, the same loading dose is repeated, followed by a maintenance infusion at a higher rate. This process, including progressively greater infusion rates, may need to be repeated until the desired end point (e.g., lowered heart rate or blood pressure) is approached. Esmolol is particularly useful in severe postoperative hypertension and is a suitable agent in situations where cardiac output, heart rate, and blood pressure are increased. The American Heart Association/American College of Cardiology guidelines recommend against using esmolol in patients already on β blocker therapy, bradycardiac patients, and decompensated heart failure patients, as the drug may compromise their myocardial function (Varon, 2008).

Acebutolol

Acebutolol (SECTRAL, others) is a β_1-selective antagonist with some intrinsic sympathomimetic and membrane-stabilizing activity.

Absorption, Fate, and Excretion. Acebutolol is well absorbed, and undergoes significant first-pass metabolism to an active metabolite, diacetolol, which accounts for most of the drug's activity. Overall bioavailability is 35-50%. The elimination $t_{1/2}$ of acebutolol typically is ~3 hours, but the $t_{1/2}$ of diacetolol is 8-12 hours; it is excreted largely in the urine. Acebutolol has lipophilic properties and crosses the blood-brain barrier. It has no negative impact on serum lipids (cholesterol, triglycerides, or HDL).

Therapeutic Uses. Acebutol has been used to treat hypertension, ventricular and atrial cardiac arrhythmias, acute myocardial infarction in high-risk patients, and Smith-Magenis syndrome. The initial dose of acebutolol in hypertension usually is 400 mg/day; it may be given as a single dose, but two divided doses may be required for adequate control of blood pressure. Optimal responses usually occur with doses of 400-800 mg per day (range, 200-1200 mg).

Bisoprolol

Bisoprolol (ZEBETA) is a highly selective β_1 receptor antagonist that does not have intrinsic sympathomimetic or membrane-stabilizing activity (McGavin and Keating, 2002). It has a higher degree of β_1-selective activity than atenolol, metoprolol, or betaxolol but less than nebivolol. It is approved for the treatment of hypertension and has been investigated in randomized, double-blind multicenter trials in combination with ACE inhibitors and diuretics in patients with moderate to severe chronic heart failure (Simon et al., 2003). All-case mortality was significantly lower with bisoprolol than placebo.

Bisoprolol generally is well tolerated; side effects include dizziness, bradycardia, hypotension, and fatigue. Bisoprolol is well absorbed following oral administration, with bioavailability of ~90%. It is eliminated by renal excretion (50%) and liver metabolism to pharmacologically inactive metabolites (50%). Bisoprolol has a plasma $t_{1/2}$ of 11-17 hours. Bisoprolol can be considered a standard treatment option when selecting a β blocker for use in combination with ACE inhibitors and diuretics in patients with stable, moderate to severe chronic heart failure and in treating hypertension (McGavin and Keating, 2002; Simon et al., 2003). It has also been used to treat arrhythmias and ischemic heart disease. Bisoprolol was associated with a 34% mortality benefit in the Cardiac Insufficiency Bisoprolol Study-II (CIBIS-II).

Betaxolol

Betaxolol (BETOPTIC, LOKREN, KERLONE, others) is a selective β_1 receptor antagonist with no partial agonist activity and slight membrane-stabilizing properties.

Absorption, Fate, and Excretion. Betaxolol is well absorbed with high bioavailability and an elimination $t_{1/2}$ of 14-22 hours.

Therapeutic Uses. Betaxolol is used to treat hypertension, angina pectoris, and glaucoma. It is usually well tolerated and side effects are mild and transient. In glaucoma it reduces intraocular pressure by reducing the production of aqueous humor in the eye.

β RECEPTOR ANTAGONISTS WITH ADDITIONAL CARDIOVASCULAR EFFECTS ("THIRD GENERATION" β BLOCKERS)

In addition to the classical non-selective and β_1-selective adrenergic-receptor antagonists, there is also a series of drugs that possess vasodilatory actions. These effects are produced through a variety of mechanisms including α_1 adrenergic receptor blockade (labetalol, carvedilol, bucindolol, bevantolol, nipradilol), increased production of NO (celiprolol, nebivolol, carteolol, bopindolol, nipradolol), β_2 agonist properties (celiprolol, carteolol, bopindolol), Ca^{2+} entry blockade (carvedilol, betaxolol, bevantolol), opening of K^+ channels (tilisolol), or antioxidant action (carvedilol) (Toda, 2003). These actions are summarized in Table 12–4 and Figure 12–9. Many third-generation β receptor antagonists are not yet available in the U.S. but have undergone clinical trials and are on the market in other countries.

Labetalol

Labetalol (NORMODYNE, TRANDATE, others) is representative of a class of drugs that act as competitive antagonists at both α_1 and β receptors. Labetalol has two optical centers, and the formulation used clinically contains equal amounts of the four diastereomers. The pharmacological properties of the drug are complex, because each isomer displays different relative activities. The properties of the mixture include selective blockade of α_1 receptors (as compared with the α_2 subtype), blockade of β_1 and β_2 receptors, partial agonist activity at β_2 receptors, and inhibition of neuronal uptake of NE (cocaine-like effect) (Chapter 8). The potency of the mixture for β receptor blockade is 5-10 fold that for α_1 receptor blockade.

The pharmacological effects of labetalol have become clearer since the four isomers were separated and tested individually. The *R,R* isomer is about four times more potent as a β receptor antagonist than is racemic labetalol and accounts for much of the β blockade produced by the mixture of isomers; it no longer is in development as a separate drug (dilevalol). As an α_1 antagonist, this isomer is < 20% as potent as the racemic mixture. The *R,S* isomer is almost devoid of both α and β blocking effects. The *S,R* isomer has almost no β blocking activity, yet is about five times more potent as an α_1 blocker than is racemic labetalol. The *S,S* isomer is devoid of β blocking activity and has a potency similar to that of racemic labetalol as an α_1 receptor antagonist. The *R,R* isomer has some intrinsic sympathomimetic activity at β_2 adrenergic receptors; this may contribute to vasodilation. Labetalol also may have some direct vasodilating capacity.

The actions of labetalol on both α_1 and β receptors contribute to the fall in blood pressure observed in patients with hypertension. α_1 Receptor blockade leads to relaxation of arterial smooth muscle and vasodilation, particularly in the upright position. The β_1 blockade also contributes to a fall in blood pressure, in part by blocking reflex sympathetic stimulation of the heart. In addition, the intrinsic sympathomimetic activity of labetalol at β_2 receptors may contribute to vasodilation.

Labetalol is available in oral form for therapy of chronic hypertension and as an intravenous formulation for use in hypertensive emergencies. Labetalol has been associated with hepatic injury in a limited number of patients. Labetalol is one of the few β adrenergic antagonists that has been recommended as treatment for acute severe hypertension (hypertensive emergency). Its hypotensive action begins within 2-5 minutes after IV administration, reaching its peak at 5-15 minutes and lasting ~2-4 hours. Heart rate is either maintained or slightly reduced and cardiac output is maintained. Labetalol reduces systemic vascular resistance without reducing total peripheral blood flow. Cerebral, renal, and coronary blood flow is maintained. It can be used in the setting of pregnancy-induced hypertensive crisis because little placental transfer occurs due to the poor lipid solubility of labetalol.

Absorption, Fate, and Excretion. Although labetalol is completely absorbed from the gut, there is extensive first-pass clearance; bioavailability is only ~20-40%, is highly variable, and may be increased by food intake. The drug is rapidly and extensively metabolized in the liver by oxidative biotransformation and glucuronidation; very little unchanged drug is found in the urine. The rate of metabolism of labetalol is sensitive to changes in hepatic blood flow. The elimination $t_{1/2}$ of the drug is ~8 hours. The $t_{1/2}$ of the *R,R* isomer of labetalol (dilevalol) is ~15 hours. Labetalol provides an interesting and challenging example of pharmacokinetic-pharmacodynamic modeling applied to a drug that is a racemic mixture of isomers with different kinetics and pharmacological actions (Donnelly and Macphee, 1991).

Carvedilol

Carvedilol (COREG) is a third-generation β receptor antagonist that has a unique pharmacological profile. It blocks β_1, β_2, and α_1 receptors similarly to labetalol, but also has antioxidant and anti-inflammatory effects (Dandona et al., 2007). It has membrane-stabilizing activity but it lacks intrinsic sympathomimetic activity. Carvedilol produces vasodilation. Additional properties (e.g., antioxidant and anti-inflammatory effects) may contribute to the beneficial effects seen in treating congestive heart failure and in its cardioprotective effects. The drug is FDA-approved for use in hypertension, congestive heart failure, and left ventricular dysfunction following MI.

Carvedilol possesses two distinct antioxidant properties: it is a chemical antioxidant that can bind to and scavenge reactive oxygen species (ROS), and it can suppress the biosynthesis of ROS and oxygen radicals. Carvedilol is extremely liphophic and is able to protect cell membranes from lipid peroxidation. It prevents low density lipoprotein (LDL) oxidation, which in turn induces the uptake of LDL into the coronary vasculature. Carvedilol also inhibits ROS-mediated loss of myocardial contractility, stress-induced hypertrophy, apoptosis, and the accumulation and activation of neutrophils. At high doses, carvedilol exerts Ca^{2+} channel-blocking activity. Carvedilol does not increase β receptor density and is not associated with high levels of inverse agonist activity (Cheng et al., 2001; Dandona et al., 2007; Keating and Jarvis, 2003).

Carvedilol has been tested in numerous double-blind, randomized studies, including the U.S. Carvedilol Heart Failure Trials Program, Carvedilol or Metoprolol European Trial (COMET) (Poole-Wilson et al., 2003), Carvedilol Prospective Randomised Cumulative Survival (COPERNICUS) trial, and the Carvedilol Post Infarct Survival Control in LV Dysfunction (CAPRICORN) trial (Cleland, 2003). These trials showed that carvedilol improves ventricular function and reduces mortality and morbidity in patients with mild to severe congestive heart failure. Several experts recommend it as the standard treatment option in this setting. In addition, carvedilol combined with conventional therapy reduces mortality and attenuates myocardial infarction. In patients with chronic heart failure, carvedilol reduces cardiac sympathetic drive, but it is not clear if blockade of α_1 receptor–mediated vasodilation is maintained over long periods of time.

Absorption, Fate, and Excretion. Carvedilol is rapidly absorbed following oral administration, with peak plasma concentrations occurring in 1-2 hours. It is highly lipophilic and thus is extensively distributed into extravascular tissues. It is > 95% protein bound and is extensively metabolized in the liver, predominantly by CYP2D6 and CYP2C9. The $t_{1/2}$ is 7-10 hours. Stereoselective first-pass metabolism results in more rapid clearance of S(–)-carvedilol than R(+)-carvedilol. No significant changes in the pharmacokinetics of carvedilol were seen in elderly patients with hypertension, and no change in dosage is needed in patients with moderate to severe renal insufficiency (Cleland, 2003; Keating and Jarvis, 2003). Because of carvedilol's extensive oxidative metabolism by the liver, its pharmacokinetics can be profoundly affected by drugs that induce or inhibit oxidation. These include the inducer, rifampin, and inhibitors such as cimetidine, quinidine, fluoxetine, and paroxetine.

Bucindolol

Bucindolol (SANDONORM) is a third-generation nonselective β adrenergic antagonist with weak α_1 adrenergic blocking properties. The intrinsic sympathomimetic activity of bucindolol may be dependent on β_1 receptors.

Bucindolol increases left ventricular systolic ejection fraction and decreases peripheral resistance, thereby reducing afterload. It increases plasma HDL cholesterol, but does not affect plasma triglycerides. A large comprehensive clinical trial, the β Blocker Evaluation of Survival Trial (BEST), was terminated early because of the inability to demonstrate a survival benefit with bucindolol versus placebo. In subsequent analyses from BEST, however, benefits have been demonstrated in discrete subgroups, including a genetically identified subgroup. An evaluation was made of the therapeutic responses to bucindolol among patients with genetic variations or polymorphisms in two adrenergic receptors: β_1 389 arg/gly and α_{2C} 322-325 WT/Del. Researchers identified three distinct genotypes that predict the effect of bucindolol: very favorable (47% of BEST patients), favorable (40%), and unfavorable (13%). In the study, patients with the very favorable genotype experienced significant improvements in clinical end points compared to placebo, including reductions in all-cause mortality, cardiovascular mortality, heart failure hospitalization, and cardiovascular hospitalization. A New Drug Application (NDA) has been filed with the FDA and is currently under review.

Bucindolol is well absorbed after oral administration, reaching maximum plasma levels in 2 hours. It is highly protein bound (87%), extensively metabolized by the liver to 5-hydroxybucindolol, and has a $t_{1/2}$ of ~8 hours.

Celiprolol

Celiprolol (SELECTOL) is a third-generation cardioselective β receptor antagonist. It has low lipid solubility and possesses weak vasodilating and bronchodilating effects attributed to partial selective β_2 agonist activity and possibly papaverine-like relaxant effects on smooth muscle (including bronchial). It also has been reported to antagonize peripheral α_2 adrenergic receptor activity, to promote NO production, and to inhibit oxidative stress. There is evidence for intrinsic sympathomimetic activity at the β_2 receptor. Celiprolol is devoid of membrane-stabilizing activity. Weak α_2 antagonistic properties are present, but are not considered clinically significant at therapeutic doses (Toda, 2003).

Celiprolol reduces heart rate and blood pressure and can increase the functional refractory period of the atrioventricular node. Oral bioavailability ranges from 30-70%, and peak plasma levels are seen at 2-4 hours. It is largely unmetabolized and is excreted unchanged in the urine and feces. Celiprolol does not undergo first-pass metabolism. The predominant mode of excretion is renal. Celiprolol is used for treatment of hypertension and angina (Felix et al., 2001; Witchitz et al., 2000).

Nebivolol

Nebivolol (BYSTOLIC) is a third-generation selective β_1 receptor antagonist with endothelial NO-mediated vasodilator activity. In addition, nebivolol has antioxidant properties and neutral to favorable effects on both carbohydrate and lipid metabolism. Nebivolol lowers blood pressure by reducing peripheral vascular resistance and significantly increases stroke volume with preservation of cardiac output and maintains systemic flow and blood flow to target organs. Nebivolol generally does not negatively affect serum lipids and may increase insulin sensitivity. These benefits are also observed in the presence of metabolic syndrome, which is often present in hypertensive patients (Gielen et al., 2006; Ignarro, 2008). Nebivolol has been approved for treatment of hypertension.

Nebivolol is administered as the racemate containing equal amounts of the *d* and *l*-enantiomers. The *d*-isomer is the active β blocking component; the l-isomer is responsible for enhancing production of NO. Nebivolol is devoid of intrinsic sympathomimetic effects as well as membrane stabilizing activity and α_1 receptor blocking properties. It is lipophilic, and concomitant administration of chlorthalidone, hydrochlorothiazide, theophylline, or digoxin with nebivolol may reduce its extent of absorption. The NO-dependent vasodilating action of nebivolol and its high β_1 adrenergic receptor selectivity likely contribute to the drug's efficacy and improved tolerability (e.g., less fatigue and sexual dysfunction) as an antihypertensive agent (deBoer et al., 2007; Gupta and Wright, 2008; Moen and Wagstaff, 2006; Rosei and Rizzoni, 2007). Metabolism occurs via CYP2D6, and the influence of polymorphisms in the CYP2D6 gene on the bioavailability and duration of nebivolol's actions is being evaluated (Lefebvre et al., 2006), as is the influence of plasma concentration of receptor selectivity.

Other β Adrenergic Receptor Antagonists. There are numerous β adrenergic receptor antagonists on the market as ophthalmologic preparations for the treatment of glaucoma or other causes of high blood pressure inside the eye (Chapter 64). These include carteolol (OCUPRESS, others), metipranolol (OPTIPRANOLOL), nipradilol (HYPADIL; not available in the U.S.), levobunolol (BETAGAN, LIQUIFILM, others), betaxolol (BETOPTIC, others), and timolol (TIMOPTIC, others) (Henness et al., 2007). The use of β adrenergic receptor antagonists in glaucoma is contraindicated in patients with asthma, COPD, sympathomatic sinus bradycardia, and cardiogenic shock.

BIBLIOGRAPHY

Abdelghany O. Arformoterol: The first nebulized long-acting beta$_2$-adrenergic agonist. *Formulary,* **2007**, *42*:99–109.

Allwood MJ, Cobbold AF, Ginsberg J. Peripheral vascular effects of noradrenaline, isopropylnoradrenaline, and dopamine. *Br Med Bull*, **1963**, *19:*132–136.

Altschuld RA, Billman GE. β_2-Adrenoceptors and ventricular fibrillation. *Pharmacol Ther*, **2000**, *88:*1–14.

Alward WL. Medical management of glaucoma. *N Engl J Med*, **1998**, *339:*1298–1307.

Andersson KE. Current concepts in the treatment of disorders of micturition. *Drugs*, **1988**, *35:*477–494.

Andersson KE, Wein AJ. Pharmacology of the lower urinary tract: Basis for current and future treatment of urinary incontinence. *Pharmacol Rev*, **2004**, *56*:581–631.

Andreka P, Aiyar N, Olson LC, et al. Bucinolol displays intrinsic sympathomimetic activity in human myocardium. *Circulation*, **2002**, *105:*2429–2434.

Andrus MR, Loyed JV. Use of β-adrenoceptor antagonists in older patients with chronic obstructive pulmonary disease and cardiovascular co-morbidity. *Drugs Aging*, **2008**, *25:*131–144.

Beduschi MC, Beduschi R, Oesterling JE. α-Blockade therapy for benign prostatic hyperplasia: From a nonselective to a more selective α_{1A}-adrenergic antagonist. *Urology*, **1998**, *51:*861–872.

β-Blocker Evaluation of Survival Trial Investigators. A trial of the β-blocker bucindolol in patients with advanced chronic heart failure. *N Engl J Med*, **2001**, *344:*1659–1667.

Bolger AP, Al-Nasser F. β-Blockers for chronic heart failure: Surviving longer but feeling better? *Int J Cardiol*, **2003**, *92:*1–8.

Bosch J. Medical treatment of portal hypertension. *Digestion*, **1998**, *59:*547–555.

Breit A, Lagace M, Bouvier M. Hetero-oligomerization between β_2 and β_3 receptors generates a β-adrenergic signaling unit with distinct funtional properties. *J Biol Chem*, **2004**, *279*:28756–28765.

Breslow MJ, Ligier B. Hyperadrenergic states. *Crit Care Med*, **1991**, *19:*1566–1579.

Bristow MR, Kantrowitz NE, Ginsburg R, Fowler MB. β-Adrenergic functions in heart muscle disease and heart failure. *J Mol Cell Cardiol*, **1985**, *17*(Suppl 2):41–52.

Brixius K, Bundkirchen A, Bölck B, et al. Nebivolol, bucindolol, metoprolol and carvedilol are devoid of intrinsic sympathomimetic activity in human myocardium. *Br J Pharmacol*, **2001**, *133:*1330–1338.

Brodde OE, Michel MC. Adrenergic and muscarinic receptors in the human heart. *Pharmacol Rev*, **1999**, *51:*651–690.

Brooks AM, Gillies WE. Ocular β-blockers in glaucoma management. Clinical pharmacological aspects. *Drugs Aging*, **1992**, *2:*208–221.

Brunton LL. A positive feedback loop contributes to the deleterious effects of angiotensin. *Proc Natl Acad Sci USA*, **2005**, *102*:14483–14484.

Cazzola M, Matera MG. Novel long acting bronchodilators for COPD and asthma. *Br J Pharmacol*, **2008**, *155*:291–299.

Cheng J, Kamiya K, Kodama I. Carvedilol: Molecular and cellular basis for its multifaceted therapeutic potential. *Cardiovasc Drug Rev*, **2001**, *19:*152–171.

Chidiac P, Hebert TE, Valiquette M, et al. Inverse agonist activity of β-adrenergic antagonists. *Mol Pharmacol*, **1994**, *45:* 490–499.

Cleland JG. β-Blockers for heart failure: Why, which, when, and where. *Med Clin North Am*, **2003**, *87:*339–371.

Coats AJS. β-adrenoceptor antagonists in elderly patients with chronic heart failure. Therapeutic potential of third generation agents. *Drugs Aging,* **2006**, *23:*93–99.

Cruickshank JM. β-Blockers and diabetes. The bad guys come good. *Cardiovasc Drugs Ther*, **2002**, *16:*457–470.

Czuriga I, Riecansky I, Bodnar J, et al. for the NEBIS Investigators Group. Comparison of the new cardioselective β-blocker nebivolol with bisoprolol in hypertension: The nebivolol, bisoprolol multicenter study (NEBIS). *Cardiovasc Drugs Ther*, **2003**, *17*:257–263.

Dandona P, Ghanim H, Brook DP. Antioxidant activity of carvedilol in cardiovascular disease. *J Hypertension,* **2007**, *25*:731–741.

deBoer RA, Voors AA, vonVeldhuisen DJ. Nebivolol: Third generation beta blockade. *Expert Opin Pharmacother,* **2007**, *8*:1539–1550.

de Groot AA, Mathy MJ, van Zwieten PA, Peters SL. Antioxidant activity of nebivolol in the rat aorta. *J Cardiovasc Pharmacol*, **2004**, *43:*148–153.

DiBari M, Marchionni N, Pahor M. β-blockers after acute myocardial infarction in elderly patients with diabetes mellitus: Time to reassess. *Drugs Aging*, **2003**, *20:*13–22.

Ding B, Abe J, Wei H, et al. A positive feedback loop of PDE3 and ICER leads to cardiomyocyte apoptosis. *Proc Natl Acad Sci USA*, **2005**, *102*:14771-14776.

Dobre D, Haarjer-Ruskamp FM, Voors AA, van Veldhuisen DJ. β adrenoceptor antagonists in elderly patients with heart failure. A critical review of their efficacy and tolerability. *Drugs Aging*, **2007**, *24*:1031–1094.

Donnelly R, Macphee GJ. Clinical pharmacokinetics and kinetic-dynamic relationships of dilevalol and labetalol. *Clin Pharmacokinet*, **1991**, *21:*95–109.

Drazen JM, O'Byrne PM. Risks of long acting beta-agonists in achieving asthma control. *N Engl J Med,* **2009,** *360:* 1671–1672.

Dunne F, Kendall MJ, Martin U. β-Blockers in the management of hypertension in patients with type 2 diabetes mellitus: Is there a role? *Drugs*, **2001**, *61:*428–435.

Dzierba AL, Sanja J. Chronic obstructive pulmonary disease in the elderly: An update on pharmacological management. *Drugs Aging,* **2009,** *26:*447–456.

Ellison KE, Gandhi G. Optimizing the use of β-adrenoceptor antagonists in coronary artery disease. *Drugs*, **2005**, *65:* 787–797.

Engelhardt S, Hein L, Wiesmann F, Lohse MJ. Progressive hypertrophy and heart failure in β_1-adrenergic receptor transgenic mice. *Proc Natl Acad Sci USA*, **1999**, *96:*7059–7064.

Fanta CH. Asthma. *N Engl J Med*, **2009,** *360:*1002–1014.

Faulds D, Hollingshead LM, Goa KL. Formoterol. A review of its pharmacological properties and therapeutic potential in reversible obstructive airways disease. *Drugs*, **1991**, *42:* 115–137.

Felix SB, Stangl V, Kieback A, et al. Acute hemodynamic effects of β-blockers in patients with severe congestive heart failure: Comparison of celiprolol and esmolol. *J Cardiovasc Pharmacol*, **2001**, *38:*666–671.

Fernandez-Lopez JA, Remesar X, Foz M, Alemany M. Pharmacological approaches for the treatment of obesity. *Drugs*, **2002**, *62:*915–944.

Fitton A, Benfield P. Dopexamine hydrochloride. A review of its pharmacodynamic and pharmacokinetic properties and therapeutic potential in acute cardiac insufficiency. *Drugs*, **1990**, *39:*308–330.

Fitton A, Sorkin EM. Sotalol. An updated review of its pharmacological properties and therapeutic use in cardiac arrhythmias. *Drugs*, **1993**, *46:*678–719.

Fleckenstein A. New insights into the mechanism of actions of amphetamines. *Annu Rev Pharmacol,* **2007,** *47:*691–698.

Forray C, Bard JA, Wetzel JM, et al. The α_1-adrenergic receptor that mediates smooth muscle contraction in human prostate has the pharmacological properties of the cloned human α 1c subtype. *Mol Pharmacol*, **1994**, *45:*703–708.

Freemantle N, Cleland J, Young P, et al. β Blockade after myocardial infarction: systematic review and meta regression analysis. *BMJ*, **1999**, *318:*1730–1737.

Fung JW, Yu CM, Kum LC, et al. Role of β-blocker therapy in heart failure and atrial fibrillation. *Cardiac Electrophysiol Rev*, **2003**, *7:*236–242.

Gauthier C, Langin D, Balligand JL. β_3 adrenoceptors in the cardiovascular system. *Trends Pharmacol Sci*, **2000**, *21:*426–431.

Galderisi M, D'Errico A. β-blockers and coronary flow reserve: The importance of a vasodilatory action. *Drugs*, **2008,** *68:*579–590.

Gazzola M, Materea MC, Donner CF. Inhaled β_2-adrenoceptor agonists. Cardiovascular safety in patients with obstructive lung disease. *Drugs,* **2005,** *65:*1595–1610.

Gerstman BB, Jolson HM, Bauer M, et al. The incidence of depression in new users of β-blockers and selected antihypertensives. *J Clin Epidemiol*, **1996**, *49:*809–815.

Gielen W, Cleopohas TJ, Agrawal R. Nevivolol: A review of its clinical and pharmacological characteristics. *Int J Clin Pharmacol Ther*, **2006,** *44:*344–357.

Giembycz MA, Kaur M, Leigh R, Newton R. A Holy Grail of asthma management: Toward understanding how long acting β_2 adrenoceptor agonist enhance the clinical efficacy of inhaled corticosteroids. *Br J Pharmacol,* **2008,** *153*:1080–1104.

Goldsmith DR, Keating GM. Budesonide/fomoterol: A review of its use in asthma. *Drugs*, **2004**, *64:*1597–1618.

Goldsmith DR, Plosker GL. Doxazosin gastrointestinal therapeutic system. A review of its use in benign prostatic hyperplasia. *Drugs,* **2005,** *65:*2037–2047.

Goldstein S. Benefits of β-blocker therapy for heart failure. *Arch Intern Med*, **2002**, *162:*641–648.

Gottlieb SS, McCarter RJ, Vogel RA. Effect of β-blockade on mortality among high-risk and low-risk patients after myocardial infarction. *N Engl J Med*, **1998**, *339:*489–497.

Grimm RH Jr. Antihypertensive therapy: taking lipids into consideration. *Am Heart J*, **1991**, *122:*910–918.

Guimarães S, Moura D. Vascular adrenoceptors: An update. *Pharmacol Rev*, **2001**, *53*:319–356.

Gupta S, Wright HM. Nebivolol: A highly selective β_1-adrenergic receptor blocker that causes vasodilation by increasing nitric oxide. *Cardiovasc Ther*, **2008,** *26*:189–202.

Hayashi Y, Maze M. α_2 Adrenoceptor agonists and anaesthesia. *Br J Anaesth,* **1993**, *71:*108–118.

Henness S, Harrison TS, Keating GM. Ocular carteolol. A review of its use in the management of glaucoma and ocular hypertension. *Drugs Aging,* **2007,** *24:*509–525.

Hollenberg SM, Kavinsky CJ, Parrillo JE. Cardiogenic shock. *Ann Intern Med*, **1999**, *131:*47–59.

Hu ZW, Shi XY, Hoffman BB. Doxuzosin inhibits proliferation and migration of human vascular smooth-muscle cells independent of α_1-adrenergic receptor antagonism. *J Cardiovasc Pharmacol*, **1998**, *31*:833–839.

Ignarro LJ. Different pharmacological properties of two enantiomers in a unique β-blocker, nebivolol. *Cardiovasc Ther,* **2008,** *26*:115–134.

Ignarro LJ, Byrns RE, Trinh K, et al. Nebivolol: A selective β_1 adrenergic receptor antagonist that relaxes vascular smooth muscle by nitric-oxide and cyclic GMP-dependent mechanisms. *Nitric Oxide*, **2002**, *7:*75–82.

Ishii Y, Nakamura K, Tsutsumi K, et al. Drug interaction between cimetidine and timolol ophthalmic solution: effect on heart rate and intraocular pressure in healthy Japanese volunteers. *J Clin Pharmacol*, **2000**, *40:*193–199.

Keating GM, Jarvis B. Carvedilol: A review of its use in chronic heart failure. *Drugs*, **2003**, *63:*1697–1741.

Kenny B, Miller A, Williamson I, et al. Evaluation of the pharmacological selectivity profile of α_1 adrenoceptor antagonists at prostatic α_1 adrenoceptors: Binding, functional and *in vivo* studies. *Br J Pharmacol*, **1996**, *118*:871–878.

Khouri A, Realini T, Fechtner RD. Use of fixed dose combination drugs for the treatment of glaucoma. *Drugs Aging*, **2007,** *24:*1007–1016.

Kühlkamp V, Bosch R, Mewis C, Seipel L. Use of β-blockers in atrial fibrillation. *Am J Cardiovasc Drugs*, **2002**, *2:*37–42.

Kyprianou N. Doxazosin and terazosin suppress prostate growth by inducing apoptosis. Clinical significance. *J Urol*, **2003**, *169:*1520–1525.

Lefebvre J, Poirier L, Poirier P, et al. The influence of CYP2D6 phenotype on the clinical response of nebivolol in patients with essential hypertension. *Br J Clin Pharmacol*, **2007**, *63:* 575–582.

Liggett SB, Tepe NM, Lorenz JN, et al. Early and delayed consequences of β_2-adrenergic receptor overexpression in mouse hearts: Critical role for expression level. *Circulation*, **2000**, *101:*1707–1714.

Lipworth BJ. Long acting β_2 adrenoceptor agonists: a smart choice for asthma? *Trends Pharmacol Sci*, **2007,** *28:*257–262.

Lefkowitz RJ, Rockman HA, Koch WJ. Catecholamines, cardiac β-adrenergic receptors, and heart failure. *Circulation*, **2000**, *101:*1634–1637.

LePor H, Williford W, Barry M, et al. The efficacy of terazosin, finasteride, or both in begign prostatic hyperplasia. *N Eng J Med*, **1996**, *335*:533–539.

Ma XL, Yue TL, Lopez BL, et al. Carvedilol, a new β adrenoreceptor blocker and free radical scavenger, attenuates myocardial ischemia–reperfusion injury in hypercholesterolemic rabbits. *J Pharmacol Exp Ther*, **1996**, *277:*128–136.

Maack C, Cremers B, Flesch M, et al. Different intrinsic activities of bucindolol, carvedilol and metoprolol in human failing myocardium. *Br J Pharmacol*, **2000**, *130:*1131–1139.

Maggioni AP, Sinagra G, Opasich C, et al. β Blockers in patients with congestive heart failure: Guided use in clinical practice investigators. Treatment of chronic heart failure with β adrenergic blockade beyond controlled clinical trials: The BRING-UP experience. *Heart*, **2003**, *89:*299–305.

Man in't Veld AJ, Van den Meiracker AH, Schalekamp MA. Do β blockers really increase peripheral vascular resistance? Review of the literature and new observations under basal conditions. *Am J Hypertens*, **1988**, *1:*91–96.

Marik PE, Iglesias J. Low-dose dopamine does not prevent acute renal failure in patients with septic shock and oliguria. NORASEPT II Study Investigators. *Am J Med*, **1999**, *107:*387–390.

Matera MG, Cazzola M. Ultra-long acting β_2-adrenoceptor agonist. An emerging therapeutic option for asthma and COPD. *Drugs,* **2007,** *67:*503–515.

McClellan KJ, Wiseman LR, Wilde MI. Midodrine. A review of its therapeutic use in the management of orthostatic hypotension. *Drugs Aging*, **1998**, *12:*76–86.

McConnell JD, Roehrborn CG, Bautista OM, et al. The long-term effect of doxazosin, finasteride, and combination therapy on the clinical progression of benign prostatic hyperplasia. *N Engl J Med*, **2003**, *349:*2387–2398.

McGavin JK, Keating GM. Bisoprolol. A review of its use in chronic heart failure. *Drugs*, **2002**, *62:*2677–2696.

McPherson GA. Current trends in the study of potassium channel openers. *Gen Pharmacol*, **1993**, *24:*275–281.

MERIT-HF Study Group. Effect of metoprolol CR/XL in chronic heart failure: Metoprolol CR/XL Randomised Intervention Trial in Congestive Heart Failure (MERIT-HF). *Lancet*, **1999**, *353:*2001–2007.

Michel MD, Vrydag W. α_1-, α_2- and β-adrenoceptors in the urinary bladder urethra and prostate. *Br J Pharmacolol*, **2006**, *147*:S88–S119.

Mignot E. Sleep, sleep disorders, and hypocretin (orexin). *Sleep Med*, **2004**, *5:*S2–S8.

Mimran A, Ducailar G. Systemic and regional haemodynamic profile of diuretics and α- and β-blockers. A review comparing acute and chronic effects. *Drugs*, **1988**, *35*(Suppl 6):60–69.

Moen MD, Wagstaff AJ. Nebivolol: A review of its use in the management of hypertension and chronic heart failure. *Drugs,* **2006,** *66:*1389–1409.

Moniotte S, Kobzik L, Feron O, et al. Upregulation of β_3-adrenoceptors and altered contractile response to inotropic amines in human failing myocardium. *Circulation*, **2001**, *103:*1649–1655.

Morimoto A, Hasegawa H, Cheng HJ, et al. Endogenous β_3-adrenoceptor activation contributes to left ventricular and cardiomyocyte dysfunction in heart failure. *Am J Physiol Heart Circ Physiol*, **2004**, *286:*H2425–H2433.

Murphy MB, Murray C, Shorten GD. Fenoldopam: A selective peripheral dopamine receptor agonist for the treatment of severe hypertension. *N Engl J Med*, **2001**, *345:*1548–1557.

Nodari S, Metra M, Dei Cas L. β-Blocker treatment of patients with diastolic heart failure and atrial hypertension. A prospective, randomized comparison of the long-term effects of atenolol vs. nebivolol. *Eur J Heart Failure*, **2003**, *5:*621–627.

Osborne NN, Wood JP, Chidlow G, et al. Effectiveness of levobetaxolol and timolol at blunting retinal ischaemia is related to their calcium and sodium blocking activities: Relevance to glaucoma. *Brain Res Bull*, **2004**, *62:*525–528.

Pearce N, Beasley R, Crane J, et al. End of the New Zealand asthma mortality epidemic. *Lancet*, **1995**, *345:*41–44.

Poole-Wilson PA, Swedberg K, Cleland JG, et al. Comparison of carvedilol and metoprolol on clinical outcomes in patients with chronic heart failure in the Carvedilol Or Metoprolol European Trial (COMET): Randomised controlled trial. *Lancet*, **2003**, *362:*7–13.

Post SR, Hammond HK, Insel PA. *β*-Adrenergic receptors and receptor signaling in heart failure. *Annu Rev Pharmacol Toxicol*, **1999**, *39:*343–360.

Prakash A, Markham A. Metoprolol: a review of its use in chronic heart failure. *Drugs*, **2000**, *60:*647–678.

Redington AE. Step one for asthma treatment: β_2-agonists or inhaled corticosteroids? *Drugs*, **2001**, *61:*1231–1238.

Reynolds NA, Lyseng-Williamson KA, Wiseman LR. Inhaled salmeterol/fluticasone propionate. A review of its use in asthma. *Drugs*, **2005,** 65:1715–1734.

Ried LD, McFarland BH, Johnson RE, Brody KK. *β*-Blockers and depression: the more the murkier? *Ann Pharmacother*, **1998**, *32:*699–708.

Robidoux J, Martin TL, Collins S. *β*-Adrenergic receptors and regulation of energy expenditure: A family affair. *Annu Rev Pharmacol Toxicol*, **2004**, *44:*297–323.

Rosei EA, Rizzoni D. Metabolic profile of nebivolol, a β-adrenoceptor antagonist with unique characteristics. *Drugs*, **2007,** *67:*1097–1107.

Rosei EA, Rizzoni D, Comini S, Boari G. Nebivolol-Lisinopril Study Group. Evaluation of the efficacy and tolerability of nebivolol versus lisinopril in the treatment of essential arterial hypertension: A randomized, multicentre, double blind study. *Blood Press Suppl*, **2003**, *1:*30–35.

Rosen SG, Clutter WE, Shah SD, et al. Direct *α*-adrenergic stimulation of hepatic glucose production in human subjects. *Am J Physiol*, **1983**, *245:*E616–E626.

Rosendorff C. *β*-Blocking agents with vasodilator activity. *J Hypertens Suppl*, **1993**, *11:*S37–S40.

Rozec B, Noireaud J, Trochu J, Gauthier C. Place of β_3-adrenoceptors among other *β*-adrenoceptor sub-types in the regulation of the cardiovascular system. *Arch Mal Coeur Vaiss*, **2003**, *96:*905–913.

Ruffolo RR Jr. The pharmacology of dobutamine. *Am J Med Sci*, **1987**, *294:*244–248.

Ruffolo RR Jr, Hieble JP. Adrenoceptor pharmacology: Urogenital applications. *Eur Urol*, **1999**, *36*(Suppl 1):17–22.

Salpeter SR. Cardioselective *β* blocker use in patients with asthma and chronic obstructive pulmonary disease: An evidence-based approach to standard of care. *Respir Med*, **2003**, *24:*564–572.

Salpeter SR, Ormiston TM, Salpeter EE. Cardioselective beta-blockers for chronic obstructive pulmonary disease. *Cochrane Database Syst Rev*, **2005,** CD003566.

Sandhu JS, Vaughan ED Jr. Combination therapy for the pharmacological management of benign prostatic hyperplasia. Rationale and treatment options. *Drugs Aging*, **2005,** *22:*901–912.

Santillo VM, Lowe F. Treatment of benign prostatic hyperplasia in patients with cardiovascular disease. *Drugs*, **2006,** *23:*795–805.

Seale JP. Whither *β*-adrenoceptor agonists in the treatment of asthma? *Prog Clin Biol Res*, **1988**, *263:*367–377.

Self T, Soberman JE, Bubla JM, Chafen CC. Cardioselective *β*-blockers in patients with asthma and concomitant heart failure or history of myocardial infarction: When do benefits outweigh risks? *J Asthma*, **2003**, *40:*839–845.

Schmid-Schoenbein G, Hugli T. A new hypothesis for microvascular inflammation in shock and multiorgan failure: Self-digestion by pancreatic enzymes. *Microcirculation*, **2005**, *12:*71–82.

Shores J, Berger KR, Murphy EA, Pyeritz RE. Progression of aortic dilatation and the benefit of long-term *β*-adrenergic blockade in Marfan's syndrome. *N Engl J Med*, **1994**, *330:*1335–1341.

Simon T, Mary-Krause M, Funck-Brentano C, et al. Bisoprolol dose-response relationship in patients with congestive heart failure: A subgroups analysis in the cardiac insufficiency bisoprolol study (CIBIS II). *Eur Heart J*, **2003**, *24:*552–559.

Singh K, Communal C, Sawyer DB, Colucci WS. Adrenergic regulation of myocardial apoptosis. *Cardiovasc Res*, **2000**, *45:*713–719.

Starke K, Gothert M, Kilbinger H. Modulation of neurotransmitter release by presynaptic autoreceptors. *Physiol Rev*, **1989**, *69:*864–989.

Suissa S, Ernst P. Optical illusions from visual data analysis: Example of the New Zealand asthma mortality epidemic. *J Clin Epidemiol*, **1997**, *50:*1079–1088.

Swanson JM, Volkow ND. Serum and brain concentrations of methylphenidate: implications for use and abuse. *Neurosci Biobehav Rev*, **2003**, *27:*615–621.

Tam SW, Worcel M, Wyllie M. Yohimbine: A clinical review. *Pharmacol Ther*, **2001**, *91:*215–243.

Tfelt-Hansen P. Efficacy of *β*-blockers in migraine. A critical review. *Cephalalgia*, **1986**, *6*(Suppl 5):15–24.

Toda N. Vasodilating *β*-adrenoceptor blockers as cardiovascular therapeutics. *Pharmacol Ther*, **2003**, *100:*215–234.

Varon J. Treatment of acute severe hypertension: current and newer agents. *Drugs*, **2008,** *68:*283–297.

Villanueva C, Balanzo J, Novella MT, et al. Nadolol plus isosorbide mononitrate compared with sclerotherapy for the prevention of variceal rebleeding. *N Engl J Med*, **1996**, *334:*1624–1629.

Wagstaff AJ, Bryson HM. Tizanidine. A review of its pharmacology, clinical efficacy and tolerability in the management of spasticity associated with cerebral and spinal disorders. *Drugs*, **1997**, *53:*435–452.

Walle T, Webb JG, Bagwell EE, et al. Stereoselective delivery and actions of *β* receptor antagonists. *Biochem Pharmacol*, **1988**, *37:*115–124.

Webers C, Beckers H, Nuijts R, Schouten J. Pharmacological management of primary open-angle glaucoma second line options and beyond. *Drugs Aging*, **2008**, *25:*729–759.

Witchitz S, Cohen-Solal A, Dartois N, et al. Treatment of heart failure with celiprolol, a cardioselective *β* blocker with *β*-2 agonist vasodilator properties. The CELICARD Group. *Am J Cardiol*, **2000**, *85:*1467–1471.

Wood JP, Schmidt KG, Melena J, et al. The *β*-adrenoceptor antagonists metipranolol and timolol are retinal neuroprotectants: Comparison with betaxolol. *Exp Eye Res*, **2003**, *76:*505–516.

Wuttke H, Rau T, Heide R, et al. Increased frequency of cytochrome P450 2D6 poor metabolizers among patients with metoprolol-associated adverse effects. *Clin Pharmacol Ther*, **2002**, *72:*429–437.

Zhu QM, Lesnick JD, Jasper JR, et al. Cardiovascular effects of rilmedidine, moxonidine and clonidine in conscious wild-type and D79N α_{2A}-adrenoreceptor transgenic mice. *Br J Pharmacol*, **1999**, *126:*1522–1530.

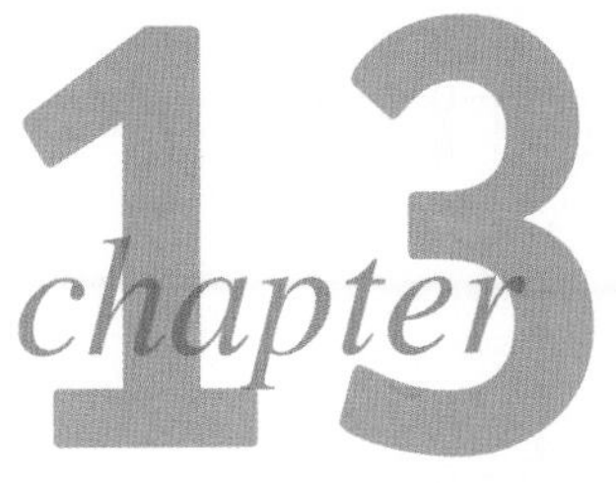

5-Hydroxytryptamine (Serotonin) and Dopamine

Elaine Sanders-Bush and
Lisa Hazelwood

5-Hydroxytryptamine (5-HT, serotonin) and dopamine (DA) are neurotransmitters in the central nervous system (CNS) and also have prominent peripheral actions. 5-HT is found in high concentrations in enterochromaffin cells throughout the GI tract, in storage granules in platelets, and broadly throughout the CNS. 5-HT regulates smooth muscle in the cardiovascular system and the GI tract and enhances platelet aggregation. The highest concentrations of DA are found in the brain; dopamine stores are also present peripherally in the adrenal medulla and the transmitter is detectable in the plexuses of the GI tract and in enteric nervous system. DA modulates peripheral vascular tone to modulate renal perfusion, heart rate, and vasoconstriction/dilation. Fourteen 5-HT receptor subtypes and five DA-receptor subtypes have been delineated by pharmacological analyses and cDNA cloning. The availability of cloned receptors has allowed the development of subtype-selective drugs and the elucidation of actions of these neurotransmitters at a molecular level. Increasingly, therapeutic goals are being achieved by drugs that target selectively one or more of the subtypes of 5-HT or DA receptors, or that act on a combination of both 5-HT and DA receptors.

5-HT and DA are widely distributed in the animal and plant kingdoms. Several important laboratory invertebrate models have serotonergic and dopaminergic systems, including the fruit fly and nematode. 5-HT and DA are considered below in separate sections.

5-HYDROXYTRYPTAMINE

History. In the 1930s, Erspamer began to study the distribution of enterochromaffin cells, which stained with a reagent for indoles. The highest concentrations were found in GI mucosa, followed by platelets and the CNS. Soon thereafter, Page and colleagues isolated and chemically characterized a vasoconstrictor substance released from platelets in clotting blood. This substance, named serotonin, was shown to be identical to the indole isolated by Erspamer. Subsequent discovery of biosynthetic and degradative pathways for 5-HT and clinical presentation of patients with carcinoid tumors of intestinal enterochromaffin cells spurred interest in 5-HT. The gross effects of 5-HT, produced in excess in malignant carcinoid, gave some indication of the physiologic and pharmacologic actions of 5-HT, as did the identification of several naturally occurring and semi-synthetic tryptamine-like substances that were hallucinogenic and induced behavioral effects similar to those observed in carcinoid patients. In the mid-1950s, the discovery that the pronounced behavioral effects of reserpine are accompanied by a profound decrease in brain 5-HT led to the proposal that serotonin may function as a neurotransmitter in the mammalian CNS.

Sources and Chemistry. 5-HT [3-(β-aminoethyl)-5-hydroxyindole] is present in vertebrates, tunicates, mollusks, arthropods, coelenterates, fruits, and nuts. It is also a component of venoms, including those of the common stinging nettle and of wasps and scorpions. Numerous synthetic or naturally occurring congeners of 5-HT have pharmacological activity (see Figure 13–1 for chemical structures). Many of the *N*- and *O*-methylated indoleamines, such as *N,N*-dimethyltryptamine, are hallucinogens. Because these compounds are behaviorally active and might be synthesized by known metabolic pathways, they have long been considered candidates for endogenous psychotomimetic substances, potentially responsible for some psychotic behaviors. Another close relative of 5-HT, melatonin (5-methoxy-*N*-acetyltryptamine), is formed by sequential *N*-acetylation and *O*-methylation (Figure 13–2). Melatonin, not to be confused with melanin, is the principal indoleamine in the pineal gland, where it may be said to constitute a pigment of the imagination. Its synthesis is controlled by external factors including environmental light. Melatonin induces pigment lightening in skin cells and suppresses ovarian functions; it also serves a role in regulating biological rhythms and shows promise in the treatment of jet lag and other sleep disturbances (Cajochen et al., 2003).

Synthesis and Metabolism of 5-HT. 5-HT is synthesized by a two-step pathway from the essential amino

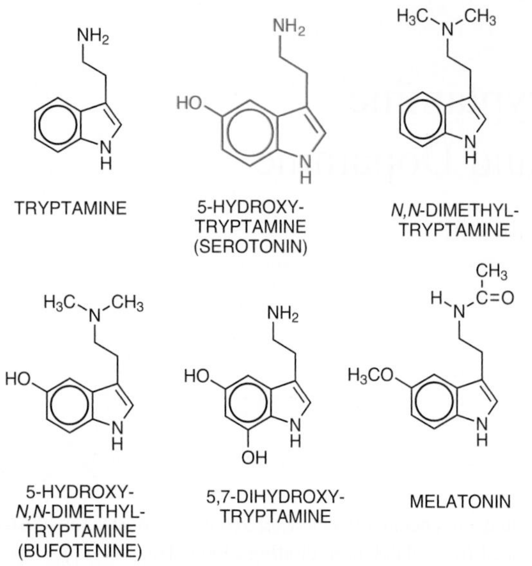

TRYPTAMINE

5-HYDROXY-TRYPTAMINE (SEROTONIN)

N,N-DIMETHYL-TRYPTAMINE

5-HYDROXY-*N,N*-DIMETHYL-TRYPTAMINE (BUFOTENINE)

5,7-DIHYDROXY-TRYPTAMINE

MELATONIN

Figure 13–1. *Structures of representative indolealkylamines.*

acid tryptophan (Figure 13–2). Tryptophan is actively transported into the brain by a carrier protein that also transports other large neutral and branched-chain amino acids. Levels of tryptophan in the brain are influenced not only by its plasma concentration but also by the plasma concentrations of other amino acids that compete for the transporter. Tryptophan hydroxylase, a mixed-function oxidase that requires molecular O_2 and a reduced pteridine cofactor for activity, is the rate-limiting enzyme in the synthetic pathway. A brain-specific isoform of tryptophan hydroxylase (TPH2) is entirely responsible for the synthesis of brain 5-HT (Walther and Bader, 2003). Human genetic studies of TPH2, fueled by discoveries of functional SNPs that alter *in vitro* enzymatic activity as well as promoter SNPs that alter expression, have focused on mood disorders, but are so far inconclusive. Unlike tyrosine hydroxylase, tryptophan hydroxylase is not regulated by end-product inhibition, although regulation by phosphorylation is common to both enzymes. Brain tryptophan hydroxylase is not generally saturated with substrate; consequently, the concentration of tryptophan in the brain influences the synthesis of 5-HT.

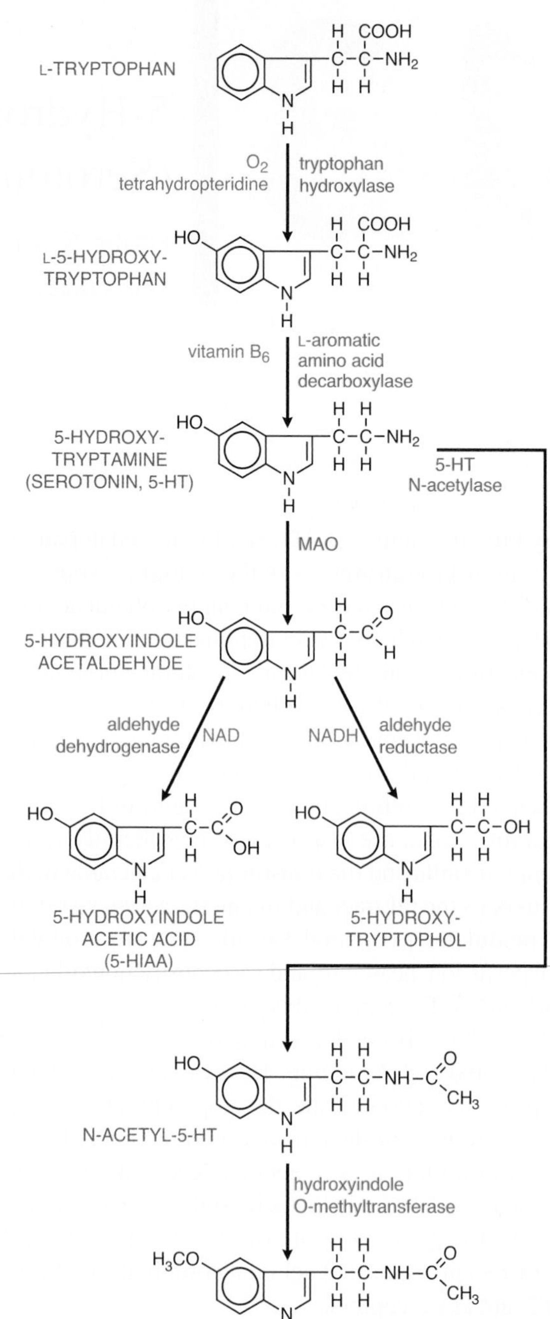

Figure 13–2. *Synthesis and inactivation of serotonin.* Enzymes are identified in red lettering, and co-factors are shown in blue.

The enzyme that converts L-5-hydroxytryptophan to 5-HT, aromatic L-amino acid decarboxylase (AADC), is widely distributed and has a broad substrate specificity. A long-standing debate about whether L-5-hydroxytryptophan decarboxylase and L-dopa decarboxylase are identical enzymes was clarified when cDNA cloning confirmed that a single gene product decarboxylates both amino acids. 5-Hydroxytryptophan is not detected in the brain because it is rapidly decarboxylated. The synthesized product, 5-HT, is accumulated in secretory granules by a vesicular monoamine transporter (VMAT2); vesicular 5-HT is released by exocytosis from serotonergic neurons. In the nervous system, the action of released 5-HT is terminated via neuronal uptake by a specific 5-HT transporter. The 5-HT transporter (SERT [SLC6A4]) is localized in the membrane of serotonergic axon terminals (where it terminates the action of 5-HT in the synapse) and in the membrane of platelets (where it takes up 5-HT from the blood). This uptake system is the means by which platelets acquire 5-HT, since they lack the enzymes required for 5-HT synthesis. The 5-HT transporter and other monoamine transporters have been cloned (Chapters 5, 8, and 12). The amine transporters are distinct from VMAT2, which concentrates amines in intracellular storage vesicles and is a nonspecific amine carrier, whereas the 5-HT transporter is specific. The 5-HT transporter is regulated by phosphorylation and subsequent internalization (for a review, see Steiner et al., 2008), providing a mechanism for dynamic regulation of serotonergic transmission.

The principal route of metabolism of 5-HT involves oxidative deamination by monoamine oxidase (MAO); the aldehyde intermediate thus formed is converted to 5-hydroxyindole acetic acid (5-HIAA) by aldehyde dehydrogenase (Figure 13–2). An alternative route, reduction of the acetaldehyde to an alcohol, 5-hydroxytryptophol, is normally insignificant. 5-HIAA is actively transported out of the brain by a process that is sensitive to the nonspecific transport inhibitor, probenecid.

Since 5-HIAA formation accounts for nearly 100% of the metabolism of 5-HT in brain, the turnover rate of brain 5-HT is estimated by measuring the ratio of 5-HIAA/5-HT. 5-HIAA from brain and peripheral sites of 5-HT storage and metabolism is excreted in the urine along with small amounts of 5-hydroxytryptophol sulfate or glucuronide conjugates. The usual range of urinary excretion of 5-HIAA by a normal adult is 2-10 mg daily. Larger amounts are excreted by patients with malignant carcinoid, providing a reliable diagnostic test for the disease. Ingestion of ethanol results in elevated amounts of $NADH_2$ (Chapter 23), which diverts 5-hydroxyindole acetaldehyde from the oxidative route to the reductive pathway (Figure 13–2) and tends to increase the excretion of 5-hydroxytryptophol and correspondingly reduce the excretion of 5-HIAA.

Of the two isoforms of MAO (A and B) (see Chapter 8 and Bortolato et al., 2008 for a review), MAO-A preferentially metabolizes 5-HT and norepinephrine; clorgyline is a specific inhibitor of this enzyme. MAO-B prefers β-phenylethylamine and benzylamine as substrates; low-dose selegiline is a relatively selective inhibitor of MAO-B. Dopamine and tryptamine are metabolized equally well by both isoforms. Neurons contain both isoforms of MAO, localized primarily in the outer membrane of mitochondria. MAO-B is the principal isoform in platelets, which contain large amounts of 5-HT.

Other minor pathways of metabolism of 5-HT, such as sulfation and *O*- or *N*-methylation, have been suggested. The latter reaction could lead to formation of an endogenous psychotropic substance, 5-hydroxy-*N,N*-dimethyltryptamine (bufotenine; Figure 13–1). However, other methylated indoleamines such as *N,N*-dimethyltryptamine and 5-methoxy-*N,N*-dimethyltryptamine are far more active hallucinogens and are more likely candidates to be endogenous psychotomimetics.

PHYSIOLOGICAL FUNCTIONS OF SEROTONIN

Multiple 5-HT Receptors

Based on data from studies of 5-HT's actions in peripheral tissues, researchers hypothesized that the multiple actions of 5-HT involved interaction with distinct 5-HT receptor subtypes. Extensive pharmacological characterization and the cloning of receptor cDNAs have confirmed this hypothesis (Barnes and Sharp, 1999; Bockaert et al., 2006). The multiple 5-HT receptor subtypes cloned comprise the largest known neurotransmitter-receptor family. The 5-HT receptor subtypes are expressed in distinct but often overlapping patterns (Palacios et al., 1990) and are coupled to different transmembrane-signaling mechanisms (Table 13–1). Most 5-HT receptors, especially the 5-HT_{2C} receptor, can activate G-proteins independently of agonists, a property known as constitutive activity (Berg et al., 2008). Four of seven currently recognized 5-HT receptor families have defined functions (described later). The 5-HT_1, 5-HT_2, and 5-HT_{4-7} receptor families are members of the superfamily of GPCRs (Chapter 3). The 5-HT_3 receptor is a ligand-gated ion channel that gates Na^+ and K^+ and has a predicted membrane topology akin to that of the nicotinic cholinergic receptor (Chapter 11).

History of 5-HT Receptor Subtypes. In 1957, Gaddum and Picarelli proposed the existence of two 5-HT receptor subtypes, *M* and *D receptors*. M receptors were believed to be located on parasympathetic nerve endings, controlling the release of acetylcholine, whereas D receptors were thought to be located on smooth muscle. Subsequent studies in both the periphery and brain were consistent with the notion of multiple subtypes of 5-HT receptors (for a review, see Sanders-Bush and Airey, 2008), now known to be members of the superfamilies of GPCRs and ligand-gated ion channel receptors. The current classification scheme (Hoyer et al., 1994) is based on pharmacological properties, second-messenger function, and deduced amino acid sequence, and includes seven subfamilies of 5-HT receptors (Table 13–1).

The radioligand-binding studies of Peroutka and Snyder (1979) provided the first definitive evidence for two distinct recognition sites for 5-HT. 5-HT_1 receptors had a high affinity for $[^3H]$5-HT, while 5-HT_2 receptors had a low affinity for $[^3H]$5-HT and a high affinity for $[^3H]$spiperone. Subsequently, high affinity for 5-HT was used as a primary criterion for classifying a receptor subtype as a member of the 5-HT_1 receptor family. This classification strategy proved to be invalid; for example, a receptor expressed in the choroid plexus was named the 5-HT_{1C} receptor because it was the third receptor shown to have a high affinity for 5-HT. However, based on its pharmacological properties, second-messenger function, and deduced amino acid sequence, the 5-HT_{1C} receptor clearly belonged to the 5-HT_2 receptor family and was subsequently renamed the 5-HT_{2C} receptor. Evidence suggests that the $5\text{-HT}_{1D\beta}$ receptor is the human

Table 13–1

Serotonin Receptor Subtypes

STRUCTURAL FAMILIES

$5\text{-}HT_1$, $5\text{-}HT_2$, $5\text{-}HT_{4-7}$: G protein–coupled receptor

$5\text{-}HT_3$: 5-HT–gated ion channel

SUBTYPE	GENE STRUCTURE	SIGNAL TRANSDUCTION	LOCALIZATION	FUNCTION	SELECTIVE AGONIST	SELECTIVE ANTAGONIST
$5\text{-}HT_{1A}$	Intronless	↓ AC	Raphe nuclei Cortex Hippocampus	Autoreceptor	8-OH-DPAT	WAY 100135
$5\text{-}HT_{1B}$[a]	Intronless	↓ AC	Subiculum Globus pallidus Substantia nigra	Autoreceptor	—	—
$5\text{-}HT_{1D}$	Intronless	↓ AC	Cranial blood vessels Globus pallidus Substantia nigra	Vasoconstriction	Sumatriptan	—
$5\text{-}HT_{1E}$	Intronless	↓ AC	Cortex Striatum	—	—	—
$5\text{-}HT_{1F}$[b]	Intronless	↓ AC	Brain and periphery	—	—	—
$5\text{-}HT_{2A}$ (D receptor)	Introns	↑ PLC and ↑ PLA_2	Platelets Smooth muscle Cerebral cortex	Aggregation Contraction Neuronal excitation	α-Methyl-5-HT, DOI, MCPP	Ketanserin LY53857 MDL 100, 907
$5\text{-}HT_{2B}$	Introns	↑ PLC	Stomach fundus	Contraction	α-Methyl-5-HT, DOI	LY53857 SB206553
$5\text{-}HT_{2C}$	Introns	↑ PLC ↑ PLA_2	Choroid plexus Hypothalamus	CSF production Neuronal excitation	α-Methyl-5-HT, DOI, MK 2.2	LY53857 SB 2022084 Mesulergine
$5\text{-}HT_3$ (M receptor)	Introns	Ligand-operated ion channel	Parasympathetic nerves Solitary tract Area postrema	Neuronal excitation	2-Methyl-5-HT	Ondansetron Tropisetron
$5\text{-}HT_4$	Introns	↑ AC	Hippocampus GI tract	Neuronal excitation	Renzapride	GR 113808
$5\text{-}HT_{5A}$	Introns	↓ AC	Hippocampus	Unknown	—	—
$5\text{-}HT_{5B}$	Introns	Unknown	—	Pseudogene	—	—
$5\text{-}HT_6$	Introns	↑ AC	Hippocampus Striatum Nucleus accumbens	Neuronal excitation	—	SB 271046
$5\text{-}HT_7$	Introns	↑ AC	Hypothalamus Hippocampus GI tract	Unknown	5-carboxamino-tryptamine	

[a]Also referred to as $5\text{-}HT_{1DB}$. [b]Also referred to as $5\text{-}HT_{1EB}$.

AC, adenylyl cyclase; PLC, phospholipase C; PLA_2; phospholipase A_2; 8-OH-DPAT, 8-hydroxy-(2-*N*,*N*-dipropylamino)-tetraline; DOI, 1-(2,5-dimethoxy-4-iodophenyl) isopropylamine; MCPP, metachlorphenylpiperazine; MK212.

homolog of the 5-HT_{1B} receptor originally characterized and subsequently cloned from rodent brain. Although the rat 5-HT_{1B} receptor and the human 5-HT_{1D} receptor show > 95% amino-acid sequence homology, they have distinct pharmacological properties. The rat 5-HT_{1B} receptor has an affinity for β adrenergic antagonists (e.g., pindolol and propranolol) that is two to three orders of magnitude higher than that of the human 5-HT_{1D} receptor. This difference appears to be due to a single amino acid difference (D→R) in the seventh transmembrane span. Many 5-HT receptor knockout mice have been created that shed light on the role of specific receptors (Table 13–2); however, most of these models cannot distinguish between developmental events versus changes related to the absence of the receptor in the adult mouse.

5-HT_1 Receptors. The 5-HT_1-receptor subfamily consists of five members, all of which preferentially couple to $G_{i/o}$ and inhibit adenylyl cyclase. The 5-HT_{1A}, 5-HT_{1B}, and 5-HT_{1D} receptor subtypes also activate a receptor-operated K^+ channel and inhibit a voltage-gated Ca^{2+} channel, a common property of receptors coupled to the pertussis toxin–sensitive G_i/G_o family. The 5-HT_{1A} receptor is found in the raphe nuclei of the brainstem, where it functions as an inhibitory, somatodendritic autoreceptor on cell bodies of serotonergic neurons (Figure 13–3). Another 5-HT_1-receptor subtype, the 5-$HT_{1D/1B}$ receptor, functions as an autoreceptor on axon terminals, inhibiting 5-HT release, as does its rat homolog, 5-HT_{1B}. 5-HT_{1D} receptors, abundantly expressed in the substantia nigra and basal ganglia, regulate the firing rate of DA-containing cells and the release of DA at axonal terminals.

5-HT_2 Receptors. The three subtypes of 5-HT_2 receptors couple to pertussis toxin–insensitive Gq/G_{11} proteins and activate phospholipase C, thereby generating two second messengers, diacylglycerol (a cofactor in the activation of PKC) and inositol trisphosphate (which mobilizes intracellular stores of Ca^{2+}). 5-HT_{2A} and 5-HT_{2C} receptors also activate phospholipase A_2, promoting the release of arachidonic acid. 5-HT_{2A} receptors are broadly distributed in the CNS, primarily in serotonergic terminal areas. High densities are found in several brain structures, including prefrontal, parietal, and somatosensory cortex, as well as in blood platelets and smooth muscle cells. 5-HT_{2A} receptors in the GI tract are thought to correspond to the D subtype of 5-HT receptor originally described by Gaddum and Picarelli (1957). 5-HT_{2B} receptors originally were found in stomach fundus, where they are abundant. The expression of 5-HT_{2B} receptors is highly restricted in the CNS. 5-HT_{2C} receptors have a very high density in the choroid plexus, an epithelial tissue that is the primary site of cerebrospinal fluid production. The 5-HT_{2C} receptor has been implicated in the control of cerebrospinal fluid production and in feeding behavior and mood. The 5-HT_{2C} receptor is the only GPCR that is regulated by RNA editing (Burns et al., 1997). Multiple 5-HT_{2C} receptor isoforms are generated by RNA editing, with alterations of three amino acids within the second intracellular loop; extensively edited isoforms have modified G protein–coupling efficiencies (Sanders-Bush et al., 2003). Splice variants of 5-HT_{2A} and 5-HT_{2C} receptors exist but do not code for functional proteins.

Table 13–2

Physiological Roles of 5-HT Receptors Defined by Phenotypes in Knockout Mice

	5-HT_{1A}	5-HT_{1B}	5-HT_{2A}	5-HT_{2B}	5-HT_{2C}	5-HT_3	5-HT_4	5-HT_{5A}	5-HT_6	5-HT_7
Anxiety	↑[a]		↓[c]							
Aggression		↑[b]								
Heart defects				Lethal[d]						
Food intake					↑[e]					
Seizure susceptibility					↑		↑[g]			
Nociception						↓[f]				
Exploratory activity								↑[h]		
Ethanol sensitivity									↓[i]	
Thermoregulation										↓[j]

Arrow indicates direction of alteration of the trait.
[a]Parks et al., 1998; [b]Saudou et al., 1994; [c]Weisstaub et al., 2007; [d]Nebigil et al., 2000; [e]Tecott et al., 1995; [f]Zeitz et al., 2002; [g]Compan et al., 2004; [h]Grailhe et al., 1999; [i]Bonasera et al., 2006; [j]Hedlund et al., 2003.

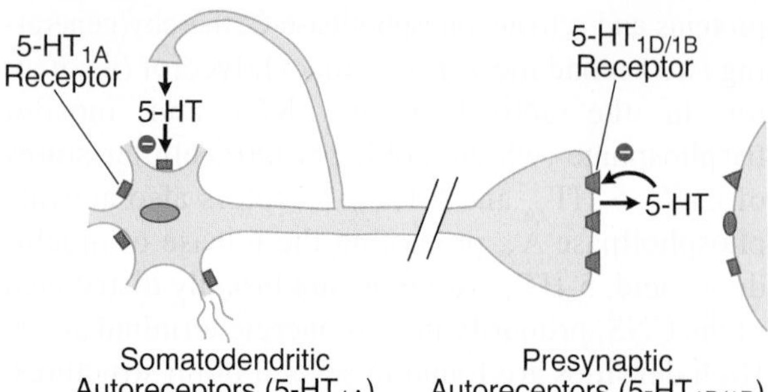

Figure 13–3. *Two classes of 5-HT autoreceptors with differential localizations.* Somatodendritic 5-HT_{1A} autoreceptors decrease raphe cell firing when activated by 5-HT released from axon collaterals of the same or adjacent neurons. The receptor subtype of the presynaptic autoreceptor on axon terminals in the forebrain has different pharmacological properties and has been classified as 5-HT_{1D} (in humans) or 5-HT_{1B} (in rodents). This receptor modulates the release of 5-HT. Postsynaptic 5-HT_1 receptors are also indicated.

5-HT_3 Receptors. The 5-HT_3 receptor is the only monoamine neurotransmitter receptor known to function as a ligand-operated ion channel. The 5-HT_3 receptor corresponds to Gaddum and Picarelli's M receptor. Activation of 5-HT_3 receptors elicits a rapidly desensitizing depolarization, mediated by the gating of cations. These receptors are located on parasympathetic terminals in the GI tract, including vagal and splanchnic afferents. In the CNS, a high density of 5-HT_3 receptors is found in the solitary tract nucleus and in the area postrema. 5-HT_3 receptors in both the GI tract and the CNS participate in the emetic response, providing a basis for the anti-emetic property of 5-HT_3 receptor antagonists. The 5-HT_3 receptor, a pentameric ligand-gated channel, belongs to the Cys-loop receptor superfamily, which includes the nicotinic cholinergic receptor and the $GABA_A$ receptor. The original, cloned 5-HT_3 receptor subunit forms functional pentameric complexes that gate cations when expressed in *Xenopus* oocytes or in cultured cells (Maricq et al., 1991). Five genes (HTR3A-E) for 5-HT_3 receptor subunits have now been cloned. Heteropentamers of the multiple gene products exhibit distinct properties and anatomical distributions (see Barnes et al., 2009).

5-HT_4 Receptors. 5-HT_4 receptors couple to G_s to activate adenylyl cyclase, leading to an increase in intracellular cyclic AMP. 5-HT_4 receptors are widely distributed throughout the body. In the CNS, the receptors are found on neurons of the superior and inferior colliculi and in the hippocampus. In the GI tract, 5-HT_4 receptors are located on neurons of the myenteric plexus and on smooth muscle and secretory cells. In the GI tract, stimulation of the 5-HT_4 receptor is thought to evoke secretion and to facilitate the peristaltic reflex. The latter effect may explain the utility of prokinetic benzamides in GI disorders (Chapter 46). Effects of pharmacological manipulation of 5-HT_4 receptors on memory and feeding in animal models suggest possible clinical applications in the future (Bockaert et al. 2008).

Additional Cloned 5-HT Receptors. Two other cloned receptors, 5-HT_6 and 5-HT_7, are linked to activation of adenylyl cyclase. Multiple splice variants of the 5-HT_7 receptor have been found, although functional distinctions are not clear. The absence of selective agonists and antagonists has foiled definitive studies of the role of the 5-HT_6 and 5-HT_7 receptors. Circumstantial evidence suggests that 5-HT_7 receptors play a role in the relaxation of smooth muscle in the GI tract and the vasculature. The atypical antipsychotic drug clozapine has a high affinity for 5-HT_6 and 5-HT_7 receptors; whether this property is related to the broader effectiveness of clozapine compared to conventional antipsychotic drugs is not known (Chapter 16). Two subtypes of the 5-HT_5 receptor have been cloned; although the 5-HT_{5A} receptor has been shown to inhibit adenylyl cyclase, functional coupling of the cloned 5-HT_{5B} receptor has not yet been described.

Actions of 5-HT in Physiological Systems

Platelets. Platelets differ from other formed elements of blood in expressing mechanisms for uptake, storage, and endocytotic release of 5-HT. 5-HT is not synthesized in platelets, but is taken up from the circulation and stored in secretory granules by active transport, similar to the uptake and storage of serotonin by serotonergic nerve terminals. Thus, Na^+-dependent transport across the surface membrane of platelets, via the 5-HT transporter, is followed by VMAT2-mediated uptake into dense core granules creating a gradient of 5-HT as high as 1000:1 with an internal concentration of 0.6 M in the dense core storage vesicles. Measuring the rate of Na^+-dependent 5-HT uptake by platelets provides a sensitive assay for 5-HT uptake inhibitors.

Main functions of platelets include adhesion, aggregation, and thrombus formation to plug holes in the endothelium; conversely, the functional integrity of the endothelium is critical for platelet action. A complex local interplay of multiple factors, including 5-HT, regulates thrombosis and hemostasis (Chapters 30 and 33). When platelets make contact with injured endothelium, they release substances that promote platelet aggregation, and secondarily, they release 5-HT (Figure 13–4). 5-HT binds to platelet 5-HT_{2A} receptors and elicits a weak aggregation response that is markedly augmented by the presence of collagen. If the damaged blood vessel is injured to a depth where vascular smooth muscle is exposed, 5-HT exerts a direct vasoconstrictor effect, thereby contributing to hemostasis, which is enhanced by locally released autocoids (thromboxane A_2, kinins, and vasoactive peptides). Conversely, 5-HT may interact with endothelial cells to stimulate production of NO and antagonize its own vasoconstrictor action, as well as the vasoconstriction produced by other locally released agents.

Cardiovascular System. The classical response of blood vessels to 5-HT is contraction, particularly in the splanchnic, renal, pulmonary,

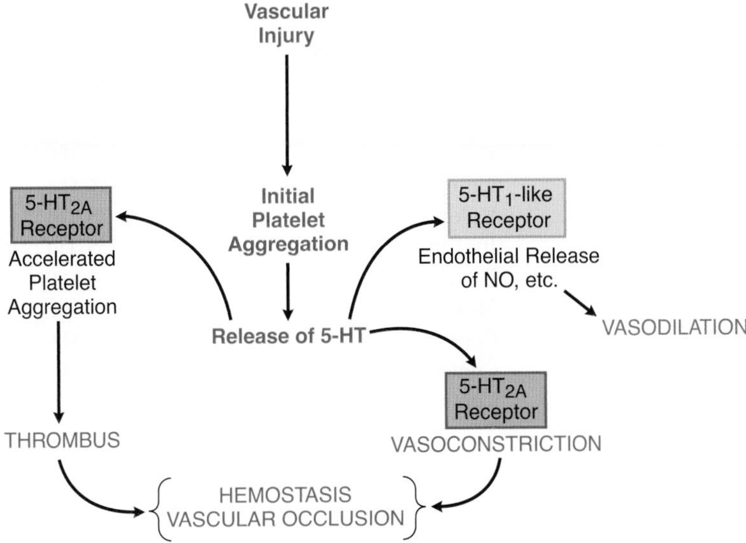

Figure 13–4. *Schematic representation of the local influences of platelet 5-HT.* The release of 5-HT stored in platelets is triggered by aggregation. The local actions of 5-HT include feedback actions on platelets (shape change and accelerated aggregation) mediated by interaction with platelet 5-HT_{2A} receptors, stimulation of NO production mediated by 5-HT_1-like receptors on vascular endothelium, and contraction of vascular smooth muscle mediated by 5-HT_{2A} receptors. These influences act in concert with many other mediators that are not shown to promote thrombus formation and hemostasis. See Chapter 30 for details of adhesion and aggregation of platelets and factors contributing to thrombus formation and blood clotting.

and cerebral vasculatures. 5-HT also induces a variety of responses by the heart that are the result of activation of multiple 5-HT receptor subtypes, stimulation or inhibition of autonomic nerve activity, or dominance of reflex responses to 5-HT (Kaumann and Levy, 2006). Thus, 5-HT has positive inotropic and chronotropic actions on the heart that may be blunted by simultaneous stimulation of afferent nerves from baroreceptors and chemoreceptors. Activation of 5-HT_3 receptors on vagus nerve endings elicits the Bezold-Jarisch reflex, causing extreme bradycardia and hypotension. The local response of arterial blood vessels to 5-HT also may be inhibitory, the result of the stimulation of endothelial NO production and prostaglandin synthesis and blockade of norepinephrine release from sympathetic nerves. On the other hand, 5-HT amplifies the local constrictor actions of norepinephrine, angiotensin II, and histamine, which reinforce the hemostatic response to 5-HT. Presumably, these constrictor effects result, at least in part, from direct action of 5-HT on vascular smooth muscle. In response to IV injection of 5-HT, these disparate effects on blood pressure may be temporally distinct.

GI Tract. Enterochromaffin cells in the gastric mucosa are the site of the synthesis and most of the storage of 5-HT in the body and are the source of circulating 5-HT. These cells synthesize 5-HT from tryptophan, by means of TPH1, and store 5-HT and other autacoids, such as the vasodilator peptide substance P and other kinins. Basal release of enteric 5-HT is augmented by mechanical stretching, such as that caused by food, and by efferent vagal stimulation. Released 5-HT enters the portal vein and is subsequently metabolized by MAO-A in the liver. 5-HT that survives hepatic oxidation may be captured by platelets or rapidly removed by the endothelium of lung capillaries and inactivated. 5-HT released from enterochromaffin cells also acts locally to regulate GI function (Gershon and Tack, 2007). Motility of gastric and intestinal smooth muscle may be either enhanced or inhibited by at least six subtypes of 5-HT receptors (Table 13–3). The stimulatory response occurs at nerve endings on longitudinal and circular enteric muscle (5-HT_4 receptors), at postsynaptic cells of the enteric ganglia (5-HT_3 and 5-HT_{1P} receptors), and by direct effects of 5-HT on the smooth-muscle cells (5-HT_{2A} receptors in intestine, 5-HT_{2B} receptors in stomach fundus). In esophagus, 5-HT acting at 5-HT_4 receptors causes either relaxation or contraction, depending on the species. Abundant 5-HT_3 receptors on vagal and other afferent neurons and on enterochromaffin cells play a pivotal role in emesis (Chapter 46). Serotonergic nerve terminals have been described in the myenteric plexus. Enteric 5-HT triggers peristaltic contraction when released in response to acetylcholine, sympathetic nerve stimulation, increases in intraluminal pressure, and lowered pH.

CNS. A multitude of brain functions are influenced by 5-HT, including sleep, cognition, sensory perception, motor activity, temperature regulation, nociception, mood, appetite, sexual behavior, and hormone secretion. All of the cloned 5-HT receptors are expressed in the brain, often in overlapping domains. Although patterns of 5-HT receptor expression in individual neurons have not been extensively defined, it is likely that multiple 5-HT receptor subtypes with similar or opposing actions are expressed in individual neurons (Bonsi et al., 2007), leading to a tremendous diversity of actions.

The principal cell bodies of 5-HT neurons are located in raphe nuclei of the brainstem and project throughout the brain and spinal cord (Chapter 14). In addition to being released at discrete synapses, release of serotonin also seems to occur at sites of axonal swelling, termed *varicosities*, which do not form distinct synaptic

Table 13–3

Some Actions of 5-HT in the Gastrointestinal Tract

SITE	RESPONSE	RECEPTOR
Enterochromaffin cells	Release of 5-HT	5-HT_3
	Inhibition of 5-HT release	5-HT_4
Enteric ganglion cells	Release of ACh	5-HT_4
(presynaptic)	Inhibition of ACh release	5-HT_{1P}, 5-HT_{1A}
Enteric ganglion cells	Fast depolarization	5-HT_3
(postsynaptic)	Slow depolarization	5-HT_{1P}
Smooth muscle, intestinal	Contraction	5-HT_{2A}
Smooth muscle, stomach fundus	Contraction	5-HT_{2B}
Smooth muscle, esophagus	Contraction	5-HT_4

ACh, acetylcholine.

contacts. 5-HT released at nonsynaptic varicosities is thought to diffuse to outlying targets, rather than acting on discrete synaptic targets. Such non-synaptic release with ensuing widespread effects is consistent with the idea that 5-HT acts as a neuromodulator as well as a neurotransmitter (Chapter 14).

Serotonergic nerve terminals contain the proteins needed to synthesize 5-HT from L-tryptophan (Figure 13–2). Newly formed 5-HT is rapidly accumulated in synaptic vesicles (through VMAT2), where it is protected from MAO. 5-HT released by nerve-impulse flow is reaccumulated into the pre-synaptic terminal by the 5-HT transporter, SERT (SLC6A4; Chapter 5). Pre-synaptic reuptake is a highly efficient mechanism for terminating the action of 5-HT released by nerve-impulse flow. MAO localized in postsynaptic elements and surrounding cells rapidly inactivates 5-HT that escapes neuronal reuptake and storage.

Electrophysiology. The physiological consequences of 5-HT release vary with the brain area and the neuronal element involved, as well as with the population of 5-HT receptor subtype(s) expressed (Bockaert et al., 2006). 5-HT has direct excitatory and inhibitory actions (Table 13–4), which may occur in the same preparation, but with distinct temporal patterns. For example, in hippocampal neurons, 5-HT elicits hyperpolarization mediated by 5-HT_{1A} receptors followed by a slow depolarization mediated by 5-HT_4 receptors.

5-HT_{1A} receptor–induced membrane hyperpolarization and reduction in input resistance results from an increase in K^+ conductance. These ionic effects, which are blocked by pertussis toxin, are independent of cAMP, suggesting that 5-HT_{1A} receptors couple, by means of $G_{\beta\gamma}$ subunits, to receptor-operated K^+ channels (Andrade et al., 1986). Somatodendritic 5-HT_{1A} receptors on raphe cells also elicit a K^+-dependent hyperpolarization. The G protein involved is pertussis toxin–sensitive, but the K^+ current apparently is different from the current elicited at postsynaptic 5-HT_{1A} receptors in the hippocampus. The precise signaling mechanism involved in inhibition of neurotransmitter release by the $5\text{-HT}_{1B/1D}$ autoreceptor at synaptic terminals is not known, although inhibition of voltage-gated Ca^{++} channels likely contributes.

Slow depolarization induced by 5-HT_{2A} receptor activation in areas such as the prefrontal cortex and nucleus accumbens involves a decrease in K^+ conductance. A second, distinct mechanism involving Ca^{2+}-activated membrane currents enhances neuronal excitability and potentiates the response to excitatory signals such as glutamate. The role of intracellular signaling cascades in these physiological actions of 5-HT_{2A} receptors has not been clearly defined. In areas where 5-HT_1 and 5-HT_{2A} receptors co-exist, the effect of 5-HT may reflect a combination of the two opposing responses: a prominent 5-HT_1 receptor–mediated hyperpolarization and an opposing 5-HT_{2A} receptor–mediated depolarization. When 5-HT_{2A} receptors are blocked, hyperpolarization is enhanced. In many cortical areas, 5-HT_{2A} receptors are localized on both GABAergic interneurons and pyramidal cells. Activation of interneurons enhances GABA (γ-aminobutyric acid) release, which secondarily slows the firing rate of pyramidal cells. Thus, there is the potential for the 5-HT_{2A} receptor to differentially regulate cortical pyramidal cells, depending on the specific target cells (interneurons versus pyramidal cells). Activation of 5-HT_{2C} receptors has been shown to depress a K^+ current, an effect that may contribute to the excitatory response. The 5-HT_4 receptor, which is coupled to activation of adenylyl cyclase, also elicits a slow neuronal depolarization mediated by a decrease in K^+ conductance. It is not clear why two distinct

Table 13–4

Electrophysiological Effects of 5-HT Receptors

SUBTYPE	RESPONSE
$5\text{-HT}_{1A,B}$	Increase K^+ conductance Hyperpolarization
$5\text{-HT}_{2A}/5\text{-HT}_{2C}$	Decrease K^+ conductance Slow depolarization
5-HT_3	Gating of Na^+, K^+ Fast depolarization
5-HT_4	Decrease K^+ conductance Slow depolarization

5-HT receptor families linked to different signaling pathways can elicit a common neurophysiological action. Yet another receptor, the 5-HT$_{1P}$ receptor, elicits a slow depolarization. This receptor, which couples to activation of adenylyl cyclase, is restricted to the enteric nervous system (Gershon and Tack, 2007). The unique pharmacological profile of the 5-HT$_{1P}$ receptor is most consistent with the 5-HT$_7$ receptor.

The fast depolarization elicited by 5-HT$_3$ receptors reflects direct gating of an ion channel intrinsic to the receptor structure itself. The 5-HT$_3$ receptor–induced inward current has the characteristics of a cation-selective, ligand-operated channel. Membrane depolarization is mediated by simultaneous increases in Na^+ and K^+ conductance, comparable to the nicotinic cholinergic receptor. 5-HT$_3$ receptors have been characterized in the CNS and in sympathetic ganglia, primary afferent parasympathetic and sympathetic nerves, and enteric neurons. The pharmacological properties of 5-HT$_3$ receptors, which are different from those of other 5-HT receptors, suggest that multiple 5-HT$_3$ receptor subtypes may exist and may correspond to different combinations of subunits (Jensen et al., 2008).

Behavior. The behavioral alterations elicited by drugs that interact with 5-HT receptors are extremely diverse. Many animal behavioral models for initial assessment of agonist and antagonist properties of drugs depend on aberrant motor or reflex responses, such as startle reflexes, hind-limb abduction, head twitches, and other stereotypical behaviors. Operant behavioral paradigms, such as drug discrimination, provide models of specific 5-HT receptor activation and are useful for exploring the action of CNS-active drugs, including agents that interact with 5-HT. For example, investigations of the mechanism of action of hallucinogenic drugs have relied heavily on drug discrimination (Winter, 2009). The following discussion focuses on animal models that may relate to pathological conditions in humans and will not attempt to cover the voluminous literature dealing with 5-HT and behavior. See King and associates (2008), Lesch and coworkers (2003), Lucki (1998), and Swerdlow and colleagues (2000) for excellent reviews on this topic.

Sleep-Wake Cycle. Control of the sleep-wake cycle is one of the first behaviors in which a role for 5-HT was identified. Following pioneering work in cats (Jouvet, 1999), many studies showed that depletion of 5-HT with *p*-chlorophenylalanine, a tryptophan hydroxylase inhibitor, elicits insomnia that is reversed by the 5-HT precursor, 5-hydroxytryptophan. Conversely, treatment with L-tryptophan or with nonselective 5-HT agonists accelerates sleep onset and prolongs total sleep time. 5-HT antagonists reportedly can increase and decrease slow-wave sleep, probably reflecting interacting or opposing roles for subtypes of 5-HT receptors. One relatively consistent finding in humans and in laboratory animals is an increase in slow-wave sleep following administration of a selective 5-HT$_{2A/2C}$-receptor antagonist such as ritanserin.

Aggression and Impulsivity. Studies in laboratory animals and in humans suggest that 5-HT serves a critical role in aggression and impulsivity. Many human studies reveal a correlation between low cerebrospinal fluid 5-HIAA and violent impulsivity and aggression. As with many effects of 5-HT, pharmacological studies of aggressive behavior in laboratory animals are not definitive, but suggest a role for 5-HT. Two genetic studies have reinforced and amplified this notion. Knockout mice lacking the 5-HT$_{1B}$ receptor exhibited extreme aggression (Saudou et al., 1994), suggesting either a role for 5-HT$_{1B}$ receptors in the development of neuronal pathways important in aggression or a direct role in the mediation of aggressive behavior. A human genetic study identified a point mutation in the gene encoding MAO-A, which was associated with extreme aggressiveness and mental retardation (Brunner et al., 1993), and this has been confirmed in knockout mice lacking MAO-A (Cases et al., 1995).

Anxiety and Depression. The effects of 5-HT–active drugs in anxiety and depressive disorders, like the effects of selective serotonin reuptake inhibitors (SSRIs), strongly suggest a role for 5-HT in the neurochemical mediation of these disorders. Mutant mice lacking the 5-HT transporter display anxiety and a "depressive-like" phenotype (Fox et al., 2007). 5-HT-related drugs with clinical effects in anxiety and depression have varied effects in classical animal models of these disorders, depending on the experimental paradigm, species, and strain. For example, the anxiolytic buspirone (Chapter 15), a partial agonist at 5-HT$_{1A}$ receptors, does not reduce anxiety in classical approach-avoidance paradigms that were instrumental in development of anxiolytic benzodiazepines. However, buspirone and other 5-HT$_{1A}$ receptor agonists are effective in other animal behavioral tests used to predict anxiolytic effects. Furthermore, studies in 5-HT$_{1A}$ receptor knockout mice suggest a role for this receptor in anxiety, and possibly depression. Agonists of certain 5-HT receptors, including 5-HT$_{2A}$ and 5-HT$_{2C}$ receptors (e.g., *m*-chlorophenylpiperazine), have anxiogenic properties in laboratory animals and in human studies. Similarly, these receptors have been implicated in the animal models of depression, such as learned helplessness.

An impressive finding in humans with depression is the abrupt reversal of the antidepressant effects of drugs such as SSRIs by manipulations that rapidly reduce the amount of 5-HT in the brain. These approaches include administration of *p*-chlorophenylalanine or a tryptophan-free drink containing large quantities of neutral amino acids (Delgado et al., 1990). Curiously, this kind of 5-HT depletion has not been shown to worsen or to induce depression in nondepressed subjects, suggesting that the continued presence of 5-HT is required to maintain the effects of these drugs. This clinical finding adds credence to somewhat less convincing neurochemical findings that suggest a role for 5-HT in the pathogenesis of depression.

Pharmacological Manipulation of the Amount of 5-HT in Tissues

A highly specific mechanism for altering synaptic availability of 5-HT is inhibition of presynaptic reaccumulation of neuronally released 5-HT. Selective serotonin reuptake inhibitors (SSRIs), such as fluoxetine (PROZAC, others), potentiate and prolong the action of 5-HT released by neuronal activity. When co-administered with L-5-hydroxytryptophan, SSRIs elicit a profound activation of serotonergic responses. SSRIs (citalopram [CELEXA], escitalopram [LEXAPRO], fluoxetine, fluvoxamine, paroxetine [PAXIL], and sertraline [ZOLOFT]) are the most widely used treatment for endogenous depression (Chapter 15). Sibutramine (MERIDIA), an inhibitor of the reuptake of 5-HT, NE, and DA, is used as an appetite suppressant in the management of obesity. The drug is converted to two active metabolites that contribute to its therapeutic effects. The relative importance of effects on single or multiple neurotransmitters in sibutramine's anti-obesity action is unclear. Sibutramine is classified as a selective serotonin/ norepinephrine reuptake inhibitor (SNRI). Other SNRIs include duloxetine (CYMBALTA; approved for depression, anxiety, peripheral neuropathy, and fibromyalgia), venlafaxine (EFFEXOR; approved for the treatment of depression, anxiety, and panic disorders), desvenlafaxine (PRISTIQ; approved for depression), and milnacipran (SAVELLA; approved for fibromyalgia).

Nonselective treatments that alter 5-HT levels include MAO inhibitors (e.g., phenelzine [NARDIL], tranylcypromine [PARNATE, others], and isocarboxazid [MARPLAN]) and reserpine. MAO inhibitors block the principal route of degradation, thereby increasing levels of 5-HT, whereas reserpine, a VMAT2 inhibitor, depletes intraneuronal stores of 5-HT. These treatments profoundly alter levels of 5-HT throughout the body. Because reserpine and MAO inhibitors also cause comparable changes in the levels of catecholamines, the drugs are of limited utility as research tools. Both agents have been used in the treatment of mental diseases: reserpine as an antipsychotic drug (Chapter 16) and MAO inhibitors as antidepressants (Chapter 15).

Experimental strategies for evaluating the role of 5-HT depend on techniques that manipulate tissue levels of 5-HT or block 5-HT receptors. Until recently, manipulation of the levels of endogenous 5-HT was the more commonly used strategy, because the actions of 5-HT receptor antagonists were poorly understood.

Tryptophan hydroxylase is the rate-limiting enzyme in 5-HT synthesis, and manipulation of its catalytic flux provides useful ways to alter 5-HT levels. A diet low in tryptophan reduces the concentration of brain 5-HT; conversely, ingestion of a tryptophan load increases levels of 5-HT in the brain. An acute decrease in brain 5-HT can be achieved by oral administration of an amino acid mixture devoid of tryptophan, a valuable tool for human studies of the role of 5-HT. In addition, administration of a tryptophan hydroxylase inhibitor causes a profound depletion of 5-HT. The most widely used selective tryptophan hydroxylase inhibitor is *p*-chlorophenylalanine, which acts irreversibly to produce long-lasting depletion of 5-HT levels with no change in levels of catecholamines.

p-Chloroamphetamine and other halogenated amphetamines promote the release of 5-HT from platelets and neurons. A rapid release of 5-HT is followed by a prolonged and selective depletion of 5-HT in brain. The mechanism of 5-HT release involves reversal of 5-HT transporter, analogous to the mechanism of the catecholamine-releasing action of amphetamine. The halogenated amphetamines are valuable experimental tools and two of them, fenfluramine and dexfenfluramine, were used clinically to reduce appetite; the once popular diet drug regimen, "fen-phen," combined fenfluramine and phentermine. Fenfluramine (PONDIMIN) and dexfenfluramine (REDUX) were withdrawn from the U.S. market in the late 1990s after reports of life-threatening heart valve disease and pulmonary hypertension associated with their use. This toxicity may be secondary to 5-HT_{2B} receptor activation (Roth, 2007). The mechanism for long-term depletion of brain 5-HT by the halogenated amphetamines remains controversial. A profound reduction in levels of 5-HT in the brain lasts for weeks and is accompanied by an equivalent loss of proteins (5-HT transporter and tryptophan hydroxylase) selectively localized in 5-HT neurons, suggesting that the halogenated amphetamines have a neurotoxic action. Despite these long-lasting biochemical deficits, neuroanatomical signs of neuronal death are not readily apparent. Another class of compounds, ring-substituted tryptamine derivatives such as 5,7-dihydroxytryptamine (Figure 13–1) produces unequivocal degeneration of 5-HT neurons. In adult animals, 5,7-dihydroxytryptamine selectively destroys serotonergic axon terminals; the remaining intact cell bodies allow eventual regeneration of axon terminals. In newborn animals, degeneration is permanent because 5,7-dihydroxytryptamine destroys serotonergic cell bodies as well as axon terminals.

5-HT RECEPTOR AGONISTS AND ANTAGONISTS

5-HT Receptor Agonists

Direct-acting 5-HT receptor agonists have widely different chemical structures, as well as diverse pharmacological properties (Table 13–5), as might be predicted from the multiplicity of 5-HT receptor subtypes. 5-HT_{1A} receptor–selective agonists have helped elucidate the functions of this receptor in the brain and have resulted in a new class of antianxiety drugs including buspirone (BUSPAR, others) and the investigational agents, gepirone and ipsapirone (Chapter 15). 5-$HT_{1B/1D}$ receptor–selective agonists, such as sumatriptan, have unique properties that result in constriction of intracranial blood vessels that are effective in the treatment of acute migraine attacks. A number of 5-HT_4 receptor–selective agonists have been developed or are being developed for the treatment of disorders of the GI tract (Chapter 46). These classes of selective 5-HT receptor agonists are discussed in more detail in the chapters that deal directly with treatment of the relevant pathological conditions.

5-HT Receptor Agonists and Migraine. Migraine headache afflicts 10-20% of the population. Although migraine is a specific neurological syndrome, the manifestations vary widely. The principal types are migraine without aura (common migraine); migraine with aura (classic migraine, which includes subclasses of migraine with typical aura, migraine with prolonged aura, migraine aura without headache, and migraine with acute-onset aura), and several rarer types. Premonitory aura may begin as long as 24 hours before the onset of pain and often is accompanied by

Table 13–5

Serotonergic Drugs: Primary Actions and Clinical Indications

RECEPTOR	ACTION	DRUG EXAMPLES	CLINICAL DISORDER
5-HT_{1A}	Partial agonist	Buspirone, ipsaperone	Anxiety, depression
5-HT_{1D}	Agonist	Sumatriptan	Migraine
$5\text{-HT}_{2A/2C}$	Antagonist	Methysergide, risperidone, ketanserin	Migraine, depression, schizophrenia
5-HT_{3}	Antagonist	Ondansetron	Chemotherapy-induced emesis
5-HT_{4}	Agonist	Cisapride	GI disorders
SERT (5-HT transporter)	Inhibitor	Fluoxetine, sertraline	Depression, obsessive-compulsive disorder, panic disorder, social phobia, post-traumatic stress disorder

photophobia, hyperacusis, polyuria, and diarrhea, and by disturbances of mood and appetite. A migraine attack may last for hours or days and be followed by prolonged pain-free intervals. The frequency of migraine attacks is extremely variable. Therapy of migraine headaches is complicated by the variable responses among and within individual patients and by the lack of a firm understanding of the pathophysiology of the syndrome. The efficacy of anti-migraine drugs varies with the absence or presence of aura, duration of the headache, its severity and intensity, and as yet undefined environmental and genetic factors (Silberstein, 2008).

The pathogenesis of migraine headache is complex, involving both neural and vascular elements (Mehrotra et al., 2008). Evidence suggesting that 5-HT is a key mediator in the pathogenesis of migraine includes:

- plasma and platelet concentrations of 5-HT vary with the different phases of the migraine attack
- urinary concentrations of 5-HT and its metabolites are elevated during most migraine attacks
- migraine may be precipitated by agents (e.g., reserpine and fenfluramine) that release 5-HT from intracellular storage sites

Consistent with the 5-HT hypothesis, 5-HT receptor agonists have become a mainstay for *acute* treatment of migraine headaches. Treatments for the *prevention* of migraines, such as β adrenergic antagonists and newer anti-epileptic drugs, have mechanisms of action that are, presumably, unrelated to 5-HT (Mehrotra et al., 2008).

5-HT_1 Receptor Agonists

The Triptans. The triptans are effective, acute anti-migraine agents. Their ability to decrease, rather than exacerbate, the nausea and vomiting of migraine is an important advance in the treatment of the condition. The selective pharmacological effects of the triptans at 5-HT_1 receptors has provided insights into the pathophysiology of migraine. Available compounds include almotriptan (AXERT), eletriptan (RELPAX), frovatriptan (FROVA), naratriptan (AMERGE), rizatriptan (MAXALT, others), sumatriptan (IMITREX, others), and zolmitriptan (ZOMIG). Sumatriptan for migraine headaches is also marketed in a fixed-dose combination with naproxen (TREXIMET).

History. Sumatriptan emerged from the first experimentally based approach to identify and develop a novel therapy for migraine. In 1972, Humphrey and colleagues initiated a project aimed at identifying novel therapeutic agents in the treatment of migraine with the goal of developing selective vasoconstrictors of the extracranial circulation, based on the theories of the etiology of migraine prevalent in the early 1970s (Humphrey et al., 1990). Sumatriptan, first synthesized in 1984, became available for clinical use in the United States in 1992; since then, several other triptans have been FDA-approved for clinical use. The second generation triptans have higher oral bioavailabilty.

Chemistry. The triptans are indole derivatives. Representative structures are given in Figure 13–5.

Pharmacological Properties. In contrast to ergot alkaloids (described later), the pharmacological effects of the triptans appear to be limited to the 5-HT_1 family of receptors, providing evidence that this receptor subclass plays an important role in the acute relief of a migraine attack. The triptans interact potently with 5-HT_{1B} and 5-HT_{1D} receptors and have a low or no affinity for other subtypes of 5-HT receptors, as well as α_1 and α_2 adrenergic, β adrenergic, dopaminergic, muscarinic cholinergic, and benzodiazepine receptors. Clinically effective doses of the triptans correlate well with their affinities for both 5-HT_{1B} and 5-HT_{1D} receptors, supporting the hypothesis that 5-HT_{1B} and/or 5-HT_{1D} receptors are the most likely receptors involved in the mechanism of action of acute anti-migraine drugs.

Mechanism of Action. There remains a controversy about the relative importance of vascular versus neurological dysfunction in migraine; thus the mechanism of the efficacy of $5\text{-HT}_{1B/1D}$ agonists in migraine is not resolved. One hypothesis implicates the capacity of these receptors to cause constriction of intracranial blood vessels including arteriovenous anastomoses. According to a prominent pathophysiological model of migraine, unknown events lead to the abnormal dilation of carotid arteriovenous anastomoses in the head and shunting of carotid arterial blood flow, producing cerebral ischemia and hypoxia. Based on this model, an effective anti-migraine agent would close the shunts and restore blood flow to the brain. Indeed,

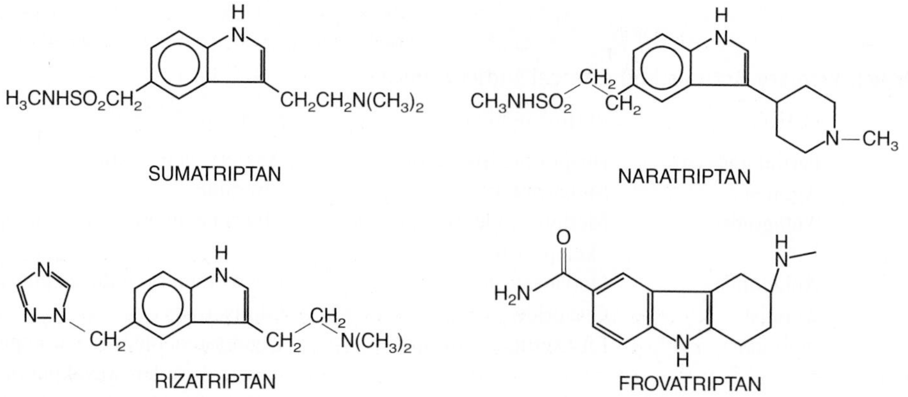

SUMATRIPTAN

NARATRIPTAN

RIZATRIPTAN

FROVATRIPTAN

Figure 13–5. *Structures of representative triptans (selective 5-HT_1 receptor agonists).*

ergotamine, dihydroergotamine, and sumatriptan share the capacity to produce this vascular effect with a pharmacological specificity that mirrors the effects of these agents on 5-HT_{1B} and 5-HT_{1D} receptor subtypes. An alternative hypothesis concerning the significance of one or more 5-HT_1 receptors in migraine pathophysiology relates to the observation that both 5-HT_{1B} and 5-HT_{1D} receptors serve as presynaptic autoreceptors, modulating neurotransmitter release from neuronal terminals (Figure 13–5). 5-HT_1 agonists may block the release of pro-inflammatory neuropeptides at the level of the nerve terminal in the perivascular space, which could account for their efficacy in the acute treatment of migraine.

Absorption, Fate, and Excretion. When given subcutaneously, sumatriptan reaches its peak plasma concentration in ~12 minutes. Following oral administration, peak plasma concentrations occur within 1-2 hours. Bioavailability following the subcutaneous route of administration is ~97%; after oral administration or nasal spray, bioavailability is only 14-17%. The elimination $t_{1/2}$ is ~1-2 hours. Sumatriptan is metabolized predominantly by MAO-A, and its metabolites are excreted in the urine.

Zolmitriptan reaches its peak plasma concentration 1.5-2 hours after oral administration. Its bioavailability is ~40% following oral ingestion. Zolmitriptan is converted to an active *N*-desmethyl metabolite, which has severalfold higher affinity for 5-HT_{1B} and 5-HT_{1D} receptors than does the parent drug. Both the metabolite and the parent drug have half-lives of 2-3 hours.

Naratriptan, administered orally, reaches its peak plasma concentration in 2-3 hours and has an absolute bioavailability of ~70%. It is the second longest acting of the triptans, having a $t_{1/2}$ of ~6 hours. Fifty percent of an administered dose of naratriptan is excreted unchanged in the urine, and ~30% is excreted as products of oxidation by CYPs.

Rizatriptan has an oral bioavailability of ~45% and reaches peak plasma levels within 1-1.5 hours after oral ingestion of tablets of the drug. An orally disintegrating dosage form has a somewhat slower rate of absorption, yielding peak plasma levels of the drug 1.6-2.5 hours after administration. The principal route of metabolism of rizatriptan is by oxidative deamination by MAO-A.

Plasma protein binding of the triptans ranges from ~14% (sumatriptan and rizatriptan) to 85% (eletriptan).

Adverse Effects and Contraindications. Rare but serious cardiac events have been associated with the administration of 5-HT_1 agonists, including coronary artery vasospasm, transient myocardial ischemia, atrial and ventricular arrhythmias, and myocardial infarction, predominantly in patients with risk factors for coronary artery disease. In general, however, only minor side effects are seen with the triptans in the acute treatment of migraine. After subcutaneous injection of sumatriptan, patients often experience irritation at the site of injection (transient mild pain, stinging, or burning sensations). The most common side effect of sumatriptan nasal spray is a bitter taste. Orally administered triptans can cause paresthesias; asthenia and fatigue; flushing; feelings of pressure, tightness, or pain in the chest, neck, and jaw; drowsiness; dizziness; nausea; and sweating.

The triptans are contraindicated in patients who have a history of ischemic or vasospastic coronary artery disease (including history of stroke or transient ischemic attacks), cerebrovascular or peripheral vascular disease, hemiplegic or basilar migraines, other significant cardiovascular diseases, or ischemic bowel diseases. Because triptans may cause an acute, usually small, increase in blood pressure, they also are contraindicated in patients with uncontrolled hypertension. Naratriptan is contraindicated in patients with severe renal or hepatic impairment. Rizatriptan should be used with caution in patients with renal or hepatic disease but is not contraindicated in such patients. Eletriptan is contraindicated in hepatic disease. Almotriptan, rizatriptan, sumatriptan, and zolmitriptan are contraindicated in patients who have taken a monoamine oxidase inhibitor within the preceding 2 weeks, and all triptans are contraindicated in patients with near-term prior exposure to ergot alkaloids or other 5-HT agonists.

Use in Treatment of Migraine. The triptans are effective in the acute treatment of migraine (with or without aura), but are not intended for use in prophylaxis of migraine. Treatment with triptans should begin as soon as possible after onset of a migraine attack. Oral dosage forms of the triptans are the most convenient to use, but they may not be practical in patients experiencing migraine-associated nausea and vomiting. Approximately 70% of individuals report significant headache relief from a 6-mg subcutaneous dose of sumatriptan. This dose may be repeated once within a 24-hour period if the first dose does not relieve the headache. An oral formulation and a nasal spray of sumatriptan also are available. The onset of action is as early as 15 minutes with the nasal spray. The recommended oral dose of sumatriptan is 25-100 mg, which may be repeated after 2 hours up to a total dose of 200 mg over a 24-hour period. When administered by nasal spray, from 5-20 mg of sumatriptan is recommended, repeatable after 2 hours up to a maximum dose of 40 mg over a 24-hour period. Zolmitriptan is given orally in a dose of 1.25-2.5 mg, which can be repeated after 2 hours, up to a maximum dose of 10 mg over 24 hours if the migraine attack persists. Naratriptan is given orally in a dose of 1-2.5 mg, which should not be repeated until 4 hours after the previous dose. The maximum dose over a 24-hour period should not exceed 5 mg. The recommended oral dose of rizatriptan is 5-10 mg. The dose can be repeated after 2 hours up to a maximum dose of 30 mg over a 24-hour period. The safety of treating more than 3 or 4 headaches over a 30-day period with triptans has not been established. No triptan should be used concurrently with (or within 24 hours of) an ergot derivative (described later) or another triptan.

Ergot and the Ergot Alkaloids. The elucidation of the constituents of ergot and their complex actions was an important chapter in the evolution of modern pharmacology, even though the very complexity of their actions limits their therapeutic uses. The pharmacological effects of the ergot alkaloids are varied and complex; in general, the effects result from their actions as partial agonists or antagonists at serotonergic, dopaminergic, and adrenergic receptors. The spectrum of effects depends on the agent, dosage, species, tissue, physiological and endocrinological state, and experimental conditions.

History. Ergot is the product of a fungus (*Claviceps purpurea*) that grows on rye and other grains. The contamination of an edible grain by a poisonous, parasitic fungus spread death for centuries. As early as 600 B.C., an Assyrian tablet alluded to a "noxious pustule in the ear of grain." Written descriptions of ergot poisoning first appeared in the Middle Ages, describing strange epidemics in which the characteristic symptom was gangrene of the feet, legs, hands, and arms. In severe cases, extremities became dry and black, and mummified limbs separated off without loss of blood. Limbs were said to be consumed by the holy fire, blackened like charcoal with agonizing burning sensations, the disease was called holy fire or St. Anthony's fire in honor of the saint at whose shrine relief was said to be obtained. The relief that followed migration to the shrine of St. Anthony was probably real, for the sufferers received a diet free of contaminated grain during their sojourn at the shrine. The symptoms of ergot poisoning were not restricted to limbs. A frequent complication of it was a dramatic abortive effect of ergot ingested during pregnancy. The active principles of ergot were isolated and chemically identified in the early 20th century.

Chemistry. The ergot alkaloids can all be considered to be derivatives of the tetracyclic compound 6-methylergoline (Table 13–6). The naturally occurring alkaloids contain a substituent in the beta configurations at position 8 and a double bond in ring D. The natural alkaloids of therapeutic interest are amide derivatives of *d*-lysergic acid. The first pure ergot alkaloid, ergotamine, was obtained in 1920, followed by the isolation of ergonovine in 1932. Numerous semi-synthetic derivatives of the ergot alkaloids have been prepared by catalytic hydrogenation of the natural alkaloids (e.g., dihydroergotamine). Another synthetic derivative, bromocriptine (2-bromo-α-ergocryptine), is used to control the secretion of prolactin, a property derived from its DA agonist effect. Other products of this series include lysergic acid diethylamide (LSD), a potent hallucinogen, and methysergide, a serotonin antagonist.

Absorption, Fate, and Excretion. The oral administration of ergotamine by itself generally results in low or undetectable systemic drug concentrations, because of extensive first-pass metabolism. The bioavailability after administration of rectal suppositories is greater. Ergotamine is metabolized in the liver by largely undefined pathways, and 90% of the metabolites are excreted in the bile. Despite a plasma $t_{1/2}$ of ~2 hours, ergotamine produces vasoconstriction that lasts for 24 hours or longer. Dihydroergotamine is eliminated more rapidly than ergotamine, presumably due to its rapid hepatic clearance.

Ergonovine and methylergonovine are rapidly absorbed after oral administration and reach peak concentrations in plasma within 60-90 minutes that are more than 10-fold those achieved with an equivalent dose of ergotamine. Although often given IV, an uterotonic effect in postpartum women can be observed within 10 minutes after oral administration of 0.2 mg of ergonovine. The $t_{1/2}$ of methylergonovine in plasma ranges between 0.5 and 2 hours.

Use in the Treatment of Migraine. The multiple pharmacological effects of ergot alkaloids have complicated the determination of their precise mechanism of action in the acute treatment of migraine. Based on the mechanism of action of sumatriptan and other $5\text{-HT}_{1B/1D}$ receptor agonists, the actions of ergot alkaloids at $5\text{-HT}_{1B/1D}$ receptors likely mediate their *acute* anti-migraine effects.

The use of ergot alkaloids for migraine should be restricted to patients having frequent, moderate migraine or infrequent, severe migraine attacks. As with other medications used to abort an attack, ergot preparations should be administered as soon as possible after the onset of a headache. GI absorption of ergot alkaloids is erratic, perhaps contributing to the large variation in patient response to these drugs. Available preparations currently in the United States include sublingual tablets of ergotamine tartrate (ERGOMAR) and a nasal spray and solution for injection of dihydroergotamine mesylate (MIGRANAL, D.H.E. 45, respectively). Ergotamine in fixed-dose combinations with caffeine is also marketed under the brand names of CAFERGOT (oral tablets) and MIGERGOT (rectal suppositories) and as generic formulations (oral tablets). The recommended dose for ergotamine tartrate is 2 mg sublingually, which can be repeated at 30-minute intervals if necessary up to a total dose of 6 mg in a 24-hour period or 10 mg a week. Dihydroergotamine mesylate injections can be given intravenously, subcutaneously, or intramuscularly. The recommended dose is 1 mg, which can be repeated after 1 hour if necessary up to a total dose of 2 mg (intravenously) or 3 mg (subcutaneously or intramuscularly) in a 24-hour period or 6 mg in a week. The dose of dihydroergotamine mesylate administered as a nasal spray is 0.5 mg (one spray) in each nostril, repeated after 15 minutes for a total dose of 2 mg (4 sprays). The safety of > 3 mg over 24 hours or 4 mg over 7 days has not been established.

Adverse Effects and Contraindications of Ergot Alkaloids. Nausea and vomiting, due to a direct effect on CNS emetic centers, occur in ~10% of patients after oral administration of ergotamine, and in

Table 13–6

Natural and Semisynthetic Ergot Alkaloids

A. AMINE ALKALOIDS AND CONGENERS

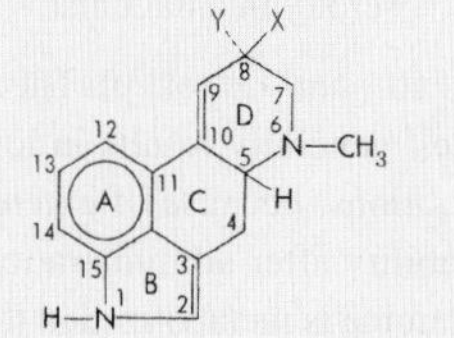

ALKALOID	X	Y
d-Lysergic acid	—COOH	—H
d-Isolysergic acid	—H	—COOH
d-Lysergic acid diethylamide (LSD)	$-C(=O)-N(CH_2CH_3)_2$	—H
Ergonovine (ergometrine)	$-C(=O)-NH-CH(CH_3)CH_2OH$	—H
Methylergonovine	$-C(=O)-NH-CH(CH_2CH_3)CH_2OH$	—H
Methysergide[a]	$-C(=O)-NH-CH(CH_2CH_3)CH_2OH$	—H
Lisuride[b]	—H	$-NH-C(=O)-N(CH_2CH_3)_2$
Lysergol	$-CH_2OH$	—H
Lergotrile[c]	$-CH_2CN$	—H
Metergoline[a,b]	$-CH_2-NH-C(=O)-O-CH_2-$phenyl	—H

B. AMINO ACID ALKALOIDS

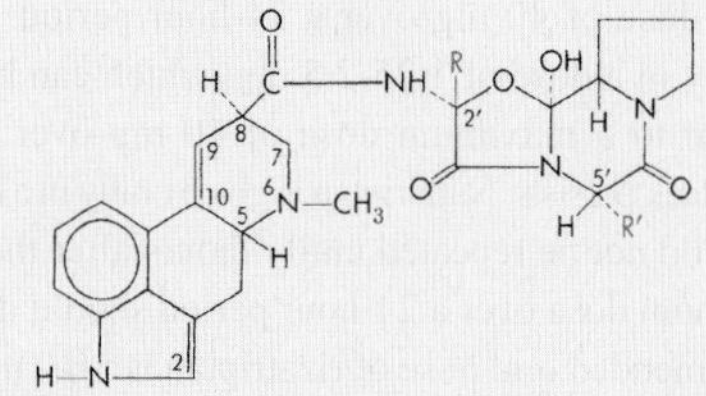

ALKALOID[d]	R(2′)	R′(5′)
Ergotamine	$-CH_3$	$-CH_2-$phenyl
Ergosine	$-CH_3$	$-CH_2CH(CH_3)_2$
Ergostine	$-CH_2CH_3$	$-CH_2-$phenyl
Ergotoxine group:		
Ergocornine	$-CH(CH_3)_2$	$-CH(CH_3)_2$
Ergocristine	$-CH(CH_3)_2$	$-CH_2-$phenyl
α-Ergocryptine	$-CH(CH_3)_2$	$-CH_2CH(CH_3)_2$
β-Ergocryptine	$-CH(CH_3)_2$	$-CH(CH_3)CH_2CH_3$
Bromocriptine[e]	$-CH(CH_3)_2$	$-CH_2CH(CH_3)_2$

[a]Contains methyl substitution at N1. [b]Contains hydrogen atoms at C9 and C10. [c]Contains chlorine atom at C2. [d]Dihydro derivatives contain hydrogen atoms at C9 and C10. [e]Contains bromine atom at C2.

about twice that number after parenteral administration. This side effect is problematic, since nausea and sometimes vomiting are part of the symptomatology of a migraine headache. Leg weakness is common, and muscle pains that occasionally are severe may occur in the extremities. Numbness and tingling of fingers and toes are other reminders of the ergotism that this alkaloid may cause. Precordial distress and pain suggestive of angina pectoris, as well as transient tachycardia or bradycardia, also have been noted, presumably as a result of coronary vasospasm induced by ergotamine. Localized edema and itching may occur in an occasional hypersensitive patient, but usually do not necessitate interruption of ergotamine therapy. In the event of acute or chronic poisoning (ergotism), treatment consists of complete withdrawal of the offending drug and symptomatic measures to maintain adequate circulation by agents such as anticoagulants, low-molecular-weight dextran, and potent vasodilator drugs such as intravenous sodium nitroprusside. Dihydroergotamine has lower potency than does ergotamine as an emetic, vasoconstrictor, and oxytocic.

Ergot alkaloids are contraindicated in women who are, or may become, pregnant because the drugs may cause fetal distress and miscarriage. Ergot alkaloids also are contraindicated in patients with peripheral vascular disease, coronary artery disease, hypertension, impaired hepatic or renal function, and sepsis. Ergot alkaloids should not be taken within 24 hours of the use of the triptans, and should not be used concurrently with other drugs that can cause vasoconstriction.

Use of Ergot Alkaloids in Postpartum Hemorrhage. All of the natural ergot alkaloids markedly increase the motor activity of the uterus. After small doses, uterine contractions are increased in force or frequency, or both, but are followed by a normal degree of relaxation. As the dose is increased, contractions become more forceful and prolonged, resting tone is dramatically increased, and sustained contracture can result. Although this characteristic precludes their use for induction or facilitation of labor, it is quite compatible with their use postpartum or after abortion to control bleeding and maintain uterine contraction. The gravid uterus is very sensitive, and small doses of ergot alkaloids can be given immediately postpartum to obtain a marked uterine response, usually without significant side effects. In current obstetric practice, ergot alkaloids are used primarily to prevent postpartum hemorrhage. Although all natural ergot alkaloids have qualitatively the same effect on the uterus, ergonovine is the most active and also is less toxic than ergotamine. For these reasons ergonovine (ERGOTRATE) and its semisynthetic derivative methylergonovine (METHERGINE, others) have replaced other ergot preparations as uterine-stimulating agents in obstetrics.

Methysergide. Methysergide (SANSERT; 1-methyl-*d*-lysergic acid butanolamide) is a congener of methylergonovine (Table 13–6). Reflecting the fickle nature of the ergot compounds, methysergide is neither a selective antagonist nor always an antagonist. It interacts with 5-HT_1 receptors, but its therapeutic effects appear primarily to reflect blockade of 5-HT_2 receptors; it blocks 5-HT_{2A} and 5-HT_{2C} receptors, but has partial agonist activity in some preparations. Although methysergide is an ergot derivative, it has only weak vasoconstrictor and oxytocic activity.

Methysergide is without benefit when given during an acute migraine attack but has been used for the prophylactic treatment of migraine and other vascular headaches, including Horton's syndrome. A potentially serious complication of prolonged treatment is inflammatory fibrosis, giving rise to various syndromes that include retroperitoneal fibrosis, pleuropulmonary fibrosis, and coronary and endocardial fibrosis. Usually the fibrosis regresses after drug withdrawal, although persistent cardiac valvular damage has been reported. Because of this danger, other drugs are preferred for the prophylactic treatment of migraine (see the earlier discussion of migraine therapy). If methysergide is used chronically, treatment should be interrupted for 3 weeks or more every 6 months. Methysergide is not available in the U.S.

D-Lysergic Acid Diethylamide (LSD). Of the many drugs that are nonselective 5-HT agonists, LSD (see structure in Table 13–6) is the most remarkable. This ergot derivative profoundly alters human behavior, eliciting perception disturbances such as sensory distortion (especially visual) and hallucinations at doses as low as 1 μg/kg. The potent, mind-altering effects of LSD explain its abuse by humans (Chapter 24), as well as the fascination of scientists with the mechanism of action of LSD.

LSD was synthesized in 1943 by Albert Hoffman, who discovered its unique properties by accidental ingestion of the drug. The chemical precursor, lysergic acid, occurs naturally in a fungus that grows on wheat and rye but is devoid of hallucinogenic actions. LSD contains an indolealkylamine moiety embedded within its structure, and early investigators postulated that it would interact with 5-HT receptors. Indeed, LSD interacts with brain 5-HT receptors as an agonist/partial agonist. LSD mimics 5-HT at 5-HT_{1A} autoreceptors on raphe cell bodies, producing a marked slowing of the firing rate of serotonergic neurons. In the raphe, LSD and 5-HT are equi-effective; however, in areas of serotonergic axonal projections (such as visual relay centers), LSD is far less effective than is 5-HT. In an animal behavioral model thought to reflect the subjective effects of abused drugs, the discriminative stimulus effects of LSD and other hallucinogenic drugs appear to be mediated by activation of 5-HT_{2A} receptors (Winter, 2009). Recent studies of 5-HT_{2A} receptor knockout mice confirm the critical role for this receptor in LSD hallucinogenic effects (González-Maeso et al., 2007). LSD also interacts potently with many other 5-HT receptors, including cloned receptors whose functions have not yet been determined. On the other hand, the hallucinogenic phenethylamine derivatives such as 1-(4-bromo-2,5-dimethoxyphenyl)-2-aminopropane are selective 5-$HT_{2A/2C}$ receptor agonists. Current theories of the mechanism of action of LSD and other hallucinogens focus on 5-HT_{2A} receptor-mediated disruption of thalamic gating with sensory overload of the cortex (Geyer and Vollenweider, 2008). Progress in understanding the unusual properties of hallucinogens are arising from clinical investigations. For example, positron emission tomography imaging studies revealed that administration of the hallucinogen psilocybin (the active component of "shrooms") mimics the pattern of brain activation found in schizophrenic patients experiencing hallucinations. Consistent with animal studies, this action of psilocybin is blocked by pretreatment with a 5-$HT_{2A/2C}$ antagonist.

8-Hydroxy-(2-N,N-Dipropylamino)-Tetraline (8-OH-DPAT). This prototypic 5-HT_{1A}-selective receptor agonist is a valuable experimental tool.

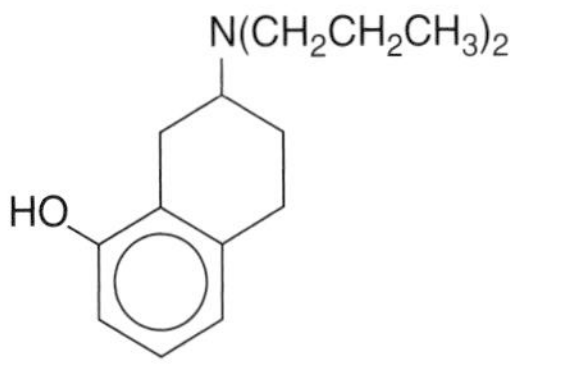

$N(CH_2CH_2CH_3)_2$

HO

8-OH-DPAT

8-OH-DPAT is considered to be a 5-HT_{1A} selective agonist. It does not interact with other members of the 5-HT_1-receptor subfamily or with 5-HT_2, 5-HT_3, or 5-HT_4 receptors, although activation of the 5-HT_7 receptor has been reported. 8-OHDPAT reduces the firing rate of raphe cells by activating 5-HT_{1A} autoreceptors and inhibits neuronal firing in terminal fields (e.g., hippocampus) by direct interaction with postsynaptic 5-HT_{1A} receptors.

Buspirone (BUSPAR, *others*). A series of long-chain arylpiperazines, such as buspirone, gepirone, and ipsapirone, are selective partial agonists at 5-HT_{1A} receptors. Other closely related arylpiperazines act as 5-HT_{1A}-receptor antagonists. Buspirone, the first clinically available drug in this series, has been effective in the treatment of anxiety (Chapter 15). Buspirone mimics the antianxiety properties of benzodiazepines but does not interact with $GABA_A$ receptors and or display the sedative and anticonvulsant properties of benzodiazepeines. The absence of sedative effects may explain why patients prefer the benzodiazepines to relieve anxiety.

m-Chlorophenylpiperazine (mCPP). The actions of mCPP *in vivo* primarily reflect activation of 5-HT_{1B} and/or 5-$HT_{2A/2C}$ receptors, although this agent is not subtype selective in radioligand-binding studies *in vitro*.

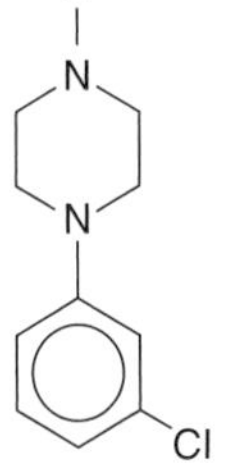

H
N
N
Cl

mCPP

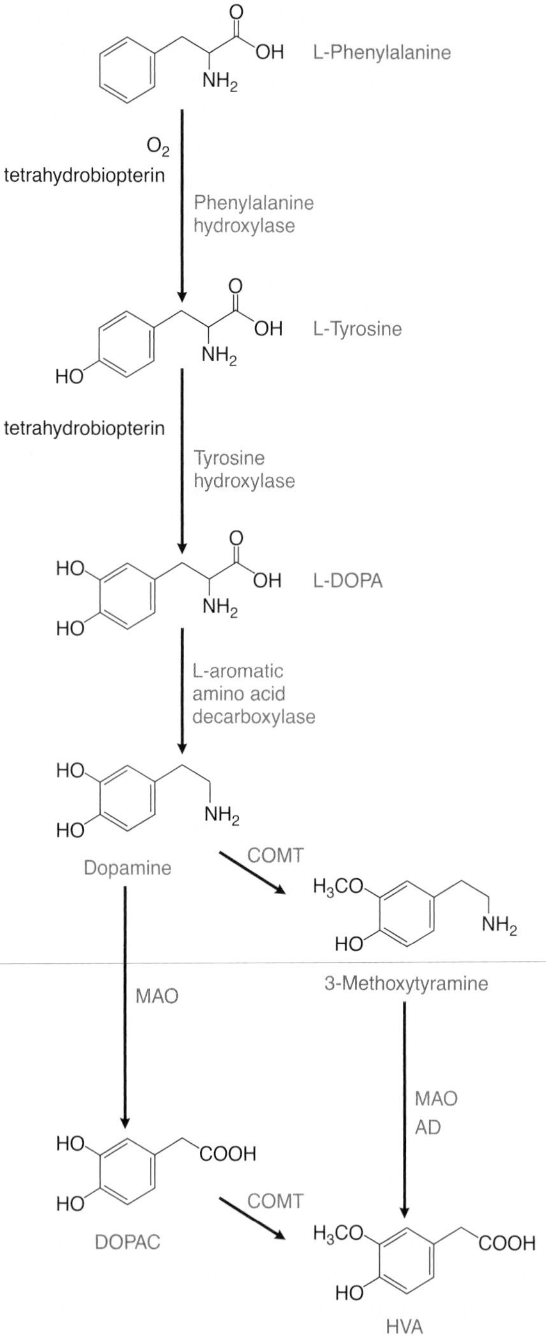

Figure 13–6. *Synthesis and inactivation of dopamine.* Enzymes are identified in blue lettering, and co-factors are shown in black letters.

(Chapter 8). Four alternatively spliced isoforms of tyrosine hydroxylase have been identified in humans, which is in contrast to many non-human primates (two isoforms) and rat (one isoform). At present, it is unclear if these various isoforms play different roles. Once generated, L-DOPA is rapidly converted to DA by AADC, the same enzyme that generates 5-HT from L-5-hydroxytryptophan. In the CNS and periphery, AADC activity is very high, and basal levels of L-DOPA cannot be readily measured. Unlike DA, L-DOPA readily crosses the blood-brain barrier and is converted to DA in the brain, which explains its utility in therapy for Parkinson disease (Chapter 22).

The neurochemical events that underlie DA neurotransmission are summarized in Figure 13–7. In dopaminergic neurons, synthesized DA is packaged into secretory vesicles (or into granules within adrenal chromaffin cells) by the vesicular monoamine transporter, VMAT2. This packaging allows DA to be stored in readily releasable aliquots and protects the transmitter from further anabolism or catabolism. By contrast, in adrenergic or noradrenergic cells, the DA is not packaged; instead, it is converted to NE by DA β-hydroxylase and, in adrenergic cells, further altered to epinephrine in cells expressing phenylethanolamine *N*-methyltransferase (Chapter 8). Synaptically released DA is subject to both transporter clearance and metabolism. The DA transporter (DAT) is not selective for DA; moreover, DA can also be cleared from the synapse by the NE transporter, NET. Reuptake of DA by the DA transporter is the primary mechanism for termination of DA action, and allows for either vesicular repackaging of transmitter or metabolism. The DA transporter is regulated by phosphorylation, offering the potential for DA to regulate its own uptake.

The DA transporter is predominantly localized perisynaptically so that DA is cleared at a distance from its release site, suggesting that high concentrations of DA are released into the synapse, thus necessitating a spatially distant transporter. In addition to clearing synaptic neurotransmitter, the DA transporter is a site of action for cocaine and methamphetamine, which have distinct mechanisms to increase extracellular DA. The DA transporter is also the molecular target for some neurotoxins, including 6-hydroxydopamine and 1-methyl-4-phenylpyridium (MPP+), the neurotoxic metabolite of 1-methyl-4-phenyl-1,2,3,6-tetrahydropyridine (MPTP). Following uptake into dopaminergic neurons, MPP+ and 6-hydroxydopamine elicit intra- and extracellular DA release, ultimately resulting in neuronal death. This selective dopaminergic degeneration mimics Parkinson disease, and serves as an animal model for this disorder.

Metabolism of DA occurs primarily by the cellular MAO enzymes localized on both pre- and postsynaptic elements. MAO acts on DA to generate an inactive aldehyde derivative by oxidative deamination (Figures 13–6 and 13-7), which is subsequently metabolized by aldehyde dehydrogenase to form 3,4-dihydroxyphenylacetic acid (DOPAC).

DOPAC can be further metabolized by catechol-*O*-methyltransferase (COMT) to form homovanillic acid (HVA). Both DOPAC and HVA, as well as DA, are excreted in the urine. Levels of DOPAC and HVA are reliable indicators of DA turnover; ratios of these metabolites to DA in cerebral spinal fluid serve as accurate representations of brain dopaminergic activity. In addition to metabolizing DOPAC, COMT also utilizes DA as a substrate to generate 3-methoxytyramine, which is subsequently converted to HVA by MAO. In humans, HVA is the principal metabolite of DA. COMT in

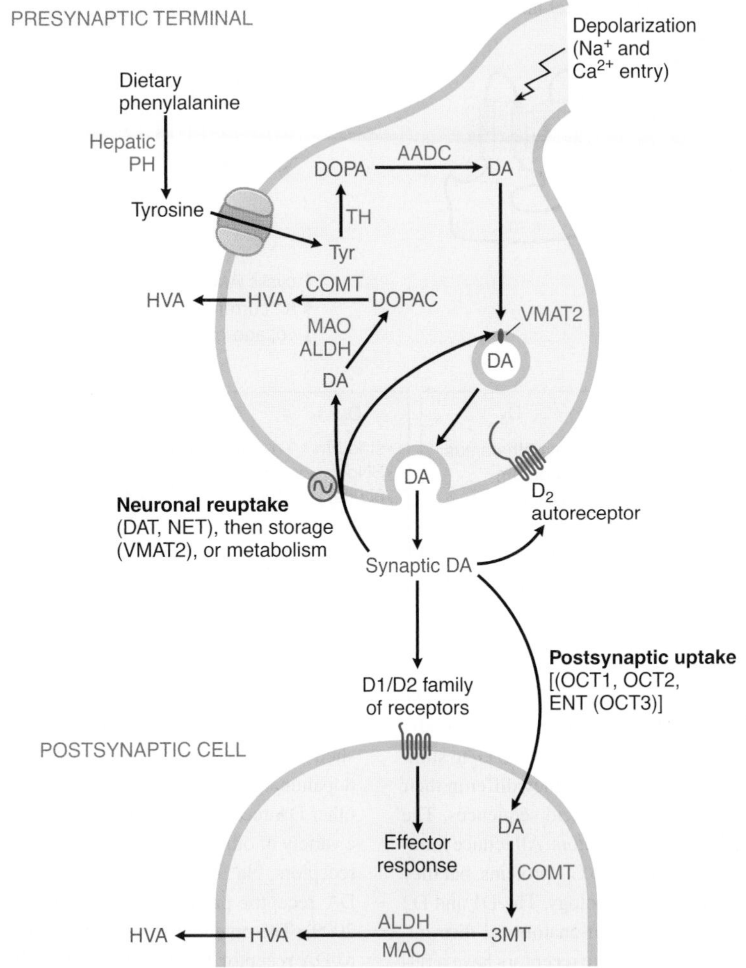

Figure 13–7. *Dopaminergic nerve terminal.* Dopamine (DA) is synthesized from tyrosine in the nerve terminal by the sequential actions of tyrosine hydrolase (TH) and aromatic amino acid decarboxylase (AADC). DA is sequestered by VMAT2 in storage granules and released by exocytosis. Synaptic DA activates presynaptic autoreceptors and postsynaptic D1 and D2 receptors. Synaptic DA may be taken up into the neuron via the DA and NE transporters (DAT, NET), or removed by postsynaptic uptake via OCT3 transporters. Cytosolic DA is subject to degradation by monoamine oxidase (MAO) and aldehyde dehydrogenase (ALDH) in the neuron, and by catechol-O-methyl tranferase (COMT) and MAO/ALDH in non-neuronal cells; the final metabolic product is homovanillic acid (HVA). See structures in Figure 13-6. PH, phenylalanine hydroxylase.

the periphery also metabolizes L-DOPA to 3-O-methyldopa, which then competes with L-DOPA for uptake into the CNS. Consequently, L-DOPA given in the treatment of Parkinson disease must be co-administered with peripheral COMT inhibitors to preserve L-DOPA and allow sufficient entry into the CNS (Chapter 22).

PHYSIOLOGICAL FUNCTIONS OF DOPAMINE

Multiple DA Receptors

Five distinct GPCRs have been cloned and determined to mediate the actions of DA (Figure 13–8). Though the cloning and classification of these receptors was initially based on mammalian studies, subsequent experimentation has revealed similar DA receptor groups in both vertebrate and invertebrate systems. The DA receptors are distinct from one another in pharmacology, amino acid sequence, distribution, and physiological function. They have been organized into two families—the D1-like and D2-like receptors—based upon their effector-coupling profile (for a recent review of DA receptors, see Rankin et al., 2009).

History of DA Receptor Subtypes. In 1971, Kebabian and Greengard determined that DA caused an increase in neostriatal cyclic AMP production, presumably by activating a DA-sensitive adenylyl cyclase enzyme. Subsequently, the DA-induced increase in cyclic AMP was attributed to a D1 receptor while a second category of DA receptors that did not raise cyclic AMP levels was termed the D2 receptor. Differences in pharmacological responsiveness gave rise to the hypothesis that there were multiple subtypes of DA

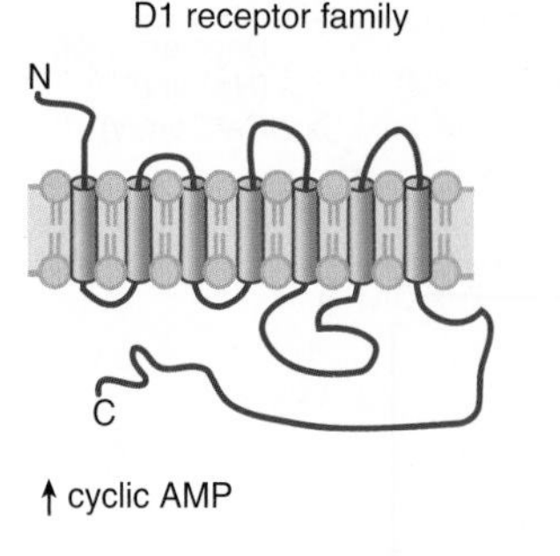

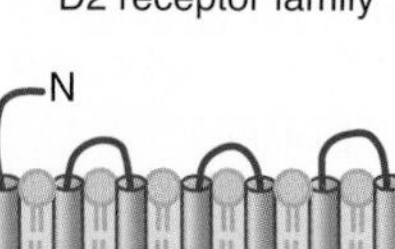

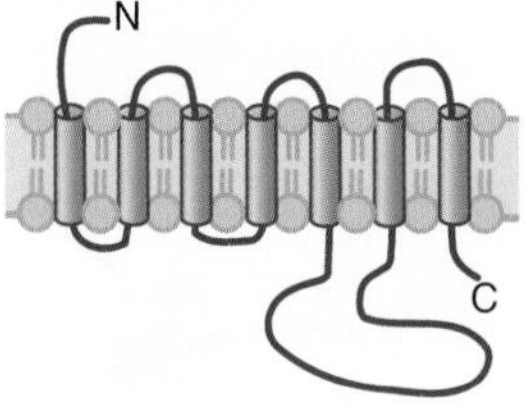

↓ cyclic AMP
↑ K^+ currents
↓ voltage-gated Ca^{2+} currents

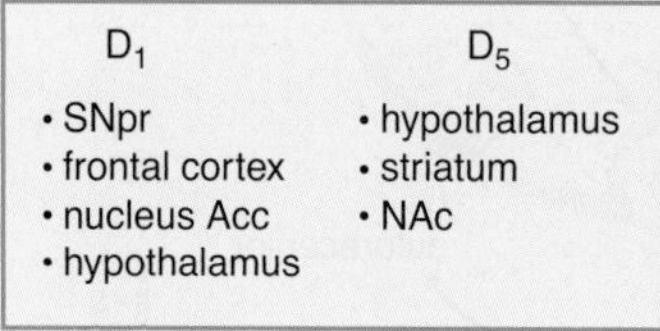

D_1	D_5
• SNpr • frontal cortex • nucleus Acc • hypothalamus	• hypothalamus • striatum • NAc

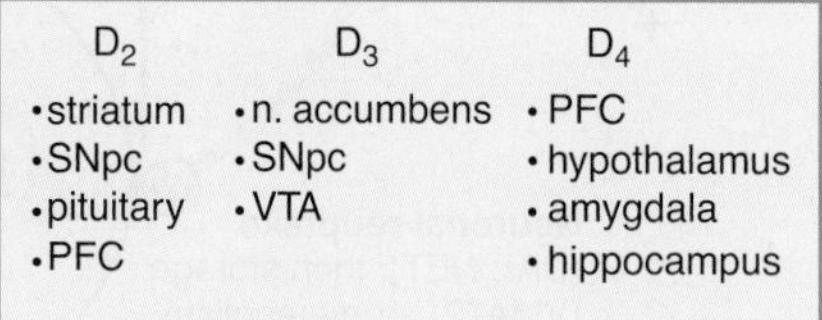

D_2	D_3	D_4
• striatum • SNpc • pituitary • PFC	• n. accumbens • SNpc • VTA	• PFC • hypothalamus • amygdala • hippocampus

Figure 13–8. *Distribution and characterization of DA receptors in the CNS.*

receptors beyond the D1 and D2. This idea proved to be correct. The D1 subfamily consists of the D_1 and D_5 receptor subtypes (initially classified as D_{1A} and D_{1B}); both are GPCRs that couple to G_s to stimulate cellular cyclic AMP production couple, but they differ in their pharmacological profiles and primary amino acid sequences. The D2 subfamily contains the D_2, D_3, and D_4 receptors. All reduce intracellular cyclic AMP production by coupling to $G_{i/o}$ proteins, but they diverge in amino acid sequence and pharmacology. The D1 and D2 families can be further differentiated by their anatomical distribution and by structural differences—the D1-like receptors have a relatively long carboxyl terminus and a short third intracellular loop.

D_1 Receptors. The D_1 receptor is the most highly conserved and the most highly expressed of the DA receptors. The highest levels of D_1 receptor protein are found within the CNS, particularly in the caudate putamen, substantia nigra pars reticulata, nucleus accumbens, hypothalamus, frontal cortex, and olfactory bulb. The D_1 receptor is also located in the kidney, retina, and cardiovascular system. Cloning reveals that the D_1 receptor lacks introns and encodes a protein that is 446 amino acids long in the human. The D_1 receptor couples primarily to $G\alpha_s$, activating the cAMP-PKA pathway. However, the neostriatum expresses the highest levels of D_1 receptor, but does not express any detectable $G\alpha_s$ protein. In this region of the brain, the D_1 receptor appears to couple to G_{olf} to increase levels of cAMP and its downstream effectors (for a review of dopaminergic signaling, see Neve et al., 2004).

Reports of D_1 receptors coupling to G_q raised the possibility that a third D1-like receptor might exist; there also are D_1-D_2 receptor heterodimers that couple to the G_q signaling cascade (Lee et al., 2004). The presence of a functionally distinct heterodimer with a unique dopaminergic pharmacology is a novel concept that could shed new light on the actions of DA and drugs acting on the dopaminergic system. In addition to forming protein complexes with other DA receptors, the D_1 receptor has been shown to interact with a variety of other proteins, including A_1 adenosine receptors, NMDA receptors, Na^+,K^+-ATPase, calnexin, and caveolin (for a review of DA receptor protein-protein interactions, see Hazelwood et al., 2009). The potential significance of these interactions with respect to DA receptor function and potential pharmacotherapies has not been fully realized.

D_2 Receptors. The D_2 receptor was the first dopamine receptor to be cloned. It is expressed throughout the brain, including the striatum, nucleus accumbens, olfactory tubercule, prefrontal cortex, amygdala, ventral tegmental area, hippocampus, hypothalamus, and substantia nigra pars compacta. Unlike the D_1 receptor, the D_2 receptor contains six introns and exists as either a long or short splice variant. The D_2 short (D_{2S}) receptor is missing 29 amino acids in the third intracellular loop that are present in the D_2 long (D_{2L}) receptor variant. The D_{2L} receptor is the more predominantly expressed variant in the brain and occurs primarily post-synaptically, where it likely regulates impulse/signal propagation (Usiello et al., 2000). The D_{2S} variant is primarily expressed pre-synaptically and likely acts to limit DA release. The D_{2S} and D_{2L} receptors have similar pharmacological properties and both function as autoreceptors, inhibiting cAMP formation by coupling to $G_{i/o}$.

D_2 receptor signaling through $G_{\beta\gamma}$ also regulates a variety of cellular functions, including inwardly rectifying K^+ channels, N-type

Ca^{2+} channels, arachidonic acid levels (via PLA_2), extracellular signal-regulated kinase, and IP_3-sensitive Ca^{2+} stores and L-type Ca^{2+} channels. The D_2 receptor has the ability to activate $G_{i/o}$ proteins independent of agonist, a property known as constitutive activity (Strange, 1999). As with the D_1 receptor, the D_2 DA receptor can also form stable complexes with other proteins, including the AMPA receptor, Na^+,K^+-ATPase, calnexin, and the DA transporter (Hazelwood et al., 2009).

D_3 Receptors. The D_3 receptor contains five introns. It is less abundant than the D_2 receptor, and is only expressed in the limbic regions of the brain. The highest levels of the D_3 receptor are found in the islands of Calleja, nucleus accumbens, substantia nigra pars compacta, and ventral tegmental area. Splice variants of the human D_3 receptor exist, but do not code functional protein products. The D_3 receptor signals through pertussis toxin-sensitive $G_{i/o}$ proteins, though not as effectively as the D_2 receptor.

D_4 Receptors. The D_4 receptor contains three introns. It is abundantly expressed in the retina, and is also found in the hypothalamus, prefrontal cortex, amygdala, hippocampus, and pituitary. D_4 is the most polymorphic of the DA receptors, containing a variable number of tandem repeats (VNTR) within the third intracellular loop (Van Tol et al., 1992). In humans, the four-repeat variant is the most common. There are several single nucleotide polymorphisms (SNPs) in the D_4 receptor, one of which results in dramatic alterations in ligand binding (Liu et al., 1996). There are associations between a seven-repeat D_4 VNTR variant and attention deficit hyperactivity disorder (see below).

D_5 Receptors. The D_5 gene, like the D_1 gene, is intronless. Pseudogenes of the D_5 receptor yield protein products with no known functional role. Like the D_4 receptor, the D_5 gene is polymorphic; several functional SNPs within the transmembrane domains alter binding properties of numerous ligands, including DA (Cravchik and Gejman, 1999). The D_5 receptor couples primarily to G_s and exhibits ligand-independent constitutive activity. The D_5 receptor also activates G_z, but the functional consequences of this interaction remain unclear. The D_5 receptor is most highly expressed in the substantia nigra, hypothalamus, striatum, cerebral cortex, nucleus accumbens, and olfactory tubercle.

Actions of DA on Physiologic Systems

Heart and Vasculature. At low concentrations, circulating DA primarily stimulates vascular D_1 receptors, causing vasodilation and reducing cardiac afterload. The net result is a decrease in blood pressure and an increase in cardiac contractility. As circulating DA concentrations rise, DA is able to activate β adrenergic receptors to further increase cardiac contractility. At very high concentrations, circulating DA activates α adrenergic receptors in the vasculature, thereby causing vasoconstriction; thus, high concentrations of DA increase blood pressure. Clinically, DA administration is used to treat severe congestive heart failure, sepsis, or cardiogenic shock. It is only administered intravenously and is not considered a long-term treatment.

Kidney. DA is a paracrine/autocrine transmitter in the kidney and binds to both D1-like and D2-like receptors. Renal DA primarily serves to increase natriuresis, though it can also increase renal blood flow and glomerular filtration. Under basal sodium conditions, DA regulates Na^+ excretion by inhibiting the activity of various Na^+ transporters, including the apical Na^+-H^+ exchanger and the basolateral Na^+,K^+-ATPase. DA can also influence the renin–angiotensin system: activation of D_1 receptors increases renin secretion, whereas DA, acting on D_3 receptors, reduces renin secretion. Abnormalities in the DA system and its receptors have been implicated in human hypertension (Jose et al., 1998). In some cases, poor regulation of natriuresis occurs due to constitutive desensitization of the D_1 receptor and uncoupling of the receptor from the signal transduction machinery. Although multiple polymorphisms exist in the DA receptors, none has been consistently associated with human hypertension.

Pituitary Gland. DA is the primary regulator of prolactin secretion from the pituitary gland. DA is released from the hypothalamus into the hypophyseal portal blood supply, directly infusing lactotrophs in the pituitary with high concentrations of DA. DA acts on lactotroph D_{2S} and D_{2L} receptors to decrease prolactin secretion (Chapter 38).

Catecholamine Release. Both D_1 and D_2 receptors modulate the release of NE and epinephrine. The D_2 receptor provides tonic inhibition of epinephrine release from chromaffin cells of the adrenal medulla, and of norepinephrine release from sympathetic nerve terminals. In contrast, the D_1 receptor responds to high-frequency DA stimulation to promote the release of catecholamines from the adrenal medulla. This D_1 receptor stimulation is thought to contribute to the "fight or flight" response.

CNS. DA in the brain projects via four main pathways (Figure 13–9)—mesolimbic, mesocortical, nigrostriatal and tuberoinfundibular—to regulate a variety of functions. The physiological processes under dopaminergic control include reward, emotion, cognition, memory, and motor activity. Dysregulation of the dopaminergic system is critical in a number of disease states, including Parkinson disease, Tourette's syndrome, bipolar depression, schizophrenia, attention-deficit hyperactivity disorder, and addiction/substance abuse.

The mesolimbic pathway is associated with reward and, less so, with learned behaviors. Dysfunction in this pathway is associated with addiction, schizophrenia, and psychoses (including bipolar depression), and learning deficits. The mesocortical pathway is important for "higher-order" cognitive functions including motivation, reward, emotion, and impulse control. It is also implicated in psychoses, including schizophrenia, and in attention-deficit hyperactivity disorder. The mesolimbic and mesocortical pathways are sometimes grouped together as mesolimbocortical. The nigrostriatal pathway is a key regulator of movement (Chapter 22). Impairments in this pathway are evident in Parkinson disease and underlie

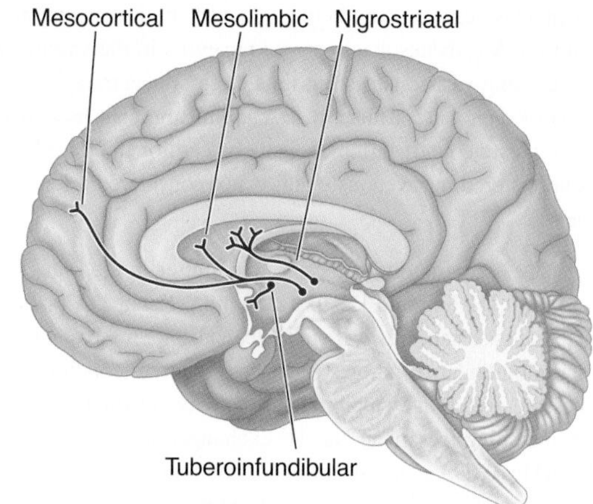

Figure 13–9. *Major DA pathways in brain.*

detrimental movement side effects associated with dopaminergic therapy, including tardive dyskinesia. DA released in the tuberoinfundibular pathway is carried by the hypophyseal blood supply to the pituitary, where it regulates prolactin secretion.

Electrophysiology. DA receptors regulate multiple distinct voltage-gated ion channels that impact firing of action potentials and neural transmission. D1-like receptor activation modulates Na^+, as well as N-, P- and L-type Ca^{2+} currents, via a PKA-dependent pathway. D2 receptors regulate K^+ currents. DA also modulates the activity of ligand-gated ion channels, including NMDA and AMPA receptors. As such, DA is not a classical excitatory or inhibitory neurotransmitter, but rather acts as a modulator of neurotransmission. A lack of subtype-specific ligands, and overlapping expression patterns, makes investigation of individual DA receptors difficult. As a consequence, most studies have investigated D1 and D2 families of receptors (with family-specific ligands) in discrete brain regions, especially the striatum and prefrontal cortex.

Dopaminergic neurons are strongly influenced by excitatory glutamate and inhibitory GABA input. In general, glutamate inputs enable burst-like firing of dopaminergic neurons, resulting in high concentrations of synaptic DA. GABA inhibition of DA neurons causes a tonic, basal level of DA release into the synapse (Goto et al., 2007). Interestingly, DA release also modulates GABA and glutamate neurons, thus providing an additional level of interaction and complexity between DA and other neurotransmitters. Strong phasic or slow tonic release of DA, and the subsequent activation of DA receptors, has differential effects on the induction of long-term potentiation (LTP) and long-term depression (LTD). In the striatum, phasic activation of DA neurons and stimulation of D1 receptors favors LTP induction, while tonic DA release with concomitant activation of both D1- and D2-like receptors favors LTD (Gerdeman et al., 2003).

Roles of DA in Behavior: Lesioning and Knockout Studies

For several decades, pharmacological agents have been used to specifically ablate dopaminergic neurons. This technique allowed functional characterization of discrete dopaminergic brain regions in animal models. More recently, the generation of knockout mice lacking specific DA receptor subtypes has furthered understanding of the dopaminergic system, from brain regions to the functional impact of individual receptors (Holmes et al., 2004; Sibley,1999). These tools, along with dopaminergic ligands, have enabled exploration of the broad-reaching effects of DA on physiological processes and behaviors.

Locomotion: Models of Parkinson Disease (PD). In the early 1980s, several young people in California developed rapid-onset parkinsonism. All of the affected individuals had injected a synthetic analog of meperidine that was contaminated with 1-methyl-4-phenyl-1,2,3, 6-tetrahydropyridine (MPTP). MPTP is metabolized by MAO-B to the neurotoxic MPP^+, which is selectively taken into dopaminergic neurons by the DA transporter. Once inside the cell, MPP^+ causes intra- and extracellular DA release, which is oxidized to form quinones and reactive oxygen species that cause in neuronal death. Because of the high specificity of MPP^+ for the DA transporter, neuronal death is largely restricted to the substantia nigra and ventral tegmental area, resulting in a phenotype remarkably similar to Parkinson's disease. 6-Hydroxydopamine (6-OHDA) is similar to MPTP in both mechanism of action and utility as an animal model. In contrast to MPTP, however, 6-OHDA does not cross the blood-brain barrier and it is not specific to dopaminergic neurons (it is also a substrate for NET, the neuronal NE transporter). Thus, in animal models of Parkinson disease, 6-OHDA must be injected intracranially and co-administered with a blocker of NET. Lesioning animals with MPTP or 6-OHDA results in tremor, grossly diminished locomotor activity, and rigidity. As with Parkinson disease, these motor deficits are alleviated with L-DOPA therapy or dopaminergic agonists. These neurotoxins are valuable tools for studying potential neuroprotective agents and novel treatment strategies, such as neural grafting and stem cell transplantation; their effects underscore the singular importance of the dopaminergic system in locomotor activity and Parkinson disease.

Other pharmacological agents are also known to alter locomotor activity via dopaminergic actions, including cocaine and amphetamine. These drugs of abuse bind to DAT and inhibit reuptake of synaptic DA. Amphetamine is a substrate for the transporter, blocks it competitively, and enters the neuron, where it displaces (releases) DA from vesicular stores, causing an efflux of DA from the neuronal cytosol into the synapse, possibly by reversal of the DA transporter. The accumulation of synaptic DA increases stimulation of DA receptors and results in heightened locomotor activity. Mice lacking DAT are hyperactive, and do not display increased locomotion in response to cocaine or amphetamine treatment.

Targeted disruption of the DA receptor genes has revealed specific information about the receptor subtypes that mediate locomotor activity. Mice lacking the D_1 receptor show generalized alterations in locomotor activity, although there is not good agreement about the specific motor phenotype. Studies with D_1 receptor knockout mice indicate that the D_1 receptor, but not the D_5 receptor, is primarily responsible for the increase in locomotor activity that occurs following administration of D1-family agonists. D_2 receptor knockout mice display marked reductions in locomotor activity, initiation of movement, and rearing behaviors. This reduction in motor activity is also present in mice that are specifically lacking only the D_{2L} receptor, indicating that the D_{2S} isoform plays a lesser role in regulation of movement and is not able to compensate for the lack of D_{2L} receptor. The D_3 and D_4 receptor knockout animals display unique locomotor alterations in response to novel environments. However, these changes may be related to novelty-seeking behavior rather than actual motor impairments.

Reward: Implications in Addiction. In general, drugs of abuse cause increased DA levels in the nucleus accumbens, an area critical for rewarded behaviors. This role for mesolimbic DA in addiction has led to numerous studies on abused drugs in DA receptor knockout mice. Studies of D_1 receptor knockout mice show a reduction in the rewarding properties of ethanol, suggesting that the rewarding and reinforcing properties of ethanol are dependent, at least in part, on the D_1 receptor. D_2 receptor knockout mice also display reduced preference for ethanol consumption. Morphine also lacks rewarding properties in D_2 knockout mice when measured by conditioned place-preference or self-administration paradigms. However, mice lacking the D_2 receptor exhibit enhanced self-administration of high doses of cocaine. These data implicate a complex and drug-specific role for the D_2 receptor in rewarding and reinforcing behaviors. The D_3 receptor, highly expressed in the limbic system, has also been implicated in the rewarding properties of several drugs of abuse. However, D_3 knockout mice display drug-associated place preference similar to wild-type mice following amphetamine or morphine administration. Recently developed D_3-selective ligands implicate a role for the D_3 receptor in motivation for drug-seeking and in drug relapse, rather than in the direct reinforcing effects of the drugs (Heidbreder, 2008).

Cognition, Learning and Memory. Mice lacking the D_1 receptor display deficits in multiple forms of memory. D_1 knockout mice have impaired spatial memory using the Morris water maze as a read-out. Deficits in prefrontal cortex-dependent working memory occur in D_1 knockout mice, in agreement with pharmacological evidence that cortical working memory can be modulated with D_1 agonists and antagonists (Williams and Castner, 2006). Amphetamine administration disrupts prepulse inhibition in wildtype animals but not in D_2 knockout animals. Prepulse inhibition is unaltered in mice lacking only the D_{2L} isoform of the receptor, indicating that the long and short isoforms of the receptor may serve different purposes in sensorimotor gating and higher order processing. These findings imply an important role for the D_2 receptor in disorders with defects in sensorimotor gating, most notably schizophrenia. Indeed, many of the antipsychotic drugs used in the treatment of schizophrenia are high affinity antagonists for the D_2 receptor.

DA Receptor Agonists and Antagonists

DA Receptor Agonists. DA receptor agonists are currently used in the treatment of PD, restless leg syndrome, and hyperprolactinemia. One of the primary limitations to the therapeutic use of dopaminergic agonists is the lack of receptor subtype selectivity, that is, stimulation of DA receptor subtypes not involved with

Table 13–7

Experimental Tools at DA Receptors

	AGONIST	ANTAGONIST
D1-like	Dihydrexidine SKF38393	SCH23390 SKF83566
D2-like	7-OH-DPAT	Sulpiride
D_3	7-OH-PIPAT	U99194 BP-897
D_4	PD168077	L-745,870
D_5	ADTN	—

the disease causes an array of unpleasant side effects. However, recent advances in receptor-ligand structure-function relationships have enabled the development of subtype-specific drugs, many of which have already proven to be useful experimental tools (Table 13–7). Some ligands can preferentially activate one downstream signaling cascade over another, a property known as functional selectivity (Urban et al., 2007). Furthermore, DA receptor activity can be modulated by drugs that bind to allosteric sites on the receptor, thereby enhancing or decreasing endogenous DA signaling in a receptor-specific manner (Schetz, 2005). All of these interactions between ligands and DA receptors can be exploited in future drug development endeavors to evoke a more specific receptor-mediated response.

DA Receptor Agonists and Parkinson Disease. Parkinson disease (PD), a neurodegenerative disorder of unknown etiology, is characterized by extensive degeneration of dopaminergic neurons within the substantia nigra, resulting in tremor, rigidity, and bradykinesia. While the principal pharmacotherapy for PD is L-DOPA, limitations to its therapeutic effects (Chapter 22) have generated intense interest in developing alternative therapies for PD, with the intent of either delaying the usage of L-DOPA or alleviating L-DOPA side effects and restoring its efficacy. One treatment strategy is the use of DA receptor agonists, which act directly on the depleted nigrostriatal dopaminergic system and have fewer undesirable side effects. DA agonists can be used in conjunction with lower doses of L-DOPA in a combined therapy approach. Two general classes of dopaminergic agonists are used in the treatment of PD: ergots and non-ergots. The pharmacological properties of these drugs are described below; their use in the management of PD is described in Chapter 22.

D1/D2 Receptor Agonists: Ergot Allkaloids. Ergot derivatives are nonselective compounds that act on several different neurotransmitter systems, including DA, 5-HT, and adrenergic receptors. In the U.S., bromocriptine (PARLODEL) and pergolide (PERMAX) are approved for the treatment of PD (see Table 13–6 for structures); however, their use has fallen out of favor because of the associated risk for serious cardiac complications. Bromocriptine is a potent D_2

receptor agonist and a weak D_1 antagonist. Pergolide is a partial agonist of D_1 receptors and a strong D2-family agonist with high affinity for both D_2 and D_3 receptor subtypes. Ergot derivatives are commonly reported to cause unpleasant side effects, including nausea, dizziness, and hallucinations. Pergolide was removed from the U.S. market as therapy for PD after it was associated with an increased risk for valvular heart disease.

Ergot Alkaloids in the Treatment of Hyperprolactinemia. Despite the contraindications for PD, ergot-based DA agonists are still used in the treatment of hyperprolactinemia. Like bromocriptine, cabergoline (DOSTINEX) is a strong agonist at D_2 receptors, and has lower affinity for D_1, 5-HT, and α adrenergic receptors. The therapeutic utility of bromocriptine and cabergoline in hyperprolactinemia is derived from their properties as DA receptor agonists: they activate D_2 receptors in the pituitary to reduce prolactin secretion. The risk of valvular heart disease in ergot therapy is associated with higher doses of drug (necessary for PD treatment), but not with the lower doses used in treating hyperprolactinemia. The use of bromocriptine and cabergoline in the management of hyperprolactinemia is described in Chapter 38.

D1/D2 Receptor Agonists (Non-Ergot Alkaloids). Apomorphine (APOKYN), a derivative of morphine, is approved for the treatment of PD. Apomorphine binds with the order of potence $D_4{>}D_2{>}D_3{>}D_5$. Apomorphine also binds with lower affinity to D_1, α-adrenergic, 5-HT_{1A}, and 5-HT_2 receptors. The therapeutic benefits of apomorphine in PD are likely due to its higher affinity and efficacy at DA receptors, especially D2-family receptors. Apomorphine is most commonly used in combination with L-DOPA to surmount the sudden "off" periods that can occur after long-term L-DOPA treatment.

Rotigotine is offered in a transdermal patch (NEUPRO) for the treatment of PD. Rotigotine preferentially binds to D_2 and D_3 receptors and has much lower affinity for D_1 receptors. In addition, rotigotine is an agonist at 5-HT_{1A} and 5-HT_2 receptors, and an antagonist at α_2 adrenergic receptors. Due to problems with patch release, rotigotine is currently not sold in the U.S., but is available in Europe.

D2 Family Receptor Agonists (Non-Ergot Alkaloids). Based on the role of DA in PD and the initial therapeutic utility of ergot compounds, more selective D2 dopaminergic agonists were developed for PD treatment. Pramipexole (MIRAPEX) and ropinirole (REQUIP) are agonists at all D2 family receptors and, notably, bind with highest affinity to the D_3 receptor subtype. Interestingly, pramipexole is reported to have neuroprotective properties when administered before MPTP or 6-OHDA in animal models of PD (Joyce and Millan, 2007); agonist activity at the D_3 receptor may be the underlying neuroprotective mechanism.

Ropinirole in the Treatment of Restless Leg Syndrome (RLS). In addition to its utility in the treatment of PD, ropinirole has also been FDA-approved as pharmacotherapy for RLS. Mild dopaminergic hypofunction has been noted in patients with RLS. Somnolence and other side effects reported for PD therapy are less pronounced in the treatment of RLS, presumably due to the lower dose required for RLS therapy.

D_4 Receptor Agonists and Attention Deficit-Hyperactivity Disorder (ADHD). The D_4 receptor is known to be significant in ADHD; an association has been reproducibly demonstrated between the seven-repeat D_4 VNTR variant and patients with ADHD. Recent preclinical testing has uncovered potential therapeutic benefits of the selective D_4 agonist, A-412997, in cognitive tasks and animal models of ADHD. Animals treated with A-412997 showed cognitive improvements well below hyperlocomotive doses and, importantly, A-412997 did not show potential for abuse at any dose tested (Woolley et al., 2008). This is in marked contrast to the currently available drug therapies for ADHD treatment that have high abuse potential. While all published studies to date are preclinical, D_4-selective agonists show significant promise for the next generation of ADHD therapy.

DA Receptor Antagonists

Just as enhancing DA neurotransmission is clinically important, inhibiting an over-active dopaminergic system can be useful. As with the DA receptor agonists, a lack of subtype-specific antagonists has limited the therapeutic utility of this group of ligands. Recent advances in defining GPCR structure, along with ligand-binding modeling, have advanced rational drug design, and selective antagonists are now available as experimental tools (Table 13–7). Many subtype-selective antagonists are in early stages of preclinical testing for therapeutic utility.

DA Receptor Antagonists and Schizophrenia. DA receptor antagonists are a mainstay in the pharmacotherapy of schizophrenia. While many neurotransmitter systems likely contribute to the complex pathology of schizophrenia (Chapter 16), DA dysfunction is considered the basis of this disorder. The DA hypothesis of schizophrenia has its origins in the characteristics of the drugs used to treat this disorder: all antipsychotic compounds used clinically have high affinity for DA receptors. Moreover, psychostimulants that increase extracellular DA levels can induce or worsen psychotic symptoms in schizophrenic patients. The advent of neuroimaging techniques for visualization of DA in human brain regions has led to new insights into the role of specific DA systems. DA hyperfunction in subcortical regions, most notably the striatum, has been associated with the positive symptoms of schizophrenia that respond well to antipsychotic treatment. In contrast, the prefrontal cortex of schizophrenic patients exhibits dopaminergic hypofunction, which has been associated with the more treatment-refractory negative/cognitive symptoms. The drugs currently used to treat schizophrenia are classified as either typical (also referred to as first generation) or atypical (second generation) antipsychotics. This nomenclature stems from the high efficacy and lack of extrapyramidal side effects observed with atypical antipsychotics. Some of the newer drugs in development do not fit into this classification scheme, including the D1-selective agonist, dihydrexidine. Dihydrexidine shows great promise to improve the refractory negative symptoms of schizophrenia, and may be especially useful in combination therapy with current antipsychotics that preferentially reduce positive symptoms by antagonizing D2 receptors (Mu et al., 2007).

Antipsychotic Agents

Typical Antipsychotics. The first antipsychotic drug used to treat schizophrenia was chlorpromazine (THORAZINE). Despite its affinity for a wide array of neurotransmitter receptors, the antipsychotic properties of chlorpromazine were attributed to its antagonism of DA receptors, especially the D_2 receptor. More D_2-selective ligands were developed to improve the antipsychotic properties, including haloperidol (HALDOL) and similar D_2-selective drugs. While all typical antipsychotics markedly improve positive symptoms, they are not very beneficial in the treatment of negative or cognitive symptoms. As promising as these drugs initially seemed, their debilitating side effects limited their utility and gave rise to the development of the next generation of antipsychotic drugs, the atypical agents.

CHLORPROMAZINE

CLOZAPINE

ARIPIPRAZOLE

Atypical Antipsychotics. This class of antipsychotic drugs originated with clozapine (FAZACLO) and is distinguished by a vastly improved side effect profile over the typical antipsychotics. The lack of extrapyramidal side effects has been attributed to a much lower affinity for the D_2 receptor compared to the typical antipsychotics. Atypical agents are also less likely to stimulate prolactin production. Clozapine has higher affinity for the D_4 receptor, which is highly expressed in the limbic system. Most atypical antipsychotics are low affinity antagonists at the D_2 receptor and high affinity antagonists or inverse agonists at the 5-HT_{2A} receptor. While the precise role of 5-HT_{2A} receptor binding in the efficacy of clozapine remains unclear, this dual DA-5-HT receptor blockade shaped the development of antipsychotics for several decades.

Aripiprazole (ABILIFY) has gained recent attention for causing even fewer side effects than earlier atypical antipsychotics. Aripiprazole diverges from the traditional atypical profile in two ways: first, it has higher affinity for D_2 receptors than for 5-HT_{2A} receptors; secondly, and perhaps more importantly, it is a partial agonist, rather than an antagonist, at D_2 receptors. As a partial agonist, aripiprazole may diminish the subcortical DA hyperfunction by competing with DA for receptor binding, while simultaneously enhancing dopaminergic neurotransmission in the prefrontal cortex by acting as an agonist. The dual mechanism afforded by a partial agonist may thus treat both the positive and negative symptoms associated with schizophrenia.

D_3 Receptor Antagonists and Drug Addiction. Although much work remains to determine clinical utility, D_3-selective antagonists show promise in the treatment of addiction (Heidbreder, 2008). This interest stems from the high expression of the D_3 receptor in the limbic system, the reward center of the brain. Animal studies of highly D_3-selective antagonists BP-897 and SB-277011A have suggested a role for the D_3 receptor in the motivation to abuse drugs and in the potential for drug-abuse relapse.

BIBLIOGRAPHY

Aloyo VJ, Berg KA, Spampinato U, et al. Current status of inverse agonism at serotonin 2A (5-HT_{2A}) and 5-HT_{2C} receptors. *Pharmacol Ther*, **2009**, *121*:160–173.

Andrade R, Malenka RC, Nicoll RA. A G protein couples serotonin and GABA-B receptors to the same channels in hippocampus. *Science*, **1986**, *234*:1261–1265.

Barnes NM, Sharp T. A review of central 5-HT receptors and their function. *Neuropharmacology*, **1999**, *38*:1083–1152.

Berg KA, Harvey JA, Spampinato U, Clarke WP. Physiological and therapeutic relevance of constitutive activity of 5-HT_{2A} and 5-HT_{2C} receptors for the treatment of depression. *Prog Brain Res*, **2008**, *172*:287–305.

Bockaert J, Claeysen S, Bécamel C, et al. Neuronal 5-HT metabotropic receptors: fine-tuning of their structure, signaling, and roles in synaptic modulation. *Cell Tissue Res*, **2006**, *326*:553–572.

Bockaert J, Claeysen S, Compan V, Dumuis A. 5-HT_4 receptors: history, molecular pharmacology and brain functions. *Neuropharmacology,* **2008**, *55*:922–931.

Bonasera SJ, Chu HM, Brennan TJ, Tecott LH. A null mutation of the serotonin 6 receptor alters acute responses to ethanol. *Neuropsychopharmacology*, **2006**, *31*:1801–1813.

Bonsi P, Cuomo D, Ding J, et al. Endogenous serotonin excites striatal cholinergic interneurons via the activation of 5-HT_{2C}, 5-HT_6, and 5-HT_7 serotonin receptors: Implications for extrapyramidal side effects of serotonin reuptake inhibitors. *Neuropsychopharmacology,* **2007**, *32*:1840–1854.

Bortolato M, Chen K, Shih JC. Monoamine oxidase inactivation: from pathophysiology to therapeutics. *Adv Drug Deliv Rev*, **2008**, *60*:1527–1533.

Brunner HC, Nelen M, Breakefield XO, et al. Abnormal behavior associated with a point mutation in the structural gene for monoamine oxidase A. *Science*, **1993**, *262*:578–580.

Burns CM, Chu H, Rueter SM, et al. Regulation of serotonin-2C receptor G-protein coupling by RNA editing. *Nature*, **1997**, *387*:303–308.

Cases O, Seif I, Grimsby J, et al. Aggressive behavior and altered amounts of brain serotonin and norepinephrine in mice lacking MAOA. *Science*, **1995**, *268*:1763–1766.

Cajochen C, Krauchi K, Wirz-Justice A. Role of melatonin in the regulation of human circadian rhythms and sleep. *J Neuroendocrinol*, **2003**, *15*:432–437.

CompanV, Zhou M, Grailhe R, et al. Attenuated response to stress and novelty and hypersensitivity to seizures in 5-HT_4 receptor knock-out mice. *J Neurosci,* **2004**, *24:*412–419.

Cravchik A, Gejman PV. Functional analysis of the human D_5 dopamine receptor missense and nonsense variants: differences in dopamine binding affinities, *Pharmacogenetics*, **1999**, *9*:199–206.

Delgado PL, Charney DS, Price LH, et al. Serotonin function and the mechanism of antidepressant action. Reversal of antidepressant-induced remission by rapid depletion of plasma tryptophan. *Arch Gen Psychiatry*, **1990**, *47*:411–418.

Fox MA, Andrews AM, Wendland JR, et al. A pharmacological analysis of mice with a targeted disruption of the serotonin transporter. *Psychopharmacology (Berl)*, **2007**, *195*:147–166.

Gaddum JH, Picarelli ZP. Two kinds of tryptamine receptors. *Br J Pharmacol*, **1957**, *12*:323–328.

Gerdeman GL, Partridge JG, Lupica CR, Lovinger DM. It could be habit forming: drugs of abuse and striatal synaptic plasticity. *Trends Neurosci*, **2003**, *26*:184–192.

Gershon MD, Tack J. The serotonin signaling system: From basic understanding to drug development for functional GI disorders. *Gastroenterology*, **2007**, *132*:397–414.

Geyer MA, Vollenweider FX. Serotonin research: Contributions to understanding psychoses. *Trends Pharmacol Sci*, **2008**, *29*:445–453.

Goto Y, Otani S, Grace AA. The Yin and Yang of dopamine release: A new perspective, *Neuropharmacology*, **2007**, *53*:583–587.

Gonzalez-Maeso J, Weisstaub NV, Zhou M, et al. Hallucinogens recruit specific cortical 5-HT_{2A} receptor-mediated signaling pathways to affect behavior. *Neuron*, **2007**, *53*:439–452.

Gray JA, Roth BL. Paradoxical trafficking and regulation of 5-HT_{2A} receptors by agonists and antagonists. *Brain Res Bull*, **2001**, *56*:441–451.

Grailhe R, Waeber C, Dulawa SC, et al. Increased exploratory activity and altered response to LSD in mice lacking the 5-HT(5A) receptor. *Neuron*, **1999**, *22*:581–591.

Hazelwood LA, Free RB, Sibley DR. Dopamine receptor-interacting proteins. In *The Dopamine Receptors* (Neve KA, ed.). Humana Press, Totowa, NJ, **2009**.

Heidbreder C. Selective antagonism at dopamine D_3 receptors as a target for drug addiction pharmacotherapy: a review of preclinical evidence. *CNS Neurol Disord Drug Targets*, **2008**, *7*:410–421.

Hedlund PB, Danielson PE, Thomas EA. No hypothermic response to serotonin in 5-HT7 receptor knockout mice. *Proc Natl Acad Sci USA*, **2003**, *100*:1375–1380.

Holmes A, Lachowicz JE, Sibley DR. Phenotypic analysis of dopamine receptor knockout mice; recent insights into the functional specificity of dopamine receptor subtypes. *Neuropharmacology*, **2004**, *47*:1117–1134.

Hornykiewicz O. Dopamine miracle: From brain homogenate to dopamine replacement. *Mov Disord*, 2002, *17*:501–508.

Hoyer D, Clarke DE, Fozard JR, *et al*. International Union of Pharmacology classification of receptors for 5-hydroxytryptamine (serotonin). *Pharmacol Rev*, **1994**, *46*:157–203.

Humphrey PP, Aperley E, Feniuk W, Perren MJ. A rational approach to identifying a fundamentally new drug for the treatment of migraine. In *Cardiovascular Pharmacology of 5-Hydroxytryptamine: Prospective Therapeutic Applications*. (Saxena PR, Wallis DI, Wouters W, Bevan P, eds.). Kluwer Academic Publishers, Dordrecht, Netherlands, **1990**, pp. 417–431.

Jensen AA, Davies PA, Bräuner-Osborne H, Krzywkowski K, 3B but which 3B? And that's just one of the questions: the heterogeneity of human 5-HT_3 receptors. *Trends Pharmacol Sci*, **2008**, *29*:437–444.

Jose PA, Eisner GM, Felder RA. Renal dopamine receptors in health and hypertension. *Pharmacol Ther*, **1998**, *80*:149–182.

Jouvet M. Sleep and serotonin: an unfinished story. *Neuropsychopharmacology*, **1999**, *21*(suppl 2):24S–27S.

Joyce JN, Millan MJ. Dopamine D3 receptor agonists for protection and repair in Parkinson's disease. *Curr Opin Pharmacol*, **2007**, *7*:100–105.

Kaumann AJ, Levy FO. 5-hydroxytryptamine receptors in the human cardiovascular system. *Pharmacol Ther*, **2006**, *111*: 674–706.

Kebabian JW, Calne DB. Multiple receptors for dopamine. *Nature*, **1979**, *277*:93–96.

Kebabian JW, Greengard P. Dopamine-sensitive adenyl cyclase: possible role in synaptic transmission. *Science*, **1971**, *174*:1346–1349.

King MV, Marsden CA, Fone KC. A role for the 5-HT_{1A}, 5-HT_4 and 5-HT_6 receptors in learning and memory. *Trends Pharmacol Sci*, **2008**, *29*:482–492.

Lee SP, So CH, Rashid AJ, et al. Dopamine D1 and D2 receptor co-activation generates a novel phospholipase C-mediated calcium signal. *J Biol Chem*, **2004**, *279*:35671–35678.

Lesch KP, Zeng Y, Reif A, Gutknecht L. Anxiety-related traits in mice with modified genes of the serotonergic pathway. *Eur J Pharmacol*, **2003**, *480*:185–204.

Liu IS, Seeman P, Sanyal S, et al. Dopamine D_4 receptor variant in Africans, D4valine194glycine, is insensitive to dopamine and clozapine: report of a homozygous individual. *Am J Med Genet*, **1996**, *61*:277–282.

Lucki I. The spectrum of behaviors influenced by serotonin. *Biol Psychiatry*, **1998**, *44*:151–162.

Maricq AV, Peterson AS, Brake AJ, et al. Primary structure and functional expression of the 5HT3 receptor, a serotonin-gated ion channel. *Science*, **1991**, *254*:432–437.

Mehrotra S, Gupta S, Chan KY, et al. Current and prospective pharmacological targets in relation to antimigraine action. *Naunyn Schmiedebergs Arch Pharmacol*, **2008**, *378*:371–394.

Meltzer HY, Huang M. In vivo actions of atypical antipsychotic drug on serotonergic and dopaminergic systems. *Prog Brain Res*, **2008**, *172*:177–197.

Mu Q, Johnson K, Morgan PS, et al. A single 20 mg dose of the full D1 dopamine agonist dihydrexidine (DAR-0100) increases prefrontal perfusion in schizophrenia. *Schizophr Res*, **2007**, *94*:332–341.

Nebigil CG, Choi DS, Dierich A. Serotonin 2B receptor is required for heart development. *Proc Natl Acad Sci USA*, **2000**, *97*:9508–9513.

Neve KA, Seamans JK, Trantham-Davidson H. Dopamine receptor signaling. *J Recept Signal Transduct Res*, **2004**, *24*:165–205.

Parks CL, Robinson PS, Sibille E, et al. Increased anxiety of mice lacking the serotonin1A receptor. *Proc Natl Acad Sci USA*, **1998**, *95*:10734–10739.

Peroutka SJ, Snyder SH. Multiple serotonin receptors: differential binding of [^{3}H]5-hydroxytryptamine, [^{3}H]lysergic acid diethylamide and [^{3}H]spiroperidol. *Mol Pharmacol*, **1979**, *16*:687–699.

Rankin ML, Hazelwood LA, Free RB, et al. Molecular pharmacology of the dopamine receptors. In *Dopamine Handbook* (al Ile, ed.). Oxford University Press, New York, **2009**.

Roth BL. Drugs and valvular heart disease. *N Engl J Med*, **2007**, *356*:6–9.

Sanders-Bush E, Airey DC. Centennial perspective: serotonin receptors. *Mol Interv,* **2008**, *8*:200–203.

Sanders-Bush E, Fentress H, Hazelwood L. Serotonin 5-HT_2 receptors: Molecular and genomic diversity. *Mol Interv*, **2003**, *3*:319–330.

Saudou F, Amara DA, Dierich A, et al. Enhanced aggressive behavior in mice lacking 5-HT1B receptor. *Science*, **1994**, *265*:1875–1878.

Schetz JA. Allosteric modulation of dopamine receptors. *Mini Rev Med Chem,* **2005**, *5*:555–561.

Sibley DR. New insights into dopaminergic receptor function using antisense and genetically altered animals. *Annu Rev Pharmacol Toxicol,* **1999**, *39*:313–341.

Silberstein SD. Treatment recommendations for migraine. *Nat Clin Pract Neurol*, **2008**, *4*:482–489.

Steiner JA, Carneiro AM, Blakely RD. Going with the flow: Trafficking-dependent and -independent regulation of serotonin transport. *Traffic,* **2008**, *9:*1393–1402.

Strange PG. Agonism and inverse agonism at dopamine D2-like receptors. *Clin Exp Pharmacol Physiol Suppl*, **1999**, *26*:S3–S9.

Swerdlow NR, Braff DL, Geyer MA. Animal models of deficient sensorimotor gating: what we know, what we think we know, and what we hope to know soon. *Behav Pharmacol*, **2000**, *11*:185–204.

Tecott LH, Sun LM, Akana SF, et al. Eating disorder and epilepsy in mice lacking 5-HT_{2C} serotonin receptors. *Nature*, **1995**, *374*:542–546.

Urban JD, Clarke WP, von Zastrow M, et al. Functional selectivity and classical concepts of quantitative pharmacology. *J Pharmacol Exp Ther,* **2007**, *320*:1–13.

Usiello A, Baik JH, Rouge-Pont F, et al. Distinct functions of the two isoforms of dopamine D2 receptors. *Nature*, **2000**, *408*:199–203.

Van Tol HH, Wu CM, Guan HC, et al. Multiple dopamine D4 receptor variants in the human population. *Nature,* **1992**, *358*:149–152.

Van Tol HH, Wu CM, Guan HC, et al. Multiple dopamine D_4 receptor variants in the human population. *Nature,* **1992**, *358*:149–152.

Walther DJ, Bader M. A unique central tryptophan hydroxylase isoform. *Biochem Pharmacol*, **2003**, *66*:1673–1680.

Walther DJ, Bader M. A unique central tryptophan hydroxlyase isoform. *Biochem Pharmacol*, **2003**, *66*:1673–1680.

Weisstaub NV, Zhou M, Lira A, et al. Cortical 5-HT2A receptor signaling modulates anxiety-like behaviors in mice. *Science,* **2006**, *313*:536–540.

Williams GV, Castner SA. Under the curve: critical issues for elucidating D1 receptor function in working memory. *Neuroscience*, **2006**, *139*:263–276.

Winter JC. Hallucinogens as discriminative stimuli in animals: LSD, phenethylamines, and tryptamines. *Psychopharmacology (Berl),* **2009**, *203*:251–263.

Woolley ML, Waters KA, Reavill C, et al. Selective dopamine D4 receptor agonist (A-412997) improves cognitive performance and stimulates motor activity without influencing reward-related behaviour in rat. *Behav Pharmacol,* **2008**, *19*:765–776.

Zeitz KP, Guy N, Malmberg AB, *et al*. The 5-HT_3 subtype of serotonin receptor contributes to nociceptive processing via a novel subset of myelinated and unmyelinated nociceptors. *J Neurosci,* **2002**, *22*:1010–1019.

Neurotransmission and the Central Nervous System

Perry B. Molinoff

Drugs that act in the central nervous system (CNS) are invaluable therapeutically. They can, e.g., relieve pain, reduce fever, suppress disordered movements, induce sleep or arousal, reduce appetite, and allay the tendency to vomit. Selectively acting drugs can be used to treat anxiety, depression, mania, or schizophrenia and do so without altering consciousness (Chapters 15 and 16). Socially acceptable stimulants and anti-anxiety agents contribute to emotional stability, relief of anxiety, and pleasure. However, the excessive use of such drugs can affect lives adversely when uncontrolled, self-administration leads to physical dependence or to toxic side effects (Chapter 24). The nonmedical self-administration of CNS-active drugs— recreational pharmacology—is widespread.

The identification of targets for drugs that affect the nervous system and behavior presents extraordinary scientific challenges. Understanding the cellular and molecular basis for the complex and varied functions of the human brain is only the beginning. Complicating the effort is the fact that a CNS-active drug may act at multiple sites with disparate and even opposing effects. In addition, many CNS disorders involve multiple brain regions and pathways, which can frustrate efforts to use a single therapeutic agent. CNS pharmacologists have two overlapping goals: to use drugs to elucidate the mechanisms that operate in the normal CNS, and to develop drugs to correct pathophysiological events in the abnormal CNS. Advances in molecular biology and neurobiology are facilitating the development of drugs that can selectively treat diseases of the CNS.

This chapter introduces guidelines and fundamental principles for the comprehensive study of drugs that affect the CNS. Specific therapeutic approaches to neurological and psychiatric disorders are discussed in Chapters 15 to 17, 21, 22, and 24. For further detail, see the specialized texts by Cooper (2003), Siegel (2006), Nestler (2009), and their associates. For detailed information on specific receptors and ion channels see the official database of the IUPHAR Committee on Receptor Nomenclature and Drug Classification.

ORGANIZATIONAL PRINCIPLES OF THE CNS

The brain is a complex assembly of interacting neurons and nuclei that regulate their own and each other's activities in a dynamic fashion, generally through chemical neurotransmission. It is useful to examine the major anatomical regions of the CNS and their associations with specific neurotransmitter systems and the effect of pharmacological agents thereon.

Cerebral Cortex. The two cerebral hemispheres constitute the largest division of the brain. Regions of the cortex are classified in several ways:

- by the modality of information processed (e.g., sensory, including somatosensory, visual, auditory, and olfactory, as well as motor and associational)
- by anatomical position (frontal, temporal, parietal, and occipital)
- by the geometric relationship between cell types in the major cortical layers ("cytoarchitectonic" classification)

The specialized functions of a cortical region arise from the interplay between connections with other regions of the cortex (corticocortical systems) and noncortical areas of the brain (subcortical systems) and a basic intracortical processing module of ~100 vertically connected cortical columns (Mountcastle, 1997). Varying numbers of adjacent columnar modules may be functionally linked into larger information-processing ensembles. The pathology of Alzheimer's disease, e.g., destroys the integrity of the columnar modules and the corticocortical connections (Chapter 22). Cortical areas termed association areas process information from primary cortical sensory regions to produce higher cortical functions such as abstract thought, memory, and consciousness. The cerebral cortices also provide supervisory integration of the autonomic nervous system and integrate somatic and vegetative functions, including those controlling the cardiovascular and gastrointestinal systems.

Limbic System. The *limbic system* is an archaic term for an assembly of brain regions (hippocampal formation, amygdaloid complex, septum, olfactory nuclei, basal ganglia, and selected nuclei of the diencephalon) grouped around the subcortical borders of the underlying brain core to which a variety of complex emotional and motivational functions have been attributed. Modern neuroscience tends to avoid this term because the ill-defined regions of the "limbic system" do not function consistently as a system. Parts of these limbic regions also participate individually in functions that can be more precisely defined. Thus, the basal ganglia or neostriatum (the *caudate nucleus, putamen, globus pallidus,* and *lentiform nucleus*) form an essential regulatory segment of the *extrapyramidal motor system* that complements the function of the pyramidal (or voluntary) motor system. Damage to the extrapyramidal system affects the ability to initiate voluntary movements and causes disorders characterized by involuntary movements, such as the tremors and rigidity of Parkinson disease or the uncontrollable limb movements of Huntington's chorea (Chapter 22). Similarly, the hippocampus may be crucial to the formation of recent memory, since this function is lost in patients with extensive bilateral damage to the hippocampus. Memory is also disrupted by Alzheimer's disease, which destroys the intrinsic structure of the hippocampus as well as parts of the frontal cortex.

Diencephalon. The *thalamus* lies in the center of the brain, beneath the cortex and basal ganglia and above the hypothalamus. The neurons of the thalamus are arranged in distinct clusters, or nuclei, which are either paired or midline structures. These nuclei act as relays between incoming sensory pathways and the cortex, between discrete regions of the thalamus and the hypothalamus, and between the basal ganglia and the association regions of the cerebral cortex. The thalamic nuclei and the basal ganglia also exert regulatory control over visceral functions; aphagia and adipsia, as well as general sensory neglect, follow damage to the corpus striatum or to selected circuits ending in the striatum. The *hypothalamus* is the principal integrating region for the autonomic nervous system and regulates body temperature, water balance, intermediary metabolism, blood pressure, sexual and circadian cycles, secretion from the adenohypophysis, sleep, and emotion.

Midbrain and Brainstem. The *mesencephalon, pons,* and *medulla oblongata* connect the cerebral hemispheres and thalamus-hypothalamus to the spinal cord. These "bridge portions" of the CNS contain most of the nuclei of the cranial nerves, as well as the major inflow and outflow tracts from the cortices and spinal cord. These regions contain the *reticular activating system*, an important but incompletely characterized region of gray matter linking peripheral sensory and motor events with higher levels of nervous integration. The major monoamine-containing neurons of the brain are found here. Together, these regions represent the points of central integration for coordination of essential reflexive acts, such as swallowing and vomiting, and those that involve the cardiovascular and respiratory systems; these areas also include the primary receptive regions for most visceral afferent sensory information. The reticular activating system is essential for the regulation of sleep, wakefulness, and level of arousal, as well as for coordination of eye movements. The fiber systems projecting from the reticular formation have been called nonspecific because the targets to which they project are relatively more diffuse in distribution than those of many other neuronal systems (e.g., specific thalamocortical projections). However, the chemically homogeneous components of the reticular system innervate targets in a coherent and functionally integrated manner despite their broad distribution.

Cerebellum. The cerebellum arises from the posterior pons behind the cerebral hemispheres. It is highly laminated and redundant in its detailed cytological organization. The lobules and folia of the cerebellum project onto specific deep cerebellar nuclei, which in turn make relatively selective projections to the motor cortex (by way of the thalamus) and to brainstem nuclei concerned with vestibular function (position-stabilization). In addition to maintaining the proper tone of antigravity musculature and providing continuous feedback during volitional movements of the trunk and extremities, the cerebellum also may regulate visceral functions (e.g., controlling heart rate, so as to maintain blood flow despite changes in posture).

Spinal Cord. The spinal cord extends from the caudal end of the medulla oblongata to the lower lumbar vertebrae. Within this mass of nerve cells and tracts, sensory information from skin, muscles, joints, and viscera is locally coordinated with motoneurons and with primary sensory relay cells that project to and receive signals from higher levels. The spinal cord is divided into anatomical segments (cervical, thoracic, lumbar, and sacral) that correspond to divisions of the peripheral nerves and spinal column (see Figure 8–1). Ascending and descending tracts of the spinal cord are located within the white matter at the perimeter of the cord, while intersegmental connections and synaptic contacts are concentrated within an H-shaped internal mass of gray matter. Sensory information flows into the dorsal cord, and motor commands exit *via* the ventral portion. The preganglionic neurons of the autonomic nervous system are found in intermediolateral columns of gray matter. Autonomic reflexes (e.g., changes in skin vasculature with alteration of temperature) can be elicited within local segments of the spinal cord, as shown by the maintenance of these reflexes after the cord has been severed.

Microanatomy of the Brain

Neurons operate either within layered structures such as the olfactory bulb, cerebral cortex, hippocampal formation, and cerebellum or in clustered groupings, defined collections of neurons that aggregate into nuclei. Specific connections between neurons within or across the macro-divisions of the brain are essential to the function of the brain. Through patterns of neuronal circuitry, individual neurons form functional ensembles to regulate the flow of information within and between the regions of the brain.

Cellular Organization of the Brain. Present understanding of the cellular organization of the CNS can be viewed from the perspective of the size, shape, location, and interconnections between neurons (Cooper et al., 2003; Shepherd, 2003).

Cell Biology of Neurons. Neurons are classified according to function (sensory, motor, or interneuron), location, the identity of the transmitter they synthesize and release or the class or classes of receptor expressed on the cell surface. Microscopic analysis of a neuron focuses on its general shape and in particular the complexity of the afferent receptive surfaces on the dendrites and cell body that receive synaptic contacts from other neurons. Neurons (Figure 14–1) exhibit the cytological characteristics of highly active secretory cells with large nuclei: large amounts of smooth and rough endoplasmic reticulum; and frequent clusters of specialized smooth endoplasmic reticulum (Golgi complex), in which secretory products of the cell are packaged into membrane-bound organelles for transport from the perikaryon to the axon or dendrites. Neurons and their cellular extensions are rich in microtubules, which support the complex cellular structure and assist in the reciprocal transport of essential macromolecules and organelles between the cell body and distant axon or dendrites. The sites of interneuronal communication in the CNS are termed *synapses* Although synapses are functionally analogous to "junctions" in the somatic motor and autonomic nervous systems, central junctions contain an array of specific proteins presumed to be the active zone for transmitter release and response (Husi et al., 2000). Like peripheral "junctions," central synapses are denoted by accumulations of tiny (50-150 nm) *synaptic vesicles*. The proteins of these vesicles have specific roles in transmitter storage, vesicle docking onto presynaptic membranes, voltage- and Ca^{2+}-dependent secretion, and recycling and restorage of released transmitter (Jahn, 2004, Murthy and Camilli, 2003; Nestler et al., 2009).

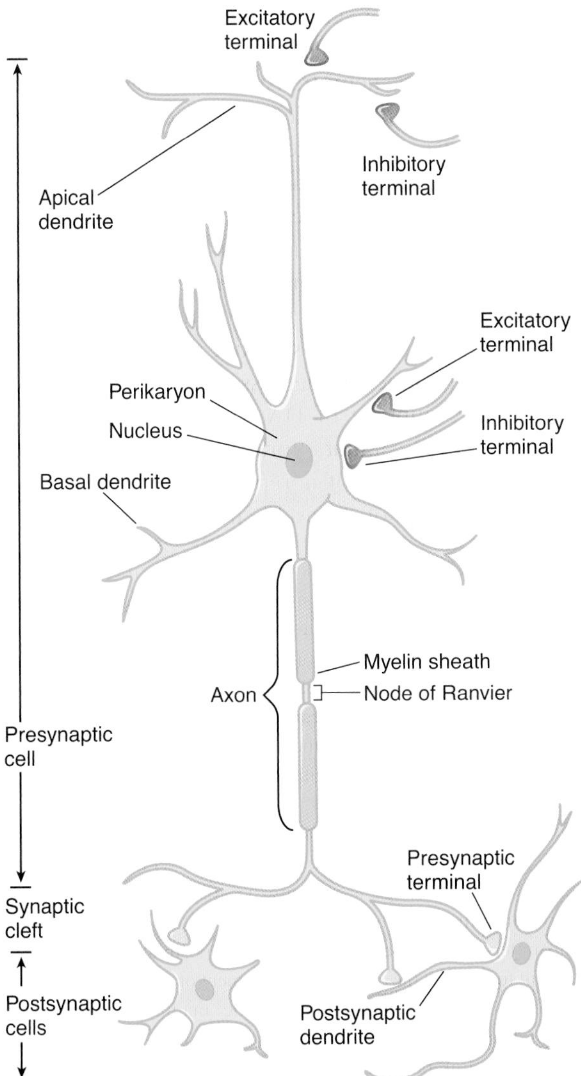

Figure 14–1. *Principal features of a typical vertebrate neuron.* Dendrites, including apical dendrites, receive synapses from presynaptic terminals. The cell body contains the nucleus and is the site of transcription and translation. The axon carries information from the perikaryon to the presynaptic terminals, which form synapses with the dendrites of other neurons. Axo-somatic synapses also occur. Many CNS-active pharmacological agents act at the presynaptic and postsynaptic membranes of the synaptic clefts, and at areas of transmitter storage near the synapses. (Adapted with permission from Kandel ER, Schwartz JH, Jessell TM (eds). *Principles of Neuroscience*, 4th ed. New York: McGraw-Hill, **2000**, p 22. Copyright © 2000 by The McGraw-Hill Companies, Inc. All rights reserved.)

Support Cells. Neurons are not the only cells in the CNS. According to most estimates, neurons are outnumbered, perhaps by an order of magnitude, by various types of support cells. These include macroglia, microglia, the cells of the vascular elements comprising the intracerebral vasculature, the cerebrospinal fluid-forming cells of the choroid plexus found within the intracerebral ventricular system, and the meninges, which cover the surface of the brain and comprise the cerebrospinal fluid-containing envelope. Macroglia are the most abundant support cells; some are categorized as *astrocytes* (cells interposed between the vasculature and the neurons, often surrounding individual compartments of synaptic complexes). Astrocytes play a variety of metabolic support roles including furnishing energy intermediates and supplementary removal of neurotransmitters following release (Pellerin and Magistretti, 2003). The *oligodendroglia*, a second prominent category of macroglia, are myelin-producing cells. Myelin, made up of multiple layers of compacted membranes, insulate segments of axons bioelectrically and permit non-decremental propagation of action potentials. Microglia are relatively uncharacterized support cells believed to be of mesodermal origin and related to the macrophage/monocyte lineage (Carson, 2002). Some microglia reside within the brain, while additional cells of this class may be recruited to the brain during periods of inflammation following either microbial infection or brain injury. The response of the brain to inflammation differs strikingly from that of other tissues (Glass et al., 2010).

Blood-Brain Barrier. Apart from exceptional instances in which drugs are introduced directly into the CNS, the concentration of an agent in the blood after oral or parenteral administration may differ substantially from its concentration in the brain. The *blood-brain barrier* (BBB) is an important boundary between the periphery and the CNS that forms a permeability barrier to the passive diffusion of substances from the bloodstream into the CNS. Evidence for the existence of the BBB is provided by the greatly diminished rate of access of many chemicals from plasma to the brain and the localization of several drug export systems in the cells that constitute the BBB (Chapter 5). An exception exists for lipophilic molecules, which diffuse fairly freely across the BBB and accumulate in the brain. This barrier is nonexistent in the peripheral nervous system, and is much less prominent in the hypothalamus and in several small, specialized organs (the circumventricular organs) lining the third and fourth ventricles of the brain: the median eminence, area postrema, pineal gland, subfornical organ, and subcommissural organ. While the BBB may impose limitations on the diffusion of macromolecules (including penicillin and pentylenetetrazol) are relatively selective antagonists of the action of GABA. Useful therapeutic effects have not yet been obtained through the use of agents that mimic GABA (such as muscimol), inhibit its active reuptake (such as 2,4-diaminobutyrate, nipecotic acid, and guvacine), or alter its turnover (such as aminooxyacetic acid).

GABA receptors have been divided into three main types: A, B, and C.

- The most prominent GABA-receptor subtype, the $GABA_A$ receptor, is a ligand-gated Cl^- ion channel, an "ionotropic receptor."
- The $GABA_B$ receptor is a GPCR.
- The $GABA_C$ receptor is a transmitter-gated Cl^- channel.

$GABA_A$ receptor subunit proteins have been well characterized due to their abundance. The receptor also has been extensively characterized as the site of action of many neuroactive drugs, notably benzodiazepines, barbiturates, ethanol, anesthetic steroids, and volatile anesthetics (Figure 14–11).

Based on sequence homology to the first reported $GABA_A$ subunit cDNAs, multiple subunits have been cloned, including 6α, 4β, and 3γ subunits. They appear to be expressed in multiple multimeric, pharmacologically distinctive combinations. In addition to these subunits, which are products of separate genes, splice variants for several subunits have been described.

The $GABA_A$ receptor is probably pentameric or tetrameric in structure with subunits that assemble together around a central pore typical for other ionotropic receptors. The major form of the $GABA_A$ receptor contains at least three different subunits α, β, and γ, with likely stoichiometry of 2α, 2β, 1γ. All three subunits are required to interact with benzodiazepines with the profile expected of a native $GABA_A$ receptor. The distribution of different subunit combinations of $GABA_A$ and their functions in the mammalian brain are summarized in Table 14–2 (Fritschy and Mohler, 1995).

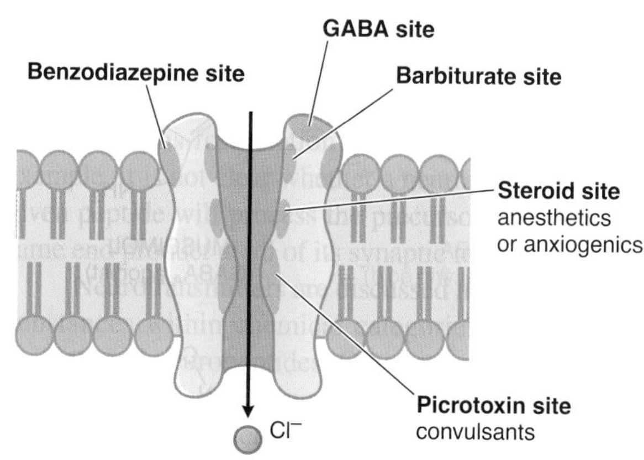

Figure 14–11. *Pharmacologic binding sites on the $GABA_A$ receptor.* (Reproduced with permission from Nestler EJ, Hyman SE, Malenka RC (eds). *Molecular Neuropharmacology*. New York: McGraw-Hill, **2000**, p 135. Copyright © 2009 by The McGraw-Hill Companies, Inc. All rights reserved.)

The $GABA_B$ or metabotropic GABA receptor interacts with G_i to inhibit adenylyl cyclase, activate K^+ channels, and reduce Ca^{2+} conductance. Presynaptic $GABA_B$ receptors function as autoreceptors, inhibiting GABA release, and may play the same role on neurons releasing other transmitters. Functional $GABA_B$ receptors are heterodimers made up of $GABA_BR_1$ and $GABA_BR_2$ subunits (Bettler et al., 2004) The $GABA_C$ receptor is less widely distributed than the A and B subtypes. GABA is more potent by an order of magnitude at $GABA_C$ than at $GABA_A$ receptors, and a number of $GABA_A$ agonists (e.g., baclofen) and modulators (e.g., benzodiazepines and barbiturates) seem not to interact with $GABA_C$ receptors. $GABA_C$

Table 14–2

Composition, Distribution, and Major Functions of $GABA_A$ Receptors

SUBUNIT COMPOSITION	LOCATION	FUNCTION	COMMENTS
α1β2γ2	Widespread GABA Neurons	Sedation, anticonvulsant activity	Adult, BZ-sensitive, reduced in drug tolerance?
α2β3γ2	Forebrain, spinal cord	Anxiety, muscle relaxant	Axon hillock in some cells, BZ-sensitive
α2β1γ1	Glia		
α3β3γ2	Cortex	Anticonvulsant activity	Embryonic and adult BZ-sensitive
α4β2γ2	Thalamus		Insensitive to agonist BZ
α4β2/3γ2	Dentate gyrus		Elevated in drug withdrawal?
α4β2δ	Thalamus	Tonic inhibition	Extrasynaptic, BZ-insensitive in adults
α4β2/3δ	Dentate gyrus		
α5β3γ2	Hippocampus CA1 Sensory Ganglia	Tonic inhibition	Extrasynaptic, BZ-insensitive
α6β2/3γ2	Cerebellar granule cells		Insensitive to agonist BZ
α6β2/3δ	Cerebellar granule cells	Tonic inhibition	Extrasynaptic, BZ-insensitive, adult
γ3, θ, ε	Little information		

BZ, benzodiazepines.

receptors are found in the retina, spinal cord, superior colliculus, and pituitary (Olsen and Betz, 2005).

Glycine. Many of the features described for the $GABA_A$ receptor family also apply to the inhibitory glycine receptor, which is prominent in the brainstem and spinal cord. Multiple subunits assemble into a variety of glycine receptor subtypes. These pharmacological subtypes are detected in brain tissue with particular neuroanatomical and neurodevelopmental profiles. As with the $GABA_A$ receptor, the complete functional significance of glycine receptor subtypes is not known. There is evidence for clustering of glycine receptors by the anchoring protein gephyrin (Sola et al., 2004). An additional role for glycine is as a co-agonist at NMDA receptors, at which both glutamate and glycine must be present for activation to occur.

Glutamate and Aspartate. Glutamate and aspartate are found in very high concentrations in brain, and both amino acids have powerful excitatory effects on neurons in virtually every region of the CNS. Their widespread distribution initially obscured their roles as transmitters, but there now is broad acceptance that glutamate and possibly aspartate are the principal fast ("classical") excitatory transmitters throughout the CNS (Bleich et al., 2003; Conn, 2003). Multiple subtypes of receptors for excitatory amino acids have been cloned, expressed, and characterized pharmacologically, based on the relative potencies of synthetic agonists and the discovery of potent and selective antagonists (Kotecha and MacDonald, 2003). Glutamate receptors are classed functionally either as ligand-gated ion channel ("ionotropic") receptors or as "metabotropic" GPCRs (Table 14–3).

Neither the precise number of subunits that assembles to generate a functional glutamate ionotropic receptor ion channel *in vivo* nor the intramembranous topography of each subunit has been established unequivocally. The ligand-gated ion channels are further classified according to the identity of agonists that selectively activate each receptor subtype, and are broadly divided into *N*-methyl-D-aspartate

Table 14–3

Classification of Glutamate and Aspartate Receptors[a]

FUNCTIONAL CLASSES	GENE FAMILIES	AGONISTS	ANTAGONISTS	
Ionotropic				
AMPA	GluR1, 2, 3, 4	AMPA Kainate (s) -5-fluorowillardine	CNQX NBQX GYK153655	
Kainate	GluR5, 6, 7 KA1, 2	Kainate ATPA	CNQX LY294486	
NMDA	NR1, 2A, 2B, 2C, 2D	Aspartate NMDA	D-AP5 2R-CPPene MK-801 Ketamine Phencyclidine D-aspartate	
Metabotropic				INTRACELLULAR SIGNALING
Group 1	mGluR1 mGluR5	3,5-DHPG, quisqalate	AIDA CBPG	↑ G_i-PLC-IP_3-Ca^{2+}
Group2	mGluR2 mGluR3	APDC, MGS0028 DCG-IV, LY354740	EGLU PCCG-4	↑ G_i-AC (↓ cAMP)
Group3	mGluR4 mGluR6 mGluR7 mGluR8	L-AP-4 L-AP4 L-AP4 L-AP4, (S)-3,4-DCPG	MAP4 MPPG LY341495	↑ G_i-AC (↓ cAMP)

[a]Glutamate is the principal agonist at both ionotropic and Metabotropic receptors for glutamate and aspartate.
CNQX, 6-Cyano-7-nitroquinoxaline-2,3-dione; NBQX, 1,2,3,4-Tetrahydro-6-nitro-2,3-dioxo-benzo[f]quinoxaline-7-sulfonamide; D-AP5, D-2-amino-5-phosphonovaleric acid; AIDA, 1-aminoindan-1,5-dicarboxylic acid; CBPG, (S)-(+)-2-(3′-carboxybicyclo(1.1.1)pentyl)-glycine; EGLU, (2S)-α-ethylglutamic acid; PCCG-4, phenylcarboxycyclopropylglycine; MAP4, (S)-amino-2-methyl-4-phosphonobutanoic acid; MPPG, (RS)-a-methyl-4-phosphonophenylglycine; AMPA, α-amino-3-hydroxy-5-methyl-4-isoxazolepropionic acid; ATPA, 2-amino-3(3-hydroxy-5-tert-butylisoxazol-4-yl)propanoic acid; NMDA, N-methyl-D-aspartate; 3,5-DHPG, 3,5-dihydroxyphenylglycine; DCG-IV, dicarboxycyclopropyl)glycine; L-AP-4, L-2-amino-4-phosphonobutiric acid; (S)-3,4-DCPG, (S)-3,4-dicarboxyphenylglycine.

(NMDA) receptors and non-NMDA receptors. The non-NMDA receptors include the α-amino-3-hydroxy-5-methyl-4-isoxazole propionic acid (AMPA), and kainic acid (KA) receptors (Table 14–3). Selective antagonists for these receptors are now available. In the case of NMDA receptors, agonists include open-channel blockers such as phencyclidine (PCP or "angel dust"), antagonists such as 5,7-dichlorokynurenic acid, which act at an allosteric glycine-binding site, and the novel antagonist ifenprodil, which may act as a closed-channel blocker. In addition, the activity of NMDA receptors is sensitive to pH and to modulation by a variety of endogenous agents including Zn^{2+}, some neurosteroids, arachidonic acid, redox reagents, and polyamines such as spermine. Additional diversity of glutamate receptors arises by alternative splicing or by single-base editing of mRNAs encoding the receptors or receptor subunits. Alternative splicing has been described for metabotropic receptors and for subunits of NMDA, AMPA, and kainate receptors. For some subunits of AMPA and kainate receptors, the RNA sequence differs from the genomic sequence in a single codon of the receptor subunit that markedly affects the Ca^{2+} permeability of the receptor channel (Conn and Pin, 1997). AMPA and kainate receptors mediate fast depolarization at glutamatergic synapses in the brain and spinal cord. NMDA receptors are involved in normal synaptic transmission, but activation of NMDA receptors is usually associated more closely with the induction of various forms of synaptic plasticity rather than with fast point-to-point signaling in the brain. AMPA or kainate receptors and NMDA receptors may be co-localized at many glutamatergic synapses.

Activation of NMDA receptors is obligatory for the induction of a type of long-term potentiation (LTP) that occurs in the hippocampus. NMDA receptors normally are blocked by Mg^{2+} at resting membrane potentials. Thus, activation of NMDA receptors requires not only binding of synaptically released glutamate, but simultaneous depolarization of the postsynaptic membrane. This is achieved by activation of AMPA/kainate receptors at nearby synapses involving inputs from different neurons. AMPA receptors also are dynamically regulated to affect their sensitivity to the synergism with NMDA. Thus, NMDA receptors may function as coincidence detectors, being activated only when there is simultaneous firing of two or more neurons. A well-characterized phenomenon involving NMDA receptors is the induction of LTP. LTP refers to a prolonged (hours to days) increase in the size of a postsynaptic response to a presynaptic stimulus of given strength. NMDA receptors also can induce long-term depression (LTD; the converse of LTP) at CNS synapses. The frequency and pattern of synaptic stimulation may dictate whether a synapse undergoes LTP or LTD (Nestler et al., 2009). It is believed that NMDA-dependent LTP and LTD reflect the insertion and internalization of AMPA receptors, possibly mediated by CaM-kinase II and calcineurin/protein phosphatase 1, respectively (Figure 14–12).

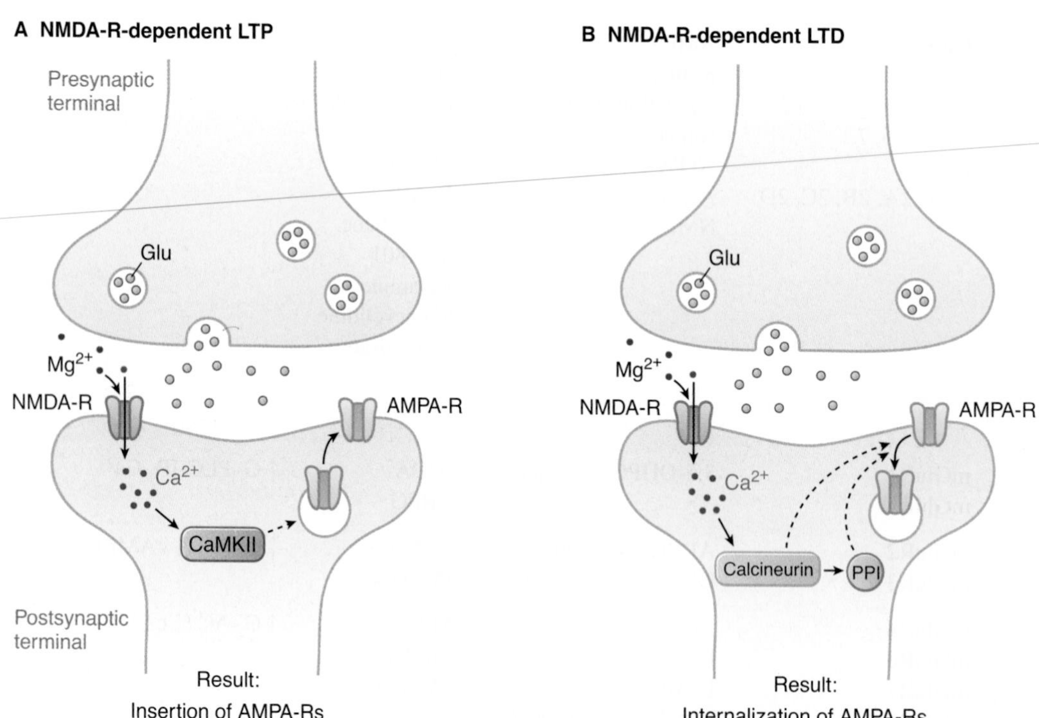

Figure 14–12. *Major forms of NMDA receptor-dependent LTP and LTD.* ***A.*** NMDA receptor-dependent LTP requires postsynaptic NMDA receptor activation leading to a rise in Ca^{2+} and activation of CaM kinase II (CaMKII). AMPA receptor insertion into the postsynaptic membrane is a major mechanism underlying LTP expression. ***B.*** NMDA receptor-dependent LTD is triggered by Ca^{2+} entry through postsynaptic NMDA receptor channels, leading to increases in the activity of the protein phosphatases calcineurin and PP1. LTD occurs when postsynaptic AMPA receptors are internalized. (Redrawn with permission from Nestler EJ, Hyman SE, Malenka RC (eds). *Molecular Neuropharmacology*. New York: McGraw-Hill, **2000**, p 132. Copyright © 2009 by The McGraw-Hill Companies, Inc. All rights reserved.)

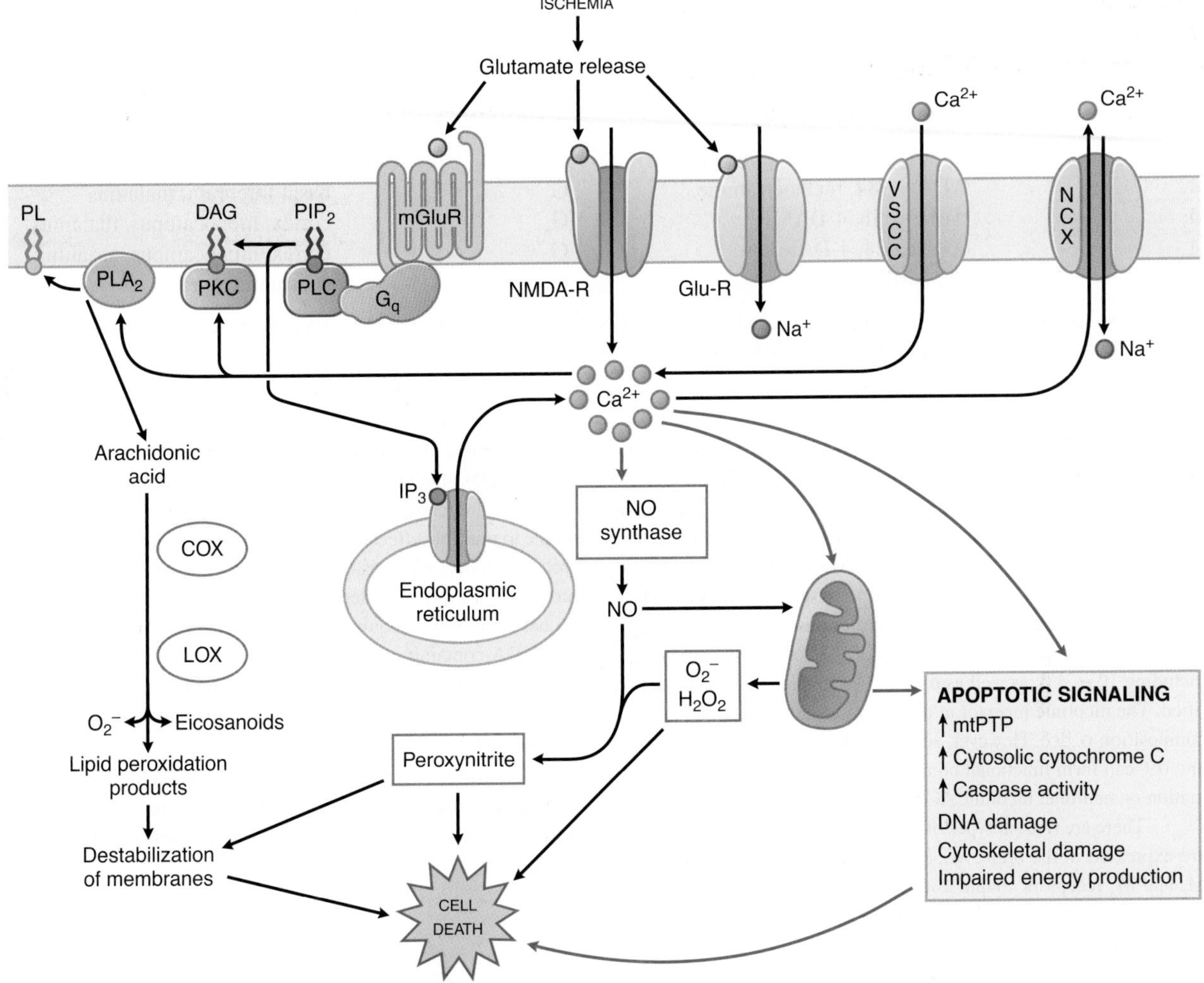

Figure 14–13. *Mechanisms contributing to neuronal injury during ischemia-reperfusion.* Several pathways contribute to excitotoxic neuronal injury in ischemia, with excess cytosolic Ca^{2+} playing a precipitating role. *DAG,* diacylglycerol; *GluR,* AMPA/kainate type of glutamate receptors; IP_3, inositol trisphosphate; *mGluR,* metabotropic glutamate receptor; *NMDA-R, N*—methyl-D-aspartate receptor; O_2^-, superoxide radical; PIP_2, phophatidyinositol 4,5-bisphosphate; PKC, protein kinase C; PL, phospholipids, PL phospholipase, VSCC, voltage-sensitive Ca^{2+} channel. COX, cyclooxygenase; LOX, lipoxygenase; NCX, NA^+/Ca^{2+} exchanger; mtPTP, mitochondrial permeability transition pore. (Reproduced with permission from Dugan LL, Kim-Han JS: Hypoxic-ischemic brain injury and oxidative stress, in Siegel GS, Albers RW, Brady S, Price D (eds): *Basic Neurochemistry: Molecular, Cellular, and Medical Aspects*, 7th ed. Burlington, MA: Elsevier Academic Press, 2006, p 564. Copyright © 2006, American Society for Neurochemistry. All rights reserved.)

Glutamate Excitotoxicity. High concentrations of glutamate lead to neuronal cell death by mechanisms that have only recently begun to be clarified (Figure 14–13). The cascade of events leading to neuronal death is thought to be triggered by excessive activation of NMDA or AMPA/kinase receptors, allowing significant influx of Ca^{2+} into neurons. Glutamate-mediated excitotoxicity may underlie the damage that occurs after ischemia or hypoglycemia in the brain, during which a massive release and impaired reuptake of glutamate in the synapse leads to excess stimulation of glutamate receptors and subsequent cell death. NMDA receptor antagonists can attenuate neuronal cell death induced by activation of these receptors (Haeberlein and Lipton, 2009). Because of their widespread distribution in the CNS, glutamate receptors have become targets for diverse therapeutic interventions. For example, a role for disordered glutamatergic transmission in the etiology of chronic neurodegenerative diseases and in schizophrenia has been postulated (Chapters 16 and 22).

Acetylcholine. Based on a non-homogeneous distribution within the CNS and the observation that peripheral cholinergic drugs could produce marked behavioral effects after central administration, many investigators addressed the possibility that ACh might also be a central neurotransmitter. In the late 1950s, Eccles and colleagues identified ACh as a neurotransmitter for the excitation of spinal cord Renshaw interneurons by the recurrent axon collaterals of spinal motoneurons. Subsequently, the capacity of ACh to elicit neuronal discharge has been replicated on scores of CNS cells (Shepherd, 2003). Eight major clusters of ACh neurons and their pathways have been characterized (Cooper et al., 2003; Nestler et al., 2009; Shepherd, 2003). For additional details, see Chapter 9.

Table 14–4

Subtypes of Muscarinic Receptors in the CNS

SUBTYPE	SELECTIVE ANTAGONISTS	G-PROTEIN FAMILY	LOCALIZATION IN THE CNS
M_1	pirenzepine, telenzepine, 4-DAMP	G_q	cortex, hippocampus, striatum
M_2	AF-Dx-384, methoctramine	G_i	basal forebrain, thalamus
M_3	darifenacin, 4-DAMP	G_q	cortex, hippocampus, thalamus
M_4	AF-Dx384, 4-DAMP	G_i	cortex, hippocampus, striatum
M_5	4-DAMP	G_q	substantia nigra

Non-selective agonists include carbachol, pilocarpine, and oxotremorine. Non-selective antagonists include atropine and scopolamine. McN-A-3436 is a selective agonist at the M_1 receptor. 4-DAMP, 4-diphenylacetoxy-N-methylpiperidine.

In most regions of the CNS, the effects of ACh result from interaction with a mixture of nicotinic and muscarinic receptors. Nicotinic ACh receptors are found in autonomic ganglia, the adrenal gland, and in the CNS. Activation by ACh results in a rapid increase in the influx of Na^+ and Ca^{2+} and subsequent depolarization. Nicotinic cholinergic receptors appear to desensitize rapidly. The receptors are composed by five heterologous subunits arranged around a central pore (see Figure 14–4). A total of 17 subunits, including 10 α, 4 β, as well as δ, ε, and γ subunits, have been identified. The nicotinic receptor at the neuromuscular junction has the composition $\alpha_2\beta\varepsilon\delta$. However, some α subunits, including α7, α8, and α9, can form functional homo-oligomers. For additional information on neuronal nicotinic ACh receptors, see Chapter 11.

There are five subtypes of muscarinic receptors, all of which are expressed in the brain. M_1, M_3, and M_5 couple to G_q while the M_2 and M_4 receptors couple to G_i (Table 14–4). Several presumptive cholinergic pathways have been proposed in addition to that of the motoneuron-Renshaw cell.

Catecholamines. The brain contains separate neuronal systems that utilize three different catecholamines—dopamine, norepinephrine, and epinephrine. Each system is anatomically distinct and serves separate, functional roles within its field of innervation (Nestler et al., 2009)

Dopamine. Although DA was originally regarded only as a precursor of NE, assays of distinct regions of the CNS revealed that the distributions of DA and NE are markedly different. In fact, more than half the CNS content of catecholamine is DA and extremely large amounts of DA are found in the basal ganglia. There are three major DA-containing pathways in the CNS (Figure 14–14):

- the nigrostriatal pathway
- the mesocortical pathway, where neurons in the ventral tegmental nucleus project to a variety of midbrain structures and to the frontal cortex
- the tuberoinfundibular pathway, which delivers DA to cells in the anterior pituitary

Initial pharmacological studies discriminated between two subtypes of DA receptors: D_1 (which couples to G_S to stimulate adenylyl cyclase) and D_2 (which couples to G_i to inhibit adenylyl cyclase). Subsequent studies identified three additional genes encoding subtypes of DA receptors: the D_5 receptor, which is related to the D_1 receptor; and the D_3 and D_4 receptors, which are part of what is called the D2 receptor family. There are also two isoforms of the D_2 receptor that differ in the predicted length of their third intracellular loops (Nestler et al., 2009). The D_1 and D_5 receptors activate the G_s-adenylyl cyclase-cyclic AMP-PKA system. The D_2 receptors couple to multiple effector systems, including inhibition of adenylyl cyclase activity, suppression of Ca^{2+} currents, and activation of K^+ currents. The effector systems to which the D_3 and D_4 receptors couple have not been unequivocally defined (Greengard, 2001) (Table 14–5). DA-containing pathways and receptors have been implicated in the pathophysiology of schizophrenia and Parkinson disease and in the side effects seen following pharmacotherapy of these disorders (Chapters 16 and 22).

Norepinephrine. There are relatively large amounts of NE within the hypothalamus and in certain parts of the limbic system, such as the central nucleus of the amygdala and the dentate gyrus of the

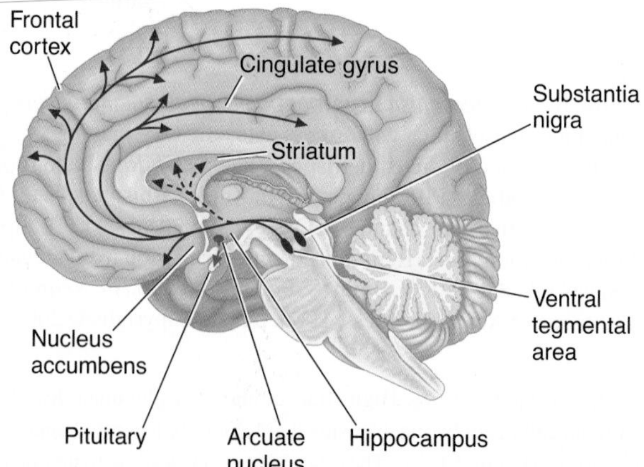

Figure 14–14. *The three major dopaminergic projections in the CNS.* 1. The mesostriatal (or nigrostriatal) pathway. Neurons in the substantia nigra pars compacta (SNc) project to the dorsal striatum (*upward dashed blue arrows*); this is the pathway that degenerates in Parkinson disease. 2. Neurons in the ventral tegmental area project to the ventral striatum (nucleus accumbens), olfactory bulb, amygdala, hippocampus, orbital and medial prefrontal cortex, and cinguate gyrus (*solid blue arrows*). 3. Neurons in the arcuate nucleus of the hypothalamus project by the tuberoinfundibular pathway in the hypothalamus, from which DA is delivered to the anterior pituitary (*red arrows*).

Table 14–5

Dopamine Receptors in the CNS

RECEPTOR	AGONISTS	ANTAGONISTS	G-PROTEIN FAMILY	AREAS OF LOCALIZATION
D_1	SKF82958 SKF81297	SCH23390 SKF83566; haloperidol	G_s	neostriatum; cerebral cortex; olfactory tubercle; nucleus accumbens
D_2	Bromocriptine, apomorphine	Raclopride, sulpiride, haloperidol	G_i	neostriatum; olfactory tubercle; nucleus accumbens
D_3	Quinpirole 7-OH-DPAT	Raclopride	G_i	nucleus accumbens; islands of Calleja
D_4		Clozapine, L-745,870, sonepiprazole	G_i	midbrain; amygdala; hippocampus; hypothalamus
D_5	SKF38393	SCH23390	G_s	

7-OH-DPAT, 7-hydroxy-N,N-di-n-propyl-2-aminotetralin.

hippocampus. However, this catecholamine also is present in significant, although lower, amounts in most brain regions. Detailed mapping studies indicate that noradrenergic neurons of the locus ceruleus innervate specific target cells in a large number of cortical, subcortical, and spinomedullary fields (Nestler et al., 2009). NE has been established as the transmitter at synapses between presumptive noradrenergic pathways and a wide variety of target neurons. For example, stimulation of the locus ceruleus depresses the spontaneous activity of target neurons in the cerebellum; this is associated with a slowly developing hyperpolarization and a decrease in membrane conductance (Aston-Jones et al., 2001; Nestler et al., 2009).

Multiple types and subtypes of adrenergic receptors (α_1, α_2, and *β*) and their subtypes have been described in the CNS; all are GPCRs (Table 14–6). As expected, β receptors couple to G_s and

Table 14–6

Adrenergic Receptors in the CNS

RECEPTOR	AGONIST	ANTAGONIST	G-PROTEIN FAMILY	AREAS OF LOCALIZATION IN THE BRAIN
α_{1A}	A61603 phenylephrine oxymetazoline	nigulpidine prazosin 5-methylurapidil	G_q	cortex, hippocampus
α_{1B}	phenylephrine oxymetazoline	spiperone prazosin (+)-cyclazosin	G_q	cortex brainstem
α_{1D}	phenylephrine oxymetazoline	A-119637 tamsulosin	G_q	cortex
α_{2A}	oxymetazoline clonidine	yohimbine; rauwolscine; bromocriptine	G_i	locus ceruleus and hippocampus
α_{2B}	clonidine dexmedetomidine	yohimbine; rauwolscine; lisuride	G_i	diencephalon
α_{2C}	clonidine	yohimbine; rauwolscine; lisuride	G_i	widely distributed
β_1	CGP 12177 prenalterol	alprenolol betaxolol metoprolol	G_s	cortex and hypothalamus
β_2	fenoterol salmeterol	propranolol ICI 118551	G_s	cerebellum, hippocampus, cortex
β_3	carazolol	carvedilol; tertalolol	? G_s	unknown

thence to adenylyl cyclase. α_1 Adrenergic receptors are coupled to G_q, resulting in stimulation of phospholipase C, and are associated predominantly with neurons. α_2 Adrenergic receptors are found on glial and vascular elements, as well as on neurons; they couple to G_i and thence to inhibition of adenylyl cyclase activity. α_1 Receptors on noradrenergic target neurons of the neocortex and thalamus respond to NE with prazosin-sensitive, depolarizing responses due to decreases in K^+ conductance. However, stimulation of α_1 receptors also can augment cyclic AMP accumulation in neocortical slices in response to concurrent stimulation of the G_s pathway, possibly an example of G_q-G_S cross-talk involving Ca^{2+}/calmodulin and/or PKC (Ostrom et al., 2003). α_2 Adrenergic receptors are prominent on noradrenergic neurons, where they presumably couple to G_i, inhibit adenylyl cyclase, and mediate a hyperpolarizing response due to enhancement of an inwardly rectifying K^+ channel. As in the periphery, α_2 receptors are located presynaptically, where they function as inhibitory autoreceptors. There is also evidence for postsynaptic α_2 receptors that modulate sympathetic tone. Effects mediated through α_2 receptors on blood pressure have been reported. It is believed, e.g., that the antihypertensive effects of the α_2 selective agonist clonidine are due to stimulation of α_2 receptors in the lower brainstem.

Epinephrine. Neurons in the CNS that contain epinephrine were recognized only after the development of sensitive enzymatic assays and immunocytochemical staining techniques for phenylethanolamine-*N*-methyltransferase, the enzyme that converts NE into epinephrine. Epinephrine-containing neurons are found in the medullary reticular formation and make restricted connections to pontine and diencephalic nuclei, eventually coursing as far rostrally as the paraventricular nucleus of the thalamus. Their physiological properties have not been unambiguously identified.

5-Hydroxytryptamine (Serotonin). In mammals, 5-HT containing neurons are found in nine nuclei lying in or adjacent to the midline (raphe) regions of the pons and upper brainstem. Cells receiving cytochemically demonstrable 5-HT input, such as the suprachiasmatic nucleus, ventrolateral geniculate body, amygdala, and hippocampus, exhibit a uniform and dense investment of serotinergic terminals.

Molecular biological approaches have led to identification of 14 distinct mammalian 5-HT receptor subtypes (Table 14–7). These subtypes exhibit characteristic ligand-binding profiles, couple to different intracellular signaling systems, exhibit subtype-specific distributions within the CNS, and mediate distinct behavioral effects of 5-HT. Most 5-HT receptors are GPCRs coupling to a variety of G-protein α subunits. The 5-HT_3 receptor, however, is a ligand-gated ion channel with structural similarity to the α-subunit of the nicotinic acetylcholine receptor. As seen with subtypes of glutamate receptors, mRNA editing has also been observed for the 5-HT_{2C} receptor (Niswender et al., 2001); the resulting isoforms differ in agonist affinity and distribution in the brain.

The family of 5-HT_1 receptors is composed of at least five receptor subtypes (Table 14–7) that are linked to inhibition of adenylyl cyclase activity or to regulation of K^+ or Ca^{2+} channels. 5-HT_{1A} Receptors are abundantly expressed on 5-HT neurons in the dorsal raphe nucleus, where they are thought to be involved in temperature regulation. They also are found in regions of the CNS associated with mood and anxiety such as the hippocampus and amygdala. Activation of 5-HT_{1A} receptors opens an inwardly rectifying K^+ conductance, which leads to hyperpolarization and neuronal inhibition. These receptors can be activated by drugs including buspirone, which is used for the treatment of anxiety and also used off-label for panic disorders. In contrast, 5-HT_{1D} receptors are activated by low concentrations ofsumatriptan, which is currently prescribed for acute management of migraine headaches (Chapters 13 and 34). The 5-HT_2 receptor class has three subtypes: 5-HT_{2A}, 5-HT_{2B}, and 5-HT_{2C}; these receptors couple to pertussis toxin-insensitive G proteins (e.g., G_q and G_{11}) and link to activation of PLC. Based on ligand binding and mRNA *in situ* hybridization patterns, 5-HT_{2A} receptors are enriched in forebrain regions such as the neocortex and olfactory tubercle, as well as in several nuclei arising from the brainstem. The 5-HT_{2C} receptor, which is very similar in sequence and pharmacology to the 5-HT_{2A} receptor, is expressed abundantly in the choroid plexus, where it may modulate cerebrospinal fluid production. Many of the effects of antidepressants are thought to be a consequence of increased stimulation of 5-HT receptors following inhibition of 5-HT reuptake by SERT. On the other hand, inhibition of 5-HT_{2c} receptors may account for the increased weight gain associated with neuroleptics used to treat schizophrenia.

5-HT_3 receptors function as ligand-gated ion channels; these receptors were first recognized in the peripheral autonomic nervous system. Within the CNS, they are expressed in the area postrema and solitary tract nucleus, where they couple to potent depolarizing responses that show rapid desensitization to continued 5-HT exposure. Actions of 5-HT at central 5-HT_3 receptors can lead to emesis and anti-nociceptive actions, and 5-HT_3 antagonists are beneficial in the management of chemotherapy-induced emesis (Chapter 46).

Within the CNS, 5-HT_4 receptors occur on neurons within the inferior and superior colliculi and in the hippocampus. Activation of 5-HT_4 receptors stimulates the G_s-adenylyl cyclase-cyclic AMP pathway. Other 5-HT receptors are less well studied in the CNS. The 5-HT_6 and 5-HT_7 receptors also couple to G_s; their affinity for clozapine may contribute to its antipsychotic efficacy (Chapter 16).

The hallucinogen lysergic acid diethylamide (LSD) is a potent partial agonist at 5-HT_2 receptors. When applied iontophoretically, LSD inhibits the firing of raphe (5-HT) neurons. The inhibitory effect of LSD on raphe neurons offers a plausible explanation for its hallucinogenic effects, namely that these effects result from depression of activity in a system that tonically inhibits visual and other sensory inputs. However, typical LSD-induced behaviors are seen in animals with destroyed raphe nuclei or after blockade of the synthesis of 5-HT by *p*-chlorophenylalanine (Aghajanian and Marek, 1999); Nichols, 2004).

Histamine. Histamine and antihistamines have long been known to produce significant effects on animal behavior. Biochemical detection of histamine synthesis by neurons and direct cytochemical localization of these neurons have defined a histaminergic system in the CNS. Most of these neurons are located in the ventral posterior hypothalamus; they give rise to long ascending and descending tracts that are typical of the patterns characteristic of other aminergic systems. Based on the presumptive central effects of histamine antagonists, the histaminergic system is thought to affect arousal, body temperature, and vascular dynamics. Four subtypes of histamine receptors have been described; all are GPCRs (Figure 14–15). H_1 receptors, the most prominent, are located on glia and vessels as well as on neurons and act to mobilize Ca^{2+} in receptive cells through the G_q-PLC pathway.

Table 14–7

5-HT Receptors in the CNS

RECEPTOR	AGONISTS	ANTAGONISTS	TRANSDUCER	LOCALIZATION
$5HT_{1A}$	8-OH-DPAT, buspirone, lisuride	WAY 100135, NAD 299	G_i	hippocampus, septum, amygdala, dorsal raphe, cortex
$5HT_{1B}$	sumatriptan, dihydroergotamine, oxymetazoline	GR-127935, ketanserin	G_i	substantia nigra, basal ganglia
$5HT_{1D}$	sumatriptan, dihydroergotamine, oxymetazoline	GR127935, methysergide, L-772405	G_i	substantia nigra, striatum, nucleus accumbens, hippocampus
$5HT_{1E}$	eletriptan, ORG-5222		G_i	
$5HT_{1F}$	LY334370, naratriptan	methysergide	G_i	dorsal raphe, hippocampus, cortex
$5HT_{2A}$	DMT, DOB, DOI, ergotamine, LSD	amoxapine, chlorpromazine, ketanserin	G_q	cortex, olfactory tubercle, claustrum
$5HT_{2B}$	cabergoline, 5-MeOT	clozapine, lisuride, LY53857	G_q	not located in the brain
$5HT_{2C}$	ergotamine, DOI, lisuride	amoxepine, fluoxetine, mesulergine	G_q	basal ganglia, choroid plexus, substantia nigra
$5HT_3$		ondansetron, granisetron	Ligand-gated channel	spinal cord, cortex, hippocampus, brainstem nuclei
$5HT_4$	cisapride, metoclopramide	GR113808, SB204070	G_s	hippocampus, nucleus accumbens striatum, substantia nigra
$5HT_{5A}$		methiothepin	G_s	cortex, hippocampus, cerebellum
$5HT_{5B}$		ergotamine, methiothepin	?G_i	habenula, hippocampal CA1
$5HT_6$	bromocriptine	methiothepin, clozapine, amiltriptyline	G_s	striatum, olfactory tubercle, cortex, hippocampus
$5HT_7$	pergolide, 5-MeOT	methiothepin, clozapine, metergoline	G_s	hypothalamus, thalamus, cortex, suprachiasmatic nucleus

8-OH-DPAT, 8-hydroxy-N,N-dipropyl-2-aminotetralin; DOB, 2,5-Dimethoxy-4-bromoamphetamine; DOI, (±)-2,5-dimethoxy-4-iodoamphetamine; DMT, N,N-dimethyltryptamine; 5-MeOT, 2-(5-methoxy-1H-indol-3-yl) ethanamine; LSD, Lysergic acid diethylamide.

H_2 receptors couple via G_S to the activation of adenylyl cyclase. H_3 receptors, which have the greatest sensitivity to histamine, are localized primarily in basal ganglia and olfactory regions in rat brain and act through G_i to inhibit adenylyl cyclase. Consequences of H_3 receptor activation remain unresolved but may include reduced Ca^{2+} influx and feedback inhibition of transmitter synthesis and release (Chapter 32). H_4 receptors are expressed on cells of hematopoietic origin: eosinophils, T cells, mast cells, basophils, and dendritic cells. H_4 receptors appear to couple to G_i and G_q and are postulated to play a role in inflammation and chemotaxis (Thurmond et al., 2004). Unlike the monoamines and amino acid transmitters, there does not appear to be an active process for reuptake of histamine after its release. Inhibition of H_1 receptors causes drowsiness, an effect that limits the use of H_1 antagonists to treat allergic reactions. The development of H_1 antagonists with low CNS penetration has reduced the incidence of these side effects.

Peptides. The discovery during the 1980s of numerous novel peptides in the CNS, each capable of regulating neuronal function, produced considerable excitement and an imposing catalog of substances as well as potential medications based upon interaction with peptide receptors (Darlison and Richter, 1999; Hökfelt et al., 2003). In addition, certain peptides previously thought to be restricted to the GI tract or to endocrine glands have been found in the CNS. Most of these peptides bind to GPCRs. Many of the effects are modulatory rather than causing direct excitation or inhibition. Myriad peptide neurotransmitters or neuromodulators have been described (Table 14–8). Relatively detailed neuronal maps are available that identify immunoreactivity to peptide-specific antisera. While some CNS peptides may function on their own, most are now thought to act primarily in concert with co-existing transmitters, both amines and amino acids.

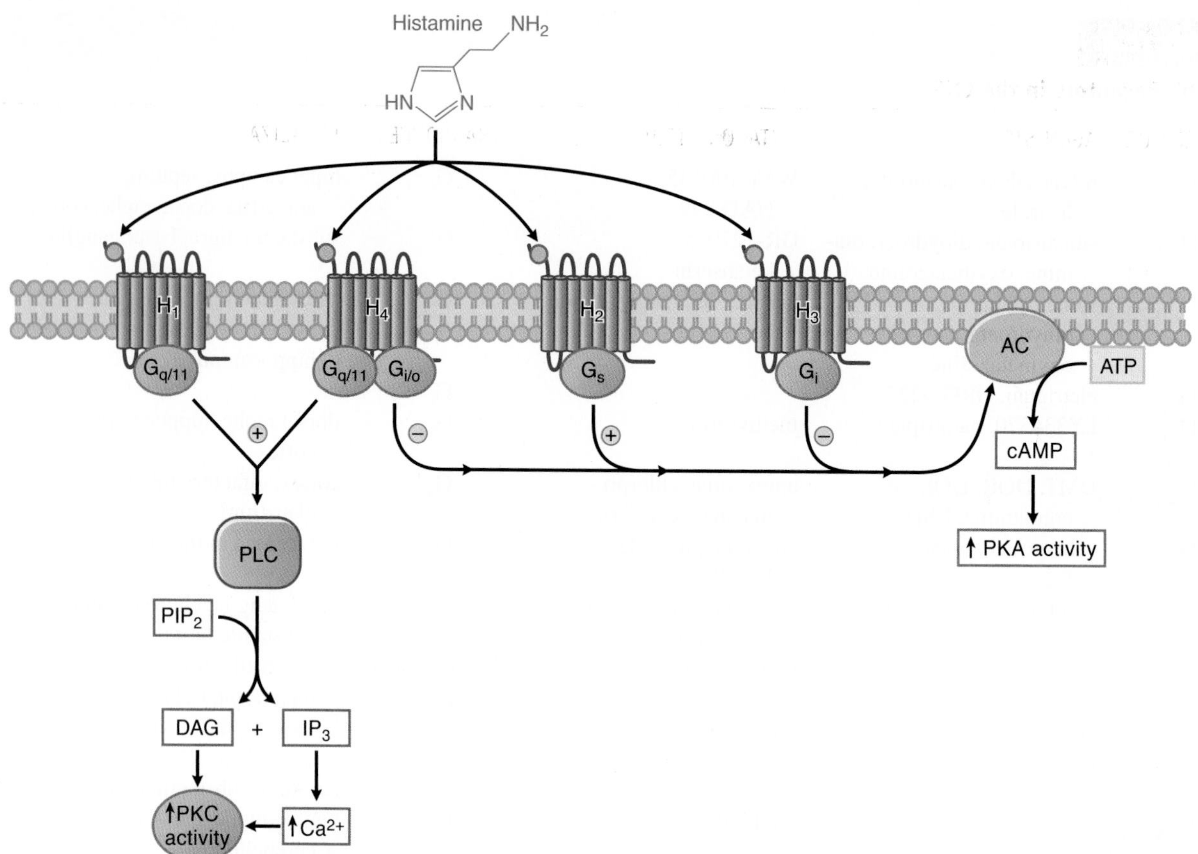

Figure 14–15. *Main signaling pathways for histamine receptors.* Histamine can couple to a variety of G protein-linked signal transduction pathways via four different receptors. The H_1 receptor and some H_4 receptors activate phosphatidylinositol turnover via $G_{q/11}$. The other receptors couple either positively (H_2 receptor) or negatively (H_3 and H_4 receptor) to adenylyl cyclase activity via G_s and $G_{i/o}$.

Neuropeptides are processed and stored in large, dense-core vesicles (LDCVs; see Figure 14–7). The peptides may be co-localized and released together with small molecule transmitters, such as a biogenic amine. Multiple peptides may be co-localized within the same neuron. As noted, some neurons may contain two or more transmitters, including peptides, and their release can be independently regulated.

In contrast to the biogenic amines or amino acids, peptide synthesis requires transcription of DNA into mRNA and translation of mRNA into protein. This takes place primarily in perikaria and the resulting peptide is then transported to nerve terminals. Single genes can, through the post-translational action of peptidases, give rise to multiple neuropeptides. For example, proteolytic processing of proopiomelanocortin (POMC) gives rise to, among other things, ACTH, α and γ MSH, β-MSH, and β-endorphin (Figure 14–16). In addition, alternative splicing of RNA transcripts may result in distinct mRNA species. For example, calcitonin and calcitonin gene-related peptide (CGRP) are derived in specific tissues from the same primary transcript.

Organization by Function. Since most peptides were identified initially on the basis of bioassays, their names reflect these biologically assayed functions (e.g., thyrotropin-releasing hormone and vasoactive intestinal polypeptide). These names become trivial when more ubiquitous distributions and additional functions are discovered. Some general integrative role might be hypothesized for widely separated neurons (and other cells) that make the same peptide. However, a more parsimonious view is that each peptide has unique messenger roles at the cellular level that are used repeatedly in biologically similar pathways within functionally distinct systems.

Most neuropeptide receptors are GPCRs. In comparison to GPCRs for smaller ligands such as biogenic amines and amino acids, the extracellular domains of neuropeptide receptors play a larger role in ligand binding. As seen with other transmitter systems, there are often multiple subtypes of receptor for the same peptide transmitter (Table 14–9). For example, there are five subtypes of receptor for somatostatin and all inhibit adenylyl cyclase through an interaction with G_i; they differ in their interaction with various somatostatin analogs. The cloning of the major members of the opioid-peptide receptors has revealed unexpected, and as yet unexplained, homologies with receptors for somatostatin, angiotensin, and other peptides. Multiple melanocortin receptors exist that respond to various peptides derived from POMC. Not surprisingly, the receptor on adrenal

Table 14–8

Examples of Neuropeptides

Calcitonin Family	Tachykinins
Calcitonin	Neurokinin A (substance A)
Calcitonin gene-related peptide (CGRP)	Neurokinin B
Hypothalamic Hormones	Neuropeptide K
Oxytocin	Substance P
Vasopressin	VIP-Glucagon Family
Hypothalamic Releasing and Inhibitory Hormones	Glucagon
Corticotropin-releasing factor (CRF or CRH)	Glucagon-like peptide (GLP-1)
Gonadotropin-releasing hormone (GnRH)	Pituitary adenylyl cyclase—activating peptide (PACAP)
Growth hormone releasing hormone (GHRH)	Vasoactive intestinal polypeptide (VIP)
Somatostatin (SST)	Some Other Peptides
Thyrotropin releasing hormone (TRH)	Agouti-related peptide (ARP)
Neuropeptide Y Family	Bombesin
Neuropeptide Y (NPY)	Bradykinin (BK)
Neuropeptide YY (PYY)	Cholecystokinin (CCK; multiple forms)
Pancreatic polypeptide (PP)	Cocaine- and amphetamine-regulated transcript (CART)
Opioid Peptides	Galanin
β-endorphin (also pituitary hormone)	Ghrelin
Dynorphin peptides	Melanin-concentrating hormone (MCH)
Leu-enkephalin	Neurotensin
Met-enkephalin	Nerve growth factor (NGF)
Pituitaty Hormones	Orexins (or Hypocretins)
Adrenocorticotropic hormone (ACTH)	Orphanin GQ (or Nociceptin) (also grouped with opioids)
α-Melanocyte-stimulating hormone (α-MSH)	
Growth hormone (GH)	
Follicle-stimulating hormone (FSH)	
β-lipotropin (β-LPH)	
Luteinizing hormone (LH)	

Modified with permission from Nestler, E.J., Hyman, S.E., and Malenka, R.C. Molecular Neuropharmacology. McGraw-Hill, New York, 2009, page 184, Table 7–1.

cortical cells responds to ACTH, while that on melanocytes responds to α-MSH. Further evidence for complexity comes from the realization that agonists at subtypes of melanocortin receptors are associated with a variety of biological effects including skin darkening (MCR1), decreased appetite (MCR3 and/or MCR4), and sexual arousal (MCR4).

Although most peptide receptors are GPCRs, exceptions do exist. The amiloride-sensitive FMRF amide (phe-met-arg-phe-amide) receptor is a peptide-gated ion channel. The large number of neuropeptides and peptide receptors has lead to increased interest in identifying therapeutic agents. Examples include experimental substance P antagonists as antidepressants or to treat anxiety, and antagonists of CRH for stress related disorders.

Comparison with Other Transmitters. Peptides differ in several important respects from the monoamine and amino acid transmitters. Peptide synthesis takes place in the rough endoplasmic reticulum. The propeptide is cleaved (processed) to the secreted form as secretory vesicles are transported from the perinuclear cytoplasm to the nerve terminal. Active mechanisms for the local synthesis of peptides have not been described; thus, peptidergic nerve terminals depend on distant sites of synthesis. As for structure-activity relationships for peptide transmitters, linear chains of amino acids can assume many conformations at their receptors, making it difficult to define the sequences and their steric relationships that are critical for activity. Until recently, it was difficult to develop non-peptidic synthetic agonists or antagonists that interact with specific peptide receptors. Such agents now are being developed for many neuropeptides (Hökfelt et al., 2003). Natural products have not been good sources of drugs that affect peptidergic transmission. Only one plant alkaloid, morphine, has been found to act selectively at peptidergic synapses. Fortunately for pharmacologists, morphine was discovered before the endorphins, or rigid

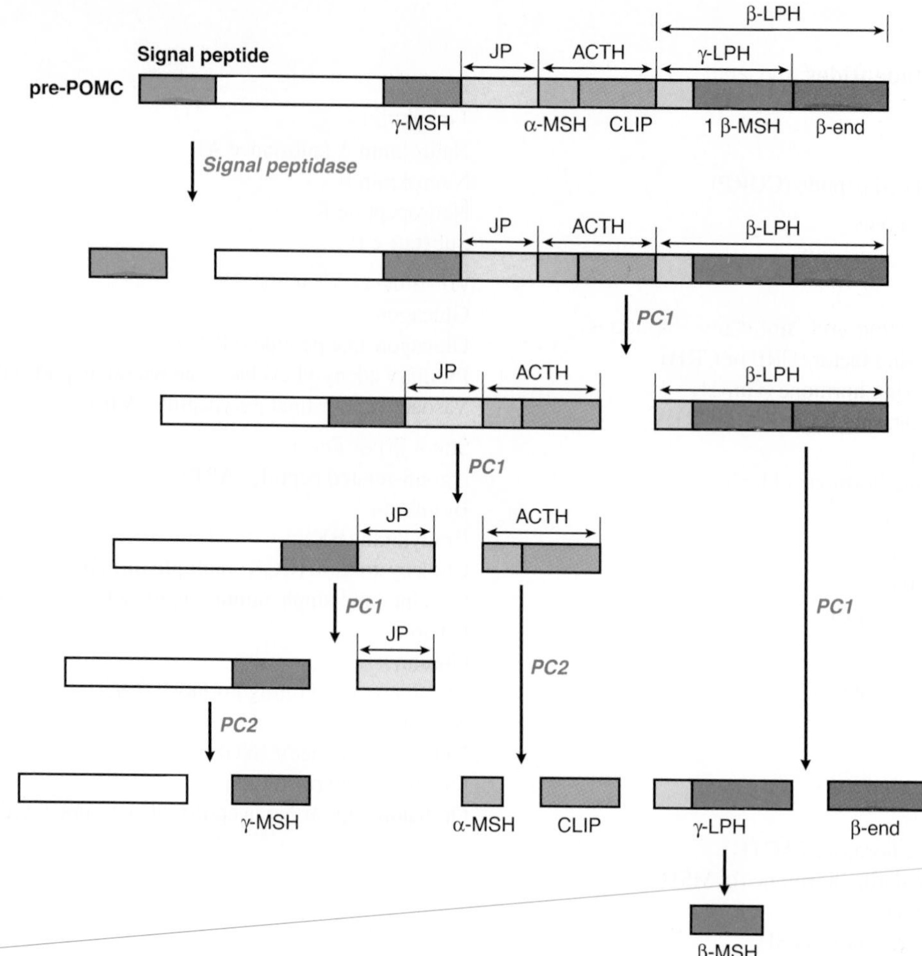

Figure 14–16. *Proteolytic processing of praopiomelanocortin (POMC).* After removal of the signal peptide from pre-POMC, the remaining propeptide undergoes endoprotolysis by prohormone convertases 1 and 2 (PC1 and PC2) at dibasic residues. PC1 liberates the bioactive peptides adrenocorticotropic hormone (ACTH), β-endorphin (β end), and γ-lipotrophic hormone (γ-LPH). PC2 cleaves ACTH into corticotrophin-like intermediate lobe peptide (CLIP) and α-melanocyte stimulating hormone (α-MSH) and also releases γ-MSH from the N-terminal portion of the propeptide. The joining peptide (JP) is the region between ACTH and γ-MSH. β-MSH is formed by cleavage of γ-LPH. Some of the resulting peptides are amidated or acetylated before they become fully active.

molecules capable of acting at peptide receptors might have been deemed impossible to develop.

Other Regulatory Substances

Cannnabinoids. Delta-9-tetrahydrocannabinol (THC) is one of several active substances in marijuana (Figure 14–17). It has dramatic short-term effects, including causing feelings of euphoria and altered sensory perception. After chronic or long-term use, withdrawal symptoms include irritability and sleep disturbances. The primary pharmacologic effects of THC follow its interaction with CB_1 receptors in the CNS and CB_2 receptors in the periphery. CB_1 receptors are found primarily in the basal ganglia, hippocampus, cerebellum, and cerebral cortex. They are also expressed in some non-neuronal cells and tissues, including leukocytes and testis. CB_2 receptors are expressed in the spleen, tonsils, bone marrow, and on peripheral blood leukocytes. The natural endogenous ligands for these receptors are arachidonic acid derivatives including anandamide and 2-arachidonyl glycerol (Figure 14–17). Both CB_1 and CB_2 receptors are linked to G_i and inhibition of adenylyl cyclase activity. Activation of CB_1 receptors results in inhibition of glutamate release. Efforts to develop CB_1 antagonists like rimonabant have focused on possible treatments for drug addiction and obesity. Efforts are also underway to develop agonists that interact with CB_1 and CB_2 receptors for the relief of pain. THC (*dronabinol,* MARINOL) is sometimes used in the control of nausea and moderate pain (Chapter 46).

Purines. Adenosine, ATP, UDP, and UTP have roles as extracellular signaling molecules (Robertson et al., 2001; Siegel et al., 2006). High concentrations of ATP are found in adrenergic storage vesicles and ATP is released along with catecholamines and the other contents

Table 14–9

Peptide transmitters and receptors

PEPTIDE	RECEPTOR	AGONISTS	EFFECTOR MECHANISM	ANTAGONISTS
Opioid	δ κ μ	DADLE, diprenorphine bremazocine, etorphine DAMGO, etorphine	↑ G_i-AC (↓ cAmp)	naltriben, naltrindole nalmefene, naltrexone diprenorphine, naltrexone
Somatostatin	SST_1 SST_2 SST_3 SST_4 SST_5	CST-17 BIM 23059 BIM 23066 CGP 23996 BIM 23313	↑ G_i-AC (↓ cAmp)	SRA880 D-Tyr8-CYN 154806 sst3-ODN-8 L-Tyr8-CYN 154806
Neurotensin	NTS1 NTS2	EISAI-1, JMV431 levocabastine	↑ G_q-PLC	SR142948A
Oxenin	OX_1 OX_2		↑ G_q-PLC	SB-410220
Tachykinin	NK_1 NK_2 NK_3	Substance P methyl ester β-{ala²}$NKA_{4\text{-}10}$ GR138676	↑ G_q-PLC	
CCK	CCK_1 CCK_2	ARL-15849, SR14613 BC-264, PBC-264	↑ G_q-PLC	FK-480, lintitript Triglumide, PD-149164
NPY	Y_1 Y_2 Y_4 Y_5		↑ G_i-AC (↓ cAmp) ↓ cAmp ↑ G_q-PLC ↑ G_i-AC (↓ cAmp)	GR231118 BIIE0246 CGP 71683A

DADLE, 2-Alanyl-Leucine enkephalin; DAMGO, 2-Ala-4-MePhe-5-Gly-enkephalin

of adrenergic storage granules. Intracellular nucleotides may also reach the cell surface by other means (Lazarowski et al., 2003), including as a consequence of cellular hypoxia or cell death, and extracellular adenosine can result from cellular release and metabolism of ATP (Jackson and Raghvendra, 2004). The concentration of ATP may greatly exceed the concentration of adenosine and, given the presence of nucleotidases, it can be difficult to unambiguously distinguish between effects of, e.g., adenosine and ATP.

Extracellular nucleotides and adenosine act on a family of purinergic receptors that is divided into two classes, P1 and P2 (Table 14–10). P1 receptors are GPCRs that interact with adenosine; two of these receptors (A_1 and A_3) couple to G_i and two (A_{2a} and A_{2b}) couple to G_s; methylxanthines antagonize A_1 and A_3 receptors. Activation of A_1 receptors is associated with inhibition of adenylyl cyclase, activation of K^+ currents, and in some instances, with activation of PLC; stimulation of A_2 receptors activates adenylyl cyclase. The P2 class includes a large number of P2X receptors that are ligand-gated ion channels and the P2Y receptors, a similarly large subclass of GPCRs that couple to G_q or G_i and their associated effectors. The $P2Y_{14}$ receptor is expressed in the CNS; it interacts with UDP-glucose and may couple to G_q. The $P2Y_{12}$ receptor is important clinically, since inhibition of this receptor in platelets inhibits platelet aggregation.

Although many of these receptors have been detected in brain, most of the current interest stems from pharmacological rather than physiological observations. Adenosine can act presynaptically throughout the cortex and hippocampal formation to inhibit the release of amine and amino acid transmitters. ATP-regulated responses have been linked pharmacologically to a variety of pathophysiological functions, including anxiety, stroke, and epilepsy. A_1 antagonists are being investigated as potential therapeutic agents to enhance awareness and learning. A_2 receptors and dopamine D_2 receptors appear to be functionally antagonistic, leading to investigation of A_{2a} antagonists as adjunctive therapy for Parkinson disease (Jacobson and Gao, 2006).

Lipid Mediators. Substances identified as physiological regulators in systems throughout the body have been examined for their roles within the CNS. Arachidonic acid, normally stored within the cell membrane as a glycerol ester, can be liberated during phospholipid hydrolysis (by pathways involving phospholipases A_2, C, and D). Phospholipases are activated via a variety of receptors (Chapter 3). Arachidonic acid can be converted to highly reactive regulators by three major enzymatic pathways (Chapter 33): cyclooxygenases (leading to prostaglandins and thromboxane), lipoxygenases

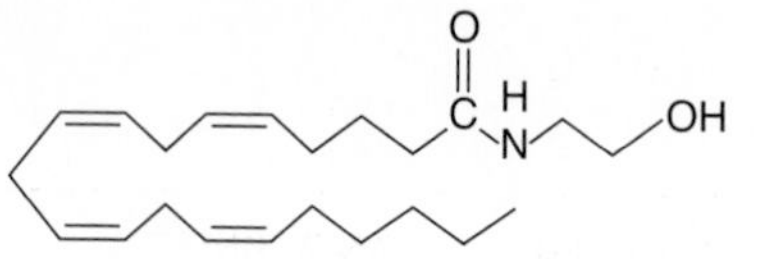

Anandamide

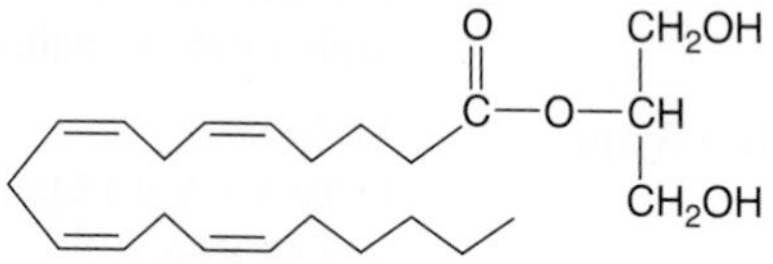

2-Arachidonylglycerol

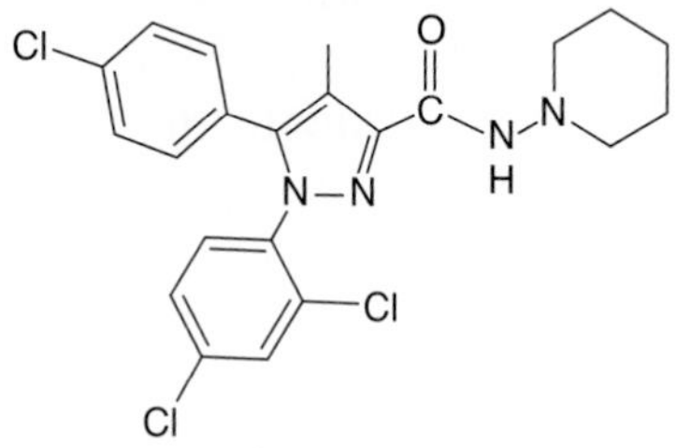

Rimonabant

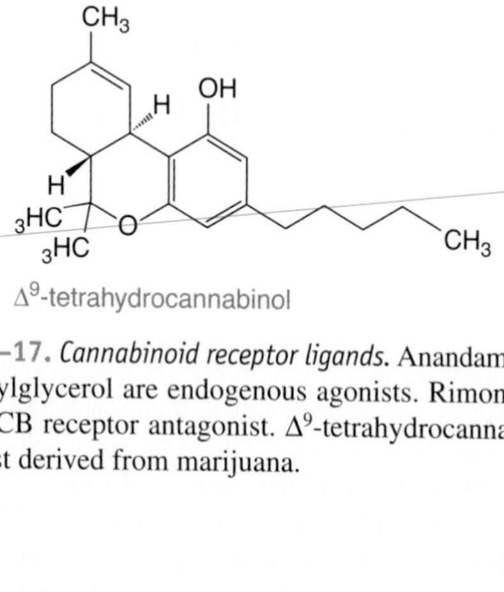

Δ^9-tetrahydrocannabinol

Figure 14–17. *Cannabinoid receptor ligands.* Anandamide and 2-arachidonylglycerol are endogenous agonists. Rimonabant is a synthetic CB receptor antagonist. Δ^9-tetrahydrocannabinol is a CB agonist derived from marijuana.

(leading to the leukotrienes and other transient catabolites of eicosatetraenoic acid), and CYPs (which are inducible and also expressed at low levels in brain). Arachidonic acid metabolites have been implicated as diffusible modulators in the CNS, possibly involved with the formation of LTP and other forms of neuronal plasticity.

Nitric Oxide and Carbon Monoxide. Nitric Oxide (NO), an important regulator of vascular and inflammatory mediation, came into focus with respect to roles in the CNS after the characterization of brain nitric oxide synthase (NOS) activities (see Chapter 3 and Boehning and Snyder, 2003). Both constitutive and inducible forms of NOS are expressed in the brain. The application of inhibitors of NOS (e.g., methylarginine and nitroarginine) and of NO donors (such as nitroprusside) suggests the involvement of NO in a host of CNS phenomena, including neurotransmitter release and enhancement of glutamate (NMDA)-mediated neurotoxicity and LTP. Neuronal NOS (nNOS) is activated following NMDA-mediated receptor mediated increases in intracellular Ca^{2+}. NO diffuses freely across membranes, acting primarily to stimulate soluble guanylyl cyclase, which catalyzes the formation of cyclic GMP. Formation of NO can also result in S-nitrosylation of cysteine residues in a variety of proteins including G proteins and ion channels. Other gases may also act as intracellular messengers. One candidate is carbon monoxide (CO), which is generated in neurons by three isoforms of hemeoxygenase (HO), isoform 2 predominating in neurons. Like NO, CO stimulates soluble guanylyl cyclase.

Cytokines. Cytokines are a large and diverse family of polypeptide regulators that are produced widely throughout the body by cells of diverse embryological origin. The effects of cytokines are regulated by the conditions imposed by other cytokines, interacting as a network with variable effects leading to synergistic, additive, or opposing actions. Tissue-produced peptides, termed *chemokines,* serve to attract immune and inflammatory cells into interstitial spaces. These special cytokines have received attention as potential regulators of nervous system inflammation (as in early stages of dementia, following infection with human immunodeficiency virus, and during recovery from traumatic injury). Some of the more conventional neuronal- and glial-derived growth-enhancing and growth-retarding factors have been identified earlier. The fact that neurons and astrocytes may be induced under some pathophysiological conditions to express cytokines or other growth factors further blurs the dividing line between neurons and glia (Campbell, 2004; Wang et al., 2002).

ACTIONS OF DRUGS IN THE CNS

Specificity and Nonspecificity of CNS Drug Actions

The effect of a drug in the CNS is considered to be specific when it affects an identifiable molecular mechanism unique to target cells that bear receptors for that drug. Conversely, a drug is regarded as being nonspecific when it produces effects at a variety of different target cells, thus affecting a diverse set of neurobiological systems. This distinction is often affected by the dose-response relationship of the drug and the cell or mechanisms under scrutiny. Even a drug that is highly specific when tested at low concentrations may exhibit nonspecific actions at higher doses. In general, the more potent a drug at its desired target, the lower the probability that it will have off-target effects. Conversely, even drugs that have a broad spectrum of activity may not act identically at all levels of the CNS. For example, sedatives, hypnotics, and general anesthetics would have very limited utility if central neurons that control the respiratory and cardiovascular systems were especially sensitive to their actions. Although relief of pain is the goal when administering an opiate, one must also contend with potential off-target effects including respiratory depression and constipation.

General (Nonspecific) CNS Depressants

This category includes the anesthetic gases and vapors, the aliphatic alcohols, and some hypnotic-sedative drugs. These agents share the capacity to depress excitable tissue at all levels of the CNS, leading to a decrease in the amount of transmitter released by the nerve impulse, as well as to general depression of postsynaptic responsiveness and ion flux. At sub-anesthetic concentrations, these agents

Table 14–10

Characteristics of Purinergic Receptors

CLASS	RECEPTOR SUBTYPE							
P1 (adenosine)	A_1	A_{2A}	A_{2B}	A_3				
Transducer	G_i	G_s	G_s	G_i				
Agonists	CPA	CGS21680		1B-MECA				
Antagonists	CPX	SCH58261	MRS-1754					
P2X (ionotropic)	$P2X_1$	$P2X_2$	$P2X_3$	$P2X_4$	$P2X_5$	$P2X_6$	$P2X_7$	
Substrate Specificity	ATP>ADP	ATP	ATP	ATP>CTP	ATP	unknown	ATP	
Antagonist	NF449	NF279	TNP-ATP	protons	PPADS	none known	Brilliant Blue G	
P2Y (metabotropic)	$P2Y_1$	$P2Y_2$	$P2Y_4$	$P2Y_6$	$P2Y_{11}$	$P2Y_{12}$	$P2Y_{13}$	$P2Y_{14}$
Transducer	G_q	G_q, G_i	G_q, G_i	G_q	G_q	G_i	G_i	G_i
Substrate specificity	ADP, ATP, ApoA	ATP=UTP	UTP>ATP	UDP	ATP>ADP	ADP	ADP	UDP-glucose[a]

[a]$P2Y_{14}$ binds UDP-glucose, UDP-galactose, and/or UDP-acetylglucosamine.
NECA is a non-selective agonist of P1 receptors.
CPA, N6-cyclopentyladenosine; CPX, 8-cyclopentyl-1,3-dipropylxanthine; 1B-MECA, N6-(3-iodobenzyl)-adenosine-5α-N-methylcarboxamide; NECA, 1-(6-amino-9H-purin-9-yl)-1-deoxy-N-ethyl-β-D-ribofuronamide; PPADS, Pyridoxalphosphate-6-azophenyl-2',4'-disulfonic acid; TNP-ATP, 2',3'-O-(2,4,6-trinitrophenyl)adenosine-5'-triphosphate.

(e.g., ethanol) can exert relatively specific effects on certain groups of neurons, which may account for differences in their behavioral effects, especially the propensity to produce dependence.

General (Nonspecific) CNS Stimulants

The drugs in this category include pentylenetetrazol and related agents that are capable of powerful excitation of the CNS, and the methylxanthines, which have a much weaker stimulant action. Stimulation may be accomplished by one of two general mechanisms: (1) blockade of inhibition or (2) direct neuronal excitation that may involve increased transmitter release or more prolonged transmitter action, as occurs when the reuptake of a released transmitter is inhibited.

Drugs That Selectively Modify CNS Function

The agents in this group may cause either depression or excitation. In some instances, a drug may produce both effects simultaneously on different systems. Some agents in this category have little effect on the level of excitability in doses that are used therapeutically. The principal classes of these CNS drugs are anticonvulsants, drugs used in treating Parkinson disease, opioid and non-opioid analgesics, appetite suppressants, anti-emetics, analgesic-antipyretics, certain stimulants, antidepressants, anti-manic and anti-psychotic agents, tranquilizers, sedatives and hypnotics, and medications employed in the treatment of Alzheimer's disease (cholinesterase inhibitors and anti-glutamate neuroprotectants). Although selectivity of action may be remarkable, a drug usually affects several CNS functions to varying degrees. When only one constellation of effects is wanted in a therapeutic situation, the remaining effects of the drug are regarded as limitations in selectivity (i.e., unwanted side effects or off-target effects). *The specificity of a drug's action is frequently overestimated. This is partly due to the fact that drugs are often identified with the effect that is implied by the class name.*

General Characteristics of CNS Drugs

Combinations of centrally acting drugs frequently are administered to therapeutic advantage (e.g., an anticholinergic drug and levodopa for Parkinson disease). However, other combinations of drugs may be detrimental because of potentially dangerous additive or mutually antagonistic effects. The effects of a CNS drug may be additive with the physiological state and the effects of other depressant and stimulant drugs. For example, anesthetics are less effective in a hyperexcitable subject than in a normal patient; the converse is true for stimulants. In general, the depressant effects of drugs from different categories are additive (e.g., the potentially fatal combination of barbiturates or benzodiazepines with ethanol), as are the effects of stimulants. Therefore, respiration depressed by morphine is further impaired by depressant drugs, while stimulant drugs can augment the excitatory effects of morphine to produce vomiting and convulsions.

Antagonism between depressants and stimulants is variable. Some instances of true pharmacological antagonism among CNS drugs are known; for example, opioid antagonists can selectively antagonize the effects of opioid analgesics. However, the antagonism exhibited between two CNS drugs is most often physiological in nature. For example, an individual whose CNS is depressed by an opiate cannot be returned entirely to normal by stimulation with caffeine.

The selective effects of drugs on specific neurotransmitter systems may be additive or competitive. The potential for drug interactions must be considered whenever such drugs are concurrently administered. To minimize such interactions, a drug-free period may be required when modifying therapy; in fact, development of desensitized and supersensitive states with prolonged therapy may limit the speed with which one drug may be halted and another started. An excitatory effect is commonly observed with low concentrations of certain depressant drugs due either to depression of inhibitory systems or to a transient increase in the release of excitatory transmitters. Examples include the stage of excitement seen during induction of general anesthesia. The excitatory phase typically occurs with low concentrations of the depressant; uniform depression ensues with increasing drug concentration. The excitatory effects can be minimized, when appropriate, by pretreatment with a depressant drug that is devoid of such effects (e.g., benzodiazepines in preanesthetic medication). Acute, excessive stimulation of the cerebrospinal axis normally is followed by depression, which is in part a consequence of neuronal fatigue and exhaustion of stores of transmitters. Postictal depression is additive with the effects of depressant drugs. Acute, drug-induced depression generally is not followed by stimulation. However, chronic drug-induced sedation or depression may be followed by prolonged hyperexcitability upon abrupt withdrawal of the medication (barbiturates or alcohol). This type of hyperexcitability can be controlled effectively by the same or another depressant drug (Chapters 17, 23, and 24).

Organization of CNS-Drug Interactions. The structural and functional properties of neurons provide a means to specify the possible sites at which drugs could interact, specifically or generally, in the CNS. In this scheme, drugs that affect neuronal energy metabolism, membrane integrity, or transmembrane ionic equilibria would be generally acting compounds. Similarly general in action would be drugs that affect molecular motors and thereby affect the transport of materials from cell bodies to nerve terminals and back. These general effects may exhibit different dose-response or time-response relationships based, e.g., on neuronal properties such as rate of firing, dependence of discharge on external stimuli or internal pacemakers, resting ionic fluxes, or axon length. In contrast, when the actions of a drug can be related to specific aspects of the metabolism, release, or function of a neurotransmitter, then the site, specificity, and mechanism of action of the drug can be defined by systematic studies of dose-response and time-response relationships.

Transmitter-dependent actions of drugs can be grouped into presynaptic and postsynaptic categories. The presynaptic category includes the events in the perikaryon and nerve terminal that regulate transmitter synthesis (including the acquisition of adequate substrates and co-factors), storage, release, and metabolism. Transmitter concentrations can be lowered by blockade of synthesis, inhibition of storage, or both. The amount of transmitter released per impulse generally is stable but may be subject to regulation. The effective concentration of transmitter may be increased by inhibition of metabolic enzymes or by blockade of re-uptake transporters. The transmitter that is released at a synapse also can exert actions on the terminal from which it was released by interacting with receptors at these sites (*autoreceptors*). Activation of presynaptic autoreceptors can inhibit or stimulate the rate of release of transmitter and thereby provide a feedback mechanism that controls the concentration of transmitter in the synaptic cleft.

The postsynaptic category includes all the events that follow release of the transmitter in the vicinity of the postsynaptic receptor. Examples include the molecular mechanisms by which receptor occupancy alters the properties of the membrane of the postsynaptic cell (shifts in membrane potential), as well as more enduring biochemical actions (e.g., changes in second messenger concentrations, protein kinase and phosphoprotein phosphatase activities, and phosphoprotein formation). Direct postsynaptic effects of drugs generally require relatively high affinity for the receptors or resistance to metabolic degradation. Each of these presynaptic or postsynaptic actions is potentially highly specific and can be envisioned as restricted to a single, chemically defined subset of CNS cells.

Convergence, Synergism, and Antagonism Result from Transmitter Interactions. Although the power of the reductionist approach to clone cDNAs for receptors or receptor subunits and to determine their properties by expression in cells that do not normally express the receptor or subunit cannot be underestimated, *the simplicity of cell culture models may not reproduce the nuances of receptor function in vivo and may divert attention from the complexity of the intact CNS*. A given neurotransmitter may interact simultaneously with all of the various isoforms of its receptor on neurons that also are under the influence of multiple other afferent pathways and their transmitters. Thus, the use of model systems to predict the behavioral or therapeutic consequences of drugs in humans may fail as a consequence of the complexity of the interactions possible, including differences between normal and diseased tissue.

CNS Drug Discovery. As is evident from the chapters to follow, a large number of agents have been developed to treat neuropsychiatric diseases. With few exceptions these agents offer primarily symptomatic improvement; few are truly disease modifying. For example, the use of L-dopa to treat Parkinson disease alleviates the symptoms effectively but the disease continues to progress. Similarly, although antipsychotics and antidepressants are often efficacious, the symptoms tend to recur. Moreover, many drugs developed to treat CNS diseases are not uniformly effective: Approximately one-third of patients with severe depression are "treatment-resistant." CNS diseases are complex, with multiple symptoms, some of which, like the negative symptoms of schizophrenia, tend to be resistant to treatment. Furthermore, the complexity of the brain and its neuronal pathways results in significant risk of side effects, even when the most biochemically selective agent is administered. Particularly disquieting side effects include tardive dyskinesias that can result from prolonged treatment with antipsychotics and the hypnotic effects of agents used for the treatment of seizure disorders.

The lack of disease-modifying treatments for CNS diseases represents a very significant unmet medical need and makes the discovery of such agents a high priority. Drug discovery is generally a high-risk/high-reward effort (Chapter 1) and CNS-active agents are no exception. Overall, the probability of success in developing a drug from the time a compound enters into clinical trials is ~10%; the success rate for CNS drugs is somewhat lower. Myriad factors contribute to the increased difficulty and reduced probability of success in efforts to develop drugs to treat CNS disease. Factors that reduce the probability of success include the complexity of neural pathways governing behavior and its pathology, and the permeability barriers that restrict access of drugs to CNS sites (including the blood-brain barrier and drug export systems; see Chapters 2 and 5). For example, a drug that affects serotinergic transmission may affect 14 5-HT receptor subtypes that are involved in a plethora of biological systems. Moreover, animal models of CNS diseases are often incompletely validated and an effect in an animal model may not be predictive of efficacy in human disease. For instance, a number of agents reduce the size of the infarct when given to animals following occlusion of the middle cerebral artery, yet none of these agents has shown positive results in human clinical trials. A number of agents that inhibit the reuptake of 5-HT and NE are effective in treating depression. In a number of animal models of depression, these agents produce an effect after a single dose, which corresponds nicely with the time course for the inhibition of neurotransmitter reuptake in experimental animals, whereas, a period of several weeks is typically required to see a therapeutic effect in humans. Given this discrepancy, one can understand the reluctance of pharmaceutical companies to invest in clinical trials of new antidepressants on the basis of effects in animal models.

Clinical trials represent another area of challenge in developing new therapies for CNS diseases. For example, testing an agent to treat depression likely requires a trial lasting 6 or more weeks and the placebo response rate may exceed 50%. Such conditions necessitate large, prolonged, and therefore expensive trials. Studies of treatments for neurodegenerative disease are even more difficult. With current diagnostic capabilities, it is difficult to detect a significant change in the rate of progression of cognitive decline in patients with Alzheimer's disease in less than a year. One way to circumvent the long time necessary to detect a biological meaningful result is through the use of surrogate markers (e.g., a decrease in serum cholesterol for improved cardiovascular morbidity and mortality). Regrettably, there are relatively few useful surrogate markers for CNS diseases.

Impact of Genomics on CNS Drug Discovery. The sequencing of the human genome has the potential to significantly change drug discovery in the CNS. Thus, genetic testing may predict the likelihood that a given individual will develop a particular disease, will respond to a particular therapy, or will suffer side effects from a particular treatment paradigm. Genetic testing may be particularly important in the case of CNS diseases, where the etiology is likely to be multigenic. Molecular approaches will likely speed development of more and improved animal models that better mimic human disease.

BIBLIOGRAPHY

Aimone JB, Deng W, Gage FH. Adult neurogenesis: integrating theories and functions. *Trends Cogn Sci*, **2010**, *14:* in press.

Alexander SPH, Mathie A, Peters JA. Guide to Receptors and Channels. *Br J Pharmacol*, **2006,** *147(s3)*: S1.

Aston-Jones G, Chen S, Zhu Y, Oshinsky ML. A neural circuit for circadian regulation of arousal. *Nat Neurosci*, **2001,** *4*:732–738.

Bettler B, Kaupmann K, Mosbacher J, Gassmann M. Molecular structure and physiological functions of $GAGA_B$ receptors. *Physiol Rev,* **2004,** 84:835–867.

Biel M, Michalakis S. Cyclic nucleotide-gated channels. *Handb Exp Pharmacol,* **2009,** *191:* 111–136.

Bleich S, Romer K, Wiltfang J, Kornhuber J. Glutamate and the glutamate receptor system: A target for drug action. *Int J Geriatr Psychiatry,* **2003,** *18*(Suppl 1):S33–S40.

Boehning D, Snyder SH. Novel neural modulators. *Annu Rev Neurosci,* **2003,** *26:*105–131.

Bourne HR, Nicoll R. Molecular machines integrate coincident synaptic signals. *Cell,* **1993,** *72*:65–75.

Burnstock G. Noradrenaline and ATP: Co-transmitters and neuromodulators. *J Physiol Pharmacol,* **1995,** *46:*365–384.

Campbell IL. Chemokines as plurifunctional mediators in the CNS: Implications for the pathogenesis of stroke. *Ernst Schering Res Found Workshop,* **2004,** *45:*31–51.

Carson MJ. Microglia as liaisons between the immune and central nervous systems: Functional implications for multiple sclerosis. *Glia,* **2002,** *40:*218–231.

Carson MJ, *et al.* Mature microglia resemble immature antigen-presenting cell. *Glia,* **1998,** *22*:72–85.

Catterall WA. Structure and function of voltage-gated ion channels. *Trends Neurosci,* **1993,** *16:*500–506.

Catterall WA, Epstein PN. Ion channels. *Diabetologia,* **1992,** *2:*S23–S33.

Clapham DE, Julius D, Montell C, Schultz G. Transient Receptor Channels. IUPHAR, **2002**. Available at: http://www.iuphar-db.org/iuphar-ic/TRPC.html. Accessed January 1, 2010.

Conn PJ. Physiological roles and therapeutic potential of metabotropic glutamate receptors. *Ann NY Acad Sci,* **2003,** *1003*:12–21.

Conn PJ, Pin JP. Pharmacology and functions of metabotropic glutamate receptors. **1997**, *Annu Rev Pharmacol Toxicol, 37:*205–237.

Cooper J, Bloom F, Roth R. *The Biochemical Basis of Neuropharmacology*. Oxford University Press, New York, **2003**.

Cowan WM, Harter DH, Kandel ER. The emergence of modern neuroscience: Some implications for neurology and psychiatry. *Annu Rev Neurosci,* **2000,** *23*:343–391.

Cowan WM, Kopnisky KL, Hyman SE. The Human Genome Project and its impact on psychiatry. *Annu Rev Neurosci,* **2002,** *25:*1–50.

Darlison MG, Richter D. Multiple genes for neuropeptides and their receptors: Co-evolution and physiology. *Trends Neurosci,* **1999,** *22*:81–88.

Fritschy JM, Mohler H. $GABA_A$ Receptor heterogeneity in the adult rat brain: differential regional and cellular distribution of seven major subunits. *J Comp Neurol*, **1995**; *359:*154–194.

Glass CK, Saijo K, Winner B, Marchetto MC, Gage FH. Mechanisms underlying inflammation in neurodegeneration. *Cell*, **2010**, *140:*918–934.

Giger RJ, Venkatesh K, Chivatakarn O, et al. Mechanisms of CNS myelin inhibition: evidence for distinct and neuronal all type specific receptor systems. *Restor Neurol Neurosci,* **2008**, *26:*97–115.

Greengard P. The neurobiology of dopamine signaling. *Biosc Rep,* **2001,** *21:*247–269.

Haeberlein SL, Lipton SA. Excitotoxicity in neurodegenerative disease *Encyc Neurosci,* **2009,** *4:*77–86.

Harmar AJ, Hills RA, Rosser EM, *et al.* IUPHAR-DB: The IUPHAR database of G protein-coupled receptors and ion channels. *Nucl Acids Res*, **2009**, *37*, D680–D685.

Herrling P. Excitatory amino acids. In, *Clinical Results with Antagonists*. Academic Press, San Diego, **1997.**

Hofmann F, Biel M, Kaupp UB. Cyclic nucleotide-modulated channels. Available at: http://www.iuphar-db.org/iuphar-ic/CNGA.html. Accessed January 1, **2010**.

Hökfelt T, Bartfai T, Bloom F. Neuropeptides: Opportunities for drug discovery. *Lancet Neurol,* **2003,** *2:*463–472.

Hökfelt T., Broberger C, Xu ZQD, *et al.* Neuropeptides-an overview. *Neuropharmacology,* **2000,** *39:*1337–1356.

Huang EJ, Reichardt LF. Neurotrophins: Roles in neuronal development and function. *Annu Rev Neurosci,* **2001,** *24:* 677–736.

Husi H, *et al.* Proteomic analysis of NMDA receptor-adhesion protein signaling complexes. *Nat Neurosci*, **2000,** *3:* 661–669.

Jackson EK, Raghvendra DK. The extracellular cyclic AMP-adenosine pathway in renal physiology. *Annu Rev Physiol,* **2004,** *66:*571–599.

Jacobson KA, Gao ZG. Adenosine receptors as therapeutic targets. *Nat Rev Drug Discov*, **2006,** *5:*247–264.

Jahn R. Principles of exocytosis and membrane fusion. *Ann NY Acad Sci,* **2004,** *1014:*170–178.

Korpi ER, Grunder G, Luddens H. Drug interactions at $GABA_A$ receptors. *Prog Neurobiol,* **2002,** *67:*113–159.

Kotecha SA, MacDonald JF. Signaling molecules and receptor transduction cascades that regulate NMDA receptor-mediated synaptic transmission. *Int Rev Neurobiol,* **2003,** *54:*51–106.

Lazarowski ER, Boucher RC, Harden TK. Mechanisms of release of nucleotides and integration of the action as P2X- and P2Y-receptor activating molecules. *Mol Pharmacol,* **2003,** *64:*785–795.

Madinier A, Bertrand N, Mossiat C, et al. Microglial involvement in neuroplastic changes following focal brain ischemia in rats. *PLoS One*, **2009**, *4:*e8101.

Marchetto MC, Winner B, Gage FH. Pluripotent stem cells in neurodegenerative and neurodevelopmental diseases. *Hum Mol Genet*, **2010**, *19:*R71–76.

Mountcastle VB. The columnar organization of the neocortex. *Brain*, **1997,** *120:*701–722.

Murthy VN, Camilli PD. Cell biology of the presynaptic terminal. *Annu Rev Neurosci,* **2003,** *26:*701–728.

Nestler EJ, Hyman SE, Malenka RC. *Molecular Neuropharmacology*. McGraw-Hill, New York, **2001, 2009**.

Nichols DE. Hallucinogens. *Pharmacol Ther,* **2004,** *101:*131–181.

Niswender CM, Herrick-Davis K, Dilley GE, *et al.* RNA editing of the human serotonin $5\text{-}HT_{2C}$ receptor, alterations in suicide and implications for serotonergic pharmacotherapy. *Neuropsychopharmacology,* **2001,** *24:*478–491.

Olsen RW, Betz H. GABA and Glycine. In, *Basic neurochemistry: molecular, cellular and medical aspects*, 7th ed. (Siegel GJ, Albers RW, Brady S, Price DD, eds.) Academic Press, Boston, **2005**, pp. 291–302.

Ostrom RS, Naugle JE, Hase M, *et al.* Angiotensin II enhances adenylyl cyclase signaling via Ca^{2+}/Calmodulin. G_q-G_s cross-talk regulates collagen production in cardiac fibroblasts. *J Biol Chem*, **2003,** *278*:24461–24468.

Pellerin L, Magistretti PJ. How to balance the brain energy budget while spending glucose differently. *J Physiol*, **2003;** *546*(Pt 2):325.

Piomelli D. The molecular logic of endocannabinoid signaling. *Nat Rev Neurosci,* **2003,** *4:*873–884.

Ralevic V, Burnstock G. Receptors for purines and pyrimidines. *Pharm Rev*, **1998**, *50:*413–492.

Ramsey IS, Delling M, Clapham DE. An introduction to TRP channels. *Annu Rev Physiol,* **2006,** *68:*619–647.

Robas N, O'Reilly M, Katugampola S, Fidock M. Maximizing serendipity: strategies for identifying ligands for orphan G-protein-coupled receptors. *Curr Opin Pharmacol,* **2003,** *3:*121–126.

Robertson SJ, Ennion SJ, Evans RJ, Edwards FA. Synaptic P2X receptors. *Curr Opin Neurobiol,* **2001,** *11:*378–386.

Shepherd GM. *The Synaptic Organization of the Brain*. Oxford University Press, New York, **2003.**

Siegel GJ, Albers RW, Brady ST, Price DL. *Basic Neurochemistry: Molecular, Cellular and Medical Aspects.* Elsevier, San Diego, **2006**.

Sola M, Bavro VN, Timmins J, *et al.* Structural basis of dynamic glycine receptor clustering by gephyrin. *EMBO J,* **2004,** *23:*2510–2519.

Thurmond RL, Desai PJ, Dunford PJ, *et al.* A potent and selective histamine H_4 receptor antagonist with antiinflammatory properties. *J Pharmacol Exp Ther*, **2004,** *309*:404–413.

Unwin N. Nicotinic acetylcholine receptor at 9Å resolution. *J Mol Biol*, **1993,** *229*:1101–1124.

Violin JD, Lefkowitz RJ. β-Arrestin-biased ligands at seven-transmembrane receptors. *Trends Pharm Sci,* **2007,** *28;* 416–422.

Wang J, Asensio VC, Campbell IL. Cytokines and chemokines as mediators of protection and injury in the central nervous system assessed in transgenic mice. *Curr Top Microbiol Immunol,* **2002,** *265*:23–48.

Yu FH, Yarov-Yarovoy V, Gutman GA, Catterall WA. Overview of molecular relationships in the voltage-gated ion channel superfamily. *Pharmacol Rev*, **2005**, *57:*387–395.

Drug Therapy of Depression and Anxiety Disorders

James M. O'Donnell and
Richard C. Shelton

Depression and anxiety disorders are the most common mental illnesses, each affecting in excess of 10-15% of the population at some time in their lives. Both anxiety and depressive disorders are amenable to pharmacological treatments that have been developed since the 1950s. With the discovery of more selective and safer drugs, the use of antidepressants and anxiolytics has moved from the domain of psychiatry to other medical specialties, including primary care. *The relative safety of the majority of commonly used antidepressants and anxiolytics notwithstanding, their optimal use requires a clear understanding of their mechanisms of action, pharmacokinetics, potential drug interactions, and the differential diagnosis of psychiatric illnesses.*

A confluence of symptoms of depression and anxiety may affect an individual patient; some of the drugs discussed here are effective in treating both disorders, suggesting common underlying mechanisms of pathophysiology and response to pharmacotherapy. In large measure, our current understanding of pathophysiological mechanisms underlying depression and anxiety has been inferred from the mechanisms of action of psychopharmacological compounds (Chapter 14). While depression and anxiety disorders comprise a wide range of symptoms, including changes in mood, behavior, somatic function, and cognition, some progress has been made in developing animal models that respond with some sensitivity and selectivity to antidepressant or anxiolytic drugs (Cryan and Holmes, 2005; Miller et al., 2010). Recent work has focused on identifying endophenotypes associated with psychiatric diseases, with the goals of understanding their underlying pathophysiology and targeting them pharmacologically (Cannon and Keller, 2006). Although animal models are useful for investigating pharmacological mechanisms of action and providing initial evidence of efficacy, the development of antidepressant and anxiolytic drugs depends on clinical trials. However, it is not uncommon for psychopharmacological agents to fail to show efficacy in clinical trials; in large measure this is due to significant placebo effects and the lack of objective and firm end points. In spite of these limitations, the last half century has seen notable advances in the discovery and development of drugs for treating depression and anxiety.

CHARACTERIZATION OF DEPRESSIVE AND ANXIETY DISORDER

Symptoms of Depression

Depression, in general, is classified as major depression (i.e., unipolar depression) or bipolar depression (i.e., manic depressive illness); bipolar depression and its treatment are discussed in Chapter 16. Lifetime risk of unipolar depression is ~15%. Females are affected twice as frequently as males (Kessler et al., 1994). Depressive episodes are characterized by depressed or sad mood, pessimistic worry, diminished interest in normal activities, mental slowing and poor concentration, insomnia or increased sleep, significant weight loss or gain due to altered eating and activity patterns, psychomotor agitation or retardation, feelings of guilt and worthlessness, decreased energy and libido, and suicidal ideation, occurring most days for a period of at least 2 weeks. In some cases, the primary complaint of patients involves somatic pain or other physical symptoms and can present a diagnostic challenge for primary care physicians. Depressive symptoms also can occur secondary to other illnesses such as hypothyroidism, Parkinson's disease, and inflammatory conditions. Further, depression often complicates the management of other medical conditions (e.g., severe trauma, cancer, diabetes, and cardiovascular disease, especially myocardial infarction) (Andrews and Nemeroff, 1994).

Depression is underdiagnosed and undertreated (Suominen et al., 1998). This is of particular concern due to the inherent risk of suicide associated with depression. Approximately 10-15% of those with severe depression attempt suicide at some time (Chen and Dilsaver, 1996). Thus, it is important that symptoms of depression be recognized and treated in a timely manner. Furthermore, the response to treatment must be assessed and decisions made regarding continued treatment with the initial drug, dose adjustment, adjunctive therapy, or alternative medication.

Symptoms of Anxiety

Anxiety disorders encompass a constellation of symptoms, and include generalized anxiety disorder, obsessive-compulsive disorder, panic disorder, post-traumatic stress disorder, separation anxiety disorder, social phobia, specific phobias, and acute stress (Atack, 2003). In general, symptoms of anxiety that lead to pharmacological treatment are those that interfere significantly with normal function. Symptoms of anxiety also are often associated with depression and other medical conditions.

Anxiety is a normal human emotion that serves an adaptive function from a psychobiological perspective. However, in the psychiatric setting, feelings of fear or dread that are unfocused (e.g., generalized anxiety disorder) or out of scale with the perceived threat (e.g., specific phobias) often require treatment. Drug treatment includes acute drug administration to manage episodes of anxiety, and chronic or repeated treatment to manage unrelieved and continuing anxiety disorders.

ANTIDEPRESSANT DRUGS

Mechanisms of Action. Many different antidepressants have established track records of efficacy for treating major depression (Millan, 2006). However, they all suffer some limitations in efficacy, since at least 20% of all depressed patients are refractory to multiple different antidepressants at adequate doses (Rush et al., 2006). The most commonly used medications, often referred to as second-generation antidepressants, are the selective serotonin reuptake inhibitors (SSRIs) and the serotonin-norepinephrine reuptake inhibitors (SNRIs), which have greater efficacy and safety compared to most older drugs (i.e., first-generation antidepressants). Relatively selective norepinephrine reuptake inhibitors also have been developed as antidepressants (e.g., maprotiline, reboxetine).

In monoamine systems, reuptake of the transmitter is the main mechanism by which neurotransmission is terminated; thus, inhibition of reuptake can enhance neurotransmission, presumably by slowing clearance of the transmitter from the synapse and prolonging the dwell-time of the transmitter in the synapse. Enhancing neurotransmission may subsequently lead to adaptive changes (described later). Reuptake inhibitors inhibit either SERT, the neuronal serotonin (5-hydroxytryptamine; 5-HT) transporter; NET, the neuronal norepinephrine (NE) transporter; or both (Figure 15–1). Similarly, the first-generation drugs, which include monoamine oxidase inhibitors (MAOIs) and tricyclic antidepressants (TCAs), also enhance monoaminergic neurotransmission: the MAOIs by inhibiting monoamine metabolism and thereby enhancing neurotransmitter storage in secretory granules, the TCAs by inhibiting 5-HT and norepinephrine reuptake. While efficacious, these first-generation agents exhibit side effects and drug and food interactions that limit their use relative to the newer drugs. Table 15–1 summarizes the actions of the most widely used antidepressants.

All drugs commonly used to treat depression share, at some level, primary effects on serotonergic or noradrenergic neurotransmitter systems (Shelton and Lester, 2006). In general, antidepressants enhance serotonergic or noradrenergic transmission, although the nature of this effect may change with chronic treatment (Shelton, 2000). The dependence of many current treatments on serotonergic or noradrenergic mechanisms is highlighted by clinical studies employing monoamine depletion strategies. For example, tryptophan depletion that acutely reduces 5-HT neurotransmission results in a relatively brisk relapse (within 5-10 hours) of the symptoms of depression in patients who had shown remission on an SSRI but not a NE reuptake inhibitor (Delgado et al., 1991). Conversely, catecholamine depletion by blocking the rate-limiting enzyme for the synthesis of NE and dopamine (DA) results in a relapse of symptoms in patients who had recently remitted on an NE reuptake inhibitor, but not an SSRI (Miller et al., 1996). Sites of interaction of antidepressant drugs with noradrenergic and serotonergic neurons are depicted in Figure 15–1.

Long-term effects of antidepressant drugs evoke adaptive or regulatory mechanisms that enhance the effectiveness of therapy. These responses include increased adrenergic or serotonergic receptor density or sensitivity, increased receptor-G protein coupling and cyclic nucleotide signaling, induction of neurotrophic factors, and increased neurogenesis in the hippocampus (Schmidt and Duman, 2007). Persistent antidepressant effects depend on the continued inhibition of 5-HT or NE transporters, or enhanced serotonergic or noradrenergic neurotransmission achieved by an alternative pharmacological mechanism. For example, chronic treatment with some antidepressants that interact directly with monoamine transporters (e.g., SSRIs, SNRIs, or NE reuptake inhibitors) reduces the expression and activity of 5-HT or NE transporters in the brain, which results in enhanced serotonergic or noradrenergic neurotransmission (Benmansour et al., 1999; Zhao et al., 2008). Compelling evidence suggests that sustained signaling via NE or 5-HT increases the

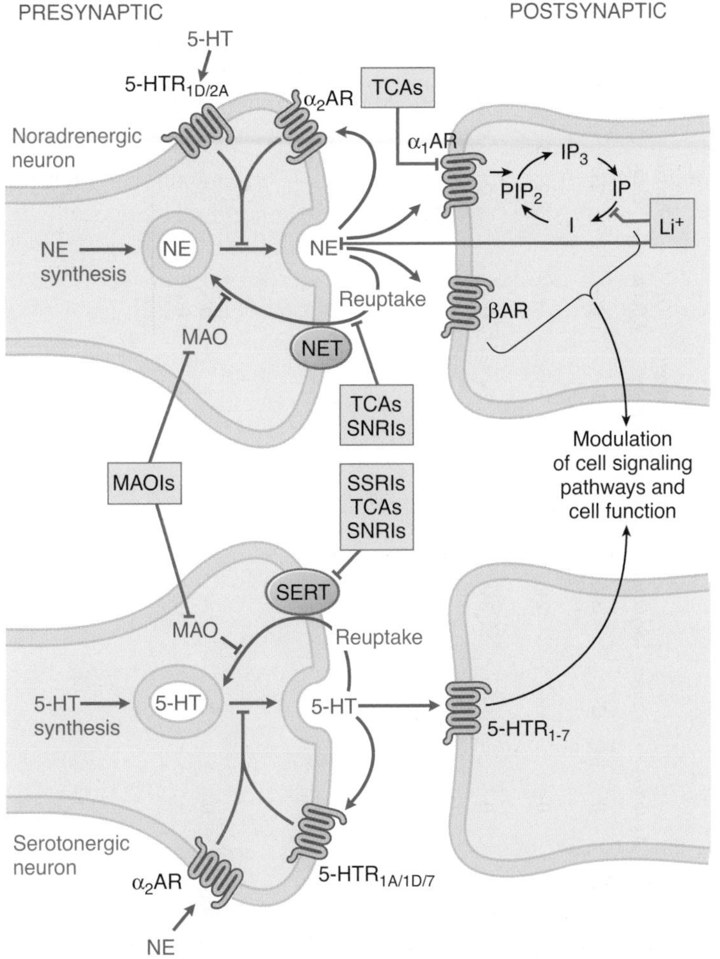

Figure 15–1. *Sites of action of antidepressants.* Schematics representing noradrenergic (top) and serotonergic (bottom) nerve terminals. SSRIs, SNRIs, and TCAs increase noradrenergic or serotonergic neurotransmission by blocking the norepinephrine or serotonergic transporter at presynaptic terminals (NET, SERT). MAOIs inhibit the catabolism of norepinephrine and serotonin. Some antidepressants such as trazodone and related drugs have direct effects on serotonergic receptors that contribute to their clinical effects. Chronic treatment with a number of antidepressants desensitizes presynaptic autoreceptors and heteroreceptors, producing long-lasting changes in monoaminergic neurotransmission. Post-receptor effects of antidepressant treatment, including modulation of GPCR signaling and activation of protein kinases and ion channels, are involved in the mediation of the long-term effects of antidepressant drugs. Note that NE and 5-HT also affect each other's neurons.

expression of specific downstream gene products, particularly brain-derived neurotrophic factor (BDNF), which appears to be related to the ultimate mechanism of action of these drugs (Sen et al., 2008). Unfortunately, neither earlier theories of monoaminergic receptor down-regulation and altered signaling nor current theories of neurogenesis and modulation of neurotrophic factors has yet led to new antidepressant treatments. Glutamate, neurokinin, corticotropin releasing hormone receptors and cyclic nucleotide phosphodiesterases may be potential targets for the development of novel antidepressant drugs (O'Donnell and Zhang, 2004; Rakofsky et al., 2009; Witkin et al., 2007; Zarate et al., 2006).

Clinical Considerations with Antidepressant Drugs

Following initiation of antidepressant drug treatment there is generally a "therapeutic lag" lasting 3-4 weeks before a measurable therapeutic response becomes evident. This is the reason that electroconvulsive therapy may be the treatment of choice for agitated, depressed patients with a high risk of suicide. Some patients may respond to antidepressant treatment sooner than 3-4 weeks; others may require > 8 weeks for an adequate response. Some symptoms respond more rapidly and are predictive of a more global response (Katz et al., 2004). Approximately two-thirds of depressed patients will show a 50% decrease in depressive symptoms over the course of an 8-week antidepressant trial; one-third will experience a complete remission with a single antidepressant (Rush et al., 2006). In general, if a patient does not respond to a given antidepressant after an 8-week trial on an adequate dose, then switching to

Table 15–1

Antidepressants: Chemical Structures, Dose and Dosage Forms, and Side Effects

NONPROPRIETARY NAME (TRADE NAME)	DOSE AND DOSAGE FORMS		AMINE EFFECTS	SIDE EFFECTS								
	Usual[a] Dose (mg/day)	*Dosage Form*		*Agitation*	*Seizures*	*Sedation*	*Hypo-tension*	*Anti-cholinergic Effects*	*GI Effects*	*Weight Gain*	*Sexual Effects*	*Cardiac Effects*
***Norepinephrine Reuptake Inhibitors:* Tertiary Amine Tricyclics**												
R_1 R_2 R_3												
Amitriptyline (ELAVIL and others) C H $C{=}CH(CH_2)_2N(CH_3)_2$	100–200	O, I	NE, 5-HT	0	2+	3+	3+	3+	0/+	2+	2+	3+
Clomipramine (ANAFRANIL) C Cl $N{-}(CH_2)_3N(CH_3)_2$	100–200	O	NE, 5-HT	0	3+	2+	2+	3+	+	2+	3+	3+
Doxepin (ADAPIN, SINEQUAN) O H $C{=}CH(CH_2)_2N(CH_3)_2$	100–200	O	NE, 5-HT	0	2+	3+	2+	2+	0-+	2+	2+	3+
Imipramine (TOFRANIL and others) C H $N{-}(CH_2)_3N(CH_3)_2$	100–200	O, I	NE, 5-HT	0/+	2+	2+	2+	2+	0/+	2+	2+	3+
(+)-Trimipramine (SURMONTIL) C H	75–200	O	NE, 5-HT	0	2+	3+	2+	3+	0/+	2+	2+	3+
***Norepinephrine Reuptake Inhibitors:* Secondary Amine Tricyclics**												
Amoxapine (ASENDIN)	200–300	O	NE, DA	0	2+	+	2+	+	0/+	+	2+	2+
Desipramine (NORPRAMIN)	100–200	O	NE	+	+	0/+	+	+	0/+	+	2+	2+

Maprotiline (LUDIOMIL)	100–150	O	NE	0/+	3+	2+	2+	2+	0/+	+	2+	2+
Nortriptyline (PAMELOR)	75–150	O	NE	0	+	+	+	+	0/+	+	2+	2+
Protriptyline (VIVACTIL)	15–40	O	NE	2+	2+	0/+	+	2+	0/+	+	2+	3+
Selective Serotonin Reuptake Inhibitors												
(±)-Citalopram (CELEXA)	20–40	O	5-HT	0/+	0	0/+	0	0	3+	0	3+	0
(+)- Escitalopram (LEXAPRO)	10–20	O	5-HT	0/+	0	0/+	0	0	3+	0	3+	0
(±)-Fluoxetine (PROZAC)	20–40	O	5-HT	+	0/+	0/+	0	0	3+	0/+	3+	0/+
Fluvoxamine (LUVOX)	100–200	O	5-HT	0	0	0/+	0	0	3+	0	3+	0
(–)-Paroxetine (PAXIL)	20–40	O	5-HT	+	0	0/+	0	0/+	3+	0	3+	0
(+)-Sertraline (ZOLOFT)	100–150	O	5-HT	+	0	0/+	0	0	3+	0	3+	0

(*Continued*)

Table 15–1

Antidepressants: Chemical Structures, Dose and Dosage Forms, and Side Effects (*continued*)

NONPROPRIETARY NAME (TRADE NAME)	DOSE AND DOSAGE FORMS		AMINE EFFECTS	SIDE EFFECTS								
	Usual[a] Dose (mg/day)	*Dosage Form*		*Agitation*	*Seizures*	*Sedation*	*Hypo-tension*	*Anti-cholinergic Effects*	*GI Effects*	*Weight Gain*	*Sexual Effects*	*Cardiac Effects*
Selective Serotonin Reuptake Inhibitors (cont.)												
(±)-Venlafaxine (EFFEXOR)	75–225	O	5-HT, NE	0/+	0	0	0	0	3+	0	3+	0/+
Atypical Antidepressants												
(–)-Atomoxetine (STRATTERA)	40–80 (children: mg/kg)	O	NE	0	0	0	0	0	0/+	0	0	0
Bupropion (WELLBUTRIN)	200–300	O	DA, ?NE	3+	4+	0	0	0	2+	0	0	0
(+)-Duloxetine (CYMBALTA)	80–100	O	NE, 5-HT	+	0	0/+	0/+	0	0/+	0/+	0/+	0/+

(±)-Mirtazapine (REMERON)	15–45	O	5-HT, NE	0	0	4+	0/+	0	0/+	0/+	0	0
Nefazodone (SERZONE)	200–400	O	5-HT	0	0	3+	0	0	2+	0/+	0/+	0/+
Trazodone (DESYREL)	150–200	O	5-HT	0	0	3+	0	0	2+	+	+	0/+
Monoamine Oxidase Inhibitors												
Phenelzine (NARDIL)	30–60	O	NE, 5-HT, DA	0/+	0	+	+	0	0/+	+	3+	0
Tranylcypromine (PARNATE)	20–30	O	NE, 5-HT, DA	2+	0	0	+	0	0/+	+	2+	0
(–)-Selegiline (ELDEPRYL)	10	O	DA, ?NE, ?5-HT	0	0	0	0	0	0	0	+	0

Note: Most of the drugs are hydrochloride salts, but SURMONTIL and LUVOX are maleates; CELEXA is a hydrobromide, and REMERON is a free-base. Selegiline is approved for early Parkinson disease, but may have antidepressant effects, especially at daily doses 20 mg, and is under investigation for administration by transdermal patch. [a]Both higher and lower doses are sometimes used, depending on an individual patient's needs and response to the drug; see the literature and FDA-approved dosage recommendations.

O, oral tablet or capsule; I, injectable; NE, norepinephrine; 5-HT, serotonin, DA, dopamine; 0, negligible; 0/+, minimal; +, mild; 2+, moderate; 3+, moderately severe; 4+, severe.

Other significant side effects for individual drugs are described in the text.

another antidepressant with a different mechanism of action is a reasonable next step (e.g., SSRI to SNRI). If a partial response has been observed, other drugs may be added to the primary SSRI or SNRI medications; these additive medications include the antidepressant drug bupropion, thyroid hormone (triiodothyronine), or an atypical antipsychotics (aripiprazole or olanzapine) (Shelton, 2007). After the successful initial treatment phase, a 6-12 month maintenance treatment phase is typical, after which the drug is gradually withdrawn. If a patient has experienced two separate episodes of major depression or is chronically depressed (i.e., > 2 years), lifelong treatment with an antidepressant is advisable. Certain psychotherapies such as cognitive behavioral therapy or behavioral activation therapy are suitable options for many patients and may reduce the risk for relapse (DeRubeis et al., 2008). Finally, in addition to electroconvulsive therapy, other non-pharmacological interventions have been developed; these include transmagnetic stimulation of the brain and deep brain stimulation (Rakofsky et al., 2009).

The challenge of management of the depressive episode through the "therapeutic lag" is compounded by the early emergence of side effects. Most of the adverse reactions are well tolerated. A significant aspect of effective management of depression is informing the patient about the time course of both the therapeutic and side effects of medications and encouraging persistence with treatment.

Another important issue in the use of antidepressants is a phenomenon known as the "switch" from a depressed episode to a manic or hypomanic episode (Goldberg and Truman, 2003), a significant challenge in managing bipolar illness. For this reason, antidepressants are not recommended as monotherapy for bipolar illness. However, patients with bipolar illness may present with major depressive episodes early in the course of their illness. SSRIs and bupropion may be somewhat less likely to induce the switch from depression to mania than antidepressants from other pharmacological classes.

A controversial issue regarding the use of all antidepressants is their relationship to suicide (Mann et al., 2006). Data establishing a clear link between antidepressant treatment and suicide are lacking. In general, for reasons of safety, suicidal patients are not enrolled in clinical trials designed to seek approval for marketing a new medication. Thus, the FDA uses "suicidality" (i.e., suicidal ideation or suicide attempts and self-injurious behavior) as a proxy for risk of suicide. The FDA has issued a "black box" warning regarding the use of SSRIs and a number of other antidepressants in children and adolescents, particularly during the early phase of treatment, due to the possibility of an association between antidepressant treatment and suicide. However, there is strong epidemiological evidence that the rate of suicide has been decreasing since the time that SSRIs were first prescribed and then gained widespread usage; these data, however, cannot demonstrate a causal relationship. An analysis of health records of over 65,000 patients undergoing different types of pharmacological treatment for depression found no suggestion of increases in suicide or suicide attempts (Simon et al., 2006). Relevant to this point is the observation that an increase in suicide occurred for children and adolescents after regulatory authorities in the U.S. and Europe issued public health warnings about a possible association between antidepressants and suicidal ideation and acts, perhaps due to a reduction in the use of antidepressants in these patient populations after the announcement (Gibbons et al., 2007). Most clinicians agree that for seriously depressed patients, the risk of not being on an effective antidepressant drug outweighs the risk of being treated with one. Of course, clinical common sense also demands that special attention be paid to potentially suicidal patients regardless of their medication status. In addition, patients and family members should be warned to look for the exacerbation of symptoms such as insomnia, agitation, anxiety, or either the onset or worsening of suicidal thoughts and behaviors, particularly early in the course of therapy.

Monoamine Oxidase Inhibitors

The first class of drugs with relatively specific antidepressant effects were the MAOIs (Hollister, 1981). Iproniazid, which was developed initially for the treatment of tuberculosis, was found to have mood-elevating effects in patients with tuberculosis. Subsequently, iproniazid was shown to inhibit MAO, leading to the development of additional MAOIs including phenelzine, isocarboxazid, and tranylcypromine. As irreversible inhibitors of both MAO-A and MAO-B, these drugs have pronounced effects on the body's ability to metabolize endogenous monoamines (e.g., 5-HT, NE, and DA) and exogenous monoamines (e.g., tyramine). The protection of exogenous monoamines leads to significant drug and food interactions. More recently, reversible and selective inhibitors of MAO-A and MAO-B have been developed (Livingston and Livingston, 1996), and these have fewer side effects and fewer interactions with food and other drugs. The MAO-B selective inhibitor selegiline is used in the treatment of Parkinson disease; selective inhibitors of MAO-A, such as moclobemide, are effective antidepressants but are not approved for use in the U.S.

Tricyclic Antidepressant and Selective Reuptake Inhibitors

The initial development of the TCAs resulted from psychopharmacological characterization of a series of structural analogs that had been developed as potential antihistamines, sedatives, analgesics, and antiparkinson drugs (Hollister, 1981). One of the compounds, imipramine, which has a phenothiazine-like structure, modified behavior in animal models. Unlike the phenothiazines, imipramine had limited efficacy in schizophrenic patients, but improved symptoms of depression. Imipramine and related TCAs became the mainstay of drug treatment of depression until the later development of the SSRIs.

TCAs with a tertiary-amine side chain, including amitriptyline, doxepin, and imipramine, inhibit both norepinephrine and serotonin uptake, while clomipramine is somewhat selective for inhibition of serotonin uptake. Chemical modification of the TCA structure led to the earliest SSRI zimelidine which, while effective, was withdrawn from the market due to serious adverse effects. Fluoxetine and fluvoxamine were the first widely used SSRIs. At the same time, selective inhibitors of norepinephrine reuptake entered clinical development; while not approved for use in the U.S. for the treatment of depression, one norepinephrine reuptake inhibitor, atomoxetine, is used for the treatment of attention deficit hyperactivity disorder. Subsequent drug development efforts focused on serotonin and norepinephrine reuptake inhibitors (SNRIs), resulting in venlafaxine and duloxetine, which lack the complex receptor pharmacology exhibited by the TCAs.

Selective Serotonin Reuptake Inhibitors

A number of SSRIs were introduced from 1984-1997, including fluoxetine, paroxetine, sertraline, citalopram, escitalopram, and fluvoxamine; the FDA has approved fluvoxamine for treatment of obsessive-compulsive disorder and social anxiety disorder, but not depression. Citalopram is labeled for use in premenstrual dysphoric disorder. All of the SSRIs show a clear improvement in safety margin compared to the TCAs and are much safer in overdose, and in clinical practice have affected a broad range of psychiatric, behavioral, and medical conditions, for which they are used, on and off label.

The SSRIs are effective in treating major depression. In typical studies, only about two-thirds of SSRI-treated patients, compared to about one-third of placebo-treated patients, exhibit a 50% reduction of depressive symptoms during a 6-8 week trial. SSRI treatment results in ~ 35% of patients enjoying a remission, as defined by a Hamilton Depression Rating Score < 7, indicative of a complete resolution of symptoms, compared to 25% of patients who experience a remission with placebo treatment (Rush et al., 2006).

In addition to use as an antidepressant, SSRIs also are anxiolytics with demonstrated efficacy in the treatment of generalized anxiety, panic, social anxiety, and obsessive-compulsive disorders. Sertraline and paroxetine also have been approved for the treatment of posttraumatic stress disorder (PTSD), although treatment of this condition remains highly challenging. SSRIs also are used for treatment of premenstrual dysphoric syndrome and for preventing vasovagal symptoms in post-menopausal women (although the SNRI venlafaxine is the most extensively studied drug for this problem).

Mechanism of Action. SERT mediates the reuptake of serotonin into the presynaptic terminal; neuronal uptake is the primary process by which neurotransmission via 5-HT is terminated (Figure 15–1). Thus, treatment with an SSRI initially blocks reuptake and results in enhanced and prolonged serotonergic neurotransmission. SSRIs used clinically are relatively selective, that is, 10-fold or more, for inhibition of SERT relative to NET (Table 15–2). Increased synaptic availability of serotonin stimulates a large number of postsynaptic 5-HT receptor subtypes, as well as somatodendritic and presynaptic terminal receptors that regulate serotonergic neuron activity and serotonin release.

SSRI treatment causes stimulation of 5-HT$_{1A}$ and 5-HT$_7$ autoreceptors on cell bodies in the raphe nucleus and of 5-HT$_{1D}$ autoreceptors on serotonergic terminals, and this reduces serotonin synthesis and release toward pre-drug levels. With repeated treatment with SSRIs, there is a gradual down-regulation and desensitization of these autoreceptor mechanisms. In addition, down-regulation of postsynaptic 5-HT$_{2A}$ receptors may contribute to antidepressant efficacy directly or by influencing the function of noradrenergic and other neurons via serotonergic heteroreceptors. Other postsynaptic 5-HT receptors likely remain responsive to increased synaptic concentrations of 5-HT and contribute to the therapeutic effects of the SSRIs.

Later-developing effects of SSRI treatment also may be important in mediating ultimate therapeutic responses. These include sustained increases in cyclic AMP signaling and phosphorylation of the nuclear transcription factor CREB, as well as increases in the expression of trophic factors such as BDNF. In addition, SSRI treatment increases neurogenesis from progenitor cells in the dentate nucleus of the hippocampus and subventricular zone (Santarelli et al., 2003). In animals models, some behavioral effects of SSRIs depend on increased neurogenesis (probably via increased expression of BDNF and its receptor TrkB), suggesting a role for this mechanism in the antidepressant effects. Recent evidence indicates the presence of neural progenitor cells in the human hippocampus, providing some support for the relevance of this mechanism to the clinical situation (Manganas et al., 2007). Further, repeated treatment with SSRIs reduces the expression of SERT, resulting in reduced clearance of released 5-HT and increased serotonergic neurotransmission. These changes in transporter expression parallel behavioral changes observed in animal models, suggesting some role for this regulatory mechanism in the late-developing effects of SsRIs (Zhao et al., 2009). These persistent behavioral changes depend on increased serotonergic neurotransmission, similar to what has been demonstrated clinically using depletion strategies (Delgado et al., 1991).

Serotonin-Norepinephrine Reuptake Inhibitors

Many older TCAs block both SERT and NET, but at a high side effect burden. Four medications with a non-tricyclic structure that inhibit the reuptake of both 5-HT and norepinephrine have been approved for use in the U.S. for treatment of depression, anxiety disorders, and pain: venlafaxine and its demethylated metabolite, desvenlafaxine; duloxetine; and milnacipran (approved only for fibromyalgia pain in the U.S.). Off-label uses include stress urinary incontinence (duloxetine), autism, binge eating disorders, hot flashes, pain syndromes, premenstrual dysphoric disorders, and posttraumatic stress disorders (venlafaxine)

The rationale behind the development of these newer agents was that targeting both SERT and NET, analogous to the effects of some TCAs, might improve overall treatment response. Meta-analyses provide some support for this hypothesis (Entsuah et al., 2001). Specifically, the remission rate for venlafaxine appears slightly better than for SSRIs in head-to-head trials. However, many

Table 15–2

Potencies of Antidepressants at the Human Transporters for Norepinephrine (NET), Serotonin (SERT), and Dopamine (DAT)

DRUG	NET	SERT	DAT	SELECTIVITY
NE Selective				NET *vs* SERT
Oxaprotiline	5	4000	4350	800
Maprotiline	11.1	5900	1000	532
Viloxazine	156	17,000	100,000	109
Nomifensine	15.6	1000	55.6	64
Desipramine	0.8	17.5	3200	22
Protriptyline	1.4	19.6	2130	14
Atomoxetine	3.5	43	1270	12
Reboxetine	7.1	58.8	11,500	8.3
Nortriptyline	4.4	18.5	1140	4.2
Amoxapine	16.1	58.5	4350	3.6
Doxepin	29.4	66.7	12,200	2.3
5-HT Selective				SERT *vs* NET
S-Citalopram	7840	1.1	>10,000	7127
R,S-Citalopram	5100	1.4	28,000	3643
Sertraline	417	0.3	25	1390
Fluvoxamine	1300	2.2	9100	591
Paroxetine	40	0.1	500	400
Fluoxetine	244	0.8	3600	305
Clomipramine	37	0.3	2200	123
Venlafaxine	1060	9.1	9100	116
Nor_1-citalopram	780	7.4	—	105
Nor_2-citalopram	1500	24	—	63
Zimelidine	9100	152	12,000	60
Trazodone	8300	160	7140	52
Imipramine	37	1.4	8300	26
Norfluoxetine	410	25	1100	16
Amitriptyline	34.5	4.3	3200	8.0
Duloxetine	11.2	1.6	—	7.0
Dothiepin	45.5	8.3	5300	5.5
Norsertraline	420	76	440	5.5
Milnacipran	200	123	—	1.6
DA Selective				DAT vs NET
Bupropion	52,600	9100	526	1000

Values shown are experimentally determined constants (K_i values, nM) for inhibiting the function of human NET, SERT, and DAT expressed in cell lines. Drugs shown include clinically used antidepressants, important metabolites, and experimental drugs not used clinically. Selectivity is defined as ratio of the relevant K_i values (SERT/NET, NET/SERT, NET/DAT). Bupropion is selective for the DAT relative to the NET and SERT. *Source:* Data are adapted from Frazer (1997), Owens et al. (1997), and Leonard and Richelson (2000).

of the studies included in the meta-analyses used a daily venlafaxine dose of 150 mg, which would have modest effects on noradrenergic neurotransmission. Duloxetine, in addition to being approved for use in the treatment of depression and anxiety, also is used for treatment of fibromyalgia and neuropathic pain associated with peripheral neuropathy.

Mechanism of Action. SNRIs inhibit both SERT and NET (Table 15–2). Depending on the drug, the dose, and the potency at each site, SNRIs cause enhanced serotonergic and/or noradrenergic neurotransmission. Similar to the action of SSRIs, the initial inhibition of SERT induces activation of 5-HT_{1A} and 5-HT_{1D} autoreceptors. This action decreases serotonergic neurotransmission by a negative feedback mechanism until these serotonergic autoreceptors are desensitized. Then, the enhanced serotonin concentration in the synapse can interact with postsynaptic 5-HT receptors.

Serotonin Receptor Antagonists

Several antagonists of the 5-HT_2 family of receptors are effective antidepressants, although most agents of this class affect other receptor classes as well. The class includes two pairs of close structural analogues, trazodone and nefazodone, as well as mirtazapine (REMERON, others) and mianserin (not marketed in the U.S.).

The efficacy of trazodone may be somewhat more limited than the SSRIs; however, low doses of trazodone (50-100 mg) have been used widely both alone and concurrently with SSRIs or SNRIs to treat insomnia. When used to treat depression, trazodone typically is started at 150 mg/day in divided doses with 50 mg increments every 3-4 days. The maximally recommended dose is 400 mg/day for outpatients and 600 mg/day for inpatients.

Both mianserin and mirtazapine are quite sedating and are treatments of choice for some depressed patients with insomnia. The recommended initial dosing of mirtazapine is 15 mg/day with a maximal recommended dose of 45 mg/day. Since the $t_{1/2}$ is 16-30 hours, the recommended interval for dose changes is no less than 2 weeks.

Mechanism of Action. The most potent pharmacological effects of trazodone are blockade of the 5-HT_2 and α_1 adrenergic receptors. Trazodone also inhibits the serotonin transporter, but is markedly less potent for this action relative to its blockade of 5-HT_{2A} receptors. Similarly, the most potent pharmacological action of nefazodone also is the blockade of the 5-HT_2 family of receptors.

Both mirtazapine and mianserin potently block histamine H_1 receptors. They also have some affinity for α_2 adrenergic receptors, which is claimed to be related to their therapeutic efficacy, but this point is questionable. Their affinities for 5-HT_{2A}, 5-HT_{2C}, and 5-HT_3 receptors are high, though less so than for histamine H_1 receptors. Both of these drugs have been shown in double-blind, placebo-controlled studies to increase the antidepressant response when combined with SSRIs compared to the action of the SSRIs alone. The exact monoamine receptor accounting for the effects of mirtazapine and mianserin is not clear, although the data from clinical trials suggest that olanzapine, aripiprazole, and quetiapine enhance the therapeutic effects of SSRIs or SNRIs, an important hint that their unique capacity to block the 5-HT_{2A} receptor is the most potent shared pharmacological action amongst these antidepressant and antipsychotic drugs.

Bupropion

Bupropion (WELLBUTRIN, others) is discussed separately because it appears to act via multiple mechanisms. It enhances both noradrenergic and dopaminergic neurotransmission via reuptake inhibition (Table 15–2); in addition, its mechanism of action may involve the presynaptic release of NE and DA (Foley et al., 2006). Bupropion is indicated for the treatment of depression, prevention of seasonal depressive disorder, and as a smoking cessation treatment (under the ZYBAN brand). Bupropion has effects on sleep EEG that are opposite those of most antidepressant drugs. Bupropion may improve symptoms of attention deficit hyperactivity disorder (ADHD) and has been used off-label for neuropathic pain and weight loss. Clinically, bupropion is widely used in combination with SSRIs to obtain a greater antidepressant response; however, there are very limited clinical data providing strong support for this practice.

Mechanism of Action. Bupropion appears to inhibit NET. It also blocks the DAT but its effects on this transporter are not particularly potent in animal studies. In addition, it has effects on VMAT2, the vesicular monoamine transporter (see Figure 8–6). The hydroxybupropion metabolite may contribute to the therapeutic effects of bupropion: this metabolite appears to have a similar pharmacology and is present in substantial levels.

Atypical Antipsychotics

In addition to their use in schizophrenia, bipolar depression, and major depression with psychotic disorders, atypical antipsychotics have gained further, off-label use for major depression without psychotic features (Jarema, 2007). In fact, both aripiprazole (ABILIFY) added to SSRIs and SNRIs and a combination of olanzapine and the SSRI fluoxetine (SYMBYAX) have been approved by the FDA for treatment-resistant major depression (i.e., following an inadequate response to at least two different antidepressants).

The initial recommended dose of aripiprazole is 2-5 mg/day with a recommended maximal dose of 15 mg/day following increments of no more than 5 mg/day every week. The olanzapine-fluoxetine combination is available in fixed-dose combinations of either 6 or 12 mg of olanzapine and 25 or 50 mg of fluoxetine. Quetiapine (SEROQUEL) may have either primary antidepressant actions on its own or adjunctive benefit for treatment-resistant depression; it is used off-label for insomnia. Quetiapine also is currently under review by the FDA for additional indications in major depression and generalized anxiety disorder.

Mechanism of Action. The mechanism of action and adverse effects of the atypical antipsychotics are described in detail in Chapter 16. The side effects seen with atypical antipsychotics in patients with schizophrenia may not exactly translate to patients with major depression, due to a predisposition toward metabolic syndrome in patients with schizophrenia. The major risks of these agents are weight gain and metabolic syndrome, a greater problem for quetiapine and olanzapine than for aripiprazole.

Tricyclic Antidepressants

Due to their potential to cause serious side effects, the TCAs generally are not used as first-line drugs for the treatment of depression. Nevertheless, these drugs have established value for the treatment of major depression (Hollister, 1981). TCAs and first-generation antipsychotics are synergistic for the treatment of psychotic depression. Tertiary amine TCAs (e.g., doxepin, amitriptyline) have been used for many years in relatively low doses for treating insomnia. In addition, because of the role of norepinephrine and serotonin in pain transmission, these drugs are commonly used to treat a variety of pain conditions.

Mechanism of Action. The inspiration for the development of both SSRIs and SNRIs derived from the appreciation that a salient pharmacological action of TCAs is antagonism of serotonin and norepinephrine transporters (Table 15–2). The antidepressant action of TCAs was discovered during clinical trials in schizophrenic patients; imipramine had little effect on psychotic symptoms but had beneficial effects on depressive symptoms (Hollister, 1981). In addition to inhibiting NET somewhat selectively (desipramine, nortriptyline, protriptyline, amoxapine) or both SERT and NET (imipramine, amitriptyline), these drugs also block other receptors (H_1, 5-HT_2, α_1, and muscarinic). Given the superior activity of clomipramine over SSRIs, some combination of these additional pharmacological actions may contribute to the therapeutic effects of TCAs. One TCA, amoxapine, also is a dopaminergic receptor antagonist; its use, unlike that of other TCAs, poses some risk for the development of extrapyramidal side effects such as tardive dyskinesia.

Monoamine Oxidase Inhibitors

MAOIs have efficacy equivalent to that of the TCAs but are rarely used because of their toxicity and major drug and food interactions (Hollister, 1981). The MAOIs approved for treatment of depression include tranylcypromine (PARNATE, others), phenelzine (NARDIL), and isocarboxazid (MARPLAN). Selegiline (EMSAM) is available as a transdermal patch and approved for use in the treatment of depression; transdermal delivery may reduce the risk for diet-associated hypertensive reactions (described later).

Mechanism of Action. The MAOIs nonselectively and irreversibly inhibit both MAO-A and MAO-B, which are located in the mitochondria and metabolize (inactivate) monoamines, including 5-HT and NE (Chapter 8). Selegiline inhibits MAO-B at lower doses, with effects on MAO-A at higher doses. Selegiline also is a reversible inhibitor of monoamine oxidase, which may reduce the potential for serious adverse drug and food interactions. While both MAO-A and MAO-B are involved in metabolizing 5-HT, only MAO-B is found in serotonergic neurons (Chapter 13).

Pharmacokinetics

The metabolism of most antidepressants is mediated by hepatic CYPs (see Table 15–3). Some antidepressants inhibit the clearance of other drugs by the CYP system, as discussed in the following section, and this possibility of drug interactions should be a significant factor in considering the choice of agents.

Selective Serotonin Reuptake Inhibitors. All of the SSRIs are orally active and possess elimination half-lives consistent with once-daily dosing (Hiemke and Hartter, 2000). In the case of fluoxetine, the combined action of the parent and the desmethyl metabolite norfluoxetine allows for a once weekly formulation (PROZAC WEEKLY). CYP2D6 is involved in the metabolism of most SSRIs and the SSRIs are at least moderately potent inhibitors of this isoenzyme (Table 15–3). This creates a significant potential for drug interaction for post-menopausal women taking the breast cancer drug and estrogen antagonist, tamoxifen (Chapter 62); the parent molecule is converted to a more active metabolite by CYP2D6, and SSRIs may inhibit this activation and diminish the therapeutic activity of tamoxifen. Since venlafaxine and desvenlafaxine are weak inhibitors of CYP2D6, these antidepressants are not contraindicated in this clinical situation. However, care should be used in combining SSRIs with drugs that are metabolized by CYPs 1A2, 2D6, 2C9, and 3A4 (e.g., warfarin, tricyclic antidepressants, paclitaxel).

Serotonin-Norepinephrine Reuptake Inhibitors. Both immediate release and extended-release (tablet or capsule) preparations of venlafaxine (EFFEXOR XR, others) produces steady state-levels of drug in plasma within 3 days. The elimination half-lives for the parent venlafaxine and its active and major metabolite desmethyl venlafaxine are 5 and 11 hours, respectively. Desmethylvenlafaxine is eliminated by hepatic metabolism and by renal excretion. Venlafaxine dose reductions are suggested for patients with renal or hepatic impairment. Duloxetine has a $t_{1/2}$ of 12 hours. Duloxetine is not recommended for those with end-stage renal disease or hepatic insufficiency.

Serotonin Receptor Antagonists. Mirtazapine has an elimination $t_{1/2}$ of 16-30 hours. Thus, dose changes are suggested no more often than 1-2 weeks. Clearance of mirtazapine is decreased in the elderly and in patients with moderate to severe renal or hepatic impairment. Pharmacokinetics and adverse effects of mirtazapine may have an enantiomer-selective component (Brockmöller et al., 2007). Steady-state trazodone is observed within 3 days following either a twice or three times daily dosing regimen. Nefazodone has a $t_{1/2}$ of only 2-4 hours; its major metabolite hydroxynefazodone has a $t_{1/2}$ of 1.5-4 hours.

Bupropion. The terminal phase of bupropion elimination has a $t_{1/2}$ of 21 hours. The elimination of bupropion involves both hepatic and renal routes. Patients with severe hepatic cirrhosis should receive a maximum dose of 150 mg every other day while consideration for a decreased dose should also be made in cases of renal impairment.

Tricyclic Antidepressants. The TCAs, or their active metabolites, have plasma exposure half-lives of 8-80 hours; this makes once-daily dosing possible for most of the compounds (Rudorfer and Potter, 1999). Steady-state concentrations occur within several days to several weeks of beginning treatment. TCAs are largely eliminated by hepatic CYPs (see Table 15–3). Determination of plasma levels may be useful in identifying patients who appear to have toxic effects and may have excessively high levels of the drug, or those in whom lack of absorption or noncompliance is suspected. Dosage adjustments of TCAs are typically made according to patient's clinical response, not based on plasma levels. Nonetheless, monitoring the plasma exposure has an important relationship to treatment response: there is a relatively narrow therapeutic window, as discussed below.

About 7% of patients metabolize TCAs slowly due to a variant CYP2D6 isoenzyme, causing a 30-fold difference in plasma concentrations among different patients given the same TCA dose. To avoid toxicity in "slow metabolizers," plasma levels should be monitored and doses adjusted downward.

Monoamine Oxidase Inhibitors. MAOIs are metabolized by acetylation, although the end products are incompletely characterized.

Table 15–3

Disposition of Antidepressants

DRUG	ELIMINATION $t_{1/2}$, (h) PARENT DRUG *(Active Metabolite)*	TYPICAL C_p (ng/mL)	PREDOMINANT CYP INVOLVED IN METABOLISM
Tricyclic Antidepressants			
Amitriptyline	16 *(30)*	100–250	2D6, 2C19, 3A3/4, 1A2
Amoxapine	8 *(30)*	200–500	
Clomipramine	32 *(70)*	150–500	
Desipramine	30	125–300	
Doxepin	18 *(30)*	150–250	
Imipramine	12 *(30)*	175–300	
Maprotiline	48	200–400	
Nortriptyline	31	60–150	
Protriptyline	80	100–250	
Trimipramine	16 *(30)*	100–300	
Selective Serotonin Reuptake Inhibitors			
R,S-Citalopram	36	75–150	3A4, 2C19
S-Citalopram	30	40–80	3A4, 2C19
Fluoxetine	53 *(240)*	100–500	2D6, 2C9
Fluvoxamine	18	100–200	2D6, 1A2, 3A4, 2C9
Paroxetine	17	30–100	2D6
Sertraline	23 *(66)*	25–50	2D6
Serotonin-Norepinephrine Reuptake Inhibitors			
Duloxetine	11	—	2D6
Venlafaxine	5 *(11)*	—	2D6, 3A4
Other Antidepressants			
Atomoxetine	5–20 (child: 3)	—	2D6, 3A3/4
Bupropion	11	75–100	2B6
Mirtazapine	16	—	2D6
Nefazodone	2–4	—	3A3/4
Reboxetine	12	—	—
Trazodone	6	800–1600	2D6

Values shown are elimination $t_{1/2}$ values for a number of clinically used antidepressant drugs; numbers in parentheses are $t_{1/2}$ values of active metabolites. Fluoxetine (2D6), fluvoxamine (1A2, 2C8, 3A3/4), paroxetine (2D6), and nefazodone (3A3/4) are potent inhibitors of CYPs; sertraline (2D6), citalopram (2C19), and venlafaxine are less potent inhibitors. Plasma concentrations are those observed at typical clinical doses. Information was obtained from manufacturers' summaries and Appendix II, which the reader should consult for important details.

A significant portion of the population (50% of the Caucasian population and an even higher percentage among Asians) are "slow acetylators" and will exhibit elevated plasma levels. The nonselective MAOIs used in the treatment of depression are irreversible (sometimes called "suicide") inhibitors; thus, it takes up to 2 weeks for MAO activity to recover, even though the parent drug is excreted within 24 hours (Livingston and Livingston, 1996). Recovery of normal enzyme function is dependent on synthesis and transport of new

MAO to monoaminergic nerve terminals. Despite this irreversible enzyme inhibition, MAOIs require daily dosing.

Adverse Effects

Selective Serotonin Reuptake Inhibitors. The SSRIs, unlike the TCAs, do not cause major cardiovascular side effects. The SSRIs are generally free of antimuscarinic side effects (dry mouth, urinary retention, confusion), do not block histamine or α adrenergic receptors, and are not sedating (Table 15–4). The favorable side effect profile of the SSRIs may lead to better patient compliance compared to that for the TCAs.

SSRIs are not free from side effects, however. Excessive stimulation of brain 5-HT_2 receptors may result in insomnia, increased anxiety, irritability, and decreased libido, effectively worsening prominent depressive symptoms. Excess activity at spinal 5-HT_2 receptors causes sexual side effects including erectile dysfunction,

Table 15–4

Potencies of Selected Antidepressants at Muscarinic, Histamine H_1, and $Alpha_1$ Adrenergic Receptors

	RECEPTOR TYPE		
DRUG	MUSCARINIC CHOLINERGIC	HISTAMINE H_1	α_1 ADRENERGIC
Amytriptyline	18	1.1	27
Amoxapine	1000	25	50
Atomoxetine	≥1000	≥1000	≥1000
Bupropion	40,000	6700	4550
R,S-Citalopram	1800	380	1550
S-Citalopram	1240	1970	3870
Clomipramine	37	31.2	39
Desipramine	196	110	130
Doxepin	83.3	0.24	24
Duloxetine	3000	2300	8300
Fluoxetine	2000	6250	5900
Fluvoxamine	24,000	>100,000	7700
Imipramine	91	11.0	91
Maprotiline	560	2.0	91
Mirtazapine	670	0.1	500
Nefazodone	11,000	21	25.6
Nortriptyline	149	10	58.8
Paroxetine	108	22,000	>100,000
Protriptyline	25	25	130
Reboxetine	6700	312	11,900
Sertraline	625	24,000	370
Trazodone	>100,000	345	35.7
Trimipramine	59	0.3	23.8
Venlafaxine	>100,000	>100,000	>100,000

Values are experimentally determined potencies (K_i values, nM) for binding to receptors that contribute to common side effects of clinically used antidepressant drugs: muscarinic cholinergic receptors (e.g., dry mouth, urinary retention, confusion), histamine H_1 receptors (sedation), and α_1 adrenergic receptors (orthostatic hypotension, sedation).
Source: Data adapted from Leonard and Richelson (2000).

anorgasmia, and ejaculatory delay; these effects may be more prominent with paroxetine (Vaswani et al., 2003). Stimulation of 5-HT_3 receptors in the CNS and periphery contributes to GI effects, which are usually limited to nausea but may include diarrhea and emesis. Some patients experience an increase in anxiety, especially with the initial dosing of SSRIs. With continued treatment, some patients also report a dullness of intellectual abilities and concentration. In addition a phenomenon of a residual "flat affect" can occur in an otherwise successful treatment with SSRIs. A number of these side effects may be difficult to distinguish from symptoms of depression.

In general, there is not a strong relationship between SSRI serum concentrations and therapeutic efficacy. This finding is not surprising given that most antidepressant studies have been conducted at doses/plasma exposures which saturate the brain SERT, consistent with the flat dose or exposure/efficacy relationships observed. Thus, dosage adjustments are based more on evaluation of clinical response and management of side effects than on measurements of plasma drug concentrations.

Sudden withdrawal of antidepressants can precipitate a withdrawal syndrome. For SSRIs or SNRIs, the symptoms of withdrawal may include dizziness, headache, nervousness, nausea, and insomnia. This withdrawal syndrome appears most intense for paroxetine and venlafaxine compared to other antidepressants due to their relatively short half-lives and, in the case of paroxetine, lack of active metabolites. On the other hand, the active metabolite of fluoxetine, norfluoxetine, has such a long $t_{1/2}$ (1-2 weeks) that few patients experience any withdrawal symptoms when discontinuing fluoxetine.

Unlike the other SSRIs, paroxetine is associated with an increased risk of congenital cardiac malformations. Epidemiological data suggest that paroxetine might increase the risk of congenital cardiac malformations when administered in the first trimester of pregnancy. Venlafaxine also is associated with an increased risk of perinatal complications. Therefore, these drugs should not be used in pregnant women; careful consideration should be given to using these mediations in women of reproductive potential, and these subjects should be advised to avoid pregnancy while they are taking the drugs.

Serotonin-Norepinephrine Reuptake Inhibitors. The SNRIs have desirable safety advantages over the TCAs (Table 15–4). SNRIs have a side effect profile similar to that of the SSRIs, including nausea, constipation, insomnia, headaches, and sexual dysfunction. The immediate release formulation of venlafaxine can induce sustained diastolic hypertension (systolic blood pressure > 90 mm Hg at consecutive weekly visits) in 10-15% of patients at higher doses; this risk is reduced with the extended-release form. This effect of venlafaxine may not be associated simply with inhibition of NET, since duloxetine does not share this side effect.

Serotonin Receptor Antagonists. The main side effects of mirtazapine, seen in >10% of the patients in clinical trials, are somnolence, increased appetite, and weight gain. A rare side effect of mirtazapine is agranulocytosis. In the 2 patients having this side effect during the pre-marketing phase in nearly 2800 patients, bone marrow function recovered when mirtazapine treatment was discontinued. Trazodone use is associated with priapism in rare instances; this should be considered a medical emergency and surgical intervention may be required. Nefazodone was voluntarily withdrawn from the market in Europe and the U.S. after rare cases of liver failure were associated with its use. Generic nefazodone is still available in the U.S.

Bupropion. At doses higher than that recommended for depression (450 mg/day), the risk of seizures increases significantly. The use of extended release formulations often blunts the maximum concentration observed after dosing and minimizes the chance of reaching drug levels associated with an increased risk of seizures.

Tricyclic Antidepressants. TCAs are potent antagonists at histamine H_1 receptors; H_1 receptor antagonism contributes to the sedative effects of TCAs (Table 15–4). Antagonism of muscarinic acetylcholine receptors contributes to cognitive dulling as well as a range of adverse effects mediated by the parasympathetic nervous system (blurred vision, dry mouth, tachycardia, constipation, difficulty urinating). Some tolerance does occur for these anticholinergic effects, which are mitigated by titration strategies to reach therapeutic doses over a reasonable period of time. Antagonism of α_1 adrenergic receptors contributes to orthostatic hypotension and sedation. Weight gain is another side effect of this class of antidepressants.

TCAs also have quinidine-like effects on cardiac conduction that can be life threatening with overdose and limit the use of TCAs in patients with coronary heart disease. This is the primary reason that no more than a one-week supply should be provided to a new patient; even during maintenance treatment, only a very limited supply should be available to the patient at any given time. Like other antidepressant drugs, TCAs also lower the seizure threshold.

Monoamine Oxidase Inhibitors. Hypertensive crisis resulting from food or drug interactions is one of the life-threatening toxicities associated with use of the MAOIs. Foods containing tyramine are a contributing factor. MAO-A within the intestinal wall and MAO-A and MAO-B in the liver normally degrade dietary tyramine. However, when MAO-A is inhibited, the ingestion of certain aged cheeses, red wines, sauerkraut, fava beans, and a variety of other tyramine-containing foods leads to accumulation of tyramine in adrenergic nerve endings and neurotransmitter vesicles and induces norepinephrine and epinephrine release. The released catecholamines stimulate postsynaptic receptors in the periphery, increasing blood pressure to dangerous levels. These episodes can be reversed by antihypertensive medications. Even when the patient is highly vigilant, dietary indiscretions or use of prescription or over-the-counter medications that contain sympathomimetic compounds may occur, resulting in a potentially life-threatening elevation of blood pressure. In comparison to tranylcypromine and isocarboxazid, the selegiline transdermal patch is better tolerated and safer. Another serious, life-threatening issue with chronic administration of MAOIs is hepatotoxicity.

MAO-A inhibitors are efficacious in treating depression. However, MAO-B inhibitors such as selegiline (with oral formulations) are effective in treating depression only when given at doses that block both MAO-A and MAO-B. Thus, these data emphasize the importance of enhancing the synaptic availability of 5-HT and NE as important mediating events for many antidepressant drugs. While not available in the U.S., reversible inhibitors of MAO-A (RIMAs, such as moclobemide) have been developed. Since these drugs are selective for MAO-A, significant MAO-B activity remains. Further, since the inhibition of MAO-A by RIMAs is reversible and competitive, as concentrations of tyramine rise, enzyme inhibition is surmounted. Thus, RIMAs produce antidepressant effects with reduced risk of tyramine-induced hypertensive crisis.

Drug Interactions

Selective Serotonin Reuptake Inhibitors. Most antidepressants, including the SSRIs, exhibit drug-drug interactions based on their routes of metabolism CYPs. Paroxetine and, to a lesser degree, fluoxetine are potent inhibitors of CYP2D6 (Hiemke and Hartter, 2000). The other SSRIs, outside of fluvoxamine, are at least moderate inhibitors of CYP2D6. This inhibition can result in disproportionate increases in plasma concentrations of drugs metabolized by CYP2D6 when doses of these drugs are increased. Fluvoxamine directly inhibits CYP1A2 and CYP2C19; fluoxetine and fluvoxamine also inhibit CYP3A4. A prominent interaction is the increase in TCA exposure that may be observed during co-administration of TCAs and SSRIs.

Another important drug-drug interaction with SSRIs occurs via a pharmacodynamic mechanism. MAOIs enhance the effects of SSRIs due to inhibition of serotonin metabolism. Administration of these drugs together can produce synergistic increases in extracellular brain serotonin, leading to the serotonin syndrome. Symptoms of the serotonin syndrome include hyperthermia, muscle rigidity, myoclonus, tremors, autonomic instability, confusion, irritability, and agitation; this can progress toward coma and death. Other drugs that may induce the serotonin syndrome include substituted amphetamines such as methylenedioxymethamphetamine (Ecstasy), which directly releases serotonin from nerve terminals. The primary treatment is stopping all serotonergic drugs, administering nonselective serotonin antagonists, and supportive measures.

Since currently available MAOIs bind irreversibly to MAO and block the enzymatic metabolism of monoaminergic neurotransmitters, SSRIs should not be started until at least 14 days following discontinuation of treatment with an MAOI; this allows for synthesis of new MAO. For all SSRIs but fluoxetine, at least 14 days should pass prior to beginning treatment with an MAOI following the end of treatment with an SSRI. Since the active metabolite norfluoxetine has a $t_{1/2}$ of 1-2 weeks, at least 5 weeks should pass between stopping fluoxetine and beginning an MAOI.

Serotonin-Norepinephrine Reuptake Inhibitors. While 14 days are suggested to elapse from ending MAOI therapy and starting venlafaxine treatment, an interval of only 7 days after stopping venlafaxine is considered safe before beginning an MAOI. Duloxetine has a similar interval to initiation following MAOI therapy, but requires only a 5-day waiting period to begin MAOI treatment after ending duloxetine. Failure to observe these required waiting periods can result in the serotonin syndrome, as noted above for SSRIs.

Serotonin Receptor Antagonists. Trazodone dosing may need to be lowered when given together with drugs that inhibit CYP3A4. Mirtazapine is metabolized by CYPs 2D6, 1A2, and 3A4, but does not potently inhibit any of these isoenzymes. Trazodone and nefazodone are weak inhibitors of serotonin uptake and should not be administered with MAOIs due to concerns about the serotonin syndrome. However, it is unclear whether these drugs appreciably block brain SERT at doses used in the treatment of depression.

Bupropion. The major route of metabolism for bupropion is CYP2B6. While there does not appear to be any evidence for metabolism by CYP2D6 and this drug is frequently administered with SSRIs, the potential for interactions with drugs metabolized by CYP2D6 should be kept in mind until the safety of the combination is firmly established.

Tricyclic Antidepressants. Drugs that inhibit CYP2D6, such as SSRIs, may increase plasma exposures of TCAs. Other drugs that may act similarly are phenothiazine antipsychotic agents, type 1C anti-arrhythmic drugs, and other drugs with antimuscarinic, antihistaminic, and α adrenergic antagonistic effects. TCAs can potentiate the actions of sympathomimetic amines and should not be used concurrently with MAOIs or within 14 days of stopping MAOIs.

Monoamine Oxidase Inhibitors. A large number of drug-drug interactions lead to contraindications for simultaneous use with MAOIs. CNS depressants including meperidine and other narcotics, alcohol, and anesthetic agents should not be used with MAOIs. Meperidine and other opioid agonists in combination with MAOIs also induce the serotonin syndrome. As discussed earlier, SSRIs and SNRIs are contraindicated in patients on MAOIs, and vice versa, to avoid the serotonin syndrome. In general, other antidepressants such as TCAs and bupropion also should be avoided in patients taking an MAOI.

Anxiolytic Drugs

A variety of agents and drug classes provide anxiolytic effects. The primary treatments for anxiety-related disorders include the SSRIs, SNRIs, benzodiazepines, the azipirone buspirone, and beta adrenergic antagonists (Atack, 2003). Historically, TCAs, particularly clomipramine, and MAOIs have been used for the treatment of some anxiety-related disorders, but their use has been supplanted by drugs with lower toxicity. Specific issues relating to mechanism of action, adverse effects, pharmacokinetics, and drug interactions are discussed earlier and in Chapters 16 and 17.

The SSRIs and the SNRI venlafaxine (discussed earlier) are well tolerated with a reasonable side effect profile; in addition to their documented antidepressant activity, they also have have anxiolytic activity with chronic treatment. The benzodiazepines are effective anxiolytics as both acute and chronic treatment. There is concern regarding their use because of their potential for dependence and abuse as well as negative effects on cognition and memory. Buspirone, like the SSRIs, is effective following chronic treatment. In acts, at least in part, via the serotonergic system, where it is a partial agonist at 5-HT_{1A} receptors. Buspirone also has antagonistic effects at dopamine D_2 receptors, but the relationship between this effect and its clinical actions is uncertain. β adrenergic antagonists, particularly those with higher lipophilicity (e.g., propranolol and nadolol) are occasionally used for performance anxiety such as fear of public speaking; their use is limited due to significant side effects such as hypotension.

The antihistamine hydroxyzine and various sedative-hypnotic agents have been used as anxiolytics, but are generally not recommended because of their side effect profiles. Hydroxyzine, which produces short-term sedation, has been used in patients that cannot use other types of anxiolytics (e.g., those with a history of drug or alcohol abuse where benzodiazepines would be avoided). Chloral hydrate has been used for situational anxiety, but there is a narrow dose range where anxiolytic effects are observed in the absence of significant sedation, and, therefore, the use of chloral hydrate is not recommended.

Clinical Considerations with Anxiolytic Drugs. The choice of pharmacological treatment for anxiety is dictated by the specific anxiety-related disorders and the clinical need for acute anxiolytic effects (Millan, 2003). Among the commonly used anxiolytics, only the benzodiazepines and β adrenergic antagonists are effective acutely; the use of β adrenergic antagonists is generally limited to treatment of situational anxiety. Chronic treatment with SSRIs, SNRIs, and buspirone is required to produce and sustain anxiolytic effects. When an immediate anxiolytic effects is desired, benzodiazepines are typically selected.

Benzodiazepines, such as alprazolam, chlordiazepoxide, clonazepam, clorazepate, diazepam, lorazepam, and oxazepam, are effective in the treatment of generalized anxiety disorder, panic disorder, and situational anxiety. In addition to their anxiolytic effects, benzodiazepines produce sedative, hypnotic, anesthetic, anticonvulsant, and muscle relaxant effects. The benzodiazepines also impair cognitive performance and memory, adversely affect motor control, and potentiate the effects of other sedatives including alcohol. The anxiolytic effects of this class of drugs are mediated by allosteric interactions with the pentameric benzodiazepine-$GABA_A$ receptor complex, in particular those $GABA_A$ receptors comprised of α2, α3, and α5 subunits (Chapters 14 and 17). The primary effect of the anxiolytic benzodiazepines is to enhance the inhibitory effects of the neurotransmitter GABA.

One area of concern regarding the use of benzodiazepines in the treatment of anxiety is the potential for habituation, dependence, and abuse. Patients with certain personality disorders or a history of drug or alcohol abuse are particularly susceptible. However, the risk of dependence must be balanced with the need for treatment, since benzodiazepines are effective in both short- and long-term treatment of patients with sustained or recurring bouts of anxiety. Further, premature discontinuation of benzodiazepines, in the absence of other pharmacological treatment, results in a high rate of relapse. Withdrawal of benzodiazepines after chronic treatment, particularly those with short durations of action, can include increased anxiety and seizures. For this reason, it is important that discontinuation be carried out in a gradual manner.

Benzodiazepines cause many adverse effects, including sedation, mild memory impairments, decreased alertness, and slowed reaction time (which may lead to accidents). Memory problems can include visual-spatial deficits, but will manifest clinically in a variety of ways, including difficulty in word-finding. Occasionally, paradoxical reactions can occur with benzodiazepines such as increases in anxiety, sometimes reaching panic attack proportions. Other pathological reactions can include irritability, aggression, or behavioral disinhibition. Amnesic reactions (i.e., loss of memory for particular periods) can also occur. Benzodiazepines should not be used in pregnant women; there have been rare reports of craniofacial defects. In addition, benzodiazepines taken prior to delivery may result in sedated, under-responsive newborns and prolonged withdrawal reactions. In the elderly, benzodiazepines increase the risk for falls and must be used cautiously. These drugs are safer than classical sedative-hypnotics in overdosage and typically are fatal only if combined with other CNS depressants.

Benzodiazepines have at least some abuse potential, although their capacity for abuse is considerably below that of other classical sedative-hypnotic agents. When these agents are abused, it is generally in a multi-drug abuse pattern. In fact, the primary reason for misuse of these agents often is failed attempts to control anxiety. Tolerance to the anxiolytic effects develops with chronic administration, with the result that some patients escalate the dose of benzodiazepines over time. Ideally, benzodiazepines should be used for short periods of time and in conjunction with other medications (e.g., SSRIs) or evidence-based psychotherapies (e.g., cognitive behavioral therapy for anxiety disorders).

SSRIs and the SNRI venlafaxine are first-line treatments for most types of anxiety disorders, except when an acute drug effect is desired; fluvoxamine is approved only for obsessive-compulsive disorder. As for their antidepressant actions, the anxiolytic effects of these drugs become manifest following chronic treatment. Other drugs with actions on serotonergic neurotransmission, including trazodone, nefazodone, and mirtazapine, also are used in the treatment of anxiety disorders. Details regarding the pharmacology of these classes of were presented earlier.

Both SSRIs and SNRIs are beneficial in specific anxiety conditions such as generalized anxiety disorder, social phobias, obsessive-compulsive disorder, and panic disorder. These effects appear to be related to the capacity of serotonin to regulate the activity of brain structures such as amygdala and locus coeruleus that are thought to be involved in the genesis of anxiety. Interestingly, the SSRIs and SNRIs often will produce some increases in anxiety in the short-term that dissipate with time. Therefore, the maxim "*start low and go slow*" is indicated with anxious patients; however, many patients with anxiety disorders ultimately will require doses that are about the same as those required for the treatment of depression. Anxious patients appear to be particularly prone to severe discontinuation reactions with certain medications such as venlafaxine and paroxetine; therefore, slow off-tapering is required.

Buspirone is used in the treatment of generalized anxiety disorder (Goodman, 2004). Like the SSRIs, buspirone requires chronic treatment for effectiveness. Also, like the SSRIs, buspirone lacks many of the other pharmacological effects of the benzodiazepines: it is not an anticonvulsant, muscle relaxant, or sedative, and it does not impair psychomotor performance or result in dependence. Buspirone is primarily effective in the treatment of generalized anxiety disorder, but not for other anxiety disorders. In fact, patients with panic disorder often note an increase in anxiety acutely following initiation of buspirone treatment; this may be the result of the fact that buspirone causes increased firing rates of the locus coeruleus, which is thought to underlie part of the pathophysiology of panic disorder.

CLINICAL SUMMARY

Mood and anxiety disorders are the most common psychiatric illnesses and are encountered frequently by clinicians in all disciplines. Depression represents a spectrum of conditions with a range of severity and a high frequency of comorbidities. Depressive conditions range from mild, self-limiting conditions to extremely severe illnesses that can include a high suicidal potential, psychosis, and serious functional impairment. Whereas the likelihood of receiving treatment for depression or anxiety has improved, problems remain with regard to duration, dosing, and adherence to treatment. Unfortunately, persons with depressive or anxiety disorders continue to suffer considerable delays in diagnosis and adequate treatment. Prominently used agents inhibit transmitter reuptake via SERT and NET.

Current antidepressant and anxiolytic treatment strategies are imperfect. Many patients have significant residual symptoms after pharmacotherapy. Fortunately, antidepressant/anxiolytic drug development is expanding beyond standard 5-HT and NE uptake inhibitors. New antidepressant medications include triple (5-HT, NE, and DA)

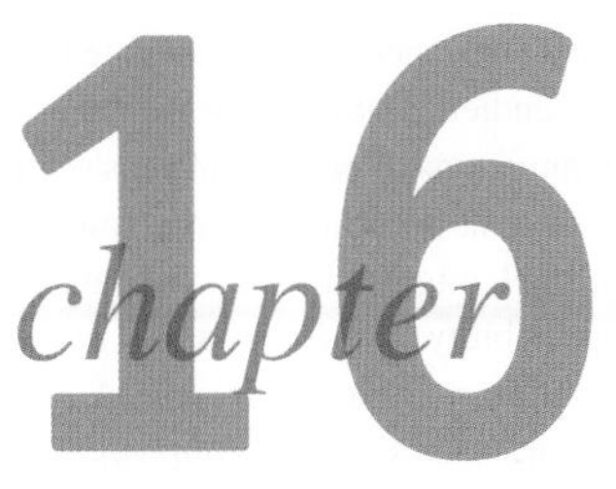

Pharmacotherapy of Psychosis and Mania

Jonathan M. Meyer

TREATMENT OF PSYCHOSIS

Psychosis is a symptom of mental illnesses characterized by a distorted or non-existent sense of reality. Psychotic disorders have different etiologies, each of which demands a unique treatment approach. Common psychotic disorders include mood disorders (major depression or mania) with psychotic features, substance-induced psychosis, dementia with psychotic features, delirium with psychotic features, brief psychotic disorder, delusional disorder, schizoaffective disorder, and schizophrenia. Schizophrenia has a worldwide prevalence of 1% and is considered the prototypic disorder for understanding the phenomenology of psychosis and the impact of antipsychotic treatment, but patients with schizophrenia exhibit features that extend beyond those seen in other psychotic illnesses. Hallucinations, delusions, disorganized speech, and disorganized or agitated behavior comprise the types of psychotic symptoms found individually, or rarely together, in all psychotic disorders, and are typically responsive to pharmacotherapy. In addition to *positive symptoms*, schizophrenia patients also suffer from *negative symptoms* (apathy, avolition, alogia), and *cognitive deficits*, particularly deficits in working memory, processing speed, social cognition, and problem solving that test 1.5-2 standard deviations below population norms (Green et al., 2004). Cognitive dysfunction is the strongest predictor of functional impairment among schizophrenia patients, yet negative symptoms and cognitive deficits show limited improvement with antipsychotic treatment (Buchanan et al., 2007). That schizophrenia is not identical to other psychoses is important for appreciating the differential impact of antipsychotic medications on psychotic symptomatology, and for understanding the rationale for non-dopaminergic antipsychotic drugs based on the underlying pathophysiology of schizophrenia (Carpenter and Koenig 2008).

The Dopamine Hypothesis. The development of our understanding of the neurobiology and pharmacotheorapy of psychoses profited from the synthesis of chlorpromazine in 1950 and of haloperidol in 1958. The DA hypothesis of psychosis derived from the fortuitous discovery of chlorpromazine's therapeutic efficacy in schizophrenia, and the subsequent elucidation by Carlsson that postsynaptic DA D_2 receptor antagonism was the common mechanism that explained antipsychotic properties. Reserpine, derived from *Rauwolfia*, exhibited antipsychotic properties by decreasing dopaminergic neurotransmission; however, unlike D_2 receptor antagonists, reserpine exerted its effects through depletion of monoamines from presynaptic nerve terminals. The dopamine theory of psychosis was reinforced by the high risk for drug-induced psychosis among substances that directly increased synaptic dopamine availability, including cocaine, amphetamines, and the Parkinson's disease treatment *L*-dopa (Carlsson, 1978).

The dopamine (DA) overactivity hypothesis has led to the development of the first therapeutic class of antipsychotic agents, now referred to as *typical* or first-generation antipsychotic drugs. These medications differed in potency, but shared the common mechanism of significant DA D_2 blockade and associated risk for extrapyramidal side effects. In the past, the term "neuroleptic" was also employed to refer to typical antipsychotic drugs, literally meaning to "take hold of the nerves" in Greek, but this has been dropped from contemporary usage (as has the term "major tranquilizer") in favor of "antipsychotic drug," a term that more accurately reflects the primary clinical use of these agents.

While the DA hypothesis is an advance over earlier conceptualizations of psychosis, it has limitations, and does not account for the cognitive deficits associated with schizophrenia that appear to be related to decreased DA signaling in the prefrontal cortex. The DA hypothesis also does not explain the psychotomimetic effects of agonists of other pathways (e.g., *d*-lysergic acid, a potent serotonin 5-HT_2 receptor agonist), or the effects of phencyclidine and ketamine, antagonists of the *N*-methyl-D-aspartate (NMDA) glutamate receptor. Advances in treatment have emerged from exploration of alternative (non-dopaminergic) mechanisms for psychosis and from experience with atypical antipsychotic agents such as clozapine. These newer antipsychotics potently antagonize the 5-HT_2 receptor, while blocking D_2 receptors less potently than older typical antipsychotic agents, resulting in the atypical clinical profile of antipsychotic efficacy with limited extrapyramidal side effects. Also promising are medications that target glutamate and 5-HT_7 receptor subtypes, receptors for γ-aminobutyric acid (GABA) and acetylcholine (both muscarinic and nicotinic), and even peptide hormone receptors (e.g., oxytocin) (Carpenter and Koenig, 2008).

Review of Relevant Pathophysiology

Not all psychosis is schizophrenia, and the pathophysiology relevant to effective schizophrenia treatment may not apply to other psychotic disorders. The effectiveness of dopamine D_2 antagonists for the positive symptoms of psychosis seen in most psychotic disorders suggests a common etiology for these symptoms related to excessive dopaminergic neurotransmission in mesolimbic dopamine pathways. In substance-induced psychotic disorders, the substance may directly increase postsynaptic DA activity through increased presynaptic neurotransmitter release (amphetamine), inhibition of presynaptic DA reuptake (methylphenidate, cocaine, and amphetamine), or increased DA availability (*L*-dopa). The NMDA antagonists phencyclidine and ketamine indirectly act to stimulate DA availability by decreasing the glutamate-mediated tonic inhibition of DA release in the mesolimbic DA pathway.

The psychoses related to delirium and dementia, particularly dementia of the Alzheimer type, may share a common etiology: the deficiency in cholinergic neurotransmission, either due to anticholinergic properties of medications (Chew et al., 2008), age- or disease-related neuronal loss, or both (Barten and Albright, 2008; Hshieh et al., 2008). Among hospitalized elderly patients, increased plasma concentrations of anticholinergic medications are directly associated with increased delirium risk (Flacker and Lipsitz, 1999); however, unlike in Alzheimer's dementia, where psychotic symptoms are directly related to cholinergic neuronal loss and may respond to acetylcholinesterase therapy, delirium may have numerous precipitants besides medication-associated anticholinergic properties, all of which require specific treatment (e.g., infection, electrolyte imbalance, metabolic derangement) in addition to removal of offending anticholinergic medications.

Schizophrenia is a neurodevelopmental disorder with complex genetics and incompletely understood pathophysiology. Certain environmental exposures confer an increased risk of developing schizophrenia, including fetal second-trimester viral and nutritional insults, birth complications, and substance abuse in the late teen or early adult years (Fanous and Kendler, 2008). Rather than being the result of a single gene defect, mutations or polymorphisms of many genes appear to contribute to the risk for schizophrenia. Implicated are genes that regulate neuronal migration and synaptogenesis (*neuregulin 1*), synaptic DA availability (*Val{108/158}Met polymorphism of catechol-O-methyltransferase,* which increases DA catabolism), glutamate and DA neurotransmission (*dystrobrevin binding protein 1 or dysbindin*, particularly with schizophrenia patients with prominent negative symptoms), nicotinic neurotransmission (*α7-receptor polymorphisms*), and cognition (*disrupted-in-schizophrenia-1*) (Porteous, 2008). Schizophrenia patients also have increased rates of genome-wide DNA microduplications termed *copy number variants* (Need et al., 2009) and *epigenetic* changes, including disruptions in DNA methylation patterns in various brain regions (Porteous, 2008). This genetic variability is consistent with the clinical disease heterogeneity, and suggests that any one specific mechanism is unlikely to account for large amounts of disease risk. In addition to increased mesolimbic DA activity related to positive symptoms, schizophrenia patients have decreased DA D_1 activity in the dorsolateral and ventromedial prefrontal cortex (PFC) that is associated with cognitive deficits and negative symptoms (Buchanan et al., 2007).

Cognitive dysfunction is the greatest predictor of poor functional outcome in schizophrenia and shows limited response to antipsychotic treatment. Experimental studies have provided new insights into the mechanisms of cognitive dysfunction. Glutamate NMDA receptor stimulation is involved in tonic inhibition of mesolimbic DA release, but facilitates mesocortical DA release (Sodhi et al., 2008). Ketamine infusion studies in animals and healthy volunteers demonstrate that decreased NMDA function results in a picture that more accurately encompasses all aspects of schizophrenia, including positive, negative, and cognitive symptoms, and social withdrawal. Several of the newer antipsychotic drugs remediate not only the positive psychotic symptoms but also the cognitive disruption induced by ketamine and other potent NMDA antagonists such as MK-801 (dizocilpine). These results have prompted the clinical investigation of agents without affinity for DA receptors, but with potent agonist properties at metabotropic glutamate receptor subtypes (Patil et al., 2007).

Review of Psychosis Pathology and the General Goals of Pharmacotherapy

Common to all psychotic disorders are positive symptoms, which may include hallucinatory behavior, disturbed thinking, and behavioral dyscontrol. For many psychotic disorders the state of psychosis is transient, and antipsychotic drugs are only administered during and shortly after periods of symptom exacerbation. Patients with delirium, dementia, mania or major depressive disorder with psychotic features, substance-induced psychoses, and brief psychotic disorder will typically receive short-term antipsychotic treatment that is discontinued after resolution of psychotic symptoms, although the duration may vary considerably based upon the etiology. In the majority of substance-induced psychoses, removal of the offending agent results in prompt improvement of psychotic symptoms with no further need for antipsychotic therapy. This may not apply to advanced Parkinson's disease patients, for whom *L*-dopa cannot be stopped and for whom ongoing antipsychotic treatment may be necessary (Chapter 22). Patients with psychosis related to mood disorders, in particular manic patients, may have antipsychotic treatment extended for several months after resolution of the psychosis, since antipsychotic medications are effective in controlling mania symptoms. Chronic psychotic symptoms in dementia patients may also be amenable to drug therapy, but potential benefits must be balanced with the documented risk of mortality and cerebrovascular events associated with the use of antipsychotic medications in this patient population (Jeste et al., 2008).

Delusional disorder, schizophrenia, and schizoaffective disorder are chronic diseases that require long-term antipsychotic treatment, although there are few reliable studies of treatment outcomes for delusional disorder patients. Individuals with monosymptomatic delusions (e.g., paranoia, marital infidelity) do not have neurocognitive dysfunction and may continue to perform work and social functions unaffected by their illness, aside from behavioral consequences related to the specific delusional belief (American Psychiatric Association, 2000). These patients often have limited or no psychiatric contact outside of mandated legal interventions, thus limiting the opportunity for clinical trials. For schizophrenia and schizoaffective disorder, the goal of antipsychotic treatment is to maximize functional recovery by decreasing the severity of positive symptoms and their behavioral influence, improving negative symptoms, decreasing social withdrawal, and remediating cognitive dysfunction. That only 15% of chronic schizophrenia patients are employed in any capacity and 11% are married has been attributed to the relatively limited effect of treatment on core negative and cognitive symptoms of the illness (Lieberman et al., 2005). Nonetheless, continuous antipsychotic treatment reduces 1-year relapse rates from 80% among unmedicated patients, to ~15%. Poor adherence to antipsychotic treatment increases relapse risk, and is often related to adverse drug events, cognitive dysfunction, substance use, and limited illness insight.

Regardless of the underlying pathology, the immediate goal of antipsychotic treatment is a decrease in acute symptoms that induce patient distress, particularly behavioral symptoms (e.g., hostility, agitation) that may present a danger to the patient or others. The dosing, route of administration, and choice of antipsychotic depend on the underlying disease state, clinical acuity, drug-drug interactions with concomitant medications, and patient sensitivity to short- or long-term adverse effects. With the exception of clozapine's superior efficacy in treatment-refractory schizophrenia (Leucht et al., 2009), neither the clinical presentation nor biomarkers predict the likelihood of response to a specific antipsychotic class or agent. As a result, avoidance of adverse effects based upon patient and drug characteristics, or exploitation of certain medication properties (e.g., sedation related to histamine H_1 or muscarinic antagonism) are the principal determinants for choosing initial antipsychotic therapy.

All commercially available antipsychotic drugs reduce dopaminergic neurotransmission (Figure 16–1). This finding implicates D_2 blockade (or, in the case of aripiprazole, modulation of DA activity) as the primary therapeutic mechanism. Chlorpromazine and other early low-potency typical antipsychotic agents are also profoundly sedating, a feature that used to be considered relevant to their therapeutic pharmacology. The development of the high-potency typical antipsychotic agent haloperidol, a drug with limited H_1 and M_1 affinity and significantly less sedative effects, and the clinical efficacy of intramuscular forms of nonsedating newer antipsychotic drugs, aripiprazole and ziprasidone, demonstrate that sedation is not necessary for antipsychotic activity, although at times desirable.

Short-Term Treatment

Delirium and Dementia. Disease variables have considerable influence on selection of antipsychotic agents. Psychotic symptoms of delirium or dementia are generally treated with low medication doses, although doses may have to be repeated at frequent intervals initially to achieve adequate behavioral control (Lacasse et al., 2006). Despite widespread clinical use, not a single antipsychotic drug has received approval for dementia-related psychosis. Moreover, all antipsychotic drugs carry warnings that they may increase mortality in this setting (Jeste et al., 2008). Because anticholinergic drug effects may worsen delirium (Hshieh et al., 2008) and dementia, high-potency typical antipsychotic drugs (e.g., haloperidol) or atypical antipsychotic agents with limited antimuscarinic properties (e.g., risperidone) are often the drugs of choice (Jeste et al., 2008; Lacasse et al., 2006).

The best-tolerated doses in dementia patients are one-fourth of adult schizophrenia doses (e.g., risperidone 0.5-1.5 mg/day), although extrapyramidal neurological symptoms (EPS), orthostasis, and sedation are particularly problematic in this patient population (Chapter 22). Significant antipsychotic benefits are usually seen in acute psychosis within 60-120 minutes after drug administration. Delirious or demented patients may be reluctant or unable to swallow tablets, so oral dissolving tablet (ODT) preparations for risperidone, aripiprazole, and olanzapine, or liquid concentrate forms of risperidone or aripiprazole, are options. The dissolving tablets adhere

Table 16–1

Chemical Structures, Dosages for Acute Psychosis and Schizophrenia Maintenance, and Metabolic Risk Profile[a]

NON-PROPRIETARY NAME (TRADE NAME) Dosage Forms	ORAL DOSAGE (mg/day)				METABOLIC SIDE EFFECTS		
	ACUTE PSYCHOSIS		MAINTENANCE				
	1ST Episode	Chronic	1ST Episode	Chronic	Weight Gain	Lipids	Glucose
Typical Antipsychotic Agents							
Phenothiazines							
Chlorpromazine (THORAZINE) ***O, S, IM***	200-600	400–800	150-600	250-750	+++	+++	++
Perphenazine (TRILAFON) ***O, S, IM***	12-50	24-48	12-48	24-60	+/–	–	–
Trifluoperazine (STELAZINE) ***O, S, IM***	5-30	10-40	2.5-20	10-30	+/–	–	–
Fluphenazine (PROLIXIN) ***O, S, IM***	2.5-15	5-20	2.5-10	5-15	+/–	–	–
Fluphenazine decanoate ***Depot IM***	Not for acute use		5-75 mg/2 wks		+/–	–	–
Other Typical Agents							
Molindone (MOBAN) ***O, S***	15-50	30-60	15-50	30-60	–	–	–
Loxapine (LOXITANE) ***O, S, IM***	15-50	30-60	15-50	30-60	+	–	–
Haloperidol (HALDOL) 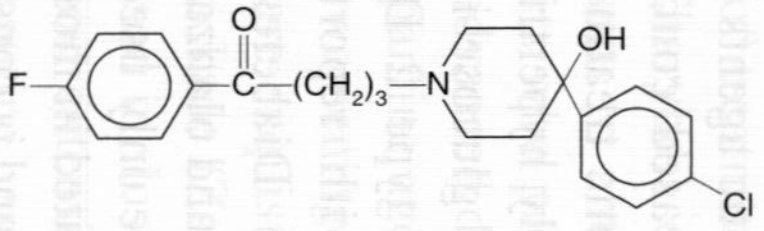 ***O, S, IM***	2.5–10	5–20	2.5–10	5–15	+/–	–	–
Haloperidol decanoate ***Depot IM***	Not for acute use		100-300 mg/month		+/–	–	–

Atypical Antipsychotic Agents							
Aripiprazole (ABILIFY) ***O, S, ODT, IM***	10–20	15–30	10–20	15–30	+/–	–	–
Asenapine (SAPHRIS, SYCREST) ***ODT***	10	10–20	10	10–20	+/–	–	–
Clozapine (CLOZARIL, FAZCLO) ***O, ODT***	200–600	400–900	200–600	300–900	++++	+++	+++
Iloperidone (FANAPT) ***O***		12–24[b]		8–16	+	+/–	+/–
Olanzapine (ZYPREXA) ***O, ODT, IM***	7.5–20	10–30	7.5–15	15–30	++++	+++	+++
Paliperidone (INVEGA) ***O***	6–9	6–12	3–9	6–15	+	+/–	+/–
Paliperidone palmitate (SUSTENNA)[c] ***Depot IM***	See note[c] on dosing				+	+/–	+/–

(*Continued*)

Table 16–1

Chemical Structures, Dosages for Acute Psychosis and Schizophrenia Maintenance, and Metabolic Risk Profile[a] (continued)

NONPROPRIETARY NAME (TRADE NAME) Dosage Forms	ORAL DOSAGE (mg/day)				METABOLIC SIDE EFFECTS		
	ACUTE PSYCHOSIS		MAINTENANCE				
	1ST Episode	Chronic	1ST Episode	Chronic	Weight Gain	Lipids	Glucose
Quetiapine (SEROQUEL, SEROQUEL XR) ***O***	200–600	400–900	200–600	300–900	+	+	+/–
Risperidone (RISPERDAL) ***O, S, ODT***	2–4	3–6	2–6	3–8	+	+/–	+/–
RISPERDAL CONSTA ***Depot IM***	Not for acute use		25–50 mg/2 wks				
Sertindole (SERDOLECT, SERLECT)[d] ***O***	4–16	12–20	12–20	12–32	+/–	–	–
Ziprasidone (GEODON, ZELDOX)[e] ***O, IM***	120–160	120–200	80–160	120–200	+/–	–	–

Dosage Forms: O, tablet; S, solution; IM, acute intramuscular; ODT, orally dissolving tablet.

[a]For further information on antipsychotic dosing in psychotic disorders, see Expert Consensus Panel for Optimizing Pharmacologic Treatment of Psychotic Disorders. The expert consensus guideline series. Optimizing pharmacologic treatment of psychotic disorders. *J Clin Psychiatry*, **2003,** *64(Suppl 12)*:2–97.
Note that doses in first-episode, younger, or antipsychotic-naïve patients are lower than for chronic schizophrenia patients. Dose in elderly schizophrenia patients is approximately 50% of that used in younger adults with schizophrenia; dosing for dementia-related psychosis is approximately 25%.

[b]Due to orthostasis risk, dose titration of iloperidone is 1 mg bid on day 1, increasing to 2, 4, 6, 8, 10, and 12 mg bid on days 2, 3, 4, 5, 6, and 7 (as needed). Safety data exist for daily doses up to 16 mg bid.

[c]Paliperidone palmitate dosing: in acute schizophrenia, deltoid IM loading doses of 234 mg at day 1 and 156 mg at day 8 provide paliperidone levels equivalent to 6 mg oral paliperidone during the first week, and peaking on day 15 at a level comparable to 12 mg oral paliperidone. No oral antipsychotic needed in first week. Maintenance IM doses can be given in deltoid or gluteus every 4 weeks after day 8. Maintenance dose options: 39, 78, 117, 156, or 234 mg every 4 weeks. Failure to give initiation doses (except for those switching from depot) will result in subtherapeutic levels for months.

[d]Not available in the U.S.

[e]Oral dose must be given with food (500 kcal) to facilitate absorption. Food increases the absorption of single doses of 20-, 40-, and 80-mg capsules by 48%, 87%, and 101%, respectively.

Table 16–2

Potencies of Antipsychotic Agents at Neurotransmitter Receptors[a]

	DOPAMINE	SEROTONIN			$5HT_{2A}/D_2$	DOPAMINE		MUSCARINIC	ADRENERGIC		HISTAMINE
	D_2	$5\text{-}HT_{1A}$	$5\text{-}HT_{2A}$	$5\text{-}HT_{2C}$	RATIO	D_1	D_4	M_1	α_{1A}	α_{2A}	H_1
Typical Agents											
Haloperidol	1.2	2100	57	4500	47	120	5.5	>10,000	12	1130	1700
Fluphenazine	0.8	1000	3.2	990	3.9	17	29	1100	6.5	310	14
Thiothixene	0.7	410	50	1360	72	51	410	>10,000	12	80	8
Perphenazine	0.8	420	5.6	130	7.4	37	40	1500	10	810	8.0
Loxapine	11	2550	4.4	13	0.4	54	8.1	120	42	150	4.9
Molindone	20	3800	>5000	10,000	>250	>10,000	>2000	>10,000	2600	1100	2130
Thioridazine	8.0	140	28	53	3.5	94	6.4	13	3.2	130	16
Chlorpromazine	3.6	2120	3.6	16	1	76	12	32	0.3	250	3.1
Atypical Agents											
Asenapine[b]	1.4	2.7	0.1	0.03	0.05	1.4	1.1	>10,000	1.2	1.2	1.0
Ziprasidone	6.8	12	0.6	13	0.1	30	39	>10,000	18	160	63
Sertindole[b]	2.7	280	0.4	0.90	0.2	12	13	>5000	1.8	640	130
Zotepine[b]	8.0	470	2.7	3.2	0.3	71	39	330	6.0	210	3.2
Risperidone	3.2	420	0.2	50	0.05	240	7.3	>10,000	5.0	16	20
Paliperidone	4.2	20	0.7	48	0.2	41	54	>10,000	2.5	4.7	19
Iloperidone	6.3	90	5.6	43	0.9	130	25	4900	0.3	160	12
Aripiprazole	1.6	6.0	8.7	22	5.0	1200	510	6800	26	74	28
Sulpiride[b]	6.4	>10,000	>10,000	>10,000	>1000	>10,000	54	>10,000	>10000	>5000	>10,000
Olanzapine	31	2300	3.7	10	0.1	70	18	2.5	110	310	2.2
Quetiapine	380	390	640	1840	2.0	990	2020	37	22	2900	6.9
Clozapine	160	120	5.4	9.4	0.03	270	24	6.2	1.6	90	1.1

[a]Data are averaged K_i values (nM) from published sources determined by competition with radioligands for binding to the indicated cloned human receptors. Data derived from receptor binding to human or rat brain tissue is used when cloned human receptor data is lacking.

[b]Not available in the U.S.

Source: NIMH Psychoactive Drug Screening Program (PDSP) K_i Database: http://pdsp.med.unc.edu/pdsp.php (Accessed June 30, 2009).

antipsychotic switching, and history of response to prior agents. Patients with refractory schizophrenia on clozapine are not good candidates for switching because they are resistant to other medications (see the definition of refractory schizophrenia later in this section).

There are many reasons for psychotic relapse or inadequate response to antipsychotic treatment in schizophrenia patients. Examples are ongoing substance use, psychosocial stressors, inherent refractory illness, and poor medication adherence. Outside of controlled settings, the problem of medication nonadherence remains a significant barrier to successful treatment, yet one that is not easily assessed. Serum drug levels can be obtained for most antipsychotic medications, but there is limited dose-response data for atypical antipsychotic agents (except for clozapine), leaving clinicians little guidance about the interpretation of antipsychotic drug levels. Even low or undetectable levels may not reflect nonadherence, but rather can be the result of genetic variation or induction of hepatic CYPs that decrease drug availability, such as the high prevalence of CYP2D6 ultrarapid metabolizers among individuals from North Africa and the Middle East. Nevertheless, the common problem of medication nonadherence among schizophrenia patients has led to the development of long-acting injectable (LAI) antipsychotic medications, often referred to as depot antipsychotics. They are more widely used in the E.U. Only < 5% of U.S. patients receive depot antipsychotic treatment. There are currently four available LAI forms in the U.S.: decanoate esters of fluphenazine and haloperidol, risperidone-impregnated microspheres, and paliperidone palmitate. Patients receiving LAI antipsychotic medications show consistently lower relapse rates compared to patients receiving comparable oral forms and may suffer fewer adverse effects. LAI risperidone and paliperidone palmitate are currently the only atypical antipsychotic agents in depot form. However, clinical trials of LAI aripiprazole and olanzapine are in progress and these agents should become available in the near future. LAI risperidone is administered as biweekly intramuscular (IM) injections of 25-50 mg. Based on extensive kinetic modeling of clinical data, paliperidone palmitate therapy in acute schizophrenia is initiated with IM deltoid loading doses of 234 mg at day 1 and 156 mg at day 8 to provide serum paliperidone levels equivalent to 6 mg oral paliperidone during the first week, obviating the need for oral antipsychotic supplementation. Serum paliperidone levels from these two injections peak on day 15 at a level comparable to 12 mg oral paliperidone. Maintenance IM doses are given in deltoid or gluteus muscle every 4 weeks after day 8. Unlike acute IM preparations or paliperidone palmitate, all other LAI antipsychotic medications require several weeks to attain therapeutic levels and months to reach steady state, necessitating the use of oral medications for the initial 4 weeks of treatment.

Lack of response to adequate antipsychotic drug doses for adequate periods of time may indicate treatment-refractory illness. Refractory schizophrenia is defined using the Kane criteria: failed 6-week trials of two separate agents and a third trial of a high-dose typical antipsychotic agent (e.g., haloperidol or fluphenazine 20 mg/day). In this patient population, response rates to typical antipsychotic agents, defined as 20% symptom reduction using standard rating scales (e.g., Positive and Negative Syndrome Scale [PANSS]), are 0%, and for any atypical antipsychotic except clozapine, are < 10% (Leucht et al., 2009). Due to the long titration involved to minimize orthostasis, and to sedation and other tolerability issues, adequate clozapine trials often require 6 months, but response rates in 26-week-long studies are consistently 60% in refractory schizophrenia patients. The therapeutic clozapine dose for a specific patient is not predictable, but various studies have found correlations between trough serum clozapine levels > 327-504 ng/mL and likelihood of clinical response. When therapeutic serum concentrations are reached, response to clozapine occurs within 8 weeks.

In addition to agranulocytosis risk that mandates routine ongoing hematological monitoring, clozapine has numerous other adverse effects. Examples are high metabolic risk, dose-dependent lowering of the seizure threshold, orthostasis, sedation, anticholinergic effects (especially constipation), and sialorrhea related to muscarinic agonism at M_4 receptors. As a result, clozapine use is limited to refractory schizophrenia patients.

Electroconvulsive therapy is considered a treatment of last resort in refractory schizophrenia and is rarely employed. Despite widespread clinical use of combining several antipsychotic agents, there is virtually no data supporting this practice, and metabolic risk increases with use of multiple antipsychotic agents (Correll et al., 2007). In one of few instances where a sound pharmacological rationale exists for combination treatment, the addition of a potent D_2 antagonist (e.g., risperidone, haloperidol) to maximally tolerated doses of clozapine (a weak D_2 blocker), the results have been decidedly mixed. That multiple antipsychotic agents ("polypharmacy") are commonly used in clinical practice attests to the limitations of current treatment. Lastly, antipsychotic drug therapy is the foundation of schizophrenia treatment, yet adequate management of schizophrenia patients requires a multimodal approach that also includes psychosocial, cognitive, and vocational rehabilitation to promote functional recovery.

Pharmacology of Antipsychotic Agents

Chemistry. In the past, the chemical structure of selected agents was informative regarding their antipsychotic activity, since most were derived from phenothiazine or butyrophenone structures. Phenothiazines have a tricyclic structure in which two benzene rings are linked by a sulfur and a nitrogen atom (Table 16–1). The chemically related thioxanthenes have a carbon in place of the nitrogen at position 10 with the R_1 moiety linked through a double bond. Substitution of an electron-withdrawing group at position 2 increases the antipsychotic efficacy of phenothiazines (e.g., chlorpromazine). The nature of the substituent at position 10 also influences pharmacological activity, and the phenothiazines and thioxanthenes can be divided into three groups on the basis of substitution at this site. Those with an aliphatic side chain include chlorpromazine and are relatively low in potency. Those with a piperidine ring in the side chain include thioridazine, which has lower EPS risk, possibly due to increased central antimuscarinic activity, but is rarely used due to concerns over QTc prolongation and risk of torsade de pointes. Several potent phenothiazine antipsychotic compounds have a piperazine group in the side chain (fluphenazine, perphenazine, and trifluoperazine) and have reduced affinity for H_1, M, and α_1 receptors. Those with a free hydroxyl can also be esterified to long-chain fatty acids to produce LAI antipsychotic medications (e.g., fluphenazine decanoate). Thioxanthenes also have aliphatic or piperazine side-chain substituents. Piperazine-substituted thioxanthenes include the high potency agent thiothixene. Since thioxanthenes have an olefinic double bond between the central-ring C10 and the side chain, geometric isomers exist. The *cis* isomers are more active. The antipsychotic phenothiazines and thioxanthenes have three carbon atoms interposed between position 10 of the central ring and the first amino nitrogen atom of the side chain at this position; the amine is always tertiary. Antihistaminic phenothiazines (e.g., promethazine) or strongly anticholinergic phenothiazines have only two carbon atoms separating the amino group from position 10 of the central ring. Metabolic *N*-dealkylation of the side chain or increasing the size of amino *N*-alkyl substituents reduces antidopaminergic and antipsychotic activity. Additional tricyclic antipsychotic agents are the benzepines, containing a 7-member central ring, of which loxapine (a dibenzoxazepine) and clozapine (a dibenzodiazepine) are available in the U.S. Clozapine-like atypical antipsychotic agents may lack a substituent on the aromatic ring (e.g., quetiapine, a dibenzothiazepine), have an analogous methyl substituent (olanzapine), or have an electron-donating substituent at position 8 (e.g., clozapine). In addition to their moderate potencies at DA receptors, clozapine-like agents interact with varying affinities at several other classes of receptors (α_1 and α_2 adrenergic, 5-HT_{1A}, 5-HT_{2A}, 5-HT_{2C}, M, H_1). The prototypical butyrophenone (phenylbutylpiperidine) antipsychotic is haloperidol, originally developed as a substituted derivative of the phenylpiperidine analgesic meperidine. An analogous compound, droperidol, is a very short-acting and highly sedating agent that was used almost exclusively for emergency sedation and anesthesia until QTc and torsade de pointes concerns substantially curtailed its use and the use of the related diphenylbutylpiperidine pimozide. Several other classes of heterocyclic compounds have antipsychotic effects, of which only the indole molindone has generated any interest due to its unusual association with modest weight loss (Sikich et al., 2008a). The enantiomeric, substituted benzamides are another group of heterocyclic compounds that are relatively selective antagonists at central D_2 receptors and have antipsychotic activity. Examples (not available in the U.S.) include sulpiride and its congener, amisulpride.

The introduction of clozapine stimulated research into agents with antipsychotic activity and low EPS risk. This search led to a series of atypical antipsychotic agents with certain pharmacological similarities to clozapine: namely lower affinity for D_2 receptors than typical antipsychotic drugs and high 5-HT_2 antagonist effects. The currently available atypical antipsychotic medications include the structurally related olanzapine, quetiapine, and clozapine; the benzisoxazoles risperidone, its active metabolite paliperidone, and iloperidone; ziprasidone (a benzisothiazolpiprazinylindolone derivative); asenapine (a dibenzo-oxepino pyrrole), and aripiprazole (a quinolinone derivative). Table 16–1.

Presently, antipsychotic agents include many different chemical structures with a range of activities at different neurotransmitter receptors (e.g., 5-HT_{2A} antagonism, 5-HT_{1A} partial agonism). As a result, structure-function relationships that were relied upon in the past have become less important. Instead, receptor-function relationships and functional assays are more clinically relevant. Aripiprazole represents a good example of how an examination of the structure provides little insight into its mechanism, which is based on dopamine partial agonism (discussed later). Detailed knowledge of receptor affinities (Table 16–2) and the functional effect at specific receptors (e.g., full, partial or inverse agonism or antagonism) can provide important insight into the therapeutic and adverse effects of antipsychotic agents. Nevertheless, there are limits. For example, it is not known which properties are responsible for clozapine's unique effectiveness in refractory schizophrenia, although many hypotheses exist. Other notable antipsychotic properties not fully explained by receptor parameters include the reduced seizure threshold, the unexpected extent of prolactin elevation for risperidone and paliperidone, the effects of antipsychotic agents on metabolic function, and the increased risk for cerebrovascular events and mortality among dementia patients (see "Adverse Effects and Drug Interactions" later in the chapter).

Mechanism of Action. While emerging data indicate that stimulation of glutamate or muscarinic receptors may confer antipsychotic properties, no clinically available effective antipsychotic is devoid of D_2 antagonistic activity. This reduction in dopaminergic neurotransmission is presently achieved through one of two mechanisms: D_2 antagonism or partial D_2 agonism, of which aripiprazole is the only current example. Another partial agonist, bifeprunox, completed clinical trials but failed to gain FDA approval.

Aripiprazole has an affinity for D_2 receptors only slightly less than DA itself, but its intrinsic activity is ~25% that of dopamine. As depicted in Figure 16–3, when dopamine is given in increasing concentrations in an *in vitro* model, 100% stimulation of the available D_2 receptors occurs (as measured by forskolin-stimulated cyclic AMP accumulation). In the absence of DA, aripiprazole produces a maximal level of D_2 activity ~25% that of DA (Burris et al., 2002). The potent D_2 antagonist haloperidol is capable of reducing dopamine's effect to zero, but when DA is incubated with increasing concentrations of aripiprazole, maximal inhibition of D_2 activity did not exceed 25% of the DA response, that is, the level of agonism provided by aripiprazole. Aripiprazole's capacity to stimulate D_2 receptors in brain areas where synaptic DA levels are limited (e.g., PFC neurons) or decrease dopaminergic activity when dopamine concentrations are high (e.g., mesolimbic cortex) is thought to be the basis for its clinical effects in schizophrenia. Evidence for its partial DA agonist properties is seen clinically as a reduction in

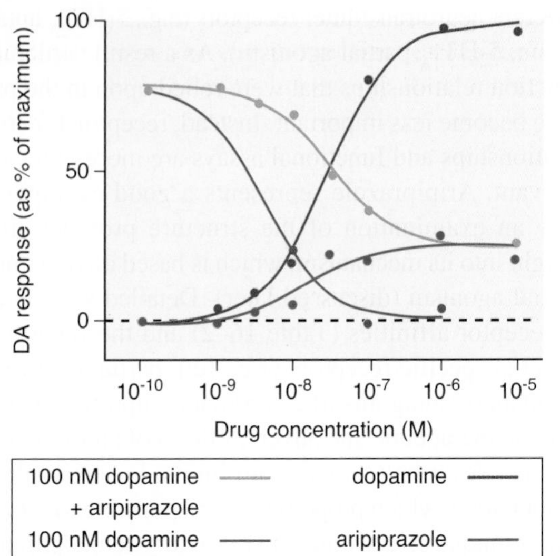

Figure 16–3. *Aripiprazole activity at D_2 receptors in the presence or absence of dopamine.* Aripiprazole is a partial D_2 agonist; thus it inhibits effects of DA and reduces stimulation at the D_2 receptor only to the extent of its own capacity as an agonist. Haloperidol, an antagonist without agonist activity, completely antagonizes D_2 receptor activation. Here, receptor activity was measured as inhibition of forskolin-induced cAMP accumulation in CHO cells transfected with human D_{2L} DNA. (Adapted from Burris et al., 2002.)

serum prolactin levels. Unlike other antipsychotic agents, in which striatal D_2 occupancy (i.e., reduction in postsynaptic D_2 signal) > 78% is associated with EPS, aripiprazole requires significantly higher D_2 occupancy levels. Even with 100% receptor occupancy, aripiprazole's intrinsic dopaminergic agonism can generate a 25% postsynaptic signal, implying a maximal 75% reduction in DA neurotransmission, below the 78% threshold that triggers EPS in most individuals, although rare reports of acute dystonia exist, primarily in antipsychotic-naïve, younger patients.

Animal models of antipsychotic activity have evolved over a half-century of antipsychotic drug development to incorporate emerging knowledge of psychosis pathophysiology. Prior to the elucidation of D_2 antagonism as a common mechanism for antipsychotic agents, early behavioral paradigms exploited known animal effects that predicted clinical efficacy. As expected, these models, including catalepsy induction and blockade of apomorphine-induced stereotypic behavior, were subsequently found to be dependent on potent D_2 receptor antagonism (Lieberman et al., 2008). Clozapine failed these early trials and was not suspected to possess antipsychotic activity until experimental human use in the mid-1960s revealed it to be an effective treatment for schizophrenia, particularly in patients who had failed other antipsychotic medications, and with virtually absent EPS risk. By 1989, the pharmacological basis for some of these atypical properties, namely clinical efficacy without EPS induction, was found to result from a significantly weaker D_2 antagonism than existing antipsychotic agents, combined with potent 5-HT_2 antagonism. Subsequent research demonstrated that 5-HT_{2A} receptor antagonism is responsible for facilitation of dopamine release in both mesocortical and nigrostriatal pathways. The behavioral pharmacology of 5-HT_{2A} antagonism and related 5-HT_{2C} and 5-HT_{1A} receptor agonism has since been characterized, and relevant animal behavioral assays developed. Clozapine possesses activity at numerous other receptors including antagonism and agonism at various muscarinic receptor subtypes and antagonism at dopamine D_4 receptors; however, subsequent D_4 antagonists that did not also have D_2 antagonism lacked antipsychotic activity. Clozapine's active metabolite, *N*-desmethylclozapine, is a potent muscarinic M_1 agonist (Li et al., 2005). Although *N*-desmethylclozapine failed clinical trials as schizophrenia monotherapy, it increased interest in cholinergic agonists as primary treatments or adjunctive cognitive enhancing medications for schizophrenia. Important targets of agents in preclinical and clinical drug development include M_1 agonism (Janowsky and Davis 2009), M_4 agonism (Chan et al., 2008), and α7- and α4β2-nicotinic receptor agonism (Buchanan et al., 2007).

The glutamate hypofunction hypothesis of schizophrenia has led to novel animal models that examine the influence of proposed antipsychotic agents, including those in clinical development with agonist properties at metabotropic glutamate receptors $mGlu_2$ and $mGlu_3$ (Patil et al., 2007) and other subtypes. Atypical antipsychotic drugs are better than typical antipsychotic medications at reversing the negative symptoms, cognitive deficits and social withdrawal induced by glutamate antagonists. At the present time, however, it is unclear whether glutamate agonist that lack direct D_2 antagonist properties will prove as effective as serotonin-dopamine antagonists for schizophrenia treatment, or whether glutamate agonist mechanisms might be more useful when combined with D_2 modulation, much in the same manner as 5-HT_{2A} antagonism. Schizophrenia patients also exhibit specific neurophysiological abnormalities. For example, a disruption in the normal processing of sensory and cognitive information is exhibited in various preconscious inhibitory processes, including deficiencies in sensorimotor gating as assessed by prepulse inhibition (PPI) of the acoustic startle reflex. PPI is the automatic suppression of startle magnitude that occurs when the louder acoustic stimulus is preceded 30-500 ms by a weaker prepulse (Swerdlow et al., 2006). In schizophrenia patients, PPI is increased more robustly with atypical than typical antipsychotic agents, and in animal models, atypical antipsychotic agents are also more effective at opposing PPI disruption from NMDA antagonists. Increased understanding of the pharmacological basis for neurophysiological deficits provides another means for developing antipsychotic treatments that are specifically effective for schizophrenia and may not necessarily apply to other forms of psychosis.

Dopamine Receptor Occupancy and Behavioral Effects. Dopaminergic projections from the midbrain terminate on septal nuclei, the olfactory tubercle and basal forebrain, the amygdala, and other structures within the temporal and prefrontal cerebral lobes and the hippocampus. The dopamine hypothesis has focused considerable attention on the mesolimbic and mesocortical systems as possible sites where antipsychotic effects are mediated. Recent research confirms that excessive dopaminergic functions in the limbic system are central to the positive symptoms of psychosis. The behavioral effects and the time course of antipsychotic response parallel the rise in D_2 occupancy and include calming of psychomotor agitation, decreased hostility, decreased social isolation, and less interference from disorganized or delusional thought processes and hallucinations.

Levels of central D_2 occupancy estimated by positron emission tomography (PET) brain imaging in patients treated with antipsychotic drugs support conclusions arising from laboratory studies that receptor occupancy predicts clinical efficacy, EPS, and serum level-clinical response relationships. Occupation of > 78% of D_2 receptors in the basal ganglia is associated with a risk of EPS across all dopamine antagonist antipsychotic agents, while occupancies in the range of 60-75% are associated with antipsychotic efficacy (Figure 16–2) (Kapur et al., 2000b). With the exception of aripiprazole, all atypical antipsychotic drugs at low doses have much greater occupancy of 5-HT_{2A} receptors (e.g., 75-99%) than typical agents (Table 16–2). Among atypical agents, clozapine has the highest ratio of 5-HT_{2A}/D_2 binding. Clozapine's D_2 occupancy 12-hours post-dose ranges from 51-63% (Kapur et al., 1999), providing evidence for its limited EPS risk. The trough D_2 occupancy for quetiapine is even lower (< 30%), but PET studies obtained 2-3 hours after dosing reveal D_2 receptor occupancies in the expected therapeutic range (54-64%), albeit transiently. Ziprasidone absorption is sensitive to the presence of food, but PET studies demonstrate that clinical efficacy occurs when D_2 occupancy exceeds 60%, which corresponds to a minimum daily dose of 120 mg (with food) (Mamo et al., 2004).

Among the typical antipsychotic drugs, receptor occupancy is best studied for haloperidol. Haloperidol has complex metabolism and is susceptible to modulation by CYP inhibitors, inducers, and CYP polymorphisms (Table 16–3), complicating the establishment of dose-response relationships in patients. Nonetheless, the use of serum levels can predict D_2 occupancy (Fitzgerald et al., 2000):

% D_2 receptor occupancy = 100 × (Plasma haloperidol ng/mL)/(0.40 ng/mL + Plasma haloperidol ng/mL)

Similar formulas also exist for several atypical antipsychotic drugs, although their plasma concentrations are rarely measured in the clinical setting.

D_3 and D_4 Receptors in the Basal Ganglia and Limbic System. The discovery that D_3 and D_4 receptors are preferentially expressed in limbic areas has led to efforts to identify selective inhibitors for these receptors that might have antipsychotic efficacy and low EPS risk. As previously noted, clozapine has modest selectivity for D_4 receptors, which are preferentially localized in cortical and limbic brain regions in relatively low abundance, and are up-regulated after repeated administration of most typical and atypical antipsychotic drugs (Tarazi et al., 2001). These receptors may contribute to clinical antipsychotic actions, but agents that are D_4 selective (e.g., sonepiprazole) or mixed D_4/5-HT_{2A} antagonists (e.g., fananserin) lack antipsychotic efficacy in clinical studies. In contrast to effects on D_2 and D_4 receptors, long-term administration of typical and atypical antipsychotic drugs does not alter D_3 receptor levels in rat forebrain regions (Tarazi et al., 2001). These findings suggest that D_3 receptors are unlikely to play a pivotal role in antipsychotic drug actions, perhaps because their avidity for endogenous DA prevents their interaction with antipsychotic agents. The subtle and atypical functional activities of cerebral D_3 receptors suggest that D_3 agonists rather than antagonists may have useful psychotropic effects, particularly in antagonizing stimulant-reward and dependence behaviors. Aripiprazole possesses affinity and intrinsic activity at D_3 receptors equivalent to that at D_2; the clinical advantage of this property is not readily apparent, although preclinical data suggest some effects on substance use.

The Role of Non-Dopamine Receptors for Atypical Antipsychotic Agents. The concept of atypicality was initially based on clozapine's absence of EPS within the therapeutic range, combined with a prominent role of 5-HT_2 receptor antagonism. As subsequent agents were synthesized using clozapine's 5-HT_2/D_2 ratio as a model, most of which possessed greater D_2 affinity and EPS risk than clozapine, there has been considerable debate on the definition of an atypical antipsychotic agent and its necessary properties. Aripiprazole in particular is problematic for the model based on ratios of 5-HT_2 to D_2, since its action as partial agonist necessitates very high D_2 affinity. Loxapine is another problematic agent for the model since its receptor pharmacology suggests atypical properties based on 5-HT_2/D_2 ratio; however, in clinical practice its use was associated with the expected higher level of EPS characteristic of typical antipsychotic drugs, perhaps related to the additive D_2 antagonist properties of the active metabolite amoxapine. These dilemmas have lead some to suggest abandonment or modification of the atypical/typical antipsychotic terminology, perhaps in lieu of the designation by generation (e.g., first, second, etc.), as is used with antibiotics, or some other organizing scheme (Gründer et al., 2009). Nonetheless, the term "atypical" persists in common usage and designates lesser (but not absent) EPS risk and other decreased effects of excessive D_2 antagonism, or more accurately, reduction in D_2-mediated neurotransmission.

The neuropharmacology and behavioral pharmacology of 5-HT_2 antagonism provide insights into the advantageous properties of medications with these effects (Marek et al., 2003). Antipsychotic agents with appreciable 5-HT_2 affinity have significant effects at both 5-HT_{2A} and 5-HT_{2C} receptors with individual medications varying in their relative potencies at each subtype (Tarazi et al., 2002). As discussed previously, atypical antipsychotic agents exhibit potent functional antagonism at both subtypes of 5-HT_2 receptors, but *in vitro* assays suggest that these effects result from inverse agonism at these G-coupled receptors.

5-HT_{2A} receptors are widely distributed, but antagonism exerts the greatest effect on prefrontal and basal ganglia DA release and midbrain noradrenergic outflow, with recent data implicating 5-HT_{2A} receptor polymorphisms in differential antidepressant response (McMahon et al., 2006). There are significant interrelationships between serotonin receptors, with evidence from animal studies that stimulation of either 5-HT_{1A} or 5-HT_{2C} receptors antagonizes the behavioral effects of 5-HT_{2A} agonists (Marek et al., 2003). This can be seen with agents that have direct effects on 5-HT_{2A} activity and also in studies of NMDA antagonists where there are opposing modulatory effects of 5-HT_{2A} and 5-HT_{2C} stimulation. By virtue of their impact on noradrenergic neurotransmission, 5-HT_{2A} antagonists

Table 16–3

Metabolism of Common Antipsychotic Drugs

AGENT	METABOLIC PATHWAYS	EFFECT OF CYP INHIBITION	EFFECT OF CYP INDUCTION
		Atypical Antipsychotic Agents	
Aripiprazole	2D6 and 3A4 convert aripiprazole to active metabolite dehydro-aripiprazole. Metabolite has longer $t_{1/2}$ (75 vs. 94 hours) and represents 40% of AUC at steady state.	2D6 PMs experience 80% ↑ in aripiprazole AUC, and 30% ↓ in metabolite AUC (net effect is 60% ↑ in AUC for active moiety). Aripiprazole $t_{1/2} \approx$ 146 hrs in PM. 2D6 inhibitors ↑ aripiprazole AUC by 112% and ↓ metabolite AUC by 35%. Ketoconazole (a potent 3A4 inhibitor) with a 15-mg single dose of aripiprazole ↑ the AUC of aripiprazole and its active metabolite by 63% and 77%, respectively.	3A4 induction ↓ maximum concentration and AUC of aripiprazole and metabolite by 70%.
Asenapine	Primarily glucuronidation (UGT 1A4), and limited oxidation via CYP 1A2, and to a lesser extent 2D6 and 3A4. No active metabolites.	Fluvoxamine, 25 mg twice daily for 8 days, ↑ C_{max} by 13% and AUC 29%. Paroxetine ↓ both C_{max} and AUC by 13%. Valproate, a UGT 1A4 inhibitor, ↑ C_{max} 2%, and ↓ AUC 1%.	Smoking had no effect on clearance or other kinetic parameters. Carbamazepine ↓ both C_{max} and AUC by 16%.
Clozapine	Multiple enzymes convert clozapine to active metabolite *N*-desmethylclozapine. The mean contributions of CYPs 1A2, 2C19, 3A4, 2C9, and 2D6 are 30%, 24%, 22%, 12%, and 6%, respectively. CYP1A2 is the most important form at low concentrations, which is in agreement with clinical findings.	Fluvoxamine ↑ C_p 5-10 fold. 2D6 inhibition may ↑ levels as much as 100%.	Loss of smoking-related 1A2 induction ↑ serum levels by 50%. Carbamazepine ↓ clozapine levels on average by 50%.

Iloperidone	2D6 and 3A4 convert iloperidone to active metabolites P88 and P95. In 2D6 EM, the $t_{1/2}$ of P88 and P95 are 26 and 23 hours, respectively; in PM, 37 and 31 hours, respectively. Only P88 has affinity for D_2. P88 accounts for 19.5% and 34.0% of total exposure in EM and PM, respectively. P95 has K_i of 3.91 nM for $5HT_{2A}$ and 4.7 nM for α_{1A}, and accounts for 48% and 25% of total exposure in EM and PM, respectively.	Ketoconazole ↑ AUC of a single 3-mg iloperidone dose and its metabolites P88 and P95 by 57%, 55%, and 35%, respectively. Fluoxetine ↑ 3-mg single dose AUC of iloperidone and P88 metabolite 2-3 fold, and P95 AUC by 50%. Paroxetine ↑ AUC of iloperidone and P88 metabolite 1.6-fold, and reduces P95 AUC by 50%. Paroxetine (8-12 mg twice daily) ↑ steady state C_{max} of iloperidone and P88 by 1.6-fold, and ↓ steady state C_{max} of P95 by 50%. Combined use ↑ steady state C_{max} of iloperidone and P88 by 1.4-fold, and ↓ steady state C_{max} of P95 1.4-fold.	Impact of 3A4 inducers not documented.
Olanzapine	Direct glucuronidation or 1A2 mediated oxidation to *N*-desmethylolanzapine (inactive).	Increase in olanzapine C_{max} following fluvoxamine is 54% in female nonsmokers and 77% in male smokers. The mean increase in olanzapine AUC is 52% and 108%, respectively.	Carbamazepine use ↑ clearance by 50%. Olanzapine C_p lower in smokers (with equal dosing).
Paliperidone	59% excreted unchanged in urine, 32% excreted as metabolites. Phase 2 metabolism accounts for no more than 10%.	Unlikely to have much of an effect.	Carbamazepine use ↓ steady state C_{max} and AUC by 37%.
Quetiapine	3A4 mediated sulfoxidation to active metabolite norquetiapine, $t_{1/2} \approx 12$ hours. Steady state mean C_{max} and AUC of norquetiapine are ~25% and ~50% of that for quetiapine.	Ketoconazole (200 mg once daily for 4 days), ↓ oral clearance of quetiapine by 84%, resulting in a 335% ↑ in maximum C_p.	Phenytoin increases clearance 5-fold.
Risperidone	2D6 converts risperidone to active metabolite 9-OH risperidone. In 2D6 PMs, half-lives are: risperidone, 20 hours; 9-OH risperidone, 30 hours	Fluoxetine and paroxetine ↑ risperidone concentration ~ 2.5 fold and 3-9 fold, respectively. Fluoxetine did not affect 9-OH risperidone conc., but paroxetine lowered 9-OH risperidone (13%). Net effect: 2D6 inhibition ↑ levels of active moiety up to 75%.	In a drug interaction study of risperidone 6 mg/day × 3 weeks, followed by 3 weeks of carbamazepine, concentration of active moieties (risperidone + 9-OH risperidone) was decreased 50%.

(Continued)

Table 16–3

Metabolism of Common Antipsychotic Drugs (continued)

	METABOLIC PATHWAYS	EFFECT OF CYP INHIBITION	EFFECT OF CYP INDUCTION
		Atypical Antipsychotic Agents	
Ziprasidone	3A4 (~1/3) Aldehyde Oxidase (~2/3)	Concomitant ketoconazole ↑ AUC by 35%	Carbamazepine ↓ AUC by 35%.
		Typical Antipsychotic Agents	
Haloperidol	Multiple CYP pathways, particularly 2D6, 3A4, and minor pathway 1A2. Only active metabolite, reduced haloperidol (formed by ketone reductase). Reduced haloperidol inhibits CYP2D6 and may be re-oxidized to the parent drug. Therapeutic serum levels not well defined; 5-20 ng/mL used as a target for dosing.	Half-life prolonged in CYP 2D6 PMs Individuals with only one functional 2D6 allele experience 2-fold greater trough serum levels, those with no functioning alleles 3-4 fold higher.	Carbamazepine and phenytoin ↑ haloperidol clearance ~32%, with ↓ C_p (mean, 47%). Discontinuation of carbamazepine ↑ C_p 2-3 fold.
Chlorpromazine	CYP2D6. Over 10 identified human metabolites, most inactive. Chlorpromazine is a moderate 2D6 inhibitor, and also induces its own metabolism. Levels drop 25-33% during weeks 1-3 of treatment.	Case report of fluoxetine-chlorpromazine interaction, but no serum level data on extent of effect.	3A4/PGP inducers (e.g., phenobarbital, carbamazepine) decrease chlorpromazine levels by ~35%. Carbamazepine discontinuation ↑ C_p (30-80%).

AUC, area under the curve; PM, poor metabolizer; EM, extensive metabolizer; $t_{1/2}$, half life; C_p, plasma concentration; C_{max}, maximum plasma concentration.
[a]May have multiphasic elimination with much longer terminal $t_{1/2}$.

pass many preclinical *in vivo* assays of antidepressant activity; conversely, 5-HT_{2C} antagonists exhibit a similar spectrum of antidepressant properties, although pure 5-HT_{2A} or 5-HT_{2C} agents are, by themselves, not effective antidepressants in human trials (Marek et al., 2003). Data also indicate that 5-HT_{2C} agonism decreases mesolimbic DA neurotransmission, a mechanism that is being explored in clinical trials of vabicaserin, a pure 5-HT_{2C} agonist. At the cellular level, stimulation of 5-HT_{2A} and 5-HT_{1A} receptors causes depolarization and hyperpolarization, respectively, of cortical pyramidal cells (Marek et al., 2003). No atypical antipsychotic agent is a potent agonist of 5-HT_{1A} receptors, but several, including clozapine, ziprasidone and aripiprazole are partial agonists. The extent to which this contributes to any clinical effect is unknown, but more potent selective 5-HT_{1A} agonists have anxiolytic effects and appear to exert procognitive effects in schizophrenia patients when added to existing antipsychotic treatment.

Based upon trials of the selective α_2 adrenergic antagonist idazoxan, researchers have postulated effects of α_2 blockade on mood, but ongoing research into this mechanism has not been promising. Risperidone is the one antipsychotic with relatively high affinity for α_2 adrenergic receptors, at which it is an antagonist; however, the clinical correlate of this unique profile is unclear. Any benefit on major depressive symptoms from low-dose risperidone augmentation of SSRI antidepressants is more likely conveyed by effects at the 5-HT_{2A} receptor, at which risperidone has > 100-fold greater potency than at α_2 adrenergic receptors.

Tolerance and Physical Dependence. As defined in Chapter 24, antipsychotic drugs are not addicting; however, tolerance to the antihistaminic and anticholinergic effects of antipsychotic agents usually develops over days or weeks. Loss of efficacy with prolonged treatment is not known to occur with antipsychotic agents; however, tolerance to antipsychotic drugs and cross-tolerance among the agents are demonstrable in behavioral and biochemical experiments in animals, particularly those directed toward evaluation of the blockade of dopaminergic receptors in the basal ganglia (Tarazi et al., 2001). This form of tolerance may be less prominent in limbic and cortical areas of the forebrain. One correlate of tolerance in striatal dopaminergic systems is the development of receptor supersensitivity (mediated by upregulation of supersensitive DA receptors) referred to as D_2^{High} receptors (Lieberman et al., 2008). These changes may underlie the clinical phenomenon of withdrawal-emergent dyskinesias and may contribute to the pathophysiology of tardive dyskinesia. This may also partly explain the ability of certain chronic schizophrenia patients to tolerate high doses of potent DA antagonists with limited EPS.

Absorption, Distribution, and Elimination. The pharmacokinetic constants for these drugs may be found in Appendix II. Table 16–3 outlines the metabolic pathways of atypical antipsychotic agents available in the U.S. and selected typical agents in common use. Most antipsychotic drugs are highly lipophilic, highly membrane- or protein-bound, and accumulate in the brain, lung, and other tissues with a rich blood supply. They also enter the fetal circulation and breast milk. Despite half-lives that may be short, the biological effects of single doses of most antipsychotic medications usually persist for at least 24 hours, permitting once-daily dosing for many agents once the patient has adjusted to initial side effects.

Elimination from the plasma may be more rapid than from sites of high lipid content and binding, notably the CNS, as evidenced by PET pharmacokinetic studies that demonstrate half-lives in the CNS that exceed those in plasma. For example, mean single-dose plasma half-lives of olanzapine and risperidone are 24.2 and 10.3 hours respectively, whereas a 50% reduction from peak striatal D_2 receptor occupancy requires 75.2 hours for olanzapine and 66.6 hours for risperidone (Tauscher et al., 2002). Similar discrepancies are seen between the time course of plasma levels and occupancy of extrastriatal D_2 and 5-HT_{2A} receptors (Tauscher et al., 2002). Metabolites of long acting injectable medications have been detected in the urine several months after drug administration was discontinued. Slow removal of drug may contribute to the typical delay of exacerbation of psychosis after stopping drug treatment. Depot decanoate esters of fluphenazine and haloperidol, paliperidone palmitate, as well as risperidone-impregnated microspheres, are absorbed and eliminated much more slowly than are oral preparations. For example, the $t_{1/2}$ of oral fluphenazine is ~20 hours while the IM decanoate ester has a $t_{1/2}$ of 14.3 days; oral haloperidol has a $t_{1/2}$ of 24-48 hours in CYP2D6-extensive metabolizers (de Leon et al., 2004), while haloperidol decanoate has a $t_{1/2}$ of 21 days (Altamura et al., 2003); paliperidone palmitate has a $t_{1/2}$ of 25-49 days compared to an oral paliperidone $t_{1/2}$ of 23 hours. Clearance of fluphenazine and haloperidol decanoate following repeated dosing can require 6-8 months. Effects of LAI *risperidone* (RISPERDAL CONSTA) are delayed for 4 weeks because of slow biodegradation of the microspheres and persist for at least 4-6 weeks after the injections are discontinued (Altamura et al., 2003). The dosing regimen recommended for starting patients on LAI paliperidone generates therapeutic levels in the first week, obviating the need for routine oral antipsychotic supplementation.

With the exception of asenapine, paliperidone and ziprasidone, all antipsychotic drugs undergo extensive phase 1 metabolism by CYPs and subsequent phase 2 glucuronidation, sulfation, and other conjugations (Table 16–3). Hydrophilic metabolites of these drugs are excreted in the urine and to some extent in the bile. Most oxidized metabolites of antipsychotic drugs are biologically inactive; a few (e.g., P88 metabolite of iloperidone, hydroxy metabolite of haloperidol 9-OH risperidone, *N*-desmethylclozapine, and dehydroaripiprazole) are active. These active metabolites may contribute to biological activity of the parent compound and complicate correlating serum drug levels with clinical effects. The active metabolite of risperidone, paliperidone (9-OH risperidone), is already the product of oxidative metabolism, and 59% is excreted unchanged in urine with a lesser amount (32%) excreted as metabolites or via phase 2 metabolism (≤ 10%). Ziprasidone's primary metabolic pathway is through the aldehyde oxidase system that is neither saturable nor inhibitable by commonly encountered xenobiotics, with ~ one-third of ziprasidone's metabolism through CYP3A4 (Meyer, 2007). Asenapine is metabolized primarily through glucuronidation (UGT4), with a minor contribution from CYP1A2. The potential for drug-drug interactions is covered in "Adverse Effects and Drug Interactions" later in the chapter.

Absorption for most agents is quite high, and concurrent administration of anticholinergic anti-parkinsonian agents does not appreciably diminish intestinal absorption. Most orally-disintegrating tablets (ODT) and liquid preparations provide similar pharmacokinetics since there is little mucosal absorption and effects depend on swallowed drug. Asenapine remains the only exception. It is only available as an ODT preparation administered sublingually, and all absorption occurs via oral mucosa, with bioavailability of 35% by this route. If swallowed, the first pass effect is > 98%, indicating that drug swallowed with oral secretions is not bioavailable. Intramuscular administration avoids much of the first-pass enteric metabolism and provides measurable concentrations in plasma within 15-30 minutes. Most agents are highly protein bound, but this protein binding may include glycoprotein sites. Kinetic studies indicate that antipsychotic drugs do not significantly displace other pre-albumin- or albumin-bound medications. Antipsychotic medications are predominantly highly lipophilic with apparent volumes of distribution as high as 20 L/kg.

Therapeutic Uses

The use of antipsychotic medications for the treatment of schizophrenia spectrum disorders, for mania treatment, and as adjunctive use for treatment-resistant major depression has been discussed previously. Antipsychotic agents are also utilized in several nonpsychotic neurological disorders and as antiemetics.

Anxiety Disorders. There are two anxiety disorders in which double-blind, placebo-controlled trials have shown benefit of adjunctive treatment with antipsychotic drugs: obsessive compulsive disorder (OCD) and post-traumatic stress disorder (PTSD). While SSRI antidepressants remain the only psychotropic medication with FDA approval for PTSD treatment, adjunctive low-dose quetiapine, olanzapine, and particularly risperidone significantly reduce the overall level of symptoms in SSRI-resistant PTSD (Bartzokis et al., 2005). OCD patients with limited response to the standard 12-week regimen of high dose SSRI also benefit from adjunctive risperidone (mean dose 2.2 mg), even in the presence of comorbid tic disorders (McDougle et al., 2000). For generalized anxiety disorder, double-blind placebo controlled clinical trials demonstrate efficacy for quetiapine as monotherapy, and for adjunctive low-dose risperidone.

Tourette's Disorder. The ability of antipsychotic drugs to suppress tics in patients with Tourette's disorder has been known for decades, and relates to reduced D_2 neurotransmission in basal ganglia sites. In prior decades, the use of low-dose, high-potency typical antipsychotic agents (e.g., haloperidol, pimozide) was the treatment of choice, but these nonpsychotic patients were extremely sensitive to the impact of DA blockade on cognitive processing speed, and on reward centers. Safety concerns regarding pimozide's QTc prolongation and increased risk for ventricular arrhythmias have large ended its clinical use. While lacking FDA approval for tic disorders, risperidone and aripiprazole have indications for child and adolescent schizophrenia and bipolar disorder (acute mania) treatment, and these agents (as well as ziprasidone) have published data supporting their use for tic suppression. Given the enormous sensitivity of preadolescent and teenage patients to antipsychotic-induced weight gain, aripiprazole has an advantage in this patient population due to somewhat lower risk for weight gain, and low risk for hyperprolactinemia or concerns over QTc effects.

Huntington's Disease. Huntington's disease is another neuropsychiatric condition, which, like tic disorders, is associated with basal ganglia pathology. DA blockade can suppress the severity of choreoathetotic movements, but is not strongly endorsed due to the risks associated of excessive DA antagonism that outweigh the marginal benefit. Inhibition of the vesicular monoamine transporter type 2 (VMAT2) with tetrabenazine has replaced DA receptor blockade in the management of chorea (Chapter 22).

Autism. Autism is a disease whose neuropathology is incompletely understood, but in some patients is associated with explosive behavioral outbursts, and aggressive or self-injurious behaviors that may be stereotypical. Risperidone has FDA approval for irritability associated with autism in child and adolescent patients ages 5-16, with common use for disruptive behavior problems in autism and other forms of mental retardation. Initial risperidone daily doses are 0.25 mg for patients weighing < 20 kg, and 0.5 mg for others, with a target dose of 0.5 mg/day in those < 20 kg weight, and 1.0 mg/day for other patients, with a range 0.5-3.0 mg/day.

Anti-emetic Use. Most antipsychotic drugs protect against the nausea- and emesis-inducing effects of DA agonists such as apomorphine that act at central DA receptors in the chemoreceptor trigger zone of the medulla. Antipsychotic drugs are effective antiemetics already at low doses. Drugs or other stimuli that cause emesis by an action on the nodose ganglion, or locally on the GI tract, are not antagonized by antipsychotic drugs, but potent piperazines and butyrophenones are sometimes effective against nausea caused by vestibular stimulation. The commonly used antiemetic phenothiazines are weak DA antagonists (e.g., prochlorperazine) without antipsychotic activity, but can be associated with EPS or akathisia.

Adverse Effects and Drug Interactions

Adverse Effects Predicted by Monoamine Receptor Affinities

Dopamine D_2 Receptor. With the exception of the D_2 partial agonist aripiprazole (and the commercially unavailable agent bifeprunox), all other antipsychotic agents possess D_2 antagonist properties, the strength of which determines the likelihood for EPS, akathisia, long-term tardive dyskinesia risk, and hyperprolactinemia. The manifestations of EPS are described in Table 16-4, along with the usual treatment approach. Acute dystonic reactions occur in the early hours and days of treatment with highest risk among younger patients (peak incidence ages 10-19), especially antipsychotic-naïve individuals, in response to abrupt decreases in nigrostriatal D_2 neurotransmission. The dystonia typically involves head and neck muscles, the tongue, and in its severest form, the oculogyric crisis, extraocular muscles, and is very frightening to the patient.

Table 16–4

Neurological Side Effects of Antipsychotic Drugs

REACTION	FEATURES	TIME OF ONSET AND RISK INFO	PROPOSED MECHANISM	TREATMENT
Acute dystonia	Spasm of muscles of tongue, face, neck, back	Time: 1-5 days. Young, antipsychotic naïve patients at highest risk	Acute DA antagonism	Anti-parkinsonian agents are diagnostic and curative[a]
Akathisia	Subjective and objective restlessness; *not* anxiety or "agitation"	Time: 5-60 days	Unknown	Reduce dose or change drug; clonazepam, propranolol more effective than anti-parkinsonian agents[b]
Parkinsonism	Bradykinesia, rigidity, variable tremor, mask facies, shuffling gait	Time: 5-30 days. Elderly at greatest risk	DA antagonism	Dose reduction; change medication; anti-parkinsonian agents[c]
Neuroleptic malignant syndrome	Extreme rigidity, fever, unstable BP, myoglobinemia; can be fatal	Time: weeks–months. Can persist for days after stopping antipsychotic	DA antagonism	Stop antipsychotic immediately; supportive care; dantrolene and bromocriptine[d]
Perioral tremor ("rabbit syndrome")	Perioral tremor (may be a late variant of parkinsonism)	Time: months or years of treatment	Unknown	Anti-parkinsonian agents often help[c]
Tardive dyskinesia	Orofacial dyskinesia; rarely widespread choreoathetosis or dystonia	Time: months, years of treatment. Elderly at 5-fold greater risk. Risk $\propto$ potency of D_2 blockade	Postsynaptic DA receptor supersensitivity, up-regulation	Prevention crucial; treatment unsatisfactory. May be reversible with early recognition and drug discontinuation

[a]Treatment: diphenhydramine 25-50 mg IM, or benztropine 1-2 mg IM. Due to long antipsychotic $t_{1/2}$, may need to repeat, or follow with oral medication.

[b]Propranolol often effective in relatively low doses (20–80 mg/day in divided doses). β_1-Selective adrenergic receptor antagonists are less effective. Non-lipophilic β adrenergic antagonists have limited CNS penetration and are of no benefit (e.g., atenolol).

[c]Use of amantadine avoids anticholinergic effects of benztropine or diphenhydramine.

[d]Despite the response to dantrolene, there is no evidence of abnormal Ca^{2+} transport in skeletal muscle; with persistent antipsychotic effects (e.g., long-acting injectable agents), bromocriptine may be tolerated in large doses (10-40 mg/day). Anti-parkinsonian agents are not effective.

Parkinsonism resembling its idiopathic form occurs when striatal D_2 occupancy exceeds 78%, and often responds to dose reduction or switching to an antipsychotic with weaker D_2 antagonism. In situations where this is neither possible nor desirable, anti-parkinsonian medication may be employed. Clinically, there is a generalized slowing and impoverishment of volitional movement (bradykinesia) with masked facies and reduced arm movements during walking. The syndrome characteristically evolves gradually over days to weeks as the risk of acute dystonia diminishes. The most noticeable signs are slowing of movements, and sometimes rigidity and variable tremor at rest, especially involving the upper extremities. "Pill-rolling" movements and other types of resting tremor (at a frequency of 3-5 Hz, as in Parkinson's disease) may be seen, although they are less prominent in antipsychotic-induced than in idiopathic parkinsonism. Bradykinesia and masked facies may be mistaken for clinical depression. Elderly patients are at greatest risk.

The treatment of acute dystonia and antipsychotic-induced parkinsonism involves the use of anti-parkinsonian agents, although dose reduction should be considered as the initial strategy for parkinsonism. Muscarinic cholinergic receptors modulate nigrostriatal DA release, with blockade increasing synaptic DA availability. Important issues in the use of anticholinergics include the negative impact on cognition and memory, peripheral antimuscarinic adverse effects (e.g., urinary retention, dry mouth, cycloplegia, etc.), and the relative risk of exacerbating tardive dyskinesia. In patients receiving chronic anticholinergic therapy, there are also short-term risks of cholinergic rebound following abrupt anticholinergic withdrawal, which may include sleep disturbance (vivid dreams, nightmares) and also increased EPS if the patient continues to receive antipsychotic treatment. For parenteral administration, diphenhydramine (25-50 mg IM) and benztropine (1-2 mg IM) are the agents most commonly used. Diphenhydramine is an antihistamine that also possesses anticholinergic properties. Benztropine combines a benzhydryl group with a tropane group to create a compound which is more anticholinergic than trihexyphenidyl but less antihistaminic than diphenhydramine. The clinical effect of a single dose lasts 5 hours, thereby requiring 2 or 3 daily doses. Dosing usually starts at 0.5-1 mg bid, with a daily maximum of 6 mg, although slightly higher doses are used in rare circumstances. The piperidine compound trihexyphenidyl was one of the first synthetic anticholinergic agents available, and replaced the belladonna alkaloids for treatment of PD in the 1940s due to its more favorable side effect profile. Trihexyphenidyl inhibits the presynaptic DA reuptake transporter, and therefore has a concomitant higher risk of abuse than the antihistamines or benztropine. Trihexyphenidyl has good GI absorption, achieving peak plasma levels in 1-2 hours, with a serum $t_{1/2}$ ~10-12 hours, generally necessitating multiple daily dosing to achieve satisfactory clinical results. The total daily dosage range is 5-15 mg, given 2-3 times a day as divided doses. Biperiden (AKINETON) is another drug in this class.

Amantadine (SYMMETREL), originally marketed as an antiviral agent toward influenza A, represents the most commonly used non-anticholinergic medication for antipsychotic-induced parkinsonism. Its mechanism of action is unclear but appears to involve presynaptic DA reuptake blockade, facilitation of DA release, postsynaptic DA agonism, and receptor modulation. These properties are sufficient to reduce symptoms of drug-induced parkinsonism, and only rarely have been reported to exacerbate psychotic symptoms. Amantadine is well absorbed after oral administration, with peak levels achieved 1-4 hours after ingestion; clearance is renal, with > 90% recovered unmetabolized in the urine. The plasma $t_{1/2}$ is 12-18 hours in healthy young adults, but is sufficiently longer in those with renal impairment and the elderly that a 50% dose reduction is recommended. Starting dosage is 100 mg orally bid in healthy adults, which may be increased to 200 mg bid. A dose of 100 mg bid yields peak plasma levels of 0.5-0.8 μg/mL and trough levels of 0.3 μg/mL. Toxicity is seen at serum levels of 1.0-5.0 μg/mL. Amantadine's primary advantage, especially in older patients, is avoidance of adverse CNS and peripheral anticholinergic effects.

Tardive dyskinesia is a situation of increased nigrostriatal dopaminergic activity as the result of postsynaptic receptor supersensitivity and up-regulation from chronically high levels of postsynaptic D_2 blockade (and possible direct toxic effects of high-potency DA antagonists). Tardive dyskinesia occurs more frequently in older patients, and the risk may be somewhat greater in patients with mood disorders than in those with schizophrenia. Its prevalence averages 15-25% in young adults treated with typical antipsychotic agents for more than a year. The annual incidence was 3-5% with typical antipsychotic drugs, with a somewhat smaller annual rate of spontaneous remission, even with continued treatment. The risk is one-fifth to one-tenth that of a atypical antipsychotic drug.

Tardive dyskinesia is characterized by stereotyped, repetitive, painless, involuntary, quick choreiform (tic-like) movements of the face, eyelids (blinks or spasm), mouth (grimaces), tongue, extremities, or trunk. There are varying degrees of slower athetosis (twisting movements), while tardive dystonia and tardive akathisia are rarely encountered as use of high-dose, high-potency typical antipsychotic medications has abated. The movements all disappear in sleep (as do many other extrapyramidal syndromes), vary in intensity over time, and are dependent on the level of arousal or emotional distress, sometimes reappearing during acute psychiatric illnesses following prolonged disappearance. The dyskinetic movements can be suppressed partially by use of a potent DA antagonist, but such interventions over time may worsen the severity, as this was part of the initial pharmacological insult. Switching patients from potent D_2 antagonists to weaker agents, especially clozapine has at times proven effective. When possible, drug discontinuation may be beneficial, but usually cannot be offered to schizophrenia patients. Trials of the antioxidant vitamin E have proved ineffective and are not recommended, especially in light of adverse cardiovascular effects from chronic vitamin E exposure.

Unlike antipsychotic-induced parkinsonism and acute dystonia, the phenomenology and treatment of *akathisia* suggests involvement of structures outside the nigrostriatal pathway. Akathisia was seen quite commonly during treatment with high doses of high potency typical antipsychotic drugs, but also can be seen with atypical agents, including those with weak D_2 affinities (e.g., quetiapine), and aripiprazole. Among the predominantly antipsychotic drug-naïve population with major depression in clinical studies with adjunctive aripiprazole, akathisia incidence was 23% using a starting dose of 5 mg, suggesting that dopaminergic partial agonism, rather than antagonism, may be etiologic for this medication (Berman et al., 2007; Marcus et al., 2008). Despite the association with D_2 blockade, akathisia does not have a robust response to antiparkinsonian drugs, so other treatment strategies must be employed, including the use of high-potency benzodiazepines (e.g., clonazepam), nonselective β blockers with good CNS penetration (e.g., propranolol), and also dose reduction, or switching to another antipsychotic agent. That clonazepam and propranolol have significant cortical activity and are ineffective for other forms of EPS, points to an extrastriatal origin for akathisia symptoms.

The rare neuroleptic malignant syndrome (NMS) resembles a very severe form of parkinsonism, with signs of autonomic instability (hyperthermia and labile pulse, blood pressure, and respiration rate), stupor, elevation of creatine kinase in serum, and sometimes myoglobinemia with potential nephrotoxicity. At its most severe, this syndrome may persist for more than a week after the offending agent is discontinued, and is associated with mortality. This reaction has been associated with various types of antipsychotic agents, but its prevalence may be greater when relatively high doses of potent agents are used, especially when they are administered parenterally. Aside from cessation of antipsychotic treatment and provision of supportive care, including aggressive cooling measures, specific pharmacological treatment is unsatisfactory, although administration of dantrolene and the dopaminergic agonist bromocriptine may be helpful. While dantrolene also is used to manage the syndrome of malignant hyperthermia induced by general anesthetics, the neuroleptic-induced form of hyperthermia probably is not associated with a defect in Ca^{2+} metabolism in skeletal muscle. There are anecdotal reports of NMS with atypical antipsychotic agents, but this syndrome is now rarely seen in its full presentation.

Hyperprolactinemia results from blockade of the pituitary actions of the tuberoinfundibular dopaminergic neurons; these neurons project from the arcuate nucleus of the hypothalamus to the median eminence, where they deliver DA to the anterior pituitary via the hypophyseoportal blood vessels. D_2 receptors on lactotropes in the anterior pituitary mediate the tonic prolactin-inhibiting action of DA. Correlations between the D_2 potency of antipsychotic drugs and prolactin elevations are excellent. With the exception of risperidone and paliperidone, atypical antipsychotic agents show limited (asenapine, iloperidone, olanzapine, quetiapine, ziprasidone) to almost no effects (clozapine, aripiprazole) on prolactin secretion.

The hyperprolactinemia from antipsychotic drugs is rapidly reversible when the drugs are discontinued. Hyperprolactinemia can directly induce breast engorgement and galactorrhea. Approximately 33% of human breast cancers are prolactin-dependent *in vitro*, a factor of potential importance if the prescription of these drugs is contemplated in a patient with previously detected breast cancer. By suppressing the secretion of gonadotropins and sex steroids, hyperprolactinemia can cause amenorrhea in women and sexual dysfunction or infertility in men. The development of amenorrhea is of concern as it represents low serum estradiol levels and ongoing risk for bone density loss. The development of amenorrhea becomes a sensitive marker for sex hormone levels, and should prompt clinical action, while asymptomatic measurable increases in serum prolactin levels do not necessarily merit any intervention. Dose reduction can be tried to decrease serum prolactin levels, but caution must be exercised to keep treatment within the antipsychotic therapeutic range. When switching from offending antipsychotic agents is not feasible, bromocriptine can be employed. There is also anecdotal evidence that aripiprazole augmentation may be effective.

All DA antagonist antipsychotic drugs possess antiemetic properties by virtue of their actions at the medullary chemoreceptor trigger zone (Figure 46–4). The D_2 partial agonists aripiprazole (and bifeprunox), however, can be associated with nausea. For aripiprazole this effect was noted in clinical trials of oral medication for acute mania, bipolar maintenance, or schizophrenia (nausea incidence 15% for aripiprazole vs. 11% for placebo; vomiting incidence 11% for aripiprazole vs. 6% for placebo), and also in studies of pediatric bipolar mania in patients ages 10-17 (nausea incidence 11%) and in acute IM trials for agitation in schizophrenia or acute mania (nausea incidence 9%). Bifeprunox possessed a level of intrinsic DA agonism that was slightly greater than that for aripiprazole (25-28%), but was significant enough to cause clinical problems with nausea and vomiting, that a 10-day titration from an initial starting dose of 0.125 mg was necessary to reach the proposed effective dosage range of 10-30 mg (Glick and Peselow, 2008).

H_1 Receptors. Central antagonism of H_1 receptors is associated with two major adverse effects: sedation and weight gain via appetite stimulation. Examples of sedating antipsychotic drugs include low-potency typical agents such as chlorpromazine and thioridazine, and the atypical agents clozapine and quetiapine. The sedating effect is easily predicted by their high H_1 receptor affinities (Table 16–2). Some tolerance to the sedative properties will develop, a fact that must be kept in mind when switching patients to nonsedating agents.

There is an extended-release quetiapine preparation available, with markedly reduced C_{max} compared to the immediate-release form. Immediate-release quetiapine generates peak serum levels > 800 ng/mL within 2 hours of ingestion, while the extended release preparation has C_{max} ~50% lower, with peak serum levels seen 4-8 hours after ingestion. In clinical practice the onset of sedation for extended-release quetiapine is delayed for at least 3 hours after oral administration, and subjectively the sedation is much less profound than with the immediate-release form (Mamo et al., 2008).

Rapid discontinuation of sedating antihistaminic antipsychotic drugs is inevitably followed by significant complaints of rebound insomnia and sleep disturbance. If discontinuation of sedating antipsychotic treatment is deemed necessary, except for emergency cessation of clozapine for agranulocytosis, the medication should be tapered slowly over 4-8 weeks, and the clinician should be prepared to utilize a sedative when the end of the titration is reached. Generous dosing of another antihistamine (hydroxyzine), or the anticholinergic antihistamine diphenhydramine are reasonable replacement sedative medications, but others can used, including benzodiazepines, non-benzodiazepine hypnotics that act at specific benzodiazepine sites (e.g., zolpidem, eszopiclone), and sedating antidepressants (e.g., trazodone). Sedation may be useful during acute psychosis, but excessive sedation can interfere with patient evaluation, may prolong emergency room and psychiatric hospital stays unnecessarily, and is poorly tolerated among elderly dementia and delirium patients, so appropriate caution must be exercised with the choice of agent and the dose.

Weight gain is a significant problem during long-term use of antipsychotic drugs and represents a major barrier to medication adherence, as well as a significant threat to the physical and emotional health of the patient. Weight gain has effectively replaced concerns over EPS as the adverse effect causing the most consternation among patients and clinicians alike. Appetite stimulation is the primary mechanism involved, with little evidence to suggest that decreased activity (due to sedation) is a main contributor to antipsychotic-related weight gain (Gothelf et al., 2002). Recent animal studies indicate that medications with significant H_1 antagonism induce appetite stimulation through effects at hypothalamic sites (Kim et al., 2007). The low-potency phenothiazine chlorpromazine, and the atypical antipsychotic drugs olanzapine and clozapine, are the agents of highest risk, but weight gain of some extent is seen with nearly all antipsychotic drugs, partly related to the fact that acutely psychotic patients may lose weight; in placebo-controlled acute schizophrenia trials, the placebo cohort inevitably loses weight (Meyer, 2001). For clozapine and olanzapine, massive weight gains of 50 kg or more are not uncommon, and mean annual weight gains of 13 kg are reported in schizophrenia clinical trials, with 20% of subjects gaining ≥ 20% of baseline weight. High-potency typical antipsychotic drugs (e.g., haloperidol, fluphenazine), and newer atypical antipsychotics asenapine, ziprasidone, and aripiprazole, are associated with mean annual weight gains < 2 kg in schizophrenia patients, with mean gains of 2.5-3 kg noted for iloperidone, risperidone, and quetiapine (Meyer, 2001). For unknown reasons, molindone is associated with modest weight loss. Younger and antipsychotic drug-naïve patients are much more sensitive to the weight gain from all antipsychotic agents, including those which appear roughly weight neutral in adult studies, leading some to conjecture that DA blockade may also play a small additive role in weight gain. 5-HT_{2C} antagonism is also thought to play an additive role in promoting weight gain for medications that possess high H_1 affinities (e.g., clozapine, olanzapine), but appears to have no effect in the absence of significant H_1 blockade, as seen with ziprasidone, a weight-neutral antipsychotic drug with extremely high 5-HT_{2C} affinity. Switching to more weight-neutral medications can achieve significant results; however, when not feasible or when unsuccessful, behavioral strategies must be employed, and should be considered for all chronically mentally ill patients given the high obesity prevalence in this patient population.

M_1 Receptors. Muscarinic antagonism is responsible for the central and peripheral anticholinergic effects of medications. Most of the atypical antipsychotic drugs, including risperidone, paliperidone, asenapine, iloperidone, ziprasidone, and aripiprazole, have no muscarinic affinity and no appreciable anticholinergic effects, while clozapine and low-potency phenothiazines have significant anticholinergic adverse effects (Table 16–2). Quetiapine has modest muscarinic affinity, but its active metabolite norquetiapine is likely responsible for anticholinergic complaints (Jensen et al., 2008). Clozapine is particularly associated with significant constipation, perhaps due to the severely ill population under treatment. Routine use of stool softeners, and repeated inquiry into bowel habits are necessary to prevent serious intestinal obstruction from undetected constipation. In general, avoidance of anticholinergic medications obviates the need to secondarily treat problems related to central or peripheral antagonism. Medications with significant anticholinergic properties should be particularly avoided in elderly patients, especially those with dementia or delirium.

α_1 Receptors. α_1 Adrenergic antagonism is associated with risk of orthostatic hypotension and can be particularly problematic for elderly patients who have poor vasomotor tone. Compared to high-potency typical agents, low-potency typical agents have significantly greater affinities for α_1 receptors and greater risk for orthostasis. While risperidone has a K_i that indicates greater α_1-adrenergic affinity than chlorpromazine, thioridazine, clozapine, and quetiapine, in clinical practice risperidone is used at 0.01-0.005 times the dosages of these medications, and thus causes a relatively lower incidence of orthostasis in non-elderly patients. Since clozapine-treated patients have few other antipsychotic options, the potent mineralocorticoid fludrocortisone is sometimes tried at the dose of 0.1 mg/day as a volume expander.

Adverse Effects Not Predicted by Monoamine Receptor Affinities

Adverse Metabolic Effects. Such effects have become the area of greatest concern during long-term antipsychotic treatment, paralleling the overall concern for high prevalence of pre-diabetic conditions and type 2 diabetes mellitus, and 2-fold greater CV mortality among patients with schizophrenia (Meyer and Nasrallah, 2009). Aside from weight gain, the two predominant metabolic adverse seen with antipsychotic drugs are dyslipidemia, primarily elevated serum triglycerides, and impairments in glycemic control.

Low-potency phenothiazines were known to elevate serum triglyceride values, but this effect was not seen with high-potency agents (Meyer and Koro, 2004). As atypical antipsychotic drugs became more widely used, significant increases in fasting triglyceride levels were noted during clozapine and olanzapine exposure, and to a lesser extent, with quetiapine (Meyer et al., 2008). Mean increases during chronic treatment of 50-100 mg/dL are common, with serum triglyceride levels exceeding 7000 mg/dL in some patients. Effects on total cholesterol and cholesterol fractions are significantly less, but show expected associations related to agents of highest risk: clozapine, olanzapine, and quetiapine. Risperidone and paliperidone have fewer effects on serum lipids, while asenapine, iloperidone, aripiprazole, and ziprasidone appear to have none (Meyer and Koro, 2004). Weight gain in general may induce deleterious lipid changes, but there is compelling evidence to indicate that antipsychotic-induced hypertriglyceridemia is a weight-independent adverse event that temporally occurs within weeks of starting an offending medication, and which similarly resolves within 6 weeks after medication discontinuation. The finding that serum triglycerides may change 70-80 mg/dL during a period when weight has changed relatively little propelled the search for adiposity-independent physiological mechanisms to explain this phenomenon.

In individuals not exposed to antipsychotic drugs, elevated fasting triglycerides are a direct consequence of insulin resistance since insulin-dependent lipases in fat cells are normally inhibited by insulin. As insulin resistance worsens, inappropriately high levels of lipolysis lead to the release of excess amounts of free fatty acids that are hepatically transformed into triglyceride particles (Smith, 2007). Elevated fasting triglyceride levels thus become a sensitive marker of insulin resistance, leading to the hypothesis that the triglyceride increases seen during antipsychotic treatment are the result of derangements in glucose-insulin homeostasis. The ability of antipsychotic drugs to induce hyperglycemia was first noted during low-potency phenothiazine treatment, with chlorpromazine occasionally exploited for this specific property as adjunctive presurgical treatment for insulinoma. As atypical antipsychotic drugs found widespread use, numerous case series documented the association of new-onset diabetes and diabetic ketoacidosis associated with treatment with atypical antipsychotic drugs, with most of cases observed during clozapine and olanzapine therapy (Jin et al., 2002, 2004). Analysis of the FDA MedWatch database found that reversibility was high upon drug discontinuation (~78%) for olanzapine- and clozapine-associated diabetes and ketoacidosis, supporting the contention of a drug effect. Comparable rates for risperidone and quetiapine were significantly lower. The mechanism by which antipsychotic drugs disrupt glucose-insulin homeostasis is not known, but recent *in vivo* animal experiments document immediate dose-dependent effects of clozapine and olanzapine on whole-body and hepatic insulin sensitivity (Houseknecht et al., 2007).

Antipsychotic-induced weight gain, and other diabetes risk factors (e.g., age, family history, gestational diabetes, obesity, race, ethnicity, smoking) all contribute to metabolic dysfunction. There may also be inherent disease-related mechanisms that increase risk for metabolic disorders among patients with schizophrenia, but the medication itself is the primary modifiable risk factor. As a result, all atypical antipsychotic drugs have a hyperglycemia warning in the drug label in the U.S., although there is essentially no evidence that asenapine, iloperidone, aripiprazole, and ziprasidone cause hyperglycemia. Use of the metabolically more benign agents is recommended for the initial treatment of all patients where long-term treatment is expected. Clinicians should obtain baseline metabolic data, including fasting glucose, lipid panel, and also waist circumference, given the known association between central obesity and future type 2 diabetes risk. Ongoing follow-up of metabolic parameters is commonly built into psychiatric charts and community mental health clinic procedures to insure that all patients receive some level of metabolic monitoring. As with weight gain, the changes in fasting glucose and lipids should prompt reevaluation of ongoing treatment, institution of measures to improve metabolic health (diet, exercise, nutritional counseling), and consideration of switching antipsychotic agents.

Adverse Cardiac Effects. Ventricular arrhythmias and sudden cardiac death (SCD) are a concern with the use of antipsychotic agents. Most of the older antipsychotic agents (e.g., thioridazine) inhibit cardiac K^+ channels, and all antipsychotic medications marketed in the U.S. carry a class label warning regarding QTc prolongation. A black box warning exists for thioridazine, mesoridazine, pimozide, IM droperidol, and IV (but not oral or IM) haloperidol due to reported cases of torsade de pointes and subsequent fatal ventricular arrhythmias (discussed next and in Chapter 29). Although the newer atypical agents are thought to have less effects on heart electrophysiology compared to the typical agents, a recent retrospective analysis found a dose-dependent increased risk for SCD among antipsychotic users of newer and older agents alike compared to antipsychotic nonusers, with a relative risk of 2 (Ray et al., 2009).

Cardiac arrhythmia is the most common etiology for SCD, but it is important to determine whether the arrhythmia is primary or secondary to structural changes related to cardiomyopathy, myocarditis, or acute myocardial infarction. Secondary ventricular arrhythmia is probably the most frequent form of fatal tachyarrhythmia, but the exact distribution of SCD deaths by etiology among antipsychotic-treated patients is unclear in the absence of large autopsy samples. The true incidence of drug-induced ventricular arrhythmia can only be estimated, due partly to underreporting, and the fact that drug-induced torsade de pointes is rarely captured with confirmatory EKG (Nielsen and Toft, 2009).

Multiple ion channels are involved in the depolarization and repolarization of cardiac ventricular cells, which are discussed in detail in Chapter 29. Myoycte depolarization is seen as the QRS complex on EKG, and is primarily mediated by ion channels that permit rapid Na^+ influx. Antagonism of these voltage-gated Na^+ channels causes QRS widening and an increase in the PR interval, with increased risk for ventricular arrhythmia. Thioridazine has been shown to inhibit Na^+ channels at high dosages, but other antipsychotic medications have not (Nielsen and Toft, 2009). Repolarization is mediated in part by K^+ efflux via two channels: the rapid I_{kr} and the slow I_{ks} channel. The I_{kr} channel is encoded by the human-ether-a-related-go-go gene (HERG), polymorphisms of which are involved in the congenital long QT syndrome associated with syncope and SCD. Many antipsychotic drugs block the I_{kr} channel to an extent comparable with that seen in congenital long QT syndrome. Antagonism of I_{kr} channels is the mechanism responsible for most cases of drug-induced QT prolongation, and is the suspected mechanism for the majority of antipsychotic-induced sudden cardiac deaths (Nielsen and Toft, 2009).

Aside from individual agents, where anecdotal and pharmacosurveillance data indicate risk for torsade de pointes (e.g., thioridazine, pimozide), most of the commonly used newer antipsychotic agents are associated with known risk for ventricular arrhythmias, including ziprasidone in overdose up to 12,000 mg. One exception is sertindole, an agent not available in the U.S. that was withdrawn in 1998 based on anecdotal reports of torsade de pointes, and then reintroduced in Europe in 2006 with strict EKG monitoring guidelines (Nielsen and Toft, 2009). Although *in vitro* data revealed sertindole's affinity for the K^+ rectifier channel, several epidemiological studies published over the past decade were unable to confirm an increased risk of sudden death due to sertindole exposure, thereby providing justification for its reintroduction. Aside from sertindole, the apparent safety of newer antipsychotic medications appears at odds with retrospective findings of SCD among antipsychotic users (Ray et al., 2009), thus confronting the clinician with contradictory information regarding antipsychotic drug-related SCD risk, and leading to conflicting clinical recommendations. Currently, there are no data that would suggest a benefit of routine EKG monitoring for prevention of SCD among antipsychotic drug users.

Other Adverse Effects. Seizure risk is an unusual adverse effect of antipsychotic drugs, with anecdotal reports of uncertain causality present for many agents. In the U.S., there is a class label warning for seizure risk on all antipsychotic agents, with reported incidences well below 1%. Among commonly used newer antipsychotic drugs, only clozapine has a dose-dependent seizure risk, with an incidence of 3-5% per year. The structurally related olanzapine had an incidence of 0.9% in premarketing studies. Seizure disorder patients who commence antipsychotic treatment must receive adequate prophylaxis, with consideration given to avoiding carbamazepine and phenytoin due to their capacity to induce CYPs and P-glycoprotein. Carbamazepine is also contraindicated during clozapine treatment due to its bone marrow effects, particularly leucopenia. Redistribution and increased spacing of doses to minimize high peak serum clozapine levels can help, but patients may eventually require antiseizure medication. Valproic acid derivatives (e.g., divalproex sodium) are often used, but will compound clozapine-associated weight gain.

Clozapine possesses a host of unusual adverse effects aside from seizure induction, the most concerning of which is agranulocytosis. Clozapine's introduction in the U.S. was based on its efficacy in refractory schizophrenia, but came with FDA-mandated CBC monitoring that is overseen by industry-created registries. Now that several generic forms of clozapine are available in addition to proprietary CLOZARIL, clinicians must verify with each manufacturer the history of prior exposure. The overall agranulocytosis incidence is slightly under 1%, with highest risk during the initial 6 months of treatment, peaking at months 2-3 and diminishing rapidly thereafter. The mechanism is immune mediated, and patients who have verifiable clozapine-related agranulocytosis should not be rechallenged. Increased risk is associated with certain HLA types and advanced age. An extensive algorithm guiding clinical response to agranulocytosis, and lesser forms of neutropenia, is available from manufacturer web sites, and must be followed, along with the current recommended CBC monitoring frequency.

While rarely used due to its risk of QTc prolongation, thioridazine is also associated with pigmentary retinopathy at daily doses ≥ 800 mg/day. Low-potency phenothiazines are associated with the development of photosensitivity, which necessitated warnings regarding sun exposure. Phenothiazines are also associated with development of a cholestatic picture on laboratory assessments (e.g., elevated alkaline phosphatase), and rarely elevations in hepatic transaminases.

Increased Mortality in Dementia Patients. Perhaps the least understood adverse effect is the increased risk for cerebrovascular events and all-cause mortality among elderly dementia patients exposed to antipsychotic medications. All antipsychotic agents carry a mortality warning in the drug label regarding their use in dementia patients. The cerebrovascular adverse event rates in 10-week dementia trials range from 0.4-0.6% for placebo to 1.3-1.5% for risperidone, olanzapine and aripiprazole (Jeste et al., 2008). The mortality warning indicates a 1.6-1.7 fold increased mortality risk for drug versus placebo. Mortality is due to heart failure, sudden death, or pneumonia. The underlying etiology for antipsychotic-related cerebrovascular and mortality risk is unknown, but the finding of virtually equivalent mortality risk for typical agents compared to atypical antipsychotic drugs (including aripiprazole) suggests an impact of reduced D_2 signaling regardless of individual antipsychotic mechanisms.

Overdose with typical antipsychotic agents is of particular concern with *low*-potency agents (e.g., chlorpromazine) due to the risk of torsades de pointes, sedation, anticholinergic effects, and orthostasis. Patients who overdose on *high*-potency typical antipsychotic drugs (e.g., haloperidiol) and the substituted benzamides are at greater risk for EPS due to the high D_2 affinity, but also must be observed for EKG changes. Overdose experience with newer agents, including ziprasidone, indicates a much lower risk for torsade de pointes ventricular arrhythmias compared to older antipsychotic medications; however, combinations of antipsychotic agents with other medications can lead to fatality, primarily through respiratory depression (Ciranni et al., 2009).

Drug-Drug Interactions. Antipsychotic agents are not significant inhibitors of CYP enzymes with a few notable exceptions (chlorpromazine, perphenazine, and thioridazine inhibit CYP 2D6) (Otani and Aoshima, 2000). The plasma half-lives of a number of these agents are altered by induction or inhibition of hepatic CYPs and by genetic polymorphisms that alter specific CYP activities (Table 16–3). While antipsychotic drugs are highly protein bound, there is no evidence of significant displacement of other protein bound medications, so dosage adjustment is not required for anticonvulsants, warfarin, or other agents with narrow therapeutic indices. With respect to drug-drug interactions, it is important to consider the effects of environmental exposures (smoking, nutraceuticals, grapefruit juice), and changes in these behaviors.

Changes in smoking status can be especially problematic for clozapine-treated patients, and will alter serum levels by 50% or more. Within 2 weeks of smoking discontinuation (e.g., hospitalization in nonsmoking environment), the absence of aryl hydrocarbons will cause upregulated CYP1A2 activity to return to baseline levels, with a concomitant rise in serum clozapine concentrations (Rostami-Hodjegan et al., 2004). For smoking patients with high serum clozapine levels, this loss of enzyme induction may result in nonlinear increases in clozapine levels, with potentially catastrophic results. Conversely, patients discharged from nonsmoking wards to the community will be expected to resume smoking behavior, with an expected 50% decrease in clozapine levels. Monitoring of serum clozapine concentrations, anticipation of changes in smoking habits, and dosage adjustment can minimize development of subtherapeutic or supratherapeutic levels.

Use in Pediatric Populations. Both risperidone and aripiprazole have indications for child and adolescent bipolar disorder (acute mania) for ages 10-17, and for adolescent schizophrenia (ages 13-17). Risperidone and aripiprazole are FDA-approved for irritability associated with autism in child and adolescent patients ages 5-16. As discussed in the sections on adverse effects, antipsychotic drug-naïve patients and younger patients are more susceptible to EPS and to weight gain. Use of the minimum effective dose can minimize EPS risk; aripiprazole and ziprasidone have the lowest risk, olanzapine the highest. Risperidone's effects on prolactin must be monitored by clinical inquiry, but long-term follow-up studies indicate some tolerance to hyperprolactinemia, with levels after 12 months of exposure significantly lower than peak levels, and close to baseline. Delayed sexual maturation was not seen in adolescents in clinical trials with risperidone, but should nevertheless be monitored.

Use in Geriatric Populations. The increased sensitivity to EPS, orthostasis, sedation, and anticholinergic effects are important issues for the geriatric population, and often dictate the choice of antipsychotic medication. Avoidance of drug-drug interactions is also important, as older patients on numerous concomitant medications have multiple opportunities for interactions. Dose adjustment can offset known drug-drug interactions, but clinicians must be attentive to changes in concurrent medications and the potential pharmacokinetic consequences. Vigilance must also be maintained for the additive pharmacodynamic effects of α_1 adrenergic, antihistaminic, and anticholinergic properties of other agents. Elderly patients have an increased risk for tardive dyskinesia and parkinsonism, with TD rates ~5-fold higher than those seen with younger patients. With typical antipsychotics, the reported annual TD incidence among elderly patients in 20-25% compared to 4-5% for younger patients. With atypical antipsychotic, the annual TD rate in elderly patients is much lower (2-3%). Increased risk for cerebrovascular events and all-cause mortality is also seen in elderly patients with dementia (see "Increased Mortality in Dementia Patients"). Compared to younger patients, antipsychotic-induced weight gain is lower in elderly patients.

Use During Pregnancy and Lactation. Antipsychotic agents carry pregnancy class B or C warnings. Human data from anecdotal case reports and manufacturer registries indicate limited or no patterns of toxicity and no consistent increased rates of malformations. Nonetheless, the use of any medication during pregnancy must be balanced by concerns over fetal impact, especially first-trimester exposure, and the mental health of the mother. Haloperidol is often cited as the agent with the best safety record based on decades of accumulated human exposure reports, but newer antipsychotic drugs, such as risperidone, have not generated any signals of concern (Viguera et al., 2009). As antipsychotic drugs are designed to cross the blood-brain barrier, all have high rates of placental passage. Placental passage ratios are estimated to be highest for olanzapine (72%), followed by haloperidol (42%), risperidone (49%), and quetiapine (24%). Neonates exposed to olanzapine, the atypical agent with highest placental passage ratio, exhibit a trend towards greater neonatal intensive care unit admission (Viguera et al., 2009). Use in lactation presents a separate set of concerns due to the low level of infant hepatic catabolic activity in the first 2 postpartum months. While breast milk presents an important source of protective antibodies for the baby, the inability of the newborn to adequately metabolize xenobiotics presents a significant risk for antipsychotic drug toxicity. The available data do not provide adequate guidance on choice of agent.

Major Drugs Available in the Class

In the U.S., atypical antipsychotic drugs have largely replaced older agents, primarily due to their more favorable EPS profile, although typical agents are widely used throughout the world. Table 16–1 describes the acute and maintenance doses for adult schizophrenia treatment based on consensus recommendations.

Acute IM forms exist for many typical antipsychotic drugs, and also for aripiprazole, ziprasidone, and olanzapine, with the latter being the most sedating due to its antihistaminic and anticholinergic properties. The standard IM doses are 9.75 mg for aripiprazole, 10 mg for olanzapine, and 20 mg for ziprasidone (Altamura et al., 2003). The 20-mg IM ziprasidone dose generates serum levels that exceed those from 160 mg/day orally, but has not been associated with reports of torsade de pointes or cardiac dysrhythmia. There are numerous LAI (long-acting injectable) formulations of typical antipsychotics, but in the U.S., the only available LAI typical agents are fluphenazine and haloperidol (as decanoate esters), with usual dosages 12.5-25 mg IM every 2 weeks and 50-200 mg (not to exceed 100 mg as the initial dose) IM monthly, respectively. Haloperidol decanoate has more predictable kinetics, while fluphenazine decanoate's serum level can increase within days after administration and induce adverse effects (Altamura et al., 2003). EPS remains a significant barrier for using these agents. LAI risperidone was studied at doses of 25, 50, and 75 mg IM biweekly, but the higher dose was found to be without increased efficacy and with greater EPS rates. Current available doses, all distributed as complete, single-dose kits, are 12.5, 25, 37.5, and 50 mg, given as a 2-mL water-based injection. LAI risperidone is impregnated into organic microspheres that require several weeks to liberate free drug. The impact of any dosage change (or missed dose) of LAI risperidone is seen 4 weeks later. LAI paliperidone has recently become available, and dosing is initiated with two loading IM deltoid injections given at days 1 (234 mg) and 8 (156 mg), followed by injections every 4 weeks starting at day 36. This loading strategy can be omitted if transitioning patients from another LAI antipsychotic, with LAI paliperidone given in lieu of the next injection, and the every 4 weeks thereafter. The package insert provides detailed information on dose equivalency with oral paliperidone, and on handling missed injections. ODT forms are available for aripiprazole, clozapine, olanzapine, and risperidone, and are the only form for asenapine. These ODT preparations are commonly used in emergency and inpatient settings where patients may be prone to cheeking or spitting out oral tablets.

Clinical Summary: Treatment of Psychosis

The pharmacological profile of newer, atypical antipsychotic drugs has expanded the uses of antipsychotic medications during the last decade to include adjunctive use for major depression and bipolar depression, with supporting data for certain anxiety disorders. Considerable debate exists over the clinical superiority touted for the newer antipsychotic drugs for the treatment of schizophrenia compared to older, typical agents. What is clear is that the more favorable therapeutic indices of newer agents (e.g., fewer neurological adverse effects) permit clinicians to avoid the effects of excessive antagonism of D_2 dopamine receptors. Aside from refractory schizophrenia, where clozapine exhibits superior effectiveness, drug choice primarily revolves around the avoidance of adverse effects, concerns regarding drug-drug interactions, and the availability of acute injectable, long-acting injectable, or orally dissolving tablet forms. Atypical antipsychotic drugs have generated considerable interest in non-dopaminergic mechanisms of action, including the useful property of 5-HT_{2A} antagonism. The greater understanding of schizophrenia pathophysiology has furthered investigation into glutamatergic and cholinergic agents, some of which have advanced to later-stage clinical trials. Knowledge of receptor binding affinities combined with neuroimaging data on CNS receptor occupancy provide a guide to gauging the risk of most adverse effects of a particular drug. However, the pathophysiology for adiposity-independent effects on glucose-insulin homeostasis seen with certain antipsychotic medications has yet to be elucidated. Given the inherent cardiometabolic risk factors common among the severely mentally ill, close medical monitoring during long-term antipsychotic therapy is considered the standard of care, regardless of the metabolic risk of the specific antipsychotic agent. Judicious use of antipsychotic drugs with more favorable risk profiles is the primary guide to medication choice.

TREATMENT OF MANIA

Mania is a period of elevated, expansive or irritable mood with co-existing symptoms of increased energy and goal-directed activity, and decreased need for sleep (discussed later). Mania represents one pole of what had been termed manic-depressive illness, but is now referred to as bipolar disorder (American Psychiatric Association, 2000). As with psychosis, mania may be induced by medications (e.g., DA agonists, antidepressants, stimulants) or substances of abuse, primarily cocaine and amphetamines, although periods of substance-induced mania should not be relied upon solely to make a diagnosis of bipolar disorder. Nonetheless, there is recognition that patients who develop antidepressant-induced mania do have a bipolar diathesis even with no prior independent history of mania, and should be followed carefully, especially if antidepressant treatment is again considered during periods of major depression.

Mania is distinguished from its less severe form, hypomania, by the fact that hypomania, by definition, does not result in functional impairment or hospitalization, and is not associated with psychotic symptoms. Patients who experience periods of hypomania and major depression have bipolar II disorder, those with mania at any time, bipolar I, and those with hypomania, but less severe forms of depression, cyclothymia (American Psychiatric Association, 2000). The prevalence of bipolar I disorder is roughly 1% of the population, and the prevalence of all forms of bipolar disorder 3-5%.

Genetics studies of bipolar disorder have yielded several loci of interest associated with disease risk and predictors of treatment response, but the data are not yet at the phase of clinical application. Unlike schizophrenia, where the biological understanding of monoamine neurotransmission has permitted synthesis of numerous effective compounds, no medication has yet been designed to treat the full spectrum of bipolar disorder based on preformed biological hypotheses of the illness, although candidate medications have passed certain *in vitro* and *in vivo* assays. Lithium carbonate was introduced fortuitously in 1949 for the treatment of mania (Cade, 1949) and approved for this purpose in the U.S. in 1970. While many classes of agents demonstrate efficacy in acute mania, including lithium, antipsychotic drugs, and certain anticonvulsants, no medication has surpassed lithium's efficacy for prophylaxis of future manic and depressive phases of bipolar disorder, and no other medication has demonstrated lithium's reduction in suicidality among bipolar patients.

Pharmacological Properties of Agents for Mania

Antipsychotic Agents. The chemistry and pharmacology of antipsychotic medications are addressed earlier in this chapter.

Anticonvulsants. The pharmacology and chemistry of the anticonvulsants with significant data for acute mania (valproic acid compounds, carbamazepine) and for bipolar maintenance (lamotrigine) are covered extensively in Chapter 21. These compounds are of diverse chemical classes, but share the common property of functional blockade of voltage-gated Na^+ channels, albeit with differing binding sites. Valproate exhibits non-specific binding to voltage-gated Na^+ channels, while carbamazepine (and its congeners) and lamotrigine have specific high affinity for the open-channel configuration of the alpha subunit (Söderpalm, 2002). These anticonvulsants have varying affinities for voltage-dependent Ca^{2+} channels, and differ in their ability to facilitate GABA-ergic (valproate) or inhibit glutamatergic neurotransmission (lamotrigine). The extent to which any of these actions is necessary for antimanic or other mood stabilizing activity is unknown, but the failure of phenytoin, gabapentin, and topiramate to be effective antimanic and mood-stabilizing medications suggests that potent blockade of voltage-gated Na^+ channels (which gabapentin and topiramate lack) is necessary but not sufficient, since phenytoin is very active at these channels.

Lithium. Lithium (Li^+) is the lightest of the alkali metals (group Ia); the salts of this monovalent cation share some characteristics with those of Na^+ and K^+. Li^+ is readily assayed in biological fluids and can be detected in brain tissue by magnetic resonance spectroscopy (Soares et al., 2000). Traces of the ion occur normally in animal tissues, but it has no known physiological role. Lithium carbonate and lithium citrate currently are used therapeutically in the U.S.

Mechanism of Action. Therapeutic concentrations of Li^+ have almost no discernible psychotropic effects in individuals without psychiatric symptoms. There are numerous molecular and cellular actions of Li^+, some of which overlap with identified properties of other mood-stabilizing agents (particularly valproate), and are discussed below. An important characteristic of Li^+ is that, unlike Na^+ and K^+, Li^+ develops a relatively small gradient across biological membranes. Although it can replace Na^+ in supporting a single action potential in a nerve cell, it is not a substrate for the Na^+ pump and therefore cannot maintain membrane potentials. It is uncertain whether therapeutic concentrations of Li^+ (0.5-1.0 mEq/L) affect the transport of other monovalent or divalent cations by nerve cells.

Hypotheses for the Mechanism of Action of Lithium, and Relationship to Anticonvulsants. Plausible hypotheses focus on lithium's impact on monoamines implicated in the pathophysiology of mood disorders, and on second-messenger and other intracellular molecular mechanisms involved in signal transduction, gene regulation, and cell survival (Quiroz et al., 2004). In animal brain tissue, lithium at concentrations of 1-10 mEq/L inhibits the depolarization-provoked and Ca^{++}-dependent release of NE and DA, but not 5-HT, from nerve terminals. Li^+ may even transiently enhance release of 5-HT, especially in the limbic system, but has limited effects on catecholamine-sensitive adenylyl cyclase activity or on the binding of ligands to monoamine receptors in brain tissue, although it does influence response of 5-HT autoreceptors to agonists (Lenox and Wang, 2003). Li^+ modifies some hormonal responses mediated by adenylyl cyclase or PLC in other tissues, including the actions of vasopressin and thyroid-stimulating hormone on their peripheral target tissues (Quiroz et al., 2004). Li^+ can inhibit the effects of receptor-blocking agents that cause supersensitivity in such systems. In part, the actions of Li^+ may reflect its ability to interfere with the activity of both stimulatory and inhibitory G proteins (G_s and G_i) by keeping them in their inactive $\alpha\beta\gamma$ trimeric state (Jope, 1999).

Considered by many as relevant for lithium's therapeutic efficacy is its inhibition of inositol monophosphatase and interference with the phosphatidylinositol pathway (Figure 16–1), leading to decreased cerebral inositol concentrations (Williams et al., 2002). Phosphatidylinositol (PI) is a membrane lipid that is phosphorylated to form phosphatidylinositol bisphosphate (PIP_2). Activated phospholipase C cleaves PIP_2 into diacylglycerol and inositol 1,4,5- trisphosphate (IP_3), with the latter stimulating Ca^{2+} release from cellular stores. IP_3 is dephosphorylated to inositol monophosphate (IP) and thence to inositol by inositol monophosphatase. Within its range of therapeutic concentrations, Li^+ uncompetitively inhibits this last step (Chapter 3), with resultant decrease in available inositol for resynthesis into PIP_2 (Shaldubina et al., 2001). The inositol depletion effect can be detected *in vivo* with magnetic resonance spectroscopy (Manji and Lenox, 2000). A recent genome-wide association study has implicated diacylglycerol kinase in the etiology of bipolar disorder, strengthening the association between Li^+ actions and PI metabolism (Baum et al., 2008). Further support for the role of inositol signaling in mania rests on the finding that valproate, and valproate derivatives, decrease intracellular inositol concentrations (Shaltiel et al., 2007). Unlike Li^+, valproate decreases inositol through inhibition of myo-inositol-1-phosphate synthase. Carbamazepine exposure in cultured sensory neurons alters the dynamic behavior of neuron growth cones, effects that are remediated through inositol supplementation, implicating inositol depletion as a mechanism underlying carbamazepine's mood stabilizing properties (Williams et al., 2002).

Stimulation of NMDA receptors results in IP_3 accumulation in primate brain, leading some to postulate that lithium's activity in the inositol pathway might also relate to glutamatergic effects (Dixon and Hokin, 1998). Subsequent experiments demonstrated the ability of acute high lithium levels to increase synaptic glutamate in mice and non-human primates, primarily through inhibition of glutamate reuptake at presynaptic nerve terminals by lowering the V_{max} of glutamate transport, but not glutamate binding to the transporter (Dixon and Hokin, 1998). The impact of supratherapeutic Li^+ on synaptic glutamate may be implicated in lithium-induced neurotoxicity during overdose; conversely, chronic Li^+ administration at therapeutic CNS concentrations results in increased glutamate uptake and increased levels of glutamate in presynaptic synaptosomes (Dixon and Hokin, 1998). This effect occurs at therapeutic Li^+ serum concentrations, leading to speculation that the neuroprotective effects of Li^+ seen in models of excitotoxic cell death may be mediated through modulation of synaptic glutamate availability (Bauer et al., 2003).

Li^+ treatment also leads to consistent decreases in the functioning of protein kinases in brain tissue, including PKC, particularly isoforms α and β (Jope, 1999; Manji and Lenox, 2000; Quiroz et al., 2004). Among other proposed antimanic or mood-stabilizing agents, this effect is also shared with valproic acid (particularly for PKC) but not with carbamazepine (Manji and Lenox, 2000). Long-term treatment of rats with lithium carbonate or valproate decreases cytoplasm-to-membrane translocation of PKC and reduces PKC stimulation–induced release of 5-HT from cerebral cortical and hippocampal tissue. Excessive PKC activation can disrupt prefrontal cortical regulation of behavior, but pretreatment of monkeys and rats with lithium carbonate or valproate blocks the impairment in working memory induced by activation of PKC in a manner also seen with the PKC inhibitor chelerythrine (Yildiz et al., 2008). The impact of Li^+ or valproate on PKC activity may secondarily alter the release of amine neurotransmitters and hormones as well as the activity of tyrosine hydroxylase (Manji and Lenox, 2000). A major substrate for cerebral PKC is the myristolated alanine-rich C-kinase substrate (MARCKS) protein, which has been implicated in synaptic and neuronal plasticity. The expression of MARCKS protein is reduced by treatment with both Li^+ and valproate, but not by carbamazepine, antipsychotic medications, or antidepressants (Watson and Lenox, 1996). This proposed mechanism of PKC inhibition has been the basis for therapeutic trials of tamoxifen, a selective estrogen receptor modulator that is also a potent centrally active PKC inhibitor (Einat et al., 2007). In acutely manic bipolar I patients, tamoxifen has shown evidence of efficacy as adjunctive treatment, and in two double-blind, placebo-controlled monotherapy trials (Yildiz et al., 2008; Zarate et al., 2007).

Both Li^+ and valproate treatment also inhibit the activity of glycogen synthase kinase-3β (GSK-3β) (Williams et al., 2002). Of relevance to mood disorders, GSK-3 inhibition increases hippocampal levels of β-catenin, a function implicated in mood stabilization (Kozikowski et al., 2007). GSK-3β has been found to regulate mood stabilizer-induced axonal growth and synaptic remodeling and to modulate brain-derived neurotrophic factor response. Mice with mutant forms of the GSK-3β gene demonstrate abnormalities of biological rhythms that are proposed endophenotypes for the circadian disruption seen in manic patients. In animal models, Li^+ induces molecular and behavioral effects comparable to that seen when one GSK-3β gene locus is inactivated. Potent and selective GSK-3β inhibitors show expected activity in mouse models of mania, thus providing further stimulus for exploring this mechanism (Kozikowski et al., 2007).

Another proposed common mechanism for the actions of Li^+ and valproate relates to reduction in arachidonic acid turnover in brain membrane phospholipids (Rao et al., 2008). Rats fed Li^+ in amounts that achieve therapeutic CNS drug levels have reduced turnover of PI (↓ 83%) and phosphatidylcholine (↓ 73%); chronic intraperitoneal valproate achieves reductions of 34% and 36%, respectively. Li^+ also decreased gene expression of PLA_2 and decreased levels of COX-2 and its products (Rapoport and Bosetti 2002).

5-HT release from presynaptic terminals is regulated by 5-HT_{1A} autoreceptors located on the cell body and 5-HT_{1B} receptors on the nerve terminal. *In vitro* electrophysiological studies suggest that Li^+ facilitates 5-HT release. Li^+ augements effects of antidepressants, and in animal models of depression, lithium's activity appears to be mediated through desensitizing actions at 5-HT_{1B} sites; Li^+ also antagonizes mouse behaviors induced by administration of selective 5-HT_{1B} agonists (Shaldubina et al., 2001).

Li^+ and valproic acid both interact with nuclear regulatory factors that affect gene expression (e.g., AP-1, AMI-1β, PEBP-2β; both agents increase expression of Bcl-2, which is associated with protection against neuronal degeneration/apoptosis (Manji and Chen, 2002).

Absorption, Distribution, and Elimination. Li^+ is absorbed readily and almost completely from the GI tract. Complete absorption occurs in ~ 8 hours, with peak plasma concentrations occurring 2-4 hours after an oral dose (Sproule, 2002). Slow-release preparations of lithium carbonate minimize early peaks in plasma concentrations, and to some extent may decrease local GI adverse effects, but the increased trough levels may increase the risk for, and the extent of, nephrogenic diabetes insipidus (Schou et al., 1982). Li^+ initially is distributed in the extracellular fluid, and gradually accumulates in various tissues; it does not bind appreciably to plasma proteins. The concentration gradient across plasma membranes is much smaller than those for Na^+ and K^+. The final volume of distribution (0.7-0.9 L/kg) approaches that of total body water and is lower than agents that are lipophilic and protein bound. Passage through the blood-brain barrier is slow, and when a steady state is achieved, the concentration of Li^+ in the cerebrospinal fluid and in brain tissue is ~ 40-50% of the concentration in plasma. The kinetics of Li^+ can be monitored in human brain with magnetic resonance spectroscopy (Soares et al., 2000).

Approximately 95% of a single dose of Li^+ is eliminated in the urine. From one- to two-thirds of an acute dose is excreted during a 6-12 hour initial phase of excretion, followed by slow excretion over the next 10-14 days (Goodnick and Schorr-Cain, 1991). The elimination $t_{1/2}$ averages 20-24 hours, obviating the need for multiple daily dosing. Once-daily dosing not only improves adherence, but is also associated with decreased polyuria (Schou et al., 1982). With repeated administration, Li^+ excretion increases during the first 5-6 days until a steady state is achieved after ~5 half-lives. When Li^+ is stopped, there is a rapid phase of renal excretion followed by a slow 10- to 14-day phase. Since 80% of the filtered Li^+ is reabsorbed by the proximal renal tubules, clearance of Li^+ by the kidney is ~ 20% of that for creatinine, 15-30 mL/min (Goodnick and Schorr-Cain 1991; Hopkins and Gelenberg 2000); this rate is somewhat lower in elderly patients (10-15 mL/min) (Juurlink et al., 2004; Tueth et al., 1998). Loading with Na^+ produces a small enhancement of Li^+ excretion, but Na^+ depletion promotes a clinically important degree of Li^+ retention. Although the pharmacokinetics of Li^+ varies considerably among subjects, the volume of distribution and clearance are relatively stable in an individual patient.

Li^+ is completely filtered, and 80% is reabsorbed in the proximal tubules (Goodnick and Schorr-Cain, 1991). Li^+ competes with Na^+ for reabsorption, and Li^+ retention can be increased by Na^+ loss related to diuretic use, or febrile, diarrheal, or other GI illness. Heavy sweating leads to a preferential secretion of Li^+ over Na^+ (Jefferson et al., 1982); however, the repletion of excessive sweating using free water without electrolytes can cause hyponatremia, and promote Li^+ retention. Thiazide diuretics deplete Na^+ and can cause significant reductions in Li^+ clearance that result in toxic levels. The K^+-sparing diuretics triamterene, spironolactone, and amiloride have modest effects on the excretion of Li^+, with concomitantly smaller increases in serum levels. Loop diuretics such as furosemide seem to have limited impact on Li^+ levels (Juurlink et al., 2004). Renal excretion can be increased by administration of osmotic diuretics or acetazolamide, but not sufficiently for the management of acute Li^+ intoxication. Through alteration of renal perfusion, some nonsteroidal anti-inflammatory agents can facilitate renal proximal tubular resorption of Li^+ and thereby increase serum concentrations (Phelan et al., 2003). This interaction appears to be particularly prominent with indomethacin, but also may occur with ibuprofen, naproxen, and COX-2 inhibitors, and possibly less so with sulindac and aspirin (Phelan et al., 2003). Angiotensin-converting enzyme inhibitors, particularly the renally cleared lisinopril, also cause Li^+ retention, with isolated reports of toxicity among stable lithium-treated patients switched from fosinopril to lisinopril (Meyer et al., 2005).

Less than 1% of ingested Li^+ leaves the human body in the feces; 4-5% is secreted in sweat (Sproule, 2002). Li^+ is secreted in saliva in concentrations about twice those in plasma, while its concentration in tears is about equal to that in plasma. As noted under "Pregnancy and Lactation" later in the chapter, Li^+ is secreted in human milk, but serum levels in breast-fed infants are ~20% that of maternal levels, and are not associated with notable behavioral effects (Viguera et al., 2007).

Serum Level Monitoring and Dose. Because of the low therapeutic index for Li^+, periodic determination of serum concentrations is crucial. Li^+ cannot be used with adequate safety in patients who cannot be tested regularly. Concentrations considered to be effective and acceptably safe are between 0.6 and 1.5 mEq/L. The range of 1.0-1.5 mEq/L is favored for treatment of acutely manic or hypomanic patients (Sproule, 2002). Somewhat lower values (0.6-1.0 mEq/L) are considered adequate and are safer for long-term prophylaxis. Serum concentrations of Li^+ have been found to follow a clear dose-effect relationship between 0.4 and 1.0 mEq/L, but with a corresponding dose-dependent rise in polyuria and tremor as indices of adverse effects. Nonetheless, patients who maintain trough levels of 0.8-1.0 mEq/L experience decreased relapse risk compared to those maintained at lower serum concentrations. There are patients who may do well with serum levels of 0.5-0.8 mEq/L, but there are no current clinical or biological predictors to permit *a priori* identification of these individuals. Individualization of serum levels is often necessary to obtain a favorable risk-benefit relationship.

The concentration of Li^+ in blood usually is measured at a trough of the daily oscillations that result from repetitive administration (i.e., from samples obtained 10-12 hours after the last oral dose of the day). Peaks can be two or three times higher at a steady state. When the peaks are reached, intoxication may result, even when concentrations in morning samples of plasma at the daily nadir are in the acceptable range of 0.6-1 mEq/L. Single daily doses generate relatively large oscillations of plasma Li^+ concentration but lower mean trough levels than with multiple daily dosing, and are associated with a reduction in the extent and risk for polyuria (Schou et al., 1982); moreover, single nightly dosing means that peak serum levels occur during sleep, so complaints regarding CNS adverse effects are minimized. While relatively uncommon, GI complaints are one compelling reason for multiple daily dosing or using delayed release Li^+ preparations, bearing in mind the increased polyuria risk from these strategies.

Therapeutic Uses

Drug Treatment of Bipolar Disorder. Treatment with Li^+ ideally is conducted in patients with normal cardiac and renal function. Occasionally, patients with severe systemic illnesses are treated with Li^+, provided that the indications are compelling, but the need for diuretics, nonsteroidal anti-inflammatory agents, or other medications that pose potential kinetic problems often precludes lithium use in those with multiple medical problems. Treatment of acute mania and the prevention of recurrences of bipolar illness in adults or adolescents are uses approved by the FDA. Li^+ is the only mood stabilizer with data on suicide reduction in bipolar patients (Cipriani et al., 2005 Goodwin et al., 2003; Tondo et al., 2001), and Li^+ also has abundant efficacy data for augmentation in unipolar depressive patients who are inadequate responders to antidepressant therapy (Bschor et al., 2002).

Drug Treatment of Mania. The modern treatment of the manic, depressive, and mixed-mood phases of bipolar disorder was revolutionized by the introduction of Li^+ in 1949, its gradual acceptance worldwide by the 1960s, and late official acceptance in the U.S. in 1970, initially for acute mania only, and later primarily for prevention of recurrences of mania. While Li^+, valproate, and carbamazepine have efficacy in acute mania, in clinical practice these are usually combined with atypical antipsychotic drugs, even in manic patients without psychotic features, due to their delayed onset of action. Li^+, carbamazepine, and valproic acid preparations are only effective with daily dosing that maintains adequate serum levels, and require serum level monitoring. Mania patients are often irritable and poorly cooperative with medication administration and phlebotomy, thus, atypical antipsychotic drugs may be the sole initial therapy, and have proven efficacy as monotherapy (Scherk et al., 2007); moreover, acute IM forms of olanzapine, ziprasidone, and aripiprazole can be used to achieve rapid control of psychosis and agitation. Benzodiazepines are often used adjunctively for agitation and sleep induction.

Li^+ is effective in acute mania, but is rarely employed as a sole treatment for reasons noted above, and because 5-7 days are required for clinical effect. A 600-mg loading dose of Li^+ can be given to hasten the time to steady state, and can also be used to predict dosage requirements based on the 24-hour serum Li^+ result, with a very high correlation coefficient ($r = 0.972$) (Cooper et al., 1973). Acutely manic patients may require higher dosages to achieve therapeutic serum levels, and downward adjustment may be necessary once the patient is euthymic. When adherence with oral capsules or tablets is an issue, the liquid Li^+ citrate can be used. Each 5 mL of lithium citrate syrup provides 8.12 mEq of Li^+, equivalent to 300 mg of lithium carbonate.

The anticonvulsant sodium valproate provides more rapid antimanic effects than Li^+, with therapeutic benefit seen within 3-5 days. The most common form of valproate in use is divalproex sodium, preferred over valproic acid due to lower incidence of GI and other adverse effects. Divalproex is initiated at 25 mg/kg once daily and titrated to effect or the desired serum concentration. Serum concentrations of 90-120 μg/mL show the best response in clinical studies (Bowden et al., 2006). With immediate release forms of valproic acid and divalproex sodium, 12-hour troughs are used to guide treatment. With the extended-release divalproex preparation, patients respond best when the 24-hour trough levels are in the high therapeutic range (Bowden et al., 2006).

Carbamazepine is effective for acute mania. Immediate release forms of carbamazepine cannot be loaded or rapidly titrated over 24 hours as with valproate due to the development of neurological adverse effects such as dizziness or ataxia, even within the therapeutic range (6-12 μg/mL) (Post et al., 2007); the extended-release form of carbamazepin was FDA-approved for acute mania in 2005. The extended-release form is better tolerated compared to older preparations, and effective as monotherapy with once-daily dosing (Weisler et al., 2006). Carbamazepine response rates are lower than those for valproate compounds or Li^+, with mean rates of 45-60% cited in the literature (Post et al., 2007). Nevertheless, certain individuals respond to carbamazepine after failing Li^+ and valproate. Initial doses are 400 mg/day, with the larger dose given at bedtime due to the sedating properties of carbamazepine. Titration proceeds by 200-mg increments every 24-48 hours based on clinical response and serum trough levels. Due to increased risk of Stevens-Johnson syndrome in Asian individuals (especially those from China, Hong Kong, Malaysia, and the Philippines where HLA-B*1502 prevalence is > 15%), HLA testing must be performed prior to treatment in populations at risk.

Lamotrigine has no role in acute mania due to the slow, extended titration necessary to minimize risk of Stevens-Johnson syndrome (Hahn et al., 2004).

Prophylactic Treatment of Bipolar Disorder. The choice of ongoing prophylaxis is determined by the need for continued antipsychotic drug use and for use of a mood-stabilizing agent. Both aripiprazole and olanzapine are effective as monotherapy for mania prophylaxis, but olanzapine use is eschewed out of concern for metabolic effects, and aripiprazole shows no benefit for prevention of depressive relapse.

In the pivotal maintenance trials, the mean end-point aripiprazole dose was 27.9 mg (Keck et al., 2007), and mean olanzapine dose 16.2 mg (Tohen et al., 2003). In 2009, LAI risperidone was also approved for bipolar maintenance treatment to be used adjunctively with Li^+ or valproate, or as monotherapy. If used as monotherapy, coverage with an oral antipsychotic is necessary for the first 4 weeks after the initial injection. When antipsychotic drugs have been employed as adjunctive agents, the optimal duration treatment is unclear, but most clinicians will continue with combination treatment for 2-4 months after the acute manic phase has been controlled. Clozapine can be beneficial in refractory mania patients as adjunctive therapy and as monotherapy (Hummel et al., 2002).

The overriding concern guiding bipolar treatment is the high recurrence rate. Individuals who experience mania have an 80-90% lifetime risk of subsequent manic episodes. As with schizophrenia, lack of insight, poor psychosocial support, and substance abuse all interfere with treatment adherence. While the anticonvulsants lamotrigine, carbamazepine, and divalproex have data supporting their use in bipolar prophylaxis, only concern has consistently been shown to reduce the risk of suicide compared to non-lithium users (Cipriani et al., 2005; Tondo et al., 2001), and compared to bipolar patients on valproate acid derivatives (Goodwin et al., 2003). Early case series and retrospective clinical literature indicated preferential benefit of valproate over concern in rapid-cycling patients, but a recent large trial failed to substantiate this effect, and found no significant differences in time to relapse between the two agents (Calabrese et al., 2005b). Based largely on subanalyses of acute mania trials, there are also claims that valproate may be superior to concern for patients experiencing mixed episodes, but the lack of prospective data from randomized trials also raises questions about the validity of these findings. Lamotrigine was effective in two large, 18-month long maintenance trials for bipolar patients whose most recent mood episode was manic or depressed, with greater effect on depressive relapse (Bowden et al., 2003; Calabrese et al., 2003). The ability to provide prophylaxis for future depressive episodes combined with data in acute bipolar depression (Hahn et al., 2004) has made lamotrigine a useful choice for bipolar treatment, given that bipolar I and II patients spend large amounts of time in depressive phases (32% and 50%, respectively) (Judd et al., 2003).

Bipolar disorder is a lifetime illness with high recurrence rates. Individuals who experience an episode of mania should be educated about the probable need for ongoing treatment. Stopping mood stabilizer therapy can be considered in patients who have experienced only one lifetime manic episode, particularly when there may have been a pharmacological precipitant (e.g., substance or antidepressant use), and who have been euthymic for extended periods. For bipolar II patients, the impact of hypomania is relatively limited, so the decision to recommend prolonged maintenance treatment with a mood stabilizer is based on clinical response and risk:benefit ratio. Discontinuation of maintenance Li^+ treatment in bipolar I patients carries a high risk of early recurrence and of suicidal behavior over a period of several months, even if the treatment had been successful for several years. Recurrence is much more rapid than is predicted by the natural history of untreated bipolar disorder, in which cycle lengths average ~1 year. This risk may be moderated by slow, gradual removal of Li^+, while rapid discontinuation should be avoided unless dictated by medical emergencies.

Other Uses of Lithium. Li^+ has been shown to be effective as adjunct therapy in treatment-resistant major depression (Bschor et al., 2002). Clinical data also support Li^+ use as monotherapy for unipolar depression. Meta-analyses indicate that lithium's benefit on suicide reduction extends to unipolar mood disorder patients (Cipriani et al, 2005; Tondo et al., 2001). While maintenance Li^+ levels of 0.6-1.0 mEq/L are used for bipolar prophylaxis, a lower range (0.4-0.8 mEq/L) is recommended for antidepressant augmentation.

Based on its neuroprotective properties, there has been consideration of Li^+ treatment for conditions associated with excitotoxic and apoptotic cell death, such as stroke and spinal cord injury, as well as in neurodegenerative disorders, including dementia of the Alzheimer type, stroke, Parkinson's disease, Huntington's disease, amyotrophic lateral sclerosis, progressive supranuclear palsy, and spinocerebellar ataxia type I (Aghdam and Barger 2007; Bauer et al., 2003; Chuang, 2004).

Interactions with Other Drugs. Interactions between Li^+ and diuretics (especially thiazides spironolactone and amiloride), angiotensin-converting enzyme inhibitors, and nonsteroidal anti-inflammatory agents have been discussed earlier. Amiloride has been used safely to reverse the syndrome of nephrogenic diabetes insipidus associated with Li^+ therapy, but requires careful monitoring and Li^+ dosage reduction to prevent lithium toxicity (Kosten and Forrest, 1986).

Adverse Effects

CNS Effects. The most common CNS effect of Li^+ in the therapeutic dose range is fine postural hand tremor, indistinguishable from essential tremor. Severity and risk for tremor are dose-dependent, with incidence ranging from 15-70%. Some tolerance may develop over time, but tremor may be sufficiently bothersome to require intervention. In addition to the avoidance of caffeine and other agents that increase tremor amplitude, therapeutic options include dose reduction (bearing in mind the increased relapse risk with lower serum Li^+ levels), or in those without contraindications for β adrenergic blockade, use of propranolol, starting at 20 mg/day in divided doses, and gradually increased until the desired clinical effect is achieved (typically at doses ≤ 160 mg/day). Valproate treatment has a similar problem, and the approach to valproate-induced tremor is identical. At peak serum (and CNS) levels, some individuals may complain of incoordination, ataxia, or slurred speech, all of which can be avoided by dosing Li^+ at bedtime. Patients may also complain of mental fatigue or cognitive dulling at higher serum Li^+ levels, but this should be carefully assessed to determine whether this reflects a true side effect or a desire to regain the mental high from hypomania.

Li^+ routinely causes EEG changes characterized by diffuse slowing, widened frequency spectrum, and potentiation with disorganization of background rhythm. Seizures have been reported in non-epileptic patients with therapeutic plasma concentrations of Li^+. Li^+ treatment has also been associated with increased risk of post-ECT confusion, and is generally tapered off prior to a course of ECT.

Li^+ (and valproate) treatment results in significant weight gain, a problem that is magnified by concurrent use of antipsychotic drugs. Mean weight gain at one year in prospective Li^+ trials ranges from −1 kg to + 4 kg, but the proportion of individuals who gain > 5% of baseline weight is 13-62% (Keck and McElroy, 2003). Although the mechanism is unclear, central appetite stimulation at hypothalamic sites is the most plausible explanation (Keck and McElroy, 2003).

Renal Effects. Long-term renal effects of Li^+ treatment are an important concern. The kidneys' ability to concentrate urine decreases during Li^+ therapy, and ~60% of individuals exposed to Li^+ experience some form of polyuria and compensatory polydipsia. The mechanism of polyuria is unclear, but the result is decreased vasopressin stimulation of renal reabsorption of water, and the clinical picture of nephrogenic diabetes insipidus. Mean 24-hour urinary volumes of 3 L/day are common among long-term Li^+ users, but Li^+ discontinuation or a switch to single daily dosing may reverse the impact on renal concentrating ability in patients with < 5 years of Li^+ exposure (Kusalic and Engelsmann, 1996). Patients exposed to multiple daily dosing or sustained- release Li^+ preparations are at greatest risk for renal effects. Renal function should be monitored with biyearly serum blood urea nitrogen and creatinine levels, calculation of estimated GFR using standard formulas (Morriss and Benjamin, 2008), and annual measurement of 24-hour urinary volume. Reassessment of Li^+ treatment, more frequent renal function tests, and possible nephrology consultation should be considered when estimated GFR is < 60 mL/min on several periodic measurements, daily urinary volume exceeds 4 L, or serum creatinine continues to rise on three separate occasions (Morriss and Benjamin, 2008).

Thyroid and Endocrine Effects. A small number of patients on Li^+ develop a benign, diffuse, nontender thyroid enlargement suggestive of compromised thyroid function, although many of these patients will have normal thyroid function. Measurable effects of Li^+ on thyroid indices are seen in a fraction of patients: 7-10% develop overt hypothyroidism (Jefferson, 2000), and 23% have subclinical disease, with women at 3-9 times greater risk (Kleiner et al., 1999). There appears to be no plateau in the incidence of hypothyroidism in studies covering up to 10 years' exposure; thus, ongoing monitoring of TSH and free T_4 is recommended throughout the course of Li^+ treatment. The development of hypothyroidism is easily treated through exogenous replacement, and is not a reason to discontinue Li^+ therapy. Rare reports of hyperthyroidism during Li^+ treatment also exist (Jefferson, 2000).

EKG Effects. The prolonged use of Li^+ causes a benign and reversible T-wave flattening in ~20% of patients and the appearance of U waves, effects unrelated to depletion of Na^+ or K^+. At therapeutic concentrations there are rare reports of Li^+-induced effects on cardiac conduction and pacemaker automaticity, effects that become pronounced during overdose and lead to sinus bradycardia, atrioventricular blocks, and possible cardiovascular compromise. Routine EKG monitoring is not recommended in younger patients, but may be considered in older patients, particularly those with a history of arrhythmia or coronary heart disease.

Skin Effects. Allergic reactions such as dermatitis, folliculitis, and vasculitis can occur with Li^+ administration. Worsening of acne vulgaris, psoriasis, and other dermatological conditions is a common problem that is usually treatable by topical measures, but in a small number may improve only upon discontinuation of Li^+. Some patients on Li^+ (and valproate) may experience alopecia; daily supplementation with a multivitamin containing at least 100 μg of selenium and 15 mg of zinc may be beneficial.

Pregnancy and Lactation. Li^+ is classified as risk category D (see Appendix I). The use of Li^+ in early pregnancy may be associated with an increase in the incidence of cardiovascular anomalies of the newborn, especially Ebstein's malformation (Freeman and Freeman, 2006). The basal risk of Ebstein's anomaly of ~1 per 20,000 live births may rise several-fold with first-trimester Li^+ exposure, but probably not above 1 per 2500. Moreover, the defect typically is detectable *in utero* by ultrasonography and often is surgically correctable after birth. Although the anticonvulsants valproic acid and carbamazepine are also pregnancy risk category D, these agents are associated with irreversible neural tube defects. In balancing the risk vs. benefit of using Li^+ in pregnancy, it is important to evaluate the risk of inadequate prophylaxis for the bipolar disorder patient, and subsequent risk that mania poses for the patient and fetus. In patients who choose to forego medication exposure during the first trimester, potentially safer treatments for acute mania include antipsychotic drugs or ECT (Dodd and Berk, 2006; Yonkers et al., 2004).

In pregnancy, maternal polyuria may be exacerbated by Li^+. Concomitant use of Li^+ with medications that waste Na^+ or a low-Na^+ diet during pregnancy can contribute to maternal and neonatal

by barbiturates and volatile anesthetics. All the benzodiazepines have similar pharmacological profiles. Nevertheless, the drugs differ in selectivity, and the clinical usefulness of individual benzodiazepines thus varies considerably.

As the dose of a benzodiazepine is increased, sedation progresses to hypnosis and then to stupor. The clinical literature often refers to the "anesthetic" effects and uses of certain benzodiazepines, but the drugs do not cause a true general anesthesia because awareness usually persists, and immobility sufficient to allow surgery cannot be achieved. However, at "preanesthetic" doses, there is amnesia for events subsequent to administration of the drug.

Although considerable attempts have been made to separate the anxiolytic actions of benzodiazepines from their sedative-hypnotic effects, distinguishing between these behaviors still is problematic. Measurements of anxiety and sedation are difficult in humans, and the validity of animal models for anxiety and sedation is uncertain. The existence of multiple benzodiazepine receptors may explain in part the diversity of pharmacological responses in different species.

Animal Models of Anxiety. In animal models of anxiety, most attention has focused on the ability of benzodiazepines to increase locomotor, feeding, or drinking behavior that has been suppressed by novel or aversive stimuli. In one paradigm, animal behaviors that previously had been rewarded by food or water are punished periodically by an electric shock. The time during which shocks are delivered is signaled by some auditory or visual cue, and untreated animals stop performing almost completely when the cue is perceived. The difference in behavioral responses during the punished and unpunished periods is eliminated by benzodiazepine receptor agonists, usually at doses that do not reduce the rate of unpunished responses or produce other signs of impaired motor function. Similarly, rats placed in an unfamiliar environment exhibit markedly reduced exploratory behavior (neophobia), whereas animals treated with benzodiazepines do not. Opioid analgesics and antipsychotic drugs do not increase suppressed behaviors, and phenobarbital and meprobamate usually do so only at doses that also reduce spontaneous or unpunished behaviors or produce ataxia.

The difference between the dose required to impair motor function and that necessary to increase punished behavior varies widely among the benzodiazepines and depends on the species and experimental protocol. Although such differences may have encouraged the marketing of some benzodiazepines as selective sedative-hypnotic agents, they have not predicted with any accuracy the magnitude of sedative effects among those benzodiazepines marketed as anxiolytic agents.

Tolerance to Benzodiazepines. Studies on tolerance in laboratory animals often are cited to support the belief that disinhibitory effects of benzodiazepines are distinct from their sedative-ataxic effects. For example, tolerance to the depressant effects on rewarded or neutral behavior occurs after several days of treatment with benzodiazepines; the disinhibitory effects of the drugs on punished behavior are augmented initially and decline after 3-4 weeks (File, 1985). Although most patients who ingest benzodiazepines chronically report that drowsiness wanes over a few days, tolerance to the impairment of some measures of psychomotor performance (e.g., visual tracking) usually is not observed. Whether tolerance develops to the anxiolytic effects of benzodiazepines remains a subject of debate. Many patients can maintain themselves on a fairly constant dose; increases or decreases in dosage appear to correspond with changes in problems or stresses. On the other hand, some patients either do not reduce their dosage when stress is relieved or steadily escalate dosage. Such behavior may be associated with the development of drug dependence (Chapter 24).

Some benzodiazepines induce muscle hypotonia without interfering with normal locomotion and can decrease rigidity in patients with cerebral palsy. In contrast to effects in animals, there is only a limited degree of selectivity in humans. Clonazepam in non-sedative doses does cause muscle relaxation, but diazepam and most other benzodiazepines do not. Tolerance occurs to the muscle relaxant and ataxic effects of these drugs.

Experimentally, benzodiazepines inhibit seizure activity induced by either pentylenetetrazol or picrotoxin, but strychnine- and maximal electroshock-induced seizures are suppressed only at doses that also severely impair locomotor activity. Clonazepam, nitrazepam, and nordazepam have more selective anticonvulsant activity than most other benzodiazepines. Benzodiazepines also suppress photic seizures in baboons and ethanol-withdrawal seizures in humans. However, the development of tolerance to the anticonvulsant effects has limited the usefulness of benzodiazepines in the treatment of recurrent seizure disorders in humans (Chapter 21).

Although analgesic effects of benzodiazepines have been observed in experimental animals, only transient analgesia is apparent in humans after intravenous administration. Such effects actually may involve the production of amnesia. Unlike barbiturates, benzodiazepines do not cause hyperalgesia.

Effects on the Electroencephalogram (EEG) and Sleep Stages. The effects of benzodiazepines on the waking EEG resemble those of other sedative-hypnotic drugs. Alpha activity is decreased, but there is an increase in low-voltage fast activity. Tolerance occurs to these effects.

Benzodiazepines decrease sleep latency, especially when first used, and diminish the number of awakenings and the time spent in stage 0 (a stage of wakefulness). Time in stage 1 (descending drowsiness) usually is decreased, and there is a prominent decrease in the time spent in slow-wave sleep (stages 3 and 4). Most benzodiazepines increase the time from onset of spindle sleep to the first burst of rapid-eye-movement (REM) sleep, and the time spent in REM sleep usually is shortened. However, the number of cycles of REM sleep usually is increased, mostly late in the sleep time. Zolpidem and zaleplon suppress REM sleep to a lesser extent than do benzodiazepines and thus may be superior to benzodiazepines for use as hypnotics (Dujardin et al., 1998).

Despite the shortening of stage 4 and REM sleep, benzodiazepine administration typically increases total sleep time, largely by increasing the time spent in stage 2 (which is the major fraction of non-REM sleep). The effect is greatest in subjects with the shortest baseline total sleep time. In addition, despite the increased number of

REM cycles, the number of shifts to lighter sleep stages (1 and 0) and the amount of body movement are diminished. Nocturnal peaks in the secretion of growth hormone, prolactin, and luteinizing hormone are not affected. During chronic nocturnal use of benzodiazepines, the effects on the various stages of sleep usually decline within a few nights. When such use is discontinued, the pattern of drug-induced changes in sleep parameters may "rebound," and an increase in the amount and density of REM sleep may be especially prominent. If the dosage has not been excessive, patients usually will note only a shortening of sleep time rather than an exacerbation of insomnia.

Although some differences in the patterns of effects exerted by the various benzodiazepines have been noted, their use usually imparts a sense of deep or refreshing sleep. It is uncertain to which effect on sleep parameters this feeling can be attributed. As a result, variations in the pharmacokinetic properties of individual benzodiazepines appear to be much more important determinants of their effects on sleep than are any potential differences in their pharmacodynamic properties.

Molecular Targets for Benzodiazepine Actions in the CNS. Benzodiazepines appear to exert most of their effects by interacting with inhibitory neurotransmitter receptors directly activated by GABA (Chapter 14). The ionotropic $GABA_A$ receptors consist of five subunits that co-assemble to form an integral chloride channel (Figure 14–11). $GABA_A$ receptors are responsible for most inhibitory neurotransmission in the CNS. Benzodiazepines act at $GABA_A$ receptors by binding directly to a specific site that is distinct from that of GABA binding. Unlike barbiturates, benzodiazepines do not activate $GABA_A$ receptors directly; rather, benzodiazepines act allosterically by modulating the effects of GABA. Benzodiazepines and GABA analogs bind to their respective sites on brain membranes with nanomolar affinity. Benzodiazepines modulate GABA binding, and GABA alters benzodiazepine binding in an allosteric fashion.

Benzodiazepines and related compounds can act as agonists, antagonists, or inverse agonists at the benzodiazepine-binding site on $GABA_A$ receptors. Agonists at the binding site increase, and inverse agonists decrease, the amount of chloride current generated by $GABA_A$-receptor activation. Agonists at the benzodiazepine binding site shift the GABA concentration-response curve to the left, whereas inverse agonists shift the curve to the right. Both these effects are blocked by antagonists at the benzodiazepine binding site. In the absence of an agonist or inverse agonist for the benzodiazepine binding site, an antagonist for this binding site does not affect $GABA_A$ receptor function. One such antagonist, flumazenil, is used clinically to reverse the effects of high doses of benzodiazepines. The behavioral and electrophysiological effects of benzodiazepines also can be reduced or prevented by prior treatment with antagonists at the GABA binding site (e.g., bicuculline).

The strongest evidence that benzodiazepines act directly on $GABA_A$ receptors comes from recombinant expression of cDNAs encoding subunits of the receptor complex, which resulted in high-affinity benzodiazepine binding sites and GABA-activated chloride conductances that were enhanced by benzodiazepine receptor agonists (Burt, 2003). The properties of the expressed receptors generally resemble those of $GABA_A$ receptors found in most CNS neurons. Each $GABA_A$ receptor is believed to consist of a pentamer of homologous subunits. Thus far 16 different subunits have been identified and classified into seven subunit families: six α, three β, three γ, and single δ, ε, π, and θ subunits. Additional complexity arises from RNA splice variants of some of these subunits (e.g., $\gamma2$ and $\alpha6$). The exact subunit structures of native GABA receptors still are unknown, but it is thought that most GABA receptors are composed of α, β, and γ subunits that co-assemble with some uncertain stoichiometry. The multiplicity of subunits generates heterogeneity in $GABA_A$ receptors and is responsible, at least in part, for the pharmacological diversity in benzodiazepine effects in behavioral, biochemical, and functional studies. Studies of cloned $GABA_A$ receptors have shown that the co-assembly of a γ subunit with α and β subunits confers benzodiazepine sensitivity to $GABA_A$ receptors (Burt, 2003). Receptors composed solely of α and β subunits produce functional $GABA_A$ receptors that also respond to barbiturates, but they neither bind nor are affected by benzodiazepines. Benzodiazepines are believed to bind at the interface between α and γ subunits, and both subunits determine the pharmacology of the benzodiazepine binding site (Burt, 2003). For example, receptors containing the $\alpha1$ subunit are pharmacologically distinct from receptors containing $\alpha2$, $\alpha3$, or $\alpha5$ subunits (Pritchett and Seeburg, 1990), reminiscent of the pharmacological heterogeneity detected with radioligand-binding studies using brain membranes. Receptors containing the $\alpha6$ subunit do not display high-affinity binding of diazepam and appear to be selective for the benzodiazepine receptor inverse agonist RO 15-4513, which has been tested as an alcohol antagonist (Lüddens et al., 1990). The subtype of γ subunit also modulates benzodiazepine pharmacology, with lower-affinity binding observed in receptors containing the $\gamma1$ subunit. Although theoretically ~1 million different $GABA_A$ receptors could be assembled from all these different subunits, constraints for the assembly of these receptors apparently limit their numbers (Sieghart et al., 1999).

An understanding of which $GABA_A$ receptor subunits are responsible for particular effects of benzodiazepines *in vivo* has emerged. The mutation to arginine of a histidine residue at position 101 of the $GABA_A$ receptor $\alpha1$ subunit renders receptors containing that subunit insensitive to the GABA-enhancing effects of diazepam (Kleingoor et al., 1993). Mice bearing these mutated subunits fail to exhibit the sedative, the amnestic, and in part the anticonvulsant effects of diazepam while retaining sensitivity to the anxiolytic, muscle-relaxant, and ethanol-enhancing effects. Conversely, mice bearing the equivalent mutation in the $\alpha2$ subunit of the $GABA_A$ receptor are insensitive to the anxiolytic effects of diazepam (Burt, 2003). The attribution of specific behavioral effects of benzodiazepines to individual receptor subunits will aid in the development of new compounds exhibiting fewer undesired side effects.

Electrophysiological studies *in vitro* have shown that the enhancement of GABA-induced chloride currents by benzodiazepines results primarily from an increase in the frequency of bursts of chloride channel opening produced by submaximal amounts of GABA (Twyman et al., 1989). Inhibitory synaptic transmission measured after stimulation of afferent fibers is potentiated by benzodiazepines at therapeutically relevant concentrations. Prolongation of spontaneous miniature inhibitory postsynaptic currents (IPSCs) by benzodiazepines also has been observed. Although sedative barbiturates also enhance such chloride currents, they do so by prolonging the duration of individual channel-opening events. Macroscopic measurements of $GABA_A$ receptor-mediated currents indicate that benzodiazepines shift the GABA concentration-response curve to the left without increasing the maximum current evoked with GABA. These findings collectively are consistent with a model in which benzodiazepines exert their major actions by increasing the gain of inhibitory neurotransmission mediated by $GABA_A$ receptors.

$GABA_A$ receptor subunits also may play roles in the targeting of assembled receptors to their proper locations in synapses. In knockout mice lacking the $\gamma2$ subunit, $GABA_A$ receptors did not localize to synapses, although they were formed and translocated to the cell surface (Essrich et al., 1998). The synaptic clustering molecule gephyrin also plays a role in receptor localization.

$GABA_A$ Receptor-Mediated Electrical Events: in vivo Properties. The remarkable safety of the benzodiazepines is likely related to the fact that their effects *in vivo* depend on the presynaptic release of GABA; in the absence of GABA, benzodiazepines have no effects on $GABA_A$ receptor function. Although barbiturates also enhance the effects of GABA at low concentrations, they directly activate GABA receptors at higher concentrations, which can lead to profound CNS depression (discussed later). Further, the behavioral and sedative effects of benzodiazepines can be ascribed in part to potentiation of GABA-ergic pathways that serve to regulate the firing of neurons containing various monoamines (Chapter 14). These neurons are known to promote behavioral arousal and are important mediators of the inhibitory effects of fear and punishment on behavior. Finally, inhibitory effects on muscular hypertonia or the spread of seizure activity can be rationalized by potentiation of inhibitory GABA-ergic circuits at various levels of the neuraxis. In most studies conducted *in vivo* or *in situ,* the local or systemic administration of benzodiazepines reduces the spontaneous or evoked electrical activity of major (large) neurons in all regions of the brain and spinal cord. The activity of these neurons is regulated in part by small inhibitory interneurons (predominantly GABA-ergic) arranged in feedback and feedforward types of circuits. The magnitude of the effects produced by benzodiazepines varies widely depending on such factors as the types of inhibitory circuits that are operating, the sources and intensity of excitatory input, and the manner in which experimental manipulations are performed and assessed. For example, feedback circuits often involve powerful inhibitory synapses on the neuronal soma near the axon hillock, which are supplied predominantly by recurrent pathways. The synaptic or exogenous application of GABA to this region increases chloride conductance and can prevent neuronal discharge by shunting currents that otherwise would depolarize the membrane of the initial segment. Accordingly, benzodiazepines markedly prolong the period after brief activation of recurrent GABA-ergic pathways during which neither spontaneous nor applied excitatory stimuli can evoke neuronal discharge; this effect is reversed by the $GABA_A$ receptor antagonist bicuculline (see Figure 14–10).

The macromolecular complex containing GABA-regulated chloride channels also may be a site of action of general anesthetics, ethanol, inhaled drugs of abuse, and certain metabolites of endogenous steroids (Whiting, 2003). Among the latter, allopregnanolone (3α-hydroxy, 5α-dihydroprogesterone) is of particular interest. This compound, a metabolite of progesterone that can be formed in the brain from precursors in the circulation and also synthesized by glial cells, produces barbiturate-like effects, including promotion of GABA-induced chloride currents and enhanced binding of benzodiazepines and GABA-receptor agonists. As with the barbiturates, higher concentrations of the steroid activate chloride currents in the absence of GABA, and its effects do not require the presence of a γ subunit in $GABA_A$ receptors expressed in transfected cells. Unlike the barbiturates, however, the steroid cannot reduce excitatory responses to glutamate (discussed later). These effects are produced very rapidly and apparently are mediated by interactions at sites on the cell surface. A congener of allopregnanolone (alfaxalone) was used previously outside the U.S. for the induction of anesthesia.

Respiration. Hypnotic doses of benzodiazepines are without effect on respiration in normal subjects, but special care must be taken in the treatment of children (Kriel et al., 2000) and individuals with impaired hepatic function, such as alcoholics (Guglielminotti et al., 1999). At higher doses, such as those used for preanesthetic medication or for endoscopy, benzodiazepines slightly depress alveolar ventilation and cause respiratory acidosis as the result of a decrease in hypoxic rather than hypercapnic drive; these effects are exaggerated in patients with chronic obstructive pulmonary disease (COPD), and alveolar hypoxia and CO_2 narcosis may result. These drugs can cause apnea during anesthesia or when given with opioids. Patients severely intoxicated with benzodiazepines only require respiratory assistance when they also have ingested another CNS-depressant drug, most commonly ethanol.

In contrast, hypnotic doses of benzodiazepines may worsen sleep-related breathing disorders by adversely affecting control of the upper airway muscles or by decreasing the ventilatory response to CO_2. The latter effect may cause hypoventilation and hypoxemia in some patients with severe COPD, although benzodiazepines may improve sleep and sleep structure in some instances. In patients with obstructive sleep apnea (OSA), hypnotic doses of benzodiazepines may decrease muscle tone in the upper airway and exaggerate the impact of apneic episodes on alveolar hypoxia, pulmonary hypertension, and cardiac ventricular load. Many clinicians consider the presence of OSA to be a contraindication to the use of alcohol or any sedative-hypnotic agent, including a benzodiazepine; caution also should be exercised with patients who snore regularly, because partial airway obstruction may be converted to OSA under the influence of these drugs. In addition, benzodiazepines may promote the appearance of episodes of apnea during REM sleep (associated with decreases in oxygen saturation) in patients recovering from a myocardial infarction; however, no impact of these drugs on survival of patients with cardiac disease has been reported.

Cardiovascular System. The cardiovascular effects of benzodiazepines are minor in normal subjects except in severe intoxication; the adverse effects in patients with obstructive sleep disorders or cardiac disease were noted above. In preanesthetic doses, all benzodiazepines decrease blood pressure and increase heart rate. With midazolam, the effects appear to be secondary to a decrease in peripheral resistance, but with diazepam, they are secondary to a decrease in left ventricular work and cardiac output. Diazepam increases coronary flow, possibly by an action to increase interstitial concentrations of adenosine, and the accumulation of this cardiodepressant metabolite also may explain the negative inotropic effects of the drug. In large doses, midazolam decreases cerebral blood flow and oxygen assimilation considerably (Nugent et al., 1982).

GI Tract. Benzodiazepines are thought by some gastroenterologists to improve a variety of "anxiety related" gastrointestinal disorders. There is a paucity of evidence for direct actions. Benzodiazepines partially protect against stress ulcers in rats, and diazepam markedly decreases nocturnal gastric secretion in humans. Other agents are considerably more effective in acid-peptic disorders (Chapter 45).

Absorption, Fate, and Excretion. The physicochemical and pharmacokinetic properties of the benzodiazepines greatly affect their clinical utility. They all have high lipid–water distribution coefficients in the non-ionized form; nevertheless, lipophilicity varies >50-fold according to the polarity and electronegativity of various substituents.

All the benzodiazepines are absorbed completely, with the exception of clorazepate; this drug is decarboxylated rapidly in gastric juice to *N*-desmethyldiazepam (nordazepam), which subsequently is absorbed completely. Drugs active at the benzodiazepine receptor may be divided into four categories based on their elimination $t_{1/2}$:

- Ultra-short-acting benzodiazepines
- Short-acting agents ($t_{1/2}$ <6 hours), including triazolam, the non-benzodiazepine zolpidem ($t_{1/2}$ ~2 hours), and eszopiclone ($t_{1/2}$ 5-6 hours)
- Intermediate-acting agents ($t_{1/2}$ 6-24 hours), including estazolam and temazepam
- Long-acting agents ($t_{1/2}$ >24 hours), including flurazepam, diazepam, and quazepam

Flurazepam itself has a short $t_{1/2}$ (~2.3 hours), but a major active metabolite, *N*-des-alkyl-flurazepam, is long-lived ($t_{1/2}$ 47-100 hours), which complicates the classification of individual benzodiazepines.

The benzodiazepines and their active metabolites bind to plasma proteins. The extent of binding correlates strongly with lipid solubility and ranges from ~70% for alprazolam to nearly 99% for diazepam. The concentration in the cerebrospinal fluid is approximately equal to the concentration of free drug in plasma. While competition with other protein-bound drugs may occur, no clinically significant examples have been reported.

The plasma concentrations of most benzodiazepines exhibit patterns that are consistent with two-compartment models (Chapter 2), but three-compartment models appear to be more appropriate for the compounds with the highest lipid solubility. Accordingly, there is rapid uptake of benzodiazepines into the brain and other highly perfused organs after intravenous administration (or oral administration of a rapidly absorbed compound); rapid uptake is followed by a phase of redistribution into tissues that are less well perfused, especially muscle and fat. Redistribution is most rapid for drugs with the highest lipid solubility. In the regimens used for nighttime sedation, the rate of redistribution sometimes can have a greater influence than the rate of biotransformation on the duration of CNS effects (Dettli, in Symposium, 1986a). The kinetics of redistribution of diazepam and other lipophilic benzodiazepines are complicated by enterohepatic circulation. The volumes of distribution of the benzodiazepines are large and in many cases are increased in elderly patients. These drugs cross the placental barrier and are secreted into breast milk.

The benzodiazepines are metabolized extensively by hepatic CYPs, particularly CYPs 3A4 and 2C19. Some benzodiazepines, such as oxazepam, are conjugated directly and are not metabolized by these enzymes (Tanaka, 1999). Erythromycin, clarithromycin, ritonavir, itraconazole, ketoconazole, nefazodone, and grapefruit juice are inhibitors of CYP3A4 (Chapter 6) and can affect the metabolism of benzodiazepines (Dresser et al., 2000). Because active metabolites of some benzodiazepines are biotransformed more slowly than are the parent compounds, the duration of action of many benzodiazepines bears little relationship to the $t_{1/2}$ of elimination of the parent drug that was administered, as noted above for flurazepam. Conversely, the rate of biotransformation of agents that are inactivated by the initial reaction is an important determinant of their duration of action; these agents include oxazepam, lorazepam, temazepam, triazolam, and midazolam.

Metabolism of the benzodiazepines occurs in three major stages. These and the relationships between the drugs and their metabolites are shown in Table 17–2.

For benzodiazepines that bear a substituent at position 1 (or 2) of the diazepine ring, the initial and most rapid phase of metabolism involves modification and/or removal of the substituent. With the exception of triazolam, alprazolam, estazolam, and midazolam, which contain either a fused triazolo or a imidazolo ring, the eventual products are *N*-desalkylated compounds that are biologically active. One such compound, nordazepam, is a major metabolite common to the biotransformation of diazepam, clorazepate, and prazepam; it also is formed from demoxepam, an important metabolite of chlordiazepoxide.

The second phase of metabolism involves hydroxylation at position 3 and also usually yields an active derivative (*e.g.*, oxazepam from nordazepam). The rates of these reactions are usually very much slower than the first stage ($t_{1/2}$ >40-50 hours) such that appreciable accumulation of hydroxylated products with intact substituents at position 1 does not occur. There are two significant exceptions to this rule: (1) small amounts of temazepine accumulate during the chronic administration of diazepam and (2) following the replacement of S with O in quazepam, most of the resulting 2-oxoquazepam is hydroxylated slowly at position 3 without removal of the *N*-alkyl group. However, only small amounts of the 3-hydroxyl derivative accumulate during chronic administration of quazepam because this compound is conjugated at an unusually rapid rate. In contrast, the *N*-desalkylflurazepam that is formed by the "minor" metabolic pathway does accumulate during quazepam administration, and it contributes significantly to the overall clinical effect.

The third major phase of metabolism is the conjugation of the 3-hydroxyl compounds, principally with glucuronic acid; the $t_{1/2}$ of these reactions usually are ~6-12 hours, and the products invariably are inactive. Conjugation is the only major route of metabolism for oxazepam and lorazepam and is the preferred pathway for temazepam because of the slower conversion of this compound to oxazepam. Triazolam and alprazolam are metabolized principally by initial hydroxylation of the methyl group on the fused triazolo ring; the absence of a chlorine residue in ring C of alprazolam slows this reaction significantly. The products, sometimes referred to as *α-hydroxylated compounds,* are quite active but are metabolized very

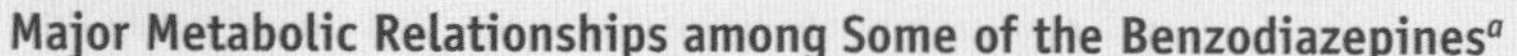

Table 17–2

Major Metabolic Relationships among Some of the Benzodiazepines[a]

		N-DESALKYLATED COMPOUNDS	3-HYDROXYLATED COMPOUNDS	
Chlordiazepoxide (I) ↘				
	Desmethyl-chlordiazepoxide (I) →	Demoxepam (L) ↓	Temazepam (I) → (⇣ Oxazepam)	G
Diazepam (L) } Clorazepate (S) } →		Nordazepam (L) →	Oxazepam (I) →	L
			Lorazepam (I) →	U
Flurazepam (S) →	*N*-Hydroxyethyl-flurazepam (S) →	*N*-Desalkylflur-azepam (L) →	3-Hydroxy derivative (I) →	C U R O
Quazepam (L) →	2-Oxo-quazepam (L) (⇢ *N*-Desalkylflurazepam) →		2-Oxo-3-hydroxy-quazepam (S) →	N I D
Estazolam (I)[b] →			3-Hydroxy derivative (S) →	A T
Triazolam (S)[b] →	α-Hydroxy-triazolam (S) →			I O
Alprazolam (I)[b] →	α-Hydroxy-alprazolam (S) →			N
Midazolam (S)[b] →	α-Hydroxy-midazolam (S) →			

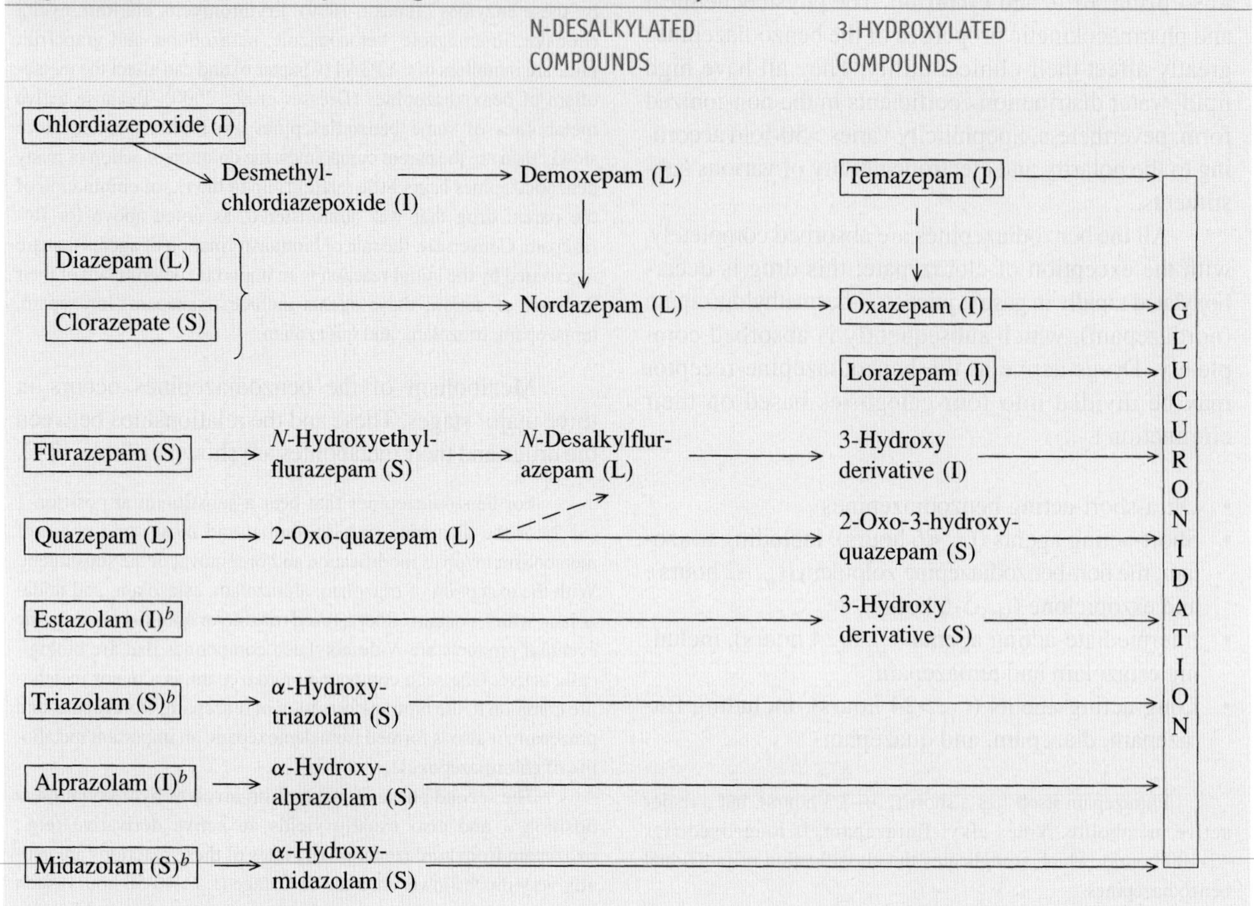

[a]Compounds enclosed in boxes are marketed in the U.S. The approximate half-lives of the various compounds are denoted in parentheses; S (short-acting), $t_{1/2}$ <6 hours; I (intermediate-acting), $t_{1/2}$ = 6-24 hours; L (long-acting), $t_{1/2}$ = >24 hours. All compounds except clorazepate are biologically active; the activity of 3-hydroxydesalkylflurazepam has not been determined. Clonazepam (not shown) is an *N*-desalkyl compound, and it is metabolized primarily by reduction of the 7-NO_2 group to the corresponding amine (inactive), followed by acetylation; its $t_{1/2}$ is 20-40 hours. [†]See text for discussion of other pathways of metabolism.

rapidly, primarily by conjugation with glucuronic acid, such that there is no appreciable accumulation of active metabolites. The fused triazolo ring in estazolam lacks a methyl group and is hydroxylated to only a limited extent; the major route of metabolism involves the formation of the 3-hydroxyl derivative. The corresponding hydroxyl derivatives of triazolam and alprazolam also are formed to a significant extent. Compared with compounds without the triazolo ring, the rate of this reaction for all three drugs is unusually swift, and the 3-hydroxyl compounds are rapidly conjugated or oxidized further to benzophenone derivatives before excretion.

Midazolam is metabolized rapidly, primarily by hydroxylation of the methyl group on the fused imidazo ring; only small amounts of 3-hydroxyl compounds are formed. The α-hydroxylated compound, which has appreciable biological activity, is eliminated with a $t_{1/2}$ of 1 hour after conjugation with glucuronic acid. Variable and sometimes substantial accumulation of this metabolite has been noted during intravenous infusion (Oldenhof et al., 1988).

The aromatic rings (A and C) of the benzodiazepines are hydroxylated only to a small extent. The only important metabolism at these sites is reduction of the 7-nitro substituents of clonazepam, nitrazepam, and flunitrazepam; the $t_{1/2}$ of these reactions are usually 20-40 hours. The resulting amines are inactive and are acetylated to varying degrees before excretion.

Because the benzodiazepines apparently do not significantly induce the synthesis of hepatic CYPs, their chronic administration usually does not result in the accelerated metabolism of other substances or of the benzodiazepines. Cimetidine and oral contraceptives inhibit *N*-dealkylation and 3-hydroxylation of benzodiazepines. Ethanol, isoniazid, and phenytoin are less effective in this regard. These reactions usually are reduced to a greater extent in elderly patients and in patients with chronic liver disease than are those involving conjugation.

Pharmacokinetics and the Ideal Hypnotic. An ideal hypnotic agent would have a rapid onset of action when taken at bedtime, a sufficiently sustained action to facilitate sleep throughout the night, and no residual action by the following morning. Among the benzodiazepines that are used commonly as hypnotic agents, triazolam theoretically fits this description most closely. Because of the slow rate of elimination of desalkylflurazepam, flurazepam (or quazepam) might seem to be unsuitable for this purpose. In practice, there appear to be some disadvantages to the use of agents that have a relatively rapid rate of disappearance, including the early-morning insomnia that is experienced by some patients and a greater likelihood of rebound insomnia on drug discontinuation (Gillin et al., 1989; Roth and Roehrs, 1992). With careful selection of dosage, flurazepam and other benzodiazepines with slower rates of elimination than triazolam can be used effectively. The biotransformation and pharmacokinetic properties of the benzodiazepines have been reviewed (Laurijssens and Greenblatt, 1996).

Therapeutic Uses

The therapeutic uses and routes of administration of individual benzodiazepines that are marketed in the U.S. are summarized in Table 17–3. Most benzodiazepines can be used interchangeably. For example, diazepam can be used for alcohol withdrawal, and most benzodiazepines work as hypnotics. In general, the therapeutic uses of a given benzodiazepine depend on its $t_{1/2}$ and may not match the FDA-approved indications. Benzodiazepines that are useful as anticonvulsants have a long $t_{1/2}$, and rapid entry into the brain is required for efficacy in treatment of status epilepticus. A short elimination $t_{1/2}$ is desirable for hypnotics, although this carries the drawback of increased abuse liability and severity of withdrawal after drug discontinuation. Anti-anxiety agents, in contrast, should have a long $t_{1/2}$ despite the drawback of the risk of neuropsychological deficits caused by drug accumulation.

Untoward Effects. At the time of peak concentration in plasma, hypnotic doses of benzodiazepines can be expected to cause varying degrees of light-headedness, lassitude, increased reaction time, motor incoordination, impairment of mental and motor functions, confusion, and anterograde amnesia. Cognition appears to be affected less than motor performance. *All of these effects can greatly impair driving and other psychomotor skills, especially if combined with ethanol.* When the drug is given at the intended time of sleep, the persistence of these effects during the waking hours is adverse. These dose-related residual effects can be insidious because most subjects underestimate the degree of their impairment. Residual daytime sleepiness also may occur, even though successful drug therapy can reduce the daytime sleepiness resulting from chronic insomnia (Dement, 1991). The intensity and incidence of CNS toxicity generally increase with age; both pharmacokinetic and pharmacodynamic factors are involved (Monane, 1992).

Other relatively common side effects of benzodiazepines are weakness, headache, blurred vision, vertigo, nausea and vomiting, epigastric distress, and diarrhea; joint pains, chest pains, and incontinence are much rarer. Anticonvulsant benzodiazepines sometimes actually increase the frequency of seizures in patients with epilepsy. The possible adverse effects of alterations in the sleep pattern are discussed later.

Adverse Psychological Effects. Benzodiazepines may cause paradoxical effects. Flurazepam occasionally increases the incidence of nightmares—especially during the first week of use—and sometimes causes garrulousness, anxiety, irritability, tachycardia, and sweating. Amnesia, euphoria, restlessness, hallucinations, sleep-walking, sleep-talking, other complex behaviors, and hypomanic behavior have been reported to occur during use of various benzodiazepines. The release of bizarre uninhibited behavior has been noted in some users, whereas hostility and rage may occur in others; collectively, these are sometimes referred to as *disinhibition* or *dyscontrol reactions*. Paranoia, depression, and suicidal ideation also occasionally may accompany the use of these agents. Such paradoxical or disinhibition reactions are rare and appear to be dose related. Because of reports of an increased incidence of confusion and abnormal behaviors, triazolam has been banned in the U.K., although the FDA declared triazolam to be safe and effective in low doses of 0.125-0.25 mg. Surveys in the U.K. after the ban found that patients did not have fewer side effects with replacement treatments (Hindmarch et al., 1993), which is consonant with controlled studies that do not support the conclusion that such reactions occur more frequently with any one benzodiazepine than with others (Jonas et al., 1992; Rothschild, 1992).

Chronic benzodiazepine use poses a risk for development of dependence and abuse (Woods et al., 1992), but not to the same extent as seen with older sedatives and other recognized drugs of abuse (Uhlenhuth et al., 1999). Abuse of benzodiazepines includes the use of flunitrazepam (rohypnol; not licensed for use in the U.S.) as a "date-rape drug" (Woods and Winger, 1997). Mild dependence may develop in many patients who have taken therapeutic doses of benzodiazepines on a regular basis for prolonged periods. Withdrawal symptoms may include temporary intensification of the problems that originally prompted their use (e.g., insomnia or anxiety). Dysphoria, irritability, sweating, unpleasant dreams, tremors, anorexia, and faintness or dizziness also may occur, especially when withdrawal of the benzodiazepine occurs abruptly (Petursson, 1994). Hence, it is prudent to taper the dosage gradually when therapy is to be discontinued. Despite their adverse effects, benzodiazepines are relatively safe drugs. Even huge doses are rarely fatal unless other drugs are taken concomitantly. Ethanol is a common contributor to deaths involving benzodiazepines, and true coma is uncommon in the absence of another CNS depressant. Although overdosage with a benzodiazepine rarely causes severe cardiovascular or respiratory depression, therapeutic doses can further compromise respiration in patients with COPD or obstructive sleep apnea (see "Respiration" earlier in the chapter).

A wide variety of serious allergic, hepatotoxic, and hematologic reactions to the benzodiazepines may occur, but the incidence is quite low; these reactions have been associated with the use of flurazepam, triazolam, and temazepam. Large doses taken just before or during labor may cause hypothermia, hypotonia, and mild respiratory

Table 17–3

Trade Names, Routes of Administration, and Therapeutic Uses of Benzodiazepines

COMPOUND (TRADE NAME)	ROUTES OF ADMINISTRATION[a]	EXAMPLES OF THERAPEUTIC USES[b]	COMMENTS	$t_{1/2}$, hours[c]	USUAL SEDATIVE-HYPNOTIC DOSAGE, mg[d]
Alprazolam (XANAX)	Oral	Anxiety disorders, agoraphobia	Withdrawal symptoms may be especially severe	12±2	—
Chlordiazepoxide (LIBRIUM, others)	Oral, IM, IV	Anxiety disorders, management of alcohol withdrawal, anesthetic premedication	Long-acting and self-tapering because of active metabolites	10±3.4	50-100, qd–qid[e]
Clonazepam (KLONOPIN)	Oral	Seizure disorders, adjunctive treatment in acute mania and certain movement disorders	Tolerance develops to anticonvulsant effects	23±5	—
Clorazepate (TRANXENE, others)	Oral	Anxiety disorders, seizure disorders	Prodrug; activity due to formation of nordazepam during absorption	2.0±0.9	3.75-20, bid–qid[e]
Diazepam (VALIUM, others)	Oral, IM, IV, rectal	Anxiety disorders, status epilepticus, skeletal muscle relaxation, anesthetic premedication	Prototypical benzodiazepine	43±13	5-10, tid–qid[e]
Estazolam (PROSOM)	Oral	Insomnia	Contains triazolo ring; adverse effects may be similar to those of triazolam	10–24	1-2
Flurazepam (DALMANE)	Oral	Insomnia	Active metabolites accumulate with chronic use	74±24	15-30
Lorazepam (ATIVAN)	Oral, IM, IV	Anxiety disorders, preanesthetic medication	Metabolized solely by conjugation	14±5	2-4
Midazolam (VERSED)	IV, IM	Preanesthetic and intraoperative medication	Rapidly inactivated	1.9±0.6	—[f]
Oxazepam (SERAX)	Oral	Anxiety disorders	Metabolized solely by conjugation	8.0±2.4	15-30, tid–qid[e]
Quazepam (DORAL)	Oral	Insomnia	Active metabolites accumulate with chronic use	39	7.5-15
Temazepam (RESTORIL)	Oral	Insomnia	Metabolized mainly by conjugation	11±6	7.5-30
Triazolam (HALCION)	Oral	Insomnia	Rapidly inactivated; may cause disturbing daytime side effects	2.9±1.0	0.125-0.25

[a]IM, intramuscular injection; IV, intravenous administration; qd, once a day; bid, twice a day; tid, three times a day; qid, four times a day. [b]The therapeutic uses are identified as examples to emphasize that most benzodiazepines can be used interchangeably. In general, the therapeutic uses of a given benzodiazepine are related to its $t_{1/2}$ and may not match the marketed indications. The issue is addressed more extensively in the text. [c]Half-life of active metabolite may differ. See Appendix II for additional information. [d]For additional dosage information, see Chapter 13 (anesthesia), Chapter 17 (anxiety), and Chapter 19 (seizure disorders). [e]Approved as a sedative-hypnotic only for management of alcohol withdrawal; doses in a nontolerant individual would be smaller. [f]Recommended doses vary considerably depending on specific use, condition of patient, and concomitant administration of other drugs.

depression in the neonate. Abuse by the pregnant mother can result in a withdrawal syndrome in the newborn.

Except for additive effects with other sedative or hypnotic drugs, reports of clinically important pharmacodynamic interactions between benzodiazepines and other drugs have been infrequent. Ethanol increases both the rate of absorption of benzodiazepines and the associated CNS depression. Valproate and benzodiazepines in combination may cause psychotic episodes. Pharmacokinetic interactions were discussed earlier.

Novel Benzodiazepine Receptor Agonists

Hypnotics in this class are commonly referred to as "Z compounds". They include zolpidem (AMBIEN), zaleplon (SONATA), zopiclone (not marketed in the U.S.), and eszopiclone (LUNESTA), which is the S(+) enantiomer of zopiclone. Although the Z compounds are structurally unrelated to each other and to benzodiazepines, their therapeutic efficacy as hypnotics is due to agonist effects on the benzodiazepine site of the $GABA_A$ receptor. Compared to benzodiazepines, Z compounds are less effective as anticonvulsants or muscle relaxants, which may be related to their relative selectivity for $GABA_A$ receptors containing the α1 subunit. Over the last decade, Z compounds have largely replaced benzodiazepines in the treatment of insomnia. Z compounds were initially promoted as having less potential for dependence and abuse than traditional benzodiazepines. However, based on post-marketing clinical experience with zopiclone and zolpidem, tolerance and physical dependence can be expected during long-term use of Z compounds, especially with higher doses (Zammit, 2009). Reports of abuse of Z compounds are on the rise world-wide (Victorri-Vigneau, 2007). Zopiclone and its isomers are classified as schedule IV drugs in the U.S. The clinical presentation of overdose with Z compounds is similar to that of benzodiazepine overdose and can be treated with the benzodiazepine antagonist flumazenil.

Zaleplon and zolpidem are effective in relieving sleep-onset insomnia. Both drugs have been approved by the FDA for use for up to 7-10 days at a time. Zaleplon and zolpidem have sustained hypnotic efficacy without occurrence of rebound insomnia on abrupt discontinuation (Mitler, 2000; Walsh et al., 2000). Zaleplon and zolpidem have similar degrees of efficacy. Zolpidem has a $t_{1/2}$ of ~2 hours, which is sufficient to cover most of a typical 8-hour sleep period, and is presently approved for bedtime use only. Zaleplon has a shorter $t_{1/2}$ ~1 hour, which offers the possibility for safe dosing later in the night, within 4 hours of the anticipated rising time. As a result, zaleplon is approved for use immediately at bedtime or when the patient has difficulty falling asleep after bedtime. Because of its short $t_{1/2}$, zaleplon has not been shown to be different from placebo in measures of duration of sleep and number of awakenings. Zaleplon and zolpidem differ in residual side effects; late-night administration of zolpidem has been associated with morning sedation, delayed reaction time, and anterograde amnesia, whereas zaleplon does not differ from placebo.

Zaleplon. Zaleplon (SONATA, generic) is a non-benzodiazepine and is a member of the pyrazolopyrimidine class of compounds.

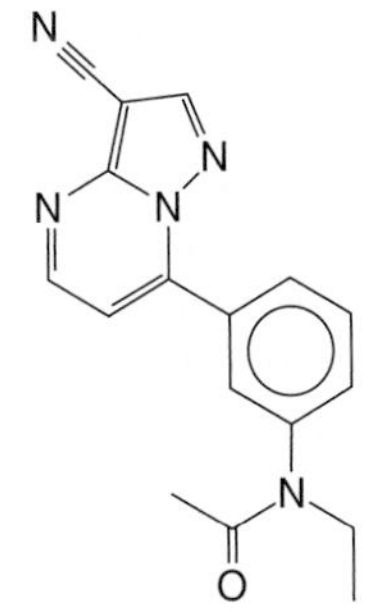

ZALEPLON

Zaleplon preferentially binds to the benzodiazepine-binding site on $GABA_A$ receptors containing the α1 receptor subunit. Zaleplon is absorbed rapidly and reaches peak plasma concentrations in ~1 hour. Its bioavailability is ~30% because of presystemic metabolism. Zaleplon has a volume of distribution of ~1.4 L/kg and plasma-protein binding of ~60%. Zaleplon is metabolized largely by aldehyde oxidase and to a lesser extent by CYP3A4. Its oxidative metabolites are converted to glucuronides and eliminated in urine. Less than 1% of zaleplon is excreted unchanged in urine. None of zaleplon's metabolites are pharmacologically active.

Zaleplon (usually administered in 5-, 10-, or 20-mg doses) has been studied in clinical trials of patients with chronic or transient insomnia (Dooley and Plosker, 2000), focusing on the drug's effects in decreasing sleep latency. Zaleplon-treated subjects with either chronic or transient insomnia have experienced shorter periods of sleep latency than have placebo-treated subjects.

Zolpidem. Zolpidem (AMBIEN, others) is a non-benzodiazepine sedative-hypnotic drug. It is classified as an imidazopyridine:

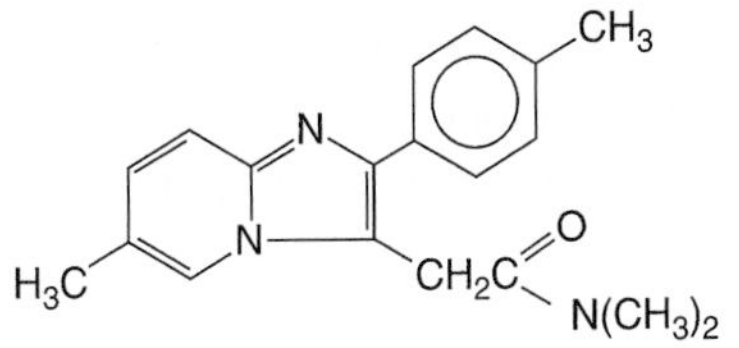

ZOLPIDEM

Although the actions of zolpidem are due to agonist effects on $GABA_A$ receptors and generally resemble those of benzodiazepines, it produces only weak anticonvulsant effects in experimental animals, and its relatively strong sedative actions appear to mask anxiolytic effects in various animal models of anxiety (Langtry and Benfield, 1990). Although chronic administration of zolpidem to rodents produces neither tolerance to its sedative effects nor signs of withdrawal when the drug is discontinued and flumazenil is injected (Perrault et al., 1992), tolerance and physical dependence have been observed with chronic administration of zolpidem to baboons (Griffiths et al., 1992). During U.S. clinical trials, withdrawal effects within 48 hours of drug discontinuation occurred at an incidence of 1% or less. Post-marketing reports of abuse, dependence, and withdrawal have been recorded.

Unlike the benzodiazepines, zolpidem has little effect on the stages of sleep in normal human subjects. The drug is as effective as benzodiazepines in shortening sleep latency and prolonging total sleep time in patients with insomnia. After discontinuation of zolpidem, the beneficial effects on sleep reportedly persist for up to 1 week (Herrmann et al., 1993), but mild rebound insomnia on the first night also has occurred. Tolerance and physical dependence develop only rarely and under unusual circumstances (Cavallaro *et al.,* 1993; Morselli, 1993). Indeed, zolpidem-induced improvement in sleep time of chronic insomniacs was sustained during as much as 6 months of treatment without signs of withdrawal or rebound after stopping the drug (Kummer et al., 1993). Nevertheless, zolpidem is approved only for the short-term treatment of insomnia. At therapeutic doses (5 to 10 mg), zolpidem infrequently produces residual daytime sedation or amnesia, and the incidence of other adverse effects (e.g., GI complaints or dizziness) also is low. As with the benzodiazepines, large overdoses of zolpidem do not produce severe respiratory depression unless other agents (e.g., ethanol) also are ingested (Garnier et al., 1994). Hypnotic doses increase the hypoxia and hypercarbia of patients with obstructive sleep apnea.

Zolpidem is absorbed readily from the GI tract; first-pass hepatic metabolism results in an oral bioavailability of ~70%, but this value is lower when the drug is ingested with food because of slowed absorption and increased hepatic blood flow. Zolpidem is eliminated almost entirely by conversion to inactive products in the liver, largely through oxidation of the methyl groups on the phenyl and imidazopyridine rings to the corresponding carboxylic acids. Its plasma $t_{1/2}$ is ~2 hours in individuals with normal hepatic blood flow or function. This value may be increased 2-fold or more in those with cirrhosis and also tends to be greater in older patients; adjustment of dosage often is necessary in both categories of patients. Although little or no unchanged zolpidem is found in the urine, elimination of the drug is slower in patients with chronic renal insufficiency largely owing to an increase in its apparent volume of distribution.

Eszopiclone. Eszopiclone (LUNESTA) is the active S(+) enantiomer of zopiclone. Eszopiclone has no structural similarity to benzodiazepines, zolpidem, or zaleplon.

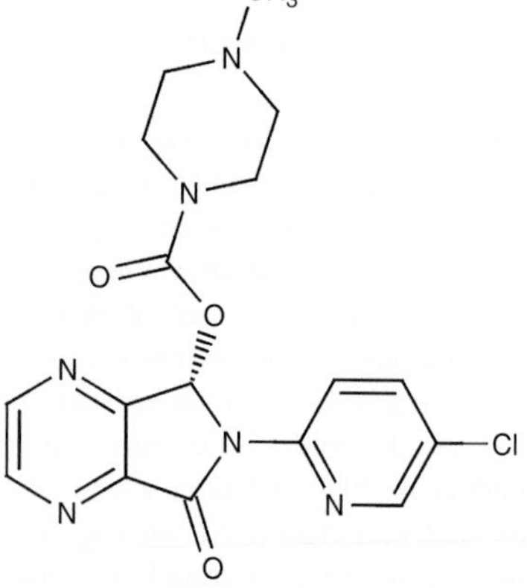

ESZOPICLONE

Eszopiclone is used for the long-term treatment of insomnia and for sleep maintenance. It is prescribed to patients who have difficulty falling asleep as well as those who experience difficulty staying asleep, and is available in 1-, 2-, or 3-mg tablets.

Eszopiclone received FDA approval based on six randomized placebo-controlled clinical trials that showed it has efficacy in treating transient (Rosenberg et al., 2005) and chronic insomnia. In the transient insomnia study subjects receiving the drug showed a decreased latency to attain sleep, increased sleep efficiency, and fewer awakenings, as measured by both polysomnography and a morning questionnaire. There were no observed psychomotor aftereffects observed the next day. Eszopiclone also possesses efficacy as a sleep aid when taken chronically, for as long as 12 months (Melton et al., 2005). All chronic studies conducted to date found that eszopiclone decreased the latency to onset of sleep. No tolerance was observed, nor were signs of serious withdrawal, such as seizures or rebound insomnia, seen upon discontinuation of the drug. However, there are such reports for zopiclone, the racemate used outside the U.S. Mild withdrawal consisting of abnormal dreams, anxiety, nausea, and upset stomach can occur (rate ≤2%). A minor reported adverse effect of eszopiclone was a bitter taste. Eszopiclone is a schedule IV controlled substance in the U.S.

Eszopiclone is absorbed rapidly after oral administration, with a bioavailability of ~80%, and shows wide distribution throughout the body. It is 50-60% bound to plasma proteins and has a $t_{1/2}$ of ~6 hours. It is metabolized by CYPs 3A4 and 2E1. Eszopiclone is believed to exert its sleep-promoting effects through its enhancement of $GABA_A$ receptor function at the benzodiazepine binding site (Hanson et al., 2008; Jia et al., 2009),

FLUMAZENIL: A BENZODIAZEPINE RECEPTOR ANTAGONIST

Flumazenil (ROMAZICON, generic), the only member of this class, is an imidazobenzodiazepine (Table 17–1) that behaves as a specific benzodiazepine receptor antagonist (Hoffman and Warren, 1993). Flumazenil binds with high affinity to specific sites on the $GABA_A$ receptor, where it competitively antagonizes the binding and allosteric effects of benzodiazepines and other ligands. Flumazenil antagonizes both the electrophysiological and behavioral effects of agonist and inverse-agonist benzodiazepines and β-carbolines. The drug is given intravenously.

In animal models, the intrinsic pharmacological actions of flumazenil have been subtle; effects resembling those of inverse agonists sometimes have been detected at low doses, whereas slight benzodiazepine-like effects often have been evident at high doses. The evidence for intrinsic activity in human subjects is even more vague, except for modest anticonvulsant effects at high doses. However, anticonvulsant effects cannot be relied on for therapeutic utility because the administration of flumazenil may precipitate seizures under certain circumstances (discussed later).

Flumazenil is available only for intravenous administration. On intravenous administration, flumazenil is eliminated almost entirely by hepatic metabolism to inactive products with a $t_{1/2}$ of ~1 hour; the duration of clinical effects usually is only 30-60 minutes. Although absorbed rapidly after oral administration, <25% of the drug reaches the systemic circulation owing to extensive first-pass hepatic metabolism; effective oral doses are apt to cause headache and dizziness.

The primary indications for the use of flumazenil are the management of suspected benzodiazepine overdose and the reversal of sedative effects produced by benzodiazepines administered during either general anesthesia or diagnostic and/or therapeutic procedures.

The administration of a series of small injections is preferred to a single bolus injection. A total of 1 mg flumazenil given over 1-3 minutes usually is sufficient to abolish the effects of therapeutic doses of benzodiazepines; patients with suspected benzodiazepine overdose should respond adequately to a cumulative dose of 1-5 mg given over 2-10 minutes; a lack of response to 5 mg flumazenil strongly suggests that a benzodiazepine is not the major cause of sedation. Additional courses of treatment with flumazenil may be needed within 20-30 minutes should sedation reappear.

Flumazenil is not effective in single-drug overdoses with either barbiturates or tricyclic antidepressants. To the contrary, the administration of flumazenil in these settings may be associated with the onset of seizures, especially in patients poisoned with tricyclic antidepressants (Spivey, 1992). Seizures or other withdrawal symptoms also may be precipitated in patients who had been taking benzodiazepines for protracted periods and in whom tolerance and/or dependence may have developed.

MELATONIN CONGENERS

Ramelteon. Ramelteon (ROZEREM) is a synthetic tricyclic analog of melatonin with the chemical name (S)-*N*-[2-(1,6,7,8-tetrahydro-2*H*-indeno[5,4-b] furan-8-yl)ethyl] propionamide. It was approved in the U.S. in 2005 for the treatment of insomnia, specifically sleep onset difficulties. Unlike other drugs licensed by the FDA for insomnia, ramelteon is not a controlled substance.

MELATONIN RAMELTEON

Mechanism of Action. Melatonin levels in the suprachiastmatic nucleus rise and fall in a circadian fashion, with concentrations increasing in the evening as an individual prepares for sleep, and then reaching a plateau and ultimately decreasing as the night progresses. Two GPCRs for melatonin, MT_1 and MT_2, are found in the suprachiasmatic nucleus, each playing a different role in sleep. Binding of agonists, such as melatonin, to MT_1 receptors promotes the onset of sleep while melatonin binding to MT_2 receptors shifts the timing of the circadian system (Liu et al., 1997). Ramelteon binds to both MT_1 and MT_2 receptors with high affinity but, unlike melatonin, it does not bind appreciably to quinone reductase 2, the structurally unrelated MT_3 receptor (Nosjean et al., 2000). Ramelteon is not known to bind to any other classes of receptors, such as nicotinic acetylcholine, neuropeptide, dopamine, or opiate receptors, or the benzodiazepine-binding site on $GABA_A$ receptors.

Clinical Pharmacology. Prescribing guidelines suggest that an 8-mg tablet be taken ~30 minutes before bedtime. Ramelteon is rapidly absorbed from the GI tract and a peak serum concentration is obtained within an hour (Hibberd and Stevenson 2004). Because of the significant first-pass metabolism that occurs after oral administration, ramelteon bioavailability is <2% (Amakye et al., 2004). In the bloodstream, ~80% of ramelteon is protein bound (Takeda Pharmaceuticals North America, 2006). The drug is largely metabolized by the hepatic CYPs 1A2, 2C, and 3A4, with $t_{1/2}$ of ~2 hours in humans. Of the four metabolites, one, M-II, acts as an agonist at MT_1 and MT_2 receptors and may contribute to the sleep-promoting effects of ramelteon.

Ramelteon is efficacious in combating both transient and chronic insomnia. Subjects given 16 or 64 mg of ramelteon in a clinical trial showed a significantly shorter latency to sleep onset, as well as increased total sleep time, compared to placebo controls (Roth et al., 2005); the drug was generally well tolerated by patients and did not impair next-day cognitive function. Ramelteon is also useful in the treatment of chronic insomnia, with no tolerance occurring in its reduction of sleep onset latency even after 6 months of drug administration (Mayer et al., 2009). Sleep latency, evaluated by polysomnography as well as by subject questionnaires, was consistently found to be shorter in patients given ramelteon compared to placebo controls (Erman et al., 2006; Zammit et al., 2007). No evidence of rebound insomnia or withdrawal effects were noted upon ramelteon withdrawal. Ramelteon appears to act by producing a phase advance of the endogenous circadian rhythm (Richardson et al., 2008).

In animals, ramelteon does not produce discriminative stimulus effects similar to those of benzodiazepine receptor agonists, and long-term administration has no effects on spontaneous or operant behaviors, motor activity or posture (France et al., 2006). In addition, ramelteon has no demonstrated positive reinforcing effects in intravenous self-administration experiments performed in rhesus monkeys and there is no indication of abuse liability in humans (Griffiths and Johnson, 2005).

BARBITURATES

The barbiturates were once used extensively as sedative-hypnotic drugs. Except for a few specialized uses, they have been largely replaced by the much safer benzodiazepines.

Chemistry. Barbituric acid is 2,4,6-trioxohexahydropyrimidine. This compound lacks central depressant activity, but the presence of alkyl or aryl groups at position 5 confers sedative-hypnotic and sometimes other activities. The general structural formula for the barbiturates and the structures of selected compounds are included in Table 17–4.

Table 17–4

Structures, Trade Names, and Major Pharmacological Properties of Selected Barbiturates

(or S=)* O=C2 ring structure: R_3–N3–C(=O)–5C(R_{5a})(R_{5b})–C(=O)–N(H)–C2(=O)

COMPOUND (TRADE NAMES)	R_3	R_{5a}	R_{5b}	DOSAGE FORMS[b]	$t_{1/2}$ (hours)	THERAPEUTIC USES	COMMENTS
Amobarbital (AMYTAL)	—H	$—C_2H_5$	$—CH_2CH_2CH(CH_3)_2$	IM, IV	10-40	Insomnia, pre-op sedation, emergency management of seizures	Only Na^+ salt administered parenterally
Butabarbital (BUTISOL, others)	—H	$—C_2H_5$	$—CH(CH_3)CH_2CH_3$	Oral	35-50	Insomnia, pre-op sedation	Redistribution shortens duration of action of single dose to 8 hours
Mephobarbital (MEBARAL)	$—CH_3$	$—C_2H_5$	—phenyl (benzene ring)	Oral	10-70	Seizure disorders, daytime sedation	Second-line anticonvulsant
Methohexital (BREVITAL)	$—CH_3$	$—CH_2CH{=}CH_2$	$—CH(CH_3)C{\equiv}CCH_2CH_3$	IV	3-5[c]	Induction and maintenance of anesthesia	Only Na^+ salt available; single dose provides 5-7 min of anesthesia[c]
Pentobarbital (NEMBUTAL)	—H	$—C_2H_5$	$—CH(CH_3)CH_2CH_2CH_3$	Oral, IM, IV, rectal	15-50	Insomnia, pre-op sedation, emergency management of seizures	Only Na^+ salt administered parenterally
Phenobarbital (LUMINAL, others)	—H	$—C_2H_5$	—phenyl (benzene ring)	Oral, IM, IV	80-120	Seizure disorders, status epilepticus, daytime sedation	First-line anti-convulsant; only Na^+ salt administered parenterally
Secobarbital (SECONAL)	—H	$—CH_2CH{=}CH_2$	$—CH(CH_3)CH_2CH_2CH_3$	Oral	15-40	Insomnia, preoperative sedation	Only Na^+ salt available
Thiopental (PENTOTHAL)	—H	$—C_2H_5$	$—CH(CH_3)CH_2CH_2CH_3$	IV	8-10[c]	Induction/maintenance of anesthesia, pre-op sedation, emergency management of seizures	Only Na^+ salt available; single dose provides brief of anesthesia[c]

[a]O except in thiopental, where it is replaced by S. [b]IM, intramuscular injection; IV, intravenous administration. [c]Value represents terminal $t_{1/2}$ due to metabolism by the liver; redistribution following parenteral administration produces effects lasting only a few minutes

The carbonyl group at position 2 takes on acidic character because of lactam–lactim ("keto"–"enol") tautomerization, which is favored by its location between the two electronegative amido nitrogens. The lactim form is favored in alkaline solution, and salts result. Barbiturates in which the oxygen at C2 is replaced by sulfur sometimes are called *thiobarbiturates*. These compounds are more lipid-soluble than the corresponding *oxybarbiturates*. In general, structural changes that increase lipid solubility decrease duration of action, decrease latency to onset of activity, accelerate metabolic degradation, and increase hypnotic potency.

Pharmacological Properties

The barbiturates reversibly depress the activity of all excitable tissues. The CNS is exquisitely sensitive, and even when barbiturates are given in anesthetic concentrations, direct effects on peripheral excitable tissues are weak. However, serious deficits in cardiovascular and other peripheral functions occur in acute barbiturate intoxication.

Central Nervous System

Sites and Mechanisms of Action on the CNS. Barbiturates act throughout the CNS; non-anesthetic doses preferentially suppress polysynaptic responses. Facilitation is diminished, and inhibition usually is enhanced. The site of inhibition is either postsynaptic, as at cortical and cerebellar pyramidal cells and in the cuneate nucleus, substantia nigra, and thalamic relay neurons, or pre-synaptic, as in the spinal cord. Enhancement of inhibition occurs primarily at synapses where neurotransmission is mediated by GABA acting at $GABA_A$ receptors.

The barbiturates exert several distinct effects on excitatory and inhibitory synaptic transmission. For example, (–)-pentobarbital potentiates GABA-induced increases in chloride conductance and depresses voltage-activated Ca^{2+} currents at similar concentrations (below 10 μM) in isolated hippocampal neurons; above 100 μM, chloride conductance is increased in the absence of GABA (French-Mullen et al., 1993). Phenobarbital is less efficacious and much less potent in producing these effects, whereas (+)-pentobarbital has only weak activity. Thus, the more selective anticonvulsant properties of phenobarbital and its higher therapeutic index may be explained by its lower capacity to depress neuronal function as compared with the anesthetic barbiturates.

The mechanisms underlying the actions of barbiturates on $GABA_A$ receptors appear to be distinct from those of either GABA or the benzodiazepines for reasons that include the following:

- Like benzodiazepines, barbiturates enhance the binding of GABA to $GABA_A$ receptors in a Cl^--dependent and picrotoxin-sensitive fashion; however, barbiturates promote (rather than reduce) the binding of benzodiazepines.
- Barbiturates potentiate GABA-induced Cl^- currents by prolonging periods during which bursts of channel opening occur rather than by increasing the frequency of these bursts, as benzodiazepines do.
- Only α and β (not γ) subunits are required for barbiturate action.
- Barbiturate-induced increases in Cl^- conductance are not affected by the deletion of the tyrosine and threonine residues in the β subunit that govern the sensitivity of $GABA_A$ receptors to activation by agonists (Amin and Weiss, 1993).

Sub-anesthetic concentrations of barbiturates also can reduce glutamate-induced depolarizations (Macdonald and McLean, 1982) (Chapter 12); only the AMPA subtypes of glutamate receptors sensitive to kainic acid (Figure 14–10) or quisqualic acid appear to be affected (Marszalec and Narahashi, 1993). At higher concentrations that produce anesthesia, pentobarbital suppresses high-frequency repetitive firing of neurons, apparently as a result of inhibiting the function of voltage-dependent, tetrodotoxin-sensitive Na^+ channels (Figure 11–4); in this case, however, both stereoisomers are about equally effective (Frenkel et al., 1990). At still higher concentrations, voltage-dependent K^+ conductances are reduced. Taken together, the findings that barbiturates activate inhibitory $GABA_A$ receptors and inhibit excitatory AMPA receptors can explain their CNS-depressant effects (Saunders and Ho, 1990).

Barbiturates can produce all degrees of depression of the CNS, ranging from mild sedation to general anesthesia. The use of barbiturates for general anesthesia is discussed in Chapter 19. Certain barbiturates, particularly those containing a 5-phenyl substituent (e.g., phenobarbital and mephobarbital), have selective anticonvulsant activity (Chapter 21). The anti-anxiety properties of the barbiturates are inferior to those exerted by the benzodiazepines.

Except for the anticonvulsant activities of phenobarbital and its congeners, the barbiturates possess a low degree of selectivity and a narrow therapeutic index. Thus, it is not possible to achieve a desired effect without evidence of general depression of the CNS. Pain perception and reaction are relatively unimpaired until the moment of unconsciousness, and in small doses, barbiturates increase reactions to painful stimuli. Hence, they cannot be relied on to produce sedation or sleep in the presence of even moderate pain.

Effects on Stages of Sleep. Hypnotic doses of barbiturates increase the total sleep time and alter the stages of sleep in a dose-dependent manner. Like the benzodiazepines, these drugs decrease sleep latency, the number of awakenings, and the durations of REM and slow-wave sleep. During repetitive nightly administration, some tolerance to the effects on sleep occurs within a few days, and the effect on total sleep time may be reduced by as much as 50% after 2 weeks of use. Discontinuation leads to rebound increases in all the parameters reported to be decreased by barbiturates.

Tolerance. Pharmacodynamic (functional) and pharmacokinetic tolerance to barbiturates can occur. The former contributes more to the decreased effect than does the latter. With chronic administration of gradually increasing doses, pharmacodynamic tolerance continues to develop over a period of weeks to months, depending on the dosage schedule, whereas pharmacokinetic tolerance reaches its peak in a few days to a week. Tolerance to the effects on mood, sedation, and hypnosis occurs more readily and is greater than that to the anticonvulsant and lethal effects; thus, as tolerance increases, the therapeutic index decreases. Pharmacodynamic tolerance to barbiturates confers cross-tolerance to all general CNS-depressant drugs, including ethanol.

Abuse and Dependence. Like other CNS depressant drugs, barbiturates are abused, and some individuals develop a dependence on them (Chapter 24). Moreover, the barbiturates may have euphoriant effects.

Peripheral Nervous Structures. Barbiturates selectively depress transmission in autonomic ganglia and reduce nicotinic excitation by choline esters. This effect may account, at least in part, for the fall in blood pressure produced by intravenous oxybarbiturates and by severe barbiturate intoxication. At skeletal neuromuscular junctions, the blocking effects of both tubocurarine and decamethonium are enhanced during barbiturate anesthesia. These actions probably result from the capacity of barbiturates at hypnotic or anesthetic concentrations to inhibit the passage of current through nicotinic cholinergic receptors. Several distinct mechanisms appear to be involved, and little stereoselectivity is evident.

Respiration. Barbiturates depress both the respiratory drive and the mechanisms responsible for the rhythmic character of respiration. The neurogenic drive is diminished by hypnotic doses but usually no more so than during natural sleep. However, neurogenic drive is essentially eliminated by a dose three times greater than that used normally to induce sleep. Such doses also suppress the hypoxic drive and, to a lesser extent, the chemoreceptor drive. At still higher doses, the powerful hypoxic drive fails. However, the margin between the lighter planes of surgical anesthesia and dangerous respiratory depression is sufficient to permit the ultra-short-acting barbiturates to be used, with suitable precautions, as anesthetic agents.

The barbiturates only slightly depress protective reflexes until the degree of intoxication is sufficient to produce severe respiratory depression. Coughing, sneezing, hiccoughing, and laryngospasm may occur when barbiturates are employed as intravenous anesthetic agents. Indeed, laryngospasm is one of the chief complications of barbiturate anesthesia.

Cardiovascular System. When given orally in sedative or hypnotic doses, barbiturates do not produce significant overt cardiovascular effects except for a slight decrease in blood pressure and heart rate such as occurs in normal sleep. In general, the effects of thiopental anesthesia on the cardiovascular system are benign in comparison with those of the volatile anesthetic agents; there usually is either no change or a fall in mean arterial pressure (Chapter 19).

Apparently, a decrease in cardiac output usually is sufficient to offset an increase in peripheral resistance, which sometimes is accompanied by an increase in heart rate. Cardiovascular reflexes are obtunded by partial inhibition of ganglionic transmission. This is most evident in patients with congestive heart failure or hypovolemic shock, whose reflexes already are operating maximally and in whom barbiturates can cause an exaggerated fall in blood pressure. Because barbiturates also impair reflex cardiovascular adjustments to inflation of the lung, positive-pressure respiration should be used cautiously and only when necessary to maintain adequate pulmonary ventilation in patients who are anesthetized or intoxicated with a barbiturate.

Other cardiovascular changes often noted when thiopental and other intravenous thiobarbiturates are administered after conventional preanesthetic medication include decreased renal and cerebral blood flow with a marked fall in CSF pressure. Although cardiac arrhythmias are observed only infrequently, intravenous anesthesia with barbiturates can increase the incidence of ventricular arrhythmias, especially when epinephrine and halothane also are present. Anesthetic concentrations of barbiturates have direct electrophysiological effects on the heart; in addition to depressing Na^+ channels, they reduce the function of at least two types of K^+ channels (Nattel et al., 1990; Pancrazio et al., 1993). However, direct depression of cardiac contractility occurs only when doses several times those required to cause anesthesia are administered, which probably contributes to the cardiovascular depression that accompanies acute barbiturate poisoning.

GI Tract. The oxybarbiturates tend to decrease the tone of the GI musculature and the amplitude of rhythmic contractions. The locus of action is partly peripheral and partly central, depending on the dose. A hypnotic dose does not significantly delay gastric emptying in humans. The relief of various GI symptoms by sedative doses is probably largely due to the central-depressant action.

Liver. The best-known effects of barbiturates on the liver are those on the microsomal drug-metabolizing system (Chapter 6), a site at which significant drug-drug interactions can occur. These effects vary with the duration of exposure to the barbiturate.

Acutely, the barbiturates combine with several CYPs and inhibit the biotransformation of a number of other drugs and endogenous substrates, such as steroids; other substrates may reciprocally inhibit barbiturate biotransformations. Drug interactions may result even when the other substances and barbiturates are oxidized by different microsomal enzyme systems.

Chronic administration of barbiturates markedly increases the protein and lipid content of the hepatic smooth endoplasmic reticulum, as well as the activities of glucuronyl transferase and CYPs 1A2, 2C9, 2C19, and 3A4. The induction of these enzymes increases the metabolism of a number of drugs and endogenous substances, including steroid hormones, cholesterol, bile salts, and vitamins K and D. This also results in an increased rate of barbiturate metabolism, which partly accounts for tolerance to barbiturates. Many sedative-hypnotics, various anesthetics, and ethanol also are metabolized by and/or induce the microsomal enzymes, and some degree of cross-tolerance therefore can occur. *Not all microsomal biotransformations of drugs and endogenous substrates are affected equally, but a convenient rule of thumb is that at maximal induction in humans, the rates are approximately doubled.* The inducing effect is not limited to the microsomal enzymes; for example, there are increases in δ-aminolevulinic acid (ALA) synthetase, a mitochondrial enzyme, and aldehyde dehydrogenase, a cytosolic enzyme. The effect of barbiturates on ALA synthetase can cause dangerous disease exacerbations in persons with intermittent porphyria.

Kidney. Severe oliguria or anuria may occur in acute barbiturate poisoning largely as a result of the marked hypotension.

Absorption, Fate, and Excretion. For sedative-hypnotic use, the barbiturates usually are administered orally (Table 17–4). Such doses are absorbed rapidly and probably completely; Na^+ salts are absorbed more rapidly than the corresponding free acids, especially from liquid formulations. The onset of action varies from 10-60 minutes, depending on the agent and the formulation, and is delayed by the presence of food in the stomach. When necessary, intramuscular injections of solutions of the Na^+ salts should be placed deeply into large muscles to avoid the pain and possible necrosis that can result at more superficial sites. The intravenous route usually is reserved for the management of status epilepticus (phenobarbital sodium) or for the induction and/or maintenance of general anesthesia (e.g., thiopental or methohexital).

Barbiturates are distributed widely, and they readily cross the placenta. The highly lipid-soluble barbiturates, led by those used to induce anesthesia, undergo redistribution after intravenous injection. Uptake into less vascular tissues, especially muscle and fat, leads to a decline in the concentration of barbiturate in the plasma and brain. With thiopental and methohexital, this results in the awakening of patients within 5-15 minutes of the injection of the usual anesthetic doses (Chapter 19).

Except for the less lipid-soluble aprobarbital and phenobarbital, nearly complete metabolism and/or conjugation of barbiturates in the liver precedes their renal excretion. The oxidation of radicals at C5 is the most important biotransformation that terminates biological activity. Oxidation results in the formation of alcohols, ketones, phenols, or carboxylic acids, which may appear in the urine as such or as glucuronic acid conjugates. In some instances (e.g., phenobarbital), *N*-glycosylation is an important metabolic pathway. Other biotransformations include *N*-hydroxylation, desulfuration of thiobarbiturates to oxybarbiturates, opening of the barbituric acid ring, and *N*-dealkylation of *N*-alkyl barbiturates to active metabolites (e.g., mephobarbital to phenobarbital). About 25% of phenobarbital and nearly all of aprobarbital are excreted unchanged in the urine. Their renal excretion can be increased greatly by osmotic diuresis and/or alkalinization of the urine.

The metabolic elimination of barbiturates is more rapid in young people than in the elderly and infants, and $t_{1/2}$ are increased during pregnancy partly because of the expanded volume of distribution. Chronic liver disease, especially cirrhosis, often increases the $t_{1/2}$ of the biotransformable barbiturates. Repeated administration, especially of phenobarbital, shortens the $t_{1/2}$ of barbiturates that are metabolized as a result of the induction of microsomal enzymes.

None of the barbiturates used for hypnosis in the U.S. appears to have an elimination $t_{1/2}$ that is short enough for elimination to be virtually complete in 24 hours (Table 17–4). However, the relationship between duration of action and $t_{1/2}$ of elimination is complicated by the fact that enantiomers of optically active barbiturates often differ in both biological potencies and rates of biotransformation. *All of these barbiturates will accumulate during repetitive administration unless appropriate adjustments in dosage are made. Furthermore, the persistence of the drug in plasma during the day favors the development of tolerance and abuse.*

Therapeutic Uses

The major uses of individual barbiturates are listed in Table 17–4. As with the benzodiazepines, the selection of a particular barbiturate for a given therapeutic indication is based primarily on pharmacokinetic considerations.

CNS Uses. Benzodiazepines and other compounds for sedation have largely replaced barbiturates. Barbiturates, especially butabarbital and phenobarbital, are used sometimes to antagonize unwanted CNS-stimulant effects of various drugs, such as ephedrine, dextroamphetamine, and theophylline, although a preferred approach is adjustment of dosage or substitution of alternative therapy for the primary agents (see Chapter 24).

Untoward Effects

After-Effects. Drowsiness may last for only a few hours after a hypnotic dose of barbiturate, but residual CNS depression sometimes is evident the following day, and subtle distortions of mood and impairment of judgment and fine motor skills may be demonstrable. For example, a 200-mg dose of secobarbital has been shown to impair performance of driving or flying skills for 10-22 hours. Residual effects also may take the form of vertigo, nausea, vomiting, or diarrhea, or sometimes may be manifested as overt excitement. The user may awaken slightly intoxicated and feel euphoric and energetic; later, as the demands of daytime activities challenge possibly impaired faculties, the user may display irritability and temper.

Paradoxical Excitement. In some persons, barbiturates produce excitement rather than depression, and the patient may appear to be inebriated. This type of idiosyncrasy is relatively common among geriatric and debilitated patients and occurs most frequently with phenobarbital and *N*-methylbarbiturates. Barbiturates may cause restlessness, excitement, and even delirium when given in the presence of pain and may worsen a patient's perception of pain.

Hypersensitivity. Allergic reactions occur, especially in persons with asthma, urticaria, angioedema, or similar conditions. Hypersensitivity reactions include localized swellings, particularly of the eyelids, cheeks, or lips, and erythematous dermatitis. Rarely, exfoliative dermatitis may be caused by phenobarbital and can prove fatal; the skin eruption may be associated with fever, delirium, and marked degenerative changes in the liver and other parenchymatous organs.

Drug Interactions. Barbiturates combine with other CNS depressants to cause severe depression; ethanol is the most frequent offender, and interactions with first-generation antihistamines also are common. Isoniazid, methylphenidate, and monoamine oxidase inhibitors also increase the CNS-depressant effects.

Barbiturates competitively inhibit the metabolism of certain other drugs; however, the greatest number of drug interactions results from induction of hepatic CYPs and the accelerated disappearance of many drugs and endogenous substances. The metabolism of vitamins D and K is accelerated, which may hamper bone mineralization and lower Ca^{2+} absorption in patients taking phenobarbital and may be responsible for the reported coagulation defects in neonates whose mothers had been taking phenobarbital. Hepatic enzyme induction enhances metabolism of endogenous steroid hormones, which may cause endocrine disturbances, as well as of oral contraceptives, which may result in unwanted pregnancy. Barbiturates also induce the hepatic generation of toxic metabolites of chlorocarbons (chloroform, trichloroethylene, carbon tetrachloride) and consequently promote lipid peroxidation, which facilitates periportal necrosis of the liver caused by these agents.

Other Untoward Effects. Because barbiturates enhance porphyrin synthesis, they are absolutely contraindicated in patients with acute intermittent porphyria or porphyria variegata. In hypnotic doses, the effects of barbiturates on the control of respiration are minor; however, in the presence of pulmonary insufficiency, serious respiratory depression may occur, and the drugs thus are contraindicated. Rapid intravenous injection of a barbiturate may cause cardiovascular collapse before anesthesia ensues, so the CNS signs of depth of anesthesia may fail to give an adequate warning of impending toxicity. Blood pressure can fall to shock levels; even slow intravenous injection of barbiturates often produces apnea and occasionally laryngospasm, coughing, and other respiratory difficulties.

Barbiturate Poisoning. The incidence of barbiturate poisoning has declined markedly, largely as a result of their decreased use as sedative-hypnotic agents. Nevertheless, poisoning with barbiturates is a significant clinical problem, and death occurs in a few percent of cases (Gary and Tresznewksy, 1983). Most of the cases are the result of deliberate attempts at suicide, but some are from accidental poisonings in children or in drug abusers. The lethal dose of barbiturate varies, but severe poisoning is likely to occur when >10 times the full hypnotic dose has been ingested at once. If alcohol or other depressant drugs also are present, the concentrations that can cause death are lower.

In severe intoxication, the patient is comatose; respiration is affected early. Breathing may be either slow or rapid and shallow. Eventually, blood pressure falls because the effect of the drug and of hypoxia on medullary vasomotor centers; depression of cardiac contractility and sympathetic ganglia also contributes. Pulmonary complications (e.g., atelectasis, edema, and bronchopneumonia) and renal failure are likely to be the fatal complications of severe barbiturate poisoning.

The treatment of acute barbiturate intoxication is based on general supportive measures, which are applicable in most respects to poisoning by any CNS depressant. Hemodialysis or hemoperfusion is necessary only rarely, and the use of CNS stimulants is contraindicated because they increase the mortality rate. If renal and cardiac functions are satisfactory, and the patient is hydrated, forced diuresis and alkalinization of the urine will hasten the excretion of phenobarbital. Measures to prevent or treat atelectasis should be taken, and mechanical ventilation should be initiated when indicated. See Chapter 4, *Drug Toxicity and Poisoning*.

In severe acute barbiturate intoxication, circulatory collapse is a major threat. Often the patient is admitted to the hospital with severe hypotension or shock, and dehydration frequently is severe. Hypovolemia must be corrected, and if necessary, the blood pressure can be supported with dopamine. Acute renal failure consequent to shock and hypoxia accounts for perhaps one-sixth of the deaths. In the event of renal failure, hemodialysis should be instituted.

MISCELLANEOUS SEDATIVE-HYPNOTIC DRUGS

Many drugs with diverse structures have been used for their sedative-hypnotic properties, including ramelteon, paraldehyde, chloral hydrate, and meprobamate. With the exception of ramelteon and meprobamate, the pharmacological actions of these drugs generally resemble those of the barbiturates: they all are general CNS depressants that can produce profound hypnosis with little or no analgesia; their effects on the stages of sleep are similar to those of the barbiturates; their therapeutic index is limited, and acute intoxication, which produces respiratory depression and hypotension, is managed similarly to barbiturate poisoning; their chronic use can result in tolerance and physical dependence; and the syndrome after chronic use can be severe and life-threatening. The properties of meprobamate bear some resemblance to those of the benzodiazepines, but the drug has a distinctly higher potential for abuse and has less selective anti-anxiety effects.

The clinical use of these agents has decreased markedly, and deservedly so. Some of them may be useful in certain settings, particularly in hospitalized patients. The chemical structures and major pharmacological properties of paraldehyde, ethchlorvynol (PLACIDYL, others), chloral hydrate (NOCTEC, others), meprobamate, glutethimide, methyprylon, and ethinamate can be found in previous editions of this book.

Paraldehyde. Paraldehyde is a polymer of acetaldehyde, basically a cyclic polyether. It has a strong odor and a disagreeable taste. Orally, it is irritating to the throat and stomach, and it is not administered parenterally because of its injurious effects on tissues. Use of paraldehyde has been discontinued in the U.S.

Chloral Hydrate. Chloral hydrate is formed by adding one molecule of water to the carbonyl group of chloral (2,2,2-trichloroacetaldehyde). Chloral hydrate may be used to treat patients with paradoxical reactions to benzodiazepines. Chloral hydrate is reduced rapidly to the active compound, trichloroethanol (CCl_3CH_2OH), largely by hepatic alcohol dehydrogenase; significant amounts of chloral hydrate are not found in the blood after its oral administration. Therefore, its pharmacological effects probably are caused by trichloroethanol. Indeed, the latter compound can exert barbiturate-like effects on $GABA_A$ receptor channels *in vitro* (Lovinger et al., 1993).

Chloral hydrate is best known in the U.S. as a literary poison, the "knock-out drops" added to a strong alcoholic beverage to produce a "Mickey Finn" or "Mickey," a cocktail given to an unwitting imbiber to render him malleable or unconscious, most famously Sam Spade in Dashiell Hammett's 1930 novel, *The Maltese Falcon*. Now that detectives drink wine rather than whiskey, this off-label use of chloral hydrate has waned.

Meprobamate. Meprobamate a *bis*-carbamate ester, was introduced as an anti-anxiety agent and this remains its only approved use in the U.S. However, it also became popular as a sedative-hypnotic drug and is discussed here mainly because of its continued use for such purposes. The question of whether the sedative and anti-anxiety actions of meprobamate differ is unanswered, and clinical proof for the efficacy of meprobamate as a selective anti-anxiety agent in humans is lacking.

The pharmacological properties of meprobamate resemble those of the benzodiazepines in a number of ways. Meprobamate can release suppressed behaviors in experimental animals at doses that cause little impairment of locomotor activity, and although it can cause widespread depression of the CNS, it cannot produce anesthesia. However, ingestion of large doses of meprobamate alone can cause severe or even fatal respiratory depression, hypotension, shock, and heart failure. Meprobamate appears to have a mild analgesic effect in patients with musculoskeletal pain, and it enhances the analgesic effects of other drugs.

Meprobamate is well absorbed when administered orally. Nevertheless, an important aspect of intoxication with meprobamate is the formation of gastric bezoars consisting of undissolved meprobamate tablets; hence treatment may require endoscopy, with mechanical removal of the bezoar. Most of the drug is metabolized in the liver, mainly to a side-chain hydroxy derivative and a glucuronide; the kinetics of elimination may depend on the dose. The $t_{1/2}$ of meprobamate may be prolonged during its chronic administration, even though the drug can induce some hepatic CYPs.

The major unwanted effects of the usual sedative doses of meprobamate are drowsiness and ataxia; larger doses produce considerable impairment of learning and motor coordination and prolongation of reaction time. Like the benzodiazepines, meprobamate enhances the CNS depression produced by other drugs.

The abuse of meprobamate has continued despite a substantial decrease in the clinical use of the drug. Carisoprodol (SOMA), a skeletal muscle relaxant whose active metabolite is meprobamate, also has abuse potential and has become a popular "street drug" (Reeves et al., 1999). Meprobamate is preferred to the benzodiazepines by subjects with a history of drug abuse. After long-term medication, abrupt discontinuation evokes a withdrawal syndrome usually characterized by anxiety, insomnia, tremors, and, frequently, hallucinations; generalized seizures occur in ~10% of cases. The intensity of symptoms depends on the dosage ingested.

Other Agents. Etomidate (AMIDATE, generic) is used in the U.S. and other countries as an intravenous anesthetic, often in combination with fentanyl. It is advantageous because it lacks pulmonary and vascular depressant activity, although it has a negative inotropic effect on the heart. Its pharmacology and anesthetic uses are described in Chapter 13. It also is used in some countries as a sedative-hypnotic drug in intensive care units, during intermittent positive-pressure breathing, in epidural anesthesia, and in other situations. Because it is administered only intravenously, its use is limited to hospital settings. The myoclonus commonly seen after anesthetic doses is not seen after sedative-hypnotic doses.

Clomethiazole has sedative, muscle relaxant, and anticonvulsant properties. It is used outside the U.S. for hypnosis in elderly and institutionalized patients, for preanesthetic sedation, and especially in the management of withdrawal from ethanol (Symposium, 1986b). Given alone, its effects on respiration are slight, and the therapeutic index is high. However, deaths from adverse interactions with ethanol are relatively frequent.

Propofol (DIPRIVAN) is a rapidly acting and highly lipophilic diisopropylphenol used in the induction and maintenance of general anesthesia (Chapter 19), as well as in the maintenance of long-term sedation. Propofol sedation is of a similar quality to that produced by midazolam. Emergence from sedation occurs quickly owing to its rapid clearance (McKeage and Perry, 2003). Propofol has found use in intensive care sedation in adults (McKeage and Perry, 2003), as well as for sedation during gastrointestinal endoscopy procedures (Heuss and Inauen, 2004) and transvaginal oocyte retrieval (Dell and Cloote, 1998). Although its mechanism of action is not understood completely, propofol is believed to act primarily through enhancement of $GABA_A$ receptor function. Effects on other ligand-gated channels and GPCRs also have been reported (Trapani et al., 2000).

Nonprescription Hypnotic Drugs. As part of the ongoing systematic review of over-the-counter (OTC) drug products, the FDA has ruled that diphenhydramine is the only antihistamine that is recognized as generally safe and effective for use in nonprescription sleep aids. Despite the prominent sedative side effects encountered during the use of doxylamine and pyrilamine, these agents subsequently were eliminated as ingredients in the OTC nighttime sleep aids marketed in the U.S.. In 2004, doxylamine regained FDA approval as an OTC sleep aid and re-entered the market as Unisom Nighttime Sleep Aid (doxylamine 25-mg tablets). With elimination $t_{1/2}$ of ~9 hours (diphenhydramine) and 10 hours (doxylamine), these antihistamines can be associated with prominent residual daytime sleepiness when taken the prior evening as a sleep aid.

MANAGEMENT OF INSOMNIA

Insomnia is one of the most common complaints in general medical practice, and its treatment is predicated on proper diagnosis. Although the precise function of sleep is not known, adequate sleep improves the quality of daytime wakefulness, and hypnotics should be used judiciously to avoid its impairment.

A number of pharmacological agents are available for the treatment of insomnia. The "perfect" hypnotic would allow sleep to occur with normal sleep architecture rather than produce a pharmacologically altered sleep pattern. It would not cause next-day effects, either of rebound anxiety or of continued sedation. It would not interact with other medications. It could be used chronically without causing dependence or rebound insomnia on discontinuation. Regular moderate exercise meets these criteria but often is not effective by itself, and many patients may not be able to exercise. However, even small amounts of exercise often are effective in promoting sleep.

Controversy in the management of insomnia revolves around two issues:

- Pharmacological versus nonpharmacological treatment
- Use of short-acting versus long-acting hypnotics

The side effects of hypnotic medications must be weighed against the sequelae of chronic insomnia, which include a 4-fold increase in serious accidents (Balter and Uhlenhuth, 1992). In addition to appropriate pharmacological treatment, the management of insomnia should correct identifiable causes, address inadequate sleep hygiene, eliminate performance anxiety related to falling asleep, provide entrainment of the biological clock so that maximum sleepiness occurs at the hour of attempted sleep, and suppress the use of alcohol and OTC sleep medications (Nino-Murcia, 1992).

Categories of Insomnia. The National Institute of Mental Health Consensus Development Conference (1984) divided insomnia into three categories:

- *Transient insomnia* lasts <3 days and usually is caused by a brief environmental or situational stressor. It may respond to attention to sleep hygiene rules. If hypnotics are prescribed, they should be used at the lowest dose and for only 2-3 nights. However, benzodiazepines given acutely before important life events, such as examinations, may result in impaired performance (James and Savage, 1984).
- *Short-term insomnia* lasts from 3 days to 3 weeks and usually is caused by a personal stressor such as illness, grief, or job problems. Again, sleep hygiene education is the first step. Hypnotics may be used adjunctively for 7-10 nights. Hypnotics are best used intermittently during this time, with the patient skipping a dose after 1-2 nights of good sleep.
- *Long-term insomnia* is insomnia that has lasted for >3 weeks; no specific stressor may be identifiable. A more complete medical evaluation is necessary in these patients, but most do not need an all-night sleep study.

Insomnia Accompanying Major Psychiatric Illnesses. The insomnia caused by major psychiatric illnesses often responds to specific pharmacological treatment for that illness. In major depressive episodes with insomnia, e.g., the selective serotonin reuptake inhibitors, which may cause insomnia as a side effect, usually will result in improved sleep because they treat the depressive syndrome. In patients whose depression is responding to the serotonin reuptake inhibitor but who have persistent insomnia as a side effect of the medication, judicious use of evening trazodone may improve sleep (Nierenberg et al., 1994), as well as augment the antidepressant effect of the reuptake inhibitor. However, the patient should be monitored for priapism, orthostatic hypotension, and arrhythmias.

Adequate control of anxiety in patients with anxiety disorders often produces adequate resolution of the accompanying insomnia. Sedative use in the anxiety disorders is decreasing because of a growing appreciation of the effectiveness of other agents, such as β adrenergic receptor antagonists (Chapter 12) for performance anxiety and serotonin reuptake inhibitors for obsessive-compulsive disorder and perhaps generalized anxiety disorder. The profound insomnia of patients with acute psychosis owing to schizophrenia or mania usually responds to dopamine-receptor antagonists (Chapters 13 and 16). Benzodiazepines often are used adjunctively in this situation to reduce agitation; their use also will result in improved sleep.

Insomnia Accompanying Other Medical Illnesses. For long-term insomnia owing to other medical illnesses, adequate treatment of the underlying disorder, such as congestive heart failure, asthma, or COPD, may resolve the insomnia.

Adequate pain management in conditions of chronic pain, including terminal cancer pain, will treat both the pain and the insomnia and may make hypnotics unnecessary.

Many patients simply manage their sleep poorly. *Adequate attention to sleep hygiene, including reduced caffeine intake, avoidance of alcohol, adequate exercise, and regular sleep and wake times, often will reduce the insomnia.*

Conditioned (Learned) Insomnia. In those who have no major psychiatric or other medical illness and in whom attention to sleep hygiene is ineffective, attention should be directed to conditioned (learned) insomnia. These patients have associated the bedroom with activities consistent with wakefulness rather than sleep. In such patients, the bed should be used only for sex and sleep. All other activities associated with waking, even such quiescent activities as reading and watching television, should be done outside the bedroom.

Sleep-State Misperception. Some patients complain of poor sleep but have been shown to have no objective polysomnographic evidence of insomnia. They are difficult to treat.

Long-Term Insomnia. Nonpharmacological treatments are important for all patients with long-term insomnia. These include education about sleep hygiene, adequate exercise (where possible), relaxation training, and behavioral-modification approaches, such as sleep-restriction and stimulus-control therapies. In sleep-restriction therapy, the patient keeps a diary of the amount of time spent in bed and then chooses a time in bed of 30-60 minutes less than this time. This induces a mild sleep debt, which aids sleep onset. In stimulus-control therapy, the patient is instructed to go to bed only when sleepy, to use the bedroom only for sleep and sex, to get up and leave the bedroom if sleep does not occur within 15-20 minutes, to return to bed again only when sleepy, to arise at the same time each morning regardless of sleep quality the preceding night, and to avoid daytime naps. Nonpharmacological treatments for insomnia have been found to be particularly effective in reducing sleep-onset latency and time awake after sleep onset (Morin et al., 1994).

Side effects of hypnotic agents may limit their usefulness for insomnia management. The use of hypnotics for long-term insomnia is problematic for many reasons. Long-term hypnotic use leads to a decrease in effectiveness and may produce rebound insomnia on discontinuance. Almost all hypnotics change sleep architecture. The barbiturates reduce REM sleep; the benzodiazepines reduce slow-wave non-REM sleep and, to a lesser extent, REM sleep. While the significance of these findings is not clear, there is an emerging consensus that slow-wave sleep is particularly important for physical restorative processes. REM sleep may aid in the consolidation of learning. The blockade of slow-wave sleep by benzodiazepines may partly account for their diminishing effectiveness over the long term, and it also may explain their effectiveness in blocking sleep terrors, a disorder of arousal from slow-wave sleep.

Long-acting benzodiazepines can cause next-day confusion, with a concomitant increase in falls, whereas shorter-acting agents can produce rebound next-day anxiety. Paradoxically, the acute amnestic effects of benzodiazepines may be responsible for the patient's subsequent report of restful sleep. Triazolam has been postulated to induce cognitive changes that blur the subjective distinction between waking and sleeping (Mendelson, 1993). Anterograde amnesia may be more common with triazolam. While the performance-disruptive effects of alcohol and diphenhydramine are reduced after napping, those of triazolam are not (Roehrs et al., 1993).

Benzodiazepines may worsen sleep apnea. Some hypersomnia patients do not feel refreshed after a night's sleep and so may ask for sleeping pills to improve the quality of their sleep. The consensus is that hypnotics should not be given to patients with sleep apnea, especially of the obstructive type, because these agents decrease upper airway muscle tone while also decreasing the arousal response to hypoxia (Robinson and Zwillich, 1989). These individuals benefit from all-night sleep studies to guide treatment.

Insomnia in Older Patients. The elderly, like the very young, tend to sleep in a *polyphasic* (multiple sleep episodes per day) pattern rather than the *monophasic* pattern characteristic of younger adults. They may have single or multiple daytime naps in addition to nighttime sleep. This pattern makes assessment of adequate sleep time difficult. Anyone who naps regularly will have shortened nighttime sleep without evidence of impaired daytime wakefulness, regardless of age. This pattern is exemplified in "siesta" cultures and probably is adaptive.

Changes in the pharmacokinetic profiles of hypnotic agents occur in the elderly because of reduced body water, reduced renal function, and increased body fat, leading to a longer $t_{1/2}$ for benzodiazepines. A dose that produces pleasant sleep and adequate daytime wakefulness during week 1 of administration may produce daytime confusion and amnesia by week 3 as the level continues to rise, particularly with long-acting hypnotics. For example, the benzodiazepine diazepam is highly lipid soluble and is excreted by the kidney. Because of the increase in body fat and the decrease in renal excretion that typically occur from age 20-80, the $t_{1/2}$ of the drug may increase 4-fold over this span.

Elderly people who are living full lives with relatively unimpaired daytime wakefulness may complain of insomnia because they are not sleeping as long as they did when they were younger. Injudicious use of hypnotics in these individuals can produce daytime cognitive impairment and so impair overall quality of life.

Once an older patient has been taking benzodiazepines for an extended period, whether for daytime anxiety or for nighttime sedation, terminating the drug can be a long, involved process. Since attempts at drug withdrawal may not be successful, it may be necessary to leave the patient on the medication, with adequate attention to daytime side effects.

Management of Patients After Long-Term Treatment with Hypnotic Agents. Patients who have been taking hypnotics for many months or even years pose a special problem (Fleming, 1993). If a benzodiazepine has been used regularly for >2 weeks, it should be tapered rather than discontinued abruptly. In some patients on hypnotics with a short $t_{1/2}$, it is easier to switch first to a hypnotic with a long $t_{1/2}$ and then to taper. The onset of withdrawal symptoms from medications with a long $t_{1/2}$ may be delayed. Consequently, the patient should be warned about the symptoms associated with withdrawal effects.

Prescribing Guidelines for the Management of Insomnia. Hypnotics that act at $GABA_A$ receptors, including the benzodiazepine hypnotics and the newer agents zolpidem, zopiclone, and zaleplon, are preferred to barbiturates because they have a greater therapeutic index, are less toxic in overdose, have smaller effects on sleep architecture, and have less abuse potential. Compounds with a shorter $t_{1/2}$ are favored in patients with sleep-onset insomnia but without significant daytime anxiety who need to function at full effectiveness during the day. These compounds also are appropriate for the elderly because of a decreased risk of falls and respiratory depression. However, the patient and physician should be aware that early-morning awakening, rebound daytime anxiety, and amnestic episodes also may occur. These undesirable side effects are more common at higher doses of the benzodiazepines.

Benzodiazepines with longer $t_{1/2}$ are favored for patients who have significant daytime anxiety and who may be able to tolerate next-day sedation but would be impaired further by rebound daytime anxiety. These benzodiazepines also are appropriate for patients receiving treatment for major depressive episodes because the short-acting agents can worsen early-morning awakening. However, longer-acting benzodiazepines can be associated with next-day cognitive impairment or delayed daytime cognitive impairment (after 2-4 weeks of treatment) as a result of drug accumulation with repeated administration.

Older agents such as barbiturates, chloral hydrate, and meprobamate should be avoided for the management of insomnia. They have high abuse potential and are dangerous in overdose.

Amakye DD, Hibberd M, Stevenson SJ. A phase I study to investigate the absolute bioavailability of a single oral dose of ramelteon (TAK-375) in healthy male subjects. *Sleep,* **2004,** *27*(Abstract Suppl):A54.

Amin J, Weiss DS. $GABA_A$ receptor needs two homologous domains of the *β*-subunit for activation by GABA but not by pentobarbital. *Nature,* **1993,** *366*:565–569.

Balter MB, Uhlenhuth EH. New epidemiologic findings about insomnia and its treatment. *J Clin Psychiatry,* **1992,** *53*(Suppl):34–39.

Burt DR. Reducing GABA receptors. *Life Sci,* **2003,** *73*:1741–1758.

Cavallaro R, Regazzetti MG, Covelli G, Smeraldi E. Tolerance and withdrawal with zolpidem. *Lancet,* **1993,** *342*:374–375.

Dell RG, Cloote AH. Patient-controlled sedation during transvaginal oocyte retrieval: An assessment of patient acceptance of patient-controlled sedation using a mixture of propofol and alfentanil. *Eur J Anaesthesiol,* **1998,** *15*:210–215.

Dement WC. Objective measurements of daytime sleepiness and performance comparing quazepam with flurazepam in two adult populations using the Multiple Sleep Latency Test. *J Clin Psychiatry,* **1991,** *52*(Suppl):31–37.

Dooley M, Plosker GL. Zaleplon: A review of its use in the treatment of insomnia. *Drugs,* **2000,** *60*:413–445.

Dresser GK, Spence JD, Bailey DG. Pharmacokinetic–pharmacodynamic consequences and clinical relevance of cytochrome P450 3A4 inhibition. *Clin Pharmacokinet,* **2000,** *38*:41–57.

Dujardin K, Guieu JD, Leconte-Lambert C, et al. Comparison of the effects of zolpidem and flunitrazepam on sleep structure and daytime cognitive functions: A study of untreated insomniacs. *Pharmacopsychiatry,* **1998,** *31*:14–18.

Erman M, Seiden D, Zammit G, et al. An efficacy, safety, and dose response study of ramelteon in patients with chronic primary insomnia. *Sleep Med,* **2006,** *7*:17–24.

Essrich C, Lorez M, Benson JA, et al. Postsynaptic clustering of major $GABA_A$ receptor subtypes requires the *γ*2 subunit and gephyrin. *Nature Neurosci,* **1998,** *1*:563–571.

File SE. Tolerance to the behavioral actions of benzodiazepines. *Neurosci Biobehav Rev,* **1985,** *9*:113–121.

Fleming JA. The difficult to treat insomniac patient. *J Psychosom Res,* **1993,** *37*(Suppl 1):45–54.

France CP, Weltman RH, Koek W, et al. Acute and chronic effects of ramelteon in rhesus monkeys (macaca mulatta): Dependence liability studies. *Behav Neurosci,* **2006,** *120*:535–541.

ffrench-Mullen JM, Barker JL, Rogawski MA. Calcium current block by (–)-pentobarbital, phenobarbital, and CHEB but not (+)-pentobarbital in acutely isolated hippocampal CA1 neurons: Comparison with effects on GABA-activated Cl^- current. *J Neurosci,* **1993,** *13*:3211–3221.

Frenkel C, Duch DS, Urban BW. Molecular actions of pentobarbital isomers on sodium channels from human brain cortex. *Anesthesiology,* **1990,** *72*:640–649.

Garnier R, Guerault E, Muzard D, et al. Acute zolpidem poisoning—analysis of 344 cases. *J Toxicol Clin Toxicol,* **1994,** *32*: 391–404.

Gary NE, Tresznewsky O. Clinical aspects of drug intoxication: Barbiturates and a potpourri of other sedatives, hypnotics, and tranquilizers. *Heart Lung,* **1983,** *12*:122–127.

Gillin JC, Spinweber CL, Johnson LC. Rebound insomnia: A critical review. *J Clin Psychopharmacol,* **1989,** *9*:161–172.

Greenblatt DJ. Benzodiazepine hypnotics: Sorting the pharmacokinetic facts. *J Clin Psychiatry,* **1991,** *52*(Suppl):4–10.

Griffiths RR, Johnson MW. Relative abuse liability of hypnotic drugs: A conceptual framework and algorithm for differentiating among compounds. *J Clin Psychiatry,* **2005,** *66*(Suppl 9): 31–41.

Griffiths RR, Sannerud CA, Ator NA, Brady JV. Zolpidem behavioral pharmacology in baboons: Self-injection, discrimination, tolerance and withdrawal. *J Pharmacol Exp Ther,* **1992,** *260*:1199–1208.

Guglielminotti J, Maury E, Alzieu M, et al. Prolonged sedation requiring mechanical ventilation and continuous flumazenil infusion after routine doses of clonazepam for alcohol withdrawal syndrome. *Intensive Care Med,* **1999,** *25*:1435–1436.

Hanson SM, Morlock EV, Satyshur KA, et al. Structural requirements for eszopiclone and zolpidem binding to the gamma-aminobutyric acid type-A ($GABA_A$) receptor are different. *J Med Chem,* **2008,** *51*:7243–7252.

Herrmann WM, Kubicki ST, Boden S, et al. Pilot controlled, double-blind study of the hypnotic effects of zolpidem in patients with chronic "learned" insomnia: Psychometric and polysomnographic evaluation. *J Int Med Res,* **1993,** *21*: 306–322.

Heuss LT, Inauen W. The dawning of a new sedative: Propofol in gastrointestinal endoscopy. *Digestion,* **2004,** *69*:20–26.

Hibberd M, Stevenson SJ. A phase-I open-label study of the absorption, metabolism, and excretion of (14C)-ramelteon (TAK-375) following a single oral dose in healthy male subjects. *Sleep,* **2004,** *27*(Abstract Suppl):A54

Hindmarch I, Fairweather DB, Rombaut N. Adverse events after triazolam substitution. *Lancet,* **1993,** *341*:55.

Hoffman, E.J., and Warren, E.W. Flumazenil: A benzodiazepine antagonist. *Clin Pharmacol,* **1993,** *12*:641–656.

Holm KJ, Goa KL. Zolpidem: An update of its pharmacology, therapeutic efficacy and tolerability in the treatment of insomnia. *Drugs,* **2000,** *59*:865–889.

James I, Savage I. Beneficial effect of nadolol on anxiety-induced disturbances of performance in musicians: A comparison with diazepam and placebo. *Am Heart J,* **1984,** *108*: 1150–1155.

Jia F, Goldstein PA, Harrison NL.The modulation of synaptic $GABA_A$ receptors in the thalamus by eszopiclone and zolpidem. *J Pharmacol Exp Ther,* **2009,** *328*:1000–1006.

Jonas JM, Coleman BS, Sheridan AQ, Kalinske RW. Comparative clinical profiles of triazolam versus other shorter-acting hypnotics. *J Clin Psychiatry,* **1992,** *53*(Suppl):19–31.

Kato K, Hirai K, Nishiyama K, et al. Neurochemical properties of ramelteon (TAK-375), a selective MT1/MT2 receptor agonist. *Neuropharmacology,* **2005,** *48*:301–310.

Kleingoor C, Wieland HA, Korpi ER, et al. Current potentiation by diazepam but not GABA sensitivity is determined by a single histidine residue. *Neuroreport,* **1993,** *4*:187–190.

Kriel RL, Cloyd JC, Pellock JM. Respiratory depression in children receiving diazepam for acute seizures: A prospective study. *Dev Med Child Neurol,* **2000,** *42*:429–430.

Kummer J, Guendel L, Linden J, et al. Long-term polysomnographic study of the efficacy and safety of zolpidem in elderly psychiatric in-patients with insomnia. *J Int Med Res,* **1993,** *21*:171–184.

Lader M, File S. The biological basis of benzodiazepine dependence. *Psychol Med,* **1987,** *17*:539–547.

Langtry HD, Benfield P. Zolpidem: A review of its pharmacodynamic and pharmacokinetic properties and therapeutic potential. *Drugs,* **1990,** *40*:291–313.

Laurijssens BE, Greenblatt DJ. Pharmacokinetic–pharmacodynamic relationships for benzodiazepines (review). *Clin Pharmacokinet*, **1996**, *30*:52–76.

Liu C, Weaver DR, Jin X, *et al*. Molecular dissection of two distinct actions of melatonin on the suprachiasmatic circadian clock. *Neuron,* **1997,** *19:*91–102.

Lovinger DM, Zimmerman SA, Levitin M, et al. Trichloroethanol potentiates synaptic transmission mediated by γ-aminobutyric acid$_A$ receptors in hippocampal neurons. *J Pharmacol Exp Ther,* **1993,** *264*:1097–1103.

Lüddens H, Pritchett DB, Köhler M, et al. Cerebellar GABA$_A$ receptor selective for a behavioural alcohol antagonist. *Nature,* **1990,** *346*:648–651.

Macdonald RL, McLean MJ. Cellular bases of barbiturate and phenytoin anticonvulsant drug action. *Epilepsia,* **1982,** *23*(Suppl 1):S7–S18.

Marszalec W, Narahashi T. Use-dependent pentobarbital block of kainate and quisqualate currents. *Brain Res,* **1993,** *608*:7–15.

Mayer G, Wang-Weigand S, Roth-Schechter B, et al. Efficacy and safety of 6-month nightly ramelteon administration in adults with chronic primary insomnia. *Sleep,* **2009,** *32:* 351–360.

McKeage K, Perry CM. Propofol: A review of its use in intensive care sedation of adults. *CNS Drugs,* **2003,** *17*:235–272.

Melton ST, Wood JM, Kirkwood CK, et al. Eszopiclone for Insomnia. *Ann Pharmacother*, **2005,** *39:*1659–1666.

Mendelson WB. Pharmacologic alteration of the perception of being awake or asleep. *Sleep,* **1993,** *16*:641–646.

Meyer BR. Benzodiazepines in the elderly. *Med Clin North Am,* **1982,** *66*:1017–1035.

Mitler MM. Nonselective and selective benzodiazepine receptor agonists—where are we today? *Sleep,* **2000,** *23*(Suppl 1): S39–S47.

Monane M. Insomnia in the elderly. *J Clin Psychiatry,* **1992,** *53*(Suppl):23–28.

Morin CM, Culbert JP, Schwartz SM. Nonpharmacological interventions for insomnia: A meta-analysis of treatment efficacy. *Am J Psychiatry,* **1994,** *151*:1172–1180.

Morselli PL. Zolpidem side effects. *Lancet,* **1993,** *342*:868–869.

National Institute of Mental Health Consensus Development Conference. Drugs and insomnia: The use of medications to promote sleep. *JAMA,* **1984,** *251*:2410–2414.

Nattel S, Wang ZG, Matthews C. Direct electrophysiological actions of pentobarbital at concentrations achieved during general anesthesia. *Am J Physiol,* **1990,** *259*:H1743–H1751.

Nierenberg AA, Adler LA, Peselow E, et al. Trazodone for antidepressant-associated insomnia. *Am J Psychiatry,* **1994,** *151*:1069–1072.

Nino-Murcia G. Diagnosis and treatment of insomnia and risks associated with lack of treatment. *J Clin Psychiatry,* **1992,** *53*(Suppl):43–47.

Nosjean O, Ferro M, Coge F, et al. Identification of the melatonin binding site MT3 as the quinone reductase 2. *J Biol Chem,* **2000,** *275:*31311–31317.

Nugent M, Artru AA, Michenfelder JD. Cerebral metabolic, vascular and protective effects of midazolam maleate: Comparison to diazepam. *Anesthesiology,* **1982,** *56*:172–176.

Oldenhof H, de Jong M, Steenhoek A, Janknegt R. Clinical pharmacokinetics of midazolam in intensive care patients, a wide interpatient variability? *Clin Pharmacol Ther,* **1988,** *43*:263–269.

Pancrazio JJ, Frazer MJ, Lynch C III. Barbiturate anesthetics depress the resting K$^+$ conductance of myocardium. *J Pharmacol Exp Ther,* **1993,** *265*:358–365.

Perrault G, Morel E, Sanger DJ, Zivkovic B. Lack of tolerance and physical dependence upon repeated treatment with the novel hypnotic zolpidem. *J Pharmacol Exp Ther,* **1992,** *263*:298–303.

Petursson H. The benzodiazepine withdrawal syndrome. *Addiction,* **1994,** *89*:1455–1459.

Pritchett DB, Seeburg PH. γ-Aminobutyric acid A receptor α5-subunit creates novel type II benzodiazepine receptor pharmacology. *J Neurochem,* **1990,** *54*:1802–1804.

Reeves RR, Carter OS, Pinkofsky HB, et al. Carisoprodol (SOMA): Abuse potential and physician unawareness. *J Addict Dis,* **1999,** *18*:51–56.

Richardson GS, Zee PC, Wang-Weigand S, et al. Circadian phase-shifting effects of repeated ramelteon administration in healthy adults. *J Clin Sleep Med*, **2008,** *4:*456–461.

Robinson RW, Zwillich CW. The effect of drugs on breathing during sleep. In, *Principles and Practice of Sleep Medicine.* (Kryger MH, Roth T, Dement WC, eds.) Saunders, Philadelphia, **1989.**

Roehrs T, Claiborue D, Knox M, Roth T. Effects of ethanol, diphenhydramine, and triazolam after a nap. *Neuropsychopharmacology,* **1993,** *9*:239–245.

Rosenberg R, Caron J, Roth T, et al. An assessment of the efficacy and safety of eszopiclone in the treatment of transient insomnia in healthy adults. *Sleep Med,* **2005,** *6:*15–22.

Roth T, Roehrs TA. Issues in the use of benzodiazepine therapy. *J Clin Psychiatry,* **1992,** *53*(Suppl):14–18.

Roth T, Stubbs C, Walsh JK. Ramelteon (TAK-375), a selective MT1/MT2-receptor agonist, reduces latency to persistent sleep in a model of transient insomnia related to a novel sleep environment. *Sleep,* **2005,** *28:*303–307.

Rothschild AJ. Disinhibition, amnestic reactions, and other adverse reactions secondary to triazolam: A review of the literature. *J Clin Psychiatry,* **1992,** *53*(Suppl):69–79.

Saunders PA, Ho IK. Barbiturates and the GABA$_A$ receptor complex. *Prog Drug Res,* **1990,** *34*:261–286.

Sieghart W, Fuchs K, Tretter V, et al. Structure and subunit composition of GABA$_A$ receptors. *Neurochem Int,* **1999,** *34*: 379–385.

Spivey WH. Flumazenil and seizures: An analysis of 43 cases. *Clin Ther,* **1992,** *14*:292–305.

Symposium (various authors). Modern hypnotics and performance. (Nicholson A, Hippius H, Rüther E, Dunbar G, eds.) *Acta Psychiatr Scand Suppl,* **1986a,** *332*:3–174.

Symposium (various authors). Chlormethiazole 25 years: Recent developments and historical perspectives. (Evans JG, Feuerlein W, Glatt MM, *et al.,* eds.) *Acta Psychiatr Scand Suppl,* **1986b,** *329*:1–198.

Takeda Pharmaceuticals North America. Rozerem prescribing information. **2006.**

Tanaka E. Clinically significant pharmacokinetic drug interactions with benzodiazepines. *J Clin Pharm Ther,* **1999,** *24*: 347–355.

Trapani G, Altomare C, Liso G, et al. Propofol in anesthesia: Mechanism of action, structure–activity relationships, and drug delivery. *Curr Med Chem,* **2000,** *7*:249–271.

Twyman RE, Rogers CJ, Macdonald RL. Differential regulation of -aminobutyric acid receptor channels by diazepam and phenobarbital. *Ann Neurol,* **1989,** *25*:213–220.

Uhlenhuth EH, Balter MB, Ban TA, Yang K. International study of expert judgment on therapeutic use of benzodiazepines and other psychotherapeutic medications: IV. Therapeutic dose dependence and abuse liability of benzodiazepines in the long-term treatment of anxiety disorders. *J Clin Psychopharmacol,* **1999,** *19*(Suppl 2):23S–29S.

Victorri-Vigneau C, Dailly E, Veyrac G, Jolliet P. Evidence of zolpidem abuse and dependence: results of the French Center for Evaluation and Information on Pharmacodependence (CEIP) network survey. *Br J Clin Pharmacol*, **2007**, *64*:198–209.

Walsh JK, Vogel GW, Schart M, et al. A five-week polysomnographic assessment of zaleplon 10 mg for the treatment of primary insomnia. *Sleep Med,* **2000,** *1*:41–49.

Whiting PJ. The $GABA_A$ receptor gene family: New opportunities for drug development. *Curr Opin Drug Discov Dev,* **2003**, *6*:648–657.

Woods JH, Katz JL, Winger G. Benzodiazepines: Use, abuse, and consequences. *Pharmacol Rev,* **1992,** *44*:151–347.

Woods JH, Winger G. Abuse liability of flunitrazepam. *J Clin Psychopharmacol,* **1997,** *17*:1S–57S.

Zammit G. Comparative tolerability of newer agents for insomnia. *Drug Safety*, **2009**, *32*:735–748.

Zammit G, Erman M, Wang-Weigand S, et al. Evaluation of the efficacy and safety of ramelteon in subjects with chronic insomnia. *J Clin Sleep Med,* **2007,** *3*:495–504.

Opioids, Analgesia, and Pain Management

Tony L. Yaksh
and Mark S. Wallace

Pain is a component of virtually all clinical pathologies, and management of pain is a primary clinical imperative. Opioids are a mainstay of pain treatment, but rational therapy may involve, depending upon the pain state, one or more drug classes, such as NSAIDs, anticonvulsants, and antidepressants. The properties of these non-opioid agents are presented in Chapters 34, 21, and 15. This chapter focuses first on the biochemical, pharmacological, and functional nature of the opioid system that defines the effects of opioids on pain processing, gastrointestinal-endocrine-autonomic functions, and reward-addiction circuits. Subsequently, the chapter presents principles that guide the use of opioid and non-opioid agents in the management of clinical pain states.

The term *opiate* refers to compounds structurally related to products found in opium, a word derived from *opos*, the Greek word for "juice," natural opiates being derived from the resin of the opium poppy, *Papaver somniferum*. Opiates include the natural plant alkaloids, such as morphine, codeine, thebaine, and many semi-synthetic derivatives. An opioid is any agent, regardless of structure, that has the functional and pharmacological properties of an opiate. Endogenous opioids, many of which are peptides, are naturally occurring ligands for opioid receptors found in animals. The term *endorphin* is used synonymously with *endogenous opioid peptides* but also refers to a specific endogenous opioid, β-endorphin. The term *narcotic* was derived from the Greek word *narkotikos*, for "benumbing" or "stupor." Although narcotic originally referred to any drug that induced narcosis or sleep, the word has become associated with opioids and is often used in a legal context to refer to a variety of substances with abuse or addictive potential.

History. The first undisputed reference to opium is found in the writings of Theophrastus in the third century B.C. Arab physicians were well-versed in the uses of opium; Arab traders introduced the drug to the Orient, where it was employed mainly for the control of dysentery. By 1680, Sydenham was lauding opium: "Among the remedies which it has pleased Almighty God to give to man to relieve his sufferings, none is so universal and so efficacious as opium."

Opium contains >20 distinct alkaloids. In 1806, Frederich Sertürner, a pharmacist's assistant, reported the isolation by crystallization of a pure substance in opium that he named morphine, after Morpheus, the Greek god of dreams. By the middle of the 19th century, the use of pure alkaloids in place of crude opium preparations began to spread throughout the medical world, an event that coincided with the development of the hypodermic syringe and hollow needle, permitting direct delivery of such water-soluble formulations "under the skin" into the body.

In addition to the remarkable beneficial effects of opioids, the side effects and addictive potential of these drugs also have been known for centuries. In the civil war in the U.S., the administration of "soldier's joy" often led to "soldier's disease," the opiate addiction brought about by medication of chronic pain states arising from war wounds. These problems stimulated a search for potent synthetic opioid analgesics free of addictive potential and other side effects. The early discovery of the synthetic product heroin by C.R. Alder Wright in 1874 was followed by its widespread utilization as a purportedly non-addictive cough suppressant and sedative. Unfortunately, heroin and all subsequent synthetic compounds that have been introduced into clinical use share the liabilities of classical opioids, including their addictive properties. However, this search for new opioid agonists led to the synthesis of opioid antagonists and compounds with mixed agonist–antagonist properties, which expanded therapeutic options and provided important tools for exploring mechanisms of opioid actions.

Until the early 1970s, the effects of morphine, heroin, and other opioids as anti-nociceptive and addictive agents, were well described, but mechanisms mediating the interaction of the opioid alkaloids with biological systems were unknown. *In vivo* and *in vitro* physiological studies investigating the pharmacology of opiate agonists, their antagonists, and cross-tolerance led to the hypothesis of three separate opioid receptors: mu (μ), kappa (κ), and delta (δ) (Martin et al., 1976). These results were paralleled by work showing multiple radioligand binding sites for opiates on brain cell membranes (Goldstein et al., 1971; Pert et al., 1973). The three-receptor hypothesis was confirmed by subsequent cloning, which indicated

Table 18–1

Actions and Selectivities of Some Opioids at μ, δ, and κ Receptors (*Continued*)

OPIOID LIGANDS	RECEPTOR TYPES		
	μ	δ	κ
Antagonists			
Naloxone[d]	– – –	–	– –
Naltrexone[d]	– – –	–	– – –
CTOP[a]	– – –		
Diprenorphine	– – –	– –	– – –
β-Funaltrexamine[a,e]	– – –	–	++
Naloxonazine	– – –	–	–
nor-Binaltorphimine	–	–	– – –
Naltrindole[b]	–	– – –	–
Naloxone benzoylhydrazone	– – –	–	–

[a]Protoypical *μ*-preferring. [b]Prototypical δ- preferring. [c]Prototypical κ- preferring. [d]Universal ligand. [e]Irreversible ligand. +, agonist; –, antagonist; P, partial agonist. The number of symbols is an indication of potency; the ratio for a given drug denotes selectivity. These values are obtained primarily from a composite overview of results obtained in vivo/in vitro animal pharmacological work and in ligand binding and activity studies and should be extrapolated to humans with caution.
Source: Reproduced with permission from Raynor et al, 1994.

extensive sequence homologies (55-58%). The greatest diversity is found in their extracellular loops. In addition, all opioid receptors possess two conserved cysteine residues in the first and second extracellular loops forming a disulfide bridge.

μ, δ, and κ opioid receptors are widely distributed and this distribution has been examined in detail using immunohistochemistry, *in situ* hybridization, and more recently by noninvasive imaging techniques. The profound and diverse effects on CNS function are consistent with the density and diverse distribution of receptors in the brain and spinal cord (Henriksen et al., 2008). In addition, these receptors are expressed in a wide variety of peripheral tissues, including vascular, cardiac, airway/lung, gut, and many resident and circulating immune/inflammatory cells (discussed subsequently).

Following the cloning of the classical opioid receptors, the G-protein coupled opiate receptor-like protein (ORL1 or NOP) was cloned based on its structural homology (48-49% identity) to other members of the opioid receptor family; it has an endogenous ligand, nociceptin/orphanin (FQ: N/OFQ) (Stevens, 2009). See Figure 18–2. Since this system does not display an opioid pharmacology (Fioravanti et al., 2008), it will not be discussed in detail in this chapter.

N/OFQ binding sites have been found to be largely in the CNS and to be densely distributed in cortical regions, ventral forebrain, hippocampus, brainstem, and spinal cord, as well as in a number of peripheral cells including basophils, endothelial cells, and macrophages.

Opiate Receptor Subtypes

The existence of three classes of opiate receptors (MOR, DOR, and KOR) is widely accepted. The opioid receptors appear early in vertebrate evolution, being already present with the appearance of jawed vertebrates. The human opiate receptors have been mapped to chromosome 1p355-33 (DOR), chromosome 8q11.23-21 (KOR), chromosome 6q25-26 (MOR), and chromosome 20q13.33 (NOR) (Dreborg et al., 2008). Low-stringency hybridization procedures have identified no opioid receptor types other than the cloned opioid receptors. Nevertheless, pharmacological studies have suggested the possible existence of at least two subtypes of each receptor. While cloning studies have not supported the existence of these subtypes as distinct classes, the modified specificity for opioid ligands may result from several underlying events.

Heterodimerization. In the membrane, opiate receptors can form both homo- and heterodimers. Dimerization can alter the pharmacological properties of the respective receptors. For example, DORs form heterodimers with both MORs and KORs. Thus, MOR-DOR and DOR-KOR heterodimers show less affinity for highly selective agonists, reduced agonist-induced receptor trafficking, and mutual synergy between receptor-selective agonists in binding to the

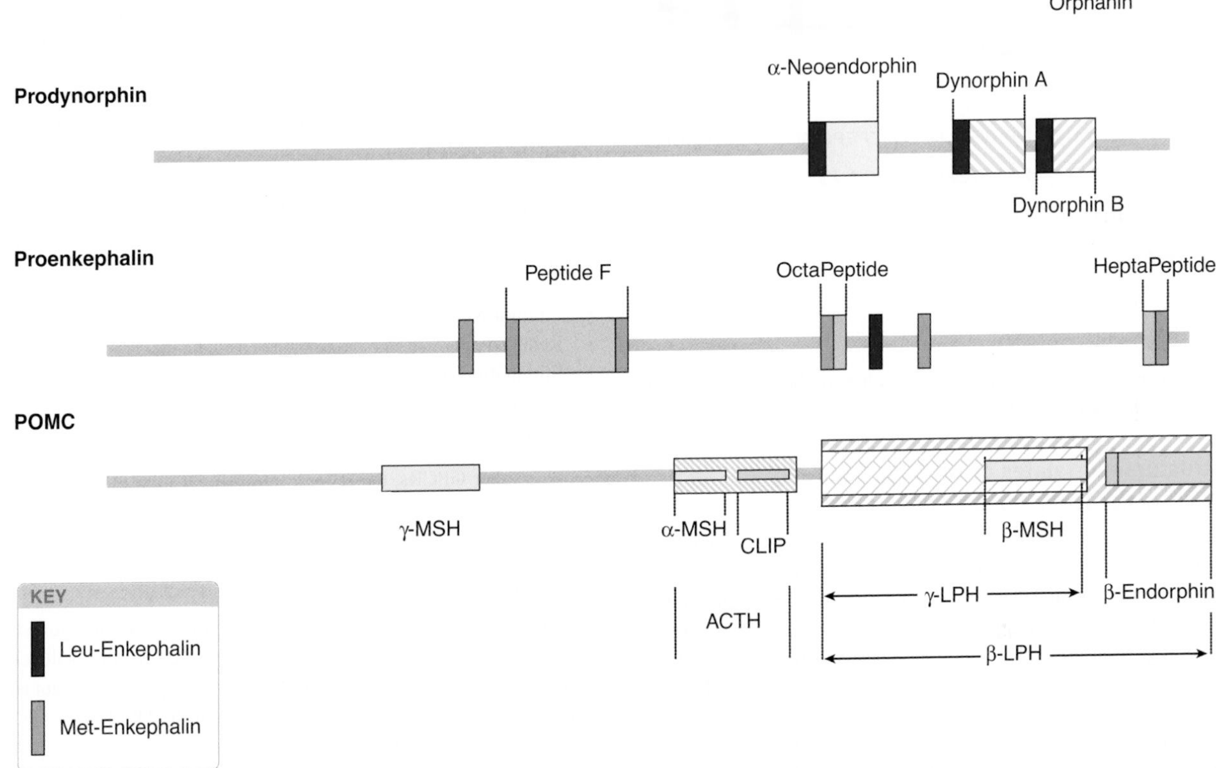

Figure 18–1. *Peptide precursors.* (Reproduced with permission from Akil et al, 1998. Copyright © Elsevier.)

respective agonists and also in the agonist-induced intracellular signaling (Gupta et al., 2006).

Alternative Splicing of Receptor RNA

Alternative splicing of receptor heteronuclear RNA (e.g., exon skipping and intron retention) is thought to play an important role in producing *in vivo* diversity within many members of the GPCR superfamily (Chapter 3). Splice variants exist within each of the three opioid receptor families, and this alternative splicing of receptor transcripts may be crucial for the diversity of opioid receptors. As an example, the human *Oprm* gene has at least two promoters, multiple exons, with many exons generating at least 11 splice variants that encode multiple morphine-binding isoforms, varying largely at their carboxy (intracellular) terminus. Given the functional importance of the intracellular components of the GPCRs, it is not surprising that significant differences exist for the receptor isoforms in terms of agonist-induced G protein activation and receptor internalization. Importantly, these splice variants have been found expressed *in vivo* (Pan, 2005).

Receptor Subtype Agonists/Antagonists

Studies on the presence and function of these receptors have depended upon the convergence between agonist/antagonist structure-activity studies and a variety of functional assays in biological and cloned receptor systems. Highly selective agonists have been developed that show specific affinity for the respective binding site and G-protein coupled reporter activation in cloned expression systems (e.g., DAMGO for MOR, DPDPE for DOR, and U-50,488, and U-69,593 for KOR) (Table 18–1). The study of the biological functions of opioid receptors *in vivo* has been aided by synthesis of selective antagonists. Among the most commonly used antagonists are cyclic analogs of somatostatin such as CTOP as a MOR antagonist, a derivative of naloxone called naltrindole as a DOR-receptor antagonist, and a bivalent derivative of naltrexone called nor-binaltorphimine (nor-BNI) as a KOR antagonist. These tools have made possible the characterization of the distribution of binding which, in conjunction with immunohistochemistry using antibodies derived from cloned receptors, has served to define the anatomical distribution of the receptors and the roles of the respective receptors in biological functions. Positron emission tomography (PET) has been used to characterize *in vivo* binding in brain with selective isotopically labeled ligands (Henriksen and Willoch, 2008). *In vivo* delivery of selective antagonists and agonists into specific brain regions has established the receptor types and anatomical distribution involved in mediating various opioid effects (see below).

Receptor Structure

Each receptor consists of an extracellular N-terminus, seven transmembrane helices, three extra- and intracellular loops, and an intracellular C-terminus characteristic of the GPCRs. The opioid receptors

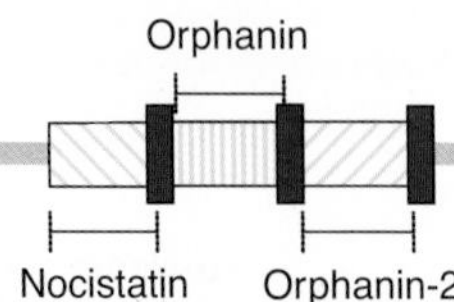

98-127 Nocistatin	MPRVRSLFQEQEEPEPGMEEAGEMEQKQLQ
130-146 Orphanin	FGGFTGARKSARKLANQ
149-165 Orphanin-2	FSEFMRQYLVLSMQSSQ

Figure 18–2. *Human pro-orphanin-derived peptides.*

also possess two conserved cysteine residues in the first and second extracellular loops, which form a disulfide bridge.

Structural Correlates of Binding/Coupling Requirements for Opiate Ligands

Opiate Receptor Structures. Studies of chimeric receptors and site-directed mutagenesis of cloned receptors have provided definitive insights into structural determinants of opioid ligand–receptor interaction. Though there is significant complexity (Kane et al., 2006), several general principles define binding and selectivity. First, all opioid receptors display a binding pocket formed by TM_3-TM_7. Second, the pocket in the respective receptor is partially covered by the extracellular loops, which together with the extracellular termini of the TM segments, provide a gate conferring selectivity, allowing ligands, particularly peptides, to be differentially accessible to the different receptor types. Thus, alkaloids (e.g., morphine) bind in the core of the transmembrane portion of the receptor, whereas large peptidyl ligands bind at the extracellular loops. As noted, it is the extracellular loops that show the greatest structural diversity across receptors. Third, selectivity has been attributed to extracellular loops: first and third for the MOR, second for the KOR, and third for the DOR (Waldhoer et al., 2004). Alkaloid antagonists are thought to bind deeper into the pocket sterically hindering conformational changes leading to a functional antagonism.

Structure-Activity Relationships. Receptor selectivity by the various opiate agonists is commonly explained in terms of the "message-address" concept (Takemori and Portoghese, 1992). Thus, elements shared by all structures (reflecting agents that bind at all sites, such as naltrexone) represent the "message," while elements associated with a ligand binding at a specific receptor represent the structural "address." The common structural features constituting the message are:

- a protonated nitrogen
- a phenolic ring (that, with the protonated nitrogen, forms tyramine)
- a hydrophobic domain

To this "message" are added a variable "linker" region and the "address" that specifies opiate receptor selectivity (Figure 18–3). Refinements of this message-linker-address model have led to the synthesis of new compounds with the predicted specificity. For the KOR and DOR, elements constituting the address have been defined. Thus, for the KOR, a second basic hydrophobic group is implicated in forming a specific salt bridge; for the DOR, a hydrophobic group such as an indole forms the address. MOR ligands such as morphine lack a common chemical moiety and thus other elements are thought to contribute to ligand specificity at that receptor (Kane et al., 2006).

Opiate Receptor Coupling to Membrane Function

Agonist binding results in conformational changes in the GPCR, initiating the G protein activation/inactivation cycle (Chapter 3). The μ, δ, and κ receptors largely couple through pertussis toxin-sensitive, G_i/G_o proteins (but occasionally to G_s or G_z). Upon receptor activation, the G_i/G_o coupling results in a large number of intracellular events, including:

- Inhibition of adenylyl cyclase activity
- Reduced opening of voltage-gated Ca^{2+} channels
- Stimulation of K^+ current though several channels including G protein-activated inwardly rectifying K^+ channels (GIRKs)
- Activation of PKC and PLC_β

As with other GPCRs, the second intracellular loop is involved in the efficacy of G-protein activation while the third loop defines the α subunit that is activated (Gether, 2000).

Regulation of Opiate Receptor Disposition

Like other GPCRs, MOR and DORs can undergo rapid agonist-mediated internalization via a classic endocytic, β-arrestin-mediated pathway, whereas KORs do not internalize after prolonged agonist exposure (Chu et al., 1997). Internalization of the MOR and DORs apparently occurs via partially distinct endocytic pathways, suggesting receptor-specific interactions with different mediators of intracellular trafficking. These processes may be induced differentially as a function of the structure of the ligand. For example, certain agonists, such as etorphine and enkephalins, cause rapid internalization of the receptor, whereas morphine does not cause MOR internalization, even though it decreases adenylyl cyclase activity equally well. In addition, a truncated receptor with normal G-protein coupling recycles constitutively from the membrane to the cytosol (Segredo et al., 1997), suggesting that activation of signal transduction and internalization are controlled by distinct molecular mechanisms. These studies also support the hypothesis that different ligands induce different conformational changes in the receptor that result in divergent intracellular events, and they may provide an explanation for differences in the spectrum of effects of various opioids.

Functional Consequences of Acute and Chronic Opiate Receptor Activation

The loss of effect with exposure to opiates occurs over short- and long-term intervals.

Desensitization. Acute agonist occupancy of the opiate receptors results in activation of the intracellular signaling outlined previously. In the face of a transient activation (minutes to hours), a phenomenon called acute tolerance or desensitization can be observed that is specific for that receptor and disappears with a time course parallel to the clearance of the agonist. Short-term desensitization probably involves phosphorylation of the receptors resulting in an uncoupling of the receptor from its G-protein and/or internalization of the receptor.

Tolerance. Sustained administration of an opiate agonist (days to weeks) leads to progressive loss of drug effect. Here tolerance refers to a decrease in the apparent effectiveness of a drug with continuous

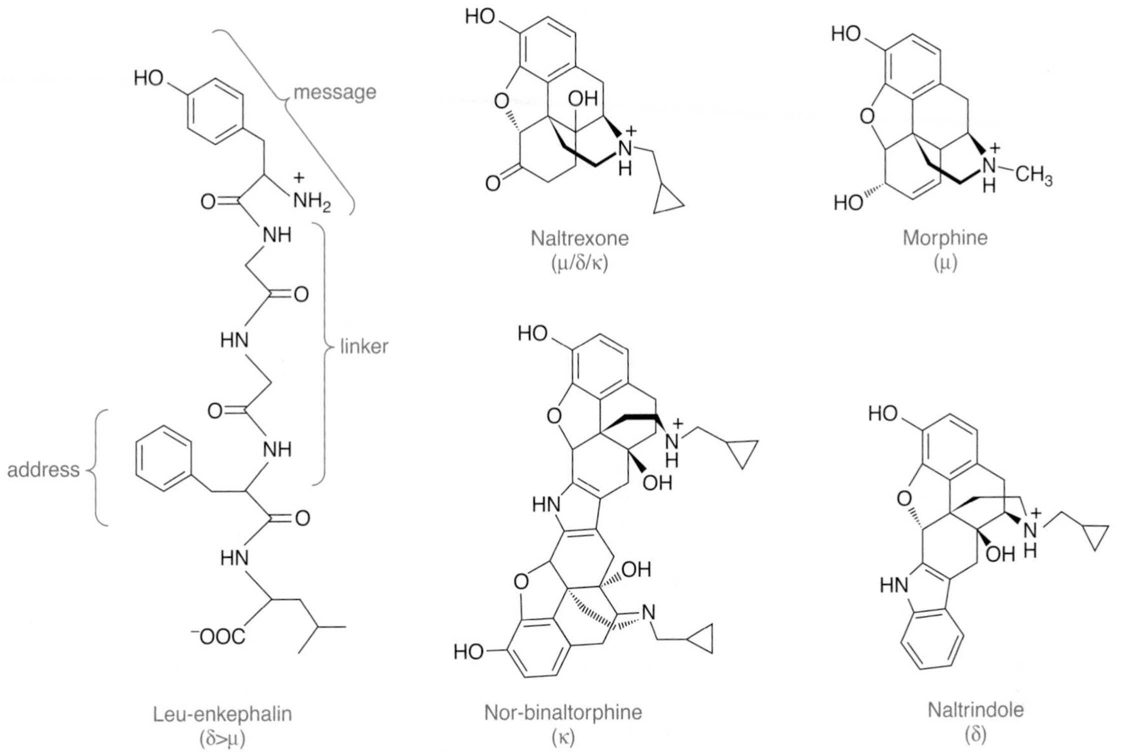

Figure 18–3. *Structural features of opioid ligands contribute to receptor selectivity.* The "message-linker-address" formulation (Takemore and Portoghese, 1992) has been refined and used to synthesize non-peptide ligands that exhibit predicted opiate receptor specificity. The ligands pictured above demonstrate some of the common (message) and variable (linker and address) features thought to contribute to ligand-receptor interactions for both opiate receptor agonists and antagonists.

or repeated agonist administration, and with the removal of the agonist disappears over several weeks. This tolerance is reflected by a reduction in the maximum achievable effect or a right shift in the dose-effect curve. This phenomenon can be manifested at the level of the intracellular cascade (e.g., reduced inhibition of adenylyl cyclase) and at the organ system level (e.g., loss of sedative and analgesic effects).

This loss of effect with persistent exposure to an opiate agonist has several key properties:

- Changes in response are time-dependent, with changes occurring over short-term (minutes to hours, as with desensitization) and long-term intervals (weeks to months).
- Tolerance to drug effect is surmountable with higher doses of the opioid.
- Tolerance is reversible over time after termination of the drug.
- Different physiological responses develop tolerance at different rates. Thus, at the organ system level, some end points show little or no tolerance development (pupillary miosis), some show moderate tolerance (constipation, emesis, analgesia, sedation), and some show rapid tolerance (euphorogenic).
- In general, opiate agonists of a given class will typically show a reduced response in a system rendered tolerant to another agent of that class (e.g., cross-tolerance between the μ agonists, such as morphine and fentanyl).

The completeness of this cross-tolerance is not consistent and forms the basis for the switching between opioid drugs used in clinical therapy. This incomplete cross-tolerance has been hypothesized to reflect small but important differences in the receptors with which the different opiates of the same class bind (Pasternak, 2005).

Dependence. During the state of tolerance, the phenomenon of dependence is observed. Dependence represents a state of adaptation manifested by receptor/drug class-specific withdrawal syndrome produced by cessation of drug exposure (e.g., by drug abstinence) or administration of an antagonist (e.g., naloxone). The withdrawal is manifested by the exaggerated appearance of enhanced signs of cellular activation. In the CNS, increased adenylyl cyclase, release of excitatory amino acids and cytokines, activation of microglia and astrocytes, and the initiation of apoptotic processes have been reported. Such indices of hyperexcitability are also noted in peripheral plexi such as are present in the GI tract and in autonomic ganglia (discussed later). At the organ system level, withdrawal is manifested by significant somatomotor and autonomic outflow (reflected by agitation, hyperalgesia, hyperthermia, hypertension, diarrhea, pupillary dilation, and release of virtually all pituitary and adrenomedullary hormones) and by affective symptoms (dysphoria, anxiety, and depression) (Kreek et al., 1998). These phenomena are considered to be highly aversive and motivate the drug recipient to make robust efforts to avoid the withdrawal state. Consistent with the receptor selectivity of the effects, the withdrawal signs observed in an animal tolerant to a given opiate can be suppressed by application of another drug from the same class.

Addiction. Addiction is a behavioral pattern characterized by compulsive use of a drug and overwhelming involvement with its procurement and use. The positive, rewarding effects of opiates are considered to be the driving component for initiating the recreational use of opiates. This positive reward property in humans and animals is subject to the development of tolerance. Given the aversive nature of withdrawal symptoms, in the dependent organism, it is not surprising that avoidance and alleviation of withdrawal symptoms may become a primary motivation for compulsive drug taking (Kreek and Koob, 1998). When the drive to acquire the drug leads to drug-seeking behaviors that occur in spite of the physical, emotional, or societal damage suffered by the drug seeker, then the obsession or compulsion to acquire and use the drug is considered to reflect an addicted state. In animals, this may be manifest by willingness to tolerate very stressful conditions to acquire drug delivery. In humans, aberrant behaviors considered to be signs of addiction include prescription forgery, stealing drugs from others, and obtaining prescription drugs from nonmedical sources; these behaviors are considered indicators of an addiction disorder. Note that drug dependence is *not* synonymous with drug addiction. Any individual who is exposed for some period to opiates will display some degree of tolerance and should the drug be removed abruptly, there will be an expression of withdrawal signs, the severity of which will depend upon the dose and duration of drug exposure. Such a condition does not itself indicate an addicted state. Thus, tolerance and dependence are physiological responses seen in all patients but are not predictors of addiction (Chapter 24). For example, cancer pain often requires prolonged treatment with high doses of opioids, leading to tolerance and dependence. Yet abuse in this setting is considered to be unusual (Foley, 1993).

Mechanisms of Tolerance/Dependence-Withdrawal

The mechanisms underlying chronic tolerance and dependence/withdrawal are controversial. Several types of events are considered to contribute.

Receptor Disposition. With chronic opiate exposure, the general consensus is that the loss of effect is not related to the density of membrane receptors. As noted, acute desensitization or receptor internalization may play a role in the initiation of chronic tolerance but is not sufficient to explain persistent changes observed with chronic exposure. Thus, morphine, unlike other μ agonists, does not promote μ receptor internalization or receptor phosphorylation and desensitization (Koch et al., 2005; von Zastrow et al., 2003). These studies suggest that receptor desensitization and down-regulation are agonist specific. Other studies of GPCRs indicate that endocytosis and sequestration of receptors do not invariably lead to receptor degradation but can also result in receptor dephosphorylation and recycling to the surface of the cell (Krupnick and Benovic, 1998). Accordingly, opioid tolerance may not be related to receptor desensitization but rather to a lack of desensitization. Agonists that rapidly internalize opioid receptors also would rapidly desensitize signaling, but this desensitization would be at least partially reset by recycling of "reactivated" opioid receptors. The lack of desensitization caused by morphine may result in prolonged receptor signaling, which even though less efficient than that observed with other agonists, would lead to further downstream cellular adaptations that increase tolerance development. The measurement of relative agonist signaling versus endocytosis (RAVE) for opioid agonists could be predictive of the potential for tolerance development (Waldhoer et al., 2004).

Adaptation of Intracellular Signaling Mechanisms in the Opioid Receptor-Bearing Neurons. Coupling of MOR to cellular effectors, such as inhibition of adenylyl cyclase, activation of inwardly rectifying K^+ channels, inhibition of Ca^{2+} currents, and inhibition of terminal release of transmitters demonstrates functional uncoupling of receptor occupancy from effector function (Williams et al., 2001). Importantly, the chronic opioid effect initiates adaptive counterregulatory change. The best example of such cellular counterregulatory processes is the rebound increase in cellular cyclic AMP levels produced by "superactivation" of adenylyl cyclase and up-regulation of the amount of enzyme. Such superactivation leads to an induction of an excitatory state mediated by an increased cation current through activation of PKA. Terminal transmitter release is thus commonly enhanced during opioid withdrawal (Bailey and Connor, 2005).

System Level Counteradaptation. In the face of chronic opiate exposure, an evident loss of drug effect is noted. An important line of speculation is that the apparent loss of inhibitory effect may reflect an enhanced excitability of the regulated link. Thus, tolerance to the analgesic action of chronically administered μ opiates may result in an activation of bulbospinal pathways that increases the excitability of spinal dorsal horn pain transmission linkages. Similarly, in the face of chronic opiate exposure, opiate receptor occupancy will lead to the activation of PKC, which can phosphorylate and, accordingly, enhance the activation of local glutamate receptors of the N-methyl-D-aspartate (NMDA) type (Chapter 14). These receptors are known to mediate a facilitated state leading to enhanced spinal pain processing. Blocking of these receptors can at least partially attenuate the loss of analgesic efficacy with continued opiate exposure (Trujillo and Akil, 1991). These system level counteradaptation hypotheses may represent mechanisms that apply to specific systems (e.g., pain modulation) but not necessarily to others (e.g., sedation or miosis) (Christie, 2008).

Differential Tolerance Development and Fractional Occupancy Requirements. An interesting problem posed in explaining tolerance relates to the differential rates of tolerance development noted earlier. Why responses such as miosis show no tolerance over extended exposure (indeed, it is considered symptomatic in drug overdose of highly tolerant patients) while analgesia and sedation are more likely to show a reduction is not clear. One possibility is that tolerance represents a functional uncoupling of some fraction of the receptor population and that different physiological end points may require activation of different fractions of their coupled receptors to produce a given physiological effect. Accordingly, it would be consistent that receptors in the miosis pathways need to activate a small fraction of their receptors, relative to those systems mediating pain control to produce a significant physiological action (e.g., the systems mediating miosis have a greater functional receptor reserve).

Effect Profile of Clinically Used Opioids

Opiates, depending upon their receptor preferences, produce a variety of effects consistent with the role played by the organ systems with which the receptors are associated. Whereas the primary clinical use of opioids is for their pain-relieving properties, opioids produce a host of other effects. This is not surprising in view of the wide distribution of opioid receptors in the brain and the periphery. Within the nervous systems, these effects range from analgesia to effects upon motivation and higher-order affect (euphoria), arousal, and a number of autonomic, hormonal, and motor processes. In the periphery, opiates can influence a variety of visceromotor systems, including those related to GI motility and smooth muscle tone. The next sections consider these class actions and their mechanisms.

Analgesia. In humans, morphine-like drugs produce analgesia, drowsiness, changes in mood, and mental clouding. When therapeutic doses of morphine are given to patients with pain, they report the pain to be less intense or entirely gone. Patients frequently report that the pain, though still present, is tolerable and that they feel more comfortable. In addition to relief of distress, some patients may experience euphoria. A significant feature of the analgesia is that it often occurs without loss of consciousness, though drowsiness commonly occurs (see "Respiration" later in the chapter). Morphine at these doses does not have anticonvulsant activity and usually does not cause slurred speech, emotional lability, or significant motor uncoordination.

When morphine in an analgesic dose is given to normal, pain-free individuals, the patients may report the drug experience to be frankly unpleasant. There may be drowsiness, difficulty in mentation, apathy, and lessened physical activity. As the dose is increased, the subjective, analgesic, and toxic effects, including respiratory depression, become more pronounced.

Specificity of Analgesic Effects. The relief of pain by morphine-like opioids is selective in that other somatosensory modalities, such as light touch, proprioception, and the sense of moderate temperatures, are unaffected. Systematic psychophysical studies have shown that low doses of morphine produce reductions in the affective but not the perceived intensity of pain whereas higher (clinically effective) doses reduced both reported perceived intensity and the affective response otherwise evoked by acute experimental pain stimuli (Price et al., 1985). In general, continuous dull pain (as generated by tissue injury and inflammation) is relieved more effectively than sharp intermittent (incident) pain, such as that associated with the movement of an inflamed joint, but with sufficient amounts of opioid it is possible to relieve even the severe piercing pain associated with acute renal or biliary colic.

Pain States and Mechanisms Underlying Different Pain States. Any meaningful discussion of the action of analgesic agents must include the appreciation that all pain is not the same and that a number of variables contribute to the patient's pain report and therefore to the effect of the analgesic. Heuristically, one may think mechanistically of pain as several distinct sets of events, described in the next sections.

Acute Nociception. Acute activation of small high-threshold sensory afferents (Aδ and C fibers) generates transient input into the spinal cord, which in turn leads to activation of neurons that project contralaterally to the thalamus and thence to the somatosensory cortex. A parallel spinofugal projection is to the medial thalamus and from there to the anterior cingulate cortex, part of the limbic system. The output produced by acutely activating this ascending system is sufficient to evoke pain reports. Examples of such stimuli include a hot coffee cup, a needle stick, or an incision.

Tissue Injury. Following tissue injury or local inflammation (e.g., local skin burn, toothache, rheumatoid joint), an ongoing pain state arises that is characterized by burning, throbbing, or aching and an abnormal pain response (hyperalgesia) and can be evoked by otherwise innocuous or mildly aversive stimuli (tepid bathwater on a sunburn; moderate extension of an injured joint). This pain typically reflects the effects of active factors (such as prostaglandins, bradykinin, cytokines, and H^+ ions, among many mediators) released into the injury site, which have the ability to activate the terminal of small high-threshold afferents (Aδ and C fibers) and to reduce the stimulus intensity required to activate these sensory afferents (peripheral sensitization). In addition, the ongoing afferent traffic initiated by the injury leads to the activation of spinal facilitatory cascades, yielding a greater output to the brain for any given input. This facilitation is thought to underlie the hyperalgesic states. Such tissue injury-evoked pain is often referred to as "nociceptive" pain (Figure 18–4)

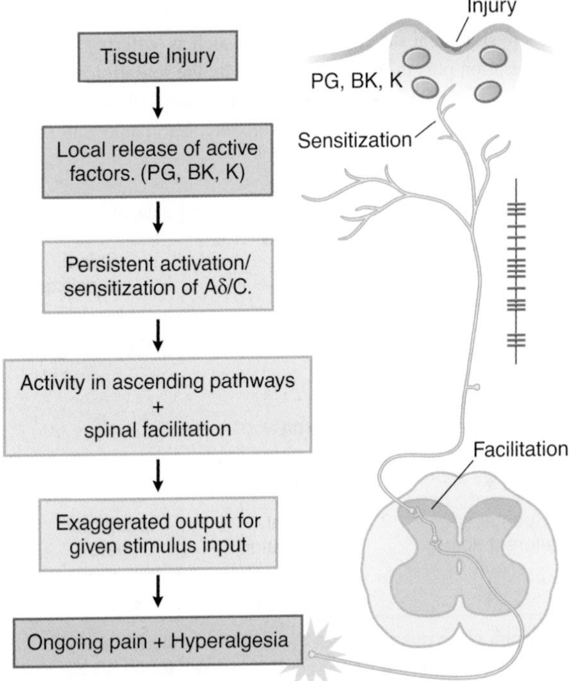

Figure 18–4. *Mechanistic flow diagram of tissue injury–evoked nociception.*

(Sorkin and Wallace, 1999). Examples of such states would be burn, post-incision, abrasion of the skin, inflammation of the joint, and musculoskeletal injury.

Nerve Injury. Injury to the peripheral nerve yields complex anatomical and biochemical changes in the nerve and spinal cord that induce spontaneous dysesthesias (shooting, burning pain) and allodynia (light touch hurts). This nerve injury pain state may not depend upon the activation of small afferents, but may be initiated by low-threshold sensory afferents (e.g., Aβ fibers). Such nerve injuries result in the development of ectopic activity arising from neuromas formed by nerve injury and the dorsal root ganglia of the injured axons as well as a dororsal horn reorganization, such that low-threshold afferent input carried by Aβ fibers evokes a pain state. This dorsal horn reorganization reflects changes in ongoing inhibition and in the excitability of dorsal horn projection neurons (Latremoliere and Woolf, 2009). Examples of such nerve injury-inducing events include nerve trauma or compression (carpal tunnel syndrome), chemotherapy (as for cancer), diabetes, and in the post-herpetic state (shingles). These pain states are said to be neuropathic (Figure 18–5). Many clinical pain syndromes, such as found in cancer, typically represent a combination of these inflammatory and neuropathic mechanisms. Although nociceptive pain usually is responsive to opioid analgesics, neuropathic pain is typically considered to respond less well to opioid analgesics (McQuay, 1988).

Sensory Versus Affective Dimensions. Information generated by a high intensity peripheral stimulus initiates activity in defined pathways that activate higher-order systems that reflect the aversive magnitude of the stimulus. This reflects the *sensory-discriminative* dimension of the pain experience (such as the ability to accurately estimate and characterize the pain state). Painful stimuli have the certain ability to generate strong emotional components that reflect a distinction between pain as a specific sensation subserved by distinct neurophysiological structures, and pain such as suffering (the original sensation plus the reactions evoked by the sensation; the *affective motivational* dimension) (Melzack and Casey, 1968). When pain does not evoke its usual responses (anxiety, fear, panic, and suffering), a patient's ability to tolerate the pain may be markedly increased, even when the capacity to perceive the sensation is relatively unaltered. It is clear, however, that alteration of the emotional reaction to painful stimuli is not the sole mechanism of analgesia. Thus, intrathecal administration of opioids can produce profound segmental analgesia without causing significant alteration of motor or sensory function or subjective effects (Yaksh, 1988).

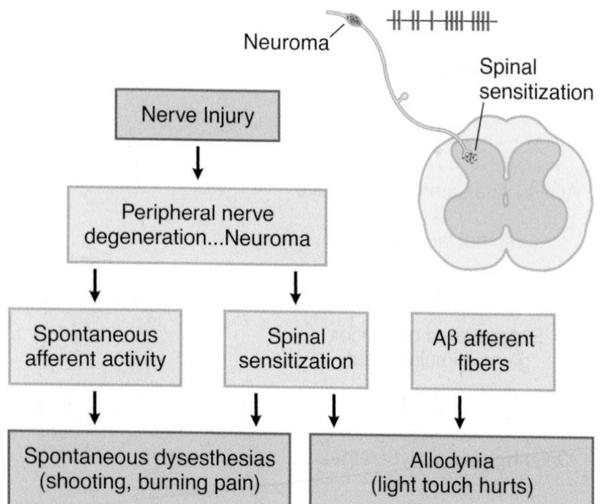

Figure 18–5. *Mechanistic flow diagram of nerve injury–evoked nociception.*

Mechanisms of Opioid-Induced Analgesia. The analgesic actions of opiates after systemic delivery are believed to represent actions in the brain, spinal cord, and in some instances in the periphery.

Supraspinal Actions. The microinjection of opiates through chronically placed microinjection cannulae targeted at specific brain sites has shown that opiate agonists will, in a manner consistent with their respective activity at a MOR, block pain behavior after delivery into a number of highly circumscribed brain regions and that these analgesic effects are naloxone reversible. The best characterized of these sites is the mesencephalic periaqueductal gray (PAG) matter. Microinjections of morphine into this region will block nociceptive responses in every species examined from rodents to primates; naloxone will reverse these effects.

Several mechanisms exist whereby opiates with an action limited to the PAG may act to alter nociceptive transmission. These are summarized in Figure 18–6. MOR agonists block release of the inhibitory transmitter GABA from tonically active PAG systems that regulate activity in projections to the medulla. PAG projections to the medulla activate medullospinal release of NE and 5-HT at the level of the spinal dorsal horn. This release can attenuate dorsal horn excitability (Yaksh, 1997). Interestingly, this PAG organization can also serve to increase excitability of dorsal raphe and locus coeruleus from which ascending serotonergic and noradrenergic projections to the limbic forebrain originate (the role of forebrain 5-HT and NE in mediating emotional tone is discussed in Chapter 15). In humans, it is not feasible to routinely access the site of action within the brain where opiates may act to alter nociceptive transmission as is done in preclinical models. However, intracerebroventricular opioids have been employed in humans for pain relief in cancer patients. Accordingly, it seems probable that the supraspinal site of opiate action in the human, as in other animal models, lies close to the ventricular lumen (Karavelis et al., 1996).

Spinal Opiate Action. A local action of opiates in the spinal cord will selectively depress the discharge of spinal dorsal horn neurons evoked by small (high-threshold) but not large (low-threshold) afferent nerve fibers. Intrathecal administration of opioids in animals ranging from mouse to human will reliably attenuate the response of the organism to a variety of somatic and visceral stimuli that otherwise evoke pain states. Specific opiate binding and receptor protein are limited for the most part to the substantia gelatinosa of the superficial dorsal horn, the region in which small, high-threshold sensory afferents show their principal termination. A significant proportion of these opiate receptors are associated with small peptidergic primary afferent C fibers and the remainder are on local dorsal horn neurons. This finding is consistent with the presence of opioid receptor protein being synthesized in and transported from small dorsal root ganglion cells.

Confirmation of the presynaptic action is provided by the observation that spinal opiates reduce the release of primary afferent

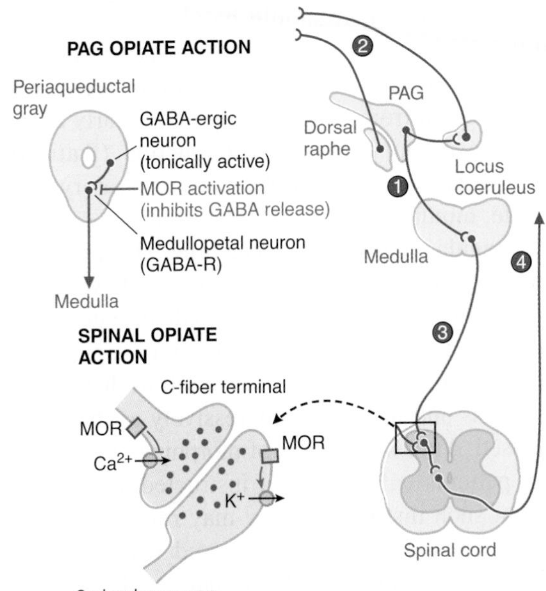

Figure 18–6. *Mechanisms of opiate action in producing analgesia.* Top left: Schematic of organization of opiate action in the periaqueductal gray. Top right: Opiate-sensitive pathways in PAG Mu opiate actions block the release of GABA from tonically active systems that otherwise regulate the projections to the medulla (1) leading to an activation of PAG outflow resulting and activation of forebrain (2) and spinal (3) monoamine receptors that regulate spinal cord projections (4) which provide sensory input to higher centers and mood.
Bottom left: Schematic of primary afferent synapse with second order dorsal horn spinal neuron, showing pre- and post-synaptic opiate receptors coupled to Ca^{2+} and K^+ channels, respectively. Opiate receptor binding is highly expressed in the superficial spinal dorsal horn (substantia gelatinosa). These receptors are located presynaptically on the terminals of small primary afferents (C fibers) and postsynaptially on second order neurons. Presynaptically, activation of MOR blocks the opening of the voltage sensitve Ca^{2+} channel, which otherwise initiates transmitter release. Postsynaptically, MOR activation enhances opening of K^+ channels, leading to hyperpolarization. Thus, an opiate agonist acting at these sites jointly serves to attenuate the afferent-evoked excitation of the second order neuron.

peptide transmitters such as substance P contained in small afferents (Yaksh et al., 1980). The presynaptic action corresponds to the ability of opiates to prevent the opening of voltage-sensitive Ca^{2+} channels, thereby preventing transmitter release. A postsynaptic action is demonstrated by the ability of opiates to block excitation of dorsal horn neurons directly evoked by glutamate, reflecting a direct activation of dorsal horn projection neurons. The activation of K^+ channels in these postsynaptic neurons, leading to hyperpolarization, is consistent with a direct postsynaptic inhibition. The joint capacity of spinal opiates to reduce the release of excitatory neurotransmitters from C fibers and to decrease the excitability of dorsal horn neurons is believed to account for the powerful and selective effect of opiates on spinal nociceptive processing. In humans, there is extensive literature indicating that a variety of opiates delivered spinally (intrathecally or epidurally) can induce a powerful analgesia that is reversed by low doses of systemic naloxone (Yaksh, 1997).

Peripheral Action. It has been a principal tenet of opiate action that these agents act "centrally." Direct application of opiates to a peripheral nerve can, in fact, produce a local anesthetic-like action at high concentrations, but this is not naloxone reversible and is believed to reflect a "nonspecific" action. Moreover, in studies examining normal animals, it can be demonstrated that the analgesic actions are limited if the agent does not readily penetrate the brain. Alternately, studies employing the direct injection of these agents into peripheral sites have demonstrated that under conditions of inflammation, where there is an increased terminal sensitivity leading to an exaggerated pain response (e.g., hyperalgesia), the local action of opiates can exert a normalizing effect upon the exaggerated thresholds. This has been demonstrated for the response to mechanical stimulation applied to inflamed paw or inflamed knee joints. In the absence of inflammation, there is no local peripheral effect. This action is believed to be mediated by opiate receptors on the peripheral terminals of small primary afferents. Local opiates in the knee joint and in the skin can reduce the firing of spontaneously active afferents observed when these tissues are inflamed. Whether the effects are uniquely on the afferent terminal, whether the opiate acts upon inflammatory cells that release products that sensitize the nerve terminal, or both, is not known (Stein and Lang, 2009).

Mood Alterations and Rewarding Properties. The mechanisms by which opioids produce euphoria, tranquility, and other alterations of mood (including rewarding properties) are complex and not entirely clear. Neural systems thought to mediate opioid reinforcement overlap with, but are distinct from, those involved in physical dependence and analgesia (Koob et al., 1988). Behavioral and pharmacological data point to a pivotal role of the mesocorticolimbic (MCL) dopamine system, a basal forebrain circuit long implicated in reward and motivation (Figure 18–7).

The mesolimbic dopamine system originates in the ventral segmental area (VTA) and projects to the nucleus accumbens (NAc) in the forebrain. Dopamine and glutamate projections from the VTA and prefrontal cortex (PFC), respectively, synapse on NAc GABAergic neurons. These cells project to the ventral pallidum (VP). In the NAc, ionotropic glutamate receptors activate, while dopamine D_2-like receptors inhibit GABAergic neurons. In general, interventions that suppress the NAc-VP GABA pathway leading to increased dopamine release are considered to be positively rewarding, supporting, for example, self-administration. Thus, dopamine delivered directly into the NAc, mimicking increased extracellular release, is powerfully reinforcing. Opiates increase DA release in the NAc, and catheterized animals will activate administration of opiates directly into their VTA and into the NAc, emphasizing the importance of that system in opiate reward. In the NAc, MORs are present postsynaptically on GABAergic neurons. The reinforcing effects of opiates in the VTA are thought to be mediated through

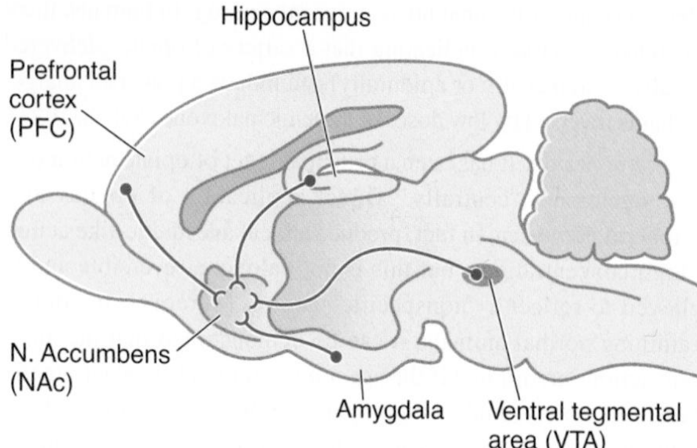

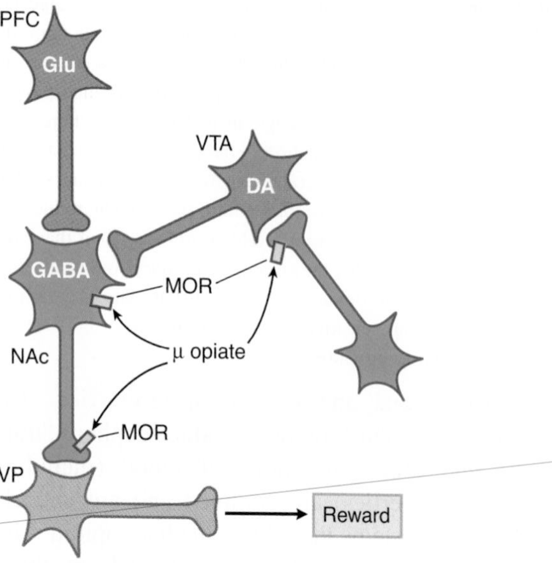

Figure 18–7. *Schematic pathways underlying rewarding properties of opiates.*
Upper panel: This saggital section of rat brain displays simplified DA and GABA inputs from the ventral tegmental area (VTA) and prefrontal cortex (PFC), respectively, into the nucleus accumbens (NAc).
Lower panel: Neurons are labeled with their primary neurotransmitters. At a cellular level, MOR agonists reduce excitability and transmitter release at the sites indicated by inhbiting Ca^{2+} influx and enhancing K^+ current (see Figure 18-6). Thus, opiate-induced inhibition in the VTA on GABA-ergic interneurons or in the NAc reduce GABA-mediated inhibition and increase outflow from the ventral pallidum (VP), which appears to correlate with a positive reinforcing state (enhanced reward).

inhibition of local GABAergic neuronal activity, which otherwise acts to inhibit DA outflow (Xi and Stein, 2002).

Respiration. Although effects on respiration are readily demonstrated, clinically significant respiratory depression rarely occurs with standard analgesic doses in the absence of other contributing variables (discussed in the next sections). It should be stressed, however, that *respiratory depression represents the primary cause of morbidity secondary to opiate therapy.* In humans, death from opiate poisoning is nearly always due to respiratory arrest or obstruction (Pattinson, 2008). Opiates depress all phases of respiratory activity (rate, minute volume, and tidal exchange) and produce irregular and aperiodic breathing. The diminished respiratory volume is due primarily to a slower rate of breathing; with toxic amounts of opioids, the rate may fall to 3-4 breaths per minute. The respiratory depression is discernible even with doses too small to disturb consciousness and increases progressively as the dose is increased. After large doses of morphine or other agonists, patients will breathe if instructed to do so, but without such instruction, they may remain relatively apneic. Thus, opioids must be used with caution in patients with asthma, COPD, cor pulmonale, decreased respiratory reserve, preexisting respiratory depression, hypoxia, or hypercapnia to avoid apnea due to a decrease in respiratory drive coinciding with an increase airway resistance. While respiratory depression is not considered to be a favorable therapeutic effect of opiates, their ability to suppress respiratory drive is used to therapeutic advantage to treat dyspnea resulting, for example, in patients with chronic obstructive pulmonary disease (COPD), where air hunger leads to extreme agitation, discomfort, and gasping; similarly, opiates find use in patients who require artificial ventilation (Clemens and Klaschik, 2007).

Mechanisms Underlying Respiratory Depression. Respiratory rate and tidal volume depend upon intrinsic rhythm generators located in the ventrolateral medulla. These systems generate a "respiratory" rhythm that is driven by afferent input reflecting the partial pressure of arterial O_2 as measured by chemosensors in the carotid and aortic bodies and CO_2 as measured by chemosensors in the brainstem. Morphine-like opioids depress respiration through MOR and DOR receptors in part by a direct depressant effect on rhythm generation, with changes in respiratory pattern and rate observed at lower doses than changes in tidal volume. A key property of opiate effects on respiration is the depression of the ventilatory response to increased CO_2. This effect is mediated by opiate depression of the excitability of brainstem chemosensory neurons. In addition to the effects on the CO_2 response, opiates will depress ventilation otherwise driven by hypoxia though an effect upon carotid and aortic body chemosensors. Importantly, with opiates, hypoxic stimulation of chemoreceptors still may be effective when opioids have decreased the responsiveness to CO_2, and inhalation of O_2 may remove the residual drive resulting from the elevated PO_2 and produce apnea (Pattinson, 2008). In addition to the effect upon respiratory rhythm and chemosensitivity, opiates can have mechanical effects on airway function by increasing chest wall rigidity and diminishing upper airway patency (Lalley, 2008).

Factors Exacerbating Opiate-Induced Respiratory Depression. A number of factors are recognized as increasing the risk of opiate-related respiratory depression even at therapeutic doses:

- *Other medications.* The combination of opiates with other depressant medications, such as general anesthetics, tranquilizers, alcohol, or sedative-hypnotics, produces additive depression of respiratory activity.
- *Sleep.* Natural sleep produces a decrease in the sensitivity of the medullary center to CO_2, and the depressant effects of morphine and sleep are at least additive. Obstructive sleep apnea is considered to be an important risk factor for increasing the likelihood of fatal respiratory depression.
- *Age.* Newborns can show significant respiratory depression and desaturation; and this may be evident in lower Apgar scores if opioids are administered parenterally to women within 2-4 hours of delivery because of transplacental passage of opioids. Elderly patients are at greater risk of depression because of reduced lung elasticity, chest wall stiffening, and decreased vital capacity.
- *Disease.* Opiates may cause a greater depressant action in patients with chronic cardiopulmonary or renal diseases because they can manifest a desensitization of their response to increased CO_2.
- *COPD.* Enhanced depression can also be noted in patients with chronic obstructive pulmonary disease (COPD) and sleep apnea secondary to diminished hypoxic drive.
- *Relief of Pain.* Because pain stimulates respiration, removal of the painful condition (as with the analgesia resulting from the therapeutic use of the opiate) will reduce the ventilatory drive and lead to apparent respiratory depression.

Sedation. Opiates can produce drowsiness and cognitive impairment. Such depression can augment respiratory impairment. These effects are most typically noted following initiation of opiate therapy or after dose incrementation. Importantly, these effects upon arousal resolve over a few days. As with respiratory depression, the degree of drug effect can be enhanced by a variety of predisposing patient factors including dementia, encephalopathies, or brain tumors as well as other depressant medications, including sleep aids, antihistamines, antidepressants, and anxiolytics (Cherny, 1996).

Different Opiates. Numerous studies have compared morphine and morphine-like opioids with respect to their ratios of analgesic to respiratory-depressant activities, and most have found that when equianalgesic doses are used, there is no significant difference. Maximal respiratory depression occurs within 5-10 minutes of intravenous administration of morphine or within 30-90 minutes of intramuscular or subcutaneous administration. Maximal respiratory depressant effects occur more rapidly with more lipid-soluble agents. After therapeutic doses, respiratory minute volume may be reduced for as long as 4-5 hours. Agents that have persistent kinetics, such as methadone, must be carefully monitored, particularly after dose incrementation.

Management of Opiate Depression. Life-threatening respiratory depression produced by any opiate agonist can be readily reversed by delivery of an opiate antagonist. Conversely, the ability to reverse the somnolent patient is considered to be indicative of an opiate-mediated effect. It is important to remember that most opiate antagonists have a relatively short duration of action as compared to an agonist such as morphine or methadone and fatal "re-narcotization" can occur if vigilance is not exercised.

Neuroendocrine Effects. The regulation of the release of hormones and factors from the pituitary is under complex regulation by opiate receptors in the hypothalamic-pituitary-adrenal (HPA) axis. Broadly considered, morphine-like opioids block the release of a large number of HPA hormones.

Sex Hormones. In males, acute opiate therapy reduces plasma cortisol, testosterone, and gonadotrophins. Inhibition of adrenal function is reflected by reduced cortisol production and reduced adrenal androgens (dehydroepiandrosterone, DHEA). In females, morphine will additionally result in lower LH and FSH release. In both males and females, chronic therapy can result in endocrinopathies, including hypogonadotrophic hypogonadism. In men, this may result in decreased libido and, with extended exposure, reduced secondary sex characteristics. In women these exposures are associated with menstrual cycle irregularities. Importantly, these changes are reversible with removal of the opiate.

The mechanisms of the opiate regulation of gonadotrophin release may reflect a direct effect upon secreting pituicytes and an indirect action, through an effect on receptors present on hypothalamic neurons, to block release of gonadotropin-releasing hormone (GnRH) and corticotropin-releasing hormone (CRH). This reduction of the releasing factors leads to reduced release of luteinizing hormone (LH), follicle-stimulating hormone (FSH), ACTH, and β-endorphin. This series of events leads to reduced circulating testosterone and cortisol. Secretion of thyrotropin is relatively unaffected.

Prolactin. Prolactin release from lactotrope cells in the anterior pituitary is under inhibitory control by dopamine released from tuberoinfundibulum neurons of the arcuate nucleus. MOR agonists act presynaptically on these dopamine-releasing terminals to inhibit DA release and thereby increase plasma prolactin.

Growth Hormone. Growth hormone (GH) is released in a pulsatile fashion from somatotrophs in the anterior pituitary. GH-releasing hormone (GHRH) neurons in the hypothalamic arcuate nucleus and inhibitory input from somatostatin (SST) cells in the periventricular nucleus regulate this. Although some opioids increase GH release, possibly by inhibiting SST release, acute morphine has little effect on plasma GH concentration (Bluet-Pajot et al., 2001).

Antidiuretic Hormone and Oxytocin. The effects of opiates on ADH and oxytocin release are complex. These hormones are synthesized in the perikarya of the magnocellular neurons in the parventricular and supraoptic nuclei of the hypothalamus and released from the posterior pituitary (Chapter 38). ADH (vasopressin) release can occur secondary to surgical stress, hypovolemia, hypotension, and low osmolarity, while oxytocin release typically is released with afferent stimuli related to the milk ejection pathway. KOR agonists inhibit the release of oxytocin and antidiuretic hormone (and cause prominent diuresis). In humans, the administration of MOR agonists has little effect or tends to produce antidiuretic effects. Morphine reduces oxytocin secretion in nursing women (Lindow et al., 1999). It should be noted that agents such as morphine may yield a hypotension secondary to histamine release and this would, by itself, promote ADH release. Based on electrophysiology and localization of opiate receptors, these effects upon vasopressin and oxytocin release may reflect both a direct effect upon terminal secretion as well as indirect effects upon dopaminergic and noradrenergic modulatory projections into the parventricular and supraoptic hypothalamus (Gimpl and Fahrenholz, 2001).

Miosis. Illumination of the pupil activates a reflex arc, which through local circuitry in the Edinger Westphal nucleus, activates parasympathetic outflow through the ciliary ganglion to the pupil, producing constriction. MOR opiates induce pupillary constriction (miosis) in the awake state and block pupillary reflex dilation during anesthesia. The parasympathetic outflow is locally regulated by GABAergic interneurons. Opiates are believed to block the GABAergic interneuron-mediated inhibition (Larson, 2008). At high doses of agonists, the miosis is marked, and pinpoint pupils are pathognomonic; however, marked mydriasis will occur with the onset of asphyxia. While some tolerance to the miotic effect develops, addicts with high circulating concentrations of opioids continue to have constricted pupils. Therapeutic doses of morphine increase accommodative power and lower intraocular tension in normal and glaucomatous eyes.

Seizures and Convulsions. In older children and adults, moderately higher doses of opiates produce EEG slowing. In the newborn, morphine has been shown to produce epileptiform activity (Young and da Silva, 2000) and occasionally seizure activity. While increased jaw and chest wall rigidity routinely occur at doses used for anesthesia induction, frank seizures and convulsions typically occur only at doses far in excess of those required to produce even profound analgesia. Myoclonus and seizures have been reported particularly in opioid tolerant patients on high doses of morphine-like opiates, including fentanyl, as encountered in hospice and terminal stages of pain therapy (Vella-Brincat and Macleod., 2007). However, seizures that are produced by some agents such as meperidine may occur at doses only moderately higher than those required for analgesia, especially in children, particularly with repeated delivery.

Several mechanisms are most certainly involved in these excitatory actions:

- *Inhibition of inhibitory interneurons.* Morphine-like drugs excite certain groups of neurons, especially hippocampal pyramidal cells, probably from inhibition of the release of GABA by interneurons (McGinty, 1988).
- *Direct stimulatory effects.* Opiates may interact with receptors coupled through both inhibitory and stimulatory G-protein, with the inhibitory coupling but not the excitatory coupling showing tolerance with continued exposure (King et al., 2005).
- *Actions mediated by non-opioid receptors.* The metabolites of several opiates have been implicated in seizure activity, notably morphine-3-glucuronide (from morphine) and normeperidine (from meperidine) (Seifert and Kenendy, 2004; Smith, 2000).

A special case is the withdrawal syndrome from an opiate-dependent state in the adult and in the infant born to an opiate-dependent mother. Withdrawal in these circumstances, either by antagonists or abstinence, can lead to prominent EEG activation, tremor, and rigidity. Approaches to the management of such activation are controversial. Re-narcotization with a tapering dose and management of symptoms with anticonvulsants and anesthetics has been suggested (Farid et al., 2008). Anticonvulsant agents may not always be effective in suppressing opioid-induced seizures (Chapter 21).

Cough. Morphine and related opioids depress the cough reflex at least in part by a direct effect on a cough center in the medulla and this can be achieved without altering the protective glottal function. There is no obligatory relationship between depression of respiration and depression of coughing, and effective antitussive agents are available that do not depress respiration (antitussives are discussed later in the chapter). Suppression of cough by such agents appears to involve receptors in the medulla that are less sensitive to naloxone (an opioid antagonist) than those responsible for analgesia (Chung and Pavord, 2008).

Cough is a protective reflex evoked by airway stimulation. It involves rapid expression of air against a transiently closed glottis. The reflex is complex, involving the central and peripheral nervous systems as well as the smooth muscle of the bronchial tree. Irritation of the bronchial mucosa causes bronchoconstriction, which in turn stimulates cough receptors (which probably represent a specialized type of stretch receptor) located in tracheobronchial passages. Afferent conduction from these receptors is via fibers in the vagus nerve; central components of the reflex probably include several mechanisms or centers that are distinct from the mechanisms involved in the regulation of respiration.

Nauseant and Emetic Effects. Nausea is the prodomal sensation that is a common feature of gastric upset that is associated with reduced gastric motility and increased secretions. Vomiting, the motor sequela of nausea, is a complex reflex characterized by simultaneous contractions of inspiratory-expiratory respiratory muscle, increased stomach pressure, relaxation of the esophageal sphincter, and retrograde reflex propulsion of gastric contents. Nausea and vomiting produced by morphine-like drugs are side-effects caused by direct stimulation of the chemoreceptor trigger zone for emesis in the area postrema of the medulla. Apomorphine is a structural analog of morphine that has no opioid action but has prominent emetogenic actions.

Nausea and vomiting are relatively uncommon in recumbent patients given therapeutic doses of morphine, but nausea occurs in ~40% and vomiting in 15% of ambulatory patients given 15 mg of the drug subcutaneously. This suggests that a vestibular component is also operative. Indeed, the nauseant and emetic effects of morphine are markedly enhanced by vestibular stimulation, and morphine and related synthetic analgesics produce an increase in vestibular sensitivity. A component of nausea is likely due to the gastric stasis that occurs postoperatively and that is exacerbated by analgesic doses of morphine (Greenwood-Van Meerveld, 2007). All clinically useful agonists produce some degree of nausea and vomiting. Careful, controlled clinical studies usually demonstrate that, in equianalgesic dosage, the incidence of such side effects is not significantly lower than that seen with morphine. Antagonists to the 5-HT3 receptor have supplanted phenothiazines and drugs used for motion sickness as the drugs of choice for the treatment of opioid-induced nausea and vomiting. Gastric prokinetic agents such as metoclopramide also are useful anti-nausea and anti-emetic drugs (Cameron et al., 2003); however, caution is warranted due to the propensity of metoclopramide to cause tardive dyskinesia (Chapter 46).

Cardiovascular System. In the supine patient, therapeutic doses of morphine-like opioids have no major effect on blood pressure or cardiac rate and rhythm. Such doses can, however, produce peripheral vasodilation, reduced peripheral resistance, and an inhibition of baroreceptor reflexes. Thus, when supine patients assume the head-up position, orthostatic hypotension and fainting may occur. The peripheral arteriolar and venous dilation produced by morphine involves several mechanisms:

- morphine-induced release of histamine from mast cells, leading to vasodilation (reveresed by naloxone only partially blocked by H_1 antagonists)
- blunting of the reflex vasoconstriction caused by increased P_{CO_2}

High doses of MOR agonists, such as fentanyl and sufentanil, used as anesthetic induction agents, have only modest effects upon hemodynamic stability, in part because they do not cause release of histamine (Monk et al., 1988).

Effects on the myocardium are not significant in normal individuals. In patients with coronary artery disease but no acute medical problems, 8-15 mg morphine administered intravenously produces a decrease in O_2 consumption, left ventricular end-diastolic pressure, and cardiac work; effects on cardiac index usually are slight. In patients with acute myocardial infarction, the cardiovascular responses to morphine may be more variable than in normal subjects, and the magnitude of changes (e.g., the decrease in blood pressure) may be more pronounced (Roth et al., 1988). Anesthetic induction doses (described later) of the MOR result in a centrally mediated increase in vagal outflow to the heart, leading to an atropine-sensitive bradycardia.

Morphine may exert its well-known therapeutic effect in the treatment of angina pectoris and acute myocardial infarction by decreasing preload, inotropy, and chronotropy, thus favorably altering determinants of myocardial O_2 consumption and helping to relieve ischemia. It is not clear whether the analgesic properties of morphine in this situation are due to the reversal of acidosis that may stimulate local acid-sensing ion channels (McCleskey and Gold, 1999) or to a direct analgesic effect on nociceptive afferents from the heart.

When administered before experimental ischemia, morphine has been shown to produce cardioprotective effects. Morphine can mimic the phenomenon of ischemic preconditioning, where a short ischemic episode paradoxically protects the heart against further ischemia. This effect appears to be mediated through receptors signaling through a mitochondrial ATP-sensitive K^+ channel in cardiac myocytes; the effect also is produced by other GPCRs signaling through Gi (Fryer et al., 2000). Some researchers suggest that opioids can be anti-arrhythmic and anti-fibrillatory during and after periods of ischemia (Fryer et al., 2000), although other data suggest that opioids can be arrhythmogenic (McIntosh et al., 1992).

Morphine-like opioids should be used with caution in patients who have decreased blood volume because these agents can aggravate hypovolemic shock. Morphine should be used with great care in patients with cor pulmonale because deaths after ordinary therapeutic doses have been reported. The concurrent use of certain phenothiazines may increase the risk of morphine-induced hypotension.

Cerebral circulation is not affected directly by therapeutic doses of opiates. However, opioid-induced respiratory depression and CO_2 retention can result in cerebral vasodilation and an increase in cerebrospinal fluid pressure. This pressure increase does not occur when PCO_2 is maintained at normal levels by artificial ventilation. Nevertheless, opioids produce changes in arousal that can obscure the clinical course of patients with head injuries.

Motor Tone. At therapeutic doses required for analgesia, opiates have little effect upon motor tone or function. However, high doses of opioids, as used for anesthetic induction, produce muscular rigidity in humans. Thus, rigidity of the chest wall and masseter severe enough to compromise respiration and intubation is not uncommon during anesthesia and routinely requires the use muscle relaxants.

Myoclonus, ranging from mild twitching to generalized spasm, is an occasional side-effect, which has been reported with all clinical opiate agonists; while it may be observed at lower therapeutic doses, it is particularly prevalent in hospice patients receiving high doses (Lyss et al., 1997). The increased muscle tone is certainly mediated by a central effect although the mechanisms of its effects are not clear. High doses of spinal opiates can increase motor tone, possibly through an inhibition of inhibitory interneurons in the ventral horn of the spinal cord. Alternately, intracranial delivery can initiate rigidity in animal models possible reflecting on increased extrapyramidal activity. As already indicated, both actions are reversed by opiate antagonists.

GI Tract. Opiates have important effects upon all aspects of GI function. It is estimated that 40-95% of patients treated with opioids develop constipation and that changes in bowel function can be demonstrated even with acute dosing (Benyamin et al., 2008). Opioid receptors are densely distributed in enteric neurons between the myenteric and submucosal plexi and on a variety of secretory cells. The more prominent expression of the action mediated by these receptors will be reviewed in the next sections. Importantly, the presence of opioids can obscure recognition of the diagnosis or clinical course in patients with acute abdominal conditions.

Esophagus. The esophageal sphincter is under control by brainstem reflexes that activate cholinergic motor neurons originating in the esophageal myenteric plexus. This system regulates passage of material from the esophagus to the stomach and prevents regurgitation; conversely, it allows relaxation in the act of emesis. Morphine inhibits lower esophageal sphincter relaxation induced by swallowing and by esophageal distension. This effect is believed to be centrally mediated, as peripherally restricted opiates such as loperamide do not alter esophageal sphincter tone (Sidhu and Triadafilopoulos, 2008).

Stomach. Movement of a meal though the stomach reflects the coordinated contractions of the antrum and the resting tone of the gastric reservoir. Relatively low doses of morphine result in an increase in tonic contracture of the antral musculature (secondary to an inhibition of local inhibitory neurons) and upper duodenum and reduced resting tone in the musculature of the gastric reservoir (secondary to inhibition of the motor neurons to the reservoir musculature), thereby prolonging gastric emptying time and increasing the likelihood of esophageal reflux. Passage of the gastric contents through the duodenum may be delayed by as much as 12 hours, and the absorption of orally administered drugs is retarded. Morphine and other agonists usually decrease secretion of hydrochloric acid, although stimulation sometimes is evident. Activation of opioid receptors on parietal cells enhances secretion, but indirect effects, including increased secretion of somatostatin from the pancreas and reduced release of acetylcholine, appear to be dominant in most circumstances (Kromer, 1988).

Intestine. Morphine reduces propulsatile activity in the small and large intestine and diminishes intestinal secretions.

Propulsatile Activity. Opiate agonists suppress local neurogenic networks that provide a rhythmic inhibition of muscle tone leading to concurrent increases in basal tone in the circular muscle of the small and large intestine. This results in enhanced high-amplitude phasic contractions, which are nonpropulsatile. The upper part of the small intestine, particularly the duodenum, is affected more than the ileum. A period of relative atony may follow the hypertonicity. The reduced rate of passage of the intestinal contents, along with reduced intestinal secretion, leads to increased water absorption, increasing viscosity of the bowel contents, and constipation. The tone of the anal sphincter is augmented greatly, and reflex relaxation in response to rectal distension is reduced. These actions, combined with inattention to the normal sensory stimuli for defecation reflex owing to the central actions of the drug, contribute to morphine-induced constipation (Wood and Galligan, 2004).

The clinical relevance of the role of the peripheral opioid receptors in regulating GI motility after systemic opioids is supported by:

- The efficacy of peripherally limited opiate agonists such as loperamide as anti-diarrheals
- The ability of peripherally limited opiate antagonists such as methylnaltrexone to reverse the constipatory actions of systemic opiate agonists

Direct delivery of opioids into the cerebral ventricles or into the spinal intrathecal space could also inhibit GI propulsive activity as long as the extrinsic innervation to the bowel is intact. Although some tolerance develops to the effects of opioids on GI motility, patients who take opioids chronically remain constipated.

Intestinal Secretions. In the presence of intestinal hypersecretion that may be associated with diarrhea, morphine-like drugs inhibit the transfer of fluid and electrolytes into the lumen by naloxone-sensitive actions on the intestinal mucosa and within the CNS (Kromer, 1988). Intestinal secretion arises from activation of enterocytes by local cholinergic submucosal plexus secretomotor neurons. Opioids act though μ/δ receptors on these secretomotor neurons to inhibit their excitatory output to the enterocytes and thereby reduce intestinal secretion.

Biliary Tract. Bile flow is regulated by the periodic contractions of the sphincter of Oddi, which is relaxed by inhibitory innervation. This inhibitory innervation is suppressed by opiates. After the subcutaneous injection of 10 mg morphine sulfate, the sphincter of Oddi constricts, and the pressure in the common bile duct may rise >10-fold within 15 minutes; this effect may persist for 2 hours or more. Fluid pressure also may increase in the gallbladder and produce symptoms that may vary from epigastric distress to typical biliary colic.

Some patients with biliary colic experience exacerbation rather than relief of pain when given opioids. Spasm of the sphincter of Oddi probably is responsible for elevations of plasma amylase and lipase that occur sometimes after morphine administration. All opioids can cause biliary spasm. Atropine only partially prevents morphine-induced biliary spasm, but opioid antagonists prevent or relieve it. Papaverine, another alkaloid of the poppy that lacks opioid activity, produces smooth muscle relaxation and is used therapeutically for GI, urethral, and biliary colic and for other nonvisceral conditions (e.g., embolism and angina pectoris) accompanied by smooth muscle spasm.

Other Smooth Muscle

Ureter and Urinary Bladder. Voiding is a highly organized response initiated by afferents activated by bladder filling and spinobulbospinal reflex arcs, which lead to contraction of the bladder and a reflex relaxation of the external urinary sphincter (Fowler et al., 2008). Morphine inhibits the urinary voiding reflex and increases the tone of the external sphincter with a resultant increase in the volume of the bladder. In animal models, this effect is mediated by MOR and DOR agonists. Stimulation of either receptor type in the brain or in the spinal cord exerts similar actions on bladder motility (Dray and Nunan, 1987). Tolerance develops to these effects of opioids on the bladder. Clinically, opiate-mediated inhibition of micturition can be of such clinical severity that catheterization sometimes is required after therapeutic doses of morphine, particularly with spinal drug administration. Importantly, in humans, the inhibition of systemic opiate effects on micturition is reversed by peripherally restricted antagonists (Rosow et al., 2007).

Uterus. If the uterus has been made hyperactive by oxytocics, morphine tends to restore the tone, frequency, and amplitude of contractions to normal.

Skin. Therapeutic doses of morphine cause dilation of cutaneous blood vessels. The skin of the face, neck, and upper thorax frequently becomes flushed. These changes may be due in part to the release of histamine and may be responsible for the sweating and some of the pruritus that commonly follow the systemic administration of morphine (described later). Histamine release probably accounts for the urticaria commonly seen at the site of injection. Though controversial, it is not blocked by naloxone and thought not to be mediated by opioid receptors. Itching is readily seen with morphine and meperidine but to a much lesser extent with oxymorphone, methadone, fentanyl, or sufentanil. This pruritus is a common and potentially disabling complication of opioid use. It can be caused by systemic as well as intraspinal injections of therapeutic doses of opioids, but it appears to be more intense after epidural or intrathecal administration (Ballantyne et al., 1988). The spinal effect, which is reversible by naloxone, may reflect a disinhibition of itch-specific neurons that have been identified in the spinal dorsal horn (Schmelz, 2002).

Immune System. The effects of opioids on the immune system are complex. Opioids modulate immune function by direct effects on cells of the immune system and indirectly through centrally mediated neuronal mechanisms (Sharp and Yaksh, 1997). The acute central immunomodulatory effects of opioids may be mediated by activation of the sympathetic nervous system; the chronic effects of opioids may involve modulation of the hypothalamic-pituitary-adrenal (HPA) axis (Mellon and Bayer, 1998).

Direct effects on immune cells may involve unique, incompletely characterized variants of the classical neuronal opioid receptors, with MOR variants being most prominent (Sharp and Yaksh, 1997). Atypical receptors could account for the fact that it has been very difficult to demonstrate significant opioid binding on immune cells despite the observance of robust functional effects. In contrast, morphine-induced immune suppression largely is abolished in knockout mice lacking the receptor gene, suggesting that the receptor is a major target of morphine's actions on the immune system (Gaveriaux-Ruff et al., 1998). A proposed mechanism for the immune suppressive effects of morphine on neutrophils is through a nitric oxide–dependent inhibition of NF-kB activation (Welters et al., 2000). Others have proposed that the induction and activation of MAP kinase also may play a role (Chuang et al., 1997).

Overall, the effects of opioids appear to be modestly immunosuppressive, and increased susceptibility to infection and tumor spread have been observed. In some situations, immune effects appear more prominent with acute administration than with chronic administration, which could have important implications for the care of the critically ill (Sharp and Yaksh, 1997). In contrast, opioids have been shown to reverse pain-induced immunosuppression and increase tumor metastatic potential in animal models (Page and Ben-Eliyahu, 1997). Therefore, opioids may either inhibit or augment immune function depending on the context in which they are used. These studies also indicate that withholding opioids in the presence of pain in immunocompromised patients actually could worsen immune function. Taken together, these studies indicate that opioid-induced immune suppression may be clinically relevant both to the treatment of severe pain and in the susceptibility of opioid addicts to infection (e.g., human immunodeficiency virus (HIV) infection and tuberculosis). Different opioid agonists also may have unique immunomodulatory properties. Better understanding of these properties eventually should help to guide the rational use of opioids in patients with cancer or at risk for infection or immune compromise.

Temperature Regulation. Opioids alter the equilibrium point of the hypothalamic heat-regulatory mechanisms such that body temperature usually falls slightly. Systematic studies have shown that MOR agonists such as alfentanil and meperidine, acting in the CNS, will result in slightly increased thresholds for sweating and significantly lower the threshold temperatures for evoking vasoconstriction and shivering (Sessler, 2008). In precipitated withdrawal, elevated body temperatures are observed, an observation consistent with the report that chronic high dosage may increase body temperature (Martin, 1983).

FUNCTIONAL OPIOID DRUG TYPES

Most of the clinically used opioid agonists presented below are relatively selective for MOR. They produce analgesia, affect mood and rewarding behavior, and alter respiratory, cardiovascular, GI, and neuroendocrine function. KOR agonists, with few exceptions (e.g., butorphanol), are not typically employed for long-term therapy since they may produce dysphoric and psychotomimetic effects. DOR agonists, while analgesic in animal models, have not found clinical utility, and NOR agonists have largely proven to lack analgesic effects. Opiates that are relatively receptor selective at lower doses will interact with additional receptor types when given at high doses. This is especially true as doses are escalated to overcome tolerance.

The mixed agonist–antagonist agents frequently interact with more than one receptor class at usual clinical doses. The actions of these drugs are particularly interesting because they may act as an agonist at one receptor and as an antagonist at another. Mixed agonist–antagonist compounds were developed with the hope that they would have less addictive potential and less respiratory depression than morphine and related drugs. In practice, however, for the same degree of analgesia, the same intensity of side effects occurs. A "ceiling effect" limiting the amount of analgesia attainable often is seen with these drugs, such as buprenorphine, which is approved for the treatment of opioid dependence. Some mixed agonist–antagonist drugs, such as pentazocine and nalorphine (not available in the U.S.), can precipitate withdrawal in opioid-tolerant patients. For these reasons, except for the sanctioned use of buprenorphine to manage opioid addiction, the clinical use of these mixed agonist–antagonist drugs is generally limited.

The dosing guidelines and duration of action for the numerous drugs that are part of opioid therapy are summarized in Table 18–2.

MORPHINE AND STRUCTURALLY RELATED AGONISTS

Even though there are many compounds with pharmacological properties similar to those of morphine, morphine remains the standard against which new analgesics are measured.

Source and Composition of Opium

Because the synthesis of morphine is difficult, the drug still is obtained from opium or extracted from poppy straw. Opium is obtained from the unripe seed capsules of the poppy plant, *Papaver somniferum*. The milky juice is dried and powdered to make powdered opium, which contains a number of alkaloids. Only a few—morphine, codeine, and papaverine—have clinical utility. These alkaloids can be divided into two distinct chemical classes, phenanthrenes and benzylisoquinolines. The principal phenanthrenes are morphine (10% of opium), codeine (0.5%), and thebaine (0.2%).

Table 18–2

Dosing Data for Clinically Employed Opioid Analgesics

DRUG	APPROXIMATE EQUI-ANALGESIC ORAL DOSE	APPROXIMATE EQUI-ANALGESIC PARENTERAL DOSE	RECOMMENDED STARTING DOSE (adults >50 kg) ORAL	RECOMMENDED STARTING DOSE (adults >50 kg) PARENTERAL	RECOMMENDED STARTING DOSE (children and adults <50 kg)[a] ORAL	RECOMMENDED STARTING DOSE (children and adults <50 kg)[a] PARENTERAL
Opioid Agonists						
Morphine[b]	30 mg q3–4h (around-the-clock dosing) 60 mg q3–4h (single dose or intermittent dosing	10 mg q3–4h	15 mg q3–4h	5 mg q3–4h	0.3 mg/kg q3–4h	0.1 mg/kg q3–4h
Codeine[c]	130 mg q3–4h	75 mg q3–4h	30 mg q3–4h	30 mg q2h (IM/SC)	1 mg/kg q3–4h[d]	Not recommended
Hydromophone (DILAUDID)[b]	7.5 mg q3–4h	1.5 mg q3–4h	4 mg q3–4h	1 mg q3–4h	0.06 mg/kg q3–4h	0.015 mg/kg q3–4h
Hydrocodone (in LORCET, LORTAB, VICODIN, others, typically with acetominophen)	30 mg q3–4h	Not available	5 mg q3–4h	Not available	0.2 mg/kg q3–4h[d]	Not available
Levorphanol	4 mg q6–8h	2 mg q6–8h	2 mg q6–8h	1 mg q6–8h	0.04 mg/kg q6–8h	0.02 mg/kg q6–8h
Meperidine (DEMEROL)	300 mg q2–3h	100 mg q3h	Not recommended	50 mg q3h	Not recommended	0.75 mg/kg q2–3h
Methadone (DOLOPHINE, others)	20 mg q6–8h	10 mg q6–8h	2.5 mg q12h	2.5 mg q12h	0.2 mg/kg q12h	0.1 mg/kg q6–8h
Oxycodone (REXICODONE, OXYCONTIN, also in PERCOCET, PERCODAN, TYLOX, others)[g]	30 mg q3–4h	Not available	5 mg q3–4h	Not available	0.2 mg/kg q3–4h[d]	Not available
Oxymorphone[b] (NUMORPHAN)	Not available	1 mg q3–4h	Not available	1 mg q3–4h	Not recommended	Not recommended
Propoxyphene (DARVON)	130 mg[e]	Not available	65 mg q4–6h[e]	Not available	Not recommended	Not recommended
Tramadol[f] (ULTRAM)	100 mg[e]	100 mg	50–100 mg q6h[e]	50–100 mg q6h[e]	Not recommended	Not recommended
Opioid Agonist–Antagonists or Partial Agonists						
Buprenorphine (BUPRENEX)	Not available	0.3–0.4 mg q6–8h	Not available	0.4 mg q6–8h	Not available	0.004 mg/kg q6–8h
Butorphanol (STADOL)	Not available	2 mg q3–4h	Not available	2 mg q3–4h	Not available	Not recommended
Nalbuphine (NUBAIN)	Not available	10 mg q3–4h	Not available	10 mg q3–4h	Not available	0.1 mg/kg q3–4h

Published tables vary in the suggested doses that are equi-analgesic to morphine. Clinical response is the criterion that must be applied for each patient; titration to clinical response is necessary. Because there is not complete cross-tolerance among these drugs, it is usually necessary to use a lower than equianalgesic dose when changing drugs and to retitrate to response. *Caution*: Recommended doses do not apply to patients with renal or hepatic insufficiency or other conditions affecting drug metabolism and kinetics. [a]*Caution*: Doses listed for patients with body weight less than 50 kg cannot be used as initial starting doses in babies less than 6 months of age. Consult the *Clinical Practice Guideline for Acute Pain Management: Operative or Medical Procedures and Trauma* section on management of pain in neonates for recommendations. [b]For morphine, hydromorphone, and oxymorphone, rectal administration is an alternate route for patients unable to take oral medications, but equianalgesic doses may differ from oral and parenteral doses because of pharmacokinetic differences. [c]Caution: Codeine doses above 65 mg often are not appropriate due to diminishing incremental analgesia with increasing doses but continually increasing constipation and other side effects. [d]Caution: Doses of aspirin and acetaminophen in combination opioid/NSAID preparations must also be adjusted to the patient's body weight. Maximum acetaminophen dose: 4 g/day in adults, 90 mg/kg/day in children. [e]Doses for moderate pain not necessarily equivalent to 30 mg oral or 10 mg parenteral morphine. [f]Risk of seizures: parenteral formulation not available in the U.S. [g]Oxycontin is an extended-release preparation containing up to 160 mg of oxycodone per tablet and recommended for use every 12 hours. It has been subject to substantial abuse. Modified from Agency for Healthcare Policy and Research, 1992.

The principal benzylisoquinolines are papaverine (1%) (a smooth muscle relaxant) and noscapine (6%).

Chemistry of Morphine and Its Congeners

The structure of morphine is shown in Figure 18–8. Many semisynthetic derivatives are made by relatively simple modifications of morphine or thebaine. Codeine is methylmorphine, the methyl substitution being on the phenolic hydroxyl group. Thebaine differs from morphine only in that both hydroxyl groups are methylated and that the ring has two double bonds (6,7; 8,14). Thebaine has little analgesic action but is a precursor of several important 14-OH compounds, such as oxycodone and naloxone. Certain derivatives of thebaine are >1000 times as potent as morphine (e.g., etorphine). Diacetylmorphine, or heroin, is made from morphine by acetylation at the 3 and 6 positions. Apomorphine, which also can be prepared from morphine, is a potent emetic and dopaminergic D1 and D2 agonist, has no opiate receptor interactions, and displays no analgesic actions (Chapters 22 and 46). Hydromorphone, oxymorphone, hydrocodone, and oxycodone also are made by modifying the morphine molecule. The structural relationships between morphine and some of its surrogates and antagonists are shown in Figure 18–8.

Structure-Activity Relationship of the Morphine-Like Opioids. In addition to morphine, codeine, and the semisynthetic derivatives of the natural opium alkaloids, a number of other structurally distinct chemical classes of drugs have pharmacological actions similar to those of morphine. Clinically useful compounds include the morphinans, benzomorphans, methadones, phenylpiperidines, and propionanilides. Although the two-dimensional representations of these chemically diverse compounds appear to be quite different, molecular models show certain common characteristics, as indicated by the heavy lines in the structure of morphine shown in Figure 18–8. Among the important properties of the opioids that can be altered by structural modification are their affinities for various types of opioid receptors, their activities as agonists versus antagonists, their lipid solubilities, and their resistance to metabolic breakdown. For example, blockade of the phenolic hydroxyl at position 3, as in codeine and heroin, drastically reduces binding to receptors; these compounds are converted *in vivo* to the potent analgesics morphine and 6-acetyl morphine, respectively.

Absorption, Distribution, Metabolism, and Excretion

Absorption. In general, the opioids are modestly absorbed from the GI tract; absorption through the rectal mucosa is adequate and a few agents (e.g., morphine, hydromorphone) are available in suppositories. The more lipophilic opioids are absorbed readily through the nasal or buccal mucosa. Those with the greatest lipid solubility also can be absorbed transdermally. Opioids, particularly morphine, have been widely used for spinal delivery to produce analgesia though a spinal action. These agents display useful transdural movement adequate to permit their use epidurally.

With most opioids, including morphine, the effect of a given dose is less after oral than after parenteral administration because of variable but significant first-pass metabolism in the liver. For example, the bioavailability of oral preparations of morphine is only ~25%. The shape of the time-effect curve also varies with the route of administration, so the duration of action often is somewhat longer with the oral route. If adjustment is made for variability of first-pass metabolism and clearance, adequate relief of pain can be achieved with oral administration of morphine. Satisfactory analgesia in cancer patients is associated with a very broad range of steady-state concentrations of morphine in plasma (16-364 ng/mL) (Neumann et al., 1982).

When morphine and most opioids are given intravenously, they act promptly. However, the more lipid-soluble compounds (e.g., fentanyl) act more rapidly than morphine after subcutaneous administration because of differences in the rates of absorption and entry into the CNS. Compared with more lipid-soluble opioids such as codeine, heroin, and methadone, morphine crosses the blood-brain barrier at a considerably lower rate.

Distribution and Metabolism. About one-third of morphine in the plasma is protein-bound after a therapeutic dose. Morphine itself does not persist in tissues, and 24 hours after the last dose, tissue concentrations are low.

The major pathway for the metabolism of morphine is conjugation with glucuronic acid. The two major metabolites formed are morphine-6-glucuronide and morphine-3-glucuronide. Small amounts of morphine-3,6-diglucuronide also may be formed. Although the 3- and 6-glucuronides are quite polar, both still can cross the blood-brain barrier to exert significant clinical effects (Christrup, 1997).

Morphine-6-glucuronide has pharmacological actions indistinguishable from those of morphine. Morphine-6-glucuronide given systemically is approximately twice as potent as morphine in animal models (Paul et al., 1989) and in humans (Osborne et al., 1988). With chronic administration, the 6-glucuronide accounts for a significant portion of morphine's analgesic actions (Osborne et al., 1988). Indeed, with chronic oral dosing, the blood levels of morphine-6-glucuronide typically exceed those of morphine. Given its greater MOR potency and its higher concentration, morphine-6-glucuronide may be responsible for most of morphine's analgesic activity in patients receiving chronic oral morphine. Morphine-6-glucuronide is excreted by the kidney. In renal failure, the levels of morphine-6-glucuronide can accumulate, perhaps explaining morphine's potency and long duration in patients with compromised renal function. In adults, the $t_{1/2}$ of morphine is ~2 hours; the $t_{1/2}$ of morphine-6-glucuronide is somewhat longer. Children achieve adult renal function values by 6 months of age. In elderly patients, lower doses of morphine are recommended based on a smaller volume of distribution (Owen et al., 1983) and the general decline in renal function in the elderly.

Morphine-3-glucuronide, another important metabolite, has little affinity for opioid receptors but may contribute to excitatory effects of morphine (Smith, 2000). N-Demethylation of morphine to normorphine is a minor metabolic pathway in humans but is more prominent in rodents (Yeh et al., 1977). N-Dealkylation also is important in the metabolism of some congeners of morphine.

Excretion. *Morphine* is eliminated by glomerular filtration, primarily as morphine-3-glucuronide; 90% of the total excretion takes place during the first day. Very little morphine is excreted unchanged. Enterohepatic circulation of morphine and its glucuronides occurs,

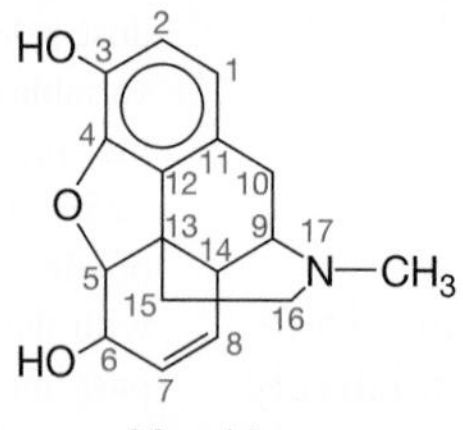

Nonproprietary name	Chemical radicals and position[a] 3	6	17	Other changes†
Morphine	—OH	—OH	—CH_3	—
Heroin	—$OCOCH_3$	—$OCOCH_3$	—CH_3	—
Hydromorphone	—OH	=O	—CH_3	(1)
Oxymorphone	—OH	=O	—CH_3	(1), (2)
Levorphanol	—OH	—H	—CH_3	(1), (3)
Levallorphan	—OH	—H	—$CH_2CH{=}CH_2$	(1), (3)
Codeine	—OCH_3	—OH	—CH_3	—
Hydrocodone	—OCH_3	=O	—CH_3	(1)
Oxycodone	—OCH_3	=O	—CH_3	(1), (2)
Nalmefene	—OH	=CH_2	—CH_2—(cyclopropyl)	(1), (2)
Nalorphine	—OH	—OH	—$CH_2CH{=}CH_2$	—
Naloxone	—OH	=O	—$CH_2CH{=}CH_2$	(1), (2)
Naltrexone	—OH	=O	—CH_2—(cyclopropyl)	(1), (2)
Buprenorphine	—OH	—OCH_3	—CH_2—(cyclopropyl)	(1), (4)
Butorphanol	—OH	—H	—CH_2—(cyclobutyl)	(1), (2), (3)
Nalbuphine	—OH	—OH	—CH_2—(cyclobutyl)	(1), (2)
Methylnaltrexone	—OH	=O	—(N)—CH_2—(cyclopropyl), N—CH_3	(1), (2)

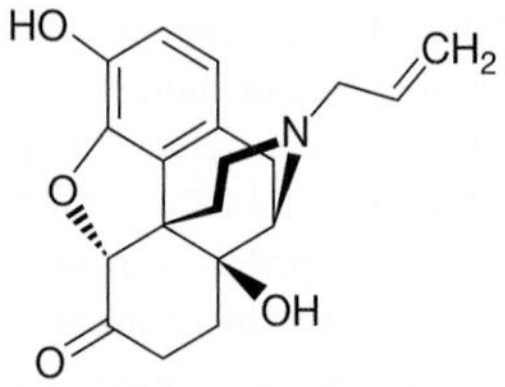

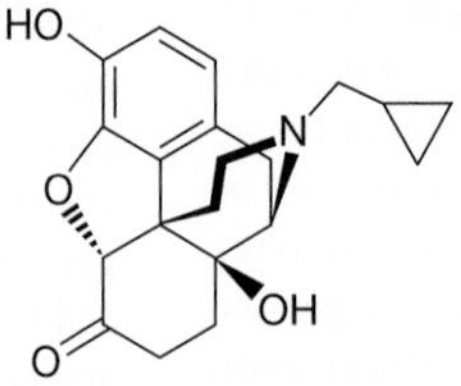

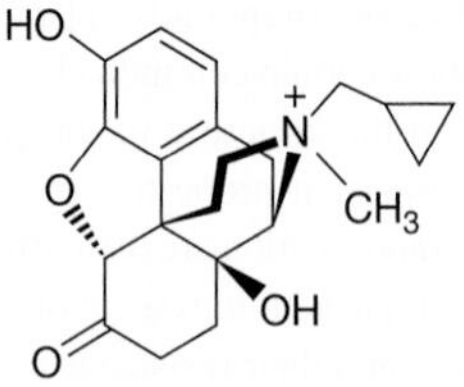

[a]The numbers 3, 6, and 17 refer to positions in the morphine molecule, as shown above. †Other changes in the morphine molecule are: (1) Single instead of double bond between C7 and C8: (2) OH added to C14: (3) No oxygen between C4 and C5: (4) *Endo*etheno bridge between C6 and C14: 1-hydroxy-1,2,2-trimethylpropyl substitution on C7.

Figure 18–8. *Structures of morphine-related opiate agonists and antagonists.*

which accounts for the presence of small amounts of morphine in feces and urine for several days after the last dose.

In contrast to morphine, codeine is ~60% as effective orally as parenterally as an analgesic and as a respiratory depressant. Codeine analogs such as levorphanol, oxycodone, and methadone have a high ratio of oral-to-parenteral potency. The greater oral efficacy of these drugs reflects lower first-pass metabolism in the liver. Once absorbed, codeine is metabolized by the liver, and its metabolites are excreted chiefly as inactive forms in the urine. A small fraction (~10%) of administered codeine is O-demethylated to morphine, and free and conjugated morphine can be found in the urine after therapeutic doses of codeine. Codeine has an exceptionally low affinity for opioid receptors, and the analgesic effect of codeine is due to its conversion to morphine. However, codeine's antitussive actions may involve distinct receptors that bind codeine itself, and codeine is commonly employed for the management of cough. The $t_{1/2}$ of codeine in plasma is 2-4 hours.

CYP2D6 catalyzes the conversion of codeine to morphine. Well-characterized genetic polymorphisms in CYP2D6 lead to the inability to convert codeine to morphine, thus making codeine ineffective as an analgesic for ~10% of the Caucasian population (Eichelbaum and Evert, 1996). Other polymorphisms (e.g., the CYP2D6*2x2 genotype) can lead to ultra-rapid metabolism and thus increased sensitivity to codeine's effects due to higher than expected serum morphine levels in 4-5% of the US population and 16-28% of North Africans, Ethiopians, and Arabs (Eichelbaum and Evert, 1996). Other variations in metabolic efficiency among ethnic groups are apparent. For example, Chinese produce less morphine from codeine than do Caucasians and also are less sensitive to morphine's effects. The reduced sensitivity to morphine may be due to decreased production of morphine-6-glucuronide (Caraco et al., 1999). Thus, it is important to consider the possibility of metabolic enzyme polymorphism in any patient who experiences toxicity or does not receive adequate analgesia from codeine or other opioid prodrugs (e.g., hydrocodone and oxycodone).

Heroin (diacetylmorphine) is rapidly hydrolyzed to 6-monoacetylmorphine (6-MAM), which in turn is hydrolyzed to morphine. Heroin and 6-MAM are more lipid soluble than morphine and enter the brain more readily. Evidence suggests that morphine and 6-MAM are responsible for the pharmacological actions of heroin. Heroin is excreted mainly in the urine largely as free and conjugated morphine.

Therapeutic Actions and Precautions

Morphine and related opioids produce a wide spectrum of unwanted effects, including respiratory depression, nausea, vomiting, dizziness, mental clouding, dysphoria, pruritus, constipation, increased pressure in the biliary tract, urinary retention, and hypotension. The bases of these effects were described earlier. Rarely, a patient may develop delirium. Increased sensitivity to pain after analgesia has worn off and between-dose withdrawal also may occur.

A number of factors may alter a patient's sensitivity to opioid analgesics, including the integrity of the blood-brain barrier. For example, when morphine is administered to a newborn infant in weight-appropriate doses extrapolated from adults, unexpectedly profound effects (analgesia and respiratory depression) may be observed. This is due to the immaturity of the blood-brain barrier in neonates. As mentioned previously, morphine is hydrophilic, so proportionately less morphine normally crosses into the CNS than with more lipophilic opioids. In neonates or when the blood-brain barrier is compromised, lipophilic opioids may give more predictable clinical results than morphine. In adults, the duration of the analgesia produced by morphine increases progressively with age; however, the degree of analgesia that is obtained with a given dose changes little. Changes in pharmacokinetic parameters only partially explain these observations. The patient with severe pain may tolerate larger doses of morphine. However, as the pain subsides, the patient may exhibit sedation and even respiratory depression as the stimulatory effects of pain are diminished.

All opioid analgesics are metabolized by the liver and should be used with caution in patients with hepatic disease because increased bioavailability after oral administration or cumulative effects may occur. Renal disease also significantly alters the pharmacokinetics of morphine, codeine, dihydrocodeine, meperidine, and propoxyphene. Although single doses of morphine are well tolerated, the active metabolite, morphine-6-glucuronide, may accumulate with continued dosing, and symptoms of opioid overdose may result (Chan and Matzke, 1987). This metabolite also may accumulate during repeated administration of codeine to patients with impaired renal function. When repeated doses of meperidine are given to such patients, the accumulation of normeperidine may cause tremor and seizures. Similarly, the repeated administration of propoxyphene may lead to naloxone-insensitive cardiac toxicity caused by the accumulation of norpropoxyphene (Chan and Matzke, 1987).

Morphine and related opioids must be used cautiously in patients with compromised respiratory function (e.g., emphysema, kyphoscoliosis, severe obesity). In patients with cor pulmonale, death has occurred after therapeutic doses of morphine. Although many patients with such conditions seem to be functioning within normal limits, they are already using compensatory mechanisms, such as increased respiratory rate. Many have chronically elevated levels of plasma CO_2 and may be less sensitive to the stimulating actions of CO_2. The further imposition of the depressant effects of opioids can be disastrous. The respiratory-depressant effects of opioids and the related capacity to elevate intracranial pressure must be considered in the presence of head injury or an already elevated intracranial pressure. While head injury *per se* does not constitute an absolute contraindication to the use of opioids, the possibility of exaggerated depression of respiration and the potential need to control ventilation of the patient must be considered. Finally, since opioids may produce mental clouding and side effects such as miosis and vomiting, which are important signs in following the clinical course of patients with head injuries, the advisability of their use must be weighed carefully against these risks.

Patients with reduced blood volume are considerably more susceptible to the vasodilating effects of morphine and related drugs, and these agents must be used cautiously in patients with hypotension from any cause.

Morphine causes histamine release, which can cause bronchoconstriction and vasodilation. Morphine has the potential to precipitate or exacerbate asthmatic attacks and should be avoided in patients with a history of asthma. Other receptor agonists associated with a lower incidence of histamine release, such as the fentanyl derivatives, may be better choices for such patients.

Aside from their ability to release histamine, opioid analgesics may evoke allergic phenomena, but a true allergic response is uncommon. The effects usually are manifested as urticaria and other types of skin rashes such as fixed eruptions; contact dermatitis in nurses and pharmaceutical workers also occurs. Wheals at the site of injection of morphine, codeine, and related drugs are likely secondary to histamine release. Anaphylactoid reactions have been reported after intravenous administration of codeine and morphine, but such reactions are rare. Such reactions may contribute to sudden death, episodes of pulmonary edema, and other complications that occur among addicts who use heroin intravenously (Chapter 24).

LEVORPHANOL

Levorphanol (LEVO-DROMORAN) is the principal available opioid agonist of the morphinan series (see structure in Figure 18–8). The D-isomer (dextrorphan) is devoid of analgesic action but has inhibitory effects at NMDA receptors.. It has affinity at the MOR, KOR, and DORs and is available for IV, IM, and PO administration. The pharmacological effects of levorphanol closely parallel those of morphine. However, clinical reports suggest that it may produce less nausea and vomiting.

Levorphanol is metabolized less rapidly than morphine and has a $t_{1/2}$ of 12-16 hours; repeated administration at short intervals may thus lead to accumulation of the drug in plasma. Other agents in this class include nalbuphine (NUBAIN, others) and butorphanol (STADOL, others), which are discussed in the section "Opioid Agonists/Antagonists and Partial Agonists" later in the chapter.

MEPERIDINE, DIPHENOXYLATE, LOPERAMIDE

The structural formulas of meperidine, a phenylpiperidine, and some of its congeners, are shown in Figure 18–9. Two important congeners are diphenoxylate and loperamide. These agents are MOR agonists with principal pharmacological effects on the CNS and neural elements in the bowel.

Meperidine

Meperidine is predominantly a MOR agonist that produces a pattern of effects similar but not identical to those already described for morphine.

Effects on Organ Systems

CNS Actions. Meperidine is a potent MOR agonist yielding strong analgesic actions. Peak respiratory depression is observed within 1 hour of intramuscular administration, and there is a return toward normal starting at ~2 hours. Like other opioids, meperidine causes pupillary constriction, increases the sensitivity of the labyrinthine apparatus, and has effects on the secretion of pituitary hormones similar to those of morphine. Meperidine sometimes causes CNS excitation, characterized by tremors, muscle twitches, and seizures; these effects are due largely to accumulation of a metabolite, normeperidine. Meperidine has well known local anesthetic properties, particularly noted after epidural administration. As with morphine, respiratory depression is responsible for an accumulation of CO_2, which in turn leads to cerebrovascular dilation, increased cerebral blood flow, and elevation of cerebrospinal fluid pressure.

Cardiovascular System. The effects of meperidine on the cardiovascular system generally resemble those of morphine, including the ability to release histamine following parenteral administration. Intramuscular administration of meperidine does not affect heart rate significantly, but intravenous administration frequently produces a marked increase in heart rate.

Smooth Muscle. Meperidine has effects on certain smooth muscles qualitatively similar to those observed with other opioids. Meperidine does not cause as much constipation as does morphine, even when given over prolonged periods of time; this may be related to its greater ability to enter the CNS, thereby producing analgesia at lower systemic concentrations. As with other opioids, clinical doses of meperidine slow gastric emptying sufficiently to delay absorption of other drugs significantly.

The uterus of a nonpregnant woman usually is mildly stimulated by meperidine. Administered before an oxytocic, meperidine does not exert any antagonistic effect. Therapeutic doses given during active labor do not delay the birth process; in fact, the frequency, duration, and amplitude of uterine contraction sometimes may be increased (Zimmer et al., 1988). The drug does not interfere with normal postpartum contraction or involution of the uterus, and it does not increase the incidence of postpartum hemorrhage. See also "Therapeutic Uses" later in the chapter.

Absorption, Distribution, Metabolism, and Excretion. Meperidine is absorbed by all routes of administration, but the rate of absorption may be erratic after intramuscular injection. The peak plasma concentration usually occurs at ~45 minutes, but the range is wide. After oral administration, only ~50% of the drug escapes first-pass metabolism to enter the circulation, and peak concentrations in plasma usually are observed in 1-2 hours.

In humans, meperidine is hydrolyzed to meperidinic acid, which in turn is partially conjugated. Meperidine also is N-demethylated to normeperidine, which then may be hydrolyzed to normeperidinic acid and subsequently conjugated. The clinical significance of the formation of normeperidine is discussed later. Meperidine is metabolized chiefly in the liver, with a $t_{1/2} \approx 3$ hours. In patients with cirrhosis, the bioavailability of meperidine is increased to as much as 80%, and the $t_{1/2}$ of both meperidine and normeperidine are prolonged. Approximately 60% of meperidine in plasma is protein bound. Only a small amount of meperidine is excreted unchanged.

Untoward Effects, Precautions, and Contraindications. The pattern and overall incidence of untoward effects that follow the use of meperidine are similar to those observed after equianalgesic doses of morphine, except that constipation and urinary retention may be less common. Patients who experience nausea and vomiting with morphine

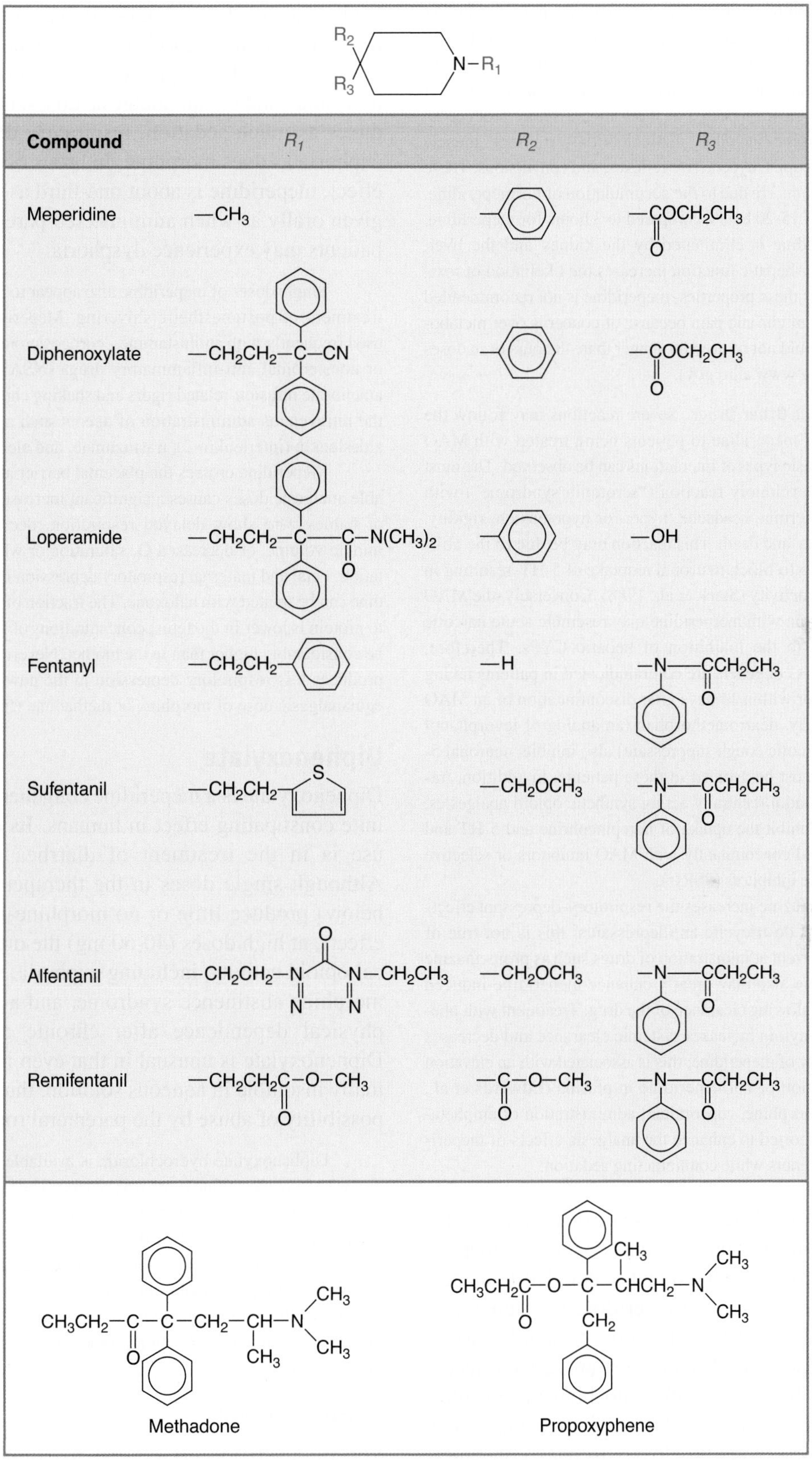

R_2, R_3, $N-R_1$

Compound	R_1	R_2	R_3
Meperidine	$-CH_3$		$-\underset{\|\atop O}{C}OCH_2CH_3$
Diphenoxylate	$-CH_2CH_2-C-CN$		$-\underset{\|\atop O}{C}OCH_2CH_3$
Loperamide	$-CH_2CH_2-C-\underset{\|\atop O}{C}-N(CH_3)_2$		$-OH$
Fentanyl	$-CH_2CH_2-$	$-H$	$-N-\underset{\|\atop O}{C}CH_2CH_3$
Sufentanil	$-CH_2CH_2-$ (S)	$-CH_2OCH_3$	$-N-\underset{\|\atop O}{C}CH_2CH_3$
Alfentanil	$-CH_2CH_2-N$ (O; N, N) $N-CH_2CH_3$	$-CH_2OCH_3$	$-N-\underset{\|\atop O}{C}CH_2CH_3$
Remifentanil	$-CH_2CH_2\underset{\|\atop O}{C}-O-CH_3$	$-\underset{\|\atop O}{C}-O-CH_3$	$-N-\underset{\|\atop O}{C}CH_2CH_3$

$CH_3CH_2-\underset{\|\atop O}{C}-C-CH_2-\underset{|\atop CH_3}{CH}-N(CH_3)(CH_3)$

Methadone

$CH_3CH_2\underset{\|\atop O}{C}-O-\underset{|\atop CH_2}{C}-\overset{CH_3\atop |}{C}HCH_2-N(CH_3)(CH_3)$

Propoxyphene

Figure 18–9. *Chemical structures of piperidine and phenylpiperidine analgesics.*

may not do so with meperidine; the converse also may be true. As with other opioids, tolerance develops to some of these effects. The contraindications generally are the same as for other opioids. In patients or addicts who are tolerant to the depressant effects of meperidine, large doses repeated at short intervals may produce an excitatory syndrome including hallucinations, tremors, muscle twitches, dilated pupils, hyperactive reflexes, and convulsions. These excitatory symptoms are due to the accumulation of normeperidine, which has a $t_{1/2}$ of 15-20 hours, compared to 3 hours for meperidine. Since normeperidine is eliminated by the kidney and the liver, decreased renal or hepatic function increases the likelihood of toxicity. As a result of these properties, meperidine is not recommended for the treatment of chronic pain because of concerns over metabolite toxicity. It should not be used for longer than 48 hours or in doses >600 mg/day (see www.ahrq.gov).

Interactions with Other Drugs. Severe reactions may follow the administration of meperidine to patients being treated with MAO inhibitors. Two basic types of interactions can be observed. The most prominent is an excitatory reaction ("serotonin syndrome") with delirium, hyperthermia, headache, hyper- or hypotension, rigidity, convulsions, coma, and death. This reaction may be due to the ability of meperidine to block neuronal reuptake of 5-HT, resulting in serotonergic overactivity (Stack et al., 1988). Conversely, the MAO inhibitor interaction with merperidine may resemble acute narcotic overdose owing to the inhibition of hepatic CYPs. Therefore, meperidine and its congeners are contraindicated in patients taking MAO inhibitors or within 14 days after discontinuation of an MAO inhibitor. Similarly, dextromethorphan (an analog of levorphanol used as a non-narcotic cough suppressant) also inhibits neuronal 5-HT uptake and must be avoided in these patients. In addition, tramadol and tapentadol (centrally acting synthetic opioid analgesics, described later) inhibit the uptake of norepinephrine and 5-HT and should not be used concomitantly with MAO inhibitors or selective serotonin reuptake inhibitors (SSRIs).

Chlorpromazine increases the respiratory-depressant effects of meperidine, as do tricyclic antidepressants; this is not true of diazepam. Concurrent administration of drugs such as promethazine or chlorpromazine also may greatly enhance meperidine-induced sedation without slowing clearance of the drug. Treatment with phenobarbital or phenytoin increases systemic clearance and decreases oral bioavailability of meperidine; this is associated with an elevation of the concentration of normeperidine in plasma (Edwards et al., 1982). As with morphine, concomitant administration of amphetamine has been reported to enhance the analgesic effects of meperidine and its congeners while counteracting sedation.

Therapeutic Uses. The major use of meperidine is for analgesia. Unlike morphine and its congeners, meperidine is not used for the treatment of cough or diarrhea. The analgesic effects of meperidine are detectable ~15 minutes after oral administration, peak in 1-2 hours, and subside gradually. The onset of analgesic effect is faster (within 10 minutes) after subcutaneous or intramuscular administration, and the effect reaches a peak in ~1 hour, corresponding closely to peak concentrations in plasma. In clinical use, the duration of effective analgesia is ~1.5-3 hours. In general, 75-100 mg meperidine hydrochloride (pethidine, DEMEROL, others) given parenterally is approximately equivalent to 10 mg morphine, and in equianalgesic doses, meperidine produces as much sedation, respiratory depression, and euphoria as does morphine. In terms of total analgesic effect, meperidine is about one-third as effective when given orally as when administered parenterally. A few patients may experience dysphoria.

Single doses of meperidine also appear to be effective in the treatment of postanesthetic shivering. Meperidine, 25-50 mg, is used frequently with antihistamines, corticosteroids, acetaminophen, or nonsteroidal anti-inflammatory drugs (NSAIDs) to prevent or ameliorate infusion-related rigors and shaking chills that accompany the intravenous administration of agents such as amphotericin B, aldesleukin (interleukin-2), trastuzumab, and alemtuzumab.

Meperidine crosses the placental barrier and even in reasonable analgesic doses causes a significant increase in the percentage of babies who show delayed respiration, decreased respiratory minute volume, or decreased O_2 saturation or who require resuscitation. Fetal and maternal respiratory depression induced by meperidine can be treated with naloxone. The fraction of drug that is bound to protein is lower in the fetus; concentrations of free drug thus may be considerably higher than in the mother. Nevertheless, meperidine produces less respiratory depression in the newborn than does an equianalgesic dose of morphine or methadone (Fishburne, 1982).

Diphenoxylate

Diphenoxylate is a meperidine congener that has a definite constipating effect in humans. Its only approved use is in the treatment of diarrhea (Chapter 46). Although single doses in the therapeutic range (see below) produce little or no morphine-like subjective effects, at high doses (40-60 mg) the drug shows typical opioid activity, including euphoria, suppression of morphine abstinence syndrome, and a morphine-like physical dependence after chronic administration. Diphenoxylate is unusual in that even its salts are virtually insoluble in aqueous solution, thus obviating the possibility of abuse by the parenteral route.

Diphenoxylate hydrochloride is available only in combination with atropine sulfate (LOMOTIL, others). The recommended daily dosage of diphenoxylate for the treatment of diarrhea in adults is 20 mg in divided doses. Diarrhea refractory to maximal doses of diphenoxylate for 10 days is unlikely to be controlled by further therapy. Difenoxin, a metabolite of diphenoxylate, has actions similar to those of the parent compound. Like diphenoxylate, difenoxin is marketed in a fixed dose with atropine (MOTOFEN) for the management of diarrhea.

Loperamide

Loperamide (IMODIUM, others), like diphenoxylate, is a piperidine derivative (Figure 18–3). It slows GI motility by effects on the circular and longitudinal muscles of the intestine, presumably as a result of its interactions with opioid receptors in the intestine. Some part of its antidiarrheal effect may be due to a reduction of gastrointestinal secretion (described earlier) (Kromer, 1988). In controlling chronic diarrhea, loperamide is as effective as diphenoxylate. In clinical studies, the most common side effect was abdominal cramps. Little tolerance develops to its constipating effect.

In human volunteers taking large doses of loperamide, concentrations of drug in plasma peak ~4 hours after ingestion; this long latency may be due to inhibition of GI motility and to enterohepatic circulation of the drug. The apparent elimination $t_{1/2}$ is 7-14 hours. Loperamide is poorly absorbed after oral administration and, in addition, apparently does not penetrate well into the brain due to the exporting activity of P-glycoprotein, which is widely expressed in the brain endothelium (Sadeque et al., 2000). Mice with deletions of one of the genes encoding the P-glycoprotein transporter have much higher brain levels and significant central effects after administration of loperamide (Schinkel et al., 1996). Inhibition of P-glycoprotein by many clinically used drugs, such as quinidine and verapamil, possibly could lead to enhanced central effects of loperamide.

In general, loperamide is unlikely to be abused parenterally because of its low solubility; large doses of loperamide given to human volunteers do not elicit pleasurable effects typical of opioids. The usual dosage is 4-8 mg/day; the daily dose should not exceed 16 mg.

FENTANYL AND CONGENERS

Fentanyl

Fentanyl is a synthetic opioid related to the phenylpiperidines (Figure 18–9). The actions of fentanyl and its congeners, sufentanil, remifentanil, and alfentanil, are similar to those of other MOR agonists. Alfentanil (ALFENTA, others) is seldom used. Fentanyl and sufentanil, are very important drugs in anesthetic practice because of their relatively short time to peak analgesic effect, rapid termination of effect after small bolus doses, minimal direct depressant effects on the myocardium, and their ability to significantly reduce the dosing requirement for the volatile agents ("MAC-sparing"; see Chapter 19). In addition to a role in anesthesia, fentanyl also is used in the management of severe pain states.

Pharmacological Properties

CNS Effects. Fentanyl and its congeners are all extremely potent analgesics and typically exhibit a very short duration of action when given parenterally. As with other opioids, nausea, vomiting, and itching can be observed. Muscle rigidity, while possible after all narcotics, appears to be more common after the high doses used in anesthetic induction. Rigidity can be treated with depolarizing or non-depolarizing neuromuscular blocking agents while controlling the patient's ventilation. Care must be taken to make sure that the patient is not simply immobilized but aware. Respiratory depression is similar to that observed with other receptor agonists, but the onset is more rapid. As with analgesia, respiratory depression after small doses is of shorter duration than with morphine but of similar duration after large doses or long infusions. As with morphine and meperidine, delayed respiratory depression also can be seen after the use of fentanyl or sufentanil, possibly owing to enterohepatic circulation. High doses of fentanyl can cause neuroexcitation and, rarely, seizure-like activity in humans (Bailey and Stanley, 1994). Fentanyl has minimal effects on intracranial pressure when ventilation is controlled and the arterial CO_2 concentration is not allowed to rise.

Cardiovascular System. Fentanyl and its derivatives decrease heart rate and mildly decrease blood pressure. However, these drugs do not release histamine and direct depressant effects on the myocardium are minimal. For this reason, high doses of fentanyl or sufentanil are commonly used as the primary anesthetic for patients undergoing cardiovascular surgery or for patients with poor cardiac function.

Absorption, Distribution, Metabolism, and Excretion. These agents are highly lipid soluble and rapidly cross the blood-brain barrier. This is reflected in the $t_{1/2}$ for equilibration between the plasma and cerebrospinal fluid of ~5 minutes for fentanyl and sufentanil. The levels in plasma and cerebrospinal fluid decline rapidly owing to redistribution of fentanyl from highly perfused tissue groups to other tissues, such as muscle and fat. As saturation of less well-perfused tissue occurs, the duration of effect of fentanyl and sufentanil approaches the length of their elimination $t_{1/2}$, 3-4 hours. Fentanyl and sufentanil undergo hepatic metabolism and renal excretion. With the use of higher doses or prolonged infusions, the drugs accumulate, these clearance mechanisms become progressively saturated, and fentanyl and sufentanil become longer acting.

Therapeutic Uses. Fentanyl citrate (SUBLIMAZE, others) and sufentanil citrate (SUFENTA, others) have widespread popularity as anesthetic adjuvants (Chapter 19). They are used commonly either intravenously, epidurally, or intrathecally. The analgesic effects of fentanyl and sufentanil are similar to those of morphine and other opioids. Fentanyl is ~100 times more potent than morphine, and sufentanil is ~1000 times more potent than morphine. The time to peak analgesic effect after intravenous administration of fentanyl and sufentanil (~5 minutes) is notably less than that for morphine and meperidine (~15 minutes). Recovery from analgesic effects also occurs more quickly. However, with larger doses or prolonged infusions, the effects of these drugs become more lasting, with durations of action becoming similar to those of longer-acting opioids (described later). Intravenous use of fentanyl and sufentanil for postoperative pain has been popular.

Epidural use of fentanyl and sufentanil for postoperative or labor analgesia has significant popularity. A combination of epidural opioids with local anesthetics permits reduction in the dosage of both components, minimizing the side effects of the local anesthetic (i.e., motor blockade) and the opioid (i.e., urinary retention, itching, and delayed respiratory depression in the case of morphine). An important caveat to their spinal use is that because of their rapid clearance, these agents at analgesic spinal doses can produce blood levels that are similar to those producing effects after systemic administration (Bernards, 2004).

The use of fentanyl and sufentanil in chronic pain treatment has become more widespread. The development of novel, minimally invasive routes of administration for fentanyl has facilitated the use of these compounds in chronic pain management. Transdermal patches (DURAGESIC, others) that provide sustained release of fentanyl for 48-72 hours are available. However, factors promoting increased absorption (e.g., fever) can lead to relative overdosage and increased side effects (see "Routes of Analgesic Drug Administration" later in the chapter). Transbuccal absorption by the use of buccal tablets, soluble buccal film, and lollypop-like lozenges permits rapid absorption and has found use in the management of acute incident pain (FENTORA, ACTIQ, ONSOLIS, others) and for the relief of breakthrough cancer pain. As fentanyl is poorly absorbed in the GI tract, the optimal absorption is though buccal absorption. Accordingly, there is little opportunity for overdosing by that route.

Remifentanil

This compound was developed in an effort to create an analgesic with a more rapid onset and predictable termination of effect. The potency of remifentanil is approximately equal to that of fentanyl. The pharmacological properties of remifentanil are similar to those of fentanyl and sufentanil. They produce similar incidences of nausea, vomiting, and dose-dependent muscle rigidity. Nausea, vomiting, itching, and headaches have been reported when remifentanil has been used for conscious analgesia for painful procedures. Intracranial pressure changes are minimal when ventilation is controlled. Seizures after remifentanil administration have been reported (Beers and Camporesi, 2004).

Absorption, Fate, and Excretion. Remifentanil has a more rapid onset of analgesic action than fentanyl or sufentanil. Analgesic effects occur within 1-1.5 minutes following intravenous administration. Peak respiratory depression after bolus doses of remifentanil occurs after 5 minutes (Patel and Spencer, 1996). Remifentanil is metabolized by plasma esterases, with a $t_{1/2}$ of 8-20 minutes (Burkle et al., 1996); thus, elimination is independent of hepatic metabolism or renal excretion. There is no prolongation of effect with repeated dosing or prolonged infusion. Age and weight can affect clearance of remifentanil, requiring that dosage be reduced in the elderly and based on lean body mass. However, neither of these conditions causes major changes in duration of effect. After 3- to 5-hour infusions of remifentanil, recovery of respiratory function can be seen within 3-5 minutes; full recovery from all effects of remifentanil is observed within 15 minutes (Glass et al., 1999). The primary metabolite, remifentanil acid, has 0.05-0.025% of the potency of the parent compound, and is excreted renally.

Therapeutic Uses. Remifentanil hydrochloride (ULTIVA) is useful for short, painful procedures that require intense analgesia and blunting of stress responses; the drug is routinely given by continuous intravenous infusion because its short duration of action makes bolus administration impractical. The titratability of remifentanil and its consistent, rapid offset make it ideally suited for short surgical procedures where rapid recovery is desirable. Remifentanil also has been used successfully for longer neurosurgical procedures, where rapid emergence from anesthesia may be important. However, in cases where postprocedural analgesia is required, remifentanil alone is a poor choice. In this situation, either a longer-acting opioid or another analgesic modality should be combined with remifentanil for prolonged analgesia, or another opioid should be used. Remifentanil is not used intraspinally because of its formulation with glycine, an inhibitory transmitter in the spinal dorsal horn.

METHADONE AND PROPOXYPHENE

Methadone

Methadone (Figure 18–9) is a long-acting MOR agonist with pharmacological properties qualitatively similar to those of morphine. The analgesic activity of methadone, a racemate, is almost entirely the result of its content of L-methadone, which is 8-50 times more potent than the D isomer. D-methadone also lacks significant respiratory depressant action and addiction liability but possesses antitussive activity.

CNS Effects. The outstanding properties of methadone are its analgesic activity, its efficacy by the oral route, its extended duration of action in suppressing withdrawal symptoms in physically dependent individuals, and its tendency to show persistent effects with repeated administration. Miotic and respiratory-depressant effects can be detected for >24 hours after a single dose; on repeated administration, marked sedation is seen in some patients. Effects on cough, bowel motility, biliary tone, and the secretion of pituitary hormones are qualitatively similar to those of morphine.

Absorption, Distribution, Metabolism, and Excretion. Methadone is absorbed well from the GI tract and can be detected in plasma within 30 minutes of oral ingestion; it reaches peak concentrations at ~4 hours. After therapeutic doses, ~90% of methadone is bound to plasma proteins. Peak concentrations occur in brain within 1-2 hours of subcutaneous or intramuscular administration, and this correlates well with the intensity and duration of analgesia. Methadone also can be absorbed from the buccal mucosa.

Methadone undergoes extensive biotransformation in the liver. The major metabolites, the results of N-demethylation and cyclization to form pyrrolidines and pyrroline, are excreted in the urine and the bile along with small amounts of unchanged drug. The amount of methadone excreted in the urine is increased when the urine is acidified. The $t_{1/2}$ of methadone is long, 15-40 hours.

Methadone appears to be firmly bound to protein in various tissues, including brain. After repeated administration, there is gradual accumulation in tissues. When administration is discontinued, low concentrations are maintained in plasma by slow release from extravascular binding sites; this process probably accounts for the relatively mild but protracted withdrawal syndrome.

Side Effects, Toxicity, Drug Interactions, and Precautions. Side effects, toxicity, and conditions that alter sensitivity, as well as the treatment of acute intoxication, are similar to those described for morphine. During long-term administration, there may be excessive sweating, lymphocytosis, and increased concentrations of prolactin, albumin, and globulins in the plasma. Rifampin and phenytoin accelerate the metabolism of methadone and can precipitate withdrawal symptoms. Unlike other opioids, methadone is associated with the prolonged QT syndrome and is additive with agents known to prolong the QT interval. Serious cardiac arrhythmias, including torsades de pointes, have been observed during treatment with methadone.

Therapeutic Uses. The primary uses of methadone hydrochloride (DOLOPHINE, others) are relief of chronic pain, treatment of opioid abstinence syndromes, and treatment of heroin users. In the U.S., prescribing methadone for abstinence syndrome and maintenance of heroin users is regulated by Federal Opioid Treatment Standards (42 CFR 8.12). The onset of analgesia occurs 10-20 minutes after parenteral administration and 30-60 minutes after oral medication. The average minimal effective analgesic concentration in blood is ~30 ng/mL (Gourlay et al., 1986). The typical oral dose is 2.5-10 mg repeated every 8-12 hours as needed depending on the severity of the pain and the response of the patient. Care must be taken when escalating the dosage because of the prolonged $t_{1/2}$ of the drug and its tendency to accumulate over a period of several days with repeated dosing. Iatrogenic overdoses have occurred during initiation of therapy and dosing titration with methadone because of too-rapid titration or the concomitant use of depressant drugs. The peak respiratory depressant effects of methadone typically occur later and persist longer than the peak analgesic effects so it is necessary to exercise vigilance and strongly caution patients against self-medicating with CNS depressants, particularly during treatment initiation and dose titration. Methadone is not used widely as an antiperistaltic agent and should not be used in labor.

Despite its longer plasma $t_{1/2}$, the duration of the analgesic action of single doses is essentially the same as that of morphine. With repeated use, cumulative effects are seen, so either lower dosages or longer intervals between doses become possible. In contrast to morphine, methadone and many of its congeners retain a considerable degree of their effectiveness when given orally. In terms of total analgesic effects, methadone given orally is ~50% as effective as the same dose administered intramuscularly; however, the oral-parenteral potency ratio is considerably lower when peak analgesic effect is considered. In equianalgesic doses, the pattern and incidence of untoward effects caused by methadone and morphine are similar.

Because of its oral bioavailability and long $t_{1/2}$, methadone has been widely implemented as a replacement modality to treat heroin dependence. Methadone, like other opiates, will produce tolerance and dependence. Thus, addicts who receive daily subcutaneous or oral therapy develop partial tolerance to the nauseant, anorectic, miotic, sedative, respiratory-depressant, and cardiovascular effects of methadone. Many former heroin users treated with oral methadone show virtually no overt behavioral effects (Mattick et al., 2009). Development of physical dependence during the long-term administration of methadone can be demonstrated following abrupt drug withdrawal or by administration of an opioid antagonist. Likewise, subcutaneous administration of methadone to former opioid addicts produces euphoria equal in duration to that caused by morphine, and its overall abuse potential is comparable with that of morphine.

Propoxyphene

Propoxyphene is structurally related to methadone (Figure 18–9). Its analgesic effect resides in the D-isomer. However, L-propoxyphene seems to have some antitussive activity. D-propoxyphene may be combined with a number of adjuvants including acetaminophen or acetylsalicylic acid. A variant on propoxyphene is formulation as the napsylate salt, which slows absorption and reduces solubility (to diminish diversion for IV delivery).

Pharmacological Actions. Although slightly less selective than morphine, propoxyphene binds primarily to μ opioid receptors and produces analgesia and other CNS effects that are similar to those seen with morphine-like opioids. It is likely that at equianalgesic doses the incidence of side effects such as nausea, anorexia, constipation, abdominal pain, and drowsiness are similar to those of codeine.

As an analgesic, propoxyphene is about one-half to two-thirds as potent as codeine given orally. A dose of 90-120 mg of propoxyphene hydrochloride administered orally would equal the analgesic effects of 60 mg of codeine, a dose that usually produces about as much analgesia as 600 mg aspirin. Combinations of propoxyphene and aspirin, like combinations of codeine and aspirin, afford a higher level of analgesia than does either agent given alone (Beaver, 1988).

Absorption, Distribution, Metabolism, and Excretion. After oral administration, concentrations of propoxyphene in plasma reach their highest values at 1-2 hours. There is great variability between subjects in the rate of clearance and the plasma concentrations that are achieved. The average $t_{1/2}$ of propoxyphene in plasma after a single dose is 6-12 hours, which is longer than that of codeine. In humans, the major route of metabolism is N-demethylation to yield norpropoxyphene. The $t_{1/2}$ of norpropoxyphene is ~30 hours, and its accumulation with repeated doses may be responsible for some of the observed toxicity (Chan and Matzke, 1987).

Toxicity. Given orally, propoxyphene is approximately one-third as potent as orally administered codeine in depressing respiration. Moderately toxic doses usually produce CNS and respiratory depression, but with still larger doses the clinical picture may be complicated by convulsions in addition to respiratory depression. Delusions, hallucinations, confusion, cardiotoxicity, and pulmonary edema also have been noted. Respiratory-depressant effects are significantly enhanced when ethanol or sedative-hypnotics are ingested concurrently. Naloxone antagonizes the respiratory-depressant, convulsant, and some of the cardiotoxic effects of propoxyphene. A second aspect of propoxyphene toxicity is liver or renal toxicity that arises when the combination medication containing acetaminophen or acetylsalicylate, respectively, is employed in conjunction with intake of those medications separately, leading to a frank overdose of these adjuvants.

Tolerance and Dependence. Very large doses (800 mg propoxyphene hydrochloride [DARVON, others] or 1200 mg of the napsylate [DARVON-N] per day) reduce the intensity of the morphine withdrawal syndrome somewhat less effectively than do 1500 mg doses of codeine. Maximal tolerated doses are equivalent to daily doses of 20-25 mg morphine given subcutaneously. The use of higher doses of propoxyphene is accompanied by untoward effects including toxic psychoses. Very large doses produce some respiratory depression in morphine-tolerant addicts, suggesting that cross-tolerance between propoxyphene and morphine is incomplete. Abrupt discontinuation of chronically administered propoxyphene hydrochloride (up to 800 mg/day given for almost 2 months) results in mild abstinence phenomena, and large oral doses (300-600 mg) produce subjective effects that are considered pleasurable by postaddicts. The drug is quite irritating when administered either intravenously or subcutaneously, so abuse by these routes results in severe damage to veins and soft tissues.

Therapeutic Uses. In 2009, the European Medicines Agency completed a review of the safety and effectiveness of dextropropoxyphene-containing medicines and concluded that the benefits do not outweigh the risks and recommended a gradual withdrawal of marketing authorization throughout the EU (European Medicines Agency, 2009). The conclusion reached by the agency included an assessment that dextropropoxyphene-containing medicines are weak painkillers with a limited effectiveness in the treatment of pain and a narrow therapeutic index. Furthermore, the agency judged acetaminophen (paracetamol) containing combinations with dextropropoxyphene to be no more effective than acetaminophen alone. In the U.S., propoxyphene has been approved for mild to moderate pain since 1957. Recently the drug has been labeled with additional warnings related to the risk of rapidly fatal effects in the event of an overdose (FDA, 2009). Thus, in the U.S., propoxyphene should not be prescribed to patients who are suicidal or have a history of suicidal ideation. In addition, higher than expected serum levels of propoxyphene should be anticipated from the concommitant administration of strong CYP3A4 inhibitors such as ritonavir, ketoconazole, itraconazole, clarithromycin, nelfinavir, nefazadone, amiodarone, amprenavir, aprepitant, diltiazem, erythromycin, fluconazole, fosamprenavir, grapefruit juice, and verapamil. Propoxphene alternatives should be considered for patients receiving a strong CYP3A4 inhibitor and others at risk for overdose, particularly those with pre-existing heart disease.

Other Opioid Agonists

Tramadol. Tramadol (ULTRAM) is a synthetic codeine analog that is a weak MOR agonist. Part of its analgesic effect is produced by inhibition of uptake of norepinephrine and serotonin. In the treatment of mild to moderate pain, tramadol is as effective as morphine or meperidine. However, for the treatment of severe or chronic pain, tramadol is less effective. Tramadol is as effective as meperidine in the treatment of labor pain and may cause less neonatal respiratory depression.

Pharmacokinetics. Tramadol is 68% bioavailable after a single oral dose and 100% available when administered intramuscularly. Its affinity for the μ opioid receptor is only 1/6000 that of morphine. However, the primary O-demethylated metabolite of tramadol is two to four times as potent as the parent drug and may account for part of the analgesic effect. Tramadol is supplied as a racemic mixture, which is more effective than either enantiomer alone. The (+)-enantiomer binds to the receptor and inhibits serotonin uptake. The (–)-enantiomer inhibits norepinephrine uptake and stimulates α_2 adrenergic receptors (Lewis and Han, 1997). Tramadol undergoes extensive hepatic metabolism by a number of pathways, including CYP2D6 and CYP3A4, as well as by conjugation with subsequent renal excretion. The rate of formation of the active metabolite is dependent on CYP2D6 and therefore is subject to both metabolic induction and inhibition. The elimination $t_{1/2}$ is 6 hours for tramadol and 7.5 hours for its active metabolite. Analgesia begins within an hour of oral dosing and peaks within 2-3 hours. The duration of analgesia is ~6 hours. The maximum recommended daily dose is 400 mg.

Side Effects and Adverse Effects. Common side effects of tramadol include nausea, vomiting, dizziness, dry mouth, sedation, and headache. Respiratory depression appears to be less than with equianalgesic doses of morphine, and the degree of constipation is less than that seen after equivalent doses of codeine (Duthie, 1998). Tramadol can cause seizures and possibly exacerbate seizures in patients with predisposing factors. While tramadol-induced analgesia is not entirely reversible by naloxone, tramadol-induced respiratory depression is reversed by naloxone. However, the use of naloxone increases the risk of seizure in patients exposed to tramadol. Misuse, diversion, physical dependence, abuse, addiction, and withdrawal have been reported in conjunction with the use of tramadol. Tramadol has been shown to reinitiate physical dependence in some patients who have previously been dependent on other opioids, thus it should be avoided in patients with a history of addiction. Precipitation of withdrawal necessitates that tramadol be tapered prior to discontinuation. Tramadol should not be used in patients taking MAO inhibitors (Lewis and Han, 1997), SSRIs, or other drugs that lower the seizure threshold (described earlier).

Tapentadol. Tapentadol (NUCYNTA) is structurally and mechanistically similar to tramadol. It displays a mild opioid activity and possesses monoamine reuptake inhibitor activity. It is considered similar to tramadol in activity, efficacy, and side-effect profile. Like tramadol, it should not be used concurrently with agents that enhance monamine activity or lower the seizure threshold, such as MAO inhibitors and SSRIs. The major pathway of tapentadol metabolism is conjugation with glucuronic acid; ~70% of the dose is excreted in urine in the conjugated form.

OPIOID AGONISTS/ANTAGONISTS AND PARTIAL AGONISTS

The drugs described in this section differ from clinically used μ opioid receptor agonists. Drugs such as nalbuphine and butorphanol are competitive MOR antagonists but exert their analgesic actions by acting as agonists at KOR receptors. Pentazocine qualitatively resembles these drugs, but it may be a weaker MOR receptor antagonist or partial agonist while retaining its KOR agonist activity. Buprenorphine, on the other hand, is a partial agonist at MOR. The stimulus for the development of mixed agonist–antagonist drugs was a desire for analgesics with less respiratory depression and addictive potential. However, the clinical use of these compounds is limited by undesirable side-effects and limited analgesic effects.

Pentazocine

Pentazocine was synthesized as part of a deliberate effort to develop an effective analgesic with little or no abuse potential. It has agonistic actions and weak opioid antagonistic activity.

Pharmacological Actions and Side Effects. The pattern of CNS effects produced by pentazocine generally is similar to that of the morphine-like opioids, including analgesia, sedation, and respiratory depression. The analgesic effects of pentazocine are due to agonistic actions at opioid receptors. Higher doses of pentazocine (60-90 mg) elicit dysphoric and psychotomimetic effects. The mechanisms responsible for these side effects are not known but might involve activation of supraspinal receptors because it has been suggested that these untoward effects may be reversible by naloxone.

The cardiovascular responses to pentazocine differ from those seen with typical receptor agonists, in that high doses cause an increase in blood pressure and heart rate. Pentazocine acts as a weak antagonist or partial agonist at opioid receptors. Pentazocine does not antagonize the respiratory depression produced by morphine. However, when given to patients dependent on morphine or other MOR agonists, pentazocine may precipitate withdrawal. Ceiling effects for analgesia and respiratory depression are observed at doses above 50-100 mg of pentazocine (Bailey and Stanley, 1994).

Therapeutic Uses. Pentazocine lactate (TALWIN) injection is indicated for the relief of moderate to severe pain and is also used as a preoperative medication and as a supplement to anesthesia. Pentazocine tablets for oral use are only available in fixed-dose combinations with acetaminophen (TALACEN, others) or naloxone (TALWIN NX). Combination of pentazocine with naloxone reduces the potential misuse of tablets as a source of injectable pentazocine by producing undesirable effects in subjects dependent on opioids. After oral ingestion, naloxone is destroyed rapidly by the liver. An oral dose of ~50 mg pentazocine results in analgesia equivalent to that produced by 60 mg of orally administered codeine.

Nalbuphine

Nalbuphine is related structurally to naloxone and oxymorphone (Figure 18–8). It is generally considered to be a KOR agonist-MOR antagonist opioid with a spectrum of effects that qualitatively resembles that of pentazocine; however, nalbuphine is considered to be less likely to produce dysphoric side effects than is pentazocine.

Pharmacological Actions and Side Effects. An intramuscular dose of 10 mg nalbuphine is equianalgesic to 10 mg morphine, with similar onset and duration of analgesic and subjective effects. Nalbuphine depresses respiration as much as do equianalgesic doses of morphine; however, nalbuphine exhibits a ceiling effect such that increases in dosage beyond 30 mg produce no further respiratory depression as well as no futher analgesia. In contrast to pentazocine and butorphanol, 10 mg nalbuphine given to patients with stable coronary artery disease does not produce an increase in cardiac index, pulmonary arterial pressure, or cardiac work, and systemic blood pressure is not significantly altered; these indices also are relatively stable when nalbuphine is given to patients with acute myocardial infarction (Roth et al., 1988); nevertheless, morphine is generally considered a first-line agent for use during acute cardiac events to relieve chest pain and anxiety. The GI effects of nalbuphine probably are similar to those of pentazocine. Nalbuphine produces few side effects at doses of 10 mg or less; sedation, sweating, and headache are the most common. At much higher doses (70 mg), psychotomimetic side effects (e.g., dysphoria, racing thoughts, and distortions of body image) can occur. Nalbuphine is metabolized in the liver and has a plasma $t_{1/2}$ of 2-3 hours. Nalbuphine is 20-25% as potent when administered orally as when given intramuscularly. No oral dosage forms are commercially available in the U.S.

Tolerance and Physical Dependence. In subjects dependent on low doses of morphine (60 mg/day), nalbuphine precipitates an abstinence syndrome. Prolonged administration of nalbuphine can produce physical dependence. The withdrawal syndrome is similar in intensity to that seen with pentazocine. The potential for abuse of parenteral nalbuphine in subjects not dependent on receptor agonists probably is similar to that for parenteral pentazocine.

Therapeutic Use. Nalbuphine hydrochloride (NUBAIN, others) is used to produce analgesia. Because it is an agonist–antagonist, administration to patients who have been receiving morphine-like opioids may create difficulties unless a brief drug-free interval is interposed. The usual adult dose is 10 mg parenterally every 3-6 hours; this may be increased to 20 mg in nontolerant individuals. A caveat: agents that act through the KOR have been reported to be relatively more effective in women than in men (Gear et al., 1999).

Butorphanol

Butorphanol is a morphinan congener with a profile of actions similar to those of pentazocine and nalbuphine: KOR agonist-MOR antagonist opioid. The structural formula of butorphanol is shown in Figure 18–8.

Therapeutic Use. In general, butorphanol tartrate (STADOL, others) is considered to be best suited for the relief of acute pain (e.g., postoperative), and because of its potential for antagonizing MOR agonists should not be used in combination. Because of its side effects on the heart, it is less useful than morphine or meperidine in patients with congestive heart failure or myocardial infarction. The usual dose is 1-4 mg of the tartrate given intramuscularly, or 0.5-2 mg given intravenously, every 3-4 hours. A nasal formulation is available and has proven to be effective in pain relief, including migraine pain. This formulation may be particularly useful for patients with severe headaches who are unresponsive to other forms of treatment.

Pharmacological Actions and Side Effects. In postoperative patients, a parenteral dose of 2-3 mg butorphanol produces analgesia and respiratory depression approximately equal to that produced by 10 mg morphine or 80-100 mg meperidine; the onset, peak, and duration of action are similar to those that follow the administration of morphine. The plasma $t_{1/2}$ of butorphanol is ~3 hours. Like pentazocine, analgesic doses of butorphanol produce an increase in pulmonary arterial pressure and in the work of the heart; systemic arterial pressure is slightly decreased (Popio et al., 1978).

The major side effects of butorphanol are drowsiness, weakness, sweating, feelings of floating, and nausea. While the incidence

syndrome in patients dependent on pentazocine, butorphanol, or nalbuphine. Naloxone produces overshoot phenomena suggestive of early acute physical dependence 6-24 hours after a single dose of an μ agonist (Heishman et al., 1989). In dependent patients, peripheral side-effects, notably reduced GI motility and constipation, can be reversed by methylnaltrexone with doses of 0.15 mg/kg subcutaneously, producing reliable bowel movements and no evidence of centrally mediated withdrawal signs (Thomas et al., 2008).

Absorption, Distribution, Metabolism, and Excretion

Although absorbed readily from the GI tract, naloxone is almost completely metabolized by the liver before reaching the systemic circulation and thus must be administered parenterally. The drug is absorbed rapidly from parenteral sites of injection and is metabolized in the liver primarily by conjugation with glucuronic acid; other metabolites are produced in small amounts. The $t_{1/2}$ of naloxone is ~1 hour, but its clinically effective duration of action can be even less.

Compared with naloxone, naltrexone retains much more of its efficacy by the oral route, and its duration of action approaches 24 hours after moderate oral doses. Peak concentrations in plasma are reached within 1-2 hours and then decline with an apparent $t_{1/2}$ of ~3 hours; this value does not change with long-term use. Naltrexone is metabolized to 6-naltrexol, which is a weaker antagonist but has a longer $t_{1/2}$, ~13 hours. Naltrexone is much more potent than naloxone, and 100 mg oral doses given to patients addicted to opioids produce concentrations in tissues sufficient to block the euphorigenic effects of 25-mg intravenous doses of heroin for 48 hours (Gonzalez and Brogden, 1988). Methylnaltrexone is handled similarly to naltrexone. It is converted to methyl-6-naltrexol isomers and is largely eliminated primarily as the unchanged drug with significant active renal secretion. The terminal disposition $t_{1/2}$ of methylnaltrexone is ~8 hours.

Therapeutic Uses

Treatment of Opioid Overdosage. Opioid antagonists, particularly naloxone, have an established use in the treatment of opioid-induced toxicity, especially respiratory depression. Its specificity is such that reversal by this agent is virtually diagnostic for the contribution of an opiate to the depression. Naloxone acts rapidly to reverse the respiratory depression associated with high doses of opioids. It should be used cautiously because it also can precipitate withdrawal in dependent subjects and cause undesirable cardiovascular side effects. By carefully titrating the dose of naloxone, it usually is possible to rapidly antagonize the respiratory-depressant actions without eliciting a fully expressed withdrawal syndrome. The duration of action of naloxone is relatively short, and it often must be given repeatedly or by continuous infusion. Opioid antagonists also have been employed effectively to decrease neonatal respiratory depression secondary to the intravenous or intramuscular administration of opioids to the mother. In the neonate, the initial dose is 10 μg/kg given intravenously, intramuscularly, or subcutaneously.

Management of Constipation. The peripherally limited antagonists such as methylnaltrexone have a very important role in the management of the constipation and the reduced GI motility present in the patient undergoing chronic opioid therapy (as for chronic pain or methadone maintenance) and have been approved by the FDA for that use. With distribution restricted to the periphery, these agents do not alter central opioid agonist actions. Worrisome reports of GI perforation in this setting are under review by FDA. Other strategies for the management of opioid-induced constipation are described in Chapter 46.

Management of Abuse Syndromes. There is considerable interest in the use of opiate antagonists such as naltrexone as an adjuvant in treating a variety of non-opioid dependency syndromes such as alcoholism (Chapters 23 and 24), where an opiate antagonist decreases the chance of relapse (Anton, 2008). Interestingly, patients with a single nucleotide polymorphism (SNP) in the MOR gene have significantly lower relapse rates to alcoholism when treated with naltrexone (Haile et al., 2008). Naltrexone is FDA-approved for treatment of alcoholism.

Trauma. The potential utility of opiate antagonists in the treatment of shock, stroke, spinal cord and brain trauma, and other disorders that may involve mobilization of endogenous opioid peptides has been reported; but opioid antagonists have failed to demonstrate neuroprotective benefits and their study in trauma has been largely abandoned (Hawryluk et al., 2008).

CENTRALLY ACTIVE ANTITUSSIVES

Cough is a useful physiological mechanism that serves to clear the respiratory passages of foreign material and excess secretions. It should not be suppressed indiscriminately. There are, however, many situations in which cough does not serve any useful purpose but may, instead, annoy the patient, prevent rest and sleep, or hinder adherence to otherwise beneficial medication regimens (e.g., angiotension-converting enzyme (ACE) inhibitor-induced cough). Chronic cough can contribute to fatigue, especially in elderly patients. In such situations, the physician should try to substitute a drug with a different side effect profile (e.g., an AT_1 antagonist in place of an ACE inhibitor) or add an antitussive agent that will reduce the frequency or intensity of the coughing (Chapters 12 and 36).

A number of drugs reduce cough as a result of their central actions, including opioid analgesics (codeine, hydrocodone, and dihydrocodeine are the opioids most commonly used to suppress cough). Cough suppression often occurs with lower doses of opioids than those needed for analgesia. A 10- or 20-mg oral dose of codeine, although ineffective for analgesia, produces a demonstrable antitussive effect, and higher doses produce even more suppression of chronic cough. A few other antitussive agents are noted below.

Dextromethorphan

Dextromethorphan (D-3-methoxy-N-methylmorphinan) is the D-isomer of the codeine analog methorphan; however, unlike the L-isomer, it has no analgesic or addictive properties and does not act through opioid receptors. The drug acts centrally to elevate the threshold for coughing. Its effectiveness in patients with pathological cough has been demonstrated in controlled studies; its potency is nearly equal to that of codeine. Compared with codeine, dextromethorphan produces fewer subjective and GI side effects (Matthys et al., 1983). In therapeutic dosages, the drug does not inhibit ciliary activity, and its antitussive effects persist for 5-6 hours. Its toxicity is low, but extremely high doses may produce CNS depression.

Sites that bind dextromethorphan with high affinity have been identified in membranes from various regions of the brain (Craviso et al., 1983). Although dextromethorphan is known to function as an NMDA-receptor antagonist, the dextromethorphan binding sites are not limited to the known distribution of NMDA receptors (Elliott et al., 1994). Thus, the mechanism by which dextromethorphan exerts its antitussive effect still is not clear.

The average adult dosage of dextromethorphan hydrobromide is 10-30 mg three to six times daily, not to exceed 120 mg daily. The drug is marketed for over-the-counter sale in liquids, syrups, capsules, soluble strips, lozenges, and freezer pops or in combinations with antihistamines, bronchodilators, expectorants, and decongestants. An extended-release dextromethorphan suspension (DELSYM) is approved for twice daily administration.

Two other antitussives not currently recognized as generally safe and effective (GRAS/E) by the FDA, carbetapentane (pentoxyverine) and caramiphen, are known to bind avidly to the dextromethorphan binding sites; codeine, levopropoxyphene, and other antitussive opioids (as well as naloxone) do not bind. Although noscapine (discussed later) enhances the affinity of dextromethorphan, it appears to interact with distinct binding sites (Karlsson et al., 1988). The relationship of these binding sites to antitussive actions is not known; however, these observations, coupled with the ability of naloxone to antagonize the antitussive effects of codeine but not those of dextromethorphan, indicate that cough suppression can be achieved by a number of different mechanisms.

Other Antitussives

Pholcodine [3-O-(2-morpholinoethyl) morphine] is used clinically in many countries outside the U.S. Although structurally related to the opioids, pholcodine has no opioid-like actions because the substitution at the 3-position is not removed by metabolism. Pholcodine is at least as effective as codeine as an antitussive; it has a long $t_{1/2}$ and can be given once or twice daily.

Benzonatate (TESSALON, others) is a long-chain polyglycol derivative chemically related to procaine and believed to exert its antitussive action on stretch or cough receptors in the lung, as well as by a central mechanism. It is available in oral capsules and the dosage is 100 mg three times daily; doses as high as 600 mg daily have been used safely.

ROUTES OF ANALGESIC DRUG ADMINISTRATION

In addition to the traditional oral and parenteral formulations for opioids, many other methods of administration have been developed in an effort to improve therapeutic efficacy while minimizing side effects. These alternative routes generally improve the ease of use of opioids and some increase patient satisfaction.

Patient-Controlled Analgesia (PCA)

With this modality, the patient has limited control of the dosing of opioid from an infusion pump programmed within tightly mandated parameters. PCA can be used for intravenous, epidural, or intrathecal administration of opioids. This technique avoids delays inherent in administration by a caregiver and generally permits better alignment between pain control and individual differences in pain perception and responsiveness to opioids. The PCA technique also gives the patient a greater sense of control over the pain. With shorter-acting opioids, serious toxicity or excessive use rarely occurs; however, caution is warranted due to the potential for serious medication errors associated with this delivery method. PCA is suitable for adults and children capable of understanding the principles involved. It is generally conceded that PCA is preferred over intramuscular injections for postoperative pain control.

Spinal Delivery

Administration of opioids into the epidural or intrathecal space provides more direct access to the first pain-processing synapse in the dorsal horn of the spinal cord. This permits the use of doses substantially lower than those required for oral or parenteral administration (Table 18–3). Systemic side effects of opoid administration thus are decreased. In postoperative pain management sustained release epidural injections are accomplished through the incorporation of morphine into a liposomal formulation (DEPODUR), providing up to 48 hours of pain relief (Hartrick and Hartrick, 2008). The management of chronic pain with spinal opiates has been addressed by the use of chronically implanted intrathecal catheters connected to subcutaneously implanted refillable pumps (Wallace and Yaksh, 2000).

Though they have important therapeutic uses, epidural and intrathecal opioids have their own dose-dependent side effects, such as pruritis, nausea, vomiting, respiratory depression, and urinary retention. Hydrophilic opioids such as morphine (DURAMORPH, others)

Table 18–3

Epidural or Intrathecal Opioids for the Treatment of Acute (Bolus) or Chronic (Infusion) Pain

DRUG	SINGLE DOSE (mg)[a]	INFUSION RATE (mg/h)[b]	ONSET (min)	DURATION OF EFFECT OF A SINGLE DOSE (h)[c]
Epidural				
Morphine	1-6	0.1-1.0	30	6-24
Meperidine	20-150	5-20	5	4-8
Methadone	1-10	0.3-0.5	10	6-10
Hydromorphone	1-2	0.1-0.2	15	10-16
Fentanyl	0.025-0.1	0.025-0.10	5	2-4
Sufentanil	0.01-0.06	0.01-0.05	5	2-4
Alfentanil	0.5-1	0.2	15	1-3
Subarachnoid (Intrathecal)				
Morphine	0.1-0.3		15	8-24+
Fentanyl	0.005-0.025		5	3-6

[a]Low doses may be effective when administered to the elderly or when injected in the thoracic region.
[b]If combining with a local anesthetic, consider using 0.0625% bupivacaine. [c]Duration of analgesia varies widely; higher doses produce longer duration. With the exception of epidural/intrathecal morphine or epidural sufentanil, all other spinal opioid use is considered to be off label.
Adapted from International Association for the Study of Pain, 1992.

have a longer residence times in the cerebrospinal fluid; as a consequence, after intrathecal or epidural morphine, delayed respiratory depression can be observed for as long as 24 hours after a bolus dose. While the risk of delayed respiratory depression is reduced with more lipophilic opioids, it is not eliminated. Extreme vigilance and appropriate monitoring are required for all opioid-naïve patients receiving intraspinal narcotics. Use of intraspinal opioids in the opioid-naïve patient is reserved for postoperative pain control in an inpatient monitored setting. Epidural administration of opioids has become popular in the management of postoperative pain and for providing analgesia during labor and delivery. Lower systemic opioid levels are achieved with epidural opioids, leading to less placental transfer and less potential for respiratory depression of the newborn (Shnider and Levinson, 1987). Many opioids and other adjuvants are commonly used for neuraxial administration in adults and children; however, the majority of agents employed have not undergone appropriate preclinical safety evaluation and approval for these clinical indications; thus, such uses are "off-label". Thus, at this time, those agents approved for spinal delivery are certain preservative-free formulations of morphine sulfate (DURAMORPH, DEPODUR, others) and sufentanil (SUFENTA). It is important to remember that the spinal route of delivery represents a novel environment wherein the neuraxis may be exposed to exceedingly high concentrations of an agent for an extended period of time and safety by another route (e.g., PO, IV) may not translate to safety after spinal delivery (Yaksh and Allen, 2004).

Patients on chronic spinal opioid therapy are less likely to experience respiratory depression. Selected patients who fail conservative therapies for chronic pain may receive intraspinal opioids chronically through an implanted programmable pump.

Analogous to the relationship between systemic opioids and NSAIDs, intraspinal narcotics often are combined with other agents that include local anesthetics, N-type Ca^{2+} channel blockers (e.g., ziconotide), α_2 adrenergic agonists, and $GABA_B$ agonists. This permits synergy between drugs with different mechanisms allowing the use of lower concentrations of both agents, minimizing side-effects and the opioid-induced complications (Wallace and Yaksh, 2000).

Local Drug Action

Opioid receptors on peripheral sensory nerves respond to locally applied opioids during inflammation (Stein, 1993). Peripheral analgesia permits the use of lower doses, applied locally, than those necessary to achieve a systemic effect. The pain relief generated by this route of delivery is limited but the technique has been demonstrated to have some efficacy in postoperative pain (Stein, 1993). Development of such compounds and expansion of clinical applications of this technique are active areas of research.

Rectal Administration

This route is an alternative for patients with difficulty swallowing or other oral pathology and who prefer a less invasive route than parenteral administration. This route is not well tolerated by most children. Onset of action is within 10 minutes. In the U.S., only morphine and hydromorphone are available in rectal suppository formulations.

Inhalation

Opioids can be delivered by nebulizer. However, this delivery method is rarely used due to erratic absorption from the lung and highly variable therapeutic effect.

Oral Transmucosal Administration

Opioids can be absorbed through the oral mucosa more rapidly than through the stomach. Bioavailability is greater owing to avoidance of first-pass metabolism, and lipophilic opioids are absorbed better by this route than are hydrophilic compounds such as morphine. A transmucosal delivery system that suspends fentanyl in a dissolvable sugar-based lollipop (ACTIQ, others) or rapidly dissolving buccal tablet (FENTORA) have been approved for the treatment of cancer pain; in this setting, transmucosal fentanyl relieves pain within 15 minutes, and patients easily can titrate the appropriate dose.

A buccal fentanyl "film" is FDA-approved for the treatment of cancer pain (ONSOLIS). The film is applied to the buccal mucosa and slowly dissolves releasing the fentanyl to cross the mucosa into the bloodstream. A New Drug Application has been filed with the FDA for a sublingual tablet (ABSTRAL, formerly RAPINYL). Transmucosal fentanyl also has been studied as a premedicant for children; however, this technique has been largely abandoned owing to undesirable side effects such as respiratory depression, sedation, nausea, vomiting, and pruritus.

Transnasal Administration

Butorphanol, a KOR agonist/MOR antagonist has been employed intranasally. A transnasal pectin-based fentanyl spray is currently in clinical trials for the treatment of cancer related pain. Administration is well tolerated and pain relief occurs within 10 minutes of delivery (Kress et al., 2009).

Transdermal and Iontophoretic Administration

Transdermal fentanyl patches are approved for use in sustained pain. The opioid permeates the skin, and a "depot" is established in the stratum corneum layer. Unlike other transdermal systems (i.e., transdermal scopolamine), anatomic position of the patch does not affect absorption. However, fever and external heat sources (heating pads, hot baths) can increase absorption of fentanyl and potentially lead to an overdose (Rose et al., 1993). This modality is well suited for cancer pain treatment because of its ease of use, prolonged duration of action, and stable blood levels (Portenoy et al., 1993). It may take up to 12 hours to develop analgesia and up to 16 hours to observe full clinical effect. Plasma levels stabilize after two sequential patch applications, and the kinetics do not appear to change with repeated applications (Portenoy et al., 1993). However, there may be a great deal of variability in plasma levels after a given dose. The plasma $t_{1/2}$ after patch removal is ~17 hours. Thus, if excessive sedation or respiratory depression is experienced, antagonist infusions may need to be maintained for an extended period. Dermatological side effects from the patches, such as rash and itching, usually are mild.

Iontophoresis is the transport of soluble ions through the skin by using a mild electric current. This technique has been employed with morphine (Ashburn et al., 1992). Unlike transdermal opioids, a drug reservoir does not build up in the skin, thus limiting the duration of both desired and undesired effects. Patient-controlled iontophoretic transdermal fentanyl systems have been developed, but none is currently marketed.

THERAPEUTIC USE OF OPIATES IN PAIN CONTROL

Management of pain is an important element in any therapeutic intervention. Failure to adequately manage pain can have important negative consequences on physiological function such as autonomic hyper-reactivity (increased blood pressure, heart rate, suppression of gastrointestinal motility, reduced secretions), reduced mobility leading to deconditioning, muscle wasting, joint stiffening, and decalcification, and can contribute to deleterious changes in the psychological state (depression, helplessness syndromes, anxiety). By many hospital accrediting organizations, and by law in many states, appropriate pain assessment and adequate pain management are considered to be standard of care, with pain being considered the "fifth vital sign."

The comments included here are only a general orientation to the principles in pain management. Extensive efforts by many individuals and organizations have resulted in the publication of many useful guidelines for the management of pain states including acute pain, cancer pain, and neuropathic pain (Table 18–4). In the case of cancer pain, adherence to standardized protocols has been shown to improve pain management

Table 18–4

Resources for Pain Management

PAIN STATE	REFERENCES
Acute and cancer pain (postoperative)	American Pain Society Recommendations for Improving the Quality of Acute and Cancer Pain Management, American Pain Society, 2005 *www.ampainsoc.org/pub/bulletin/fal05/inno1.htm* Guidelines for the Management of Cancer Pain in Adults and Children, American Pain Society, 2005 *www.guideline.gov/summary/summary.aspx?ss=15* Principles of Analgesic Use in the Treatment of Acute Pain and Cancer Pain, American Pain Society, 2008 *www.ampainsoc.org/pub/principles.htm*
Neuropathic	Pharmacologic Management of Neuropathic Pain: Evidence-Based Recommendations, International Association for the Study of Pain, 2007 *www.guideline.gov/summary/summary.aspx?ss=15* European Federation of Neurologic Societies Guidelines on Pharmacologic Treatment of Neuropathic Pain, European Federation of Neurologic Societies, 2007 *www.guideline.gov/summary/summary.aspx?ss=15; www.efns.org*

Source: Dworkin et al., 2007.

significantly (Du Pen et al., 1999). The next sections provide guidelines for rational drug selection, discuss routes of administration other than the standard oral and parenteral methods, and outline general principles for the use of opioids in acute and chronic pain states.

Guidelines for Opiate Dosing

Whereas the World Health Organization three-step ladder was initially targeted at the treatment of cancer pain, it is accepted practice to use this three-step ladder to treat chronic noncancer pain (Table 18–5). The three-step ladder encourages the use of more conservative therapies before initiating opioid therapy. However, in the presence of severe pain, the opioids should be considered sooner rather than later.

Numerous societies and agencies have published guidelines for the use of strong opioids in treating pain, including the American Academy of Pain Medicine, the American Pain Society, the Federation of State Medical Boards (FSMB), and the Drug Enforcement Agency. While slightly different in particulars, all guidelines to date share the criteria established by the FSMB (Table 18–6).

Table 18–5

World Health Organization Analgesic Ladder[a]

Step 1 Mild to Moderate Pain

Non-opioid ± adjuvant agent

- Acetaminophen or an NSAID should be used, unless contraindicated. Adjuvant agents are those that enhance analgesic efficacy, treat concurrent symptoms that exacerbate pain, and/or provide independent analgesic activity for specific types of pain.

Step 2 Mild to Moderate Pain or Pain Uncontrolled after Step 1

Short-acting opioid as required ± non-opioid around the clock (ATC) ± adjuvant agent

- Morphine, oxycodone, or hydromorphone should be added to acetaminophen or an NSAID for maximum flexibility of opioid dose.

Step 3 Moderate to Severe Pain or Pain Uncontrolled after Step 2

Sustained release/long-acting opioid ATC or continuous infusion + short-acting opioid as required ± non-opioid ± adjuvant agent

- Sustained release oxycodone, morphine, oxymorphone or transdermal fentanyl is indicated.

[a]http://www.who.int/cancer/palliative/painladder/en/

Guidelines for the oral and parenteral dosing of commonly used opioids are presented in Table 18–2. *Tables such as those presented here are only guidelines.* They are typically constructed with the use of these agents in the management of acute (e.g., postoperative) pain in opioid-naive patients. A number of factors will contribute to the dosing requirement (described in subsequent sections).

Methadone is considered separately in Table 18–7 as updated safety information has emerged more recently. In 2006, the FDA notified health care professionals of reports of death and life-threatening adverse events, such as respiratory depression and cardiac arrhythmias in patients receiving methadone. Methadone is thought to be involved in about one-third of all prescription opioid-related deaths, exceeding hydrocodone and oxycodone, despite being prescribed one-tenth as often. This has led to revisions in the labeled dosing recommendations.

Variables Modifying the Therapeutic Response to Opiates

There is substantial individual variability in responses to opioids. A standard intramuscular dose of 10 mg morphine sulfate will relieve severe pain adequately in only 2 of 3 patients. The minimal effective analgesic concentration for opioids, such as morphine, meperidine (pethidine), alfentanil, and sufentanil, varies among patients by factors of 5–10 (Woodhouse and Mather, 2000). Adjustments will have to be made based on clinical response. Appropriate therapeutics typically involve undertaking a treatment strategy that most efficiently addresses the pain state, minimizes the potential for undesired drug effects, and accounts for the variables that can influence an individual patient's response to opiate analgesia.

Pain Intensity. Increased pain intensity may require titrating doses to produce acceptable analgesia with tolerable side effects.

Type of Pain State. Systems underlying a pain state may be broadly categorized as being mediated by events secondary to injury and inflammation and by injury to the sensory afferent or nervous system. Neuropathic conditions may be less efficaciously managed by opiates than pain secondary to tissue injury and inflammation. Such pain states are more efficiently managed by combination treatment modalities.

Acuity and Chronicity of Pain. The pain state in any given clinical condition is not typically constant and will vary over time. In chronic pain states, the daily course of the pain may fluctuate, e.g., being greater in the morning hours or upon awakening. Arthritic states display flares that are associated with an exacerbated pain condition. Changes in the magnitude of pain occur during the daily routine resulting in "breakthrough pain" during episodic events such as

Table 18–6

Guidelines for the Use of Opioids to Treat Chronic Pain

- *Evaluation of the patient*: A complete medical history and physical must be conducted and documented in the medical record.
- *Treatment plan*: The treatment plan should state objectives that are used to determine treatment success.
- *Informed consent and agreement*: The physician should discuss the risks, benefits, and alternatives to chronic opioid therapy with the patient. Many practitioners have developed an "opioid contract" that outlines the responsibilities of the physician and the patient for continued prescription of controlled substances.
- *Periodic review*: At reasonable intervals, the patient should be seen by the physician to review the course of treatment and document results of consultation, diagnostic, testing, laboratory results, and the success of treatment.
- *Consultation*: The physician should refer the patient for consultation when appropriate.
- *Documentation/medical records*: The physician should keep actual and complete medical records that include: (a) medical history and physical examination; (b) diagnostic, therapeutic, and laboratory results; (c) evaluations and consultations; (d) treatment objectives; (e) discussion of risks and benefits; (f) treatment; (g) medications including date, type, dosage, and quantity prescribed; (h) instructions and agreements; and (i) periodic reviews.
- *Compliance with controlled substances law and regulations*: To prescribe, dispense or administer controlled substances, the physician must be licensed in the state and comply with applicable state and federal regulations.

dressing changes (incident pain). These examples emphasize the need for individualized management of increased or decreased pain levels with baseline analgesic dosing supplemented with the use of short-acting "rescue" medications as required. In the face of ongoing severe pain, analgesics should be dosed in continuous or "around-the-clock" fashion rather than on an as-needed basis. This provides more consistent analgesic levels and avoids unnecessary suffering (Vashi et al., 2005).

Opioid Tolerance. Chronic exposure to one opiate agonist typically leads to a reduction in the efficacy of other opiate agonists. The degree of tolerance can be remarkable. For example, 10 mg of an oral opioid (such as morphine) is considered a high dose for a treatment-naïve individual whereas 100 mg IV may produce only minor sedation in severely tolerant individual.

Patient Physical State and Genetic Variables. Codeine, hydrocodone, and oxycodone are weak analgesic prodrugs that are metabolized into the much more effective analgesic drugs morphine, hydromorphone, and oxymorphone, respectively, by CYP2D6 (Supernaw, 2001). The analgesic properties of morphine, hydromorphone, oxymorphone, propoxyphene, and fentanyl are largely due to their direct influence on opioid receptors and do not require additional metabolism, although the first metabolite of propoxyphene, norpropoxyphene, is also an effective analgesic with a very long $t_{1/2}$. CYP2D6 activity is genetically diminished in 7% of whites, 3% of blacks, and 1% of Asians (Eichelbaum and Gross, 1990); rendering oxycodone, hydrocodone, and codeine relatively ineffective analgesics in these "poor metabolizers" and potentially toxic for "ultra-rapid" metabolizers.

The activity of CYP2D6 is inhibited by selective serotonin reuptake inhibitors, including fluoxetine, fluvoxamine, paroxetine, sertraline, and bupropion, medications that are commonly administered to pain patients. The CYP2D6 inhibition resulting from these interacting medications may render opioids less effective as analgesics in some patients. Whereas diminished activity of the CYP2D6 isoenzyme will lead to less efficacy of prodrug opioids, the opposite occurs with methadone. Although methadone is primarily metabolized through the CYP3A4 isoenzyme, genetic polymorphisms involving deficiencies in the CYP2C9, CYP2CI9, and CYP2D6 isoenzymes may lead to surprisingly high methadone plasma concentrations resulting in overdose.

Opioids are highly protein bound and factors such as plasma pH may dramatically change binding. In addition, α_1-acid glycoprotein (AAG) is an acute-phase reactant protein that is elevated in cancer patients and has a high affinity for basic drugs such as methadone and meperidine. Morphine and meperidine should be avoided in patients with renal impairment since morphine-6-glucuronide (a metabolite of morphine) and normeperidine (a metabolite of meperidine) are excreted by the kidney and will accumulate and lead to toxicity. Other states that may increase the risk of adverse effects of the opioids include chronic obstructive pulmonary disease, sleep apnea, dementia, benign prostratic hypertrophy, unstable gait, and pretreatment constipation.

Table 18–7

Oral Morphine to Methadone Conversion Guidelines

	CONVERSION RATIOS		
DAILY MORPHINE DOSE(mg/24 h, ORALLY)	MORPHINE (oral)	:	METHADONE (oral)
< 100	3	:	1
101-300	5	:	1
301-600	10	:	1
601-800	12	:	1
801-1000	15	:	1
> 1001	20	:	1

Routes of Administration Available. The aim in chronic pain states is to prefer to employ the least invasive routes of drug administration, which include oral, buccal, or transdermal delivery. IV routes are more useful in perioperative in-hospital pain management and during end-of-life care. Patients with chronic pain states where side effects from systemic drug exposure are intolerable and are candidates for spinal drug delivery; however, this may require surgery for indwellng catheterization and pump placement.

Dose Selection/Titration. The conservative approach to the initiation of chronic opioid therapy suggests starting with low doses that may be incremented on the basis of the pharmacokinetics of the drug. In chronic pain states, the aim would be the use of long-acting medications to permit once or twice daily dosing (e.g., controlled release formulations or methadone). Such agents reach steady-state slowly. Rapid incrementation is to be avoided and rescue medication should be made available for breakthrough pain during initial dosing titration.

Opiate Rotation. Opioid rotation is the practice of changing to a different opioid when the patient either fails to achieve benefit or side effects are reached before analgesia is sufficient. In a retrospective review, it was found that the first opioid prescribed was effective for 36% of patients, was stopped because of side effects in 30%, and was stopped for ineffectiveness in 34% (Quang-Cantagrel et al., 2000). Of the remaining patients, the second opioid prescribed after the failure of the first was effective in 31%, the third in 40%, the fourth in 56%, and the fifth in 14%. Thus, if it is necessary to change the opioid prescription because of intolerable side effects or ineffectiveness, the cumulative percentage of efficacy increases with each new opioid tested. Failure or intolerance of one opioid cannot necessarily predict the patient's response or acceptance to another. Practically, opioid rotation involves incrementing the dose of a given opioid, e.g. morphine, to one limited by side-effect and insufficient analgesia. At this point an alternate opioid medication at an equieffective dose may be substituted for the first medication. Agents typically involved in such rotation sequences are various oral opioids such as morphine, methadone, dilaudid, and oxycodone and the fentanyl patch systems. Care must be taken to titrate the doses and monitor the patient closely during such drug transitions.

Combination Therapy. In general, the use of combinations of drugs with the same pharmacological kinetic profile is not warranted (e.g., morphine plus methadone). Nor if the drugs have overlapping targets and opposing effects (e.g., combining a MOR agonist with an agent having mixed agonist/antagonist properties). On the other hand, certain opiate combinations are useful. For example, in a chronic pain state with periodic incident or breakthrough pain, the patient might receive a slow-release formulation of morphine for baseline pain relief and the acute incident pain may be managed with a rapid-onset/short-lasting formulation such as buccal fentanyl.

For inflammatory or nociceptive pain, it is routinely recommended that opioids be combined with other analgesic agents, such as NSAIDs or acetaminophen. In this way, one can take advantage of the analgesic effects produced by the adjuvant and minimize the dose requirement of the opioid. In some situations, NSAIDs can provide analgesia equal to that produced by 60 mg codeine. The analgesic synergism between opioids and aspirin-like drugs is discussed below and in Chapter 34. In the case of neuropathic pain, other drug classes may be useful in combination with the opiate. For example, antidepressants that block amine reuptake, such as amitriptyline or duloxetine, and anticonvulsants such as gabapentin, may enhance the analgesic effect and may be synergistic in some pain states. Different classes of drug may have distinguishable efficacy in different models of pain processing (Table 18–8).

The "opioid-sparing" strategy is the backbone of the "analgesic ladder" for pain management proposed by the World Health Organization. Weaker opioids can be supplanted by stronger opioids in cases of moderate and severe pain. Antidepressants such as duloxetine and amitriptyline are used in the treatment of chronic neuropathic pain but have limited intrinsic analgesic actions in acute pain. However, antidepressants may enhance morphine-induced analgesia (Levine et al., 1986).

NON-ANALGESIC THERAPEUTIC USES OF OPIOIDS

Dyspnea

Morphine is used to alleviate the dyspnea of acute left ventricular failure and pulmonary edema, and the response to intravenous morphine may be dramatic. The mechanism underlying this relief is not clear. It may involve an alteration of the patient's reaction to impaired respiratory function and an indirect reduction of the work of the heart owing to reduced fear and apprehension. However, it is more probable that the major benefit is due to cardiovascular effects, such as decreased peripheral resistance and an increased capacity of the peripheral and splanchnic vascular compartments. Nitroglycerin, which also causes vasodilation, may be superior to morphine in this condition (Hoffman and Reynolds, 1987). In patients with normal blood gases but severe breathlessness owing to chronic obstruction of airflow ("pink puffers"), dihydrocodeine, 15 mg orally before exercise, reduces the feeling of breathlessness and increases exercise tolerance (Johnson et al., 1983). Nonetheless, opioids generally are contraindicated in pulmonary edema unless severe pain also is present.

Anesthetic Adjuvants

High doses of opioids, notably fentanyl and sufentanil, are widely used as the primary anesthetic agents in many surgical procedures. They have powerful "MAC-sparing" effects', e.g., they reduce the concentrations of volatile anesthetic otherwise required to produce an adequate anesthetic depth. Although respiration is so depressed that physical assistance is required, patients can retain consciousness. Therefore, when using opioids as the primary anesthetic agent, it is important to use in conjunction with an agent that results in unconsciousness and produces amnesia such as the benzodiazepines or low concentrations of volatile anesthetics. High doses of opiate also result in prominent rigidity of the chest wall and masseters requiring concurrent treatment with muscle relaxants to permit intubations and ventilation.

TREATMENT OF ACUTE OPIOID TOXICITY

Acute opioid toxicity may result from clinical overdosage, accidental overdosage, or attempts at suicide. Occasionally, a delayed type of toxicity may occur from

Table 18–8

Summary of Drug Target and Site of Action of Common Drug Classes and Relative Efficacy by Pain State

DRUG CLASS (REPRESENTATIVE AGENTS IN PARENTHESES)	DRUG ACTION	SITE OF ACTION[a]	RELATIVE EFFICACY IN PAIN STATES[b]
NSAIDs (ibuprofen, aspirin acetominophen)	Nonspecific COX inhibitors	Peripheral and spinal	Tissue injury >> acute stimuli = nerve injury = 0 (Hamza and Dionne, 2009, Svensson and Yaksh, 2002)
COX 2 inhibitor (celecoxib)	COX2-selective inhibitor	Peripheral and spinal	Tissue injury >> acute stimuli = nerve injury = 0 (Hamza and Dionne, 2009)
Opioids (morphine)	μ receptor agonist	Supraspinal and spinal	Tissue injury = acute stimuli ≥ nerve injury > 0 (see this chapter)
Anticonvulsants (gabapentin)	Na^+ channel block, $\alpha_2\delta$ subunit of Ca^{2+} channel	Supraspinal and spinal	Nerve injury > tissue injury = acute stimuli = 0 (Lai et al., 2004; Taylor, 2009)
Tricyclic antidepressants (amitryptiline)	Inhibit uptake of 5-HT/NE	Supraspinal and spinal	Nerve injury ≥ tissue injury >> acute stimuli = 0 (Mochizucki, 2004)

[a]Studies based on local delivery in preclinical models, e.g., intracranial microinjection or intraventricular injections, lumbar intrathecal delivery or topical/sq application at injury site. [b]Pain states are defined by preclinical models: acute: hot plate/tail flick/acute mechanical compression; tissue injury: intraplantar injections of irritants, focal thermal injury; nerve injury: compression/ligation of sciatic nerve or its branches or of nerve roots; systemic delivery of chemotherapeutics. See Mogil, 2009.

the injection of an opioid into chilled skin areas or in patients with low blood pressure and shock. The drug is not fully absorbed, and therefore, a subsequent dose may be given. When normal circulation is restored, an excessive amount may be absorbed suddenly. It is difficult to define the exact amount of any opioid that is toxic or lethal to humans. Recent experiences with methadone indicate that in nontolerant individuals, serious toxicity may follow the oral ingestion of 40-60 mg. Older literature suggests that in the case of morphine, a normal, opiate-naïve, pain-free adult is not likely to die after oral doses <120 mg or to have serious toxicity with <30 mg parenterally.

Symptoms and Diagnosis

The patient who has taken an overdose of an opioid usually is stuporous or, if a large overdose has been taken, may be in a profound coma. The respiratory rate will be very low, or the patient may be apneic, and cyanosis may be present. As respiratory exchange decreases, blood pressure, at first likely to be near normal, will fall progressively. If adequate oxygenation is restored early, the blood pressure will improve; if hypoxia persists untreated, there may be capillary damage, and measures to combat shock may be required. The pupils will be symmetrical and pinpoint in size; however, if hypoxia is severe, they may be dilated. Urine formation is depressed. Body temperature falls, and the skin becomes cold and clammy. The skeletal muscles are flaccid, the jaw is relaxed, and the tongue may fall back and block the airway. Frank convulsions occasionally may be noted in infants and children. When death occurs, it is nearly always from respiratory failure. Even if respiration is restored, death still may occur as a result of complications that develop during the period of coma, such as pneumonia or shock. Noncardiogenic pulmonary edema is seen commonly with opioid poisoning. It probably is not due to contaminants or to anaphylactic reactions, and it has been observed after toxic doses of morphine, methadone, propoxyphene, and pure heroin.

The triad of coma, pinpoint pupils, and depressed respiration strongly suggests opioid poisoning. The finding of needle marks suggestive of addiction further supports the diagnosis. Mixed poisonings, however, are not uncommon. Examination of the urine and gastric contents for drugs may aid in diagnosis, but the results usually become available too late to influence treatment.

Treatment

The first step is to establish a patent airway and ventilate the patient. Opioid antagonists can produce dramatic reversal of the severe respiratory depression, and the antagonist naloxone is the treatment of choice. However, care should be taken to avoid precipitating withdrawal in dependent patients, who may be extremely sensitive to antagonists. The safest approach is to dilute the standard naloxone dose (0.4 mg) and slowly administer it intravenously, monitoring arousal and respiratory function. With care, it usually is possible to reverse the respiratory depression without precipitating a major withdrawal syndrome. If no response is seen with the first dose, additional doses can be given. Patients should be observed for rebound increases in sympathetic nervous system activity, which may result in cardiac arrhythmias and pulmonary edema. For reversing opioid poisoning in children, the initial dose of naloxone is 0.01 mg/kg. If no effect is seen after a total dose of 10 mg, one can reasonably question the accuracy of the diagnosis. Pulmonary edema sometimes associated with opioid overdosage may be countered by positive-pressure respiration. Tonic-clonic seizures, occasionally seen as part of the toxic syndrome with meperidine, propoxyphene, and tramadol, are ameliorated by treatment with naloxone.

The presence of general CNS depressants does not prevent the salutary effect of naloxone, and in cases of mixed intoxications, the situation will be improved largely owing to antagonism of the respiratory-depressant effects of the opioid. However, some evidence indicates that naloxone and naltrexone also may antagonize some of the depressant actions of sedative-hypnotics. One need not attempt to restore the patient to full consciousness. The duration of action of the available antagonists is shorter than that of many opioids; hence patients can slip back into coma. This is particularly important when the overdosage is due to methadone. The depressant effects of these drugs may persist for 24-72 hours, and fatalities have occurred as a result of premature discontinuation of naloxone. In cases of overdoses of these drugs, a continuous infusion of naloxone should be considered. Toxicity owing to overdose of pentazocine and other opioids with mixed actions may require higher doses of naloxone.

CLINICAL SUMMARY

Opioid analgesics provide symptomatic relief of pain, but the underlying disease remains. The clinician must weigh the benefits of this relief against any potential risk to the patient, which may be quite different in an acute compared with a chronic disease.

In acute problems, opioids will reduce the intensity of pain. However, physical signs (such as abdominal rigidity with an acute abdomen) generally will remain. Relief of pain can facilitate history taking and examination in the emergency room, and the patient's ability to tolerate diagnostic procedures. In most cases analgesics should not be withheld for fear of obscuring the progression of underlying disease.

The problems that arise in the relief of pain associated with chronic conditions are more complex. Repeated daily administration of opioid analgesics eventually will produce tolerance and some degree of physical dependence. The degree will depend on the particular drug, the frequency of administration, the quantity administered, the genetic predisposition, and the psychosocial status of the patient. The decision to control any chronic symptom, especially pain, by the repeated administration of an opioid must be made carefully. When pain is due to chronic nonmalignant disease, conservative measures using non-opioid drugs should be tried before resorting to the opioids. Such measures include the use of NSAIDs, local nerve blocks, antidepressant drugs, electrical stimulation, acupuncture, hypnosis, and behavioral modification.

Selected subpopulations of chronic nonmalignant pain patients can clearly be maintained adequately on opioids for extended periods of time. Careful patient selection is important before starting chronic opioid therapy. All patients should have a risk assessment for drug abuse, diversion, and noncompliance using a validated assessment questionnaire. Chronic pain patients at a higher risk of abuse should not necessarily be denied opioids; however, these patients will require a higher level of monitoring (i.e., random urine drug testing, limited supplies, pill counting) and perhaps referral to a specialist in pain or addiction to assist with therapy.

In the usual doses, morphine-like drugs relieve suffering by altering the emotional component of the painful experience, as well as by producing analgesia. Control of pain, especially chronic pain, must include attention to both psychological factors and the social impact of the illness that sometimes play dominant roles in determining the suffering experienced by the patient. The physician must consider the substantial variabilities in patients' capacities to tolerate pain and in their responses to opioids. Some clinicians, out of an exaggerated concern for the possibility of inducing addiction, tend to prescribe initial doses of opioids that are too small or given too infrequently to alleviate pain and then respond to the patient's continued complaints with an even more exaggerated concern about drug dependence despite the high probability that the request for more drug is only the expected consequence of the inadequate dosage initially prescribed. Infants and children probably are more apt to receive inadequate treatment for pain than are adults owing to communication challenges, physician's lack of familiarity with appropriate pain assessment methodologies in this population, and inexperience with the use of strong opioids in children. If an illness or procedure causes pain for an adult, there is no reason to assume that it will produce less pain for a child (Yaster and Deshpande, 1988).

Pain of Terminal Illness and Cancer Pain

Opioids are not indicated in all cases of terminal illness, but the analgesia, tranquility, and even euphoria afforded by the use of opioids can make the final days of life far less distressing for the patient and family. Although physical dependence and tolerance may develop, this possibility should not prevent physicians from fulfilling their primary obligation to ease the patient's discomfort. The physician should not wait until the pain becomes agonizing; no patient should ever wish for death because of a physician's reluctance to use adequate amounts of effective opioids. This sometimes may entail the regular use of opioid analgesics in substantial doses. Such patients, while they may be physically dependent, are not "addicts" even though they may need large doses on a regular basis. Physical dependence is not equivalent to addiction (Chapter 24).

Most clinicians who are experienced in the management of chronic pain associated with malignant disease or terminal illness recommend that a baseline long-acting opioid be administered around the clock so that pain is continually under control and patients do not dread its return (Foley, 1993). For breakthrough pain episodes, a fast-onset, short-acting opioid can be administered. Less drug is needed to prevent the recurrence of pain than to relieve it initially. Morphine remains the opioid of choice in most of these situations, and the route and dose should be adjusted to the needs of the individual patient. Oral morphine is adequate in most situations. Sustained-release preparations of oral morphine and oxycodone are available that can be administered at 8-, 12-, or 24-hour intervals (morphine) or 8- to 12-hour intervals (oxycodone); thus, superior control of pain often can be achieved with fewer side effects using the same daily dose; a decrease in the fluctuation of plasma concentrations of morphine may be partially responsible.

Constipation is an exceedingly common problem when opioids are used, and the use of stool softeners and laxatives should be initiated early; newer modalities include the use of peripheral opiate antagonists such as methylnaltrexone. Amphetamines have demonstrable mood-elevating and analgesic effects, enhance opioid-induced analgesia, and can reverse opioid induced sedation. However, not all terminal patients require the euphoriant effects of amphetamine, and some experience side effects, such as anorexia. Controlled studies demonstrate no superiority of oral heroin over oral morphine. Similarly, after adjustment is made for potency, parenteral heroin is not superior to morphine in terms of analgesia, effects on mood, or side effects (Sawynok, 1986). Although tolerance does develop to oral opioids, many patients obtain relief from the same dosage for weeks or months. In cases where one opioid loses effectiveness, switching to another may provide better pain relief. "Cross-tolerance" among opioids exists, but clinically and experimentally, cross-tolerance among related receptor agonists is not complete. The reasons for this are not clear but may relate to differences between agonists in receptor-binding characteristics and subsequent cellular signaling interactions.

When oral opioids and other analgesics are no longer satisfactory, subcutaneous or intravenous opioids, nerve blocks, or neurolysis may be required if the nature of the disease permits. Epidural or intrathecal administration of opioids may be useful when administration of opioids by usual routes no longer yields adequate relief of pain.

BIBLIOGRAPHY

Agency for Health Care Policy and Research. *Acute Pain Management in Infants, Children, and Adolescents: Operative and Medical Procedures*. No. 92-0020. U.S. Dept. of Health and Human Services, Rockville, MD, **1992a**.

Agency for Health Care Policy and Research. *Acute Pain Management: Operative or Medical Procedures and Trauma. No.* 92-0032. U.S. Dept. of Health and Human Services, Rockville, MD, **1992b**.

Agency for Health Care Policy and Research. Management of Cancer Pain. No. 94-0592. U.S. Dept. of Health and Human Services, Rockville, MD, **1994**.

Akil H, Owens C, Gutstein H, et al. Endogenous opioids: Overview and current issues. *Drug Alcohol Depend,* **1998**, *51*:127–140.

Akil H, Watson SJ, Young E, et al. Endogenous opioids: Biology and function. *Annu Rev Neurosci,* **1984**, *7*:223–255.

Amir S. Anaphylactic shock: Catecholamine actions in the responses to opioid antagonists. *Prog Clin Biol Res,* **1988**, *264*:265–274.

Anton RF. Naltrexone for the management of alcohol dependence. *N Engl J Med,* **2008**, *359*:715–721.

Ashburn MA, Stephen RL, Ackerman E, et al. Iontophoretic delivery of morphine for postoperative analgesia. *J Pain Symptom Manage,* **1992**, *7*:27–33.

Atkinson RL. Opioid regulation of food intake and body weight in humans. *Fed Proc,* **1987**, *46*:178–182.

Bailey CP, Connor M. Opioids: Cellular mechanisms of tolerance and physical dependence. *Curr Opin Pharmacol,* **2005**, *5*:60–68.

Bailey PL, Stanley TH. *Intravenous opioid anesthetics*. In, *Anesthesia*, 4th ed. (Miller RD, ed.) Churchill Livingstone, New York, **1994**, pp. 291–387.

Ballantyne JC, Loach AB, Carr DB. Itching after epidural and spinal opiates. *Pain,* **1988**, *33*:149–160.

Beaver WT. Impact of non-narcotic oral analgesics on pain management. *Am J Med,* **1988**, *84*:3–15.

Beers R, Camporesi E. Remifentanil update: Clinical science and utility. *CNS Drugs,* **2004**, *18*:1085–1104.

Benedetti F, Amanzio M. The neurobiology of placebo analgesia: From endogenous opioids to cholecystokinin. *Prog Neurobiol,* **1997**, *52*:109–125.

Benyamin R, Trescot AM, Datta S, et al. Opioid complications and side effects. *Pain Physician,* **2008**, *11*:S105–S120.

Bernards CM. Recent insights into the pharmacokinetics of spinal opioids and the relevance to opioid selection. *Curr Opin Anaesthesiol,* **2004**, *17*:441–447.

Bluet-Pajot MT, Tolle V, Zizzari P, et al. Growth hormone secretagogues and hypothalamic networks. *Endocrine,* **2001**, *14*:1–8.

Boas RA, Villiger JW. Clinical actions of fentanyl and buprenorphine. The significance of receptor binding. *Br J Anaesth,* **1985**, *57*:192–196.

Boysen K, Hertel S, Chraemmer-Jorgensen B, *et al.* Buprenorphine antagonism of ventilatory depression following fentanyl anaesthesia. *Acta Anaesthesiol Scand,* **1988**, *32*:490–492.

Burkle H, Dunbar S, Van Aken H. Remifentanil: A novel, short-acting, mu-opioid. *Anesth Analg,* **1996**, *83*:646–651.

Cameron D, Gan TJ. Management of postoperative nausea and vomiting in ambulatory surgery. *Anesthesiol Clin North Am,* **2003**, *21*:347–365.

Caraco Y, Sheller J, Wood AJ. Impact of ethnic origin and quinidine coadministration on codeine's disposition and pharmacodynamic effects. *J Pharmacol Exp Ther,* **1999**, *290*:413–422.

Chan GL, Matzke GR. Effects of renal insufficiency on the pharmacokinetics and pharmacodynamics of opioid analgesics. *Drug Intell Clin Pharm,* **1987**, *21*:773–783.

Cherny NI. Opioid analgesics: Comparative features and prescribing guidelines. *Drugs,* **1996**, *51*:713–737.

Christie MJ. Cellular neuroadaptations to chronic opioids: Tolerance, withdrawal and addiction. *Br J Pharmacol,* **2008**, *154*:384–396.

Christrup LL. Morphine metabolites. *Acta Anaesthesiol Scand,* **1997**, *41*:116–122.

Chu P, Murray S, Lissin D, von Zastrow M. Delta and kappa opioid receptors are differentially regulated by dynamin-dependent endocytosis when activated by the same alkaloid agonist. *J Biol Chem,* **1997**, *272*:27124–27130.

Chuang LF, Killam KF Jr, Chuang RY. Induction and activation of mitogen-activated protein kinases of human lymphocytes as one of the signaling pathways of the immunomodulatory effects of morphine sulfate. *J Biol Chem,* **1997**, *272*: 26815–26817.

Chung KF, Pavord ID. Prevalence, pathogenesis, and causes of chronic cough. *Lancet,* **2008**, *371*:1364–1374.

Clemens KE, Klaschik E. Symptomatic therapy of dyspnea with strong opioids and its effect on ventilation in palliative care patients. *J Pain Symptom Manage,* **2007**, *33*:473–481.

Craviso GL, Musacchio JM. High-affinity dextromethorphan binding sites in guinea pig brain. II. Competition experiments. *Mol Pharmacol,* **1983**, *23*:629–640.

Dixon R, Howes J, Gentile J, et al. Nalmefene: Intravenous safety and kinetics of a new opioid antagonist. *Clin Pharmacol Ther,* **1986**, *39*:49–53.

Dray A, Nunan L. Supraspinal and spinal mechanisms in morphine-induced inhibition of reflex urinary bladder contractions in the rat. *Neuroscience,* **1987**, *22*:281–287.

Dreborg S, Sundstrom G, Larsson TA, Larhammar D. Evolution of vertebrate opioid receptors. *Proc Natl Acad Sci USA,* **2008**, *105*:15487–15492.

Drolet G, Dumont EC, Gosselin I, et al. Role of endogenous opioid system in the regulation of the stress response. *Prog Neuropsychopharmacol Biol Psychiatry,* **2001**, *25*:729–741.

Duce MA, Hernande LF. Origins of the hypodermic syringe and local anesthesia. Their influence on hernia surgery. *Hernia,* **1999**, *3*:103–106.

Du Pen SL, Du Pen AR, Polissar N, et al. Implementing guidelines for cancer pain management: Results of a randomized controlled clinical trial. *J Clin Oncol,* **1999**, *17*:361–370.

Duthie DJ. Remifentanil and tramadol. *Br J Anaesth,* **1998**, *81*:51–57.

Dworkin RH, Backonja M, Rowbotham MC, et al. Advances in neuropathic pain: Diagnosis, mechanisms, and treatment recommendations. *Arch Neurol,* **2003**, *60*:1524–1534.

Edwards DJ, Svensson CK, Visco JP, Lalka D. Clinical pharmacokinetics of pethidine: 1982. *Clin Pharmacokinet,* **1982**, *7*: 421–433.

Eichelbaum M, Evert B. Influence of pharmacogenetics on drug disposition and response. *Clin Exp Pharmacol Physiol,* **1996**, *23*:983–985.

Eichelbaum M, Gross AS. The genetic polymorphism of debrisoquine/sparteine metabolism—clinical aspects. *Pharmacol Ther,* **1990**, *46*:377–394.

Elliott K, Hynansky A, Inturrisi CE. Dextromethorphan attenuates and reverses analgesic tolerance to morphine. *Pain,* **1994**, *59*:361–368.

Evans CJ, Keith DE Jr., Morrison H, et al. Cloning of a delta opioid receptor by functional expression. *Science,* **1992**, *258*: 1952–1955.

Faden AI. Role of thyrotropin-releasing hormone and opiate receptor antagonists in limiting central nervous system injury. *Adv Neurol,* **1988**, *47*:531–546.

Farid WO, Dunlop SA, Tait RJ, Hulse GK. The effects of maternally administered methadone, buprenorphine and naltrexone on offspring: Review of human and animal data. *Curr Neuropharmacol,* **2008**, *6*:125–150.

Fichna J, Janecka A, Costentin J, Do Rego JC. The endomorphin system and its evolving neurophysiological role. *Pharmacol Rev,* **2007**, *59*:88–123.

Fioravanti B, Vanderah TW. The ORL-1 receptor system: Are there opportunities for antagonists in pain therapy? *Curr Top Med Chem,* **2008**, *8*:1442–1451.

Fishburne JI. Systemic analgesia during labor. *Clin Perinatol,* **1982**, *9*:29–53.

Foley KM. Opioid analgesics in clinical pain management. In, BOOK TITLE NEEDED. (Herz A, ed.) Springer-Verlag, Berlin, **1993**, pp. 693–743.

Fowler CJ, Griffiths D, de Groat WC. The neural control of micturition. *Nat Rev Neurosci,* **2008**, *9*:453–466.

France CR, al'Absi M, Ring C, et al. Nociceptive flexion reflex and pain rating responses during endogenous opiate blockade with naltrexone in healthy young adults. *Biol Psychol,* **2007**, *75*:95–100.

Fryer RM, Hsu AK, Nagase H, Gross GJ. Opioid-induced cardioprotection against myocardial infarction and arrhythmias: Mitochondrial versus sarcolemmal ATP-sensitive potassium channels. *J Pharmacol Exp Ther,* **2000**, *294*:451–457.

Fudala PJ, Johnson RE, Bunker E. Abrupt withdrawal of buprenorphine following chronic administration. *Clin Pharmacol Ther*, **1989**.

Gaveriaux-Ruff C, Matthes HW, Peluso J, Kieffer BL. Abolition of morphine-immunosuppression in mice lacking the mu-opioid receptor gene. *Proc Natl Acad Sci USA,* **1998**, *95*: 6326–6330.

Gear RW, Miaskowski C, Gordon NC, et al. The kappa opioid nalbuphine produces gender- and dose-dependent analgesia and antianalgesia in patients with postoperative pain. *Pain,* **1999**, *83*:339–345.

Gether U. Uncovering molecular mechanisms involved in activation of G protein-coupled receptors. *Endocr Rev,* **2000**, *21*: 90–113.

Gimpl G, Fahrenholz F. The oxytocin receptor system: structure, function, and regulation. *Physiol Rev,* **2001**, *81*:629–683.

Glass PS, Gan TJ, Howell S. A review of the pharmacokinetics and pharmacodynamics of remifentanil. *Anesth Analg,* **1999**, *89*:S7–S14.

Goldstein A, Lowney LI, Pal BK. Stereospecific and nonspecific interactions of the morphine congener levorphanol in subcellular fractions of mouse brain. *Proc Natl Acad Sci USA*, **1971**, *68:*1742–1747.

Gonzalez JP, Brogden RN. Naltrexone. A review of its pharmacodynamic and pharmacokinetic properties and therapeutic efficacy in the management of opioid dependence. *Drugs,* **1988**, *35*:192–213.

Gourlay GK, Cherry DA, Cousins MJ. A comparative study of the efficacy and pharmacokinetics of oral methadone and morphine in the treatment of severe pain in patients with cancer. *Pain,* **1986**, *25*:297–312.

Greenwood-Van Meerveld B. Emerging drugs for postoperative ileus. *Expert Opin Emerg Drugs,* **2007**, *12*:619–626.

Gupta A, Decaillot FM, Devi LA. Targeting opioid receptor heterodimers: strategies for screening and drug development. *Aaps J,* **2006**, *8*:E153–E159.

Haile CN, Kosten TA, Kosten TR. Pharmacogenetic treatments for drug addiction: alcohol and opiates. *Am J Drug Alcohol Abuse,* **2008**, *34*:355–381.

Hamza M, Dionne RA. Mechanisms of non-opioid analgesics beyond cyclooxygenase enzyme inhibition. *Curr Mol Pharmacol,* **2009**, *2*:1–14.

Hartrick CT, Hartrick KA. Extended-release epidural morphine (DepoDur): Review and safety analysis. *Expert Rev Neurother,* **2008**, *8*:1641–1648.

Hawryluk GWJ, Rowland J, Kwon BK, et al. Protection and repair of the injured spinal cord: a review of completed, ongoing, and planned clinical trials for acute spinal cord injury. *Neurosurg Focus*, **2008**, *25*:E14.

Heishman SJ, Stitzer ML, Bigelow GE, Liebson IA. Acute opioid physical dependence in postaddict humans: Naloxone dose effects after brief morphine exposure. *J Pharmacol Exp Ther,* **1989**, *248*:127–134.

Henriksen G, Willoch F. Imaging of opioid receptors in the central nervous system. *Brain,* **2008**, *131*:1171–1196.

Hoffman JR, Reynolds S. Comparison of nitroglycerin, morphine and furosemide in treatment of presumed pre-hospital pulmonary edema. *Chest,* **1987**, *92*:586–593.

Hook V, Funkelstein L, Lu D, et al. Proteases for processing proneuropeptides into peptide neurotransmitters and hormones. *Annu Rev Pharmacol Toxicol,* **2008**, *48*:393–423.

Hughes J, Smith TW, Kosterlitz HW, et al. Identification of two related pentapeptides from the brain with potent opiate agonist activity. *Nature,* **1975**, *258*:577–580. International Association for the Study of Pain. *Management of Acute Pain: A Practical Guide*. IASP Publications, Seattle, WA, **1992**.

Johnson MA, Woodcock AA, Geddes DM. Dihydrocodeine for breathlessness in "pink puffers." *Br Med J (Clin Res Ed),* **1983**, *286*:675–677.

Kane BE, Svensson B, Ferguson DM. Molecular recognition of opioid receptor ligands. *AAPS J,* **2006**, *8*:E126–E137.

Karavelis A, Foroglou G, Selviaridis P, Fountzilas G. Intraventricular administration of morphine for control of intractable cancer pain in 90 patients. *Neurosurgery,* **1996**, *39*:57–61; discussion 61–52.

Karlsson MO, Dahlstrom B, Neil A. Characterization of high-affinity binding sites for the antitussive [3H]noscapine in guinea pig brain tissue. *Eur J Pharmacol,* **1988**, *145*: 195–203.

King T, Ossipov MH, Vanderah TW, et al. Is paradoxical pain induced by sustained opioid exposure an underlying mechanism of opioid antinociceptive tolerance? *Neurosignals,* **2005**, *14*:194–205.

Koch T, Widera A, Bartzsch K, et al. Receptor endocytosis counteracts the development of opioid tolerance. *Mol Pharmacol,* **2005**, *67*:280–287.

Koob GF, Bloom FE. Cellular and molecular mechanisms of drug dependence. *Science,* **1988**, *242*:715–723.

Kreek MJ, Koob GF. Drug dependence: Stress and dysregulation of brain reward pathways. *Drug Alcohol Depend,* **1998**, *51*:23–47.

Kreek MJ, LaForge KS, Butelman E. Pharmacotherapy of addictions. *Nat Rev Drug Discov,* **2002**, *1*:710–726.

Kress HG, Oronska A, Kaczmarek Z, et al. Efficacy and tolerability of intranasal fentanyl spray 50 to 200 µg for breakthrough pain in patients with cancer: A phase III, multinational, randomized, double-blind, placebo-controlled, crossover trial with a 10-month, open-label extension treatment period. *Clin Ther,* **2009**, *31*:1177–1191.

Kromer W. Endogenous and exogenous opioids in the control of gastrointestinal motility and secretion. *Pharmacol Rev,* **1988**, *40*:121–162.

Krupnick JG, Benovic JL. The role of receptor kinases and arrestins in G protein-coupled receptor regulation. *Annu Rev Pharmacol Toxicol,* **1998**, *38*:289–319.

Lai J, Porreca F, Hunter JC, Gold MS. Voltage-gated sodium channels and hyperalgesia. *Annu Rev Pharmacol Toxicol,* **2004**, *44*:371–397.

Lalley PM. Opioidergic and dopaminergic modulation of respiration. *Respir Physiol Neurobiol,* **2008**, *164*:160–167.

Larson MD. Mechanism of opioid-induced pupillary effects. *Clin Neurophysiol,* **2008**, *119*:1358–1364.

Latremoliere A, Woolf CJ. Central sensitization: A generator of pain hypersensitivity by central neural plasticity. *J Pain,* **2009**, *10*:895–926.

Levine JD, Gordon NC, Smith R, McBryde R. Desipramine enhances opiate postoperative analgesia. *Pain,* **1986**, *27*: 45–49.

Lewis KS, Han NH. Tramadol: A new centrally acting analgesic. *Am J Health Syst Pharm,* **1997**, *54*:643–652.

Lindow SW, Hendricks MS, Nugent FA, et al. Morphine suppresses the oxytocin response in breast-feeding women. *Gynecol Obstet Invest,* **1999**, *48*:33–37.

Lyss AP, Portenoy RK. Strategies for limiting the side effects of cancer pain therapy. *Semin Oncol,* **1997**, *24*:S16-28–34.

Martin WR. Pharmacology of opioids. *Pharmacol Rev,* **1983**, *35*:283–323.

Martin WR, Eades CG, Thompson JA, et al. The effects of morphine- and nalorphine- like drugs in the nondependent and morphine-dependent chronic spinal dog. *J Pharmacol Exp Ther,* **1976**, *197*:517–532.

Matthys H, Bleicher B, Bleicher U. Dextromethorphan and codeine: Objective assessment of antitussive activity in patients with chronic cough. *J Int Med Res,* **1983**, *11*:92–100.

Mattick RP, Breen C, Kimber J, Davoli M. Methadone maintenance therapy versus no opioid replacement therapy for opioid dependence. *Cochrane Database Syst Rev,* **2009**, CD002209.

McCleskey EW, Gold MS. Ion channels of nociception. *Annu Rev Physiol,* **1999**, *61*:835–856.

McGinty JF. What we know and still need to learn about opioids in the hippocampus. *NIDA Res Monogr,* **1988**, *82*:1–11.

McIntosh M, Kane K, Parratt J. Effects of selective opioid receptor agonists and antagonists during myocardial ischaemia. *Eur J Pharmacol,* **1992**, *210*:37–44.

McQuay H.J. Pharmacological treatment of neuralgic and neuropathic pain. *Cancer Surv,* **1988**, *7*:141–159.

Mellon RD, Bayer BM. Evidence for central opioid receptors in the immunomodulatory effects of morphine: Review of potential mechanism(s) of action. *J Neuroimmunol,* **1998**, *83*: 19–28.

Melzack R, Casey KL. *Sensory, Motivational and Central Control Determinants of Pain: A New Conceptual Model*. Thomas, Springfield, IL, **1968**.

Meng F, Xie GX, Thompson RC, et al. Cloning and pharmacological characterization of a rat kappa opioid receptor. *Proc Natl Acad Sci USA,* **1993**, *90*:9954–9958.

Mochizucki D. Serotonin and noradrenaline reuptake inhibitors in animal models of pain. *Hum Psychopharmacol,* **2004**, *19(suppl 1)*:S15–A19.

Mogil JS.Animal models of pain: progress and challenges. *Nat Rev Neurosci,* **2009,** *10*:283–294.

Monk JP, Beresford R, Ward A. Sufentanil. A review of its pharmacological properties and therapeutic use. *Drugs,* **1988**, *36*:286–313.

Moulin DE, Clark AJ, Gilron I, et al. Pharmacological management of chronic neuropathic pain—consensus statement and guidelines from the Canadian Pain Society. *Pain Res Manage,* **2007**, *12*:13–21.

Neumann PB, Henriksen H, Grosman N, Christensen CB. Plasma morphine concentrations during chronic oral administration in patients with cancer pain. *Pain,* **1982**, *13*:247–252.

Osborne R, Joel S, Trew D, Slevin M. Analgesic activity of morphine-6-glucuronide. *Lancet,* **1988**, *1*:828.

Owen JA, Sitar DS, Berger L, et al. Age-related morphine kinetics. *Clin Pharmacol Ther,* **1983**, *34*:364–368.

Page GG, Ben-Eliyahu S. The immune-suppressive nature of pain. *Semin Oncol Nurs,* **1997**, *13*:10–15.

Pan YX. Diversity and complexity of the mu opioid receptor gene: Alternative pre-mRNA splicing and promoters. *DNA Cell Biol,* **2005**, *24*:736–750.

Pasternak GW. Molecular biology of opioid analgesia. *J Pain Symptom Manage,* **2005**, *29*:S2–S9.

Patel SS, Spencer CM. Remifentanil. *Drugs,* **1996**, *52*:417–427; discussion 428.

Pattinson KT. Opioids and the control of respiration. *Br J Anaesth,* **2008**, *100*:747–758.

Paul D, Standifer KM, Inturrisi CE, Pasternak GW. Pharmacological characterization of morphine-6 beta-glucuronide, a very potent morphine metabolite. *J Pharmacol Exp Ther,* **1989**, *251*:477–483.

Pert CB, Snyder SH. Opiate receptor: Demonstration in nervous tissue. *Science,* **1973**, *179*:1011–1014.

Popio KA, Jackson DH, Ross AM, et al.Hemodynamic and respiratory effects of morphine and butorphanol. *Clin Pharmacol Ther,* **1978**, *23*:281–287.

Portenoy RK, Southam MA, Gupta SK, et al. Transdermal fentanyl for cancer pain. Repeated dose pharmacokinetics. *Anesthesiology,* **1993**, *78*:36–43.

Portoghese PS. Bivalent ligands and the message-address concept in the design of selective opioid receptor antagonists. *Trends Pharmacol Sci,* **1989**, *10*:230–235.

Price DD, Von der Gruen A, Miller J, et al. A psychophysical analysis of morphine analgesia. *Pain,* **1985**, *22*:261–269.

Quang-Cantagrel ND, Wallace MS, Magnuson SK. Opioid substitution to improve the effectiveness of chronic noncancer pain control: A chart review. *Anesth Analg,* **2000**, *90*: 933–937.

Raynor K, Kong H, Chen Y, et al. Pharmacological characterization of the cloned kappa-, delta-, and mu-opioid receptors. *Mol Pharmacol,* **1994**, *45*:330–334.

Rose PG, Macfee MS, Boswell MV. Fentanyl transdermal system overdose secondary to cutaneous hyperthermia. *Anesth Analg,* **1993**, *77*:390–391.

Rosow CE, Gomery P, Chen TY, et al. Reversal of opioid-induced bladder dysfunction by intravenous naloxone and methylnaltrexone. *Clin Pharmacol Ther,* **2007**, *82*:48–53.

Roth A, Keren G, Gluck A, et al. Comparison of nalbuphine hydrochloride versus morphine sulfate for acute myocardial infarction with elevated pulmonary artery wedge pressure. *Am J Cardiol,* **1988**, *62*:551–555.

Sadeque AJ, Wandel C, He H, et al. Increased drug delivery to the brain by P-glycoprotein inhibition. *Clin Pharmacol Ther,* **2000**, *68*:231–237.

Sawynok J. The therapeutic use of heroin: A review of the pharmacological literature. *Can J Physiol Pharmacol,* **1986**, *64*:1–6.

Schinkel AH, Wagenaar E, Mol CA, van Deemter L. P-glycoprotein in the blood-brain barrier of mice influences the brain penetration and pharmacological activity of many drugs. *J Clin Invest,* **1996**, *97*:2517–2524.

Schmelz M. Itch—mediators and mechanisms. *J Dermatol Sci,* **2002**, *28*:91–96.

Segredo V, Burford NT, Lameh J, Sadee W. A constitutively internalizing and recycling mutant of the mu-opioid receptor. *J Neurochem,* **1997**, *68*:2395–2404.

Seifert CF, Kennedy S. Meperidine is alive and well in the new millennium: Evaluation of meperidine usage patterns and frequency of adverse drug reactions. *Pharmacotherapy,* **2004**, *24*:776–783.

Sessler DI. Temperature monitoring and perioperative thermoregulation. *Anesthesiology,* **2008**, *109*:318–338.

Sharp B, Yaksh T. Pain killers of the immune system. *Nat Med,* **1997**, *3*:831–832.

Shnider SM, Levinson G. *Anesthesia for Obstetrics*. Lippincott Williams & Wilkins, Baltimore, **1987**.

Sidhu AS, Triadafilopoulos G. Neuro-regulation of lower esophageal sphincter function as treatment for gastroesophageal reflux disease. *World J Gastroenterol,* **2008**, *14*:985–990.

Smith MT. Neuroexcitatory effects of morphine and hydromorphone: Evidence implicating the 3-glucuronide metabolites. *Clin Exp Pharmacol Physiol,* **2000**, *27*:524–528.

Sorkin LS, Wallace MS. Acute pain mechanisms. *Surg Clin North Am,* **1999**, *79*:213–229.

Stack CG, Rogers P, Linter SP. Monoamine oxidase inhibitors and anaesthesia. A review. *Br J Anaesth,* **1988**, *60*:222–227.

Stein C. Peripheral mechanisms of opioid analgesia. *Anesth Analg,* **1993**, *76*:182–191.

Stein C, Lang LJ. Peripheral mechanisms of opioid analgesia. *Curr Opin Pharmacol,* **2009**, *9*:3–8.

Stevens CW. The evolution of vertebrate opioid receptors. *Front Biosci,* **2009**, *14*:1247–1269.

Supernaw RB. CYP2D6 and the efficacy of codeine and codeine-like drugs. *Am J Pain Manage,* **2001**, *11*:30–31.

Svensson CI, Yaksh TL. The spinal phospholipase-cyclooxygenase-prostanoid cascade in nociceptive processing. *Annu Rev Pharmacol Toxicol,* **2002**, *42*:553–583.

Takemori AE, Portoghese PS. Selective naltrexone-derived opioid receptor antagonists. *Annu Rev Pharmacol Toxicol,* **1992**, *32*:239–269.

Taylor CP. Mechanisms of analgesia by gabapentin and pregabalin—calcium channel alpha2-delta [Cavalpha2-delta] ligands. *Pain,* **2009**, *142*:13–16.

Thomas J, Karver S, Cooney GA, et al. Methylnaltrexone for opioid-induced constipation in advanced illness. *N Engl J Med,* **2008**, *358*:2332–2343.

Thompson RC, Mansour A, Akil H, Watson SJ. Cloning and pharmacological characterization of a rat mu opioid receptor. *Neuron,* **1993**, *11*:903–913.

Trujillo KA, Akil H. Inhibition of morphine tolerance and dependence by the NMDA receptor antagonist MK-801. *Science,* **1991**, *251*:85–87.

Vashi V, Harris S, El-Tahtawy A, et al. Clinical pharmacology and pharmacokinetics of once-daily hydromorphone hydrochloride extended-release capsules. *J Clin Pharmacol,* **2005**, *45*:547–554.

Vella-Brincat J, Macleod AD. Adverse effects of opioids on the central nervous systems of palliative care patients. *J Pain Palliat Care Pharmacother,* **2007**, *21*:15–25.

von Zastrow M, Svingos A, Haberstock-Debic H, Evans C. Regulated endocytosis of opioid receptors: cellular mechanisms and proposed roles in physiological adaptation to opiate drugs. *Curr Opin Neurobiol,* **2003**, *13*:348–353.

Waldhoer M, Bartlett SE, Whistler JL. Opioid receptors. *Annu Rev Biochem,* **2004**, *73*:953–990.

Wallace M, Yaksh TL. Long-term spinal analgesic delivery: a review of the preclinical and clinical literature. *Reg Anesth Pain Med,* **2000**, *25*:117–157.

Wallenstein SL, Kaiko RF, Rogers AG, Houde RW. Crossover trials in clinical analgesic assays: studies of buprenorphine and morphine. *Pharmacotherapy,* **1986**, *6*:228–235.

Welters ID, Menzebach A, Goumon Y, *et al.* Morphine inhibits NF-kappaB nuclear binding in human neutrophils and monocytes by a nitric oxide-dependent mechanism. *Anesthesiology,* **2000**, *92*:1677–1684.

Williams JT, Christie MJ, Manzoni O. Cellular and synaptic adaptations mediating opioid dependence. *Physiol Rev,* **2001**, *81*:299–343.

Wood JD, Galligan JJ. Function of opioids in the enteric nervous system. *Neurogastroenterol Motil,* **2004**, *16(suppl 2)*:17–28.

Woodhouse A, Mather LE. The minimum effective concentration of opioids: a revisitation with patient controlled analgesia fentanyl. *Reg Anesth Pain Med,* **2000**, *25*:259–267.

Xi ZX, Stein EA. GABAergic mechanisms of opiate reinforcement. *Alcohol Alcohol,* **2002**, *37*:485–494.

Yaksh TL. CNS mechanisms of pain and analgesia. *Cancer Surv,* **1988**, *7*:5–28.

Yaksh TL. Pharmacology and mechanisms of opioid analgesic activity. *Acta Anaesthesiol Scand,* **1997**, *41*:94–111.

Yaksh TL, Allen JW. The use of intrathecal midazolam in humans: A case study of process. *Anesth Analg,* **2004**, *98*: 1536–1545.

Yaksh TL, Jessell TM, Gamse R, et al. Intrathecal morphine inhibits substance P release from mammalian spinal cord in vivo. *Nature,* **1980**, *286*:155–157.

Yaster M, Deshpande JK. Management of pediatric pain with opioid analgesics. *J Pediatr,* **1988**, *113*:421–429.

Yeh SY, Gorodetzky CW, Krebs HA. Isolation and identification of morphine 3- and 6-glucuronides, morphine 3,6-diglucuronide, morphine 3-ethereal sulfate, normorphine, and normorphine 6-glucuronide as morphine metabolites in humans. *J Pharm Sci,* **1977**, *66*:1288–1293.

Yoburn BC, Luke MC, Pasternak GW, Inturrisi CE. Upregulation of opioid receptor subtypes correlates with potency changes of morphine and DADLE. *Life Sci,* **1988**, *43*:1319–1324.

Young GB, da Silva OP. Effects of morphine on the electroencephalograms of neonates: A prospective, observational study. *Clin Neurophysiol,* **2000**, *111*:1955–1960.

Zadina JE, Hackler L, Ge LJ, Kastin AJ. A potent and selective endogenous agonist for the mu-opiate receptor. *Nature,* **1997**, *386*:499–502.

Zimmer EZ, Divon MY, Vadasz A. Influence of meperidine on fetal movements and heart rate beat-to-beat variability in the active phase of labor. *Am J Perinatol,* **1988**, *5*: 197–200.

asthmaticus with halothane and intractable angina with epidural local anesthetics, should not obscure this critical point that permeates the training and practice of the specialty. Hence, administration of general anesthesia, as well as the development of new anesthetic agents and physiologic monitoring technology, has been driven by three general objectives:

1. *Minimizing the potentially deleterious direct and indirect effects of anesthetic agents and techniques.*
2. *Sustaining physiologic homeostasis during surgical procedures* that may involve major blood loss, tissue ischemia, reperfusion of ischemic tissue, fluid shifts, exposure to a cold environment, and impaired coagulation.
3. *Improving postoperative outcomes* by choosing techniques that block or treat components of the surgical stress response, which may lead to short- or long-term sequelae.

Hemodynamic Effects of General Anesthesia. The most prominent physiological effect of anesthesia induction, associated with the majority of both intravenous and inhalational agents, is a decrease in systemic arterial blood pressure. The causes include direct vasodilation, myocardial depression, or both; a blunting of baroreceptor control; and a generalized decrease in central sympathetic tone. Agents vary in the magnitude of their specific effects (described later in the chapter), but in all cases the hypotensive response is enhanced by underlying volume depletion or preexisting myocardial dysfunction. Even anesthetics that show minimal hypotensive tendencies under normal conditions (e.g., etomidate and ketamine) must be used with caution in trauma victims, in whom intravascular volume depletion is being compensated by intense sympathetic discharge. Smaller-than-normal anesthetic dosages are employed in patients presumed to be sensitive to hemodynamic effects of anesthetics.

Respiratory Effects of General Anesthesia. Airway maintenance is essential following induction of anesthesia, as nearly all general anesthetics reduce or eliminate both ventilatory drive and the reflexes that maintain airway patency. Therefore, ventilation generally must be assisted or controlled for at least some period during surgery. The gag reflex is lost, and the stimulus to cough is blunted. Lower esophageal sphincter tone also is reduced, so both passive and active regurgitation may occur. Endotracheal intubation, introduced by Kuhn in the early 1900s, has been a major reason for a decline in the number of aspiration deaths during general anesthesia. Muscle relaxation is valuable during the induction of general anesthesia where it facilitates management of the airway, including endotracheal intubation. Neuromuscular blocking agents commonly are used to effect such relaxation (Chapter 11), reducing the risk of coughing or gagging during laryngoscopic-assisted instrumentation of the airway, and thus reducing the risk of aspiration prior to secure placement of an endotracheal tube. Alternatives to an endotracheal tube include a facemask and a laryngeal mask, an inflatable mask placed in the oropharynx forming a seal around the glottis. The choice of airway management is based on the type of procedure and characteristics of the patient.

Hypothermia. Patients commonly develop hypothermia (body temperature $< 36°C$) during surgery. The reasons for the hypothermia include low ambient temperature, exposed body cavities, cold intravenous fluids, altered thermoregulatory control, and reduced metabolic rate. General anesthetics lower the core temperature set point at which thermoregulatory vasoconstriction is activated to defend against heat loss. Furthermore, vasodilation produced by both general and regional anesthesia offsets cold-induced peripheral vasoconstriction, thereby redistributing heat from central to peripheral body compartments, leading to a decline in core temperature (Sessler, 2000). Metabolic rate and total body oxygen consumption decrease with general anesthesia by ~30%, reducing heat generation.

Even small drops in body temperatures may lead to an increase in perioperative morbidity, including cardiac complications, wound infections, and impaired coagulation. Prevention of hypothermia has emerged as a major goal of anesthetic care. Modalities to maintain normothermia include using warm intravenous fluids, heat exchangers in the anesthesia circuit, forced-warm-air covers, and new technology involving water-filled garments with microprocessor feedback control to a core temperature set point.

Nausea and Vomiting. Nausea and vomiting in the postoperative period continue to be significant problems following general anesthesia and are caused by an action of anesthetics on the chemoreceptor trigger zone and the brainstem vomiting center, which are modulated by serotonin (5-HT), histamine, acetylcholine (ACh), and dopamine (DA). The 5-HT_3-receptor antagonists, ondansetron and dolasetron (Chapters 13 and 46), are very effective in suppressing nausea and vomiting. Common treatments also include droperidol, metoclopramide, dexamethasone, and avoidance of N_2O. The use of propofol as an induction agent and the nonsteroidal anti-inflammatory drug ketorolac as a substitute for opioids may decrease the incidence and severity of postoperative nausea and vomiting.

Other Emergence and Postoperative Phenomena. Hypertension and tachycardia are common as the sympathetic nervous system regains its tone and is enhanced by pain. Myocardial ischemia can appear or markedly worsen during emergence in patients with coronary artery disease. Emergence excitement occurs in 5-30% of patients and is characterized by tachycardia, restlessness, crying, moaning, and thrashing. A variety of neurologic signs, including delirium, spasticity, hyperreflexia, and Babinski sign, are often manifest in the patient emerging from anesthesia. Postanesthesia shivering occurs frequently because of core hypothermia. A small dose of meperidine (12.5 mg) lowers the shivering trigger temperature and effectively stops the activity. The incidence of all of these emergence phenomena is greatly reduced when opioids and α_2 agonists (dexmedetomidine) are employed as part of the intraoperative regimen.

Airway obstruction may occur during the postoperative period because residual anesthetic effects continue to partially obtund consciousness and reflexes (especially in patients who normally snore or who have sleep apnea). Strong inspiratory efforts against a closed glottis can lead to negative-pressure pulmonary edema. Pulmonary function is reduced postoperatively following all types of anesthesia and surgery, and hypoxemia may occur. Hypertension can be prodigious, often requiring aggressive treatment.

Pain control can be complicated in the immediate postoperative period. The respiratory suppression associated with opioids can be problematic among postoperative patients who still have a substantial residual anesthetic effect. Patients can alternate between states of excruciating pain to somnolence with airway obstruction, all in a matter of moments. The nonsteroidal anti-inflammatory agent ketorolac (30-60 mg intravenously) frequently is effective, and the development of injectable cyclooxygenase-2 inhibitors (Chapter 34) holds promise for analgesia without respiratory depression. In addition, regional anesthetic techniques are an important part of a perioperative multimodal approach that employs local anesthetic wound infiltration; epidural, spinal, and plexus blocks; and nonsteroidal anti-inflammatory drugs, opioids, α_2 adrenergic receptor agonists, and NMDA-receptor antagonists. Patient-controlled administration of intravenous and epidural analgesics makes use of small, computerized pumps activated on demand but programmed with safety limits to prevent overdose. The agents used are opioids (frequently morphine) by the intravenous route, and an opioid, local anesthetic, or both by the epidural route. These techniques have revolutionized postoperative pain management, can be continued for hours or days, and promote ambulation and improved bowel function until oral pain medications are initiated.

ACTIONS AND MECHANISMS OF GENERAL ANESTHETICS

The Anesthetic State

General anesthetics are a structurally diverse class of drugs that produce a common end point—a behavioral state referred to as *general anesthesia*. In the broadest sense, general anesthesia can be defined as a global but reversible depression of CNS function resulting in the loss of response to and perception of all external stimuli. While this definition is appealing in its simplicity, it is not useful for two reasons: First, it is inadequate because anesthesia is not simply a deafferented state; e.g., amnesia is an important aspect of the anesthetic state. Second, not all general anesthetics produce identical patterns of deafferentation. Barbiturates, e.g., are very effective at producing amnesia and loss of consciousness, but are not effective as analgesics.

An alternative way of defining the anesthetic state is to consider it as a collection of "component" changes in behavior or perception. The components of the anesthetic state include:

- *amnesia*
- *immobility* in response to noxious stimulation
- *attenuation of autonomic responses* to noxious stimulation
- *analgesia*
- *unconsciousness*

It is important to remember that general anesthesia is useful only insofar as it facilitates the performance of surgery or other noxious procedures. The performance of surgery usually requires an immobilized patient who does not have an excessive autonomic response to surgery (blood pressure and heart rate) and who has amnesia for the procedure. Indeed, if an anesthetic produces profound amnesia, it can be difficult in principle to determine if it also produces either analgesia or unconsciousness.

Measurement of Anesthetic Potency

The potency of general anesthetic agents usually is measured by determining the concentration of general anesthetic that prevents movement in response to surgical stimulation. For inhalational anesthetics, anesthetic potency is measured in MAC units, with 1 MAC defined as the minimum alveolar concentration that prevents movement in response to surgical stimulation in 50% of subjects.

The strengths of MAC as a measurement are that:

- alveolar concentrations can be monitored continuously by measuring end-tidal anesthetic concentration using infrared spectroscopy or mass spectrometry
- it provides a direct correlate of the free concentration of the anesthetic at its site(s) of action in the CNS
- it is a simple-to-measure end point that reflects an important clinical goal

End points other than immobilization also can be used to measure anesthetic potency. For example, the ability to respond to verbal commands (MAC_{awake}) and the ability to form memories also have been correlated with alveolar anesthetic concentration. Interestingly, verbal response and memory formation both are suppressed at a fraction

Table 19–1

Properties of Inhalational Anesthetic Agents

ANESTHETIC AGENT	MAC[a] (vol %)	MAC_{AWAKE}[b] (vol %)	EC_{50}[c] FOR SUPPRESSION OF MEMORY (vol %)	VAPOR PRESSURE (mm Hg at 20°C)	PARTITION COEFFICIENT AT 37°C Blood:Gas	Brain:Blood	Fat:Blood	RECOVERED AS METABOLITES (%)
Halothane	0.75	0.41	—	243	2.3	2.9	51	20
Isoflurane	1.2	0.4	0.24	250	1.4	2.6	45	0.2
Enflurane	1.6	0.4	—	175	1.8	1.4	36	2.4
Sevoflurane	2	0.6	—	160	0.65	1.7	48	3
Desflurane	6	2.4	—	664	0.45	1.3	27	0.02
Nitrous oxide	105	60.0	52.5	Gas	0.47	1.1	2.3	0.004
Xenon	71	32.6	—	Gas	0.12	—	—	0

[a]MAC (minimum alveolar concentration) values are expressed as vol %, the percentage of the atmosphere that is anesthetic. A value of MAC greater than 100% means that hyperbaric conditions would be required.
[b]MAC_{awake} is the concentration at which appropriate responses to commands are lost.
[c]EC_{50} is the concentration that produces memory suppression in 50% of patients. —, Not available.

of MAC. Furthermore, the ratio of the anesthetic concentrations required to produce amnesia and immobility vary significantly among different inhalational anesthetic agents (nitrous oxide versus isoflurane) (Table 19–1), suggesting that anesthetic agents may produce these behavioral end points through different cellular and molecular mechanisms. The potency of intravenous anesthetic agents is somewhat more difficult to measure; we lack methods to measure blood or plasma anesthetic concentration continuously, and we cannot determine the free concentration of the drug at its site of action. Generally, the potency of intravenous agents is defined as the free plasma concentration (at equilibrium) that produces loss of response to surgical incision (or other end points) in 50% of subjects.

Mechanisms of Anesthesia

The molecular and cellular mechanisms by which general anesthetics produce their effects have remained one of the great mysteries of pharmacology. For most of the 20th century, it was theorized that all anesthetics act by a common mechanism (the unitary theory of anesthesia). The leading unitary theory was that anesthesia is produced by perturbation of the physical properties of cell membranes. This thinking was based largely on the observation that the anesthetic potency of a gas correlated with its solubility in olive oil. This correlation, referred to as the Meyer-Overton rule, was interpreted as implicating the lipid bilayer as the likely target of anesthetic action. Clear exceptions to the Meyer-Overton rule have now been noted (Franks, 2006). For example, inhalational and intravenous anesthetics can be enantioselective in their action as anesthetics (etomidate, steroids, isoflurane). The fact that enantiomers with identical physical properties have unique actions indicates that properties other than bulk solubility are important in determining anesthetic action. Consequently, the lipid theory of anesthesia has largely been discarded (Franks, 2006). This realization has focused thinking on identification of specific protein binding sites for anesthetics.

A substantial body of work indicates that an anesthetic agent produces different components of the anesthetic state by means of actions at different anatomic loci in the nervous system and may produce these component effects through different cellular and molecular actions. Moreover, increasing evidence supports the hypothesis that different anesthetic agents produce specific components of anesthesia by actions at different molecular targets. Given these insights, the unitary theory of anesthesia has been largely discarded.

Cellular Mechanisms of Anesthesia. General anesthetics produce two important physiologic effects at the cellular level.

First, the inhalational anesthetics can hyperpolarize neurons. This may be an important effect on neurons serving a pacemaker role and on pattern-generating circuits. It also may be important in synaptic communication, since reduced excitability in a postsynaptic neuron may diminish the likelihood that an action potential will be initiated in response to neurotransmitter release.

Second, at anesthetizing concentrations, both inhalational and intravenous anesthetics have substantial effects on synaptic transmission and much smaller effects on action-potential generation or propagation.

The inhalational anesthetics inhibit excitatory synapses and enhance inhibitory synapses in various preparations. These effects likely are produced by both pre- and postsynaptic actions of the inhalational anesthetics. The inhalational anesthetic isoflurane clearly can inhibit neurotransmitter release, while the small reduction in presynaptic action potential amplitude produced by isoflurane (3% reduction at MAC concentration) substantially inhibits neurotransmitter release (Wu et al., 2004b). The latter effect occurs because the reduction in the presynaptic action potential is amplified into a much larger reduction in presynaptic Ca^{2+} influx, which in turn is amplified into an even greater reduction in transmitter release. This effect may account for the majority of the reduction in transmitter release by inhalational anesthetics at some excitatory synapses. Inhalational anesthetics also can act postsynaptically, altering the response to released neurotransmitter. These actions are thought to be due to specific interactions of anesthetic agents with neurotransmitter receptors.

The intravenous anesthetics produce a narrower range of physiological effects. Their predominant actions are at the synapse, where they have profound and relatively specific effects on the postsynaptic response to released neurotransmitter. Most of the intravenous agents act predominantly by enhancing inhibitory neurotransmission, whereas ketamine predominantly inhibits excitatory neurotransmission at glutamatergic synapses.

Molecular Actions of General Anesthetics. A variety of ligand-gated ion channels, receptors and signal transduction proteins are modulated by general anesthetics. Of these, the strongest evidence for a direct effect of anesthetics exists for the $GABA_A$ and NMDA receptors and the two-pore K^+ channels, as described later in this section.

Chloride channels gated by the inhibitory $GABA_A$ receptors (Chapters 14 and 17) are sensitive to clinical concentrations of a wide variety of anesthetics, including the halogenated inhalational agents and many intravenous agents (propofol, barbiturates, etomidate, and neurosteroids). At clinical concentrations, general anesthetics increase the sensitivity of the $GABA_A$ receptor to GABA, thus enhancing inhibitory neurotransmission and depressing nervous system activity. The action of anesthetics on the $GABA_A$ receptor probably is mediated by binding of the anesthetics to specific sites on the $GABA_A$-receptor protein, since point mutations of the receptor can eliminate the effects of the anesthetic on ion channel function (Rudolph and Antkowiak, 2004). Judging from the capacity of mutations in various regions (and subunits) of the $GABA_A$ receptor to selectively affect the actions of various anesthetics, there likely are specific binding sites for at least several classes of anesthetics (Belelli et al., 1997). Notably, none of the general anesthetics competes with GABA for its binding site on the receptor. The capacity of propofol and etomidate to inhibit the response to noxious stimuli is mediated by a specific site on the β_3 subunit of the $GABA_A$ receptor, whereas the sedative effects of these anesthetics are mediated by the same site on the β_2 subunit (Reynolds et al., 2003). These results indicate that two components of anesthesia *can* be mediated by $GABA_A$ receptors. For anesthetics other than propofol and etomidate, which components of anesthesia *are* produced by actions on $GABA_A$ receptors remains a matter of conjecture.

Structurally related to the $GABA_A$ receptors are other ligand-gated ion channels including glycine receptors and neuronal nicotinic acetylcholine receptors. Glycine receptors may play a role in mediating inhibition by anesthetics of responses to noxious stimuli. Clinical concentrations of inhalational anesthetics enhance the capacity of glycine to activate glycine-gated chloride channels (glycine receptors), which play an important role in inhibitory neurotransmission in the spinal cord and brainstem. Propofol, neurosteroids, and barbiturates also potentiate glycine-activated currents, whereas etomidate and ketamine do not. Subanesthetic concentrations of the inhalational anesthetics inhibit some classes of neuronal nicotinic acetylcholine receptors (Violet et al., 1997). However, these actions do not appear to mediate anesthetic immobilization (Eger et al., 2002); rather, neuronal nicotinic receptors could mediate other components of anesthesia such as analgesia or amnesia.

The only general anesthetics that do not have significant effects on $GABA_A$ or glycine receptors are ketamine, nitrous oxide, cyclopropane, and xenon. These agents inhibit a different type of ligand-gated ion channel, the *N*-methyl-D-aspartate (NMDA) receptor (Chapter 14). NMDA receptors are glutamate-gated cation channels that are somewhat selective for calcium and are involved in long-term modulation of synaptic responses (long-term potentiation) and glutamate-mediated neurotoxicity. Ketamine inhibits NMDA receptors by binding to the phencyclidine site on the NMDA-receptor protein, and the NMDA receptor is thought to be the principal molecular target for ketamine's anesthetic actions. Nitrous oxide (Jevtovic-Todorovic et al., 1998), cyclopropane (Raines et al., 2001), and xenon (de Sousa et al., 2000) are potent and selective inhibitors of NMDA-activated currents, suggesting that these agents also may produce unconsciousness by means of actions on NMDA receptors.

Inhalational anesthetics have two other known molecular targets that may mediate some of their actions. Halogenated inhalational anesthetics activate some members of a class of K^+ channels known as two-pore domain channels (Patel et al., 1999); other two-pore domain channel family members are activated by xenon, nitrous oxide, and cyclopropane (Franks, 2006). These channels are located in both pre-synaptic and post-synaptic sites. The post-synaptic channels are important in setting the resting membrane potential of neurons and may be the molecular locus through which these agents hyperpolarize neurons. Activation of pre-synaptic channels can lead to hyperpolarization of the pre-synaptic terminal, thereby reducing neurotransmitter release. Modulation of neurotransmitter release can also be modulated by interaction of anesthetics with the molecular machinery involved in neurotransmitter release. The action of inhalational anesthetics requires a protein complex (syntaxin, SNAP-25, synaptobrevin) involved in synaptic neurotransmitter release (van Swinderen et al., 1999). These molecular interactions may explain, in part, the capacity of inhalational anesthetics to cause presynaptic inhibition in the hippocampus and could contribute to the amnesic effect of inhalational anesthetics.

Anatomic Sites of Anesthetic Action. In principle, general anesthetics could interrupt nervous system function at myriad levels, including peripheral sensory neurons, the spinal cord, the brainstem, and the cerebral cortex. Delineation of the precise anatomic sites of action is difficult because many anesthetics diffusely inhibit electrical activity in the CNS. For example, isoflurane at 2 MAC can cause electrical silence in the brain. However, *in vitro* studies show that specific cortical pathways exhibit markedly different sensitivities to both inhalational and intravenous anesthetics (MacIver and Roth, 1988), suggesting that anesthetics produce specific components of the anesthetic state through actions at specific sites in the CNS. Consistent with this possibility, inhalational anesthetics produce immobilization in response to a surgical incision (the end point used in determining MAC) by action on the spinal cord (Rampil, 1994). Given that amnesia or unconsciousness cannot result from anesthetic actions in the spinal cord, one concludes that different components of anesthesia are produced at different sites in the CNS. Indeed, recent studies show that the sedative effects of pentobarbital and propofol (GABA-ergic anesthetics) are mediated by $GABA_A$ receptors in the tuberomammillary nucleus (Nelson et al., 2002), and the sedative effects of the intravenous anesthetic dexmedetomidine (an α_2 adrenergic receptor agonist) are produced by actions in the locus ceruleus (Mizobe et al., 1996). These findings suggest that the sedative actions of some anesthetics share the neuronal pathways involved in endogenous sleep.

Functional imaging studies of the awake and anesthetized brain have revealed that most anesthetics cause, with some exceptions, a global reduction in cerebral metabolic rate (CMR) and in cerebral blood flow (CBF); agent-specific effects on CMR and CBF will be described later in the chapter. A consistent feature of general anesthesia is a suppression of metabolism in the thalamus (Alkire et al., 2008). This is not surprising given the demonstration that inhalational anesthetics depress the excitability of thalamic neurons. The thalamus serves as a major relay by which sensory input from the periphery ascends to the cortex. Suppression of thalamic activity might isolate the cortex from ascending input. Thus, the thalamus may serve as a switch between the awake and anesthetized states (Franks, 2008). In addition, general anesthesia results in the suppression of activity in specific regions of the cortex, including the mesial parietal cortex, posterior cingulate cortex, precuneus, and inferior parietal cortex. Of interest is the recent observation that electrical activity in the cortex is suppressed before that in the thalamus. This suggests that it is cortical suppression that, via the corticothalamic fibers, leads to thalamic suppression, thereby making the cortex the primary target of anesthetics (Alkire et al., 2008). However, the temporal relationships between thalamus and cortical activity (and deactivation) under general anesthesia need further clarification before the relative importance of each site to anesthetic induced loss of consciousness is known (Franks, 2008).

The similarities between natural sleep and the anesthetized state suggest that anesthetics might also modulate endogenous sleep regulating pathways, which include ventrolateral preoptic (VLPO) and tuberomammillary nuclei. VLPO projects inhibitory GABA-ergic fibers to ascending arousal nuclei, which in turn project to the cortex, forebrain, and subcortical areas; release of histamine, 5-HT, orexin, NE, and ACh mediate wakefulness (Sanders and Maze, 2007). Intravenous and inhalational agents with activity at $GABA_A$ receptors can increase the inhibitory effects of VLPO, thereby suppressing consciousness. Dexmedetomidine, an α_2 agonist, also increases VLPO-mediated inhibition by suppressing the inhibitory effect of locus ceruleus neurons on VLPO (Sanders et al., 2007). Finally, both intravenous and inhalational anesthetics depress hippocampal neurotransmission (Kendig et al., 1991), a probable locus for their amnestic effects.

Summary. Current evidence supports the view that most intravenous general anesthetics act predominantly through $GABA_A$ receptors and perhaps through some interactions with other ligand-gated ion channels such as NMDA receptors and two-pore K^+ channels. The halogenated inhalational agents have a variety of molecular targets, consistent with their status as complete (all components) anesthetics. Nitrous oxide, ketamine, and xenon constitute a third category of general anesthetics that are likely to produce unconsciousness by inhibition of the NMDA receptor and/or activation of two-pore-domain K^+ channels.

PARENTERAL ANESTHETICS

Pharmacokinetic Principles

Parenteral anesthetics are small, hydrophobic, substituted aromatic or heterocyclic compounds (Figure 19–1). Hydrophobicity is the key factor governing their pharmacokinetics. After a single intravenous bolus, these drugs preferentially partition into the highly perfused and lipophilic tissues of the brain and spinal cord where they produce anesthesia within a single circulation

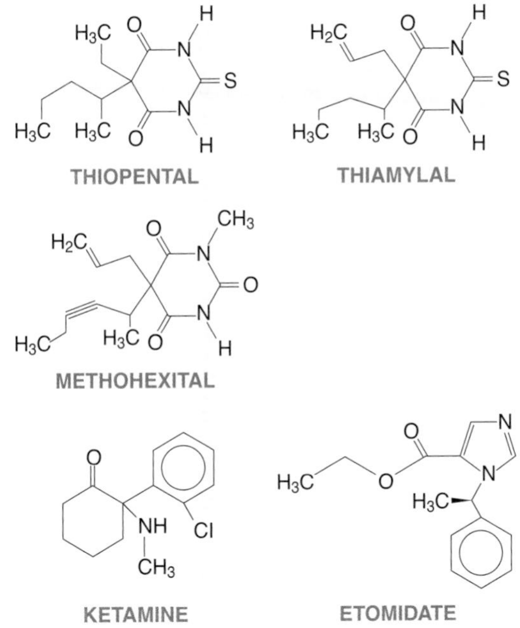

THIOPENTAL THIAMYLAL

METHOHEXITAL

KETAMINE ETOMIDATE

Figure 19–1. *Structures of some parenteral anesthetics.*

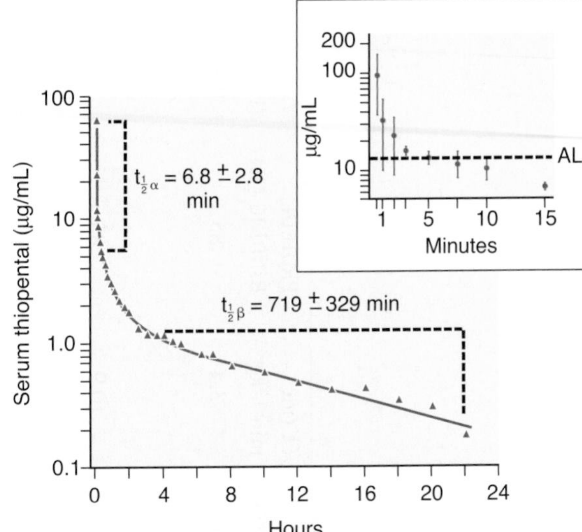

Figure 19–2. *Thiopental serum levels after a single intravenous induction dose.* Thiopental serum levels after a bolus can be described by two time constants, $t_{1/2}\alpha$ and $t_{1/2}\beta$. The initial fall is rapid ($t_{1/2\alpha}$<10 min) and is due to redistribution of drug from the plasma and the highly perfused brain and spinal cord into less well-perfused tissues such as muscle and fat. During this redistribution phase, serum thiopental concentration falls to levels at which patients awaken (AL, awakening level; *see* inset—the average thiopental serum concentration in 12 patients after a 6-mg/kg intravenous bolus of thiopental). Subsequent metabolism and elimination is much slower and is characterized by a half-life ($t_{1/2}$ β) of more than 10 hours. (Adapted with permission from Burch PG, and Stanski DR, The role of metabolism and protein binding in thiopental anesthesia. *Anesthesiology*, **1983**, *58*:146–152. Copyright Lippincott Williams & Wilkins. http://lww.com.)

time. Subsequently blood levels fall rapidly, resulting in drug redistribution out of the CNS back into the blood. The anesthetic then diffuses into less perfused tissues such as muscle and viscera, and at a slower rate into the poorly perfused but very hydrophobic adipose tissue. Termination of anesthesia after single boluses of parenteral anesthetics primarily reflects redistribution out of the CNS rather than metabolism (Figure 19–2). After redistribution, anesthetic blood levels fall according to a complex interaction between the metabolic rate and the amount and lipophilicity of the drug stored in the peripheral compartments. Thus, parenteral anesthetic half-life are "context-sensitive," and the degree to which a $t_{1/2}$ is contextual varies greatly from drug to drug, as might be predicted based on their differing hydrophobicities and metabolic clearances (Table 19–2 and Figure 19–3). For example, after a single bolus of thiopental, patients usually emerge from anesthesia within 10 minutes; however, a patient may require more than a day to awaken from a prolonged thiopental infusion.

Most individual variability in sensitivity to parenteral anesthetics can be accounted for by pharmacokinetic factors. For example, in patients with lower cardiac output, the relative perfusion of the brain and the fraction of anesthetic dose delivered to the brain are higher; thus, patients in septic shock or with cardiomyopathy usually require lower doses of anesthetic. The elderly also typically require a smaller anesthetic dose, primarily because of a smaller initial volume of distribution. As described later in the chapter, similar principles govern the pharmacokinetics of the hydrophobic inhalational anesthetics, with the added complexity of drug uptake by inhalation.

SPECIFIC PARENTERAL AGENTS

Barbiturates

Chemistry and Formulations. Barbiturates are derivatives of barbituric acid (2,4,6-trioxohexahydropyrimidine), with either an oxygen or a sulfur at the 2-position (Figure 19–1). The three barbiturates most commonly used in clinical anesthesia are sodium thiopental, thiamylal, and methohexital. Sodium thiopental (PENTOTHAL, others) has been used most frequently for inducing anesthesia. Thiamylal (SURITAL) is licensed in the U.S. only for veterinary use. Barbiturates are supplied as racemic mixtures despite enantioselectivity in their anesthetic potency. Barbiturates are formulated as the sodium salts with 6% sodium carbonate and

Table 19–2

Pharmacological Properties of Parenteral Anesthetics

DRUG	FORMULATION	IV INDUCTION DOSE (mg/kg)	MINIMAL HYPNOTIC LEVEL (μg/mL)	INDUCTION DOSE DURATION (min)	$t_{1/2}\beta$ (HOURS)	*CL* (mL · min^{-1} · kg^{-1})	PROTEIN BINDING (%)	V_{SS} (L/kg)
Thiopental	25 mg/mL in aqueous solution + 1.5 mg/mL Na_2CO_3; pH = 10–11	3-5	15.6	5-8	12.1	3.4	85	2.3
Methohexital	10 mg/mL in aqueous solution + 1.5 mg/mL Na_2CO_3; pH = 10–11	1-2	10	4-7	3.9	10.9	85	2.2
Propofol	10 mg/mL in 10% soybean oil, 2.25% glycerol, 1.2% egg PL, 0.005% EDTA or 0.025% Na-MBS; pH = 4.5–7	1.5-2.5	1.1	4-8	1.8	30	98	2.3
Etomidate	2 mg/mL in 35% PG; pH = 6.9	0.2-0.4	0.3	4-8	2.9	17.9	76	2.5
Ketamine	10, 50, or 100 mg/mL in aqueous solution; pH = 3.5–5.5	0.5-1.5	1	10-15	3.0	19.1	27	3.1

$t_{1/2}\beta$, β phase half-life; *CL*, clearance; V_{ss}, volume of distribution at steady state; EDTA, ethylenediaminetetraacetic acid; Na-MBS, Na-metabisulfite; PG, propylene glycol; PL, phospholipid.

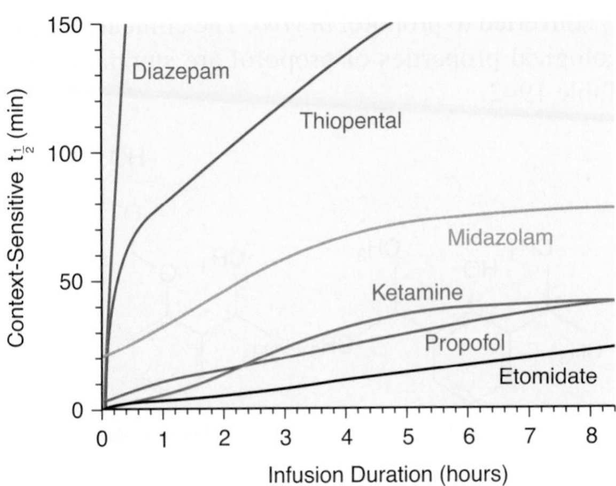

Figure 19–3. *Context-sensitive half-time of general anesthetics.* The duration of action of single intravenous doses of anesthetic/hypnotic drugs is similarly short for all and is determined by redistribution of the drugs away from their active sites (see Figure 19–2). However, after prolonged infusions, drug half-lives and durations of action are dependent on a complex interaction between the rate of redistribution of the drug, the amount of drug accumulated in fat, and the drug's metabolic rate. This phenomenon has been termed the *context-sensitive half-time*; that is, the $t_{1/2}$ of a drug can be estimated only if one knows the context—the total dose and over what time period it has been given. Note that the half-times of some drugs such as etomidate, propofol, and ketamine increase only modestly with prolonged infusions; others (e.g., diazepam and thiopental) increase dramatically. (Reproduced with permission from Reves JG, Glass PSA, Lubarsky DA, et al: Intravenous anesthetics, in Miller RD et al, (eds): *Miller's Anesthesia*, 7th ed. Philadelphia: Churchill Livingstone, 2010, p 718. Copyright © Elsevier.)

reconstituted in water or isotonic saline to produce 2.5% (thiopental), 2% (thiamylal), or 1% (methohexital) alkaline solutions ($10 \leq pH \leq 11$). *Mixing barbiturates with drugs in acidic solutions during anesthetic induction can result in precipitation of the barbiturate as the free acid; thus, standard practice is to delay the administration of other drugs until the barbiturate has cleared the intravenous tubing.*

Dosages and Clinical Use. Recommended intravenous dosing for parenteral anesthetics in a healthy young adult is given in Table 19–2.

The typical induction dose (3-4 mg/kg) of thiopental produces unconsciousness in 10-30 seconds with a peak effect in 1 minute and duration of anesthesia of 5-8 minutes. Neonates and infants usually require a higher induction dose (5-8 mg/kg), whereas elderly and pregnant patients require less (1-3 mg/kg) (Gin et al., 1997). Dosage calculation based on lean body mass reduces individual variation in dosage requirements. Doses can be reduced by 10-50% after premedication with benzodiazepines, opiates, or α_2 adrenergic agonists, because of their additive hypnotic effect (Nishina et al., 1994; Short et al., 1991; Wang et al., 1996). Thiamylal is approximately equipotent with and in all aspects similar to thiopental. Methohexital (BREVITAL) is 3-fold more potent but otherwise similar to thiopental in onset and duration of action. Thiopental and thiamylal produce little to no pain on injection; methohexital elicits mild pain. Veno-irritation can be reduced by injection into larger non-hand veins and by prior intravenous injection of lidocaine (0.5-1 mg/ kg). For induction of pediatric patients without IV access, any of the three drugs can be given off-label per rectum at ~ 10-fold the IV dose.

Pharmacokinetics and Metabolism. Pharmacokinetic parameters for parenteral anesthetics are given in Table 19–2. As already discussed, the principal mechanism limiting anesthetic duration after single doses is redistribution of these hydrophobic drugs from the brain to other tissues. However, after multiple doses or infusions, the duration of action of the barbiturates varies considerably depending on their clearances.

Methohexital differs from the other two intravenous barbiturates in its much more rapid clearance; thus, it accumulates less during prolonged infusions. Because of their slow elimination and large volumes of distribution, prolonged infusions or very large doses of thiopental and thiamylal can produce unconsciousness lasting several days. Even single induction doses of thiopental and to a lesser degree methohexital can produce psychomotor impairment lasting up to 8 hours (Beskow et al., 1995). Propofol has largely supplanted methohexital for outpatient procedures that require a rapid return to an alert state (see "Propofol" later in the chapter).

All three barbiturates are primarily eliminated by hepatic metabolism and renal excretion of inactive metabolites; a small fraction of thiopental undergoes desulfuration to the longer-acting hypnotic pentobarbital. In patients with cirrhosis, a larger volume of distribution combined with a reduction in clearance can result in prolongation of the clinical action of barbiturates. These drugs are highly protein bound (Table 19–2). Hepatic disease or other conditions that reduce serum protein concentration will increase the initial free concentration and hypnotic effect of an induction dose; this is noted in patients with advanced cirrhosis in whom the protein synthesis capacity of the liver is greatly compromised.

Side Effects

Nervous System. Barbiturates suppress the EEG and can produce burst suppression of the EEG. They reduce the cerebral metabolic rate, as measured by cerebral O_2 consumption ($CMRO_2$), in a dose-dependent manner. Induction doses of thiopental reduce $CMRO_2$ by 25-30%, with a maximal decrease of 55% occurring at two to five times that dose (Stullken et al., 1977). As a consequence of the decrease in $CMRO_2$, cerebral blood flow and intracranial pressure are similarly reduced.

Because it markedly lowers cerebral metabolism, thiopental has been used as a protectant against cerebral ischemia; however, the large doses required and the subsequent prolonged sedation have precluded its use clinically for this purpose. Thiopental also reduces intraocular pressure. Presumably in part due to their CNS depressant activity, barbiturates are effective anticonvulsants. Thiopental in particular is a proven medication in the treatment of status epilepticus. Methohexital can increase ictal activity, and seizures have been described in patients who received doses sufficient to produce burst suppression of the EEG (Todd et al., 1984). This property makes methohexital a good choice for anesthesia in patients who undergo electroconvulsive therapy.

Cardiovascular System. The anesthetic barbiturates produce dose-dependent decreases in blood pressure. The effect is due primarily to vasodilation, particularly venodilation, and to a lesser degree to a direct decrease in cardiac contractility. Typically, heart rate increases as a compensatory response to a lower blood pressure, although barbiturates also blunt the baroreceptor reflex. Thiopental maintains the ratio of myocardial O_2 supply to demand in patients with coronary artery disease within a normal blood pressure range.

Hypotension can be severe in patients with an impaired ability to compensate for venodilation such as those with hypovolemia, cardiomyopathy, valvular heart disease, coronary artery disease, cardiac tamponade, or β adrenergic blockade. None of the barbiturates has been shown to be arrhythmogenic.

Respiratory System. Barbiturates are respiratory depressants. Induction doses of thiopental decrease minute ventilation and tidal volume, with a smaller and inconsistent decrease in respiratory rate (Grounds et al., 1987). Reflex responses to hypercarbia and hypoxia are diminished by anesthetic barbiturates (Hirshman et al., 1975); and at higher doses or in the presence of other respiratory depressants such as opiates, apnea can result. With the exception of uncommon anaphylactoid reactions, these drugs have little effect on bronchomotor tone (Kingston and Hirshman, 1984). Compared to propofol, barbiturates produce a higher incidence of wheezing in asthmatics, attributed to histamine release from mast cells, during induction of anesthesia (Pizov et al., 1995).

Other Side Effects. Short-term administration of barbiturates has no clinically significant effect on the hepatic, renal, or endocrine systems. A single induction dose of thiopental does not alter tone of the gravid uterus, but may produce mild transient depression of newborn activity. True allergies to barbiturates are rare; however, direct drug-induced histamine release is occasionally seen (Sprung et al., 1997).

Barbiturates can induce fatal attacks of porphyria in patients with acute intermittent or variegate porphyria and are contraindicated in such patients. The abnormal synthesis of protoporphyrin (important in hemoglobin production) results in excess porphobilinogen. Barbiturates induce aminolevulinic acid synthase, an enzyme responsible for phophobilinogen synthesis. This leads to excessive porphobilinogen levels and can precipitate acute porphyric crises that are manifested by severe abdominal pain, nausea, vomiting, psychiatric disorders, and neurologic abnormalities.

Methohexital can produce pain on injection to a greater degree than thiopental. Inadvertent intra-arterial injection of thiobarbiturates can induce a severe inflammatory and potentially necrotic reaction that can threaten limb survival. Methohexital and to a lesser degree other barbiturates can produce excitatory symptoms on induction such as cough, hiccup, muscle tremors, twitching, and hypertonus.

Unlike inhalational anesthetics and succinylcholine, barbiturates and all other parenteral anesthetics apparently do not trigger malignant hyperthermia (Rosenberg et al., 1997).

Propofol

Propofol is the most commonly used parenteral anesthetic in the U.S. Fospropofol is a prodrug form that is converted to propofol *in vivo*. The clinical pharmacological properties of propofol are summarized in Table 19–2.

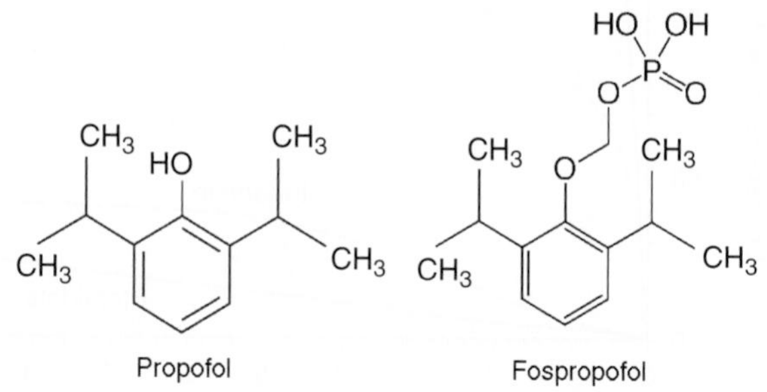

Propofol

Fospropofol

Chemistry and Formulations. The active ingredient in propofol, 2,6-diisopropylphenol, is an oil at room temperature and insoluble in aqueous solutions. Propofol is formulated for IV administration as a 1% (10 mg/mL) emulsion in 10% soybean oil, 2.25% glycerol, and 1.2% purified egg phosphatide. In the U.S., disodium EDTA (0.05 mg/mL) or sodium metabisulfite (0.25 mg/mL) is added to inhibit bacterial growth. Nevertheless, significant bacterial contamination of open containers has been associated with serious patient infections; propofol should be administered within 4 hours of its removal from sterile packaging; unused drug should be discarded.

The lipid emulsion formulation of propofol is associated with significant pain on injection and hyperlipidemia. A new aqueous formulation of propofol, fospropofol, which is not associated with these adverse effects, has recently been approved for use for sedation in patients undergoing diagnostic procedures. Fospropofol, which itself is inactive, is a phosphate ester prodrug of propofol that is hydrolyzed by endothelial alkaline phosphatases to yield propofol, phosphate, and formaldehyde. The formaldehyde is rapidly converted to formic acid, which then is metabolized by tetrahydrofolate dehydrogenase to CO_2 and water (Fechner et al., 2008).

Dosage and Clinical Use. The induction dose of propofol (DIPRIVAN, others) in a healthy adult is 2-2.5 mg/kg and it has an onset and duration of anesthesia similar to thiopental (Table 19–2). As with barbiturates, dosages should be reduced in the elderly and in the presence of other sedatives and increased in young children. Because of its reasonably short elimination $t_{1/2}$, propofol often is used for maintenance of anesthesia as well as for induction. For short procedures, small boluses (10-50% of the induction dose) every 5 minutes or as needed are effective. An infusion of propofol produces a more stable drug level (100-300 μg/kg per minute) and is better suited for longer-term anesthetic maintenance. Infusion rates should be tailored to patient response and the levels of other hypnotics. Sedating doses of propofol are 20-50% of those required for general anesthesia. However, even at these lower doses, caregivers should be vigilant and prepared for all of the side effects of propofol discussed below, particularly airway obstruction and apnea.

Fospropofol produces dose-dependent sedation and can be administered in otherwise healthy individuals at 2-8 mg/kg intravenously (delivered either as a bolus or by a short infusion over 5-10 min). The optimum dose for sedation is ~6.5 mg/kg. This results in a loss of consciousness in ~10 minutes. The duration of the sedative effect is ~45 min.

Pharmacokinetics and Metabolism. The pharmacokinetics of propofol are governed by the same principles that apply to barbiturates. Onset and duration of anesthesia after a single bolus are similar to thiopental. Recovery after multiple doses or continuous infusion has been shown to be much faster after propofol than after thiopental or even methohexital. Propofol has a context-sensitive $t_{1/2}$ of ~10 min with an infusion lasting 3 hours and ~40 minutes for infusions lasting up to 8 hours (Figure 19–3). Propofol's shorter duration of action after infusion can be explained by its very high clearance, coupled with the slow diffusion of drug from the peripheral to the central compartment (Figure 19–3). The rapid clearance of propofol explains the more rapid emergence from anesthesia in comparison to barbiturates; this facilitates a more rapid discharge from the recovery room.

Propofol is metabolized in the liver by conjugation to sulfate and glucunoride to less active metabolites that are renally excreted; however, its clearance exceeds hepatic blood flow, and anhepatic metabolism, particularly in the lungs and kidneys, has been demonstrated (Veroli et al., 1992). In patients with moderate cirrhosis, the volume of distribution of propofol is increased significantly. However, terminal elimination $t_{1/2}$ and emergence from propofol anesthesia is not substantially different from healthy patients (Servin et al., 1990). Propofol is highly protein bound, and its pharmacokinetics, like those of the barbiturates, may be affected by conditions that alter serum protein levels.

Clearance of propofol is reduced in the elderly; given that the central volume of distribution of propofol is also reduced, the required dose of propofol for both induction and maintenance of anesthesia may be decreased. In neonates, propofol clearance is also reduced (Allegaert et al., 2007). Infusion of propofol in neonates therefore has the potential for substantial accumulation and a consequent delay in emergence from anesthesia or sedation. By contrast, in young children, a more rapid clearance in combination with a larger central volume may necessitate larger doses of propofol for induction and maintenance of anesthesia (Kataria et al., 1994).

The $t_{1/2}$ for hydrolysis of fospropofol is 8 min. Fospropofol has a small volume of distribution and a terminal $t_{1/2}$ ~46 min. The currently published pharmacokinetic data on fospropofol were derived using an analytical method that has now been shown to be inaccurate; correct pharmacokinetic data are not yet available (Fechner et al., 2008).

Pharmacology and Side Effects

Nervous System. The sedation and hypnotic actions of propofol are mediated by its action on $GABA_A$ receptors; agonism at these receptors results in an increased chloride conduction and hyperpolarization of neurons. Propofol suppresses the EEG, and in sufficient doses, can produce burst suppression of the EEG. Propofol decreases $CMRO_2$, cerebral blood flow, and intracranial and intraocular pressures by about the same amount as thiopental. Like thiopental, propofol has been used in patients at risk for cerebral ischemia; however, no human outcome studies have been performed to determine its efficacy as a neuroprotectant. Excitatory phenomena, such as choreiform movements and opisthotonus, have been observed after propofol injection with the same frequency as that seen with thiopental but less than with methohexital. These movements, which are transient, are *not* associated with seizure activity. Results from studies on the anticonvulsant effects of propofol have been mixed; some data even suggest it has proconvulsant activity when combined with other drugs. However, propofol has been shown to suppress seizure activity in experimental models and has been used for the treatment of status epilepticus in humans (Parviainen et al., 2007).

Cardiovascular System. Propofol produces a dose-dependent decrease in blood pressure that is significantly greater than that produced by thiopental. The fall in blood pressure can be explained by both vasodilation and possibly mild depression of myocardial contractility. Propofol appears to blunt the baroreceptor reflex and reduce sympathetic nerve activity (Ebert and Muzi, 1994). As with thiopental, propofol should be used with caution in patients at risk for or intolerant of decreases in blood pressure; these include patients with significant blood loss and hypovolemia.

Respiratory System. At equipotent doses, propofol produces a slightly greater degree of respiratory depression than thiopental (Blouin et al., 1991). Patients given propofol should be monitored to ensure adequate oxygenation and ventilation. Propofol appears to be less likely than barbiturates to provoke bronchospasm and may be the induction agent of choice in asthmatics (Pizov et al., 1995). The bronchodilator properties of propofol may be attenuated by the metabisulfite preservative in some propofol formulations (Brown et al., 2001).

Other Side Effects. Propofol has no clinically significant effects on hepatic, renal, or endocrine organ systems. Unlike thiopental, propofol does not have an anti-analgesic effect. It has a significant anti-emetic action. Propofol elicits pain on injection that can be reduced with lidocaine and the use of larger arm and antecubital veins. Propofol provokes anaphylactoid reactions at about the same low frequency as thiopental; the histamine release (in the absence of anaphylactic or anaphylactoid reactions) that occurs with thiopental administration is greater than that with propofol. Although propofol does cross placental membranes, it is considered safe for use in pregnant women; like thiopental, propofol only transiently depresses activity in the newborn (Abboud et al., 1995). Propofol does not trigger malignant hyperthermia.

A rare but potentially fatal complication, termed propofol infusion syndrome (PRIS), has been described primarily in prolonged, higher-dose infusions of propofol in young or head-injured patients. The syndrome is characterized by metabolic acidosis, hyperlipidemia, rhabdomyolysis, and an enlarged liver. While the precise mechanisms by which PRIS occurs are not clear, alterations in mitochondrial metabolism and electron transport chain function have been described (Kam and Cardone, 2007).

The side-effect profile of fospropofol is similar to that of propofol. Fospropofol's slower onset of sedation (due to the need for hydrolysis of the prodrug) results in a lower incidence of hypotension, respiratory depression, apnea, and loss of airway patency. Nonetheless, unintended deep levels of sedation can occur with fospropofol, and the drug should therefore be used only by individuals who can maintain an adequate airway and support cardiorespiratory function.

Whether fospropofol can also cause PRIS is not currently known (Fechner et al., 2008). A metabolic byproduct of fospropofol is formic acid. This is degraded to CO_2 and water by tetrahydrofolate dehydrogenase, an enzyme that requires folate as a co-factor. In patients who have a folate deficiency, there is a theoretical risk of formic acid accumulation; to date, such an adverse event has not been reported.

Etomidate

Etomidate is a substituted imidazole that is supplied as the active d-isomer (Figure 19–1). Etomidate is poorly soluble in water and is formulated as a 2 mg/mL solution in 35% propylene glycol. An aqueous solution of etomidate using sulfobutyl ether-7β-cyclodextrin as a solubilizing agent has been developed; this formulation is not currently available for clinical use in the U.S.. Unlike thiopental, etomidate does not induce precipitation of neuromuscular blockers or other drugs frequently given during anesthetic induction. Etomidate's clinical pharmacological properties are listed in Table 19–2.

Dosage and Clinical Use. Etomidate (AMIDATE, others) is primarily used for anesthetic induction of patients at risk for hypotension.

Induction doses of etomidate (0.2-0.6 mg/kg) have a rapid onset and short duration of action (Table 19–2) and are accompanied by a high incidence of pain on injection and myoclonic movements. Lidocaine effectively reduces the pain of injection, while myoclonic movements can be reduced by premedication with either benzodiazepines or opiates. These myoclonic movements, which are similar to seizures, are not associated with convulsive activity on the EEG. Etomidate is pharmacokinetically suitable for off-label infusion for anesthetic maintenance (10 μg/kg per minute) or sedation (5 μg/kg per minute); however, long-term infusions are not recommended (see below, under "Respiratory and Other Side Effects"). Etomidate also may be given rectally (6.5 mg/kg) with an onset of ~5 minutes.

Pharmacokinetics and Metabolism. An induction dose of etomidate has a rapid onset; redistribution limits the duration of action (Table 19–2). Metabolism occurs in the liver, primarily to inactive compounds. Elimination is both renal (78%) and biliary (22%). Compared to thiopental, the duration of action of etomidate increases less with repeated doses (Figure 19–3). The plasma protein binding of etomidate is high but less than that of barbiturates and propofol (Table 19–2).

Side Effects

Nervous System. Etomidate produces hypnosis and has no analgesic effects. The effects of etomidate on cerebral blood flow, metabolism, and intracranial and intraocular pressures are similar to those of thiopental (without dropping mean arterial blood pressure) (Modica and Tempelhoff, 1992). Etomidate has been used as a protectant against cerebral ischemia; however, animal studies have failed to show a consistent beneficial effect (Drummond et al., 1995), and no controlled human trials have been performed. Etomidate produces increased EEG activity in epileptogenic foci and has been associated with seizures (Ebrahim et al., 1986).

Cardiovascular System. Cardiovascular stability after induction is a major advantage of etomidate over either barbiturates or propofol. Induction doses of etomidate typically produce a small increase in heart rate and little or no decrease in blood pressure or cardiac output Etomidate has little effect on coronary perfusion pressure while reducing myocardial O_2 consumption (Kettler et al., 1974). Thus, of all induction agents, etomidate is best suited to maintain cardiovascular stability in patients with coronary artery disease, cardiomyopathy, cerebral vascular disease, or hypovolemia.

Respiratory and Other Side Effects. The degree of respiratory depression due to etomidate appears to be less than that due to thiopental. Like methohexital, etomidate may induce hiccups but does not significantly stimulate histamine release. Despite minimal cardiac and respiratory effects, etomidate does have two major drawbacks. Etomidate has been associated with nausea and vomiting. The drug also inhibits adrenal biosynthetic enzymes required for the production of cortisol and some other steroids. Single induction doses of etomidate may mildly and transiently reduce cortisol levels but no significant differences in outcome after short-term administration have been found, even for variables specifically known to be associated with adrenocortical suppression (Wagner et al., 1984). Thus, while etomidate is not recommended for long-term infusion, it appears safe for anesthetic induction and has some unique advantages in patients prone to hemodynamic instability. A rapidly metabolized and ultra-short-acting analog, methoxycarbonyl-etomidate, has been developed that retains the favorable pharmacological properties of etomidate but does not produce adrenocortical suppression after bolus dosing (Cotton and Claing, 2009).

Ketamine

Ketamine is an arylcyclohexylamine, a congener of phencyclidine (Figure 19–1). Clinical pharmacokinetic data for ketamine appear in Table 19–2.

Ketamine is supplied as a mixture of the R+ and S- isomers even though the S- isomer is more potent with fewer side effects. Although more lipophilic than thiopental, ketamine is water soluble and available as 10-, 50-, and 100-mg/mL solutions in sodium chloride plus the preservative benzethonium chloride.

Dosage and Clinical Use. Ketamine (KETALAR, others) has unique properties that make it useful for anesthetizing patients at risk for hypotension and bronchospasm and for certain pediatric procedures. However, significant side effects limit its routine use. Ketamine rapidly produces a hypnotic state quite distinct from that of other anesthetics. Patients have profound analgesia, unresponsiveness to commands, and amnesia, but may have their eyes open, move their limbs involuntarily, and breathe spontaneously. This cataleptic state has been termed *dissociative anesthesia*. The administration of ketamine has been shown to reduce the development of tolerance to long-term opioid use. Low-dose ketamine infusion for this purpose has been advocated in patients who have developed significant tolerance to opioids (Himmelseher and Durieux, 2005).

Ketamine typically is administered intravenously but also is effective by intramuscular, oral, and rectal routes. The induction doses are 0.5-1.5 mg/kg IV, 4-6 mg/kg IM, and 8-10 mg/kg PR. Onset of action after an intravenous dose is similar to that of the other parenteral anesthetics, but the duration of anesthesia of a single dose is longer (Table 19–2). For anesthetic maintenance, ketamine occasionally is continued as an infusion (25-100 μg/kg per minute). Ketamine does not elicit pain on injection or true excitatory behavior as described for methohexital, although involuntary movements produced by ketamine can be mistaken for anesthetic excitement.

Pharmacokinetics and Metabolism. The onset and duration of an induction dose of ketamine are determined by the same distribution/redistribution mechanisms operant for all the other parenteral anesthetics.

Ketamine is hepatically metabolized to norketamine, which has reduced CNS activity; norketamine is further metabolized and excreted in urine and bile. Ketamine has a large volume of distribution and rapid clearance that make it suitable for continuous infusion without the lengthening in duration of action seen with thiopental (Table 19–2 and Figure 19–3). Protein binding is much lower with ketamine than with the other parenteral anesthetics (Table 19–2).

Side Effects

Nervous System. Ketamine has indirect sympathomimetic activity and can support blood pressure on anesthetic induction in patients who are at risk of developing significant hypotension. Ketamine's behavioral effects are distinct from those of other anesthetics. The ketamine-induced cataleptic state is accompanied by nystagmus with pupillary dilation, salivation, lacrimation, and spontaneous limb movements with increased overall muscle tone. Although ketamine does not produce the classic anesthetic state, patients are amnestic and unresponsive to painful stimuli. Ketamine produces profound analgesia, a distinct advantage over other parenteral anesthetics.

Unlike other parenteral anesthetics, ketamine increases cerebral blood flow and intracranial pressure (ICP) with minimal alteration of cerebral metabolism. The racemic mixture of ketamine can increase cerebral metabolic rate (CMR) and cerebral blood flow (CBF), particularly in the anterior cingulate and frontal cortex, thalamus, and putamen (Langsjo et al., 2004). S ketamine produces similar changes in CBF and CMR whereas R+ ketamine reduces both CMR and CBF (Vollenweider et al., 1997). These properties of ketamine have raised a concern that ICP can increase in patients with compromised intracranial compliance. However, ketamine does not increase ICP in patients with intracranial hypertension (Bourgoin et al., 2005). Moreover, the effects of ketamine on CBF can be readily attenuated by the simultaneous administration of sedative hyponotics (propofol, midazolam, barbiturates). In aggregate, the available data suggest that the contraindication of ketamine in patients with intracranial pathology or cerebral ischemia needs re-evaluation (Himmelseher et al., 2005).

In some studies, ketamine increased intraocular pressure, and its use for induction of patients with open eye injuries is controversial (Whitacre and Ellis, 1984). The effects of ketamine on seizure activity appear mixed, without either strong pro- or anticonvulsant activity. Emergence delirium, characterized by hallucinations, vivid dreams, and delusions, is a frequent complication of ketamine that can result in serious patient dissatisfaction and can complicate postoperative management. Delirium symptoms are most frequent in the first hour after emergence and appear to occur less frequently in children. Benzodiazepines reduce the incidence of emergence delirium (Dundee and Lilburn, 1978).

Cardiovascular System. Unlike other anesthetics, induction doses of ketamine typically increase blood pressure, heart rate, and cardiac output. The cardiovascular effects are indirect and are most likely mediated by inhibition of both central and peripheral catecholamine reuptake. Ketamine has direct negative inotropic and vasodilating activity, but these effects usually are overwhelmed by the indirect sympathomimetic action (Pagel et al., 1992). Thus, ketamine is a useful drug, along with etomidate, for patients at risk for hypotension during anesthesia. While not arrhythmogenic, ketamine increases myocardial O_2 consumption and is not an ideal drug for patients at risk for myocardial ischemia.

Respiratory System. The respiratory effects of ketamine are perhaps the best indication for its use. Induction doses of ketamine produce small and transient decreases in minute ventilation, but respiratory depression is less severe than with other general anesthetics. Ketamine is a potent bronchodilator due to its indirect sympathomimetic activity and perhaps some direct bronchodilating activity. Thus, ketamine is particularly well-suited for anesthetizing patients at high risk for bronchospasm. Increased salivation that attends ketamine administration can be effectively prevented by anticholinergic agents such as glycopyrrolate.

Summary of Parenteral Anesthetics

Parenteral anesthetics are the most common drugs used for anesthetic induction of adults. Their lipophilicity, coupled with the relatively high perfusion of the brain and spinal cord, results in rapid onset and short duration after a single bolus dose. However, these drugs ultimately accumulate in fatty tissue, prolonging recovery if multiple doses are given, particularly for drugs with lower rates of clearance. Each anesthetic has its own unique set of properties and side effects (Table 19–3). Propofol and thiopental are the two most commonly used parenteral agents. Propofol is advantageous for procedures where rapid return to a preoperative mental status is desirable. Thiopental has a long-established track record of safety. Etomidate usually is reserved for patients at risk for hypotension and/or myocardial ischemia. Ketamine is best suited for patients with asthma or for children undergoing short, painful procedures.

INHALATIONAL ANESTHETICS

Introduction

A wide variety of gases and volatile liquids can produce anesthesia. The structures of the currently used inhalational anesthetics are shown in Figure 19–4. One of the troublesome properties of the inhalational anesthetics is their low safety margin. The inhalational anesthetics have therapeutic indices (LD_{50}/ED_{50}) that range from 2 to 4, making these among the most dangerous drugs in clinical use.

The toxicity of these drugs is largely a function of their side effects, and each of the inhalational anesthetics has a unique side-effect profile. Hence, the selection of an inhalational anesthetic often is based on matching a patient's pathophysiology with drug side-effect profiles. The specific adverse effects of each of

Table 19–3

Some Pharmacological Effects of Parenteral Anesthetics[a]

DRUG	CBF	CMR_{O_2}	ICP	MAP	HR	CO	RR	$\dot{V}_E$
Thiopental	---	---	---	-	+	-	-	--
Etomidate	---	---	---	0	0	0	-	-
Ketamine	++	0	++	+	++	+	0	0
Propofol	---	---	---	--	+	-	--	---

ABBREVIATIONS: CBF, cerebral blood flow; CMR_{O_2}, cerebral oxygen consumption; ICP, intracranial pressure; MAP, mean arterial pressure; HR, heart rate; CO, cardiac output; RR, respiratory rate; V_E, minute ventilation.

[a]Typical effects of a single induction dose in humans; *see* text for references. Qualitative scale from --- to +++ = slight, moderate, or large decrease or increase, respectively; 0 indicates no significant change.

the inhalational anesthetics are emphasized in the following sections.

Table 19–1 lists the widely varying physical properties of the inhalational agents in clinical use. These properties are important because they govern the pharmacokinetics of the inhalational agents. Ideally, an inhalational agent would produce a rapid induction of anesthesia and a rapid recovery following discontinuation.

Pharmacokinetic Principles

The inhalational agents are some of the very few pharmacological agents administered as gases. The fact that these agents behave as gases rather than as liquids requires that different pharmacokinetic constructs be used in analyzing their uptake and distribution.

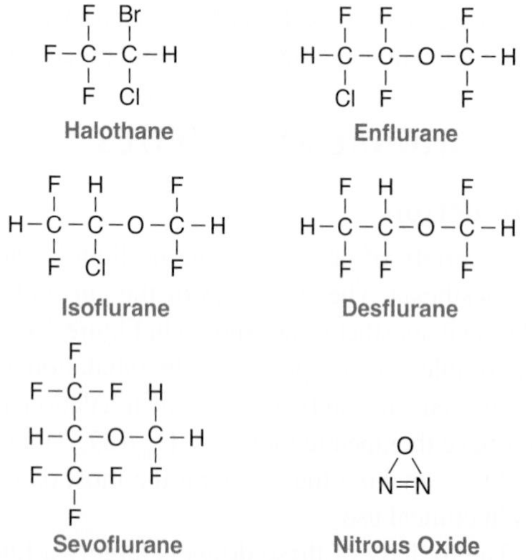

It is essential to understand that inhalational anesthetics distribute between tissues (or between blood and gas) such that equilibrium is achieved when the partial pressure of anesthetic gas is equal in the two tissues. When a person has breathed an inhalational anesthetic for a sufficiently long time that all tissues are equilibrated with the anesthetic, the partial pressure of the anesthetic in all tissues will be equal to the partial pressure of the anesthetic in inspired gas. Note, however, that while the partial pressure of the anesthetic may be equal in all tissues, the concentration of anesthetic in each tissue will be different. Indeed, anesthetic partition coefficients are defined as the ratio of anesthetic concentration in two tissues when the partial pressures of anesthetic are equal in the two tissues. Blood:gas, brain:blood, and fat:blood partition coefficients for the various inhalational agents are listed in Table 19–1. These partition coefficients show that inhalational anesthetics are more soluble in some tissues (e.g., fat) than they are in others (e.g., blood), and that there is significant range in the solubility of the various inhalational agents in such tissues.

In clinical practice, one can monitor the equilibration of a patient with anesthetic gas. Equilibrium is achieved when the partial pressure in inspired gas is equal to the partial pressure in end-tidal (alveolar) gas. In other words, equilibrium is the point at which there is no *net* uptake of anesthetic from the alveoli into the blood. For inhalational agents that are not very soluble in blood or any other tissue, equilibrium is achieved quickly, as illustrated for nitrous oxide in Figure 19–5. If an agent is more soluble in a tissue such as fat, equilibrium may take many hours to reach. This occurs

```
    F  Br                 F  F     F
    |  |                  |  |     |
 F—C—C—H              H—C—C—O—C—H
    |  |                  |  |     |
    F  Cl                 Cl F     F
  Halothane              Enflurane

    F  H     F            F  H     F
    |  |     |            |  |     |
 H—C—C—O—C—H          H—C—C—O—C—H
    |  |     |            |  |     |
    F  Cl    F            F  F     F
  Isoflurane             Desflurane

      F
      |
   F—C—F  H
      |     |
   H—C—O—C—H                O
      |     |               / \
   F—C—F  F                N=N
      |
      F
  Sevoflurane            Nitrous Oxide
```

Figure 19–4. *Structures of inhalational general anesthetics.* Note that all inhalational general anesthetic agents except nitrous oxide and halothane are ethers, and that fluorine progressively replaces other halogens in the development of the halogenated agents. All structural differences are associated with important differences in pharmacological properties.

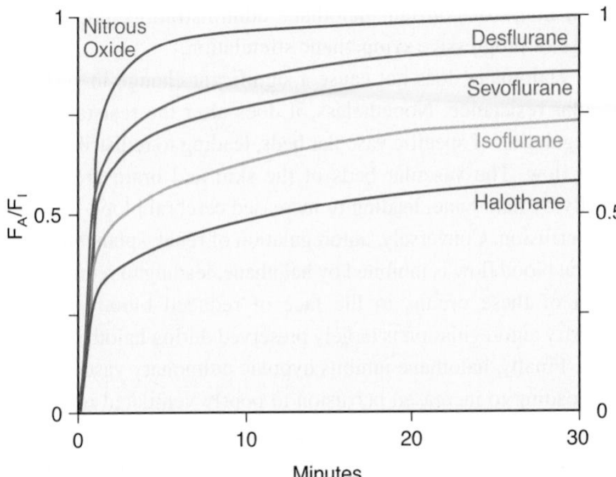

Figure 19–5. *Uptake of inhalational general anesthetics.* The rise in end-tidal alveolar (F_A) anesthetic concentration toward the inspired (F_I) concentration is most rapid with the least soluble anesthetics, nitrous oxide and desflurane, and slowest with the most soluble anesthetic, halothane. All data are from human studies. (Reproduced with permission from Eger EI, II: Inhaled anesthetics: Uptake and distribution, in Miller RD et al, (eds): *Miller's Anesthesia*, 7th ed. Philadelphia: Churchill Livingstone, 2010, p 540. Copyright © Elsevier.)

because fat represents a huge anesthetic reservoir that will be filled only slowly because of the modest blood flow to fat. This is illustrated by the slow approach of halothane alveolar partial pressure to inspired partial pressure of halothane in Figure 19–5.

In considering the pharmacokinetics of anesthetics, one important parameter is the speed of anesthetic induction. Anesthesia is produced when anesthetic partial pressure in brain is equal to or greater than MAC. Because the brain is well perfused, anesthetic partial pressure in brain becomes equal to the partial pressure in alveolar gas (and in blood) over the course of several minutes. Therefore, anesthesia is achieved shortly after alveolar partial pressure reaches MAC. While the rate of rise of alveolar partial pressure will be slower for anesthetics that are highly soluble in blood and other tissues, this limitation on speed of induction can be overcome largely by delivering higher inspired partial pressures of the anesthetic.

Elimination of inhalational anesthetics is largely the reverse process of uptake. For agents with low blood and tissue solubility, recovery from anesthesia should mirror anesthetic induction, regardless of the duration of anesthetic administration. For inhalational agents with high blood and tissue solubility, recovery will be a function of the duration of anesthetic administration. This occurs because the accumulated amounts of anesthetic in the fat reservoir will prevent blood (and therefore alveolar) partial pressures from falling rapidly. Patients will be arousable when alveolar partial pressure reaches MAC_{awake}, a partial pressure somewhat lower than MAC (Table 19–1).

Halothane

Halothane is 2-bromo-2-chloro-1,1,1-trifluoroethane (Figure 19–4). Halothane is a volatile liquid at room temperature and must be stored in a sealed container. Because halothane is a light-sensitive compound that also is subject to spontaneous breakdown, it is marketed in amber bottles with thymol added as a preservative. Mixtures of halothane with O_2 or air are neither flammable nor explosive.

Pharmacokinetics. Halothane has a relatively high blood:gas partition coefficient and high fat:blood partition coefficient (Table 19–1). Induction with halothane therefore is relatively slow, and the alveolar halothane concentration remains substantially lower than the inspired halothane concentration for many hours of administration. Because halothane is soluble in fat and other body tissues, it will accumulate during prolonged administration. Therefore, the speed of recovery from halothane is lengthened as a function of duration of administration.

Approximately 60-80% of halothane taken up by the body is eliminated unchanged by the lungs in the first 24 hours after its administration. A substantial amount of the halothane not eliminated in exhaled gas is biotransformed by hepatic CYPs. The major metabolite of halothane is trifluoroacetic acid, which is formed by removal of bromine and chlorine ions. Trifluoroacetic acid, bromine, and chlorine all can be detected in the urine. Trifluoroacetylchloride, an intermediate in oxidative metabolism of halothane, can trifluoroacetylate several proteins in the liver. An immune reaction to these altered proteins may be responsible for the rare cases of fulminant halothane-induced hepatic necrosis. A minor reductive pathway accounts for ~1% of halothane metabolism that generally is observed only under hypoxic conditions.

Clinical Use. Halothane, introduced in 1956, was the first modern, halogenated inhalational anesthetic used in clinical practice. It is a potent agent that usually is used for maintenance of anesthesia. It is not pungent and is therefore well tolerated for inhalation induction of anesthesia. This is most commonly done in children, in whom preoperative placement of an intravenous catheter can be difficult. Anesthesia is produced by halothane at end-tidal concentrations of 0.7-1%. The use of halothane in the U.S. has diminished substantially in the past decade because of the introduction of newer inhalational agents with better pharmacokinetic and side-effect profiles. Halothane continues to be extensively used in children because it is well tolerated for inhalation induction and because the serious side effects appear to be diminished in children. Halothane has a low cost and therefore is still widely used in developing countries.

Side Effects

Cardiovascular System. The most predictable side effect of halothane is a dose-dependent reduction in arterial blood pressure. Mean arterial pressure typically decreases ~20-25% at MAC concentrations of halothane. This reduction in blood pressure is primarily the result of direct myocardial depression leading to reduced cardiac output (Figure 19–6). Myocardial depression is thought to result from attenuation of depolarization-induced intracellular calcium transients. Halothane-induced hypotension usually is accompanied by either bradycardia or a normal heart rate. Attenuation of baroreceptor reflex function decreases the chronotropic and inotropic responses to a reduction in blood pressure (Constant et al., 2004). Heart rate can be increased during halothane anesthesia by exogenous catecholamine or by sympathoadrenal stimulation. Halothane-induced reductions in blood pressure and heart rate generally disappear after several hours of constant halothane administration, presumably because of progressive sympathetic stimulation.

Halothane does not cause a significant change in systemic vascular resistance. Nonetheless, it does alter the resistance and autoregulation of specific vascular beds, leading to redistribution of blood flow. The vascular beds of the skin and brain are dilated directly by halothane, leading to increased cerebral blood flow and skin perfusion. Conversely, autoregulation of renal, splanchnic, and cerebral blood flow is inhibited by halothane, leading to reduced perfusion of these organs in the face of reduced blood pressure. Coronary autoregulation is largely preserved during halothane anesthesia. Finally, halothane inhibits hypoxic pulmonary vasoconstriction, leading to increased perfusion to poorly ventilated regions of the lung and an increased alveolar:arterial O_2 gradient.

Halothane also has significant effects on cardiac rhythm. Sinus bradycardia and atrioventricular rhythms occur frequently during halothane anesthesia but usually are benign. These rhythms result mainly from a direct depressive effect of halothane on sinoatrial node discharge. Halothane also can sensitize the myocardium to the arrhythmogenic effects of epinephrine (Sumikawa et al., 1983). Premature ventricular contractions and sustained ventricular tachycardia can be observed during halothane anesthesia when exogenous administration or endogenous adrenal production elevates plasma epinephrine levels.

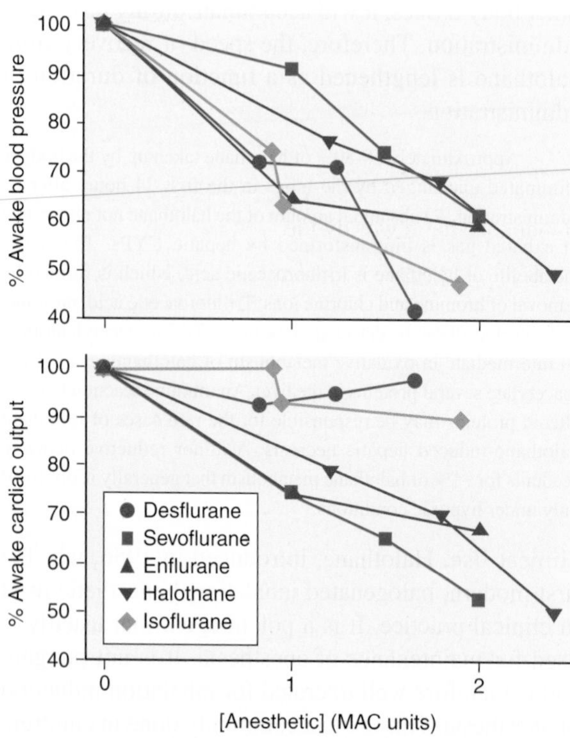

Figure 19–6. ***Influence of inhalational general anesthetics on the systemic circulation.*** While all of the inhalational anesthetics reduce systemic blood pressure in a dose-related manner (*top*), the lower figure shows that cardiac output is well preserved with isoflurane and desflurane, and therefore that the causes of hypotension vary with the agent. (Data from Bahlman et al., 1972; Calverley et al., 1978; Cromwell et al., 1971; Stevens et al., 1971; Weiskopf et al., 1991).

Respiratory System. Spontaneous respiration is rapid and shallow during halothane anesthesia. The decreased alveolar ventilation results in an elevation in arterial CO_2 tension from 40 mm Hg to >50 mm Hg at 1 MAC (Figure 19–7). The elevated CO_2 does not provoke a compensatory increase in ventilation, because halothane causes a concentration-dependent inhibition of the ventilatory response to CO_2. This action of halothane is thought to be mediated by depression of central chemoceptor mechanisms. Halothane also inhibits peripheral chemoceptor responses to arterial hypoxemia. Thus, neither hemodynamic (tachycardia and hypertension) nor ventilatory responses to hypoxemia are observed during halothane anesthesia, making it prudent to monitor arterial O_2 directly. Halothane also is an effective bronchodilator (Yamakage, 1992) and has been effectively used as a treatment of last resort in patients with status asthmaticus (Gold and Helrich, 1970).

Nervous System. Halothane dilates the cerebral vasculature, increasing cerebral blood flow and cerebral blood volume. This can result in an increase in intracranial pressure, especially in patients with space-occupying intracranial masses, brain edema, or preexisting intracranial hypertension. Halothane attenuates autoregulation of cerebral blood flow in a dose-dependent manner. Hence, cerebral blood flow can increase even with a modest reduction in arterial pressure. With a reduction of arterial pressure that is below the lower limit of autoregulation, cerebral blood flow can decrease significantly. Halothane suppresses cerebral metabolism and cerebral metabolic rate is decreased.

Muscle. Halothane causes some relaxation of skeletal muscle by its central depressant effects. Halothane also potentiates the actions of non-depolarizing muscle relaxants (curariform drugs; Chapter 11), increasing both their duration of action and the magnitude of their effect. Halothane and the other halogenated inhalational anesthetics can trigger malignant hyperthermia, a syndrome characterized by

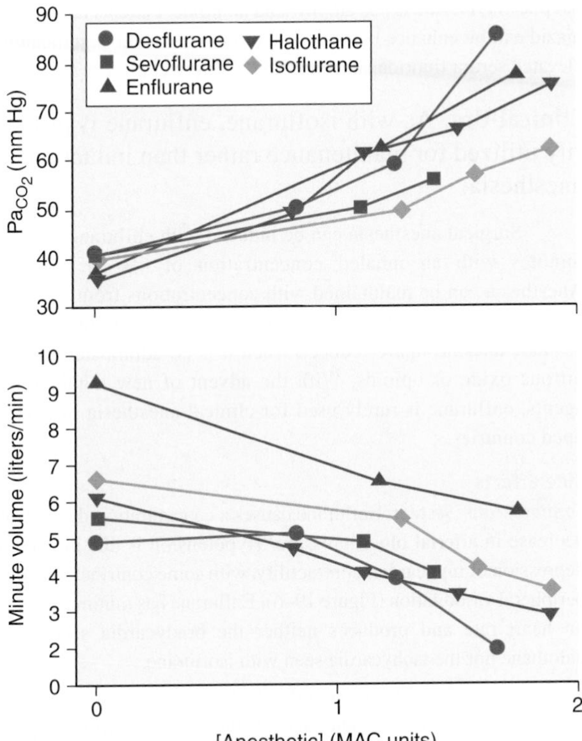

Figure 19–7. *Respiratory effects of inhalational anesthetics.* Spontaneous ventilation with all of the halogenated inhalational anesthetics reduces minute volume of ventilation in a dose-dependent manner (*lower panel*). This results in an increased arterial carbon dioxide tension (*top panel*). Differences among agents are modest. (Data from Calverley et al., 1978; Doi and Ikeda, 1987; Fourcade et al., 1971; Lockhart et al., 1991; Munson et al., 1966.)

severe muscle contraction, rapid development of hyperthermia, and a massive increase in metabolic rate in genetically susceptible patients. This syndrome frequently is fatal and is treated by immediate discontinuation of the anesthetic and administration of dantrolene.

Uterine smooth muscle is relaxed by halothane. This is a useful property for manipulation of the fetus (version) in the prenatal period and for delivery of retained placenta postnatally. However, halothane inhibits uterine contractions during parturition, prolonging labor and increasing blood loss, and therefore is not used as an analgesic or anesthetic for labor and vaginal delivery.

Kidney. Patients anesthetized with halothane usually produce a small volume of concentrated urine. This is the consequence of halothane-induced reduction of renal blood flow and glomerular filtration rate, which may be reduced by 40-50% at 1 MAC. Halothane-induced changes in renal function are fully reversible and are not associated with long-term nephrotoxicity.

Liver and GI Tract. Halothane reduces splanchnic and hepatic blood flow as a consequence of reduced perfusion pressure, as discussed above. This reduced blood flow has not been shown to produce detrimental effects on hepatic or GI function.

Halothane can produce fulminant hepatic necrosis in a small number of patients. This syndrome generally is characterized by fever, anorexia, nausea, and vomiting, developing several days after anesthesia and can be accompanied by a rash and peripheral eosinophilia. There is a rapid progression to hepatic failure, with a fatality rate of ~50%. This syndrome occurs in ~1 in 10,000 patients receiving halothane and is referred to as *halothane hepatitis* (Study, 1966). Current thinking is that halothane hepatitis is the result of an immune response to hepatic proteins that become trifluoroacetylated as a consequence of halothane metabolism (see the "Pharmacokinetics" section for halothane earlier in the chapter).

Isoflurane

Isoflurane (FORANE, others) is 1-chloro-2,2,2-trifluoroethyl difluoromethyl ether (Figure 19–4). It is a volatile liquid at room temperature and is neither flammable nor explosive in mixtures of air or oxygen.

Pharmacokinetics. Isoflurane has a blood:gas partition coefficient substantially lower than that of halothane or enflurane (Table 19–1). Consequently, induction with isoflurane and recovery from isoflurane are faster than with halothane. Changes in anesthetic depth also can be achieved more rapidly with isoflurane than with halothane or enflurane.

More than 99% of inhaled isoflurane is excreted unchanged by the lungs. Approximately 0.2% of absorbed isoflurane is metabolized by CYP2E1. This small amount of isoflurane degradation products produced is insufficient to produce any renal, hepatic, or other organ toxicity. Isoflurane does not appear to be a mutagen, teratogen, or carcinogen.

Clinical Use. Isoflurane is a commonly used inhalational anesthetic worldwide.

It is typically used for maintenance of anesthesia *after induction* with other agents because of its pungent odor, but induction of anesthesia can be achieved in < 10 minutes with an inhaled concentration of 3% isoflurane in O_2; this concentration is reduced to 1-2% (~1-2 MAC) for maintenance of anesthesia. The use of other drugs such as opioids or nitrous oxide reduces the concentration of isoflurane required for surgical anesthesia.

Side Effects

Cardiovascular System. Isoflurane produces a concentration-dependent decrease in arterial blood pressure. Unlike halothane, cardiac output is well maintained with isoflurane, and hypotension is the result of decreased systemic vascular resistance (Figure 19–6). Isoflurane produces vasodilation in most vascular beds, with particularly pronounced effects in skin and muscle. Isoflurane is a potent coronary vasodilator, simultaneously producing increased coronary blood flow and decreased myocardial O_2 consumption. In theory, this makes isoflurane a particularly safe anesthetic to use for patients with ischemic heart disease. Concern that isoflurane might produce myocardial ischemia by inducing "coronary steal" has not been substantiated in animal and human studies. Isoflurane significantly attenuates baroreceptor function. Patients anesthetized with isoflurane generally have mildly elevated heart rates as a compensatory response to reduced blood pressure; however, rapid changes in isoflurane concentration can produce both transient tachycardia and hypertension due to isoflurane-induced sympathetic stimulation.

Respiratory System. Isoflurane produces concentration-dependent depression of ventilation. Patients spontaneously breathing isoflurane have a normal respiration rate but a reduced tidal volume, resulting in a marked reduction in alveolar ventilation and an increase in arterial CO_2 tension (Figure 19–7). Isoflurane is particularly effective at depressing the ventilatory response to hypercapnia and hypoxia (Hirshman et al., 1977). While isoflurane is an effective bronchodilator, it also is an airway irritant and can stimulate airway reflexes during induction of anesthesia, producing coughing and laryngospasm.

Nervous System. Isoflurane dilates the cerebral vasculature, producing increased cerebral blood flow; this vasodilating activity is less than that of either halothane or enflurane (Drummond et al., 1983). There is a modest risk of an increase in intracranial pressure in patients with preexisting intracranial hypertension. Isoflurane reduces cerebral metabolic O_2 consumption in a dose dependent manner. At 1.5-2.0 MAC, isoflurane produces burst suppression of the EEG and reduces cerebral metabolic rate by ~50%. The modest effects of isoflurane on cerebral blood flow can be reversed readily by hyperventilation (McPherson et al., 1989).

Muscle. Isoflurane produces some relaxation of skeletal muscle by its central effects. It also enhances the effects of both depolarizing and non-depolarizing muscle relaxants. Isoflurane is more potent than halothane in its potentiation of neuromuscular blocking agents. Like other halogenated inhalational anesthetics, isoflurane relaxes uterine smooth muscle and is not recommended for analgesia or anesthesia for labor and vaginal delivery.

Kidney. Isoflurane reduces renal blood flow and glomerular filtration rate, resulting in a small volume of concentrated urine. Changes in renal function observed during isoflurane anesthesia are rapidly reversed, with no long-term renal sequelae or toxicities.

Liver and Gastrointestinal Tract. Splanchnic and hepatic blood flows are reduced with increasing doses of isoflurane as systemic arterial pressure decreases. Liver function tests are minimally affected by isoflurane, with no reported incidence of hepatic toxicity.

Enflurane

Enflurane (ETHRANE, others) is 2-chloro-1,1,2-trifluoroethyl difluoromethyl ether (Figure 19–4).

It is a clear, colorless liquid at room temperature with a mild, sweet odor. Like other inhalational anesthetics, it is volatile and must be stored in a sealed bottle. It is nonflammable and non-explosive in mixtures of air or oxygen.

Pharmacokinetics. Because of its relatively high blood:gas partition coefficient, induction of anesthesia and recovery from enflurane are relatively slow (Table 19–1).

Enflurane is metabolized to a modest extent, with 2-8% of absorbed enflurane undergoing oxidative metabolism in the liver by CYP2E1. Fluoride ions are a by-product of enflurane metabolism, but plasma fluoride levels are low and nontoxic. Patients taking isoniazid exhibit enhanced metabolism of enflurane with significantly elevated serum fluoride concentrations (Mazze et al., 1982).

Clinical Use. As with isoflurane, enflurane is primarily utilized for maintenance rather than induction of anesthesia.

Surgical anesthesia can be induced with enflurane in < 10 minutes with an inhaled concentration of 4% in oxygen. Anesthesia can be maintained with concentrations from 1.5-3%. As with other anesthetics, the enflurane concentrations required to produce anesthesia are reduced when it is co-administered with nitrous oxide or opioids. With the advent of new inhalational agents, enflurane is rarely used for clinical anesthesia in developed countries.

Side Effects

Cardiovascular System. Enflurane causes a concentration-dependent decrease in arterial blood pressure. Hypotension is due in part to depression of myocardial contractility, with some contribution from peripheral vasodilation (Figure 19–6). Enflurane has minimal effects on heart rate and produces neither the bradycardia seen with halothane nor the tachycardia seen with isoflurane.

Respiratory System. The respiratory effects of enflurane are similar to those of halothane. Spontaneous ventilation with enflurane produces a pattern of rapid, shallow breathing. Minute ventilation is markedly decreased, and a Pa_{CO2} of 60 mm Hg can be seen with 1 MAC of enflurane (Figure 19–7). Enflurane produces a greater depression of the ventilatory responses to hypoxia and hypercarbia than do either halothane or isoflurane (Hirshman et al., 1977). Enflurane, like other inhalational anesthetics, is an effective bronchodilator.

Nervous System. Enflurane is a cerebral vasodilator and thus can increase intracranial pressure in some patients. Like other inhalational anesthetics, enflurane reduces cerebral metabolic O_2 consumption. Enflurane has an unusual property of producing electrical seizure activity. High concentrations of enflurane or profound hypocarbia during enflurane anesthesia result in a characteristic high-voltage, high-frequency electroencephalographic (EEG) pattern that progresses to spike-and-dome complexes. The spike-and-dome pattern can be punctuated by frank seizure activity that may or may not be accompanied by peripheral motor manifestations of seizure activity. The seizures are self-limited and are not thought to produce permanent damage. Epileptic patients are not particularly susceptible to enflurane-induced seizures. Nonetheless, enflurane generally is not used in patients with seizure disorders.

Muscle. Enflurane produces significant skeletal muscle relaxation in the absence of muscle relaxants. It also significantly enhances the effects of non-depolarizing muscle relaxants. As with other inhalational agents, enflurane relaxes uterine smooth muscle. It is not widely used for obstetric anesthesia.

Kidney. Like other inhalational anesthetics, enflurane reduces renal blood flow, glomerular filtration rate, and urinary output. These effects are rapidly reversed upon drug discontinuation. Enflurane metabolism produces significant plasma levels of fluoride ions (20-40 μmol) and can produce transient urinary-concentrating defects following prolonged administration (Mazze et al., 1977). There is scant evidence of long-term nephrotoxicity following enflurane use, and it is safe to use in patients with renal impairment, provided that the depth of enflurane anesthesia and the duration of administration are not excessive.

Liver and GI Tract. Enflurane reduces splanchnic and hepatic blood flow in proportion to reduced arterial blood pressure. Enflurane does not appear to alter liver function or to be hepatotoxic.

Desflurane

Desflurane (SUPRANE) is difluoromethyl 1-fluoro-2,2,2-trifluoromethyl ether (Figure 19–4). It is a highly volatile liquid at room temperature (vapor pressure = 681 mm Hg) and thus must be stored in tightly sealed bottles.

Delivery of a precise concentration of desflurane requires the use of a specially heated vaporizer that delivers pure vapor that then is diluted appropriately with other gases (O_2, air, or N_2O). Desflurane is nonflammable and non-explosive in mixtures of air or oxygen.

Pharmacokinetics. Desflurane has a very low blood:gas partition coefficient (0.42) and also is not very soluble in fat or other peripheral tissues (Table 19–1). For this reason, the alveolar (and blood) concentration rapidly rises to the level of inspired concentration.

Indeed, within 5 minutes of administration, the alveolar concentration reaches 80% of the inspired concentration. This provides for a very rapid induction of anesthesia and for rapid changes in depth of anesthesia following changes in the inspired concentration. Emergence from anesthesia also is very rapid with desflurane. The time to awakening following desflurane is shorter than with halothane or sevoflurane and usually does not exceed 5-10 minutes in the absence of other sedative agents (La Colla et al., 2007).

Desflurane is metabolized to a minimal extent, and > 99% of absorbed desflurane is eliminated unchanged through the lungs. A small amount of absorbed desflurane is oxidatively metabolized by hepatic CYPs. Virtually no fluoride ions are detectable in serum after desflurane administration, but low concentrations of trifluoroacetic acid are found in serum and urine (Koblin et al., 1988).

Clinical Use. Desflurane is a widely used anesthetic for outpatient surgery because of its rapid onset of action and rapid recovery. The drug irritates the tracheobronchial tree and can provoke coughing, salivation, and bronchospasm. Anesthesia therefore usually is induced with an intravenous agent, with desflurane subsequently administered for maintenance of anesthesia. Maintenance of anesthesia usually requires inhaled concentrations of 6-8% (~1 MAC). Lower concentrations of desflurane are required if it is co-administered with nitrous oxide or opioids.

Side Effects

Cardiovascular System. Desflurane, like all inhalational anesthetics, causes a concentration-dependent decrease in blood pressure. Desflurane has a very modest negative inotropic effect and produces hypotension primarily by decreasing systemic vascular resistance (Eger, 1994) (Figure 19–6). Thus, cardiac output is well preserved during desflurane anesthesia, as is blood flow to the major organ beds (splanchnic, renal, cerebral, and coronary). Marked increases in heart rate often are noted during induction of desflurane anesthesia and during abrupt increases in the delivered concentration of desflurane. This transient tachycardia results from desflurane-induced stimulation of the sympathetic nervous system (Ebert and Muzi, 1993). Unlike some inhalational anesthetics, the hypotensive effects of desflurane do not wane with increasing duration of administration.

Respiratory System. Similarly to halothane and enflurane, desflurane causes a concentration-dependent increase in respiratory rate and a decrease in tidal volume. At low concentrations (< 1 MAC) the net effect is to preserve minute ventilation. At desflurane concentrations > 1 MAC, minute ventilation is markedly depressed, resulting in elevated arterial CO_2 tension (Pa_{CO_2}) (Figure 19–7). Patients spontaneously breathing desflurane at concentrations > 1.5 MAC will have extreme elevations of $Paco_2$ and may become apneic. Desflurane, like other inhalational agents, is a bronchodilator. However, it also is a strong airway irritant, and can cause coughing, breath-holding, laryngospasm, and excessive respiratory secretions. *Because of its irritant properties, desflurane is not used for induction of anesthesia.*

Nervous System. Desflurane decreases cerebral vascular resistance and cerebral metabolic O_2 consumption. Burst suppression of the EEG is achieved with ~ 2 MAC desflurane; at this level, $CMRO_2$ is reduced by ~ 50%. Under conditions of normocapnia and normotension, desflurane produces an increase in cerebral blood flow and can increase intracranial pressure in patients with poor intracranial compliance. The vasoconstrictive response to hypocapnia is preserved during desflurane anesthesia, and increases in intracranial pressure thus can be prevented by hyperventilation.

Muscle. Desflurane produces direct skeletal muscle relaxation as well as enhancing the effects of non-depolarizing and depolarizing neuromuscular blocking agents (Caldwell et al., 1991).

Kidney. Consistent with its minimal metabolic degradation, desflurane has no reported nephrotoxicity.

Liver and GI Tract. Desflurane is not known to affect liver function tests or to cause hepatotoxicity.

Desflurane and Carbon Monoxide. Inhaled anesthetics are administered via a circle system circuit that permits unidirectional flow of gas. This systems permits rebreathing of exhaled gases that contain CO_2. To prevent rebreathing of CO_2 (which can lead to hypercarbia), CO_2 absorbers are incorporated into the anesthesia delivery circuits. These CO_2 absorbers contained either $Ca(OH)_2$ or $Ba(OH)_2$ and smaller quantities of more potent alkalis, NaOH and KOH. Interaction of inhaled anesthetics with these strong alkalis results in the formation of CO. The amount of CO produced is insignificant as long as the CO_2 absorbent is sufficiently hydrated. With almost complete dessication of the CO_2 absorbents, substantial quantities of CO can be produced. This effect is greatest with desflurane and can be prevented by the use of well-hydrated, fresh CO_2 absorbent.

Sevoflurane

Sevoflurane (ULTANE, others) is fluoromethyl 2,2,2-trifluoro-1-[trifluoromethyl]ethyl ether (Figure 19–4).

It is a clear, colorless, volatile liquid at room temperature and must be stored in a sealed bottle. It is

anesthesia (Rasmussen et al., 2006). Xenon is well tolerated in patients of advanced age. No long-term side effects from xenon anesthesia have been reported.

Effects on Organ Systems

Cardiovascular System. Xenon has minimal effects on cardiovascular function. Arterial pressure, unlike the situation with other anesthetic agents, is well maintained. Left ventricular contractility is not affected and heart rate and systemic vascular resistance are essentially unchanged. Autonomic function is better maintained under xenon anesthesia than under anesthesia with propofol and inhaled anesthetics (Hanss et al., 2006). Even in patients with significant cardiac disease, xenon maintains a favorable profile (Lockwood et al., 2006).

Respiratory System. Under xenon anesthesia, respiratory rate is reduced slightly. However, an increase in tidal volume maintains minute ventilation, indicating that there is minimal respiratory depression. An increase in airway pressure does occur; this has been attributed to the greater density and viscosity of xenon (compared to oxygen) and not due to changes in bronchomotor tone (Baumert et al., 2002).

Central Nervous System. Like other anesthetic agents, xenon reduces cerebral metabolism by 25-30%. This reduction in metabolism is accompanied by a corresponding reduction in cerebral blood flow. Consequently, xenon is not expected to increase intracranial pressure.

Liver, Kidney, and GI Tract. Xenon is an inert agent and does not undergo metabolism. Hepatic or renal toxicity with its use have not been reported.

ANESTHETIC ADJUNCTS

A general anesthetic is rarely given as the sole agent. Anesthetic adjuncts usually are used to augment specific components of anesthesia, permitting lower doses of general anesthetics with fewer side effects. Because they are such an integral part of general anesthetic drug regimens, their use as anesthetic adjuncts is described briefly here. The detailed pharmacology of each drug is covered in other chapters.

Benzodiazepines

While benzodiazepines (Chapter 17) can produce anesthesia similar to that of barbiturates, they are more commonly used for sedation rather than general anesthesia because prolonged amnesia and sedation may result from anesthetizing doses. As adjuncts, benzodiazepines are used for anxiolysis, amnesia, and sedation prior to induction of anesthesia or for sedation during procedures not requiring general anesthesia. The benzodiazepine most frequently used in the perioperative period is midazolam followed distantly by diazepam (VALIUM, others), and lorazepam (ATIVAN, others).

Midazolam is water soluble and typically is administered intravenously but also can be given orally, intramuscularly, or rectally; oral midazolam is particularly useful for sedation of young children. Midazolam produces minimal venous irritation as opposed to diazepam and lorazepam, which are formulated in propylene glycol and are painful on injection, sometimes producing thrombophlebitis. Midazolam has the pharmacokinetic advantage, particularly over lorazepam, of being more rapid in onset and shorter in duration of effect. Sedative doses of midazolam (0.01-0.05 mg/kg intravenously) reach peak effect in ~2 minutes and provide sedation for ~30 minutes. Elderly patients tend to be more sensitive to and have a slower recovery from benzodiazepines (Jacobs et al., 1995); thus, titration to the desired effect of smaller doses in this age group is prudent. Midazolam is hepatically metabolized with a clearance (6-11 mL/min per kg), similar to that of methohexital and ~20 and 7 times higher than those of diazepam and lorazepam, respectively. Either for prolonged sedation or for general anesthetic maintenance, midazolam is more suitable for infusion than are other benzodiazepines, although its duration of action does significantly increase with prolonged infusions (Figure 19–3). Benzodiazepines reduce both cerebral blood flow and metabolism but at equi-anesthetic doses are less potent in this respect than are barbiturates. They are effective anticonvulsants and sometimes are given to treat status epilepticus. Benzodiazepines modestly decrease blood pressure and respiratory drive, occasionally resulting in apnea. Thus, blood pressure and respiratory rate should be monitored in patients sedated with intravenous benzodiazepines.

α_2 Adrenergic Agonists. Dexmedetomidine (PRECEDEX) is an imidazole derivative that is a highly selective α_2 adrenergic receptor agonist (Kamibayashi and Maze, 2000). Dexmedetomidine is FDA-approved for short-term (< 24 hours) sedation of critically ill adults and sedation prior to and/or during surgical or other medical procedures in non-intubated patients. Activation of the α_{2A} adrenergic receptor by dexmedetomidine produces both sedation and analgesia, but does not reliably provide general anesthesia, even at maximal doses (Lakhlani et al., 1997).

Dexmedetomidine is a sedative-hypnotic that provides analgesia with little respiratory depression and, in most patients, a tolerable decrease in blood pressure and heart rate. The drug is likely to be increasingly used for sedation and as an anesthetic adjunct.

The most common side effects of dexmedetomidine include hypotension and bradycardia, both of which are attributed to decreased catecholamine release by activation peripherally and in the CNS of the α_{2A} receptor (Lakhlani et al., 1997). Nausea and dry mouth also are common untoward reactions. At higher drug concentrations, the α_{2B} subtype is activated, resulting in hypertension and a further decrease in heart rate and cardiac output. Dexmedetomidine has the very useful property of producing sedation and analgesia with minimal respiratory depression (Belleville et al., 1992); thus, it is particularly valuable in sedation of patients who are not endotracheally intubated and mechanically ventilated. The sedation produced by dexmedetomidine has been noted to be more akin to natural sleep, with patients relatively easy to arouse (Hall et al., 2000). However, dexmedetomidine does not appear to provide reliable amnesia and additional agents may need to be employed if lack of recall is desirable.

Dexmedetomidine is supplied as an aqueous solution of the hydrochloride salt and should be diluted in normal saline to a final concentration of 4 μg/mL for intravenous delivery, the only approved route of administration. The recommended loading dose is 1 μg/kg given over 10 minutes, followed by infusion at a rate of 0.2-0.7 μg/kg per hour. Reduced doses should be considered in patients with risk factors for severe hypotension. The distribution and terminal half-lives are 6 minutes and 2 hours, respectively. Dexmedetomidine is highly protein bound and is primarily hepatically metabolized; the glucuronide and methyl conjugates are excreted in the urine.

Analgesics

With the exception of ketamine, neither parenteral nor currently available inhalational anesthetics are effective analgesics. Thus, analgesics typically are administered with general anesthetics to reduce anesthetic requirement and minimize hemodynamic changes produced by painful stimuli. Nonsteroidal anti-inflammatory drugs, COX-2 inhibitors, and acetaminophen (Chapter 34) sometimes provide adequate analgesia for minor surgical procedures. However, opioids are the primary analgesics used during the perioperative period because of the rapid and profound analgesia they produce.

Fentanyl (SUBLIMAZE, others), sufentanil (SUFENTA, others), alfentanil (ALFENTA, others), remifentanil (ULTIVA), meperidine (DEMEROL, others), and morphine are the major parenteral opioids used in the perioperative period. The primary analgesic activity of each of these drugs is produced by agonist activity at μ-opioid receptors. Their order of potency (relative to morphine) is: sufentanil (1000 ×), remifentanil (300 ×), fentanyl (100 ×), alfentanil (15 ×), morphine (1 ×), and meperidine (0.1 ×). These agents are discussed in more detail in Chapter 18.

The choice of a perioperative opioid is based primarily on duration of action, since, at appropriate doses, all produce similar analgesia and side effects. Remifentanil has an ultrashort duration of action (~10 minutes) and accumulates minimally with repeated doses or infusion; it is particularly well suited for procedures that are briefly painful, but for which little analgesia is required postoperatively. Single doses of fentanyl, alfentanil, and sufentanil all have similar intermediate durations of action (30, 20, and 15 minutes, respectively), but recovery after prolonged administration varies considerably. Fentanyl's duration of action lengthens the most with infusion, sufentanil's much less so, and alfentanil's the least. Except for remifentanil, all of the above-mentioned opioids are metabolized in the liver, followed by renal and biliary excretion of the metabolites. Remifentanil is hydrolyzed by tissue and plasma esterases. Given its rapid elimination, termination of the effects of remifentanil can result in significant pain in the surgical patient. Consequently, longer-acting opiates are often given prior to discontinuation of remifentanil.

During the perioperative period, opioids often are given at induction to preempt responses to predictable painful stimuli (e.g., endotracheal intubation and surgical incision). Subsequent doses either by bolus or infusion are titrated to the surgical stimulus and the patient's hemodynamic response. Marked decreases in respiratory rate and heart rate with much smaller reductions in blood pressure are seen to varying degrees with all opioids. Muscle rigidity that can impair ventilation sometimes accompanies larger doses of opioids. The incidence of sphincter of Oddi spasm is increased with all opioids, although morphine appears to be more potent in this regard (Hahn et al., 1988). The frequency and severity of nausea, vomiting, and pruritus after emergence from anesthesia are increased by all opioids to about the same degree. A useful side effect of meperidine is its capacity to reduce shivering, a common problem during emergence from anesthesia (Pauca et al., 1984); other opioids are not as efficacious against shivering, perhaps due to less κ receptor agonism. Finally, opioids often are administered intrathecally and epidurally for management of acute and chronic pain (Chapter 18). Neuraxial opioids with or without local anesthetics can provide profound analgesia for many surgical procedures; however, respiratory depression and pruritus usually limit their use to major operations.

Neuromuscular Blocking Agents

The practical aspects of the use of neuromuscular blockers as anesthetic adjuncts are briefly described here. The detailed pharmacology of this drug class is presented in Chapter 11.

Depolarizing (e.g., succinylcholine) and non-depolarizing muscle relaxants (e.g., vecuronium) often are administered during the induction of anesthesia to relax muscles of the jaw, neck, and airway and thereby facilitate laryngoscopy and endotracheal intubation. Barbiturates will precipitate when mixed with muscle relaxants and should be allowed to clear from the intravenous line prior to injection of a muscle relaxant. Following induction, continued muscle relaxation is desirable for many procedures to aid surgical exposure and to provide additional insurance of immobility. Of course, muscle relaxants are not by themselves anesthetics and should not be used in lieu of adequate anesthetic depth. The action of non-depolarizing muscle relaxants usually is antagonized, once muscle paralysis is no longer desired, with an acetylcholinesterase inhibitor such as neostigmine or edrophonium (Chapter 10) combined with a muscarinic receptor antagonist (e.g., glycopyrrolate or atropine; Chapter 9) to offset the muscarinic activation resulting from esterase inhibition. Other than histamine release by some agents, non-depolarizing muscle relaxants used in this manner have few side effects. However, succinylcholine has multiple serious side effects (bradycardia, hyperkalemia, and severe myalgia) including induction of malignant hyperthermia in susceptible individuals.

ANESTHETIC CYTOPROTECTION AND TOXICITY

The conventional view of general anesthesia is that anesthetics produce a reversible loss of consciousness and that CNS function returns to basal levels upon termination of anesthesia and recovery of consciousness. Recent data, however, have cast doubt upon this notion. Exposure of rodents to anesthetic agents during the period of synaptogenesis (within the first 10 days post birth) results in widespread neurodegeneration in the developing brain (Jevtovic-Todorovic et al., 2003). This neuronal injury, which is apoptotic in nature, results in disturbed electrophysiologic function and cognitive dysfunction in adolescent and adult rodents that were exposed to anesthetics during the neonatal period. A variety of agents, including isoflurane, propofol, midazolam, nitrous oxide, and thiopental, manifest this toxicity (Patel and Sun, 2009).

Although the etiology is not clear, $GABA_A$ agonism and NMDA receptor antagonism play a role. In particular, the combination of a $GABA_A$ agonist and NMDA receptor antagonist produce the greatest toxicity. Until the occurrence of this neurotoxicity during brain development has been established in pre-clinical studies, its relevance to the use of anesthetics in humans will not be clear. To date, there are no data to suggest that the provision of anesthesia to neonates and infants undergoing surgery produces any neurotoxicity. Ongoing clinical trials in humans should clarify this within the next few years.

By contrast, anesthetics reduce ischemic injury to a variety of tissues, including the brain and heart. This protective effect is robust and results in better functional outcomes in comparison to ischemic injury that occurs in unanesthetized awake subjects. With respect to ischemic injury of the brain, anesthetics (inhalational agents, propofol, barbiturates, ketamine, lidocaine, midazolam) suppress excitotoxic injury produced by excessive glutamate release, reduce inflammation, and promote pro-survival signaling (Head et al., 2007). In addition, exposure to anesthesia results in the activation of plasmalemmal and mitochondrial ATP-dependent K^+ channels, activation of signal transduction pathways (NO synthase, MAP kinases), and protein synthesis that render the brain less vulnerable to subsequent ischemic injury. In a similar fashion, volatile anesthetics and, under some conditions, propofol and barbiturates, reduce myocardial ischemia-reperfusion injury (Frassdorf et al., 2009). The molecular mechanisms leading to cardiac protection by volatile anesthetics involve activation of "classical" preconditioning signaling pathways (e.g., GPCRs, endothelial NO synthase, survival protein kinases, PKC, reactive oxygen species, ATP-dependent K^+ channels, and the mitochondrial permeability transition pore) (Hausenloy and Scorrano, 2007). Propofol and barbiturates may induce specific components of the "classical" pathways involved in cardiac protection; however, there is debate as to whether these agents are truly protective or injurious to the ischemic myocardium (Frassdorf et al., 2009).

Therapeutic Gases

OXYGEN

Oxygen (O_2) is essential to life. Hypoxia is a life-threatening condition in which oxygen delivery is inadequate to meet the metabolic demands of the tissues. Since oxygen delivery is the product of blood flow and oxygen content, hypoxia may result from alterations in tissue perfusion, decreased oxygen tension in the blood, or decreased oxygen-carrying capacity. In addition, hypoxia may result from restricted oxygen transport from the microvasculature to cells or impaired utilization within the cell. An inadequate supply of oxygen ultimately results in the cessation of aerobic metabolism and oxidative phosphorylation, depletion of high-energy compounds, cellular dysfunction, and death.

Normal Oxygenation

Oxygen makes up 21% of air, which at sea level represents a partial pressure of 21 kPa (158 mm Hg). While the fraction (percentage) of O_2 remains constant regardless of atmospheric pressure, the partial pressure of O_2 (Po_2) decreases with lower atmospheric pressure. Since the partial pressure drives the diffusion of O_2, ascent to elevated altitude reduces the uptake and delivery of oxygen to the tissues. Conversely, increases in atmospheric pressure (e.g., hyperbaric therapy or breathing at depth) raise the Po_2 in inspired air and increase gas uptake. As the air is delivered to the distal airways and alveoli, the Po_2 decreases by dilution with CO_2 and water vapor and by uptake into the blood.

Under ideal conditions, when ventilation and perfusion are well matched, the alveolar Po_2 will be ~14.6 kPa (110 mm Hg). The corresponding alveolar partial pressures of water and CO_2 are 6.2 kPa (47 mm Hg) and 5.3 kPa (40 mm Hg), respectively. Under normal conditions, there is complete equilibration of alveolar gas and capillary blood, and the Po_2 in end-capillary blood is typically within a fraction of a kPa of that in the alveoli. In some diseases, the diffusion barrier for gas transport may be increased, or, during exercise, when high cardiac output reduces capillary transit time, full equilibration may not occur, and the alveolar–end-capillary Po_2 gradient may be increased.

The Po_2 in arterial blood, however, is further reduced by venous admixture (shunt), the addition of mixed venous blood from the pulmonary artery, which has a Po_2 of ~5.3 kPa (40 mm Hg). Together, the diffusional barrier, ventilation–perfusion mismatches, and the shunt fraction are the major causes of the alveolar-to-arterial oxygen gradient, which is normally 1.3-1.6 kPa (10-12 mm Hg) when air is breathed and 4.0-6.6 kPa (30-50 mm Hg) when 100% oxygen is breathed.

Oxygen is delivered to the tissue capillary beds by the circulation and again follows a gradient out of the blood and into cells. Tissue extraction of oxygen typically reduces the Po_2 of venous blood by an additional 7.3 kPa (55 mm Hg). Although the Po_2 at the site of cellular oxygen utilization—the mitochondria—is not known, oxidative phosphorylation can continue at a Po_2 of only a few mm Hg.

In the blood, oxygen is carried primarily in chemical combination with hemoglobin and is to a small extent dissolved in solution. The quantity of oxygen combined with hemoglobin depends on the Po_2, as illustrated by the sigmoidal oxyhemoglobin dissociation curve (Figure 19–8). Hemoglobin is ~98% saturated with oxygen when air is breathed under normal circumstances, and it binds 1.3 mL of oxygen per gram when fully saturated. The steep slope of this curve with falling Po_2 facilitates unloading of oxygen from hemoglobin at the tissue level and reloading when desaturated mixed venous blood arrives at the lung. Shifting of the curve to the right with increasing temperature, increasing Pco_2, and decreasing pH, as is found in metabolically active tissues, lowers the oxygen saturation for the same Po_2 and thus delivers additional oxygen where and when it is most needed. However, the flattening of the curve with higher Po_2 indicates that increasing blood Po_2 by inspiring oxygen-enriched mixtures can increase the amount of oxygen carried by hemoglobin only minimally. Further increases in blood oxygen content can occur only by increasing the amount of oxygen dissolved in plasma. Because of the low solubility of oxygen (0.226 mL/L per kPa or 0.03 mL/L per mm Hg at 37°C), breathing 100% oxygen can increase the amount of oxygen dissolved in blood by only 15 mL/L, less than one-third of normal metabolic demands. However, if the inspired Po_2 is increased to 3 atm (304 kPa) in a hyperbaric chamber, the amount of dissolved oxygen is sufficient to meet normal metabolic demands even in the absence of hemoglobin (Table 19–4).

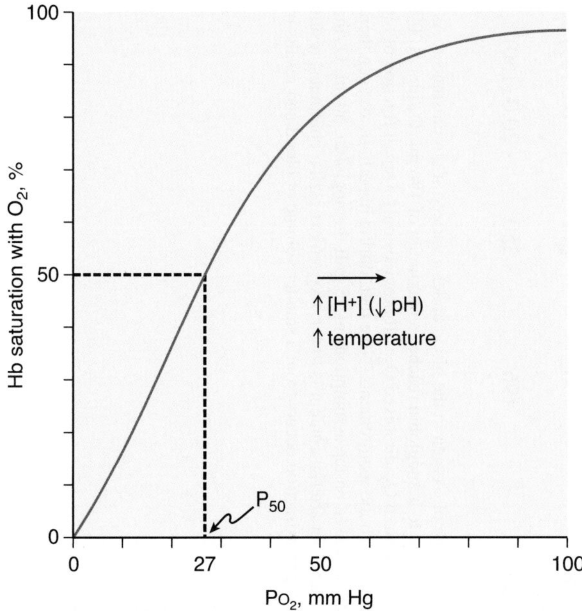

Figure 19–8. *Oxyhemoglobin dissociation curve for whole blood.* The relationship between Po_2 and hemoglobin (Hb) saturation is shown. The P_{50}, or the Po_2 resulting in 50% saturation, is indicated as well. An increase in temperature or a decrease in pH (as in working muscle) shifts this relationship to the right, reducing the hemoglobin saturation at the same Po_2 and thus aiding in the delivery of oxygen to the tissues.

Oxygen Deprivation

An understanding of the causes and effects of oxygen deficiency is necessary for the rational therapeutic use of the gas. *Hypoxia* is the term used to denote insufficient oxygenation of the tissues. *Hypoxemia* generally implies a failure of the respiratory system to oxygenate arterial blood.

Pulmonary Mechanisms of Hypoxemia. Classically, there are five causes of hypoxemia: low inspired oxygen fraction (FI_{O_2}), increased diffusion barrier, hypoventilation, ventilation–perfusion mismatch, and shunt or venous admixture.

Low FI_{O_2} is a cause of hypoxemia only at high altitude or in the event of equipment failure, such as a gas blender malfunction or a mislabeled compressed-gas tank. An increase in the barrier to diffusion of oxygen within the lung is rarely a cause of hypoxemia in a resting subject, except in end-stage parenchymal lung disease. Both these problems may be alleviated with administration of supplemental oxygen, the former by definition and the latter by increasing the gradient driving diffusion.

Hypoventilation causes hypoxemia by reducing the alveolar Po_2 in proportion to the buildup of CO_2 in the alveoli. During hypoventilation, there is decreased delivery of oxygen to the alveoli, whereas its removal by the blood remains the same, causing its alveolar concentration to fall. The opposite occurs with carbon dioxide. This is described by the alveolar gas equation:

$$PA_{O_2} = PI_{O_2} - (PA_{CO_2}/R)$$

where PA_{O_2} and PA_{CO_2} are the alveolar partial pressures of oxygen and carbon dioxide, PI_{O_2} is the partial pressure of oxygen in the inspired gas, and R the respiratory quotient.

Under normal conditions, breathing room air at sea level (corrected for the partial pressure of water vapor), the PI_{O_2} is ~ 20 kPa (150 mm Hg), the PA_{CO_2} ~ 5.3 kPa (40 mm Hg), R is 0.8, and thus the PA_{O_2} is normally around 13.3 kPa (100 mm Hg). It would require

Table 19–4

The Carriage of Oxygen in Blood[a]

ARTERIAL Po_2	ARTERIAL O_2 CONTENT (mL O_2/L)			MIXED VENOUS Po_2	MIXED VENOUS O_2 CONTENT (mL O_2/L)			
kPa (mmHg)	DISSOLVED	BOUND TO HEMOGLOBIN	TOTAL	kPa (mmHg)	DISSOLVED	BOUND TO HEMOGLOBIN	TOTAL	EXAMPLES
4.0 (30)	0.9	109	109.9	2.7 (20)	0.6	59	59.6	High altitude; respiratory failure breathing air
12.0 (90)	2.7	192	194.7	5.5 (41)	1.2	144	145.2	Normal person breathing air
39.9 (300)	9.0	195	204	5.9 (44)	1.3	153	154.3	Normal person breathing 50% O_2
79.7 (600)	18	196	214	6.5 (49)	1.5	163	164.5	Normal person breathing 100% O_2
239 (1800)	54	196	250	20.0 (150)	4.5	196	200.5	Normal person breathing hyperbaric O_2

[a]This table illustrates the carriage of oxygen in the blood under a variety of circumstances. As arterial O_2 tension increases, the amount of dissolved O_2 increases in direct proportion to the Po_2, but the amount of oxygen bound to hemoglobin reaches a maximum of 196 mL O_2/liter (100% saturation of hemoglobin at 15 g/dL). Further increases in O_2 content require increases in dissolved oxygen. At 100% inspired O_2, dissolved O_2 still provides only a small fraction of total demand. Hyperbaric oxygen therapy is required to increase the amount of dissolved oxygen to supply all or a large part of metabolic requirements. Note that, during hyperbaric oxygen therapy, the hemoglobin in the mixed venous blood remains fully saturated with O_2. The figures in this table are approximate and are based on the assumptions of 15 g/dL hemoglobin, 50 mL O_2/liter whole-body oxygen extraction, and constant cardiac output. When severe anemia is present, arterial Po_2 remains the same, but arterial content is lower; oxygen extraction continues, resulting in lower O_2 content and tension in mixed venous blood. Similarly, as cardiac output falls significantly, the same oxygen extraction occurs from a smaller volume of blood and results in lower mixed venous oxygen content and tension.

substantial hypoventilation, with the PA_{CO_2} rising to over 9.8 kPa (72 mm Hg), to cause the PA_{O_2} to fall below 7.8 kPa (60 mm Hg). This cause of hypoxemia is readily prevented by administration of even small amounts of supplemental O_2.

Shunt and $\dot{V}/\dot{Q}$ mismatch are related causes of hypoxemia but with an important distinction in their responses to supplemental oxygen. Optimal gas exchange occurs when blood flow ($\dot{Q}$) and ventilation ($\dot{V}$) are matched quantitatively. However, regional variations in $\dot{V}/\dot{Q}$ matching typically exist within the lung, particularly in the presence of lung disease. As ventilation increases relative to blood flow, the alveolar Po_2 (PA_{O_2}) increases; because of the flat shape of the oxyhemoglobin dissociation curve at high Po_2 (Figure 19–8), this increased PA_{O_2} does not contribute much to the oxygen content of the blood. Conversely, as the $\dot{V}/\dot{Q}$ ratio falls and perfusion increases relative to ventilation, the PA_{O_2} of the blood leaving these regions falls relative to regions with better matched ventilation and perfusion. Since the oxyhemoglobin dissociation curve is steep at these lower Po_2 values, the oxygen saturation and content of the pulmonary venous blood falls significantly. At the extreme of low $\dot{V}/\dot{Q}$ ratios, there is no ventilation to a perfused region, and a pure shunt results; thus the blood leaving the region has the same low Po_2 and high PA_{CO_2} as mixed venous blood.

The deleterious effect of $\dot{V}/\dot{Q}$ mismatch on arterial oxygenation is a direct result of the asymmetry of the oxyhemoglobin dissociation curve. Adding supplemental oxygen generally will make up for the fall in PA_{O_2} in low $\dot{V}/\dot{Q}$ units and thereby improve arterial oxygenation. However, since there is no ventilation to units with pure shunt, supplemental oxygen will not be effective in reversing hypoxemia from this cause. Because of the steep oxyhemoglobin dissociation curve at low Po_2, even moderate amounts of pure shunt will cause significant hypoxemia despite oxygen therapy (Figure 19–9). For the same reason, factors that decrease mixed venous Po_2, such as decreased cardiac output or increased O_2 consumption, enhance the hypoxemic effects of mismatch and shunt.

Nonpulmonary Causes of Hypoxia. In addition to failure of the respiratory system to oxygenate the blood adequately, a number of other factors can contribute to hypoxia at the tissue level. These may be divided into categories of O_2 delivery and O_2 utilization. Oxygen delivery decreases globally when cardiac output falls or locally when regional blood flow is compromised, such as from a vascular occlusion (e.g., stenosis, thrombosis, or microvascular occlusion) or increased downstream pressure (e.g., compartment syndrome, venous stasis, or venous hypertension). Decreased O_2-carrying capacity of the blood likewise will reduce oxygen delivery, such as occurs with anemia, CO poisoning, or hemoglobinopathy. Finally, hypoxia may occur when transport of O_2 from the capillaries to the tissues is decreased (edema) or utilization of the O_2 by the cells is impaired (CN^- toxicity).

Effects of Hypoxia. There has been a considerable increase in our understanding of the cellular and biochemical changes that occur after acute and chronic hypoxia. Regardless of the cause, hypoxia produces a marked alteration in gene expression, mediated in part by hypoxia inducible factor-1α (Brahimi-Horn and Pouyssegur, 2009). Ultimately, hypoxia results in the cessation of aerobic metabolism, exhaustion of high-energy intracellular stores, cellular dysfunction, and death. The time course of cellular demise depends on the tissue's relative metabolic requirements, O_2 and energy stores, and anaerobic capacity. Survival times (the time from the onset of circulatory arrest to significant organ dysfunction) range from 1-2 minutes in the cerebral cortex to around 5 minutes in the heart and 10 minutes in the kidneys and liver, with the potential for some degree of recovery if reperfused. Revival times (the duration of hypoxia beyond which recovery is no longer possible) are ~4 to 5 times longer. Less severe degrees of hypoxia have progressive physiological

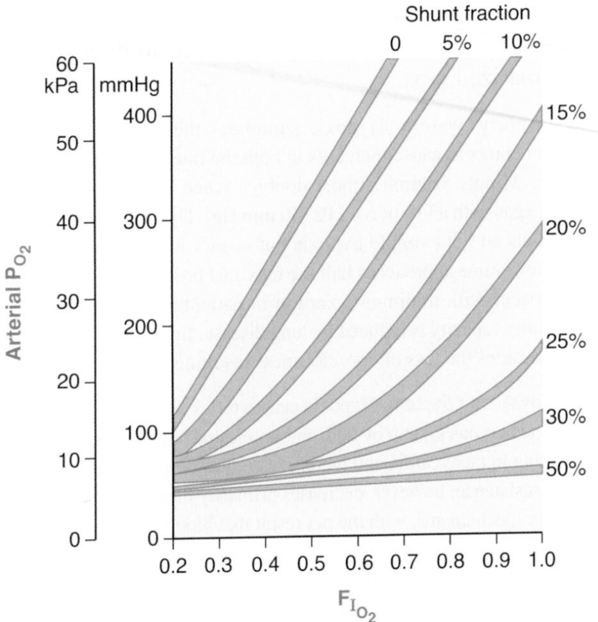

Figure 19–9. *Effect of shunt on arterial oxygenation.* The iso-shunt diagram shows the effect of changing inspired oxygen concentration on arterial oxygenation in the presence of different amounts of pure shunt. As shunt fraction increases, even an inspired oxygen fraction (FI_{O_2}) of 1.0 is ineffective at increasing the arterial Po_2. This estimation assumes hemoglobin (Hb) 10-14 g/dL, arterial Pco_2 3.3-5.3 kPa (25-40 mm Hg), and an arterial–venous (a–v) O_2 content difference of 5 mL/100 mL. (Redrawn from Benatar SR, Hewlett AM, Nunn JF. The use of iso-shunt lines for control of oxygen therapy. *Br J Anaesth*, **1973**, *45*:711–718, with permission. Copyright © The Board of Management and Trustees of the British Journal of Anaesthesia. Reproduced with permission of Oxford University Press/British Journal of Anaesthesia.)

effects on different organ systems (Nunn, 2005b). Responses of individual organ systems to hypoxia are summarized next.

Respiratory System. Hypoxia stimulates the carotid and aortic baroreceptors to cause increases in both the rate and depth of ventilation. Minute volume almost doubles when normal individuals inspire gas with a Po_2 of 6.6 kPa (50 mm Hg). Dyspnea is not always experienced with simple hypoxia but occurs when the respiratory minute volume approaches half the maximal breathing capacity; this may occur with minimum exertion in patients in whom maximal breathing capacity is reduced by lung disease. In general, little warning precedes the loss of consciousness resulting from hypoxia.

Cardiovascular System. Hypoxia causes reflex activation of the sympathetic nervous system by both autonomic and humoral mechanisms, resulting in tachycardia and increased cardiac output. Peripheral vascular resistance, however, decreases primarily through local autoregulatory mechanisms, with the net result that blood pressure generally is maintained unless hypoxia is prolonged or severe. In contrast to the systemic circulation, hypoxia causes pulmonary vasoconstriction and hypertension, an extension of the normal regional vascular response that matches perfusion with ventilation to optimize gas exchange in the lung (hypoxic pulmonary vasoconstriction).

CNS. The CNS is least able to tolerate hypoxia. Hypoxia is manifest initially by decreased intellectual capacity and impaired judgment and psychomotor ability. This state progresses to confusion and restlessness and ultimately to stupor, coma, and death as the arterial Po_2 decreases below 4-5.3 kPa (30-40 mm Hg). Victims often are unaware of this progression.

Cellular and Metabolic Effects. When the mitochondrial Po_2 falls below ~ 0.13 kPa (1 mm Hg), aerobic metabolism stops, and the less efficient anaerobic pathways of glycolysis become responsible for the production of cellular energy. End products of anaerobic metabolism, such as lactic acid, are released into the circulation in measurable quantities. Energy-dependent ion pumps slow, and transmembrane ion gradients dissipate. Intracellular concentrations of Na^+, Ca^{2+}, and H^+ increase, finally leading to cell death. The time course of cellular demise depends on the relative metabolic demands, oxygen storage capacity, and anaerobic capacity of the individual organs. Restoration of perfusion and oxygenation prior to hypoxic cell death paradoxically can result in an accelerated form of cell injury (ischemia–reperfusion syndrome), which is thought to result from the generation of highly reactive oxygen free radicals.

Adaptation to Hypoxia. Long-term hypoxia results in adaptive physiological changes; these have been studied most thoroughly in persons exposed to high altitude. Adaptations include increased numbers of pulmonary alveoli, increased concentrations of hemoglobin in blood and myoglobin in muscle, and a decreased ventilatory response to hypoxia. Short-term exposure to high altitude produces similar adaptive changes. In susceptible individuals, however, acute exposure to high altitude may produce *acute mountain sickness*, a syndrome characterized by headache, nausea, dyspnea, sleep disturbances, and impaired judgment progressing to pulmonary and cerebral edema. Mountain sickness is treated with rest and analgesics when mild or supplemental oxygen, descent to lower altitude, or an increase in ambient pressure when more severe. Acetazolamide (a carbonic anhydrase inhibitor) and dexamethasone also may be helpful. The syndrome usually can be avoided by a slow ascent to altitude, adequate hydration, and prophylactic use of acetazolamide or dexamethasone.

Certain aspects of fetal and newborn physiology are strongly reminiscent of adaptation mechanisms found in hypoxia-tolerant animals (Mortola, 1999), including shifts in the oxyhemoglobin dissociation curve (fetal hemoglobin), reductions in metabolic rate and body temperature (hibernation-like mode), reductions in heart rate and circulatory redistribution (as in diving mammals), and redirection of energy utilization from growth to maintenance metabolism. These adaptations probably account for the relative tolerance of the fetus and neonate to both chronic (uterine insufficiency) and short-term hypoxia.

Oxygen Inhalation

Physiological Effects of Oxygen Inhalation. Oxygen inhalation is used primarily to reverse or prevent the development of hypoxia; other consequences usually are minor. However, when O_2 is breathed in excessive amounts or for prolonged periods, secondary physiological changes and toxic effects can occur.

Respiratory System. Inhalation of O_2 at 1 atm or above causes a small degree of respiratory depression in normal subjects, presumably as a result of loss of tonic chemoreceptor activity. However, ventilation typically increases within a few minutes of O_2 inhalation because of a paradoxical increase in the tension of CO_2 in tissues. This increase results from the increased concentration of oxyhemoglobin in venous blood, which causes less efficient removal of carbon dioxide from the tissues.

In a small number of patients whose respiratory center is depressed by long-term retention of CO_2, injury, or drugs, ventilation is maintained largely by stimulation of carotid and aortic chemoreceptors, commonly referred to as the *hypoxic drive*. The provision of too much oxygen can depress this drive, resulting in respiratory acidosis. In these cases, supplemental oxygen should be titrated carefully to ensure adequate arterial saturation. If hypoventilation results, then mechanical ventilatory support with or without tracheal intubation should be provided.

Expansion of poorly ventilated alveoli is maintained in part by the nitrogen content of alveolar gas; nitrogen is poorly soluble and thus remains in the airspaces while oxygen is absorbed. High oxygen concentrations delivered to poorly ventilated lung regions dilute the nitrogen content and can promote absorption atelectasis, occasionally resulting in an increase in shunt and a paradoxical worsening of hypoxemia after a period of oxygen administration.

Cardiovascular System. Aside from reversing the effects of hypoxia, the physiological consequences of oxygen inhalation on the cardiovascular system are of little significance. Heart rate and cardiac output are slightly reduced when 100% O_2 is breathed; blood pressure changes little. While pulmonary arterial pressure changes little in normal subjects with oxygen inhalation, elevated pulmonary artery pressures in patients living at high altitude who have chronic hypoxic pulmonary hypertension may reverse with oxygen therapy or return to sea level. In particular, in neonates with congenital heart disease and left-to-right shunting of cardiac output, oxygen supplementation must be regulated carefully because of the risk of further reducing pulmonary vascular resistance and increasing pulmonary blood flow.

Metabolism. Inhalation of 100% O_2 does not produce detectable changes in O_2 consumption, CO_2 production, respiratory quotient, or glucose utilization.

Oxygen Administration

Oxygen is supplied as a compressed gas in steel cylinders, and a purity of 99% is referred to as *medical grade*. Most hospitals have oxygen piped from insulated liquid oxygen containers to areas of frequent use. For safety, oxygen cylinders and piping are color-coded (green in the U.S.), and some form of mechanical indexing of valve connections is used to prevent the connection of other gases to oxygen systems. Oxygen concentrators, which employ molecular sieve, membrane, or electrochemical technologies, are available for low-flow home use. Such systems produce 30-95% oxygen depending on the flow rate.

Oxygen is delivered by inhalation except during extracorporeal circulation, when it is dissolved directly into the circulating blood. Only a closed delivery system with an airtight seal to the patient's airway and complete separation of inspired from expired gases can precisely control $F_{I_{O_2}}$. In all other systems, the actual delivered $F_{I_{O_2}}$ will depend on the ventilatory pattern (i.e., rate, tidal volume, inspiratory–expiratory time ratio, and inspiratory flow) and delivery system characteristics.

Low-Flow Systems. Low-flow systems, in which the oxygen flow is lower than the inspiratory flow rate, have a limited ability to raise the $F_{I_{O_2}}$ because they depend on entrained room air to make up the balance of the inspired gas. The $F_{I_{O_2}}$ of these systems is extremely sensitive to small changes in the ventilatory pattern. Nasal cannulae—small, flexible prongs that sit just inside each naris—deliver oxygen at 1-6 L/min. The nasopharynx acts as a reservoir for storing the oxygen, and patients may breathe through either the mouth or nose as long as the nasal passages remain patent. These devices typically deliver 24-28% $F_{I_{O_2}}$ at 2-3 L/min. Up to 40% $F_{I_{O_2}}$ is possible at higher flow rates, although this is poorly tolerated for more than brief periods because of mucosal drying. The simple face mask, a clear plastic mask with side holes for clearance of expiratory gas and inspiratory air entrainment, is used when higher concentrations of oxygen delivered without tight control are desired. The maximum $F_{I_{O_2}}$ of a face mask can be increased from around 60% at 6-15 L/min to > 85% by adding a 600- to 1000-mL reservoir bag. With this partial rebreathing mask, most of the inspired volume is drawn from the reservoir, avoiding dilution by entrainment of room air.

High-Flow Systems. The most commonly used high-flow oxygen delivery device is the Venturi-style mask, which uses a specially designed mask insert to entrain room air reliably in a fixed ratio and thus provides a relatively constant $F_{I_{O_2}}$ at relatively high flow rates. Typically, each insert is designed to operate at a specific oxygen flow rate, and different inserts are required to change the $F_{I_{O_2}}$. Lower delivered $F_{I_{O_2}}$ values use greater entrainment ratios, resulting in higher total (oxygen plus entrained air) flows to the patient, ranging from 80 L/min for 24% $F_{I_{O_2}}$ to 40 L/min at 50% $F_{I_{O_2}}$. While these flow rates are much higher than those obtained with low-flow devices, they still may be lower than the peak inspiratory flows for patients in respiratory distress, and thus the actual delivered O_2 concentration may be lower than the nominal value. Oxygen nebulizers, another type of Venturi-style device, provide patients with humidified oxygen at 35-100% $F_{I_{O_2}}$ at high flow rates. Finally, oxygen blenders provide high inspired oxygen concentrations at very high flow rates. These devices mix high-pressure compressed air and oxygen to achieve any concentration of O_2 from 21-100% at flow rates of up to 100 L/min. These same blenders are used to provide control of $F_{I_{O_2}}$ for ventilators, CPAP/BiPAP machines, oxygenators, and other devices with similar requirements. Again, despite the high flows, the delivery of high $F_{I_{O_2}}$ to an individual patient also depends on maintaining a tight-fitting seal to the airway and/or the use of reservoirs to minimize entrainment of diluting room air.

Monitoring of Oxygenation. Monitoring and titration are required to meet the therapeutic goal of oxygen therapy and to avoid complications and side effects. Although cyanosis is a physical finding of substantial clinical importance, it is not an early, sensitive, or reliable index of oxygenation. Cyanosis appears when ~5 g/dL of deoxyhemoglobin is present in arterial blood, representing an oxygen saturation of ~67% when a normal amount of hemoglobin (15 g/dL) is present. However, when anemia lowers the hemoglobin to 10 g/dL, then cyanosis does not appear until the arterial blood saturation has decreased to 50%. Invasive approaches for monitoring oxygenation include intermittent laboratory analysis of arterial or mixed venous blood gases and placement of intravascular cannulae capable of continuous measurement of oxygen tension. The latter method, which relies on fiber-optic oximetry, is used frequently for the continuous measurement of mixed venous hemoglobin saturation as an index of tissue extraction of oxygen, usually in critically ill patients.

Noninvasive monitoring of arterial oxygen saturation can be achieved using transcutaneous pulse oximetry, in which oxygen saturation is measured from the differential absorption of light by oxyhemoglobin and deoxyhemoglobin and the arterial saturation determined from the pulsatile component of this signal. Application is simple, and calibration is not required. Pulse oximetry measures hemoglobin saturation and not P_{O_2}. It is not sensitive to increases in P_{O_2} that exceed levels required to saturate the blood fully. Pulse oximetry is very useful for monitoring the adequacy of oxygenation during procedures requiring sedation or anesthesia, rapid evaluation and monitoring of potentially compromised patients, and titrating oxygen therapy in situations where toxicity from oxygen or side effects of excess oxygen are of concern. Near infrared spectroscopy (NIRS) is a noninvasive technique being used to monitor oxygen content in the cerebral cortex. Unlike pulse oximetry NIRS measures all reflected light in both pulsatile arterial blood and nonpulsatile venous blood, the primary compartment in the cerebral vascular bed. NIRS is useful to monitor cerebral oxygenation in surgical procedures involving cardiopulmonary bypass and circulatory arrest (Guarracino, 2008).

Complications of Oxygen Therapy. Administration of supplemental oxygen is not without potential complications. In addition to the potential to promote absorption atelectasis and depress ventilation (discussed earlier), high flows of dry oxygen can dry out and irritate mucosal surfaces of the airway and the eyes, as well as decrease mucociliary transport and clearance of secretions. Humidified oxygen thus should be used when prolonged therapy (>1 hour) is required. Finally, any oxygen-enriched atmosphere constitutes a fire hazard, and appropriate precautions must be taken both in the operating room and for patients on oxygen at home.

It is important to realize that hypoxemia still can occur despite the administration of supplemental oxygen. Furthermore, when supplemental oxygen is administered, desaturation occurs at a later time after airway obstruction or hypoventilation, potentially delaying the detection of these critical events. Therefore, whether or not oxygen is administered to a patient at risk for these problems, it is essential that both O_2 saturation and adequacy of ventilation be assessed frequently.

Therapeutic Uses of Oxygen

Correction of Hypoxia. The primary therapeutic use of oxygen is to correct hypoxia. Hypoxia is most commonly a manifestation of an underlying disease, and administration of oxygen thus should be viewed as temporizing therapy. Efforts must be directed at correcting the cause of the hypoxia. For example, airway obstruction is unlikely to respond to an increase in inspired oxygen tension without relief of the obstruction. More important, while hypoxemia owing to hypoventilation after a narcotic overdose can be improved with supplemental oxygen administration, the patient remains at risk for respiratory failure if ventilation is not increased through stimulation, narcotic reversal, or mechanical ventilation. Hypoxia resulting from most pulmonary diseases can be alleviated at least partially by administration of oxygen, allowing time for definitive therapy to reverse the primary process. Thus, administration of oxygen is basic and important treatment for all forms of hypoxia.

Reduction of Partial Pressure of an Inert Gas. Since nitrogen constitutes some 79% of ambient air, it also is the predominant gas in most gas-filled spaces in the body. In situations such as bowel distension from obstruction or ileus, intravascular air embolism, or pneumothorax, it is desirable to reduce the volume of air-filled spaces. Since nitrogen is relatively insoluble, inhalation of high concentrations of oxygen (and thus low concentrations of nitrogen) rapidly lowers the total-body partial pressure of nitrogen and provides a substantial gradient for the removal of nitrogen from gas spaces. Administration of oxygen for air embolism is additionally beneficial because it helps to relieve localized hypoxia distal to the vascular obstruction. In the case of *decompression sickness*, or *bends*, lowering the inert gas tension in blood and tissues by oxygen inhalation prior to or during a barometric decompression reduces the supersaturation that occurs after decompression so that bubbles do not form. If bubbles do form in either tissues or the vasculature, administration of oxygen is based on the same rationale as that described for gas embolism.

Hyperbaric Oxygen Therapy. Oxygen can be administered at greater than atmospheric pressure in hyerbaric chambers (Thom, 2009). Clinical uses of hyperbaric oxygen therapy include the treatment of trauma, burns, radiation damage, infections, non-healing ulcers, skin grafts, spasticity, and other neurological conditions. Hyperbaric chambers can withstand pressures that range from 200 to 600 kPa (2-6 atm), although inhaled oxygen tension that exceeds 300 kPa (3 atm) rarely is used. Chambers range from single-person units to multiroom establishments housing complex medical equipment.

Hyperbaric oxygen therapy has two components: increased hydrostatic pressure and increased O_2 pressure. Both factors are necessary for the treatment of decompression sickness and air embolism. The hydrostatic pressure reduces bubble volume, and the absence of inspired nitrogen increases the gradient for elimination of nitrogen and reduces hypoxia in downstream tissues. Increased oxygen pressure at the tissue is the primary therapeutic goal for other indications for hyperbaric O_2. A small increase in Po_2 in ischemic areas enhances the bactericidal activity of leukocytes and increases angiogenesis. Repetitive brief exposures to hyperbaric oxygen may enhance therapy for chronic refractory osteomyelitis, osteoradionecrosis, crush injury, or the recovery of compromised skin and tissue grafts. Increased O_2 tension can be bacteriostatic and useful in the treatment for the spread of infection with *Clostridium perfringens* and clostridial myonecrosis (gas gangrene).

Hyperbaric oxygen may be useful in generalized hypoxia. In CO poisoning, hemoglobin (Hb) and myoglobin become unavailable for O_2 binding because of the high affinity of these proteins for CO. Affinity for CO is ~250 times greater than the affinity for O_2; thus, an alveolar concentration of CO = 0.4 mm Hg (1/250th that of alveolar O_2, which is ~100 mm Hg), will compete equally with O_2 for binding sites on Hb. High Po_2 facilitates competition of O_2 for Hb binding sites as CO is exchanged in the alveoli. In addition, hyperbaric O_2 increases the availability of dissolved O_2 in the blood (Table 19–4). In a randomized clinical trial (Weaver et al., 2002), hyperbaric O_2 decreased the incidence of long- and short-term neurological sequelae after CO intoxication. The occasional use of hyperbaric oxygen in cyanide poisoning has a similar rationale. Hyperbaric oxygen may be useful in severe short-term anemia since sufficient oxygen can be dissolved in the plasma at 3 atm to meet metabolic demand. Such treatment must be limited because oxygen toxicity depends on increased Po_2, not on the oxygen content of the blood.

Adverse effects of hyperbaric oxygen therapy include middle ear barotrauma, CNS toxicity, seizures, lung toxicity, and aspiration pneumonia. Contraindications to hyperbaric oxygen therapy include pneumothorax and concurrent doxorubicin, bleomycin, or disulfiram therapy. Relative contraindications include respiratory tract infections, severe obstructive lung disease, fever, seizure disorders, optic neuritis, pregnancy, concurrent steroid use, and claustrophobia.

Oxygen Toxicity

Oxygen is used in cellular energy production and is crucial for cellular metabolism. However, oxygen also has deleterious actions at the cellular level. Oxygen toxicity may result from increased production of hydrogen peroxide and reactive agents such as superoxide anion, singlet oxygen, and hydroxyl radicals that attack and damage lipids, proteins, and other macromolecules, especially those in biological membranes. A number of factors limit the toxicity of oxygen-derived reactive agents, including enzymes such as superoxide dismutase, glutathione peroxidase, and catalase, which scavenge toxic oxygen by-products, and reducing agents such as iron, glutathione, and ascorbate. These factors, however, are insufficient to limit the destructive actions of oxygen when patients are exposed to high concentrations over an extended time period. Tissues show differential sensitivity to oxygen toxicity, which is likely the result of differences in both their production of reactive compounds and their protective mechanisms.

Respiratory Tract. The pulmonary system is usually the first to exhibit toxicity, a function of its continuous exposure to the highest oxygen tensions in the body. Subtle changes in pulmonary function can occur within 8-12 hours of exposure to 100% O_2. Increases in capillary permeability, which will increase the alveolar/arterial oxygen gradient and ultimately lead to further hypoxemia, and decreased pulmonary function can be seen after only 18 hours of exposure (Clark, 1988). Serious injury and death, however, require much longer exposures. Pulmonary damage is directly related to the inspired oxygen tension, and concentrations of < 0.5 atm appear to be safe over long time periods. The capillary endothelium is the most sensitive tissue of the lung. Endothelial injury results in loss of surface area from interstitial edema and leaks into the alveoli.

Decreases of inspired oxygen concentrations remain the cornerstone of therapy for oxygen toxicity. Tolerance also may play a role in protection from oxygen toxicity; animals exposed briefly to high O_2 tensions are subsequently more resistant to toxicity. Sensitivity in humans also can be altered by preexposure to both high and low O_2 concentrations (Clark, 1988). These studies strongly suggest that changes in alveolar surfactant and cellular levels of antioxidant enzymes play a role in protection from oxygen toxicity.

Nervous System. Retinopathy of prematurity (ROP) is an eye disease in premature infants involving abnormal vascularization of the developing retina that can result from oxygen toxicity or relative hypoxia (Lutty et al., 2006). Retinal changes can progress to blindness and are likely caused by fibrovascular proliferation. Central nervous system problems are rare, and toxicity occurs only under hyperbaric conditions where exposure exceeds 200 kPa (2 atm). Symptoms include seizures and visual changes, which resolve when oxygen tension is returned to normal. Increased inspired oxygen concentrations are often administered to patients who have sustained acute ischemic central nervous system injury. In premature neonates and those who have sustained in utero asphyxia, hyperoxia and hypocapnia are associated with worse neurologic outcomes (Klinger et al., 2005). Similarly, in preclinical studies, resuscitation from cardiac arrest with high inspired oxygen concentrations leads to worse outcomes (Balan et al., 2006). These data indicate that oxygen therapy should be titrated to maintain an acceptable Po_2 and that hyperoxemia should be avoided (Sola, 2008).

CARBON DIOXIDE

Transfer and Elimination of CO_2

Carbon dioxide is produced by metabolism at approximately the same rate as O_2 is consumed. At rest, this value is ~3 mL/kg per minute, but it may increase dramatically with exercise. CO_2 diffuses readily from the cells into the blood, where it is carried partly as bicarbonate ion (HCO_3^-), partly in chemical combination with hemoglobin and plasma proteins, and partly in solution at a partial pressure of ~6 kPa (46 mm Hg) in mixed venous blood. CO_2 is transported to the lung, where it is normally exhaled at the rate it is produced, leaving a partial pressure of ~5.2 kPa (40 mm Hg) in the alveoli and in arterial blood. An increase in PCO_2 results in a respiratory acidosis and may be due to decreased ventilation or the inhalation of CO_2, whereas an increase in ventilation results in decreased PCO_2 and a respiratory alkalosis. Since CO_2 is freely diffusible, the changes in blood PCO_2 and pH soon are reflected by intracellular changes in PCO_2 and pH.

Effects of Carbon Dioxide

Alterations in PCO_2 and pH have widespread effects in the body, particularly on respiration, circulation, and the CNS. Complete discussions of these and other effects are found in textbooks of respiratory physiology (Nunn, 2005a).

Respiration. CO_2 is a rapid, potent stimulus to ventilation in direct proportion to the inspired CO_2. Inhalation of 10% carbon dioxide can produce minute volumes of 75 L/min in normal individuals. CO_2 stimulates breathing by acidifying central chemoreceptors and the peripheral carotid bodies (Guyenet, 2008). Elevated Pco_2 causes bronchodilation, whereas hypocarbia causes constriction of airway smooth muscle; these responses may play a role in matching pulmonary ventilation and perfusion (Duane et al., 1979).

Circulation. The circulatory effects of CO_2 result from the combination of its direct local effects and its centrally mediated effects on the autonomic nervous system. The direct effect of CO_2 on the heart, diminished contractility, results from pH changes and a decreased myofilament Ca^{2+} responsiveness (van den Bos et al., 1979). The direct effect on systemic blood vessels results in vasodilation. CO_2 causes widespread activation of the sympathetic nervous system and an increase in the plasma concentrations of epinephrine, norepinephrine, angiotensin, and other vasoactive peptides. The results of sympathetic nervous system activation generally are opposite to the local effects of carbon dioxide. The sympathetic effects consist of increases in cardiac contractility, heart rate, and vasoconstriction (Chapter 12).

The balance of opposing local and sympathetic effects, therefore, determines the total circulatory response to CO_2. The net effect of CO_2 inhalation is an increase in cardiac output, heart rate, and blood pressure. In blood vessels, however, the direct vasodilating actions of CO_2 appear more important, and total peripheral resistance decreases when the PCO_2 is increased. CO_2 also is a potent coronary vasodilator. Cardiac arrhythmias associated with increased PCO_2 are due to the release of catecholamines.

Hypocarbia results in opposite effects: decreased blood pressure and vasoconstriction in skin, intestine, brain, kidney, and heart. These actions are exploited clinically in the use of hyperventilation to diminish intracranial hypertension.

CNS. Hypercarbia depresses the excitability of the cerebral cortex and increases the cutaneous pain threshold through a central action. This central depression has therapeutic importance. For example, in patients who are hypoventilating from narcotics or anesthetics, increasing Pco_2 may result in further CNS depression, which in turn may worsen the respiratory depression. This positive-feedback cycle can have lethal consequences. The inhalation of high concentrations of carbon dioxide (~50%) produces marked cortical and subcortical depression of a type similar to that produced by anesthetic agents.

Methods of Administration. CO_2 is marketed in gray metal cylinders as the pure gas or as CO_2 mixed with oxygen. It usually is administered at a concentration of 5-10% in combination with O_2 by means of a face mask. Another method for the temporary administration of CO_2 is by rebreathing, such as from an anesthesia breathing circuit when the soda lime canister is bypassed or from something as simple as a paper bag. A potential safety issue exists in that tanks containing carbon dioxide plus oxygen are the same color as those containing 100% CO_2. When tanks containing CO_2 and O_2 have been used inadvertently where a fire hazard exists (e.g., in the presence of electrocautery during laparoscopic surgery), explosions and fires have resulted.

Therapeutic Uses. CO_2 is used for insufflation during endoscopic procedures (e.g., laparoscopic surgery) because it is highly soluble and does not support combustion. Inadvertent gas emboli thus are dissolved and eliminated more easily by the respiratory system. CO_2 can be used to flood the surgical field during cardiac surgery. Because of its density, carbon dioxide displaces the air surrounding the open heart so that any gas bubbles trapped in the heart are carbon dioxide rather than insoluble nitrogen (Nadolny and Svensson, 2000). Similarly, CO_2 is used to de-bubble cardiopulmonary bypass and extracorporeal membrane oxygenation (ECMO) circuits. It is used to adjust pH during cardiopulmonary bypass procedures when a patient is cooled.

Hypocarbia, with its attendant respiratory alkalosis, still has some uses in anesthesia. It constricts cerebral vessels, decreasing brain size slightly, and thus may facilitate the performance of neurosurgical operations. While short-term hypocarbia is effective for this purpose, sustained hypocarbia has been associated with worse outcomes in patients with head injury (Muizelaar et al., 1991). Consequently, hypocarbia should be instituted with a clearly defined indication and normocarbia should be re-established as soon the indication for hypocabia no longer applies.

NITRIC OXIDE

Nitric oxide (NO) is a free-radical gas long known as an air pollutant and a potential toxin. NO is now known as a critical endogenous cell-signaling molecule with an increasing number of potential therapeutic applications.

Endogenous NO is produced from L-arginine by a family of enzymes called NO synthases (neural, inducible and endothelial). NO is both an intra-cellular and a cell-cell messenger implicated in a wide range of physiological and pathophysiological events in numerous cell types, including the cardiovascular, immune, and nervous systems. NO activates the soluble guanylyl cyclase, increasing cellular cyclic GMP (Chapter 3). In the vasculature, basal release of NO produced by endothelial cells is a primary determinant of resting vascular tone; NO causes vasodilation when synthesized in response to shear stress or a variety of vasodilating agents (Chapter 27). It also inhibits platelet aggregation and adhesion. Impaired NO production has been implicated in diseases such as atherosclerosis, hypertension, cerebral and coronary vasospasm, and ischemia–reperfusion injury. In the immune system, NO serves as an effector of macrophage-induced cytotoxicity, and overproduction of NO is a mediator of inflammation. In neurons, NO acts as a mediator of long-term potentiation, cytotoxicity resulting from N-methyl-D-aspartate (NMDA), and non-adrenergic non-cholinergic neurotransmission; NO has been implicated in mediating central nociceptive pathways (Chapters 8 and 18).

NO is rapidly inactivated in the circulation by oxyhemoglobin and by the reaction of NO with the heme iron, leading to the formation of nitrosyl-hemoglobin. Small quantities of methemoglobin are also produced and these are converted to the ferrous form of heme iron by cytochrome b5 reductase. The majority of inhaled NO is excreted in the urine in the form of nitrate. Rapid withdrawal of NO can result in a rebound increase in pulmonary pressure; gradual withdrawal should minimize rebound phenomena (Griffiths and Evans, 2005).

Therapeutic Uses. NO when inhaled selectively dilates the pulmonary vasculature with minimal systemic cardiovascular effects due to its rapid inactivation by oxyhemoglobin in the pulmonary circulation (Cooper, 1999). Ventilation–perfusion matching is preserved or improved by NO because inhaled NO is distributed only to ventilated areas of the lung and dilates only those vessels directly adjacent to the ventilated alveoli. Thus, inhaled NO decreases elevated pulmonary artery pressure and pulmonary vascular resistance and often improves oxygenation. The dose of NO that is required for an improvement in oxygenation is lower than that required for a reduction in pulmonary pressure (Griffiths and Evans, 2005).

Inhaled NO (iNO) has potential as a therapy for numerous diseases associated with increased pulmonary vascular resistance. In patients with adult respiratory distress syndrome (ARDS), iNO is more often used to improve oxygenation rather than reducing pulmonary pressure. NO does improve oxygenation but this effect is transient. Moreover, the use of iNO therapy is not associated with either a reduction in the duration of mechanical ventilation or in morbidity or mortality (Taylor et al., 2004). iNO-mediated reductions in pulmonary pressure have prompted its use in patients with pulmonary hypertension in other clinical settings. Transient reduction in pulmonary pressure have been reported in patients undergoing cardiac surgery (Winterhalter et al., 2008) and pulmonary transplantation (Ardehali et al., 2001). Although transient physiologic improvements do occur, long-term outcome is essentially unchanged (Meade et al., 2003). Several small studies and case reports have suggested potential benefits of inhaled NO in a variety of conditions, including pulmonary hypertension and right heart failure associated with orthotopic heart transplantation, weaning from cardiopulmonary bypass in adult and congenital heart disease patients, ventricular assist device placement, primary pulmonary hypertension, pulmonary embolism, acute chest syndrome in sickle-cell patients, congenital diaphragmatic hernia, high-altitude pulmonary edema, and lung transplantation (Haddad et al., 2000). Larger prospective, randomized studies for these disease conditions either have not yet been performed or have failed to confirm any changes in outcome.

Inhaled NO is FDA-approved for only one indication, persistent pulmonary hypertension of the newborn (Mourani et al., 2004). A recent systematic review of the available data in neonates has shown that in very sick neonates with poor oxygenation, iNO does improve oxygenation but it does not improve mortality, reduce the incidence of bronchopulmonary dysplasia that is common in this population, or reduce the incidence of brain injury (Hintz et al., 2007, Su and Chen, 2008). Whether there are subsets of patients who may have a favorable response to iNO remains to be determined.

Diagnostic Uses. Inhaled NO also is used in several diagnostic applications. Inhaled NO can be used during cardiac catheterization to safely and selectively evaluate the pulmonary vasodilating capacity of patients with heart failure and infants with congenital heart disease. Inhaled NO also is used to determine the diffusion capacity (DL) across the alveolar–capillary unit. NO is more effective than carbon dioxide in this regard because of its greater affinity for hemoglobin and its higher water solubility at body temperature (Haddad et al., 2000).

NO is produced from the nasal passages and from the lungs of normal human subjects and can be detected in exhaled gas. The measurement of fractional exhaled NO (FeNO) is a noninvasive marker for airway inflammation with utility in the assessment of respiratory tract diseases including asthma, respiratory tract infection and chronic lung diseases (Taylor et al., 2006).

Toxicity. Administered at low concentrations (0.1-50 ppm), inhaled NO appears to be safe and without significant side effects. Pulmonary toxicity can occur with levels higher than 50-100 ppm. In the context of NO as an atmospheric pollutant, the Occupational Safety and Health Administration places the 7-hour exposure limit at 50 ppm. Part of the toxicity of NO may be related to its further oxidation to nitrogen dioxide (NO_2) in the presence of high concentrations of O_2. Even low concentrations of NO_2 (2 ppm) have been shown to be highly toxic in animal models, with observed changes in lung histopathology, including loss of cilia, hypertrophy, and focal hyperplasia in the epithelium of terminal bronchioles. It is important, therefore, to keep NO_2 formation during NO therapy at a low level. This can be achieved by the administration of NO at a site in the respiratory circuit as close to the patient as possible and timing the delivery of NO to inspiration. Laboratory studies have suggested potential additional toxic effects of chronic low doses of inhaled NO, including surfactant inactivation and the formation of peroxynitrite by interaction with superoxide. Nitric oxide and peroxynitrite have been implicated in cellular mechanisms of oxygen toxicity in the lung and central nervous system (Allen et al., 2009). The ability of NO to inhibit or alter the function of a number of iron- and heme-containing proteins, including cyclooxygenase, lipoxygenases, and oxidative cytochromes, as well as its interactions with ADP-ribosylation, suggests a need for further investigation of the toxic potential of NO under therapeutic conditions (Haddad et al., 2000).

The development of methemoglobinemia is a significant complication of inhaled NO at higher concentrations, and rare deaths have been reported with overdoses of NO. The blood content of methemoglobin, however, generally will not increase to toxic levels with appropriate use of inhaled NO. Methemoglobin concentrations should be monitored intermittently during NO inhalation (Haddad et al., 2000).

Inhaled NO can inhibit platelet function and has been shown to increase bleeding time in some clinical studies, although bleeding complications have not been reported.

In patients with impaired function of the left ventricle, NO has a potential to further impair left ventricular performance by dilating the pulmonary circulation and increasing the blood flow to the left ventricle, thereby increasing left atrial pressure and promoting pulmonary edema formation. Careful monitoring of cardiac output, left atrial pressure, or pulmonary capillary wedge pressure is important in this situation.

Despite these concerns, there are limited reports of inhaled NO-related toxicity in humans. The most important requirements for safe NO inhalation therapy include:

- continuous measurement of NO and NO_2 concentrations using either chemiluminescence or electrochemical analyzers
- frequent calibration of monitoring equipment
- intermittent analysis of blood methemoglobin levels
- the use of certified tanks of NO
- administration of the lowest NO concentration required for therapeutic effect

Methods of Administration. Courses of treatment of patients with inhaled NO are highly varied, extending from 0.1 to 40 ppm in dose and for periods of a few hours to several weeks in duration. The minimum effective inhaled NO concentration should be determined for each patient to minimize the chance for toxicity. Given that sensitivity to NO can vary in the patient during the course of administration, the determination of dose response relationship on a frequent basis should assist in the titration of the optimum dose of NO. Commercial NO systems are available that will accurately deliver inspired NO concentrations between 0.1 and 80 ppm and simultaneously measure NO and NO_2 concentrations. A constant inspired concentration of NO is obtained by administering NO in nitrogen to the inspiratory limb of the ventilator circuit in either a pulse or continuous mode. While inhaled NO may be administered to spontaneously breathing patients by a closely fitting mask, it usually is delivered during mechanical ventilation. Nasal prong administration is being employed in therapeutic trials of home administration for treatment of primary pulmonary hypertension (Griffiths et al., 2005).

HELIUM

Helium (He) is an inert gas whose low density, low solubility, and high thermal conductivity provide the basis for its medical and diagnostic uses. Helium is produced by separation from liquefied natural gas and is supplied in brown cylinders. Helium can be mixed with oxygen and administered by mask or endotracheal tube. Under hyperbaric conditions, it can be substituted for the bulk of other gases, resulting in a mixture of much lower density that is easier to breathe.

The primary uses of helium are in pulmonary function testing, the treatment of respiratory obstruction, laser airway surgery, as a label in imaging studies, and for diving at depth. The determinations of residual lung volume, functional residual capacity, and related lung volumes require a highly diffusible nontoxic gas that is insoluble and does not leave the lung by the bloodstream so that, by dilution, the lung volume can be measured. Helium is well suited to these needs. A breath of a known concentration of helium is given, and the concentration of helium is measured in the mixed expired gas, allowing calculation of the other pulmonary volumes.

Pulmonary gas flow normally is laminar. With increased flow rates or a narrowed flow pathway, a component of pulmonary gas flow becomes turbulent. Helium can be added to oxygen to reduce turbulence due to airway obstruction since the density of helium is less than that of air and the viscosity of helium is greater than that of air. Addition of helium reduces the Reynolds number of the mixture (the Reynolds number is proportional to density and inversely proportional to viscosity), thereby reducing turbulence. Mixtures of helium and oxygen reduce the work of breathing. The utility of helium/oxygen mixtures is limited by the fact that oxygenation often accompanies airway obstruction. The need for increased inspired O_2 concentration limits the fraction of helium that can be used. Furthermore, even though helium reduces the Reynolds number of the gas mixture, the viscosity of helium is greater than that of air, and the increased viscosity increases the resistance to flow according to Poiseuille's law, whereby flow is inversely proportional to viscosity.

Helium has high thermal conductivity, making it useful during laser surgery on the airway. This more rapid conduction of heat away from the point of contact of the laser beam reduces the spread of tissue damage and the likelihood that the ignition point of flammable materials in the airway will be reached. Its low density improves the flow through the small endotracheal tubes typically used in such procedures. However, its use for this purpose is rare.

Laser-polarized helium is used as an inhalational contrast agent for pulmonary magnetic resonance imaging. Optical pumping of hyperpolarized helium increases the signal from the gas in the lung to permit detailed imaging of the airways and inspired airflow patterns (Hopkins et al., 2007).

Hyperbaric Applications. The depth and duration of diving activity are limited by oxygen toxicity, inert gas (nitrogen) narcosis, and nitrogen supersaturation when decompressing. Oxygen toxicity is a problem with prolonged exposure to compressed air at 500 kPa (5 atm) or more. This problem can be minimized by dilution of oxygen with helium, which lacks narcotic potential even at very high pressures and is quite insoluble in body tissues. This low solubility reduces the likelihood of bubble formation after decompression, which therefore can be achieved more rapidly. The low density of helium also reduces the work of breathing in the otherwise dense hyperbaric atmosphere. The lower heat capacity of helium also decreases respiratory heat loss, which can be significant when diving at depth.

HYDROGEN SULFIDE

Hydrogen sulfide (H_2S), which has a characteristic rotten egg smell, is a colorless, flammable, water-soluble gas that is primarily considered a toxic agent due to its ability to inhibit mitochondrial respiration through blockade of cytochrome c oxidase. Recent research has demonstrated that H_2S in low quantities may have the potential to limit cell death (Lefer, 2007). Inhibition of respiration is potentially toxic; however, if depression of respiration occurs in a controlled manner, it may allow non-hibernating species exposed to inhaled H_2S to enter a state akin to suspended animation (i.e., a slowing of cellular activity to a point where metabolic processes are inhibited but not terminal) and thereby increase tolerance to stress. H_2S also may cause activation of ATP-dependent K^+ channels, cause vasodilation properties, and serve as a free radical scavenger. H_2S has been shown to protect against whole-body hypoxia, lethal hemorrhage, and ischemia-reperfusion injury in various organs including the kidney, lung, liver, and heart. Currently, effort is underway for development of gas-releasing molecules that could deliver H_2S and other therapeutic gases to diseased tissue (Bannenberg and Vieira, 2009). Though H_2S has clinical potential, further verification in preclinical models is necessary as is more information regarding the route of delivery, timing, formulation, and concentration of H_2S.

BIBLIOGRAPHY

Abboud TK, Zhu J, Richardson M, et al. Intravenous propofol vs thiamylal-isoflurane for caesarean section, comparative maternal and neonatal effects. *Acta Anaesthesiol Scand*, **1995**, *39*:205–209.

Alkire MT, Hudetz AG, Tononi G. Consciousness and anesthesia. *Science*, **2008**, *322*:876–880.

Allegaert K, Peeters MY, Verbesselt R, et al. Inter-individual variability in propofol pharmacokinetics in preterm and term neonates. *Br J Anaesth*, **2007**, *99*:864–870.

Allen BW, Demchenko IT, Piantadosi CA. Two faces of nitric oxide: Implications for cellular mechanisms of oxygen toxicity. *J Appl Physiol*, **2009**, *106*:662–667.

Ardehali A, Laks H, Levine M, *et al*. A prospective trial of inhaled nitric oxide in clinical lung transplantation. *Transplantation*, **2001**, *72*:112–115.

Bahlman SH, Eger EI, Holsey MJ, et al. The cardiovascular effects of halolthane in man during spontaneous ventitation. *Anesthesiology*, **1972**, *36*:494–502.

Balan IS, Fiskum G, Hazelton J, et al. Oximetry-guided reoxygenation improves neurological outcome after experimental cardiac arrest. *Stroke*, **2006**, *37*:3008–3013.

Bannenberg GL, Vieira HL. Therapeutic applications of the gaseous mediators carbon monoxide and hydrogen sulfide. *Expert Opin Ther Pat*, **2009**, *19*:663–682.

Baumert JH, Reyle-Hahn M, Hecker K, et al. Increased airway resistance during xenon anaesthesia in pigs is attributed to physical properties of the gas. *Br J Anaesth*, **2002**, *88*:540–545.

Belelli D, Lambert JJ, Peters JA, et al. The interaction of the general anesthetic etomidate with the gamma-aminobutyric acid type A receptor is influenced by a single amino acid. *Proc Natl Acad Sci USA*, **1997**, *94*:11031–11036.

Belleville JP, Ward DS, Bloor BC, Maze M. Effects of intravenous dexmedetomidine in humans. I. Sedation, ventilation, and metabolic rate. *Anesthesiology*, **1992**, *77*:1125–1133.

Beskow A, Werner O, Westrin P. Faster recovery after anesthesia in infants after intravenous induction with methohexital instead of thiopental. *Anesthesiology*, **1995**, *83*:976–979.

Blouin RT, Conard PF, Gross JB. Time course of ventilatory depression following induction doses of propofol and thiopental. *Anesthesiology*, **1991**, *75*:940–944.

Bourgoin A, Albanese J, Leone M, et al. Effects of sufentanil or ketamine administered in target-controlled infusion on the cerebral hemodynamics of severely brain-injured patients. *Crit Care Med*, **2005**, *33*:1109–1113.

Brahimi-Horn MC, Pouyssegur J. HIF at a glance. *J Cell Sci*, **2009**, *122*:1055–1057.

Brown RH, Greenberg RS, Wagner EM. Efficacy of propofol to prevent bronchoconstriction: Effects of preservative. *Anesthesiology*, **2001**, *94*:851–855; discussion 856A.

Burch PG, Stanski DR. The role of metabolism and protein binding in thiopental anesthesia. *Anesthesiology*, **1983**, *58*:146–152.

Caldwell JE, Laster MJ, Magorian T, et al. The neuromuscular effects of desflurane, alone and combined with pancuronium or succinylcholine in humans. *Anesthesiology*, **1991**, *74*: 412–418.

Calverley RK, Smith NT, Jone CW. et al. Ventilatory and cardiovascular effects of enflurane anesthesia during spontaneous ventilation in man. *Anesth Analog*, **1978**, *57*:610–618.

Calverley RK, Smith NT, Prys-Roberts C. et al. Cardiovascular effects of enflurane during controlled ventilation in man. *Anesth Analog*, **1978**, *57*:619–628.

Clark JM. Pulmonary limits of oxygen tolerance in man. *Exp Lung Res*, **1988**, *14(suppl)*:897–910.

Constant I, Laude D, Hentzgen E, Murat I. Does halothane really preserve cardiac baroreflex better than sevoflurane? A noninvasive study of spontaneous baroreflex in children anesthetized with sevoflurane versus halothane. *Anesth Analg*, **2004**, *99*:360–369, table of contents.

Cooper CE. Nitric oxide and iron proteins. *Biochim Biophys Acta*, **1999**, *1411*:290–309.

Cotton M, Claing A. G protein-coupled receptors stimulation and the control of cell migration. *Cell Signal*, **2009**, *21*:1045–1053.

Cromwell TH, Stevens WC, Eger EI, et al. The cardiovascular effects of compound 469 (Forane) during spontaneous ventilation and CO_2 challenge in man. *Anesthesiology*, **1971**, *35*:17–25.

de Sousa SL, Dickinson R, Lieb WR, Franks NP. Contrasting synaptic actions of the inhalational general anesthetics isoflurane and xenon. *Anesthesiology*, **2000**, *92:*1055 –1066.

Doi M, Ikeda K. Respiratory effects of Sevoflurane *Anesth Analog*, **1987**, *66*:241–244.

Doi M, Ikeda K. Respiratory effects of sevoflurane. *Anesth Analg*, **1987**, *66*:241–244.

Drummond JC, Cole DJ, Patel PM, Reynolds LW. Focal cerebral ischemia during anesthesia with etomidate, isoflurane, or thiopental: A comparison of the extent of cerebral injury. *Neurosurgery*, **1995**, *37*:742–748; discussion 748–749.

Drummond JC, Todd MM, Toutant SM, Shapiro HM. Brain surface protrusion during enflurane, halothane, and isoflurane anesthesia in cats. *Anesthesiology*, **1983**, *59*:288–293.

Duane SF, Weir EK, Stewart RM, Niewoehner DE. Distal airway responses to changes in oxygen and carbon dioxide tensions. *Respir Physiol*, **1979**, *38*:303–311.

Dundee JW, Lilburn JK. Ketamine-iorazepam. Attenuation of psychic sequelae of ketamine by lorazepam. *Anaesthesia*, **1978**, *33*:312–314.

Ebert TJ, Muzi M. Sympathetic hyperactivity during desflurane anesthesia in healthy volunteers. A comparison with isoflurane. *Anesthesiology*, **1993**, *79*:444–453.

Ebert TJ, Muzi M. Propofol and autonomic reflex function in humans. *Anesth Analg*, **1994**, *78*:369–375.

Ebrahim ZY, DeBoer GE, Luders H, et al. Effect of etomidate on the electroencephalogram of patients with epilepsy. *Anesth Analg*, **1986**, *65*:1004–1006.

Eger EI II. New inhaled anesthetics. *Anesthesiology*, **1994**, *80*:906–922.

Eger EI II, Gong D, Xing Y, et al. Acetylcholine receptors and thresholds for convulsions from flurothyl and 1,2-dichlorohexafluorocyclobutane. *Anesth Analg*, **2002**, *95*:1611–1615, table of contents.

Eger EI II, Koblin DD, Bowland T, et al. Nephrotoxicity of sevoflurane versus desflurane anesthesia in volunteers. *Anesth Analg*, **1997**, *84*:160–168.

Fang F, Guo TZ, Davies MF, Maze M. Opiate receptors in the periaqueductal gray mediate analgesic effect of nitrous oxide in rats. *Eur J Pharmacol*, **1997**, *336*:137–141.

Fatheree RS, Leighton BL. Acute respiratory distress syndrome after an exothermic Baralyme-sevoflurane reaction. *Anesthesiology*, **2004**, *101*:531–533.

Fechner J, Schwilden H, Schuttler J. Pharmacokinetics and pharmacodynamics of GPI 15715 or fospropofol (Aquavan injection)—a water-soluble propofol prodrug. *Handb Exp Pharmacol*, **2008**, 253–266.

Fourcade HE, Stevens WC, Larson CP, et al. The ventilatory effects of Forane, a new inhaled anesthetic. *Anesthesiology*, **1971**, *35*:26–31.

Franks NP. Molecular targets underlying general anaesthesia. *Br J Pharmacol*, **2006**, *147(suppl 1)*:S72–S81.

Franks NP. General anaesthesia: From molecular targets to neuronal pathways of sleep and arousal. *Nat Rev Neurosci*, **2008**, *9*:370–386.

Franks NP, Honore E. The TREK K2P channels and their role in general anaesthesia and neuroprotection. *Trends Pharmacol Sci*, **2004**, *25*:601–608.

Frassdorf J, De Hert S, Schlack W. Anaesthesia and myocardial ischaemia/reperfusion injury. *Br J Anaesth*, **2009**, *103*:89–98.

Gin T, Mainland P, Chan MT, Short TG. Decreased thiopental requirements in early pregnancy. *Anesthesiology*, **1997**, *86*: 73–78.

Gold MI, Helrich M. Pulmonary mechanics during general anesthesia: V. Status asthmaticus. *Anesthesiology*, **1970**, *32*: 422–428.

Griffiths MJ, Evans TW. Inhaled nitric oxide therapy in adults. *N Engl J Med*, **2005**, *353*:2683–2695.

Grounds RM, Maxwell DL, Taylor MB, et al. Acute ventilatory changes during i.v. induction of anaesthesia with thiopentone or propofol in man. Studies using inductance plethysmography. *Br J Anaesth*, **1987**, *59*:1098–1102.

Guarracino F. Cerebral monitoring during cardiovascular surgery. *Curr Opin Anaesthesiol*, **2008**, *21*:50–54.

Guyenet PG. The 2008 Carl Ludwig Lecture: Retrotrapezoid nucleus, CO_2 homeostasis, and breathing automaticity. *J Appl Physiol*, **2008**, *105*:404–416.

Haddad E, Lowson SM, Johns RA, Rich GF. Use of inhaled nitric oxide perioperatively and in intensive care patients. *Anesthesiology*, **2000**, *92*:1821–1825.

Hahn M, Baker R, Sullivan S. The effect of four narcotics on cholecystokinin octapeptide stimulated gallbladder contraction. *Aliment Pharmacol Ther*, **1988**, *2*:129–134.

Hall JE, Uhrich TD, Barney JA, et al. Sedative, amnestic, and analgesic properties of small-dose dexmedetomidine infusions. *Anesth Analg*, **2000**, *90*:699–705.

Hanaki C, Fujii K, Morio M, Tashima T. Decomposition of sevoflurane by sodalime. *Hiroshima J Med Sci*, **1987**, *36*: 61–67.

Hanss R, Bein B, Turowski P, et al. The influence of xenon on regulation of the autonomic nervous system in patients at high risk of perioperative cardiac complications. *Br J Anaesth*, **2006**, *96*:427–436.

Hausenloy DJ, Scorrano L. Targeting cell death. *Clin Pharmacol Ther*, **2007**, *82*:370–373.

Head BP, Patel HH, Tsutsumi YM, et al. Caveolin-1 expression is essential for N-methyl-D-aspartate receptor-mediated Src and extracellular signal-regulated kinase 1/2 activation and protection of primary neurons from ischemic cell death. *FASEB J*, **2008**, *22*: 828–840.

Himmelseher S, Durieux ME. Revising a dogma: Ketamine for patients with neurological injury? *Anesth Analg*, **2005**, *101*:524–534, table of contents.

Hintz SR, Van Meurs KP, Perritt R, et al. Neurodevelopmental outcomes of premature infants with severe respiratory failure enrolled in a randomized controlled trial of inhaled nitric oxide. *J Pediatr*, **2007**, *151*:16–22.e3.

Hirshman CA, McCullough RE, Cohen PJ, Weil JV. Hypoxic ventilatory drive in dogs during thiopental, ketamine, or pentobarbital anesthesia. *Anesthesiology*, **1975**, *43*: 628–634.

Hirshman CA, McCullough RE, Cohen PJ, Weil JV. Depression of hypoxic ventilatory response by halothane, enflurane and isoflurane in dogs. *Br J Anaesth*, **1977**, *49*:957–963.

Hopkins SR, Levin DL, Emami K, et al. Advances in magnetic resonance imaging of lung physiology. *J Appl Physiol*, **2007**, *102*:1244–1254.

Jacobs JR, Reves JG, Marty J, et al. Aging increases pharmacodynamic sensitivity to the hypnotic effects of midazolam. *Anesth Analg*, **1995**, *80*:143–148.

Jevtovic-Todorovic V, Beals J, Benshoff N, Olney JW. Prolonged exposure to inhalational anesthetic nitrous oxide kills neurons in adult rat brain. *Neuroscience*, **2003**, *122*:609–616.

Jevtovic-Todorovic V, Todorovic SM, Mennerick S, et al. Nitrous oxide (laughing gas) is an NMDA antagonist, neuroprotectant and neurotoxin. *Nat Med*, **1998**, *4*:460–463.

Kam PC, Cardone D. Propofol infusion syndrome. *Anaesthesia*, **2007**, *62*:690–701.

Kamibayashi T, Maze M. Clinical uses of alpha2-adrenergic agonists. *Anesthesiology*, **2000**, *93*:1345–1349.

Kataria BK, Ved SA, Nicodemus HF, et al. The pharmacokinetics of propofol in children using three different data analysis approaches. *Anesthesiology*, **1994**, *80*:104–122.

Kendig JJ, MacIver MB, Roth SH. Anesthetic actions in the hippocampal formation. *Ann NY Acad Sci*, **1991**, *625*:37–53.

Kettler D, Sonntag H, Donath U, et al. [Haemodynamics, myocardial mechanics, oxygen requirement and oxygenation of the human heart during induction of anaesthesia with etomidate (author's transl)]. *Anaesthesist*, **1974**, *23*:116–121.

Kharasch ED, Armstrong AS, Gunn K, et al. Clinical sevoflurane metabolism and disposition. II. The role of cytochrome P450 2E1 in fluoride and hexafluoroisopropanol formation. *Anesthesiology*, **1995**, *82*:1379–1388.

Kingston HG, Hirshman CA. Perioperative management of the patient with asthma. *Anesth Analg*, **1984**, *63*:844–855.

Klinger G, Beyene J, Shah P, Perlman M. Do hyperoxaemia and hypocapnia add to the risk of brain injury after intrapartum asphyxia? *Arch Dis Child Fetal Neonatal Ed*, **2005**, *90*: F49–F52.

Koblin DD, Eger EI II, Johnson BH, et al. I-653 resists degradation in rats. *Anesth Analg*, **1988**, *67*:534–538.

La Colla L, Albertin A, La Colla G, Mangano A. Faster wash-out and recovery for desflurane vs sevoflurane in morbidly obese patients when no premedication is used. *Br J Anaesth*, **2007**, *99*:353–358.

Lakhlani PP, MacMillan LB, Guo TZ, et al. Substitution of a mutant alpha2a-adrenergic receptor via "hit and run" gene targeting reveals the role of this subtype in sedative, analgesic, and anesthetic-sparing responses in vivo. *Proc Natl Acad Sci USA*, **1997**, *94*:9950–9955.

Langsjo JW, Salmi E, Kaisti KK, et al. Effects of subanesthetic ketamine on regional cerebral glucose metabolism in humans. *Anesthesiology*, **2004**, *100*:1065–1071.

Lefer DJ. A new gaseous signaling molecule emerges: Cardioprotective role of hydrogen sulfide. *Proc Natl Acad Sci USA*, **2007**, *104*:17907–17908.

Lockhart SH, Rampil IJ, Yasuda N, et al. Depression of ventilation by desflurane in humans. *Anesthesiology*, **1991**, *74*:484–488.

Lockwood GG, Franks NP, Downie NA, et al. Feasibility and safety of delivering xenon to patients undergoing coronary artery bypass graft surgery while on cardiopulmonary bypass: Phase I study. *Anesthesiology*, **2006**, *104*:458–465.

Lutty GA, Chan-Ling T, Phelps DL, et al. Proceedings of the Third International Symposium on Retinopathy of Prematurity: An update on ROP from the lab to the nursery (November 2003, Anaheim, California). *Mol Vis*, **2006**, *12*:532–580.

Lynch C III, Baum J, Tenbrinck R. Xenon anesthesia. *Anesthesiology*, **2000**, *92*:865–868.

MacIver MB, Roth SH. Inhalation anaesthetics exhibit pathway-specific and differential actions on hippocampal synaptic responses in vitro. *Br J Anaesth*, **1988**, *60*:680–691.

Mazze RI, Callan CM, Galvez ST, et al. The effects of sevoflurane on serum creatinine and blood urea nitrogen concentrations: A retrospective, twenty-two-center, comparative evaluation of renal function in adult surgical patients. *Anesth Analg*, **2000**, *90*:683–688.

Mazze RI, Calverley RK, Smith NT. Inorganic fluoride nephrotoxicity: prolonged enflurane and halothane anesthesia in volunteers. *Anesthesiology*, **1977**, *46*:265–271.

Mazze RI, Woodruff RE, Heerdt ME. Isoniazid-induced enflurane defluorination in humans. *Anesthesiology*, **1982**, *57*:5–8.

McPherson RW, Briar JE, Traystman RJ. Cerebrovascular responsiveness to carbon dioxide in dogs with 1.4% and 2.8% isoflurane. *Anesthesiology*, **1989**, *70*:843–850.

Meade MO, Granton JT, Matte-Martyn A, et al. A randomized trial of inhaled nitric oxide to prevent ischemia-reperfusion injury after lung transplantation. *Am J Respir Crit Care Med*, **2003**, *167*:1483–1489.

Mizobe T, Maghsoudi K, Sitwala K, et al. Antisense technology reveals the alpha2A adrenoceptor to be the subtype mediating the hypnotic response to the highly selective agonist, dexmedetomidine, in the locus coeruleus of the rat. *J Clin Invest*, **1996**, *98*:1076–1080.

Modica PA, Tempelhoff R. Intracranial pressure during induction of anaesthesia and tracheal intubation with etomidate-induced EEG burst suppression. *Can J Anaesth*, **1992**, *39*:236–241.

Mortola JP. How newborn mammals cope with hypoxia. *Respir Physiol*, **1999**, *116*:95–103.

Mourani PM, Ivy DD, Gao D, Abman SH. Pulmonary vascular effects of inhaled nitric oxide and oxygen tension in bronchopulmonary dysplasia. *Am J Respir Crit Care Med*, **2004**, *170*:1006–1013.

Muizelaar JP, Marmarou A, Ward JD, et al. Adverse effects of prolonged hyperventilation in patients with severe head injury: a randomized clinical trial. *J Neurosurg*, **1991**, *75*:731–739.

Munson ES, Larson CP Jr, Babad AA, et al. The effects of halothane, fluroxene and cyclopropane on ventilation; a comparative study in man. *Anesthesiology*, **1966**, *27*:716–728.

Nadolny EM, Svensson LG. Carbon dioxide field flooding techniques for open heart surgery: monitoring and minimizing potential adverse effects. *Perfusion*, **2000**, *15*:151–153.

Nelson LE, Guo TZ, Lu J, et al. The sedative component of anesthesia is mediated by GABA(A) receptors in an endogenous sleep pathway. *Nat Neurosci*, **2002**, *5*:979–984.

Nishina K, Mikawa K, Maekawa N, et al. Clonidine decreases the dose of thiamylal required to induce anesthesia in children. *Anesth Analg*, **1994**, *79*:766–768.

Nunn JF. Carbon dioxide. In, *Nunn's Applied Respiratory Physiology*. Butterworth-Heineman, Oxford, **2005a**.

Nunn JF. *Hypoxia*. In, *Nunn's Applied Respiratory Physiology*. Butterworth-Heineman, Oxford, **2005b**.

Pagel PS, Kampine JP, Schmeling WT, Warltier DC. Ketamine depresses myocardial contractility as evaluated by the preload recruitable stroke work relationship in chronically instrumented dogs with autonomic nervous system blockade. *Anesthesiology*, **1992**, *76*:564–572.

Parviainen I, Kalviainen R, Ruokonen E. Propofol and barbiturates for the anesthesia of refractory convulsive status epilepticus: Pros and cons. *Neurol Res*, **2007**, *29*:667–671.

Patel AJ, Honore E, Lesage F, et al. Inhalational anesthetics activate two-pore-domain background K+ channels. *Nat Neurosci*, **1999**, *2*:422–426.

Patel P, Sun L. Update on neonatal anesthetic neurotoxicity: Insight into molecular mechanisms and relevance to humans. *Anesthesiology*, **2009**, *110*:703–708.

Pauca AL, Savage RT, Simpson S, Roy RC. Effect of pethidine, fentanyl and morphine on post-operative shivering in man. *Acta Anaesthesiol Scand*, **1984**, *28*:138–143.

Pizov R, Brown RH, Weiss YS, et al. Wheezing during induction of general anesthesia in patients with and without asthma. A randomized, blinded trial. *Anesthesiology*, **1995**, *82*: 1111–1116.

Raines DE, Claycomb RJ, Scheller M, Forman SA. Nonhalogenated alkane anesthetics fail to potentiate agonist actions on two ligand-gated ion channels. *Anesthesiology*, **2001**, *95*:470–477.

Rampil IJ. Anesthetic potency is not altered after hypothermic spinal cord transection in rats. *Anesthesiology*, **1994**, *80*: 606–610.

Rasmussen LS, Schmehl W, Jakobsson J. Comparison of xenon with propofol for supplementary general anaesthesia for knee replacement: a randomized study. *Br J Anaesth*, **2006**, *97*:154–159.

Reynolds DS, Rosahl TW, Cirone J, et al. Sedation and anesthesia mediated by distinct GABA(A) receptor isoforms. *J Neurosci*, **2003**, *23*:8608–8617.

Rooke GA, Choi JH, Bishop MJ. The effect of isoflurane, halothane, sevoflurane, and thiopental/nitrous oxide on respiratory system resistance after tracheal intubation. *Anesthesiology*, **1997**, *86*:1294–1299.

Rosenberg H, Fletcher JE, Seitman D. Pharmacogenetics. In: *Clinical Anesthesia*, Lippincott-Raven, Philadelphia, **1997**.

Rudolph U, Antkowiak B. Molecular and neuronal substrates for general anaesthetics. *Nat Rev Neurosci*, **2004**, *5*:709–720.

Sanders RD, Maze M. Alpha2-adrenoceptor agonists. *Curr Opin Invest Drugs*, **2007**, *8*:25–33.

Sawamura S, Kingery WS, Davies MF, et al. Antinociceptive action of nitrous oxide is mediated by stimulation of noradrenergic neurons in the brainstem and activation of [alpha]2B adrenoceptors. *J Neurosci*, **2000**, *20*:9242–9251.

Servin F, Cockshott ID, Farinotti R, et al. Pharmacokinetics of propofol infusions in patients with cirrhosis. *Br J Anaesth*, **1990**, *65*:177–183.

Sessler DI. Perioperative heat balance. *Anesthesiology*, **2000**, *92*:578–596.

Short TG, Galletly DC, Plummer JL. Hypnotic and anaesthetic action of thiopentone and midazolam alone and in combination. *Br J Anaesth*, **1991**, *66*:13–19.

Sola A. Oxygen for the preterm newborn: One infant at a time. *Pediatrics*, **2008**, *121*:1257.

Sprung J, Schoenwald PK, Schwartz LB. Cardiovascular collapse resulting from thiopental-induced histamine release. *Anesthesiology*, **1997**, *86*:1006–1007.

Stevens WC, Cromwell TH, Halsey MJ, et al. The cardiovascular effects of a new inhalation anesthetic, Forane, in human volunteers at constant arterial carbon dioxide tension. *Anesthesiology*, **1971**, *35*:8–16.

Study SotNH. Summary of the National Halothane Study. Possible association between halothane anesthesia and postoperative hepatic necrosis. *JAMA*, **1966**, *197*:775–788.

Stullken EH, Milde JH, Michenfelder JD, et al. The nonlinear responses of cerebral metabolism to low concentrations of halothane, enflurane, isoflurane, and thiopental. *Anesthesiology*, **1977**, *46*:28–34.

Su PH, Chen JY. Inhaled nitric oxide in the management of preterm infants with severe respiratory failure. *J Perinatol*, **2008**, *28*:112–116.

Sumikawa K, Ishizaka N, Suzaki M. Arrhythmogenic plasma levels of epinephrine during halothane, enflurane, and pentobarbital anesthesia in the dog. *Anesthesiology*, **1983**, *58*: 322–325.

Taylor DR, Pijnenburg MW, Smith AD, De Jongste JC. Exhaled nitric oxide measurements: Clinical application and interpretation. *Thorax*, **2006**, *61*:817–827.

Taylor RW, Zimmerman JL, Dellinger RP, et al. Low-dose inhaled nitric oxide in patients with acute lung injury: A randomized controlled trial. *JAMA*, **2004**, *291*:1603–1609.

Thom SR. Oxidative stress is fundamental to hyperbaric oxygen therapy. *J Appl Physiol*, **2009**, *106*:988–995.

Todd MM, Drummond JC, U HS. The hemodynamic consequences of high-dose methohexital anesthesia in humans. *Anesthesiology*, **1984**, *61*:495–501.

van den Bos GC, Drake AJ, Noble MI. The effect of carbon dioxide upon myocardial contractile performance, blood flow and oxygen consumption. *J Physiol*, **1979**, *287*:149–161.

van Swinderen B, Saifee O, Shebester L, et al. A neomorphic syntaxin mutation blocks volatile-anesthetic action in *Caenorhabditis elegans*. *Proc Natl Acad Sci USA*, **1999**, *96*: 2479–2484.

Veroli P, O'Kelly B, Bertrand F, et al. Extrahepatic metabolism of propofol in man during the anhepatic phase of orthotopic liver transplantation. *Br J Anaesth*, **1992**, *68*:183–186.

Violet JM, Downie DL, Nakisa RC, et al. Differential sensitivities of mammalian neuronal and muscle nicotinic acetylcholine receptors to general anesthetics. *Anesthesiology*, **1997**, *86*:866–874.

Vollenweider FX, Leenders KL, Oye I, et al. Differential psychopathology and patterns of cerebral glucose utilisation produced by (S)- and (R)-ketamine in healthy volunteers using positron emission tomography (PET). *Eur Neuropsychopharmacol*, **1997**, *7*:25–38.

Wagner RL, White PF, Kan PB, et al. Inhibition of adrenal steroidogenesis by the anesthetic etomidate. *N Engl J Med*, **1984**, *310*:1415–1421.

Wang LP, Hermann C, Westrin P. Thiopentone requirements in adults after varying pre-induction doses of fentanyl. *Anaesthesia*, **1996**, *51*:831–835.

Weaver LK, Hopkins RO, Chan KJ, et al. Hyperbaric oxygen for acute carbon monoxide poisoning. *N Engl J Med*, **2002**, *347*:1057–1067.

Weiskopf RB, Cahalan MK, Eger EI, et al. Cardiovascular actions of desflurane in normocarbic volunteers. *Anesth Analog*, **1991**, *73*:143–156.

Whitacre MM, Ellis PP. Outpatient sedation for ocular examination. *Surv Ophthalmol*, **1984**, *28*:643–652.

Winterhalter M, Simon A, Fischer S, et al. Comparison of inhaled iloprost and nitric oxide in patients with pulmonary hypertension during weaning from cardiopulmonary bypass in cardiac surgery: A prospective randomized trial. *J Cardiothorac Vasc Anesth*, **2008**, *22*:406–413.

Wu J, Previte JP, Adler E, et al. Spontaneous ignition, explosion, and fire with sevoflurane and barium hydroxide lime. *Anesthesiology*, **2004a**, *101*:534–537.

Wu XS, Sun JY, Evers AS, et al. Isoflurane inhibits transmitter release and the presynaptic action potential. *Anesthesiology*, **2004b**, *100*:663–670.

Yamakage M. Direct inhibitory mechanisms of halothane on canine tracheal smooth muscle contraction. *Anesthesiology*, **1992**, *77*:546–553.

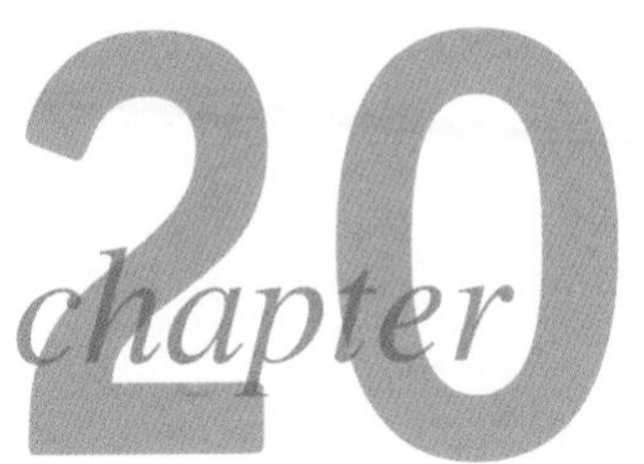

Local Anesthetics

William A. Catterall and
Kenneth Mackie

Local anesthetics bind reversibly to a specific receptor site within the pore of the Na^+ channels in nerves and block ion movement through this pore. When applied locally to nerve tissue in appropriate concentrations, local anesthetics can act on any part of the nervous system and on every type of nerve fiber, reversibly blocking the action potentials responsible for nerve conduction. Thus, a local anesthetic in contact with a nerve trunk can cause both sensory and motor paralysis in the area innervated. These effects of clinically relevant concentrations of local anesthetics are reversible with recovery of nerve function and no evidence of damage to nerve fibers or cells in most clinical applications.

History. The first local anesthetic, cocaine, was serendipitously discovered to have anesthetic properties in the late 19th century. Cocaine occurs in abundance in the leaves of the coca shrub (*Erythroxylon coca*). For centuries, Andean natives have chewed an alkali extract of these leaves for its stimulatory and euphoric actions. Cocaine was first isolated in 1860 by Albert Niemann. He, like many chemists of that era, tasted his newly isolated compound and noted that it caused a numbing of the tongue. Sigmund Freud studied cocaine's physiological actions, and Carl Koller introduced cocaine into clinical practice in 1884 as a topical anesthetic for ophthalmological surgery. Shortly thereafter, Halstead popularized its use in infiltration and conduction block anesthesia.

Chemistry and Structure-Activity Relationship. Cocaine is an ester of benzoic acid and the complex alcohol 2-carbomethoxy, 3-hydroxy-tropane (Figure 20–1). Because of its toxicity and addictive properties (Chapter 24), a search for synthetic substitutes for cocaine began in 1892 with the work of Einhorn and colleagues, resulting in the synthesis of procaine, which became the prototype for local anesthetics for nearly half a century. The most widely used agents today are procaine, lidocaine, bupivacaine, and tetracaine.

The typical local anesthetics contain hydrophilic and hydrophobic moieties that are separated by an intermediate ester or amide linkage (Figure 20–1). A broad range of compounds containing these minimal structural features can satisfy the requirements for action as local anesthetics. The hydrophilic group usually is a tertiary amine but also may be a secondary amine; the hydrophobic moiety must be aromatic. The nature of the linking group determines some of the pharmacological properties of these agents. For example, local anesthetics with an ester link are hydrolyzed readily by plasma esterases.

The structure-activity relationship and the physicochemical properties of local anesthetics have been reviewed by Courtney and Strichartz (1987). Hydrophobicity increases both the potency and the duration of action of the local anesthetics; association of the drug at hydrophobic sites enhances the partitioning of the drug to its sites of action and decreases the rate of metabolism by plasma esterases and hepatic enzymes. In addition, the receptor site for these drugs on Na^+ channels is thought to be hydrophobic (see *Mechanism of Action*), so that receptor affinity for anesthetic agents is greater for more hydrophobic drugs. Hydrophobicity also increases toxicity, so that the therapeutic index is decreased for more hydrophobic drugs.

Molecular size influences the rate of dissociation of local anesthetics from their receptor sites. Smaller drug molecules can escape from the receptor site more rapidly. This characteristic is important in rapidly firing cells, in which local anesthetics bind during action potentials and dissociate during the period of membrane repolarization. Rapid binding of local anesthetics during action potentials causes the frequency- and voltage-dependence of their action.

Mechanism of Action. Local anesthetics act at the cell membrane to prevent the generation and the conduction of nerve impulses. Conduction block can be demonstrated in squid giant axons from which the axoplasm has been removed.

Local anesthetics block conduction by decreasing or preventing the large transient increase in the permeability of excitable membranes to Na^+ that normally is produced by a slight depolarization of the membrane (Chapters 8, 11, and 14) (Strichartz and Ritchie, 1987). This action of local anesthetics is due to their direct interaction with voltage-gated Na^+ channels. As the anesthetic action progressively develops in a nerve, the threshold for electrical excitability gradually increases, the rate of rise of the action potential declines, impulse

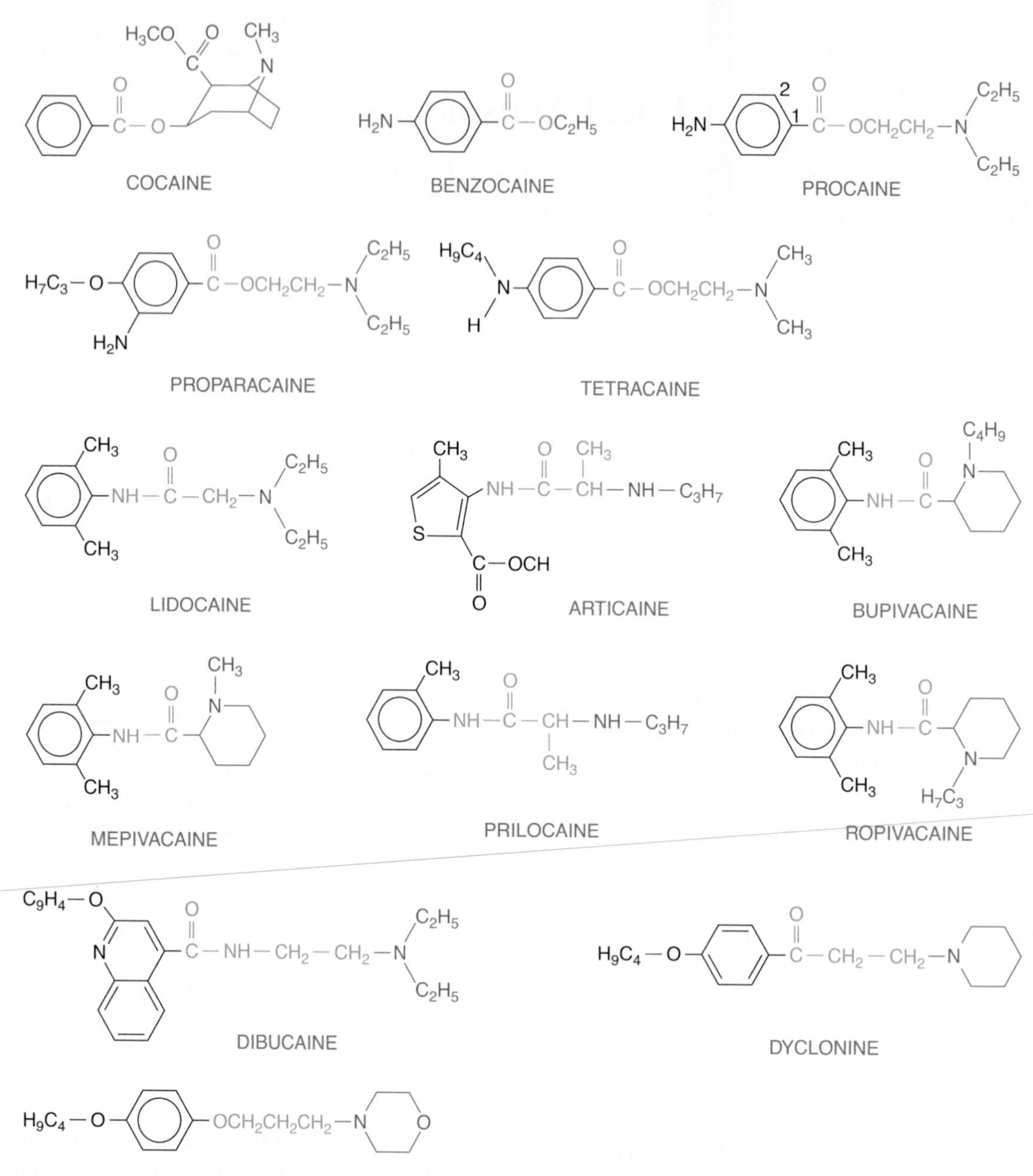

Figure 20–1. *Structural formulas of selected local anesthetics.* Most local anesthetics consist of a hydrophobic (aromatic) moiety (black), a linker region (orange), and a substituted amine (hydrophilic region, in red). The structures above are grouped by the nature of the linker region. Procaine is a prototypic ester-type local anesthetic; esters generally are well hydrolyzed by plasma esterases, contributing to the relatively short duration of action of drugs in this group. Lidocaine is a prototypic amide-type local anesthetic; these structures generally are more resistant to clearance and have longer durations of action. There are exceptions, including benzocaine (poorly water soluble; used only topically) and the structures with a ketone, an amidine, and an ether linkage. Chloroprocaine has a chlorine atom on C2 of the aromatic ring of procaine.

conduction slows, and the safety factor for conduction decreases. These factors decrease the probability of propagation of the action potential, and nerve conduction eventually fails.

Local anesthetics can bind to other membrane proteins (Butterworth and Strichartz, 1990). In particular, they can block K^+ channels (Strichartz and Ritchie, 1987). However, since the interaction of local anesthetics with K^+ channels requires higher concentrations of drug, blockade of conduction is not accompanied by any large or consistent change in resting membrane potential.

Quaternary analogs of local anesthetics block conduction when applied internally to perfused giant axons of squid but are relatively ineffective when applied externally. These observations suggest that the site at which local anesthetics act, at least in their charged form, is accessible only from the inner surface of the membrane (Narahashi and Frazier, 1971; Strichartz and Ritchie, 1987). Therefore, local anesthetics applied externally first must cross the membrane before they can exert a blocking action.

Although a variety of physicochemical models have been proposed to explain how local anesthetics achieve conduction block (Courtney and Strichartz, 1987), it now is generally accepted that the major mechanism of action of these drugs involves their interaction with one or more specific binding sites within the Na^+ channel (Butterworth and Strichartz, 1990). The Na^+ channels of the mammalian brain are complexes of glycosylated proteins with an aggregate molecular size in excess of 300,000 Da; the individual subunits are designated α (260,000 Da) and β_1 to β_4 (33,000-38,000 Da). The large α subunit of the Na^+ channel contains four homologous domains (I-IV); each domain is thought to consist of six transmembrane segments in α-helical conformation (S1-S6; Figure 20–2) and an additional, membrane-reentrant pore (*P*) loop. The Na^+-selective transmembrane pore of the channel presumably resides in the center of a nearly symmetrical structure formed by the four homologous domains. The voltage dependence of channel opening is hypothesized to reflect conformational changes that result from the movement of "gating charges" within the voltage-sensor module of the sodium channel in response to changes in the transmembrane potential. The gating charges are located in the S4 transmembrane helix; the S4 helices are both hydrophobic and positively charged, containing lysine or arginine residues at every third position. It is postulated that these residues move perpendicular to the plane of the membrane under the influence of the transmembrane potential, initiating a series of conformational changes in all four domains, which leads to the open state of the channel (Figure 20–2) (Catterall, 2000; Yu et al., 2005).

The transmembrane pore of the Na^+ channel is thought to be surrounded by the S5 and S6 transmembrane helices and the short membrane-associated segments between them that form the *P* loop. Amino acid residues in these short segments are the most critical determinants of the ion conductance and selectivity of the channel.

After it opens, the Na^+ channel inactivates within a few milliseconds due to closure of an inactivation gate. This functional gate is formed by the short intracellular loop of protein that connects homologous domains III and IV (Figure 20–2). This loop folds over the intracellular mouth of the transmembrane pore during the process of inactivation and binds to an inactivation gate "receptor" formed by the intracellular mouth of the pore.

Amino acid residues important for local anesthetic binding are found in the S6 segments in domains I, III, and IV (Ragsdale et al., 1994; Yarov-Yarovoy et al., 2002). Hydrophobic amino acid residues near the center and the intracellular end of the S6 segment may interact directly with bound local anesthetics (Figure 20–3). Experimental mutation of a large hydrophobic amino acid residue (isoleucine) to a smaller one (alanine) near the extracellular end of this segment creates a pathway for access of charged local anesthetic drugs from the extracellular solution to the receptor site. These findings place the local anesthetic receptor site within the intracellular half of the transmembrane pore of the Na^+ channel, with part of its structure contributed by amino acids in the S6 segments of domains I, III, and IV.

Frequency- and Voltage-Dependence of Local Anesthetic Action. The degree of block produced by a given concentration of local anesthetic depends on how the nerve has been stimulated and on its resting membrane potential. Thus, a resting nerve is much less sensitive to a local anesthetic than one that is repetitively stimulated; higher frequency of stimulation and more positive membrane potential cause a greater degree of anesthetic block. These frequency- and voltage-dependent effects of local anesthetics occur because the local anesthetic molecule in its charged form gains access to its binding site within the pore only when the Na^+ channel is in an open state and because the local anesthetic binds more tightly to and stabilizes the inactivated state of the Na^+ channel (Butterworth and Strichartz, 1990; Courtney and Strichartz, 1987). Local anesthetics exhibit these properties to different extents depending on their pK_a, lipid solubility, and molecular size. In general, the frequency dependence of local anesthetic action depends critically on the rate of dissociation from the receptor site in the pore of the Na^+ channel. A high frequency of stimulation is required for rapidly dissociating drugs so that drug binding during the action potential exceeds drug dissociation between action potentials. Dissociation of smaller and more hydrophobic drugs is more rapid, so a higher frequency of stimulation is required to yield frequency-dependent block. Frequency-dependent block of ion channels is most important for the actions of antiarrhythmic drugs (Chapter 29).

Differential Sensitivity of Nerve Fibers to Local Anesthetics. Although there is great individual variation, for most patients treatment with local anesthetics causes the sensation of pain to disappear first, followed by loss of the sensations of temperature, touch, deep pressure, and finally motor function (Table 20–1). Classical experiments with intact nerves showed that the δ wave in the compound action potential, which represents slowly conducting, small-diameter myelinated fibers, was reduced more rapidly and at lower concentrations of cocaine than was the α wave, which represents rapidly conducting, large-diameter fibers (Gasser and Erlanger, 1929). In general, autonomic fibers, small

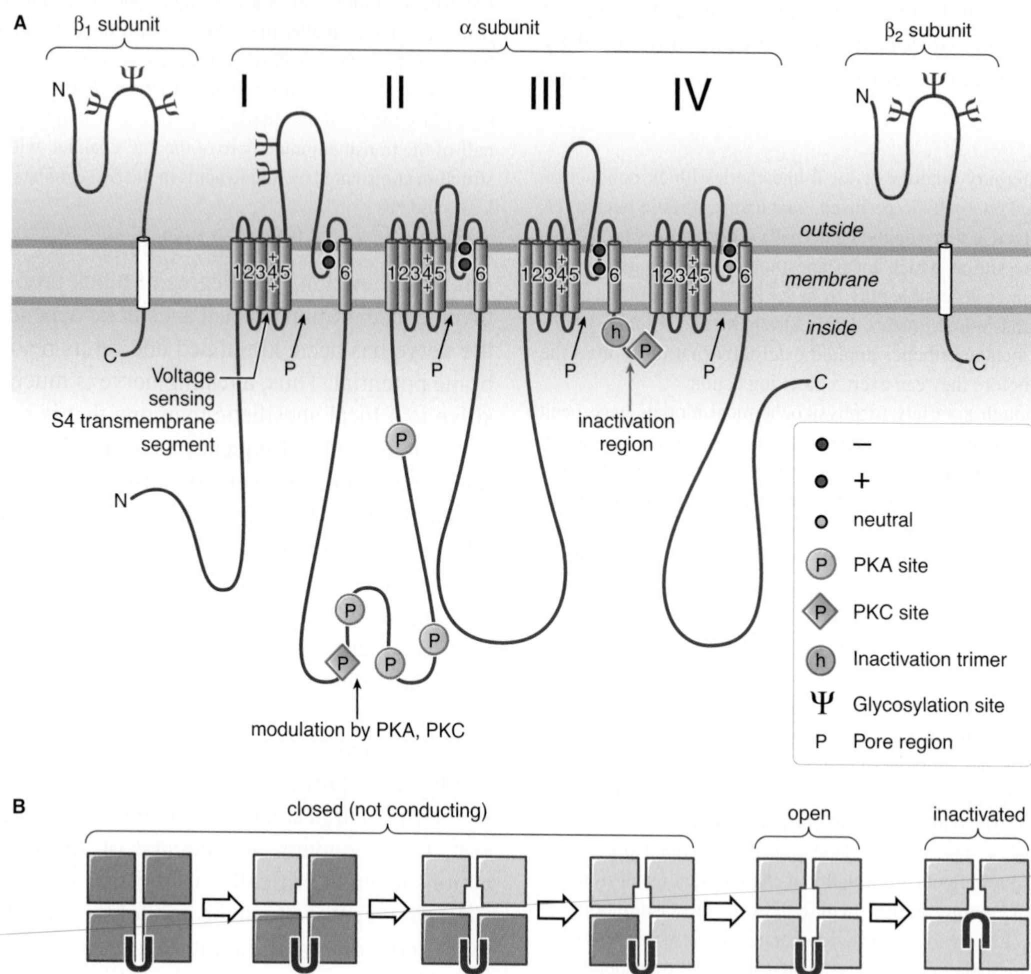

B

closed (not conducting)

open

inactivated

Figure 20–2. *Structure and function of voltage-gated Na^+ channels. **A***. A two-dimensional representation of the α (center), β_1 (left), and β_2 (right) subunits of the voltage-gated Na^+ channel from mammalian brain. The polypeptide chains are represented by continuous lines with length approximately proportional to the actual length of each segment of the channel protein. Cylinders represent regions of transmembrane α helices. ψ indicates sites of demonstrated N-linked glycosylation. Note the repeated structure of the four homologous domains (I-IV) of the α subunit. **Voltage Sensing**. The S4 transmembrane segments in each homologous domain of the α subunit serve as voltage sensors. (+) represents the positively charged amino acid residues at every third position within these segments. Electrical field (negative inside) exerts a force on these charged amino acid residues, pulling them toward the intracellular side of the membrane; depolarization allows them to move outward. **Pore**. The S5 and S6 transmembrane segments and the short membrane-associated loop between them (*P* loop) form the walls of the pore in the center of an approximately symmetrical square array of the four homologous domains (see panel ***B***). The amino acid residues indicated by circles in the *P* loop are critical for determining the conductance and ion selectivity of the Na^+ channel and its ability to bind the extracellular pore-blocking toxins tetrodotoxin and saxitoxin. **Inactivation**. The short intracellular loop connecting homologous domains III and IV serves as the inactivation gate of the Na^+ channel. It is thought to fold into the intracellular mouth of the pore and occlude it within a few milliseconds after the channel opens. Three hydrophobic residues (isoleucine–phenylalanine–methionine; IFM) at the position marked **h** appear to serve as an inactivation particle, entering the intracellular mouth of the pore and binding therein to an inactivation gate receptor there. **Modulation**. The gating of the Na^+ channel can be modulated by protein phosphorylation. Phosphorylation of the inactivation gate between homologous domains III and IV by PKC slows inactivation. Phosphorylation of sites in the intracellular loop between homologous domains I and II by either PKC or PKA reduces Na^+ channel activation. (Adapted from Catterall, 2000, with permission.Copyright © Elsevier.). ***B***. The four homologous domains of the Na^+ channel α subunit are illustrated as a square array, as viewed looking down on the membrane. The sequence of conformational changes that the Na^+ channel undergoes during activation and inactivation is diagrammed. Upon depolarization, each of the four homologous domains sequentially undergoes a conformational change to an activated state. After all four domains have activated, the Na^+ channel can open. Within a few milliseconds after opening, the inactivation gate between domains III and IV closes over the intracellular mouth of the channel and occludes it, preventing further ion conductance (see Catterall, 2000).

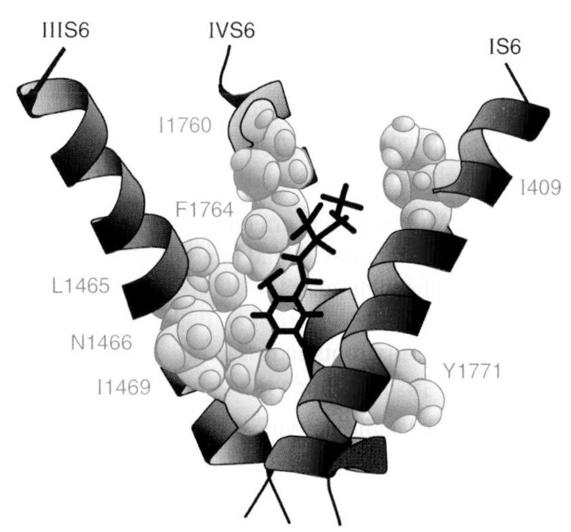

Figure 20–3. *The local anesthetic receptor site. **A**.* A drawing of the pore structure of a bacterial K^+ channel (KcsA), which is related to the sodium channel. The KcsA channel has two transmembrane segments, analogous to the S5 and S6 segments of sodium channels. The S6-like segment forms the walls of the inner pore while the *P* loop forms the narrow ion selectivity filter at its extracellular (top) end. Four separate KcsA subunits form the pore in their center; only two of the subunits are shown here. ***B***. A structural model of the local anesthetic receptor site. The S6 segments from domains I, III, and IV of the sodium channel α subunit are illustrated, based on the structure of the KcsA channel (panel ***A***). The amino acid residues in these three transmembrane segments that contribute to the local anesthetic receptor site are indicated in single letter code and are presented in space-filling representation (light blue). An etidocaine molecule (black) is illustrated bound in the receptor site. Substitutions of the light blue residues with alanine reduce the affinity for local anesthetic block of sodium channels. It therefore is likely that the side chains of these amino acid residues contact bound local anesthetics in their receptor site. I1760 and I409 likely form the outer boundary of the local anesthetic receptor site. Mutations of I1760 allow drug access to the receptor site from the extracellular side. (This figure was originally published in the Journal of Biological Chemistry. Yarov-Yarovoy V, McPhee JC, Idsvoog D, Pate C, Scheuer T, Catterall WA: Role of amino acid resides in transmembrane segments IS6 and IIS6 of the Na^+ channel alpha subunit in voltage-dependent gating and drug block. *J Biol Chem* 2002:277, 35393. © the American Society for Biochemistry and Molecular Biology.)

unmyelinated C fibers (mediating pain sensations), and small myelinated Aδ fibers (mediating pain and temperature sensations) are blocked before the larger myelinated Aγ, Aβ, and Aα fibers (mediating postural, touch, pressure, and motor information) (Raymond and Gissen, 1987). *The differential rate of block exhibited by fibers mediating different sensations is of considerable practical importance in the use of local anesthetics.*

The precise mechanisms responsible for this apparent specificity of local anesthetic action on pain fibers are not known, but several factors may contribute. The initial hypothesis from the classical work on intact nerves was that sensitivity to local anesthetic block increases with decreasing fiber size, consistent with high sensitivity for pain sensation mediated by small fibers and low sensitivity for motor function mediated by large fibers (Gasser and Erlanger, 1929). However, when nerve fibers are dissected from nerves to allow direct measurement of action potential generation, no clear correlation of the concentration dependence of local anesthetic block with fiber diameter is observed (Fink and Cairns, 1984; Franz and Perry, 1974; Huang et al., 1997). Therefore, it is unlikely that the fiber size *per se* determines the sensitivity to local anesthetic block under steady-state conditions. However, the spacing of nodes of Ranvier increases with the size of nerve fibers. Because a fixed number of nodes must be blocked to prevent conduction, small fibers with closely spaced nodes of Ranvier may be blocked more rapidly during treatment of intact nerves, because the local anesthetic reaches a critical length of nerve more rapidly (Franz and Perry, 1974). Differences in tissue barriers and location of smaller C fibers and Aδ fibers in nerves also may influence the rate of local anesthetic action.

Effect of pH. Local anesthetics tend to be only slightly soluble as unprotonated amines. Therefore, they generally are marketed as water-soluble salts, usually hydrochlorides. Inasmuch as the local anesthetics are weak bases (typical pK_a values range from 8-9), their hydrochloride salts are mildly acidic. This property increases the stability of the local anesthetic esters and the catecholamines added as vasoconstrictors. Under usual conditions of administration, the pH of the local anesthetic solution rapidly equilibrates to that of the extracellular fluids.

Although the unprotonated species of the local anesthetic is necessary for diffusion across cellular membranes, it is the cationic such as methylparaben that may provoke an allergic reaction (Covino, 1987). Local anesthetic preparations containing a vasoconstrictor also may elicit allergic responses due to the sulfite added as an antioxidant for the catecholamine/vasoconstrictor.

Metabolism of Local Anesthetics. The metabolic fate of local anesthetics is of great practical importance, because their toxicity depends largely on the balance between their rates of absorption and elimination. As noted earlier, the rate of absorption of many anesthetics can be reduced considerably by the incorporation of a vasoconstrictor agent in the anesthetic solution. However, the rate of degradation of local anesthetics varies greatly, and this is a major factor in determining the safety of a particular agent. Since toxicity is related to the free concentration of drug, binding of the anesthetic to proteins in the serum and to tissues reduces the concentration of free drug in the systemic circulation, and consequently reduces toxicity. For example, in intravenous regional anesthesia of an extremity, about half of the original anesthetic dose still is tissue-bound 30 minutes after the restoration of normal blood flow (Arthur, 1987).

Some of the common local anesthetics (e.g., tetracaine) are esters. They are hydrolyzed and inactivated primarily by a plasma esterase, probably plasma cholinesterase. The liver also participates in hydrolysis of local anesthetics. Since spinal fluid contains little or no esterase, anesthesia produced by the intrathecal injection of an anesthetic agent will persist until the local anesthetic agent has been absorbed into the circulation.

The amide-linked local anesthetics are, in general, degraded by the hepatic CYPs the initial reactions involving *N*-dealkylation and subsequent hydrolysis (Arthur, 1987). However, with prilocaine, the initial step is hydrolytic, forming *o*-toluidine metabolites that can cause methemoglobinemia. The extensive use of amide-linked local anesthetics in patients with severe hepatic disease requires caution. The amide-linked local anesthetics are extensively (55-95%) bound to plasma proteins, particularly α_1-acid glycoprotein. Many factors increase (e.g., cancer, surgery, trauma, myocardial infarction, smoking, and uremia) or decrease (e.g., oral contraceptives) the level of this glycoprotein, thereby changing the amount of anesthetic delivered to the liver for metabolism and thus influencing systemic toxicity. Age-related changes in protein binding of local anesthetics also occur. The neonate is relatively deficient in plasma proteins that bind local anesthetics and thereby is more susceptible to toxicity. Plasma proteins are not the sole determinant of local anesthetic availability. Uptake by the lung also may play an important role in the distribution of amide-linked local anesthetics in the body. Reduced cardiac output slows delivery of the amide compounds to the liver, reducing their metabolism and prolonging their plasma half-lives.

COCAINE

Chemistry. Cocaine, an ester of benzoic acid and methylecgonine, occurs in abundance in the leaves of the coca shrub. Ecgonine is an amino alcohol base closely related to tropine, the amino alcohol in atropine. It has the same fundamental structure as the synthetic local anesthetics (Figure 20–1).

Pharmacological Actions and Preparations. The clinically desired actions of cocaine are the blockade of nerve impulses, as a consequence of its local anesthetic properties, and local vasoconstriction, secondary to inhibition of local NE reuptake. Toxicity and its potential for abuse have steadily decreased the clinical uses of cocaine. Its high toxicity is due to reduced catecholamine uptake in both the central and peripheral nervous systems. Its euphoric properties are due primarily to inhibition of catecholamine uptake, particularly DA, in the CNS. Other local anesthetics do not block the uptake of NE and do not produce the sensitization to catecholamines, vasoconstriction, or mydriasis characteristic of cocaine. Currently, cocaine is used primarily for topical anesthesia of the upper respiratory tract, where its combination of both vasoconstrictor and local anesthetic properties provide anesthesia and shrinking of the mucosa. Cocaine hydrochloride is provided as a 1%, 4%, or 10% solution for topical application. For most applications, the 1% or 4% preparation is preferred to reduce toxicity. Because of its abuse potential, cocaine is listed as a schedule II controlled substance by the U.S. Drug Enforcement Agency.

LIDOCAINE

Lidocaine (XYLOCAINE, others), an aminoethylamide (Figure 20–1), is the prototypical amide local anesthetic.

Pharmacological Actions. Lidocaine produces faster, more intense, longer-lasting, and more extensive anesthesia than does an equal concentration of procaine. Lidocaine is an alternative choice for individuals sensitive to ester-type local anesthetics.

Absorption, Fate, and Excretion. Lidocaine is absorbed rapidly after parenteral administration and from the GI and respiratory tracts. Although it is effective when used without any vasoconstrictor, epinephrine decreases the rate of absorption, such that the toxicity is decreased and the duration of action usually is prolonged. In addition to preparations for injection, lidocaine is formulated for topical, opthalmic, mucosal, and transdermal use.

A lidocaine transdermal patch (LIDODERM) is used for relief of pain associated with postherpetic neuralgia. An oral patch (DENTIPATCH) is available for application to accessible mucous membranes of the mouth prior to superficial dental procedures. The combination of lidocaine (2.5%) and prilocaine (2.5%) in an occlusive dressing (EMLA, others) is used as an anesthetic prior to venipuncture, skin graft harvesting, and infiltration of anesthetics into genitalia. Lidocaine in combination with tetracaine (PLIAGLIS) in a formulation that generates a "peel" is approved for topical local analgesia prior to superficial dermatological procedures such as filler injections and laser-based treatments. Lidocaine in combination with tetracaine is marketed in a formulation that generates heat upon exposure to air (SYNERA), which is used prior to venous access and superficial dermatological procedures such as excision, electrodessication, and shave biopsy of skin lesions. The mild warming is intended to increase skin temperature by up to 5°C for the purpose of enhancing delivery of local anesthetic into the skin.

Lidocaine is dealkylated in the liver by CYPs to monoethylglycine xylidide and glycine xylidide, which can be metabolized further to monoethylglycine and xylidide. Both monoethylglycine xylidide and glycine xylidide retain local anesthetic activity. In humans, ~75% of the xylidide is excreted in the urine as the further metabolite 4-hydroxy-2, 6-dimethylaniline (Arthur, 1987).

Toxicity. The side effects of lidocaine seen with increasing dose include drowsiness, tinnitus, dysgeusia, dizziness, and twitching. As the dose increases, seizures, coma, and respiratory depression and arrest will occur. Clinically significant cardiovascular depression usually occurs at serum lidocaine levels that produce marked CNS effects. The metabolites monoethylglycine xylidide and glycine xylidide may contribute to some of these side effects.

Clinical Uses. Lidocaine has a wide range of clinical uses as a local anesthetic; it has utility in almost any application where a local anesthetic of intermediate duration is needed. Lidocaine also is used as an antiarrhythmic agent (Chapter 29).

BUPIVACAINE

Pharmacological Actions. Bupivacaine (MARCAINE, SENSORCAINE, others), is a widely used amide local anesthetic; its structure is similar to that of lidocaine except that the amine-containing group is a butyl piperidine (Figure 20–1). Bupivacaine is a potent agent capable of producing prolonged anesthesia. Its long duration of action plus its tendency to provide more sensory than motor block has made it a popular drug for providing prolonged analgesia during labor or the postoperative period. By taking advantage of indwelling catheters and continuous infusions, bupivacaine can be used to provide several days of effective analgesia.

Toxicity. Bupivacaine is more cardiotoxic than equi-effective doses of lidocaine. Clinically, this is manifested by severe ventricular arrhythmias and myocardial depression after inadvertent intravascular administration. Although lidocaine and bupivacaine both rapidly block cardiac Na^+channels during systole, bupivacaine dissociates much more slowly than does lidocaine during diastole, so a significant fraction of Na^+ channels at physiological heart rates remains blocked with bupivacaine at the end of diastole (Clarkson and Hondeghem, 1985). Thus, the block by bupivacaine is cumulative and substantially more than would be predicted by its local anesthetic potency. At least a portion of the cardiac toxicity of bupivacaine may be mediated centrally, as direct injection of small quantities of bupivacaine into the medulla can produce malignant ventricular arrhythmias (Thomas et al., 1986). Bupivacaine-induced cardiac toxicity can be very difficult to treat, and its severity is enhanced by coexisting acidosis, hypercarbia, and hypoxemia.

OTHER SYNTHETIC LOCAL ANESTHETICS

The number of synthetic local anesthetics is so large that it is impractical to consider them all here. Some local anesthetic agents are too toxic to be given by injection. Their use is restricted to topical application to the eye (Chapter 64), the mucous membranes, or the skin (Chapter 65). Many local anesthetics are suitable, however, for infiltration or injection to produce nerve block; some of these also are useful for topical application. The main categories of local anesthetics are given in the following discussion; agents are listed alphabetically. See Figure 20–1 for their structures.

Local Anesthetics Suitable for Injection

Articaine. Articaine (SEPTOCAINE) is approved in the U.S. for dental and periodontal procedures. Although it is an amide local anesthetic, it also contains an ester, whose hydrolysis terminates its action. Thus, articaine exhibits a rapid onset (1-6 minutes) and duration of action of ~1 hour.

Chloroprocaine. Chloroprocaine (NESACAINE, others) is a chlorinated derivative of procaine. Its major assets are its rapid onset and short duration of action and its reduced acute toxicity due to its rapid metabolism (plasma $t_{1/2}$ ~25 seconds). Enthusiasm for its use has been tempered by reports of prolonged sensory and motor block after epidural or subarachnoid administration of large doses. This toxicity appears to have been a consequence of low pH and the use of sodium metabisulfite as a preservative in earlier formulations. There are no reports of neurotoxicity with newer preparations of chloroprocaine, which contain calcium EDTA as the preservative, although these preparations also are not recommended for intrathecal administration. A higher than expected incidence of muscular back pain following epidural anesthesia with 2-chloroprocaine has also been reported (Stevens et al., 1993). This back pain is thought to be due to tetany in the paraspinus muscles, which may be a consequence of Ca^{2+} binding by the EDTA included as a preservative; the incidence of back pain appears to be related to the volume of drug injected and its use for skin infiltration.

Mepivacaine. Mepivacaine (CARBOCAINE, POLOCAINE, others) is an intermediate-acting amino amide. Its pharmacological properties are similar to those of lidocaine. Mepivacaine, however, is more toxic to the neonate and thus is not used in obstetrical anesthesia. The increased toxicity of mepivacaine in the neonate is related to ion trapping of this agent because of the lower pH of neonatal blood and the pK_a of mepivacaine rather than to its slower metabolism in the neonate. It appears to have a slightly higher therapeutic index in adults than does lidocaine. Its onset of action is similar to that of lidocaine and its duration slightly longer (~20%) than that of lidocaine in the absence of a co-administered vasoconstrictor. Mepivacaine is not effective as a topical anesthetic.

Prilocaine. Prilocaine (CITANEST) is an intermediate-acting amino amide. It has a pharmacological profile similar to that of lidocaine. The primary differences are that it causes little vasodilation and thus can be used without a vasoconstrictor, and its increased volume of distribution reduces its CNS toxicity, making it suitable for intravenous regional blocks (described later). The use of prilocaine is largely limited to dentistry because the drug is unique among the local anesthetics in its propensity to cause methemoglobinemia. This effect is a consequence of the metabolism of the aromatic ring to *o*-toluidine. Development of methemoglobinemia is dependent on the total dose administered, usually appearing after a dose of 8 mg/kg. If necessary, it can be treated by the intravenous administration of methylene blue (1-2 mg/kg). Methemoglobinemia following prilocaine has limited its use in obstetrical anesthesia, because it amount of cream that can be applied and area of skin covered. These mixtures must not be used on mucous membranes or abraded skin, as rapid absorption across these surfaces may result in systemic toxicity.

Infiltration Anesthesia

Infiltration anesthesia is the injection of local anesthetic directly into tissue without taking into consideration the course of cutaneous nerves. Infiltration anesthesia can be so superficial as to include only the skin. It also can include deeper structures, including intra-abdominal organs, when these too are infiltrated.

The duration of infiltration anesthesia can be approximately doubled by the addition of epinephrine (5 μg/mL) to the injection solution; epinephrine also decreases peak concentrations of local anesthetics in blood. *Epinephrine-containing solutions should not, however, be injected into tissues supplied by end arteries—for example, fingers and toes, ears, the nose, and the penis. The resulting vasoconstriction may cause gangrene.* For the same reason, epinephrine should be avoided in solutions injected intracutaneously. Since epinephrine also is absorbed into the circulation, its use should be avoided in those for whom adrenergic stimulation is undesirable.

The local anesthetics used most frequently for infiltration anesthesia are lidocaine (0.5-1%), procaine (0.5-1%), and bupivacaine (0.125-0.25%). When used without epinephrine, up to 4.5 mg/kg of lidocaine, 7 mg/kg of procaine, or 2 mg/kg of bupivacaine can be employed in adults. When epinephrine is added, these amounts can be increased by one-third.

The advantage of infiltration anesthesia and other regional anesthetic techniques is that it can provide satisfactory anesthesia without disrupting normal bodily functions. The chief disadvantage of infiltration anesthesia is that relatively large amounts of drug must be used to anesthetize relatively small areas. This is no problem with minor surgery. When major surgery is performed, however, the amount of local anesthetic that is required makes systemic toxic reactions likely. The amount of anesthetic required to anesthetize an area can be reduced significantly and the duration of anesthesia increased markedly by specifically blocking the nerves that innervate the area of interest. This can be done at one of several levels: subcutaneously, at major nerves, or at the level of the spinal roots.

Field Block Anesthesia

Field block anesthesia is produced by subcutaneous injection of a solution of local anesthetic in order to anesthetize the region distal to the injection. For example, subcutaneous infiltration of the proximal portion of the volar surface of the forearm results in an extensive area of cutaneous anesthesia that starts 2-3 cm distal to the site of injection. The same principle can be applied with particular benefit to the scalp, the anterior abdominal wall, and the lower extremity.

The drugs, concentrations, and doses recommended are the same as for infiltration anesthesia. The advantage of field block anesthesia is that less drug can be used to provide a greater area of anesthesia than when infiltration anesthesia is used. Knowledge of the relevant neuroanatomy obviously is essential for successful field block anesthesia.

Nerve Block Anesthesia

Injection of a solution of a local anesthetic into or about individual peripheral nerves or nerve plexuses produces even greater areas of anesthesia than do the techniques already described. Blockade of mixed peripheral nerves and nerve plexuses also usually anesthetizes somatic motor nerves, producing skeletal muscle relaxation, which is essential for some surgical procedures. The areas of sensory and motor block usually start several centimeters distal to the site of injection. Brachial plexus blocks are particularly useful for procedures on the upper extremity and shoulder. Intercostal nerve blocks are effective for anesthesia and relaxation of the anterior abdominal wall. Cervical plexus block is appropriate for surgery of the neck. Sciatic and femoral nerve blocks are useful for surgery distal to the knee. Other useful nerve blocks prior to surgical procedures include blocks of individual nerves at the wrist and at the ankle, blocks of individual nerves such as the median or ulnar at the elbow, and blocks of sensory cranial nerves.

There are four major determinants of the onset of sensory anesthesia following injection near a nerve:

- proximity of the injection to the nerve
- concentration and volume of drug
- degree of ionization of the drug
- time

Local anesthetic is never intentionally injected into the nerve, as this would be painful and could cause nerve damage. Instead, the anesthetic agent is deposited as close to the nerve as possible. Thus the local anesthetic must diffuse from the site of injection into the nerve, where it acts. The rate of diffusion is determined chiefly by the concentration of the drug, its degree of ionization (ionized local anesthetic diffuses more slowly), its hydrophobicity, and the physical characteristics of the tissue surrounding the nerve. Higher concentrations of local anesthetic will provide a more rapid onset of peripheral nerve block. The utility of higher concentrations, however, is limited by systemic toxicity and by direct neural toxicity of concentrated local anesthetic solutions. For a given concentration, local anesthetics with lower pK_a values tend to have a more rapid onset of action because more drug is uncharged at neutral pH. For example, the onset of action of lidocaine occurs in ~3 minutes; 35% of lidocaine is in the basic form at pH 7.4. In contrast, the onset of action of bupivacaine requires ~15 minutes; only 5-10% of bupivacaine is uncharged at this pH. Increased hydrophobicity might be expected to speed onset by increased penetration into nerve tissue. However, it also will increase binding in tissue lipids. Furthermore, the more hydrophobic local anesthetics also are more potent (and toxic) and thus must be used at lower concentrations, decreasing the concentration gradient for diffusion. Tissue factors also play a role in determining the rate of onset of anesthetic effects. The amount of connective tissue that must be penetrated can be significant in a nerve plexus compared to isolated nerves and can slow or even prevent adequate diffusion of local anesthetic to the nerve fibers.

Duration of nerve block anesthesia depends on the physical characteristics of the local anesthetic used and the presence or absence of vasoconstrictors. Especially important physical characteristics are lipid solubility and protein binding. Local anesthetics can be broadly divided into three categories:

- those with a short (20-45 minutes) duration of action in mixed peripheral nerves, such as procaine
- those with an intermediate (60-120 minutes) duration of action, such as lidocaine and mepivacaine

- those with a long (400-450 minutes) duration of action, such as bupivacaine, ropivacaine, and tetracaine

Block duration of the intermediate-acting local anesthetics such as lidocaine can be prolonged by the addition of epinephrine (5 μg/mL). The degree of block prolongation in peripheral nerves following the addition of epinephrine appears to be related to the intrinsic vasodilatory properties of the local anesthetic and thus is most pronounced with lidocaine.

The types of nerve fibers that are blocked when a local anesthetic is injected about a mixed peripheral nerve depend on the concentration of drug used, nerve-fiber size, internodal distance, and frequency and pattern of nerve-impulse transmission (see above, sections on *Frequency and Voltage-Dependence* and *Differential Sensitivity*). Anatomical factors are similarly important. A mixed peripheral nerve or nerve trunk consists of individual nerves surrounded by an investing epineurium. The vascular supply usually is centrally located. When a local anesthetic is deposited about a peripheral nerve, it diffuses from the outer surface toward the core along a concentration gradient (DeJong, 1994; Winnie et al., 1977). Consequently, nerves in the outer mantle of the mixed nerve are blocked first. These fibers usually are distributed to more proximal anatomical structures than are those situated near the core of the mixed nerve and often are motor. If the volume and concentration of local anesthetic solution deposited about the nerve are adequate, the local anesthetic eventually will diffuse inward in amounts adequate to block even the most centrally located fibers. Lesser amounts of drug will block only nerves in the mantle and the smaller and more sensitive central fibers. Furthermore, since removal of local anesthetics occurs primarily in the core of a mixed nerve or nerve trunk, where the vascular supply is located, the duration of blockade of centrally located nerves is shorter than that of more peripherally situated fibers.

The choice of local anesthetic and the amount and concentration administered are determined by the nerves and the types of fibers to be blocked, the required duration of anesthesia, and the size and health of the patient. For blocks of 2-4 hours, lidocaine (1-1.5%) can be used in the amounts recommended earlier (see "Infiltration Anesthesia"). Mepivacaine (up to 7 mg/kg of a 1-2% solution) provides anesthesia that lasts about as long as that from lidocaine. Bupivacaine (2-3 mg/kg of a 0.25-0.375% solution) can be used when a longer duration of action is required. Addition of 5 μg/mL epinephrine slows systemic absorption and therefore prolongs duration and lowers the plasma concentration of the intermediate-acting local anesthetics.

Peak plasma concentrations of local anesthetics depend on the amount injected, the physical characteristics of the local anesthetic, whether epinephrine is used, the rate of blood flow to the site of injection, and the surface area exposed to local anesthetic. This is of particular importance in the safe application of nerve block anesthesia, since the potential for systemic reactions is related to peak free serum concentrations. For example, peak concentrations of lidocaine in blood following injection of 400 mg without epinephrine for intercostal nerve blocks average 7 μg/mL; the same amount of lidocaine used for block of the brachial plexus results in peak concentrations in blood of ~3 μg/mL (Covino and Vassallo, 1976). Therefore, the amount of local anesthetic that can be injected must be adjusted according to the anatomical site of the nerve(s) to be blocked to minimize untoward effects. Addition of epinephrine can decrease peak plasma concentrations by 20-30%. Multiple nerve blocks (e.g., intercostal block) or blocks performed in vascular regions require reduction in the amount of anesthetic that can be given safely, because the surface area for absorption or the rate of absorption is increased.

Intravenous Regional Anesthesia (Bier's Block)

This technique relies on using the vasculature to bring the local anesthetic solution to the nerve trunks and endings. In this technique, an extremity is exsanguinated with an Esmarch (elastic) bandage, and a proximally located tourniquet is inflated to 100-150 mm Hg above the systolic blood pressure. The Esmarch bandage is removed, and the local anesthetic is injected into a previously cannulated vein. Typically, complete anesthesia of the limb ensues within 5-10 minutes. Pain from the tourniquet and the potential for ischemic nerve injury limits tourniquet inflation to 2 hours or less. However, the tourniquet should remain inflated for at least 15-30 minutes to prevent toxic amounts of local anesthetic from entering the circulation following deflation. Lidocaine, 40-50 mL (0.5 mL/kg in children) of a 0.5% solution without epinephrine is the drug of choice for this technique. For intravenous regional anesthesia in adults using a 0.5% solution without epinephrine, the dose administered should not exceed 4 mg/kg. A few clinicians prefer prilocaine (0.5%) over lidocaine because of its higher therapeutic index. The attractiveness of this technique lies in its simplicity. Its primary disadvantages are that it can be used only for a few anatomical regions, sensation (pain) returns quickly after tourniquet deflation, and premature release or failure of the tourniquet can produce toxic levels of local anesthetic (e.g., 50 mL of 0.5% lidocaine contains 250 mg of lidocaine). For the last reason and because its longer durations of action offer no advantage, the more cardiotoxic local anesthetic, bupivacaine, is not recommended for this technique. Intravenous regional anesthesia is used most often for surgery of the forearm and hand, but can be adapted for the foot and distal leg.

Spinal Anesthesia

Spinal anesthesia follows the injection of local anesthetic into the cerebrospinal fluid (CSF) in the lumbar space. For a number of reasons, including the ability to produce anesthesia of a considerable fraction of the body with a dose of local anesthetic that produces negligible plasma levels, spinal anesthesia remains one of the most popular forms of anesthesia. In most adults, the spinal cord terminates above the second lumbar vertebra; between that point and the termination of the thecal sac in the sacrum, the lumbar and sacral roots are bathed in CSF. Thus, in this region there is a relatively large volume of CSF within which to inject drug, thereby minimizing the potential for direct nerve trauma.

A brief discussion of the physiological effects of spinal anesthesia relating to the pharmacology of the local anesthetics used is presented here. See more specialized texts (e.g., Cousins et al., 2008) for additional details.

Physiological Effects of Spinal Anesthesia. Most of the physiological side effects of spinal anesthesia are a consequence of the sympathetic blockade produced by local anesthetic block of the sympathetic fibers in the spinal nerve roots. A thorough understanding of these physiological effects is necessary for the safe and successful application of spinal anesthesia. Although some of them may be deleterious and require treatment, others can be beneficial for the patient or can improve operating conditions. Most sympathetic fibers leave the spinal cord between T1 and L2 (Chapter 8, Figure 8–1). Although local anesthetic is injected below these levels in the lumbar portion of the dural sac, cephalad spread of the local anesthetic occurs with all but the smallest volumes injected. This cephalad spread is of considerable importance in the practice of spinal anesthesia and potentially is under the control of numerous variables, of which patient position and baricity (density of the drug relative to the density of the CSF) are the most important (Greene, 1983). The degree of sympathetic block is related to the height of sensory anesthesia; often the level of sympathetic blockade is several spinal segments higher, since the preganglionic sympathetic fibers are more sensitive to low concentrations of local anesthetic. The effects of sympathetic blockade involve both the actions (now partially unopposed) of the parasympathetic nervous system and the response of the unblocked portion of the sympathetic nervous system. Thus, as the level of sympathetic block ascends, the actions of the parasympathetic nervous system are increasingly dominant, and the compensatory mechanisms of the unblocked sympathetic nervous system are diminished. As most sympathetic nerve fibers leave the cord at T1 or below, few additional effects of sympathetic blockade are seen with cervical levels of spinal anesthesia. The consequences of sympathetic blockade will vary among patients as a function of age, physical conditioning, and disease state. Interestingly, sympathetic blockade during spinal anesthesia appears to be minimal in healthy children.

Clinically, the most important effects of sympathetic blockade during spinal anesthesia are on the cardiovascular system. At all but the lowest levels of spinal blockade, some vasodilation will occur. Vasodilation is more marked on the venous than on the arterial side of the circulation, resulting in blood pooling in the venous capacitance vessels. This reduction in circulating blood volume is well tolerated at low levels of spinal anesthesia in healthy patients. With an increasing level of block, this effect becomes more marked and venous return becomes gravity-dependent. If venous return decreases too much, cardiac output and organ perfusion decline precipitously. Venous return can be increased by a modest (10-15 degree) head-down tilt or by elevating the legs. At high levels of spinal blockade, the cardiac accelerator fibers, which exit the spinal cord at T1-T4, will be blocked. This is detrimental in patients dependent on elevated sympathetic tone to maintain cardiac output (e.g., during congestive heart failure or hypovolemia), and it also removes one of the compensatory mechanisms available to maintain organ perfusion during vasodilation. Thus, as the level of spinal block ascends, the rate of cardiovascular compromise can accelerate if not carefully observed and treated. Sudden asystole also can occur, presumably because of loss of sympathetic innervation in the continued presence of parasympathetic activity at the sinoatrial node (Caplan et al., 1988). In the usual clinical situation, blood pressure serves as a surrogate marker for cardiac output and organ perfusion. Treatment of hypotension usually is warranted when the blood pressure decreases to ~30% of *resting* values. Therapy is aimed at maintaining brain and cardiac perfusion and oxygenation. To achieve these goals, administration of oxygen, fluid infusion, manipulation of patient position, and the administration of vasoactive drugs are all options. In practice, patients typically are administered a bolus (500-1000 mL) of fluid prior to the administration of spinal anesthesia in an attempt to prevent some of the deleterious effects of spinal blockade. Since the usual cause of hypotension is decreased venous return, possibly complicated by decreased heart rate, drugs with preferential venoconstrictive and chronotropic properties are preferred. For this reason, ephedrine, 5-10 mg intravenously, often is the drug of choice. In addition to the use of ephedrine to treat deleterious effects of sympathetic blockade, direct-acting α_1 adrenergic receptor agonists such as phenylephrine (Chapter 12) can be administered either by bolus or continuous infusion.

A beneficial effect of spinal anesthesia partially mediated by the sympathetic nervous system is on the intestine. Sympathetic fibers originating from T5-L1 inhibit peristalsis; thus, their blockade produces a small, contracted intestine. This, together with a flaccid abdominal musculature, produces excellent operating conditions for some types of bowel surgery. The effects of spinal anesthesia on the respiratory system mostly are mediated by effects on the skeletal musculature. Paralysis of the intercostal muscles will reduce a patient's ability to cough and clear secretions, which may produce dyspnea in patients with bronchitis or emphysema. Respiratory arrest during spinal anesthesia is seldom due to paralysis of the phrenic nerves or to toxic levels of local anesthetic in the CSF of the fourth ventricle; it is much more likely to be due to medullary ischemia secondary to hypotension.

Pharmacology of Spinal Anesthesia. Currently in the U.S., the drugs most commonly used in spinal anesthesia are lidocaine, tetracaine, and bupivacaine. Procaine occasionally is used for diagnostic blocks when a short duration of action is desired. The choice of local anesthetic is primarily determined by the desired duration of anesthesia. General guidelines are to use lidocaine for short procedures, bupivacaine for intermediate to long procedures, and tetracaine for long procedures. As mentioned earlier, the factors contributing to the distribution of local anesthetics in the CSF have received much attention because of their importance in determining the height of block. The most important pharmacological factors include the amount, and possibly the volume, of drug injected and its baricity. The speed of injection of the local anesthesia solution also may affect the height of the block, just as the position of the patient can influence the rate of distribution of the anesthetic agent and the height of blockade achieved (described in the next section). For a given preparation of local anesthetic, administration of increasing amounts leads to a fairly predictable increase in the level of block attained. For example, 100 mg of lidocaine, 20 mg of bupivacaine, or 12 mg of tetracaine usually will result in a T4 sensory block. More complete tables of these relationships can be found in standard anesthesiology texts. Epinephrine often is added to spinal anesthetics to increase the duration or intensity of block. Epinephrine's effect on duration of block is dependent on the technique used to measure duration. A commonly used measure of block duration is the length of time it takes for the block to recede by two dermatomes from the maximum height of the block, while a second is the duration of block at some specified level, typically L1. In most studies, addition of 200 μg of epinephrine to tetracaine solutions prolongs the duration of block by both measures. However, addition of epinephrine to lidocaine or bupivacaine does not affect the first measure of duration, but does prolong the block at lower levels. In different clinical situations, one or the other measure of anesthesia duration may be more relevant, and this must be kept in mind when deciding whether to add epinephrine to spinal local anesthetics. The mechanism of action of vasoconstrictors in prolonging spinal anesthesia is uncertain. It has been hypothesized that these agents decrease spinal cord blood flow, decreasing clearance of local anesthetic from the CSF, but this has not been convincingly demonstrated. Epinephrine and other α-adrenergic agonists have been shown to decrease nociceptive transmission in the spinal cord, and studies in genetically modified mice suggest that α_{2A} adrenergic receptors play a principal role in this response (Stone et al., 1997). Such actions may contribute to the beneficial effects of epinephrine, clonidine, and dexmedetomidine when these agents are added to spinal local anesthetics.

Drug Baricity and Patient Position. The baricity of the local anesthetic injected will determine the direction of migration within the dural sac. Hyperbaric solutions will tend to settle in the dependent portions of the sac, while hypobaric solutions will tend to migrate in the opposite direction. Isobaric solutions usually will stay in the vicinity where they were injected, diffusing slowly in all directions. Consideration of the patient position during and after the performance of the block and the choice of a local anesthetic of the appropriate baricity is crucial for a successful block during some surgical procedures. Lidocaine and bupivacaine are marketed in both isobaric and hyperbaric preparations, and if desired, can be diluted with sterile, preservative-free water to make them hypobaric.

Complications of Spinal Anesthesia. Persistent neurological deficits following spinal anesthesia are extremely rare. Thorough evaluation of a suspected deficit should be performed in collaboration with a neurologist. Neurological sequelae can be both immediate and late. Possible causes include introduction of foreign substances (such as disinfectants or talc) into the subarachnoid space, infection, hematoma, or direct mechanical trauma. Aside from drainage of an abscess or hematoma, treatment usually is ineffective; thus, avoidance and careful attention to detail while performing spinal anesthesia are necessary.

High concentrations of local anesthetic can cause irreversible block. After administration, local anesthetic solutions are diluted rapidly, quickly reaching nontoxic concentrations. However, there are several reports of transient or longer-lasting neurological deficits following lidocaine spinal anesthesia, particularly with 5% lidocaine (i.e., 180 mmol) in 7.5% glucose (Zaric and Pace, 2009). Spinal anesthesia sometimes is regarded as contraindicated in patients with pre-existing disease of the spinal cord. No experimental evidence exists to support this hypothesis. Nonetheless, it is prudent to avoid spinal anesthesia in patients with progressive diseases of the spinal cord. However, spinal anesthesia may be very useful in patients with fixed, chronic spinal cord injury.

A more common sequela following any lumbar puncture, including spinal anesthesia, is a postural headache with classic features. The incidence of headache decreases with increasing age of the patient and decreasing needle diameter. Headache following lumbar puncture must be thoroughly evaluated to exclude serious complications such as meningitis. Treatment usually is conservative, with bed rest and analgesics. If this approach fails, an epidural blood patch with the injection of autologous blood can be performed; this procedure usually is successful in alleviating postdural puncture headaches, although a second blood patch may be necessary. If two epidural blood patches are ineffective in relieving the headache, the diagnosis of postdural puncture headache should be reconsidered. Intravenous caffeine (500 mg as the benzoate salt administered over 4 hours) also has been advocated for the treatment of postdural puncture headache; however, the efficacy of caffeine is less than that of a blood patch, and relief usually is transient.

Evaluation of Spinal Anesthesia. Spinal anesthesia is a safe and effective technique, especially during surgery involving the lower abdomen, the lower extremities, and the perineum. It often is combined with intravenous medication to provide sedation and amnesia. The physiological perturbations associated with low spinal anesthesia often have less potential harm than those associated with general anesthesia. The same does not apply for high spinal anesthesia. The sympathetic blockade that accompanies levels of spinal anesthesia adequate for mid- or upper-abdominal surgery, coupled with the difficulty in achieving visceral analgesia, is such that equally satisfactory and safer operating conditions can be realized by combining the spinal anesthetic with a "light" general anesthetic or by the administration of a general anesthetic and a neuromuscular blocking agent.

Epidural Anesthesia

Epidural anesthesia is administered by injecting local anesthetic into the epidural space—the space bounded by the ligamentum flavum posteriorly, the spinal periosteum laterally, and the dura anteriorly. Epidural anesthesia can be performed in the sacral hiatus (caudal anesthesia) or in the lumbar, thoracic, or cervical regions of the spine. Its current popularity arises from the development of catheters that can be placed into the epidural space, allowing either continuous infusions or repeated bolus administration of local anesthetics. The primary site of action of epidurally administered local anesthetics is on the spinal nerve roots. However, epidurally administered local anesthetics also may act on the spinal cord and on the paravertebral nerves.

The selection of drugs available for epidural anesthesia is similar to that for major nerve blocks. As for spinal anesthesia, the choice of drugs to be used during epidural anesthesia is dictated primarily by the duration of anesthesia desired. However, when an epidural catheter is placed, short-acting drugs can be administered repeatedly, providing more control over the duration of block. Bupivacaine, 0.5-0.75%, is used when a long duration of surgical block is desired. Due to enhanced cardiotoxicity in pregnant patients, the 0.75% solution is not approved for obstetrical use. Lower concentrations—0.25%, 0.125%, or 0.0625%—of bupivacaine, often with 2 μg/mL of fentanyl added, frequently are used to provide analgesia during labor. They also are useful preparations for providing postoperative analgesia in certain clinical situations. Lidocaine 2% is the most frequently used intermediate-acting epidural local anesthetic. Chloroprocaine, 2% or 3%, provides rapid onset and a very short duration of anesthetic action. However, its use in epidural anesthesia has been clouded by controversy regarding its potential ability to cause neurological complications if the drug is accidentally injected into the subarachnoid space (discussed earlier). The duration of action of epidurally administered local anesthetics frequently is prolonged, and systemic toxicity decreased, by addition of epinephrine. Addition of epinephrine also makes inadvertent intravascular injection easier to detect and modifies the effect of sympathetic blockade during epidural anesthesia.

For each anesthetic agent, a relationship exists between the volume of local anesthetic injected epidurally and the segmental level of anesthesia achieved. For example, in 20- to 40-year-old, healthy, nonpregnant patients, each 1-1.5 mL of 2% lidocaine will give an additional segment of anesthesia. The amount needed decreases with increasing age and also decreases during pregnancy and in children.

The concentration of local anesthetic used determines the type of nerve fibers blocked. The highest concentrations are used when sympathetic, somatic sensory, and somatic motor blockade are required. Intermediate concentrations allow somatic sensory anesthesia without muscle relaxation. Low concentrations will block only preganglionic sympathetic fibers. As an example, with bupivacaine these effects might be achieved with concentrations of 0.5%, 0.25%, and 0.0625%, respectively. The total amounts of drug that can be injected with safety at one time are approximately those mentioned earlier in the chapter under "Nerve Block Anesthesia" and "Infiltration Anesthesia." Performance of epidural anesthesia requires a greater degree of skill than does spinal anesthesia. The technique of epidural anesthesia and the volumes, concentrations, and types of drugs used are described in detail in standard texts on regional anesthesia (e.g., Cousins et al., 2008).

A significant difference between epidural and spinal anesthesia is that the dose of local anesthetic used can produce high concentrations in blood following absorption from the epidural space. Peak concentrations of lidocaine in blood following injection of 400 mg (without epinephrine) into the lumbar epidural space average 3-4 μg/mL; peak concentrations of bupivacaine in blood average 1 μg/mL after the lumbar epidural injection of 150 mg. Addition of epinephrine (5 μg/mL) decreases peak plasma concentrations by ~25%. Peak blood concentrations are a function of the total dose of drug administered rather than the concentration or volume of solution following epidural injection (Covino and Vassallo, 1976). The risk of inadvertent intravascular injection is increased in epidural anesthesia, as the epidural space contains a rich venous plexus.

Another major difference between epidural and spinal anesthesia is that there is no zone of differential sympathetic blockade with epidural anesthesia; thus, the level of sympathetic block is close to the level of sensory block. Because epidural anesthesia does not result in the zones of differential sympathetic blockade observed during spinal anesthesia, cardiovascular responses to epidural anesthesia might be expected to be less prominent. In practice this is not the case; the potential advantage of epidural anesthesia is offset by the cardiovascular responses to the high concentration of anesthetic in blood that occurs during epidural anesthesia. This is most apparent when, as is often the case, epinephrine is added to the epidural injection. The resulting concentration of epinephrine in blood is sufficient to produce significant β_2 adrenergic receptor-mediated vasodilation. As a consequence, blood pressure decreases, even though cardiac output increases due to the positive inotropic and chronotropic effects of epinephrine (Chapter 12). The result is peripheral hyperperfusion and hypotension. Differences in cardiovascular responses to equal levels of spinal and epidural anesthesia also are observed when a local anesthetic such as lidocaine is used without epinephrine. This may be a consequence of the direct effects of high concentrations of lidocaine on vascular smooth muscle and the heart. The magnitude of the differences in responses to equal sensory levels of spinal and epidural anesthesia varies, however, with the local anesthetic used for the epidural injection (assuming no epinephrine is used). For example, local anesthetics such as bupivacaine, which are highly lipid soluble, are distributed less into the circulation than are less lipid-soluble agents such as lidocaine.

High concentrations of local anesthetics in blood during epidural anesthesia are especially important when this technique is used to control pain during labor and delivery. Local anesthetics cross the placenta, enter the fetal circulation, and at high concentrations may cause depression of the neonate. The extent to which they do so is determined by dosage, acid-base status, the level of protein binding in both maternal and fetal blood, placental blood flow, and solubility of the agent in fetal tissue. These concerns have been lessened by the trend toward using more dilute solutions of bupivacaine for labor analgesia.

Epidural and Intrathecal Opiate Analgesia. Small quantities of opioid injected intrathecally or epidurally produce segmental analgesia (Yaksh and Rudy, 1976). This observation led to the clinical use of spinal and epidural opioids during surgical procedures and for the relief of postoperative and chronic pain (Cousins and Mather, 1984). As with local anesthesia, analgesia is confined to sensory nerves that enter the spinal cord dorsal horn in the vicinity of the injection. Presynaptic opioid receptors inhibit the release of substance P and other neurotransmitters from primary afferents, while postsynaptic opioid receptors decrease the activity of certain dorsal horn neurons in the spinothalamic tracts (Willcockson et al., 1986; see also Chapters 8 and 18). Since conduction in autonomic, sensory, and motor nerves is not affected by the opioids, blood pressure, motor function, and non-nociceptive sensory perception typically are not influenced by spinal opioids. The volume-evoked micturition reflex is inhibited, as manifested by urinary retention. Other side effects include pruritus, nausea, and vomiting in susceptible individuals. Delayed respiratory depression and sedation, presumably from cephalad spread of opioid within the CSF, occur infrequently with the doses of opioids currently used.

Spinally administered opioids by themselves do not provide satisfactory anesthesia for surgical procedures. Thus, opioids have found the greatest use in the treatment of postoperative and chronic pain. In selected patients, spinal or epidural opioids can provide excellent analgesia following thoracic, abdominal, pelvic, or lower extremity surgery without the side effects associated with high doses of systemically administered opioids. For post-operative analgesia, spinally administered morphine, 0.2-0.5 mg, usually will provide 8-16 hours of analgesia. Placement of an epidural catheter and repeated boluses or an infusion of opioid permits an increased duration of analgesia. Many opioids have been used epidurally. Morphine, 2-6 mg, every 6 hours, commonly is used for bolus injections, while fentanyl, 20-50 μg/hour, often combined with bupivacaine, 5-20 mg/hour, is used for infusions. For cancer pain, repeated doses of epidural opioids can provide analgesia of several months' duration. The dose of epidural morphine, e.g., is far less than the dose of systemically administered morphine that would be required to provide similar analgesia. This reduces the complications that usually accompany the administration of high doses of systemic opioids, particularly sedation and constipation. Unfortunately, as with systemic opioids, tolerance will develop to the analgesic effects of epidural opioids, but this usually can be managed by increasing the dose.

BIBLIOGRAPHY

Arthur GR. Pharmacokinetics. In, *Local Anesthetics*. (Strichartz GR, ed.) *Handbook of Experimental Pharmacology*, vol. 81. Springer-Verlag, Berlin, **1987**, pp. 165–186.

Butterworth J, Oxford G. Local Anesthetics: A New Hydrophilic Pathway for Drug-receptor Reaction. *Anesthesiology*, **2009**, *111*:12–14.

Butterworth JF IV, Strichartz GR. Molecular mechanisms of local anesthesia: A review. *Anesthesiology*, **1990**, *72:*711–734.

Caplan RA, Ward RJ, Posner K, Cheney FW. Unexpected cardiac arrest during spinal anesthesia: A closed claims analysis of predisposing factors. *Anesthesiology*, **1988,** *68:*5–11.

Carpenter RL, Mackey DC. Local anesthetics. In, *Clinical Anesthesia*, 2nd ed. (Barash PG, Cullen BF, Stoelting RK, eds.) Lippincott, Philadelphia, **1992**, pp. 509–541.

Catterall WA. From ionic currents to molecular mechanisms: the structure and function of voltage-gated sodium channels. *Neuron*, **2000**, *26:*13–25.

Charnet P, Labarca C, Leonard RJ, *et al*. An open-channel blocker interacts with adjacent turns of α-helices in the nicotinic acetylcholine receptor. *Neuron*, **1990,** *4:*87–95.

Clarkson CW, Hondeghem LM. Mechanism for bupivacaine depression of cardiac conduction: Fast block of sodium channels during the action potential with slow recovery from block during diastole. *Anesthesiology*, **1985,** *62:* 396–405.

Courtney KR, Strichartz GR. Structural elements which determine local anesthetic activity. In, *Local Anesthetics*. (Strichartz GR, ed.) *Handbook of Experimental Pharmacology*, vol. 81. Springer-Verlag, Berlin, **1987**, pp. 53–94.

Cousins MJ, Bridenbaugh PO, Carr DB, Horlocker TT, eds. *Neural Blockade in Clinical Anesthesia and Management of Pain*, 4th ed. Lippincott-Raven, Philadelphia, **2008**.

Cousins MJ, Mather LE. Intrathecal and epidural administration of opioids. *Anesthesiology*, **1984**, *61:*276–310.

Covino BG. Toxicity and systemic effects of local anesthetic agents. In, *Local Anesthetics*. (Strichartz GR, ed.) *Handbook of Experimental Pharmacology*, vol. 81. Springer-Verlag, Berlin, **1987**, pp. 187–212.

Covino BG, Vassallo HG. *Local Anesthetics: Mechanisms of Action and Clinical Use*. Grune & Stratton, New York, **1976**.

DeJong RH. *Local Anesthetics*. Mosby, St. Louis, **1994**.

Fink BR, Cairns AM. Differential slowing and block of conduction by lidocaine in individual afferent myelinated and unmyelinated axons. *Anesthesiology*, **1984**, *60:*111–120.

Franz DN, Perry RS. Mechanisms for differential block among single myelinated and nonmyelinated axons by procaine. *J Physiol*, **1974**, *236:*193–210.

Garfield JM, Gugino L. Central effects of local anesthetics. In, *Local Anesthetics*. (Strichartz GR, ed.) *Handbook of Experimental Pharmacology*, vol. 81. Springer-Verlag, Berlin, **1987**, pp. 253–284.

Gasser HS, Erlanger J. The role of fiber size in the establishment of a nerve block by pressure or cocaine. *Am J Physiol*, **1929**, *88:*581–591.

Gintant GA, Hoffman BF. The role of local anesthetic effects in the actions of antiarrhythmic drugs. In, *Local Anesthetics*. (Strichartz GR, ed.) *Handbook of Experimental Pharmacology*, vol. 81. Springer-Verlag, Berlin, **1987**, pp. 213–251.

Greene NM. Uptake and elimination of local anesthetics during spinal anesthesia. *Anesth Analg*, **1983**, *62:*1013–1024.

Huang JH, Thalhammer JG, Raymond SA, Strichartz GR. Susceptibility to lidocaine of impulses in different somatosensory fibers of rat sciatic nerve. *J Pharmacol Exp Ther*, **1997**, *292:*802–811.

McClure JH. Ropivacaine. *Br J Anaesth*, **1996**, *76:*300–307.

Narahashi T, Frazier DT. Site of action and active form of local anesthetics. *Neurosci Res (NY)*, **1971**, *4:*65–99.

Neher E, Steinbach JH. Local anesthetics transiently block currents through single acetylcholine-receptor channels. *J Physiol*, **1978**, *277:*153–176.

Ragsdale DR, McPhee JC, Scheuer T, Catterall WA. Molecular determinants of state-dependent block of Na^+ channels by local anesthetics. *Science*, **1994**, *265:*1724–1728.

Raymond SA, Gissen AJ. Mechanism of differential nerve block. In, *Local Anesthetics*. (Strichartz GR, ed.) *Handbook of Experimental Pharmacology*, vol. 81. Springer-Verlag, Berlin, **1987,** pp. 95–164.

Ritchie JM. Tetrodotoxin and saxitoxin and the sodium channels of excitable tissues. *Trends Pharmacol Sci*, **1980**, *1:*275–279.

Ritchie JM, Greengard P. On the mode of action of local anesthetics. *Annu Rev Pharmacol*, **1966**, *6:*405–430.

Stevens RA, Urmey WF, Urquhart BL, Kao TC. Back pain after epidural anesthesia with chloroprocaine. *Anesthesiology*, **1993**, *78:*492–497.

Stommel EW, Watters MR. Marine neurotoxins: Ingestible toxins. *Curr Treat Options Neurol*, **2004**, *6:*105–114.

Stone LS, MacMillan LB, Kitto KF, *et al*. The α_{2a} adrenergic receptor subtype mediates spinal analgesia evoked by α_2 agonists and is necessary for spinal adrenergic-opioid synergy. *J Neurosci*, **1997**, *17:*7157–7165.

Strichartz GR, Ritchie JM. The action of local anesthetics on ion channels of excitable tissues. In, *Local Anesthetics*. (Strichartz GR, ed.) *Handbook of Experimental Pharmacology*, vol. 81. Springer-Verlag, Berlin, **1987**, pp. 21–53.

Terlau H, Heinemann SH, Ståhmer W, *et al*. Mapping the site of block by tetrodotoxin and saxitoxin of sodium channel II. *FEBS Lett*, **1991**, *293:*93–96.

Thomas RD, Behbehani MM, Coyle DE, Denson DD. Cardiovascular toxicity of local anesthetics: an alternative hypothesis. *Anesth Analg*, **1986**, *65:*444–450.

Willcockson WS, Kim J, Shin HK, *et al*. Actions of opioid on primate spinothalamic tract neurons. *J Neurosci*, **1986**, *6:*2509–2520.

Winnie AP, Tay CH, Patel KP, *et al*. Pharmacokinetics of local anesthetics during plexus blocks. *Anesth Analg*, **1977**, *56:* 852–861.

Yaksh TL, Rudy TA. Analgesia mediated by a direct spinal action of narcotics. *Science*, **1976**, *192:*1357–1358.

Yarov-Yarovoy V, McPhee JC, Idsvoog D, *et al*. Role of amino acid residues in transmembrane segments IS6 and IIS6 of the sodium channel α subunit in voltage-dependent gating and drug block. *J Biol Chem*, **2002**, *277:*35393–35401.

Yu F, Yarov-Yarovoy V, Gutman GA, Catterall WA. Overview of molecular relationships in the voltage-gated ion channel superfamily. *Pharmacol Rev*, **2005**, *57:*387–395.

Zaric D, Pace NL. Transient neurological symptoms (TNS) following spinal anesthesia with lidocaine versus other local anesthetics. *Cochrane Database Syst Rev*, **2009**, *2:* CD003006.

Zipf HF, Dittmann EC. General pharmacological effects of local anesthetics. In, *Local Anesthetics*, vol. 1. *International Encyclopedia of Pharmacology and Therapeutics*, Sect. 8. (Lechat P, ed.) Pergamon Press, Oxford, **1971**, pp. 191–238.

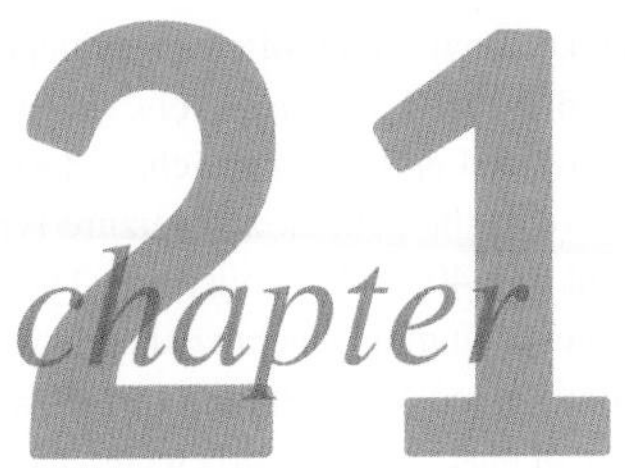

Pharmacotherapy of the Epilepsies

James O. McNamara

The epilepsies are common and frequently devastating disorders, affecting ~2.5 million people in the U.S. alone. More than 40 distinct forms of epilepsy have been identified. Epileptic seizures often cause transient impairment of consciousness, leaving the individual at risk of bodily harm and often interfering with education and employment. Therapy is symptomatic in that available drugs inhibit seizures, but neither effective prophylaxis nor cure is available. Compliance with medication is a major problem because of the need for long-term therapy together with unwanted effects of many drugs.

The mechanisms of action of anti-seizure drugs fall into three major categories.

1. The first mechanism is to limit the sustained, repetitive firing of neurons, an effect mediated by promoting the inactivated state of voltage-activated Na^+ channels.
2. A second mechanism appears to involve enhanced γ-aminobutyric acid (GABA)–mediated synaptic inhibition, an effect mediated either by a presynaptic or postsynaptic action. Drugs effective against the most common forms of epileptic seizures, partial and secondarily generalized tonic-clonic seizures, appear to work by one of these two mechanisms.
3. Drugs effective against absence seizure, a less common form of epileptic seizure, work by a third mechanism, inhibition of voltage-activated Ca^{2+} channels responsible for T-type Ca^{2+} currents.

Although many treatments are available, much effort is being devoted to elucidating the genetic causes and the cellular and molecular mechanisms by which a normal brain becomes epileptic, insights that promise to provide molecular targets for both symptomatic and preventive therapies.

TERMINOLOGY AND EPILEPTIC SEIZURE CLASSIFICATION

The term *seizure* refers to a transient alteration of behavior due to the disordered, synchronous, and rhythmic firing of populations of brain neurons. The term *epilepsy* refers to a disorder of brain function characterized by the periodic and unpredictable occurrence of seizures. Seizures can be "non-epileptic" when evoked in a normal brain by treatments such as electroshock or chemical convulsants, or "epileptic" when occurring without evident provocation. Pharmacological agents in current clinical use inhibit seizures, and thus are referred to as anti-seizure drugs. Whether any of these prevent the development of epilepsy (epileptogenesis) is uncertain.

Seizures are thought to arise from the cerebral cortex, and not from other central nervous system (CNS) structures such as the thalamus, brainstem, or cerebellum. Epileptic seizures have been classified into *partial* seizures, those beginning focally in a cortical site, and *generalized* seizures, those that involve both hemispheres widely from the outset (Commission on Classification and Terminology, 1981). The behavioral manifestations of a seizure are determined by the functions normally served by the cortical site at which the seizure arises. For example, a seizure involving motor cortex is associated with clonic jerking of the body part controlled by this region of cortex. A *simple* partial seizure is associated with preservation of consciousness. A *complex* partial seizure is associated with impairment of consciousness. The majority of complex partial seizures originate from the temporal lobe. Examples of generalized seizures include absence, myoclonic, and tonic-clonic. The type of epileptic seizure is one determinant of the drug selected for therapy. More detailed information is presented in Table 21–1.

Apart from this epileptic seizure classification, an additional classification specifies epileptic syndromes, which refer to a cluster of symptoms frequently occurring together and include seizure types, etiology, age of onset, and other factors (Commission on Classification and Terminology, 1989). More than 50 distinct epileptic syndromes have been identified and categorized into partial versus generalized epilepsies. The partial epilepsies may consist of any of the partial seizure types (Table 21–1) and account for roughly 60% of all epilepsies. The etiology commonly consists of a lesion in some part of the cortex, such as a tumor, developmental malformation, or damage due to trauma or stroke. Such lesions often are evident on brain magnetic resonance imaging (MRI). Alternatively, the etiology may be genetic. The generalized epilepsies are characterized most commonly by one or more of the generalized seizure types listed in Table 21–1 and account for ~40% of all epilepsies. The etiology is usually genetic. The most common generalized epilepsy is referred to as juvenile myoclonic epilepsy, accounting for ~10% of all epileptic syndromes. The age of onset is in the early teens, and the condition is characterized by myoclonic, tonic-clonic, and often absence seizures. Like most of the generalized-onset epilepsies, juvenile myoclonic epilepsy is a complex genetic disorder that is probably due to inheritance of multiple susceptibility genes; there is a familial clustering of cases, but the pattern of inheritance is not

Table 21–1

Classification of Epileptic Seizures

SEIZURE TYPE	FEATURES	CONVENTIONAL ANTI-SEIZURE DRUGS	RECENTLY DEVELOPED ANTI-SEIZURE DRUGS
Partial Seizures			
Simple partial	Diverse manifestations determined by the region of cortex activated by the seizure (e.g., if motor cortex representing left thumb, clonic jerking of left thumb results; if somatosensory cortex representing left thumb, paresthesia of left thumb results), lasting approximating 20-60 seconds. *Key feature is preservation of consciousness.*	Carbamazepine, phenytoin, valproate	Gabapentin, lacosamide, lamotrigine, levetiracetam, rufinamide, tiagabine, topiramate, zonisamide
Complex partial	Impaired consciousness lasting 30 seconds to 2 minutes, often associated with purposeless movements such as lip smacking or hand wringing.		
Partial with secondarily generalized tonic-clonic seizure	Simple or complex partial seizure evolves into a tonic-clonic seizure with loss of consciousness and sustained contractions (tonic) of muscles throughout the body followed by periods of muscle contraction alternating with periods of relaxation (clonic), typically lasting 1-2 minutes	Carbamazepine, phenobarbital, phenytoin, primidone, valproate	
Generalized Seizures			
Absence seizure	Abrupt onset of impaired consciousness associated with staring and cessation of ongoing activities typically lasting less than 30 seconds.	Ethosuximide, valproate, clonazepam	Lamotrigine
Myoclonic seizure	A brief (perhaps a second), shocklike contraction of muscles that may be restricted to part of one extremity or may be generalized.	Valproate, clonazepam	Levetiracetam
Tonic-clonic seizure	As described earlier in table for partial with secondarily generalized tonic-clonic seizures except that it is not preceded by a partial seizure.	Carbamazepine, phenobarbital, phenytoin, primidone, valproate	Lamotrigine, levetiracetam, topiramate

mendelian. The classification of epileptic syndromes guides clinical assessment and management, and in some instances, selection of anti-seizure drugs.

NATURE AND MECHANISMS OF SEIZURES AND ANTI-SEIZURE DRUGS

Partial Epilepsies

More than a century ago, John Hughlings Jackson, the father of modern concepts of epilepsy, proposed that seizures were caused by "occasional, sudden, excessive, rapid and local discharges of gray matter," and that a generalized convulsion resulted when normal brain tissue was invaded by the seizure activity initiated in the abnormal focus. This insightful proposal provided a valuable framework for thinking about mechanisms of partial epilepsy. The advent of the electroencephalogram (EEG) in the 1930s permitted the recording of electrical activity from the scalp of humans with epilepsy and demonstrated that the epilepsies are disorders of neuronal excitability.

The pivotal role of synapses in mediating communication among neurons in the mammalian brain suggested that defective synaptic function might lead to a seizure. That is, a reduction of inhibitory synaptic activity or enhancement of excitatory synaptic activity might be expected to trigger a seizure; pharmacological studies of seizures support this notion. The neurotransmitters mediating the bulk of synaptic transmission in the mammalian brain are amino acids, with γ-aminobutyric acid (GABA) and glutamate being the principal inhibitory and excitatory neurotransmitters, respectively (Chapter 14). Pharmacological studies disclosed that *antagonists* of the $GABA_A$ receptor or *agonists* of different glutamate-receptor subtypes (NMDA, AMPA, or kainic acid) (Chapter 14) trigger seizures in experimental animals in vivo. Conversely, pharmacological agents that enhance GABA-mediated synaptic inhibition suppress seizures in diverse models. Glutamate-receptor antagonists also inhibit seizures in diverse models, including seizures evoked by electroshock and chemical convulsants such as pentylenetetrazol.

Such studies support the idea that pharmacological regulation of synaptic function can regulate the propensity for seizures and provide a framework for electrophysiological analyses aimed at elucidating the role of both synaptic and nonsynaptic mechanisms in seizures and epilepsy. Progress in techniques has fostered the progressive refinement of the analysis of seizure mechanisms from the EEG to populations of neurons (field potentials) to individual neurons to individual synapses and individual ion channels on individual neurons. Beginning in the mid-1960s, cellular electrophysiological studies of epilepsy focused on elucidating the mechanisms underlying the depolarization shift (DS), the intracellular correlate of the "interictal spike" (Figure 21–1). The interictal (or between-seizures) spike is a sharp waveform recorded in the EEG of patients with epilepsy; it is asymptomatic in that it is accompanied by no overt change in the patient's behavior. The location of the interictal spike helps localize the brain region from which seizures originate in a given patient. The DS consists of a large depolarization of the neuronal membrane associated with a burst of action potentials. In most cortical neurons, the DS is generated by a large excitatory synaptic current that can be enhanced by activation of voltage-gated intrinsic membrane currents. Although the mechanisms generating the DS are increasingly understood, it remains unclear whether the interictal spike triggers a seizure, inhibits a seizure, or is an epiphenomenon with respect to seizure occurrence in an epileptic brain. While these questions remain unanswered, the study of the mechanisms of DS generation set the stage for inquiry into the cellular mechanisms of a seizure.

During the 1980s, various *in vitro* models of seizures were developed in isolated brain slice preparations, in which many synaptic connections are preserved. Electrographic events with features similar to those recorded during seizures *in vivo* have been produced in hippocampal slices by multiple methods, including altering ionic constituents of media bathing the brain slices (McNamara, 1994) such as low Ca^{2+}, zero Mg^{2+}, or elevated K^+. The accessibility and experimental control provided by these preparations has permitted mechanistic investigations into the induction of seizures. Analyses of multiple *in vitro* models confirmed the importance of synaptic function for initiating a seizure, demonstrating that subtle (e.g., 20%) reductions of inhibitory synaptic function could lead to epileptiform activity and that activation of excitatory synapses could be pivotal in seizure initiation. Other important factors were identified, including the volume of the extracellular space as well as intrinsic properties of a neuron, such as voltage-gated ion channels (e.g., K^+, Na^+, and Ca^{2+} channels) (Traynelis and Dingledine, 1988). Identification of these diverse synaptic and nonsynaptic factors controlling seizures *in vitro* provides potential pharmacological targets for regulating seizure susceptibility *in vivo*.

Additional studies have centered on understanding the mechanisms by which a normal brain is transformed into an epileptic brain. Some common forms of partial epilepsy arise months to years after cortical injury sustained as a consequence of stroke, trauma, or other factors. An effective prophylaxis administered to patients at high risk would be highly desirable. The drugs described in this chapter provide symptomatic therapy; that is, the drugs inhibit seizures in patients with epilepsy. No effective anti-epileptogenic agent has been identified.

Understanding the mechanisms of epileptogenesis in cellular and molecular terms should provide a framework for development of novel therapeutic approaches. The availability of animal models provides an opportunity to investigate the underlying mechanisms.

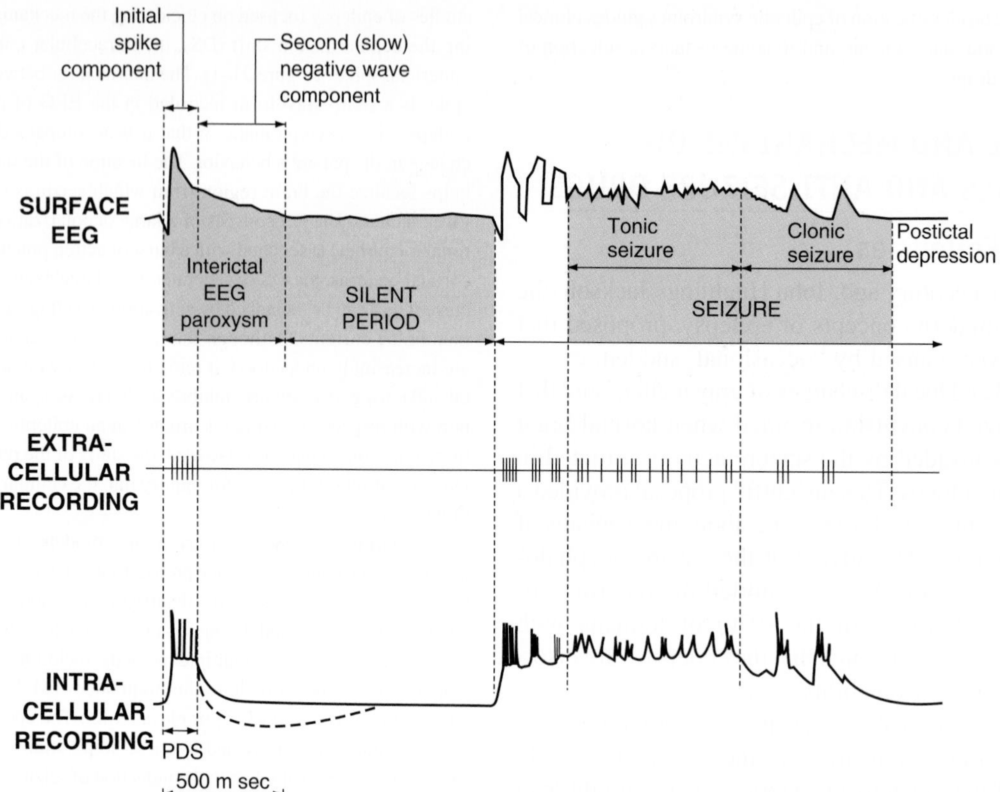

Figure 21–1. *Relations among cortical EEG, extracellular, and intracellular recordings in a seizure focus induced by local application of a convulsant agent to mammalian cortex.* The extracellular recording was made through a high-pass filter. Note the high-frequency firing of the neuron evident in both extracellular and intracellular recording during the paroxysmal depolarization shift (PDS). (Modified with permission from Ayala GF, Dichter M, Gumnit RJ, et al. Genesis of epileptic interictal spikes. New knowledge of cortical feedback systems suggests a neurophysiological explanation of brief paroxysms. *Brain Res*, **1973**, *52*:1–17. Copyright © Elsevier.)

One model, termed "kindling," is induced by periodic administration of brief, low-intensity electrical stimulation of the amygdala or other limbic structures. Initial stimulations evoke a brief electrical seizure recorded on the EEG without behavioral change, but repeated (e.g., 10-20) stimulations result in progressive intensification of seizures, culminating in tonic-clonic seizures. Once established, the enhanced sensitivity to electrical stimulation persists for the life of the animal. Despite the exquisite propensity to intense seizures, spontaneous seizures or a truly epileptic condition do not occur until 100-200 stimulations have been administered. The ease of control of kindling induction (i.e., stimulations administered at the investigator's convenience), its graded onset, and the ease of quantitating epileptogenesis (number of stimulations required to evoke tonic-clonic seizures) simplify experimental study. In mice, deletion of the gene encoding the receptor tyrosine kinase, TrkB, prevents epileptogenesis in the kindling model (He et al., 2004), which advances TrkB and its downstream signaling pathways as attractive targets for developing small molecule inhibitors for prevention of epilepsy or its progression.

Additional models are produced by induction of continuous seizures for hours ("status epilepticus"), with the inciting agent being a chemoconvulsant, such as kainic acid or pilocarpine, or sustained electrical stimulation. The fleeting episode of status epilepticus is followed weeks later by the onset of spontaneous seizures, an intriguing parallel to the scenario of complicated febrile seizures in young children preceding the emergence of spontaneous seizures years later. In contrast to the limited or absent neuronal loss characteristic of the kindling model, overt destruction of hippocampal neurons occurs in the status epilepticus models, reflecting aspects of hippocampal sclerosis observed in humans with severe limbic seizures. Indeed, the discovery that complicated febrile seizures precede and presumably are the cause of hippocampal sclerosis in young children (VanLandingham et al., 1998) establishes yet another commonality between these models and the human condition.

Several questions arise with respect to these models. What transpires during the latent period between status epilepticus and emergence of spontaneous seizures that causes the epilepsy? Might an anti-epileptogenic agent that was effective in one of these models be effective in other models?

Important insights into the mechanisms of action of drugs that are effective against partial seizures have emerged in the past two decades (Rogawski and Loscher, 2004). These insights largely have come from electrophysiological studies of relatively simple *in vitro* models, such as neurons isolated from the mammalian CNS and maintained in primary culture. The experimental control and accessibility provided by these models—together with careful attention to clinically relevant concentrations of the drugs—led to clarification of their mechanisms. Although it is difficult to prove unequivocally that a given drug effect observed *in vitro* is both necessary and sufficient to inhibit a seizure in an animal or humans *in vivo*, there is an excellent likelihood that the putative mechanisms identified do in fact underlie the clinically relevant anti-seizure effects. Table 21–2 summarizes putative mechanisms of action of anti-seizure drugs.

Electrophysiological analyses of individual neurons during a partial seizure demonstrate that the neurons undergo depolarization and fire action potentials at high frequencies (Figure 21–1). This pattern of neuronal firing is characteristic of a seizure and is uncommon during physiological neuronal activity. Thus, selective inhibition of this pattern of firing would be expected to reduce seizures with minimal unwanted effects. Carbamazepine, lamotrigine, phenytoin, and valproic acid inhibit high-frequency firing at concentrations

Table 21–2

Proposed Mechanisms of Action of Anti-Seizure Drugs

MOLECULAR TARGET AND ACTIVITY	DRUG	CONSEQUENCES OF ACTION
Na^+ channel modulators that:		
enhance fast inactivation	PHT, CBZ, LTG, FBM, OxCBZ, TPM, VPA	• block action potential propagation • stabilize neuronal membranes • ↓ neurotransmitter release, focal firing, and seizure spread
enhance slow inactivation	LCM	• ↑ spike frequency adaptation • ↓ AP bursts, focal firing, and seizure spread • stabilize neuronal membrane
Ca^{2+} channel blockers	ESM, VPA, LTG	• ↓ neurotransmitter release (N- & P-types) • ↓ slow-depolarization (T-type) and spike-wave discharges
$\alpha 2\delta$ ligands	GBP, PGB	• modulate neurotransmitter release
$GABA_A$ receptor allosteric modulators	BZDs, PB, FBM, TPM, CBZ, OxCBZ	• ↑ membrane hyperpolarization and seizure threshold • ↓ focal firing BZDs—attenuate spike-wave discharges PB, CBZ, OxCBZ—aggravate spike-wave discharges
GABA uptake inhibitors/ GABA-transaminase inhibitors	TGB, VGB	• ↑ extrasynaptic GABA levels and membrane hyperpolarization • ↓ focal firing • aggravate spike-wave discharges
NMDA receptor antagonists	FBM	• ↓ slow excitatory neurotransmission • ↓ excitatory amino acid neurotoxicity • delay epileptogenesis
AMPA/kainate receptor antagonists	PB, TPM	• ↓ fast excitatory neurotransmission and focal firing
Enhancers of HCN channel activity	LTG	• buffers large hyperpolarizing and depolarizing inputs • suppresses action potential initiation by dendritic inputs
SV2A protein ligand	LEV	• unknown; may decrease transmitter release
Inhibitors of brain carbonic anhydrase	ACZ, TPM, ZNS	• ↑ HCN-mediated currents • ↓ NMDA-mediated currents • ↑ GABA-mediated inhibition

ACZ, acetazolamide; BZDs, benzodiazepines; CBZ, carbamazepine; FBM, felbamate; GBP, gabapentin; LEV, levetiracetam; LCM, lacosamide; LTG, Lamotrigine; OxCBZ, oxcarbazepine; PB, phenobarbital; PGB, pregagalin; PHT, phenytoin; TGB, tiagabine; TPM, topiramate; VGB, vigabatrin; VPA, valproic acid; ZNA, zonisamide. Modified with permission from Leppik IE, Kelly KM, deToledo-Morrell L et al. Basic research in epilepsy and aging. *Epilepsy Res*, **2006**, 68 (Suppl 1): 21. Copyright© Elsevier.

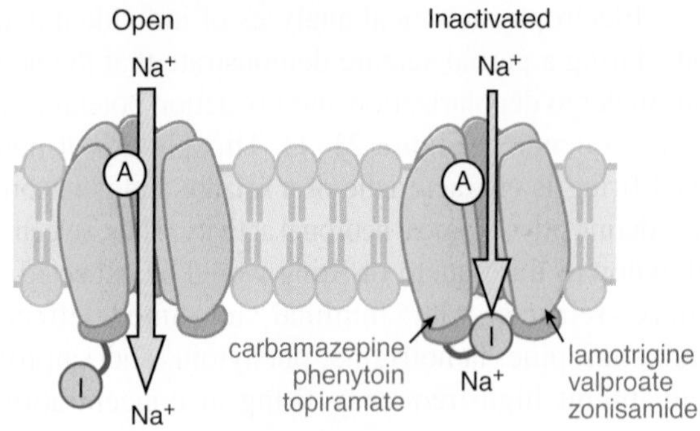

Figure 21–2. *Anti-seizure drug-enhanced Na^+ channel inactivation.* Some anti-seizure drugs (shown in blue text) prolong the inactivation of the Na^+ channels, thereby reducing the ability of neurons to fire at high frequencies. Note that the inactivated channel itself appears to remain open, but is blocked by the inactivation gate **I**. A, activation gate.

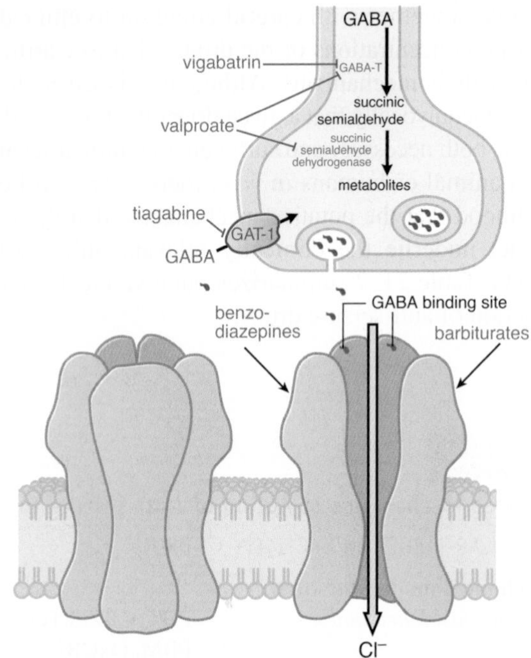

Figure 21–3. *Enhanced GABA synaptic transmission.* In the presence of GABA, the $GABA_A$ receptor (structure on left) is opened, allowing an influx of $C1^-$, which in turn increases membrane polarization (Chapter 14). Some anti-seizure drugs (show in larger blue text) act by reducing the metabolism of GABA. Others act at the $GABA_A$ receptor, enhancing $C1^-$ influx in response to GABA. As outlined in the text, gabapentin acts presynaptically to promote GABA release; its molecular target is currently under investigation. ⬊ GABA molecules, GABA-T, GABA transaminase; GAT-1, GABA transporter.

known to be effective at limiting seizures in humans (Rogawski and Loscher, 2004). Inhibition of the high-frequency firing is thought to be mediated by reducing the ability of Na^+ channels to recover from inactivation (Figure 21–2). That is, depolarization-triggered opening of the Na^+ channels in the axonal membrane of a neuron is required for an action potential; after opening, the channels spontaneously close, a process termed *inactivation*. This inactivation is thought to cause the refractory period, a short time after an action potential during which it is not possible to evoke another action potential. Upon recovery from inactivation, the Na^+ channels are again poised to participate in another action potential. Because firing at a slow rate permits sufficient time for Na^+ channels to recover from inactivation, inactivation has little or no effect on low-frequency firing. However, reducing the rate of recovery of Na^+ channels from inactivation would limit the ability of a neuron to fire at high frequencies, an effect that likely underlies the effects of carbamazepine, lamotrigine, phenytoin, topiramate, valproic acid, and zonisamide against partial seizures.

Insights into mechanisms of seizures suggest that enhancing GABA-mediated synaptic inhibition would reduce neuronal excitability and raise the seizure threshold. Several drugs are thought to inhibit seizures by regulating GABA-mediated synaptic inhibition through an action at distinct sites of the synapse (Rogawski and Loscher, 2004). The principal postsynaptic receptor of synaptically released GABA is termed the $GABA_A$ receptor (Chapters 14 and 17). Activation of the $GABA_A$ receptor inhibits the postsynaptic cell by increasing the inflow of Cl^- ions into the cell, which tends to hyperpolarize the neuron. Clinically relevant concentrations of both benzodiazepines and barbiturates enhance $GABA_A$ receptor–mediated inhibition through distinct actions on the $GABA_A$ receptor (Figure 21–3), and this enhanced inhibition probably underlies the effectiveness of these compounds against partial and tonic-clonic seizures in humans. At higher concentrations, such as might be used for status epilepticus, these drugs also can inhibit high-frequency firing of action potentials. A second mechanism of enhancing GABA-mediated synaptic inhibition is thought to underlie the anti-seizure mechanism of tiagabine; tiagabine inhibits the GABA transporter, GAT-1, and reduces neuronal and glial uptake of GABA (Rogawski and Loscher, 2004).

Generalized-Onset Epilepsies: Absence Seizures

In contrast to partial seizures, which arise from localized regions of the cerebral cortex, generalized-onset seizures arise from the reciprocal firing of the thalamus and cerebral cortex (Huguenard and McCormick, 2007). Among the diverse forms of generalized seizures, absence seizures have been studied most intensively. The striking synchrony in appearance of generalized seizure discharges in widespread areas of neocortex led to the idea that a structure in the thalamus and/or brainstem (the "centrencephalon") synchronized these seizure discharges. Focus on the thalamus in particular emerged from the demonstration that low-frequency stimulation of midline thalamic structures triggered EEG rhythms in the cortex similar to spike-and-wave discharges characteristic of absence seizures. Intra-cerebral electrode recordings from humans subsequently demonstrated the presence of thalamic and neocortical involvement in the spike-and-wave discharge of absence seizures.

Many of the structural and functional properties of the thalamus and neocortex that lead to the generalized spike-and-wave discharges have been elucidated (Huguenard and McCormick, 2007).

The EEG hallmark of an absence seizure is generalized spike-and-wave discharges at a frequency of 3 per second (3 Hz). These bilaterally synchronous spike-and-wave discharges, recorded locally from electrodes in both the thalamus and the neocortex, represent oscillations between the thalamus and neocortex. A comparison of EEG and intracellular recordings reveals that the EEG spikes are associated with the firing of action potentials and the following slow wave with prolonged inhibition. These reverberatory, low-frequency rhythms are made possible by a combination of factors, including reciprocal excitatory synaptic connections between the neocortex and thalamus as well as intrinsic properties of neurons in the thalamus (Huguenard and McCormick, 2007). One intrinsic property of thalamic neurons that is pivotally involved in the generation of the 3-Hz spike-and-wave discharges is a particular type of Ca^{2+} current, the low threshold ("T-type") current. T-type Ca^{2+} channels are activated at a much more negative membrane potential (hence "low threshold") than most other voltage-gated Ca^{2+} channels expressed in the brain. T-type currents are much larger in many thalamic neurons compared to neurons outside the thalamus. Indeed, bursts of action potentials in thalamic neurons are mediated by activation of the T-type currents. T-type currents amplify thalamic membrane potential oscillations, with one oscillation being the 3-Hz spike-and-wave discharge of the absence seizure. Importantly, the principal mechanism by which anti–absence-seizure drugs (ethosuximide, valproic acid) are thought to act is by inhibition of the T-type Ca^{2+} channels (Figure 21–4) (Rogawski and Loscher, 2004). Thus, inhibiting voltage-gated ion channels is a common mechanism of action among anti-seizure drugs, with anti–partial-seizure drugs inhibiting voltage-activated Na^+ channels and anti–absence-seizure drugs inhibiting voltage-activated Ca^{2+} channels.

Genetic Approaches to the Epilepsies

Genetic causes contribute to a wide diversity of human epilepsies. Genetic causes are solely responsible for

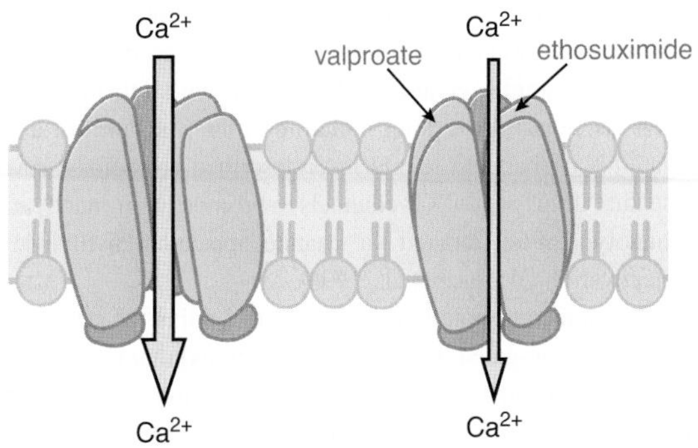

Figure 21–4. *Anti-seizure drug-induced reduction of current through T-type Ca^{2+} channels.* Some anti-seizure drugs (shown in blue text) reduce the flow of Ca^{2+} through T-type Ca^{2+} channels thus reducing the pacemaker current that underlies the thalamic rhythm in spikes and waves seen in generalized absence seizures.

rare forms inherited in an autosomal dominant or autosomal recessive manner. Genetic causes also are mainly responsible for more common forms such as juvenile myoclonic epilepsy (JME) or childhood absence epilepsy (CAE), the majority of which are likely due to inheritance of two or more susceptibility genes. Genetic determinants also may contribute some degree of risk to epilepsies caused by injury of the cerebral cortex.

Enormous progress has been made in understanding the genetics of mammalian epilepsy. Mutant genes have been identified for a number of symptomatic epilepsies, in which the epilepsy is a manifestation of the underlying neurodegenerative disease. Because most patients with epilepsy are neurologically normal, elucidating the mutant genes underlying familial epilepsy in otherwise normal individuals is of particular interest; this has led to the identification of 25 distinct genes implicated in distinct idiopathic epilepsy syndromes that account for < 1% of all of the human epilepsies. Interestingly, almost all of the mutant genes encode voltage- or ligand-gated ion channels (Reid et al., 2008). Mutations have been identified in Na^+, K^+, Ca^{2+}, and Cl^- channels, in channels gated by GABA and acetylcholine, and most recently, in intracellular Ca^{2+} release channels (RyR2) activated by Ca^{2+}. The genotype-phenotype correlations of these genetic syndromes are complex; the same mutation in one channel can be associated with divergent clinical syndromes ranging from simple febrile seizures to intractable seizures with intellectual decline. Conversely, clinically indistinguishable epilepsy syndromes have been associated with mutation of distinct genes. The implication of genes encoding ion channels in familial epilepsy is particularly interesting because episodic disorders involving other organs also result from mutations of these genes. For example, episodic disorders of the heart (cardiac arrhythmias), skeletal muscle (periodic paralyses), cerebellum (episodic ataxia), vasculature (familial hemiplegic migraine), and other organs all have been linked to mutations in genes encoding components of voltage-gated ion channels (Ptacek and Fu, 2001).

The cellular electrophysiological consequences of these mutations can inform on the mechanisms of seizures and anti-seizure drugs. For example, generalized epilepsy with febrile seizures (GEFS+) is caused by a point mutation in the β subunit of a voltage-gated Na^+ channel (*SCN1B*). As described previously, several anti-seizure drugs act on Na^+ channels to promote their inactivation; the phenotype of the mutated Na^+ channel appears to involve defective inactivation (Wallace et al., 1998).

Spontaneous mutations in *SCN1A (*encoding the α subunit of the major voltage-gated Na^+ channel in neurons) that result in truncations and presumed loss of Na^+ channel function have been identified in a subset of infants with a catastrophic severe myoclonic epilepsy of infancy. An intriguing clue as to how this genotype may lead to an epileptic phenotype has emerged from the study of *SCN1A* knock-out mice (Yu et al., 2006). Heterozygote mice have only one functional allele and provide a mouse model of this epileptic syndrome. Because activation of voltage-gated Na^+ channels depolarizes and activates a neuron, it seemed odd that a loss of function mutation of *SCN1A* would result in increased excitability of networks of neurons and epilepsy. This led to the discovery of impaired firing of inhibitory interneurons, but not excitatory principal neurons, in *SCN1A* heterozygous mice (Yu et al., 2006). These findings suggest that loss of function mutations of *SCN1A* may cause epilepsy as a consequence of reduced firing of inhibitory interneurons. Because interneurons effect inhibition by releasing GABA, this suggests that drugs acting to enhance GABA-mediated inhibition may be effective anticonvulsants in *SCN1A* mutant mice and infants with these mutations. Consistent with this hypothesis, preliminary findings reveal that an experimental anti-seizure drug that increases the duration of $GABA_A$ receptor channel open times (Quilichini et al., 2006) was beneficial in children with severe myoclonic epilepsy of infancy (Chiron, 2007). If confirmed, this would provide the first instance of rational use of anti-seizure drugs in that insight into the cellular mechanism of the epilepsy would guide selection of drugs acting by a given mechanism.

ANTI-SEIZURE DRUGS: GENERAL CONSIDERATIONS

History. The first anti-epileptic drug was bromide, which was used in the late 19th century. Phenobarbital was the first synthetic organic agent recognized as having anti-seizure activity. Its usefulness, however, was limited to generalized tonic-clonic seizures, and to a lesser degree, simple and complex partial seizures. It had no effect on absence seizures. Merritt and Putnam developed the electroshock seizure test in experimental animals to screen chemical agents for anti-seizure effectiveness; in the course of screening a variety of drugs, they discovered that diphenylhydantoin (later renamed phenytoin) suppressed seizures in the absence of sedative effects. The electroshock seizure test is extremely valuable, because drugs that are effective against tonic hind limb extension induced by electroshock generally have proven to be effective against partial and tonic-clonic seizures in humans. Another screening test, seizures induced by the chemoconvulsant pentylenetetrazol, is most useful in identifying drugs that are effective against myoclonic seizures in humans. These screening tests are still used. The chemical structures of most of the drugs introduced before 1965 were closely related to phenobarbital. These included the hydantoins and the succinimides. Between 1965 and 1990, the chemically distinct structures of the benzodiazepines, an iminostilbene (carbamazepine), and a branched-chain carboxylic acid (valproic acid) were introduced, followed in the 1990s by a phenyltriazine (lamotrigine), a cyclic analog of GABA (gabapentin), a sulfamate-substituted monosaccharide (topiramate), a nipecotic acid derivative (tiagabine), and a pyrrolidine derivative (levetiracetam).

Therapeutic Aspects. The ideal anti-seizure drug would suppress all seizures without causing any unwanted effects. Unfortunately, the drugs used currently not only fail to control seizure activity in some patients, but frequently cause unwanted effects that range in severity from minimal impairment of the CNS to death from aplastic anemia or hepatic failure. In 2009, all manufacturers of anti-seizure drugs were required to update their product labeling to include a warning about an increased risk of suicidal thoughts or actions and to develop information targeted at helping patients understand this risk. The risk applies to all anti-seizure drugs used for any indication. Details are online at the FDA website.

The clinician who treats patients with epilepsy is faced with the task of selecting the appropriate drug or combination of drugs that best controls seizures in an individual patient at an acceptable level of untoward effects. As a general rule, complete control of seizures can be achieved in up to 50% of patients, while another 25% can be improved significantly. The degree of success varies as a function of seizure type, cause, and other factors.

To minimize toxicity, treatment with a single drug is preferred. If seizures are not controlled with the initial agent at adequate plasma concentrations, substitution of a second drug is preferred to the concurrent administration of another agent. However, multiple-drug therapy may be required, especially when two or more types of seizure occur in the same patient.

Measurement of drug concentrations in plasma facilitates optimizing anti-seizure medication, especially when therapy is initiated, after dosage adjustments, in the event of therapeutic failure, when toxic effects appear, or when multiple-drug therapy is instituted. However, clinical effects of some drugs do not correlate well with their concentrations in plasma, and recommended concentrations are only guidelines for therapy. The ultimate therapeutic regimen must be determined by clinical assessment of effect and toxicity.

The individual agents are introduced in the next sections, followed by a discussion of some general principles of the drug therapy of the epilepsies.

HYDANTOINS

Phenytoin

Phenytoin (diphenylhydantoin; DILANTIN, others) is effective against all types of partial and tonic-clonic seizures but not absence seizures. Properties of other hydantoins (ethotoin, PEGANONE) are described in previous editions of this book.

History. Phenytoin was first synthesized in 1908 by Biltz, but its anticonvulsant activity was not discovered until 1938. In contrast to the earlier accidental discovery of the anti-seizure properties of bromide and phenobarbital, phenytoin was the product of a search among nonsedative structural relatives of phenobarbital for agents capable of suppressing electroshock convulsions in laboratory animals. It was introduced for the treatment of epilepsy in the same year. Since this agent is not a sedative in ordinary doses, it established that anti-seizure drugs need not induce drowsiness and encouraged the search for drugs with selective anti-seizure action.

PHENYTOIN

Structure-Activity Relationship. A 5-phenyl or other aromatic substituent appears essential for activity against generalized tonic-clonic seizures. Alkyl substituents in position 5 contribute to sedation, a property absent in phenytoin. The carbon 5 position permits asymmetry, but there appears to be little difference in activity between isomers.

Pharmacological Effects

Central Nervous System. Phenytoin exerts anti-seizure activity without causing general depression of the CNS. In toxic doses, it may produce excitatory signs and at lethal levels a type of decerebrate rigidity.

The most significant effect of phenytoin is its ability to modify the pattern of maximal electroshock seizures. The characteristic tonic phase can be abolished completely, but the residual clonic seizure may be exaggerated and prolonged. This seizure-modifying action is observed with many other anti-seizure drugs that are effective against generalized tonic-clonic seizures. By contrast, phenytoin does not inhibit clonic seizures evoked by pentylenetetrazol.

Mechanism of Action. Phenytoin limits the repetitive firing of action potentials evoked by a sustained depolarization of mouse spinal cord neurons maintained *in vitro* (McLean and Macdonald, 1986a). This effect is mediated by a slowing of the rate of recovery of voltage-activated Na^+ channels from inactivation, an action that is both voltage- (greater effect if membrane is depolarized) and use-dependent. These effects of phenytoin are evident at concentrations in the range of therapeutic drug levels in cerebrospinal fluid (CSF) in humans, which correlate with the free (or unbound) concentration of phenytoin in the serum. At these concentrations, the effects on Na^+ channels are selective, and no changes of spontaneous activity or responses to iontophoretically applied GABA or glutamate are detected. At concentrations 5- to 10-fold higher, multiple effects of phenytoin are evident, including reduction of spontaneous activity and enhancement of responses to GABA; these effects may underlie some of the unwanted toxicity associated with high levels of phenytoin.

Pharmacokinetic Properties. Phenytoin is available in two types of oral formulations that differ in their pharmacokinetics: rapid-release and extended-release forms. Once-daily dosing is possible only with the extended-release formulations, and due to differences in dissolution and other formulation-dependent factors, the plasma phenytoin level may change when converting from one formulation to another. Confusion also can arise because different formulations can include either phenytoin or phenytoin sodium. Therefore, comparable doses can be approximated by considering "phenytoin equivalents," but serum level monitoring is also necessary to assure therapeutic safety.

The pharmacokinetic characteristics of phenytoin are influenced markedly by its binding to serum proteins, by the nonlinearity of its elimination kinetics, and by its metabolism by hepatic CYPs (Table 21–3). Phenytoin is extensively bound (~90%) to serum proteins, mainly albumin. Small variations in the percentage of phenytoin that is bound dramatically affect the absolute amount of free (active) drug; increased proportions of free drug are evident in the neonate, in patients with hypoalbuminemia, and in uremic patients. Some agents can compete with phenytoin for binding sites on plasma proteins and increase free phenytoin at the time the new drug is added to the regimen. However, the effect on free phenytoin is only short-lived and usually does not cause clinical complications unless inhibition of phenytoin metabolism also occurs. For example, valproate competes for protein binding sites *and* inhibits phenytoin metabolism, resulting in marked and sustained increases in free phenytoin. Measurement of free rather than total phenytoin permits direct assessment of this potential problem in patient management.

Phenytoin is one of the few drugs for which the rate of elimination varies as a function of its concentration (i.e., the rate is nonlinear). The plasma $t_{1/2}$ of phenytoin ranges between 6 and 24 hours at plasma concentrations below 10 μg/mL but increases with higher concentrations; as a result, plasma drug concentration increases disproportionately as dosage is

Table 21–3

Interactions of Anti-Seizure Drugs with Hepatic Microsomal Enzymes

	INDUCES		INHIBITS		METABOLIZED BY	
DRUG	CYP	UGT	CYP	UGT	CYP	UGT
Carbamazepine	2C9/3A	Yes			1A2/2C8 2C9/3A4	No
Ethosuximide	No	No	No	No	?	?
Gabapentin	No	No	No	No	No	No
Lacosamide	No	No	No	No	2C19	?
Lamotrigine	No	Yes	No	No	No	Yes
Levetiracetam	No	No	No	No	No	No
Oxcarbazepine	3A4/5	Yes	2C19	Weak	No	Yes
Phenobarbital	2C/3A	Yes	Yes	No	2C9/19	No
Phenytoin	2C/3A	Yes	Yes	No	2C9/19	No
Pregabalin	No	No	No	No	No	No
Primidone	2C/3A	Yes	Yes	No	2C9/19	No
Rufinamide	3A4	2C9/19	No	?	No	Yes
Tiagabine	No	No	No	No	3A4	No
Topiramate	No	No	2C19	No		
Valproate	No	No	2C9	Yes	2C9/19	Yes
Vigabatrin	No	No	No	No	No	No
Zonisamide	No	No	No	No	3A4	Yes

CYP, cytochrome P450; UGT, uridine diphosphate-glucuronosyltransferase.

increased, even with small adjustments for levels near the therapeutic range.

The majority (95%) of phenytoin is metabolized in the hepatic endoplasmic reticulum by CYP2C9/10 and to a lesser extent CYP2C19 (Table 21–3). The principal metabolite, a parahydroxyphenyl derivative, is inactive. Because its metabolism is saturable, other drugs that are metabolized by these enzymes can inhibit the metabolism of phenytoin and increase its plasma concentration. Conversely, the degradation rate of other drugs that are substrates for these enzymes can be inhibited by phenytoin; one such drug is warfarin, and addition of phenytoin to a patient receiving warfarin can lead to bleeding disorders (Chapter 30). An alternative mechanism of drug interactions arises from phenytoin's ability to induce diverse CYPs (Chapter 6); co-administration of phenytoin and medications metabolized by these enzymes can lead to an increased degradation of such medications. Of particular note in this regard are oral contraceptives, which are metabolized by CYP3A4; treatment with phenytoin can enhance the metabolism of oral contraceptives and lead to unplanned pregnancy. The potential teratogenic effects of phenytoin underscore the importance of attention to this interaction. Carbamazepine, oxcarbazepine, phenobarbital, and primidone also can induce CYP3A4 and likewise might increase degradation of oral contraceptives.

The low water solubility of phenytoin hindered its intravenous use and led to production of fosphenytoin, a water-soluble prodrug. *Fosphenytoin* (CEREBYX, others) is converted into phenytoin by phosphatases in liver and red blood cells with a $t_{1/2}$ of 8-15 minutes. Fosphenytoin is extensively bound (95-99%) to human plasma proteins, primarily albumin. This binding is saturable and fosphenytoin displaces phenytoin from protein-binding sites. Fosphenytoin is useful for adults with partial or generalized seizures when intravenous or intramuscular administration is indicated.

Toxicity. The toxic effects of phenytoin depend on the route of administration, the duration of exposure, and the dosage.

When fosphenytoin, the water-soluble prodrug, is administered intravenously at an excessive rate in the emergency treatment of status epilepticus, the most notable toxic signs are cardiac arrhythmias with or without hypotension, and/or CNS depression. Although cardiac toxicity occurs more frequently in older patients and in those with known cardiac disease, it also can develop in young, healthy patients. These complications can be minimized by administering fosphenytoin at a rate of < 150 mg of phenytoin sodium equivalents per minute. Acute oral overdosage results primarily in signs referable to the cerebellum and vestibular system; high doses have been associated with marked cerebellar atrophy. Toxic effects associated with chronic treatment also are primarily dose-related cerebellar-vestibular effects but also include other CNS effects, behavioral changes, increased frequency of seizures, GI symptoms, gingival hyperplasia, osteomalacia, and megaloblastic anemia. Hirsutism is an annoying untoward effect in young females. Usually, these phenomena can be diminished by proper adjustment of dosage. Serious adverse effects, including those on the skin, bone marrow, and liver, probably are manifestations of drug allergy. Although rare, they necessitate withdrawal of the drug. Moderate elevation of the plasma concentrations of hepatic transaminases sometimes are observed; since these changes are transient and may result in part from induced synthesis of the enzymes, they do not necessitate withdrawal of the drug.

Gingival hyperplasia occurs in ~20% of all patients during chronic therapy and is probably the most common manifestation of phenytoin toxicity in children and young adolescents. It may be more frequent in those individuals who also develop coarsened facial features. The overgrowth of tissue appears to involve altered collagen metabolism. Toothless portions of the gums are not affected. The condition does not necessarily require withdrawal of medication and can be minimized by good oral hygiene.

A variety of endocrine effects have been reported. Inhibition of release of anti-diuretic hormone (ADH) has been observed in patients with inappropriate ADH secretion. Hyperglycemia and glycosuria appear to be due to inhibition of insulin secretion. Osteomalacia, with hypocalcemia and elevated alkaline phosphatase activity, has been attributed to both altered metabolism of vitamin D and the attendant inhibition of intestinal absorption of Ca^{2+}. Phenytoin also increases the metabolism of vitamin K and reduces the concentration of vitamin K–dependent proteins that are important for normal Ca^{2+} metabolism in bone. This may explain why the osteomalacia is not always ameliorated by the administration of vitamin D.

Hypersensitivity reactions include morbilliform rash in 2-5% of patients and occasionally more serious skin reactions, including Stevens-Johnson syndrome and toxic epidermal necrolysis. Systemic lupus erythematosus and potentially fatal hepatic necrosis have been reported rarely. Hematological reactions include neutropenia and leukopenia. A few cases of red-cell aplasia, agranulocytosis, and mild thrombocytopenia also have been reported. Lymphadenopathy, resembling Hodgkin's disease and malignant lymphoma, is associated with reduced immunoglobulin A (IgA) production. Hypoprothrombinemia and hemorrhage have occurred in the newborns of mothers who received phenytoin during pregnancy; vitamin K is effective treatment or prophylaxis.

Plasma Drug Concentrations. A good correlation usually is observed between the total concentration of phenytoin in plasma and its clinical effect. Thus, control of seizures generally is obtained with total concentrations above 10 μg/mL, while toxic effects such as nystagmus develop at total concentrations around 20 μg/mL. Control of seizures generally is obtained with free phenytoin concentrations of 0.75-1.25 μg/mL.

Drug Interactions. Concurrent administration of any drug metabolized by CYP2C9 or CYP2C10 can increase the plasma concentration of phenytoin by decreasing its rate of metabolism (Table 21–3). Carbamazepine, which may enhance the metabolism of phenytoin, causes a well-documented *decrease* in phenytoin concentration. Conversely, phenytoin reduces the concentration of carbamazepine. Interaction between phenytoin and phenobarbital is variable.

Therapeutic Uses

Epilepsy. Phenytoin is one of the more widely used anti-seizure agents, and it is effective against partial and tonic-clonic but not absence seizures. The use of phenytoin and other agents in the therapy of epilepsies is discussed further at the end of this chapter. Phenytoin preparations differ significantly in bioavailability and rate of absorption. In general, patients should consistently be treated with the same drug from a single manufacturer. However, if it becomes necessary to temporarily switch between products, care should be taken to select a therapeutically equivalent product and patients should be monitored for loss of seizure control or onset of new toxicities.

Other Uses. Trigeminal and related neuralgias occasionally respond to phenytoin, but carbamazepine may be preferable. The use of phenytoin in the treatment of cardiac arrhythmias is discussed in Chapter 29.

ANTI-SEIZURE BARBITURATES

The pharmacology of the barbiturates as a class is described in Chapter 17; discussion in this chapter is limited to phenobarbital. Use of other long-acting barbiturates (e.g., mephobarbital, MEBARAL) for therapy of the epilepsies is described in previous editions of this book.

Phenobarbital

Phenobarbital (LUMINAL, others) was the first effective organic anti-seizure agent. It has relatively low toxicity, is inexpensive, and is still one of the more effective and widely used drugs for this purpose.

Structure-Activity Relationship. The structural formula of phenobarbital (5-phenyl-5-ethylbarbituric acid) is shown in Chapter 17. The structure-activity relationships of the barbiturates have been studied extensively. Maximal anti-seizure activity is obtained when one substituent at carbon 5 position is a phenyl group. The 5,5-diphenyl derivative has less anti-seizure potency than does phenobarbital, but it is virtually devoid of hypnotic activity. By contrast, 5,5-dibenzyl barbituric acid causes convulsions.

Anti-Seizure Properties. Most barbiturates have anti-seizure properties. However, only some of these agents, such as phenobarbital, exert maximal anti-seizure action at doses below those required for hypnosis, which determines their clinical utility as anti-seizure agents. Phenobarbital is active in most anti-seizure tests in animals but is relatively nonselective. It inhibits tonic hind limb extension in the maximal electroshock model, clonic seizures evoked by pentylenetetrazol, and kindled seizures.

Mechanism of Action. The mechanism by which phenobarbital inhibits seizures likely involves potentiation of synaptic inhibition through an action on the $GABA_A$ receptor. Intracellular recordings of mouse cortical or spinal cord neurons demonstrated that phenobarbital enhances responses to iontophoretically applied GABA.

These effects have been observed at therapeutically relevant concentrations of phenobarbital. Analyses of single channels in outside-out patches isolated from mouse spinal cord neurons demonstrated that phenobarbital increased the $GABA_A$ receptor–mediated current by increasing the duration of bursts of $GABA_A$ receptor–mediated currents without changing the frequency of bursts (Twyman et al., 1989). At levels exceeding therapeutic concentrations, phenobarbital also limits sustained repetitive firing; this may underlie some of the anti-seizure effects of higher concentrations of phenobarbital achieved during therapy of status epilepticus.

Pharmacokinetic Properties. Oral absorption of phenobarbital is complete but somewhat slow; peak concentrations in plasma occur several hours after a single dose. It is 40-60% bound to plasma proteins and bound to a similar extent in tissues, including brain. Up to 25% of a dose is eliminated by pH-dependent renal excretion of the unchanged drug; the remainder is inactivated by hepatic microsomal enzymes, principally CYP2C9, with minor metabolism by CYP2C19 and CYP2E1. Phenobarbital induces uridine diphosphate-glucuronosyltransferase (UGT) enzymes as well as the CYP2C and CYP3A subfamilies. Drugs metabolized by these enzymes can be more rapidly degraded when co-administered with phenobarbital; importantly, oral contraceptives are metabolized by CYP3A4.

Toxicity. Sedation, the most frequent undesired effect of phenobarbital, is apparent to some extent in all patients upon initiation of therapy, but tolerance develops during chronic medication. Nystagmus and ataxia occur at excessive dosage. Phenobarbital can produce irritability and hyperactivity in children, and agitation and confusion in the elderly.

Scarlatiniform or morbilliform rash, possibly with other manifestations of drug allergy, occurs in 1-2% of patients. Exfoliative dermatitis is rare. Hypoprothrombinemia with hemorrhage has been observed in the newborns of mothers who have received phenobarbital during pregnancy; vitamin K is effective for treatment or prophylaxis. As with phenytoin, megaloblastic anemia that responds to folate and osteomalacia that responds to high doses of vitamin D occur during chronic phenobarbital therapy of epilepsy. Other adverse effects of phenobarbital are discussed in Chapter 17.

Plasma Drug Concentrations. During long-term therapy in adults, the plasma concentration of phenobarbital averages 10 μg/mL per daily dose of 1 mg/kg; in children, the value is 5-7 μg/mL per 1 mg/kg. Although a precise relationship between therapeutic results and concentration of drug in plasma does not exist, plasma concentrations of 10-35 μg/mL are usually recommended for control of seizures.

The relationship between plasma concentration of phenobarbital and adverse effects varies with the development of tolerance. Sedation, nystagmus, and ataxia usually are absent at concentrations below 30 μg/mL during long-term therapy, but adverse effects may be apparent for several days at lower concentrations when therapy is initiated or whenever the dosage is increased. Concentrations > 60 μg/mL may be associated with marked intoxication in the nontolerant individual.

Since significant behavioral toxicity may be present despite the absence of overt signs of toxicity, the tendency to maintain patients, particularly children, on excessively high doses of phenobarbital should be resisted. The plasma phenobarbital concentration should be increased above 30-40 μg/mL only if the increment is adequately tolerated and only if it contributes significantly to control of seizures.

Drug Interactions. Interactions between phenobarbital and other drugs usually involve induction of the hepatic CYPs by phenobarbital (see Table 21–3 and Chapters 6 and 17). The interaction between phenytoin and phenobarbital is variable. Concentrations of phenobarbital in plasma may be elevated by as much as 40% during concurrent administration of valproic acid.

Therapeutic Uses. Phenobarbital is an effective agent for generalized tonic-clonic and partial seizures. Its efficacy, low toxicity, and low cost make it an important agent for these types of epilepsy. However, its sedative effects and its tendency to disturb behavior in children have reduced its use as a primary agent. It is not effective for absence seizures.

IMINOSTILBENES

Carbamazepine

Carbamazepine (TEGRETOL, CARBATROL, others) was initially approved in the U.S. for use as an anti-seizure agent in 1974. It has been employed since the 1960s for the treatment of trigeminal neuralgia. It is now considered to be a primary drug for the treatment of partial and tonic-clonic seizures.

Chemistry. Carbamazepine is related chemically to the tricyclic antidepressants. It is a derivative of iminostilbene with a carbamyl group at the 5 position; this moiety is essential for potent anti-seizure activity.

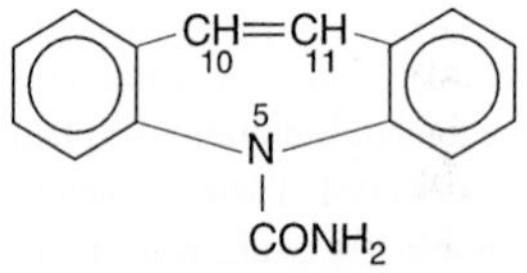

CH=CH (10, 11); N (5); $CONH_2$

CARBAMAZEPINE

Pharmacological Effects. Although the effects of carbamazepine in animals and humans resemble those of phenytoin in many ways, the two drugs exhibit important differences. Carbamazepine has been found to produce therapeutic responses in manic-depressive patients, including some in whom lithium carbonate is not effective. Further, carbamazepine has anti-diuretic effects that are sometimes associated with increased concentrations of anti-diuretic hormone (ADH) in plasma. The mechanisms responsible for these effects of carbamazepine are not clearly understood.

Mechanism of Action. Like phenytoin, carbamazepine limits the repetitive firing of action potentials evoked by a sustained depolarization of mouse spinal cord or cortical neurons maintained *in vitro* (McLean and Macdonald, 1986a). This appears to be mediated by a slowing of the rate of recovery of voltage-activated Na^+ channels from inactivation. These effects of carbamazepine are evident at concentrations in the range of therapeutic drug levels in CSF in humans. The effects of carbamazepine are selective at these concentrations, in that there are no effects on spontaneous activity or on responses to iontophoretically applied GABA or glutamate. The carbamazepine metabolite, 10,11-epoxycarbamazepine, also limits sustained repetitive firing at therapeutically relevant concentrations, suggesting that this metabolite may contribute to the anti-seizure efficacy of carbamazepine.

Pharmacokinetic Properties. The pharmacokinetics of carbamazepine are complex. They are influenced by its limited aqueous solubility and by the ability of many anti-seizure drugs, including carbamazepine itself, to increase their conversion to active metabolites by hepatic oxidative enzymes (Table 21–3).

Carbamazepine is absorbed slowly and erratically after oral administration. Peak concentrations in plasma usually are observed 4-8 hours after oral ingestion, but may be delayed by as much as 24 hours, especially following the administration of a large dose. The drug distributes rapidly into all tissues. Approximately 75% of carbamazepine binds to plasma proteins and concentrations in the CSF appear to correspond to the concentration of free drug in plasma.

The predominant pathway of metabolism in humans involves conversion to the 10,11-epoxide. This metabolite is as active as the parent compound in various animals, and its concentrations in plasma and brain may reach 50% of those of carbamazepine, especially during the concurrent administration of phenytoin or phenobarbital. The 10,11-epoxide is metabolized further to inactive compounds, which are excreted in the urine principally as glucuronides. Carbamazepine also is inactivated by conjugation and hydroxylation. Hepatic CYP3A4 is primarily responsible for biotransformation of carbamazepine. Carbamazepine induces CYP2C, CYP3A, and UGT, thus enhancing the metabolism of drugs degraded by these enzymes. Of particular importance in this regard are oral contraceptives, which are also metabolized by CYP3A4.

Toxicity. Acute intoxication with carbamazepine can result in stupor or coma, hyperirritability, convulsions, and respiratory depression. During long-term therapy, the more frequent untoward effects of the drug include drowsiness, vertigo, ataxia, diplopia, and blurred vision. The frequency of seizures may increase, especially with overdosage. Other adverse effects include nausea, vomiting, serious hematological toxicity (aplastic anemia, agranulocytosis), and hypersensitivity reactions (dangerous skin reactions, eosinophilia, lymphadenopathy, splenomegaly). A late complication of therapy with carbamazepine is retention of water, with decreased osmolality and concentration of Na^+ in plasma, especially in elderly patients with cardiac disease.

Some tolerance develops to the neurotoxic effects of carbamazepine, and they can be minimized by gradual increase in dosage or adjustment of maintenance dosage. Various hepatic or pancreatic abnormalities have been reported during therapy with carbamazepine, most commonly a transient elevation of hepatic transaminases in plasma in 5-10% of patients. A transient, mild leukopenia occurs in ~10% of patients during initiation of therapy and usually resolves within the first 4 months of continued treatment; transient thrombocytopenia also has been noted. In ~2% of patients, a persistent leukopenia may develop that requires withdrawal of the drug. The initial concern that aplastic anemia might be a frequent complication of long-term therapy with carbamazepine has not materialized. In most cases, the administration of multiple drugs or the presence of another underlying disease has made it difficult to establish a causal relationship. The prevalence of aplastic anemia appears to be ~1 in 200,000 patients who are treated with the drug. It is not clear whether monitoring of hematological function can avert the development of irreversible aplastic anemia. Although carbamazepine is carcinogenic in rats, it is not known to be carcinogenic in humans. Possible teratogenic effects are discussed later in the chapter.

Plasma Drug Concentrations. There is no simple relationship between the dose of carbamazepine and concentrations of the drug in plasma. Therapeutic concentrations are reported to be 6-12 μg/mL, although considerable variation occurs. Side effects referable to the CNS are frequent at concentrations above 9 μg/mL.

Drug Interactions. Phenobarbital, phenytoin, and valproate may increase the metabolism of carbamazepine by inducing CYP3A4; carbamazepine may enhance the biotransformation of phenytoin. Concurrent administration of carbamazepine may lower concentrations of valproate, lamotrigine, tiagabine, and topiramate. Carbamazepine reduces both the plasma concentration and therapeutic effect of haloperidol. The metabolism of carbamazepine may be inhibited by propoxyphene, erythromycin, cimetidine, fluoxetine, and isoniazid.

Therapeutic Uses. Carbamazepine is useful in patients with generalized tonic-clonic and both simple and complex partial seizures (Table 21–1). When it is used, renal and hepatic function and hematological parameters should be monitored. The therapeutic use of carbamazepine is discussed further at the end of this chapter.

Carbamazepine is the primary agent for treatment of trigeminal and glossopharyngeal neuralgias. It is also effective for lightning-type ("tabetic") pain associated with bodily wasting. Most patients with neuralgia benefit initially, but only 70% obtain continuing relief. Adverse effects require discontinuation of medication in 5-20% of patients. The therapeutic range of plasma concentrations for anti-seizure therapy serves as a guideline for its use in neuralgia. Carbamazepine is also used in the treatment of bipolar affective disorders, as discussed further in Chapter 16.

Oxcarbazepine

Oxcarbazepine (TRILEPTAL, others) (10,11-dihydro-10-oxocarbamazepine) is a keto analog of carbamazepine.

Oxcarbazepine is a prodrug that is almost immediately converted to its main active metabolite, a 10-monohydroxy derivative, which is inactivated by glucuronide conjugation and eliminated by renal excretion.

Its mechanism of action is similar to that of carbamazepine. Oxcarbazepine is a less potent enzyme inducer than carbamazepine. Substitution of oxcarbazepine for carbamazepine is associated with increased levels of phenytoin and valproic acid, presumably because of reduced induction of hepatic enzymes. Oxcarbazepine does not induce the hepatic enzymes involved in its own degradation. Although oxcarbazepine does not appear to reduce the anticoagulant effect of warfarin, it does induce CYP3A and thus reduces plasma levels of steroid oral contraceptives. It has been approved for monotherapy or adjunct therapy for partial seizures in adults, as monotherapy for partial seizures in children ages 4-16, and as adjunctive therapy in children 2 years of age and older with epilepsy.

SUCCINIMIDES

Ethosuximide

Ethosuximide (ZARONTIN, others) is a primary agent for the treatment of absence seizures.

Structure-Activity Relationship. The structure-activity relationship of the succinimides is in accord with that for other anti-seizure classes. Methsuximide (CELONTIN) has phenyl substituents and is more active against maximal electroshock seizures. It is no longer in common use. Discussion of its properties can be found in previous editions of this book. Ethosuximide, with alkyl substituents, is the most active of the succinimides against seizures induced by pentylenetetrazol and is the most selective for absence seizures.

Pharmacological Effects. The most prominent characteristic of ethosuximide at nontoxic doses is protection against clonic motor seizures induced by pentylenetetrazol. By contrast, at nontoxic doses ethosuximide does not inhibit tonic hind limb extension of electroshock seizures or kindled seizures. This profile correlates with efficacy against absence seizures in humans.

Mechanism of Action. Ethosuximide reduces low threshold Ca^{2+} currents (T-type currents) in thalamic neurons (Coulter et al., 1989). The thalamus plays an important role in generation of 3-Hz spike-and-wave rhythms typical of absence seizures (Huguenard and McCormick, 2007). Neurons in the thalamus exhibit large-amplitude T-type currents that underlie bursts of action potentials and likely play an important role in thalamic oscillatory activity such as 3-Hz spike-and-wave activity. At clinically relevant concentrations, ethosuximide inhibits the T-type current, as is evident in voltage-clamp recordings of acutely isolated, ventrobasal thalamic neurons from rats and guinea pigs. Ethosuximide reduces this current without modifying the voltage dependence of steady-state inactivation or the time course of recovery from inactivation. By contrast, succinimide derivatives with convulsant properties do not inhibit this current. Ethosuximide does not inhibit sustained repetitive firing or enhance GABA responses at clinically relevant concentrations. Inhibition of T-type currents likely is the mechanism by which ethosuximide inhibits absence seizures.

Pharmacokinetic Properties. Absorption of ethosuximide appears to be complete, with peak concentrations in plasma within ~3 hours after a single oral dose. Ethosuximide is not significantly bound to plasma proteins; during long-term therapy, its concentration in the CSF is similar to that in plasma. The apparent volume of distribution averages 0.7 L/kg.

Approximately 25% of the drug is excreted unchanged in the urine. The remainder is metabolized by hepatic microsomal enzymes, but whether CYPs are responsible is unknown. The major metabolite, the hydroxyethyl derivative, accounts for ~40% of administered drug, is inactive, and is excreted as such and as the glucuronide in the urine. The plasma $t_{1/2}$ of ethosuximide averages between 40 and 50 hours in adults and ~30 hours in children.

Toxicity. The most common dose-related side effects are gastrointestinal complaints (nausea, vomiting, and anorexia) and CNS effects (drowsiness, lethargy, euphoria, dizziness, headache, and hiccough). Some tolerance to these effects develops. Parkinson-like symptoms and photophobia also have been reported. Restlessness, agitation, anxiety, aggressiveness, inability to concentrate, and other behavioral effects have occurred primarily in patients with a prior history of psychiatric disturbance.

Urticaria and other skin reactions, including Stevens-Johnson syndrome, as well as systemic lupus erythematosus, eosinophilia, leukopenia, thrombocytopenia, pancytopenia, and aplastic anemia also have been attributed to the drug. The leukopenia may be transient despite continuation of the drug, but several deaths have resulted from bone marrow depression. Renal or hepatic toxicity has not been reported.

Plasma Drug Concentrations. During long-term therapy, the plasma concentration of ethosuximide averages ~2 μg/mL per daily dose of 1 mg/kg. A plasma concentration of 40-100 μg/mL usually is required for satisfactory control of absence seizures.

Therapeutic Uses. Ethosuximide is effective against absence seizures but not tonic-clonic seizures.

An initial daily dose of 250 mg in children (3-6 years old) and 500 mg in older children and adults is increased by 250-mg increments at weekly intervals until seizures are adequately controlled or toxicity intervenes. Divided dosage is required occasionally to prevent nausea or drowsiness associated with once-daily dosing. The usual maintenance dose is 20 mg/kg per day. Increased caution is required if the daily dose exceeds 1500 mg in adults or 750-1000 mg in children. The therapeutic use of ethosuximide is discussed further at the end of the chapter.

VALPROIC ACID

The anti-seizure properties of valproic acid (DEPAKENE, others) were discovered serendipitously when it was employed as a vehicle for other compounds that were being screened for anti-seizure activity.

$$\begin{matrix} CH_3CH_2CH_2 \diagdown \\ \quad\quad\quad\quad CHCOOH \\ CH_3CH_2CH_2 \diagup \end{matrix}$$

VALPROIC ACID

Chemistry. Valproic acid (*n*-dipropylacetic acid) is a simple branched-chain carboxylic acid. Certain other branched-chain carboxylic acids have potencies similar to that of valproic acid in antagonizing pentylenetetrazol-induced convulsions. However, increasing the number of carbon atoms to nine introduces marked sedative properties. Straight-chain carboxylic acids have little or no activity.

Pharmacological Effects. Valproic acid is strikingly different from phenytoin or ethosuximide in that it is effective in inhibiting seizures in a variety of models. Like phenytoin and carbamazepine, valproate inhibits tonic hind limb extension in maximal electroshock seizures and kindled seizures at nontoxic doses. Like ethosuximide, valproic acid at subtoxic doses inhibits clonic motor seizures induced by pentylenetetrazol. Its efficacy in diverse models parallels its efficacy against absence as well as partial and generalized tonic-clonic seizures in humans.

Mechanism of Action. Valproic acid produces effects on isolated neurons similar to those of phenytoin and ethosuximide (Table 21–2). At therapeutically relevant concentrations, valproate inhibits sustained repetitive firing induced by depolarization of mouse cortical or spinal cord neurons (McLean and Macdonald, 1986b). The action is similar to that of both phenytoin and carbamazepine and appears to be mediated by a prolonged recovery of voltage-activated Na^+ channels from inactivation. Valproic acid does not modify neuronal responses to iontophoretically applied GABA. In neurons isolated from the nodose ganglion, valproate also produces small reductions of T-type Ca^{2+} currents (Kelly et al., 1990) at clinically relevant but slightly higher concentrations than those that limit sustained repetitive firing; this effect on T-type currents is similar to that of ethosuximide in thalamic neurons (Coulter et al., 1989). Together, these actions of limiting sustained repetitive firing and reducing T-type currents may contribute to the effectiveness of valproic acid against partial and tonic-clonic seizures and absence seizures, respectively.

Another potential mechanism that may contribute to valproate's anti-seizure actions involves metabolism of GABA. Although valproate has no effect on responses to GABA, it does increase the amount of GABA that can be recovered from the brain after the drug is administered to animals. *In vitro*, valproate can stimulate the activity of the GABA synthetic enzyme, glutamic acid decarboxylase, and inhibit GABA degradative enzymes, GABA transaminase and succinic semialdehyde dehydrogenase. Thus far it has been difficult to relate the increased GABA levels to the anti-seizure activity of valproate.

Pharmacokinetic Properties. Valproic acid is absorbed rapidly and completely after oral administration. Peak concentration in plasma is observed in 1-4 hours, although this can be delayed for several hours if the drug is administered in enteric-coated tablets or is ingested with meals.

The apparent volume of distribution for valproate is ~0.2 L/kg. Its extent of binding to plasma proteins is usually ~90%, but the fraction bound is reduced as the total concentration of valproate is increased through the therapeutic range. Although concentrations of valproate in CSF suggest equilibration with free drug in the blood, there is evidence for carrier-mediated transport of valproate both into and out of the CSF.

The vast majority of valproate (95%) undergoes hepatic metabolism, with < 5% excreted unchanged in urine. Its hepatic metabolism occurs mainly by UGT enzymes and β-oxidation. Valproate is a substrate for CYP2C9 and CYP2C19, but metabolism by these enzymes accounts for a relatively minor portion of its elimination. Some of the drug's metabolites, notably 2-propyl-2-pentenoic acid and 2-propyl-4-pentenoic acid, are nearly as potent anti-seizure agents as the parent compound; however, only the former (2-en-valproic acid) accumulates in plasma and brain to a potentially significant extent. The $t_{1/2}$ of valproate is ~15 hours but is reduced in patients taking other anti-epileptic drugs.

Toxicity. The most common side effects are transient GI symptoms, including anorexia, nausea, and vomiting in ~16% of patients. Effects on the CNS include sedation, ataxia, and tremor; these symptoms occur infrequently and usually respond to a decrease in dosage. Rash, alopecia, and stimulation of appetite have been observed occasionally and weight gain has been seen with chronic valproic acid treatment in some patients. Valproic acid has several effects on hepatic function. Elevation of hepatic transaminases in plasma is observed in up to 40% of patients and often occurs asymptomatically during the first several months of therapy.

A rare complication is a fulminant hepatitis that is frequently fatal (Dreifuss et al., 1989). Pathological examination reveals a microvesicular steatosis without evidence of inflammation or hypersensitivity reaction. Children below 2 years of age with other medical conditions who were given multiple anti-seizure agents were especially likely to suffer fatal hepatic injury. At the other extreme, there were no deaths reported for patients over the age of 10 years who received only valproate. Acute pancreatitis and hyperammonemia also have been frequently associated with the use of valproic acid. Valproic acid can also produce teratogenic effects such as neural tube defects.

Plasma Drug Concentrations. Valproate plasma concentrations associated with therapeutic effects are ~30-100 μg/mL. However, there is a poor correlation between the plasma concentration and efficacy. There appears to be a threshold at ~30-50 μg/mL; this is the concentration at which binding sites on plasma albumin begin to become saturated.

Drug Interactions. Valproate primarily inhibits the metabolism of drugs that are substrates for CYP2C9, including phenytoin and phenobarbital. Valproate also inhibits UGT and thus inhibits the metabolism of lamotrigine and lorazepam. A high proportion of valproate is bound to albumin, and the high molar concentrations of valproate in the clinical setting result in valproate's displacing phenytoin and other drugs from albumin. With respect to phenytoin in particular, valproate's inhibition of the drug's metabolism is exacerbated by

explain lamotrigine's actions on partial and secondarily generalized seizures. However, as mentioned in the subsequent "Therapeutic Use" section, lamotrigine is effective against a broader spectrum of seizures than phenytoin and carbamazepine, suggesting that lamotrigine may have actions in addition to regulating recovery from inactivation of Na^+ channels. The mechanisms underlying its broad spectrum of actions are incompletely understood. One possibility involves lamotrigine's inhibition of glutamate release in rat cortical slices treated with veratridine, a Na^+ channel activator, raising the possibility that lamotrigine inhibits synaptic release of glutamate by acting at Na^+ channels themselves.

Pharmacokinetics. Lamotrigine is completely absorbed from the gastrointestinal tract and is metabolized primarily by glucuronidation. The plasma $t_{1/2}$ of a single dose is 24-30 hours. Administration of phenytoin, carbamazepine, or phenobarbital reduces the $t_{1/2}$ and plasma concentrations of lamotrigine. Conversely, addition of valproate markedly increases plasma concentrations of lamotrigine, likely by inhibiting glucuronidation. Addition of lamotrigine to valproic acid produces a reduction of valproate concentrations by ~25% over a few weeks. Concurrent use of lamotrigine and carbamazepine is associated with increases of the 10,11-epoxide of carbamazepine and clinical toxicity in some patients.

Therapeutic Use. Lamotrigine is useful for monotherapy and add-on therapy of partial and secondarily generalized tonic-clonic seizures in adults and Lennox-Gastaut syndrome in both children and adults. Lennox-Gastaut syndrome is a disorder of childhood characterized by multiple seizure types, mental retardation, and refractoriness to anti-seizure medication.

Lamotrigine monotherapy in newly diagnosed partial or generalized tonic-clonic seizures is equivalent to carbamazepine or phenytoin, monotherapy (Brodie et al., 1995; Steiner et al., 1999). A double-blind, placebo-controlled trial of addition of lamotrigine to existing anti-seizure drugs further demonstrated effectiveness of lamotrigine against tonic-clonic seizures and drop attacks in children with the Lennox-Gastaut syndrome (Motte et al., 1997). Lamotrigine was also found to be superior to placebo in a double-blind study of children with newly diagnosed absence epilepsy (Frank et al., 1999).

Patients who are already taking a hepatic enzyme–inducing anti-seizure drug (such as carbamazepine, phenytoin, phenobarbital, or primidone, but not valproate) should be given lamotrigine initially at 50 mg/day for 2 weeks. The dose is increased to 50 mg twice per day for 2 weeks and then increased in increments of 100 mg/day each week up to a maintenance dose of 300-500 mg/day divided into two doses. For patients taking valproate in addition to an enzyme-inducing anti-seizure drug, the initial dose should be 25 mg every other day for 2 weeks, followed by an increase to 25 mg/day for 2 weeks; the dose then can be increased by 25-50 mg/day every 1-2 weeks up to a maintenance dose of 100-150 mg/day divided into two doses.

Toxicity. The most common adverse effects are dizziness, ataxia, blurred or double vision, nausea, vomiting, and rash when lamotrigine was added to another anti-seizure drug. A few cases of Stevens-Johnson syndrome and disseminated intravascular coagulation have been reported. The incidence of serious rash in pediatric patients (~0.8%) is higher than in the adult population (0.3%).

Levetiracetam

Levetiracetam (KEPPRA, others) is a pyrrolidine, the racemically pure S-enantiomer of α-ethyl-2-oxo-1-pyrrolidineacetamide and is FDA-approved for adjunctive therapy for myoclonic, partial-onset, and primary generalized tonic-clonic seizures in adults and children as young as 4 years old.

LEVETIRACETAM

Pharmacological Effects and Mechanism of Action. Levetiracetam exhibits a novel pharmacological profile insofar as it inhibits partial and secondarily generalized tonic-clonic seizures in the kindling model, yet is ineffective against maximum electroshock- and pentylenetetrazol-induced seizures, findings consistent with clinical effectiveness against partial and secondarily generalized tonic-clonic seizures. The mechanism by which levetiracetam exerts these anti-seizure effects is unknown. No evidence for an action on voltage-gated Na^+ channels or either GABA- or glutamate-mediated synaptic transmission has emerged. The correlation between binding affinity of levetiracetam analogs and their potency toward audiogenic seizures suggests that a synaptic vesicle protein, SV2A, mediates the anticonvulsant effects of levetiracetam (Rogawski and Bazil, 2008). Uncertainty as to the function of SV2A limits insights into how binding of levetiracetam to SV2A might affect cellular function or neuronal excitability.

Pharmacokinetics. Levetiracetam is rapidly and almost completely absorbed after oral administration and is not bound to plasma proteins. Ninety-five percent of the drug and its inactive metabolite are excreted in the urine, 65% of which is unchanged drug; 24% of the drug is metabolized by hydrolysis of the acetamide group. It neither induces nor is a high-affinity substrate for CYP isoforms or glucuronidation enzymes and thus is devoid of known interactions with other anti-seizure drugs, oral contraceptives, or anticoagulants.

Therapeutic Use. Double-blind, placebo-controlled trials of adults with either refractory partial seizures or uncontrolled generalized tonic-clonic seizures associated with idiopathic generalized epilepsy revealed that addition of levetiracetam to other anti-seizure medications was superior to placebo. Levetiracetam also has efficacy as adjunctive therapy for refractory generalized myoclonic seizures (Andermann et al., 2005). Insufficient evidence is available about its use as monotherapy for partial or generalized epilepsy.

Toxicity. Levetiracetam is well tolerated. The most frequently reported adverse effects are somnolence, asthenia, and dizziness.

Tiagabine

Tiagabine (GABITRIL) is a derivative of nipecotic acid and approved by the FDA as adjunct therapy for partial seizures in adults.

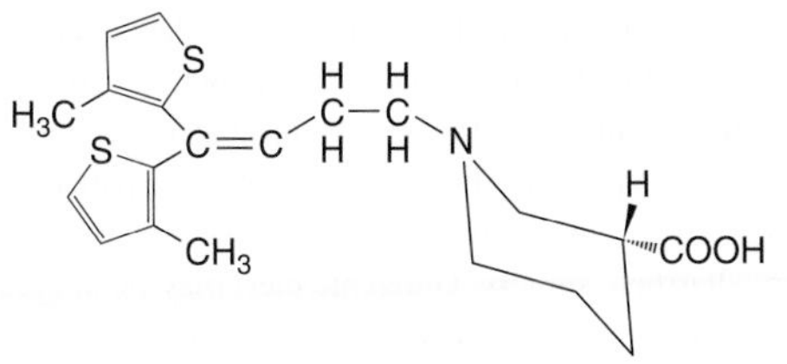

TIAGABINE

Pharmacological Effects and Mechanism of Action. Tiagabine inhibits the GABA transporter, GAT-1, and thereby reduces GABA uptake into neurons and glia. In CA1 neurons of the hippocampus, tiagabine increases the duration of inhibitory synaptic currents, findings consistent with prolonging the effect of GABA at inhibitory synapses through reducing its reuptake by GAT-1. Tiagabine inhibits maximum electroshock seizures and both limbic and secondarily generalized tonic-clonic seizures in the kindling model, results suggestive of clinical efficacy against partial and tonic-clonic seizures. Paradoxically, tiagabine has been associated with the occurrence of seizures in patients without epilepsy and off-label use of the drug is discouraged.

Pharmacokinetics. Tiagabine is rapidly absorbed after oral administration, extensively bound to serum or plasma proteins, and metabolized mainly in the liver, predominantly by CYP3A. Its $t_{1/2}$ of ~8 hours is shortened by 2-3 hours when co-administered with hepatic enzyme–inducing drugs such as phenobarbital, phenytoin, or carbamazepine.

Therapeutic Use. Double-blind, placebo-controlled trials have established tiagabine's efficacy as add-on therapy of refractory partial seizures with or without secondary generalization. Its efficacy as monotherapy for newly diagnosed or refractory partial and generalized epilepsy has not been established.

Toxicity. The principal adverse effects include dizziness, somnolence, and tremor; they appear to be mild to moderate in severity and appear shortly after initiation of therapy. Tiagabine and other drugs that enhance effects of synaptically released GABA can facilitate spike-and-wave discharges in animal models of absence seizures. Case reports suggest that tiagabine treatment of patients with a history of spike-and-wave discharges causes exacerbations of their EEG abnormalities. Thus, tiagabine may be contraindicated in patients with generalized absence epilepsy.

Topiramate

Topiramate (TOPAMAX, others) is a sulfamate-substituted monosaccharide that is FDA-approved as initial monotherapy (in patients at least 10 years old) and as adjunctive therapy (for patients as young as 2 years of age) for partial-onset or primary generalized tonic-clonic seizures, for Lennox-Gastaut syndrome in patients 2 years of age and older, and for migraine headache prophylaxis in adults.

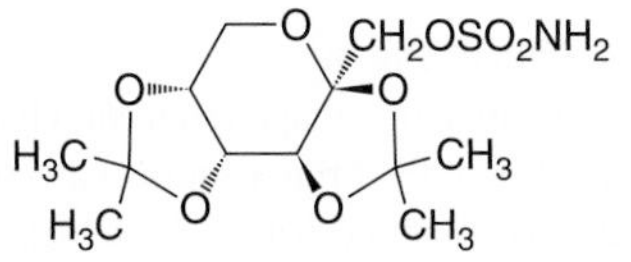

TOPIRAMATE

Pharmacological Effects and Mechanisms of Action. Topiramate reduces voltage-gated Na^+ currents in cerebellar granule cells and may act on the inactivated state of the channel similar to phenytoin. In addition, topiramate activates a hyperpolarizing K^+ current, enhances postsynaptic $GABA_A$-receptor currents, and limits activation of the AMPA-kainate-subtype(s) of glutamate receptor. Topiramate is a weak carbonic anhydrase inhibitor. Topiramate inhibits maximal electroshock and pentylenetetrazol-induced seizures as well as partial and secondarily generalized tonic-clonic seizures in the kindling model, findings predictive of a broad spectrum of anti-seizure actions clinically.

Pharmacokinetics. Topiramate is rapidly absorbed after oral administration, exhibits little (10-20%) binding to plasma proteins, and is mainly excreted unchanged in the urine. The remainder undergoes metabolism by hydroxylation, hydrolysis, and glucuronidation with no single metabolite accounting for > 5% of an oral dose. Its $t_{1/2}$ is ~1 day. Reduced estradiol plasma concentrations occur with concurrent topiramate, suggesting the need for higher doses of oral contraceptives when coadministered with topiramate.

Therapeutic Use. A double-blind study revealed topiramate to be equivalent to valproate and carbamazepine in children and adults with newly diagnosed partial and primary generalized epilepsy (Privitera et al., 2003). Additional studies disclosed topiramate to be effective as monotherapy for refractory partial epilepsy (Sachdeo et al., 1997) and refractory generalized tonic-clonic seizures (Biton et al., 1999). Topiramate also was found to be significantly more effective than placebo against both drop attacks and tonic-clonic seizures in patients with Lennox-Gastaut syndrome (Sachdeo et al., 1999).

Toxicity. Topiramate is well tolerated. The most common adverse effects are somnolence, fatigue, weight loss, and nervousness. It can precipitate renal calculi, which is most likely due to inhibition of carbonic anhydrase. Topiramate has been associated with cognitive impairment and patients may complain about a change in the taste of carbonated beverages.

Felbamate

Felbamate (FELBATOL) is a dicarbamate that was approved by the FDA for partial seizures in 1993. An association between felbamate and aplastic anemia in at least 10 cases resulted in a recommendation by the FDA and the manufacturer for the immediate withdrawal of most patients from treatment with this drug. Postmarketing experience revealed an association between felbamate exposure and liver failure.

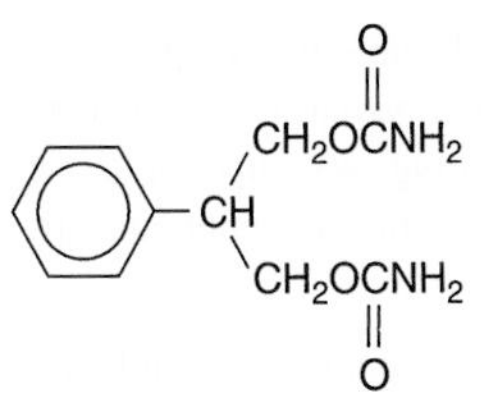

FELBAMATE

Pharmacological Effects and Mechanisms of Action. Felbamate is effective in both the maximal electroshock and pentylenetetrazol seizure models. Clinically relevant concentrations of felbamate inhibit NMDA-evoked responses and potentiate GABA-evoked responses in whole-cell, voltage-clamp recordings of cultured rat hippocampal neurons (Rho et al., 1994). This dual action on excitatory and inhibitory transmitter responses may contribute to the wide spectrum of action of the drug in seizure models.

Therapeutic Use. An active control, randomized, double-blind protocol demonstrated the efficacy of felbamate in patients with poorly controlled partial and secondarily generalized seizures (Sachdeo et al., 1992). Felbamate also reduced seizures in patients with Lennox-Gastaut syndrome (Felbamate Study Group in Lennox-Gastaut Syndrome, 1993). The clinical efficacy of this compound, which inhibits responses to NMDA and potentiates those to GABA, underscores the potential value of additional anti-seizure agents with similar mechanisms of action.

Zonisamide

Zonisamide (ZONEGRAN, others) is a sulfonamide derivative that is FDA approved as adjunctive therapy of partial seizures in adults.

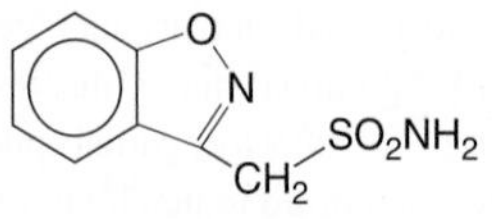

ZONISAMIDE

Pharmacological Effects and Mechanism of Action. Zonisamide inhibits the T-type Ca^{2+} currents. In addition, zonisamide inhibits the sustained, repetitive firing of spinal cord neurons, presumably by prolonging the inactivated state of voltage-gated Na^+ channels in a manner similar to actions of phenytoin and carbamazepine.

Zonisamide inhibits tonic hind limb extension evoked by maximal electroshock and inhibits both partial and secondarily generalized seizures in the kindling model, results predictive of clinical effectiveness against partial and secondarily generalized tonic-clonic seizures. Zonisamide does not inhibit minimal clonic seizures induced by pentylenetetrazol, suggesting that the drug will not be effective clinically against myoclonic seizures.

Pharmacokinetics. Zonisamide is almost completely absorbed after oral administration, has a long $t_{1/2}$ (~63 hours), and is ~40% bound to plasma protein. Approximately 85% of an oral dose is excreted in the urine, principally as unmetabolized zonisamide and a glucuronide of sulfamoylacetyl phenol, which is a product of metabolism by CYP3A4. Phenobarbital, phenytoin, and carbamazepine decrease the plasma concentration/dose ratio of zonisamide, whereas lamotrigine increases this ratio. Conversely, zonisamide has little effect on the plasma concentrations of other anti-seizure drugs.

Therapeutic Use. Double-blind, placebo-controlled studies of patients with refractory partial seizures demonstrated that addition of zonisamide to other drugs was superior to placebo. There is insufficient evidence for its efficacy as monotherapy for newly diagnosed or refractory epilepsy.

Toxicity. Overall, zonisamide is well tolerated. The most common adverse effects include somnolence, ataxia, anorexia, nervousness, and fatigue. Approximately 1% of individuals develop renal calculi during treatment with zonisamide, which may relate to its ability to inhibit carbonic anhydrase. Post-marketing experience indicates that zonisamide can cause metabolic acidosis in some patients. Patients with predisposing conditions (e.g., renal disease, severe respiratory disorders, diarrhea, surgery, ketogenic diet) may be at greater risk. The risk of zonisamide-induced metabolic acidosis also appears to be more frequent and severe in younger patients. Measurement of serum bicarbonate prior to initiating therapy and periodically thereafter, even in the absence of symptoms, is recommended.

Lacosamide

Lacosamide (VIMPAT) is a functionalized amino acid that was approved by the FDA in 2008 as adjunctive therapy for partial-onset seizures in patients 17 years of age and older. An injectable formulation is available for short term use when oral administration is not feasible.

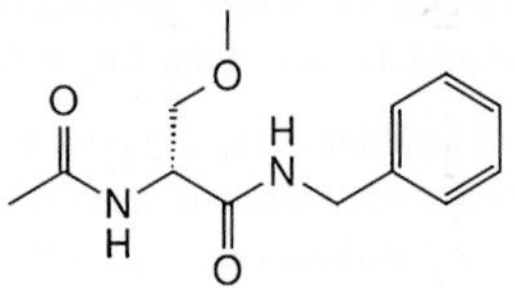

LACOSAMIDE

Pharmacological Effects and Mechanism of Action. Lacosamide enhances slow inactivation of voltage-gated Na^+ channels and limits sustained repetitive firing, the neuronal firing pattern characteristic of partial seizures. Lacosamide also binds collapsin response mediator protein 2 (crmp-2), a phosphoprotein involved in neuronal differentiation and axon outgrowth. Its anti-seizure mechanism of action is more likely mediated by its enhancing slow inactivation of Na^+ channels.

Therapeutic Use. Double-blind, placebo-controlled studies of adults with refractory partial seizures demonstrated that addition of lacosamide to other drugs was superior to placebo.

Rufinamide

Rufinamide (BANZEL) is a triazole derivative structurally unrelated to other marketed anti-epileptic drugs. It was approved by the FDA in 2008 for adjunctive treatment of seizures associated with Lennox-Gastaut syndrome in children 4 years and older and adults.

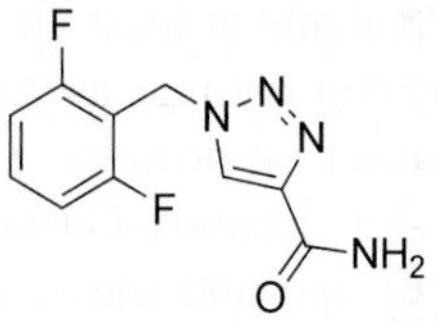

RUFINAMIDE

Pharmacological Effects and Mechanism of Action. Rufinamide enhances slow inactivation of voltage gated Na^+ channels and limits sustained repetitive firing, the firing pattern characteristic of partial seizures. Whether this is the mechanism by which rufinamide suppresses seizures is presently unclear.

Therapeutic Use. A double-blind, placebo-controlled study of children with Lennox-Gastaut syndrome demonstrated that rufinamide reduced tonic-atonic seizure frequency to a greater extent than placebo.

Vigabatrin

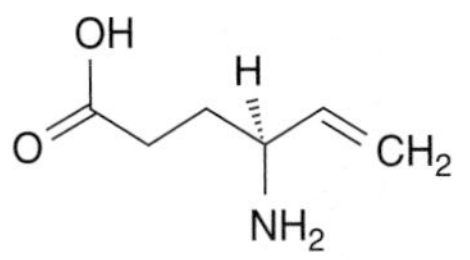

VIGABATRIN

Vigabatrin (SABRIL) was approved by the FDA in 2009 as adjunctive therapy of refractory partial complex seizures in adults. In addition, vigabatrin is designated as an orphan drug for treatment of infantile spasms (described in the subsequent "Therapeutic Use" section). Due to progressive and permanent bilateral vision loss, vigabatrin must be reserved for patients who have failed several alternative therapies; its availability is restricted under the conditions of the SHARE special distribution program.

Pharmacological Effects and Mechanism of Action. Vigabatrin is a structural analog of GABA that irreversibly inhibits the major degradative enzyme for GABA, GABA-transaminase, thereby leading to increased concentrations of GABA in the brain. Its mechanism of action is thought to involve enhancement of GABA-mediated inhibition.

Therapeutic Use. A 2-week, randomized, single masked clinical trial of vigabatrin for infantile spasms in children < 2 years old revealed time- and dose-dependent increases in responders, evident as freedom from spasms for 7 consecutive days. The subset of children in whom infantile spasms were caused by tuberous sclerosis was particularly responsive to vigabatrin.

Acetazolamide

Acetazolamide, the prototype for the carbonic anhydrase inhibitors, is discussed in Chapter 25. Its anti-seizure actions have been discussed in previous editions of this textbook. Although it is sometimes effective against absence seizures, its usefulness is limited by the rapid development of tolerance. Adverse effects are minimal when it is used in moderate dosage for limited periods.

GENERAL PRINCIPLES AND CHOICE OF DRUGS FOR THE THERAPY OF THE EPILEPSIES

Early diagnosis and treatment of seizure disorders with a single appropriate agent offers the best prospect of achieving prolonged seizure-free periods with the lowest risk of toxicity. An attempt should be made to determine the cause of the epilepsy with the hope of discovering a correctable lesion, either structural or metabolic. The drugs commonly used for distinct seizure types are listed in Table 21–1. The efficacy combined with the unwanted effects of a given drug determine which particular drug is optimal for a given patient.

The first decision to make is whether and when to initiate treatment (French and Pedley, 2008). For example, it may not be necessary to initiate anti-seizure therapy after an isolated tonic-clonic seizure in a healthy young adult who lacks a family history of epilepsy and who has a normal neurological exam, a normal EEG, and a normal brain MRI scan. The odds of seizure recurrence in the next year (15%) are similar to the risk of a drug reaction sufficiently severe to warrant discontinuation of medication (Bazil and Pedley, 1998). On the other hand, a similar seizure occurring in an individual with a positive family history of epilepsy, an abnormal neurological exam, an abnormal EEG, and an abnormal MRI carries a risk of recurrence approximating 60%, odds that favor initiation of therapy.

Unless extenuating circumstances such as status epilepticus exist, only monotherapy should be initiated. Initial dosing should target steady-state plasma drug concentrations within at least the lower portion of the range associated with clinical efficacy. At the same time the initial dose should be as low as possible to minimize dose-related adverse effects. Dosage is increased at appropriate intervals as required for control of seizures or as limited by toxicity. Such adjustment should be assisted by monitoring of drug concentrations in plasma. Compliance with a properly selected, single drug in maximal tolerated dosage results in complete control of seizures in ~50% of patients. If a seizure occurs despite optimal drug levels, the physician should assess the presence of potential precipitating factors such as sleep deprivation, a concurrent febrile illness, or drugs (e.g., large amounts of caffeine or over-the-counter medications that can lower the seizure threshold).

If compliance has been confirmed yet seizures persist, another drug should be substituted. Unless serious adverse effects of the drug dictate otherwise, dosage always should be reduced gradually to minimize risk of seizure recurrence. In the case of partial seizures in adults, the diversity of available drugs permits selection of a second drug that acts by a different mechanism (see Table 21–2). Among previously untreated patients, 47% became seizure free with the first drug and an additional 14% became seizure free with a second or third drug (Kwan and Brodie, 2000).

If therapy with a second single drug also is inadequate, combination therapy is warranted. This decision should not be taken lightly, because most patients obtain optimal seizure control with fewest unwanted effects when taking a single drug. Nonetheless, some patients will not be controlled adequately without the simultaneous use of two or more anti-seizure agents. No properly controlled studies have systematically compared one particular drug combination with another. The chances of complete control with this approach are not high; Kwan and Brodie (2000), found that epilepsy was controlled by treatment with two drugs in only 3% of patients. It seems wise to select two drugs that act by distinct mechanisms (e.g., one that promotes Na^+ channel inactivation and another that enhances GABA-mediated synaptic inhibition). Side effects of each drug and the potential drug interactions also should be considered. As specified in Table 21–3, many of these drugs induce expression of CYPs and thereby impact the metabolism of themselves and/or other drugs (Table 21–3).

Essential to optimal management of epilepsy is the filling out of a seizure chart by the patient or a relative. Frequent visits to the physician may be necessary early in the period of treatment, since hematological and other possible side effects may require a change in medication. Long-term follow-up with neurological examinations and possibly EEG and neuroimaging studies is appropriate. Most crucial for successful management is patient adherence to the drug regimen; noncompliance is the most frequent cause for failure of therapy with anti-seizure drugs.

Measurement of plasma drug concentration at appropriate intervals greatly facilitates the initial adjustment of dosage to minimize dose-related adverse effects without sacrificing seizure control. Periodic monitoring during maintenance therapy can also detect noncompliance. Knowledge of plasma drug concentrations can be especially helpful during multiple-drug therapy. If toxicity occurs, monitoring helps to identify the particular drug(s) responsible and can guide adjustment of dosage.

Duration of Therapy

Once initiated, anti-seizure drugs are typically continued for at least 2 years. Tapering and discontinuing therapy should be considered, if the patient is seizure free after 2 years.

Factors associated with high risk for recurrent seizures following discontinuation of therapy include EEG abnormalities, known structural lesions, abnormalities on neurological exam, and history of frequent seizures or medically refractory seizures prior to control. Conversely, factors associated with low risk for recurrent seizures include idiopathic epilepsy, normal EEG, onset in childhood, and seizures easily controlled with a single drug. The risk of recurrent seizures ranges from 12-66% (French and Pedley, 2008). Typically 80% of recurrences will occur within 4 months of discontinuing therapy. The clinician and patient must weigh the risk of recurrent seizure and the associated potential deleterious consequences (e.g., loss of driving privileges) against the various implications of continuing medication including cost, unwanted effects, implications of diagnosis of epilepsy, etc. Medications should be tapered slowly over a period of several months.

Simple and Complex Partial and Secondarily Generalized Tonic-Clonic Seizures

The efficacy and toxicity of carbamazepine, phenobarbital, and phenytoin for treatment of partial and secondarily generalized tonic-clonic seizures in adults have been examined in a double-blind prospective study (Mattson et al., 1985). Carbamazepine and phenytoin were the most effective agents. The choice between carbamazepine and phenytoin required assessment of toxic effects of each drug. Decreased libido and impotence were associated with all three drugs (carbamazepine 13%, phenobarbital 16%, and phenytoin 11%). In direct comparison with valproate, carbamazepine provided superior control of complex partial seizures (Mattson et al., 1992). With respect to adverse effects, carbamazepine was more commonly associated with skin rash, but valproate was more commonly associated with tremor and weight gain. Overall, the data demonstrated that carbamazepine and phenytoin are preferable for treatment of partial seizures, but phenobarbital and valproic acid are also efficacious.

Control of secondarily generalized tonic-clonic seizures did not differ significantly with carbamazepine, phenobarbital, or phenytoin (Mattson et al., 1985). Valproate was as effective as carbamazepine for control of secondarily generalized tonic-clonic seizures (Mattson et al., 1992). Since secondarily generalized tonic-clonic seizures usually coexist with partial seizures, these data indicate that among drugs introduced before 1990, carbamazepine and phenytoin are the first-line drugs for these conditions.

One key issue confronting the treating physician is choosing the optimal drug for initiating treatment in new onset epilepsy. At first glance, this issue may appear unimportant because ~50% of newly diagnosed patients become seizure free with the first drug, whether old or new drugs are used (Kwan and Brodie, 2000). However, responsive patients typically receive the initial drug for several years, underscoring the importance of proper drug selection. Among the drugs available before 1990, phenytoin, carbamazepine, and phenobarbital induce hepatic CYPs, thereby complicating use of multiple anti-seizure drugs as well as impacting metabolism of oral contraceptives, warfarin, and many other drugs. These drugs also enhance metabolism of endogenous compounds including gonadal steroids and vitamin D, potentially impacting reproductive function and bone density. By contrast, most of the newer drugs have little if any effect on the CYPs. Factors arguing against use of recently introduced drugs include higher costs and less clinical experience with the compounds.

Ideally, a prospective study would systematically compare newly introduced anti-seizure drugs with drugs available before 1990 in a study design adjusting dose as needed and observing responses for extended periods of time (e.g., 2 years or more), in much the same manner as that used when comparing the older anti-seizure drugs with one another as described earlier (Mattson et al., 1985).

Unfortunately, such a study has not been performed. Many of the studies referenced in description of newer drugs did compare a new with an older anti-seizure drug, but study design did not permit declaring a clearly superior drug; moreover, differences in study design and patient populations preclude comparing a new drug with multiple older drugs or with other new drugs. The use of recently introduced anti-seizure drugs for newly diagnosed epilepsy was analyzed by subcommittees of the American Academy of Neurology and the American Epilepsy Society (French et al., 2004a; French et al., 2004b); the authors concluded that available evidence supported the use of gabapentin, lamotrigine, and topiramate for newly diagnosed partial or mixed seizure disorders. None of these drugs, however, has been approved by the FDA for either of these indications. Insufficient evidence was available on the remaining newly introduced drugs to permit meaningful assessment of their effectiveness for this indication.

Absence Seizures

Ethosuximide and valproate are considered equally effective in the treatment of absence seizures (Mikati and Browne, 1988). Between 50% and 75% of newly diagnosed patients are free of seizures following therapy with either drug. If tonic-clonic seizures are present or emerge during therapy, valproate is the agent of first choice. French and others concluded that available evidence indicates that lamotrigine is also effective for newly diagnosed absence epilepsy despite the fact that lamotrigine is not approved for this indication by the FDA.

Myoclonic Seizures

Valproic acid is the drug of choice for myoclonic seizures in the syndrome of juvenile myoclonic epilepsy, in which myoclonic seizures often coexist with tonic-clonic and absence seizures. Levetiracetam also has demonstrated efficacy as adjunctive therapy for refractory generalized myoclonic seizures.

Febrile Convulsions

Two to four percent of children experience a convulsion associated with a febrile illness. From 25-33% of these children will have another febrile convulsion. Only 2-3% become epileptic in later years, a 6-fold increase in risk compared with the general population. Several factors are associated with an increased risk of developing epilepsy: preexisting neurological disorder or developmental delay, a family history of epilepsy, or a complicated febrile seizure (i.e., the febrile seizure lasted > 15 minutes, was one-sided, or was followed by a second seizure in the same day). If all of these risk factors are present, the risk of developing epilepsy is ~10%.

The increased risk of developing epilepsy or other neurological sequelae led many physicians to prescribe anti-seizure drugs prophylactically after a febrile seizure. Uncertainties regarding the efficacy of prophylaxis for reducing epilepsy combined with substantial side effects of phenobarbital prophylaxis (Farwell et al., 1990) argue against the use of chronic therapy for prophylactic purposes (Freeman, 1992). For children at high risk of developing recurrent febrile seizures and epilepsy, rectally administered diazepam at the time of fever may prevent recurrent seizures and avoid side effects of chronic therapy.

Seizures in Infants and Young Children

Infantile spasms with *hypsarrhythmia* (abnormal inter-ictal high amplitude slow waves and multifocal asynchronous spikes on EEG) are refractory to the usual anti-seizure agents. Corticotropin or the glucocorticoids are commonly used and repository corticotropin (H.P. ACTHAR GEL) was designated as an orphan drug for this purpose in 2003. A randomized study found vigabatrin (γ-vinyl GABA; SABRIL) to be efficacious in comparison to placebo (Appleton et al., 1999). Constriction of visual fields has been reported in a high percentage of patients treated with vigabatrin (Miller et al., 1999). The potential for progressive and permanent vision loss has resulted in vigabatrin being labeled with a black-box warning and marketed under a restrictive distribution program. The drug received orphan drug status for the treatment of infantile spasms in the U.S. in 2000 (and was FDA-approved in 2009 as adjunctive therapy for adults with refractory complex partial seizures). Ganaxolone also has been designated as an orphan drug since 1994 for the treatment of infantile spasms and completed a phase II clinical trial for uncontrolled partial-onset seizures in adults in 2009.

The Lennox-Gastaut syndrome is a severe form of epilepsy which usually begins in childhood and is characterized by cognitive impairments and multiple types of seizures including tonic-clonic, tonic, atonic, myoclonic, and atypical absence seizures. Addition of lamotrigine to other anti-seizure drugs resulted in improved seizure control in comparison to placebo in a double-blind trial (Motte et al., 1997), demonstrating lamotrigine to be an effective and well-tolerated drug for this treatment-resistant form of epilepsy. Felbamate also was found to be effective for seizures in this syndrome, but the occasional occurrence of aplastic anemia and hepatic failure have limited its use (French et al., 1999). Topiramate has also been demonstrated to be effective for Lennox-Gastaut syndrome (Sachdeo et al., 1999).

Status Epilepticus and Other Convulsive Emergencies

Status epilepticus is a neurological emergency. Mortality for adults approximates 20% (Lowenstein and Alldredge, 1998). The goal of treatment is rapid termination of behavioral and electrical seizure activity; the longer the episode of status epilepticus is untreated, the more difficult it is to control and the greater the risk of permanent brain damage. Critical to the management is a clear plan, prompt treatment with effective drugs in adequate doses, and attention to hypoventilation and hypotension. Since hypoventilation may result from high doses of drugs used for treatment, it may be necessary to assist respiration temporarily. Drugs should be administered by the intravenous route only. Because of slow and unreliable absorption, the intramuscular route has no place in treatment of status epilepticus. To assess the optimal initial drug regimen, a double-blind, multicenter trial compared four intravenous treatments: diazepam followed by phenytoin; lorazepam; phenobarbital; and phenytoin alone (Treiman et al., 1998). The treatments had similar efficacies, with success rates ranging from 44-65%. Lorazepam alone was significantly better than phenytoin alone. No significant differences were found with respect to recurrences or adverse reactions.

Anti-Seizure Therapy and Pregnancy

Use of anti-seizure drugs has diverse implications of great importance for the health of women. Issues include interactions with oral contraceptives, potential teratogenic effects, and effects on vitamin K metabolism in pregnant women (Pack, 2006). Guidelines for the care of women with epilepsy have been published by the American Academy of Neurology (Morrell, 1998).

The effectiveness of oral contraceptives appears to be reduced by concomitant use of anti-seizure drugs. The failure rate of oral contraceptives is 3.1/100 years in women receiving anti-seizure drugs compared to a rate of 0.7/100 years in non-epileptic women. One attractive explanation of the increased failure rate is the increased rate of oral contraceptive metabolism caused by anti-seizure drugs that induce hepatic enzymes (Table 21–2); particular caution is needed with anti-seizure drugs that induce CYP3A4.

Teratogenicity. Epidemiological evidence suggests that anti-seizure drugs have teratogenic effects (Pack, 2006). These teratogenic effects add to the deleterious consequences of oral contraceptive failure. Infants of epileptic mothers are at 2-fold greater risk of major congenital malformations than offspring of non-epileptic mothers (4-8% compared to 2-4%). These malformations include congenital heart defects, neural tube defects, cleft lip, cleft palate, and others. Inferring causality from the associations found in large epidemiological studies with many uncontrolled variables can be hazardous, but a causal role for anti-seizure drugs is suggested by association of congenital defects with higher concentrations of a drug or with polytherapy compared to monotherapy. Phenytoin, carbamazepine, valproate, lamotrigine, and phenobarbital all have been associated with teratogenic effects. Newer anti-seizure drugs have teratogenic effects in animals but whether such effects occur in humans is yet uncertain. One consideration for a woman with epilepsy who wishes to become pregnant is a trial free of anti-seizure drug; monotherapy with careful attention to drug levels is another alternative. Polytherapy with toxic levels should be avoided. Folate supplementation (0.4 mg/day) has been recommended by the U.S. Public Health Service for all women of childbearing age to reduce the likelihood of neural tube defects, and this is appropriate for epileptic women as well.

Anti-seizure drugs that induce CYPs have been associated with vitamin K deficiency in the newborn, which can result in a coagulopathy and intracerebral hemorrhage. Treatment with vitamin K_1, 10 mg/day during the last month of gestation, has been recommended for prophylaxis.

BIBLIOGRAPHY

Andermann E., Andermann F, Meyvisch P, *et al.* Seizure control with levetiracetam in juvenile myoclonic epilepsies. *Epilepsia*, **2005**, *46(suppl 8)*:205.

Appleton RE, Peters AC, Mumford JP, Shaw DE. Randomised, placebo-controlled study of vigabatrin as first-line treatment of infantile spasms. *Epilepsia*, **1999**, *40:*1627–1633.

Bazil CW, Pedley TA. Advances in the medical treatment of epilepsy. *Annu Rev Med*, **1998**, *49:*135–162.

Biton V, Montouris GD, Ritter F, *et al.* A randomized, placebo-controlled study of topiramate in primary generalized tonic-clonic seizures: Topiramate YTC Study Group. *Neurology*, **1999**, *52:*1330–1337.

Brodie MJ, Richens A, Yuen AW. Double-blind comparison of lamotrigine and carbamazepine in newly diagnosed epilepsy. UK Lamotrigine/Carbamazepine Monotherapy Trial Group. *Lancet*, **1995,** *345:*476–479.

Chadwick DW, Anhut H, Grenier MJ, *et al.* A double-blind trial of gabapentin monotherapy for newly diagnosed partial seizures: International Gabapentin Monotherapy Study Group 945-77. *Neurology*, **1998**, *51:*1282–1288.

Chiron C. Stiripentol. *Neurotherapeutics*, **2007**, *4*:123–125.

Commission on Classification and Terminology of the International League Against Epilepsy. Proposal for revised clinical and electroencephalographic classification of epileptic seizures. *Epilepsia*, **1981,** *22:*489–501.

Commission on Classification and Terminology of the International League Against Epilepsy. Proposal for revised classification of epilepsies and epileptic syndromes. *Epilepsia*, **1989**, *30:*389–399.

Coulter DA, Huguenard JR, Prince DA. Characterization of ethosuximide reduction of low-threshold calcium current in thalamic neurons. *Ann Neurol*, **1989**, *25:*582–593.

Dreifuss FE, Langer DH, Moline KA, Maxwell JE. Valproic acid hepatic fatalities. II. U. S. experience since 1984. *Neurology*, **1989**, *39:*201–207.

Farwell JR, Lee YJ, Hirtz DG, *et al.* Phenobarbital for febrile seizures—effects on intelligence and on seizure recurrence. *N Engl J Med*, **1990**, *322:*364–369.

Felbamate Study Group in Lennox-Gastaut Syndrome. Efficacy of felbamate in childhood epileptic encephalopathy (Lennox-Gastaut syndrome). *N Engl J Med*, **1993**, *328:*29–33.

Field MJ, Cox PJ, Stott E, *et al.* Identification of the α_2-δ-1 subunit of voltage-dependent calcium channels as a molecular target for pain mediating the analgesic actions of pregablain. *Proc Natl Acad Sci USA,* **2006**, *103:*17537–17542

Frank LM, Enlow T, Holmes GL, *et al.* Lamictal (lamotrigine) monotherapy for typical absence seizure in children. *Epilepsia*, **1999,** *40:*973–979.

Freeman JM. The best medicine for febrile seizures. *N Engl J Med*, **1992**, *327:*1161–1163.

French JA, Kanner AM, Bautista J, *et al.* Efficacy and tolerability of the new antiepileptic drugs. I. Treatment of new-onset epilepsy: Report of the TTA and QSS subcommittees of the American Academy of Neurology and American Epilepsy Society. *Neurology*, **2004a,** *62:*1252–1260.

French JA, Kanner AM, Bautista J, *et al.* Efficacy and tolerability of the new antiepileptic drugs. II. Treatment of refractory epilepsy: Report of the TTA and QSS subcommittees of the American Academy of Neurology and the American Epilepsy Society. *Neurology*, **2004b**, *62:*1261–1273.

French JA, Kugler AR, Robbins JL, Knapp L. Dose-response trial of pregabalin adjunctive therapy in patiens with partial seizures. *Neurology*, **2003**, *60:*1631–1637.

French JA, Pedley TA. Initial management of epilepsy. *N Engl J Med*, **2008**, *359*:166–176.

French J, Smith M, Faught E, Brown L. Practice advisory: The use of felbamate in the treatment of patients with intractable epilepsy. Report of the Quality Standards Subcommittee of the American Academy of Neurology and the American Epilepsy Society. *Neurology*, **1999**, *52:*1540–1545.

Gee NS, Brown JP, Dissanayake VU, *et al.* The novel anticonvulsant drug, gabapentin (Neurontin) binds to the 2 subunit of a calcium channel. *J Biol Chem*, **1996**, *271*:5768–5776

He XP, Kotloski R, Nef S, *et al.* Conditional deletion of TrkB but not BDNF prevents epileptogenesis in the kindling model. *Neuron*, **2004**, *43:*31–42.

Huguenard JR, McCormick DA. Thalamic synchrony and dynamic regulation of global forebrain oscillations. Trends Neurosci, **2007** *30*:350–356.

Kelly KM, Gross RA, Macdonald RL. Valproic acid selectively reduces the low-threshold (T) calcium current in rat nodose neurons. *Neurosci Lett*, **1990**, *116:*233–238.

Kwan P, Brodie MJ. Early identification of refractory epilepsy. *N Engl J Med*, **2000**, *342:*314–319.

Lowenstein DH, Alldredge BK. Status epilepticus. *N Engl J Med*, **1998**, *338:*970–976.

Macdonald RL, Greenfield LJ Jr. Mechanisms of action of new antiepileptic drugs. *Curr Opin Neurol*, **1997**, *10:*121–128.

Mattson RH, Cramer JA, Collins JF, *et al.* Comparison of carbamazepine, phenobarbital, phenytoin, and primidone in partial and secondarily generalized tonic-clonic seizures. *N Engl J Med*, **1985**, *313:*145–151.

Mattson RH, Cramer JA, Collins JF. A comparison of valproate with carbamazepine for the treatment of complex partial seizures and secondarily generalized tonic-clonic seizures in adults. The Department of Veterans Affairs Epilepsy Cooperative Study No. 264 Group. *N Engl J Med*, **1992**, *327:*765–771.

McLean MJ, Macdonald RL. Carbamazepine and 10,11-epoxycarbamazepine produce use- and voltage-dependent limitation of rapidly firing action potentials of mouse central neurons in cell culture. *J Pharmacol Exp Ther*, **1986a**, *238:*727–738.

McLean MJ, Macdonald RL. Sodium valproate, but not ethosuximide, produces use- and voltage-dependent limitation of high-frequency repetitive firing of action potentials of mouse central neurons in cell culture. *J Pharmacol Exp Ther*, **1986b**, *237:*1001–1011.

McNamara JO. Cellular and molecular basis of epilepsy. *J Neurosci*, **1994**, *14:*3413–3425.

Mikati MA, Browne TR. Comparative efficacy of antiepileptic drugs. *Clin Neuropharmacol*, **1988**, *11:*130–140.

Miller NR, Johnson MA, Paul SR, *et al.* Visual dysfunction in patients receiving vigabatrin: clinical and electrophysiologic findings. *Neurology*, **1999**, *53:*2082–2087.

Morrell MJ. Guidelines for the care of women with epilepsy. *Neurology*, **1998**, *51:*S21–S27.

Motte J, Trevathan E, Arvidsson JF, *et al.* Lamotrigine for generalized seizures associated with the Lennox-Gastaut syndrome. Lamictal Lennox-Gastaut Study Group. *N Engl J Med*, **1997**, *337:*1807–1812.

Pack AM. Therapy insight: Clinical management of pregnant women with epilepsy. *Nat Clin Prac Neurol*, **2006**, *2:* 190–200.

Privitera MD, Brodie MJ, Mattson RH, *et al.* Topiramate, carbamazepine and valproate monotherapy: Double-blind comparison in newly diagnosed epilepsy. *Acta Neurol Scand*, **2003**, *107:*165–175.

Ptacek LJ, Fu YH. Channelopathies: Episodic disorders of the nervous system. Epilepsia, **2001**;*42(suppl 5)*:35–43.

Quilichini PP, *et al.* Stiripentol, a putative antiepileptic drug, enhances the duration of opening of GABA-A receptor channels. *Epilepsia* **2006**, *47*:704–716.

Reid CA, Berkovic SF, Petrou S. Mechanisms of human inherited epilepsies. *Prog Neurobiol*, **2008**, Oct 5. (Epub ahead of print.)

Rho JM, Donevan SD, Rogawski MA. Mechanism of action of the anticonvulsant felbamate: Opposing effects on *N*-methyl-D-aspartate and $GABA_A$ receptors. *Ann Neurol*, **1994**, *35:* 229–234.

Rogawski MA, Bazil CW. New molecular targets for antiepileptic drugs: $_2$, SV2A, and K_v7/KCNQ/M potassium channels. *Curr Neurol Neurosci Rep*, **2008**, *8*:345–352

Rogawski MA, Löscher W. The neurobiology of antiepileptic drugs. *Nat Rev Neurosci,* **2004**, *5*:553–564,

Sachdeo RC, Glauser TA, Ritter F, *et al.* A double-blind, randomized trial of topiramate in Lennox-Gastaut syndrome: Topiramate YL Study Group. *Neurology*, **1999**, *52:*1882–1887.

Sachdeo RC, Kramer LD, Rosenberg A, Sachdeo S. Felbamate monotherapy: controlled trial in patients with partial onset seizures. *Ann Neurol*, **1992**, *32:*386–392.

Sachdeo RC, Leroy RF, Krauss GL, *et al.* Tiagabine therapy for complex partial seizures: A dose-frequency study. The Tiagabine Study Group. *Arch Neurol*, **1997**, *54:*595–601.

Sivenius J, Kalviainen R, Ylinen A, *et al.* Double-blind study of gabapentin in the treatment of partial seizures. *Epilepsia*, **1991,** *32:*539–542.

Steiner T J, Dellaportas CI, Findley LS, *et al.* Lamotrigine monotherapy in newly diagnosed untreated epilepsy: A double-blind comparison with phenytoin. *Epilepsia*, **1999**, *40:*601–607.

Traynelis SF, Dingledine R. Potassium-induced spontaneous electrographic seizures in the rat hippocampal slice. *J Neurophysiol*, **1988**, *59:*259–276.

Treiman DM, Meyers PD, Walton NY, *et al.* A comparison of four treatments for generalized convulsive status epilepticus. Veterans Affairs Status Epilepticus Cooperative Study Group. *N Engl J Med*, **1998**, *339:*792–798.

Twyman RE, Rogers CJ, Macdonald RL. Differential regulation of γ-aminobutyric acid receptor channels by diazepam and phenobarbital. *Ann Neurol*, **1989**, *25:*213–220.

VanLandingham KE, Heinz ER, Cavazos JE, Lewis DV. Magnetic resonance imaging evidence of hippocampal injury after prolonged focal febrile convulsions. *Ann Neurol*, **1998**, *43:*413–426.

Wallace RH, Wang DW, Singh R, *et al.* Febrile seizures and generalized epilepsy associated with a mutation in the Na^+-channel β1 subunit gene *SCN1B*. *Nat Genet*, **1998**, *19:*366–370.

Yu FH, et al. Reduced sodium current in GABAergic interneurons in a mouse model of severe myoclonic epilepsy in infancy. *Nat Neurosci,* **2006**, *9*:1142–1149.

Xie X, Lancaster B, Peakman T, Garthwaite J. Interaction of the antiepileptic drug lamotrigine with recombinant rat brain type IIA Na^+ channels and with native Na^+ channels in rat hippocampal neurones. *Pflugers Arch*, **1995**, *430:*437–446.

Treatment of Central Nervous System Degenerative Disorders

David G. Standaert
and Erik D. Roberson

Neurodegenerative disorders are characterized by progressive and irreversible loss of neurons from specific regions of the brain. Prototypical neurodegenerative disorders include Parkinson disease (PD) and Huntington's disease (HD), where loss of neurons from structures of the basal ganglia results in abnormalities in the control of movement; Alzheimer's disease (AD), where the loss of hippocampal and cortical neurons leads to impairment of memory and cognitive ability; and amyotrophic lateral sclerosis (ALS), where muscular weakness results from the degeneration of spinal, bulbar, and cortical motor neurons.

As a group, these disorders are relatively common and represent a substantial medical and societal problem. They are primarily disorders of later life, developing in individuals who are neurologically normal, although childhood-onset forms of each of the disorders are recognized. PD is observed in more than 1% of individuals over the age of 65 (Tanner, 1992), whereas AD affects as many as 10% of the same population (Evans et al., 1989). HD, which is a genetically determined autosomal dominant disorder, is less frequent in the population as a whole but affects, on average, 50% of each generation in families carrying the gene. ALS also is relatively rare but often leads rapidly to disability and death (Kurtzke, 1982).

Currently available therapies for neurodegenerative disorders alleviate the disease symptoms but do not alter the underlying neurodegenerative process. Symptomatic treatment for PD, where the neurochemical deficit produced by the disease is well defined, is, in general, relatively successful, and a number of effective agents are available. The available symptomatic treatments for AD, HD, and ALS are much more limited in effectiveness. On the horizon are pharmacological treatments aimed at preventing or retarding progression of neurodegeneration. A wide range of such disease-modifying approaches hold the promise to transform the approach to both the diagnosis and the treatment of neurodegenerative disorders.

SELECTIVE VULNERABILITY AND NEUROPROTECTIVE STRATEGIES

Selective Vulnerability. A striking feature of neurodegenerative disorders is the exquisite specificity of the disease processes for particular types of neurons. For example, in PD there is extensive destruction of the dopaminergic neurons of the substantia nigra, whereas neurons in the cortex and many other areas of the brain are unaffected. In contrast, neural injury in AD is most severe in the hippocampus and neocortex, and even within the cortex, the loss of neurons is not uniform but varies dramatically in different functional regions (Arnold et al., 1991). Even more striking is the observation that in HD the mutant gene responsible for the disorder is expressed throughout the brain and in many other organs, yet the pathological changes are most prominent in the neostriatum (Landwehrmeyer et al., 1995). In ALS, there is loss of spinal motor neurons and the cortical neurons that provide their descending input (Tandan and Bradley, 1985). The diversity of these patterns of neural degeneration suggests that the process of neural injury results from the interaction of genetic and environmental influences with the intrinsic physiological characteristics of the affected populations of neurons. The intrinsic factors may include susceptibility to excitotoxic injury, regional variation in capacity for oxidative metabolism, and the production of toxic free radicals as by-products of cellular metabolism. New neuroprotective agents may target the factors that convey selective vulnerability.

Genetics and Environment. Each of the major neurodegenerative disorders may be familial in nature. HD is exclusively familial; it is transmitted by autosomal dominant inheritance, and the molecular mechanism of the genetic defect has been defined. Nevertheless, environmental factors importantly influence the age of onset and rate of progression of HD symptoms. PD, AD, and ALS are mostly sporadic without clear pattern of inheritance. But for each there are well-recognized genetic forms. For example, there are both dominant (*α-synuclein, LRRK2*) and recessive (*parkin, DJ-1, PINK1*) gene mutations that may give rise to PD (Farrer, 2006). In AD, mutations in the genes coding for the amyloid precursor protein (APP) and proteins known as the presenilins (involved in APP processing) lead to inherited forms of the disease (Selkoe and Podlisny, 2002). Mutations in the gene coding for copper-zinc superoxide dismutase (*SOD1*) account for about 2% of the cases of adult-onset ALS (Boillée et al., 2006). Several other less common mutations have also been described.

In addition to these monogenic forms of neurodegenerative disease, there are also genetic risk factors that influence the probability of disease onset and modify the phenotype. For example, the apolipoprotein E (apo E) genotype constitutes an important risk factor for AD. Three distinct isoforms of this protein exist. Although all isoforms carry out their primary role in lipid metabolism equally well, individuals who are homozygous for the apoE4 allele ("4/4") have a much higher lifetime risk of AD than do those homozygous for the apoE2 allele ("2/2"). The mechanism by which the apoE4 protein increases the risk of AD is not exactly known. ApoE4 probably has multiple effects, some of which are mediated through altering *β*-amyloid (Aβ) aggregation or processing, and some of which that are Aβ-independent (Mahley et al., 2006).

Environmental factors including infectious agents, environmental toxins, and acquired brain injury have been proposed in the etiology of neurodegenerative disorders. The role of infection is best documented in the cases of PD that developed following the epidemic of encephalitis lethargica (Von Economo's encephalitis) in the early part of the 20th century. Most contemporary cases of PD are not preceded by encephalitis, and there is no convincing evidence for an infectious contribution to HD, AD, or ALS. Traumatic brain injury has been suggested as a trigger for neurodegenerative disorders, and in the case of AD there is some evidence to support this view (Cummings et al., 1998). At least one toxin, *N*-methyl-4-phenyl-1,2,3,6-tetrahydropyridine (MPTP), can induce a condition closely resembling PD (Langston et al., 1983). More recently, evidence has linked pesticide exposure with PD (Costello et al., 2009). Exposure of soldiers to neurotoxic chemicals has been implicated in ALS (as part of "Gulf War syndrome") (Golomb, 2008). While these examples illustrate the potential of environmental factors to influence neurodegenerative disease, it is clear that the causes identified so far are too few to account for more than a small minority of the cases. Further progress in understanding the causes of neurodegenerative disorders will require a deeper understanding of the interactions between genetic predisposition and environmental factors, an area that is just beginning to be explored.

Common Cellular Mechanisms of Neurodegeneration. Despite their varied phenotypes, the neurodegenerative disorders share some common features. For example, misfolded and aggregated proteins are found in every major neurodegenerative disorder: alpha-synuclein, in PD; amyloid-β (Aβ) and tau in AD; huntingtin in HD; and SOD and TDP-43 in ALS. The accumulation of misfolded proteins may result from either genetic mutations producing abnormal structure, or from impaired cellular clearance. Age-related decline in the ability to clear misfolded proteins may be an important predisposing factor, and strategies to augment the clearance of misfolded proteins are being studied as potential therapies.

The term *excitotoxicity* describes the neural injury that results from the presence of excess glutamate in the brain. Glutamate is used as a neurotransmitter by many different neural systems and is believed to mediate most excitatory synaptic transmission in the mammalian brain (see Table 14–3). Although glutamate is required for normal brain function, the presence of excessive amounts of glutamate can lead to excitotoxic cell death (see Figure 14–13). The destructive effects of glutamate are mediated by glutamate receptors, particularly those of the *N*-methyl-D-aspartate (NMDA) type. Excitotoxic injury contributes to the neuronal death that occurs in acute processes such as stroke and head trauma (Choi and Rothman, 1990). The role of excitotoxicity is less certain in the chronic neurodegenerative disorders; nevertheless, regional and cellular differences in susceptibility to excitotoxic injury, conveyed, e.g., by differences in types of glutamate receptors, may contribute to selective vulnerability. This has led to the development of glutamate antagonists as neuroprotective therapies, with two such agents (memantine and riluzole, described later) currently in clinical use.

Aging is associated with a progressive impairment in the capacity of neurons for oxidative metabolism, perhaps in part because of a progressive accumulation of mutations in the mitochondrial genome. A consequence of impaired oxidative capacities is the production of reactive compounds such as hydrogen peroxide and oxygen radicals. Unchecked, these reactive species can lead to DNA damage, peroxidation of membrane lipids, and neuronal death. This has led to pursuit of drugs that can enhance cellular metabolism (such as the mitochondrial cofactor coenzyme Q_{10}) and anti-oxidant strategies as treatments to prevent or retard degenerative diseases (Beal, 2005).

Parkinson Disease (PD)

Clinical Overview. Parkinsonism is a clinical syndrome consisting of four cardinal features:

- bradykinesia (slowness and poverty of movement)
- muscular rigidity
- resting tremor (which usually abates during voluntary movement)
- an impairment of postural balance leading to disturbances of gait and falling

The most common form of parkinsonism is idiopathic PD, first described by James Parkinson in 1817 as *paralysis agitans,* or the "shaking palsy." The pathological hallmark of PD is the loss of the pigmented, dopaminergic neurons of the substantia nigra pars compacta, with the appearance of intracellular inclusions known as *Lewy bodies*. Progressive loss of dopamine (DA) containing neurons is a feature of normal aging; however, most people do not lose the 70-80% of dopaminergic neurons required to cause symptomatic PD. Without treatment, PD progresses over 5-10 years to a rigid, akinetic state in which patients are incapable of caring for themselves. Death frequently results from complications of immobility, including aspiration pneumonia or pulmonary embolism. The availability of effective pharmacological treatment has radically altered the prognosis of PD; in most cases, good functional mobility can be maintained for many years. Life expectancy of adequately treated patients is increased substantially, but overall mortality remains higher than that of the general population. In addition, while DA neuron loss is the most prominent feature of the disease, the disorder affects a wide range of other brain structures, including the brainstem, hippocampus, and cerebral cortex (Braak and Del Tredici, 2008). This pathology is likely responsible for the "non-motor" features of PD, which include sleep disorders, depression, and memory impairment. As treatments for the motor features have improved, these non-motor aspects have become important sources of disability for patients (Langston, 2006).

It is important to recognize that several disorders other than idiopathic PD also may produce parkinsonism, including some relatively rare neurodegenerative disorders, stroke, and intoxication with DA-receptor antagonists. Drugs that may cause parkinsonism include antipsychotics such as haloperidol and thorazine (Chapter 16) and anti-emetics such as prochloperazine and metoclopramide (Chapter 46). Although a complete discussion of the clinical diagnosis of parkinsonism exceeds the scope of this chapter, the distinction between idiopathic PD and other causes of parkinsonism is important because parkinsonism arising from other causes usually is refractory to all forms of treatment.

Pathophysiology. The dopaminergic deficit in PD arises from a loss of the neurons in the substantia nigra pars compacta that provide innervation to the striatum (caudate and putamen). The current understanding of the pathophysiology of PD is based on the finding that the striatal DA content is reduced in excess of 80%. This paralleled the loss of neurons from the substantia nigra, suggesting that replacement of DA could restore function (Cotzias et al., 1969; Hornykiewicz, 1973). These fundamental observations led to an extensive investigative effort to understand the metabolism and actions of DA and to learn how a deficit in DA gives rise to the clinical features of PD. We now have a model of the function of the basal ganglia that, while incomplete, is still useful.

Dopamine Synthesis, Metabolism, and Receptors. DA, a catecholamine, is synthesized in the terminals of dopaminergic neurons from tyrosine and stored, released, and metabolized by processes described in Chapter 13 and summarized in Figure 22–1. The actions of DA in the brain are mediated by a family of DA-receptor proteins. Two types of DA receptors were identified in the mammalian brain using pharmacological techniques: D_1 receptors, which stimulate the synthesis of the intracellular second messenger cyclic AMP; and D_2 receptors, which inhibit cyclic AMP synthesis as well as suppress Ca^{2+} currents and activate receptor-operated K^+ currents. More recently, genetic studies revealed at least five distinct DA receptors (D_1-D_5) (Chapter 13). All the DA receptors are G protein–coupled receptors (GPCRs) (Chapter 3). The D_1 and D_5 proteins have a long intracellular carboxy-terminal tail and are members of the class defined pharmacologically as D_1; they stimulate the formation of cyclic AMP and phosphatidyl inositol hydrolysis. The D_2, D_3, and D_4 receptors share a large third intracellular loop and are of the D_2 class. They decrease cyclic AMP formation and modulate K^+ and Ca^{2+} currents. Each of the five DA receptor proteins has a distinct anatomical pattern of expression in the brain. The D_1 and D_2 proteins are abundant in the striatum and are the most important receptor sites with regard to the causes and treatment of PD. The D_4 and D_5 proteins are largely extrastriatal, whereas D_3 expression is low in the caudate and putamen but more abundant in the nucleus accumbens and olfactory tubercle.

Neural Mechanism of Parkinsonism. Considerable effort has been devoted to understanding how the loss of dopaminergic input to the neurons of the neostriatum gives rise to the clinical features of PD (for review, see Albin et al., 1989; Mink and Thach, 1993; and Wichmann and DeLong, 1993). The basal ganglia can be viewed as a modulatory side loop that regulates the flow of information from the cerebral cortex to the motor neurons of the spinal cord (Figure 22–2). The neostriatum is the principal input structure of the basal ganglia and receives excitatory glutamatergic input from many areas of the cortex. Most neurons within the striatum are projection neurons that innervate other basal ganglia structures. A small but important

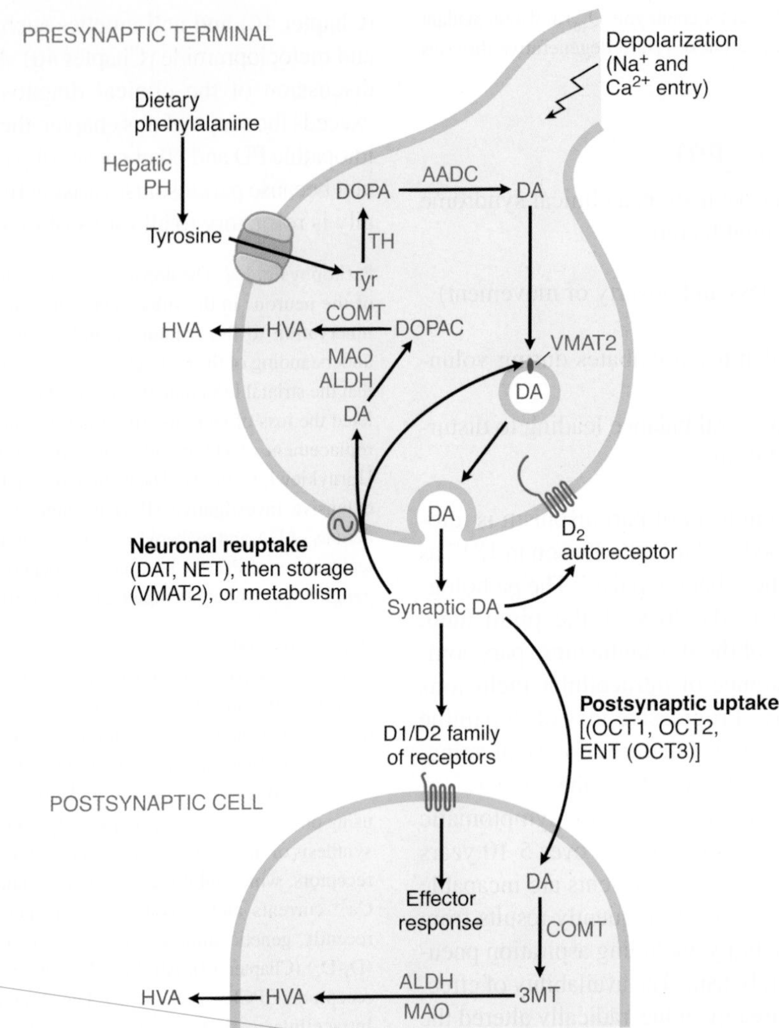

Figure 22–1. *Dopaminergic nerve terminal.* Dopamine (DA) is synthesized from tyrosine in the nerve terminal by the sequential actions of tyrosine hydrolase (TH) and aromatic amino acid decarboxylase (AADC). DA is sequestered by VMAT2 in storage granules and released by exocytosis. Synaptic DA activates presynaptic autoreceptors and postsynaptic D1 and D2 receptors. Synaptic DA may be taken up into the neuron via the DA and NE transporters (DAT, NET), or removed by postsynaptic uptake via OCT3 transporters. Cytosolic DA is subject to degradation by monoamine oxidase (MAO) and aldehyde dehydrogenase (ALDH) in the neuron, and by catechol-O-methyl tranferase (COMT) and MAO/ALDH in non-neuronal cells; the final metabolic product is homovanillic acid (HVA). See structures in Figure 22-4. PH, phenylalanine hydroxylase.

subgroup of striatal neurons consists of interneurons that connect neurons within the striatum but do not project beyond its borders. Acetylcholine (ACh) and neuropeptides are used as transmitters by these striatal interneurons.

The outflow of the striatum proceeds along two distinct routes, termed the *direct* and *indirect pathways.* The direct pathway is formed by neurons in the striatum that project directly to the output stages of the basal ganglia, the substantia nigra pars reticulata (SNpr) and the globus pallidus interna (GPi); these, in turn, relay to the ventroanterior and ventrolateral thalamus, which provides excitatory input to the cortex. The neurotransmitter of both links of the direct pathway is γ-aminobutyric acid (GABA), which is inhibitory, so that the net effect of stimulation of the direct pathway at the level of the striatum is to increase the excitatory outflow from the thalamus to the cortex. The indirect pathway is composed of striatal neurons that project to the globus pallidus externa (GPe). This structure, in turn, innervates the subthalamic nucleus (STN), which provides outflow to the SNpr and GPi output stage. As in the direct pathway, the first two links—the projections from striatum to GPe and GPe to STN—use the inhibitory transmitter GABA; however, the final link—the projection from STN to SNpr and GPi—is an excitatory glutamatergic pathway. Thus, the net effect of stimulating the indirect pathway at the level of the striatum is to reduce the excitatory outflow from the thalamus to the cerebral cortex.

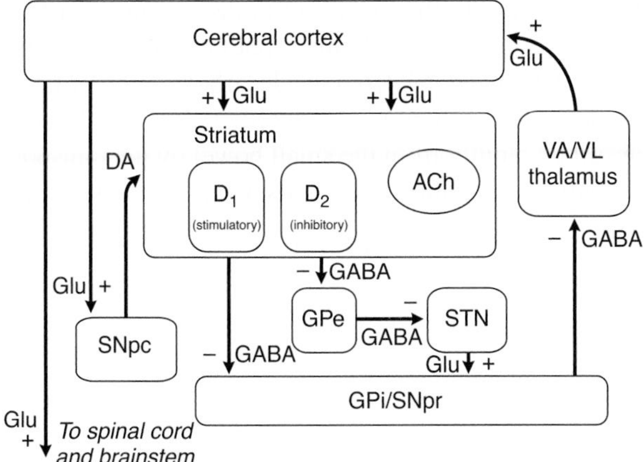

Figure 22–2. *Schematic wiring diagram of the basal ganglia.* The striatum is the principal input structure of the basal ganglia and receives excitatory glutamatergic input from many areas of cerebral cortex. The striatum contains projection neurons expressing predominantly D_1 or D_2 dopamine receptors, as well as interneurons that use ACh as a neurotransmitter. Outflow from the striatum proceeds along two routes. The direct pathway, from the striatum to the substantia nigra pars reticulata (SNpr) and globus pallidus interna (GPi), uses the inhibitory transmitter GABA. The indirect pathway, from the striatum through the globus pallidus externa (GPe) and the subthalamic nucleus (STN) to the SNpr and GPi, consists of two inhibitory GABAergic links and one excitatory glutamatergic projection (Glu). The substantia nigra pars compacta (SNpc) provides dopaminergic innervation to the striatal neurons, giving rise to both the direct and indirect pathways, and regulates the relative activity of these two paths. The SNpr and GPi are the output structures of the basal ganglia and provide feedback to the cerebral cortex through the ventroanterior and ventrolateral nuclei of the thalamus (VA/VL).

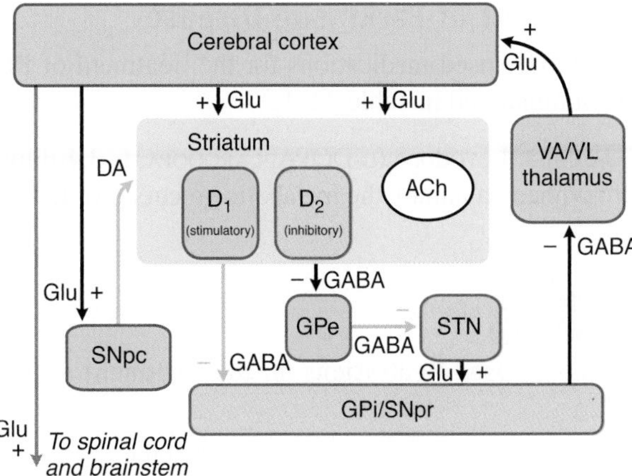

Figure 22–3. *The basal ganglia in Parkinson disease.* The primary defect is destruction of the dopaminergic neurons of the SNpc. The striatal neurons that form the direct pathway from the striatum to the SNpr and GPi express primarily the *excitatory* D_1 DA receptor, whereas the striatal neurons that project to the GPe and form the indirect pathway express the *inhibitory* D_2 dopamine receptor. Thus, loss of the dopaminergic input to the striatum has a differential effect on the two outflow pathways; the direct pathway to the SNpr and GPi is less active (*structures in purple*), whereas the activity in the indirect pathway is increased (*structures in red*). The net effect is that neurons in the SNpr and GPi become more active. This leads to increased inhibition of the VA/VL thalamus and reduced excitatory input to the cortex. Light blue lines indicate primary pathways with reduced activity. (See legend to Figure 22–2 for definitions of anatomical abbreviations.)

The key feature of this model of basal ganglia function, which accounts for the symptoms observed in PD as a result of loss of dopaminergic neurons, is the differential effect of DA on the direct and indirect pathways (Figure 22–3). The dopaminergic neurons of the substantia nigra pars compacta (SNpc) innervate all parts of the striatum; however, the target striatal neurons express distinct types of DA receptors. The striatal neurons giving rise to the direct pathway express primarily the *excitatory* D_1 dopamine receptor protein, whereas the striatal neurons forming the indirect pathway express primarily the *inhibitory* D_2 type. Thus, DA released in the striatum tends to increase the activity of the direct pathway and reduce the activity of the indirect pathway, whereas the depletion that occurs in PD has the opposite effect. The net effect of the reduced dopaminergic input in PD is to increase markedly the inhibitory outflow from the SNpr and GPi to the thalamus and reduce excitation of the motor cortex.

There are several limitations of this model of basal ganglia function (Parent and Cicchetti, 1998): The anatomical connections are considerably more complex than envisioned originally. In addition, many of the pathways involved use not just one, but several neurotransmitters. For example, the neuropeptides substance P and dynorphin are found predominantly in striatal neurons making up the direct pathway, whereas most of the indirect pathway neurons express enkephalin. These transmitters are expected to have slow modulatory effects on signaling, in contrast to the rapid effects of glutamate and GABA, but the functional significance of these modulatory effects remains unclear. Nevertheless, the model is useful and has important implications for the rational design and use of pharmacological agents in PD. First, it suggests that to restore the balance of the system through stimulation of DA receptors, the complementary effect of actions at both D_1 and D_2 receptors, as well as the possibility of adverse effects that may be mediated by D_3, D_4, or D_5 receptors, must be considered. Second, it explains why replacement of DA is not the only approach to the treatment of PD. Drugs that inhibit cholinergic receptors have long been used for treatment of parkinsonism. Although their mechanisms of action are not completely understood, their effect is likely mediated at the level of the striatal projection neurons, which normally receive cholinergic input from striatal cholinergic interneurons. Only few clinically useful drugs for parkinsonism are presently available based on actions through GABA and glutamate receptors, even though both have crucial roles in the circuitry of the basal ganglia. However, they represent a promising avenue for drug development (Hallet and Standaert, 2004).

Treatment of Parkinson Disease

Commonly used medications for the treatment of PD are summarized in Table 22–1.

Levodopa. Levodopa (L-DOPA, LARODOPA, L-3,4-dihydroxyphenylalanine), the metabolic precursor of DA, is the single most effective agent in the treatment of PD. Levodopa is itself largely inert; both its therapeutic and adverse effects result from the decarboxylation of levodopa to DA. When administered orally, levodopa is absorbed rapidly from the small bowel by the transport system for aromatic amino acids. Concentrations of the

Table 22–1

Commonly Used Medications for the Treatment of Parkinson Disease

AGENT	TYPICAL INITIAL DOSE	DAILY DOSE RANGE	COMMENTS
Levodopa Formulations			
Carbidopa/levodopa	25 mg carbidopa + 100 mg levodopa ("25/100" tablet), 2-3x daily	200-1200 mg levodopa	
Carbidopa/levodopa sustained-release	50 mg carbidopa + 200 mg levodopa ("50/200 sustained-release" tablet) 2x daily	200-1200 mg levodopa	Bioavailability 75% of immediate-release form
Carbidopa-levodopa orally disintegrating tablets (PARCOPA)	25 mg carbidopa + 100 mg levodopa ("25/100" tablet), 2-3x daily	200-1200 mg levodopa	
COMT Inhibitors			
Entacapone	200 mg with each dose of levodopa/carbidopa	600-2000 mg	
Tolcapone	100 mg with carbidopa/levodopa	100-300 mg	May be hepatotoxic. Use only in patients not responding satisfactorily to other treatments. Requires monitoring of liver function
Carbidopa/levodopa/entacapone	12.5 mg carbidopa + 50 mg levodopa + 200 mg entacapone (STALEVO 50), 3x daily	150-1200 mg levodopa	
DA Agonists			
Apomorphine	2 mg subcutaneous	6-18 mg subcutaneous	Trimethobenzamide is used to reduce nausea when initiating therapy
Bromocriptine	1.25 mg	2.5-15 mg daily	Ergot; long-term use is associated with cardiac valve fibrosis
Pramipexole	0.125 mg 3x daily	1.5-4.5 mg	
Ropinirole	0.25 mg 3x daily	1.5-24 mg	
Ropinirole sustained-release	2 mg per day	2-24 mg	
MAO Inhibitors			
Rasagiline	1 mg daily	0.5-1 mg	
Selegiline	5 mg 2x daily	2.5-10 mg	
Other Medications			
Trihexyphenidyl HCl	1 mg 2x daily	2-15 mg	
Amantadine	100 mg 2x daily	100-200 mg	

drug in plasma usually peak between 0.5 and 2 hours after an oral dose. The $t_{1/2}$ in plasma is short (1-3 hours). The rate and extent of absorption of levodopa depends on the rate of gastric emptying, the pH of gastric juice, and the length of time the drug is exposed to the degradative enzymes of the gastric and intestinal mucosa. Competition for absorption sites in the small bowel from dietary amino acids also may have a marked effect on the absorption of levodopa; administration of levodopa with high-protein meals delays absorption and reduces peak plasma concentrations. Entry of the drug into the CNS across the blood-brain barrier also is mediated by a membrane transporter for aromatic amino acids, and competition between dietary protein and levodopa may occur at this level. In the brain, levodopa is converted to DA by decarboxylation primarily within the presynaptic terminals of dopaminergic neurons in the stratium. The DA produced is responsible for the therapeutic effectiveness of the drug in PD; after release, it is either transported back into dopaminergic terminals by the presynaptic uptake mechanism or metabolized by the actions of MAO and catechol-*O*-methyltransferase (COMT) (Figure 22–4).

In clinical practice, levodopa is almost always administered in combination with a peripherally acting inhibitor of aromatic L-amino acid decarboxylase, such as carbidopa or benserazide (available outside the U.S.), drugs that do not penetrate well into the CNS. If levodopa is administered alone, the drug is largely decarboxylated by enzymes in the intestinal mucosa and other peripheral sites so that relatively little unchanged drug reaches the cerebral circulation and probably <1% penetrates the CNS. In addition, DA release into the circulation by peripheral conversion of levodopa produces undesirable effects, particularly nausea. Inhibition of peripheral decarboxylase markedly increases the fraction of administered levodopa that remains unmetabolized and available to cross the blood-brain barrier (Figure 22–5) and reduces the incidence of GI side effects.

In most individuals, a daily dose of 75 mg carbidopa is sufficient to prevent the development of nausea. For this reason, the most commonly prescribed form of carbidopa/levodopa (SINEMET, ATAMET, others) is the 25/100 form, containing 25 mg carbidopa and 100 mg levodopa. With this formulation, dosage schedules of three or more tablets daily provide acceptable inhibition of decarboxylase in most individuals. Occasionally, individuals will require larger doses of carbidopa to minimize gastrointestinal side effects, and administration of supplemental carbidopa (LODOSYN) may be beneficial. Carbidopa/levodopa is also available in an orally disintegrating tablet (PARCOPA). This may be useful in patients with swallowing difficulty, although it is important to note that levodopa is not absorbed through the oral mucosa, and must still be delivered to the small intestine for absorption. Thus, the time to onset of action of PARCOPA is not appreciably different from that of standard oral formulations.

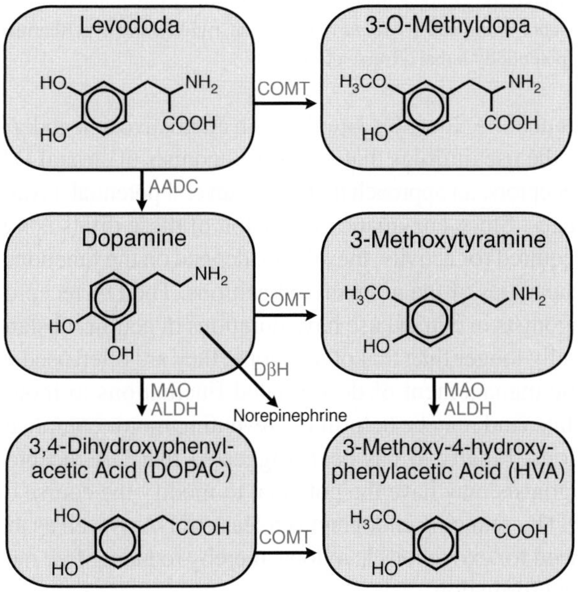

Figure 22–4. *Metabolism of levodopa (L-DOPA).* ALDH, aldehyde dehydrogenase; COMT, catechol-*O*-methyltransferase; DβH, dopamine *β*-hydroxylase; AADC, aromatic L-amino acid decarboxylase; MAO, monoamine oxidase.

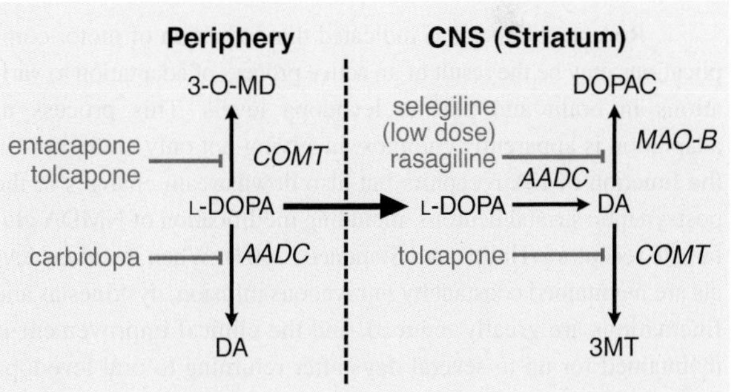

Figure 22–5. *Pharmacological preservation of L-DOPA and striatal dopamine.* The principal site of action of inhibitors of catechol-*O*-methyltransferase (COMT) (such as tolcapone and entacapone) is in the peripheral circulation. They block the *O*-methylation of levodopa (L-DOPA) and increase the fraction of the drug available for delivery to the brain. Tolcapone also has effects in the CNS. Inhibitors of MAO-B, such as low-dose selegiline and rasagiline, will act within the CNS to reduce oxidative deamination of DA, thereby enhancing vesicular stores. AADC, aromatic L-amino acid decarboxylase; DA, dopamine; DOPAC, 3,4-dihydroxyphenylacetic acid; MAO, monoamine oxidase; 3MT, 3-methoxyltyramine; 3-O-MD, 3-O-methyl DOPA

Levodopa therapy can have a dramatic effect on all the signs and symptoms of PD. Early in the course of the disease, the degree of improvement in tremor, rigidity, and bradykinesia may be nearly complete. In early PD, the duration of the beneficial effects of levodopa may exceed the plasma lifetime of the drug, suggesting that the nigrostriatal DA system retains some capacity to store and release DA. A principal limitation of the long-term use of levodopa therapy is that with time this apparent "buffering" capacity is lost, and the patient's motor state may fluctuate dramatically with each dose of levodopa, a condition described as *motor complications* of levodopa. A common problem is the development of the "wearing off" phenomenon: each dose of levodopa effectively improves mobility for a period of time, perhaps 1-2 hours, but rigidity and akinesia return rapidly at the end of the dosing interval. Increasing the dose and frequency of administration can improve this situation, but this often is limited by the development of dyskinesias, excessive and abnormal involuntary movements. Dyskinesias are observed most often when the plasma levodopa concentration is high, although in some individuals dyskinesias or dystonia may be triggered when the level is rising or falling. These movements can be as uncomfortable and disabling as the rigidity and akinesia of PD. In the later stages of PD, patients may fluctuate rapidly between being "off," having no beneficial effects from their medications, and being "on" but with disabling dyskinesias, a situation called the *on/off phenomenon.*

Recent evidence has indicated that induction of motor complications may be the result of an active process of adaptation to variations in brain and plasma levodopa levels. This process of adaptation is apparently complex, involving not only alterations in the function of DA receptors but also downstream changes in the postsynaptic striatal neurons, including modification of NMDA glutamate receptors (Hallett and Standaert, 2004). When levodopa levels are maintained constant by intravenous infusion, dyskinesias and fluctuations are greatly reduced, and the clinical improvement is maintained for up to several days after returning to oral levodopa dosing (Mouradian et al., 1990). A sustained-release formulation consisting of carbidopa/levodopa in an erodable wax matrix (SINEMET CR) has been marketed in an attempt to produce more stable plasma levodopa levels than can be obtained with oral administration of standard carbidopa/levodopa formulations. This formulation is helpful in some cases, but absorption of the sustained-release formulation is not entirely predictable. Other approaches to more continuous delivery of levodopa, including gel and transdermal formulations, are under study.

An important unanswered question regarding the use of levodopa in PD is whether this medication alters the course of the underlying disease or merely modifies the symptoms. A recent randomized trial has provided evidence that levodopa does not have an adverse effect on the course of the underlying disease, but has also confirmed that high doses of levodopa are associated with early onset of dyskinesias (Fahn et al., 2004). Most practitioners have adopted a pragmatic approach, using levodopa only when the symptoms of PD cause functional impairment and other treatments are inadequate or not well tolerated.

In addition to motor complications and nausea, several other adverse effects may be observed with levodopa treatment. A frequent and troubling adverse effect is the induction of hallucinations and confusion, especially in elderly patients or in patients with preexisting cognitive dysfunction. This adverse effect often limits the ability to treat parkinsonian symptoms adequately. Conventional antipsychotic agents, such as the phenothiazines, are effective against levodopa-induced psychosis but may cause marked worsening of parkinsonism, probably through actions at the D_2 DA receptor. An alternative approach has been to use "atypical" antipsychotic agents (Chapter 16). However, not all of these are equally useful in this setting, and some of the "atypical" agents may nevertheless worsen PD symptoms. The two drugs which appear to be most effective and best tolerated in patients with advanced PD are clozapine and quetiapine (Friedman and Factor, 2000).

Peripheral decarboxylation of levodopa and release of DA into the circulation may activate vascular DA receptors and produce orthostatic hypotension. Administration of levodopa with nonspecific inhibitors of MAO, such as phenelzine and tranylcypromine, markedly accentuates the actions of levodopa and may precipitate life-threatening hypertensive crisis and hyperpyrexia; nonspecific MAO inhibitors always should be discontinued at least 14 days before levodopa is administered (note that this prohibition does not include the MAO-B subtype-specific inhibitors selegiline and rasagiline (AZILECT), which, as discussed later, are often administered safely in combination with levodopa). Abrupt withdrawal of levodopa or other dopaminergic medications may precipitate the *neuroleptic malignant syndrome* of confusion, rigidity, and hyperthermia, a potentially lethal adverse effect.

Dopamine-Receptor Agonists. An alternative to levodopa is the use of drugs that are direct agonists of striatal DA receptors, an approach that offers several potential advantages. Since enzymatic conversion of these drugs is not required for activity, they do not depend on the functional capacities of the nigrostriatal neurons. The DA receptor agonists in clinical use have durations of action substantially longer than that of levodopa; they are often used in the management of dose-related fluctuations in motor state, and may be helpful in preventing motor complications. Finally, it has been suggested that DA receptor agonists may have the potential to modify the course of PD by reducing endogenous release of DA as well as the need for exogenous levodopa, thereby reducing free radical formation.

Two orally administered DA receptor agonists are commonly used for treatment of PD: ropinirole (REQUIP) and pramipexole (MIRAPEX).

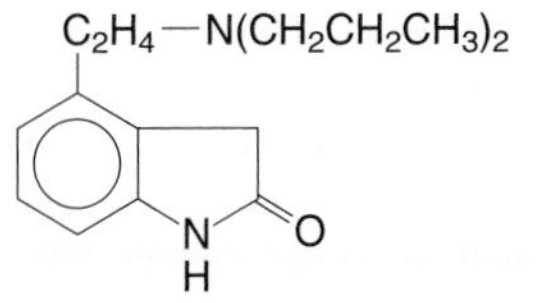

$C_2H_4{-}N(CH_2CH_2CH_3)_2$

ROPINIROLE

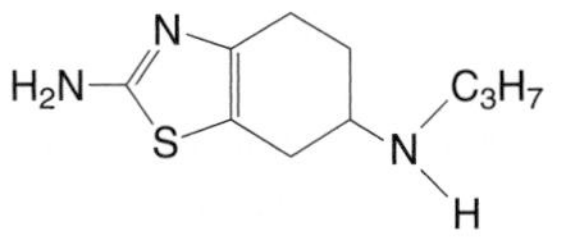

PRAMIPEXOLE

These agents are better tolerated and have largely replaced the older agents (e.g., bromocriptine, pergolide), which have to be titrated more slowly. Pergolide was withdrawn from the U.S. market in 2007 because of cardiac valve fibrosis. Ropinirole and pramipexole have selective activity at D_2 class sites (specifically at the D_2 and D_3 receptor) and little or no activity at D_1 class sites. Both are well absorbed orally and have similar therapeutic actions. Like levodopa, they can relieve the clinical symptoms of PD. The duration of action of the DA agonists (8-24 hours) often is longer than that of levodopa (6-8 hours), and they are particularly effective in the treatment of patients who have developed on/off phenomena. Ropinirole is also available in a once-daily sustained release formulation (REQUIP XL), which is more convenient and may reduce adverse effects related to intermittent dosing. Both pramipexole and ropinirole may produce hallucinosis or confusion, similar to that observed with levodopa, and may cause nausea and orthostatic hypotension. They should be initiated at low dose and titrated slowly to minimize these effects. The DA agonists, as well as levodopa itself, are also associated with fatigue and somnolence. The somnolence in some cases may be quite severe, and several instances of sudden attacks of irresistible sleepiness leading to motor vehicle accidents have been reported (Frucht et al., 1999). Although an uncommon complication, it is prudent to advise patients of this possibility and to switch to another agent when somnolence is an issue.

Apomorphine. Apomorphine (APOKYN) is a dopaminergic agonist that can be administered by subcutaneous injection. It has high affinity for D_4 receptors; moderate affinity for D_2, D_3, D_5, and adrenergic α_{1D}, α_{2B}, and α_{2C} receptors; and low affinity for D_1 receptors. Apomorphine has been used in Europe for many years and is FDA-approved as a "rescue therapy" for the acute intermittent treatment of "off" episodes in patients with a fluctuating response to dopaminergic therapy.

Apomorphine has the same side effects as discussed earlier for the oral DA agonists. In addition, apomorphine is highly emetogenic and requires pre- and post-treatment anti-emetic therapy. Oral trimethobenzamide (TIGAN), at a dose of 300 mg three times daily, should be started 3 days prior to the initial dose of apomorphine and continued at least during the first 2 months of therapy. Profound hypotension and loss of consciousness have occurred when apomorphine was administered with ondansetron; hence, the concomitant use of apomorphine with antiemetic drugs of the 5-HT_3 antagonist class is contraindicated. Other potentially serious side effects of apomorphine include QT prolongation, injection-site reactions, and the development of a pattern of abuse characterized by increasingly frequent dosing leading to hallucinations, dyskinesia, and abnormal behavior. Because of these potential adverse effects, use of apomorphine is appropriate only when other measures, such as oral DA agonists or COMT inhibitors, have failed to control the "off" episodes. Apomorphine therapy should be initiated with a 2-mg test dose in a setting where the patient can be monitored carefully. If tolerated, it can be titrated slowly up to a maximum dosage of 6 mg. For effective control of symptoms, patients may require three or more injections daily.

Catechol-O-Methyltransferase (COMT) Inhibitors. Drugs for the treatment of PD include inhibitors of the enzyme COMT, which, together with MAO, metabolizes levodopa and DA. COMT transfers a methyl group from the donor *S*-adenosyl-L-methionine, producing the pharmacologically inactive compounds 3-*O*-methyl DOPA (from levodopa) and 3-methoxytyramine (from DA; Figure 22–5). When levodopa is administered orally, nearly 99% of the drug is metabolized and does not reach the brain. Most is converted by aromatic L-amino acid decarboxylase (AADC) to DA, which causes nausea and hypotension. Addition of an AADC inhibitor such as carbidopa reduces the formation of DA but increases the fraction of levodopa that is methylated by COMT. The principal therapeutic action of the COMT inhibitors is to block this peripheral conversion of levodopa to 3-*O*-methyl DOPA, increasing both the plasma $t_{1/2}$ of levodopa as well as the fraction of each dose that reaches the CNS.

Two COMT inhibitors presently are available for this use in the United States, tolcapone (TASMAR) and entacapone (COMTAN). In double-blind clinical trials, both agents significantly reduced the "wearing off" symptoms in patients treated with levodopa/carbidopa (Parkinson Study Group, 1997). The two drugs differ only in their pharmacokinetic properties and adverse effects: tolcapone has a relatively long duration of action, allowing for administration two to three times a day, and appears to act by both central and peripheral inhibition of COMT. Entacapone has a short duration of action (2 hours) and usually is administered simultaneously with each dose of levodopa/carbidopa. The action of entacapone is attributable principally to peripheral inhibition of COMT. The common adverse effects of these agents are similar to those of levodopa/carbidopa alone and include nausea, orthostatic hypotension, vivid dreams, confusion, and hallucinations. An important adverse effect associated with tolcapone is hepatotoxicity. Up to 2% of the patients treated have increased serum alanine aminotransferase and aspartate transaminase; and at least three fatal cases of fulminant hepatic failure in patients taking tolcapone have been observed, leading to addition of a black box warning to the label. At present, tolcapone should be used only in patients who have not responded to other therapies and with appropriate monitoring for hepatic injury. Entacapone has not been associated with hepatotoxicity and requires no special monitoring. Entacapone also is available in fixed-dose combinations with levodopa/carbidopa (STALEVO).

Selective MAO-B Inhibitors. Two isoenzymes of MAO oxidize monoamines. While both isoenzymes (MAO-A and MAO-B) are present in the periphery and inactivate monoamines of intestinal origin, the isoenzyme MAO-B is the predominant form in the striatum and is responsible for most of the oxidative metabolism of DA in the brain. Two selective MAO-B inhibitors are used for the treatment of PD: selegiline (ELDEPRYL, EMSAM, ZELAPAR) and rasagiline (AZILECT). When used at recommended doses, these agents selectively inactivate MAO-B through irreversible inhibition of the enzyme (Elmer and Bertoni, 2008). Both agents exert modest beneficial effects on the symptoms of PD. The basis of this efficacy is presumed to be the inhibition of breakdown of DA in the striatum. Unlike nonspecific inhibitors of MAO (such as phenelzine, tranylcypromine, and isocarboxazid), selective MAO-B inhibitors do not substantially inhibit the peripheral metabolism of catecholamines and can be taken safely with levodopa. These agents also do not exhibit the "cheese effect," the potentially lethal potentiation of catecholamine action observed when patients on nonspecific MAO inhibitors ingest indirectly acting sympathomimetic amines such as the tyramine found in certain cheeses and wine.

Selegiline has been used for many years as a symptomatic treatment for PD and is generally well tolerated in younger patients with early or mild PD. In patients with more advanced PD or underlying cognitive impairment, selegiline may accentuate the adverse motor and cognitive effects of levodopa therapy. Metabolites of selegiline include amphetamine and methamphetamine, which may cause anxiety, insomnia, and other adverse symptoms. Recently, selegiline has become available in an orally disintegrating tablet (ZELEPAR) as well as a transdermal patch (EMSAM). Both of these delivery routes are intended to reduce hepatic first-pass metabolism and limit the formation of the amphetamine metabolites.

Unlike selegiline, rasagiline does not give rise to undesirable amphetamine metabolites. In randomized controlled clinical trials, rasagiline monotherapy was effective in early PD. Adjunctive therapy significantly reduced levodopa-related "wearing off" symptoms in advanced PD.

A consequence of the inhibition of MAO-B in the brain is a reduction in the overall catabolism of DA, which may reduce the formation of potentially toxic free radicals. This observation has led to studies which have examined the question of whether MAO-B inhibition can alter the rate of neurodegeneration in PD. The potential protective role of selegiline in idiopathic PD was evaluated in several multicenter randomized trials; although there was some evidence supporting a neuroprotective effect, the outcomes were obscured by the difficulty of distinguishing long-term neuroprotective effects from short-term symptomatic effects (Parkinson Study Group, 1993; Yacoubian and Standaert, 2008). A more recent study, using a different design, has produced more convincing data suggesting a neuroprotective effect of rasagiline (Olanow, 2008).

Although selective MAO-B inhibitors are generally well tolerated, drug interactions can be troublesome. Similar to the nonspecific MAO inhibitors, selegiline can lead to the development of stupor, rigidity, agitation, and hyperthermia when administered with the analgesic meperidine. Although the mechanics, of this interaction is uncertain, selegiline or rasagiline should not be given in combination with meperidine. Adverse effects have been reported from coadministration of MAO-B inhibitors with tricyclic antidepressants or with serotonin-reuptake inhibitors. However, interactions with antidepressants are uncommon, and many patients do take these combinations of medications without apparent adverse interaction; nonetheless, concomitant administration of selegiline or rasagiline with serotonergic drugs should be done with caution, especially in patients on high doses of serotonin-reuptake inhibitors.

Muscarinic Receptor Antagonists. Antagonists of muscarinic acetylcholine receptors were used widely for the treatment of PD before the discovery of levodopa. The biological basis for the therapeutic actions of anticholinergics is not completely understood. They may act within the neostriatum through the receptors that normally mediate the response to intrinsic cholinergic innervation of this structure, which arises primarily from cholinergic striatal interneurons. Several muscarinic cholinergic receptors have been cloned (Chapters 9 and 14); like the DA receptors, these are GPCRs. Five subtypes of muscarinic receptors exist. All five subtypes are probably present in the striatum, although each one has a distinct distribution (Hersch et al., 1994). Anticholinergic drugs currently used in the treatment of PD include trihexyphenidyl (2-4 mg three times per day), benztropine mesylate (1-4 mg two times per day), and diphenhydramine hydrochloride (25-50 mg three or four times per day). Diphenhydramine also is a histamine H_1 antagonist (Chapter 32).

All of these drugs have relatively modest antiparkinsonian activity and are only used in the treatment of early PD or as an adjunct to dopamimetic therapy. Adverse effects result from their anticholinergic properties. Most troublesome are sedation and mental confusion. Other side effects are constipation, urinary retention, and blurred vision through cycloplegia. All anticholinergic drugs must be used with caution in patients with narrow-angle glaucoma (Chapter 65).

Amantadine. Amantadine (SYMMETREL), an antiviral agent used for the prophylaxis and treatment of influenza A (Chapter 58), has antiparkinsonian activity. Amantadine appears to alter DA release in the striatum, has anticholinergic properties, and blocks NMDA glutamate receptors. However, it is not well understood which of amantadine's pharmacological effects are responsible for its antiparkinsonian actions. In any case, the effects of amantadine in PD are modest. It is used as initial therapy of mild PD. It also may be helpful as an adjunct in patients on levodopa with dose-related fluctuations and dyskinesias. The antidyskinetic properties of amantadine have been attributed to actions at NMDA receptors (Hallett and Standaert, 2004), although the closely related NMDA receptor antagonist memantine (discussed later) does not seem to have this effect.

Amantadine is usually administered at a dose of 100 mg twice a day and is well tolerated. Dizziness, lethargy, anticholinergic effects, and sleep disturbance, as well as nausea and vomiting, have been observed occasionally, but even when present, these effects are mild and reversible.

Neuroprotective Treatments for Parkinson Disease. It would be desirable to identify a treatment that modifies the progressive degeneration that underlies PD rather than simply controlling the symptoms. Current research strategies are based on the disease mechanisms described earlier (e.g., energy metabolism, oxidative stress, environmental triggers, and excitotoxicity) and on discoveries related to the genetics of PD (Yacoubian and Standaert, 2008). Several studies have examined the potential neuroprotective effects of existing medications. In a randomized controlled trial, levodopa did not worsen the disease state. Some benefits persisted for several weeks after treatment was stopped, but whether this was truly a "neuroprotective" effect remains uncertain (Fahn et al., 2004).

Two trials have attempted to examine the effect of pramipexole or ropinirole on neurodegeneration in PD (Parkinson Study Group, 2002; Whone et al., 2003). Both trials observed that in patients treated with either one of these agonists, there was a reduced rate of loss of markers of dopaminergic neurotransmission measured by brain imaging compared with a similar group of patients treated with levodopa. These intriguing data should be viewed cautiously, particularly because there is considerable uncertainty about the relationship of the imaging results techniques used and the true rate of neurodegeneration (Albin and Frey, 2003).

Inhibition of MAO-B in the brain reduces the overall catabolism of DA, which may decrease the formation of potentially toxic free radicals and consequently the rate of neurodegeneration in PD. The protective role of selegiline in idiopathic PD was evaluated in several multicenter randomized trials. Unfortunately, distinguishing long-term neuroprotective effects from short-term symptomatic effects was difficult in the earlier studies (Parkinson Study Group, 1993; Yacoubian and Standaert, 2008). A different study design showed more convincingly a neuroprotective effect of rasagiline (2008).

Another strategy under study is the use of compounds that augment cellular energy metabolism such coenzyme Q10, a cofactor required for the mitochondrial electron-transport chain. A small study has demonstrated that this drug is well tolerated in PD and has suggested that coenzyme Q10 may slow the course of the disease (Shults et al., 2002). A much larger study is in progress. Therapies directly targeting the molecules which are implicated in the pathogenesis of PD are still in a nascent stage, and may require unconventional delivery strategies such as gene therapy (Lewis and Standaert, 2008).

Clinical Summary. Pharmacological treatment of PD should be tailored to the individual patient. Drug therapy is not obligatory in early PD; many patients can be managed for a time with exercise and lifestyle interventions. For patients with mild symptoms, MAO-B inhibitors, amantadine, or (in younger patients) anticholinergics are reasonable choices. In most patients, treatment with a dopaminergic drug, either levodopa or a DA agonist, is eventually required. Large controlled clinical trials provide convincing evidence for a reduced rate of motor fluctuation in patients in which DA agonists are used as initial treatment. This benefit was, however, accompanied by an increased rate of adverse effects, especially somnolence and hallucinations (Parkinson Study Group, 2000; Rascol et al., 2000). Practitioners prefer DA agonist as initial therapy in younger patients in order to reduce the occurrence of motor complications. In older patients or those with substantial comorbidity, levodopa/carbidopa is generally better tolerated.

ALZHEIMER'S DISEASE (AD)

Clinical Overview. The brain region most vulnerable to neuronal dysfunction and cell loss in AD is the medial temporal lobe, including entorhinal cortex and hippocampus. Typical early AD symptoms are due to dysfunction of these structures resulting in anterograde episodic memory loss: repeated questions, misplaced items, missed appointments, and forgotten details of daily life. A typical patient presents with memory dysfunction that is noticeable by the patient and/or family members, but not severe enough to impair daily function. Because current diagnostic criteria for AD require the presence of dementia (i.e., cognitive impairments sufficient to reduce function), these patients are generally given a diagnosis of mild cognitive impairment (MCI). Patients with MCI progress at a rate of about 10% per year to AD (Petersen et al., 2005), although not all MCI patients will develop AD. The decline in both cognitive and functional capacity follows a course of gradual but relentless progression in AD, spreading to involve other cognitive domains including visuospatial and executive function. The later stages of the disease are characterized by increasing dependence and progression toward the akinetic-mute state that typifies end-stage neurologic disease. Death, most often from a complication of immobility such as pneumonia or pulmonary embolism, usually ensues within 6-12 years of onset.

At present, the diagnosis of AD is based on the clinical assessment of the patient. Structural neuroimaging and appropriate laboratory tests are used to exclude other disorders that may mimic AD. In the near future, laboratory measures to specifically identify AD, including analysis of biomarkers such as CSF or serum factors, genetic testing, and molecular or functional neuroimaging, are likely to be incorporated into AD diagnostic criteria to enhance the sensitivity of diagnosis, especially at early stages of the disease (Dubois et al., 2007). A direct antemortem confirmatory test currently does not exist.

Genetics. Mutations in three genes have been identified as causes of autosomal dominant, early-onset AD: *APP*, which encodes amyloid-β precursor protein, and *PSEN1* and *PSEN2*, encoding presenilin 1 and 2. All three genes are involved in the production of amyloid-β peptides (Aβ). Aβ is generated by sequential proteolytic cleavage of APP by two enzymes, β-secretase and γ-secretase; the presenilins form the catalytic core of γ-secretase. The genetic evidence, combined with the fact that Aβ accumulates in the brain in the form of soluble oligomers and amyloid plaques, and is toxic when applied to neurons, forms the basis for the amyloid hypothesis of AD pathogenesis (Tanzi and Bertram, 2005).

Autosomal-dominant cases of AD are quite rare, but there is also a significant genetic component to the more common, sporadic, late-onset cases of AD. Many genes have been identified as having alleles that increase AD risk (Bertram et al., 2007). By far the most important of these is *APOE*, which encodes the lipid carrier protein apolipoprotein E (apoE) (Raber et al., 2004). Individuals inheriting the ε4 allele of *APOE* have a more than 3-fold higher risk of developing AD. While they make up less than one-fourth of the population, they account for more than half of all AD cases. Several clinical trials have shown a different response rate between apoE4-carriers and noncarriers, suggesting an important potential pharmacogenetic influence of apoE genotype on the choice of therapy. However, at this point genetic testing for apoE status is not a routine part of the clinical evaluation for AD.

Pathophysiology. The pathological hallmarks of AD are amyloid plaques, which are extracellular accumulations of Aβ, and intracellular neurofibrillary tangles composed of the microtubule-associated protein tau (Figure 22–6). While the development of amyloid plaques is an early and invariant feature of AD, tangle burden accrues over time in a manner that correlates more closely with the development of cognitive impairment. The current consensus is that Aβ accumulation is an upstream event that triggers tau pathology, resulting in impaired neuronal function and cell loss. In autosomal dominant AD, Aβ accumulates due to mutations that cause its overproduction. The cause of high cerebral Aβ levels in late-onset sporadic AD is unclear but is likely caused by impaired clearance rather than overproduction.

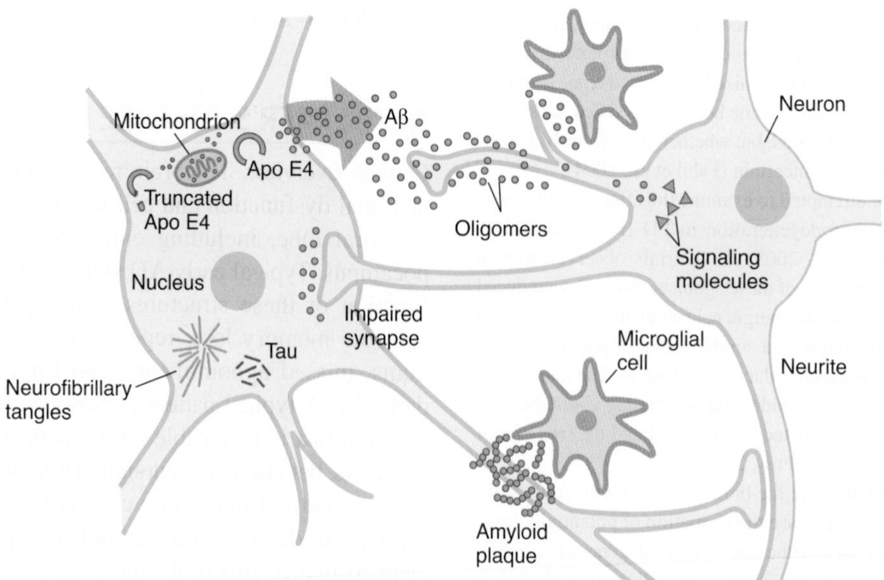

Figure 22–6. *Molecular and cellular processes presumed to participate in AD pathogenesis.* (From Roberson ED, Mucke L. 100 years and counting: Prospects for defeating Alzheimer's disease. *Science*, 2006, 314:781–784. Reprinted with permission from AAAS.)

Aggregation of Aβ is an important event in AD pathogenesis. While plaques consist of highly ordered fibrils of Aβ, it appears that soluble Aβ oligomers, perhaps as small as dimers, are more highly pathogenic. Tau also aggregates to form the paired helical filaments that make up neurofibrillary tangles. Post-translational modifications of tau including phosphorylation, proteolysis, and other changes cause loss of tau's normal functions and increase its propensity to aggregate. Mechanisms by which Aβ and tau induce neuronal dysfunction and death may include direct impairment of synaptic transmission and plasticity, excitotoxicity, oxidative stress, and neuroinflammation. The factors underlying the selective vulnerability of particular cortical neurons to the pathological effects of AD are not known.

Neurochemistry. The most striking neurochemical disturbance in AD is a deficiency of acetylcholine. The anatomical basis of the cholinergic deficit is atrophy and degeneration of subcortical cholinergic neurons, particularly those in the basal forebrain (nucleus basalis of Meynert) that provide cholinergic innervation to the cerebral cortex. The selective deficiency of ACh in AD, as well as the observation that central cholinergic antagonists such as atropine can induce a confusional state that bears some resemblance to the dementia of AD, has given rise to the "cholinergic hypothesis," which proposes that a deficiency of ACh is critical in the genesis of the AD symptoms (Perry, 1986). Although viewing AD as a "cholinergic deficiency syndrome" akin to the "dopaminergic deficiency syndrome" of PD provides a useful framework, it is important to note that the deficit in AD is far more complex. AD involves multiple neurotransmitter systems, including glutamate, 5-HT, and neuropeptides, and there is destruction of not only cholinergic neurons but also the cortical and hippocampal targets that receive cholinergic input.

Treatment of Alzheimer's Disease

At present, no disease-modifying therapy for AD is available. While aggressive attempts to develop drugs targeting Aβ, tau, apoE, and other molecules involved in AD pathogenesis are underway (Roberson and Mucke, 2006), current treatment is aimed at alleviating symptoms.

Treatment of Cognitive Symptoms. Augmentation of the cholinergic transmission is currently the mainstay of AD treatment. Three drugs, donepezil, rivastigmine, and galantamine, are widely used for this purpose; a fourth, tacrine, was the first drug approved to treat AD but is rarely used now because it has much more extensive side effects compared to the newer agents (Table 22–2). All four agents are reversible antagonists of cholinesterases, enzymes that act to limit cholinergic neurotransmission by catalyzing the cleavage of acetylcholine in the synaptic cleft into choline and acetate (Chapter 10). Cholinesterase inhibitors are the usual first-line therapy for symptomatic treatment of cognitive impairments in mild or moderate AD. These agents have a beneficial, albeit quite modest, effect on cognition in clinical AD studies (Birks, 2006). They are also widely used to treat other neurodegenerative diseases with cholinergic deficits, including dementia with Lewy bodies (Bhasin et al., 2007) and vascular dementia (Kavirajan and Schneider, 2007). In addition, they are sometimes used in MCI, where they may also have symptomatic benefit but do not slow the conversion to AD (Raschetti et al., 2007). The drugs are usually well tolerated, with the most common side effects being GI distress, muscle cramping, and abnormal dreams. Because of their cholinergic and

Table 22–2

Cholinesterase Inhibitors Used for the Treatment of Alzheimer's Disease

	DONEPEZIL	RIVASTIGMINE	GALANTAMINE	TACRINE[a]
Brand name	ARICEPT	EXELON, generic	RAZADYNE, generic	COGNEX
Enzymes inhibited[b]	AChE	AChE, BuChE	AChE	AChE, BuChE
Mechanism	Noncompetitive	Noncompetitive	Competitive	Noncompetitive
Typical maintenance dose[c]	10 mg once daily	9.5 mg/24h (transdermal) 3-6 mg twice daily (oral)	8-12 mg twice daily (immediate-release) 16-24 mg/day (extended-release)	20 mg, four times daily
FDA-approved indications	Mild–severe AD	Mild–moderate AD, Mild–moderate PDD[d]	Mild–moderate AD	Mild–moderate AD
Metabolism[e]	CYP2D6, CYP3A4	Esterases	CYP2D6, CYP3A4	CYP1A2

[a]Tacrine was the first cholinesterase inhibitor approved for the treatment of AD, but is now rarely used because of hepatotoxicity and adverse effects. [b]AChE (acetylcholinesterase) is the major cholinesterase in the brain; BuChE (butyrylcholinesterase) is a serum and hepatic cholinesterase that is upregulated in AD brain. [c] Typical starting doses are one-half of the maintenance dose and are given for the first month of therapy. [d] PDD, Parkinson disease dementia. [e] Drugs metabolized by CYP2D6 and CYP3A4 are subject to increased serum levels when co-administered with drugs known to inhibit these enzymes, such as ketoconazole and paroxetine. Similarly, tacrine levels are increased by co-administration with the CYP1A2 inhibitors theophylline, cimetidine, and fluvoxamine.

potentially vagotonic properties, they should be used with caution in patients with bradycardia or syncope.

Memantine (NAMENDA) is used either as an adjunct or an alternative to cholinesterase inhibitors in AD, and is also commonly used to treat other neurodegenerative dementias. Memantine is a noncompetitive antagonist of the NMDA-type glutamate receptor. It interacts with the Mg^{2+} binding site of the channel to prevent excessive activation while sparing normal function (Lipton, 2007). Memantine significantly reduces the rate of clinical deterioration in patients with moderate to severe AD (Raina et al., 2008). Whether this is due to a true disease-modifying effect, possibly reduced excitotoxicity, or to a symptomatic effect of the drug is unclear. Adverse effects of memantine include headache or dizziness, but are usually mild and reversible. The drug is excreted by the kidneys, and dosage should be reduced in patients with severe renal impairment.

Treatment of Behavioral Symptoms. In addition to cognitive decline, behavioral and psychiatric symptoms in dementia (BPSD) are common, particularly in middle stages of the disease. These symptoms, including irritability and agitation, paranoia and delusional thinking, wandering, anxiety, and depression, are a major source of caregiver distress and often precipitate nursing home placement. Treatment can be difficult, and nonpharmacological approaches should generally be first-line (Beier, 2007; Sink et al., 2005).

A variety of pharmacological options are also available. In addition to their effects on cognitive measures, both cholinesterase inhibitors and memantine reduce some BPSD (Maidment et al., 2008; Trinh et al., 2003). However, their effects are modest, and they do not treat some of the most troublesome symptoms, such as agitation (Howard et al., 2007). Furthermore, because most AD patients are already treated with these drugs, other options are often needed when behavioral symptoms emerge.

Atypical antipsychotics, such as risperidone, olanzapine, and quetiapine (Chapter 16), are the most efficacious therapy for agitation and psychosis in AD. Risperdone and olanzapine are effective, but their use is often limited by adverse effects, including parkinsonism, sedation, and falls (Schneider et al., 2006). In addition, the use of atypical antipsychotics in elderly patients with dementia-related psychosis has been associated with a higher risk of stroke and overall mortality (Douglas and Smeeth, 2008; Schneider et al., 2005), leading the FDA to order inclusion of a boxed warning in the prescribing information for all drugs in this class. Unfortunately, there are few effective alternatives.

Mood stabilizers (Chapter 16) have been the focus of several trials for BPSD. Carbamazepine has shown some benefit in small trials but carries numerous risks in the elderly, especially the potential for drug-drug interactions. There is little evidence of benefit from valproic acid. Lithium is of considerable interest given its ability to inhibit glycogen synthase kinase, which is implicated in AD pathogenesis, but clinical trial results are limited and concerns persist about the narrow therapeutic window in elderly patients. Benzodiazepines (Chapter 17) can be used for occasional control of acute agitation, but are not recommended for long-term management because of their adverse effects on cognition and other risks in the elderly population. The typical antipsychotic haloperidol (Chapter 16) may be useful for aggression, but sedation and extrapyramidal symptoms limit its use to control of acute episodes.

Antidepressants (Chapter 15) can be useful for BPSD, particularly when depression or anxiety contribute. Because of the adverse anticholinergic effects of tricyclic agents, serotonergic antidepressants are favored. These agents are generally well tolerated. Trazodone has modest benefits, but for the most part, selective serotonin reuptake inhibitors (SSRIs) are the preferred class of drugs.

Clinical Summary. The typical AD patient presenting in early stages of disease should probably be treated with a cholinesterase inhibitor. Patients and families should be counseled that a realistic goal of therapy is to induce a temporary reprieve from progression, or at least a reduction in the rate of decline, rather than long-term recovery of cognition. As the disease progresses, memantine can be added to the regimen. Behavioral symptoms are often treated with a serotonergic antidepressant or, if they are severe enough to warrant the risk of higher mortality, an atypical antipsychotic. Eliminating drugs likely to aggravate cognitive impairments, particularly anticholinergics, benzodiazepines, and other sedative/hypnotics, from the patient's regimen is another important aspect of AD pharmacotherapy.

HUNTINGTON'S DISEASE (HD)

Clinical Features. HD is a dominantly inherited disorder characterized by the gradual onset of motor incoordination and cognitive decline in midlife. Symptoms develop insidiously, either as a movement disorder manifest by brief, jerk-like movements of the extremities, trunk, face, and neck (chorea) or as personality changes or both. Fine-motor incoordination and impairment of rapid eye movements are early features. Occasionally, especially when the onset of symptoms occurs before age 20, choreic movements are less prominent; instead, bradykinesia and dystonia predominate. As the disorder progresses, the involuntary movements become more severe, dysarthria and dysphagia develop, and balance is impaired. The cognitive disorder manifests first as slowness of mental processing and difficulty in organizing complex tasks. Memory is impaired, but affected persons rarely lose their memory of family, friends, and the immediate situation. Such persons often become irritable, anxious, and depressed. Less frequently, paranoia and delusional states are manifest. The outcome of HD is invariably fatal; over a course of 15-30 years, the affected person becomes totally disabled and unable to communicate, requiring full-time care; death ensues from the complications of immobility (Shoulson, 1992).

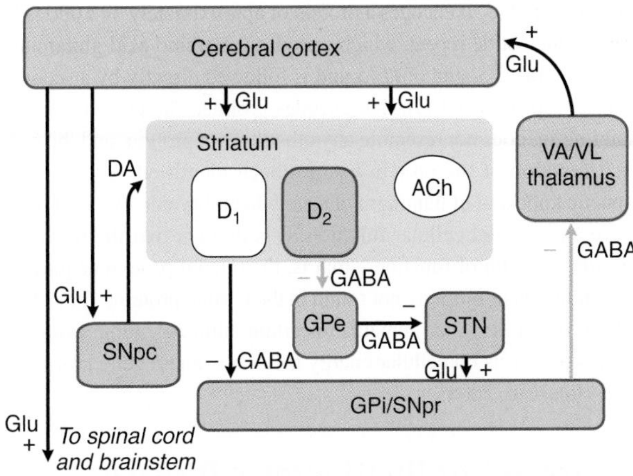

Figure 22–7. *The basal ganglia in Huntington's disease.* HD is characterized by loss of neurons from the striatum. The neurons that project from the striatum to the GPe and form the indirect pathway are affected earlier in the course of the disease than those which project to the GPi. This leads to a loss of inhibition of the GPe. The increased activity in this structure, in turn, inhibits the STN, SNpr, and GPi, resulting in a loss of inhibition to the VA/VL thalamus and increased thalamocortical excitatory drive. Structures in purple have reduced activity in HD, whereas structures in purple have increased activity. Light blue line indicate primary pathways of reduced activity. (See legend to Figure 22–2 for definitions of anatomical abbreviations.)

Pathology and Pathophysiology. HD is characterized by prominent neuronal loss in the striatum (caudate/putamen) of the brain (Vonsattel et al., 1985). Atrophy of these structures proceeds in an orderly fashion, first affecting the tail of the caudate nucleus and then proceeding anteriorly from mediodorsal to ventrolateral. Other areas of the brain also are affected, although much less severely; morphometric analyses indicate that there are fewer neurons in cerebral cortex, hypothalamus, and thalamus. Even within the striatum, the neuronal degeneration of HD is selective. Interneurons and afferent terminals are largely spared, whereas the striatal projection neurons (the medium spiny neurons) are severely affected. This leads to large decreases in striatal GABA concentrations, whereas SST and DA concentrations are relatively preserved (Ferrante et al., 1987).

Selective vulnerability also appears to underlie the most conspicuous clinical feature of HD, the development of chorea. In most adult-onset cases, the medium spiny neurons that project to the GPi and SNpr (the indirect pathway) appear to be affected earlier than those projecting to the GPe (the direct pathway; Figure 22–5) (Albin et al., 1992). The disproportionate impairment of the indirect pathway increases excitatory drive to the neocortex, producing involuntary choreiform movements (Figure 22–7). In some individuals, rigidity rather than chorea is the predominant clinical feature; this is especially common in juvenile-onset cases. Here, the striatal neurons giving rise to both the direct and indirect pathways are impaired to a comparable degree.

Genetics. HD is an autosomal dominant disorder with nearly complete penetrance. The average age of onset is between 35 and 45 years, but the range varies from as early as age 2 to as late as the middle 80s. Although the disease is inherited equally from mother and father, more than 80% of those developing symptoms before age 20 inherit the defect from the father. This is an example of *anticipation,* or the tendency for the age of onset of a disease to decline with each succeeding generation, which also is observed in other neurodegenerative diseases with similar genetic mechanisms. Known homozygotes for HD show clinical characteristics identical to the typical HD heterozygote, indicating that the unaffected chromosome does not attenuate the disease symptomatology. Until the discovery of the genetic defect responsible for HD, *de novo* mutations causing HD were thought to be unusual; but it is now clear that the disease can arise from unaffected parents, especially when one carries an "intermediate allele," as described in the next paragraph.

The discovery of the genetic mutation responsible for HD was the product of an arduous 10-year, multi-investigator collaborative effort. In 1993, a region near the end of the short arm of chromosome 4 was found to contain a polymorphic $(CAG)_n$ trinucleotide repeat that was significantly expanded in all individuals with HD (Huntington's Disease Collaborative Research Group, 1993). The expansion of this trinucleotide repeat is the genetic alteration responsible for HD. The CAG repeat is unstable, and may expand during the DNA synthesis associated with meiosis. This is particularly common during spermatogenesis, and accounts for the phenomenon of anticipation. The range of CAG repeat length in normal individuals is between 9 and 34 triplets, with a median repeat length on normal chromosomes of 19. The repeat length in HD varies from 40 to over 100. Repeat lengths of 35-39 represent intermediate alleles; some of these individuals develop HD late in life, whereas others are not affected. Repeat length is correlated inversely with age of onset. The younger the age of onset, the higher the probability of a large repeat number. This correlation is most powerful in individuals with onset before age 30; with onset above age 30, the correlation is weaker. Thus, repeat length cannot serve as an adequate predictor of age of onset in most individuals. Several other neurodegenerative diseases also arise through expansion of a CAG repeat, including hereditary spinocerebellar ataxias and Kennedy's disease, a rare inherited disorder of motor neurons.

Selective Vulnerability. The mechanism by which the expanded trinucleotide repeat leads to the clinical and pathological features of HD is unknown. The HD mutation lies within a large gene (10 kilobases) designated *IT15*. It encodes a protein of approximately 348,000 DA. The trinucleotide repeat, which encodes the amino acid glutamine, occurs at the 5′5' end of *IT15* and is followed directly by a second, shorter repeat of $(CCG)_n$ that encodes proline. The protein, named huntingtin, does not resemble any other known protein, and the normal function of the protein has not been identified. Mice with a genetic knockout of huntingtin die early in embryonic life, so it must have an essential cellular function. It is thought that the mutation results in a gain of function—that is, the mutant protein acquires a new function or property not found in the normal protein. The nature of the function gained remains uncertain, although some evidence points to effects on cellular energy metabolism and gene transcription (Imarisio, 2008).

Treatment of Huntington's Disease

Symptomatic Treatment. Treatment for symptomatic HD emphasizes the selective use of medications (Shoulson, 1992). None of the currently available medications slows the progression of the disease. HD patients are frequently very sensitive to side effects of medications. Treatment is needed for patients who are depressed, irritable, paranoid, excessively anxious, or psychotic. Depression can be treated effectively with standard antidepressant drugs with the caveat that drugs with substantial anticholinergic profiles can exacerbate chorea. Fluoxetine (Chapter 15) is effective treatment for both the depression and the irritability manifest in symptomatic HD. Carbamazepine (Chapter 21) also has been found to be effective for depression. Paranoia, delusional states, and psychosis are treated with antipsychotic drugs, but usually at lower doses than those used in primary psychiatric disorders (Chapter 16). These agents also reduce cognitive function and impair mobility and thus should be used in the lowest doses possible and should be discontinued when the psychiatric symptoms resolve. In individuals with predominantly rigid HD, clozapine, quetiapine (Chapter 16), or carbamazepine may be more effective for treatment of paranoia and psychosis.

The movement disorder of HD *per se* only rarely justifies pharmacological therapy. For those with large-amplitude chorea causing frequent falls and injury, tetrabenazine (XENAZINENITOMAN) has recently become available in the U.S. for the treatment of chorea associated with HD. Tetrabenazine, and the related drug reserpine, are inhibitors of the vesicular monoamine transporter 2 (VMAT2), and cause presynaptic depletion of catecholamines. Tetrabenazine is a reversible inhibitor; inhibition by reserpine is irreversible and may lead to long-lasting effects. Both drugs may cause hypotension and depression with suicidality; the shorter duration of effect of tetrabenazine greatly simplifies the clinical management. Antipsychotic agents also can be used, but these often do not improve overall function because they decrease fine motor coordination and increase rigidity. Many HD patients exhibit worsening of involuntary movements as a result of anxiety or stress. In these situations, judicious use of sedative or anxiolytic benzodiazepines can be very helpful. In juvenile-onset cases where rigidity rather than chorea predominates, DA agonists have had variable success in the improvement of rigidity. These individuals also occasionally develop myoclonus and seizures that can be responsive to clonazepam, valproic acid, and other anticonvulsants (Chapter 21).

Clinical Summary. HD is an autosomal dominant disorder caused by mutations in the *IT15* gene that encodes huntingtin. The gene defect leads to progressive motor and cognitive symptoms. At present there is no effective treatment for the primary disorder, although antidepressant and antipsychotic medications may be useful to control specific symptoms and catecholamine depleting agents may be useful to control the motor features of the disease.

AMYOTROPHIC LATERAL SCLEROSIS (ALS)

Clinical Features and Pathology. ALS (or Lou Gehrig's disease) is a disorder of the motor neurons of the ventral horn of the spinal cord (lower motor neurons) and the cortical neurons that provide their afferent input (upper motor neurons). The disorder is characterized by rapidly progressive weakness, muscle atrophy and fasciculations, spasticity, dysarthria, dysphagia, and respiratory compromise. Sensory, autonomic, and oculomotor function is generally spared. While it was previously thought that higher cortical function was also unaffected, many ALS patients exhibit behavioral changes and cognitive dysfunction, and there is clinical, genetic, and neuropathological overlap between ALS and frontotemporal dementia spectrum disorders (Strong et al., 2009). ALS usually is progressive and fatal. Most patients die of respiratory compromise and pneumonia after 2-3 years, although some individuals have a more indolent course and survive for many years. The pathology of ALS corresponds closely to the clinical features: There is prominent loss of the spinal and brainstem motor neurons that project to striated muscles (although the oculomotor neurons are spared), as well as loss of the large pyramidal motor neurons in layer V of motor cortex, which are the origin of the descending corticospinal tracts.

Etiology. About 10% of ALS cases are familial (FALS), usually with an autosomal dominant pattern of inheritance. Most of the mutations responsible have not been identified, but an important subset of FALS patients are families with a mutation in the gene for the enzyme SOD1 (Rosen et al., 1993). Mutations in this protein account for about 20% of cases of FALS. Most of the mutations are alterations of single amino acids, but more than 30 different alleles have been found in different kindreds. Transgenic mice expressing mutant human *SOD1* develop a progressive degeneration of motor neurons that closely mimics the human disease, providing an important animal model for research and pharmaceutical trials. Interestingly, many of the mutations of *SOD1* that can cause disease do not reduce the capacity of the enzyme to perform its primary function, the catabolism of superoxide radicals. Thus, as may be the case in HD, mutations in *SOD1* may confer a toxic "gain of function," the precise nature of which is unclear.

More recently, mutations in the *TARDBP* gene encoding TAR DNA-binding protein (TDP-43) and in the *FUS/TLS* gene have been identified as causes of FALS (Lagier-Tourenne and Cleveland, 2009). Both TDP-43 and FUS/TLS bind DNA and RNA, and regulate transcription and alternative splicing.

More than 90% of ALS cases are sporadic. Of these, a few are caused by *de novo* mutations in *SOD1*, *TDP-43*, *FUS/TLS*, or other genes, but for the majority of sporadic cases the etiology remains unclear. Possible pathogenic mechanisms underlying sporadic ALS include autoimmunity, excitotoxicity, free radical toxicity, and viral infection (Rothstein, 2009), although none is well supported by available data. There is evidence that glutamate reuptake may be abnormal in the disease, leading to accumulation of glutamate and excitotoxic injury (Rothstein et al., 1992). The only currently approved therapy for ALS, riluzole, is based on these observations (Brooks, 2009).

Treatment of ALS

Riluzole. Riluzole (2-amino-6-[trifluoromethoxy] benzothiazole; RILUTEK) is an agent with complex actions in the nervous system (Doble, 1996; Zarate and Manji, 2008).

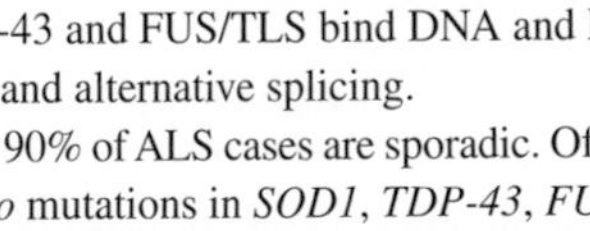

F_3C—O—[benzothiazole]—NH_2

RILUZOLE

Riluzole is absorbed orally and is highly protein bound. It undergoes extensive metabolism in the liver by both CYP–mediated hydroxylation and glucuronidation. Its $t_{1/2}$ is about 12 hours. *In vitro* studies have shown that riluzole has both presynaptic and postsynaptic effects. It inhibits glutamate release, but it also blocks postsynaptic NMDA- and kainate-type glutamate receptors and inhibits voltage-dependent Na^+ channels. Some of the effects of riluzole *in vitro* are blocked by pertussis toxin, implicating the drug's interaction with an as yet-unidentified G protein–coupled receptor (GPCR). In clinical trials riluzole has modest but genuine effects on the survival of patients with ALS.

Meta-analyses of the available trials indicate that riluzole extends survival by 2-3 months (Miller et al., 2007). The recommended dose is 50 mg twice daily, taken 1 hour before or 2 hours after a meal. Riluzole usually is well tolerated, although nausea or diarrhea may occur. Rarely, riluzole may produce hepatic injury with elevations of serum transaminases, and periodic monitoring of these is recommended. Although the magnitude of the effect of riluzole on ALS is small, it represents a significant therapeutic milestone in the treatment of a disease refractory to all previous treatments.

Symptomatic Therapy of ALS: Spasticity. Spasticity is an important component of the clinical features of ALS and the feature most amenable to present forms of treatment. Spasticity often leads to considerable pain and discomfort and further reduces mobility, which already is compromised by weakness. *Spasticity* is defined as an increase in muscle tone characterized by an initial resistance to passive displacement of a limb at a joint, followed by a sudden relaxation (the so-called clasped-knife phenomenon). Spasticity results from loss of descending inputs to the spinal motor neurons, and the character of the spasticity depends on which nervous system pathways are affected (Sheean, 2008). Whole repertoires of movement can be generated directly at the spinal cord level; it is beyond the scope of this chapter to describe these in detail. The monosynaptic tendon-stretch reflex is the simplest of the spinal mechanisms contributing to spasticity. Primary Ia afferents from muscle spindles, activated when the muscle is stretched rapidly, synapse directly on motor neurons going to the stretched muscle, causing it to contract and resist the movement. A collateral of the primary Ia afferent synapses on a "Ia-coupled interneuron" that inhibits the motor neurons innervating the antagonist of the stretched muscle, allowing contraction of the muscle to be unopposed. Upper motor neurons from the cerebral cortex (the pyramidal neurons) suppress spinal reflexes and the lower motor neurons indirectly by activating the spinal cord inhibitory interneuron pools (Figure 22–8).

The pyramidal neurons use glutamate as a neurotransmitter. When the pyramidal influences are removed, the reflexes are released from inhibition and become more active, leading to hyperreflexia. Other descending pathways from the brainstem, including the rubro-, reticulo-, and vestibulospinal pathways and the descending catecholamine pathways, also influence spinal reflex activity. When just the pyramidal pathway is affected, extensor tone in the legs and flexor tone in the arms are increased. When the vestibulospinal and catecholamine pathways are impaired, increased flexion of all extremities is observed, and light cutaneous stimulation can lead to disabling whole-body spasms. In ALS, pyramidal pathways are impaired with relative preservation of the other descending pathways, resulting in hyperactive deep-tendon reflexes, impaired fine motor coordination, increased extensor tone in the legs, and increased flexor tone in the arms. The gag reflex often is overactive as well.

The best agent for the symptomatic treatment of spasticity in ALS is baclofen (LIORESAL), a $GABA_B$ receptor agonist. Initial doses

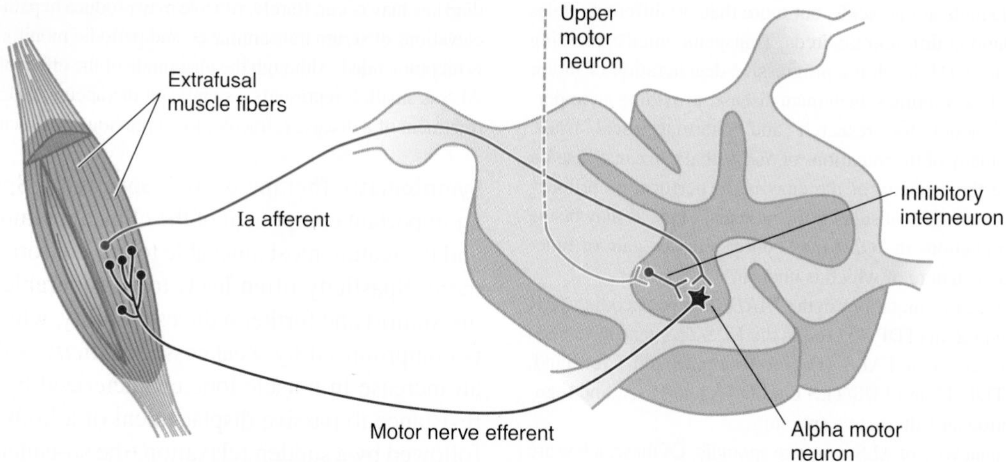

Figure 22–8. *Monosynaptic muscle stretch reflex with descending control via inhibitory interneurons.* Primary Ia afferents (green) from muscle spindles, activated when the muscle is stretched rapidly, synapse directly on motor neurons (blue) going to the stretched muscle, causing it to contract and resist the movement. Pyramidal upper motor neurons (aqua) from the cerebral cortex suppress spinal reflexes and the lower motor neurons indirectly by activating the spinal cord inhibitory interneuron pools (red). When the pyramidal influences are removed, the reflexes are released from inhibition and become more active, leading to hyperreflexia and spasticity. Baclofen acts to restore the lost inhibition by stimulating postsynaptic GABA receptors. Tizanidine acts presynaptically to stimulate GABA release from spinal cord inhibitory interneuron.

of 5-10 mg/day are recommended, which can be increased to as much as 200 mg/day if necessary. If weakness occurs, the dose should be lowered. Alternatively, baclofen can be delivered directly into the space around the spinal cord using a surgically implanted pump and an intrathecal catheter. This approach minimizes the adverse effects of the drug, especially sedation, but it carries the risk of potentially life-threatening CNS depression. Moreover, abrupt withdrawal of intrathecal baclofen can cause rebound spasticity, rhabdomyolitis, multi-organ failure, and even death. Intrathecal baclofen should be used only by physicians trained in delivering chronic intrathecal therapy.

Tizanidine (ZANAFLEX) is an agonist of α_2 adrenergic receptors in the CNS. It reduces muscle spasticity and is assumed to act by increasing presynaptic inhibition of motor neurons. Tizanidine is primarily used in the treatment of spasticity in multiple sclerosis or after stroke, but it also may be effective in patients with ALS. Treatment should be initiated at a low dose of 2-4 mg at bedtime and titrated upward gradually. Drowsiness, asthenia, and dizziness may limit the dose that can be administered. Benzodiazepines (Chapter 17) such as clonazepam (KLONIPIN) are effective antispasticity agents, but they may contribute to respiratory depression in patients with advanced ALS. Dantrolene (DANTRIUM) also is approved in the U.S. for the treatment of muscle spasm. In contrast to the other agents discussed, dantrolene acts directly on skeletal muscle fibers, impairing Ca^{2+} release from the sarcoplasmic reticulum. Because it can exacerbate muscular weakness, it is not used in ALS but is effective in treating spasticity associated with stroke or spinal cord injury and in treating malignant hyperthermia (Chapter 8). Dantrolene may cause hepatotoxicity, so it is important to monitor liver associated enzymes before and during therapy with the drug.

Clinical Summary. ALS is a progressive degenerative disease of spinal motor neurons leading to weakness and eventually paralysis. It is the most rapidly progressive of the common neurodegenerative disorders and often is fatal within 2-3 years of onset. The only therapy established to alter the course of ALS is the drug riluzole, which acts through inhibition of glutamate release as well as other mechanisms. The effect of this treatment is modest, prolonging survival by a few months.

BIBLIOGRAPHY

Albin RL, Frey KA. Initial agonist treatment of Parkinson's disease: A critique. *Neurology*, **2003**, *60*:390–394.

Albin RL, Reiner A, Anderson KD, et al. Preferential loss of striato-external pallidal projection neurons in presymptomatic Huntington's disease. *Ann Neurol,* **1992**, *31*:425–430.

Albin RL, Young AB, Penney JB. The functional anatomy of basal ganglia disorders. *Trends Neurosci,* **1989**, *12*: 366–375.

Arnold SE, Hyman BT, Flory J, et al. The topographical and neuroanatomical distribution of neurofibrillary tangles and neuritic plaques in the cerebral cortex of patients with Alzheimer's disease. *Cereb Cortex,* **1991**, *1*:103–116.

Baldwin CM, Keating GM. Rotigotine transdermal patch: A review of its use in the management of Parkinson's disease. *CNS Drugs*, **2007**, *21*:1039–1055.

Beal MF. Mitochondria take center stage in aging and neurodegeneration. *Ann Neurol*, **2005**, *58*:495–505.

Beier MT. Treatment strategies for the behavioral symptoms of Alzheimer's disease: Focus on early pharmacologic intervention. *Pharmacotherapy*, **2007**, *27*:399–411.

Bertram L, McQueen MB, Mullin, et al. Systematic meta-analyses of Alzheimer disease genetic association studies: The AlzGene database. *Nat Genet*, **2007**, *39*:17–23.

Bhasin M, Rowan E, Edwards K, McKeith I. Cholinesterase inhibitors in dementia with Lewy bodies: A comparative analysis. *Int J Geriatr Psychiatry*, **2007**, *22*:890–895.

Birks J. Cholinesterase inhibitors for Alzheimer's disease. *Cochrane Database Syst Rev*, **2006**, CD005593.

Boillée S, Van de Velde C, Cleveland DW. ALS: A disease of motor neurons and their nonneuronal neighbors. *Neuron,* **2006**, *52*:39–59.

Braak H, Del Tredici K. Invited article: Nervous system pathology in sporadic Parkinson disease. *Neurology*, **2008**, *70*:1916–1925.

Brooks BR. Managing amyotrophic lateral sclerosis: Slowing disease progression and improving patient quality of life. *Ann Neurol*, **2009**, *65(suppl 1)*:S17–S23.

Choi DW, Rothman SM. The role of glutamate neurotoxicity in hypoxic-ischemic neuronal death. *Annu Rev Neurosci,* **1990**, *13*:171–182.

Costello S, Cockburn M, Bronstein J, et al. Parkinson's disease and residential exposure to maneb and paraquat from agricultural applications in the central valley of California. *Am J Epidemiol*, **2009**, *169*:919–926.

Cotzias GC, Papavasiliou PS, Gellene R. Modification of Parkinsonism: Chronic treatment with L-DOPA. *N Engl J Med,* **1969**, *280*:337–345.

Cummings JL, Vinters HV, Cole GM, Khachaturian ZS. Alzheimer's disease: Etiologies, pathophysiology, cognitive reserve, and treatment opportunities. *Neurology,* **1998**, *51*:S2–S17.

Doble A. The pharmacology and mechanism of action of riluzole. *Neurology*, **1996**, *47*:S233–S241.

Douglas IJ, Smeeth L. Exposure to antipsychotics and risk of stroke: self controlled case series study. *BMJ*, **2008**, *337*:a1227.

Dubois B, Feldman HH, Jacova C, et al. Research criteria for the diagnosis of Alzheimer's disease: Revising the NINCDS-ADRDA criteria. *Lancet Neurol*, **2007**, *6*:734–746.

Elmer LW, Bertoni JM. The increasing role of monoamine oxidase type B inhibitors in Parkinson's disease therapy. *Expert Opin Pharmacother*, **2008**, *9*:2759–2772.

Evans DA, Funkenstein HH, Albert MS, et al. Prevalence of Alzheimer's disease in a community population of older persons: Higher than previously reported. *JAMA,* **1989**, *262*:2551–2556.

Fahn S, Oakes D, Shoulson I, et al. Levodopa and the progression of Parkinson's disease. *N Engl J Med*, **2004**, *351*:2498–2508.

Farrer MJ. Genetics of Parkinson disease: paradigm shifts and future prospects. *Nat Rev Genet*, **2006**, *7*:306–318.

Ferrante RJ, Kowall NW, Beal MF, et al. Morphologic and histochemical characteristics of a spared subset of striatal neurons in Huntington's disease. *J Neuropathol Exp Neurol,* **1987**, *46*:12–27.

Friedman JH, Factor SA. Atypical antipsychotics in the treatment of drug-induced psychosis in Parkinson's disease. *Mov Disord,* **2000**, *15*:201–211.

Frucht S, Rogers JG, Greene PE, et al. Falling asleep at the wheel: Motor vehicle mishaps in persons taking pramipexole and ropinirole. *Neurology,* **1999**, *52*:1908–1910.

Golomb BA. Acetylcholinesterase inhibitors and Gulf War illnesses. *Proc Natl Acad Sci USA*, **2008**, *105*:4295–4300.

Hallett PJ, Standaert DG. Rationale for and use of NMDA receptor antagonists in Parkinson's disease. *Pharmacol Ther*, **2004,** *102*:155–174.

Hersch SM, Gutekunst CA, Rees HD, et al. Distribution of m1-m4 muscarinic receptor proteins in the rat striatum: Light and electron microscopic immunocytochemistry using subtype-specific antibodies. *J Neurosci,* **1994**, *14*:3351–3363.

Hornykiewicz O. Dopamine in the basal ganglia: Its role and therapeutic indications (including the clinical use of L-DOPA). *Br Med Bull,* **1973**, *29*:172–178.

Howard RJ, Juszczak E, Ballard CG, et al. Donepezil for the treatment of agitation in Alzheimer's disease. *N Engl J Med,* **2007**, *357*:1382–1392.

Huntington's Disease Collaborative Research Group. A novel gene containing a trinucleotide repeat that is expanded and unstable on Huntington's disease chromosomes. *Cell,* **1993**, *72*:971–983.

Imarisio S, Carmichael J, Korolchuk V, et al. Huntington's disease: From pathology and genetics to potential therapies. *Biochem J*, **2008,** *412*:191–209.

Kavirajan H, Schneider LS. Efficacy and adverse effects of cholinesterase inhibitors and memantine in vascular dementia: A meta-analysis of randomised controlled trials. *Lancet Neurol*, **2007**, *6*:782–792.

Kurtzke JF. Epidemiology of amyotrophic lateral sclerosis. In, *Human Motor Neuron Diseases.* (Rowland LP, ed.) *Advances in Neurology,* vol. 36. Raven Press, New York, **1982**, pp. 281–302.

Lagier-Tourenne C, Cleveland DW. Rethinking ALS: The FUS about TDP-43. *Cell*, **2009**, *136*:1001–1004.

Landwehrmeyer GB, McNeil SM, Dure LS, et al. Huntington's disease gene: Regional and cellular expression in brain of normal and affected individuals. *Ann Neurol,* **1995**, *37*: 218–230.

Lang AE, Lozano AM. Parkinson's disease. First of two parts. *N Engl J Med,* **1998**, *339*:1044–1053.

Langston JW. The Parkinson's complex: Parkinsonism is just the tip of the iceberg. *Ann Neurol*, **2006**, *59*:591–596.

Langston JW, Ballard P, Tetrud JW, Irwin I. Chronic Parkinsonism in humans due to a product of meperidine-analog synthesis. *Science,* **1983**, *219*:979–980.

Lewis TB, Standaert DG. Design of clinical trials of gene therapy in Parkinson disease. *Exp Neurol*, **2008**, *209*:41–47.

Lipton SA. Pathologically activated therapeutics for neuroprotection. *Nat Rev Neurosci*, **2007**, *8*:803–808.

Mahley RW, Weisgraber KH, Huang Y. Apolipoprotein E4: A causative factor and therapeutic target in neuropathology, including Alzheimer's disease. *Proc Natl Acad Sci USA*, **2006**, *103*:5644–5651.

Maidment ID, Fox CG, Boustani M, et al. Efficacy of memantine on behavioral and psychological symptoms related to dementia: A systematic meta-analysis. *Ann Pharmacother*, **2008**, *42*:32–38.

Miller RG, Mitchell JD, Lyon M, Moore DH. Riluzole for amyotrophic lateral sclerosis (ALS)/motor neuron disease (MND). *Cochrane Database Syst Rev*, **2007**, CD001447.

Mink JW, Thach WT. Basal ganglia intrinsic circuits and their role in behavior. *Curr Opin Neurobiol,* **1993**, *3*:950–957.

Mouradian MM, Heuser IJ, Baronti F, Chase TN. Modification of central dopaminergic mechanisms by continuous levodopa therapy for advanced Parkinson's disease. *Ann Neurol,* **1990**, *27*:18–23.

Olanow CW, Hauser RA, Jankovic J, et al. A randomized, double-blind, placebo-controlled, delayed start study to assess rasagiline as a disease modifying therapy in Parkinson's disease (the ADAGIO study): Rationale, design, and baseline characteristics. *Mov Disord*, **2008**, *23*:2194–2201.

Parent A, Cicchetti F. The current model of basal ganglia organization under scrutiny. *Mov Disord,* **1998**, *13*:199–202.

Parkinson Study Group. Effects of tocopherol and deprenyl on the progression of disability in early Parkinson's disease. *N Engl J Med,* **1993**, *328*:176–183.

Parkinson Study Group. Entacapone improves motor fluctuations in levodopa-treated Parkinson's disease patients. *Ann Neurol,* **1997**, *42*:747–755. Published erratum appears in *Ann Neurol,* **1998**, *44*:292.

Parkinson Study Group. Pramipexole vs. levodopa as initial treatment for Parkinson's disease: A randomized, controlled trial. *JAMA,* **2000,** *284*:1931–1938.

Parkinson Study Group. Dopamine transporter imaging to asses the effects of pramipexole vs levodopa on Parkinson disease progression. *JAMA*, **2002**, *287*:1653–1661.

Perry EK. The cholinergic hypothesis—ten years on. *Br Med Bull*, **1986**, *42*:63–69.

Petersen RC, Thomas RG, Grundman M, et al. Vitamin E and donepezil for the treatment of mild cognitive impairment. *N Engl J Med*, **2005**, *352*:2379–2388.

Raber J, Huang Y, Ashford JW. ApoE genotype accounts for the vast majority of AD risk and AD pathology. *Neurobiol Aging*, **2004**, *25*:641–650.

Raina P, Santaguida P, Ismaila A, et al. Effectiveness of cholinesterase inhibitors and memantine for treating dementia: Evidence review for a clinical practice guideline. *Ann Intern Med*, **2008**, *148*:379–397.

Raschetti R, Albanese E, Vanacore N, Maggini M. Cholinesterase inhibitors in mild cognitive impairment: A systematic review of randomised trials. *PLoS Med*, **2007**, *4*:e338.

Rascol O, Brooks DJ, Korczyn AD, et al. A five-year study of the incidence of dyskinesia in patients with early Parkinson's disease who were treated with ropinirole or levodopa. 056 Study Group. *N Engl J Med,* **2000**, *342*: 1484–1491.

Roberson ED, Mucke L. 100 years and counting: Prospects for defeating Alzheimer's disease. *Science*, **2006**, *314*:781–784.

Rosen DR, Siddique T, Patterson D, et al. Mutations in Cu/Zn superoxide dismutase gene are associated with familial amyotrophic lateral sclerosis. *Nature,* **1993**, *362*:59–62. Published erratum appears in *Nature,* **1993**, *364*:362.

Rothstein JD. Current hypotheses for the underlying biology of amyotrophic lateral sclerosis. *Ann Neurol*, **2009**, *65*(Suppl 1): S3–S9.

Rothstein JD, Marin LJ, Kuncl RW. Decreased glutamate transport by the brain and spinal cord in amyotrophic lateral sclerosis. *N Engl J Med,* **1992**, *326*:1464–1468.

Schneider LS, Dagerman KS, Insel P. Risk of death with atypical antipsychotic drug treatment for dementia: Meta-analysis of randomized placebo-controlled trials. *JAMA,* **2005**, *294*:1934–1943.

Schneider LS, Tariot PN, Dagerman KS, et al. Effectiveness of atypical antipsychotic drugs in patients with Alzheimer's disease. *N Engl J Med*, **2006**, *355*:1525–1538.

Selkoe DJ, Podlisny MB. Deciphering the genetic basis of Alzheimer's disease. *Annu Rev Genomics Hum Genet,* **2002**, *3*:67–99.

Sheean G. Neurophysiology of spasticity. In, *Upper Motor Neurone Syndrome and Spasticity: Clinical Management and Neurophysiology,* 2nd ed. (Barnes MP, Johnson GR, eds.) Cambridge University Press, Cambridge, England, **2008**, pp. 9–63.

Shoulson I. Huntington's disease. In, *Diseases of the Nervous System: Clinical Neurobiology.* (Asbury AK, McKhann GM, McDonald WI, eds.) Saunders, Philadelphia, **1992**, pp. 1159–1168.

Shults CW, Oakes D, Kieburtz K, et al. Effects of coenzyme Q10 in early Parkinson disease: Evidence of slowing of the functional decline. *Arch Neurol*, **2002**, *59*:1541–1550.

Sink KM, Holden KF, Yaffe K. Pharmacological treatment of neuropsychiatric symptoms of dementia: A review of the evidence. *JAMA*, **2005**, *293*:596–608.

Strong MJ, Grace GM, Freedman M, et al. Consensus criteria for the diagnosis of frontotemporal cognitive and behavioural syndromes in amyotrophic lateral sclerosis. *Amyotroph Lateral Scler,* **2009**, DOI: 10.1080/17482960802654364.

Tandan R, Bradley WG. Amyotrophic lateral sclerosis: 2. Etiopathogenesis. *Ann Neurol,* **1985**, *18*:419–431.

Tanner CM. Epidemiology of Parkinson's disease. *Neurol Clin,* **1992**, *10*:317–329.

Tanzi R, Bertram L. Twenty years of the Alzheimer's disease amyloid hypothesis: A genetic perspective. *Cell*, **2005**, *120*: 545–555.

Trinh NH, Hoblyn J, Mohanty S, Yaffe K. Efficacy of cholinesterase inhibitors in the treatment of neuropsychiatric symptoms and functional impairment in Alzheimer disease: A meta-analysis. *JAMA*, **2003**, *289*:210–216.

Vonsattel JP, Myers RH, Stevens TJ, et al. Neuropathological classification of Huntington's disease. *J Neuropathol Exp Neurol,* **1985**, *44*:559–577.

Whone AL, Watts RL, Stoessl AJ, et al. Slower progression of Parkinson's disease with ropinirole versus levodopa: The REAL-PET study. *Ann Neurol*, **2003**, *54*:93–101.

Wichmann T, DeLong MR. Pathophysiology of parkinsonian motor abnormalities. *Adv Neurol,* **1993**, *60*:53–61.

Yacoubian TA, Standaert DG. Targets for neuroprotection in Parkinson's disease. *Biochim Biophys Acta*, **2008**, DOI: 10.1016/j.bbadis.2008.09.009.

Zarate CA, Manji HK. Riluzole in psychiatry: A systematic review of the literature. *Expert Opin Drug Metab Toxicol*, **2008**, *4*:1223–1234.

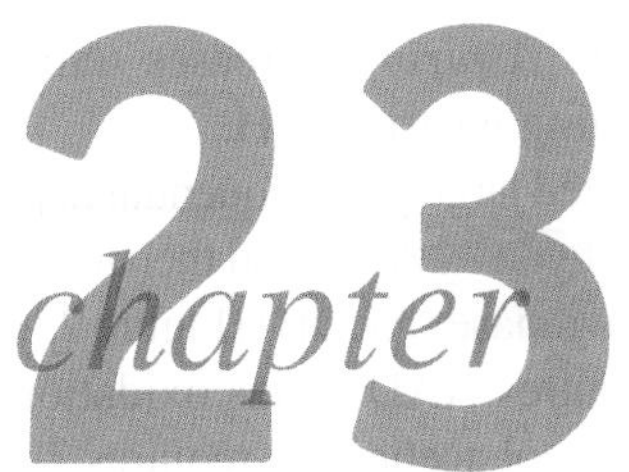

Ethanol and Methanol

Marc A. Schuckit

The two-carbon alcohol ethanol (CH_3CH_2OH), or beverage alcohol, is one of the most versatile drugs known to man, with multiple direct effects on a diverse range of neurochemical systems. Produced in nature, rewarding in its effects, and easy to manufacture, it has been taken by humans since the beginning of recorded history, is consumed by a large majority of people in the Western world, and is likely to contribute to more morbidity, mortality, and public health costs than all of the illicit drugs combined. Yet most pharmacologists, pharmacists, and healthcare providers receive only minimal education about ethanol and the mechanisms through which it contributes to such diverse pathology.

This chapter presents an overview of the effects of ethanol on various physiological systems, then focuses on the mechanisms of ethanol's effects in the central nervous system (CNS) as the basis for understanding the rewards, disease processes, and treatments for ethanol-related conditions. First, it is worthwhile to recount the history of the human use of alcoholic beverages.

Human Consumption of Ethanol: A Brief History. The use of alcoholic beverages has been documented since at least 10,000 BC (Hanson, 1995). By about 3000 BC, the Greeks, Romans, and inhabitants of Babylon continued to incorporate ethanol into religious festivals, while also using these beverages for pleasure, to facilitate socialization, as a source of nutrition, and as part of medicinal practices. The role of ethanol in society continued through biblical times, with beverage alcohol incorporated into most religions, and occupying a central role in daily life. Over the last 2000 years, alcoholic beverages have been identified in most cultures, including pre-Columbian America in ~200 AD, and the Islamic world in the 700s.

Whiskey was invented in ~1400 in Ireland and rapidly increased in popularity; champagne was developed in France in 1670. In 1690, the English government enacted a law encouraging the consumption of distilled spirits, and the production of gin subsequently increased from about 0.5 million gallons in 1685 to 5 million by 1727 and 18 million gallons by the early 1800s.

The dangers of heavy consumption of beverage alcohol have been recognized by almost all cultures, with most stressing the importance of moderation. Despite these warnings, problems with ethanol are as ancient as the pattern of use of this beverage itself, and were noted early on in India, Greece, and Rome. The increase in use of ethanol in the 1800s, along with industrialization and need for a more dependable work force, contributed to the development of more widespread organized efforts to discourage drunkenness. The subsequent temperance movements set the stage for the prohibition against drinking instituted in the U.S. in 1920. In 1933, the long tradition of the use of alcohol, as well as the large minority of the population who favored the availability of alcoholic beverages, resulted in the repeal of the constitutional amendment enacting prohibition.

Beverage alcohol has widespread use in today's society, with an average age of first use of ~15 years in most Western countries. Almost two-thirds of women and as many as 80% of men in these countries have consumed alcoholic beverages, with one-half to two-thirds reporting alcohol consumption within the past year (Faden, 2006). The highest quantities and frequencies of drinking are usually observed in the late teens to early 20s, and in the U.S., the average adult consumes alcoholic beverages containing the equivalent of 2.2 gallons (8.3 L) of absolute alcohol per year. Among drinkers, as many as half have had a temporary alcohol-related problem such as missing school or work, alcohol-related amnesia (blackouts), or operating a motor vehicle after consuming alcohol. More severe repetitive problems with alcohol (known as abuse and dependence) have a lifetime risk in men of almost 20% and in women of 10-15% (Hasin et al., 2007). The annual costs associated with heavy drinking and associated problems have been estimated to be $185 billion in the U.S. in recent years, and this drug contributes to 100,000 deaths per year in the U.S. alone, including as many as 20,000 alcohol-related fatal car accidents annually (Harwood et al., 1999; Rehm et al., 2007). Thus, the delivery of optimal medical care in modern times is greatly affected by the use of beverage alcohol, with this drug adversely affecting many body systems, interacting with medications and other drugs, and responsible for a great deal of the healthcare dollar.

Ethanol Consumption. Compared with other drugs, surprisingly large amounts of alcohol are required for physiological effects, resulting in its consumption more as a food than a drug. The alcohol content of beverages typically ranges from 4-6% (volume/volume) for beer, 10-15% for wine, and 40% and higher for distilled spirits methanol is taken along with ethanol. As little as 15 mL of methanol can produce toxicity, including blindness, with doses in excess of 70 mL capable of producing death. Methanol poisoning consists of headache, GI distress, and pain (partially related to pancreatic injury), difficulty breathing, restlessness, and blurred vision associated with hyperemic optic disks. Severe metabolic acidosis can develop due to the accumulation of formic acid, and the respiratory depression can be severe, especially in the context of coma. The visual disturbances associated with methanol intoxication are a prominent part of the picture, and occur as a consequence of injury to ganglion cells of the retina by the metabolite, formic acid, with subsequent inflammation, atrophy, and potential bilateral blindness. The clinical picture can also include necrosis of the pancreas.

Genetic Variation in Ethanol Metabolism. The enzymes involved in ethanol metabolism (Figure 23–1) are mainly ADH and ALDH, and secondarily, catalase and CYP2E1. Several of these enzymes have genetic variants that alter alcohol metabolism and susceptibility to its effects.

The genetics of the ADH isoforms are important for understanding risk factors for severe repetitive ethanol problems. The three relevant forms are ADH1A, 1B, and 1C (genes on chromosome 4 q22). These class I ADHs have K_m<34 mmol (0.15 g/dL) and are responsible for 70% of the ethanol metabolizing capacity at BECs of 22 mM (i.e., ~0.10 g/dL) (Edenberg et al., 2006). These ADH forms are the rate-limiting step in ethanol metabolism, reducing the blood ethanol concentrations by ~4-5 mM (0.015-0.020 g/dL) per hour, the approximate levels of alcohol resulting from the consumption of one standard drink.

The ADH1A gene has no polymorphisms known to significantly affect the rate of alcohol metabolism. The ADH1B gene has a polymorphism, ADH1B*2, with arginine 47 replaced by histidine to produce a variant form of ADH with a 40-fold higher V_{max} than ADH1B. This polymorphism is seen in 30-45% of Chinese, Japanese, and Koreans, less than 10% of most Europeans, but in 50-90% of Russians and Jews (Edenberg et al., 2006). The potential faster metabolism of ethanol may result in a transient slightly higher blood level of acetaldehyde and is reported to be associated with a lower risk for heavy drinking and ethanol-related problems. A second polymorphism for ADH1B, ADH1B*3 (arginine 269 replaced by cysteine), has a 30-fold higher V_{max}. ADHIB*3 is seen in about 30% of Africans and also is associated with lower risk of heavy drinking and ethanol problems.

A third ADH gene found in the chromosome 4q22 cluster, ADH1C, exhibits two polymorphisms in high linkage disequilibrium, the γ1 and γ2 forms. The V_{max} of γ1 is twice that of γ2, and this ADH1C*1 allele is hypothesized to be associated with a slightly faster metabolism of ethanol and/or a higher level of acetaldehyde. The independent effects of ADH1C*1 and ADH1B*2 alleles are difficult to determine. The ADH cluster on chromosome 4 also contains class II ADHs with K_m = 34 mM (~0.15 g/dL). The class II forms contribute about 30% of the ethanol metabolizing capacity noted above. There are polymorphisms hypothesized to be associated with the alcoholism risk, but less information is known about these forms (Luo et al., 2007).

Other systems also contribute to the metabolism of ethanol to acetaldehyde including via catalase (Kuo et al., 2008). In addition, at higher BELs, the microsomal ethanol metabolizing system (MEOS) is important, especially CYP2E1, but also CYPs1A2 and 3A4. Variations of the CYP2E1 gene located on chromosome 10 have been hypothesized to relate to the level of sensitivity or reaction to the ethanol observed in the brain.

Acetaldehyde is produced from the breakdown of ethanol at the rate of approximately one standard drink per hour. As shown in Figure 23–1, the acetaldehyde is then rapidly broken down through the actions of ALDH2, primarily in the mitochondria of liver cells. The actions of ALDH2, a phase 2 enzyme (Chapter 6), are important because low levels of acetaldehyde may be perceived as rewarding and stimulating, while high blood levels of this substance produce severe adverse reactions that can include vomiting, diarrhea, and unstable blood pressure (Husemoen et al., 2008). There is a mutation in the ALDH2 gene (12q24), ALDH2*2 (resulting from a substitution of glycine 487 with lysine). Homozygotes with a nonfunctional ALDH2*2 occur in 5-10% of Japanese, Chinese, and Korean individuals, for whom severe adverse reactions occur after consumption of one drink or less. Consequently, their risk for severe repetitive heavy drinking is close to zero. This reaction operates through the same mechanism that occurs with drinking after taking the ALDH2 inhibitor, disulfiram. Heterozygotes for this polymorphism (ALDH2*2, 2*1) make up 30-40% of Asian individuals who, after consuming ethanol experience a facial flush and an enhanced sensitivity to beverage alcohol, but who do not necessarily report an overall adverse response to the drug (Wall and Ehlers, 1995). The heterozygotes tend to drink lower quantities of ethanol than the general population, although repeated intake may relate to an enhanced risk for adverse ethanol-related organ damage (including esophageal cancer and, perhaps, pancreatitis), possibly associated with higher acetaldehyde levels. While additional ALDH mutations occur, less is known about potential associations between these polymorphisms and the risk from alcohol.

EFFECTS OF ETHANOL ON PHYSIOLOGICAL SYSTEMS

William Shakespeare described the acute pharmacological effects of imbibing ethanol in the Porter scene (act 2, scene 3) of *Macbeth*. The Porter, awakened from an alcohol-induced sleep by Macduff, explains three effects of alcohol and then wrestles with a fourth effect that combines the contradictory aspects of soaring overconfidence with physical impairment:

Porter: . . . and drink, sir, is a great provoker of three things.

Macduff: What three things does drink especially provoke?

Porter: Marry, sir, nose-painting [*cutaneous vasodilation*], sleep [*CNS depression*], and urine [*a consequence of the inhibition of antidiuretic hormone (vasopressin) secretion, exacerbated by volume loading*]. Lechery, sir, it provokes and unprovokes: it provokes the desire but it takes away the performance. Therefore much drink may be said to be an equivocator with lechery: it makes him and it mars him; it sets him on and it takes him off; it persuades him and disheartens him, makes him stand to and not stand to [*the imagination desires what the corpus cavernosum cannot deliver*]; in conclusion, equivocates him in a sleep, and, giving him the lie, leaves him.

More recent research has added details to Shakespeare's enumeration—see the bracketed additions to the Porter's words in the preceding paragraph and the section on organ systems later in the chapter—but the most noticeable consequences of the recreational use of ethanol still are well summarized by the gregarious and garrulous Porter, whose delighted and devilish demeanor demonstrates a frequently observed influence of modest concentrations of ethanol on the CNS. The sections that follow detail ethanol's effects on physiological systems.

Central Nervous System

Although the public often views alcoholic drinks as stimulating, ethanol primarily is a CNS depressant. Ingestion of moderate amounts of ethanol, like that of other depressants such as barbiturates and benzodiazepines, can have anti-anxiety actions and produce behavioral disinhibition at a wide range of dosages. Individual signs of intoxication vary from expansive and vivacious affect to uncontrolled mood swings and emotional outbursts that may have violent components. With more severe intoxication, CNS function generally is impaired, and a condition of general anesthesia ultimately prevails. However, there is little margin between the anesthetic actions and lethal effects (usually owing to respiratory depression).

About 10% of alcohol drinkers progress to levels of consumption that are physically and socially detrimental. Chronic abuse is accompanied by tolerance, dependence, and craving for the drug (*see* Tolerance, Dependence, and Chronic Ethanol Use, and Chapter 24). Alcoholism is characterized by compulsive use despite clearly deleterious social and medical consequences. Alcoholism is a progressive illness, and brain damage from chronic alcohol abuse contributes to the deficits in cognitive functioning and judgment seen in alcoholics. Alcoholism is a leading cause of dementia in the U.S. (Oslin et al., 1998). Chronic alcohol abuse results in shrinkage of the brain owing to loss of both white and gray matter (Kril and Halliday, 1999). The frontal lobes are particularly sensitive to damage by alcohol, and the extent of damage is determined by the amount and duration of alcohol consumption, with older alcoholics being more vulnerable than younger ones (Pfefferbaum et al., 1998). It is important to note that ethanol itself is neurotoxic, and although malnutrition or vitamin deficiencies probably play roles in complications of alcoholism such as Wernicke's encephalopathy and Korsakoff's psychosis, most of the alcohol-induced brain damage in Western countries is due to alcohol itself. In addition to loss of brain tissue, alcohol abuse also reduces brain metabolism (as determined by positron-emission tomography), and this hypometabolic state rebounds to a level of increased metabolism during detoxification. The magnitude of decrease in metabolic state is determined by the number of years of alcohol use and the age of the patients (Volkow et al., 1994).

Table 23–1

Impact of Ethanol on Key Neurochemical Systems

NEUROTRANSMITTER SYSTEM	EFFECTS
$GABA_A$	GABA release, ↑ receptor density
NMDA	Inhibition of postsynaptic NMDA receptors; with chronic use, up-regulation
DA	↑ Synaptic DA, ↑ effects on ventral tegmentum/nucleus accumbens reward
ACTH	↑ CNS and blood levels of ACTH
Opioid	Release of β endorphins, activation of μ receptors
5-HT	↑ in 5-HT synaptic space
Cannabinoid	↑ CB1 activity → changes in DA, GABA, glutamate activity

Actions of Ethanol on Neurochemical Pathways and Signaling. Ethanol affects almost all brain systems. The changes across neurochemical pathways occur simultaneously and the alterations often interact. An additional complication in describing CNS effects is the rapid adaptation to ethanol observed in the brain, with the result that the acute effects of the first dose of ethanol are often the opposite of the neurochemical consequences from repeated administration and those observed during falling blood ethanol levels and withdrawal syndromes (Schuckit, 2006b).

Alcohol perturbs the balance between excitatory and inhibitory influences in the brain, resulting in anxiolysis, ataxia, and sedation. This is accomplished by either enhancing inhibitory or antagonizing excitatory neurotransmission. Ethanol likely produces its effects by simultaneously altering the functioning of a number of proteins that can affect neuronal excitability (Table 23–1). A key issue has been to identify proteins that determine neuronal excitability and are sensitive to ethanol at the concentrations (5-20 mM) that produce behavioral effects. Many of the prominent effects are on ligand-gated and voltage-gated ion channels and GPCR systems.

Ion Channels. The primary mediators of inhibitory neurotransmission in the brain are the ligand-gated γ-aminobutyric acid A ($GABA_A$) receptors, whose function is markedly enhanced by a number of classes of sedative, hypnotic, and anesthetic agents, including barbiturates, benzodiazepines, and volatile anesthetics (Chapter 14). Substantial data implicate the $GABA_A$ receptor as an important target for the *in vivo* actions of ethanol. Stimulation of this multi-subunit, ligand-gated Cl^- channel system contributes to feelings of sleepiness, muscle relaxation, and the acute anticonvulsant properties associated with all GABA-boosting drugs (Krystal et al.,

2006). Acutely, ethanol results in GABA release; chronic heavy use alters the pattern of expression of genes impacting on $GABA_A$ subunits. Intoxication with ethanol can be viewed as a GABA-rich state, and withdrawal phenomena are related in part to $GABA_A$ activity deficiencies. Several $GABA_A$ receptor gene polymorphisms correlate with a predisposition toward heavy drinking and alcohol use disorders (Dick et al., 2006a,b).

The nicotinic ACh receptor is also sensitive to the effects of ethanol. Drinking acutely increases ACh in the ventral tegmental area, with a subsequent increase in DA in the nucleus accumbens (Joslyn et al., 2008). Varenicline, a partial agonist at the $\alpha_4\beta_2$ subtype of the nicotininc ACh receptor (Chapter 11), decreases ethanol-seeking behavior and ethanol consumption in a rodent model, similar to its actions to effects on nicotine dependence (Steensland et al., 2007). Effects of ethanol on these receptors may be particularly important because there is an association between nicotine exposure (smoking) and alcohol consumption in humans. Furthermore, several studies indicate that nicotine increases alcohol consumption in animal models (Smith et al., 1999).

Excitatory ionotropic glutamate receptors are divided into the *N*-methyl-D-aspartate (NMDA) and non-NMDA receptor classes, with the latter consisting of kainate- and AMPA-receptor subtypes (see Chapter 14). Ethanol inhibits the function of the NMDA- and kainate-receptor subtypes; AMPA receptors are largely resistant to alcohol (Carta et al., 2003). As with the $GABA_A$ receptors, phosphorylation of the glutamate receptor can modulate sensitivity to ethanol.

A number of other types of channels are sensitive to alcohol at concentrations routinely achieved *in vivo*. Ethanol enhances the activity of large conductance, Ca^{2+}-activated K^+ channels in neurohypophyseal terminals (Dopico et al., 1999), perhaps contributing to the reduced release of oxytocin and vasopressin after ethanol consumption. Ethanol inhibits N- and P/Q-type Ca^{2+} channels in a manner that can be antagonized by channel phosphorylation by PKA (Solem et al., 1997). BK (Maxi-K, slo1) channels also are a target for alcohol action (Davies et al., 2003). G protein-gated inwardly rectifying K^+ channels (GIRK or Kir channels) can be activated by the $\beta\gamma$ subunits of the G_i/G_o family, by PIP_2, and, via a different mechanism, by alcohols. Small alcohols bind to a hydrophobic binding pocket on GIRKs, leading to channel activation via stabilization of the open conformation (Aryal et al., 2009).

Other Neurotransmitter Systems. Dopamine-related systems have central importance regarding the feelings of reward and craving associated with all intoxicating substances (Koob and Kreek, 2007). Of special importance are alterations in DA activity in the ventral tegmental and related areas, especially the nucleus accumbens, which are likely to play a major role in feelings of euphoria and reward. Acute alcohol results in an increase in synaptic DA; repeated administration is associated with changes in both D_2 and D_4 receptors that may be important in the perpetuation of alcohol use as well as in relapse (Voronin et al., 2008).

The impact of ethanol on dopaminergic pathways is closely linked to changes in stress-related systems. These changes are hypothesized to relate to reinforcement from beverage alcohol and other drugs of abuse, as well as withdrawal symptoms and negative moods related to problems with regulation of the DA-rich brain reward systems. Dopaminergic activity in the nucleus accumbens is affected by multiple types of opioid receptors, and acute ethanol causes the release of β endorphins (Job et al., 2007). These actions subsequently activate μ opioid receptors in the ventral tegmentum and nucleus accumbens, with associated release of DA. Thus, many of the effects of alcohol on reward systems, and changes in how the CNS reacts to ethanol (including sensitization), may relate to alterations in opioid systems (Pastor and Aragon, 2006).

The acute administration of ethanol is associated with a significant increase in 5-HT in the synaptic space; continued use of ethanol produces an up-regulation of 5-HT receptors. Lower levels of 5-HT in the synapse, perhaps related to a more rapid reuptake by the 5-HT transporter, is associated with higher levels of alcohol intake and, potentially, lower levels of intensity of reaction to beverage alcohol (Barr et al., 2005). Changes in DA systems are likely to relate to alterations in 5-HT as well.

Cannabinoid receptors, especially CB_1 encoded by the gene CNR1, are also affected by ethanol (Hutchinson et al., 2008; Perra et al., 2008). CB_1 is a GPCR that is densely represented in the ventral tegmentum, nucleus accumbens, and prefrontal cortex. Activation of CB_1 occurs with acute ethanol administration and affects the release of DA, GABA, and glutamate, and reward circuits of the brain. Antagonists of CB_1 receptors, such as rimonabant, may block the effect of ethanol on dopaminergic systems.

Protein Kinases and Signaling Enzymes. Knockout mice lacking the γ isoform of PKC display reduced effects of ethanol measured behaviorally and a loss of enhancement by ethanol of GABA's effects measured *in vitro* (Harris et al., 1995). Intracellular signal-transduction cascades, such as MAPK, tyrosine kinases, and neurotrophic factor receptors, also are thought to be affected by ethanol (Valenzuela and Harris, 1997). Translocation of PKC and PKA between subcellular compartments also is sensitive to alcohol (Constantinescu et al., 1999).

Ethanol enhances the activities of several isoforms of adenylyl cyclase, with AC7 being the most sensitive (Tabakoff and Hoffman, 1998). This promotes increased production of cyclic AMP and thus increased activity of PKA. Ethanol's actions appear to be mediated by activation of G_s and promotion of the interaction between G_s and adenylyl cyclase.

Ethanol Consumption and CNS Function. There are a series of relatively common and temporary effects of ethanol with relatively high prevalence rates reflecting changes in the GABA system that are generally caused by CNS depressants. Large doses of ethanol can interfere with encoding of memories, producing anterograde amnesias, commonly referred to as *alcoholic blackouts*; affected individuals are unable to recall all or part of experiences during the period of heavy intake. At even 2-3 drinks, ethanol consumption can produce disturbances in sleep architecture, with frequent awakenings and restless sleep; high doses are associated with vivid and disturbing dreams late as a consequence of earlier suppression of night rapid eye movement dream state at higher blood ethanol levels. Perhaps reflecting the effect of ethanol on respirations as well as the muscle-relaxant effects of this drug, heavier drinking can be associated with sleep apnea, especially in older alcohol-dependent subjects (Sakurai et al., 2007). The transient CNS effects of heavy ethanol consumption that produce a hangover—the "next morning" syndrome of headache, thirst, nausea, and cognitive impairment—contribute to much time lost from work and school, and may reflect mechanisms similar to mild alcohol withdrawal, dehydration, and/or mild acidosis (Stephens et al., 2008).

Chronic heavy drinking reportedly increases the probability of developing a more permanent cognitive deficit often referred to as *alcoholic dementia*. However, the signs of cognitive deficits and brain atrophy observed soon after a heavy drinking period often reverse over the subsequent several weeks to months following abstinence (Bartsch et al., 2007). The thiamine depletion that can accompany heavy ethanol consumption contributes to Wernicke-Korsakoff syndromes; however, the ataxia and ophalmoparesis of Wernicke's, and the severe anterograde and retrograde amnesias of Korsakoff's, are seen in <<1% of chronic alcohol-dependent individuals. Additional severe neurological syndromes associated with chronic heavy use of alcohol include cerebellar degeneration with associated atrophy of the cerebellar vermis (seen in ~1% of alcoholics), and a peripheral neuropathy (observed in ~10% of alcoholics) (Alexander-Kaufman et al., 2007; Peters et al., 2006). The specific mechanisms associated with damage to the cerebellum and peripheral nerves have not been definitively identified.

Heavy doses of ethanol over multiple days or weeks are also associated with several temporary but disturbing "alcohol-induced" psychiatric syndromes (Schuckit, 2006a). As many as 40% of alcohol-dependent humans develop severe alcohol-related depressive symptoms that can include temporary suicidal thoughts and behaviors. Similarly, a range of anxiety conditions, including those characterized by panic attacks and generalized anxiety, are likely in a large minority of alcohol-dependent individuals during the withdrawal syndrome. Perhaps 3% of alcohol-dependent men and women report experiencing temporary auditory hallucinations and paranoid delusions that resemble schizophrenia beginning during periods of heavy intoxication; all of these psychiatric syndromes are likely to markedly improve within several days to a month of abstinence, with residual mild symptoms continuing to diminish thereafter. While no definitive data on the mechanisms for these alcohol-induced psychiatric conditions are available, it is logical to assume that alcohol-related changes in CNS pathways (NE and 5-HT levels, the balance between $GABA_A$ and NMDA receptor activity, dopaminergic activity) may operate here in a manner similar to those seen in depression, anxiety, and schizophrenic disorders.

Cardiovascular System

Ethanol intake greater than three standard drinks per day elevates the risk for heart attacks and bleeding-related strokes (Hvidtfeldt et al., 2008). Indeed, vascular-related diseases are among the leading causes of early death in alcohol-dependent individuals. The risk includes a 6-fold increased risk for coronary artery disease, a heightened risk for cardiac arrhythmias, and an elevated rate of congestive heart failure. The causes are complex and observations are complicated by certain positive effects of small amounts of ethanol.

Serum Lipoproteins and Cardiovascular Effects. In most countries, the risk of mortality due to coronary heart disease (CHD) is correlated with a high dietary intake of saturated fat and elevated serum cholesterol levels. France is an exception to this rule, with relatively low mortality from CHD despite the consumption of high quantities of saturated fats (the "French paradox"). Epidemiological studies suggest that widespread wine consumption (20-30 g ethanol per day) is one of the factors conferring a cardioprotective effect, with 1-3 drinks per day resulting in a 10-40% decreased risk of coronary heart disease compared with abstainers. In contrast, daily consumption of greater amounts of alcohol leads to an increased incidence of non-coronary causes of cardiovascular failure, such as arrhythmias, cardiomyopathy, and hemorrhagic stroke, offsetting the beneficial effects of alcohol on coronary arteries; that is, alcohol has a J-shaped dose-mortality curve. Reduced risks for CHD are seen at intakes as low as one-half drink per day (Libby et al., 2007). Young women and others at low risk for heart disease derive little benefit from light to moderate alcohol intake, whereas those of both sexes who are at high risk and who may have had a myocardial infarction clearly benefit. Data based on a number of prospective, cohort, cross-cultural, and case-control studies in diverse populations consistently reveal lower rates of angina pectoris, myocardial infarction, and peripheral artery disease in those consuming light (1-20 g/day) to moderate (21-40 g/day) amounts of alcohol.

One possible mechanism by which alcohol could reduce the risk of CHD is through its effects on blood lipids. Changes in plasma lipoprotein levels, particularly increases in high-density lipoprotein (HDL; Chapter 31), have been associated with the protective effects of ethanol. HDL binds cholesterol and returns it to the liver for elimination or reprocessing, decreasing tissue cholesterol levels. Ethanol-induced increases in HDL-cholesterol thus could antagonize cholesterol accumulation in arterial walls, lessening the risk of infarction. Approximately half the risk reduction associated with ethanol consumption is explained by changes in total HDL levels (Langer et al., 1992). HDL is found as two subfractions, named HDL_2 and HDL_3. Increased levels of HDL_2 (and possibly also HDL_3) are associated with reduced risk of myocardial infarction. Levels of both subfractions are increased following alcohol consumption and decrease when alcohol consumption ceases. Apolipoproteins A-I and A-II are constituents of HDL. Increased levels of both apolipoproteins A-I and A-II are associated with individuals who are daily heavy drinkers. In contrast, there are reports of decreased serum apolipoprotein(a) levels following acute alcohol consumption. Elevated apolipoprotein(a) levels have been associated with an increased risk for the development of atherosclerosis.

All forms of alcoholic beverages confer cardio-protection. A variety of alcoholic beverages increase HDL levels while decreasing the risk of myocardial infarction. The flavonoids found in red wine (and purple grape juice) may have an additional antiatherogenic role by protecting low-density lipoprotein (LDL) from oxidative damage. Oxidized LDL has been implicated in several steps of atherogenesis (Chapter 31). Another way in which alcohol consumption conceivably could play a cardioprotective role is by altering factors involved in blood clotting. Alcohol consumption elevates the levels of tissue plasminogen activator, a clot-dissolving enzyme (Chapter 30), decreasing the likelihood of clot formation. Decreased fibrinogen concentrations seen following ethanol consumption also could be cardioprotective (Rimm et al., 1999), and epidemiological studies have linked the moderate consumption of ethanol to an inhibition of platelet activation (Rubin, 1999).

Should abstainers from alcohol be advised to consume ethanol in moderate amounts? The answer is *no*. There have been no randomized clinical trials to test the efficacy of daily alcohol use in reducing rates of coronary heart disease and mortality, and it is inappropriate for physicians to advocate alcohol ingestion solely to prevent heart disease. Many abstainers avoid alcohol because of a family history of alcoholism or for other health reasons, and it is imprudent to suggest that they begin drinking. Other lifestyle changes or medical treatments should be encouraged if patients are at risk for the development of CHD.

Hypertension. Heavy alcohol use can raise diastolic and systolic blood pressure. Studies indicate a positive, nonlinear association between alcohol use and hypertension that is unrelated to age, education, smoking status, or the use of oral contraceptives. Consumption above 30 g alcohol per day (more than 2 standard drinks) is associated with a 1.5-2.3 mm Hg rise in diastolic and systolic blood pressure.

The prevalence of hypertension attributable to excess alcohol consumption is not known, but studies suggest a range of 5-11%. The prevalence probably is higher for men than for women because of higher alcohol consumption by men. A reduction in or cessation of alcohol use in heavy drinkers may reduce the need for antihypertensive medication or reduce the blood pressure to the normal range. A safe amount of alcohol consumption for hypertensive patients who are light drinkers (1-2 drinks per occasion and less than 14 drinks per week) has not been determined. Factors to consider are a personal history of ischemic heart disease, a history of binge drinking, or a family history of alcoholism or of cerebrovascular accident. Hypertensive patients with any of these risk factors should abstain from alcohol use.

Cardiac Arrhythmias. Alcohol has a number of pharmacological effects on cardiac conduction, including prolongation of the QT interval, prolongation of ventricular repolarization, and sympathetic stimulation. Atrial arrhythmias associated with chronic alcohol use include supraventricular tachycardia, atrial fibrillation, and atrial flutter. Some 15-20% of idiopathic cases of atrial fibrillation may be induced by chronic ethanol use (Libby et al., 2007). Ventricular tachycardia may be responsible for the increased risk of unexplained sudden death that has been observed in persons who are alcohol-dependent (Kupari and Koskinen, 1998). During continued alcohol use, treatment of these arrhythmias may be more resistant to cardioversion, digoxin, or Ca^{2+} channel blocking agents. Patients with recurrent or refractory atrial arrhythmias should be questioned carefully about alcohol use.

Cardiomyopathy. Ethanol is known to have dose-related toxic effects on both skeletal and cardiac muscle. Numerous studies have shown that alcohol can depress cardiac contractility and lead to cardiomyopathy. Echocardiography demonstrates global hypokinesis. Approximately half of all patients with idiopathic cardiomyopathy are alcohol-dependent. Although the clinical signs and symptoms of idiopathic and alcohol-induced cardiomyopathy are similar, alcohol-induced cardiomyopathy has a better prognosis if patients are able to stop drinking. Women are at greater risk of alcohol-induced cardiomyopathy than are men (Urbano–Marquez et al., 1995). Since 40-50% of persons with alcohol-induced cardiomyopathy who continue to drink die within 3-5 years, abstinence remains the primary treatment.

Stroke. Clinical studies indicate an increased incidence of hemorrhagic and ischemic stroke in persons who drink more than 40-60 g alcohol per day (Hansagi et al., 1995). Many cases of stroke follow prolonged binge drinking, especially when stroke occurs in younger patients. Proposed etiological factors include:

- alcohol-induced cardiac arrhythmias and associated thrombus formation
- high blood pressure from chronic alcohol consumption and subsequent cerebral artery degeneration
- acute increases in systolic blood pressure and alterations in cerebral artery tone
- head trauma

The effects on hemostasis, fibrinolysis, and blood clotting are variable and could prevent or precipitate acute stroke (Numminen et al., 1996). The effects of alcohol on the formation of intracranial aneurysms are controversial, but the statistical association disappears when one controls for tobacco use and gender (Qureshi et al., 1998).

Skeletal Muscle

Alcohol has a number of effects on skeletal muscle. Chronic, heavy, daily alcohol consumption is associated with decreased muscle strength, even when adjusted for other factors such as age, nicotine use, and chronic illness. Heavy doses of alcohol also can cause irreversible damage to muscle, reflected by a marked increase in the activity of creatine kinase in plasma.

Muscle biopsies from heavy drinkers also reveal decreased glycogen stores and reduced pyruvate kinase activity (Vernet et al., 1995). Approximately 50% of chronic heavy drinkers have evidence of type II fiber atrophy. These changes correlate with reductions in muscle protein synthesis and serum carnosinase activities (Wassif et al., 1993). Most patients with chronic alcoholism show electromyographical changes, and many show evidence of a skeletal myopathy similar to alcoholic cardiomyopathy.

Body Temperature

Ingestion of ethanol causes a feeling of warmth because alcohol enhances cutaneous and gastric blood flow. Increased sweating also may occur. Heat, therefore, is lost more rapidly, and the internal body temperature falls. After consumption of large amounts of ethanol, the central temperature-regulating mechanism becomes depressed, and the fall in body temperature may become pronounced. The action of alcohol in lowering body temperature is greater and more dangerous when the ambient environmental temperature is low. Studies of deaths from hypothermia suggest that alcohol is a major risk factor in these events. Patients with ischemic limbs secondary to peripheral vascular disease are particularly susceptible to cold damage.

Diuresis

Alcohol inhibits the release of vasopressin (antidiuretic hormone) from the posterior pituitary gland, resulting in enhanced diuresis. The volume loading that accompanies imbibing complements the diuresis that occurs as a result of reduced vasopressin secretion.

Alcoholics have less urine output than do control subjects in response to a challenge dose with ethanol, suggesting that tolerance develops to the diuretic effects of ethanol (Collins et al., 1992). Alcoholics withdrawing from alcohol exhibit increased vasopressin release and a consequent retention of water, as well as dilutional hyponatremia.

Gastrointestinal System

Esophagus. Alcohol frequently is either the primary etiologic factor or one of multiple causal factors associated with esophageal dysfunction. Ethanol also is associated with the development of esophageal reflux, Barrett's esophagus, traumatic rupture of the esophagus, Mallory-Weiss tears, and esophageal cancer.

When compared with nonalcoholic nonsmokers, alcohol-dependent patients who smoke have a 10-fold increased risk of developing cancer of the esophagus. There is little change in esophageal function at low blood alcohol concentrations, but at higher blood alcohol concentrations, a decrease in peristalsis and decreased lower esophageal sphincter pressure occur. Patients with chronic reflux esophagitis may respond to proton pump inhibitors and abstinence from alcohol.

Stomach. Heavy alcohol use can disrupt the gastric mucosal barrier and cause acute and chronic gastritis. Ethanol appears to stimulate gastric secretions by exciting sensory nerves in the buccal and gastric mucosa and promoting the release of gastrin and histamine. Beverages containing more than 40% alcohol also have a direct toxic effect on gastric mucosa. While these effects are seen most often in chronic heavy drinkers, they can occur after moderate and short-term alcohol use. The diagnosis may not be clear because many patients have normal endoscopic examinations and upper gastrointestinal radiographs. Clinical symptoms include acute epigastric pain that is relieved with antacids or histamine H_2 receptor blockers.

Alcohol is not thought to play a role in the pathogenesis of peptic ulcer disease. Unlike acute and chronic gastritis, peptic ulcer disease is not more common in alcoholics. Nevertheless, alcohol exacerbates the clinical course and severity of ulcer symptoms. It appears to act synergistically with *Helicobacter pylori* to delay healing (Lieber, 1997). Acute bleeding from the gastric mucosa, while uncommon, can be a life-threatening emergency. Upper GI bleeding is associated more commonly with esophageal varices, traumatic rupture of the esophagus, and clotting abnormalities.

Intestines. Many alcoholics have chronic diarrhea as a result of malabsorption in the small intestine (Addolorato et al., 1997). The major symptom is frequent loose stools. The rectal fissures and *pruritus ani* that frequently are associated with heavy drinking probably are related to chronic diarrhea. The diarrhea is caused by structural and functional changes in the small intestine (Papa et al., 1998); the intestinal mucosa has flattened villi, and digestive enzyme levels often are decreased. These changes frequently are reversible after a period of abstinence. Treatment is based on replacing essential vitamins and electrolytes, slowing transit time with an agent such as loperamide, and abstaining from all alcoholic beverages. Patients with severe magnesium deficiencies (serum Mg^{2+} < 1 mEq/L) or symptomatic patients (a positive Chvostek's sign or asterixis) should receive 1 g $MgSO_4$ intravenously or intramuscularly every 4 hours until the serum $[Mg^{2+}] > 1$ mEq/L.

Pancreas. Heavy alcohol use is the most common cause of both acute and chronic pancreatitis in the U.S. While pancreatitis has been known to occur after a single episode of heavy alcohol use, prolonged heavy drinking is common in most cases. Acute alcoholic pancreatitis is characterized by the abrupt onset of abdominal pain, nausea, vomiting, and increased levels of serum or urine pancreatic enzymes. Computed tomography is being used increasingly for diagnostic testing. While most attacks are not fatal, hemorrhagic pancreatitis can develop and lead to shock, renal failure, respiratory failure, and death. Management usually involves intravenous fluid replacement—often with nasogastric suction—and opioid pain medication. The etiology of acute pancreatitis probably is related to a direct toxic metabolic effect of alcohol on pancreatic acinar cells.

Two-thirds of patients with recurrent alcoholic pancreatitis will develop chronic pancreatitis. Chronic pancreatitis is treated by replacing the endocrine and exocrine deficiencies that result from pancreatic insufficiency. The development of hyperglycemia often requires insulin for control of blood-sugar levels (Chapter 43). Pancreatic enzyme capsules containing lipase, amylase, and proteases may be necessary to treat malabsorption (Chapter 46).

Liver. Ethanol produces a constellation of dose-related deleterious effects in the liver (Fickert and Zatloukal, 2000). The primary effects are fatty infiltration of the liver, hepatitis, and cirrhosis. Because of its intrinsic toxicity, alcohol can injure the liver in the absence of dietary deficiencies (Lieber, 2000). The accumulation of fat in the liver is an early event and can occur in normal individuals after the ingestion of relatively small amounts of ethanol. This accumulation results from inhibition of both the tricarboxylic acid cycle and the oxidation of fat, in part owing to the generation of excess NADH produced by the actions of ADH and ALDH (Figure 23–1).

Fibrosis, resulting from tissue necrosis and chronic inflammation, is the underlying cause of alcoholic cirrhosis. Normal liver tissue is replaced by fibrous tissue. Alcohol can affect stellate cells in the liver directly; chronic alcohol use is associated with transformation of stellate cells into collagen-producing, myofibroblast-like cells, resulting in deposition of collagen around terminal hepatic venules (Lieber, 2000). The histological hallmark of alcoholic cirrhosis is the formation of Mallory bodies, which are thought to be related to an altered intermediate cytoskeleton (Denk et al., 2000).

A number of molecular mechanisms for alcoholic cirrhosis have been proposed. In nonhuman primate models, alcohol alters phospholipid peroxidation. Ethanol decreases phosphatidylcholine levels in hepatic mitochondria, a change associated with decreased oxidase activity and O_2 consumption. Cytokines, such as transforming growth factor β and tumor necrosis factor α, can increase rates of fibrinogenesis and fibrosis in the liver. Acetaldehyde is thought to have a number of adverse effects, including depletion of glutathione (Lieber, 2000), depletion of vitamins and trace metals, and decreased transport and secretion of proteins owing to inhibition of tubulin polymerization. Acetaminophen-induced hepatic toxicity (Chapters 4, 6, and 34) has been associated with alcoholic cirrhosis as a result of alcohol-induced increases in microsomal production of toxic acetaminophen metabolites (Whitcomb and Block, 1994). Liver failure secondary to cirrhosis and resulting in impaired clearance of toxins such as ammonia also may contribute to alcohol-induced hepatic encephalopathy. Ethanol also appears to increase intracellular free hydroxy-ethyl radical formation.

Vitamins and Minerals

The almost complete lack of protein, vitamins, and most other nutrients in alcoholic beverages predisposes those who consume large quantities of alcohol to nutritional deficiencies. Alcoholics often present with these deficiencies owing to decreased intake, decreased absorption, or impaired utilization of nutrients. The peripheral neuropathy, Korsakoff's psychosis, and Wernicke's encephalopathy seen in alcoholics probably are caused by deficiencies of the B complex of vitamins (particularly thiamine), although direct toxicity produced by alcohol itself has not been ruled out (Harper, 1998). Chronic alcohol abuse decreases the dietary intake of retinoids and carotenoids and enhances the metabolism of retinol by the induction of degradative enzymes (Lieber, 2000). Retinol and ethanol compete for metabolism by ADH; vitamin A supplementation therefore should be monitored carefully in alcoholics when they are consuming alcohol to avoid retinol-induced hepatotoxicity. The chronic consumption of alcohol inflicts an oxidative stress on the liver owing to the generation of free radicals, contributing to ethanol-induced liver injury. The antioxidant effects of α-tocopherol (vitamin E) may ameliorate some of this ethanol-induced toxicity in the liver. Plasma levels of α-tocopherol often are reduced in myopathic alcoholics compared with alcoholic patients without myopathy.

Chronic alcohol consumption has been implicated in osteoporosis (Chapter 44). The reasons for this decreased bone mass remain unclear, although impaired osteoblastic activity has been implicated. Acute administration of ethanol produces an initial reduction in serum parathyroid hormone (PTH) and Ca^{2+} levels, followed by a rebound increase in PTH that does not restore Ca^{2+} levels to normal. Alcohol-induced osteopenia improves with abstinence (Alvisa-Negrin J, et al., 2009). Since vitamin D requires hydroxylation in the liver for activation, alcohol-induced liver damage can indirectly affect the role of vitamin D in the intestinal and renal absorption of Ca^{2+}.

Sexual Function

Despite the widespread belief that alcohol can enhance sexual activities, the opposite effect is generally noted. Many drugs of abuse, including alcohol, have disinhibiting effects that may lead initially to increased libido.

Both acute and chronic alcohol use can lead to impotence in men. Increased blood alcohol concentrations lead to decreased sexual arousal, increased ejaculatory latency, and decreased orgasmic pleasure. The incidence of impotence may be as high as 50% in patients with chronic alcoholism. Additionally, many chronic alcoholics develop testicular atrophy and decreased fertility. The mechanism involved in this is complex and likely involves altered hypothalamic function and a direct toxic effect of alcohol on Leydig cells. Gynecomastia is associated with alcoholic liver disease and is related to increased cellular response to estrogen and to accelerated metabolism of testosterone.

Sexual function in alcohol-dependent women is less clearly understood. Many female alcoholics complain of decreased libido, decreased vaginal lubrication, and menstrual cycle abnormalities. Their ovaries often are small and without follicular development. Some data suggest that fertility rates are lower for alcoholic women. The presence of comorbid disorders such as anorexia nervosa or bulimia can aggravate the problem. The prognosis for patients who abstain is favorable in the absence of significant hepatic or gonadal failure (O'Farrell et al., 1997).

Hematological and Immunological Effects

Chronic alcohol use is associated with a number of anemias. Microcytic anemia can occur because of chronic blood loss and iron deficiency. Macrocytic anemias and increases in mean corpuscular volume are common and may occur in the absence of vitamin deficiencies. Normochromic anemias also can occur owing to effects of chronic illness on hematopoiesis. In the presence of severe liver disease, morphological changes can include the development of burr cells, schistocytes, and ringed sideroblasts. Alcohol-induced sideroblastic anemia may respond to vitamin B_6 replacement (Wartenberg, 1998). Alcohol use also is associated with reversible thrombocytopenia, although platelet counts under 20,000/mm^3 are rare. Bleeding is uncommon unless there is an alteration in vitamin K_1–dependent clotting factors (Chapter 30); proposed mechanisms have focused on platelet trapping in the spleen and marrow.

Alcohol also affects granulocytes and lymphocytes (Schirmer et al., 2000). Effects include leukopenia, alteration of lymphocyte subsets, decreased T-cell mitogenesis, and changes in immunoglobulin production. These disorders may play a role in alcohol-related liver disease. In some patients, depressed leukocyte migration into inflamed areas may account in part for the poor resistance of alcoholics to some types of infection (e.g., *Klebsiella* pneumonia, listeriosis, and tuberculosis). Alcohol consumption also may alter the distribution and function of lymphoid cells by disrupting cytokine regulation, in particular that involving interleukin 2 (IL-2). Alcohol appears to play a role in the development of infection with the human immunodeficiency virus-1 (HIV). *In vitro* studies with human lymphocytes suggest that alcohol can suppress CD4 T-lymphocyte function and concanavalin A–stimulated IL-2 production and enhance *in vitro* replication of HIV. Moreover, persons who abuse alcohol have higher rates of high-risk sexual behavior.

ACUTE ETHANOL INTOXICATION

Signs of intoxication typical of CNS depression are seen in most people following 2-3 drinks, with the most prominent effect seen at the times of peak BEL, ~30-60 minutes following consumption on an empty stomach. These symptoms include an initial feeling of stimulation (perhaps due to inhibition of CNS inhibitory systems), giddiness, muscle relaxation, and impaired judgment. Higher blood levels (~80 mg/dL or ~17 mM) are associated with slurred speech, incoordination, unsteady gait, and potential impairments of attention; levels between 80 and 200 mg/dL (~17-43 mM) are associated with more intense mood lability, and greater cognitive deficits, potentially accompanied by aggressiveness, and anterorgrade amnesia (an alcoholic blackout) (Schuckit, 2009c). Blood ethanol levels >200 mg/dL can produce nystagmus and unwanted falling asleep; levels of 300 mg/dL (~65 mM) and higher can produce failing vital signs, coma, and death. All of these symptoms are likely to be exacerbated and occur at a lower BEC when ethanol is taken along with other CNS depressants (e.g., diazepam or similar benzodiazepines), or with any drug or medication for which sleepiness and incoordination are likely.

An increased reaction time, diminished fine motor control, impulsivity, and impaired judgment become evident when the concentration of ethanol in the blood is 20-30 mg/dL. More than 50% of persons are grossly intoxicated by a concentration of 150 mg/dL. In fatal cases, the average concentration is about 400 mg/dL, although alcohol-tolerant individuals often can withstand comparable blood alcohol levels. The definition of intoxication varies by state and country. In the U.S., most states set the ethanol level defined as intoxication at 80 mg/dL. There is increasing evidence that lowering the limit to 50-80 mg/dL can reduce motor vehicle injuries and fatalities significantly. While alcohol can be measured in saliva, urine, sweat, and blood, measurement of levels in exhaled air remains the primary method of assessing the level of intoxication.

Many factors, such as body weight and composition and the rate of absorption from the GI tract, determine the concentration of ethanol in the blood after ingestion of a given amount of ethanol. On average, the ingestion of 3 standard drinks (42 g ethanol) on an empty stomach results in a maximum blood concentration of 67-92 mg/dL in men. After a mixed meal, the maximal blood concentration from three drinks is 30-53 mg/dL in men. Concentrations of alcohol in blood will be higher in women than in men consuming the same amount of alcohol because, on average, women are smaller than men, have less body water per unit of weight into which ethanol can distribute, and have less gastric ADH activity than men. For individuals with normal hepatic function, ethanol is metabolized at a rate of one standard drink every 60-90 minutes.

The characteristic signs and symptoms of alcohol intoxication are well known. Nevertheless, an erroneous diagnosis of drunkenness may occur with patients who appear inebriated but who have not ingested ethanol. Diabetic coma, e.g., may be mistaken for severe alcoholic intoxication. Drug intoxication, cardiovascular accidents, and skull fractures also may be confused with alcohol intoxication. The odor of the breath of a person who has consumed ethanol is due not to ethanol vapor but to impurities in alcoholic beverages. Breath odor in a case of suspected intoxication can be misleading because there can be other causes of breath odor similar to that after alcohol consumption. Blood alcohol levels are necessary to confirm the presence or absence of alcohol intoxication (Schuckit, 2006b).

The treatment of acute alcohol intoxication is based on the severity of respiratory and CNS depression. Acute alcohol intoxication can be a medical emergency, and a number of young people die every year from this disorder. Patients who are comatose and who exhibit evidence of respiratory depression should be intubated to protect the airway and to provide ventilatory assistance (see Chapter 4). The stomach may be lavaged, but care must be taken to prevent pulmonary aspiration of the return flow. Since ethanol is freely miscible with water, ethanol can be removed from blood by hemodialysis (Schuckit, 2006b).

Acute alcohol intoxication is not always associated with coma, and careful observation is the primary treatment. Usual care involves observing the patient in the emergency room for 4-6 hours while the patient metabolizes the ingested ethanol. Blood alcohol levels will be reduced by ~15 mg/dL per hour. During this period, some individuals may display extremely violent behavior. Sedatives and antipsychotic agents have been employed to quiet such patients. Great care must be taken, however, when using sedatives to treat patients who have ingested an excessive amount of another CNS depressant, such as, ethanol, because of synergistic effects.

CLINICAL USES OF ETHANOL

Dehydrated alcohol may be injected in close proximity to nerves or sympathetic ganglia to relieve the long-lasting pain related to trigeminal neuralgia, inoperable carcinoma, and other conditions. Epidural, subarachnoid, and lumbar paravertebral injections of ethanol also have been employed for inoperable pain. For example, lumbar paravertebral injections of ethanol may destroy sympathetic ganglia and thereby produce vasodilation, relieve pain, and promote healing of lesions in patients with vascular disease of the lower extremities.

Systemically administered ethanol is confined to the treatment of poisoning by methyl alcohol and ethylene glycol. The ingestion results in formation of methanol's metabolites, formaldehyde and formic acid (Figure 23–1). Formic acid causes nerve damage; its effects on the retina and optic nerve can cause blindness. Treatment consists of sodium bicarbonate to combat acidosis, hemodialysis, and the administration of ethanol, which slows formate production by competing with methanol for metabolism by alcohol dehydrogenase.

The use of alcohol to treat patients in alcohol withdrawal or obstetrical patients with premature contractions is no longer recommended (Chapter 24).

TOLERANCE, DEPENDENCE, AND CHRONIC ETHANOL USE

Tolerance is defined as a reduced behavioral or physiological response to the same dose of ethanol (Chapter 24). There is a marked acute tolerance that is detectable soon after administration of ethanol. Acute tolerance can be demonstrated by measuring behavioral impairment at the same BELs on the ascending limb of the absorption phase of the BEL–time curve (minutes after ingestion of alcohol) and on the descending limb of the curve as BELs are lowered by metabolism (one or more hours after ingestion). Behavioral impairment and subjective feelings of intoxication are much greater at a given BEL on the ascending than on the descending limb. There also is a chronic tolerance that develops in the long-term heavy drinker. In contrast to acute tolerance, chronic tolerance often has a metabolic component owing to induction of alcohol-metabolizing enzymes.

Physical dependence is demonstrated by the elicitation of a withdrawal syndrome when alcohol consumption is terminated. The symptoms and severity are determined by the amount and duration of alcohol consumption and include sleep disruption, autonomic nervous system (sympathetic) activation, tremors, and in severe cases, seizures. In addition, two or more days after withdrawal, some individuals experience *delirium tremens,* characterized by hallucinations, delirium, fever, and tachycardia. Delirium tremens can be fatal. Another aspect of dependence is craving and drug-seeking behavior, often termed *psychological dependence*.

Ethanol tolerance and physical dependence are studied readily in animal models. Strains of mice with genetic differences in tolerance and dependence have been characterized, and a search for the relevant genes and ethanol-sensitive microRNAs is under way (Miranda et al., 2010). Neurobiological mechanisms of tolerance and dependence are not understood completely, but chronic alcohol consumption results in changes in synaptic and intracellular signaling likely owing to changes in gene expression. Most of the systems that are acutely affected by ethanol also are affected by chronic exposure, resulting in an adaptive or maladaptive response that can cause tolerance and dependence (see Table 23–1). In particular, chronic actions of ethanol likely require changes in signaling by glutamate and GABA receptors and down-stream signaling pathways. The increase in NMDA-receptor function after chronic alcohol ingestion could contribute to the CNS hyperexcit-ability and neurotoxicity seen during ethanol withdrawal. Arginine vasopressin, acting on V_1 receptors, maintains tolerance to ethanol in laboratory animals even after chronic ethanol administration has ceased (Hoffman et al., 1990).

The neurobiological basis of the switch from controlled, volitional alcohol use to compulsive and uncontrolled addiction remains obscure. Impairment of the dopaminergic reward system and the resulting increase in alcohol consumption in an attempt to regain activation of the system is a possibility. In addition, the prefrontal cortex is particularly sensitive to damage from alcohol abuse and influences decision making and emotion, processes clearly compromised in the alcoholic (Pfefferbaum et al., 1998). Thus, impairment of executive function in cortical regions by chronic alcohol consumption may be responsible for some of the lack of judgment and control that is expressed as obsessive alcohol consumption. The loss of brain volume and impairment of function seen in the chronic alcoholic is at least partially reversible by abstinence but will worsen with continued drinking. Early diagnosis and treatment of alcoholism are important in limiting the brain damage that promotes the progression to severe addiction.

Etiology of Alcohol Use Disorders and the Role of Genes

A wide range of social, cultural, interpersonal, and biological factors combine to contribute to the risk for heavier drinking and alcohol use disorders (Schuckit, 2009b). The initial decision to consume alcohol is predominantly a response to the environment and culture in which one lives. Environmental and cultural factors that contribute to alcohol use include stress, expectations regarding the effects alcohol is likely to produce, drinking patterns within one's culture and peer group, availability of alcohol, and attitudes toward drunkenness. These nonbiological forces contribute to perhaps 70-80% of the initial decision to drink and at least 40% of the transition from drinking to alcohol-related problems and alcohol use disorders. Correspondingly, ~60% of the susceptibility to alcohol use disorders results from heritable factors (Table 23–2).

The search for the genes and alleles responsible for alcoholism is complicated by the polygenetic nature of the disease and the general difficulty in defining multiple genes responsible for complex diseases. As noted earlier in the chapter, polymorphisms in the enzymes of ethanol metabolism seem to explain why some populations (mainly Asian) are protected from alcoholism. This has been attributed to genetic differences in alcohol- and aldehyde-metabolizing enzymes. Specifically, genetic variants of ADH that exhibit high activity and variants of ALDH that exhibit low activity protect against heavy drinking, probably because alcohol consumption by individuals who have these variants results in accumulation of acetaldehyde, which produces a variety of unpleasant effects (Li, 2000).

Table 23–2

Genes for Intermediate Phenotypes Affecting Risk for Alcohol Use Disorder

PHENOTYPE	GENES
Facial flush after drinking	ALDH2 ADH1B, ADH1C
Impulsivity and disinhibition	GABRA2 ADH4 CHRM2 DRD2, DRD4
Low level of response to ethanol	GABRA1, GABRA6 5HTT promoter KCNMA1 CHRN cluster

In contrast to these protective genetic variants, there are few consistent data about genes responsible for increased risk for alcoholism. A genetic mechanism associated with an enhanced risk for both alcohol and other drug use disorders operates through the intermediate characteristic (or phenotype) of impulsivity and disinhibition (King et al., 2004). The identified polymorphisms include two variations of the $GABA_A$ receptors (Dick et al., 2006a,b), a variation in ADH4 hypothesized to be related to personality characteristics (Edenberg et al., 2006), and a muscarinic cholinergic receptor gene, CHRM2 (Jones et al., 2006).

Another phenotype related to an enhanced risk for alcohol use disorders (but not other drug use disorders) is associated with a low level of response (perhaps reflecting low sensitivity) to ethanol (Schuckit, 2009b). The need for higher amounts of ethanol to achieve the desired effects may contribute to the decision to drink more per occasion, which in turn leads to altered expectations of the effects of beverage alcohol, an enhanced probability of selecting heavier-drinking peers, as well as problematic approaches to dealing with stress (Schuckit et al., 2008). To date, genetic contributions to the level of response have been tentatively identified for two $GABA_A$ subunits (Dick et al., 2006a,b), a polymorphism in the promoter region of the 5-HT transporter that is associated with lower levels of 5-HT in the synaptic space (Barr et al., 2005), a polymorphism of the K^+ channel-related KCNMA1 (Schuckit et al., 2005), and a variant nicotinic Ach receptor that is also related to an increased risk for heavy smoking and related consequences (Joslyn et al., 2008). Antisocial alcoholism has been linked with polymorphisms of several 5-HT receptors (Ducci et al, 2009). Polymorphisms in dopaminergic and opioid systems and in genes that correlate with a predisposition to bipolar disorder, schizophrenia, and several anxiety disorders may also contribute to a general vulnerability to a range of substance abuse disorders.

TERATOGENIC EFFECTS: FETAL ALCOHOL SYNDROME

Children born to alcoholic mothers display a common pattern of distinct dysmorphology known as *fetal alcohol syndrome* (FAS) (Jones and Smith, 1973; Lemoine et al., 1968). The diagnosis of FAS typically is based on the observance of a triad of abnormalities in the newborn, including:

- a cluster of craniofacial abnormalities
- CNS dysfunction
- pre- and/or postnatal stunting of growth

Hearing, language, and speech disorders also may become evident as the child ages (Church and Kaltenbach, 1997). Children who do not meet all the criteria for a diagnosis of FAS still may show physical and mental deficits consistent with a partial phenotype,

metabolites of the drug, especially diethylthiomethylcarbamate, behave as suicide-substrate inhibitors of ALDH *in vitro*. These metabolites reach significant concentrations in plasma following the administration of disulfiram (Johansson, 1992).

The ingestion of alcohol by individuals previously treated with disulfiram gives rise to marked signs and symptoms of acetaldehyde poisoning. Within 5-10 minutes, the face feels hot and soon afterward becomes flushed and scarlet in appearance. As the vasodilation spreads over the whole body, intense throbbing is felt in the head and neck, and a pulsating headache may develop. Respiratory difficulties, nausea, copious vomiting, sweating, thirst, chest pain, considerable hypotension, orthostatic syncope, marked uneasiness, weakness, vertigo, blurred vision, and confusion are observed. The facial flush is replaced by pallor, and the blood pressure may fall to shock levels.

Alarming reactions may result from the ingestion of even small amounts of alcohol in persons being treated with disulfiram. The use of disulfiram as a therapeutic agent thus is not without danger, and it should be attempted only under careful medical and nursing supervision. Patients must be warned that as long as they are taking disulfiram, the ingestion of alcohol in any form will make them sick and may endanger their lives. Patients must learn to avoid disguised forms of alcohol, as in sauces, fermented vinegar, cough syrups, and even after-shave lotions and back rubs.

The drug never should be administered until the patient has abstained from alcohol for at least 12 hours. In the initial phase of treatment, a maximal daily dose of 500 mg is given for 1-2 weeks. Maintenance dosage then ranges from 125-500 mg daily depending on tolerance to side effects. Unless sedation is prominent, the daily dose should be taken in the morning, the time when the resolve not to drink may be strongest. Sensitization to alcohol may last as long as 14 days after the last ingestion of disulfiram because of the slow rate of restoration of ALDH (Johansson, 1992).

Disulfiram and/or its metabolites can inhibit many enzymes with crucial sulfhydryl groups, and it thus has a wide spectrum of biological effects. It inhibits hepatic CYPs and thereby interferes with the metabolism of phenytoin, chlordiazepoxide, barbiturates, warfarin, and other drugs.

Disulfiram by itself usually is innocuous, but it may cause acneform eruptions, urticaria, lassitude, tremor, restlessness, headache, dizziness, a garlic-like or metallic taste, and mild GI disturbances. Peripheral neuropathies, psychosis, and ketosis also have been reported.

Other Agents

Ondansetron, a 5-HT$_3$-receptor antagonist and antiemetic drug (Chapters 13 and 46), reduces alcohol consumption in laboratory animals and currently is being tested in humans. Preliminary findings suggest that ondansetron is effective in the treatment of early-onset alcoholics, who respond poorly to psychosocial treatment alone, although the drug does not appear to work well in other types of alcoholics. Ondansetron administration lowers the amount of alcohol consumed, particularly by drinkers who consume fewer than 10 drinks per day (Sellers et al., 1994). It also decreases the subjective effects of ethanol on 6 of 10 scales measured, including the desire to drink (Johnson et al., 1993), while at the same time not having any effect on the pharmacokinetics of ethanol.

Topiramate, a drug used for treating seizure disorders (Chapter 21), appears useful for treating alcohol dependence. Compared with the placebo group, patients taking topiramate achieved more abstinent days and a lower craving for alcohol (Johnson et al., 2003). The mechanism of action of topiramate is not well understood but is distinct from that of other drugs used for the treatment of dependence (e.g., opioid antagonists), suggesting that it may provide a new and unique approach to pharmacotherapy of alcoholism.

BIBLIOGRAPHY

Abel EL. An update on incidence of FAS: FAS is not an equal opportunity birth defect. *Neurotoxicol Teratol,* **1995**, *17*: 437–443.

Abel EL, Sokol RJ. Incidence of fetal alcohol syndrome and economic impact of FAS-related anomalies. *Drug Alcohol Depend,* **1987**, *19*:51–70.

Addolorato, Montalto M, Capristo E, et al. Influence of alcohol on gastrointestinal motility: Lactulose breath hydrogen testing in orocecal transit time in chronic alcoholics, social drinkers, and teetotaler subjects. *Hepatogastroenterology,* **1997**, *44*:1076–1081.

Alexander-Kaufman K, Harper C, Wilice P, et al. Cerebellar vermis proteome of chronic alcoholic individuals. *Alcohol Clin Exp Res,* **2007**, *31*:1286–1296

Alvisa-Negrin J, Gonzalez-Reimers E, Santolaria-Fernandez F, et al. Osteopenia in alcoholics: Effect of alcohol abstinence. *Alcohol Alcoholism,* **2009**, *44*:468–475.

Anton R, Moak D, Waid R, et al. Naltrexone and cognitive behavioral therapy for the treatment of outpatient alcoholics: Results of a placebo-controlled trial. *Am J Psychiatry,* **1999**, *156*:1758–1764.

Aryal P, Dvir H, Choe S, Slesinger P. A Diserete Alcohol Binding Pocket Involved in GIRK Channel Activation. *Nat Neurosci,* **2009**, *12*:988–995.

Baer, S, Barr HM, Bookstein, FL, et al. Prenatal alcohol exposure and family history of alcoholism in the etiology of adolescent alcohol problems. *J Stud Alcohol,* **1998**, *59*:533–543.

Besson J, Aeby F, Kasas A, et al. Combined efficacy of acamprosate and disulfiram in the treatment of alcoholism: A controlled study. *Alcohol Clin Exp Res,* **1998**, *22*:573–579.

Barr CS, Newman T, Lindell S, et al. Interaction between serotonin transporter gene variation and rearing condition in alcohol preference and consumption in female primates. *Arch Gen Psychiatry,* **2005**, *61*:1146–1152.

Bartsch AJ, Homola G, Biller A, et al. Manifestations of early brain recovery associated with abstinence from alcoholism. *Brain,* **2007**, *130*:36–47.

Carta M, Ariwodola OJ, Weiner JL, and Valenzuela CF. Alcohol potently inhibits the kainite receptor-dependent excitatory drive of hippocampal interneurons. *Proc Natl Acad Sci USA,* **2003**, *100*:6813–6818.

Church MW, Kaltenbach JA. Hearing, speech, language, and vestibular disorders in the fetal alcohol syndrome: A literature review. *Alcohol Clin Exp Res,* **1997**, *21*:495–512.

Collins GB, Brosnihan KB, Zuti RA, et al. Neuroendocrine, fluid balance, and thirst responses to alcohol in alcoholics. *Alcohol. Clin Exp Res,* **1992**, *16*:228–233.

Constantinescu A, Diamond I, Gordon AS. Ethanol-induced translocation of cAMP-dependent protein kinase to the nucleus: Mechanism and functional consequences. *J Biol Chem,* **1999**, *274*:26985–26991.

Davies AG, Pierce-Shimomura JT, Kim H, et al. A central role of the BK potassium channel in behavioral responses to ethanol in *C. elegans*. *Cell,* **2003**, *115*:655–666.

Denk H, Stumptner C, Zatloukal K. Mallory bodies revisited. *J Hepatol,* **2000**, *32*:689–702.

Dick DM, Bierut L, Hinrichs A, et al. The role of GABRA2 in risk for conduct disorder and alcohol and drug dependence across developmental stages. *Behav Genet,* **2006a**, *36*:577–590.

Dick DM, Plunkett J, Wetherill LF, et al. Association between GABRA1 and drinking behaviors in the Collaborative Study on the Genetics of Alcoholism sample. *Alcohol Clin Exp Res,* **2006b**, *30*:1101–1110.

Dopico AM, Chu B, Lemos, JR, Treistman SN. Alcohol modulation of calcium-activated potassium channels. *Neurochem Int,* **1999**, *35*:103–106.

Ducci F, Enoch M, Yuan Q et al. HTR3B is associated with alcoholism with antisocial behavior and alpha EEG power—an intermediate phenotype for alcoholism and co-morbid behaviors. Alcohol, **2009**, *43*:73–84.

Edenberg HJ, Xuei X, Chen HJ, et al. Association of alcohol dehydrogenase genes with alcohol dependence: a comprehensive analysis. *Hum Mol Genet,* **2006**, *15*:1539–1549.

Erstad BL, Cotugno CL. Management of alcohol withdrawal. *Am J Health Syst Pharm,* **1995**, *52*:697–709.

Faden VB. Trends in initiation of alcohol use in the United States 1975 to 2003. *Alcohol Clin Exp Res,* **2006**, *30*:1011–1022

Fickert P, Zatloukal K. Pathogenesis of alcoholic liver disease. In, *Handbook of Alcoholism.* (Zernig G, Saria A, Kurz M, and O'Malley S, eds.) CRC Press, Boca Raton, FL, **2000**, pp. 317–323.

Garbutt JC, West SL, Carey TS, et al. Pharmacological treatment of alcohol dependence: A review of the evidence. *JAMA,* **1999**, *281*:1318–1325.

Goldschmidt L, Richardson GA, Stoffer DS, et al. Prenatal alcohol exposure and academic achievement at age six: A nonlinear fit. *Alcohol Clin Exp Res,* **1996**, *20*:763–770.

Hansagi H, Romelsjo A, Gerhardsson de Verdier M, *et al.* Alcohol consumption and stroke mortality: 20-year follow-up of 15,077 men and women. *Stroke,* **1995**, *26*:1768–1773.

Harper C. The neuropathology of alcohol-specific brain damage, or does alcohol damage the brain? *J Neuropathol Exp Neurol,* **1998**, *57*:101–110.

Harris RA, McQuilkin SJ, Paylor R, et al. Mutant mice lacking the γ isoform of protein kinase C show decreased behavioral actions of ethanol and altered function of γ-aminobutyrate type A receptors. *Proc Natl Acad Sci USA,* **1995**, *92*:3658–3662.

Hanson DJ. *Preventing Alcohol Abuse: Alcohol, Culture, and Control*. Westport, CT: Praeger, **1995**.

Hartzler B, Fromme K. Fragmentary blackouts: Their etiology and effect on alcohol expectancies. *Alcohol Clin Exp Res,* **2003**, *27*:628–637.

Harwood HJ, Fountain D, Livermore G. Economic cost of alcohol and drug abuse in the United States, 1992: A report. *Addiction,* **1999**, *94*:631–635.

Hasin DS, Stinson FS, Ogburn E, et al. Prevalence, correlates, disability, and comorbidity of DSM-IV alcohol abuse and dependence in the United States. *Arch Gen Psychiatry,* **2007**, *64*:830–842.

Hoffman PL, Ishizawa H, Giri PR, et al. The role of arginine vasopressin in alcohol tolerance. *Ann Med,* **1990**, *22*:269–274.

Husemoen LL, Fenger M, Friedrich N, et al. The association of ADH and ALDH gene variants with alcohol drinking habits and cardiovascular disease risk factors. *Alcohol Clin Exp Res,* **2008**;*32*:1984–1991.

Hutchison KE, Haughey H, Niculescu M, et al. The incentive salience of alcohol: Translating the effects of genetic variant in CNR1. *Arch Gen Psychiatry,* **2008**, *65*:841–850.

Hvidtfeldt UA, Frederiksen ME, Thygesen LC, et al. Incidence of cardiovascular and cerebrovascular disease in Danish men and women with a prolonged heavy alcohol intake. *Alcohol Clin Exp Res,* **2008**, *32*:1920–1924.

Jacobson JL, Jacobson SW, and Sokol RJ. Increased vulnerability to alcohol-related birth defects in the offspring of mothers over 30. *Alcohol Clin Exp Res,* **1996**, *20*:359–363.

Johansson B. A review of the pharmacokinetics and pharmacodynamics of disulfiram and its metabolites. *Acta Psychiatr Scand Suppl,* **1992**, *369*:15–26.

Johnson BA, Ait-Daoud N, Bowden CL, *et al.* Oral topiramate for treatment of alcohol dependence: A randomized, controlled trial. *Lancet,* **2003**, *361*:1677–1685.

Johnson BA, Campling GM, Griffiths P, Cowen PJ. Attenuation of some alcohol-induced mood changes and the desire to drink by 5-HT_3 receptor blockade: A preliminary study in healthy male volunteers. *Psychopharmacology (Berl.),* **1993**, *112*:142–144.

Jones KL, Smith DW. Recognition of the fetal alcohol syndrome in early infancy. *Lancet,* **1973**, *2*:999–1001.

Job MO, Tang A, Hall FS, et al. Mu opioid receptor regulation of ethanol-induced dopamine response in the ventral striatum: Evidence of genotype specific sexual dimorphic epistasis. *Biol Psychiatry,* **2007**, *62*:627–634.

Jones KA, Porjesz B, Almasy L, et al. A cholinergic receptor gene (CHRM2) affects event-related oscillations. *Behav Genet,* **2006**, *36*:627–639.

Joslyn G, Brush G, Robertson M, et al. Chromosome 15q25.1 genetic markers associated with level of response to alcohol in humans. *Proc Natl Acad Sci USA,* **2008**, *105*:20368–20373.

King SM, Iacono WG, McGue J. Childhood externalizing and internalizing psychopathology in the prediction of early substance use. *Addiction,* **2004**, *99*:1548–1559.

Koob G, Kreek MJ. Stress, dysregulation of drug reward pathways, and the transition to drug dependence. *Am J Psychiatry,* **2007**, *164*:1149–1159.

Kril JJ, Halliday GM. Brain shrinkage in alcoholics: A decade on and what have we learned? *Prog Neurobiol,* **1999**, *58*: 381–387.

Krystal JH, Staley J, Mason G, et al. γ-aminobutyric acid Type A receptors and alcoholism: Intoxication, dependence, vulnerability, and treatment. *Arch Gen Psychiatry,* **2006**, *63*:957–968.

Kuo P, Kalsi G, Prescott C, et al. Association of ADH and ALDH genes with alcohol dependence in the Irish affected sib pair study of alcohol dependence (IASPSAD) sample. *Alcohol Clin Exp Res,* **2008**, *32*:785–795.

Kupari M, Koskinen P. Alcohol, cardiac arrhythmias, and sudden death. In, *Alcohol and Cardiovascular Diseases.* (Goode, J., ed.) Wiley, New York, **1998**, p. 68.

Langer RD, Criqui MH, Reed DM. Lipoproteins and blood pressure as biological pathways for effect of moderate alcohol consumption on coronary heart disease. *Circulation,* **1992**, *85*:910–915.

Lemoine P, Harousseau H, Borteyru JP, Menuet JC. Les enfants de perents alcooliques: Anomalies observees. A propos de 127 cas. *Quest Medicale,* **1968**, *25*:476–482.

Lewohl JM, Wilson WR, Mayfield RD, et al. G protein–coupled inwardly rectifying potassium channels are targets of alcohol action. *Nature Neurosci,* **1999**, *2*:1084–1090.

Li TK. Pharmacogenetics of responses to alcohol and genes that influence alcohol drinking. *J Stud Alcohol,* **2000**, *61*:5–12.

Libby P, et al, eds. Braunwald's *Heart Disease: A Textbook of Cardiovascular Medicine,* 8th ed. Saunders, Philadelphia, **2007**.

Lieber CS. Alcohol and the liver: Metabolism of alcohol and its role in hepatic and extrahepatic diseases. *Mt Sinai J Med,* **2000**, *67*:84–94.

Lieber CS. Gastric ethanol metabolism and gastritis: Interactions with other drugs, *Helicobacter pylori,* and antibiotic therapy (1957–1997): A review. *Alcohol Clin Exp Res,* **1997**, *21*:1360–1366.

Luo X, Kranzler H, Zuo L, et al. Personality traits of aggreeableness and extraversion are associated ADH4 variation. *Biol Psychiatry,* **2007**, *61*:599–608.

Lushine KA, Harris CR, Holger JS. Methanol ingestion: Prevention of toxic sequelae after massive ingestion. *J Emerg Med,* **2003**, *24*:433–436.

Mason BJ, Salvato FR, Williams LD, et al. A double-blind, placebo-controlled study of oral nalmefene for alcohol dependence. *Arch Gen Psychiatry,* **1999**, *56*:719–724.

Mattson SN, Riley EP, Jernigan TL, et al. Fetal alcohol syndrome: A case report of neuropsychological, MRI, and EEG assessment of two children. *Alcohol Clin Exp Res,* **1992**, *16*:1001–1003.

Mehta AK, and Ticku MK. An update on $GABA_A$ receptors. *Brain Res. Brain Res Rev,* **1999**, *29*:196–217.

Miranda R, Pietrzykowski A, Tang Y et al. MicroRNAs: master regulators of ethanol abuse and toxicity? *Alcohol Clin Exp Res,* **2010**, *34*:575–587.

Numminen H, Hillborn M, Juvela S. Platelets, alcohol consumption, and onset of brain infarction. *J Neurol Neurosurg Psychiatry,* **1996**, *61*:376–380.

O'Farrell TJ, Choquette KA, Cutter HS, Birchler GR. Sexual satisfaction and dysfunction in marriages of male alcoholics: Comparison with nonalcoholic maritally conflicted and nonconflicted couples. *J Stud Alcohol,* **1997**, *58*:91–99.

Oslin D, Atkinson RM, Smith DM, Hendrie H. Alcohol-related dementia: Proposed clinical criteria. *Int J Geriatr Psychiatry,* **1998**, *13*:203–212.

Pastor R, Aragon CMG. The role of opioid receptor subtypes in the development of behavioral sensitization to ethanol. *Neuropsychopharmacology,* **2006**, *31*:1489–1499.

Papa A, Tursi A, Cammarota G, et al. Effect of moderate and heavy alcohol consumption on intestinal transit time. *Panminerva Med,* **1998**, *40*:183–185.

Perra S, Pillolla G, Luchicchi A, et al. Alcohol inhibits spontaneous activity of basolateral amygdala projection neurons in the rat: Involvement of the endocannabinoid system. *Alcohol Clin Exp Res,* **2008**, *32*:443–449.

Peters TJ, Kotowicz J, Nyka W, et al. Treatment of alcoholic polyneuropathy with vitamin B complex: A randomized controlled trial. *Alcohol Alcohol,* **2006**, *41*:636–642.

Pfefferbaum A, Sullivan EV, Rosenbloom MJ, et al. A controlled study of cortical gray matter and ventricular changes in alcoholic men over a 5-year interval. *Arch Gen Psychiatry,* **1998**, *55*:905–912.

Qureshi AI, Suarez JI, Parekh PD, et al. Risk factors for multiple intracranial aneurysms. *Neurosurgery,* **1998**, *43*:22–26.

Rehm J, Gnam W, Popova S, et al. The costs of alcohol, illegal drugs, and tobacco in Canada, 2002. *J Studies Alcohol Drugs,* **2007**, *68*:886–895.

Rimm EB, Williams P, Fosher K, et al. Moderate alcohol intake and lower risk of coronary heart disease: Meta-analysis of effects on lipids and haemostatic factors. *BMJ,* **1999**, *319*:1523–1528.

Rubin R. Effect of ethanol on platelet function. *Alcohol Clin Exp Res,* **1999**, *23*:1114–1118.

Sakurai S, Cui R, Tanigawa T, et al. Alcohol consumption before sleep is associated with severity of sleep-disordered breathing among professional Japanese truck drivers. *Alcohol Clin Exp Res,* **2007**, *31*:2053–2058.

Schenker S, Montalvo R. Alcohol and the pancreas. *Recent Dev Alcohol,* **1998**, *14*:41–65.

Schirmer M, Widerman C, Konwalinka G. Immune system. In, *Handbook of Alcoholism.* (Zernig G, Saria A, Kurz M, and O'Malley S, eds.) CRC Press, Boca Raton, FL, **2000**, pp. 225–230.

Schuckit MA. Comorbidity between substance use disorders and psychiatric conditions. *Addiction,* **2006a**, *101*:76–88.

Schuckit MA. *Drug and Alcohol Abuse: Clinical Guide to Diagnosis and Treatment,* 4th ed. Plenum Press, New York, **1995**.

Schuckit MA. *Drug and Alcohol Abuse: A Clinical Guide to Diagnosis and Treatment,* 6th ed. Springer, New York, **2006b**.

Schuckit MA. Alcohol use disorders. *The Lancet,* **2009a**, *373*: 492–501.

Schuckit MA. An overview of genetic influences in alcoholism. *J Substance Abuse Treat,* **2009b**, *36*:S5–S14.

Schuckit MA. Alcohol-related disorders. In, *Kaplan & Sadock's Comprehensive Textbook of Psychiatry.* (Sadock BJ, Sadock VA, Ruiz P, eds.) Wolters Kluwer, Lippincott Williams & Wilkins, **2009c**.

Schuckit MA, Smith TL, Trim R, et al. Testing the level of response to alcohol-based model of heavy drinking and alcohol problems in offspring from the San Diego Prospective Study. *J Stud Alcohol Drugs,* **2008**, *69*:571–579.

Schuckit MA, Smith TL. The relationships of a family history of alcohol dependence, a low level of response to alcohol and six domains of life functioning to the development of alcohol use disorders. *J Stud Alcohol,* **2000**, *61*:827–835.

Sellers EM, Toneatto T, Romach MK, et al. Clinical efficacy of the $5\text{-}HT_3$ antagonist ondansetron in alcohol abuse and dependence. *Alcohol Clin Exp Res,* **1994**, *18*:879–885.

Smith BR, Horan JT, Gaskin S, Amit Z. Exposure to nicotine enhances acquisition of ethanol drinking by laboratory rats in a limited access paradigm. *Psychopharmacology (Berl.),* **1999**, *142*:408–412.

Steensland P, Simms JA, Holgate J, et al. Varenicline, an $\alpha_4\beta_2$ nicotinic acetylcholine receptor partial agonist, selectively decreases ethanol consumption and seeking. *Proc Natl Acad Sci USA,* **2007**, *104*:12518–12523.

Stephens R, Ling J, Heffernan TJ, et al. A review of the literature on the cognitive effects of alcohol hangover. *Alcohol Alcohol,* **2008**, *43*:163–170.

Solem M, McMahon T, Messing RO. Protein kinase A regulates inhibition of N- and P/Q-type calcium channels by ethanol in PC12 cells. *J Pharmacol Exp Ther,* **1997**, *282*: 1487–1495.

Tabakoff B, Hoffman PL. Adenylyl cyclases and alcohol. *Adv. Second Messenger Phosphoprotein Res,* **1998**, *32*:173–193.

Urbano-Marquez A, Estruch R, Fernandez-Sola J, et al. The greater risk of alcoholic cardiomyopathy and myopathy in women compared with men. *JAMA,* **1995**, *274*:149–154.

Valenzuela CF, Harris, RA. Alcohol: Neurobiology. In, *Substance Abuse: A Comprehensive Textbook.* (Lowinson, JH, Ruiz P, Millman, RB, Langrod JB, eds.) Williams & Wilkins, Baltimore, **1997**, pp. 119–142.

Voronin K, Randall P, Myrick H, et al. Aripiprazole effects on alcohol consumption and subjective reports in a clinical laboratory paradigm: Possible influence of self-control. *Alcohol Clin Exp Res*, **2008**, *32*:1954–1961.

Vernet M, Cadefau JA, Balaque A, et al. Effect of chronic alcoholism on human muscle glycogen and glucose metabolism. *Alcohol Clin Exp Res,* **1995**, *19*:1295–1299.

Volkow ND, Wang GJ, Hitzemann R, et al. Recovery of brain glucose metabolism in detoxified alcoholics. *Am J Psychiatry,* **1994**, *151*:178–183.

Wall TL, Ehlers CL. Genetic influences affecting alcohol use among Asians. *Alcohol Health Res World,* **1995**, *19*:184–189.

Wartenberg AA. Management of common medical problems. In, *Principles of Addiction Medicine,* 2d ed. (Graham AW and Shultz TK, eds.) American Society of Addiction Medicine, Chevy Chase, MD, **1998**, pp. 731–740.

Wassif WS, Preedy VR, Summers B, et al. The relationship between muscle fibre atrophy factor, plasma carnosinase activities, and muscle RNA and protein composition in chronic alcoholic myopathy. *Alcohol Alcohol,* **1993**, *28*:325–331.

Whitcomb DC, Block GD. Association of acetaminophen hepatotoxicity with fasting and ethanol use. *JAMA,* **1994**, *272*: 1845–1850.

Wilde MI, Wagstaff AJ. Acamprosate: A review of its pharmacology and clinical potential in the management of alcohol dependence after detoxification. *Drugs,* **1997**, *53*: 1038–1053.

Drug Addiction

Charles P. O'Brien

The terminology used in discussing drug dependence, abuse, and addiction has long been confusing. Confusion stems from the fact that repeated use of certain prescribed medications can produce neuroplastic changes resulting in two distinctly abnormal states. The first is *dependence*, sometimes called "physical" dependence, produced when there is progressive pharmacological adaptation to the drug resulting in tolerance. In the tolerant state, repeating the same dose of drug produces a smaller effect. If the drug is abruptly stopped, a withdrawal syndrome ensues in which the adaptive responses are now unopposed by the drug. Thus, withdrawal symptoms are opposite to the original drug effects. The appearance of withdrawal symptoms is the cardinal sign of "physical" dependence. As thus defined, dependence can occur with the use of opioids, β blockers, antidepressants, benzodiazepines, and stimulants, even when these agents are used as prescribed for therapeutic purposes. The state of "physical" dependence is a normal response, easily treatable by tapering the drug dose, and is not in itself a sign of addiction.

The second abnormal state that can be produced by repeated drug use occurs in only a minority of those who initiate drug use. It leads progressively to compulsive, out-of-control drug use. Unfortunately, in 1987 the American Psychiatric Association (APA) chose to use the word "dependence" when defining the state of uncontrolled drug use more commonly known as *addiction*. The word "addiction" was at that time considered pejorative and thus to be avoided. The result, over the last two decades, is that confusion has developed between dependence as a normal response and dependence as addiction. The newest version of the *Diagnostic and Statistical Manual of Mental Disorders* (DSM-V) due to be released in 2012 will correct this confusion.

This distinction between dependence and addiction is important because patients with pain sometimes are deprived of adequate opioid medication simply because they have shown evidence of tolerance or they exhibit withdrawal symptoms if the analgesic medication is stopped or reduced abruptly.

Modern neuroscience has greatly increased our understanding of the phenomenology of addiction. Using animal models as well as human brain imaging studies and clinical observations, addiction can be defined fundamentally as a form of maladaptive memory. It begins with the administration of substances (e.g., cocaine) or behaviors (e.g., the thrill of gambling) that directly and intensely activate brain reward circuits. Activation of these circuits motivates normal behavior and most humans simply enjoy the experience without being compelled to repeat it. For some (~16% of those who try cocaine) the experience produces strong conditioned associations to environmental cues that signal the availability of the drug or the behavior. Thus, reflexive activation of reward circuits becomes involuntary and with a very rapid onset. The cues acquire strong salience that overwhelms other behaviors. The individual becomes drawn into compulsive repetition of the experience focusing on the immediate pleasure despite negative long-term consequences and neglect of important social responsibilities. Of course, underlying this behavior are poorly understood changes in neural circuits (Kalivas and O'Brien, 2008).

The framers of DSM-V are strongly motivated to devise a classification well-grounded in neuroscientific evidence. Unfortunately, complex psychiatric disorders still have no proven genetic basis nor are there reliable biomarkers of these disorders. Thus, the plan is to make DSM-V a flexible document that can be further revised as reliable, replicated data are developed.

Origins of Substance Dependence

The chronic, relapsing nature of addiction fulfills criteria for a chronic disease (McLellan et al., 2000), but because of the voluntary component at initiation, the disease concept is controversial. Most of those who initiate drug use do not progress to become addicts. Many variables operate simultaneously to influence the likelihood that a beginning drug user will lose control and develop an addiction. These variables can be organized into three categories: agent (drug), host (user), and environment (Table 24–1).

Agent (Drug) Variables. Drugs vary in their capacity to produce immediate good feelings in the user. Drugs that reliably produce intensely pleasant feelings (euphoria) are more likely to be taken repeatedly. *Reinforcement* refers to the capacity of drugs to produce effects that make the user wish to take them again. The more strongly reinforcing a drug is, the greater is the likelihood that the drug will be abused.

Table 24–1

Multiple Simultaneous Variables Affecting Onset and Continuation of Drug Abuse and Addiction

Agent (drug)
Availability
Cost
Purity/potency
Mode of administration
Chewing (absorption *via* oral mucous membranes)
Gastrointestinal
Intranasal
Subcutaneous and intramuscular
Intravenous
Inhalation
Speed of onset and termination of effects (pharmacokinetics: combination of agent and host)
Host (user)
Heredity
Innate tolerance
Speed of developing acquired tolerance
Likelihood of experiencing intoxication as pleasure
Metabolism of the drug (nicotine and alcohol data already available)
Psychiatric symptoms
Prior experiences/expectations
Propensity for risk-taking behavior
Environment
Social setting
Community attitudes
Peer influence, role models
Availability of other reinforcers (sources of pleasure or recreation)
Employment or educational opportunities
Conditioned stimuli: environmental cues become associated with drugs after repeated use in the same environment

Reinforcing properties of a drug can be measured reliably in animals. Generally, animals such as rats or monkeys equipped with intravenous catheters connected to lever-regulated pumps will work to obtain injections of the same drugs in roughly the same order of potency that humans will. Thus, medications can be screened for their potential for abuse in humans by the use of animal models. Other drugs such as ethanol can be self-administered by the oral route by experimental animals. Animals can also model relapse to drug-taking in humans. For example, rats learn to drink alcohol in preference to water. If alcohol availability is removed, the animals go through withdrawal. They will restart ("relapse" to) alcohol drinking if presented with cues previously associated with alcohol availability or if given mild stress (foot shock).

Reinforcing properties of drugs are associated with their capacity to increase neuronal activity in critical brain areas (Chapter 14). Cocaine, amphetamine, ethanol, opiates, cannabinoids, and nicotine all reliably increase extracellular fluid dopamine (DA) levels in the ventral striatum, specifically the nucleus accumbens region. In experimental animals, usually rats, brain microdialysis permits sampling of extracellular fluid while the animals are freely moving or receiving drugs. Smaller increases in DA in the nucleus accumbens also are observed when the rat is presented with sweet foods or a sexual partner. In contrast, drugs that block DA receptors generally produce bad feelings, i.e., dysphoric effects. Neither animals nor humans will take such drugs spontaneously. Despite strong correlative findings, a causal relationship between DA and euphoria/dysphoria has not been established, and other findings emphasize additional roles of serotonin (5-HT), glutamate, norepinephrine (NE), endogenous opioids, and γ-aminobutyric acid (GABA) in mediating the reinforcing effects of drugs.

The abuse liability of a drug is enhanced by rapidity of onset because effects that occur soon after administration are more likely to initiate the chain of events that leads to loss of control over drug-taking. The pharmacokinetic variables that influence the time it takes a drug to reach critical receptor sites in the brain are explained in more detail in Chapter 2. The history of cocaine use illustrates the changes in abuse liability of the same compound, depending on the form and the route of administration.

When coca leaves are chewed, cocaine is absorbed slowly through the buccal mucosa. This method produces low cocaine blood levels and correspondingly low levels in the brain. The mild stimulant effects produced by the chewing of coca leaves have a gradual onset, and this practice has produced few, if any, behavior problems despite use over thousands of years by natives of the Andes mountains. Beginning in the late 19th century, scientists isolated cocaine hydrochloride from coca leaves and refined the technology for extraction of pure cocaine. Cocaine could be taken in higher doses by oral ingestion (GI absorption) or by absorption through the nasal mucosa, producing higher cocaine levels in the blood and a more rapid onset of stimulation. Subsequently, it was found that a solution of cocaine hydrochloride could be administered intravenously, giving a more rapid onset of stimulatory effects. Each newly available cocaine preparation that provided greater speed of onset and an increment in blood level was paralleled by a greater likelihood of addiction. In the 1980s, the availability of cocaine to the American public was increased further with the invention of crack cocaine. Crack, sold illegally and at a low price ($1-3 per dose), is alkaloidal cocaine (free base), which can be readily vaporized by heating. Simply inhaling the vapors produces blood levels comparable to those resulting from intravenous cocaine owing to the large surface area for absorption into the pulmonary circulation following inhalation. The cocaine-containing blood then enters the left side of the heart and reaches the cerebral circulation without dilution by the systemic circulation. Thus, inhalation of crack cocaine is much more addictive than chewing, drinking, or sniffing cocaine. Inhalation, with rapid attainment of effective drug levels in the brain, also is the preferred route for users of nicotine and cannabis.

Although the drug variables are important, they do not fully explain the development of addiction. Most people who experiment with drugs of high addictive potential (addiction liability) do not intensify their drug use and lose control. The risk for developing addiction among those who try nicotine is about twice that for those who try cocaine (Table 24–2). This does not imply that the pharmacological addiction liability of nicotine is twice that of cocaine. Rather, there are other variables listed in the categories of host factors and environmental conditions that influence the development of addiction.

Table 24–2

Dependence among Users 1990–1992

AGENT	EVER USED* %	ADDICTION %	RISK OF ADDICTION %
Tobacco	75.6	24.1	31.9
Alcohol	91.5	14.1	15.4
Illicit drugs	51.0	7.5	14.7
Cannabis	46.3	4.2	9.1
Cocaine	16.2	2.7	16.7
Stimulants	15.3	1.7	11.2
Anxiolytics	12.7	1.2	9.2
Analgesics	9.7	0.7	7.5
Psychedelics	10.6	0.5	4.9
Heroin	1.5	0.4	23.1
Inhalants	6.8	0.3	3.7

*The ever-used and addiction percentages are those of the general population. The risk of addiction is specific to the drug indicated and refers to the percentage who met criteria for addiction among those who reported having used the agent at least once (i.e., each value in column 4 was obtained by expressing the number in column 3 as a percentage of the number in column 2, subject to errors of rounding). *Source:* Anthony et al., 1994.

Host (User) Variables. In general, effects of drugs vary among individuals. Even blood levels can show wide variation when the same dose of a drug on a milligram-per-kilogram basis is given to different people. Polymorphism of genes that encode enzymes involved in absorption, metabolism, and excretion and in receptor-mediated responses may contribute to the different degrees of reinforcement or euphoria observed among individuals (Chapters 6 and 7).

Children of alcoholics show an increased likelihood of developing alcoholism, even when adopted at birth and raised by nonalcoholic parents. The studies of genetic influences in this disorder show only an *increased risk* for developing alcoholism, not a 100% determinism, consistent with a polygenic disorder that has multiple determinants. Even identical twins, who share the same genetic endowment, do not have 100% concordance when one twin is alcoholic. However, the concordance rate for identical twins is much higher than that for fraternal twins. The abuse of alcohol and other drugs tends to have some familial characteristics, suggesting that common mechanisms may be involved.

Innate tolerance to alcohol as measured by level of response to alcohol administered under experimental conditions may represent a biological trait that contributes to the development of alcoholism (Chapter 23). While innate tolerance increases vulnerability to alcoholism, impaired metabolism may *protect* against it. See Chapter 23 for a discussion of the genetic variation common in Asian populations that results in facial flushing and reduced alcohol intake or no alcohol intake in those homozygous for the gene variant. Similarly, individuals who inherit a gene associated with slow nicotine metabolism may experience unpleasant effects when beginning to smoke and reportedly have a lower probability of becoming nicotine dependent.

Psychiatric disorders constitute another category of host variables. Drugs may produce immediate, subjective effects that relieve preexisting symptoms. People with anxiety, depression, insomnia, or even subtle symptoms such as shyness may find, on experimentation or by accident, that certain drugs give them relief. However, the apparent beneficial effects are transient, and repeated use of the drug may lead to tolerance and eventually compulsive, uncontrolled drug use. While psychiatric symptoms are seen commonly in drug abusers presenting for treatment, most of these symptoms begin *after* the person starts abusing drugs. Thus, drugs of abuse appear to produce more psychiatric symptoms than they relieve.

Environmental Variables. Initiating and continuing illegal drug use appear to be influenced significantly by societal norms and peer pressure. Taking drugs may be seen initially as a form of rebellion against authority. In some communities, drug users and drug dealers are role models who seem to be successful and respected; thus, young people emulate them. There also may be a paucity of other options for pleasure, diversion, or income. These factors are particularly important in communities where educational levels are low and job opportunities scarce.

Pharmacological Phenomena

Tolerance. While abuse and addiction are complex conditions combining the many variables outlined earlier, there are a number of relevant pharmacological phenomena that occur independent of social and psychological dimensions. First are the changes in the way the body responds to a drug with repeated use. *Tolerance*, the most common response to repetitive use of the same drug, can be defined as the reduction in response to the drug after repeated administrations. Figure 24–1 shows an idealized dose-response curve for an administered drug. As the dose of the drug increases, the observed effect of the drug increases. With repeated use of the drug, however, the curve shifts to the right (tolerance). Thus, a higher dose is required to produce the same effect that was once obtained at a lower dose. Diazepam, e.g., typically produces sedation at doses of 5-10 mg in a first-time user, but those who repeatedly use it to produce a kind of "high" may become tolerant to doses of several hundreds of milligrams; some abusers have had documented tolerance to >1000 mg/day. As outlined in Table 24–3, there are many forms of tolerance likely arising through multiple mechanisms.

Table 24–3

Types of Tolerance

Types of Tolerance
Innate (pre-existing sensitivity or insensitivity)
Acquired
Pharmacokinetic (dispositional or metabolic)
Pharmacodynamic
Learned tolerance
Behavioral
Conditioned
Acute tolerance
Reverse tolerance (sensitization)
Cross-tolerance

Tolerance to some drug effects develops much more rapidly than to other effects of the same drug. For example, tolerance develops rapidly to the euphoria produced by opioids such as heroin, and addicts tend to increase their dose in order to re-experience that elusive "high." In contrast, tolerance to the gastrointestinal effects of opioids develops more slowly. The discrepancy between tolerance to euphorigenic effects (rapid) and tolerance to effects on vital functions (slow), such as respiration and blood pressure, can lead to potentially fatal overdoses in sedative abusers trying to re-experience the euphoria they recall from earlier use.

Innate tolerance refers to genetically determined lack of sensitivity to a drug that is observed the first time that the drug is administered. Innate tolerance was discussed earlier as a host variable that influences the development of addiction. See Chapter 23 for discussion of the inheritance of level of response to ethanol.

Acquired tolerance can be divided into three major types: pharmacokinetic, pharmacodynamic, and learned tolerance, and includes acute, reverse, and cross-tolerance (Table 24–3).

Pharmacokinetic or *dispositional tolerance* refers to changes in the distribution or metabolism of a drug after repeated administrations such that a given dose produces a lower blood concentration than the same dose did on initial exposure. The most common mechanism is an increase in the rate of metabolism of the drug. For example, barbiturates stimulate the production of higher levels of hepatic CYPs, causing more rapid removal and breakdown of barbiturates from the circulation. Since the same enzymes metabolize many other drugs, they too are metabolized more quickly. This results in a decrease in their plasma levels as well and a reduction in their therapeutic effects.

Pharmacodynamic tolerance refers to adaptive changes that have taken place within systems affected by the drug so that response to a given concentration of the drug is reduced. Examples include drug-induced changes in receptor density or efficiency of receptor coupling to signal-transduction pathways (Chapters 3 and 14).

Learned tolerance refers to a reduction in the effects of a drug owing to compensatory mechanisms that are acquired by past experiences. One type of learned tolerance is called *behavioral tolerance.* This simply describes the skills that can be developed through repeated experiences with attempting to function despite a state of mild to moderate intoxication. A common example is learning to walk a straight line despite the motor impairment produced by alcohol intoxication. This probably involves both acquisition of motor skills and the learned awareness of one's deficit, causing the person to walk more carefully. At higher levels of intoxication, behavioral tolerance is overcome, and the deficits are obvious.

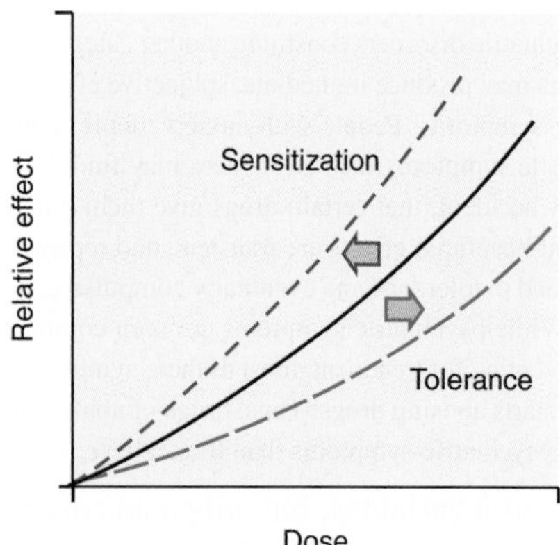

Figure 24–1. *Shifts in a dose-response curve with tolerance and sensitization.* With tolerance, there is a shift of the curve to the right such that doses higher than initial doses are required to achieve the same effects. With sensitization, there is a leftward shift of the curve such that for a given dose, there is a greater effect than seen after the initial dose.

Conditioned tolerance (situation-specific tolerance) develops when environmental cues such as sights, smells, or situations consistently are paired with the administration of a drug. When a drug affects homeostatic balance by producing sedation and changes in blood pressure, pulse rate, gut activity, and so on, there is usually a reflexive counteraction or adaptation in the direction of maintaining the status quo. If a drug always is taken in the presence of specific environmental cues (e.g., smell of drug preparation and sight of syringe), these cues begin to predict the effects of the drug, and the adaptations begin to occur even before the drug reaches its sites of action. If the drug always is preceded by the same cues, the adaptive response to the drug will be learned, and this will prevent the full manifestation of the drug's effects (tolerance). This mechanism of conditioned tolerance production follows classical (pavlovian) principles of learning and results in drug tolerance under circumstances where the drug is "expected." When the drug is received under novel or "unexpected" circumstances, conditioned tolerance does not occur, and drug effects are enhanced.

The term *acute tolerance* refers to rapid tolerance developing with repeated use on a single occasion, such as in a "binge." For example, cocaine often is used in a binge, with repeated doses over one to several hours, sometimes longer, producing a decrease in response to subsequent doses of cocaine during the binge. This is the opposite of *sensitization*, observed with an intermittent dosing schedule, described in the next section.

Sensitization. With stimulants such as cocaine or amphetamine, *reverse tolerance*, or *sensitization*, can occur. This refers to an increase in response with repetition of the same dose of the drug. Sensitization results in a shift to the left of the dose-response curve (Figure 24–1). For example, with repeated daily administration to rats of a dose of cocaine that produces increased motor activity, the effect increases over several days, even though the dose remains constant. A conditioned response also can be a part of sensitization to cocaine. Simply putting a rat into a cage where cocaine is expected or giving a placebo injection after several days of receiving cocaine under the same circumstances produces an increase in motor activity as though cocaine actually were given, i.e., a conditioned response. Sensitization, in contrast to acute tolerance during a binge, requires a longer interval between doses, usually ~1 day.

Sensitization has been studied in rats equipped with microdialysis cannulas for monitoring extracellular DA (Kalivas and Duffy, 1990) (Figure 24–2). The initial response to 10 mg/kg of cocaine administered intraperitoneally is an increase in measured DA levels. After seven daily injections, the DA increase is significantly greater than on the first day, and the behavioral response also is greater. Figure 24–2 also provides an example of a conditioned response (learned drug effect): injection of saline produced both an increase in DA levels and an increase in behavioral activity when administered 3 days after cocaine injections had stopped. Little research on sensitization has been conducted in human subjects, but the results suggest that the phenomenon can occur. It has been postulated that stimulant psychosis results from a sensitized response after long intermittent periods of use.

Cross-tolerance occurs when repeated use of a drug in a given category confers tolerance not only to that drug but also to other drugs in the same structural and mechanistic category. Understanding cross-tolerance is important in the medical management of persons dependent on any drug. *Detoxification* is a form of treatment for drug dependence that involves giving gradually decreasing doses of the drug to prevent withdrawal symptoms, thereby weaning the patient from the drug of dependence (see "Detoxification" later in the chapter). Detoxification can be accomplished with any medication in the same category as the initial drug of dependence. For example, users of heroin also are tolerant to other opioids. Thus, the detoxification of heroin-dependent patients can be accomplished with any medication that activates opioid receptors.

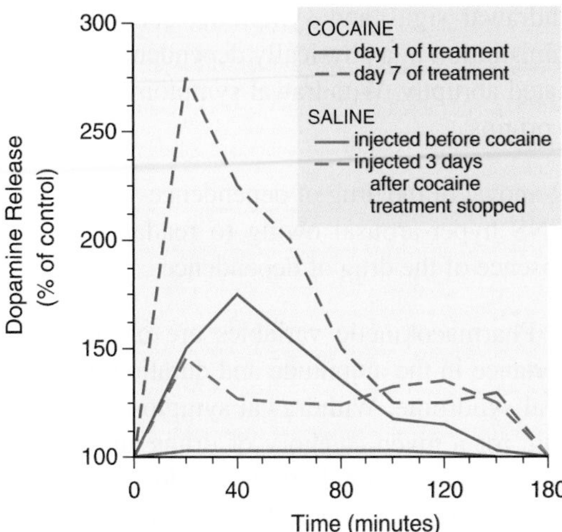

Figure 24–2. *Cocaine-induced changes in CNS dopamine release.* Dopamine was measured in the extracellular fluid of the nucleus accumbens of rats after daily injections of cocaine (10 mg/kg, i.p.). The first injection of cocaine produced a modest increase and the last, after 7 days, produced a much greater increase in dopamine release. The first saline injection produced no effect on dopamine levels, whereas the second, given 3 days after 7 days of cocaine injections, produced a significant rise in dopamine, presumably due to conditioning. (Adapted from Kalivas and Duffy, 1990.)

Physical Dependence

Physical dependence is a state that develops as a result of the adaptation (tolerance) produced by a resetting of homeostatic mechanisms in response to repeated drug use. Drugs can affect numerous systems that previously were in equilibrium; these systems find a new balance in the presence of inhibition or stimulation by a specific drug. A person in this adapted or physically dependent state requires continued administration of the drug to maintain normal function. If administration of the drug is stopped abruptly, there is another imbalance, and the affected systems again must go through a process of readjusting to a new equilibrium without the drug.

Withdrawal Syndrome. The appearance of a withdrawal syndrome when administration of the drug is terminated is the only actual evidence of physical dependence.

Withdrawal signs and symptoms occur when drug administration in a physically dependent person is terminated abruptly. Withdrawal symptoms have at least two origins:

- Removal of the drug of dependence
- CNS hyper-arousal owing to readaptation to the absence of the drug of dependence

Pharmacokinetic variables are of considerable importance in the amplitude and duration of the withdrawal syndrome. Withdrawal symptoms are characteristic for a given category of drugs and tend to be opposite to the original effects produced by the drug before tolerance developed. Thus, abrupt termination of a drug (such as an opioid agonist) that produces miotic (constricted) pupils and slow heart rate will produce a withdrawal syndrome including dilated pupils and tachycardia. Tolerance, physical dependence, and withdrawal are all biological phenomena. They are the natural consequences of drug use and can be produced in experimental animals and in any human being who takes certain medications repeatedly. These symptoms in themselves do not imply that the individual is involved in misuse or addictive behavior. This form of dependence should not be confused with addiction (compulsive drug-taking). *Patients who take medicine for appropriate medical indications and in correct dosages still may show tolerance, physical dependence, and withdrawal symptoms if the drug is stopped abruptly rather than gradually.* For example, a hypertensive patient receiving a β adrenergic receptor blocker such as metoprolol may have a good therapeutic response, but if the drug is stopped abruptly, the patient may experience a withdrawal syndrome consisting of rebound increased blood pressure temporarily higher than that prior to beginning the medication. This response is thought to be due to adaptive synthesis of β receptors that, in sudden the absence of antagonist, facilitate an excessive β adrenergic response in cardiac cells.

Medical addict is a term used to describe a patient in treatment for a medical disorder who has become "addicted" to the available prescribed drugs; the patient begins taking them in excessive doses, out of control. An example would be a patient with chronic pain, anxiety, or insomnia who begins using the prescribed medication more often than directed by the physician. If the physician restricts the prescriptions, the patient may begin seeing several doctors without the knowledge of the primary physician. Such patients also may visit emergency rooms for the purpose of obtaining additional medication. This scenario is very uncommon, considering the large number of patients who receive medications capable of producing tolerance and physical dependence. *Fear of producing such medical addicts results in needless suffering among patients with pain,* because physicians needlessly limit appropriate medications. Tolerance and physical dependence are inevitable consequences of chronic treatment with opioids and certain other drugs, but tolerance and physical dependence by themselves do not imply "addiction."

CLINICAL ISSUES

The treatment of physical dependence will be discussed with reference to the specific drug of abuse and dependence problems characteristic to each category: CNS depressants, including alcohol and other sedatives; nicotine and tobacco; opioids; psychostimulants, such as amphetamine and cocaine; cannabinoids; psychedelic drugs; and inhalants (volatile solvents, nitrous oxide, and ethyl ether). Abuse of combinations of drugs across these categories is common. Alcohol is so widely available that it is combined with practically all other categories. Some combinations reportedly are taken because of their interactive effects. An example is the combination of heroin and cocaine ("speedball"), which will be described with the opioid category. Alcohol and cocaine is another very common combination. When confronted with a patient exhibiting signs of overdose or withdrawal, the physician must be aware of these possible combinations because each drug may require specific treatment.

CNS Depressants

Ethanol. Experimentation with ethanol is almost universal, and a high proportion of users find the experience pleasant. More than 90% of American adults report experience with ethanol (commonly called "alcohol"), and ~70% report some level of current use. The lifetime prevalence of alcohol use disorders (alcoholism) in men is almost 20% and in women is 10-15% (Hasin et al., 2007). This drug is discussed more fully in Chapter 23. Ethanol is classified as a depressant because it indeed produces sedation and sleep. However, the initial effects of alcohol, particularly at lower doses, often are perceived as stimulation owing to a suppression of inhibitory systems. Those who perceive only sedation from alcohol generally choose not to drink when evaluated in a test procedure (de Wit et al., 1989).

Alcohol impairs recent memory and, in high doses, produces the phenomenon of "blackouts": the drinker has no memory of his or her behavior while intoxicated. The effects of alcohol on memory are unclear, but evidence suggests that reports from patients about their reasons for drinking and their behavior during a binge are not reliable. Alcohol-dependent persons often say that they drink to relieve anxiety or depression. When allowed to drink under observation, however, alcoholics typically become more dysphoric as drinking continues

(Mendelson and Mello, 1979), thus not supporting the idea that alcoholics drink to relieve tension.

Tolerance, Physical Dependence, and Withdrawal. Mild intoxication by alcohol is familiar to almost everyone, but the symptoms vary among individuals. Some simply experience motor incoordination and sleepiness. Others initially become stimulated and garrulous. As the blood level increases, the sedating effects increase, with eventual coma and death occurring at high alcohol levels. The initial sensitivity (innate tolerance) to alcohol varies greatly among individuals and is related to family history of alcoholism (Wilhelmsen et al., 2003). Experience with alcohol can produce greater tolerance (acquired tolerance) such that extremely high blood levels (300-400 mg/dL) can be found in alcoholics who do not appear grossly sedated. In these cases, the lethal dose does not increase proportionately to the sedating dose, and thus the margin of safety (therapeutic index) is decreased.

Heavy consumers of alcohol not only acquire tolerance but also inevitably develop a state of physical dependence. This often leads to drinking in the morning to restore blood alcohol levels diminished during the night. Eventually, they may awaken during the night and take a drink to avoid the restlessness produced by falling alcohol levels. The alcohol-withdrawal syndrome (Table 24–4) generally depends on the size of the average daily dose and usually is "treated" by resumption of alcohol ingestion. Withdrawal symptoms are experienced frequently but usually are not severe or life-threatening until they occur in conjunction with other problems, such as infection, trauma, malnutrition, or electrolyte imbalance. In the setting of such complications, the syndrome of delirium tremens becomes likely.

Alcohol addiction produces cross-tolerance to other sedatives such as benzodiazepines. This tolerance is operative in abstinent alcoholics, but while the alcoholic is drinking, the sedating effects of alcohol add to those of other sedatives, making the combination more dangerous. This is particularly true for benzodiazepines, which are relatively safe in overdose when given alone but potentially are lethal in combination with alcohol.

The chronic use of alcohol and other sedatives is associated with the development of depression (McLellan et al., 1979), and the risk of suicide among alcoholics is one of the highest of any diagnostic category. Cognitive deficits have been reported in alcoholics tested while sober. These deficits usually improve after weeks to months of abstinence. More severe recent memory impairment is associated with specific brain damage caused by nutritional deficiencies common in alcoholics (e.g., thiamine deficiency).

Alcohol is toxic to many organ systems. As a result, the medical complications of alcohol abuse and dependence include liver disease, cardiovascular disease, endocrine and GI effects, and malnutrition, in addition to the CNS dysfunctions outlined earlier. Ethanol readily crosses the placental barrier, producing the fetal alcohol syndrome, a major cause of mental retardation (Chapter 23).

Pharmacological Interventions.

Detoxification. A patient who presents in a medical setting with an alcohol-withdrawal syndrome should be considered to have a potentially lethal condition. Although most mild cases of alcohol withdrawal never come to medical attention, severe cases require general evaluation; attention to hydration and electrolytes; vitamins, especially high-dose thiamine; and a sedating medication that has cross-tolerance with alcohol. To block or diminish the symptoms described in Table 24–4, a short-acting benzodiazepine such as oxazepam can be used at a dose of 15-30 mg every 6-8 hours according to the stage and severity of withdrawal; some authorities recommend a long-acting benzodiazepine unless there is demonstrated liver impairment. Anticonvulsants such as carbamazepine have been shown to be effective in alcohol withdrawal, although they appear not to relieve subjective symptoms as well as benzodiazepines. After medical evaluation, uncomplicated alcohol withdrawal can be treated effectively on an outpatient basis. When there are medical problems, a history of seizures, or simultaneous dependence on other drugs, hospitalization is required.

Pharmacotherapy. Detoxification is only the first step of treatment. Complete abstinence is the objective of long-term treatment, and this is accomplished mainly by behavioral approaches. Medications that aid in the prevention of relapse are under development. Disulfiram (ANTABUSE; Chapter 23) has been useful in some programs that focus behavioral efforts on ingestion of the medication. Disulfiram blocks aldehyde dehydrogenase, the second step in ethanol metabolism, resulting in the accumulation of acetaldehyde, which produces an unpleasant flushing reaction when alcohol is ingested. Knowledge of this unpleasant reaction helps the patient to resist taking a drink. Although quite effective pharmacologically, disulfiram has not been found to be effective in controlled clinical trials because so many patients failed to ingest the medication.

Naltrexone (REVIA; Chapter 23), an opioid receptor antagonist that blocks the reinforcing properties of alcohol, is FDA-approved as an adjunct in the treatment of alcoholism. Chronic administration of naltrexone resulted in a decreased rate of relapse to alcohol drinking in the majority of published double-blind clinical trials (Pettinati et al., 2006). It works best in combination with behavioral treatment programs that encourage adherence to medication and abstinence from alcohol. A depot preparation with a duration of 30 days (VIVITROL) was approved by the FDA in 2006; it greatly improves medication adherence, the major problem with the use of medications in alcoholism.

Table 24–4

Alcohol Withdrawal Syndrome

Alcohol Withdrawal Syndrome
Alcohol craving
Tremor, irritability
Nausea
Sleep disturbance
Tachycardia
Hypertension
Sweating
Perceptual distortion
Seizures (6-48 hours after last drink)
Visual (and occasionally auditory or tactile) hallucinations (12-48 hours after last drink)
Delirium tremens (48-96 hours after last drink; rare in uncomplicated withdrawal)
Severe agitation
Confusion
Fever, profuse sweating
Tachycardia
Nausea, diarrhea
Dilated pupils

A significant development in identifying a potential endophenotype of alcoholism has grown out of the clinical experience with naltrexone. Animal studies have demonstrated that alcohol causes the release of endogenous opioids in brain reward systems and the disinhibition or activation of DA neurons, a condition common to all drugs of abuse. Blocking opioid receptors prevents this dopaminergic effect and results in less stimulation or reward from alcohol (Ray and Hutchison, 2007). A functional allele of the gene for the μ opioid receptor that naltrexone blocks has been associated with alcohol stimulation and with good response to naltrexone treatment among alcoholics (Anton et al., 2006).

Acamprosate (CAMPRAL), another FDA-approved medication for alcoholism (Mason, 2003), is a competitive inhibitor of the *N*-methyl-D-aspartate (NMDA)–type glutamate receptor. The drug appears to normalize the dysregulated neurotransmission associated with chronic ethanol intake and thereby to attenuate one of the mechanisms that lead to relapse (Chapter 23).

Benzodiazepines. Benzodiazepines are among the most commonly prescribed medications worldwide; they are used mainly for the treatment of anxiety disorders and insomnia (Chapters 15 and 17). Considering their widespread use, intentional abuse of prescription benzodiazepines is relatively uncommon. When a benzodiazepine is taken for up to several weeks, there is little tolerance and no difficulty in stopping the medication when the condition no longer warrants its use. After several months, the proportion of patients who become tolerant increases, and reducing the dose or stopping the medication produces withdrawal symptoms (Table 24–5).

It can be difficult to distinguish withdrawal symptoms from the reappearance of the anxiety symptoms for which the benzodiazepine was prescribed initially. Some patients may increase their dose over time because tolerance definitely develops to the sedative effects. Many patients and their physicians, however, contend that anti-anxiety benefits continue to occur long after tolerance to the sedating effects. Moreover, these patients continue to take the medication for years according to medical directions without increasing their dose and are able to function very effectively as long as they take the benzodiazepine. The degree to which tolerance develops to the anxiolytic effects of benzodiazepines is a subject of controversy. There is, however, good evidence that significant tolerance does not develop to all benzodiazepine actions because some effects of acute doses on memory persist in patients who have taken benzodiazepines for years. According to a task force that reviewed the issues and published guidelines on the proper medical use of benzodiazepines (American Psychiatric Association, 1990), intermittent use only when symptoms occur retards the development of tolerance and therefore is preferable to daily use. Patients with a history of alcohol- or other drug-abuse problems have an increased risk for the development of benzodiazepine abuse and should rarely, if ever, be treated with benzodiazepines on a chronic basis.

While relatively few patients who receive benzodiazepines for medical indications abuse their medication, there are individuals who specifically seek benzodiazepines for their ability to produce a "high." Among these abusers, there are differences in drug popularity; benzodiazepines that have a rapid onset, such as diazepam and alprazolam, tend to be the most desirable. The drugs may be obtained by simulating a medical condition and deceiving physicians or simply through illicit channels. Unsupervised use can lead to self-administration of large doses and therefore tolerance to the benzodiazepine's sedating effects. For example, while 5-20 mg/day of diazepam is a typical dose for a patient receiving prescribed medication, abusers may take over 1000 mg/day and not appear grossly sedated.

Abusers may combine benzodiazepines with other drugs to increase the effect. For example, it is part of the "street lore" that taking diazepam 30 minutes after an oral dose of methadone will produce an augmented high not obtainable with either drug alone.

While there is some illicit use of benzodiazepines as a primary drug of abuse, most of the unsupervised use seems to be by abusers of other drugs who are attempting to self-medicate the side effects or withdrawal effects of their primary drug of abuse. Thus, cocaine addicts often take diazepam to relieve the irritability and agitation produced by cocaine binges, and opioid addicts find that diazepam and other benzodiazepines relieve some of the anxiety symptoms of opioid withdrawal when they are unable to obtain their preferred drug.

Pharmacological Interventions. If patients receiving long-term benzodiazepine treatment by prescription wish to stop their medication, the process may take months of gradual dose reduction. Withdrawal symptoms (Table 24–5) may occur during this outpatient detoxification, but in most cases the symptoms are mild. If anxiety symptoms return, a non-benzodiazepine such as buspirone may be prescribed, but this agent usually is less effective than benzodiazepines for treatment of anxiety in these patients. Some authorities recommend transferring the patient to a long $t_{1/2}$ benzodiazepine during detoxification; others recommend the anticonvulsants carbamazepine and phenobarbital. Controlled studies comparing different treatment regimens are lacking. Since patients who have been on low doses of benzodiazepines for years usually have no adverse effects, the physician and patient should decide jointly whether detoxification and possible transfer to a new anxiolytic are worth the effort.

The specific benzodiazepine receptor antagonist flumazenil has been found useful in the treatment of overdose and in reversing the effects of long-acting benzodiazepines used in anesthesia. It has been used experimentally in the treatment of persistent withdrawal symptoms after cessation of long-term benzodiazepine treatment.

Table 24–5

Benzodiazepine Withdrawal Symptoms

Following moderate dose usage
- Anxiety, agitation
- Increased sensitivity to light and sound
- Paresthesias, strange sensations
- Muscle cramps
- Myoclonic jerks
- Sleep disturbance
- Dizziness

Following high-dose usage
- Seizures
- Delirium

Deliberate abusers of high doses of benzodiazepines usually require inpatient detoxification. Frequently, benzodiazepine abuse is part of a combined dependence involving alcohol, opioids, and cocaine. Detoxification can be a complex clinical pharmacological problem requiring knowledge of the pharmacokinetics of each drug. The patient's history may be unreliable not simply because of lying but also because the patient frequently does not *know* the true identity or dose of drugs purchased on the street. Medication for detoxification should not be prescribed by the "cookbook" approach but by careful titration and patient observation. The withdrawal syndrome from diazepam, e.g., may not become evident until the patient develops a seizure in the second week of hospitalization. One approach to complex detoxification is to focus on the CNS-depressant drug and temporarily hold the opioid component constant with a low dose of methadone. Opioid detoxification can begin later. A long-acting benzodiazepine such as diazepam or clorazepate (TRANXENE, others) or a long-acting barbiturate such as phenobarbital can be used to block the sedative withdrawal symptoms. The phenobarbital dose should be determined by a series of test doses and subsequent observations to determine the level of tolerance. Most complex detoxifications can be accomplished using this phenobarbital loading-dose strategy (Robinson et al., 1981).

After detoxification, the prevention of relapse requires a long-term outpatient rehabilitation program similar to the treatment of alcoholism. No specific medications have been found to be useful in the rehabilitation of sedative abusers; but, of course, specific psychiatric disorders such as depression or schizophrenia, if present, require appropriate medications.

Barbiturates and Older Sedatives. The use of barbiturates and older non-benzodiazepine sedating medications (e.g., meprobamate, glutethimide, chloral hydrate) has declined greatly in recent years owing to the increased safety and to the efficacy of the benzodiazepines and the newer agents zolpidem, eszopiclone, zaleplon, and ramelteon (Chapters 15 and 17). Abuse problems with barbiturates resemble those seen with benzodiazepines in many ways. Treatment of abuse and addiction should be handled similarly to interventions for the abuse of alcohol and benzodiazepines. Because drugs in this category frequently are prescribed as hypnotics for patients complaining of insomnia, physicians should be aware of the problems that can develop when the hypnotic agent is withdrawn. Insomnia rarely should be treated with medication as a primary disorder except when produced by short-term stressful situations. Insomnia often is a symptom of an underlying chronic problem, such as depression or respiratory dysfunction, or may be due simply to a change in sleep requirements with age. Prescription of sedative medications, however, can change the physiology of sleep with subsequent tolerance to these medication effects. When the sedative is stopped, there is a rebound effect with worsened insomnia. This medication-induced insomnia requires detoxification by gradual dose reduction.

Nicotine

The basic pharmacology of nicotine and agents for smoking cessation are discussed in Chapter 11. Because nicotine provides the reinforcement for cigarette smoking, the most common cause of preventable death and disease in the U.S., it is arguably the most dangerous dependence-producing drug. The dependence produced by nicotine can be extremely durable, as exemplified by the high failure rate among smokers who try to quit. Although >80% of smokers express a desire to quit, only 35% try to stop each year, and fewer than 5% are successful in unaided attempts to quit (American Psychiatric Association, 2000).

Cigarette (nicotine) addiction is influenced by multiple variables. Nicotine itself produces reinforcement; users compare nicotine to stimulants such as cocaine or amphetamine, although its effects are of lower magnitude. While there are many casual users of alcohol and cocaine, few individuals who smoke cigarettes smoke a small enough quantity (≤5 cigarettes per day) to avoid dependence. Nicotine is absorbed readily through the skin, mucous membranes, and lungs. The pulmonary route produces discernible CNS effects in as little as 7 seconds. Thus, each puff produces some discrete reinforcement. With 10 puffs per cigarette, the one-pack-per-day smoker reinforces the habit 200 times daily. The timing, setting, situation, and preparation all become associated repetitively with the effects of nicotine.

Nicotine has both stimulant and depressant actions. The smoker feels alert, yet there is some muscle relaxation. Nicotine activates the nucleus accumbens reward system in the brain; increased extracellular DA has been found in this region after nicotine injections in rats. Nicotine affects other systems as well, including the release of endogenous opioids and glucocorticoids.

There is evidence for tolerance to the subjective effects of nicotine. Smokers typically report that the first cigarette of the day after a night of abstinence gives the "best" feeling. Smokers who return to cigarettes after a period of abstinence may experience nausea if they return immediately to their previous dose. Persons naive to the effects of nicotine will experience nausea at low nicotine blood levels, and smokers will experience nausea if nicotine levels are raised above their accustomed levels.

Negative reinforcement refers to the benefits obtained from the termination of an unpleasant state. In dependent smokers, the urge to smoke correlates with a low blood nicotine level, as though smoking were a means to achieve a certain nicotine level and thus avoid withdrawal symptoms. Some smokers even awaken during the night to have a cigarette, which ameliorates the effect of low nicotine blood levels that could disrupt sleep. If the nicotine level is maintained artificially by a slow intravenous infusion, the number of cigarettes smoked and in the number of puffs decrease. Thus, smokers may be smoking to achieve the reward of nicotine effects, to avoid the pain of nicotine withdrawal, or most likely a combination of the two. Nicotine withdrawal symptoms are listed in Table 24–6.

crosses the blood-brain barrier quickly, and is deacetylated to the active metabolites 6-monoacetyl morphine and morphine. After the intense euphoria, which lasts from 45 seconds to several minutes, there is a period of sedation and tranquility ("on the nod") lasting up to an hour. The effects of heroin wear off in 3-5 hours, depending on the dose. Experienced users may inject two to four times per day. Thus, the heroin addict is constantly oscillating between being "high" and feeling the sickness of early withdrawal (Figure 24–4). This produces many problems in the homeostatic systems regulated at least in part by endogenous opioids. For example, the hypothalamic-pituitary-gonadal axis and the hypothalamic-pituitary-adrenal axis are abnormal in heroin addicts. Women on heroin have irregular menses, and men have a variety of sexual performance problems. Mood also is affected. Heroin addicts are relatively docile and compliant after taking heroin, but during withdrawal, they become irritable and aggressive.

Based on patient reports, tolerance develops early to the euphoria-producing effects of opioids. There also is tolerance to the respiratory depressant, analgesic, sedative, and emetic properties. Heroin users tend to increase their daily dose, depending on their financial resources and the availability of the drug. If a supply is available, the dose can be increased progressively 100 times. Even in highly tolerant individuals, the possibility of overdose remains if tolerance is exceeded. Overdose is likely to occur when potency of the street sample is unexpectedly high or when the heroin is mixed with a far more potent opioid, such as fentanyl (SUBLIMAZE, others).

Addiction to heroin or other short-acting opioids produces behavioral disruptions and usually becomes incompatible with a productive life. There is a significant risk for opioid abuse and dependence among physicians and other health care workers who have access to potent opioids, tempting them toward unsupervised experimentation. Physicians often begin by assuming that they can manage their own dose, and they may rationalize their behavior based on the beneficial effects of the drug. Over time, however, the typical unsupervised opioid user loses control, and behavioral changes are observed by family and co-workers. Apart from the behavioral changes and the risk of overdose, especially with very potent opioids, chronic use of opioids is relatively nontoxic.

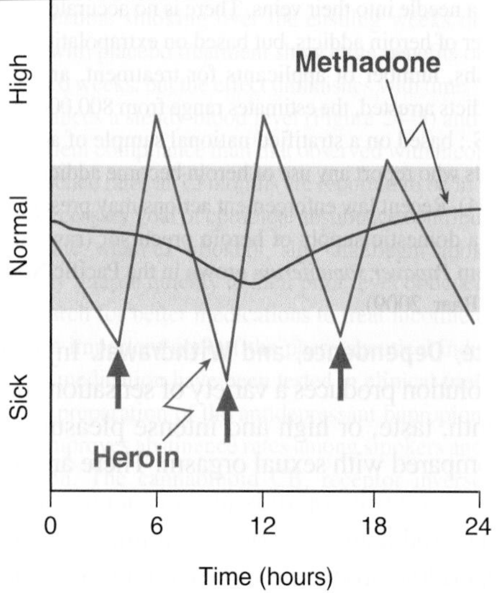

Figure 24–4. *Differences in responses to heroin and methadone.* A person who injects heroin (↑) several times per day oscillates (red line) between being sick and being high. In contrast, the typical methadone patient (purple line) remains in the "normal" range (indicated in blue) with little fluctuation after dosing once per day. The ordinate values represent the subject's mental and physical state, not plasma levels of the drug.

Opioids frequently are used in combinations with other drugs. A common combination is heroin and cocaine ("speedball"). Users report an improved euphoria because of the combination, and there is evidence of an interaction, because cocaine reduces the signs of opiate withdrawal, and heroin may reduce the irritability seen in chronic cocaine users.

The mortality rate for street heroin users is very high. Early death comes from involvement in crime to support the habit; from the uncertain dose, purity, and even identity of what is purchased on the street; and from serious infections associated with nonsterile drugs and sharing of injection paraphernalia. Heroin users commonly acquire bacterial infections producing skin abscesses; endocarditis; pulmonary infections, especially tuberculosis; and viral infections producing hepatitis C and acquired immune deficiency syndrome (AIDS).

As with other addictions, the first stage of treatment addresses physical dependence and consists of detoxification (Kosten and O'Conner, 2003). The opioid-withdrawal syndrome (Table 24–7) is very unpleasant but not life-threatening. It begins within 6-12 hours after the last dose of a short-acting opioid and as long as 72-84 hours after a very long-acting opioid medication. Heroin addicts go through early stages of this syndrome frequently when heroin is scarce or expensive. Some therapeutic communities as a matter of policy elect not to treat withdrawal so that the addict can experience the suffering while being given group support. The duration and intensity of the syndrome are related to the clearance of the individual drug. Heroin withdrawal is brief (5-10 days) and intense. Methadone withdrawal is slower in onset and lasts longer. Protracted withdrawal also is likely to be longer with methadone. (See more detailed discussions of protracted withdrawal under "Long-Term Management" later in the chapter.)

Table 24–7

Characteristics of Opioid Withdrawal

SYMPTOMS	SIGNS
Regular withdrawal	
Craving for opioids	Pupillary dilation
Restlessness, irritability	Sweating
Increased sensitivity to pain	Piloerection ("gooseflesh")
Nausea, cramps	Tachycardia
Muscle aches	Vomiting, diarrhea
Dysphoric mood	Increased blood pressure
Insomnia, anxiety	Yawning
	Fever
Protracted withdrawal	
Anxiety	Cyclic changes in weight, pupil size, respiratory center sensitivity
Insomnia	
Drug craving	

Pharmacological Interventions. Opioid withdrawal signs and symptoms can be treated by three different approaches. The first and most commonly used approach depends on cross-tolerance and consists of transfer to a prescription opioid medication and then gradual dose reduction. The same principles of detoxification apply as for other types of physical dependence. It is convenient to change the patient from a short-acting opioid such as heroin to a long-acting one such as methadone. Detoxification and subsequent maintenance of opiate dependence with methadone is specifically limited to accredited opioid treatment programs (OTPs) and is regulated by Federal Opioid Treatment Standards. The initial dose of methadone is typically 20-30 mg. This is a test dose to determine the level needed to reduce observed withdrawal symptoms. The first day's total dose then can be calculated depending on the response and then reduced by 20% per day during the course of detoxification.

A second approach to detoxification involves the use of oral clonidine (CATAPRES, others), a medication approved only for the treatment of hypertension. Clonidine is an α_2 adrenergic agonist that decreases adrenergic neurotransmission from the locus ceruleus. Many of the autonomic symptoms of opioid withdrawal such as nausea, vomiting, cramps, sweating, tachycardia, and hypertension result from the loss of opioid suppression of the locus ceruleus system during the abstinence syndrome. Clonidine, acting upon distinct receptors but by cellular mechanisms that mimic opioid effects, can alleviate many of the symptoms of opioid withdrawal, but not the generalized aches and opioid craving. When using clonidine to treat withdrawal, the dose must be titrated according to the stage and severity of withdrawal, beginning with 0.2 mg orally; postural hypotension is commonly a side effect. A similar drug, lofexidine (currently in clinical trials in the U.S.), has greater selectivity for α_{2A} adrenergic receptors and is associated with less of the hypotension that limits the usefulness of clonidine in this setting.

A third method of treating opioid withdrawal involves activation of the endogenous opioid system without medication. The techniques proposed include acupuncture and several methods of CNS activation using transcutaneous electrical stimulation. While attractive theoretically, this has not yet been found to be practical. Rapid antagonist-precipitated opioid detoxification under general anesthesia has received considerable publicity because it promises detoxification in several hours while the patient is unconscious and not experiencing withdrawal discomfort. A mixture of medications has been used, but morbidity and mortality as reported in the lay press are unacceptable, with no demonstrated advantage in long-term outcome (Collins et al., 2005).

Long-Term Management. If patients are simply discharged from the hospital after withdrawal from opioids, there is a high probability of a quick return to compulsive opioid use. Addiction is a chronic disorder that requires long-term treatment. Numerous factors influence relapse. One factor is that the withdrawal syndrome does not end in 5-7 days. There are subtle signs and symptoms often called the *protracted withdrawal syndrome* (Table 24–7) that persist for up to 6 months. Physiological measures tend to oscillate as though a new set point were being established; during this phase, outpatient drug-free treatment has a low probability of success, even when the patient has received intensive prior treatment while protected from relapse in a residential program.

The most successful treatment for heroin addiction consists of stabilization on methadone in accordance with state and federal regulations. Patients who relapse repeatedly during drug-free treatment can be transferred directly to methadone without requiring detoxification. The dose of methadone must be sufficient to prevent withdrawal symptoms for at least 24 hours. The introduction of buprenorphine, a partial agonist at μ opioid receptors (Chapter 18), represents a major change in the treatment of opiate addiction. This drug produces minimal withdrawal symptoms when discontinued and has a low potential for overdose, a long duration of action, and the ability to block heroin effects. Treatment can take place in a qualified physician's private office rather than in a special center, as required for methadone. When taken sublingually, buprenorphine (SUBUTEX) is active, but it also has the potential to be dissolved and injected (abused). A buprenorphine-naloxone combination (SUBOXONE) is also available. When taken orally (sublingually), the naloxone moiety is not effective, but if the patient abuses the medication by injecting, the naloxone will block or diminish the subjective high that could be produced by buprenorphine alone.

Agonist or Partial-Agonist Maintenance. Patients receiving methadone or buprenorphine will not experience the ups and downs produced by heroin (Figure 24–4). Drug craving diminishes and may disappear. Neuroendocrine rhythms eventually are restored (Kreek et al., 2002). Because of cross-tolerance (from methadone to heroin), patients who inject street heroin report a reduced effect from usual heroin doses. This cross-tolerance effect is dose-related, so higher methadone maintenance doses result in less illicit opioid use, as determined by random urine testing. Buprenorphine, as a partial agonist, has a ceiling effect at ~16 mg of the sublingual tablet equaling no more than 60 mg methadone. If the patient has a higher level of physical dependence, a full agonist (methadone) must be used. Patients become tolerant to the sedating effects of methadone and can attend school or function in a job. Opioids also have a persistent, mild, stimulating effect noticeable after tolerance to the sedating effect, such that reaction time is quicker and vigilance is increased while on a stable dose of methadone.

Antagonist Treatment. Another pharmacological option is opioid antagonist treatment. Naltrexone (REVIA, others; Chapter 18) is an antagonist with a high affinity for the μ opioid receptor (MOR); it will competitively block the effects of heroin or other MOR agonists. Naltrexone has almost no agonist effects of its own and will not satisfy craving or relieve protracted withdrawal symptoms. For these reasons, naltrexone treatment does not appeal to the average heroin addict, but it can be used after detoxification for patients with high motivation to remain opioid-free. Physicians, nurses, and pharmacists who have frequent access to opioid drugs make excellent candidates for this treatment approach. A depot formulation of naltrexone that provides 30 days of medication after a single injection (VIVITROL) has been approved for the treatment of alcoholism. This formulation eliminates the necessity of daily pill-taking and prevent relapse when the recently detoxified patient leaves a protected environment.

Cocaine and Other Psychostimulants

Cocaine. More than 23 million Americans have used cocaine at some time. Although chronic use and use by high school students has declined, the number of frequent users (at least weekly) has remained steady since 1991 at ~600,000. Not all users become addicts, and the variables that influence this risk are discussed at the beginning of this chapter. A key factor is the widespread availability of relatively inexpensive cocaine in the alkaloidal form (free base, "crack") suitable for smoking and in the hydrochloride powder form suitable for nasal or intravenous use. Drug abuse in men occurs about twice as frequently as in women. However, free basing is particularly common in young women of child-bearing age, who may use cocaine in this manner as commonly as do men.

The reinforcing effects of cocaine and cocaine analogs correlate best with their effectiveness in blocking the transporter that recovers DA from the synapse. This leads to increased DA concentrations at critical brain sites (Ritz et al., 1987). However, cocaine also blocks both NE and 5-HT reuptake, and chronic use of cocaine leads to reductions in the neurotransmitter metabolites 3-methoxy-4 hydroxyphenethyleneglycol (MOPEG or MHPG) and 5-hydroxyindoleacetic acid (5-HIAA).

The general pharmacology and medicinal use of cocaine as a local anesthetic are discussed in Chapter 20. Cocaine produces a dose-dependent increase in heart rate and blood pressure accompanied by increased arousal, improved performance on tasks of vigilance and alertness, and a sense of self-confidence and well-being. Higher doses produce euphoria, which has a brief duration and often is followed by a desire for more drug. Repeated doses may lead to involuntary motor activity, stereotyped behavior, and paranoia. Irritability and increased risk of violence are found among heavy chronic users. The $t_{1/2}$ of cocaine in plasma is ~50 minutes, but inhalant (crack) users typically desire more cocaine after 10-30 minutes. Intranasal and intravenous uses also result in a high of shorter duration than would be predicted by plasma cocaine levels, suggesting that a declining plasma concentration is associated with termination of the high and resumption of cocaine seeking. This theory is supported by positron-emission tomographic imaging studies using ^{11}C-labeled cocaine, which show that the time course of subjective euphoria parallels the accumulation and decline of the drug in the corpus striatum (Volkow et al., 2003).

The major route for cocaine metabolism involves hydrolysis of each of its two ester groups. Benzoylecgonine, produced on loss of the methyl group, represents the major urinary metabolite and can be found in the urine for 2-5 days after a binge. As a result, the benzoylecgonine test is a valid method for detecting cocaine use; the metabolite remains detectable in the urine of heavy users for up to 10 days. Cocaine frequently is used in combination with other drugs, as discussed previously. Ethanol is frequently abused with cocaine, as it reduces the irritability induced by cocaine. Dual addiction to alcohol and cocaine is common. When cocaine and alcohol are taken concurrently, cocaine may be transesterified to cocaethylene, which is equipotent to cocaine in blocking DA reuptake (Hearn et al., 1991).

Addiction is the most common complication of cocaine abuse. Intranasal users can continue intermittent use for years. Others become compulsive users despite elaborate methods to maintain control. In general, stimulants tend to be abused much more irregularly than opioids, nicotine, and alcohol. Binge use is very common, and a binge may last hours to days, terminating only when supplies of the drug are exhausted.

Toxicity. Other risks of cocaine, beyond the potential for addiction, include cardiac arrhythmias, myocardial ischemia, myocarditis, aortic dissection, cerebral vasoconstriction, and seizures. Death from trauma also is associated with cocaine use. Cocaine may induce premature labor and abruptio placentae (Chasnoff et al., 1989). The developmental abnormalities reported in infants born to cocaine users may be the result of cocaine effects as well as multiple other factors (the infant's prematurity, multiple-drug and alcohol exposure, and inadequate pre- and postnatal care).

Cocaine has been reported to produce a prolonged and intense orgasm if taken prior to intercourse, and users often indulge in compulsive and promiscuous sexual activity. However, chronic cocaine use reduces sexual drive. Chronic use is also associated with psychiatric disorders, including anxiety, depression, and psychosis, and while some of these disorders undoubtedly existed prior to addiction, many are likely attributable to the drug (McLellan et al., 1979).

Tolerance, Dependence, and Withdrawal. Sensitization, a consistent finding in animal studies of cocaine and other stimulants, is produced by intermittent use and typically is manifested as behavioral hyperactivity. In human cocaine users, the euphoric effect typically is not subject to sensitization. On the contrary, most experienced users become desensitized and, over time, require more cocaine to obtain euphoria, i.e., tolerance develops. In the laboratory, tolerance is rapidly induced by repeated administration of the same dose in one session (tachyphylaxis). Sensitization may involve conditioning (Figure 24–2). Cocaine users often report a strong response on seeing cocaine before it is administered, consisting of physiological arousal and increased drug craving with concomitant activation of brain limbic structures (Childress et al., 1999). Sensitization in humans has been linked to paranoid, psychotic manifestations of cocaine use (Satel et al., 1991). Since cocaine typically is used intermittently, even heavy users go through frequent periods of withdrawal or "crash." The symptoms of withdrawal seen in users admitted to hospitals are listed in Table 24–8. Careful studies of cocaine users during withdrawal show gradual diminution of these symptoms over 1-3 weeks (Weddington et al., 1990). Residual depression, often seen after cocaine withdrawal, should be treated with antidepressant agents if it persists (Chapter 15).

Pharmacological Interventions. Since cocaine withdrawal is generally mild, treatment of withdrawal symptoms usually is not required. The major problem in treatment is not detoxification but helping the patient to resist the urge to resume compulsive cocaine use. Rehabilitation programs involving individual and group psychotherapy based on the principles of Alcoholics Anonymous, and behavioral treatments based

Table 24–8

Cocaine Withdrawal Symptoms and Signs

Cocaine Withdrawal Symptoms and Signs
Dysphoria, depression
Sleepiness, fatigue
Cocaine craving
Bradycardia

on reinforcing cocaine-free urine tests, result in significant improvement in the majority of cocaine users (Alterman et al., 1994; Higgins et al., 1994). Nonetheless, there is great interest in finding a medication that can aid in the rehabilitation of cocaine addicts.

Numerous medications have been tried in placebo-controlled clinical trials with cocaine addicts, but no medication has yet consistently improved upon the results of behavior therapy alone. Animal models suggest that enhancing GABAergic inhibition can reduce reinstatement of cocaine self-administration, and a controlled clinical trial of topiramate (TOPAMAX) showed a significant reduction in cocaine use. Topiramate also reduced the relapse rate in alcoholics, prompting current studies in patients dually dependent on cocaine and alcohol. Baclofen (LIORESAL, others), a $GABA_B$ agonist, was found in a single-site trial to reduce relapse in cocaine addicts, but was not effective in a multisite trial. A different approach was taken using modafinil (PROVIGIL), a medication that increases alertness and is approved for the treatment of narcolepsy. This medication was found to reduce the euphoria produced by cocaine and to relieve cocaine withdrawal symptoms. Modafinil is currently being tested in clinical trials of cocaine, methamphetamine, alcohol, and other substance abuse disorders. A novel approach to cocaine addiction employs a vaccine that produces cocaine-binding antibodies. Preliminary studies showed some success in reducing cocaine use. Larger trials are in progress. For now, behavioral therapy remains the treatment of choice, with medication indicated for specific co-existing disorders such as depression.

Amphetamine and Related Agents. Subjective effects similar to those of cocaine are produced by amphetamine, dextroamphetamine, methamphetamine, phenmetrazine, methylphenidate, and diethylpropion. Amphetamines increase synaptic DA, NE, and 5-HT primarily by stimulating pre-synaptic release rather than by blockade of reuptake, as is the case with cocaine. Intravenous or smoked methamphetamine produces an abuse/dependence syndrome similar to that of cocaine, although clinical deterioration may progress more rapidly. In animal studies, methamphetamine in doses comparable with those used by human abusers produces neurotoxic effects, as reflected by histologic changes in dopaminergic and serotonergic neurons.

Methamphetamine can be synthesized from ephedrine in small, clandestine laboratories. Methamphetamine addiction has become a major public health problem, particularly in the western half of the U.S. Behavioral and medical treatments for methamphetamine addiction are similar to those used for cocaine. Until recently, ephedrine was a widely available nonprescription stimulant (a "wake-up" pill). Oral stimulants, such as those prescribed in a weight-reduction program, have short-term efficacy because of tolerance development. Only a small proportion of patients introduced to these appetite suppressants subsequently exhibits dose escalation or drug-seeking from various physicians; such patients may meet diagnostic criteria for abuse or addiction.

Caffeine. Caffeine, a mild stimulant, is the most widely used psychoactive drug in the world. It is present in soft drinks, coffee, tea, cocoa, chocolate, and numerous prescription and over-the-counter drugs. It mildly increases NE and DA release and enhances neural activity in numerous brain areas. Caffeine is absorbed from the digestive tract and is distributed rapidly throughout all tissues and easily crosses the placental barrier. Many of caffeine's effects are believed to occur by means of competitive antagonism at adenosine receptors; as a methylxanthine, caffeine also inhibits cyclic nucleotide phosphodiesterases. Adenosine is a neuromodulator that influences a number of functions in the CNS, as is cyclic AMP (Chapter 14). The mild sedating effects that occur when adenosine activates particular adenosine-receptor subtypes can be antagonized by caffeine.

Tolerance occurs rapidly to the stimulating effects of caffeine. Thus, a mild withdrawal syndrome has been produced in controlled studies by abruptly discontinuing the intake of as little as one to two cups of coffee per day. Caffeine withdrawal consists of feelings of fatigue and sedation. With higher doses, headaches and nausea have been reported during withdrawal; vomiting is rare (Silverman et al., 1992). Although a withdrawal syndrome can be demonstrated, few caffeine users report loss of control of caffeine intake or significant difficulty in reducing or stopping caffeine, if desired (Dews et al., 1999). Thus, caffeine is not listed in the category of addicting stimulants (American Psychiatric Association, 2000).

Cannabinoids (Marijuana)

The cannabis plant has been cultivated for centuries both for the production of hemp fiber and for its presumed medicinal and psychoactive properties. The smoke from burning cannabis contains many chemicals, including 61 different cannabinoids that have been identified. One of these, Δ-9-tetrahydrocannabinol (Δ-9-THC), produces most of the characteristic pharmacological effects of smoked marijuana.

Marijuana is the most commonly used illegal drug in the U.S. Surveys over the period 2006-2009 report that ~32% of highschool seniors have tied marijuana, down from a high of 51% in 1974, but up from 22% in 1992 (Johnston et al., 2010).

Cannabinoid receptors CB_1 (mainly CNS) and CB_2 (peripheral) have been identified and cloned. An arachidonic acid derivative, anandamide, has been proposed as an endogenous ligand for CB receptors. While the physiological function of these receptors and their endogenous ligands are incompletely understood, they are likely to have important functions because they are dispersed widely with high densities in the cerebral cortex, hippocampus, striatum, and cerebellum (Iversen, 2003). Specific CB_1 antagonists have been developed and tested in controlled clinical trials. One of these, rimonabant, was found to reduce relapse in cigarette smokers and to produce weight loss in obese patients; however, its development has been abandoned because of depressive and neurologic side effects.

The pharmacological effects of Δ-9-THC vary with the dose, route of administration, experience of the user, vulnerability to psychoactive effects, and setting of use. Intoxication with marijuana produces changes in mood, perception, and motivation, but the effect most frequently sought is the "high" and "mellowing out." This effect is described as different from the high produced by a stimulant or opiate. Effects vary with dose, but typically last ~2 hours. During the high, cognitive functions, perception, reaction time, learning, and memory are impaired. Coordination and tracking behavior may be impaired for several hours beyond the perception of the high, with obvious implications for the operation of a motor vehicle and performance in the workplace or at school.

Marijuana also produces complex behavioral changes such as giddiness and increased hunger. There are unsubstantiated claims of increased pleasure from sex and increased insight during a marijuana high. Unpleasant reactions such as panic or hallucinations and even acute psychosis may occur; several surveys indicate that 50-60% of marijuana users have reported at least one anxiety experience. These reactions are seen commonly with higher doses and with oral ingestion rather than smoked marijuana, because smoking permits the titration of dose according to the effects. While there is no convincing evidence that marijuana can produce a lasting schizophrenia-like syndrome, association studies suggest a correlation of early marijuana use with an increased risk of later developing schizophrenia. Numerous clinical reports suggest that marijuana use may precipitate a recurrence of psychosis in people with a history of schizophrenia.

One of the most controversial of the reputed effects of marijuana is the production of an "amotivational syndrome." This syndrome is not an official diagnosis, but it has been used to describe young people who drop out of social activities and show little interest in school, work, or other goal-directed activity. When heavy marijuana use accompanies these symptoms, the drug often is cited as the cause, even though there are no data that demonstrate a causal relationship between marijuana smoking and these behavioral characteristics. There is no evidence that marijuana damages brain cells or produces any permanent functional changes, although there are animal data indicating impairment of maze learning that persists for weeks after the last dose. These findings are consistent with clinical reports of gradual improvement in mental state after cessation of chronic high-dose marijuana use.

Marijuana has medicinal effects, including antiemetic properties that relieve side effects of anticancer chemotherapy. It also has muscle-relaxing effects, anticonvulsant properties, and the capacity to reduce the elevated intraocular pressure of glaucoma. These medical benefits come at the cost of the psychoactive effects that often impair normal activities. Thus, there is no clear advantage of marijuana over conventional treatments for any of these indications (Joy et al., 1999). An oral capsule containing Δ-9-THC (dronabinol; MARINOL, others) is approved for anorexia associated with weight loss in patients with HIV infection and for cancer chemotherapy-induced nausea and vomiting. With the cloning of cannabinoid receptors, the discovery of endogenous ligands, and the synthesis of specific agonists and antagonists, it is likely that new orally effective medications will be developed without the undesirable properties of smoked marijuana and without the deleterious effects of inhaling smoke particles and the chemical products of high-temperature combustion.

Tolerance, Dependence, and Withdrawal. Tolerance to most of the effects of marijuana can develop rapidly after only a few doses, but also disappears rapidly (Martin et al., 2004). Tolerance to large doses persists in experimental animals for long periods after cessation of drug use. Withdrawal symptoms and signs typically are not seen in clinical populations. In fact, few patients ever seek treatment for marijuana addiction. Human subjects develop a withdrawal syndrome when they receive regular oral doses of the agent (Table 24–9). This syndrome, however, is only seen clinically in persons who use marijuana on a daily basis and then suddenly stop.

Pharmacological Interventions. Marijuana abuse and addiction have no specific treatments. Heavy users may suffer from accompanying depression and thus may respond to antidepressant medication, but this should be decided on an individual basis considering the severity of the affective symptoms after the marijuana effects have dissipated. The residual drug effects may continue for several weeks. The CB_1 receptor antagonist rimonabant has been reported to block the acute effects of smoked marijuana, but development of this drug has been halted due to safety concerns (discussed under "Pharmacological Interventions" in the nicotine section earlier in the chapter).

Psychedelic Agents

Perceptual distortions that include hallucinations, illusions, and disorders of thinking such as paranoia can be produced by toxic doses of many drugs. These phenomena also may follow withdrawal from toxic sedatives such as alcohol. There are, however, certain drugs that have as their primary effect the production of disturbances of perception, thought, or mood at low doses with minimal effects on memory and orientation. These are commonly called *hallucinogenic drugs*, but their

Table 24–9

Marijuana Withdrawal Syndrome
Restlessness
Irritability
Mild agitation
Insomnia
Sleep EEG disturbance
Nausea, cramping

use does not always result in frank hallucinations. In the late 1990s, the use of "club drugs" at all-night dance parties became popular. Such drugs include methylenedioxymethamphetamine (MDMA, "ecstasy"), lysergic acid diethylamide (LSD), phencyclidine (PCP), and ketamine (KETALAR). They often are used in association with illegal sedatives such as flunitrazepam (ROHYPNOL) or γ-hydroxybutyrate (GHB). The latter drug has the reputation of being particularly effective in preventing memory storage, and has been implicated in "date rapes."

While psychedelic effects can be produced by a variety of different drugs, there are two main categories of psychedelic compounds, indoleamines and phenethylamines. The indoleamine hallucinogens include LSD, N,N-dimethyltryptamine (DMT), and psilocybin. The phenethylamines include mescaline, dimethoxymethylamphetamine (DOM), methylenedioxyamphetamine (MDA), and MDMA. Both groups have a relatively high affinity for 5-HT_2 receptors (Chapter 13), but they differ in their affinity for other subtypes of 5-HT receptors. There is a good correlation between the relative affinity of these compounds for 5-HT_2 receptors and their potency as hallucinogens in humans (Titeler et al., 1988). The 5-HT_2 receptor is further implicated in the mechanism of hallucinations by the observation that antagonists of that receptor, such as ritanserin, are effective in blocking the behavioral and electrophysiological effects of hallucinogenic drugs in animal models. However, LSD interacts with many receptor subtypes at nanomolar concentrations, and it is not possible to attribute the psychedelic effects to any single 5-HT receptor subtype (Peroutka, 1994).

LSD. LSD is the most potent hallucinogenic drug and produces significant psychedelic effects with a total dose of as little as 25-50 μg. This drug is > 3000 times more potent than mescaline. LSD is sold on the illicit market in a variety of forms. A popular contemporary system involves postage stamp-sized papers impregnated with varying doses of LSD (50-300 μg or more). While most street samples sold as LSD actually contain LSD, samples of mushrooms and other botanicals sold as sources of psilocybin and other psychedelics have a low probability of containing the advertised hallucinogen.

The effects of hallucinogenic drugs are variable, even in the same individual on different occasions. LSD is absorbed rapidly after oral administration, with effects beginning at 40-60 minutes, peaking at 2-4 hours, and gradually returning to baseline over 6-8 hours. At a dose of 100 μg, LSD produces perceptual distortions and sometimes hallucinations; mood changes, including elation, paranoia, or depression; intense arousal; and sometimes a feeling of panic. Signs of LSD ingestion include pupillary dilation, increased blood pressure and pulse, flushing, salivation, lacrimation, and hyperreflexia. Visual effects are prominent. Colors seem more intense, and shapes may appear altered. The subject may focus attention on unusual items such as the pattern of hairs on the back of the hand.

A "bad trip" usually consists of severe anxiety, although at times it is marked by intense depression and suicidal thoughts. Visual disturbances usually are prominent. The bad trip from LSD may be difficult to distinguish from reactions to anticholinergic drugs and phencyclidine. There are no documented toxic fatalities from LSD use, but fatal accidents and suicides have occurred during or shortly after intoxication. Prolonged psychotic reactions lasting 2 days or more may occur after the ingestion of a hallucinogen. Schizophrenic episodes may be precipitated in susceptible individuals, and there is some evidence that chronic use of these drugs is associated with the development of persistent psychotic disorders (McLellan et al., 1979).

Claims about the potential of psychedelic drugs for enhancing psychotherapy and for treating addictions and other mental disorders have not been supported by controlled treatment outcome studies. Consequently, there is no current indication for these drugs as medications.

Tolerance, Physical Dependence, and Withdrawal. Frequent, repeated use of psychedelic drugs is unusual, and thus tolerance is not commonly seen. Tolerance does develop to the behavioral effects of LSD after three or four daily doses, but no withdrawal syndrome has been observed. Cross-tolerance among LSD, mescaline, and psilocybin has been demonstrated in animal models.

Pharmacological Intervention. Because of the unpredictability of psychedelic drug effects, any use carries some risk. Dependence and addiction do not occur, but users may require medical attention because of "bad trips." Severe agitation may respond to diazepam (20 mg orally). "Talking down" by reassurance also is effective and is the management of first choice. Antipsychotic medications (Chapter 16) may intensify the experience and thus are not indicated.

A particularly troubling after-effect of the use of LSD and similar drugs is the occasional occurrence of episodic visual disturbances. These originally were called "flashbacks" and resembled the experiences of prior LSD trips. Flashbacks belong to an official diagnostic category called the *hallucinogen persisting perception disorder* (HPPD; American Psychiatric Association, 1994). The symptoms include false fleeting perceptions in the peripheral fields, flashes of color, geometric pseudohallucinations, and positive afterimages (Abraham and Aldridge, 1993). The visual disorder appears stable in half the cases and represents an apparently permanent alteration of the visual system. Precipitants include stress, fatigue, emergence into a dark environment, marijuana, antipsychotic agents, and anxiety states.

MDMA ("Ecstasy") and MDA. MDMA and MDA are phenylethylamines that have stimulant as well as psychedelic effects. MDMA became popular during the 1980s on college campuses because of testimonials that it enhances insight and self-knowledge. It was recommended by some psychotherapists as an aid to the process of therapy, although no controlled data exist to support this contention. Acute effects are dose-dependent and include feelings of energy, altered sense of time, and pleasant sensory experiences with enhanced perception. Negative effects include tachycardia, dry mouth, jaw clenching, and muscle aches. At higher doses, visual hallucinations, agitation, hyperthermia, and panic attacks have been reported. A typical oral dose is one or two 100-mg tablets and lasts 3-6 hours, although dosage and potency of street samples are variable (~100 mg per tablet).

MDA and MDMA produce degeneration of serotonergic nerve cells and axons in rats. While nerve degeneration has not been demonstrated in humans, the cerebrospinal fluid of chronic MDMA users has low levels of serotonin metabolites (Ricaurte et al., 2000). Thus, there is possible neurotoxicity with no evidence that the claimed benefits of MDMA actually occur.

Phencyclidine (PCP). PCP deserves special mention because of its widespread availability and because its pharmacological effects are different from those of the psychedelics such as LSD. PCP was developed originally as an anesthetic in the 1950s and later was abandoned because of a high frequency of postoperative delirium with hallucinations. It was classified as a dissociative anesthetic because, in the anesthetized state, the patient remains conscious with staring gaze, flat facies, and rigid muscles. PCP became a drug of abuse in the 1970s, first in an oral form and then in a smoked version enabling a better regulation of the dose. The effects of PCP have been observed in normal volunteers under controlled conditions. As little as 50 μg/kg produces emotional withdrawal, concrete thinking, and bizarre responses to projective testing. Catatonic posturing also is produced and resembles that of schizophrenia. Abusers taking higher doses may appear to be reacting to hallucinations and may exhibit hostile or assaultive behavior. Anesthetic effects increase with dosage; stupor or coma may occur with muscular rigidity, rhabdomyolysis, and hyperthermia. Intoxicated patients in the emergency room may progress from aggressive behavior to coma, with elevated blood pressure and enlarged nonreactive pupils.

PCP binds with high affinity to sites located in the cortex and limbic structures, resulting in blocking of *N*-methyl-D-aspartate (NMDA)–type glutamate receptors (Chapter 14). LSD and other psychedelics do not bind to NMDA receptors. There is evidence that NMDA receptors are involved in ischemic neuronal death caused by high levels of excitatory amino acids; as a result, there is interest in PCP analogs that block NMDA receptors but with fewer psychoactive effects. Both PCP and ketamine ("Special K"), another "club drug," produce similar effects by altering the distribution of the neurotransmitter glutamate.

Tolerance, Dependence, and Withdrawal. PCP is reinforcing in monkeys, as evidenced by self-administration patterns that produce continuous intoxication. Humans tend to use PCP intermittently, but a small fraction may use it daily. Tolerance to the behavioral effects of PCP develops in animals, but this has not been studied systematically in humans. Signs of a PCP withdrawal syndrome have been observed in monkeys after interruption of daily access to the drug, and include somnolence, tremor, seizures, diarrhea, piloerection, bruxism, and vocalizations.

Pharmacological Intervention. Overdose must be treated by life support because there is no antagonist of PCP effects and no proven way to enhance excretion, although acidification of the urine has been proposed. PCP coma may last 7-10 days. The agitated or psychotic state produced by PCP can be treated with diazepam. Prolonged psychotic behavior requires antipsychotic medication. Because of the anticholinergic activity of PCP, antipsychotic agents with significant anticholinergic effects such as chlorpromazine should be avoided.

Inhalants

Abused inhalants consist of many different categories of chemicals that are volatile at room temperature and produce abrupt changes in mental state when inhaled. Examples include toluene (from model airplane glue), kerosene, gasoline, carbon tetrachloride, amyl nitrite, and nitrous oxide. There are characteristic patterns of response for each substance. Solvents such as toluene typically are used by children. The material usually is placed in a plastic bag and the vapors inhaled. After several minutes of inhalation, dizziness and intoxication occur. Aerosol sprays containing fluorocarbon propellants are another source of solvent intoxication. Prolonged exposure or daily use may result in damage to several organ systems. Clinical problems include cardiac arrhythmias, bone marrow depression, cerebral degeneration, and damage to liver, kidney, and peripheral nerves. Death occasionally has been attributed to inhalant abuse, probably from cardiac arrhythmias, especially accompanying exercise or upper airway obstruction.

Amyl nitrite produces dilation of smooth muscle, has been used in the past for the treatment of angina, and continues to be available by prescription as a component of cyanide antidote kits and for certain diagnostic procedures. It is a yellow, volatile, flammable liquid with a fruity odor. In recent years, amyl nitrite and butyl nitrite have been used to relax smooth muscle and enhance orgasm, particularly by male homosexuals. These agents are commercially available as room deodorizers and can produce a feeling of "rush," flushing, and dizziness. Adverse effects include palpitations, postural hypotension, and headache progressing to loss of consciousness.

Anesthetic gases such as nitrous oxide and halothane sometimes are used as intoxicants by medical personnel. Nitrous oxide also is abused by food-service employees because it is supplied for use as a propellant in disposable aluminum mini tanks for whipping cream canisters. Nitrous oxide produces euphoria and analgesia and then loss of consciousness. Compulsive use and chronic toxicity are reported rarely, but there are obvious risks of overdose (coma) and chronic use (neuropathy) associated with the abuse of this anesthetic.

CLINICAL SUMMARY

The management of drug abuse and addiction must be individualized according to the drugs involved and the associated psychosocial problems of the individual patient. An understanding of the pharmacology of the drug or combination of drugs ingested by the patient is essential to rational and effective treatment. This may be a matter of urgency for the treatment of overdose or for the detoxification of a patient who is experiencing withdrawal symptoms. It must be recognized, however, that the treatment of the underlying addictive disorder requires months or years of rehabilitation. The behavior patterns encoded in memory during thousands of prior drug ingestions do not disappear with detoxification from the drug, even after a typical 28-day inpatient rehabilitation program. Long periods of outpatient treatment are necessary. There probably will be periods of relapse and remission. While complete abstinence is the preferred goal, in reality, most patients are at risk to resume drug-seeking behavior and require one or more periods of retreatment. Maintenance medication can be effective in some circumstances, such as methadone, buprenorphine, or naltrexone for opioid dependence, and disulfiram, naltrexone, or acamprosate for alcoholism. The process can best be compared to the treatment of other chronic disorders such as diabetes, asthma, or hypertension. Long-term medication may be necessary, and cures are not likely. When viewed in the context of chronic disease, the available treatments for addiction are quite successful in that the majority of patients improve, but improvement does not necessarily persist after treatment has ceased (McLellan et al., 2000; O'Brien, 1994).

Long-term treatment is accompanied by improvements in physical status as well as in mental, social, and occupational function. Unfortunately, there is general pessimism in the medical community about the benefits of treatment such that most of the therapeutic effort is directed at the complications of addiction, such as pulmonary, cardiac, and hepatic disorders. Prevention of these complications can be accomplished by addressing the underlying addictive disorder.

BIBLIOGRAPHY

Abraham HD, Aldridge AM. Adverse consequences of lysergic acid diethylamide. *Addiction*, **1993,** *88:*1327–1334.

Alterman AI, O'Brien CP, McLellan AT, et al. Effectiveness and costs of inpatient versus day hospital cocaine rehabilitation. *J Nerv Ment Dis*, **1994,** *182:*157–163.

American Psychiatric Association. *Benzodiazepine Dependence, Toxicity, and Abuse: A Task Force Report of the American Psychiatric Association.* APA, Washington, DC, **1990.**

American Psychiatric Association. *Diagnostic and Statistical Manual of Mental Disorders*, 4th ed. (DSM IV). APA, Washington, DC, **1994.**

American Psychiatric Association. *Diagnostic and Statistical Manual of Mental Disorder,* 4th Ed. (DSM-IV-TR), APA, Washington, DC, **2000**, 265.

Anthony JC, Warner LA, Kessler KC. Comparative epidemiology of dependence on tobacco, alcohol, controlled substances and the inhalants: Basic findings from the national comorbidity survey. *Exp Clin Psychopharmacol*, **1994,** *2:*244–268.

Anton RA, O'Malley SS, Ciraulo DA, et al. Combined pharmacotherapies and behavioral interventions for alcohol dependence, The COMBINE study: a randomized controlled trial. *JAMA*, **2006,** *295*:2003–2017.

Baer A. Discovery of opium poppies has law officers concerned. OPB News, August 12, 2009. http://news.opb.org/article/5606-discovery-opium-poppies-has-law-officers-concerned/. Accessed November **2009**.

Behavioral interventions for alcohol dependence, the COMBINE study: A randomized controlled trial. *JAMA*, **2006,** *295:* 2003–2017.

Benowitz NL, Porchet H, Sheiner L, Jacob P III. Nicotine absorption and cardiovascular effects with smokeless tobacco use: Comparison with cigarettes and nicotine gum. *Clin Pharmacol Ther*, **1988,** *44:*23–28.

Chasnoff IJ, Griffith DR, MacGregor S, et al. Temporal patterns of cocaine use in pregnancy: Perinatal outcome. *JAMA*, **1989,** *261*:1741–1744.

Childress AR, Mozley PD, McElgin W, et al. Limbic activation during cue-induced cocaine craving. *Am J Psychiatry*, **1999,** *156:*11–18.

Collins ED, Kleber HD, Whittington RA, et al. Anesthesia-assisted vs buprenorphine- or clonidine-assisted heroin detoxification and naltrexone induction: A randomized trial. *JAMA*, **2005**, *294*:903–913.

de Wit H, Pierri J, Johanson CE. Assessing individual differences in alcohol preference using a cumulative dosing procedure. *Psychopharmacology*, **1989,** *98:*113–119.

Dews PB, Curtis GL, Hanford KJ, O'Brien CP. The frequency of caffeine withdrawal in a population-based survey and in a controlled, blinded pilot experiment. *J Clin Pharmacol*, **1999,** *39:*1221–1232.

Hasin DS, Stinson FS, Ogburn E, et al. Prevalence, correlates, disability, and comorbidity of DSM-IV alcohol abuse and dependence in the United States: Results from the National Epidemiologic Survey on Alcohol and Related Conditions. *Arch Gen Psychiatry,* **2007,** *64:*830–842.

Hearn WL, Flynn DD, Hime GW, et al. Cocaethylene: A unique cocaine metabolite displays high affinity for the dopamine transporter. *J Neurochem*, **1991,** *56:*698–701.

Higgins ST, Budney AJ, Bickel WK, et al. Outpatient behavioral treatment for cocaine dependence: One-year outcome. Presented at College on Problems of Drug Dependence 56th annual meeting, Palm Beach, **1994.**

Iversen L. Cannabis and the brain. *Brain*, **2003,** *126:*1252–1270.

Johnston LD, Bachman JG, O'Malley PM. *Monitoring the future: questionnaire responses from the nation's high school seniors 2009*. University of Michigan, *Ann Arbor*, **2010**.

Joy JE, Watson SJ, Benson JA, Institute of Medicine. *Marijuana and Medicine: Assessing the Science Base.* National Academy Press, Washington, DC, **1999.**

Kalivas PW, Duffy P. Effect of acute and daily cocaine treatment on extracellular dopamine in the nucleus accumbens. *Synapse*, **1990,** *5:*48–58.

Kalivas PW, O'Brien C. Drug addiction as a pathology of staged neuroplasticity. *Neuropsychopharmacology*, **2008**, *33:*166–180.

Kalix P. Pharmacological properties of the stimulant khat. *Pharmacol Ther*, **1990,** *48:*397–416.

Kosten TA, O'Conner PG. Management of drug and alcohol withdrawal. *N Engl J Med*, **2003,** *348:*1786–1795.

Kreek MJ. Rationale for maintenance pharmacotherapy of opiate dependence. In, *Addictive States.* (O'Brien CP, Jaffe JH, eds.) Raven Press, New York, **1992,** pp. 205–230.

Kreek MJ, LaForge KS, Butelman E. Pharmacotherapy of addictions. *Nature Rev Drug Discov*, **2002,** *1*:710–726.

Martin BR, Sim-Selley LJ, Selley DE. Signaling pathways involved in the development of cannabinoid tolerance. *Trends Pharmacol Sci*, **2004,** *25:*325–330.

Mason BJ. Acamprosate and naltrexone treatment for alcohol dependence: An evidence-based risk benefits assessment. *Eur Neuropsychopharmacol*, **2003,** *13:*469–475.

McLellan AT, Lewis DC, O'Brien CP, Kleber HD. Drug dependence, a chronic medical illness: Implications for treatment, insurance, and outcomes evaluation. *JAMA*, **2000,** *13:*1689–1695.

McLellan AT, Woody GE, O'Brien CP. Development of psychiatric illness in drug abusers: Possible role of drug preference. *N Engl J Med*, **1979,** *301:*1310–1314.

Mendelson JH, Mello NK. Medical progress: Biologic concomitants of alcoholism. *N Engl J Med*, **1979,** *301:*912–921.

O'Brien CP. Treatment of alcoholism as a chronic disorder. *EXS*, **1994**, *71*:349–359.

Peroutka SJ. 5-Hydroxytryptamine receptor interactions of *d*-lysergic acid diethylamide. In, *50 Years of LSD: Current status and Perspectives of Hallucinogens.* (Pletscher A, Ladewig D, eds.) Parthenon Publishing, New York, **1994,** pp. 19–26.

Pettinati HM, O'Brien CP, Rabinowitz AR, et al. The status of naltrexone in the treatment of alcohol dependence: Specific effects of heavy drinking. *J Clin Psychopharmacol*, **2006**, *26:*610–615.

Ray LA, Hutchison KE. Effects of naltrexone on alcohol sensitivity and genetic moderators of medication response: A double-blind placebo-controlled study. *Arch Gen Psychiatry*, **2007**; *64:*1069–1077.

Ricaurte GA, McCann UD, Szabo Z, Scheffel U. Toxicodynamics and long-term toxicity of the recreational drug, 3,4-methylenedioxymethamphetamine (MDMA, "ecstasy"). *Toxicol Lett*, **2000,** *112–113:*143–146.

Ritz MC, Lamb RJ, Goldberg SR, Kuhar MJ. Cocaine receptors on dopamine transporters are related to self-administration of cocaine. *Science*, **1987,** *237:*1219–1223.

Robinson GM, Sellers EM, Janecek E. Barbiturate and hypnosedative withdrawal by a multiple oral phenobarbital loading dose technique. *Clin Pharmacol Ther*, **1981,** *30:*71–76.

Satel SL, Southwick SM, Gawin FH. Clinical features of cocaine-induced paranoia. *Am J Psychiatry*, **1991,** *148:*495–498.

Silverman K, Evans SM, Strain EC, Griffiths RR. Withdrawal syndrome after the double-blind cessation of caffeine consumption. *N Engl J Med*, **1992,** *327*:1109–1114.

Srivastava ED, Russell MA, Feyerabend C, et al. Sensitivity and tolerance to nicotine in smokers and nonsmokers. *Psychopharmacology*, **1991,** *105:*63–68.

Titeler M, Lyon RA, Glennon RA. Radioligand binding evidence implicates the brain 5-HT_2 receptor as a site of action for LSD and phenylisopropylamine hallucinogens. *Psychopharmacology*, **1988,** *94:*213–216.

Trujillo KA, Akil H. Inhibition of morphine tolerance and dependence by the NMDA receptor antagonist MK-801. *Science*, **1991,** *251:*85–87.

Volkow ND, Fowler JS, Wang GJ. The addicted human brain: insights from imaging studies. *J Clin Invest* **2003,** *111:*1444–1451.

Weddington WW, Brown BS, Haertzen CA, et al. Changes in mood, craving, and sleep during short-term abstinence reported by male cocaine addicts. A controlled residential study. *Arch Gen Psychiatry*, **1990,** *47:*861–868.

Wilhelmsen KC, Schuckit M, Smith TL. The search for genes related to a low-level response to alcohol determined by alcohol challenges. *Alcohol Clin Exp Res*, **2003,** *27:*1041–1047.

Williams KE, Reeves KR, Billing CB, et al. A double-blind study evaluating the long-term safety of varenicline for smoking cessation. *Curr Med Res Opin,* **2007**, *23*:793–801.

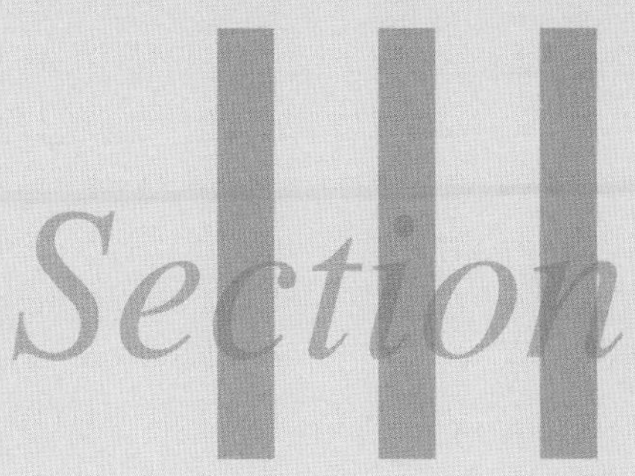

MODULATION OF CARDIOVASCULAR FUNCTION

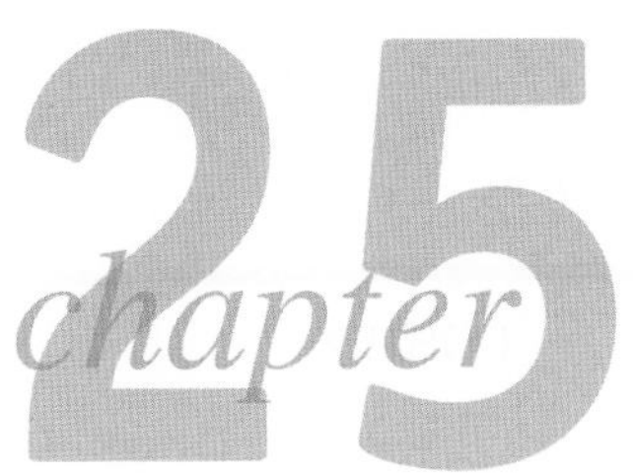

Regulation of Renal Function and Vascular Volume

Robert F. Reilly and Edwin K. Jackson

What engineer, wishing to regulate the composition of the internal environment of the body on which the function of every bone, gland, muscle, and nerve depends, would devise a scheme that operated by throwing the whole thing out 16 times a day and rely on grabbing from it, as it fell to earth, only those precious elements which he wanted to keep?

Homer Smith, *From Fish to Philosopher*

As the philosophizing physiologist, Homer Smith, noted, the kidney filters the extra cellular fluid volume across the renal glomeruli an average of 16 times a day, and the renal nephrons precisely regulate the fluid volume of the body and its electrolyte content via processes of secretion and reabsorption. Disease states such as hypertension, heart failure, renal failure, nephrotic syndrome, and cirrhosis may disrupt this balance. Diuretics increase the rate of urine flow and Na^+ excretion and are used to adjust the volume and/or composition of body fluids in these disorders. Precise regulation of body fluid osmolality is also essential. It is controlled by a finely tuned homeostatic mechanism that operates by adjusting both the rate of water intake and the rate of solute-free water excretion by the kidneys—that is, water balance. Abnormalities in this homeostatic system can result from genetic diseases, acquired diseases, or drugs and may cause serious and potentially life-threatening deviations in plasma osmolality.

This chapter first describes renal anatomy and physiology, then introduces diuretics with regard to chemistry, mechanism of action, site of action, effects on urinary composition, and effects on renal hemodynamics, and finally, integrates diuretic pharmacology with a discussion of mechanisms of edema formation and the role of diuretics in clinical medicine. Specific therapeutic applications of diuretics are presented in Chapters 27 (hypertension) and 28 (heart failure).

The second half of this chapter describes the physiological mechanisms that regulate plasma osmolality and factors that perturb those mechanisms, and examines pharmacological approaches for treating disorders of water balance.

RENAL ANATOMY AND PHYSIOLOGY

The basic urine-forming unit of the kidney is the nephron, which consists of a filtering apparatus, the glomerulus, connected to a long tubular portion that reabsorbs and conditions the glomerular ultrafiltrate. Each human kidney is composed of ~1 million nephrons. The nomenclature for segments of the tubular portion of the nephron has become increasingly complex as renal physiologists have subdivided the nephron into shorter and shorter named segments. These subdivisions were based initially on the axial location of the segments but increasingly have been based on the morphology of the epithelial cells lining the various nephron segments. Figure 25–1 illustrates subdivisions of the nephron.

Glomerular Filtration. In the glomerular capillaries, a portion of plasma water is forced through a filter that has three basic components: the fenestrated capillary endothelial cells, a basement membrane lying just beneath the endothelial cells, and the filtration slit diaphragms formed by epithelial cells that cover the basement membrane on its urinary space side. Solutes of small size flow with filtered water (solvent drag) into the urinary (Bowman's) space, whereas formed elements and macromolecules are retained by the filtration barrier. For each nephron unit, the rate of filtration (single-nephron glomerular filtration rate [SNGFR]) is a function of the hydrostatic pressure in the glomerular capillaries (P_{GC}), the hydrostatic pressure in Bowman's space (which can be equated with pressure in the proximal tubule, P_T), the mean colloid osmotic pressure in the glomerular capillaries (Π_{GC}), the colloid osmotic pressure in the proximal tubule (Π_T), and the ultra-filtration coefficient (K_f), according to the equation

$$\text{SNGFR} = K_f[(p_{GC} - p_T) - (\Pi_{GC} - \Pi_T)] \quad (25\text{-}1)$$

If $P_{GC} - P_T$ is defined as the transcapillary hydraulic pressure difference (ΔP), and if Π_T is negligible (as it usually is because little protein is filtered), then

$$\text{SNGFR} = K_f(\Delta P - \Pi_{GC}) \quad (25\text{-}2)$$

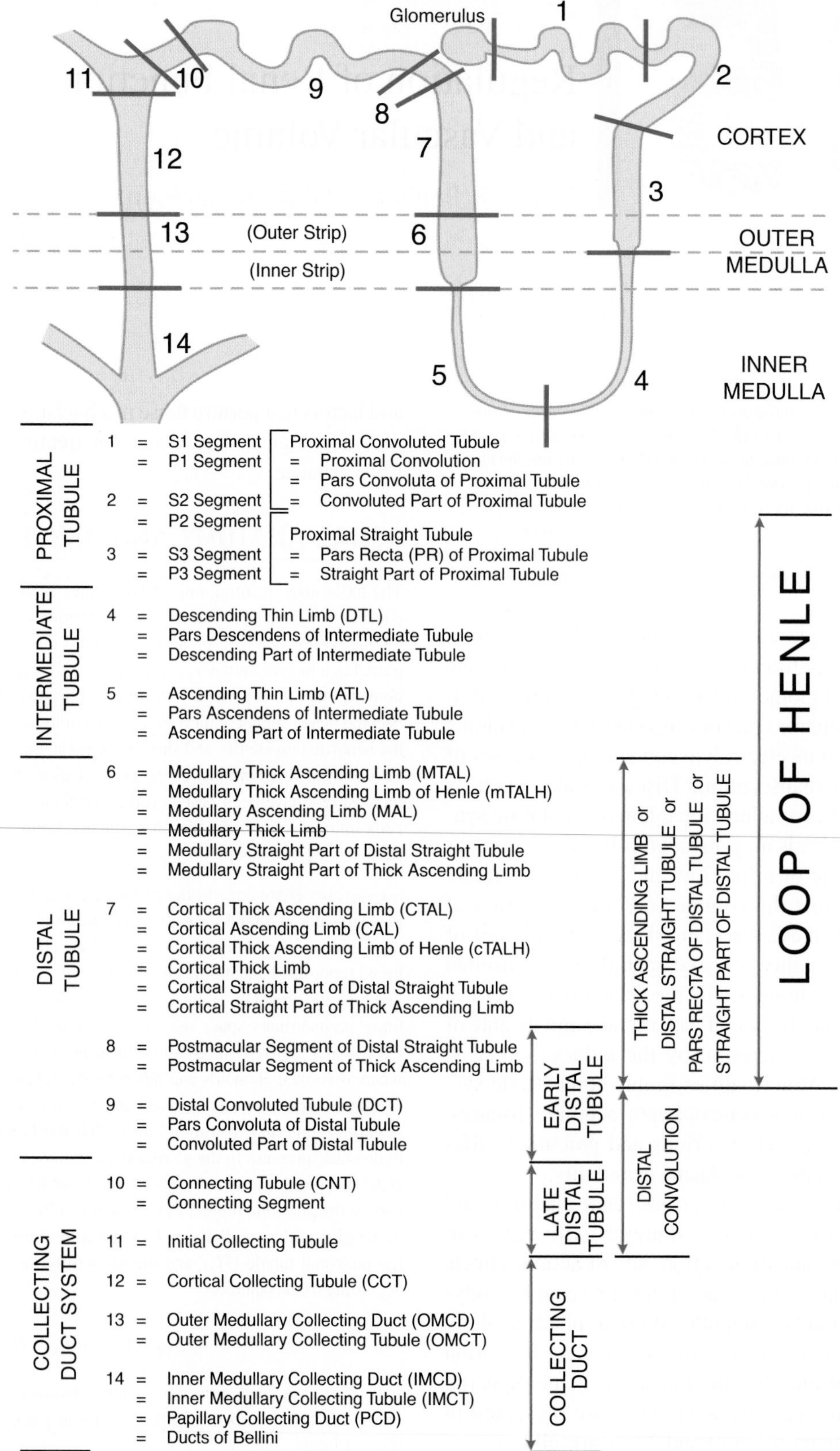

Figure 25–1. *Anatomy and nomenclature of the nephron.*

This latter equation succinctly expresses the three major determinants of SNGFR. However, each of these three determinants can be influenced by a number of other variables. K_f is determined by the physicochemical properties of the filtering membrane and by the surface area available for filtration. ΔP is determined primarily by the arterial blood pressure and by the proportion of the arterial pressure that is transmitted to the glomerular capillaries. This is governed by the relative resistances of preglomerular and postglomerular vessels. Π_{GC} is determined by two variables, the concentration of protein in the arterial blood entering the glomerulus and the single-nephron blood flow (Q_A). Q_A influences Π_{GC} because as blood transverses the glomerular capillary bed, filtration concentrates proteins in the capillaries, causing Π_{GC} to rise with distance along the glomerular bed. When Q_A is high, this effect is reduced; however, when Q_A is low, Π_{GC} may increase to the point that $\Pi_{GC} = \Delta P$, and filtration ceases (a condition known as *filtration equilibrium*).

Overview of Nephron Function. The kidney is designed to filter large quantities of plasma, reabsorb substances that the body must conserve, and leave behind and/or secrete substances that must be eliminated. The two kidneys in humans produce together ~120 mL of ultrafiltrate per minute, yet only 1 mL/min of urine is produced. Therefore, >99% of the glomerular ultrafiltrate is reabsorbed at a staggering energy cost. The kidneys consume 7% of total-body oxygen intake despite the fact that the kidneys make up only 0.5% of body weight.

The proximal tubule is contiguous with Bowman's capsule and takes a tortuous path until finally forming a straight portion that dives into the renal medulla. Based on the morphology of the epithelial cells lining the tubule, the proximal tubule has been subdivided into S1, S2, and S3 segments. Normally, ~65% of filtered Na^+ is reabsorbed in the proximal tubule, and since this part of the tubule is highly permeable to water, reabsorption is essentially isotonic.

Between the outer and inner strips of the outer medulla, the tubule abruptly changes morphology to become the descending thin limb (DTL), which penetrates the inner medulla, makes a hairpin turn, and then forms the ascending thin limb (ATL). At the juncture between the inner and outer medulla, the tubule once again changes morphology and becomes the thick ascending limb, which is made up of three segments: a medullary portion (MTAL), a cortical portion (CTAL), and a postmacular segment. Together the proximal straight tubule, DTL, ATL, MTAL, CTAL, and postmacular segment are known as the *loop of Henle*. The DTL is highly permeable to water, yet its permeability to NaCl and urea is low. In contrast, the ATL is permeable to NaCl and urea but is impermeable to water. The thick ascending limb actively reabsorbs NaCl but is impermeable to water and urea. Approximately 25% of filtered Na^+ is reabsorbed in the loop of Henle, mostly in the thick ascending limb, which has a large reabsorptive capacity.

The thick ascending limb passes between the afferent and efferent arterioles and makes contact with the afferent arteriole by means of a cluster of specialized columnar epithelial cells known as the *macula densa*. The macula densa is strategically located to sense concentrations of NaCl leaving the loop of Henle. If the concentration of NaCl is too high, the macula densa sends a chemical signal (perhaps adenosine or ATP) to the afferent arteriole of the same nephron, causing it to constrict. This, in turn, causes a reduction in P_{GC} and Q_A and decreases SNGFR. This homeostatic mechanism, known as *tubuloglomerular feedback* (TGF), serves to protect the organism from salt and volume wasting. Besides mediating the TGF response, the macula densa also regulates renin release from the adjacent juxtaglomerular cells in the wall of the afferent arteriole.

Approximately 0.2 mm past the macula densa, the tubule changes morphology once again to become the distal convoluted tubule (DCT). The postmacular segment of the thick ascending limb and the distal convoluted tubule often are referred to as the *early distal tubule*. Like the thick ascending limb, the DCT actively transports NaCl and is impermeable to water. Since these characteristics impart the ability to produce a dilute urine, the thick ascending limb and the DCT are collectively called the *diluting segment of the nephron*, and the tubular fluid in the DCT is hypotonic regardless of hydration status. However, unlike the thick ascending limb, the DCT does not contribute to the countercurrent-induced hypertonicity of the medullary interstitium (described later in this section). There are marked species differences in transporter expression in the DCT. The DCT has been subdivided into DCT1 and DCT2. DCT1 expresses the thiazide-sensitive NaCl co-transporter but does not express genes involved in transepithelial Ca^{2+} transport such as the Ca^{2+} entry channel, TRPV5, and the Na^+/Ca^{2+} exchanger. DCT2 expresses Ca^{2+} transport proteins and amiloride-sensitive epithelial Na^+ channels.

The collecting duct system (connecting tubule + initial collecting tubule + cortical collecting duct + outer and inner medullary collecting ducts—segments 10–14 in Figure 25–1) is an area of fine control of ultrafiltrate composition and volume. It is here that final adjustments in electrolyte composition are made, a process modulated by the adrenal steroid aldosterone. In addition, antidiuretic hormone modulates permeability of this part of the nephron to water.

The more distal portions of the collecting duct pass through the renal medulla, where the interstitial fluid is markedly hypertonic. In the absence of ADH, the collecting duct system is impermeable to water, and a dilute urine is excreted. In the presence of ADH, the collecting duct system is permeable to water, so water is reabsorbed. The movement of water out of the tubule is driven by the steep concentration gradient that exists between tubular fluid and medullary interstitium.

The hypertonicity of the medullary interstitium plays a vital role in the ability of mammals and birds to concentrate urine, and therefore is a key adaptation necessary for living in a terrestrial environment. This is accomplished by a combination of the unique topography of the loop of Henle and the specialized permeability features of the loop's subsegments. Although the precise mechanisms giving rise to the medullary hypertonicity have remained elusive, the "passive countercurrent multiplier hypothesis" is an intuitively attractive model that is qualitatively accurate. According to this hypothesis, the process begins with active transport in the thick ascending limb, which concentrates NaCl in the interstitium of the outer medulla. Since this segment of the nephron is impermeable to water, active transport in the ascending limb dilutes the tubular fluid. As the dilute fluid passes into the collecting-duct system, water is extracted if, and only if, ADH is present. Since the cortical and outer medullary collecting ducts have a low permeability to urea, urea is concentrated in the tubular fluid. The inner medullary collecting duct, however, is permeable to urea, so urea diffuses into the

7. As water and solutes accumulate in the intercellular space, hydrostatic pressure increases, thus providing a driving force for bulk water flow. Bulk water flow carries solute (solute convection) out of the intercellular space into the interstitial space and, finally, into the peritubular capillaries. The movement of fluid into peritubular capillaries is governed by the same Starling forces that determine transcapillary fluid movement for any capillary bed.

Mechanism of Organic Acid and Organic Base Secretion. The kidney is a major organ involved in the elimination of organic chemicals from the body. Organic molecules may enter the renal tubules by glomerular filtration of molecules not bound to plasma proteins or may be actively secreted directly into tubules. The proximal tubule has a highly efficient transport system for organic acids and an equally efficient but separate transport system for organic bases. Current models for these secretory systems are illustrated in Figure 25–4. Both systems are powered by the sodium pump in the basolateral membrane, involve secondary and tertiary active transport, and use a facilitated-diffusion step. There are at least nine different organic acid and five different organic base transporters; the precise roles that these transporters play in organic acid and base transport remain ill defined (Dresser et al., 2001). A family of organic anion transporters (OATs) countertransport organic anions with dicarboxylates (Figure 25–4A). OATs most likely exist as α-helical dodecaspans connected by short segments of ~10 or fewer amino acids, except for large interconnecting stretches of amino acids between helices 1 and 2 and helices 6 and 7 (Eraly et al., 2004); see Chapter 5.

Renal Handling of Specific Anions and Cations. Reabsorption of Cl^- generally follows reabsorption of Na^+. In segments of the tubule with low-resistance tight junctions (i.e., "leaky" epithelium), such as the proximal tubule and thick ascending limb, Cl^- movement can occur paracellularly. With regard to transcellular Cl^- flux, Cl^- crosses the luminal membrane by antiport with formate and oxalate (proximal tubule), symport with Na^+/K^+ (thick ascending limb), symport with Na^+ (DCT), and antiport with HCO_3^- (collecting-duct system). Cl^- crosses the basolateral membrane by symport with K^+ (proximal tubule and thick ascending limb), antiport with Na^+/HCO_3^- (proximal tubule), and Cl^- channels (thick ascending limb, DCT, collecting-duct system).

Eighty to ninety percent of filtered K^+ is reabsorbed in the proximal tubule (diffusion and solvent drag) and thick ascending limb (diffusion) largely through the paracellular pathway. In contrast, the DCT and collecting-duct system secrete variable amounts of K^+ by a conductive (channel-mediated) pathway. Modulation of the rate of K^+ secretion in the collecting-duct system, particularly by aldosterone, allows urinary K^+ excretion to be matched with dietary intake. The transepithelial potential difference (V_T), lumen-positive in the thick ascending limb and lumen-negative in the collecting-duct system, provides an important driving force for K^+ reabsorption and secretion, respectively.

Most of the filtered Ca^{2+} (~70%) is reabsorbed by the proximal tubule by passive diffusion through a paracellular route. Another 25% of filtered Ca^{2+} is reabsorbed by the thick ascending limb in part by a paracellular route driven by the lumen-positive V_T and in part by active transcellular Ca^{2+} reabsorption modulated by parathyroid hormone (PTH; see Chapter 44). Most of the remaining Ca^{2+} is reabsorbed in DCT by a transcellular pathway. The transcellular pathway in the thick ascending limb and DCT involves passive Ca^{2+} influx across the luminal membrane through Ca^{2+} channels (TRPV5), followed by Ca^{2+} extrusion across the basolateral membrane by a Ca^{2+}-ATPase. Also, in DCT and CNT, Ca^{2+} crosses the basolateral membrane by Na^+-Ca^{2+} exchanger (antiport).

Inorganic phosphate (P_i) is largely reabsorbed (80% of filtered load) by the proximal tubule. The Na^+-P_i symporter uses the free energy of the Na^+ electrochemical gradient to transport P_i into

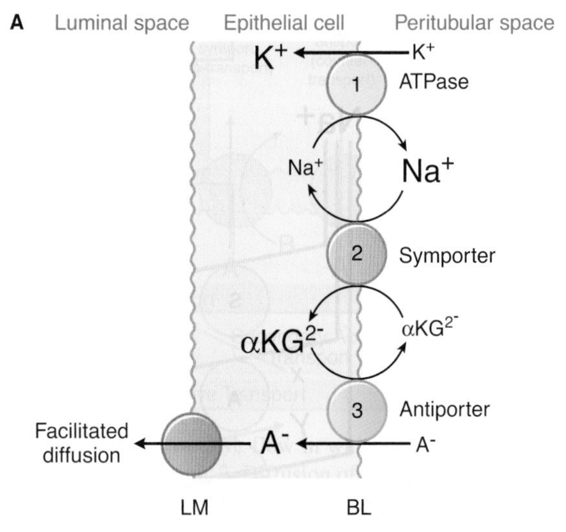

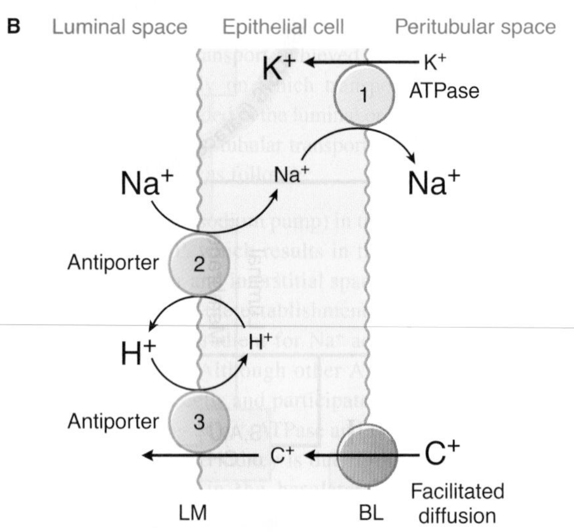

Figure 25–4. ***Mechanisms of organic acid (A) and organic base (B) secretion in the proximal tubule.*** The numbers 1, 2, and 3 refer to primary, secondary, and tertiary active transport. A^-, organic acid [anion]; C^+, organic base [cation]; αKG^{2-}, α-ketoglutarate but also other dicarboxylates. BL and LM indicate basolateral and luminal membranes, respectively.

the cell. The Na^+-P_i symporter is inhibited by PTH. P_i exits the basolateral membrane down its electrochemical gradient by a poorly understood transport system.

Only 20-25% of Mg^{2+} is reabsorbed in the proximal tubule, and only 5% is reabsorbed by the DCT and collecting-duct system. The bulk of Mg^{2+} is reabsorbed in the thick ascending limb by a paracellular pathway driven by the lumen-positive V_T. However, transcellular movement of Mg^{2+} also may occur with basolateral exit by Na^+-Mg^{2+} antiport or an Mg^{2+}-ATPase.

The renal tubules play an extremely important role in the reabsorption of HCO_3^- and secretion of protons (tubular acidification) and thus participate critically in the maintenance of acid-base balance. These processes are described in the section on carbonic anhydrase inhibitors.

PRINCIPLES OF DIURETIC ACTION

By definition, diuretics are drugs that increase the rate of urine flow; however, clinically useful diuretics also increase the rate of Na^+ excretion (natriuresis) and of an accompanying anion, usually Cl^-. NaCl in the body is the major determinant of extracellular fluid volume, and most clinical applications of diuretics are directed toward reducing extracellular fluid volume by decreasing total-body NaCl content. A sustained imbalance between dietary Na^+ intake and Na^+ loss is incompatible with life. A net positive Na^+ balance would result in volume overload with pulmonary edema, and a net negative Na^+ balance would result in volume depletion and cardiovascular collapse. Although continued diuretic administration causes a sustained net deficit in total-body Na^+, the time course of natriuresis is finite because renal compensatory mechanisms bring Na^+ excretion in line with Na^+ intake, a phenomenon known as *diuretic braking*. These compensatory, or braking, mechanisms include activation of the sympathetic nervous system, activation of the rennin–angiotensin–aldosterone axis, decreased arterial blood pressure (which reduces pressure natriuresis), renal epithelial cell hypertrophy, increased renal epithelial transporter expression, and perhaps alterations in natriuretic hormones such as atrial natriuretic peptide (Ellison, 1999). This is shown in Figure 25–5.

Historically, the classification of diuretics was based on a mosaic of ideas such as site of action (loop diuretics), efficacy (high-ceiling diuretics), chemical structure (thiazide diuretics), similarity of action with other diuretics (thiazide-like diuretics), and effects on K^+ excretion (K^+-sparing diuretics). However, since the mechanism of action of each of the major classes of diuretics is now well understood, a classification scheme based on mechanism of action is used in this chapter.

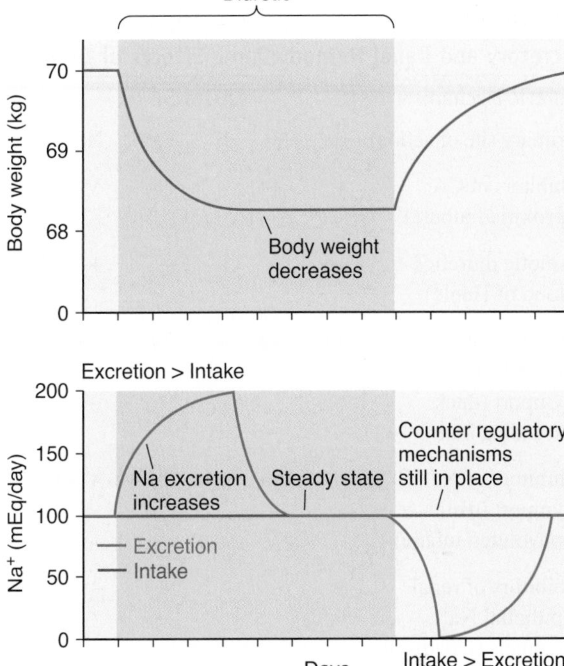

Figure 25–5. *Changes in extracellular fluid volume and weight with diuretic therapy.* The period of diuretic administration is shown in the shaded box along with its effects on body weight in the upper part of the figure and Na^+ excretion in the lower half of the figure. Initially, when Na^+ excretion exceeds intake, body weight and extracellular fluid volume (ECFV) decrease. Subsequently, a new steady state is achieved where Na^+ intake and excretion are equal but at a lower ECFV and body weight. This results from activation of the renin-angiotensin-aldosterone system (RAAS) and sympathetic nervous system (SNS), "the braking phenomenon." When the diuretic is discontinued, body weight and ECFV rise during a period where Na^+ intake exceeds excretion. A new steady state is then reached as stimulation of the RAAS and SNS wane.

Diuretics not only alter the excretion of Na^+ but also may modify renal handling of other cations (e.g., K^+, H^+, Ca^{2+}, and Mg^{2+}), anions (e.g., Cl^-, HCO_3^-, and $H_2PO_4^-$), and uric acid. In addition, diuretics may alter renal hemodynamics indirectly. Table 25–1 gives a comparison of the general effects of the major diuretic classes.

INHIBITORS OF CARBONIC ANHYDRASE

Acetazolamide (DIAMOX, others) is the prototype of a class of agents that have limited usefulness as diuretics but have played a major role in the development of fundamental concepts of renal physiology and pharmacology.

Table 25–1

Excretory and Renal Hemodynamic Effects of Diuretics[a]

Diuretic Mechanism	CATIONS					ANIONS			URIC ACID		RENAL HEMODYNAMICS			
(Primary site of action)	Na^+	K^+	H^{+b}	Ca^{2+}	Mg^{2+}	Cl^-	HCO_3^-	$H_2PO_4^-$	*Acute*	*Chronic*	RBF	GFR	FF	TGF
Inhibitors of CA (proximal tubule)	+	++	–	NC	V	(+)	++	++	I	–	–	–	NC	+
Osmotic diuretics (loop of Henle)	++	+	I	+	++	+	+	+	+	I	+	NC	–	I
Inhibitors of Na^+-K^+-$2Cl^-$ symport (thick ascending limb)	++	++	+	++	++	++	+[c]	+[c]	+	–	V(+)	NC	V(–)	–
Inhibitors of Na^+-Cl^- symport (distal convoluted tubule)	+	++	+	V(–)	V(+)	+	+[c]	+[c]	+	–	NC	V(–)	V(–)	NC
Inhibitors of renal epithelial Na^+ channels (late distal tubule, collecting duct)	+	–	–	–	–	+	(+)	NC	I	–	NC	NC	NC	NC
Antagonists of mineralocorticoid receptors (late distal tubule, collecting duct)	+	–	–	I	–	+	(+)	I	I	–	NC	NC	NC	NC

[a]Except for uric acid, changes are for acute effects of diuretics in the absence of significant volume depletion, which would trigger complex physiological adjustments. [b]H^+, titratable acid and NH_4^+. [c]In general, these effects are restricted to those individual agents that inhibit carbonic anhydrase. However, there are notable exceptions in which symport inhibitors increase bicarbonate and phosphate (e.g., metolazone, bumetanide).

++, +, (+),–, NC, V, V(+), V(–) and I indicate marked increase, mild to moderate increase, slight increase, decrease, no change, variable effect, variable increase, variable decrease, and insufficient data, respectively. For cations and anions, the indicated effects refer to absolute changes in fractional excretion.

RBF, renal blood flow; GFR, glomerular filtration rate; FF, filtration fraction; TGF, tubuloglomerular feedback; CA, carbonic anhydrase.

Chemistry. When sulfanilamide was introduced as a chemotherapeutic agent, metabolic acidosis was recognized as a side effect. This observation led to the demonstration that sulfanilamide is an inhibitor of carbonic anhydrase. Subsequently, an enormous number of sulfonamides were synthesized and tested for their ability to inhibit carbonic anhydrase; of these compounds, acetazolamide has been studied most extensively. There are three orally administered carbonic anhydrase inhibitors—acetazolamide, dichlorphenamide (not marketed in the U.S.), and methazolamide. The common molecular motif of available carbonic anhydrase inhibitors is an unsubstituted sulfonamide moiety (Table 25–2).

Mechanism and Site of Action. Proximal tubular epithelial cells are richly endowed with the zinc metalloenzyme carbonic anhydrase, which is found in the luminal and basolateral membranes (type IV carbonic anhydrase, an enzyme tethered to the membrane by a glycosylphosphatidylinositol linkage), as well as in the cytoplasm (type II carbonic anhydrase). Carbonic anhydrase plays a key role in $NaHCO_3$ reabsorption and acid secretion.

In the proximal tubule, the free energy in the Na^+ gradient established by the basolateral Na^+ pump is used by an Na^+-H^+ antiporter (also referred to as an Na^+-H^+ exchanger [NHE]) in the luminal membrane to transport H^+ into the tubular lumen in exchange for Na^+ (Figure 25–6). In the lumen, H^+ reacts with filtered HCO_3^- to form H_2CO_3, which decomposes rapidly to CO_2 and water in the presence of carbonic anhydrase in the brush border. Normally, the reaction occurs slowly, but carbonic anhydrase reversibly accelerates this reaction several thousand times. CO_2 is lipophilic and rapidly diffuses across the luminal membrane into the

Table 25–2

Inhibitors of Carbonic Anhydrase

DRUG	STRUCTURE	RELATIVE POTENCY	ORAL AVAILABILITY	$t_{1/2}$ (HOURS)	ROUTE OF ELIMINATION
Acetazolamide (DIAMOX)	CH_3CONH, S, SO_2NH_2; N—N	1	~100%	6-9	R
Dichlorphenamide (DARAMIDE)	SO_2NH_2; Cl, SO_2NH_2; Cl	30	ID	ID	ID
Methazolamide (GLAUCTABS)	CH_3CON, S, SO_2NH_2; N—N; H_3C	>1; <10	~100%	~14	~25%, ~75% M

Abbreviations: R, renal excretion of intact drug; M, metabolism; ID, insufficient data.

epithelial cell, where it reacts with water to form H_2CO_3, a reaction catalyzed by cytoplasmic carbonic anhydrase (Figure 25–6). Continued operation of the Na^+-H^+ antiporter maintains a low proton concentration in the cell, so H_2CO_3 ionizes spontaneously to form H^+ and HCO_3^-, creating an electrochemical gradient for HCO_3^- across the basolateral membrane. The electrochemical gradient for HCO_3^- is used by an Na^+-HCO_3^- symporter (also referred to as the Na^+-HCO_3^- co-transporter [NBC]) in the basolateral membrane to transport $NaHCO_3$ into the interstitial space. The net effect of this process is transport of $NaHCO_3$ from the tubular lumen to the interstitial space, followed by movement of water (isotonic reabsorption). Removal of water concentrates Cl^- in the tubular lumen, and consequently, Cl^- diffuses down its concentration gradient into the interstitium by the paracellular pathway.

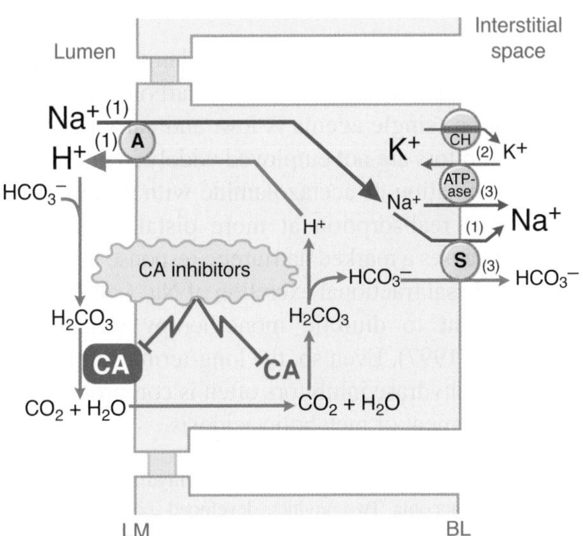

Figure 25–6. *$NaHCO_3$ reabsorption in proximal tubule and mechanism of diuretic action of carbonic anhydrase inhibitors.* The actual reaction catalyzed by carbonic anhydrase is $OH^- + CO_2 \rightarrow HCO_3^-$; however, $H_2O \rightarrow OH^- + H^+$, and $HCO_3^- + H^+ \rightarrow H_2CO_3$, so the net reaction is $H_2O + CO_2 \rightarrow H_2CO_3$. Numbers in parentheses indicate stoichiometry. A, antiporter; S, symporter; CH, ion channel; BL, basolateral membrane; LM, luminal membrane.

Carbonic anhydrase inhibitors potently inhibit (IC_{50} for acetazolamide is 10 n*M*) both the membrane-bound and cytoplasmic forms of carbonic anhydrase, resulting in nearly complete abolition of $NaHCO_3$ reabsorption in the proximal tubule. Studies with a high-molecular-weight carbonic anhydrase inhibitor that inhibits only luminal enzyme because of limited cellular permeability indicate that inhibition of both membrane-bound and cytoplasmic pools of carbonic anhydrase contributes to the diuretic activity of carbonic anhydrase inhibitors. Because of the large excess of carbonic anhydrase in proximal tubules, a high percentage of enzyme activity must be inhibited before an effect on electrolyte excretion is observed. Although the proximal tubule is the major site of action of carbonic anhydrase inhibitors, carbonic anhydrase also is involved in secretion of titratable acid in the collecting duct system (a process that involves a proton pump); therefore, the collecting duct system is a secondary site of action for this class of drugs.

Effects on Urinary Excretion. Inhibition of carbonic anhydrase is associated with a rapid rise in urinary HCO_3^- excretion to ~35% of filtered load. This, along with inhibition of titratable acid and NH_4^+ secretion in the collecting-duct system, results in an increase in urinary pH to ~8 and development of a metabolic acidosis.

However, even with a high degree of inhibition of carbonic anhydrase, 65% of HCO_3^- is rescued from excretion by poorly understood mechanisms that may involve carbonic anhydrase-independent HCO_3^- reabsorption at downstream sites. Inhibition of the transport mechanism described in the preceding section results in increased delivery of Na^+ and Cl^- to the loop of Henle, which has a large reabsorptive capacity and captures most of the Cl^- and a portion of the Na^+. Thus only a small increase in Cl^- excretion occurs, HCO_3^- being the major anion excreted along with the cations Na^+ and K^+. The fractional excretion of Na^+ may be as much as 5%, and the fractional excretion of K^+ can be as much as 70%. The increased excretion of K^+ is in part secondary to increased delivery of Na^+ to the distal nephron. The mechanism by which increased distal Na^+ delivery enhances K^+ excretion is described in the section on inhibitors of Na^+ channels.

Other mechanisms contributing to enhanced K^+ excretion include flow-dependent enhancement of K^+ secretion by the collecting duct, nonosmotic vasopressin release, and activation of the renin-angiotensin-aldosterone axis. Carbonic anhydrase inhibitors increase phosphate excretion (mechanism unknown) but have little or no effect on Ca^{2+} or Mg^{2+} excretion. The effects of carbonic anhydrase inhibitors on renal excretion are self-limiting, probably because the resulting metabolic acidosis decreases the filtered load of HCO_3^- to the point that the uncatalyzed reaction between CO_2 and water is sufficient to achieve HCO_3^- reabsorption. Studies in rabbits show that the K_i for luminal carbonic anhydrase inhibition in outer medulla is increased >100-fold over the concentration required in control tubules. These results suggest that acidosis induces a conformational change in the protein making it less sensitive to inhibition by acetazolamide (Tsuroka, 1998).

Effects on Renal Hemodynamics. By inhibiting proximal reabsorption, carbonic anhydrase inhibitors increase delivery of solutes to the macula densa. This triggers TGF, which increases afferent arteriolar resistance and reduces renal blood flow (RBF) and glomerular filtration rate (GFR).

Other Actions. Carbonic anhydrase is present in a number of extrarenal tissues, including the eye, gastric mucosa, pancreas, central nervous system (CNS), and erythrocytes. Carbonic anhydrase in the ciliary processes of the eye mediates formation of large amounts of HCO_3^- in aqueous humor. Inhibition of carbonic anhydrase decreases the rate of formation of aqueous humor and consequently reduces intraocular pressure. Acetazolamide frequently causes paresthesias and somnolence, suggesting an action of carbonic anhydrase inhibitors in the CNS. The efficacy of acetazolamide in epilepsy is due in part to the production of metabolic acidosis; however, direct actions of acetazolamide in the CNS also contribute to its anticonvulsant action. Owing to interference with carbonic anhydrase activity in erythrocytes, carbonic anhydrase inhibitors increase CO_2 levels in peripheral tissues and decrease CO_2 levels in expired gas. Large doses of carbonic anhydrase inhibitors reduce gastric acid secretion, but this has no therapeutic application. Acetazolamide causes vasodilation by opening vascular Ca^{2+}-activated K^+ channels; however, the clinical significance of this effect is unclear.

Absorption and Elimination. Carbonic anhydrase inhibitors are avidly bound by carbonic anhydrase, and accordingly, tissues rich in this enzyme will have higher concentrations of carbonic anhydrase inhibitors following systemic administration. See Table 25–2 for structures and pharmacokinetic data.

Toxicity, Adverse Effects, Contraindications, Drug Interactions. Serious toxic reactions to carbonic anhydrase inhibitors are infrequent; however, these drugs are sulfonamide derivatives and, like other sulfonamides, may cause bone marrow depression, skin toxicity, sulfonamide-like renal lesions, and allergic reactions in patients hypersensitive to sulfonamides. With large doses, many patients exhibit drowsiness and paresthesias. Most adverse effects, contraindications, and drug interactions are secondary to urinary alkalinization or metabolic acidosis, including:

- diversion of ammonia of renal origin from urine into the systemic circulation, a process that may induce or worsen hepatic encephalopathy (the drugs are contraindicated in patients with hepatic cirrhosis)
- calculus formation and ureteral colic owing to precipitation of calcium phosphate salts in an alkaline urine
- worsening of metabolic or respiratory acidosis (the drugs are contraindicated in patients with hyperchloremic acidosis or severe chronic obstructive pulmonary disease)
- reduction of the urinary excretion rate of weak organic bases

Therapeutic Uses. Although acetazolamide is used for treatment of edema, the efficacy of carbonic anhydrase inhibitors as single agents is low, and carbonic anhydrase inhibitors are not employed widely in this regard. The combination of acetazolamide with diuretics that block Na^+ reabsorption at more distal sites in the nephron causes a marked natriuretic response in patients with low basal fractional excretion of Na^+ (<0.2%) who are resistant to diuretic monotherapy (Knauf and Mutschler, 1997). Even so, the long-term usefulness of carbonic anhydrase inhibitors often is compromised by the development of metabolic acidosis.

The major indication for carbonic anhydrase inhibitors is open-angle glaucoma. Two products developed specifically for this use are dorzolamide (TRUSOPT, others) and brinzolamide (AZOPT), which are available only as ophthalmic drops. Carbonic anhydrase inhibitors also may be employed for secondary glaucoma and preoperatively in acute angle-closure glaucoma to lower intraocular pressure before surgery (Chapter 64). Acetazolamide also is used for the treatment of epilepsy (Chapter 21). The rapid development of tolerance, however, may limit the usefulness of carbonic anhydrase inhibitors for epilepsy.

Acetazolamide can provide symptomatic relief in patients with *high-altitude illness* or *mountain sickness*; however, it is more appropriate to give acetazolamide as a prophylactic measure. Acetazolamide also is useful in patients with familial periodic paralysis. The mechanism for the beneficial effects of acetazolamide in altitude sickness and familial periodic paralysis is not clear, but it may be related to the induction of a metabolic acidosis. Other off-label clinical uses include the treatment of dural ectasia in individuals with Marfan syndrome, of sleep apnea, and of idiopathic intracranial hypertension. Finally, carbonic anhydrase inhibitors can be useful for correcting a metabolic alkalosis, especially one caused by diuretic-induced increases in H^+ excretion.

OSMOTIC DIURETICS

Osmotic diuretics are agents that are freely filtered at the glomerulus, undergo limited reabsorption by the renal tubule, and are relatively inert pharmacologically. Osmotic diuretics are administered in doses large enough to increase significantly the osmolality of plasma and tubular fluid. Table 25–3 lists four osmotic diuretics—glycerin (OSMOGLYN), isosorbide, mannitol (OSMITROL, others), and urea (currently not available in the U.S.).

Mechanism and Site of Action. For many years it was thought that osmotic diuretics act primarily in the proximal tubule as nonreabsorbable solutes that limit the osmosis of water into the interstitial space and thereby reduce luminal Na^+ concentration to the point that net Na^+ reabsorption ceases. Although early micropuncture studies supported this concept, subsequent studies suggested that this mechanism, while operative, may be of only secondary importance and that the major site of action of osmotic diuretics is the loop of Henle.

By extracting water from intracellular compartments, osmotic diuretics expand extracellular fluid volume, decrease blood viscosity, and inhibit renin release. These effects increase RBF, and the increase in renal medullary blood flow removes NaCl and urea from the renal medulla, thus reducing medullary tonicity. Under some circumstances, prostaglandins may contribute to the renal vasodilation and medullary washout induced by osmotic diuretics. A reduction in medullary tonicity causes a decrease in the extraction of water from the DTL, which in turn limits the concentration of NaCl in the tubular fluid entering the ATL. This latter effect diminishes the passive reabsorption of NaCl in the ATL. In addition, the marked ability of osmotic diuretics to inhibit Mg^{2+} reabsorption, a cation that is reabsorbed mainly in the thick ascending limb, suggests that osmotic diuretics also interfere with transport processes in the thick ascending limb. The mechanism of this effect is unknown.

In summary, osmotic diuretics act both in proximal tubule and loop of Henle, with the latter being the primary site of action. Also, osmotic diuretics probably act by an osmotic effect in the tubules and by reducing medullary tonicity.

Table 25–3

Osmotic Diuretics

DRUG	STRUCTURE	ORAL AVAILABILITY	$t_{1/2}$ (HOURS)	ROUTE OF ELIMINATION
Glycerin (OSMOGLYN)	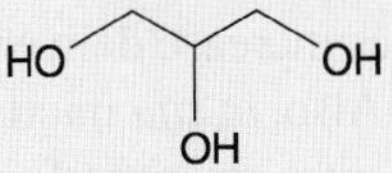 HO, OH, OH	Orally active	0.5-0.75	~80% M ~20% U
Isosorbide (ISMOTIC)	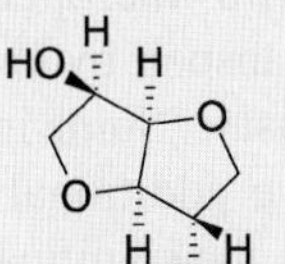 H, HO, H, O, O, H, H, OH	Orally active	5-9.5	R
Mannitol (OSMITROL)	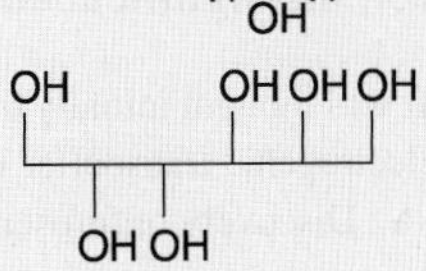 OH, OH OH OH, OH OH	Negligible	0.25-1.7[a]	~80% R ~20% M + B
Urea (UREAPHIL)	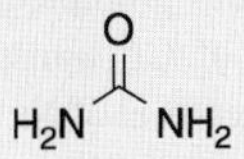 O, H_2N, NH_2	Negligible	ID	R

[a]In renal failure, 6–36. *Abbreviations:* R, renal excretion of intact drug; M, metabolism; B, excretion of intact drug into bile; U, unknown pathway of elimination; ID, insufficient data.

Effects on Urinary Excretion. Osmotic diuretics increase urinary excretion of nearly all electrolytes, including Na^+, K^+, Ca^{2+}, Mg^{2+}, Cl^-, HCO_3^-, and phosphate.

Effects on Renal Hemodynamics. Osmotic diuretics increase RBF by a variety of mechanisms. Osmotic diuretics dilate the afferent arteriole, which increases P_{GC}, and dilute the plasma, which decreases Π_{GC}. These effects would increase GFR were it not for the fact that osmotic diuretics also increase P_T. In general, superficial SNGFR is increased, but total GFR is little changed.

Absorption and Elimination. Pharmacokinetic data on the osmotic diuretics are listed in Table 25–3. Glycerin and isosorbide can be given orally, whereas mannitol and urea must be administered intravenously.

Toxicity, Adverse Effects, Contraindications, and Drug Interactions. Osmotic diuretics are distributed in the extracellular fluid and contribute to the extracellular osmolality. Thus, water is extracted from intracellular compartments, and the extracellular fluid volume becomes expanded. In patients with heart failure or pulmonary congestion, this may cause frank pulmonary edema. Extraction of water also causes hyponatremia, which may explain the common adverse effects, including headache, nausea, and vomiting. On the other hand, loss of water in excess of electrolytes can cause hypernatremia and dehydration. Osmotic diuretics are contraindicated in patients who are anuric owing to severe renal disease. Urea may cause thrombosis or pain if extravasation occurs, and it should not be administered to patients with impaired liver function because of the risk of elevation of blood ammonia levels. Both mannitol and urea are contraindicated in patients with active cranial bleeding. Glycerin is metabolized and can cause hyperglycemia.

Therapeutic Uses. One use for mannitol is in the treatment of dialysis disequilibrium syndrome. Too rapid a removal of solutes from the extracellular fluid by hemodialysis results in a reduction in the osmolality of extracellular fluid. Consequently, water moves from the extracellular compartment into the intracellular compartment, causing hypotension and CNS symptoms (headache, nausea, muscle cramps, restlessness, CNS depression, and convulsions). Osmotic diuretics increase the osmolality of the extracellular fluid compartment and thereby shift water back into the extracellular compartment.

By increasing the osmotic pressure of plasma, osmotic diuretics extract water from the eye and brain. All osmotic diuretics are used to control intraocular pressure during acute attacks of glaucoma and for short-term reductions in intraocular pressure both preoperatively and postoperatively in patients who require ocular surgery. Also, mannitol and urea are used to reduce cerebral edema and brain mass before and after neurosurgery.

INHIBITORS OF Na^+-K^+-$2Cl^-$ SYMPORT (LOOP DIURETICS, HIGH-CEILING DIURETICS)

Drugs in this group of diuretics inhibit activity of the Na^+-K^+-$2Cl^-$ symporter in the thick ascending limb of the loop of Henle; hence these diuretics also are referred to as *loop diuretics*. Although the proximal tubule reabsorbs ~65% of filtered Na^+, diuretics acting only in the proximal tubule have limited efficacy because the thick ascending limb has a great reabsorptive capacity and reabsorbs most of the rejectate from the proximal tubule. Diuretics acting predominantly at sites past the thick ascending limb also have limited efficacy because only a small percentage of the filtered Na^+ load reaches these more distal sites. In contrast, inhibitors of Na^+-K^+-$2Cl^-$ symport in thick ascending limb are highly efficacious, and for this reason, they sometimes are called *high-ceiling diuretics*. The efficacy of inhibitors of Na^+-K^+-$2Cl^-$ symport in the thick ascending limb of the loop of Henle is due to a combination of two factors: (1) approximately 25% of the filtered Na^+ load normally is reabsorbed by the thick ascending limb, and (2) nephron segments past the thick ascending limb do not possess the reabsorptive capacity to rescue the flood of rejectate exiting the thick ascending limb.

Chemistry. Inhibitors of Na^+-K^+-$2Cl^-$ symport are a chemically diverse group (Table 25–4). Only furosemide (LASIX, others), bumetanide (BUMEX, others), ethacrynic acid (EDECRIN, others), and torsemide (DEMADEX, others) are available currently in the U.S. Furosemide and bumetanide contain a sulfonamide moiety. Ethacrynic acid is a phenoxyacetic acid derivative and torsemide is a sulfonylurea.

Mechanism and Site of Action. Inhibitors of Na^+-K^+-$2Cl^-$ symport act primarily in the thick ascending limb. Micropuncture of the DCT demonstrates that loop diuretics increase delivery of solutes out of the loop of Henle. Also, *in situ* microperfusion of the loop of Henle and *in vitro* microperfusion of CTAL indicate inhibition of transport by low concentrations of furosemide in the perfusate. Some inhibitors of Na^+-K^+-$2Cl^-$ symport may have additional effects in the proximal tubule; however, the significance of these effects is unclear.

It was thought initially that Cl^- was transported by a primary active electrogenic transporter in the luminal membrane independent of Na^+. Discovery of furosemide-sensitive Na^+-K^+-$2Cl^-$ symport in other tissues prompted a more careful investigation of the Na^+ dependence of Cl^- transport in isolated perfused rabbit CTAL. Scrupulous removal of Na^+ from the luminal perfusate demonstrated the dependence of Cl^- transport on Na^+.

It is now well accepted that flux of Na^+, K^+, and Cl^- from the lumen into epithelial cells in thick ascending limb is mediated by an

Table 25–4

Inhibitors of Na^+–K^+–$2Cl^-$ Symport (Loop Diuretics, High-Ceiling Diuretics)

DRUG	STRUCTURE	RELATIVE POTENCY	ORAL AVAILABILITY	$t_{1/2}$ (HOURS)	ROUTE OF ELIMINATION
Furosemide (LASIX)	Cl, NH-CH_2, O, H_2NO_2S, COOH	1	~60%	~1.5	~65% R, ~35% M[b]
Bumetanide (BUMEX)	NH-CH_2-CH_2-CH_2-CH_3, O, H_2NO_2S, COOH	40	~80%	~0.8	~62% R, ~38% M
Ethacrynic acid (EDECRIN)	O, Cl, Cl, O, H_3C-H_2C-C-C, O-CH_2-C-OH, CH_2	0.7	~100%	~1	~67% R, ~33% M
Torsemide (DEMADEX)	H, N, N, H_3C, CH_3, O_2S – NH — C – NH – CH, O, CH_3	3	~80%	~3.5	~20% R, ~80% M
Axosemide[a]	Cl, NH-CH_2, S, N, N, H_2NO_2S, N–N, H	1	~12%	~2.5	~27% R, 63% M
Piretanide[a]	N, O, H_2NO_2S, COOH	3	~80%	0.6-1.5	~50% R, ~50% M
Tripamide[a]	Cl, H, H, CONH – N, H_2NO_2S, H, H	ID	ID	ID	ID

[a]Not available in the United States. [b]For furosemide, metabolism occurs predominantly in the kidney. *Abbreviations:* R, renal excretion of intact drug; M, metabolism; ID, insufficient data.

Na^+-K^+-$2Cl^-$ symporter (Figure 25–7). This symporter captures free energy in the Na^+ electrochemical gradient established by the basolateral Na^+ pump and provides for "uphill" transport of K^+ and Cl^- into the cell. K^+ channels in the luminal membrane (called ROMK) provide a conductive pathway for the apical recycling of this cation, and basolateral Cl^- channels (called CLC-Kb) provide a basolateral exit mechanism for Cl^-. Luminal membranes of epithelial cells in thick ascending limb have a large conductive pathway (channels) for K^+; therefore, apical membrane voltage is determined by the equilibrium potential for K^+ (E_K) and is hyperpolarized. In contrast, the basolateral membrane has a large conductive pathway (channels) for Cl^-, so the basolateral membrane voltage is less negative than E_K;

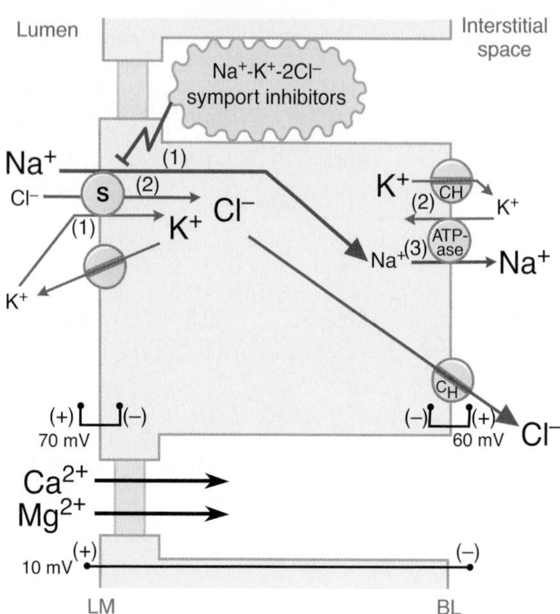

Figure 25–7. *NaCl reabsorption in thick ascending limb and mechanism of diuretic action of Na⁺-K⁺-2Cl symport inhibitors.* Numbers in parentheses indicate stoichiometry. Designated voltages are the potential differences across the indicated membrane or cell. The mechanisms illustrated here apply to the medullary, cortical, and postmacular segments of the thick ascending limb. S, symporter; CH, ion channel; BL, basolateral membrane; LM, luminal membrane.

that is, conductance for Cl^- depolarizes the basolateral membrane. Hyperpolarization of the luminal membrane and depolarization of the basolateral membrane result in a transepithelial potential difference of ~10 mV, with the lumen positive with respect to the interstitial space. This lumen-positive potential difference repels cations (Na^+, Ca^{2+}, and Mg^{2+}) and thereby provides an important driving force for the paracellular flux of these cations into the interstitial space.

Inhibitors of Na^+-K^+-$2Cl^-$ symport bind to the Na^+-K^+-$2Cl^-$ symporter in the thick ascending limb and block its function, bringing salt transport in this segment of the nephron to a virtual standstill. The molecular mechanism by which this class of drugs blocks the Na^+-K^+-$2Cl^-$ symporter is unknown, but evidence suggests that these drugs attach to the Cl^- binding site located in the symporter's transmembrane domain (Isenring and Forbush, 1997). Inhibitors of Na^+-K^+-$2Cl^-$ symport also inhibit Ca^{2+} and Mg^{2+} reabsorption in the thick ascending limb by abolishing the transepithelial potential difference that is the dominant driving force for reabsorption of these cations.

Na^+-K^+-$2Cl^-$ symporters are an important family of transport molecules found in many secretory and absorbing epithelia. The rectal gland of the dogfish shark is a particularly rich source of the protein, and a cDNA encoding an Na^+-K^+-$2Cl^-$ symporter was isolated from a cDNA library obtained from the dogfish shark rectal gland by screening with antibodies to the shark symporter (Xu et al., 1994). Molecular cloning revealed a deduced amino acid sequence of 1191 residues containing 12 putative membrane-spanning domains flanked by long N and C termini in the cytoplasm. Expression of this protein resulted in Na^+-K^+-$2Cl^-$ symport that was sensitive to bumetanide. The shark rectal gland Na^+-K^+-$2Cl^-$ symporter cDNA was used subsequently to screen a human colonic cDNA library, and this provided Na^+-K^+-$2Cl^-$ symporter cDNA probes from this tissue. These latter probes were used to screen rabbit renal cortical and renal medullary libraries, which allowed cloning of the rabbit renal Na^+-K^+-$2Cl^-$ symporter (Payne and Forbush, 1994). This symporter is 1099 amino acids in length, is 61% identical to the dogfish shark secretory Na^+-K^+-$2Cl^-$ symporter, has 12 predicted transmembrane helices, and contains large N- and C-terminal cytoplasmic regions. Subsequent studies demonstrated that Na^+-K^+-$2Cl^-$ symporters are of two varieties (Kaplan et al., 1996). The "absorptive" symporter (called *ENCC2, NKCC2*, or *BSCl*) is expressed only in the kidney, is localized to the apical membrane and subapical intracellular vesicles of the thick ascending limb, and is regulated by cyclic AMP/PKA (Obermüller et al., 1996; Plata et al., 1999). At least six different isoforms of the absorptive symporter are generated by alternative mRNA splicing (Mount et al., 1999), and alternative splicing of the absorptive symporter determines the dependency of transport on K^+ (Plata et al., 2001). The "secretory" symporter (called *ENCC3, NKCCl*, or *BSC2*) is a "housekeeping" protein that is expressed widely and, in epithelial cells, is localized to the basolateral membrane. The affinity of loop diuretics for the secretory symporter is somewhat less than for the absorptive symporter (e.g., 4-fold difference for bumetanide). A model of Na^+-K^+-$2Cl^-$ symport has been proposed based on ordered binding of ions to the symporter (Lytle et al., 1998). Mutations in genes coding for the absorptive Na^+-K^+-$2Cl^-$ symporter, the apical K^+ channel, the basolateral Cl^- channel, or the chloride channel subunit Barttin are causes of Bartter syndrome (inherited hypokalemic alkalosis with salt wasting and hypotension) (Simon and Lifton, 1998).

Effects on Urinary Excretion. Owing to blockade of the Na^+-K^+-$2Cl^-$ symporter, loop diuretics increase urinary Na^+ and Cl^- excretion profoundly (i.e., up to 25% of the filtered Na^+ load). Abolition of the transepithelial potential difference also results in marked increases in Ca^{2+} and Mg^{2+} excretion. Given in excessive amounts, loop diuretics can lead to dehydration and electrolyte depletion. Some (e.g., furosemide) but not all (e.g., bumetanide) sulfonamide-based loop diuretics have weak carbonic anhydrase–inhibiting activity. Drugs with carbonic anhydrase–inhibiting activity increase urinary excretion of HCO_3^- and phosphate. The mechanism by which inhibition of carbonic anhydrase increases phosphate excretion is not known. All inhibitors of Na^+-K^+-$2Cl^-$ symport increase urinary K^+ and titratable acid excretion. This effect is due in part to increased Na^+ delivery to the distal tubule. The mechanism by which increased distal Na^+ delivery enhances K^+ and H^+ excretion is discussed in the section on Na^+ channel inhibitors. Other mechanisms contributing to enhanced K^+ and H^+ excretion include flow-dependent enhancement of ion secretion by the collecting duct,

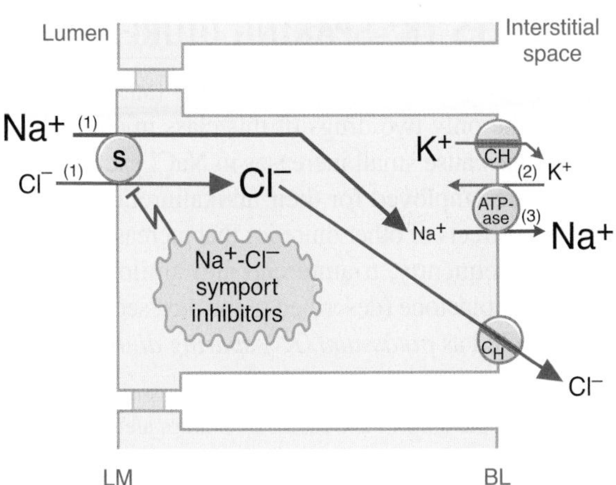

Figure 25–9. *NaCl reabsorption in distal convoluted tubule and mechanism of diuretic action of Na^+-Cl^- symport inhibitors.* Numbers in parentheses indicate stoichiometry. S, symporter; CH, ion channel; BL, basolateral membrane; LM, luminal membrane.

diuresis. However, since the DCT is not involved in the mechanism that generates a hypertonic medullary interstitium, thiazide diuretics do not alter the kidney's ability to concentrate urine during hydropenia.

Effects on Renal Hemodynamics. In general, inhibitors of Na^+-Cl^- symport do not affect RBF and only variably reduce GFR owing to increases in intratubular pressure. Since thiazides act at a point past the macula densa, they have little or no influence on TGF.

Other Actions. Thiazide diuretics may inhibit cyclic nucleotide phosphodiesterases, mitochondrial O_2 consumption, and renal uptake of fatty acids; however, these effects are not clinically significant.

Absorption and Elimination. Pharmacokinetic parameters of Na^+-Cl^- symport inhibitors are listed in Table 25–5.

Note the wide range of half-lives for this class of drugs. Sulfonamides are organic acids and therefore are secreted into the proximal tubule by the organic acid secretory pathway. Since thiazides must gain access to the tubular lumen to inhibit the Na^+-Cl^- symporter, drugs such as probenecid can attenuate the diuretic response to thiazides by competing for transport into proximal tubule. However, plasma protein binding varies considerably among thiazide diuretics, and this parameter determines the contribution that filtration makes to tubular delivery of a specific thiazide.

Toxicity, Adverse Effects, Contraindications, Drug Interactions. Thiazide diuretics rarely cause CNS (e.g., vertigo, headache, paresthesias, xanthopsia, and weakness), GI (e.g., anorexia, nausea, vomiting, cramping, diarrhea, constipation, cholecystitis, and pancreatitis), hematological (e.g., blood dyscrasias), and dermatological (e.g., photosensitivity and skin rashes) disorders. The incidence of erectile dysfunction is greater with Na^+-Cl^- symport inhibitors than with several other antihypertensive agents (e.g., β adrenergic receptor antagonists, Ca^{2+}-channel blockers, or angiotensin converting enzyme inhibitors) (Grimm et al., 1997), but usually is tolerable. As with loop diuretics, most serious adverse effects of thiazides are related to abnormalities of fluid and electrolyte balance. These adverse effects include extracellular volume depletion, hypotension, hypokalemia, hyponatremia, hypochloremia, metabolic alkalosis, hypomagnesemia, hypercalcemia, and hyperuricemia. Thiazide diuretics have caused fatal or near-fatal hyponatremia, and some patients are at recurrent risk of hyponatremia when rechallenged with thiazides.

Thiazide diuretics also decrease glucose tolerance, and latent diabetes mellitus may be unmasked during therapy. Recent concerns have also been raised in randomized prospective blood-pressure lowering trials regarding an increased incidence of type II diabetes mellitus compared to other antihypertensive agents such as angiotensin-converting enzyme inhibitors and angiotensin receptor blockers. The mechanism of impaired glucose tolerance is not completely understood but appears to involve reduced insulin secretion and alterations in glucose metabolism. Hyperglycemia may be related in some way to K^+ depletion, in that hyperglycemia is reduced when K^+ is given along with the diuretic. In addition to contributing to hyperglycemia, thiazide-induced hypokalemia impairs its antihypertensive effect and cardiovascular protection (Franse et al., 2000) afforded by thiazides in patients with hypertension. Thiazide diuretics also may increase plasma levels of LDL cholesterol, total cholesterol, and total triglycerides. Thiazide diuretics are contraindicated in individuals who are hypersensitive to sulfonamides.

With regard to drug interactions, thiazide diuretics may diminish the effects of anticoagulants, uricosuric agents used to treat gout, sulfonylureas, and insulin and may increase the effects of anesthetics, diazoxide, digitalis glycosides, lithium, loop diuretics, and vitamin D. The effectiveness of thiazide diuretics may be reduced by NSAIDs, nonselective or selective COX-2 inhibitors, and bile acid sequestrants (reduced absorption of thiazides). Amphotericin B and corticosteroids increase the risk of hypokalemia induced by thiazide diuretics.

A potentially lethal drug interaction warranting special emphasis is that involving thiazide diuretics and quinidine. Prolongation of the QT interval by quinidine can lead to the development of polymorphic ventricular tachycardia (torsades de pointes) owing to triggered activity originating from early after-depolarizations (Chapter 29). Torsades de pointes may deteriorate into fatal ventricular fibrillation. Hypokalemia increases the risk of quinidine-induced torsades de pointes, and thiazide diuretics cause hypokalemia. Thiazide diuretic–induced K^+ depletion may account for many cases of quinidine-induced torsades de pointes. In addition, alkalinization of the urine by thiazides increases the systemic exposure to quinidine by reducing its elimination.

Therapeutic Uses. Thiazide diuretics are used for the treatment of edema associated with heart (congestive heart failure), liver (hepatic cirrhosis), and renal (nephrotic syndrome, chronic renal failure, and acute glomerulonephritis) disease. With the possible exceptions of metolazone and indapamide, most thiazide diuretics are ineffective when the GFR is <30-40 mL/min.

Thiazide diuretics decrease blood pressure in hypertensive patients by increasing the slope of the renal pressure-natriuresis relationship (Figure 26–7), and thiazide diuretics are used widely for the treatment of hypertension either alone or in combination with other antihypertensive drugs (Chapter 28). In this regard, thiazide diuretics are inexpensive, as efficacious as other classes of antihypertensive agents, and well tolerated. Thiazides can be administered once daily, do not require dose titration, and have few contraindications. Moreover, thiazides have additive or synergistic effects when combined with other classes of antihypertensive agents. A common dose for hypertension is 25 mg/day of hydrochlorothiazide or the dose equivalent of another thiazide. The ALLHAT study (ALLHAT Officers and Coordinators for the ALLHAT Collaborative Research Group, 2002) provides strong evidence that thiazide diuretics are the best initial therapy for uncomplicated hypertension, a conclusion endorsed by the Joint National Committee on Prevention, Detection, Evaluation, and Treatment of High Blood Pressure (Chobanian et al., 2003) (Chapter 27). Studies also suggest that the antihypertensive response to thiazides is influenced by polymorphisms in the angiotensin-converting enzyme and α-adducin genes (Sciarrone et al., 2003).

Thiazide diuretics, which reduce urinary Ca^{2+} excretion, sometimes are employed to treat Ca^{2+} nephrolithiasis and may be useful for treatment of osteoporosis (Chapter 44). Thiazide diuretics also are the mainstay for treatment of nephrogenic diabetes insipidus, reducing urine volume by up to 50%. Although it may seem counterintuitive to treat a disorder of increased urine volume with a diuretic, thiazides reduce the kidney's ability to excrete free water. They do so by increasing proximal tubular water reabsorption (secondary to volume contraction) and by blocking the ability of the distal convoluted tubule to form dilute urine. This latter effect results in an increase in urine osmolality. Since other halides are excreted by renal processes similar to those for Cl^-, thiazide diuretics may be useful for the management of Br^- intoxication.

INHIBITORS OF RENAL EPITHELIAL Na^+ CHANNELS (K^+-SPARING DIURETICS)

Triamterene (DYRENIUM) and amiloride (MIDAMOR, others) are the only two drugs of this class in clinical use. Both drugs cause small increases in NaCl excretion and usually are employed for their antikaliuretic actions to offset the effects of other diuretics that increase K^+ excretion. Consequently, triamterene and amiloride, along with spironolactone (described in the next section), often are classified as *potassium (K^+)-sparing diuretics.*

Chemistry. Amiloride is a pyrazinoylguanidine derivative, and triamterene is a pteridine (Table 25–6). Both drugs are organic bases and are transported by the organic base secretory mechanism in proximal tubule.

Mechanism and Site of Action. Available data suggest that triamterene and amiloride have similar mechanisms of action, which is illustrated in Figure 25–10.

Principal cells in the late distal tubule and collecting duct have, in their luminal membranes, epithelial Na^+ channels that provide a conductive pathway for Na^+ entry into the cell down the electrochemical gradient created by the basolateral Na^+ pump. The higher permeability of the luminal membrane for Na^+ depolarizes the luminal membrane but not the basolateral membrane, creating a lumen-negative transepithelial potential difference. This transepithelial voltage provides an important driving force for the secretion of K^+ into the lumen by K^+ channels (ROMK) in the luminal membrane. Carbonic anhydrase inhibitors, loop diuretics, and thiazide diuretics increase Na^+ delivery to the late distal tubule and collecting duct, a situation that often is associated with increased K^+ and H^+ excretion. It is likely that the elevation in luminal Na^+ concentration in distal nephron induced by such diuretics augments depolarization

Table 25–6

Inhibitors of Renal Epithelial Na^+ Channels (K^+-Sparing Diuretics)

DRUG	STRUCTURE	RELATIVE POTENCY	ORAL AVAILABILITY	$t_{1/2}$ (HOURS)	ROUTE OF ELIMINATION
Amiloride (DYRENIUM)	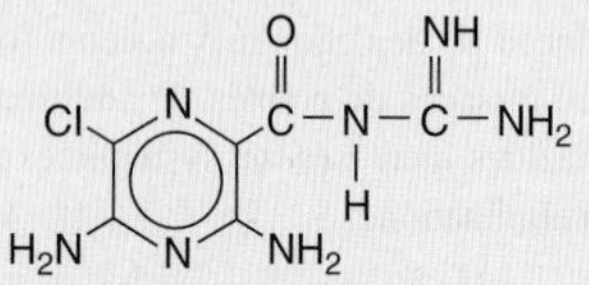	1	15–25%	~21	R
Triamterene (MIDAMOR)	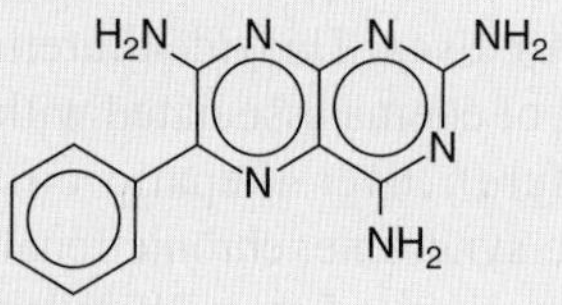	0.1	~50%	~4	M

Abbreviations: R, renal excretion of intact drug; M, metabolism; however, triamterene is transformed into an active metabolite that is excreted in the urine.

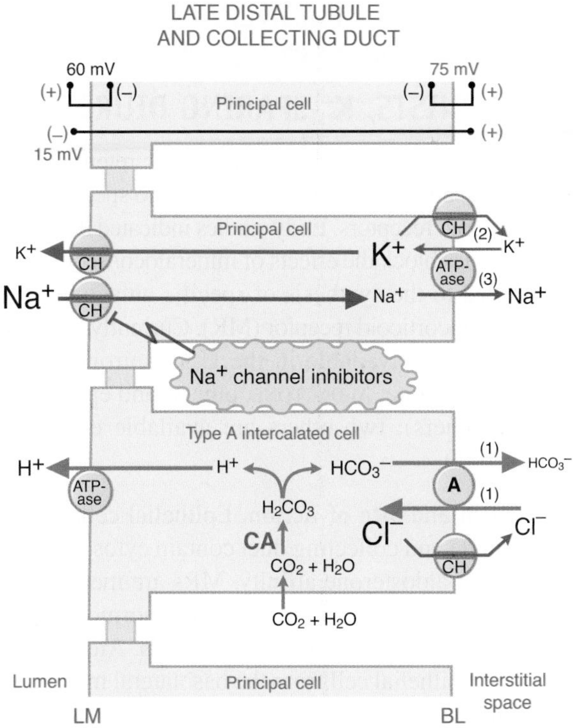

Figure 25–10. *Na^+ reabsorption in late distal tubule and collecting duct and mechanism of diuretic action of epithelial Na^+-channel inhibitors.* Cl^- reabsorption (not shown) occurs both paracellularly and transcellularly, and the precise mechanism of Cl^- transport appears to be species-specific. Numbers in parentheses indicate stoichiometry. Designated voltages are the potential differences across the indicated membrane or cell. A, antiporter; CH, ion channel; CA, carbonic anhydrase; BL, basolateral membrane; LM, luminal membrane.

of the luminal membrane and thereby enhances the lumen-negative V_T, which facilitates K^+ excretion. In addition to principal cells, the collecting duct also contains type A intercalated cells that mediate H^+ secretion into the tubular lumen. Tubular acidification is driven by a luminal H^+-ATPase (proton pump), and this pump is aided by partial depolarization of the luminal membrane. The luminal H^+-ATPase is of the vacuolar-type and is distinct from the gastric H^+-K^+-ATPase that is inhibited by drugs such as omeprazole. However, increased distal Na^+ delivery is not the only mechanism by which diuretics increase K^+ and H^+ excretion. Activation of the renin-angiotensin-aldosterone axis by diuretics also contributes to diuretic-induced K^+ and H^+ excretion, as discussed later in the section on mineralocorticoid antagonists.

Considerable evidence indicates that amiloride blocks epithelial Na^+ channels in the luminal membrane of principal cells in late distal tubule and collecting duct. The amiloride-sensitive Na^+ channel (called *ENaC*) consists of three subunits (α, β, and γ) (Kleyman et al., 1999). Although the α subunit is sufficient for channel activity, maximal Na^+ permeability is induced when all three subunits are coexpressed in the same cell, probably forming a tetrameric structure consisting of two α subunits, one β subunit, and one γ subunit. Studies in *Xenopus* oocytes expressing ENaC suggest that triamterene and amiloride bind ENaC by similar mechanisms. The K_i of amiloride for ENaC is submicromolar, and molecular studies identified critical domains in ENaC that participate in amiloride binding (Kleyman et al., 1999). Liddle syndrome is an autosomal dominant form of low-renin, volume-expanded hypertension that is due to mutations in the β or γ subunits, leading to increased basal ENaC activity.

Effects on Urinary Excretion. Since the late distal tubule and collecting duct have a limited capacity to reabsorb solutes, Na^+ channel blockade in this part of the nephron only mildly increases Na^+ and Cl^- excretion rates (~2% of filtered load). Blockade of Na^+ channels hyperpolarizes the luminal membrane, reducing the lumen-negative transepithelial voltage. Since the lumen-negative potential difference normally opposes cation reabsorption and facilitates cation secretion, attenuation of the lumen-negative voltage decreases K^+, H^+, Ca^{2+}, and Mg^{2+} excretion rates. Volume contraction may increase reabsorption of uric acid in the proximal tubule; hence chronic administration of amiloride and triamterene may decrease uric acid excretion.

Effects on Renal Hemodynamics. Amiloride and triamterene have little or no effect on renal hemodynamics and do not alter TGF.

Other Actions. Amiloride, at concentrations higher than needed to elicit therapeutic effects, also blocks the Na^+-H^+ and Na^+-Ca^{2+} antiporters and inhibits Na^+, K^+-ATPase.

Absorption and Elimination. Pharmacokinetic data for amiloride and triamterene are listed in Table 25–6.

Amiloride is eliminated predominantly by urinary excretion of intact drug. Triamterene is metabolized extensively to an active metabolite, 4-hydroxytriamterene sulfate, and this metabolite is excreted in urine. The pharmacological activity of 4-hydroxytriamterene sulfate is comparable with that of the parent drug. Therefore, triamterene toxicity may be enhanced in both hepatic disease (decreased metabolism of triamterene) and renal failure (decreased urinary excretion of active metabolite).

Toxicity, Adverse Effects, Contraindications, Drug Interactions. The most dangerous adverse effect of renal Na^+-channel inhibitors is hyperkalemia, which can be life-threatening. Consequently, amiloride and triamterene are contraindicated in patients with hyperkalemia, as well as in patients at increased risk of developing hyperkalemia (e.g., patients with renal failure, patients receiving other K^+-sparing diuretics, patients taking angiotensin-converting enzyme inhibitors, or patients taking K^+ supplements). Even NSAIDs can increase the likelihood of hyperkalemia in patients receiving Na^+-channel inhibitors.

Pentamidine and high-dose trimethoprim are used often to treat *Pneumocystis jirovecii* pneumonia in patients with acquired immune deficiency syndrome (AIDS). Because these compounds are weak inhibitors of ENaC, they too may cause hyperkalemia. Risk with trimethoprim is related to both the dosage employed and the underlying level of renal function. It was first reported with high-dose therapy (200 mg/kg/day) in 1983. Subsequent reports of hyperkalemia occurred in HIV-infected patients with normal renal function on high doses of the drug. In one series of 30 such patients, 50% developed a serum K^+ concentration >5.0 mEq/L and 10% >6.0 mEq/L. In a prospective study of otherwise healthy outpatients, the frequency was lower with a serum K^+ concentration >5.5 mEq/L in only 6%. Within 3-10 days after onset of treatment, 10-21% of patients develop a K^+ concentration >5.5 mEq/L (Perazella, 2000). Risk factors for severe hyperkalemia are older age, high-dose therapy, renal impairment, hypoaldosteronism, and treatment with other drugs that impair renal K^+ excretion (e.g., NSAIDs and ACE inhibitors). Serum K^+ concentration should be monitored after 3-4 days of trimethoprim treatment especially in those at increased risk. Likewise, routine monitoring of the serum K^+ level is essential in patients receiving K^+-sparing diuretics. Cirrhotic patients are prone to megaloblastosis because of folic acid deficiency, and triamterene, a weak folic acid antagonist, may increase the likelihood of this adverse event. Triamterene also can reduce glucose tolerance and induce photosensitization and has been associated with interstitial nephritis and renal stones. Both drugs can cause CNS, GI, musculoskeletal, dermatological, and hematological adverse effects. The most common adverse effects of amiloride are nausea, vomiting, diarrhea, and headache; those of triamterene are nausea, vomiting, leg cramps, and dizziness.

Therapeutic Uses. Because of the mild natriuresis induced by Na^+-channel inhibitors, these drugs seldom are used as sole agents in treatment of edema or hypertension. Rather, their major utility is in combination with other diuretics; indeed, each is marketed in a fixed-dose combination with a thiazide: triamterene/hydrochlorothiazide (DYAZIDE, MAXZIDE, others), amiloride/hydrochlorothiazide (generic).

Co-administration of an Na^+-channel inhibitor augments the diuretic and antihypertensive response to thiazide and loop diuretics. More important, the ability of Na^+-channel inhibitors to reduce K^+ excretion tends to offset the kaliuretic effects of thiazide and loop diuretics; consequently, the combination of an Na^+-channel inhibitor with a thiazide or loop diuretic tends to result in normal plasma K^+ values. Liddle syndrome can be treated effectively with Na^+-channel inhibitors. Approximately 5% of people of African origin carry a *T594M* polymorphism in the β subunit of ENaC, and amiloride is particularly effective in lowering blood pressure in patients with hypertension who carry this polymorphism (Baker et al., 2002). Aerosolized amiloride has been shown to improve mucociliary clearance in patients with cystic fibrosis. By inhibiting Na^+ absorption from the surfaces of airway epithelial cells, amiloride augments hydration of respiratory secretions and thereby improves mucociliary clearance. Amiloride also is useful for lithium-induced nephrogenic diabetes insipidus because it blocks Li^+ transport into collecting tubule cells.

ANTAGONISTS OF MINERALOCORTICOID RECEPTORS (ALDOSTERONE ANTAGONISTS, K^+-SPARING DIURETICS)

Mineralocorticoids cause salt and water retention and increase K^+ and H^+ excretion by binding to specific mineralocorticoid receptors. Early studies indicated that some spirolactones block the effects of mineralocorticoids; this finding led to the synthesis of specific antagonists for the mineralocorticoid receptor (MR). Currently, two MR antagonists are available in the U.S., spironolactone (a 17-spirolactone; ALDACTONE, others) and eplerenone (INSPRA, others); two others are available elsewhere (Table 25–7).

Mechanism and Site of Action. Epithelial cells in late distal tubule and collecting duct contain cytosolic MRs with a high aldosterone affinity. MRs are members of the superfamily of receptors for steroid hormones, thyroid hormones, vitamin D, and retinoids. Aldosterone enters the epithelial cell from the basolateral membrane and binds to MRs; the MR-aldosterone complex translocates to the nucleus, where it binds to specific sequences of DNA (hormone-responsive elements) and thereby regulates the expression of multiple gene products called *aldosterone-induced proteins* (AIPs). Consequently, transepithelial NaCl transport is enhanced, and the lumen-negative transepithelial voltage is increased. The latter effect increases the driving force for K^+ and H^+ secretion into the tubular lumen.

The discovery of gene mutation responsible for rare monogenic diseases that cause hypertension such as Liddle syndrome and apparent mineralocorticoid excess helped clarify how aldosterone regulates Na^+ transport in the distal nephron (Figure 25–11). Mutations in the carboxy-terminal PY motif of either the β or γ subunits of ENaC are associated with Liddle syndrome. The PY motif is an area involved in protein-protein interaction. The PY motif of ENaC interacts with the ubiquitin ligase Nedd4-2, a protein that ubiquitinates ENaC. This then results in internalization of ENaC and proteasome-mediated degradation. Subsequent studies revealed that Nedd4-2 is phosphorylated and inactivated by SGK1 (serum and glucocorticoid-stimulated kinase) and that SGK1 is up-regulated after ~30 minutes by aldosterone. By tracing back the pathophysiologic mechanism of Liddle syndrome, one of the mechanisms whereby aldosterone acts in the collecting duct was identified. Aldosterone up-regulates SGK1, which phosphorylates and inactivates Nedd4-2. As a result, ENaC is not ubiquitinated and removed from the membrane, thereby increasing Na^+ reabsorption. When the mineralocorticoid receptor was cloned and tested *in vitro* it was noted to have equal affinity for mineralocorticoid and glucocorticoids. It had been assumed that the mineralocorticoid receptor would have specificity for mineralocorticoids, but surprisingly this was not the case. Given that glucocorticoids circulate at 100- to 1000-fold

Table 25–7

Mineralocorticoid Receptor Antagonists (Aldosterone Antagonists, Potassium-Sparing Diuretics)

DRUG	STRUCTURE	ORAL AVAILABILITY	$t_{1/2}$ (HOURS)	ROUTE OF ELIMINATION
Spironolactone (ALDACTONE)		~65%	~1.6	M
Canrenone[a]		ID	~16.5	M
Potassium canrenoate[a]		ID	ID	M
Eplerenone (INSPRA)		ID	~5	M

[a]Not available in United States. M, metabolism; ID, insufficient data.

higher concentration than mineralocorticoids, it was unclear how mineralocorticoids would ever bind to their receptor. The mineralocorticoid receptor would be predominantly occupied by glucocorticoids. This mystery was solved with the cloning of the enzyme type II 11-β-hydroxysteroid dehydrogenase (HSD). Mineralocorticoid target tissues expresses type II 11-β-HSD, which converts cortisol to the inactive cortisone. This allows mineralocorticoids to bind to the receptor. The type II 11-β-HSD enzyme is genetically absent in the inherited disorder of apparent mineralocorticoid excess.

Drugs such as spironolactone and eplerenone competitively inhibit the binding of aldosterone to the MR. Unlike the MR-aldosterone complex, the MR-spironolactone complex is not able to induce the synthesis of AIPs. Since spironolactone and eplerenone block biological effects of aldosterone, these agents also are referred to as *aldosterone antagonists*.

MR antagonists are the only diuretics that do not require access to the tubular lumen to induce diuresis.

Effects on Urinary Excretion. The effects of MR antagonists on urinary excretion are very similar to those induced by renal epithelial Na^+-channel inhibitors. However, unlike Na^+-channel inhibitors, the clinical efficacy of MR antagonists is a function of endogenous aldosterone levels. The higher the endogenous

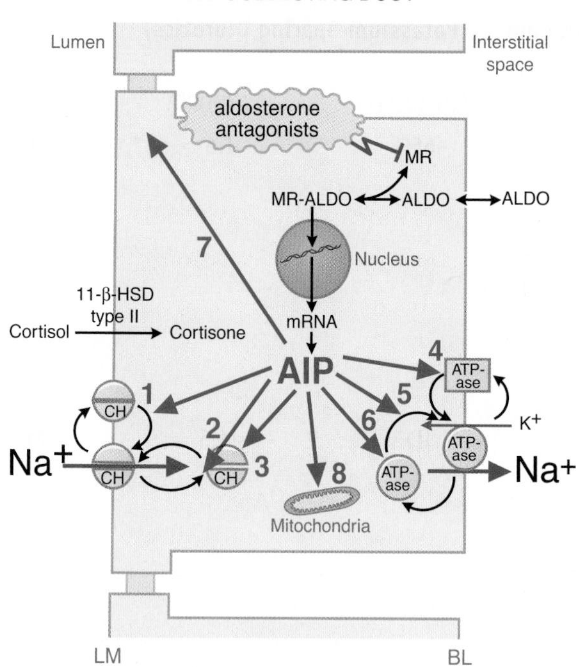

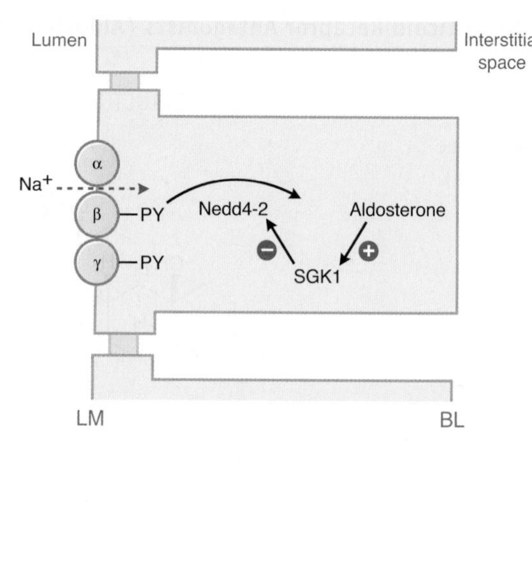

Figure 25–11. *Effects of aldosterone on late distal tubule and collecting duct and diuretic mechanism of aldosterone antagonists.* **A.** Cortisol also has affinity for the mineralocorticoid receptor (MR), but is inactivated in the cell by 11-β-hydroxysteroid dehydrogenase (HSD) type II. **B.** Serum and glucorticoid-regulated kinase (SGK)-1 is upregulated after ~30 minutes by aldosterone. SGK-1 phosphorylates and inactivates Nedd4-2 a ubiquitin-protein ligase that acts on ENaC, leading to its degradation. Phosphorylated Nedd4-2 no longer interacts with the PY motif of ENaC. As a result, the protein is not ubiquitinated and remains in the membrane, the end result of which is increased Na^+ entry into the cell. 1. Activation of membrane-bound Na^+ channels. 2. Na^+ channel (ENaC) removal from the membrane is inhibited. 3. *De novo* synthesis of Na^+ channels. 4. Activation of membrane-bound Na^+,K^+- ATPase. 5. Redistribution of Na^+,K^+-ATPase from cytosol to membrane. 6. *De novo* synthesis of Na^+,K^+-ATPase. 7. Changes in permeability of tight junctions. 8. Increased mitochondrial production of ATP. AIP, aldosterone-induced proteins; ALDO, aldosterone; MR, mineralocorticoid receptor; CH, ion channel; BL, basolateral membrane; LM, luminal membrane.

aldosterone level, the greater the effects of MR antagonists on urinary excretion.

Effects on Renal Hemodynamics. MR antagonists have little or no effect on renal hemodynamics and do not alter TGF.

Other Actions. Spironolactone has some affinity toward progesterone and androgen receptors and thereby induces side effects such as gynecomastia, impotence, and menstrual irregularities. Owing to the 9,11-epoxide group, eplerenone has very low affinity for progesterone and androgen receptors (<1% and <0.1%, respectively) compared with spironolactone. High spironolactone concentrations were reported to interfere with steroid biosynthesis by inhibiting steroid hydroxylases (e.g., CYPs 11A1, 11B1, 11B2, and C21; see Chapters 40 and 41). These effects have limited clinical relevance.

Absorption and Elimination. Spironolactone is absorbed partially (~65%), is metabolized extensively (even during its first passage through the liver), undergoes enterohepatic recirculation, is highly protein bound, and has a short $t_{1/2}$ (~1.6 hours). The $t_{1/2}$ is prolonged to 9 hours in patients with cirrhosis.

Spironolactone undergoes metabolism by both deacylation and dethioacetylation to a variety of metabolites with prolonged $t_{1/2}$; of these, 7α thiomethyl spirononlactone is the primary active metabolite.

Although not available in the U.S., canrenone and the K^+ salt of canrenoate also are in clinical use. Canrenoate is not active *per se* but is converted to canrenone. Eplerenone has good oral availability and is eliminated primarily by metabolism by CYP3A4 to inactive metabolites, with a $t_{1/2}$ of ~5 hours.

Toxicity, Adverse Effects, Contraindications, Drug Interactions. As with other K^+-sparing diuretics, MR antagonists may cause life-threatening hyperkalemia. Indeed, hyperkalemia is the principal risk of MR antagonists. Therefore, these drugs are contraindicated in patients with hyperkalemia and in those at increased risk of developing hyperkalemia either because of disease or administration of other medications. MR antagonists also can induce metabolic acidosis in cirrhotic patients.

Salicylates may reduce the tubular secretion of canrenone and decrease diuretic efficacy of spironolactone, and spironolactone may alter the clearance of digitalis glycosides. Owing to its affinity for other steroid receptors, spironolactone may cause gynecomastia, impotence, decreased libido, hirsutism, deepening of the voice, and menstrual irregularities. Spironolactone also may induce diarrhea, gastritis, gastric bleeding, and peptic ulcers (the drug is contraindicated in patients with peptic ulcers). CNS adverse effects include drowsiness, lethargy, ataxia, confusion, and headache. Spironolactone may cause skin rashes and, rarely, blood dyscrasias. Breast cancer has occurred in patients taking spironolactone chronically (cause and effect not established), and high doses of spironolactone are associated with malignant tumors in rats. Whether or not therapeutic spironolactone doses can induce malignancies remains an open question. Strong inhibitors of CYP3A4 may increase plasma levels of eplerenone, and such drugs should not be administered to patients taking eplerenone, and vice versa. Other than hyperkalemia and GI disorders, the rate of adverse events for eplerenone is similar to that of placebo (Pitt et al., 2003).

Therapeutic Uses. As with other K^+-sparing diuretics, spironolactone often is coadministered with thiazide or loop diuretics in the treatment of edema and hypertension, and spironolactone in combination with hydrochlorothiazide (ALDACTAZIDE, others) is marketed. Such combinations result in increased mobilization of edema fluid while causing lesser perturbations of K^+ homeostasis. Spironolactone is particularly useful in the treatment of resistant hypertension due to primary hyperaldosteronism (adrenal adenomas or bilateral adrenal hyperplasia) and of refractory edema associated with secondary aldosteronism (cardiac failure, hepatic cirrhosis, nephrotic syndrome, and severe ascites). Spironolactone is considered the diuretic of choice in patients with hepatic cirrhosis. Spironolactone, added to standard therapy, substantially reduces morbidity and mortality (Pitt et al., 1999) and ventricular arrhythmias (Ramires et al., 2000) in patients with heart failure (Chapter 28).

Clinical experience with eplerenone is less than that with spironolactone. Eplerenone appears to be a safe and effective antihypertensive drug (Ouzan et al., 2002). It is somewhat more specific for the MR and therefore the incidence of progesterone-related adverse effects (e.g., gynecomastia) is lower than with spironolactone. In patients with acute myocardial infarction complicated by left ventricular systolic dysfunction, addition of eplerenone to optimal medical therapy significantly reduces morbidity and mortality (Pitt et al., 2003).

INHIBITORS OF THE NONSPECIFIC CATION CHANNEL: ATRIAL NATRIURETIC PEPTIDES

The inner medullary collecting duct (IMCD) is a major site of action of natriuretic peptides. Although five different natriuretic peptides exist, only four are relevant with respect to human physiology: atrial natriuretic peptide (ANP), brain natriuretic peptide (BNP), C-type natriuretic peptide (CNP), and urodilatin. ANP and BNP are produced by the heart in response to wall stretch, CNP is of endothelial and renal cell origin, while urodilatin is found in urine and acts as a paracrine regulator of Na^+ transport (Lee and Burnett, 2007). Human recombinant ANP (carperitide, available only in Japan) and BNP (nesiritide [NATRECOR]) are currently available therapeutic agents of this class.

Mechanism and Site of Action. The IMCD is the final site along the nephron where Na^+ is reabsorbed. Up to 5% of the filtered Na^+ load can be reabsorbed here. Na^+ enters the IMCD cell across the apical membrane down an electrochemical gradient through Na^+ channels and exits via the Na^+/K^+-ATPase (Figure 25–12). Two types of Na^+

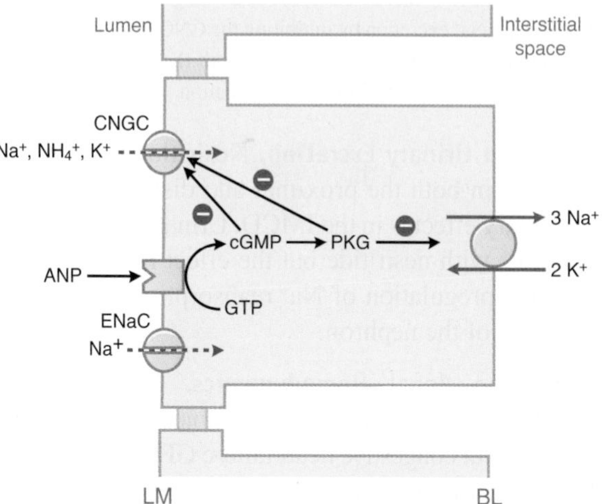

Figure 25–12. *Inner medullary collecting duct (IMCD) Na^+ transport and its regulation.* Na^+ enters the IMCD cell in one of two ways. The first is via ENaC, and the second is through a cyclic nucleotide gated nonspecific cation channel (CNGC) that transports Na^+, K^+, and NH_4^+ and is gated by cyclic GMP. Na^+ then exits the cell via the Na^+, K^+-ATPase. It is the CNGC that is the primary pathway for Na^+ entry, and is inhibited by natriuretic peptides. Atrial natriuretic peptides (ANP) bind to surface receptors (natriuretic peptide receptors A, B, and C). The A and B receptors are isoforms of particulate guanylate cyclase that catalyze the conversion of GTP to cyclic GMP. Cyclic GMP inhibits the CNGC directly, and indirectly through PKG. PKG activation also inhibits Na^+ exit via the Na^+, K^+-ATPase.

channels are expressed in IMCD. The first is an amiloride-sensitive, 28pS, nonselective, cyclic nucleotide gated cation (CNG) channel. This channel is highly selective for cations over anions, has equal permeability for Na^+ and K^+, and is inhibited by cGMP, PKG, PKC, ATP, and atrial natriuretic peptides via their capacity to stimulate membrane-bound guanylyl cyclase activity and elevate cellular cGMP. Its open probability is increased by rises in intracellular Ca^{2+} concentration. CNG channels are expressed in all nephron segments with the possible exception of the thin limb of Henle's loop. The second type of Na^+ channel expressed in the IMCD is the low-conductance 4 pS highly-selective Na^+ channel ENaC. It appears that the majority of Na^+ reabsorption in the IMCD is mediated via the CNG channel.

ANP has a 17 amino acid core ring and a cysteine bridge. It is produced in the cardiac atria in response to wall stretch. It binds to the natriuretic peptide receptor (NPR) A and increases intracellular cyclic GMP resulting in inhibition of the CNG channel and natriuresis. It also inhibits production of renin and aldosterone. BNP is produced in the ventricle, also binds to the NPR-A receptor and acts in a similar fashion as ANP. CNP binds to the NPR-B receptor and increases cGMP in vascular smooth muscle and mediates vasodilation. Urodilatin arises from the same precursor molecule as ANP but has four additional amino acids at the N terminus. It binds with lower affinity than ANP to the NPR-B receptor and has effects in glomeruli and IMCD. As a result of these effects, natriuretic peptides have been utilized to treat congestive heart failure. Human recombinant ANP (carperitide) is available in Japan but not yet in the U.S., where human recombinant BNP (nesiritide) is available. Urodilatin (ularitide) remains in preclinical trials in the U.S. and Europe. Only the use of nesiritide is discussed in the following sections. Nesiritide effects renal Na^+ excretion by inhibiting the CNG nonspecific-cation channel, as well as through inhibiting both the renin-angiotensin-aldosterone system and endothelin production.

Effects on Urinary Excretion. Nesiritide inhibits Na^+ transport in both the proximal and distal nephron but its primary effect is in the IMCD. Urinary Na^+ excretion increases with nesiritide but the effect may be attenuated by upregulation of Na^+ reabsorption in upstream segments of the nephron.

Effects on Renal Hemodynamics. GFR increases administered nesiritide in normal subjects, but in treated patients with congestive heart failure GFR may increase, decrease, or remain unchanged.

Other Actions. Administration of nesiritide decreases systemic and pulmonary resistances and left ventricular filling pressure, and induces a secondary increase in cardiac output. In one study, mean arterial pressure, pulmonary capillary wedge pressure, and right atrial pressure declined 17%, 48%, and 56%, respectively. Declines in blood pressure with administration are dose related.

Elimination. Natriuretic peptides are administered intravenously and have short $t_{1/2}$ values. Nesiritide has a distribution $t_{1/2}$ of 2 minutes and a mean terminal $t_{1/2}$ of 18 minutes. Its volume of distribution is small, 0.19 L/kg. It is cleared via three mechanisms: binding to the NPR-C receptor, degradation via a neutral endopeptidase, and renal excretion. There is no need to adjust the dose for renal insufficiency.

Toxicity, Adverse Effects, Contraindications, Drug Interactions. There are concerns about adverse renal effects and reports of increased short-term mortality in patients treated with nesiritide. Increases in serum creatinine concentration may be related to decreases in extracellular fluid volume, higher doses of diuretics used, decreases in blood pressure, and activation of the renin-angiotensin-aldosterone system. The Vasodilation in the Management of Acute CHF (VAMC) trial showed no increased risk with low or moderate doses of diuretics but an increased risk with high-dose diuretics (>160 mg furosemide), rising with increasing doses. The risk of hypotension was 4.4% and lasted an average of 2.2 hours. Oral ACE inhibitors may increase the risk of hypotension with nesiritide. Data on whether 30-day mortality is increased by nesiritide are conflicting. There are no data to suggest that nesiritide reduces mortality in the short term or long term in patients with acute decompensated CHF.

Therapeutic Uses. Use of nesiritide should be limited to patients with acutely decompensated CHF with shortness of breath at rest; the drug should not be used in place of diuretics. Nesiritide reduces symptoms and improves hemodynamic parameters in those with dyspnea at rest who are not hypotensive. Nesiritide is available for administration as a continuous intravenous infusion; there is little experience with administering nesiritide for longer than 48 hours.

CLINICAL USE OF DIURETICS

Site and Mechanism of Diuretic Action. An understanding of the sites and mechanisms of action of diuretics enhances comprehension of the clinical aspects of diuretic pharmacology. Figure 25–13 provides an overview of the sites and mechanisms of actions of diuretics. Much of the pharmacology of diuretics can be deduced from this figure.

Mechanism of Edema Formation. A complex set of interrelationships (Figure 25–14) exists among the cardiovascular system, kidneys, CNS (Na^+ appetite, thirst regulation), and tissue capillary beds (distribution of extracellular fluid volume [ECFV]), so perturbations at one of these sites can affect all other sites. A primary law of the kidney is that Na^+ excretion is a steep function of mean arterial blood pressure (MABP), such that small increases in MABP cause marked increases in Na^+ excretion (Guyton, 1991). Over any given time interval, the net change in total-body Na^+ (either positive or negative) is simply the dietary Na^+ intake minus the urinary excretion rate minus other losses (e.g., sweating, fecal losses, and vomiting). When a net positive Na^+ balance occurs, the Na^+ concentration in the extracellular fluid (ECF) will increase, stimulating water intake (thirst) and reducing urinary water output

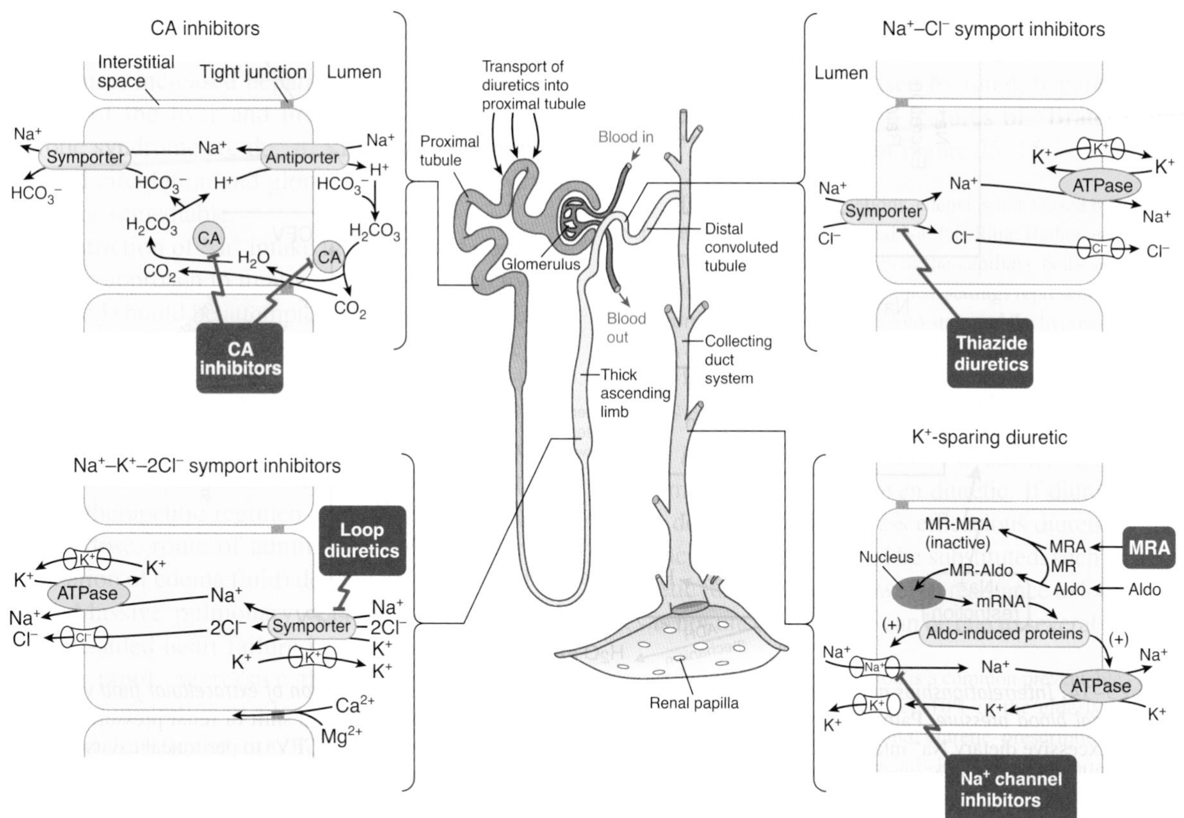

Figure 25–13. *Summary of the site and mechanism of action of diuretics.* Three important features of this summary figure are worth special note. 1. Transport of solute across epithelial cells in all nephron segments involves highly specialized proteins, which for the most part are apical and basolateral membrane integral proteins. 2. Diuretics target and block the action of epithelial proteins involved in solute transport. 3. The site and mechanism of action of a given class of diuretics are determined by the specific protein inhibited by the diuretic. CA, carbonic anhydrase; MR, mineralocorticoid receptor; MRA, mineralocorticoid receptor antagonist; Aldo, aldosterone.

(by ADH release). Opposite changes occur during a net negative Na^+ balance.

Changes in water intake and output adjust ECFV toward normal, thereby expanding or contracting total ECFV. Total ECFV is distributed among many body compartments; however, since ECF volume on the arterial side of the circulation pressurizes the arterial tree, it is this fraction of ECFV that determines MABP, and it is this fraction of ECFV that is "sensed" by the cardiovascular system and kidneys. Since MABP is a major determinant of Na^+ output, a closed loop is established (Figure 25–14). This loop cycles until net Na^+ accumulation is zero; i.e., in the long run, Na^+ intake must equal Na^+ loss.

The preceding discussion implies that three fundamental types of perturbations contribute to venous congestion and/or edema formation:

1. A shift to the right in the renal pressure-natriuresis relationship (e.g., chronic renal failure) causes reduced Na^+ excretion for any level of MABP. If all other factors remain constant, this would increase total-body Na^+, ECFV, and MABP. The additional ECFV would be distributed throughout various body compartments according to the state of cardiac function and prevailing Starling forces and would predispose toward venous congestion and/or edema. Even so, in the absence of any other predisposing factors for venous congestion and/or edema, a rightward shift in the renal pressure-natriuresis curve generally causes hypertension with only a slight (usually immeasurable) increase in ECFV. As elucidated by Guyton (1991), ECFV expansion triggers a series of events: expanded ECFV → augmented cardiac output → enhanced vascular tone (i.e., total-body autoregulation) → increased total peripheral resistance → elevated MABP → pressure natriuresis → reduction of ECFV and cardiac output toward normal. Most likely, a

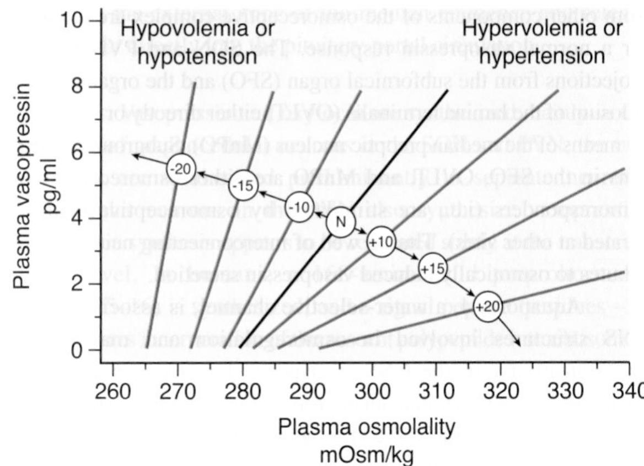

Figure 25–18. *Interactions between osmolality and hypovolemia/hypotension.* Numbers in circles refer to percentage increase (+) or decrease (–) in blood volume or arterial blood pressure. N indicates normal blood volume/blood pressure. (Reprinted by permission from Macmillan Publishers Ltd: Robertson GL, Shelton RL, Athar S: The osmoregulation of vasopressin. *Kidney Internat 10*:25, 1976. Copyright © 1976.)

known, and the vasopressin response to hypovolemia or hypotension serves as a mechanism to stave off cardiovascular collapse during periods of severe blood loss and/or hypotension. Hemodynamic regulation of vasopressin secretion does not disrupt osmotic regulation; rather, hypovolemia/hypotension alters the set point and slope of the plasma osmolality-plasma vasopressin relationship (Figure 25–18).

Neuronal pathways that mediate hemodynamic regulation of vasopressin release are different from those involved in osmoregulation. Baroreceptors in left atrium, left ventricle, and pulmonary veins sense blood volume (filling pressures), and baroreceptors in carotid sinus and aorta monitor arterial blood pressure. Nerve impulses reach brainstem nuclei predominantly through the vagal trunk and glossopharyngeal nerve; these signals are relayed to the solitary tract nucleus, then to the A_1-noradrenergic cell group in the caudal ventrolateral medulla, and finally to the SON and PVN.

Hormones and Neurotransmitters. Vasopressin-synthesizing magnocellular neurons have a large array of receptors on both perikarya and nerve terminals; therefore, vasopressin release can be accentuated or attenuated by chemical agents acting at both ends of the magnocellular neuron. Also, hormones and neurotransmitters can modulate vasopressin secretion by stimulating or inhibiting neurons in nuclei that project, either directly or indirectly, to the SON and PVN. Because of these complexities, results of any given investigation may depend critically on route of administration of the agent and on the experimental paradigm. In many cases, the precise mechanism by which a given agent modulates vasopressin secretion is either unknown or controversial, and the physiological relevance of the modulation of vasopressin secretion by most hormones and neurotransmitters is unclear.

Nonetheless, several agents are known to stimulate vasopressin secretion, including acetylcholine (by nicotinic receptors), histamine (by H_1 receptors), dopamine (by both D_1 and D_2 receptors), glutamine, aspartate, cholecystokinin, neuropeptide Y, substance P, vasoactive intestinal polypeptide, prostaglandins, and angiotensin II (AngII). Inhibitors of vasopressin secretion include atrial natriuretic peptide, γ-aminobutyric acid, and opioids (particularly dynorphin *via* κ receptors). The affects of AngII have received the most attention. AngII, applied directly to magnocellular neurons in the SON and PVN, increases neuronal excitability; when applied to the MnPO, AngII indirectly stimulates magnocellular neurons in the SON and PVN. In addition, AngII stimulates angiotensin-sensitive neurons in the OVLT and SFO (circumventricular nuclei lacking a blood-brain barrier) that project to the SON/PVN. Thus, AngII synthesized in the brain and circulating AngII may stimulate vasopressin release. Inhibition of the conversion of AngII to AngIII blocks AngII-induced vasopressin release, suggesting that AngIII is the main effector peptide of the brain renin-angiotensin system controlling vasopressin release (Reaux et al., 2001).

Pharmacological Agents. A number of drugs alter urine osmolality by stimulating or inhibiting vasopressin secretion. In some cases the mechanism by which a drug alters vasopressin secretion involves direct effects on one or more CNS structures that regulate vasopressin secretion. In other cases vasopressin secretion is altered indirectly by the effects of a drug on blood volume, arterial blood pressure, pain, or nausea. In most cases the mechanism is not known. Stimulators of vasopressin secretion include vincristine, cyclophosphamide, tricyclic antidepressants, nicotine, epinephrine, and high doses of morphine. Lithium, which inhibits the renal effects of vasopressin, also enhances vasopressin secretion. Inhibitors of vasopressin secretion include ethanol, phenytoin, low doses of morphine, glucocorticoids, fluphenazine, haloperidol, promethazine, oxilorphan, and butorphanol. Carbamazepine has a renal action to produce antidiuresis in patients with central diabetes insipidus but actually inhibits vasopressin secretion by a central action.

BASIC PHARMACOLOGY OF VASOPRESSIN

Vasopressin Receptors. Cellular vasopressin effects are mediated mainly by interactions of the hormone with the three types of receptors, V_{1a}, V_{1b}, and V_2. The V_{1a} receptor is the most widespread subtype of vasopressin receptor; it is found in vascular smooth muscle, adrenal gland, myometrium, bladder, adipocytes, hepatocytes, platelets, renal medullary interstitial cells, vasa recta in the renal microcirculation, epithelial cells in the renal cortical collecting-duct, spleen, testis, and many CNS structures. V_{1b} receptors have a more limited distribution and are found in the anterior pituitary, several brain regions, pancreas, and adrenal medulla. V_2 receptors are located predominantly in principal cells of the renal collecting-duct system but also are present on epithelial cells in thick ascending limb and on vascular endothelial cells. Although originally defined by pharmacological criteria, vasopressin receptors now are defined by their primary amino acid sequences. The cloned vasopressin receptors are typical heptahelical GPCRs. Manning and co-workers (1999) synthesized novel hypotensive vasopressin peptide agonists that do not interact with V_{1a}, V_{1b}, or V_2 receptors and may stimulate a putative vasopressin vasodilatory receptor.

Two additional putative receptors for vasopressin have been cloned. A vasopressin-activated Ca^{2+}-mobilizing receptor with one transmembrane domain binds vasopressin and increases intracellular Ca^{2+} (Serradeil-Le Gal et al., 2002). A dual AngII-vasopressin heptahelical receptor activates adenylyl cyclase in response to both AngII and vasopressin (Serradeil-Le Gal et al., 2002). The physiological roles of these putative vasopressin receptors are unclear.

V_1 Receptor-Effector Coupling. Figure 25–19 summarizes the current model of V_1 receptor-effector coupling. Vasopressin binding to V_1 receptors activates the G_q-PLC-IP_3 pathway, thereby mobilizing intracellular Ca^{2+} and activating PKC, ultimately causing biological effects that include immediate responses (e.g., vasoconstriction, glycogenolysis, platelet aggregation, and ACTH release) and growth responses in smooth muscle cells. Other effects of V_1-receptor activation may be mediated by stimulation of small G proteins, activation of PLD and PLA_2, and activation of V_1-sensitive Ca^{2+} influx. Some effects of V_1-receptor activation are secondary to synthesis of prostaglandins and epoxyeicosatrienoic acids (Chapter 33).

V_2 Receptor-Effector Coupling. Principal cells in renal collecting duct have V_2 receptors on their basolateral membranes that couple to G_S to stimulate adenylyl cyclase activity (Figure 25–20) when vasopressin binds to V_2 receptors. The resulting increase in cellular cyclic AMP and PKA activity triggers an increased rate of

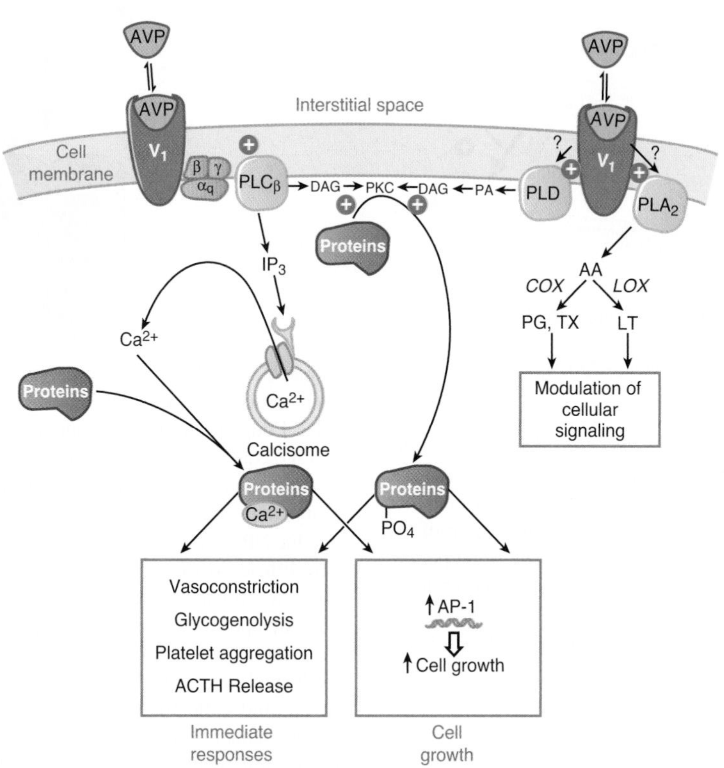

Figure 25–19. *Mechanism of V_1 receptor-effector coupling.* Binding of 8-arginine vasopressin (AVP) to V_1 vasopressin receptors (V_1) stimulates several membrane-bound phospholipases. Stimulation of the G_q-PLC_β pathway results in IP_3 formation, mobilization of intracellular Ca^{2+}, and activation of PKC. Activation of V_1 receptors also causes influx of extracellular Ca^{2+} by an unknown mechanism. PKC and Ca^{2+}/calmodulin-activated protein kinases phosphorylate cell-type-specific proteins leading to cellular responses. A further component of the AVP response derives from the production of eicosanoids secondary to the activation of PLA_2; the resulting mobilization of arachidonic acid (AA) provides substrate for eicosanoid synthesis by the cyclooxygenase (COX) and lipoxygenase (LOX) pathways, leading to local production of prostaglandins (PG), thromboxanes (TX), and leukotrienes (LT), which may activate a variety of signaling pathways, including those linked to G_S and G_q. Biological effects mediated by the V_1 receptor include vasoconstriction, glycogenolysis, platelet aggregation, ACTH release, and growth of vascular smooth muscle cells. The effects of vasopressin on cell growth involve transcriptional regulation by the FOS/JUN AP-1 transcription complex.

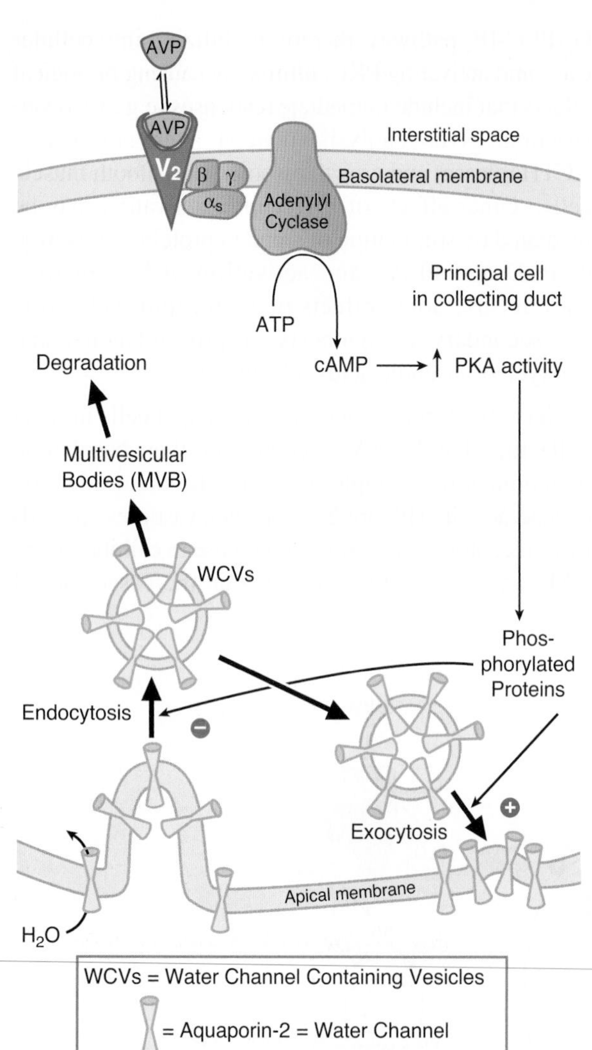

Figure 25–20. *Mechanism of V_2 receptor-effector coupling.* Binding of vasopressin (AVP) to the V_2 receptor activates the G_S-adenylyl cyclase-cAMP-PKA pathway and shifts the balance of aquaporin 2 trafficking toward the apical membrane of the principal cell of the collecting duct, thus enhancing water permeability. Although phosphorylation of serine 256 of aquaporin 2 is involved in V_2 receptor signaling, other proteins located both in the water channel-containing vesicles and the apical membrane of the cytoplasm also may be involved.

insertion of water channel-containing vesicles (WCVs) into the apical membrane and a decreased rate of endocytosis of WCVs from the apical membrane (Snyder et al., 1992). Distribution of WCVs between the cytosolic compartment and apical membrane compartment is thus shifted in favor of the apical membrane compartment (Nielsen et al., 1999). Because WCVs contain preformed functional water channels (aquaporin 2), their net shift into apical membranes in response to V_2-receptor stimulation greatly increases water permeability of the apical membrane (see Figures 25–20 and 25–21).

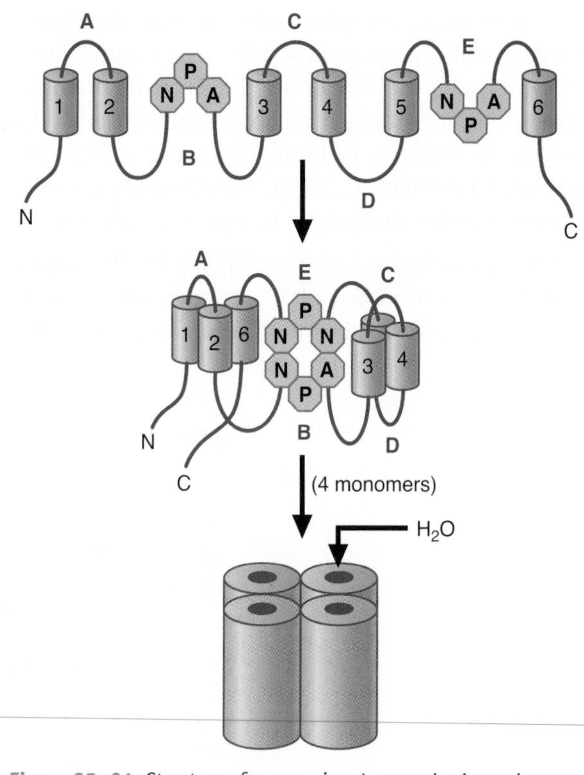

Figure 25–21. *Structure of aquaporins.* Aquaporins have six transmembrane domains, and the NH_2 and COOH termini are intracellular. Loops B and E each contain an asparagine-proline-alanine (NPA) sequence. Aquaporins fold with transmembrane domains 1, 2, and 6 in close proximity and transmembrane domains 3, 4 and 5 in juxtaposition. The long B and E loops dip into the membrane, and the NPA sequences align to create a pore through which water can diffuse. Most likely aquaporins form a tetrameric oligomer. At least seven aquaporins are expressed at distinct sites in the kidney. Aquaporin 1, abundant in the proximal tubule and descending thin limb, is essential for concentration of urine. Aquaporin 2, exclusively expressed in the principal cells of the connecting tubule and collecting duct, is the major vasopressin-regulated water channel. Aquaporin 3 and aquaporin 4 are expressed in the basolateral membranes of collecting-duct principal cells and provide exit pathways for water reabsorbed apically by aquaporin 2. Aquaporin 7 is in the apical brush border of the straight proximal tubule. Aquaporins 6 to 8 are also expressed in kidney; their functions remain to be clarified. Vasopressin regulates water permeability of the collecting duct by influencing the trafficking of aquaporin 2 from intracellular vesicles to the apical plasma membrane (Figure 25–20). AVP-induced activation of the cAMP-PKA pathway also enhances expression of aquaporin 2 mRNA and protein; chronic dehydration thus causes up-regulation of aquaporin 2 and water transport in the collecting duct.

For maximum concentration of urine, large amounts of urea must be deposited in the interstitium of the inner medulla. It is not surprising, therefore, that V_2-receptor activation also increases urea permeability by 400% in the terminal portions of the inner medullary collecting duct. V_2 receptors increase urea permeability by activating a vasopressin-regulated urea transporter (termed *VRUT, UT1*, or *UT-A1*), most likely by PKA-induced phosphorylation (Sands, 2003). Kinetics of vasopressin-induced water and urea permeability differ, and vasopressin-induced regulation of VRUT does not entail vesicular trafficking to the plasma membrane (Inoue et al., 1999).

In addition to increasing water permeability of the collecting duct and urea permeability of the inner medullary collecting duct, V_2-receptor activation also increases Na^+ transport in thick ascending limb and collecting duct. Increased Na^+ transport in thick ascending limb is mediated by three mechanisms that affect the Na^+-K^+-$2Cl^-$ symporter: rapid phosphorylation of the symporter, translocation of the symporter into the luminal membrane, and increased expression of symporter protein (Ecelbarger et al., 2001). Enhanced Na^+ transport in collecting duct is mediated by increased expression of subunits of the epithelial Na^+ channel (Ecelbarger et al., 2001). The multiple mechanisms by which vasopressin increases water reabsorption are summarized in Figure 25–22.

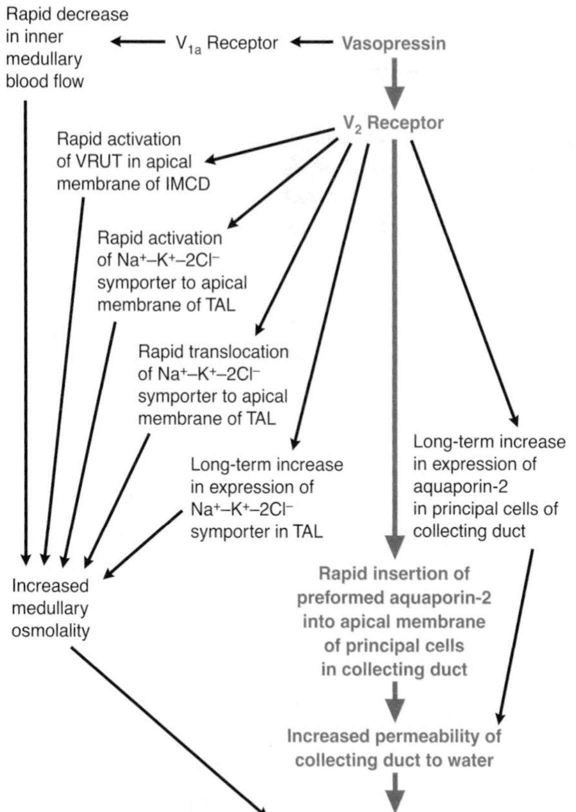

Figure 25–22. *Mechanisms by which vasopressin increases the renal conservation of water.* Red and black arrows denote major and minor pathways, respectively. IMCD, inner medullary collecting duct; TAL, thick ascending limb; VRUT, vasopressin-regulated urea transporter.

Renal Actions of Vasopressin. Several sites of vasopressin action in kidney involve both V_1 and V_2 receptors (Bankir, 2001). V_1 receptors mediate contraction of mesangial cells in the glomerulus and contraction of vascular smooth muscle cells in vasa recta and efferent arteriole. V_1-receptor-mediated reduction of inner medullary blood flow contributes to the maximum concentrating capacity of the kidney (Franchini and Cowley, 1996) (Figure 25–22). V_1 receptors also stimulate prostaglandin synthesis by medullary interstitial cells. Since PGE_2 inhibits adenylyl cyclase in collecting duct, stimulation of prostaglandin synthesis by V_1 receptors may counterbalance V_2-receptor-mediated antidiuresis. V_1 receptors on principal cells in cortical collecting duct may inhibit V_2-receptor-mediated water flux by activation of PKC. V_2 receptors mediate the most prominent response to vasopressin, which is increased water permeability of the collecting duct. Indeed, vasopressin can increase water permeability in collecting duct at concentrations as low as 50 fM. Thus, V_2-receptor-mediated effects of vasopressin occur at concentrations far lower than are required to engage V_1-receptor-mediated actions. This differential sensitivity may not be due to differences in receptor affinities because cloned rat V_{1a} and V_2 receptors have similar affinities for vasopressin (K_d = 0.7 and 0.4 nM, respectively) but rather may be due to differential amplification of their signal-transduction pathways.

The collecting-duct system is critical for water conservation. By the time tubular fluid arrives at the cortical collecting duct, it has been rendered hypotonic by the upstream diluting segments of the nephron that reabsorb NaCl without reabsorbing water. In the well-hydrated subject, plasma osmolality is in the normal range, concentrations of vasopressin are low, the entire collecting duct is relatively impermeable to water, and the urine is dilute. Under conditions of dehydration, plasma osmolality is increased, concentrations of vasopressin are elevated, and the collecting duct becomes permeable to water. The osmotic gradient between dilute tubular urine and hypertonic renal interstitial fluid (which becomes progressively more hypertonic in deeper regions of the renal medulla) provides for osmotic flux of water out of the collecting duct. The final osmolality of urine may be as high as 1200 mOsm/kg in humans, and a significant saving of solute-free water thus is possible.

Other renal actions mediated by V_2 receptors include increased urea transport in inner medullary collecting duct and increased Na^+ transport in thick ascending limb; both effects contribute to the urine-concentrating ability of the kidney (Figure 25–22). V_2 receptors also increase Na^+ transport in cortical collecting duct (Ecelbarger et al., 2001), and this may synergize with aldosterone to enhance Na^+ reabsorption during hypovolemia.

Pharmacological Modification of the Antidiuretic Response to Vasopressin. Nonsteroidal anti-inflammatory drugs (NSAIDs), particularly indomethacin, enhance the antidiuretic response to vasopressin. Since prostaglandins attenuate antidiuretic responses to vasopressin and NSAIDs inhibit prostaglandin synthesis, reduced prostaglandin production probably accounts for potentiation of vasopressin's antidiuretic response. Carbamazepine and chlorpropamide also enhance antidiuretic effects of vasopressin by unknown mechanisms. In rare instances, chlorpropamide can induce water intoxication.

A number of drugs inhibit the antidiuretic actions of vasopressin. Lithium is of particular importance because of its use in the treatment of manic-depressive disorders. Acutely, Li^+ appears to reduce V_2-receptor-mediated stimulation of adenylyl cyclase. Also, Li^+ increases plasma levels of parathyroid hormone, a partial antagonist to vasopressin. In most patients, the antibiotic demeclocycline attenuates the antidiuretic effects of vasopressin, probably owing to decreased accumulation and action of cyclic AMP.

Nonrenal Actions of Vasopressin. Vasopressin and related peptides are ancient hormones in evolutionary terms, and they are found in species that do not concentrate urine. Thus, it is not surprising that vasopressin has nonrenal actions in mammals.

Cardiovascular System. The cardiovascular effects of vasopressin are complex, and vasopressin's role in physiological situations is ill-defined. Vasopressin is a potent vasoconstrictor (V_1 receptor-mediated), and resistance vessels throughout the circulation may be affected. Vascular smooth muscle in the skin, skeletal muscle, fat, pancreas, and thyroid gland appear most sensitive, with significant vasoconstriction also occurring in GI tract, coronary vessels, and brain. Despite the potency of vasopressin as a direct vasoconstrictor, vasopressin-induced pressor responses in vivo are minimal and occur only with vasopressin concentrations significantly higher than those required for maximal antidiuresis. To a large extent, this is due to circulating vasopressin actions on V_1 receptors to inhibit sympathetic efferents and potentiate baroreflexes. In addition, V_2 receptors cause vasodilation in some blood vessels.

A large body of data supports the conclusion that vasopressin helps to maintain arterial blood pressure during episodes of severe hypovolemia/hypotension. At present, there is no convincing evidence for a role of vasopressin in essential hypertension in humans (Kawano et al., 1997).

The effects of vasopressin on heart (reduced cardiac output and heart rate) are largely indirect and result from coronary vasoconstriction, decreased coronary blood flow, and alterations in vagal and sympathetic tone. In humans, vasopressin effects on coronary blood flow can be demonstrated easily, especially if large doses are employed. The cardiac actions of the hormone are of more than academic interest. Some patients with coronary insufficiency experience angina even in response to the relatively small amounts of vasopressin required to control diabetes insipidus, and vasopressin-induced myocardial ischemia has led to severe reactions and even death.

CNS. It is likely that vasopressin plays a role as a neurotransmitter and/or neuromodulator. Vasopressin may participate in the acquisition of certain learned behaviors, in the development of some complex social processes, and in the pathogenesis of specific psychiatric diseases such as depression. However, the physiological/ pathophysiological relevance of these findings is controversial, and some actions of vasopressin on memory and learned behavior may be due to visceral autonomic effects. Many studies support a physiological role for vasopressin as a naturally occurring antipyretic factor. Although vasopressin can modulate CNS autonomic systems controlling heart rate, arterial blood pressure, respiration rate, and sleep patterns, the physiological significance of these actions is unclear. Finally, ACTH secretion is enhanced by vasopressin released from parvicellular neurons in the PVN and secreted into pituitary portal capillaries from axon terminals in the median eminence. Although vasopressin is not the principal corticotropin-releasing factor, vasopressin may provide for sustained activation of the hypothalamic-pituitary-adrenal axis during chronic stress. CNS effects of vasopressin appear to be mediated predominantly by V_1 receptors.

Blood Coagulation. Activation of V_2 receptors by desmopressin or vasopressin increases circulating levels of procoagulant factor VIII and of von Willebrand factor. These effects are mediated by extrarenal V_2 receptors (Bernat et al., 1997). Presumably, vasopressin stimulates secretion of von Willebrand factor and of factor VIII from storage sites in vascular endothelium. However, since release of von Willebrand factor does not occur when desmopressin is applied directly to cultured endothelial cells or to isolated blood vessels, intermediate factors are likely to be involved.

Other Nonrenal Effects of Vasopressin. At high concentrations, vasopressin stimulates smooth muscle contraction in uterus (by oxytocin receptors) and GI tract (by V_1 receptors). Vasopressin is stored in platelets, and activation of V_1 receptors stimulates platelet aggregation. Also, activation of V_1 receptors on hepatocytes stimulates glycogenolysis. The physiological significance of these effects of vasopressin in not known.

VASOPRESSIN RECEPTOR AGONISTS AND ANTAGONISTS

A number of vasopressin-like peptides occur naturally (Table 25–8). All are nonapeptides, contain cysteine residues in positions 1 and 6, have an intramolecular disulfide bridge between the two cysteine residues (essential for agonist activity), have additional conserved amino acids in positions 5, 7, and 9 (asparagine, proline, and glycine, respectively), contain a basic amino acid in position 8, and are amidated on the carboxyl terminus. In all mammals except swine, the neurohypophyseal peptide is 8-arginine vasopressin, and the terms vasopressin, arginine vasopressin (AVP), and antidiuretic hormone (ADH) are used interchangeably.

The chemical structure of oxytocin is closely related to that of vasopressin: oxytocin is [Ile^3, Leu^8]AVP. Oxytocin binds to specific oxytocin receptors on myoepithelial cells in mammary gland and on

Table 25–8

Vasopressin Receptor Agonists

	A	W	X	Y	Z
I. NATURALLY OCCURRING VASOPRESSIN-LIKE PEPTIDES					
A. *Vertebrates*					
1. Mammals					
Arginine vasopressin[a] (AVP) (humans and other mammals)	NH_2	Tyr	Phe	Gln	Arg
Lypressin[a] (pigs, marsupials)	NH_2	Tyr	Phe	Gln	Lys
Phenypressin (macropodids)	NH_2	Phe	Phe	Gln	Arg
2. Nonmammalian vertebrates					
Vasotocin	NH_2	Tyr	Ile	Gln	Arg
B. *Invertebrates*					
1. Arginine conopressin (*Conus striatus*)	NH_2	Ile	Ile	Arg	Arg
2. Lysine conopressin (*Conus geographicus*)	NH_2	Phe	Ile	Arg	Lys
3. Locust subesophageal ganglia peptide	NH_2	Leu	Ile	Thr	Arg
II. SYNTHETIC VASOPRESSIN PEPTIDES					
A. *V_1-selective agonists*					
1. V_{1a}-selective: [Phe[2], Ile[3], Orn[8]] AVP	NH_2	Phe	Ile	Gln	Orn
2. V_{1b}-selective: Deamino [D-3-(3′-pyridyl)-Ala[2]]AVP	H	D-3-(3′-pyridyl)-Ala[2]	Phe	Gln	Arg
B. *V_2-selective agonists*					
1. Desmopressin[a] (DDAVP)	H	Tyr	Phe	Gln	D-Arg
2. Deamino[Val[4], D-Arg[8]]AVP	H	Tyr	Phe	Val	D-Arg
III. NONPEPTIDE AGONIST					
A. *OPC-51803*					

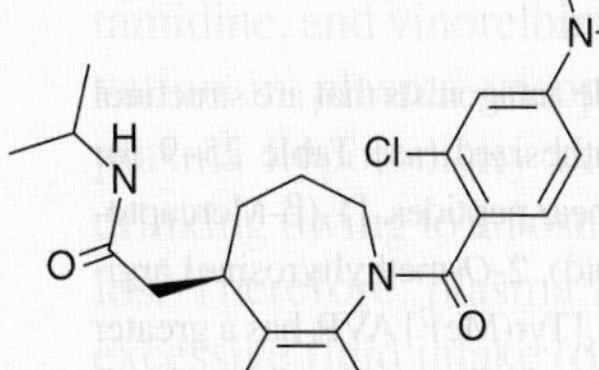

[a]Available for clinical use.

smooth muscle cells in the uterus, causing milk ejection and uterine contraction, respectively. Inasmuch as vasopressin and oxytocin are structurally similar, it is not surprising that vasopressin and oxytocin agonists and antagonists can bind to each other's receptors. Therefore, most of the available peptide vasopressin agonists and antagonists have some affinity for oxytocin receptors; at high doses, they may block or mimic the effects of oxytocin.

Many vasopressin analogs were synthesized with the goal of increasing duration of action and selectivity for vasopressin receptor subtypes (V_1 versus V_2 vasopressin receptors, which mediate pressor responses and antidiuretic responses, respectively). Deamination at position 1 increases duration of action and increases

Therefore, Li^+ should be considered for use only in patients with symptomatic SIADH who cannot be controlled by other means or in whom tetracyclines are contraindicated (e.g., patients with liver disease). It is important to stress that the majority of patients with SIADH do not require therapy because plasma Na^+ stabilizes in the range of 125-132 m*M*; such patients usually are asymptomatic. Only when symptomatic hypotonicity ensues, generally when plasma Na^+ levels drop below 120 m*M*, should therapy with demeclocycline be initiated. Since hypotonicity, which causes an influx of water into cells with resulting cerebral swelling, is the cause of symptoms, the goal of therapy is simply to increase plasma osmolality toward normal. For a more complete description of the diagnosis and treatment of SIADH, see Robertson (2001).

Other Water-Retaining States. In patients with congestive heart failure, cirrhosis, or nephrotic syndrome, *effective* blood volume often is reduced, and hypovolemia frequently is exacerbated by the liberal use of diuretics. Since hypovolemia stimulates vasopressin release, patients may become hyponatremic owing to vasopressin-mediated retention of water. The development of potent orally active V_2 receptor antagonists and specific inhibitors of water channels in the collecting duct has provided a new therapeutic strategy not only in patients with SIADH but also in the more common setting of hyponatremia in patients with heart failure, liver cirrhosis, and nephrotic syndrome, as discussed in the next section.

CLINICAL PHARMACOLOGY OF VASOPRESSIN PEPTIDES

Agonists

Therapeutic Uses. Two antidiuretic peptides are available for clinical use in the U.S.:

- Vasopressin (synthetic 8-L-arginine vasopressin; PITRESSIN, others) is available as a sterile aqueous solution; it may be administered subcutaneously, intramuscularly, or intranasally.
- Desmopressin acetate (synthetic 1-deamino-8-D-argi-nine vasopressin; DDAVP, others) is available as a sterile aqueous solution packaged for intravenous or subcutaneous injection, in a solution for intranasal administration with either a nasal spray pump or rhinal tube delivery system, and in tablets for oral administration.

The therapeutic uses of vasopressin and its congeners can be divided into two main categories according to the type of vasopressin receptor involved.

V_1 receptor-mediated therapeutic applications are based on the rationale that V_1 receptors cause GI and vascular smooth muscle contraction. V_1 receptor-mediated GI smooth muscle contraction has been used to treat postoperative ileus and abdominal distension and to dispel intestinal gas before abdominal roentgenography to avoid interfering gas shadows. V_1 receptor-mediated vasoconstriction of the splanchnic arterial vessels reduces blood flow to the portal system and, thereby, attenuates pressure and bleeding in esophageal varices (Burroughs, 1998). Although endoscopic variceal banding ligation is the treatment of choice for bleeding esophageal varices, V_1 receptor agonists have been used in an emergency setting until endoscopy can be performed (Vlavianos and Westaby, 2001). Simultaneous administration of nitroglycerin with V_1 receptor agonists may attenuate the cardiotoxic effects of V_1 agonists while enhancing their beneficial splanchnic effects. Also, V_1 receptor agonists have been used during abdominal surgery in patients with portal hypertension to diminish the risk of hemorrhage during the procedure. Finally, V_1 receptor-mediated vasoconstriction has been used to reduce bleeding during acute hemorrhagic gastritis, burn wound excision, cyclophosphamide-induced hemorrhagic cystitis, liver transplant, cesarean section, and uterine myoma resection.

The applications of V_1 receptor agonists can be accomplished with vasopressin; however, the use of vasopressin for all these indications is no longer recommended because of significant adverse reactions. Terlipressin (LUCASSIN) is preferred for bleeding esophageal varices because of increased safety compared with vasopressin (Vlavianos and Westaby, 2001) and is designated as an orphan drug for this use. Moreover, terlipressin is effective in patients with hepatorenal syndrome, particularly when combined with albumin (Ortega et al., 2002). Terlipressin has been granted priority review, orphan drug status, and fast-track designation by the FDA for type I hepatorenal syndrome.

Vasopressin levels in patients with vasodilatory shock are inappropriately low, and such patients are extraordinarily sensitive to the pressor actions of vasopressin. The combination of vasopressin and norepinephrine is superior to norepinephrine alone in the management of catecholamine-resistant vasodilatory shock. However, recent clinical trials show that, in comparison to catecholamines alone, addition of vasopressin does not improve outcomes in either cardiac arrest or septic shock.

V_2 receptor-mediated therapeutic applications are based on the rationale that V_2 receptors cause water conservation and release of blood coagulation factors. Central but not nephrogenic DI can be treated with V_2 receptor agonists, and polyuria and polydipsia usually are well controlled by these agents. Some patients experience transient DI (e.g., in head injury or surgery in the area of the pituitary); however, therapy for most patients with DI is lifelong. Desmopressin is the drug of choice for the vast majority of patients, and numerous clinical trials demonstrated the efficacy and tolerability of desmopressin in both adults and children.

The duration of effect from a single intranasal dose is from 6-20 hours; twice-daily administration is effective in most patients. There is considerable variability in the intranasal dose of desmopressin required to maintain normal urine volume, and the dosage must be tailored individually. The usual intranasal dosage in adults is 10-40 μg daily either as a single dose or divided into two or three doses. In view of the high cost of the drug and the importance of avoiding water intoxication, the schedule of administration should be adjusted to the minimal amount required. An initial dose of 2.5 μg can be used, with therapy first directed toward control of nocturia. An equivalent or higher morning dose controls daytime polyuria in most patients, although a third dose occasionally may be needed in the afternoon. In some patients, chronic allergic rhinitis or other nasal pathology may preclude reliable peptide absorption following nasal administration. Oral administration of desmopressin in doses 10-20 times the intranasal dose provides adequate desmopressin blood levels to control polyuria. Subcutaneous administration of 1-2 μg daily of desmopressin also is effective in central DI.

Vasopressin has little, if any, place in the long-term therapy of DI because of its short duration of action and V_1 receptor-mediated side effects. Vasopressin can be used as an alternative to desmopressin in the initial diagnostic evaluation of patients with suspected DI and to control polyuria in patients with DI who recently have undergone surgery or experienced head trauma. Under these circumstances, polyuria may be transient, and long-acting agents may produce water intoxication.

An additional V_2 receptor-mediated therapeutic application is the use of desmopressin in bleeding disorders (Mannucci, 1997). In most patients with type I von Willebrand's disease (vWD) and in some with type IIn vWD, desmopressin will elevate von Willebrand factor and shorten bleeding time. However, desmopressin generally is ineffective in patients with types IIa, IIb, and III vWD. Desmopressin may cause a marked transient thrombocytopenia in individuals with type IIb vWD and is contraindicated in such patients. Desmopressin also increases factor VIII levels in patients with mild to moderate hemophilia A. Desmopressin is not indicated in patients with severe hemophilia A, those with hemophilia B, or those with factor VIII antibodies. Using a test dose of nasal spray, the response of any given patient with type I vWD or hemophilia A to desmopressin should be determined at the time of diagnosis or 1-2 weeks before elective surgery to assess the extent of increase in factor VIII or von Willebrand factor. Desmopressin is employed widely to treat the hemostatic abnormalities induced by uremia. In patients with renal insufficiency, desmopressin shortens bleeding time and increases circulating levels of factor VIII coagulant activity, factor VIII-related antigen, and ristocetin cofactor. It also induces the appearance of larger von Willebrand factor multimers. Desmopressin is effective in some patients with liver cirrhosis-induced or drug-induced (e.g., heparin, hirudin, and antiplatelet agents) bleeding disorders. Desmopressin, given intravenously at a dose of 0.3 μg/kg, increases factor VIII and von Willebrand factor for > 6 hours. Desmopressin can be given at intervals of 12-24 hours depending on the clinical response and severity of bleeding. Tachyphylaxis to desmopressin usually occurs after several days (owing to depletion of factor VIII and von Willebrand factor storage sites) and limits its usefulness to preoperative preparation, postoperative bleeding, excessive menstrual bleeding, and emergency situations.

Another V_2 receptor-mediated therapeutic application is the use of desmopressin for primary nocturnal enuresis. Bedtime administration of desmopressin intranasal spray or tablets provides a high response rate that is sustained with long-term use, that is safe, and that accelerates the cure rate. Finally, desmopressin has been found to relieve post-lumbar puncture headache probably by causing water retention and thereby facilitating rapid fluid equilibration in the CNS.

Pharmacokinetics. When vasopressin and desmopressin are given orally, they are inactivated quickly by trypsin, which cleaves the peptide bond between amino acids 8 and 9.

Inactivation by peptidases in various tissues (particularly liver and kidney) results in a plasma $t_{1/2}$ of vasopressin of 17-35 minutes. Following intramuscular or subcutaneous injection, antidiuretic effects of vasopressin last 2-8 hours. The plasma $t_{1/2}$ of desmopressin has two components, a fast component (~8 min) and a slow component (30-117 min). Only 3% and 0.15%, respectively, of intranasally and orally administered desmopressin is absorbed.

Toxicity, Adverse Effects, Contraindications, Drug Interactions. Most adverse effects are mediated through V_1 receptor activation on vascular and GI smooth muscle; consequently, such adverse effects are much less common and less severe with desmopressin than with vasopressin.

After injection of large doses of vasopressin, marked facial pallor owing to cutaneous vasoconstriction is observed commonly. Increased intestinal activity is likely to cause nausea, belching, cramps, and an urge to defecate. Most serious, however, is the effect on the coronary circulation. Vasopressin should be administered only at low doses and with extreme caution in individuals suffering from vascular disease, especially coronary artery disease. Other cardiac complications include arrhythmia and decreased cardiac output. Peripheral vasoconstriction and gangrene were encountered in patients receiving large doses of vasopressin.

The major V_2 receptor-mediated adverse effect is water intoxication, which can occur with desmopressin or vasopressin. In this regard, many drugs, including carbamazepine, chlorpropamide, morphine, tricyclic antidepressants, and NSAIDs, can potentiate the antidiuretic effects of these peptides. Several drugs such as Li^+, demeclocycline, and ethanol can attenuate the antidiuretic response to desmopressin. Desmopressin and vasopressin should be used cautiously in disease states in which a rapid increase in extracellular water may impose risks (e.g., in angina, hypertension, and heart failure) and should not be used in patients with acute renal failure. Patients receiving desmopressin to maintain hemostasis should be advised to reduce fluid intake. Also, it is imperative that these peptides not be administered to patients with primary or psychogenic polydipsia because severe hypotonic hyponatremia will ensue.

Table 25–9

Vasopressin Receptor Antagonists *(Continued)*

C. *V_2-selective antagonists (cont.)*

OPC-31260 (mozavaptan)[c]

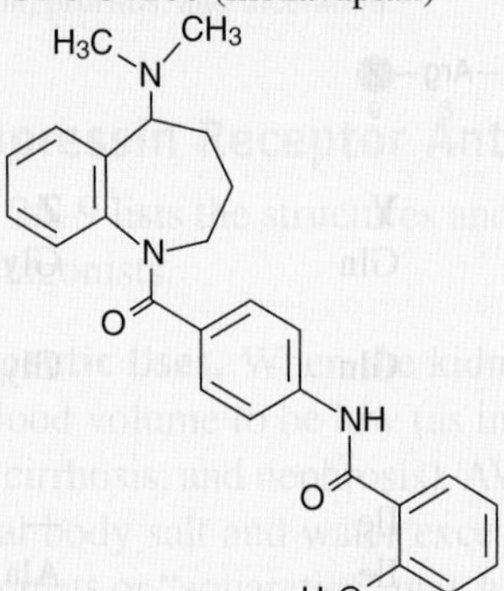

OPC-41061 (tolvaptan)[c]

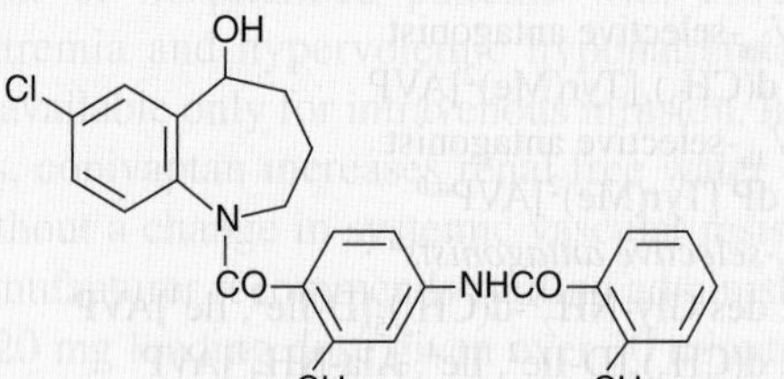

D. *V_{1a}-/V_2-selective antagonists*

YM-471

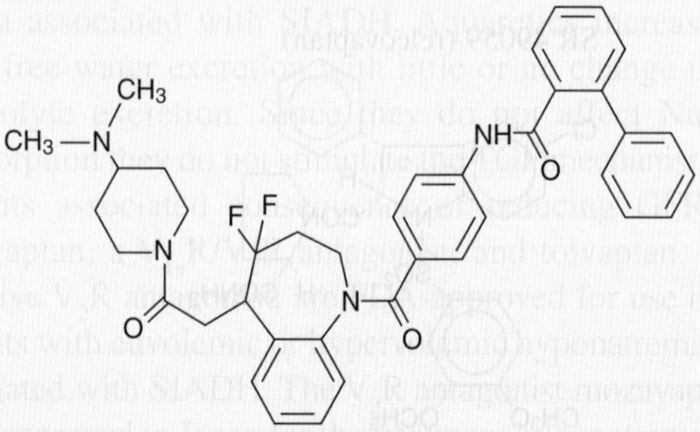

YM 087 (conivaptan)[c]

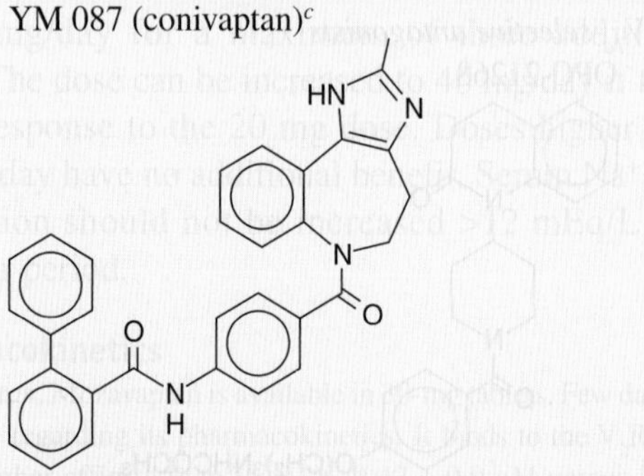

JTV-605

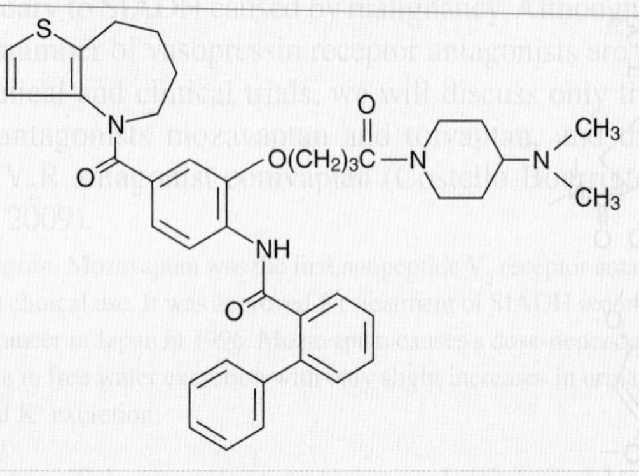

CL-385004

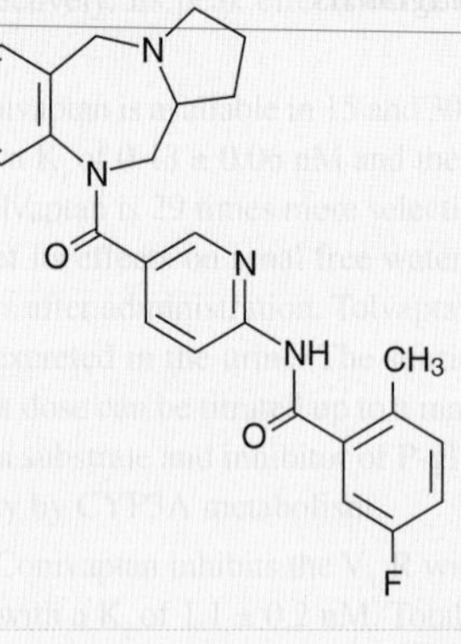

[a]Also blocks V_{1a} receptor, [b] $(H_3C)_2C<$ rather than $H_2C(CH_2-CH_2)_2C<$

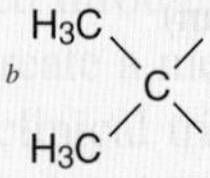

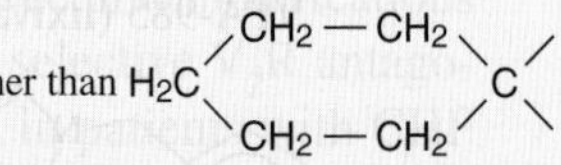

V_2 antagonistic activity in rats; however, antagonistic activity may be less or nonexistent in other species. Also, with prolonged infusion may exhibit significant agonist activity. [c]Available for clinical use.

adverse effects listed for tolvaptan are GI effects, hyperglycemia, and pyrexia. Less common are cerebrovascular accident, deep vein thrombosis, disseminated intravascular coagulation, intracardiac thrombus, ventricular fibrillation, urethral hemorrhage, vaginal hemorrhage, pulmonary embolism, respiratory failure, diabetic ketoacidosis, ischemic colitis, increaese in prothrombin time and rhabdomyolysis.

Conivaptan. Conivaptan is metabolized by CYP3A4 and as a result is associated with a variety of drug-drug interactions. It should not be administered in patients receiving ketoconazole, itraconazole, ritonavir, indinavir, clarithromycin, or other strong CYP3A4 inhibitors. Conivaptan increases levels of simvastatin, digoxin, amlodipine, and midazolam. It is not known to interact with warfarin or prolong the QT_c interval. Due to multiple drug-drug interactions conivaptan is no longer being developed for chronic long-term oral use. The most common adverse effect of conivaptan is an infusion site reaction. The manufacturer recommends that the drug only be infused into large veins and that infusion sites be changed daily. Other adverse effects have included headache, hypertnesion, hypotension, hypokalemia, and pyrexia.

Future Directions in Vasopressin Analogs

Nonpeptide vasopressin receptor antagonists and agonists are being developed for a wide range of clinical indications, including for V_{1a}-selective antagonists: dysmenorrhea, preterm labor, and Raynaud's syndrome; for V_{1b}-selective antagonists: stress-related disorders, anxiety, depression, ACTH-secreting tumors, and Cushing's syndrome; for V_2-selective and V_{1a}/V_2-selective antagonists: heart failure, SIADH, cirrhosis, hyponatremia, brain edema, nephrotic syndrome, diabetic nephropathy, and glaucoma; and for V_2-selective agonists: central DI, nocturnal enuresis, nocturnal polyuria, and urinary incontinence (Wong and Verbalis, 2001).

Preliminary data support several of the indications mentioned earlier for vasopressin receptor antagonists and agonists. Relcovaptan (SR 49059) is a V_{1a}-selective antagonist that has efficacy in primary dysmenorrhea (Brouard et al., 2000), and nelivaptan (SSR 149415) is a V_{1b}-selective antagonist that demonstrates anxiolytic activity in animal models of stress (Griebel et al., 2002). Aquaretics are drugs that increase free-water clearance with minimal effects on electrolyte excretion. The V_2-selective antagonist lixivaptan (VPA-985) is an effective aquaretic in patients with hyponatremia of various etiologies (Wong et al., 2003). In contrast, the V_2-selective agonist OPC-51803 has strong antidiuretic effects in animals and is being developed for central DI, nocturnal enuresis, and urinary incontinence (Nakamura et al., 2003). It is likely that more nonpeptide vasopressin receptor antagonists and agonists will become available clinically in the near future.

BIBLIOGRAPHY

Agarwal R, Gorski JC, Sundblad K, Brater DC. Urinary protein binding does not affect response to furosemide in patients with nephrotic syndrome. *J Am Soc Nephrol*, **2000**, *11*:1100–1105.

Agre P, Konozo D. Aquaporin water channels: Molecular mechanisms for human disease. *FEBS Lett*, **2003**, *555*:72–78.

ALLHAT Officers and Coordinators for the ALLHAT Collaborative Research Group. Major outcomes in high-risk hypertensive patients randomized to angiotensin-converting enzyme inhibitor or calcium channel blocker vs. diuretic: The Antihypertensive and Lipid-Lowering Treatment to Prevent Heart Attack Trial (ALLHAT). *JAMA*, **2002**, *288*:2981–2997.

Bachmann S, Velazquez H, Obermuller N, et al. Expression of the thiazide-sensitive Na–Cl cotransporter by rabbit distal convoluted tubule cells. *J Clin Invest*, **1995**, *96*:2510–2514.

Baker EH, Duggal A, Dong Y, et al. Amiloride, a specific drug for hypertension in black people with *T594M* variant? *Hypertension*, **2002**, *40*:13–17.

Bankir L. Antidiuretic action of vasopressin: Quantitative aspects and interaction between V_{1a} and V_2 receptor-mediated effects. *Cardiovasc Res*, **2001**, *51*(suppl.):372–390.

Bernat A, Hoffmann T, Dumas A, et al. V_2 receptor antagonism of DDAVP-induced release of hemostatic factors in conscious dogs. *J Pharmacol Exp Ther*, **1997**, *282*:597–602.

Brater DC. Clinical pharmacology of loop diuretics. *Drugs*, **1991**, *41*:14–22.

Brater DC. Diuretic therapy. *N Engl J Med*, **1998**, *339*:387–395.

Brouard R, Bossmar T, Fournie-Lloret D, et al. Effect of SR49059, an orally active V_{1a} vasopressin receptor antagonist, in the prevention of dysmenorrhea. *Int J Obstet Gynecol*, **2000**, *107*:614–619.

Burroughs AK. Pharmacological treatment of acute variceal bleeding. *Digestion*, **1998**, *59*:28–36.

Chobanian A, Bakris G, Black R, et al., and National High Blood Pressure Education Program Coordinating Committee. Seventh report of the Joint National Committee on Prevention, Detection, Evaluation and Treatment of High Blood Pressure. *Hypertension*, **2003**, *42*:1206–1252.

Costello-Boerrigter LC, Boerrigter G, Burnett JC. Pharmacology of vasopressin antagonists. *Heart Failure Rev*, **2009**, 75–82.

Dresser MJ, Leabman MK, Giacomini KM. Transporters involved in the elimination of drugs in the kidney: Organic anion transporters and organic cation transporters. *J Pharm Sci*, **2001**, *90*:397–421.

Ecelbarger CA, Kim GH, Wade JB, Knepper MA. Regulation of the abundance of renal sodium transporters and channels by vasopressin. *Exp Neurol*, **2001**, *171*:227–234.

Ellison DH. Diuretic resistance: Physiology and therapeutics. *Semin Nephrol*, **1999**, *19*:581–597.

Eraly SA, Bush KT, Sampogna RV, et al. The molecular pharmacology of organic anion transporters: From DNA to FDA? *Mol Pharmacol*, **2004**, *65*:479–487.

Faris R, Flather M, Purcell H, et al. Current evidence supporting the role of diuretics in heart failure: A meta-analysis of randomised, controlled trials. *Int J Cardiol*, **2002**, *82*:149–158.

Ferguson JA, Sundblad KJ, Becker PK, et al. Role of duration of diuretic effect in preventing sodium retention. *Clin Pharmacol Ther*, **1997**, *62*:203–208.

Franchini KG, Cowley AW Jr. Renal cortical and medullary blood flow responses during water restriction: Role of vasopressin. *Am J Physiol*, **1996**, *270*:R1257–R1264.

Franse LV, Pahor M, Di Bari M, et al. Hypokalemia associated with diuretic use and cardiovascular events in the Systolic Hypertension in the Elderly Program. *Hypertension*, **2000**, *35*:1025–1030.

Gamba G, Saltzberg SN, Lombardi M, et al. Primary structure and functional expression of a cDNA encoding the thiazide-sensitive, electroneutral sodium–chloride cotransporter. *Proc Natl Acad Sci USA*, **1993**, *90*:2749–2753.

Gottlieb SS, Brater DC, Thomas I, et al. BG9719 (CVT-124), an A_1 adenosine receptor antagonist, protects against the decline in renal function observed with diuretic therapy. *Circulation*, **2002**, *105*:1348–1353.

Griebel G, Simiand J, Serradeil-Le Gal C, et al. Anxiolytic- and anti-depressant-like effects of the nonpeptide vasopressin V_{1b} receptor agonist SSR149415 suggest an innovative approach for the treatment of stress-related disorders. *Proc Natl Acad Sci USA*, **2002**, *99*:6370–6375.

Grimm RH Jr, Grandits GA, Prineas RJ, et al. Long-term effects on sexual function of five antihypertensive drugs and nutritional hygienic treatment in hypertensive men and women. Treatment of Mild Hypertension Study (TOMHS). *Hypertension*, **1997**, *29*:8–14.

Guyton AC. Blood pressure control: Special role of the kidneys and body fluids. *Science*, **1991**, *252*:1813–1816.

Inoue T, Terris J, Ecelbarger CA, et al. Vasopressin regulates apical targeting of aquaporin-2 but not of UT1 urea transporter in renal collecting duct. *Am J Physiol*, **1999**, *276*:F559–F566.

Isenring P, Forbush B III. Ion and bumetanide binding by the Na–K–Cl cotransporter: Importance of transmembrane domains. *J Biol Chem*, **1997**, *272*:24556–24562.

Kaplan MR, Mount DB, Delpire E. Molecular mechanisms of NaCl cotransport. *Annu Rev Physiol*, **1996**, *58*:649–668.

Kawano Y, Matsuoka H, Nishikimi T, et al. The role of vasopressin in essential hypertension: Plasma levels and effects of the V_1 receptor antagonist OPC-21268 during different dietary sodium intakes. *Am J Hypertens*, **1997**, *10*:1240–1244.

Kim GH, Masilamani S, Turner R, et al. The thiazide-sensitive Na–Cl cotransporter is an aldosterone-induced protein. *Proc Natl Acad Sci USA*, **1998**, *95*:14552–14557.

Kleyman, T.R., Sheng, S., Kosari, F., and Kieber-Emmons, T. Mechanisms of action of amiloride: A molecular prospective. *Semin Nephrol*, **1999**, *19*:524–532.

Knauf H, Mutschler E. Sequential nephron blockade breaks resistance to diuretics in edematous states. *J Cardiovasc Pharmacol*, **1997**, *29*:367–372.

Kovacs L, Robertson GL. Syndrome of inappropriate antidiuresis. *Endocrinol Metab Clin North Am*, **1992**, *21*:859–875.

Krum H, Nolly H, Workman D, et al. Efficacy of eplerenone added to renin–angiotensin blockade in hypertensive patients. *Hypertension*, **2002**, *40*:117–123.

Kuan CJ, Herzer WA, Jackson EK. Cardiovascular and renal effects of blocking A_1 adenosine receptors. *J Cardiovasc Pharmacol*, **1993**, *21*:822–828.

Lane PH, Tyler LD, Schmitz PG. Chronic administration of furosemide augments renal weight and glomerular capillary pressure in normal rats. *Am J Physiol*, **1998**, *275*:F230–F234.

Lee CYW, Burnett JC Jr. Natriuretic peptides and therapeutic applications. *Heart Fail Rev*, **2007**, *12*:131–142.

Lytle C, McManus TJ, Haas M. A model of Na–K–2Cl cotransport based on ordered ion binding and glide symmetry. *Am J Physiol*, **1998**, *274*:C299–C309.

Manning M, Stoev S, Cheng LL, et al. Discovery and design of novel vasopressin hypotensive peptide agonists. *J Recept Signal Transduct Res*, **1999**, *19*:631–644.

Mannucci PM. Desmopressin (DDAVP) in the treatment of bleeding disorders: The first 20 years. *Blood*, **1997**, *90*: 2515–2521.

Mount DB, Baekgaard A, Hall AE, et al. Isoforms of the Na^+–K^+–2Cl cotransporter in murine TAL: I. Molecular characterization and intrarenal localization. *Am J Physiol*, **1999**, *276*:F347–F358.

Nakamura S, Hirano T, Yamamura Y, et al. Effects of OPC-51803, a novel, nonpeptide vasopressin V_2-receptor agonist, on micturition frequency in Brattleboro and aged rats. *J Pharmacol Sci*, **2003**, *93*:484–488.

Nakamura S, Yamamura Y, Itoh S, et al. Characterization of a novel nonpeptide vasopressin V_2-receptor agonist, OPC-51803, in cells transfected human vasopressin receptor subtypes. *Br J Pharmacol*, **2000**, *129*:1700–1706.

Nielsen S, Kwon TH, Christensen BM, et al. Physiology and patho-physiology of renal aquaporins. *J Am Soc Nephrol*, **1999**, *10*:647–663.

Nishimoto G, Zelenina M, Li D, et al. Arginine vasopressin stimulates phosphorylation of aquaporin-2 in rat renal tissue. *Am J Physiol*, **1999**, *276*:F254–F259.

Obermuller N, Bernstein P, Velazquez H, *et al*. Expression of the thiazide-sensitive Na–Cl cotransporter in rat and human kidney. *Am J Physiol*, **1995**, *269*:F900–F910.

Obermuller N, Kunchaparty S, Ellison DH, Bachmann S. Expression of the Na–K–2Cl cotransporter by macula densa and thick ascending limb cells of rat and rabbit nephron. *J Clin Invest*, **1996**, *98*:635–640.

Ortega R, Ginès P, Uriz J, et al. Terlipressin therapy with and without albumin for patients with hepatorenal syndrome: Results of a prospective, nonrandomized study. *Hepatology*, **2002**, *36*:941–948.

Ouzan J, Perault C, Lincoff AM, et al. The role of spironolactone in the treatment of patients with refractory hyper-tension. *Am J Hypertens*, **2002**, *15*:333–339.

Payne JA, Forbush B III. Alternatively spliced isoforms of the putative renal Na–K–Cl cotransporter are differentially distributed within the rabbit kidney. *Proc Natl Acad Sci USA*, **1994**, *91*:4544–4548.

Perazella MA. Trimethoprim-induced hyperkalemia. *Drug Safety*, **2000**, *22*:227–236.

Pitt B, Remme W, Zannad F, et al. for the Eplerenone Post-Acute Myocardial Infarction Heart Failure Efficacy and Survival Study Investigators. Eplerenone, a selective aldosterone blocker, in patients with left ventricular dysfunction after myocardial infarction. *N Engl J Med*, **2003**, *348*:1309–1321.

Pitt B, Zannad F, Remme W, et al., for the Randomized Aldactone Evaluation Study Investigators. The effect of spironolactone on morbidity and mortality in patients with severe heart failure. Randomized Aldactone Evaluation Study Investigators. *N Engl J Med*, **1999**, *341*:709–717.

Plata C, Meade P, Hall A, et al. Alternatively spliced isoform of apical Na^+–K^+–Cl^- cotransporter gene encodes a furosemide-sensitive Na^+–Cl^- cotransporter. *Am J Physiol Renal Physiol*, **2001**, *280*:F574–F582.

Plata C, Mount DB, Rubio V, et al. Isoforms of the Na–K–2Cl cotransporter in murine TAL: II. Functional characterization and activation by cAMP. *Am J Physiol*, **1999**, *276*:F359–F366.

Plotkin MD, Kaplan MR, Verlander JW, et al. Localization of the thiazide-sensitive Na–Cl cotransporter *rTSCl* in the rat kidney. *Kidney Int*, **1996**, *50*:174–183.

Ramires, F.J., Mansur, A., Coelho, O., et al. Effect of spironolactone on ventricular arrhythmias in congestive heart failure secondary to idiopathic dilated or to ischemic cardiomyopathy. *Am J Cardiol*, **2000**, *85*:1207–1211.

Reaux A, Fournie-Zaluski MC, Llorens-Cortes C. Angiotensin III: A central regulator of vasopressin release and blood pressure. *Trends Endocrinol Metab*, **2001**, *12*:157–162.

Rejnmark L, Vestergaard P, Pedersen AR, et al. Dose-effect relations of loop and thiazide diuretics on calcium homeostasis: A randomized, double-blinded, Latin-square, multiple cross-over study in postmenopausal osteopenic women. *Eur J Clin Invest*, **2003**, *33*:41–50.

Robertson GL. Regulation of vasopressin secretion. In, *The Kidney: Physiology and Pathophysiology*, vol. 2, 2nd ed. (Seldin DW, Giebisch G, eds.) Raven Press, New York, **1992**, pp. 1595–1613.

Robertson GL. Antidiuretic hormone, normal and disordered function. *Endocrinol Metab Clin North Am*, **2001**, *30*: 671–694.

Robertson GL, Athar S, Shelton RL. Osmotic control of vasopressin function. In, *Disturbances in Body Fluid Osmolality*. (Andreoli TE, Grantham JJ, Rector FC, eds.) American Physiological Society, Bethesda, MD, **1977**, pp. 125–148.

Sands JM. Molecular mechanisms of urea transport. *J Membrane Biol*, **2003**, *191*:149–163.

Sciarrone MT, Stella P, Barlassina C, et al. ACE and α-adducin polymorphism as markers of individual response to diuretic therapy. *Hypertension*. **2003**, *41*:398–403.

Serradeil-Le Gal C, Wagnon J, Simiand J, et al. Characterization of (2*S*,4*R*)-1-[5-chloro-1-[2,4-dimethoxyphenyl)sulfonyl]-3-(2-methoxyphenyl)-2-oxo-2,3-dihydro-1H-indol-3-yl]-4-hydroxy-*N,N*-dimethyl-2-pyrrolidine carboxamide (SSR149415), a selective and orally active vasopressin V_{1b} receptor antagonist. *J Pharmacol Exp Ther*, **2002**, *300*:1122–1130.

Simon DB, Lifton RP. Mutations in Na(K)Cl transporters in Gitleman's and Bartter's syndromes. *Curr Opin Cell Biol*, **1998**, *10*:450–454.

Snyder HM, Noland TD, Breyer MD. cAMP-dependent protein kinase mediates hydro-osmotic effect of vasopressin in collecting duct. *Am J Physiol*, **1992**, *263*:C147–C153.

Takeda M, Yoshitomi K, Imai M. Regulation of Na^+–$3HCO_3^-$ cotransport in rabbit proximal convoluted tubule via adenosine A_1 receptor. *Am J Physiol*, **1993**, *265*:F511–F519.

Tsuruoka S, Schwartz GJ. HCO_3^- absorption in rabbit outer medullary collecting duct: Role of luminal carbonic anhydrase. *Am J Physiol,* **1998**, *274*:F139–F147.

van Buren M, Bijlsma JA, Boer P, et al. Natriuretic and hypotensive effect of adenosine-1 blockade in essential hypertension. *Hypertension*, **1993**, *22*:728–734.

Velazquez H, Bartiss A, Bernstein P, Ellison DH. Adrenal steroids stimulate thiazide-sensitive NaCl transport by rat renal distal tubules. *Am J Physiol*, **1996**, *270*:F211–F219.

Vlavianos P, Westaby D. Management of acute variceal haemorrhage. *Eur J Gastroenterol Hepatol*, **2001**, *13*:335–342.

Weinberger MH, Roniker B, Krause SL, Weiss RJ. Eplerenone, a selective aldosterone blocker, in mild to moderate hypertension. *Am J Hypertens*, **2002**, *15*:709–716.

Wells T. Vesicular osmometers, vasopressin secretion and aquaporin-4: A new mechanism for osmoreception? *Mol Cell Endocrinol*, **1998**, *136*:103–107.

White WB, Carr AA, Krause S, et al. Assessment of the novel selective aldosterone blocker eplerenone using ambulatory and clinical blood pressure in patients with systemic hypertension. *Am J Cardiol*, **2003**, *92*:38–42.

Wong F, Blei AT, Blendis LM, Thuluvath PJ. A vasopressin receptor antagonist (VPA-985) improves serum sodium concentration in patients with hyponatremia: A multicenter, randomized, placebo-controlled trial. *Hepatology*, **2003**, *37*: 182–191.

Wong LL, Verbalis JG. Vasopressin V_2 receptor antagonists. *Cardiovasc Res*, **2001**, *51*:391–402.

Xu JC, Lytle C, Zhu TT, et al. Molecular cloning and functional expression of the bumetanide-sensitive Na–K–Cl cotransporter. *Proc Natl Acad Sci USA*, **1994**, *91*:2201–2205.

Yancy CY. Benefit-risk assessment of nesiritide in the treatment of acute decompensated heart failure. *Drug Safety,* **2007**, *30*:765–781.

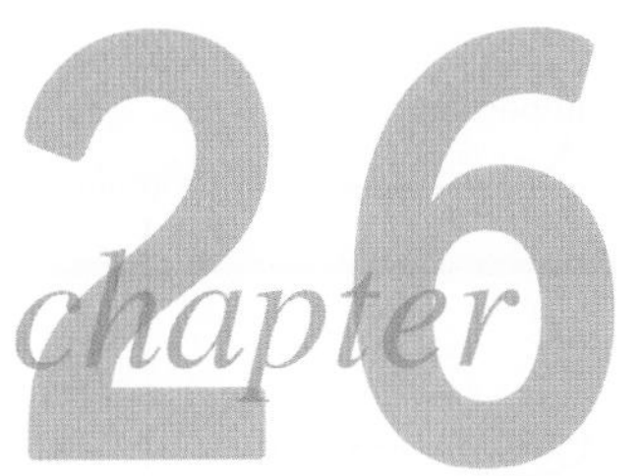

Renin and Angiotensin

Randa Hilal-Dandan

The renin–angiotensin system (RAS) participates significantly in the pathophysiology of hypertension, congestive heart failure, myocardial infarction, and diabetic nephropathy. This realization has led to a thorough exploration of the RAS and the development of new approaches for inhibiting its actions. This chapter discusses the biochemistry, molecular and cellular biology, and physiology of the RAS; the pharmacology of drugs that interrupt the RAS; and the clinical utility of inhibitors of the RAS. Therapeutic applications of drugs covered in this chapter are also discussed in Chapters 27 and 28.

THE RENIN–ANGIOTENSIN SYSTEM

History. In 1898, Tiegerstedt and Bergman found that crude saline extracts of the kidney contained a pressor substance that they named *renin*. In 1934, Goldblatt and his colleagues demonstrated that constriction of the renal arteries produced persistent hypertension in dogs. In 1940, Braun-Menéndez and his colleagues in Argentina and Page and Helmer in the U.S. reported that renin was an enzyme that acted on a plasma protein substrate to catalyze the formation of the actual pressor material, a peptide, that was named *hypertensin* by the former group and *angiotonin* by the latter. These two terms persisted for nearly 20 years until it was agreed to rename the pressor substance *angiotensin* and to call the plasma substrate *angiotensinogen*. In the mid-1950s, two forms of angiotensin were recognized, a decapeptide (angiotensin I [AngI]) and an octapeptide (angiotensin II [AngII]) formed by proteolytic cleavage of AngI by an enzyme termed *angiotensin-converting enzyme* (ACE). The octapeptide was shown to be the more active form, and its synthesis in 1957 by Schwyzer and by Bumpus made the material available for intensive study.

It was later shown that the kidneys are important for aldosterone regulation and that angiotensin potently stimulates the production of aldosterone in humans. Moreover, renin secretion increased with depletion of Na^+. Thus, the RAS came to be recognized as a mechanism to stimulate aldosterone synthesis and secretion and an important homeostatic mechanism in the regulation of blood pressure and electrolyte composition.

In the early 1970s, polypeptides were discovered that either inhibited the formation of AngII or blocked AngII receptors. These inhibitors revealed important physiological and pathophysiological roles for the RAS and inspired the development of a new and broadly efficacious class of antihypertensive drugs: the orally active ACE inhibitors. Studies with ACE inhibitors uncovered roles for the RAS in the pathophysiology of hypertension, heart failure, vascular disease, and renal failure. Selective and competitive antagonists of AngII receptors were developed that yielded losartan, the first orally active, highly selective, and potent nonpeptide AngII receptor antagonist. Subsequently, many other AngII receptor antagonists have been developed. Recently aliskiren, a direct renin inhibitor, was approved for antihypertensive therapy (see Chapter 27).

Components of the Renin–Angiotensin System

Overview. AngII, the most active angiotensin peptide, is derived from angiotensinogen in two proteolytic steps. First, renin, an enzyme released from the kidneys, cleaves the decapeptide AngI from the amino terminus of angiotensinogen (renin substrate). Then, ACE removes the carboxy-terminal dipeptide of AngI to produce the octapeptide AngII. These enzymatic steps are summarized in Figure 26–1. AngII acts by binding to two heptahelical GPCRs, AT_1 and AT_2.

The understanding of the RAS has expanded in recent years. The current view of the RAS also includes a local (tissue) RAS, alternative pathways for AngII synthesis (ACE independent), formation of other biologically active angiotensin peptides (AngIII, AngIV, Ang[1–7]), and additional angiotensin binding receptors (angiotensin subtypes 1, 2, and 4 [AT_1, AT_2, AT_4]; Mas) that participate in cell growth differentiation, hypertrophy, inflammation, fibrosis, and apoptosis. All components of the RAS are described in detail in a later section.

Renin. Renin is the major determinant of the rate of AngII production. It is synthesized, stored, and secreted by exocytosis into the

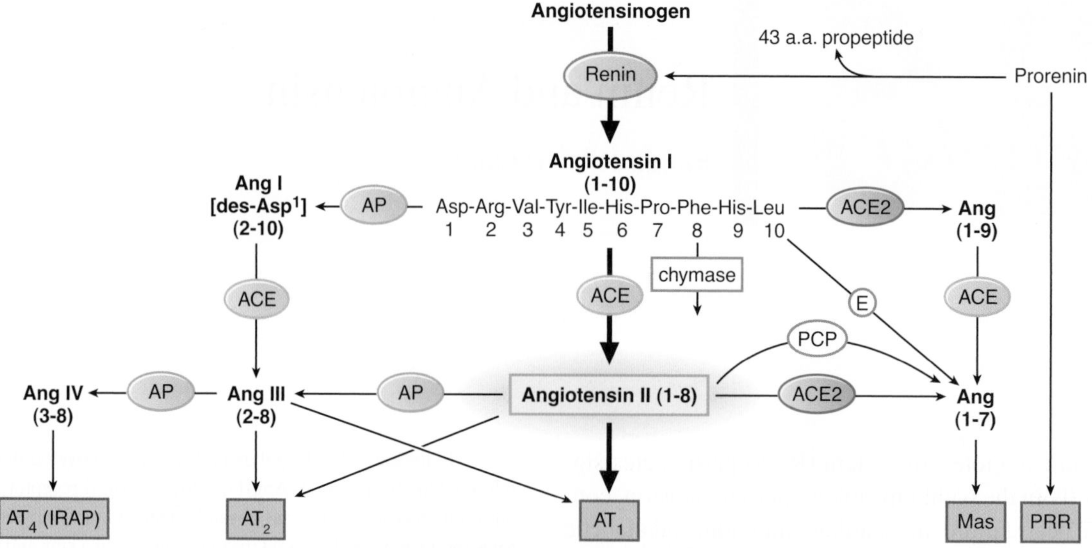

Figure 26–1. *Components of the RAS.* The heavy arrows show the classical pathway, and the light arrows indicate alternative pathways. ACE, angiotensin-converting enzyme; Ang, angiotensin; AP, aminopeptidase; E, endopeptidases; IRAP, insulin-regulated amino peptidases; PCP, prolylcarboxylpeptidase; PRR, (pro)renin receptor. Receptors involved: AT_1, AT_2, Mas, AT_4, and PRR. *Exposure of the active site of renin can also occur non-proteolytically; see text and Figure 26-3.

renal arterial circulation by the granular juxtaglomerular cells (Figure 26–2) located in the walls of the afferent arterioles that enter the glomeruli. Renin is an aspartyl protease that cleaves the bond between residues 10 and 11 at the amino terminus of angiotensinogen to generate AngI. The active form of renin is a glycoprotein that contains 340 amino acids. It is synthesized as a preproenzyme of 406 amino acid residues that is processed to prorenin. Prorenin is proteolytically activated by proconvertase 1 or cathepsin B enzymes that remove 43 amino acids (propeptide) from its amino terminus to uncover the active site of renin (Figure 26–3). The active site of renin is located in a cleft between the two homologous lobes of the enzyme. Nonproteolytic activation of prorenin, central to the activation of local (tissue) RAS, occurs when prorenin binds to the prorenin/renin ((pro)renin) receptor, resulting in conformational changes that unfold the propeptide and expose the active catalytic site of the enzyme. (Danser et al., 2005). Both renin and prorenin are stored in the juxtaglomerular cells and, when released, circulate in the blood. The concentration of prorenin in the circulation is ~10-fold greater than that of the active enzyme. The $t_{1/2}$ of circulating renin is ~15 minutes.

Control of Renin Secretion. The secretion of renin from juxtaglomerular cells is controlled predominantly by three pathways (Figure 26–2):

- the macula densa pathway
- the intrarenal baroreceptor pathway
- the β_1 adrenergic receptor pathway

The first mechanism is the *macula densa pathway*. The macula densa lies adjacent to the juxtaglomerular cells and is composed of specialized columnar epithelial cells in the wall of that portion of the cortical thick ascending limb that passes between the afferent and efferent arterioles of the glomerulus. A change in NaCl reabsorption by the macula densa results in the transmission to nearby juxtaglomerular cells of chemical signals that modify renin release. Increases in NaCl flux across the macula densa inhibit renin release, whereas decreases in NaCl flux stimulate renin release. ATP, adenosine, and prostaglandins modulate the macula densa pathway. ATP and adenosine are released when NaCl transport increases ATP acts on P2Y receptors to inhibit renin release. Adenosine acts via the A_1 adenosine receptor to inhibit renin release. Prostaglandins (PGE_2, PGI_2) are released when NaCl transport decreases and stimulate renin release through enhancing cyclic AMP formation. Prostaglandin production is stimulated by inducible cyclooxygenase-2 (COX-2). COX-2 and neuronal nitric oxide synthase (nNOS) participate in the mechanism of macula densa–stimulated renin release. The expression of COX-2 and nNOS is upregulated by chronic dietary Na^+ restriction; selective inhibition of either COX-2 or nNOS inhibits renin release. The nNOS/NO pathway, in part, may mediate increases in COX-2 expression induced by a low-Na^+ diet; however, COX-2 expression in the macula densa is not attenuated in nNOS knockout mice, which suggests that other mechanisms can compensate for nNOS in the regulation of COX-2.

Regulation of the macula densa pathway is more dependent on the luminal concentration of Cl^- than Na^+. NaCl transport into the macula densa is mediated by the Na^+–K^+–$2Cl^-$ symporter (Figure 26–2B), and the half-maximal concentrations of Na^+ and Cl^- required for transport via this symporter are 2-3 and 40 mEq/L, respectively. Because the luminal concentration of Na^+ at the macula densa usually is much greater than the level required for half-maximal transport, physiological variations in luminal Na^+ concentrations at the macula densa have little effect on renin release (i.e., the symporter remains saturated with respect to Na^+). On the other hand, physiological changes in Cl^- concentrations (20-60 mEq/L) at the macula densa profoundly affect macula densa–mediated renin release.

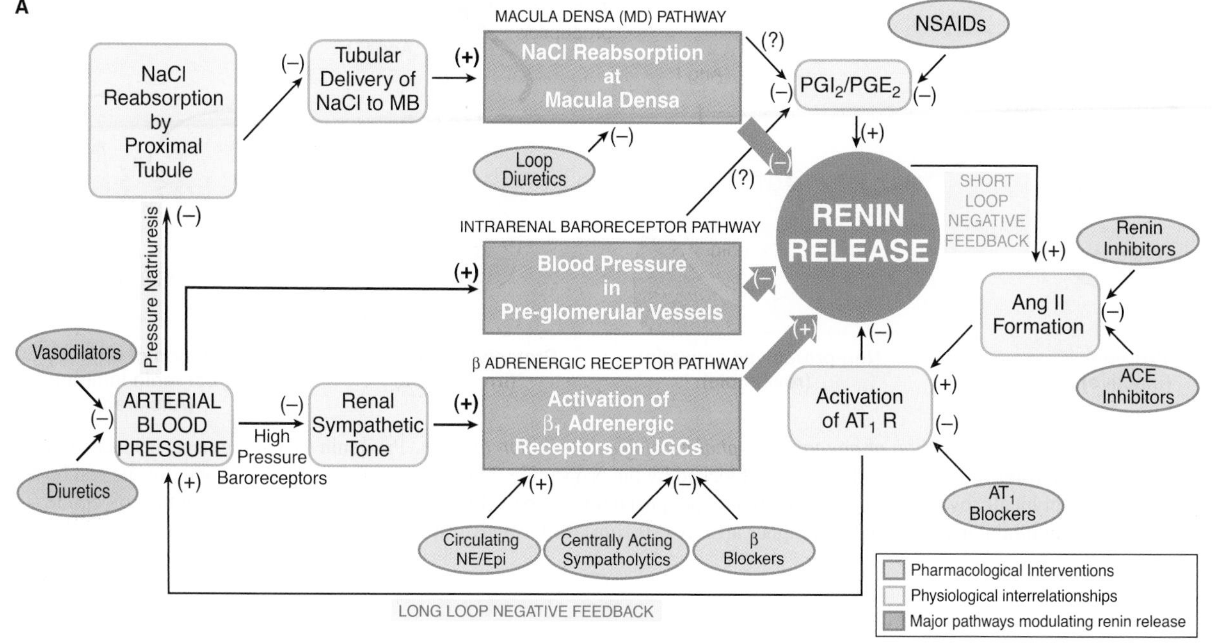

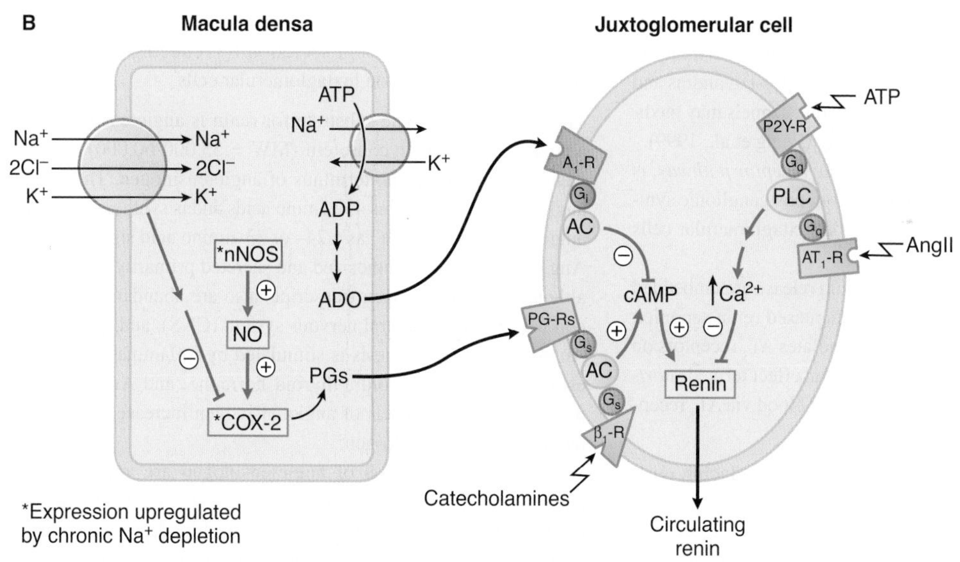

Figure 26–2. *A*. Schematic portrayal of the three major physiological pathways regulating renin release. *See* text for details. MD, macula densa; PGI_2/PGE_2 prostaglandins I_2 and E_2; NSAIDs, nonsteroidal antiinflammatory drugs; Ang II, angiotensin II: ACE, angiotensin-converting enzyme. AT_1 R, angiotensin subtype 1 receptor; NE/Epi, norepinephrine/epinephrine; JGCs, juxtaglomerular cells. *B*. Mechanisms by which the macula densa regulates renin release. Changes in tubular delivery of NaCl to the macula densa cause appropriate signals to be conveyed to the juxtaglomerular cells. Sodium depletion upregulates nNOS and COX-2 in the macula densa to enhance production of prostaglandins (PGs). PGs and catecholamines stimulate cyclic AMP production and thence renin release from the juxtaglomerular cells. Increased NaCl transport depletes ATP and increases adenosine (ADO) levels. Adenosine diffuses to the juxtaglomerular cells and inhibits cyclic AMP production and renin release via G_i-coupled A_1 receptors. Increased NaCl transport in the macula densa augments the efflux of ATP, which may inhibit renin release directly by binding to P2Y receptors and activating the G_q-PLC-IP_3-Ca^{2+} pathway in juxtaglomerular cells. Circulating AngII also inhibits renin release on juxtaglomerular cells via G_q-coupled AT_1 receptors.

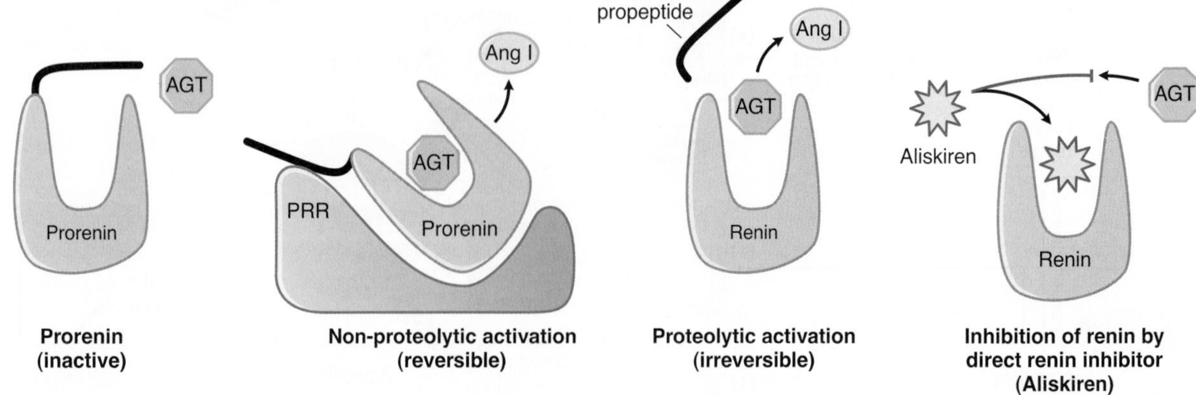

Figure 26-3. *Biological activation of prorenin and pharmacological inhibition of renin.* Pro-renin (black segment) is inactive; accessibility of angiotensinogen (AGT) to the active is blocked by the propeptide (black segment). The blocked catalytic site can be activated non-proteolytically by the binding of prorenin to the (pro) renin receptor (PRR) or by proteolytic removal of the propeptide. The competitive renin inhibitor, aliskiren, has a higher affinity (~0.1μm) for the active site of renin than does AGT (~1 μm).

The second mechanism controlling renin release is the *intrarenal baroreceptor pathway*. Increases and decreases in blood pressure or renal perfusion pressure in the preglomerular vessels inhibit and stimulate renin release, respectively. The immediate stimulus to secretion is believed to be reduced tension within the wall of the afferent arteriole. The release of renal prostaglandins and biomechanical coupling via stretch-activated ion channels may mediate in part the intrarenal baroreceptor pathway (Wang et al., 1999).

The third mechanism, the *β adrenergic receptor pathway*, is mediated by the release of norepinephrine from postganglionic sympathetic nerves; activation of β_1 receptors on juxtaglomerular cells enhances renin secretion.

The three mechanisms regulating renin release are embedded in a feedback regulation (Figure 26–2A). Increased renin secretion enhances the formation of AngII, which stimulates AT_1 receptors on juxtaglomerular cells to inhibit renin release, an effect termed *short-loop negative feedback*. AngII increases arterial blood via AT_1 receptors; this effect inhibits renin release by:

- activating high-pressure baroreceptors, thereby reducing renal sympathetic tone
- increasing pressure in the preglomerular vessels
- reducing NaCl reabsorption in the proximal tubule (pressure natriuresis), which increases tubular delivery of NaCl to the macula densa

The inhibition of renin release owing to AngII-induced increases in blood pressure has been termed *long-loop negative feedback*.

The physiological pathways regulating renin release are influenced by arterial blood pressure, dietary salt intake, and a number of pharmacological agents (Figure 26–2A). Loop diuretics stimulate renin release by decreasing arterial blood pressure and by blocking the reabsorption of NaCl at the macula densa. *Nonsteroidal anti-inflammatory drugs* (NSAIDs; see Chapter 34) inhibit prostaglandin synthesis and thereby decrease renin release. ACE inhibitors, angiotensin receptor blockers (ARBs), and renin inhibitors interrupt both the short- and long-loop negative feedback mechanisms and therefore increase renin release. Increasing cyclic AMP in the juxtaglomerular cells stimulates renin. Centrally acting sympatholytic drugs (see Chapter 12), as well as β adrenergic receptor antagonists, decrease renin secretion by reducing activation of β adrenergic receptors on juxtaglomerular cells.

Angiotensinogen. The substrate for renin is angiotensinogen, an abundant globular glycoprotein (MW = 55,000-60,000). AngI is cleaved from the amino terminus of angiotensinogen. The human angiotensinogen contains 452 amino acids and is synthesized as preangiotensinogen, which has a 24– or 33–amino acid signal peptide. Angiotensinogen is synthesized and secreted primarily by the liver, although angiotensinogen transcripts also are abundant in fat, certain regions of the central nervous system (CNS), and the kidneys. Angiotensinogen synthesis is stimulated by inflammation, insulin, estrogens, glucocorticoids, thyroid hormone, and AngII. During pregnancy, plasma levels of angiotensinogen increase several-fold owing to increased estrogen.

Circulating levels of angiotensinogen are approximately equal to the K_m of renin for its substrate (~1 μM). Consequently, the rate of AngII synthesis, and therefore blood pressure, can be influenced by changes in angiotensinogen levels. For instance, knockout mice lacking angiotensinogen are hypotensive, and there is a progressive relationship among the number of copies of the angiotensinogen gene, plasma levels of angiotensinogen, and arterial blood pressure. Oral contraceptives containing estrogen increase circulating levels of angiotensinogen and can induce hypertension. A missense mutation in the angiotensinogen gene (a methionine to threonine at position 235 of angiotensinogen) that increases plasma levels of angiotensinogen is associated with essential and pregnancy-induced hypertension (Sethi et al., 2003). Angiotensinogen shares sequence homologies that have anti-angiogenic properties with the serpin protein family (Célérier et al., 2002).

Angiotensin-Converting Enzyme (ACE, Kininase II, Dipeptidyl Carboxypeptidase). ACE is an ectoenzyme and glycoprotein with an apparent molecular weight of 170,000. Human ACE contains 1277 amino acid residues and has two homologous domains, each with a catalytic site and a Zn^{2+}-binding region. ACE has a large amino-terminal extracellular domain, a short carboxyl-terminal intracellular domain, and a 17–amino acid hydrophobic region that anchors the ectoenzyme to the cell membrane. ACE is rather nonspecific and cleaves dipeptide units from substrates with diverse amino acid sequences. Preferred substrates have only one free carboxyl group in the carboxyl-terminal amino acid, and proline must not be the penultimate amino acid; thus, the enzyme does not degrade AngII. ACE is identical to kininase II, the enzyme that inactivates bradykinin and other potent vasodilator peptides. Although slow conversion of AngI to AngII occurs in plasma, the very rapid metabolism that occurs *in vivo* is due largely to the activity of membrane-bound ACE present on the luminal surface of endothelial cells throughout the vascular system.

The *ACE* gene contains an insertion/deletion polymorphism in intron 16 that explains 47% of the phenotypic variance in serum ACE levels. The deletion allele, associated with higher levels of serum ACE and increased metabolism of bradykinin, may confer an increased risk of hypertension, cardiac hypertrophy, atherosclerosis, and diabetic nephropathy (Hadjadj et al., 2001) but may be protective against Alzheimer's disease (Sayed-Tabatabaei et al., 2006; Castrop et al., 2010).

Angiotensin-Converting Enzyme 2. Two groups independently discovered a novel ACE-related carboxypeptidase, now termed *ACE2* (Donoghue et al., 2000; Tipnis et al., 2000). Human ACE2 is 805 amino acids in length with a short putative signal sequence. ACE2 contains a single catalytic domain that is 42% identical to the two catalytic domains of ACE. ACE2 cleaves one amino acid from the carboxyl terminal to convert AngI to Ang(1–9) and AngII to Ang(1–7). AngII is the preferred substrate for ACE2 with 400-fold higher affinity than AngI. The physiological significance of ACE2 is still uncertain; it may serve as a counter-regulatory mechanism to oppose the effects of ACE. ACE2 regulates the levels of AngII and limits its effects by converting it to Ang(1–7), which binds to Mas receptors and elicits vasodilator and anti-proliferative responses (Varagic et al., 2008). ACE2 is not inhibited by the standard ACE inhibitors and has no effect on bradykinin. In animals, reduced expression of ACE2 is associated with hypertension, defects in cardiac contractility, and elevated levels of AngII (Crackower et al., 2002). Overexpression of the ACE2 gene prevents AngII-induced cardiac hypertrophy in hypertensive rats (Huentelman et al., 2005). ACE2 also serves as a receptor for the SARS coronavirus (Li et al., 2003).

Angiotensin Peptides. When given intravenously, AngI is rapidly converted to AngII. However, AngI *per se* is less than 1% as potent as AngII on smooth muscle, the heart, and the adrenal cortex. Angiotensin III (AngIII), also called Ang(2–8), can be formed either by the action of aminopeptidase on AngII or by the action of ACE on Ang(2–10). AngII and AngIII cause qualitatively similar effects. AngII and AngIII stimulate aldosterone secretion with equal potency; however, AngIII is only 25% and 10% as potent as AngII in elevating blood pressure and stimulating the adrenal medulla, respectively.

Ang(1-7) is formed by multiple pathways (Figure 26–1). AngI can be converted to Ang(1–7) by endopeptidases. AngII can be converted to Ang(1–7) by prolylcarboxypeptidase (Ferrario et al., 1997). ACE2 converts AngI to Ang(1–9) and AngII to Ang(1–7); ACE metabolizes Ang(1-9) to Ang(1–7). In animal models, Ang(1–7) opposes many of the effects of AngII: it induces vasodilation, promotes NO production, potentiates the vasodilatory effects of bradykinin, and inhibits AngII-induced activation of ERK1/2; it has anti-angiogenic, anti-proliferative, and anti-thrombotic effects; and is cardioprotective in cardiac ischemia and heart failure. The effects of Ang(1–7) are mediated by a specific Mas receptor. The *Mas* proto-oncogene encodes an orphan G protein–coupled receptor (Santos et al., 2008; Varagic et al., 2008). Ferrario and colleagues (1997) proposed that Ang(1–7) serves to counterbalance the actions of AngII, which may depend on ACE-AngII/ACE2-Ang(1–7) activity ratio (Santos et al. 2008). ACE inhibitors increase tissue and plasma levels of Ang(1–7), both because AngI levels are increased and diverted away from AngII formation (Figure 26–1) and because ACE contributes to the plasma clearance of Ang(1–7). AT_1 receptor blockade boosts the levels of AngII that is converted to Ang(1–7) by ACE2.

Angiotensin IV (AngIV), also called Ang(3–8), is formed from AngIII through the catalytic action of aminopeptidase M and has potent effects on memory and cognition. Central and peripheral actions of AngIV are mediated through specific AT_4 receptors identified as insulin-regulated amino peptidases (IRAPs). AngIV binding to AT_4 receptors inhibits the catalytic activity of IRAPs and enables accumulation of various neuropeptides linked to memory potentiation. Other actions include renal vasodilation, natriuresis, neuronal differentiation, hypertrophy, inflammation, and extracellular matrix remodeling (Ruiz-Ortega et al., 2007). Analogs of angiotensin IV are being developed for their therapeutic potential in cognition in Alzheimer disease or head injury (Albiston et al., 2007).

Angiotensinases. These include aminopeptidases, endopeptidases, carboxypeptidases, and other peptidases that degrade and inactivate angiotensin peptides; none is specific.

Local (Tissue) Renin–Angiotensin Systems. The traditional view of the RAS as classical endocrine system is oversimplified. The modern view of the RAS also includes the local (tissue) RAS. Local (tissue) RAS is an AngII-producing system that is being recognized for its role in hypertrophy, inflammation, remodeling, and apoptosis. Activation of (tissue) RAS and local AngII production require the binding of renin or prorenin to the specific (pro)renin receptor (PRR), located on cell surfaces. In this regard, it is important to distinguish between *extrinsic* and *intrinsic* local RAS:

Extrinsic Local RAS. ACE is present on the luminal face of vascular endothelial cells throughout the circulation, and circulating renin of renal origin can be taken up by the arterial wall and by other tissues (Danser et al., 1994).

Intrinsic Local RAS. Many tissues—including the brain, pituitary, blood vessels, heart, kidney, and adrenal gland—express mRNAs for renin, angiotensinogen, and/or ACE, and various cells cultured from these tissues produce renin, angiotensinogen, ACE, and angiotensins I, II, and III. Thus, it appears that local RASs exist independently of the renal/hepatic-based system and may influence vascular, cardiac, and renal function and structure (Paul et al., 2006).

The (Pro)Renin Receptor. The PRR is the functional receptor, located on the cell surface, that binds prorenin and renin with high affinity (K_D ~6 and 20 nM, respectively) and specificity (Batenburg and Danser, 2008). Human PRR is a 350–amino acid protein that shares no homology with any membrane protein. The PRR gene is located in the locus p11.4 of the X chromosome and is named ATP6ap2 (ATPase-associated protein). Knockout of the PRR gene is lethal. In humans, mutations in the PRR gene are associated with mental retardation and epilepsy, suggesting an important role in cognition, brain development, and survival (Nguyen and Danser, 2008; Ramser et al., 2005). Prorenin and renin also bind to mannose-6-phosphate receptor (M6P), an insulin-like growth factor II receptor that functions as a clearance receptor.

Binding of (pro)renin to PRR enhances the catalytic activity of renin by 4-5 fold and induces non-proteolytic activation of prorenin (Figure 26-3). Bound, activated (pro)renin catalyzes the conversion of angiotensinogen to AngI, which is subsequently converted to AngII by ACE located on the cell surface. Locally produced AngII binds to AT_1 receptors and activates intracellular signaling events that regulate cell growth, collagen deposition, fibrosis, inflammation, and apoptosis (Nguyen and Danser, 2008).

The binding of (pro)renin to PRR also induces AngII-independent signaling events that include activation of ERK1/2, p38, tyrosine kinases, TGF-β gene expression, and plasminogen activator inhibitor type 1 (PAI-1). These signaling pathways are not blocked by ACE inhibitors or AT_1 receptor antagonists and are reported to contribute to fibrosis, nephrosis, and organ damage (Kaneshiro et al., 2007; Nguyen and Danser, 2008; see Figure 26-4). PRR is abundant in the heart, brain, eye, adrenals, placenta, adipose tissue, liver, and kidneys. Overexpression of the human PRR in transgenic animals increases plasma aldosterone levels in the absence of changes in plasma renin levels and induces hypertension and nephropathy. Rats overexpressing PRR exhibit increased expression of COX-2 in the macula densa and develop proteinuria and glomerulosclerosis that increase with aging (Kaneshiro et al., 2006; Kaneshiro et al., 2007).

Prorenin is no longer considered the inactive precursor of renin. Prorenin is capable of activating local (tissue) RAS and AngII-dependent and independent events that may contribute to organ damage. Circulating plasma concentrations of prorenin are 10-fold higher than renin in healthy subjects but are elevated to 100-fold in diabetic patients and are associated with increased risk of nephropathy, renal fibrosis, and retinopathy (Danser and Deinum, 2005; Nguyen and Danser, 2008). The interaction of prorenin with PRR has become a target for therapeutic interventions.

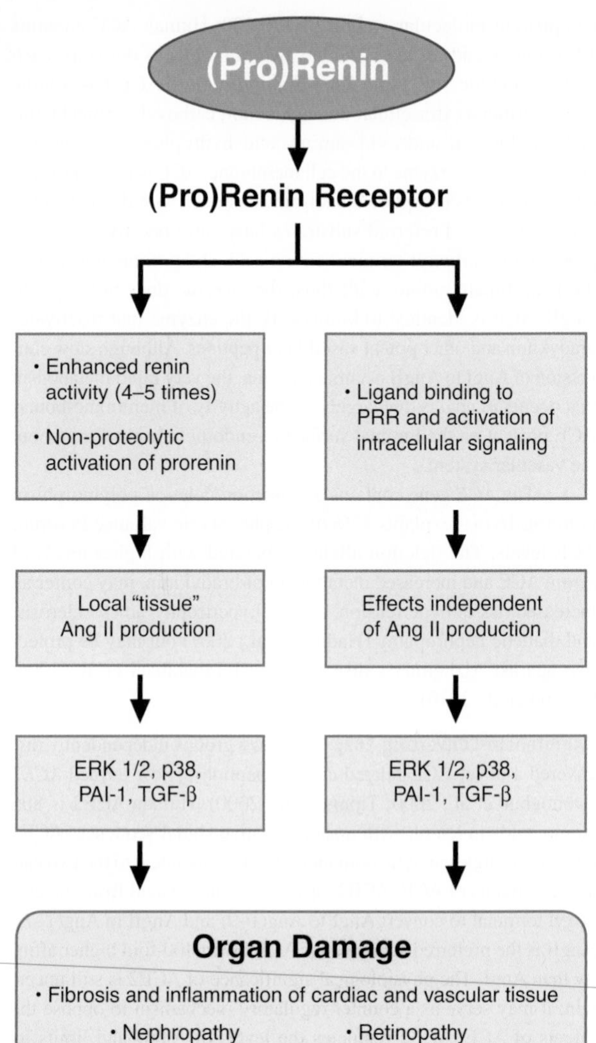

Figure 26-4. *Ang II-dependent and Ang II-independent actions of prorenin.* See text for details.

Alternative Pathways for Angiotensin Biosynthesis. Angiotensinogen may be converted to AngI or directly to AngII by cathepsin G and tonin. Other enzymes that convert AngI to AngII include cathepsin G, chymostatin-sensitive AngII-generating enzyme, and heart chymase. Chymase contributes to the local tissue conversion of AngI to AngII, particularly in the heart and kidneys (Paul et al., 2006).

Angiotensin Receptors. AngII and AngIII couple to specific GPCRs designated AT_1 and AT_2 (de Gasparo et al., 2000). The AT_1 receptor has a 10,000-fold higher affinity for losartan (and related biphenyl tetrazole derivatives) than the AT_2 receptor. The AT_1 receptor (359 amino acids) and the AT_2 receptor (363 amino acids) share 34% sequence homology.

Most of the known biological effects of AngII are mediated by the AT_1 receptor. The AT_1 receptor gene contains a polymorphism (A-to-C transversion in position 1166) associated with hypertension, hypertrophic cardiomyopathy, and coronary artery vasoconstriction. Moreover, the C allele synergizes with the ACE deletion allele with regard to increased risk of coronary artery disease (Álvarez et al., 1998). Preeclampsia is associated with the development of agonistic auto-antibodies against the AT_1 receptor (Wallukat et al., 1999).

Functional roles for the AT_2 receptors are less well defined, but they may counterbalance many of the effects of the AT_1 receptors by having antiproliferative, proapoptotic, vasodilatory, natriuretic, and antihypertensive effects (Jones et al., 2008; Carey et al., 2001). The AT_2 receptor is distributed widely in fetal tissues, but its distribution is more restricted in adults. Although the AT_2 receptor generally is conceptualized as a cardiovascular protective receptor, its overexpression and activation may contribute to myocyte hypertrophy and cardiac fibrosis (D'Amore et al., 2005; Ichihara et al., 2001). Expression of AT_2 receptors is upregulated in cardiovascular diseases, including heart failure, cardiac fibrosis, and ischemic heart disease; however, the significance of increased AT_2 receptor expression is unclear (Jones et al., 2008).

The Mas receptor mediates the effects of Ang(1–7), which include vasodilation and anti-proliferation. Deletion of the *Mas* gene in transgenic mice reveals cardiac dysfunction (Santos et al., 2008).

The AT_4 receptor (IRAP; see Figure 26-2) mediates the effects of AngIV. This receptor is a single transmembrane protein (1025 amino acids) that co-localizes with the glucose transporter GLUT4. AT_4 receptors are detectable in a number of tissues, such as heart, vasculature, adrenal cortex, and brain regions processing sensory and motor functions (Chai et al., 2004).

Angiotensin Receptor–Effector Coupling. AT_1 receptors activate a large array of signal-transduction systems to produce effects that vary with cell type and that are a combination of primary and secondary responses. AT_1 receptors couple to several heterotrimeric G proteins, including G_q, $G_{12/13}$, and G_i. In most cell types, AT_1 receptors couple to G_q to activate the PLCβ–IP_3–Ca^{2+} pathway. Secondary to G_q activation, activation of PKC, PLA_2, and PLD and eicosanoid production, as well as activation of Ca^{2+}-dependent and MAP kinases and the Ca^{2+}–calmodulin–dependent activation of NOS may occur. Activation of G_i may occur and will reduce the activity of adenylyl cyclase, lowering cellular cyclic AMP content; however, there also is evidence for $G_q \rightarrow G_s$ cross-talk such that activation of the AT_1–G_q–PLC pathway enhances cyclic AMP production (Meszaros et al., 2000; Epperson et al., 2004). The βγ subunits of G_i and activation of $G_{12/13}$ lead to activation of tyrosine kinases and small G proteins such as Rho. Ultimately, the JAK/STAT pathway may be activated and a variety of transcriptional regulatory factors induced. By these mechanisms, angiotensin influences the expression of a host of gene products relating to cell growth and the production of components of the extracellular matrix. AT_1 receptors also stimulate the activity of a membrane-bound NADH/NADPH oxidase that generates reactive oxygen species (ROS). ROS may contribute to biochemical effects (activation of MAP kinase, tyrosine kinase, and phosphatases; inactivation of NO; and expression of monocyte chemoattractant protein-1) and physiological effects (acute effects on renal function, chronic effects on blood pressure, and vascular hypertrophy and inflammation) (Mehta and Griendling, 2007; Higuchi et al., 2007). The relative importance of these myriad signal-transduction pathways in mediating biological responses to AngII is tissue specific. The presence of other receptors may alter the response to AT_1 receptor activation. For example, AT_1 receptors heterodimerize with bradykinin B_2 receptors, a process that enhances AngII sensitivity in preeclampsia (AbdAlla et al., 2002).

Less is known about AT_2 receptor–effector coupling. Signaling from AT_2 receptors is mediated by G protein-dependent and independent pathways. Consequences of AT_2 receptor activation include activation of phosphoprotein phosphatases, K^+ channels, synthesis of NO and cyclic GMP, bradykinin production, and inhibition of Ca^{2+} channel functions (Jones et al., 2008). AT_2 receptors may possess constitutive activity. Overexpression of AT_2 receptors has been reported to induce NO production in vascular smooth muscle cells and hypertrophy in cardiac myocytes through an intrinsic activity of the AT_2 receptor independent of angiotensin binding (D'Amore et al., 2005; Jones et al., 2008). Homo-oligomerization of AT_2 receptors also has been reported to induce apoptosis (Miura et al., 2005). The AT_2 receptor may bind directly to and antagonize the AT_1 receptor (AbdAlla et al., 2001) and can form heterodimers with the bradykinin B_2 receptor to enhance NO production (Abadir, 2006).

Functions and Effects of the Renin–Angiotensin System

The main effects of AngII on the cardiovascular system include:

- rapid pressor response
- slow pressor response
- vascular and cardiac hypertrophy and remodeling

Modest increases in plasma concentrations of AngII acutely raise blood pressure; on a molar basis, AngII is ~40 times more potent than NE (see Chapter 12); the EC_{50} of AngII for acutely raising arterial blood pressure is ~0.3 nM. When a single moderate dose of AngII is injected intravenously, systemic blood pressure begins to rise within seconds, peaks rapidly, and returns to normal within minutes (Figure 26–5). This *rapid pressor response* to AngII is due to a swift increase in total peripheral resistance—a response that helps to maintain arterial blood pressure in the face of an acute hypotensive challenge (e.g., blood loss or vasodilation). Although AngII increases cardiac contractility directly (via opening voltage-gated Ca^{2+} channels in cardiac myocytes) and increases heart rate indirectly (via facilitation of sympathetic tone, enhanced adrenergic neurotransmission, and adrenal catecholamine release), the rapid increase in arterial blood pressure activates a baroreceptor reflex that decreases sympathetic tone and increases vagal tone. Thus, depending on the physiological

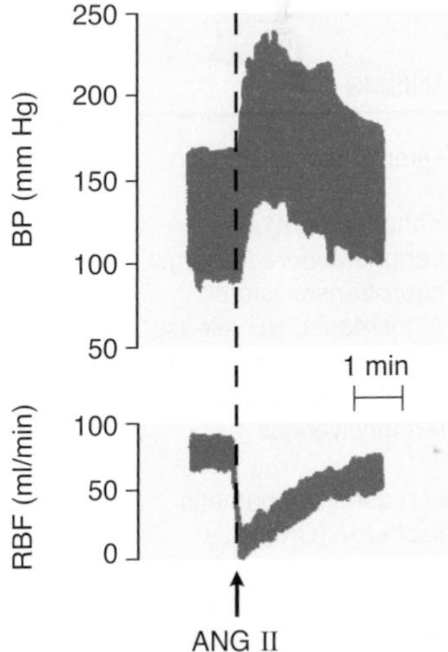

Figure 26–5. *Effect of a bolus intravenous injection of AngII (0.05 μg/kg) on arterial blood pressure (BP) and renal blood flow (RBF) in a conscious dog.* (Reproduced with permission, from Zimmerman BG. Absence of adrenergic mediation of agonist response to [Sar[1],Ala[8]] angiotensin II in conscious normotensive and hypertensive dogs. *Clin Sci*, 1979, 57:71–81. © the Biochemical Society.)

state, AngII may increase, decrease, or not change cardiac contractility, heart rate, and cardiac output. Changes in cardiac output therefore contribute little, if at all, to the rapid pressor response induced by AngII.

AngII also causes a *slow pressor response* that helps to stabilize arterial blood pressure over the long term. A continuous infusion of initially subpressor doses of AngII gradually increases arterial blood pressure, with the maximum effect requiring days to achieve. This slow pressor response probably is mediated by a decrement in renal excretory function that shifts the renal pressure–natriuresis curve to the right (see the next section). AngII stimulates the synthesis of endothelin-1 and superoxide anion, which may contribute to the slow pressor response.

In addition to its effects on arterial blood pressure, AngII stimulates remodeling of the cardiovascular system, causing hypertrophy of vascular and cardiac cells and increased synthesis and deposition of collagen by cardiac fibroblasts.

Mechanisms by Which Angiotensin II Increases Total Peripheral Resistance. AngII increases total peripheral resistance (TPR) via direct and indirect effects on blood vessels (Figure 26–6).

Rapid Pressor Response

Direct Vasoconstriction. AngII constricts precapillary arterioles and, to a lesser extent, postcapillary venules by activating AT_1 receptors located on vascular smooth muscle cells and stimulating the G_q–PLC–IP_3–Ca^{2+} pathway. AngII has differential effects on vascular beds. Direct vasoconstriction is strongest in the kidneys (Figure 26–5) and somewhat less in the splanchnic vascular bed; blood flow in these regions falls sharply when AngII is infused. AngII-induced vasoconstriction is much less in vessels of the brain and still weaker in

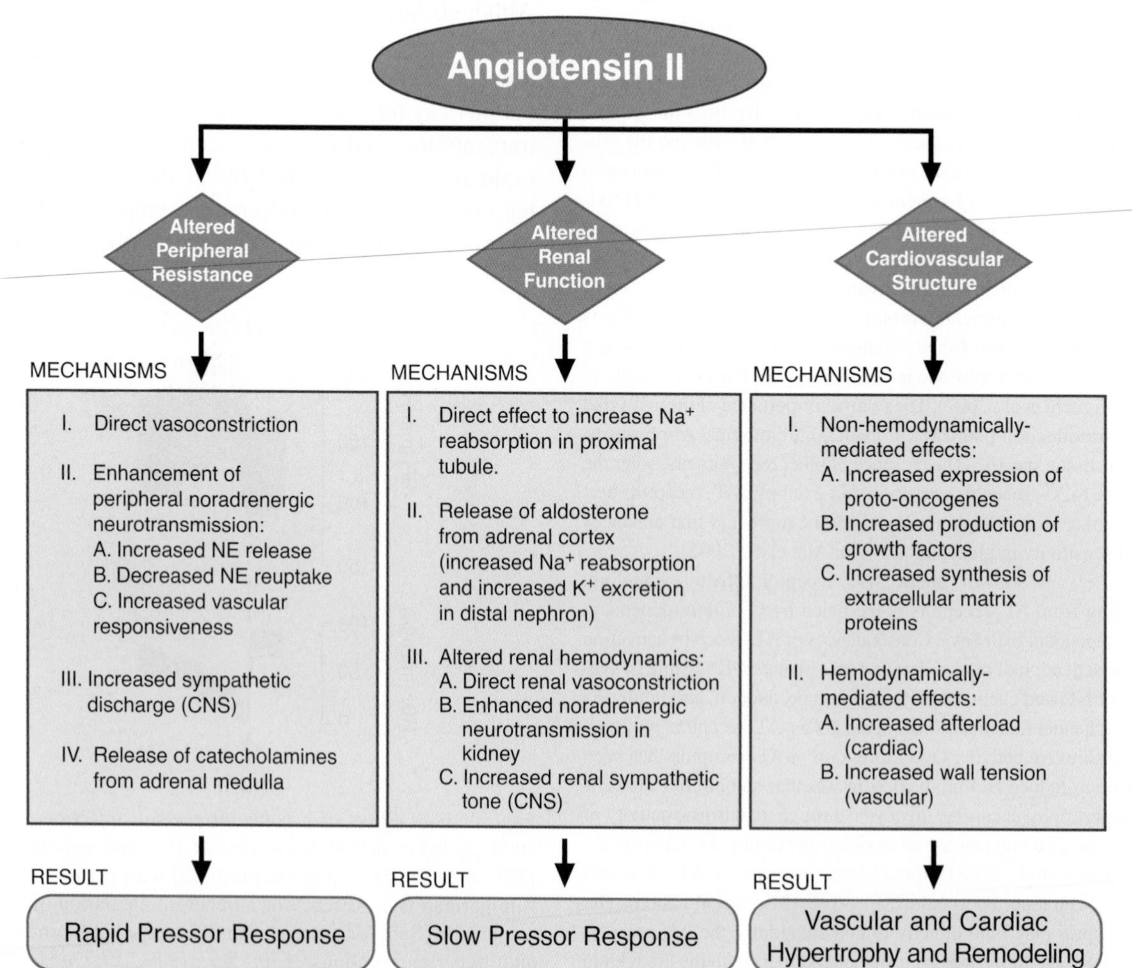

Figure 26–6. *Summary of the three major effects of AngII and the mechanisms that mediate them.* NE, norepinephrine.

those of the lung and skeletal muscle. Nevertheless, high circulating concentrations of AngII may decrease cerebral and coronary blood flow.

Enhancement of Peripheral Noradrenergic Neurotransmission. AngII augments norepinephrine release from sympathetic nerve terminals by inhibiting the reuptake of norepinephrine into nerve terminals and by enhancing the vascular response to NE (see Chapter 12). High concentrations of the peptide stimulate ganglion cells directly.

Effects on the CNS. Small amounts of AngII infused into the vertebral arteries cause an increase in arterial blood pressure. This response—mediated by increased sympathetic outflow—reflects effects of the hormone on circumventricular nuclei that are not protected by a blood-brain barrier (e.g., area postrema, subfornical organ, organum vasculosum of the lamina terminalis). Circulating AngII also attenuates baroreceptor-mediated reductions in sympathetic discharge, thereby increasing arterial pressure. The CNS is affected both by bloodborne AngII and by AngII formed within the brain, where it may serve as a neurotransmitter. The brain contains all components of the RAS. In addition to increasing sympathetic tone, AngII also causes a centrally mediated dipsogenic (thirst) effect and enhances the release of vasopressin from the neurohypophysis.

Release of Catecholamines from the Adrenal Medulla. AngII stimulates the release of catecholamines from the adrenal medulla by depolarizing chromaffin cells.

Slow Pressor Response

Alteration of Renal Function. AngII has pronounced effects on renal function, reducing the urinary excretion of Na^+ and water while increasing the excretion of K^+. The overall effect of AngII on the kidneys is to shift the renal pressure–natriuresis curve to the right (Figure 26–7).

Direct Effects of Angiotensin II on Na^+ Reabsorption in the Renal Tubules. Very low concentrations of AngII stimulate Na^+/H^+ exchange in the proximal tubule—an effect that increases Na^+, Cl^-, and bicarbonate reabsorption. Approximately 20-30% of the bicarbonate handled by the nephron may be affected by this mechanism. AngII also increases the expression of the Na^+–glucose symporter in the proximal tubule (Bautista et al., 2004). Paradoxically, at high concentrations, AngII may inhibit Na^+ transport in the proximal tubule. AngII also directly stimulates the Na^+–K^+–$2Cl^-$ symporter in the thick ascending limb. The proximal tubule secretes angiotensinogen, and the connecting tubule releases renin, so a paracrine tubular RAS may contribute to Na^+ reabsorption.

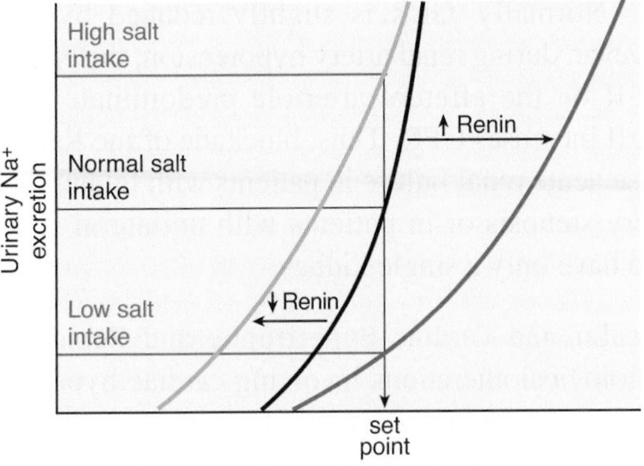

Figure 26–7. *Pressure-natriuresis curve: effects of Na^+ intake on renin release (AngII formation) and arterial blood pressure.* Inhibition of the renin-angiotensin system will cause a large drop in blood pressure in Na^+-depleted individuals. (Modified with permission from Jackson EK, Branch RA, et al: Physiological functions of the renal prostaglandin, renin, and kalikrein systems, in Seldin DW, Giebisch GH, eds: *The Kidney: Physiology and Pathophysiology*, Vol 1. Philadelphia: Lippincott Williams & Wilkins, 1985, p 624. http://lww.com.)

Release of Aldosterone from the Adrenal Cortex. AngII stimulates the zona glomerulosa of the adrenal cortex to increase the synthesis and secretion of aldosterone, and augments responses to other stimuli (e.g., ACTH, K^+). Increased output of aldosterone is elicited by concentrations of AngII that have little or no acute effect on blood pressure. Aldosterone acts on the distal and collecting tubules to cause retention of Na^+ and excretion of K^+ and H^+. The stimulant effect of AngII on aldosterone synthesis and release is enhanced under conditions of hyponatremia or hyperkalemia and is reduced when concentrations of Na^+ and K^+ in plasma are altered in the opposite directions.

Altered Renal Hemodynamics. AngII reduces renal blood flow and renal excretory function by directly constricting the renal vascular smooth muscle, by enhancing renal sympathetic tone (a CNS effect), and by facilitating renal adrenergic transmission (an intrarenal effect). AngII-induced vasoconstriction of preglomerular microvessels is enhanced by endogenous adenosine owing to signal-transduction systems activated by AT_1 and the adenosine A_1 receptor (Hansen et al., 2003).

AngII influences glomerular filtration rate (GFR) by means of several mechanisms:

- constriction of the afferent arterioles, which reduces intraglomerular pressure and tends to reduce GFR
- contraction of mesangial cells, which decreases the capillary surface area within the glomerulus available for filtration and also tends to decrease GFR
- constriction of efferent arterioles, which increases intraglomerular pressure and tends to increase GFR

Normally, GFR is slightly reduced by AngII; however, during renal artery hypotension, the effects of AngII on the efferent arteriole predominate so that AngII increases GFR. Thus, blockade of the RAS may cause acute renal failure in patients with bilateral renal artery stenosis or in patients with unilateral stenosis who have only a single kidney.

Vascular and Cardiac Hypertrophy and Remodeling. Pathological alterations involving cardiac hypertrophy and remodeling increase morbidity and mortality. These morbid changes in cardiovascular structure are due to increased migration, proliferation (hyperplasia), and hypertrophy of cells, as well as to increased extracellular matrix. The cells involved include vascular smooth muscle cells, cardiac myocytes, and fibroblasts. In this regard, AngII:

- stimulates the migration, proliferation, and hypertrophy of vascular smooth muscle cells
- increases extracellular matrix production by vascular smooth muscle cells
- causes hypertrophy of cardiac myocytes
- increases extracellular matrix production by cardiac fibroblasts

These effects of AngII are mediated by acting directly on cells to induce the expression of specific proto-oncogenes (c-*fos*, c-*jun*, c-*myc*, and *egr*-1) that alter the expression of growth factors such as basic FGF, PDGF, and TGF- β. In addition, AngII alters extracellular matrix formation and degradation indirectly by increasing aldosterone.

Hemodynamically Mediated Effects of Angiotensin II on Cardiovascular Structure. In addition to the direct cellular effects of AngII on cardiovascular structure, changes in cardiac preload (volume expansion owing to Na^+ retention) and afterload (increased arterial blood pressure) probably contribute to cardiac hypertrophy and remodeling. Arterial hypertension also contributes to hypertrophy and remodeling of blood vessels.

Role of the RAS in Long-Term Maintenance of Arterial Blood Pressure Despite Extremes in Dietary Na^+ Intake. Arterial blood pressure is a major determinant of Na^+ excretion. This is illustrated graphically by plotting urinary Na^+ excretion versus mean arterial blood pressure (Figure 26–7), a plot known as the *renal pressure–natriuresis curve*. Over the long term, Na^+ excretion must equal Na^+ intake; therefore, the set point for long-term levels of arterial blood pressure can be obtained as the intersection of a horizontal line representing Na^+ intake with the renal pressure–natriuresis. As illustrated in Figure 26–7, the RAS plays a major role in maintaining a constant set point for long-term levels of arterial blood pressure despite extreme changes in dietary Na^+ intake. When dietary Na^+ intake is low, renin release is stimulated, and AngII acts on the kidneys to shift the renal pressure–natriuresis curve to the right. Conversely, when dietary Na^+ is high, renin release is inhibited, and the withdrawal of AngII shifts the renal pressure–natriuresis curve to the left. When modulation of the RAS is blocked by drugs, changes in salt intake markedly affect long-term levels of arterial blood pressure.

Other Effects of the RAS. Expression of the RAS is required for the development of normal kidney morphology, particularly the maturational growth of the renal papilla (Niimura et al., 1995). AngII causes a marked anorexigenic effect and weight loss, and high circulating levels of AngII may contribute to the anorexia, wasting, and cachexia of heart failure (Brink et al., 1996).

Angiotensin and Vascular Disease

The RAS induces vascular disease by multiple mechanisms, including directly and indirectly (via aldosterone): stimulating vascular smooth muscle cell migration, proliferation, and extracellular matrix production; increasing the release of plasminogen activator inhibitor type 1 and enhancing the expression of monocyte chemoattractant protein 1; augmenting the expression of adhesion proteins (e.g., ICAM-1, integrins, and osteopontin) in vascular cells; and stimulating the production of inflammatory chemokines and cytokines that enhance the migration of inflammatory cells (Schmieder et al., 2007). AngII markedly accelerates the development of atherosclerosis in apolipoprotein E–deficient mice (Weiss et al., 2001), an animal model of atherosclerosis.

INHIBITORS OF THE RENIN–ANGIOTENSIN SYSTEM

Clinical interest focuses on developing inhibitors of the RAS. Three types of inhibitors are utilized therapeutically (Figure 26–8):

- ACE inhibitors (ACEIs)
- angiotensin receptor blockers (ARBs)
- direct renin inhibitors (DRIs)

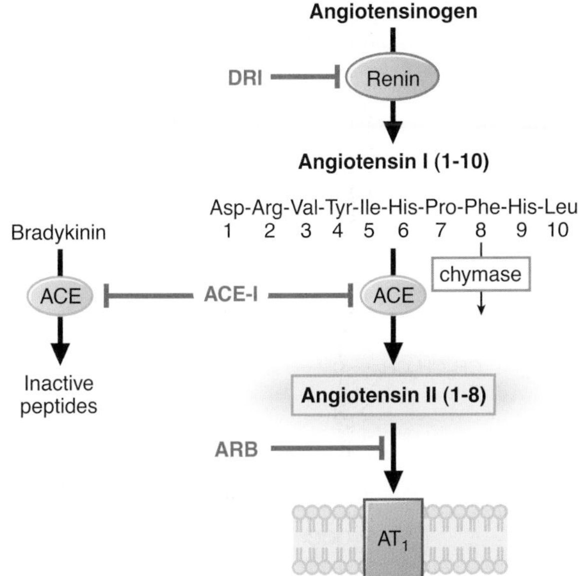

Figure 26-8. *Inhibitors of the RAS.* ACE-I, angiotensin-converting enzyme inhibitor; ARB, angiotensin receptor blocker; DRI, direct renin inhibitor.

Angiotensin-Converting Enzyme Inhibitors

History. In the 1960s, Ferreira and colleagues found that the venoms of pit vipers contain factors that intensify vasodilator responses to bradykinin. These bradykinin-potentiating factors are a family of peptides that inhibit kininase II, an enzyme that inactivates bradykinin. Erdös and coworkers established that ACE and kininase II are the same enzyme, which catalyzes both the synthesis of AngII and the destruction of bradykinin. Based on these findings, the nonapeptide teprotide (snake venom peptide that inhibits kininase II and ACE) was later synthesized and tested in human subjects. It lowered blood pressure in many patients with essential hypertension and exerted beneficial effects in patients with heart failure.

The orally effective ACE inhibitor *captopril* was developed by a rational approach that involved analysis of the inhibitory action of teprotide, inference about the action of ACE on its substrates, and analogy with carboxypeptidase A, which was known to be inhibited by D-benzylsuccinic acid. Ondetti, Cushman, and colleagues argued that inhibition of ACE might be produced by succinyl amino acids that corresponded in length to the dipeptide cleaved by ACE. This led to the synthesis of a series of carboxy alkanoyl and mercapto alkanoyl derivatives that are potent competitive inhibitors of ACE. Most active was captopril (Vane, 1999).

Pharmacological Effects in Normal Laboratory Animals and Humans. The effect of ACE inhibitors on the RAS is to inhibit the conversion of AngI to the active AngII. Inhibition of AngII production will lower blood pressure and enhance natriuresis. ACE is an enzyme with many substrates, and inhibition of ACE may also induce effects unrelated to reducing the levels of AngII. ACE inhibitors increase bradykinin levels and bradykinin stimulates prostaglandin biosynthesis; both may contribute to the pharmacological effects of ACE inhibitors. ACE inhibitors increase by 5-fold the circulating levels of the natural stem cell regulator *N*-acetyl-seryl-aspartyl-lysyl-proline, which may contribute to the cardioprotective effects of ACE inhibitors (Rhaleb et al., 2001). In addition, ACE inhibitors will increase renin release and the rate of formation of AngI by interfering with both short- and long-loop negative feedbacks on renin release (Figure 26–2A). Accumulating AngI is directed down alternative metabolic routes, resulting in the increased production of vasodilator peptides such as Ang(1–7). In healthy, Na^+-replete animals and humans, a single oral dose of an ACE inhibitor has little effect on systemic blood pressure, but repeated doses over several days cause a small reduction in blood pressure. By contrast, even a single dose of these inhibitors lowers blood pressure substantially in normal subjects depleted of Na^+ (Figure 26-7).

Clinical Pharmacology. ACE inhibitors can be classified into three broad groups based on chemical structure: (1) sulfhydryl-containing ACE inhibitors structurally related to captopril; (2) dicarboxyl-containing ACE inhibitors structurally related to enalapril (e.g., lisinopril, benazepril, quinapril, moexipril, ramipril, trandolapril, perindopril); and (3) phosphorus-containing ACE inhibitors structurally related to fosinopril. Many ACE inhibitors are ester-containing prodrugs that are 100-1000 times less potent but have a better oral bioavailability than the active molecules. Currently, 11 ACE inhibitors are available for clinical use in the U.S. (Figure 26–9). They differ with regard to potency, whether ACE inhibition is primarily a direct effect of the drug itself or the effect of an active metabolite, and pharmacokinetics.

With the exceptions of fosinopril and spirapril (which display balanced elimination by the liver and kidneys), ACE inhibitors are cleared predominantly by the kidneys. Impaired renal function significantly diminishes the plasma clearance of most ACE inhibitors, and dosages of these drugs should be reduced in patients with renal impairment. *Elevated plasma renin activity renders patients hyperresponsive to ACE inhibitor–induced hypotension, and initial dosages of all ACE inhibitors should be reduced in patients with high plasma levels of renin (e.g., patients with heart failure and salt-depleted patients).*

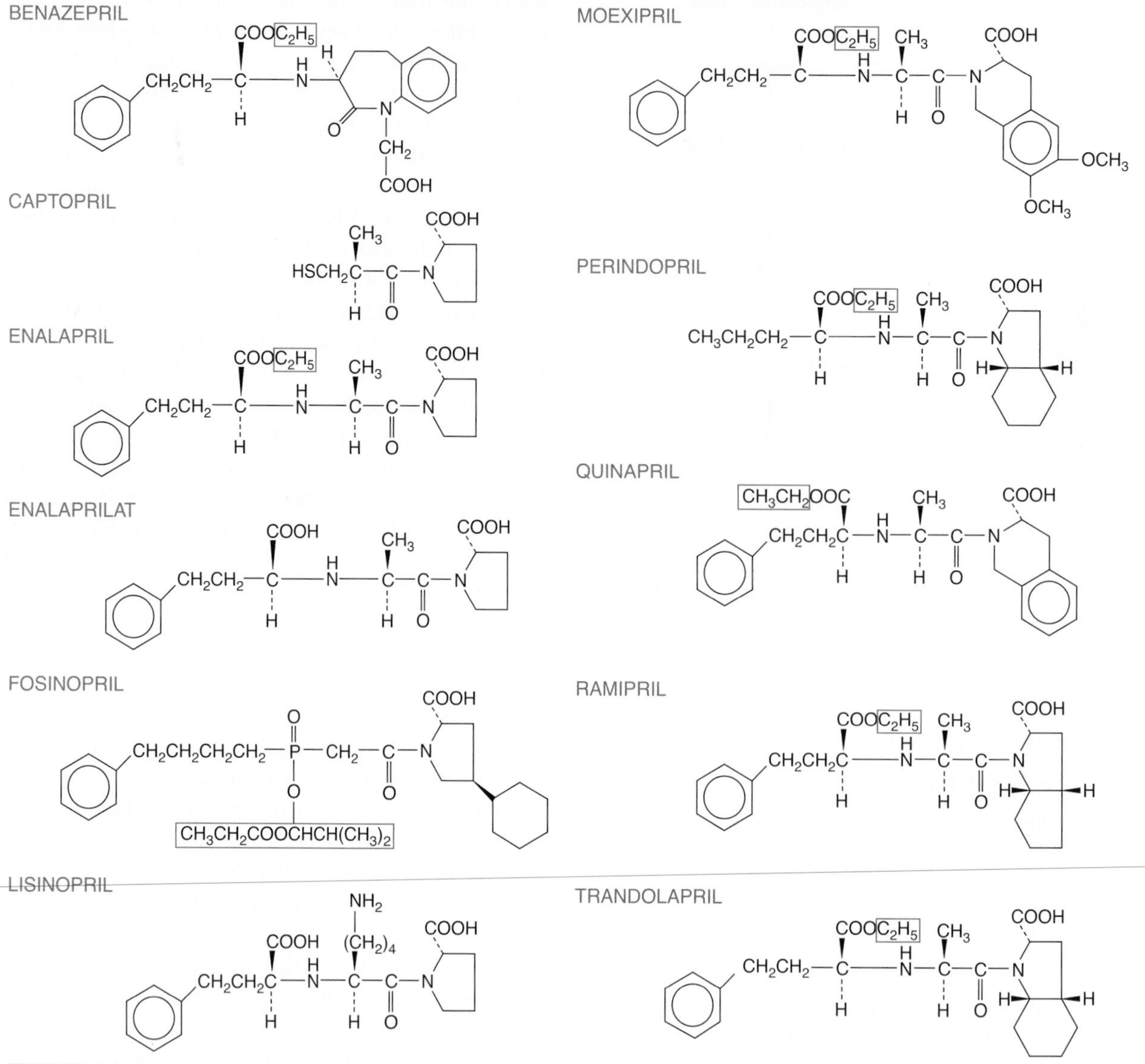

BENAZEPRIL

MOEXIPRIL

CAPTOPRIL

PERINDOPRIL

ENALAPRIL

QUINAPRIL

ENALAPRILAT

FOSINOPRIL

RAMIPRIL

LISINOPRIL

TRANDOLAPRIL

Figure 26–9. *Chemical structures of selected ACE inhibitors.* Captopril, lisinopril, and enalaprilat are active molecules. Benazepril, enalapril, fosinopril, moexipril, perindopril, quinapril, ramipril, and trandolapril are relatively inactive until converted to their corresponding diacids. The structures enclosed within red boxes are removed by esterases and replaced with a hydrogen atom to form the active molecule *in vivo* (e.g., enalapril to enalaprilat or ramipril to ramiprilat).

All ACE inhibitors block the conversion of AngI to AngII and have similar therapeutic indications, adverse-effect profiles, and contraindications. Although captopril and enalapril are indistinguishable with regard to antihypertensive efficacy and safety, the Quality-of-Life Hypertension Study Group reported that captopril may have a more favorable effect on quality of life (Testa et al., 1993). Because hypertension usually requires lifelong treatment, quality-of-life issues are an important consideration in comparing antihypertensive drugs. ACE inhibitors differ markedly in tissue distribution, and it is possible that this difference could be exploited to inhibit some local (tissue) RAS while leaving others relatively intact.

Captopril (CAPOTEN, others). Captopril, the first ACE inhibitor to be marketed, is a potent ACE inhibitor with a K_i of 1.7 nM. It is the only ACE inhibitor approved for use in the U.S. that contains a sulfhydryl moiety. Given orally, captopril is absorbed rapidly and has a bioavailability ~75%. Bioavailability is reduced by 25-30% with food, so captopril should be given 1 hour before meals. Peak concentrations in plasma occur within an hour, and the drug is cleared rapidly with a $t_{1/2}$ ~2 hours. Most of the drug is eliminated in urine, 40-50% as captopril and the rest as captopril disulfide dimers and captopril–cysteine disulfide. The oral dose of captopril ranges from 6.25-150 mg two to three times daily, with 6.25 mg three times daily or 25 mg twice daily being appropriate for the initiation of therapy for heart failure or hypertension, respectively. Most patients should not receive daily doses in excess of 150 mg, although the maximum labeled dose for heart failure is 450 mg/day.

Enalapril (VASOTEC, others). Enalapril maleate is a prodrug that is hydrolyzed by esterases in the liver to produce the active dicarboxylic acid, enalaprilat. Enalaprilat is a highly potent inhibitor of ACE with a K_i of 0.2 nM. Although it also contains a "proline surrogate," enalaprilat differs from captopril in that it is an analog of a tripeptide rather than of a dipeptide. Enalapril is absorbed rapidly when given orally and has an oral bioavailability of ~60% (not reduced by food). Although peak concentrations of enalapril in plasma occur within an hour, enalaprilat concentrations peak only after 3-4 hours. Enalapril has a $t_{1/2}$ ~1.3 hours, but enalaprilat, because of tight binding to ACE, has a plasma $t_{1/2}$ of ~11 hours. Nearly all the drug is eliminated by the kidneys as either intact enalapril or enalaprilat. The oral dosage of enalapril ranges from 2.5-40 mg daily (single or divided dose), with 2.5 and 5 mg daily being appropriate for the initiation of therapy for heart failure and hypertension, respectively.

Enalaprilat (VASOTEC INJECTION, others). Enalaprilat is not absorbed orally but is available for intravenous administration when oral therapy is not appropriate. For hypertensive patients, the dosage is 0.625-1.25 mg given intravenously over 5 minutes. This dosage may be repeated every 6 hours.

Lisinopril (PRINIVIL, ZESTRIL, others). Lisinopril is the lysine analog of enalaprilat; unlike enalapril, lisinopril itself is active. *In vitro*, lisinopril is a slightly more potent ACE inhibitor than is enalaprilat. Lisinopril is absorbed slowly, variably, and incompletely (~30%) after oral administration (not reduced by food); peak concentrations in plasma are achieved in ~7 hours. It is cleared as the intact compound by the kidney, and its $t_{1/2}$ in plasma is ~12 hours. Lisinopril does not accumulate in tissues. The oral dosage of lisinopril ranges from 5-40 mg daily (single or divided dose), with 5 and 10 mg daily being appropriate for the initiation of therapy for heart failure and hypertension, respectively. A daily dose of 2.5 mg and close medical supervision is recommended for patients with heart failure who are hyponatremic or have renal impairment.

Benazepril (LOTENSIN, others). Cleavage of the ester moiety by hepatic esterases transforms benazepril, a prodrug, into benazeprilat, an ACE inhibitor that *in vitro* is more potent than captopril, enalaprilat, or lisinopril. Benazepril is absorbed rapidly but incompletely (37%) after oral administration (only slightly reduced by food). Benazepril is nearly completely metabolized to benazeprilat and to the glucuronide conjugates of benazepril and benazeprilat, which are excreted into both the urine and bile; peak concentrations of benazepril and benazeprilat in plasma are achieved in 0.5-1 hour and 1-2 hours, respectively. Benazeprilat has an effective plasma $t_{1/2}$ of 10-11 hours. With the exception of the lungs, benazeprilat does not accumulate in tissues. The oral dosage of benazepril ranges from 5-80 mg daily (single or divided dose).

Fosinopril (MONOPRIL, others). Fosinopril is the only ACE inhibitor approved for use in the U.S. that contains a phosphinate group that binds to the active site of ACE. Cleavage of the ester moiety by hepatic esterases transforms fosinopril, a prodrug, into fosinoprilat, an ACE inhibitor that *in vitro* is more potent than captopril yet less potent than enalaprilat. Fosinopril is absorbed slowly and incompletely (36%) after oral administration (rate but not extent reduced by food). Fosinopril is largely metabolized to fosinoprilat (75%) and to the glucuronide conjugate of fosinoprilat. These are excreted in both the urine and bile; peak concentrations of fosinoprilat in plasma are achieved in ~3 hours. Fosinoprilat has an effective plasma $t_{1/2}$ of ~11.5 hours; its clearance is not significantly altered by renal impairment. The oral dosage of fosinopril ranges from 10-80 mg daily (single or divided dose). The initial dose is reduced to 5 mg daily in patients with Na^+ or water depletion or renal failure.

Trandolapril (MAVIK, others). An oral dose of trandolapril is absorbed without reduction by food and produces plasma levels of trandolapril (10% bioavailability) and trandolaprilat (70% bioavailability). Trandolaprilat is ~8 times more potent than trandolapril as an ACE inhibitor. Trandolapril is metabolized to trandolaprilat and to inactive metabolites (mostly glucuronides of trandolapril and deesterification products), and these are recovered in the urine (33%, mostly trandolaprilat) and feces (66%). Peak concentrations of trandolaprilat in plasma are achieved in 4-10 hours. Trandolaprilat displays biphasic elimination kinetics with an initial $t_{1/2}$ of ~10 hours (the major component of elimination), followed by a more prolonged $t_{1/2}$ (owing to slow dissociation of trandolaprilat from tissue ACE). Plasma clearance of trandolaprilat is reduced by both renal and hepatic insufficiency. The oral dosage ranges from 1-8 mg daily (single or divided dose). The initial dose is 0.5 mg in patients who are taking a diuretic or who have renal impairment, and 2 mg for African-Americans.

Quinapril (ACCUPRIL, others). Cleavage of the ester moiety by hepatic esterases transforms quinapril, a prodrug, into quinaprilat, an ACE inhibitor that *in vitro* is about as potent as benazeprilat. Quinapril is absorbed rapidly (peak concentrations are achieved in 1 hour), and the rate, but not extent, of oral absorption (60%) may be reduced by food (delayed peak). Quinaprilat and other minor metabolites of quinapril are excreted in the urine (61%) and feces (37%). Peak concentrations of quinaprilat in plasma are achieved in ~2 hours. Conversion of quinapril to quinaprilat is reduced in patients with diminished liver function. The initial $t_{1/2}$ of quinaprilat is ~2 hours; a prolonged terminal $t_{1/2}$ ~25 hours may be due to high-affinity binding of the drug to tissue ACE. The oral dosage of quinapril ranges from 5-80 mg daily (single or divided dose).

Ramipril (ALTACE, others). Cleavage of the ester moiety by hepatic esterases transforms ramipril into ramiprilat, an ACE inhibitor that *in vitro* is about as potent as benazeprilat and quinaprilat. Ramipril is absorbed rapidly (peak concentrations are achieved in 1 hour), and the rate but not extent of its oral absorption (50-60%) is reduced by food. Ramipril is metabolized to ramiprilat and to inactive metabolites (glucuronides of ramipril and ramiprilat and the diketopiperazine ester and acid) that are excreted predominantly by the kidneys. Peak concentrations of ramiprilat in plasma are achieved in ~3 hours. Ramiprilat displays triphasic elimination kinetics with half-lives of 2-4 hours, 9-18 hours, and >50 hours. This triphasic elimination is due to extensive distribution to all tissues (initial $t_{1/2}$), clearance of free ramiprilat from plasma (intermediate $t_{1/2}$), and dissociation of ramiprilat from tissue ACE (long terminal $t_{1/2}$). The oral dosage of ramipril ranges from 1.25-20 mg daily (single or divided dose).

Moexipril (UNIVASC, others). Moexipril is another prodrug whose antihypertensive activity is almost entirely due to its deesterified effective. Once ACE inhibitors are stopped, the cough disappears, usually within 4 days.

Hyperkalemia. Significant K^+ retention is rarely encountered in patients with normal renal function. However, ACE inhibitors may cause hyperkalemia in patients with renal insufficiency or diabetes or in patients taking K^+-sparing diuretics, K^+ supplements, β receptor blockers, or NSAIDs.

Acute Renal Failure. AngII, by constricting the efferent arteriole, helps to maintain adequate glomerular filtration when renal perfusion pressure is low. Inhibition of ACE can induce acute renal insufficiency in patients with bilateral renal artery stenosis, stenosis of the artery to a single remaining kidney, heart failure, or volume depletion owing to diarrhea or diuretics.

Fetopathic Potential. The fetopathic effects may be due in part to fetal hypotension. Once pregnancy is diagnosed, it is imperative that ACE inhibitors be discontinued as soon as possible.

Skin Rash. ACE inhibitors occasionally cause a maculopapular rash that may itch, but that may resolve spontaneously or with antihistamines. Although initially attributed to the presence of the sulfhydryl group in captopril, a rash also may occur with other ACE inhibitors, albeit less frequently.

Angioedema. In 0.1-0.5% of patients, ACE inhibitors induce a rapid swelling in the nose, throat, mouth, glottis, larynx, lips, and/or tongue. Once ACE inhibitors are stopped, angioedema disappears within hours; meanwhile, the patient's airway should be protected, and if necessary, epinephrine, an antihistamine, and/or a glucocorticoid should be administered. African-Americans have a 4.5 times greater risk of ACE inhibitor–induced angioedema than Caucasians (Brown et al., 1996). Although rare, angioedema of the intestine (visceral angioedema) characterized by emesis, watery diarrhea, and abdominal pain also has been reported.

Other Side Effects. Extremely rare but reversible side effects include *dysgeusia* (an alteration in or loss of taste), *neutropenia* (symptoms include sore throat and fever), *glycosuria* (spillage of glucose into the urine in the absence of hyperglycemia), and *hepatotoxicity.*

Drug Interactions. Antacids may reduce the bioavailability of ACE inhibitors; capsaicin may worsen ACE inhibitor–induced cough; NSAIDs, including aspirin, may reduce the antihypertensive response to ACE inhibitors; and K^+-sparing diuretics and K^+ supplements may exacerbate ACE inhibitor–induced hyperkalemia. ACE inhibitors may increase plasma levels of digoxin and lithium and may increase hypersensitivity reactions to allopurinol.

NON-PEPTIDE ANGIOTENSIN II RECEPTOR ANTAGONISTS

History. Attempts to develop therapeutically useful AngII receptor antagonists date to the early 1970s, and these initial endeavors concentrated on angiotensin peptide analog. Saralasin, 1-sarcosine, 8-isoleucine AngII, and other 8-substituted angiotensins were potent AngII receptor antagonists but were of no clinical value because of lack of oral bioavailability and unacceptable partial agonist activity.

A breakthrough came in the early 1980s with the synthesis and testing of a series of imidazole-5-acetic acid derivatives that attenuated pressor responses to AngII in rats. Two compounds, S-8307 and S-8308, were found to be highly specific, albeit very weak, non-peptide AngII receptor antagonists that were devoid of partial agonist activity. Through a series of stepwise modifications, the orally active, potent, and selective non-peptide AT_1 receptor antagonist losartan was developed (Timmermans et al., 1993) and approved for clinical use in the U.S. in 1995. Since then, six additional AT_1 receptor antagonists (Figure 26–10) have been approved. Although these AT_1 receptor antagonists are devoid of partial agonist activity, structural modifications as minor as a methyl group can transform a potent antagonist into an agonist (Perlman et al., 1997).

Pharmacological Effects. The AngII receptor blockers bind to the AT_1 receptor with high affinity and are more than 10,000-fold selective for the AT_1 receptor over the AT_2 receptor. The rank-order affinity of the AT_1 receptor for ARBs is candesartan = olmesartan > irbesartan = eprosartan > telmisartan = valsartan = EXP 3174 (the active metabolite of losartan) > losartan. Although binding of ARBs to the AT_1 receptor is competitive, the inhibition by ARBs of biological responses to AngII often is insurmountable (the maximal response to AngII cannot be restored in the presence of the ARB regardless of the concentration of AngII added to the experimental preparation).

The mechanism of insurmountable antagonism by ARBs may be due to slow dissociation kinetics of the compounds from the AT_1 receptor; however, a number of other factors may contribute, such as ARB-induced receptor internalization and alternative binding sites for ARBs on the AT_1 receptor (McConnaughey et al., 1999). Insurmountable antagonism has the theoretical advantage of sustained receptor blockade even with increased levels of endogenous ligand and with missed doses of drug. Whether this advantage translates into an enhanced clinical performance remains to be determined.

ARBs potently and selectively inhibit most of the biological effects of AngII (Timmermans et al., 1993; Csajka et al., 1997), including AngII–induced (1) contraction of vascular smooth muscle, (2) rapid pressor responses, (3) slow pressor responses, (4) thirst, (5) vasopressin release, (6) aldosterone secretion, (7) release of adrenal catecholamines, (8) enhancement of noradrenergic neurotransmission, (9) increases in sympathetic tone, (10) changes in renal function, and (11) cellular hypertrophy and hyperplasia. ARBs reduce arterial blood pressure in animals with renovascular and genetic hypertension, as well as in transgenic animals overexpressing the renin gene. ARBs, however, have little effect on arterial blood pressure in animals with low-renin hypertension (e.g., rats with hypertension induced by NaCl and deoxycorticosterone).

Do ARBs have therapeutic efficacy equivalent to that of ACE inhibitors? Although both classes of drugs block the RAS, they differ in several important aspects:

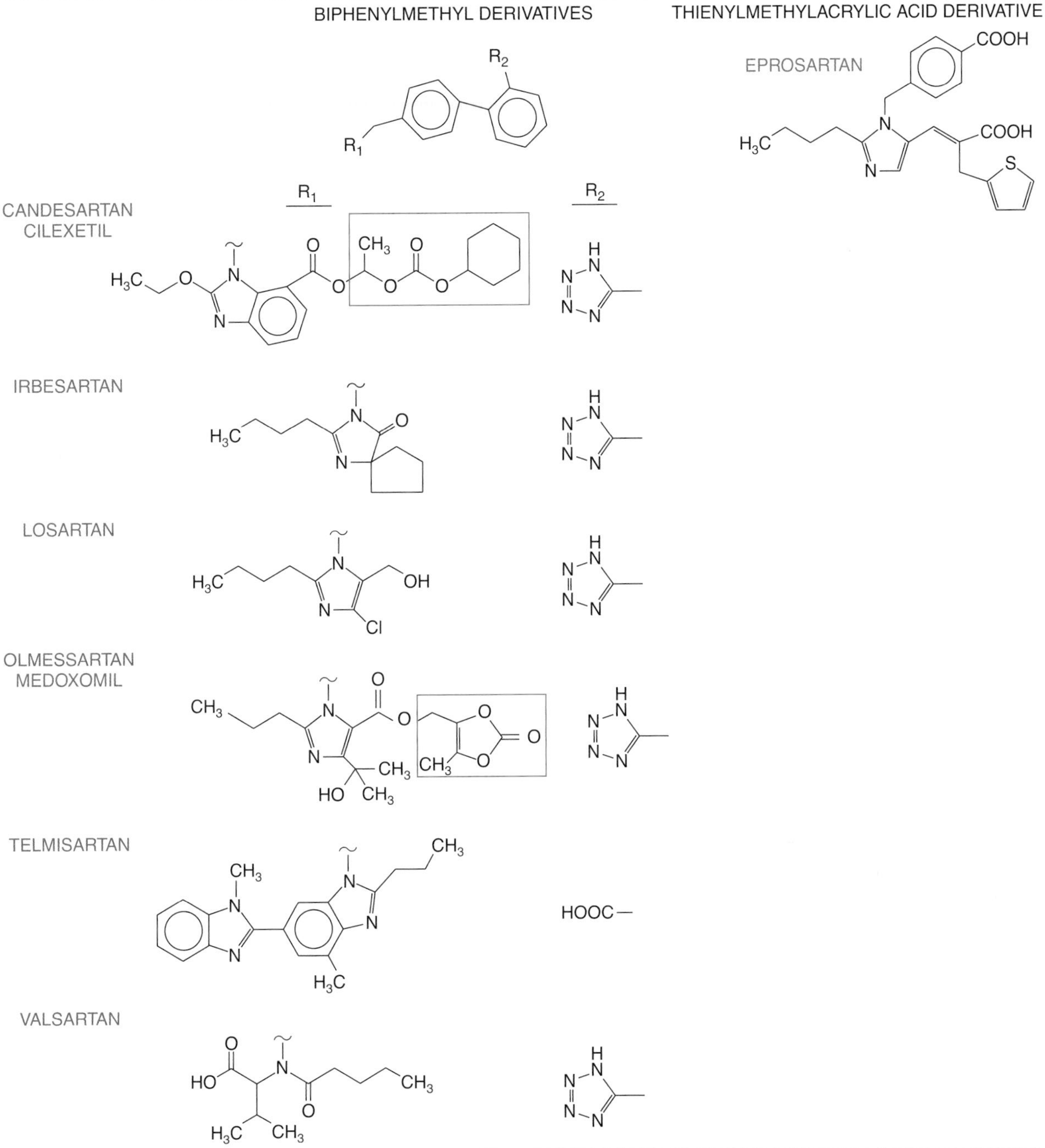

Figure 26–10. ***AngII receptor antagonists.*** Structures within red boxes are removed by esterases and replaced with a hydrogen atom to form the active molecule *in vivo*. "~" indicates point of attachment to biphenyl core.

- *ARBs reduce activation of AT_1 receptors more effectively than do ACE inhibitors.* ACE inhibitors reduce the biosynthesis of AngII by the action of ACE, but do not inhibit alternative non-ACE AngII-generating pathways. ARBs block the actions of AngII via the AT_1 receptor regardless of the biochemical pathway leading to AngII formation.

- In contrast to ACE inhibitors, *ARBs permit activation of AT_2 receptors.* ACE inhibitors increase renin release, but block the conversion of AngI to AngII. ARBs also stimulate renin release; however, with ARBs, this translates into a several-fold increase in circulating levels of AngII. Because ARBs block AT_1 receptors, this increased level of AngII is available to activate AT_2 receptors.

(75-300 mg) reductions in blood pressure. Aliskiren is as effective as ACE inhibitors (ramipril), ARBs (losartan, irbesartan, valsartan), and hydrochlorothiazide (HCTZ) in lowering blood pressure in patients with mild-to-moderate hypertension (Oparil et al., 2007; Sanoski, 2009). Aliskiren also is as effective as lisinopril in lowering blood pressure in patients with severe hypertension (Strasser et al., 2007). The long $t_{1/2}$ of aliskiren allows its antihypertensive effects to be sustained for several days following termination of therapy (Oh et al., 2007).

Many short-term studies indicate that the effect of aliskiren in combination with ACE inhibitors, ARBs, and HCTZ is additive in lowering blood pressure. The antihypertensive effects of aliskiren in monotherapy and in combination therapy were evaluated in patients with mild-to-moderate hypertension. In these studies, supplementing aliskiren to ramipril, irbesartan, valsartan, or HCTZ induced additional decreases in systolic and diastolic blood pressure that were larger than that induced by any of the drugs alone. PRA is inhibited by aliskiren but significantly elevated with ramipril, irbesartan, and HCTZ (Table 26-1). Co-administration of aliskiren with ramipril, irbesartan, or HCTZ neutralized the increase in plasma renin activity to baseline levels (Staessen, 2006; Sanoski, 2009). Because plasma renin levels correlate with the capacity to generate AngII, the ability of aliskiren to neutralize plasma renin in combination therapy may contribute to better control of blood pressure than monotherapy.

The antihypertensive effect of aliskiren is significantly augmented in combination with HCTZ (Oparil et al., 2007). Fixed-dose combinations of aliskiren/HCTZ are marketed for antihypertensive therapy (Baldwin and Plosker, 2009).

Therapeutic Uses of Aliskiren in End-Organ Damage. The ability of aliskiren to inhibit the increased PRA caused by ACE inhibitors and ARBs theoretically provides a more comprehensive blockade of the RAS and may limit activation of the local (tissue) RAS (Table 26-1). Studies are ongoing to address whether aliskiren provides better protection against end-organ damage in cardiovascular and renal diseases.

The ALLAY trial (Aliskiren in Left Ventricular Hypertrophy trial) compared the effect of aliskiren with losartan on left ventricular hypertrophy as a marker of end-organ damage. Both aliskiren and losartan were equivalent in reducing blood pressure and decreasing left ventricular mass, but there was no additional reduction in left ventricular mass with combination therapy (Solomon et al., 2009).

The ALOFT trial (Aliskiren Observation of Heart Failure Treatment) indicated that aliskiren was beneficial when added to ACE inhibitors in heart failure treatment (McMurray et al., 2008). Patients received aliskiren or placebo in addition to standard heart failure treatment (ACE inhibitors, ARBs, β blockers), and the primary outcome measured was changes in N-terminal proB type natriuretic peptide (BNP). Aliskiren caused a significant decrease in plasma BNP levels, urinary BNP, and aldosterone levels, indicating favorable neurohormonal effects of aliskiren in heart failure when added to standard therapy. A follow-up SPHERE trial (Aliskiren Trial to Mediate Outcome Prevention in Heart Failure) will address long-term outcome in heart failure patients.

The AVOID trial (Aliskiren in Evaluation of Proteinuria I Diabetes Trial) reported aliskiren to be renoprotective in patients with hypertension and type 2 diabetes. Patients were on the maximal dose of losartan for 3 months before adding aliskiren or placebo for 6 months. At the end of the study period, patients taking aliskiren had their mean urinary albumin-to-creatinine ratio significantly decreased by 20%, and the decrease was 50% or more in 24.7% of patients compared with placebo. The renoprotective effects of aliskiren were independent of blood pressure–lowering effects

Table 26–1

Effects of Anti-hypertensive Agents on Components of the RAS

	DIRECT RENIN INHIBITORS	ACE-INHIBITORS	ARBs	DIURETICS	Ca^{2+} CHANNEL BLOCKERS	β BLOCKERS
PRC	↑	↑	↑	↑	↔	↓
PRA	↓	↑	↑	↑	↔	↓
Ang I	↓	↑	↑	↑	↔	↓
Ang II	↓	↓	↑	↑	↔	↓
ACE	↔	↓	↔			
Bradykinin	↔	↑	↔			
AT_1 receptors	↔	↔	inhibition			
AT_2 receptors	↔	↔	stimulation			

PRC, plasma renin concentration; PRA, plasma renin activity; ACE, angiotensin converting enzyme; ARB, angiotensin receptor blocker.

(Parving et al., 2008). The long-term ALTITUDE study (Aliskiren Trial in Type 2 Diabetes Using Cardio-Renal Endpoints) is in progress to assess if aliskiren will reduce cardiovascular and renal morbidity and mortality when added to ACE inhibitors and ARBs. The study is expected to end in 2011 (Parving et al., 2009).

Aliskiren is an effective antihypertensive agent that is well tolerated in monotherapy and combination therapy. It has cardioprotective and renoprotective effects in combination therapy; however, long-term advantages still need to be established. Aliskiren is recommended in patients who are intolerant to other antihypertensive therapies or for use in combination with other drugs for further blood pressure control.

Adverse Events. Aliskiren is well tolerated, and adverse events are mild or comparable to placebo with no gender difference. Adverse effects include mild gastrointestinal symptoms such as diarrhea observed at high doses (600 mg daily), abdominal pain, dyspepsia, and gastroesophageal reflux; headache; nasopharyngitis; dizziness; fatigue; upper-respiratory tract infection; back pain; angiodema; and cough (cough was much less common than with ACE inhibitors). Other adverse effects reported for aliskiren that were slightly increased compared with placebo include rash, hypotension, hyperkalemia in diabetics on combination therapy, elevated uric acid, renal stones, and gout. Like other RAS inhibitors, aliskiren is not recommended in pregnancy.

Drug Interactions. Aliskiren does not interact with drugs that interact with CYPs. Aliskiren reduces absorption of furosemide by 50%. Irbesartan reduces the C_{max} of aliskiren by 50%. Aliskiren plasma levels are increased by drugs, such as ketoconazole, atorvastatin, and cyclosporine, that inhibit P-glycoprotein.

Pharmacological Lowering of Blood Pressures Alters Components of the RAS

The renin-angiotensin system responds to alterations in blood pressure with compensatory changes (Figure 26-2). Thus, pharmacological agents that lower blood pressure will alter the feedback loops that regulate the RAS and cause changes in the levels and activities of the system's components. These changes are summarized in Table 26-1.

BIBLIOGRAPHY

Abadir PM, Periasamy A, Carey RM, et al. Angiotensin II type 2 receptor-bradykinin B2 receptor functional heterodimerization. *Hypertension,* **2006**, *48:*316–322.

AbdAlla S, Lother H, Abdel-tawab AM, Quitterer U. The angiotensin II AT_2 receptor is an AT_1 receptor antagonist. *J Biol Chem,* **2001**, *276:*39721–39726.

AbdAlla S, Lother H, El Massiery A, Quitterer U. Increased AT_1 receptor heterodimers in preeclampsia mediate enhanced angiotensin II responsiveness. *Nature Med,* **2002**, *7:* 1003–1009.

ACE Inhibitor Myocardial Infarction Collaborative Group. Indications for ACE inhibitors in the early treatment of acute myocardial infarction: Systematic overview of individual data from 100,000 patients in randomized trials. *Circulation,* **1998**, *97:*2202–2212.

Albiston AL, Peck GR, Yeatman HR, et al. Therapeutic targeting of insulin-regulated aminopeptidase: Heads and tails? *Pharmacol Ther,* **2007**, *116:*417–427.

Álvarez R, Reguero JR, Batalla A, et al. Angiotensin-converting enzyme and angiotensin II receptor 1 polymorphisms: Association with early coronary disease. *Cardiovasc Res,* **1998**, *40:*375–379.

Baldwin CM, Plosker GL. Aliskiren/hydrochlorothiazide combination: In mild to moderate hypertension. *Drugs,* **2009**, *69:* 833–841.

Batenburg W, Danser AJ. Prorenin and the (pro)renin receptor: Binding kinetics, signalling and interaction with aliskiren. *J Renin Angiotensin Aldosterone Syst,* **2008**, *9:*181–184.

Bautista R, Manning R, Martinez F, et al. Antiotensin II–dependent increased expression of Na^+–glucose cotransporter in hypertension. *Am J Physiol Renal Physiol,* **2004**, *286:*F127–F133.

Borghi C, Bacchelli S, Esposti DD, et al. Effects of the administration of an angiotensin-converting enzyme inhibitor during the acute phase of myocardial infarction in patients with arterial hypertension. SMILE Study Investigators. Survival of Myocardial Infarction Long-Term Evaluation. *Am J Hypertens,* **1999**, *12:*665–672.

Brenner BM, Zagrobelny J. Clinical renoprotection trials involving angiotensin II–receptor antagonists and angiotensin-converting-enzyme inhibitors. *Kidney Int,* **2003**, *63*(suppl)*:* S77–S85.

Brink M, Wellen J, Delafontaine P. Angiotensin II causes weight loss and decreases circulating insulin-like growth factor I in rats through a pressor-independent mechanism. *J Clin Invest,* **1996**, *97:*2509–2516.

Brown NJ, Ray WA, Snowden M, Griffin MR. Black Americans have an increased rate of angiotensin converting enzyme inhibitor–associated angioedema. *Clin Pharmacol Ther,* **1996**, *60:*8–13.

Carey RM, Howell NL, Jin X-H, Siragy HM. Angiotensin type 2 receptor–mediated hypotension in angiotensin type 1 receptor–blocked rats. *Hypertension,* **2001**, *38:*1272–1277.

Castrop H, Hocherl K, Kurtz A, et al. Physiology of Kidney Renin. *Physiol Rev,* **2010**, *90:*607–673.

Célérier J, Cruz A, Lamandé N, et al. Angiotensin and its cleaved derivatives inhibit angiogenesis. *Hypertension,* **2002**, *39:* 224–228.

Chai SY, Fernando R, Peck G, et al. The angiotensinIV/AT_4 receptor. *Cell Mol Life Sci,* **2004**, *6:*2728–2737.

Cohn JN, Tognoni G. A randomized trial of the angiotensin-receptor blocker valsartan in chronic heart failure. *N Engl J Med,* **2001**, *345:*1667–1675.

Crackower MA, Sarao R, Oudit GY, et al. Angiotensin-converting enzyme 2 is an essential regulator of heart function. *Nature,* **2002**, *417:*822–828.

Csajka, C, Buclin T, Brunner HR, Biollaz J. Pharmacokinetic–pharmacodynamic profile of angiotensin II receptor antagonists. *Clin Pharmacokinet,* **1997**, *32:*1–29.

Dahlöf B, Devereux RB, Kjeldsen SE, et al., for the LIFE Study Group. Cardiovascular morbidity and mortality in the Losartan Intervention For Endpoint reduction in hypertension study

(LIFE): A randomized trial against atenolol. *Lancet*, **2002**, *359*:995–1003.

D'Amore A, Black MJ, Thomas WG. The angiotensin II type 2 receptor causes constitutive growth of cardiomyocytes and does not antagonize angiotensin II type 1 receptor-mediated hypertrophy. *Hypertension,* **2005**, *46:*1347–1354.

Danser AH, Deinum J. Renin, prorenin and the putative (pro)renin receptor. *Hypertension,* **2005**, *46:*1069–1076.

Danser AH, van Kats JP, Admiraal PJ, et al. Cardiac renin and angiotensins: Uptake from plasma versus *in situ* synthesis. *Hypertension*, **1994**, *24:*37–48.

de Gasparo M, Catt KJ, Inagami T, et al. International union of pharmacology: XXIII. The angiotensin II receptors. *Pharmacol Rev*, **2000**, *52:*415–472.

Donoghue M, Hsieh F, Baronas E, et al. A novel angiotensin-converting enzyme–related carboxypeptidase (ACE2) converts angiotensin I to angiotensin(1–9). *Circ Res*, **2000**, *87:*E1–E9.

Epperson S, Gustafsson AB, Gonzalez AM, et al. Pharmacology of G-protein-linked signaling in cardiac fibroblasts. In: Villarreal FJ, ed. *Interstitial Fibrosis and Heart Failure*. Springer, New York, **2004**, pp. 83–97.

EURopean trial On reduction of cardiac events with Perindopril in stable coronary Artery disease (EUROPA) Investigators. Efficacy of perindopril in reduction of cardiovascular events among patients with stable coronary artery disease: Randomised, double-blind, placebo-controlled, multicentre trial (the EUROPA study). *Lancet*, **2003**, *362:*782–788.

Ferrario CM, Chappell MC, Tallant EA, et al. Counterregulatory actions of angiotensin-(1–7). *Hypertension*, **1997**, *30:*535–541.

Granger CB, McMurray JJ, Yusuf S, et al., for the CHARM Investigators and Committees. Effects of candesartan in patients with chronic heart failure and reduced left-ventricular systolic function intolerant to angiotensin-converting-enzyme inhibitors: The CHARM-alternative trial. *Lancet*, **2003**, *362:*772–776.

Hadjadj S, Belloum R, Bouhanick B, et al. Prognostic value of angiotensin-I converting enzyme *I/D* polymorphism for nephropathy in type 1 diabetes mellitus: A prospective study. *J Am Soc Nephrol*, **2001**, *12*:541–549.

Hansen PB, Hashimoto S, Briggs J, Schnermann J. Attenuated renovascular constrictor responses to angiotensin II in adenosine 1 receptor knockout mice. *Am J Physiol Regul Integr Comp Physiol*, **2003**, *285:*R44–R49.

Heart Outcomes Prevention Study Investigators. Effects of an angiotensin-converting-enzyme inhibitor ramipril on cardiovascular events in high-risk patients. The Heart Outcomes Prevention Evaluation Study Investigators. *New Engl J Med*, **2000**, *342*:145–153 (published erratum appears in *New Engl J Med*, **2000**, *342:*478).

Higuchi S, Ohtsu H, Suzuki H, et al. Angiotensin II signal transduction through the AT1 receptor: Novel insights into mechanisms and pathophysiology. *Clin Sci*, **2007**, *112:*417–428.

Huentelman MJ, Grobe JL, Vazquez J, et al. Protection from angiotensin II-induced cardiac hypertrophy and fibrosis by systemic lentiviral delivery of ACE2 in rats. *Exp Physiol*, **2005**, *90:*783–790.

Ichihara S, Senbonmatsu T, Price E Jr, et al. Angiotensin II type 2 receptor is essential for left ventricular hypertrophy and cardiac fibrosis in chronic angiotensin II–induced hypertension. *Circulation*, **2001**, *104:*346–351.

Jones E, Vinh A, McCarthy CA, et al. AT2 receptors: Functional relevance in cardiovascular disease. *Pharmacol Ther,* **2008**, *120:*292–316.

Kaneshiro Y, Ichihara A, Sakoda M, et al. Slowly progressive, angiotensin II-independent glomerulosclerosis in human (pro)renin receptor-transgenic rats. *J Am Soc Nephrol,* **2007**, *18*:1789–1795.

Kaneshiro Y, Ichihara A, Takemitsu T, et al. Increased expression of cyclooxygenase-2 in the renal cortex of human prorenin receptor gene-transgenic rats. *Kidney Int,* **2006**,*70:*641–646.

Krämer C, Sunkomat J, Witte J, et al. Angiotensin II receptor-independent antiinflammatory and angiaggregatory properties of losartan: Role of the active metabolite EXP3179. *Circ Res*, **2002**, *90*:770–776.

Lage SG, Kopel L, Medeiros CCJ, et al. Angiotensin II contributes to arterial compliance in congestive heart failure. *Am J Physiol Heart Circ Physiol*, **2002**, *283:*H1424–H1429.

Lang RM, Elkayam U, Yellen LG, et al. Comparative effects of losartan and enalapril on exercise capacity and clinical status in patients with heart failure. The Losartan Pilot Exercise Study Investigators. *J Am Coll Cardiol*, **1997**, *30*: 983–991.

Levy PJ, Yunis C, Owen J, et al. Inhibition of platelet aggregability by losartan in essential hypertension. *Am J Cardiol*, **2000**, *86*:1188–1192.

Li W, Moore MJ, Vasilieva N, et al. Angiotensin-converting enzyme 2 is a functional receptor for the SARS coronavirus. *Nature*, **2003**, *426:*450–454.

Madrid AH, Bueno MG, Rebollo JMG, et al. Use of irbesartan to maintain sinus rhythm in patients with long-lasting persistent atrial fibrillation: A prospective and randomized study. *Circulation*, **2002**, *106:*331–336.

Maggioni AP, Anand I, Gottlieb SO, et al., on behalf of the ValHeFT Investigators. Effects of valsartan on morbidity and mortality in patients with heart failure not receiving angiotensin-converting enzyme inhibitors. *J Am Coll Cardiol*, **2002**, *40*:1414–1421.

McConnaughey MM, McConnaughey JS, Ingenito AJ. Practical considerations of the pharmacology of angiotensin receptor blockers. *J Clin Pharmacol*, **1999**, *39:*547–559.

McMurray JJ, Ostergren J, Swedberg K, et al., for the CHARM Investigators and Committees. Effects of candesartan in patients with chronic heart failure and reduced left-ventricular systolic function taking angiotensin-converting-enzyme inhibitors: The CHARM-added trial. *Lancet*, **2003**, *362:* 767–771.

McMurray JJ, Pitt B, Latini R, et al. Effects of the oral direct renin inhibitor aliskiren in patients with symptomatic heart failure. *Circ Heart Fail,* **2008**, *1:*17–24.

Mehta PK, Griendling KK. Angiotensin II cell signaling: Physiological and pathological effects in the cardiovascular system. *Am J Physiol Cell Physiol,* **2007**, 292*:*C82–C97.

Meszaros JG, Gonzalez AM, Endo-Mochizuki Y, et al. Identification of G protein–coupled signaling pathways in cardiac fibro-blasts: Cross-talk between G_q and G_s. *Am J Physiol*, **2000**, *278:*154–162.

Miura S, Karnik SS, Saku K. Constitutively active homo-oligomeric angiotensin II type 2 receptor induces cell signaling independent of receptor conformation and ligand stimulation. *J Biol Chem*, **2005**, *280:*18237–18244.

Nguyen G, Danser AH. Prorenin and (pro)renin receptor: A review of available data from in vitro studies and experimental models in rodents. *Exp Physiol,* **2008**, *93:*557–563.

Niimura F, Labosky PA, Kakuchi J, et al. Gene targeting in mice reveals a requirement for angiotensin in the development and maintenance of kidney morphology and growth factor regulation. *J Clin Invest,* **1995**, *96:*2947–2954.

Nussberger J, Wuerzner G, Jensen C, et al. Angiotensin II suppression in humans by the orally active renin inhibitor Aliskiren (SPP100): Comparison with enalapril. *Hypertension,* **2002**, *39:*E1–E8.

Oh BH, Mitchell J, Herron JR, et al. Aliskiren, an oral renin inhibitor, provides dose-dependent efficacy and sustained 24-hour blood pressure control in patients with hypertension. *J Am Coll Cardiol,* **2007**, *49:*1157–1163.

ONTARGET Investigators. Telmisartan, ramipril, or both in patients at high risk for vascular events. *N Engl J Med,* **2008**, *358:*1547–1559.

Oparil S, Yarows SA, Patel S, et al. Efficacy and safety of combined use of aliskiren and valsartan in patients with hypertension: A randomised, double-blind trial. *Lancet,* **2007**, *370:* 221–229.

Parving HH, Brenner BM, McMurray JJ, et al. Aliskiren Trial in Type 2 Diabetes Using Cardio-Renal Endpoints (ALTITUDE): Rationale and study design. *Nephrol Dial Transplant,* **2009**, *24:*1663–1671.

Parving HH, Persson F, Lewis JB, et al. Aliskiren combined with losartan in type 2 diabetes and nephropathy. *N Engl J Med,* **2008**, *358:*2433–2246.

Paul M, Poyan Mehr A, Kreutz R. Physiology of local renin-angiotensin systems. *Physiol Rev,* **2006**, *86:*747–803.

Perlman S, Costa-Neto CM, Miyakawa AA, et al. Dual agonistic and antagonistic property of nonpeptide angiotensin AT_1 ligands: Susceptibility to receptor mutations. *Mo. Pharmacol,* **1997**, *51:*301–311.

Pfeffer MA, McMurray JJ, Velazquez EJ, et al., for the Valsartan in Acute Myocardial Infarction Trial Investigators. Valsartan, captopril, or both in myocardial infarction complicated by heart failure, left ventricular dysfunction, or both. *New Engl J Med,* **2003**, *349:*1893–1906.

Pilz BE, Shagdarsuren M, Wellner A, et al., Aliskiren, a human renin inhibitor, ameliorates cardiac and renal damage in double-transgenic rats. *Hypertension,* **2005**, *46:*569–576.

Pitt B, Poole-Wilson PA, Segal R, et al., on behalf of the ELITE II investigators. Effect of losartan compared with captopril on mortality in patients with symptomatic heart failure: Randomized trial—the Losartan Heart Failure Survival Study ELITE II. *Lancet,* **2000**, *355:*1582–1587.

Pitt B, Segal R, Martinez FA, et al. Randomised trial of losartan versus captopril in patients over 65 with heart failure (Evaluation of Losartan in the Elderly study, ELITE). *Lancet,* **1997**, *349:*747–752.

Ramser J, Abidi FE, Burckle CA, et al. A unique exonic splice enhancer mutation in a family with X-linked mental retardation and epilepsy points to a novel role of the renin receptor. *Hum Mol Genet,* **2005**, *14:*1019–1027.

Rhaleb N-E, Peng H, Yang X-P, et al. Long-term effect of *N*-acetyl-seryl-aspartyl-lysly-proline on left ventricular collagen deposition in rats with two-kidney, one-clip hypertension. *Circulation,* **2001**, *103:*3136–3141.

Ruggenenti P, Cravedi P, Remuzzi G. The RAAS in the pathogenesis and treatment of diabetic nephropathy. *Nat Rev Nephrol,* **2010**, in press.

Ruiz-Ortega M, Esteban V, Egido J. The regulation of the inflammatory response through nuclear factor-κB pathway by angiotensin IV extends the role of the renin angiotensin system in cardiovascular disease. *Trends Cardiovasc Med,* **2007**, *17:*19–25.

Sanoski CA. Aliskiren: An oral direct renin inhibitor for the treatment of hypertension. *Pharmacotherapy,* **2009**, *29:*193–212.

Santos RA, Ferreira AJ, Simões ESAC. Recent advances in the angiotensin-converting enzyme 2-angiotensin(1-7)-Mas axis. *Exp Physiol,* **2008**, *93:*519–527.

Sayed-Tabatabaei FA, Oostra BA, Isaacs A, et al. *ACE* Polymorphisms. *Circ Res,* **2006**, *98:*1123–1133.

Schmieder RE, Hilgers KF, Schlaich MP, et al. Renin-angiotensin system and cardiovascular risk. *Lancet,* **2007**, *369:*1208–1219.

Schneider AW, Kalk JF, Klein CP. Effect of losartan, an angiotensin II receptor antagonist, on portal pressure in cirrhosis. *Hepatology,* **1999**, *29:*334–339.

Sethi AA, Nordestgaard BG, Gronholdt M-LM, et al. Angiotensinogen single nucleotide polymorphisms, elevated blood pressure, and risk of cardiovascular disease. *Hypertension,* **2003**, *41:*1202–1211.

Solomon SD, Appelbaum E, Manning WJ, et al. Effect of the direct renin inhibitor aliskiren, the angiotensin receptor blocker losartan, or both on left ventricular mass in patients with hypertension and left ventricular hypertrophy. *Circulation,* **2009**, *119:*530–537.

Staessen JA, Li Y, Richart T. Oral renin inhibitors. *Lancet,* **2006**, *368:*1449–1456.

Steen VD, Medsger TA Jr. Long-term outcomes of scleroderma renal crisis. *Ann Intern Med,* **2000**, *17:*600–603.

Strasser RH, Puig JG, Farsang C, et al. A comparison of the tolerability of the direct renin inhibitor aliskiren and lisinopril in patients with severe hypertension. *J Hum Hypertens,* **2007**, *21:*780–787.

Testa MA, Anderson RB, Nackley JF, et al. Quality of life and anti-hypertensive therapy in men: A comparison of captopril with enalapril. *New Engl J Med,* **1993**, *328:*907–913.

Timmermans PBMWM, Wong PC, Chiu AT, et al. Angiotensin II receptors and angiotensin II receptor antagonists. *Pharmacol Rev,* **1993**, *45:*205–251.

Tipnis SR, Hooper NM, Hyde R, et al. A human homolog of angiotensin-converting enzyme: Cloning and functional expression as a captopril-insensitive carboxypeptidase. *J Biol Chem,* **2000**, *275:*33238–33243.

Vaidyanathan S, Jarugula V, Dieterich HA, et al. Clinical pharmacokinetics and pharmacodynamics of aliskiren. *Clin Pharmacokinet,* **2008**, *47:*515–531.

Vane JR. The history of inhibitors of angiotensin converting enzyme. *J Physiol Pharmacol,* **1999**, *50:*489–498.

Varagic J, Trask AJ, Jessup JA, et al. New angiotensins. *J Mol Med,* **2008**, *86:*663–671.

Viberti G, Wheeldon NM, for the MicroAlbuminuria Reduction with VALsartan (MARVAL) study investigators. Microalbuminuria reduction with valsartan in patients with type 2 diabetes mellitus: A blood pressure–independent effect. *Circulation,* **2002**, *106:*672–678.

Wallukat G, Homuth V, Fischer T, et al. Patients with preeclampsia develop agonistic autoantibodies against the angiotensin AT_1 receptor. *J Clin Invest*, **1999**, *103:*945–952.

Wang J-L, Cheng H-F, Harris RC. Cyclooxygenase-2 inhibition decreases renin content and lowers blood pressure in a model of renovascular hypertension. *Hypertension*, **1999**, *34:*96–101.

Weiss D, Kools JJ, Taylor WR. Angiotensin II–induced hypertension accelerates the development of atherosclerosis in ApoE-deficient mice. *Circulation*, **2001**, *103:*448–454.

Wood JM, Maibaum J, Rahuel J, et al. Structure-based design of aliskiren, a novel orally effective renin inhibitor. *Biochem Biophys Res Commun*, **2003**, *308:*698–705.

Wood JM, Schnell CR, Cumin F, et al. Aliskiren, a novel, orally effective renin inhibitor, lowers blood pressure in marmosets and spontaneously hypertensive rats. *J Hypertens*, **2005**, *23:*417–426.

Zimmerman BG. Absence of adrenergic mediation of agonist response to [Sar^1,Ala^8]angiotensin II in conscious normotensive and hypertensive dogs. *Clin Sci*, **1979**, *57:*71–81.

Zuanetti G, Latini R, Maggioni AP, et al. Effect of the ACE inhibitor lisinopril on mortality in diabetic patients with acute myocardial infarction: Data from the GISSI-3 study. *Circulation*, **1997**, *96:*4239–4245.

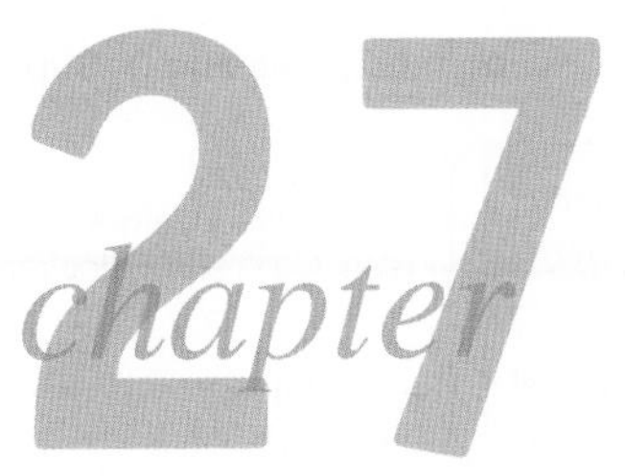

Treatment of Myocardial Ischemia and Hypertension

Thomas Michel and
Brian B. Hoffman

PATHOPHYSIOLOGY OF ISCHEMIC HEART DISEASE

Angina pectoris, the primary symptom of ischemic heart disease, is caused by transient episodes of myocardial ischemia that are due to an imbalance in the myocardial oxygen supply–demand relationship. This imbalance may be caused by an increase in myocardial oxygen demand (which is determined by heart rate, ventricular contractility, and ventricular wall tension) or by a decrease in myocardial oxygen supply (primarily determined by coronary blood flow, but occasionally modified by the oxygen-carrying capacity of the blood) or sometimes by both (Figure 27–1). Because blood flow is inversely proportional to the fourth power of the artery's luminal radius, the progressive decrease in vessel radius that characterizes coronary atherosclerosis can impair coronary blood flow and lead to symptoms of angina when myocardial O_2 demand increases, as with exertion (so-called typical angina pectoris). In some patients, anginal symptoms may occur without any increase in myocardial O_2 demand, but rather as a consequence of an abrupt reduction in blood flow, as might result from coronary thrombosis (unstable angina) or localized vasospasm (variant or Prinzmetal angina). Regardless of the precipitating factors, the sensation of angina is similar in most patients. Typical angina is experienced as a heavy, pressing substernal discomfort (rarely described as a "pain"), often radiating to the left shoulder, flexor aspect of the left arm, jaw, or epigastrium. However, a significant minority of patients note discomfort in a different location or of a different character. Women, the elderly, and diabetics are more likely to experience myocardial ischemia with atypical symptoms. In most patients with typical angina, whose symptoms are provoked by exertion, the symptoms are relieved by rest or by administration of sublingual nitroglycerin.

Angina pectoris is a common symptom, affecting more than 9 million Americans (Rosamond et al., 2008). Angina pectoris may occur in a stable pattern over many years or may become unstable, increasing in frequency or severity and even occurring at rest. In typical stable angina, the pathological substrate is usually fixed atherosclerotic narrowing of an epicardial coronary artery, on which exertion or emotional stress superimposes an increase in myocardial O_2 demand. In variant angina, focal or diffuse coronary vasospasm episodically reduces coronary flow. Patients also may display a mixed pattern of angina with the addition of altered vessel tone on a background of atherosclerotic narrowing. In most patients with unstable angina, rupture of an atherosclerotic plaque, with consequent platelet adhesion and aggregation, decreases coronary blood flow. Superimposed thrombosis may lead to the complete abrogation of blood flow. Atherosclerotic plaques with thinner fibrous caps appear to be more "vulnerable" to rupture.

Myocardial ischemia also may be *silent*, with electrocardiographic, echocardiographic, or radionuclide evidence of ischemia appearing in the absence of symptoms. While some patients have only silent ischemia, most patients who have silent ischemia have symptomatic episodes as well. The precipitants of silent ischemia appear to be the same as those of symptomatic ischemia. We now know that the *ischemic burden* (i.e., the total time a patient is ischemic each day) is greater in many patients than was recognized previously. In most trials, the agents that are efficacious in typical angina also are efficacious in reducing silent ischemia. β Adrenergic

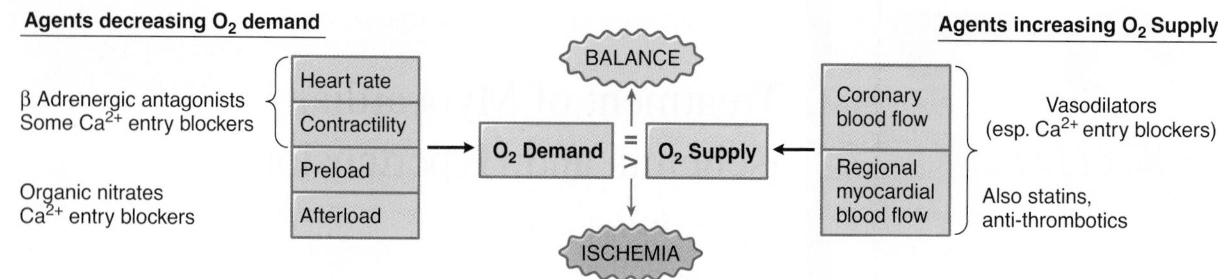

Figure 27–1. *Pharmacological modification of the major determinants of myocardial O_2 supply.* When myocardial O_2 requirements exceed O_2 supply, an ischemic episode results. This figure shows the primary hemodynamic sites of actions of pharmacological agents that can reduce O_2 demand (*left side*) or enhance O_2 supply (*right side*). Some classes of agents have multiple effects. Stents, angioplasty, and coronary bypass surgery are mechanical interventions that increase O_2 supply. Both pharmacotherapy and mechanotherapy attempt to restore a dynamic balance between O_2 demand and O_2 supply.

receptor antagonists appear to be more effective than the Ca^{2+} channel blockers in the prevention of episodes. Therapy directed at abolishing all silent ischemia has not been shown to be of additional benefit over conventional therapy.

This section describes the principal pharmacological agents used in the treatment of angina. The major drugs are nitrovasodilators, *β* adrenergic receptor antagonists (see Chapter 12), and Ca^{2+} channel antagonists. These anti-anginal agents improve the balance of myocardial O_2 supply and O_2 demand, increasing supply by dilating the coronary vasculature and/or decreasing demand by reducing cardiac work (Figure 27–1).

Other drugs also have efficacy in treatment of both stable and unstable angina, including antiplatelet agents (see Chapters 30) as well as statins (HMG CoA-reductase inhibitors) (see Chapter 31), which may have a role in stabilizing the vulnerable plaque. A new class of medications that appears to be effective in treatment of angina is exemplified by ranolazine (RANEXA) (Wilson et al., 2009), which has been approved for treatment of chronic angina. The mechanisms whereby ranolazine exerts its anti-anginal effect are incompletely understood, but the drug appears to exert direct effects on cardiac myocyte Na^+ channels (Hasenfuss and Maier 2008; Nash and Nash 2008).

Increasing the cardiac extraction of O_2 from the blood has not been a practical therapeutic goal. Drugs used in typical angina function principally by reducing myocardial O_2 demand by decreasing heart rate, myocardial contractility, and/or ventricular wall stress. By contrast, the principal therapeutic goal in unstable angina is to increase myocardial blood flow; strategies include the use of antiplatelet agents and *heparin* to reduce intracoronary thrombosis, often accompanied by efforts to restore flow by mechanical means, including percutaneous coronary interventions using coronary stents, or (less commonly) emergency coronary bypass surgery. The principal therapeutic aim in variant or Prinzmetal angina is to prevent coronary vasospasm.

Anti-anginal agents may provide prophylactic or symptomatic treatment, but *β* adrenergic receptor antagonists also reduce mortality apparently by decreasing the incidence of sudden cardiac death associated with myocardial ischemia and infarction. The chronic use of organic nitrate vasodilators, which are highly efficacious in treatment of angina, is not associated with improvements in cardiac mortality, and some investigators have suggested that chronic use of nitroglycerin may have adverse cardiovascular effects (Parker, 2004). It is unclear whether the new anti-anginal agent ranolazine may have beneficial effects on cardiovascular mortality, but this drug does appear to have salutary effects on glucose metabolism (Morrow et al., 2009).

The treatment of cardiac risk factors can reduce the progression or even lead to the regression of atherosclerosis. *Aspirin* is used routinely in patients with myocardial ischemia, and daily aspirin use reduces the incidence of clinical events (Gibbons et al., 2003). Other antiplatelet agents such as oral clopidogrel and intravenous anti-integrin drugs such as abciximab, tirofiban, and eptifibatide have been shown to reduce morbidity in patients with angina who undergo coronary artery stenting (Yeghizarians et al., 2000). Lipid-lowering drugs such as the statins reduce mortality in patients with hypercholesterolemia with or without known coronary artery disease (Libby et al., 2002). Angiotensin-converting enzyme

(ACE) inhibitors (see Chapter 26) also reduce mortality in patients with coronary disease (Yusuf et al., 2000) and are particularly recommended for patients when there is concomitant impairment of cardiac systolic function (Gibbons et al., 2003).

Coronary artery bypass surgery and percutaneous coronary interventions such as angioplasty and coronary artery stent deployment can complement pharmacological treatment. In some subsets of patients, percutaneous or surgical revascularization may have a survival advantage over medical treatment alone. Intracoronary drug delivery using drug-eluting coronary stents represents an intersection of mechanical and pharmacological approaches in the treatment of coronary artery disease. Novel therapies that modify the expression of vascular or myocardial cell genes eventually may become an important part of the therapy of ischemic heart disease.

ORGANIC NITRATES

These agents are prodrugs that are sources of nitric oxide (NO). NO activates the soluble isoform of guanylyl cyclase, thereby increasing intracellular levels of cyclic GMP. In turn, cyclic GMP promotes the dephosphorylation of the myosin light chain and the reduction of cystolic Ca^{2+} and leads to the relaxation of smooth muscle cells in a broad range of tissues. The NO-dependent relaxation of vascular smooth muscle leads to vasodilation; NO-mediated guanylyl cyclase activation inhibits platelet aggregation and relaxes smooth muscle in the bronchi and GI tract (Murad, 1996).

The broad biological response to nitrovasodilators reflects the existence of endogenous NO-modulated regulatory pathways. The endogenous synthesis of NO in humans is catalyzed by a family of NO synthases that oxidize the amino acid L-arginine to form NO, plus L-citrulline as a co-product. There are three distinct mammalian NO synthase isoforms termed *nNOS*, *eNOS*, and *iNOS* (see Chapter 3), and they are involved in processes as diverse as neurotransmission, vasomotion, and immunomodulation. In several vascular disease states, pathways of endogenous NO-dependent regulation appear to be deranged (reviewed in Dudzinski et al., 2006).

History. Nitroglycerin was first synthesized in 1846 by Sobrero, who observed that a small quantity placed on the tongue elicited a severe headache. The explosive properties of nitroglycerin also were soon noted, and control of this unstable compound for military and industrial use was not realized until Alfred Nobel devised a process to stabilize the nitroglycerin and patented a specialized detonator in 1863. The vast fortune that Nobel accrued from the nitroglycerin detonator patent provided the funds later used to establish the Nobel prizes. In 1857, T. Lauder Brunton of Edinburgh administered *amyl nitrite*, a known vasodepressor, by inhalation and noted that anginal pain was relieved within 30- 60 seconds. The action of amyl nitrite was transitory, however, and the dosage was difficult to adjust. Subsequently, William Murrell surmised that the action of nitroglycerin mimicked that of amyl nitrite and established the use of sublingual nitroglycerin for relief of the acute anginal attack and as a prophylactic agent to be taken prior to exertion. The empirical observation that organic nitrates could dramatically and safely alleviate the symptoms of angina pectoris led to their widespread acceptance by the medical profession. Indeed, Alfred Nobel himself was prescribed nitroglycerin by his physicians when he developed angina in 1890. Basic investigations defined the role of NO in both the vasodilation produced by nitrates and endogenous vasodilation. The importance of NO as a signaling molecule in the cardiovascular system and elsewhere was recognized by the awarding of the 1998 Nobel Prize in medicine/physiology to the pharmacologists Robert Furchgott, Louis Ignarro, and Ferid Murad.

Chemistry. Organic nitrates are polyol esters of nitric acid, whereas organic nitrites are esters of nitrous acid (Table 27–1). Nitrate esters ($—C—O—NO_2$) and nitrite esters (—C—O—NO) are characterized by a sequence of carbon–oxygen–nitrogen, whereas nitro compounds possess carbon–nitrogen bonds ($C—NO_2$). Thus glyceryl trinitrate is not a nitro compound, and it is erroneously called nitroglycerin; however, this nomenclature is both widespread and official. Amyl nitrite is a highly volatile liquid that must be administered by inhalation and is of limited therapeutic utility. Organic nitrates of low molecular mass (such as nitroglycerin) are moderately volatile, oily liquids, whereas the high-molecular-mass nitrate esters (e.g., erythrityl tetranitrate, isosorbide dinitrate, and isosorbide mononitrate) are solids. In the pure form (without an inert carrier such as lactose), nitroglycerin is explosive. The organic nitrates and nitrites, collectively termed *nitrovasodilators*, must be metabolized (reduced) to produce gaseous NO, which appears to be the active principle of this class of compounds. Nitric oxide gas also can be directly administered by inhalation (Bloch et al., 2007).

Pharmacological Properties

Mechanism of Action. Nitrites, organic nitrates, nitroso compounds, and a variety of other nitrogen oxide–containing substances (including *nitroprusside;* see later in the chapter) lead to the formation of the reactive gaseous free radical NO and related NO-containing compounds. Nitric oxide gas also may be administered by inhalation. The exact mechanism(s) of denitration of the organic nitrates to liberate NO remains an active area of investigation (Chen et al., 2002).

Phosphorylation of the myosin light chain regulates the maintenance of the contractile state in smooth muscle. NO can activate guanylyl cyclase, increase the cellular level of cyclic GMP, activate PKG, and modulate the activities of cyclic nucleotide phosphodiesterases (PDEs 2, 3, and 5) in a variety of cell types. In smooth muscle, the net result is reduced phosphorylation of myosin light chain, reduced Ca^{2+} concentration in the cytosol, and relaxation. One important

Table 27–1

Organic Nitrates Available for Clinical Use

NONPROPRIETARY NAMES AND TRADE NAMES	CHEMICAL STRUCTURE	PREPARATIONS, USUAL DOSES, AND ROUTES OF ADMINISTRATION[a]
Nitroglycerin (glyceryl trinitrate; NITRO-BID, NITROSTAT, NITROL, NITRO-DUR, others)	$H_2C—O—NO_2$ / $HC—O—NO_2$ / $H_2C—O—NO_2$	T: 0.3-0.6 mg as needed S: 0.4 mg per spray as needed C: 2.5-9 mg 2-4 times daily B: 1 mg every 3-5 h O: 2.5-5 cm, topically to skin every 4-8 h D: 1 disc (2.5-15 mg) for 12-16 h per day IV: 10-20 μg/min; increments of 10 μg/min to a maximum of 400 μg/min
Isosorbide dinitrate (ISORDIL, SORBITRATE, DILATRATE-SR, others)	H_2C / $HC—O—NO_2$ / O / CH / HC / O / $O_2N—O—CH$ / CH_2	T: 2.5-10 mg every 2-3 h T(C): 5-10 mg every 2-3 h T(O): 5-40 mg every 8 h C: 40-80 mg every 12 h
Isosorbide-5-mononitrate (IMDUR, ISMO, others)	H_2C / $HC—O—NO_2$ / O / CH / HC / O / H—O—CH / CH_2	T: 10-40 mg twice daily C: 60-120 mg daily

[a]B, buccal (transmucosal) tablet; C, sustained-release capsule or tablet; D, transdermal disc or patch; IV, intravenous injection; O, ointment; S, lingual spray; T, tablet for sublingual use; T(C), chewable tablet; T(O), oral tablet or capsule.

consequence of the NO-mediated increase in intracellular cyclic GMP is the activation of PKG, which catalyzes the phosphorylation of various proteins in smooth muscle. Another important target of this kinase is the myosin light-chain phosphatase, which is activated on binding PKG and leads to dephosphorylation of the myosin light chain and thereby promotes vasorelaxation and smooth muscle relaxation in many other tissues.

The pharmacological and biochemical effects of the nitrovasodilators appear to be identical to those of an endothelium-derived relaxing factor now known to be NO. Although the soluble isoform of guanylyl cyclase remains the most extensively characterized molecular "receptor" for NO, it is increasingly clear that NO also forms specific adducts with thiol groups in proteins and with reduced glutathione to form nitrosothiol compounds with distinctive biological properties (Stamler et al., 2001). Mitochondrial aldehyde dehydrogenase has been shown to catalyze the reduction of nitroglycerin to yield bioactive NO metabolites (Chen et al., 2002), providing a potentially important clue to the biotransformation of organic nitrates in intact tissues. The regulation and pharmacology of eNOS have been reviewed (Dudzinski et al., 2006).

Cardiovascular Effects Hemodynamic Effects. The nitrovasodilators promote relaxation of vascular smooth muscle. Low concentrations of nitroglycerin preferentially dilate veins more than arterioles. This venodilation decreases venous return, leading to a fall in left and right ventricular chamber size and end-diastolic pressures, but usually results in little change in systemic vascular resistance. Systemic arterial pressure may fall slightly, and heart rate is unchanged or may increase slightly in response to a decrease in blood pressure. Pulmonary vascular resistance and cardiac output are slightly reduced. Doses of nitroglycerin that do not alter systemic arterial pressure may still produce arteriolar dilation in the face and neck, resulting in a facial flush, or dilation of meningeal arterial vessels, causing headache. The molecular basis for the differential response of arterial versus venous tissues to nitroglycerin remains incompletely understood.

Higher doses of organic nitrates cause further venous pooling and may decrease arteriolar resistance as well, thereby decreasing systolic and diastolic blood pressure and cardiac output and causing pallor, weakness, dizziness, and activation of compensatory sympathetic reflexes. The reflex tachycardia and peripheral arteriolar vasoconstriction tend to restore systemic vascular resistance; this is superimposed on sustained venous pooling. Coronary blood flow may increase transiently as a result of coronary vasodilation but may decrease subsequently if cardiac output and blood pressure decrease sufficiently.

In patients with autonomic dysfunction and an inability to increase sympathetic outflow (multiple-system atrophy and pure autonomic failure are the most common forms, much less commonly seen in the autonomic dysfunction associated with diabetes), the fall in blood pressure consequent to the venodilation produced by nitrates cannot be compensated. In these clinical contexts, nitrates may reduce arterial pressure and coronary perfusion pressure significantly, producing potentially life-threatening hypotension and even aggravating angina. The appropriate therapy in patients with orthostatic angina and normal coronary arteries is to correct the orthostatic hypotension by expanding volume (*fludrocortisone* and a high-sodium diet), to prevent venous pooling with fitted support garments, and to carefully titrate use of oral vasopressors. Because patients with autonomic dysfunction occasionally may have coexisting coronary artery disease, the coronary anatomy should be defined before therapy is undertaken.

Effects on Total and Regional Coronary Blood Flow. Myocardial ischemia is a powerful stimulus to coronary vasodilation, and regional blood flow is adjusted by autoregulatory mechanisms. In the presence of atherosclerotic coronary artery narrowing, ischemia distal to the lesion stimulates vasodilation; if the stenosis is severe, much of the capacity to dilate is used to maintain resting blood flow. When demand increases, further dilation may not be possible. After demonstration of direct coronary artery vasodilation in experimental animals, it became generally accepted that nitrates relieved anginal pain by dilating coronary arteries and thereby increasing coronary blood flow. In the presence of significant coronary stenoses, there is a disproportionate reduction in blood flow to the subendocardial regions of the heart, which are subjected to the greatest extravascular compression during systole; organic nitrates tend to restore blood flow in these regions toward normal.

The hemodynamic mechanisms responsible for these effects are not entirely clear. Most hypotheses have focused on the ability of organic nitrates to cause dilation and prevent vasoconstriction of large epicardial vessels without impairing autoregulation in the small vessels, which are responsible for ~90% of the overall coronary vascular resistance. The vessel diameter is an important determinant of the response to nitroglycerin; vessels >200 μm in diameter are highly responsive, whereas those >100 μm respond minimally. Experimental evidence in patients undergoing coronary bypass surgery indicates that nitrates do have a relaxant effect on large coronary vessels. Collateral flow to ischemic regions also is increased. Moreover, analyses of coronary angiograms in humans have shown that sublingual nitroglycerin can dilate epicardial stenoses and reduce the resistance to flow through such areas (Brown et al., 1981; Feldman et al., 1981). The resulting increase in blood flow would be distributed preferentially to ischemic myocardial regions as a consequence of vasodilation induced by autoregulation. An important indirect mechanism for a preferential increase in subendocardial blood flow is the nitroglycerin-induced reduction in intracavitary systolic and diastolic pressures that oppose blood flow to the subendocardium (see below). To the extent that organic nitrates decrease myocardial requirements for O_2 (see the next section), the increased blood flow in ischemic regions could be balanced by decreased flow in nonischemic areas, and an overall increase in coronary artery blood flow need not occur. Dilation of cardiac veins may improve the perfusion of the coronary microcirculation. Such redistribution of blood flow to subendocardial tissue is *not* typical of all vasodilators. *Dipyridamole*, e.g., dilates resistance vessels nonselectively by distorting autoregulation and is ineffective in patients with typical angina.

In patients with angina owing to coronary artery spasm, the ability of organic nitrates to dilate epicardial coronary arteries, and particularly regions affected by spasm, may be the primary mechanism by which they are of benefit.

Effects on Myocardial O_2 Requirements. By their effects on the systemic circulation, the organic nitrates also can reduce myocardial O_2 demand. The major determinants of myocardial O_2 consumption include left ventricular wall tension, heart rate, and myocardial contractility. Ventricular wall tension is affected by a number of factors that may be considered under the categories of preload and afterload. *Preload* is determined by the diastolic pressure that distends the ventricle (ventricular end-diastolic pressure). Increasing end-diastolic volume augments the ventricular wall tension (by the law of Laplace, tension is proportional to pressure times radius). Increasing venous capacitance with nitrates decreases venous return to the heart, decreases ventricular end-diastolic volume, and thereby decreases O_2

consumption. An additional benefit of reducing preload is that it increases the pressure gradient for perfusion across the ventricular wall, which favors subendocardial perfusion. *Afterload* is the impedance against which the ventricle must eject. In the absence of aortic valvular disease, afterload is related to peripheral resistance. Decreasing peripheral arteriolar resistance reduces afterload and thus myocardial work and O_2 consumption.

Organic nitrates decrease both preload and afterload as a result of respective dilation of venous capacitance and arteriolar resistance vessels. Organic nitrates do not appear to significantly alter the inotropic or chronotropic state of the heart, although NO synthesized by cardiac myocytes and fibroblasts may play a role in the modulation of cyclic nucleotide metabolism and may thereby alter autonomic responses (Gustafsson and Brunton, 2002). Because nitrates affect several of the primary determinants of myocardial O_2 demand, their net effect usually is to decrease myocardial O_2 consumption. In addition, an improvement in the lusitropic state of the heart may be seen with more rapid early diastolic filling. This may be secondary to the relief of ischemia rather than primary, or it may be due to a reflex increase in sympathetic activity. Nitrovasodilators also increase cyclic GMP in platelets, with consequent inhibition of platelet function (Loscalzo, 2001) and decreased deposition of platelets in animal models of arterial wall injury (Lam et al., 1988). While this may contribute to their anti-anginal efficacy, the effect appears to be modest and in some settings may be confounded by the potential of nitrates to alter the pharmacokinetics of heparin, reducing its anti-thrombotic effect.

When nitroglycerin is injected or infused directly into the coronary circulation of patients with coronary artery disease, anginal attacks (induced by electrical pacing) are not aborted even when coronary blood flow is increased. However, sublingual administration of nitroglycerin does relieve anginal pain in the same patients. Furthermore, venous phlebotomy that is sufficient to reduce left ventricular end-diastolic pressure can mimic the beneficial effect of nitroglycerin.

Patients can exercise for considerably longer periods after the administration of nitroglycerin. Nevertheless, with or without nitroglycerin, angina occurs at the same value of the *triple product* (aortic pressure × heart rate × ejection time, which is roughly proportional to myocardial consumption of O_2). The observation that angina occurs at the same level of myocardial O_2 consumption suggests that the beneficial effects of nitroglycerin result from reduced cardiac O_2 demand rather than an increase in the delivery of O_2 to ischemic regions of myocardium. However, these results do not preclude the possibility that a favorable redistribution of blood flow to ischemic subendocardial myocardium may contribute to relief of pain in a typical anginal attack, nor do they preclude the possibility that direct coronary vasodilation may be the major effect of nitroglycerin in situations where vasospasm compromises myocardial blood flow.

Mechanism of Relief of Symptoms of Angina Pectoris. The ability of nitrates to dilate epicardial coronary arteries, even in areas of atherosclerotic stenosis, is modest, and the preponderance of evidence continues to favor a reduction in myocardial work, and thus in myocardial O_2 demand, as their primary effect in chronic stable angina.

Paradoxically, high doses of organic nitrates may reduce blood pressure to such an extent that coronary flow is compromised; reflex tachycardia and adrenergic enhancement of contractility also occur. These effects may override the beneficial action of the drugs on myocardial O_2 demand and can aggravate ischemia. Additionally, sublingual nitroglycerin administration may produce bradycardia and hypotension, probably owing to activation of the Bezold-Jarisch reflex.

Other Effects. The nitrovasodilators act on almost all smooth muscle tissues. Bronchial smooth muscle is relaxed irrespective of the preexisting tone. The muscles of the biliary tract, including those of the gallbladder, biliary ducts, and sphincter of Oddi, are effectively relaxed. Smooth muscle of the GI tract, including that of the esophagus, can be relaxed and its spontaneous motility decreased by nitrates both *in vivo* and *in vitro*. The effect may be transient and incomplete *in vivo*, but abnormal "spasm" frequently is reduced. Indeed, many incidences of atypical chest pain and "angina" are due to biliary or esophageal spasm, and these too can be relieved by nitrates. Similarly, nitrates can relax ureteral and uterine smooth muscle, but these responses are of uncertain clinical significance.

Absorption, Fate, and Excretion. More than a century after the first use of organic nitrates to treat angina pectoris, their biotransformation remains the subject of active investigation. Studies in the 1970s suggested that nitroglycerin is reductively hydrolyzed by hepatic glutathione–organic nitrate reductase. More recent studies have implicated a mitochondrial aldehyde dehydrogenase enzyme in the biotransformation of nitroglycerin (Chen et al., 2002). Other enzymatic and nonenzymatic pathways also may contribute to the biotransformation of nitrovasodilators. Despite uncertainties about the quantitative importance of the various pathways involved in nitrovasodilator metabolism, the pharmacokinetic properties of nitroglycerin and isosorbide dinitrate have been studied in some detail (Parker and Parker, 1998).

Preparations

Nitroglycerin. In humans, peak concentrations of nitroglycerin are found in plasma within 4 minutes of sublingual administration; the drug has a $t_{1/2}$ of 1-3 minutes. The onset of action of nitroglycerin may be even more rapid if it is delivered as a sublingual spray rather than as a sublingual tablet. Glyceryl dinitrate metabolites, which have about one-tenth the vasodilator potency, appear to have half-lives of ~40 minutes.

Isosorbide Dinitrate. The major route of metabolism of isosorbide dinitrate in humans appears to be by enzymatic denitration followed by glucuronide conjugation. Sublingual administration produces maximal plasma concentrations of the drug by 6 minutes, and the fall in concentration is rapid ($t_{1/2}$ of ~45 minutes). The primary initial metabolites, isosorbide-2-mononitrate and isosorbide-5-mononitrate, have longer half-lives (3-6 hours) and are presumed to *contribute to the therapeutic efficacy of the drug.*

Isosorbide-5-Mononitrate. This agent is available in tablet form. It does not undergo significant first-pass metabolism and so has excellent bioavailability after oral administration. The mononitrate has a significantly longer $t_{1/2}$ than does isosorbide dinitrate and has been formulated as a plain tablet and as a sustained-release preparation; both have longer durations of action than the corresponding dosage forms of isosorbide dinitrate.

Inhaled NO. Nitric oxide gas administered by inhalation appears to exert most of its therapeutic effects on the pulmonary vasculature because of the rapid inactivation of NO by hemoglobin in the blood. The selective pulmonary vasodilation observed when NO is administered by inhalation has formed the basis for the widespread use of inhaled NO to treat pulmonary hypertension in hypoxemic neonates, where inhaled NO has been shown to significantly reduce morbidity and mortality (Bloch et al., 2007). The efficacy of inhaled NO in adults for other clinical situations that are characterized by elevated pulmonary vascular pressures (acute lung injury and primary pulmonary hypertension, among other disease states) has not yet been established, and therapies using inhaled NO remain under active investigation.

Correlation of Plasma Concentrations of Drug and Biological Activity. Intravenous administration of nitroglycerin or long-acting organic nitrates in anesthetized animals produces the same transient (1-4 minutes) decrease in blood pressure. Because denitration markedly reduces the activity of the organic nitrates, their rapid clearance from blood indicates that the transient duration of action under these conditions correlates with the concentrations of the parent compounds. The rate of hepatic denitration is characteristic of each nitrate and is influenced by hepatic blood flow or the presence of hepatic disease. In experimental animals, injection of moderate amounts of organic nitrates into the portal vein results in little or no vasodepressor activity, indicating that a substantial fraction of drug can be inactivated by first-pass metabolism in the liver (isosorbide mononitrate is an exception).

Tolerance

Sublingual organic nitrates should be taken at the time of an anginal attack or in anticipation of exercise or stress. Such intermittent treatment provides reproducible cardiovascular effects. However, frequently repeated or continuous exposure to high doses of organic nitrates leads to a marked attenuation in the magnitude of most of their pharmacological effects. The magnitude of tolerance is a function of dosage and frequency of use.

Tolerance may result from a reduced capacity of the vascular smooth muscle to convert nitroglycerin to NO, *true vascular tolerance*, or to the activation of mechanisms extraneous to the vessel wall, *pseudotolerance* (Münzel et al., 1995). Multiple mechanisms have been proposed to account for nitrate tolerance, including volume expansion, neurohumoral activation, cellular depletion of sulfhydryl groups, and the generation of free radicals (Parker and Parker, 1998). Inactivation of mitochondrial aldehyde dehydrogenase, an enzyme implicated in biotransformation of nitroglycerin, is seen in models of nitrate tolerance (Sydow et al., 2004), potentially associated with oxidative stress (Parker, 2004). A reactive intermediate formed during the generation of NO from organic nitrates may itself damage and inactivate the enzymes of the activation pathway; tolerance could involve endothelium-derived reactive oxygen species (Münzel et al., 1995; Parker 2004). Clinical data relating to the ability of agents that modify the renin–angiotensin–aldosterone system to prevent nitrate tolerance are contradictory (Parker and Parker, 1998). Important to the interpretation of clinical trials, factors that may influence the ability of such modification to prevent nitrate tolerance include the dose, whether the ACE inhibitors or angiotensin receptor antagonists were administered prior to the initiation of nitrates, and the tissue specificity of the agent. Despite experimental evidence that depletion of sulfhydryl groups may lead to impaired biotransformation of nitrates to NO and thereby result in nitrate tolerance, experimental results to date with sulfhydryl donors have been disappointing. Other changes that are observed in the setting of nitroglycerin tolerance include an enhanced response to vasoconstrictors such as angiotensin II (AngII), serotonin, and phenylephrine. Administration of nitroglycerin is associated with plasma volume expansion, which may be reflected by a decrease in hematocrit. Although diuretic therapy with hydrochlorothiazide can improve a patient's exercise duration, appropriately designed crossover trials have failed to demonstrate an effect of diuretics on nitrate tolerance (Parker et al., 1996).

A more effective approach to restoring responsiveness is to interrupt therapy for 8-12 hours each day, which allows the return of efficacy. It is usually most convenient to omit dosing at night in patients with exertional angina either by adjusting dosing intervals of oral or buccal preparations or by removing cutaneous nitroglycerin. However, patients whose anginal pattern suggests its precipitation by increased left ventricular filling pressures (i.e., occurring in association with orthopnea or paroxysmal nocturnal dyspnea) may benefit from continuing nitrates at night and omitting them during a quiet period of the day. Tolerance also has been seen with isosorbide-5-mononitrate; an eccentric twice-daily dosing schedule appears to maintain efficacy (Parker and Parker, 1998).

While these approaches appear to be effective, some patients develop an increased frequency of nocturnal angina when a nitrate-free interval is employed using nitroglycerin patches; such patients may require another class of anti-anginal agent during this period. Tolerance is not universal, and some patients develop only partial tolerance. The problem of anginal rebound during nitrate-free intervals is especially problematic in the treatment of unstable angina with intravenous nitroglycerin. As tolerance develops, increasing doses are required to achieve the same therapeutic effects; eventually, despite dose escalation, the drug loses efficacy.

A special form of nitroglycerin tolerance is observed in individuals exposed to nitroglycerin in the manufacture of explosives. If protection is inadequate, workers may experience severe headaches, dizziness, and postural weakness during the first several days of employment. Tolerance then develops, but headache and other symptoms may reappear after a few days away from the job—the "Monday disease." The most serious effect of chronic exposure is a form of organic nitrate dependence. Workers without demonstrable organic vascular disease have been reported to have an increase in the incidence of acute coronary syndromes during the 24-72-hour periods away from the work environment (Parker et al., 1995). Coronary and digital arteriospasm during withdrawal and its relaxation by nitroglycerin also have been demonstrated radiographically. Because of the potential problem of nitrate dependence, it seems prudent not to withdraw nitrates abruptly from a patient who has received such therapy chronically.

Toxicity and Untoward Responses

Untoward responses to the therapeutic use of organic nitrates are almost all secondary to actions on the cardiovascular system. Headache is common and can be severe. It usually decreases over a few days if treatment is continued and often can be controlled by decreasing the dose. Transient episodes of dizziness, weakness, and other manifestations associated with postural hypotension may develop, particularly if the patient is standing immobile, and may progress occasionally to loss of consciousness, a reaction that appears to be accentuated by alcohol. It also may be seen with very low doses of nitrates in patients with autonomic dysfunction. Even in severe nitrate syncope, positioning and other measures that facilitate venous return are the only therapeutic measures required. All the organic nitrates occasionally can produce drug rash.

Interaction of Nitrates with PDE5 Inhibitors. Erectile dysfunction is a frequently encountered problem whose risk factors parallel those of coronary artery disease. Thus many men desiring therapy for erectile dysfunction already may be receiving (or may require, especially if they increase physical activity) anti-anginal therapy. The combination of sildenafil and other phosphodiesterase 5 (PDE5) inhibitors with organic nitrate vasodilators can cause extreme hypotension.

Cells in the corpus cavernosum produce NO during sexual arousal in response to nonadrenergic, noncholinergic neurotransmission (Burnett et al., 1992). NO stimulates the formation of cyclic GMP, which leads to relaxation of smooth muscle of the corpus cavernosum and penile arteries, engorgement of the corpus cavernosum, and erection. The accumulation of cyclic GMP can be enhanced by inhibition of the cyclic GMP–specific PDE5 family. Sildenafil (VIAGRA, REVATIO) and congeners inhibit PDE5 and have been demonstrated to improve erectile function in patients with erectile dysfunction. Not surprisingly, PDE5 inhibitors have assumed the status of widely used recreational drugs. Since the introduction of sildenafil, two additional PDE5 inhibitors have been developed for use in therapy of erectile dysfunction. Tadalafil (CIALIS, ADCIRCA) and vardenafil (LEVITRA) share similar therapeutic efficacy and side-effect profiles with sildenafil; tadalafil has a longer time to onset of action and a longer therapeutic $t_{1/2}$ than the other PDE5 inhibitors. Sildenafil has been the most thoroughly characterized of these compounds, but all three PDE5 inhibitors are contraindicated for patients taking organic nitrate vasodilators, and the PDE5 inhibitors should be used with caution in patients taking α or β adrenergic receptor antagonists (see Chapter 12).

The side effects of sildenafil and other PDE5 inhibitors are largely predictable on the basis of their effects on PDE5. Headache, flushing, and rhinitis may be observed, as well as dyspepsia owing to relaxation of the lower esophageal sphincter. Sildenafil and vardenafil also weakly inhibit PDE6, the enzyme involved in photoreceptor signal transduction (Chapters 3 and 64), and can produce visual disturbances, most notably changes in the perception of color hue or brightness. In addition to visual disturbances, sudden one-sided hearing loss has also been reported. Tadalafil inhibits PDE11, a widely distributed PDE isoform, but the clinical importance of this effect is not clear. The most important toxicity of all these PDE5 inhibitors is hemodynamic. When given alone to men with severe coronary artery disease, these drugs have modest effects on blood pressure, producing >10% fall in systolic, diastolic, and mean systemic pressures and in pulmonary artery systolic and mean pressures (Herrmann et al., 2000). However, sildenafil, tadalafil, and vardenafil all have a significant and potentially dangerous interaction with organic nitrates, the therapeutic actions of which are mediated via their conversion to NO with resulting increases in cyclic GMP. In the presence of a PDE5 inhibitor, nitrates cause profound increases in cyclic GMP and can produce dramatic reductions in blood pressure. Compared with controls, healthy male subjects pretreated with sildenafil or the other PDE5 inhibitors exhibit a much greater decrease in systolic blood pressure when treated with sublingual glyceryl trinitrate, and in many subjects a fall of more than 25 mm Hg was detected. This drug class toxicity is the basis for the warning that PDE5 inhibitors should not be prescribed to patients receiving any form of nitrate (Cheitlin et al., 1999) and dictates that patients should be questioned about the use of PDE5 inhibitors within 24 hours before nitrates are administered. A period of longer than 24 hours may be needed following administration of a PDE5 inhibitor for safe use of nitrates, especially with tadalafil because of its prolonged $t_{1/2}$. In the event that patients develop significant hypotension following combined administration of sildenafil and a nitrate, fluids and α-adrenergic receptor agonists, if needed, should be used for support (Cheitlin et al., 1999). These same hemodynamic responses to PDE5 inhibition also may underlie the efficacy of sildenafil in the treatment of patients with primary pulmonary hypertension, in whom chronic treatment with the drug appears to result in enhanced exercise capacity associated with a decrease in pulmonary vascular resistance (Tsai and Kass, 2009). PDE5 inhibitors also are being studied in patients with congestive heart failure and cardiac hypertrophy (see Chapter 28).

Sildenafil, tadalafil, and vardenafil are metabolized via CYP3A4, and their toxicity may be enhanced in patients who receive other substrates of this enzyme, including macrolide and imidazole antibiotics, some statins, and antiretroviral agents (see individual chapters and Chapter 6). PDE5 inhibitors also may prolong cardiac repolarization by blocking the I_{Kr}. Although these interactions and effects are important clinically, the overall incidence and profile of adverse events observed with PDE5 inhibitors, when used without nitrates, are consistent with the expected background frequency of the same events in the treated population. In patients with coronary artery disease whose exercise capacity indicates that sexual activity is unlikely to precipitate angina and who are not currently taking nitrates, the use of PDE5 inhibitors can be considered. Such therapy needs to be individualized, and appropriate warnings must be given about the risk of toxicity if nitrates are taken subsequently for angina; this drug interaction may persist for approximately 24 hours for sildenafil and vardenafil and for considerably longer with tadalafil. Alternative non-nitrate anti-anginal therapy, such as β adrenergic receptor antagonists, should be used during these time periods (Cheitlin et al., 1999).

Therapeutic Uses

Angina. Diseases that predispose to angina should be treated as part of a comprehensive therapeutic program with the primary goal being to prolong life. Conditions such as hypertension, anemia, thyrotoxicosis, obesity, heart failure, cardiac arrhythmias, and acute anxiety can precipitate anginal symptoms in many patients. Patients should be counseled to stop smoking, lose weight, and maintain a low-fat, high-fiber diet; hypertension and hyperlipidemia should be corrected; and daily aspirin (or clopidogrel if aspirin is not tolerated) (see Chapter 30) should be prescribed. Exposure to sympathomimetic agents (e.g., those in nasal decongestants and other sources) probably should be avoided. The use of drugs that modify the perception of pain is a poor approach to the treatment of angina because the underlying myocardial ischemia is not relieved.

Table 27–1 lists the preparations and dosages of the nitrites and organic nitrates. The rapidity of onset, the duration of action, and the likelihood of developing tolerance are related to the method of administration.

Sublingual Administration. Because of its rapid action, long-established efficacy, and low cost, nitroglycerin is the most useful drug of the organic nitrates given sublingually. The onset of action is within 1-2 minutes, but the effects are undetectable by 1 hour after administration. An initial dose of 0.3 mg nitroglycerin often relieves pain within 3 minutes. Absorption may be limited in patients with dentures or with dry mouths. Nitroglycerin tablets are stable but should be dispensed in glass containers and protected from moisture, light, and extremes of temperature. Active tablets usually produce a burning sensation under the tongue, but the absence of this sensation does not reliably predict loss of activity; elderly patients especially may be unable to detect the burning sensation. Anginal pain may be prevented when the drug is used prophylactically immediately prior to exercise or stress. The smallest effective dose should be prescribed. Patients should be instructed to seek medical attention immediately if three tablets taken over a 15-minute period do not relieve a sustained attack because this situation may be indicative of myocardial infarction (MI), unstable angina, or another cause of the pain. Patients also should be advised that there is no virtue in trying to avoid taking sublingual nitroglycerin for anginal pain. Other nitrates that can be taken sublingually do not appear to be longer acting than nitroglycerin because their half-lives depend only on the rate at which they are delivered to the liver. They are no more effective than nitroglycerin and often are more expensive.

Oral Administration. Oral nitrates often are used to provide prophylaxis against anginal episodes in patients who have more than occasional angina. They must be given in sufficient dosage to provide effective plasma levels after first-pass hepatic degradation. Low doses (e.g., 5-10 mg isosorbide dinitrate) are no more effective than placebo in decreasing the frequency of anginal attacks or increasing exercise tolerance. Higher doses of either isosorbide dinitrate (e.g., 20 mg or more orally every 4 hours) or sustained-release preparations of nitroglycerin decrease the frequency of anginal attacks and improve exercise tolerance. Effects peak at 60-90 minutes and last for 3-6 hours. Under these circumstances, the activities of less potent metabolites also may contribute to the therapeutic effect. Chronic oral administration of isosorbide dinitrate (120-720 mg daily) results in persistence of the parent compound and higher plasma concentrations of metabolites. However, these doses are more likely to cause troublesome side effects and lead to tolerance. Administration of isosorbide mononitrate (typically starting at 20 mg) once or twice daily (in the latter case, with the doses administered 7 hours apart) is efficacious in the treatment of chronic angina, and once-daily dosing or an eccentric twice-daily dosing schedule can minimize the development of tolerance.

Cutaneous Administration. Application of nitroglycerin ointment can relieve angina, prolong exercise capacity, and reduce ischemic ST-segment depression with exercise for 4 hours or more. Nitroglycerin ointment (2%) is applied to the skin (2.5-5 cm) as it is squeezed from the tube and then spread in a uniform layer; the dosage must be adjusted for each patient. Effects are apparent within 30-60 minutes (although absorption is variable) and last for 4-6 hours. The ointment is particularly useful for controlling nocturnal angina, which commonly develops within 3 hours after the patient goes to sleep. Transdermal nitroglycerin disks use a nitroglycerin-impregnated polymer (bonded to an adhesive bandage) that permits gradual absorption and a continuous plasma nitrate concentration over 24 hours. The onset of action is slow, with peak effects occurring at 1-2 hours. To avoid tolerance, therapy should be interrupted for at least 8 hours each day. With this regimen, long-term prophylaxis of ischemic episodes often can be attained.

Transmucosal or Buccal Nitroglycerin. This formulation is inserted under the upper lip above the incisors, where it adheres to the gingiva and dissolves gradually in a uniform manner. Hemodynamic effects are seen within 2-5 minutes, and it is therefore useful for short-term prophylaxis of angina. Nitroglycerin continues to be released into the circulation for a prolonged period, and exercise tolerance may be enhanced for up to 5 hours.

Congestive Heart Failure. The utility of nitrovasodilators to relieve pulmonary congestion and to increase cardiac output in congestive heart failure is addressed in Chapter 28.

Unstable Angina Pectoris and Non-ST-Segment–Elevation Myocardial Infarction. The term *unstable angina pectoris* has been used to describe a broad spectrum of clinical entities characterized by an acute or subacute worsening in a patient's anginal symptoms. The variable prognosis of unstable angina no doubt reflects the broad range of clinical entities subsumed by the term. More recently, efforts have been directed toward identifying patients with unstable angina on the basis of their risks for subsequent adverse outcomes such as MI or death. The term *acute coronary syndrome* has been useful in this context: Common to most clinical presentations of acute coronary syndrome is disruption of a coronary plaque, leading to local platelet aggregation and thrombosis at the arterial wall, with subsequent partial or total occlusion of the vessel. There is some variability in the pathogenesis of unstable angina, with gradually progressive atherosclerosis accounting for some cases of new-onset exertional angina. Less commonly, vasospasm in minimally atherosclerotic coronary vessels may account for some cases where rest angina has not been preceded by symptoms of exertional angina. For the most part, the pathophysiological principles that underlie therapy for exertional angina—which are directed at decreasing myocardial oxygen *demand*—have limited efficacy in the treatment of acute coronary syndromes characterized by an insufficiency of myocardial oxygen (blood) *supply*.

Notably, the degree of coronary stenosis correlates poorly with the likelihood of plaque rupture. Drugs that reduce myocardial O_2 consumption by reducing ventricular preload (nitrates) or by reducing heart rate and ventricular contractility (using β adrenergic receptor antagonists) are efficacious, but additional therapies are directed at the atherosclerotic plaque itself and the consequences (or prevention) of its rupture. As discussed later, these therapies include combinations of:

- anti-platelet agents, including aspirin and thioenopyridines such as clopidogrel or prasugrel
- anti-thrombin agents such as heparin and the thrombolytics
- anti-integrin therapies that directly inhibit platelet aggregation mediated by glycoprotein (GP)IIb/IIIa
- mechano-pharmacological approaches with percutaneously deployed intracoronary stents
- coronary bypass surgery for selected patients

Along with nitrates and β adrenergic receptor antagonists, antiplatelet agents represent the cornerstone of therapy for acute coronary syndrome (Hillis and Lange, 2009). Aspirin (see later in the chapter) inhibits platelet aggregation and improves survival (Yeghiazarians et al., 2000). Heparin (either unfractionated or low-molecular-weight) also appears to reduce angina and prevent infarction. These and related agents are discussed in detail in Chapters 34 and 30. Anti-integrin agents directed against the platelet integrin GPIIb/IIIa (including abciximab, tirofiban, and eptifibatide) are effective in combination with heparin, as discussed later. Nitrates are useful both in reducing vasospasm and in reducing myocardial O_2 consumption by decreasing ventricular wall stress. Intravenous administration of nitroglycerin allows high concentrations of drug to be attained rapidly. Because nitroglycerin is degraded rapidly, the dose can be titrated quickly and safely using intravenous administration. If coronary vasospasm is present, intravenous nitroglycerin is likely to be effective, although the addition of a Ca^{2+} channel blocker may be required to achieve complete control in some patients. Because of the potential risk of profound hypotension, nitrates should be withheld and alternate anti-anginal therapy administered if patients have consumed a PDE5 inhibitor within 24 hours (discussed earlier).

Acute Myocardial Infarction. Therapeutic maneuvers in MI are directed at reducing the size of the infarct, preserving or retrieving viable tissue by reducing the O_2 demand of the myocardium, and preventing ventricular remodeling that could lead to heart failure.

Nitroglycerin is commonly administered to relieve ischemic pain in patients presenting with MI, but evidence that nitrates improve mortality in MI is sparse. Because they reduce ventricular preload through vasodilation, nitrates are effective in relief of pulmonary congestion. A decreased ventricular preload should be avoided in patients with right ventricular infarction because higher right-sided heart filling pressures are needed in this clinical context. Nitrates are relatively contraindicated in patients with systemic hypotension. According to the American Heart Association/American College of Cardiology (AHA/ACC) guidelines, "nitrates should not be used if hypotension limits the administration of β blockers, which have more powerful salutary effects" (Antman et al., 2004).

Because the proximate cause of MI is intracoronary thrombosis, reperfusion therapies are critically important, employing, when possible, direct percutaneous coronary interventions (PCIs) for acute MI, usually using drug-eluting intracoronary stents (Antman et al., 2004). Thrombolytic agents are administered at hospitals where emergency PCI is not performed, but outcomes are better with direct PCI than with thrombolytic therapy (Antman et al., 2004) (see discussion of thrombolytic and antiplatelet therapies in Chapter 30).

Variant (Prinzmetal) Angina. The large coronary arteries normally contribute little to coronary resistance. However, in variant angina, coronary constriction results in reduced blood flow and ischemic pain. Multiple mechanisms have been proposed to initiate vasospasm, including endothelial cell injury. Whereas long-acting nitrates alone are occasionally efficacious in abolishing episodes of variant angina, additional therapy with Ca^{2+} channel blockers usually is required. Ca^{2+} channel blockers, but not nitrates, have been shown to influence mortality and the incidence of MI favorably in variant angina; they should generally be included in therapy.

Ca^{2+} CHANNEL ANTAGONISTS

Voltage-sensitive Ca^{2+} channels (L-type or slow channels) mediate the entry of extracellular Ca^{2+} into smooth muscle and cardiac myocytes and sinoatrial (SA) and atrioventricular (AV) nodal cells in response to electrical depolarization. In both smooth muscle and cardiac myocytes, Ca^{2+} is a trigger for contraction, albeit by different mechanisms. Ca^{2+} channel antagonists, also called *Ca^{2+} entry blockers*, inhibit Ca^{2+} channel function. In vascular smooth muscle, this leads to relaxation, especially in arterial beds. These drugs also may produce negative inotropic and chronotropic effects in the heart.

History. The work in the 1960s of Fleckenstein, Godfraind, and their colleagues led to the concept that drugs can alter cardiac and smooth muscle contraction by blocking the entry of Ca^{2+} into myocytes. Godfraind and associates showed that the effect of the diphenylpiperazine analoges in preventing agonist-induced vascular smooth muscle contraction could be overcome by raising the concentration of Ca^{2+} in the extracellular medium (Godfraind et al., 1986).

Hass and Hartfelder reported in 1962 that verapamil, a coronary vasodilator, possessed negative inotropic and chronotropic effects that were not seen with other vasodilatory agents, such as nitroglycerin. In 1967, Fleckenstein suggested that the negative inotropic effect resulted from inhibition of excitation–contraction coupling and that the mechanism involved reduced movement of Ca^{2+} into cardiac myocytes. Verapamil was the first clinically available calcium-channel blocker; it is a congener of papaverine. Many other calcium entry blockers with a wide range of structures are now available. Other compounds, such as nifedipine and diltiazem, also were shown to block the movement of Ca^{2+} through the cardiac myocyte Ca^{2+} channel, or the slow channel (see Chapter 29), and thereby alter the plateau phase of the cardiac action potential. Subsequently, drugs in several chemical classes have been shown to alter cardiac and smooth muscle contraction by blocking or "antagonizing" the entry of Ca^{2+} through channels in the myocyte membrane.

Chemistry. The multiple Ca^{2+} channel antagonists that are approved for clinical use in the U.S. have diverse chemical structures. Clinically used Ca^{2+} channel antagonists include the phenylalkylamine compound verapamil, the benzothiazepine diltiazem, and numerous dihydropyridines, including nifedipine, amlodipine, felodipine, isradipine, nicardipine, nisoldipine, and nimodipine. The structures and specificities of several of these drugs are shown in Table 27–2. Although these drugs are commonly grouped together as "calcium channel blockers," there are fundamental differences among verapamil, diltiazem, and the dihydropyridines, especially with respect to pharmacological characteristics, drug interactions, and toxicities.

Mechanisms of Action. An increased concentration of cytosolic Ca^{2+} causes increased contraction in both cardiac and vascular smooth muscle cells. The entry of extracellular Ca^{2+} is more important in initiating the contraction of cardiac myocytes (Ca^{2+}-induced Ca^{2+} release). The release of Ca^{2+} from intracellular storage sites also contributes to contraction of vascular smooth muscle, particularly in some vascular beds. Cytosolic Ca^{2+} concentrations can be increased by diverse contractile stimuli in vascular smooth muscle cells. Many hormones and autocoids increase Ca^{2+} influx through so-called receptor-operated channels, whereas increases in external concentrations of K^+ and depolarizing electrical stimuli increase Ca^{2+} influx through voltage-sensitive, or "potential operated," channels. The Ca^{2+} channel antagonists produce their effects by binding to the α_1 subunit of the L-type Ca^{2+} channels and reducing Ca^{2+} flux through the channel. The vascular and cardiac effects of some of the Ca^{2+} channel blockers are summarized in the next section and in Table 27–2.

Voltage-sensitive channels contain domains of homologous sequence that are arranged in tandem within a single large subunit. In addition to the major channel-forming subunit (termed α_1), Ca^{2+} channels contain several other associated subunits (termed α_2, β, γ, and δ) (Schwartz, 1992). Voltage-sensitive Ca^{2+} channels have been divided into at least three subtypes based on their conductances and sensitivities to voltage (Schwartz, 1992; Tsien et al., 1988). The channels best characterized to date are the L, N, and T subtypes. Only the L-type channel is sensitive to the dihydropyridine Ca^{2+} channel blockers. All approved Ca^{2+} channel blockers bind to the α_1 subunit of the L-type Ca^{2+} channel, which is the main pore-forming unit of the channel. This ~250,000-Da subunit is associated with a disulfide-linked $\alpha_2\delta$ subunit of ~140,000 Da and a smaller intracellular β subunit. The α_1 subunits share a common topology of four homologous domains, each of which is composed of six putative transmembrane segments (S1–S6). The α_2, δ, and β subunits modulate the α_1 subunit (see Figure 14–2). The phenylalkylamine Ca^{2+} channel blocker verapamil binds to transmembrane segment 6 of domain IV (IVS6), the benzothiazepine Ca^{2+} channel blocker diltiazem

Table 27–2

Ca^{2+} Channel Blockers: Chemical Structures and Some Relative Cardiovascular Effects[a]

CHEMICAL STRUCTURE Generic name (trade name)	VASODILATION (CORONARY FLOW)	SUPPRESSION OF CARDIAC CONTRACTILITY	SUPPRESSION OF AUTOMATICITY (SA NODE)	SUPPRESSION OF CONDUCTION (AV NODE)
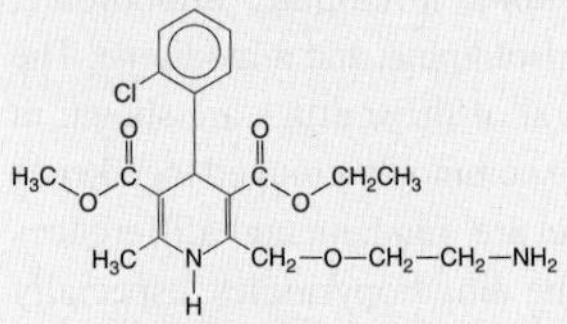 Amlodipine (NORVASC, others)	5	1	1	0
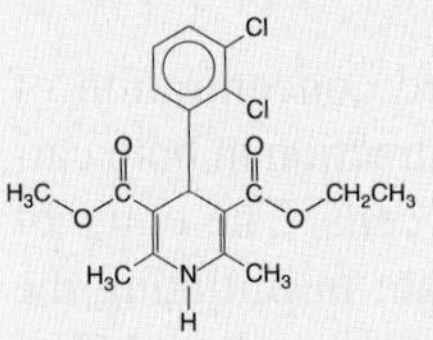 Felodipine (PLENDIL, others)	5	1	1	0
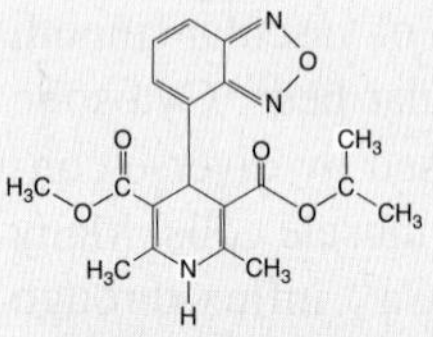 Isradipine (DYNACIRC, others)	NR	NR	NR	NR
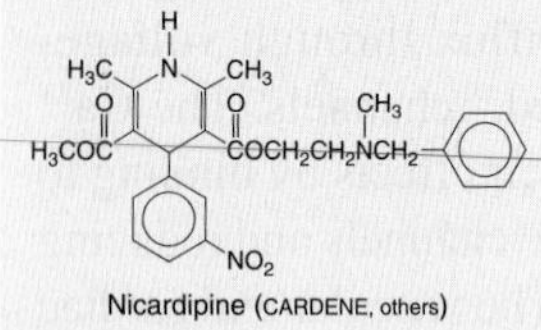 Nicardipine (CARDENE, others)	5	0	1	0
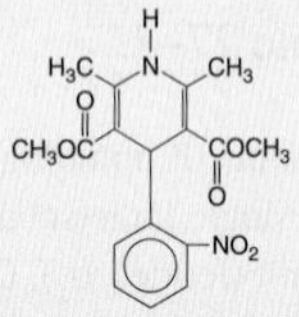 Nifedipine (ADALAT, PROCARDIA, others)	5	1	1	0
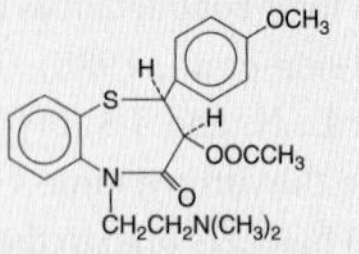 Diltiazem (CARDIZEM, DILACOR-XR, others)	3	2	5	4
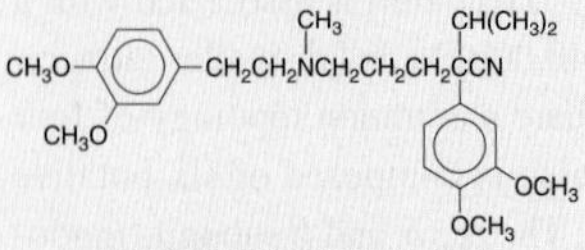 Verapamil (CALAN, ISOPTIN, others)	4	4	5	5

[a]Relative effects are ranked from *no effect* (0) to *prominent* (5). NR, not ranked. (Modified from Julian, 1987; Taira, 1987.)

binds to the cytoplasmic bridge between domain III (IIIS) and domain IV (IVS), and the dihydropyridine Ca^{2+} channel blockers (nifedipine and several others) bind to transmembrane segments of both domains III and IV. These three separate receptor sites are linked allosterically.

Pharmacological Properties

Cardiovascular Effects. Actions in Vascular Tissue. Although there is some involvement of Na^+ currents, depolarization of vascular smooth muscle cells depends primarily on the influx of Ca^{2+}. At least three distinct mechanisms may be responsible for contraction of vascular smooth muscle cells. First, voltage-sensitive Ca^{2+} channels open in response to depolarization of the membrane, and extracellular Ca^{2+} moves down its electrochemical gradient into the cell. After closure of Ca^{2+} channels, a finite period of time is required before the channels can open again in response to a stimulus. Second, agonist-induced contractions that occur without depolarization of the membrane result from stimulation of the G_q–PLC–IP_3 pathway, resulting in the release of intracellular Ca^{2+} from the sarcoplasmic reticulum (Chapter 3). This receptor-mediated release of intracellular Ca^{2+} may trigger further influx of extracellular Ca^{2+}. Third, receptor-operated Ca^{2+} channels allow the entry of extracellular Ca^{2+} in response to receptor occupancy.

An increase in cytosolic Ca^{2+} results in enhanced binding of Ca^{2+} to calmodulin. The Ca^{2+}–calmodulin complex in turn activates myosin light-chain kinase, with resulting phosphorylation of the myosin light chain. Such phosphorylation promotes interaction between actin and myosin and leads to contraction of smooth muscle. Ca^{2+} channel antagonists inhibit the voltage-dependent Ca^{2+} channels in vascular smooth muscle at significantly lower concentrations than are required to interfere with the release of intracellular Ca^{2+} or to block receptor-operated Ca^{2+} channels. All Ca^{2+} channel blockers relax arterial smooth muscle, but they have a less pronounced effect on most venous beds and hence do not affect cardiac preload significantly.

Actions in Cardiac Cells. The mechanisms involved in excitation–contraction coupling in the cardiac muscle differ from those in vascular smooth muscle in that a portion of the two inward currents is carried by Na^+ through the fast channel in addition to that carried by Ca^{2+} through the slow channel. Within the cardiac myocyte, Ca^{2+} binds to troponin, relieving the inhibitory effect of troponin on the contractile apparatus and permitting a productive interaction of actin and myosin, leading to contraction. Thus, Ca^{2+} channel blockers can produce a negative inotropic effect. Although this is true of all classes of Ca^{2+} channel blockers, the greater degree of peripheral vasodilation seen with the dihydropyridines is accompanied by a sufficient baroreflex-mediated increase in sympathetic tone to overcome the negative inotropic effect. Diltiazem also may inhibit mitochondrial Na^+–Ca^{2+} exchange (Schwartz, 1992).

In the SA and AV nodes, depolarization largely depends on the movement of Ca^{2+} through the slow channel. The effect of a Ca^{2+} channel blocker on AV conduction and on the rate of the sinus node pacemaker depends on whether or not the agent delays the recovery of the slow channel (Schwarz, 1992). Although nifedipine reduces the slow inward current in a dose-dependent manner, it does not affect the rate of recovery of the slow Ca^{2+} channel. The channel blockade caused by nifedipine and related dihydropyridines also shows little dependence on the frequency of stimulation. At doses used clinically, nifedipine does not affect conduction through the AV node. In contrast, verapamil not only reduces the magnitude of the Ca^{2+} current through the slow channel but also decreases the rate of recovery of the channel. In addition, channel blockade caused by verapamil (and to a lesser extent by diltiazem) is enhanced as the frequency of stimulation increases, a phenomenon known as *frequency dependence* or *use dependence*. Verapamil and diltiazem depress the rate of the sinus node pacemaker and slow AV conduction; the latter effect is the basis for their use in the treatment of supraventricular tachyarrhythmias (see Chapter 29). Bepridil, like verapamil, inhibits both slow inward Ca^{2+} current and fast inward Na^+ current. It has a direct negative inotropic effect. Its electrophysiological properties lead to slowing of the heart rate, prolongation of the AV nodal effective refractory period, and importantly, prolongation of the QTc interval. Particularly in the setting of hypokalemia, the last effect can be associated with *torsades de pointes*, a potentially lethal ventricular arrhythmia (see Chapter 29).

Hemodynamic Effects. All the Ca^{2+} channel blockers approved for clinical use decrease coronary vascular resistance and can lead to an increase in coronary blood flow. The dihydropyridines are more potent vasodilators *in vivo* and *in vitro* than verapamil, which is more potent than diltiazem. The hemodynamic effects of these agents vary depending on the route of administration and the extent of left ventricular dysfunction.

Nifedipine given intravenously increases forearm blood flow with little effect on venous pooling; this indicates a selective dilation of arterial resistance vessels. The decrease in arterial blood pressure elicits sympathetic reflexes, with resulting tachycardia and positive inotropy. Nifedipine also has direct negative inotropic effects *in vitro*. However, nifedipine relaxes vascular smooth muscle at significantly lower concentrations than those required for prominent direct effects on the heart. Thus, arteriolar resistance and blood pressure are lowered, contractility and segmental ventricular function are improved, and heart rate and cardiac output are increased modestly. After oral administration of nifedipine, arterial dilation increases peripheral blood flow; venous tone does not change.

The other dihydropyridines—amlodipine, felodipine, isradipine, nicardipine, nisoldipine, nimodipine, and clevidipine— share many of the cardiovascular effects of nifedipine.

Amlodipine is a dihydropyridine that has a slow absorption and a prolonged effect. With a plasma $t_{1/2}$ of 35-50 hours, plasma levels and effect increase over 7-10 days of daily administration of a constant dose. Amlodipine produces both peripheral arterial vasodilation and coronary dilation, with a hemodynamic profile similar to that of nifedipine. However, there is less reflex tachycardia with amlodipine, possibly because the long $t_{1/2}$ produces minimal peaks and troughs in plasma concentrations (van Zwieten and Pfaffendorf, 1993). Felodipine may have even greater vascular specificity than does nifedipine or amlodipine. At concentrations producing vasodilation, there is no negative inotropic effect. Like nifedipine, felodipine indirectly activates the sympathetic nervous system, leading to an increase in heart rate. Nicardipine has anti-anginal properties similar to those of nifedipine and may have selectivity for coronary vessels. Isradipine also produces the typical peripheral vasodilation seen with other dihydropyridines, but because of its inhibitory effect on the SA node, little or no rise in heart rate is seen. This inhibitory effect does not extend to the cardiac myocytes, however, because no cardiodepressant effect is seen.

Despite the negative chronotropic effect, isradipine appears to have little effect on the AV node, so it may be used in patients with AV block or combined with a β adrenergic receptor antagonist. In general, because of their lack of myocardial depression and, to a greater or lesser extent, lack of negative chronotropic effect, dihydropyridines are less effective as monotherapy in stable angina than are verapamil, diltiazem, or a β adrenergic receptor antagonist. Nisoldipine is more than 1000 times more potent in preventing contraction of human vascular smooth muscle than in preventing contraction of human cardiac muscle *in vitro*, suggesting a high degree of vascular selectivity (Godfraind et al., 1992). Although nisoldipine has a short elimination $t_{1/2}$, a sustained-release preparation that is efficacious as an anti-anginal agent has been developed. Nimodipine has high lipid solubility and was developed as an agent to relax the cerebral vasculature. It is effective in inhibiting cerebral vasospasm and has been used primarily to treat patients with neurological defects associated with cerebral vasospasm after subarachnoid hemorrhage.

Clevidipine is a novel dihydropyridine L-type Ca^{2+} channel blocker—available for intravenous administration—that has a very rapid ($t_{1/2}$ ~2 minutes) onset and offset of action. It is metabolized by esterases in blood, similar to the fate of esmolol. Clevidipine preferentially affects arterial smooth muscle compared to targeting veins or the heart. It may be useful in controlling blood pressure in severe or perioperative hypertension when oral therapy is not possible or desirable. Infusions are typically started at a rate of 1-2 μg/kg/min and titrated to the desired effect on blood pressure. Cumulative experience with the drug in clinical settings is relatively limited.

Verapamil is a less potent vasodilator *in vivo* than are the dihydropyridines. Like dihydropyridines, verapamil causes little effect on venous resistance vessels at concentrations that produce arteriolar dilation. With doses of verapamil sufficient to produce peripheral arterial vasodilation, there are more direct negative chronotropic, dromotropic, and inotropic effects than with the dihydropyridines. Intravenous verapamil causes a decrease in arterial blood pressure owing to a decrease in vascular resistance, but the reflex tachycardia is blunted or abolished by the direct negative chronotropic effect of the drug. This intrinsic negative inotropic effect is partially offset by both a decrease in afterload and the reflex increase in adrenergic tone. Thus, in patients without congestive heart failure, ventricular performance is not impaired and actually may improve, especially if ischemia limits performance. In contrast, in patients with congestive heart failure, intravenous verapamil can cause a marked decrease in contractility and left ventricular function. Oral administration of verapamil reduces peripheral vascular resistance and blood pressure, often with minimal changes in heart rate. The relief of pacing-induced angina seen with verapamil is due primarily to a reduction in myocardial oxygen demand.

Intravenous administration of diltiazem can result initially in a marked decrease in peripheral vascular resistance and arterial blood pressure, which elicits a reflex increase in heart rate and cardiac output. Heart rate then falls below initial levels because of the direct negative chronotropic effect of the agent. Oral administration of diltiazem decreases both heart rate and mean arterial blood pressure. While diltiazem and verapamil produce similar effects on the SA and AV nodes, the negative inotropic effect of diltiazem is more modest.

The effects of Ca^{2+} channel blockers on diastolic ventricular relaxation (the lusitropic state of the ventricle) are complex. The direct effect of several of these agents, especially when given into the coronary arteries, is to impair relaxation (Walsh and O'Rourke, 1985). Clinical studies suggest an improvement in peak left ventricular filling rates when verapamil, nifedipine, nisoldipine, or nicardipine are given systemically, but one must be cautious in extrapolating this change in filling rates to enhancement of relaxation. Because ventricular relaxation is so complex, the effect of even a single agent may be pleiotropic. If reflex stimulation of sympathetic tone increases cyclic AMP levels in myocytes, increased lusitropy will result that may outweigh a direct negative lusitropic effect. Likewise, a reduction in afterload will improve the lusitropic state. In addition, if ischemia is improved, the negative lusitropic effect of asymmetrical left ventricular contraction will be reduced. The sum total of these effects in any given patient cannot be determined *a priori*. Thus, caution should be exercised in the use of Ca^{2+} channel blockers for this purpose; the ideal is to determine the end result objectively before committing the patient to therapy.

Absorption, Fate, and Excretion. Although the absorption of these agents is nearly complete after oral administration, their bioavailability is reduced, in some cases markedly, by first-pass hepatic metabolism. The effects of these drugs are evident within 30-60 minutes of an oral dose, with the exception of the more slowly absorbed and longer-acting agents amlodipine, isradipine, and felodipine. Sustained-release forms of the Ca^{2+} channel blockers are used clinically to reduce the number of daily doses needed to maintain therapeutic drug levels, and in the case of nifedipine, sustained-release forms of the drug appear to mitigate the reflex tachycardia sometimes seen following oral administration. Intravenous administration of diltiazem or verapamil leads to a rapid therapeutic response.

These agents all are bound extensively to plasma proteins (70-98%); their elimination half-lives vary widely and range from 1.3-64 hours. During repeated oral administration, bioavailability and $t_{1/2}$ may increase because of saturation of hepatic metabolism. The bioavailability of some of these drugs may be increased by grapefruit juice, likely through inhibition of enzyme CYP3A4 expressed in the small bowel. A major metabolite of diltiazem is desacetyldiltiazem, which has about one-half of diltiazem's potency as a vasodilator. *N*-Demethylation of verapamil results in production of norverapamil, which is biologically active but much less potent than the parent compound. The $t_{1/2}$ of norverapamil is ~10 hours. The metabolites of the dihydropyridines are inactive or weakly active. In patients with hepatic cirrhosis, the bioavailabilities and half-lives of the Ca^{2+} channel blockers may be increased, and dosage should be decreased accordingly. The half-lives of these agents also may be longer in older patients. Except for diltiazem and nifedipine, all the Ca^{2+} channel blockers are administered as racemic mixtures (Abernethy and Schwartz, 1999).

Toxicity and Untoward Responses. The profile of adverse reactions to the Ca^{2+} channel blockers varies among the drugs in this class. Patients receiving immediate-release capsules of nifedipine develop headache, flushing, dizziness, and peripheral edema. However, short-acting formulations of nifedipine are not appropriate in the long-term treatment of angina or hypertension. Dizziness and flushing are much less of a problem with the sustained-release formulations and with the dihydropyridines having a long $t_{1/2}$ and relatively constant concentrations of drug in plasma. Peripheral edema may occur in some patients with Ca^{2+} channel blockers but is not the result of generalized fluid retention; it most likely results from increased hydrostatic pressure in the lower extremities owing to precapillary dilation and reflex postcapillary constriction (Epstein and Roberts, 2009). Some other adverse effects of these drugs are due to actions in nonvascular smooth muscle. Contraction of the lower esophageal sphincter is inhibited by the Ca^{2+} channel blockers. For example, Ca^{2+} channel blockers can cause or aggravate gastroesophageal reflux. Constipation is a common side effect of verapamil, but it occurs less frequently with other Ca^{2+} channel blockers. Urinary retention is a rare adverse effect. Uncommon adverse effects include rash and elevations of liver enzymes. Worsened myocardial ischemia has been observed with nifedipine (Egstrup and Andersen, 1993). Worsening of angina was observed in patients with an angiographically demonstrable coronary collateral circulation. The worsening of angina may have resulted from excessive hypotension and decreased coronary perfusion, selective coronary vasodilation in nonischemic regions of the myocardium in a setting where vessels perfusing ischemic regions were already maximally dilated (i.e., coronary steal), or an increase in O_2 demand owing to increased sympathetic tone and excessive tachycardia. In a study of monotherapy with an immediate-release formulation of nisoldipine, the dihydropyridine was not superior to placebo and was associated with a trend toward an increased incidence of serious adverse events, a process termed *proischemia* (Waters, 1991).

Although bradycardia, transient asystole, and exacerbation of heart failure have been reported with verapamil, these responses usually have occurred after intravenous administration of verapamil in patients with disease of the SA node or AV nodal conduction disturbances or in the presence of β blockade. The use of intravenous verapamil with an intravenous β adrenergic receptor antagonist is contraindicated because of the increased propensity for AV block and/or severe depression of ventricular function. Patients with ventricular dysfunction, SA or AV nodal conduction disturbances, and systolic blood pressures below 90 mm Hg should not be treated with verapamil or diltiazem, particularly intravenously. Some Ca^{2+} channel antagonists can cause an increase in the concentration of digoxin in plasma, although toxicity from the cardiac glycoside rarely develops. The use of verapamil to treat digitalis toxicity thus is contraindicated; AV nodal conduction disturbances may be exacerbated.

Several studies have raised concerns about the long-term safety of short-acting nifedipine (Opie et al., 2000). The proposed mechanism for this adverse effect lies in abrupt vasodilation with reflex sympathetic activation. There does not appear to be either significant reflex tachycardia or long-term adverse outcomes from treatment with sustained-release forms of nifedipine or with the dihydropyridine Ca^{2+} blockers such as amlodipine or felodipine, which have more favorable (slower) pharmacokinetics.

Important drug–drug interactions may be encountered with Ca^{2+} channel blockers. Verapamil blocks the P-glycoprotein drug transporter. Both the renal and hepatic disposition of digoxin occurs via this transporter. Accordingly, verapamil inhibits the elimination of digoxin and other drugs that are cleared from the body by the P-glycoprotein (see Chapter 5). When used with quinidine, Ca^{2+} channel blockers may cause excessive hypotension, particularly in patients with idiopathic hypertrophic subaortic stenosis.

Therapeutic Uses

Variant Angina. Variant angina results from reduced blood flow (a consequence of transient localized vasoconstriction) rather than increased oxygen demand. Controlled clinical trials have demonstrated efficacy of the Ca^{2+} channel blocking agents for the treatment of variant angina (Gibbons et al., 2003). These drugs can attenuate ergonovine-induced vasospasm in patients with variant angina, which suggests that protection in variant angina is due to coronary dilation rather than to alterations in peripheral hemodynamics.

Table 27–3

Recommended Drug Therapy for Angina in Patients with Other Medical Conditions

CONDITION	RECOMMENDED TREATMENT (AND ALTERNATIVES) FOR ANGINA	DRUGS TO AVOID
Medical Conditions		
Systemic hypertension	β receptor antagonists (Ca^{2+} channel antagonists)	
Migraine or vascular headaches	β receptor antagonists (Ca^{2+} channel antagonists)	
Asthma or chronic obstructive pulmonary disease with bronchospasm	Verapamil or diltiazem	β receptor antagonists
Hyperthyroidism	β receptor antagonists	
Raynaud's syndrome	Long-acting, slow-release Ca^{2+} antagonists	β receptor antagonists
Insulin-dependent diabetes mellitus	β receptor antagonists (particularly if prior MI) or long-acting, slow-release Ca^{2+} channel antagonists	
Non-insulin-dependent diabetes mellitus	β receptor antagonists or long-acting, slow-release Ca^{2+} channel antagonists	
Depression	Long-acting, slow-release Ca^{2+} channel antagonists	β receptor antagonists
Mild peripheral vascular disease	β receptor antagonists or Ca^{2+} channel antanogists	
Severe peripheral vascular disease with rest ischemia	Ca^{2+} channel antagonists	β receptor antagonists
Cardiac Arrhythmias and Conduction Abnormalities		
Sinus bradycardia	Dihydropyridine Ca^{2+} channel antagonists	β receptor antagonists, diltiazem, verapamil
Sinus tachycardia (not due to heart failure)	β receptor antagonists	
Supraventricular tachycardia	Verapamil, diltiazem, or β receptor antagonists	
Atrioventricular block	Dihydropyridine Ca^{2+} channel antagonists	β receptor antagonists, diltiazem, verapamil
Rapid atrial fibrillation (with digitalis)	Verapamil, diltiazem, or β receptor antagonists	
Ventricular arrhythmias	β receptor antagonists	
Left Ventricular Dysfunction		
Congestive heart failure		
Mild (LVEF ≥40%)	β receptor antagonists	
Moderate to severe (LVEF <40%)	Amlodipine or felodipine (nitrates)	
Left-sided valvular heart disease		
Mild aortic stenosis	β receptor antagonists	
Aortic insufficiency	Long-acting, slow-release dihydropyridines	
Mitral regurgitation	Long-acting, slow-release dihydropyridines	
Mitral stenosis	β receptor antagonists	
Hypertrophic cardiomyopathy	β receptor antagonists, non-dihydropyridine Ca^{2+} channel antagonists	Nitrates, dihydropyridine Ca^{2+} channel antagonists

MI, myocardial infarction; LVEF, left ventricular ejection fraction. (Gibbons RJ, Chatterjee K, Daley J, Douglas JS, Fihn SD, Gardin JM, Grunwald MA, Levy D, Lytle BW, O'Rourke RA, Schafer WP, Williams SV. ACC/AHA/ACP-ASIM. Guidelines for the management of patients with chronic stable angina: a report of the American College of Cardiology/ American Heart Association Task Force on Practice Guidelines (Committee on the Management of Patients With Chronic Stable Angina). *J Am Coll Cardiol* 1999; 33:2092–197. Copyright © 1999 by the American College of Cardiology Foundation.)

Combination Therapy and New Anti-Anginal Drugs. Because the different categories of anti-anginal agents have different mechanisms of action, it has been suggested that combinations of these agents would allow the use of lower doses, increasing effectiveness and reducing the incidence of side effects. However, despite the predicted advantages, combination therapy rarely achieves this potential and may be accompanied by serious side effects. The new anti-anginal agent ranolazine elicits its therapeutic effects by different and incompletely understood mechanisms that distinguish this new drug from the "classical" classes of anti-anginal drugs (organic nitrates, β adrenergic blockers and Ca^{2+} channel blockers). Some studies have suggested that ranolazine may have additional efficacy in combination with other anti-anginal agents (Chaitman et al., 2004), and the effects of ranolazine on cardiac arrhythmias and glucose metabolism may identify indications for this drug independent of its role as an anti-anginal agent (Morrow et al., 2009). Indeed, most of the anti-anginal drugs have broader indications in cardiovascular therapeutics, including (among others): β blockers for treatment of hypertension, arrhythmias, and heart failure; dihydropyridine calcium channel blockers in treatment of hypertension and heart failure; and diltiazem and verapamil to treat cardiac arrhythmias and hypertension. Table 27–3 shows some of the important indications and contraindications for use of anti-anginal agents in the context of other disease states.

Nitrates and β Adrenergic Receptor Antagonists. The concurrent use of organic nitrates and β adrenergic receptor antagonists can be very effective in the treatment of typical exertional angina. The additive efficacy primarily is a result of the blockade by one drug of a reflex effect elicited by the other. β Adrenergic receptor antagonists can block the baroreceptor-mediated reflex tachycardia and positive inotropic effects that are sometimes associated with nitrates, whereas nitrates, by increasing venous capacitance, can attenuate the increase in left ventricular end-diastolic volume associated with β receptor blockade. Concurrent administration of nitrates also can alleviate the increase in coronary vascular resistance associated with blockade of β adrenergic receptors.

Ca^{2+} Channel Blockers and β Receptor Antagonists. Because there is a proven mortality benefit from the use of β adrenergic receptor antagonists in patients with heart disease, this class of drugs represents the first line of therapy. However, when angina is not controlled adequately by a β receptor antagonist plus nitrates, additional improvement sometimes can be achieved by the addition of a Ca^{2+} channel blocker, especially if there is a component of coronary vasospasm. The differences among the chemical classes of Ca^{2+} channel blockers can lead to important adverse or salutary drug interactions with β receptor antagonists. If the patient already is being treated with maximal doses of verapamil or diltiazem, it is difficult to demonstrate any additional benefit of β receptor blockade, and excessive bradycardia, heart block, or heart failure may ensue. However, in patients treated with a dihydropyridine such as nifedipine or with nitrates, substantial reflex tachycardia often limits the effectiveness of these agents. A β receptor antagonist may be a helpful addition in this situation, resulting in a lower heart rate and blood pressure with exercise. The efficacy of amlodipine is improved by combination with a β adrenergic receptor antagonist. However, in the Total Ischaemic Burden European Trial (TIBET), which compared the effects of atenolol, a sustained-release form of nifedipine, and their combination on exercise parameters and ambulatory ischemia in patients with mild angina, there were no differences between the agents, either singly or in combination, on any of the measured ischemic parameters (Fox et al., 1996). On the other hand, in studies of patients with more severe but still stable angina, atenolol and propranolol were shown to be superior to nifedipine, and the combination of propranolol and nifedipine was more effective than a β receptor antagonist alone.

Relative contraindications to the use of β receptor antagonists for treatment of angina—bronchospasm, Raynaud's syndrome, or Prinzmetal angina—may lead to a choice to initiate therapy with a Ca^{2+} channel blocker. Fluctuations in coronary tone are important determinants of variant angina. It is likely that episodes of increased tone, such as those precipitated by cold and by emotion, superimposed on fixed disease have a role in the variable anginal threshold seen in some patients with otherwise chronic stable angina. Increased coronary tone also may be important in the anginal episodes occurring early after MI and after coronary angioplasty, and it probably accounts for those patients with unstable angina who respond to dihydropyridines. Atherosclerotic arteries have abnormal vasomotor responses to a number of stimuli (Dudzinski et al., 2006), including exercise, other forms of sympathetic activation, and cholinergic agonists; in such vessels, stenotic segments actually may become more severely stenosed during exertion. This implies that the normal exercise-induced increase in coronary flow is lost in atherosclerosis. Similar exaggerated vascular contractile responses are seen in hyperlipidemia, even before anatomical evidence of atherosclerosis develops. Because of this, coronary vasodilators (nitrates and/or Ca^{2+} channel blockers) are an important part of the therapeutic program in the majority of patients with ischemic heart disease.

Ca^{2+} Channel Blockers and Nitrates. In severe exertional or vasospastic angina, the combination of a nitrate and

a Ca^{2+} channel blocker may provide additional relief over that obtained with either type of agent alone. Because nitrates primarily reduce preload, whereas Ca^{2+} channel blockers reduce afterload, the net effect on reduction of O_2 demand should be additive. However, excessive vasodilation and hypotension can occur. The concurrent administration of a nitrate and nifedipine has been advocated in particular for patients with exertional angina with heart failure, the sick-sinus syndrome, or AV nodal conduction disturbances, but excessive tachycardia may be seen.

Ca^{2+} Channel Blockers, β Receptor Antagonists, and Nitrates. In patients with exertional angina that is not controlled by the administration of two types of antianginal agents, the use of all three may provide improvement, although the incidence of side effects increases significantly. The dihydropyridines and nitrates dilate epicardial coronary arteries, the dihydropyridines decrease afterload, the nitrates decrease preload, and the *β* receptor antagonists decrease heart rate and myocardial contractility. Therefore, there is theoretical, and sometimes real, benefit with their combination, although adverse drug interactions may lead to clinically important events. For example, combining verapamil or diltiazem with a *β* receptor antagonist greatly increases the risk of conduction system and left ventricular dysfunction–related side effects and should be undertaken only with extreme caution and only if no other alternatives exist.

ANTI-PLATELET, ANTI-INTEGRIN, AND ANTI-THROMBOTIC AGENTS

Aspirin reduces the incidence of MI and death in patients with unstable angina. In addition, low doses of aspirin appear to reduce the incidence of MI in patients with chronic stable angina. Aspirin, given in doses of 160-325 mg at the onset of treatment of MI, reduces mortality in patients presenting with unstable angina. The addition of the thioenopyridine clopidogrel to aspirin therapy reduces mortality in patients with acute coronary syndromes (Hillis and Lange, 2009); a related thioenopyridine, prasugrel, has been approved for treatment of acute coronary syndromes (Wiviott et al., 2007). Heparin, in its unfractionated form and as low-molecular-weight heparin, also reduces symptoms and prevents infarction in unstable angina (Yeghiazarians et al., 2000). Thrombin inhibitors, such as hirudin or bivalirudin, directly inhibit even clot-bound thrombin, are not affected by circulating inhibitors, and function independently of antithrombin III. Thrombolytic agents, on the other hand, are of no benefit in unstable angina (Yeghiazarians et al., 2000). Intravenous inhibitors of the platelet GPIIb/IIIa receptor (abciximab, tirofiban, and eptifibatide) are effective in preventing the complications of PCIs and in the treatment of some patients presenting with acute coronary syndromes (Hillis and Lange, 2009).

TREATMENT OF CLAUDICATION AND PERIPHERAL VASCULAR DISEASE

Most patients with peripheral vascular disease also have coronary artery disease, and the therapeutic approaches for peripheral and coronary arterial diseases overlap. Mortality in patients with peripheral vascular disease is most commonly due to cardiovascular disease (Regensteiner and Hiatt, 2002), and treatment of coronary disease remains the central focus of therapy. Many patients with advanced peripheral arterial disease are more limited by the consequences of peripheral ischemia than by myocardial ischemia. In the cerebral circulation, arterial disease may be manifest as stroke or transient ischemic attacks. The painful symptoms of peripheral arterial disease in the lower extremities (claudication) typically are provoked by exertion, with increases in skeletal muscle O_2 demand exceeding blood flow impaired by proximal stenoses. When flow to the extremities becomes critically limiting, peripheral ulcers and rest pain from tissue ischemia can become debilitating.

Most of the therapies shown to be efficacious for treatment of coronary artery disease also have a salutary effect on progression of peripheral artery disease (Hirsch et al., 2005). Reductions in cardiovascular morbidity and mortality in patients with peripheral arterial disease have been documented with anti-platelet therapy using aspirin, clopidogrel, or ticlopidine, administration of ACE inhibitors, and treatment of hyperlipidemia (Regensteiner and Hiatt, 2002). Interestingly, neither intensive treatment of diabetes mellitus nor antihypertensive therapy appears to alter the progression of symptoms of claudication. Other risk factor and lifestyle modifications remain cornerstones of therapy for patients with claudication: Physical exercise, rehabilitation, and smoking cessation have proven efficacy. Drugs used specifically in the treatment of lower-extremity claudication include pentoxifylline and cilostozol (Hiatt, 2001). Pentoxifylline is a methylxanthine derivative that is called a *rheologic modifier* for its effects on increasing the deformability of red blood cells. However, the effects of pentoxifylline on lower-extremity claudication appear to be modest. Cilostazol is an inhibitor of PDE3 and promotes accumulation of intracellular cyclic AMP in many cells, including blood platelets. Cilostazol-mediated increases in cyclic AMP inhibit platelet aggregation and promote vasodilation. The drug is metabolized by CYP3A4 and has important drug interactions with other drugs metabolized via this pathway (see Chapter 6). Cilostazol treatment improves symptoms of claudication but has no effect on cardiovascular mortality.

As a PDE3 inhibitor, cilostazol is in the same drug class as milrinone, which had been used orally as an inotropic agent for patients with heart failure. Milrinone therapy was associated with an increase in sudden cardiac death, and the oral form of the drug was withdrawn from the market. Concerns about several other inhibitors of PDE3 (inamrinone, flosequinan) followed. Cilostazol, therefore, is labeled as being contraindicated in patients with heart failure, although it is not clear that cilostazol itself leads to increased mortality in such patients. Cilostazol has been reported to increase nonsustained ventricular tachycardia; headache is the most common side effect. Other treatments for claudication, including naftidrofuryl, propionyl levocarnitine, and prostaglandins, have been explored in clinical trials, and there is some evidence that some of these therapies may be efficacious.

MECHANO-PHARMACOLOGICAL THERAPY: DRUG-ELUTING ENDOVASCULAR STENTS

Intracoronary stents can ameliorate angina and reduce adverse events in patients with acute coronary syndromes. However, the long-term efficacy of intracoronary stents is limited by subacute luminal restenosis within the stent, which occurs in a substantial minority of patients. The pathways that lead to "in-stent restenosis" are complex, but smooth muscle proliferation within the lumen of the stented artery is a common pathological finding. Local antiproliferative therapies at the time of stenting have been explored over many years, and the development of drug-eluting stents has had an important impact on clinical practice (Moses et al., 2003; Stone et al., 2004). Two drugs are currently being used in intravascular stents: paclitaxel and sirolimus. Paclitaxel is a tricyclic diterpene that inhibits cellular proliferation by binding to and stabilizing polymerized microtubules. Sirolimus is a hydrophobic macrolide that binds to the cytosolic immunophilin FKBP12; the FKBP12–sirolimus complex inhibits the mammalian kinase target of rapamycin (mTOR), thereby inhibiting cell cycle progression (see Chapter 60). Paclitaxel and sirolimus differ markedly in their mechanisms of action but share common chemical properties as hydrophobic small molecules. Differences in the intracellular targets of these two drugs are associated with marked differences in their distribution in the vascular wall (Levin et al., 2004). Stent-induced damage to the vascular endothelial cell layer can lead to thrombosis; patients typically are treated with antiplatelet agents, including clopidogrel (for up to 6 months) and aspirin (indefinitely), sometimes in conjunction with intravenous heparin and/or GPIIb/IIIa inhibitors administered at the time of the revascularization procedure. The inhibition of cellular proliferation by paclitaxel and sirolimus not only affects vascular smooth muscle cell proliferation but also attenuates the formation of an intact endothelial layer within the stented artery. Therefore, antiplatelet therapy (typically with clopidogrel) is continued for several months after intracoronary stenting with drug-eluting stents. The rate of restenosis with drug-eluting stents is reduced markedly compared with "bare metal" stents, and the ongoing development of mechanopharmacological approaches likely will lead to novel approaches in intravascular therapeutics.

An important caveat in the use of drug-eluting stents is that stent thrombosis can occur even many months after placement of the stent, sometimes temporally associated with discontinuation of antiplatelet therapy with clopidogrel (Hillis and Lange, 2009). Long-term therapy with clopidogrel added to lifelong therapy with aspirin may be considered for many patients with drug-eluting stents; such long-term therapy carries an increased risk of bleeding. In some patients, the risk-benefit ratio between bare metal and drug-eluting stents may lead to the choice of a bare metal stent. The relative efficacy, morbidity, and morbidity of percutaneous coronary revascularization versus surgical coronary artery bypass grafting are topics of active investigation and debate, well beyond the scope of this chapter. Mechano-pharmaclogical therapies influence this important ongoing discussion.

THERAPY OF HYPERTENSION

Hypertension is the most common cardiovascular disease. The prevalence of hypertension increases with advancing age; for example, about 50% of people between the ages of 60 and 69 years old have hypertension, and the prevalence is further increased beyond age 70 (Chobanian et al., 2003).

Elevated arterial pressure causes pathological changes in the vasculature and hypertrophy of the left ventricle. As a consequence, hypertension is the principal cause of stroke; a major risk factor for coronary artery disease and its attendant complications, MI and sudden cardiac death; and a major contributor to cardiac failure, renal insufficiency, and dissecting aneurysm of the aorta.

Hypertension is defined conventionally as a sustained increase in blood pressure ≥140/90 mm Hg, a criterion that characterizes a group of patients whose risk of hypertension-related cardiovascular disease is high enough to merit medical attention. Actually, the risk of both fatal and nonfatal cardiovascular disease in adults is lowest with systolic blood pressures of <120 mm Hg and diastolic BP <80 mm Hg; these risks increase progressively with higher systolic and diastolic blood pressures. Recognition of this continuously increasing risk provides a simple definition of hypertension (Chobanian et al., 2003) (Table 27–4). Although many of the clinical trials classify the severity of hypertension by diastolic pressure, progressive elevations of systolic pressure are similarly predictive of adverse cardiovascular events; at every level of diastolic pressure, risks are greater with higher levels of systolic blood pressure. Indeed, beyond age 50 years, systolic blood pressure predicts outcome better than diastolic blood pressure. Systolic blood pressure tends to rise disproportionately greater in the elderly due to decreased compliance in blood vessels associated with aging and atherosclerosis. Isolated systolic hypertension (sometimes defined as systolic BP >140-160 mm Hg with diastolic BP <90 mm Hg) is largely confined to people older than 60 years of age.

At very high blood pressures (systolic ≥210 mm Hg and/or diastolic ≥120 mm Hg), a subset of patients develops fulminant arteriopathy characterized by endothelial injury and a marked proliferation of cells in the intima, leading to intimal thickening and ultimately to arteriolar occlusion. This is the pathological basis of the syndrome of immediately life-threatening hypertension, which is associated with rapidly progressive microvascular occlusive disease in the kidney (with renal failure), brain (hypertensive encephalopathy), congestive heart failure, and pulmonary edema. These patients typically require in-hospital management on an emergency basis for prompt lowering of blood pressure. Interestingly, isolated retinal changes with papilledema in an otherwise asymptomatic patient with very high blood pressure (formerly called "malignant hypertension") may benefit from a more gradual lowering of blood pressure over days rather than hours.

Table 27–4

Criteria for Hypertension in Adults

	BLOOD PRESSURE (mm Hg)	
CLASSIFICATION	SYSTOLIC	DIASTOLIC
Normal	<120	and <80
Prehypertension	120-139	or 80-89
Hypertension, stage 1	140-159	or 90-99
Hypertension, stage 2	≥160	or ≥100

The presence of pathological changes in certain target organs heralds a worse prognosis than the same level of blood pressure in a patient lacking these findings. Consequently, retinal hemorrhages, exudates, and papilledema in the eyes indicate a far worse short-term prognosis for a given level of blood pressure. Left ventricular hypertrophy defined by electrocardiogram, or more sensitively by echocardiography, is associated with a substantially worse long-term outcome that includes a higher risk of sudden cardiac death. The risk of cardiovascular disease, disability, and death in hypertensive patients also is increased markedly by concomitant cigarette smoking, diabetes, or elevated low-density lipoprotein; the coexistence of hypertension with these risk factors increases cardiovascular morbidity and mortality to a degree that is compounded by each additional risk factor. Because the purpose of treating hypertension is to decrease cardiovascular risk, other dietary and pharmacological interventions may be required to treat these conditions.

Pharmacological treatment of patients with hypertension decreases morbidity and mortality from cardiovascular disease. Effective antihypertensive therapy markedly reduces the risk of strokes, cardiac failure, and renal insufficiency due to hypertension. However, reduction in risk of MI may be less impressive.

Principles of Antihypertensive Therapy. Nonpharmacological therapy is an important component of treatment of all patients with hypertension. In some stage 1 hypertensives (see Table 27–4), blood pressure may be adequately controlled by a combination of weight loss (in overweight individuals), restricting sodium intake, increasing aerobic exercise, and moderating consumption of alcohol. These lifestyle changes, though difficult for many to implement, may facilitate pharmacological control of blood pressure in patients whose responses to lifestyle changes alone are insufficient.

Arterial pressure is the product of cardiac output and peripheral vascular resistance. Drugs lower blood pressure by actions on peripheral resistance, cardiac output, or both. Drugs may decrease the cardiac output by inhibiting myocardial contractility or by decreasing ventricular filling pressure. Reduction in ventricular filling pressure may be achieved by actions on the venous tone or on blood volume via renal effects. Drugs can decrease peripheral resistance by acting on smooth muscle to cause relaxation of resistance vessels or by interfering with the activity of systems that produce constriction of resistance vessels (e.g., the sympathetic nervous system, the renin–angiotensin system [RAS]). In patients with isolated systolic hypertension, complex hemodynamics in a rigid arterial system contribute to increased blood pressure; drug effects may be mediated by changes in peripheral resistance but also via effects on large artery stiffness (Franklin, 2000). Antihypertensive drugs can

Table 27–5

Classification of Antihypertensive Drugs by Their Primary Site or Mechanism of Action

Diuretics (Chapter 25)

1. Thiazides and related agents (hydrochlorothiazide, chlorthalidone, chlorothiazide, indapamide, methylclothiazide, metolazone)
2. Loop diuretics (furosemide, bumetanide, torsemide, ethacrynic acid)
3. K^+-sparing diuretics (amiloride, triamterene, spironolactone)

Sympatholytic drugs (Chapter 12)

1. β receptor antagonists (metoprolol, atenolol, betaxolol, bisoprolol, carteolol, esmolol, nadolol, nebivolol, penbutolol, pindolol, propranolol, timolol)
2. α receptor antagonists (prazosin, terazosin, doxazosin, phenoxybenzamine, phentolamine)
3. Mixed α-β receptor antagonists (labetalol, carvedilol)
4. Centrally acting adrenergic agents (methyldopa, clonidine, guanabenz, guanfacine)
5. Adrenergic neuron blocking agents (guanadrel, reserpine)

Ca^{2+} channel blockers (verapamil, diltiazem, nisoldipine, felodipine, nicardipine, isradipine, amlodipine, clevidipine, nifedipine[a])

Angiotensin-converting enzyme inhibitors (Chapter 26; captopril, enalapril, lisinopril, quinapril, ramipril, benazepril, fosinopril, moexipril, perindopril, trandolapril)

AngII receptor antagonists (Chapter 26; losartan, candesartan, irbesartan, valsartan, telmisartan, eprosartan, olmesartan)

Direct Renin Inhibitor (*Chapter 26*; aliskiren)

Vasodilators

1. Arterial (hydralazine, minoxidil, diazoxide, fenoldopam)
2. Arterial and venous (nitroprusside)

[a]Extended-release nifedipine is approved for hypertension.

be classified according to their sites or mechanisms of action (Table 27–5).

The hemodynamic consequences of long-term treatment with antihypertensive agents (Table 27–6) provide a rationale for potential complementary effects of concurrent therapy with two or more drugs. The simultaneous use of drugs with similar mechanisms of action and hemodynamic effects often produces little additional benefit. However, concurrent use of drugs from different classes is a strategy for achieving effective control of blood pressure while minimizing dose-related adverse effects.

It generally is not possible to predict the responses of individuals with hypertension to any specific drug. For example, for some antihypertensive drugs, on average about two-thirds of patients will have a meaningful clinical response, whereas about one-third of patients will not respond to the same drug. Racial origin and age may have modest influence on the likelihood of a favorable response to a particular class of drugs. There is considerable interest in identifying genetic variation to improve selection of antihypertensive drugs in individual patients. Polymorphisms in a number of genes involved in the metabolism of antihypertensive drugs have been identified, for example in the CYP family (phase I metabolism) and in phase II metabolism, such as catechol-*O*-methyltransferase (see Chapters 6 and 7). While these polymorphisms change the pharmacokinetics of specific drugs, it is not clear that there will be substantial differences in efficacy given the dose range available clinically for these drugs. Consequently, identification of polymorphisms that influence pharmacodynamic responses to antihypertensive drugs are of considerable interest. Polymorphisms influencing the actions of a number of classes of antihypertensive drugs, including ACE inhibitors and diuretics, have been identified; so far, individual genes have not been found to have a major impact on pharmacodynamic responses. Genome-wide scanning may lead to identification of novel genes that are more clinically significant. Likewise, treatment may benefit from an increased understanding of the molecular and genetic bases of hypertension (Charchar et al., 2008; Shih and O'Connor, 2008).

DIURETICS

An early strategy for the management of hypertension was to alter Na^+ balance by restriction of salt in the diet. Pharmacological alteration of Na^+ balance became practical with the development of the orally active thiazide diuretics (see Chapter 25). These and related diuretic agents have antihypertensive effects when used

Table 27–6

Hemodynamic Effects of Long-Term Administration of Antihypertensive Agents

	HEART RATE	CARDIAC OUTPUT	TOTAL PERIPHERAL RESISTANCE	PLASMA VOLUME	PLASMA RENIN ACTIVITY
Diuretics	↔	↔	↓	–↓	↑
Sympatholytic agents					
Centrally acting	–↓	–↓	↓	–↑	–↓
Adrenergic neuron blockers	–↓	↓	↓	↑	–↑
α receptor antagonists	–↑	–↑	↓	–↑	↔
β receptor antagonists					
No ISA	↓	↓	–↓	–↑	↓
ISA	↔	↔	↓	–↑	–↓
Arteriolar vasodilators	↑	↑	↓	↑	↑
Ca^{2+} channel blockers	↓ or ↑	↓ or ↑	↓	–↑	–↑
ACE inhibitors	↔	↔	↓	↔	↑
AT_1 receptor antagonists	↔	↔	↓	↔	↑
Renin inhibitor	↔	↔	↓	↔	↓ (but [renin] ↑)

↑, increased; ↓, decreased; –↑, increased or no change; –↓, decreased or no change; ↔, unchanged. ACE, angiotensin-converting enzyme; AT_1, the type 1 receptor for angiotensin II; ISA, intrinsic sympathomimetic activity.

alone, and they enhance the efficacy of virtually all other antihypertensive drugs. On account of these considerations, coupled with the very large favorable experience with diuretics in randomized trials in patients with hypertension, this class of drugs remains very important in the treatment of hypertension.

The exact mechanism for reduction of arterial blood pressure by diuretics is not certain. The initial action of these drugs decreases extracellular volume by interacting with a thiazide-sensitive NaCl co-transporter (NCC; gene symbol SLC12A3) expressed in the distal convoluted tubule in the kidney, enhancing Na^+ excretion in the urine, and leading to a fall in cardiac output. However, the hypotensive effect is maintained during long-term therapy due to decreased vascular resistance; cardiac output returns to pretreatment values and extracellular volume returns almost to normal due to compensatory responses such as activation of the RAS. The explanation for the long-term vasodilation induced by these drugs is unknown. Thiazides directly promote vasodilation in isolated arteries *in vitro*. On the other hand, there is suggestive evidence that vasodilation may occur as an indirect consequence of action of the drugs on the kidneys (Ellison and Loffing, 2009).

Hydrochlorothiazide may open Ca^{2+}-activated K^+ channels, leading to hyperpolarization of vascular smooth muscle cells, which leads in turn to closing of L-type Ca^{2+} channels and lower probability of opening, resulting in decreased Ca^{2+} entry and reduced vasoconstriction. Hydrochlorothiazide also inhibits vascular carbonic anhydrase, which hypothetically may alter smooth-cell systolic pH and thereby cause opening of Ca^{2+}-activated K^+ channels with the consequences noted above (Pickkers et al., 1999). The relevance of these findings—largely assessed *in vitro*—to the observed antihypertensive effects of thiazides is speculative. The major action of these drugs on SLC12A3—expressed predominantly in the distal convoluted tubules and not in vascular smooth muscle or the heart—has contributed to repeated suggestions that these drugs decrease peripheral resistance as an indirect effect of negative sodium balance. That thiazides lose efficacy in treating hypertension in patients with co-existing renal insufficiency is compatible with this hypothesis. Moreover, carriers of rare functional mutations in SLC12A3 that decrease renal Na^+ reabsorption have lower blood pressure than appropriate controls (Ji et al., 2008); in a sense, this is an experiment of nature that may mimic the therapeutic effect of thiazides. Nonetheless, sorting out direct versus indirect actions of thiazides in promoting decreased peripheral resistance requires further experimental testing (Ellison and Loffing, 2009).

Benzothiadiazines and Related Compounds

Benzothiadiazines ("thiazides") and related diuretics are the most frequently used class of antihypertensive agents in the U.S. Following the discovery of *chlorothiazide*, a number of oral diuretics were developed that have an arylsulfonamide structure and block the NaCl co-transporter. Some of these are not benzothiadiazines but have structural features and molecular functions that are similar to the original benzothiadiazine compounds; consequently, they are designated as members of the thiazide class of diuretics. For example, chlorthalidone, one of the non-benzothiadiazines, is widely used in the treatment of hypertension, as is indapamide.

Regimen for Administration of the Thiazide-Class Diuretics in Hypertension. Because members of the thiazide class have similar pharmacological effects, they generally have been viewed as interchangeable with appropriate adjustment of dosage (see Chapter 25). However, the pharmacokinetics and pharmacodynamics of these drugs may differ, so they may not necessarily have the same clinical efficacy in treating hypertension (Carter et al., 2004). Indeed, there has been renewed debate about whether or not this group of diuretics should be considered as a class in terms of capacity to lower blood pressure and also decrease adverse clinical events due to hypertension (Sicca, 2006).

A direct comparison using 24-hour ambulatory blood pressure monitoring suggested that the antihypertensive efficacy of chlorthalidone is more favorable than that of hydrochlorothiazide (Ernst et al., 2006). Interestingly, the differences were primarily due to greater antihypertensive efficacy during the night and not with routine daytime office measurements of blood pressure. It is possible that the greater effect at night arises on account of the much longer $t_{1/2}$ of chlorthalidone (>24 hours) compared to hydrochlorothiaze (several hours). In light of the considerable clinical trial data supporting the capacity of chlorthalidone to diminish adverse cardiovascular events—in comparison to that available for currently used low doses of hydrochlorothiazide—there is a growing concern that chlorthalidone may be an underutilized drug in hypertensives requiring a diuretic.

When a thiazide-class diuretic is utilized as the sole antihypertensive drug (monotherapy), its dose-response curve for lowering blood pressure in patients with hypertension should be kept in mind. Antihypertensive effects can be achieved in many patients with as little as 12.5 mg daily of chlorthalidone or hydrochlorothiazide. Furthermore, when used as monotherapy, the maximal daily dose of thiazide-class diuretics usually should not exceed 25 mg of hydrochlorothiazide or chlorthalidone (or equivalent). Even though more diuresis can be achieved with higher doses of these diuretics, some evidence suggests that doses higher than this are not generally more efficacious in lowering blood pressure in patients with normal renal function. For example, a large study comparing 25 and 50 mg of hydrochlorothiazide daily in an elderly population did not show a greater decrease in blood pressure with the larger dose (Medical Research Council Working Party, 1987). However, these conclusions are based on conventional rather than ambulatory blood pressure measurements. Other studies suggest that low doses of hydrochlorothiazide have inadequate effects on blood pressure when monitored in this more detailed manner (Lacourcière et al., 1995). In summary, recent critical attention has been focused on whether low doses of hydrochlorothiazide are as efficacious as low doses of chlorthalidone and whether low doses of hydrochlorothiazide are efficacious as monotherapy in protecting against the cardiovascular complications of hypertension. Relatively low doses of either thiazide are not at the top of the dose-response curve for adverse effects such as K^+ wasting and inhibition of uric acid excretion, emphasizing the importance of knowledge about the dose-response relationships for both beneficial and adverse effects.

In the clinical trials of antihypertensive therapy in the elderly that demonstrated the best outcomes in cardiovascular morbidity and mortality, 25 mg of hydrochlorothiazide or chlorthalidone was the maximum dose given; if this dose did not achieve the target blood pressure reduction, treatment with a second drug was initiated (SHEP Cooperative Research Group, 1991; Dahlöf et al., 1991; Medical Research Council Working Party, 1992). With respect to safety, a case-control study (Siscovick et al., 1994) found a dose-dependent increase in the occurrence of sudden death at doses of hydrochlorothiazide >25 mg daily. This finding supports the hypothesis proposed by the Multiple Risk Factor Intervention Trial Research Group (1982), suggesting that increased cardiovascular mortality is associated with higher diuretic doses. Taken together, clinical studies indicate that if adequate blood pressure reduction is not achieved with the 25-mg daily dose of hydrochlorothiazide or chlorthalidone, a second drug should be added rather than increasing the dose of diuretic. There is some concern that thiazide diuretics, especially at higher doses and in the absence of K^+-sparing diuretics or K^+ supplements, may increase the risk of sudden death. However, their overall therapeutic benefits are well established.

Urinary K^+ loss can be a problem with thiazides. ACE inhibitors and angiotensin receptor antagonists will attenuate diuretic-induced loss of K^+ to some degree, and this is a consideration if a second drug is required to achieve further blood pressure reduction beyond that attained with the diuretic alone. Because the diuretic and hypotensive effects of these drugs are greatly enhanced when they are given in combination, care should be taken to initiate combination therapy with low doses of each of these drugs. Administration of ACE inhibitors or angiotensin receptor antagonists together with other K^+-sparing agents or with K^+ supplements requires great caution; combining K^+-sparing agents with each other or with K^+ supplementation can cause potentially dangerous hyperkalemia in some patients.

In contrast to the limitation on the dose of thiazide-class diuretics used as monotherapy, the treatment of severe hypertension that is unresponsive to three or more drugs may require larger doses of the thiazide-class diuretics. Indeed, hypertensive patients may become

promotes endothelial cell dependent vasodilation via activation of the NO pathway (Pedersen and Cockcroft, 2006).

Pharmacological Effects. The β adrenergic blockers vary in their selectivity for the β_1 receptor subtype, presence of partial agonist or intrinsic sympathomimetic activity, and vasodilating capacity. Despite these differences, all of the β receptor antagonists are effective as antihypertensive agents. However, these differences do influence the clinical pharmacokinetics and spectrum of adverse effects of the various drugs. Drugs without intrinsic sympathomimetic activity produce an initial reduction in cardiac output and a reflex-induced rise in peripheral resistance, generally with no net change in arterial pressure. In patients who respond with a reduction in blood pressure, peripheral resistance gradually returns to pretreatment values or less. Generally, persistently reduced cardiac output and possibly decreased peripheral resistance accounts for the reduction in arterial pressure. Drugs with intrinsic sympathomimetic activity produce lesser decreases in resting heart rate and cardiac output; the fall in arterial pressure correlates with a fall in vascular resistance below pretreatment levels, possibly because of stimulation of vascular β_2 receptors that mediate vasodilation.

The clinical significance, if any, of these differences is uncertain. However, there is increasing concern that some β receptor blockers, particularly atenolol, may have less efficacy as monotherapy for hypertension than some other drug classes in terms of decreasing risk of adverse cardiovascular consequences of hypertension, particularly due to stroke and coronary artery disease (Carlberg et al., 2004; Kaplan, 2008; Pedersen and Cockcroft, 2009). Particular interest has focused on evidence suggesting that atenolol-based therapy may not lower central (aortic) blood pressure as effectively as it appears when conventionally measured in the brachial artery using a standard arm cuff (CAFE Investigators, 2006). However, teasing out the comparative efficacy of the various classes of antihypertensive drugs represents a complex undertaking. Results of a detailed meta-analysis of 147 randomized trials of blood pressure reduction showed that, regardless of blood pressure before treatment, lowering systolic blood pressure by 10 mm Hg or diastolic blood pressure by 5 mm Hg using any of the main classes of antihypertensive drugs significantly reduces coronary events and stroke without an increase in nonvascular mortality (Law et al., 2009).

Adverse Effects and Precautions. The adverse effects of β adrenergic blocking agents are discussed in Chapter 12. These drugs should be avoided in patients with reactive airway disease (asthma) or with SA or AV nodal dysfunction or in combination with other drugs that inhibit AV conduction, such as verapamil. The risk of hypoglycemic reactions may be increased in diabetics taking insulin. β Receptor antagonists without intrinsic sympathomimetic activity increase concentrations of triglycerides in plasma and lower those of HDL cholesterol without changing total cholesterol concentrations. β receptor blocking agents with intrinsic sympathomimetic activity have little or no effect on blood lipids or increase HDL cholesterol. The long-term consequences of these effects are unknown.

Sudden discontinuation of β adrenergic blockers can produce a withdrawal syndrome that is likely due to upregulation of β receptors during blockade, causing enhanced tissue sensitivity to endogenous catecholamines; this can exacerbate the symptoms of coronary artery disease. The result, especially in active patients, can be rebound hypertension. Thus, β adrenergic blockers should not be discontinued abruptly except under close observation; dosage should be tapered gradually over 10-14 days prior to discontinuation.

NSAIDs such as *indomethacin* can blunt the antihypertensive effect of propranolol and probably other β receptor antagonists. This effect may be related to inhibition of vascular synthesis of prostacyclin, as well as to retention of Na^+ (Beckmann et al., 1988).

Epinephrine. can produce severe hypertension and bradycardia when a nonselective β antagonist is present. The hypertension is due to the unopposed stimulation of α adrenergic receptors when vascular β_2 receptors are blocked; the bradycardia is the result of reflex vagal stimulation. Such paradoxical hypertensive responses to β receptor antagonists have been observed in patients with hypoglycemia or pheochromocytoma, during withdrawal from *clonidine*, following administration of epinephrine as a therapeutic agent, or in association with the illicit use of cocaine.

Therapeutic Uses. The β receptor antagonists provide effective therapy for all grades of hypertension. Despite marked differences in their pharmacokinetic properties, the antihypertensive effect of all the β blockers is of sufficient duration to permit once- or twice-daily administration. Populations that tend to have a lesser antihypertensive response to β blocking agents include the elderly and African-Americans. However, intraindividual differences in antihypertensive efficacy are generally much larger than statistical evidence of differences between racial or age-related groups. Consequently, these observations should not discourage the use of these drugs in individual patients in groups reported to be less responsive.

The β receptor antagonists usually do not cause retention of salt and water, and administration of a diuretic is not necessary to avoid edema or the development of tolerance. However, diuretics do have additive antihypertensive effects when combined with β blockers. The combination of a β receptor antagonist, a diuretic, and a vasodilator is effective for patients who require a third drug. β receptor antagonists are highly preferred drugs for hypertensive patients with conditions such as MI, ischemic heart disease, or congestive heart failure. However, for other hypertensive patients, enthusiasm for their early use in treatment has diminished, as noted earlier.

α_1 Adrenergic Receptor Antagonists

The availability of drugs that selectively block α_1 adrenergic receptors without affecting α_2 adrenergic receptors adds another group of antihypertensive agents. The pharmacology of these drugs is discussed in detail in Chapter 12. Prazosin, terazosin, and doxazosin are the agents that are available for the treatment of hypertension.

Pharmacological Effects. Initially, α_1 adrenergic receptor antagonists reduce arteriolar resistance and increase venous capacitance; this causes a sympathetically mediated reflex increase in heart rate and plasma renin activity. During long-term therapy, vasodilation persists, but cardiac output, heart rate, and plasma renin activity return to normal. Renal blood flow is unchanged during therapy with an α_1 receptor antagonist. The α_1 adrenergic blockers cause a variable amount of postural hypotension, depending on the plasma volume. Retention of salt and water occurs in many patients during continued administration, and this attenuates the postural hypotension. α_1 Receptor antagonists reduce plasma concentrations of triglycerides and total LDL cholesterol and increase HDL cholesterol. These potentially favorable effects on lipids persist when a thiazide-type diuretic is given concurrently. The long-term consequences of these small, drug-induced changes in lipids are unknown.

Adverse Effects. The use of doxazosin as monotherapy for hypertension increased the risk for developing congestive heart failure (ALLHAT Officers, 2002). This may be a class effect that represents an adverse effect of all of the α_1 receptor antagonists. However, this interpretation of the outcome of the ALLHAT study is controversial.

A major precaution regarding the use of the α_1 receptor antagonists for hypertension is the so-called first-dose phenomenon, in which symptomatic orthostatic hypotension occurs within 30-90 minutes (or longer) of the initial dose of the drug or after a dosage increase. This effect may occur in up to 50% of patients, especially in patients who are already receiving a diuretic or an α receptor antagonist. After the first few doses, patients develop a tolerance to this marked hypotensive response.

Therapeutic Uses. α_1 Receptor antagonists are not recommended as monotherapy for hypertensive patients primarily as a consequence of the ALLHAT study. Consequently, they are used primarily in conjunction with diuretics, β blockers, and other antihypertensive agents. β Receptor antagonists enhance the efficacy of the α_1 blockers. α_1 Receptor antagonists are not the drugs of choice in patients with pheochromocytoma, because a vasoconstrictor response to epinephrine can still result from activation of unblocked vascular α_2 adrenergic receptors. α_1 Receptor antagonists are attractive drugs for hypertensive patients with benign prostatic hyperplasia, because they also improve urinary symptoms.

COMBINED α_1 AND β ADRENERGIC RECEPTOR ANTAGONISTS

Labetalol (see Chapter 12) is an equimolar mixture of four stereoisomers. One isomer is an α_1 antagonist (like prazosin), another is a nonselective β antagonist with partial agonist activity (like pindolol), and the other two isomers are inactive. Because of its capacity to block α_1 adrenergic receptors, labetalol given intravenously can reduce blood pressure sufficiently rapidly to be useful for the treatment of hypertensive emergencies. Labetalol has efficacy and adverse effects that would be expected with any combination of β and α_1 receptor antagonists; it also has the disadvantages that are inherent in fixed-dose combination products: the extent of α-receptor antagonism compared to β receptor antagonism is somewhat unpredictable and varies from patient to patient.

Carvedilol (see Chapters 12) is a β receptor antagonist with α_1 receptor antagonist activity. The drug has been approved for the treatment of hypertension and symptomatic heart failure. The ratio of α_1 to β receptor antagonist potency for carvedilol is approximately 1:10. Carvedilol undergoes oxidative metabolism and glucuronidation in the liver; the oxidative metabolism occurs via CYP2D6. Carvedilol reduces mortality in patients with congestive heart failure associated with systolic dysfunction when used as an adjunct to therapy with diuretics and ACE inhibitors. It should not be given to those patients with decompensated heart failure who are dependent on sympathetic stimulation. As with labetalol, the long-term efficacy and side effects of carvedilol in hypertension are predictable based on its properties as a β and α_1 adrenergic receptor antagonist.

Nebivolol is a β_1 selective adrenergic antagonist that also promotes vasodilatation; rather than blocking α_1 receptors, nebivolol augments arterial smooth muscle relaxation via NO (Veverka et al., 2006). In addition, nebivolol has agonist activity at β_3 receptors, although the clinical significance of this effect is not known.

Methyldopa

Methyldopa is a centrally acting antihypertensive agent. It is a prodrug that exerts its antihypertensive action via an active metabolite. Although used frequently as an antihypertensive agent in the past, methyldopa's significant adverse effects limit its current use largely to treatment of hypertension in pregnancy, where it has a record for safety.

Methyldopa (α-methyl-3,4-dihydroxy-L-phenylalanine), an analog of 3,4-dihydroxyphenylalanine (DOPA), is metabolized by the L-aromatic amino acid decarboxylase in adrenergic neurons to α-methyldopamine, which then is converted to α-methylnorepinephrine. α-Methylnorepinephrine is stored in the secretory vesicles of adrenergic neurons, substituting for norepinephrine (NE) itself. Consequently, when the adrenergic neuron discharges its neurotransmitter, α-methylnorepinephrine is released instead of norepinephrine. α-Methylnorepinephrine acts in the central nervous system (CNS) to inhibit adrenergic neuronal outflow from the brainstem and probably acts as an agonist at presynaptic α_2 adrenergic receptors in the brainstem, attenuating NE release and thereby reducing the output of vasoconstrictor adrenergic signals to the peripheral sympathetic nervous system.

Absorption, Metabolism, and Excretion. Because methyldopa is a prodrug that is metabolized in the brain to the active form, its concentration in plasma has less relevance for its effects than that for many other drugs. Peak concentrations in plasma occur after 2-3 hours. The drug is eliminated with a $t_{1/2}$ of ~2 hours. Methyldopa is excreted in the urine primarily as the sulfate conjugate (50-70%) and as the parent drug (25%). The remaining fraction is excreted as other metabolites, including methyldopamine, methylnorepinephrine, and *O*-methylated products of these catecholamines. The $t_{1/2}$ of methyldopa is prolonged to 4-6 hours in patients with renal failure.

In spite of its rapid absorption and short $t_{1/2}$, the peak effect of methyldopa is delayed for 6-8 hours, even after intravenous administration, and the duration of action of a single dose is usually about 24 hours; this permits once- or twice-daily dosing. The discrepancy between the effects of methyldopa and the measured concentrations of the drug in plasma is most likely related to the time required for transport into the CNS, conversion to the active metabolite storage of α-methylnorepinephrine and its subsequent release in the vicinity of relevant α_2 receptors in the CNS. This is a good example of the potential for a complex relationship between a drug's pharmacokinetics and its pharmacodynamics. Patients with renal failure are more sensitive to the antihypertensive effect of methyldopa, but it is not known if this is due to alteration in excretion of the drug or to an increase in transport into the CNS.

Adverse Effects and Precautions. Methyldopa produces sedation that is largely transient. A diminution in psychic energy may persist in some patients, and depression occurs occasionally. Methyldopa may produce dryness of the mouth. Other adverse effects include diminished libido, parkinsonian signs, and hyperprolactinemia that may become sufficiently pronounced to cause gynecomastia and galactorrhea. Methyldopa may precipitate severe bradycardia and sinus arrest.

Methyldopa also produces some adverse effects that are not related to its pharmacological action. Hepatotoxicity, sometimes associated with fever, is an uncommon but potentially serious toxic effect of methyldopa. At least 20% of patients who receive methyldopa for a year develop a positive Coombs test (antiglobulin test) that is due to autoantibodies directed against the Rh antigen on erythrocytes. The development of a positive Coombs test is not necessarily an indication to stop treatment with methyldopa; 1-5% of these patients will develop a hemolytic anemia that requires prompt discontinuation of the drug. The Coombs test may remain positive for as long as a year after discontinuation of methyldopa, but the hemolytic anemia usually resolves within a matter of weeks. Severe hemolysis may be attenuated by treatment with glucocorticoids. Adverse effects that are even more rare include leukopenia, thrombocytopenia, red cell aplasia, lupus erythematosus–like syndrome, lichenoid and granulomatous skin eruptions, myocarditis, retroperitoneal fibrosis, pancreatitis, diarrhea, and malabsorption.

Therapeutic Uses. Methyldopa is a preferred drug for treatment of hypertension during pregnancy based on its effectiveness and safety for both mother and fetus. The usual initial dose of methyldopa is 250 mg twice daily, and there is little additional effect with doses >2 g/day. Administration of a single daily dose of methyldopa at bedtime minimizes sedative effects, but administration twice daily is required for some patients.

Clonidine, Guanabenz, and Guanfacine

The detailed pharmacology of the α_2 adrenergic agonists clonidine, *guanabenz*, and *guanfacine* is discussed in Chapter 12. These drugs stimulate the α_{2A} subtype of α_2 adrenergic receptors in the brainstem, resulting in a reduction in sympathetic outflow from the CNS (Macmillan et al., 1996). The decrease in plasma concentrations of NE is correlated directly with the hypotensive effect (Goldstein et al., 1985). Patients who have had a spinal cord transection above the level of the sympathetic outflow tracts do not display a hypotensive response to clonidine. At doses higher than those required to stimulate central α_{2A} receptors, these drugs can activate α_2 receptors of the α_{2B} subtype on vascular smooth muscle cells (MacMillan et al., 1996). This effect accounts for the initial vasoconstriction that is seen when overdoses of these drugs are taken, and may be responsible for the loss of therapeutic effect that is observed with high doses. A major limitation in the use of these drugs is the paucity of information about their efficacy in reducing the risk of cardiovascular consequences of hypertension.

Pharmacological Effects. The α_2 adrenergic agonists lower arterial pressure by an effect on both cardiac output and peripheral resistance. In the supine position, when the sympathetic tone to the vasculature is low, the major effect is to reduce both heart rate and stroke volume; however, in the upright position, when sympathetic outflow to the vasculature is normally increased, these drugs reduce vascular resistance. This action may lead to postural hypotension. The decrease in cardiac sympathetic tone leads to a reduction in myocardial contractility and heart rate that could promote congestive heart failure in susceptible patients.

Adverse Effects and Precautions. Many patients experience annoying and sometimes intolerable adverse effects with these drugs. Sedation and xerostomia are prominent adverse effects. The xerostomia may be accompanied by dry nasal mucosa, dry eyes, and parotid gland swelling and pain. Postural hypotension and erectile dysfunction may be prominent in some patients. Clonidine may produce a lower incidence of dry mouth and sedation when given transdermally, perhaps because high peak concentrations are avoided. Less common CNS side effects include sleep disturbances with vivid dreams or nightmares, restlessness, and depression. Cardiac effects related to the sympatholytic action of these drugs include symptomatic bradycardia and sinus arrest in patients with dysfunction of the SA node and AV block in patients with AV nodal disease or in patients taking other drugs that depress AV conduction. Some 15-20% of patients who receive transdermal clonidine may develop contact dermatitis.

Sudden discontinuation of clonidine and related α_2 adrenergic agonists may cause a withdrawal syndrome consisting of headache, apprehension, tremors, abdominal pain, sweating, and tachycardia. The arterial blood pressure may rise to levels above those that were present prior to treatment, but the syndrome may occur in the absence of an overshoot in pressure. Symptoms typically occur 18-36 hours after the drug is stopped and are associated with increased sympathetic discharge, as evidenced by elevated plasma and urine concentrations of catecholamines. The exact incidence of the withdrawal syndrome is not known, but it is likely dose related and more dangerous in patients with poorly controlled hypertension. Rebound hypertension also has been seen after discontinuation of transdermal administration of clonidine (Metz et al., 1987).

Treatment of the withdrawal syndrome depends on the urgency of reducing the arterial blood pressure. In the absence of life-threatening target organ damage, patients can be treated by restoring the use of clonidine. If a more rapid effect is required, *sodium nitroprusside* or a combination of an α and β adrenergic blocker is appropriate. β Adrenergic blocking agents should not be used alone in this setting, because they may accentuate the hypertension by allowing unopposed α adrenergic vasoconstriction caused by activation of the sympathetic nervous system and elevated circulating catecholamines.

Because perioperative hypertension has been described in patients in whom clonidine was withdrawn the night before surgery, surgical patients who are being treated with an α_2 adrenergic agonist either should be switched to another drug prior to elective surgery or should receive their morning dose and/or transdermal clonidine prior to the procedure. All patients who receive one of these drugs should be warned of the potential danger of discontinuing the drug abruptly, and patients suspected of being noncompliant with medications should not be given α_2 adrenergic agonists for hypertension.

Adverse drug interactions with α_2 adrenergic agonists are rare. Diuretics predictably potentiate the hypotensive effect of these drugs. Tricyclic antidepressants may inhibit the antihypertensive effect of clonidine, but the mechanism of this interaction is not known.

Therapeutic Uses. The CNS effects are such that this class of drugs is not a leading option for monotherapy of hypertension. Indeed, there is no fixed place for these drugs in the treatment of hypertension. They effectively lower blood pressure in some patients who have not responded adequately to combinations of other agents. Enthusiasm for these drugs is diminished by the relative absence of evidence demonstrating reduction in risk of adverse cardiovascular events.

Clonidine has been used in hypertensive patients for the diagnosis of pheochromocytoma. The lack of suppression of the plasma concentration of NE to >500 pg/mL 3 hours after an oral dose of 0.3 mg of clonidine suggests the presence of such a tumor. A modification of this test, wherein overnight urinary excretion of NE and epinephrine is measured after administration of a 0.3-mg dose of clonidine at bedtime, may be useful when results based on plasma NE concentrations are equivocal. Other uses for α_2 adrenergic agonists are discussed in Chapters 12, 13, and 23.

Guanadrel

Guanadrel specifically inhibits the function of peripheral postganglionic adrenergic neurons. The structure of guanadrel, which contains the strongly basic guanidine group, is:

GUANADREL

Locus and Mechanism of Action. Guanadrel is an exogenous false neurotransmitter that is accumulated, stored, and released like NE but is inactive at adrenergic receptors. The drug reaches its site of action by active transport into the neuron by the same transporter that is responsible for the reuptake of NE (see Chapter 8). In the neuron, guanadrel is concentrated within the adrenergic storage vesicle, where it replaces NE. During chronic administration, guanadrel acts as a "false neurotransmitter": It is present in storage vesicles, depletes the normal transmitter, and can be released by stimuli that normally release NE, but is inactive at adrenergic receptors. This replacement of NE with an inactive transmitter is probably the principal mechanism of action of guanadrel. Because guanadrel can promote NE release from pheochromocytomas, it is contraindicated in those patients.

Pharmacological Effects. Essentially all of the therapeutic and adverse effects of guanadrel result from functional sympathetic blockade. The antihypertensive effect is achieved by a reduction in peripheral vascular resistance that results from inhibition of α receptor–mediated vasoconstriction. Consequently, arterial pressure is reduced modestly in the supine position when sympathetic activity is usually low, but the pressure can fall to a greater extent during situations in which reflex sympathetic activation is an important mechanism for maintaining arterial pressure, particularly when standing.

Absorption, Distribution, Metabolism, and Excretion. Because guanadrel must be transported into and accumulate in adrenergic neurons, the maximum effect on blood pressure is not seen until 4-5 hours. The $t_{1/2}$ of the pharmacological effect of guanadrel is determined by the drug's persistence in this neuronal pool and is probably at least 10 hours.

Adverse Effects. Guanadrel produces undesirable effects that are related to sympathetic blockade. Symptomatic hypotension during standing, exercise, ingestion of alcohol, or in hot weather is the result of the lack of sympathetic compensation for these stresses. A general feeling of fatigue and lassitude is partially, but not entirely, related to postural hypotension. Sexual dysfunction usually presents as delayed or retrograde ejaculation. Diarrhea also may occur.

Because guanadrel is actively transported to its site of action, drugs that block or compete for the catecholamine transporter on the presynaptic membrane will inhibit the effect of guanadrel. Such drugs include the tricyclic antidepressants *cocaine*, *chlorpromazine*, *ephedrine*, *phenylpropanolamine*, and *amphetamine* (see Chapter 8).

Therapeutic Uses. Because of the availability of a number of drugs that lower blood pressure without producing similar adverse effects, guanadrel is used very rarely; the drug is no longer marketed in the U.S. The usual starting dose is 10 mg daily, and side effects can be minimized by not exceeding 20 mg daily.

Reserpine

Reserpine was the first drug that was found to interfere with the function of the sympathetic nervous system in humans, and its use began the modern era of effective pharmacotherapy of hypertension.

Reserpine is an alkaloid extracted from the root of *Rauwolfia serpentina*, a climbing shrub indigenous to India. Ancient Hindu Ayurvedic writings describe medicinal uses of the plant; Sen and Bose described its use in the Indian biomedical literature. However, rauwolfia alkaloids were not used in western medicine until the mid-1950s.

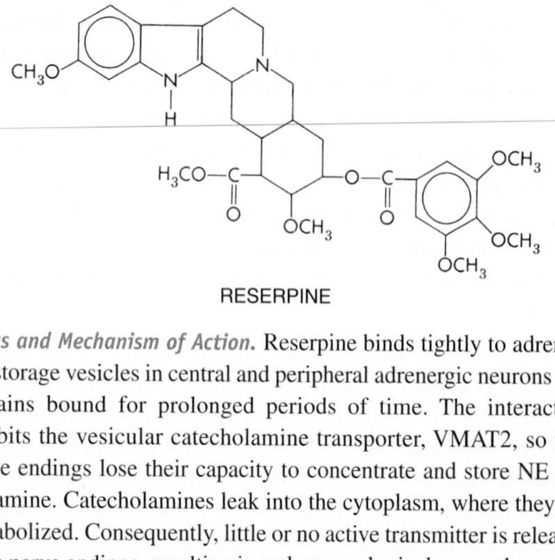

CH_3O N H N H_3CO—C O OCH_3 O—C O OCH_3 OCH_3 OCH_3

RESERPINE

Locus and Mechanism of Action. Reserpine binds tightly to adrenergic storage vesicles in central and peripheral adrenergic neurons and remains bound for prolonged periods of time. The interaction inhibits the vesicular catecholamine transporter, VMAT2, so that nerve endings lose their capacity to concentrate and store NE and dopamine. Catecholamines leak into the cytoplasm, where they are metabolized. Consequently, little or no active transmitter is released from nerve endings, resulting in a pharmacological sympathectomy. Recovery of sympathetic function requires synthesis of new storage vesicles, which takes days to weeks after discontinuation of the drug. Because reserpine depletes amines in the CNS as well as in the peripheral adrenergic neuron, it is probable that its antihypertensive effects are related to both central and peripheral actions.

Pharmacological Effects. Both cardiac output and peripheral vascular resistance are reduced during long-term therapy with reserpine.

Absorption, Metabolism, and Excretion. Few data are available on the pharmacokinetic properties of reserpine because of the lack of an assay capable of detecting low concentrations of the drug or its metabolites. Reserpine that is bound to isolated storage vesicles cannot be removed by dialysis, indicating that the binding is not in equilibrium with the surrounding medium. Because of the irreversible nature of reserpine binding, the amount of drug in plasma is unlikely to bear any consistent relationship to drug concentration at the site of action. Free reserpine is entirely metabolized; none of the parent drug is excreted unchanged.

Toxicity and Precautions. Most adverse effects of reserpine are due to its effect on the CNS. Sedation and inability to concentrate or perform complex tasks are the most common adverse effects. More serious is the occasional psychotic depression that can lead to suicide. Depression usually appears insidiously over many weeks or months and may not be attributed to the drug because of the delayed and gradual onset of symptoms. Reserpine must be discontinued at the first sign of depression; reserpine-induced depression may last several months after the drug is discontinued. The risk of depression is likely dose related. Depression appears to be uncommon, but not unknown, with doses of 0.25 mg/day or less. The drug should never be given to patients with a history of depression. Other adverse effects include nasal stuffiness and exacerbation of peptic ulcer disease, which is uncommon with small oral doses.

Therapeutic Uses. With the availability of newer drugs that are both effective and well tolerated, the use of reserpine has diminished because of its CNS side effects. Nonetheless, there has been some recent interest in using reserpine at low doses, in combination with diuretics, in the treatment of hypertension, especially in the elderly. Reserpine is used once daily with a diuretic, and several weeks are necessary to achieve a maximum effect. The daily dose should be limited to 0.25 mg or less, and as little as 0.05 mg/day may be efficacious when a diuretic is also used. One advantage of reserpine is that it is considerably less expensive than other antihypertensive drugs; thus, it is still used in developing nations.

Metyrosine

Metyrosine (DEMSER) is (–)-α-methyl-L-tyrosine. Metyrosine inhibits tyrosine hydroxylase, the enzyme that catalyzes the conversion of tyrosine to DOPA and the rate-limiting step in catecholamine biosynthesis (see Chapter 8). At a dose of 1-4 g/day, metyrosine decreases catecholamine biosynthesis by 35-80% in patients with pheochromocytoma. The maximal decrease in synthesis occurs only after several days and may be assessed by measurements of urinary catecholamines and their metabolites.

Metyrosine is used as an adjuvant to phenoxybenzamine and other α adrenergic blocking agents for the management of pheochromocytoma and in the preoperative preparation of patients for resection of pheochromocytoma. Metyrosine carries a risk of crystalluria, which can be minimized by maintaining a daily urine volume of >2 L. Other adverse effects include orthostatic hypotension, sedation, extrapyramidal signs, diarrhea, anxiety, and psychic disturbances. Doses must be titrated carefully to achieve significant inhibition of catecholamine biosynthesis and yet minimize these substantive side effects.

Ca^{2+} CHANNEL ANTAGONISTS

Ca^{2+} channel blocking agents are an important group of drugs for the treatment of hypertension. The general pharmacology of these drugs is presented earlier in this chapter. The basis for their use in hypertension comes from the understanding that hypertension generally is the result of increased peripheral vascular resistance. Because contraction of vascular smooth muscle is dependent on the free intracellular concentration of Ca^{2+}, inhibition of transmembrane movement of Ca^{2+} through voltage-sensitive Ca^{2+} channels can decrease the total amount of Ca^{2+} that reaches intracellular sites. Indeed, all of the Ca^{2+} channel blockers lower blood pressure by relaxing arteriolar smooth muscle and decreasing peripheral vascular resistance (Weber, 2002). As a consequence of a decrease in peripheral vascular resistance, the Ca^{2+} channel blockers evoke a baroreceptor-mediated sympathetic discharge. In the case of the dihydropyridines, tachycardia may occur from the adrenergic stimulation of the SA node; this response is generally quite modest except when the drug is administered rapidly. Tachycardia is typically minimal to absent with verapamil and diltiazem because of the direct negative chronotropic effect of these two drugs. Indeed, the concurrent use of a β receptor antagonist drug may magnify negative chronotropic effects of these drugs or cause heart block in susceptible patients. Consequently, the concurrent use of β receptor antagonists with either verapamil or diltiazem may be problematic.

Ca^{2+} channel blockers are effective when used alone or in combination with other drugs for the treatment of hypertension; this view has been strengthened by a number of recent large clinical trials (Dahlöf et al., 2005; Jamerson et al., 2008).

Oral administration of nifedipine as an approach to urgent reduction of blood pressure has been abandoned. Sublingual administration does not achieve the maximum plasma concentration any more quickly than does oral administration. Moreover, in the absence of deleterious consequences of high arterial pressure, data do not support the rapid lowering of blood pressure. There is no place in the treatment of hypertension for the use of nifedipine or other dihydropyridine Ca^{2+} channel blockers with short half-lives when administered in a standard (immediate-release) formulation, because of the oscillation in blood pressure and concurrent surges in sympathetic reflex activity within each dosage interval. As noted earlier, parenteral administration of the novel dihydropyridine clevidipine may be useful in treating severe or perioperative hypertension.

Compared with other classes of antihypertensive agents, there may be a greater frequency of achieving blood pressure control with Ca^{2+} channel blockers as monotherapy in elderly subjects and in African-Americans, population groups in which the low renin status is more prevalent. However, intrasubject variability is more important than relatively small differences between population groups. Ca^{2+} channel blockers are effective in lowering blood pressure and decreasing cardiovascular events in the elderly with isolated systolic hypertension (Staessen et al., 1997). Indeed, these drugs may be a preferred treatment in patients with isolated systolic hypertension.

ANGIOTENSIN-CONVERTING ENZYME INHIBITORS

Angiotensin II is an important regulator of cardiovascular function (see Chapter 26). The ability to reduce levels of AngII with orally effective inhibitors of ACE represents an important advance in the treatment of hypertension. Captopril was the first such agent to be developed for the treatment of hypertension. Since then, enalapril, lisinopril, quinapril, ramipril, benazepril, moexipril, fosinopril, trandolapril, and perindopril also have become available. These drugs have proven to be very useful for the treatment of hypertension because of their efficacy and their very favorable profile of adverse effects, which enhances patient adherence. Chapter 26 presents the pharmacology of ACE inhibitors in detail.

The ACE inhibitors appear to confer a special advantage in the treatment of patients with diabetes, slowing the development and progression of diabetic glomerulopathy. They also are effective in slowing the progression of other forms of chronic renal disease, such as glomerulosclerosis, and many of these patients also have hypertension. An ACE inhibitor is the preferred initial agent in these patients. Patients with hypertension and ischemic heart disease are candidates for treatment with ACE inhibitors; administration of ACE inhibitors in the immediate post-MI period has been shown to improve ventricular function and reduce morbidity and mortality (see Chapter 28).

The endocrine consequences of inhibiting the biosynthesis of AngII are of importance in a number of facets of hypertension treatment. Because ACE inhibitors blunt the rise in aldosterone concentrations in response to Na^+ loss, the normal role of aldosterone to oppose diuretic-induced natriuresis is diminished. Consequently, ACE inhibitors tend to enhance the efficacy of diuretic drugs. This means that even very small doses of diuretics may substantially improve the antihypertensive efficacy of ACE inhibitors; conversely, the use of high doses of diuretics together with ACE inhibitors may lead to excessive reduction in blood pressure and to Na^+ loss in some patients.

The attenuation of aldosterone production by ACE inhibitors also influences K^+ homeostasis. There is only a very small and clinically unimportant rise in serum K^+ when these agents are used alone in patients with

expression of hypoxia-inducible factor (HIF-1) and downstream targets of HIF in vascular smooth muscle cells (Knowles et al., 2004). However, the relationship between these pharmacological effects and the clinical consequence of use of hydralazine are unclear. In addition, hydralazine has been found to induce DNA demethylation (Arce et al., 2006).

The drug does not relax venous smooth muscle. Hydralazine-induced vasodilation is associated with powerful stimulation of the sympathetic nervous system, likely due to baroreceptor-mediated reflexes, which results in increased heart rate and contractility, increased plasma renin activity, and fluid retention; all of these effects tend to counteract the antihypertensive effect of hydralazine.

Pharmacological Effects. Most of the effects of hydralazine are confined to the cardiovascular system. The decrease in blood pressure after administration of hydralazine is associated with a selective decrease in vascular resistance in the coronary, cerebral, and renal circulations, with a smaller effect in skin and muscle. Because of preferential dilation of arterioles over veins, postural hypotension is not a common problem; hydralazine lowers blood pressure similarly in the supine and upright positions.

Absorption, Metabolism, and Excretion. Hydralazine is well absorbed through the gastrointestinal tract, but the systemic bioavailability is low (16% in fast acetylators and 35% in slow acetylators). Hydralazine is *N*-acetylated in the bowel and/or the liver. The $t_{1/2}$ of hydralazine is 1 hour, and systemic clearance of the drug is ~50 mL/kg/min.

The rate of acetylation is genetically determined; about half of the U.S. population acetylates rapidly, and half do so slowly. The acetylated compound is inactive; thus, the dose necessary to produce a systemic effect is larger in fast acetylators. Because the systemic clearance exceeds hepatic blood flow, extrahepatic metabolism must occur. Indeed, hydralazine rapidly combines with circulating α-keto acids to form hydrazones, and the major metabolite recovered from the plasma is hydralazine pyruvic acid hydrazone. This metabolite has a longer $t_{1/2}$ than hydralazine, but it does not appear to be very active. Although the rate of acetylation is an important determinant of the bioavailability of hydralazine, it does not play a role in the systemic elimination of the drug, probably because the hepatic clearance is so high that systemic elimination is principally a function of hepatic blood flow.

The peak concentration of hydralazine in plasma and the peak hypotensive effect of the drug occur within 30-120 minutes of ingestion. Although its $t_{1/2}$ in plasma is about an hour, the duration of the hypotensive effect of hydralazine can last as long as 12 hours. There is no clear explanation for this discrepancy.

Toxicity and Precautions. Two types of adverse effects occur after the use of hydralazine. The first, which are extensions of the pharmacological effects of the drug, include headache, nausea, flushing, hypotension, palpitations, tachycardia, dizziness, and angina pectoris. Myocardial ischemia can occur on account of increased O_2 demand induced by the baroreceptor reflex-induced stimulation of the sympathetic nervous system. Following parenteral administration to patients with coronary artery disease, the myocardial ischemia may be sufficiently severe and protracted to cause frank MI. For this reason, parenteral administration of hydralazine is not advisable in hypertensive patients with coronary artery disease, hypertensive patients with multiple cardiovascular risk factors, or older patients. In addition, if the drug is used alone, there may be salt retention with development of high-output congestive heart failure. When combined with a β adrenergic receptor blocker and a diuretic, hydralazine is better tolerated, although adverse effects such as headache are still commonly described and may necessitate discontinuation of the drug.

The second type of adverse effect is caused by immunological reactions, of which the drug-induced lupus syndrome is the most common. Administration of hydralazine also can result in an illness that resembles serum sickness, hemolytic anemia, vasculitis, and rapidly progressive glomerulonephritis. The mechanism of these autoimmune reactions is unknown, although it has been suggested that the drug's capacity to promote DNA demethylation may be involved (Arce et al., 2006).

The drug-induced lupus syndrome usually occurs after at least 6 months of continuous treatment with hydralazine, and its incidence is related to dose, sex, acetylator phenotype, and race. In one study, after 3 years of treatment with hydralazine, drug-induced lupus occurred in 10% of patients who received 200 mg daily, 5% who received 100 mg daily, and none who received 50 mg daily (Cameron and Ramsay, 1984). The incidence is four times higher in women than in men, and the syndrome is seen more commonly in Caucasians than in African-Americans. The rate of conversion to a positive antinuclear antibody test is faster in slow acetylators than in rapid acetylators, suggesting that the native drug or a nonacetylated metabolite is responsible. However, because the majority of patients with positive antinuclear antibody tests do not develop the drug-induced lupus syndrome, hydralazine need not be discontinued unless clinical features of the syndrome appear. These features are similar to those of other drug-induced lupus syndromes and consist mainly of arthralgia, arthritis, and fever. Pleuritis and pericarditis may be present, and pericardial effusion can occasionally cause cardiac tamponade. Discontinuation of the drug is all that is necessary for most patients with the hydralazine-induced lupus syndrome, but symptoms may persist in a few patients, and administration of corticosteroids may be necessary.

Hydralazine also can produce a pyridoxine-responsive polyneuropathy. The mechanism appears to be related to the ability of hydralazine to combine with pyridoxine to form a hydrazone. This side effect is very unusual with doses ≤200 mg/day.

Therapeutic Uses. Hydralazine is no longer a first-line drug in the treatment of hypertension on account of its relatively unfavorable adverse-effect profile. The drug is marketed as a combination pill containing isosorbide dinitrate (BiDil) that is used for the treatment of heart failure (see Chapter 28). Hydralazine may have utility in the treatment of some patients with severe hypertension, can be part of evidence-based therapy in patients with congestive heart failure (in combination with nitrates for patients who cannot tolerate ACE inhibitors or AT_1 receptor antagonists), and may be useful in the treatment of hypertensive emergencies in pregnant women (especially preeclampsia). Hydralazine should be used with the great caution in elderly patients and in hypertensive patients with coronary artery disease because of the possibility of precipitation of myocardial ischemia due to reflex tachycardia. The usual oral dosage of hydralazine is 25-100 mg twice daily. Off-label twice-daily administration is as effective as administration four times a day for control of blood pressure, regardless of acetylator phenotype. The maximum recommended dose of hydralazine is 200 mg/day to minimize the risk of drug-induced lupus syndrome.

K_{ATP} Channel Openers: Minoxidil

The discovery in 1965 of the hypotensive action of minoxidil was a significant advance in the treatment of hypertension, because the drug has proven to be efficacious in patients with the most severe and drug-resistant forms of hypertension.

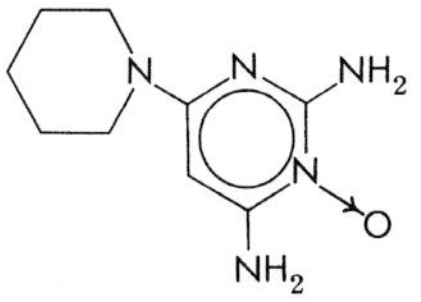

MINOXIDIL

Locus and Mechanism of Action. Minoxidil is not active *in vitro* but must be metabolized by hepatic sulfotransferase to the active molecule, minoxidil *N-O* sulfate; the formation of this active metabolite is a minor pathway in the metabolic disposition of minoxidil. Minoxidil sulfate relaxes vascular smooth muscle in isolated systems where the parent drug is inactive. Minoxidil sulfate activates the ATP-modulated K^+ channel. By opening K^+ channels in smooth muscle and thereby permitting K^+ efflux, it causes hyperpolarization and relaxation of smooth muscle (Leblanc et al., 1989).

Pharmacological Effects. Minoxidil produces arteriolar vasodilation with essentially no effect on the capacitance vessels; the drug resembles hydralazine and diazoxide in this regard. Minoxidil increases blood flow to skin, skeletal muscle, the gastrointestinal tract, and the heart more than to the CNS. The disproportionate increase in blood flow to the heart may have a metabolic basis, in that administration of minoxidil is associated with a reflex increase in myocardial contractility and in cardiac output. The cardiac output can increase markedly, as much as 3- to 4-fold. The principal determinant of the elevation in cardiac output is the action of minoxidil on peripheral vascular resistance to enhance venous return to the heart; by inference from studies with other drugs, the increased venous return probably results from enhancement of flow in the regional vascular beds, with a fast time constant for venous return to the heart (Ogilvie, 1985). The adrenergically mediated increase in myocardial contractility contributes to the increased cardiac output but is not the predominant causal factor.

The effects of minoxidil on the kidney are complex. Minoxidil is a renal artery vasodilator, but systemic hypotension produced by the drug occasionally can decrease renal blood flow. Renal function usually improves in patients who take minoxidil for the treatment of hypertension, especially if renal dysfunction is secondary to hypertension (Mitchell et al., 1980). Minoxidil is a very potent stimulator of renin secretion; this effect is mediated by a combination of renal sympathetic stimulation and activation of the intrinsic renal mechanisms for regulation of renin release.

Discovery of K^+_{ATP} channels in a variety of cell types and in mitochondria is prompting consideration of K^+_{ATP} channel modulators as therapeutic agents in myriad cardiovascular diseases (Pollesello and Mebazaa, 2004) and may provide explanations for some of the effects of minoxidil noted in the previous section. Various K^+_{ATP} channels possess different regulatory sulfonylurea receptor subunits and thus exhibit tissue-specific responses. Recent studies suggest that certain actions of K^+_{ATP} channel openers can be influenced by hypercholesterolemia and by concurrent administration of sulfonylurea hypoglycemic agents (Miura and Miki, 2003).

Absorption, Metabolism, and Excretion. Minoxidil is well absorbed from the GI tract. Although peak concentrations of minoxidil in blood occur 1 hour after oral administration, the maximal hypotensive effect of the drug occurs later, possibly because formation of the active metabolite is delayed.

The bulk of the absorbed drug is eliminated by hepatic metabolism; ~20% is excreted unchanged in the urine. The major metabolite of minoxidil is the glucuronide conjugate at the *N*-oxide position in the pyrimidine ring. This metabolite is less active than minoxidil, but it persists longer in the body. The extent of biotransformation of minoxidil to its active metabolite, minoxidil *N-O* sulfate, has not been evaluated in humans. Minoxidil has a plasma $t_{1/2}$ of 3-4 hours, but its duration of action is 24 hours or occasionally even longer. It has been proposed that persistence of minoxidil in vascular smooth muscle is responsible for this discrepancy. However, without knowledge of the pharmacokinetic properties of the active metabolite, an explanation for the prolonged duration of action cannot be given.

Adverse Effects and Precautions. The adverse effects of minoxidil can be severe and are divided into three major categories: fluid and salt retention, cardiovascular effects, and hypertrichosis.

Retention of salt and water results from increased proximal renal tubular reabsorption, which is in turn secondary to reduced renal perfusion pressure and to reflex stimulation of renal tubular α adrenergic receptors. Similar antinatriuretic effects can be observed with the other arteriolar dilators (e.g., diazoxide and hydralazine). Although administration of minoxidil causes increased secretion of renin and aldosterone, this is not an important mechanism for retention of salt and water in this case. Fluid retention usually can be controlled by the administration of a diuretic. However, thiazides may not be sufficiently efficacious, and it may be necessary to use a loop diuretic, especially if the patient has any degree of renal dysfunction. Retention of salt and water in patients taking minoxidil may be profound, requiring large doses of loop diuretics to prevent edema formation.

The cardiac consequences of the baroreceptor-mediated activation of the sympathetic nervous system during minoxidil therapy are similar to those seen with hydralazine; there is an increase in heart rate, myocardial contractility, and myocardial O_2 consumption. Thus, myocardial ischemia can be induced by minoxidil in patients with coronary artery disease. The cardiac sympathetic responses are attenuated by concurrent administration of a β adrenergic blocker. The adrenergically induced increase in renin secretion also can be ameliorated by a β receptor antagonist or an ACE inhibitor, with enhancement of blood pressure control.

The increased cardiac output evoked by minoxidil has particularly adverse consequences in those hypertensive patients who have left ventricular hypertrophy and diastolic dysfunction. Such poorly compliant ventricles respond suboptimally to increased volume loads, with a resulting increase in left ventricular filling pressure. This probably is a major contributor to the increased pulmonary artery pressure seen with minoxidil (and hydralazine) therapy in hypertensive patients and is compounded by the retention of salt and water caused by minoxidil. Cardiac failure can result from minoxidil therapy in such patients; the potential for this complication can be reduced but not prevented by effective diuretic therapy. Pericardial effusion is an uncommon but serious complication of minoxidil. Although more commonly described in patients with cardiac and renal failure, pericardial effusion can occur in patients with normal cardiovascular and renal function. Mild and asymptomatic pericardial effusion is not an indication for discontinuing minoxidil, but the situation should be monitored closely to avoid progression to tamponade. Effusions usually clear when the drug is discontinued but can recur if treatment with minoxidil is resumed.

Flattened and inverted T waves frequently are observed in the electrocardiogram following the initiation of minoxidil treatment. These are not ischemic in origin and are seen with other drugs that activate K^+ channels. These drugs accelerate myocardial repolarization, shorten the refractory period, and one of them, *pinacidil*, lowers the ventricular fibrillation threshold and increases spontaneous ventricular fibrillation in the setting of myocardial ischemia (Chi et al., 1990). The effect of minoxidil on the refractory period and ischemic ventricular fibrillation has not been investigated; whether or not such findings enhance the risk of ventricular fibrillation in human myocardial ischemia is unknown.

Hypertrichosis occurs in patients who receive minoxidil for an extended period and is probably a consequence of K^+ channel activation. Growth of hair occurs on the face, back, arms, and legs and is particularly offensive to women. Frequent shaving or depilatory agents can be used to manage this problem. Topical minoxidil (ROGAINE) is marketed over-the-counter for the treatment of male pattern baldness and hair thinning and loss on the top of the head in women. The topical use of minoxidil also can cause measurable cardiovascular effects in some individuals.

Other side effects of the drug are rare and include rashes, Stevens-Johnson syndrome, glucose intolerance, serosanguineous bullae, formation of antinuclear antibodies, and thrombocytopenia.

Therapeutic Uses. Systemic minoxidil is best reserved for the treatment of severe hypertension that responds poorly to other antihypertensive medications, especially in male patients with renal insufficiency (Campese, 1981). It has been used successfully in the treatment of hypertension in both adults and children. Minoxidil should never be used alone; it must be given concurrently with a diuretic to avoid fluid retention and with a sympatholytic drug (usually a β receptor antagonist) to control reflex cardiovascular effects. The drug usually is administered either once or twice a day, but some patients may require more frequent dosing for adequate control of blood pressure. The initial daily dose of minoxidil may be as little as 1.25 mg, which can be increased gradually to 40 mg in one or two daily doses.

Sodium Nitroprusside

Although sodium nitroprusside has been known since 1850 and its hypotensive effect in humans was described in 1929, its safety and usefulness for the short-term control of severe hypertension were not demonstrated until the mid-1950s. Several investigators subsequently demonstrated that sodium nitroprusside also was effective in improving cardiac function in patients with left ventricular failure (see Chapter 28).

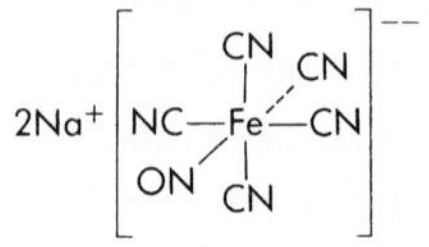

$$2Na^+ \left[\begin{array}{c} CN \quad CN \\ NC-Fe-CN \\ ON \quad CN \end{array} \right]^{--}$$

SODIUM NITROPRUSSIDE

Locus and Mechanism of Action. Nitroprusside is a nitrovasodilator that acts by releasing NO. NO activates the guanylyl cyclase–cyclic GMP–PKG pathway, leading to vasodilation (Linder et al., 2005), mimicking the production of NO by vascular endothelial cells, which is impaired in many hypertensive patients (Ramchandra et al., 2005). The mechanism of release of NO is not clear and likely involves both enzymatic and nonenzymatic pathways (Feelisch, 1998). Tolerance develops to *nitroglycerin* but not to nitroprusside (Fung, 2004). The pharmacology of the organic nitrates, including nitroglycerin, was presented earlier.

Pharmacological Effects. Nitroprusside dilates both arterioles and venules, and the hemodynamic response to its administration results from a combination of venous pooling and reduced arterial impedance. In subjects with normal left ventricular function, venous pooling affects cardiac output more than does the reduction of afterload; cardiac output tends to fall. In contrast, in patients with severely impaired left ventricular function and diastolic ventricular distention, the reduction of arterial impedance is the predominant effect, leading to a rise in cardiac output (see Chapter 28).

Sodium nitroprusside is a nonselective vasodilator, and regional distribution of blood flow is little affected by the drug. In general, renal blood flow and glomerular filtration are maintained, and plasma renin activity increases. Unlike minoxidil, hydralazine, diazoxide, and other arteriolar vasodilators, sodium nitroprusside usually causes only a modest increase in heart rate and an overall reduction in myocardial O_2 demand.

Absorption, Metabolism, and Excretion. Sodium nitroprusside is an unstable molecule that decomposes under strongly alkaline conditions or when exposed to light. The drug must be protected from light and given by continuous intravenous infusion to be effective. Its onset of action is within 30 seconds; the peak hypotensive effect occurs within 2 minutes, and when the infusion of the drug is stopped, the effect disappears within 3 minutes.

The metabolism of nitroprusside by smooth muscle is initiated by its reduction, which is followed by the release of cyanide and then NO (Bates et al., 1991). Cyanide is further metabolized by liver rhodanase to form thiocyanate, which is eliminated almost entirely in the urine. The mean elimination $t_{1/2}$ for thiocyanate is 3 days in patients with normal renal function, and it can be much longer in patients with renal insufficiency.

Therapeutic Uses. Sodium nitroprusside is used primarily to treat hypertensive emergencies but also can be used in many situations when short-term reduction of cardiac preload and/or afterload is desired. Nitroprusside has been used to lower blood pressure during acute aortic dissection; improve cardiac output in congestive heart failure, especially in hypertensive patients with pulmonary edema that does not respond to other treatment (see Chapter 28); and decrease myocardial oxygen demand after acute MI. In addition, nitroprusside is used to induce controlled hypotension during anesthesia in order to reduce bleeding in surgical procedures. In the treatment of acute aortic dissection, it is important to administer a β adrenergic receptor antagonist with nitroprusside, because reduction of blood pressure with nitroprusside alone can increase the rate of rise in pressure in the aorta as a result of increased myocardial contractility, thereby enhancing propagation of the dissection.

Sodium nitroprusside is available in vials that contain 50 mg. The contents of the vial should be dissolved in 2-3 mL of 5% dextrose in water. Addition of this solution to 250-1000 mL of 5% dextrose in water produces a concentration of 50-200 μg/mL. Because the compound decomposes in light, only fresh solutions should be used, and the bottle should be covered with an opaque wrapping. The drug must be administered as a controlled continuous infusion, and the patient must be closely observed. The majority of hypertensive patients respond to an infusion of 0.25-1.5 μg/kg/min. Higher rates of infusion are necessary to produce controlled hypotension in normotensive patients under surgical anesthesia. Patients who are receiving other antihypertensive medications usually require less nitroprusside to lower blood pressure. If infusion rates of 10 μg/kg/min do not produce adequate reduction of blood pressure within 10 minutes, the rate of administration of nitroprusside should be reduced to minimize potential toxicity.

Toxicity and Precautions. The short-term adverse effects of nitroprusside are due to excessive vasodilation, with hypotension and the consequences thereof. Close monitoring of blood pressure and the use of a continuous variable-rate infusion pump will prevent an excessive hemodynamic response to the drug in the majority of cases.

Less commonly, toxicity may result from conversion of nitroprusside to cyanide and thiocyanate. Toxic accumulation of cyanide leading to severe lactic acidosis usually occurs when sodium nitroprusside is infused at a rate >5 μg/kg/min but also can occur in some patients receiving doses ~2 μg/kg/min for a prolonged period. The limiting factor in the metabolism of cyanide appears to be the availability of sulfur-containing substrates in the body (mainly thiosulfate). The concomitant administration of sodium thiosulfate can prevent accumulation of cyanide in patients who are receiving higher-than-usual doses of sodium nitroprusside; the efficacy of the drug is unchanged (Schulz, 1984). The risk of thiocyanate toxicity increases when sodium nitroprusside is infused for more than 24-48 hours, especially if renal function is impaired. Signs and symptoms of thiocyanate toxicity include anorexia, nausea, fatigue, disorientation, and toxic psychosis. The plasma concentration of thiocyanate should be monitored during prolonged infusions of nitroprusside and should not be allowed to exceed 0.1 mg/mL. Rarely, excessive concentrations of thiocyanate may cause hypothyroidism by inhibiting iodine uptake by the thyroid gland. In patients with renal failure, thiocyanate can be removed readily by hemodialysis.

Nitroprusside can worsen arterial hypoxemia in patients with chronic obstructive pulmonary disease because the drug interferes with hypoxic pulmonary vasoconstriction and therefore promotes mismatching of ventilation with perfusion.

Diazoxide. Diazoxide was used in the treatment of hypertensive emergencies but fell out of favor at least in part due to the risk of marked falls in blood pressure when large bolus doses of the drug were used. Other drugs are now preferred for parenteral administration in the control of hypertension. Diazoxide also is administered orally (PROGLYCEM) to treat patients with various forms of hypoglycemia (see Chapter 43).

NONPHARMACOLOGICAL THERAPY OF HYPERTENSION

Nonpharmacological approaches to the treatment of hypertension may be sufficient in patients with modestly elevated blood pressure. Such approaches also can augment the effects of antihypertensive drugs in patients with more marked initial elevations in blood pressure. The indications and efficacy of various lifestyle modifications in hypertension are reviewed in a summary statement from the Joint National Committee (Chobanian et al., 2003).

- Reduction in body weight for people who are modestly overweight or frankly obese may be useful (Horvath et al., 2008).
- Restricting sodium consumption lowers blood pressure in some patients. The Dietary Approaches to

Stop Hypertension (DASH) diet may be particularly useful (Champagne, 2006).

- For some patients, restriction of ethanol intake to modest levels may lower blood pressure.
- Increased physical activity may improve control of hypertension.

SELECTION OF ANTIHYPERTENSIVE DRUGS IN INDIVIDUAL PATIENTS

Choice of antihypertensive drugs for individual patients may be complex; there are many sources of influence that modify therapeutic decisions. While results derived from randomized controlled clinical trials are the optimal foundation for rational therapeutics, it may be difficult to sort through the multiplicity of results and address how they apply to an individual patient. While therapeutic guidelines can be useful in reaching appropriate therapeutic decisions, it often is difficult for clinicians to apply guidelines at the point of care, and guidelines often do not provide enough information about recommended drugs. In addition, intense marketing of specific drugs to both clinicians and patients may confound optimal decision making. Moreover, persuading patients to continue taking sometimes expensive drugs for an asymptomatic disease is a challenge. Clinicians may be reluctant to prescribe and patients reluctant to consume the number of drugs that may be necessary to adequately control blood pressure. For these and other reasons, perhaps one-half of patients being treated for hypertension have not achieved therapeutic goals in blood pressure lowering.

Choice of an antihypertensive drug should be driven by the likely benefit in an individual patient, taking into account concomitant diseases such as diabetes mellitus, problematic adverse effects of specific drugs, and cost.

National guidelines (Chobaniry et al, 2003) recommend diuretics as preferred initial therapy for most patients with uncomplicated stage 1 hypertension (Table 27–4) who are unresponsive to nonpharmacological measures. Patients also are commonly treated with other drugs: β-receptor antagonists, ACE inhibitors/AT_1-receptor antagonists, and Ca^{2+} channel blockers. Patients with uncomplicated stage 2 hypertension will likely require the early introduction of a diuretic and another drug from a different class. Subsequently, doses can be titrated upward and additional drugs added to achieve goal blood pressures (blood pressure <140/90 mm Hg in uncomplicated patients). Some of these patients may require four different drugs to reach the goal.

An important and high-risk group of patients with hypertension are those with compelling indications for specific drugs on account of other underlying serious cardiovascular disease (heart failure, post-MI, or with high risk for coronary artery disease), chronic kidney disease, or diabetes (Chobanian et al., 2003). For example, a hypertensive patient with congestive heart failure ideally should be treated with a diuretic, β receptor antagonist, ACE inhibitor/AT_1-receptor antagonist, and (in selected patients) spironolactone because of the benefit of these drugs in congestive heart failure, even in the absence of hypertension (see Chapter 28). Similarly, ACE inhibitors/AT_1-receptor antagonists should be first-line drugs in the treatment of diabetics with hypertension in view of these drugs' well-established benefits in diabetic nephropathy.

Other patients may have less serious underlying diseases that could influence choice of antihypertensive drugs. For example, a hypertensive patient with symptomatic benign prostatic hyperplasia might benefit from having an α_1 receptor antagonist as part of his or her therapeutic program, because α_1 antagonists are efficacious in both diseases. Similarly, a patient with recurrent migraine attacks might particularly benefit from use of a β receptor antagonist because a number of drugs in this class are efficacious in preventing migraine attacks. On the other hand, in pregnant hypertensives, some drugs that are otherwise little used (methyldopa) may be preferred and popular drugs (ACE inhibitors) avoided on account of concerns about safety.

Patients with isolated systolic hypertension (systolic blood pressure >160 mm Hg and diastolic blood pressure <90 mm Hg) benefit particularly from diuretics and also from Ca^{2+} channel blockers and ACE inhibitors. These should be first-line drugs in these patients in terms of efficacy, but compelling indications as noted earlier need to be taken into account.

These considerations apply to patients with hypertension that need treatment to reduce long-term risk, not patients in immediately life-threatening settings due to hypertension. While there are very limited clinical trial data, clinical judgment favors rapidly lowering blood pressure in patients with life-threatening complications of hypertension, such as patients with hypertensive encephalopathy or pulmonary edema due to severe hypertension. However, rapid reduction in blood pressure has considerable risks for the patients; if blood pressure is decreased too quickly or extensively, cerebral blood flow may diminish due to adaptations in the cerebral circulation that protect the brain from the sequelae of very high blood pressures. The temptation

Pharmacotherapy of Congestive Heart Failure

Bradley A. Maron
and Thomas P. Rocco

Congestive heart failure (CHF) is responsible for more than half a million deaths annually in the U.S., carries a 1-year mortality rate of more than 50% in patients with advanced forms of the condition, and is responsible for nearly $27 billion annually in healthcare costs (Binanay et al., 2005). Fortunately, substantive advances in CHF pharmacotherapy have altered clinical practice by shifting the paradigm of its management from exclusively symptom palliation to modification of disease progression and, in some cases, an expectation of prolonged survival.

In the past, drug therapies targeted the endpoints of this syndrome: volume overload (congestion) and myocardial dysfunction (pump failure). As a consequence, diuretics and cardiac glycosides dominated the medical management of CHF for more than 40 years. These drugs remain effective for symptom relief and in stabilizing patients with hemodynamic decompensation but do not improve long-term survival. The contemporary focus of CHF as a disorder of circulatory hemodynamics, pathologic cardiac remodeling, and increased arrhythmogenic instability has translated into the development of novel pharmacotherapies that reduce CHF-associated morbidity and mortality rates. Before discussing the clinical pharmacology of CHF in specific, it is useful to establish a pathophysiologic framework through which its treatment is approached.

Defining Congestive Heart Failure. The onset and progression of clinically evident CHF from left ventricular (LV) systolic dysfunction follows a pathophysiologic sequence in response to an initial insult to myocardial dysfunction. A reduction in forward cardiac output leads to expanded activation of the sympathetic nervous system and the renin–angiotensin–aldosterone axis that, together, maintain perfusion of vital organs by increasing LV preload, stimulating myocardial contractility, and increasing arterial tone. Acutely, these mechanisms sustain cardiac output by allowing the heart to operate at elevated end-diastolic volumes, while peripheral vasoconstriction promotes regional redistribution of the cardiac output to the central nervous system, coronary, and renal vascular beds.

Unfortunately, however, these compensatory mechanisms over time propagate disease progression. Intravascular volume expansion increases diastolic and systolic wall stress that disrupts myocardial energetics and causes pathologic LV hypertrophy. By increasing LV afterload, peripheral arterial vasoconstriction also adversely affects diastolic ventricular wall stress, thereby increasing myocardial O_2 demand. Finally, neurohumoral effectors such as norepinephrine (NE) and angiotensin II (AngII) are associated with myocyte apoptosis, abnormal myocyte gene expression, and pathologic changes in the extracellular matrix that increase LV stiffness (Villarreal, 2005).

In clinical practice, the term CHF describes a final common pathway for the expression of myocardial dysfunction. While some emphasize the clinical distinction between systolic versus diastolic heart failure, many patients demonstrate dysfunction in both contractile performance and ventricular relaxation/filling. Indeed, these physiologic processes are interrelated; for example, the rate and duration of LV diastolic filling are directly influenced by impairment in systolic contractile performance. Despite inherent difficulties in creating a singular description to encompass the diverse pathophysiologic mechanisms that result in CHF (e.g., myocardial infarction (MI), viral myocarditis), the following definitions are useful for establishing a conceptual framework to describe this clinical syndrome:

Congestive heart failure is the pathophysiologic state in which the heart is unable to pump blood at a rate commensurate with the requirements of metabolizing tissues, or can do so only from an elevated filling pressure (Braunwald and Bristow, 2000).

Heart failure is a complex of symptoms—fatigue, shortness of breath, and congestion—that are related to the inadequate perfusion of tissue during exertion and often to the retention of fluid. Its primary cause is an impairment of the heart's ability to fill or empty the left ventricle properly (Cohn, 1996).

From these definitions, one may consider CHF as a condition in which failure of the heart to provide adequate forward output at normal end-diastolic filling pressures results in a clinical syndrome of decreased exercise tolerance with pulmonary and systemic venous congestion. Numerous cardiovascular comorbidities are associated with CHF, including coronary artery disease, MI, and sudden cardiac death.

PHARMACOLOGIC TREATMENT OF HEART FAILURE

The abnormalities of myocardial structure and function that characterize CHF are often irreversible. These changes narrow the end-diastolic volume range that is compatible with normal cardiac function. Although CHF is predominately a chronic disease, subtle changes to an individual's hemodynamic status (e.g., increased circulating volume from high dietary sodium intake, increased systemic blood pressure from medication nonadherence) often provoke an acute clinical decompensation.

Not surprisingly, therefore, CHF therapy has for many years utilized diuretics to control volume overload and subsequent worsening in LV function. Other proven pharmacotherapies target ventricular wall stress, the renin–angiotensin–aldosterone axis, and the sympathetic nervous system to decrease pathologic ventricular remodeling, attenuate disease progression, and improve survival in selected patients with severe CHF and low LV ejection fraction. Figure 28–1 provides an overview of the sites of action for major drug classes commonly used in clinical practice. Note that these therapies largely improve cardiac hemodynamics and function through preload reduction, afterload reduction, and enhancement of inotropy (i.e., myocardial contractility). In addition, pharmacotherapeutics that target peripheral and coronary vascular function are receiving increased attention as potential participants in the comprehensive management of CHF patients.

Diuretics

Diuretics remain central in the pharmacologic management of congestive symptoms in patients with CHF. The pharmacologic properties of these agents are presented in detail in Chapter 25. Their importance (and frequency of use) in CHF management reflects the deleterious downstream effects of volume expansion on increased LV end-diastolic volume, an intermediate step in the development of elevated right-heart pressure, pulmonary venous congestion, and peripheral edema (Hillege et al., 2000).

Diuretics reduce extracellular fluid volume and ventricular filling pressure (or "preload"). Because CHF patients often operate on a "plateau" phase of the *Frank-Starling* curve (Figure 28–2), incremental preload reduction occurs under these conditions without a reduction in cardiac output. Sustained natriuresis and/or a rapid decline in intravascular volume, however, may "push" one's profile leftward on the Frank-Starling curve, resulting in an unwanted decrease in cardiac output. In this way, excessive diuresis is counterproductive secondary to reciprocal neurohormonal *overactivation* from volume depletion (McCurley et al., 2004). For this reason, it is preferable to avoid diuretics in patients with asymptomatic LV dysfunction and to only administer the minimal dose required to maintain euvolemia in those patients symptomatic from hypervolemia. Despite the efficacy of loop or thiazide diuretics in controlling congestive symptoms and improving exercise capacity, their use is not associated with a reduction in CHF mortality.

Dietary Sodium Restriction. All patients with clinically significant LV dysfunction, regardless of symptom status, should be advised to limit dietary sodium intake to 2-3 g/day. More stringent salt restriction is seldom necessary and may be counterproductive, as it can lead to hyponatremia, hypokalemia, and hypochloremic metabolic alkalosis when combined with loop diuretic administration.

Loop Diuretics. Of the loop diuretics currently available, furosemide (LASIX, others), bumetanide (BUMEX, others), and torsemide (DEMADEX, others) are widely used in the treatment of CHF. Due to the increased risk of ototoxicity, ethacrynic acid (EDECRIN) is recommended only for patients with sulfonamides allergies or who are intolerant to alternative options.

Loop diuretics inhibit a specific ion transport protein, the Na^+-K^+-$2Cl^-$ symporter on the apical membrane of renal epithelial cells in the ascending limb of the loop of Henle to increase Na^+ and fluid delivery to

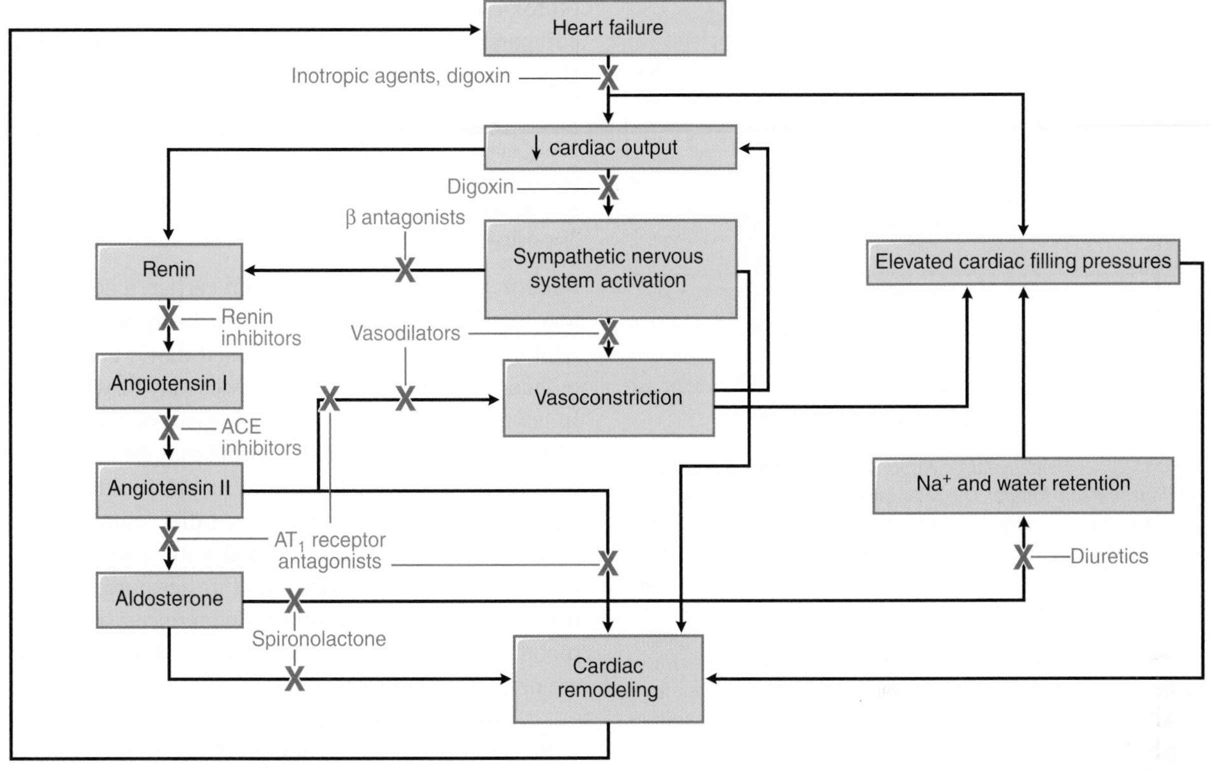

Figure 28–1. *Pathophysiologic mechanisms of heart failure and major sites of drug action.* Congestive heart failure is accompanied by compensatory neurohormonal responses, including activation of the sympathetic nervous and renin–angiotensin–aldosterone axis. Increased ventricular afterload, due to systemic vasoconstriction and chamber dilation, causes depression in systolic function. In addition, increased afterload and the direct effects of angiotensin and norepinephrine on the ventricular myocardium cause pathologic remodeling characterized by progressive chamber dilation and loss of contractile function. Key congestive heart failure medications and their targets of action are presented. ACE, angiotensin-converting enzyme; AT_1 receptor, type 1 angiotensin receptor.

distal nephron segments (see Chapter 25). These drugs also enhance K^+ secretion, particularly in the presence of elevated aldosterone levels, as is typical in CHF.

The bioavailability of orally administered furosemide ranges from 40-70%. High drug concentrations often are required to initiate diuresis in patients with worsening symptoms or in those with impaired gastrointestinal absorption, as may occur in severely hypervolemic patients with CHF-induced gut edema (Gottlieb, 2004). In contrast, the oral bioavailabilities of bumetanide and torsemide are >80%, and as a result, these agents are more consistently absorbed but are financially more costly.

Furosemide and bumetanide are short-acting drugs, and rebound Na^+ retention that occurs with sub-steady state drug levels make ≥2/day dosing an acceptable treatment strategy when using these agents, provided adequate monitoring of daily body weight and blood electrolyte level monitoring is possible.

Thiazide Diuretics. Monotherapy with thiazide diuretics (DIURIL, HYDRODIURIL, others) has a limited role in CHF. However, combination therapy with loop diuretics is often effective in those refractory to loop diuretics alone. Thiazide diuretics act on the Na^+Cl^- cotransporter in the distal convoluted tubule (see Chapter 25) and are associated with a greater degree K^+ wasting per fluid volume reduction when compared to loop diuretics (Gottlieb, 2004).

K^+-Sparing Diuretics. K^+-sparing diuretics (see Chapter 25) inhibit apical membrane Na^+-conductance channels in renal epithelial cells (e.g., amiloride, triamterene) or are mineralocorticoid (e.g., aldosterone) receptor antagonists (e.g., canrenone [not commercially available in the U.S.], spironolactone, and eplerenone). Collectively, these agents are weak diuretics, but have historically been used to achieve volume reduction with limited K^+ and Mg^{2+} wasting. The beneficial role of aldosterone receptor blockers on survival in CHF is discussed later.

Diuretics in Clinical Practice. The majority of CHF patients will require chronic administration of a loop diuretic to maintain euvolemia. In patients with clinically

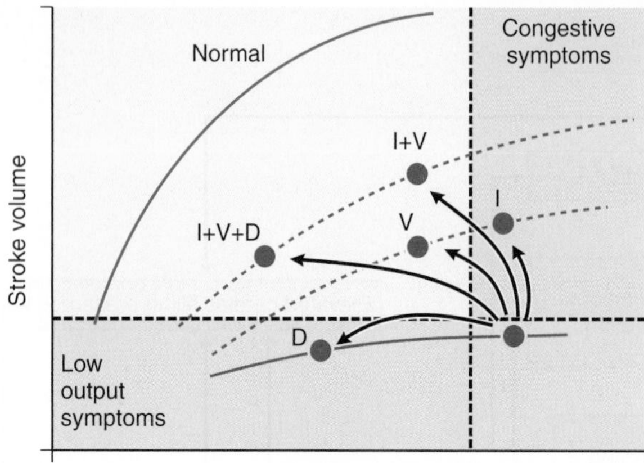

Figure 28–2. *Hemodynamic responses to pharmacologic interventions in heart failure.* The relationships between diastolic filling pressure (preload) and stroke volume (ventricular performance) are illustrated for a normal heart (*green line*; the Frank-Starling relationship) and for a patient with heart failure due to predominant systolic dysfunction (*red line*). Note that positive inotropic agents (I), such as cardiac glycosides or dobutamine, move patients to a higher ventricular function curve (*lower dashed line*), resulting in greater cardiac work for a given level of ventricular filling pressure. Vasodilators (V), such as angiotensin-converting enzyme (ACE) inhibitors or nitroprusside, also move patients to improved ventricular function curves while reducing cardiac filling pressures. Diuretics (D) improve symptoms of congestive heart failure by moving patients to lower cardiac filling pressures along the same ventricular function curve.

evident fluid retention, furosemide typically is started at a dose of 40 mg once or twice daily, and the dosage is increased until an adequate diuresis is achieved. A larger initial dose may be necessary in patients with advanced CHF and azotemia. Serum electrolytes and renal function are monitored frequently in these patients or in those for whom a rapid diuresis is necessary. If present, hypokalemia from therapy may be corrected by oral or intravenous K^+ supplementation or by the addition of a K^+-sparing diuretic. When appropriate, diuretics are decreased to the minimum effective concentration for maintaining euvolemia.

Diuretics in the Decompensated Patient. In patients with decompensated CHF warranting hospital admission, repetitive intravenously administered boluses or a constant infusion titrated to achieve a desired response may be needed to provide expeditious (and reliable) diuresis (Dormans et al., 1996). One advantage to intravenous infusion is that sustained natriuresis is achieved as a consequence of consistently elevated drug levels within the lumen of the renal tubules. In addition, the risk of ototoxicity is reduced by continuous infusion when compared to repetitive, intermittent intravenous dosing (Lahav et al., 1992).

A typical continuous furosemide infusion is initiated with a 40-mg bolus injection followed by a constant rate of 10 mg/h, with uptitration as necessary. If renal perfusion is reduced, drug efficacy may be enhanced by co-administration of drugs that increase cardiac output (e.g., *dobutamine*).

Diuretic Resistance. As mentioned earlier, a compensatory increase in renal tubular Na^+ reabsorption may prevent effective diuresis when dosed daily; as a result, reduction of diuretic dosing intervals may be warranted. In advanced CHF, invasive assessment of intracardiac filling pressures and cardiac output may be required to distinguish between low intravascular volume from aggressive diuresis versus low cardiac output states, although both states are aligned with lower diuretic delivery and drug efficacy. Furthermore, edema, decreased bowel-wall motility, and reduced splanchnic blood flow impair absorption and may delay or attenuate peak diuretic effect.

Atherosclerotic renal artery disease is associated with reduced renal perfusion pressures to levels below that necessary for adequate drug delivery. In patients with reduced renal arterial perfusion pressure (e.g., renal artery stenosis or low cardiac output), AngII-mediated efferent glomerular arteriole tone is important for preservation of normal glomerular filtration pressure. Angiotensin-converting enzyme (ACE) inhibitors or AT_1 receptor antagonists in combination with loop diuretics may, therefore, be met with a decline in creatinine clearance that is associated with low diuretic delivery and decreased drug efficacy (Ellison, 1999). Other common causes of diuretic resistance are listed in Table 28–1.

Metabolic Consequences of Diuretic Therapy. The side effects of diuretics are discussed in Chapter 25. With regard to diuretic use in CHF, the most important adverse sequelae of diuretics are electrolyte abnormalities, including hyponatremia, hypokalemia, and hypochloremic metabolic alkalosis. The clinical importance (or even existence) of significant Mg^{2+} deficiency with chronic diuretic use is controversial (Bigger, 1994).

Adenosine A_1 Receptor Antagonists. Adenosine A_1 receptor antagonists may provide a renal protective therapeutic strategy for enhanced volume loss in decompensated CHF. Adenosine is secreted from the macula densa in the renal arteriole in response to diuretic-induced increases in Na^+ and Cl^- tubular flow concentrations. This results in increased Na^+ resorption, a volume-loss counterregulatory mechanism (see Chapter 26). Na^+ reabsorption, in addition to adenosine-induced renal

Table 28–1

Causes of Diuretic Resistance in Heart Failure

Noncompliance with medical regimen; excess dietary Na^+ intake
Decreased renal perfusion and glomerular filtration rate due to:
Excessive vascular volume depletion and hypotension due to aggressive diuretic or vasodilator therapy
Decline in cardiac output due to worsening heart failure, arrhythmias, or other primary cardiac causes
Selective reduction in glomerular perfusion pressure following initiation (or dose increase) of ACE-inhibitor therapy
Nonsteroidal anti-inflammatory drugs
Primary renal pathology (e.g., cholesterol emboli, renal artery stenosis, drug-induced interstitial nephritis, obstructive uropathy)
Reduced or impaired diuretic absorption due to gut wall edema and reduced splanchnic blood flow

arteriole vasoconstriction, appears responsible (in part) for the development of complications common to the use of diuretics in decompensated CHF patients, particularly prerenal azotemia. The role of adenosine in the macula densa and juxtaglomerular (granular) cells (see Figure 26–2) suggests other effects of A_1 antagonists on the renin-angiotensin system.

As an example of the use of A_1 antagonists, the administration of *KW-3902* (ROLOFYLLINE) (30 mg) to patients with decompensated CHF already treated with loop diuretics is associated with increased volume reduction, improved renal function, and lower diuretic dosing, as compared to placebo (Givertz et al., 2007). Favorable effects on urine output and renal function also have been observed in similar patients with the A_1 receptor antagonist *BG9179* (NAXIFYLLINE) (Gottlieb et al., 2002). A large clinical trial failed to show significant benefits of rolofylline in patients with CHF, and clinical development of the drug was stopped in 2009. No A_1 antagonists are currently marketed in the U.S.

Aldosterone Antagonists and Clinical Outcome

LV systolic dysfunction deceases renal blood flow and results in overactivation of the renin–angiotensin–aldosterone axis and may increase circulating plasma aldosterone levels in CHF to 20-fold above normal (Figure 28–3). The pathophysiologic effects of hyperaldosteronemia are diverse (Table 28–2) and extend beyond Na^+ and fluid retention; importantly, however, the precise mechanism by which aldosterone receptor blockade improves outcome in CHF remains unresolved (Weber, 2004).

In the Randomized Aldactone Evaluation Study, CHF patients with low LV ejection fraction receiving spironolactone (25 mg/day) had a significant (~30%) reduction in mortality (from progressive heart failure or sudden cardiac death) and fewer CHF-related hospitalizations compared with the placebo group (Pitt et al., 1999). Treatment was well tolerated overall; most notably, however, 10% of men reported gynecomastia and 2% of all patients developed severe hyperkalemia (>6.0 mEq/L) on spironolactone (Pitt et al., 1999). Data from this and other clinical studies (Pitt et al., 2003) suggest that *despite* maximum ACE inhibition, clinically important aldosterone levels are still achieved in CHF. This may account for the beneficial effects observed in these trials where aldosterone-receptor antagonists were used in combination with ACE inhibitor therapy. Combination therapy in those with renal impairment, however, increases the probability of drug-induced hyperkalemia.

The role of aldosterone antagonists in patients with asymptomatic LV dysfunction or in those with minimal CHF-associated symptoms has not been established.

Vasodilators

The rationale for oral vasodilator drugs in the pharmacotherapy of CHF derives from experience with parenterally administered *phentolamine* and *nitroprusside* in patients with advanced disease and elevated systemic vascular resistance (Cohn and Franciosa, 1977). Although numerous vasodilators have since been developed that improve CHF symptoms, only the *hydralazine–isosorbide dinitrate* combination, ACE inhibitors, and AT_1 receptor blockers (ARBs) demonstrably improve survival. The therapeutic use of vasodilators in the treatment of hypertension and myocardial ischemia is considered in detail in Chapter 27. This chapter will focus on the uses for some of these same vasodilator drugs in the treatment of CHF. Table 28–3 summarizes properties of vasodilators commonly used to treat CHF.

Nitrovasodilators. Nitrovasodilators are nitric oxide (NO) donors that activate soluble guanylate cyclase in vascular smooth muscle cells, leading to vasodilation. The mechanism underlying the variable response profiles to nitrovasodilators in different vascular beds remains controversial; e.g., nitroglycerin preferentially induces epicardial coronary artery vasodilation. Furthermore, the mechanisms by which nitrovasodilators are converted to their active forms *in vivo* depend on the particular agent. Unlike nitroprusside, which is converted to $NO^{\bullet}$ by cellular reducing agents such as glutathione, nitroglycerin and other organic nitrates undergo a more complex enzymatic biotransformation

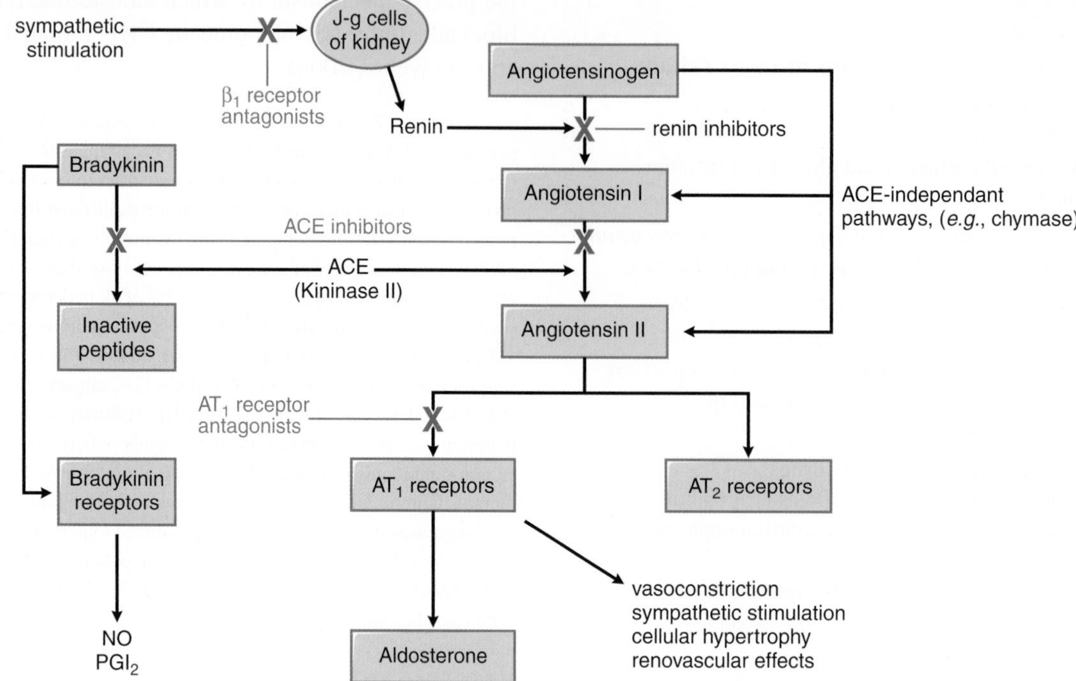

Figure 28–3. *The renin–angiotensin–aldosterone axis.* Renin, excreted in response to β adrenergic stimulation of the juxtaglomerular (J-g) cells of the kidney, cleaves plasma angiotensinogen to produce angiotensin I. Angiotensin-converting enzyme (ACE) catalyzes the conversion of angiotensin I to angiotensin II (AngII). Most of the known biologic effects of AngII are mediated by the type 1 angiotensin (AT_1) receptor. In general, the AT_2 receptor appears to counteract the effects of AngII that are mediated by activation of the AT_1 pathway. AngII also may be formed through ACE-independent pathways. These pathways, and possibly incomplete inhibition of tissue ACE, may account for persistence of Ang II in patients treated with ACE inhibitors. ACE inhibition decreases bradykinin degradation, thus enhancing its levels and biologic effects, including the production of NO and PGI_2. Bradykinin may mediate some of the biological effects of ACE inhibitors.

Table 28–2

Potential Roles of Aldosterone in the Pathophysiology of Heart Failure

MECHANISM	PATHOPHYSIOLOGIC EFFECT
Increased Na^+ and water retention	Edema, elevated cardiac filling pressures
K^+ and Mg^{2+} loss	Arrhythmogenesis and risk of sudden cardiac death
Reduced myocardial NE uptake	Potentiation of NE affects: myocardial remodeling and arrhythmogenesis
Reduced baroreceptor sensitivity	Reduced parasympathetic activity and risk of sudden cardiac death
Myocardial fibrosis, fibroblast proliferation	Remodeling and ventricular dysfunction
Alterations in Na^+ channel expression	Increased excitability and contractility of cardiac myocytes

to NO• or bioactive *S*-nitrosothiols. The activities of specific enzyme(s) and cofactor(s) required for this biotransformation appear to differ by target organ and even by different vasculature beds within a particular organ (Münzel et al., 2005).

Organic Nitrates. As discussed in Chapter 27, organic nitrates are available in a number of formulations that include rapid-acting nitroglycerin tablets or spray for sublingual administration, short-acting oral agents such as isosorbide dinitrate (ISORDIL, others), long-acting oral agents such as isosorbide mononitrate (ISMO, others), topical preparations such as nitroglycerin ointment and transdermal patches, and intravenous nitroglycerin. These preparations are relatively safe and effective; specifically, their principal action in CHF is reducing LV filling pressure. This occurs, in part, by augmentation of peripheral venous capacitance that results in preload reduction. Additional effects of organic nitrates include pulmonary and systemic vascular resistance

Table 28–3

Vasodilator Drugs Used to Treat Heart Failure

DRUG CLASS	EXAMPLES	MECHANISM OF VASODILATING ACTION	PRELOAD REDUCTION	AFTERLOAD REDUCTION
Organic nitrates	Nitroglycerin, isosorbide dinitrate	NO-mediated vasodilation	+++	+
NO donors	Nitroprusside	NO-mediated vasodilation	+++	+++
ACE inhibitors	Captopril, enalapril, lisinopril	Inhibition of AngII generation, ↓ BK degradation	++	++
Ang II receptor blockers	Losartan, candesartan	AT_1 receptors blockade	++	++
PDE inhibitors	Milrinone, inamrinone	Inhibition of cyclic AMP degradation	++	++
K^+ channel agonist	Hydralazine	Unknown	+	+++
	Minoxidil	Hyperpolarization of vascular smooth muscle cells	+	+++
α_1 antagonists	Doxazosin, prazosin	Selective α_1 adrenergic receptor blockade	+++	++
Nonselective α antagonists	Phentolamine	Nonselective α adrenergic receptor blockade	+++	+++
β/α_1 antagonists	Carvedilol, labetalol	Selective α_1 adrenergic receptor blockade	++	++
Ca^{2+} channel blockers	Amlodipine, nifedipine, felodipine	Inhibition of L-type Ca^{2+} channels	+	+++
β agonists	Isoproterenol	Stimulation of vascular β_2 adrenergic receptors	+	++

Ang II, angiotensin II; AT_1, type 1 angiotensin II receptor; NO, nitric oxide; ACE, angiotensin converting enzyme; PDE, cyclic nucleotide phosphodiesterase; BK, bradykinin.

reduction, particularly at higher doses, and epicardial coronary artery vasodilation for which systolic and diastolic ventricular function is enhanced by increased coronary blood flow. Collectively, these beneficial physiologic effects translate into improved exercise capacity and CHF-symptom reduction. However, these drugs do not substantially influence systemic vascular resistance, and pharmacologic tolerance greatly limits their utility over time. For these reasons and others, organic nitrates are not commonly used alone; rather, a number of trials have shown that when used together, selected organic nitrates increase the clinical effectiveness of other vasodilators, such as *hydralazine*, resulting in a sustained improvement in hemodynamics.

Nitrate tolerance. *Nitrate tolerance may limit the long-term effectiveness of these drugs in the treatment of CHF. Blood nitrate levels may be permitted to fall to negligible levels for at least 6-8 hours each day* (see Chapter 27). The timing of nitrate withdrawal symptoms, if present, may be useful, however, for developing an appropriate drug-dosing schedule. Patients with recurrent orthopnea or paroxysmal nocturnal dyspnea, e.g., might benefit from nighttime nitrate use. Likewise, co-treatment with hydralazine (e.g., isosorbide dinitrate and hydralazine [BIDIL]) may decrease nitrate tolerance by an antioxidant effect that attenuates superoxide formation, thereby increasing the bioavailable NO levels (Münzel et al., 1996).

Parenteral Vasodilators

Sodium Nitroprusside. Sodium nitroprusside (NITROPRESS, others) is a direct NO donor and potent vasodilator that is effective in reducing both ventricular filling pressure and systemic vascular resistance. The downstream beneficial physiologic effects of afterload reduction in CHF are outlined in Figure 28–4. Onset to

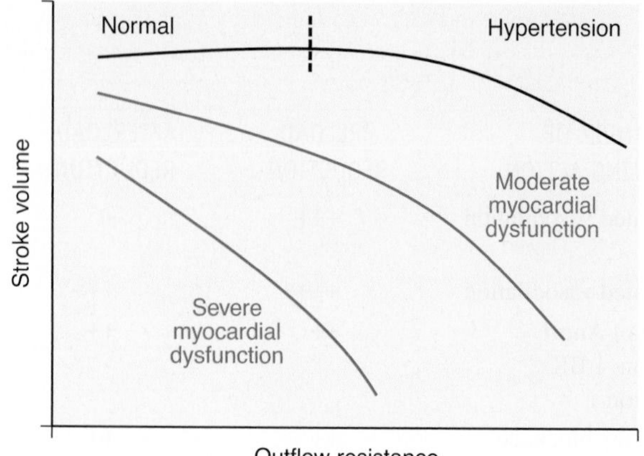

Figure 28–4. *Relationship between ventricular outflow resistance and stroke volume in patients with systolic ventricular dysfunction.* An increase in ventricular outflow resistance, a principal determinant of afterload, has little effect on stroke volume in normal hearts, as illustrated by the relatively flat curve. In contrast, in patients with systolic ventricular dysfunction, an increase in outflow resistance often is accompanied by a sharp decline in stroke volume. With more severe ventricular dysfunction, this curve becomes steeper. Because of this relationship, a reduction in systemic vascular resistance (one component of outflow resistance) in response to an arterial vasodilator may markedly increase stroke volume in patients with severe myocardial dysfunction. The resultant increase in stroke volume may be sufficient to offset the decrease in systemic vascular resistance, thereby preventing a fall in systemic arterial pressure. (Adapted with permission from Cohn and Franciosa, 1977. Copyright © Massachusetts Medical Society. All rights reserved.)

activation of sodium nitroprusside is rapid (2-5 minutes), and the drug is quickly metabolized to NO, properties that afford easy titration to achieve the desired hemodynamic effect.

Nitroprusside is particularly effective in treating critically ill patients with CHF who have elevated systemic vascular resistance or mechanical complications that follow acute MI (e.g., mitral regurgitation or ventricular septal defect-induced left-to-right shunts). As with other vasodilators, the most common adverse side effect of nitroprusside is hypotension. In general, nitroprusside initiation in patients with severe CHF results in increased cardiac output and a parallel increase in renal blood flow, improving both glomerular filtration and diuretic effectiveness. However, excessive reduction of systemic arterial pressure may limit or prevent an increase in renal blood flow in patients with more severe LV contractile dysfunction.

Cyanide produced during the biotransformation of nitroprusside is rapidly metabolized by the liver to thiocyanate, which is then renally excreted. Thiocyanate and/or cyanide toxicity is uncommon but may occur in the setting of hepatic or renal failure, or following prolonged periods of high-dose drug infusion (see Chapter 27 for details). Typical symptoms include unexplained abdominal pain, mental status changes, convulsions, and lactic acidosis. Methemoglobinemia is another unusual complication and is due to the oxidation of hemoglobin by NO•.

Intravenous Nitroglycerin. Intravenous nitroglycerin, like nitroprusside, is a vasoactive NO donor that is commonly used in the intensive care unit setting. Unlike nitroprusside, nitroglycerin is relatively selective for venous capacitance vessels, particularly at low infusion rates. In CHF, intravenous nitroglycerin is most commonly used in the treatment of LV dysfunction due to an acute myocardial ischemia. Parenteral nitroglycerin also is used in the treatment of nonischemic cardiomyopathy when expeditious LV filling pressure reduction is desired. At higher infusion rates, this drug also may decrease systemic arterial resistance, although this effect is less predictable. Nitroglycerin therapy may be limited by headache and nitrate tolerance; tolerance may be partially offset by increasing the dosage. Administration requires the use of an infusion pump capable of controlling the rate of administration.

Hydralazine. Hydralazine is a direct vasodilator that has long been in clinical use, yet its precise mechanism of action is poorly understood. The effects of this agent are not mediated through recognized neurohumoral systems, and its mechanism of action at the cellular level in vascular smooth muscle is uncertain. Lack of mechanistic understanding not with standing, hydralazine is an effective antihypertensive drug (see Chapter 27), particularly when combined with agents that blunt compensatory increases in sympathetic tone and salt and water retention. In CHF, hydralazine reduces right and left ventricular afterload by reducing pulmonary and systemic vascular resistance. This results in an augmentation of forward stroke volume and a reduction in ventricular wall stress in systole. Hydralazine also appears to have moderate "direct" positive inotropic activity in cardiac muscle independent of its afterload-reducing effects. Hydralazine is effective in reducing renal vascular resistance and in increasing renal blood flow to a greater degree than are most other vasodilators, with the exception of ACE inhibitors. For this reason, hydralazine often is used in CHF patients with renal dysfunction intolerant of ACE-inhibitor therapy.

The landmark Veterans Administration Cooperative Vasodilator-Heart Failure Trial I (V-HeFT I) demonstrated that combination therapy with isosorbide dinitrate and hydralazine (a pill containing these two compounds in combination is marketed as BiDil) reduces CHF mortality in patients with systolic dysfunction (Cohn et al., 1986). In V-HeFT I, the mortality benefit was agent specific: the α_1 receptor antagonist *prazosin* offered no advantage over placebo when compared with isosorbide plus hydralazine.

Hydralazine provides additional hemodynamic improvement for patients with advanced CHF (with or without nitrates) already treated with conventional doses of an ACE inhibitor, digoxin, and diuretics (Cohn, 1994). The hypothesis that hydralazine-mediated antioxidant effects benefit CHF patients at elevated risk for vascular endothelial dysfunction is supported by the African-American Heart Failure Trial, in which isosorbide dinitrate-hydralazine substantially decreased all-cause mortality in self-described black patients, a group associated with impaired vascular endothelial function and diminished bioavailable levels of NO when compared to white counterparts (Taylor et al., 2007).

There are several important considerations for hydralazine use. First, ACE inhibitors appear to be superior to hydralazine for mortality reduction in severe CHF. Second, side effects requiring dose adjustment of hydralazine withdrawal are common. In V-HeFT I, e.g., only 55% of patients were taking full doses of both hydralazine and isosorbide dinitrate after 6 months. The lupus-like side effects associated with hydralazine are relatively uncommon and may be more likely to occur in selected patients with the "slow-acetylator" phenotype (see Chapter 27). Finally, hydralazine is a medication taken three or four times daily, and adherence may be difficult for CHF patients, who are often prescribed multiple medications concurrently.

The oral bioavailability and pharmacokinetics of hydralazine are not altered significantly in CHF, unless severe hepatic congestion or hypoperfusion is present. Intravenous hydralazine is available but provides little practical advantage over oral formulations except for urgent use in pregnant patients. In these individuals, hydralazine is often used owing to contraindications that exist for use of most other vasodilators in pregnancy. Hydralazine is typically started at a dose of 10-25 mg three or four times per day and uptitrated to a maximum of 100 mg three or four times daily, as tolerated. At total daily doses >200 mg, hydralazine is associated with an increased risk of lupus-like effects.

Targeting Neurohormonal Regulation: The Renin–Angiotensin–Aldosterone Axis and Vasopressin Antagonists

Renin–Angiotensin–Aldosterone Axis Antagonists. The renin–angiotensin–aldosterone axis plays a central role in the pathophysiology of CHF (Figure 28–3). AngII is a potent arterial vasoconstrictor and an important mediator of Na^+ and water retention through its effects on glomerular filtration pressure and aldosterone secretion. AngII also modulates neural and adrenal medulla catecholamine release, is arrhythmogenic, promotes vascular hyperplasia and myocardial hypertrophy, and induces myocyte death. Consequently, reduction of the effects of AngII constitutes a cornerstone of CHF management (Weber, 2004).

ACE inhibitors suppress AngII (and aldosterone) production, decrease sympathetic nervous system activity, and potentiate the effects of diuretics in CHF. However, AngII levels frequently return to baseline values following chronic treatment with ACE inhibitors (see Chapter 26), due in part to AngII production via ACE-independent enzymes. The sustained clinical effectiveness of ACE inhibitors despite this AngII "escape" suggests that alternate mechanisms contribute to the clinical benefits of ACE inhibitors in CHF. ACE is identical to kininase II, which degrades bradykinin and other kinins that stimulate production of NO, cyclic GMP, and vasoactive eicosanoids. These oppose AngII-induced vascular smooth muscle cell and cardiac fibroblasts proliferation and inhibit unfavorable extracellular matrix deposition.

ACE inhibitors are preferential arterial vasodilators. ACE-inhibitor–mediated decreases in LV afterload result in increased stroke volume and cardiac output; ultimately, the magnitude of these effects is associated with the observed change in mean arterial pressure. Heart rate typically is unchanged with treatment, often despite decreases in systemic arterial pressure, a response that probably is a consequence of decreased sympathetic nervous system activity from ACE inhibition.

Most clinical actions of AngII, including its deleterious effects in CHF, are mediated through the AT_1 angiotensin receptor, whereas AT_2 receptor activation appears to counterbalance the downstream biologic effects of AT_1 receptor stimulation. Owing to enhanced target specificity, AT_1 receptor antagonists more efficiently block the effects of AngII than do ACE inhibitors. In addition, the elevated level of circulating AngII that occurs secondary to AT_1 receptor blockade results in a relative increase in AT_2 receptor activation. Unlike ACE inhibitors, AT_1 blockers do not influence bradykinin metabolism (see the next section).

Angiotensin-Converting Enzyme Inhibitors. The first orally administered ACE inhibitor, captopril (CAPOTEN, others), was introduced in 1977. Since then, six additional ACE inhibitors—enalapril (VASOTEC, others), ramipril (ALTACE, others), lisinopril (PRINIVIL, ZESTRIL, others), quinapril (ACCUPRIL, others), trandolapril (MAVIK, others) and fosinopril (MONOPRIL, others) have been FDA-approved for the treatment of CHF. Data from numerous clinical trials involving well over 100,000 patients support ACE inhibition in the management of CHF of any severity, including those with asymptomatic LV dysfunction.

ACE-inhibitor therapy typically is initiated at a low dose (e.g., 6.25 mg of captopril, 5 mg of lisinopril) to avoid iatrogenic hypotension, particularly in the setting of volume contraction. Hypotension following drug administration usually can be reversed by intravascular volume expansion, but, of course, this may be counterproductive in symptomatic CHF patients. Therefore, it is reasonable to consider initiation of these drugs while congestive symptoms are present. ACE-inhibitor doses customarily are increased over several days in hospitalized patients or over weeks in ambulatory patients, with careful observation of blood pressure, serum electrolytes, and serum creatinine levels.

If possible, drug doses are targeted in practice to match those affording maximum clinical benefit in controlled trials: captopril, 50 mg three times daily (Pfeffer et al., 1992); enalapril, 10 mg twice daily (SOLVD Investigators, 1992; Cohn et al., 1991); lisinopril, 10 mg once daily (GISSI-3, 1994); and ramipril, 5 mg twice daily (AIRE Study Investigators, 1993). If an adequate clinical response is not achieved at these doses, further increases, as tolerated, may be effective (Packer et al., 1999).

In CHF patients with decreased renal blood flow, ACE inhibitors, unlike nitrosovasodilators, impair autoregulation of glomerular perfusion pressure, reflecting their selective effect on efferent (over afferent) arteriolar tone (Kittleson et al., 2003). In the event of acute renal failure or a decrease in the glomerular filtration rate by >20%, ACE-inhibitor dosing should be reduced or the drug discontinued. Rarely, renal function impairment following drug initiation is indicative of bilateral renal artery stenosis.

ACE-Inhibitor Side Effects. Elevated bradykinin levels from ACE inhibition are associated with angioedema, a potentially life-threatening drug side effect. If this occurs, immediate and permanent cessation of *all* ACE inhibitors is indicated. Angioedema may occur at any time over the course of ACE inhibitor therapy. A characteristic, dry cough from the same mechanism is common; in this case, substitution of an AT_1 receptor antagonist for the ACE inhibitor often is curative. A small rise in serum K^+ levels is common with ACE-inhibitor use. This increase may be substantial, however, in patients with renal impairment or in diabetic patients with type IV renal tubular acidosis. Mild hyperkalemia is best managed by institution of a low-potassium diet but may require drug dose adjustment. The inability to implement ACE inhibitors as a consequence of cardiorenal side effects (e.g., excessive hypotension, progressive renal insufficiency, hyperkalemia) is itself a poor prognostic indicator in the CHF patient (Kittleson et al., 2003).

ACE Inhibitors and Survival in CHF. A number of randomized, placebo-controlled clinical trials have demonstrated that ACE inhibitors improve survival in patients with CHF due to systolic dysfunction, independent of etiology. For example, ACE inhibitors prevent mortality and the development of clinically significant LV dysfunction after acute MI (Pfeffer et al., 1992; Konstam et al., 1992; St. John Sutton et al., 1994). This occurs through attenuation or prevention of increased LV end-diastolic and end-systolic volumes, and the decline in LV ejection fraction that is central to the natural history of AMI. ACE inhibitors appear to confer these benefits by preventing postinfarction-associated adverse ventricular remodeling.

The Cooperative North Scandinavian Enalapril Survival Study (CONSENSUS Trial Study Group 1987) demonstrated a 40% mortality reduction after 6 months of enalapril therapy in severe CHF, while others have shown that enalapril also improves survival in patients with mild-to-moderate CHF (SOLVD Investigators, 1992). Furthermore, across the spectrum of CHF severity, when compared with other vasodilators, ACE inhibitors appear superior in reducing mortality (Fonarow et al., 1992). In asymptomatic patients with LV dysfunction, ACE inhibitors slow the development of symptomatic CHF.

AT_1 Receptor Antagonists. Activation of the AT_1 receptor mediates most of the deleterious effects of AngII that are described earlier. AT_1-receptor antagonism, in turn, largely obviates AngII "escape" and substantially decreases the probability of developing bradykinin-mediated side effects associated with ACE inhibition. Importantly, however, although rare, angioedema has been reported with AT_1-receptor antagonist use. Therefore, caution is still warranted when prescribing these agents to patients with a history of ACE-inhibitor–associated angioedema.

AT_1 receptor blockers (ARBs) are effective antihypertensives, and their influence on mortality in acute or chronic CHF from systolic dysfunction after acute MI is akin to that of ACE-inhibitor therapy (Konstam et al., 2005; Dickstein et al., 2002; White et al., 2005). Owing to their favorable side-effect profile, ARBs are an excellent alternative in CHF patients intolerant of ACE inhibitors (Pitt et al., 1997; Doggrell, 2005). Interestingly, age >75 years may increase the probability of developing clinically significant hypotension, renal dysfunction, and hyperkalemia (White et al., 2005).

The role of combination ACE-inhibitor and ARB therapy in the treatment of CHF remains unresolved. Although preliminary studies suggested that combined therapy with candesartan and enalapril, e.g., favorably affected cardiovascular hemodynamics, LV remodeling, and neurohormonal profile compared to therapy with either agent alone (McKelvie et al., 1999), subsequent trials have been unable to demonstrate an incremental mortality benefit from combination therapy despite a significant reduction in CHF-associated hospitalizations (McMurray et al., 2003).

Based on the hypothesis that ARB efficacy is at least in part a consequence of reduced circulating aldosterone levels, combined treatment with aldosterone receptor inhibition has been explored. Combination therapy is associated with a significant increase in LV ejection fraction and quality of life scores in patients with CHF from systolic dysfunction treated for 1 year with candesartan (8 mg daily) and spironolactone (25 mg daily) compared to those treated with candesartan alone (Chan et al., 2007). Others have corroborated the beneficial effects of combined therapy on LV remodeling, 6-minute walk distance, and functional capacity (Kum et al., 2008). The beneficial effects of dual therapy are provocative but must be weighed against the increased likelihood for inducing hyperkalemia, hypotension, and elevated elective treatment withdrawal rates reported in some trials. Data regarding mortality benefit attendant to combination therapy are not available at present.

In CHF from impaired diastolic relaxation (i.e., preserved LV ejection fraction), the role of AT_1 receptor antagonists is unresolved. These drugs do not appear to improve mortality or echocardiographic indices of diastolic relaxation but are associated with fewer CHF hospitalizations (Yusuf et al., 2003; Solomon et al., 2007; Massie et al., 2008). Some have suggested that ARB-induced improvement in arteriolar flow reserve may be protective in patients with diastolic CHF, although this hypothesis remains speculative at present (Kamezaki et al., 2007).

Direct Renin Inhibitors. There is accumulating scientific and clinical evidence to suggest that maximal pharmacologic ACE inhibition alone is insufficient for optimal attenuation of AngII-induced cardiovascular dysfunction in patients with CHF. Several molecular mechanisms have been ascribed to explain this hypothesis (Abassi et al., 2009), including:

- the presence of ACE-independent pathways that facilitate AngI conversion to AngII
- the activation of ACE homologues (e.g., ACE2) that are insensitive to conventional ACE-I therapy
- the suppression of the negative feedback effect exerted by AngI on renin secretion in the kidney

For these reasons, inhibition of renin has pharmacotherapeutic objectives for enhanced suppression of AngII synthesis in CHF.

Renin-mediated conversion of angiotensinogen to AngI is the first and rate-limiting step in the biochemical cascade that generates AngII and aldosterone (see Figures 26–1 and 28–3). The first generation of orally administered direct renin inhibitors was studied in the 1980s and was designed for the treatment of hypertension, but the broader use of these agents was hampered by the drugs' suboptimal efficacy, reflecting, at least in part, their limited bioavailability (Staessen et al., 2006). Aliskiren (TEKTURNA, RASILEZ) is the first orally administered direct renin inhibitor to obtain FDA approval for use in clinical practice. The pharmocokinetic advantages of aliskiren over earlier direct renin inhibitor prototypes include an increased bioavailability (2.7%) and a long plasma $t_{1/2}$ (~23 hour). Pilot clinical trials in humans established that aliskiren induces a concentration-dependent decrease in plasma renin activity and AngI and AngII levels that was associated with a decrease in systemic blood pressure without significant reflex tachycardia. The pharmacology of aliskiren is presented in more detail in Chapter 26.

The effect of aliskiren on blood pressure is the most thoroughly evaluated cardiovascular treatment endpoint. Several small studies have concluded that aliskiren is superior to placebo or to an ARB for monotherapy of mild-to-moderate hypertension (Sanoski, 2009). Aliskiren also appears to exert beneficial effects on myocardial remodeling by decreasing LV mass in hypertensive patients, suggesting that, similar to observations in ACE inhibitor or ARB therapy, direct renin inhibition may attenuate hypertension-induced end-organ damage (Solomon et al., 2009). Collectively, these observations provide evidence that aliskiren-mediated reductions in plasma renin activity and circulating levels of AngII may have salutary effects on the cardiovascular system in hypertension, thus opening the door for investigation of this therapy in patients with CHF.

The safety profile of aliskiren in CHF was established recently by the Aliskiren Observation of Heart Failure Treatment (ALOFT) trial (McMurray et al., 2008). Aliskiren (150 mg/day) add-on therapy to a β receptor antagonist and an ACE inhibitor or ARB was not associated with a significant increase in hypotension or hyperkalemia in a study cohort that mainly included symptomatic CHF patients with a low LV ejection fraction (~30%). Results from this trial also demonstrated that compared with placebo, aliskiren significantly decreased plasma *N*-terminal-proBNP levels, a clinically useful neurohumoral biomarker of active CHF. These findings affirm that inhibition of renin activity is an important potential target for improving symptoms and functional capacity in CHF. However, aliskiren has not yet been studied in sufficiently powered randomized-controlled clinical trials designed to analyze the efficacy of this drug in treatment of CHF.

Vasopressin Receptor Antagonists. Neurohumoral dysregulation in CHF extends beyond the renin–angiotensin–aldosterone axis to include abnormal arginine vasopressin (AVP) secretion, resulting in the perturbation of fluid balance, among various additional pathophysiogic effects. In response to 1) serum hypertonicity-induced activation of anterior pituitary osmoreceptors and 2) a perceived drop in blood pressure detected by baroreceptors in the carotid artery, aortic arch, and left atrium, AVP is secreted into the systemic circulation (Arai et al., 2007). The physiology and pharmacology of vasopressin are presented in Chapter 25.

The active form of AVP is a 9–amino acid peptide that interacts with three receptor subtypes: V_{1a}, V_{1b}, and V_2 (see Chapter 25). The AVP-V_2 receptor interaction on the basolateral membrane of the renal collecting ducts stimulates *de novo* synthesis of aquaporin-2 water channels that mediate free water reabsorption, thereby impairing diuresis and, ultimately, correcting plasma hypertonicity. Additional cell signaling pathways important in the pathophysiology of CHF include vasoconstriction, cell hypertrophy, and increased platelet aggregation mediated by activation of V_{1a} receptors in vascular smooth muscle cells and cardiac myocytes. In addition, AngII-mediated activation of centrally located AT_1 receptors is associated with increased AVP levels in

CHF and may represent one mechanism by which the use of AT_1-receptor antagonists are effective in the clinical management of these patients.

LV systolic dysfunction can be associated with hypervasopressinemia. Numerous observational and case-controlled studies have reported AVP levels nearly 2-fold above normal in CHF patients (Finley et al., 2008). The mechanisms to account for dysregulated AVP synthesis in CHF may involve impaired atrial stretch receptor sensitivity, normally a counterregulatory mechanism for AVP secretion, and increased adrenergic tone (Bristow et al., 2005). These probably do not fully explain the relationship between CHF and AVP levels; e.g., elevated levels of AVP have been observed in *asymptomatic* patients with significantly decreased LV function, calling into question the attributable role of sympathetically mediated adrenergic tone as a cause of hypervasopressinemia (Francis et al., 1990).

In addition, there is evidence to suggest that CHF is a disease of abnormal *responsiveness* to vasopressin rather than one of excessive vasopressin production alone. For example, vasopressin infusion in CHF patients decreases cardiac output and stroke volume and causes an exaggerated increase in systemic vascular resistance and pulmonary capillary wedge pressure (Finley et al., 2008). In turn, V_2 antagonists attenuate the adverse pathophysiologic effects of hypervasopressinemia by decreasing capillary wedge pressure, right atrial pressure, and pulmonary artery systolic blood pressure (Udelson et al., 2008). These agents also restore and maintain normal serum sodium levels in decompensated CHF patients, but their long-term use has not yet been convincingly linked to a decrease in CHF-associated symptoms or mortality (Gheorghiade et al., 2004).

Generally, trials designed to measure the effect of vasopressin-receptor antagonists have used agents selective for the V_2 receptor, although some drugs with both V_2 and V_{1a} receptor affinity also have been studied. Tolvaptan (SAMSCA), which preferentially binds the V_2 receptor over the V_{1a} receptor (receptor affinity ~29:1), is perhaps the most widely tested vasopressin receptor antagonist in patients with CHF and also is approved for hyponatremia. Due to the risk of overly rapid correction of hyponatremia causing osmotic demyelination, tolvaptan should be started only in a hospital setting where Na^+ levels can be monitored closely and possible drug interactions mediated by CYP and P-gp can be considered (black box warning). Conivaptan, used mainly for the treatment of hyponatremia rather than for CHF *per se*, differs from tolvaptan in that it may be intravenously administered, demonstrates high affinity for both V_2- and V_{1a}-vasopressin receptors, and has a $t_{1/2}$ that is nearly twice as long.

In the randomized, placebo-controlled EVEREST trial, the effect of tolvaptan (30 mg/day) in addition to standard therapy on immediate symptom improvement was assessed in patients administered the drug <48 hours into hospitalization for CHF (Gheorghiade et al., 2007). Data from this study substantiated that from the others, indicating that AVP antagonists decrease body weight, self-reported dypsnea, and physician-assessed peripheral edema, rales, and fatigue after a short course of therapy (<7 days). Long-term outcomes (survival, hospitalizations) were not significantly different from placebo. The identification of a CHF subgroup that stands to benefit most from AVP antagonists, in addition to the preferred agent and therapy duration, are questions of ongoing clinical investigation.

β Adrenergic Receptor Antagonists

Sympathetic nervous system activation in CHF supports circulatory function by enhancing contractility (inotropy), augmenting ventricular relaxation and filling (lusitropy), and increasing heart rate (chronotropy). For many years, pharmacologic approaches to CHF treatment targeted drugs with sympathomimetic properties. This reflected the viewpoint that CHF is fundamentally a disorder of impaired stroke volume and cardiac output. For example, CHF symptom relief from short-term *dobutamine* and *dopamine* use in patients with ventricular dysfunction led to the belief that long-term sympathomimetic use would further improve clinical outcome. Under this model, the use of β receptor antagonists was believed to be counterproductive; however, the reverse appears to be the case. Long-term sympathomimetic use is associated with increased CHF mortality rates, whereas a survival benefit is associated with chronic administration of β receptor antagonists. Initially, clinical investigation of β receptor antagonists in the treatment of CHF encountered skepticism, but reports beginning in the early 1990s demonstrated that β antagonists (e.g., *metoprolol*) improve symptoms, exercise tolerance, and are measures of LV function over several months in idiopathic dilated cardiomyopathy patients with CHF (Waagstein et al., 1993; Gottlieb et al., 1998; Swedberg, 1993; Bristow, 2000). Serial echocardiographic measurements in CHF patients indicate that a decrease in systolic function occurs immediately after initiation of a β antagonist treatment, but this recovers and improves beyond baseline over the ensuing 2-4 months (Hall et al., 1995). This trend may be due to attenuation or prevention of the β receptor–mediated adverse effects of catecholamines on the myocardium (Eichhorn and Bristow, 1996).

Mechanism of Action. The mechanisms by which β receptor antagonists influence outcome in CHF patients are not fully delineated. By preventing myocardial ischemia without significantly influencing serum electrolytes, β receptor antagonists probably influence mortality, in part, by decreasing the frequency of unstable tachyarrhythmias to which CHF patients are particularly prone. In addition, these agents may influence survival by favorably affecting LV geometry, specifically by decreasing LV chamber size and increasing LV ejection fraction. Through inhibition of sustained sympathetic nervous system activation, these agents prevent or delay progression of myocardial contractile dysfunction by inhibiting maladaptive proliferative cell signaling in the myocardium, reducing catecholamine-induced cardiomyocyte toxicity, and decreasing myocyte apoptosis (Communal et al., 1998; Bisognano et al., 2000). β Receptor antagonists may also induce positive LV remodeling by decreasing oxidative stress in the myocardium (Sawyer and Colucci, 2000).

Metoprolol. Metoprolol (LOPRESSOR, TOPROL XL, others) is a β_1-selective receptor antagonist. The short-acting form of this drug has a drug elimination $t_{1/2}$ of ~6 hours, and therefore appropriate dosing is three to four times daily. Conversely, the extended-release formulation is sufficiently dosed once daily.

A number of clinical trials have demonstrated the beneficial effects of β-antagonist therapy in CHF. In the Metoprolol Randomized Intervention Trial in Congestive Heart Failure (MERIT-HF Study Group 1999), patients with low LV ejection fraction and severe CHF receiving metoprolol succinate (target dose, 200 mg/day) received a 34% all-cause mortality benefit, an effect attributable to reductions in sudden death and death from worsening CHF. Despite the high target drug dose, the majority of patients achieved this therapeutic goal.

Carvedilol. Carvedilol (COREG, others) is a nonselective β receptor antagonist and α_1-selective antagonist that is FDA approved for the management of mild-to-severe CHF.

The U.S. Carvedilol Trial randomized patients with symptomatic but compensated CHF (New York Heart Association [NYHA] classes II to IV) and low LV ejection fraction to receive carvedilol or placebo (Packer et al., 1996). Carvedilol (25 mg twice daily) was associated with a 65% reduction in all-cause mortality that was independent of age, sex, CHF etiology, or LV ejection fraction. The mortality benefit and improvement in LV ejection fraction was carvedilol concentration dependent (Bristow et al., 1996). Exercise capacity (e.g., 6-minute walk test) did not improve with carvedilol, however, but therapy did appear to slow the progression of CHF in a subgroup of patients with good exercise capacity and mild symptoms at baseline (Colucci et al., 1996).

In the Carvedilol Post Infarct Survival Control in LV Dysfunction Trial (Dargie, 2001), patients with recent MI (3-21 days prior to enrollment) and impaired LV systolic function were randomized to carvedilol (25 mg twice daily) or placebo. Patients with symptomatic CHF and those with asymptomatic LV dysfunction were included. Although there was no difference in the primary endpoint of all-cause mortality, carvedilol therapy was associated with a significant reduction in the combined endpoint of all-cause mortality and nonfatal MI. At the opposite end of the spectrum, patients with symptomatic CHF at rest or with minimal exertion and impaired LV systolic function were randomized to carvedilol versus placebo in the Carvedilol Prospective Randomized Cumulative Survival Study (Packer et al., 2002b). Consistent with previous trials, there was a 35% decrease in all-cause mortality. Although the patients included in the trial had established CHF, it merits emphasis that the placebo group mortality at 1 year was ~18%, a finding suggestive that the patient cohort was not representative of patients with advanced CHF.

Clinical Use of β Adrenergic Receptor Antagonists in Heart Failure

Data from more than 15,000 patients with mild-to-moderate chronic CHF enrolled in various clinical trials have established that β receptor antagonists improve disease-associated symptoms, hospitalization, and mortality. Accordingly, β antagonists are recommended for use in patients with an LV ejection fraction <35% and NYHA class II or III symptoms in conjunction with an ACE inhibitor or AT_1 receptor antagonist, and diuretics as required to palliate symptoms. Interpretation of these and other clinical guidelines should, however, consider the following areas of uncertainty.

The role of β receptor antagonists in severe CHF or under circumstances of an acute clinical decompensation is not yet clear. Likewise, the utility of β blockade in patients with asymptomatic LV dysfunction has not been systematically evaluated. The marked heterogeneous pharmacologic characteristics (e.g., receptor selectivity, pharmacokinetics) of specific agents within this general drug class, as discussed in Chapter 12, play a key role in predicting the overall efficacy of a particular β receptor antagonist.

β receptor antagonist therapy is customarily initiated at very low doses, generally less than one-tenth of the final target dose, and titrated cautiously upward. Even when initiated properly, a tendency to retain fluid exists that may require diuretic dose adjustment. Insufficient evidence exists to support the unrestricted administration of β receptor antagonists in patients with severe (NYHA class IIIB and IV), new-onset, or acutely decompensated CHF.

Cardiac Glycosides

The English botanist, chemist, and physician Sir William Withering is credited with the first published observation in 1785 that *digitalis purpurea*, a derivative of the purple foxglove flower, could be used for the treatment of "cardiac dropsy," or congestive heart failure. The benefits of cardiac glycosides in CHF have been extensively studied (Eichhorn and Gheorghiade, 2002) and are generally attributed to:

- Inhibition of the plasma membrane Na^+, K^+-ATPase in myocytes
- A positive inotropic effect on the failing myocardium
- Suppression of rapid ventricular rate response in CHF-associated atrial fibrillation
- Regulation of downstream deleterious effects of sympathetic nervous system overactivation

Mechanism of the Positive Inotropic Effect. With each cardiac myocyte depolarization, Na^+ and Ca^{2+} ions shift into the intracellular space (Figure 28–5). Ca^{2+} that enters the cell via the L-type Ca^{2+} channel during depolarization triggers the release of stored intracellular Ca^{2+} from the sarcoplasmic reticulum via the ryanodine receptor (RyR). This Ca^{2+}-induced Ca^{2+} release increases the level of cytosolic Ca^{2+} available for interaction with myocyte contractile proteins, ultimately increasing myocardial contraction force. During myocyte repolarization and relaxation, cellular Ca^{2+} is re-sequestered by the sarcoplasmic reticular Ca^{2+}-ATPase and is removed from the cell by the Na^+Ca^{2+} exchanger and, to a much lesser extent, by the sarcolemmal Ca^{2+}-ATPase.

Cardiac glycosides bind and inhibit the phosphorylated (α subunit of the sarcolemmal Na^+,K^+-ATPase and thereby decreasing Na^+ extrusion and increasing cytosolic [Na^+]. This decreases the transmembrane Na^+ gradient that drives Na^+–Ca^{2+} exchange during myocyte repolarization. As a consequence, less Ca^{2+} is removed from the cell and more Ca^{2+} is accumulated in the sarcoplasmic reticulum (SR) by SERCA2. This increase in releasable Ca^{2+} (from the SR) is the mechanism by which cardiac glycosides

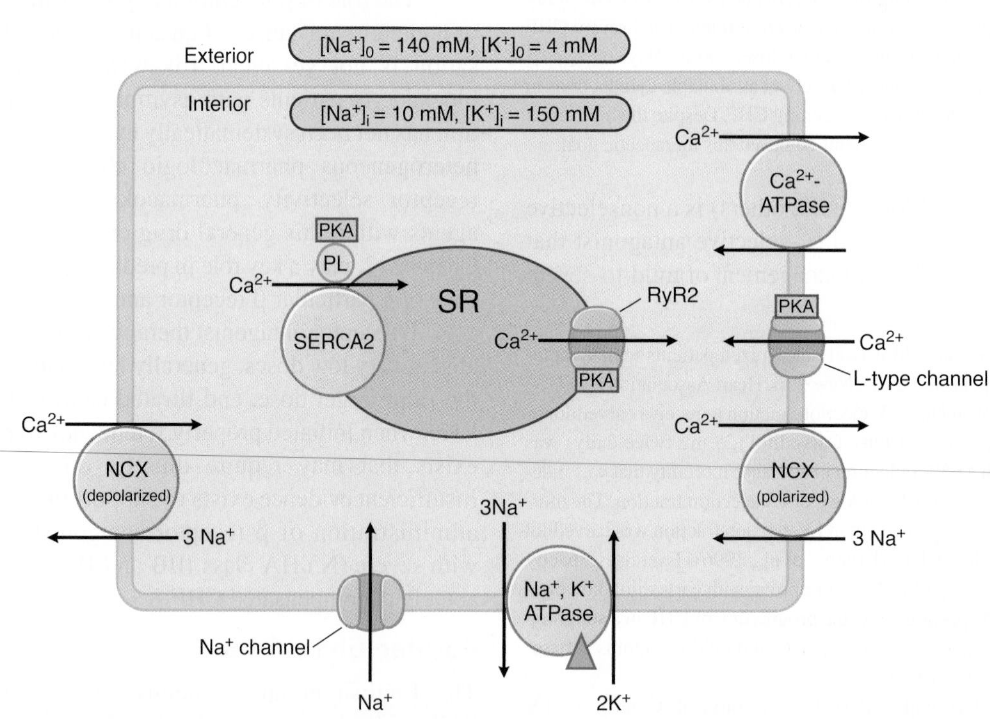

Figure 28–5. *Sarcolemmal exchange of Na^+ and Ca^{2+} during cell depolarization and repolarization.* Na^+ and Ca^{2+} enter the cardiac myocyte via the Na^+ channel and the L-type Ca^{2+} channel during each cycle of membrane depolarization, triggering the release, through the ryanodine receptor (RyR), of larger amounts of Ca^{2+} from internal stores in the sarcoplasmic reticulum (SR). The resulting increase in intracellular Ca^{2+} interacts with troponin C and activates interactions between actin and myosin that result in sarcomere shortening. The electrochemical gradient for Na^+ across the sarcolemma is maintained by active transport of Na^+ out of the cell by the sarcolemmal Na^+,K^+-ATPase. The bulk of cytosolic Ca^{2+} is pumped back into the SR by a Ca^{2+}-ATPase, SERCA2. The remainder is removed from the cell by either a sarcolemmal Ca^{2+}-ATPase or a high-capacity Na^+-Ca^{2+} exchanger, NCX. NCX exchanges 3 Na^+ for every Ca^{2+}, using the electrochemical potential of Na^+ to drive Ca^{2+} extrusion. The direction of Na^+-Ca^{2+} exchange may reverse briefly during depolarization, when the electrical gradient across the sarcolemma is transiently reversed. β adrenergic agonists and PDE inhibitors, by increasing intracellular cyclic AMP levels, activate PKA, which phosphorylates phospholamban (PL), the α subunit of the L-type Ca^{2+} channel, and regulatory components of the RyR, as well as TnI, the inhibitory subunit of troponin (not shown). As a result, the probabilities of opening of the L-type Ca^{2+} channel and the RyR2 Ca^{2+} channel are doubled; SERCA2 is uninhibited and accumulates Ca^{2+} into the SR faster, more avidly, and to a higher concentration; and relaxation occurs at slightly higher $[Ca^{2+}]_i$ due to slightly reduced sensitivity of the troponin complex to Ca^{2+}. The net effect of these phosphorylations is a positive inotropic effect: *a faster rate of tension development to a higher level of tension, followed by a faster rate of relaxation.* ▲ indicates site of cardiac glycoside binding. See the text for the mechanism of positive inotropic effect of cardiac glycosides.

enhance myocardial contractility. Elevated extracellular K^+ levels (i.e., hyperkalemia) cause dephosphorylation of the ATPase α subunit, altering the site of action of the most commonly used cardiac glycoside, *digoxin*, and thereby reducing the drug's binding and effect.

Electrophysiologic Actions. At therapeutic serum or plasma concentrations (i.e., 1-2 ng/mL), digoxin decreases automaticity and increases the maximal diastolic resting membrane potential in atrial and atrioventricular (AV) nodal tissues. This occurs via increases in vagal tone and sympathetic nervous system activity inhibition. In addition, digoxin prolongs the effective refractory period and decreases conduction velocity in AV nodal tissue. Collectively, these may contribute to sinus bradycardia, sinus arrest, prolongation of AV conduction, or high-grade AV block. At higher concentrations, cardiac glycosides may increase sympathetic nervous system activity that influences cardiac tissue automaticity, change associated with the genesis of atrial and ventricular arrhythmias. Increased intracellular Ca^{2+} loading and sympathetic tone increases the spontaneous (phase 4) rate of diastolic depolarization as well as promoting delayed afterdepolarization; together, these decrease the threshold for generation of a propagated action potential and predisposes to malignant ventricular arrhythmias (see Chapter 29).

Regulation of Sympathetic Nervous System Activity. Sympathetic nervous system overactivation in CHF occurs, in part, from aberrant arterial baroreflex responses to low cardiac output. Specifically, a decline in baroreflex response to blood pressure results in a decline in baroreflex-mediated tonic suppression of CNS-directed sympathetic activity. This cascade contributes to the sustained elevation in plasma NE, renin, and vasopressin (Ferguson et al., 1989). Cardiac glycosides favorably influence carotid baroreflex responsiveness to changes in carotid sinus pressure (Wang et al., 1990). In patients with moderate-to-advanced CHF, cardiac glycoside infusion increases forearm blood flow and cardiac index and decreased heart rate. There is clinical evidence to suggest that digoxin decreases centrally mediated sympathetic nervous system tone, although the mechanism to explain this is unresolved (Ferguson et al., 1989).

Pharmacokinetics. The elimination $t_{1/2}$ for digoxin is 36-48 hours in patients with normal or near-normal renal function, permitting once-daily dosing. Near steady-state blood levels are achieved ~7 days after initiation of maintenance therapy. Digoxin is excreted by the kidney, and increases in cardiac output or renal blood flow from vasodilator therapy or sympathomimetic agents may increase renal digoxin clearance, necessitating adjustment of daily maintenance doses. The volume of distribution and drug clearance rate are both decreased in elderly patients.

Despite renal clearance, digoxin is not removed effectively by hemodialysis due to the drug's large (4-7 L/kg) volume of distribution. The principal tissue reservoir is skeletal muscle and not adipose tissue, and thus dosing should be based on estimated lean body mass. Most digoxin tablets average 70-80% oral bioavailability; however, ~10% of the general population harbors the enteric bacterium *Eubacterium lentum*, which inactivates digoxin and thus may account for drug tolerance that is observed in some patients. Liquid-filled capsules of digoxin (LANOXICAPS) have a higher bioavailability than do tablets (LANOXIN); thus, the drug requires dosage adjustment if a patient is switched from one delivery form to the other. Digoxin is available for intravenous administration, and maintenance doses can be given intravenously when oral dosing is inappropriate. Digoxin administered intramuscularly is erratically absorbed, causes local discomfort, and usually is unnecessary. A number of clinical conditions may alter the pharmacokinetics of digoxin or patient susceptibility to the toxic manifestations of this drug. For example, chronic renal failure decreases the volume of distribution of digoxin and therefore requires a decrease in maintenance dosage of the drug. In addition, drug interactions that may influence circulating serum digoxin levels include several commonly used cardiovascular medications such as verapamil, amiodarone, propafenone, and spironolactone. The rapid administration of Ca^{2+} increases the risk of inducing malignant arrhythmias in patients already treated with digoxin. Electrolyte disturbances, especially hypokalemia, acid–base imbalances, and one's form of underlying heart disease also may alter a patient's susceptibility to digoxin side effects.

Maximal increase in LV contractility becomes apparent at serum digoxin levels ~1.4 ng/mL (1.8 nmol) (Kelly and Smith, 1992). The neurohormonal benefits of digoxin, however, may occur between 0.5-1 ng/mL. In turn, higher serum concentrations are not associated with incrementally increased clinical benefit. Moreover, there are data to suggest that the risk of death is greater with increasing serum concentrations, even at values within the traditional therapeutic range, and therefore many advocate maintaining digoxin levels <1 ng/mL.

Clinical Use of Digoxin in Heart Failure. Data from contemporary clinical trials have re-characterized the utility of cardiac glycosides, once first-line agents, in CHF, especially in patients with normal sinus rhythm (as opposed to atrial fibrillation).

Digoxin discontinuation in clinically stable patients with mild-to-moderate CHF from LV systolic dysfunction worsened symptoms and decreased maximal treadmill exercise (Uretsky et al., 1993; Packer et al., 1993). However, eventhough digoxin may decrease CHF-associated hospitalizations in patients with severe forms of the disease, drug use does not reduce all-cause mortality. Overall, digoxin use usually is limited to CHF patients with LV systolic dysfunction in atrial fibrillation or to patients in sinus rhythm who remain symptomatic despite maximal therapy with ACE inhibitors and β adrenergic receptor antagonists. The latter agents are viewed as first-line therapies because of their proven mortality benefit.

Digoxin Toxicity. The incidence and severity of digoxin toxicity have declined substantially in the past 2 decades as a consequence of alternative drugs available for the treatment of supraventricular arrhythmias in CHF, increased understanding of digoxin pharmacokinetics, improved serum digoxin level monitoring, and identification of important interactions between digoxin and other commonly co-administered drugs. Nevertheless, the recognition of digoxin toxicity remains an important consideration in the differential diagnosis of arrhythmias, and neurologic or gastrointestinal symptoms in patients receiving cardiac glycosides. An antidote, digoxin immune Fab (DIGIBIND, DIGIFAB), is available to treat toxicity.

Among the more common electrophysiologic manifestations of digoxin toxicity are ectopic beats originating from the AV junction or ventricle, first-degree AV block, abnormally slow ventricular rate response to atrial fibrillation, or an accelerated AV junctional pacemaker. When present, only dosage adjustment and appropriate monitoring are usually necessary. Sinus bradycardia, sinoatrial arrest or exit block, and second- or third-degree AV conduction delay requiring atropine or temporary ventricular pacing are uncommon. Unless in the setting of high-degree AV block, potassium administration should be considered for patients with evidence of increased AV junctional or ventricular automaticity even if serum K^+ levels are in the normal range. Lidocaine or phenytoin, which have minimal effects on AV conduction, may be used for the treatment of digoxin-induced ventricular arrhythmias that threaten hemodynamic compromise (see Chapter 29). Electrical cardioversion carries an increased risk of inducing severe rhythm disturbances in patients with overt digitalis toxicity and should be used with particular caution. Note, too, that inhibition of the Na^+,K^+-ATPase activity of skeletal muscle can cause hyperkalemia. An effective antidote for life-threatening digoxin (or digitoxin) toxicity is available in the form of anti-digoxin immunotherapy. Purified Fab fragments from ovine anti-digoxin antisera (DIGIBIND) are usually dosed by the estimated total dose of digoxin ingested in order to achieve a fully neutralizing effect. For a more comprehensive review of the treatment of digitalis toxicity, see Kelly and Smith (1992).

β Adrenergic and Dopaminergic Agonists

In the setting of severely decompensated CHF from reduced cardiac output, the principal focus of initial therapy is to increase myocardial contractility. Dopamine and dobutamine are positive inotropic agents most often used to accomplish this. These drugs provide short-term circulatory support in advanced CHF via stimulation of cardiac myocyte dopamine (D_1) and β adrenergic receptors that stimulate the G_s-adenylyl cyclase-cyclic AMP–PKA pathway. The catalytic subunit of PKA phosphorylates a number of substrates that enhance Ca^{+2}-dependent myocardial contraction and accelerate relaxation (Figure 28–5). Isoproterenol, epinephrine, and norepinephrine are useful in certain circumstances but have little role in routine CHF management. Indeed, inotropic agents that elevate cardiac cell cyclic AMP are consistently associated with increased risks of hospitalization and death, particularly in patients with NYHA class IV. At the cellular level, enhanced cyclic AMP levels have been associated with apoptosis (Brunton, 2005; Yan et al., 2007). The basic pharmacology of adrenergic agonists is discussed in Chapter 12.

Dopamine. Dopamine is an endogenous catecholamine with only limited utility in the treatment of most patients with cardiogenic circulatory failure. The pharmacologic and hemodynamic effects of dopamine are concentration dependent. *Low doses* (≤2 μg/kg lean body mass/min) induces cyclic AMP–dependent vascular smooth muscle vasodilation. In addition, activation of D_2 receptors on sympathetic nerves in the peripheral circulation at these concentrations also inhibits NE release and reduces α adrenergic stimulation of vascular smooth muscle, particularly in splanchnic and renal arterial beds. Therefore, low-dose dopamine infusion often is used to increase renal blood flow and thereby maintain an adequate glomerular filtration rate in hospitalized CHF patients with impaired renal function refractory to diuretics. Dopamine also exhibits a pro-diuretic effect directly on renal tubular epithelial cells that contributes to volume reduction.

At *intermediate* infusion rates (2-5 μg/kg/min), dopamine directly stimulates cardiac α receptors and vascular sympathetic neurons that enhance myocardial contractility and neural NE release. At *higher* infusion rates (5-15 μg/kg/min), α adrenergic receptor stimulation–mediated peripheral arterial and venous constriction occurs. This may be desirable in patients with critically reduced arterial pressure or in those with circulatory failure from severe vasodilation (e.g., sepsis, anaphylaxis). However, high-dose dopamine infusion has little role in the treatment of patients with primary cardiac contractile dysfunction; in this setting, increased vasoconstriction will lead to increased afterload and worsening of LV performance. Tachycardia, which is more pronounced with dopamine than with dobutamine, may actually provoke ischemia (and ischemia-induced malignant arrhythmias) in patients with coronary artery disease.

Dobutamine. Dobutamine is the β agonist of choice for the management of CHF patients with systolic dysfunction. In the formulation available for clinical use, dobutamine is a racemic mixture that stimulates both $β_1$ and $β_2$ receptor subtypes. In addition, the (–) enantiomer is an agonist for α adrenergic receptors, whereas the (+) enantiomer is a weak, partial agonist. At infusion rates that result in a positive inotropic effect in humans, the $β_1$ adrenergic effect in the myocardium predominates. In the vasculature, the α adrenergic agonist effect of the (–) enantiomer appears to be offset by the (+) enantiomer and vasodilating effects of $β_2$ receptor stimulation. Thus, the principal hemodynamic effect of dobutamine is an increase in stroke volume from positive inotropy, although β_2 receptor activation may cause a decrease in systemic vascular resistance and, therefore, mean arterial pressure. Despite increases in cardiac output, there is relatively little chronotropic effect.

Continuous dobutamine infusions are typically initiated at 2-3 μg/kg/min without a loading dose and uptitrated until the desired hemodynamic response is achieved. Pharmacologic tolerance may limit infusion efficacy beyond 4 days, and, therefore, addition or substitution with a class III PDE inhibitor may be necessary to maintain adequate circulatory support. The major side effects of dobutamine are tachycardia and supraventricular or ventricular arrhythmias, which may require a reduction in dosage. Recent β receptor antagonist use is a common cause of blunted clinical responsiveness to dobutamine.

Phosphodiesterase Inhibitors. The cyclic AMP–PDE inhibitors decrease cellular cyclic AMP degradation, resulting in elevated levels of cyclic AMP in cardiac and smooth muscle myocytes. The physiologic effects of this are positive myocardial inotropism and dilation of resistance and capacitance vessels. Collectively, therefore, PDE inhibition improves cardiac output through ionotropy and by decreasing preload and afterload (thus giving rise to the term *inodilator*). The clinical application of early-generation PDE inhibitors (e.g., theophylline, caffeine) is limited by low cardiovascular specificity and an unfavorable side-effect profile, whereas inamrinone, milrinone, and other more recently developed PDE inhibitors are preferred.

Inamrinone and Milrinone. Parenteral formulations of inamrinone (previously named amrinone) and milrinone are approved for short-term circulation support in advanced CHF. Both drugs are bipyridine derivatives and are selective PDE3 inhibitors, the cyclic GMP–inhibited cyclic AMP–PDE. These drugs directly stimulate myocardial contractility and accelerate myocardial relaxation. In addition, they cause balanced arterial and venous dilation with a consequent fall in systemic and pulmonary vascular resistances and left and right-heart filling pressure. As a result of its effect on LV contractility, the increase in cardiac output from milrinone is superior to that from nitroprusside, despite comparable reductions in systemic vascular resistance. Conversely, the arterial and venodilatory effects of milrinone are greater than those of dobutamine at concentrations that produce similar increases in cardiac output.

Parenteral administration of inamrinone and milrinone in patients with CHF from systolic dysfunction should be initiated with a loading dose followed by continuous infusion. For inamrinone, a 0.75-mg/kg bolus injection administered over 2-3 minutes is typically followed by a 2-20-μg/kg/min infusion. The loading dose of milrinone is ordinarily 50 μg/kg, and the continuous infusion rate ranges from 0.25-1 μg/kg/min. The elimination half-lives of inamrinone and milrinone in normal individuals are 2-3 hours and 0.5-1 hour, respectively, but are nearly doubled in patients with severe CHF. Clinically significant thrombocytopenia occurs in ~10% of those receiving inamrinone but is rare with milrinone. Because of enhanced selectivity for PDE3, short $t_{1/2}$, and favorable side-effect profile, milrinone is the agent of choice among currently available PDE inhibitors for *short-term*, parenteral inotropic support. However, vasodilation-mediated reductions in mean arterial pressure are one practical barrier to milrinone administration in patients with marginal systemic arterial blood pressure from low cardiac output.

Sildenafil. In contrast to inamrinone and milrinone, sildenafil (REVATIO) inhibits PDE5, which is the most common PDE isoform in lung tissue. This characteristic of PDE5 likely accounts for the enhanced pulmonary artery specificity observed with sildenafil use. In fact, until recently, the primary clinical application of sildenafil in CHF has mainly been limited to those with isolated right ventricular systolic failure from pulmonary artery hypertension. However, recently published reports suggest that sildenafil favorably influences exercise capacity and right-heart hemodynamics in patients with pulmonary hypertension from LV systolic dysfunction as well (Lewis et al., 2007). Preclinical experimental models also have raised the possibility that PDE5 inhibition is directly cardioprotective via attenuation of adrenergic stimulation-induced myocardial contraction and by suppressing pressure-overload mediated myocardial hypertrophy and attendant ventricular dysfunction (Kass et al., 2007). The pharmacology of PDE5 inhibitors is presented in Chapter 27.

Chronic Positive Inotropic Therapy

Several orally administered agents with combined inotropic and vasodilator properties are available for clinical use. Although improvements in CHF symptoms, functional status, and hemodynamic profile have been reported, the effect of long-term therapy on mortality is disappointing. In fact, the dopaminergic agonist ibopamine; PDE inhibitors milrinone, inamrinone, and vesnarinone; and pimobendan are associated with increased mortality (Hampton et al., 1997; Packer et al., 1991; Cohn et al., 1998). At present, digoxin remains the only oral inotropic agent available for CHF patient use.

Continuous or intermittent outpatient therapy with intravenous dobutamine or milrinone, administered by a portable or home-based infusion pump through a central venous catheter, is available for end-stage CHF patients with symptoms refractory to optimized medical therapy.

Diastolic Heart Failure

Data from population studies suggest that up to 40% of CHF patients have preserved LV systolic function. The pathogenesis of diastolic CHF includes structural and functional abnormalities of the ventricle(s) that are associated with impaired ventricular relaxation and LV distensibility. These abnormalities are reflected in the

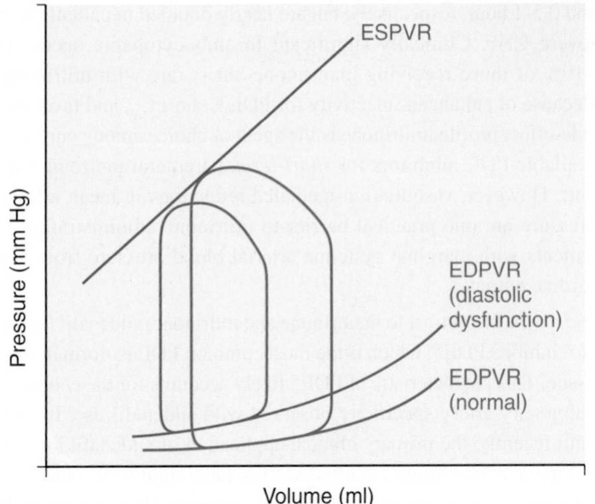

Figure 28–6. *Pressure-volume relationships in normal heart and heart with diastolic dysfunction.* Normal P-V loo (green) based on normal end diastolic pressure-volume relationship (EDPVR). P-V loop with diastolic dysfunction is shown in red. ESPVR, end-systolic pressure– volume relationship.

LV pressure–volume relationship during diastole, which is shifted upward and to the left relative to normal subjects (Figure 28–6). Consonant with the definition of CHF outlined earlier in this chapter, the diagnosis of diastolic CHF is made when the LV is unable to maintain adequate cardiac output without filling at an abnormally elevated end-diastolic filling pressure.

In patients with *primary* diastolic dysfunction, the myocardial abnormality that accounts for abnormal filling is intrinsic to the myocardium; e.g., by infiltrative disorders including cardiac amyloidosis, hemochromatosis, sarcoidosis, and rarer conditions such as endomyocardial fibrosis and Fabry's disease. Although not a disease of myocardium infiltration, clinically evident CHF may occur despite intact LV systolic function in familial hypertrophic cardiomyopathy.

Secondary diastolic dysfunction occurs as a consequence of excessive preload (e.g., renal failure), excessive afterload (e.g., systemic hypertension), or changes in LV geometry that occur in response to chronically abnormal loading conditions. Diastolic CHF also is observed in patients with long-standing epicardial coronary artery or pericardial disease. The prevalence of secondary diastolic dysfunction is higher in women and with advanced age. Reported annual mortality rates for diastolic CHF are 5-8%, although this range likely represents an underestimation (Jones et al., 2004).

Patients with diastolic CHF are typically dependent on preload to maintain adequate cardiac output. Although hypervolemic patients generally benefit from careful intravascular volume reduction, this should be accomplished gradually and treatment goals reassessed frequently. Maintaining synchronous atrial contraction (or at least ventricular rate response control) helps to maintain adequate LV filling during the latter phase of diastole and is therefore a paramount goal in the management of CHF from diastolic dysfunction. Evaluation and treatment of predisposing conditions to impaired diastolic function, such as myocardial ischemia and poorly controlled systemic hypertension, are fundamental to the overall pharmacotherapeutic strategy of this complex form of CHF.

Future Therapies: Targeting Vascular Dysfunction in Congestive Heart Failure from Systolic Dysfunction

Vascular dysfunction is an established component of the CHF syndrome and has evolved into a novel pharmacotherapeutic target for the clinical management of patients with this disease (Varin et al., 2000) (Figure 28–7). Contemporary scientific observations suggest that the blood vessel is a dynamic structure integral to normal myocardial function. This represents a paradigm shift away from the traditional perspective that blood vessels are conduit "tubes" necessary only for blood transport. Elevated levels of oxidant, nitrosative, and other forms of inflammatory stress observed in patients with CHF may impair vascular reactivity by disruption of normal vasodilatory cell signaling pathways (Erwin et al., 2005; Doehner et al., 2001). The precise mechanism by which impaired vascular reactivity is aligned with the progressive natural history of CHF is unresolved; when present, however, vascular dysfunction is associated with decreased exercise tolerance and a poorer clinical outcome. For example, hyperaldosteronism due to overactivation of the renin–angiotensin–aldosterone axis in the setting of LV dysfunction adversely affects both endothelium-dependent and endothelium-independent vascular reactivity (Leopold et al., 2007, Maron et al., 2009) enfothelium XO-I zenthine oxidase inhibitor vascular reactivity. This process is in part mediated by increased levels of reactive oxygen species, decreased endogenous levels of antioxidant enzymes, and decreased levels of bioavailable NO (Leopold et al., 2007; Farquharson and Struthers, 2000). As discussed previously, the undesirable effects of hyperaldosteronism on vascular dysfunction are attenuated clinically by aldosterone receptor blockade, resulting in significantly decreased CHF-associated morbidity and mortality (Pitt et al., 1999).

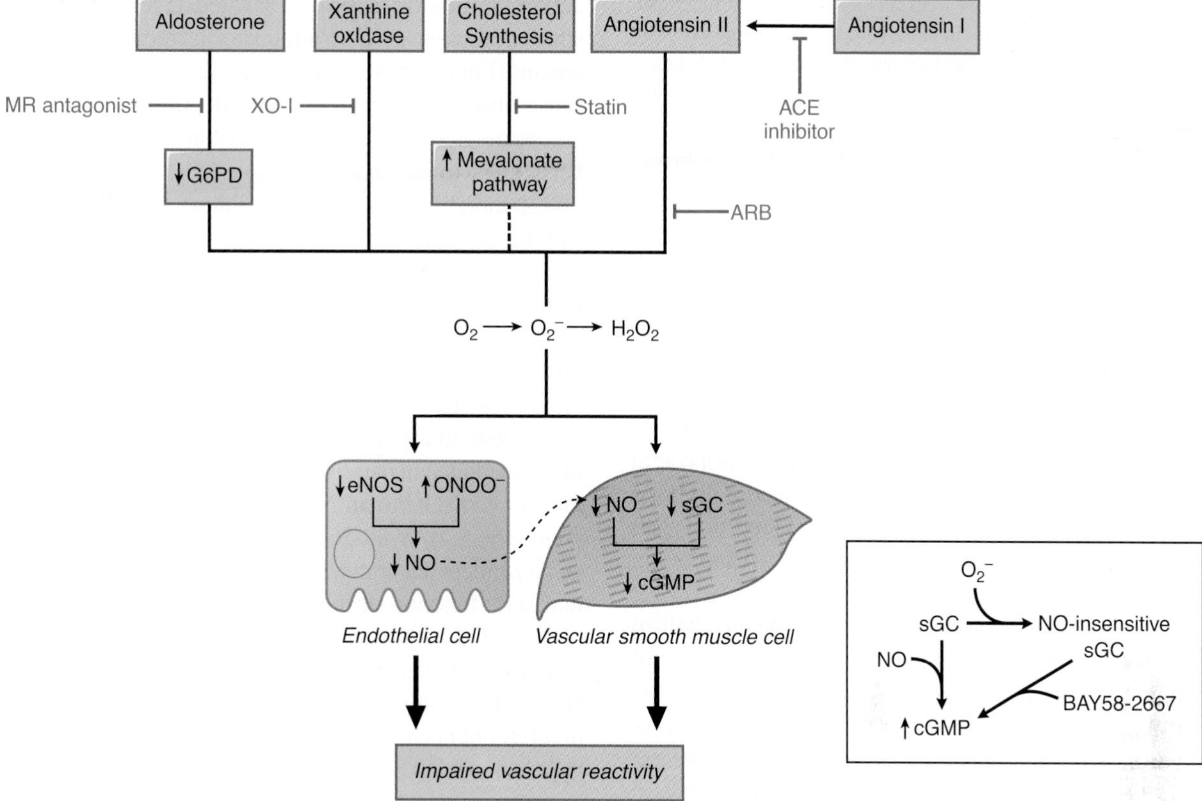

Figure 28–7. *Preserving normal vascular reactivity is a target of evolving priority in the treatment of patients with chronic congestive heart failure.* Increased levels of reactive oxygen species (ROS), including superoxide (O_2^-) and hydrogen peroxide (H_2O_2) that are generated in both endothelial cells (EC) and vascular smooth muscle cells (VSMC) impair key cell signaling pathways necessary for normal vascular function. Specifically, hyperaldosterone-induced decreased antioxidant enzyme activity in EC, such as glucose-6-phosphate dehydrogenase (G6PD), results in increased ROS formation (Leopold *et al.,* 2007). Likewise, increased xanthine oxidase (XO) activity, AT_1 receptor activation, and upregulation of signaling pathways associated with cholesterol metabolism create a cellular environment favorable for ROS formation. In EC, elevated levels of ROS impair vascular reactivity, in part, by decreasing endothelial nitric oxide synthase (eNOS) activity and increasing peroxynitrite ($ONOO^-$) formation to decrease bioavailable nitric oxide (NO) levels. In VSMC, oxidant stress decreases NO levels and impairs soluble guanylyl cyclase (sGC) sensitivity to NO, thereby decreasing cyclic GMP levels that are necessary for normal VSMC relaxation. Mineralacorticoid (MR)-receptor antagonists, XO inhibitors (XO-I), HMG-coA–reductase inhibitors (statin), AT_1 receptor blockers (ARBs), and angiotensin-converting enzyme (ACE) inhibitors block various cellular reactions associated with elevated levels of ROS and impaired vascular reactivity. The BAY compounds (e.g., BAY 58-2667; *figure inset*), in turn, are a novel group of direct sGC activators that increase enzyme activity despite oxidant stress-induced sGC modifications that convert the enzyme to an NO-insensitive state. XO-I, xanthine oxidase inhibitor.

Xanthine Oxidase and Vascular Dysfunction. Xanthine oxidase (XO) is necessary for normal purine metabolism and catalyzes the oxidation of hypoxanthine to xanthine and xanthine to uric acid in a reaction that generates superoxide. Elevated levels of uric acid are associated with clinically evident CHF (Hare et al., 2008). For example, epidemiologic data support a positive, graded association between impaired exercise capacity and circulating uric acid levels (Doehner et al., 2001). Although the myocardium is rich in XO, vascular endothelial cells also contain high concentrations of XO, an observation that ultimately lead to the hypothesis that increased XO-generated superoxide impairs vascular reactivity in CHF patients (Hare et al., 2008).

Early studies suggested allopurinol (300 mg/day), an XO inhibitor, effectively decreases generation of free oxygen radicals and improves peripheral arterial vasodilation and blood flow in hyperuricemic patients with mild-to-moderate CHF from systolic dysfunction (Doehner et al., 2002). Interestingly, probenecid, which decreases circulating urate levels by enhancing its elimination rather than by inhibiting XO activity, has not been shown to influence vascular reactivity. In patients with advanced CHF, allopurinol-induced serum uric acid level reduction (over 24 weeks) is associated with functional class improvement, but only in those with baseline serum uric acid levels >9.5 mg/dL. Overall, randomized, placebo-controlled clinical trials examining the long-term efficacy of allopurinol therapy in CHF are sparse, and active investigation in this area continues.

Statins and Vascular Dysfunction. HMG-CoA (3-hydroxy-3-methyl-glutaryl–coenzyme A) reductase catalyzes the formation of L-mevalonic acid, a key biochemical precursor in the cholesterol synthesis pathway (Goldstein and Brown, 1990). Current evidence suggests a role of crosstalk between mevalonate metabolism and cell signaling pathways involved in inflammation and oxidant stress. In this way, HMG-CoA reductase inhibitors, or "statins", may exert beneficial cardiovascular effects beyond their original intent of low-density lipoprotein reduction; specifically, statins are associated with positive LV remodeling, increased arteriolar blood flow, and decreased circulating platelet aggregation (Liao et al., 2005).

Intermediate byproducts of mevalonate metabolism (i.e., isopenylated proteins that upregulate activation of Rho, RAS, and other G proteins) are linked to impaired vascular function by increasing levels of oxidant stress and decreasing bioavailable NO levels (Hernandez-Perera et al., 1998). Statins inhibit these intermediary pathways and appear to restore endothelium-dependent (Feron et al., 2001) and endothelium-independent vascular function (Drexler et al., 1993). The pharmacology of the statins and other cholesterol-lowering agents is presented in Chapter 31.

A large number of population studies have demonstrated a favorable effect of statin therapy on outcome in CHF. For example, one retrospective analysis of ischemic- and non-ischemic cardiomyopathy patients with CHF reported a significant reduction in mortality in those treated with a statin for 1 year compared to case-matched patients treated only with standard medical therapy (Horwich et al., 2004). Others have suggested that statins delay CHF in at-risk patients with ischemic heart disease (Kjekshus et al., 1997). Unfortunately, there is a paucity of sufficiently powered prospective, randomized, placebo-controlled clinical trials demonstrating a favorable effect of statin therapy on outcome in patients with CHF. Overall, the evidence in support of statin use in CHF (of either ischemic or non-ischemic etiologies) is primarily based on observational clinical data. The clinical indications for statin therapy in CHF, preferred drug isoform, and optimal drug concentration, for example, remain undefined.

Direct Activators of Soluble Guanylyl Cyclase. Soluble guanylyl cyclase (sGC) is an enzyme that catalyzes the conversion of guanosine triphosphate to cyclic GMP, a second messenger necessary for normal vascular smooth muscle cell relaxation (Koesling, 1999). Under physiologic conditions, NO is the primary biologically active stimulator of sGC. Elevated levels of oxidant stress deactivate sGC through various molecular mechanisms. For example, aldosterone levels comparable to those observed in patients with decompensated CHF are associated with increased oxidant stress that converts sGC to an NO-insensitive state (Maron et al., 2009), thereby disrupting vasodilatory signaling necessary for normal vascular function.

Organic nitrates, which promote sGC activation by increasing bioavailable NO levels, are subject to pharmacologic tolerance that complicates long-term drug use, dosing, and administration frequency (see the organic nitrates section in Chapter 27). Although the precise mechanism to explain this phenomenon is unknown, it is likely mediated in part by elevated levels of oxidant stress that convert sGC to an NO-insensitive state. BAY compounds (e.g., BAY 58-2667 [cinaciguat]) activate sGC by an NO-independent mechanism, thereby promoting normal sGC function despite conditions of oxidant stress (Stasch et al., 2006). Data from preclinical CHF studies in animals have validated these beneficial molecular effects. In healthy humans, BAY compound administration has not been associated with severe side effects, but hypotension and headache have been reported. Likewise in humans, circulating plasma drug concentrations are decreased to clinically insignificant levels ≤30 minutes after infusion termination (Frey et al., 2008).

The utility of BAY 58-2667 in the clinical management of patients with CHF is a topic of ongoing investigation, although early published reports suggest potential for the use of this novel drug class. In a group of patients with acutely decompensated CHF, BAY 58-2667 responders demonstrated a significant decrease in pulmonary capillary wedge pressure, mean right atrial pressure, mean pulmonary artery pressure, pulmonary vascular resistance, and systemic vascular resistance. Cardiac output was significantly increased as well (Lapp et al., 2009). The potential mainstream application of BAY 58-2667 (and other similar compounds) is currently under evaluation in larger clinical trials. Nevertheless, these preliminary observations are encouraging and may expose sustained sGC activity despite enzyme insensitivity to NO$^{\bullet}$ as a promising therapeutic target for CHF patients.

CLINICAL SUMMARY

Congestive heart failure is a chronic and usually progressive illness instigated by a primary myocardial insult that impairs myocardial structure and function. Treatment (Figure 28–8) ideally begins with *prevention* of cardiac dysfunction via the identification and remediation of risk factors that predispose individuals to the development of structural heart disease. For example, because coronary artery disease is the most common

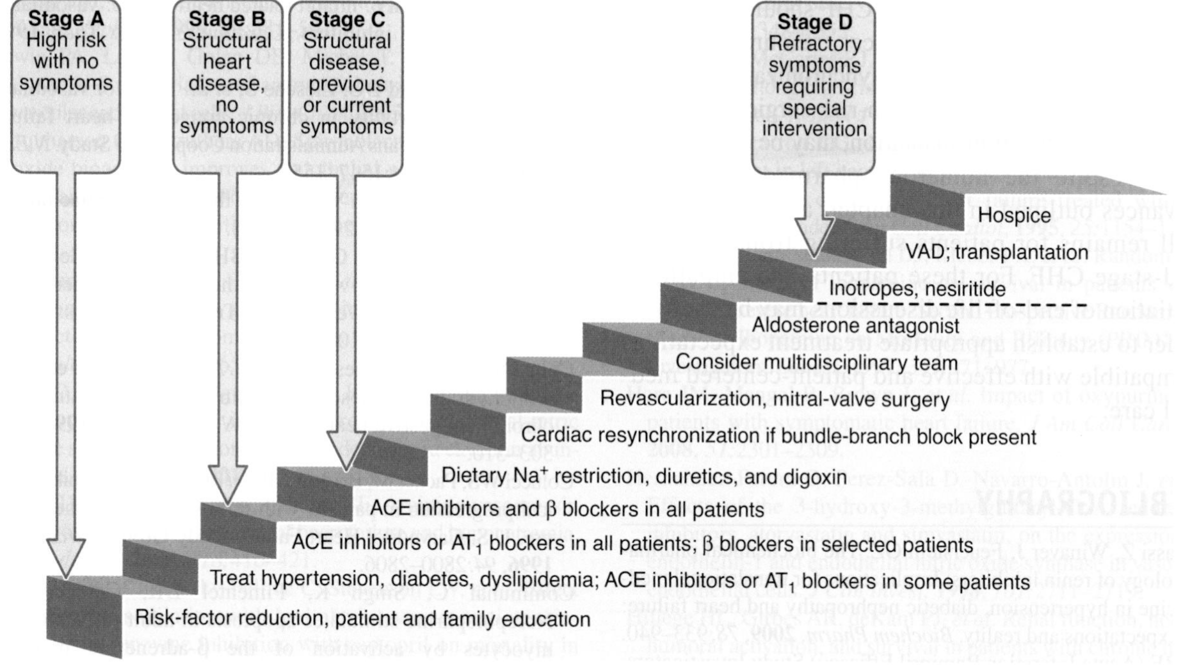

Figure 28–8. *Stages of heart failure.* (Reproduced with permission from Jessup and Brozena, 2003. Copyright © Massachusetts Medical Society. All rights reserved.)

etiology of LV systolic dysfunction, public health tactics to address strategies for prevention of MI through lipid lowering, blood pressure control, and smoking cessation are critical for effective CHF primary prevention.

In asymptomatic patients with LV dysfunction or impaired diastolic dysfunction, neurohormonal compensatory mechanisms that support cardiovascular function are activated, but, paradoxically, further disease progression. Indeed, treatment in this clinical stage is directed at attenuation of sustained neurohormonal activation, with individualized regimens of β adrenergic receptor blockers and ACE inhibitors or AT_1 receptor antagonists.

In most cases, there is unwanted progression to clinically evident CHF, indicating the development of significantly abnormal cardiovascular hemodynamics. Treatment goals in these patients include symptom relief and prevention of disease progression. This may be achieved with diuretics, load-reducing agents, and renin–angiotensin–aldosterone axis antagonists.

Symptomatic patients with hemodynamic decompensation require hospitalization, because oral diuretic and vasodilator therapy alone often are inadequate to reestablish euvolemia and adequate peripheral perfusion. Parenteral vasodilator and inotropic agents are administered parenterally to restore forward cardiac output and to reverse Na^+ and water retention. Effective treatment of these patients often is complicated by concurrent renal insufficiency and hypotension, despite evidence of persistently elevated intracardiac filling pressures. In this setting, selection of parenteral agents guided by data obtained from an indwelling pulmonary artery catheter may prove useful.

Consider as an example the clinical scenario in which a decompensated CHF patient presents with normal systemic vascular resistance. In this case, afterload reduction may be contraindicated in the short term and treatment with a parenteral agent such as dobutamine may be preferable. The risk attendant to treatment with sympathomimetic drugs is related to the increase in myocardial O_2 consumption that may occur; this is of particular concern in patients with left-heart failure that occurs as a direct consequence of myocardial ischemia. This clinical quandary has become less common in the era of aggressive myocardial revascularization; when it is encountered, coadministration of dobutamine with parenteral nitroglycerin may be necessary.

In CHF patients who are persistently symptomatic or hemodynamically unstable, referral to a specialized tertiary center with expertise in the evaluation

Konstam MA, Rousseau MF, Kronenberg MW, *et al.* Effects of the angiotensin converting enzyme inhibitor enalapril on the long-term progression of left ventricular dysfunction in patients with heart failure. Studies of Left Ventricular Dysfunction (SOLVD) Investigators. *Circulation*, **1992**, *86:*431–438.

Krikler DM. The foxglove, "The old woman from Shropshire" and William Withering. *J Am Coll Cardiol*, **1985**, *5*(A)*:*3A–9A.

Kum LC, Yip GW, Lee PW, *et al.* Comparison of angiotensin-converting enzyme inhibitor alone and in combination with irbesartan for the treatment of heart failure. *Int J Cardiol*, **2008**, *125:*16–21.

Lahav M, Regev A, Ra'anani P, Theodor E. Intermittent administration of furosemide versus continuous infusion preceded by a loading dose for congestive heart failure. *Chest*, **1992**, *102:*725–731.

Lapp H, Mitrovic V, Franz N, *et al.* Cinaciguat (BAY 58-2667) improves cardiopulmonary hemodynamics in patients with acute decompensated heart failure. *Circulation*, **2009**, *119:* 2781–2788.

Leopold JA, Dam A, Maron BA, *et al.* Aldosterone impairs vascular reactivity by decreasing glucose-6-phosphate dehydrogenase activity. *Nat Med*, **2007**, *13:*189–197.

Lewis GD, Lachmann J, Camuso J, *et al.* Sildenafil improves exercise hemodynamics and oxygen uptake in patients with systolic heart failure. *Circulation*, **2007**, *115:*59–66.

Liao JK. Effects of statins on 3-hydroxy-3-methylglutaryl coenzyme A reductase inhibition beyond low-density lipoprotein cholesterol. *Am J Cardiol,* **2005**, *96:*24F–33F.

Maron BA, Zhang YY, Handy DE, *et al.* Aldosterone increases oxidant stress to impair guanylyl cyclase activity by cysteinyl thiol oxidation in vascular smooth muscle cells. *J Biol Chem*, **2009**, *284:*7665–7672.

Massie BM, Carson PE, McMurray JJ, *et al.* Irbesartan in patients with heart failure and preserved ejection fraction. *N Engl J Med,* **2008**, *359:*2456–2467.

McCurley JM, Hanlon SU, Wei SK, *et al.* Furosemide and the progression of left ventricular dysfunction in experimental heart failure. *J Am Coll Cardiol*, **2004**, *44:*1301–1307.

McKelvie RS, Yusuf S, Pericak D, *et al.* Comparison of candesartan, enalapril, and their combination in congestive heart failure: Randomized evaluation of strategies for left ventricular dysfunction (RESOLVD) pilot study. The RESOLVD Pilot Study Investigators. *Circulation*, **1999**, *100:*1056–1064.

McMurray JJ, Ostergren J, Swedberg K, *et al.* Effects of candesartan in patients with chronic heart failure and reduced left-ventricular systolic function taking angiotensin-converting-enzyme inhibitors: The CHARM-Added trial. *Lancet*, **2003**, *362:*767–771.

McMurray JJ, Pitt B, Latini R, *et al.* Effects of the oral direct renin inhibitor aliskiren in patients with symptomatic heart failure. *Circ Heart Fail*, **2008,** *1:*17–24.

MERIT-HF Study Group. Effect of metoprolol CR/XL in chronic heart failure: Metoprolol CR/XL Randomised Intervention Trial in Congestive Heart Failure (MERIT-HF). *Lancet*, **1999**, *353:*2001–2007.

Münzel T, Daiber A, Mülsch A. Explaining the phenomenon of nitrate tolerance. *Circ Res*, **2005**, *97*:618–628.

Münzel T, Kurz S, Rajagopalan S, *et al.* Hydralazine prevents nitroglycerin tolerance by inhibiting activation of a membrane-bound NADH oxidase. A new action for an old drug. *J Clin Invest,* **1996**, *98:*1465–1470.

Packer M, Bristow MR, Cohn JN, *et al.* The effect of carvedilol on morbidity and mortality in patients with chronic heart failure. U.S. Carvedilol Heart Failure Study Group. *N Engl J Med,* **1996**, *334:*1349–1355.

Packer M, Carver JR, Rodeheffer RJ, *et al.* Effect of oral milrinone on mortality in severe chronic heart failure. PROMISE Study Research Group. *N Engl J Med,* **1991**, *325:*1468–1475.

Packer M, Fowler MB, Roecker EB, *et al.* Carvedilol Prospective Randomized Cumulative Survival (COPERNICUS) Study Group. Effects of carvedilol on morbidity of patients with severe chronic heart failure: Results of the carvedilol prospective randomized cumulative survival (COPERNICUS) study. *Circulation*, **2002**, *106:*2194–2199.

Packer M, Gheorghiade M, Young JB, *et al.* Withdrawal of digoxin from patients with chronic heart failure treated with angiotensin-converting-enzyme inhibitors. RADIANCE Study. *N Engl J Med,* **1993**, *329:*1–7.

Packer M, Poole-Wilson PA, Armstrong PW, *et al.* Comparative effects of low and high doses of the angiotensin converting enzyme inhibitor, lisinopril, on morbidity and mortality in chronic heart failure. Assessment of Treatment with Lisinopril and Survival (ATLAS) Study Group. *Circulation*, **1999**, *100:*2312–2318.

Pfeffer MA, Braunwald E, Moye LA, *et al.* Effect of captopril on mortality and morbidity in patients with left ventricular dysfunction after myocardial infarction. Results of the Survival And Ventricular Enlargement trial. The SAVE Investigators. *N Engl J Med,* **1992**, *327:*669–677.

Pitt B, Remme W, Zannad F, *et al.*, and the Eplerenone Post-Acute Myocardial Infarction Heart Failure Efficacy and Survival Study Investigators. Eplerenone, a selective aldosterone blocker, in patients with left ventricular dysfunction after myocardial infarction. *N Engl J Med,* **2003**, *348:* 1309–1321.

Pitt B, Segal R, Martinez FA, *et al.* Randomised trial of losartan versus captopril in patients over 65 with heart failure (Evaluation of Losartan in the Elderly Study, ELITE). *Lancet*, **1997**, *349:*747–752.

Pitt B, Zannad F, Remme WJ, *et al.* The effect of spironolactone on morbidity and mortality in patients with severe heart failure. Randomized Aldactone Evaluation Study Investigators. *N Engl J Med,* **1999**, *341:*709–717.

Sanoski CA. Aliskiren: An oral direct renin inhibitor for the treatment of hypertension. *Pharmacotherapy*, **2009**, *29:*193–212.

Sawyer DB, Colucci WS. Mitochondrial oxidative stress in heart failure: "Oxygen wastage" revisited. *Circ Res*, **2000**, *86:* 119–120.

Solomon SD, Appelbaum E, Manning WJ, *et al.* Effect of the direct renin inhibitor aliskiren, the angiotensin receptor blocker losartan, or both on left ventricular mass in patients with hypertension and left ventricular hypertrophy. *Circulation*, **2009**, *119:*530–537.

Solomon SD, Janardhanan R, Verma A, *et al.* Effect of angiotensin receptor blockade and antihypertensive drugs on diastolic function in patients with hypertension and diastolic dysfunction: A randomized trial. *Lancet*, **2007**, *369:*2079–2087.

St. John Sutton M, Pfeffer MA, Plappert T, *et al.* Quantitative two-dimensional echocardiographic measurements are major predictors of adverse cardiovascular events after acute myocardial infarction. The protective effects of captopril. *Circulation*, **1994**, *89:*68–75.

Staessen JA, Li Y, Richart T. Oral renin inhibitors. *Lancet,* **2006**, *368*:1449–1456.

Stasch JP, Schmidt PM, Nedvetsky PI, *et al*. Targeting the heme-oxidized nitric oxide receptor for selective vasodilatation of diseased blood vessels. *J Clin Invest*, **2006**, *116:*2552–2561.

Studies On Left Ventricular Dysfunction (SOLVD) Investigators. Effect of enalapril on mortality and the development of heart failure in asymptomatic patients with reduced left ventricular ejection fractions. *N Engl J Med,* **1992**, *327:685–691.*

Swedberg K. Initial experience with β blockers in dilated cardiomyopathy. *Am J Cardiol,* **1993**, *71:*30C–38C.

Taylor AL, Ziesche S, Yancy CW, *et al*. Early and sustained benefit on event-free survival and heart failure hospitalization from fixed-dose combination of isosorbide dinitrate/hydralazine: Consistency across subgroups in the African-American Heart Failure Trial. *Circulation*, **2007**, *115:*1747–1753.

Udelson JE, Orlandi C, Ouyang J, *et al*. Acute hemodynamic effects of tolvaptan, a vasopressin V_2 receptor blocker, in patients with symptomatic heart failure and systolic dysfunction: An international, multicenter, randomized, placebo-controlled trial. *J Am Coll Cardiol*, **2008**, *52:*1540–1545.

Uretsky BF, Young JB, Shahidi FE, *et al*. Randomized study assessing the effect of digoxin withdrawal in patients with mild to moderate chronic congestive heart failure: Results of the PROVED trial. PROVED Investigative Group. *J Am Coll Cardiol*, **1993**, *22:*955–962.

Varin R, Mulder P, Tamion F, *et al.* Improvement of endothelial function by chronic angiotensin-converting enzyme inhibition in heart failure: Role of nitric oxide, prostanoids, oxidant stress, and bradykinin. *Circulation,* **2000**, *27:*351–356.

Villarreal F, ed. *Interstitial Fibrosis in Heart Failure*. Springer, New York, **2005.**

Waagstein F, Bristow MR, Swedberg K, *et al*. Beneficial effects of metoprolol in idiopathic dilated cardiomyopathy. Metoprolol in Dilated Cardiomyopathy (MDC) Trial Study Group. *Lancet*, **1993**, *342:*1441–1446.

Wang W, Chen JS, Zucker IH. Carotid sinus baroreceptor sensitivity in experimental heart failure. *Circulation*, **1990**, *81:*1959–1966.

Weber KT. Efficacy of aldosterone receptor antagonism in heart failure: Potential mechanisms. *Curr Heart Fail Rep,* **2004**, *1:*51–56.

White HD, Aylward PE, Huang Z, *et al*. Mortality and morbidity remain high despite captopril and/or Valsartan therapy in elderly patients with left ventricular systolic dysfunction, heart failure, or both after acute myocardial infarction: Results from the Valsartan in Acute Myocardial Infarction Trial (VALIANT). *Circulation*, **2005**, *112:*3391–3399.

Yan C, Ding B, Shishido T, Chang-Hoon Woo C-H, *et al*. Activation of extracellular signal-regulated kinase 5 reduces cardiac apoptosis and dysfunction via inhibition of a phosphodiesterase 3A/inducible cAMP early repressor feedback loop. *Circ Res*, **2007**, *100:*510–519.

Yusuf S, Pfeffer M, Swedberg K, *et al*. CHARM Investigators and Committees. Effects of candesartan in patients with chronic heart failure and preserved left ventricular ejection fraction: The CHARM-Preserved trial. *Lancet*, **2003**, *362:* 777–781.

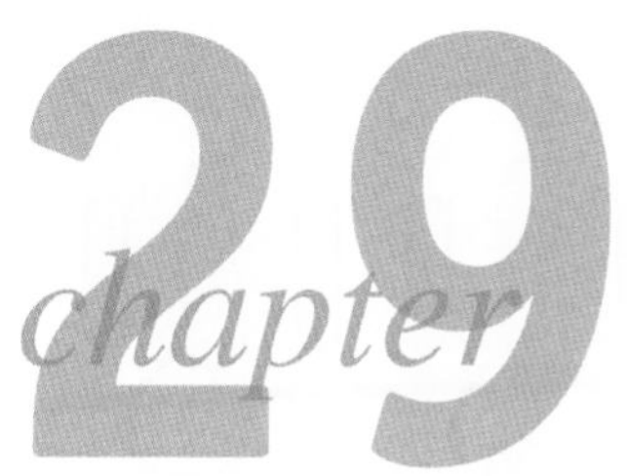

Anti-Arrhythmic Drugs

Kevin J. Sampson and
Robert S. Kass

Cardiac cells undergo depolarization and repolarization to form cardiac action potentials ~60 times/minute. The shape and duration of each action potential are determined by the activity of ion channel protein complexes in the membranes of individual cells, and the genes encoding most of these proteins now have been identified. Thus, each heartbeat results from the highly integrated electrophysiologic behavior of multiple proteins on multiple cardiac cells. Ion channel function can be perturbed by inherited mutation/polymorphism, acute ischemia, sympathetic stimulation, or myocardial scarring to create abnormalities of cardiac rhythm, or arrhythmias. Available anti-arrhythmic drugs suppress arrhythmias by blocking flow through specific ion channels or by altering autonomic function. An increasingly sophisticated understanding of the molecular basis of normal and abnormal cardiac rhythm may lead to identification of new targets for anti-arrhythmic drugs and perhaps improved therapies.

Arrhythmias can range from incidental, asymptomatic clinical findings to life-threatening abnormalities. Mechanisms underlying cardiac arrhythmias have been identified in cellular and animal experiments. In some human arrhythmias, precise mechanisms are known, and treatment can be targeted specifically against those mechanisms. In other cases, mechanisms can be only inferred, and the choice of drugs is based largely on the results of prior experience. Anti-arrhythmic drug therapy can have two goals: termination of an ongoing arrhythmia or prevention of an arrhythmia. Unfortunately, anti-arrhythmic drugs not only help to control arrhythmias but also can cause them, especially during long-term therapy. Thus, prescribing anti-arrhythmic drugs requires that precipitating factors be excluded or minimized, that a precise diagnosis of the type of arrhythmia (and its possible mechanisms) be made, that the prescriber has reason to believe that drug therapy will be beneficial, and that the risks of drug therapy can be minimized.

PRINCIPLES OF CARDIAC ELECTROPHYSIOLOGY

The flow of ions across cell membranes generates the currents that make up cardiac action potentials. The factors that determine the magnitude of individual currents and their modulation by drugs can be explained at the cellular and molecular levels (Priori et al., 1999; Nerbonne and Kass, 2005). However, the action potential is a highly integrated entity wherein changes in one current almost inevitably produce secondary changes in other currents. Most anti-arrhythmic drugs affect more than one ion current, and many exert ancillary effects such as modification of cardiac contractility or autonomic nervous system function. Thus, anti-arrhythmic drugs usually exert multiple actions and can be beneficial or harmful in individual patients (Roden, 1994; Priori et al., 1999).

The Cardiac Cell at Rest: a K^+-permeable membrane

Ions move across cell membranes in response to electrical and concentration gradients, not through the lipid bilayer but through specific ion channels or transporters. The normal cardiac cell at rest maintains a transmembrane potential ~80-90 mV negative to the exterior; this gradient is established by pumps, especially the Na^+, K^+-ATPase, and fixed anionic charges within cells. There are both an electrical and a concentration gradient that would move Na^+ ions into resting cells (Figure 29–1). However, Na^+ channels, which allow Na^+ to move along this gradient, are closed at negative transmembrane potentials, so Na^+ does not enter normal resting cardiac cells. In contrast, a specific type of K^+ channel protein (the inward rectifier channel) is in an open conformation at negative potentials. Hence, K^+ can move through these channels across the cell membrane at negative potentials in response to either electrical or concentration gradients (Figure 29–1). For each individual ion, there is an equilibrium potential E_x at which there is no net driving force for

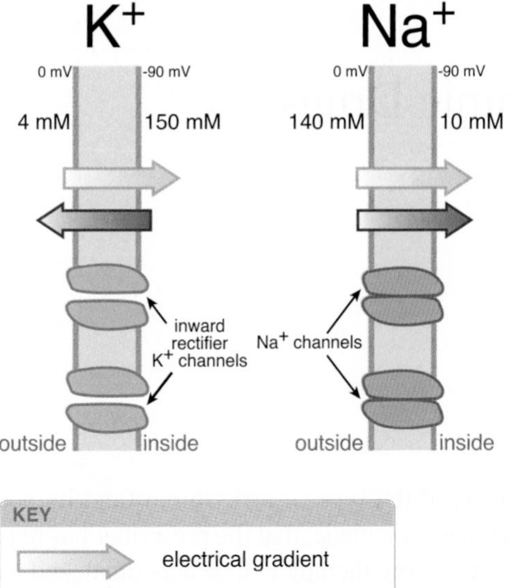

Figure 29–1. *Electrical and chemical gradients for K^+ and Na^+ in a resting cardiac cell.* Inward rectifier K^+ channels are open (*left*), allowing K^+ ions to move across the membrane and the transmembrane potential to approach E_K. In contrast, Na^+ does not enter the cell despite a large net driving force because Na^+ channel proteins are in the closed conformation (*right*) in resting cells.

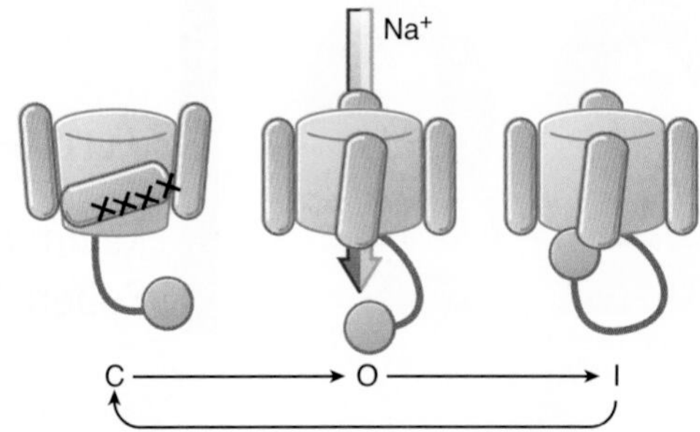

Figure 29–2. *Voltage dependent conformational changes determine current flow through Na^+ channels.* At hyperpolarized potentials, the channel is in a closed conformation and no current can flow (*left*). As depolarization begins, the pore opens, allowing conduction (*middle*). And finally, as depolarization is maintained, an intracellular particle blocks current flow, making the channel non-conducting in this inactivated state (*right*).

the ion to move across the membrane. E_x can be calculated using the Nernst equation:

$$E_x = -\ (RT/FZ_x)\ \ln([x]_i/[x]_o)$$

where Z_x is the valence of the ion, T is the absolute temperature, R is the gas constant, F is Faraday's constant, $[x]_o$ is the extracellular concentration of the ion, and $[x]_i$ is the intracellular concentration. For typical values for K^+, $[K]_o = 4$ mM and $[K]_i = 140$ mM, the calculated K^+ equilibrium potential E_K is –94 mV. There is thus no net force driving K^+ ions into or out of a cell when the transmembrane potential is –94 mV, which is close to the resting potential. If $[K]_o$ is elevated to 10 mM, as might occur in diseases such as renal failure or myocardial ischemia, the calculated E_K rises to –70 mV. In this situation, there is excellent agreement between changes in theoretical E_K owing to changes in $[K]_o$ and the actual measured transmembrane potential, indicating that the normal cardiac cell at rest is permeable to K^+ (because inward rectifier channels are open) and that $[K]_o$ is the major determinant of resting potential.

The Cardiac Action Potential

Transmembrane current through voltage-gated ion channels is the primary determinant of cardiac action potential morphology and duration. Channels are macromolecular complexes consisting of a pore-forming α subunit, as well as β subunits and further accessory proteins. These channels are transmembrane proteins consisting of a voltage-sensing domain, a selectivity filter, a conducting pore, and often an inactivating particle. In response to changes in local transmembrane potential, ion channels undergo conformational changes allowing for, or preventing, the flow of ions through the conducting pore along their electrochemical gradient (Figure 29–2).

To initiate an action potential, a cardiac myocyte at rest is depolarized above a threshold potential, usually via gap junctions by a neighboring myocyte. Upon membrane depolarization, Na^+ channel proteins change conformation from the "closed" (resting) state to the "open" (conducting) state (Figure 29–2), allowing up to 10^7 Na^+ ions/sec to enter each cell and moving the transmembrane potential toward E_{Na} (+65 mV). This surge of Na^+ ions lasts only about a millisecond, after which the Na^+ channel protein rapidly changes conformation from the "open" state to an "inactivated," non-conducting state (Figure 29–2). The maximum upstroke slope of phase 0 (dV/dt_{max}, or V_{max}) of the action potential (Figure 29–3) is largely governed by Na^+ current and plays a role in the conduction velocity of a propagating action potential. Under normal conditions, Na^+ channels, once inactivated, cannot reopen until they reassume the closed conformation. However, a small population of Na^+ channels may continue to open during the action potential plateau in some cells (Figure 29–3), providing further inward current. Certain mutations in the cardiac isoform of the Na^+ channel can further increase the number of channels that do not properly inactivate, thereby prolonging the action potential, and cause one form of the congenital long QT syndrome (Keating and Sanguinetti, 2001). In general, however, as the cell membrane repolarizes, the negative membrane potential moves Na^+ channel proteins from inactivated to "closed" conformations. The relationship between Na^+ channel availability and transmembrane potential is an important determinant of conduction and refractoriness in many cells, as discussed in the following discussion.

The changes in transmembrane potential generated by the inward Na^+ current produce, in turn, a series of openings (and in some cases subsequent inactivation) of other channels (Figure 29–3). For example, when a cell is depolarized by the Na^+ current, "transient outward" K^+ channels quickly change conformation to enter an open, or conducting, state; because the transmembrane potential at the end of phase 0 is positive to E_K, the opening of transient outward channels results in an outward, or repolarizing, K^+ current

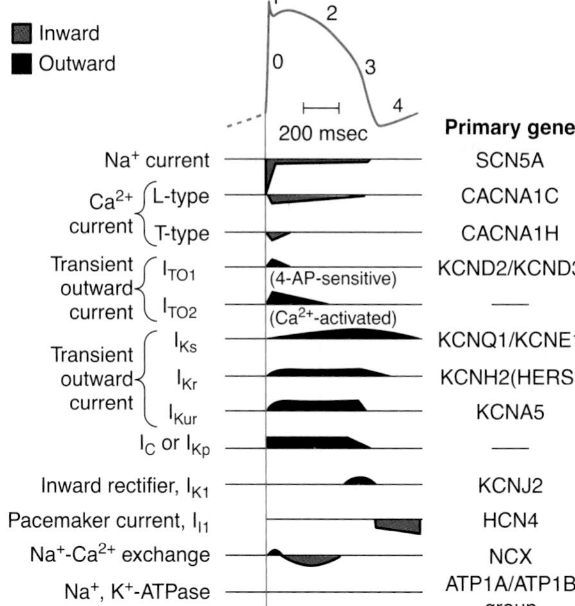

Figure 29–3. *The relationship between an action potential from the conducting system and the time course of the currents that generate it.* The current magnitudes are not to scale; the Na^+ current is ordinarily 50 times larger than any other current, although the portion that persists into the plateau (phase 2) is small. Multiple types of Ca^{2+} current, transient outward current (I_{TO}), and delayed rectifier (I_K) have been identified. Each represents a different channel protein, usually associated with ancillary (function-modifying) subunits. 4-AP (4-aminopyridine) is a widely used *in vitro* blocker of K^+ channels. I_{TO2} may be a Cl^- current in some species. Components of I_K have been separated on the basis of how rapidly they activate: slowly (I_{Ks}), rapidly (I_{Kr}), or ultra-rapidly (I_{Kur}). The voltage-activated, time-independent current may be carried by Cl^- (I_{Cl}) or K^+ (I_{Kp}, *p* for plateau). The genes encoding the major pore-forming proteins have been cloned for most of the channels shown here and are included in the right-hand column. The righthand column lists the primary genes that code for the various ion channels and transporters.

(termed I_{TO}), which contributes to the phase 1 "notch" seen in action potentials from these tissues. Transient outward K^+ channels, like Na^+ channels, inactivate rapidly. During the phase 2 plateau of a normal cardiac action potential, inward, depolarizing currents, primarily through Ca^{2+} channels, are balanced by outward, repolarizing currents primarily through K^+ ("delayed-rectifier") channels. Delayed-rectifier currents (collectively termed I_K) increase with time, whereas Ca^{2+} currents inactivate (and so decrease with time); as a result, cardiac cells repolarize (phase 3) several hundred milliseconds after the initial Na^+ channel opening. Mutations in the genes encoding repolarizing K^+ channels are responsible for the most common forms of the congenital long QT syndrome (Nerbonne and Kass, 2005). Identification of these specific channels has allowed more precise characterization of the pharmacologic effects of anti-arrhythmic drugs. A common mechanism whereby drugs prolong cardiac action potentials and provoke arrhythmias is inhibition of a specific delayed-rectifier current, I_{Kr}, generated by expression of the *human ether-a-go-go–related gene* (*HERG*). The ion channel protein generated by *HERG* expression differs from other ion channels in important structural features that make it much more susceptible to drug block; understanding these structural constraints is an important first step to designing drugs lacking I_{Kr}-blocking properties (Mitcheson et al., 2000). Avoiding I_{Kr}/*HERG* channel block has become a major issue in the development of new anti-arrhythmic drugs (Roden, 2004).

Action Potential Heterogeneity in the Heart

The diversity of action potentials seen throughout different regions of the heart plays a role in understanding the pharmacologic profiles of anti-arrhythmic drugs. This general description of the action potential and the currents that underlie it must be modified for certain cell types (Figure 29–4), primarily due to variability in the expression of ion channels and electrogenic ion transport pumps. In the ventricle, action potential duration (APD) and shape vary across the wall of each chamber, as well as apico-basally (Figure 29–4). In the neighboring His–Purkinje system, action potentials are characterized by a more hyperpolarized plateau potential and prolongation of the action potential due to divergent ion channel expression and differences in intercellular Ca^{2+} handling (Dun and Boyden, 2008). Atrial cells have short action potentials, probably because I_{TO} is larger, and an additional repolarizing K^+ current, activated by the neurotransmitter acetylcholine, is present. As a result, vagal stimulation further shortens atrial action potentials. Cells of the sinus and atrioventricular (AV) nodes lack substantial Na^+ currents, and depolarization is achieved by the movement of Ca^{2+} across the membrane. In addition, these cells, as well as cells from the conducting system, normally display the phenomenon of spontaneous diastolic, or phase 4 depolarization and thus spontaneously reach threshold for regeneration of action potentials. The rate of spontaneous firing usually is fastest in sinus node cells, which therefore serve as the natural pacemaker of the heart. Several ionic channels and transport pumps underlie pacemaker currents in the heart. One of the pacemaking currents responsible for this automaticity is generated via specialized K^+ channels, the hyperpolarization-activated cyclic nucleotide-gated (HCN) channels that are permeable to both potassium and sodium (Cohen and Robinson, 2006). Another major mechanism responsible for automaticity is the repetitive spontaneous Ca^{2+} release from the sarcoplasmic reticulum (SR), a specialized endoplasmic reticulum found in striated muscle cells (Vinogradova and Lakatta, 2009). The rise in cytosolic Ca^{2+} causes membrane depolarizations when Ca^{2+} is extruded from the cell via the electrogenic Na-Ca exchanger (NCX). In addition, sinus node cells lack inward rectifier K^+ currents that are primarily responsible for protecting working myocardium against spontaneous membrane depolarizations.

Molecular biologic and electrophysiologic techniques have refined the description of ion channels important for the normal functioning of cardiac cells and have identified channels that may be particularly important under pathologic conditions. For example, the transient outward and delayed-rectifier currents actually result from multiple ion channel subtypes (Tseng and Hoffman, 1989; Sanguinetti and Jurkiewicz, 1990) (Figure 29–3).

MECHANISMS OF CARDIAC ARRHYTHMIAS

When the normal sequence of impulse initiation and propagation is perturbed, an arrhythmia occurs. Failure of impulse initiation, in the sinus node, may result in slow heart rates (bradyarrhythmias), whereas failure in the normal propagation of action potentials from atrium to ventricle results in dropped beats (commonly referred to as heart block) that usually reflect an abnormality in either the AV node or the His–Purkinje system. These abnormalities may be caused by drugs (Table 29–1) or by structural heart disease; in the latter case, permanent cardiac pacing may be required.

Abnormally rapid heart rhythms (tachyarrhythmias) are common clinical problems that may be treated with anti-arrhythmic drugs. Three major underlying mechanisms have been identified: enhanced automaticity, triggered automaticity, and re-entry. These often are interrelated mechanisms, as the first two often serve to initiate re-entry.

Enhanced Automaticity

Enhanced automaticity may occur in cells that normally display spontaneous diastolic depolarization—the sinus and AV nodes and the His–Purkinje system. β Adrenergic stimulation, hypokalemia, and mechanical stretch of cardiac muscle cells increase phase 4 slope and so accelerate pacemaker rate, whereas acetylcholine reduces pacemaker rate both by decreasing phase 4 slope and through hyperpolarization (making the maximum diastolic potential more negative). In addition, automatic behavior may occur in sites that ordinarily lack spontaneous pacemaker activity; for example, depolarization of ventricular cells (e.g., by ischemia) may produce "abnormal" automaticity. When impulses propagate from a region of enhanced normal or abnormal automaticity to excite the rest of the heart, more complex arrhythmias may result from the induction of functional re-entry.

Afterdepolarizations and Triggered Automaticity

Under some pathophysiologic conditions, a normal cardiac action potential may be interrupted or followed by an abnormal depolarization (Figure 29–6). If this abnormal depolarization reaches threshold, it may, in turn, give rise to secondary upstrokes that can propagate and create abnormal rhythms. These abnormal secondary upstrokes occur only after an initial normal, or "triggering," upstroke and so are termed *triggered rhythms*.

Two major forms of triggered rhythms are recognized. In the first case, under conditions of intracellular or sarcoplasmic reticulum Ca^{2+} overload (e.g., myocardial ischemia, adrenergic stress, digitalis intoxication, heart failure), a normal action potential may be followed by a *delayed afterdepolarization* (DAD; Figure 29–6A). If this afterdepolarization reaches threshold, a secondary triggered beat or beats may occur. DAD amplitude is increased *in vitro* by rapid pacing, and clinical arrhythmias thought to correspond to DAD-mediated triggered beats are more frequent when the underlying cardiac rate is rapid (Priori et al., 1999). DADs are also responsible for exercise-induced ventricular tachycardia in congenital CPVT syndrome caused by mutations in RyR channels (Knollmann and Roden, 2008). In the second type of triggered activity, the key abnormality is marked prolongation of the cardiac action potential. When this occurs, phase 3 repolarization may be interrupted by an *early afterdepolarization* (EAD; Figure 29–6B). EAD-mediated triggering *in vitro* and clinical arrhythmias are most common when the underlying heart rate is slow, extracellular K^+ is low, and certain drugs that prolong APD (antiarrhythmics and others) are present. EAD-related triggered upstrokes probably reflect inward current through Na^+ or Ca^{2+} channels. EADs are induced much more readily in Purkinje cells than in epicardial or endocardial cells. When cardiac repolarization is markedly prolonged, polymorphic ventricular tachycardia with a long QT interval, known as the *torsades de pointes* syndrome, may occur. This arrhythmia is thought to be caused by EADs, which trigger functional re-entry (discussed in the following discussion) owing to heterogeneity of APDs across the ventricular wall (Priori et al., 1999). Congenital long QT syndrome, a disease in which torsades de pointes is common, can most often be caused by mutations in the genes encoding the Na^+ channels or the channels underlying the repolarizing currents I_{Kr} and I_{Ks} (Nerbonne and Kass, 2005).

Re-entry

Re-entry occurs when a cardiac impulse travels in a path such as to return to its original site and reactivate the original site and self-perpetuate rapid activation independent of the normal sinus node conduction. This abnormal activation path (or re-entrant circuit) requires anisotropic conduction slowing (or failure) due to either an anatomic or functional barrier.

Anatomically Defined Re-entry. Re-entry can occur when impulses propagate by more than one pathway

Table 29–1

Drug-Induced Cardiac Arrhythmias

ARRHYTHMIA	DRUG	LIKELY MECHANISM	TREATMENT*	CLINICAL FEATURES
Sinus bradycardia AV block	Digoxin	↑Vagal tone	Antidigoxin antibodies Temporary pacing	Atrial tachycardia may also be present
Sinus bradycardia AV block	Verapamil Diltiazem	Ca^{2+} channel block	Ca^{2+} Temporary pacing	
Sinus bradycardia AV block	β Blockers Clonidine Methyldopa	Sympatholytic	Isoproterenol Temporary pacing	
Sinus tachycardia Any other tachycardia	β Blocker withdrawal	Upregulation of β receptors with chronic therapy; β blocker withdrawal ⇒ ↑ β effects	β Blockade	Hypertension, angina also possible
↑ Ventricular rate in atrial flutter	Quinidine Flecainide Propafenone	Conduction slowing in atrium, with enhanced (quinidine) or unaltered AV conduction	AV nodal blockers	QRS complexes often widened at fast rates
↑ Ventricular rate in atrial fibrillation in patients with WPW syndrome	Digoxin Verapamil	↓ accessory pathway refractoriness	IV procainamide DC cardioversion	Ventricular rate can exceed 300 beats/min
Multifocal atrial tachycardia	Theophylline	↑ intracellular Ca^{2+} and DADs	Withdraw theophylline ?Verapamil	Often in advanced lung disease
Polymorphic VT with ↑ QT interval (torsades de pointes)	Quinidine Sotalol Procainamide Disopyramide Dofetilide Ibutilide "Noncardioactive" drugs (see text) Amiodarone (rare)	EAD-related triggered activity	Cardiac pacing Isoproterenol Magnesium	Hypokalemia, bradycardia frequent Related to ↑ plasma concentrations, except for quinidine
Frequent or difficult to terminate VT ("incessant" VT)	Flecainide Propafenone Quinidine (rarer)	Conduction slowing in re-entrant circuits	Na^+ bolus reported effective in some cases	Most often in patients with advanced myocardial scarring
Atrial tachycardia with AV block; ventricular bigeminy, others	Digoxin	DAD-related triggered activity (± ↑ vagal tone)	Antidigoxin antibodies	Co-existence of abnormal impulses with abnormal sinus or AV nodal function
Ventricular fibrillation	Inappropriate use of IV verapamil	Severe hypotension and/or myocardial ischemia	Cardiac resuscitation (DC cardioversion)	Misdiagnosis of VT as PSVT and inappropriate use of verapamil

*In each of these cases, recognition and withdrawal of the offending drug(s) are mandatory. AV, atrioventricular; DAD, delayed afterdepolarization; DC, direct current; EAD, early afterdepolarization; IV, intravenous; PSVT, paroxysmal supraventricular tachycardia; VT, ventricular tachycardia; WPW, Wolff–Parkinson–White supraventricular tachycardia; ↑, increase; ↓, decrease; ?, unclear.

Table 29–2

A Mechanistic Approach to Anti-Arrhythmic Therapy

ARRHYTHMIA	COMMON MECHANISM	ACUTE THERAPY[a]	CHRONIC THERAPY[a]
Premature atrial, nodal, or ventricular depolarizations	Unknown	None indicated	None indicated
Atrial fibrillation	Disorganized "functional" re-entry Continual AV node stimulation and irregular, often rapid, ventricular rate	1. Control ventricular response: AV node block[b] 2. Restore sinus rhythm: DC cardioversion	1. Control ventricular response: AV nodal block[b] 2. Maintain normal rhythm: K^+ channel block, Na^+ channel block, Na^+ channel block with $\tau_{recovery}$ >1 second
Atrial flutter	Stable re-entrant circuit in the right atrium Ventricular rate often rapid and irregular	Same as atrial fibrillation	Same as atrial fibrillation AV nodal blocking drugs especially desirable to avoid ↑ ventricular rate Ablation in selected cases[c]
Atrial tachycardia	Enhanced automaticity, DAD-related automaticity, or re-entry in atrium	Same as atrial fibrillation	Same as atrial fibrillation Ablation of tachycardia "focus"[c]
AV nodal reentrant tachycardia (PSVT)	Re-entrant circuit within or near AV node	*Adenosine AV nodal block Less commonly: ↑ vagal tone (digitalis, edrophonium, phenylephrine)	*AV nodal block Flecainide Propafenone *Ablation[c]
Arrhythmias associated with WPW syndrome: 1. AV re-entry (PSVT)	Re-entry (Figure 29–7)	Same as AV nodal reentry	K^+ channel block Na^+ channel block with $\tau_{recovery}$ >1 second *Ablation[c]
2. Atrial fibrillation with atrioventricular conduction via accessory pathway	Very rapid rate due to nondecremental properties of accessory pathway	*DC cardioversion *Procainamide	K^+ channel block Na^+ channel block with $\tau_{recovery}$ >1 second (AV nodal blockers can be harmful)
VT in patients with remote myocardial infarction	Re-entry near the rim of the healed myocardial infarction	Lidocaine Amiodarone Procainamide DC cardioversion	*ICD[d] Amiodarone K^+ channel block Na^+ channel block
VT in patients without structural heart disease	DADs triggered by ↑ sympathetic tone	Adenosine[e] Verapamil[e] β Blockers[e] DC cardioversion	Verapamil[e] β Blockers[e]
VF	Disorganized reentry	*DC cardioversion Lidocaine Amiodarone Procainamide Pacing	*ICD[d] Amiodarone K^+ channel block Na^+ channel block
Torsades de pointes, congenital or acquired; (often drug related)	EAD-related triggered activity	Magnesium Isoproterenol	β Blockade Pacing

*Indicates treatment of choice. [a]Acute drug therapy is administered intravenously; chronic therapy implies long-term oral use. [b]AV nodal block can be achieved clinically by adenosine, Ca^{2+} channel block, β adrenergic receptor blockade, or increased vagal tone (a major anti-arrhythmic effect of digitalis glycosides). [c]Ablation is a procedure in which tissue responsible for the maintenance of a tachycardia is identified by specialized recording techniques and then selectively destroyed, usually by high-frequency radio waves delivered through a catheter placed in the heart. [d]ICD, implanted cardioverter–defibrillator: a device that can sense VT or VF and deliver pacing and/or cardioverting shocks to restore normal rhythm. [e]These may be harmful in reentrant VT and so should be used for acute therapy only if the diagnosis is secure. DAD, delayed afterdepolarization; EAD, early afterdepolarization; WPW, Wolff–Parkinson–White syndrome; PSVT, paroxysmal supraventricular tachycardia; VT, ventricular tachycardia; VF, ventricular fibrillation.

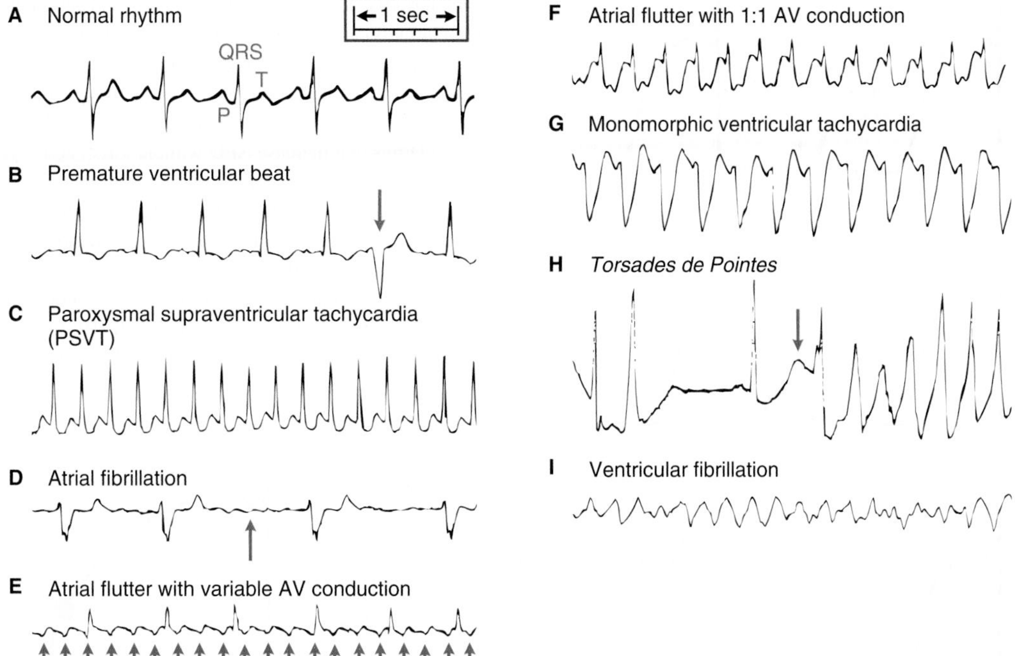

Figure 29–9. *ECGs showing normal and abnormal cardiac rhythms.* The P, QRS, and T waves in normal sinus rhythm are shown in panel ***A***. Panel ***B*** shows a premature beat arising in the ventricle (*arrow*). Paroxysmal supraventricular tachycardia (PSVT) is shown in panel ***C***; this most likely is re-entry using an accessory pathway (see Figure 29–7) or re-entry within or near the atrioventricular (AV) node. In atrial fibrillation (panel ***D***), there are no P waves, and the QRS complexes occur irregularly (and at a slow rate in this example); electrical activity between QRS complexes shows small undulations (*arrow*) corresponding to fibrillatory activity in the atria. In atrial flutter (panel ***E***), the atria beat rapidly, ~250 beats/minute (*arrows*) in this example, and the ventricular rate is variable. If a drug that slows the rate of atrial flutter is administered, 1:1 AV conduction (panel ***F***) can occur. In monomorphic ventricular tachycardia (VT, panel ***G***), identical wide QRS complexes occur at a regular rate, 180 beats/min. The electrocardiographic features of the torsades de pointes syndrome (panel ***H***) include a very long QT interval (>600 ms in this example, *arrow*) and ventricular tachycardia in which each successive beat has a different morphology (polymorphic VT). Panel ***I*** shows the disorganized electrical activity characteristic of ventricular fibrillation.

Drugs may slow automatic rhythms by altering any of the four determinants of spontaneous pacemaker discharge (Figure 29–10):

- decrease phase 4 slope
- increase threshold potential
- increase maximum diastolic potential
- increase APD

Adenosine and acetylcholine may increase maximum diastolic potential, and β receptor antagonists (see Chapter 12) may decrease phase 4 slope. Blockade of Na^+ or Ca^{2+} channels usually results in altered threshold, and blockade of cardiac K^+ channels prolongs the action potential.

Anti-arrhythmic drugs may block arrhythmias owing to DADs or EADs by two major mechanisms:

- inhibition of the development of afterdepolarizations
- interference with the inward current (usually through Na^+ or Ca^{2+} channels), which is responsible for the upstroke

Thus, arrhythmias owing to digitalis-induced DADs may be inhibited by verapamil (which blocks the development of DAD by reducing Ca^{2+} influx into the cell, thereby decreasing sarcoplasmic reticulum Ca^{2+} load and the likelihood of spontaneous Ca^{2+} release from the sarcoplasmic reticulum) or by quinidine (which blocks Na^+ channels, thereby elevating the threshold required to produce the abnormal upstroke). Similarly, two approaches are used in arrhythmias related to EAD-triggered beats (Tables 29–1 and 29–2). EADs can be inhibited by shortening APD; in practice, heart rate is accelerated by isoproterenol infusion or by pacing. Triggered beats arising from EADs can be inhibited by Mg^{2+}, without normalizing repolarization *in vitro* or QT interval, through mechanisms that are not well understood. In patients with a congenitally prolonged QT interval, torsades de pointes often occurs with adrenergic stress; therapy includes β adrenergic blockade (which does not shorten the QT interval) as well as pacing.

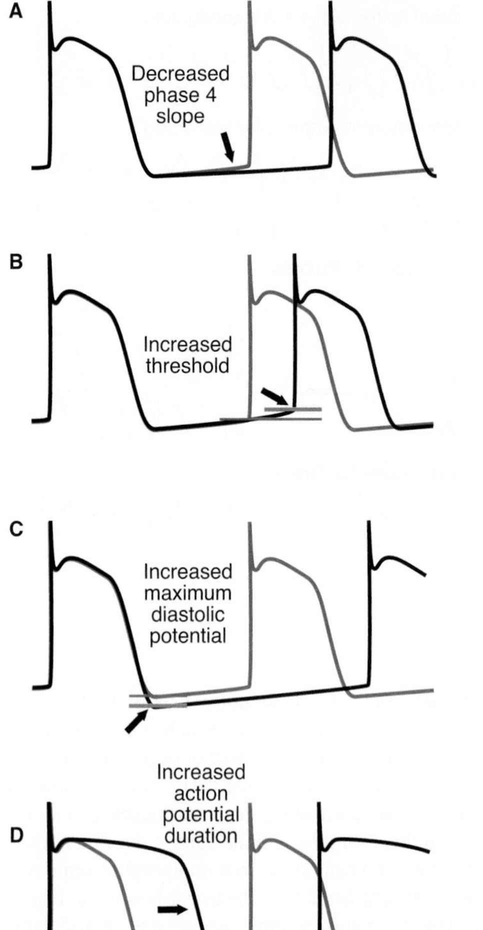

Figure 29–10. *Four ways to reduce the rate of spontaneous discharge.* The blue horizontal line represents threshold potential.

In anatomically determined re-entry, drugs may terminate the arrhythmia by blocking propagation of the action potential. Conduction usually fails in a "weak link" in the circuit. In the example of the WPW-related arrhythmia described earlier, the weak link is the AV node, and drugs that prolong AV nodal refractoriness and slow AV nodal conduction, such as Ca^{2+} channel blockers, β adrenergic receptor antagonists, or digitalis glycosides, are likely to be effective. On the other hand, slowing conduction in functionally determined re-entrant circuits may change the pathway without extinguishing the circuit. In fact, slow conduction generally promotes the development of re-entrant arrhythmias, whereas the most likely approach for terminating functionally determined re-entry is prolongation of refractoriness (Task Force, 1991). In atrial and ventricular myocytes, refractoriness can be prolonged by delaying the recovery of Na^+ channels from inactivation. Drugs that act by blocking Na^+ channels generally shift the voltage dependence of recovery from block (Figure 29–5B) and so prolong refractoriness (Figure 29–11).

Drugs that increase APD without direct action on Na^+ channels (e.g., by blocking delayed-rectifier currents) also will prolong refractoriness (Figure 29–11). Particularly in sinoatrial or AV nodal tissues, Ca^{2+} channel blockade prolongs refractoriness. Drugs that interfere with cell–cell coupling also theoretically should increase refractoriness in multicellular preparations; amiodarone may exert this effect in diseased tissue (Levine et al., 1988). Acceleration of conduction in an area of slow conduction also could inhibit re-entry; lidocaine may exert such an effect, and peptides that suppress

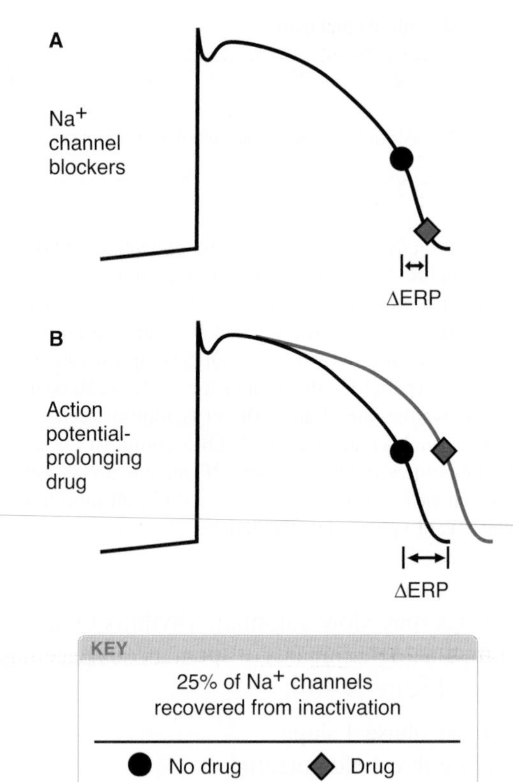

Figure 29–11. *Two ways to increase refractoriness.* In this figure, the black dot indicates the point at which a sufficient number of Na^+ channels (an arbitrary 25%; see Figure 29–5B) have recovered from inactivation to allow a premature stimulus to produce a propagated response in the absence of a drug. Block of Na^+ channels (***A***) shifts voltage dependence of recovery (see Figure 29–5B) and so delays the point at which 25% of channels have recovered (*red diamond*), prolonging refractoriness. Note that if the drug also dissociates slowly from the channel (see Figure 29–12), refractoriness in fast-response tissues actually can extend beyond full repolarization ("postrepolarization refractoriness"). Drugs that prolong the action potential (***B***) also will extend the point at which an arbitrary percentage of Na^+ channels have recovered from inactivation, even without directly interacting with Na^+ channels. ERP, effective refractory period.

experimental arrhythmias by increasing gap junction conductance have been described.

State-Dependent Ion Channel Block

Recent advances have elucidated the structural and molecular determinants of ion channel permeation and drug block. This information has begun to play an increasing role in analyzing the actions of available and new anti-arrhythmic compounds (MacKinnon, 2003). A key concept is that ion channel–blocking drugs bind to specific sites on the ion channel proteins to modify function (e.g., decrease current) and that the affinity of the ion channel protein for the drug on its target site will vary as the ion channel protein shuttles among functional conformations (or ion channel "states"; see Figure 29–2). Physicochemical characteristics, such as molecular weight and lipid solubility, are important determinants of state-dependent binding. State-dependent binding has been studied most extensively in the case of Na^+ channel–blocking drugs. Most useful agents of this type block open and/or inactivated Na^+ channels and have very little affinity for channels in the resting state. Most Na^+ channel blockers bind to a local anesthetic binding site in the pore of Nav1.5, and drug affinity is reduced with mutation to critical residues in the pore (Fozzard et al., 2005). Thus, with each action potential, drugs bind to Na^+ channels and block them, and with each diastolic interval, drugs dissociate, and the block is released.

As illustrated in Figure 29–12, the dissociation rate is a key determinant of steady-state block of Na^+ channels. When heart rate increases, the time available for dissociation decreases, and steady-state Na^+ channel block increases. The rate of recovery from block also slows as cells are depolarized, as in ischemia. This explains the finding that Na^+ channel blockers depress Na^+ current, and hence conduction, to a greater extent in ischemic tissues than in normal tissues. Open versus inactivated-state block also may be important in determining the effects of some drugs. Increased APD, which results in a relative increase in time spent in the inactivated state, may increase block by drugs that bind to inactivated channels, such as lidocaine or amiodarone.

The rate of recovery from block often is expressed as a time constant ($\tau_{recovery}$, the time required for ~63% of an exponentially determined process to be complete; Courtney, 1987). In the case of drugs such as lidocaine, $\tau_{recovery}$ is so short ($\ll$1 s) that recovery from block is very rapid, and substantial Na^+ channel block occurs only in rapidly driven tissues, particularly in ischemia. Conversely, drugs such as flecainide have such long $\tau_{recovery}$ values (>10 s) that roughly the same number of Na^+ channels is blocked during systole and diastole. As a result, marked slowing of conduction occurs even in normal tissues at normal rates.

Classifying Anti-Arrhythmic Drugs

Classifying drugs by common electrophysiologic properties emphasizes the connection between basic electrophysiologic actions and anti-arrhythmic effects (Vaughan Williams, 1992). To the extent that the clinical actions of drugs can be predicted from their basic electrophysiologic properties, such classification schemes have merit. However, as each compound is

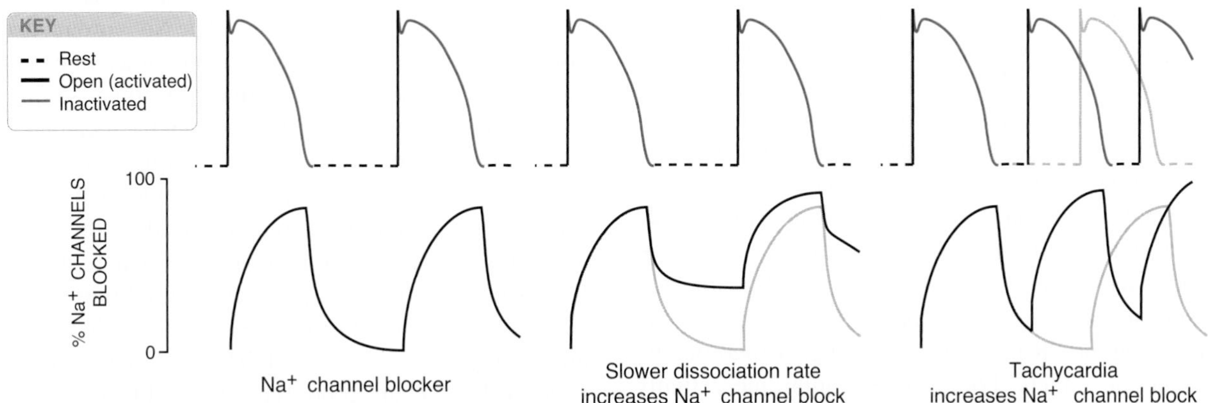

Figure 29–12. *Recovery from block of Na^+ channels during diastole.* This recovery is the critical factor determining extent of steady-state Na^+ channel block. Na^+ channel blockers bind to (and block) Na^+ channels in the open and/or inactivated states, resulting in phasic changes in the extent of block during the action potential. As shown in the *middle* panel, a decrease in the rate of recovery from block increases the extent of block. Different drugs have different rates of recovery, and depolarization reduces the rate of recovery. The *right* panel shows that increasing heart rate, which results in relatively less time spent in the rest state, also increases the extent of block. (Modified from Roden et al., 1993, with permission from Wiley-Blackwell Publishing.)

better characterized in a range of *in vitro* and *in vivo* test systems, it becomes apparent that differences in pharmacologic effects occur even among drugs that share the same classification, some of which may be responsible for the observed clinical differences in responses to drugs of the same broad "class" (Table 29–3). An alternative way of approaching anti-arrhythmic therapy is to classify arrhythmia mechanisms and then to target drug therapy to the electrophysiologic mechanism most likely to terminate or prevent the arrhythmia (Task Force, 1991) (Table 29–2). Most recently, a genetic framework of arrhythmia mechanisms has been suggested as a new approach for classifying anti-arrhythmic drug therapy (Knollmann and Roden, 2008).

Na^+ Channel Block. The extent of Na^+ channel block depends critically on heart rate and membrane potential, as well as on drug-specific physicochemical characteristics that determine $\tau_{recovery}$ (Figure 29–12). The following description applies when Na^+ channels are blocked (i.e., at rapid heart rates in diseased tissue with a rapid-recovery drug such as lidocaine or even at normal rates in normal tissues with a slow-recovery drug such as flecainide). When Na^+ channels are blocked, threshold for excitability is decreased (i.e., greater membrane depolarization is required to open enough Na^+ channels to overcome K^+ currents at the resting membrane potential and elicit an action potential). This change in threshold probably contributes to the clinical findings that Na^+ channel blockers tend to increase both pacing threshold and the energy required to defibrillate the fibrillating heart (Echt et al., 1989). These deleterious effects may be important if anti-arrhythmic drugs are used in patients with pacemakers or implanted defibrillators. Na^+ channel block decreases conduction velocity in non-nodal tissue and increases QRS duration. Usual doses of flecainide prolong QRS intervals by 25% or more during normal rhythm, whereas lidocaine increases QRS intervals only at very fast heart rates. Drugs with $\tau_{recovery}$ values greater than 10 s (e.g., flecainide) also tend to prolong the PR interval; it is not known whether this represents additional Ca^{2+} channel block (see "Ca^{2+} Channel Block") or block of fast-response tissue in the region of the AV node. Drug effects on the PR interval also are highly modified by autonomic effects. For example, quinidine actually tends to shorten the PR interval largely as a result of its vagolytic properties. Action potential duration either is unaffected or shortened by Na^+ channel block; some Na^+ channel–blocking drugs do prolong cardiac action potentials but by other mechanisms, usually K^+ channel block (Table 29–3).

By increasing threshold, Na^+ channel block decreases automaticity (Figure 29–10B) and can inhibit triggered activity arising from DADs or EADs. Many Na^+ channel blockers also decrease phase 4 slope (Figure 29–10A). In anatomically defined re-entry, Na^+ channel blockers may decrease conduction sufficiently to extinguish the propagating re-entrant wavefront. However, as described earlier, conduction slowing owing to Na^+ channel block may exacerbate re-entry. Block of Na^+ channels also shifts the voltage dependence of recovery from inactivation (Figure 29–5B) to more negative potentials, thereby tending to increase refractoriness. Thus, whether a given drug exacerbates or suppresses re-entrant arrhythmias depends on the balance between its effects on refractoriness and on conduction in a particular re-entrant circuit. Lidocaine and mexiletine have short $\tau_{recovery}$ values and are not useful in atrial fibrillation or flutter, whereas quinidine, flecainide, propafenone, and similar agents are effective in some patients. Many of these agents owe part of their anti-arrhythmic activity to blockade of K^+ channels.

Late Na^+ Channel Current Block. The long QT syndrome variant 3 (LQT3) is characterized by late inward Na^+ current caused by defects in the inactivation of the cardiac isoform of the Na^+ channel. This late current prolongs the APD and predisposes to arrhythmia. Many drugs with local anesthetic effects, including mexiletine, preferentially block this late current and can be used to successfully treat LQT3 patients. The lessons learned from LQT3 have led to a better understanding of blocking late Na^+ current, which may be a more common pathologic condition than previously thought. Recently, a number of animal models of heart failure have been shown to have a similar increase in late Na^+ current, and consequently late Na^+ blockade is an attractive candidate for anti-arrhythmic drugs in this setting. Interestingly, recent studies have shown the local anesthetic late current blockade is not unique to selective Na^+ channel blockers and other drugs bind to the same binding site, including commonly used β adrenergic antagonists (including propranolol) and an anti-anginal therapeutic (ranolazine), preferentially inhibiting late current, which may in turn play a role in their anti-arrhythmic utility in both LQT3 and heart failure patients (Fredj et al., 2006; Bankston and Kass, 2010).

Na^+ Channel–Blocker Toxicity. Conduction slowing in potential re-entrant circuits can account for toxicity of drugs that block the Na^+ channel (Table 29–1). For example, Na^+ channel block decreases conduction velocity and hence slows atrial flutter rate. Normal AV

Quinidine metabolism is induced by drugs such as *phenobarbital* and phenytoin (Data et al., 1976). In patients receiving these agents, very high doses of quinidine may be required to achieve therapeutic concentrations. If therapy with the inducing agent is then stopped, quinidine concentrations may rise to very high levels, and its dosage must be adjusted downward. Cimetidine and verapamil also elevate plasma quinidine concentrations, but these effects usually are modest.

Sotalol. Sotalol (BETAPACE, BETAPACE AF) is a nonselective β adrenergic receptor antagonist that also prolongs cardiac action potentials by inhibiting delayed-rectifier and possibly other K^+ currents (Hohnloser and Woosley, 1994). Sotalol is prescribed as a racemate; the L-enantiomer is a much more potent β adrenergic receptor antagonist than the D-enantiomer, but the two are equipotent as K^+ channel blockers. Its structure is shown below:

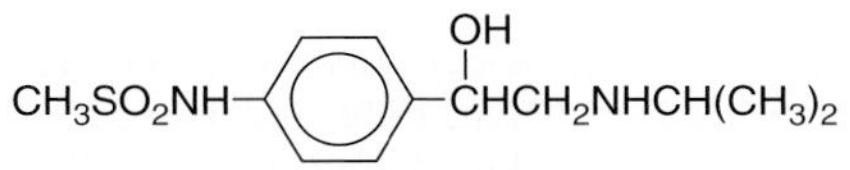

CH_3SO_2NH–C₆H₄–$CH(OH)CH_2NHCH(CH_3)_2$

SOTALOL

In the U.S., sotalol is an orphan drug approved for use in patients with both ventricular tachyarrhythmias (BETAPACE) and atrial fibrillation or flutter (BETAPACE AF). Clinical trials suggest that it is at least as effective as most Na^+ channel blockers in ventricular arrhythmias (Mason, 1993).

Sotalol prolongs APD throughout the heart and QT interval on the ECG. It decreases automaticity, slows AV nodal conduction, and prolongs AV refractoriness by blocking both K^+ channels and β adrenergic receptors, but it exerts no effect on conduction velocity in fast-response tissue. Sotalol causes EADs and triggered activity *in vitro* and can cause torsades de pointes, especially when the serum K^+ concentration is low. Unlike the situation with quinidine, the incidence of torsades de pointes (1.5-2% incidence) seems to depend on the dose of sotalol; indeed, torsades de pointes is the major toxicity with sotalol overdose. Occasional cases occur at low dosages, often in patients with renal dysfunction, because sotalol is eliminated by renal excretion of unchanged drug. The other adverse effects of sotalol therapy are those associated with β receptor blockade (see earlier in this chapter and Chapter 12).

Vernakalant. Vernakalant (RSD1235, proposed tradename KYNAPID) is an investigational inhibitor of several ion channels that are preferentially expressed in the atria, in particular the ultra-rapidly activating delayed-rectifier K^+ current (I_{Kur} encoded by Kv1.5). To a lesser extent, it also blocks the rapidly activating delayed-rectifier K^+ current (I_{Kr}), the transient outward K^+ current (I_{to}), the Na^+ current, and the L-type Ca^{2+} current. Vernakalant selectively prolongs the atrial refractory period without significantly affecting ventricular refractoriness.

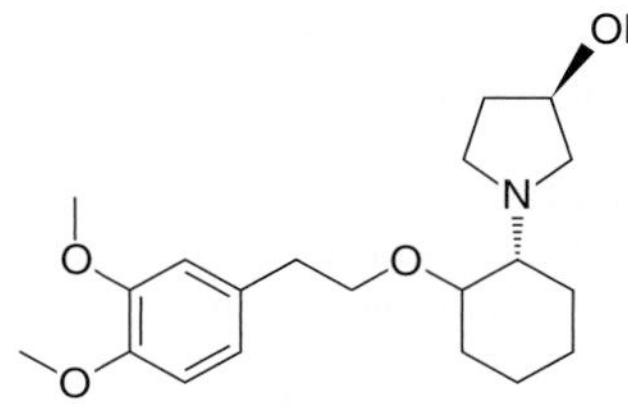

VERNAKALANT

Vernakalant is effective for converting atrial fibrillation of short duration to sinus rhythm (Roy et al., 2008). Vernakalant (3 mg/kg) is administered as a 10-minute infusion, followed by a second infusion of 2 mg/kg 15 minutes later if AF is not terminated. Vernakalant is not effective in converting long-duration AF (>7 days) or atrial flutter. The intravenous formulation of vernakalant was recommended for approval by an FDA advisory committee in 2008, but the drug has not received FDA approval at the time of this printing. An oral formulation is currently in clinical trials for the maintenance of sinus rhythm in patients with chronic atrial fibrillation. Vernakalant seems to have little or no proarrhythmic effects, with no reported cases of torsades de pointes in phase II and III studies.

Vernakalant is metabolized by rapidly by CYP2D6 to one major and inactive metabolite (RSD1385) via 4-O-demethylation (Mao et al., 2009). There appears to be little difference in C_{max} between extensive and poor 2D6 metabolizers after single-dose IV administration. However, average $t_{1/2}$ of vernakalant was much longer in two poor metabolizers (8.5 hours) than in 10 extensive metabolizers (2.7 hours). This profound difference in $t_{1/2}$ will be important if vernakalant is used chronically to prevent atrial fibrillation.

BIBLIOGRAPHY

Akiyama T, Pawitan Y, Greenberg H, et al. Increased risk of death and cardiac arrest from encainide and flecainide in patients after non-Q-wave acute myocardial infarction in the Cardiac Arrhythmia Suppression Trial. The CAST Investigators. *Am J Cardiol*, **1991**, *68*:1551–1555.

Amiodarone Trials Meta-Analysis Investigators. Effect of prophylactic amiodarone on mortality after acute myocardial infarction and in congestive heart failure—Meta-analysis of individual data from 6500 patients in randomised trials. *Lancet*, **1997**, *350*:1417–1424.

Anderson JL, Gilbert EM, Alpert BL, et al. Prevention of symptomatic recurrences of paroxysmal atrial fibrillation in patients initially tolerating antiarrhythmic therapy: A multicenter, double-blind, crossover study of flecainide and placebo with transtelephonic monitoring. Flecainide Supraventricular Tachycardia Study Group. *Circulation*, **1989**, *80*:1557–1570.

Anderson JL, Rodier HE, Green LS. Comparative effects of β-adrenergic blocking drugs on experimental ventricular fibrillation threshold. *Am J Cardiol*, **1983**, *51*:1196–1202.

Balser JR, Nuss HB, Orias DW, et al. Local anesthetics as effectors of allosteric gating: Lidocaine effects on inactivation-deficient rat skeletal muscle Na channels. *J Clin Invest*, **1996**, *98*:2874–2886.

Bankston JR, Kass RS. Molecular determinants of local anesthetic action of beta-blocking drugs: Implications for management of long QT syndrome variant 3. *J Mol Cell Cardiol*, **2010**, *48*:246–253.

Bean BP. Two kinds of calcium channels in canine atrial cells. Differences in kinetics, selectivity, and pharmacology. *J Gen Physiol*, **1985**, *86*:1–30.

Bennett PB, Woosley RL, Hondeghem LM. Competition between lidocaine and one of its metabolites, glycylxylidide, for cardiac sodium channels. *Circulation*, **1988**, *78*:692–700.

Biaggioni I, Killian TJ, Mosqueda-Garcia R, et al. Adenosine increases sympathetic nerve traffic in humans. *Circulation*, **1991**, *83*:1668–1675.

Brown MJ, Brown DC, Murphy MB. Hypokalemia from β_2-receptor stimulation by circulating epinephrine. *N Engl J Med*, **1983**, *309*:1414–1419.

Campbell RW. Mexiletine. *N Engl J Med*, **1987**, *316*:29–34.

Cardiac Arrhythmia Suppression Trial II Investigators. Effect of the antiarrhythmic agent moricizine on survival after myocardial infarction. *N Engl J Med*, **1992**, *327*:227–233.

CAST Investigators. Preliminary report: Effect of encainide and flecainide on mortality in a randomized trial of arrhythmia suppression after myocardial infarction. *N Engl J Med*, **1989**, *321*:406–412.

Clyne CA, Estes NA III, Wang PJ. Moricizine. *N Engl J Med*, **1992**, *327*:255–260.

Cohen IS, Robinson RB. Pacemaker currents and automatic rhythms: Toward a molecular understanding. *Handb Exp Pharmacol*, **2006**, *171*:41–71.

Connolly SJ. Evidence-based analysis of amiodarone efficacy and safety. *Circulation*, **1999**, *100*:2025–2034.

Courtney KR. Progress and prospects for optimum antiarrhythmic drug design. *Cardiovasc Drugs Ther*, **1987**, *1*:117–123.

Crijns HJ, van Gelder IC, Lie KI. Supraventricular tachycardia mimicking ventricular tachycardia during flecainide treatment. *Am J Cardiol*, **1988**, *62*:1303–1306.

Data JL, Wilkinson GR, Nies AS. Interaction of quinidine with anticonvulsant drugs. *N Engl J Med*, **1976**, *294*:699–702.

DiFrancesco D. Pacemaker mechanisms in cardiac tissue. *Annu Rev Physiol*, **1993**, *55*:455–472.

Dorian P, Cass D, Schwartz B, et al. Amiodarone as compared with lidocaine for shock-resistant ventricular fibrillation. *N Engl J Med*, **2002**, *346*:884–890.

Dun W, Boyden PA. The Purkinje cell; 2008 style. *J Mol Cell Cardiol*, **2008**, *45*:617–624.

Dusman RE, Stanton MS, Miles WM, et al. Clinical features of amiodarone-induced pulmonary toxicity. *Circulation*, **1990**, *82*:51–59.

Echizen H, Vogelgesang B, Eichelbaum M. Effects of D, L-verapamil on atrioventricular conduction in relation to its stereoselective first-pass metabolism. *Clin Pharmacol Ther*, **1985**, *38*:71–76.

Echt DS, Black JN, Barbey JT, et al. Evaluation of antiarrhythmic drugs on defibrillation energy requirements in dogs: Sodium channel block and action potential prolongation. *Circulation*, **1989**, *79*:1106–1117.

Follmer CH, Colatsky TJ. Block of delayed rectifier potassium current, I_K, by flecainide and E-4031 in cat ventricular myocytes. *Circulation*, **1990**, *82*:289–293.

Fozzard HA, Lee PJ, Lipkind GM. Mechanism of local anesthetic drug action on voltage-gated sodium channels. *Curr Pharm Des*, **2005**, *11*:2671–2686.

Fredj S, Sampson KJ, Lui H, Kass RS. Molecular basis of ranolazine block of LQT-3 mutant sodium channels: Evidence for site of action. *Br J Pharmacol*, **2006**, *148*:16–24.

Frishman WH, Murthy S, Strom JA. Ultra-short-acting β-adrenergic blockers. *Med Clin North Am*, **1988**, *72*:359–372.

Fromm MF, Kim RB, Stein CM, et al. Inhibition of P-glycoprotein-mediated drug transport: A unifying mechanism to explain the interaction between digoxin and quinidine. *Circulation*, **1999**, *99*:552–557.

Funck-Brentano C, Kroemer HK, Lee JT, Roden DM. Propafenone. *N Engl J Med*, **1990**, *322*:518–525.

Grace AA, Camm J. Quinidine. *N Engl J Med*, **1998**, *338*:35–45.

Gross AS, Mikus G, Fischer C, et al. Stereoselective disposition of flecainide in relation to sparteine/debrisoquine metaboliser phenotype. *Br J Clin Pharmacol*, **1989**, *28*:555–566.

Henthorn RW, Waldo AL, Anderson JL, et al. Flecainide acetate prevents recurrence of symptomatic paroxysmal supraventricular tachycardia. The Flecainide Supraventricular Tachycardia Study Group. *Circulation*, **1991**, *83*:119–125.

Herbette LG, Trumbore M, Chester DW, Katz AM. Possible molecular basis for the pharmacokinetics and pharmacodynamics of three membrane-active drugs: Propranolol, nimodipine and amiodarone. *J Mol Cell Cardiol*, **1988**, *20*:373–378.

Hilliard FA, Steele DS, Laver D, et al. Flecainide inhibits arrhythmogenic Ca^{2+} waves by open state block of ryanodine receptor Ca^{2+} release channels and reduction of Ca^{2+} spark mass. *J Mol Cell Cardiol*, **2010**, *48*:293-301.

Hine LK, Laird N, Hewitt P, Chalmers TC. Meta-analytic evidence against prophylactic use of lidocaine in acute myocardial infarction. *Arch Intern Med*, **1989**, *149*:2694–2698.

Hohnloser SH, Woosley RL. Sotalol. *N Engl J Med*, **1994**, *331*:31–38.

Ikeda N, Singh BN, Davis LD, Hauswirth O. Effects of flecainide on the electrophysiologic properties of isolated canine and rabbit myocardial fibers. *J Am Coll Cardiol*, **1985**, *5*:303–310.

ISIS-4 Collaborative Group. ISIS-4: A randomised factorial trial assessing early oral captopril, oral mononitrate, and intravenous magnesium sulphate in 58,050 patients with suspected acute myocardial infarction. ISIS-4 (Fourth International Study of Infarct Survival) Collaborative Group. *Lancet*, **1995**, *345*:669–685.

Kessler KM, Kissane B, Cassidy J, et al. Dynamic variability of binding of antiarrhythmic drugs during the evolution of acute myocardial infarction. *Circulation*, **1984**, *70*:472–478.

Knollmann BC, Roden DM. A genetic framework for improving arrhythmia therapy. *Nature*, **2008**, *451*:929–936.

Kowey PR, Levine JH, Herre JM, et al. Randomized, double-blind comparison of intravenous amiodarone and bretylium in the treatment of patients with recurrent, hemodynamically destabilizing ventricular tachycardia or fibrillation. The Intravenous Amiodarone Multicenter Investigators Group. *Circulation*, **1995**, *92*:3255–3263.

Krapivinsky G, Gordon EA, Wickman K, et al. The G protein–gated atrial K+ channel I_{KACh} is a heteromultimer of two inwardly rectifying K+-channel proteins. *Nature*, **1995**, *374*: 135–141.

Kroemer HK, Turgeon J, Parker RA, Roden DM. Flecainide enantiomers: Disposition in human subjects and electrophysiologic actions in vitro. *Clin Pharmacol Ther*, **1989**, *46*:584–590.

Kurokawa J, Suzuki T, Furukawa T. New aspects for the treatment of cardiac diseases based on the diversity of functional controls on cardiac muscles: Acute effects of female hormones on cardiac ion channels and cardiac repolarization. *J Pharmacol Sci*, **2009**, *109*:334–340.

Lee JH, Rosen MR. Use-dependent actions and effects on transmembrane action potentials of flecainide, encainide, and ethmozine in canine Purkinje fibers. *J Cardiovasc Pharmacol*, **1991**, *18*:285–292.

Lee JT, Kroemer HK, Silberstein DJ, et al. The role of genetically determined polymorphic drug metabolism in the beta-blockade produced by propafenone. *N Engl J Med*, **1990**, *322*:1764–1768.

Lerman BB, Belardinelli L. Cardiac electrophysiology of adenosine: Basic and clinical concepts. *Circulation*, **1991**, *83*:1499–1509.

Levine JH, Moore EN, Kadish AH, et al. Mechanisms of depressed conduction from long-term amiodarone therapy in canine myocardium. *Circulation*, **1988**, *78*:684–691.

Levy S, Azoulay S. Stories about the origin of quinquina and quinidine. *J Cardiovasc Electrophysiol*, **1994**, *5*:635–636.

Lie KI, Wellens HJ, van Capelle FJ, Durrer D. Lidocaine in the prevention of primary ventricular fibrillation: A double-blind, randomized study of 212 consecutive patients. *N Engl J Med*, **1974**, *291*:1324–1326.

Lima JJ, Boudoulas H, Blanford M. Concentration-dependence of disopyramide binding to plasma protein and its influence on kinetics and dynamics. *J Pharmacol Exp Ther*, **1981**, *219*: 741–747.

MacKinnon R. Potassium channels. *FEBS Lett*, **2003**, *555*: 62–65.

Mao ZL, Wheeler JJ, Clohs L, et al. Pharmacokinetics of novel atrial-selective antiarrhythmic agent vernakalant hydrochloride injection (RSD1235): Influence of CYP2D6 expression and other factors. *J Clin Pharmacol*, **2009**, *49*:17–29.

Mason JW. A comparison of seven antiarrhythmic drugs in patients with ventricular tachyarrhythmias. Electrophysiologic Study versus Electrocardiographic Monitoring Investigators. *N Engl J Med*, **1993**, *329*:452–458.

Mason JW. Amiodarone. *N Engl J Med*, **1987**, *316*:455–466.

Mitcheson JS, Chen J, Lin M, et al. A structural basis for drug-induced long QT syndrome. *Proc Natl Acad Sci USA*, **2000**, *97*:12329–12333.

Mohamed U, Napolitano C, Prioiri SG. Molecular and electrophysiological basis of catecholaminergic polymorphic ventricular tachycardia. *J Cardiovasc Electrophysiol*, **2007**, *18*: 791–797.

Morady F, Scheinman MM, Desai J. Disopyramide. *Ann Intern Med*, **1982**, *96*:337–343.

Murray KT. Ibutilide. *Circulation*, **1998**, *97*:493–497.

Myerburg RJ, Kessler KM, Cox MM, et al. Reversal of proarrhythmic effects of flecainide acetate and encainide hydrochloride by propranolol. *Circulation*, **1989**, *80*:1571–1579.

Napolitano C, Bloise R, Priori S. Gene-specific therapy for inherited arrhythmogenic diseases. *Pharmacol Ther*, **2006**, *100*:1–13.

Nerbonne JM, Kass RS. Molecular physiology of cardiac repolarization. *Physiol Rev*, **2005**, *85*:1205–1253.

Nies AS, Shand DG, Wilkinson GR. Altered hepatic blood flow and drug disposition. *Clin Pharmacokinet*, **1976**, *1*:135–155.

Patel C, Yan GX, Kowey PR. Dronedarone. *Circulation*, **2009**, *120*:636–644.

Podrid PJ, Schoeneberger A, Lown B. Congestive heart failure caused by oral disopyramide. *N Engl J Med*, **1980**, *302*: 614–617.

Priori SG, Barhanin J, Hauer RN, et al. Genetic and molecular basis of cardiac arrhythmias: Impact on clinical management. Study Group on Molecular Basis of Arrhythmias of the Working Group on Arrhythmias of the European Society of Cardiology. *Eur Heart J*, **1999**, *20*:174–195.

Roden DM. Antiarrhythmic drugs: Past, present and future. *J Cardiovasc Electrophysiol*, **2003**, *14*:1389–1396.

Roden DM. Current status of class III antiarrhythmic drug therapy. *Am J Cardiol*, **1993**, *72*:44B–49B.

Roden DM. Drug-induced prolongation of the QT interval. *N Engl J Med*, **2004**, *350*:1013–1022.

Roden DM. Risks and benefits of antiarrhythmic therapy. *N Engl J Med*, **1994**, *331*:785–791.

Roden DM, Echt DS, Lee JT, Murray KT. Clinical pharmacology of antiarrhythmic agents. In: Josephson ME, ed. *Sudden Cardiac Death*. Blackwell Scientific, London, **1993**, pp. 182–185.

Roden DM, Woosley RL. Drug therapy: Flecainide. *N Engl J Med*, **1986**, *315*:36–41.

Roy D, Pratt CM, Torp-Pedersen C, et al. Vernakalant hydrochloride for rapid conversion of atrial fibrillation: A phase 3, randomized, placebo-controlled trial. *Circulation*, **2008**, *117*: 1518–1525.

Roy D, Talajic M, Dorian P, et al. Amiodarone to prevent recurrence of atrial fibrillation. Canadian Trial of Atrial Fibrillation Investigators. *N Engl J Med*, **2000**, *342*:913–920.

Ruskin JN. The Cardiac Arrhythmia Suppression Trial (CAST). *N Engl J Med*, **1989**, *321*:386–388.

Sanguinetti MC, Jurkiewicz NK. Two components of cardiac delayed rectifier K+ current: Differential sensitivity to block by class III antiarrhythmic agents. *J Gen Physiol*, **1990**, *96*: 195–215.

Sanguinetti MC, Jurkiewicz NK, Scott A, Siegl PK. Isoproterenol antagonizes prolongation of refractory period by the class III antiarrhythmic agent E-4031 in guinea pig myocytes: Mechanism of action. *Circ Res*, **1991**, *68*:77–84.

Schwartz PJ, Priori SG, Napolitano C. Long QT syndrome. In: Zipes DP, Jalife J, eds. *Cardiac Electrophysiology: From Cell to Bedside*, 3rd ed. Saunders, Philadelphia, **2000**, pp. 615–640.

Singer DE. Anticoagulation for atrial fibrillation: Epidemiology informing a difficult clinical decision. *Proc Assoc Am Phys*, **1996**, *108*:29–36.

Singh BN. Advantages of beta blockers versus antiarrhythmic agents and calcium antagonists in secondary prevention after myocardial infarction. *Am J Cardiol*, **1990**, *66*:9C–20C.

Smith TW. Digitalis: Mechanisms of action and clinical use. *N Engl J Med*, **1988**, *318*:358–365.

Stewart RB, Bardy GH, Greene HL. Wide complex tachycardia: Misdiagnosis and outcome after emergent therapy. *Ann Intern Med*, **1986**, *104*:766–771.

Sung RJ, Shapiro WA, Shen EN, et al. Effects of verapamil on ventricular tachycardias possibly caused by reentry, automaticity, and triggered activity. *J Clin Invest*, **1983**, *72*:350–360.

Task Force of the Working Group on Arrhythmias of the European Society of Cardiology. The Sicilian gambit: A new approach to the classification of antiarrhythmic drugs based on their actions on arrhythmogenic mechanisms. *Circulation*, **1991**, *84*:1831–1851.

Torp-Pedersen C, Moller M, Bloch-Thomsen PE, et al. Dofetilide in patients with congestive heart failure and left ventricular dysfunction. Danish Investigations of Arrhythmia and Mortality on Dofetilide Study Group. *N Engl J Med*, **1999**, *341*:857–865.

Tseng GN, Hoffman BF. Two components of transient outward current in canine ventricular myocytes. *Circ Res*, **1989**, *64*: 633–647.

Tzivoni D, Banai S, Schuger C, et al. Treatment of torsade de pointes with magnesium sulfate. *Circulation*, **1988**, *77*: 392–397.

Vaughan Williams EM. Classifying antiarrhythmic actions: By facts or speculation. *J Clin Pharmacol*, **1992**, *32*:964–977.

Vinogradova TM, Lakatta EG. Regulation of basal and reserve cardiac pacemaker function by interactions of cAMP-mediated PKA-dependent Ca^{2+} cycling with surface membrane channels. *J Mol Cell Cardiol*, **2009**, *47*:456–474.

Wang ZG, Pelletier LC, Talajic M, Nattel S. Effects of flecainide and quinidine on human atrial action potentials: Role of rate-dependence and comparison with guinea pig, rabbit, and dog tissues. *Circulation*, **1990**, *82*:274–283.

Watanabe H, Chopra N, Laver D, et al. Flecainide prevents catecholaminergic polymorphic ventricular tachycardia in mice and humans. *Nat Med*, **2009**, *15*:380–383.

Weiss JN, Nademanee K, Stevenson WG, Singh B. Ventricular arrhythmias in ischemic heart disease. *Ann Intern Med*, **1991**, *114*:784–797.

Wenckebach KF. Cinchona derivates in the treatment of heart disorders. *JAMA*, **1923**, *81*:472–474.

Woods KL, Fletcher S. Long-term outcome after intravenous magnesium sulphate in suspected acute myocardial infarction: The second Leicester Intravenous Magnesium Intervention Trial (LIMIT-2). *Lancet*, **1994**, *343*:816–819.

Woosley RL, Drayer DE, Reidenberg MM, et al. Effect of acetylator phenotype on the rate at which procainamide induces antinuclear antibodies and the lupus syndrome. *N Engl J Med*, **1978**, *298*:1157–1159.

Blood Coagulation and Anticoagulant, Fibrinolytic, and Antiplatelet Drugs

Jeffrey I. Weitz

The physiological systems that control the fluidity of blood are both complex and elegant. Blood must remain fluid within the vasculature and yet clot quickly when exposed to subendothelial surfaces at sites of vascular injury. When intravascular thrombi form, rapid activation of the fibrinolytic system restores fluidity. Under normal circumstances, a delicate balance between coagulation and fibrinolysis prevents both thrombosis and hemorrhages. Alteration of this balance in favor of coagulation results in thrombosis.

Composed of platelet aggregates, fibrin, and trapped red blood cells, thrombi can form in arteries or veins. Because of the predominance of platelets and fibrin in thrombi, anti-thrombotic drugs used to treat thrombosis include antiplatelet drugs, which inhibit platelet activation or aggregation, anticoagulants, which attenuate fibrin formation, and fibrinolytic agents, which degrade fibrin. These agents have very different mechanisms of action, but because they target key steps in clot formation, all anti-thrombotic drugs increase the risk of bleeding. With these drugs, toxicity typically represents an extension of the therapeutic effects. The more potent the agent, the greater the risk of bleeding.

This chapter reviews the agents commonly used for controlling blood fluidity, including:

- The parenteral anticoagulant heparin and its derivatives, which activate a natural inhibitor of coagulant proteases
- The coumarin anticoagulants, which block multiple steps in the coagulation cascade
- Fibrinolytic agents, which degrade thrombi
- Antiplatelet agents, including aspirin, thienopyridines, and glycoprotein (GP) IIb/IIIa inhibitors

In addition, some of the newer anti-thrombotic drugs in advanced stages of development also are described.

OVERVIEW OF HEMOSTASIS: PLATELET FUNCTION, BLOOD COAGULATION, AND FIBRINOLYSIS

Hemostasis is the cessation of blood loss from a damaged vessel. Platelets first adhere to macromolecules in the subendothelial regions of the injured blood vessel, where they become activated. Adherent platelets release substances that activate nearby platelets, thereby recruiting them to the site of injury. Activated platelets then aggregate to form the primary hemostatic plug.

In addition to triggering platelet adhesion and activation, vessel wall injury also exposes tissue factor (TF), which initiates the coagulation system. Platelets support and enhance activation of the coagulation system by providing a surface onto which clotting factors assemble and by releasing stored clotting factors. This results in a burst of thrombin (factor IIa) generation. Thrombin then converts fibrinogen to fibrin, which reinforces the platelet aggregate and anchors it to the vessel wall. In addition, because it serves as a potent platelet agonist, thrombin also amplifies platelet activation and aggregation.

Later, as wound healing occurs, the platelet aggregates and fibrin clots are degraded. The processes of platelet aggregation and blood coagulation are summarized in Figures 30–1 and 30–2 (see also the animation on this book's website). The pathway of clot removal, fibrinolysis, is shown in Figure 30–3, along with sites of action of fibrinolytic agents.

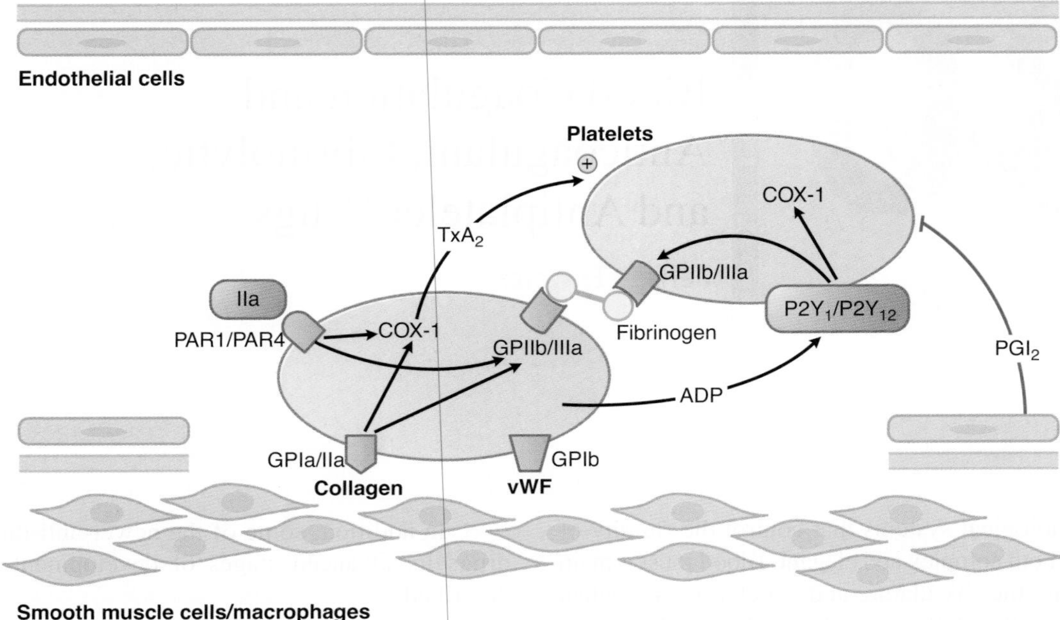

Figure 30–1. *Platelet adhesion and aggregation.* GPIa/IIa and GPIb are platelet receptors that bind to collagen and von Willebrand factor (vWF), causing platelets to adhere to the subendothelium of a damaged blood vessel. PAR1 and PAR4 are protease-activated receptors that respond to thrombin (IIa); $P2Y_1$ and $P2Y_{12}$ are receptors for ADP; when stimulated by agonists, these receptors activate the fibrinogen-binding protein GPIIb/IIIa and cyclooxygenase-1 (COX-1) to promote platelet aggregation and secretion. Thromboxane A_2 (TxA_2) is the major product of COX-1 involved in platelet activation. Prostaglandin I_2 (prostacyclin, PGI_2), synthesized by endothelial cells, inhibits platelet activation.

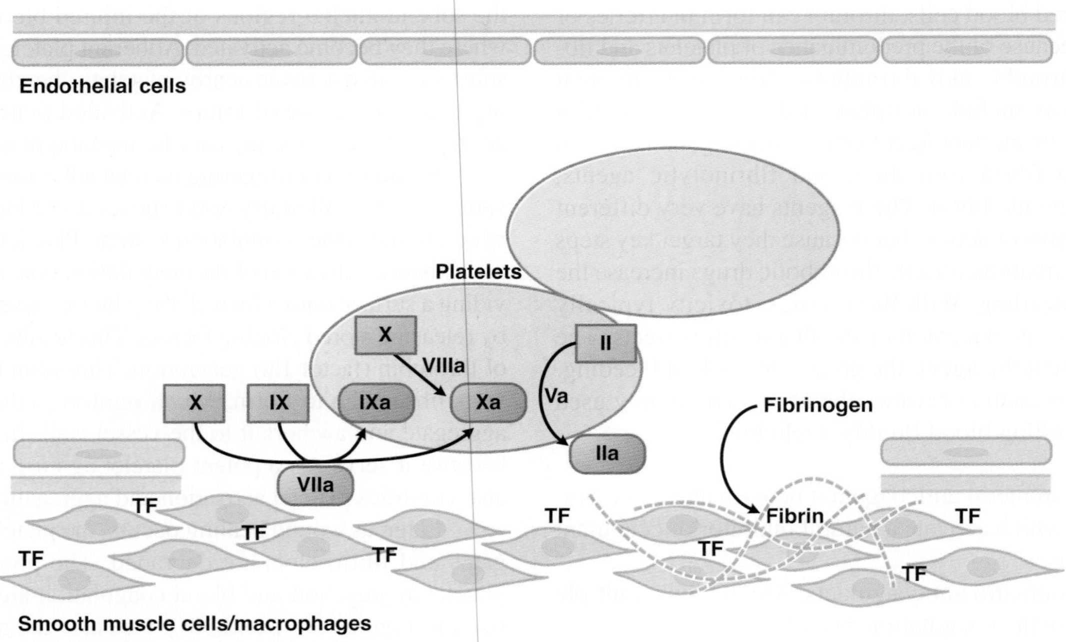

Figure 30–2. *Major reactions of blood coagulation.* Shown are interactions among proteins of the "extrinsic" (tissue factor and factor VII), "intrinsic" (factors IX and VIII), and "common" (factors X, V, and II) coagulation pathways that are important *in vivo*. Boxes enclose the coagulation factor zymogens (indicated by Roman numerals); the rounded boxes represent the active proteases. TF, tissue factor. Activated coagulation factors are followed by the letter "a": II, prothrombin; IIa, thrombin.

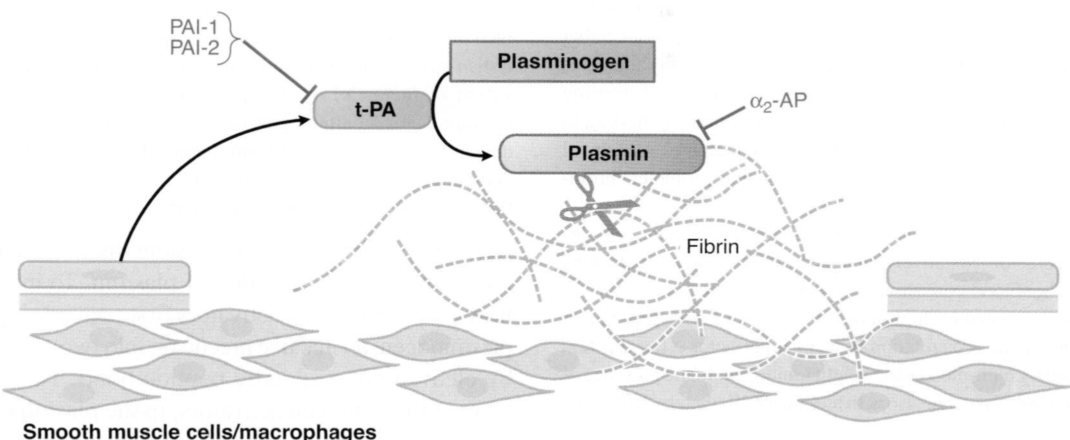

Figure 30–3. *Fibrinolysis.* Endothelial cells secrete tissue plasminogen activator (t-PA) at sites of injury. t-PA binds to fibrin and converts plasminogen to plasmin, which digests fibrin. Plasminogen activator inhibitors-1 and -2 (PAI-1, PAI-2) inactivate t-PA; α_2-antiplasmin (α_2-AP) inactivates plasmin

Coagulation involves a series of zymogen activation reactions, as shown in Figure 30–2 (Mann et al., 2003). At each stage, a precursor protein, or *zymogen,* is converted to an active protease by cleavage of one or more peptide bonds in the precursor molecule. The components at each stage include a protease from the preceding stage, a zymogen, a non-enzymatic protein cofactor, Ca^{2+}, and an organizing surface that is provided by a phospholipid emulsion *in vitro* or by activated platelets *in vivo*. The final protease generated is thrombin.

Conversion of Fibrinogen to Fibrin. Fibrinogen, a 340,000-Da protein, is a dimer, each half of which consists of three pairs of polypeptide chains (designated Aα, Bβ, and γ). Disulfide bonds covalently link the chains and the two halves of the molecule together. Thrombin converts fibrinogen to fibrin monomers by releasing fibrinopeptide A (a 16–amino acid fragment) and fibrinopeptide B (a 14–amino acid fragment) from the amino termini of the Aα and Bβ chains, respectively. Removal of the fibrinopeptides creates new amino termini, which fit into pre-formed holes on other fibrin monomers to form a fibrin gel, which is the end point of *in vitro* tests of coagulation (see "Coagulation *in vitro*"). Initially, the fibrin monomers are bound to each other non-covalently. Subsequently, factor XIII, a transglutaminase that is activated by thrombin, catalyzes interchain covalent cross-links between adjacent fibrin monomers, which enhance the strength of the clot.

Structure of Coagulation Factors. In addition to factor XIII, the coagulation factors include factors II (prothrombin), VII, IX, X, XI, XII, and prekallikrein. A stretch of about 200 amino acid residues at the carboxyl-termini of each of these zymogens exhibits homology to trypsin and contains the active site of the proteases. In addition, 9-12 glutamate residues near the amino termini of factors II, VII, IX, and X are converted to γ-carboxyglutamate (Gla) residues during their biosynthesis in the liver. The Gla residues bind Ca^{2+} and are necessary for the coagulant activities of these proteins.

Nonenzymatic Protein Cofactors. Factors V and VIII, which are homologous 350,000-Da proteins, serve as cofactors. Factor VIII circulates in plasma bound to von Willebrand factor, while factor V not only circulates in plasma but also is stored in platelets in a partially activated form. Platelets release this stored factor V when they are activated. Thrombin cleaves factors V and VIII to yield activated cofactors (factors Va and VIIIa) that have at least 50 times greater procoagulant activity than their nonactivated counterparts.

Factors Va and VIIIa serve as cofactors by binding to the surface of activated platelets, where they act as receptors for factors Xa and IXa, respectively. The activated cofactors also help localize prothrombin and factor X, the respective substrates for these enzymes, on the activated platelet surface. Assembly of these coagulation factor complexes increases the catalytic efficiency of factors Xa and IXa by $\sim 10^9$-fold.

TF is a non-enzymatic lipoprotein cofactor; it initiates coagulation by enhancing the catalytic efficiency of VIIa. Not normally present on blood-contacting cells, TF is constitutively expressed on the surface of subendothlial smooth muscle cells and fibroblasts, which are exposed when the vessel wall is damaged. Lipid-rich cores of atherosclerotic plaques also are rich in TF, which explains why atherosclerotic plaque disruption often triggers the formation of a superimposed thrombus that can occlude the lumen of the vessel.

When exposed to stimuli such as endotoxin, tumor necrosis factor, or interleukin-1, monocytes also express TF on their surface. Circulating TF-bearing monocytes and membrane fragments derived from them, known as microparticles, contribute to thrombosis. In response to inflammatory stimuli or products of coagulation, such as thrombin, endothelial cells express adhesion molecules, which tether these monocytes and microparticles onto their surface. This augments coagulation by delivering more TF to sites of injury. TF-bearing monocytes and microparticles also home to thrombi by binding to P-selectin expressed on the surface of activated platelets. Additional TF from these sources maintains coagulation and promotes thrombus expansion.

Another plasma protein, high-molecular-weight kininogen, also serves as a cofactor. Negatively charged surfaces, such as catheters, stents, and other blood-contacting medical devices, activate factor XII in a reaction enhanced by high-molecular-weight kininogen. Factor XIIa then propagates coagulation by activating factor XI, a reaction also enhanced by high-molecular-weight kininogen. In the presence of activated platelets, thrombin also activates factor XI, thereby bypassing factor XIIa.

Activation of Prothrombin. By cleaving two peptide bonds on prothrombin, factor Xa converts it to thrombin. In the presence of factor Va, a negatively charged phospholipid surface, and Ca^{2+}, factor Xa activates prothrombin with 10^9-fold greater efficiency. The maximal rate of activation only occurs when prothrombin and factor Xa contain Gla residues, which endow them with the capacity to bind to phospholipids. Artificial mixtures of anionic phospholipids substitute for activated platelets in laboratory tests of coagulation. However, activated platelets not only provide a surface for coagulation factor assembly but also release factor Va, which may be more important than circulating factor Va for thrombin generation.

Initiation of Coagulation. Under most circumstances, TF exposed at sites of vessel wall injury initiates coagulation via the extrinsic pathway. The small amount of factor VIIa circulating in plasma binds subendothelial TF and the TF-factor VIIa complex, then activates factors X and IX (Figure 30–2). In the absence of TF, factor VIIa has minimal activity. When bound to TF in the presence of anionic phospholipids and Ca^{2+}, the activity of factor VIIa increases about 30,000-fold.

The intrinsic pathway is initiated *in vitro* when factor XII, prekallikrein, and high-molecular-weight kininogen interact with kaolin, glass, or another surface to generate small amounts of factor XIIa. Activation of factor XI to factor XIa and factor IX to factor IXa follows. Factor IXa then activates factor X in a reaction accelerated by factor VIIIa, anionic phospholipids, and Ca^{2+}. Optimal thrombin generation depends on the formation of this factor IXa complex because it activates factor X more efficiently than the TF-factor VIIa complex. The bleeding that occurs in hemophiliacs who are deficient in factor IX or factor VIII highlights the importance of the factor IXa–factor VIIIa complex in thrombin generation.

Activation of factor XII is not essential for hemostasis, as evidenced by the fact that patients deficient in factor XII, prekallikrein, or high-molecular-weight kininogen do not have excessive bleeding. Factor XI deficiency is associated with a variable and usually mild bleeding disorder. The mechanism responsible for factor XI activation *in vivo* is unknown. Activation may occur through feedback activation of factor XI by thrombin. Alternatively, factor XIIa may activate factor XI after injury to the vessel wall because there is evidence that RNA released from damaged cells activates factor XII and administration of RNA-degrading enzymes to mice attenuates thrombus formation after arterial injury.

Fibrinolysis. The fibrinolytic system dissolves intravascular fibrin through the action of plasmin. To initiate fibrinolysis, plasminogen activators first convert single-chain plasminogen, an inactive precursor, into two-chain plasmin by cleavage of a specific peptide bond. There are two distinct plasminogen activators; tissue plasminogen activator (t-PA) and urokinase plasminogen activator (u-PA), or simply urokinase. Although both activators are synthesized by endothelial cells, t-PA predominates under most conditions and drives intravascular fibrinolysis. In contrast, synthesis of u-PA mainly occurs in response to inflammatory stimuli, and u-PA promotes extravascular fibrinolysis.

The fibrinolytic system is regulated such that unwanted fibrin thrombi are removed, while fibrin in wounds is preserved to maintain hemostasis (Lijnen and Collen, 2001). t-PA is released from endothelial cells in response to various stimuli, including the stasis that occurs when thrombi occlude vessels. Released t-PA is rapidly cleared from blood or inhibited by plasminogen activator inhibitor-1 (PAI-1) and, to a lesser extent, plasminogen activator inhibitor-2 (PAI-2); t-PA thus exerts little effect on circulating plasminogen in the absence of fibrin. α_2-antiplasmin rapidly inhibits any plasmin that is generated. However, when fibrin is present, t-PA binds to it, as does plasminogen. The catalytic efficiency of t-PA activation of plasminogen increases over 300-fold in the presence of fibrin, which promotes plasmin generation on its surface. Plasmin then degrades the fibrin.

Plasminogen and plasmin bind to lysine residues on fibrin via five loop-like regions near their amino termini, which are known as kringle domains. To inactivate plasmin, α_2-antiplasmin binds to the first of these kringle domains and then blocks the active site of plasmin. Because the kringle domains are occupied when plasmin binds to fibrin, plasmin on the fibrin surface is protected from inhibition by α_2-antiplasmin and can digest the fibrin. Once the fibrin clot undergoes degradation, α_2-antiplasmin rapidly inhibits any plasmin that escapes from this local milieu. To prevent premature clot lysis, factor XIIIa mediates the covalent cross-linking of small amounts of α_2-antiplasmin onto fibrin.

When thrombi occlude major arteries or veins, therapeutic doses of plasminogen activators sometimes are administered to degrade the fibrin and rapidly restore blood flow. In high doses, these plasminogen activators promote the generation of so much plasmin that the inhibitory controls are overwhelmed. Plasmin is a relatively nonspecific protease; it not only digests fibrin but also degrades other plasma proteins, including several coagulation factors. Reduction in the levels of these coagulation proteins impairs the capacity for thrombin generation, which can contribute to bleeding. In addition, unopposed plasmin tends to dissolve fibrin in hemostatic plugs as well as that in pathological thrombi, a phenomenon that also increases the risk of bleeding. Therefore, fibrinolytic drugs can be toxic, producing hemorrhage as their major side effect. The pathway of fibrinolysis and sites of pharmacological perturbation are summarized in Figure 30–3.

Coagulation in vitro. Whole blood normally clots in 4-8 minutes when placed in a glass tube. Clotting is prevented if a chelating agent such as ethylenediaminetetraacetic acid (EDTA) or citrate is added to bind Ca^{2+}. Recalcified plasma normally clots in 2-4 minutes. The clotting time after recalcification is shortened to 26-33 seconds by the addition of negatively-charged phospholipids and a particulate substance, such as kaolin (aluminum silicate) or celite (diatomaceous earth), which activates factor XII; the measurement of this is termed the *activated partial thromboplastin time* (aPTT). Alternatively, recalcified plasma clots in 12-14 seconds after addition of "thromboplastin" (a mixture of TF and phospholipids); the measurement of this is termed the *prothrombin time* (PT).

Two pathways of coagulation are recognized. An individual with a prolonged aPTT and a normal PT is considered to have a defect in the *intrinsic coagulation pathway* because all of the components of the aPTT test (except kaolin or celite) are intrinsic to the plasma. A patient with a prolonged PT and a normal aPTT has a defect in the *extrinsic coagulation pathway* because thromboplastin is extrinsic to the plasma. Prolongation of both the aPTT and the PT suggests a defect in a *common pathway*.

Natural Anticoagulant Mechanisms. Platelet activation and coagulation do not normally occur within an intact blood vessel (Edelberg et al., 2001). Thrombosis is prevented by several regulatory mechanisms that require a healthy vascular endothelium. Nitric oxide and prostacyclin (PGI_2) are synthesized by endothelial cells and released into the blood (Chapter 33). These substances induce vasodilation and inhibit platelet activation and subsequent aggregation.

Antithrombin is a plasma protein that inhibits coagulation enzymes of the intrinsic and common pathways (see "Mechanism of Action"). Heparan sulfate proteoglycans synthesized by endothelial cells enhance the activity of antithrombin by ~1000-fold. Another regulatory system involves protein C, a plasma zymogen that is homologous to factors II, VII, IX, and X; its activity depends on the binding of Ca^{2+} to Gla residues within its amino-terminal domain. Thrombin activates protein C, but the efficiency of this reaction increases by several orders of magnitude when thrombin binds to thrombomodulin, its receptor on the surface of endothelial cells (Esmon, 2003). Protein C binds to another endothelial cell receptor, endothelial protein C receptor (EPCR), which presents protein C to the thrombin–thrombomodulin complex for activation. Activated protein C then dissociates from EPCR and, in combination with protein S, its non-enzymatic Gla-containing cofactor, activated protein C degrades factors Va and VIIIa. Without these activated cofactors, the rates of activation of prothrombin and factor X are greatly diminished. Therefore, activated protein C downregulates thrombin generation (Esmon, 2006). Deficiency of protein C or protein S is associated with an increased risk of pathological thrombus formation and tissue necrosis associated with the use of warfarin (see the "Warfarin" section, later in the chapter).

With antithrombin requiring endogenous heparan sulfate for its full activity and protein C requiring activation by thrombomodulin-bound thrombin, the effects of both of these natural anticoagulants are localized to the vicinity of intact endothelial cells. Tissue factor pathway inhibitor (TFPI), a natural anticoagulant found in the lipoprotein fraction of plasma, also regulates thrombin generation by inhibiting TF-bound factor VIIa in a two-step fashion. TFPI first binds and inhibits factor Xa, and this binary complex then inhibits factor VIIa. Therefore, factor Xa regulates its own generation through this mechanism. TFPI also can localize on the endothelial cell surface by binding to heparan sulfate proteoglycans.

PARENTERAL ANTICOAGULANTS

Heparin and Its Derivatives

Biochemistry. Heparin, a glycosaminoglycan found in the secretory granules of mast cells, is synthesized from UDP-sugar precursors as a polymer of alternating D-glucuronic acid and *N*-acetyl-D-glucosamine residues (Sugahara and Kitagawa, 2002).

About 10-15 glycosaminoglycan chains, each containing 200-300 saccharide units, are attached to a core protein and yield a proteoglycan with a molecular mass of 750-1,000 kDa. The glycosaminoglycan then undergoes a series of modifications, which include the following: *N*-deacetylation and *N*-sulfation of glucosamine residues, epimerization of D-glucuronic acid to L-iduronic acid, *O*-sulfation of iduronic and glucuronic acid residues at the C2 position, and *O*-sulfation of glucosamine residues at the C3 and C6 positions. Each of these modifications is incomplete, yielding a variety of oligosaccharide structures. After transport of the heparin proteoglycan to mast cell granules, an endo-β-D-glucuronidase slowly degrades the glycosaminoglycan chains to fragments of 5-30 kDa (mean, ~15 kDa, corresponding to ~40 saccharide units).

Source. Heparin is commonly extracted from porcine intestinal mucosa, which is rich in mast cells, and preparations may contain small amounts of other glycosaminoglycans. Despite the heterogeneity in composition among different commercial preparations of heparin, their biological activities are similar (~150 USP units/mg). A USP unit reflects the quantity of heparin that prevents 1 mL of citrated sheep plasma from clotting for 1 hour after the addition of 0.2 mL of 1% $CaCl_2$. Although North American heparin manufacturers have traditionally quantified heparin potency in USP units, European manufacturers measure potency with an anti-factor Xa assay. This assay involves monitoring the activity of factor Xa added to human citrated plasma with a synthetic factor Xa–directed substrate that changes color when cleaved by the enzyme. The higher the heparin concentration in the sample, the less the residual factor Xa activity detected. To determine heparin potency, residual factor Xa activity in the sample is compared with that detected in controls containing known concentrations of an international heparin standard. When assessed this way, heparin potency is expressed in international units per mg.

Effective October 1, 2009, the new USP unit dose has been harmonized to the international unit dose. Contamination of heparin with oversulfated chondroitin sulfate, a non-heparin glycosaminoglycan, prompted this shift because this contaminant eludes detection with the USP assay but not with the anti-factor Xa assay. As a result, the new USP unit dose is less potent than the old USP unit dose by ~10%, and heparin doses using the new USP units will have to increase slightly to achieve the same level of anticoagulation. This likely is of little or no clinical consequence for subcutaneous administration, due to the low and variable bioavailability of heparin when administered by this route. However, for intravenous administration, dosing adjustments and more frequent monitoring of aPTT may be necessary.

Heparin Derivatives. Derivatives of heparin in current use include low-molecular-weight heparins (LMWHs) and fondaparinux. The features that distinguish these derivatives from heparin are outlined in Table 30–1. Several LMWH preparations are marketed (e.g., dalteparin [FRAGMIN], enoxaparin [LOVENOX], tinzaparin [INNOHEP]), but all are fragments of heparin ranging in molecular weight from 1-10 kDa (mean ~5 kDa, ~17 saccharide units). LMWH preparations differ from heparin and, to a lesser extent, from each other in their pharmacokinetic properties. The potency of LMWH is assessed with anti-factor Xa assays, which use an international LMWH standard for reference purposes.

In contrast to heparin and LMWHs, which are biologicals derived from animal tissues, fondaparinux (ARIXTRA) is a synthetic five-saccharide analog of a natural pentasaccharide sequence that is found in heparin and LMWHs and mediates their interaction with antithrombin. Fondaparinux has unique pharmacokinetic properties that distinguish it from LMWH. The potency of fondaparinux also is assessed with an anti-Xa assay.

Mechanism of Action. Heparin, LMWHs, and fondaparinux have no intrinsic anticoagulant activity. Instead, these agents bind to antithrombin and accelerate the rate at which it inhibits various coagulation proteases. Antithrombin is a glycosylated, single-chain polypeptide composed of 432 amino acid residues (Olson and Chuang, 2002). Synthesized in the liver, antithrombin circulates in plasma at an approximate concentration of 2.6 μM. Antithrombin inhibits activated coagulation factors involved in the intrinsic and common pathways but has relatively little activity against factor VIIa. Antithrombin is a "suicide substrate" for these proteases; inhibition occurs when the protease attacks a specific Arg–Ser peptide bond in the reactive center loop of antithrombin and becomes trapped as a stable 1:1 complex.

Table 30–1

Comparison of the Features of Heparin, LMWH, and Fondaparinux

FEATURES	HEPARIN	LMWH	FONDAPARINUX
Source	Biological	Biological	Synthetic
Molecular weight (Da)	15,000	5000	1500
Target	Xa and IIa	Xa and IIa	Xa
Bioavailability (%)	30	90	100
$t_{1/2}$ *(h)*	1	4	17
Renal excretion	No	Yes	Yes
Antidote effect	Complete	Partial	None
Thrombocytopenia	<5%	<1%	<1%

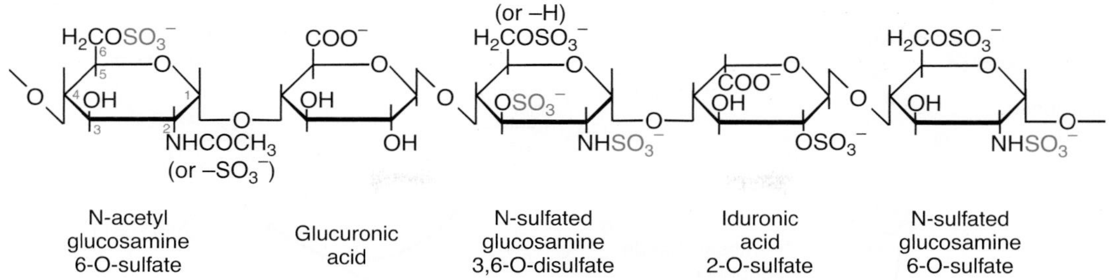

Figure 30–4. *The antithrombin-binding pentasaccharide structure of heparin.* Sulfate groups required for binding to antithrombin are indicated in red.

Heparin binds to antithrombin via a specific pentasaccharide sequence that contains a 3-*O*-sulfated glucosamine residue (Figure 30–4). This structure occurs on ~30% of heparin molecules and is less abundant on endogenous heparan sulfate molecules. Other glycosaminoglycans (e.g., dermatan sulfate, chondroitin-4-sulfate, and chondroitin-6-sulfate) lack the antithrombin-binding structure and do not activate antithrombin.

Pentasaccharide binding to antithrombin induces a conformational change in antithrombin that renders its reactive site more accessible to the target protease (Figure 30–5).

This conformational change accelerates the rate of factor Xa inhibition by at least two orders of magnitude but has no effect on the rate of thrombin inhibition. To enhance the rate of thrombin inhibition by antithrombin, heparin serves as a catalytic template to which both the inhibitor and the protease bind. Only heparin molecules composed of 18 or more saccharide units (molecular weight >5400 Da) are of sufficient length to bridge antithrombin and thrombin together. With a mean molecular weight of 15,000 Da, most of the chains of heparin are long enough to serve this role. Consequently, by definition, heparin catalyzes the rates of factor Xa and thrombin to a similar extent, as expressed by an anti-factor Xa to anti-factor IIa (thrombin) ratio of 1:1. In contrast, at least half of LMWH molecules (mean molecular weight of 5000 Da, ~17 saccharide units) are too short to provide this bridging function and have no effect on the rate of thrombin inhibition by antithrombin. Because these shorter molecules still induce the conformational change in antithrombin that accelerates inhibition of factor Xa, LMWHs have greater anti-factor Xa activity than anti-IIa activity, and the ratio ranges from 3:1 to 2:1 depending on the preparation. Fondaparinux, an analog of the pentasaccharide sequence in heparin or LMWHs that mediates their interaction with antithrombin, has only anti-factor Xa activity because it is too short to bridge antithrombin to thrombin (Figure 30–5).

Heparin, LMWHs, and fondaparinux act in a catalytic fashion. After binding to antithrombin and promoting the formation of covalent complexes between antithrombin and target proteases, the heparin, LMWH, or fondaparinux dissociates from the complex and can then catalyze other antithrombin molecules.

When the concentration of heparin in plasma is 0.1-1 units/mL, thrombin, factor IXa, and factor Xa are inhibited rapidly ($t_{1/2}$ <0.1 second) by antithrombin. This effect prolongs both the aPTT (discussed earlier) and the thrombin time (i.e., the time required for plasma to clot when exogenous thrombin is added); the PT is affected to a lesser degree. Factor Xa bound to platelets in the prothrombinase complex and thrombin bound to fibrin are both protected from inhibition by antithrombin in the presence of heparin or LMWH. Thus, heparin and LMWHs may promote the inhibition of factor Xa and thrombin only after they have diffused away from these binding sites.

Platelet factor 4, a cationic protein released from the α granules during platelet activation, binds heparin and prevents it from interacting with antithrombin. This phenomenon may limit the activity of heparin in the vicinity of platelet-rich thrombi. Because LMWH and fondaparinux have a lower affinity for platelet factor 4, these agents may retain their activity in the vicinity of such thrombi to a greater extent than heparin.

Miscellaneous Pharmacological Effects. High doses of heparin can interfere with platelet aggregation and thereby prolong the bleeding time. In contrast, LMWHs and fondaparinux have little effect on platelets. It is unclear to what extent the antiplatelet effect of heparin contributes to the hemorrhagic complications of treatment with the drug. Heparin "clears" lipemic plasma *in vivo* by causing the release of lipoprotein lipase into the circulation. Lipoprotein lipase hydrolyzes triglycerides to glycerol and free fatty acids. The clearing of lipemic plasma may occur at concentrations of heparin below those necessary to produce an anticoagulant effect. Rebound hyperlipemia may occur after heparin administration is stopped.

Clinical Use. Heparin, LMWH, and fondaparinux can be used to initiate treatment of venous thrombosis and pulmonary embolism because of their rapid onset of action (Hirsh et al., 2001). An oral vitamin K antagonist, such as warfarin, usually is started concurrently, and the heparin or heparin derivative is continued for at least 5 days to allow warfarin to achieve its full therapeutic

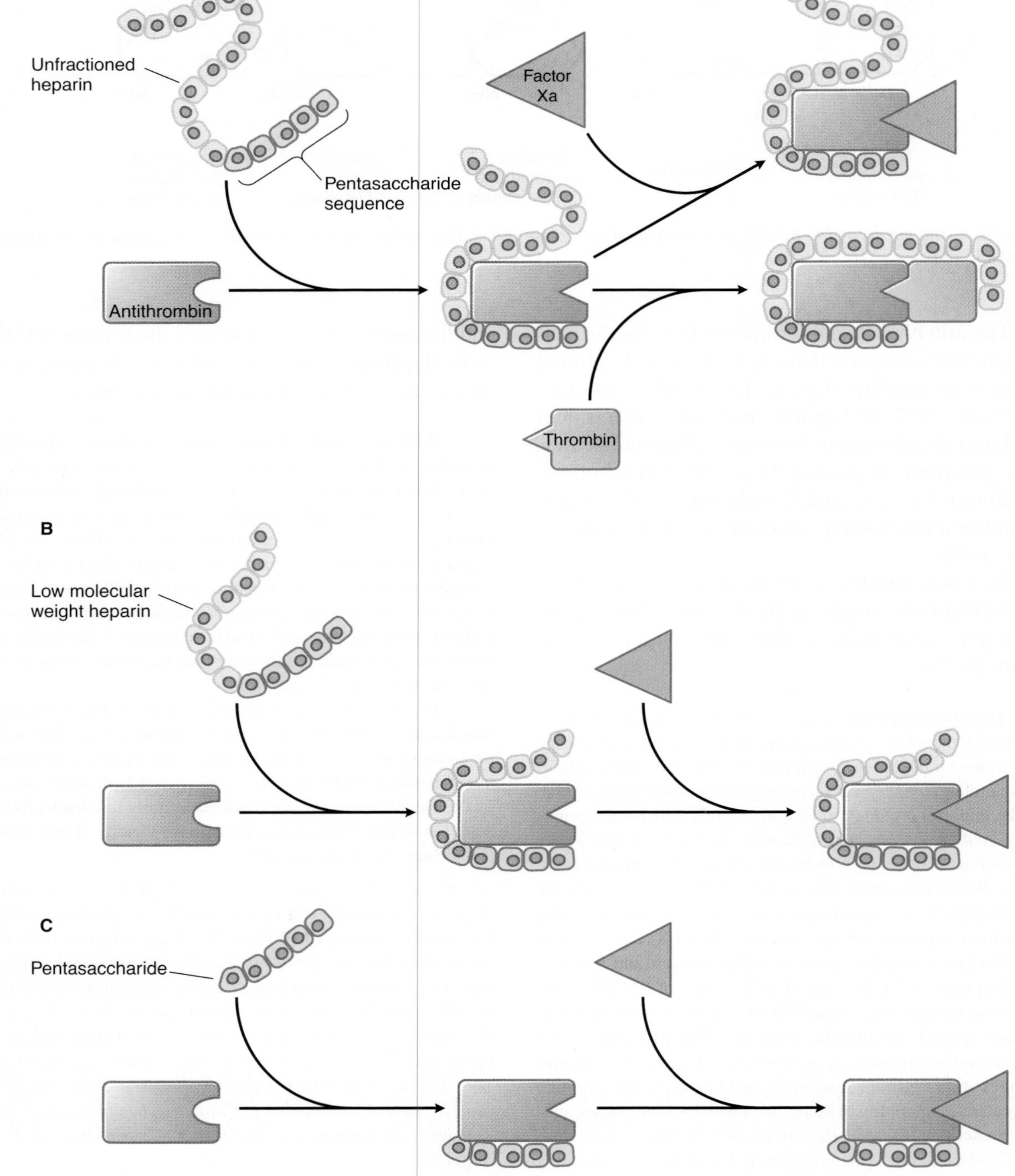

Figure 30–5. *Mechanism of action of heparin, low-molecular-weight heparin (LMWH), and fondaparinux, a synthetic pentasaccharide.* ***A.*** Heparin binds to antithrombin via its pentasaccharide sequence. This induces a conformational change in the reactive center loop of antithrombin that accelerates its interaction with factor Xa. To potentiate thrombin inhibition, heparin must simultaneously bind to antithrombin and thrombin. Only heparin chains composed of at least 18 saccharide units (molecular weight ~5,400 Da) are of sufficient length to perform this bridging function. With a mean molecular weight of 15,000 Da, virtually all of the heparin chains are long enough to do this. ***B.*** LMWH has greater capacity to potentiate factor Xa inhibition by antithrombin than thrombin because at least half of the LMWH chains (mean molecular weight 4,500-5,000 Da) are too short to bridge antithrombin to thrombin. ***C.*** The pentasaccharide accelerates only factor Xa inhibition by antithrombin; the pentasaccharide is too short to bridge antithrombin to thrombin.

effect (see the warfarin "Clinical Use" and "Monitoring Anticoagulant Therapy" sections later in the chapter). Heparin, LMWH, or fondaparinux also can be used in the initial management of patients with unstable angina or acute myocardial infarction. For most of these indications, LMWHs and fondaparinux have replaced continuous heparin infusions because of their pharmacokinetic advantages, which permit subcutaneous administration once or twice daily in fixed or weight-adjusted doses without coagulation monitoring. By contrast, full-dose heparin usually requires continuous intravenous infusion and frequent aPTT monitoring to ensure that a therapeutic level of anticoagulation has been achieved.

Because they do not require routine laboratory monitoring, LMWHs or fondaparinux can be used for out-of-hospital management of patients with venous thrombosis or pulmonary embolism, an approach that reduces healthcare expenditures. Patients who develop these disorders due to cancer often are treated with long-term LMWH instead of warfarin because nausea and vomiting from chemotherapy, involvement of the liver with cancer, and poor venous access can render therapy with warfarin problematic.

Heparin and LMWH are used during coronary balloon angioplasty with or without stent placement to prevent thrombosis. Fondaparinux is not used in this setting because of the risk of catheter thrombosis, a complication caused by catheter-induced activation of factor XII; longer heparin molecules are better than shorter ones for blocking this process. Cardiopulmonary bypass circuits also activate factor XII, which can cause clotting of the oxygenator. Heparin remains the agent of choice for surgery requiring cardiopulmonary bypass because it blocks this process and because the heparin can rapidly be neutralized with protamine sulfate after the procedure. Heparin also is used to treat selected patients with disseminated intravascular coagulation. While low-dose heparin, LMWH, or fondaparinux regimens all are effective, subcutaneous administration of low-dose heparin remains the recommended regimen for the prevention of post-operative deep venous thrombosis (DVT) and pulmonary embolism in patients undergoing major abdominothoracic surgery or who are at risk of developing thromboembolic disease. Specific recommendations for heparin use have been reviewed (Geerts et al., 2008).

In contrast to warfarin, heparin, LMWH, and fondaparinux do not cross the placenta and have not been associated with fetal malformations; therefore, these are the drugs of choice for anticoagulation during pregnancy. LMWH or fondaparinux is used most often in this setting because these agents need only be given once daily by subcutaneous injection. In addition, the risk of heparin-induced thrombocytopenia or osteoporosis is lower with LMWHs or fondaparinux than with heparin. Heparin, LMWH, and fondaparinux do not appear to increase fetal mortality or prematurity. If possible, the drugs should be discontinued 24 hours before delivery to minimize the risk of postpartum bleeding.

Absorption and Pharmacokinetics. Heparin, LMWHs, and fondaparinux are not absorbed through the GI mucosa and therefore must be given parenterally. Heparin is given by continuous intravenous infusion, intermittent infusion every 4-6 hours, or subcutaneous injection every 8-12 hours. Heparin has an immediate onset of action when given intravenously. In contrast, there is considerable variation in the bioavailability of heparin given subcutaneously, and the onset of action is delayed 1-2 hours. LMWH and fondaparinux are absorbed more uniformly after subcutaneous injection.

The $t_{1/2}$ of heparin in plasma depends on the dose administered. When doses of 100, 400, or 800 units/kg of heparin are injected intravenously, the half-lives of the anticoagulant activities are approximately 1, 2.5, and 5 hours, respectively (see Appendix II for pharmacokinetic data). Heparin appears to be cleared and degraded primarily by the reticuloendothelial system; a small amount of undegraded heparin also appears in the urine. LMWHs and fondaparinux have longer biological half-lives than heparin, 4-6 hours and ~17 hours, respectively. Because these smaller heparin fragments are cleared almost exclusively by the kidneys, the drugs can accumulate in patients with renal impairment, which can lead to bleeding. Both LMWH and fondaparinux are contraindicated in patients with a creatinine clearance <30 mL/min. In addition, fondaparinux is contraindicated in patients with body weight <50 kg undergoing hip fracture, hip replacement, knee replacement surgery, or abdominal surgery.

Administration and Monitoring. Full-dose heparin therapy usually is administered by continuous intravenous infusion. Treatment of venous thromboembolism is initiated with a fixed-dose bolus injection of 5000 units or with a weight-adjusted bolus, followed by 800-1600 units/hour delivered by an infusion pump. Therapy routinely is monitored by measuring the aPTT. The therapeutic range for heparin is considered to be that which is equivalent to a plasma heparin level of 0.3-0.7 units/mL, as determined with an anti-factor Xa assay (Hirsh et al., 2001). The aPTT value that corresponds to this range varies depending on the reagent and instrument used to perform the assay. An aPTT two to three times the normal mean aPTT value generally is assumed to be therapeutic; however, values in this range obtained with some aPTT assays may overestimate the amount of circulating heparin and therefore be subtherapeutic. The risk of recurrence of thromboembolism is greater in patients who do not achieve a therapeutic level of anticoagulation within the first 24 hours. Initially, the aPTT should be measured and the infusion rate adjusted every 6 hours; dose adjustments may be aided by use of nomograms; weight-based nomograms appear to outperform those that used fixed doses (Hirsh et al., 2001). Once a steady dosage schedule has been established in a stable patient, daily laboratory monitoring usually is sufficient.

Very high doses of heparin are required to prevent coagulation during cardiopulmonary bypass. The aPTT is infinitely prolonged over the dosage range used. A less sensitive coagulation test, such as the activated clotting time, is employed to monitor therapy in this situation. Because the activated clotting time can be performed in a point-of-care fashion, patients undergoing coronary angioplasty also typically have their heparin therapy monitored this way.

For therapeutic purposes, heparin also can be administered subcutaneously on a twice-daily basis. A total daily dose of ~35,000 units administered as divided doses every 8-12 hours usually is sufficient to achieve an aPTT of twice the control value (measured midway between doses). Monitoring generally is unnecessary once a steady dosage schedule is established. For low-dose heparin therapy (to prevent DVT and thromboembolism in hospitalized medical or surgical patients), a subcutaneous dose of 5000 units is given two to three times daily. Laboratory monitoring of heparin administered in this way usually is unnecessary because low-dose regimens have negligible effects on the aPTT.

LMWH preparations include Enoxaparin (LOVENOX), dalteparin (FRAGMIN), tinzaparin (INNOHEP, others), ardeparin (NORMIFLO), nadroparin (FRAXIPARINE, others), and reviparin (CLIVARINE) (the latter three are not available in the U.S. currently). These agents differ considerably in composition, and one cannot assume that two preparations that have similar anti-factor Xa activity will have equivalent antithrombotic effects. The more predictable pharmacokinetic properties of LMWH, however, permit administration in a fixed or weight-adjusted dosage regimen once or twice daily by subcutaneous injection.

Because LMWHs produce a relatively predictable anticoagulant response, monitoring is not done routinely. Patients with renal impairment may require monitoring with an anti-factor Xa assay because this condition may prolong the $t_{1/2}$ and slow the elimination of LMWHs. Obese patients and children given LMWHs also may require monitoring. Specific dosage recommendations for various LMWH preparations may be obtained from the manufacturer's literature.

Fondaparinux (ARIXTRA) is administered by subcutaneous injection, reaches peak plasma levels in 2 hours, and is excreted in the urine ($t_{1/2}$ ~17 h). It should not be used in patients with renal failure. Because it does not interact significantly with blood cells or plasma proteins other than antithrombin, fondaparinux can be given once a day at a fixed dose without coagulation monitoring. Fondaparinux appears to be much less likely than heparin or LMWH to trigger the syndrome of heparin-induced thrombocytopenia (see later in the chapter). Fondaparinux is approved for thromboprophylaxis in patients undergoing hip or knee surgery or surgery for hip fracture (Buller et al., 2003) and in general medical or surgical patients. It also can be used for initial therapy in patients with pulmonary embolism or DVT.

Idraparinux, a hypermethylated version of fondaparinux, underwent phase III clinical testing. This drug has a $t_{1/2}$ of 80 hours and is given subcutaneously on a once-weekly basis. To overcome the lack of an antidote, a biotin moiety was added to idraparinux to generate idrabiotaparinux, which can be neutralized with intravenous avidin. Ongoing phase III clinical trials are comparing idrabiotaparinux with warfarin for treatment of pulmonary embolism or for stroke prevention in patients with atrial fibrillation. Idraparinux, idrabiotaparinus, and avidin are not available for routine clinical use.

Heparin Resistance. The dose of heparin required to produce a therapeutic aPTT varies due to differences in the concentrations of heparin-binding proteins in plasma, such as histidine-rich glycoprotein, vitronectin, and large multimers of von Willebrand factor and platelet factor 4; these proteins competitively inhibit binding of heparin to antithrombin. Some patients do not achieve a therapeutic aPTT unless very high doses of heparin (>50,000 units/day) are administered. Such patients may have "therapeutic" concentrations of heparin in plasma at the usual dose when measured using an anti-factor Xa assay. This "pseudo" heparin resistance occurs because these patients have short aPTT values prior to treatment, as a result of increased concentrations of factor VIII. Other patients may require large doses of heparin because of accelerated clearance of the drug, as may occur with massive pulmonary embolism. Patients with inherited antithrombin deficiency ordinarily have 40-60% of the usual plasma concentration of this inhibitor and respond normally to intravenous heparin. However, acquired antithrombin deficiency, where concentrations may be <25% of normal, may occur in patients with hepatic cirrhosis, nephrotic syndrome, or disseminated intravascular coagulation; large doses of heparin may not prolong the aPTT in these individuals.

Because LMWHs and fondaparinux exhibit reduced binding to plasma proteins other than antithrombin, heparin resistance rarely occurs with these agents. For this reason, routine coagulation monitoring is unnecessary. Occasional patients, particularly those with underlying cancer, develop recurrent thrombosis despite therapeutic doses of a LMWH. Anti-factor Xa assays often are subtherapeutic in these patients, and higher doses of LMWH are needed to achieve a therapeutic response.

Toxicity and Adverse Events

Bleeding. Bleeding is the primary untoward effect of heparin. Major bleeding occurs in 1-5% of patients treated with intravenous heparin for venous thromboembolism (Hirsh et al., 2001). The incidence of bleeding is somewhat less in patients treated with LMWH for this indication. Although the risk of bleeding appears to increase with higher total daily doses of heparin and with the degree of prolongation of the aPTT, these correlations are weak, and patients can bleed with aPTT values that are within the therapeutic range. Often an underlying cause for bleeding is present, such as recent surgery, trauma, peptic ulcer disease, or platelet dysfunction.

The anticoagulant effect of heparin disappears within hours of discontinuation of the drug. Mild bleeding due to heparin usually can be controlled without the administration of an antagonist. If life-threatening hemorrhage occurs, the effect of heparin can be reversed quickly by the intravenous infusion of *protamine sulfate,* a mixture of basic polypeptides isolated from salmon sperm. Protamine binds tightly to heparin and thereby neutralizes its anticoagulant effect. Protamine also interacts with platelets, fibrinogen, and other plasma proteins and may cause an anticoagulant effect of its own. Therefore, one should give the minimal amount of protamine required to neutralize the heparin present in the plasma. This amount is approximately 1 mg of protamine for every 100 units of heparin remaining in the patient; protamine (up to a maximum of 50 mg) is given intravenously at a slow rate (over 10 minutes).

Protamine is used routinely to reverse the anticoagulant effect of heparin after cardiac surgery and other vascular procedures. Anaphylactic reactions occur in about 1% of patients with diabetes mellitus who have received protamine-containing insulin (*NPH insulin* or *protamine zinc insulin*), but untoward reactions are not limited to this group. A less common reaction consisting of pulmonary vasoconstriction, right ventricular dysfunction, systemic hypotension, and transient neutropenia also may occur after protamine administration.

Protamine only binds long heparin molecules. Therefore, protamine only partially reverses the anticoagulant activity of LMWHs and has no effect on that of fondaparinux. Because the long heparin molecules account for the anti-factor IIa activity of LMWH, protamine completely reverses this activity. In contrast, protamine only partially reverses the anti-factor Xa activity of LMWH, which is mediated by shorter heparin molecules. The very short molecules of fondaparinux do not bind protamine. Therefore, fondaparinux lacks a specific antidote.

Heparin-Induced Thrombocytopenia. Heparin-induced thrombocytopenia (platelet count <150,000/mL or a 50% decrease from the pretreatment value) occurs in ~0.5% of medical patients 5-10 days after initiation of therapy with heparin (Warkentin, 2007). Although the incidence may be lower, thrombocytopenia also occurs with LMWHs and fondaparinux, and platelet counts should be monitored. Thrombotic complications that can be life-threatening or lead to amputation occur in about one-half of the affected heparin-treated patients and may precede the onset of thrombocytopenia. The incidence of heparin-induced thrombocytopenia and thrombosis is higher in surgical patients than in medical patients. Women are twice as likely as men to develop this condition.

Venous thromboembolism occurs most commonly, but arterial thromboses causing limb ischemia, myocardial infarction, and stroke also occur. Bilateral adrenal hemorrhage, skin lesions at the site of subcutaneous heparin injection, and a variety of systemic reactions may accompany heparin-induced thrombocytopenia. The development of IgG antibodies against complexes of heparin with platelet factor 4 (or, rarely, other chemokines) appears to cause all of these reactions. These complexes activate platelets by binding to FcγIIa receptors, which results in platelet aggregation, release of more platelet factor 4, and thrombin generation. The antibodies also may trigger vascular injury by binding to platelet factor 4 attached to endogenous heparan sulfate on the endothelium.

Heparin, LMWH, and fondaparinux should be discontinued immediately if unexplained thrombocytopenia or any of the clinical manifestations mentioned above occur 5 or more days after beginning therapy, regardless of the dose or route of administration. The onset of heparin-induced thrombocytopenia may occur earlier in patients who have received heparin within the previous 3-4 months and have residual circulating antibodies. The diagnosis of heparin-induced thrombocytopenia can be confirmed by a heparin-dependent platelet activation assay or an assay for antibodies that react with heparin/platelet factor 4 complexes. Because thrombotic complications may occur after cessation of therapy, an alternative anticoagulant such as lepirudin, argatroban (see the next section), or fondaparinux should be administered to patients with heparin-induced thrombocytopenia. LMWH preparations should be avoided, because these drugs often cross-react with heparin in heparin-dependent antibody assays. In contrast, fondaparinux does not cross-react with these heparin-dependent antibodies, and, although large clinical trials are lacking, fondaparinux has been used successfully in patients with heparin-induced thrombocytopenia. Warfarin may precipitate venous limb gangrene or multicentric skin necrosis in patients with heparin-induced thrombocytopenia and should not be used until the thrombocytopenia has resolved and the patient is adequately anticoagulated with another agent.

Other Toxicities. Abnormalities of hepatic function tests occur frequently in patients who are receiving heparin or LMWHs. Mild elevations of the activities of hepatic transaminases in plasma occur without an increase in bilirubin levels or alkaline phosphatase activity. Osteoporosis resulting in spontaneous vertebral fractures can occur, albeit infrequently, in patients who have received full therapeutic doses of heparin (>20,000 units/day) for extended periods (e.g., 3-6 months). The risk of osteoporosis is lower with LMWHs or fondaparinux than it is with heparin. Heparin can inhibit the synthesis of aldosterone by the adrenal glands and occasionally causes hyperkalemia, even when low doses are given. Allergic reactions to heparin (other than thrombocytopenia) are rare.

Other Parenteral Anticoagulants

Lepirudin. Lepirudin (REFLUDAN) is a recombinant derivative (Leu^1-Thr^2-63-desulfohirudin) of hirudin, a direct thrombin inhibitor present in the salivary glands of the medicinal leech. Lepirudin is a 65–amino acid polypeptide that binds tightly to both the catalytic site and the extended substrate recognition site (exosite I) of thrombin. It is approved in the U.S. for treatment of patients with heparin-induced thrombocytopenia.

Lepirudin is administered intravenously at a dose adjusted to maintain the aPTT at 1.5-2.5 times the median of the laboratory's normal range for aPTT. The drug is excreted by the kidneys and has a $t_{1/2}$ of ~1.3 hours. Lepirudin should be used cautiously in patients with renal failure because it can accumulate and cause bleeding in these patients. Patients may develop antibodies against hirudin that occasionally prolong the $t_{1/2}$ and cause a paradoxical increase in the aPTT; therefore, daily monitoring of the aPTT is recommended. There is no antidote for lepirudin.

Desirudin. Desirudin (IPRIVASK) is a recombinant derivative of hirudin that differs only by the lack of a sulfate group on Tyr^{63}.

Desirudin is indicated for the prophylaxis of DVT in patients undergoing elective hip replacement surgery. The recommended dose is 15 mg every 12 hours by subcutaneous injection. It is eliminated by the kidney; the $t_{1/2}$ is ~2 hours following subcutaneous administration. Similar to lepirudin, the drug should be used cautiously in patients with decreased renal function, and serum creatinine and aPTT should be monitored daily.

Bivalirudin. Bivalirudin (ANGIOMAX) is a synthetic, 20–amino acid polypeptide that directly inhibits thrombin by a mechanism similar to that of lepirudin.

Bivalirudin contains the sequence Phe[1]–Pro[2]–Arg[3]–Pro[4], which occupies the catalytic site of thrombin, followed by a tetraglycine linker and a hirudin-like sequence that binds to exosite I. Thrombin slowly cleaves the Arg[3]–Pro[4] peptide bond and thus regains activity.

Bivalirudin is administered intravenously and is used as an alternative to heparin in patients undergoing coronary angioplasty or cardiopulmonary bypass surgery. Patients with heparin-induced thrombocytopenia or a history of this disorder also can be given bivalirudin instead of heparin during coronary angioplasty. The $t_{1/2}$ of bivalirudin in patients with normal renal function is 25 minutes; dosage reductions are recommended for patients with moderate or severe renal impairment.

Argatroban. Argatroban, a synthetic compound based on the structure of l-arginine, binds reversibly to the catalytic site of thrombin.

Argatroban is administered intravenously and has an immediate onset of action. Its $t_{1/2}$ is 40-50 minutes. Argatroban is metabolized by hepatic CYPs and is excreted in the bile; therefore, dosage reduction is required for patients with hepatic insufficiency. The dosage is adjusted to maintain an aPTT of 1.5-3 times the baseline value. Argatroban can be used as an alternative to lepirudin for prophylaxis or treatment of patients with, or at risk of developing, heparin-induced thrombocytopenia. In addition to prolonging the aPTT, argatroban also prolongs the PT, which can complicate the transitioning of patients from argatroban to warfarin. A chromogenic factor X assay can be used instead of the PT to monitor warfarin in these patients.

Drotrecogin Alfa. Drotrecogin alfa (XIGRIS) is a recombinant form of human activated protein C that inhibits coagulation by proteolytic inactivation of factors Va and VIIIa. It also has anti-inflammatory effects (Esmon, 2003).

A 96-hour continuous infusion of drotrecogin alfa decreases mortality in adult patients who are at high risk for death from severe sepsis if given within 48 hours of the onset of organ dysfunction (e.g., shock, hypoxemia, oliguria). The major adverse effect is bleeding.

Antithrombin. Antithrombin (ATRYN) is a recombinant form of human antithrombin produced from the milk of genetically modified goats. It is approved as an anticoagulant for patients with hereditary antithrombin deficiency undergoing surgical procedures.

ORAL ANTICOAGULANTS

Warfarin

History. Following the report of a hemorrhagic disorder in cattle that resulted from the ingestion of spoiled sweet clover silage, Campbell and Link, in 1939, identified the hemorrhagic agent as bishydroxycoumarin (dicoumarol). In 1948, a more potent synthetic congener was introduced as an extremely effective rodenticide; the compound was named *warfarin* as an acronym derived from the name of the patent holder, Wisconsin Alumni Research Foundation (WARF). Warfarin's potential as a therapeutic anticoagulant was recognized but not widely accepted, partly due to fear of unacceptable toxicity. However, in 1951, an army inductee uneventfully survived an attempted suicide with massive doses of a preparation of warfarin intended for rodent control. Since then, these anticoagulants have become a mainstay for prevention of thromboembolic disease.

Chemistry. Numerous anticoagulants have been synthesized as derivatives of 4-hydroxycoumarin and of the related compound, indan-1,3-dione (Figure 30–6). Only the coumarin derivatives are widely used; the 4-hydroxycoumarin residue, with a nonpolar carbon substituent at the position 3, is the minimal structural requirement for activity. This carbon is asymmetrical in warfarin (and in *phenprocoumon* and *acenocoumarol*). The R- and S-enantiomers differ in anticoagulant potency, metabolism, elimination, and interactions with other drugs. Commercial preparations of these anticoagulants are racemic mixtures. No advantage of administering a single enantiomer has been established.

Mechanism of Action. The oral anticoagulants are antagonists of vitamin K (see the section on "Vitamin K," later). Coagulation factors II, VII, IX, and X and the

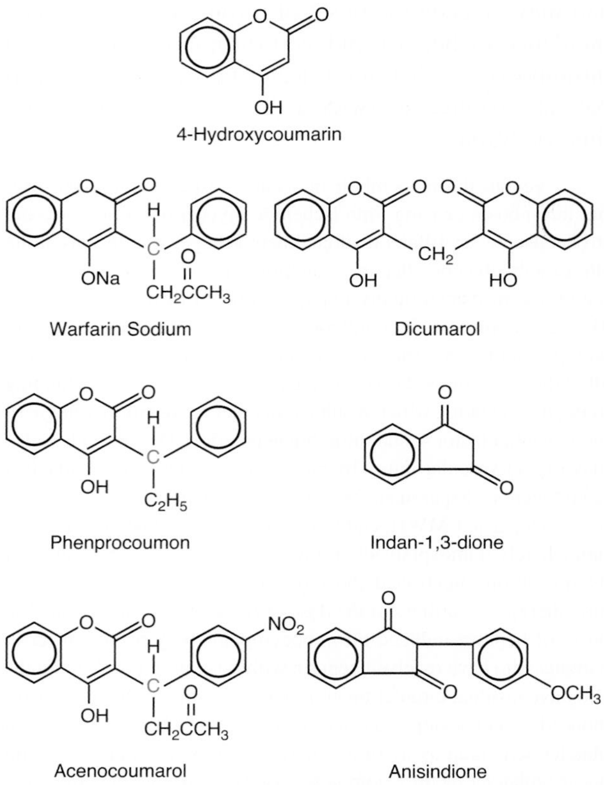

4-Hydroxycoumarin

Warfarin Sodium

Dicumarol

Phenprocoumon

Indan-1,3-dione

Acenocoumarol

Anisindione

Figure 30–6. *Structural formulas of the vitamin K antagonists.* 4-Hydroxycoumarin and indan-1,3-dione are the parent molecules from which the vitamin K antagonists are derived. The asymmetrical carbon atoms in the coumarins are shown in red.

anticoagulant proteins C and S are synthesized mainly in the liver and are biologically inactive unless 9-13 of the amino-terminal glutamate residues are carboxylated to form the Ca^{2+}-binding Gla residues. This reaction of the descarboxy precursor protein requires CO_2, O_2, and reduced vitamin K and is catalyzed by γ-glutamyl carboxylase (Figure 30–7). Carboxylation is directly coupled to the oxidation of vitamin K to its corresponding epoxide.

Reduced vitamin K must be regenerated from the epoxide for sustained carboxylation and synthesis of biologically competent proteins. The enzyme that catalyzes this, vitamin K epoxide reductase (VKOR), is inhibited by therapeutic doses of warfarin. Vitamin K (but not vitamin K epoxide) also can be converted to the corresponding hydroquinone by a second reductase, DT-diaphorase. This enzyme requires high concentrations of vitamin K and is less sensitive to coumarin drugs, which may explain why administration of sufficient vitamin K can counteract even large doses of oral anticoagulants.

Therapeutic doses of warfarin decrease by 30-50% the total amount of each vitamin K-dependent coagulation factor made by the liver; in addition, the secreted molecules are under-carboxylated, resulting in diminished biological activity (10-40% of normal). Congenital deficiencies of the procoagulant proteins to these levels cause mild bleeding disorders. Vitamin K antagonists have no effect on the activity of fully carboxylated molecules in the circulation. Thus, the time required for the activity of each factor in plasma to reach a new steady state after therapy is initiated or adjusted depends on its individual rate of clearance. The approximate $t_{1/2}$ (in hours) are as follows: factor VII, 6; factor IX, 24; factor X, 36; factor II, 50; protein C, 8; and protein S, 30. Because of the long $t_{1/2}$ of some of the coagulation factors, in particular factor II, the full anti-thrombotic effect of warfarin is not achieved for several days, even though the PT may be prolonged soon after administration due to the more rapid reduction of factors with a shorter $t_{1/2}$, in particular factor VII. There is no obvious selectivity of the effect of warfarin on any particular vitamin K-dependent coagulation factor, although the anti-thrombotic benefit and the hemorrhagic risk of therapy may be correlated

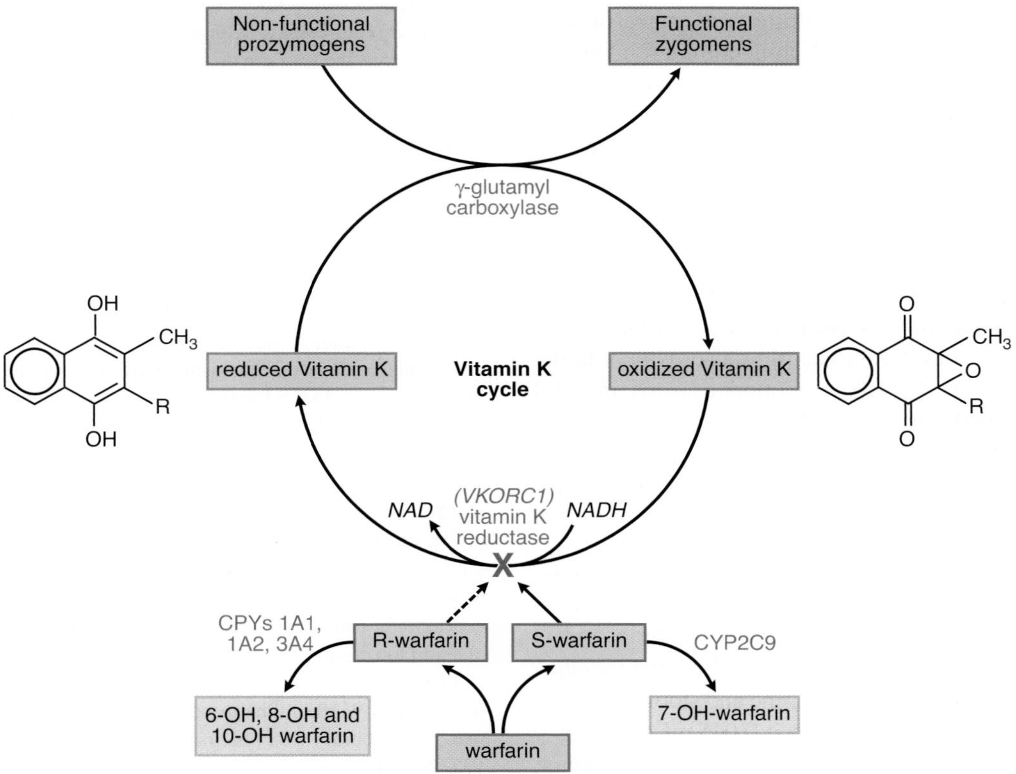

Figure 30–7. *The vitamin K cycle and mechanism of action of warfarin.* In the racemic mixture of S- and R-enantiomers, S-warfarin is more active. By blocking vitamin K epoxide reductase encoded by the *VKORC1* gene, warfarin inhibits the conversion of oxidized vitamin K epoxide into its reduced form, vitamin K hydroquinone. This inhibits vitamin K-dependent γ-carboxylation of factors II, VII, IX, and X because reduced vitamin K serves as a cofactor for a γ-glutamyl carboxylase that catalyzes the γ-carboxylation process, thereby converting prozymogens to zymogens capable of binding Ca^{2+} and interacting with anionic phospholipid surfaces. S-warfarin is metabolized by *CYP2C9*. Common genetic polymorphisms in this enzyme can influence warfarin metabolism. Polymorphisms in the C1 subunit of vitamin K reductase (VKORC1) also can affect the susceptibility of the enzyme to warfarin-induced inhibition, thereby influencing warfarin dosage requirements.

with the functional level of prothrombin, and to a lesser extent, factor X (Zivelin et al., 1993).

Dosage. The usual adult dosage of warfarin is 2-5 mg/day for 2-4 days, followed by 1-10 mg/day as indicated by measurements of the international normalized ratio (INR), a value derived from the patient's PT (see the functional definition of INR in the section on "Laboratory Monitoring"). As indicated later, common genetic polymorphisms render patients more or less sensitive to warfarin. A lower initial dose should be given to patients with an increased risk of bleeding, including the elderly. Warfarin usually is administered orally; age correlates with increased sensitivity to the drug. Warfarin also can be given intravenously without modification of the dose. Intramuscular injection is not recommended because of the risk of hematoma formation.

Absorption. The bioavailability of warfarin is nearly complete when the drug is administered orally, intravenously, or rectally. Bleeding has occurred from repeated skin contact with solutions of warfarin used as a rodenticide. However, different commercial preparations of warfarin tablets vary in their rate of dissolution, and this causes some variation in the rate and extent of absorption. Food in the GI tract also can decrease the rate of absorption. Warfarin usually is detectable in plasma within 1 hour of its oral administration, and concentrations peak in 2-8 hours.

Distribution. Warfarin is almost completely (99%) bound to plasma proteins, principally albumin, and the drug distributes rapidly into a volume equivalent to the albumin space (0.14 L/kg). Concentrations in fetal plasma approach the maternal values, but active warfarin is not found in milk (unlike other coumarins and indandiones). Therefore, warfarin can safely be administered to nursing mothers.

Biotransformation and Elimination. Warfarin is administered as a racemic mixture of S- and R-warfarin. S-warfarin is 3-5 fold more potent than R-warfarin and is metabolized principally by CYP2C9. Inactive metabolites of warfarin are excreted in urine and stool. The average rate of clearance from plasma is 0.045 $mL/min^{-1} \cdot kg^{-1}$. The $t_{1/2}$ varies (25-60 hours), with a mean of ~40 hours; the duration of action of warfarin is 2-5 days.

Polymorphisms in two genes, *CYP2C9* and *VKORC1* (vitamin K epoxide reductase complex, subunit 1) account for most of the genetic contribution to the variability in warfarin response. *CYP2C9* variants affect warfarin pharmacokinetics, whereas *VKORC1* variants affect warfarin pharmacodynamics. Common variations in the *CYP2C9* gene (designated *CYP2C9*2* and **3*), encode an enzyme with decreased activity, and thus are associated with higher drug concentrations and reduced warfarin dose requirements. At least one variant allele of *CYP2C9*2* or *CYP2C9*3* is present in ~25% of European-Americans, but these variants are relatively uncommon in African-American and Asian populations (Table 30–2). Heterozygosity for *CYP2C9*2* or **3* decreases the dose of warfarin required for anticoagulation by approximately 20-30% compared with "wild type" individuals (*CYP2C9*1/*1*). Homozygosity for *CYP2C9*2* or **3* can decrease the warfarin dose requirement by approximately 50-70%. Generally, the **3* allele has a greater effect than the *2 allele.

Consistent with decreased warfarin dose requirements, subjects who carry at least one copy of a *CYP2C9* variant allele appear to have an increased risk of bleeding. Thus, compared with individuals with no variant alleles, carriers of *CYP2C9*2* and *CYP2C9*3* have relative risks of bleeding of 1.91 and 1.77, respectively.

VKORC1 reduces vitamin K epoxide to vitamin K hydroquinone (see Figure 30–7) and is the target of coumarin anticoagulants, such as warfarin. Several genetic variations in *VKORC1* are in strong linkage disequilibrium and have been designated haplotypes A and B (or non-A). *VKORC1* variants are more prevalent than those of *CYP2C9*. The prevalence of *VKORC1* genetic variants is higher in Asians, followed by European-Americans and African-Americans. Polymorphism in *VKORC1* explains ~30% of the variability in warfarin dose requirements. Compared with *VKORC1* non-A/non-A homozygotes, the warfarin dose requirement is decreased by ~25% in heterozygotes and ~50% in A/A homozygotes.

The clinical relevance of these genetic polymorphisms remains uncertain. The goal of warfarin therapy is to maintain a patient within a target INR range, most often an INR value between 2 and 3. The risk of serious bleeding increases with INR values >4 and is highest during initiation of warfarin therapy. Variations in *VKORC1* have a greater effect than *CYP2C9* variants on warfarin responses early in therapy. Patients with *VKORC1* haplotype A have significantly higher INR values in the first week of warfarin therapy than non-A homozygotes; those with one or two *VKORC1* haplotype A alleles achieve a therapeutic INR more rapidly and are more likely to have an INR >4 than patients with two non-A alleles. Both the *VKORC1* haplotype and *CYP2C9* genotype have a significant effect on the warfarin dose after the first 2 weeks of therapy.

Based on evidence that genetic variations affect warfarin dose requirements and responses to therapy, the FDA amended the prescribing information for warfarin in 2007 to indicate that lower warfarin initiation doses be considered for patients with *CYP2C9* and *VKORC1* genetic variations. Efforts to facilitate the rational incorporation of genetic information into patient care have included the development of a warfarin dosing algorithm and point-of-care methods for *CYP2C9* and *VKORC1* genotyping. In a study of more than 4000 patients, the International Warfarin Pharmacogenetics Consortium (2009) compared the accuracy of a pharmacogenetic algorithm that included *VKORC1* and *CYP2C9* genotypes with two conventional clinical approaches: one based on clinical information to adjust the initial dose, and the other using a fixed-dose approach. The pharmacogenetic algorithm predicted the warfarin dose significantly better than the other two approaches. Moreover, the pharmacogenetic algorithm significantly improved the dose prediction for patients who required either high or low doses of warfarin (<21 mg/week or >49 mg/week).

Genetic variation clearly affects warfarin dose requirements and predilection to toxicity. Table 30–2 summarizes the effect of

Table 30–2

Frequencies of *CYP2C9* Genotypes and *VKORC1* Haplotypes in Different Populations and Their Effect on Warfarin Dose Requirements

GENOTYPE/ HAPLOTYPE	FREQUENCY (%) CAUCASIANS	AFRICAN AMERICANS	ASIANS	DOSE REDUCTION COMPARED WITH WILD-TYPE (%)
CYP2C9				
*1/*1	70	90	95	—
*1/*2	17	2	0	22
*1/*3	9	3	4	34
*2/*2	2	0	0	43
*2/*3	1	0	0	53
*3/*3	0	0	1	76
VKORC1				
Non-A/Non-A	37	82	7	—
Non-A/A	45	12	30	26
A/A	18	6	63	50

Source: Ghimire and Stein, 2009.

currently known genetic factors on warfarin dose requirements. However, it is not clear whether genotyping patients and modifying warfarin therapy accordingly will improve the quality of anticoagulation as determined by such clinically important outcomes as time to therapeutic INR, time spent within the target INR range, and rates of serious bleeding. Large randomized controlled trials comparing genotype-based therapy with standard care are under way to define the clinical impact of incorporating genetic information into clinical practice.

Drug and Other Interactions. The list of drugs and other factors that may affect the action of oral anticoagulants is prodigious and expanding (Hirsh et al., 2003). Any substance or condition is potentially dangerous if it alters:

- The uptake or metabolism of the oral anticoagulant or vitamin K
- The synthesis, function, or clearance of any factor or cell involved in hemostasis or fibrinolysis
- The integrity of any epithelial surface

Patients must be educated to report the addition or deletion of any medication, including nonprescription drugs and food supplements.

Some of the more commonly described factors that cause a decreased effect of oral anticoagulants include:

- Reduced absorption of drug caused by binding to cholestyramine in the GI tract
- Increased volume of distribution and a short $t_{1/2}$ secondary to hypoproteinemia, as in nephrotic syndrome
- Increased metabolic clearance of drug secondary to induction of hepatic enzymes, especially CYP2C9, by barbiturates, carbamazepine, or rifampin
- Ingestion of large amounts of vitamin K-rich foods or supplements
- Increased levels of coagulation factors during pregnancy

The PT can be shortened in any of these cases.

Frequently cited interactions that enhance the risk of hemorrhage in patients taking oral anticoagulants include decreased metabolism due to CYP2C9 inhibition by amiodarone, azole antifungals, cimetidine, clopidogrel, cotrimoxazole, disulfiram, fluoxetine, isoniazid, metronidazole, sulfinpyrazone, tolcapone, or zafirlukast, and displacement from protein binding sites caused by loop diuretics or valproate. Relative deficiency of vitamin K may result from inadequate diet (e.g., postoperative patients on parenteral fluids), especially when coupled with the elimination of intestinal flora by antimicrobial agents. Gut bacteria synthesize vitamin K and are an important source of this vitamin. Consequently, antibiotics can cause excessive PT prolongation in patients adequately controlled on warfarin. In addition to an effect on reducing intestinal flora, cephalosporins containing heterocyclic side chains also inhibit steps in the vitamin K cycle. Low concentrations of coagulation factors may result from impaired hepatic function, congestive heart failure, or hypermetabolic states, such as hyperthyroidism; generally, these conditions increase the prolongation of the PT. Serious interactions that do not alter the PT include inhibition of platelet function by agents such as *aspirin* and gastritis or frank ulceration induced by anti-inflammatory drugs. Agents may have more than one effect; e.g., clofibrate increases the rate of turnover of coagulation factors and inhibits platelet function. Elderly patients are more sensitive to oral anticoagulants.

Resistance to Warfarin. Some patients require >20 mg/day of warfarin to achieve a therapeutic INR. These patients often have excessive vitamin K intake from the diet or parenteral supplementation. Noncompliance and laboratory error are other causes of apparent warfarin resistance. There have been reported a few patients with hereditary warfarin resistance, in whom very high plasma concentrations of warfarin are associated with minimal depression of vitamin K-dependent coagulation factor biosynthesis; mutations in the *VKORC1* gene have been identified in some of these patients (Rost et al., 2004).

Sensitivity to Warfarin. Approximately 10% of patients require <1.5 mg/day of warfarin to achieve an INR of 2-3. As indicated earlier, these patients often possess variant alleles of *CYP2C9* or variant *VKORC1* haplotypes, which affect the pharmacokinetics or pharmacodynamics of warfarin, respectively (Daly and King, 2003).

Toxicities

Bleeding. Bleeding is the major toxicity of warfarin (Hirsh et al., 2003). The risk of bleeding increases with the intensity and duration of anticoagulant therapy, the use of other medications that interfere with hemostasis, and the presence of a potential anatomical source of bleeding. Especially serious episodes involve sites where irreversible damage may result from compression of vital structures (e.g., intracranial, pericardial, nerve sheath, spinal cord) or from massive internal blood loss that may not be diagnosed rapidly (e.g., gastrointestinal, intraperitoneal, retroperitoneal).

Although the reported incidence of major bleeding episodes varies considerably, it is generally <3% per year in patients treated with a target INR of 2-3. The risk of intracranial hemorrhage increases dramatically with an INR >4, especially in older patients. In a large outpatient anticoagulation clinic, the most common factors associated with a transient elevation of the INR to a value >6 were use of a new medication known to potentiate warfarin (e.g., acetaminophen), advanced malignancy, recent diarrheal illness, decreased oral intake, and taking more warfarin than prescribed (Hylek et al., 1998). Patients must be informed of the signs and symptoms of bleeding, and laboratory monitoring should be done at frequent intervals during intercurrent illnesses or any changes of medication or diet.

If the INR is above the therapeutic range but <5 and the patient is not bleeding or in need of a surgical procedure, warfarin can be discontinued temporarily and restarted at a lower dose once the INR is within the therapeutic range (Hirsh et al., 2003). If the INR is ≥5, vitamin K_1 (phytonadione, MEPHYTON, AQUAMEPHYTON) can be given orally at a dose of 1-2.5 mg (for 5≤ INR ≤9) or 3-5 mg (for INR >9). These doses of oral vitamin K_1 generally cause the INR to fall substantially within 24-48 hours without rendering the patient resistant to further warfarin therapy. Higher doses or parenteral administration may be required if more rapid correction of the INR is necessary. The effect of vitamin K_1 is delayed for at least several hours because reversal of anticoagulation requires synthesis of fully carboxylated coagulation factors. If immediate hemostatic competence is necessary because of serious bleeding or profound warfarin overdosage (INR >20), adequate concentrations of vitamin K-dependent coagulation factors can be restored by transfusion of fresh frozen plasma (10-20 mL/kg), supplemented with 10 mg of vitamin K_1, given by slow intravenous infusion. Transfusion of plasma may need to be repeated because the transfused factors (particularly factor VII) are cleared from the circulation more rapidly than the residual oral anticoagulant. Concentrates containing three or four of the vitamin K-dependent clotting factors are available in some countries; these rapidly restore the INR to normal. Vitamin K_1 administered intravenously carries the risk of anaphylactoid reactions and therefore should be used cautiously and administered slowly. Patients who receive high doses of vitamin K_1 may become unresponsive to warfarin for several days, but heparin can be used if continued anticoagulation is required.

Birth Defects. Administration of warfarin during pregnancy causes birth defects and abortion. A syndrome characterized by nasal hypoplasia and stippled epiphyseal calcifications that resemble chondrodysplasia punctata may result from maternal ingestion of warfarin during the first trimester. Central nervous system abnormalities have been reported following exposure during the second and third trimesters. Fetal or neonatal hemorrhage and intrauterine death may occur, even when maternal PT values are in the therapeutic range. Vitamin K antagonists should not be used during pregnancy, but as indicated in the previous section, heparin, LMWH, or fondaparinux can be used safely in this circumstance.

Skin Necrosis. Warfarin-induced skin necrosis is a rare complication characterized by the appearance of skin lesions 3-10 days after treatment is initiated. The lesions typically are on the extremities, but adipose tissue, the penis, and the female breast also may be involved. Lesions are characterized by widespread thrombosis of the microvasculature and can spread rapidly, sometimes becoming necrotic and requiring disfiguring débridement or occasionally amputation. Because protein C has a shorter $t_{1/2}$ than do the other vitamin K-dependent coagulation factors (except factor VII), its functional activity falls more rapidly in response to the initial dose of vitamin K antagonist. It has been proposed that the dermal necrosis is a manifestation of a temporal imbalance between the anticoagulant protein C and one or more of the procoagulant factors and is exaggerated in patients who are partially deficient in protein C or protein S. However, not all patients with heterozygous deficiency of protein C or protein S develop skin necrosis when treated with warfarin, and patients with normal activities of these proteins also can be affected. Morphologically similar lesions can occur in patients with vitamin K deficiency.

Other Toxicities. A reversible, sometimes painful, blue-tinged discoloration of the plantar surfaces and sides of the toes that blanches with pressure and fades with elevation of the legs (purple toe syndrome) may develop 3-8 weeks after initiation of therapy with warfarin; cholesterol emboli released from atheromatous plaques have been implicated as the cause. Other infrequent reactions include alopecia, urticaria, dermatitis, fever, nausea, diarrhea, abdominal cramps, and anorexia.

Warfarin can precipitate the syndromes of venous limb gangrene and multicentric skin necrosis when given to patients with heparin-induced thrombocytopenia who are not receiving a parenteral anticoagulant (Warkentin, 2003). Other anticoagulant agents, such as lepirudin, argatroban, or fondaparinux should be continued until the heparin-induced thrombocytopenia has resolved (see "Heparin toxicities," earlier in the chapter).

Clinical Use. Vitamin K antagonists are used to prevent the progression or recurrence of acute DVT or pulmonary embolism following an initial course of heparin. They also are effective in preventing venous thromboembolism in patients undergoing orthopedic or gynecological surgery, recurrent coronary ischemia in patients with acute myocardial infarction, and systemic embolization in patients with prosthetic heart valves or chronic atrial fibrillation. Specific recommendations for oral anticoagulant use for these and other indications have been reviewed (Geerts et al., 2008).

Prior to initiation of therapy, laboratory tests are used in conjunction with the history and physical examination to uncover hemostatic defects that might make the use of vitamin K antagonists more dangerous (e.g., congenital coagulation factor deficiency, thrombocytopenia, hepatic or renal insufficiency, vascular abnormalities). Thereafter, the INR calculated from the patient's PT is used to monitor the extent of anticoagulation and compliance. Therapeutic INR ranges for various clinical indications have been established empirically and reflect dosages that reduce the morbidity from thromboembolic disease while minimally increasing the risk of serious hemorrhage. For most indications, the target INR is 2-3. A higher target INR (e.g., 2.5-3.5) generally is recommended for patients with high-risk mechanical prosthetic heart valves (Hirsh et al., 2003).

For treatment of acute venous thromboembolism, heparin, LMWH, or fondaparinux usually is continued for at least 5 days after warfarin therapy is begun and until the INR is in the therapeutic range on 2 consecutive days. This overlap allows for adequate depletion of the vitamin K-dependent coagulation factors with long $t_{1/2}$, especially factor II. Frequent INR measurements are indicated at the onset of therapy to guard against excessive anticoagulation in the unusually sensitive patient. The testing interval can be lengthened gradually to weekly and then monthly for patients on long-term therapy whose test results have been stable.

Monitoring Anticoagulant Therapy: The INR (International Normalized Ratio). To monitor therapy, a blood sample is obtained, and the PT is determined along with that of a sample of normal pooled plasma. Formerly, the results were reported as a simple ratio of the two PT values. However, this ratio can vary widely depending on the thromboplastin reagent and the instrument used to initiate and detect clot formation. The PT is prolonged when the functional levels of fibrinogen, factor V, or the vitamin K-dependent factors II, VII, or X are decreased. Reduced levels of factor IX or proteins C or S have no effect on the PT. PT measurements are converted to INR measurements by the following equation:

$$\text{INR} = \left(\frac{\text{PT}_{\text{pt}}}{\text{PT}_{\text{ref}}}\right)^{\text{ISI}}$$

where INR = international normalized ratio

ISI = international sensitivity index

The ISI value, supplied by the manufacturer of the test regent, indicates the relative sensitivity of the PT (determined from a given batch of thromboplastin) to decreases in the vitamin K-dependent coagulation factors in comparison with a World Health Organization human thromboplastin standard. Reagents with lower ISI values are more sensitive to the effects of vitamin K antagonists (i.e., the PT is prolonged to a greater extent in comparison with that obtained with a less-sensitive reagent having a higher ISI). Ideally, the ISI value of each batch of thromboplastin should be confirmed in each clinical laboratory using a set of reference plasmas to control for local variables of sample handling and instrumentation.

The INR does not provide a reliable indication of the degree of anticoagulation in patients with the lupus anticoagulant, in whom the PT and other phospholipid-dependent coagulation tests are prolonged at baseline. In these patients, a chromogenic factor X assay or the prothrombin-proconvertin time assay may be used to monitor therapy (Moll and Ortel, 1997).

Other Vitamin K Antagonists

Phenprocoumon and Acenocoumarol. These agents generally are not available in the U.S. but are prescribed in the E.U. and elsewhere.

Phenprocoumon (MARCUMAR) has a longer plasma $t_{1/2}$ (5 days) than warfarin, as well as a somewhat slower onset of action and a longer duration of action (7-14 days). It is administered in daily maintenance doses of 0.75-6 mg. By contrast, acenocoumarol (SINTHROME) has a shorter $t_{1/2}$ (10-24 hours), a more rapid effect on the PT, and a shorter duration of action (2 days). The maintenance dose is 1-8 mg daily.

Indandione Derivatives. Anisindione (MIRADON) is available for clinical use in some countries. It is similar to warfarin in its kinetics of action but offers no clear advantages and may have a higher frequency of untoward effects. Phenindione (DINDEVAN) still is available in some countries. Serious hypersensitivity reactions, occasionally fatal, can occur within a few weeks of starting therapy with this drug, and its use can no longer be recommended.

Rodenticides. Bromadiolone, brodifacoum, diphenadione, chlorophacinone, and pindone are long-acting agents (prolongation of the PT may persist for weeks). They are of interest because they sometimes are agents of accidental or intentional poisoning. In this setting, reversal of the coagulopathy can require very large doses of vitamin K (i.e., >100 mg/day) for weeks or months.

NEW ORAL ANTICOAGULANTS

Dabigatran Etexilate (PRADAXA, PRADAX). A novel oral anticoagulant, dabigatran etexilate is a prodrug that is rapidly converted to dabigatran, which reversibly blocks the active site of thrombin.

The drug has oral bioavailability of ~6%, a peak onset of action in 2 hours, and a plasma $t_{1/2}$ of 12-14 hours. When given in fixed doses, dabigatran etexilate produces such a predictable anticoagulant response that routine coagulation monitoring is unnecessary.

Dabigatran etexilate is approved in the E.U. and Canada for prevention of venous thromboembolism after elective hip or knee replacement surgery. It is not yet available in the U.S. In phase III trials, dabigatran etexilate was non-inferior to warfarin for treatment of patients with venous thromboembolism (Schulman et al., 2009) and superior to warfarin for stroke prevention in patients with atrial fibrillation (Connolly et al., 2009). Therefore, this drug represents a promising alternative to warfarin for patients who require long-term anticoagulation.

Rivaroxaban (XARELTO). An oral factor Xa inhibitor, rivaroxaban has 80% oral bioavailability, a peak onset of action in 3 hours, and a plasma $t_{1/2}$ of 7-11 hours.

About one-third of the drug is excreted unchanged in the urine, the remainder is metabolized by the liver, and inactive metabolites are excreted in the urine or feces. This drug is given in fixed doses and does not require coagulation monitoring. Like dabigatran etexilate, rivaroxaban also is approved in the E.U. and Canada for thromboprophylaxis after hip or knee replacement surgery. Rivaroxaban is not available in the U.S. Ongoing trials are comparing rivaroxaban with warfarin for treatment of venous thromboembolism and stroke prevention in patients with atrial fibrillation.

Other New Agents. Other new oral anticoagulants include apixaban, edoxaban, betrixaban, YM150, and TAK-442, which are oral factor Xa inhibitors, and AZD0837, which is an oral thrombin inhibitor. Apixaban and edoxaban are currently undergoing phase III clinical evaluation.

FIBRINOLYTIC DRUGS

The fibrinolytic pathway is summarized by Figure 30–3. The action of fibrinolytic agents is best understood in conjunction with an understanding of the characteristics of the physiological components.

Plasminogen. Plasminogen is a single-chain glycoprotein of 791 amino acids; it is converted to an active protease by cleavage at Arg^{560}.

Plasminogen's five kringle domains mediate the binding of plasminogen (or plasmin) to carboxyl-terminal lysine residues in partially degraded fibrin; this enhances fibrinolysis. A plasma carboxypeptidase termed *thrombin-activatable fibrinolysis inhibitor* (TAFI) can remove these lysine residues and thereby attenuate fibrinolysis. The lysine binding kringle domains of plasminogen are located between amino acids 80 and 165, and they also promote formation of complexes of plasmin with α_2-antiplasmin, the major physiological plasmin inhibitor. Plasminogen concentrations in human plasma average 2 μM. A plasmin-degraded form of plasminogen termed *lys-plasminogen* binds to fibrin with higher affinity than intact plasminogen.

α_2-Antiplasmin. α_2-Antiplasmin, a glycoprotein of 452 amino acid residues, forms a stable complex with plasmin, thereby inactivating it.

Plasma concentrations of α_2-antiplasmin (1 μM) are sufficient to inhibit about 50% of potential plasmin. When massive activation of plasminogen occurs, the inhibitor is depleted, and free plasmin causes a "systemic lytic state" in which hemostasis is impaired. In this state, fibrinogen is degraded and fibrinogen degradation products impair fibrin polymerization and therefore increase bleeding from wounds. α_2-Antiplasmin inactivates plasmin nearly instantaneously, as long as the first kringle domain on plasmin is unoccupied by fibrin or other antagonists, such as *aminocaproic acid* (see "Inhibitors of Fibrinolysis" section).

Streptokinase. Streptokinase (STREPTASE) is a 47,000-Da protein produced by β-hemolytic streptococci. It has no intrinsic enzymatic activity but forms a stable, noncovalent 1:1 complex with plasminogen. This produces a conformational change that exposes the active site on plasminogen that cleaves Arg^{560} on free plasminogen to form plasmin.

Since the advent of newer agents, streptokinase is rarely used clinically for fibrinolysis. It currently is not marketed in the U.S.

Tissue Plasminogen Activator. t-PA is a serine protease of 527 amino acid residues. It is a poor plasminogen activator in the absence of fibrin (Lijnen and Collen, 2001). t-PA binds to fibrin via its finger domain and second lysine-binding kringle domain and activates fibrin-bound plasminogen several hundredfold more rapidly than it activates plasminogen in the circulation. The finger domain is homologous to a similar site on fibronectin, whereas the lysine binding kringle domain is homologous to the kringle domains on plasminogen.

Because it has little activity except in the presence of fibrin, physiological t-PA concentrations of 5-10 ng/mL do not induce systemic plasmin generation. During therapeutic infusions of t-PA, however, when concentrations rise to 300-3000 ng/mL, a systemic lytic state can occur. Clearance of t-PA primarily occurs by hepatic metabolism, and its $t_{1/2}$ is ~5 min. t-PA is effective in lysing thrombi during treatment of acute myocardial infarction or acute ischemic stroke.

t-PA (alteplase, ACTIVASE) is produced by recombinant DNA technology. The currently recommended ("accelerated") regimen for coronary thrombolysis is a 15-mg intravenous bolus, followed by 0.75 mg/kg of body weight over 30 minutes (not to exceed 50 mg) and 0.5 mg/kg (up to 35 mg accumulated dose) over the following hour. Recombinant variants of t-PA now are available (reteplase, RETAVASE and tenecteplase, TNKASE). They differ from native t-PA by having longer plasma half-lives that allow convenient bolus dosing; reteplase is administered in two bolus doses given 30 minutes apart, while tenecteplase requires only a single bolus. In contrast to t-PA and reteplase, tenecteplase is relatively resistant to inhibition by PAI-1. Despite these apparent advantages, these agents are similar to t-PA in efficacy and toxicity (GUSTO III Investigators, 1997).

Hemorrhagic Toxicity of Thrombolytic Therapy. The major toxicity of all thrombolytic agents is hemorrhage, which results from two factors: 1) the lysis of fibrin in hemostatic plugs at sites of vascular injury, and 2) the systemic lytic state that results from systemic plasmin generation, which produces fibrinogenolysis and degradation of other coagulation factors (especially factors V and VIII).

The contraindications to fibrinolytic therapy are listed in Table 30–3. Patients with these conditions should not receive such treatment.

If heparin is used concurrently with t-PA, serious hemorrhage will occur in 2-4% of patients. Intracranial hemorrhage is by far the most serious problem. Hemorrhagic stroke occurs with all regimens and is more common when heparin is used. In several large studies, t-PA was associated with an excess of hemorrhagic strokes of about 0.3% of treated patients. Based on the data of three large trials involving almost 100,000 patients, the efficacies of t-PA and streptokinase in treating myocardial infarction are essentially identical. Both agents reduce death and reinfarction by ~30% in regimens containing aspirin. With good evidence that primary coronary angioplasty with or without stent placement, when feasible, is superior to thrombolytic therapy, the use of fibrinolytic therapy has decreased. Fibrinolytic therapy remains the treatment of choice for patients with acute ischemic stroke who present within 3 hours of symptom onset.

Inhibitors of Fibrinolysis

Aminocaproic Acid. Aminocaproic acid (AMICAR, generic) is a lysine analog that competes for lysine binding sites on plasminogen and plasmin, blocking the interaction of plasmin with fibrin. Aminocaproic acid is thereby a potent inhibitor of fibrinolysis and can reverse states that are associated with excessive fibrinolysis. The main problem with its use is that thrombi that form during treatment with the drug are not lysed. For example, in patients with hematuria, ureteral obstruction by clots may lead to renal failure after treatment with aminocaproic acid. Aminocaproic acid has been used to reduce bleeding after prostatic surgery or after tooth extractions in hemophiliacs. Use of aminocaproic acid to treat a variety of other bleeding disorders has been unsuccessful, either because of limited benefit or because of thrombosis (e.g., after subarachnoid hemorrhage).

Aminocaproic acid is absorbed rapidly after oral administration, and 50% is excreted unchanged in the urine within 12 hours. For intravenous use, a loading dose of 4-5 g is given over 1 hour, followed by an infusion of 1-1.25 g/hour until bleeding is controlled. No more than 30 g should be given in a 24-hour period. Rarely, the drug causes myopathy and muscle necrosis.

Tranexamic Acid. Tranexamic acid (CYKLOKAPRON, LYSTEDA) is a lysine analog that, like aminocaproic acid, competes for lysine binding sites on plasminogen and plasmin, thus blocking their interaction with fibrin. Tranexamic acid can be used for the same

Table 30–3

Absolute and Relative Contraindications to Fibrinolytic Therapy

Absolute Contraindications

- Prior intracranial hemorrhage
- Known structural cerebral vascular lesion
- Known malignant intracranial neoplasm
- Ischemic stroke within 3 months
- Suspected aortic dissection
- Active bleeding or bleeding diathesis (excluding menses)
- Significant closed-head trauma or facial trauma within 3 months

Relative Contraindications

- Uncontrolled hypertension (systolic blood pressure >180 mm Hg or diastolic blood pressure >110 mm Hg)
- Traumatic or prolonged CPR or major surgery within 3 weeks
- Recent (within 2-4 weeks) internal bleeding
- Noncompressible vascular punctures
- For streptokinase: prior exposure (more than 5 days ago) or prior allergic reaction to streptokinase
- Pregnancy
- Active peptic ulcer
- Current use of warfarin and INR >1.7

CPR, cardiopulmonary resuscitation; INR, international normalized ratio.

indications as aminocaproic acid and can be given intravenously or orally.

Like aminocaproic acid, tranexamic acid is excreted in the urine and dose reductions are necessary in patients with renal impairment. The FDA approved oral tranexamic acid tablets for treatment of heavy menstrual bleeding in 2009. When used for this indication, tranexamic acid usually is given at a dose of 1 g four times a day for 4 days.

ANTIPLATELET DRUGS

Platelets provide the initial hemostatic plug at sites of vascular injury. They also participate in pathological thromboses that lead to myocardial infarction, stroke, and peripheral vascular thromboses. Potent inhibitors of platelet function have been developed in recent years. These drugs act by discrete mechanisms; thus, in combination, their effects are additive or even synergistic. Their availability has led to a revolution in cardiovascular medicine, whereby angioplasty and vascular stenting of lesions now are feasible with low rates of restenosis and thrombosis when effective platelet inhibition is employed. The sites of pharmacological intervention by the various antiplatelet drugs are highlighted in Figure 30–8.

Aspirin. Processes including thrombosis, inflammation, wound healing, and allergy are modulated by oxygenated metabolites of arachidonate and related polyunsaturated fatty acids that are collectively termed *eicosanoids*. Interference with the synthesis of eicosanoids is the basis for the effects of many therapeutic agents, including analgesics, anti-inflammatory drugs, and anti-thrombotic agents (see Chapters 33 and 34).

In platelets, the major cyclooxygenase product is TxA_2 (thromboxane A_2), a labile inducer of platelet aggregation and a potent vasoconstrictor. Aspirin blocks production of TxA_2 by acetylating a serine residue near the active site of platelet cyclooxygenase-1 (COX-1), the enzyme that produces the cyclic endoperoxide precursor of TxA_2. Because platelets do not synthesize new proteins, the action of aspirin on platelet COX-1 is permanent, lasting for the life of the platelet (7-10 days). Thus, repeated doses of aspirin produce a cumulative effect on platelet function.

Complete inactivation of platelet COX-1 is achieved with a daily aspirin dose of 75 mg. Therefore, aspirin is maximally effective as an anti-thrombotic agent at doses much lower than those required for other actions of the drug. Numerous trials indicate that aspirin, when used as an anti-thrombotic drug, is maximally effective at doses of 50-320 mg/day (Antithrombotic Trialists' Collaboration, 2002; Patrono et al., 2004). Higher doses do not improve efficacy; moreover, they potentially are less efficacious because of inhibition of prostacyclin production, which can be largely spared by using lower doses of aspirin. Higher doses also increase toxicity, especially bleeding.

Other NSAIDs that are reversible inhibitors of COX-1 have not been shown to have anti-thrombotic efficacy and in fact may even interfere with low-dose aspirin regimens (see Chapters 33 and 34 for details).

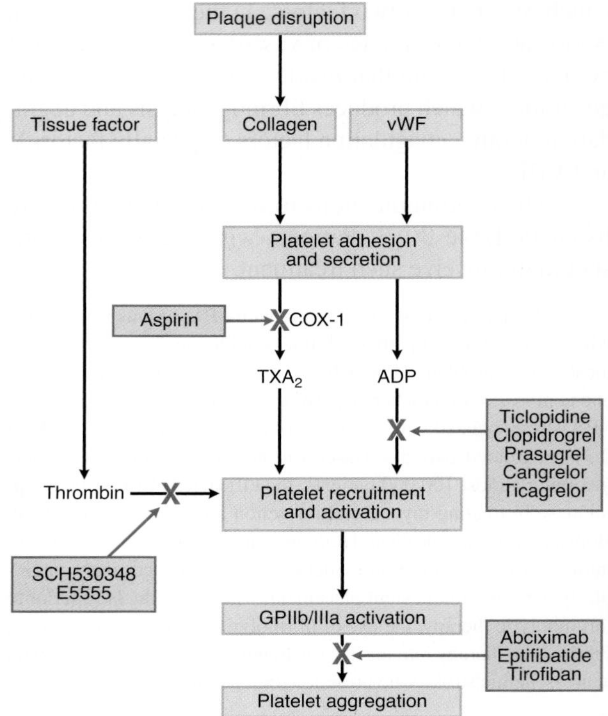

Figure 30–8. *Sites of action of antiplatelet drugs.* Aspirin inhibits thromboxane A_2 (TxA_2) synthesis by irreversibly acetylating cyclooxygenase-1 (COX-1). Reduced TxA_2 release attenuates platelet activation and recruitment to the site of vascular injury. Ticlopidine, clopidogrel, and prasugrel irreversibly block $P2Y_{12}$, a key ADP receptor on the platelet surface; cangrelor and ticagrelor are reversible inhibitors of $P2Y_{12}$. Abciximab, eptifibatide, and tirofiban inhibit the final common pathway of platelet aggregation by blocking fibrinogen and von Willebrand factor (vWF) from binding to activated glycoprotein (GP) IIb/IIIa. SCH530348 and E5555 inhibit thrombin-mediated platelet activation by targeting protease-activated receptor-1 (PAR-1), the major thrombin receptor on platelets.

Dipyridamole. Dipyridamole (PERSANTINE, others) interferes with platelet function by increasing the cellular concentration of cyclic AMP. This effect is mediated by inhibition of cyclic nucleotide phosphodiesterases and/or by blockade of uptake of adenosine, which acts at adenosine A_2 receptors to stimulate platelet adenylyl cyclase and thence cellular cyclic AMP. Dipyridamole is a vasodilator that, in combination with warfarin, inhibits embolization from prosthetic heart valves. The drug has little or no benefit as an anti-thrombotic agent.

In trials in which a regimen of dipyridamole plus aspirin was compared with aspirin alone, dipyridamole provided no additional beneficial effect (Antithrombotic Trialists' Collaboration, 2002). Two studies suggest that dipyridamole plus aspirin reduces strokes in patients with prior strokes or transient ischemic attacks (Diener et al., 1996). A formulation containing 200 mg of dipyridamole, in an extended-release form, and 25 mg of aspirin (AGGRENOX) is available. A recent study comparing this combination with clopidogrel for secondary prevention in patients with stroke or transient ischemic attacks showed no advantage of dipyridamole plus aspirin.

Ticlopidine (TICLID, others). Platelets contain two purinergic receptors, $P2Y_1$ and $P2Y_{12}$; both are GPCRs for ADP. The ADP-activated platelet $P2Y_1$ receptor couples to the G_q–PLC–IP_3–Ca^{2+} pathway and induces a shape change and aggregation. The $P2Y_{12}$ receptor couples to G_i and, when activated by ADP, inhibits adenylyl cyclase, resulting in lower levels of cyclic AMP and thereby less cyclic AMP–dependent inhibition of platelet activation. Based on pharmacological studies, it appears that both receptors must be stimulated to result in platelet activation (Jin and Kunapuli, 1998), and inhibition of either receptor is sufficient to block platelet activation. Ticlopidine is a thienopyridine prodrug (Figure 30–9) that inhibits the $P2Y_{12}$ receptor.

Ticlopidine is converted to the active thiol metabolite by a hepatic CYP (Savi et al., 2000). It is rapidly absorbed and highly bioavailable. It permanently inhibits the $P2Y_{12}$ receptor by forming a disulfide bridge between the thiol on the drug and a free cysteine residue in the extracellular region of the receptor, and thus has a prolonged effect. Like aspirin, it has a short $t_{1/2}$ but a long duration of action, which has been termed "hit-and-run pharmacology" (Hollopeter et al., 2001). Maximal inhibition of platelet aggregation is not seen until 8-11 days after starting therapy. The usual dose is 250 mg twice daily. Loading doses of 500 mg sometimes are given to achieve a more rapid onset of action. Inhibition of platelet aggregation persists for a few days after the drug is stopped.

Adverse Effects. The most common side effects are nausea, vomiting, and diarrhea. The most serious is severe neutropenia (absolute neutrophil count <500/μL), which occurred in 2.4% of stroke patients given the drug during premarketing clinical trials. Fatal agranulocytosis with thrombopenia has occurred within the first 3 months of therapy; therefore, frequent blood counts should be obtained during the first few months of therapy, with immediate discontinuation of therapy should cell counts decline. Platelet counts also should be monitored, as thrombocytopenia has been reported. Rare cases of thrombotic thrombocytopenic purpura-hemolytic uremic syndrome (TTP-HUS) have been associated with ticlopidine, with a reported incidence of 1 in 1600-4800 patients when the drug is used after cardiac stenting; the mortality associated

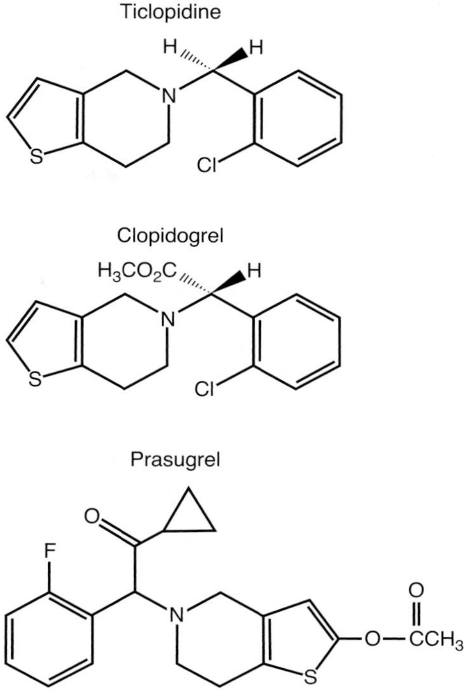

Ticlopidine

Clopidogrel

H_3CO_2C

Prasugrel

Figure 30–9. *Structures of ticlopidine, clopidogrel, and prasugrel.*

with these cases is reported to be as high as 18-57% (Bennett et al., 2000). Remission of TTP has been reported when the drug is stopped (Quinn and Fitzgerald, 1999).

Therapeutic Uses. Ticlopidine has been shown to prevent cerebrovascular events in secondary prevention of stroke and is at least as good as aspirin in this regard (Patrono et al., 1998). Because ticlopidine is associated with life-threatening blood dyscrasias and a relatively high rate of TTP, it has largely been replaced by clopidogrel.

Clopidogrel (PLAVIX). Clopidogrel is closely related to ticlopidine (Figure 30–9). Clopidogrel also is an irreversible inhibitor of platelet $P2Y_{12}$ receptors but is more potent and has a more favorable toxicity profile than ticlopidine, with thrombocytopenia and leukopenia occurring only rarely (Bennett et al., 2000). Clopidogrel is a prodrug with a slow onset of action.

The usual dose is 75 mg/day with or without an initial loading dose of 300 or 600 mg. The drug is somewhat better than aspirin in the secondary prevention of stroke, and the combination of clopidogrel plus aspirin is superior to aspirin alone for prevention of recurrent ischemia in patients with unstable angina. The superiority of the combination suggests that the actions of the two drugs are synergistic, as might be expected from their distinct mechanisms of action. Clopidogrel is used with aspirin after angioplasty and coronary stent implantation, and this combination should be continued for at least 4-6 weeks in patients with a bare metal stent and for at least 1 year in those with a drug-eluting stent. The FDA-approved indications for clopidogrel are to reduce the rate of stroke, myocardial infarction, and death in patients with recent myocardial infarction or stroke, established peripheral arterial disease, or acute coronary syndrome.

There is wide inter-individual variability in the capacity of clopidogrel to inhibit ADP-induced platelet aggregation, and some patients are designated resistant to the antiplatelet effects of the drug. This variability reflects, at least in part, genetic polymorphisms in the CYPs involved in the metabolic activation of clopidogrel, most importantly *CYP2C19*. Clopidogrel-treated patients with the loss-of-function *CYP2C19*2* allele exhibit reduced platelet inhibition compared with those with the wild-type *CYP2C19*1* allele and experience a higher rate of cardiovascular events (see Table 30–2). Even patients with the reduced-function *CYP2C19*3, *4,* or **5* alleles may derive less benefit from clopidogrel than those with the full-function *CYP2C19*1* allele. Concomitant administration of proton pump inhibitors, which are inhibitors of *CYP2C19*, with clopidogrel, produces a small reduction in the inhibitory effects of clopidogrel on ADP-induced platelet aggregation. The extent to which this interaction increases the risk of cardiovascular events remains controversial. Although *CYP3A4* also contributes to the metabolic activation of clopidogrel, polymorphisms in this enzyme do not appear to influence clopidogrel responsiveness. However, a small study in patients undergoing percutaneous coronary interventions revealed that atorvastatin, a competitive inhibitor of *CYP3A4*, reduced the inhibitory effect of clopidogrel on ADP-induced platelet aggregation. The impact of this interaction on clinical outcomes is unknown.

The observation that genetic polymorphisms that affect clopidogrel metabolism influence clinical outcomes raises the possibilities that pharmacogenetic profiling may be useful to identify clopidogrel-resistant patients and that point-of-care assessment of the extent of clopidogrel-induced platelet inhibition may help detect patients at higher risk for subsequent cardiovascular events. It is unknown whether administration of higher doses of clopidogrel to such patients will overcome this resistance.

Prasugrel (EFFIENT or EFIENT). The newest member of the thienopyridine class, prasugrel (Figure 30–9) also is a prodrug that requires metabolic activation. However, its onset of action is more rapid than that of ticlopidine or clopidogrel, and prasugrel produces greater and more predictable inhibition of ADP-induced platelet aggregation.

These characteristics reflect the rapid and complete absorption of prasugrel from the gut and its more efficient activation pathways. Virtually all of the absorbed prasugrel undergoes activation; by comparison, only 15% of absorbed clopidogrel undergoes metabolic activation, with the remainder inactivated by esterases.

Because the active metabolites of prasugrel and the other thienopyridines bind irreversibly to the $P2Y_{12}$ receptor, these drugs have a prolonged effect after discontinuation. This can be problematic if patients require urgent surgery. Such patients are at increased risk for bleeding unless the thienopyridine is stopped at least 5 days prior to the procedure.

Prasugrel was compared with clopidogrel in patients with acute coronary syndromes scheduled to undergo a coronary intervention. The incidence of cardiovascular death, myocardial infarction, and stroke was significantly lower with prasugrel than with clopidogrel mainly reflecting a reduction in the incidence of nonfatal myocardial infarction. The incidence of stent thrombosis also was lower with prasugrel than with clopidogrel. However, these advantages were at the expense of significantly higher rates of fatal and life-threatening bleeding. Because patients with a history of a prior stroke or transient ischemic attack are at particularly high risk of bleeding, the drug is contraindicated in those with a history of cerebrovascular disease. Caution is required if prasugrel is used in patients weighing <60 kg or in those with renal impairment. After a loading dose of 60 mg, prasugrel is given once daily at a dose of 10 mg. Patients >75 years of age or weighing <60 kg may do better with a daily prasugrel dose of 5 mg.

In contrast to their effect on the bioactivation of clopidogrel, *CYP2C19* polymorphisms appear to be less important determinants of the activation of prasugrel. There is no association between the loss-of-function allele and decreased platelet inhibition or increased rates of cardiovascular events with prasugrel. Therefore, prasugrel may be a reasonable alternative to clopidogrel in patients with the loss-of-function *CYP2C19* allele.

Glycoprotein IIb/IIIa Inhibitors. Glycoprotein IIb/IIIa is a platelet-surface integrin, which is designated $\alpha_{IIb}\beta_3$ by the integrin nomenclature. There are about 80,000 copies of this dimeric glycoprotein on the platelet surface. Glycoprotein IIb/IIIa is inactive on resting platelets but undergoes a conformational transformation when platelets are activated by platelet agonists such as thrombin, collagen, or TxA_2. This transformation endows glycoprotein IIb/IIIa with the capacity to serve as a receptor for fibrinogen and von Willebrand factor, which anchor platelets to foreign surfaces and to each other, thereby mediating aggregation. Inhibition of binding to this receptor blocks platelet aggregation induced by any agonist. Thus, inhibitors of this receptor are potent antiplatelet agents that act by a mechanism distinct from that of aspirin or the thienopyridine platelet inhibitors. Three agents are approved for use at present, and their features are highlighted in Table 30–4.

Abciximab. Abciximab (REOPRO) is the Fab fragment of a humanized monoclonal antibody directed against the $\alpha_{IIb}\beta_3$ receptor. It also binds to the vitronectin receptor on platelets, vascular endothelial cells, and smooth muscle cells.

The antibody is administered to patients undergoing percutaneous angioplasty for coronary thromboses, and when used in conjunction with aspirin and heparin, has been shown to prevent restenosis, recurrent myocardial infarction, and death. The unbound antibody is cleared from the circulation with a $t_{1/2}$ of about 30 minutes, but antibody remains bound to the $\alpha_{IIb}\beta_3$ receptor and inhibits platelet aggregation as measured *in vitro* for 18-24 hours after infusion is stopped. It is given as a 0.25-mg/kg bolus followed by 0.125 μg/kg/min for 12 hours or longer.

Adverse Effects. The major side effect of abciximab is bleeding, and the contraindications to its use are similar to those for the fibrinolytic

Table 30–4

Features of GPIIb/IIIa Antagonists

FEATURE	ABCIXIMAB	EPTIFIBATIDE	TIROFIBAN
Description	Fab fragment of humanized mouse monoclonal antibody	Cyclical KGD-containing heptapeptide	Nonpeptidic RGD-mimetic
Specific for GPIIb/IIIa	No	Yes	Yes
Plasma $t_{1/2}$	Short (min)	Long (2.5 h)	Long (2.0 h)
Platelet-bound $t_{1/2}$	Long (days)	Short (sec)	Short (sec)
Renal clearance	No	Yes	Yes

KGD, Lysine - Glycine - Aspartate; RGD, Arginine - Glycine - Aspartate.

agents listed in Table 30–3. The frequency of major hemorrhage in clinical trials varies from 1-10%, depending on the intensity of anticoagulation with heparin. Thrombocytopenia with a platelet count <50,000 occurs in about 2% of patients and may be due to development of neo-epitopes induced by bound antibody. Since the duration of action is long, if major bleeding or emergent surgery occurs, platelet transfusions can reverse the aggregation defect because free antibody concentrations fall rapidly after cessation of infusion. Readministration of antibody has been performed in a small number of patients without evidence of decreased efficacy or allergic reactions. The expense of the antibody limits its use.

Eptifibatide. Eptifibatide (INTEGRILIN) is a cyclic peptide inhibitor of the fibrinogen binding site on $\alpha_{IIb}\beta_3$. It is administered intravenously and blocks platelet aggregation.

Eptifibatide is given as a bolus of 180 μg/kg followed by 2 μg/kg/min for up to 96 hours. It is used to treat acute coronary syndrome and for angioplastic coronary interventions. In the latter case, myocardial infarction and death have been reduced by ~20%. Although the drug has not been compared directly to abciximab, it appears that its benefit is somewhat less than that obtained with the antibody, perhaps because eptifibatide is specific for $\alpha_{IIb}\beta_3$ and does not react with the vitronectin receptor. The duration of action of the drug is relatively short, and platelet aggregation is restored within 6-12 hours after cessation of infusion. Eptifibatide generally is administered in conjunction with aspirin and heparin.

Adverse Effects. The major side effect is bleeding, as is the case with abciximab. The frequency of major bleeding in trials was about 10%, compared with ~9% in a placebo group, which included heparin. Thrombocytopenia has been seen in 0.5-1% of patients.

Tirofiban. *Tirofiban* (AGGRASTAT) is a nonpeptide, small-molecule inhibitor of $\alpha_{IIb}\beta_3$ that appears to have a mechanism of action similar to eptifibatide. Tirofiban has a short duration of action and has efficacy in non-Q-wave myocardial infarction and unstable angina. Reductions in death and myocardial infarction have been ~20% compared to placebo, results similar to those with eptifibatide.

Side effects also are similar to those of eptifibatide. The agent is specific to $\alpha_{IIb}\beta_3$ and does not react with the vitronectin receptor. Meta-analysis of trials using $\alpha_{IIb}\beta_3$ inhibitors suggests that their value in antiplatelet therapy after acute myocardial infarction is limited (Boersma et al., 2002). Tirofiban is administered intravenously at an initial rate of 0.4 μg/kg/min for 30 minutes, and then continued at 0.1 mg/kg/min for 12-24 hours after angioplasty or atherectomy. It is used in conjunction with heparin.

Newer Antiplatelet Agents

New agents in advanced stages of development include cangrelor and ticagrelor (BRILINTA), direct-acting reversible $P2Y_{12}$ antagonists, and SCH530348 and E5555, orally active inhibitors of the protease-activated receptor-1 (PAR-1), the major thrombin receptor on platelets.

Cangrelor. Cangrelor is an adenosine analog that binds reversibly to $P2Y_{12}$ and inhibits its activity. The drug has a $t_{1/2}$ of 3-6 minutes and is given intravenously as a bolus followed by an infusion. When stopped, platelet function recovers within 60 minutes. Recent trials comparing cangrelor with placebo during coronary interventions or comparing cangrelor with clopidogrel after such procedures revealed little or no advantages of cangrelor.

Ticagrelor. Ticagrelor is an orally active, reversible inhibitor of $P2Y_{12}$. The drug is given twice daily and not only has a more rapid onset and offset of action than clopidogrel, but also produces greater and more predictable inhibition of ADP-induced platelet aggregation. When compared with clopidogrel in patients with acute coronary syndromes (Wallentin et al., 2009), ticagrelor produced a greater reduction in cardiovascular death, myocardial infarction, and stroke at 1 year than clopidogrel did. This difference reflected a significant reduction in both cardiovascular death and myocardial infarction with ticagrelor. Rates of stroke were similar with ticagrelor and clopidogrel, and there were no differences in rates of major bleeding. When minor bleeding was added to the major bleeding results, however, ticagrelor showed an increase relative to clopidogrel. Although not yet approved, ticagrelor is the first new antiplatelet drug to demonstrate a reduction in cardiovascular death compared with clopidogrel in patients with acute coronary syndromes.

SCH530348. SCH530348 an orally active inhibitor of PAR-1, is under investigation as an adjunct to aspirin or aspirin plus clopidogrel. Two large phase III trials are under way. E5555, a second oral PAR-1 antagonist, is earlier in development.

THE ROLE OF VITAMIN K

Vitamin K is essential in both mammals and photosynthetic organisms. In certain photosynthetic bacteria, vitamin K is a cofactor in the photosynthetic electron-transport system; in green plants, vitamin K_1 is a component of photosystem I, the membrane-bound, macromolecular light-sensitive complex. Green plants are a nutritional source of vitamin K for humans, in whom vitamin K is an essential cofactor in the γ-carboxylation of multiple glutamate residues of several clotting factors and anticoagulant proteins. The vitamin K-dependent formation of Gla residues permits the appropriate interactions of clotting factors, Ca^{2+}, and membrane phospholipids and modulator proteins (Figures 30–1, 30–2, and 30–3). Vitamin K antagonists (coumarin derivatives; Figure 30–6) block Gla (γ-carboxyglutamate) formation and thereby inhibit clotting; excess vitamin K_1 can reverse the effects of these oral anticoagulants.

History. In 1929, Dam observed that chickens fed inadequate diets developed a deficiency disease characterized by spontaneous bleeding and reduced prothrombin in the blood. Subsequently, Dam and coworkers (1935, 1936) found that the condition could be alleviated rapidly by feeding an unidentified fat-soluble substance, named *vitamin K* (*Koagulation* vitamin) by Dam. Independently, Almquist and Stokstad (1935) performed similar work. Quick and coworkers (1935) observed a coagulation defect in jaundiced individuals that was due to a decrease in the plasma concentration of prothrombin. In the same year, Hawkins and Whipple reported that animals with biliary fistulas were likely to develop excessive bleeding. Subsequently, Hawkins and Brinkhous (1936) showed that this, too, was due to a deficiency in prothrombin and that the condition could be relieved by the feeding of bile salts. The culmination of these studies came with the demonstration by Butt and coworkers (1938) and Warner and associates (1938) that combination therapy with vitamin K and bile salts was effective in the treatment of the hemorrhagic diathesis of jaundice. Thus, the relationship between vitamin K, adequate hepatic function, and the physiological mechanisms operating in the normal clotting of blood was established.

Chemistry and Occurrence. Vitamin K activity is associated with at least two distinct natural substances, designated as vitamin K_1 and vitamin K_2. Vitamin K_1, or *phytonadione* (also referred to as *phylloquinone*), is 2-methyl-3-phytyl-1,4-naphthoquinone; it is found in plants and is the only natural vitamin K available for therapeutic use. Vitamin K_2 actually is a series of compounds (the *menaquinones*) in which the phytyl side chain of phytonadione has been replaced by a side chain built up of 2-13 prenyl units. Considerable synthesis of menaquinones occurs in Gram-positive bacteria; indeed, intestinal flora synthesize the large amounts of vitamin K contained in human and animal feces (Bentley and Meganathan, 1982). Depending on the bioassay system used, menadione is at least as active on a molar basis as phytonadione.

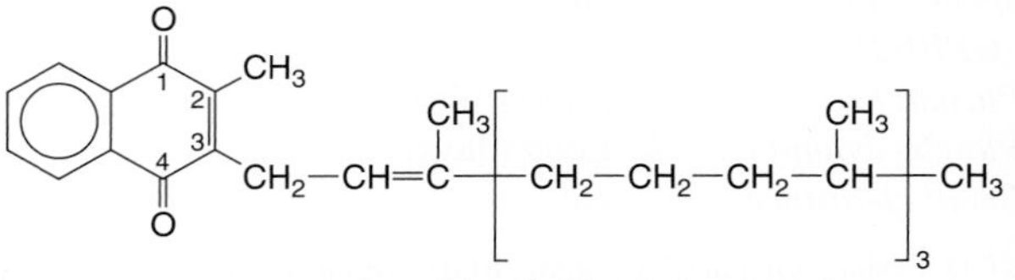

PHYTONADIONE (vitamin K_1, phylloquinone)

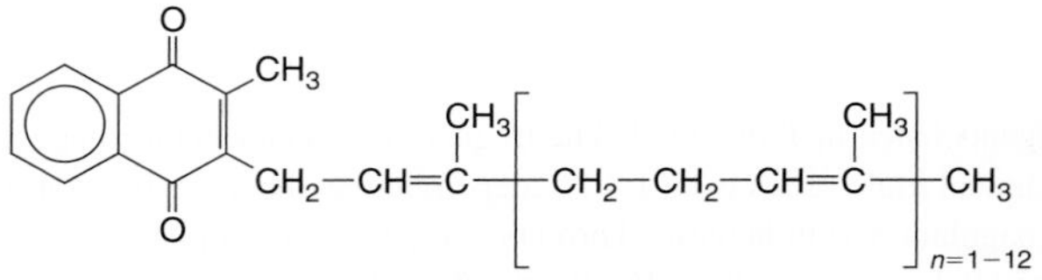

MENAQUINONE (vitamin K_2) series

Physiological Functions and Pharmacological Actions. In animals and humans, phytonadione and menaquinones promote the biosynthesis of: the Gla forms of factors II (prothrombin), VII, IX, and X; anticoagulant proteins C and S; protein Z (a cofactor to the inhibitor of Xa); the bone Gla protein osteocalcin; the matrix Gla protein; the growth arrest–specific protein 6 (Gas6); and four transmembrane monospans of unknown function (Brown et al., 2000; Broze, 2001; Kulman et al., 2001).

Figure 30–7 summarizes the coupling of the vitamin K cycle with glutamate carboxylation. Vitamin K, as KH_2, the reduced vitamin K hydroquinone, is an essential cofactor for γ-glutamyl carboxylase (Rishavy et al., 2004). Using KH_2, O_2, CO_2, and the glutamate-containing substrate, the enzyme forms a Gla protein and concomitantly, the 2,3-epoxide of vitamin K. A coumarin-sensitive 2,3-epoxide reductase regenerates KH_2. The γ-glutamyl carboxylase and epoxide reductase are integral membrane proteins of the endoplasmic reticulum and seem to function as a multicomponent system that may include the chaperone protein, calumenin, which reportedly inhibits γ-carboxylation (Wajih et al., 2004). Two natural mutations in γ-glutamyl carboxylase lead to bleeding disorders (Mutucumarana et al., 2003). With respect to proteins affecting blood coagulation, these reactions occur in the liver, but γ-carboxylation of glutamate also occurs in lung, bone, and other cell types. Vitamin K epoxide reductase recently has been cloned (Rost et al., 2004; Li et al., 2004).

The γ-carboxylation reaction is aided by the grouping of glutamate residues in a *Gla domain* (~45 residues in clotting factors) near the amino terminus of the nascent substrate protein; the reaction is guided by an adjacent propeptide (18-28 amino acids) that interacts with the carboxylase. In the case of the vitamin K-dependent clotting proteins, the Gla domain is ~45 residues long, and 9-13 glutamates are γ-carboxylated in the primary sequence of the Gla domain, C-terminal to the propeptide. The Glu→Gla conversion enables the factors to interact well with Ca^{2+} and thence with phospholipids of platelet membranes, positioning the factors in the proper conformations for interacting with their substrates and modulators. In the absence of vitamin K (or in the presence of a coumarin derivative), newly synthesized vitamin K-dependent clotting factors lack Gla residues and are inactive because the molecular conformations needed for their interactions are not achieved.

Human Requirements. The human requirement for vitamin K has not been defined precisely. In patients made vitamin K deficient by a starvation diet and antibiotic therapy for 3-4 weeks, the minimum daily requirement is estimated to be 0.03 μg/kg of body weight (Frick, 1967) and possibly as high as 1 μg/kg, which is approximately the recommended intake for adults (70 μg/day).

Symptoms of Deficiency. The chief clinical manifestation of vitamin K deficiency is an increased tendency to bleed (see the discussion of hypoprothrombinemia in the section on "Oral Anticoagulants," earlier in the chapter). Ecchymoses, epistaxis, hematuria, GI bleeding, and postoperative hemorrhage are common; intracranial hemorrhage may occur. Hemoptysis is uncommon. The discovery of a vitamin K-dependent protein in bone suggests that the fetal bone abnormalities associated with the administration of oral anticoagulants during the first trimester of pregnancy ("fetal warfarin syndrome") may be related to a deficiency of the vitamin.

Considerable evidence indicates a role for vitamin K in adult skeletal maintenance and the prevention of osteoporosis. Low concentrations of the vitamin are associated with deficits in bone mineral density and fractures; vitamin K supplementation increases the carboxylation state of osteocalcin and also improves bone mineral density, but the relationship of these two effects is unclear (Feskanich et al., 1999). Bone mineral density in adults is not changed by therapeutic use of vitamin K antagonists (Rosen et al., 1993), but new bone formation may be affected.

Toxicity. Phytonadione and the menaquinones are nontoxic to animals, even when given at 500 times the recommended daily allowance. However, menadione and its derivatives (synthetic forms of vitamin K) have been implicated in producing hemolytic anemia and kernicterus in neonates, especially in premature infants (Diploma and Ritchie, 1997). For this reason, menadione should not be used as a therapeutic form of vitamin K.

Absorption, Fate, and Excretion. The mechanism of intestinal absorption of compounds with vitamin K activity varies with their solubility. In the presence of bile salts, phytonadione and the menaquinones are adequately absorbed from the intestine, almost entirely by way of the lymph. Phytonadione is absorbed by an energy-dependent, saturable process in proximal portions of the small intestine; menaquinones are absorbed by diffusion in the distal portions of the small intestine and in the colon. Following absorption, phytonadione is incorporated into chylomicrons in close association with triglycerides and lipoproteins. In a large survey, plasma phytonadione and triglyceride concentration were well correlated (Sadowski et al., 1989). The extremely low phytonadione levels in newborns may be partly related to very low plasma lipoprotein concentrations at birth and may lead to an underestimation of vitamin K tissue stores. After absorption, phytonadione and menaquinones are concentrated in the liver, but the concentration of phytonadione declines rapidly. Menaquinones, produced in the lower bowel, are less biologically active than phytonadione due to their long side chain. Very little vitamin K accumulates in other tissues.

Phytonadione is metabolized rapidly to more polar metabolites, which are excreted in the bile and urine. The major urinary metabolites result from shortening of the side chain to five or seven carbon atoms, yielding carboxylic acids that are conjugated with glucuronate prior to excretion.

Apparently, there is only modest storage of vitamin K in the body. Under circumstances in which lack of bile interferes with absorption of vitamin K, hypoprothrombinemia develops slowly over several weeks.

Therapeutic Uses. Vitamin K is used therapeutically to correct the bleeding tendency or hemorrhage associated with its deficiency. Vitamin K deficiency can result from inadequate intake, absorption, or utilization of the vitamin, or as a consequence of the action of a vitamin K antagonist.

Phytonadione (AQUAMEPHYTON, KONAKION, MEPHYTON, generic) is available as tablets and in a dispersion with buffered polysorbate and propylene glycol (KONAKION) or polyoxyethylated fatty acid derivatives and dextrose (AQUAMEPHYTON). KONAKION is administered only intramuscularly. AQUAMEPHYTON may be given by any route; however, oral or subcutaneous injection is preferred because severe reactions resembling anaphylaxis have followed its intravenous administration.

Inadequate Intake. After infancy, hypoprothrombinemia due to dietary deficiency of vitamin K is extremely rare: The vitamin is present in many foods and also is synthesized by intestinal bacteria. Occasionally, the use of a broad-spectrum antibiotic may itself produce a hypoprothrombinemia that responds readily to small doses of vitamin K and reestablishment of normal bowel flora. Hypoprothrombinemia can occur in patients receiving prolonged intravenous alimentation. It is recommended to give 1 mg of phytonadione per week (the equivalent of about 150 μg/day) to patients on total parenteral nutrition.

Hypoprothrombinemia of the Newborn. Healthy newborn infants show decreased plasma concentrations of vitamin K-dependent clotting factors for a few days after birth, the time required to obtain an adequate dietary intake of the vitamin and to establish a normal intestinal flora. In premature infants and in infants with hemorrhagic disease of the newborn, the concentrations of clotting factors are particularly depressed. The degree to which these changes reflect true vitamin K deficiency is controversial. Measurements of non-γ-carboxylated prothrombin suggest that vitamin K deficiency occurs in about 3% of live births (Shapiro et al., 1986).

Hemorrhagic disease of the newborn has been associated with breast-feeding; human milk has low concentrations of vitamin K (Haroon et al., 1982). In addition, the intestinal flora of breast-fed infants may lack microorganisms that synthesize the vitamin (Keenan et al., 1971). Commercial infant formulas are supplemented with vitamin K.

In the neonate with hemorrhagic disease of the newborn, the administration of vitamin K raises the concentration of these clotting factors to the level normal for the newborn infant and controls the bleeding tendency within about 6 hours. The routine administration of 1 mg phytonadione intramuscularly at birth is required by law in the U.S. This dose may have to be increased or repeated if the mother has received anticoagulant or anticonvulsant drug therapy or if the infant develops bleeding tendencies. Alternatively, some clinicians treat mothers who are receiving anticonvulsants with oral vitamin K prior to delivery (20 mg/day for 2 weeks) (Vert and Deblay, 1982).

Inadequate Absorption. Vitamin K is poorly absorbed in the absence of bile. Thus, hypoprothrombinemia may be associated with either intrahepatic or extrahepatic biliary obstruction or a severe defect in the intestinal absorption of fat from other causes.

Biliary Obstruction or Fistula. Bleeding that accompanies obstructive jaundice or biliary fistula responds promptly to the administration of vitamin K. Oral phytonadione administered with bile salts is both safe and effective and should be used in the care of the jaundiced patient, both preoperatively and postoperatively. In the absence of significant hepatocellular disease, the prothrombin activity of the blood rapidly returns to normal. If oral administration is not feasible, a parenteral preparation should be used. The usual dose is 10 mg/day of vitamin K.

The treatment of a patient during hemorrhage requires transfusion of fresh blood or reconstituted fresh plasma. Vitamin K also should be given. If biliary obstruction has caused hepatic injury, the response to vitamin K may be poor.

Malabsorption Syndromes. Among the disorders that result in inadequate absorption of vitamin K from the intestinal tract are cystic fibrosis, sprue, Crohn's disease and enterocolitis, ulcerative colitis, dysentery, and extensive resection of bowel. Because drugs that greatly reduce the bacterial population of the bowel are used frequently in many of these disorders, the availability of the vitamin may be further reduced. Moreover, dietary restrictions also may limit the availability of the vitamin. For immediate correction of the deficiency, parenteral therapy should be used.

Inadequate Utilization. Hepatocellular disease may be accompanied or followed by hypoprothrombinemia. Hepatocellular damage also may be secondary to long-lasting biliary obstruction. In these conditions, the damaged parenchymal cells may not be able to produce the vitamin K-dependent clotting factors, even if excess vitamin is available. However, if an inadequate secretion of bile salts is contributing to the syndrome, some benefit may be obtained from the parenteral administration of 10 mg of phytonadione daily. Paradoxically, the administration of large doses of vitamin K or its analogs in an attempt to correct the hypoprothrombinemia associated with severe hepatitis or cirrhosis actually may result in a further depression of the concentration of prothrombin. The mechanism for this action is unknown.

Drug- and Venom-Induced Hypoprothrombinemia. Anticoagulant drugs such as warfarin and its congeners act as competitive antagonists of vitamin K and interfere with the hepatic biosynthesis of Gla-containing clotting factors. The treatment of bleeding caused by oral anticoagulants is discussed earlier in this chapter. Vitamin K may be of help in combating the bleeding and hypoprothrombinemia that follow the bite of the tropical American pit viper or other species whose venom destroys or inactivates prothrombin.

CLINICAL SUMMARY

A variety of anticoagulant, fibrinolytic, and antiplatelet agents are available and are among the most widely used drugs. Heparin and LMWHs are commonly used to treat venous thromboembolism, unstable angina, and acute myocardial infarction; these agents also are used to prevent thrombosis during coronary angioplasty and for certain other high-risk indications. The major toxicities of heparin are bleeding and the syndrome of heparin-induced thrombocytopenia, which often precipitates venous or arterial thrombosis. Direct thrombin inhibitors, such as lepirudin, bivalirudin, and argatroban, are indicated for patients with heparin-induced thrombocytopenia.

Warfarin and other vitamin K antagonists are used to prevent the progression or recurrence of acute venous thromboembolism following an initial course of heparin. They also decrease the incidence of systemic embolization in patients with atrial fibrillation or prosthetic heart valves. Warfarin has a narrow therapeutic index drug and is associated with more than 200 drug-drug and drug-food interactions. Over- and under-dosing are associated with serious consequences, including thrombosis or major bleeding in a significant number of patients. Warfarin also produces fetal abnormalities when given during pregnancy. New oral anticoagulants that target thrombin or factor Xa hopefully will replace warfarin in the future. These drugs have the potential to streamline care because they can be given in fixed doses without coagulation monitoring.

Fibrinolytic agents, such as t-PA or its derivatives, reduce the mortality of acute myocardial infarction and are used in situations in which angioplasty is not readily available. Fibrinolytic therapy also is used for patients with acute ischemic stroke.

Antiplatelet agents, including aspirin, clopidogrel, prasugrel, and glycoprotein IIb/IIIa inhibitors, are used to prevent thrombosis after coronary angioplasty and in the secondary prevention of myocardial infarction and stroke. Bleeding is the major toxicity of the antiplatelet agents. Newer antiplatelet drugs that directly target the ADP or thrombin receptor on platelets are in advanced stages of development. These more potent antiplatelet drugs may produce more bleeding, highlighting the inevitable link between the efficacy and toxicity of anti-thrombotic drugs.

BIBLIOGRAPHY

Almquist HJ, Stokstad CLR. Hemorrhagic chick disease of dietary origin. *J Biol Chem,* **1935,** *111:*105–113.

Andersen HR, Nielsen TT, Rasmussen K, *et al.* DANAMI-2 Investigators. A comparison of coronary angioplasty with fibrinolytic therapy in acute myocardial infarction. *N Engl J Med,* **2003,** *349:*733–742.

Antithrombotic Trialists' Collaboration. Collaborative meta-analysis of randomised trials of antiplatelet therapy for prevention of death, myocardial infarction, and stroke in high risk patients. *BMJ*, **2002,** *324:*71–86. Erratum in: *BMJ*, **2002,** *324:*141.

Bennett CL, Connors JM, Carwile JM, *et al*. Thrombotic thrombocytopenic purpura associated with clopidogrel. *N Engl J Med*, **2000,** *342:*1773–1777.

Bentley R, Meganathan R. Biosynthesis of vitamin K (menaquinone) in bacteria. *Microbiol Rev,* **1982,** *46:*241–280.

Blackmer AB, Oertel MD, Valgus JM. Fondaparinux and the management of heparin-induced thrombocytopenia: The journey continues. *Ann Pharmacother*, **2009**, *43:*1636–1646.

Blick SK, Orman JS, Wagstaff AJ, *et al.* Fondaparinux sodium: A review of its use in the management of acute coronary syndromes. *Am J Cardiovasc Drugs*, **2008**, *8:*113–125.

Boersma E, Harrington RA, Moliterno DJ, *et al.* Platelet glycoprotein IIb/IIIa inhibitors in acute coronary syndromes: A meta-analysis of all major randomised clinical trials. *Lancet*, **2002,** *359:*189–198. Erratum in: *Lancet*, **2002,** *359:*2120.

Brown MA, Stenberg LM, Persson U, Stenflo J. Identification and purification of vitamin K-dependent proteins and peptides with monoclonal antibodies specific for γ-carboxyglutamyl (Gla) residues. *J Biol Chem,* **2000,** *275:*19795–19802.

Broze G Jr. Protein Z-dependent regulation of coagulation. *Thromb Haemost,* **2001,** *86:*1–13.

Buller HR, Davidson BL, Decousus H, *et al.* Matisse Investigators. Subcutaneous fondaparinux versus intravenous unfractionated heparin in the initial treatment of pulmonary embolism. *N Engl J Med*, **2003,** *349:*1695–1702. Erratum in: *N Engl J Med*, **2004,** *350:*423.

Butenas S, Orfeo T, Mann KG. Tissue factor in coagulation: Which? Where? When? *Arterioscler Thromb Vasc Biol*, **2009**, *29:*1989–1996.

Butt HR, Snell AM, Osterberg AE. The use of vitamin K and bile in treatment of hemorrhagic diathesis in cases of jaundice. *Proc Staff Meet Mayo Clin,* **1938,** *13:*74–80.

Connolly SJ, Ezekowitz MD, Yusuf S, *et al.* Dabigatran versus warfarin in patients with atrial fibrillation. *N Engl J Med*, **2009,** *361:*1139–1151.

Daly AK, King BP. Pharmacogenetics of oral anticoagulants. *Pharmacogenetics*, **2003,** *13:*247–252.

Dam H, Schønheyder F. The antihaemorrhagic vitamin of the chick. *Nature,* **1935,** *135:*652–653.

Dam H, Schønheyder F, Tage-Hansen E. Studies on the mode of action of vitamin K. *Biochem J,* **1936,** *30:*1075–1079.

Diener HC, Cunha L, Forbes C, *et al*. European Stroke Prevention Study. 2. Dipyridamole and acetylsalicylic acid in the secondary prevention of stroke. *J Neurol Sci*, **1996,** *143:*1–13.

Diploma JR, Ritchie DM. Vitamin toxicity. *Annu Rev Pharmacol Toxicol,* **1997,** *17:*133–148.

Edelberg JM, Christie PD, Rosenberg RD. Regulation of vascular bed-specific prothrombotic potential. *Circ Res*, **2001,** *89:*117–124.

Esmon CT. Inflammation and the activated protein C anticoagulant pathway. *Semin Thromb Hemost*, **2006**, *32:*49–60.

Esmon CT. The protein C pathway. *Chest*, **2003,** *124*(suppl): 26S–32S.

Feskanich D, Weber P, Willett WC, *et al.* Vitamin K intake and hip fractures in women: A prospective study. *Am J Clin Nutr,* **1999,** *69:*74–79.

Fifth Organization to Assess Strategies in Acute Ischemic Syndromes Investigators, Yusuf S, Mehta SR, *et al.* Comparison of fondaparinux and enoxaparin in acute coronary syndromes. *N Engl J Med,* **2006**, *354*:1464–1470.

Frick PG, Riedler G, Brögli H. Dose response and minimal daily requirement for vitamin K in man. *J Appl Physiol,* **1967,** *23:*387–389.

Geerts WH, Bergqvist D, Pineo GF, *et al*. Prevention of venous thromboembolism: American College of Chest Physicians Evidence-Based Clinical Practice Guidelines (8th edition). *Chest*, **2008**, *133*(6 suppl):381S–453S.

Ghimire LV, Stein CM. Warfarin pharmacogenetics, Goodman and Gilman Online; www.accessmedicine.com/updatesContent.aspx?aid=1001507, accessed June 10, 2010.

Grines CL, Serruys S, O'Neill WW. Fibrinolytic therapy: Is it a treatment of the past? *Circulation*, **2003**, *107:*2538–2542.

GUSTO III (The Global Use of Strategies to Open Occluded Coronary Arteries) Investigators. A comparison of reteplase with alteplase for acute myocardial infarction. *N Engl J Med*, **1997,** *337:*1118–1123.

Haroon Y, Shearer MJ, Rahim S, *et al*. The content of phylloquinone (vitamin K_1) in human milk, cows' milk, and infant formula foods determined by high-performance liquid chromatography. *J Nutr,* **1982,** *112:*1105–1117.

Hawkins WB, Brinkhous KM. Prothrombin deficiency as the cause of bleeding in bile fistula dogs. *J Exp Med,* **1936,** *63:*795–801.

Hirsh J, Anand SS, Halperin JL, Fuster V. Guide to anticoagulant therapy. Heparin: A statement for healthcare professionals from the American Heart Association. *Circulation*, **2001,** *103:*2994–3018.

Hirsh J, Fuster V, Ansell J, Halperin JL. American Heart Association/American College of Cardiology Foundation guide to warfarin therapy. *Circulation*, **2003,** *107:*1692–1711.

Hollopeter G, Jantzen HM, Vincent D, *et al*. Identification of the platelet ADP receptor targeted by antithrombotic drugs. *Nature*, **2001,** *409:*202–207.

Hylek EM, Heiman H, Skates SJ, *et al*. Acetaminophen and other risk factors for excessive warfarin anticoagulation. *JAMA,* **1998,** *279:*657–662.

International Warfarin Pharmacogenetics Consortium, Klein TE, Altman RB, *et al.* Estimation of the warfarin dose with clinical and pharmacogenetic data. *N Engl J Med*, **2009**, *360*:753–764.

Jin J, Kunapuli SP. Coactivation of two different G protein-coupled receptors is essential for ADP-induced platelet aggregation. *Proc Natl Acad Sci U S A*, **1998,** *95:*8070–8074.

Keeley EC, Boura JA, Grines CL. Primary angioplasty versus intravenous thrombolytic therapy for acute myocardial infarction: A quantitative review of 23 randomised trials. *Lancet*, **2003**, *361*:13–20.

Keenan WJ, Jewett T, Glueck HI. Role of feeding and vitamin K in hypoprothrombinemia of the newborn. *Am J Dis Child,* **1971,** *121:*271–277.

Kulman JD, Harris JE, Xie L, Davie EW. Identification of two novel transmembrane γ-carboxyglutamic acid proteins expressed broadly in fetal and adult tissues. *Proc Natl Acad Sci U S A*, **2001,** *98:*1370–1375.

Li T, Chang CY, Jin DY, *et al*. Identification of the gene for vitamin K epoxide reductase. *Nature*, **2004,** *427:*541–544.

Lijnen HR, Collen D. Fibrinolysis and the control of hemostasis. In: Stamatoyannopoulos G, Majerus PW, Perlmutter RM,

Varmus H, eds. *The Molecular Basis of Blood Diseases,* 3rd ed. WB Saunders Co., Philadelphia, **2001,** pp. 740–763.

Mackman N, Taubman M. Tissue factor: Past, present, and future. *Arterioscler Thromb Vasc Biol*, **2009**, *29*:1986–1988.

Mann KG, Butenas S, Brummel K. The dynamics of thrombin formation. *Arterioscler Thromb Vasc Biol*, **2003,** *23:*17–25.

McClain MR, Palomaki GE, Piper M, *et al.* A rapid-ACCE review of CYP2C9 and VKORC1 alleles testing to inform warfarin dosing in adults at elevated risk for thrombotic events to avoid serious bleeding. *Genet Med*, **2008,** *10:*89–98.

Moll S, Ortel TL. Monitoring warfarin therapy in patients with lupus anticoagulants. *Ann Intern Med*, **1997,** *127:*177–185.

Mutucumarana VP, Acher F, Straight DL, *et al.* A conserved region of human vitamin K-dependent carboxylase between residues 398 and 404 is important for its interaction with the glutamate substrate. *J Biol Chem,* **2003,** *278:*46488–46493.

Olson ST, Chuang YJ. Heparin activates antithrombin anticoagulant function by generating new interaction sites (exosites) for blood clotting proteinases. *Trends Cardiovasc Med*, **2002,** *12:*331–338.

Patrono C, Bachmann F, Baigent C, *et al.* European Society of Cardiology. Expert consensus document on the use of antiplatelet agents. The task force on the use of antiplatelet agents in patients with atherosclerotic cardiovascular disease of the European Society of Cardiology. *Eur Heart J*, **2004,** *25:*166–181.

Porto I, Giubilato S, DeMaria GL, *et al.* Platelet P2Y12 receptor inhibition by thienopyridines: Status and future. *Expert Opin Investig Drugs,* **2009**, *18:*1317–1332.

Quick AJ, Stanley-Brown M, Bancroft FW. A study of the coagulation defect in hemophilia and in jaundice. *Am J Med Sci,* **1935,** *190:*501–511.

Rieder MJ, Reiner AP, Gage BF, *et al.* Effect of VKORC1 haplotypes on transcriptional regulation and warfarin dose. *N Engl J Med,* **2005**, *352*:2293–2295.

Rishavy MA, Pudota BN, Hallgren KW, *et al.* A new model for vitamin K-dependent carboxylation: The catalytic base that deprotonates vitamin K hydroquinone is not Cys but an activated amine. *Proc Natl Acad Sci U S A,* **2004,** *101:*13732–13737.

Rosen HN, Maitland LA, Suttie JW, *et al.* Vitamin K and maintenance of skeletal integrity in adults. *Am J Med*, **1993,** *94:*62–68.

Rost S, Fregin A, Ivaskevicius V, *et al.* Mutations in VKORC1 cause warfarin resistance and multiple coagulation factor deficiency type 2. *Nature*, **2004,** *427:*537–541.

Sacco RL, Diener HC, Yusuf S, *et al.* Aspirin and extended-release dipyridamole versus clopidogrel for recurrent stroke. *N Engl J Med*, **2008**, *359:*1238–1251.

Sadowski JA, Hood SJ, Dallal GE, Garry PJ. Phylloquinone in plasma from elderly and young adults: Factors influencing its concentration. *Am J Clin Nutr,* **1989,** *50:*100–108.

Sanderson S, Emery J, Higgins J. CYP2C9 gene variants, drug dose, and bleeding risk in warfarin-treated patients: A HuGEnet systematic review and meta-analysis. *Genet Med*, **2005**, *7:*97–104.

Savi P, Pereillo JM, Uzabiaga MF, *et al*. Identification and biological activity of the active metabolite of clopidogrel. *Thromb Haemost*, **2000,** *84:*891–896.

Schulman S, Kearon C, Kakkar AK, *et al.* Dabigatran versus warfarin in the treatment of acute venous thromboembolism. *N Engl J Med*, **2009**, December 6 [Epub ahead of print].

Schwarz UI, Ritchie MD, Bradford Y, *et al.* Genetic determinants of response to warfarin during initial anticoagulation. *N Engl J Med*, **2008**, *358:*999–1008.

Shantsila E, Lip GY, Chong BH. Heparin-induced thrombocytopenia. A contemporary clinical approach to diagnosis and management. *Chest*, **2009**, *135:*1651–1664.

Shapiro AD, Jacobson LJ, Armon ME, *et al.* Vitamin K deficiency in the newborn infant: Prevalence and perinatal risk factors. *J Pediatr,* **1986,** *109:*675–680.

Sugahara K, Kitagawa H. Heparin and heparan sulfate biosynthesis. *IUBMB Life,* **2002,** *54:*163–175.

Vert P, Deblay MF. Hemorrhagic disorders in infants of epileptic mothers. In: Janz D, Bossi L, Daum M, *et al.*, eds. *Epilepsy, Pregnancy, and the Child*. Raven Press, New York, **1982,** pp. 387–388.

Wajih N, Sane DC, Hutson SM, Wallin R. The inhibitory effect of calumenin on the vitamin K-dependent γ-carboxylation system. Characterization of the system in normal and warfarin-resistant rats. *J Biol Chem,* **2004,** *279:*25276–25283.

Wallentin L, Becker RC, Budaj A, *et al.* Ticagrelor versus clopidogrel in patients with acute coronary syndromes. *N Engl J Med,* **2009**, *361:*1045–1057.

Warkentin TE. Heparin-induced thrombocytopenia. *Hematol Oncol Clin North Am,* **2007**, *21*:589–607.

Warner ED, Brinkhous KM, Smith HP. Bleeding tendency of obstructive jaundice: Prothrombin deficiency and dietary factors. *Proc Soc Exp Biol Med,* **1938,** *37:*628–630.

Yusuf S, Zhao F, Mehta SR, *et al.* Clopidogrel in Unstable Angina to Prevent Recurrent Events Trial Investigators. Effects of clopidogrel in addition to aspirin in patients with acute coronary syndromes without ST-segment elevation. *N Engl J Med*, **2001,** *345:*494–502.

Zivelin A, Rao LV, Rapaport SI. Mechanism of the anticoagulant effect of warfarin as evaluated in rabbits by selective depression of individual procoagulant vitamin K-dependent clotting factors. *J Clin Invest*, **1993,** *92:*2131–2140.

Drug Therapy for Hypercholesterolemia and Dyslipidemia

Thomas P. Bersot

Hyperlipidemia is a major cause of atherosclerosis and atherosclerosis-induced conditions, such as coronary heart disease (CHD), ischemic cerebrovascular disease, and peripheral vascular disease. Although the incidence of these atherosclerosis-related cardiovascular disease (CVD) events has declined in the U.S., these conditions cause morbidity or mortality in a majority of middle-aged or older adults and account for about one-third of all deaths of persons in this age range. The incidence and absolute number of annual events will likely increase over the next decade because of the epidemic of obesity and the aging of the U.S. population. Dyslipidemias, including hyperlipidemia (hypercholesterolemia) and low levels of high-density-lipoprotein cholesterol (HDL-C), are major causes of increased atherogenic risk; both genetic disorders and lifestyle (sedentary behavior and diets high in calories, saturated fat, and cholesterol) contribute to the dyslipidemias seen in countries around the world. For many individuals, alterations in lifestyle have a far greater potential for reducing vascular disease risk and at a lower cost than drug therapy. When pharmacotherpy is indicated, providers can choose from multiple agents with proven efficacy.

Recognition that dyslipidemia is a risk factor has led to the development of drugs that modify cholesterol levels. This chapter focuses on the following classes of drugs:

- 3-hydroxy-3-methylglutaryl–coenzyme A (HMG-CoA) reductase inhibitors—the statins
- Bile acid–binding resins
- Nicotinic acid (*niacin*)
- Fibric acid derivatives
- The cholesterol absorption inhibitor *ezetimibe*

These drugs provide benefit in patients across the entire spectrum of cholesterol levels, primarily by reducing levels of low-density-lipoprotein cholesterol (LDL-C).

In early well-controlled clinical trials employing drug regimens that reduce LDL-C levels moderately (30-40%), fatal and nonfatal CHD events and strokes were reduced by as much as 30-40% (Grundy et al., 2004b). Clinical trial data support extending lipid-modifying therapy to high-risk patients whose major lipid risk factor is a reduced plasma level of HDL-C, even if their LDL-C level does not meet the existing threshold values for initiating hypolipidemic drug therapy (Grundy et al., 2004b). In patients with low HDL-C and average LDL-C levels, appropriate drug therapy reduced CHD endpoint events by 20-35% (Heart Protection Study Collaborative Group, 2002). Because two-thirds of patients with CHD in the U.S. have low HDL-C levels (<40 mg/dL in men, <50 mg/dL in women), it is important to include low-HDL-C patients in management guidelines for dyslipidemia, even if their LDL-C levels are in the normal range (Bersot et al., 2003).

Severe hypertriglyceridemia (i.e., triglyceride levels of >1000 mg/dL) requires therapy to prevent pancreatitis. It is unclear whether hypertriglyceridemia is an independent risk factor for developing atherothrombotic CVD (Sarwar et al., 2007). Moderately elevated triglyceride levels (150-400 mg/dL) are of concern because they often occur as part of the metabolic syndrome, which includes insulin resistance, obesity, hypertension, low HDL-C levels, a procoagulant state, and substantially increased risk of CVD. The atherogenic dyslipidemia in patients with the metabolic syndrome also is characterized by lipid-depleted LDL (sometimes referred to as "small, dense LDL") (Grundy et al., 2004a). The metabolic syndrome affects ~25% of adults and is common in CVD patients; hence, identification of moderate hypertriglyceridemia in a patient, even if the total cholesterol level is normal, should trigger an evaluation to identify insulin-resistant patients with this disorder.

PLASMA LIPOPROTEIN METABOLISM

Lipoproteins are macromolecular assemblies that contain lipids and proteins. The lipid constituents include free and esterified cholesterol, triglycerides, and phospholipids. The protein components, known as apolipoproteins or apoproteins, provide structural stability to the lipoproteins and also may function as ligands in lipoprotein–receptor interactions or as cofactors in enzymatic processes that regulate lipoprotein metabolism. In all spherical lipoproteins, the most water-insoluble lipids (cholesteryl esters and triglycerides) are core components, and the more polar, water-soluble components (apoproteins, phospholipids, and unesterified cholesterol) are located on the surface. The major classes of lipoproteins and a number of their properties are summarized in Table 31–1.

Table 31–2 describes apoproteins that have well-defined roles in plasma lipoprotein metabolism. These apolipoproteins include apolipoprotein (apo) A-I, apoA-II, apoA-IV, apoA-V, apoB-100, apoB-48, apoC-I, apoC-II, apoC-III, apoE, and apo(a). Except for apo(a), the lipid-binding regions of all apoproteins contain amphipathic helices that interact with the polar, hydrophilic lipids (such as surface phospholipids) and with the aqueous plasma environment in which the lipoproteins circulate. Differences in the non–lipid-binding regions determine the functional specificities of the apolipoproteins.

Chylomicrons. Chylomicrons are synthesized from the fatty acids of dietary triglycerides and cholesterol absorbed from the small intestine by epithelial cells. Fat-soluble vitamins also are incorporated into chylomicrons after absorption.

Chylomicrons, the largest plasma lipoproteins, are the only lipoproteins that float to the top of a tube of plasma that has been allowed to stand undisturbed for 12 hours. The buoyancy of chylomicrons reflects their high fat content (98-99%), of which 85% is from fatty acids of dietary triglycerides. In chylomicrons, the ratio of triglycerides to cholesterol is ~10 or greater. In normolipidemic individuals, chylomicrons are present in plasma for 3-6 hours after a fat-containing meal has been ingested. After a fast of 10-12 hours, no chylomicrons remain.

Intestinal cholesterol and plant sterol absorption is mediated by Niemann-Pick C1–Like 1 protein (NPC1L1), which appears to be the target of ezetimibe, a cholesterol absorption inhibitor (Davis and Altmann, 2009). Plant sterols, unlike cholesterol, are not normally esterified and incorporated into chylomicrons. Two ATP-binding cassette (ABC) half-transporters, ABCG5 and ABCG8, which reside on the apical plasma membrane of enterocytes, channel plant sterols back into the intestinal lumen, preventing their assimilation into the body. Patients with the autosomal recessive disorder sitosterolemia have mutations in either of the genes that encode ABCG5 and ABCG8. As a result, they absorb unusually large amounts of plant sterols, fail to excrete dietary sterols into the bile, and thus accumulate plant sterols in the blood and tissues; this accumulation is associated with tendon and subcutaneous xanthomas and a markedly increased risk of premature CHD.

Triglyceride synthesis is regulated by diacylglycerol transferase in many tissues. After their synthesis in the endoplasmic reticulum, triglycerides are transferred by *microsomal triglyceride transfer protein* (MTP) to the site where newly synthesized apoB-48 is available to form chylomicrons.

The apolipoproteins of chylomicrons include some that are synthesized by intestinal epithelial cells (apoB-48, apoA-I, and apoA-IV), and others acquired from HDL (apoE and apoC-I, C-II, and C-III) after chylomicrons have been secreted into the lymph and enter the plasma (Table 31–2). The apoB-48 of chylomicrons is one of two forms of apoB present in lipoproteins. ApoB-48, synthesized only by intestinal epithelial cells, is unique to chylomicrons. ApoB-100 is synthesized by the liver and incorporated into VLDL and intermediate-density lipoproteins (IDL) and LDL, which are products of VLDL catabolism. The apparent molecular weight of apoB-48 is 48% that of apoB-100, which accounts for the name "apoB-48." The amino acid sequence of apoB-48 is identical to the first 2152 of the 4536 residues of apoB-100. An RNA-editing mechanism unique to the intestine accounts for the premature termination of the translation of the apoB-100 mRNA. ApoB-48 lacks the portion of the sequence of apoB-100 that allows apoB-100 to bind to the LDL receptor, so apoB-48 functions primarily as a structural component of chylomicrons.

Dietary cholesterol is esterified by the type 2 isozyme of acyl coenzyme A:cholesterol acyltransferase (ACAT-2). ACAT-2 is found in the intestine and in the liver, where cellular free cholesterol is esterified before triglyceride-rich lipoproteins [chylomicrons and very-low-density lipoproteins (VLDL)] are assembled. In the intestine, ACAT-2 regulates the absorption of dietary cholesterol and thus may be a potential pharmacological target for reducing blood cholesterol levels.

Table 31–1

Characteristics of Plasma Lipoproteins

LIPOPROTEIN CLASS	DENSITY (g/mL)	MAJOR LIPID CONSTITUENT	TG:CHOL RATIO	SIGNIFICANT APOPROTEINS	SITE OF SYNTHESIS	MECHANISM(S) OF CATABOLISM
Chylomicrons and remnants	<<1.006	Dietary triglycerides and cholesterol	10:1	B-48, E, A-I, A-IV, C-I, C-II, C-III	Intestine	Triglyceride hydrolysis by LPL, apoE-mediated remnant uptake by liver
VLDL	<1.006	"Endogenous" or hepatic triglycerides	5:1	B-100, E, C-I, C-II, C-III	Liver	Triglyceride hydrolysis by LPL
IDL	1.006-1.019	Cholesteryl esters and "endogenous" triglycerides	1:1	B-100, E, C-II, C-III	Product of VLDL catabolism	50% converted to LDL mediated by HL; 50% apoE-mediated uptake by liver
LDL	1.019-1.063	Cholesteryl esters	NS	B-100	Product of VLDL catabolism	ApoB-100–mediated uptake by LDL receptor (~75% in liver)
HDL	1.063-1.21	Phospholipids, cholesteryl esters	NS	A-I, A-II, E, C-I, C-II, C-III	Intestine, liver, plasma	Complex: transfer of cholesteryl ester to VLDL and LDL; uptake of HDL cholesterol by hepatocytes
Lp(a)	1.05-1.09	Cholesteryl esters	NS	B-100, apo(a)	Liver	Unknown

apo, apolipoprotein; CHOL, cholesterol; HDL, high-density lipoproteins; IDL, intermediate-density lipoproteins; Lp(a), lipoprotein(a); LDL, low-density lipoproteins; NS, not significant (triglyceride is <5% of LDL and HDL); TG, triglyceride; VLDL, very-low-density lipoproteins; HL, hepatic lipase; LPL, lipoprotein lipase.

increasing triglyceride- and cholesterol-rich remnant lipoproteins in the plasma (type III hyperlipoproteinemia).

During the initial hydrolysis of chylomicron triglycerides by LPL, apoA-I and phospholipids are shed from the surface of chylomicrons and remain in the plasma. This is one mechanism by which nascent (precursor) HDL are generated. Chylomicron remnants are not precursors of LDL, but the dietary cholesterol delivered to the liver by remnants increases plasma LDL levels by reducing LDL receptor-mediated catabolism of LDL by the liver.

Very-Low-Density Lipoproteins. VLDL are produced in the liver when triglyceride production is stimulated by an increased flux of free fatty acids or by increased *de novo* synthesis of fatty acids by the liver. VLDL particles are 40-100 nm in diameter and are large enough to cause plasma turbidity, but unlike chylomicrons, do not float spontaneously to the top of a tube of undisturbed plasma.

ApoB-100, apoE, and apoC-I, C-II, and C-III are synthesized constitutively by the liver and incorporated into VLDL (Table 31–2). If triglycerides are not available to form VLDL, the newly synthesized apoB-100 is degraded by hepatocytes. Triglycerides are synthesized in the endoplasmic reticulum, and along with other lipid constituents, are transferred by MTP to the site in the endoplasmic reticulum where newly synthesized apoB-100 is available to form nascent (precursor) VLDL. Small amounts of apoE and the C apoproteins are incorporated into nascent particles within the liver before secretion, but most of these apoproteins are acquired from plasma HDL after the VLDL are secreted by the liver.

ApoA-V modulates plasma triglyceride levels, possibly by several mechanisms: inhibition of hepatic VLDL triglyceride production and secretion, promoting LPL-mediated hydrolysis of chylomicrons and VLDL triglycerides, and facilitating hepatic uptake of triglyceride-rich lipoproteins and their remnants (Wong and Ryan, 2007). ApoA-V is produced solely by the liver, and despite its very low plasma concentration (~0.1% of the concentration of apoA-I), profoundly affects plasma triglyceride levels in mice and humans.

Without MTP, hepatic triglycerides cannot be transferred to apoB-100. As a consequence, patients with dysfunctional MTP fail to make any of the apoB-containing lipoproteins (VLDL, IDL, or LDL). MTP also plays a key role in the synthesis of chylomicrons in the intestine, and mutations of MTP that result in the inability of triglycerides to be transferred to either apoB-100 in the liver or apoB-48 in the intestine prevent VLDL and chylomicron production and cause the genetic disorder abetalipoproteinemia. Experimental compounds that interfere with MTP function reduce triglyceride levels but cause hepatic steatosis that has precluded their use in humans. New approaches to MTP inhibition are under study (Hussain and Bakillah, 2008).

Plasma VLDL is then catabolized by LPL in the capillary beds in a process similar to the lipolytic processing of chylomicrons (Figure 31–1). When triglyceride hydrolysis is nearly complete, the VLDL remnants, usually termed IDL, are released from the capillary endothelium and reenter the circulation. ApoB-100 containing small VLDL and IDL (VLDL remnants), which have a $t_{1/2}$ <30 minutes, have two potential fates. About 40-60% are cleared from the plasma by the liver via interaction with LDL receptors and LRP, which recognize ligands (apoB-100 and apoE) on the remnants. LPL and HL convert the remainder of the IDL to LDL by removal of additional triglycerides. The C apoproteins, apoE, and apoA-V redistribute to HDL. *Virtually all LDL particles in the plasma are derived from VLDL.*

ApoE plays a major role in the metabolism of triglyceride-rich lipoproteins (chylomicrons, chylomicron remnants, VLDL, and IDL). About half of the apoE in the plasma of fasting subjects is associated with triglyceride-rich lipoproteins, and the other half is a constituent of HDL. About three-fourths of the apoE in plasma is synthesized by the liver; brain and macrophages synthesize the bulk of the remainder. In transgenic mice, overexpression of apoE by macrophages inhibits hypercholesterolemia-induced atherogenesis. Three alleles of the apoE gene (designated ε2, ε3, and ε4) occur with a frequency of ~8%, 77%, and 15%, respectively, and code for the three major forms of apoE: E2, E3, and E4. Consequently, there are three homozygous apoE phenotypes (E2/2, E3/3, and E4/4) and three heterozygous phenotypes (E2/3, E2/4, and E3/4). Approximately 60% of the human population is homozygous for apoE3. Single amino acid substitutions result from genetic polymorphisms in the apoE gene. ApoE2, with a cysteine at residue 158, differs from apoE3, which has arginine at this site. ApoE3, with a cysteine at residue 112, differs from apoE4, which has arginine at this site. These single amino acid differences affect both receptor binding and lipid binding of the three apoE isoforms. Both apoE3 and apoE4 can bind to the LDL receptor, but apoE2 binds much less effectively, and as a consequence causes the remnant lipoprotein dyslipidemia of type III hyperlipoproteinemia.

Low-Density Lipoproteins. Virtually all of the LDL particles in the circulation are derived from VLDL. The LDL particles have a $t_{1/2}$ of 1.5-2 days, which accounts for the higher plasma concentration of LDL than of VLDL and IDL. In subjects without hypertriglyceridemia, two-thirds of plasma cholesterol is found in the LDL.

Plasma clearance of LDL particles is mediated primarily by LDL receptors; a small component is mediated by nonreceptor clearance mechanisms. The most common cause of autosomal dominant hypercholesterolemia involves mutations of the LDL receptor gene.

More than 900 mutations of the LDL receptor gene have been identified in association with defective or absent LDL receptors that cause high levels of plasma LDL and familial hypercholesterolemia.

ApoB-100, the primary apoprotein of LDL, is the ligand that binds LDL to its receptor. Residues 3000-3700 in the carboxyl-terminal sequence are critical for binding. Mutations in this region disrupt binding and also are a cause of autosomal dominant hypercholesterolemia (familial defective apoB-100). A third disorder causing autosomal dominant hypercholesterolemia is caused by gain of function mutations in the gene encoding PCSK9, a serine protease that destroys LDL receptors in the liver (Horton et al., 2007). Autosomal recessive hypercholesterolemia closely resembles familial hypercholesterolemia but is not caused by LDL receptor mutations.

The liver expresses a large complement of LDL receptors and removes ~75% of all LDL from the plasma. Consequently, manipulation of hepatic LDL receptor gene expression is a most effective way to modulate plasma LDL-C levels. Thyroxine and estrogen enhance LDL receptor gene expression, which explains their LDL-C–lowering effects.

The most effective dietary alteration (decreased consumption of saturated fat and cholesterol) and pharmacological treatment (statins) for hypercholesterolemia act by enhancing hepatic LDL receptor expression. Regulation of LDL receptor expression is part of a complex process by which cells regulate their free cholesterol content. This regulatory process is mediated by transcription factors called *sterol regulatory element binding proteins* (SREBPs) and SREBP *cleavage activating protein* (Scap) (Radhakrishnan et al., 2008). Scap is both a sensor of cholesterol content in the endoplasmic reticulum (ER) and an escort of SREBPs from the ER to the Golgi apparatus. In the Golgi apparatus, SREBPs undergo proteolytic cleavage, and a dimer of the amino-terminal domain, transported by importin β, translocates to the nucleus, where it activates expression of the LDL receptor gene and of other genes encoding enzymes involved in cholesterol biosynthesis. Increased ER cholesterol content binds Scap, precluding Scap from escorting SREBP to the Golgi apparatus for processing and ultimately from reaching the nucleus.

LDL becomes atherogenic when modified by oxidation (Witztum and Steinberg, 2001), a required step for LDL uptake by the scavenger receptors of macrophages. This process leads to foam-cell formation in arterial lesions. At least two scavenger receptors (SRs) are involved (SR-AI/II and CD36). Knocking out either receptor in transgenic mice retards the uptake of oxidized LDL by macrophages. Expression of the two receptors is regulated differently: SR-AI/II appears to be expressed more in early atherogenesis, and CD36 expression is greater as foam cells form during lesion progression. Despite the large body of evidence implicating oxidation of LDL as a requisite step during atherogenesis, controlled clinical trials have not unequivocally demonstrated the efficacy of antioxidant vitamins in preventing vascular disease.

High-Density Lipoproteins. The metabolism of HDL is complex because of the multiple mechanisms by which HDL particles are modified in the plasma compartment. ApoA-I is the major HDL apoprotein, and its plasma concentration is a more powerful inverse predictor of CHD risk than is the HDL-C level (Mahley et al., 2008). ApoA-I synthesis is required for normal production of HDL. Mutations in the apoA-I gene that cause HDL deficiency are variable in their clinical expression and often are associated with accelerated atherogenesis. Conversely, overexpression of apoA-I in transgenic mice protects against experimentally induced atherogenesis.

Mature HDL can be separated by ultracentrifugation into HDL_2 (d = 1.063-1.125 g/mL), which are larger, more cholesterol-rich lipoproteins (70-100 Å in diameter), and HDL_3 (d = 1.125-1.21 g/mL), which are smaller particles (50-70 Å in diameter). In addition, two major subclasses of mature HDL particles in the plasma can be differentiated by their content of the major HDL apoproteins, apoA-I and apoA-II (Movva and Rader, 2008). Epidemiologic evidence in humans suggests that apoA-II may be atheroprotective (Birjmohun et al., 2007; Movva and Rader, 2008).

Lipoprotein particles may be distinguished by their electrophoretic mobities: mature HDL particles have α mobility; LDL particles show β mobility. The precursor of most of the α-migrating plasma HDL is a discoidal particle containing apoA-I and phospholipid, called pre-β1 HDL because of its pre-β1 electrophoretic mobility. Pre-β1 HDL are synthesized by the liver and the intestine, and they also arise when surface phospholipids and apoA-I of chylomicrons and VLDL are lost as the triglycerides of these lipoproteins are hydrolyzed. Discoidal pre-β1 HDL can then acquire free unesterified cholesterol from the cell membranes of tissues, such as arterial wall macrophages. Two macrophage membrane transporters, ABCA1 and ABCG1, promote the efflux of cholesterol from macrophages of humans studied *in vivo*. Prior studies in vitro suggested that another transport protein, class B, type I scavenger receptor (SR-BI) facilitates cholesterol egress from macrophages to HDL, but *in vivo* studies in humans do not support an important role for SR-BI in this process (Wang et al., 2007). However, SR-BI in the liver facilitates the uptake of cholesteryl esters from HDL without internalizing and degrading the lipoproteins.

The membrane transporter ABCA1 facilitates the transfer of free cholesterol from cells to HDL (Attie, 2007). When ABCA1 is defective, the acquisition of cholesterol by HDL is greatly diminished, and HDL levels are markedly reduced because poorly lipidated nascent HDL are metabolized rapidly. Loss-of-function mutations of ABCA1 cause the defect observed in

Tangier disease, a genetic disorder characterized by extremely low levels of HDL and cholesterol accumulation in the liver, spleen, tonsils, and neurons of peripheral nerves. Transgenic animals overexpressing ABCA1 in the liver and macrophages have elevated plasma levels of HDL and apoA-I and reduced susceptibility to atherosclerosis (Van Eck et al., 2006).

After free cholesterol is acquired by the pre-β1 HDL, it is esterified by lecithin:cholesterol acyltransferase. The newly esterified and nonpolar cholesterol moves into the core of the discoidal HDL. As the cholesteryl ester content increases, the HDL particle becomes spherical and less dense. These newly formed spherical HDL particles (HDL_3) further enlarge by accepting more free cholesterol, which is in turn esterified by lecithin:cholesterol acyltransferase. In this way, HDL_3 are converted to HDL_2, which are larger and less dense than HDL_3.

As the cholesteryl ester content of the HDL_2 increases, the cholesteryl esters of these particles begin to be exchanged for triglycerides derived from any of the triglyceride-containing lipoproteins (chylomicrons, VLDL, remnant lipoproteins, and LDL). This exchange is mediated by the cholesteryl ester transfer protein (CETP), and in humans accounts for the removal of about two-thirds of the cholesterol associated with HDL. The transferred cholesterol subsequently is metabolized as part of the lipoprotein into which it was transferred. Treatments that target CETP and the ABC transporters have yielded equivocal results in humans. While CETP inhibitors effectively reduce LDL, they also appear to paradoxically increase the frequency of adverse cardiovascular events (angina, revascularization, myocardial infarction, heart failure, and death) (Tall, 2007; Tall et al, 2008).

The triglyceride that is transferred into HDL_2 is hydrolyzed in the liver by HL, a process that regenerates smaller, spherical HDL_3 particles that recirculate and acquire additional free cholesterol from tissues containing excess free cholesterol. HL activity is regulated and modulates HDL-C levels. Both androgens and estrogens affect HL gene expression, but with opposite effects. Androgens increase HL activity, which accounts for the lower HDL-C values observed in men than in women. Estrogens reduce HL activity, but their impact on HDL-C levels in women is substantially less than that of androgens on HDL-C levels in men. HL appears to have a pivotal role in regulating HDLC levels, as HL activity is increased in many patients with low HDL-C levels.

HDL are protective lipoproteins that decrease the risk of CHD; thus, high levels of HDL are desirable. This protective effect may result from the participation of HDL in reverse cholesterol transport, the process by which excess cholesterol is acquired from cells and transferred to the liver for excretion. HDL also may protect against atherogenesis by mechanisms not directly related to reverse cholesterol transport. These functions include putative anti-inflammatory, antioxidative, platelet anti-aggregatory, anticoagulant, and profibrinolytic activities (deGoma et al., 2008).

Lipoprotein(a). Lipoprotein(a) [Lp(a)] is composed of an LDL particle that has a second apoprotein in addition to apoB-100 (Mahley et al., 2008). The second apoprotein, apo(a), is attached to apoB-100 by at least one disulfide bond and does not function as a lipid-binding apoprotein. Apo(a) of Lp(a) is structurally related to plasminogen and appears to be atherogenic by interfering with fibrinolysis of thrombi on the surfaces of plaques.

HYPERLIPIDEMIA AND ATHEROSCLEROSIS

Despite a 59% decline in the death rate from CHD between 1950 and 1999, deaths from CVD accounted for 36.3% of the 2.4 million deaths in the U.S. during 2004. Most of these deaths were caused by atherosclerosis, which is responsible for more deaths than cancer, accidents, chronic lung disease, and diabetes combined. Two-thirds of atherosclerosis deaths were due to CHD. About 82% of CHD deaths occurred in individuals >65 years of age. Among the 18% dying prematurely (<65 years), 80% died during their first CHD event. Among those dying of sudden cardiac death, 50% of the men and 64% of the women had previously been asymptomatic (American Heart Association, 2003).

These statistics illustrate the importance of identifying and managing risk factors for CHD. *The major conventional risk factors are elevated LDL-C, reduced HDL-C, cigarette smoking, hypertension, type 2 diabetes mellitus, advancing age, and a family history of premature CHD events (men <55 years; women <65 years) in a first-degree relative.* Control of the modifiable risk factors is especially important in preventing premature CHD. Observational studies suggest that modifiable risk factors account for 85% of excess risk (risk over and above that of individuals with optimal risk-factor profiles) for premature CHD. The presence of one or more conventional risk factors in 90% of patients with CHD belies claims that a large percentage of CHD is not attributable to conventional risk factors. When total cholesterol levels are below 160 mg/dL, CHD risk is markedly attenuated, even in the presence of additional risk factors. This pivotal role of hypercholesterolemia in atherogenesis gave rise to the almost universally accepted cholesterol-diet-CHD hypothesis: elevated plasma cholesterol levels cause CHD; diets rich in saturated (animal) fat and cholesterol raise cholesterol levels; and lowering cholesterol levels reduces CHD risk. Although the relationship between cholesterol, diet, and CHD was recognized nearly 50 years ago, proof that cholesterol lowering was safe and prevented CHD death required extensive epidemiological studies and clinical trials.

Epidemiological Studies. Epidemiological studies have demonstrated the importance of the relationship between excess saturated fat consumption and elevated cholesterol levels. Reducing the consumption of dietary saturated fat and cholesterol is the cornerstone of population-based approaches to the management of hypercholesterolemia. In addition, it is clearly established that the higher the cholesterol level, the higher the CHD risk. However, very high cholesterol levels (values >300 mg/dL) account for only 5-10% of CHD events. In fact, one-third of CHD events occur in persons with total cholesterol levels between 150 and 200 mg/dL (Castelli, 2001). The challenge is how to identify and treat the 20% of individuals with cholesterol levels between 150 and 200 mg/dL who will develop CHD.

Clinical Trials. Studies of the efficacy of cholesterol lowering began in the 1960s, and the results of the earliest trials showed that modest reductions in total cholesterol and LDL-C were associated with reductions in fatal and nonfatal CHD events but not total mortality. It was not until the advent of a more efficacious class of cholesterol-lowering drugs, the statins, that cholesterol-reduction therapy was finally proven to prevent CHD events and reduce total mortality. Patients benefit regardless of gender, age (above or below 75 years of age), baseline lipid values, or whether they have a prior history of vascular disease or type 2 diabetes mellitus (Cholesterol Treatment Trialists' Collaborators, 2008; Cholesterol Treatment Trialists' Collaborators, 2005). Stroke risk is reduced by statin therapy, too, despite the rather weak relationship between total cholesterol and LDL-C levels. Statin therapy is effective in preventing first and subsequent atherothrombotic strokes. Evidence of a benefit or harm of statin therapy in patients with a prior hemorrhagic stroke is sparse and requires additional studies. Available studies suggest caution when considering statin therapy for a patient with hemorrhagic stroke (Amarenco and Labreuche, 2009).

Results of the clinical trials employing statins demonstrate benefit without offsetting adverse effects, and the benefit is proportionate to the extent of the reduction of LDL-C level. Moderate doses of statins that lower LDL-C levels by about 40% reduce cardiovascular events by about one-third (Cholesterol Treatment Trialists' Collaborators, 2005). More intensive regimens that lower LDL-C by 45-50% reduce CVD events by as much as 50% (Cannon et al., 2006).

National Cholesterol Education Program (NCEP) Guidelines for Assessing Risk

The existing NCEP Adult Treatment Panel (ATP) III guidelines were formulated in 2001 and updated in 2004 (Grundy et al., 2004b). The key features of the update include abandoning the concept of a threshold LDL-C level that must be exceeded before initiating cholesterol-lowering drug therapy in CHD or CHD equivalent patients; adopting a new target LDL-C level (<70 mg/dL) for very high-risk patients; and employing a "standard statin dose" (a dosage sufficient to lower LDL-C by 30-40%) as a minimum therapy when initiating cholesterol-lowering therapy with statins (Grundy et al., 2004b) (Table 31–3). Subsequently, new information from clinical trials and new information about risk assessment has led to a need for a new revision, ATP IV, which is currently in progress. The new ATP IV guidelines are expected to be published in 2010. Revisions that are likely to be included in the ATP IV guidelines are described in the following discussion.

Risk Assessment. The intensity of treatment of dyslipidemia is based on the severity of a patient's risk. The risk of sustaining a heart attack or stroke or of developing heart failure in the U.S. is striking. Before death, two-thirds of men and one-half of all women will be affected (Lloyd-Jones et al., 2009). Because of this very high prevalence, it is important that all adults ≥20 years and high-risk children undergo an assessment of their risk of developing CVD (Daniels et al., 2008; The Expert Panel, 2002).

Patients at greatest risk of developing an atherothrombotic CVD event are those who have had a prior event (myocardial infarction, acute coronary syndrome, transient ischemic attack, stroke, or claudication) or who are at high risk because of type 2 diabetes mellitus. These subjects are at very high risk and require intensive management of plasma lipids (Table 31–3). Other subjects who have not had a prior CVD event require assessment of plasma lipid levels and the other major CVD risk factors to determine if treatment to reduce lipid-related risk is necessary.

Lipid levels (total cholesterol, triglycerides, LDL-C, HDL-C, and non-HDL-C) and glucose concentration should be measured following a fasting period of 10-12 hours. The LDL-C should be calculated [total cholesterol – (HDL-C) – (triglycerides/5) = LDL-C] and not measured by any of the "direct" techniques (Mora et al., 2009). Non-HDL-C is derived as follows: total cholesterol – HDL-C = non-HDL-C. The classification of plasma lipid values is shown in Table 31–4.

Measurement of apoA-I and apoB afford better risk prediction of lipid-related risk than LDL-C and HDL-C. However, lack of an established national reference laboratory for quality control of these apolipoprotein assays has precluded formal adoption of apoA-I and apoB measurements by the NCEP thus far (Contois et al., 2009; Sniderman, 2009; Sniderman and Marcovina, 2006). Despite this, targets for apoB levels have been established by the American Diabetes Association for the management of patients with type 2 diabetes mellitus (Brunzell et al., 2008).

Measurements of lipoprotein fraction concentrations, their subfractions, and lipoprotein particle diameters also are widely available, but it is not clear that these tests add to the ability to predict risk

Table 31–3

Treatment Based on LDL-C Levels (2004 Revision of NCEP Adult Treatment Panel III Guidelines)

RISK CATEGORY	LDL-C GOAL (mg/dL)	NON-HDL-C GOAL (mg/dL)	THERAPEUTIC LIFESTYLE CHANGE	THRESHOLD FOR DRUG THERAPY (mg/dL)
Very high risk Atherosclerosis-induced CHD plus one of: • multiple risk factors • diabetes mellitus • a poorly controlled single factor • acute coronary syndrome • metabolic syndrome	<70[a]	<100	No threshold (initiate change)	No threshold (initiate therapy)
High risk CHD or CHD equivalent	<100[a]	<130	No threshold	No threshold
Moderately high risk 2+ risk factors 10-year risk: <10–20%	<130 (optional <100)	<160	No threshold	≥130 (100-129)[b]
Moderate risk 2+ risk factors 10-year risk <10%	<130	<160	No threshold	>160
0–1 risk factor	<160	<160	No threshold	≥190 (optional: 160–189)[c]

[a]If pretreatment LDL-C is near or below LDL-C goal value, then a statin dose sufficient to lower LDL-C by 30-40% should be prescribed.
[b]Patients in this category include those with a 10-year risk of 10-20% and one of the following: age >60 years, three or more risk factors, a severe risk factor, triglycerides >200 mg/dL and HDL-C <40 mg/dL, metabolic syndrome, highly sensitive C-reactive protein (CRP) >3 mg/L, and coronary calcium score (age/gender adjusted) >75th percentile.
[c]Patients include those with any severe single risk factor, multiple major risk factors, 10-year risk >8%.
After attaining the LDL-C goal, additional therapy may be necessary to reach the non-HDL-C goal. CHD, coronary heart disease; CHD equivalent, peripheral vascular disease, abdominal aortic aneurysm, symptomatic carotid artery disease, >20% 10-year CHD risk, or diabetes mellitus; HDL-C, high-density-lipoprotein cholesterol; LDL-C, low-density-lipoprotein cholesterol; NCEP, National Cholesterol Education Program.

based on measurements of levels of cholesterol or apoA-I and apoB (Mora, 2009).

In addition to plasma lipid levels and a fasting glucose level, each subject requires an evaluation to assess the presence or absence of the other major CVD risk factors: age, a family history of premature CVD event, smoking, hypertension, type 2 diabetes mellitus, and obesity (Table 31–5). There are a host of additional novel risk factors that are being evaluated to determine if they will improve current risk prediction assessment schemes based on lipid levels and the established major CVD risk factors (Table 31–5). Thus far, routine use of any of these novel risk factors has not been shown to improve risk prediction (Folsom et al., 2006; Lloyd-Jones and Tian, 2006). However, in certain primary prevention patients, two of the recently described risk factors, C-reactive protein (CRP) and assessment of the extent of coronary calcification, may improve risk assessment beyond that based on the traditional major risk factors (Tables 31–3 and 31–5).

Using the values for levels of total cholesterol and HDL-C and the results of the assessment for the other major CHD risk factors, the next step is to calculate a person's risk of having a CHD event over the next 10 years. Risk prediction tables based on observational studies conducted by the Framingham Heart Study are used to calculate this 10-year risk. This approach to risk assessment was adopted by the NCEP, but in the 2001 ATP III guidelines, the risk prediction model predicted only the 10-year risk of having a fatal or nonfatal myocardial infarction. However, the same risk factors that are associated with development of myocardial infarction also promote other CVD events, including stroke, transient ischemic attack, peripheral vascular disease, and heart failure. Furthermore, many patients who develop acute coronary syndrome do not sustain a myocardial infarction because of thrombolytic therapy and revascularization procedures (angioplasty and bypass graft surgery). Because cholesterol-lowering therapy is beneficial to prevent CVD events in patients with any of these manifestations of CVD, it became apparent that it would be useful for primary care physicians to be able to predict a patient's risk of developing any one of these manifestations of CVD, not just CHD. New general CVD 10-year risk prediction tables are now available from the Framingham Heart Study (D'Agostino et al., 2008; Wickramasinghe et al., 2009) (Table 31–6). Ten-year risk calculated with the general CVD tables will exceed 10-year risk calculated using the CHD tables from the ATP III guidelines.

Table 31–4

Classification of Plasma Lipid Levels (mg/dL)[a]

Total cholesterol	
<200	Desirable
200-239	Borderline high
≥240	High
HDL-C	
<40	Low (consider <50 mg/dL as low for women)
>60	High
LDL-C	
<70	Optimal for very high risk (minimal goal for CHD equivalent patients)
<100	Optimal
100-129	Near optimal
130-159	Borderline high
160-189	High
≥190	Very high
Triglycerides	
<150	Normal
150-199	Borderline high
200-499	High
≥500	Very high

[a]2001 National Cholesterol Education Program guidelines. HDL-C, high-density-lipoprotein cholesterol; LDL-C, low-density-lipoprotein cholesterol. From The Expert Panel, 2002.

Table 31–5

Risk Factors for Coronary Heart Disease[a]

Age
Male >45 years of age or female >55 years of age
Family history of premature CHD
A first-degree relative (male <55 years of age or female <65 years of age when the first CHD clinical event occurs)
Current cigarette smoking
Defined as smoking within the preceding 30 days
Hypertension
Blood pressure ≥140/90 or use of antihypertensive medication, irrespective of blood pressure
Low HDL-C
<40 mg/dL (consider <50 mg/dL as "low" for women)
Obesity[b]
Body mass index >25 kg/m^2 and waist circumference >40 inches (men) or >35 inches (women)
Type 2 diabetes mellitus

[a]Diabetes mellitus is considered to be a CHD-equivalent disorder; therefore, the lipid management of diabetes patients is the same as that for patients with established vascular disease (American Diabetes Association, 1999).

[b]Obesity was returned to the list of CHD risk factors in 1998, although it was not included as a risk factor in the 2001 NCEP guidelines (Pi-Sunyer et al., 1998). CHD, coronary heart disease; HDL-C, high-density-lipoprotein cholesterol. From The Expert Panel, 2002.

Once the 10-year risk has been calculated, the patient's category of risk can be assigned using Table 31–3. This establishes treatment goals for LDL-C and non-HDL-C as well as thresholds for initiating drug therapy. Because CVD, diabetes mellitus, and obesity are so prevalent, diet and exercise assessment and advice are appropriate for everyone and should not depend on an arbitrary threshold value for LDL-C for implementation. Ten-year risk assessment is recognized as the guideline-mandated method for managing dyslipidemia. Unfortunately, only about 50% of physicians correctly assess their patient's risk, and 30% of adults nationwide are not being screened (Christian et al., 2006; Kuklina et al., 2009). Many high-risk patients are not being recognized and treated prior to developing clinical CHD. Among the nearly 75,000 patients admitted to 541 U.S. hospitals between 2000 and 2006 with first-ever episodes of acute coronary syndrome, only 14% were taking a cholesterol-lowering drug (Sachdeva et al., 2009).

NCEP Guidelines for Treatment: Managing Patients with Dyslipidemia

Current NCEP guidelines focus on identifying levels of risk factors associated with increased risk of a CHD event. Primary prevention involves management of risk factors to prevent a first-ever CHD event. Secondary prevention patients are those who have had a prior CHD event and whose risk factors are treated most aggressively. Recently, the concept of primordial prevention has been applied to CHD prevention (Lloyd-Jones et al., 2010). The strategy is to prevent the development of risk factors rather than treating already established risk factors. Primordial prevention is a population-based approach that targets smoking, weight management, physical activity, healthy eating habits, cholesterol and glucose levels, and blood pressure. Goals for each of these risk factors have been set for adults and children. Including children is important because adverse health behaviors are learned in childhood (Lloyd-Jones et al., 2010).

The primordial prevention guidelines include 150 minutes/week of moderate-intensity exercise (walking 20-30 minutes/day. Dietary recommendations

Table 31–6

Assessing 10-Year Risk of CVD Events[a]

MEN

RISK FACTORS AND CVD POINTS

POINTS	AGE	HDL (mg/dL)	TOTAL CHOLESTEROL (mg/dL)	SBP NOT TREATED (mm Hg)	SBP TREATED (mm Hg)	SMOKER	DIABETIC
–2		60+		<120			
–1		50-59			0		
0	30-34	45-49	<160	120-129	<120	No	No
1		35-44	160-199	130-139			
2	35-39	<35	200-239	140-159	120-129		
3			240-279	160+	130-139		Yes
4			280+		140-159	Yes	
5	40-44				160+		
6	45-49						
7							
8	50-54						
9							
10	55-59						
11	60-64						
12	65-69						
13							
14	70-74						
15	75+						

ESTIMATED CVD RISK

POINTS	RISK	POINTS	RISK	POINTS	RISK
≤–3	<1%	5	3.9%	13	15.6%
–2	1.1%	6	4.7%	14	18.4%
–1	1.4%	7	5.6%	15	21.6%
0	1.6%	8	6.7%	16	25.3%
1	1.9%	9	7.9%	17	29.4%
2	2.3%	10	9.4%	18+	>30%
3	2.8%	11	11.2%		
4	3.3%	12	13.2%		

(Continued)

include reducing total calories from fat to <30% and saturated fat to <7% to avoid trans fat; consuming <300 mg of cholesterol/day, a variety of oily fish twice a week or more often, and oils/foods rich in α-linolenic acid (canola, flaxseed, and soybean oils; flaxseed; and walnuts); and restricting sugary beverages to <36 oz/week for a person consuming 2000 Kcal daily.

The patient-based approach to manage dyslipidemia is designed for primary and secondary prevention, requires a risk assessment as described earlier (Table 31–6), and focuses on lowering LDL-C and non-HDL-C (Grundy et al., 2004b). Non-lipid risk factors, if present, should be treated appropriately (Table 31–5). For patients with elevated levels of total cholesterol, non-HDL-C, LDL-C, or triglycerides, or reduced HDL-C values, further treatment is based on the patient's risk-factor status (Table 31–5), LDL-C and non-HDL-C levels (Table 31–3), and calculation of the general CHD Framingham risk score (Table 31–6) of primary prevention patients with two or more risk factors.

All patients who meet the criteria for lipid-lowering therapy should receive instruction about therapeutic lifestyle change. Dietary

Table 31–6

Assessing 10-Year Risk of CVD Events[a] (*continued*)

WOMEN

RISK FACTORS AND CVD POINTS

POINTS	AGE	HDL (mg/dL)	TOTAL CHOLESTEROL (mg/dL)	SBP NOT TREATED (mm Hg)	SBP TREATED (mm Hg)	SMOKER	DIABETIC
≤ −3				<120			
−2		60+					
−1		50-59			<120		
0	30-34	45-49	<160	120-129		No	No
1		35-44	160-199	130-139			
2	35-39	<35		140-149	120-129		
3			200-239		130-139	Yes	
4	40-44		240-279	150-159			Yes
5	45-49		280+	160+	140-149		
6					150-159		
7	50-54				160+		
8	55-59						
9	60-64						
10	65-69						
11	70-74						
12	75+						

ESTIMATED CVD RISK

POINTS	RISK	POINTS	RISK	POINTS	RISK
≤−2	<1%	6	3.3%	14	11.7%
−1	1.0%	7	3.9%	15	13.7%
0	1.2%	8	4.5%	16	15.9%
1	1.5%	9	5.3%	17	18.5%
2	1.7%	10	6.3%	18	21.5%
3	2.0%	11	7.3%	19	24.8%
4	2.4%	12	8.6%	20	28.5%
5	2.8%	13	10.0%	21+	>30%

[a]D'Agostino *et al.*, 2008. CVD, cardiovascular disease; HDL, high-density lipoproteins; SBP, systolic blood pressure.
Reproduced, with permission, from D'Agostino RB Sr, Vasan RS, Pencina MJ et al. General cardiovascular risk profile for use in primary care: The Framingham Heart Study. *Circulation*, **2008**, *117*:743–753.

restrictions include <7% of calories from saturated and trans fatty acids, <200 mg of cholesterol daily, up to 20% of calories from monounsaturated fatty acids, up to 10% of calories from polyunsaturated fat, and total fat calories ranging between 25% and 35% of all calories. Two oily fish meals/week are especially important for post–myocardial infarction patients to provide a substantial reduction in the risk of sudden cardiac death. Patients with CHD or a CHD equivalent (symptomatic peripheral or carotid vascular disease, abdominal aortic aneurysm, >20% 10-year CHD risk, or diabetes mellitus) should immediately start appropriate lipid-lowering drug therapy irrespective of their baseline LDL-C level. Patients without CHD or CHD equivalent should be managed with lifestyle advice (diet, exercise, weight management) for 3-6 months before drug therapy is implemented.

Before drug therapy is initiated, secondary causes of hyperlipidemia should be excluded. Most secondary causes (Table 31–7) can be excluded by ascertaining the patient's medication history and by measuring serum creatinine, liver function tests, fasting glucose, and thyroid-stimulating hormone levels. Treatment of the disorder causing secondary dyslipidemia may preclude the necessity of treatment with hypolipidemic drugs.

Arterial Wall Biology and Plaque Stability

More effective lipid-lowering agents and a better understanding of atherogenesis have helped to prove that

Table 31–7

Secondary Causes of Dyslipidemia

DISORDER	MAJOR LIPID EFFECT
Diabetes mellitus	Triglycerides > cholesterol; low HDL-C
Nephrotic syndrome	Triglycerides usually > cholesterol
Alcohol use	Triglycerides > cholesterol
Contraceptive use	Triglycerides > cholesterol
Estrogen use	Triglycerides > cholesterol
Glucocorticoid excess	Triglycerides > cholesterol
Hypothyroidism	Cholesterol > triglycerides
Obstructive liver disease	Cholesterol > triglycerides

HDL-C, high-density-lipoprotein cholesterol.

aggressive lipid-lowering therapy has beneficial effects beyond those obtained by simply decreasing lipid deposition in the arterial wall. Aggressive lipid lowering results only in very small increases in lumen diameter but promptly decreases acute coronary events (Cannon et al., 2004). Lesions causing <60% occlusion are responsible for more than two-thirds of the acute events. Aggressive lipid-lowering therapy may prevent acute events through positive effects on the arterial wall; it corrects endothelial dysfunction, corrects abnormal vascular reactivity (spasm), and increases plaque stability.

Atherosclerotic lesions containing a large lipid core, large numbers of macrophages, and a poorly formed fibrous cap are prone to plaque rupture and acute thrombosis. Aggressive lipid lowering appears to alter plaque architecture, resulting in less lipid, fewer macrophages, and a larger collagen and smooth muscle cell–rich fibrous cap. Stabilization of plaque susceptibility to thrombosis appears to be a direct result of LDL-C lowering or an indirect result of changes in cholesterol and lipoprotein metabolism or arterial wall biology (see "Potential Cardioprotective Effects Other Than LDL Lowering,"later in the chapter).

Whom and When to Treat?

Large-scale trials with statins have provided new insights into which patients with dyslipidemia should be treated and when treatment should be initiated.

Gender. Both men and women with or without a prior vascular disease event benefit from lipid-lowering therapy (Heart Protection Study Collaborative Group, 2002; Ridker et al., 2008). Statins, rather than hormone-replacement therapy, now are the recommended first-line drug therapy for lowering lipids and preventing CHD events in postmenopausal women. This recommendation reflects the increased CHD morbidity in older women with established CHD who were treated with hormone-replacement therapy (see Chapter 40).

Age. Age >45 years in men and >55 years in women is considered to be a CHD risk factor. The statin trials have shown that patients >65 years of age benefit from therapy as much as do younger patients. In fact, in those >70 years, the reduction of absolute mortality is stunning compared with individuals 55 years of age (Afilalo et al., 2008; Diamond and Kaul, 2008). Old age *per se* is not a reason to refrain from initiating drug therapy in an otherwise healthy person.

Cerebrovascular Disease Patients. In most observational studies, plasma cholesterol levels correlate positively with the risk of ischemic stroke. In clinical trials, statins reduced stroke and transient ischemic attacks in patients with and without CHD (Amarenco and Labreuche, 2009).

Peripheral Vascular Disease Patients. Statins prevent CHD events and may improve walking distance in patients with peripheral vascular disease (Aung et al., 2007).

Hypertensive Patients and Smokers. The relative risk reduction for coronary events in statin trials of hypertensive patients is similar to that in subjects without hypertension (Franz et al., 2008). Relative risk is reduced more in smokers in statin clinical trials than in nonsmokers (Cheung et al., 2004).

Type 2 Diabetes Mellitus. Patients with type 2 diabetes benefit very significantly from aggressive lipid lowering (see "Treatment of Type 2 Diabetes Patients," later in the chapter) (Cholesterol Treatment Trialists' Collaborators, 2008; Heart Protection Study Collaborative Group, 2003).

Post–Myocardial Infarction or Revascularization Patients. As soon as CHD is diagnosed, it is essential to begin lipid-lowering therapy (NCEP guidelines: LDL-C goal <70 mg/dL for very high-risk patients) (Grundy et al., 2004b). Compliance with drug therapy is greatly enhanced if treatment is initiated in the hospital. Statin therapy administered prior to angioplasty reduces the requirement for procedures related to myocardial infarction risk and the need for repeat revascularization (Ebrahimi et al., 2008; Zhang et al. 2010). Statin therapy also improves the long-term outcome after bypass surgery.

Can Cholesterol Levels Be Lowered Too Much? Are there total and LDL cholesterol levels below which adverse health consequences begin to increase? Observational studies initially were confusing. In the U.S. and western Europe, low cholesterol levels were associated with an increase in noncardiac mortality from chronic pulmonary disease, chronic liver disease, cancer (many primary sites), and hemorrhagic stroke; subsequent data indicate that it is the noncardiac diseases that cause the low plasma cholesterol levels and not the reverse. One exception may be hemorrhagic stroke. In the Multiple Risk Factor Intervention Trial (MRFIT), hemorrhagic stroke occurred more frequently in hypertensive patients with total cholesterol levels <160 mg/dL; however, the increased incidence of hemorrhagic stroke was more than offset by reduced CHD risk due to the low cholesterol levels. A recent meta-analysis of statin efficacy in preventing recurrent stroke found an increase in the risk of subsequent hemorrhagic stroke among patients with a prior hemorrhagic stroke who also received a statin. However, the risk of atherothrombotic stroke was reduced in proportion to the degree of cholesterol lowering by statin therapy (Amarenco and Labreuche, 2009).

Abetalipoproteinemia and hypobetalipoproteinemia, two rare disorders associated with extremely low total cholesterol levels, are instructive because affected individuals have reduced CHD risk and no increase in noncardiac mortality. Patients who are homozygous for the mutations that cause these disorders have total cholesterol levels <50 mg/dL and triglyceride levels <25 mg/dL. With the advent of more efficacious cholesterol-lowering agents, it has been possible to test the benefits and risks of lowering LDL-C levels <50 mg/dL (Ridker et al., 2008). Lower LDL-C levels translate into greater reductions in clinical events without any increase in adverse events.

Treatment of Type 2 Diabetes Patients

Diabetes mellitus is an independent predictor of high risk for CHD. CHD morbidity is two to four times higher in patients with diabetes than in nondiabetics. Glucose control is essential but provides only minimal benefit with respect to CHD prevention. Aggressive treatment of diabetic dyslipidemia through diet, weight control, and drugs is critical in reducing risk.

Diabetic dyslipidemia usually is characterized by high triglycerides, low HDL-C, and moderate elevations of total cholesterol and LDL-C. In fact, diabetics without diagnosed CHD have the same level of risk as nondiabetics with established CHD. Thus, the dyslipidemia treatment guidelines for diabetic patients are the same as for patients with CHD, irrespective of whether the diabetic patient has had a CHD event (The Expert Panel, 2002). The American Diabetes Association recommends new lipid therapy targets for diabetics. In addition to targets for LDL-C and non-HDL-C, two targets for total plasma apoB were established based on the level of CVD risk (Brunzell et al., 2008).

Clinical trials with statins have clearly established that total and vascular disease mortality are reduced in diabetics as a consequence of prevention of CVD events (Cholesterol Treatment Trialists' Collaborators, 2008). A recently completed trial comparing statin therapy to statin plus fenofibrate therapy will provide the first outcome data for statin plus fibrate combination therapy in type 2 diabetes patients (Ginsberg et al., 2007).

Metabolic Syndrome

There is an increased CHD risk associated with the insulin-resistant, prediabetic state described under the rubric of "metabolic syndrome." This syndrome consists of a constellation of five CHD risk factors (Table 31–8).

Of the five risk factors, abdominal obesity is defined by ethnic-specific values of abdominal waist circumference (Alberti et al., 2009). An alternative to assessing the five criteria that identify the metabolic syndrome is to determine the ratio of the concentrations of fasting triglycerides divided by the HDL-C. Values >3.5 predict insulin resistance as effectively as meeting the criteria for diagnosing metabolic syndrome (McLaughlin et al., 2005). The prevalence of metabolic syndrome among patients with premature vascular disease may be as high as 50%. Treatment should focus on weight loss and increased physical activity, because being overweight or obese usually precludes optimal risk factor reduction. Specific treatment of increased LDL-C, non-HDL-C, and triglyceride levels and low HDL-C levels also should be undertaken.

Table 31–8

Clinical Identification of the Metabolic Syndrome

RISK FACTOR	DEFINING LEVEL
Abdominal obesity[a]	Waist circumference[b]
Men	>102 cm (>40 in)
Women	>88 cm (>35 in)
Triglycerides	≥150 mg/dL
HDL-C	
Men	<40 mg/dL
Women	<50 mg/dL
Blood pressure	≥130/≥85 mm Hg
Fasting glucose	>100 mg/dL[b]

The 2001 National Cholesterol Education Program (NCEP) guidelines define the metabolic syndrome as the presence of three or more of these risk factors.

[a]Overweight and obesity are associated with insulin resistance and the metabolic syndrome. However, the presence of abdominal obesity is more highly correlated with the metabolic risk factors than is an elevated body mass index. Therefore, the simple measurement of waist circumference is recommended to identify the body weight component of the metabolic syndrome.

[b]Some male patients can develop multiple metabolic risk factors when the waist circumference is only marginally increased (e.g., 94-102 cm [37-39 inches]). Such patients may have a strong genetic contribution to insulin resistance, and like men with categorical increases in waist circumference, they should benefit from changes in life habits. There is ethnic variation in the values of waist circumference that define abdominal obesity (Alberti *et al.*, 2009). HDL-C, high-density-lipoprotein cholesterol. From The Expert Panel, 2002.

Treatment of Hypertriglyceridemia

There is increased CHD risk associated with the presence of triglyceride levels >150 mg/dL. Three categories of hypertriglyceridemia are recognized (Table 31–4), and treatment is recommended based on the degree of elevation. Weight loss, increased exercise, and alcohol restriction are important for all hypertriglyceridemic patients. The LDL-C goal should be ascertained based on each patient's risk factors or CHD status (Table 31–3). If triglycerides remain >200 mg/dL after the LDL-C goal is reached, further reduction in triglycerides may be achieved by increasing the dose of a statin or of niacin. Combination therapy (statin plus niacin or statin plus fibrate) may be required, but caution is necessary with these combinations to avoid myopathy (see "Statins in Combination with Other Lipid-Lowering Drugs," later in the chapter).

Treatment of Low HDL-C. The most frequent risk factor for premature CHD is low HDL-C. In men with angiographically documented CHD, ~60% have HDL-C levels of <35 mg/dL and only 25% have LDL-C >160 mg/dL. In older men with CHD, 38% have HDL-C levels <35 mg/dL and two-thirds have HDL-C <40 mg/dL. Subjects with "normal" cholesterol levels of <200 mg/dL but with low HDL-C (<40 mg/dL) have as much CHD risk as subjects with higher total cholesterol levels (230-260 mg/dL) and more normal HDL-C (40-49 mg/dL). In a recent study of CHD patients admitted to hospitals with acute coronary syndrome between 2000 and 2006, low HDL-C levels were clearly documented as the most prevalent lipid-related risk factor (Sachdeva et al., 2009). In clinical trials employing statins to lower LDL-C, the level of HDL-C has been documented to substantially moderate risk (Jafri et al., 2009).

In patients with low HDL-C, the total cholesterol:HDL-C ratio is a particularly useful predictor of CHD risk (Bersot, 2003). Observational studies suggest that a favorable ratio is ≤3.5 and a ratio of >4.5 is associated with increased risk (Table 31–9). However, results of a *post hoc* analysis of the relationship between HDL-C levels and treatment benefit of statin therapy suggest that there is substantial additional benefit associated with a total cholesterol:HDL-C ratio <3 (Barter et al., 2007). American men, who are a high-risk group, have a typical ratio of ~4.5. Patients with low HDL-C may have what are considered to be "normal" total and LDL cholesterol levels; however, because of their low HDL-C levels, such patients may be at high risk based on the total cholesterol:HDL-C ratio (e.g., a total cholesterol, 180 mg/dL; HDL-C, 30 mg/dL; ratio, 6). A desirable total cholesterol level in low-HDL-C patients may be considerably lower than 200 mg/dL, especially because low-HDL-C patients also may have moderately elevated triglycerides, which may reflect increased levels of atherogenic remnant lipoproteins. Patients with average or low LDL-C, low HDL-C, and high total cholesterol:HDL-C ratios have benefitted from treatment (Barter et al., 2007).

The treatment of low HDL-C patients focuses on lowering LDL-C to the target level based on the patient's risk factor or CHD status (Table 31–3) *and* a reduction of VLDL cholesterol (estimated by dividing the plasma triglyceride level by 5) to <30 mg/dL to reach the target for non-HDL-C. Satisfactory treatment results are a ratio of total cholesterol:HDL-C ≤3.5 (Table 3–9). Patients with total cholesterol:HDL-C ratios >4.5 are at risk even if their "non-HDL-C" levels (LDL-C and VLDL cholesterol) are at the goal values recommended by the 2001 NCEP guidelines. Consequently, it is useful to base treatment of patients with low HDL-C levels on both LDL-C and non-HDL-C levels plus the total cholesterol:HDL-C ratio (Tables 31–3 and 31–8) (Bersot et al., 2003).

DRUG THERAPY OF DYSLIPIDEMIA

Statins

The statins are the most effective and best-tolerated agents for treating dyslipidemia. These drugs are competitive inhibitors of HMG-CoA reductase, which

Table 31–9

Guidelines Based on LDL-C and Total Cholesterol:HDL-C Ratio for Treatment of Low HDL-C Patients[a]

	GOALS			LIFESTYLE CHANGE INITIATED FOR			DRUG THERAPY INITIATED FOR		
RISK CATEGORY	LDL-C		TC:HDL-C	LDL-C		TC:HDL-C	LDL-C		TC:HDL-C
CHD or equivalent	<100	and	<3.5	≥100	or	≥3.5	≥100	or	≥3.5
2+ risk factors	<130	and	<4.5	≥130	or	≥4.5	≥130	or	≥6.0
0–1 risk factor	<160	and	<5.5	≥160	or	≥5.5	≥160	or	≥7.0

CHD, coronary heart disease; HDL-C, high-density-lipoprotein cholesterol; LDL-C, low-density-lipoprotein cholesterol; TC, total cholesterol.
[a]Units for LDL-C: mg/dL

catalyzes an early, rate-limiting step in cholesterol biosynthesis. Higher doses of the more potent statins (e.g., atorvastatin, simvastatin, and rosuvastatin) also can reduce triglyceride levels caused by elevated VLDL levels. Some statins also are indicated for raising HDL-C levels, although the clinical significance of these effects on HDL-C remains to be proven.

Multiple well-controlled clinical trials have documented the efficacy and safety of simvastatin, pravastatin, lovastatin, atorvastatin, and rosuvastatin in reducing fatal and nonfatal CHD events, strokes, and total mortality (Cholesterol Treatment Trialists' Collaborators, 2005; Ridker et al., 2008). Rates of adverse events in statin trials were the same in the placebo groups and in the groups receiving the drug.

History. Statins were isolated from a mold, *Penicillium citrinum*, and identified as inhibitors of cholesterol biosynthesis in 1976 by Endo and colleagues. Subsequent studies by Brown and Goldstein established that statins act by inhibiting HMG-CoA reductase. The first statin studied in humans was *compactin*, renamed *mevastatin*, which demonstrated the therapeutic potential of this class of drugs. Alberts and colleagues at Merck developed the first statin approved for use in humans, lovastatin (formerly known as mevinolin), which was isolated from *Aspergillus terreus*. Six other statins are also available. Pravastatin and simvastatin are chemically modified derivatives of lovastatin (Figure 31–2). Atorvastatin, *fluvastatin*, *rosuvastatin*, and *pitavastatin* are structurally distinct synthetic compounds.

A yeast that grows on rice, *monascus purpureus*, produces a series of compounds, one of which, monacolin K, is an inhibitor of HMG-CoA reductase and is chemically identical to lovastatin. OTC preparations, known as red yeast rice, contain monacolin K. As with many nutraceuticals, content of the active principle may vary, and such preparations should be used with great caution.

Chemistry. The structural formulas of the original statin (mevastatin) and the seven statins currently available in the U.S. are shown in

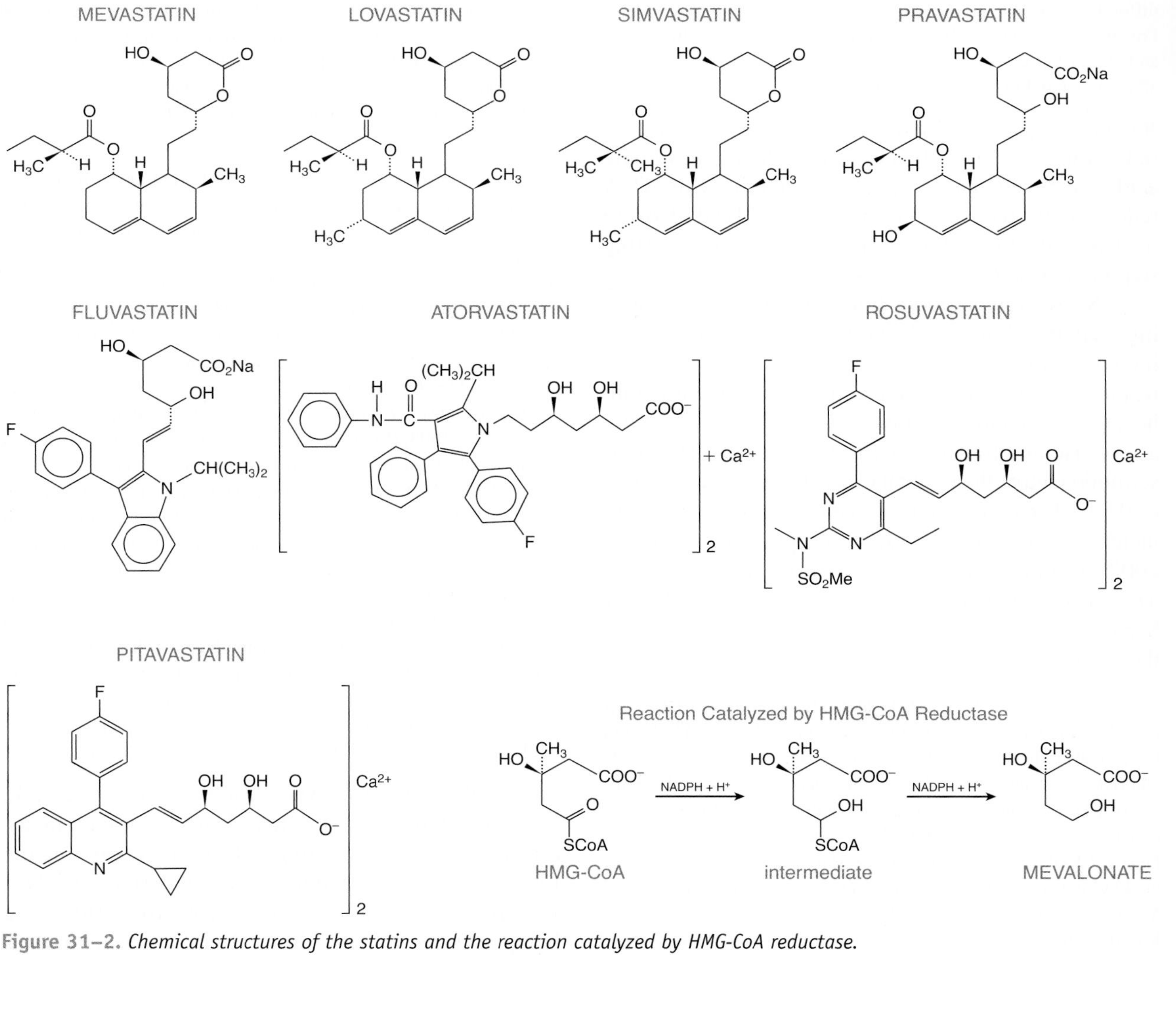

MEVASTATIN

LOVASTATIN

SIMVASTATIN

PRAVASTATIN

FLUVASTATIN

ATORVASTATIN

ROSUVASTATIN

PITAVASTATIN

Reaction Catalyzed by HMG-CoA Reductase

HMG-CoA → (NADPH + H⁺) → intermediate → (NADPH + H⁺) → MEVALONATE

Figure 31–2. *Chemical structures of the statins and the reaction catalyzed by HMG-CoA reductase.*

Figure 31–2 along with the reaction (conversion of HMG-CoA to mevalonate) catalyzed by HMG-CoA reductase, the enzyme they competitively inhibit. The statins possess a side group that is structurally similar to HMG-CoA. Mevastatin, lovastatin, simvastatin, and pravastatin are fungal metabolites, and each contains a hexahydronaphthalene ring. Lovastatin differs from mevastatin in having a methyl group at carbon 3. There are two major side chains. One is a methylbutyrate ester (lovastatin and pravastatin) or a dimethylbutyrate ester (simvastatin). The other contains a hydroxy acid that forms a six-membered analog of the intermediate compound in the HMG-CoA reductase reaction. Fluvastatin, atorvastatin, rosuvastatin, and pitavastatin are entirely synthetic compounds containing a heptanoic acid side chain that forms a structural analog of the HMG-CoA intermediate. As a result of their structural similarity to HMG-CoA, statins are reversible competitive inhibitors of the enzyme's natural substrate, HMG-CoA. The inhibition constant (K_i) of the statins is ~1nM; the dissociation constant of HMG-CoA is three orders of magnitude higher.

Lovastatin and simvastatin are lactone prodrugs that are modified in the liver to active hydroxy acid forms. Because they are lactones, they are less soluble in water than are the other statins, a difference that appears to have little if any clinical significance. Pravastatin (an acid in the active form), fluvastatin (sodium salt), and atorvastatin, rosuvastatin, and pitavastatin (calcium salts), are all administered in the active, open-ring form.

Mechanism of Action. Statins exert their major effect—reduction of LDL levels—through a mevalonic acid–like moiety that competitively inhibits HMG-CoA reductase. By reducing the conversion of HMG-CoA to mevalonate, statins inhibit an early and rate-limiting step in cholesterol biosynthesis.

Statins affect blood cholesterol levels by inhibiting hepatic cholesterol synthesis, which results in increased expression of the LDL receptor gene. In response to the reduced free cholesterol content within hepatocytes, membrane-bound SREBPs are cleaved by a protease and translocated to the nucleus. The transcription factors then bind the sterol-responsive element of the LDL receptor gene, enhancing transcription and increasing the synthesis of LDL receptors (Horton et al., 2002). Degradation of LDL receptors also is reduced. The greater number of LDL receptors on the surface of hepatocytes results in increased removal of LDL from the blood, thereby lowering LDL-C levels.

Some studies suggest that statins also can reduce LDL levels by enhancing the removal of LDL precursors (VLDL and IDL) and by decreasing hepatic VLDL production. Because VLDL remnants and IDL are enriched in apoE, a statin-induced increase in the number of LDL receptors, which recognize both apoB-100 and apoE, enhances the clearance of these LDL precursors. The reduction in hepatic VLDL production induced by statins is thought to be mediated by reduced synthesis of cholesterol, a required component of VLDL. This mechanism also likely accounts for the triglyceride-lowering effect of statins and may account for the reduction (~25%) of LDL-C levels in patients with homozygous familial hypercholesterolemia treated with 80 mg of atorvastatin or simvastatin.

Triglyceride Reduction by Statins. Triglyceride levels >250 mg/dL are reduced substantially by statins, and the percent reduction achieved is similar to the percent reduction in LDL-C. Accordingly, hypertriglyceridemic patients taking the highest doses of the most potent statins experience a 35-45% reduction in LDL-C and a similar reduction in fasting triglyceride levels (Hunninghake et al., 2004). The efficacy of triglyceride lowering by pitavastatin in patients with baseline triglyceride levels >250 mg/dL is currently unknown.

Effect of Statins on HDL-C Levels. Most studies of patients treated with statins have systematically excluded patients with low HDL-C levels. In studies of patients with elevated LDL-C levels and gender-appropriate HDL-C levels (40-50 mg/dL for men; 50-60 mg/dL for women), an increase in HDL-C of 5-10% was observed, irrespective of the dose or statin employed. However, in patients with reduced HDL-C levels (<35 mg/dL), statins may differ in their effects on HDL-C levels. Simvastatin, at its highest dose of 80 mg, increases HDL-C and apoA-I levels more than a comparable dose of atorvastatin (Crouse et al., 2000). In preliminary studies of patients with hypertriglyceridemia and low HDL-C, rosuvastatin appears to raise HDL-C levels by as much as 15-20% (Hunninghake et al., 2004). More studies are needed to ascertain whether the effects of statins on HDL-C in patients with low HDL-C levels are clinically significant.

Effects of Statins on LDL-C Levels. Statins lower LDL-C by 20-55%, depending on the dose and statin used. In large trials comparing the effects of the various statins, equivalent doses appear to be 5 mg of simvastatin = ~15 mg of lovastatin = ~15 mg of pravastatin = ~40 mg of fluvastatin (Pedersen and Tobert, 1996), 20 mg of simvastatin = ~10 mg of atorvastatin (Jones et al., 1998) (Crouse III et al., 1999), and 20 mg of atorvastatin = 10 mg of rosuvastatin (Jones et al., 2003). Analysis of dose-response relationships for all statins demonstrates that the efficacy of LDL-C lowering is log-linear; LDL-C is reduced by ~6% (from baseline) with each doubling of the dose (Jones et al., 1998; Pedersen and Tobert, 1996). Maximal effects on plasma cholesterol levels are achieved within 7-10 days.

Table 31–10 provides information on the statin doses required to reduce LDL-C by 20-55%. *The fractional reductions achieved with the various doses are the same regardless of the absolute value of the baseline LDL-C level.* The statins are effective in almost all patients with high LDL-C levels. The exception is patients with homozygous familial hypercholesterolemia, who have very attenuated responses to the usual doses of statins because both alleles of the LDL receptor gene code for dysfunctional LDL receptors; the partial response in these patients is due to a reduction in hepatic VLDL synthesis associated with the inhibition of HMG-CoA reductase–mediated cholesterol synthesis. Statin therapy does not reduce Lp(a) levels.

Potential Cardioprotective Effects Other Than LDL Lowering. Although the statins clearly exert their major effects on CHD by lowering LDL-C and improving the lipid profile as reflected in plasma cholesterol levels, a multitude of potentially cardioprotective effects are being ascribed to these drugs (Liao, 2005). However,

Table 31–10

Dose (mg) of Statins Required to Achieve Various Reductions in Low-Density-Lipoprotein Cholesterol from Baseline

	20-25%	26-30%	31-35%	36-40%	41-50%	51-55%
Atorvastatin	—	—	10	20	40	80
Fluvastatin	20	40	80			
Lovastatin	10	20	40	80		
Pitavastatin		1	2	4		
Pravastatin	10	20	40			
Rosuvastatin	—	—	—	5	10	20, 40
Simvastatin	—	10	20	40	80	

the mechanisms of action for non–lipid-lowering roles of statins have not been established, and it is not known whether these potential pleiotropic effects represent a class-action effect, differ among statins, or are biologically or clinically relevant. Until these questions are resolved, selection of a specific statin should not be based on any one of these effects. Nevertheless, the potential importance of the non-lipid roles of statins merits discussion.

Statins and Endothelial Function. A variety of studies have established that the vascular endothelium plays a dynamic role in vasoconstriction/relaxation. Hypercholesterolemia adversely affects the processes by which the endothelium modulates arterial tone. Statin therapy enhances endothelial production of the vasodilator nitric oxide, leading to improved endothelial function. Statin therapy improves endothelial function independent of changes in plasma cholesterol levels.

Statins and Plaque Stability. The vulnerability of plaques to rupture and thrombosis is of greater clinical relevance than the degree of stenosis they cause (Corti et al., 2003). Statins affect plaque stability in a variety of ways. They inhibit monocyte infiltration into the artery wall and inhibit macrophage secretion of matrix metalloproteinases *in vitro*. The metalloproteinases degrade extracellular matrix components and thus weaken the fibrous cap of atherosclerotic plaques.

Statins also appear to modulate the cellularity of the artery wall by inhibiting proliferation of smooth muscle cells and enhancing apoptosis. It is debatable whether these effects would be beneficial or harmful if they occurred *in vivo*. Reduced proliferation of smooth muscle cells and enhanced apoptosis could retard initial hyperplasia and restenosis, but they also could weaken the fibrous cap and destabilize the lesion. Interestingly, statin-induced suppression of cell proliferation and the induction of apoptosis have been extended to tumor biology. The effects of statins on isoprenoid biosynthesis and protein phenylation associated with reduced synthesis of the cholesterol precursor mevalonate may alter the development of malignancies (Li et al., 2003; Wong et al., 2002).

Statins and Inflammation. Appreciation of the importance of inflammatory processes in atherogenesis is growing, and statins may have an anti-inflammatory role. Statins decreased the risk of CHD and levels of CRP (an independent marker for inflammation and high CHD risk) independently of cholesterol lowering (Libby and Aikawa, 2003; Libby and Ridker, 2004). Body weight and the metabolic syndrome are associated with elevated levels of highly sensitive CRP, leading some to suggest that the CRP may simply be a marker of obesity and insulin resistance (Pearson et al., 2003). It remains to be determined whether the CRP is simply a marker of inflammation or if it contributes to the pathogenesis of atherosclerosis. The clinical utility of measuring CRP with "highly sensitive" assays appears to be limited to those primary prevention subjects with a moderate (10-20%) 10-year risk of sustaining a CHD event. Values of highly sensitive CRP >3 mg/L suggest that such patients should be managed as secondary prevention patients (Pearson et al., 2003).

Statins and Lipoprotein Oxidation. Oxidative modification of LDL appears to play a key role in mediating the uptake of lipoprotein cholesterol by macrophages and in other processes, including cytotoxicity within lesions. Statins reduce the susceptibility of lipoproteins to oxidation both *in vitro* and *ex vivo*.

Statins and Coagulation. The most compelling evidence of a non–lipid-lowering effect of a statin is the rosuvastatin-mediated reduction in venous thromboembolic events, a prespecified endpoint, in JUPITER. This trial demonstrated a 43% reduction in venous thromboembolic events in patients treated with rosuvastatin, 20 mg daily, compared with placebo during a median follow-up period of 1.9 years (Glynn et al., 2009). Statins reduce platelet aggregation and reduce the deposition of platelet thrombi. In addition, the different statins have variable effects on fibrinogen levels. Elevated plasma fibrinogen levels are associated with an increase in the incidence of CHD.

Absorption, Metabolism, and Excretion

Absorption from the Small Intestine. After oral administration, intestinal absorption of the statins is variable (30-85%). All the statins, except simvastatin and lovastatin, are administered in the β-hydroxy acid form, which is the form that inhibits HMG-CoA reductase. Simvastatin and lovastatin are administered as inactive lactones that must be transformed in the liver to their respective β-hydroxy acids, simvastatin acid (SVA) and lovastatin acid (LVA). There is extensive first-pass hepatic uptake of all statins, mediated primarily by the organic anion transporter OATP1B1 (see Chapter 5).

Due to extensive first-pass hepatic uptake, systemic bioavailability of the statins and their hepatic metabolites varies between 5% and 30% of administered doses. The metabolites of all statins, except fluvastatin and pravastatin, have some HMG-CoA reductase inhibitory activity (Bellosta et al., 2004). Under steady-state conditions, small amounts of the parent drug and its metabolites produced in the liver can be found in the systemic circulation. After the lactones of simvastatin and lovastatin are transformed in the liver to SVA and LVA, small amounts of these active inhibitors of HMG-CoA reductase, as well as small amounts of the lactone forms, can be found in the systemic circulation. In the plasma, >95% of statins and their metabolites are protein bound, with the exception of pravastatin and its metabolites, which are only 50% bound (Schachter, 2005).

After an oral dose, plasma concentrations of statins peak in 1-4 hours. The $t_{1/2}$ of the parent compounds are 1-4 hours, except in the case of atorvastatin and rosuvastatin, which have half-lives of ~20 hours, and simvastatin with a $t_{1/2}$ ~12 hours (Ieiri et al., 2007). The longer $t_{1/2}$ of atorvastatin and rosuvastatin may contribute to their greater cholesterol-lowering efficacy (Corsini et al., 1999). The liver biotransforms all statins, and more than 70% of statin metabolites are excreted by the liver, with subsequent elimination in the feces (Bellosta et al., 2004). Inhibition by other drugs of OATP1B1, which transports several statins into hepatocytes, and inhibition or induction of CYP3A4 by a variety of pharmacological agents provide rationales for drug-drug interactions involving statins (Shitara and Sugiyama, 2006).

Adverse Effects and Drug Interactions

Hepatotoxicity. Initial post-marketing surveillance studies of the statins revealed an elevation in hepatic transaminase to values greater than three times the upper limit of normal, with an incidence as great as 1%. The incidence appeared to be dose related. However, in the placebo-controlled outcome trials in which 10- to 40-mg doses of simvastatin, lovastatin, fluvastatin, atorvastatin, pravastatin, or rosuvastatin were used, the incidence of 3-fold elevations in hepatic transaminases was 1-3% in the active drug treatment groups and 1.1% in placebo patients (Law et al., 2006; Ridker et al., 2008). No cases of liver failure occurred in these trials. Although serious hepatotoxicity is rare, 30 cases of liver failure associated with statin use were reported to the FDA between 1987 and 2000, a rate of about one case per million person-years of use (Law et al., 2006). It is therefore reasonable to measure alanine aminotransferase (ALT) at baseline and thereafter when clinically indicated.

Observational studies and a prospective trial suggest that transaminase elevations in patients with nonalcoholic fatty liver disease and hepatitis C are not at risk of statin-induced liver toxicity (Alqahtani and Sanchez, 2008; Chalasani et al., 2004; Lewis et al., 2007; Norris et al., 2008). This is important, as many insulin-resistant patients are affected by nonalcoholic fatty liver disease and have elevated transaminases. As insulin resistance is associated with increased CVD risk, insulin-resistant patients, especially those with type 2 diabetes mellitus, benefit from lipid-lowering therapy with statins (Cholesterol Treatment Trialists' Collaborators, 2008). It is reassuring that these patients with elevated transaminases can safely take statins.

Myopathy. The major adverse effect associated with statin use is myopathy (Wilke et al., 2007). Between 1987 and 2001, the FDA recorded 42 deaths from rhabdomyolysis induced by statins (excluding *cerivastatin*, which has been withdrawn from the market worldwide). This is a rate of one death per million prescriptions (30-day supply). In the statin trials described earlier (under "Hepatotoxicity"), rhabdomyolysis occurred in eight active drug recipients versus five placebo subjects. Among active drug recipients, 0.17% had CK values exceeding 10 times the upper limit of normal; among placebo-treated subjects, the incidence was 0.13%. Only 13 out of 55 drug-treated subjects and 4 out of 43 placebo subjects with greater than 10-fold elevations of CK reported any muscle symptoms (Law et al., 2006).

The risk of myopathy and rhabdomyolysis increases in proportion to statin dose and plasma concentrations. Consequently, factors inhibiting statin catabolism are associated with increased myopathy risk, including advanced age (especially >80 years of age), hepatic or renal dysfunction, perioperative periods, multi-system disease (especially in association with diabetes mellitus), small body size, and untreated hypothyroidism (Pasternak et al., 2002; Thompson et al., 2003). Concomitant use of drugs that diminish statin catabolism or interfere with hepatic uptake is associated with myopathy and rhabdomyolysis in 50-60% of all cases (Law and Rudnicka, 2006; Thompson et al., 2003). Thus, avoiding these drug interactions should reduce myopathy and rhabdomyolysis by about one-half (Law and Rudnicka, 2006). The most common statin interactions occurred with fibrates, especially *gemfibrozil* (38%), *cyclosporine* (4%), *digoxin* (5%), *warfarin* (4%), macrolide antibiotics (3%), *mibefradil* (2%), and azole antifungals (1%) (Thompson et al., 2003). Other drugs that increase the risk of statin-induced myopathy include niacin (rare), HIV protease inhibitors, *amiodarone*, and *nefazodone* (Pasternak et al., 2002).

There are a variety of pharmacokinetic mechanisms by which these drugs increase myopathy risk when administered concomitantly with statins. Gemfibrozil, the drug most commonly associated with statin-induced myopathy, inhibits both uptake of the active hydroxy acid forms of statins into hepatocytes by OATP1B1 and interferes with the transformation of most statins by glucuronidases (Prueksaritanont et al., 2002a; Prueksaritanont et al., 2002b; Prueksaritanont et al., 2002c). Primarily due to inhibition of OATP1B1-mediated hepatic uptake, co-administration of gemfibrozil nearly doubles the plasma concentration of the statin hydroxy acids (Neuvonen et al., 2006). Other fibrates, especially fenofibrate, do not interfere with the glucuronidation of statins and pose less risk of myopathy when used in combination with statin therapy. (For reviews of statin interactions with other drugs, see Bellosta et al., 2004 and Neuvonen et al., 2006). Concomitant therapy with simvastatin, 80 mg daily, and fenofibrate, 160 mg daily, results in no clinically significant pharmacokinetic interaction (Bergman et al., 2004). Similar results were obtained in a study of low-dose rosuvastatin, 10 mg daily, plus fenofibrate, 67 mg three times a day. When statins are administered with niacin, the myopathy probably is caused by an enhanced inhibition of skeletal muscle cholesterol synthesis (a pharmacodynamic interaction).

Drugs that interfere with statin oxidation are those metabolized primarily by CYP3A4 and include certain macrolide antibiotics (e.g., *erythromycin*); azole antifungals (e.g., *itraconazole*); cyclosporine; nefazodone, a phenylpiperazine antidepressant; HIV protease inhibitors; and amiodarone (Alsheikh-Ali and Karas, 2005; Bellosta et al., 2004; Corsini, 2003). These pharmacokinetic interactions are associated with increased plasma concentrations of statins and their active metabolites. Atorvastatin, lovastatin, and simvastatin are primarily metabolized by CYPs 3A4 and 3A5. Fluvastatin is mostly (50-80%) metabolized by CYP2C9 to inactive metabolites, but CYP3A4 and CYP2C8 also contribute to its metabolism. Pravastatin, however, is not metabolized to any appreciable extent by the CYP system and is excreted unchanged in the urine. Pravastatin, fluvastatin, and rosuvastatin are not extensively metabolized by CYP3A4. Pravastatin and fluvastatin may be less likely to cause myopathy when used with one of the predisposing drugs. However, because cases of myopathy have been reported with both drugs, the benefits of combined therapy with any statin should be carefully weighed against the risk of myopathy. Although rosuvastatin is not transformed to any appreciable extent by oxidation, cases of myopathy have been reported, particularly in association with concomitant use of gemfibrozil (Schneck et al., 2004). Experience with pitavastatin is limited. There are no data regarding myopathy and rhabdomyolysis that might be associated with its use.

Despite the rarity of 10-fold elevations of CK, many patients complain of muscle aches (myalgias) while taking statins. It is unclear if such myalgias are caused by taking a statin. In one clinical trial involving 20,000 subjects randomized to simvastatin (40 mg daily) or placebo, it was observed over the 5 years of the study that one-third of patients complained of myalgia at least once, whether the active drug or the placebo was being taken (Heart Protection Study Collaborative Group, 2002).

Replacing vitamin D in patients with a vitamin D deficiency reportedly reduces statin-associated myalgias and improves statin tolerance (Ahmed et al., 2009). The observation needs to be confirmed, but it is potentially significant because vitamin D deficiency is associated with myopathy, insulin resistance, and increased incidence of CVD (Lee et al., 2008).

Pregnancy. *The safety of statins during pregnancy has not been established.* Women wishing to conceive should not take statins. During their childbearing years, women taking statins should use highly effective contraception (see Chapter 40). Nursing mothers also are advised to avoid taking statins.

Therapeutic Uses. Each statin has a low recommended starting dose that reduces LDL-C by 20-30%. Dyslipidemic patients frequently remain on their initial dose, are not titrated to achieve their target LDL-C level, and thus remain undertreated. For this reason, it is advisable to start each patient on a dose that will achieve the patient's target goal for LDL-C lowering. For example, a patient with a baseline LDL-C of 150 mg/dL and a goal of 100 mg/dL requires a 33% reduction in LDL-C and should be started on a dose expected to provide it (Table 31–10).

Hepatic cholesterol synthesis is maximal between midnight and 2:00 A.M. Thus, statins with $t_{1/2}$ ≤4 hours (all but atorvastatin and rosuvastatin) should be taken in the evening.

The initial recommended dose of lovastatin (MEVACOR) is 20 mg and is slightly more effective if taken with the evening meal than if it is taken at bedtime, although bedtime dosing is preferable to missing doses. The dose of lovastatin may be increased every 3-6 weeks up to a maximum of 80 mg/day. The 80-mg dose is slightly (2-3%) more effective if given as 40 mg twice daily. Lovastatin, at 20 mg, is marketed in combination with 500, 750, or 1000 mg of extended-release niacin (ADVICOR). Few patients are appropriate candidates for this fixed-dose combination (see the section on "Nicotinic Acid," later in the chapter).

The approved starting dose of simvastatin (ZOCOR) for most patients is 20 mg at bedtime unless the required LDL-C reduction exceeds 45% or the patient is a high-risk secondary prevention patient, in which case a 40-mg starting dose is indicated. The maximal dose is 80 mg, and the drug should be taken at bedtime. In patients taking cyclosporine, fibrates, or niacin, the daily dose should not exceed 20 mg. Simvastatin, 20 mg, is marketed in combination with 500, 750, or 1000 mg of extended-release niacin (SIMCOR). See the section on "Nicotinic Acid."

Pravastatin (PRAVACHOL) therapy is initiated with a 20- or 40-mg dose that may be increased to 80 mg. This drug should be taken at bedtime. Because pravastatin is a hydroxy acid, bile-acid sequestrants will bind it and reduce its absorption. Practically, this is rarely a problem because the resins should be taken before meals and pravastatin should be taken at bedtime. Pravastatin also is marketed in combination with buffered aspirin (PRAVIGARD). The small advantage of combining these two drugs should be weighed against the disadvantages inherent in fixed-dose combinations.

The starting dose of fluvastatin (LESCOL) is 20 or 40 mg, and the maximum is 80 mg/day. Like pravastatin, it is administered as a hydroxy acid and should be taken at bedtime, several hours after ingesting a bile-acid sequestrant (if the combination is used).

Atorvastatin (LIPITOR) has a long $t_{1/2}$, which allows administration of this statin at any time of the day. The starting dose is 10 mg, and the maximum is 80 mg/day. Atorvastatin is marketed in combination with the Ca^{2+}-channel blocker amlodipine (CADUET) for patients with hypertension or angina as well as hypercholesterolemia. The physician should weigh any advantage of combination against the associated risks and disadvantages.

Rosuvastatin (CRESTOR) is available in doses ranging between 5 and 40 mg. It has a $t_{1/2}$ of 20-30 hours and may be taken at any time of day. Because experience with rosuvastatin is limited, treatment should be initiated with 5-10 mg daily, increasing stepwise, if needed, until the incidence of myopathy is better defined. If the combination of gemfibrozil with rosuvastatin is used, the dose of rosuvastatin should not exceed 10 mg.

Pitavastatin (LIVALO) is available in doses of 1, 2, and 4 mg. There is very limited post-marketing experience with this drug. Gemfibrozil reduces clearance of pitavastatin and raises blood concentrations; consequently, gemfibrozil should be used cautiously, if at all, in combination with pitavastatin.

The choice of statins should be based on efficacy (reduction of LDL-C) and cost. Three drugs (lovastatin, simvastatin, and pravastatin) have been used safely in clinical trials involving thousands of subjects for 5 or more years. The documented safety records of these statins should be considered, especially when initiating therapy in younger patients. Once drug treatment is initiated, it is almost always lifelong. Baseline determinations of ALT and repeat testing at 3-6 months are recommended. If ALT is normal after the initial 3-6 months, then it need not be repeated more than once every 6-12 months. Measurements of CK are not routinely necessary unless the patient also is taking a drug that enhances the risk of myopathy. Because myopathy may develop months to years after the start of combined therapy, it is unlikely that routine monitoring for the accompanying rise in CK will consistently herald the onset, even if monitoring is performed every 3-4 months.

Statin Use by Children. Some statins have been approved for use in children with heterozygous familial hypercholesterolemia. Atorvastatin, lovastatin, and simvastatin are indicated for children ≥11 years. Pravastatin is approved for children ≥8 years.

Statins in Combination with Other Lipid-Lowering Drugs. Statins, in combination with the bile acid–binding resins *cholestyramine* and *colestipol*, produce 20-30% greater reductions in LDL-C than can be achieved with statins alone. Preliminary data indicate that *colesevelam hydrochloride* plus a statin lowers LDL-C by 8-16% more than statins alone. Niacin also can enhance the effect of statins, but the occurrence of myopathy increases when statin doses >25% of maximum (e.g., 20 mg of simvastatin or atorvastatin) are used with niacin. The combination of a fibrate (*clofibrate*, gemfibrozil, or fenofibrate) with a statin is particularly useful in patients with hypertriglyceridemia and high LDL-C levels. This combination increases the risk of myopathy but usually is safe with a fibrate at its usual maximal dose and a statin at no more than 25% of its maximal dose. Fenofibrate, which is least likely to interfere with statin metabolism, appears to be the safest fibrate to use with statins (Prueksaritanont et al., 2002b). Triple therapy with resins, niacin, and statins can reduce LDL-C by up to 70%. Vytorin, a fixed combination of simvastatin (10, 20, 40, or 80 mg) and ezetimibe (10 mg), decreased LDL-C levels by up to 60% at 24 weeks.

Bile-Acid Sequestrants

The two established bile-acid sequestrants or resins (cholestyramine and colestipol) are among the oldest of the hypolipidemic drugs, and they are probably the safest, because they are not absorbed from the intestine. These resins also are recommended for patients 11-20 years of age. Because statins are so effective as monotherapy, the resins are most often used as second agents if statin therapy does not lower LDL-C levels sufficiently. When used with a statin, cholestyramine and colestipol usually are prescribed at submaximal doses. Maximal doses can reduce LDL-C by up to 25% but are associated with unacceptable gastrointestinal side effects (bloating and constipation) that limit compliance. Colesevelam is a newer bile-acid sequestrant that is prepared as an anhydrous gel and taken as a tablet or as a powder that is mixed with water and taken as an oral suspension. It lowers LDL-C by 18% at its maximum dose. The safety and efficacy of colesevelam have not been studied in pediatric patients or pregnant women.

CHOLESTYRAMINE

COLESTIPOL

COLESEVELAM

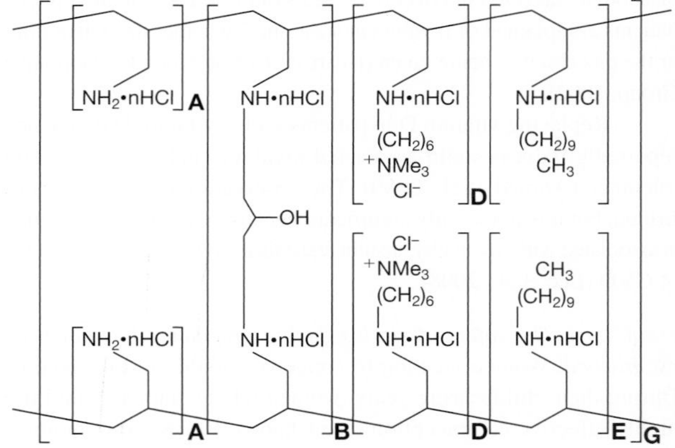

KEY
A = Primary Amines
B = Cross-linked Amines
D = Quaternary Ammonium Alkylated Amines
E = Decyalkylated Amines
n = Fraction of Protonated Amines
G = Extended Polymeric Network

Figure 31–3. *Structures of cholestyramine, colestipol, and colesevelam.*

Chemistry. Cholestyramine and colestipol (Figure 31–3) are anion-exchange resins. Cholestyramine, a polymer of styrene and divinylbenzene with active sites formed from trimethylbenzylammonium groups, is a quaternary amine. Colestipol, a copolymer of diethylenetriamine and 1-chloro-2,3-epoxypropane, is a mixture of tertiary and quaternary diamines. Cholestyramine and colestipol are hygroscopic powders administered as chloride salts and are insoluble in water. Colesevelam is a polymer, poly(allylamine hydrochloride), cross-linked with epichlorohydrin and alkylated with 1-bromodecane and (6-bromohexyl)-trimethylammonium bromide; it is a hydrophilic gel and insoluble in water.

Mechanism of Action. The bile-acid sequestrants are highly positively charged and bind negatively charged bile acids. Because of their large size, the resins are not absorbed, and the bound bile acids are excreted in the stool. Because more than 95% of bile acids are normally reabsorbed, interruption of this process depletes the pool of bile acids, and hepatic bile-acid synthesis increases. As a result, hepatic cholesterol content declines, stimulating the production of LDL receptors, an effect similar to that of statins. The increase in hepatic LDL receptors increases LDL clearance and lowers LDL-C levels, but this effect is partially offset by the enhanced cholesterol synthesis caused by upregulation of HMG-CoA reductase. Inhibition of reductase activity by a statin substantially increases the effectiveness of the resins.

The resin-induced increase in bile-acid production is accompanied by an increase in hepatic triglyceride synthesis, which is of consequence in patients with significant hypertriglyceridemia (baseline triglyceride level >250 mg/dL). In such patients, bile-acid sequestrant therapy may cause striking increases in triglyceride levels. Use of colesevelam to lower LDL-C levels in hypertriglyceridemic patients should be accompanied by frequent (every 1-2 weeks) monitoring of fasting triglyceride levels until the triglyceride level is stable, or the use of colesevelam in these patients should be avoided.

Effects on Lipoprotein Levels. The reduction in LDL-C by resins is dose dependent. Doses of 8-12 g of cholestyramine or 10-15 g of colestipol are associated with 12-18% reductions in LDL-C. Maximal doses (24 g of cholestyramine, 30 g of colestipol) may reduce LDL-C by as much as 25% but will cause gastrointestinal side effects that are poorly tolerated by most patients. One to two weeks is sufficient to attain maximal LDL-C reduction by a given resin dose. In patients with normal triglyceride levels, triglycerides may increase transiently and then return to baseline. HDL-C levels increase 4-5%. Statins plus resins or niacin plus resins can reduce LDL-C by as much as 40-60%. Colesevelam, in doses of 3-3.75 g, reduces LDL-C levels by 9-19%.

Adverse Effects and Drug Interactions. The resins are generally safe, as they are not systemically absorbed. Because they are administered as chloride salts, rare instances of hyperchloremic acidosis have been reported. Severe hypertriglyceridemia is a contraindication to the use of cholestyramine and colestipol because these resins increase triglyceride levels. At present, there are insufficient data on the effect of colesevelam on triglyceride levels.

Cholestyramine and colestipol both are available as a powder that must be mixed with water and drunk as a slurry. The gritty sensation is unpleasant to patients initially but can be tolerated. Colestipol is available in a tablet form that reduces the complaint of grittiness but not the gastrointestinal symptoms. Colesevelam is available as a hard capsule that absorbs water and creates a soft, gelatinous material that allegedly minimizes the potential for gastrointestinal irritation.

Patients taking cholestyramine and colestipol complain of bloating and dyspepsia. These symptoms can be substantially reduced if the drug is completely suspended in liquid several hours before ingestion (e.g., evening doses can be mixed in the morning and refrigerated; morning doses can be mixed the previous evening and refrigerated). Constipation may occur but sometimes can be prevented by adequate daily water intake and psyllium, if necessary. Colesevelam may be less likely to cause the dyspepsia, bloating, and constipation observed in patients treated with cholestyramine or colestipol.

Cholestyramine and colestipol bind and interfere with the absorption of many drugs, including some thiazides, *furosemide*, *propranolol*, L-*thyroxine*, digoxin, warfarin, and some of the statins. The effect of cholestyramine and colestipol on the absorption of most drugs has not been studied. For this reason, it is wise to administer all drugs either 1 hour before or 3-4 hours after a dose of cholestyramine or colestipol. Colesevelam does not appear to interfere with the absorption of fat-soluble vitamins or of drugs such as digoxin, lovastatin, warfarin, *metoprolol*, *quinidine*, and *valproic acid*. The maximum concentration and the AUC of sustained-release *verapamil* are reduced by 31% and 11%, respectively, when the drug is co-administered with colesevelam. The effect of colesevelam on the absorption of other drugs has not been tested, but it seems prudent to recommend that patients take other medications 1 hour before or 3-4 hours after a dose of colesevelam.

Preparations and Use. Cholestyramine resin (QUESTRAN, others) is available in bulk (with scoops that measure a 4-g dose) or in individual packets of 4 g. Additional flavorings are added to increase palatability. The "light" preparations contain artificial sweeteners rather than sucrose. Colestipol hydrochloride (COLESTID, others) is available in bulk, in individual packets containing 5 g of colestipol, or as 1-g tablets.

Resins should never be taken in the dry form. The powdered forms of cholestyramine (4 g/dose) and colestipol (5 g/dose) are either mixed with a fluid (water or juice) and drunk as a slurry or mixed with crushed ice in a blender. Ideally, patients should take the resins before breakfast and before supper, starting with one scoop or packet twice daily, and increasing the dosage after several weeks or longer as needed and as tolerated. Patients generally will not take more than two doses (scoops or packets) twice a day.

Colesevelam hydrochloride (WELCHOL) is available as a solid tablet containing 0.625 g of colesevelam and as a powder in packets of 3.75 g or 1.875 g. The starting dose is either three tablets taken twice daily with meals or all six tablets taken with a meal. The tablets should be taken with a liquid. The maximum daily dose is seven tablets (4.375 g). The powder in the packets is first suspended in 4-8 oz of water and should be taken with meals. Dosing of the packet containing 3.75 g is once daily; the packet containing 1.875 g is taken twice daily.

Niacin (Nicotinic Acid)

Niacin, *nicotinic acid* (pyridine-3-carboxylic acid), one of the oldest drugs used to treat dyslipidemia, favorably affects virtually all lipid parameters.

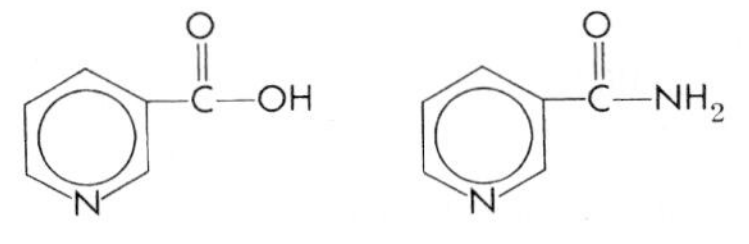

NICOTINIC ACID NICOTINAMIDE

Niacin is a water-soluble B-complex vitamin that functions as a vitamin only after its conversion to NAD or NADP, in which it occurs as an amide. Both niacin and its amide may be given orally as a source of niacin for its functions as a vitamin, but only niacin affects lipid levels. The hypolipidemic effects of niacin require larger doses than are required for its vitamin effects. Niacin is the best agent available for increasing HDL-C (30-40%); it also lowers triglycerides by 35-45% (as effectively as fibrates and the more effective statins) and reduces LDL-C levels by 20-30%. Niacin also is the only lipid-lowering drug that reduces Lp(a) levels significantly. Despite its salutary effect on lipids, niacin has side effects that limit its use (see "Adverse Effects," later in the chapter).

Mechanism of Action. In adipose tissue, niacin inhibits the lipolysis of triglycerides by hormone-sensitive lipase, which reduces transport of free fatty acids to the liver and decreases hepatic triglyceride synthesis. Niacin and related compounds (e.g., 5-methylpyrazine-2-carboxylic-4-oxide, *acipimox*) may exert their effects on lipolysis by inhibiting adipocyte adenylyl cyclase. A GPCR for niacin has been identified and designated as GPR109A; it couples to G_i (Wise et al., 2003); its mRNA is highly expressed in the adipose tissue and spleen, sites of high-affinity nicotinic acid binding (Lorenzen et al., 2001). Acting on this receptor, niacin stimulates the G_i–adenylyl cyclase pathway in adipocytes, inhibiting cyclic AMP production and decreasing hormone-sensitive lipase activity, triglyceride lipolysis, and release of free fatty acids. Niacin also may inhibit a rate-limiting enzyme of triglyceride synthesis, diacylglycerol acyltransferase-2 (Ganji et al., 2004).

In the liver, niacin reduces triglyceride synthesis by inhibiting both the synthesis and esterification of fatty acids, effects that increase apoB degradation. Reduction of triglyceride synthesis reduces hepatic VLDL production, which accounts for the reduced LDL levels. Niacin also enhances LPL activity, which promotes the clearance of chylomicrons and VLDL triglycerides. Niacin raises HDL-C levels by decreasing the fractional clearance of apoA-I in HDL rather than by enhancing HDL synthesis. This effect is due to a reduction in the hepatic clearance of HDL-apoA-I, but not of cholesteryl esters, thereby increasing the apoA-I content of plasma and augmenting reverse cholesterol transport. In macrophages, niacin stimulates expression of the scavenger receptor CD36 and the cholesterol exporter ABCA1. The net effect of niacin on monocytic cells ("foam cells") is HDL-mediated reduction of cellular cholesterol content (Rubic et al., 2004).

Effects on Plasma Lipoprotein Levels. Regular or crystalline niacin in doses of 2-6 g/day reduces triglycerides by 35-50%; the maximal effect occurs within 4-7 days. Reductions of 25% in LDL-C levels are possible with doses of 4.5-6 g/day, but 3-6 weeks are required for maximal effect. HDL-C increases less in patients with low HDL-C levels (<35 mg/dL) than in those with higher levels.

Absorption, Fate, and Excretion. The pharmacological doses of regular (crystalline) niacin used to treat dyslipidemia are almost completely absorbed, and peak plasma concentrations (up to 0.24 mmol) are achieved within 30-60 minutes. The $t_{1/2}$ is about 60 minutes, which accounts for the necessity of dosing two to three times daily. At lower doses, most niacin is taken up by the liver; only the major metabolite, nicotinuric acid, is found in the urine. At higher doses, a greater proportion of the drug is excreted in the urine as unchanged nicotinic acid.

Adverse Effects. Two of niacin's side effects, flushing and dyspepsia, limit patient compliance. The cutaneous effects include flushing and pruritus of the face and upper trunk, skin rashes, and acanthosis nigricans. Flushing and associated pruritus are prostaglandin mediated. Flushing is worse when therapy is initiated or the dosage is increased but ceases in most patients after 1-2 weeks of a stable dose. Taking an aspirin each day alleviates the flushing in many patients. Flushing recurs if only one or two doses are missed, and the flushing is more likely to occur when niacin is consumed with hot beverages (coffee, tea) or with ethanol-containing beverages. Flushing is minimized if therapy is initiated with low doses (100-250 mg twice daily) and if the drug is taken after breakfast or supper. Dry skin, a frequent complaint, can be dealt with by using skin moisturizers, and acanthosis nigricans can be dealt with by using lotions or creams containing *salicylic acid*. Dyspepsia and rarer episodes of nausea, vomiting, and diarrhea are less likely to occur if the drug is taken after a meal. Patients with any history of peptic ulcer disease should not take niacin because it can reactivate ulcer disease.

The most common, medically serious side effects are hepatotoxicity, manifested as elevated serum transaminases, and hyperglycemia. Both regular (crystalline) niacin and sustained-release niacin, which was developed to reduce flushing and itching, have been reported to cause severe liver toxicity. An extended-release niacin (NIASPAN) appears to be less likely to cause severe hepatotoxicity, perhaps simply because it is administered once daily instead of more frequently. The incidence of flushing and pruritus with this preparation is not substantially different from that with regular niacin. Severe hepatotoxicity is more likely to occur when patients take more than 2 g of sustained-release, over-the-counter preparations. Affected patients experience flu-like fatigue and weakness. Usually, aspartate transaminase and ALT are elevated, serum albumin levels decline, and total cholesterol and LDL-C levels decline substantially. In fact, reductions in LDL-C of 50% or more in a patient taking niacin should be viewed as a sign of niacin toxicity.

In patients with diabetes mellitus, niacin should be used cautiously because niacin-induced insulin resistance can cause severe hyperglycemia. Niacin use in patients with diabetes mellitus often mandates a change to insulin therapy. In a study of patients with type 2 diabetes taking niaspan, 4% stopped taking the drug because of inadequate glycemic control (Grundy et al., 2002). If niacin is prescribed for patients with known or suspected diabetes, blood glucose levels should be monitored at least weekly until proven to be stable. Niacin also elevates uric acid levels and may reactivate gout. A history of gout is a relative contraindication for niacin use. Rarer reversible side effects include toxic amblyopia and toxic maculopathy. Atrial tachyarrhythmias and atrial fibrillation have been reported, more commonly in elderly patients. *Niacin, at doses used in humans, has been associated with birth defects in experimental animals and should not be taken by pregnant women.*

Therapeutic Use. Niacin is indicated for hypertriglyceridemia and elevated LDL-C; it is especially useful in patients with both hypertriglyceridemia and low HDL-C levels. There are two commonly available forms of niacin. Crystalline niacin (immediate-release or regular) refers to niacin tablets that dissolve quickly after ingestion. Sustained-release niacin refers to preparations that continuously release niacin for 6-8 hours after ingestion. NIASPAN is the only preparation of niacin that is FDA-approved for treating dyslipidemia and that requires a prescription.

Crystalline niacin tablets are available over the counter in a variety of strengths from 50- to 500-mg tablets. To minimize the flushing and pruritus, it is best to start with a low dose (e.g., 100 mg twice daily taken after breakfast and supper). The dose may be increased stepwise every 7 days by 100-200 mg to a total daily dose of 1.5-2 g. After 2-4 weeks at this dose, transaminases, serum albumin, fasting glucose, and uric acid levels should be measured. Lipid levels should be checked and the dose increased further until the desired effect on plasma lipids is achieved. After a stable dose is attained, blood should be drawn every 3-6 months to monitor for the various toxicities.

Because concurrent use of niacin and a statin can cause myopathy, the statin should be administered at no more than 25% of its maximal dose. Patients also should be instructed to discontinue therapy if flu-like muscle aches occur. Routine measurement of CK in patients taking niacin and statins does not assure that severe myopathy will be detected before onset of symptoms, as patients have developed myopathy after several years of concomitant use of niacin with a statin.

Over-the-counter, sustained-release niacin preparations and NIASPAN are effective up to a total daily dose of 2 g. All doses of sustained-release niacin, but particularly doses above 2 g/day, have been reported to cause hepatotoxicity, which may occur soon after beginning therapy or after several years of use (Knopp et al., 2009). The potential for severe liver damage should preclude use of OTC preparations in most patients, including those who have taken an equivalent dose of crystalline niacin safely for many years and are considering switching to a sustained-release preparation. NIASPAN may be less likely to cause hepatotoxicity.

Fibric Acid Derivatives: PPAR Activators

History. In 1962, Thorp and Waring reported that ethyl chlorophenoxyisobutyrate lowered lipid levels in rats. In 1967, the ester form (clofibrate) was approved for use in the U.S. and became the most widely prescribed hypolipidemic drug. Its use declined dramatically, however, after the World Health Organization (WHO) reported that, despite a 9% reduction in cholesterol levels, clofibrate treatment did not reduce fatal cardiovascular events, although nonfatal infarcts were reduced. Total mortality was significantly greater in the clofibrate group. The increased mortality was due to multiple causes, including cholelithiasis. Interpretation of these negative results was clouded by failure to analyze the data according to the intention-to-treat principle. A later analysis demonstrated that the apparent increase in noncardiac mortality did not persist in the clofibrate-treated patients after discontinuation of the drug (Heady et al., 1992). Clofibrate use was virtually abandoned after publication of the results of the 1978 WHO trial. Clofibrate as well as two other fibrates, gemfibrozil and fenofibrate, remain available in the U.S.

Two subsequent trials involving only men have reported favorable effects of gemfibrozil therapy on fatal and nonfatal cardiac events without an increase in morbidity or mortality (Frick et al., 1987; Rubins et al., 1999). A third trial of men and women reported fewer events in a subgroup characterized by high triglyceride and low HDL-C levels (Haim et al., 1999).

Chemistry. Clofibrate, the prototype of the fibric acid derivatives, is the ethyl ester of *p*-chlorophenoxyisobutyrate. Gemfibrozil is a nonhalogenated phenoxypentanoic acid and thus is distinct from the halogenated fibrates. A number of fibric acid analogs (e.g., fenofibrate, *bezafibrate*, *ciprofibrate*) have been developed and are used in Europe and elsewhere (see Figure 31–4 for their structural formulas).

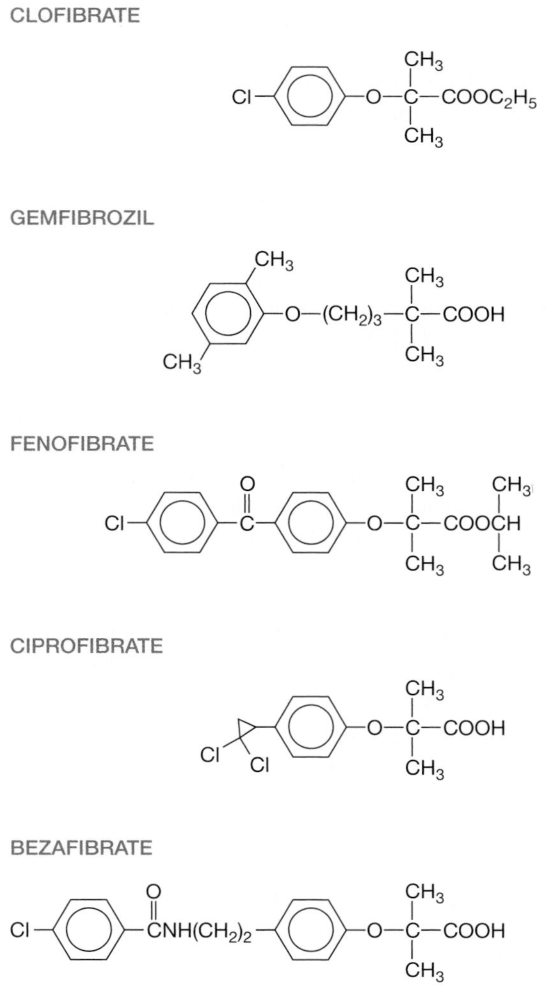

CLOFIBRATE

GEMFIBROZIL

FENOFIBRATE

CIPROFIBRATE

BEZAFIBRATE

Figure 31–4. *Structures of the fibric acids.*

Mechanism of Action. Despite extensive studies in humans, the mechanisms by which fibrates lower lipoprotein levels, or raise HDL levels, remain unclear. Recent studies suggest that many of the effects of these compounds on blood lipids are mediated by their interaction with peroxisome proliferator-activated receptors (PPARs) (Kersten et al., 2000), which regulate gene transcription. Three PPAR isotypes (α, β, and γ) have been identified. Fibrates bind to PPARα, which is expressed primarily in the liver and brown adipose tissue and to a lesser extent in kidney, heart, and skeletal muscle. Fibrates reduce triglycerides through PPARα-mediated stimulation of fatty acid oxidation, increased LPL synthesis, and reduced expression of apoC-III. An increase in LPL would enhance the clearance of triglyceride-rich lipoproteins. A reduction in hepatic production of apoC-III, which serves as an inhibitor of lipolytic processing and receptor-mediated clearance, would enhance the clearance of VLDL. Fibrate-mediated increases in HDL-C are due to PPARα stimulation of apoA-I and apoA-II expression, which increases HDL levels. Fenofibrate is more effective than gemfibrozil at increasing HDL levels.

LDL levels rise in many patients treated with gemfibrozil, especially those with hypertriglyceridemia. However, LDL levels are unchanged or fall in others, especially those whose triglyceride levels are not elevated or who are taking a second-generation agent, such as fenofibrate, bezafibrate, or ciprofibrate. The decrease in LDL levels may be due in part to changes in the cholesterol and triglyceride contents of LDL that are mediated by CETP; such changes can alter the affinity of LDL for the LDL receptor. There also is evidence that a PPARα-mediated increase in hepatic SREBP-1 production enhances hepatic expression of LDL receptors (Kersten et al., 2000). Lastly, fibrates reduce the plasma concentration of small, dense, more easily oxidized LDL particles (Vakkilainen et al., 2003).

Most of the fibric acid agents have potential antithrombotic effects, including inhibition of coagulation and enhancement of fibrinolysis. These salutary effects also could alter cardiovascular outcomes by mechanisms unrelated to any hypolipidemic activity.

Effects on Lipoprotein Levels. The effects of the fibric acid agents on lipoprotein levels differ widely, depending on the starting lipoprotein profile, the presence or absence of a genetic hyperlipoproteinemia, the associated environmental influences, and the specific fibrate used.

Patients with type III hyperlipoproteinemia (dysbetalipoproteinemia) are among the most sensitive responders to fibrates (Mahley and Rall, 2008). Elevated triglyceride and cholesterol levels are dramatically lowered, and tuberoeruptive and palmar xanthomas may regress completely. Angina and intermittent claudication also improve.

In patients with mild hypertriglyceridemia (e.g., triglycerides <400 mg/dL), fibrate treatment decreases triglyceride levels by up to 50% and increases HDL-C concentrations by about 15%; LDL-C levels may be unchanged or increase. The second-generation agents, such as fenofibrate, bezafibrate, and ciprofibrate, lower VLDL levels to a degree similar to that produced by gemfibrozil, but they also are more likely to decrease LDL levels by 15-20%. In patients with more marked hypertriglyceridemia (e.g., 400-1000 mg/dL), a similar fall in triglycerides occurs, but LDL increases of 10-30% are seen frequently. Normotriglyceridemic patients with heterozygous familial hypercholesterolemia usually experience little change in LDL levels with gemfibrozil; with the other fibric acid agents, reductions as great as 20% may occur in some patients.

Fibrates usually are the drugs of choice for treating severe hypertriglyceridemia and the chylomicronemia syndrome. While the primary therapy is to remove alcohol and as much fat from the diet as possible, fibrates help both by increasing triglyceride clearance and decreasing hepatic triglyceride synthesis. In patients with chylomicronemia syndrome, fibrate maintenance therapy and a low-fat diet keep triglyceride levels well below 1000 mg/dL and thus prevent episodes of pancreatitis.

In a 5-year study of hyperlipidemic men, gemfibrozil reduced total cholesterol by 10% and LDL-C by 11%, raised HDL-C levels by 11%, and decreased triglycerides by 35% (Frick et al., 1987). Overall, there was a 34% decrease in the sum of fatal plus nonfatal cardiovascular events without any effect on total mortality. No increased incidence of gallstones or cancers was observed. Subgroup analysis suggested that the greatest benefit occurred in the subjects with the highest levels of VLDL or combined VLDL and LDL and in those with the lowest HDL-C levels (<35 mg/dL). Gemfibrozil may have affected the outcome by influencing platelet function, coagulation factor synthesis, or LDL size. In a recent secondary prevention trial, gemfibrozil reduced fatal and nonfatal CHD events by 22% despite a lack of effect on LDL-C levels. HDL-C levels increased by 6%, which may have contributed to the favorable outcome.

Absorption, Fate, and Excretion. All of the fibrate drugs are absorbed rapidly and efficiently (>90%) when given with a meal but less efficiently when taken on an empty stomach. The ester bond is hydrolyzed rapidly, and peak plasma concentrations are attained within 1-4 hours. More than 95% of these drugs in plasma are bound to protein, nearly exclusively to albumin. The $t_{1/2}$ of fibrates differ significantly, ranging from 1.1 hours (gemfibrozil) to 20 hours (fenofibrate). The drugs are widely distributed throughout the body, and concentrations in liver, kidney, and intestine exceed the plasma level. Gemfibrozil is transferred across the placenta. The fibrate drugs are excreted predominantly as glucuronide conjugates; 60-90% of an oral dose is excreted in the urine, with smaller amounts appearing in the feces. Excretion of these drugs is impaired in renal failure, although excretion of gemfibrozil is less severely compromised in renal insufficiency than is excretion of other fibrates. The use of fibrates is contraindicated in patients with renal failure.

Adverse Effects and Drug Interactions. Fibric acid compounds usually are well tolerated. Side effects may occur in 5-10% of patients but most often are not sufficient to cause discontinuation of the drug. Gastrointestinal side effects occur in up to 5% of patients. Other side effects are reported infrequently and include rash, urticaria, hair loss, myalgias, fatigue, headache, impotence, and anemia. Minor increases in liver transaminases and alkaline phosphatase have been reported. Clofibrate, bezafibrate, and fenofibrate have been reported to potentiate the action of oral anticoagulants, in part by displacing them from their binding sites on albumin. Careful monitoring of the prothrombin time and reduction in dosage of the anticoagulant may be appropriate when treatment with a fibrate is begun.

A myopathy syndrome occasionally occurs in subjects taking clofibrate, gemfibrozil, or fenofibrate and may occur in up to 5% of patients treated with a combination of gemfibrozil and higher doses of statins. To diminish the risk of myopathy, statin doses should be reduced when combination therapy of a statin plus a fibrate is employed. Several drug interactions may contribute to this adverse response. Gemfibrozil inhibits hepatic uptake of statins by OATP1B1. Gemfibrozil also competes for the same glucuronosyl transferases that metabolize most statins. As a consequence, levels of both drugs may be increased when they are co-administered (Prueksaritanont et al., 2002b; Prueksaritanont et al., 2002c). Patients taking this combination should be instructed to be aware of the potential symptoms and should be followed at 3-month intervals with careful history and determination of CK values until a stable pattern is established. Patients taking fibrates with rosuvastatin should be followed especially closely even if low doses (5-10 mg) of rosuvastatin are employed until there is more experience with and knowledge of the safety of this specific combination. Fenofibrate is glucuronidated by enzymes that are not involved in statin glucuronidation. Thus, fenofibrate-statin combinations are less likely to cause myopathy than combination therapy with gemfibrozil and statins.

All of the fibrates increase the lithogenicity of bile. Clofibrate use has been associated with increased risk of gallstone formation.

Renal failure is a relative contraindication to the use of fibric acid agents, as is hepatic dysfunction. Combined statin-fibrate therapy should be avoided in patients with compromised renal function. Gemfibrozil should be used with caution and at a reduced dosage to treat the hyperlipidemia of renal failure. *Fibrates should not be used by children or pregnant women.*

Therapeutic Use. Clofibrate is available for oral administration. The usual dose is 2 g/day in divided doses. This compound is little used but may be useful in patients who do not tolerate gemfibrozil or fenofibrate. Gemfibrozil (LOPID) usually is administered as a 600-mg dose taken twice a day, 30 minutes before the morning and evening meals. Fenofibrate is available in two different formulations. The first preparation developed is the dimethylethyl ester of fenofibric acid, which is poorly water soluble and poorly absorbed. After uptake by the liver, this compound is hydrolyzed to produce fenofibric acid, which is the active moiety. Recently, a choline salt of fenofibric acid that is highly soluble in water and readily absorbed was developed. The effects of both formulations, however, are similar with respect to changes in plasma lipid concentrations (Grundy et al., 2005; Jones et al., 2009). The dimethylethyl ester preparations of fenofibric acid include TRICOR and LOFIBRA. The tricor brand of fenofibrate is available in tablets of 48 and 145 mg. The usual daily dose is 145 mg. Generic fenofibrate (LOFIBRA) is available in capsules containing 67, 134, and 200 mg. TRICOR, 145 mg, and LOFIBRA, 200 mg, are equivalent doses. The choline salt of fenofibric acid (TRILIPIX) is available in capsules of 135 and 45 mg. TRILIPIX, 135 mg, is equivalent to TRICOR, 145 mg, and LOFIBRA, 200 mg. Choline fenofibrate is indicated for combination therapy with statins (Jones et al., 2009). Fibrates are the drugs of choice for treating hyperlipidemic subjects with type III hyperlipoproteinemia as well as subjects with severe hypertriglyceridemia (triglycerides >1000 mg/dL) who are at risk for pancreatitis. Fibrates appear to have an important role in subjects with high triglycerides and low HDL-C levels associated with the metabolic syndrome or type 2 diabetes mellitus (Robins, 2001). When fibrates are used in such patients, the LDL levels need to be monitored; if LDL levels rise, the addition of a low dose of a statin may be needed. Many experts now treat such patients first with a statin (Heart Protection Study Collaborative Group, 2003) and then add a fibrate, based on the reported benefit of gemfibrozil therapy. However, statin-fibrate combination therapy has not been evaluated in outcome studies (American Diabetes Association, 2004). If this combination is used, there should be careful monitoring for myopathy.

Ezetimibe and the Inhibition of Dietary Cholesterol Uptake

Ezetimibe is the first compound approved for lowering total and LDL-C levels that inhibits cholesterol absorption by enterocytes in the small intestine. It lowers LDL-C levels by ~20% and is used primarily as adjunctive therapy with statins.

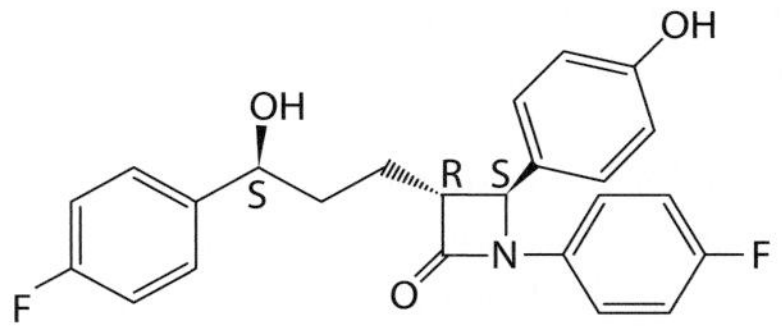

OH OH S R S N F O F

EZETIMIBE

History. Ezetimibe (SCH58235) was developed by pharmaceutical chemists studying inhibition of intestinal ACAT. Several compounds were found to inhibit cholesterol absorption, but by inhibiting intestinal cholesterol transport rather than ACAT.

Mechanism of Action. Ezetimibe inhibits luminal cholesterol uptake by jejunal enterocytes, by inhibiting the transport protein NPC1L1 (Altmann et al., 2004; Davis et al., 2004).

In wild-type mice, ezetimibe inhibits cholesterol absorption by about 70%; in NPC1L1 knockout mice, cholesterol absorption is 86% lower than in wild-type mice, and ezetimibe has no effect on cholesterol absorption (Altmann et al., 2004). Ezetimibe does not affect intestinal triglyceride absorption. In human subjects, ezetimibe reduced cholesterol absorption by 54%, precipitating a compensatory increase in cholesterol synthesis that can be inhibited with a cholesterol synthesis inhibitor such as a statin (Sudhop et al., 2002). There also is a substantial reduction of plasma levels of plant sterols (campesterol and sitosterol concentrations are reduced by 48% and 41%, respectively), indicating that ezetimibe also inhibits intestinal absorption of plant sterols.

The consequence of inhibiting intestinal cholesterol absorption is a reduction in the incorporation of cholesterol into chylomicrons. The reduced cholesterol content of chylomicrons diminishes the delivery of cholesterol to the liver by chylomicron remnants. The diminished remnant cholesterol content may decrease atherogenesis directly, as chylomicron remnants are very atherogenic lipoproteins. In experimental animal models of remnant dyslipidemia, ezetimibe profoundly diminished diet-induced atherosclerosis (Davis et al., 2001a).

Reduced delivery of intestinal cholesterol to the liver by chylomicron remnants stimulates expression of the hepatic genes regulating LDL receptor expression and cholesterol biosynthesis. The greater expression of hepatic LDL receptors enhances LDL-C clearance from the plasma. Indeed, ezetimibe reduces LDL-C levels by 15-20% (Gagné et al., 2002; Knopp et al., 2003).

Combination Therapy (Ezetimibe plus Statins). The maximal efficacy of ezetimibe for lowering LDL-C is 15-20% when used as monotherapy (Knopp et al., 2003). This reduction is equivalent to, or less than, that attained with 10- to 20-mg doses of most statins. Consequently, the role of ezetimibe as monotherapy of patients with elevated LDL-C levels appears to be limited to the small group of statin-intolerant patients.

The actions of ezetimibe are complementary to those of statins. Statins, which inhibit cholesterol biosynthesis, increase intestinal cholesterol absorption (Miettinen and Gylling, 2003). Ezetimibe, which inhibits intestinal cholesterol absorption, enhances cholesterol biosynthesis by as much as 3.5 times in experimental animals (Davis et al., 2001b). Dual therapy with these two classes of drugs prevents both the enhanced cholesterol synthesis induced by ezetimibe and the increase in cholesterol absorption induced by statins. This combination provides additive reductions in LDL-C levels irrespective of the statin employed (Ballantyne et al., 2004; Ballantyne et al., 2003; Melani et al., 2003).

A combination tablet containing ezetimibe, 10 mg, and various doses of simvastatin (10, 20, 40, and 80 mg) has been approved (VYTORIN). At the highest simvastatin dose (80 mg), plus ezetimibe (10 mg), average LDL-C reduction was 60%, which is greater than can be attained with any statin as monotherapy (Feldman et al., 2004). Despite the robust laboratory-based efficacy of this combination, the clinical cardiovascular benefits remain controversial when the combination is compared to effects of statins alone (Kastelein et al., 2008; Mitka, 2009).

Absorption, Fate, and Excretion. Ezetimibe is highly water insoluble, precluding studies of its bioavailability. After ingestion, it is glucuronidated in the intestinal epithelium and absorbed and then enters an enterohepatic recirculation (Patrick et al., 2002). Pharmacokinetic studies indicate that about 70% is excreted in the feces and about 10% in the urine (as a glucuronide conjugate) (Patrick et al., 2002). Bile-acid sequestrants inhibit absorption of ezetimibe, and the two agents should not be administered together. Otherwise, no significant drug interactions have been reported.

Adverse Effects and Drug Interactions. Other than rare allergic reactions, specific adverse effects have not been observed in patients taking ezetimibe. The safety of ezetimibe during pregnancy has not been established. With doses of ezetimibe sufficient to increase exposure 10-150 times compared with a 10-mg dose in humans, fetal skeletal abnormalities were noted in rats and rabbits. *Since all statins are contraindicated in pregnant and nursing women, combination products containing ezetimibe and a statin should not be used by women in childbearing years in the absence of contraception.*

Therapeutic Use. Ezetimibe (ZETIA) is available as a 10-mg tablet that may be taken at any time during the day, with or without food. Ezetimibe may be taken with any medication other than bile-acid sequestrants, which inhibit its absorption.

CLINICAL SUMMARY

Patients with any type of dyslipidemia (e.g., elevated levels of cholesterol, low levels of HDL-C with or without hypercholesterolemia, or moderately elevated triglyceride levels with low HDL-C levels) are at risk of developing atherosclerosis-induced vascular disease. Maintaining ideal body weight, eating a diet low in saturated fat and cholesterol, and regular exercise are the cornerstones of managing dyslipidemia. In the absence of vascular disease, type 2 diabetes mellitus, or metabolic syndrome, adoption of these behaviors will alleviate the need for cholesterol-lowering medications in many subjects. Following assessment of their future risk for a vascular disease event, patients should be treated to achieve target lipid values. In virtually every type of dyslipidemic patient, statins have been proven to reduce the risk of subsequent CHD events and nonhemorrhagic stroke. For this reason, statin therapy should be the first-line choice when choosing between classes of lipid-lowering agents.

A second principle is to treat with statin doses adequate to reduce the patient's lipid values to goal levels. Most patients are not adequately treated and do not reach goal values. Safety is greatly enhanced if doctors discuss with their patients the rare but serious side effects of hepatotoxicity and rhabdomyolysis with associated renal failure.

Finally, patients with low HDL-C levels may not receive the maximum benefit of lipid-lowering therapy as prescribed by the ATP III guidelines based on levels of LDL-C or non-HDL-C. For this reason, treatment of patients with low HDL-C levels should be based on both LDL-C levels and the ratio of total cholesterol:HDL-C (Table 31–9).

BIBLIOGRAPHY

Afilalo J, Duque G, Steele R, *et al.* Statins for secondary prevention in elderly patients: A hierarchical bayesian meta-analysis. *J Am Coll Cardiol,* **2008,** *51:*37–45.

Ahmed W, Khan N, Glueck CJ, *et al.* Low serum 25 (OH) vitamin D levels (<32 ng/mL) are associated with reversible myositis-myalgia in statin-treated patients. *Transl Res,* **2009,** *153:*11–16.

Alberti KGMM, Eckel RH, Grundy SM, *et al.* Harmonizing the metabolic syndrome: A joint interim statement of the International Diabetes Federation Task Force on Epidemiology and Prevention; National Heart, Lung, and Blood Institute;

American Heart Association; World Heart Federation; International Atherosclerosis Society; and International Association for the Study of Obesity. *Circulation,* **2009,** *120:*1640–1645.

Alqahtani SA, Sanchez W. Statins are safe for the treatment of hypercholesterolemia in patients with chronic liver disease. *Gastroenterology,* **2008,** *135:*702–704.

Alsheikh-Ali AA, Karas RH. Adverse events with concomitant amiodarone and statin therapy. *Prev Cardiol,* **2005,** *8:*95–97.

Altmann SW, Davis HR Jr, Zhu L-J, *et al.* Niemann-Pick C1 like 1 protein is critical for intestinal cholesterol absorption. *Science,* **2004,** *303:*1201–1204.

Amarenco P, Labreuche J. Lipid management in the prevention of stroke: Review and updated meta-analysis of statins for stroke prevention. *Lancet Neurol,* **2009,** *8:*453–463.

American Diabetes Association. Dyslipidemia management in adults with diabetes. *Diabetes Care,* **2004,** *27*(suppl 1): S68–S71.

American Heart Association (AHA). *Heart Disease and Stroke Statistics—2004 Update*. Dallas, TX, AHA, **2003**.

Attie AD. ABCA1: At the nexus of cholesterol, HDL and atherosclerosis. *Trends Biochem Sci,* **2007,** *32:*172–179.

Aung PP, Maxwell H, Jepson RG, *et al.* Lipid-lowering for peripheral arterial disease of the lower limb. *Cochrane Database Syst Rev,* **2007,** *4:*CD000123.

Baigent C, Landry M. Study of Heart and Renal Protection (SHARP). *Kidney Int,* **2003,** *63*(suppl 84):S207–S210.

Ballantyne CM, Blazing MA, King TR, *et al.* Efficacy and safety of *ezetimibe* co-administered with *simvastatin* compared with *atorvastatin* in adults with hypercholesterolemia. *Am J Cardiol,* **2004,** *93:*1487–1494.

Ballantyne CM, Houri J, Notarbartolo A, *et al.* Effect of ezetimibe coadministered with atorvastatin in 628 patients with primary hypercholesterolemia: A prospective, randomized, double-blind trial. *Circulation,* **2003,** *107:*2409–2415.

Barter P, Gotto AM, LaRosa JC, *et al.* HDL cholesterol, very low levels of LDL cholesterol, and cardiovascular events. *N Engl J Med,* **2007,** *357:*1301–1310.

Bellosta S, Paoletti R, Corsini A. Safety of statins. Focus on clinical pharmacokinetics and drug interactions. *Circulation,* **2004,** *109:*III-50–III-57.

Bergman AJ, Murphy G, Burke J, *et al.* Simvastatin does not have a clinically significant pharmacokinetic interaction with fenofibrate in humans. *J Clin Pharmacol,* **2004,** *44:*1054–1062.

Bersot TP, Pépin GM, Mahley RW. Risk determination of dyslipidemia in populations characterized by low levels of high-density lipoprotein cholesterol. *Am Heart J,* **2003,** *146:* 1052–1060.

Birjmohun RS, Dallinga-Thie GM, Kuivenhoven JA, *et al.* Apolipoprotein A-II is inversely associated with risk of future coronary artery disease. *Circulation,* **2007,** *116:*2029–2035.

Bradford RH, Shear CL, Chremos AN, *et al.* Expanded Clinical Evaluation of Lovastatin (EXCEL) Study results. I. Efficacy in modifying plasma lipoproteins and adverse event profile in 8245 patients with moderate hypercholesterolemia. *Arch Intern Med,* **1991,** *151:*43–49.

Brown BG, Cheung MC, Lee AC, *et al.* Antioxidant vitamins and lipid therapy. End of a long romance? *Arterioscler Thromb Vasc Biol,* **2002,** *22:*1535–1546.

Brown RJ, Rader DJ. Lipases as modulators of atherosclerosis in murine models. *Curr Drug Targets,* **2007,** *8:*1307–1319.

Brunzell JD, Davidson M, Furberg CD, *et al.* Lipoprotein management in patients with cardiometabolic risk. Consensus statement from the American Diabetes Association and the American College of Cardiology Foundation. *Diabetes Care,* **2008,** *31:*811–822.

Cannon CP, Braunwald E, McCabe CH, et al. Intensive versus moderate lipid lowering with statins after acute coronary syndromes. *N Engl J Med,* **2004,** *350:*1495–1504.

Cannon CP, Steinberg BA, Murphy SA, *et al.* Meta-analysis of cardiovascular outcomes trials comparing intensive versus moderate statin therapy. *J Am Coll Cardiol,* **2006,** *48:*438–445.

Castelli WP. Making practical sense of clinical trial data in decreasing cardiovascular risk. *Am J Cardiol,* **2001,** *88*(suppl):16F–20F.

Chalasani N, Aljadhey H, Kesterson J, *et al.* Patients with elevated liver enzymes are not at higher risk for statin hepatotoxicity. *Gastroenterology,* **2004,** *126:*1287–1292.

Chen Z, Peto R, Collins R, *et al.* Serum cholesterol concentration and coronary heart disease in population with low cholesterol concentrations. *Br Med J,* **1991,** *303:*276–282.

Cheung BMY, Lauder IJ, Lau C-P, Kumana CR. Meta-analysis of large randomized controlled trials to evaluate the impact of statins on cardiovascular outcomes. *Br J Clin Pharmacol,* **2004,** *57:*640–651.

Cholesterol Treatment Trialists' (CTT) Collaborators. Efficacy and safety of cholesterol-lowering treatment: Prospective meta-analysis of data from 90 056 participants in 14 randomised trials of statins. *Lancet,* **2005,** *366:*1267–1278.

Cholesterol Treatment Trialists' (CTT) Collaborators. Efficacy of cholesterol-lowering therapy in 18 686 people with diabetes in 14 randomised trials of statins: A meta-analysis. *Lancet,* **2008,** *371:*117–125.

Christian AH, Mills T, Simpson SL, Mosca L. Quality of cardiovascular disease preventive care and physician/practice characteristics. *J Gen Intern Med,* **2006,** *21:*231–237.

Christians U, Jacobsen W, Floren LC. Metabolism and drug interactions of 3-hydroxy-3-methylglutaryl coenzyme A reductase inhibitors in transplant patients: Are the statins mechanistically similar? *Pharmacol Ther,* **1998,** *80:*1–34.

Contois JH, McConnell JP, Sethi AA, *et al.* Apolipoprotein B and cardiovascular disease risk: Position statement from the AACC Lipoproteins and Vascular Diseases Division Working Group on Best Practices. *Clin Chem,* **2009,** *55:*407–419.

Corsini A. The safety of HMG-CoA reductase inhibitors in special populations at high cardiovascular risk. *Cardiovasc Drugs Ther,* **2003,** *17:*265–285.

Corsini A, Bellosta S, Baetta R, *et al.* New insights into the pharmacodynamic and pharmacokinetic properties of statins. *Pharmacol Ther,* **1999,** *84:*413–428.

Crouse JR III, Frolich J, Ose L, *et al.* Effects of high doses of *simvastatin* and *atorvastatin* on high-density lipoprotein cholesterol and apolipoprotein A-I. *Am J Cardiol,* **1999,** *83:* 1476–1477.

Crouse JR, Kastelein J, Isaacsohn J, *et al.* A large, 36 week study of the HDL-C raising effects and safety of simvastatin versus atorvastatin [abstract]. *Atherosclerosis,* **2000,** *151*:8–9.

D'Agostino RB Sr, Grundy S, Sullivan LM, Wilson P, for the C. H. D. Risk Prediction Group. Validation of the Framingham coronary heart disease prediction scores: Results of a multiple ethnic groups investigation. *JAMA,* **2001,** *286:*180–187.

D'Agostino RB Sr, Vasan RS, Pencina MJ, *et al.* General cardiovascular risk profile for use in primary care: The Framingham Heart Study. *Circulation,* **2008,** *117:*743–753.

Daniels SR, Greer FR, and the Committee on Nutrition. Lipid screening and cardiovascular health in childhood. *Pediatrics,* **2008,** *122:*198–208.

Davis HR Jr, Altmann SW. Niemann–Pick C1 Like 1 (NPC1L1) an intestinal sterol transporter. *Biochim Biophys Acta,* **2009,** *1791:*679–683.

Davis HR Jr, Compton DS, Hoos L, Tetzloff G. Ezetimibe, a potent cholesterol absorption inhibitor, inhibits the development of atherosclerosis in apoE knockout mice. *Arterioscler Thromb Vasc Biol,* **2001a,** *21:*2032–2038.

Davis HR Jr, Pula KK, Alton KB, *et al.* The synergistic hypercholesterolemic activity of the potent cholesterol absorption inhibitor, ezetimibe, in combination with 3-hydroxy-3-methylglutaryl coenzyme A reductase inhibitors in dogs. *Metabolism,* **2001b,** *50:*1234–1241.

Davis HR Jr, Zhu L-J, Hoos LM, *et al.* Niemann-Pick C1 Like 1 (NPC1L1) is the intestinal phytosterol and cholesterol transporter and a key modulator of whole-body cholesterol homeostasis. *J Biol Chem,* **2004,** *279:*33586–33592.

deGoma EM, deGoma RL, Rader DJ. Beyond high-density lipoprotein cholesterol levels: Evaluating high-density lipoprotein function as influenced by novel therapeutic approaches. *J Am Coll Cardiol,* **2008,** *51:*2199–2211.

Diamond GA, Kaul S. Prevention and treatment: A tale of two strategies. *J Am Coll Cardiol,* **2008,** *51:*46–48.

Ebrahimi R, Saleh J, Toggart E, *et al.* Effect of preprocedural statin use on procedural myocardial infarction and major cardiac adverse events in percutaneous coronary intervention: A meta-analysis. *J Invasive Cardiol,* **2008,** *20:*292–295.

Feldman T, Koren M, Insull W Jr, *et al.* Treatment of high-risk patients with *ezetimibe* plus *simvastatin* co-administration versus *simvastatin* alone to attain National Cholesterol Education Program Adult Treatment Panel III low-density lipoprotein cholesterol goals. *Am J Cardiol,* **2004,** *93:*1481–1486.

Folsom AR, Chambless LE, Ballantyne CM, *et al.* An assessment of incremental coronary risk prediction using C-reactive protein and other novel risk markers: The Atherosclerosis Risk in Communities Study. *Arch Intern Med,* **2006,** *166:*1368–1373.

Franz HM, Lionel P, Simon SKT, *et al.* Impact of systemic hypertension on the cardiovascular benefits of statin therapy—A meta-analysis. *Am J Cardiol,* **2008,** *101:*319–325.

Frick MH, Elo O, Haapa K, *et al.* Helsinki Heart Study: Primary-prevention trial with gemfibrozil in middle-aged men with dyslipidemia. Safety of treatment, changes in risk factors, and incidence of coronary heart disease. *N Engl J Med,* **1987,** *317:*1237–1245.

Gagné C, Bays HE, Weiss SR, *et al.* Efficacy and safety of *ezetimibe* added to ongoing statin therapy for treatment of patients with primary hypercholesterolemia. *Am J Cardiol,* **2002,** *90:*1084–1091.

Ganji SH, Tavintharan S, Zhu D, *et al.* Niacin noncompetitively inhibits DGAT2 but not DGAT1 activity in HepG2 cells. *J Lipid Res,* **2004,** *45:*1835–1845.

Ginsberg HN, Bonds DE, Lovato LC, *et al.* Evolution of the lipid trial protocol of the Action to Control Cardiovascular Risk in Diabetes (ACCORD) trial. *Am J Cardiol,* **2007,** *99*(suppl): 56i–67i.

Glynn RJ, Danielson E, Fonseca FAH, *et al.* A randomized trial of rosuvastatin in the prevention of venous thromboembolism. *N Engl J Med,* **2009,** *360:*1851–1861.

Grundy SM, Brewer HB Jr, Cleeman JI, et al. Definition of metabolic syndrome. Report of the National Heart, Lung, and Blood Institute/American Heart Association conference on scientific issues related to definition. *Circulation,* **2004a,** *109:*433–438.

Grundy SM, Cleeman JI, Merz CNB, *et al.* Implications of recent clinical trials for the National Cholesterol Education Program Adult Treatment Panel III guidelines. *Circulation,* **2004b,** *110:*227–239.

Grundy SM, Vega GL, McGovern ME, *et al.* Efficacy, safety, and tolerability of once-daily niacin for the treatment of dyslipidemia associated with type 2 diabetes: Results of the assessment of diabetes control and evaluation of the efficacy of niaspan trial. *Arch Intern Med,* **2002,** *162:*1568–1576.

Grundy SM, Vega GL, Yuan Z, *et al.* Effectiveness and tolerability of simvastatin plus fenofibrate for combined hyperlipidemia (the SAFARI trial). *Am J Cardiol,* **2005,** *95:*462–468.

Haim M, Benderly M, Brunner D, *et al.* Elevated serum triglyceride levels and long-term mortality in patients with coronary heart disease. The Bezafibrate Infarction Prevention (BIP) registry. *Circulation,* **1999,** *100:*475–482.

Heady JA, Morris JN, Oliver MF. WHO clofibrate/cholesterol trial: Clarifications. *Lancet,* **1992,** *340:*1405–1406.

Heart Protection Study Collaborative Group. MRC/BHF Heart Protection Study of cholesterol lowering with simvastatin in 20 536 high-risk individuals: A randomised placebo-controlled trial. *Lancet,* **2002,** *360:*7–22.

Heart Protection Study Collaborative Group. MRC/BHF Heart Protection Study of cholesterol-lowering with simvastatin in 5963 people with diabetes: A randomised placebo-controlled trial. *Lancet,* **2003,** *361:*2005–2016.

Horton JD, Cohen JC, Hobbs HH. Molecular biology of PCSK9: Its role in LDL metabolism. *Trends Biochem Sci,* **2007,** *32:*71–77.

Hunninghake DB, Stein EA, Bays HE, *et al.* Rosuvastatin improves the atherogenic and atheroprotective lipid profiles in patients with hypertriglyceridemia. *Coron Artery Dis,* **2004,** *15:*115–123.

Hussain MM, Bakillah A. New approaches to target microsomal triglyceride transfer protein. *Curr Opin Lipidol,* **2008,** *19:*572–578.

Ieiri I, Suwannakul S, Maeda K, *et al.* SLCO1B1 (OATP1B1, an uptake transporter) and ABCG2 (BCRP, an efflux transporter) variant alleles and pharmacokinetics of pitavastatin in healthy volunteers. *Clin Pharmacol Ther,* **2007,** *82:*541–547.

Jafri H, Alsheikh-Ali AA, Karas RH. Abstract 1423: Statin therapy does not reduce the increased cardiovascular risk associated with low levels of high-density lipoprotein cholesterol: Evidence from randomized controlled trials. *Circulation,* **2009,** *120:*S500.

Jones P, Kafonek S, Laurora I, Hunninghake D. Comparative dose efficacy study of *atorvastatin* versus *simvastatin, pravastatin, lovastatin,* and *fluvastatin* in patients with hypercholesterolemia (the CURVES study). *Am J Cardiol,* **1998,** *81:*582–587.

Jones PH, Davidson MH, Goldberg AC, *et al.* Efficacy and safety of fenofibric acid in combination with a statin in patients with mixed dyslipidemia: Pooled analysis of three phase 3, 12-week randomized, controlled studies. *J Clin Lipidol,* **2009,** *3:*125–137.

Jones PH, Davidson MH, Stein EA, *et al.* Comparison of the efficacy and safety of *rosuvastatin* versus *atorvastatin, simvastatin,* and *pravastatin* across doses (STELLAR trial). *Am J Cardiol,* **2003,** *92:*152–160.

Kastelein JJ, et al. Simvarstatin with or without ezetimibe in familial hypercholesterolemia. *N Eng Jimed,* **2008,** *358*:1431–1443.

Kersten S, Desvergne B, Wahli W. Roles of PPARs in health and disease. *Nature,* **2000,** *405:*421–424.

Knopp RH, Dujovne CA, Le Beaut A, *et al.* Evaluation of the efficacy, safety, and tolerability of ezetimibe in primary hypercholesterolaemia: A pooled analysis from two controlled phase III clinical studies. *Int J Clin Pract,* **2003,** *57:*363–368.

Knopp RH, Retzlaff BM, Fish B, *et al.* The SLIM Study: Slo-Niacin(r) and Atorvastatin Treatment of Lipoproteins and Inflammatory Markers in combined hyperlipidemia. *J Clin Lipidol,* **2009,** *3:*167–178.

Kuklina EV, Yoon PW, Keenan NL. Trends in high levels of low-density lipoprotein cholesterol in the United States, 1999-2006. *JAMA,* **2009,** *302:*2104–2110.

Law M, Rudnicka AR. Statin safety: A systematic review. *Am J Cardiol,* **2006,** *97*(suppl):52C–60C.

Lee JH, O'Keefe JH, Bell D, *et al.* Vitamin D deficiency: An important, common, and easily treatable cardiovascular risk factor? *J Am Coll Cardiol,* **2008,** *52:*1949–1956.

Lewis JH, Mortensen ME, Zweig S, et al. Efficacy and safety of high-dose pravastatin in hypercholesterolemic patients with well-compensated chronic liver disease: Results of a prospective, randomized, double-blind, placebo-controlled, multicenter trial. *Hepatology,* **2007,** *46:*1453–1463.

Li HY, Appelbaum FR, Willman CL, *et al.* Cholesterol-modulating agents kill acute myeloid leukemia cells and sensitize them to therapeutics by blocking adaptive cholesterol responses. *Blood,* **2003,** *101:*3628–3634.

Liao JK. Effects of statins on 3-hydroxy-3-methylglutaryl coenzyme A reductase inhibition beyond low-density lipoprotein cholesterol. *Am J Cardiol,* **2005,** *96*(suppl):24F–33F.

Libby P, Aikawa M. Mechanisms of plaque stabilization with statins. *Am J Cardiol,* **2003,** *91*(suppl):4B–8B.

Libby P, Ridker PM. Inflammation and atherosclerosis: Role of C-reactive protein in risk assessment. *Am J Med,* **2004,** *116:*9S–16S.

Lillis AP, Van Duyn LB, Murphy-Ullrich JE, Strickland DK. LDL receptor-related protein 1: Unique tissue-specific functions revealed by selective gene knockout studies. *Physiol Rev,* **2008,** *88:*887–918.

Lipid Research Clinics Program. The Lipid Research Clinics Coronary Primary Prevention Trial results. II. The relationship of reduction in incidence of coronary heart disease to cholesterol lowering. *JAMA,* **1984,** *251:*365–374.

Liu J, Hong Y, D'Agostino RB Sr, et al. Predictive value for the Chinese population of the Framingham CHD risk assessment tool compared with the Chinese Multi-provincial Cohort Study. *JAMA,* **2004,** *291:*2591–2599.

Lloyd-Jones D, Adams R, Carnethon M, *et al.* Heart disease and stroke statistics 2009 update: A report from the American Heart Association Statistics Committee and Stroke Statistics Subcommittee. *Circulation,* **2009,** *119:*e21–e181.

Lloyd-Jones DM, Hong Y, Labarthe D, *et al.* Defining and setting national goals for cardiovascular health promotion and disease reduction. The American Heart Association's strategic impact goal through 2020 and beyond. *Circulation,* **2010,** *121:*586–613.

Lloyd-Jones DM, Nam B-H, D'Agostino RB Sr, et al. Parental cardiovascular disease as a risk factor for cardiovascular disease in middle-aged adults. A prospective study of parents and offspring. *JAMA,* **2004,** *291:*2204–2211.

Lloyd-Jones DM, Tian L. Predicting cardiovascular risk: So what do we do now? *Ann Intern Med,* **2006,** *166:*1342–1344.

Lorenzen A, Stannek C, Lang H, *et al.* Characterization of a G protein-coupled receptor for nicotinic acid. *Mol Pharmacol,* **2001,** *59:*349–357.

Mahley RW, Weisgraber KH, Bersot TP. Disorders of lipid metabolism. In: Kronenberg HM, Melmed S, Polonsky KS, Larsen PR, eds. *Williams Textbook of Endocrinology,* 11th ed., Philadelphia, Saunders, **2008,** pp. 1589–1653.

McLaughlin T, Reaven G, Abbasi F, *et al.* Is there a simple way to identify insulin-resistant individuals at increased risk of cardiovascular disease? *Am J Cardiol,* **2005,** *96:*399–404.

Melani L, Mills R, Hassman D, *et al.* Efficacy and safety of ezetimibe coadministered with pravastatin in patients with primary hypercholesterolemia: A prospective, randomized, double-blind trial. *Eur Heart J,* **2003,** *24:*717–728.

Miettinen TA, Gylling H. Synthesis and absorption markers of cholesterol in serum and lipoproteins during a large dose of statin treatment. *Eur J Clin Invest,* **2003,** *33:*976–982.

Mitka M. Amid lingering questions, FDA reprieves LDL cholesterol-lowering medication. *JAMA,* **2009,** *301*:813-815.

Mora S. Advanced lipoprotein testing and subfractionation are not (yet) ready for routine clinical use. *Circulation,* **2009,** *119:*2396–2404.

Mora S, Rifai N, Buring JE, Ridker PM. Comparison of LDL cholesterol concentrations by Friedewald calculation and direct measurement in relation to cardiovascular events in 27 331 women. *Clin Chem,* **2009,** *55:*888–894.

Movva R, Rader DJ. Laboratory assessment of HDL heterogeneity and function. *Clin Chem,* **2008,** *54:*788–800.

Murabito JM, Pencina MJ, Nam B-H, *et al.* Sibling cardiovascular disease as a risk factor for cardiovascular disease in middle-aged adults. *JAMA,* **2005,** *294:*3117–3123.

Neuvonen PJ, Niemi M, Backman JT. Drug interactions with lipid-lowering drugs: Mechanisms and clinical relevance. *Clin Pharmacol Ther,* **2006,** *80:*565–581.

Norris W, Paredes AH, Lewis JH. Drug-induced liver injury in 2007. *Curr Opin Gastroenterol,* **2008,** *24:*287–297.

Pasternak RC, Smith SC Jr, Bairey-Merz CN, *et al.* ACC/AHA/NHLBI clinical advisory on the use and safety of statins. *Circulation,* **2002,** *106:*1024–1028.

Patrick JE, Kosoglou T, Stauber KL, *et al.* Disposition of the selective cholesterol absorption inhibitor ezetimibe in healthy male subjects. *Drug Metab Disp,* **2002,** *30:*430–437.

Pearson TA, Mensah GA, Alexander RW, *et al.* Markers of inflammation and cardiovascular disease. Application to clinical and public health practice. A statement for healthcare professionals from the Centers for Disease Control and Prevention and the American Heart Association. *Circulation,* **2003,** *107:*499–511.

Pedersen TR, Tobert JA. Benefits and risks of HMG-CoA reductase inhibitors in the prevention of coronary heart disease. A reappraisal. *Drug Saf,* **1996,** *14:*11–24.

Pennacchio LA, Olivier M, Hubacek JA, *et al.* An apolipoprotein influencing triglycerides in humans and mice revealed by comparative sequencing. *Science,* **2001,** *294:*169–173.

Prueksaritanont T, Subramanian R, Fang X, *et al.* Glucuronidation of statins in animals and humans: A novel mechanism of statin lactonization. *Drug Metab Disp,* **2002a,** *30:*505–512.

Prueksaritanont T, Tang C, Qiu Y, et al. Effects of fibrates on metabolism of statins in human hepatocytes. *Drug Metab Disp,* **2002b,** *30:*1280–1287.

Prueksaritanont T, Zhao JJ, Ma B, *et al.* Mechanistic studies on metabolic interactions between gemfibrozil and statins. *J Pharmacol Exp Ther,* **2002c,** *301:*1042–1051.

Radhakrishnan A, Goldstein JL, McDonald JG, Brown MS. Switch-like control of SREBP-2 transport triggered by small changes in ER cholesterol: A delicate balance. *Cell Metab,* **2008,** *8:*512–521.

Ridker PM, Danielson E, Fonseca FAH, *et al.* Rosuvastatin to prevent vascular events in men and women with elevated C-reactive protein. *N Engl J Med,* **2008,** *359:*2195–2207.

Robins SJ. Targeting low high-density lipoprotein cholesterol for therapy: Lessons from the Veterans Affairs High-Density Lipoprotein Intervention Trial. *Am J Cardiol,* **2001,** *88*(suppl): 19N–23N.

Rubic T, Trottmann M, Lorenz RL. Stimulation of CD36 and the key effector of reverse cholesterol transport ATP-binding cassette A1 in monocytoid cells by niacin. *Biochem Pharmacol,* **2004,** *67:*411–419.

Rubins HB, Robins SJ, Collins D, *et al.* Gemfibrozil for the secondary prevention of coronary heart disease in men with low levels of high-density lipoprotein cholesterol. *N Engl J Med,* **1999,** *341:*410–418.

Sachdeva A, Cannon CP, Deedwania PC, *et al.* Lipid levels in patients hospitalized with coronary artery disease: An analysis of 136,905 hospitalizations in Get With The Guidelines. *Am Heart J,* **2009,** *157:*111–117.

Sarwar N, Danesh J, Eiriksdottir G, *et al.* Triglycerides and the risk of coronary heart disease: 10 158 incident cases among 262 525 participants in 29 Western prospective studies. *Circulation,* **2007,** *115:*450–458.

Schachter M. Chemical, pharmacokinetic and pharmacodynamic properties of statins: An update. *Fundam Clin Pharmacol,* **2005,** *19:*117–125.

Schneck DW, Birmingham BK, Zalikowski JA, *et al.* The effect of gemfibrozil on the pharmacokinetics of rosuvastatin. *Clin Pharmacol Ther,* **2004,** *75:*455–463.

Shitara Y, Sugiyama Y. Pharmacokinetic and pharmacodynamic alterations of 3-hydroxy-3-methylglutaryl coenzyme A (HMG-CoA) reductase inhibitors: Drug–drug interactions and interindividual differences in transporter and metabolic enzyme functions. *Pharmacol Ther,* **2006,** *112:*71–105.

Shlipak MG, Simon JA, Vittinghoff E, *et al.* Estrogen and progestin, lipoprotein(a), and the risk of recurrent coronary heart disease events after menopause. *JAMA,* **2000,** *283:*1845–1852.

Sniderman A. Targets for LDL-lowering therapy. *Curr Opin Lipidol,* **2009,** *20:*282–287.

Sniderman AD, Marcovina SM. Apolipoprotein A1 and B. *Clin Lab Med,* **2006,** *26:*733–750.

Staffa JA, Chang J, Green L. Cerivastatin and reports of fatal rhabdomyolysis. *N Engl J Med,* **2002,** *346:*539–540.

Steinberg D, Witztum JL. Is the oxidative modification hypothesis relevant to human atherosclerosis? Do the antioxidant trials conducted to date refute the hypothesis? *Circulation,* **2002,** *105:*2107–2111.

Sudhop T, Lütjohann D, Kodal A, *et al.* Inhibition of intestinal cholesterol absorption by ezetimibe in humans. *Circulation,* **2002,** *106:*1943–1948.

Tall AR. CETP inhibitors to increase HDL cholesterd levels. *Engl J Med,* **2007**, *356*:1364–1366.

Tall AR, Yvan-Charvet L, Terasaka N, *et al.* HDL, ABC transporters, and cholesterol efflux: Implications for the treatment of atherosclerosis. *Cell Metabol,* **2008,** *7:*365–375.

Tamai O, Matsuoka H, Itabe H, *et al.* Single LDL apheresis improves endothelium-dependent vasodilatation in hypercholesterolemic humans. *Circulation,* **1997,** *95:*76–82.

The Expert Panel. Third Report of the National Cholesterol Education Program (NCEP) Expert Panel on Detection, Evaluation, and Treatment of High Blood Cholesterol in Adults (Adult Treatment Panel III). Final report. *Circulation,* **2002,** *106:*3143–3421.

Thompson PD, Clarkson P, Karas RH. Statin-associated myopathy. *JAMA,* **2003,** *289:*1681–1690.

Thompson PD, Clarkson PM, Rosenson RS. An assessment of statin safety by muscle experts. *Am J Cardiol,* **2006,** *97*(suppl): 69C–76C.

Vakkilainen J, Steiner G, Ansquer J-C, *et al.* Relationships between low-density lipoprotein particle size, plasma lipoproteins, and progression of coronary artery disease. The Diabetes Atherosclerosis Intervention Study (DAIS). *Circulation,* **2003,** *107:*1733–1737.

Van Eck M, Singaraja RR, Ye D, et al. Macrophage ATP-binding cassette transporter A1 overexpression inhibits atherosclerotic lesion progression in low-density lipoprotein receptor knockout mice. *Arterioscler Thromb Vasc Biol,* **2006,** *26:*929–934.

Wang X, Collins HL, Ranalletta M, *et al.* Macrophage ABCA1 and ABCG1, but not SR-BI, promote macrophage reverse cholesterol transport in vivo. *J Clin Invest,* **2007,** *117:* 2216–2224.

Wickramasinghe SR, DeFilippis AP, Lloyd-Jones DM, Blumenthal RS. A convenient tool to profile patients for generalized cardiovascular disease risk in primary care. *Am J Cardiol,* **2009,** *103:*1174–1177.

Wilke RA, Lin D, Roden D, et al. Identifying genetic risk factors for serious adverse drug reactions. *Nat Rev Drug Discov*, **2007**, *6*:904–916.

Williams JK, Sukhova GK, Herrington DM, Libby P. Pravastatin has cholesterol-lowering independent effects on the artery wall of atherosclerotic monkeys. *J Am Coll Cardiol,* **1998,** *31:*684–691.

Wise A, Foord SM, Fraser NJ, *et al.* Molecular identification of high and low affinity receptors for nicotinic acid. *J Biol Chem,* **2003,** *278:*9869–9874.

Witztum JL, Steinberg D. The oxidative modification hypothesis of atherosclerosis: Does it hold for humans? *Trends Cardiovasc Med,* **2001,** *11:*93–102.

Wong K, Ryan RO. Characterization of apolipoprotein A-V structure and mode of plasma triacylglycerol regulation. *Curr Opin Lipidol,* **2007,** *18:*319–324.

Wong WW-L, Dimitroulakos J, Minden MD, Penn LZ. HMG-CoA reductase inhibitors and the malignant cell: The statin family of drugs as triggers of tumor-specific apoptosis. *Leukemia,* **2002,** *16:*508–519.

Yusuf S. Two decades of progress in preventing vascular disease. *Lancet,* **2002,** *360:*2–3.

Zhang Z-J, Cheng Q, Jiang G-X, Marroquin OC. Statins in prevention of repeat revascularization after percutaneous coronary intervention—A meta-analysis of randomized clinical trials. *Pharmacol Res,* **2010,** *61*:316–320.

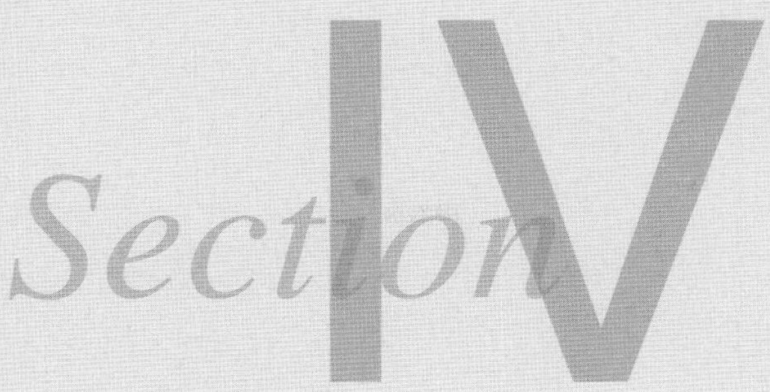

Inflammation, Immunomodulation, and Hematopoiesis

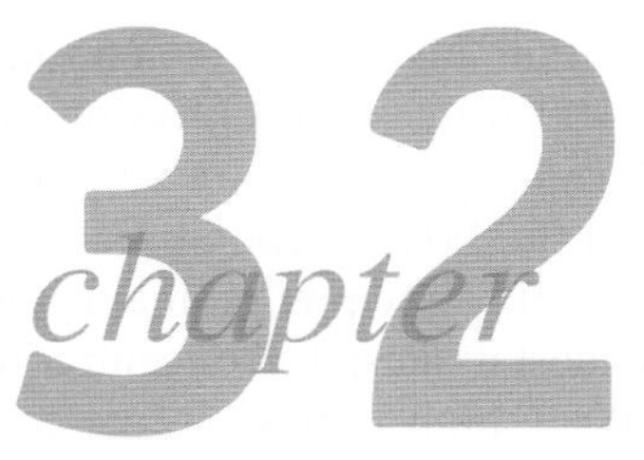

Histamine, Bradykinin, and Their Antagonists

Randal A. Skidgel, Allen P. Kaplan, and Ervin G. Erdös

The biogenic amine, histamine, is a major mediator of inflammation, anaphylaxis, and gastric acid secretion; in addition, histamine plays a role in neurotransmission. Our understanding of the physiological and pathophysiological roles of histamine has been enhanced by the development of subtype-specific receptor antagonists and by the cloning of four receptors for histamine. Competitive antagonists of H_1 receptors have diverse actions and are used therapeutically in treating allergies, urticaria, anaphylactic reactions, nausea, motion sickness, insomnia, and some symptoms of asthma. Antagonists of the H_2 receptor are effective in reducing gastric acid secretion. The peptide, bradykinin, has cardiovascular effects similar to those of histamine and plays prominent roles in inflammation and nociception.

This chapter presents the physiology and pathophysiology of histamine and kinins and the pharmacology of the antagonists that inhibit responses to these mediators.

HISTAMINE

History. The history of histamine (β-aminoethylimidazole) parallels that of acetylcholine (ACh). Both were chemically synthesized before their biological significance was recognized; they were first detected as uterine stimulants in, and isolated from, extracts of ergot, where they proved to be contaminants derived from bacterial action (Dale, 1953).

Dale and Laidlaw subjected histamine to intensive pharmacological study (Dale, 1953), discovering that it stimulated a host of smooth muscles and had an intense vasodepressor action. Importantly, they observed that when a sensitized animal was injected with a normally inert protein, the immediate responses closely resembled those of poisoning by histamine. These observations anticipated by many years the finding that endogenous histamine contributes to immediate hypersensitivity reactions and to responses to cellular injury. Best and colleagues (1927) isolated histamine from fresh samples of liver and lung, thereby establishing it as a natural constituent of mammalian tissues, hence the name *histamine* after the Greek word for tissue, *histos*. The presence of histamine in tissue extracts delayed the acceptance of the discovery of some peptide and protein hormones (e.g., gastrin) until the technology for separating the naturally occurring substances was sufficiently advanced (Grossman, 1966).

Lewis and colleagues (Lewis, 1927) proposed that a substance with the properties of histamine ("H substance") was liberated from the cells of the skin by injurious stimuli, including the reaction of antigen with antibody. We now know that endogenous histamine plays a role in the immediate allergic response and is an important regulator of gastric acid secretion. More recently, a role for histamine as a modulator of neurotransmitter release in the central and peripheral nervous systems has emerged.

Early suspicions that histamine acts through more than one receptor have been borne out by the elucidation of four classes of receptors, designated H_1 (Ash and Schild, 1966), H_2 (Black et al., 1972), H_3 (Arrang et al., 1987), and H_4 (Leurs et al., 2009). H_1 receptors are blocked selectively by the classical "antihistamines." Second-generation H_1 antagonists are collectively referred to as *nonsedating antihistamines*. The term *third generation* has been applied to some recently developed antihistamines, such as active metabolites of first- or second-generation antihistamines that are not further metabolized (e.g., cetirizine derived from hydroxyzine or fexofenadine from terfenadine) or to antihistamines that have additional therapeutic effects. However, the Consensus Group on New-Generation Antihistamines concluded that none of the currently available antihistamines can be classified as true third-generation drugs, defined as lacking in cardiotoxicity, drug-drug interactions, and CNS effects or with possible additional beneficial effects (e.g., anti-inflammatory) (Holgate et al., 2003). The discovery of H_2 antagonists and their ability to inhibit gastric secretion has contributed greatly to the resurgence of interest in histamine in biology and clinical medicine (Chapter 45). H_3 receptors were discovered as presynaptic autoreceptors on histamine-containing neurons that mediate feedback inhibition of the release and synthesis of histamine. The development of selective H_3 receptor agonists and antagonists has led to an increased understanding of the importance of H_3 receptors in histaminergic neurons *in vivo*. None of these H_3 agonists or antagonists has yet emerged as a therapeutic agent (Sander et al., 2008). The H_4 receptor is most similar to the H_3 receptor but is expressed in cells of hematopoietic lineage; the availability of H_4-specific antagonists with anti-inflammatory properties should help to define the biological roles of the H_4 receptor (Thurmond et al., 2008).

Chemistry. Histamine is a hydrophilic molecule consisting of an imidazole ring and an amino group connected by two methylene groups. The pharmacologically active form is the monocationic Nγ–H tautomer, which is the charged form of the species depicted in Figure 32–1 (Ganellin and Parsons, 1982). H_3 and H_4 receptors have a much higher affinity for histamine than H_1 and H_2 receptors, and the four histamine receptors can be activated differently by analogs of histamine (Venable and Thurmond, 2006) (Figure 32–1 and Table 32–1). The specificities of histamine analogs were re-evaluated after the discovery of the H_4 receptor. Thus, 4-methylhistamine and dimaprit, originally classified as H_2 receptors (Black et al., 1972), are full H_4 agonists with a ~100-fold higher affinity for the H_4 receptor. A number of H_3 agonists also are weaker agonists of the H_4 receptor (Lim et al., 2005; Venable and Thurmond, 2006).

Distribution and Biosynthesis of Histamine

Distribution. Histamine is widely, if unevenly, distributed throughout the animal kingdom and is present in many venoms, bacteria, and plants. Almost all mammalian tissues contain histamine in amounts ranging from <1 to >100 μg/g. Concentrations in plasma and other body fluids generally are very low, but human cerebrospinal fluid (CSF) contains significant amounts. The mast cell is the predominant storage site for histamine in most tissues; the concentration of histamine is particularly high in tissues that contain large numbers of mast cells, such as skin, bronchial mucosa, and intestinal mucosa.

Synthesis, Storage, and Metabolism. Histamine is formed by the decarboxylation of the amino acid histidine by the enzyme L-histidine decarboxylase (Figure 32-2), found in every mammalian tissue that contains histamine. The chief site of histamine storage in most tissues is the mast cell; in the blood, it is the basophil. These cells synthesize histamine and store it in secretory granules.

At the secretory granule pH of ~5.5, histamine is positively charged and ionically complexed with negatively charged acidic groups on other granule constituents, primarily proteases and heparin or chondroitin sulfate proteoglycans. The turnover rate of

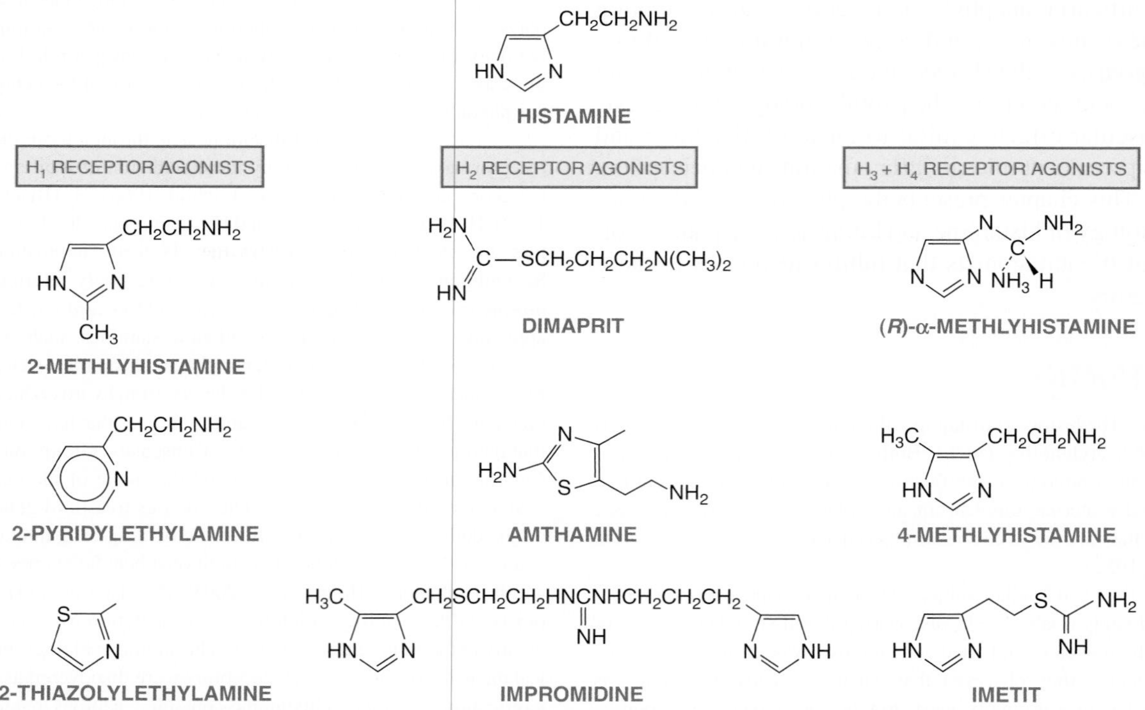

Figure 32–1. *Structure of histamine and some H_1, H_2, H_3, and H_4 agonists-* Dimaprit and 4-methylhistamine, originally identified as specific H_2 agonists, have a much higher affinity for the H_4 receptor; 4-methylhistamine is the most specific available H_4 agonist, with ~10-fold higher affinity than dimaprit, a partial H_4 agonist. Impromidine is among the most potent H_2 agonists but also is an antagonist at H_1 and H_3 receptors and a partial agonist at H_4 receptors. (*R*)-α-Methylhistamine and imetit are high-affinity agonists of H_3 receptors and lower-affinity full agonists at H_4 receptors.

Table 32–1

Characteristics of Histamine Receptors

	H_1	H_2	H_3*	H_4
Size (amino acids)	487	359	329-445	390
G protein coupling (second messengers)	$G_{q/11}$ (↑ Ca^{2+}; ↑ NO and ↑ cGMP)	G_s (↑ cAMP)	$G_{i/o}$ (↓ cAMP; ↑ MAP kinase)	$G_{i/o}$ (↓ cAMP; ↑ Ca^{2+})
Distribution	Smooth muscle, endothelial cells, CNS	Gastric parietal cells, cardiac muscle, mast cells, CNS	CNS: presynaptic	Cells of hematopoietic origin
Representative agonist	2-CH_3-histamine	Amthamine	(*R*)-α-CH_3-histamine	4-CH_3-histamine
Representative antagonist	Chlorpheniramine	Ranitidine	Tiprolisant	JNJ7777120

cAMP, cyclic AMP; cGMP, cyclic GMP; CNS, central nervous system; NO, nitric oxide.
*At least 20 alternately spliced H_3 isoforms have been detected at the mRNA level. Eight of these isoforms, ranging in size from 329-445 residues, were found to be functionally competent by binding or signaling assays (see Esbenshade et al., 2008)

histamine in secretory granules is slow, and when tissues rich in mast cells are depleted of their histamine stores, it may take weeks before concentrations return to normal levels. Non–mast cell sites of histamine formation include the epidermis, the gastric mucosa, neurons within the CNS, and cells in regenerating or rapidly growing tissues. Turnover is rapid at these non–mast cell sites because the histamine is released continuously rather than stored. Non–mast cell sites of histamine production contribute significantly to the daily excretion of histamine metabolites in the urine. Because L-histidine decarboxylase is an inducible enzyme, the histamine-forming capacity at such sites is subject to regulation. Histamine that is ingested or formed by bacteria in the gastrointestinal (GI) tract does not contribute to the body's stores; rather, it is rapidly metabolized, and the metabolites are eliminated in the urine.

There are two major paths of histamine metabolism in humans (Figure 32–2). The more important is ring methylation to form *N*-methylhistamine, catalyzed by histamine-*N*-methyltransferase, which is distributed widely. Most of the *N*-methylhistamine formed is then converted to *N*-methylimidazole acetic acid by monoamine oxidase (MAO), and this reaction can be blocked by MAO inhibitors (Chapters 8, 15, and 22). Alternatively, histamine may undergo oxidative deamination catalyzed mainly by the nonspecific enzyme diamine oxidase, yielding imidazole acetic acid, which is then converted to imidazole acetic acid riboside. These metabolites have little or no activity and are excreted in the urine. Measurement of *N*-methylhistamine in urine affords a more reliable index of histamine production than assessment of histamine itself. Artifactually elevated levels of histamine in urine arise from genitourinary tract bacteria that can decarboxylate histidine. In addition, the metabolism of histamine appears to be altered in patients with mastocytosis such that determination of histamine metabolites is a more sensitive diagnostic indicator of the disease than histamine.

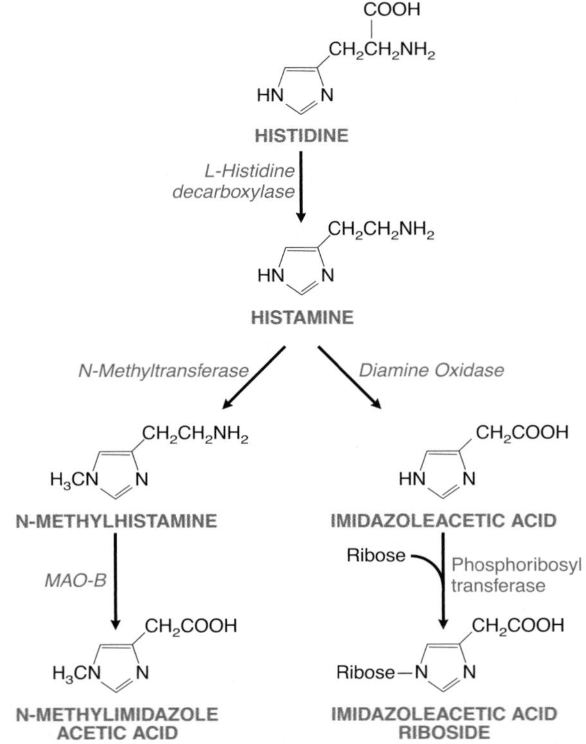

Figure 32–2. *Pathways of histamine synthesis and metabolism in humans.* Histamine is synthesized from histidine by decarboxylation. Histamine is metabolized via two pathways, predominantly by methylation of the ring followed by oxidative deamination (left side of figure), and secondarily by oxidative deamination and then conjugation with ribose.

Release and Functions of Endogenous Histamine

Histamine has important physiological roles. After its release from storage granules as a result of the interaction of antigen with immunoglobulin E (IgE) antibodies on the mast cell surface, histamine plays a central role in immediate hypersensitivity and allergic responses. The actions of histamine on bronchial smooth muscle and blood vessels account for many of the symptoms of the allergic response. In addition, some drugs act directly on mast cells to release histamine, causing untoward effects. Histamine has a major role in regulating gastric acid secretion and also modulates neurotransmitter release.

Role in Allergic Responses. The principal target cells of immediate hypersensitivity reactions are mast cells and basophils (Schwartz, 1994). As part of the allergic response to an antigen, IgE antibodies are generated and bind to the surfaces of mast cells and basophils via specific high-affinity F_c receptors. This receptor, FcεRI, consists of α, β, and two γ chains (Chapter 35). Atopic individuals develop IgE antibodies to commonly inhaled antigens. This is a heritable trait, conferring a predilection to rhinitis, asthma, and atopic dermatitis.

Antigen bridges the IgE molecules and via FcεRI activates signaling pathways in mast cells or basophils involving tyrosine kinases and subsequent phosphorylation of multiple protein substrates within 5-15 seconds of contact with antigen. Protein kinases implicated include the *Src*-related kinases Lyn and Syk. Prominent among the phosphorylated proteins are the β and γ subunits of FcεRI, itself, and phospholipase C (PLC)γ_1 and PLCγ_2, with consequent production of inositol trisphosphate (IP_3) and mobilization of intracellular Ca^{2+} (Chapter 3). These events trigger the exocytosis of the contents of secretory granules.

Release of Other Autacoids. The release of histamine only partially explains the biological effects that ensue from immediate hypersensitivity reactions because a broad spectrum of other inflammatory mediators is released on mast cell activation.

Stimulation of IgE receptors also activates phospholipase A_2 (PLA_2), leading to the production of a host of mediators, including platelet-activating factor (PAF) and metabolites of arachidonic acid such as leukotrienes C_4 and D_4, which contract the smooth muscles of the bronchial tree (Chapters 33 and 36). Kinins also are generated during some allergic responses. Thus, the mast cell secretes a variety of inflammatory mediators in addition to histamine, each contributing to the major symptoms of the allergic response (see below).

Regulation of Mediator Release. The wide variety of mediators released during the allergic response can explain the ineffectiveness of drug therapy focused on a single mediator. Agents that act at muscarinic or α-adrenergic receptors increase the release of mediators, an effect of little clinical significance. Epinephrine and related drugs that act through β_2 adrenergic receptors increase cellular cyclic AMP and thereby inhibit the secretory activities of mast cells. However, the beneficial effects of β adrenergic agonists in allergic states such as asthma are due mainly to relaxing bronchial smooth muscle (Chapters 12 and 36).

Histamine Release by Drugs, Peptides, Venoms, and Other Agents. Many compounds, including a large number of therapeutic agents, stimulate the release of histamine from mast cells directly and without prior sensitization. Responses of this sort are most likely to occur following intravenous injections of certain categories of substances, particularly organic bases such as amides, amidines, quaternary ammonium compounds, pyridinium compounds, piperidines, and alkaloids (Rothschild, 1966). Tubocurarine, succinylcholine, morphine, some antibiotics, radiocontrast media, and certain carbohydrate plasma expanders also may elicit the response. The phenomenon is one of clinical concern, and may account for unexpected anaphylactoid reactions. For example, vancomycin-induced *red-man syndrome,* involving hypotension and flushing in the upper body and face, may be mediated through histamine release.

In addition to therapeutic agents, certain experimental compounds stimulate the release of histamine as their dominant pharmacological characteristic. The archetype is the polybasic substance known as *compound 48/80*. This is a mixture of low-molecular-weight polymers of *p*-methoxy-*N*-methylphenethylamine, of which the hexamer is most active.

Basic polypeptides often are effective histamine releasers, and over a limited range, their potency generally increases with the number of basic groups. For example, bradykinin is a poor histamine releaser, whereas kallidin (Lys-bradykinin) and substance P, with more positively charged amino acids, are more active. Some venoms, such as that of the wasp, contain potent histamine-releasing peptides (Johnson and Erdös, 1973). Polymyxin B also is very active. Basic polypeptides released upon tissue injury constitute pathophysiological stimuli to secretion for mast cells and basophils.

Within seconds of the intravenous injection of a histamine liberator, human subjects experience a burning, itching sensation. This effect, most marked in the palms of the hand and in the face, scalp, and ears, is soon followed by a feeling of intense warmth. The skin reddens, and the color rapidly spreads over the trunk. Blood pressure falls, the heart rate accelerates, and the subject usually complains of headache. After a few minutes, blood pressure recovers, and crops of hives usually appear on the skin. Colic, nausea, hypersecretion of acid, and moderate bronchospasm also frequently occur. The effect becomes less intense with successive injections as the mast cell stores of histamine are depleted. Histamine liberators do not deplete tissues of non–mast cell histamine.

Mechanism of Histamine-Releasing Agents. Histamine-releasing substances activate the secretory responses of mast cells and basophils by causing a rise in intracellular Ca^{2+}. Some are ionophores and directly facilitate the entry of Ca^{2+} into the cell; others, such as neurotensin, act on specific G protein–coupled receptors (GPCRs). In contrast, the precise mechanism by which basic secretagogues (e.g., substance P, mastoparan, kallidin, compound 48/80, and polymyxin B) release histamine still is unclear. These agents can directly activate G_i proteins after being taken up by the cell (Ferry et al., 2002), but more recent evidence indicates the involvement of a cell-surface GPCR in the *Mas*-related gene family or integrin-associated protein CD47 coupled to G_i (Sick et al., 2009). The downstream effectors appear to be $\beta\gamma$ subunits released from $G\alpha_i$, which activate the PLCβ–IP_3–Ca^{2+} pathway. Antigen–IgE complexes lead to mobilization of stored Ca^{2+} and activation of isoforms of PLCγ, as described in "Role in Allergic Responses."

Histamine Release by Other Means. Clinical conditions related to histamine release include cold, cholinergic, and solar urticaria. Some of these involve specific secretory responses of the mast cells and cell-fixed IgE. However, nonspecific cellular damage from any cause can release histamine. The redness and urticaria that follow scratching of the skin is a familiar example.

Increased Proliferation of Mast Cells and Basophils and Gastric Carcinoid Tumors. In urticaria pigmentosa (cutaneous mastocytosis), mast cells aggregate in the upper corium and give rise to pigmented cutaneous lesions that sting when stroked. In systemic mastocytosis, overproliferation of mast cells also is found in other organs. Patients with these syndromes suffer a constellation of signs and symptoms attributable to excessive histamine release, including urticaria, dermographism, pruritus, headache, weakness, hypotension, flushing of the face, and a variety of GI effects, such as diarrhea or peptic ulceration. Episodes of mast cell activation with attendant systemic histamine release are precipitated by a variety of stimuli, including exertion, insect stings, exposure to heat, and exposure to drugs that release histamine directly or to which patients are allergic. In myelogenous leukemia, excessive numbers of basophils are present in the blood, raising its histamine content to high levels that may contribute to chronic pruritus. Gastric carcinoid tumors secrete histamine, which is responsible for episodes of vasodilation as part of the patchy "geographical" flush.

Gastric Acid Secretion. Histamine acting at H_2 receptors is a powerful gastric secretagogue, evoking a copious secretion of acid from parietal cells (see Figure 45–1); it also increases the output of pepsin and intrinsic factor. The secretion of gastric acid from parietal cells also is caused by stimulation of the vagus nerve and by the enteric hormone gastrin. However, histamine undoubtedly is the dominant physiological mediator of acid secretion; blockade of H_2 receptors not only antagonizes acid secretion in response to histamine but also inhibits responses to gastrin and vagal stimulation. (For regulation of gastric acid secretion and the clinical utility of H_2 antagonists, see Chapter 45.)

Central Nervous System. There is substantial evidence that histamine functions as a neurotransmitter in the CNS. Histamine-containing neurons control both homeostatic and higher brain functions, including regulation of the sleep-wake cycle, circadian and feeding rhythms, immunity, learning, memory, drinking, and body temperature (see Haas et al., 2008). However, knockout animals lacking histamine or its receptors exhibit only subtle defects unless challenged, and no human disease has yet been directly linked to dysfunction of the brain histamine system. Histamine, histidine decarboxylase, enzymes that metabolize histamine, and H_1, H_2, and H_3 receptors are distributed widely but non-uniformly in the CNS (see Haas et al., 2008). H_1 receptors are associated with both neuronal and non-neuronal elements (e.g., glia, blood cells, vessels) and are concentrated in regions that control neuroendocrine function, behavior, and nutritional state. Distribution of H_2 receptors is more consistent with histaminergic projections than H_1 receptors, suggesting that they mediate many of the postsynaptic actions of histamine. H_3 receptors also are heterogeneously concentrated in areas known to receive histaminergic projections, consistent with their function as presynaptic autoreceptors. Histamine inhibits appetite and increases wakefulness via H_1 receptors, explaining sedation by classical antihistamines (Haas et al., 2008).

Pharmacological Effects

Receptor–Effector Coupling and Mechanisms of Action. Histamine receptors are GPCRs (Leurs et al., 2009; Haas et al., 2008; Thurmond et al., 2008) (Table 32–1). H_1 receptors couple to $G_{q/11}$ and activate the PLC–IP_3–Ca^{2+} pathway and its many possible sequelae, including activation of PKC, Ca^{2+}–calmodulin–dependent enzymes (eNOS and various protein kinases), and PLA_2. H_2 receptors link to G_s to activate the adenylyl cyclase–cyclic AMP–PKA pathway, whereas H_3 and H_4 receptors couple to $G_{i/o}$ to inhibit adenylyl cyclase and decrease cellular cyclic AMP. Activation of H_3 receptors also can activate MAP kinase and inhibit the Na^+/H^+ exchanger, and activation of H_4 receptors mobilizes stored Ca^{2+} in some cells (Leurs et al., 2009; Haas et al., 2008; Thurmond et al., 2008; Esbenshade et al., 2008). Armed with this information, knowledge of the cellular expression of H receptor subtypes, and an understanding of the differentiated functions of a particular cell type, one can predict a cell's response to histamine. Of course, in a physiological setting, a cell is exposed to a myriad of hormones simultaneously, and significant interactions may occur between signaling pathways, such as the $G_q \rightarrow G_s$ cross-talk described in a number of systems (Meszaros et al., 2000). Furthermore, the differential expression of H receptor subtypes on neighboring cells and the unequal sensitivities of H receptor–effector response pathways can cause parallel and opposing cellular responses to occur together, complicating interpretation of the overall response of a tissue. For example, activation of H_1 receptors on vascular endothelium stimulates the Ca^{2+}-mobilizing pathway (G_q–PLC–IP_3) and activates eNOS to produce nitric oxide (NO), which diffuses to nearby smooth muscle cells to increase cyclic GMP and cause relaxation. Stimulation of H_1 receptors on smooth muscle also will mobilize Ca^{2+} but cause contraction, whereas activation of H_2 receptors on the same smooth muscle cell will link via G_s to enhanced cyclic AMP accumulation, activation of PKA, and thence to relaxation.

The existence of multiple histamine receptors was predicted by the studies of Ash and Schild (1966) and Black and colleagues (1972) a generation before the cloning of histamine receptors. Similarly, heterogeneity of H_3 receptors, predicted by kinetic and radioligand-binding studies, has been confirmed by cloning, which revealed H_3 isoforms differing in the third intracellular loop, transmembrane helices 6 and 7, and C-terminal tail, and in their capacity to couple G_i, inhibit adenylyl cyclase, and activate MAP kinase. Molecular cloning studies also identified the H_4 receptor.

As Figure 32–1 and Table 32–1 indicate, the pharmacological definition of H_1, H_2, and H_3 receptors is clear because relatively specific agonists and antagonists are available. However, the H_4 receptor exhibits 35-40% homology to isoforms of the H_3 receptor, and the two were harder to distinguish pharmacologically because many high-affinity H_3 ligands also interact with H_4 receptors. Several non-imidazole compounds that are more selective H_3 antagonists have been developed (Sander et al., 2008), and there are now several selective H_4 antagonists (Leurs et al., 2009; Venable and Thurmond, 2006). 4-Methylhistamine and dimaprit, previously identified as specific H_2 agonists (Black et al., 1972), are actually more potent H_4 agonists (Venable and Thurmond, 2006).

H_1 and H_2 Receptors. H_1 and H_2 receptors are distributed widely in the periphery and in the CNS. Histamine can exert local or widespread effects on smooth muscles and glands. It causes itching and stimulates secretion from nasal mucosa. It contracts many smooth muscles, such as those of the bronchi and gut, but markedly relaxes others, including those in small blood vessels. Histamine also is a potent stimulus of gastric acid secretion (see "Gastric Acid Secretion"). Other, less prominent effects include formation of edema and stimulation of sensory nerve endings. Bronchoconstriction and contraction of the gut are mediated by H_1 receptors. Gastric secretion results from the activation of H_2 receptors and, accordingly, can be inhibited by H_2 receptor antagonists. Some responses, such as vascular dilation, are mediated by both H_1 and H_2 receptor stimulation.

H_3 and H_4 Receptors. H_3 receptors are expressed mainly in the CNS (Arrang et al., 1987), especially in the basal ganglia, hippocampus, and cortex. H_3 receptors function as autoreceptors on histaminergic neurons, much like presynaptic α_2 receptors, inhibiting histamine release and modulating the release of other neurotransmitters. Because H_3 receptors have high constitutive activity, histamine release is tonically inhibited, and inverse agonists will thus reduce receptor activation and increase histamine release from histaminergic neurons. H_3 agonists promote sleep; thus, H_3 antagonists promote wakefulness. H_4 receptors primarily are found in cells of hematopoietic origin such as eosinophils, dendritic cells, mast cells, monocytes, basophils, and T cells but has also been detected in the GI tract, dermal fibroblasts, CNS, and primary sensory afferent neurons (Leurs et al., 2009). Activation of H_4 receptors in some of these cell types has been associated with induction of cellular shape change, chemotaxis, secretion of cytokines and upregulation of adhesion molecules, suggesting that H_4 antagonists may be useful inhibitors of allergic and inflammatory responses (Thurmond et al., 2008.

Effects on Histamine Release. H_2 receptor stimulation increases cyclic AMP and leads to feedback inhibition of histamine release from mast cells and basophils, whereas activation of H_3 and H_4 receptors has the opposite effect by decreasing cellular cyclic AMP (Oda et al., 2000). Activation of presynaptic H_3 receptors also inhibits histamine release from histaminergic neurons.

Histamine Toxicity from Ingestion. Histamine is the toxin in food poisoning from spoiled scombroid fish such as tuna (Morrow et al., 1991). The high histidine content combines with a large bacterial capacity to decarboxylate histidine, generating a lot of histamine. Ingestion of the fish causes severe nausea, vomiting, headache, flushing, and sweating. Histamine toxicity, manifested by headache and other symptoms, also can follow red wine consumption in persons with a diminished ability to degrade histamine. The symptoms of histamine poisoning can be suppressed by H_1 antagonists.

Cardiovascular System. Histamine characteristically dilates resistance vessels, increases capillary permeability, and lowers systemic blood pressure. In some vascular beds, histamine constricts veins, contributing to the extravasation of fluid and edema formation upstream in capillaries and postcapillary venules.

Vasodilation. This is the most important vascular effect of histamine in humans. Vasodilation involves both H_1 and H_2 receptors distributed throughout the resistance vessels in most vascular beds; however, quantitative differences are apparent in the degree of dilation that occurs in various beds. Activation of either the H_1 or H_2

receptor can elicit maximal vasodilation, but the responses differ. H_1 receptors have a higher affinity for histamine and cause Ca^{2+}-dependent activation of eNOS in endothelial cells; NO diffuses to vascular smooth muscle, increasing cyclic GMP (Table 32–1) and causing relaxation that results in a relatively rapid and short-lived vasodilation. By contrast, activation of H_2 receptors on vascular smooth muscle stimulates the cyclic AMP–PKA pathway, causing dilation that develops more slowly and is more sustained. As a result, H_1 antagonists effectively counter small dilator responses to low concentrations of histamine but only blunt the initial phase of larger responses to higher concentrations of the amine. In addition, there is a variable distribution of H_1 receptors on vascular smooth muscle, resulting in direct vasoconstrictor responses in vein, skin, and skeletal muscle and in larger coronary arteries.

Increased "Capillary" Permeability. Histamine's effect on small vessels results in efflux of plasma protein and fluid into the extracellular spaces and an increase lymph flow, causing edema. H_1 receptors on endothelial cells are the major mediators of this response; the role of H_2 receptors is uncertain.

Increased permeability results from histamine activation of H_1 receptors on postcapillary venules. This contracts the endothelial cells, disrupts interendothelial junctions, and exposes the basement membrane, which is freely permeable to plasma proteins and fluid. The gaps between endothelial cells also may permit passage of circulating cells recruited to tissues during the mast cell response. Recruitment of circulating leukocytes is enhanced by H_1 receptor–mediated expression of adhesion molecules (e.g., P-selectin) on endothelial cells (Thurmond et al., 2008).

Triple Response of Lewis. If histamine is injected intradermally, it elicits a characteristic phenomenon known as the *triple response* (Lewis, 1927). This consists of:

- a localized red spot extending for a few millimeters around the site of injection that appears within a few seconds and reaches a maximum in ~1 minute
- a brighter red flush, or "flare," extending ~1 cm beyond the original red spot and developing more slowly
- a wheal that is discernible in 1-2 minutes and occupies the same area as the original small red spot at the injection site.

The initial red spot results from the direct vasodilating effect of histamine (H_1 receptor–mediated NO production), the flare is due to histamine-induced stimulation of axon reflexes that cause vasodilation indirectly, and the wheal reflects histamine's capacity to increase capillary permeability (edema formation).

Constriction of Larger Vessels. Histamine tends to constrict larger blood vessels, in some species more than in others. In rodents, the effect extends to the arterioles and may overshadow dilation of the finer blood vessels, leading to an elevation in blood pressure. As noted earlier, H_1 receptor–mediated constriction may occur in some veins and in conduit coronary arteries.

Heart. Histamine affects both cardiac contractility and electrical events directly. It increases the force of contraction of both atrial and ventricular muscle by promoting the influx of Ca^{2+}, and it speeds heart rate by hastening diastolic depolarization in the sinoatrial (SA) node. It also directly slows atrioventricular (AV) conduction to increase automaticity and, in high doses, can elicit arrhythmias. The slowed AV conduction involves mainly H_1 receptors, while the other effects are largely attributable to H_2 receptors and cyclic AMP accumulation. The direct cardiac effects of histamine given intravenously are overshadowed by baroreceptor reflexes due to reduced blood pressure.

Histamine Shock. Histamine given in large doses or released during systemic anaphylaxis causes a profound and progressive fall in blood pressure. As the small blood vessels dilate, they trap large amounts of blood, their permeability increases, and plasma escapes from the circulation. Resembling surgical or traumatic shock, these effects diminish effective blood volume, reduce venous return, and greatly lower cardiac output.

Extravascular Smooth Muscle. Histamine directly contracts or, more rarely, relaxes various extravascular smooth muscles. Contraction is due to activation of H_1 receptors on smooth muscle to increase intracellular Ca^{2+} (in contrast to intact vessels, where endothelium-derived NO causes vasodilation; see "Vasodilation"), and relaxation is mainly due to activation of H_2 receptors. Responses vary widely among species and even among humans. Bronchial smooth muscle of guinea pigs is exquisitely sensitive. Minute doses of histamine also will evoke intense bronchoconstriction in patients with bronchial asthma and certain other pulmonary diseases, but in normal humans, the effect is much less. Although the spasmogenic influence of H_1 receptors is dominant in human bronchial muscle, H_2 receptors with dilator function also are present. Thus, histamine-induced bronchospasm *in vitro* is potentiated slightly by H_2 blockade. In asthmatic subjects in particular, histamine-induced bronchospasm may involve an additional reflex component that arises from irritation of afferent vagal nerve endings (Nadel and Barnes, 1984).

The uterus of some species is contracted by histamine; in the human uterus, gravid or not, the response is negligible. Responses of intestinal muscle also vary with species and region, but the classical effect is contraction. Bladder, ureter, gallbladder, iris, and many other smooth muscle preparations are affected little or inconsistently by histamine.

Peripheral Nerve Endings: Pain, Itch, and Indirect Effects. Histamine stimulates various nerve endings and sensory effects. In the epidermis, it causes itch; in the dermis, it evokes pain, sometimes accompanied by itching. Stimulant actions on nerve endings, including autonomic afferents and efferents, contribute to the "flare" component of the triple response and to indirect effects of histamine on the bronchi and other organs. In the periphery, neuronal receptors for histamine are generally of the H_1 type (see Rocha e Silva, 1978; Ganellin and Parsons, 1982).

Clinical Uses

The practical application of histamine is limited to use as a diagnostic agent, such as to assess nonspecific bronchial hyperreactivity in asthmatics or as a positive control injection during allergy skin testing.

H_1 RECEPTOR ANTAGONISTS

History. Antihistamine activity was first demonstrated by Bovet and Staub in 1937 with one of a series of amines with a phenolic ether moiety. The substance 2-isopropyl-5-methylphenoxy-ethyl-diethyl-amine protected guinea pigs against several lethal doses of histamine but was too toxic for clinical use. By 1944, Bovet and his colleagues had described *pyrilamine maleate*, an effective histamine antagonist of this category. The discovery of the highly effective diphenhydramine and *tripelennamine* soon followed (Ganellin and Parsons, 1982). In the 1980s, nonsedating H_1 histamine receptor antagonists were developed for treatment of allergic diseases. Despite success in blocking allergic responses to histamine, the H_1 antihistamines failed to inhibit a number of other responses, notably gastric acid secretion. The discovery of H_2 receptors and H_2 antagonists by Black and colleagues provided a new class of agents that antagonized histamine-induced acid secretion (Black et al., 1972). The pharmacology of these drugs (e.g., *cimetidine, famotidine*) is described in Chapter 45.

Pharmacological Properties

Chemistry. All the available H_1 receptor "antagonists" are actually inverse agonists (see Chapter 3) that reduce constitutive activity of the receptor and compete with histamine (Haas et al., 2008): Whereas histamine binding to the receptor induces a fully active conformation, antihistamine binding yields an inactive conformation. At the tissue level, the effect seen is proportional to receptor occupancy by the antihistamine. Like histamine, many H_1 antagonists contain a substituted ethylamine moiety.

$$-\overset{|}{\underset{|}{C}}-\overset{|}{\underset{|}{C}}-N\langle$$

Unlike histamine, which has a primary amino group and a single aromatic ring, most H_1 antagonists have a tertiary amino group linked by a two-or three-atom chain to two aromatic substituents and conform to the general formula

$$\begin{matrix}Ar_1 \\ Ar_2\end{matrix}\rangle X-\overset{|}{\underset{|}{C}}-\overset{|}{\underset{|}{C}}-N\langle$$

where Ar is aryl and X is a nitrogen or carbon atom or a —C—O— ether linkage to the β-aminoethyl side chain. Sometimes the two aromatic rings are bridged, as in the tricyclic derivatives, or the ethylamine may be part of a ring structure (Figure 32–3) (Ganellin and Parsons, 1982).

Mechanism of Action. Most H_1 antagonists have similar pharmacological actions and therapeutic applications. Their effects are largely predictable from knowledge of the consequences of the activation of H_1 receptors by histamine.

Effects on Physiological Systems.

Smooth Muscle. H_1 antagonists inhibit most of the effects of histamine on smooth muscles, especially the constriction of respiratory smooth muscle. For example, a small dose of histamine causes death by asphyxia in guinea pigs, yet the animal may survive a hundred lethal doses of histamine if given an H_1 antagonist. In the same species, striking protection also is afforded against anaphylactic bronchospasm. This is not so in humans, where allergic bronchoconstriction appears to be caused by a variety of alternative mediators, such as leukotrienes (Chapter 33).

H_1 antagonists inhibit both the vasoconstrictor effects of histamine and, to a degree, the more rapid vasodilator effects mediated by activation of H_1 receptors on endothelial cells (synthesis/release of NO and other mediators). Residual vasodilation is due to H_2 receptors on smooth muscle; administration of an H_2 antagonist suppresses the effect. The efficacy of the histamine antagonists on histamine-induced changes in systemic blood pressure parallels these vascular effects.

Capillary Permeability. H_1 antagonists strongly block the increased capillary permeability and formation of edema and wheal caused by histamine.

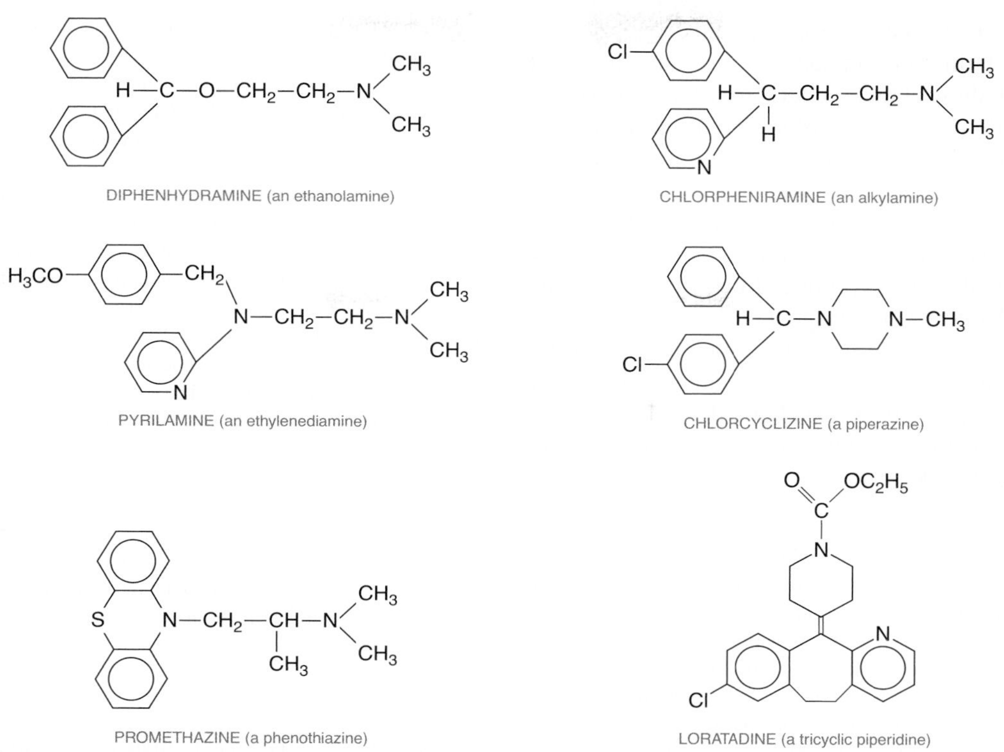

DIPHENHYDRAMINE (an ethanolamine)

CHLORPHENIRAMINE (an alkylamine)

PYRILAMINE (an ethylenediamine)

CHLORCYCLIZINE (a piperazine)

PROMETHAZINE (a phenothiazine)

LORATADINE (a tricyclic piperidine)

Figure 32–3. *Representative H_1 antagonists.*

Flare and Itch. H_1 antagonists suppress the action of histamine on nerve endings, including the flare component of the triple response and the itching caused by intradermal injection.

Exocrine Glands. H_1 antagonists do not suppress gastric secretion; they do inhibit histamine-evoked salivary, lacrimal, and other exocrine secretions, but with variable success. However, the antimuscarinic properties of many H_1 antagonists may contribute to lessened secretion in cholinergically innervated glands and reduce ongoing secretion in, e.g., the respiratory tree. Nasal sprays of some H_1 antagonists can be used to treat allergic rhinitis.

Immediate Hypersensitivity Reactions: Anaphylaxis and Allergy. During hypersensitivity reactions, histamine is one of the many potent autacoids released (see "Release of Other Autacoids"), and its relative contribution to the ensuing symptoms varies widely with species and tissue. The protection afforded by H_1 antagonists thus also varies accordingly. In humans, edema formation and itch are effectively suppressed. Other effects, such as hypotension, are less well antagonized. This may be explained by the participation of other types of H receptors and by effects of other mast cell mediators, chiefly eicosanoids (Thurmond et al., 2008; Campbell and Falck, 2007) (Chapter 25). Bronchoconstriction is reduced little, if at all.

Central Nervous System. The first-generation H_1 antagonists can both stimulate and depress the CNS. Stimulation occasionally is encountered in patients given conventional doses; they become restless, nervous, and unable to sleep. Central excitation also is a striking feature of overdose, which commonly results in convulsions, particularly in infants. Central depression, on the other hand, usually accompanies therapeutic doses of the older H_1 antagonists. Diminished alertness, slowed reaction times, and somnolence are common manifestations. Patients vary in their susceptibility and responses to individual drugs. The ethanolamines (e.g., diphenhydramine; Figure 32–3) are particularly prone to causing sedation. Because of the sedation that occurs with first-generation antihistamines, these drugs cannot be tolerated or used safely by many patients except at bedtime. Even then, patients may experience an antihistamine "hangover" in the morning, resulting in sedation with or without psychomotor impairment (Simons, 2003). Whether tolerance to such adverse effects results from protracted use when administered in divided doses to patients with chronic urticarial syndromes is unclear (Richardson et al., 2002). Thus, the development of second-generation "nonsedating" antihistamines was an important advance that allowed their general use. These newer H_1 antagonists do not cross the blood-brain barrier appreciably. Their sedative effects are similar to those of placebo.

Many antipsychotic agents are H_1 and H_2 receptor antagonists, but it is unclear whether this property plays a role in the anti-psychotic effects of these agents. The atypical anti-psychotic agent *clozapine* is an effective H_1 antagonist and a weak H_3 antagonist but an H_4 receptor agonist in the rat. The H_1 antagonist activity of typical and atypical antipsychotic drugs is responsible for the effect of these agents to cause weight gain (see Haas et al., 2008).

Anticholinergic Effects. Many of the first-generation H_1 antagonists tend to inhibit responses to ACh that are mediated by muscarinic receptors and may be manifest during clinical use (see below). Some H_1 antagonists also can be used to treat motion sickness (Chapters 9 and 46). Because *scopolamine* potently prevents motion sickness, the anticholinergic properties of H_1 antagonists may be largely responsible for this effect. Indeed, promethazine has perhaps the strongest muscarinic-blocking activity among these agents and is the most effective H_1 antagonist in combating motion sickness. The second-generation H_1 antagonists have no effect on muscarinic receptors.

Local Anesthetic Effect. Some H_1 antagonists have local anesthetic activity, and a few are more potent than procaine. Promethazine (phenergan) is especially active. However, the concentrations required for this effect are much higher than those that antagonize histamine's interactions with its receptors.

Absorption, Distribution, and Elimination. The H_1 antagonists are well absorbed from the GI tract. Following oral administration, peak plasma concentrations are achieved in 2-3 hours, and effects usually last 4-6 hours; however, some of the drugs are much longer acting (Table 32–2).

Studies of the metabolic fate of the older H_1 antagonists are limited. Diphenhydramine, given orally, reaches a maximal concentration in the blood in ~2 hours, remains there for another 2 hours, then falls exponentially with a plasma elimination $t_{1/2}$ of ~4-8 hours. The drug is distributed widely throughout the body, including the CNS. Little, if any, is excreted unchanged in the urine; most appears there as metabolites. Other first-generation H_1 antagonists can be eliminated in much the same way (see Paton and Webster, 1985). Peak concentrations of these drugs in the skin may persist after plasma levels have declined. Thus, inhibition of "wheal and flare" responses to the intradermal injection of histamine or allergen can persist for ≥36 hours after treatment, even when the concentration in plasma is low.

Like other extensively metabolized drugs, H_1 antagonists are eliminated more rapidly by children than by adults and more slowly in those with severe liver disease. H_1-receptor antagonists also induce hepatic CYPs and thus may facilitate their own metabolism (Paton and Webster, 1985).

The second-generation H_1 antagonist loratadine is absorbed rapidly from the GI tract and metabolized in the liver to an active metabolite by CYPs (Chapter 6). Consequently, metabolism of loratadine can be affected by other drugs that compete for the P450 enzymes. Two other second-generation H_1 antagonists that were marketed previously, *terfenadine* and *astemizole*, also were converted by CYPs to active metabolites. Both of these drugs were found in rare cases to induce a potentially fatal arrhythmia, *torsades de pointes*, when their metabolism was impaired, such as by liver disease or drugs that inhibit the CYP3A family (Chapter 29). This led to the withdrawal of terfenadine and astemizole from the market in 1998 and 1999, respectively. The active metabolite of terfenadine, fexofenadine, is its replacement. Fexofenadine lacks the toxic side effects of terfenadine, is not sedating, and retains the anti-allergic properties of the parent compound (Meeves and Appajosyula, 2003). Another antihistamine developed using this strategy is *desloratadine*, an active metabolite of loratadine. Cetirizine, loratadine, and fexofenadine are all well absorbed and are excreted mainly in the unmetabolized form. Cetirizine and loratadine are excreted primarily into the urine, whereas fexofenadine is excreted primarily in the feces. Levocetirizine represents the active enantiomer of cetirizine.

Therapeutic Uses

H_1 antagonists have an established place in the symptomatic treatment of various immediate hypersensitivity reactions. The central properties of some of the drugs also are of therapeutic value for suppressing motion sickness or for sedation.

Allergic Diseases. H_1 antagonists are most useful in acute types of allergy that present with symptoms of rhinitis, urticaria, and conjunctivitis. Their effect is confined to the suppression of symptoms attributable to the histamine released by the antigen-antibody reaction. In bronchial asthma, histamine antagonists have limited efficacy and are not used as sole therapy (Chapter 36). In the treatment of systemic anaphylaxis, where autacoids other than histamine are important, the mainstay of therapy is *epinephrine;* histamine antagonists have only a subordinate and adjuvant role. The same is true for severe angioedema, in which laryngeal swelling constitutes a threat to life.

Other allergies of the respiratory tract are more amenable to therapy with H_1 antagonists. The best results are obtained in seasonal rhinitis and conjunctivitis (hay fever, pollinosis), in which these drugs relieve the sneezing, rhinorrhea, and itching of eyes, nose, and throat. A gratifying response is obtained in most patients, especially at the beginning of the season when pollen counts are low; however, the drugs are less effective when the allergens are most abundant, when exposure to them is prolonged, and when nasal congestion is prominent. Nasal sprays or topical ophthalmic preparations of antihistamines such as levocabastine (discontinued in the

Table 32–2

Preparations and Dosage of Representative H_1 Receptor Antagonists[a]

CLASS AND NONPROPRIETARY NAME	TRADE NAME	DURATION OF ACTION, HOURS[b]	PREPARATIONS[c]	SINGLE DOSE (ADULT)
First-Generation Agents				
Tricyclic Dibenzoxepins				
Doxepin HCl	SINEQUAN	6-24	O, L, T	10-150 mg
Ethanolamines				
Carbinoxamine maleate	RONDEC,[f] others	3-6	O, L	4-8 mg
Clemastine fumarate	TAVIST, others	12	O, L	1.34-2.68 mg
Diphenhydramine HCl	BENADRYL, others	12	O, L, I, T	25-50 mg
Dimenhydrinate[e]	DRAMAMINE, others	4-6	O, L, I	50-100 mg
Ethylenediamines				
Pyrilamine maleate	POLY–HISTINE-D[f]	4-6	O, L, T	25-50 mg
Tripelennamine HCl	PBZ	4-6	O	25-50 mg, 100 mg (SR)
Tripelennamine citrate	PBZ	4-6	L	37.5-75 mg
Alkylamines				
Chlorpheniramine maleate	CHLOR-TRIMETON, others	24	O, L, I	4 mg 8-12 mg (SR) 5-20 mg (I)
Brompheniramine maleate	BROMPHEN, others	4-6	O, L, I	4 mg 8-12 mg (SR) 5-20 mg (I)
Piperazines				
Hydroxyzine HCl	ATARAX, others	6-24	O, L, I	25-100 mg
Hydroxyzine pamoate	VISTARIL	6-24	O, L	25-100 mg
Cyclizine HCl	MAREZINE	4-6	O	50 mg
Cyclizine lactate	MAREZINE	4-6	I	50 mg
Meclizine HCl	ANTIVERT, others	12-24	O	12.5-50 mg
Phenothiazines				
Promethazine HCl	PHENERGAN, others	4-6	O, L, I, S	12.5-50 mg
Piperidines				
Cyproheptadine HCl[g]	PERIACTIN	4-6	O, L	4 mg
Phenindamine tartrate	NOLAHIST	4-6	O	25 mg
Second-Generation Agents				
Tricyclic				
Dibenzoxepins	PATANOL	6-8	T	One drop/eye
Olopatadine HCl	PATANASE	6-8	T	Two sprays/nostril
Alkylamines				
Acrivastine[d]	SEMPREX-D[f]	6-8	O	8 mg
Piperazines				
Cetirizine HCl[d]	ZYRTEC	12-24	O	5-10 mg
Levocetirizine HCl	XYZAL	12-24	O	2.5-5 mg

(Continued)

Table 32–2

Preparations and Dosage of Representative H_1 Receptor Antagonists[a] (*Continued*)

CLASS AND NONPROPRIETARY NAME	TRADE NAME	DURATION OF ACTION, HOURS[b]	PREPARATIONS[c]	SINGLE DOSE (ADULT)
Phthalazinones				
Azelastine HCl[d]	ASTELIN	12-24	T	Two sprays/nostril
Piperidines				
Levocabastine HCl	LIVOSTIN	6-12	T	One drop/eye
Ketotifen fumarate	ZADITOR	8-12	T	One drop/eye
Loratadine	CLARITIN	24	O, L	10 mg
Desloratadine	CLARINEX, AERIUS	24	O	5 mg
Ebastine	EBASTEL	24	O	10-20 mg
Mizolastine	MIZOLLEN	24	O	10 mg
Fexofenadine HCl	ALLEGRA, TELFAST	12-24	O	60-180 mg

HCl, hydrochloride.
[a]For a discussion of phenothiazines, see Chapter 16.
[b]The duration of action of H_1 antihistamines by objective assessment of suppression of histamine- or allergen-induced symptoms is longer than might be expected from measurement of plasma concentrations or terminal elimination $t_{1/2}$ values. For a more complete discussion, see Simons, 2003.
[c]Preparations are designated as follows: O, oral solids; L, oral liquids; I, injection; S, suppository; SR, sustained release; T, topical. Many H_1 receptor antagonists also are available in preparations that contain multiple drugs.
[d]Has mild sedating effects.
[e]Dimenhydrinate is a combination of diphenhydramine and 8-chlorotheophylline in equal molecular proportions.
[f]Trade-name drug also contains other medications.
[g]Also has anti-serotonin properties.

U.S.), azelastine (ASTELIN, ASTEPRO, nasal spray; OPTIVAR, ophthalmic drops), emedastine (EMADINE, drops), epinastine (ELESTAT, drops), ketotifen (ZADITOR, drops), and olopatadine (PATANOL, drops; PATANASE, spray) are effective in allergic conjunctivitis and rhinitis. H_1 antihistamines have been investigated for potential anti-inflammatory properties because histamine releases inflammatory cytokines and eicosanoids, increases expression of endothelial adhesion molecules, and activates the pro-inflammatory transcription factor NF-κB (Holgate et al., 2003; Thurmond et al., 2008). Although H_1 antihistamines do exhibit a variety of anti-inflammatory effects *in vitro* and in animal models, in many cases the doses required are higher than those normally achieved therapeutically, and clinical effectiveness has not been proven (Holgate et al., 2003; Thurmond et al., 2008). Rupatadine is a second-generation H_1 antagonist (available in many countries outside the U.S.) that also blocks receptors for the inflammatory phospholipid, PAF (Mullol et al., 2008). Although rupatadine appears to have broader anti-inflammatory effects than other antihistamines, the clinical relevance of these properties is unclear.

Certain allergic dermatoses respond favorably to H_1 antagonists. The benefit is most striking in acute urticaria. Chronic urticaria can be less responsive but also may require higher doses than has been approved for rhinitis (Siebenhaar et al., 2009; Kaplan, 2002). Furthermore, the combined use of H_1 and H_2 antagonists sometimes is effective when therapy with an H_1 antagonist alone has failed. Angioedema also responds to treatment with H_1 antagonists, but the paramount importance of epinephrine in the severe attack must be re-emphasized, especially in life-threatening laryngeal edema (Chapter 12). In this setting, it may be appropriate to also administer an H_1 antagonist intravenously.

H_1 antagonists have a place in the treatment of pruritus. Some relief may be obtained in many patients with atopic and contact dermatitis (although topical corticosteroids are more effective) and in such diverse conditions as insect bites and poison ivy. Pruritus without an allergic basis sometimes responds to antihistamine therapy. However, the possibility of producing allergic dermatitis with local application of H_1 antagonists must be recognized. The urticarial and edematous lesions of serum sickness respond to H_1 antagonists, but fever and arthralgia often do not.

Many drug reactions attributable to allergic phenomena respond to therapy with H_1 antagonists, particularly those characterized by itch, urticaria, and angioedema. However, explosive release of histamine generally calls for treatment with epinephrine, with H_1 antagonists being accorded a subsidiary role. Nevertheless, prophylactic treatment with an H_1 antagonist may reduce symptoms to a tolerable level when a drug known to be a histamine liberator is to be given.

Common Cold. H_1 antagonists are without value in combating the common cold. The weak anticholinergic effects of the older agents may tend to lessen rhinorrhea, but this drying effect may do more harm than good, as may their tendency to induce somnolence.

Motion Sickness, Vertigo, and Sedation. Scopolamine, the muscarinic antagonist, given orally, parenterally, or transdermally, is the most effective drug for the prophylaxis and treatment of motion sickness. Some H_1 antagonists are useful for milder cases and have fewer adverse effects. These drugs include dimenhydrinate and the piperazines (e.g., cyclizine, meclizine). Promethazine, a phenothiazine, is more potent and more effective; its additional antiemetic properties may be of value in reducing vomiting, but its pronounced sedative action usually is disadvantageous. Whenever possible, the various drugs should be administered ~1 hour before the anticipated motion. Treatment after the onset of nausea and vomiting rarely is beneficial.

Some H_1 antagonists, notably dimenhydrinate and meclizine, often are of benefit in vestibular disturbances such as Meniere's disease and in other types of true vertigo. Only promethazine is useful in treating the nausea and vomiting subsequent to chemotherapy or radiation therapy for malignancies; however, other, more effective anti-emetic drugs (e.g., 5-HT_3 antagonists) are available (Chapter 46). Diphenhydramine can reverse the extrapyramidal side effects caused by phenothiazines (Chapter 16).

The tendency of some H_1 receptor antagonists to produce somnolence has led to their use as hypnotics. H_1 antagonists, principally diphenhydramine, often are present in various proprietary over-the-counter remedies for insomnia. Although these drugs generally are ineffective in the recommended doses, some sensitive individuals may derive benefit. The sedative and mild anti-anxiety activities of hydroxyzine contribute to its use as a weak anxiolytic.

Adverse Effects. The most frequent side effect in first-generation H_1 antagonists is sedation. Although sedation may be a desirable adjunct in the treatment of some patients, it may interfere with the patient's daytime activities. Concurrent ingestion of alcohol or other CNS depressants produces an additive effect that impairs motor skills. Other untoward central actions include dizziness, tinnitus, lassitude, incoordination, fatigue, blurred vision, diplopia, euphoria, nervousness, insomnia, and tremors.

The next most frequent side effects involve the digestive tract and include loss of appetite, nausea, vomiting, epigastric distress, and constipation or diarrhea. Taking the drug with meals may reduce their incidence. H_1 antagonists such as cyproheptadine may increase appetite and cause weight gain. Other side effects, owing to the antimuscarinic actions of some first-generation H_1 antagonists, include dryness of the mouth and respiratory passages (sometimes inducing cough), urinary retention or frequency, and dysuria. These effects are not observed with second-generation H_1 antagonists.

Drug allergy may develop when H_1 antagonists are given orally but occurs more commonly after topical application. Allergic dermatitis is not uncommon; other hypersensitivity reactions include drug fever and photosensitization. Hematological complications, such as leukopenia, agranulocytosis, and hemolytic anemia, are very rare. Because H_1 antihistamines cross the placenta, caution is advised for women who are or may become pregnant. Several antihistamines (e.g., azelastine, hydroxyzine, fexofenadine) had teratogenic effects in animal studies, whereas others (e.g., chlorpheniramine, diphenhydramine, cetirizine, loratadine) did not (see Simons, 2003). Antihistamines can be excreted in small amounts in breast milk, and first-generation antihistamines taken by lactating mothers may cause symptoms such as irritability, drowsiness, or respiratory depression in the nursing infant (Simons, 2003). Because H_1 antagonists interfere with skin tests for allergy, they must be withdrawn well before such tests are performed.

In acute poisoning with H_1 antagonists, their central excitatory effects constitute the greatest danger. The syndrome includes hallucinations, excitement, ataxia, incoordination, athetosis, and convulsions. Fixed, dilated pupils with a flushed face, together with sinus tachycardia, urinary retention, dry mouth, and fever, lend the syndrome a remarkable similarity to that of atropine poisoning. Terminally, there is deepening coma with cardiorespiratory collapse and death usually within 2-18 hours. Treatment is along general symptomatic and supportive lines.

Pediatric and Geriatric Indications and Problems. Although little clinical testing has been done, second-generation antihistamines are recommended for elderly patients (>65 years of age), especially those with impaired cognitive function, because of the sedative and anticholinergic effects of first-generation drugs. Therapy should be approached cautiously, possibly at reduced dosages, because of the greater likelihood of compromised renal and hepatic function in these patients, which can reduce drug elimination.

First-generation antihistamines are not recommended for use in children because their sedative effects can impair learning and school performance. The second-generation drugs loratadine, desloratadine, fexofenadine, cetirizine, levocetirizine, and azelastine (intranasal) have been approved by the FDA for use in children and are available in appropriate lower-dose formulations (e.g., chewable or rapidly dissolving tablets, syrup).

Use of over-the-counter cough and cold medicines (containing mixtures of antihistamines, decongestants, antitussives, expectorants) in young children has been associated with serious side effects and deaths (Kuehn, 2008). In 2008, the FDA recommended that they not be used in children <2 years of age, and drug manufacturers affiliated with the Consumer Healthcare Products Association voluntarily re-labeled products "do not use" for children <4 years of age. The FDA is reviewing the safety of these medicines in children aged 2-11 years.

Available H_1 Antagonists. Summarized below are the therapeutic side effects of a number of H_1 antagonists, grouped by their chemical structures. Representative preparations are listed in Table 32–2.

Dibenzoxepin Tricyclics (Doxepin). Doxepin, the only drug in this class, is marketed as a tricyclic antidepressant (Chapter 16). It also is one of the most potent H_1 antagonists and has significant H_2 antagonist activity, but this does not translate into greater clinical effectiveness. It can cause drowsiness and is associated with anticholinergic effects. Doxepin is better tolerated by patients with depression than those who are not depressed, where even small doses (e.g., 20 mg) may cause disorientation and confusion.

Ethanolamines (Prototype: Diphenhydramine). These drugs possess significant antimuscarinic activity and have a pronounced tendency to induce sedation. About half of those treated acutely with conventional doses experience somnolence. The incidence of GI side effects, however, is low with this group.

Ethylenediamines (Prototype: Pyrilamine). These include some of the most specific H_1 antagonists. Although their central effects are relatively feeble, somnolence occurs in a fair proportion of patients. GI side effects are quite common.

Alkylamines (Prototype: Chlorpheniramine). These are among the most potent H_1 antagonists. The drugs are less prone to produce drowsiness and are more suitable for daytime use, but a significant proportion of patients do experience sedation. Side effects involving CNS stimulation are more common than with other groups.

First-Generation Piperazines. The oldest member of this group, chlorcyclizine, has a more prolonged action and produces a comparatively low incidence of drowsiness. Hydroxyzine is a long-acting compound that is used widely for skin allergies; its considerable CNS-depressant activity may contribute to its prominent anti-pruritic action. Cyclizine and meclizine have been used primarily to counter motion sickness, although promethazine and diphenhydramine are more effective (as is the antimuscarinic scopolamine; see "H_1 Antihistamines").

Second-Generation Piperazines (Cetirizine). Cetirizine is the only drug in this class. It has minimal anticholinergic effects. It also has negligible penetration into the brain but is associated with a somewhat higher incidence of drowsiness than the other second-generation H_1 antagonists. The active enantiomer levocetirizine has slightly greater potency and may be used at half the dose with less resultant sedation.

Phenothiazines (Prototype: Promethazine). Most drugs of this class are H_1 antagonists and also possess considerable anticholinergic activity. Promethazine, which has prominent sedative effects, and its many congeners are used primarily for their antiemetic effects (Chapter 37).

First-Generation Piperidines (Cyproheptadine, Phenindamine). Cyproheptadine uniquely has both antihistamine and anti-serotonin activity. Cyproheptadine and phenindamine cause drowsiness and also have significant anticholinergic effects and can increase appetite.

Second-Generation Piperidines (Prototype: Terfenadine). Terfenadine and astemizole were withdrawn from the market. Current drugs in this class include loratadine, desloratadine, and fexofenadine. These agents are highly selective for H_1 receptors, lack significant anticholinergic actions, and penetrate poorly into the CNS. Taken together, these properties appear to account for the low incidence of side effects of piperidine antihistamines.

H_2 RECEPTOR ANTAGONISTS

The pharmacology and clinical utility of H_2 antagonists to inhibit gastric acid secretion are described in Chapter 45.

THE HISTAMINE H_3 RECEPTOR AND ITS ANTAGONISTS

The H_3 receptor was characterized as a novel G_i-coupled receptor using (R)-α-methylhistamine, a selective H_3 agonist, and thioperamide, an antagonist (Arrang et al., 1987). The cloning of its cDNA revealed it to be a GPCR with low sequence identity (~20%) to H_1 and H_2 receptors (Lovenberg et al., 1999). Further studies on the H_3 receptor uncovered a variety of functional isoforms resulting from alternative splicing, many within a pseudo-intron in the third intracellular loop that may control constitutive activity (Arrang et al., 2007); this, combined with the influence of cell type, signaling pathway, and interspecies differences, yields H_3 receptors with a variety of binding and signaling properties (Esbenshade et al., 2008).

H_3 receptors are presynaptic autoreceptors on histaminergic neurons that originate in the tuberomammillary nucleus in the hypothalamus and project throughout the CNS, most prominently to the hippocampus, amygdala, nucleus accumbens, globus pallidus, striatum, hypothalamus, and cortex (Haas et al., 2008; Sander et al., 2008). The activated H_3 receptor depresses neuronal firing at the level of cell bodies/dendrites and decreases histamine release from depolarized terminals. Thus, H_3 agonists decrease histaminergic transmission, and antagonists increase it. H_3 receptors also are presynaptic heteroreceptors on a variety of neurons in brain and peripheral tissues, and their activation inhibits release from noradrenergic, serotoninergic, GABA-ergic, cholinergic, and glutamatergic neurons, as well as pain-sensitive C fibers. H_3 receptors in the brain have significant constitutive activity in the absence of agonist, which varies according to splicing isoform, cell type, and signaling pathway stimulated; consequently, inverse agonists will activate these neurons.

In the enterochromaffin-like cells of the stomach, H_3 receptors inhibit gastrin-induced release of histamine and, therefore, decrease HCl secretion mediated by H_2 receptors, but the effect is not large enough to warrant development of therapeutic agents. H_3 agonists decrease tachykinin release from capsaicin-sensitive C-fiber terminals and thereby reduce capsaicin-induced plasma extravasation and are antinociceptive. H_3 agonists also depress exaggerated catecholamine release in the heart (e.g., during ischemia).

By blocking H_3 autoreceptors on histaminergic neurons and H_3 heteroreceptors on other neurons, H_3 antagonists/inverse agonists have a wide range of central effects; for example, they promote wakefulness, improve cognitive function (e.g., enhance memory, learning, and attention), and reduce food intake (Esbenshade et al., 2008; Sander et al., 2008). As a result, there is considerable interest in developing H_3 antagonists for possible treatment of sleeping disorders, attention-deficit hyperactivity disorder (ADHD), epilepsy, cognitive impairment, schizophrenia, obesity, neuropathic pain, and Alzheimer's disease (Esbenshade et al., 2008; Sander et al., 2008). However, this task is complicated by the heterogeneity in receptor isoforms and signaling pathways, varying levels of constitutive H_3 activity, species differences in ligand affinities, and the effects of H_3 antagonists/inverse agonists on the release of neurotransmitters in addition to histamine (e.g., DA, ACh, NE, GABA, glutamate, and substance P) (Sander et al., 2008; Esbenshade et al., 2008). Although drug development is focused on inverse agonists to block basal and agonist-stimulated H_3 activity, it is not yet clear that such drugs will necessarily be clinically superior to neutral antagonists.

Thioperamide was the first "specific" H_3 antagonist/inverse agonist available experimentally, but it turned out to be equally effective on the H_4 receptor. A number of other imidazole derivatives have been developed as H_3 antagonists, including clobenpropit, ciproxifan, and proxyfan. However, the imidazole group can bind to and inhibit CYPs, reduce bioavailability in and penetration into the CNS, and enhance binding to H_4 receptors, prompting efforts to develop more selective H_3-receptor antagonists using non-imidazole-based structures. This has resulted in the generation of numerous antagonists/inverse agonists representing a remarkably broad variety of structural classes (Sander et al., 2008; Esbenshade et al., 2008). Although none is approved for clinical use, several non-imidazole H_3 antagonists/inverse agonists are in phase II clinical trials for treating epilepsy, narcolepsy and other sleep disorders, cognitive impairment, Alzheimer's disease, schizophrenia, and ADHD; these include tiprolisant (BF2.649), GSK189254, GSK239512, JNJ-17216498, and MK0249.

THE HISTAMINE H_4 RECEPTOR AND ITS ANTAGONISTS

The discovery of a fourth histamine receptor with a unique pharmacology and distribution has further expanded the search for new drugs based on histamine function in inflammation (Leurs et al., 2009; Thurmond et al., 2008). The H_4 receptor has the highest homology with the H_3 receptor and binds many H_3 ligands, especially those with imidazole rings, although sometimes with different effects. For example, thioperamide is an effective inverse agonist at both H_3 and H_4 receptors, whereas H_3 inverse agonist clobenpropit is a partial agonist of the H_4 receptor; impentamine (an H_3 agonist) and iodophenpropit (an H_3 inverse agonist) are both neutral H_4 antagonists (Lim et al., 2005).

Because the H_4 receptor is expressed on cells with inflammatory or immune functions (see the discussion earlier), there is great interest in developing H_4 antagonists to treat various inflammatory conditions (Thurmond et al., 2008). Indeed, H_4 receptors can mediate histamine-induced chemotaxis, induction of cell shape change, secretion of cytokines, and upregulation of adhesion molecules. For example, the H_4 receptor likely accounts for early reports of histamine-dependent eosinophil chemotaxis, which was independent of H_1 receptors and inhibited by H_2 receptors (Clark et al., 1977). The presence of H_4 receptors in the CNS and animal studies with H_4 agonists and antagonists also have indicated a role for this receptor in pruritus and neuropathic pain (Leurs et al., 2009). The first selective H_4 antagonist, JNJ7777120, exhibits ~1000-fold selectivity over other H receptors, has acceptable oral bioavailability, and has *in vivo* activity; however, its short $t_{1/2}$ (~0.8 hour) limits its potential clinical usefulness. In addition to derivatives of the benzimidazole JNJ7777120, promising H_4 antagonists have been developed using several different scaffolds, including methylpiperazine-substituted 2-quinoxalinones, quinazolines, and aminopyrimidines (Leurs et al., 2009). Although these are high-affinity ligands, relatively high doses are required for significant anti-inflammatory effects *in vivo*, possibly due to either their pharmacokinetic properties or competition with endogenous histamine, which also has a high affinity for the receptor (Leurs et al., 2009). No H_4 antagonists have yet been tested in clinical trials.

CLINICAL SUMMARY: ANTI-HISTAMINES

H_1 Antihistamines. These medications are used widely in the treatment of allergic disorders. H_1 antihistamines are most effective in relieving the symptoms of seasonal rhinitis and conjunctivitis (e.g., sneezing; rhinorrhea; itching of the eyes, nose, and throat). In bronchial asthma, they have limited beneficial effects and are not useful as sole therapy. H_1 antagonists are useful adjuncts to epinephrine in the treatment of systemic anaphylaxis or severe angioedema. Certain allergic dermatoses, such as acute urticaria, respond favorably to H_1 antagonists, which help to relieve the itch in atopic or contact dermatitis but have no effect on the rash. Physical and chronic urticaria may require increased dosage to counter the levels of skin histamine generated (Siebenhaar et al., 2009).

Side effects are most prominent with first-generation H_1 antihistamines (e.g., diphenhydramine, chlorpheniramine, doxepin, hydroxyzine), which cross the blood-brain barrier and cause sedation. Some of the first-generation H_1 receptor antagonists also have anticholinergic properties that can be responsible for symptoms such as dryness of the mouth and respiratory passages, urinary retention or frequency, and dysuria. The second-generation drugs (e.g., levocetirizine, cetirizine, loratadine, desloratadine, fexofenadine) are largely devoid of these side effects because they do not penetrate the CNS and do not have antimuscarinic properties. Thus, they usually are the drugs of choice for the treatment of allergic disorders.

The significant sedative effects of some first-generation antihistamines have led to their use in treating insomnia, although better drugs are available. Some first-generation H_1 antagonists (e.g., dimenhydrinate, cyclizine, meclizine, and promethazine) can prevent motion sickness, although scopolamine is more effective. Antiemetic effects of these H_1 antihistamines can be beneficial in treating vertigo or postoperative emesis.

Many H_1 antihistamines are metabolized by CYPs. Thus, inhibitors of CYP activity, such as macrolide antibiotics (e.g., erythromycin) or imidazole antifungals (e.g., ketoconazole) can increase H_1 antihistamine levels, leading to toxicity. Some newer antihistamines, such as cetirizine, fexofenadine, levocabastine, and acrivastine, are not subject to these drug interactions.

Caution should be used in treating pregnant or lactating women with certain H_1 antihistamines, especially first-generation drugs, because of their possible teratogenic effects or symptomatic effects on infants resulting from secretion of the drug into breast milk. Cetirizine and loratadine are preferred if H_1 antihistamines are required, but if they are not effective, diphenhydramine can be used safely in pregnant (but not breast-feeding) women.

H_2 Antihistamines. These drugs (e.g., cimetidine, ranitidine) primarily are used to inhibit gastric acid secretion in the treatment of GI disorders (Chapter 45).

H_3 and H_4 Antihistamines. Although specific H_3 and H_4 receptor antagonists have been developed, no drugs have been approved for clinical use. Based on the functions of H_3 receptors in the CNS, H_3 antagonists have potential in the treatment of sleeping disorders, ADHD, epilepsy, cognitive impairment, schizophrenia, obesity, neuropathic pain, and Alzheimer's disease. Because of the unique localization and function of H_4 receptors, H_4 antagonists are promising candidates to treat inflammatory conditions such as allergic rhinitis, asthma, rheumatoid arthritis, and possibly pruritus and neuropathic pain.

BRADYKININ, KALLIDIN, AND THEIR ANTAGONISTS

Tissue damage, allergic reactions, viral infections, and other inflammatory events activate a series of proteolytic reactions that generate bradykinin and kallidin in the circulation or tissues. Kinin metabolites released by basic carboxypeptidases, formerly considered inactive degradation products, are agonists of a receptor (B_1) that differs from that of intact kinins (B_2). B_1 receptor expression is induced by tissue injury or inflammation. These peptides contribute to inflammatory responses as autacoids that act locally to produce pain, vasodilation, and increased vascular permeability but can also have beneficial effects, for example in the heart, kidney, and circulation. Much of their activity is due to stimulation of the release of potent mediators such as prostaglandins, NO, or endothelium-derived hyperpolarizing factor (EDHF). Although both B_1 and B_2 receptors are referred to as "bradykinin" receptors, this term properly applies only to the B_2 receptor; the B_1 receptor binds des-Arg metabolites of the kinins (Figure 32–4). These B receptors for kinins must not be confused with β receptors for catecholamines. Current efforts to develop potent non-peptide B_1 and B_2 antagonists may open novel avenues for therapeutic intervention in chronic inflammatory conditions.

History. In the 1920s and 1930s, Frey, Kraut, and Werle characterized a hypotensive substance in urine and found a similar material in saliva, plasma, and a variety of tissues. The pancreas also was a rich source, so they named this material *kallikrein* after a Greek synonym for that organ, *kallikréas*. By 1937, Werle, Götze, and Keppler had established that kallikreins generate a pharmacologically active substance from an inactive precursor present in plasma; the active substance, *kallidin*, proved to be a polypeptide cleaved from a plasma globulin termed *kallidinogen* (see Werle, 1970).

Interest in the field intensified when Rocha e Silva, Beraldo, and associates reported that trypsin and certain snake venoms acted on plasma globulin to produce a substance that lowered blood pressure and caused a slowly developing contraction of the gut (Rocha e Silva et al., 1949; Beraldo and Andrade, 1997). Because of this slow response, they named the substance *bradykinin*, a term derived from the Greek words *bradys*, meaning "slow," and *kinein*, meaning "to move." In 1960, the nonapeptide bradykinin was isolated by Elliott and coworkers and synthesized by Boissonnas and associates. Shortly thereafter, kallidin was found to be a decapeptide bradykinin with an additional lysine residue at the amino terminus. These peptides, except for Lys^1, have identical chemical structures (Table 32–3) and quite similar pharmacological properties. For the whole group, the generic term *kinins* has been adopted. The kinins have short half-lives because they are destroyed by plasma and tissue enzymes originally called *kininase I* and *kininase II*. Kininase I releases a single C-terminal amino acid; kininase II releases a dipeptide (Skidgel and Erdös, 1998). Kininase II is identical to angiotensin-converting enzyme (ACE) (Yang et al., 1970).

Ferreira and colleagues (1970) reported the isolation of a bradykinin-potentiating factor from the venom of the Brazilian snake *Bothrops jararaca*. Ondetti and colleagues (1971) subsequently determined the structure of a peptide from the venom that inhibited ACE and lowered blood pressure when given intravenously to hypertensive patients. Synthetic ACE inhibitors, administered orally (Chapter 26), now are widely used in the treatment of hypertension, diabetic nephropathy, congestive heart failure, and after myocardial infarction (Pfeffer and Frolich, 2006).

Regoli and Barabé (1980) divided the kinin receptors into B_1 and B_2 classes based on the rank order of potency of kinin analogs, and this was validated at the molecular level by cloning of the B_1 and B_2 receptors (Bhoola et al., 1992; Hess, 1997). A primary feature that distinguishes peptide ligands of the B_1 and B_2 receptors is the presence of a C-terminal Arg residue; intact kinins (bradykinin and kallidin) are agonists of the B_2 receptor, whereas their des-Arg forms ([des-Arg^9]-bradykinin and [des-Arg^{10}]-kallidin) are agonists for the B_1 receptor. First-generation B_2 kinin–receptor antagonists were developed in the mid-1980s (Stewart, 2004), followed by second- and third-generation blockers. These antagonists revealed the role of kinins in the therapeutic effects of ACE/kininase II inhibitors and have led to increased acceptance of the importance of kinins. Studies involving B_1 and B_2 receptor knockout mice (Hess, 1997; Pesquero and Bader, 2006; Jiang et al., 2009) have furthered our understanding of the role of bradykinin in the regulation of cardiovascular homeostasis and inflammatory processes.

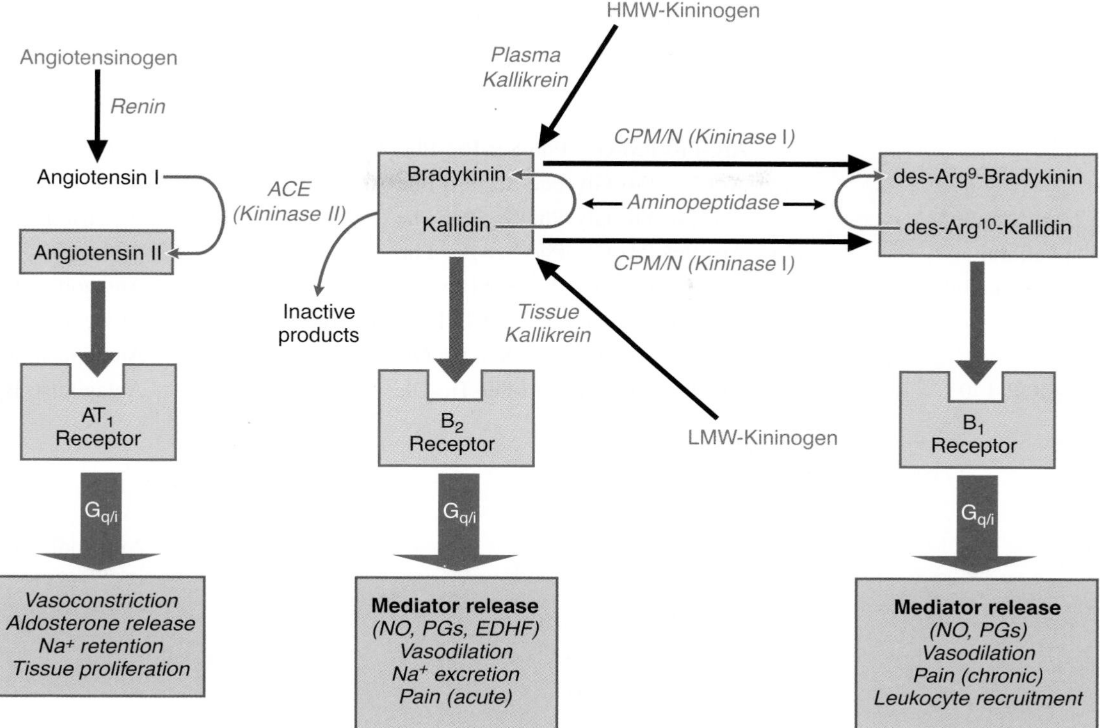

Figure 32–4. *Synthesis and receptor interactions of active peptides generated by the kallikrein-kinin and renin-angiotensin systems.* Bradykinin is generated by the action of *plasma* kallikrein on high-molecular-weight (HMW) kininogen, whereas kallidin (Lys[1]-bradykinin) is released by the hydrolysis of low-molecular-weight (LMW) kininogen by *tissue* kallikrein. Kallidin and bradykinin are the natural ligands of the B_2 receptor but can be converted to corresponding agonists of the B_1 receptor by removal of the C-terminal Arg by kininase I–type enzymes: the plasma membrane–bound carboxypeptidase M (CPM) or soluble plasma carboxypeptidase N (CPN). Kallidin or [des-Arg[10]]-kallidin can be converted to the active peptides bradykinin or to [des-Arg[9]]-bradykinin by aminopeptidase cleavage of the N-terminal Lys residue. In a parallel fashion, the inactive decapeptide angiotensin I is generated by the action of renin on the plasma substrate angiotensinogen. By removal of the C-terminal His–Leu dipeptide, angiotensin-converting enzyme (ACE) generates the active peptide angiotensin II (AngII). These two systems have opposing effects. AngII is a potent vasoconstrictor that also causes aldosterone release and Na^+ retention via activation of the AT_1 receptor; bradykinin is a vasodilator that stimulates Na^+ excretion by activating the B_2 receptor. ACE generates active AngII and, at the same time, inactivates bradykinin and kallidin; thus, its effects are prohypertensive, and ACE inhibitors are effective antihypertensive agents. The B_2 receptor mediates most of bradykinin's effects under normal circumstances, whereas synthesis of the B_1 receptor is induced by inflammatory mediators in inflammatory conditions. Both B_1 and B_2 receptors couple through G_q to activate PLC and increase intracellular Ca^{2+}; the physiological response depends on receptor distribution on particular cell types and occupancy by agonist peptides. For instance, on endothelial cells, activation of B_2 receptors results in Ca^{2+}–calmodulin–dependent activation of eNOS and generation of NO, which causes cyclic GMP accumulation and relaxation in neighboring smooth muscle cells. However, in endothelial cells under inflammatory conditions, B_1 receptor stimulation results in prolonged NO production via G_i and MAP kinase-dependent activation of iNOS expression. On smooth muscle cells, activation of kinin receptors coupling through G_q results in an increased $[Ca^{2+}]_i$ and contraction. B_1 and B_2 receptors also can couple through G_i to activate PLA_2, causing the release of arachidonic acid and the local generation of prostanoids (PGs) and other metabolites such as endothelium-derived hyperpolarizing factor (EDHF). Kallikrein also plays a role in the intrinsic blood coagulation pathway (see Chapter 30).

The Endogenous Kallikrein–Kininogen–Kinin System

Synthesis of Kinins. Bradykinin is a nonapeptide; kallidin, a decapeptide containing an additional N-terminal lysine, is sometimes referred to as *lysyl-bradykinin* (Table 32–3). The two peptides are cleaved from α_2 globulins termed *kininogens* (Figure 32–4). There are two kininogens: high-molecular-weight (HMW) kininogen and low-molecular-weight (LMW) kininogen. A number of serine proteases will generate kinins, but the highly specific proteases that release bradykinin

Table 32–3

Structure of Kinin Agonists and Antagonists

NAME	STRUCTURE	FUNCTION
Bradykinin	Arg-Pro-Pro-Gly-Phe-Ser-Pro-Phe-Arg	Agonist, B_2
Kallidin	Lys-Arg-Pro-Pro-Gly-Phe-Ser-Pro-Phe-Arg	Agonist, B_2
[des-Arg^9]-bradykinin	Arg-Pro-Pro-Gly-Phe-Ser-Pro-Phe	Agonist, B_1
[des-Arg^{10}]-kallidin	Lys-Arg-Pro-Pro-Gly-Phe-Ser-Pro-Phe	Agonist, B_1
des-Arg^{10}-[Leu^9]-kallidin	Lys-Arg-Pro-Pro-Gly-Phe-Ser-Pro-Leu	Antagonist, B_1
NPC-349	[D-Arg]-Arg-Pro-Hyp-Gly-Thi-Ser-D-Phe-Thi-Arg	Antagonist, B_2
HOE-140	[D-Arg]-Arg-Pro-Hyp-Gly-Thi-Ser-Tic-Oic-Arg	Antagonist, B_2
[des-Arg^{10}]-HOE-140	[D-Arg]-Arg-Pro-Hyp-Gly-Thi-Ser-Tic-Oic	Antagonist, B_1
FR173657	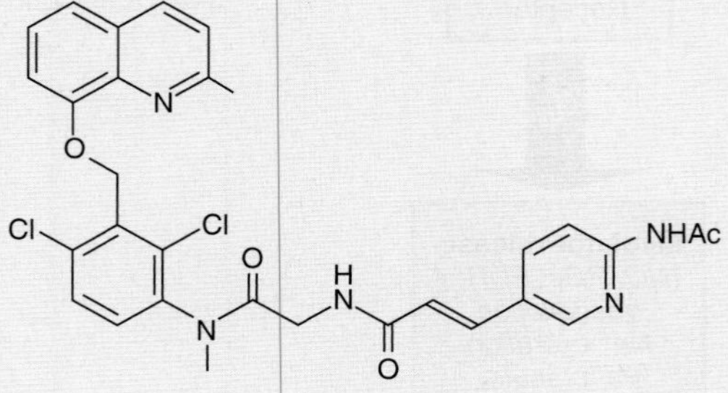	Antagonist, B_2
FR190997	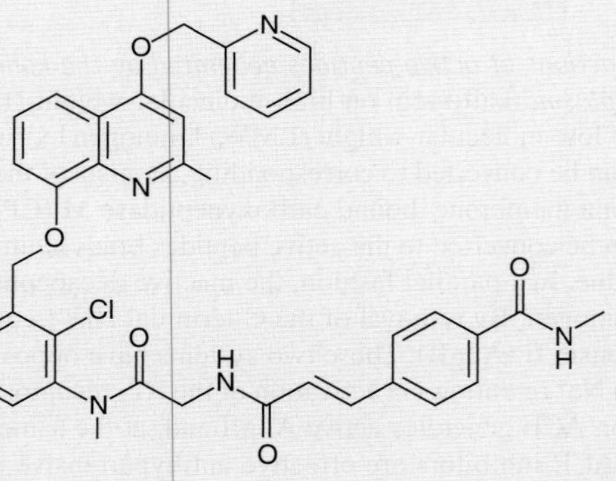	Agonist, B_2
SSR240612	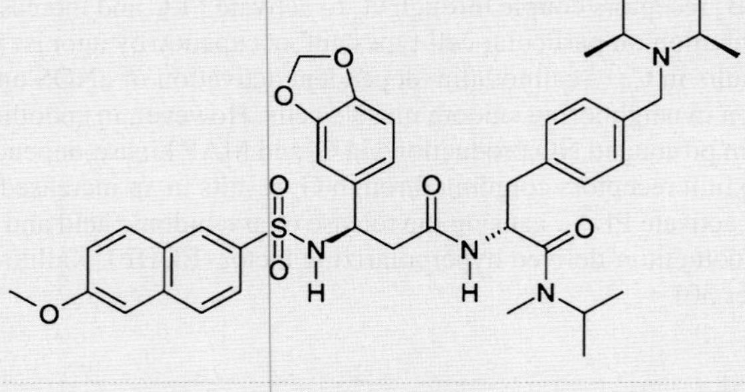	Antagonist, B_1

ABBREVIATIONS: Hyp, *trans*-4-hydroxy-Pro; Thi, *β*-(2-thienyl)-Ala; Tic, [D]-1,2,3,4-tetrahydroisoquinolin-3-yl-carbonyl; Oic, (3as,7as)-octahydroindol-2-yl-carbonyl.

and kallidin from the kininogens are termed *kallikreins* (see "Kallikreins").

Kallikreins. Bradykinin and kallidin are cleaved from HMW or LMW kininogens by plasma or tissue kallikrein, respectively (Figure 32–4). Plasma kallikrein and tissue kallikrein are distinct enzymes that are activated by different mechanisms (Bhoola et al., 1992).

Plasma prekallikrein is an inactive protein of ~88,000 Da that complexes with its substrate, HMW kininogen (Mandle et al., 1976). The ensuing proteolytic cascade is restrained by the protease inhibitors present in plasma. Among the most important of these are the inhibitor of the activated first component of complement (C1-INH) and α_2 macroglobulin. Under experimental conditions, the kallikrein–kinin system is activated by the binding of factor XII, also known as *Hageman factor*, to negatively charged surfaces. Factor XII, a protease that is common to both the kinin and the intrinsic coagulation cascades (Chapter 30), undergoes autoactivation (Silverberg et al., 1980) and, in turn, activates prekallikrein. Importantly, kallikrein further activates factor XII, thereby exerting a positive feedback on the system. *In vivo*, factor XII may not undergo autoactivation on binding to endothelial cells. Instead, the binding of the HMW kininogen–prekallikrein heterodimer to a multiprotein-receptor complex on endothelial cells leads to activation of the prekallikrein-HMW kininogen complex (but not free prekallikrein) by heat shock protein 90 (Joseph et al., 2002) and by a lysosomal enzyme designated *prolylcarboxypeptidase*, which also is present on endothelial cell membranes (Schmaier, 2008). Kallikrein activates factor XII, cleaves HMW kininogen, and activates prourokinase (Schmaier, 2008; Kaplan et al., 2002; Colman, 1999). Human tissue kallikrein is a member of a large multigene family of 15 members with high sequence identity that are clustered at chromosome 19q13.4 (Emami and Diamandis, 2007). Only the classical (or "true") tissue kallikrein, hK1, generates kinins from kininogen. Another member, hK3, better known as the prostate-specific antigen (PSA), is an important marker in diagnosing prostate cancer, and several other family members are promising tumor biomarkers (Emami and Diamandis, 2007).

Compared with plasma kallikrein, tissue kallikrein is a smaller protein (29,000 Da). It is synthesized as a preproprotein in the epithelial cells or secretory cells in several tissues, including salivary glands, pancreas, prostate, and distal nephron. Tissue kallikrein also is expressed in human neutrophils. It acts locally near its sites of origin. The synthesis of tissue prokallikrein is controlled by a number of factors, including aldosterone in the kidney and salivary gland and androgens in certain other glands. The secretion of the tissue prokallikrein also may be regulated; *for example,* its secretion from the pancreas is enhanced by stimulation of the vagus nerve. The activation of tissue prokallikrein to kallikrein requires proteolytic cleavage to remove a 7–amino acid propeptide (Takada et al., 1985).

Kininogens. The two substrates for the kallikreins, HMW kininogen and LMW kininogen, are derived from a single gene by alternative splicing. The HMW kininogen contains 626 amino acid residues: The N-terminal "heavy chain" sequence (362 amino acids) consists of domains 1-3, followed by 9 residue bradykinin sequence (domain 4), connected to a C-terminal "light chain" sequence (255 amino acids) containing domains D5 and D6. LMW kininogen is identical to domains 1-4 of HMW kininogen but is distinguished by its short C-terminal light chain (Takagaki et al., 1985). HMW kininogen is cleaved by plasma and tissue kallikrein to yield bradykinin and kallidin, respectively. LMW kininogen is a substrate only of tissue kallikrein, and the product is kallidin. The kininogens also inhibit cysteine proteinases and thrombin binding and have anti-adhesive and profibrinolytic properties.

Metabolism of Kinins. The decapeptide kallidin is about as active as the nonapeptide bradykinin, even without conversion to bradykinin, which occurs when the N-terminal lysine residue is removed by an aminopeptidase (Skidgel and Erdös, 1998) (Figure 32–4). The nonapeptide has the minimal effective structure for standard responses on B_2 receptors (Figure 32–4 and Table 32–3).

The kinins have an evanescent existence—their $t_{1/2}$ in plasma is only ~15 seconds, and some 80-90% of the kinins may be destroyed in a single passage through the pulmonary vascular bed. Plasma concentrations of bradykinin are difficult to measure because inadequate inhibition of kininogenases or kininases in the blood can lead to artifactual formation or degradation of bradykinin during blood collection. When care is taken to inhibit these processes, the reported physiological concentrations of bradykinin in blood are in the picomolar range.

The principal catabolizing enzyme in the lung and other vascular beds is kininase II, or ACE (Figure 32–4) (Chapter 26). Removal of the C-terminal dipeptide by ACE or neutral endopeptidase 24.11 (neprilysin) inactivates kinins (Skidgel and Erdös, 1998) (Figure 32–5). A slower-acting enzyme, carboxypeptidase N (lysine carboxypeptidase, kininase I), releases the C-terminal arginine residue, producing [desArg^9]-bradykinin or [des-Arg^{10}]-kallidin (Table 32–3 and Figures 32–4 and 32–5), which are potent B_1 receptor agonists that no longer bind B_2 receptors (Bhoola et al., 1992; Skidgel and Erdös, 1998). Carboxypeptidase N is expressed constitutively in blood plasma, where its level is ~10^{-7} M (Skidgel and Erdös, 1998; Skidgel and Erdös, 2007). Carboxypeptidase M, which also cleaves basic C-terminal amino acids, is a widely distributed plasma membrane–bound enzyme (Skidgel and Erdös, 1998). The recently established crystal structures of the active subunit of carboxypeptidases N and M revealed an overall similarity with unique features consistent with their different localizations and functions (Skidgel and Erdös, 2007). A familial carboxypeptidase N deficiency, due to mutations in the active subunit, causes low plasma levels of this enzyme and is associated with angioedema or urticaria (Skidgel and Erdös, 2007; Matthews et al., 2004). Finally, aminopeptidase P can cleave the N-terminal arginine, rendering bradykinin inactive and susceptible to cleavage by dipeptidyl peptidase IV (Figure 32–5).

Kinin Receptors. The B_1 and B_2 kinin receptors are both GPCRs, sharing 36% amino acid sequence identity (Hess, 1997; Leeb-Lundberg et al., 2005).

The classical bradykinin B_2 receptor is constitutively expressed in most normal tissues, where it selectively binds intact bradykinin and kallidin (Table 32–3 and Figure 32–4) and mediates the majority of their effects. The B_1 receptor is activated by the des-Arg metabolites of bradykinin and kallidin produced by the actions of carboxypeptidases N and M (Table 32–3 and Figures 32–4 and 32–5). Interestingly, carboxypeptidase M and the B_1 receptor

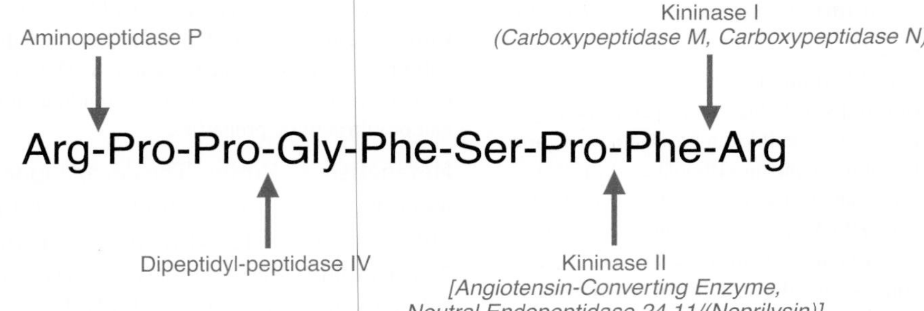

Figure 32–5. *Schematic diagram of the degradation of bradykinin.* Arrows denote the primary cleavage sites in bradykinin. Bradykinin and kallidin are inactivated *in vivo* primarily by kininase II [angiotensin-converting enzyme (ACE)]. Neutral endopeptidase 24.11 (neprilysin), cleaves bradykinin and kallidin at the same Pro–Phe bond as ACE and also is classified as a kininase II–type enzyme. In addition, aminopeptidase P can inactivate bradykinin by hydrolyzing the N-terminal Arg^1–Pro^2 bond, leaving bradykinin susceptible to further degradation by dipeptidyl peptidase IV. Bradykinin and kallidin are converted to their respective des-Arg^9 or des-Arg^{10} metabolites by kininase I–type carboxypeptidases M and N. Unlike the parent peptides, these kinin metabolites are potent ligands for B_1 kinin receptors but not B_2 kinin receptors.

interact on the cell surface to form an efficient signaling complex; disruption of this interaction decreases the efficiency of generation and delivery of des-Arg-kinin agonist to the B_1 receptor and reduces subsequent B_1 signaling (Zhang et al., 2008). B_1 receptors are normally absent or expressed at low levels in most tissues. B_1 receptor expression is upregulated by tissue injury and inflammation and by cytokines, endotoxins, and growth factors (Bhoola et al., 1992; Leeb-Lundberg et al., 2005). Carboxypeptidase M expression also is increased by cytokines (Sangsree et al., 2003), to such a degree that B_1 receptor effects may predominate over B_2 effects.

The B_2 receptor activates PLA_2 and PLC via interaction with distinct G proteins. Kinin-induced PLC activation through G_q activates the IP_3–Ca^{2+} pathway, stimulating PKC activity and also enhancing NO synthesis by eNOS/NOS3. Bradykinin activates the pro-inflammatory transcription factor NF-κB through $G\alpha_q$ and βγ subunits and also activates the MAP kinase pathway. Coupling of activated B_2 receptors to G_i leads to PLA_2 activation and the liberation of arachidonate from membrane-bound phospholipids, which is converted to a variety of derivatives, including inflammatory mediators and vasodilator epoxyeicosatrienoic acids (EETs) and prostacyclin (Campbell and Falck, 2007; Leeb-Lundberg et al., 2005) (Chapter 33).

B_1 receptors also couple through G_q and G_i to activate many of the same signal transduction pathways as the B_2 receptor (Leeb-Lundberg et al., 2005). However, B_1 receptor activation enhances NO production by stimulation of the inducible nitric oxide synthase (iNOS) rather than eNOS (Zhang et al., 2007). The B_1 and B_2 receptors also differ in their time courses of downregulation; the B_2 receptor response is rapidly desensitized, whereas the B_1 response is not. This likely is due to modification at a Ser/Thr-rich cluster present in the C-terminal tail of the B_2 receptor that is not conserved in the B_1 receptor sequence (Leeb-Lundberg et al., 2005).

Because B_2 receptors are distributed widely and couple to several G proteins, receptor agonists are employed frequently as tools to activate and study signal transduction pathways in a variety of cells. The antagonist icatibant (HOE-140) is commonly used to prove that cellular responses are mediated by B_2 receptors. Nevertheless, blocking increased signaling through the B_2 receptor does not necessarily indicate enhanced kinin generation because some proteases (e.g., kallikrein) can activate the B_2 receptor directly, and this also is blocked by HOE-140 (Biyashev et al., 2006).

Activation of the angiotensin AT_2 receptor results in responses (e.g., vasodilation) that oppose those of the activated angiotensin AT_1 receptor (e.g., vasoconstriction) (Chapter 26); this can be mediated in part by cross-talk through activation of B_2 receptors (Widdop et al., 2003).

Functions and Pharmacology of Kallikreins and Kinins

The availability of specific kinin-receptor antagonists and the generation of B_1 and B_2 receptor knockout mice have advanced our understanding of the roles of the kinins (Leeb-Lundberg et al., 2005; Pesquero and Bader, 2006). Antagonists currently are being investigated in diverse areas such as pain, inflammation, chronic inflammatory diseases and the cardiovascular system. That the beneficial effects of ACE inhibitor therapy rests in part on enhancing bradykinin activity (e.g., on the heart, kidney, blood pressure; see Chapter 26) demonstrates the complexities in interpreting bradykinin's actions.

Systems Pharmacology of Kinins

Pain. The kinins are powerful algesic agents that cause an intense burning pain when applied to the exposed base of a blister. Bradykinin excites primary sensory neurons and provokes the release of neuropeptides such as substance P, neurokinin A, and calcitonin gene–related peptide. Although there is overlap, B_2 receptors generally mediate acute bradykinin algesia, whereas the pain of chronic inflammation appears to involve increased numbers and activation of B_1 receptors.

Inflammation. Kinins participate in a variety of inflammatory conditions. Plasma kinins increase permeability in the microcirculation, acting on the small venules to cause disruption of the inter-endothelial junctions. This, together with an increased hydrostatic pressure gradient, causes edema. Edema, coupled with stimulation of nerve endings, results in a "wheal and flare" response to intradermal injection.

In hereditary angioedema, bradykinin is formed, and there is depletion of the upstream components of the kinin cascade during episodes of swelling, laryngeal edema, and abdominal pain. B_1 receptors on inflammatory cells (e.g., macrophages) can elicit production of the inflammatory mediators IL-1 and TNF-α (Bhoola et al., 1992). Kinin levels are increased in a number of chronic inflammatory diseases and may be significant in gout, disseminated intravascular coagulation, inflammatory bowel disease, rheumatoid arthritis, or asthma. Kinins also may contribute to the skeletal changes seen in chronic inflammatory states. Kinins stimulate bone resorption through B_1 and possibly B_2 receptors, perhaps by osteoblast-mediated osteoclast activation (Chapter 44).

Respiratory Disease. The kinins have been implicated in allergic airway disorders such as asthma and rhinitis (Abraham et al., 2006). Inhalation or intravenous injection of kinins causes bronchospasm in asthmatic patients but not in normal individuals. This bradykinin-induced bronchoconstriction is blocked by anticholinergic agents but not by antihistamines or cyclooxygenase inhibitors. Similarly, nasal challenge with bradykinin is followed by sneezing and glandular secretions in patients with allergic rhinitis. A B_2 receptor antagonist improved pulmonary function in patients with severe asthma and reduced nasal symptoms in allergic rhinitis (Abraham et al., 2006).

Cardiovascular System. In experimental animals and humans, infusion of bradykinin causes vasodilation and lowers blood pressure. Bradykinin causes vasodilation by activating its B_2 receptor on endothelial cells, resulting in the generation of NO, prostacyclin, and a hyperpolarizing EET that is a CYP-derived metabolite of arachidonic acid (Campbell et al., 1996). In B_2 antagonist–treated animals or B_2 receptor knockout mice, basal blood pressure is normal; however, these animals have an exaggerated blood pressure response to salt loading or activation of the renin–angiotensin system. These data suggest that the endogenous kallikrein–kinin system plays a minor role in the regulation of normal blood pressure, but it may be important in hypertensive states. Urinary kallikrein concentrations are decreased in individuals with high blood pressure (Margolius, 1995).

The kallikrein–kinin system is cardioprotective, as revealed by studies showing that many of the beneficial effects of ACE inhibitors on heart function are attributable to enhancement of bradykinin effects, such as their anti-proliferative activity or ability to increase glucose uptake in tissue (Pfeffer and Frolich, 2006; Henriksen et al., 1999; Heitsch, 2003). Bradykinin contributes to the beneficial effect of preconditioning to protect the heart against ischemia and reperfusion injury. Bradykinin also stimulates tissue plasminogen activator (tPA) release from the vascular endothelium (Leeb-Lundberg et al., 2005) and may contribute to the endogenous defense against some cardiovascular events, such as myocardial infarction and stroke. Stimulation of either B_1 or B_2 receptors produces cardioprotective effects after myocardial infarction (Leeb-Lundberg et al., 2005; Heitsch, 2003; Jiang et al., 2009).

Kidney. Renal kinins act in a paracrine manner to regulate urine volume and composition (Saitoh et al., 1995). Kallikrein is synthesized and secreted by the connecting cells of the distal nephron. Tissue kininogen and kinin receptors are present in the cells of the collecting duct. Like other vasodilators, kinins increase renal blood flow. Bradykinin also causes natriuresis by inhibiting sodium reabsorption at the cortical collecting duct. Treatment with mineralocorticoids, ACE inhibitors, and neutral endopeptidase (neprilysin) inhibitors increases renal kallikrein.

Other Effects. Many initial discoveries in the kallikrein– kinin system were made using a bioassay measuring isotonic contractions of the isolated rat uterus in estrus, which is especially sensitive to kinins. Kinins promote dilation of the fetal pulmonary artery, closure of the ductus arteriosus, and constriction of the umbilical vessels, all of which occur in the transition from fetal to neonatal circulation. The kallikrein–kinin system also functions in many other areas in the body, serving to mediate edema formation and smooth muscle contraction. Kinins also affect the CNS, disrupting the blood-brain barrier and allowing increased CNS penetration.

Potential Therapeutic Uses. Bradykinin contributes to many of the effects of the ACE inhibitors (Figure 32–4; see the history section under "Bradykinin, Kallidin, and Their Antagonists"). *Aprotinin*, a kallikrein and plasmin inhibitor, has been administered to patients undergoing coronary bypass to minimize bleeding and blood requirements (see "Kallikrein Inhibitors", below). Based on the pro-inflammatory and algesic effects of kinins, B_1 and B_2 receptor antagonists are being tested for the treatment of inflammatory conditions and certain types of pain (Abraham et al., 2006; Campos et al., 2006).

Kallikrein Inhibitors

Aprotinin (TRASYLOL) is a natural proteinase inhibitor obtained for commercial purposes from bovine lung and is identical to Kunitz's pancreatic trypsin inhibitor (Waxler and Rabito, 2003). Aprotinin inhibits mediators of the inflammatory response, fibrinolysis, and thrombin generation following cardiopulmonary bypass surgery, including kallikrein and plasmin. Administration of aprotinin reduces requirements for blood products in patients undergoing coronary artery bypass grafting (Waxler and Rabito, 2003). Recent retrospective meta-analyses and a prospective multicenter trial linked aprotinin use with higher mortality and renal morbidity (Dietrich, 2009). Although there is controversy regarding the validity of these conclusions, the manufacturer has withdrawn the drug from the market (Dietrich, 2009); it remains available through a special investigational treatment protocol. Ecallantide (DX-88), a synthetic plasma kallikrein inhibitor, inhibits acute episodes of angioedema in patients with hereditary angioedema (Schneider et al., 2007).

Bradykinin and the Effects of ACE Inhibitors. ACE inhibitors are widely used in the treatment of hypertension, and they reduce mortality in patients with diabetic nephropathy, left ventricular dysfunction, previous myocardial infarction, or coronary artery disease (Pfeffer and Frohlich, 2006). ACE inhibitors block the conversion of Ang I to Ang II, a potent vasoconstrictor and growth promoter (Figure 32–4) (Chapter 25). Studies with the kinin B_2 antagonist HOE-140 demonstrate that bradykinin also contributes to many of the protective effects of ACE inhibitors. For example, administration of HOE-140 in animal models attenuates the favorable effects of ACE inhibitors on blood pressure, myocardial infarct size, and ischemic preconditioning. Bradykinin receptor antagonism also attenuates blood pressure lowering by acute ACE inhibition in humans (Gainer et al., 1998). These effects may result not only from decreased degradation of bradykinin by ACE but also from induction of enhanced receptor sensitivity by ACE inhibitors (Marcic et al., 1999; Biyashev et al., 2006).

A rare side effect of ACE inhibitors is angioedema, which may occur shortly after initiating therapy. This is a class effect of ACE inhibitors and may be connected to the inhibition of kinin metabolism by ACE (Slater et al., 1988). ACE inhibitor–associated angioedema is more common in blacks than in Caucasians. A common side effect of ACE inhibitors is a chronic, nonproductive cough that dissipates when the drug is stopped. The finding that angiotensin AT_1 receptor antagonists do not cause cough supports the role of bradykinin in this effect, but the mechanism has not been clearly defined.

Bradykinin also may contribute to the effects of the AT_1-receptor antagonists. During AT_1 receptor blockade, Ang II concentrations increase, which enhances signaling through the unopposed AT_2 subtype receptor, causing an increase in renal bradykinin concentrations (Widdop et al., 2003).

A new class of antihypertensive agent was developed to inhibit two major kinin-degrading enzymes, ACE and neprilysin, and the added inhibition of bradykinin metabolism was expected to enhance therapeutic effectiveness. In phase III clinical trials, the prototype drug omapatrilat was an effective antihypertensive agent but was associated with a 3-fold higher incidence of angioedema than with an ACE inhibitor alone, causing withdrawal of the drug.

Kinin Receptor Antagonists. The substitution of a D-Phe for Pro at position 7 in bradykinin conferred weak antagonist activity at the B_2 receptor and blocked the action of ACE. The addition of an N-terminal, D-Arg substitution of hydroxyproline in position 3 and thienylalanine at positions 5 and 8 resulted in the first useful and potent B_2 antagonist with *in vivo* activity (NPC-349; Table 32–3) (Stewart, 2004). However, this antagonist had a short $t_{1/2}$ owing to enzymatic degradation by carboxypeptidase N *in vivo*, which converted it into a B_1 antagonist. Based on NPC-349, the longer-acting selective B_2 receptor antagonist HOE-140 (*icatibant*) was developed by substituting synthetic amino acids at positions 7 [*D*-tetrahydroisoquinoline-3-carboxylic acid (Tic)] and 8 [octahydroindole-2-carboxylic acid (Oic)] (Table 32–3). Icatibant (FIRAZYR) has been approved in the E.U. for treatment of acute episodes of swelling in patients with hereditary angioedema (Bork et al., 2008). It is administered by subcutaneous injection.

Orally active non-peptide receptor antagonists would be preferable for therapeutic use. The first of these for the B_2 receptor, WIN64338, had significant muscarinic cholinergic activity. In animals, a newer, more specific non-peptide B_2 antagonist, FR173657 (Table 32–3), decreased bradykinin-induced edema, hypotension, pain, bronchoconstriction, and inflammatory responses (Leeb-Lundberg et al., 2005; Abraham et al., 2006). This has led to increased interest by the drug industry and the generation of several new non-peptide B_2 antagonists with good oral bioavailability and *in vivo* stability and activity (Leeb-Lundberg et al., 2005; Abraham et al., 2006). On the other hand, synthetic B_2 receptor agonists (such as FR190997; Table 32–3) may be cardioprotective. Synthetic small-molecule bradykinin agonists or antagonists would not necessarily bind to the same regions of the B_2 receptor as the peptide (Heitsch, 2003).

Peptide antagonists of the B_1 receptor include des-Arg^{10}-[Leu^8]-kallidin and [des-Arg^{10}]-HOE-140 (Table 32–3), among others (Campos et al., 2006). More recently, several non-peptide B_1 antagonists with *in vivo* activity have been developed (Campos et al., 2006; Feng et al., 2008); the most promising of these is SSR240612 (Table 32–3), which is orally active and inhibits inflammation and neuropathic pain in animal studies. None has yet been tested clinically.

CLINICAL SUMMARY: KININS

Aprotinin (TRASYLOL), the potent inhibitor of kallikrein and other serine proteases, has been employed clinically to reduce blood loss in patients undergoing coronary artery bypass surgery, but unfavorable survival statistics in retrospective and prospective studies have resulted in its discontinuation (Dietrich, 2009).

Because kinins and [des-Arg]-kinins enhance pain and inflammation via activation of the two kinin receptors, B_2 and B_1, antagonists may be useful in treating inflammatory diseases. A peptide-based B_2 receptor antagonist, icatibant (FIRAZYR), has been approved in the E.U. for treatment of acute episodes of swelling in patients with hereditary angioedema (Bork et al., 2008).

ACE inhibitors are widely used drugs in the treatment of hypertension, congestive heart failure, and diabetic nephropathy, and they reduce mortality in patients with a variety of cardiovascular risk factors (Chapter 26). One effect of ACE inhibitors is to prevent the degradation of bradykinin. Because bradykinin, by activating its B_2 receptor, is responsible for many of the beneficial cardioprotective effects of ACE inhibitors, the search is on to find a suitable stable B_2 agonist for clinical evaluation. A major problem for such applications is to establish a safe therapeutic window between potentially protecting the heart and avoiding pro-inflammatory stimulation (Heitsch, 2003).

BIBLIOGRAPHY

Abraham WM, Scuri M, Farmer SG. Peptide and non-peptide bradykinin receptor antagonists: Role in allergic airway disease. *Eur J Pharmacol,* **2006**, *533:*215–221.

Arrang JM, Garbarg M, Lancelot JC, et al. Highly potent and selective ligands for histamine H_3-receptors. *Nature*, **1987**, *327:*117–123.

Arrang JM, Morisset S, Gbahou F. Constitutive activity of the histamine H3 receptor. *Trends Pharmacol Sci,* **2007**, *28:*350–357.

Ash ASF, Schild HO. Receptors mediating some actions of histamine. *Br J Pharmacol*, **1966**, *27*:427–439.

Beraldo WT, Andrade SP. Discovery of bradykinin and the kallikrein-kinin system. In: Farmer SG, ed. *The Kinin System.* San Diego, Academic Press, **1997**, pp. 1–8.

Best CH, Dale HH, Dudley JW, Thorpe WV. The nature of the vasodilator constituents of certain tissue extract. *J Physiol*, **1927**, *62:*397–417.

Bhoola KD, Figueroa CD, Worthy K. Bioregulation of kinins: Kallikreins, kininogens, and kininases. *Pharmacol Rev*, **1992**, *44:*1–80.

Biyashev D, Tan F, Chen Z, et al. Kallikrein activates bradykinin B2 receptors in absence of kininogen. *Am J Physiol Heart Circ Physiol,* **2006**, *290:*H1244–H1250.

Black JW, Duncan WA, Durant CJ, et al. Definition and antagonism of histamine H_2-receptors. *Nature*, **1972**, *236:*385–390.

Bork K, Yasothan U, Kirkpatrick P. Icatibant. *Nat Rev Drug Discov,* **2008**, *7*:801–802.

Campbell WB, Falck JR. Arachidonic acid metabolites as endothelium-derived hyperpolarizing factors. *Hypertension,* **2007**, *49*:590–596.

Campbell WB, Gebremedhin D, Pratt PF, Harder DR. Identification of epoxyeicosatrienoic acids as endothelium-derived hyper-polarizing factors. *Circ Res*, **1996**, *78:*415–423.

Campos MM, Leal PC, Yunes RA, Calixto JB. Non-peptide antagonists for kinin B1 receptors: New insights into their therapeutic potential for the management of inflammation and pain. *Trends Pharmacol Sci,* **2006**, *27*:646–651.

Clark RA, Sandler JA, Gallin JI, Kaplan AP. Histamine modulation of eosinophil migration. *J Immunol,* **1977**, *118:* 137–145.

Colman RW. Biologic activities of the contact factors in vivo—Potentiation of hypotension, inflammation, and fibrinolysis, and inhibition of cell adhesion, angiogenesis and thrombosis. *Thromb Haemost*, **1999,** *82:*1568–1577.

Dale HH. *Adventures in Pharmacology*. London, Pergamon Press, **1953**.

Dietrich W. Aprotinin: 1 year on. *Curr Opin Anaesthesiol,* **2009**, *22:*121–127.

Emami N, Diamandis EP. New insights into the functional mechanisms and clinical applications of the kallikrein-related peptidase family. *Mol Oncol,* **2007**, *1*:269–287.

Esbenshade TA, Browman KE, Bitner RS, et al. The histamine H3 receptor: An attractive target for the treatment of cognitive disorders. *Br J Pharmacol,* **2008**, *154:*1166–1181.

Feng DM, DiPardo RM, Wai JM, et al. A new class of bradykinin B1 receptor antagonists with high oral bioavailability and minimal PXR activity. *Bioorg Med Chem Lett,* **2008**, *18:*682–687.

Ferreira SH, Bartelt DC, Greene LJ. Isolation of bradykinin-potentiating peptides from *Bothrops jararaca* venom. *Biochemistry*, **1970**, *9:*2583–2593.

Ferry X, Brehin S, Kamel R, Landry Y. G protein–dependent activation of mast cell by peptides and basic secretagogues. *Peptides*, **2002**, *23:*1507–1515.

Gainer JV, Morrow JD, Loveland A, et al. Effect of bradykinin-receptor blockade on the response to angiotensin-converting-enzyme inhibitor in normotensive and hypertensive subjects. *N Engl J Med*, **1998**, *339:*1285–1292.

Grossman ML. Some notes on the history of gastrin. In: Grossman ML, ed. *Gastrin*. Berkeley, CA, University of California Press, **1966**, pp. 1–7.

Haas HL, Sergeeva OA, Selbach O. Histamine in the nervous system. *Physiol Rev,* **2008**, *88:*1183–1241.

Heitsch H. The therapeutic potential of bradykinin B_2 receptor agonists in the treatment of cardiovascular disease. *Expert Opin Invest Drugs*, **2003**, *12:*759–770.

Henriksen EJ, Jacob S, Kinnick TR, et al. ACE inhibition and glucose transport in insulin resistant muscle: Roles of bradykinin and nitric oxide. *Am J Physiol,* **1999**, *277:* R332–R336.

Hess JF. Molecular pharmacology of kinin receptors. In: Farmer SG, ed. *The Kinin System*. San Diego, Academic Press, **1997**, pp. 45–55.

Holgate ST, Canonica GW, Simons FE, et al. Consensus Group on New-Generation Antihistamines (CONGA): Present status and recommendations. *Clin Exp Allergy*, **2003**, *33:*1305–1324.

Jiang X, Carretero OA, Shesely EG, et al. The kinin B1 receptor contributes to the cardioprotective effect of angiotensin-converting enzyme inhibitors and angiotensin receptor blockers in mice. *Exp Physiol,* **2009**, *94:*322–329.

Johnson AR, Erdös EG. Release of histamine from mast cells by vasoactive peptides. *Proc Soc Exp Biol Med*, **1973**, *142:*1252–1256.

Joseph K, Tholanikunnel BG, Kaplan AP. Heat shock protein 90 catalyzes activation of the prekallikrein-kininogen complex in the absence of factor XII. *Proc Natl Acad Sci U S A,* **2002**, *99:*896–900.

Kaplan AP. Clinical practice. Chronic urticaria and angioedema. *N Engl J Med,* **2002**, *346:*175–179.

Kaplan AP, Joseph K, Silverberg M. Pathways for bradykinin formation and inflammatory disease. *J Allergy Clin Immunol,* **2002**, *109:*195–209.

Kuehn BM. Debate continues over the safety of cold and cough medicines for children. *JAMA,* **2008**, *300:*2354–2356.

Leeb-Lundberg LM, Marceau F, Muller-Esterl W, et al. International union of pharmacology. XLV. Classification of the kinin receptor family: From molecular mechanisms to pathophysiological consequences. *Pharmacol Rev,* **2005**, *57:*27–77.

Leurs R, Chazot PL, Shenton FC, et al. Molecular and biochemical pharmacology of the histamine H4 receptor. *Br J Pharmacol,* **2009**, *157:*14–23.

Lewis T. *The Blood Vessels of the Human Skin and Their Responses*. London, Shaw and Sons, **1927**.

Lim HD, van Rijn RM, Ling P, et al. Evaluation of histamine H_1-, H_2-, and H_3-receptor ligands at the human histamine H_4 receptor: Identification of 4-methylhistamine as the first potent and selective H_4 receptor agonist. *J Pharmacol Exp Ther,* **2005**, *314:*1310–1321.

Lovenberg TW, Roland BL, Wilson SJ, et al. Cloning and functional expression of the human histamine H_3 receptor. *Mol Pharmacol*, **1999**, *55:*1101–1105.

Mandle RJ, Colman RW, Kaplan AP. Identification of prekallikrein and high-molecular-weight kininogen as a complex in human plasma. *Proc Natl Acad Sci U S A,* **1976**, *73:* 4179–4183.

Marcic B, Deddish PA, Jackman HL, Erdös EG. Enhancement of bradykinin and resensitization of its B_2 receptor. *Hypertension*, **1999**, *33:*835–843.

Margolius HS. Theodore Cooper Memorial Lecture. Kallikreins and kinins: Some unanswered questions about system characteristics and roles in human disease. *Hypertension*, **1995**, *26:*221–229.

Matthews KW, Mueller-Ortiz SL, Wetsel RA. Carboxypeptidase N: A pleiotropic regulator of inflammation. *Mol Immunol,* **2004**, *40:*785–793.

Meeves SG, Appajosyula S. Efficacy and safety profile of fexofenadine HCL: A unique therapeutic option in H_1-receptor antagonist treatment. *J Allergy Clin Immunol*, **2003**, *112:*S29–S37.

Meszaros JG, Gonzalez AM, Endo-Mochizuki Y, et al. Identification of G protein–coupled pathways in cardiac fibroblasts: Cross-talk between G_q and G_s. *Am J Physiol*, **2000**, *278:*C154–C162.

Morrow JD, Margolies GR, Rowland J, Roberts LJ II. Evidence that histamine is the causative toxin of scombroid-fish poisoning. *N Engl J Med*, **1991**, *324:*716–720.

Mullol J, Bousquet J, Bachert C, et al. Rupatadine in allergic rhinitis and chronic urticaria. *Allergy,* **2008**, *63*(suppl): 5–28.

Nadel JA, Barnes PJ. Autonomic regulation of the airways. *Annu Rev Med*, **1984**, *35:*451–467.

Oda T, Morikawa N, Saito Y, et al. Molecular cloning and characterization of a novel type of histamine receptor preferentially expressed in leukocytes. *J Biol Chem*, **2000**, *275:* 36781–36786.

Ondetti MA, Williams NJ, Sabo EF, et al. Angiotensin-converting enzyme inhibitors from the venom of *Bothrops jararaca:* Isolation, elucidation of structure, and synthesis. *Biochemistry*, **1971**, *10:*4033–4039.

Paton DM, Webster DR. Clinical pharmacokinetics of H_1-receptor antagonists (the antihistamines). *Clin Pharmacokinet*, **1985,** *10:*477–497.

Pesquero JB, Bader M. Genetically altered animal models in the kallikrein-kinin system. *Biol Chem,* **2006**, *387:*119–126.

Pfeffer MA, Frohlich ED. Improvements in clinical outcomes with the use of angiotensin-converting enzyme inhibitors: Cross-fertilization between clinical and basic investigation. *Am J Physiol Heart Circ Physiol,* **2006**, *291:*H2021–H2025.

Regoli D, Barabe J. Pharmacology of bradykinin and related kinins. *Pharmacol Rev,* **1980**, *32*:1–46.

Richardson GS, Roehrs TA, Rosenthal L, et al. Tolerance to daytime sedative effects of H_1 antihistamines. *J Clin Psychopharmacol,* **2002**, *22*:511–515.

Rocha e Silva M, ed. *Histamine and Anti-Histaminics: Chemistry, Metabolism and Physiological and Pharmacological Actions.* In: *Handbook of Experimental Pharmacology*, Vol. 18, Pt. 2. Berlin, Springer-Verlag, **1978**.

Rocha e Silva M, Beraldo WT, Rosenfeld G. Bradykinin, a hypotensive and smooth muscle stimulating factor released from plasma globulin by snake venoms and by trypsin. *Am J Physiol*, **1949,** *156:*261–273.

Rothschild AM. Histamine release by basic compounds. In: Rocha e Silva M, ed. *Histamine and Anti-Histamines. Handbook of Experimental Pharmacology*, Vol 18. Berlin, Springer-Verlag, **1966**, pp. 386–430.

Saitoh S, Scicli AG, Peterson E, Carretero OA. Effect of inhibiting renal kallikrein on prostaglandin E_2, water, and sodium excretion. *Hypertension*, **1995**, *25:*1008–1013.

Sander K, Kottke T, Stark H. Histamine H3 receptor antagonists go to clinics. *Biol Pharm Bull,* **2008**, *31:*2163–2181.

Sangsree S, Brovkovych V, Minshall RD, Skidgel RA. Kininase I-type carboxypeptidases enhance nitric oxide production in endothelial cells by generating bradykinin B_1 receptor agonists. *Am J Physiol Heart Circ Physiol,* **2003**, *284:* H1959–H1968.

Schmaier AH. Assembly, activation, and physiologic influence of the plasma kallikrein/kinin system. *Int Immunopharmacol,* **2008**, *8*:161–165.

Schneider L, Lumry W, Vegh A, et al. Critical role of kallikrein in hereditary angioedema pathogenesis: A clinical trial of ecallantide, a novel kallikrein inhibitor. *J Allergy Clin Immunol,* **2007**, *120:*416–422.

Schwartz LB. Mast cells: Function and contents. *Curr Opin Immunol*, **1994**, *6:*91–97.

Sick E, Niederhoffer N, Takeda K, et al. Activation of CD47 receptors causes histamine secretion from mast cells. *Cell Mol Life Sci,* **2009**, *66:*1271–1282.

Siebenhaar F, Degener F, Zuberbier T, et al. High-dose desloratadine decreases wheal volume and improves cold provocation thresholds compared with standard-dose treatment in patients with acquired cold urticaria: A randomized, placebo-controlled, crossover study. *J Allergy Clin Immunol,* **2009**, *123:*672–679.

Silverberg M, Dunn JT, Garen L, Kaplan AP. Autoactivation of human Hageman factor. Demonstration utilizing a synthetic substrate. *J Biol Chem,* **1980**, *255:*7281–7286.

Simons SER. Antihistamines. In: Adkinson J, Franklin N, Younginger JW, et al., eds. *Middelton's Allergy: Principles and Practice*, 6th ed. Philadelphia, Mosby, **2003**, pp. 834–869.

Skidgel RA, Erdös EG. Enzymatic degradation of bradykinin. In: Said SI, ed. *Pro-inflammatory and Antiinflammatory Peptides*. New York, Marcel Dekker, **1998**, pp. 459–516.

Skidgel RA, Erdös EG. Structure and function of human plasma carboxypeptidase N, the anaphylatoxin inactivator. *Int Immunopharmacol,* **2007**, *7:*1888–1899.

Slater EE, Merrill DD, Guess HA, et al. Clinical profile of angioedema associated with angiotensin-converting enzyme inhibition. *JAMA*, **1988**, *260:*967–970.

Stewart JM. Bradykinin antagonists: Discovery and development. *Peptides,* **2004**, *25:*527–532.

Takada Y, Skidgel RA, Erdös EG. Purification of human urinary prokallikrein. Identification of the site of activation by the metalloproteinase thermolysin. *Biochem J,* **1985**, *232:*851–858.

Takagaki Y, Kitamura N, Nakanishi S. Cloning and sequence analysis of cDNAs for human high molecular weight and low molecular weight prekininogens: Primary structures of two human prekininogens. *J Biol Chem*, **1985**, *260:*8601–8609.

Thurmond RL, Gelfand EW, Dunford PJ. The role of histamine H1 and H4 receptors in allergic inflammation: The search for new antihistamines. *Nat Rev Drug Discov,* **2008**, *7:*41–53.

Waxler B, Rabito SF. Aprotinin: A serine protease inhibitor with therapeutic actions: Its interaction with ACE inhibitors. *Curr Pharm Des*, **2003**, *9:*777–787.

Werle E. Discovery of the most important kallikreins and kallikrein inhibitors. In: Erdös EG, ed. *Bradykinin, Kallidin and Kallikrein.* In: *Handbook of Experimental Pharmacology*, Vol. 25. Berlin, Springer-Verlag, **1970**, pp. 1–6.

Widdop RE, Jones ES, Hannan RE, Gaspari TA. Angiotensin AT_2 receptors: Cardiovascular hope or hype? *Br J Pharmacol*, **2003**, *140:*809–824.

Yang HYT, Erdös EG, Levin Y. A dipeptidyl carboxypeptidase that converts angiotensin I and inactivates bradykinin. *Biochim Biophys Acta*, **1970**, *214:*374–376.

Zhang X, Tan F, Zhang Y, Skidgel RA. Carboxypeptidase M and kinin B1 receptors interact to facilitate efficient B1 signaling from B2 agonists. *J Biol Chem,* **2008**, *283:*7994–8004.

Zhang Y, Brovkovych V, Brovkovych S, et al. Dynamic receptor-dependent activation of inducible nitric-oxide synthase by ERK-mediated phosphorylation of Ser745. *J Biol Chem,* **2007**, *282:*32453–32461.

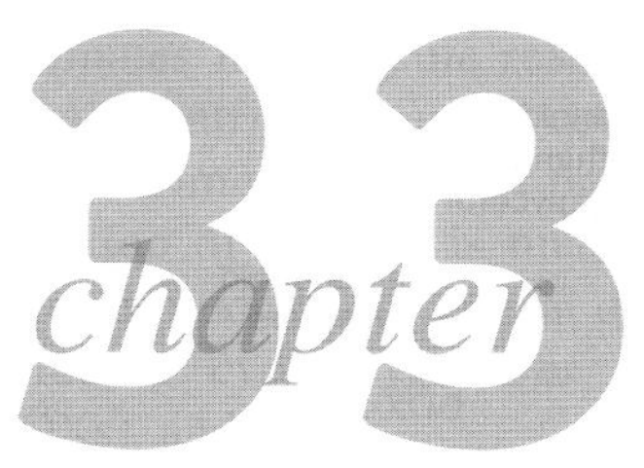

Lipid-Derived Autacoids: Eicosanoids and Platelet-Activating Factor

Emer M. Smyth, Tilo Grosser, and Garret A. FitzGerald

Membrane lipids supply the substrate for the synthesis of eicosanoids and platelet-activating factor (PAF). Eicosanoids—arachidonate metabolites, including prostaglandins (PGs), prostacyclin (PGI_2), thromboxane A_2 (TxA_2), *leukotrienes* (LTs), lipoxins, and hepoxilins—are not stored but are produced, by most cells, when a variety of physical, chemical, and hormonal stimuli activate acyl hydrolases that make arachidonate available. Membrane glycerophosphocholine derivatives can be modified enzymatically to produce PAF. PAF is formed by a smaller number of cell types, principally leukocytes, platelets, and endothelial cells. Eicosanoids and PAF lipids contribute to inflammation, smooth muscle tone, hemostasis, thrombosis, parturition, and gastrointestinal secretion. Several classes of drugs, most notably aspirin, the traditional non-steroidal anti-inflammatory agents (tNSAIDs), and the specific inhibitors of cyclooxygenase-2 (COX-2), such as the coxibs, owe their principal therapeutic effects to blockade of eicosanoid formation. To understand the therapeutic potential of selective inhibitors of eicosanoid synthesis and action, we must first review the synthesis, metabolism, and mechanism of action of eicosanoids and PAF.

EICOSANOIDS

History. In 1930, Kurzrok and Lieb, two American gynecologists, observed that strips of uterine myometrium relax or contract when exposed to semen. Subsequently, Goldblatt in England and von Euler in Sweden reported independently on smooth muscle-contracting and vasodepressor activities in seminal fluid and accessory reproductive glands. In 1935, von Euler identified the active material as a lipid-soluble acid, which he named *prostaglandin*, inferring its origin in the prostatic gland. Samuelsson, Bergström, and their colleagues elucidated the structures of prostaglandin E_1 (PGE_1) and prostaglandin $F_1\alpha$ ($PGF_1\alpha$) in 1962. In 1964, Bergström and coworkers, and van Dorp and associates, independently achieved biosynthesis of PGE_2 from arachidonic acid (AA). Discovery of TxA_2, PGI_2, and the LTs followed. Vane, Smith, and Willis reported that aspirin and NSAIDs act by inhibiting prostaglandin biosynthesis (Vane, 1971). This remarkable period of discovery linked the Nobel Prize of von Euler in 1970 to that of Bergström, Samuelsson, and Vane in 1982.

PGs, LTs, and related compounds are called *eicosanoids*, from the Greek *eikosi* ("twenty"). Precursor essential fatty acids contain 20 carbons and three, four, or five double bonds: 8,11,14-eicosatrienoic acid (dihomo-γ-linolenic acid), 5,8,11,14-eicosatetraenoic acid [AA; Figure 33–1], and 5,8,11,14,17-eicosapentaenoic acid (EPA). In humans, AA, the most abundant precursor, is either derived from dietary linoleic acid (9,12-octadecadienoic acid) or ingested directly as a dietary constituent. EPA is a major constituent of oils from fatty fish such as salmon.

Biosynthesis. Biosynthesis of eicosanoids is limited by the availability of substrate and depends primarily on the release of AA, esterified in the *sn*-2 domain of cell membrane phospholipids, or other complex lipids, to the eicosanoid-synthesizing enzymes by acyl hydrolases, most notably phospholipase A_2 (PLA_2). Chemical and physical stimuli activate the Ca^{2+}-dependent translocation of group IV_A cytosolic PLA_2 ($cPLA_2$), which has a high affinity for AA, to the membrane, where it hydrolyzes the *sn*-2 ester bond of membrane phospholipids (particularly phosphatidylcholine and phosphatidylethanolamine), releasing arachidonate. Multiple additional PLA_2 isoforms (secretory [s] and Ca^{2+}-independent [i] forms) have been characterized. Under nonstimulated conditions, AA liberated by $iPLA_2$ is reincorporated into cell membranes, so there is negligible eicosanoid biosynthesis. Although $cPLA_2$

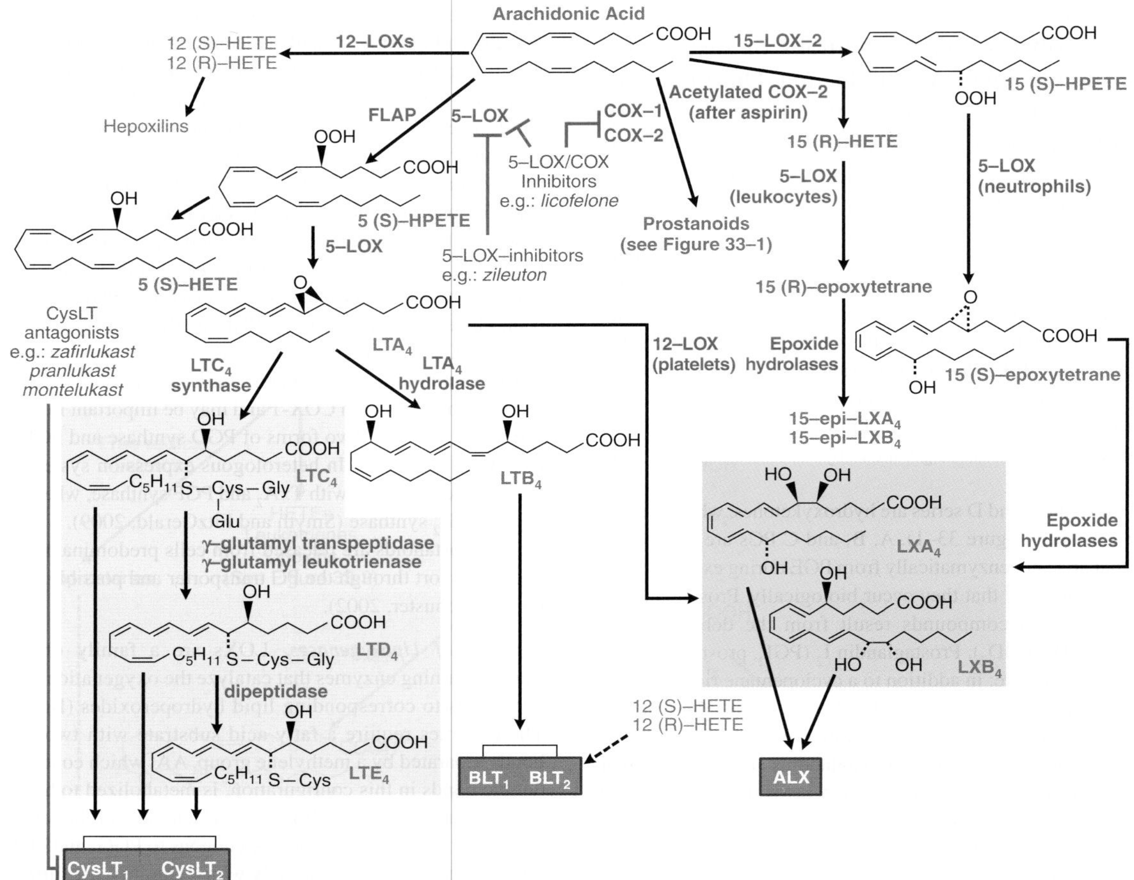

Figure 33–2. *Lipoxygenase pathways of arachidonic acid metabolism.* 5-LOX-activating protein (FLAP) presents arachidonic acid to 5-LOX, leading to the generation of the LTs. CysLTs are shaded in *gray*. Lipoxins (*shaded in orange*) are products of cellular interaction via a 5-LOX–12-LOX pathway or via a 15-LOX–5-LOX pathway. Biological effects are transduced via membrane-bound receptors (*blue boxes*). The *dashed line* indicates putative ligand–receptor interactions. Zileuton inhibits 5-LOX but not the COX pathways (expanded in Figure 33–1). Dual 5-LOX–COX inhibitors interfere with both pathways. CysLT antagonists prevent activation of the CysLT1 receptor. See the text for abbreviations.

dehydration of 5-HPETE to an unstable 5,6-epoxide known as LTA_4. LTA_4 is transformed into bioactive eicosanoids by multiple pathways depending on the cellular context: transformation by LTA_4 hydrolase to a 5,12-dihydroxyeicosatetraenoic acid known as *LTB_4*; conjugation with GSH by LTC_4 synthase, in eosinophils, monocytes, and mast cells, to form LTC_4; and extracellular metabolism of the peptide moiety of LTC_4, leading to the removal of glutamic acid and subsequent cleavage of glycine, to generate LTD_4 and LTE_4, respectively (Peters-Golden and Henderson, 2007). LTC_4, LTD_4, and LTE_4, the *cysteinyl leukotrienes* (CysLTs), were known originally as the *slow-reacting substance of anaphylaxis* (SRS-A), first described >60 years ago. LTB_4 and LTC_4 are actively transported out of the cell.

At least two isoforms of 15-LOX exists, 15-LOX-1 and 15-LOX-2. The former prefers linoleic acid as a substrate and forms 15(*S*)-hydroxyoctadecadienoic acid, whereas the latter uses AA to generate 15(*S*)-HETE. Platelet-type 12*(S)*-LOX generates 12(*S*)-HETE from AA, whereas the leukocyte isozyme can synthesize both 12- and 15-HETE and often is referred to as *12/15-LOX*. 12*(S)*-LOX can further metabolize LTA_4, the primary product of the 5-LOX pathway, to form the *lipoxins* LXA_4 and LXB_4. These mediators also can arise through 5-LOX metabolism of 15-HETE. 15(*R*)-HETE, derived from aspirin-acetylated COX-2, can be further transformed in leukocytes by 5-LOX to the *epilipoxins* 15-epi-LXA_4 or 15-epi-LXB_4, the so-called aspirin-triggered lipoxins (Brink et al., 2003). 12-HETE also can undergo a catalyzed molecular rearrangement to epoxyhydroxyeicosatrienoic acids called *hepoxilins*. Two additional groups of lipid mediators, the *resolvins* and *protectins*, may be generated from EPA and DHA, through the sequential action of aspirin-acetylated COX-2 and 5- or 15-LOX (Serhan et al., 2008).

The epidermal LOXs [12(*R*)-LOX, 15-LOX-2, and eLOX-3] are distinct from "conventional" enzymes in their substrate preferences and products (Furstenberger et al., 2007). Although the roles of epidermal LOXs in normal skin function are not clear, they may be relevant for skin barrier function and adipocyte differentiation. Epidermal accumulation of 12(*R*)-HETE is a feature of psoriasis and ichthyosis. Inhibitors of 12(*R*)-LOX are under investigation for the treatment of these proliferative skin disorders.

Products of CYPs. Multiple CYPs can metabolize AA (Capdevila and Falck, 2002). The epoxyeicosatrienoic acids (EETs), formed by CYP epoxygenases, primarily CYP2C and CYP2J in humans, have been a primary focus of research. Four regioisomers (14,15-; 11,12-; 8,9-; and 5,6-EETs), each containing a mixture of the (*R,S*) and (*S,R*) enantiomers, are formed in a CYP isoform–specific manner. EETs are synthesized in endothelial cells, where they function as endothelium-derived hyperpolarizing factors (EDHFs), particularly in the coronary circulation (Campbell and Falck, 2007). Their biosynthesis can be altered by pharmacological, nutritional, and genetic factors that affect CYP expression (see Chapter 6). CYP hydroxylases (primarily CYPs 4A, 4F) generate hydroxyeicosatetraenoic acids (16-, 17-, 18-, 19-, or 20-HETE), with 20-HETE being the principle product CYP-derived AA metabolite in vascular smooth muscle cells. 20-HETE is generated in response to smooth muscle cell stretch or to vasoactive agents, including angiotensin II (AngII).

EETs are metabolized by numerous pathways. The corresponding biologically less active (or inactive) dihydroxyeicosatrienoic acids (DHETs) are formed by epoxide hydrolases (EHs), whereas lysolipid acylation results in incorporation of EETs and DHETs into cellular phospholipids, where they can be stored. Inhibitors of EHs currently are under investigation. Glutathione conjugation and oxidation by COX and CYPs generate a series of glutathione conjugates, epoxyprostaglandins, diepoxides, tetrahydrofuran (THF) diols, and epoxyalcohols, whose biological relevance is not known. Similarly, 20-HETE can be converted by the COX pathway to the 20-hydroxy PGs. Intracellular fatty acid–binding proteins (FABPs) may bind EETs and DHETs differentially, thus modulating their metabolism, activities, and targeting.

Other Pathways. In addition to enzymatic formation of eicosanoids, several families of eicosanoid isomers are generated at significant concentrations *in vivo* by non-enzymatic free radical catalyzed oxidation of AA. The best characterized of these isoeicosanoids are the F_2-isoprostanes (F_2-IsoPs) (Lawson et al., 1999; Fam and Morrow, 2003; Milne et al., 2008). Unlike PGs, these compounds are initially formed esterified in phospholipids, after which they are hydrolyzed to their free form by phospholipases, including PAF acetylhydrolase (Stafforini et al., 2006), which then circulate and are metabolized and excreted into urine. Their production is not inhibited *in vivo* by inhibitors of COX-1 or COX-2, but their formation is suppressed by antioxidants. The $PGF_{2\alpha}$ isomer, 8-iso-$PGF_{2\alpha}$, was the first F_2-IsoP to be identified. Measuring levels of these compounds in plasma and urine is considered the most accurate method to assess oxidative stress status *in vivo*, and increased levels are found in a large number of clinical conditions. Isoprostanes correlate with cardiovascular risk factors, but their use as predictors of coronary events remains an area of active investigation. Of particular interest is the recent finding that levels of F_2-IsoPs predict 30-day outcome in acute coronary syndrome (LeLeiko et al., 2009).

In addition to F_2-IsoPs, other PG-like isomers, including D_2/E_2-IsoPs, isothromboxanes, and isolevuglandins (alternatively termed isoketals), are also formed *in vivo* by non-enzymatic oxidation of AA (Brame et al., 2004). Isoleukotrienes are also generated non-enzymatically. Because several isoprostanes can activate prostanoid receptors, it has been speculated that they may contribute to the pathophysiology of inflammatory responses in a manner insensitive to COX inhibitors.

In the brain, the endocannabinoids arachidonylethanolamide (anandamide) and 2-arachidonoylglycerol are endogenous ligands of cannabinoid receptors (Bisogno, 2008). They mimic several pharmacological effects of Δ9-tetrahydrocannabinol, the active principle of *Cannabis sativa* preparations such as hashish and marijuana, including inhibition of adenylyl cyclase, inhibition of L-type Ca^{2+} channels, analgesia, and hypothermia. Several pathways have been proposed, but the prevalent one for biosynthesis *in vivo* remains unclarified. Conversion of anandamide and 2-arachidonylglycerol by COX-2 generates PG-ethanolamides (prostamides) and PG-glyceryl esters (Woodward et al., 2008); their biological significance remains to be clarified.

Inhibitors of Eicosanoid Biosynthesis. A number of the biosynthetic steps just described can be inhibited by drugs. Inhibition of PLA_2 decreases the release of the precursor fatty acid and thus the synthesis of all its metabolites. Because PLA_2 is activated by Ca^{2+} and calmodulin, it may be inhibited by drugs that reduce the availability of Ca^{2+}. *Glucocorticoids* also inhibit PLA_2, but they appear to do so indirectly by inducing the synthesis of a group of proteins termed *annexins* (formerly *lipocortins*) that modulate PLA_2 activity (see Chapter 42). Glucocorticoids also downregulate induced expression of COX-2 but not of COX-1. Aspirin and tNSAIDs originally were found to prevent the synthesis of PGs from AA in tissue homogenates (Vane, 1971). It is now known that these drugs inhibit the COX, but not the POX, moieties of both PG G/H synthases, and thus the formation of their downstream prostanoid products. In addition, these drugs do not inhibit LOXs and may cause increased formation of LTs by shunting of substrate to the LOX pathway. LTs may contribute to the GI side effects associated with NSAIDs. Dual inhibitors of the COX and 5-LOX pathways, in particular *licofelone,* are under investigation (Kulkarni and Singh, 2007). However, the exact interplay between these enzyme families remains to be defined.

COX-1 and COX-2 differ in their sensitivity to inhibition by certain anti-inflammatory drugs (Grosser et al., 2006). This observation has led to the recent development of selective inhibitors of COX-2, including the coxibs (see Chapter 34). It was hypothesized that these drugs would have therapeutic advantages over tNSAIDs, many of which are non-selective for COX-1/2. COX-2 is the predominant COX at sites of inflammation, whereas COX-1 is the major source of cytoprotective PGs in the GI tract. Two randomized trials of selective COX-2 inhibitors reported their superiority in GI safety over tNSAID comparators. However, there now is compelling evidence that COX-2 inhibitors confer a spectrum of cardiovascular hazards comprised of myocardial infarction, stroke, systemic and pulmonary hypertension, congestive heart failure, and sudden cardiac death (Grosser et al., 2006). Mechanistically, this hazard can be explained by suppression of cardioprotective COX-2-derived PGs, especially PGI_2, a general restraint on endogenous stimuli—including platelet COX-1-derived TxA_2—for platelet activation, vascular proliferation and remodeling, hypertension, atherogenesis, and cardiac function.

Compounds that preferentially and selectively inhibit the downstream enzymes that metabolize PGH_2 have been considered for some time. For example, agents that inhibit TxA_2 synthase might block platelet aggregation and induce vasodilation. Indeed, such drugs block TxA_2 production *in vitro* and *in vivo;* however, they have been disappointing in clinical development, perhaps owing to activation of the TxA_2 receptor by accumulated PGH_2 precursor. Given the problems associated with COX-2 inhibitors, there has been intense interest in developing drugs that might conserve the efficacy of COX-2 selectivity while shedding the cardiovascular risk. Microsomal prostaglandin E synthase-1 (mPGES-1), which catalyzes the isomerization of the COX product-PGH_2 into PGE_2, has emerged as a drug target (Samuelsson et al., 2007). The differential cardiovascular impact of mPGES-1 versus COX-2 inhibition in humans currently is unknown. However, deletion of mPGES-1 does not accelerate the response to a thrombogenic stimulus *in vivo* in rodents, in contrast to either selective inhibition of COX-2 or deletion of the IP, the I prostanoid receptor for PGI_2 (Cheng et al., 2006b). Indeed, deletion of mPGES-1 depresses systemic production of PGE_2 and augments biosynthesis of PGI_2 by rediversion of the intermediate COX product PGH_2 to PGI synthase. It currently is unclear what contribution elevated PGI_2 makes to the impact on mPGES-1 inhibition and whether this shift in substrate will be seen with pharmacological inhibitors in humans.

Because LTs mediate inflammation, efforts have focused on development of LT-receptor antagonists and selective inhibitors of the LOXs. *Zileuton*, an inhibitor of 5-LOX, and selective CysLT-receptor antagonists (*zafirlukast, pranlukast*, and *montelukast*) have established efficacy in the treatment of mild to moderate asthma (see Chapter 36). These treatments remain, however, less effective than inhaled corticosteroids. A common polymorphism in the gene for LTC_4 synthase that correlates with increased LTC_4 generation is associated with aspirin-intolerant asthma and with the efficacy of anti-LT therapy (Kanaoka and Boyce, 2004). Interestingly, although polymorphisms in the genes encoding 5-LOX or FLAP do not appear to be linked to asthma, studies have demonstrated an association of these genes with myocardial infarction, stroke, and atherosclerosis (Peters-Golden and Henderson, 2007); thus, inhibition of LT biosynthesis may be useful in the prevention of cardiovascular disease.

Eicosanoid Catabolism. Most eicosanoids are efficiently and rapidly inactivated. About 95% of infused PGE_2 (but not PGI_2) is inactivated during one passage through the pulmonary circulation. Broadly speaking, the enzymatic catabolic reactions are of two types: a relatively rapid initial step, catalyzed by widely distributed PG-specific enzymes, wherein PGs lose most of their biological activity, and a second step in which these metabolites are oxidized, probably by enzymes identical to those responsible for the β and ω oxidation of fatty acids (Figure 33–3). The initial step is the oxidation of the 15-OH group to the corresponding ketone by PG 15-OH dehydrogenase (PGDH) (Tai et al., 2002). Two types of 15-PGDHs have been identified. Type I, an NAD^+-dependent enzyme, is the predominant form involved in eicosanoid catabolism. There is little circulating PGDH activity; thus, it is likely that metabolism first requires active transport to the intracellular space. The 15-keto compound then is reduced to the 13,14-dihydro derivative, a reaction catalyzed by PG Δ^{13}-reductase. This enzyme is identical to the LTB_4 12-hydroxydehydrogenase (see the discussion later). Subsequent steps consist of β and ω oxidation of the PG side chains, giving rise to polar dicarboxylic acids in the case of PGEs, which then are excreted in the urine as major metabolites (Figure 33–1); these reactions occur primarily in the liver.

Unlike PGE_2, PGD_2 initially is reduced *in vivo* to the F-ring PG, 9α11β-PGF_2, which possesses significant biological activity. Subsequently, this compound undergoes metabolism similar to that of other eicosanoids (Figure 33–3). TxA_2 breaks down non-enzymatically ($t_{1/2}$ = 30 seconds) into the chemically stable but biologically inactive thromboxane B_2 (TxB_2), which then is further metabolized by 11-hydroxy TxB_2 dehydrogenase to generate 11-dehydro-TxB_2 or by β oxidation to form 2,3-dinor-TxB_2 (Figure 33–3).

The degradation of PGI_2 ($t_{1/2}$ = 3 minutes) apparently begins with its spontaneous hydrolysis in blood to 6-keto-$PGF_{1\alpha}$. The metabolism of this compound in humans involves the same steps as those for PGE_2 and $PGF_{2\alpha}$.

The degradation of LTC_4 occurs in the lungs, kidney, and liver. The initial steps involve its conversion to LTE_4. LTC_4 also may be inactivated by oxidation of its cysteinyl sulfur to a sulfoxide. In leukocytes, LTB_4 is inactivated principally by oxidation by members of the CYP4F subfamily. Conversion to 12-oxo-LTB_4 by LTB 12-OH dehydrogenase (see the discussion earlier) is a key pathway in tissues other than leukocytes.

Pharmacological Properties of Eicosanoids

The eicosanoids show numerous and diverse effects in biological systems. This discussion highlights those that are thought to be the most important.

Mechanism of Action. The eicosanoids function through activation of specific cell surface receptors that couple to intracellular second-messenger systems to modulate cellular activity.

Prostaglandin Receptors. PGs activate membrane receptors locally near their sites of formation. The diversity of their effects is explained to a large extent by their interaction with a diverse family of distinct receptors (Table 33–1). Eicosanoid receptors interact with G_s, G_i, and G_q to modulate the activities of adenylyl cyclase and phospholipase C (see Chapter 3). Single gene products have been identified for the receptors for PGI_2 (the IP), $PGF_{2\alpha}$ (the FP), and TxA_2 (the TP). Four distinct PGE_2 receptors (EP_{1-4}) and two PGD_2 receptors (DP_1 and DP_2—also known as $CRTH_2$) have been cloned. Additional isoforms

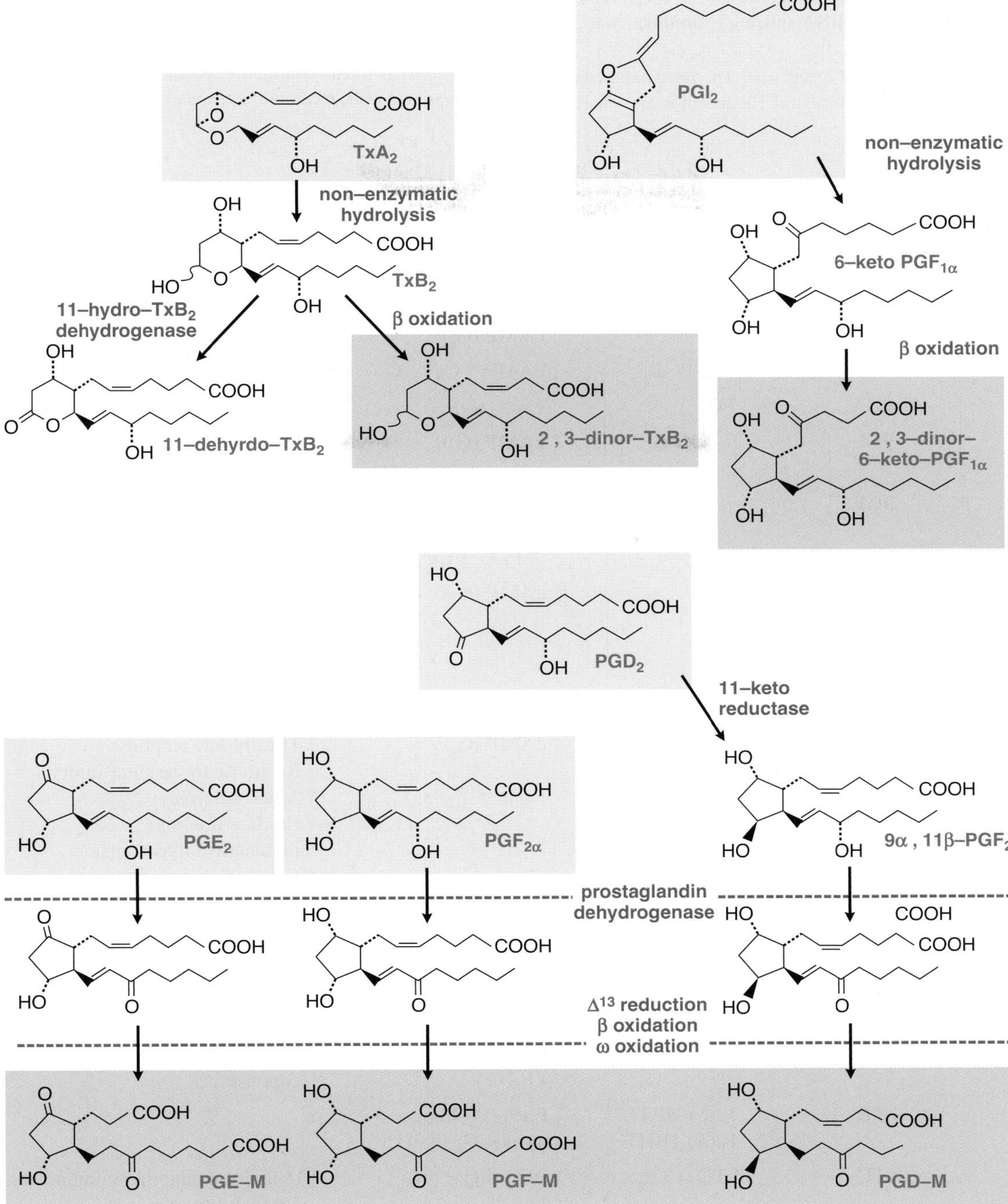

Figure 33–3. *Major pathways of prostanoid degradation.* Active metabolites are shaded in *gray*. Major urinary metabolites are shaded in *orange*. The *red dashed lines* indicate reactions that use common enzymatic processes. M, metabolite. See the text for other abbreviations.

of the TP (α and β), FP (A and B), and EP_3 (I-VI, e, f) receptors can arise through differential mRNA splicing (Narumiya et al., 1999; Smyth et al., 2009).

Cell Signaling Pathways and Expression. The prostanoid receptors appear to derive from an ancestral EP receptor and share high homology. Phylogenetic comparison of this family reveals three subclusters: The first consists of the relaxant receptors EP_2, EP_4, IP, and DP_1, which increase cellular cyclic AMP generation; the second consists of the contractile receptors EP_1, FP, and TP, which increase cytosolic levels of Ca^{2+}; and a third, consisting only of EP_3,

Table 33–1

Eicosanoid Receptors

RECEPTOR	PRIMARY LIGAND	SECONDARY LIGAND	PRIMARY COUPLING	MAJOR PHENOTYPE IN KNOCKOUT MICE
DP_1	PGD_2		↑ cAMP (G_s)	↓ Allergic asthma
DP_2/$CHRT_2$	PGD_2	15d-PGJ_2	↓ cAMP, ↑ Ca^{2+}_i (G_i)	↑ or ↓ Allergic airway inflammation
EP_1	PGE_2	PGI_2	↑ Ca^{2+}_i (G_q)	↓ Response of colon to carcinogens
EP_2	PGE_2		↑ cAMP (G_s)	Impaired ovulation and fertilization Salt-sensitive hypertension
EP_3 I-VI, e, f	PGE_2		↓ cAMP, ↑ Ca^{2+}_i (G_i); ↑ cAMP (G_s); ↑ PLC, ↑ Ca^{2+}_i (G_q)	Resistance to pyrogens ↓ Acute cutaneous inflammation
EP_4	PGE_2		↑ cAMP (G_s)	Patent ductus arteriosus ↓ Bone mass/density in aged mice ↑ Bowel inflammatory response ↓ Colon carcinogenesis
$FP_{A,B}$	$PGF_{2\alpha}$	IsoPs	↑ PLC, ↑ Ca^{2+}_i (G_q)	Failure of parturition
IP	PGI_2	PGE_2	↑ cAMP (G_s)	↑ Thrombotic response ↓ Response to vascular injury ↑ Atherosclerosis ↑ Cardiac fibrosis Salt-sensitive hypertension ↓ Joint inflammation
$TP_{\alpha,\beta}$	TxA_2	IsoPs	↑ PLC, ↑ Ca^{2+}_i (G_q, G_i, $G_{12/13}$, G_{16}); ↑ Rho, ↑ ERK activation (G_q, $G_{12/13}$, G_{16})	↑ Bleeding time ↓ Response to vascular injury ↓ Atherosclerosis ↑ Survival after cardiac allograft
BLT_1	LTB_4		↑ Ca^{2+}_i, ↓ cAMP (G_{16}, G_i)	Some suppression of inflammatory response
BLT_2	LTB_4	12(*S*)-HETE 12(*R*)-HETE	↑ Ca^{2+}_i (G_q-like, G_i-like, G_z-like)	?
$CysLT_1$	LTD_4	LTC_4/LTE_4	↑ PLC, ↑ Ca^{2+}_i (G_q)	↓ Innate and adaptive immune vascular permeability response ↑ Pulmonary inflammatory and fibrotic response
$CysLT_2$	LTC_4/LTD_4	LTE_4	↑ PLC, ↑ Ca^{2+}_i (G_q)	↓ Pulmonary inflammatory and fibrotic response

This table lists the major classes of eicosanoid receptors and their signaling characteristics. Splice variants for EP_3, TP, and FP are indicated. Major phenotypes in knockout mouse models are listed. Ca^{2+}_i, cytosolic Ca^{2+}; cAMP, cyclic AMP; PLC, phospholipase C (activation leads to increased cellular inositol phosphate and diacylglycerol generation and increased Ca^{2+}_i); IsoPs, isoprostanes; 15d-PGJ_2, 15-deoxy-$\Delta^{12,14}$-PGJ_2; DP_2 is a member of the fMLP-receptor superfamily; fMLP, formyl-methionyl-leucyl-phenylalanine. See the text for other abbreviations.

can couple to both elevation of intracellular calcium and a decrease in cyclic AMP. The DP_2 receptor is an exception and is unrelated to the other prostanoid receptors; rather, it is a member of the formyl-methionyl-leucyl-phenylalanine (fMLP)-receptor superfamily (Table 33–1).

TP_α and TP_β receptors couple via G_q and several other G proteins, to activate the PLC–IP_3–Ca^{2+} pathway (Figure 33–4). Activation of TP receptors also may activate or inhibit adenylyl cyclase via G_s (TP_α) or G_i (TP_β), respectively, and signal via G_q, $G_{12/13}$, and G_{16}, to stimulate small G protein–signaling pathways, including ERK and Rho. TP is expressed in platelets, vasculature, lung, kidney, heart, thymus, and spleen. The TP_α apparently is the sole isoform expressed in platelets (see Smyth and FitzGerald, 2009). Recognized differences between the splice variants are limited to G protein activation and receptor regulation in heterologous *in vitro* expression systems.

IP couples with G_s to stimulate adenylyl cyclase activity. It is expressed in many tissues and cells, including human kidney, lung, spine, liver, vasculature, and heart.

DP_1 also couples with adenylyl cyclase through G_s. It is the least abundant of the prostanoid receptors, with expression in mouse ileum, lung, stomach, and uterus. In humans, several subtypes of leukocytes express DP_1, including eosinophils, basophils, monocytes, dendritic cells, and T lymphocytes. DP_1 also is expressed in the central nervous system (CNS), where it appears to be limited specifically to the leptomeninges and the vasculature. DP_2 couples with the G_q–PLC–IP_3 pathway to increase intracellular Ca^{2+} (Figure 33-4). Its mRNA is found in many human tissues (brain, heart, thymus, spleen, liver, and intestine). DP_2 is expressed on mast cells, T lymphocytes (Th2 but not Th1), basophils, and eosinophils (Kim and Luster, 2007).

EP_2 and EP_4 receptors activate adenylate cyclase via G_s. The EP_2 receptor is expressed at much lower levels in most tissues and can be induced in response to inflammatory stimuli, suggesting distinct roles for these two G_s-coupled EP receptors. The EP_1 receptor, via an unclassified G protein, can activate the PLC–IP_3–Ca^{2+} pathway. All human EP_3 isoforms can activate G_i to inhibit adenylyl cyclase; however, certain isoforms can activate G_s or $G_{12/13}$. EP_1 and EP_2

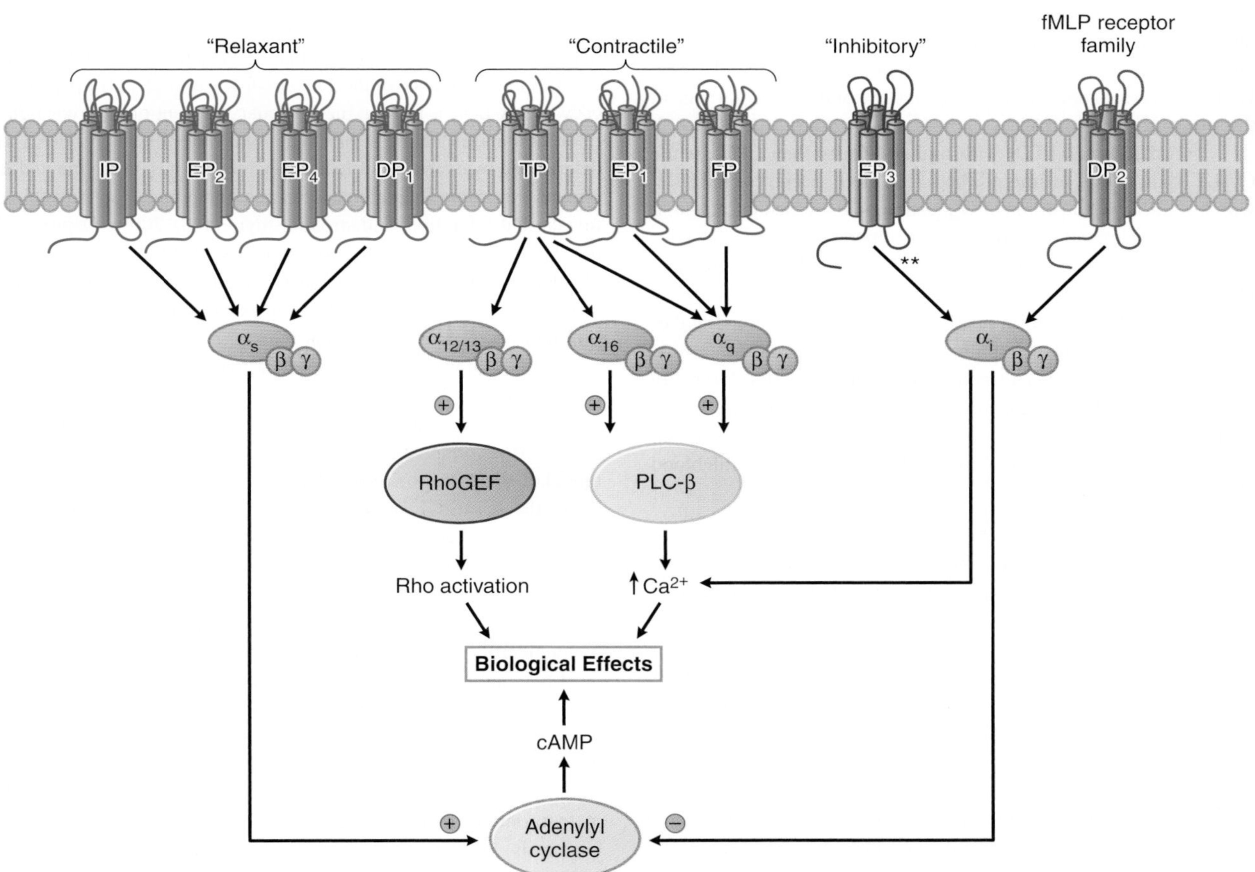

Figure 33–4. *Prostanoid receptors and their primary signaling pathways.* Prostanoid receptors are members of the heptaspanning, G protein–coupled receptor superfamily. The terms "relaxant," "contractile," and "inhibitory" refer to the phylogenetic characterization of their primary effects. **All EP_3 isoforms couple through G_i, but some can also activate G_s or $G_{12/13}$ pathways. See the text for additional details.

receptors have limited distribution compared with the distribution of EP_3 and EP_4 receptors.

FP_A and FP_B receptors couple via G_q–PLC–IP_3 to mobilize cellular Ca^{2+} and activate PKC. In addition, stimulation of FP activates Rho kinase, leading to the formation of actin stress fibers, phosphorylation of p125 focal adhesion kinase, and cell rounding. The FP receptor is expressed in kidney, heart, lung, stomach, and eye; it is most abundant in the corpus luteum, where its expression pattern varies during the estrus cycle.

Leukotriene and Lipoxin Receptors. Several receptors for the LTs and lipoxins have been identified (Peters-Golden and Henderson, 2007) (Table 33–1). Two receptors exist for both LTB_4 (BLT_1 and BLT_2) and the cysteinyl leukotrienes ($CysLT_1$ and $CysLT_2$). A receptor that binds lipoxin, ALX, is identical to the fMLP-1 receptor; the nomenclature now reflects LXA_4 as a natural and potent ligand (Chiang et al., 2006).

Cell Signaling Pathways and Expression. Phylogenetic comparison reveals two clusters of LT/lipoxin receptors: the chemoattractant receptors (BLT_1, BLT_2, and ALX), which also contain the DP_2 receptor for PGD_2, and the $CysLT_1$ and $CysLT_2$ receptors. All are G protein–coupled receptors (GPCRs) and couple with G_q and other G proteins (Table 33–1), depending on the cellular context. The BLT_1 is expressed predominantly in leukocytes, thymus, and spleen, whereas BLT_2, the low-affinity receptor for LTB_4, is found in spleen, leukocytes, ovary, liver, and intestine. BLT_2 binds 12(*S*)- and 12(*R*)-HETE with reasonable affinity, although the biological relevance of this observation is not clear.

$CysLT_1$ binds LTD_4 with higher affinity than LTC_4, while $CysLT_2$ shows equal affinity for both LTs. Both receptors bind LTE_4 with low affinity. Activation of G_q, leading to increased intracellular Ca^{2+}, is the primary signaling pathway reported. Studies also have placed G_i downstream of $CysLT_2$. $CysLT_1$ is expressed in lung and intestinal smooth muscle, spleen, and peripheral blood leukocytes, whereas $CysLT_2$ is found in heart, spleen, peripheral blood leukocytes, adrenal medulla, and brain.

Responses to ALX-receptor activation vary with cell type. In human neutrophils, AA release is stimulated, whereas Ca^{2+} mobilization is blocked; in monocytes, LXA_4 stimulates Ca^{2+} mobilization. The ALX receptor is expressed in lung, peripheral blood leukocytes, and spleen.

Other Agents. Other AA metabolites (e.g., isoprostanes, epoxyeicosatrienoic acids, hepoxilins) have potent biological activities, and there is evidence for distinct receptors for some of these substances. Some isoprostanes appear to act as incidental ligands at the TP (Audoly et al., 2000), which may be important in the pathology of cardiovascular disease. Others activate the FP (Kunapuli et al., 1997). Certain eicosanoids, most notably 15-deoxy-$\Delta^{12,14}$-PGJ_2 (15d-PGJ_2), a dehydration product of PGD_2, have been reported as endogenous ligands for a family of nuclear receptors called peroxisome proliferator–activated receptors (PPARs) that regulate lipid metabolism and cellular proliferation and differentiation. However, their affinities for PPARs are significantly lower than for cell surface receptors, raising doubt about the physiological relevance of the ligand–receptor interaction. *in vitro* 15d-PGJ_2 can bind PPARγ, but the quantities formed *in vivo* are orders of magnitude lower than those necessary for PPAR activation (Bell-Parikh et al., 2003). Specific receptors for the HETEs and EETs have been proposed but not yet isolated.

Endogenous Prostaglandins, Thromboxanes, and Leukotrienes: Functions in Physiological and Pathological Processes

The widespread biosynthesis and myriad of pharmacological actions of eicosanoids are reflected in their complex physiology and pathophysiology. The development of mice with targeted disruptions of genes regulating eicosanoid biosynthesis and eicosanoid receptors has revealed unexpected roles for these autacoids and has clarified hypotheses about their function (Austin and Funk, 1999; Narumiya and FitzGerald, 2001; Matsuoka and Narumiya, 2007; Smyth and FitzGerald, 2009).

Platelets. Platelet aggregation leads to activation of membrane phospholipases, with the release of AA and consequent eicosanoid biosynthesis. In human platelets, TxA_2 and 12-HETE are the two major eicosanoids formed, although eicosanoids from other sources (e.g., PGI_2 derived from vascular endothelium) also affect platelet function. A naturally occurring mutation in the first intracellular loop of the TP receptor is associated with a mild bleeding diathesis and resistance of platelet aggregability to TP agonists (Hirata et al., 1994). The importance of the TxA_2 pathway is evident from the efficacy of low-dose aspirin in the secondary prevention of myocardial infarction and ischemic stroke. The total biosynthesis of TxA_2, as determined by excretion of its urinary metabolites, is augmented in clinical syndromes of platelet activation, including unstable angina, myocardial infarction, and stroke (Smyth et al., 2009). Deletion of the TP receptor in the mouse prolongs bleeding time, renders platelets unresponsive to TP agonists, modifies their response to collagen but not to ADP, and blunts the response to vasopressors and the proliferative response to vascular injury.

PGI_2 inhibits platelet aggregation and disaggregates preformed clumps. Deficiency of the IP receptor in disease-free mice does not alter platelet aggregation significantly *ex vivo,* although increased responsiveness to thrombin was evident in a mouse model of atherosclerosis (Smyth and FitzGerald, 2009). Augmented biosynthesis of PGI_2 in syndromes of platelet activation serves to constrain the effects platelet agonists, vasoconstrictors, and stimuli to platelet activation. However, PGI_2 does limit platelet activation by TxA_2 *in vivo*, reducing the thrombotic response to vascular injury (Cheng et al., 2002). The increased incidence of myocardial infarction and stroke in patients receiving selective inhibitors of COX-2, most parsimoniously explained by inhibition of COX-2-dependent PGI_2 formation, supports this concept (Grosser et al., 2006b).

Low concentrations of PGE_2 activate the EP_3 receptor, leading to platelet aggregation (Fabre, 2001). Deletion of the EP_3 in mice leads to an increased bleeding tendency and decreased susceptibility to thromboembolism. Deletion of mPGES-1 did not affect thrombogenesis *in vivo,* probably due to substrate rediversion and augmented formation of PGI_2 (Cheng et al., 2006b).

Vascular Tone. Because of their short $t_{1/2}$, prostanoids do not circulate and generally are considered not to impact directly on systemic vascular tone. They may, however, modulate vascular tone locally at their sites of biosynthesis or through renal or other indirect effects. PGI_2, the major arachidonate metabolite released from the vascular endothelium, is derived primarily from COX-2 in humans (Catella-Lawson et al., 1999; McAdam et al., 1999). PGI_2 generation and release is regulated by shear stress and by both vasoconstrictor and vasodilator autacoids. Deletion of the IP in mice augments vascular proliferation, remodeling, atherogenesis, and hypertension, while PGI synthase polymorphisms have been associated with essential hypertension and myocardial infarction (Smyth and FitzGerald, 2009). PGI_2 limits pulmonary hypertension induced by hypoxia and systemic hypertension induced by AngII and lowers pulmonary resistance in patients with pulmonary hypertension.

Deficiency of EP_1 or EP_4 receptors reduces resting blood pressure in male mice; EP_1-receptor deficiency is associated with elevated renin–angiotensin activity. Both EP_2 and EP_4 receptor–deficient animals develop hypertension in response to a high-salt diet, reflecting the importance of PGE_2 in maintenance of renal blood flow and salt excretion. PGI_2 and PGE_2 are implicated in the hypotension associated with septic shock. PGs also may play a role in the maintenance of placental blood flow. Although conflicting data exist, it appears that loss of mPGES-1 in mice is less likely than loss of COX-2 to alter blood pressure (Smyth et al., 2009).

COX-2-derived PGE_2, via the EP_4 receptor, maintains the ductus arteriosus patent until birth, when reduced PGE_2 levels (a consequence of increased PGE_2 metabolism) permit closure. (Coggins et al., 2002). The tNSAIDs induce closure of a patent ductus in neonates (see Chapter 34). Contrary to expectation, animals lacking the EP_4 receptor die with a patent ductus during the perinatal period (Table 33–1) because the mechanism for control of the ductus *in utero*, and its remodeling at birth, is absent.

Endogenous biosynthesis of EETs is increased in human syndromes of hypertension. An analog of 11,12-EET abrogated the enhanced renal microvascular reactivity to AngII associated with hypertension (Imig et al., 2001), and blood pressure is lower in mice deficient in soluble EH (Sinal et al., 2000); these findings suggest that EH enzyme may be a potential pharmacological target for hypertension. Much indirect evidence suggests the existence of EET receptors, although none has been cloned.

Inflammatory Vascular Disease. Studies with knockout mice strongly implicate prostanoids in the development of atherogenesis and abdominal aortic aneurism; both inflammatory cardiovascular diseases (Smyth et al., 2009; Smyth and FitzGerald, 2009). Suppression of TxA_2 biosynthesis, as well as antagonism or deletion of the TP, retards atherogenesis in mice. Deletion of the FP receptor reduces blood pressure and retards atherogenesis, coincident with reduced renin. Conversely, PGI_2 appears atheroprotective and also limits vascular proliferative and remodeling responses. In humans, an arginine^{212} to cysteine substitution in the fifth intracellular loop of the IP, which disrupts IP signaling, co-segregated with increased cardiovascular risk in a recent study (Arehart et al., 2008), concordant with a role for this prostanoid in modifying human cardiovascular disease.

The role of PGE_2 effects on inflammatory cardiovascular disease is less clear. Deletion of mPGES-1 does not accelerate the response to a thrombogenic stimulus *in vivo* in rodents (in contrast to either selective inhibition of COX-2 or deletion of the IP (Cheng et al., 2006b) but does retard atherogenesis in fat-fed hyperlipidemic mice (Wang et al., 2006). It is unclear, however, whether this results from loss of PGE_2 or because of concomitant elevations in PGI_2 biosynthesis. Deletion, or selective inhibition, of COX-2, but not inhibition of COX-1, decreases abdominal aortic aneurism formation in hyperlipidemic mice (King et al., 2006). Similar results were seen in mPGES-1-deficient mice (Wang et al., 2008), although, again, it is unclear to what extent rediversion to biosynthesis of other prostanoids (e.g., PGI_2) contributes.

There is growing evidence for a role of the LTs in cardiovascular disease (Peters-Golden and Henderson, 2007). Although conflicting data have been reported in animal studies, human genetic studies have demonstrated a link between cardiovascular disease and polymorphisms in the LT biosynthetic enzymes and FLAP.

Lung. A complex mixture of autacoids is released when sensitized lung tissue is challenged by the appropriate antigen. COX-derived bronchodilator (PGE_2) and bronchoconstrictor (e.g., $PGF_{2\alpha}$, TxA_2, PGD_2) substances are released. IP deletion in mice exaggerates features of acute and chronic experimental asthma, including increased bronchial hyperresponsiveness. Inhaled iloprost (a PGI_2 analog) suppresses the cardinal features of asthma in mice via inhibition of airway dendritic cell function.

Polymorphisms in the genes for PGD_2 synthase and the TP receptor have been associated with asthma in humans. Deletion of either DP_1 or DP_2 in mice suggests an important role of this prostanoid in asthma (and in other allergic responses), although contradictory findings in DP_2-deficient mice suggest significant complexity in the function of PGD_2 in airway inflammation (Pettipher et al., 2007).

The CysLTs probably dominate during allergic constriction of the airway (Drazen, 1999). Deficiency of 5-LOX leads to reduced influx of eosinophils in airways and attenuates bronchoconstriction. Furthermore, unlike COX inhibitors and histaminergic antagonists, CysLT-receptor antagonists and 5-LOX inhibitors are effective in the treatment of human asthma (see "Inhibitors of Eicosanoid Biosynthesis"). The relatively slow LT metabolism in lung contributes to the long-lasting bronchoconstriction that follows challenge with antigen and may be a factor in the high bronchial tone that is observed in asthmatic patients in periods between acute attacks (see Chapter 36).

Kidney. Long-term use of all COX inhibitors is limited by the development of hypertension, edema, and congestive heart failure in a significant number of patients. PGE_2, along with PGI_2, apparently derived from COX-2, plays a critical role in maintaining renal blood flow and salt excretion, whereas there is some evidence that the COX-1-derived vasoconstrictor TxA_2 may play a counterbalancing role. Biosynthesis of PGE_2 and PGI_2 is increased by factors that reduce renal blood flow (e.g., stimulation of sympathetic nerves; AngII).

Bartter's syndrome is an autosomal recessive trait that is manifested as hypokalemic metabolic alkalosis. The syndrome results from inappropriate renal salt absorption caused primarily by dysfunctional mutations in the Na^+–K^+–$2Cl^-$ co-transporter NKCC2, a target of loop diuretics in the ascending thick limb of the loop of Henle (Simon et al., 1996) (see Chapter 25). The syndrome also can result from dysfunctional alterations in proteins whose activities can limit NKCC2 function: the K^+ channel ROMK2 (Kir1.1) that recycles K^+ into the tubular fluid; the basolateral membrane Cl^- channel, ClC–Kb; and Barttin, the integral membrane protein that forms the α-subunit of the ClC–Kb heteromer (O'Shaughnessy and Karet, 2004). The antenatal variant of Bartter's syndrome, owing to dysfunctional ROMK2, also is known as *hyperprostaglandin E syndrome*. The elevated PGE_2 may exacerbate the symptoms of salt and water loss. The relationship between dysfunctional ROMK2 and elevated PGE_2 synthesis is not clear. However, in patients with antenatal Bartter's syndrome, inhibition of COX-2 ameliorates many of the clinical symptoms (Nüsing et al., 2001).

Inflammatory and Immune Responses. PGs and LTs are synthesized in response to a host of stimuli that elicit inflammatory and immune responses, and contribute significantly to inflammation and immunity (Tilley et al., 2001; Brink et al., 2003; Kim and Luster, 2007). Prostanoids generally promote acute inflammation, although there are some exceptions, such as the inhibitory actions of PGE_2 on mast cell activation (see "Inflammation and Immunity"). Data from animals deficient in either COX-1 or COX-2 yield conflicting results depending on the inflammatory model used, perhaps reflecting the contribution of both isozymes to inflammation. Deletion of mPGES markedly reduced inflammation in several mouse models.

LTs are potent mediators of inflammation. Deletion of either 5-LOX or FLAP reduces inflammatory responses. Generation of BLT_1-deficient mice confirms the role of LTB_4 in chemotaxis, adhesion, and recruitment of leukocytes to inflamed tissues (Toda et al., 2002). Increased vascular permeability resulting from innate and adaptive immune challenges is offset in mice deficient in $CysLT_1$ or LTC_4 synthase (Kanaoka and Boyce, 2004) (Table 33–1). Deletion either of LTC_4 synthase (and thus loss of CysLT biosynthesis) or $CysLT_2$ reduced chronic pulmonary inflammation and fibrosis in response to bleomycin. In contrast, absence of $CysLT_1$ led to an exaggerated response. These findings demonstrate a role for $CysLT_2$ in promoting, and an unexpected role for $CysLT_1$ in counteracting, chronic inflammation.

Heart. Studies suggest a role for COX-2 in cardiac function (Smyth et al., 2009). PGI_2 and PGE_2, acting on the IP or the EP_3, respectively (Dowd et al., 2001; Shinmura et al., 2005), protect against oxidative injury in cardiac tissue. IP deletion augments myocardial ischemia/reperfusion injury and both mPGES-1 deletion (Degousee et al., 2008) and cardiomyocyte specific deletion of the EP_4 (Qian et al., 2008) exacerbate the decline in cardiac function after experimental myocardial infarction. COX-2-derived TxA_2 contributed to oxidant stress, isoprostane generation, and activation of the TP, and also possibly the FP, to increase cardiomyocyte apoptosis and fibrosis in a model of heart failure (Zhang et al., 2003). Selective deletion of COX-2 in cardiomyocytes results in mild heart failure and a predisposition to arrhythmogenesis.

Reproduction and Parturition. Studies with knockout mice confirm a role for PGs in reproduction and parturition (Smyth and FitzGerald, 2009). COX-1-derived $PGF_{2\alpha}$ appears important for luteolysis, consistent with delayed parturition in mice deficient in COX-1. Subsequent upregulation of COX-2 generates prostanoids, including $PGF_{2\alpha}$ and TxA_2, that are important in the final stages of parturition. Mice lacking both COX-1 and oxytocin undergo normal parturition, demonstrating the critical interplay between $PGF_{2\alpha}$ and oxytocin in onset of labor. EP_2 receptor–deficient mice demonstrate a preimplantation defect (Table 33–1), which likely underlies some of the breeding difficulties seen in COX-2 knockouts.

Cancer. Pharmacological inhibition or genetic deletion of COX-2 restrains tumor formation in models of colon, breast, lung, and other cancers. Large human epidemiological studies report that the incidental use of NSAIDs is associated with significant reductions in relative risk for developing these and other cancers (Harris et al., 2005). PGE_2 has been implicated as the primary pro-oncogenic prostanoid in multiple studies. The pro- and anti-oncogenic roles of other prostanoids remain under investigation, with TxA_2 emerging as another likely COX-2-derived pro-carcinogenic mediator. Studies in mice lacking EP_1, EP_2, and EP_4 reduce disease in multiple carcinogenesis models. EP_3, in contrast, may even play a protective role in some cancers. Three randomized controlled trials of COX-2 inhibitors reported a significant reduction in the reoccurrence of adenomas in patients receiving either celecoxib or rofecoxib compared to placebo (Bertagnolli, 2007), while polymorphisms in COX-2 have been associated with an increased risk of colon and other cancers. In mouse mammary tissue, COX-2 is pro-oncogenic (Liu et al., 2001), whereas aspirin use is associated with a reduced risk of breast cancer in women, especially for hormone receptor–positive tumors (Terry et al., 2004). Despite the emphasis on COX-2, studies support a role for both COX enzymes in pro-oncogenic processes, and it remains untested whether selective COX-2 inhibitors will prove superior to nonselective NSAIDs for the prevention or treatment of human cancer. The CysLT and LTB_4 receptors also are implicated in cancer, raising interest in the use of LT inhibitors/antagonists in chemoprevention/therapy.

Pharmacological Effects

Cardiovascular System. Prostanoids do not circulate and thus do not directly impact systemic vascular tone. They may, however, modulate local vascular tone at the site of their formation and affect systemic blood pressure through their renal actions, including changes of tone of the efferent arteriole. In most vascular beds, PGE_2, PGI_2, and PGD_2 elicit vasodilation and a drop in blood pressure (Smyth and FitzGerald, 2009). PGE_2 can cause vasoconstriction through activation of the EP_1 and EP_3. Infusion of PGD_2 in humans results in flushing, nasal stuffiness, and hypotension. Local subcutaneous release of PGD_2 contributes to dilation of the vasculature in the skin, which causes facial flushing associated with niacin treatment in humans (Cheng et al., 2006a). Subsequent formation of F-ring metabolites from PGD_2 may result in hypertension. PGI_2 relaxes vascular smooth muscle, causing hypotension and reflex tachycardia on intravenous administration. Responses to $PGF_{2\alpha}$ vary with species and vascular bed; it is a potent constrictor of both pulmonary arteries and veins in humans. Blood pressure is increased by $PGF_{2\alpha}$ in some experimental animals, owing to venoconstriction; however, in humans, $PGF_{2\alpha}$ does not alter blood pressure. TxA_2 is a potent vasoconstrictor. It contracts vascular smooth muscle *in vitro* and is a vasoconstrictor in the whole animal and in isolated vascular beds.

Cardiac output generally is increased by infusion of PGs of the E and F series. Weak, direct inotropic effects have been noted in various isolated preparations. In the intact animal, however, increased force of contraction and increased heart rate are, in large measure, a reflex consequence of a fall in total peripheral resistance. Animal studies suggest direct cardioprotective effects of PGI_2 and PGE_2 (Smyth et al., 2009).

LTC_4 and LTD_4 can constrict or relax isolated vascular smooth muscle preparations, depending on the concentrations used and the vascular bed (Brink et al., 2003). Hypotension in humans may result partly from a decrease in intravascular volume and also from decreased cardiac contractility secondary to a marked LT-induced reduction in coronary blood flow. Although LTC_4 and LTD_4 have little effect on most large arteries or veins, coronary arteries and distal segments of the pulmonary artery are contracted by nanomolar concentrations of these agents. The renal vasculature is resistant to this constrictor action, but the mesenteric vasculature is not. LTC_4 and LTD_4 act in the microvasculature to increase permeability of postcapillary venules; they are approximately 1,000-fold more potent than histamine in this regard. At higher concentrations, LTC_4 and LTD_4 can constrict arterioles and reduce exudation of plasma. Vascular smooth muscle proliferation can be promoted by 12S-HETE and 20-HETE.

EETs cause vasodilation in a number of vascular beds by activating the large conductance Ca^{2+}-activated K^+ channels of smooth muscle cells, thereby hyperpolarizing the smooth muscle and causing relaxation. EETs likely also function as endothelium-derived hyperpolarizing factors (EDHFs), particularly in the coronary circulation (Campbell and Falck, 2007). In contrast to EETs, 20-HETE inhibits large conductance Ca^{2+}-activated K^+ channels, resulting in depolarization of the vascular smooth muscle cell, Ca^{2+} entry, and potent vasoconstriction (Kroetz and Xu, 2005). Evidence supports the role of 20-HETE in the regulation of vascular tone, particularly in renal autoregulation.

Isoprostanes usually are vasoconstrictors, although there are examples of vasodilation in preconstricted vessels.

Platelets. Low concentrations of PGE_2, via the EP_3, enhance platelet aggregation. In contrast, higher concentrations of PGE_2, acting via the IP or possibly the G_s-coupled EP_2 or EP_4, inhibit platelet aggregation (Smyth et al., 2009). Both PGI_2 and PGD_2 inhibit the aggregation of human platelets *in vitro*, through cyclic AMP–dependent deactivation of myosin light-chain kinase.

Mature platelets express only COX-1. Megakaryocytes and immature platelet forms, released in clinical conditions of accelerated platelet turnover, also express COX-2 (Rocca et al., 2002), but its role in platelet development and function has yet to be elucidated. TxA_2, the major product of COX-1 in platelets, induces platelet shape change, through G_{12}/G_{13}-mediated Rho/Rho-kinase-dependent regulation of myosin light-chain phosphorylation, and aggregation through G_q-dependent activation of PKC. Perhaps more importantly, TxA_2 amplifies the signal for other, more potent platelet agonists, such as thrombin and ADP (FitzGerald, 1991). The actions of TxA_2 on platelets are restrained by its short $t_{1/2}$ (~30 seconds), by rapid TP desensitization, and by endogenous inhibitors of platelet function, including NO and PGI_2, which inhibits platelet aggregation by all recognized agonists. The biological importance of 12-HETE formation is poorly understood, although deletion of the platelet 12-LOX augments ADP-induced platelet aggregation and AA-induced sudden death in mice. Some isoprostanes increase the response of platelets to pro-aggregatory agonists *in vitro*.

Inflammation and Immunity. Eicosanoids play a major role in the inflammatory and immune responses, as reflected by the clinical usefulness of the NSAIDs. While LTs generally are pro-inflammatory and lipoxins anti-inflammatory, prostanoids can exert both kinds of activity. A more complete description of inflammation is outlined in Chapter 34.

COX-2 is the major source of prostanoids formed during and after an inflammatory response, although COX-1 also contributes. PGE_2 and PGI_2 are the predominant pro-inflammatory prostanoids, as a result of increased vascular permeability and blood flow in the inflamed region. TxA_2 can increase platelet–leukocyte interaction. Prostanoids, especially PGD_2, also contribute to resolution of inflammation. PGs generally inhibit lymphocyte function and proliferation, suppressing the immune response (Rocca et al., 2002). PGE_2 depresses the humoral antibody response by inhibiting the differentiation of B lymphocytes into antibody-secreting plasma cells. PGE_2 acts on T lymphocytes to inhibit mitogen-stimulated proliferation and lymphokine release by sensitized cells. PGE_2 and TxA_2 also may play a role in T lymphocyte development by regulating apoptosis of immature thymocytes (Tilley et al., 2001). PGD_2, a major product of mast cells, is a potent leukocyte chemoattractant (Pettipher et al., 2007), primarily through the DP_2. Activation of the DP_2 promotes chemotaxis and activation of T_H2 lymphocytes, eosinophils, and basophils. The PGD_2 degradation product, 15d-PGJ_2, also may activate eosinophils via the DP_2. PDG_2-mediated polarization of T cells to the T_H2 phenotype is DP_1-mediated. A counterregulatory role for DP_1 in leukocyte activation has been proposed, although complementary functions for the two receptors have been reported. The precise interplay between DP_1 and DP_2 *in vivo* remains to be clarified.

LTB_4 is a potent activator and chemotactic agent for neutrophils, T lymphocytes, eosinophils, monocytes, dendritic cells, and possibly also mast cells (Kim and Luster, 2007). These effects are primarily BLT_1 receptor-mediated and, although BLT_2 expression has been reported in eosinophils, mast cells, and dendritic cells, its contribution to LBT_4 function is unclear. LTB_4 stimulates the aggregation of eosinophils and promotes degranulation and the generation of superoxide. LTB_4 promotes adhesion of neutrophils to vascular endothelial cells and their transendothelial migration and stimulates synthesis of pro-inflammatory cytokines from macrophages and lymphocytes. Mast cell–generated LTB_4 also may contribute significantly to T lymphocyte migration.

The CysLTs are chemotaxins for eosinophils and monocytes through activation of the $CysLT_1$ receptor. They also induce cytokine generation in eosinophils, mast cells, and dendritic cells. A distinct set of cytokines are produced through activation of mast cell $CysLT_1$ and $CysLT_2$. At higher concentrations, these LTs also promote eosinophil adherence, degranulation, cytokine or chemokine release, and oxygen radical formation. In addition, CysLTs contribute to inflammation by increasing endothelial permeability, thus promoting migration of inflammatory cells to the site of inflammation.

Lipoxins have diverse effects on leukocytes, including activation of monocytes and macrophages and inhibition of neutrophil, eosinophil, and lymphocyte activation (McMahon and Godson, 2004). Both lipoxin A and B inhibit natural killer cell cytotoxicity.

Smooth Muscle. PGs also contract or relax smooth muscles in tissues outside the vasculature. The LTs contract most smooth muscles.

Bronchial and Tracheal Muscle. In general, TxA_2, $PGF_{2\alpha}$, and PGD_2 contract, and PGE_2 and PGI_2 relax, bronchial and tracheal muscle. PGD_2 appear to be the primary bronchoconstrictor prostanoid of relevance in humans. Roughly 10% of people given aspirin or tNSAIDs develop bronchospasm. This appears attributable to a shift in AA metabolism to LT formation, as reflected by an increase in urinary LTE_4 in response to aspirin challenge in such individuals. This substrate diversion appears to involve COX-1; such patients do not develop bronchospasm when treated with selective inhibitors of COX-2. The CysLTs are bronchoconstrictors in many species, including humans (Brink et al., 2003). These LTs act principally on smooth muscle in the airways and are a thousand times more potent than histamine both *in vitro* and *in vivo*. They also stimulate bronchial mucus secretion and cause mucosal edema.

PGI_2 causes bronchodilation in most species; human bronchial tissue is particularly sensitive, and PGI_2 antagonizes bronchoconstriction induced by other agents.

Uterus. Strips of nonpregnant human uterus are contracted by $PGF_{2\alpha}$ and TxA_2 but are relaxed by PGEs. Sensitivity to the contractile response is most prominent before menstruation, whereas relaxation is greatest at midcycle. Uterine strips obtained at hysterectomy from pregnant women are contracted by $PGF_{2\alpha}$ and by low concentrations of PGE_2. PGE_2, together with oxytocin, is essential for the onset of parturition. PGI_2 and high concentrations of PGE_2 produce relaxation. The intravenous infusion of PGE_2 or $PGF_{2\alpha}$ to pregnant women produces a dose-dependent increase in uterine tone and in the frequency and intensity of rhythmic uterine contractions. PGEs and PGFs are used to terminate pregnancy. Uterine responsiveness to PGs increases as pregnancy progresses but remains smaller than the response to oxytocin.

Gastrointestinal Muscle. PGEs and PGFs stimulate contraction of the main longitudinal muscle from stomach to colon. PG endoperoxides, TxA_2, and PGI_2 also produce contraction but are less active. Circular muscle generally relaxes in response to PGE_2 and contracts in response to $PGF_{2\alpha}$. The LTs have potent contractile effects. PGs reduce transit time in the small intestine and colon. Diarrhea, cramps, and reflux of bile have been noted in response to oral PGE; these are common side effects (along with nausea and vomiting) in patients given PGs for abortion. PGEs and PGFs stimulate the movement of water and electrolytes into the intestinal lumen. Such effects may underlie the watery diarrhea that follows their oral or parenteral administration. By contrast, PGI_2 does not induce diarrhea; indeed, it prevents that provoked by other PGs.

PGE_2 appears to contribute to the water and electrolyte loss in cholera, a disease that is somewhat responsive to therapy with tNSAIDs.

Gastric and Intestinal Secretions. In the stomach, PGE_2 and PGI_2 contribute to increased mucus secretion (*cytoprotection*), reduced acid secretion, and reduced pepsin content. These effects result from their vasodilatory properties and probable direct effects on secretory cells. PGE_2 and its analogs also inhibit gastric damage caused by a variety of ulcerogenic agents and promote healing of duodenal and gastric ulcers (see Chapter 45). Although COX-1 may be the dominant source of such cytoprotective PGs under physiological conditions, COX-2 predominates during ulcer healing. Selective inhibitors of COX-2 and deletion of the enzyme delay ulcer healing in rodents, but the impact of COX-2 inhibitors in humans is unclear. CysLTs, by constricting gastric blood vessels and enhancing production of pro-inflammatory cytokines, may contribute to the gastric damage.

Kidney. Renal prostanoids, especially PGE_2 and PGI_2, but also $PGF_{2\alpha}$ and TxA_2, perform complex and intricate functions in the kidney (Hao and Breyer, 2007). Both the renal medulla and cortex synthesize prostanoids, although substantially more are generated in the medulla. COX-2-derived PGE_2 and PGI_2 increase medullary blood flow and inhibit tubular sodium reabsorption. Expression of medullary COX-2 is increased during high salt intake. COX-1-derived products promote salt excretion in the collecting ducts. Cortical COX-2-derived PGE_2 and PGI_2 increase renal blood flow and glomerular filtration through their local vasodilating effects, actions that may be particularly relevant to maintaining renal function in marginally functioning kidneys and volume-contracted states. An added layer of complexity is evident from the increased expression of cortical COX-2 expression during low dietary salt intake. Through the action of PGE_2, and also possibly PGI_2, this results in increased renin release, leading to sodium retention and elevated blood pressure.

TxA_2, generated at low levels in the normal kidney, has potent vasoconstrictor effects that reduce renal blood flow and glomerular filtration rate. Infusion of $PGF_{2\alpha}$ causes both natriuresis and diuresis. Conversely, $PGF_{2\alpha}$ may activate the renin–angiotensin system, contributing to elevated blood pressure.

There is substantial evidence for a role of the CYP epoxygenase products in regulating renal function, although their exact role in the human kidney remains unclear. Both 20-HETE and the EETs are generated in renal tissue. 20-HETE constricts the renal arteries, while EETs mediate vasodilation and natriuresis.

Eye. Although $PGF_{2\alpha}$ induces constriction of the iris sphincter muscle, its overall effect in the eye is to decrease intraocular pressure (IOP) by increasing the aqueous humor outflow of the eye via the uveoscleral and trabecular meshwork pathway. A variety of FP receptor agonists have proven effective in the treatment of open-angle glaucoma, a condition associated with the loss of COX-2 expression in the pigmented epithelium of the ciliary body (see Chapter 64).

CNS. Although effects have been reported following injection of several PGs into discrete brain areas, the best established biologically active mediators are PGE_2 and PGD_2. The induction of fever by a range of endogenous and exogenous pyrogens appears to be mediated by PGE_2 (Smyth and FitzGerald, 2009). The hypothalamus regulates the body temperature set point, which is elevated by endogenous pyrogens such as interleukin (IL)-1β, IL-6, tumor necrosis factor-α (TNF-α), and interferons. The initial phase of the thermoregulatory response to pyrogens is thought to be mediated by ceramide release in neurons of the preoptic area in the anterior hypothalamus, while the late response is mediated by coordinate induction of COX-2 and mPGES-1 in the endothelium of blood vessels in the preoptic hypothalamic area to form PGE_2. PGE_2 can cross the blood-brain barrier and acts on EP_3, and perhaps EP_1, on thermosensitive neurons. This triggers the hypothalamus to elevate body temperature by promoting an increase in heat generation and a decrease in heat loss. Exogenous $PGF_{2\alpha}$ and PGI_2 induce fever but do not contribute to the pyretic response. PGD_2 and TxA_2 do not induce fever. PGD_2 also appears to act on arachnoid trabecular cells in the basal forebrain to mediate an increase in extracellular adenosine that, in turn, facilitates induction of sleep.

COX-2-derived prostanoids also have been implicated in several CNS degenerative disorders (e.g, Alzheimer's disease, Parkinson disease; see Chapter 22), although the therapeutic efficacy of blocking their synthesis or action remains to be established.

Pain. Inflammatory mediators, including LTs and PGs, increase the sensitivity of nociceptors and potentiate pain perception. Both PGE_2, through the EP_1 and EP_4, and PGI_2, via the IP, reduce the threshold to stimulation of nociceptors, causing "peripheral sensitization". Centrally, both COX-1 and COX-2 are expressed in the spinal cord under basal conditions and release PGs in response to peripheral pain stimuli. PGE_2, and perhaps also PGD_2, PGI_2, and $PGF_{2\alpha}$, can increase excitability in pain transmission neuronal pathways in the spinal cord, causing hyperalgesia and allodynia. Hyperalgesia also is produced by LTB_4. The release of these eicosanoids during the inflammatory process thus serves as an amplification system for the pain mechanism. The role of PGE_2 and PGI_2 in inflammatory pain is discussed in more detail in Chapter 34.

Endocrine System. A number of endocrine tissues respond to PGs. In several species, the systemic administration of PGE_2 increases circulating concentrations of adrenocorticotropic hormone (ACTH), growth hormone, prolactin, and gonadotropins. Other effects include stimulation of steroid production by the adrenals, stimulation of insulin release, and thyrotropin-like effects on the thyroid. The critical role of $PGF_{2\alpha}$ in parturition relies on its ability to induce an oxytocin-dependent decline in progesterone levels. PGE_2 works as part of a positive-feedback loop to induce oocyte maturation required for fertilization during and after ovulation.

LOX metabolites also have endocrine effects. 12-HETE stimulates the release of aldosterone from the adrenal cortex and mediates a portion of the aldosterone release stimulated by AngII, but not that which occurs in response to ACTH.

Bone. PGs are strong modulators of bone metabolism. COX-1 is expressed in normal bone, while COX-2 is upregulated in certain settings, such as inflammation and during mechanical stress. PGE_2 stimulates bone formation by increasing osteoblastogenesis. Bone resorption also is mediated via PGE_2, through activation of osteoclasts.

Therapeutic Uses

Inhibitors and Antagonists. As a consequence of the important and diverse physiological roles of eicosanoids, mimicking their effects with stable agonists, inhibiting eicosanoid formation, and antagonizing eicosanoid receptors produce therapeutically useful responses. As outlined earlier in "Inhibitors of Eicosanoid Biosynthesis" and in Chapter 34, the nonselective tNSAIDs, and those with selective COX-2 inhibition, are used widely as anti-inflammatory drugs, whereas low-dose aspirin is employed frequently for cardioprotection. LT antagonists are useful clinically in the treatment of asthma, and FP agonists are used in the treatment of open-angle glaucoma (Chapter 64). EP agonists are used to induce labor and to ameliorate gastric irritation owing to tNSAIDs.

There are as of yet no potent selective antagonists of prostanoid receptors in clinical use. TP antagonists were abandoned as antiplatelet agents when it seemed like they would confer nothing superior to aspirin. Now that the clinical implications of suppressing PGI_2 are recognized, the partial suppression by even low doses of aspirin may confer an advantage on TP antagonists, as may blockade of receptor activation by unconventional ligands such as oxidized lipids. DP_1 antagonists may be useful in offsetting the facial flushing associated with niacin. Orally active antagonists of LTC_4 and D_4, which block the $CysLT_1$ receptor, are used in the treatment of mild to moderately severe asthma (see Chapter 36). Their effectiveness in patients with aspirin-induced asthma also has been shown.

The use of eicosanoids or eicosanoid derivatives themselves as therapeutic agents is limited in part because systemic administration of prostanoids frequently is associated with significant adverse effects and because of their short $t_{1/2}$ in the circulation. Despite these limitations, however, several prostanoids are of clinical utility in the following situations.

Therapeutic Abortion. The ability of PGEs, PGFs, and their analogs, to terminate pregnancy at any stage by promoting uterine contractions has been adapted to common clinical use. When given early in pregnancy, their action as abortifacients may be variable and often incomplete and accompanied by adverse effects. PGs appear, however, to be of value in missed abortion and molar gestation, and they have been used widely for the induction of midtrimester abortion. Dinoprostone, a synthetic preparation of PGE_2, is approved for inducing abortion in the second trimester of pregnancy, for missed abortion, for cervical ripening prior to induction of labor, and for managing benign hydatidiform moles. Several studies have shown that systemic or intravaginal administration of the PGE_1 analog misoprostol in combination with mifepristone (RU486) or methotrexate is highly effective in the termination of early pregnancy. An analog of $PGF_{2\alpha}$, carboprost tromethamine, is used to induce second-trimester abortions and to control postpartum hemorrhage that is not responding to conventional methods.

PGE_2 or $PGF_{2\alpha}$ can induce labor at term. However, they may have more value when used to facilitate labor by promoting ripening and dilation of the cervix.

Gastric Cytoprotection. The capacity of several PG analogs to suppress gastric ulceration is a property of therapeutic importance. Misoprostol (CYTOTEC), a PGE_1 analog, is approved for prevention of NSAID-induced gastric ulcers. It is about as effective as the proton pump inhibitor omeprazole (Chapter 45).

Impotence. PGE_1 (alprostadil), given as an intracavernous injection (CAVERJECT, EDEX) or urethral suppository (MUSE) is a second-line treatment of erectile dysfunction. The erection lasts for 1-3 hours and is sufficient for sexual intercourse. PGE_1 has been superseded largely by the use of phosphodiesterase 5 (PDE5) inhibitors, such as sildenafil, tadalafil, and vardenafil (see Chapters 27 and 28).

Maintenance of Patent Ductus Arteriosus. The ductus arteriosus in neonates is highly sensitive to vasodilation by PGE_1. Maintenance of a patent ductus may be important hemodynamically in some neonates with congenital heart disease. PGE_1 (alprostadil, PROSTIN VR PEDIATRIC) is highly effective for palliative, but not definitive, therapy to maintain temporary patency until surgery can be performed. Apnea is observed in ~10% of neonates treated, particularly those who weigh <2 kg at birth.

Pulmonary Hypertension. Primary pulmonary hypertension is a rare idiopathic disease that mainly affects young adults. It leads to right-sided heart failure and frequently is fatal. Long-term therapy with PGI_2 (prostacyclin; epoprostenol, FLOLAN), via continuous intravenous infusion, improves symptoms and can delay or preclude the need for lung or heart-lung transplantation in a number of patients. Epoprostenol also has been used successfully to treat portopulmonary hypertension that arises secondary to liver disease, again with a goal of facilitating ultimate transplantation (Krowka et al., 1999). Several PGI_2 analogs with longer $t_{1/2}$ have been developed and used clinically. Iloprost can be inhaled (VENTAVIS) or delivered by intravenous administration (not available in the U.S.). Treprostinil (REMODULN) ($t_{1/2}$ ~4 hours) may be delivered by continuous subcutaneous or intravenous infusion.

Glaucoma. Latanoprost, a stable, long-acting $PGF_{2\alpha}$ derivative, was the first prostanoid used for glaucoma. The success of latanoprost has stimulated development of similar prostanoids with ocular hypotensive effects, and bimatoprost and travoprost are now available. These drugs act as agonists at the FP receptor and are administered as ophthalmic drops (Chapter 64).

PLATELET-ACTIVATING FACTOR

History. In 1971, Henson demonstrated that a soluble factor released from leukocytes caused platelets to aggregate. Benveniste and his coworkers characterized the factor as a polar lipid and named it *platelet-activating factor*. During this period, Muirhead described an antihypertensive polar renal lipid (APRL) produced by interstitial cells of the renal medulla that proved to be identical to PAF. Hanahan and coworkers then synthesized acetyl glyceryl ether phosphorylcholine (AGEPC) and determined that this phospholipid had chemical and biological properties identical to those of PAF. Independent determination of the structures of PAF and APRL showed them to be structurally identical to AGEPC. The commonly accepted name for this substance is platelet-activating factor; however, its actions extend far beyond platelets.

Chemistry and Biosynthesis. PAF is 1-*O*-alkyl-2-acetyl-*sn*-glycero-3-phosphocholine.

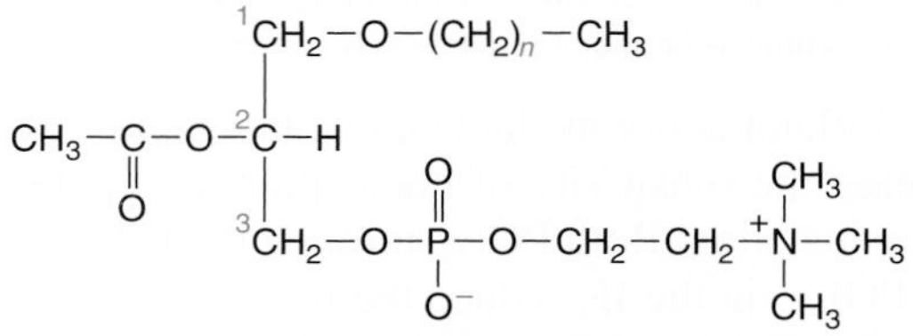

$$
\begin{array}{l}
{}^{1}CH_2{-}O{-}(CH_2)_n{-}CH_3 \\
CH_3{-}\underset{\|}{\overset{}{C}}{-}O{-}{}^{2}C{-}H \quad (C{=}O) \\
{}^{3}CH_2{-}O{-}P(=O)(O^-){-}O{-}CH_2{-}CH_2{-}\overset{+}{N}(CH_3)_3
\end{array}
$$

PLATELET-ACTIVATING FACTOR (n = 11 to 17)

PAF contains a long-chain alkyl group joined to the glycerol backbone in an ether linkage at position 1 and an acetyl group at position 2. PAF actually represents a family of phospholipids because the alkyl group at position 1 can vary in length from 12-18 carbon atoms. In human neutrophils, PAF consists predominantly of a mixture of the 16- and 18-carbon ethers, but its composition may change when cells are stimulated. The family is expanded by unregulated oxidative production to PAF-like lipids whose mode of action is analogous to PAF (Stafforini et al., 2003).

Analogous to the eicosanoids, PAF is not stored in cells but is synthesized in response to stimulation. The major pathway, termed the remodeling pathway, of PAF generation involves the precursor 1-*O*-alkyl-2-acyl-glycerophosphocholine, a lipid found in high concentrations in the membranes of many types of cells. The 2-acyl substituents include AA. PAF is synthesized from this substrate in two steps (Figure 33–5). The first involves the action of PLA_2, the initiating enzyme for eicosanoid biosynthesis, with the formation of 1-*O*-alkyl-2-lyso-glycerophosphocholine (lyso-PAF) and a free fatty acid (usually AA) (Prescott et al., 2000; Honda et al., 2002; Stafforini et al., 2003). Eicosanoid and PAF biosynthesis thus is closely coupled, and deletion of $cPLA_2$ in mice leads to an almost complete loss of both eicosanoid and PAF generation. The second, rate-limiting step is performed by the acetyl-coenzyme-A-lyso-PAF acetyltransferase. PAF synthesis also can occur *de novo*; a phosphocholine substituent is transferred to alkyl acetyl glycerol by a distinct lyso-glycerophosphate acetyl-coenzyme-A transferase. This pathway may contribute to physiological levels of PAF for normal cellular functions. The synthesis of PAF may be stimulated during antigen–antibody reactions or by a variety of agents, including chemotactic peptides, thrombin, collagen, and other autacoids; PAF also can stimulate its own formation. Both the phospholipase and acetyltransferase are Ca^{2+}-dependent enzymes; thus, PAF synthesis is regulated by the availability of Ca^{2+}.

The inactivation of PAF is catalyzed by PAF acetylhydrolyases (PAF-AHs) (McIntyre et al., 2009) (Figure 33–5). This is a family of four related Ca^{2+}-independent phospholipases A_2 that show marked specificity for phospholipids with short acyl chains at the *sn*-2 position. Two PAF-AHs, which are group VII enzymes, are commonly known as plasma PAF-AH (or lipoprotein-associated PLA_2) and liver type II PAF-AH. The remaining two are known as type I and II intracellular PAF-AH. PAF is inactivated by PAF-AH-catalyzed hydrolysis of the acetyl group, generating Lyso-PAF, which is then converted to a 1-*O*-alkyl-2-acyl-glycerophosphocholine by an acyltransferase.

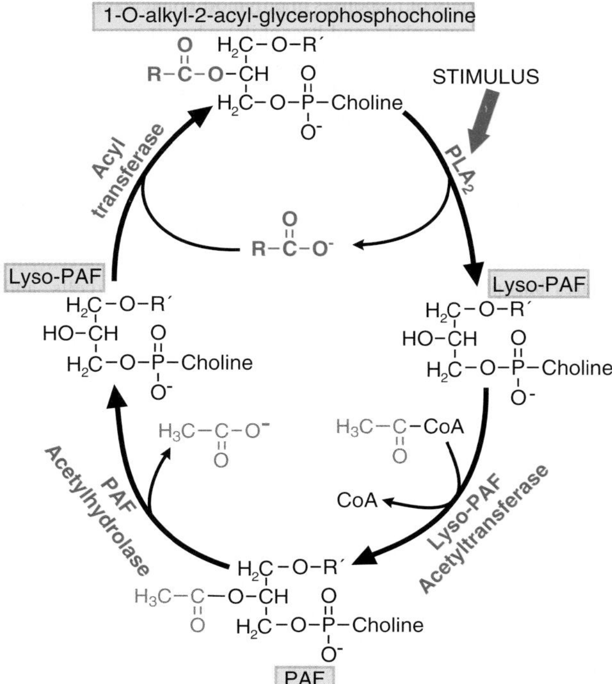

Figure 33–5. *Synthesis and degradation of platelet-activating factor (PAF).* $RCOO^-$ is a mixture of fatty acids but is enriched in arachidonic acid that may be metabolized to eicosanoids. CoA, coenzyme A.

PAF is synthesized by platelets, neutrophils, monocytes, mast cells, eosinophils, renal mesangial cells, renal medullary cells, and vascular endothelial cells. Depending on cell type, PAF can either remain cell associated or be secreted. For example, PAF is released from monocytes but retained by leukocytes and endothelial cells. In endothelial cells, PAF is displayed on the surface for juxtacrine signaling and stimulates adherent leukocytes (Honda et al., 2002).

In addition to these enzymatic routes, PAF-like molecules can be formed from the oxidative fragmentation of membrane phospholipids (oxPLs) (Stafforini et al., 2003). These compounds are increased in settings of oxidant stress, such as cigarette smoking, and differ structurally from PAF in that they contain a fatty acid at the *sn*-1 position of glycerol joined through an ester bond and various short-chain acyl groups at the *sn*-2 position. oxPLs mimic the structure of PAF closely enough to bind to its receptor (see "Mechanism of Action of PAF") and elicit the same responses. Unlike the synthesis of PAF, which is highly controlled, oxPL production is unregulated; degradation by PAF-AH, therefore, is necessary to suppress the toxicity of oxPLs. Levels of plasma PAF-AH are increased in colon cancer, cardiovascular disease, and stroke (Prescott et al., 2002), and polymorphisms have been associated with altered risk of cardiovascular events (Ninio et al., 2004). A common missense mutation in Japanese people is associated disproportionately with more severe asthma.

Mechanism of Action of PAF. Extracellular PAF exerts its actions by stimulating a specific GPCR (Honda et al., 2002). The PAF receptor's strict recognition requirements, including a specific head group and specific atypical *sn*-2 residue, also are met by oxPLs. The PAF receptor couples to activation of the PLC-IP_3–Ca^{2+} pathway and to inhibition of adenylyl cyclase, via G_q and G_i respectively. Activation of phospholipases A_2, C, and D give rise to second messengers. These include AA-derived PGs, TxA_2, or LTs, which may function as extracellular mediators of the effects of PAF. In addition, p38 MAP kinase is activated downstream of PAF-receptor coupling to G_q, while ERK activation can occur through a number of pathways, including coupling to G_q, G_o, or $G_{\beta\gamma}$ or via transactivation of the epidermal growth factor receptor, leading to NF-κB activation (Stafforini et al., 2003). Thus, the PAF receptor couples to a variety of downstream signaling cascades in a cell-dependent manner.

PAF exerts many of its important pro-inflammatory actions without leaving its cell of origin. For example, PAF is synthesized in a regulated fashion by endothelial cells stimulated by inflammatory mediators. This PAF is presented on the surface of the endothelium, where it activates the PAF receptor on juxtaposed cells, including platelets, polymorphonuclear leukocytes, and monocytes, and acts cooperatively with P selectin to promote adhesion (Prescott et al., 2000). This function of PAF is important for orchestrating the interaction of platelets and circulating inflammatory cells with the inflamed endothelium.

FitzGerald GA. Mechanisms of platelet activation: Thromboxane A2 as an amplifying signal for other agonists. *Am J Cardiol,* **1991,** *68*:11B–15B.

FitzGerald GA, Loll P. COX in a crystal ball: Current status and future promise of prostaglandin research. *J Clin Invest,* **2001,** *107*:1335–1337.

Furstenberger G, Epp N, Eckl KM, et al. Role of epidermis-type lipoxygenases for skin barrier function and adipocyte differentiation. *Prostaglandins Other Lipid Mediat,* **2007,** *82*:128–134.

Grosser T, Fries S, Fitzgerald GA. Biological basis for the cardiovascular consequences of COX-2 inhibition: Therapeutic challenges and opportunities. *J Clin Invest,* **2006,** *116*:4–15.

Hao CM, Breyer MD. Physiologic and pathophysiologic roles of lipid mediators in the kidney. *Kidney Int,* **2007,** *71*:1105–1115.

Harris RE, Beebe-Donk J, Doss H, Burr Doss D. Aspirin, ibuprofen, and other non-steroidal anti-inflammatory drugs in cancer prevention: A critical review of non-selective COX-2 blockade (review). *Oncol Rep,* **2005,** *13*:559–583.

Hirata T, Kakizuka A, Ushikubi F, et al. Arg60 to Leu mutation of the human thromboxane A2 receptor in a dominantly inherited bleeding disorder. *J Clin Invest,* **1994,** *94*:1662–1667.

Honda Z, Ishii S, Shimizu T. Platelet-activating factor receptor. *J Biochem,* **2002,** *131*:773–779.

Imig JD, Zhao X, Falck JR, et al. Enhanced renal microvascular reactivity to angiotensin II in hypertension is ameliorated by the sulfonimide analog of 11,12-epoxyeicosatrienoic acid. *J Hypertens,* **2001,** *19*:983–992.

Ishii S, Nagase T, Shimizu T. Platelet-activating factor receptor. *Prostaglandins Other Lipid Mediat,* **2002,** *68–69*:599–609.

Ishii S, Shimizu T. Platelet-activating factor (PAF) receptor and genetically engineered PAF receptor mutant mice. *Prog Lipid Res,* **2000,** *39*:41–82.

Kanaoka Y, Boyce JA. Cysteinyl leukotrienes and their receptors: Cellular distribution and function in immune and inflammatory responses. *J Immunol,* **2004,** *173*:1503–1510.

Kim N, Luster AD. Regulation of immune cells by eicosanoid receptors. *ScientificWorldJournal,* **2007,** *7*:1307–1328.

King VL, Trivedi DB, Gitlin JM, et al. Selective cyclooxygenase-2 inhibition with celecoxib decreases angiotensin II-induced abdominal aortic aneurysm formation in mice. *Arterioscler Thromb Vasc Biol,* **2006,** *26*:1137–1143.

Kroetz DL, Xu F. Regulation and inhibition of arachidonic acid omega-hydroxylases and 20-HETE formation. *Annu Rev Pharmacol Toxicol,* **2005,** *45*:413–438.

Krowka MJ, Frantz RP, McGoon MD, et al. Improvement in pulmonary hemodynamics during intravenous epoprostenol (prostacyclin): A study of 15 patients with moderate to severe portopulmonary hypertension. *Hepatology,* **1999,** *30*:641–648.

Kulkarni SK, Singh VP. Licofelone—A novel analgesic and anti-inflammatory agent. *Curr Top Med Chem,* **2007,** *7*:251–263.

Kunapuli P, Lawson JA, Rokach J, et al. Functional characterization of the ocular prostaglandin f2alpha (PGF2alpha) receptor. Activation by the isoprostane, 12-iso-PGF2alpha. *J Biol Chem,* **1997,** *272*:27147–27154.

Lawson JA, Rokach J, FitzGerald GA. Isoprostanes: Formation, analysis and use as indices of lipid peroxidation in vivo. *J Biol Chem,* **1999,** *274*:24441–24444.

LeLeiko RM, Vaccari CS, Sola S, et al. Usefulness of elevations in serum choline and free F(2)-isoprostane to predict 30-day cardiovascular outcomes in patients with acute coronary syndrome. *Am J Cardiol,* **2009,** *104*:638–643.

Liu CH, Chang SH, Narko K, et al. Overexpression of cyclooxygenase-2 is sufficient to induce tumorigenesis in transgenic mice. *J Biol Chem,* **2001,** *276*:18563–18569.

Lopez-Novoa JM. Potential role of platelet activating factor in acute renal failure. *Kidney Int,* **1999,** *55*:1672–1682.

Matsuoka T, Narumiya S. Prostaglandin receptor signaling in disease. *ScientificWorldJournal,* **2007,** *7*:1329–1347.

McAdam BF, Catella-Lawson F, Mardini IA, et al. Systemic biosynthesis of prostacyclin by cyclooxygenase (COX)-2: The human pharmacology of a selective inhibitor of COX-2. *Proc Natl Acad Sci U S A,* **1999,** *96*:272–277.

McIntyre TM, Prescott SM, Stafforini DM. The emerging roles of PAF acetylhydrolase. *J Lipid Res,* **2009,** *50*(suppl): S255–S259.

McMahon B, Godson C. Lipoxins: Endogenous regulators of inflammation. *Am J Physiol Renal Physiol,* **2004,** *286*:F189–F201.

Milne GL, Yin H, Morrow JD. Human biochemistry of the isoprostane pathway. *J Biol Chem,* **2008,** *283*:15533–15537.

Narumiya S, FitzGerald GA. Genetic and pharmacological analysis of prostanoid receptor function. *J Clin Invest,* **2001,** *108*:25–30.

Ninio E, Tregouet D, Carrier JL, et al. Platelet-activating factor-acetylhydrolase and PAF-receptor gene haplotypes in relation to future cardiovascular event in patients with coronary artery disease. *Hum Mol Genet,* **2004,** *13*:1341–1351.

Nüsing RM, Reinalter SC, Peters M, et al. Pathogenetic role of cyclooxygenase-2 in hyperprostaglandin E syndrome/antenatal Bartter syndrome: Therapeutic use of the cyclooxygenase-2 inhibitor nimesulide. *Clin Pharmacol Ther,* **2001,** *70*:384–390.

O'Shaughnessy KM, Karet FE. Salt handling and hypertension. *J Clin Invest,* **2004,** *113*:1075–1081.

Peters-Golden M, Henderson WR Jr. Leukotrienes. *N Engl J Med,* **2007,** *357*:1841–1854.

Pettipher R, Hansel TT, Armer R. Antagonism of the prostaglandin D2 receptors DP1 and CRTH2 as an approach to treat allergic diseases. *Nat Rev Drug Discov,* **2007,** *6*:313–325.

Prescott SM, McIntyre TM, Zimmerman GA, et al. Sol Sherry lecture in thrombosis: Molecular events in acute inflammation. *Arterioscler Thromb Vasc Biol,* **2002,** *22*:727–733.

Prescott SM, Zimmerman GA, Stafforini DM, et al. Platelet-activating factor and related lipid mediators. *Annu Rev Biochem,* **2000,** *69*:419–445.

Qian JY, Harding P, Liu Y, et al. Reduced cardiac remodeling and function in cardiac-specific EP4 receptor knockout mice with myocardial infarction. *Hypertension,* **2008,** *51*: 560–566.

Rocca B, Secchiero P, Ciabattoni G, et al. Cyclooxygenase-2 expression is induced during human megakaryopoiesis and characterizes newly formed platelets. *Proc Natl Acad Sci U S A,* **2002,** *99*:7634–7639.

Salomon RG, Subbanagounder G, O'Neil J, et al. Levuglandin E2-protein adducts in human plasma and vasculature. *Chem Res Toxicol,* **1997**, *10*:536–545.

Samuelsson B, Morgenstern R, Jakobsson PJ. Membrane prostaglandin E synthase-1: A novel therapeutic target. *Pharmacol Rev,* **2007,** *59*:207–224.

Schuster VL. Prostaglandin transport. *Prostaglandins Other Lipid Mediat,* **2002,** *68–69*:633–647.

Serhan CN, Chiang N, Van Dyke TE. Resolving inflammation: Dual anti-inflammatory and pro-resolution lipid mediators. *Nat Rev Immunol,* **2008,** *8*:349–361.

Shinmura K, Tamaki K, Sato T, et al. Prostacyclin attenuates oxidative damage of myocytes by opening mitochondrial ATP-sensitive K+ channels via the EP3 receptor. *Am J Physiol Heart Circ Physiol,* **2005,** *288*:H2093–H2101.

Simon DB, Karet FE, Hamdan JM, et al. Bartter's syndrome, hypokalaemic alkalosis with hypercalciuria, is caused by mutations in the Na-K-2Cl cotransporter NKCC2. *Nat Genet,* **1996,** *13*:183–188.

Sinal CJ, Miyata M, Tohkin M, et al. Targeted disruption of soluble epoxide hydrolase reveals a role in blood pressure regulation. *J Biol Chem,* **2000,** *275*:40504–40510.

Smith WL, DeWitt DL, Garavito RM. Cyclooxygenases: Structural, cellular, and molecular biology. *Annu Rev Biochem,* **2000,** *69*:145–182.

Smith WL, Langenbach R. Why there are two cyclooxygenase isozymes. *J Clin Invest,* **2001,** *107*:1491–1495.

Smyth EM, FitzGerald GA. Prostaglandin mediators. In: Bradshaw RA, Dennis EA, eds. *Handbook of Cell Signaling*. Elsevier, **2009.**

Smyth EM, Grosser T, Wang M, et al. Prostanoids in health and disease. *J Lipid Res,* **2009,** *50*(suppl):S423–S428.

Stafforini DM. Biology of platelet-activating factor acetylhydrolase (PAF-AH, lipoprotein associated phospholipase A2). *Cardiovasc Drugs Ther,* **2009,** *23*:73–83.

Stafforini DM, McIntyre TM, Zimmerman GA, et al. Platelet-activating factor, a pleiotrophic mediator of physiological and pathological processes. *Crit Rev Clin Lab Sci,* **2003,** *40*: 643–672.

Stafforini DM, Sheller JR, Blackwell TS, et al. Release of free F2-isoprostanes from esterified phospholipids is catalyzed by intracellular and plasma platelet-activating factor acetylhydrolases. *J Biol Chem,* **2006,** *281*:4616–4623.

Tai HH, Ensor CM, Tong M, et al. Prostaglandin catabolizing enzymes. *Prostaglandins Other Lipid Mediat,* **2002,** *68–69*: 483–493.

Terry MB, Gammon MD, Zhang FF, et al. Association of frequency and duration of aspirin use and hormone receptor status with breast cancer risk. *JAMA,* **2004,** *291*:2433–2440.

Tilley SL, Coffman TM, Koller BH. Mixed messages: Modulation of inflammation and immune responses by prostaglandins and thromboxanes. *J Clin Invest,* **2001,** *108*:15–23.

Toda A, Yokomizo T, Shimizu T. Leukotriene B4 receptors. *Prostaglandins Other Lipid Mediat,* **2002,** *68–69*:575–585.

Vane JR. Inhibition of prostaglandin synthesis as a mechanism of action for aspirin-like drugs. *Nat New Biol,* **1971,** *231*: 232–235.

Wang M, Lee E, Song W, et al. Microsomal prostaglandin E synthase-1 deletion suppresses oxidative stress and angiotensin II-induced abdominal aortic aneurysm formation. *Circulation,* **2008,** *117*:1302–1309.

Wang M, Zukas AM, Hui Y, et al. Deletion of microsomal prostaglandin E synthase-1 augments prostacyclin and retards atherogenesis. *Proc Natl Acad Sci U S A,* **2006,** *103*:14507–14512.

Woodward DF, Carling RW, Cornell CL, et al. The pharmacology and therapeutic relevance of endocannabinoid derived cyclo-oxygenase (COX)-2 products. *Pharmacol Ther,* **2008,** *120*:71–80.

Zhang Z, Vezza R, Plappert T, et al. COX-2-dependent cardiac failure in Gh/tTG transgenic mice. *Circ Res,* **2003,** *92*:1153–1161.

Zimmerman GA, McIntyre TM, Prescott SM, Stafforini DM. The platelet-activating factor signaling system and its regulators in syndromes of inflammation and thrombosis. *Crit Care Med* **2002,** *30*(suppl):S294–S301.

Anti-Inflammatory, Antipyretic, and Analgesic Agents; Pharmacotherapy of Gout

Tilo Grosser, Emer Smyth, and Garret A. FitzGerald

This chapter describes the nonsteroidal anti-inflammatory drugs (NSAIDs) used to treat inflammation, pain, and fever and the drugs used for hyperuricemia and gout.

Most currently available traditional NSAIDs (tNSAIDs) act by inhibiting the prostaglandin (PG) G/H synthase enzymes, colloquially known as the cyclooxygenases (COXs; see Chapter 33). The inhibition of cyclooxygenase-2 (COX-2) is thought to mediate, in large part, the antipyretic, analgesic, and anti-inflammatory actions of tNSAIDs, while the simultaneous inhibition of cyclooxygenase-1 (COX-1) largely but not exclusively accounts for unwanted adverse effects in the GI tract. Selective inhibitors of COX-2 (celecoxib, etoricoxib, lumiracoxib) are a subclass of NSAIDs that are also discussed. Aspirin, which irreversibly acetylates COX, is discussed, along with several structural subclasses of tNSAIDs, including propionic acid derivatives (ibuprofen, naproxen), acetic acid derivatives (indomethacin), and enolic acids (piroxicam), all of which compete in a reversible manner with the arachidonic acid (AA) substrate at the active site of COX-1 and COX-2. Acetaminophen (paracetamol) is a weak anti-inflammatory drug; it is effective as an antipyretic and analgesic agent at typical doses that partly inhibit COXs. Acetaminophen has fewer GI side effects than the tNSAIDs.

History. The history of aspirin provides an interesting example of the translation of a compound from the realm of herbal folklore to contemporary therapeutics. The use of willow bark and leaves to relieve fever has been attributed to Hippocrates but was most clearly documented by Edmund Stone in a 1763 letter to the president of The Royal Society. Similar properties were attributed to potions from meadowsweet (*Spiraea ulmaria*), from which the name aspirin is derived. Salicin was crystallized in 1829 by Leroux, and Pina isolated salicylic acid in 1836. In 1859, Kolbe synthesized salicylic acid, and by 1874, it was being produced industrially. It soon was being used for rheumatic fever, gout, and as a general antipyretic. However, its unpleasant taste and adverse GI effects made it difficult to tolerate for more than short periods. In 1899, Hoffmann, a chemist at Bayer Laboratories, sought to improve the adverse-effect profile of salicylic acid (which his father was taking with difficulty for arthritis). Hoffmann came across the earlier work of the French chemist, Gerhardt, who had acetylated salicylic acid in 1853, apparently ameliorating its adverse-effect profile, but without improving its efficacy, and therefore abandoned the project. Hoffmann resumed the quest, and Bayer began testing acetylsalicylic acid (ASA) in animals by 1899—the first time that a drug was tested on animals in an industrial setting—and proceeded soon thereafter to human studies and the marketing of aspirin.

Acetaminophen was first used in medicine by von Mering in 1893. However, it gained popularity only after 1949, when it was recognized as the major active metabolite of both acetanilide and phenacetin. Acetanilide is the parent member of this group of drugs. It was introduced into medicine in 1886 under the name antifebrin by Cahn and Hepp, who had discovered its antipyretic action accidentally. However, acetanilide proved to be excessively toxic. A number of chemical derivatives were developed and tested. One of the more satisfactory of these was phenacetin. It was introduced into therapy in 1887 and was extensively employed in analgesic mixtures until it was implicated in analgesic-abuse nephropathy, hemolytic anemia, and bladder cancer; it was withdrawn in the 1980s. Discussion of its pharmacology can be found in earlier editions of this textbook.

Inflammation, Pain, and Fever

Inflammation. The inflammatory process is the response to an injurious stimulus. It can be evoked by a wide variety of noxious agents (e.g., infections, antibodies, physical injuries). The ability to mount an inflammatory response is essential for survival in the face of environmental pathogens and injury; in some situations and diseases, the inflammatory response may be exaggerated and sustained without apparent benefit and even with severe adverse consequences. No matter what the initiating stimulus, the classic inflammatory symptoms include calor (warmth), dolor (pain), rubor (redness), and tumor (swelling). The inflammatory response is characterized mechanistically by a transient local vasodilation and increased capillary permeability, infiltration of leukocytes and phagocytic cells, and tissue degeneration and fibrosis.

Many molecules are involved in the promotion and resolution of the inflammatory process (Nathan, 2002). Histamine was one of the first identified mediators of the inflammatory process. Although several H_1 histamine receptor antagonists are available, they are useful only for the treatment of vascular events in the early transient phase of inflammation (see Chapter 32). Bradykinin and 5-hydroxytryptamine (serotonin, 5-HT) also may play a role, but their antagonists ameliorate only certain types of inflammatory response (see Chapter 32). Leukotrienes (LTs) exert pro-inflammatory actions and LT-receptor antagonists (montelukast and zafirlukast) and have been approved for the treatment of asthma (see Chapters 33 and 36). Another lipid autacoid, platelet-activating factor (PAF), has been implicated as an important mediator of inflammation; however, inhibitors of PAF synthesis and PAF-receptor antagonists have proven disappointing in the treatment of inflammation (see Chapter 33).

Prostanoid biosynthesis is significantly increased in inflamed tissue. Inhibitors of the COXs, which depress prostanoid formation, are effective and widely used anti-inflammatory agents, highlighting the general role of prostanoids as pro-inflammatory mediators. The rapid induction of COX-2 in inflamed tissue and infiltrating cells provided a rationale for the development of selective COX-2 inhibitors for treatment of inflammation (see Chapter 33). Although COX-2 is the major source of pro-inflammatory prostanoids, COX-1 also contributes (McAdam et al., 2000). Both COX isozymes are expressed in circulating inflammatory cells *ex vivo,* and COX-1 accounts for ~10-15% of the PG formation induced by lipopolysaccharide in volunteers. Impaired inflammatory responses have been reported in both COX-1- and COX-2-deficient mouse models, although they diverge in time course and intensity (Langenbach et al., 1999; Ballou et al., 2000; Yu et al., 2005). Human data are compatible with the concept that COX-1-derived products play a dominant role in the initial phase of an acute inflammatory response, while COX-2 is upregulated within several hours.

Prostaglandin E_2 (PGE_2) and prostacyclin (PGI_2) are the primary prostanoids that mediate inflammation. They increase local blood flow, vascular permeability, and leukocyte infiltration through activation of their respective receptors, EP_2 and IP (see Table 33–1 and Figure 33–4). PGD_2, a major product of mast cells, contributes to inflammation in allergic responses, particularly in the lung. Activation of its DP_1 receptor increases perfusion and vascular permeability and promotes T_H2 cell differentiation. PGD_2 also can activate mature T_H2 cells and eosinophils via its DP_2 receptor (Pettipher et al., 2007). DP_2 antagonists may prove useful in the treatment of airway inflammation.

Activation of endothelial cells plays a key role in "targeting" circulating cells to inflammatory sites. Cell adhesion occurs by recognition of cell-surface glycoproteins and carbohydrates on circulating cells due to the augmented expression of adhesion molecules on resident cells. Thus, endothelial activation results in leukocyte adhesion as the leukocytes recognize newly expressed L- and P-selectin; other important interactions include those of endothelial-expressed E-selectin with sialylated Lewis X and other glycoproteins on the leukocyte surface and endothelial intercellular adhesion molecule (ICAM)-1 with leukocyte integrins.

The recruitment of inflammatory cells to sites of injury also involves the concerted interactions of several types of soluble mediators. These include the complement factor C5a, PAF, and the eicosanoid LTB_4 (see Chapter 33). All can act as chemotactic agonists. Several cytokines also play essential roles in orchestrating the inflammatory process, especially tumor necrosis factor (TNF) (Dempsey et al., 2003) and interleukin-1 (IL-1) (O'Neill, 2008). They are secreted by monocytes, macrophages, adipocytes, and other cells. Working in concert with each other and various cytokines and growth factors (such as IL-6, IL-8, and granulocyte-macrophage colony-stimulating factor [GM-CSF]; see Chapters 32, 33, and 35), they induce gene expression and protein synthesis—including expression of COX-2, adhesion molecules, and acute-phase proteins—in a variety of cells to mediate and promote inflammation.

TNF is composed of two closely related proteins: mature TNF (TNF-α) and lymphotoxin (TNF-β), both of which are recognized by the TNF receptors, a 75-kd type 1 receptor and a 55-kd type 2 receptor (Dempsey et al., 2003). TNF-α blockers (see Chapter 35) are used to treat inflammatory conditions, including rheumatoid arthritis, juvenile idiopathic arthritis, psoriasis and psoriatic arthritis, ankylosing spondylitis, and Crohn's disease. TNF-α blockers fall into the category of disease-modifying anti-rheumatic drugs (DMARDs) because they reduce the disease activity of rheumatoid arthritis and retard the progression of arthritic tissue destruction. NSAIDs generally are not considered DMARDs.

IL-1 comprises two distinct polypeptides (IL-1α and IL-1β) that bind to an 80-kd IL-1 receptor type 1 and a 68-kd IL-1 receptor type 2, which are present on different cell types (O'Neill, 2008). Plasma IL-1 levels are increased in patients with active inflammation. A naturally occurring IL-1 receptor antagonist (IL-1ra) competes with IL-1 for receptor binding and blocks IL-1 activity *in vitro* and *in vivo*. IL-1ra often is found in high levels in patients with various infections or inflammatory conditions and may act to limit the extent of an inflammatory response. Clinical studies suggest that the administration of a recombinant form of human IL-1ra (anakinra; see Chapter 35) antagonizes IL-1 action at its receptor and thereby inhibits the progression of structural damage associated with active rheumatoid arthritis and other inflammatory conditions. Canakinumab (ILARIS) is an IL-1β monoclonal antibody recently approved for two forms of the cryopyrin-associated periodic syndrome: familial cold auto-inflammatory syndrome and Muckle-Wells syndrome (see Chapter 35).

Other cytokines and growth factors (e.g., IL-2, IL-6, IL-8, GM-CSF) contribute to manifestations of the inflammatory response. The concentrations of many of these factors are increased in the synovia of patients with inflammatory arthritis. Glucocorticoids interfere with the synthesis and actions of cytokines, such as IL-1 or TNF-α (see Chapter 35). Although some of the actions of these cytokines are accompanied by the release of PGs and thromboxane A_2 (TxA_2), COX inhibitors appear to block only their pyrogenic effects. In addition, many of the actions of the PGs are inhibitory to the immune response, including suppression of the function of helper T cells and B cells and inhibition of the production of IL-1 (see Chapter 33). Other cytokines and growth factors counter the effects and initiate resolution of inflammation. These include transforming growth factor β_1 (TGF-β_1), which increases extracellular matrix formation and acts as an immunosuppressant; IL-10, which decreases cytokine and PGE_2 formation by inhibiting monocytes; and interferon gamma (IFN-γ), which possesses myelosuppressive activity and inhibits collagen synthesis and collagenase production by macrophages.

Many cytokines, including IL-1 and TNF-α, have been found in the rheumatoid synovium. Rheumatoid arthritis appears to be an autoimmune disease driven largely by activated T cells, giving rise to T cell–derived cytokines, such as IL-1 and TNF-α. Activation of B cells and the humoral response also are evident, although most of the antibodies generated are immunoglobulins G of unknown specificity, apparently elicited by polyclonal activation of B cells rather than from a response to a specific antigen (Brennan and McInnes, 2008).

Pain. Nociceptors, peripheral terminals of primary afferent fibers that sense pain, can be activated by various stimuli, such as heat, acids, or pressure. Inflammatory mediators released from non-neuronal cells during tissue injury increase the sensitivity of nociceptors and potentiate pain perception. Some of the main components of this inflammatory "mélange" are bradykinin, H^+, neurotransmitters such as serotonin and ATP, neutrophins (nerve growth factor), LTs, and PGs. Cytokines appear to liberate PGs and some of the other mediators. Neuropeptides, such as substance P and calcitonin gene-related peptide (CGRP), also may be involved in eliciting pain (see Chapter 18).

PGE_2 and PGI_2 reduce the threshold to stimulation of nociceptors, causing *peripheral sensitization* (Lopshire and Nicol, 1998; Pulichino et al., 2006). Thus, PGE_2 promotes—probably via its receptors, EP_1 and EP_4—the phosphorylation of transient receptor potential V_1 and other ion channels on nociceptors and increases their terminal membrane excitability. Reversal of peripheral sensitization is thought to represent the mechanistic basis for the peripheral component of the analgesic activity of NSAIDs. NSAIDs also have important central actions in the spinal cord and brain. Both COX-1 and COX-2 are expressed in the spinal chord under basal conditions and release PGs in response to peripheral pain stimuli (Vanegas and Schaible, 2001). Centrally active PGE_2 and perhaps also PGD_2, PGI_2, and $PGF_{2\alpha}$ contribute to *central sensitization*, an increase in excitability of spinal dorsal horn neurons that causes hyperalgesia and allodynia in part by disinhibition of glycinergic pathways (Reinold et al., 2005).

Basal COX-2, expressed in both neurons and glia cells, contributes to central sensitization in the early phase of peripheral inflammation. COX-2 is upregulated widely in the spinal chord within a few hours to contribute to prolonged central sensitization (Samad et al., 2001). A role for COX-1 in nociception has been implicated by COX-1–deleted mice, which show increased tolerance to pain stimuli (Ballou et al., 2000). This isoform is predominant in neurons of dorsal root ganglia. Central sensitization reflects the plasticity of the nociceptive system that is invoked by injury. This usually is reversible within hours to days following adequate responses of the nociceptive system (e.g., in postoperative pain). However, chronic inflammatory diseases may cause persistent modification of the architecture of the nociceptive system, which may lead to long-lasting changes in its responsiveness. These mechanisms contribute to chronic pain.

Fever. Regulation of body temperature requires a delicate balance between the production and loss of heat; the hypothalamus regulates the set point at which body temperature is maintained. This set point is elevated in fever, reflecting an infection, or resulting from tissue damage, inflammation, graft rejection, or malignancy. These conditions all enhance formation of cytokines such as IL-1β, IL-6, TNF-α, and interferons, which act as endogenous pyrogens. The initial phase of the thermoregulatory response to such pyrogens is thought to be mediated by ceramide release in neurons of the preoptic area in the anterior hypothalamus (Sanchez-Alavez et al., 2006). The late response is mediated by coordinate induction of COX-2 and microsomal PGE synthase-1 (mPGES-1) in the endothelium of blood vessels in the preoptic hypothalamic area to form PGE_2 (Engblom et al., 2003). PGE_2 can cross the blood-brain barrier and acts on EP_3 and perhaps EP_1 receptors on thermosensitive neurons. This triggers the hypothalamus to elevate body temperature by promoting an increase in heat generation and a decrease in heat loss. NSAIDs suppress this response by inhibiting PGE_2 synthesis.

NONSTEROIDAL ANTI-INFLAMMATORY DRUGS

NSAIDs traditionally are grouped by their chemical characteristics. Following the development of the selective COX-2 inhibitors, the classification into tNSAIDs, which inhibit both COX-1 and COX-2, and COX-2–selective NSAIDs, emerged. Initially, only agents designed specifically for the purpose of COX-2–selective inhibition—colloquially termed the coxibs—were attributed to the group of COX-2–selective NSAIDs. However, some older NSAIDs (e.g., diclofenac, meloxicam, nimesulide) show a degree of selectivity for COX-2 that is similar to that of the first coxib, celecoxib. Thus, these drugs might better be classified as COX-2–selective NSAIDs, although this is not, as yet, commonplace (Figure 34–1). Other classifications of NSAIDs were developed based on $t_{1/2}$, such as those with a shorter (<6 hours) or longer (>10 hours) $t_{1/2}$ (Figure 34–1).

Most NSAIDs are competitive, reversible, active site inhibitors of the COX enzymes. However, aspirin (ASA) acetylates the isozymes and inhibits them irreversibly; thus, aspirin often is distinguished from the tNSAIDs. Similarly, acetaminophen, which is antipyretic

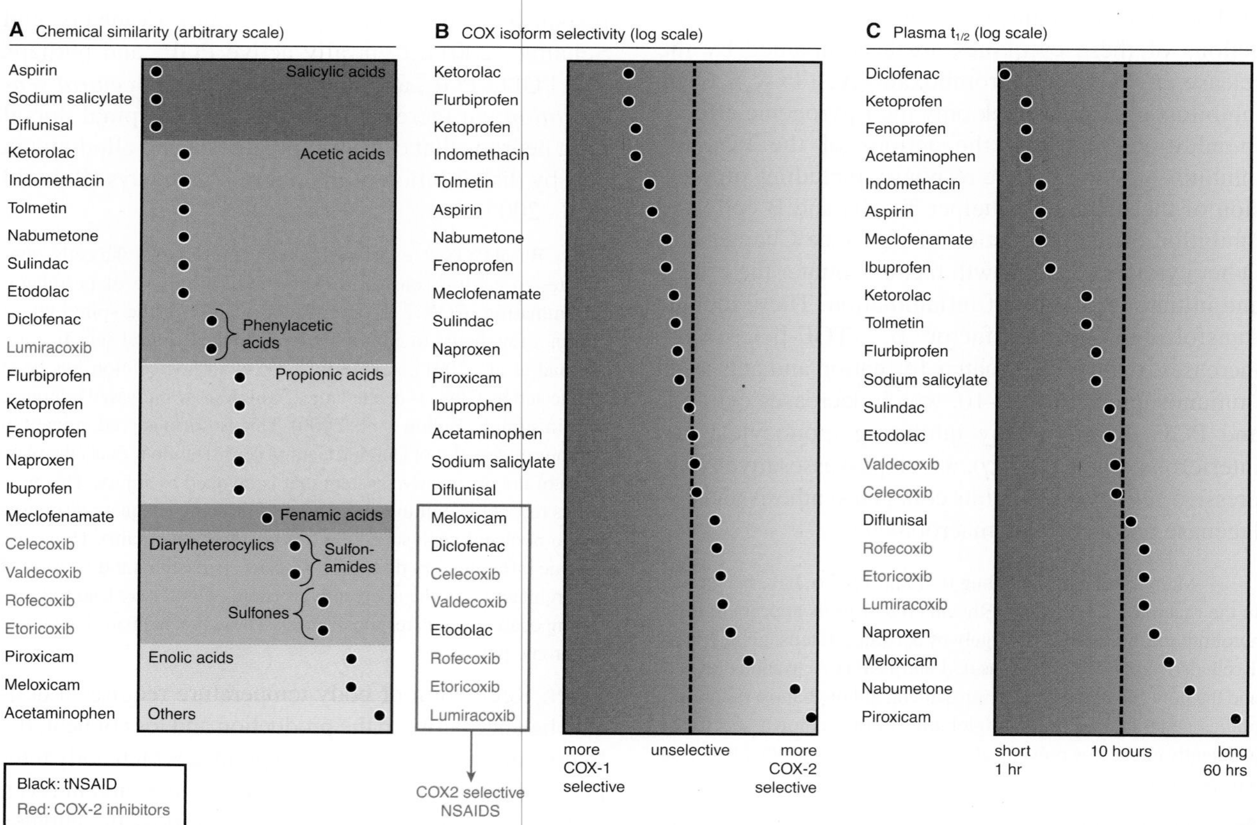

Figure 34–1. *Classification of NSAIDs by chemical similarity* (panel A), *cyclooxygenase (COX) isoform selectivity* (panel B), *and plasma* $t_{1/2}$ (panel C). The COX selectivity chart is plotted from data published in Warner et al., 1999, and FitzGerald and Patrono, 2001. tNSAIDs, traditional nonsteroidal anti-inflammatory drugs.

and analgesic but largely devoid of anti-inflammatory activity, also is conventionally segregated from the group, despite sharing many properties with tNSAIDs relevant to its clinical action *in vivo*.

Chemistry. NSAIDs are a chemically heterogeneous group of compounds, which nevertheless share certain therapeutic actions and adverse effects. The class includes derivatives of salicylic acid (e.g., aspirin, diflusinal), propionic acid (e.g., naproxen, ibuprofen, flurbiprofen, ketoprofen), acetic acid (e.g., indomethacin, etodolac, diclofenac, ketorolac), enolic acid (e.g., piroxicam, phenylbutazone), fenamic acid (e.g., mefenamic acid, meclofenamic acid), alkanones (nabumetone), and diaryl heterocyclic compounds (e.g., celecoxib, valdecoxib, rofecoxib, etoricoxib) (Figure 34–1).

The vast majority of tNSAID compounds are organic acids with relatively low pK_a values (Figure 34–1). Even the non-acidic parent drug nabumetone is converted to an active acetic acid derivative *in vivo*. As organic acids, the compounds generally are well absorbed orally, highly bound to plasma proteins, and excreted either by glomerular filtration or by tubular secretion. They also accumulate in sites of inflammation, where the pH is lower, potentially confounding the relationship between plasma concentrations and duration of drug effect. Most COX-2–selective NSAIDs are diaryl heterocyclic compounds with a relatively bulky side group, which aligns with a large side pocket in the AA binding channel of COX-2 but hinders its optimal orientation in the smaller binding channel of COX-1 (Figure 34–2) (Smith et al., 2000). Both tNSAIDs and the COX-2–selective NSAIDs generally are hydrophobic drugs, a feature that allows them to access the hydrophobic arachidonate binding channel and results in shared pharmacokinetic characteristics. Again, aspirin and acetaminophen are exceptions to this rule.

Mechanism of Action

Cyclooxygenase Inhibition. The principal therapeutic effects of NSAIDs derive from their ability to inhibit PG production. The first enzyme in the PG synthetic pathway is COX, also known as PG G/H synthase. This enzyme converts AA to the unstable intermediates PGG_2 and PGH_2 and leads to the production of the prostanoids, TxA_2, and a variety of PGs (see Chapter 33).

There are two forms of COX, COX-1 and COX-2. COX-1, expressed constitutively in most cells, is the dominant (but not exclusive) source of prostanoids for housekeeping functions, such as gastric epithelial cytoprotection and hemostasis. Conversely, COX-2, induced by cytokines, shear stress, and tumor promoters, is the more important source of prostanoid formation in inflammation and perhaps in cancer (see Chapter 33). However, both enzymes contribute to the generation of autoregulatory and homeostatic prostanoids, and both can contribute to prostanoid formation in syndromes of human inflammation and pain (see "Inflammation and Pain" at the beginning of this chapter). Importantly, COX-1 is expressed as the dominant, constitutive isoform in gastric epithelial cells and is thought to be the major source of cytoprotective PG formation. Inhibition of COX-1 at this site is thought to account largely for the gastric adverse events that complicate therapy with tNSAIDs, thus providing the rationale for the development of NSAIDs specific for inhibition of COX-2 (FitzGerald and Patrono, 2001).

Aspirin and NSAIDs inhibit the COX enzymes and PG production; they do not inhibit the lipoxygenase (LOX) pathways of AA metabolism and hence do not suppress LT formation (see Chapter 33). Glucocorticoids suppress the induced expression of

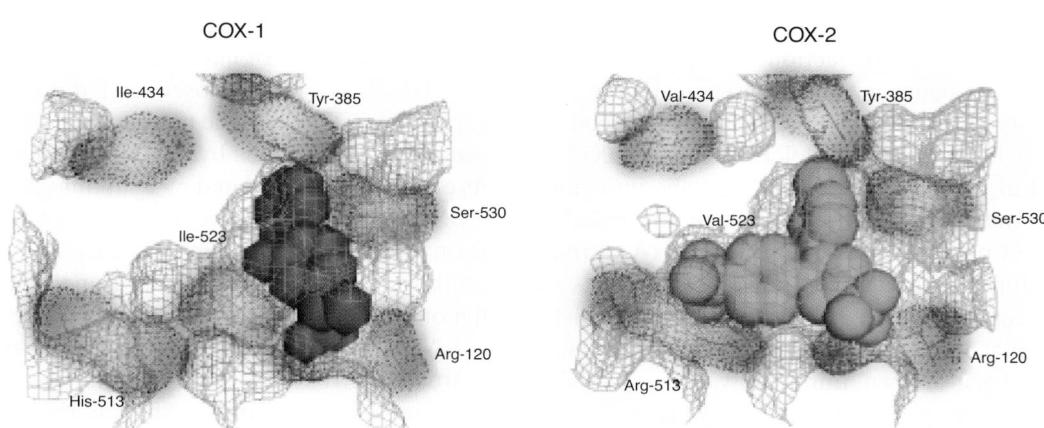

Figure 34–2. *Structural basis for cyclooxygenase-2 (COX-2)-selective inhibition.* The active centers of COX-1 and COX-2 are shown crystallized with the nonselective inhibitor flurbiprofen (COX-1) (Picot et al., 1994) and the experimental COX-2 inhibitor SC-558 (Kurumbail et al., 1996). The active center of COX-2 is characterized by a larger side pocket, which can accommodate molecules with bulkier side chains than COX-1. (Courtesy of Dr. Vineet Sangar.)

COX-2, and thus COX-2–mediated PG production. They also inhibit the action of PLA_2, which releases AA from the cell membrane. These effects contribute to the anti-inflammatory actions of glucocorticoids (see Chapter 35).

At higher concentrations, NSAIDs also are known to reduce production of superoxide radicals, induce apoptosis, inhibit the expression of adhesion molecules, decrease NO synthase, decrease pro-inflammatory cytokines (e.g., TNF-α, IL-1), modify lymphocyte activity, and alter cellular membrane functions *in vitro*. However, there are differing opinions as to whether any of these actions might contribute to the anti-inflammatory activity of NSAIDs (Vane and Botting, 1998) at the concentrations attained during clinical dosing. The hypothesis that their anti-inflammatory actions in humans derive solely from COX inhibition alone has not been rejected based on current evidence.

Observational studies suggest that acetaminophen, which is a very weak anti-inflammatory agent at the typical dose of 1000 mg, is associated with a reduced incidence of GI adverse effects compared to tNSAIDs. At this dose, acetaminophen inhibits both COXs by ~50%. The ability of acetaminophen to inhibit the enzyme is conditioned by the peroxide tone of the immediate environment (Boutaud et al., 2002). This may partly explain the poor anti-inflammatory activity of acetaminophen, because sites of inflammation usually contain increased concentrations of leukocyte-generated peroxides.

Irreversible Cyclooxygenase Inhibition by Aspirin. Aspirin covalently modifies COX-1 and COX-2, irreversibly inhibiting COX activity. This is an important distinction from all the NSAIDs because the duration of aspirin's effects is related to the turnover rate of COXs in different target tissues. The duration of effect of non-aspirin NSAIDs, which inhibit the active sites of the COX enzymes competitively, relates to the time course of drug disposition. The importance of enzyme turnover in recovery from aspirin action is most notable in platelets, which, being anucleate, have a markedly limited capacity for protein synthesis. Thus, the consequences of inhibition of platelet COX-1 (COX-2 is expressed in megakaryocytes and perhaps immature platelet forms) last for the lifetime of the platelet. Inhibition of platelet COX-1–dependent TxA_2 formation therefore is cumulative with repeated doses of aspirin (at least as low as 30 mg/day) and takes ~8-12 days—the platelet turnover time—to recover fully once therapy has been stopped. Importantly, even a partially recovered platelet pool—just a few days after the last aspirin dose—may afford recovery of sufficient hemostatic integrity for some types of elective surgery to be performed. However, such a partial platelet function also may predispose noncompliant patients to thrombotic events.

COXs are configured such that the active site is accessed by the AA substrate via a hydrophobic channel. Aspirin acetylates serine 529 of COX-1, located high up in the hydrophobic channel. Interposition of the bulky acetyl residue prevents the binding of AA to the active site of the enzyme and thus impedes the ability of the enzyme to make PGs. Aspirin acetylates a homologous serine at position 516 in COX-2. Although covalent modification of COX-2 by aspirin also blocks the COX activity of this isoform, an interesting property not shared by COX-1 is that acetylated COX-2 synthesizes 15(*R*)-hydroxyeicosatetraenoic acid [15(*R*)-HETE]. This may be metabolized, at least *in vitro*, by 5-LOX to yield 15-epi-lipoxin A4, which has potent anti-inflammatory properties (see Chapter 33). Repeated doses of aspirin that acutely do not completely inhibit platelet COX-1–derived TxA_2 can exert a cumulative effect with complete blockade. This has been shown in randomized trials for doses as low as 30 mg/day. However, most of the clinical trials demonstrating cardioprotection from low-dose aspirin have used doses in the range of 75-81 mg/day.

The unique sensitivity of platelets to inhibition by such low doses of aspirin is related to their presystemic inhibition in the portal circulation before aspirin is deacetylated to salicylate on first pass through the liver (Pedersen and FitzGerald, 1984). In contrast to aspirin, salicylic acid has no acetylating capacity. It is a weak, reversible, competitive inhibitor of COX. Salicylic acid derivates, rather than the acid, are available for clinical use. The lack of acetylation often is used as justification to prefer trisalicylate or salsalate over aspirin in presurgical patients. High doses of salicylate inhibit the activation of NFκB *in vitro*, but the relevance of this property to the concentrations attained *in vivo* is not clear (Yin et al., 1998). Salicylic acid also may inhibit the expression of COX-2 by interfering with the binding of CCAAT/enhancer binding protein (C/EBP) β transcription factor to the COX-2 promoter (Cieslik et al., 2002). This was observed *in vitro* at concentrations of salicylic acid that are attained in humans.

Selective Inhibition of Cyclooxygenase-2. The therapeutic use of the tNSAIDs is limited by their poor GI tolerability. Chronic users are prone to experience GI irritation in ≤20% of cases. Following the discovery of COX-2, it was proposed that the constitutively expressed COX-1 was the predominant source of cytoprotective PGs formed by the GI epithelium. Because its expression is regulated by cytokines and mitogens, COX-2 was thought to be the dominant source of PG formation in inflammation and cancer. Thus, selective inhibitors of COX-2 were developed based on the hypothesis that they would afford efficacy similar to tNSAIDs with better GI tolerability (FitzGerald and Patrono, 2001). Six COX-2 inhibitors specifically designed for such purpose, the coxibs, were initially approved for use in the U.S. or E.U.: celecoxib, rofecoxib, valdecoxib and its prodrug parecoxib, etoricoxib, and lumiracoxib. Most coxibs have been either severely restricted in their use or withdrawn from the market in view of their adverse event profile. Celecoxib

(CELEBREX) currently is the only COX-2 inhibitor licensed for use in the U.S.

The relative degree of selectivity for COX-2 inhibition is lumiracoxib = etoricoxib > valdecoxib = rofecoxib >> celecoxib (Figure 34–1). Although there were differences in relative hierarchies, depending on whether screens were performed using recombinantly expressed enzymes, cells, or whole-blood assays, most tNSAIDs expressed similar selectivity for inhibition of the two enzymes. Some compounds, conventionally thought of as tNSAIDs—diclofenac, meloxicam, and nimesulide (not available in the U.S.)—exhibit selectivity for COX-2 that is close to that of celecoxib *in vitro* (Figure 34–1) (Warner et al., 1999; FitzGerald and Patrono, 2001). Indeed, meloxicam achieved approval in some countries as a selective inhibitor of COX-2. Thus, selectivity for COX-2 should not be viewed as an absolute category; the isoform selectivity for COX-2 (just like selectivity for β_1 adrenergic receptors) is a continuous rather than a discreet variable, as illustrated in Figure 34–1.

Absorption, Distribution, and Elimination

Absorption. Most NSAIDs are rapidly absorbed following oral ingestion, and peak plasma concentrations usually are reached within 2-3 hours. All COX-2–selective NSAIDs are well absorbed, but peak concentrations are achieved with lumiracoxib and etoricoxib in ~1 hour compared to 2-4 hours with the other agents. The poor aqueous solubility of most NSAIDs often is reflected by a less than proportional increase in area under the curve (AUC) of plasma concentration–time curves, due to incomplete dissolution, when the dose is increased. Food intake may delay absorption and sometimes decreases systemic availability (i.e., fenoprofen, sulindac). Antacids, commonly prescribed to patients on NSAID therapy, variably delay, but rarely reduce, absorption. Most interaction studies performed with proton pump inhibitors suggest that relevant changes in NSAID kinetics are unlikely. Little information exists regarding the absolute oral bioavailability of many NSAIDs, as solutions suitable for intravenous administration often are not available. Some compounds (e.g., diclofenac, nabumetone) undergo first-pass or presystemic elimination. Acetaminophen is metabolized to a small extent during absorption. Aspirin begins to acetylate platelets within minutes of reaching the presystemic circulation.

Distribution. Most NSAIDs are extensively bound to plasma proteins (95-99%), usually albumin. Plasma protein binding often is concentration dependent (i.e., naproxen, ibuprofen) and saturable at high concentrations. Conditions that alter plasma protein concentration may result in an increased free drug fraction with potential toxic effects. Highly protein bound NSAIDs have the potential to displace other drugs, if they compete for the same binding sites. Most NSAIDs are distributed widely throughout the body and readily penetrate arthritic joints, yielding synovial fluid concentrations in the range of half the plasma concentration (i.e., ibuprofen, naproxen, piroxicam). Some substances yield synovial drug concentrations similar to (i.e., indomethacin), or even exceeding (i.e., tolmetin), plasma concentrations. Most NSAIDs achieve sufficient concentrations in the CNS to have a central analgesic effect. Celecoxib is particularly lipophilic, so it accumulates in fat and is readily transported into the CNS. Lumiracoxib is more acidic than other COX-2–selective NSAIDs, which may favor its accumulation at sites of inflammation. Multiple NSAIDs are marketed in formulations for topical application on inflamed or injured joints. However, direct transport of topically applied NSAIDs into inflamed tissues and joints appears to be minimal, and detectable concentrations in synovial fluid of some agents (i.e., diclofenac) following topical use are primarily attained via dermal absorption and systemic circulation.

Elimination. Plasma $t_{1/2}$ varies considerably among NSAIDs. For example, ibuprofen, diclofenac, and acetaminophen have relatively rapid elimination ($t_{1/2}$ of 1-4 hours), while piroxicam has a $t_{1/2}$ of ~50 hours at steady state that can increase to up to 75 hours in the elderly. Published estimates of the $t_{1/2}$ of COX-2–selective NSAIDs vary (2-6 hours for lumiracoxib, 6-12 hours for celecoxib, and 20-26 hours for etoricoxib). However, peak plasma concentrations of lumiracoxib at marketed doses considerably exceed those necessary to inhibit COX-2, suggesting an extended pharmacodynamic $t_{1/2}$. Hepatic biotransformation and renal excretion is the principal route of elimination of the majority of NSAIDs. Some have active metabolites (e.g., fenbufen, nabumetone, meclofenamic acid, sulindac). Elimination pathways frequently involve oxidation or hydroxylation (Table 34–1). Acetaminophen, at therapeutic doses, is oxidized only to a small fraction to form traces of the highly reactive metabolite, *N*-acetyl-*p*-benzoquinone imine (NAPQI). When overdosed (usually >10 g of acetaminophen), however, the principal metabolic pathways are saturated, and hepatotoxic NAPQI concentrations can be formed (see Chapters 4 and 6). Rarely, other NSAIDs also may be complicated by hepatotoxicity (e.g., diclofenac, lumiracoxib). Several NSAIDs or their metabolites are glucuronidated or otherwise conjugated. In some cases, such as the propionic acid derivatives naproxen and ketoprofen, the glucuronide metabolites can hydrolyze back to form the active parent drug when the metabolite is not removed efficiently due to renal insufficiency or competition for renal excretion with other drugs. This may prolong elimination of the NSAID significantly. NSAIDs usually are not removed by hemodialysis due to their extensive plasma protein binding; salicylic acid is an exemption to this rule. In general, NSAIDs are not recommended in the setting of advanced hepatic or renal disease due to their adverse pharmacodynamic effects.

Therapeutic Uses

All NSAIDs, including selective COX-2 inhibitors, are antipyretic, analgesic, and anti-inflammatory, with the exception of acetaminophen, which is antipyretic and analgesic but is largely devoid of anti-inflammatory activity.

Inflammation. NSAIDs find their chief clinical application as anti-inflammatory agents in the treatment of musculoskeletal disorders, such as rheumatoid arthritis and osteoarthritis. In general, NSAIDs provide mostly symptomatic relief from pain and inflammation associated with the disease and are not considered to be DMARDs. A number of NSAIDs are approved for the treatment of ankylosing spondylitis and gout. The use of NSAIDs for mild arthropathies, together with rest

Table 34–1

Classification and Comparison of Nonsteroidal Analgesics

CLASS/DRUG (SUBSTITUTION)	PHARMACOKINETICS		DOSING[d]		COMMENTS	COMPARED TO ASPIRIN
Salicylates						
Aspirin (acetyl ester)	Peak C_p[a] Protein binding Metabolites[b] $t_{1/2}$[c], therapeutic $t_{1/2}$, toxic dose	1 hour 80-90% Salicyluric acid 2-3 hours 15-30 hours	Antiplatelet Pain/fever Rheumatic fever Children	40-80 mg/day 325-650 mg every 4-6 hours 1 g every 4-6 hours 10 mg/kg every 4-6 hours	Permanent platelet COX-1 inhibition (acetylation) Main side effects: GI, increased bleeding time, hypersensitivity Avoid in children with acute febrile illness	
Diflunisal (defluoro-phenyl)	Peak C_p Protein binding Metabolites $t_{1/2}$	2-3 hours 99% Glucuronide 8-12 hours	250-500 mg every 8-12 hours		Not metabolized to salicylic acid Competitive COX inhibitor Excreted into breast milk	Analgesic and anti-inflammatory effects 4-5 times more potent Antipyretic effect weaker Fewer platelet and GI side effects
Para-aminophenol derivative						
Acetaminophen	Peak C_p Protein binding Metabolites $t_{1/2}$	30-60 minutes 20-50% Glucuronide conjugates (60%); sulfuric acid conjugates (35%) 2 hours	10-15 mg/kg every 4 hours (maximum of 5 doses/24 hours)		Weak nonspecific inhibitor at common doses Potency may be modulated by peroxides Overdose leads to production of toxic metabolite and liver necrosis	Analgesic and antipyretic effects equivalent Anti-inflammatory, GI, and platelet effects less than aspirin at 1000 mg/day
Acetic acid derivatives						
Indomethacin (methylated indole)	Peak C_p Protein binding Metabolites $t_{1/2}$	1-2 hours 90% *O*-demethylation (50%); unchanged (20%) 2.5 hours	25 mg 2-3 times/day; 75-100 mg at night		Side effects (3-50% of patients): frontal headache, neutropenia, thrombocytopenia; 20% discontinue therapy	10-40× more potent; intolerance limits dose

Sulindac (sulfoxide prodrug)	Peak C_p	1-2 hours; 8 hours for sulfide metabolite; extensive enterohepatic circulation	150-200 mg twice/day		20% suffer GI side effects; 10% get CNS side effects	Efficacy comparable
	Metabolites	Sulfone and conjugates (30%); sulindac and conjugates (25%)				
	$t_{1/2}$	7 hours; 18 hours for metabolite				
Etodolac (pyranocarboxylic acid)	Peak C_p	1 hour	200-400 mg 3-4 times/day		Some COX-2 selectivity *in vitro*	100 mg etodolac has similar efficacy to 650 mg of aspirin, but may be better tolerated
	Protein binding	99%				
	Metabolites	Hepatic metabolites				
	$t_{1/2}$	7 hours				
Tolmetin (heteroaryl acetate derivative)	Peak C_p	20-60	400-600 mg 3 times/day for children (anti-inflammatory)	20 mg/kg/day in 3-4 divided doses	Food delays and decreases peak absorption May persist longer in synovial fluid to give a biological efficacy longer than its plasma $t_{1/2}$	Efficacy similar; 25-40% develop side effects; 5-10% discontinue drug
	Protein binding	99%				
	Metabolites	Oxidized to carboxylic acid/other derivatives, then conjugated				
	$t_{1/2}$	5 hours				
Ketorolac (pyrrolizine carboxylate)	Peak C_p	30-60	<65 years: 20 mg (orally), then 10 mg every 4-6 hours (not to exceed 40 mg/24 hours); >65 years: 10 mg every 4-6 hours (not to exceed 40 mg/24 hours)		Commonly given parenterally (60 mg IM followed by 30 mg every 6 hours, or 30 mg IV every 6 hours) Available as ocular preparation (0.25%); 1 drop every 6 hours	Potent analgesic, poor anti-inflammatory
	Protein binding	99%				
	Metabolites	glucuronide conjugate (90%)				
	$t_{1/2}$	4-6 hours				
Diclofenac (phenylacetate derivatives)	Peak C_p	2-3 hours	50 mg 3 times/day or 75 mg twice/day		Available as topical gel, ophthalmic solution, and oral tablets combined with misoprostol First-pass effect; oral bioavailability, 50%	More potent; 20% develop side effects, 2% discontinue use, 15% develop elevated liver enzymes
	Protein binding	99%				
	Metabolites	Glucuronide and sulfide (renal 65%, bile 35%)				
	$t_{1/2}$	1-2 hours				

(*Continued*)

Table 34–1

Classification and Comparison of Nonsteroidal Analgesics (*Continued*)

CLASS/DRUG (SUBSTITUTION)	PHARMACOKINETICS		DOSING[d]		COMMENTS	COMPARED TO ASPIRIN
Fenamates (*N*-phenyl-anthranilates)						
Mefenamic acid	Peak C_p Protein binding Metabolites $t_{1/2}$	2-4 hours High Conjugates of 3-hydroxy and 3-carboxyl metabolites (20% recovered in feces) 3-4 hours	500-mg load, then 250 mg every 6 hours		Isolated cases of hemolytic anemia May have some central action	Efficacy similar; GI side effects (25%)
Meclofenamate	Peak C_p Protein binding Metabolites $t_{1/2}$	0.5-2 hours 99% Hepatic metabolism; fecal and renal excretion 2-3 hours	50-100 mg 4-6/day (maximum of 400 mg/day)			Efficacy similar; GI side effects (25%)
Flufenamic acid	*Not available in the U.S.*					
Propionic acid derivatives					Intolerance of one does not preclude use of another propionate derivative	Usually better tolerated
Ibuprofen	Peak C_p Protein binding Metabolites $t_{1/2}$	15-30 minutes 99% Conjugates of hydroxyl and carboxyl metabolites 2-4 hours	Analgesia Anti-inflammatory	200-400 mg every 4-6 hours 300 mg/6-8 hours or 400-800 mg 3-4 times/day	10-15% discontinue due to adverse effects Children's dosing Antipyretic: 5-10 mg/kg every 6 hours (max: 40 mg/kg/day) Anti-inflammatory: 20-40 mg/kg/day in 3-4 divided doses	Equipotent

Naproxen	Peak C_p Protein binding Metabolites $t_{1/2}$	1 hour 99% (less in elderly) 6-demethyl and other metabolites 14 hours	250 mg 4 times/day or 500 mg twice/day Children: anti-inflammatory	5 mg/kg twice/day	Peak anti-inflammatory effects may not be seen until 2-4 weeks of use Decreased protein binding and delayed excretion increase risk of toxicity in elderly	More potent *in vitro;* usually better tolerated; variably prolonged $t_{1/2}$ may afford cardioprotection in some individuals
Fenoprofen	Peak C_p Protein binding Metabolites $t_{1/2}$	2 hours 99% Glucuronide, 4-OH metabolite 2 hours	200 mg 4-6 times/day; 300-600 mg 3-4 times/day			15% experience side effects; few discontinue use
Ketoprofen	Peak C_p Protein binding Metabolites $t_{1/2}$	1-2 hours 98% Glucuronide conjugates 2 hours	Analgesia Anti-inflammatory	25 mg 3-4 times/day 50-75 mg 3-4 times/day		30% develop side effects (usually GI, usually mild)
Flurbiprofen	Peak C_p Protein binding Metabolites $t_{1/2}$	1-2 hours 99% Hydroxylates and conjugates 6 hours	200-300 mg/day in 2-4 divided doses		Available as a 0.03% ophthalmic solution	
Oxaprozin	Peak C_p Protein binding Major metabolites $t_{1/2}$	3-4 hours 99% Oxidates and glucuronide conjugates 40-60 hours	600-1800 mg/day		Long $t_{1/2}$ allows for daily administration; slow onset of action; inappropriate for fever/acute analgesia	
Enolic acid derivatives						
Piroxicam	Peak C_p Protein binding Metabolites $t_{1/2}$	3-5 hours 99% Hydroxylates and then conjugated 45-50 hours	20 mg/day		May inhibit activation of neutrophils, activity of proteoglycanase, collagenases	Equipotent; perhaps better tolerated 20% develop side effects; 5% discontinue drug

(*Continued*)

Table 34–1

Classification and Comparison of Nonsteroidal Analgesics (*Continued*)

CLASS/DRUG (SUBSTITUTION)	PHARMACOKINETICS		DOSING[d]	COMMENTS	COMPARED TO ASPIRIN
Meloxicam	Peak C_p Protein binding Metabolites $t_{1/2}$	5-10 hours 99% Hydroxylation 15-20 hours	7.5-15 mg/day		Some COX-2 selectivity, especially at lower doses
Nabumetone (naphthyl alkanone)	Peak C_p Protein binding Major metabolites $t_{1/2}$	3-6 hours 99% *O*-demethylation, then conjugation 24 hours	500-1000 mg 1-2 times/day	A prodrug, rapidly metabolized to 6-methoxy-2-naphthyl acetic acid; pharmacokinetics reflect active compound	Shows some COX-2 selectivity (active metabolite does not) Fewer GI side effects than many NSAIDs
Diaryl heterocyclic NSAIDs *(COX-2 selective)*				Evidence for cardiovascular adverse events	Decrease in GI side effects and in platelet effects
Celecoxib [diaryl substituted pyrazone; (sulfonamide derivative)]	Peak C_p Protein binding Metabolites $t_{1/2}$	2-4 hours 97% Carboxylic acid and glucuronide conjugates 6-12 hours	100 mg 1-2 times/day	Substrate for CYP2C9; inhibitor of CYP2D6 Coadministration with inhibitors of CYP2C9 or substrates of CYP2D6 should be done with caution	See the text for an overview of COX-2 inhibitors
Parecoxib Etoricoxib Lumaricoxi	*Not approved for use in the U.S.*				

[a]Time to peak plasma drug concentration (C_p) after a single dose. In general, food delays absorption but does not decrease peak concentration. [b]The majority of NSAIDs undergo hepatic metabolism, and the metabolites are excreted in the urine. Major metabolites or disposal pathways are listed. [c]Typical $t_{1/2}$ is listed for therapeutic doses; if $t_{1/2}$ is much different with the toxic dose, this is also given. [d]Limited dosing information given. For additional information, refer to the text and product information literature. Additional references can be found in earlier editions of this textbook. CNS, central nervous system; COX, cyclooxygenase; GI, gastrointestinal; IM, intramuscularly; IV, intravenously.

and physical therapy, generally is effective. When the symptoms are limited either to trouble sleeping because of pain or significant morning stiffness, a single NSAID dose given at night may suffice. Patients with more debilitating disease may not respond adequately to full therapeutic doses of NSAIDs and may require aggressive therapy with second-line agents. Substantial inter- and intraindividual differences in clinical response have been noted.

Pain. When employed as analgesics, these drugs usually are effective only against pain of low to moderate intensity, such as dental pain. Although their maximal efficacy is generally much less than the opioids, NSAIDs lack the unwanted adverse effects of opiates in the CNS, including respiratory depression and the potential for development of physical dependence. Coadministration of NSAIDs can reduce the opioid dose needed for sufficient pain control and reduce the likelihood of adverse opioid effects. NSAIDs do not change the perception of sensory modalities other than pain. They are particularly effective when inflammation has caused peripheral and/or central sensitization of pain perception. Thus, postoperative pain or pain arising from inflammation, such as arthritic pain, is controlled well by NSAIDs, whereas pain arising from the hollow viscera usually is not relieved. An exception to this is menstrual pain. The release of PGs by the endometrium during menstruation may cause severe cramps and other symptoms of primary dysmenorrhea; treatment of this condition with NSAIDs has met with considerable success (Marjoribanks et al., 2003). Not surprisingly, the selective COX-2 inhibitors such as rofecoxib and etoricoxib also are efficacious in this condition. NSAIDs are commonly used as first-line therapy to treat migraine attacks and can be combined with second-line drugs, such as the triptans (e.g., TREXIMET, which is a fixed-dose combination of naproxen and sumatriptan), or with antiemetics to aid relief of the associated nausea. NSAIDs lack efficacy in neuropathic pain.

Fever. Antipyretic therapy is reserved for patients in whom fever in itself may be deleterious and for those who experience considerable relief when fever is lowered. Little is known about the relationship between fever and the acceleration of inflammatory or immune processes; it may at times be a protective physiological mechanism. The course of the patient's illness may be obscured by the relief of symptoms and the reduction of fever by the use of antipyretic drugs. NSAIDs reduce fever in most situations, but not the circadian variation in temperature or the rise in response to exercise or increased ambient temperature. Comparative analysis of the impact of tNSAIDs and selective COX-2 inhibitors suggests that COX-2 is the dominant source of PGs that mediate the rise in temperature evoked by bacterial lipopolysaccharide (LPS) administration (McAdam et al., 1999). This is consistent with the antipyretic clinical efficacy of both subclasses of NSAIDs. It seems logical to select an NSAID with rapid onset for the management of fever associated with minor illness in adults.

Fetal Circulatory System. PGs have long been implicated in the maintenance of patency of the ductus arteriosus, and indomethacin, ibuprofen, and other tNSAIDs have been used in neonates to close the inappropriately patent ductus. Conversely, infusion of PGE_2 maintains ductal patency after birth. Both COX-1 and COX-2 appear to participate in maintaining patency of the ductus arteriosus in fetal lambs (Clyman et al., 1999), while in mice COX-2 appears to play the dominant role (Loftin et al., 2002). It is not known which isoform or isoforms are involved in maintaining patency of the fetal ductus *in utero* in humans.

In mice, PGE_2 maintains a low ductal smooth muscle cell tone via the G_s-coupled receptor EP_4 that increases intracellular cyclic AMP. In the late gestational period, pulmonary expression of an enzyme that eliminates PGE_2 from the bloodstream, PG 15-OH dehydrogenase (PGDH), is rapidly upregulated (Coggins et al., 2002). At birth, PGE_2 blood concentrations are dramatically reduced by pulmonary PGDH and by additional exposure of circulating PGE_2 to this enzyme with the increase of pulmonary blood flow. Due to reduced EP_4 signaling, intracellular cyclic AMP concentrations in the ductus arteriosus drop, and vasodilating effects are outweighed by vasoconstrictor signals, which initiate remodeling. However, surprisingly little information about the human ductal physiology exists, and a role for PGDH remains to be established in humans.

Cardioprotection. Ingestion of aspirin prolongs bleeding time. For example, a single 325-mg dose of aspirin approximately doubles the mean bleeding time of normal persons for 4-7 days. This effect is due to irreversible acetylation of platelet COX and the consequent inhibition of platelet function until sufficient numbers of new, unmodified platelets are released from megakaryocytes. It is the permanent and complete suppression of platelet TxA_2 formation that is thought to underlie the cardioprotective effect of aspirin. Aspirin reduces the risk of serious vascular events in high-risk patients (e.g., those with previous myocardial infarction) by 20-25%. Low-dose (<100 mg/day) aspirin, which is relatively (but not exclusively) selective for COX-1, is as effective as higher doses (e.g., 325 mg/day) but is associated with a lower risk for GI adverse events.

However, low-dose aspirin is not risk free. Placebo-controlled trials reveal that aspirin increases the incidence of serious GI bleeds, reflecting suppression not just of platelet thromboxane, but also reduction of gastroepithelial PGE_2 and PGI_2. It also increases the incidence of intracranial bleeds. Although benefit from aspirin outweighs these risks in the case of secondary prevention of cardiovascular disease, the issue is much more nuanced in patients who have never had a serious atherothrombotic event (primary prevention); here, prevention of myocardial infarction by aspirin is numerically balanced by the serious GI bleeds it precipitates (Patrono et al., 2005).

Given their relatively short $t_{1/2}$ and reversible COX inhibition, most other tNSAIDs are not thought to afford cardioprotection, a view supported by most epidemiological analyses (García Rodríguez et al., 2004). Data suggest that cardioprotection is lost when combining low-dose aspirin with ibuprofen. An exception in some individuals may be naproxen. Although there is considerable between-person variation, a small study suggests that platelet inhibition might be anticipated throughout the dosing interval in some, but not all, individuals on naproxen (Capone et al., 2005). Epidemiological evidence of cardioprotection is less impressive; it suggests an ~10% reduction in myocardial infarction, compared to 20-25% with low-dose aspirin (Antithrombotic Trialists' Collaboration, 2002). This would fit with heterogeneity of response to naproxen. Reliance on prescription databases may have constrained the ability of this approach to address the question with precision. In the Alzheimer's Disease Anti-inflammatory Prevention Trial (ADAPT Research Group, 2008), naproxen was associated with a higher rate of cardiac events than celecoxib. Hence, naproxen should not be used as a substitute for aspirin for cardioprotection. COX-2–selective NSAIDs are devoid of antiplatelet activity, as mature platelets do not express COX-2.

Other Clinical Uses

Systemic Mastocytosis. Systemic mastocytosis is a condition in which there are excessive mast cells in the bone marrow, reticuloendothelial system, GI system, bones, and skin. In patients with systemic mastocytosis, PGD_2, released from mast cells in large amounts, has been found to be the major mediator of severe episodes of flushing, vasodilation, and hypotension; this PGD_2 effect is resistant to antihistamines. The addition of aspirin or ketoprofen has provided relief (Worobec, 2000). However, aspirin and tNSAIDs can cause degranulation of mast cells, so blockade with H_1 and H_2 histamine receptor antagonists should be established before NSAIDs are initiated.

Niacin Tolerability. Large doses of niacin (nicotinic acid) effectively lower serum cholesterol levels, reduce low-density lipoprotein, and raise high-density lipoprotein (see Chapter 31). However, niacin is tolerated poorly because it induces intense facial flushing. This flushing is mediated largely by release of PGD_2 from the skin, which can be inhibited by treatment with aspirin (Jungnickel et al., 1997), and would be susceptible to inhibition of PGD synthesis, or antagonism of its DP_1 receptor.

Bartter Syndrome. Bartter syndrome includes a series of rare disorders (frequency ≤1/100,000 persons) characterized by hypokalemic, hypochloremic metabolic alkalosis with normal blood pressure and hyperplasia of the juxtaglomerular apparatus. Fatigue, muscle weakness, diarrhea, and dehydration are the main symptoms. Distinct variants are caused by mutations in a Na^+-K^+-$2Cl^-$ co-transporter, an apical ATP-regulated K^+ channel, a basolateral Cl^- channel, a protein (barttin) involved in co-transporter trafficking, and the extracellular Ca^{2+}-sensing receptor. Renal COX-2 is induced, and biosynthesis of PGE_2 is increased. Treatment with indomethacin, combined with potassium repletion and spironolactone, is associated with improvement in the biochemical derangements and symptoms. Selective COX-2 inhibitors also have been used (Guay-Woodford, 1998).

Cancer Chemoprevention. Chemoprevention of cancer is an area in which the potential use of aspirin and/or NSAIDs is under active investigation. Epidemiological studies suggested that frequent use of aspirin is associated with as much as a 50% decrease in the risk of colon cancer (Kune et al., 2007). Similar observations have been made with NSAID use in this and other cancers (Harris et al., 2005). NSAIDs have been used in patients with familial adenomatous polyposis (FAP), an inherited disorder characterized by multiple adenomatous colon polyps developing during adolescence and the inevitable occurrence of colon cancer by the sixth decade.

Studies in small numbers of patients over short periods of follow-up have shown a decrease in the polyp burden with the use of sulindac, celecoxib, or rofecoxib (Steinbach et al., 2000; Cruz-Correa et al., 2002; Hallak et al., 2003). Celecoxib is approved as an adjunct to endoscopic surveillance and surgery in FAP based on superiority in a short-term, placebo-controlled trial for polyp prevention/regression. However, more recently, the Adenoma Prevention with Celecoxib (APC) Trial showed a significant reduction in the incidence of adenomatous polyps in patients with a history of colorectal adenomas at high doses of celecoxib (200 mg twice a day and 400 mg twice a day versus placebo) (Bertagnolli et al., 2009). The trial was prematurely terminated because of a 2.5 times increase in cardiovascular risk for patients taking 200 mg twice a day of celecoxib and a 3.4 times increase in risk for patients taking 400 mg twice a day (Solomon et al., 2005). Similarly, the Prevention of colorectal Sporadic Adenomatous Polyps (PreSAP) trial found a reduction of polyps at a single daily dose of 400 mg of celecoxib (Arber et al., 2006), which was offset by an increase in cardiovascular risk (Solomon et al., 2006). Finally, the APPROVe trial of 25 mg of rofecoxib showed a reduction in the incidence of adenomatous polyps (Baron et al., 2006) and an increase in cardiovascular adverse events (Bresalier et al., 2005; Baron et al., 2008) that led to the termination of the trial and to rofecoxib's withdrawal from the market. Controlled evidence is not available to determine if selective COX-2 inhibitors differ from non-COX-2–selective tNSAIDs or aspirin in the extent of adenomatous colorectal polyp reduction in patients with FAP. Likewise, it is unknown whether there is even a clinical benefit from the reduction. Increased expression of COX-2 has been reported in multiple epithelial tumors, and in some cases, the degree of expression has been related to prognosis. Deletion or inhibition of COX-2 dramatically inhibits polyp formation in mouse genetic models of polyposis coli. Although the phenotypes in these models do not completely recapitulate the human disease, deletion of COX-1 had a similar effect. Speculation as to how the two COXs might interact in tumorigenesis includes the possibility that products of COX-1 might induce expression of COX-2. However, the nature of this interaction is poorly understood, as are its therapeutic consequences.

Alzheimer's Disease. Observational studies have suggested that NSAID use, in particular ibuprofen, is associated with lower risk of developing Alzheimer's disease. However, more recent prospective studies, including a randomized, controlled clinical trial comparing celecoxib, naproxen, and placebo (ADAPT Research Group, 2008), did not find a significant reduction in Alzheimer's dementia with the use of NSAIDs.

Adverse Effects of NSAID Therapy

Common adverse events that complicate therapy with aspirin and NSAIDs are outlined in Table 34–2. Age generally is correlated with an increased probability of developing serious adverse reactions to NSAIDs, and caution is warranted in choosing a lower starting dose for elderly patients. NSAIDs are labeled with a black box warning related to cardiovascular risks and are specifically contraindicated following coronary artery bypass graft (CABG) surgery.

Gastrointestinal. The most common symptoms associated with these drugs are gastrointestinal, including anorexia, nausea, dyspepsia, abdominal pain, and diarrhea. These symptoms may be related to the induction of gastric or intestinal ulcers, which is estimated to occur in 15-30% of regular users. Ulceration may range from small superficial erosions to full-thickness perforation of the muscularis mucosa. There may be single or multiple ulcers, and ulceration may be uncomplicated or complicated by bleeding, perforation, or obstruction. Blood loss can be gradual, leading to anemia over time, or acute and life-threatening. The risk is further increased in those with *Helicobacter pylori* infection, heavy alcohol consumption, or other risk factors for mucosal injury, including the concurrent use of glucocorticoids. Although there is a perception that tNSAIDs vary considerably in their tendency to cause erosions and ulcers, this is based on overview analyses of small and heterogeneous studies, often at single doses of individual tNSAIDs.

Large-scale comparative studies of tNSAIDs have not been performed, and there is no reliable information on which to assess the comparative likelihood of GI ulceration on anti-inflammatory doses of aspirin versus tNSAIDs. Thus, most information is derived from the use of surrogate markers or from epidemiological data sets and suggests that the relative risk for serious adverse GI events is elevated about 3-fold in tNSAID users compared to non-users. Epidemiological studies suggest that combining low-dose aspirin (for cardioprotection) with other NSAIDs synergistically increases the likelihood of GI adverse events (see "Drug Interactions"). Similarly, the combination of multiple tNSAIDs and high dosage of a single tNSAIDs (including inappropriately high dosage in the elderly) has been found to raise the risk for ulcer complications by 7- and 9-fold, respectively. Age >70 years alone increases the likelihood of complications almost 6-fold. The risk of ulcer complications is increased in patients with past uncomplicated (6-fold) or complicated ulcers (13-fold), or concurrent drug therapy including

Table 34–2

Common and Shared Side Effects of NSAIDs

SYSTEM	MANIFESTATIONS
GI	Abdominal pain
	Nausea
	Diarrhea
	Anorexia
	Gastric erosions/ulcers[a]
	Anemia[a]
	GI hemorrhage[a]
	Perforation/obstruction[a]
Platelets	Inhibited platelet activation[a]
	Propensity for bruising[a]
	Increased risk of hemorrhage[a]
Renal	Salt and water retention
	Edema, worsening of renal function in renal/cardiac and cirrhotic patients
	Decreased effectiveness of antihypertensive medications
	Decreased effectiveness of diuretic medications
	Decreased urate excretion (especially with aspirin)
	Hyperkalemia
Cardiovascular	Closure of ductus arteriosus
	Myocardial infarction[b]
	Stroke[b]
	Thrombosis[b]
CNS	Headache
	Vertigo
	Dizziness
	Confusion
	Hyperventilation (salicylates)
Uterus	Prolongation of gestation
	Inhibition of labor
Hypersensitivity	Vasomotor rhinitis
	Angioneurotic edema
	Asthma
	Urticaria
	Flushing
	Hypotension
	Shock

[a]Side effects decreased with COX-2-selective NSAIDs. [b]With the exception of low-dose aspirin.

warfarin (12-fold), glucocorticoids (4-fold), or selective serotonin reuptake inhibitors (SSRIs; 3-fold) (Gabriel et al., 1991; Dalton et al., 2003; García Rodríguez and Barreales Tolosa, 2007).

COX-2–selective NSAIDs were originally designed for a niche indication, to improve treatment safety for patients at high risk for GI complications requiring chronic tNSAIDs—a population of <5% of tNSAID users (Dai et al., 2005). Prescription behavior changed over time, however, and more than one-third of patients at the lowest risk for GI events received a COX-2 inhibitor in 2002. Paradoxically, the incidence of GI adverse events had been falling sharply in the population prior to the introduction of the coxibs—which were developed to reduce the risk of serious GI complication, perhaps reflecting a move away from use of high-dose aspirin as an anti-inflammatory drug strategy. All selective COX-2 inhibitors are less prone to induce endoscopically visualized gastric ulcers than equally efficacious doses of tNSAIDs (Deeks et al., 2002). A more detailed discussion on this topic can be found in the prior edition of this textbook.

Gastric damage by NSAIDs can be brought about by at least two distinct mechanisms (see Chapter 33). Inhibition of COX-1 in gastric epithelial cells depresses mucosal cytoprotective PGs, especially PGI_2 and PGE_2. These eicosanoids inhibit acid secretion by the stomach, enhance mucosal blood flow, and promote the secretion of cytoprotective mucus in the intestine. Inhibition of PGI_2 and PGE_2 synthesis may render the stomach more susceptible to damage and can occur with oral, parenteral, or transdermal administration of aspirin or NSAIDs. There is some evidence that COX-2 also contributes to constitutive formation of these PGs by human gastric epithelium; products of COX-2 certainly contribute to ulcer healing in rodents (Mizuno et al., 1997). This may partly reflect an impairment of angiogenesis by the inhibitors (Jones et al., 1999). Indeed, coincidental deletion or inhibition of both COX-1 and COX-2 seems necessary to replicate NSAID-induced gastropathy in mice, and there is some evidence for gastric pathology in the face of prolonged inhibition or deletion of COX-2 alone (Sigthorsson et al., 2002). Another mechanism by which NSAIDs or aspirin may cause ulceration is by local irritation from contact of orally administered drug with the gastric mucosa. Local irritation allows backdiffusion of acid into the gastric mucosa and induces tissue damage. However, the incidence of GI adverse events is not significantly reduced by formulations that reduce drug contact with the gastric mucosa, such as enteric coating or efferent solutions, suggesting that the contribution of direct irritation to the overall risk is minor. It also is possible that enhanced generation of LOX products (e.g., LTs) contributes to ulcerogenicity in patients treated with NSAIDs.

Co-administration of the PGE_1 analog, misoprostol, or proton pump inhibitors (PPIs) in conjunction with NSAIDs can be beneficial in the prevention of duodenal and gastric ulceration (Rostom et al., 2002).

Several groups have attached NO–donating moieties to NSAIDs and to aspirin in the hope of reducing the incidence of adverse events. Benefit might be attained by abrogation of the inhibition of angiogenesis by tNSAIDs during ulcer healing, as observed in rodents (Ma et al., 2002); however, the clinical benefit of this strategy remains to be established. Similarly, LTs may accumulate in the presence of COX inhibition, and there is some evidence in rodents that combined LOX-COX inhibition may be a useful strategy.

Cardiovascular. COX-2–selective NSAIDs were developed to improve the GI safety of anti-inflammatory therapy in patients at elevated risk for GI complications. However, placebo-controlled trials with three structurally distinct compounds—celecoxib, valdecoxib (withdrawn), and rofecoxib (withdrawn)—revealed an increase in the incidence of myocardial infarction, stroke, and thrombosis (Bresalier et al., 2005; Nussmeier et al., 2005; Solomon et al., 2006). The risk appears to also extend to those of the older tNSAIDs, which are quite selective for COX-2, such as diclofenac, meloxicam, and nimesulide (Grosser et al., 2006). Regulatory agencies in the U.S, E.U., and Australia have concluded that all NSAIDs have the potential to increase the risk of heart attack and stroke.

The cardiovascular hazard is plausibly explained by the depression of COX-2-dependent prostanoids formed in vasculature and kidney (Grosser et al., 2006). Vascular PGI_2 constrains the effect of prothrombotic and atherogenic stimuli, and renal PGI_2 and PGE_2 formed by COX-2 contribute to arterial pressure homeostasis (see Chapter 33). Genetic deletion of the PGI_2 receptor, IP, in mice augments the thrombotic response to endothelial injury, accelerates experimental atherogenesis, increases vascular proliferation, and adds to the effect of hypertensive stimuli (Cheng et al., 2002; Egan et al., 2004; Kobayashi et al., 2004; Cheng et al., 2006). Genetic deletion or inhibition of COX-2 accelerates the response to thrombotic stimuli and raises blood pressure. Together, these mechanisms would be expected to alter the cardiovascular risk of humans, as COX-2 inhibition in humans depresses PGI_2 synthesis (Catella-Lawson et al., 1999; McAdam et al., 1999). Indeed, a human mutation of the IP, which disrupts its signaling, is associated with increased cardiovascular risk (Arehart et al., 2008).

Patients at increased risk of cardiovascular disease or thrombosis are likely to be particularly prone to cardiovascular adverse events while on NSAIDs. This includes patients with rheumatoid arthritis, as the relative risk of myocardial infarction is increased in these patients compared to patients with osteoarthritis or no arthritis. The risk appears to be conditioned by factors influencing drug exposure, such as dose, $t_{1/2}$, degree of COX-2 selectivity, potency, and treatment duration. Thus, the lowest possible dose should be prescribed for the shortest possible period. NSAIDs with selectivity for COX-2 should be reserved for patients at high risk for GI complications.

Blood Pressure, Renal, and Renovascular Adverse Events. NSAIDs and COX-2 inhibitors have been associated with renal and renovascular adverse events. NSAIDs have little effect on renal function or blood pressure in normal human subjects. However, in patients with congestive heart failure, hepatic cirrhosis, chronic kidney disease, hypovolemia, and other states of activation of the sympathoadrenal or renin–angiotensin systems, PG formation becomes crucial in model systems and in humans. NSAIDs are associated with loss of the

PG-induced inhibition of both the reabsorption of Cl^- and the action of antidiuretic hormone, leading to the retention of salt and water.

Experiments in mice that attribute the generation of vasodilator PGs (PGE_2 and PGI_2) to COX-2 raise the likelihood that the incidence of hypertensive complications (either new onset or worsened control) induced by NSAIDs in patients may correlate with the degree of inhibition of COX-2 in the kidney and the selectivity with which it is attained (Qi et al., 2002). Deletion of receptors for both PGI_2 and PGE_2 elevate blood pressure in mice, mechanistically integrating hypertension with a predisposition to thrombosis. Although this hypothesis has never been addressed directly, epidemiological studies suggest hypertensive complications occur more commonly in patients treated with coxibs than with tNSAIDs.

NSAIDs promote reabsorption of K^+ as a result of decreased availability of Na^+ at distal tubular sites and suppression of the PG-induced secretion of renin. The latter effect may account in part for the usefulness of NSAIDs in the treatment of Bartter syndrome (see "Bartter Syndrome").

Analgesic Nephropathy. Analgesic nephropathy is a condition of slowly progressive renal failure, decreased concentrating capacity of the renal tubule, and sterile pyuria. Risk factors are the chronic use of high doses of combinations of NSAIDs and frequent urinary tract infections. If recognized early, discontinuation of NSAIDs permits recovery of renal function.

Pregnancy and Lactation. In the hours before parturition, there is induction of myometrial COX-2 expression, and levels of PGE_2 and $PGF_{2\alpha}$ increase markedly in the myometrium during labor (Slater et al., 2002). Prolongation of gestation by NSAIDs has been demonstrated in model systems and in humans. Some NSAIDs, particularly indomethacin, have been used off-label to terminate preterm labor. However, this use is associated with closure of the ductus arteriosus and impaired fetal circulation *in utero*, particularly in fetuses older than 32 weeks' gestation. COX-2–selective inhibitors have been used off-label as tocolytic agents; this use has been associated with stenosis of the ductus arteriosus and oligohydramnios. Finally, the use of NSAIDs and aspirin late in pregnancy may increase the risk of postpartum hemorrhage. Therefore, pregnancy, especially close to term, is a relative contraindication to the use of all NSAIDs. In addition, their use must be weighed against potential fetal risk, even in cases of premature labor, and especially in cases of pregnancy-induced hypertension (Duley et al., 2004).

Hypersensitivity. Certain individuals display hypersensitivity to aspirin and NSAIDs, as manifested by symptoms that range from vasomotor rhinitis, generalized urticaria, and bronchial asthma to laryngeal edema, bronchoconstriction, flushing, hypotension, and shock. Aspirin intolerance is a contraindication to therapy with any other NSAID because cross-sensitivity can provoke a life-threatening reaction reminiscent of anaphylactic shock. Despite the resemblance to anaphylaxis, this reaction does not appear to be immunological in nature.

Although less common in children, this cross-sensitivity may occur in 10-25% of patients with asthma, nasal polyps, or chronic urticaria and in 1% of apparently healthy individuals. It is provoked by even low doses (<80 mg) of aspirin and apparently involves COX inhibition. Cross-sensitivity extends to other salicylates, structurally dissimilar NSAIDs, and rarely acetaminophen (see "Adverse Effects" in the "Acetaminophen" section). Treatment of aspirin hypersensitivity is similar to that of other severe hypersensitivity reactions, with support of vital organ function and administration of epinephrine. Aspirin hypersensitivity is associated with an increase in biosynthesis of LTs, perhaps reflecting diversion of AA to LOX metabolism. Indeed, results in a small number of patients suggest that blockade of 5-LOX with the drug zileuton or off-label use of the LT-receptor antagonists may ameliorate the symptoms and signs of aspirin intolerance, albeit incompletely.

Aspirin Resistance. All forms of treatment failure with aspirin have been collectively called *aspirin resistance*. Although this has attracted much attention, there is little information concerning the prevalence of a stable, aspirin-specific resistance or the precise mechanisms that might convey this "resistance." Genetic variants of COX-1 that co-segregate with resistance have been described, but the relation to clinical outcome is not clear.

Reye's Syndrome. Due to the possible association with Reye's syndrome, aspirin and other salicylates are contraindicated in children and young adults <20 years of age with viral illness–associated fever. Reye's syndrome, a severe and often fatal disease, is characterized by the acute onset of encephalopathy, liver dysfunction, and fatty infiltration of the liver and other viscera (Glasgow and Middleton, 2001). The etiology and pathophysiology are not clear, nor is it clear whether a causal relationship between aspirin and Reye's syndrome exists (Schror, 2007). However, the epidemiologic evidence for an association between aspirin use and Reye's syndrome seemed sufficiently compelling that labeling of aspirin and aspirin-containing medications to indicate Reye's syndrome as a risk in children was first mandated in 1986 and extended to bismuth subsalicylate in 2004. Since then, the use of aspirin in children has declined dramatically, and Reye's syndrome has almost disappeared. Acetaminophen has not been implicated in Reye's syndrome and is the drug of choice for antipyresis in children, teens, and young adults.

Concomitant NSAIDs and Low-Dose Aspirin. Many patients combine either tNSAIDs or COX-2 inhibitors with "cardioprotective," low-dose aspirin. Epidemiological studies suggest that this combination therapy increases significantly the likelihood of GI adverse events over either class of NSAID alone.

Prior occupancy of the active site of platelet COX-1 by the commonly consumed tNSAID ibuprofen impedes access of aspirin to its target Ser 529 and prevents irreversible inhibition of platelet function (Catella-Lawson et al., 2001). Epidemiological studies have provided conflicting data as to whether this adversely impacts clinical outcomes, but they generally are constrained by the use of prescription databases to examine an interaction between two drug groups commonly obtained without prescription. Evidence in support of this interaction has been observed in comparing ibuprofen-treated patients with and without aspirin in two coxib outcome studies (CLASS and TARGET), but the trials were not powered to address this question definitively. In theory, this interaction should not occur with selective COX-2 inhibitors, because mature human platelets lack COX-2. However, the GI safety advantage of NSAIDs selective for COX-2 is lost when they are combined with low-dose aspirin.

Drug Interactions

Angiotensin-converting enzyme (ACE) inhibitors act, at least partly, by preventing the breakdown of kinins that stimulate PG production. Thus, it is logical that NSAIDs might attenuate the effectiveness of ACE inhibitors by blocking the production of vasodilator and natriuretic PGs. Due to hyperkalemia, the combination of NSAIDs and ACE inhibitors also can produce marked bradycardia leading to syncope, especially in the elderly and in patients with hypertension, diabetes mellitus, or ischemic heart disease. Corticosteroids and SSRIs may increase the frequency or severity of GI complications when combined with NSAIDs. NSAIDs may augment the risk of bleeding in patients receiving warfarin both because almost all tNSAIDs suppress normal platelet function temporarily during the dosing interval and because some NSAIDs also increase warfarin levels by interfering with its metabolism; thus, concurrent administration should be avoided. Many NSAIDs are highly bound to plasma proteins and thus may displace other drugs from their binding sites. Such interactions can occur in patients given salicylates or other NSAIDs together with warfarin, sulfonylurea hypoglycemic agents, or methotrexate; the dosage of such agents may require adjustment to prevent toxicity. Patients taking lithium should be monitored because certain NSAIDs (e.g., piroxicam) can reduce the renal excretion of this drug and lead to toxicity, while others can decrease lithium levels (e.g., sulindac).

Pediatric and Geriatric Indications and Problems

Therapeutic Uses in Children. Therapeutic indications for NSAID use in children include fever, mild pain, postoperative pain, and inflammatory disorders, such as juvenile arthritis and Kawasaki disease. Inflammation associated with cystic fibrosis has emerged as a potential indication for pediatric NSAID use (Konstan et al., 1995); however, concern about GI adverse effects has limited NSAID use for this indication. The choice of drugs for children is considerably restricted; only drugs that have been extensively tested in children should be used (acetaminophen, ibuprofen, and naproxen).

Kawasaki Disease. Aspirin generally is avoided in pediatric populations due to its potential association with Reye's syndrome (see "Reye's Syndrome"). However, high doses of aspirin (30-100 mg/kg/day) are used to treat children during the acute phase of Kawasaki disease, followed by low-dose antiplatelet therapy in the subacute phase. Aspirin is thought to reduce the likelihood of aneurysm formation as a consequence of the vasculitis particularly in the coronary arteries. Small randomized studies did not conclusively show whether aspirin adds benefit beyond the standard treatment of Kawasaki disease with intravenous immunoglobulin (Baumer et al., 2006).

Pharmacokinetics in Children. Despite the recognition that age-dependent differences in gastric emptying time, plasma protein binding capacity and oxidative liver metabolism affect NSAID pharmacokinetics in children, dosing recommendations frequently are based on extrapolation of pharmacokinetic data from adults. The majority of pharmacokinetic studies that were performed in children involved patients >2 years of age, which often provide insufficient data for dose selection in younger infants. For example, the pharmacokinetics of the most commonly used NSAID in children, acetaminophen, differ substantially between the neonatal period and older children or adults. The systemic bioavailability of rectal acetaminophen formulations in neonates and preterm babies is higher than in older patients. Acetaminophen clearance is reduced in preterm neonates probably due to their immature glucuronide conjugation system (sulphatation is the principal route of biotransformation at this age). Therefore, acetaminophen dosing intervals need to be extended (8-12 hours) or daily doses reduced to avoid accumulation and liver toxicity. Aspirin elimination also is delayed in neonates and young infants compared to adults bearing the risk of accumulation.

Disease also may affect NSAID disposition in children. For example, ibuprofen plasma concentrations are reduced and clearance increased (~80%) in children with cystic fibrosis. This probably is related to the GI and hepatic pathologies associated with this disease. Aspirin's kinetics are markedly altered during the febrile phase of rheumatic fever or Kawasaki vasculitis. The reduction in serum albumin associated with these conditions causes an elevation of the free salicylate concentration, which may saturate renal excretion and result in salicylate accumulation to toxic levels. In addition to dose reduction, monitoring of the free drug may be warranted in these situations.

Pharmacokinetics in the Elderly. Physiological changes in absorption, distribution, and elimination in aging patients can be expected to affect the pharmacokinetics of most drugs, including NSAIDs. Coincident diseases may further complicate the prediction of the response to the drug. The clearance of many NSAIDs is reduced in the elderly due to changes in hepatic metabolism. Particularly NSAIDs with a long $t_{1/2}$ and primarily oxidative metabolism (i.e., piroxicam, tenoxicam, celecoxib) have elevated plasma concentrations in elderly patients. For example, plasma concentrations after the same dose of celecoxib may rise up to 2-fold higher in patients >65 years of age than in patients <50 years of age (U.S. Food and Drug Administration, 2001), warranting careful dose adjustment. The capacity of plasma albumin to bind drugs is diminished in older patients and may result in higher concentrations of unbound NSAIDs. Free naproxen concentrations, e.g., are markedly increased in older patients, although total plasma concentrations essentially are unchanged. The higher susceptibility of older patients to GI complications may be due to both a reduction in gastric mucosal defense and to elevated total and/or free NSAID concentrations. Generally, it is advisable to start most NSAIDs at a low dosage in the elderly and increase the dosage only if the therapeutic efficacy is insufficient.

SPECIFIC PROPERTIES OF INDIVIDUAL NSAIDS

General properties shared by tNSAIDs (including aspirin and acetaminophen) and COX-2–selective NSAIDs were considered in the preceding section, "Nonsteroidal Anti-Inflammatory Drugs." In the following section, important characteristics of individual substances are discussed. NSAIDs are grouped by their chemical similarity (Figure 34–1).

ASPIRIN AND OTHER SALICYLATES

Despite the introduction of many new drugs, aspirin is still the most widely consumed analgesic, antipyretic, and anti-inflammatory agent and is the standard for the comparison and evaluation of the others. Aspirin is the most common household analgesic; yet, because the drug is so generally available, the possibility of misuse and serious toxicity probably is underappreciated, and it remains a cause of fatal poisoning in children.

Chemistry. Salicylic acid (orthohydroxybenzoic acid) is so irritating that it can only be used externally; therefore various derivatives of this acid have been synthesized for systemic use. These comprise two large classes, namely esters of salicylic acid obtained from substitutions within the carboxyl group and salicylate esters of organic acids, in which the carboxyl group is retained and substitution is made in the hydroxyl group. For example, aspirin is an ester of acetic acid. In addition, there are sodium, magnesium, and choline salts of salicylic acid. The chemical relationships can be seen from the structural formulas shown in Figure 34–3. Substitutions on the carboxyl or hydroxyl groups change the potency or toxicity of salicylates. The ortho position of the hydroxyl group is an important feature for the action of the salicylates. The effects of simple substitutions on the benzene ring have been studied extensively. A difluorophenyl derivative, diflunisal, also is available for clinical use.

Mechanism of Action

Salicylates generally act by virtue of their content of salicylic acid. The effects of aspirin are largely caused by its capacity to acetylate proteins, as described in "Irreversible Cyclooxygenase Inhibition by Aspirin," although high concentrations of aspirin result in therapeutic plasma concentrations of salicylic acid. In addition to their effect on PG biosynthesis (see the NSAIDs section and Chapter 33), the mechanism of action of the salicylates in rheumatic disease also may involve effects on other cellular and immunological processes in mesenchymal and connective tissues. Attention has been directed to the capacity of salicylates to suppress a variety of antigen–antibody reactions. These include the inhibition of antibody production, of antigen–antibody aggregation, and of antigen-induced release of histamine. Salicylates also induce a nonspecific stabilization of

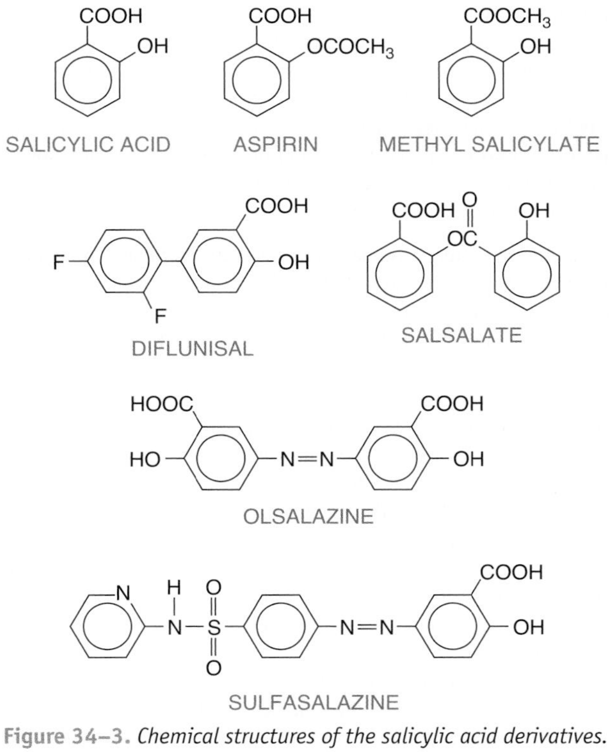

COOH OH — SALICYLIC ACID
COOH $OCOCH_3$ — ASPIRIN
$COOCH_3$ OH — METHYL SALICYLATE
F F COOH OH — DIFLUNISAL
COOH O OC OH — SALSALATE
HOOC HO N=N COOH OH — OLSALAZINE
N H N O S O N=N COOH OH — SULFASALAZINE

Figure 34–3. *Chemical structures of the salicylic acid derivatives.*

capillary permeability during immunological insults. The concentrations of salicylates needed to produce these effects are high, and the relationship of these effects to the anti-rheumatic efficacy of salicylates is not clear. Salicylates also can influence the metabolism of connective tissue, and these effects may be involved in their anti-inflammatory action. For example, salicylates can affect the composition, biosynthesis, or metabolism of connective tissue mucopolysaccharides in the ground substance that provides barriers to the spread of infection and inflammation.

Absorption, Distribution, and Elimination

Absorption. Orally ingested salicylates are absorbed rapidly, partly from the stomach but mostly from the upper small intestine. Appreciable concentrations are found in plasma in <30 minutes; after a single dose, a peak value is reached in ~1 hour and then declines gradually. The rate of absorption is determined by many factors, particularly the disintegration and dissolution rates of the tablets administered, the pH at the mucosal surface, and gastric emptying time.

Salicylate absorption occurs by passive diffusion primarily of undissociated salicylic acid or ASA across GI membranes and hence is influenced by gastric pH. Even though salicylate is more ionized as the pH is increased, a rise in pH also increases the solubility of salicylate and thus dissolution of the tablets. The overall effect is to enhance absorption. As a result, there is little meaningful difference between the rates of absorption of sodium salicylate, aspirin, and the numerous buffered preparations of salicylates. The presence of food delays absorption of salicylates. Rectal absorption of salicylate usually is slower than oral absorption and is incomplete and inconsistent.

Salicylic acid is absorbed rapidly from the intact skin, especially when applied in oily liniments or ointments, and systemic poisoning has occurred from its application to large areas of skin. Methyl salicylate likewise is speedily absorbed when applied cutaneously; however, its GI absorption may be delayed many hours, making gastric lavage effective for removal even in poisonings that present late after oral ingestion.

Distribution. After absorption, salicylates are distributed throughout most body tissues and transcellular fluids, primarily by pH-dependent passive processes. Salicylates are transported actively by a low-capacity, saturable system out of the cerebrospinal fluid (CSF) across the choroid plexus. The drugs readily cross the placental barrier.

The volume of distribution of usual doses of aspirin and sodium salicylate in normal subjects averages ~170 mL/kg of body weight; at high therapeutic doses, this volume increases to ~500 mL/kg because of saturation of binding sites on plasma proteins. Ingested aspirin mainly is absorbed as such, but some enters the systemic circulation as salicylic acid after hydrolysis by esterases in the GI mucosa and liver. Aspirin can be detected in the plasma only for a short time as a result of hydrolysis in plasma, liver, and erythrocytes; for example, 30 minutes after a dose of 0.65 g, only 27% of the total plasma salicylate is in the acetylated form. Methyl salicylate also is hydrolyzed rapidly to salicylic acid, mainly in the liver.

Roughly 80-90% of the salicylate in plasma is bound to proteins, especially albumin, at concentrations encountered clinically; the proportion of the total that is bound declines as plasma concentrations increase. Hypoalbuminemia, as may occur in rheumatoid arthritis, is associated with a proportionately higher level of free salicylate in the plasma. Salicylate competes with a variety of compounds for plasma protein binding sites; these include thyroxine, triiodothyronine, penicillin, phenytoin, sulfinpyrazone, bilirubin, uric acid, and other NSAIDs such as naproxen. Aspirin is bound to a more limited extent; however, it acetylates human plasma albumin *in vivo* by reaction with the ε-amino group of lysine and may change the binding of other drugs to albumin. Aspirin also acetylates hormones, DNA, and hemoglobin and other proteins.

Elimination. The biotransformation of salicylates takes place in many tissues, but particularly in the hepatic endoplasmic reticulum and mitochondria. The three chief metabolic products are salicyluric acid (the glycine conjugate), the ether or phenolic glucuronide, and the ester or acyl glucuronide. In addition, a small fraction is oxidized to gentisic acid (2,5-dihydroxybenzoic acid) and to 2,3-dihydroxybenzoic and 2,3,5-trihydroxybenzoic acids; gentisuric acid, the glycine conjugate of gentisic acid, also is formed.

Salicylates are excreted in the urine as free salicylic acid (10%), salicyluric acid (75%), salicylic phenolic (10%) and acyl glucuronides (5%), and gentisic acid (<1%). However, excretion of free salicylates is extremely variable and depends on the dose and the urinary pH. In alkaline urine, >30% of the ingested drug may be eliminated as free salicylate, whereas in acidic urine, this may be as low as 2%.

The plasma $t_{1/2}$ for aspirin is ~20 minutes, and for salicylate is 2-3 hours at antiplatelet doses, rising to 12 hours at usual anti-inflammatory doses. The $t_{1/2}$ of salicylate may be as long as 15-30 hours at high therapeutic doses or when there is intoxication. This dose-dependent elimination is the result of the limited capacity of the liver to form salicyluric acid and the phenolic glucuronide, resulting in a larger proportion of unchanged drug being excreted in the urine at higher doses.

Salicylate metabolism shows high intersubject variability due to the variable contribution of different metabolic pathways. Women frequently exhibit higher plasma concentrations, perhaps due to lower intrinsic esterase activity and gender differences in hepatic metabolism. Salicylate clearance is reduced and salicylate exposure is significantly increased in the elderly (see "Pharmacokinetics in the Elderly"). The plasma concentration of salicylate is increased by conditions that decrease glomerular filtration rate or reduce proximal tubule secretion, such as renal disease or the presence of inhibitors that compete for the transport system (e.g., probenecid). Changes in urinary pH also have significant effects on salicylate excretion. For example, the clearance of salicylate is about four times as great at pH 8 as at pH 6, and it is well above the glomerular filtration rate at pH 8. High rates of urine flow decrease tubular reabsorption, whereas the opposite is true in oliguria. In case of an overdose, hemodialysis and hemofiltration techniques remove salicylic acid effectively from the circulation.

Monitoring of Plasma Salicylate Concentrations. Aspirin is one of the NSAIDs for which plasma salicylate can provide a means to monitor therapy and toxicity. Intermittent analgesic–antipyretic doses of aspirin typically produce plasma aspirin levels of <20 μg/mL and plasma salicylate levels of <60 μg/mL. The daily ingestion of anti-inflammatory doses of 4-5 g of aspirin produces plasma salicylate levels in the range of 120-350 μg/mL. Optimal anti-inflammatory effects for patients with rheumatic diseases require plasma salicylate concentrations of 150-300 μg/mL. Significant adverse effects can be seen at levels of >300 μg/mL. At lower concentrations, the drug clearance is nearly constant (despite the fact that saturation of metabolic capacity is approached) because the fraction of drug that is free, and thus available for metabolism or excretion, increases as binding sites on plasma proteins are saturated. The total concentration of salicylate in plasma is therefore a relatively linear function of dose at lower concentrations. At higher concentrations, however, as metabolic pathways of disposition become saturated, small increments in dose can disproportionately increase plasma salicylate concentration. Failure to anticipate this phenomenon can lead to toxicity.

Therapeutic Uses

Systemic Uses. The dose of salicylate depends on the condition being treated.

The analgesic–antipyretic dose of aspirin for adults is 324-1000 mg orally every 4-6 hours. The anti-inflammatory doses of aspirin recommended for arthritis, spondyloarthropathies, and systemic lupus erythematosus (SLE) range from 3-4 g/day in divided doses. Salicylates are contraindicated for fever associated with viral infection in children (see "Reye's Syndrome"); for nonviral etiologies, 40-60 mg/kg/day given in six divided doses every 4 hours is recommended. The maximum recommended daily dose of aspirin for adults and children >12 years or older is 4 g. The rectal administration of aspirin suppositories may be preferred in infants or when the oral route is unavailable. Although aspirin is regarded as the standard against which other drugs should be compared for the treatment of rheumatoid arthritis, many clinicians favor the use of other NSAIDs perceived to have better GI tolerability, even though this perception remains untested by randomized clinical trials. Salicylates suppress clinical signs and improve tissue inflammation in acute rheumatic fever. Much of the possible subsequent tissue damage, such as cardiac lesions and other visceral involvement, however, is unaffected by salicylate therapy.

Other salicylates available for systemic use include salsalate (salicylsalicylic acid), which is hydrolyzed to salicylic acid during and after absorption, and magnesium salicylate (tablets; DOAN'S, MOMEMTUM, others). A combination of choline salicylate and magnesium salicylate (choline magnesium–trisalicylate) also is available.

Diflunisal is a difluorophenyl derivative of salicylic acid that is not converted to salicylic acid *in vivo*. Diflunisal is more potent than aspirin in anti-inflammatory tests in animals and appears to be a competitive inhibitor of COX. However, it is largely devoid of antipyretic effects, perhaps because of poor penetration into the CNS. The drug has been used primarily as an analgesic in the treatment of osteoarthritis and musculoskeletal strains or sprains; in these circumstances, it is about three to four times more potent than aspirin. The usual initial dose is 1000 mg, followed by 500 mg every 8-12 hours. For rheumatoid arthritis or osteoarthritis, 250-1000 mg/day is administered in two divided doses; maintenance dosage should not exceed 1.5 g/day. Diflunisal produces fewer auditory side effects (see "Ototoxic Effects") and appears to cause fewer and less intense GI and antiplatelet effects than does aspirin.

Local Uses. Mesalamine (5-aminosalicylic acid) is a salicylate that is used for its local effects in the treatment of inflammatory bowel disease (see Chapter 47, especially Figure 47–4). The drug as an immediate-release formulation would not be effective orally because it is poorly absorbed and is inactivated before reaching the lower intestine. However, oral formulations that deliver drug to the lower intestine—mesalamine formulated in a pH-sensitive, polymer-coated, delayed-release tablet (ASACOL, LIALDA); an extended-release mesalamine capsule (APRISO); and olsalazine (sodium azodisalicylate, a dimer of 5-aminosalicylate linked by an azo bond; DIPENTUM)—are efficacious in the treatment of inflammatory bowel disease (in particular, ulcerative colitis). Mesalamine is available as a rectal enema (ROWASA, others) for treatment of mild to moderate ulcerative colitis, proctitis, and proctosigmoiditis and as a rectal suppository (CANASA) for the treatment of active ulcerative proctitis. Sulfasalazine (salicylazosulfapyridine; AZULFIDINE, others) contains mesalamine linked covalently to sulfapyridine, and balsalazide (COLAZAL, others) contains mesalamine linked to the inert carrier molecule 4-aminobenzoyl-β-alanine. Both drugs are absorbed poorly after oral administration and cleaved to the active moiety by bacteria in the colon. Sulfasalazine and olsalazine have been used in the treatment of rheumatoid arthritis and ankylosing spondylitis. Some over-the-counter medications to relieve indigestion and diarrhea agents contain bismuth subsalicylate (PEPTO-BISMOL, others) and have the potential to cause salicylate intoxication, particularly in children.

The keratolytic action of free salicylic acid is employed for the local treatment of warts, corns, fungal infections, and certain types of eczematous dermatitis. After treatment with salicylic acid, tissue cells swell, soften, and desquamate. Methyl salicylate (oil of wintergreen) is a common ingredient of ointments and deep-heating liniments used in the management of musculoskeletal pain; it also is available in herbal medicines and as a flavoring agent. The cutaneous application of methyl salicylate can result in pharmacologically active, and even toxic, systemic salicylate concentrations and has been reported to increase prothrombin time in patients receiving warfarin.

Adverse Effects

Respiration. Salicylates increase O_2 consumption and CO_2 production (especially in skeletal muscle) at anti-inflammatory doses; these effects are a result of uncoupling oxidative phosphorylation. The increased production of CO_2 stimulates respiration (mainly by an increase in depth of respiration with only a slight increase in rate). The increased alveolar ventilation balances the increased CO_2 production, and thus plasma CO_2 tension (PCO_2) does not change or may decrease slightly. Salicylates also stimulate the respiratory center directly in the medulla. Respiratory rate and depth increases, the Pco_2 falls, and primary respiratory alkalosis ensues. Both mechanisms can occur in parallel, although the stimulation of ventilation after initiation of therapy is predominantly driven by the increase in the metabolic rate, and direct effects of salicylates on the central nervous respiratory center contribute later at higher steady-state concentrations.

Acid–Base and Electrolyte Balance and Renal Effects. Therapeutic doses of salicylate produce definite changes in the acid–base balance and electrolyte pattern. Compensation for the initial event, respiratory alkalosis (see "Respiration" in the aspirin section), is achieved by increased renal excretion of bicarbonate, which is accompanied by increased Na^+ and K^+ excretion; plasma bicarbonate is thus lowered, and blood pH returns toward normal. This is the stage of compensatory renal acidosis. This stage is most often seen in adults given intensive salicylate therapy and seldom proceeds further unless toxicity ensues (see "Salicylate Intoxication"). Salicylates can cause retention of salt and water, as well as acute reduction of renal function in patients with congestive heart failure, renal disease, or hypovolemia. Although long-term use of salicylates alone rarely is associated with nephrotoxicity, the prolonged and excessive ingestion of analgesic mixtures containing salicylates in combination with other NSAIDs can produce papillary necrosis and interstitial nephritis (see "Analgesic Nephropathy").

Cardiovascular Effects. Low doses of aspirin (≤100 mg daily) are used widely for their cardioprotective effects. At high therapeutic doses (≥3 g daily), as might be given for acute rheumatic fever, salt and water retention can lead to an increase (≤20%) in circulating plasma volume and decreased hematocrit (via a dilutional effect). There is a tendency for the peripheral vessels to dilate because of a direct effect on vascular smooth muscle. Cardiac output and work are increased. Those with carditis or compromised cardiac function may not have sufficient cardiac reserve to meet the increased demands, and congestive cardiac failure and pulmonary edema can occur. High doses of salicylates can produce noncardiogenic pulmonary edema, particularly in older patients who ingest salicylates regularly over a prolonged period.

GI Effects. The ingestion of salicylates may result in epigastric distress, nausea, and vomiting. Salicylates also may cause gastric ulceration, exacerbation of peptic ulcer symptoms (heartburn, dyspepsia), GI hemorrhage, and erosive gastritis. These effects occur primarily with acetylated salicylates (i.e., aspirin). Because nonacetylated salicylates lack the ability to acetylate COX and thereby irreversibly inhibit its activity, they are weaker inhibitors than aspirin.

Aspirin-induced gastric bleeding sometimes is painless and, if unrecognized, may lead to iron-deficiency anemia. The daily ingestion of anti-inflammatory doses of aspirin (3-4 g) results in an average fecal blood loss of between 3 and 8 mL/day, as compared with ~0.6 mL/day in untreated subjects. Gastroscopic examination of aspirin-treated subjects often reveals discrete ulcerative and hemorrhagic lesions of the gastric mucosa; in many cases, multiple hemorrhagic lesions with sharply demarcated areas of focal necrosis are observed.

Hepatic Effects. Salicylates can cause hepatic injury, usually in patients treated with high doses of salicylates that result in plasma concentrations of >150 μg/mL. The injury is not an acute effect; rather, the onset characteristically occurs after several months of treatment. The majority of cases occur in patients with connective tissue disorders. There usually are no symptoms, simply an increase in serum levels of hepatic transaminases, but some patients note right upper quadrant abdominal discomfort and tenderness. Overt jaundice is uncommon. The injury usually is reversible upon discontinuation of salicylates. However, the use of salicylates is contraindicated in patients with chronic liver disease. Considerable evidence, as discussed earlier in "Reye's Syndrome," implicates the use of salicylates as an important factor in the severe hepatic injury and encephalopathy observed in Reye's syndrome. Large doses of salicylates may cause hyperglycemia and glycosuria and deplete liver and muscle glycogen.

Uricosuric Effects. The effects of salicylates on uric acid excretion are markedly dependent on dose. Low doses (1 or 2 g/day) may decrease urate excretion and elevate plasma urate concentrations; intermediate doses (2 or 3 g/day) usually do not alter urate excretion. Large doses (>5 g/day) induce uricosuria and lower plasma urate levels; however, such large doses are tolerated poorly. Even small doses of salicylate can block the effects of probenecid and other uricosuric agents that decrease tubular reabsorption of uric acid.

Effects on the Blood. Irreversible inhibition of platelet function is the mechanism underlying the cardioprotective effect of aspirin (see "Concomitant NSAIDs and Low-Dose Aspirin"). If possible, aspirin therapy should be stopped at least 1 week before surgery; however, preoperative aspirin often is recommended prior to carotid artery stenting, carotid endarterectomy, infrainguinal arterial bypass, and PCI procedures. Patients with severe hepatic damage, hypoprothrombinemia, vitamin K deficiency, or hemophilia should avoid aspirin because the inhibition of platelet hemostasis can result in hemorrhage. Care also should be exercised in the use of aspirin during long-term treatment with oral anticoagulant agents because of the combined danger of prolongation of bleeding time coupled with blood loss from the gastric mucosa. On the other hand, aspirin is used widely for the prophylaxis of thromboembolic disease, especially in the coronary and cerebral circulation, and is coupled frequently with oral anticoagulants in patients with bioprosthetic or mechanical heart valves (see Chapter 30).

Salicylates ordinarily do not alter the leukocyte or platelet count, the hematocrit, or the hemoglobin content. However, doses of 3-4 g/day markedly decrease plasma iron concentration and shorten erythrocyte survival time. Aspirin can cause a mild degree of hemolysis in individuals with a deficiency of glucose-6-phosphate dehydrogenase. As noted earlier (see "Cardiovascular Effects"), high doses (>3 g/day) can expand plasma volume and decrease hematocrit by dilution.

Endocrine Effects. Long-term administration of salicylates decreases thyroidal uptake and clearance of iodine, but increases O_2 consumption and the rate of disappearance of thyroxine and triiodothyronine from the circulation. These effects probably are caused by the competitive displacement by salicylate of thyroxine and triiodothyronine from transthyretin and the thyroxine-binding globulin in plasma (see Chapter 39).

Ototoxic Effects. Hearing impairment, alterations of perceived sounds, and tinnitus commonly occur during high-dose salicylate therapy. Tinnitus, historically used as an index of exceeding the acceptable plasma concentration in patients, is not a reliable guide; thus, surveillance for this symptom is no substitute for periodic monitoring of serum salicylate levels. Ototoxic symptoms sometimes are observed at low doses, and no threshold plasma concentration exists. Symptoms usually resolve within 2 or 3 days after withdrawal of the drug. Ototoxic symptoms are caused by increased labyrinthine pressure or an effect on the hair cells of the cochlea, perhaps secondary to vasoconstriction in the auditory microvasculature. As most competitive COX inhibitors are not associated with hearing loss or tinnitus, a direct effect of salicylic acid rather than suppression of PG synthesis is likely.

Salicylates and Pregnancy. Infants born to women who ingest salicylates for long periods may have significantly reduced birth weights. When administered during the third trimester, there also is an increase in perinatal mortality, anemia, antepartum and postpartum hemorrhage, prolonged gestation, and complicated deliveries; thus, its use during this period should be avoided. As mentioned earlier in "Pregnancy and Lactation," administration of NSAIDs during the third trimester of pregnancy also can cause premature closure of the ductus arteriosus. The use of aspirin has been advocated for the treatment of women at high risk of preeclampsia, but it is estimated that treatment of 90 women is required to prevent one case of preeclampsia (Villar et al., 2004).

Local Irritant Effects. Salicylic acid is irritating to skin and mucosa and destroys epithelial cells.

Drug Interactions. The plasma concentration of salicylates generally is little affected by other drugs, but concurrent administration of aspirin lowers the concentrations of indomethacin, naproxen, ketoprofen, and fenoprofen, at least in part by displacement from plasma proteins. Important adverse interactions of aspirin with warfarin, sulfonylureas, and methotrexate are mentioned earlier in "Drug Interactions." Other interactions of aspirin include the antagonism of spironolactone-induced natriuresis and the blockade of the active transport of penicillin from CSF to blood. Magnesium-aluminum hydroxide antacids can alkalize the urine enough to increase salicylic acid clearance significantly and reduce steady-state concentrations. Conversely, discontinuation of antacid therapy can increase plasma concentrations to toxic levels.

Salicylate Intoxication

Salicylate poisoning or serious intoxication often occurs in children and sometimes is fatal. CNS effects, intense hyperpnea, and hyperpyrexia are prominent symptoms. Salicylate intoxication should be seriously considered in any young child with coma, convulsions, or cardiovascular collapse. The fatal dose varies with the preparation of salicylate. Death has followed use of 10-30 g of sodium salicylate or aspirin in adults, but much larger amounts (130 g of aspirin in one case) have been ingested without a fatal outcome. The lethal dose of methyl salicylate (also known as oil of wintergreen, sweet birch oil, gaultheria oil, betula oil) is considerably less than that of sodium salicylate. As little as a taste of methyl salicylate by children <6 years of age and >4 mL (4.7 g) of methyl salicylate by children ≥6 years of age may cause severe systemic toxicity and warrants referral to an emergency department. Symptoms of poisoning by methyl salicylate differ little from those described earlier for aspirin in "Adverse Effects." The drug's odor can be detected easily on the breath and in the urine and vomitus. Poisoning by salicylic acid differs only in the increased prominence of GI symptoms due to the marked local irritation. Mild chronic salicylate intoxication is called *salicylism*. When fully developed, the syndrome includes headache, dizziness, tinnitus, difficulty hearing, dimness of vision, mental confusion, lassitude, drowsiness, sweating, thirst, hyperventilation, nausea, vomiting, and occasionally diarrhea.

Neurological Effects. In high doses, salicylates have toxic effects on the CNS, consisting of stimulation (including convulsions) followed by depression. Confusion, dizziness, tinnitus, high-tone deafness, delirium, psychosis, stupor, and coma may occur. Salicylates induce nausea and vomiting, which result from stimulation of sites that are accessible from the CSF, probably in the medullary chemoreceptor trigger zone. In humans, centrally induced nausea and vomiting often appear at plasma salicylate concentrations of ~270 μg/mL, but these same effects may occur at much lower plasma levels as a result of local gastric irritation.

Respiration. The respiratory effects of salicylates contribute to the serious acid–base balance disturbances that characterize poisoning by this class of compounds. Salicylates stimulate respiration indirectly by uncoupling of oxidative phosphorylation and directly by stimulation of the respiratory center in the medulla (see "Respiration" in the aspirin section). Uncoupling of oxidative phosphorylation also leads to excessive heat production, and salicylate toxicity is associated with hyperthermia, particularly in children. Marked hyperventilation occurs when the level approaches 500 μg/mL. However, should salicylate toxicity be associated with the co-administration of a barbiturate or opioid, then central respiratory depression will prevent hyperventilation, and the salicylate-induced uncoupling of oxidative phosphorylation will be associated with a marked increase in plasma Pco_2 and respiratory acidosis. Prolonged exposure to high doses of salicylates leads to depression of the medulla, with central respiratory depression and circulatory collapse, secondary to vasomotor depression. Because enhanced CO_2 production continues, respiratory acidosis ensues. Respiratory failure is the usual cause of death in fatal cases of salicylate poisoning. Elderly patients with chronic salicylate intoxication often develop noncardiogenic pulmonary edema, which is considered an indication for hemodialysis.

Acid–Base Balance and Electrolytes. As described earlier in "Acid–Base and Electrolyte Balance and Renal Effects" in the aspirin section, high therapeutic doses of salicylate are associated with a primary respiratory alkalosis and compensatory renal acidosis. Subsequent changes in acid–base status generally occur only when toxic doses of salicylates are ingested by infants and children or occasionally after large doses in adults. The phase of primary respiratory alkalosis rarely is recognized in children with salicylate toxicity. They usually present in a state of mixed respiratory and renal acidosis, characterized by a decrease in blood pH, a low plasma bicarbonate concentration, and normal or nearly normal plasma Pco_2. Direct salicylate-induced depression of respiration prevents adequate respiratory hyperventilation to match the increased peripheral production of CO_2. Consequently, plasma Pco_2 increases and blood pH decreases. Because the concentration of bicarbonate in plasma already is low due to increased renal bicarbonate excretion, the acid–base status at this stage essentially is an uncompensated respiratory acidosis. Superimposed, however, is a true metabolic acidosis caused by accumulation of acids as a

Management of Acetaminophen Overdose. Acetaminophen overdose constitutes a medical emergency (Heard, 2008). Severe liver damage occurs in 90% of patients with plasma concentrations of acetaminophen >300 μg/mL at 4 hours or 45 μg/mL at 15 hours after the ingestion of the drug. Minimal hepatic damage can be anticipated when the drug concentration is <120 μg/mL at 4 hours or 30 μg/mL at 12 hours after ingestion. The Rumack-Matthew nomogram relates the plasma levels of acetaminophen and time after ingestion to the predicted risk of liver injury (Rumack et al., 1981).

Early diagnosis and treatment of acetaminophen overdose is essential to optimize outcome. Perhaps 10% of poisoned patients who do not receive specific treatment develop severe liver damage; 10-20% of these eventually die of hepatic failure despite intensive supportive care. Activated charcoal, if given within 4 hours of ingestion, decreases acetaminophen absorption by 50-90% and is the preferred method of gastric decontamination. Gastric lavage generally is not recommended.

N-acetylcysteine (NAC) (MUCOMYST, ACETADOTE) is indicated for those at risk of hepatic injury. NAC therapy should be instituted in suspected cases of acetaminophen poisoning before blood levels become available, with treatment terminated if assay results subsequently indicate that the risk of hepatotoxicity is low. NAC functions by detoxifying NAPQI. It both repletes GSH stores and may conjugate directly with NAPQI by serving as a GSH substitute. There is some evidence that in cases of established acetaminophen toxicity, NAC may protect against extrahepatic injury by its anti-oxidant and anti-inflammatory properties. Even in the presence of activated charcoal, there is ample absorption of NAC, and neither should activated charcoal be avoided nor NAC administration be delayed because of concerns of a charcoal-NAC interaction. Adverse reactions to NAC include rash (including urticaria, which does not require drug discontinuation), nausea, vomiting, diarrhea, and rare anaphylactoid reactions. An oral loading dose of 140 mg/kg is given, followed by the administration of 70 mg/kg every 4 hours for 17 doses. Where available, the intravenous loading dose is 150 mg/kg by intravenous infusion in 200 mL of 5% dextrose over 60 minutes, followed by 50 mg/kg by intravenous infusion in 500 mL of 5% dextrose over 4 hours, then 100 mg/kg by intravenous infusion in 1000 mL of 5% dextrose over 16 hours.

In addition to NAC therapy, aggressive supportive care is warranted. This includes management of hepatic and renal failure if they occur and intubation if the patient becomes obtunded. Hypoglycemia can result from liver failure, and plasma glucose should be monitored closely. Fulminant hepatic failure is an indication for liver transplantation, and a liver transplant center should be contacted early in the course of treatment of patients who develop severe liver injury despite NAC therapy.

ACETIC ACID DERIVATIVES

Indomethacin

Indomethacin (INDOCIN, others), a methylated indole derivative, was introduced in 1963 and is indicated for the treatment of moderate to severe rheumatoid arthritis, osteoarthritis, and acute gouty arthritis; ankylosing spondylitis; and acute painful shoulder. Although indomethacin is still used clinically, mainly as a steroid-sparing agent, toxicity and the availability of safer alternatives have limited its use. Indomethacin is available in an injectable form for the closure of patent ductus arteriosus.

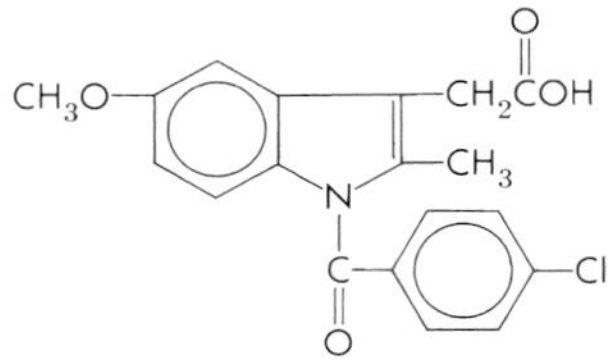

INDOMETHACIN

Mechanism of Action. Indomethacin is a more potent nonselective inhibitor of the COXs than is aspirin; it also inhibits the motility of polymorphonuclear leukocytes, depresses the biosynthesis of mucopolysaccharides, and may have a direct, COX-independent vasoconstrictor effect. Indomethacin has prominent anti-inflammatory and analgesic–antipyretic properties similar to those of the salicylates.

Absorption, Distribution, and Elimination. Oral indomethacin has excellent bioavailability. Peak concentrations occur 1-2 hours after dosing (Table 34–1). The concentration of the drug in the CSF is low, but its concentration in synovial fluid is equal to that in plasma within 5 hours of administration. There is enterohepatic cycling of the indomethacin metabolites and probably of indomethacin itself. The $t_{1/2}$ in plasma is variable, perhaps because of enterohepatic cycling, but averages ~2.5 hours.

Therapeutic Uses. Indomethacin is estimated to be ~20 times more potent than aspirin. A high rate of intolerance limits the long-term analgesic use of indomethacin. Likewise, it is not commonly used as an analgesic or antipyretic unless the fever has been refractory to other agents (e.g., Hodgkin's disease). When tolerated, indomethacin often is more effective than aspirin.

Indomethacin is FDA approved for closure of persistent patent ductus arteriosus in premature infants who weigh between 500 and 1750 g, who have a hemodynamically significant patent ductus arteriosus, and in whom other supportive maneuvers have been attempted. The regimen involves intravenous administration of 0.1-0.25 mg/kg every 12 hours for three doses, with the course repeated one time if necessary. Successful closure can be expected in >70% of neonates treated. The principal limitation of treating neonates is renal toxicity, and therapy is interrupted if the output of urine falls to <0.6 mL/kg/hr. Renal failure, enterocolitis, thrombocytopenia, or hyperbilirubinemia are contraindications to the use of indomethacin. Treatment with indomethacin also may decrease the incidence and severity of intraventricular hemorrhage in low-birth-weight neonates (Ment et al., 1994).

Adverse Effects and Drug Interactions. A very high percentage (35-50%) of patients receiving usual therapeutic doses of indomethacin experience untoward symptoms, and ~20% must discontinue its use because of the side effects. GI adverse events are common and can be fatal; elderly patients are at significantly greater risk. Diarrhea may occur and sometimes is associated with ulcerative lesions of the bowel. Acute pancreatitis has been reported, as have rare, but potentially fatal, cases of hepatitis. The most frequent CNS effect (indeed, the most common side effect) is severe frontal headache, occurring in 25-50% of patients who take the drug for long periods. Dizziness, vertigo, light-headedness, and mental confusion may occur. Seizures have been reported, as have severe depression, psychosis, hallucinations, and suicide. Caution is advised when administering indomethacin to elderly patients or to those with underlying epilepsy, psychiatric disorders, or Parkinson's disease, because they are at greater risk for the development of serious CNS adverse effects. Hematopoietic reactions include neutropenia, thrombocytopenia, and rarely aplastic anemia.

The total plasma concentration of indomethacin plus its inactive metabolites is increased by concurrent administration of probenecid, but indomethacin does not interfere with the uricosuric effect of probenecid. Indomethacin antagonizes the natriuretic and antihypertensive effects of furosemide and thiazide diuretics and blunts the antihypertensive effect of β-receptor antagonists, AT_1-receptor antagonists, and ACE inhibitors.

Sulindac

Sulindac (CLINORIL, others) is a congener of indomethacin, which was developed in an attempt to find a less toxic but effective alternative (see Haanen, 2001).

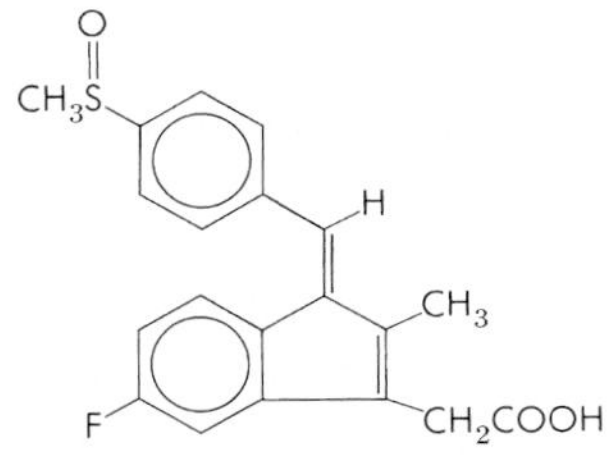

SULINDAC

Mechanism of Action. Sulindac is a prodrug and appears to be either inactive or relatively weak *in vitro*. The active sulfide metabolite is >500 times more potent than sulindac as an inhibitor of COX but less than half as potent as indomethacin. The early notion that gastric or intestinal mucosa is not directly exposed to high concentrations of active drug after oral administration of sulindac provided an initial rationale for the claim that sulindac results in a lower incidence of GI toxicity than indomethacin. However, this notion ignores the fact that the mucosa of the GI tract is directly exposed to circulating levels of active drug and no advantage of sulindac over non-indomethacin NSAIDs has materialized in clinical practice. Similarly, early clinical studies suggesting that sulindac, in contrast to other NSAIDs, did not alter renal PG levels and therefore might avoid the association with hypertension in susceptible individuals, have been discredited (Kulling et al., 1995). *In short, the same precautions that apply to other NSAIDs regarding patients at risk for GI toxicity, cardiovascular risk, and renal impairment also apply to sulindac.*

Absorption, Distribution, and Elimination. The metabolism and pharmacokinetics of sulindac are complex. About 90% of the drug is absorbed in humans after oral administration (Table 34–1). Peak concentrations of sulindac in plasma are attained within 1-2 hours, while those of the sulfide metabolite occur ~8 hours after oral administration. Sulindac undergoes two major biotransformations. It is oxidized to the sulfone and then reversibly reduced to the sulfide, the active metabolite. The sulfide is formed largely by the action of bowel microflora on sulindac excreted in the bile. All three compounds are found in comparable concentrations in human plasma. The $t_{1/2}$ of sulindac itself is ~7 hours, but the active sulfide has a $t_{1/2}$ as long as 18 hours. Sulindac and its metabolites undergo extensive enterohepatic circulation, and all are bound highly to plasma protein. Little of the sulfide (or of its conjugates) is found in urine. The principal components excreted in the urine are the sulfone and its conjugates, which account for nearly 30% of an administered dose; sulindac and its conjugates account for ~20%. Up to 25% of an oral dose may appear as metabolites in the feces.

Therapeutic Uses. Sulindac has been used mainly for the treatment of rheumatoid arthritis, osteoarthritis, ankylosing spondylitis, tendonitis, bursitis, acute painful shoulder, and the pain of acute gout. Its analgesic and anti-inflammatory effects are comparable to those achieved with aspirin. The most common dosage for adults is 150-200 mg twice a day. A use proposed for sulindac is to prevent colon cancer in patients with familial adenomatous polyposis (see "Cancer Chemoprevention").

Adverse Effects. Although the incidence of toxicity is lower than with indomethacin, untoward reactions to sulindac are common. The typical NSAID GI side effects are seen in nearly 20% of patients. CNS side effects as described earlier for indomethacin in "Adverse Effects and Drug Interactions" are seen in ≤10% of patients. Rash and pruritus occur in 5% of patients. Transient elevations of hepatic transaminases in plasma are less common.

Etodolac

Therapeutic Uses. Etodolac is an acetic acid derivative with some degree of COX-2 selectivity (Figure 34–1). Thus, at anti-inflammatory doses, the frequency of gastric irritation may be less than with other tNSAIDs (Warner et al., 1999). A single oral dose (200-400 mg) of etodolac provides postoperative analgesia that typically lasts for 6-8 hours. Etodolac also is effective in the treatment of osteoarthritis, rheumatoid arthritis, and mild to moderate pain, and the drug appears to be uricosuric. Sustained-release preparations are available, allowing once-a-day administration.

Adverse Effects. Etodolac appears to be relatively well tolerated. About 5% of patients who have taken the drug for ≤1 year discontinue treatment because of side effects, which include GI intolerance, rashes, and CNS effects.

Tolmetin

Therapeutic Uses. Tolmetin (TOLECTIN, others), a heteroaryl acetic acid derivative, is approved in the U.S. for the treatment of osteoarthritis, rheumatoid arthritis, and juvenile rheumatoid arthritis; it also has been used in the treatment of ankylosing spondylitis. Accumulation of the drug in synovial fluid begins within 2 hours and persists for ≤8 hours after a single oral dose. It appears to be approximately equivalent in efficacy to moderate doses of aspirin, in recommended doses (200-600 mg three times/day). The maximum recommended dose is 1.8 g/day, typically given in divided doses with meals, milk, or antacids to lessen abdominal discomfort. However, peak plasma concentrations and bioavailability are reduced when the drug is taken with food. Tolmetin possesses typical tNSAID properties and side effects.

Adverse Effects. Side effects occur in 25-40% of patients who take tolmetin, and 5-10% discontinue use of the drug. GI side effects are the most common (15%), and gastric ulceration has been observed. CNS side effects similar to those seen with indomethacin and aspirin occur, but they are less common and less severe.

Ketorolac

Ketorolac, a heteroaryl acetic acid derivative, is a potent analgesic but only a moderately effective anti-inflammatory drug.

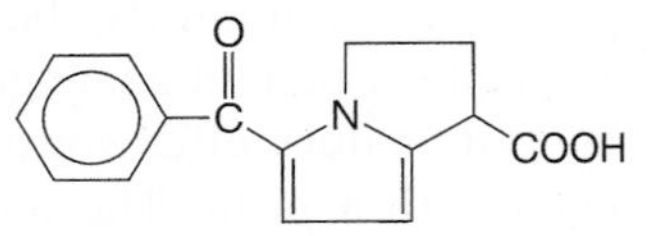

KETOROLAC

Therapeutic Uses. The use of ketorolac is limited to ≤5 days for acute pain requiring opioid-level analgesia and can be administered intramuscularly, intravenously, or orally. Like other NSAIDs, aspirin sensitivity is a contraindication to the use of ketorolac. Typical doses are 30-60 mg (intramuscular), 15-30 mg (intravenous), and 10-20 mg (oral). Ketorolac has a rapid onset of action and a short duration of action. It is widely used in postoperative patients, but it should not be used for routine obstetric analgesia. Topical (ophthalmic) ketorolac (ACULAR, others) is FDA approved for the treatment of seasonal allergic conjunctivitis and postoperative ocular inflammation after cataract extraction and after corneal refractive surgery. The pharmacology of ketorolac has been reviewed (Buckley and Brogden, 1990).

Adverse Effects. Side effects at usual oral doses include somnolence, dizziness, headache, GI pain, dyspepsia, nausea, and pain at the site of injection. The black box warning for ketorolac stresses the possibility of serious adverse GI, renal, bleeding, and hypersensitivity reactions from the use of this potent NSAID analgesic. Patients receiving greater than recommended doses or concomitant NSAID therapy and those at the extremes of age appear to be particularly at risk.

Nabumetone

Nabumetone is the prodrug of 6-methoxy-2-naphthylacetic acid; thus it is a weak inhibitor of COX *in vitro* but a potent COX inhibitor *in vivo*.

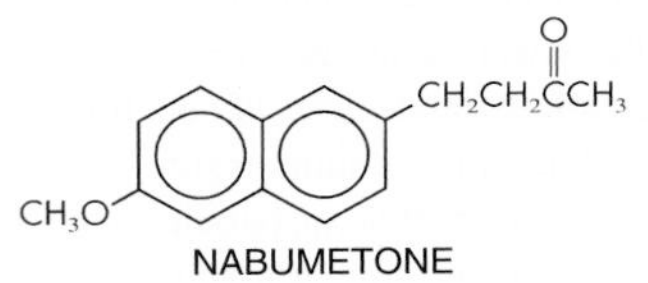

NABUMETONE

Therapeutic Uses. Nabumetone is an anti-inflammatory agent approved in 1991 for use in the U.S. It has been reviewed (Davies, 1997). Clinical trials with nabumetone have indicated substantial efficacy in the treatment of rheumatoid arthritis and osteoarthritis, with a relatively low incidence of side effects. The dose typically is 1000 mg given once daily. The drug also has off-label use in the short-term treatment of soft-tissue injuries.

Absorption, Distribution, and Elimination. Nabumetone is absorbed rapidly and is converted in the liver to one or more active metabolites, principally 6-methoxy-2-naphthylacetic acid, a potent nonselective inhibitor of COX. This metabolite, inactivated by *O*-demethylation in the liver, is then conjugated before excretion and is eliminated with a $t_{1/2}$ of ~24 hours.

Common Adverse Effects. Nabumetone is associated with crampy lower abdominal pain and diarrhea, but the incidence of GI ulceration appears to be lower than with other tNSAIDs, although randomized, controlled studies directly comparing tolerability and clinical outcomes have not been performed. Other side effects include rash, headache, dizziness, heartburn, tinnitus, and pruritus.

Diclofenac

Diclofenac, a phenylacetic acid derivative, is among the most commonly used NSAIDs in the E.U. (McNeely and Goa, 1999). It is marketed as a potassium salt (ZIPSOR, others) for oral administration, as an epolamine form (FLECTOR) for transdermal administration, and as a sodium salt for topical (SOLARAZE gel; VOLTAREN ophthalmic drops, others) or oral (VOLTAREN, VOLTAREN-XR, others) administration.

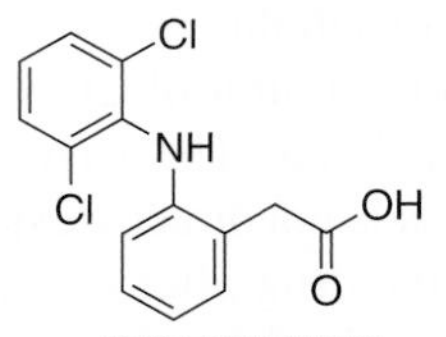

DICLOFENAC

Mechanism of Action. Diclofenac has analgesic, antipyretic, and anti-inflammatory activities. Its potency is substantially greater than that of indomethacin, naproxen, or several other tNSAIDs. The selectivity of diclofenac for COX-2 resembles that of celecoxib. In addition, diclofenac appears to reduce intracellular concentrations of free AA in leukocytes, perhaps by altering its release or uptake.

Absorption, Distribution, and Elimination. Diclofenac has rapid absorption, extensive protein binding, and a $t_{1/2}$ of 1-2 hours (Table 34–1). The short $t_{1/2}$ makes it necessary to dose diclofenac considerably higher than would be required to inhibit COX-2 fully at peak plasma concentrations to afford inhibition throughout the dosing interval. There is a substantial first-pass effect, such that only ~50% of diclofenac is available systemically. The drug accumulates in synovial fluid after oral administration, which may explain why its duration of therapeutic effect is considerably longer than its plasma $t_{1/2}$. Diclofenac is metabolized in the liver by a member of the CYP2C subfamily to 4-hydroxydiclofenac, the principal metabolite, and other hydroxylated forms; after glucuronidation and sulfation, the metabolites are excreted in the urine (65%) and bile (35%).

Therapeutic Uses. Diclofenac is approved in the U.S. for the long-term symptomatic treatment of rheumatoid arthritis, osteoarthritis, ankylosing spondylitis, pain, primary dysmenorrhea, and acute migraine. Four oral formulations are available: immediate-release tablets (CATAFLAM, others) and capsules (ZIPSOR), delayed-release tablets [VOLTAREN, VOLTAROL (U.K.), others], extended-release tablets (VOLTAREN-XR, others), and a powder for oral solution (CAMBIA). The usual daily oral dosage is 100-200 mg, given in several divided doses. For migraine, one packet of powder (50 mg) dissolved in 1-2 oz of water is administered. Diclofenac for topical use is available as a gel (VOLTAREN) and as a transdermal patch (FLECTOR); systemically active concentrations released from these preparations are thought to contribute more to symptom relief than direct transport through the skin into the inflamed tissue. Diclofenac also is available in combination with misoprostol, a PGE_1 analog (ARTHROTEC). This combination retains the efficacy of diclofenac while reducing the frequency of GI ulcers and erosions. In addition, an ophthalmic solution of diclofenac (VOLTAREN, others) is available for treatment of postoperative inflammation following cataract extraction and postoperative pain and photophobia following corneal refractive surgery.

Adverse Effects. Diclofenac produces side effects (particularly GI) in ~20% of patients, and ~2% of patients discontinue therapy as a result. The incidence of serious GI adverse effects did not differ between diclofenac and the COX-2–selective inhibitors, celecoxib (Juni et al., 2002) and etoricoxib (Cannon et al., 2006), likely because diclofenac exhibits a degree of COX-2 selectivity that is similar to that of celecoxib. The drug carries the same black box warning as all other tNSAIDs regarding cardiovascular events. Hypersensitivity reactions have occurred following topical application.

Modest elevation of hepatic transaminases in plasma occurs in 5-15% of patients. Although usually moderate, transaminase values may increase more than 3-fold in a small percentage of patients. The elevations usually are reversible. Another member of this phenylacetic acid family of NSAIDs, bromfenac, was withdrawn from the market because of its association with severe, irreversible liver injury in some patients. Bromfenac was re-licensed in the U.S. in 2005 as an ophthalmic solution (XIBROM) for postoperative ocular inflammation and pain following cataract extraction. The structurally similar nepafenac (NEVANAC) was licensed as an ophthalmic in the same year for the same indication. Lumiracoxib, another diclofenac analog (see the following section), was withdrawn from the market in several countries due to liver toxicity. Transaminases should be measured during the first 8 weeks of therapy with diclofenac, and the drug should be discontinued if abnormal values persist or if other signs or symptoms develop. Other untoward responses to diclofenac include CNS effects, rashes, allergic reactions, fluid retention, edema, and renal function impairment. The drug is not recommended for children, nursing mothers, or pregnant women. Consistent with its preference for COX-2, and unlike ibuprofen, diclofenac does not interfere with the antiplatelet effect of aspirin (Catella-Lawson et al., 2001).

Lumiracoxib

Lumiracoxib is an analog of diclofenac; it differs only by an additional methyl group and one fluorine substitution for chlorine. Lumiracoxib has greater COX-2 selectivity *in vitro* than any of the currently available coxibs. Its structural similarity to diclofenac is thought to account for their common hepatic adverse event profiles that may occur via a mechanism independent from COX inhibition. Lumiracoxib's potency is similar to that of naproxen. It is used at daily doses of 100 or 200 mg for osteoarthritis and 400 mg for acute pain. Lumiracoxib is not approved in the U.S., and marketing authorization was revoked in 2007 in many countries following reports of serious liver toxicity. Refer to earlier editions of this text for further details.

PROPIONIC ACID DERIVATIVES

Ibuprofen, the most commonly used tNSAID in the U.S., was the first member of the propionic acid class of NSAIDs to come into general use and is available without a prescription in the U.S. Naproxen, also available without prescription, has a longer but variable $t_{1/2}$, making twice-daily administration feasible (and perhaps once daily in some individuals). Oxaprozin also has a long $t_{1/2}$ and may be given once daily. Figure 34–4 shows the chemical structures of propionic acid derivatives.

Mechanism of Action. Propionic acid derivatives are nonselective COX inhibitors with the effects and side effects common to other tNSAIDs. Although there is considerable variation in their potency as COX inhibitors, this is not of obvious clinical consequence. Some of the propionic acid derivatives, particularly naproxen, have prominent inhibitory effects on leukocyte function, and some data suggest that naproxen may have slightly better efficacy with regard to analgesia and relief of morning stiffness. This suggestion of benefit accords with the clinical pharmacology of naproxen that suggests that some but not all individuals dosed with 500 mg twice daily sustain platelet inhibition throughout the dosing interval.

Therapeutic Uses. Ibuprofen, naproxen, flurbiprofen, fenoprofen, ketoprofen, and oxaprozin, are available in the U.S. Several additional agents in this class, including fenbufen, carprofen, pirprofen, indobufen, and tiaprofenic acid, are in use or under study in other countries.

Propionic acid derivatives are approved for use in the symptomatic treatment of rheumatoid arthritis and osteoarthritis. Some also are approved for pain, ankylosing spondylitis, acute gouty arthritis, tendinitis, bursitis, and migraine and for primary dysmenorrhea. Small clinical studies suggest that the propionic acid

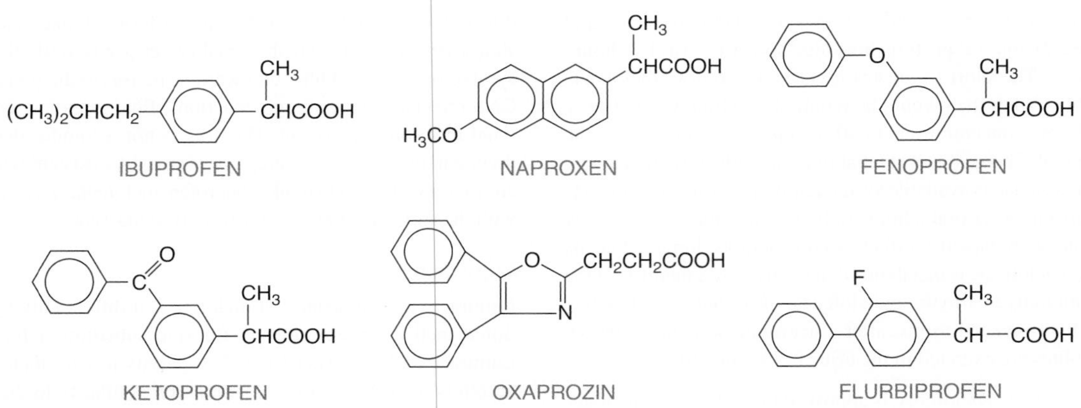

Figure 34–4. *Chemical structures of propionic acid derivatives.*

derivatives are comparable in efficacy to aspirin for the control of the signs and symptoms of rheumatoid arthritis and osteoarthritis, perhaps with improved tolerability.

Drug Interactions. Ibuprofen also has been shown to interfere with the antiplatelet effects of aspirin (see "Concomitant NSAIDs and Low-Dose Aspirin"). There also is evidence for a similar interaction between aspirin and naproxen. Propionic acid derivatives have not been shown to alter the pharmacokinetics of the oral hypoglycemic drugs or warfarin.

Ibuprofen

Absorption, Distribution, and Elimination. Ibuprofen is absorbed rapidly, bound avidly to protein, and undergoes hepatic metabolism (90% is metabolized to hydroxylate or carboxylate derivatives) and renal excretion of metabolites. The $t_{1/2}$ is ~2 hours. Slow equilibration with the synovial space means that its anti-arthritic effects may persist after plasma levels decline. In experimental animals, ibuprofen and its metabolites readily cross the placenta.

Therapeutic Uses. Ibuprofen [ADVIL, MOTRIN IB, BRUFEN (U.K.), ANADIN ULTRA (U.K.), others] is supplied as tablets, capsules, caplets, and gelcaps containing 50-800 mg; as oral drops; and as an oral suspension. Dosage forms containing ≤200 mg are available without a prescription. Ibuprofen is licensed for marketing in fixed-dose combinations with antihistamines, decongestants, oxycodone (COMBUNOX, others), and hydrocodone (REPREXAIN, IBUDONE, VICOPROFEN, others). An injectable formulation for closure of patent ductus (ibuprofen lysine; NEOPROFEN) has been licensed since 2006, and an injectable formulation for pain that was initially approved in 1974, CALDOLOR, was licensed by the FDA in 2009 for in-hospital use.

Doses of ≤800 mg four times daily can be used in the treatment of rheumatoid arthritis and osteoarthritis, but lower doses often are adequate. The usual dose for mild to moderate pain, such as that of primary dysmenorrhea, is 400 mg every 4-6 hours as needed. For pain or fever, intravenous ibuprofen is administered at a dose of 100-800 mg over 30 minutes every 4-6 hours. Ibuprofen has been reviewed (Davies, 1998a; Rainsford, 2003).

Adverse Effects. Ibuprofen is thought to be better tolerated than aspirin and indomethacin and has been used in patients with a history of GI intolerance to other NSAIDs. Nevertheless, 5-15% of patients experience GI side effects.

Epidemiological studies suggest that the relative risk of myocardial infarction is unaltered by ibuprofen or perhaps slightly increased but is considerably less than the risk from COX-2–selective inhibitors. Other adverse effects of ibuprofen have been reported less frequently. They include thrombocytopenia, rashes, headache, dizziness, blurred vision, and in a few cases, toxic amblyopia, fluid retention, and edema. Patients who develop ocular disturbances should discontinue the use of ibuprofen. Ibuprofen can be used occasionally by pregnant women; however, the concerns apply regarding third-trimester effects, including delay of parturition. Excretion into breast milk is thought to be minimal, so ibuprofen also can be used with caution by women who are breastfeeding.

Naproxen

Naproxen (ALEVE, NAPROSYN, others) is supplied as tablets, delayed-release tablets, controlled-release tablets, gelcaps, and caplets containing 200-750 mg of naproxen or naproxen sodium and as an oral suspension. Dosage forms containing ≤200 mg are available without a prescription. Naproxen is licensed for marketing in fixed-dose combinations with pseudoephedrine (ALEVE-D SINUS & COLD, others) and sumatriptan (TREXIMET) and is co-packaged with lansoprazole (PREVACID NAPRAPAC). Naproxen holds more FDA-approved indications than other tNSAIDs. It is indicated for juvenile and rheumatoid arthritis, osteoarthritis, ankylosing spondylitis, pain, primary dysmenorrhea, tendonitis, bursitis, and acute gout. The pharmacological properties and therapeutic uses of naproxen have been reviewed (Davies and Anderson, 1997b).

Absorption, Distribution, and Elimination. Naproxen is absorbed fully when administered orally. Food delays the rate but not the extent of absorption. Peak concentrations in plasma occur within 2-4 hours and are somewhat more rapid after the administration of naproxen sodium. Absorption is accelerated by the concurrent administration of sodium bicarbonate but delayed by magnesium oxide or aluminum hydroxide. Naproxen also is absorbed rectally but more slowly than after oral administration. The $t_{1/2}$ of naproxen in plasma is variable. About 14 hours in the young, it may increase about 2-fold in the elderly because of age-related decline in renal function (Table 34–1).

Metabolites of naproxen are excreted almost entirely in the urine. About 30% of the drug undergoes 6-demethylation, and most of this metabolite, as well as naproxen itself, is excreted as the glucuronide or other conjugates.

Naproxen is almost completely (99%) bound to plasma proteins after normal therapeutic doses. Naproxen crosses the placenta and appears in the milk of lactating women at ~1% of the maternal plasma concentration.

Common Adverse Effects. Epidemiological studies suggest that the relative risk of myocardial infarction may be reduced by ~10% by naproxen, compared to a reduction of 20-25% by aspirin. This is consistent with its long $t_{1/2}$, which may result in complete and persistent platelet inhibition in some patients. However, increased rates of cardiovascular events also have been reported (see the "Cardioprotection" and "Cardiovascular" sections). Typical GI adverse effects with naproxen occur at approximately the same frequency as with indomethacin and other tNSAIDs but perhaps with less severity. CNS side effects range from drowsiness, headache, dizziness, and sweating to fatigue, depression, and ototoxicity. Less common reactions include pruritus and a variety of dermatological problems. A few instances of jaundice, impairment of renal function, angioedema, thrombocytopenia, and agranulocytosis have been reported.

Other Propionic Acid Derivatives

Fenoprofen. The pharmacological properties and therapeutic uses of fenoprofen (NALFON 200, others) have been reviewed (Brogden et al., 1981). Oral doses of fenoprofen are readily but incompletely (85%) absorbed (Table 34–1). The concomitant administration of antacids does not seem to alter the concentrations that are achieved. The GI side effects of fenoprofen are similar to those of ibuprofen or naproxen and occur in ~15% of patients.

Ketoprofen. A more potent S-enantiomer is available in Europe (Barbanoj et al., 2001). In addition to COX inhibition, ketoprofen may stabilize lysosomal membranes and antagonize the actions of bradykinin. It is unknown if these actions are relevant to its efficacy in humans. Ketoprofen is conjugated with glucuronic acid in the liver, and the conjugate is excreted in the urine (Table 34–1). Patients with impaired renal function eliminate the drug more slowly. Approximately 30% of patients experience mild GI side effects with ketoprofen, which are decreased if the drug is taken with food or antacids.

Flurbiprofen. Flurbiprofen is available as tablets (ANSAID, others) and as an ophthalmic solution (OCUFEN, others) indicated for intraoperative miosis. The pharmacological properties, therapeutic indications, and adverse effects of orally administered flurbiprofen are similar to those of other anti-inflammatory derivatives of propionic acid (Table 34–1) and have been reviewed (Davies, 1995).

Oxaprozin. Oxaprozin (DAYPRO, others) has similar pharmacological properties, adverse effects, and therapeutic uses to those of other propionic acid derivatives (Davies, 1998b). However, its pharmacokinetic properties differ considerably. Peak plasma levels are not achieved until 3-6 hours after an oral dose, while its $t_{1/2}$ of 40-60 hours allows for once-daily administration.

THE FENAMATES

Mefenamic acid and meclofenamate are *N*-substituted phenylanthranilic acids. The pharmacological properties of the fenamates are those of typical tNSAIDs, and therapeutically, they have no clear advantages over others in the class.

Available Preparations and Therapeutic Uses. The fenamates include mefenamic, meclofenamic, and flufenamic acids. Mefenamic acid [PONSTEL, PONSTAN (U.K.), DYSMAN (U.K.)] and meclofenamate sodium have mostly been used in the short-term treatment of pain in soft-tissue injuries, dysmenorrhea, and rheumatoid and osteoarthritis; flufenamic acid is not licensed for use in the U.S. These drugs are not recommended for use in children or pregnant women.

Common Adverse Effects. Approximately 25% of users develop GI side effects at therapeutic doses. Roughly 5% of patients develop a reversible elevation of hepatic transaminases. Diarrhea, which may be severe and associated with steatorrhea and inflammation of the bowel, also is relatively common. Autoimmune hemolytic anemia is a potentially serious but rare side effect.

ENOLIC ACIDS (OXICAMS)

The oxicam derivatives are enolic acids that inhibit COX-1 and COX-2 and have anti-inflammatory, analgesic, and antipyretic activity. In general, they are nonselective COX inhibitors, although one member (meloxicam) shows modest COX-2 selectivity comparable to celecoxib in human blood *in vitro* and was approved as a COX-2–selective NSAID in some countries. The oxicam derivatives are similar in efficacy to aspirin, indomethacin, or naproxen for the long-term treatment of rheumatoid arthritis or osteoarthritis. Controlled trials comparing GI tolerability with aspirin have not been performed. The main advantage suggested for these compounds is their long $t_{1/2}$, which permits once-a-day dosing.

Piroxicam

The pharmacological properties and therapeutic uses of piroxicam (FELDENE, others) have been reviewed (Guttadauria, 1986).

Mechanism of Action. Piroxicam can inhibit activation of neutrophils, apparently independently of its ability to inhibit COX; hence, additional modes of anti-inflammatory action have been proposed, including inhibition of proteoglycanase and collagenase in cartilage.

Absorption, Distribution, and Elimination. Piroxicam is absorbed completely after oral administration and undergoes enterohepatic recirculation; peak concentrations in plasma occur within 2-4 hours (Table 34–1). Food may delay absorption. Estimates of the $t_{1/2}$ in plasma have been variable; the average is ~50 hours.

After absorption, piroxicam is extensively (99%) bound to plasma proteins. Concentrations in plasma and synovial fluid are similar at steady state (e.g., after 7-12 days). Less than 5% of the drug is excreted into the urine unchanged. The major metabolic transformation in humans is hydroxylation of the pyridyl ring (predominantly by an isozyme of the CYP2C subfamily), and this inactive metabolite and its glucuronide conjugate account for ~60% of the drug excreted in the urine and feces.

Therapeutic Uses. Piroxicam is approved in the U.S. for the treatment of rheumatoid arthritis and osteoarthritis. Due to its slow onset of action and delayed attainment of steady state, it is less suited for acute analgesia but has been used to treat acute gout. The usual daily dose is 20 mg, and because of the long $t_{1/2}$, steady-state blood levels are not reached for 7-12 days.

Adverse Events. Approximately 20% of patients experience side effects with piroxicam, and ~5% of patients discontinue use because of these effects. In 2007, the European Medicines Agency reviewed the safety of orally administered piroxicam and concluded that its benefits outweigh its risks, but advised it should no longer be used first-line, nor should it be used for the treatment of acute (short-term) pain and inflammation. Piroxicam was singled out for special review because of signals that it is associated with more GI and serious skin reactions than other nonselective NSAIDs.

Meloxicam

Therapeutic Uses. Meloxicam (MOBIC, others) is FDA-approved for use in osteoarthritis. It has been reviewed (Davies and Skjodt, 1999; Fleischmann et al., 2002). The recommended dose for meloxicam is 7.5-15 mg once daily.

Adverse Events. On average, meloxicam demonstrates ~10-fold COX-2 selectivity in *ex vivo* assays. However, this is quite variable, and a clinical advantage or hazard has yet to be established for the drug. Indeed, even with surrogate markers, the relationship to dose is nonlinear. There is significantly less gastric injury compared to piroxicam (20 mg/day) in subjects treated with 7.5 mg/day of meloxicam, but the advantage is lost with a dosage of 15 mg/day.

Other Oxicams

A number of other oxicam derivatives are under study or in use outside the U.S. These include several prodrugs of piroxicam (ampiroxicam, droxicam, and pivoxicam), which have been designed to reduce GI irritation. However, as with sulindac, any theoretical diminution in gastric toxicity associated with administration of a prodrug is offset by gastric COX-1 inhibition from active drug circulating systemically. Other oxicams under study or in use outside the U.S. include lornoxicam, cinnoxicam, sudoxicam, and tenoxicam. The efficacy and toxicity of these drugs are similar to those of piroxicam. Lornoxicam is unique among the enolic acid derivatives in that it has a rapid onset of action and a relatively short $t_{1/2}$ (3-5 hours).

PYRAZOLON DERIVATIVES

This group of drugs includes phenylbutazone, oxyphenbutazone, antipyrine, aminopyrine, and dipyrone; currently, only antipyrine eardrops are available for human use in the U.S. These drugs were used clinically for many years but have essentially been abandoned because of their propensity to cause irreversible agranulocytosis. Dipyrone was reintroduced in the E.U. a decade ago because epidemiological studies suggested that the risk of adverse effects was similar to that of acetaminophen and lower than that of aspirin. However, the use of dipyrone remains limited. The pyrazolone derivatives are discussed in previous editions of this book and may be accessed on the G&G website.

DIARYL HETEROCYCLIC COX-2–SELECTIVE NSAIDS

The first COX-2–selective NSAIDs were diaryl heterocyclic coxibs. Celecoxib is the only such compound still approved in the U.S. Etoricoxib is approved in several countries; rofecoxib and valdecoxib were withdrawn worldwide and have been discussed in previous editions. Parecoxib is a water soluble, injectable prodrug of valdecoxib marketed for treatment of acute pain in several countries. Lumiracoxib, a structural analog of the phenylacetic acid derivative diclofenac, also is not available in the U.S. and has been discussed earlier (see "Lumiracoxib").

Chemistry. Most members of the diaryl heterocyclic family of selective COX-2 inhibitors consist of a central 1,2-diaryl heterocyclic moiety. Celecoxib is a diaryl substituted pyrazole compound; valdecoxib is a diaryl substituted isoxazol derivative. Valdecoxib was made water soluble for parenteral use (parecoxib) by coupling propionic acid via an amide group to its sulfonamide moiety. Etoricoxib is slightly different; it is a monoaryl substituted bipyridine, which results in a three-ring configuration that is superimposable onto the diaryl heterocyclic pharmacophore. Celecoxib, valdecoxib, and its prodrug parecoxib contain a sulfonamide moiety that bares the risk for cross-reactivity in patients with sulfonamide hypersensitivity and, thus, must be avoided in such patients. Etoricoxib has a methylsulfonyl group that is thought to be free of such risk.

Mechanism of Action. Compounds with higher affinity for COX-2 than COX-1 were identified in screens of combinatorial libraries. Subsequent crystallography revealed a hydrophobic pocket in the substrate binding channel of COX-2, which is absent in COX-1 (Figure 34–2). Thus, selective inhibitors of COX-2 are molecules with side chains—the third ring—that fit within this hydrophobic pocket but are too large to block COX-1 with equally high affinity. There is considerable difference in response to the coxibs among individuals (Fries et al., 2006), and it is not known how the degree of selectivity may relate to either efficacy or adverse effect profile, although it seems likely to be related to both. No controlled clinical trials comparing outcomes among the coxibs have been performed. Several tNSAIDs (e.g., nimesulide, diclofenac, meloxicam) exhibit relative selectivity for COX-2 inhibition in whole blood assays that resembles that of celecoxib (FitzGerald and Patrono, 2001; Brune and Hinz, 2004).

Therapeutic Uses. All COX-2–selective NSAIDs have been shown to afford relief from postextraction dental pain and to afford dose-dependent relief from inflammation in osteoarthritis and rheumatoid arthritis. The European Medicines Agency advises that these medicines should not be used in patients with ischemic heart disease or stroke and that prescribers should exercise caution when using selective COX-2 inhibitors in patients with risk factors for heart disease such as hypertension, hyperlipidemia, diabetes, smoking, or peripheral arterial disease. As for all NSAIDs, the agency advises the lowest effective dose for the shortest possible duration of treatment.

Celecoxib

Celecoxib (CELEBREX) was approved for marketing in the U.S. in 1998. Details of its pharmacology have been reviewed (Davies et al., 2000).

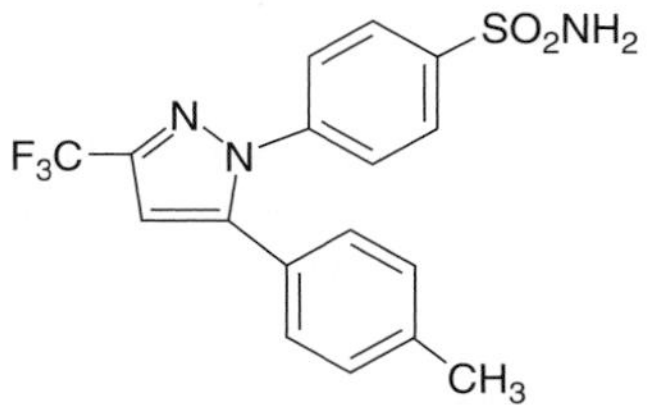

CELECOXIB

Absorption, Distribution, and Elimination. The bioavailability of oral celecoxib is not known, but peak plasma levels occur at 2-4 hours after the dose is taken. The elderly (≥65 years of age) may have up to 2-fold higher peak concentrations and AUC values than younger patients (≤55 years of age). Celecoxib is bound extensively to plasma proteins. Little drug is excreted unchanged; most is excreted as carboxylic acid and glucuronide metabolites in the urine and feces. The elimination $t_{1/2}$ is ~11 hours. The drug commonly is given once or twice per day during chronic treatment. Renal insufficiency is associated with a modest, clinically insignificant decrease in plasma concentration. Celecoxib has not been studied in patients with severe renal insufficiency. Plasma concentrations are increased by ~40% and 180% in patients with mild and moderate hepatic impairment, respectively, and dosages should be reduced by at least 50% in patients with moderate hepatic impairment. Celecoxib is metabolized predominantly by CYP2C9. Although not a substrate, celecoxib is an inhibitor of CYP2D6. Clinical vigilance is necessary during co-administration of drugs that are known to inhibit CYP2C9 and drugs that are metabolized by CYP2D6. For example, celecoxib inhibits the metabolism of metoprolol and can result in its accumulation.

Therapeutic Uses. Celecoxib is approved in the U.S. for the management of acute pain in adults, for the treatment of osteoarthritis, rheumatoid arthritis, juvenile rheumatoid arthritis, ankylosing spondylitis, and primary dysmenorrhea. The recommended dose for treating osteoarthritis is 200 mg/day as a single dose or divided as two 100-mg doses. In the treatment of rheumatoid arthritis, the recommended dose is 100-200 mg twice per day. In the light of its cardiovascular hazard, physicians are advised to use the lowest possible dose for the shortest possible time. Current evidence does not support use of celecoxib as a first choice among the tNSAIDs. Celecoxib also is approved for the chemoprevention of polyposis coli; however, placebo-controlled trials revealed a dose-dependent increase in myocardial infarction and stroke (Solomon et al., 2006).

Adverse Effects. Placebo-controlled trials have established that celecoxib confers a risk of myocardial infarction and stroke and this appears to relate to dose and the underlying risk of cardiovascular disease that anteceded drug administration. Effects attributed to inhibition of PG production in the kidney—hypertension and edema—occur with nonselective COX inhibitors and also with celecoxib. Studies in mice and some epidemiological evidence suggest that the likelihood of patients' developing hypertension while on NSAIDs reflects the degree of inhibition of COX-2 and the selectivity with which it is attained. Indeed, the prevalence of hypertension is higher in patients taking etoricoxib than diclofenac, consistent with the greater selectivity for inhibition of COX-2 of the former drug (Cannon et al., 2006; Laime et al., 2007). Thus, the risk of thrombosis, hypertension, and accelerated atherogenesis are mechanistically integrated. The coxibs should be avoided in patients prone to cardiovascular or cerebrovascular disease. None of the coxibs has established superior efficacy over tNSAIDs. Celecoxib carries the same cardiovascular and GI black box warning as tNSAIDs. Although selective COX-2 inhibitors do not interact to prevent the antiplatelet effect of aspirin, it now is thought that they lose their GI advantage over a tNSAID alone when used in conjunction with aspirin. Experience with selective COX-2 inhibitors in patients who exhibit aspirin hypersensitivity is limited, and caution should be observed.

Parecoxib

Parecoxib is the only COX-2–selective NSAID administered by injection and has been shown to be an effective analgesic for the peri-operative period when patients are unable to take oral medication. It is not widely available, and clinical experience is limited.

Absorption, Distribution, and Elimination. Parecoxib is absorbed rapidly (~15 minutes after intramuscular injection) and converted (15-50 minutes) by deoxymethylation to valdecoxib, the active drug (Table 34–1). Valdecoxib undergoes extensive hepatic metabolism by CYPs 3A4 and 2C9 and non–CYP-dependent glucuronidation. It is a weak inhibitor of CYP2C9 and a weak to moderate inhibitor of CYP2C19. The metabolites of valdecoxib are excreted in the urine. The $t_{1/2}$ is ~7-8 hours but can be significantly prolonged in the elderly or those with hepatic impairment, with subsequent drug accumulation.

Therapeutic Uses. Parecoxib (DYNASTAT) is available in Germany and Australia, but not in the U.K. or U.S., for management of acute pain, including moderate to severe postsurgical pain. It is supplied as a lyophilized powder equivalent to 20 or 40 mg parecoxib to be reconstituted with sterile saline for injection.

Adverse Effects. The cardiovascular risk of parecoxib and valdecoxib was detected in two postoperative pain management trials of high-risk patients (Grosser et al., 2006). Patients undergoing coronary bypass graft (CABG) surgery were initially treated intravenously with parecoxib or placebo and then switched to oral valdecoxib or placebo. The majority of cardiovascular events occurred within days of treatment initiation in these populations, who were subject to acute hemostatic activation after bypass surgery. Clinical studies suggest that cardiovascular complications attributable to COX-2–selective NSAIDs is proportional to baseline cardiovascular risk and to the duration of drug exposure (Grosser et al., 2006). All NSAIDs and celecoxib carry a black box warning contraindicating their use for pain following CABG surgery.

Life-threatening skin reactions (including toxic epidermal necrolysis, Stevens-Johnson syndrome, and erythema multiforme) have been reported in association with valdecoxib, which contains a sulfonamide group. The risk of hypersensitivity or skin reactions applies also to parecoxib. The drug must be discontinued at the first sign of rash, mucosal lesion, or any other sign of hypersensitivity. This additional hazard renders valdecoxib an unlikely therapeutic choice.

Etoricoxib

Etoricoxib is a COX-2–selective inhibitor with selectivity second only to that of lumiracoxib.

Absorption, Distribution, and Elimination. Etoricoxib is incompletely (~80%) absorbed and has a long $t_{1/2}$ of ~20-26 hours (Table 34–1). It is extensively metabolized before excretion. Small studies suggest that those with moderate hepatic impairment are prone to drug accumulation, and the dosing interval should be adjusted. Renal insufficiency does not affect drug clearance.

Therapeutic Uses. Etoricoxib (ARCOXIA) is approved in some countries (not in U.S.) as a once-daily medicine for symptomatic relief in the treatment of osteoarthritis, rheumatoid arthritis, and acute gouty arthritis, as well as for the short-term treatment of musculoskeletal pain, postoperative pain, and primary dysmenorrhea (Patrignani et al., 2003).

Common Adverse Effects. In keeping with other coxibs, etoricoxib shows decreased GI injury as assessed endoscopically. The European regulatory agency concluded that etoricoxib, along with other coxibs, increased the risk of heart attack and stroke; the agency specifically restricted its use in patients with uncontrolled hypertension.

Rofecoxib

Rofecoxib (VIOXX) was introduced in 1999. Details of its pharmacodynamics, pharmacokinetics, therapeutic efficacy, and toxicity have been reviewed (Davies et al., 2003). Based on interim analysis of data from the Adenomatous Polyp Prevention on Vioxx (APPROVe) study, which showed a significant (2-fold) increase in the incidence of serious thromboembolic events in subjects receiving 25 mg of rofecoxib relative to placebo (Bresalier et al., 2005), rofecoxib was withdrawn from the market worldwide in 2004.

OTHER NONSTEROIDAL ANTI-INFLAMMATORY DRUGS

Apazone (Azapropazone)

Apazone is a tNSAID that has anti-inflammatory, analgesic, and antipyretic activity and is a potent uricosuric agent. It is available in E.U. but not in U.S. Some of its efficacy may arise from its capacity to inhibit neutrophil migration, degranulation, and superoxide production.

Apazone has been used for the treatment of rheumatoid arthritis, osteoarthritis, ankylosing spondylitis, and gout but usually is restricted to cases where other tNSAIDs have failed. Typical doses are 600 mg three times per day for acute gout. Once symptoms have abated, or for non-gout indications, typical dosage is 300 mg three to four times per day. Clinical experience to date suggests that apazone is well tolerated. Mild GI side effects (nausea, epigastric pain, dyspepsia) and rashes occur in ~3% of patients, while CNS effects (headache, vertigo) are reported less frequently. Precautions appropriate to other nonselective COX inhibitors also apply to apazone.

Nimesulide

Nimesulide is a sulfonanilide compound available in Europe that demonstrates COX-2 selectivity similar to celecoxib in whole-blood assays. Additional effects include inhibition of neutrophil activation, decrease in cytokine production, decrease in degradative enzyme production, and possibly activation of glucocorticoid receptors (Bennett, 1999).

Nimesulide is administered orally in doses ≤100 mg twice daily as an anti-inflammatory, analgesic, and antipyretic. Its use in the E.U. is limited to ≤15 days due to the risk of hepatotoxicity.

CLINICAL SUMMARY: NSAIDs

Both tNSAIDs and COX-2–selective NSAIDs have anti-inflammatory, analgesic, and antipyretic activity by virtue of inhibition of PG biosynthesis. Selective inhibitors of COX-2 were developed to reduce GI adverse effects but have never been shown to exhibit an efficacy advantage over tNSAIDs, and most have been eliminated from the market due to cardiovascular and hepatic toxicities. Choice and dosing of an NSAID are usually guided by multiple considerations, including the therapeutic indication, patient age, coincident diseases or allergies, the drug's safety and interaction profile, and cost considerations. Drugs with more rapid onset of action and shorter duration of action (sometimes marketed as rapid release or liquid formulations that facilitate absorption) probably are preferable for fever accompanying minor viral illnesses, pain after minor musculoskeletal injuries, or headache, whereas a longer duration of action may be preferable for management of postoperative or arthritic pain.

The choice among tNSAIDs for the treatment of chronic arthritic conditions such as rheumatoid arthritis largely is empirical. Substantial differences in response have been noted among individuals treated with the same tNSAID and within an individual treated with different tNSAIDs, even when the drugs are structurally related. It is reasonable to give a drug for a week or two as a therapeutic trial and to continue it if the response is satisfactory. Initially, all patients should be asked about previous hypersensitivity to aspirin or any member of the NSAID class. Thereafter, low doses of the chosen agent should be prescribed to determine initial patient tolerance. Older patients may require lower doses than younger patients to reduce the risk of toxicity. Regulatory agencies stress use of the lowest effective dose for the shortest possible duration of treatment. Alterations in dosing may take several days (>3-4 $t_{1/2}$) to translate into clinically detectable changes. Delayed distribution into the synovial compartment may extend this interval. Indeed, some NSAIDs that are short lived in plasma are sustained in synovial fluid and may afford sufficient relief even when administered at intervals longer than their plasma $t_{1/2}$ time. If the patient does not achieve therapeutic benefit from one NSAID, another may be tried. For mild arthropathies, the scheme outlined earlier in this paragraph, together with rest and physical therapy, probably will be sufficiently effective. When the patient has sleeping problems because of pain or morning stiffness, a larger proportion of the daily dose may be given at night. However, patients with more debilitating disease may not respond adequately, prompting the initiation of more aggressive therapy with disease-modifying anti-rheumatic drugs (see below). The experience in children is limited to a small number of drugs, which are dosed by age and body weight.

Some adverse effects may manifest in the first weeks of therapy; however, the risk of gastric ulceration and bleeding accumulates with the duration of dosing. Combination therapy with more than one NSAID is to be avoided. A number of risk factors for GI complications have been determined in epidemiological studies. Patients at high risk for GI complications should be prescribed a gastroprotective agent. These patients also are potential candidates for a COX-2–selective NSAID.

Placebo-controlled trials have established that selective inhibition of COX-2 confers an increased risk of heart attack and stroke. The likelihood of hazard would be expected to be related to selectivity attained *in vivo*, dose, potency and duration of action, and duration of dosing, as well as the underlying cardiovascular risk profile of an individual patient. It seems likely that some of the older drugs with COX-2 selectivity (e.g., diclofenac) may closely resemble celecoxib. The cardiovascular hazard from both celecoxib and rofecoxib, the two inhibitors for which data are available from placebo-controlled trials lasting >1 year, appeared to increase with chronicity of dosing. This is consistent with a mechanism-based acceleration of atherogenesis directly via inhibition of PGI_2 and indirectly due to the rise in blood pressure consequent to inhibition of COX-2-derived PGE_2 and PGI_2. Similarly, the increased risk conferred by rofecoxib has been shown to dissipate slowly, if at all, in the year after drug cessation. If a COX-2–selective inhibitor is prescribed, it should be used at the lowest possible dose for the shortest period of time.

Patients at risk of cardiovascular disease or prone to thrombosis should not be treated with COX-2-selective NSAIDs. Small absolute risks of thrombosis attributable to these drugs may interact geometrically with small absolute risks from genetic variants like factor V Leiden or concomitant therapies, such as anovulant oral contraceptives. Some tNSAIDs (ibuprofen, naproxen) have been shown to interfere with the antiplatelet activity of low-dose aspirin, and aspirin's cardioprotective effect may be diminished in patients who take low-dose aspirin and a tNSAID concomitantly. The administration of immediate-release (not enteric-coated) aspirin should be separated from the dose of tNSAID to avoid the interaction. For example, ibuprofen should not be taken within 30 minutes of the ingestion of low-dose aspirin and low-dose aspirin should not be ingested within 8 hours of a dose of ibuprofen. Patients at high risk for cardiovascular events should preferentially use analgesics that do not interfere with platelet action.

DISEASE-MODIFYING ANTI-RHEUMATIC DRUGS

Rheumatoid arthritis is an autoimmune disease that affects ~1% of the population. The pharmacological management of rheumatoid arthritis includes symptomatic relief through the use of NSAIDs. However, although they have anti-inflammatory effects, NSAIDs have minimal, if any effect on progression of joint deformity. DMARDs (disease-modifying anti-rheumatic drugs), on the other hand, reduce the disease activity of rheumatoid arthritis and retard the progression of arthritic tissue destruction. DMARDs include a diverse group of small molecule non-biologicals and biological agents (mainly antibodies or binding proteins), as summarized in Table 34–3.

Treatment with single non-biological DMARDs can achieve remission or at least a state of very low disease activity in a large number of rheumatoid arthritis patients (Saag et al., 2008). Combinations of non-biological DMARDs (e.g., methotrexate + sulfasalazine, methotrexate + hydroxychloroquine, methotrexate + leflunomide, methotrexate + sulfasalazine + hydroxychloroquine) are indicated for patients with moderate or high disease activity or prolonged disease duration or for those who fail to respond to a single compound. Biological DMARDs remain reserved for patients

Table 34–3

Disease-Modifying Anti-Rheumatic Drugs

DRUG	CLASS OR ACTION	REFERENCE (CHAPTER NUMBER)
Small molecules		
Methotrexate	Anti-folate	61
Leflunomide	Pyrimidine synthase inhibitor	61
Hydroxychloroquine	Anti-malarial	49
Minocycline	5-lipoxygenase inhibitor, tetracycline antibiotic	33, 55
Sulfasalazine	Salicylate	34, 47
Azathioprine	Purine synthase inhibitor	61
Cyclosporine	Calcineurin inhibitor	35
Cyclophosphamide	Alkylating agent	61
Biologicals		
Adalimumab	Ab, TNF-α antagonist	35
Golimumab	Ab, TNF-α antagonist	35
Infliximab	IgG-TNF receptor fusion protein (anti-TNF)	35
Certolizumab	Fab fragment toward TNF-α	35
Abatacept	T-cell co-stimulation inhibitor (binds B7 protein on antigen-presenting cell)	35
Rituximab	Ab toward CD20 (cytotoxic toward B cells)	62
Anakinra	IL-1-receptor antagonist	35, 62

IL, interleukin; TNF, tumor necrosis factor.

with persistent moderate or high disease activity and indicators of poor prognosis such as functional impairment, radiographic bony erosions, extra-articular disease, and rheumatoid factor positivity. Therapy is tailored to the individual patient, and the use of these agents must be weighed against their potentially serious adverse effects. The combination of NSAIDs with these agents is common.

Short-term glucocorticoids often are used to bring the level of inflammation quickly under control. Glucocorticoids are not suitable for long-term use because of adrenal suppression. The older agents (gold, penicillamine) have unclear mechanisms of action and tend to have slight efficacy and significant side effects. Their pharmacology is described in more detail in previous editions of this book.

PHARMACOTHERAPY OF GOUT

Gout results from the precipitation of urate crystals in the tissues and the subsequent inflammatory response (Terkeltaub et al., 2006). Acute gout usually causes an exquisitely painful distal monoarthritis, but it also can cause joint destruction, subcutaneous deposits (tophi), and renal calculi and damage. Gout affects ~0.5-1% of the population of Western countries. Once considered a disease of kings and the rich, gout is no respecter of class and is found at all socioeconomic strata. Indeed, gout is the most common form of inflammatory arthritis in the elderly.

The pathophysiology of gout is understood incompletely. Hyperuricemia, while a prerequisite, does not inevitably lead to gout. Uric acid, the end product of purine metabolism, is relatively insoluble compared to its hypoxanthine and xanthine precursors, and normal serum urate levels (~5 mg/dL, or 0.3 mM) approach the limit of solubility. In most patients with gout, hyperuricemia arises from underexcretion rather than overproduction of urate. Mutations of one of the renal urate transporters, URAT-1, are associated with hypouricemia (Enomoto et al., 2002); the uricosuric effect of benzbromarone and probenecid can be explained by inhibition of this transporter. Urate tends to crystallize as monosodium urate in colder or more acidic conditions. Monosodium urate crystals activate monocytes/macrophages via the Toll-like receptor pathway mounting an innate immune response. This results in the secretion of cytokines, including IL-1β and TNF-α; endothelial activation; and attraction of neutrophils to the site of inflammation (Terkeltaub et al., 2006). Neutrophils secrete inflammatory mediators that lower the local pH and lead to further urate precipitation.

The aims of treatment are to:

- decrease the symptoms of an acute attack
- decrease the risk of recurrent attacks
- lower serum urate levels

The substances available for these purposes are:

- drugs that relieve inflammation and pain (NSAIDs, colchicine, glucocorticoids)
- drugs that prevent inflammatory responses to crystals (colchicine and NSAIDs)
- drugs that act by inhibition of urate formation (allopurinol, febuxostat) or to augment urate excretion (probenecid)

NSAIDs have been discussed earlier. Glucocorticoids are discussed in Chapter 42. This section focuses on colchicine, allopurinol, febuxostat and the uricosuric agents probenecid and benzbromarone.

Colchicine

Colchicine is one of the oldest available therapies for acute gout. Plant extracts containing colchicine were used for joint pain in the sixth century. Colchicine is considered second-line therapy because it has a narrow therapeutic window and a high rate of side effects, particularly at higher doses. There no longer is a role for colchicine in the treatment of primary biliary cirrhosis, psoriasis, or Behçet's disease.

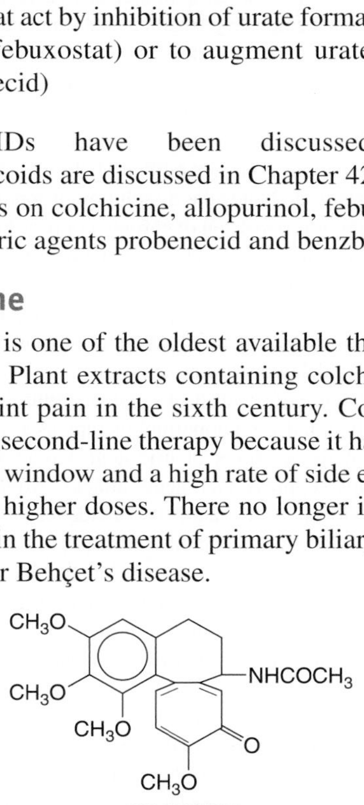

CH_3O CH_3O CH_3O $-NHCOCH_3$ O CH_3O

COLCHICINE

Mechanism of Action. Colchicine exerts a variety of pharmacological effects, but how these occur or how they relate to its activity in gout is not well understood. Its structure-activity relationship has been discussed (Levy et al., 1991). It has antimitotic effects, arresting cell division in G_1 by interfering with microtubule and spindle formation (an effect shared with vinca alkaloids). This effect is greatest on cells with rapid turnover (e.g., neutrophils, GI epithelium). Colchicine may alter neutrophil motility in *ex vivo* assays (Levy et al., 1991). Experimental data suggest that colchicine decreases the crystal-induced secretion of chemotactic factors and superoxide anions by activated neutrophils. It also limits neutrophil adhesion to endothelium by modulating the expression of endothelial adhesion molecules. Higher concentrations inhibit IL-1β processing and release from neutrophils *in vitro*.

Colchicine inhibits the release of histamine-containing granules from mast cells, the secretion of insulin from pancreatic β cells, and the movement of melanin granules in melanophores. These processes also may involve interference with the microtubular system, but whether this occurs at clinically relevant concentrations is questionable.

Colchicine also exhibits a variety of other pharmacological effects. It lowers body temperature, increases the sensitivity to central depressants, depresses the respiratory center, enhances the response to sympathomimetic agents, constricts blood vessels, and induces hypertension by central vasomotor stimulation. It enhances GI activity by neurogenic stimulation but depresses it by a direct effect, and alters neuromuscular function.

Absorption, Distribution, and Elimination. The absorption of oral colchicine is rapid but variable. Peak plasma concentrations occur 0.5-2 hours after dosing. In plasma, 50% of colchicine is protein bound. The formation of colchicine-tubulin complexes in many tissues contributes to its large volume of distribution. There is significant enterohepatic circulation. The exact metabolism of colchicine in humans is unknown, but *in vitro* studies indicate that it may undergo oxidative demethylation by CYP3A4. Indeed, other CYP3A4 substrates, such as cimetidine, have been associated with an increase in colchicine plasma $t_{1/2}$ and the emergence of colchicine toxicity. The drug is contraindicated in patients with hepatic or renal impairment requiring concomitant therapy with CYP3A4 or *P*-glycoprotein inhibitors. Only 10-20% is excreted in the urine, although this increases in patients with liver disease. The kidney, liver, and spleen also contain high concentrations of colchicine, but it apparently is largely excluded from heart, skeletal muscle, and brain. The plasma $t_{1/2}$ of colchicine is ~9 hours, but the drug can be detected in leukocytes and in the urine for at least 9 days after a single intravenous dose.

Therapeutic Uses. A minimum of 3 days, but preferably 7 or 14 days, should elapse between courses of gout treatment with colchicine to avoid cumulative toxicity. Patients with hepatic or renal disease and dialysis patients should receive reduced doses and/or less frequent therapy. Great care should be exercised in prescribing colchicine for elderly patients, for whom the dose should be based on renal function. For those with cardiac, renal, hepatic, or GI disease, NSAIDs or glucocorticoids may be preferred.

Acute Gout. Colchicine dramatically relieves acute attacks of gout. It is effective in roughly two-thirds of patients if given within 24 hours of attack onset. Pain, swelling, and redness abate within 12 hours and are completely gone within 48-72 hours. In the past, the typical dosing regimen was 0.6 mg each hour until pain was relieved or diarrhea developed; the typical course of therapy ranged from 4-8 mg. The new regimen approved by the FDA in 2009 for adults recommends a total of only two doses taken 1 hour apart: 1.2 mg (two tablets) at the first sign of a gout flare followed by 0.6 mg (one tablet) 1 hour later. The dose must be adjusted in patients exposed to inhibitors of *P*-glycoprotein or CYP3A4 within the previous 14 days.

Prevention of Acute Gout. The main off-label indication for colchicine is in the prevention of recurrent gout, particularly in the early stages of antihyperuricemic therapy. The typical dose for prophylaxis is 0.6 mg taken orally 3 or 4 days/wk for patients who have <1 attack per year, 0.6 mg daily for patients who have >1 attack per year, and 0.6 mg two or three times daily for patients who have severe attacks. The dose must be decreased for patients with impaired renal function.

Familial Mediterranean Fever. The administration of daily colchicine is useful for the prevention of attacks of familial Mediterranean fever and prevention of amyloidosis, which may complicate this disease. The dose for adults and children >12 years of age is 1.2-2.4 mg daily. The dose for patients as young as 4 years is reduced on the basis of age.

Adverse Effects. Exposure of the GI tract to large amounts of colchicine and its metabolites via enterohepatic circulation and the rapid rate of turnover of the GI mucosa may explain why the GI tract is particularly susceptible to colchicine toxicity. Nausea, vomiting, diarrhea, and abdominal pain are the most common untoward effects and the earliest signs of impending colchicine toxicity. Drug administration should be discontinued as soon as these symptoms occur. There is a latent period, which is not altered by dose or route of administration, of several hours or more between the administration of the drug and the onset of symptoms. A dosing study required as part of FDA approval demonstrated that one dose initially and a single additional dose after 1 hour was much less toxic than traditional hourly dosing for acute gout flares. Acute intoxication causes hemorrhagic gastropathy. Intravenous colchicine was previously used to treat acute gouty arthritis; however, this route obviates early GI side effects that can be a harbinger of serious systemic toxicity. The FDA suspended the U.S. marketing of all injectable dosage forms of colchicine in 2008. Other serious side effects of colchicine therapy include myelosuppression, leukopenia, granulocytopenia, thrombopenia, aplastic anemia, and rhabdomyolysis. Life-threatening toxicities are associated with administration of concomitant therapy with *P*-glycoprotein or CYP3A4 inhibitors.

Allopurinol

Allopurinol inhibits xanthine oxidase and prevents the synthesis of urate from hypoxanthine and xanthine. Allopurinol is used to treat hyperuricemia in patients with gout and to prevent it in those with hematological malignancies about to undergo chemotherapy (acute tumor lysis syndrome). Even though underexcretion rather than overproduction is the underlying defect in most gout patients, allopurinol remains effective therapy.

History. Allopurinol initially was synthesized as a candidate antineoplastic agent but was found to lack antineoplastic activity. Subsequent testing showed it to be an inhibitor of xanthine oxidase that was useful clinically for the treatment of gout.

Chemistry. Allopurinol is an analog of hypoxanthine. Its active metabolite, oxypurinol, is an analog of xanthine.

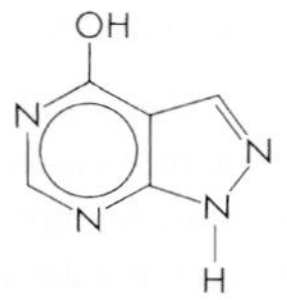

OH N N N N H

ALLOPURINOL

Mechanism of Action. Both allopurinol and its primary metabolite, oxypurinol (alloxanthine), inhibit xanthine oxidase and reduce urate production. Allopurinol competitively inhibits xanthine oxidase at low concentrations and is a noncompetitive inhibitor at high concentrations. Allopurinol also is a substrate for xanthine oxidase; the product of this reaction, oxypurinol, also is a noncompetitive inhibitor of the enzyme. The formation of oxypurinol, together with its long persistence in tissues, is responsible for much of the pharmacological activity of allopurinol.

In the absence of allopurinol, the dominant urinary purine is uric acid. During allopurinol treatment, the urinary purines include hypoxanthine, xanthine, and uric acid. Because each has its independent solubility, the concentration of uric acid in plasma is reduced and purine excretion increased, without exposing the urinary tract to an excessive load of uric acid. Despite their increased concentrations during allopurinol therapy, hypoxanthine and xanthine are efficiently excreted, and tissue deposition does not occur. There is a small risk of xanthine stones in patients with a very high urate load before allopurinol therapy, which can be minimized by liberal fluid intake and alkalization of the urine with sodium bicarbonate, potassium citrate, or citrate combinations such as modified Shohl's solution.

Allopurinol facilitates the dissolution of tophi and prevents the development or progression of chronic gouty arthritis by lowering the uric acid concentration in plasma below the limit of its solubility. The formation of uric acid stones virtually disappears with therapy, which prevents the development of nephropathy. Once significant renal injury has occurred, allopurinol cannot restore renal function but may delay disease progression.

The incidence of acute attacks of gouty arthritis may increase during the early months of allopurinol therapy as a consequence of mobilization of tissue stores of uric acid. Co-administration of colchicine helps suppress such acute attacks. After reduction of excess tissue stores of uric acid, the incidence of acute attacks decreases and colchicine can be discontinued.

In some patients, the allopurinol-induced increase in excretion of oxypurines is less than the reduction in uric acid excretion; this disparity primarily is a result of re-utilization of oxypurines and feedback inhibition of *de novo* purine biosynthesis.

Absorption, Distribution, and Elimination. Allopurinol is absorbed relatively rapidly after oral ingestion, and peak plasma concentrations are reached within 60-90 minutes. About 20% is excreted in the feces in 48-72 hours, presumably as unabsorbed drug, and 10-30% is excreted unchanged in the urine. The remainder undergoes metabolism, mostly to oxypurinol apparently by the catalytic activity of aldehyde oxidoreductase. Oxypurinol is excreted slowly in the urine by glomerular filtration, counterbalanced by some tubular reabsorption. The plasma $t_{1/2}$ of allopurinol and oxypurinol is ~1-2 hours and ~18-30 hours (longer in those with renal impairment), respectively. This allows for once-daily dosing and makes allopurinol the most commonly used antihyperuricemic agent.

Allopurinol and its active metabolite oxypurinol are distributed in total tissue water, with the exception of brain, where their concentrations are about one-third of those in other tissues. Neither compound is bound to plasma proteins. The plasma concentrations of the two compounds do not correlate well with therapeutic or toxic effects. The clinical pharmacology of allopurinol and its metabolite have been reviewed (Day et al., 2007).

Drug Interactions. Allopurinol increases the $t_{1/2}$ of probenecid and enhances its uricosuric effect, while probenecid increases the clearance of oxypurinol, thereby increasing dose requirements of allopurinol.

Allopurinol inhibits the enzymatic inactivation of mercaptopurine and its derivative azathioprine by xanthine oxidase. Thus, when allopurinol is used concomitantly with oral mercaptopurine or azathioprine, dosage of the antineoplastic agent must be reduced to one-fourth to one-third of the usual dose (see Chapters 35 and 61). This is of importance when treating gout in the transplant recipient. The risk of bone marrow suppression also is increased when allopurinol is administered with cytotoxic agents that are not metabolized by xanthine oxidase, particularly cyclophosphamide.

Allopurinol also may interfere with the hepatic inactivation of other drugs, including warfarin. Although the effect is variable, increased monitoring of prothrombin activity is recommended in patients receiving both medications.

It remains to be established whether the increased incidence of rash in patients receiving concurrent allopurinol and ampicillin should be ascribed to allopurinol or to hyperuricemia. Hypersensitivity reactions have been reported in patients with compromised renal function, especially those who are receiving a combination of allopurinol and a thiazide diuretic. The concomitant administration of allopurinol and theophylline leads to increased accumulation of an active metabolite of theophylline, 1-methylxanthine; the concentration of theophylline in plasma also may be increased (see Chapter 36).

Therapeutic Uses. Allopurinol (ZYLOPRIM, ALOPRIM, others) is available for oral and intravenous use. Oral therapy provides effective therapy for primary and secondary gout, hyperuricemia secondary to malignancies, and calcium oxalate calculi. Intravenous therapy is indicated for hyperuricemia secondary to cancer chemotherapy for patients unable to tolerate oral therapy.

Allopurinol is contraindicated in patients who have exhibited serious adverse effects or hypersensitivity reactions to the medication and in nursing mothers and children, except those with malignancy or certain inborn errors of purine metabolism (e.g., Lesch-Nyhan syndrome). Allopurinol generally is used in complicated hyperuricemia post-transplantation, to prevent acute tumor lysis syndrome, or in patients with hyperuricemia post-transplantation. If necessary, it can be used in conjunction with a uricosuric agent such as probenecid.

The goal of therapy is to reduce the plasma uric acid concentration to <6 mg/dL (<360 μmol/L). In the management of gout, it is customary to antecede allopurinol therapy with colchicine and to avoid starting allopurinol during an acute attack. Fluid intake should be sufficient to maintain daily urinary volume of >2 L; slightly alkaline urine is preferred. An initial daily dose of 100 mg in patients with estimated glomerular filtration rates >40 mg/min is increased by 100-mg increments at weekly intervals according to the antihyperuricemic effect achieved. Plasma uric acid concentration <6 mg/dL (<360 μmol/L) are attained in less than half of the patients on 300 mg/day, the most commonly prescribed dose. Achieving sufficient reduction of uric acid serum levels may require 400-600 mg/day. Those with hematological malignancies may need up to 800 mg/day beginning 2-3 days before the start of chemotherapy. Interindividual variability in drug response is high. Daily doses >300 mg should be divided. Dosage must be reduced in patients in proportion to the reduction in glomerular filtration (e.g., 300 mg/day if creatinine clearance is >90 mL/min, 200 mg/day if creatinine clearance is between 60 and 90 mL/min, 100 mg/day if creatinine clearance is 30-60 mL/min, and 50-100 mg/day if creatinine clearance is <30 mL/min) (Terkeltaub, 2003).

The usual daily dose in children with secondary hyperuricemia associated with malignancies is 150-300 mg, depending on age.

Allopurinol also is useful in lowering the high plasma concentrations of uric acid in patients with Lesch-Nyhan syndrome and thereby prevents the complications resulting from hyperuricemia; there is no evidence that it alters the progressive neurological and behavioral abnormalities that are characteristic of the disease.

Adverse Effects. Allopurinol generally is well tolerated, but the drug occasionally induces drowsiness. The most common adverse effects are hypersensitivity reactions that may manifest after months or years of therapy. Serious hypersensitivity reactions preclude further use of the drug.

The cutaneous reaction caused by allopurinol is predominantly a pruritic, erythematous, or maculopapular eruption, but occasionally the lesion is urticarial or purpuric. Rarely, toxic epidermal necrolysis or Stevens-Johnson syndrome occurs, which can be fatal. The risk for Stevens-Johnson syndrome is limited primarily to the first 2 months of treatment. Because the rash may precede severe hypersensitivity reactions, patients who develop a rash should discontinue allopurinol. If indicated, desensitization to allopurinol can be carried out starting at 10-25 μg/day, with the drug diluted in oral suspension and doubled every 3-14 days until the desired dose is reached. This is successful in approximately half of patients (Terkeltaub, 2003). Oxypurinol has orphan drug status and is available for compassionate use in the U.S. for patients intolerant of allopurinol.

Fever, malaise, and myalgias also may occur. Such effects are noted in ~3% of patients with normal renal function and more frequently in those with renal impairment. Transient leukopenia or leukocytosis and eosinophilia are rare reactions that may require cessation of therapy. Hepatomegaly and elevated levels of transaminases in plasma and progressive renal insufficiency also may occur.

Febuxostat

Febuxostat is a novel xanthine oxidase inhibitor that was recently approved for treatment of hyperuricemia in patients with gout (Pascual et al., 2009).

Chemistry. Febuxostat is a two-ring molecule with substituted phenyl and thiazole rings.

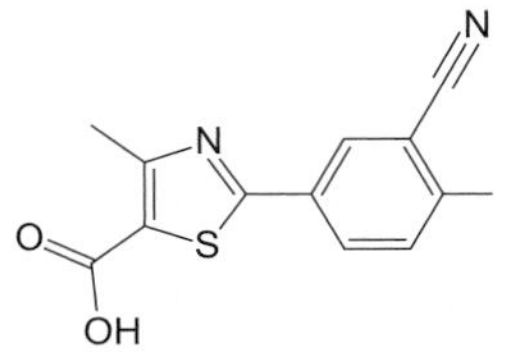

N
N
O
S
OH
FEBUXOSTAT

Mechanism of Action. Febuxostat is a non-purine inhibitor of xanthine oxidase. While oxypurinol, the active metabolite of allopurinol, inhibits the reduced form of the enzyme, febuxostat forms a stable complex with both the reduced and oxidized enzyme and inhibits catalytic function in both states.

Absorption, Distribution, and Elimination. Febuxostat is rapidly absorbed with maximum plasma concentrations between 1-1.5 hours post-dose. The absorption of radiolabeled compound was estimated to be at least 49%, however, the absolute bioavailability is unknown. Magnesium hydroxide and aluminum hydroxide delay absorption ~1 hour. Food reduces absorption slightly, but has no clinically significant effect on the reduction of serum uric acid concentration. Febuxostat is highly plasma protein bound and has a volume of distribution of 50 L. It is extensively metabolized by oxidation by CYPs 1A2, 2C8, and 2C9 and non-CYP enzymes conjugation via UGTs 1A1, 1A3, 1A9 and 2B7. The relative contribution of each metabolic route is not known. The oxidation of the isobutyl side chain leads to the formation of four pharmacologically active hydroxy metabolites, all of which occur in plasma at markedly lower concentrations than febuxostat. Febuxostat has a $t_{1/2}$ of 5-8 hours and is eliminated by both hepatic and renal pathways. Mild to moderate renal or hepatic impairment does not affect its elimination kinetics relevantly.

Therapeutic Use. Febuxostat (ULORIC; ADNEURIC [EUROPE]) is approved for hyperuric patients with gout attacks, but not recommended for treatment of asymptomatic hyperuricemia. It is available in 40 and 80-mg oral tablets. Three randomized controlled clinical trials that compared febuxostat with allopurinol showed that 40 mg/day febuxostat lowered serum uric acid to similar levels as 300 mg/day allopurinol. More patients reached the target concentration of 6.0 mg/dL (360 μmol/L) on 80 mg/day febuxostat than on 300 mg/day allopurinol (Becker et al., 2005a; Becker et al., 2005b; Schumacher et al., 2008). Thus, therapy should be initiated with 40 mg/day and the dose increased if the target serum uric acid concentration is not reached within 2 weeks.

Common Adverse Events. The most common adverse reactions in clinical studies were liver function abnormalities, nausea, joint pain, and rash. Liver function should be monitored periodically. An increase in gout flares was frequently observed after initiation of therapy, due to reduction in serum uric acid levels resulting in mobilization of urate from tissue deposits. Concurrent prophylactic treatment with an NSAID or colchicine is usually required. There was also a numerically higher rate of myocardial infarction and stroke in patients on febuxostat than on allopurinol. It is currently unknown whether there is a causal relationship between the cardiovascular events and febuxostat therapy or whether these were due to chance. The FDA has imposed as a condition for approval that a prospective study designed to assess the drug's cardiovascular safety be performed. Meanwhile patients should be monitored for cardiovascular complications.

Drug Interactions. Plasma levels of drugs that are metabolized by xanthine oxidase (e.g., theophylline, mercaptopurine, azathioprine) can be expected to increase—possibly to toxic levels—when administered concurrently with febuxostat, although drug interaction studies with these drugs have not been conducted. Thus, febuxostat is contraindicated in patients on azathioprine, mercaptopurine, or theophylline. Based on *in vitro* studies, interactions between febuxostat and CYP inhibitors are likely, but interactions studies have not been performed in humans.

Rasburicase

Rasburicase (ELITEK) is a recombinant urate oxidase that catalyzes the enzymatic oxidation of uric acid into the soluble and inactive metabolite allantoin. It has been shown to lower urate levels more effectively than allopurinol (Bosly et al., 2003). It is indicated for the initial management of elevated plasma uric acid levels in pediatric patients with leukemia, lymphoma, and solid tumor malignancies who are receiving anticancer therapy expected to result in tumor lysis and significant hyperuricemia.

Produced by a genetically modified *Saccharomyces cerevisiae* strain, the therapeutic efficacy may be hampered by the production of antibodies against the drug. Hemolysis in glucose-6-phosphate dehydrogenase (G6PD)-deficient patients, methemoglobinemia, acute renal failure, and anaphylaxis have been associated with the use of rasburicase. Other frequently observed adverse reactions include vomiting, fever, nausea, headache, abdominal pain, constipation, diarrhea, and mucositis. Rasburicase causes enzymatic degradation of the uric acid in blood samples, and special handling is required to prevent spuriously low values for plasma uric acid in patients receiving the drug. The recommended dose of rasburicase is 0.15 mg/kg or 0.2 mg/kg as a single daily dose for 5 days, with chemotherapy initiated 4-24 hours after infusion of the first rasburicase dose.

Uricosuric Agents

Uricosuric agents increase the rate of excretion of uric acid. In humans, urate is filtered, secreted, and reabsorbed by the kidneys. Reabsorption predominates, such that the net the amount excreted usually is ~10% of that filtered. Reabsorption is mediated by an organic anion transporter family member, URAT-1, which can be inhibited. A number of other organic acid transporters, may also participate in urate exchange at the basolateral membrane of proximal tubule epithelial cells (Terkeltaub et al., 2006).

URAT-1 exchanges urate for either an organic anion such as lactate or nicotinate or less potently for an inorganic anion such as chloride. The monocarboxylate metabolite of the anti-tuberculous drug pyrazinamide, an organic anion, is a potent stimulator of urate reuptake. Uricosuric drugs such as probenecid, sulfinpyrazone, benzbromarone, and losartan compete with urate for the transporter, thereby inhibiting its reabsorption via the urate–anion exchanger system. However, transport is bidirectional, and depending on dosage, some drugs, including salicylates, may either decrease or increase the excretion of uric acid. Decreased excretion usually occurs at a low dosage, while increased excretion is observed at a higher dosage. Not all agents show this phenomenon, and one uricosuric drug may either add to or inhibit the action of another.

Two mechanisms for a drug-induced decrease in urinary excretion of urate have been advanced; they are not mutually exclusive. The first presumes that the small secretory movement of urate is inhibited by very low concentrations of the drug. Higher concentrations may inhibit urate reabsorption in the usual manner. The second proposal suggests that the urate-retaining anionic drug gains access to the intracellular fluid by an independent mechanism and promotes reabsorption of urate across the brush border by anion exchange.

There also are two mechanisms by which one drug may nullify the uricosuric action of another. First, the drug may inhibit the secretion of the uricosuric agent, thereby denying it access to its site of action, the luminal aspect of the brush border. Second, the inhibition of urate secretion by one drug may counterbalance the inhibition of urate reabsorption by the other.

Many compounds have incidental uricosuric activity by acting as exchangeable anions, but only probenecid is prescribed routinely for this purpose. Sulfinpyrazone has been withdrawn from the U.S. market (see the previous edition of this book for the pharmacology of sulfinpyrazone). Benzbromarone is an alternative uricosuric agent that is available in the E.U. Conversely, a number of drugs and toxins cause retention of urate; these have been reviewed elsewhere (Maalouf et al., 2004). The angiotensin II–receptor antagonist, losartan, has a modest uricosuric effect and may be an option for those who are intolerant to probenecid and are hypertensive.

Probenecid.

Probenecid is a highly lipid-soluble benzoic acid derivative (pK_a 3.4).

$CH_3CH_2CH_2$ / $CH_3CH_2CH_2$ >NSO_2–C_6H_4–COOH

PROBENECID

Mechanism of Action

Inhibition of Organic Acid Transport. The actions of probenecid are confined largely to inhibition of the transport of organic acids across epithelial barriers. When tubular secretion of a substance is inhibited, its final concentration in the urine is determined by the degree of filtration, which in turn is a function of binding to plasma protein, and by the degree of reabsorption. The significance of each of these factors varies widely with different compounds. Usually, the end result is decreased tubular secretion of the compound, leading to decreased urinary and increased plasma concentration. Probenecid inhibits the reabsorption of uric acid by organic anion transporters, principally URAT-1. Uric acid is the only important endogenous compound whose excretion is known to be increased by probenecid. The uricosuric action of probenecid is blunted by the co-administration of salicylates.

Inhibition of Transport of Miscellaneous Substances. Probenecid inhibits the tubular secretion of a number of drugs, such as methotrexate and the active metabolite of clofibrate. It inhibits renal secretion of the inactive glucuronide metabolites of NSAIDs such as naproxen, ketoprofen, and indomethacin, and thereby can increase their plasma concentrations.

Inhibition of Monoamine Transport to CSF. Probenecid inhibits the transport of 5-hydroxyindoleacetic acid (5-HIAA) and other acidic metabolites of cerebral monoamines from the CSF to the plasma. The transport of drugs such as penicillin G also may be affected.

Inhibition of Biliary Excretion. Probenecid depresses the biliary secretion of certain compounds, including the diagnostic agents indocyanine green and bromosulfophthalein (BSP). It also decreases the biliary secretion of rifampin, leading to higher plasma concentrations.

Absorption, Distribution, and Elimination. Probenecid is absorbed completely after oral administration. Peak concentrations in plasma are reached in 2-4 hours. The $t_{1/2}$ of the drug in plasma is dose dependent and varies from <5 hours to >8 hours over the therapeutic range. Between 85% and 95% of the drug is bound to plasma albumin. The 5-15% of unbound drug is cleared by glomerular filtration. The majority of the drug is secreted actively by the proximal tubule. The high lipid solubility of the undissociated form results in virtually complete absorption by backdiffusion unless the urine is markedly alkaline. A small amount of probenecid glucuronide appears in the urine. It also is hydroxylated to metabolites that retain their carboxyl function and have uricosuric activity.

Therapeutic Uses (Gout). Probenecid [PROBALAN, BENURYL (U.K.)] is marketed for oral administration. The starting dose is 250 mg twice daily, increasing over 1-2 weeks to 500-1000 mg twice daily. Probenecid increases urinary urate levels. Liberal fluid intake therefore should be maintained throughout therapy to minimize the risk of renal stones. Probenecid should not be used in gouty patients with nephrolithiasis or with overproduction of uric acid. Concomitant colchicine or NSAIDs are indicated early in the course of therapy to avoid precipitating an attack of gout, which may occur in ≤20% of gouty patients treated with probenecid alone.

Combination with Penicillin. Probenecid was developed for the purpose of delaying the excretion of penicillin. Higher doses of probenecid are used as an adjuvant to prolong penicillin concentrations. This dosing method usually is confined to those being treated for gonorrhea or neurosyphilis infections or to cases in which penicillin resistance may be an issue (see Chapter 53).

Common Adverse Effects. Probenecid is well tolerated. Approximately 2% of patients develop mild GI irritation. The risk is increased at higher doses, and caution should be used in those with a history of peptic ulcer. It is ineffective in patients with renal insufficiency and should be avoided in those with creatinine clearance of <50 mL/min. Hypersensitivity reactions usually are mild and occur in 2-4% of patients. Serious hypersensitivity is extremely rare. The appearance of a rash during the concurrent administration of probenecid and penicillin G presents the physician with an awkward diagnostic dilemma. Substantial overdosage with probenecid results in CNS stimulation, convulsions, and death from respiratory failure.

Benzbromarone

Benzbromarone is a potent uricosuric agent that is used in Europe. It was withdrawn from the market in Europe in 2003, but was registered again with restrictions in some countries in 2004. Hepatotoxicity has been reported in conjunction with its use. The drug is absorbed readily after oral ingestion, and peak concentrations in blood are achieved in ~4 hours. It is metabolized to monobromine and dehalogenated derivatives, both of which have uricosuric activity, and is excreted primarily in the bile. The uricosuric action is blunted by aspirin or sulfinpyrazone. No paradoxical retention of urate has been observed. It is a potent and reversible inhibitor of the urate–anion exchanger in the proximal tubule. As the micronized powder, it is effective in a single daily dose of 40-80 mg. It is effective in patients with renal insufficiency and may be prescribed to patients who are either allergic or refractory to other drugs used for the treatment of gout. Preparations that combine allopurinol and benzbromarone are more effective than either drug alone in lowering serum uric acid levels, in spite of the fact that benzbromarone lowers plasma levels of oxypurinol, the active metabolite of allopurinol.

CLINICAL SUMMARY: TREATMENT OF GOUT

Gout is an inflammatory response to the precipitation of monosodium urate crystals in tissues. Although distal joints are typically affected, deposition of crystals can principally occur in any tissue and present as tophaceous gout or urate nephropathy if crystallization is localized in the renal medulla.

Treatment of Acute Gout. Acute gouty arthritis resolves spontaneously within a few days to several weeks. Anti-inflammatory therapy with NSAIDs, colchicines, and intra-articular or systemic glucocorticoids alleviates symptoms more quickly. The IL-1β antagonist, anakinra, is under investigation for this indication.

Several NSAIDs reportedly are effective in the treatment of acute gout, particularly if treatment is initiated within 24 hours of symptom onset. When effective, NSAIDs should be given at relatively high doses for 3-4 days and then tapered for a total of 7-10 days. Indomethacin, naproxen, sulindac, celecoxib, and etoricoxib all have been found to alleviate inflammatory symptoms, although the first three are the only NSAIDs that have received FDA approval for the treatment of gout. Aspirin is not used because it can inhibit urate excretion at low doses, and through its uricosuric actions, can increase the risk of renal calculi at higher doses. In addition, aspirin can inhibit the actions of uricosuric agents. Likewise, apazone should not be used in acute gout because of the concern that its uricosuric effects may promote nephrolithiasis.

Glucocorticoids give rapid relief within hours of therapy. Systemic therapy is initiated with high doses that are then tapered rapidly (e.g., prednisone 30-60 mg/day for 3 days, then tapered over 10-14 days), depending on the size and number of affected joints. Intra-articular glucocorticoids are useful if only a few joints are involved and septic arthritis has been ruled out. Further information on these agents is available in Chapter 42.

Colchicine is thought to alleviate inflammation rapidly through multiple mechanisms, including the inhibition of neutrophil chemotaxis and activation. Symptoms resolve usually within 2-3 days, but adverse GI events are frequent, and toxicity may include bone marrow depression. The therapeutic index of colchicine is narrow—especially in the elderly.

Prevention of Recurrent Attacks. Recurrent attacks of gout can be prevented with the use of NSAIDs or colchicine (e.g., 0.6 mg daily or on alternate days). These agents are used early in the course of uricosuric therapy when mobilization of urate is associated with a temporary increase in the risk of acute gouty arthritis.

Antihyperuricemic Therapy. Isolated hyperuricemia is not necessarily an indication for therapy, as not all of these patients develop gout. Persistently elevated uric acid levels, complicated by recurrent gouty arthritis, nephropathy, or subcutaneous tophi, can be lowered by allopurinol or febuxostat, which inhibit the formation of urate, or by uricosuric agents. Some physicians recommend measuring 24-hour urinary urate levels in patients who are on a low-purine diet to distinguish underexcretors from overproducers. However, tailored and empirical therapies have similar outcomes (Terkeltaub, 2003).

Probenecid and other uricosuric agents increase the rate of uric acid excretion by inhibiting its tubular reabsorption. They compete with uric acid for organic acid transporters, primarily URAT-1, which mediate urate exchange in the proximal tubule. Certain drugs, particularly thiazide diuretics (see Chapter 25) and immunosuppressant agents (especially cyclosporine) may impair urate excretion and thereby increase the risk of gout attacks. Probenecid generally is well tolerated but causes mild GI irritation in some patients. Other uricosuric agents, sulfinpyrazone and benzbromarone, are not available in the U.S.

Rasburicase lowers urate levels by enzymatic oxidation of uric acid into the soluble and inactive metabolite allantoin. It is approved for management of hyperuricemia in children secondary to malignancies. Routine use for hyperuricemia in adults would be limited by the risk of antibody development to uricase, which may result in hypersensitivity. A pegylated uricase form is under development.

BIBLIOGRAPHY

ADAPT Research Group. Cognitive function over time in the Alzheimer's Disease Anti-inflammatory Prevention Trial (ADAPT): Results of a randomized, controlled trial of naproxen and celecoxib. *Arch Neurol,* **2008,** *65*:896–905.

Antithrombotic Trialists' Collaboration. Collaborative meta-analysis of randomised trials of antiplatelet therapy for prevention of death, myocardial infarction, and stroke in high risk patients. *BMJ,* **2002,** *324*:71–86.

Arber N, Eagle CJ, Spicak J, et al. Celecoxib for the prevention of colorectal adenomatous polyps. *N Engl J Med,* **2006,** *355*:885–895.

Arehart E, Stitham J, Asselbergs FW, et al. Acceleration of cardiovascular disease by a dysfunctional prostacyclin receptor mutation: Potential implications for cyclooxygenase-2 inhibition. *Circ Res,* **2008,** *102*:986–993.

Ballou LR, Botting RM, Goorha S, et al. Nociception in cyclooxygenase isozyme-deficient mice. *Proc Natl Acad Sci U S A,* **2000,** *97*:10272–10276.

Barbanoj, MJ, Antonijoan RM, Gich I. Clinical pharmacokinetics of dexketoprofen. *Clin Pharmacokinet,* **2001,** *40*:245–262.

Baron JA, Sandler RS, Bresalier RS, et al. A randomized trial of rofecoxib for the chemoprevention of colorectal adenomas. *Gastroenterology,* **2006,** *131*:1674–1682.

Baron JA, Sandler RS, Bresalier RS, et al. Cardiovascular events associated with rofecoxib: Final analysis of the APPROVe trial. *Lancet,* **2008,** *372*:1756–1764.

Baumer JH, Love SJ, Gupta A, et al. Salicylate for the treatment of Kawasaki disease in children. *Cochrane Database Syst Rev,* **2006,** (4):CD004175.

Becker MA, Schumacher HR Jr, Wortmann RL, et al. Febuxostat, a novel nonpurine selective inhibitor of xanthine oxidase: A twenty-eight-day, multicenter, phase II, randomized, double-blind, placebo-controlled, dose-response clinical trial examining safety and efficacy in patients with gout. *Arthritis Rheum,* **2005a,** *52*:916–923.

Becker MA, Schumacher HR Jr, Wortmann RL, et al. Febuxostat compared with allopurinol in patients with hyperuricemia and gout. *N Engl J Med,* **2005b,** *353*:2450–2461.

Bennett A. Overview of nimesulide. *Rheumatology,* 1999, *38*(suppl):1–3.

Bertagnolli MM, Eagle CJ, Zauber AG, et al. Five-year efficacy and safety analysis of the Adenoma Prevention with Celecoxib Trial. *Cancer Prev Res (Phila Pa),* **2009,** *2*:310–321.

Bombardier C, Laine L, Reicin A, et al. Comparison of upper gastrointestinal toxicity of rofecoxib and naproxen in patients with rheumatoid arthritis. VIGOR Study Group. *N Engl J Med,* **2000,** *343*:1520–1528, 2 p following 1528.

Bosly A, Sonet A, Pinkerton CR, et al. Rasburicase (recombinant urate oxidase) for the management of hyperuricemia in patients with cancer: Report of an international compassionate use study. *Cancer,* **2003,** *98*:1048–1054.

Boutaud O, Aronoff DM, Richardson JH, et al. Determinants of the cellular specificity of acetaminophen as an inhibitor of prostaglandin H(2) synthases. *Proc Natl Acad Sci U S A,* **2002,** *99*:7130–7135.

Brennan FM, McInnes IB. Evidence that cytokines play a role in rheumatoid arthritis. *J Clin Invest,* **2008,** *118*:3537–3545.

Bresalier RS, Sandler RS, Quan H, et al. Cardiovascular events associated with rofecoxib in a colorectal adenoma chemoprevention trial. *N Engl J Med,* **2005,** *352*:1092–1102.

Brogden RN, Heel RC, Speight TM, Avery GS. Fenbufen: A review of its pharmacological properties and therapeutic use in rheumatic diseases and acute pain. *Drugs,* **1981,** *21*:1–22.

Brune K, Hinz B. Selective cyclooxygenase-2 inhibitors: Similarities and differences. *Scand J Rheumatol,* **2004,** *33*:1–6.

Buckley MM, Brogden RN. Ketorolac. A review of its pharmacodynamic and pharmacokinetic properties, and therapeutic potential. *Drugs,* **1990,** *39*:86–109.

Cannon CP, Curtis SP, FitzGerald GA, et al. Cardiovascular outcomes with etoricoxib and diclofenac in patients with osteoarthritis and rheumatoid arthritis in the Multinational Etoricoxib and Diclofenac Arthritis Long-term (MEDAL) programme: A randomised comparison. *Lancet,* **2006,** *368*: 1771–1781.

Capone ML, Sciulli MG, Tacconelli S, et al. Pharmacodynamic interaction of naproxen with low-dose aspirin in healthy subjects. *J Am Coll Cardiol,* **2005,** *45*:1295–1301.

Catella-Lawson F, McAdam B, Morrison BW, et al. Effects of specific inhibition of cyclooxygenase-2 on sodium balance, hemodynamics, and vasoactive eicosanoids. *J Pharmacol Exp Ther,* **1999,** *289*:735–741.

Catella-Lawson F, Reilly MP, Kapoor SC, et al. Cyclooxygenase inhibitors and the antiplatelet effects of aspirin. *N Engl J Med,* **2001,** *345*:1809–1817.

Chandrasekharan NV, Dai H, Roos KL, et al. COX-3, a cyclooxygenase-1 variant inhibited by acetaminophen and other analgesic/antipyretic drugs: Cloning, structure, and expression. *Proc Natl Acad Sci U S A,* **2002,** *99*:13926–13931.

Cheng Y, Austin SC, Rocca B, et al. Role of prostacyclin in the cardiovascular response to thromboxane A2. *Science,* **2002,** *296*:539–541.

Cheng Y, Wang M, Yu Y, et al. Cyclooxygenases, microsomal prostaglandin E synthase-1, and cardiovascular function. *J Clin Invest,* **2006,** *116*:1391–1399.

Cieslik K, Zhu Y, Wu KK. Salicylate suppresses macrophage nitric-oxide synthase-2 and cyclo-oxygenase-2 expression by inhibiting CCAAT/enhancer-binding protein-beta binding via a common signaling pathway. *J Biol Chem,* **2002,** *277*: 49304–49310.

Clyman RI, Hardy P, Waleh N, et al. Cyclooxygenase-2 plays a significant role in regulating the tone of the fetal lamb ductus arteriosus. *Am J Physiol,* **1999,** *276*(3 pt 2):R913–R921.

Coggins KG, Latour A, Nguyen MS, et al. Metabolism of PGE2 by prostaglandin dehydrogenase is essential for remodeling the ductus arteriosus. *Nat Med,* **2002,** *8*:91–92.

Cruz-Correa M, Hylind LM, Romans KE, et al. Long-term treatment with sulindac in familial adenomatous polyposis: A prospective cohort study. *Gastroenterology,* **2002,** *122*: 641–645.

Dai C, Stafford RS, Alexander GC. National trends in cyclooxygenase-2 inhibitor use since market release: Nonselective diffusion of a selectively cost-effective innovation. *Arch Intern Med,* **2005,** *165*:171–177.

Dalton SO, Johansen C, Mellemkjaer L, et al. Use of selective serotonin reuptake inhibitors and risk of upper gastrointestinal tract bleeding: A population-based cohort study. *Arch Intern Med,* **2003,** *163*:59–64.

Davies NM. Clinical pharmacokinetics of flurbiprofen and its enantiomers. *Clin Pharmacokinet,* **1995,** *28*:100–114.

Davies NM. Clinical pharmacokinetics of ibuprofen. The first 30 years. *Clin Pharmacokinet,* **1998a,** *34*:101–154.

Davies NM. Clinical pharmacokinetics of nabumetone. The dawn of selective cyclo-oxygenase-2 inhibition? *Clin Pharmacokinet,* **1997,** *33*:404–416.

Davies NM. Clinical pharmacokinetics of oxaprozin. *Clin Pharmacokinet,* **1998b,** *35*:425–436.

Davies NM, Anderson KE. Clinical pharmacokinetics of diclofenac. Therapeutic insights and pitfalls. *Clin Pharmacokinet,* **1997a,** *33*:184–213.

Davies NM, Anderson KE. Clinical pharmacokinetics of naproxen. *Clin Pharmacokinet,* **1997b,** *32*:268–293.

Davies NM, McLachlan AJ, Day RO, Williams KM. Clinical pharmacokinetics and pharmacodynamics of celecoxib: a selective cyclo-oxygenase-2 inhibitor. *Clin Pharmacokinet,* **2000,** *38*:225–242.

Davies NM, Skjodt NM. Clinical pharmacokinetics of meloxicam. A cyclo-oxygenase-2 preferential nonsteroidal anti-inflammatory drug. *Clin Pharmacokinet,* **1999,** *36*: 115–126.

Davies NM, Teng XW, Skjodt NM. Pharmacokinetics of rofecoxib: A specific cyclo-oxygenase-2 inhibitor. *Clin Pharmacokinet,* **2003,** *42*:545–556.

Day RO, Graham GG, Hicks M, et al. Clinical pharmacokinetics and pharmacodynamics of allopurinol and oxypurinol. *Clin Pharmacokinet,* **2007,** *46*:623–644.

Deeks JJ, Smith LA, Bradley MD. Efficacy, tolerability, and upper gastrointestinal safety of celecoxib for treatment of osteoarthritis and rheumatoid arthritis: Systematic review of randomised controlled trials. *BMJ,* **2002,** *325*:619.

Dempsey PW, Doyle SE, He JQ, Cheng G. The signaling adaptors and pathways activated by TNF superfamily. *Cytokine Growth Factor Rev,* **2003,** *14*:193–209.

Duley L, Henderson-Smart DJ, Knight M, King JF. Antiplatelet agents for preventing pre-eclampsia and its complications. *Cochrane Database Syst Rev,* **2004,** (1):CD004659.

Egan KM, Lawson JA, Fries S, et al. COX-2-derived prostacyclin confers atheroprotection on female mice. *Science,* **2004,** *306*:1954–1957.

Engblom D, Saha S, Engström L, et al. Microsomal prostaglandin E synthase-1 is the central switch during immune-induced pyresis. *Nat Neurosci,* **2003,** *6*:1137–1138.

Enomoto A, Kimura H, Chairoungdua A, et al. Molecular identification of a renal urate anion exchanger that regulates blood urate levels. *Nature,* **2002,** *417*:447–452.

Farkouh ME, Kirshner H, Harrington RA, et al. Comparison of lumiracoxib with naproxen and ibuprofen in the Therapeutic Arthritis Research and Gastrointestinal Event Trial (TARGET), cardiovascular outcomes: Randomised controlled trial. *Lancet,* **2004,** *364*:675–684.

FitzGerald GA, Patrono C. The coxibs, selective inhibitors of cyclooxygenase-2. *N Engl J Med,* **2001,** *345*:433–442.

Fleischmann R, Iqbal I, Slobodin G. Meloxicam. *Expert Opin Pharmacother,* **2002,** *3*:1501–1512.

Fries S, Grosser T, Price TS, et al. Marked interindividual variability in the response to selective inhibitors of cyclooxygenase-2. *Gastroenterology,* **2006,** *130*:55–64.

Gabriel SE, Jaakkimainen L, Bombardier C. Risk for serious gastrointestinal complications related to use of nonsteroidal anti-inflammatory drugs. A meta-analysis. *Ann Intern Med,* **1991,** *115*:787–796.

García Rodríguez LA, Barreales Tolosa L. Risk of upper gastrointestinal complications among users of traditional NSAIDs and COXIBs in the general population. *Gastroenterology,* **2007,** *132*:498–506.

García Rodríguez LA, Varas-Lorenzo C, Maguire A, González-Pérez A. Nonsteroidal antiinflammatory drugs and the risk of myocardial infarction in the general population. *Circulation,* **2004,** *109*:3000–3006.

Glasgow JF, Middleton B. Reye syndrome—Insights on causation and prognosis. *Arch Dis Child,* **2001,** *85*:351–353.

Grosser T, Fries S, FitzGerald GA. Biological basis for the cardiovascular consequences of COX-2 inhibition: therapeutic challenges and opportunities. *J Clin Invest,* **2006,** *116*:4–15.

Guay-Woodford LM. Bartter syndrome: Unraveling the pathophysiologic enigma. *Am J Med,* **1998,** *105*:151–161.

Guttadauria M. The clinical pharmacology of piroxicam. *Acta Obstet Gynecol Scand Suppl,* **1986,** *138*:11–13.

Haanen C. Sulindac and its derivatives: A novel class of anticancer agents. *Curr Opin Investig Drugs,* **2001,** *2*:677–683.

Hallak A, Alon-Baron L, Shamir R, et al. Rofecoxib reduces polyp recurrence in familial polyposis. *Dig Dis Sci,* **2003,** *48*:1998–2002.

Harris RE, Beebe-Donk J, Doss H, Burr Doss D, et al. Aspirin, ibuprofen, and other non-steroidal anti-inflammatory drugs in cancer prevention: A critical review of non-selective COX-2 blockade (review). *Oncol Rep,* **2005,** *13*:559–583.

Heard KJ. Acetylcysteine for acetaminophen poisoning. *N Engl J Med,* **2008,** *359*:285–292.

Jones MK, Wang H, Peskar BM, et al. Inhibition of angiogenesis by nonsteroidal anti-inflammatory drugs: Insight into mechanisms and implications for cancer growth and ulcer healing. *Nat Med,* **1999,** *5*:1418–1423.

Jungnickel PW, Maloley PA, Vander Tuin EL, et al. Effect of two aspirin pretreatment regimens on niacin-induced cutaneous reactions. *J Gen Intern Med,* **1997,** *12*:591–596.

Juni P, Rutjes AW, Dieppe PA. Are selective COX 2 inhibitors superior to traditional non steroidal anti-inflammatory drugs? *BMJ,* **2002,** *324*:1287–1288.

Kobayashi T, Tahara Y, Matsumoto M, et al. Roles of thromboxane A(2) and prostacyclin in the development of atherosclerosis in apoE-deficient mice. *J Clin Invest,* **2004,** *114*:784–794.

Konstan MW, Byard PJ, Hoppel CL, Davis PB. Effect of high-dose ibuprofen in patients with cystic fibrosis. *N Engl J Med,* **1995,** *332*:848–854.

Kulling PE, Backman EA, Skagius AS, Beckman EA. Renal impairment after acute diclofenac, naproxen, and sulindac overdoses. *J Toxicol Clin Toxicol,* **1995,** *33*:173–177.

Kune GA, Kune S, Watson LF. Colorectal cancer risk, chronic illnesses, operations and medications: Case control results from the Melbourne Colorectal Cancer Study. 1988. *Int J Epidemiol,* **2007,** *36*:951–957.

Kurumbail RG, Stevens AM, Gierse JK, et al. Structural basis for selective inhibition of cyclooxygenase-2 by anti-inflammatory agents. *Nature,* **1996,** *384*:644–648.

Laine L, Curtis SP, Cryer B, et al. Assessment of upper gastrointestinal safety of etoricoxib and diclofenac in patients with osteoarthritis and rheumatoid arthritis in the Multinational Etoricoxib and Diclofenac Arthritis Long-term (MEDAL) programme: A randomised comparison. *Lancet,* **2007,** *369*:465–473.

Langenbach R, Loftin CD, Lee C, Tiano H. Cyclooxygenase-deficient mice. A summary of their characteristics and susceptibilities to inflammation and carcinogenesis. *Ann N Y Acad Sci,* **1999,** *889*:52–61.

Levy M, Spino M, Read SE. Colchicine: A state-of-the-art review. *Pharmacotherapy,* **1991,** *11*:196–211.

Loftin CD, Trivedi DB, Langenbach R. Cyclooxygenase-1-selective inhibition prolongs gestation in mice without adverse effects on the ductus arteriosus. *J Clin Invest,* **2002,** *110*: 549–557.

Lopshire JC, Nicol GD. The cAMP transduction cascade mediates the prostaglandin E2 enhancement of the capsaicin-elicited current in rat sensory neurons: Whole-cell and single-channel studies. *J Neurosci,* **1998,** *18*:6081–6092.

Ma L, del Soldato P, Wallace JL. Divergent effects of new cyclooxygenase inhibitors on gastric ulcer healing: Shifting the angiogenic balance. *Proc Natl Acad Sci U S A,* **2002,** *99*:13243–13247.

Maalouf NM, Cameron MA, Moe OW, Sakhaee K. Novel insights into the pathogenesis of uric acid nephrolithiasis. *Curr Opin Nephrol Hypertens,* **2004,** *13*:181–189.

Marjoribanks J, Proctor ML, Farquhar C. Nonsteroidal anti-inflammatory drugs for primary dysmenorrhoea. *Cochrane Database Syst Rev,* **2003,** (4):CD001751.

McAdam BF, Catella-Lawson F, Mardini IA, et al. Systemic biosynthesis of prostacyclin by cyclooxygenase (COX)-2: The human pharmacology of a selective inhibitor of COX-2. *Proc Natl Acad Sci U S A,* **1999,** *96*:272–277.

McAdam BF, Mardini IA, Habib A, et al. Effect of regulated expression of human cyclooxygenase isoforms on eicosanoid and isoeicosanoid production in inflammation. *J Clin Invest,* **2000,** *105*:1473–1482.

McNeely W, Goa KL. Diclofenac-potassium in migraine: A review. *Drugs,* **1999,** *57*:991–1003.

Ment LR, Oh W, Ehrenkranz RA, et al. Low-dose indomethacin therapy and extension of intraventricular hemorrhage: A multicenter randomized trial. *J Pediatr,* **1994,** *124*:951–955.

Mizuno H, Sakamoto C, Matsuda K, et al. Induction of cyclooxygenase 2 in gastric mucosal lesions and its inhibition by the specific antagonist delays healing in mice. *Gastroenterology,* **1997,** *112*:387–397.

Nathan C. Points of control in inflammation. *Nature,* **2002,** *420*:846–852.

Nussmeier NA, Whelton AA, Brown MT, et al. Complications of the COX-2 inhibitors parecoxib and valdecoxib after cardiac surgery. *N Engl J Med,* **2005,** *352*:1081–1091.

O'Malley GF. Emergency department management of the salicylate-poisoned patient. *Emerg Med Clin North Am,* **2007,** *25*:333–346; abstract viii.

O'Neill LA. The interleukin-1 receptor/Toll-like receptor superfamily: 10 years of progress. *Immunol Rev,* **2008,** *226*:10–18.

Ouellet M, Percival MD. Mechanism of acetaminophen inhibition of cyclooxygenase isoforms. *Arch Biochem Biophys,* **2001,** *387*:273–280.

Pascual E, Sivera F, Yasothan U, Kirkpatrick P. Febuxostat. *Nat Rev Drug Discov,* **2009,** *8*:191–192.

Patrignani P, Capone ML, Tacconelli S. Clinical pharmacology of etoricoxib: A novel selective COX2 inhibitor. *Expert Opin Pharmacother,* **2003,** *4*:265–284.

Patrono C, García Rodríguez LA, Landolfi R, Baigent C. Low-dose aspirin for the prevention of atherothrombosis. *N Engl J Med,* **2005,** *353*:2373–2383.

Pedersen AK, FitzGerald GA. Dose-related kinetics of aspirin. Presystemic acetylation of platelet cyclooxygenase. *N Engl J Med,* **1984,** *311*:1206–1211.

Pettipher R, Hansel TT, Armer R. Antagonism of the prostaglandin D2 receptors DP1 and CRTH2 as an approach to treat allergic diseases. *Nat Rev Drug Discov,* **2007,** *6*:313–325.

Picot D, Loll PJ, Garavito RM. The X-ray crystal structure of the membrane protein prostaglandin H2 synthase-1. *Nature,* **1994,** *367*:243–249.

Pulichino AM, Rowland S, Wu T, et al. Prostacyclin antagonism reduces pain and inflammation in rodent models of hyperalgesia and chronic arthritis. *J Pharmacol Exp Ther,* **2006,** *319*: 1043–1050.

Qi Z, Hao CM, Langenbach RI, et al. Opposite effects of cyclooxygenase-1 and -2 activity on the pressor response to angiotensin II. *J Clin Invest,* **2002,** *110*:61–69.

Rainsford KD. Discovery, mechanisms of action and safety of ibuprofen. *Int J Clin Pract Suppl,* **2003,** (135):3–8.

Reinold H, Ahmadi S, Depner UB, et al. Spinal inflammatory hyperalgesia is mediated by prostaglandin E receptors of the EP2 subtype. *J Clin Invest,* **2005,** *115*:673–679.

Rostom A, Dube C, Wells G, et al. Prevention of NSAID-induced gastroduodenal ulcers. *Cochrane Database Syst Rev,* **2002,** (4):CD002296.

Rumack BH, Peterson RC, Koch GG, Amara IA. Acetaminophen overdose. 662 cases with evaluation of oral acetylcysteine treatment. *Arch Intern Med,* **1981,** *141*(3 Spec No.):380–385.

Saag KG, Teng GG, Patkar NM, et al. American College of Rheumatology 2008 recommendations for the use of non-biologic and biologic disease-modifying antirheumatic drugs in rheumatoid arthritis. *Arthritis Rheum,* **2008,** *59*: 762–784.

Samad TA, Moore KA, Sapirstein A, et al. Interleukin-1beta-mediated induction of Cox-2 in the CNS contributes to inflammatory pain hypersensitivity. *Nature,* **2001,** *410*:471–475.

Sanchez-Alavez M, Tabarean IV, Behrens MM, Bartfai T. Ceramide mediates the rapid phase of febrile response to IL-1beta. *Proc Natl Acad Sci U S A,* **2006,** *103*: 2904–2908.

Schnitzer TJ, Burmester GR, Mysler E, et al. Comparison of lumiracoxib with naproxen and ibuprofen in the Therapeutic Arthritis Research and Gastrointestinal Event Trial (TARGET), reduction in ulcer complications: Randomised controlled trial. *Lancet,* **2004,** *364*:665–674.

Schror K. Aspirin and Reye syndrome: A review of the evidence. *Paediatr Drugs,* **2007,** *9*:195–204.

Schumacher HR Jr, Becker MA, Wortmann RL, et al. Effects of febuxostat versus allopurinol and placebo in reducing serum urate in subjects with hyperuricemia and gout: A 28-week, phase III, randomized, double-blind, parallel-group trial. *Arthritis Rheum,* **2008,** *59*:1540–1548.

Schworer H, Ramadori G. Treatment of acute gouty arthritis with the 5-hydroxytryptamine antagonist ondansetron. *Clin Investig,* **1994,** *72*:811–813.

Sigthorsson G, Simpson RJ, Walley M, et al. COX-1 and 2, intestinal integrity, and pathogenesis of nonsteroidal anti-inflammatory drug enteropathy in mice. *Gastroenterology,* **2002,** *122*:1913–1923.

Silverstein FE, Faich G, Goldstein JL, et al. Gastrointestinal toxicity with celecoxib vs nonsteroidal anti-inflammatory drugs for osteoarthritis and rheumatoid arthritis: The CLASS study: A randomized controlled trial. Celecoxib Long-term Arthritis Safety Study. *JAMA,* **2000,** *284*:1247–1255.

Singh G, Fort JG, Goldstein JL, et al. Celecoxib versus naproxen and diclofenac in osteoarthritis patients: SUCCESS-I Study. *Am J Med,* **2006,** *119*:255–266.

Slater DM, Zervou S, Thornton S. Prostaglandins and prostanoid receptors in human pregnancy and parturition. *J Soc Gynecol Investig,* **2002,** *9*:118–124.

Smith WL, DeWitt DL, Garavito RM. Cyclooxygenases: Structural, cellular, and molecular biology. *Annu Rev Biochem,* **2000,** *69*:145–182.

Solomon SD, McMurray JJ, Pfeffer MA, et al. Cardiovascular risk associated with celecoxib in a clinical trial for colorectal adenoma prevention. *N Engl J Med,* **2005,** *352*: 1071–1080.

Solomon SD, Pfeffer MA, McMurray JJ, et al. Effect of celecoxib on cardiovascular events and blood pressure in two trials for the prevention of colorectal adenomas. *Circulation,* **2006,** *114*:1028–1035.

Steinbach G, Lynch PM, Phillips RK, et al. The effect of celecoxib, a cyclooxygenase-2 inhibitor, in familial adenomatous polyposis. *N Engl J Med,* **2000,** *342*:1946–1952.

Terkeltaub R, Bushinsky DA, Becker MA. Recent developments in our understanding of the renal basis of hyperuricemia and the development of novel antihyperuricemic therapeutics. *Arthritis Res Ther,* **2006,** *8*(suppl):S4.

Terkeltaub RA. Clinical practice. Gout. *N Engl J Med,* **2003,** *349*:1647–1655.

U.S. Food and Drug Administration. COX-2 Selective and Non-Selective Non-Steroidal Anti-Inflammatory Drugs, updated 03/03/2010. Available at: www.fda.gov/drugs/drugsafety/postmarketdrugsafetyinformationforpatientsandproviders/ucm103420.htm, accessed July 30, 2010.

Vane JR, Botting RM. Mechanism of action of nonsteroidal anti-inflammatory drugs. *Am J Med,* **1998,** *104*:2S–8S; discussion 21S–22S.

Vanegas H, Schaible HG. Prostaglandins and cyclooxygenases in the spinal cord. *Prog Neurobiol,* **2001,** *64*:327–363.

Veys EM. 20 years' experience with ketoprofen. *Scand J Rheumatol Suppl,* **1991,** *90*(suppl):1–44.

Villar J, Abalos E, Nardin JM, et al. Strategies to prevent and treat preeclampsia: Evidence from randomized controlled trials. *Semin Nephrol,* **2004,** *24*:607–615.

Warner TD, Giuliano F, Vojnovic I, et al. Nonsteroid drug selectivities for cyclo-oxygenase-1 rather than cyclo-oxygenase-2 are associated with human gastrointestinal toxicity: A full in vitro analysis. *Proc Natl Acad Sci U S A,* **1999,** *96*: 7563–7568.

Worobec AS. Treatment of systemic mast cell disorders. *Hematol Oncol Clin North Am,* **2000,** *14*:659–687, vii.

Yin MJ, Yamamoto Y, Gaynor RB. The anti-inflammatory agents aspirin and salicylate inhibit the activity of I(kappa)B kinase-beta. *Nature,* **1998,** *396*:77–80.

Yu Y, Cheng Y, Fan J, et al. Differential impact of prostaglandin H synthase 1 knockdown on platelets and parturition. *J Clin Invest,* **2005,** *115*:986–995.

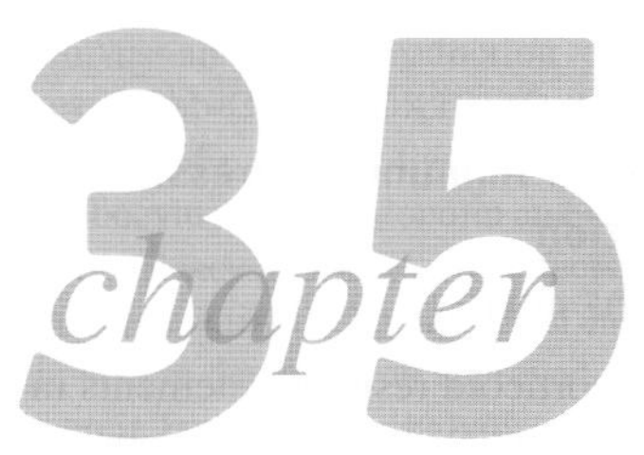

Immunosuppressants, Tolerogens, and Immunostimulants

Alan M. Krensky, William M. Bennett, and Flavio Vincenti

THE IMMUNE RESPONSE

The immune system evolved to discriminate self from nonself. Multicellular organisms were faced with the problem of destroying infectious invaders (microbes) or dysregulated self (tumors) while leaving normal cells intact. These organisms responded by developing a robust array of receptor-mediated sensing and effector mechanisms broadly described as innate and adaptive. Innate, or natural, immunity is primitive, does not require priming, and is of relatively low affinity, but is broadly reactive. Adaptive, or learned, immunity is antigen specific, depends on antigen exposure or priming, and can be of very high affinity. The two arms of immunity work closely together, with the innate immune system being most active early in an immune response and adaptive immunity becoming progressively dominant over time. The major effectors of innate immunity are complement, granulocytes, monocytes/macrophages, natural killer cells, mast cells, and basophils. The major effectors of adaptive immunity are B and T lymphocytes. B lymphocytes make antibodies; T lymphocytes function as helper, cytolytic, and regulatory (suppressor) cells. These cells are important in the normal immune response to infection and tumors but also mediate transplant rejection and auto-immunity. Immunoglobulins (antibodies) on the B-lymphocyte surface are receptors for a large variety of specific structural conformations. In contrast, T lymphocytes recognize antigens as peptide fragments in the context of self major histocompatibility complex (MHC) antigens (called human leukocyte antigens [HLAs] in humans) on the surface of antigen-presenting cells, such as dendritic cells, macrophages, and other cell types expressing MHC class I (HLA-A, -B, and -C) and class II antigens (HLA-DR, -DP, and -DQ) in humans. Once activated by specific antigen recognition via their respective clonally restricted cell-surface receptors, both B and T lymphocytes are triggered to differentiate and divide, leading to release of soluble mediators (cytokines, lymphokines) that perform as effectors and regulators of the immune response.

The impact of the immune system in human disease is enormous. Developing vaccines against emerging infectious agents such as human immunodeficiency virus (HIV) and Ebola virus is among the most critical challenges facing the research community. Immune system–mediated diseases are significant medical problems. Immunological diseases are growing at epidemic proportions that require aggressive and innovative approaches to develop new treatments. These diseases include a broad spectrum of auto-immune diseases, such as rheumatoid arthritis, type I diabetes mellitus, systemic lupus erythematosus, and multiple sclerosis (MS); solid tumors and hematological malignancies; infectious diseases; asthma; and various allergic conditions. Furthermore, one of the great therapeutic opportunities for the treatment of many disorders is organ transplantation. However, immune system–mediated graft rejection remains the single greatest barrier to widespread use of this technology. An improved understanding of the immune system has led to the development of new therapies to treat immune system–mediated diseases.

This chapter briefly reviews drugs used to modulate the immune response in three ways: immunosuppression, tolerance, and immunostimulation. Four major classes of immunosuppressive drugs are discussed: glucocorticoids (Chapter 42), calcineurin inhibitors, antiproliferative and antimetabolic agents (Chapter 61), and antibodies. The "holy grail" of immunomodulation is other immunosuppressive agents to prevent and treat transplant rejection. High-dose pulses of intravenous methylprednisolone sodium succinate (SOLU-MEDROL, others) are used to reverse acute transplant rejection and acute exacerbations of selected auto-immune disorders. Glucocorticoids also are efficacious for treatment of graft-versus-host disease in bone-marrow transplantation. Glucocorticoids are routinely used to treat auto-immune disorders such as rheumatoid and other arthritides, systemic lupus erythematosus, systemic dermatomyositis, psoriasis and other skin conditions, asthma and other allergic disorders, inflammatory bowel disease, inflammatory ophthalmic diseases, auto-immune hematological disorders, and acute exacerbations of MS (see "Multiple Sclerosis"). In addition, glucocorticoids limit allergic reactions that occur with other immunosuppressive agents and are used in transplant recipients to block first-dose cytokine storm caused by treatment with muromonab-CD3 and to a lesser extent ATG (see "Antithymocyte Globulin").

Toxicity. Unfortunately, the extensive use of steroids often results in disabling and life-threatening adverse effects. These effects include growth retardation in children, avascular necrosis of bone, osteopenia, increased risk of infection, poor wound healing, cataracts, hyperglycemia, and hypertension (Chapter 42). The advent of combined glucocorticoid/calcineurin inhibitor regimens has allowed reduced doses or rapid withdrawal of steroids, resulting in lower steroid-induced morbidities.

Calcineurin Inhibitors

Perhaps the most effective immunosuppressive drugs in routine use are the calcineurin inhibitors, cyclosporine and tacrolimus, which target intracellular signaling pathways induced as a consequence of T cell–receptor activation. Although they are structurally unrelated (Figure 35-1) and bind to distinct (albeit related) molecular targets, they inhibit normal T-cell signal transduction essentially by the same mechanism (Figure 35–2). Cyclosporine and tacrolimus do not act *per se* as immunosuppressive agents. Instead, these drugs bind to an immunophilin (cyclophilin for cyclosporine [see "Cyclosporine"] or FKBP-12 for tacrolimus [see "Tacrolimus"]), resulting in subsequent interaction with calcineurin to block its phosphatase activity. Calcineurin-catalyzed dephosphorylation is required for movement of a component of the nuclear factor of activated T lymphocytes (NFAT) into the nucleus (Figure 35–2). NFAT, in turn, is required to induce a number of cytokine genes, including that for interleukin-2 (IL-2), a prototypic T-cell growth and differentiation factor.

Tacrolimus. Tacrolimus (PROGRAF, FK506) is a macrolide antibiotic produced by *Streptomyces tsukubaensis* (Goto et al., 1987). Because of perceived slightly greater efficacy and ease of blood level monitoring, tacrolimus has become the preferred calcineurin inhibitor in most transplant centers (Ekberg et al., 2008).

Mechanism of Action. Like cyclosporine, tacrolimus inhibits T-cell activation by inhibiting calcineurin. Tacrolimus binds to an intracellular protein, FK506-binding protein–12 (FKBP-12), an immunophilin structurally related to cyclophilin. A complex of tacrolimus-FKBP-12, Ca^{2+}, calmodulin, and calcineurin then forms, and calcineurin phosphatase activity is inhibited. As described for cyclosporine and depicted in Figure 35–2, the inhibition of phosphatase activity prevents dephosphorylation and nuclear translocation of NFAT and inhibits T-cell activation. Thus, although the intracellular receptors differ, cyclosporine and tacrolimus target the same pathway for immunosuppression.

Disposition and Pharmacokinetics. Tacrolimus is available for oral administration as capsules (0.5, 1, and 5 mg) and as a solution for injection (5 mg/mL). Immunosuppressive activity resides primarily in the parent drug. Because of intersubject variability in pharmacokinetics, individualized dosing is required for optimal therapy. Whole blood, rather than plasma, is the most appropriate sampling compartment to describe tacrolimus pharmacokinetics. For tacrolimus, the trough drug level seems to correlate better with clinical events than it does for cyclosporine. Target concentrations in most centers are 10-15 ng/mL in the early preoperative period and 100-200 ng/mL 3 months after transplantation. Gastrointestinal absorption is incomplete and variable. Food decreases the rate and extent of absorption. Plasma protein binding of tacrolimus is 75-99%, involving primarily albumin and α_1-acid glycoprotein. The $t_{1/2}$ of tacrolimus is ~12 hours. Tacrolimus is extensively metabolized in the liver by CYP3A; at least some of the metabolites are active. The bulk of excretion of the parent drug and metabolites is in the feces. Less than 1% of administered tacrolimus is excreted unchanged in the urine.

Therapeutic Uses. Tacrolimus is indicated for the prophylaxis of solid-organ allograft rejection in a manner similar to cyclosporine (see "Cyclosporine") and is used off label as rescue therapy in patients with rejection episodes despite "therapeutic" levels of cyclosporine.

Recommended initial oral doses are 0.2 mg/kg/day for adult kidney transplant patients, 0.1-0.15 mg/kg/day for adult liver transplant patients, 0.075 mg/kg/day for adult heart transplant patients, and 0.15-0.2 mg/kg/day for pediatric liver transplant patients in two divided doses 12 hours apart. These dosages are intended to achieve typical blood trough levels in the 5- to 20-ng/mL range.

Toxicity. Nephrotoxicity, neurotoxicity (e.g., tremor, headache, motor disturbances, seizures), GI complaints, hypertension, hyperkalemia, hyperglycemia, and diabetes all are associated with tacrolimus use. As with cyclosporine, nephrotoxicity is limiting. Tacrolimus has a negative effect on pancreatic islet β cells, and glucose intolerance and diabetes mellitus are well-recognized complications of tacrolimus-based immunosuppression. As with other immunosuppressive agents,

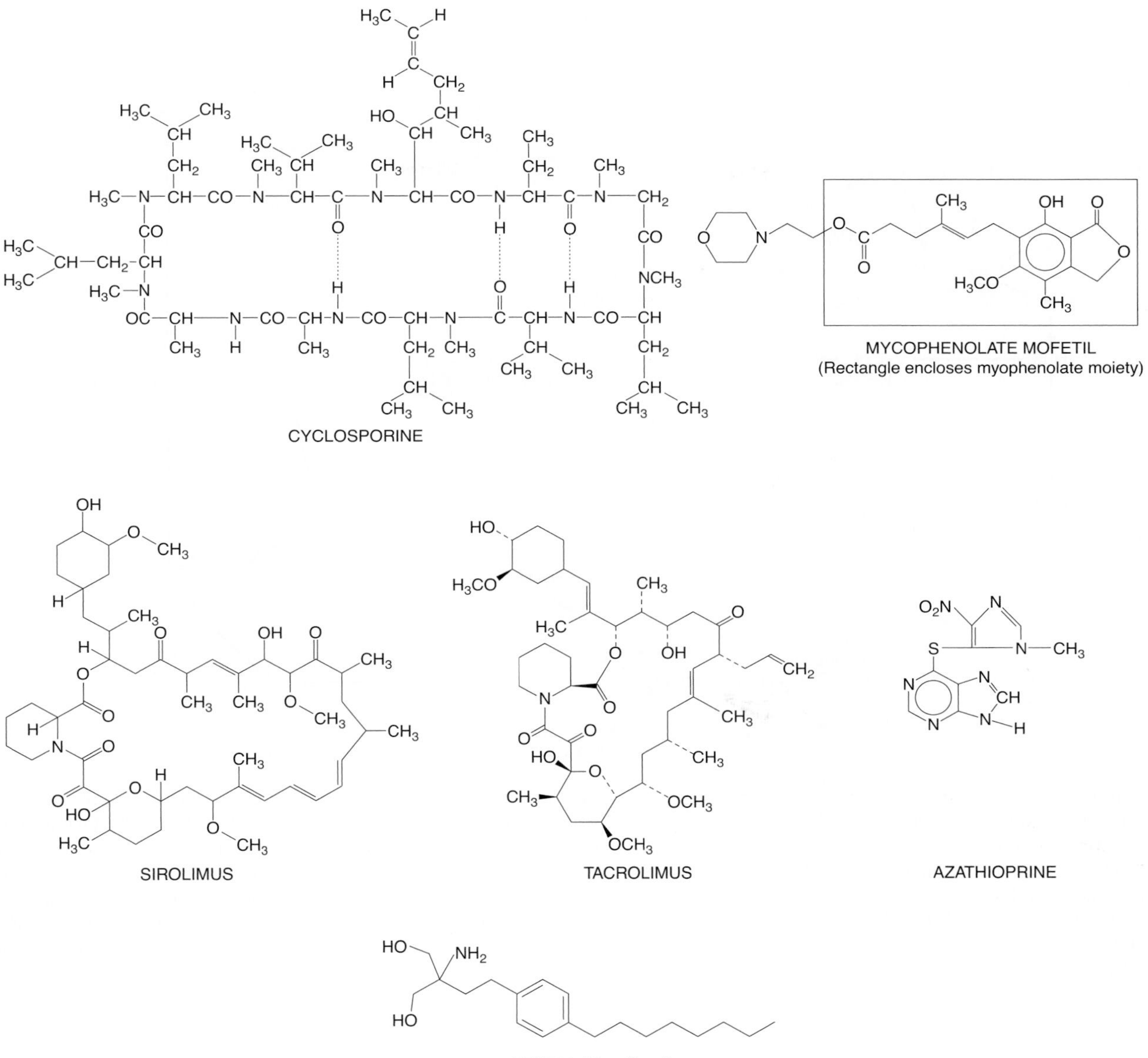

CYCLOSPORINE

MYCOPHENOLATE MOFETIL
(Rectangle encloses myophenolate moiety)

SIROLIMUS

TACROLIMUS

AZATHIOPRINE

FTY720 (Fingolimod)

Figure 35–1. *Chemical structures of immunosuppressive drugs.*

there is an increased risk of secondary tumors and opportunistic infections. Notably, tacrolimus does not adversely affect uric acid or LDL cholesterol. Diarrhea and alopecia are commonly noted in patients on concomitant mycophenolate therapy.

Drug Interactions. Because of its potential for nephrotoxicity, tacrolimus blood levels and renal function should be monitored closely, especially when tacrolimus is used with other potentially nephrotoxic drugs. Co-administration with cyclosporine results in additive or synergistic nephrotoxicity; therefore, a delay of at least 24 hours is required when switching a patient from cyclosporine to tacrolimus. Because tacrolimus is metabolized mainly by CYP3A, the potential interactions described in the following section for cyclosporine also apply for tacrolimus.

Cyclosporine

Chemistry. Cyclosporine (cyclosporin A), a cyclic polypeptide of 11 amino acids, is produced by the fungus *Beauveria nivea*. Because cyclosporine is lipophilic and highly hydrophobic, it is formulated for clinical administration using castor oil or other strategies to ensure solubilization.

Mechanism of Action. Cyclosporine suppresses some humoral immunity but is more effective against T cell–dependent immune

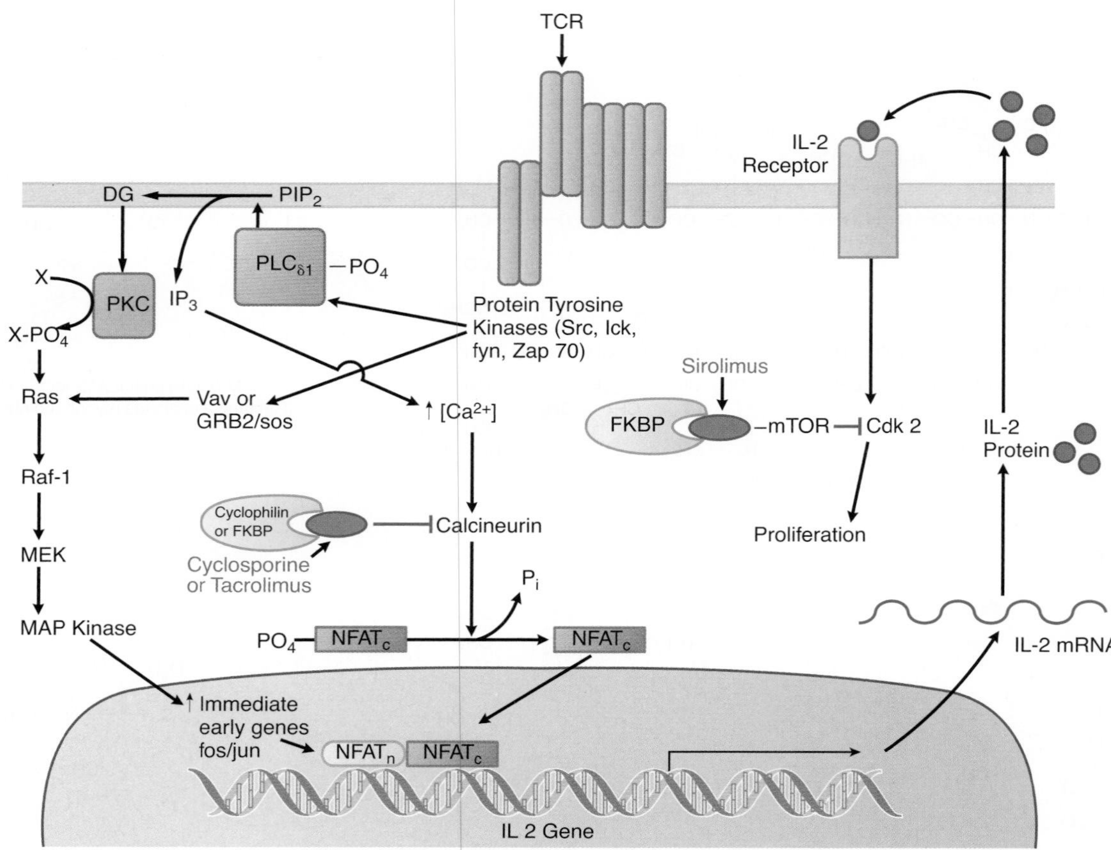

Figure 35–2. *Mechanisms of action of cyclosporine, tacrolimus, and sirolimus on T lymphocytes.* Both cyclosporine and tacrolimus bind to immunophilins (cyclophilin and FK506-binding protein [FKBP], respectively), forming a complex that binds the phosphatase calcineurin and inhibits the calcineurin-catalyzed dephosphorylation essential to permit movement of the nuclear factor of activated T cells (NFAT) into the nucleus. NFAT is required for transcription of interleukin-2 (IL-2) and other growth- and differentiation-associated cytokines (lymphokines). Sirolimus (rapamycin) works at a later stage in T-cell activation, downstream of the IL-2 receptor. Sirolimus also binds FKBP, but the FKBP-sirolimus complex binds to and inhibits the mammalian target of rapamycin (mTOR), a kinase involved in cell-cycle progression (proliferation). TCR, T-cell receptor. (From Pattison et al., 1997, with permission. Copyright © Lippincott Williams & Wilkins. http://lww.com.)

mechanisms such as those underlying transplant rejection and some forms of auto-immunity. It preferentially inhibits antigen-triggered signal transduction in T lymphocytes, blunting expression of many lymphokines, including IL-2, and the expression of anti-apoptotic proteins. Cyclosporine forms a complex with cyclophilin, a cytoplasmic-receptor protein present in target cells (Figure 35-2). This complex binds to calcineurin, inhibiting Ca^{2+}-stimulated dephosphorylation of the cytosolic component of NFAT (Schreiber and Crabtree, 1992). When cytoplasmic NFAT is dephosphorylated, it translocates to the nucleus and complexes with nuclear components required for complete T-cell activation, including transactivation of IL-2 and other lymphokine genes. Calcineurin phosphatase activity is inhibited after physical interaction with the cyclosporine/cyclophilin complex. This prevents NFAT dephosphorylation such that NFAT does not enter the nucleus, gene transcription is not activated, and the T lymphocyte fails to respond to specific antigenic stimulation. Cyclosporine also increases expression of transforming growth factor β (TGF-β), a potent inhibitor of IL-2–stimulated T-cell proliferation and generation of cytotoxic T lymphocytes (CTLs) (Khanna et al., 1994).

Disposition and Pharmacokinetics. Cyclosporine can be administered intravenously or orally. The intravenous preparation (SANDIMMUNE, others) is provided as a solution in an ethanol-polyoxyethylated castor oil vehicle that must be further diluted in 0.9% sodium chloride solution or 5% dextrose solution before injection. The oral dosage forms include soft gelatin capsules and oral solutions. Cyclosporine supplied in the original soft gelatin capsule is absorbed slowly, with 20-50% bioavailability. A modified microemulsion formulation (NEORAL) has become the most widely used preparation. It has more uniform and slightly increased bioavailability compared to the original formulation. It is provided as 25-mg and 100-mg soft gelatin capsules and a 100-mg/mL oral solution. Because the original and microemulsion formulations are not bioequivalent, they cannot be used interchangeably without supervision by a physician and monitoring of drug concentrations in plasma. Generic preparations of both NEORAL and SANDIMMUNE, now widely available, are bioequivalent by FDA criteria. When switching between formulations, increased surveillance is recommended to ensure that drug levels remain in the therapeutic range. This need for increased monitoring is based on anecdotal experience rather than validated differences. *Because* SANDIMMUNE *and* NEORAL *differ in terms of their pharmacokinetics and definitely are not bioequivalent, their generic versions cannot be used interchangeably*. This has been a source of confusion to pharmacists and patients. Transplant units need to educate patients that SANDIMMUNE and its generics are not the same as NEORAL and its generics, such that one preparation cannot be substituted for another without risk of inadequate immunosuppression or increased toxicity.

Blood is most conveniently sampled before the next dose (a C_0 or trough level). Although convenient to obtain, C_0 concentrations do not reflect the area under the drug concentration curve (AUC) as a measure of cyclosporine exposure in individual patients. As a practical solution to this problem and to better measure the overall exposure of a patient to the drug, it has been proposed that levels be taken 2 hours after a dose administration (so-called C_2 levels) (Cole et al., 2003). Some studies have shown a better correlation of C_2 with the AUC, but no single time point can simulate the exposure as measured by more frequent drug sampling. In complex patients with delayed absorption, such as diabetics, the C_2 level may underestimate the peak cyclosporine level obtained, and in others who are rapid absorbers, the C_2 level may have peaked before the blood sample is drawn. In practice, if a patient has clinical signs or symptoms of toxicity, or if there is unexplained rejection or renal dysfunction, a pharmacokinetic profile can be used to estimate that person's exposure to the drug. Many clinicians, particularly those caring for transplant patients some time after the transplant, monitor cyclosporine blood levels only when a clinical event (e.g., renal dysfunction or rejection) occurs. In that setting, either a C_0 or C_2 level helps to ascertain whether inadequate immunosuppression or drug toxicity is present. As described above, cyclosporine absorption is incomplete following oral administration and varies with the individual patient and the formulation used. The elimination of cyclosporine from the blood generally is biphasic, with a terminal $t_{1/2}$ of 5-18 hours (Noble and Markham, 1995). After intravenous infusion, clearance is ~5-7 mL/min/kg in adult recipients of renal transplants, but results differ by age and patient populations. For example, clearance is slower in cardiac transplant patients and more rapid in children. Thus, the intersubject variability is so large that individual monitoring is required.

After oral administration of cyclosporine (as NEORAL), the time to peak blood concentrations is 1.5-2 hours (Noble and Markham, 1995). Administration with food delays and decreases absorption. High- and low-fat meals consumed within 30 minutes of administration decrease the AUC by ~13% and the maximum concentration by 33%. This makes it imperative to individualize dosage regimens for outpatients.

Cyclosporine is distributed extensively outside the vascular compartment. After intravenous dosing, the steady-state volume of distribution reportedly is as high as 3-5 L/kg in solid-organ transplant recipients.

Only 0.1% of cyclosporine is excreted unchanged in urine. Cyclosporine is extensively metabolized in the liver by CYP3A and to a lesser degree by the GI tract and kidneys. At least 25 metabolites have been identified in human bile, feces, blood, and urine. All of the metabolites have reduced biological activity and toxicity compared to the parent drug. Cyclosporine and its metabolites are excreted principally through the bile into the feces, with ~6% being excreted in the urine. Cyclosporine also is excreted in human milk. In the presence of hepatic dysfunction, dosage adjustments are required. No adjustments generally are necessary for dialysis or renal failure patients.

Therapeutic Uses. Clinical indications for cyclosporine are kidney, liver, heart, and other organ transplantation; rheumatoid arthritis; and psoriasis. Its use in dermatology is discussed in Chapter 65. Cyclosporine generally is recognized as the agent that ushered in the modern era of organ transplantation, increasing the rates of early engraftment, extending kidney graft survival, and making cardiac and liver transplantation possible. Cyclosporine usually is combined with other agents, especially glucocorticoids and either azathioprine or mycophenolate and, most recently, sirolimus.

The dose of cyclosporine varies, depending on the organ transplanted and the other drugs used in the specific treatment protocol(s). The initial dose generally is not given before the transplant because of the concern about nephrotoxicity. Especially for renal transplant patients, therapeutic algorithms have been developed to delay cyclosporine or tacrolimus introduction until a threshold renal function has been attained. The amount of the initial dose and reduction to maintenance dosing is sufficiently variable that no specific recommendation is provided here. Dosing is guided by signs of rejection (too low a dose), renal or other toxicity (too high a dose), and close monitoring of blood levels. Great care must be taken to differentiate renal toxicity from rejection in kidney transplant patients. Ultrasound-guided allograft biopsy is the best way to assess the reason for renal dysfunction. Because adverse reactions have been ascribed more frequently to the intravenous formulation, this route of administration is discontinued as soon as the patient can take the drug orally.

In rheumatoid arthritis, cyclosporine is used in severe cases that have not responded to methotrexate. Cyclosporine can be combined with methotrexate, but the levels of both drugs must be monitored closely. In psoriasis, cyclosporine is indicated for treatment of adult immunocompetent patients with severe and disabling disease for whom other systemic therapies have failed. Because of its mechanism of action, there is a theoretical basis for the use of cyclosporine in a variety of other T cell–mediated diseases. Cyclosporine reportedly is effective in Behçet's acute ocular syndrome, endogenous uveitis, atopic dermatitis, inflammatory bowel disease, and nephrotic syndrome, even when standard therapies have failed.

Toxicity. The principal adverse reactions to cyclosporine therapy are renal dysfunction and hypertension; tremor, hirsutism, hyperlipidemia, and gum hyperplasia also are frequently encountered. Hypertension occurs in ~50% of renal transplant and almost all cardiac transplant patients. Hyperuricemia may lead to worsening of gout, increased P-glycoprotein activity, and hypercholesterolemia. Nephrotoxicity occurs in the majority of patients and is the major reason for cessation or modification of therapy (Nankivell et al., 2003). Recent reviews of calcineurin inhibitor nephrotoxicity are available (Burdmann et al., 2003). Combined use of calcineurin inhibitors and glucocorticoids is particularly diabetogenic, although this apparently is more problematic in patients treated with tacrolimus (see "Tacrolimus" section earlier). Especially at risk are obese patients, African-American or Hispanic transplant recipients, or those with a family history of type II diabetes or obesity. Cyclosporine, as opposed to tacrolimus, is more likely to produce elevations in LDL cholesterol (Artz et al., 2003).

Drug Interactions. Cyclosporine interacts with a wide variety of commonly used drugs, and close attention must be paid to drug interactions. Any drug that affects microsomal enzymes, especially CYP3A, may impact cyclosporine blood concentrations.

Substances that inhibit this enzyme can decrease cyclosporine metabolism and increase blood concentrations. These include Ca^{2+} channel blockers (e.g., verapamil, nicardipine), antifungal agents (e.g., fluconazole, ketoconazole), antibiotics (e.g., erythromycin), glucocorticoids (e.g., methylprednisolone), HIV-protease inhibitors (e.g., indinavir), and other drugs (e.g., allopurinol, metoclopramide). Grapefruit juice inhibits CYP3A and the P-glycoprotein multidrug efflux pump and should be minimized by patients taking cyclosporine because these effects can increase cyclosporine blood concentrations. In contrast, drugs that induce CYP3A activity can increase cyclosporine metabolism and decrease blood concentrations. Such drugs include antibiotics (e.g., nafcillin, rifampin), anticonvulsants (e.g., phenobarbital, phenytoin), and others (e.g., octreotide, ticlopidine). In general, close monitoring of cyclosporine blood levels and the levels of other drugs is required when such combinations are used.

Interactions between cyclosporine and sirolimus (also see "Drug Interactions" in the sirolimus section) have led to the recommendation that administration of the two drugs be separated by time. Sirolimus aggravates cyclosporine-induced renal dysfunction, while cyclosporine increases sirolimus-induced hyperlipidemia and myelosuppression. Other drug interactions of concern include additive nephrotoxicity when cyclosporine is co-administered with nonsteroidal anti-inflammatory drugs (NSAIDs) and other drugs that cause renal dysfunction; elevation of methotrexate levels when the two drugs are co-administered; and reduced clearance of other drugs, including prednisolone, digoxin, and statins.

ISATX247. This is a new oral semisynthetic structural analog of cyclosporine. The cyclosporine molecule is modified at the first amino acid residue. It is more potent on a weight basis than cyclosporine *in vitro* for calcineurin inhibition. Some preclinical studies show reduced nephrotoxicity, and thus the drug is in clinical development as a primary immunosuppressive drug. Phase 2 clinical trials are in process and thus far show similar or less nephrotoxicity with less frequent glucose intolerance compared to tacrolimus-treated patients (Vincenti and Kirk, 2008).

Janus Kinase Inhibitors/CP-690550. Cytokine receptors are enticing targets for modulation by new small immunosuppressive molecules. Janus kinase (JAK) inhibitors are a class of drugs that inhibit important cytoplasmic tyrosine kinases that are involved in cell signaling. The molecule CP-690550 currently is in clinical trials. As an immunosuppressive drug, this compound inhibits JAK3, which is found primarily on hematopoietic cells. In preclinical studies, this JAK3 inhibitor has been tolerated without nephrotoxicity, malignancy, or other important side effects. To date, all studies have shown non-inferiority with other standard immunosuppressive regimens (Vincenti and Kirk, 2008).

Protein Kinase C Inhibitors/AEB071. Various isoforms of PKC are important mediators in signaling pathways distal to the T-cell receptor and co-stimulators. AEB071 is a low-molecular-weight compound that blocks T-cell activation by inhibition of PKC, thus producing immunosuppression by a different mechanism than calcineurin inhibitors. Clinical studies are ongoing. Early trials using PKC inhibitors in combination with calcineurin inhibitors (CNIs) followed by discontinuation of the CNI had to be stopped because acute rejections occurred when the CNIs were discontinued (Vincenti and Kirk, 2008).

Anti-Proliferative and Antimetabolic Drugs

Sirolimus

Sirolimus (rapamycin; RAPAMUNE) is a macrocyclic lactone (Figure 35–1) produced by *Streptomyces hygroscopicus*.

Mechanism of Action. Sirolimus inhibits T-lymphocyte activation and proliferation downstream of the IL-2 and other T-cell growth factor receptors (Figure 35–2). Like cyclosporine and tacrolimus, therapeutic action of sirolimus requires formation of a complex with an immunophilin, in this case FKBP-12. However, the sirolimus–FKBP-12 complex does not affect calcineurin activity. It binds to and inhibits a protein kinase, designated mTOR, which is a key enzyme in cell-cycle progression. Inhibition of mTOR blocks cell-cycle progression at the $G_1 \rightarrow S$ phase transition. In animal models, sirolimus not only inhibits transplant rejection, graft-versus-host disease, and a variety of auto-immune diseases, but its effect also lasts several months after discontinuing therapy, suggesting a tolerizing effect (see "Tolerance") (Groth et al., 1999). A newer indication for sirolimus is the avoidance of calcineurin inhibitors, even when patients are stable, to protect kidney function (Flechner et al., 2008).

Disposition and Pharmacokinetics. After oral administration, sirolimus is absorbed rapidly and reaches a peak blood concentration within ~1 hour after a single dose in healthy subjects and within ~2 hours after multiple oral doses in renal transplant patients. Systemic availability is ~15%, and blood concentrations are proportional to doses between 3 and 12 mg/m^2. A high-fat meal decreases peak blood concentration by 34%; sirolimus therefore should be taken consistently either with or without food, and blood levels should be monitored closely. About 40% of sirolimus in plasma is protein bound, especially to albumin. The drug partitions into formed elements of blood, with a blood-to-plasma ratio of 38 in renal transplant patients. Sirolimus is extensively metabolized by CYP3A4 and is transported by P-glycoprotein. Seven major metabolites have been identified in whole blood. Metabolites also are detectable in feces and urine, with the bulk of total excretion being in feces. Although some of its metabolites are active, sirolimus itself is the major active component in whole blood and contributes >90% of the immunosuppressive effect. The blood $t_{1/2}$ after multiple doses in stable renal transplant patients is 62 hours (Zimmerman and Kahan, 1997). A loading dose of three times the maintenance dose will provide nearly steady-state concentrations within 1 day in most patients.

Therapeutic Uses. Sirolimus is indicated for prophylaxis of organ transplant rejection usually in combination with a reduced dose of calcineurin inhibitor and glucocorticoids. In patients experiencing or at high risk for calcineurin inhibitor–associated nephrotoxicity, sirolimus has been used with glucocorticoids and mycophenolate to avoid permanent renal damage. Sirolimus dosing regimens are relatively complex with blood levels generally targeted between 5-15 ng/mL. It is recommended that the daily maintenance dose be reduced by approximately one-third in patients with hepatic impairment (Watson et al., 1999). Sirolimus also has been incorporated into stents to inhibit local cell proliferation and blood vessel occlusion.

Toxicity. The use of sirolimus in renal transplant patients is associated with a dose-dependent increase in serum cholesterol and triglycerides that may require treatment. Although immunotherapy with sirolimus *per se* is not nephrotoxic, patients treated with cyclosporine plus sirolimus have impaired renal function compared to patients treated with cyclosporine and either azathioprine or placebo. Sirolimus also may prolong delayed graft function in deceased donor kidney transplants, presumably because of its antiproliferative action (Smith et al., 2003). Renal function therefore must be monitored closely in such patients. Lymphocele, a known surgical complication associated with renal transplantation, is increased in a dose-dependent fashion by sirolimus, requiring close postoperative follow-up. Other adverse effects include anemia, leukopenia, thrombocytopenia, mouth ulcer, hypokalemia, proteinuria, and GI effects. Delayed wound healing may occur with sirolimus use. As with other immunosuppressive agents, there is an increased risk of neoplasms, especially lymphomas, and infections. Sirolimus is not recommended in liver and lung transplants due to the risk of hepatic artery thrombosis and bronchial anastomotic dehiscence, respectively.

Drug Interactions. Because sirolimus is a substrate for CYP3A4 and is transported by P-glycoprotein, close attention to interactions with other drugs that are metabolized or transported by these proteins is required. As noted above, cyclosporine and sirolimus interact, and their administration should be separated by time. Dose adjustment may be required when sirolimus is co-administered with diltiazem or rifampin. Dose adjustment apparently is not required when sirolimus is co-administered with acyclovir, digoxin, glyburide, nifedipine, norgestrel/ethinyl estradiol, prednisolone, or trimethoprim–sulfamethoxazole. This list is incomplete, and blood levels and potential drug interactions must be monitored closely.

Everolimus

Everolimus [40-*O*-(2-hydroxyethyl)-rapamycin] is closely related chemically and clinically to sirolimus but has distinct pharmacokinetics. The main difference is a shorter $t_{1/2}$ and thus a shorter time to achieve steady-state concentrations of the drug. Dosage on a milligram per kilogram basis is similar to that of sirolimus. Aside from the shorter $t_{1/2}$, no studies have compared everolimus with sirolimus in standard immunosuppressive regimens (Eisen et al., 2003). As with sirolimus, the combination of a calcineurin inhibitor and an mTOR inhibitor produces worse renal function at 1 year than does calcineurin inhibitor therapy alone, suggesting a drug interaction between the mTOR inhibitors and the calcineurin inhibitors that enhances toxicity and reduces rejection. The toxicity of everolimus and the drug interactions reported to date seem to be the same as with sirolimus.

Azathioprine

Azathioprine (IMURAN, others) is a purine antimetabolite. It is an imidazolyl derivative of 6-mercaptopurine (see Figure 61–11).

Mechanism of Action. Following exposure to nucleophiles such as glutathione, azathioprine is cleaved to 6-mercaptopurine, which in turn is converted to additional metabolites that inhibit *de novo* purine synthesis (Chapter 61). A fraudulent nucleotide, 6-thio-IMP, is converted to 6-thio-GMP and finally to 6-thio-GTP, which is incorporated into DNA. Cell proliferation thereby is inhibited, impairing a variety of lymphocyte functions. Azathioprine appears to be a more potent immunosuppressive agent than 6-mercaptopurine, which may reflect differences in drug uptake or pharmacokinetic differences in the resulting metabolites.

Disposition and Pharmacokinetics. Azathioprine is well absorbed orally and reaches maximum blood levels within 1-2 hours after administration. The $t_{1/2}$ of azathioprine is ~10 minutes, while that of its metabolite, 6-mercaptopurine, is ~1 hour. Other metabolites have a $t_{1/2}$ of up to 5 hours. Blood levels have limited predictive value because of extensive metabolism, significant activity of many different metabolites, and high tissue levels attained. Azathioprine and mercaptopurine are moderately bound to plasma proteins and are partially dialyzable. Both are rapidly removed from the blood by oxidation or methylation in the liver and/or erythrocytes. Renal clearance has little impact on biological effectiveness or toxicity.

Therapeutic Uses. Azathioprine was first introduced as an immunosuppressive agent in 1961, helping to make allogeneic kidney transplantation possible. It is indicated as an adjunct for prevention of organ transplant rejection and in severe rheumatoid arthritis. Although the dose of azathioprine required to prevent organ rejection and minimize toxicity varies, 3-5 mg/kg/day is the usual starting dose. Lower initial doses (1 mg/kg/day) are used in treating rheumatoid arthritis. Complete blood count and liver function tests should be monitored.

Toxicity. The major side effect of azathioprine is bone marrow suppression, including leukopenia (common), thrombocytopenia (less common), and/or anemia (uncommon). Other important adverse effects include increased susceptibility to infections (especially varicella and herpes simplex viruses), hepatotoxicity, alopecia, GI toxicity, pancreatitis, and increased risk of neoplasia.

Drug Interactions. Xanthine oxidase, an enzyme of major importance in the catabolism of azathioprine metabolites, is blocked by allopurinol. If azathioprine and allopurinol are used concurrently, the azathioprine dose must be decreased to 25-33% of the usual dose; it is best not to use these two drugs together. Adverse effects resulting from co-administration of azathioprine with other myelosuppressive agents or angiotensin-converting enzyme inhibitors include leukopenia, thrombocytopenia, and anemia as a result of myelosuppression.

Mycophenolate Mofetil

Mycophenolate mofetil (MMF; CELL-CEPT) is the 2-morpholinoethyl ester of mycophenolic acid (MPA).

Mechanism of Action. MMF is a prodrug that is rapidly hydrolyzed to the active drug, MPA, a selective, noncompetitive, reversible inhibitor of inosine monophosphate dehydrogenase (IMPDH), an important enzyme in the *de novo* pathway of guanine nucleotide synthesis. B and T lymphocytes are highly dependent on this pathway for cell proliferation, while other cell types can use salvage pathways; MPA therefore selectively inhibits lymphocyte proliferation and functions, including antibody formation, cellular adhesion, and migration.

Disposition and Pharmacokinetics. MMF undergoes rapid and complete metabolism to MPA after oral or intravenous administration. MPA, in turn, is metabolized to the inactive phenolic glucuronide MPAG. The parent drug is cleared from the blood within a few minutes. The $t_{1/2}$ of MPA is ~16 hours. Negligible (<1%) amounts of MPA are excreted in the urine. Most (87%) is excreted in the urine as MPAG. Plasma concentrations of MPA and MPAG are increased in patients with renal insufficiency. In early renal transplant patients (<40 days after transplant), plasma concentrations of MPA after a single dose of MMF are about half of those found in healthy volunteers or stable renal transplant patients.

Therapeutic Uses. MMF is indicated for prophylaxis of transplant rejection, and it typically is used in combination with glucocorticoids and a calcineurin inhibitor but not with azathioprine. Combined treatment with sirolimus is possible, although potential drug interactions necessitate careful monitoring of drug levels.

For renal transplants, 1 g is administered orally or intravenously (over 2 hours) twice daily (2 g/day). A higher dose, 1.5 g twice daily (3 g/day), may be recommended for African-American renal transplant patients and all liver and cardiac transplant patients. MMF is increasingly used off label in systemic lupus.

Toxicity. The principal toxicities of MMF are gastrointestinal and hematologic. These include leukopenia, pure red cell aplasia, diarrhea, and vomiting. There also is an increased incidence of some infections, especially sepsis associated with cytomegalovirus; progressive multifocal leukoencephalopathy also has been reported in conjunction with the administration of MMF. Tacrolimus in combination with MMF has been associated with activation of polyoma viruses such as BK virus, which can cause interstitial nephritis difficult to distinguish from acute rejection (Hirsch et al., 2002). Excessive immunosuppression is suspected to be responsible for this adverse effect, not necessarily this widely used drug combination. The use of mycophenolate in pregnancy is associated with congenital anomalies and increased risk of pregnancy loss. Women of childbearing potential taking mycophenolate must use effective contraception.

Drug Interactions. Potential drug interactions between MMF and several other drugs commonly used by transplant patients have been studied. There appear to be no untoward effects produced by combination therapy with cyclosporine, trimethoprim–sulfamethoxazole, or oral contraceptives. Unlike cyclosporine, tacrolimus delays elimination of MMF by impairing the conversion of MPA to MPAG. This may enhance GI toxicity. Co-administration with antacids containing aluminum or magnesium hydroxide leads to decreased absorption of MMF; thus, these drugs should not be administered simultaneously. MMF should not be administered with cholestyramine or other drugs that affect enterohepatic circulation. Such agents decrease plasma MPA concentrations, probably by binding free MPA in the intestines. Acyclovir and ganciclovir may compete with MPAG for tubular secretion, possibly resulting in increased concentrations of both MPAG and the antiviral agents in the blood, an effect that may be compounded in patients with renal insufficiency.

A delayed-release tablet form of MPA (MYFORTIC) also is available. It does not release MPA under acidic conditions (pH <5) such as in the stomach but is highly soluble in neutral pH present in the intestine. The enteric coating results in a delay in the time to reach maximum MPA concentrations and may improve GI tolerability, although data are sparse and not convincing (Darji et al., 2008).

Other Anti-Proliferative and Cytotoxic Agents. Many of the cytotoxic and antimetabolic agents used in cancer chemotherapy (Chapter 61) are immunosuppressive due to their action on lymphocytes and other cells of the immune system. Other cytotoxic drugs that have been used off label as immunosuppressive agents include methotrexate, cyclophosphamide, thalidomide (THALOMID), and chlorambucil (LEUKERAN). Methotrexate is used for treatment of graft-versus-host disease, rheumatoid arthritis, psoriasis, and some cancers. Cyclophosphamide and chlorambucil are used in leukemia and lymphomas and a variety of other malignancies. Cyclophosphamide also is FDA approved for childhood nephrotic syndrome and is used widely for treatment of severe systemic lupus erythematosus and other vasculitides such as Wegener's granulomatosis. Leflunomide (ARAVA, others) is a pyrimidine-synthesis inhibitor indicated for the treatment of adults with rheumatoid arthritis (Prakash and Jarvis, 1999). This drug has found increasing empirical use in the treatment of polyomavirus nephropathy seen in immunosuppressed renal transplant recipients. There are no controlled studies showing efficacy compared with control patients treated with only withdrawal or reduction of immunosuppression alone in BK virus nephropathy. The drug inhibits dihydroorotate dehydrogenase in the *de novo* pathway of pyrimidine synthesis. It is hepatotoxic and can cause fetal injury when administered to pregnant women.

Fingolimod (FTY720). This is the first agent in a new class of small molecules, sphingosine-1-phosphate receptor (S1P-R) agonists (Figure 35–1). This S1P receptor prodrug reduces recirculation of lymphocytes from the lymphatic system to the blood and peripheral tissues, including inflammatory lesions and organ grafts.

Therapeutic Uses. The drug has not been as effective as standard regimens in phase III trials, and further drug development has been limited (Vincenti and Kirk, 2008).

Mechanism of Action. Unlike other immunosuppressive agents, FTY720 acts via "lymphocyte homing." It specifically and reversibly sequesters host lymphocytes into the lymph nodes and Peyer's patches and thus away from the circulation. This protects the graft from T cell–mediated attack. Although FTY720 sequesters lymphocytes, it does not impair either T- or B-cell functions. FTY720 is phosphorylated by sphingosine kinase-2, and the FTY720-phosphate product is a potent agonist of S1P receptors. Altered lymphocyte traffic induced by FTY720 clearly results from its effect on S1P receptors.

Toxicity. Lymphopenia, the most common side effect of FTY720, is predicted from its pharmacological effect and is fully reversible upon drug discontinuation. Of greater concern is the negative chronotropic effect of FTY720 on the heart, which has been observed with the first dose in up to 30% of patients. In most patients, the heart rate returns to baseline within 48 hours, with the remainder returning to baseline thereafter.

Biological Immunosuppression Antibodies and Fusion Receptor Protein

Both polyclonal and monoclonal antibodies against lymphocyte cell-surface antigens are widely used for prevention and treatment of organ transplant rejection. Polyclonal antisera are generated by repeated injections of human thymocytes (ATG) or lymphocytes (antilymphocyte globulin, ALG) into animals such as horses, rabbits, sheep, or goats and then purifying the serum immunoglobulin fraction. Although highly effective immunosuppressive agents, these preparations vary in efficacy and toxicity from batch to batch. The advent of hybridoma technology to produce monoclonal antibodies was a major advance in immunology (Kohler and Milstein, 1975). It now is possible to make essentially unlimited amounts of a single antibody of a defined specificity (Figure 35–3). These monoclonal reagents

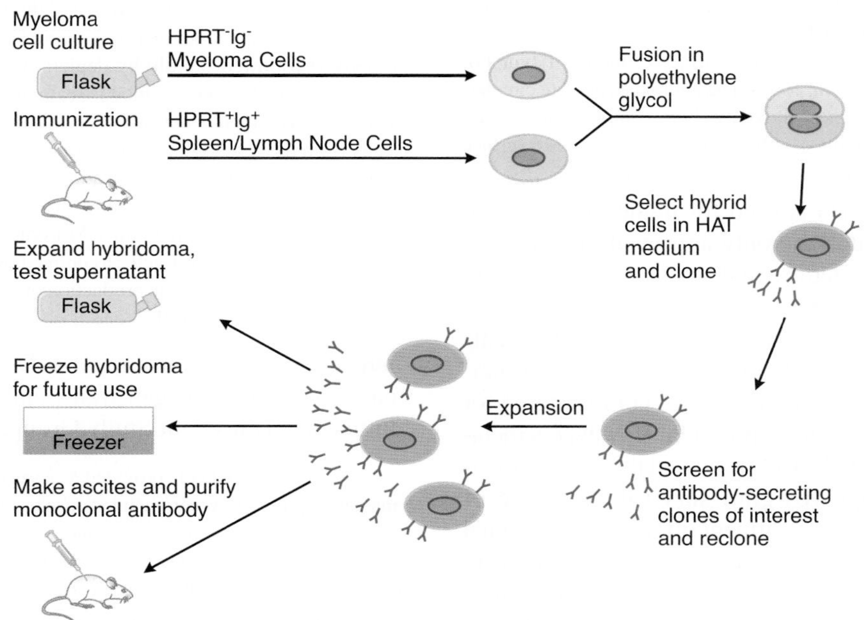

Figure 35–3. *Generation of monoclonal antibodies.* Mice are immunized with the selected antigen, and spleen or lymph node is harvested and B cells separated. These B cells are fused to a suitable B-cell myeloma that has been selected for its inability to grow in medium supplemented with hypoxanthine, aminopterin, and thymidine (HAT). Only myelomas that fuse with B cells can survive in HAT-supplemented medium. The hybridomas expand in culture. Those of interest based on a specific screening technique are then selected and cloned by limiting dilution. Monoclonal antibodies can be used directly as supernatants or ascites fluid experimentally but are purified for clinical use. HPRT, hypoxanthine–guanine phosphoribosyl transferase. (Reproduced with permission from Krensky A.M. and Clayberger C. Transplantation immunobiology. In, *Pediatric Nephrology*, 5th ed. (Avner E.D., Harmon W.E., Niauder P., eds) Lippincott Williams & Wilkins, Philadelphia, 2004. (http://lww.com).)

have overcome the problems of variability in efficacy and toxicity seen with the polyclonal products, but they are more limited in their target specificity.

The first-generation murine monoclonal antibodies have been replaced by newer humanized or fully human monoclonal antibodies that lack antigenicity, have a prolonged $t_{1/2}$, and can be mutagenized to alter their affinity to Fc receptors. Another class of biological agents being developed for both auto-immunity and transplantation are fusion receptor proteins. These agents usually consist of the ligand-binding domains of receptors bound to the Fc region of an immunoglobulin (usually IgG_1) to provide a longer $t_{1/2}$. Examples of such agents include abatacept (CTLA4-Ig) and belatacept (a second-generation CTLA4-Ig), discussed later in "Co-stimulatory Blockade." Thus, polyclonal and monoclonal antibodies as well as fusion receptor proteins have a place in immunosuppressive therapy.

Antithymocyte Globulin

ATG is a purified gamma globulin from the serum of rabbits immunized with human thymocytes (Regan et al., 1999). It is provided as a sterile, freeze-dried product for intravenous administration after reconstitution with sterile water.

Mechanism of Action. ATG contains cytotoxic antibodies that bind to CD2, CD3, CD4, CD8, CD11a, CD18, CD25, CD44, CD45, and HLA class I and II molecules on the surface of human T lymphocytes (Bourdage and Hamlin, 1995). The antibodies deplete circulating lymphocytes by direct cytotoxicity (both complement and cell mediated) and block lymphocyte function by binding to cell surface molecules involved in the regulation of cell function.

Therapeutic Uses. ATG is used for induction immunosuppression, although the only approved indication is in the treatment of acute renal transplant rejection in combination with other immunosuppressive agents (Mariat et al., 1998). Antilymphocyte-depleting agents (THYMOGLOBULIN, ATGAM, and OKT3) have been neither rigorously tested in clinical trials nor registered for use as induction immunosuppression. However, a meta-analysis (Szczech et al., 1997) showed that antilymphocyte induction improves graft survival. A course of antithymocyte-globulin treatment often is given to renal transplant patients with delayed graft function to avoid early treatment with the nephrotoxic calcineurin inhibitors and thereby aid in recovery from ischemic reperfusion injury. The recommended dose for acute rejection of renal grafts is 1.5 mg/kg/day (over 4-6 hours) for 7-14 days. Mean T-cell counts fall by day 2 of therapy. ATG also is used for acute rejection of other types of organ transplants and for prophylaxis of rejection (Wall, 1999).

Toxicity. Polyclonal antibodies are xenogeneic proteins that can elicit major side effects, including fever and chills with the potential for hypotension. Premedication with corticosteroids, acetaminophen, and/or an antihistamine and administration of the antiserum by slow infusion (over 4-6 hours) into a large-diameter vessel minimize such reactions. Serum sickness and glomerulonephritis can occur; anaphylaxis is a rare event. Hematologic complications include leukopenia and thrombocytopenia. As with other immunosuppressive agents, there is an increased risk of infection and malignancy, especially when multiple immunosuppressive agents are combined. No drug interactions have been described; anti-ATG antibodies develop, although they do not limit repeated use.

Monoclonal Antibodies

Anti-CD3 Monoclonal Antibodies. Antibodies directed at the ε chain of CD3, a trimeric molecule adjacent to the T-cell receptor on the surface of human T lymphocytes, have been used with considerable efficacy since the early 1980s in human transplantation. The original mouse IgG_{2a} antihuman CD3 monoclonal antibody, muromonab-CD3 (OKT3, ORTHOCLONE OKT3), still is used to reverse glucocorticoid-resistant rejection episodes (Cosimi et al., 1981).

Mechanism of Action. Muromonab-CD3 binds to the ε chain of CD3, a monomorphic component of the T-cell receptor complex involved in antigen recognition, cell signaling, and proliferation. Antibody treatment induces rapid internalization of the T-cell receptor, thereby preventing subsequent antigen recognition. Administration of the antibody is followed rapidly by depletion and extravasation of a majority of T cells from the bloodstream and peripheral lymphoid organs such as lymph nodes and spleen. This absence of detectable T cells from the usual lymphoid regions is secondary both to complement activation-induced cell death and to margination of T cells onto vascular endothelial walls and redistribution of T cells to nonlymphoid organs such as the lungs. Muromonab-CD3 also reduces function of the remaining T cells, as defined by lack of IL-2 production and great reduction in the production of multiple cytokines, perhaps with the exception of IL-4 and IL-10.

Therapeutic Uses. Muromonab-CD3 is indicated for treatment of acute organ transplant rejection (Ortho Multicenter Transplant Study Group, 1985).

Muromonab-CD3 is provided as a sterile solution containing 5 mg per ampule. The recommended dose is 5 mg/day (in adults; less for children) in a single intravenous bolus (<1 minute) for 10-14 days. Antibody levels increase over the first 3 days and then plateau. Circulating T cells disappear from the blood within minutes of administration and return within ~1 week after termination of therapy. Repeated use of muromonab-CD3 results in the immunization of the patient against the mouse determinants of the antibody, which can neutralize and prevent its immunosuppressive efficacy. Thus, repeated treatment with the muromonab-CD3 or other mouse monoclonal antibodies generally is contraindicated. The use of muromonab-CD3 for induction and rejection therapy has diminished substantially in the past 5 years because of its toxicity and the availability of ATG.

Toxicity. The major side effect of anti-CD3 therapy is the "cytokine release syndrome" (Ortho Multicenter Transplant Study Group, 1985). The syndrome typically begins 30 minutes after infusion of the antibody (but can occur later) and may persist for hours. Antibody binding to the T-cell receptor complex combined with Fc receptor–mediated cross-linking is the basis for the initial activating properties of this agent. The syndrome is associated with and attributed to increased serum levels of cytokines (including tumor necrosis factor-α [TNF-α], IL-2, IL-6, and interferon-γ [IFN-γ]), which are released by activated T cells and/or monocytes. In several studies, the production of TNF-α has been shown to be the major cause of the toxicity (Herbelin et al., 1995). The symptoms usually are worst with the first dose; frequency and severity decrease with subsequent doses. Common clinical manifestations include high fever, chills/rigor, headache, tremor, nausea, vomiting, diarrhea, abdominal pain, malaise, myalgias, arthralgias, and generalized weakness. Less common complaints include skin reactions and cardiorespiratory and central nervous system (CNS) disorders, including aseptic meningitis. Potentially fatal pulmonary edema, acute respiratory distress syndrome, cardiovascular collapse, cardiac arrest, and arrhythmias have been described.

Administration of glucocorticoids before the injection of muromonab-CD3 prevents the release of cytokines, reduces first-dose reactions considerably, and now is a standard procedure. Volume status of patients also must be monitored carefully before therapy; steroids and other premedications should be given, and a fully competent resuscitation facility must be immediately available for patients receiving their first several doses of this therapy.

Other toxicities associated with anti-CD3 therapy include anaphylaxis and the usual infections and neoplasms associated with immunosuppressive therapy. "Rebound" rejection has been observed when muromonab-CD3 treatment is stopped. Anti-CD3 therapies may be limited by anti-idiotypic or antimurine antibodies in the recipient.

Currently, muromomab-CD3 rarely is used in transplantation. It has been replaced by ATG and alemtuzumab.

New-Generation Anti-CD3 Antibodies. Recently, genetically altered anti-CD3 monoclonal antibodies have been developed that are "humanized" to minimize the occurrence of anti-antibody responses and mutated to prevent binding to Fc receptors (Friend et al., 1999). The rationale for developing this new generation of anti-CD3 monoclonal antibodies is that they could induce selective immunomodulation in the absence of toxicity associated with conventional anti-CD3 monoclonal antibody therapy. In initial clinical trials, a humanized anti-CD3 monoclonal antibody that does not bind to Fc receptors reversed acute renal allograft rejection without causing the first-dose cytokine-release syndrome. Clinical efficacy of these agents in auto-immune diseases is being evaluated (Herold et al., 2002).

It is not clear whether any of the new generation of anti-CD3s will be developed for use in transplantation.

Anti-IL-2 Receptor (Anti-CD25) Antibodies. Daclizumab (ZENAPAX), a humanized murine complementarity-determining region (CDR)/human IgG_1 chimeric monoclonal antibody, and basiliximab (SIMULECT), a murine-human chimeric monoclonal antibody, have been produced by recombinant DNA technology (Wiseman and Faulds, 1999). The composite daclizumab antibody consists of human (90%) constant domains of IgG_1 and variable framework regions of the Eu myeloma antibody and murine (10%) CDR of the anti-Tac antibody.

Mechanism of Action. Daclizumab has a somewhat lower affinity but a longer $t_{1/2}$ (20 days) than basiliximab. The exact mechanism of action of the anti-CD25 mAbs is not completely understood but likely results from the binding of the anti-CD25 mAbs to the IL-2 receptor on the surface of activated, but not resting, T cells (Vincenti et al., 1998; Amlot et al., 1995).

Significant depletion of T cells does not appear to play a major role in the mechanism of action of these mAbs. However, other mechanisms of action may mediate the effect of these antibodies. In a study of daclizumab-treated patients, there was a moderate decrease in circulating lymphocytes staining with 7G7, a fluorescein-conjugated antibody that binds a different α-chain epitope than that recognized and bound by daclizumab (Vincenti et al., 1998). Similar results were obtained in studies with basiliximab (Amlot et al., 1995). These findings indicate that therapy with the anti IL-2R mAbs results in a relative decrease of the expression of the α chain, either from depletion of coated lymphocytes or modulation of the α chain secondary to decreased expression or increased shedding. There also is recent evidence that the β chain may be downregulated by the anti-CD25 antibody. Recent evidence suggests that T-regulatory cells are transiently depleted during anti-CD25 therapy (Bluestone et al., 2008).

Therapeutic Uses. Anti–IL-2-receptor monoclonal antibodies are used for prophylaxis of acute organ rejection in adult patients. There are two anti–IL-2R preparations for use in clinical transplantation: daclizumab and basiliximab (Vincenti et al., 1998).

In phase III trials, daclizumab was administered in five doses (1 mg/kg given intravenously over 15 minutes in 50-100 mL of normal saline) starting immediately preoperatively, and subsequently at biweekly intervals. The $t_{1/2}$ of daclizumab was 20 days, resulting in saturation of the IL-2Rα on circulating lymphocytes for up to 120 days after transplantation. In these trials, daclizumab was used with maintenance immunosuppressive regimens (cyclosporine, azathioprine, and steroids; cyclosporine and steroids). Subsequently, daclizumab was successfully used with a maintenance triple-therapy regimen—either with cyclosporine or tacrolimus, steroids, and MMF substituting for azathioprine (Pescovitz et al., 2003). In phase III trials, basiliximab was administered in a fixed dose of 20 mg preoperatively and on days 0 and 4 after transplantation (Kahan et al., 1999). This regimen of basiliximab resulted in a concentration of ≥0.2 μg/mL, sufficient to saturate IL-2R on circulating lymphocytes for 25-35 days after transplantation.

The $t_{1/2}$ of basiliximab was 7 days. In the phase III trials, basiliximab was used with a maintenance regimen consisting of cyclosporine and prednisone. In one randomized trial, basiliximab was found to be safe and effective when used in a maintenance regimen consisting of cyclosporine, MMF, and prednisone (Lawen et al., 2000).

There presently is no marker or test to monitor the effectiveness of anti–IL-2R therapy. Saturation of an α chain on circulating lymphocytes during anti–IL-2R mAb therapy does not predict rejection. The duration of IL-2R blockade by basiliximab was similar in patients with or without acute rejection episodes (34 ± 14 days versus 37 ± 14 days, mean ± SD) (Kovarik et al., 1999). In another daclizumab trial, patients with acute rejection were found to have circulating and intragraft lymphocytes with saturated IL-2R (Vincenti et al., 2001). A possible explanation is that those patients who reject despite anti–IL-2R blockade do so through a mechanism that bypasses the IL-2 pathway due to cytokine–cytokine receptor redundancy (i.e., IL-7, IL-15).

Toxicity. No cytokine-release syndrome has been observed with these antibodies, but anaphylactic reactions can occur. Although lymphoproliferative disorders and opportunistic infections may occur, as with the depleting antilymphocyte agents, the incidence ascribed to anti-CD25 treatment appears remarkably low. No significant drug interactions with anti–IL-2-receptor antibodies have been described (Hong and Kahan, 1999).

Alemtuzumab. Alemtuzumab (CAMPATH) is a humanized mAb that has been approved for use in chronic lymphocytic leukemia. The antibody targets CD52, a glycoprotein expressed on lymphocytes, monocytes, macrophages, and natural killer cells; thus, the drug causes extensive lympholysis by inducing apoptosis of targeted cells. It has achieved some use in renal transplantation because it produces prolonged T- and B-cell depletion and allows drug minimization. Large controlled studies of efficacy or safety are not available. Although short-term results are promising, further clinical experience is needed before alemtuzumab is accepted into the clinical armamentarium for transplantation.

Anti-TNF Reagents. TNF has been implicated in the pathogenesis of several immune-mediated intestinal, skin, and joint diseases. For example, patients with rheumatoid arthritis have elevated levels of TNF-α in their joints, while patients with Crohn's disease have elevated levels of TNF-α in their stools. As a result, a number of anti-TNF agents have been developed for the treatment of these disorders.

Infliximab (REMICADE) is a chimeric anti–TNF-α monoclonal antibody containing a human constant region and a murine variable region. It binds with high affinity to TNF-α and prevents the cytokine from binding to its receptors.

In one trial, infliximab plus methotrexate improved the signs and symptoms of rheumatoid arthritis more than methotrexate alone. Patients with active Crohn's disease who had not responded to other immunosuppressive therapies also improved when treated with infliximab, including those with Crohn's-related fistulae. Infliximab is approved in the U.S. for treating the symptoms of rheumatoid arthritis and is typically used in combination with methotrexate in patients who do not respond to methotrexate alone. Infliximab also is approved for treatment of symptoms of moderate to severe Crohn's disease in patients who have failed to respond to conventional therapy and in treatment to reduce the number of draining fistulae in Crohn's disease patients (Chapter 47). Other FDA-approved indications include ankylosing spondylitis, plaque psoriasis, psoriatic arthritis, and ulcerative colitis. About one of six patients receiving infliximab experiences an infusion reaction characterized by fever, urticaria, hypotension, and dyspnea within 1-2 hours after antibody administration. The development of antinuclear antibodies, and rarely a lupus-like syndrome, has been reported after treatment with infliximab.

Although not a monoclonal antibody, etanercept (ENBREL) is mechanistically related to infliximab because it also targets TNF-α. Etanercept contains the ligand-binding portion of a human TNF-α receptor fused to the Fc portion of human IgG_1, and binds to TNF-α and prevents it from interacting with its receptors. It is approved in the U.S. for treatment of the symptoms of rheumatoid arthritis in patients who have not responded to other treatments, as well as for treatment of ankylosing spondylitis, plaque psoriasis, polyarticular juvenile idiopathic arthritis, and psoriatic arthritis. Etanercept can be used in combination with methotrexate in patients who have not responded adequately to methotrexate alone. Injection-site reactions (i.e., erythema, itching, pain, or swelling) have occurred in more than one-third of etanercept-treated patients.

Adalimumab (HUMIRA) is another anti-TNF product for intravenous use. This recombinant human IgG_1 monoclonal antibody was created by phage display technology and is approved for use in rheumatoid arthritis, ankylosing spondylitis, Crohn's disease, juvenile idiopathic arthritis, plaque psoriasis, and psoriatic arthritis.

Toxicity. *All anti-TNF agents (i.e., infliximab, etanercept, adalimumab) increase the risk for serious infections, lymphomas, and other malignancies.* For example, fatal hepatosplenic T-cell lymphomas have been reported in adolescent and young adult patients with Crohn's disease treated with infliximab in conjunction with azathioprine or 6-mercaptopurine.

IL-1 Inhibition

Plasma IL-1 levels are increased in patients with active inflammation (Moltó and Olivé, 2009; see also Chapter 34). In addition to the naturally occurring IL-1 receptor antagonist (IL-1RA), several IL-1 receptor antagonists are in development and a few have been approved for clinical use. Anakinra is an FDA-approved recombinant, non-glycosylated form of human IL-1RA for the management of joint disease in rheumatoid arthitis. It can be used alone or in combination with anti-TNF agents such as etanercept (ENBREL), infliximab (REMICADE), or adalimumab (HUMIRA). Canakinumab (ILARIS) is an IL-1β monoclonal antibody approved by the FDA in June 2009 for Cryoprin-associated periodic syndromes (CAPS), a group of rare inherited inflammatory diseases associated with overproduction of IL-1 that includes Familial Cold Autoinflammatory and Muckle-Wells Syndromes (Lachmann et al., 2009). Canakinumab is also being evaluated for use in chronic obstructive pulmonary disease (Church et al., 2009). Rilonacept (IL-1 TRAP) is another IL-1 blocker (a fusion protein that binds IL-1) that is now being evaluated in a phase 3 study for gout (Terkeltaub et al., 2009). IL-1 is an inflammatory mediator of joint pain associated with elevated uric acid crystals.

Lymphocyte Function–Associated Antigen-1 (LFA-1) Inhibition

Efalizumab. (RAPTIVA) is a humanized IgG_1 mAb targeting the CD11a chain of lymphocyte function–associated antigen-1 (LFA-1). Efalizumab binds to LFA-1 and prevents the LFA-1–intercellular adhesion molecule (ICAM) interaction to block T-cell adhesion, trafficking, and activation.

Pretransplant therapy with anti-CD11a prolonged survival of murine skin and heart allografts and monkey heart allografts (Nakakura et al., 1996). A randomized, multicenter trial of a murine anti–ICAM-1 mAb (enlimomab) failed to reduce the rate of acute rejection or to improve delayed graft function of cadaveric renal transplants (Salmela et al., 1999). This may have been due to either the murine nature of the mAb or the redundancy of the ICAMs. Efalizumab also is approved for use in patients with psoriasis. In a phase I/II open-label, dose-ranging, multidose, multicenter trial, efalizumab (dose, 0.5 mg/kg or 2 mg/kg) was administered subcutaneously for 12 weeks after renal transplantation (Vincenti et al., 2001; Vincenti et al., 2007). Both doses of efalizumab decreased the incidence of acute rejection. Pharmacokinetic and pharmacodynamic studies showed that efalizumab produced saturation and 80% modulation of CD11a within 24 hours of therapy. In a subset of 10 patients who received the higher dose efalizumab (2 mg/kg) with full-dose cyclosporine, MMF, and steroids, three patients developed post-transplant lymphoproliferative diseases. Progressive multifocal leukoencephalopathy (PML) also has occurred during therapy with efalizumab. Although efalizumab appears to be an effective immunosuppressive agent, it may be best used in a lower dose and with an immunosuppressive regimen that spares calcineurin inhibitors. Several trials are being conducted with efalizumab in renal, liver, and islet cell transplantation.

Alefacept

(AMEVIVE) is a human LFA-3-IgG1 fusion protein. The LFA-3 portion of alefacept binds to CD2 on T lymphocytes, blocking the interaction between LFA-3 and CD2 and interfering with T-cell activation. Alefacept is FDA approved for use in psoriasis.

Treatment with alefacept has been shown to produce a dose-dependent reduction in T-effector memory cells (CD45, RO+) but not in naïve cells (CD45, RA+). This effect has been related to its efficacy in psoriatic disease and is of significant interest in transplantation because T-effector memory cells have been associated with co-stimulation blockade resistant and depletional induction-resistant rejection. Alefacept will delay rejection in non-human primate (NHP) cardiac transplantation and has recently been shown to have synergistic potential when used with co-stimulation blockade and/or sirolimus-based regimens in NHPs (Vincenti and Kirk, 2008). A phase II randomized, open-label, parallel-group, multicenter study to assess the safety and efficacy of maintenance therapy with alefacept in kidney transplant recipients currently is under way.

Targeting B Cells

Most of the advances in transplantation can be attributed to drugs designed to inhibit T-cell responses. As a result, T cell–mediated acute rejection has been become much less of a problem, while B cell–mediated responses such as antibody-mediated rejection and other effects of donor-specific antibodies have become more evident. Thus, several agents, both biologicals and small molecules with B-cell specific effects now are being considered for development in transplantation, including humanized monoclonal antibodies to CD20 and inhibitors of the two B cell–activation factors BLYS and APRIL and their respective receptors.

TOLERANCE

Immunosuppression has concomitant risks of opportunistic infections and secondary tumors. Therefore, the ultimate goal of research on organ transplantation and auto-immune diseases is to induce and maintain immunological tolerance, the active state of antigen-specific nonresponsiveness (Krensky and Clayberger, 1994). Tolerance, if attainable, would represent a true cure for conditions discussed earlier in this section without the side effects of the various immunosuppressive therapies. The calcineurin inhibitors prevent tolerance induction in some, but not all, preclinical models (Van Parijs and Abbas, 1998). In these same model systems, sirolimus does not prevent tolerance and may even promote tolerance induction (Li et al., 1998). Several other promising approaches are being evaluated in clinical trials. Because they remain experimental, they are discussed only briefly here.

Co-stimulatory Blockade. Induction of specific immune responses by T lymphocytes requires two signals: an antigen-specific signal via the T-cell receptor and a co-stimulatory signal provided by the interaction of molecules such as CD28 on the T lymphocyte and CD80 and CD86 on the antigen-presenting cell (Figure 35–4; Khoury et al., 1999).

In preclinical studies, inhibition of the co-stimulatory signal has been shown to induce tolerance (Weaver et al., 2008). Experimental approaches to inhibit co-stimulation include a

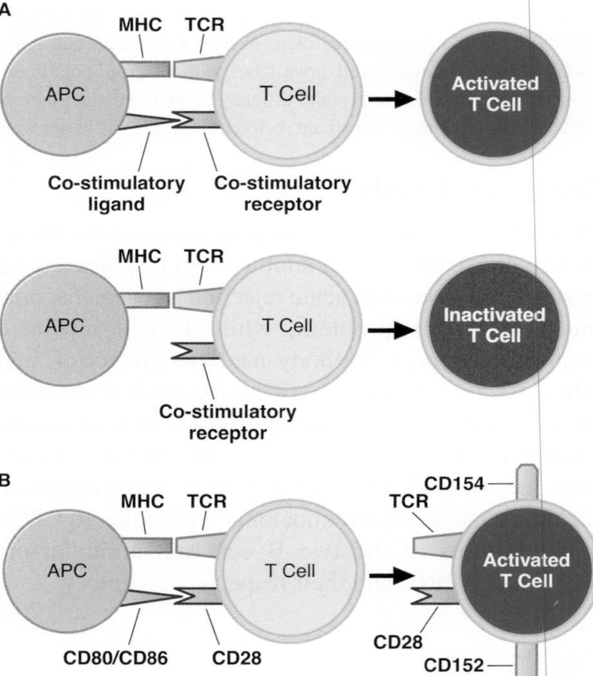

Figure 35–4. *Co-stimulation.* ***A.*** Two signals are required for T-cell activation. Signal 1 is via the T-cell receptor (TCR), and signal 2 is via a co-stimulatory receptor–ligand pair. Both signals are required for T-cell activation. Signal 1 in the absence of signal 2 results in an inactivated T cell. ***B.*** One important co-stimulatory pathway involves CD28 on the T cell and B7-1 (CD80) and B7-2 (CD86) on the antigen-presenting cell (APC). After a T cell is activated, it expresses additional co-stimulatory molecules. CD152 is CD40 ligand, which interacts with CD40 as a co-stimulatory pair. CD154 (CTLA4) interacts with CD80 and CD86 to dampen or downregulate an immune response. Antibodies against CD80, CD86, and CD152 are being evaluated as potential therapeutic agents. CTLA4-Ig, a chimeric protein consisting of part of an immunoglobulin molecule and part of CD154, also has been tested as a therapeutic agent. (Adapted with permission from Clayberger, C., and Krensky, A.M. Mechanisms of allograft rejection. In, *Immunologic Renal Diseases*. (Nielson, E.G., and Couser, W.G., eds) Lippincott-Raven, Philadelphia, 2001. (http://lww.com).)

recombinant fusion protein molecule, CTLA4-Ig, and anti-CD80 and/or anti-CD86 mAbs. The antibodies h1F1 and h3D1 are humanized anti-CD80 and anti-CD86 mAbs, respectively. *In vitro*, h1F1 and h3D1 block CD28-dependent T-cell proliferation and decrease mixed lymphocyte reactions. These mAbs must be used in tandem, because either CD80 or CD86 is sufficient to stimulate T cells via CD28. In nonhuman primates, anti-CD80 and anti-CD86 mAbs were proven effective in renal transplantation, either as monotherapy or in combination with steroids or cyclosporine (Weaver et al., 2008), but did not induce durable tolerance. A phase I study of h1F1 and h3D1 in renal transplant recipients was performed in patients receiving maintenance therapy consisting of cyclosporine, MMF, and steroids (Vincenti, 2002). Although the results of this study showed that h1F1 and h3D1 are relatively safe and possibly effective, clinical development was not further pursued.

CTLA4-Ig (abatacept) contains the binding region of CTLA4, which is a CD28 homolog, and the constant region of the human IgG_1. CTLA4-Ig competitively inhibits CD28. Numerous animal studies have confirmed the efficacy of CTLA4-Ig in inhibiting alloimmune responses, resulting in successful organ transplantation. More recently, CTLA4-Ig was shown to be effective in the treatment of rheumatoid arthritis. However, CTLA4-Ig was less effective when utilized in nonhuman primate models of renal transplantation. Belatacept (LEA29Y) (Figure 35–5) is a second-generation CTLA4-Ig with two amino acid substitutions. Belatacept has higher affinity for CD80 (2-fold) and CD86 (4-fold), yielding a 10-fold increase in potency *in vitro* as compared to CTLA4-Ig. Preclinical renal transplant studies in nonhuman primates showed that belatacept did not induce tolerance but did prolong graft survival.

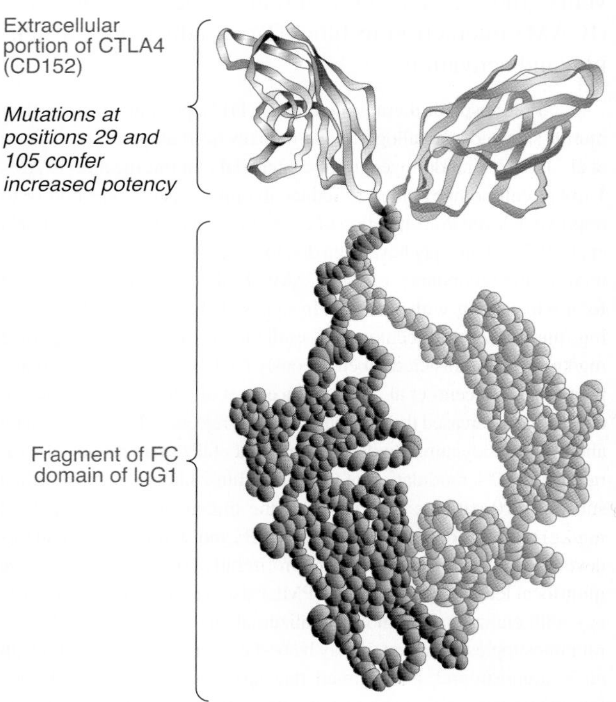

Figure 35–5. *Structure of belatacept, a CLTA4Ig congener.* For details, see the text and Figure 35–4.

In a large phase II clinical trial, belatacept was administered intravenously initially every 2 weeks then every 4 or 8 weeks without calcineurin inhibitors and compared to a cyclosporine-based regimen (Vincenti et al., 2005). Belatacept showed comparable efficacy to cyclosporine but was associated with better renal function. Recent reports from phase III trials show similar results to phase II except that the more intense regimen was no more efficacious than the lower intensity regimen but was associated with more infections and post-transplant lymphoproliferative disease (PTLD) (Emamaullee et al., 2009). Because of the risk of PTLD, EBV negative patients should not be treated with belatacept. Belatacept may be approved for maintenance biologic therapy in renal transplantation soon.

A second co-stimulatory pathway involves the interaction of CD40 on activated T cells with CD40 ligand (CD154) on B cells, endothelium, and/or antigen-presenting cells (Figure 35–4). Among the purported activities of anti-CD154 antibody treatment is the blockade of B7 expression induced by immune activation. Two humanized anti-CD154 monoclonal antibodies have been used in clinical trials in renal transplantation and auto-immune diseases. The development of these antibodies, however, is on hold because of associated thromboembolic events. An alternative approach to block the CD154-CD40 pathway is to target CD40 with monoclonal antibodies. These antibodies are undergoing trials in non-Hodgkin's lymphoma but are also likely to be developed for auto-immunity and transplantation.

Donor Cell Chimerism

Another promising approach is induction of chimerism (co-existence of cells from two genetic lineages in a single individual) by any of a variety of protocols that first dampen or eliminate immune function in the recipient with ionizing radiation, drugs such as cyclophosphamide, and/or antibody treatment and then provide a new source of immune function by adoptive transfer (transfusion) of bone marrow or hematopoietic stem cells (Starzl et al., 1997). Upon reconstitution of immune function, the recipient no longer recognizes new antigens provided during a critical period as "nonself." Such tolerance is long lived and is less likely to be complicated by the use of calcineurin inhibitors. Although the most promising approaches in this arena have been therapies that promote the development of mixed or macrochimerism, in which substantial numbers of donor cells are present in the circulation, some microchimerization approaches also have shown promise in the development of long-term unresponsiveness.

Soluble HLA

In the pre-cyclosporine era, blood transfusions were shown to be associated with improved outcomes in renal transplant patients (Opelz and Terasaki, 1978). These findings gave rise to donor-specific transfusion protocols that improved outcomes (Opelz et al., 1997). After the introduction of cyclosporine, however, these effects of blood transfusions disappeared, presumably due to the efficacy of this drug in blocking T-cell activation. Nevertheless, the existence of tolerance-promoting effects of transfusions is irrefutable. It is possible that this effect is due to HLA molecules on the surface of cells or in soluble forms. Recently, soluble HLA and peptides corresponding to linear sequences of HLA molecules have been shown to induce immunological tolerance in animal models via a variety of mechanisms (Murphy and Krensky, 1999).

Antigens

Specific antigens provided in a variety of forms (generally as peptides) induce immunological tolerance in preclinical models of diabetes mellitus, arthritis, and MS. Clinical trials of such approaches are under way. The past decade has witnessed a revolution in our understanding of the basis of immune tolerance. It is now well established that antigen/MHC complex binding to the T cell–receptor/CD3 complex coupled with soluble and membrane-bound co-stimulatory signals initiates a cascade of signaling events that lead to productive immunity. In addition, the immune response is regulated by a number of negative signaling events that control cell survival and expansion. *In vitro* and preclinical *in vivo* studies have demonstrated that one can selectively inhibit immune responses to specific antigens without the associated toxicity of established immunosuppressive therapies (Van Parijs and Abbas, 1998). With these insights comes the promise of specific immune therapies to treat the vast array of immune disorders from auto-immunity to transplant rejection. These new therapies will take advantage of a combination of drugs that target the primary T-cell receptor–mediated signal, either by blocking cell-surface receptor interactions or inhibiting early signal transduction events. The drugs will be combined with therapies that effectively block co-stimulation to prevent cell expansion and differentiation of those cells that have engaged antigen while maintaining a non-inflammatory milieu.

IMMUNOSTIMULATION

General Principles

In contrast to immunosuppressive agents that inhibit the immune response in transplant rejection and auto-immunity, a few immunostimulatory drugs have been developed with applicability to infection, immunodeficiency, and cancer. Problems with such drugs include systemic (generalized) effects at one extreme or limited efficacy at the other.

Immunostimulants

Levamisole. Levamisole (ERGAMISOL) was synthesized originally as an anthelmintic but appears to "restore" depressed immune function of B lymphocytes, T lymphocytes, monocytes, and macrophages. Its only clinical indication was as adjuvant therapy with 5-fluorouracil after surgical resection in patients with Dukes' stage C colon cancer (Moertel et al., 1990). Because of its risk for fatal agranulocytosis, levamisole was withdrawn from the U.S. market in 2005.

Thalidomide. Thalidomide (THALOMID) is best known for the severe, life-threatening birth defects it caused when administered to pregnant women. For this reason, it is available only under a restricted distribution program and can be prescribed only by specially registered physicians who understand the risk of teratogenicity if thalidomide is used during pregnancy. *Thalidomide should never be taken by women who are pregnant or who could become pregnant while taking the drug.* Nevertheless, it is indicated for the treatment of patients with erythema nodosum leprosum (Chapter 56) and multiple myeloma. In addition, it has orphan drug status for mycobacterial infections, Crohn's disease, HIV-associated wasting, Kaposi sarcoma, lupus, myelofibrosis, brain malignancies, leprosy, graft-versus-host disease, and aphthous ulcers.

Its mechanism of action is unclear (see Figure 62–4). Reported immunological effects vary substantially under different conditions. For example, thalidomide has been reported to decrease circulating TNF-α in patients with erythema nodosum leprosum but to increase it in patients who are HIV seropositive. Alternatively, it has been suggested that the drug affects angiogenesis (Paravar and Lee, 2008). The anti–TNF-α effect has led to its evaluation as a treatment for severe, refractory rheumatoid arthritis.

Lenalidomide. Lenalidomide (REVLIMID), 3-(4-amino-1-oxo 1, 3-dihydro-2H-isoindol-2-yl) piperidine-2,6-dione, is a thalidomide analog with immunomodulatory and anti-angiogenic properties. Lenalidomide is FDA approved for the treatment of patients with transfusion-dependent anemia due to low- or intermediate risk myelodysplastic syndromes associated with a deletion 5q cytogenetic abnormality with or without additional cytogenetic abnormalities.

The usual starting dose is 10 mg/day. Because lenalidomide causes significant neutropenia and thrombocytopenia in almost all patients, patients have to be closely monitored with weekly blood counts and lenalidomide dose adjusted according to the labeling information. Lenalidomide also is associated with a significant risk for deep vein thrombosis. Lenalidomide carries the same risk of teratogenicity as thalidomide, and pregnancy has to be avoided. Lenalidomide's availability is limited to a special distribution program administered by the manufacturer.

Bacillus Calmette-Guérin (BCG). Live BCG (TICE BCG, THERACYS) is an attenuated, live culture of the bacillus of Calmette and Guérin strain of *Mycobacterium bovis* that induces a granulomatous reaction at the site of administration. By unclear mechanisms, this preparation is active against tumors and is indicated for the treatment and prophylaxis of carcinoma *in situ* of the urinary bladder and for prophylaxis of primary and recurrent stage Ta and/or T1 papillary tumors after transurethral resection (Patard et al., 1998). Adverse effects include hypersensitivity, shock, chills, fever, malaise, and immune complex disease.

Recombinant Cytokines

Interferons. Although interferons (α, β, and γ) initially were identified by their antiviral activity, these agents also have important immunomodulatory activities (Ransohoff, 1998). The interferons bind to specific cell-surface receptors that initiate a series of intracellular events: induction of certain enzymes, inhibition of cell proliferation, and enhancement of immune activities, including increased phagocytosis by macrophages and augmentation of specific cytotoxicity by T lymphocytes.

Recombinant IFN-α-2b (INTRON A) is obtained from *Escherichia coli* by recombinant expression. It is a member of a family of naturally occurring small proteins with molecular weights of 15,000-27,600 Da, produced and secreted by cells in response to viral infections and other inducers. IFN-α-2b is indicated in the treatment of a variety of tumors, including hairy cell leukemia, malignant melanoma, follicular lymphoma, and AIDS-related Kaposi sarcoma (Sinkovics and Horvath, 2000). It also is indicated for infectious diseases, chronic hepatitis B, and condylomata acuminata. In addition, it is supplied in combination with ribavirin (REBETRON) for treatment of chronic hepatitis C in patients with compensated liver function not treated previously with IFN-α-2b or who have relapsed after IFN-α-2b therapy (Lo Iacono et al., 2000).

Flu-like symptoms, including fever, chills, and headache, are the most common adverse effects after IFN-α-2b administration. Adverse experiences involving the cardiovascular system (e.g., hypotension, arrhythmias, and rarely cardiomyopathy and myocardial infarction) and CNS (e.g., depression, confusion) are less frequent side effects. All α interferons carry a boxed warning regarding development of pulmonary hypertension.

IFN-γ-1b (ACTIMMUNE) is a recombinant polypeptide that activates phagocytes and induces their generation of oxygen metabolites that are toxic to a number of microorganisms. It is indicated to reduce the frequency and severity of serious infections associated with chronic granulomatous disease and to delay the time to progression in severe malignant osteopetrosis. IFN-γ-1b is not effective and may increase mortality in patients with idiopathic pulmonary fibrosis. Adverse reactions include fever, headache, rash, fatigue, GI distress, anorexia, weight loss, myalgia, and depression.

IFN-β-1a (AVONEX, REBIF), a 166–amino acid recombinant glycoprotein, and IFN-β-1b (BETASERON), a 165–amino acid recombinant protein, have antiviral and immunomodulatory properties. They are FDA-approved for the treatment of relapsing MS to reduce the frequency of clinical exacerbations (see "Multiple Sclerosis"). The mechanism of their action in MS is unclear. Flu-like symptoms (e.g., fever, chills, myalgia) and injection-site reactions have been common adverse effects.

Further discussion of the use of these and other interferons in the treatment of viral diseases can be found in Chapter 58.

Interleukin-2. Human recombinant IL-2 (aldesleukin, PROLEUKIN; des-alanyl-1, serine-125 human IL-2) is produced by recombinant DNA technology in *E. coli* (Taniguchi and Minami, 1993). This recombinant form differs from native IL-2 in that it is not glycosylated, has no amino-terminal alanine, and has a serine substituted for the cysteine at amino acid 125 (Doyle et al., 1985). The potency of the preparation is represented in International Units in a lymphocyte proliferation assay such that 1.1 mg of recombinant IL-2 protein equals 18 million IU. Aldesleukin has the following *in vitro* biological activities of native IL-2: enhancement of lymphocyte proliferation and growth of IL-2-dependent cell lines, enhancement of lymphocyte-mediated cytotoxicity and killer cell activity, and induction of IFN-γ activity (Whittington and Faulds, 1993). *In vivo* administration of aldesleukin in animals produces multiple immunological effects in a dose-dependent manner. Cellular immunity is profoundly activated with lymphocytosis, eosinophilia, thrombocytopenia, and release of multiple cytokines (e.g., TNF, IL-1, IFN-γ). Aldesleukin is indicated for the treatment of adults with metastatic renal cell carcinoma and melanoma.

Administration of aldesleukin has been associated with serious cardiovascular toxicity resulting from capillary leak syndrome, which involves loss of vascular tone and leak of plasma proteins and fluid into the extravascular space. Hypotension, reduced organ perfusion, and death may occur. An increased risk of disseminated infection due to impaired neutrophil function also has been associated with aldesleukin treatment.

Immunization

Immunization may be active or passive. Active immunization involves stimulation with an antigen to develop immunological defenses against a future exposure. Passive immunization involves administration of preformed antibodies to an individual who is already exposed or is about to be exposed to an antigen.

Vaccines. Active immunization, vaccination, involves administration of an antigen as a whole, killed (inactivated) organism; attenuated (live) organism; or a specific protein or peptide constituent of an organism. Booster doses often are required, especially when killed organisms are used as the immunogen. In the U.S., vaccination has sharply curtailed or practically eliminated a variety of major infections, including diphtheria, measles, mumps, pertussis, rubella, tetanus, *Haemophilus influenzae* type b, and pneumococcus.

Although most vaccines have targeted infectious diseases, a new generation of vaccines may provide complete or limited protection from specific cancers or auto-immune diseases. Because T cells optimally are activated by peptides and co-stimulatory ligands that are present on antigen-presenting cells (APCs), one approach for vaccination has consisted of immunizing patients with APCs expressing a tumor antigen. The first generation of anticancer vaccines used whole cancer cells or tumor-cell lysates as a source of antigen in combination with various adjuvants, relying on host APCs to process and present tumor-specific antigens (Sinkovics and Horvath, 2000). These anticancer vaccines resulted in occasional clinical responses and are being tested in prospective clinical trials. Second-generation anticancer vaccines utilized specific APCs incubated *ex vivo* with antigen or transduced to express antigen and subsequently reinfused into patients. In laboratory animals, immunization with dendritic cells previously pulsed with MHC class I–restricted peptides derived from tumor-specific antigens led to pronounced antitumor cytotoxic T-lymphocyte responses and protective tumor immunity (Tarte and Klein, 1999). Finally, multiple studies have demonstrated the efficacy of DNA vaccines in small- and large-animal models of infectious diseases and cancer (Lewis and Babiuk, 1999). The advantage of DNA vaccination over peptide immunization is that it permits generation of entire proteins, enabling determinant selection to occur in the host without having to restrict immunization to patients bearing specific HLA alleles. However, a safety concern about this technique is the potential for integration of the plasmid DNA into the host genome, possibly disrupting important genes and thereby leading to phenotypic mutations or carcinogenicity. A final approach to generate or enhance immune responses against specific antigens consists of infecting cells with recombinant viruses that encode the protein antigen of interest. Different types of viral vectors that can infect mammalian cells, such as vaccinia, avipox, lentivirus, adenovirus, or adenovirus-associated virus, have been used.

Immune Globulin. Passive immunization is indicated when an individual is deficient in antibodies because of a congenital or acquired immunodeficiency, when an individual with a high degree of risk is exposed to an agent and there is inadequate time for active immunization (e.g., measles, rabies, hepatitis B), or when a disease is already present but can be ameliorated by passive antibodies (e.g., botulism, diphtheria, tetanus). Passive immunization may be provided by several different products (Table 35–2). Nonspecific immunoglobulins or highly specific immunoglobulins may be provided based on the indication. The protection provided usually lasts 1-3 months. Immune globulin is derived from pooled plasma of adults by an alcohol-fractionation procedure. It contains largely IgG (95%) and is indicated for antibody-deficiency disorders, exposure to infections such as hepatitis A and measles, and specific immunological diseases such as immune thrombocytopenic purpura and Guillain-Barré syndrome. In contrast, specific immune globulins ("hyperimmune") differ from other immune globulin preparations in that donors are selected for high titers of the desired antibodies.

Table 35–2

Selected Immune Globulin Preparations

GENERIC NAME	COMMON SYNONYMS	ORIGIN	BRAND NAME
Antithymocyte globulin	ATG	Rabbit	THYMOGLOBULIN
Botulism immune globulin intravenous	BIG-IV	Human	BABYBIG
Cytomegalovirus immune globulin intravenous	CMV-IGIV	Human	CYTOGAM
Hepatitis B immune globulin	HBIG	Human	HEPAGAM B, HYPERHEP B S/D, NABI-HB
Immune globulin intramuscular	Gamma globulin, IgG, IGIM	Human	GAMASTAN S/D
Immune globulin intravenous	IVIG	Human	CARIMUNE NF, FLEBOGAMMA 5%, GAMMAGARD LIQUID, GAMUNEX, IVEEGAM EN, OCTAGAM, PRIVIGEN
Immune globulin subcutaneous	IGSC	Human	VIVAGLOBIN
Lymphocyte immune globulin	ALG, antithymocyte globulin (equine), ATG (equine)	Equine	ATGAM
Rabies immune globulin	RIG	Human	HYPERRAB S/D, IMOGAM RABIES–HT
Rho(D) immune globulin intramuscular	Rho[D] IGIM	Human	HYPERRHO S/D, RHOGAM
Rho(D) immune globulin intravenous	Rho[D] IGIV	Human	RHOPHYLAC, WINRHO SDF
Rho(D) immune globulin microdose	Rho[D] IG microdose	Human	HYPERRHO S/D MICRODOSE, MICRHOGAM
Tetanus immune globulin	TIG	Human	BAYTET
Vaccinia immune globulin intravenous	VIGIV	Human	Generic

Specific immune globulin preparations are available for hepatitis B, rabies, tetanus, varicella-zoster, cytomegalovirus, botulism, and respiratory syncytial virus. Rho(D) immune globulin is a specific hyperimmune globulin for prophylaxis against hemolytic disease of the newborn due to Rh incompatibility between mother and fetus. All such plasma-derived products carry the theoretical risk of transmission of infectious disease.

Rho(D) Immune Globulin. The commercial forms of Rho(D) immune globulin (Table 35–2) consist of IgG containing a high titer of antibodies against the Rh(D) antigen on the surface of red blood cells. All donors are carefully screened to reduce the risk of transmitting infectious diseases. Fractionation of the plasma is performed by precipitation with cold alcohol followed by passage through a viral clearance system (Bowman, 1998).

Mechanism of Action. Rho(D) immune globulin binds Rho antigens, thereby preventing sensitization (Peterec, 1995). Rh-negative women may be sensitized to the "foreign" Rh antigen on red blood cells via the fetus at the time of birth, miscarriage, ectopic pregnancy, or any transplacental hemorrhage. If the women go on to have a primary immune response, they will make antibodies to Rh antigen that can cross the placenta and damage subsequent fetuses by lysing red blood cells. This syndrome, called hemolytic disease of the newborn, is life-threatening. The form due to Rh incompatibility is largely preventable by Rho(D) immune globulin.

Therapeutic Use. Rho(D) immune globulin is indicated whenever fetal red blood cells are known or suspected to have entered the circulation of an Rh-negative mother unless the fetus is known to also be Rh negative. The drug is given intramuscularly. The $t_{1/2}$ of circulating immunoglobulin is ~21-29 days.

Toxicity. Injection-site discomfort and low-grade fever have been reported. Systemic reactions are extremely rare, but myalgia, lethargy, and anaphylactic shock have been reported. As with all plasma-derived products, there is a theoretical risk of transmission of infectious diseases.

Intravenous Immunoglobulin (IVIG). In recent years, indications for the use of IVIG have expanded beyond replacement therapy for agammaglobulinemia and other immunodeficiencies to include a variety of bacterial and viral infections, and an array of auto-immune and inflammatory diseases as diverse as thrombocytopenic purpura, Kawasaki disease, and auto-immune skin, neuromuscular, and neurological diseases.

Although the mechanism of action of IVIG in immune modulation remains largely unknown, proposed mechanisms include modulation of expression and function of Fc receptors on leukocytes and endothelial cells, interference with complement activation and cytokine production, provision of anti-idiotypic antibodies (Jerne's network theory), and effects on the activation and effector function of T and B lymphocytes. Although IVIG is effective in many autoimmune diseases, its spectrum of efficacy and appropriate dosing (especially duration of therapy) are unknown. Additional controlled studies of IVIG are needed to identify proper dosing, cost-benefit, and quality-of-life parameters.

A CASE STUDY: IMMUNOTHERAPY FOR MULTIPLE SCLEROSIS

Clinical Features and Pathology. MS is a demyelinating inflammatory disease of the CNS white matter that displays a triad of pathogenic symptoms: mononuclear cell infiltration, demyelination, and scarring (gliosis). The peripheral nervous system is uninvolved. The disease, which may be episodic or progressive, occurs in early to middle adulthood with prevalence increasing from late adolescence to 35 years of age and then declining. MS is roughly 3-fold more common in females than in males and occurs mainly in higher latitudes of the temperate climates. Epidemiologic studies suggest a role for environmental factors in the pathogenesis of MS; despite many suggestions, associations with infectious agents have proven inconclusive, even though several viruses can cause similar demyelinating diseases in laboratory animals and humans. A stronger linkage is the genetic one: people of northern European ancestry have a higher susceptibility to MS, and studies in twins and siblings suggest a strong genetic component of susceptibility to MS.

Specifically, MS is a complex genetic disease in which multiple allelic variants lead to disease susceptibility. Although there is long-range linkage disequilibrium in the MHC region, HLA-DR2 clearly is associated with risk of developing MS ($p = 10^{-228}$), as is HLA-B*4402. Genome-wide association studies have identified predominantly immune-related variants associated with disease risk, including the IL-2RA chain ($p = 10^{-27}$), IL-7R chain ($p = 10^{-20}$), CLEC16A ($p = 10^{-15}$), CD58 (LFA-3, $p = 10^{-10}$), and CD226 ($p = 10^{-8}$) (IMSGC, 2007; IMSGC, 2008; Hafler, 2008). It is estimated that >200 common allelic variants will be uncovered as genome-wide association studies become properly powered. Interestingly, these variants are strikingly common among the different auto-immune diseases.

There also is substantial evidence of an autoimmune component to MS: in MS patients, there are activated T cells that are reactive to different myelin antigens, including myelin basic protein (MBP). In addition, there is evidence for the presence of autoantibodies to myelin oligodendrocyte glycoprotein (MOG) and to MBP that can be eluted from the CNS plaque tissue, although it appears unlikely that high-affinity auto-antibodies are present in the circulation. These antibodies may act with pathogenic T cells to produce some of the cellular pathology of MS. The neurophysiological result is altered conduction (both positive and negative) in myelinated fibers within the CNS (cerebral white matter, brain stem, cerebellar tracts, optic nerves, spinal cord); some alterations appear to result from exposure of voltage-dependent K^+ channels that normally are covered by myelin.

Attacks are classified by type and severity and likely correspond to specific degrees of CNS damage and pathological processes. Thus, physicians refer to relapsing-remitting MS (the form in 85% of younger patients), secondary progressive MS (progressive neurological deterioration following a long period of relapsing-remitting disease), and primary progressive MS (~15% of patients, wherein deterioration with relatively little inflammation is apparent at onset). De Jager and Hafler (2007) have reviewed current concepts of the etiology, natural history, and current therapy of MS.

Pharmacotherapy for MS. Specific therapies are aimed at resolving acute attacks, reducing recurrences and exacerbations, and slowing the progression of disability (Table 35–3). Nonspecific therapies focus on maintaining function and quality of life. For acute attacks, pulse glucocorticoids often are employed (typically, 1 g/day of methylprednisolone administered intravenously for 3-5 days). There is no evidence that tapered doses of oral prednisone are useful or even desirable.

For reducing the recurrence of relapsing-remitting attacks, immunomodulatory therapies are approved: β-1 interferons [IFN-β-1a, IFN-β-1b], and glatiramer acetate (GA; COPAXONE). The interferons suppress the proliferation of T lymphocytes, inhibit their movement into the CNS from the periphery, and shift the cytokine profile from pro- to anti-inflammatory types.

Random polymers that contain amino acids commonly used as MHC anchors and T cell–receptor contact residues have been proposed as possible "universal APLs (altered peptide ligands)." GA is a random-sequence polypeptide consisting of four amino acids [alanine (A), lysine (K), glutamate (E), and tyrosine (Y) at a molar ratio of A:K:E:Y of 4.5:3.6:1.5:1] with an average length of 40-100 amino acids. Directly labeled GA binds efficiently to different murine H2 I-A molecules, as well as to their human counterparts, the MHC class II DR molecules, but does not bind MHC class II DQ or MHC class I molecules *in vitro*. In phase III clinical trials, GA, administered subcutaneously to patients with relapsing-remitting MS, decreased the rate of exacerbations by ~30% (De Jager and Hafler, 2007). *In vivo* administration of GA induces highly cross-reactive $CD4^+$ T cells that are immune deviated to secrete Th2 cytokines and prevents the appearance of new lesions detectable by magnetic resonance imaging. This represents one of the first successful uses of an agent that ameliorates auto-immune disease by altering signals through the T cell–receptor complex.

For relapsing-remitting attacks and for secondary progressive MS, the alkylating agent cyclophosphamide (De Jager and Hafler, 2007) and the anthracenedione-derivative mitoxantrone (NOVANTRONE, others) currently are used in patients refractory to other immunomodulators. These agents, primarily used for cancer chemotherapy, have significant toxicities (see Chapter 61 for structures and pharmacology). Although cyclophosphamide in patients with MS may not be limited by an accumulated dose exposure, mitoxantrone generally can be tolerated only up to an accumulated dose of 100-140 mg/m^2 (Crossley, 1984). However, because decreases in left-ventricular ejection fraction (LVEF) and frank congestive heart failure have occurred in patients who have received <100 mg/m^2, the FDA now recommends that LVEF be evaluated before initiating therapy, prior to each dose, and annually after patients have finished treatment to detect late-occurring cardiac toxicity. The utility of interferon therapy in patients with secondary progressive MS is unclear. In primary progressive MS, with no discrete attacks and less observed inflammation, suppression of inflammation seems to be less helpful. A minority of patients at this stage will respond to high doses of glucocorticoids. Table 35–3 summarizes current immunomodulatory therapies for MS.

Table 35–3

Pharmacotherapy of Multiple Sclerosis

THERAPEUTIC AGENT	BRAND NAME (DOSE, REGIMEN)	INDICATIONS	RESULTS	MECHANISM OF ACTION
IFN-β-1a	AVONEX (30 μg, IM, weekly) REBIFF (22 or 44 μg, SC, 3 times weekly)	Treatment of RRMS	Reduction of relapses by one-third Reduction of new MRI T2 lesions and the volume of enlarging T2 lesions Reduction in the number and volume of Gd-enhancing lesions Slowing of brain atrophy	Acts on blood-brain barrier by interfering with T-cell adhesion to the endothelium by binding VLA-4 on T cells or by inhibiting the T-cell expression of MMP Reduction in T cell activation by interfering with HLA class II and co-stimulatory molecules B7/CD28 and CD40:CD40L Immune deviation of Th2 over Th1 cytokine profile
IFN-β-1b	BETASERON (0.25 mg, SC, every other day after 6-week titration)	Treatment of RRMS	Same as IFN-β-1a, above	Same as IFN-β-1a, above
Glatiramer acetate	COPAXONE (20 mg, SC, daily)	Treatment of RRMS	Reduction of relapses by one-third Reduction in the number and volume of Gd-enhancing lesions	Induces T-helper type 2 cells that enter the CNS; mediates bystander suppression at sites of inflammation
Mitoxantrone	NOVANTRONE, generic (12 mg/m^2, as short [5–15 minute] IV infusion every 3 months)	Worsening forms of RRMS SPMS	Reduction in relapses by 67% Slowed progression on EDSS, ambulation index, and MRI disease activity	Intercalates DNA (see Chapter 61) Suppresses cellular and humoral immune response

EDSS, Expanded Disability Status Scale, a neurologic assessment scale for MS pathology. Gd, gadolinium, used in Gd-enhanced MRI to assess the number and size of inflammatory brain lesions; IFN, interferon; IM, intramuscularly; IV, intravenously; MMP, matrix metalloprotease; MS, multiple sclerosis; RRMS, relapsing-remitting MS; SC, subcutaneously; SPMS, secondary progressive MS; MRI, magnetic resonance imaging.

Each of the agents mentioned in this section has side effects and contraindications that may be limiting: infections (for glucocorticoids), hypersensitivity and pregnancy (for immunomodulators), and prior anthracycline/anthracenedione use, mediastinal irradiation, or cardiac disease (mitoxantrone). With all of these agents, it is clear that the earlier they are used, the more effective they are in preventing disease relapses. What is not clear is whether any of these agents will prevent or diminish the later onset of secondary progressive disease, which causes the more severe form of disability. Given the fluctuating nature of this disease, only long-term studies lasting decades will answer this question.

A number of other new immunomodulatory therapies have either recently been approved by the FDA or are completing phase III trials. The monoclonal antibody, natalizumab (TYSABRI), directed against the adhesion molecule α_4 integrin, antagonizes interactions with integrin heterodimers containing α_4 integrin, such as $\alpha_4\beta_1$ integrin that is expressed on the surface of activated lymphocytes and monocytes. Preclinical data suggest that an interaction of $\alpha_4\beta_1$ integrin with vascular-cellular adhesion molecule (VCAM)-1 is critical for T-cell trafficking from the periphery into the CNS (Steinman, 2004); thus, blocking this interaction would hypothetically inhibit disease exacerbations. Phase III clinical trials demonstrated a significant decrease in the number of new lesions as determined by magnetic resonance imaging and clinical attacks in MS patients receiving natalizumab (Polman et al., 2006). Postmarketing use of natalizumab has been associated with the development of progressive multifocal leukoencephalopathy, and availability has been limited to a special distribution program (TOUCH) administered by the manufacturer. Monoclonal antibodies directed against the IL-2 receptor and against CD52 (alemtuzumab; CAMPATH) are also in phase III clinical trials. The pharmacotherapy of MS has been reviewed by De Jager and Hafler (2007); the utility of immunotherapy for auto-immune diseases has been reviewed by Steinman (2004).

CLINICAL SUMMARY

Most transplant centers employ some combination of immunosuppressive drugs with antilymphocyte induction therapy with either a monoclonal or polyclonal antibody agent. Maintenance immunosuppression consists of a calcineurin inhibitor (cyclosporine or tacrolimus), glucocorticoids, and an antimetabolite (azathioprine or mycophenolate). Mycophenolate has largely replaced azathioprine as part of the standard immunosuppressive regimen after transplantation. At present, a number of centers are conducting trials with new drug combinations including either cyclosporine or tacrolimus in combination with glucocorticoids and mycophenolate, with or without antibody-induction therapy or fingolimod with cyclosporine. Sirolimus is being used to limit exposure to the nephrotoxic calcineurin inhibitors, while steroid avoidance or minimization strategies are used increasingly. Newer immunosuppressive agents are providing more effective control of rejection and permitting transplantation to become an accepted procedure with a number of different organs, including kidney, liver, pancreas, and heart. The apparent effectiveness of new drug combinations has resulted in a resurgence of interest in reducing or avoiding glucocorticoids and calcineum inhibitors.

BIBLIOGRAPHY

Akalin E, Ames S, Sehgal V, et al. Intravenous immunoglobulin and thymoglobulin facilitate kidney transplantation in complement-dependent cytotoxicity B-cell and blow cytometry T- or B-cell crossmatch-positive patients. *Transplantation*, **2003**, *76*:1444–1447.

Amlot PL, Rawlings E, Fernando ON, et al. Prolonged action of chimeric interleukin-2 receptor (CD25) monoclonal antibody used in cadaveric renal transplantation. *Transplantation*, **1995**, *60*:748–756.

Artz MA, Boots JMM, Ligtenberg G, et al. Improved cardiovascular risk profile and renal function in renal transplant patients after randomized conversion from cyclosporine to tacrolimus. *J Am Soc Nephrol*, **2003**, *14*:1880–1888.

Auphan N, DiDonato JA, Rosette C, et al. Immunosuppression by glucocorticoids: Inhibition of NF-κB activity through induction of I κB synthesis. *Science*, **1995**, *270*:286–290.

Bluestone JA, Liu W, Yabu JM, et al. The effect of costimulatory and interleukin 2 receptor blockade on regulatory T cells in renal transplantation. *Am J Transplant,* **2008**, *8*:2086–2096.

Bourdage JS, Hamlin DM. Comparative polyclonal antithymocyte globulin and antilymphocyte/antilymphoblast globulin anti-CD antigen analysis by flow cytometry. *Transplantation*, **1995**, *59*:1194–1200.

Bowman JM. RhD hemolytic disease of the newborn. *N Engl J Med*, **1998**, *339*:1775–1777.

Burdmann E, Yu L, Andoh T, et al. Calcineurin inhibitors and sirolimus. In: DeBroe ME, Porter GA, Bennett WM, Verpooten GA, eds. *Clinical Nephrotoxins: Renal Injury from Drugs and Chemicals,* 2nd ed. Dordrecht, Kluwer, **2003**.

Church LD, Mcdermott MF. Canakinumab, a fully-human mAb against IL-1 beta for the potential treatment of inflammatory disorders. *Curr Opin Mol Ther*, **2009,** *11*:81–89.

Cole E, Maham N, Cardella C, et al. Clinical benefits of Neoral C2 monitoring in the long-term management of renal transplant recipients. *Transplantation*, **2003**, *75:*2086–2090.

Cosimi AB, Burton RC, Colvin RB, et al. Treatment of acute renal allograft rejection with OKT3 monoclonal antibody. *Transplantation*, **1981**, *32*:535–539.

Darji P, Vijayaraghavan R, Thiagarajan MN, et al. Conversion from mycophenolate mofetil to enteric-coated mycophenolate sodium in renal transplant recipients with gastrointestinal tract disorders. *Transplant Proc*, **2008**, *40*:2262–2267.

DeJager PL, Hafler DA. 2007. New therapeutic approaches for multiple sclerosis. *Ann Rev Med,* **2007**, *58*:417–432.

Doyle MV, Lee MT, Fong S. Comparison of the biological activities of human recombinant interleukin-2 (125) and native inter-leukin-2. *J Biol Response Mod*, **1985**, *4*:96–109.

Eisen HJ, Tuzcu EM, Dorent R, et al., for the RAD B253 Study Group. Everolimus for the prevention of allograft rejection and vasculopathy in cardiac-transplant recipients. *N Engl J Med*, **2003**, *349*:847–858.

Ekberg H, Tedesco-Silva H, Demirbas A, et al. Reduced exposure to calcineurin inhibitors in renal transplantation. *N Engl J Med,* **2007**, *357*:2562–2575.

Emamaullee J, Toso C, Merani S, Shapiro AM. Costimulatory blockade with belatacept in clinical and experimental transplantation-a review. *Expert Opin Biol Ther*, **2009**, *9*:789–796.

Flechner SM, Kobashigawa J, Klintmalm G. Calcineurin inhibitor-sparing regimens in solid organ transplantation: Focus on improving renal function and nephrotoxicity. *Clin Transplant*, **2008**, *22*:1–15.

Friend PJ, Hale G, Chatenoud L, et al. Phase I study of an engineered aglycosylated humanized CD3 antibody in renal transplant rejection. *Transplantation*, **1999**, *68*:1632–1637.

Goto T, Kino T, Hatanaka H, et al. Discovery of FK-506, a novel immunosuppressant isolated from *Streptomyces tsukubaensis. Transplant Proc*, **1987**, *19*:4–8.

Groth CG, Backman L, Morales JM, et al. Sirolimus (rapamycin)-based therapy in human renal transplantation: Similar efficacy and different toxicity compared with cyclosporine. Sirolimus European Renal Transplant Study Group. *Transplantation*, **1999**, *67*:1036–1042.

Hafler JP, Maier LM, Cooper JD, et al., for the International Multiple Sclerosis Genetics Consortium (IMSGC). CD226 Gly307Ser association with multiple autoimmune diseases. *Genes Immun,* 2008 Oct 30 [Epub ahead of print].

Herbelin A, Chatenoud L, Roux-Lombard P, et al. *In vivo* soluble tumor necrosis factor receptor release in OKT3-treated patients. Differential regulation of TNF-sR55 and TNF-sR75. *Transplantation*, **1995**, *59*:1470–1475.

Herold KC, Hagopian W, Auger JA, et al. Anti-CD3 monoclonal antibody in new-onset type 1 diabetes mellitus. *N Engl J Med*, **2002**, *346*:1692–1698.

Hirsch HH, Knowles W, Dickenmann M, et al. Prospective study of polyomavirus type BK replication and nephropathy in renal-transplant recipients. *N Engl J Med,* **2002**, *347*:488–496.

Hong JC, Kahan BD. Use of anti-CD25 monoclonal antibody in combination with rapamycin to eliminate cyclosporine treatment during the induction phase of immunosuppression. *Transplantation*, **1999**, *68*:701–704.

Hong JC, Kahan BD. Immunosuppressive agents in organ transplantation: Past, present, and future. *Semin Nephrol*, **2000**, *20*:108–125.

Howard RJ, Condie RM, Sutherland DE, et al. The use of antilymphoblast globulin in the treatment of renal allograft rejection: A double-blind, randomized study. *Transplantation*, **1997**, *24*:419–423.

International Multiple Sclerosis Genetic Consortium, Hafler DA, Compston A, et al. Risk alleles for multiple sclerosis identified by a genomewide study. *N Engl J Med,* **2007**, *357*:851–862.

International Multiple Sclerosis Genetics Consortium (IMSGC). Refining genetic associations in multiple sclerosis. *Lancet Neurol,* **2008**, *7*:567–569.

Kahan BD, Julian BA, Pescovitz MD, et al. Sirolimus reduces the incidence of acute rejection episodes despite lower cyclosporine doses in Caucasian recipients of mismatched primary renal allografts: A phase II trial. Rapamune Study Group. *Transplantation*, **1999**, *68*:1526–1532.

Khanna A, Li B, Stenzel KH, Suthanthiran M. Regulation of new DNA synthesis in mammalian cells by cyclosporine. Demonstration of a transforming growth factor beta-dependent mechanism of inhibition of cell growth. *Transplantation*, **1994**, *57*:577–582.

Khoury S, Sayegh MH, Turka LA. Blocking costimulatory signals to induce transplantation tolerance and prevent autoimmune disease. *Int Rev Immunol*, **1999**, *18*:185–199.

Kohler G, Milstein C. Continuous cultures of fused cells secreting antibody of predefined specificity. *Nature*, **1975**, *256*:495–497.

Kovarik JM, Kahan BD, Rajagopalan PR, et al. Population pharmacokinetics and exposure-response relationships for basiliximab in kidney transplantation. The U.S. Simulect Renal Transplant Study Group. *Transplantation*, **1999**, *68*:1288–1294.

Krensky AM, Clayberger C. Prospects for induction of tolerance in renal transplantation. *Pediatr Nephrol*, **1994**, *8*:772–779.

Lachmann HJ, Kone-Paut I, Kuemmerle-Deschner JB, et al. Canakinumab in CAPS Study Group. Use of canakinumab in the cryopyrin-associated periodic syndrome. *N Eng J Med*, **2009**, *360*:2416–2425.

Lawen J, Davies E, Morad F, et al. Basiliximab (Simulect) is safe and effective in combination with triple therapy of Neoral, steroids and CellCept in renal transplant patients. *Transplantation*, **2000**, *69*:S260.

Lewis PJ, Babiuk L A. DNA vaccines: A review. *Adv Virus Res*, **1999**, *54*:129–188.

Li Y, Zheng XX, Li XC, et al. Combined costimulation blockade plus rapamycin but not cyclosporine produces permanent engraftment. *Transplantation*, **1998**, *66*:1387–1388.

Lo Iacono O, Castro A, Diago M, et al. Interferon alfa-2b plus ribavirin for chronic hepatitis C patients who have not responded to interferon monotherapy. *Aliment Pharmacol Ther*, **2000**, *14:*463–469.

Mariat C, Alamartine E, Diab N, et al. Randomized prospective study comparing low-dose OKT3 to low-dose ATG for the treatment of acute steroid-resistant rejection episodes in kidney transplant recipients. *Transplant Int*, **1998**, *11*:231–236.

Moertel CG, Fleming TR, Macdonald JS, et al. Levamisole and fluorouracil for adjuvant therapy of resected colon carcinoma. *N Engl J Med*, **1990**, *322*:352–358.

Monaco AP. A new look at polyclonal antilymphocyte antibodies in clinical transplantation. *Graft*, **1999**, *2*:S2–S5.

Moltó A, Olivé A. Anti-IL-1 molecules: New comers and new indications. *Joint Bone Spine*, **2010**, *77*:102–107.

Murphy B, Krensky AM. HLA-derived peptides as novel immunomodulatory therapeutics. *J Am Soc Nephrol*, **1999**, *10*:1346–1355.

Nakakura EK, Shorthouse RA, Zheng B, et al. Long-term survival of solid organ allografts by brief anti-lymphocyte function-associated antigen-1 monoclonal antibody monotherapy. *Transplantation*, **1996**, *62*:547–552.

Nankivel BJ, Borrows RJ, Fung CL, et al. The natural history of chronic allograft nephropathy. *N Engl J Med,* **2003**, *349*: 2326–2333.

Noble S, Markham A. Cyclosporin. A review of the pharmacokinetic properties, clinical efficacy and tolerability of a microemulsion-based formulation (Neoral). *Drugs*, **1995**, *50*: 924–941.

Opelz G, Terasaki PI. Improvement of kidney-graft survival with increased numbers of blood transfusions. *N Engl J Med*, **1978**, *299*:799–803.

Opelz G, Vanrenterghem Y, Kirste G, et al. Prospective evaluation of pretransplant blood transfusions in cadaver kidney recipients. *Transplantation*, **1997**, *63*:964–967.

Ortho Multicenter Transplant Study Group. A randomized clinical trial of OKT3 monoclonal antibody for acute rejection of cadaveric renal transplants. *N Engl J Med*, **1985**, *313*: 337–342.

Paravar T, Lee DJ. Thalidomide: Mechanism of action. *Int Rev Immunol,* **2008**, *27*:111–135.

Patard JJ, Saint F, Velotti F, et al. Immune response following intravesical bacillus Calmette-Guérin instillations in superficial bladder cancer: A review. *Urol Res*, **1998**, *26*:155–159.

Pattison JM, Sibley RK, Krensky AM. Mechanisms of allograft rejection. In: Neilson EG, Couser WG, eds. *Immunologic Renal Diseases*. Philadelphia, Lippincott-Raven, **1997**, pp. 331–354.

Pescovitz MD, Bumgardner GL, Gaston RS, et al. Addition of daclizumab to mycophenolate mofetil, cyclosporine, and steroids in renal transplantation: Pharmacokinetics, safety, and efficacy. *Clin Transplant*, **2003**, *17*:511–517.

Peterec SM. Management of neonatal Rh disease. *Clin Perinatol*, **1995**, *22*:561–592.

Polman CH, O'Connor PW, Havrdova E, et al. A randomized, placebo-controlled trial of natalizumab for relapsing multiple sclerosis. *N Engl J Med,* **2006**, *354*:899–910.

Prakash A, Jarvis B. Leflunomide: A review of its use in active rheumatoid arthritis. *Drugs*, **1999**, *58*:1137–1164.

Ransohoff RM. Cellular responses to interferons and other cytokines: The JAK-STAT paradigm. *N Engl J Med*, **1998**, *338*:616–618.

Regan JF, Campbell K, Van Smith L, et al. Sensitization following Thymoglobulin and Atgam rejection therapy as determined with a rapid enzyme-linked immunosorbent assay. US Thymoglobulin Multi-Center Study Group. *Transplant Immunol*, **1999**, *7*:115–121.

Salmela K, Wramner L, Ekberg H, et al. A randomized multicenter trial of the anti-ICAM-1 monoclonal antibody (enlimomab) for the prevention of acute rejection and delayed onset of graft function in cadaveric renal transplantation: A report of the European Anti-ICAM-1 Renal Transplant Study Group. *Transplantation*, **1999**, *67*:729–736.

Schreiber SL, Crabtree GR. The mechanism of action of cyclosporin A and FK506. *Immunol Today*, **1992**, *13*:136–142.

Sinkovics JG, Horvath JC. Vaccination against human cancers [review]. *Int J Oncol*, **2000**, *16*:81–96.

Smith KD, Wrenshall LE, Nicosia RF, et al. Delayed graft function and case nephropathy associated with tacrolimus plus rapamycin use. *J Am Soc Nephrol*, **2003**, *14*:1037–1045.

Starzl TE, Demetris AJ, Murase N, et al. Chimerism after organ transplantation. *Curr Opin Nephrol Hypertens*, **1997**, *6*: 292–298.

Steinman L. Immune therapy for autoiummune diseases. *Science*, **2004**, *305*:212–216.

Suthanthiran M, Morris RE, Strom TB. Immunosuppressants: Cellular and molecular mechanisms of action. *Am J Kidney Dis*, **1996**, *28*:159–172.

Szczech LA, Berlin JA, Aradhye S, et al. Effect of antilymphocyte induction therapy on renal allograft survival: A meta-analysis. *J Am Soc Nephrol*, **1997**, *8*:1771–1777.

Taniguchi T, Minami Y. The IL-2/IL-2 receptor system: A current overview. *Cell*, **1993**, *73*:5–8.

Tarte K, Klein B. Dendritic cell-based vaccine: A promising approach for cancer immunotherapy. *Leukemia*, **1999**, *13*: 653–663.

Terkeltaub R, Sundy JS, Schumacher HR, et al. The interleukin 1 inhibitor rilonacept in treatment of chronic gouty arthritis: results of a placebo-controlled, monosequence crossover, non-randomised, single-blind pilot study. *Ann Rheum Dis*, **2009**, *68*:1613–1617.

Van Parijs L, Abbas AK. Homeostasis and self-tolerance in the immune system: Turning lymphocytes off. *Science*, **1998**, *280*:243–248.

Vincenti F, Kirk AD. What's next in the pipeline. *Am J Transplant,* **2008**, *8:*1972–1981.

Vincenti F, Kirkman R, Light S, et al. Interleukin-2-receptor blockade with daclizumab to prevent acute rejection in renal transplantation. Daclizumab Triple Therapy Study Group. *N Engl J Med*, **1998**, *338*:161–165.

Vincenti F, Larsen C, Durrbach A, et al. Costimulation blockade with belatacept in renal transplantation. *N Engl J Med,* **2005**, *353:*770–781.

Vincenti F, Mendez R, Pescovitz M, et al. A phase I/II randomized open-label multicenter trial of efalizumab, a humanized anti-CD11a, anti-LFA-1 in renal transplantation. *Am J Transplant,* **2007**, *7*:1770–1777.

Vincenti F, Mendez R, Rajagopalan PR, et al. A phase I/II trial of anti-CD11a monoclonal antibody in renal transplantation. *Am J Transplant*, **2001**, *1*(suppl):276.

Vincenti F, Schena FP, Paraskevas S, et al. A randomized, multicenter study of steroid avoidance, early steroid withdrawal or standard steroid therapy in kidney transplant recipients. *Am J Transplant,* **2008**, *8*:307–316.

Vo AA, Lukovsky M, Toyoda M, et al. Rituximab and intravenous immune globulin for densensitization during renal transplantation. *N Engl J Med,* **2008**, *359*:242–251.

Wall WJ. Use of antilymphocyte induction therapy in liver transplantation. *Liver Transplant Surg,* **1999**, *5*:S64–S70.

Watson CJ, Friend PJ, Jamieson NV, et al. Sirolimus: A potent new immunosuppressant for liver transplantation. *Transplantation,* **1999**, *67*:505–509.

Weaver TA, Charafeddine AH, Kirk AD. Costimulation blockade: Towards clinical application. *Front Biosci,* **2008**, *13*:2120–2139.

Whittington R, Faulds D. Interleukin-2. A review of its pharmacological properties and therapeutic use in patients with cancer. *Drugs*, **1993**, *46*:446–514.

Wiseman LR, Faulds D. Daclizumab: A review of its use in the prevention of acute rejection in renal transplant recipients. *Drugs*, **1999**, *58*:1029–1042.

Zachary AA, Montgomery RA, Ratner LE, et al. Specific and durable elimination of antibody to donor HLA antigens in renal-transplant patients. *Transplantation*, **2003**, *76*:1519–1525.

Zimmerman JJ, Kahan BD. Pharmacokinetics of sirolimus in stable renal transplant patients after multiple oral dose administration. *J Clin Pharmacol*, **1997**, *37*:405–415.

chapter 36 Pulmonary Pharmacology

Peter J. Barnes

INTRODUCTION

Pulmonary pharmacology concerns understanding how drugs act on the lung and the pharmacological therapy of pulmonary diseases. Much of pulmonary pharmacology is concerned with the effects of drugs on the airways and the therapy of airway obstruction, particularly asthma and chronic obstructive pulmonary disease (COPD), which are among the most common chronic diseases in the world. Both asthma and COPD are characterized by chronic inflammation of the airways, although there are marked differences in inflammatory mechanisms and response to therapy between these diseases (Barnes, 2008b). After a brief introduction to asthma and COPD, this chapter discusses the pharmacotherapy of obstructive airways disease, particularly bronchodilators, which act mainly by reversing airway smooth muscle contraction, and anti-inflammatory drugs, which suppress the inflammatory response in the airways. This chapter focuses on the pulmonary pharmacology of β_2 agonists and corticosteroids; the basic pharmacology of these classes of agents is presented elsewhere (Chapters 12 and 42). In presenting the details of pharmacotherapy of asthma and COPD, the chapter also covers the physiology and molecular pathology surrounding these conditions, deriving knowledge of the diseases by assessing their responses to various classes of drugs.

This chapter also discusses other drugs used to treat obstructive airway diseases, such as mucolytics and respiratory stimulants, and covers the drug therapy of cough, the most common respiratory symptom, as well as drugs used to treat pulmonary hypertension. Drugs used in the treatment of lung infections, including tuberculosis (Chapter 56), are covered elsewhere.

MECHANISMS OF ASTHMA

Asthma is a chronic inflammatory disease of the airways that is characterized by activation of mast cells, infiltration of eosinophils, and T helper 2 (T_H2) lymphocytes (Figure 36–1) (Barnes, 2008b). Mast cell activation by allergens and physical stimuli releases bronchoconstrictor mediators, such as histamine, leukotriene D_4, and prostaglandin D_2, which cause bronchoconstriction, microvascular leakage, and plasma exudation (Chapters 32 and 33). Increased numbers of mast cells in airway smooth muscle are a characteristic of asthma. Many of the symptoms of asthma are due to airway smooth muscle contraction, and therefore bronchodilators are important as symptom relievers. Whether airway smooth muscle is intrinsically abnormal in asthma is not clear, but increased contractility of airway smooth muscle may contribute to airway hyperresponsiveness, the physiological hallmark of asthma. The mechanism of chronic inflammation in asthma is still not well understood. It may initially be driven by allergen exposure, but it appears to become autonomous so that asthma is essentially incurable. The inflammation may be orchestrated by dendritic cells that regulate T_H2 cells that drive eosinophilic inflammation and also IgE formation by B lymphocytes. Airway epithelium plays an important role through the release of multiple inflammatory mediators and through the release of growth factors in an attempt to repair the damage caused by inflammation. The inflammatory process in asthma is mediated through the release of >100 inflammatory mediators (Barnes et al., 1998a). Complex cytokine networks, including chemokines and growth factors, play important roles in orchestrating the inflammation process (Barnes, 2008a).

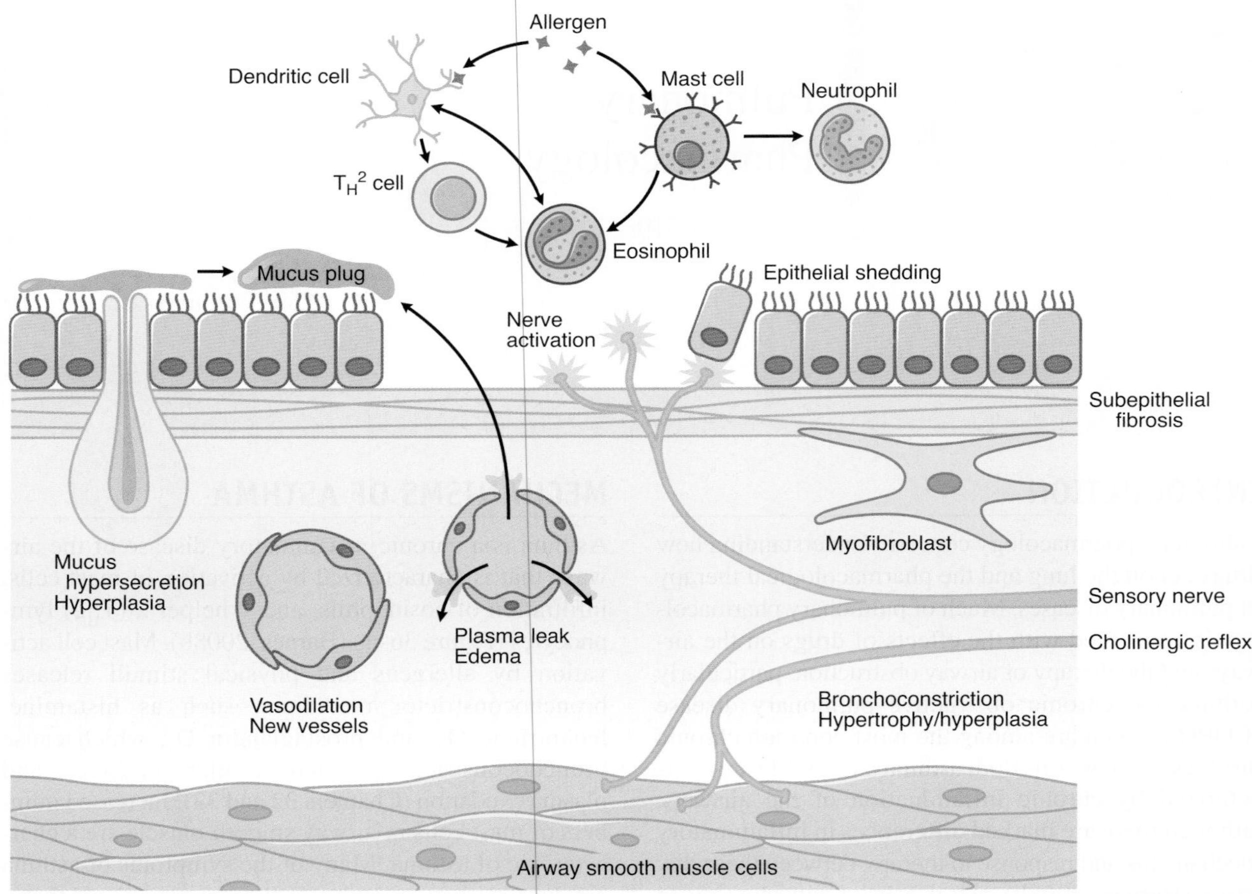

Figure 36–1. *Cellular mechanisms of asthma.* Myriad inflammatory cells are recruited and activated in the airways, where they release multiple inflammatory mediators, which can also arise from structural cells. These mediators lead to bronchoconstriction, plasma exudation and edema, vasodilation, mucus hypersecretion, and activation of sensory nerves. Chronic inflammation leads to structural changes, including subepithelial fibrosis (basement membrane thickening), airway smooth muscle hypertrophy and hyperplasia, angiogenesis, and hyperplasia of mucus-secreting cells.

Chronic inflammation may lead to structural changes in the airways, including an increase in the number and size of airway smooth muscle cells, blood vessels, and mucus-secreting cells. A characteristic histological feature of asthma is collagen deposition (fibrosis) below the basement membrane of the airway epithelium (Figure 36–1). This appears to be the result of eosinophilic inflammation and is found even at the onset of asthmatic symptoms. The complex inflammation of asthma is suppressed by corticosteroids in most patients, but even if asthma is well controlled, the inflammation and symptoms return if corticosteroids are discontinued. Asthma usually starts in early childhood, then may disappear during adolescence and reappear in adulthood. It is characterized by variable airflow obstruction and typically shows a good therapeutic response to bronchodilators and corticosteroids. Asthma severity usually does not change, so that patients with mild asthma rarely progress to severe asthma and patients with severe asthma usually have this from the onset, although some patients, particularly with late-onset asthma, show a progressive loss of lung function like patients with COPD. Patients with severe asthma may have a pattern of inflammation more similar to COPD and are characterized by reduced responsiveness to corticosteroids (Wenzel and Busse, 2007).

MECHANISMS OF CHRONIC OBSTRUCTIVE PULMONARY DISEASE

Chronic obstructive pulmonary disease involves inflammation of the respiratory tract with a pattern that differs from that of asthma. In COPD, there is a predominance of neutrophils, macrophages, and cytotoxic

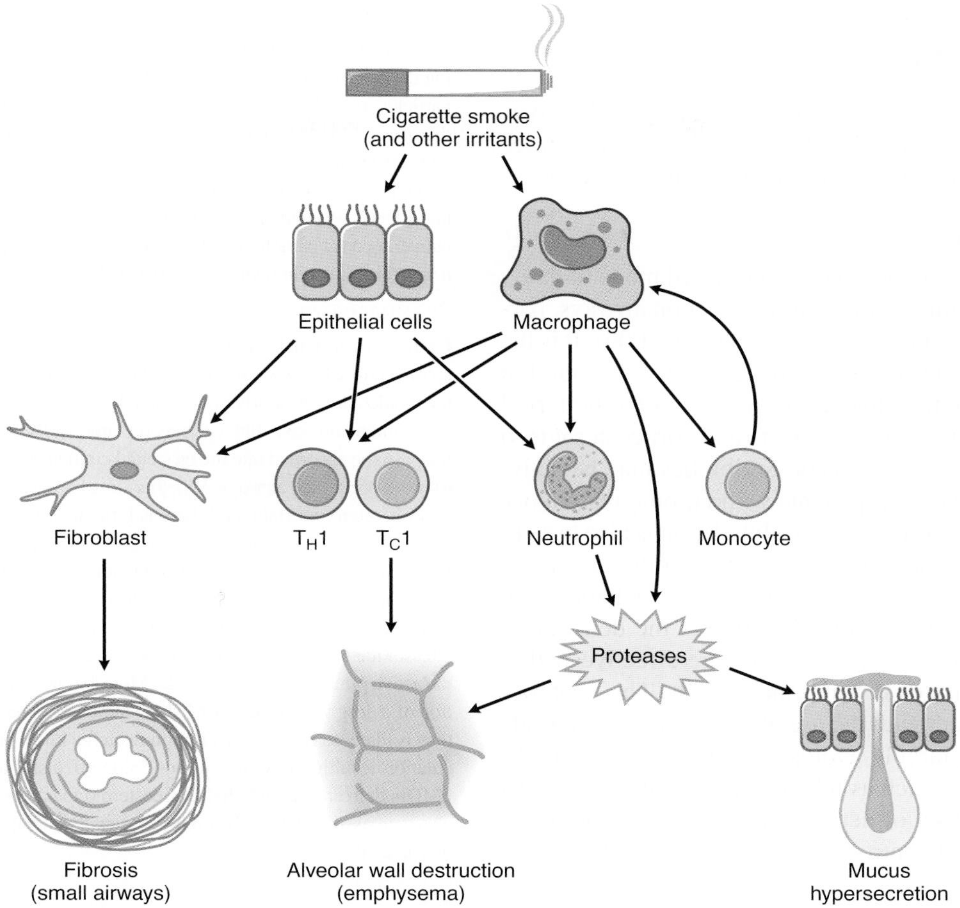

Figure 36–2. *Cellular mechanisms in chronic obstructive pulmonary disease.* Cigarette smoke and other irritants activate epithelial cells and macrophages in the lung to release mediators that attract circulating inflammatory cells, including monocytes (which differentiate to macrophages within the lung), neutrophils, and T lymphocytes (T_H1 and T_C1 cells). Fibrogenic factors released from epithelial cells and macrophages lead to fibrosis of small airways. Release of proteases results in alveolar wall destruction (emphysema) and mucus hypersecretion (chronic bronchitis).

T-lymphocytes (Tc1 cells). The inflammation predominantly affects small airways, resulting in progressive small airway narrowing and fibrosis (chronic obstructive bronchiolitis) and destruction of the lung parenchyma with destruction of the alveolar walls (emphysema) (Figure 36–2) (Barnes, 2008b). These pathological changes result in airway closure on expiration, leading to air trapping and hyperinflation, particularly on exercise (dynamic hyperinflation). This accounts for shortness of breath on exertion and exercise limitation that are characteristic symptoms of COPD.

Bronchodilators reduce air trapping by dilating peripheral airways and are the mainstay of treatment in COPD. In contrast to asthma, the airflow obstruction of COPD tends to be progressive. The inflammation in the peripheral lung of COPD patients is mediated by multiple inflammatory mediators and cytokines, although the pattern of mediators differs from that of asthma (Barnes, 2004; Barnes, 2008a). In marked contrast to asthma, the inflammation in COPD patients is largely corticosteroid resistant, and there are currently no effective anti-inflammatory treatments for this disease. In addition to pulmonary disease, many patients with COPD have systemic manifestations (skeletal muscle wasting, weight loss, depression, osteoporosis, anemia) and comorbid diseases (ischemic heart disease, hypertension, congestive heart failure, diabetes) (Barnes and Celli, 2009). Whether these are due to spillover of inflammatory mediators from the lung or due to common causal mechanisms (such as smoking) is not yet clear, but it may be important to treat the systemic components in the overall management of COPD.

ROUTES OF DRUG DELIVERY TO THE LUNGS

Drugs may be delivered to the lungs by oral or parenteral routes and also by inhalation. The choice depends on the drug and on the respiratory disease.

Inhaled Route

Inhalation (Figure 36–3) is the preferred mode of delivery of many drugs with a direct effect on airways, particularly for asthma and COPD (Berger, 2009). It is the only way to deliver some drugs such as cromolyn sodium and anticholinergic drugs and is the preferred route of delivery for β_2 agonists and corticosteroids to reduce systemic side effects. Antibiotics may be delivered by inhalation in patients with chronic respiratory sepsis (e.g., in cystic fibrosis). Inhalation is also used to facilitate systemic drug delivery in other diseases (e.g., to avoid daily injections with insulin; see Chapter 43). The major advantage of inhalation is the delivery of drug to the airways in doses that are effective with a much lower risk of systemic side effects. This is particularly important with the use of inhaled corticosteroids (ICS), which largely avoids systemic side effects. In addition, drugs such as inhaled bronchodilators have a more rapid onset of action than when taken orally so that more rapid control of symptoms is possible.

Particle Size

The size of particles for inhalation is of critical importance in determining the site of deposition in the respiratory tract. The optimum size for particles to settle in the airways is 2-5 μm mass median aerodynamic diameter (MMAD). Larger particles settle out in the upper airways, whereas smaller particles remain suspended and are therefore exhaled. There is increasing interest in delivering drugs to small airways, particularly in COPD and severe asthma (Sturton et al., 2008). This involves delivering drug particles of ~1 μm MMAD, which is now possible using drugs formulated in hydrofluoroalkane (HFA) propellant.

Pharmacokinetics

Of the total drug delivered, only 10-20% enters the lower airways with a conventional pressurized metered-dose inhaler (pMDI). The fate of the inhaled drug is poorly understood. Drugs are absorbed from the airway lumen and have direct effects on target cells of the airway. Drugs may also be absorbed into the bronchial circulation and then distributed to more peripheral airways. Whether drugs are metabolized in the airways is often uncertain, and there is little understanding of the factors that may influence local absorption and metabolism of inhaled drugs. Drugs with higher molecular weights tend to be retained to a greater extent in the airways. Nevertheless, several drugs have greater therapeutic efficacy when given by the inhaled route. The inhaled corticosteroid ciclesonide is a prodrug activated by esterases in the respiratory tract to the active principle des-ciclesonide. More extensive pulmonary distribution of a drug with a smaller MMAD increases alveolar deposition and thus is likely to increase absorption from the lungs into the general circulation resulting in more systemic side effects. Thus, although HFA pMDIs deliver more inhaled corticosteroid to smaller airways, there is also increased systemic absorption, so that the therapeutic ratio may not be changed.

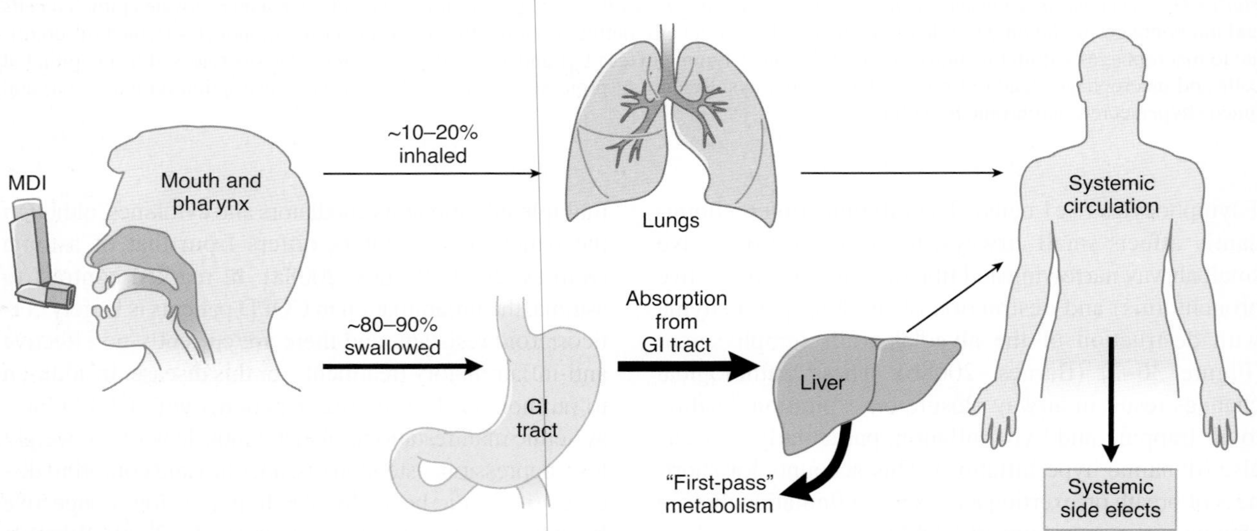

Figure 36–3. *Schematic representation of the deposition of inhaled drugs (e.g., corticosteroids, β_2 agonists).* Inhalation therapy deposits drugs directly, but not exclusively, in the lungs. Distribution between lungs and oropharynx depends mostly on the particle size and the efficiency of the delivery method. Most material will be swallowed and absorbed, entering systemic circulation after undergoing the first-pass effect in the liver. Some drug will also be absorbed into the systemic circulation from the lungs. Use of a large-volume spacer will reduce the amount of drug deposited on oropharynx, thereby reducing amount swallowed and absorbed from GI tract, thus limiting systemic effects. MDI, metered-dose inhaler.

Delivery Devices

Several ways of delivering inhaled drugs are possible (Virchow et al., 2008).

Pressurized Metered-Dose Inhalers. Drugs are propelled from a canister with the aid of a propellant, previously with a chlorofluorocarbon (Freon) but now replaced by a hydrofluoroalkane (HFA) that is "ozone friendly." These devices are convenient, portable, and typically deliver 100-400 doses of drug. It is necessary to coordinate inhalation with activation of the device, so it is important that patients are taught to use these devices correctly. Many patients find this difficult despite instruction.

Spacer Chambers. Large-volume spacer devices between the pMDI and the patient reduce the velocity of particles entering the upper airways and the size of the particles by allowing evaporation of liquid propellant. This reduces the amount of drug that impinges on the oropharynx and increases the proportion of drug inhaled into the lower airways. The need for careful coordination between activation and inhalation is also reduced because the pMDI can be activated into the chamber and the aerosol subsequently inhaled from the one-way valve. Perhaps the most useful application of spacer chambers is in the reduction of the oropharyngeal deposition of inhaled corticosteroids and the consequent reduction in the local side effects of these drugs. Large volume spacers also reduce the systemic side effects of drugs because less is deposited in the oropharynx, and therefore swallowed. It is the swallowed fraction of the drug absorbed from the GI tract that makes the greatest contribution to the systemic fraction. This is of particular importance in the use of certain inhaled steroids, such as beclomethasone dipropionate, which can be absorbed from the GI tract. Spacer devices are also useful in delivering inhaled drugs to small children who are not able to use a pMDI. Children as young as 3 years of age are able to use a spacer device fitted with a face mask.

Dry Powder Inhalers. Drugs may also be delivered as a dry powder using devices that scatter a fine powder dispersed by air turbulence on inhalation. These devices may be preferred by some patients (Chan, 2006) because careful coordination is not as necessary as with the pMDI, but some patients find that the dry powder is an irritant. Children <7 years of age find it difficult to use a dry powder inhaler (DPI) because they may not be able to generate sufficient inspiratory flow. DPIs have been developed to deliver peptides and proteins, such as insulin (e.g., EXUBERA, AFRESA), systemically.

Nebulizers. Two types of nebulizer are available. Jet nebulizers are driven by a stream of gas (air or oxygen), whereas ultrasonic nebulizers use a rapidly vibrating piezo-electric crystal and thus do not require a source of compressed gas. The nebulized drug may be inspired during tidal breathing, and it is possible to deliver much higher doses of drug compared with pMDI. Nebulizers are therefore useful in treating acute exacerbations of asthma and COPD, for delivering drugs when airway obstruction is extreme (e.g., in severe COPD), for delivering inhaled drugs to infants and small children who cannot use the other inhalation devices, and for giving drugs such as antibiotics when relatively high doses must be delivered. Small handheld nebulizers (soft mist inhalers) are now also available.

Oral Route

Drugs for treatment of pulmonary diseases may also be given orally. The oral dose is much higher than the inhaled dose required to achieve the same effect (typically by a ratio of ~20:1), so that systemic side effects are more common. *When there is a choice of inhaled or oral route for a drug (e.g., β_2 agonist or corticosteroid), the inhaled route is always preferable, and the oral route should be reserved for the few patients unable to use inhalers (e.g., small children, patients with physical problems such as severe arthritis of the hands).* Theophylline is ineffective by the inhaled route and therefore must be given systemically. Corticosteroids may have to be given orally for parenchymal lung diseases (e.g., in interstitial lung diseases), although it may be possible in the future to deliver such drugs into alveoli using specially designed inhalation devices with a small particle size.

Parenteral Route

The intravenous route should be reserved for delivery of drugs in the severely ill patient who is unable to absorb drugs from the GI tract. Side effects are generally frequent due to the high plasma concentrations.

BRONCHODILATORS

Bronchodilator drugs relax constricted airway smooth muscle *in vitro* and cause immediate reversal of airway obstruction in asthma *in vivo*. They also prevent bronchoconstriction (and thereby provide bronchoprotection). Three main classes of bronchodilator are in current clinical use:

- β_2 Adrenergic agonists (sympathomimetics)
- Theophylline (a methylxanthine)
- Anticholinergic agents (muscarinic receptor antagonists)

Drugs such as cromolyn sodium, which prevent bronchoconstriction, have no direct bronchodilator action and are ineffective once bronchoconstriction has occurred. Anti-leukotrienes (leukotriene receptor antagonists and 5′-lipoxygenase inhibitors) have a small bronchodilator effect in some asthmatic patients and appear to prevent bronchoconstriction. Corticosteroids, although gradually improving airway obstruction, have no direct effect on contraction of airway smooth muscle and are not therefore considered to be bronchodilators.

β_2 ADRENERGIC AGONISTS

Inhaled β_2 agonists are the bronchodilator treatment of choice in asthma because they are the most effective bronchodilators and have minimal side effects when used correctly. Systemic, short-acting, and nonselective β agonists, such as isoproterenol (isoprenaline) or metaproterenol, should only be used as a last resort.

Chemistry. The development of β_2 agonists is based on substitutions in the catecholamine structure of norepinephrine and epinephrine (Chapter 12). The catechol ring consists of hydroxyl groups in the 3 and 4 positions of the benzene ring (Figure 36–4). Norepinephrine

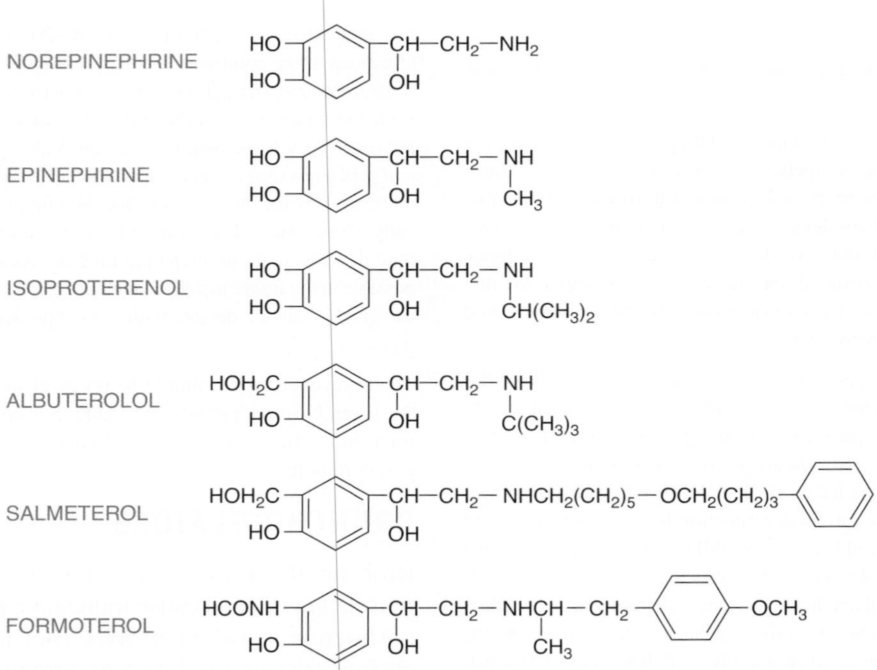

NOREPINEPHRINE

EPINEPHRINE

ISOPROTERENOL

ALBUTEROLOL

SALMETEROL

FORMOTEROL

Figure 36–4. *Chemical structure of some adrenergic agonists showing development from catecholamines by substitutions on the catechol nucleus and side chain.*

differs from epinephrine only in the terminal amine group; in general, further modification at this site confers β receptor selectivity. Further substitution of the terminal amine resulted in β_2 receptor selectivity, as in albuterol (salbutamol) and terbutaline. Exogenous catecholamines are rapidly metabolized by catechol-*O*-methyl transferase (COMT), which methylates in the 3-hydroxyl position, and accounts for the short duration of action of catecholamines. Modification of the catechol ring, as in albuterol and terbutaline, prevents this degradation and therefore prolongs the effect. Catecholamines are also broken down in sympathetic nerve terminals and in the GI tract by monoamine oxidase (MAO), which cleaves the side chain. Isoproterenol, which is a substrate for MAO, is metabolized in the gut, making absorption variable. Substitution in the amine group confers resistance to MAO and ensures reliable absorption. Many other β_2-selective agonists have now been introduced and, although there may be differences in potency, there are no clinically significant differences in selectivity. Inhaled β_2-selective drugs in current clinical use (apart from rimiterol [not available in the U.S.] that is broken down by COMT) have a similar duration of action (3-6 hours). The inhaled long-acting inhaled β_2 agonists salmeterol and formoterol have a much longer duration of effect, providing bronchodilation and bronchoprotection for >12 hours (Kips and Pauwels, 2001). Formoterol has a bulky substitution in the aliphatic chain and has a moderate lipophilicity, which appears to keep the drug in the membrane close to the receptor, so it behaves as a slow-release drug. Salmeterol has a long aliphatic chain, and its long duration may be due to binding within the receptor binding cleft ("exosite") that anchors the drug in the binding cleft. Once-daily β_2 agonists, such as indacaterol, with a duration of action >24 hours, are now in development (Cazzola and Matera, 2008).

Mode of Action

Occupation of β_2 receptors by agonists results in the activation of the G_s-adenylyl cyclase-cAMP-PKA pathway, resulting in phosphorylative events leading to bronchial smooth muscle relaxation (Figure 36–5). β Agonists produce bronchodilation by directly stimulating β_2 receptors in airway smooth muscle, and *in vitro* relax human bronchi and lung strips (indicating an effect on peripheral airways). *In vivo* there is a rapid decrease in airway resistance. β_2 Receptors have been localized to airway smooth muscle of all airways by direct receptor binding techniques and autoradiographic mapping studies.

The molecular mechanisms by which β agonists induce relaxation of airway smooth muscle include:

- Lowering of $[Ca^{2+}]_i$ concentration by active removal of Ca^{2+} from the cytosol into intracellular stores and out of the cell
- Acute inhibition of the PLC-IP_3 pathway and its mobilization of cellular Ca^{2+} (prolonged use can upregulate expression of $PLC_{\beta 1}$)
- Inhibition of myosin light chain kinase activation
- Activation of myosin light chain phosphatase
- Opening of a large conductance Ca^{2+}-activated K^+ channel (K_{Ca}), which repolarizes the smooth muscle cell and may stimulate the sequestration of Ca^{2+} into intracellular stores. β_2 Receptors may also couple to K_{Ca} via G_s so that relaxation of airway smooth muscle may occur independently of an increase in cAMP.

Several actions of β_2 agonists are mediated not by PKA but by other cAMP-regulated proteins, such as the exchange protein activated by cAMP (EPAC) (Holz et al., 2006). β_2 Agonists act as *functional antagonists* and reverse bronchoconstriction irrespective of

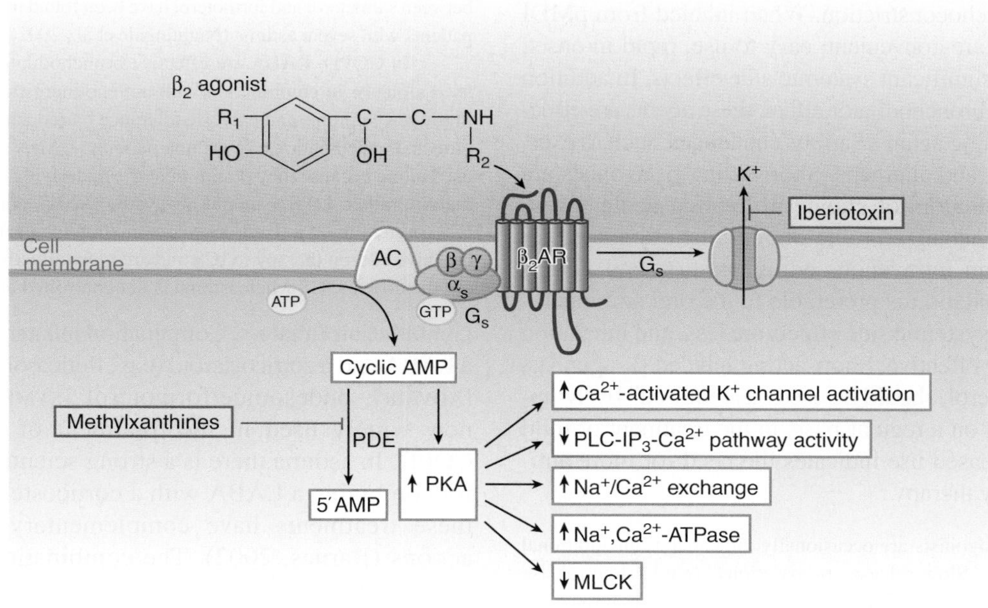

Figure 36–5. *Molecular actions of β_2 agonists to induce relaxation of airway smooth muscle cells.* Activation of β_2 receptors (β_2AR) results in activation of adenylyl cyclase (AC) via a stimulatory G protein (G_s), leading to an increase in intracellular cyclic AMP and activation of PKA. PKA phosphorylates a variety of target substrates, resulting in opening of Ca^{2+}-activated K^+ channels (K_{Ca}), thereby facilitating hyperpolarization, decreased phosphoinositide (PI) hydrolysis, increased Na^+/Ca^{2+} exchange, increased Na^+,Ca^{2+}- ATPase activity, and decreased myosin light chain kinase (MLCK) activity. β_2 Receptors may also couple to K_{Ca} via G_s. PDE, cyclic nucleotide phosphodiesterase.

the contractile agent. This is an important property for the treatment of asthma because many bronchoconstrictor mechanisms (neurotransmitters and mediators) are likely to be contributory. In COPD the major mechanism of action is likely to be reduction of cholinergic neural bronchoconstriction.

β_2 Receptors are localized to several different airway cells, where they may have additional effects. Thus, β_2 agonists may cause bronchodilation *in vivo* not only via a direct action on airways smooth muscle, but also indirectly by inhibiting the release of bronchoconstrictor mediators from inflammatory cells and of bronchoconstrictor neurotransmitters from airway nerves. These mechanisms include:

- Prevention of mediator release from isolated human lung mast cells (via β_2 receptors).
- Prevention of microvascular leakage and thus the development of bronchial mucosal edema after exposure to mediators, such as histamine and leukotriene D_4.
- Increase in *mucus secretion* from submucosal glands and *ion transport* across airway epithelium; these effects may enhance mucociliary clearance, and thereby reverse the defective clearance found in asthma.
- Reduction in *neurotransmission* in human airway cholinergic nerves by an action at presynaptic β_2 receptors to inhibit acetylcholine release. This may contribute to their bronchodilator effect by reducing reflex cholinergic bronchoconstriction.

Although these additional effects of β_2 agonists may be relevant to the prophylactic use of these drugs against various challenges, their rapid bronchodilator action is probably attributable to a direct effect on airway smooth muscle.

Anti-Inflammatory Effects

Whether β_2 agonists have anti-inflammatory effects in asthma is controversial. The inhibitory effects of β_2 agonists on mast cell mediator release and microvascular leakage are clearly anti-inflammatory, suggesting that β_2 agonists may modify *acute* inflammation. However, β_2 agonists do not appear to have a significant inhibitory effect on the *chronic* inflammation of asthmatic airways, which is suppressed by corticosteroids. This has now been confirmed by several biopsy and bronchoalveolar lavage studies in patients with asthma who are taking regular β_2 agonists (including long-acting inhaled β_2 agonists), that demonstrate no significant reduction in the number or activation in inflammatory cells in the airways, in contrast to resolution of the inflammation that occurs with ICS. This may be related to the fact that effects of β_2 agonists on macrophages, eosinophils, and lymphocytes are rapidly desensitized.

Clinical Use

Short-Acting β_2 Agonists. Inhaled short-acting β_2 agonists are the most widely used and effective bronchodilators in the treatment of asthma due to their functional antagonism of bronchoconstriction. When inhaled from pMDI or DPI, they are convenient, easy to use, rapid in onset, and without significant systemic side effects. In addition to their acute bronchodilator effect, these agents are effective in protecting against various challenges, such as exercise, cold air, and allergens. Short-acting β_2 agonists are the bronchodilators of choice in treating acute severe asthma. The nebulized route of administration is easier and safer than intravenous administration and just as effective. Inhalation is preferable to the oral administration because systemic side effects are less, and inhalation may be more effective. Short-acting inhaled β_2 agonists, such as albuterol, should be used "as required" by symptoms and not on a regular basis in the treatment of mild asthma; increased use indicates the need for more anti-inflammatory therapy.

Oral β_2 agonists are occasionally indicated as an additional bronchodilator. Slow-release preparations (e.g., slow-release albuterol and bambuterol [a prodrug that slowly releases terbutaline but is not commercially available in the U.S.]) may be indicated in nocturnal asthma; however, these agents are less useful than inhaled β agonists because of an increased risk of side effects. Several short-acting β_2 agonists are available. With the exception of rimiterol (which retains the catechol ring structure and is therefore susceptible to rapid enzymatic degradation), they are resistant to uptake and enzymatic degradation by COMT and MAO. There is little to choose between the various short-acting β_2 agonists currently available; all are usable by inhalation and orally, have a similar duration of action (~3-4 hours; less in severe asthma), and similar side effects. Differences in β_2 selectivity have been claimed but are not clinically important. Drugs in clinical use include albuterol (salbutamol), levalbuterol, metaproterenol, terbutaline, as well as several not available in the U.S., fenoterol, tulobuterol, rimiterol, and pirbuterol.

Long-Acting Inhaled β_2 Agonists. The long-acting inhaled β_2 agonists (LABA) salmeterol, formoterol, and arformoterol have proved to be a significant advance in asthma and COPD therapy. These drugs have a bronchodilator action of >12 hours and also protect against bronchoconstriction for a similar period (Kips and Pauwels, 2001). They improve asthma control (when given twice daily) compared with regular treatment with short-acting β_2 agonists (four to six times daily).

Tolerance to the bronchodilator effect of formoterol and the bronchoprotective effects of formoterol and salmeterol have been demonstrated, but this is a small loss of protection that does not appear to be progressive and is of doubtful clinical significance. Although both drugs have a similar duration of effect in clinical studies, there are differences. Formoterol has a more rapid onset of action and is an almost full agonist, whereas salmeterol is a partial agonist with a slower onset of action. These differences might confer a theoretical advantage for formoterol in more severe asthma, whereas it may also make it more likely to induce tolerance. However, no significant clinical differences between salmeterol and formoterol have been found in the treatment of patients with severe asthma (Nightingale et al., 2002).

In COPD, LABA are effective bronchodilators that may be used alone or in combination with anticholinergics or ICS. LABA improve symptoms and exercise tolerance by reducing both air trapping and exacerbations. In asthma patients, LABA should never be used alone because they do not treat the underlying chronic inflammation; rather, LABA should always be used in combination with ICS (preferably in a fixed-dose combination inhaler). LABA are an effective add-on therapy to ICS and are more effective than increasing the dose of ICS when asthma is not controlled at low doses.

Combination Inhalers. Combination inhalers that contain a LABA and a corticosteroid (e.g., fluticasone/salmeterol [ADVAIR], budesonide/formoterol [SYMBICORT]) are now widely used in the treatment of asthma and COPD. In asthma there is a strong scientific rationale for combining a LABA with a corticosteroid because these treatments have complementary synergistic actions (Barnes, 2002). The combination inhaler is more convenient for patients, simplifies therapy, and improves compliance with ICS because the patients perceive clinical benefit, but there may be an additional advantage because delivering the two drugs in the same inhaler ensures they are delivered simultaneously to the same cells in the airways, allowing the beneficial molecular interactions between LABA and corticosteroids to occur. It is likely that these inhalers will become the preferred therapy for all patients with persistent asthma. These combination inhalers are also more effective in COPD patients than LABA and ICS alone, but the mechanisms accounting for this beneficial interaction are less well understood than in patients with asthma.

Recently, a combination inhaler that contains formoterol and budesonide was shown to be more effective for relieving acute symptoms than either terbutaline or formoterol alone, suggesting that the inhaled corticosteroids may also be contributing to the benefit (Rabe et al., 2006). This may make it possible to control asthma with a single inhaler both for maintenance and relief of symptoms.

Stereoselective β_2 Agonists. Albuterol is a racemic mixture of active *R*- and inactive *S*-isomers. Animal studies suggest that the *S*-isomer may increase airway responsiveness, providing a rationale for the development of *R*-albuterol (levalbuterol). Although the *R*-isomer is more potent than racemic *R/S*-albuterol in some studies, careful dose responses show no advantage in terms of efficacy and no evidence that the *S*-albuterol is detrimental in asthmatic patients (Lotvall et al., 2001). Because levalbuterol is more expensive than normally used racemic albuterol, this therapy has no clear clinical advantage (Barnes, 2006b). Stereoselective formoterol (*R*, *R*-formoterol, arformoterol) has now been developed as a nebulized solution but also appears to offer no clinical advantage over racemic formoterol (Madaan, 2009).

β_2 Receptor Polymorphisms. Several single nucleotide polymorphisms and haplotypes of the human β_2 adrenergic receptor gene (*ADRβ2*), which affect the structure of β_2 receptors, have been described. The common variants are $Gly^{16}Arg$ and $Gln^{27}Glu$, which have *in vitro* effects on receptor desensitization, but clinical studies have shown inconsistent effects on the bronchodilator responses to short- and long-acting β_2 agonists (Hawkins et al., 2008). Some studies have shown that patients with the common homozygous $Arg^{16}Arg$ variant have more frequent adverse effects and a poorer response to short-acting β_2 agonists than heterozygotes or $Gly^{16}Gly$ homozygotes, but overall these differences are small, and there appears to be no clinical value in measuring *ADRβ2* genotype. No differences have been found with responses to LABA between these genotypes (Bleecker et al., 2007).

Side Effects. Unwanted effects are dose related and due to stimulation of extrapulmonary β receptors (Table 36–1 and Chapter 12). Side effects are not common with inhaled therapy but quite common with oral or intravenous administration.

- *Muscle tremor* due to stimulation of β_2 receptors in skeletal muscle is the most common side effect. It may be more troublesome with elderly patients and so is a more frequent problem in COPD patients.
- *Tachycardia* and *palpitations* are due to reflex cardiac stimulation secondary to peripheral vasodilation, from direct stimulation of atrial β_2 receptors (human heart has a relatively high proportion of β_2 receptors; see Chapter 12), and possibly also from stimulation of myocardial β_1 receptors as the doses of β_2 agonist are increased. These side effects tend to disappear with continued use of the drug, reflecting the development of tolerance. There can be a dose-related prolongation of the corrected QT interval (QTc).
- *Hypokalemia* is a potentially serious side effect. This is due to β_2 receptor stimulation of potassium entry into skeletal muscle, which may be secondary to a rise in insulin secretion. Hypokalemia might be serious in the presence of hypoxia, as in acute asthma, when there may be a predisposition to cardiac arrhythmias (Chapter 29). In practice, however, significant arrhythmias after nebulized β_2 agonists are rarely observed in acute asthma or COPD patients.
- *Ventilation-perfusion(V/Q) mismatch* due to pulmonary vasodilation in blood vessels previously constricted by hypoxia, resulting in the shunting of blood to poorly ventilated areas and a fall in arterial oxygen tension. Although in practice the effect of β_2 agonists on Pao_2 is usually very small (<5 mm Hg fall), occasionally in severe COPD it can be large, although it may be prevented by giving additional inspired oxygen (O_2).
- *Metabolic* effects (increase in free fatty acid, insulin, glucose, pyruvate, and lactate) are usually seen only after large systemic doses.

Table 36–1

Side Effects of β_2 Agonists

- Muscle tremor (direct effect on skeletal muscle β_2 receptors)
- Tachycardia (direct effect on atrial β_2 receptors, reflex effect from increased peripheral vasodilation via β_2 receptors)
- Hypokalemia (direct β_2 effect on skeletal muscle uptake of K^+)
- Restlessness
- Hypoxemia (increased $\dot{V}/\dot{Q}$ mismatch due to reversal of hypoxic pulmonary vasoconstriction)

Tolerance. Continuous treatment with an agonist often leads to tolerance (desensitization, subsensitivity), which may be due to down-regulation of the receptor (Chapter 12). For this reason there have been many studies of bronchial β receptor function after prolonged therapy with β_2 agonists. Tolerance of non-airway β_2 receptor–mediated responses, such as tremor and cardiovascular and metabolic responses, is readily induced in normal and asthmatic subjects. Tolerance of human airway smooth muscle to β_2 agonists *in vitro* has been demonstrated, although the concentration of agonist necessary is high and the degree of desensitization is variable. In normal subjects, bronchodilator tolerance is not a consistent finding after high-dose inhaled albuterol. In asthmatic patients tolerance to the bronchodilator effects of β_2 agonists has not usually been found. However, tolerance develops to the bronchoprotective effects of β_2 agonists, and this is more marked with indirect bronchoconstrictors that activate mast cells (e.g., adenosine, allergen, and exercise) than with direct bronchoconstrictors, such as histamine and methacholine. The reason for the relative resistance of airway smooth muscle β_2 responses to desensitization remains uncertain but may reflect the large receptor reserve: >90% of β_2 receptors may be lost without any reduction in the relaxation response. The high level of *ADRβ2 expression* in airway smooth muscle compared with peripheral lung may also contribute to the resistance to tolerance because a high rate of β receptor synthesis is likely. In addition, the expression of GRK2, which phosphorylates and inactivates occupied β_2 receptors, is very low in airway smooth muscle (McGraw and Liggett, 1997). By contrast there is no receptor reserve in inflammatory cells, GRK2 expression is high, and tolerance to β_2 agonists rapidly develops at these sites.

Experimental studies have shown that corticosteroids prevent the development of tolerance in airway smooth muscle, and prevent and reverse the fall in pulmonary β receptor density (Mak et al., 1995). However, ICS fail to prevent the tolerance to the bronchoprotective effect of inhaled β_2 agonists, possibly because they do not reach airway smooth muscle in a high enough concentration.

Long-Term Safety. Because of a possible relationship between adrenergic drug therapy and the rise in asthma deaths in several countries during the early 1960s, doubts were cast on the long-term safety of β agonists. A causal relationship between β agonist use and mortality has never been firmly established, although in retrospective studies this would not be possible. A particular β_2 agonist, fenoterol, was linked to the rise in asthma deaths in New Zealand in the early 1990s because significantly more of the fatal cases were prescribed fenoterol than the case-matched control patients. An epidemiological study examined the links between drugs prescribed for asthma and death or near death from asthma attacks, based on computerized records of prescriptions. There was a marked increase in the risk of death with high doses of all inhaled β_2 agonists (Spitzer et al., 1992). The risk was greater with fenoterol, but when the dose is adjusted to the equivalent dose for albuterol, there is no significant difference in the risk for these two drugs. The link between high β_2 agonist usage and increased asthma mortality does not prove a causal association because patients with more severe and poorly controlled asthma, who are more likely to have an increased risk of fatal attacks, are more likely to be using higher doses of β_2 agonist inhalers and less likely to be using effective anti-inflammatory treatment. Indeed, in the patients who used regular inhaled steroids there was a significant reduction in risk of death (Suissa et al., 2000).

Regular use of inhaled β_2 agonists has also been linked to increased asthma morbidity. Regular use of fenoterol was associated with worse asthma control and a small increase in airway hyperresponsiveness compared with patients using fenoterol "on demand" for symptom control over a 6-month period (Sears et al., 1990). However, this was not found in a study with regular albuterol (Dennis et al., 2000). There is some evidence that regular inhaled β_2 agonists may increase allergen-induced asthma and sputum eosinophilia (Mcivor et al., 1998). A possible mechanism is that β_2 agonists upregulate expression of $PLC_{\beta 1}$, resulting in augmentation of the bronchoconstrictor responses to cholinergic agonists and mediators (McGraw et al., 2003). Short-acting inhaled β_2 agonists should only be used on demand for symptom control, and if they are required frequently (more than three times weekly), an ICS is needed.

The safety of LABA in asthma remains controversial. A large study of the safety of salmeterol showed an excess of respiratory deaths and near deaths in patients prescribed salmeterol, but these deaths occurred mainly in African Americans living in inner cities who were not taking ICS (Nelson et al., 2006). Similar data have also raised concerns about formoterol. This may be predictable because LABA do not treat the underlying chronic inflammation of asthma. However, concomitant treatment with ICS appears to obviate such risk, so it is recommended that LABA should only be used when ICS are also prescribed (preferably in the form of a combination inhaler so that the LABA can never be taken without the inhaled corticosteroids) (Jaeschke et al., 2008). All LABA approved in the U.S. carry a black box warning cautioning against overuse. Studies are underway to examine their long-term safety profile, especially in children with asthma. There are less safety concerns with LABA use in COPD. No major adverse effects were reported in a large study over 3 years in COPD patients and in several other studies (Calverley et al., 2007; Rodrigo et al., 2008).

Future Developments

β_2 Agonists will continue to be the bronchodilators of choice for asthma in the foreseeable future because they are effective in all patients and have few or no side effects when used in low doses. It would be difficult to find a bronchodilator that improves on the efficacy and safety of inhaled β_2 agonists. Although some concerns have been expressed about the long-term effects of short-acting inhaled β_2 agonists, when used as required for symptom control, inhaled β_2 agonists appear safe. Use of large doses of inhaled β_2 agonists indicates poor asthma control; such patients should be assessed and appropriate controller medication used. LABA are a very useful option for long-term control in asthma and COPD. In asthma patients LABA should probably only be used if the patient is receiving concomitant ICS. There is little advantage to be gained by improving β_2 receptor selectivity because most of the side effects of these agents are due to β_2 receptor stimulation (muscle tremor, tachycardia, hypokalemia). Several once daily inhaled β_2 agonists, such as indacaterol and carmoterol, are now in clinical development (Cazzola and Matera, 2008).

METHYLXANTHINES

Methylxanthines, such as theophylline, which are related to caffeine, have been used in the treatment of asthma since 1930, and theophylline is still widely used in developing countries because it is inexpensive. Theophylline became more useful with the availability of rapid plasma assays and the introduction of reliable slow-release preparations. However, the frequency of side effects and the relative low efficacy of theophylline have led to reduced use in many countries because inhaled β_2 agonists are far more effective as bronchodilators and ICS have a greater anti-inflammatory effect. In patients with severe asthma and COPD it still remains a very useful drug, however.

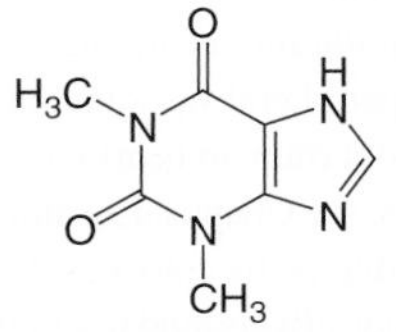

H_3C O H N N N N O CH_3

THEOPHYLLINE

Chemistry. Theophylline is a methylxanthine similar in structure to the common dietary xanthines caffeine and theobromine. Several substituted derivatives have been synthesized, but only two appear to have any advantage over theophylline: the 3-propyl derivative, enprofylline, which is more potent as a bronchodilator and may have fewer toxic effects because it does not antagonize adenosine receptors; and doxofylline (7-[1,3-dioxalan-2-ylmethyl] theophylline), a novel methylxanthine available in some countries (Dini and Cogo, 2001). Doxofylline, which has a dioxolane group at position 7, has an inhibitory effect on phosphodiesterases (PDEs) similar to that of theophylline but is less active as an adenosine antagonist and may have a more favorable side-effect profile. Many salts of theophylline have also been marketed; the most common is aminophylline, which is the ethylenediamine salt used to increase its solubility at neutral pH. Other salts either do not have any advantage (e.g., oxtriphylline [choline theophyllinate]) or are virtually inactive (e.g., acepifylline). Thus, theophylline remains the major methylxanthine in clinical use.

Mechanism of Action. The mechanisms of action of theophylline are still uncertain. In addition to its bronchodilator action, theophylline has many nonbronchodilator effects that may be relevant to its effects in asthma and COPD (Figure 36–6). Many of these molecular effects are seen only at high concentrations that exceed the therapeutic range, however. Several molecular mechanisms of action have been proposed:

- *Inhibition of phosphodiesterases.* Theophylline is a nonselective PDE inhibitor, but the degree of inhibition is relatively

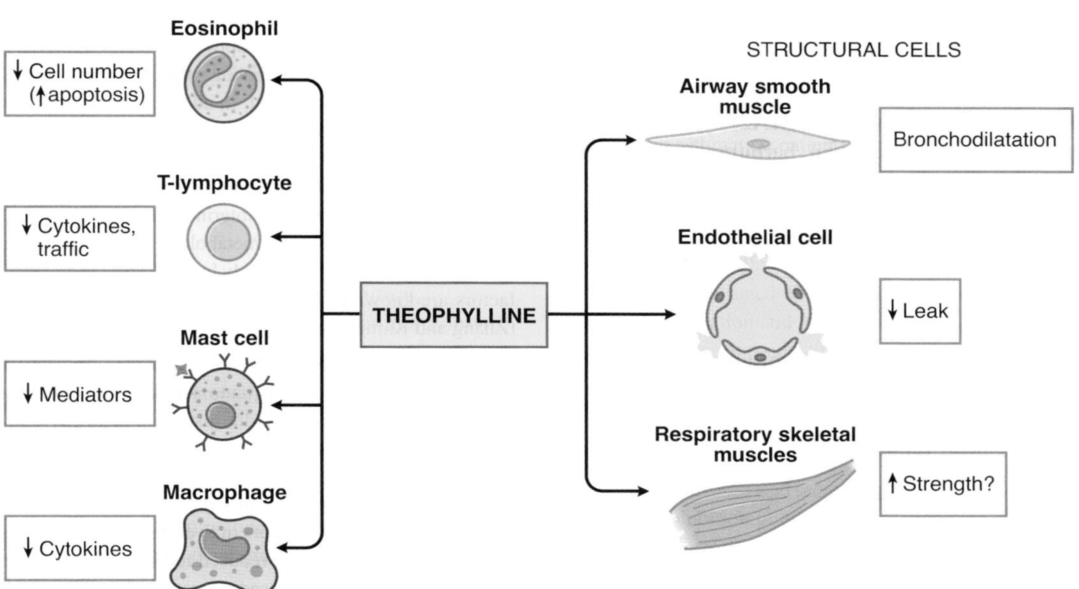

Figure 36–6. *Theophylline affects multiple cell types in the airway.*

minimal at concentrations of theophylline that are within the so-called therapeutic range. PDE inhibition and the concomitant elevation of cellular cAMP and cyclic guanosine monophosphate (cGMP) almost certainly account for the bronchodilator action of theophylline, but PDE inhibition is unlikely to account for the nonbronchodilator effects of theophylline that are seen at lower concentrations. Inhibition of PDE should lead to synergistic interaction with β agonists through an increase in cAMP (Figure 36–5), but this has not been convincingly demonstrated in clinical studies. Several isoenzyme families of PDE have now been recognized and those important in smooth muscle relaxation include PDE3, PDE4, and PDE5. Theophylline is a weak inhibitor of all PDE isoenzymes.

- *Adenosine receptor antagonism.* Theophylline antagonizes adenosine receptors at therapeutic concentrations. Adenosine causes bronchoconstriction in airways from asthmatic patients by releasing histamine and leukotrienes. Adenosine antagonism is unlikely to account for the anti-inflammatory effects of theophylline but may be responsible for serious side effects, including cardiac arrhythmias and seizures through the antagonism of A_1 receptors. Of interest may be the adenosine A_{2B} receptor on mast cells, which is activated by adenosine in asthmatic patients (Wilson, 2008).
- *Interleukin-10 release.* IL-10 has a broad spectrum of anti-inflammatory effects, and there is evidence that its secretion is reduced in asthma. IL-10 release is increased by theophylline, and this effect may be mediated via inhibition of PDE activities, although this has not been seen at the low doses that are effective in asthma (Oliver et al., 2001).
- *Effects on gene transcription.* Theophylline prevents the translocation of the pro-inflammatory transcription factor NF-κB into the nucleus, potentially reducing the expression of inflammatory genes in asthma and COPD. Inhibition of NF-κB appears to be due to a protective effect against the degradation of the inhibitory protein I-κBα (Ichiyama et al., 2001). However, these effects are seen at high concentrations and may be mediated by inhibition of PDE.
- *Effects on apoptosis.* Prolonged survival of granulocytes due to a reduction in apoptosis may be important in perpetuating chronic inflammation in asthma (eosinophils) and COPD (neutrophils). Theophylline promotes apoptosis in eosinophils and neutrophils *in vitro*. This is associated with a reduction in the anti-apoptotic protein Bcl-2 (Chung et al., 2000). This effect is not mediated via PDE inhibition, but in neutrophils may be mediated by antagonism of adenosine A_{2A} receptors (Yasui et al., 2000). Theophylline also induces apoptosis in T lymphocytes, reducing their survival; this effect appears to be mediated via PDE inhibition (Ohta and Yamashita, 1999).
- *Histone deacetylase activation.* Recruitment of histone deacetylase-2 (HDAC2) by glucocorticoid receptors switches off inflammatory genes. Therapeutic concentrations of theophylline activate HDAC, thereby enhancing the anti-inflammatory effects of corticosteroids (Cosio et al., 2004; Ito et al., 2002). This mechanism is independent of PDE inhibition or adenosine receptor antagonism and appears to be mediated by inhibition of PI3-kinase-δ, which is activated by oxidative stress (Marwick et al., 2009). The anti-inflammatory effects of theophylline are inhibited by a HDAC inhibitor, trichostatin A. Low doses of theophylline increase HDAC activity in bronchial biopsies of asthmatic patients and correlate with the reduction in eosinophil numbers in the biopsy.
- *Other effects.* Several other effects of theophylline have been described, including an increase in circulating catecholamines, inhibition of calcium influx into inflammatory cells, inhibition of prostaglandin effects, and antagonism of tumor necrosis

is the first drug to demonstrate clear anti-inflammatory effects; thus, theophylline may have a role in preventing progression of this disease (Culpitt et al., 2002).

MUSCARINIC CHOLINERGIC ANTAGONISTS

Chemical antagonism of the effects of acetylcholine at muscarinic receptors in the lung for the relief of asthma is not a new idea. *Datura* stramonium (jimson weed) and related species of the nightshade family contain a mixture of muscarinic antagonists (atropine, hyoscyamine, scopolamine) and were smoked for relief of asthma two centuries ago. Subsequently, the purified plant alkaloid atropine was introduced for treating asthma. Due to the significant side effects of atropine, particularly drying of secretions, less soluble quaternary compounds, such as atropine methylnitrate and ipratropium bromide, have been developed. These compounds are topically active and are not significantly absorbed from the respiratory or GI tracts. The basic pharmacology of the antimuscarinic agents is presented in Chapter 9.

Mode of Action

These agents are competitive antagonists of ACh binding to muscarinic cholinergic receptors; thus these drugs block the effects of endogenous ACh at muscarinic receptors, including the direct constrictor effect on bronchial smooth muscle mediated via the M_3-G_q-PLC-IP_3-Ca^{2+} pathway (Chapter 3). Their predicted efficacy stems from the role played by the parasympathetic nervous system in regulating bronchomotor tone. Multiple and diverse stimuli cause reflex increases in parasympathetic activity that contribute to bronchoconstriction. The effects of ACh on the respiratory system include not only bronchoconstriction but also increased tracheobronchial secretion and stimulation of the chemoreceptors of the carotid and aortic bodies. Thus antimuscarinic drugs might be expected to antagonize these effects of acetylcholine. One complicating factor studied in animal models is that myriad inflammatory mediators involved in the pathogenesis of asthma and COPD may also induce components of muscarinic responsiveness, such as $G\alpha_q$ and rho, and contribute to hyperresponsiveness of the airway (Chiba et al., 2008). Thus, the contractility of bronchial smooth muscle and antagonism of muscarinic responsiveness could be moving targets in asthma and COPD.

Basic research is demonstrating that the muscarinic agonists are not functionally equivalent, however. Recent research has focused on the differential capacity of muscarinic antagonists to act as antagonists, as inverse agonists inhibiting the constitutive activity of the M_3 receptor, and as modulators of upregulation of M_3 receptor expression (Casarosa et al., 2009). Such differences may have clinical relevance for long-term use of these compounds, where tolerance and withdrawal/rebound could be major issues. In this regard, a long-term study of tiotropium demonstrates no loss of its capacity for bronchodilation over 4 years (Tashkin et al., 2008).

In animals and man there is a small degree of resting bronchomotor tone that is probably due to tonic vagal nerve impulses that release acetylcholine in the vicinity of airway smooth muscle because it can be blocked by anticholinergic drugs. Acetylcholine may also be released from other airway cells, including epithelial cells (Wessler and Kirkpatrick, 2008). The synthesis of acetylcholine in epithelial cells is increased by inflammatory stimuli (such as TNF-α), which increase the expression of choline acetyltransferase, which could contribute to cholinergic effects in airway diseases. Muscarinic receptors are expressed in airway smooth muscle of small airways that do not appear to be innervated by cholinergic nerves; these receptors may be a mechanism of cholinergic narrowing in peripheral airways that could be relevant in COPD, responding to locally synthesized, non-neuronal ACh.

Myriad mechanical, chemical, and immunological stimuli elicit reflex bronchoconstriction via vagal pathways, and cholinergic pathways may play an important role in regulating acute bronchomotor responses in animals. These observations suggested that cholinergic mechanisms might underlie airway hyperresponsiveness and acute bronchoconstrictor responses in asthma, with the implication that anticholinergic drugs would be effective bronchodilators. These drugs may afford protection against acute challenge by sulfur dioxide, inert dusts, cold air, and emotional factors, but they are less effective against antigen challenge, exercise, and fog. This is not surprising because anticholinergic drugs will only inhibit reflex ACh-mediated bronchoconstriction and have no blocking effect on the *direct* effects of inflammatory mediators, such as histamine and leukotrienes, on bronchial smooth muscle. Furthermore, cholinergic antagonists probably have little or no effect on mast cells, microvascular leak, or the chronic inflammatory response.

Theoretically, anticholinergics may reduce airway mucus secretion and reduce mucus clearance, but this is generally not observed in clinical studies. Oxitropium bromide (not available in the U.S.) in high doses reduces mucus hypersecretion in patients with COPD with chronic bronchitis.

Clinical Use. In asthmatic patients, anticholinergic drugs are less effective as bronchodilators than β_2 agonists and offer less efficient protection against bronchial challenges. These drugs may be more effective in older patients with asthma in whom there is an element of fixed airway obstruction. Anticholinergics are currently used as an additional bronchodilator in asthmatic patients not controlled on a LABA. Nebulized anticholinergic drugs are effective in acute severe asthma but less effective than β_2 agonists. Nevertheless, in the acute and chronic treatment of asthma, anticholinergic drugs may have an additive effect with β_2 agonists and should therefore be considered

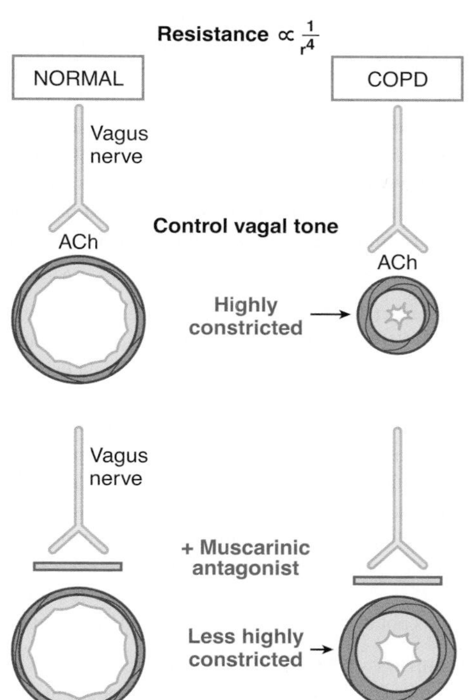

Figure 36–7. *Anticholinergic drugs inhibit vagally mediated airway tone, thereby producing bronchodilation.* This effect is small in normal airways but is greater in airways of patients with chronic obstructive pulmonary disease (COPD), which are structurally narrowed and have higher resistance to airflow because airway resistance is inversely related to the fourth power of the radius (r). ACh, acetylcholine.

when control of asthma is not adequate with nebulized β_2 agonists. A muscarinic antagonist should be considered when there are problems with theophylline or when inhaled β_2 agonists cause a troublesome tremor in elderly patients.

In COPD, anticholinergic drugs may be as effective as or even superior to β_2 agonists. Their relatively greater effect in COPD than in asthma may be explained by an inhibitory effect on vagal tone, which, although not necessarily increased in COPD, may be the only reversible element of airway obstruction and one that is exaggerated by geometric factors in the narrowed airways of COPD patients (Figure 36–7). Anticholinergic drugs reduce air trapping and improve exercise tolerance in COPD patients.

Therapeutic Choices. Ipratropium bromide (ATROVENT, others) is available as a pMDI and nebulized preparation. The onset of bronchodilation is relatively slow and is usually maximal 30-60 minutes after inhalation, but may persist for 6-8 hours. It is usually given by MDI three to four times daily on a regular basis, rather than intermittently for symptom relief, in view of its slow onset of action.

Oxitropium bromide (not available in the U.S.) is a quaternary anticholinergic bronchodilator that is similar to ipratropium bromide in terms of receptor blockade. It is available in higher doses by inhalation and may therefore have a more prolonged effect. Thus, it may be useful in some patients with nocturnal asthma.

Combination inhalers of an anticholinergic and β_2 agonist, such as ipratropium/albuterol (COMBIVENT, DUONEB, others), are popular, particularly among patients with COPD. Several studies have demonstrated additive effects of these two drugs, thus providing an advantage over increasing the dose of β_2 agonist in patients who have side effects.

Tiotropium bromide is a long-acting anticholinergic drug that is suitable for once-daily dosing as a DPI (SPIRIVA) or via a soft mist mini-nebulizer device (not available in the U.S.) (Barr et al., 2006). Tiotropium binds to all muscarinic receptor subtypes but dissociates very slowly from M_3 and M_1 receptors, giving it a degree of kinetic receptor selectivity for these receptors compared with M_2 receptors, from which it dissociates more rapidly. Thus, compared with ipratropium, tiotropium is less likely to antagonize M_2-mediated inhibition of ACh release (the resulting increase in ACh could counteract the blockade of M_3 receptor–mediated bronchoconstriction) (Chapter 9). It is an effective bronchodilator in patients with COPD and is more effective than ipratropium four times daily without any loss of efficacy over a 1-year treatment period. Over a 4-year period, tiotropium improves lung function and health status and reduces exacerbations and all-cause mortality, although there is no effect on disease progression (Tashkin et al., 2008). As a result, tiotropium is becoming the bronchodilator of choice for COPD patients.

Adverse Effects. Inhaled anticholinergic drugs are generally well tolerated. On stopping inhaled anticholinergics, a small rebound increase in airway responsiveness has been described, but the clinical relevance of this is uncertain. Systemic side effects after ipratropium bromide and tiotropium bromide are uncommon during normal clinical use because there is little systemic absorption. Because cholinergic agonists can stimulate *mucus secretion,* there has been concern that anticholinergics may reduce secretion and lead to more viscous mucus. However, ipratropium bromide, even in high doses, has no detectable effect on mucociliary clearance in either normal subjects or in patients with airway disease. A significant unwanted effect is the unpleasant *bitter taste* of inhaled ipratropium, which may contribute to poor compliance. Nebulized ipratropium bromide may precipitate *glaucoma* in elderly patients due to a direct effect of the nebulized drug on the eye. This may be prevented by nebulization with a mouthpiece rather than a face mask. Reports of *paradoxical bronchoconstriction* with ipratropium bromide, particularly when given by nebulizer, were largely explained as effects of the hypotonic nebulizer solution and by antibacterial additives, such as benzalkonium chloride and ethylenediaminetetraacetic acid (EDTA). This problem has not been described with tiotropium. Occasionally, bronchoconstriction may occur with ipratropium bromide given by MDI. It is possible that this is due to blockade of prejunctional M_2 receptors on airway cholinergic nerves that normally inhibit acetylcholine release. Tiotropium causes dryness of the mouth in 10-15% of patients, but this usually disappears during continued therapy. Urinary retention is occasionally seen in elderly patients.

Future Developments. Anticholinergics are the bronchodilators of choice in COPD and therefore have a growing market. Several long-acting muscarinic antagonists are now in clinical development, including glycopyrrolate and aclidinium (Cazzola, 2009; Hansel et al., 2005). Dual-action drugs that are both muscarinic antagonists and β_2 agonist (MABA) are also in clinical development (Ray and Alcaraz, 2009).

NOVEL CLASSES OF BRONCHODILATORS

Several new classes of bronchodilator are under development, but it is difficult to foresee a more effective bronchodilator than a LABA for asthma and a long-acting anticholinergic for COPD. Inventing new classes of bronchodilators has been difficult; several agents have had problems with vasodilator side effects because they relaxed vascular smooth muscle to a greater extent than airway smooth muscle. Nonetheless, there are several classes of bronchodilators under development, as described next.

Magnesium Sulfate. Increasing evidence indicates that magnesium sulfate ($MgSO_4$) is useful as an additional bronchodilator in patients with acute severe asthma. Intravenous or nebulized $MgSO_4$ benefits adults and children with severe exacerbations (forced expiratory volume in 1 second [FEV_1] <30% of predicted value), giving improvement in lung function when added to nebulized β_2 agonist and a reduction in hospital admissions (Mohammed and Goodacre, 2007). The treatment is cheap and well tolerated, although the clinical benefit appears small. Side effects include flushing and nausea but are usually minor. Magnesium sulfate appears to act as a bronchodilator and may reduce cytosolic Ca^{2+} concentrations in airway smooth muscle cells. The concentration of magnesium is lower in serum and erythrocytes of asthmatic patients than in normal controls and correlates with airway hyperresponsiveness (Emelyanov et al., 1999), although the improvement in acute severe asthma after magnesium does not correlate with plasma concentrations. More studies are needed before intravenous and inhaled $MgSO_4$ are routinely recommended for the management of acute severe asthma. There are too few studies in acute exacerbations of COPD to make any firm recommendation (Skorodin et al., 1995).

K^+ Channel Openers. K^+ channels are involved in recovery of excitable cells after depolarization and are important in stabilization of cells. K^+ channel openers such as cromakalim or levcromakalim (the *levo*-isomer of cromakalim) open ATP-dependent K^+ channels in smooth muscle, leading to membrane hyperpolarization and relaxation of airway smooth muscle (Black et al., 1990). This suggests that K^+ channel activators may be useful as bronchodilators (Pelaia et al., 2002). Clinical studies in asthma, however, have been disappointing, with no bronchodilation or protection against bronchoconstrictor challenges. The cardiovascular side effects of these drugs (postural hypotension, flushing) limit the oral dose; furthermore, inhaled formulations are problematic. New developments include K^+ channel openers that open Ca^{2+}-activated large conductance K^+ channels (maxi-K channels) that are also opened by β_2 agonists; these drugs may be better tolerated. Maxi-K channel openers also inhibit mucus secretion and cough, and they may be of particular value in the treatment of COPD.

Atrial Natriuretic Peptides. Atrial natriuretic peptide (ANP) activates membrane-bound guanylyl cyclase and increases cellular cyclic GMP, leading to bronchodilation by mechanisms similar to those of NO on smooth muscle (Chapter 3). ANP and the related peptide urodilatin are bronchodilators in asthma and give effects comparable to those of β_2 agonists (Angus et al., 1993; Fluge et al., 1999). Because ANP and congeners work via a mechanism distinct from that of β_2 agonists, they may give additional bronchodilation that may be useful in acute severe asthma when β_2 receptor function might be impaired.

Vasoactive Intestinal Polypeptide Analogs. Vasoactive intestinal polypeptide (VIP) is a 28 amino acid peptide that binds to two GPCRs, $VPAC_1$ and $VPAC_2$, both of which couple primarily to G_s to stimulate the adenylyl cyclase-cAMP-PKA pathway leading to relaxation of smooth muscle. VIP is a potent dilator of human airway smooth muscle *in vitro* but is not effective in patients because it is rapidly metabolized (plasma $t_{1/2}$ ~2 minutes); in addition, VIP causes vasodilator side effects. More stable analogs of VIP, such as Ro 25-1533, which selectively stimulates VIP receptors in airway smooth muscle (via the $VPAC_2$ receptor), have been synthesized. Inhaled Ro 25-1533 has a rapid bronchodilator effect in asthmatic patients but is not as prolonged as formoterol (Linden et al., 2003).

Other Inhibitors of Smooth Muscle Contraction. Agents that inhibit the contractile machinery of airway smooth muscle, including rho kinase inhibitors, inhibitors of myosin light chain kinase, and myosin inhibitors, are also in development. Because these agents also cause vasodilation, it will be necessary to administer them by inhalation.

CORTICOSTEROIDS

Corticosteroids are used in the treatment of several inflammatory lung diseases. Oral corticosteroids were introduced for the treatment of asthma shortly after their discovery in the 1950s and remain the most effective controller therapy available for asthma. However, their considerable side effects have prompted considerable research into discovering new or related agents that retain the beneficial action on airways without the adverse effects. The introduction of ICS (inhaled corticosteroids), initially as a way of reducing the requirement for oral steroids, has revolutionized the treatment of chronic asthma (Barnes et al., 1998b). Because asthma is a chronic inflammatory disease, ICS are considered as first-line therapy in all but the mildest of patients. In marked contrast, ICS are much less effective in COPD and should only be used in patients with severe disease who have frequent exacerbations. Oral corticosteroids remain the mainstay of treatment of several other pulmonary diseases, such as sarcoidosis, interstitial lung diseases, and pulmonary eosinophilic syndromes. The general pharmacology of corticosteroids is presented in Chapter 42.

Chemistry. The adrenal cortex secretes cortisol (hydrocortisone) and, by modification of its structure, it was possible to develop derivatives, such as prednisone, prednisolone, and dexamethasone, with enhanced corticosteroid effects but with reduced mineralocorticoid activity (Chapter 42). These derivatives with potent glucocorticoid actions were effective in asthma when given systemically but had no anti-asthmatic activity when given by inhalation. Further substitution in the 17α ester position resulted in steroids with high topical activity, such as beclomethasone dipropionate, triamcinolone, flunisolide, budesonide, and fluticasone propionate, which are potent in the skin (dermal blanching test) and were later found to have significant anti-asthma effects when given by inhalation (Figure 36–8).

Mechanism of Action. Corticosteroids enter target cells and bind to glucocorticoid receptors (GR) in the cytoplasm (Chapter 42). There is only one type of GR that binds corticosteroids and no evidence for the existence of subtypes that might mediate different aspects of corticosteroid action (Barnes, 2006a). The steroid-GR complex moves into the nucleus, where it binds to specific sequences on the upstream regulatory elements of certain target genes, resulting in increased (or rarely, decreased) transcription of the gene, with subsequent increased (or decreased) synthesis of the gene products. GR may also interact with protein transcription factors and coactivator molecules in the nucleus and thereby influence the synthesis of certain proteins independently of any direct interaction with DNA. The repression of transcription factors, such as activator protein-1 (AP-1) and NF-κB, is likely to account for many of the anti-inflammatory effects of steroids in asthma. In particular, corticosteroids reverse the activating effect of these pro-inflammatory transcription factors on histone acetylation by recruiting HDAC2 to inflammatory genes that have been activated through acetylation of associated histones (Figure 36–9). GRs are acetylated when corticosteroids are bound and bind to DNA in this acetylated state as dimers, whereas the acetylated GR has to be deacetylated by HDAC2 in order to interact with inflammatory genes and NF-κB (Ito et al., 2006).

There may be additional mechanisms that are also important in the anti-inflammatory actions of corticosteroids. Corticosteroids have potent inhibitory effects on MAP kinase signaling pathways through the induction of MKP-1, which may inhibit the expression of multiple inflammatory genes (Clark, 2003).

Anti-Inflammatory Effects in Asthma. The mechanisms of action of corticosteroids in asthma are still poorly understood, but their efficacy is most likely related to their anti-inflammatory properties. Corticosteroids have widespread effects on gene transcription, increasing the transcription of several anti-inflammatory genes and suppressing transcription of many inflammatory genes. Steroids have inhibitory effects on many inflammatory and structural cells that are activated in asthma and prevent the recruitment of inflammatory cells into the airways (Figure 36–10). Studies of bronchial biopsies in asthma have demonstrated a reduction in the number and activation of inflammatory cells in the epithelium and submucosa after regular ICS, together with a healing of the damaged epithelium. Indeed, in patients with mild asthma the inflammation may be completely resolved after inhaled steroids.

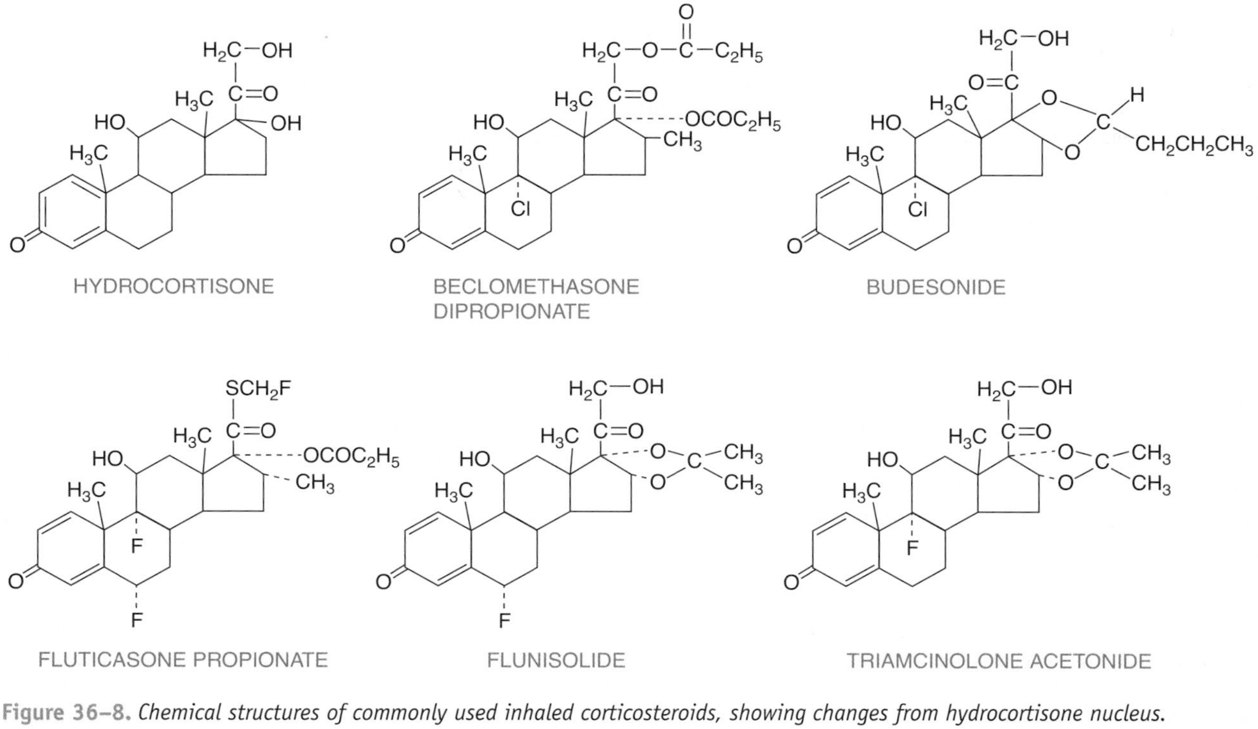

HYDROCORTISONE
BECLOMETHASONE DIPROPIONATE
BUDESONIDE
FLUTICASONE PROPIONATE
FLUNISOLIDE
TRIAMCINOLONE ACETONIDE

Figure 36–8. *Chemical structures of commonly used inhaled corticosteroids, showing changes from hydrocortisone nucleus.*

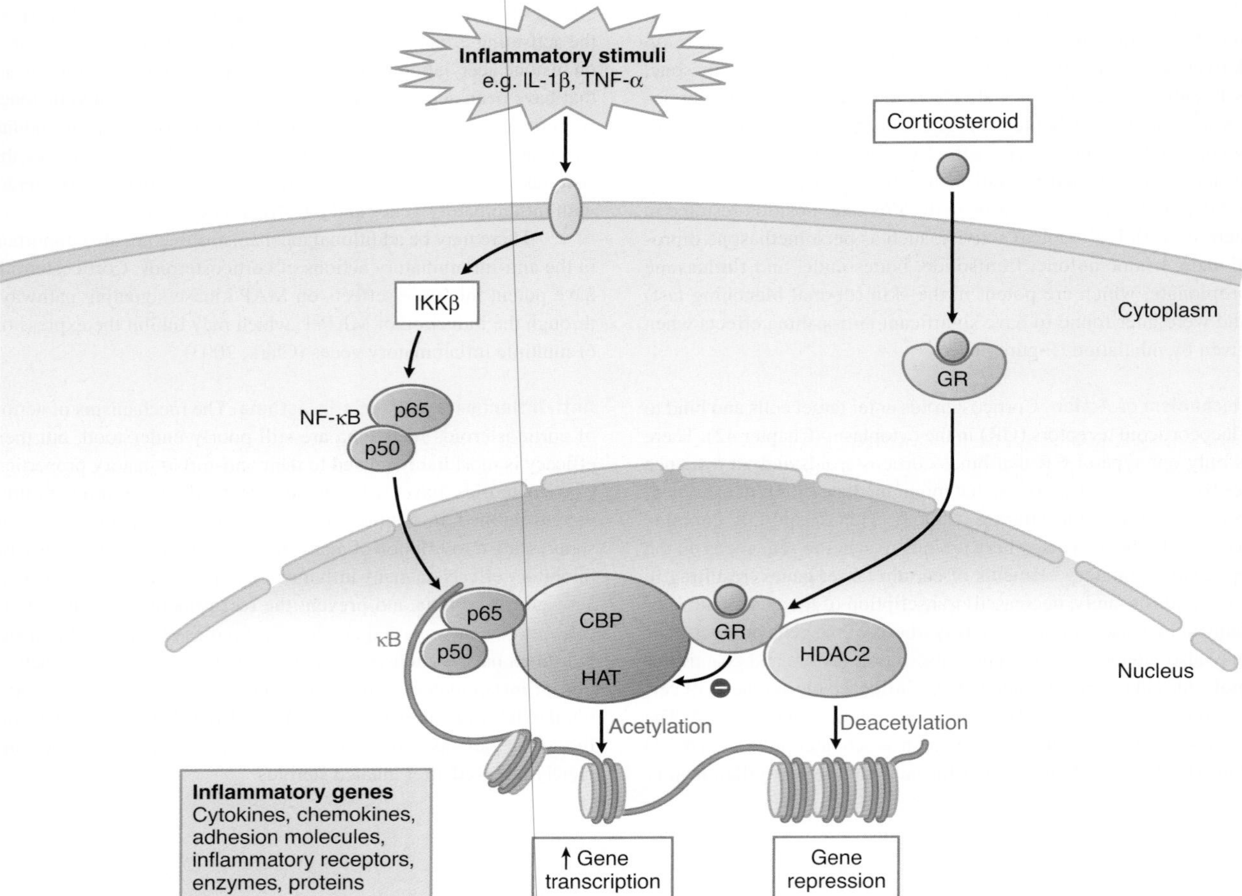

Figure 36–9. *Mechanism of anti-inflammatory action of corticosteroids in asthma.* Inflammatory genes are activated by inflammatory stimuli (IL-1β, TNF-α, etc.), resulting in activation of IKKβ (inhibitor of I-κB kinase-β), which activates the transcription factor nuclear factor κB (NF-κB). A dimer of p50 and p65 NF-κB proteins translocates to the nucleus and binds to specific κB recognition sites and also to coactivators, such as CREB-binding protein (CBP), which have intrinsic histone acetyltransferase (HAT) activity. This results in acetylation of core histones and consequent increased expression of genes encoding multiple inflammatory proteins. Cytosolic glucocorticoid receptors (GR) bind corticosteroids; the receptor-ligand complexes translocate to the nucleus and bind to coactivators to inhibit HAT activity in two ways: directly and, more importantly, by recruiting histone deacetylase-2 (HDAC2), which reverses histone acetylation, leading to the suppression of activated inflammatory genes.

Steroids potently inhibit the formation of cytokines (e.g., IL-1, IL-3, IL-4, IL-5, IL-9, IL-13, TNF-α, and granulocyte-macrophage colony-stimulating factor, GM-CSF) that are secreted in asthma by T-lymphocytes, macrophages, and mast cells. Corticosteroids also decrease eosinophil survival by inducing apoptosis. Corticosteroids inhibit the expression of multiple inflammatory genes in airway epithelial cells, probably the most important action of ICS in suppressing asthmatic inflammation. Corticosteroids also prevent and reverse the increase in vascular permeability due to inflammatory mediators in animal studies and may therefore lead to resolution of airway edema. Steroids have a direct inhibitory effect on mucus glycoprotein secretion from airway submucosal glands, as well as indirect inhibitory effects by down-regulation of inflammatory stimuli that stimulate mucus secretion.

Corticosteroids have no direct effect on contractile responses of airway smooth muscle; improvement in lung function after ICS is presumably due to an effect on the chronic airway inflammation and airway hyperresponsiveness. A single dose of ICS has no effect on the early response to allergen (reflecting their lack of effect on mast cell mediator release) but inhibits the late response (which may be due to an effect on macrophages, eosinophils, and airway wall edema) and also inhibits the increase in airway hyperresponsiveness.

ICS have rapid anti-inflammatory effects, reducing airway hyperresponsiveness and inflammatory mediator concentrations in sputum within a few hours (Erin et al., 2008). However, it may take several weeks or months to achieve maximal effects on airway hyperresponsiveness, presumably reflecting the slow healing of the damaged inflamed airway. It is important to recognize that

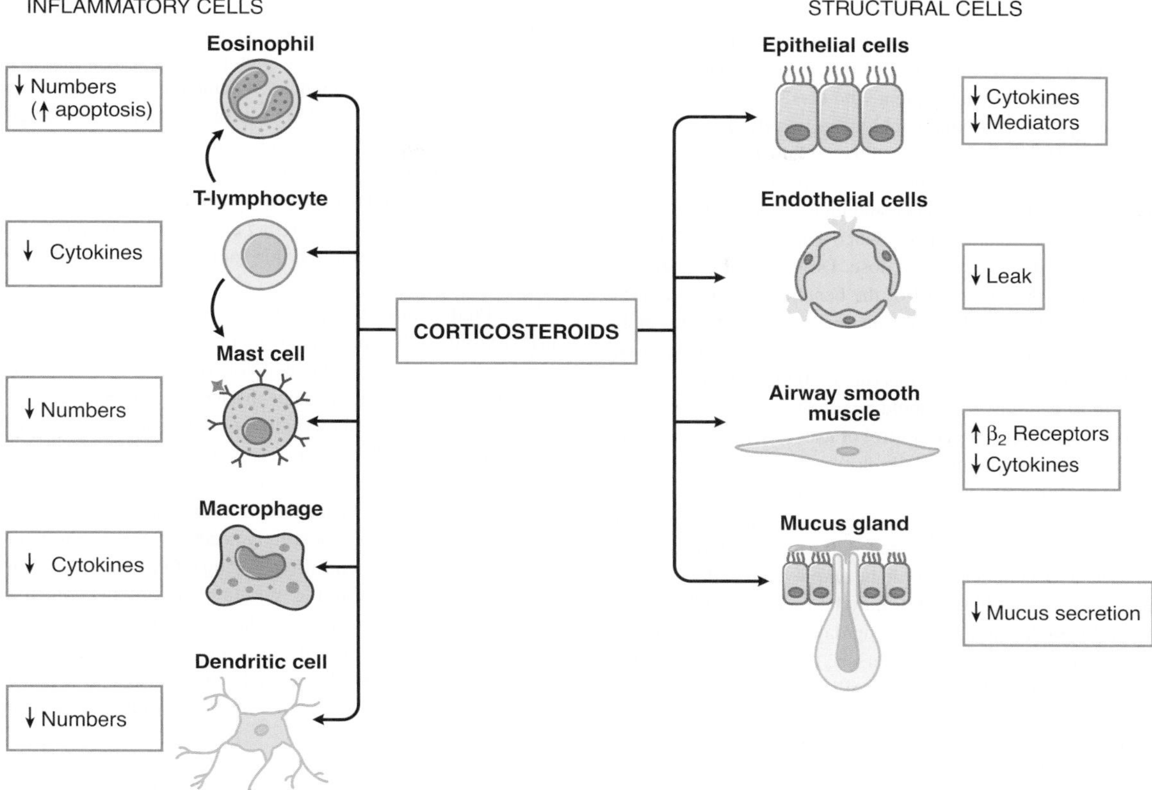

Figure 36–10. *Effect of corticosteroids on inflammatory and structural cells in the airways.*

corticosteroids *suppress* inflammation in the airways but do not cure the underlying disease. When steroids are withdrawn there is a recurrence of the same degree of airway hyperresponsiveness, although in patients with mild asthma it may take several months to return.

Effect on β_2 Adrenergic Responsiveness. Corticosteroids increase β adrenergic responsiveness, but whether this is relevant to their effect in asthma is uncertain. Steroids potentiate the effects of β agonists on bronchial smooth muscle and prevent and reverse β receptor desensitization in airways *in vitro* and *in vivo* (Barnes, 2002; Giembycz et al., 2008). At a molecular level, corticosteroids increase the transcription of the β_2 receptor gene in human lung *in vitro* and in the respiratory mucosa *in vivo* and also increase the stability of its messenger RNA. They also prevent or reverse uncoupling of β_2 receptors to G_s. In animal systems, corticosteroids prevent downregulation of β_2 receptors.

β_2 Agonists also enhance the action of GR, resulting in increased nuclear translocation of liganded GR receptors and enhancing the binding of GR to DNA. This effect has been demonstrated in sputum macrophages of asthmatic patients after an ICS and inhaled LABA (Usmani et al., 2005). This suggests that β_2 agonists and corticosteroids enhance each other's beneficial effects in asthma therapy.

Pharmacokinetics. The pharmacokinetics of oral corticosteroids are described in Chapter 42. The pharmacokinetics of inhaled corticosteroids are important in relation to systemic effects (Barnes et al., 1998b). The fraction of steroid that is inhaled into the lungs acts locally on the airway mucosa but may be absorbed from the airway and alveolar surface. Thus, a portion of an inhaled dose reaches the systemic circulation. Furthermore, the fraction of inhaled steroid that is deposited in the oropharynx is swallowed and absorbed from the gut. The absorbed fraction may be metabolized in the liver (first-pass metabolism) before reaching the systemic circulation (Figure 36–3). The use of a spacer chamber reduces oropharyngeal deposition and therefore reduces systemic absorption of ICS, although this effect is minimal in corticosteroids with a high first-pass metabolism. Mouth rinsing and discarding the rinse have a similar effect, and this procedure should be used with high-dose dry powder steroid inhalers with which spacer chambers cannot be used.

Beclomethasone dipropionate and ciclesonide are prodrugs that release the active corticosteroid after the ester group is cleaved by esterases in the lung. Ciclesonide is available as a MDI (ALVESCO) for asthma and as a nasal spray for allergic rhinitis (OMNARIS). Budesonide and fluticasone propionate have a greater first-pass metabolism than beclomethasone dipropionate and are therefore less likely to produce systemic effects at high inhaled doses.

Inhaled Corticosteroids in Asthma. Inhaled corticosteroids are recommended as first-line therapy for all patients with persistent asthma. They should be started in any patient who needs to use a β_2 agonist inhaler for symptom control more than twice weekly. They are effective in mild, moderate, and severe asthma and in children as well as adults (Barnes et al., 1998b). Although it was recommended that ICS be initiated at a relatively high dose and then the dose reduced once control was achieved, there is no evidence that this is more effective than starting with the maintenance dose. Dose-response studies for ICS are relatively flat, with most of the benefit derived from doses <400 μg beclomethasone dipropionate or equivalent (Adams et al., 2008). However, some patients (with relative corticosteroid resistance) may benefit from higher doses (up to 2000 μg/day).

For most patients, ICS should be used twice daily, a regimen that improves compliance once control of asthma has been achieved (which may require four-times daily dosing initially or a course of oral steroids if symptoms are severe). Administration once daily of some steroids (e.g., budesonide, mometasone, and ciclesonide) is effective when doses ≤400 μg are needed. If a dose >800 μg daily via pMDI is used, a spacer device should be employed to reduce the risk of oropharyngeal side effects. ICS may be used in children in the same way as in adults; at doses ≤400 μg/day there is no evidence of significant growth suppression (Pedersen, 2001). The dose of ICS should be the minimal dose that controls asthma; once control is achieved, the dose should be slowly reduced (Hawkins et al., 2003). Nebulized corticosteroids (e.g., budesonide) are useful in the treatment of small children who are not able to use other inhaler devices.

Inhaled Corticosteroids in Chronic Obstructive Pulmonary Disease. Patients with COPD occasionally respond to steroids, and these patients are likely to have concomitant asthma. Corticosteroids have no objective short-term benefit on airway function in patients with true COPD, although these agents often produce subjective benefit because of their euphoric effect. Corticosteroids do not appear to have any significant anti-inflammatory effect in COPD; there appears to be an active resistance mechanism, which may be explained by impaired activity of HDAC2 as a result of oxidative stress (Barnes, 2009). ICS have no effect on the progression of COPD, even when given to patients with presymptomatic disease; additionally, ICS have no effect on mortality (Calverley et al., 2007; Yang et al., 2007). ICS reduce the number of exacerbations in patients with severe COPD (FEV_1 <50% predicted) who have frequent exacerbations and are recommended in these patients, although there is debate about whether these effects are due to inappropriate analysis of the data (Suissa et al., 2008). Oral corticosteroids are used to treat acute exacerbations of COPD, but the effect is very small (Niewoehner et al., 1999).

Patients with cystic fibrosis, which involves inflammation of the airways, are also resistant to high doses of ICS.

Systemic Steroids. Intravenous steroids are indicated in acute asthma if lung function is <30% predicted and in patients who show no significant improvement with nebulized β_2 agonist. Hydrocortisone is the steroid of choice because it has the most rapid onset (5-6 hours after administration), compared with 8 hours with prednisolone. The required dose is uncertain; it is common to give hydrocortisone 4 mg/kg initially, followed by a maintenance dose of 3 mg/kg every 6 hours. Methylprednisolone is also available for intravenous use, but there is no evidence that the high doses previously used (1 g) are more effective. Intravenous therapy is usually given until a satisfactory response is obtained, and then oral prednisolone may be substituted. Oral prednisolone (40-60 mg) has a similar effect to intravenous hydrocortisone and is easier to administer. A high dose of inhaled fluticasone propionate (2000 μg daily) is as effective as a course of oral prednisolone in controlling acute exacerbations of asthma in a family practice setting and in children in an emergency department setting, although this route of delivery is more expensive (Levy et al., 1996; Manjra et al., 2000).

Prednisolone and prednisone are the most commonly used oral steroids. Clinical improvement with oral steroids may take several days; the maximal beneficial effect is usually achieved with 30-40 mg prednisone daily, although a few patients may need 60-80 mg daily to achieve control of symptoms. The usual maintenance dose is ~10-15 mg/day. Short courses of oral steroids (30-40 mg prednisolone daily for 1-2 weeks) are indicated for exacerbations of asthma; the dose may be tapered over 1 week after the exacerbation is resolved (the taper is not strictly necessary after a short course of therapy, but patients find it reassuring). Oral steroids are usually given as a single dose in the morning because this coincides with the normal diurnal increase in plasma cortisol and produces less adrenal suppression than if given in divided doses or at night. Alternate-day treatment has the advantage of less adrenal suppression, although in many patients control of asthma is not optimal on this regimen.

Adverse Effects. Corticosteroids inhibit ACTH and cortisol secretion by a negative feedback effect on the pituitary gland (Chapter 42). Hypothalamic-pituitary-adrenal (HPA) axis suppression depends on dose and usually only occurs with doses of prednisone >7.5-10 mg/day. Significant suppression after short courses of corticosteroid therapy is not usually a problem, but prolonged suppression may occur after several months or years. *Steroid doses after prolonged oral therapy must be reduced slowly.* Symptoms of "steroid withdrawal syndrome" include lassitude, musculoskeletal pains, and, occasionally, fever. HPA suppression with inhaled steroids is usually seen only when the daily inhaled dose exceeds 2000 μg beclomethasone dipropionate or its equivalent daily.

Side effects of long-term oral corticosteroid therapy include fluid retention, increased appetite, weight gain, osteoporosis, capillary fragility, hypertension, peptic ulceration, diabetes, cataracts, and psychosis. Their frequency tends to increase with age. Very occasionally adverse reactions (such as anaphylaxis) to intravenous hydrocortisone have been described, particularly in aspirin-sensitive asthmatic patients.

The incidence of systemic side effects after ICS is an important consideration, particularly in children (Barnes et al., 1998b) (Table 36–4). Initial studies suggested that adrenal suppression occurred only with inhaled doses >1500-2000 μg/day. More sensitive measurements of systemic effects include indices of bone metabolism, such as serum osteocalcin and urinary pyridinium cross-links, and in children, knemometry, which may be increased with inhaled doses as low as 400 μg/day beclomethasone dipropionate in some patients. The clinical relevance of these measurements is not yet clear, however. Nevertheless, it is important to reduce the likelihood of systemic effects by using the lowest dose of inhaled steroid

Table 36–4

Side Effects of Inhaled Corticosteroids

Local side effects
Dysphonia
Oropharyngeal candidiasis
Cough
Systemic side effects
Adrenal suppression and insufficiency
Growth suppression
Bruising
Osteoporosis
Cataracts
Glaucoma
Metabolic abnormalities (glucose, insulin, triglycerides)
Psychiatric disturbances (euphoria, depression)
Pneumonia

needed to control the asthma, and by use of a large-volume spacer to reduce oropharyngeal deposition.

Several systemic effects of inhaled steroids have been described and include dermal thinning and skin capillary fragility (relatively common in elderly patients after high-dose inhaled steroids). Other side effects, such as cataract formation and osteoporosis, are reported but often in patients who are also receiving courses of oral steroids. There has been particular concern about the use of inhaled steroids in children because of growth suppression (Pedersen, 2001). Most studies have been reassuring that doses ≤400 μg/day have not been associated with impaired growth; on the contrary, there may even be a growth spurt as asthma is better controlled. There is some evidence that use of high-dose ICS is associated with cataract and glaucoma, but it is difficult to dissociate the effects of ICS from the effects of courses of oral steroids that these patients usually require.

ICS may have *local side effects* due to the deposition of inhaled steroid in the oropharynx. The most common problem is hoarseness and weakness of the voice (dysphonia) due to atrophy of the vocal cords following laryngeal deposition of steroid; it may occur in up to 40% of patients and is noticed particularly by patients who need to use their voices during their work (lecturers, teachers, and singers). Throat irritation and coughing after inhalation are common with MDI and appear to be due to additives because these problems are not usually seen if the patient switches to a DPI. There is no evidence for atrophy of the lining of the airway. Oropharyngeal candidiasis occurs in ~5% of patients. There is no evidence for increased lung infections, including tuberculosis, in patients with asthma. Growing evidence suggests that high doses of ICS increase the risk of pneumonia in patients with COPD (Singh et al., 2009); although this is reported with high doses of fluticasone propionate, a similar increase in pneumonia has not been found with budesonide, which may be explained by its lower systemic effects (Sin et al., 2009).

It may be difficult to extrapolate systemic side effects of corticosteroids using data from normal subjects. In asthmatic patients, systemic absorption form the lung is reduced, presumably because of reduced and more central deposition of the inhaled drug in more severe patients (Brutsche et al., 2000; Harrison et al., 2001); most of the inhaled drug deposits in larger airways, thereby limiting effects in the smaller airways where inflammation is also found, especially in patients with severe asthma. Corticosteroid MDIs with HFA propellants produce smaller aerosol particles and may have a more peripheral deposition, making them useful in treating patients with more severe asthma.

Therapeutic Choices. Numerous ICS are now available including beclomethasone dipropionate (QVAR), triamcinolone, flunisolide (AEROBID), budesonide (PULMICORT, others), fluticasone hemihydrate (AEROSPAN), fluticasone propionate (FLOVENT), mometasone furoate (ASMANEX), and ciclesonide (ALVESCO). All are equally effective as antiasthma drugs, but there are differences in their pharmacokinetics: Budesonide, fluticasone, mometasone, and ciclesonide have a lower oral bioavailability than beclomethasone dipropionate because they are subject to greater first-pass hepatic metabolism; this results in reduced systemic absorption from the fraction of the inhaled drug that is swallowed (Derendorf et al., 2006) and thus reduced adverse effects. At high doses (>1000 μg), budesonide and fluticasone propionate have less systemic effects than beclomethasone dipropionate and triamcinolone, and they are preferred in patients who need high doses of ICS and in children. Ciclesonide is another choice; it is a prodrug that is converted to the active metabolite by esterases in the lung, giving it a low oral bioavailability and a high therapeutic index (Manning et al., 2008).

When doses of inhaled steroid exceed 800 μg beclomethasone dipropionate or equivalent daily, a large volume spacer is recommended to reduce oropharyngeal deposition and systemic absorption in the case of beclomethasone dipropionate. All currently available ICS are absorbed from the lung into the systemic circulation, so that some systemic absorption is inevitable. However, the amount of drug absorbed does not appear to have clinical effects in doses of <800 μg beclomethasone dipropionate equivalent. Although there are potency differences among corticosteroids, there are relatively few comparative studies, partly because dose comparison of corticosteroids is difficult due to their long time course of action and the relative flatness of their dose-response curves. Triamcinolone and flunisolide appear to be the least potent, with beclomethasone dipropionate and budesonide approximately of equal potency; fluticasone propionate is approximately twice as potent as beclomethasone dipropionate.

Future Developments. Early treatment with ICS in both adults and children may give a greater improvement in lung function than if treatment is delayed (O'Byrne et al., 2006), likely reflecting the fact that corticosteroids are able to modify the underlying inflammatory process and prevent structural changes (fibrosis, smooth muscle hyperplasia, etc.) in the airway that occur as a result of chronic inflammation. ICS are currently recommended for patients with persistent asthmatic symptoms. There is evidence for airway inflammation in patients with episodic asthma, but at present ICS are recommended only when there are chronic symptoms (e.g., need for an inhaled β_2 agonist more than twice a week).

New corticosteroids with fewer systemic effects would be desirable. Corticosteroids that are rapidly metabolized in the airways ("soft steroids"), such as butixocort and tipredane, proved disappointing in clinical trials; they are probably metabolized too rapidly to achieve sufficient concentration and duration to cause an anti-inflammatory effect. There is a search for corticosteroids that are metabolized rapidly in the circulation after absorption from the lungs. The anti-inflammatory actions of corticosteroids may be mediated via different molecular mechanisms from side effects (which are endocrine and metabolic actions of corticosteroids). It has been possible to develop corticosteroids that dissociate the DNA-binding effect of corticosteroids (which mediates most of the adverse effects) from the inhibitory effect on transcription factors such as NF-κB (which mediates much of the anti-inflammatory effect). Such "dissociated steroids" or selective glucocorticoid receptor agonists (SEGRAs) should, theoretically, retain anti-inflammatory activity but have a reduced risk of adverse effects; achieving this separation of desired and adverse effects is difficult *in vivo* (Schacke et al., 2007). Nonsteroidal SEGRAs are now in development.

Corticosteroid resistance is a major barrier to effective therapy in patients with severe asthma, in asthmatic patients who smoke, and in patients with COPD and cystic fibrosis (Barnes and Adcock, 2009). "Steroid-resistant" asthma is thought to be due to reduced anti-inflammatory actions of corticosteroids. Major strides have been made in understanding the molecular mechanisms for this corticosteroid resistance and in the development of therapies that have the potential to reverse this resistance and restore steroid responsiveness.

Cromones

Cromolyn sodium (sodium cromoglycate) is a derivative of khellin, an Egyptian herbal remedy and was found to protect against allergen challenge without any bronchodilator effect. A structurally related drug, *nedocromil* sodium, which has a similar pharmacological profile to cromolyn, was subsequently developed. Although cromolyn was popular in the past because of its good safety profile, its use has sharply declined with the more widespread use of the more effective ICS, particularly in children. Neither cromolyn nor nedocromil is available in the U.S. for respiratory indications. For further information, consult earlier editions of this text.

MEDIATOR ANTAGONISTS

Many inflammatory mediators have been implicated in asthma and COPD, suggesting that inhibition of synthesis or receptors of these mediators may be beneficial (Barnes, 2004; Barnes et al., 1998a). However, specific inhibitors have been largely disappointing in both asthma and COPD treatment. Both H_1 antihistamines and anti-leukotrienes have been applied to airway disease, but their added benefit over β_2 agonists and corticosteroids is slight. The variability in patient response to anti-leukotriene agents may focus our attention on the roles of leukotriene synthesis, action, and metabolism to some, but not all, asthmatic disease.

Antihistamines. Histamine mimics many of the features of asthma and is released from mast cells in acute asthmatic responses, suggesting that antihistamines may be useful in asthma therapy. There is little evidence that histamine H_1 receptor antagonists provide any useful clinical benefit, as demonstrated by a meta-analysis (van Ganse et al., 1997). Newer antihistamines, including cetirizine and azelastine, have some beneficial effects, but this may be unrelated to H_1 receptor antagonism. Antihistamines are not recommended in the routine management of asthma.

Anti-leukotrienes. There is considerable evidence that cysteinyl-leukotrienes (LTs) are produced in asthma and that they have potent effects on airway function, inducing bronchoconstriction, airway hyperresponsiveness, plasma exudation, mucus secretion, and eosinophilic inflammation (Figure 36–11; also see Chapter 33 and Peters-Golden and Henderson, 2007). These data suggested that blocking the leukotriene pathways with leukotriene modifiers could be useful in the treatment of asthma, leading to the development of 5′-lipoxygenase (5-LO) enzyme inhibitors (of which zileuton [ZYFLO] is the only drug marketed) and several antagonists of the cys-LT_1 receptor, including montelukast (SINGULAIR), zafirlukast (ACCOLATE), and pranlukast (not available in the U.S.).

Clinical Studies. Anti-leukotrienes have been intensively investigated in clinical studies (Calhoun, 2001). Leukotriene antagonists inhibit the bronchoconstrictor effect of inhaled LTD_4 in normal and asthmatic volunteers, and they also inhibit bronchoconstriction induced by a variety of challenges, including allergen, exercise, and cold air, by approximately 50%. With aspirin challenge, in aspirin-sensitive asthmatic patients, there is almost complete inhibition of the response (Szczeklik and Stevenson, 2003). Similar results have been obtained with the 5-LO inhibitor zileuton. This suggests there may be no advantage in blocking LTB_4 in addition to cysteinyl-LTs, in treating asthma. These drugs are active by oral administration, possibly an important advantage in chronic treatment.

In patients with mild to moderate asthma, anti-leukotrienes cause a significant improvement in lung function and asthma

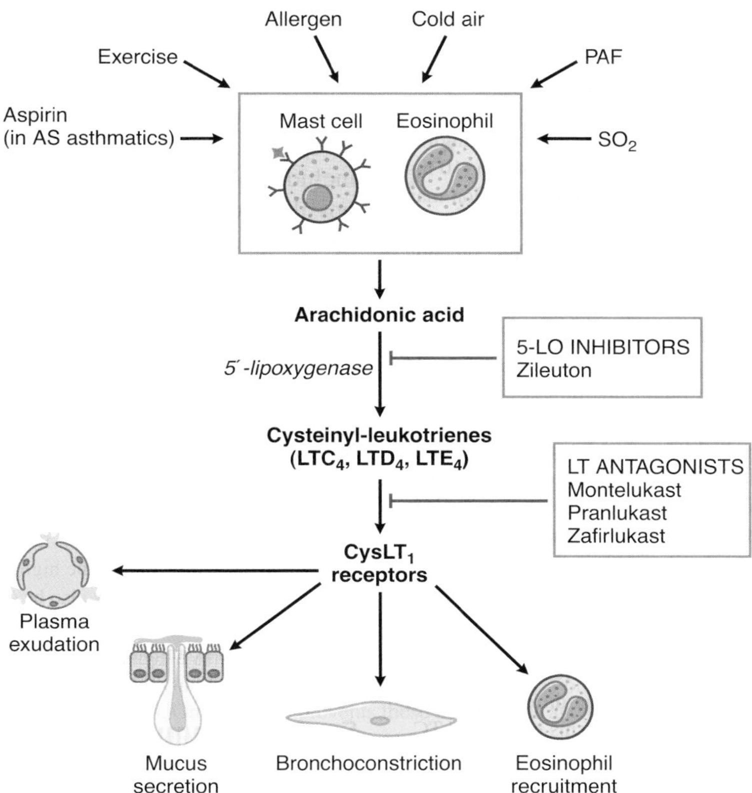

Figure 36–11. *Effects of cysteinyl-leukotrienes on the airways and their inhibition by anti-leukotrienes.* AS, aspirin sensitive; 5-LO, 5′-lipoxygenase; LT, leukotriene; PAF, platelet-activating factor.

symptoms, with a reduction in the use of rescue inhaled β_2 agonists. Several studies show evidence for a bronchodilator effect, with an improvement in baseline lung function, suggesting that leukotrienes are contributing to the baseline bronchoconstriction in asthma, although this varies among patients. However, anti-leukotrienes are considerably less effective than inhaled corticosteroids in the treatment of mild asthma and cannot be considered the treatment of first choice (Ducharme, 2003). Anti-leukotrienes are indicated as an add-on therapy in patients who are not well controlled on ICS. The added benefit is small, equivalent to doubling the dose of ICS, and less effective than adding a LABA (Ducharme et al., 2006).

In patients with severe asthma who are not controlled on high doses of ICS and LABA, anti-leukotrienes do not appear to provide any additional benefit (Robinson et al., 2001). Theoretically, anti-leukotrienes should be of particular value in patients with aspirin-sensitive asthma because they block the airway response to aspirin challenge; however, their benefit is no greater here than in other types of asthma (Dahlen et al., 2002). Anti-leukotrienes are effective in preventing exercise-induced asthma, with efficacy similar to that of LABA (Coreno et al., 2000). Anti-leukotrienes also have a weak effect in rhinitis that may be additive with the effects of an antihistamine (Nathan, 2003).

Studies have demonstrated weak anti-inflammatory effects of anti-leukotrienes in reducing eosinophils in sputum and biopsies (Minoguchi et al., 2002), but this is much less marked than with ICS and there is no additional anti-inflammatory effect when added to an ICS (O'Sullivan et al., 2003). Anti-leukotrienes therefore appear to act mainly as anti-bronchoconstrictor drugs, and they are clearly less broadly effective than β_2 agonists because they antagonize only one of several bronchoconstrictor mediators.

In COPD, Cys-LTs are not elevated in exhaled breath condensate, and cys-LT1 receptor antagonists have no role in the therapy of COPD (Barnes, 2004). By contrast, LTB_4, a potent neutrophil chemoattractant, is elevated in COPD, indicating that 5-LO inhibitors that inhibit LTB_4 synthesis may have some potential benefit by reducing neutrophil inflammation. However, a pilot study failed to indicate any clear benefit of a 5-LO inhibitor in COPD patients (Gompertz and Stockley, 2002).

Adverse Effects. Zileuton, zafirlukast, and montelukast are all associated with rare cases of hepatic dysfunction; thus liver-associated enzymes should be monitored. Several cases of Churg-Strauss syndrome have been associated with the use of zafirlukast and montelukast. Churg-Strauss syndrome is a very rare vasculitis that may affect the heart, peripheral nerves, and kidney and is associated with increased circulating eosinophils and asthma. It is uncertain whether the reported cases are due to a reduction in oral or inhaled corticosteroid dose or are a direct effect of the drug. Cases of Churg-Strauss syndrome have been described in patients on anti-leukotrienes who

IL-4 and IL-13, which determine IgE synthesis (Figure 36–12), has so far proved to be ineffective in clinical studies.

TNF-α may play a key role in amplifying airway inflammation, through the activation of NF-κB, AP-1, and other transcription factors. TNF-α production is increased in asthma and COPD, and it may be associated with the cachexia and weight loss that occur in some patients with severe COPD. In COPD patients and in patients with severe asthma, anti-TNF-α blocking antibodies have been ineffective, at the expense of increasing infections and malignancies (Rennard et al., 2007; Wenzel et al., 2009).

Chemokine Receptor Antagonists. Many chemokines are involved in asthma and COPD and play a key role in recruitment of inflammatory cells, such as eosinophils, neutrophils, macrophages, and lymphocytes into the lungs. Chemokine receptors are attractive targets because they are hepta-spanning membrane proteins; small molecule inhibitors are now in development (Donnelly and Barnes, 2006; Viola and Luster, 2008). In asthma, CCR3 antagonists, which should block eosinophil recruitment into the airways, are the most favored target, but several small molecule CCR3 antagonists have failed in development because of toxicity. In COPD, CXCR2 antagonists, which prevent neutrophil and monocyte chemotaxis due to CXC chemokines such as CXCL1 and CXCL8, have been effective in animal models of COPD and in neutrophilic inflammation in normal subjects, and are now in clinical trials in COPD patients.

Protease Inhibitors

Several proteolytic enzymes are involved in the chronic inflammation of airway diseases. Mast cell tryptase has several effects on airways, including increasing responsiveness of airway smooth muscle to constrictors, increasing plasma exudation, potentiating eosinophil recruitment, and stimulating fibroblast proliferation. Some of these effects are mediated by activation of the proteinase-activated receptor PAR2. Tryptase inhibitors have so far proved to be disappointing in clinical studies.

Proteases are involved in the degradation of connective tissue in COPD, particularly enzymes that break down elastin fibers, such as neutrophil elastase and matrix metalloproteinases (MMP), which are involved in emphysema. Neutrophil elastase inhibitors have been difficult to develop, and there are no positive clinical studies in COPD patients. MMP9 appears to be the predominant elastolytic enzyme in emphysema, and several selective inhibitors are now in development.

New Anti-Inflammatory Drugs

Phosphodiesterase Inhibitors. The preservation and elevation of cellular cyclic AMP in inflammatory cells often reduces cell activation and release of inflammatory mediators. PDE4 is the predominant PDE isoform in inflammatory cells, including mast cells, eosinophils, neutrophils, T lymphocytes, macrophages, and structural cells such as sensory nerves and epithelial cells (Houslay et al., 2005), suggesting that PDE4 inhibitors could be useful as an anti-inflammatory treatment in both asthma and COPD. In animal models of asthma, PDE4 inhibitors reduce eosinophil infiltration and responses to allergen, whereas in COPD they are effective against smoke-induced inflammation and emphysema. Several PDE4 inhibitors have been tested clinically, but with disappointing results; their usefulness has been limited by side effects, particularly nausea, vomiting, headaches, and diarrhea. In COPD, an oral PDE4 inhibitor, roflumilast, has some effect in reducing exacerbations and improving lung function, but side effects also limit its efficacy (Fabbri et al., 2009). Of the four subfamilies of PDE4, PDE4D is the major form whose inhibition is associated vomiting; inhibition of PDE4B is important for anti-inflammatory effects. Thus, selective PDE4B inhibitors may have a greater therapeutic index. Inhaled PDE4 inhibitors to reduce systemic absorption and adverse responses have proved to be ineffective. PDE5 inhibitors are vasodilators that are used in the treatment of pulmonary hypertension.

NF-κB Inhibitors. NF-κB plays an important role in the orchestration of chronic inflammation (Figure 36–9); many of the inflammatory genes that are expressed in asthma and COPD are regulated by this transcription factor (Barnes and Karin, 1997). This has prompted a search for specific blockers of these transcription factors. NF-κB is naturally inhibited by the inhibitory protein IκB, which is degraded after activation by specific kinases. Small molecule inhibitors of the IB kinase IKK2 (or IKKβ) are in clinical development (Karin et al., 2004; Kishore et al., 2003). These drugs may be of particular value in COPD, where corticosteroids are largely ineffective. However, there are concerns that inhibition of NF-κB may cause side effects such as increased susceptibility to infections, which has been observed in gene disruption studies when components of NF-κB are inhibited.

Mitogen-Activated Protein Kinase Inhibitors. There are three major MAP kinase pathways, and there is increasing recognition that these pathways are involved in chronic inflammation (Delhase et al., 2000). There has been particular interest in the p38 MAP kinase pathway that is blocked by a novel class of drugs, such as SB203580 and RWJ67657. These drugs inhibit the synthesis of many inflammatory cytokines, chemokines, and inflammatory enzymes (Cuenda and Rousseau, 2007). The p38 MAPK inhibitors are in development for the treatment of asthma (they inhibit T_H2 cytokine synthesis) and for COPD (they inhibit neutrophilic inflammation and signaling of inflammatory cytokines and chemokines). However, clinical studies have revealed marked adverse effects and toxicities; inhaled delivery is being explored.

Mucoregulators

Many pharmacological agents may influence the secretion of mucus in the airways, but there are few drugs that have demonstrably useful clinical effects on mucus hypersecretion (Rogers and Barnes, 2006). Mucus hypersecretion occurs in chronic bronchitis, COPD, cystic fibrosis, and asthma. In chronic bronchitis, mucus hypersecretion is related to chronic irritation by cigarette smoke and may involve neural mechanisms and the activation of neutrophils to release enzymes such as neutrophil elastase and proteinase-3 that have powerful stimulatory effects on mucus secretion. Mast cell–derived chymase is also a potent mucus secretagogue. This suggests that several classes of drugs may be developed to control mucus hypersecretion.

A major problem in assessing the effects of drugs on mucus hypersecretion is the difficulty in accurately quantifying airway mucus production, quality, and clearance. Several current drugs for airway disease might affect mucus production. Systemic anticholinergic drugs appear to reduce mucociliary clearance, but this is not observed with either ipratropium bromide or tiotropium bromide, presumably reflecting their poor absorption from the respiratory tract. β_2 Agonists increase mucus production and mucociliary clearance and have been shown to increase ciliary beat frequency *in vitro*. Because inflammation leads to mucus hypersecretion, anti-inflammatory treatments should reduce mucus hypersecretion; ICS are very effective in reducing increased mucus production in asthma.

Sensory nerves and neuropeptides are important in the secretory activities of the submucosal gland (which predominates in proximal airways) and goblet cell (more notable in peripheral airways). Opioids and K^+ channel openers inhibit mucus secretion mediated via sensory neuropeptide release; peripherally acting opioids may be developed to control mucus hypersecretion due to irritants in the future (Rogers, 2002).

Mucolytics

Several agents can reduce the viscosity of sputum *in vitro*. One group are derivatives of cysteine that reduce the disulfide bridges that bind glycoproteins to other proteins such as albumin and secretory IgA. These drugs also act as antioxidants and may therefore reduce airway inflammation. Only *N*-acetylcysteine (MUCOMYST, others) is available in the U.S.; carbocysteine, methylcysteine, erdosteine, and bromhexine are available elsewhere. Orally administered, these agents are relatively well tolerated, but clinical studies in chronic bronchitis, asthma, and bronchiectasis have been disappointing. A systematic review of several small studies showed a small benefit in terms of reducing exacerbations, with most of the benefit from *N*-acetylcysteine; whether this relates to the mucolytic activity of *N*-acetylcysteine or to its action as an antioxidant is unclear (Poole and Black, 2001). A large controlled study of oral *N*-acetylcysteine in COPD patients showed no effect in disease progress or in preventing exacerbations, although there was some benefit in the patients not treated with inhaled corticosteroids (Decramer et al., 2005), as confirmed in a subsequent study of carbocysteine in COPD patients not treated with other medications (Zheng et al., 2008). *N*-acetylcysteine is not currently recommended for COPD management.

DNAse (dornase alfa, PULMOZYME) reduces mucus viscosity in sputum of patients with cystic fibrosis and is indicated if there is significant symptomatic and lung function improvement after a trial of therapy (Henke and Ratjen, 2007). There is no evidence that dornase alfa is effective in COPD or asthma, however.

The epidermal growth factor receptor (EGFR) plays a critical role in airway mucus secretion from goblet cells and submucosal glands and appears to mediate the mucus secretory response to several secretagogues, including oxidative stress, cigarette smoke, inflammatory cytokines, and activated TLRs (Burgel and Nadel, 2004). Small molecule inhibitors of EGFR kinase, such as gefitinib and erlotinib, have been developed for use as anticancer therapies and are currently being assessed as treatments for mucus hypersecretion in COPD patients.

Expectorants

Expectorants are oral drugs that are supposed to enhance the clearance of mucus. Although expectorants were once commonly prescribed, there is little or no objective evidence for their efficacy. Such drugs are often emetics that are given in sub-emetic doses on the basis that gastric irritation may stimulate an increase in mucus clearance via a reflex mechanism. However, there is no good evidence for this assumption. Lacking evidence for their efficacy, the FDA has removed most expectorants from the market in a review of over-the-counter drugs. With the exception of guaifenesin, no agents are approved as expectorants in the U.S. In patients who find it difficult to clear mucus, adequate hydration and inhalation of steam may be of some benefit.

ANTITUSSIVES

Despite the fact that cough is a common symptom of airway disease, its mechanisms are poorly understood, and current treatment is unsatisfactory (Pavord and Chung, 2008). Viral infections of the upper respiratory tract are the most common cause of cough; postviral cough is usually self-limiting and commonly patient-medicated. Their wide use notwithstanding, over-the-counter cough medications are largely ineffective (Dicpinigaitis, 2009a). Because cough is a defensive reflex, its suppression may be inappropriate in bacterial lung infection. Before treatment with antitussives, it is important to identify underlying causal mechanisms that may require therapy.

Whenever possible, treat the underlying cause, not the cough. Asthma commonly presents as cough, and the cough will usually respond to ICS. A syndrome characterized by cough in association with sputum eosinophilia but no airway hyperresponsiveness and termed *eosinophilic bronchitis* also responds to ICS (Birring et al., 2003). Nonasthmatic cough does not respond to ICS but sometimes responds to anticholinergic therapy. The cough associated with postnasal drip of sinusitis responds to antibiotics (if warranted), nasal decongestants, and intranasal steroids. The cough associated with ACE inhibitors (in ~15% of patients treated) responds to lowering the dose or withdrawal of the drug and substitution of an AT_1 receptor antagonist (Chapter 26). Gastroesophageal reflux is a common cause of cough through a reflex mechanism and occasionally as a result of acid aspiration into the lungs. This cough may respond to suppression of gastric acid with an H_2 receptor antagonist or a proton pump inhibitor (Chapter 45), although even large doses may not always be effective (Chang et al., 2006). Some patients have a chronic cough with no obvious cause, and this chronic idiopathic cough may be due to airway sensory neural hyperesthesia (Haque et al., 2005).

Opiates. Opiates have a central mechanism of action on μ opioid receptors in the medullary cough center, but there is some evidence that they may have additional peripheral action on cough receptors in the proximal airways. Codeine and pholcodine (not available in the U.S.) are commonly used, but there is little evidence that they are clinically effective, particularly on postviral cough; in addition, they are associated with sedation and constipation (Dicpinigaitis, 2009a). Morphine and methadone are effective but indicated only for intractable cough associated with bronchial carcinoma. A peripherally acting opioid agonist, 443C81, does not appear to be effective for cough.

Dextromethorphan. Dextromethorphan is a centrally active *N*-methyl-D-aspartate (NMDA) receptor antagonist. It may also antagonize opioid receptors. Despite the fact that it is in numerous over-the-counter cough suppressants and used commonly to treat cough, it is poorly effective. In children with acute nocturnal cough, it is not significantly different from placebo in reducing cough

(Dicpinigaitis, 2009a). It can cause hallucinations at higher doses and has significant abuse potential.

Benzonatate. (TESSALON, others), a local anesthetic, acts peripherally by anesthetizing the stretch receptors located in the respiratory passages, lungs, and pleura. By dampening the activity of these receptors, benzonatate may reduce the cough reflex at its source. The recommended dose is 100 mg, three times/day, and up to 600 mg/day, if needed. Although clinical studies shortly after its approval showed some efficacy, benzonatate, 200 mg, was not effective in suppressing experimentally-induced cough in a recent clinical trial (Dicpinigaitis et al., 2009b). Side effects include dizziness and dysphagia. Seizures and cardiac arrest have occurred following an acute ingestion. Severe allergic reactions have been reported in patients allergic to para-aminobenzoic acid, a metabolite of benzonatate.

Other Drugs. Several other drugs reportedly have small benefits in protecting against cough challenges or in reducing cough in pulmonary diseases (Dicpinigaitis, 2009a). These drugs include moguisteine (not available in the U.S.), which acts peripherally and appears to open ATP-sensitive K^+ channels; baclofen, a $GABA_B$-selective agonist; and theobromine, a naturally occurring methylxanthine. Although the expectorant guaifenesin is not typically known as a cough suppressant, it is significantly better than placebo in reducing acute viral cough and inhibits cough-reflex sensitivity in patients with upper respiratory tract infections (Dicpinigaitis et al., 2009b).

Novel Antitussives. There is clearly a need to develop new more effective therapies for cough, particularly drugs that act peripherally in order to avoid sedation. There are close analogies between chronic cough and sensory hyperesthesia, so new therapies are likely to arise from pain research (Barnes, 2007).

Transient Receptor Potential V1 Antagonists. TRPV1 (previously called the vanilloid receptor) is a member of the transient receptor potential (TRP) family of ion channels activated by capsaicin, H^+, and bradykinin, all of which are potent tussive agents. TRPV1 antagonists block cough induced by capsaicin and bradykinin and are effective in some models of cough (McLeod et al., 2008). A side effect of these drugs is loss of temperature regulation and hyperthermia, which has prevented clinical development.

Transient Receptor Potential A1 Antagonists. TRPA1 is emerging as a more promising novel target for antitussives. This channel is activated by oxidative stress and many irritants and may be sensitized by inflammatory cytokines (Taylor-Clark et al., 2009). Several selective TRPA1 antagonists are now in development.

DRUGS FOR DYSPNEA AND VENTILATORY CONTROL

Drugs for Dyspnea

Bronchodilators should reduce breathlessness in patients with airway obstruction. Chronic oxygen may have a beneficial effect, but in a few patients dyspnea may be extreme. Drugs that reduce breathlessness may also depress ventilation in parallel and may therefore be dangerous in severe asthma and COPD. Some patients show a beneficial response to dihydrocodeine and diazepam; however, these drugs must be used with great caution because of the risk of ventilatory depression. Slow-release morphine tablets may also be helpful in COPD patients with extreme dyspnea (Currow and Abernethy, 2007). Nebulized morphine may also reduce breathlessness in COPD and could act in part on opioid receptors in the lung. Nebulized furosemide has some efficacy in treating dyspnea from a variety of causes, but the evidence is not yet sufficiently convincing to recommend this as routine therapy (Newton et al., 2008).

Ventilatory Stimulants

Several classes of drug stimulate ventilation and are indicated when ventilatory *drive* is inadequate. Nikethamide and ethamivan were originally introduced as respiratory stimulants, but effective doses are close to those causing convulsions so the use of these agents has ceased. More selective respiratory stimulants have been developed and are indicated if ventilation is impaired as a result of overdose with sedatives, in postanesthetic respiratory depression, and in idiopathic hypoventilation. Respiratory stimulants are rarely indicated in COPD because respiratory drive is already maximal and further stimulation of ventilation may be counterproductive because of the increase in energy expenditure caused by the drugs.

Doxapram (DOPRAM, others). At low doses (0.5 mg/kg IV), doxapram stimulates carotid chemoreceptors; at higher doses it stimulates medullary respiratory centers. Its effect is transient; thus, intravenous infusion (0.3-3 mg/kg per minute) is needed for sustained effect. Unwanted effects include nausea, sweating, anxiety, and hallucinations. At higher doses, increased pulmonary and systemic pressures may occur. Both the kidney and the liver participate in the clearance of doxapram, which should be used with caution if hepatic or renal function is impaired. In COPD, the infusion of doxapram is restricted to 2 hours. The use of doxapram to treat ventilatory failure in COPD has now largely been replaced by noninvasive ventilation (Greenstone and Lasserson, 2003).

Almitrine. Almitrine bismesylate is a piperazine derivative that appears to selectively stimulate peripheral chemoreceptors and is without central actions (Winkelmann et al., 1994). It is ineffective in patients with surgically removed carotid bodies. Almitrine stimulates ventilation only when there is hypoxia. Long-term use of almitrine is associated with peripheral neuropathy, limiting its availability in most countries.

Acetazolamide. The carbonic anhydrase inhibitor acetazolamide (Chapter 25) induces metabolic acidosis and thereby stimulates ventilation, but it is not widely used because the metabolic imbalance it produces may be detrimental in the face of respiratory acidosis. It has a very small beneficial effect in respiratory failure in COPD patients (Jones and Greenstone, 2001). The drug has proved useful in prevention of high altitude sickness (Basnyat and Murdoch, 2003).

Naloxone. Naloxone is a competitive opioid antagonist that is indicated only if ventilatory depression is due to overdose of opioids.

Flumazenil. Flumazenil is a benzodiazepine receptor antagonist that can reverse respiratory depression due to overdose of benzodiazepines (Gross et al., 1996).

PHARMACOTHERAPY OF PULMONARY ARTERIAL HYPERTENSION

Pulmonary arterial hypertension (PAH) is characterized by vascular proliferation and remodeling of small pulmonary arteries, resulting in a progressive increase in pulmonary vascular resistance, which may lead to right heart failure and death (Morrell et al., 2009). PAH involves dysfunction of pulmonary vascular endothelial and smooth muscle cells and their interplay and results from an imbalance in vasoconstrictor and vasodilator mediators.

Vasodilators are the mainstay of drug therapy for PAH (Barnes and Liu, 1995). However, the vasodilators used to treat systemic hypertension are problematic: they lower systemic blood pressure, which may result in reduced pulmonary perfusion. Calcium channel blockers, such as nifedipine, are poorly effective, but a few patients may benefit. There have been important advances in the development of more selective pulmonary vasodilators, based on a better understanding of the pathophysiology of PAH (McLaughlin et al., 2009). In PAH, there is an increase in the vasoconstrictor mediators endothelin-1, thromboxane A_2, and serotonin, and a decrease in the vasodilating mediators prostacyclin (PGI_2), NO, and VIP (Figure 36–13) (Humbert et al., 2004). Therapies aim at antagonizing the vasoconstrictive mediators and enhancing vasodilation. Because different classes of vasodilators work through different mechanisms, it may be possible to increase efficacy while reducing adverse effects by using combinations of agents from different classes in therapy of PAH.

Primary (idiopathic and familial) pulmonary hypertension (PPAH), where there is no identifiable cause, is uncommon. Most cases of pulmonary hypertension are associated with connective tissue disorders, such as systemic sclerosis, or they are secondary to hypoxic lung diseases, such as interstitial lung disease and COPD, where chronic hypoxia leads to hypoxic pulmonary vasoconstriction. Secondary pulmonary hypertension in COPD rarely requires specific therapy. In secondary pulmonary hypertension due to chronic hypoxia, the initial treatment is correction of hypoxia using supplementary O_2 therapy, including ambulatory oxygen, with the aim of increasing O_2 saturation to >90%. Right heart failure is treated initially with diuretics. Anticoagulants are indicated for the treatment of pulmonary hypertension secondary to chronic thromboembolic disease, but they may also be indicated for patients with severe pulmonary hypertension who have an increased risk of venous thrombosis.

Prostacyclin. Prostacyclin (PGI_2; Epoprostenol) is produced by endothelial cells in the pulmonary circulation and directly relaxes pulmonary vascular smooth muscle cells by increasing intracellular cyclic AMP concentrations (see Chapter 33). Reduced prostacyclin production in PAH has led to the therapeutic use of epoprostenol and other stable prostacyclin derivatives (Gomberg-Maitland and Olschewski, 2008). Functionally and physiologically, PGI_2 opposes the effects of TXA_2.

Intravenous epoprostenol (FLOLAN, others) is effective in lowering pulmonary arterial pressures, improving exercise performance, and prolonging survival in PPAH. Because of its short plasma $t_{1/2}$, prostacyclin must be administered by continuous intravenous infusion using an infusion pump. Common side effects are headache, flushing, diarrhea, nausea, and jaw pain. Continuous intravenous infusion is inconvenient and very expensive. This has led to the development of more stable prostacyclin analogs. Treprostinil (REMODULIN) is given by continuous subcutaneous infusion or as an inhalation (TYVASO), consisting of four daily treatment sessions with nine breaths per session. Oral beraprost sodium appears to be somewhat less effective and its effect seems to diminish after 3 months of therapy, so it has not been approved in most countries. Iloprost (VENTAVIS) is a stable analog that is given by inhalation, but it needs to be given by nebulizer six to nine times daily. It is associated with the vasodilator side effects of prostacyclin, including syncope. It may also cause cough and bronchoconstriction because it sensitizes airway sensory nerves.

Endothelin Receptor Antagonists

Endothelin-1 (ET-1) is a potent pulmonary vasoconstrictor that is produced in increased amounts in PAH. ET-1 contracts vascular smooth muscle cells and causes proliferation mainly via ET_A receptors. ET_B receptors mediate the release of prostacyclin and NO from endothelial cells. Several endothelin antagonists are now on the market for the treatment of PPAH (see Chapter 26).

Bosentan (TRACLEER) was the first ET antagonist developed and is a antagonist of both ET_A and ET_B receptors. Several long-term clinical trials have now established the efficacy of oral bosentan in reducing symptoms and improving mortality in PPAH. Starting dose is 62.5 mg twice daily for 4 weeks, then increasing to the maintenance dose of 125 mg twice daily. The drug is generally well tolerated. Adverse effects include abnormal liver function tests, anemia, headaches, peripheral edema, and nasal congestion. Given the risk of serious liver injury, liver aminotransferases should be monitored monthly. A class effect is a risk of testicular atrophy and infertility; bosentan is potentially teratogenic.

Ambrisentan (LETAIRIS) is selective ET_A receptor antagonist. It is given orally once daily at a dose of 5-10 mg. The theoretical advantage of blocking only ET_A receptors is that ET_B receptors may continue to stimulate release of PGI_2 and NO, giving a greater therapeutic effect. However, its clinical efficacy is similar to that of bosentan, as are its adverse effects. Use of ambrisentan also requires monthly monitoring of liver aminotransferases. *Sitaxsentan* (not available in the U.S.) is similar to ambrisentan but may be less likely to cause liver dysfunction.

Phosphodiesterase 5 Inhibitors

Nitric oxide activates soluble guanylate cyclase to increase cyclic GMP, which is hydrolyzed to 5′GMP by PDE5 (Chapter 27). Elevation of cGMP in smooth muscle causes relaxation (Chapter 3),

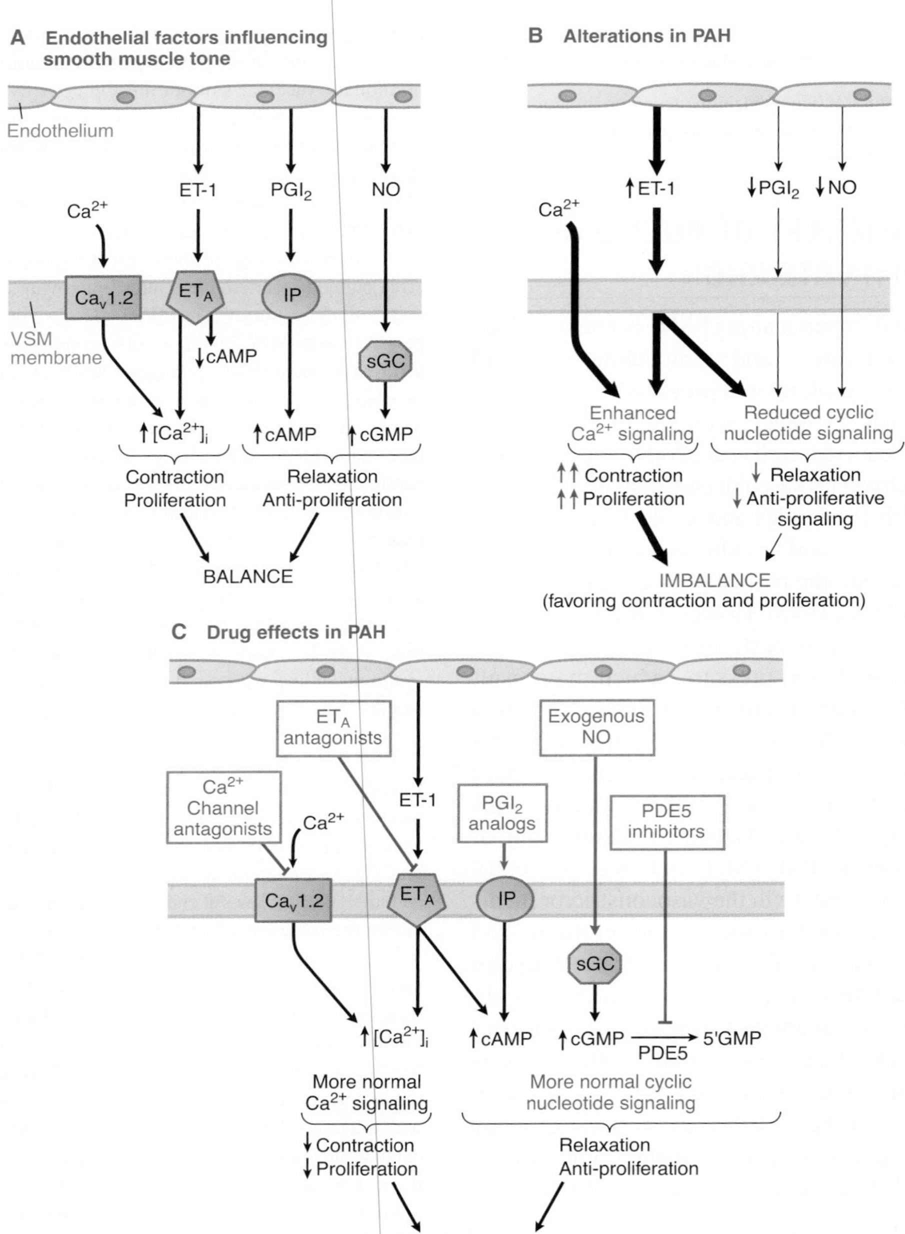

Figure 36–13. *Interactions of endothelium and vascular smooth muscle in pulmonary artery hypertension (PAH).* **A.** In normal pulmonary artery, there is a balance between constrictor and relaxant influences that may be viewed as competition between Ca^{2+} signaling pathways and cyclic nucleotide signaling pathways in vascular smooth muscle (VSM). Endothelin (ET-1) binds to the ET_A receptor on VSM cells and activates the G_q-PLC-IP_3 pathway to increase cytosolic Ca^{2+}; ET-1 may also couple to G_i to inhibit cyclic AMP (cAMP) production. In depolarizing VSM cells, Ca^{2+} may enter via the L-type Ca^{2+} channel ($Ca_v1.2$). Endothelial cells also produce relaxant factors, prostacyclin (PGI_2) and NO. NO stimulates the soluble guanylyl cyclase (cGC), causing accumulation of cyclic GMP (cGMP) in VSM cells; PGI_2 binds to the IP prostanoid receptor and stimulates the G_s-adenylyl cyclase pathway to enhance cAMP accumulation; elevation of these cyclic nucleotides promotes VSM relaxation (see Chapter 3). **B.** In PAH, ET-1 production is enhanced, production of PGI_2 and NO is reduced, and the balance is shifted toward constriction and proliferation of vascular smooth muscle. **C.** In treating PAH, ET_A receptor antagonists can reduce the constrictor effects of ET-1, and Ca^{2+} channel antagonists can further reduce Ca^{2+}-dependent contraction. Exogenous PGI_2 and NO can be supplied to promote vasodilation (relaxation of VSM); inhibition of PDE5 can enhance the relaxant effect of NO by inhibiting the degradation of cGMP, thereby promoting intracellular accumulation of cGMP and relaxation of VSM. Thus, these drugs can reduce Ca^{2+} signaling and enhance cyclic nucleotide signaling, restoring the balance between the forces of contraction/proliferation and relaxation/anti-proliferation. Remodeling and deposition of extracellular matrix by adjacent fibroblasts is influenced positively and negatively by the same contractile and relaxant signaling pathways, respectively.

which the inhibition of PDE5 prolongs and accentuates. In the pulmonary bed, inhibition of PDE5 induces vasodilation.

Sildenafil. Sildenafil (REVATIO) is a selective PDE5 inhibitor that is given at a dose (20 mg three time daily orally) that is lower than used for erectile dysfunction (100 mg; Chapter 27). It is effective in lowering pulmonary resistance and improving exercise tolerance in patients with PAH. Side effects include headache, flushing, dyspepsia, and visual disturbances.

Tadalafil. Tadalafil (ADCIRCA) has a longer duration of action than sildenafil so may be suitable for once-daily dosing. It is approved for World Health Organization group 1 PAH to improve exercise ability.

BIBLIOGRAPHY

Adams NP, Bestall JC, Jones P, et al. Fluticasone at different doses for chronic asthma in adults and children. *Cochrane Database Syst Rev*, **2008**, CD003534.

Angus RM, Mecallaum MJA, Hulks G, Thomson NC. Bronchodilator, cardiovascular and cyclic guanylyl monophosphate response to high dose infused atrial natriuretic peptide in asthma. *Am Rev Respir Dis*, **1993**, *147*:1122–1125.

Avila PC. Does anti-IgE therapy help in asthma? Efficacy and controversies. *Annu Rev Med*, **2007**, *58*:185–203.

Back M. Functional characteristics of cysteinyl-leukotriene receptor subtypes. *Life Sci*, **2002**, *71*:611–622.

Barnes PJ. Scientific rationale for combination inhalers with a long-acting β2-agonists and corticosteroids. *Eur Respir J*, **2002**, *19*:182–191.

Barnes PJ. Theophylline: New perspectives on an old drug. *Am J Respir Crit Care Med*, **2003**, *167*:813–818.

Barnes PJ. Mediators of chronic obstructive pulmonary disease. *Pharm Rev*, **2004**, *56*:515–548.

Barnes PJ. How corticosteroids control inflammation. *Br J Pharmacol*, **2006a**, *148*:245–254.

Barnes PJ. Treatment with (R)-albuterol has no advantage over racemic albuterol. *Am J Respir Crit Care Med*, **2006b**, *174*:969–972.

Barnes PJ. The problem of cough and development of novel antitussives. *Pulm Pharmacol Ther*, **2007**, *20*:416–422.

Barnes PJ. Cytokine networks in asthma and chronic obstructive pulmonary disease. *J Clin Invest*, **2008a**, *118*: 3546–3556.

Barnes PJ. Immunology of asthma and chronic obstructive pulmonary disease. *Nat Immunol Rev*, **2008b**, *8*: 183–192.

Barnes PJ. Role of HDAC2 in the pathophysiology of COPD. *Ann Rev Physiol*, **2009**, *71*:451–464.

Barnes PJ, Adcock IM. Glucocorticoid resistance in inflammatory diseases. *Lancet*, **2009**, *342*:1905–1917.

Barnes PJ, Celli BR. Systemic manifestations and comorbidities of COPD. *Eur Respir J*, **2009**, *33*:1165–1185.

Barnes PJ, Chung KF, Page CP. Inflammatory mediators of asthma: an update. *Pharmacol Rev*, **1998a**, *50*:515–596.

Barnes PJ, Karin M. Nuclear factor-κB: A pivotal transcription factor in chronic inflammatory diseases. *N Engl J Med*, **1997**, *336*:1066–1071.

Barnes PJ, Liu S-F. Regulation of pulmonary vascular tone. *Pharmacol Rev*, **1995**, *47*:87–131.

Barnes PJ, Pedersen S, Busse WW. Efficacy and safety of inhaled corticosteroids: An update. *Am J Respir Crit Care Med*, **1998b**, *157*: S1–S53.

Barr RG, Bourbeau J, Camargo CA, Ram FS. Tiotropium for stable chronic obstructive pulmonary disease: A meta-analysis. *Thorax*, **2006**, *61*: 854–862.

Barr RG, Rowe BH, Camargo CA Jr. Methylxanthines for exacerbations of chronic obstructive pulmonary disease: Meta-analysis of randomised trials. *BMJ*, **2003**, *327*: 643.

Basnyat B, Murdoch DR. High-altitude illness. *Lancet*, **2003**, *361*: 1967–1974.

Bateman ED, Hurd SS, Barnes PJ, et al. Global strategy for asthma management and prevention: GINA executive summary. *Eur Respir J*, **2008**, *31*:143–178.

Berger W. Aerosol devices and asthma therapy. *Curr Drug Deliv*, **2009**, *6*: 38–49.

Birring SS, Berry M, Brightling CE, Pavord, ID. Eosinophilic bronchitis: Clinical features, management and pathogenesis. *Am J Respir Med*, **2003**, *2*:169–173.

Black JL, Armour CL, Johnson PRA, et al. The action of a potassium channel activator BRL 38227 (lemakalim) on human airway smooth muscle. *Am Rev Respir Dis*, **1990**, *142*:1384–1389.

Bleecker ER, Postma DS, Lawrance RM, et al. Effect of ADRB2 polymorphisms on response to longacting beta2-agonist therapy: A pharmacogenetic analysis of two randomised studies. *Lancet*, **2007**, *370*:2118–2125.

Brenner MR, Berkowitz R, Marshall N, Strunk RC. Need for theophylline in severe steroid-requiring asthmatics. *Clin Allergy*, **1988**, *18*:143–150.

Broide DH. Immunomodulation of allergic disease. *Annu Rev Med*, **2009**, *60*:279–291.

Brutsche MH, Brutsche IC, Munawar M, et al. Comparison of pharmacokinetics and systemic effects of inhaled fluticasone propionate in patients with asthma and healthy volunteers: A randomised crossover study. *Lancet,* **2000**, *356*:556–561.

Burgel PR, Nadel JA. Roles of epidermal growth factor receptor activation in epithelial cell repair and mucin production in airway epithelium. *Thorax*, **2004**, *59*:992–996.

Calhoun WJ. Anti-leukotrienes for asthma. *Curr Opin Pharmacol*, **2001**, *1*:230–234.

Calverley PM, Anderson JA, Celli B, et al. Salmeterol and fluticasone propionate and survival in chronic obstructive pulmonary disease. *N Engl J Med*, **2007**, *356*:775–789.

Casarosa P, Kiechle T, Sieger P, *et al.* The constitutive activity of the human muscarinic M3 receptor unmasks differences in the pharmacology of anticholinergics. *J Pharmacol Exp Ther,* **2009** December 24 (Epub ahead of print).

Cazzola M. Aclidinium bromide, a novel long-acting muscarinic M3 antagonist for the treatment of COPD. *Curr Opin Investig Drugs*, **2009**, *10*:482–490.

Cazzola M, Matera MG. Novel long-acting bronchodilators for COPD and asthma. *Br J Pharmacol*, **2008**, *155*:291–299.

Chan HK. Dry powder aerosol delivery systems: Current and future research directions. *J Aerosol Med*, **2006**, *19*:21–27.

Chang AB, Lasserson TJ, Gaffney J, et al. Gastro-oesophageal reflux treatment for prolonged non-specific cough in children and adults. *Cochrane Database Syst Rev*, **2006**, CD004823.

Chiba Y, Shinozaki K, Ueno A, *et al.* Increased expression of $G\alpha_q$ protein in bronchial smooth muscle of mice with allergic bronchial asthma. *J Smooth Muscle Res,* **2008**, *44*:95–100.

Chung IY, Nam-Kung EK, Lee NM, et al. The downregulation of bcl-2 expression is necessary for theophylline-induced apoptosis of eosinophil. *Cell Immunol*, **2000**, *203*:95–102.

Clark AR. MAP kinase phosphatase 1: A novel mediator of biological effects of glucocorticoids? *J Endocrinol*, **2003**, *178*:5–12.

Coreno A, Skowronski M, Kotaru C, McFadden ER Jr. Comparative effects of long-acting beta2-agonists, leukotriene receptor antagonists, and a 5-lipoxygenase inhibitor on exercise-induced asthma. *J Allergy Clin Immunol*, **2000**, *106*:500–506.

Cosio BG, Iglesias A, Rios A, et al. Low-dose theophylline enhances the anti-inflammatory effects of steroids during exacerbations of chronic obstructive pulmonary disease. *Thorax*, **2009**, *64*:424–429.

Cosio BG, Tsaprouni L, Ito K, et al. Theophylline restores histone deacetylase activity and steroid responses in COPD macrophages. *J Exp Med*, **2004**, *200*:689–695.

Cox L, Platts-Mills TA, Finegold I, et al. American Academy of Allergy, Asthma & Immunology/American College of Allergy, Asthma and Immunology Joint Task Force Report on omalizumab-associated anaphylaxis. *J Allergy Clin Immunol*, **2007**, *120*:1373–1377.

Cuenda A, Rousseau S. p38 MAP-kinases pathway regulation, function and role in human diseases. *Biochim Biophys Acta*, **2007**, *1773*:1358–1375.

Culpitt SV, de Matos C, Russell RE, et al. Effect of theophylline on induced sputum inflammatory indices and neutrophil chemotaxis in COPD. *Am J Resp Crit Care Med*, **2002**, *165*: 1371–1376.

Currow DC, Abernethy AP. Pharmacological management of dyspnoea. *Curr Opin Support Palliat Care*, **2007**, *1*:96–101.

Dahlen SE, Malmstrom K, Nizankowska E, et al. Improvement of aspirin-intolerant asthma by montelukast, a leukotriene antagonist: a randomized, double-blind, placebo-controlled trial. *Am J Respir Crit Care Med*, **2002**, *165*:9–14.

Decramer M, Rutten-van Mölken M, Dekhuijzen PN, et al. Effects of N-acetylcysteine on outcomes in chronic obstructive pulmonary disease (Bronchitis Randomized on NAC Cost-Utility Study, BRONCUS): A randomised placebo-controlled trial. *Lancet*, **2005**, *365*:1552–1560.

Delhase M, Li N, Karin M. Kinase regulation in inflammatory response. *Nature*, **2000**, *406*:367–368.

Dennis SM, Sharp SJ, Vickers MR, et al. Regular inhaled salbutamol and asthma control: The TRUST randomised trial. *Lancet*, **2000**, *355*:1675–1679.

Derendorf H, Nave R, Drollmann A, et al. Relevance of pharmacokinetics and pharmacodynamics of inhaled corticosteroids to asthma. *Eur Respir J*, **2006**, *28*:1042–1050.

Dicpinigaitis PV. Currently available antitussives. *Pulm Pharmacol Ther*, **2009a**, *22*:148–151.

Dicpinigaitis PV, Gayle YE, Solomon G, Gilbert RD. Inhibition of cough-reflex sensitivity by benzonatate and guaifenesin in acute viral cough. *Respir Med*, **2009b**, *103*:902–906.

Dini FL, Cogo R. Doxofylline: A new generation xanthine bronchodilator devoid of major cardiovascular adverse effects. *Curr Med Res Opin*, **2001**, *16*:258–268.

Donnelly LE, Barnes PJ. Chemokine receptors as therapeutic targets in chronic obstructive pulmonary disease. *Trends Pharmacol Sci*, **2006**, *27*: 546–553.

Ducharme FM. Inhaled glucocorticoids versus leukotriene receptor antagonists as single agent asthma treatment: Systematic review of current evidence. *BMJ*, **2003**, *326*:621–624.

Ducharme FM, Lasserson TJ, Cates CJ. Long-acting beta2-agonists versus anti-leukotrienes as add-on therapy to inhaled corticosteroids for chronic asthma. *Cochrane Database Syst Rev*, **2006**, CD003137.

Duffy N, Walker P, Diamantea F, et al. Intravenous aminophylline in patients admitted to hospital with non-acidotic exacerbations of chronic obstructive pulmonary disease: A prospective randomised controlled trial. *Thorax*, **2005**, *60*:713–717.

Emelyanov A, Fedoseev G, Barnes PJ. Reduced intracellular magnesium concentrations in asthmatic subjects. *Eur Respir J*, **1999**, *13*:38–40.

Erin EM, Zacharasiewicz AS, Nicholson GC, et al. Rapid anti-inflammatory effect of inhaled ciclesonide in asthma: A randomised, placebo-controlled study. *Chest*, **2008**, *134*: 740–745.

Evans DJ, Taylor DA, Zetterstrom O, et al. A comparison of low-dose inhaled budesonide plus theophylline and high-dose inhaled budesonide for moderate asthma. *N Engl J Med*, **1997**, *337*:1412–1418.

Fabbri LM, Calverley PM, Izquierdo-Alonso JL, *et al.* Roflumilast in moderate-to-severe chronic obstructive pulmonary disease treated with long-acting bronchodilators: Two randomised clinical trials. *Lancet*, **2009**, *374*:695–703.

Flood-Page P, Swenson C, Faiferman I, et al. A study to evaluate safety and efficacy of mepolizumab in patients with moderate persistent asthma. *Am J Respir Crit Care Med*, **2007**, *176*:1062–1071.

Fluge T, Forssmann WG, Kunkel G, et al. Bronchodilation using combined urodilatin-albuterol administration in asthma: A randomized, double-blind, placebo-controlled trial. *Eur J Med Res*, **1999**, *4*:411–415.

Giembycz MA, Kaur M, Leigh R, Newton R. A Holy Grail of asthma management: Toward understanding how long-acting beta(2)-adrenoceptor agonists enhance the clinical efficacy of inhaled corticosteroids. *Br J Pharmacol*, **2008**, *153*:1090–1104.

Gomberg-Maitland M, Olschewski H. Prostacyclin therapies for the treatment of pulmonary arterial hypertension. *Eur Respir J*, **2008**, *31*:891–901.

Gompertz S, Stockley RA. A randomized, placebo-controlled trial of a leukotriene synthesis inhibitor in patients with COPD. *Chest*, **2002**, *122*:289–294.

Greenstone M, Lasserson TJ. Doxapram for ventilatory failure due to exacerbations of chronic obstructive pulmonary disease. *Cochrane Database Syst Rev*, **2003**, CD000223.

Gross JB, Blouin RT, Zandsberg S, et al. Effect of flumazenil on ventilatory drive during sedation with midazolam and alfentanil. *Anesthesiology*, **1996**, *85*:713–720.

Haldar P, Brightling CE, Hargadon B, et al. Mepolizumab and exacerbations of refractory eosinophilic asthma. *N Engl J Med*, **2009**, *360*:973–984.

Hansel TT, Kharitonov SA, Donnelly LE, et al. A selective inhibitor of inducible nitric oxide synthase inhibits exhaled breath nitric oxide in healthy volunteers and asthmatics. *FASEB J*, **2003**, *17*:1298–1300.

Hansel TT, Neighbour H, Erin EM, et al. Glycopyrrolate causes prolonged bronchoprotection and bronchodilatation in patients with asthma. *Chest*, **2005**, *128*:1974–1979.

Haque RA, Usmani OS, Barnes, PJ. Chronic idiopathic cough: a discrete clinical entity? *Chest*, **2005**, *127*:1710–1713.

Harrison TW, Wisniewski A, Honour J, Tattersfield AE. Comparison of the systemic effects of fluticasone propionate and budesonide given by dry powder inhaler in healthy and asthmatic subjects. *Thorax*, **2001**, *56*:186–191.

Hawkins G, McMahon AD, Twaddle S, et al. Stepping down inhaled corticosteroids in asthma: Randomised controlled trial. *BMJ*, **2003**, *326*:1115.

Hawkins GA, Weiss ST, Bleecker ER. Clinical consequences of ADRbeta2 polymorphisms. *Pharmacogenomics*, **2008**, *9*:349–358.

Henke MO, Ratjen F. Mucolytics in cystic fibrosis. *Paediatr Respir Rev*, **2007**, *8*:24–29.

Hobbs AJ, Higgs A, Moncada S. Inhibition of nitric oxide synthase as a potential therapeutic target. *Ann Rev Pharmacol Toxicol*, **1999**, *39*:191–220.

Holz GG, Kang G, Harbeck M, *et al.* Cell physiology of cAMP sensor Epac. *J Physiol*, **2006**, *577*:5–15.

Houslay MD, Schafer P, Zhang KY. Keynote review: Phosphodiesterase-4 as a therapeutic target. *Drug Discov Today*, **2005**, *10*:1503–1519.

Humbert M, Sitbon O, Simonneau G. Treatment of pulmonary arterial hypertension. *N Engl J Med*, **2004**, *351*:1425–1436.

Ichiyama T, Hasegawa S, Matsubara T, et al. Theophylline inhibits NF-κB activation and IκBα degradation in human pulmonary epithelial cells. *Naunyn Schmiedebergs Arch Pharmacol*, **2001**, *364*:558–561.

Ito K, Lim S, Caramori G, *et al.* A molecular mechanism of action of theophylline: Induction of histone deacetylase activity to decrease inflammatory gene expression. *Proc Natl Acad Sci USA*, **2002**, *99*:8921–8926.

Ito K, Yamamura S, Essilfie-Quaye S, et al. Histone deacetylase 2-mediated deacetylation of the glucocorticoid receptor enables NF-κB suppression. *J Exp Med*, **2006**, *203*: 7–13.

Jaeschke R, O'Byrne PM, Mejza F, et al. The safety of long-acting beta-agonists among patients with asthma using inhaled corticosteroids: Systematic review and metaanalysis. *Am J Respir Crit Care Med*, **2008**, *178*:1009–1016.

Jones PW, Greenstone M. Carbonic anhydrase inhibitors for hypercapnic ventilatory failure in chronic obstructive pulmonary disease. *Cochrane Database Syst Rev*, **2001**, CD002881.

Karin M, Yamamoto Y, Wang QM. The IKK NF-kappa B system: A treasure trove for drug development. *Nat Rev Drug Discov*, **2004**, *3*:17–26.

Kidney J, Dominguez M, Taylor PM, et al. Immunomodulation by theophylline in asthma: Demonstration by withdrawal of therapy. *Am J Resp Crit Care Med*, **1995**, *151*:1907–1914.

Kips JC, Pauwels RA. Long-acting inhaled β2-agonist therapy in asthma. *Am J Respir Crit Care Med*, **2001**, *164*:923–932.

Kirkham P, Rahman I. Oxidative stress in asthma and COPD: antioxidants as a therapeutic strategy. *Pharmacol Ther*, **2006**, *111*:476–494.

Kishore N, Sommers C, Mathialagan S, et al. A selective IKK-2 inhibitor blocks NF-κB-dependent gene expression in IL-1β stimulated synovial fibroblasts. *J Biol Chem*, **2003**, *277*: 13840–13847.

Larche M, Akdis CA, Valenta R. Immunological mechanisms of allergen-specific immunotherapy. *Nat Rev Immunol*, **2006**, *6*:761–771.

Leckie MJ, ten Brincke A, Khan J, et al. Effects of an interleukin-5 blocking monoclonal antibody on eosinophils, airway hyperresponsiveness and the late asthmatic response. *Lancet*, **2000**, *356*:2144–2148.

Levy ML, Stevenson C, Maslen T. Comparison of short courses of oral prednisolone and fluticasone propionate in the treatment of adults with acute exacerbations of asthma in primary care. *Thorax*, **1996**, *51*:1087–1092.

Lim S, Jatakanon A, Gordon D, et al. Comparison of high dose inhaled steroids, low dose inhaled steroids plus low dose theophylline, and low dose inhaled steroids alone in chronic asthma in general practice. *Thorax*, **2000**, *55*:837–841.

Lim S, Tomita K, Carramori G, et al. Low-dose theophylline reduces eosinophilic inflammation but not exhaled nitric oxide in mild asthma. *Am J Resp Crit Care Med*, **2001**, *164*:273–276.

Linden A, Hansson L, Andersson A, et al. Bronchodilation by an inhaled VPAC(2) receptor agonist in patients with stable asthma. *Thorax*, **2003**, *58*:217–221.

Lotvall J, Palmqvist M, Arvidsson P, et al. The therapeutic ratio of R-albuterol is comparable with that of RS-albuterol in asthmatic patients. *J Allergy Clin Immunol*, **2001**, *108*:726–731.

Madaan A. Arformoterol tartrate in the treatment of bronchoconstriction in patients with chronic obstructive pulmonary disease. *Drugs Today (Barc)*, **2009**, *45*:3–9.

Mak JCW, Nishikawa M, Shirasaki H, et al. Protective effects of a glucocorticoid on down-regulation of pulmonary β_2-adrenergic receptors *in vivo*. *J Clin Invest*, **1995**, *96*:99–106.

Manjra AI, Price J, Lenney W, et al. Efficacy of nebulized fluticasone propionate compared with oral prednisolone in children with an acute exacerbation of asthma. *Resp Med*, **2000**, *94*:1206–1214.

Manning P, Gibson PG, Lasserson TJ. Ciclesonide versus other inhaled steroids for chronic asthma in children and adults. *Cochrane Database Syst Rev*, **2008**, CD007031.

Marwick JA, Caramori G, Stevenson CC, et al. Inhibition of PI3Kδ restores glucocorticoid function in smoking-induced airway inflammation in mice. *Am J Respir Crit Care Med*, **2009**, *179*:542–548.

McGraw DW, Almoosa KF, Paul RJ, et al. Antithetic regulation by β-adrenergic receptors of Gq receptor signaling via phospholipase C underlies the airway β-agonist paradox. *J Clin Invest*, **2003**, *112*:619–626.

McGraw DW, Liggett SB. Heterogeneity in beta-adrenergic receptor kinase expression in the lung accounts for cell-specific desensitization of the beta2- adrenergic receptor. *J Biol Chem*, **1997**, *272*:7338–7344.

Mcivor RA, Pizzichini E, Turner MO, et al. Potential masking effects of salmeterol on airway inflammation in asthma. *Am J Respir Crit Care Med*, **1998**, *158*:924–930.

McLaughlin VV, Archer SL, Badesch DB, et al. ACCF/AHA 2009 expert consensus document on pulmonary hypertension. *J Am Coll Cardiol*, **2009**, *53*:1573–1619.

McLeod RL, Correll CC, Jia Y, Anthes JC. TRPV1 antagonists as potential antitussive agents. *Lung*, **2008** (*186 suppl 1*): S59–S65.

Minoguchi K, Kohno Y, Minoguchi H, et al. Reduction of eosinophilic inflammation in the airways of patients with asthma using montelukast. *Chest*, **2002**, *121*:732–738.

Mohammed S, Goodacre S. Intravenous and nebulised magnesium sulphate for acute asthma: Systematic review and meta-analysis. *Emerg Med J*, **2007**, *24*:823–830.

Morrell NW, Adnot S, Archer SL, *et al.* Cellular and molecular basis of pulmonary arterial hypertension. *J Am Coll Cardiol*, **2009**, *54*:S20–S31.

Nathan RA. Pharmacotherapy for allergic rhinitis: A critical review of leukotriene receptor antagonists compared with other treatments. *Ann Allergy Asthma Immunol*, **2003**, *90*:182–190.

Nathani N, Little MA, Kunst H, et al. Churg-Strauss syndrome and leukotriene antagonist use: A respiratory perspective. *Thorax*, **2008**, *63*:883–888.

Nelson HS, Weiss ST, Bleecker ER, et al. The Salmeterol Multicenter Asthma Research Trial: A comparison of usual pharmacotherapy for asthma or usual pharmacotherapy plus salmeterol. *Chest*, **2006**, *129*:15–26.

Newton PJ, Davidson PM, Macdonald P, et al. Nebulized furosemide for the management of dyspnea: Does the evidence support its use? *J Pain Symptom Manage*, **2008**, *36*:424–441.

Niewoehner DE, Erbland ML, Deupree RH, et al. Effect of systemic glucocorticoids on exacerbations of chronic obstructive pulmonary disease. *N Engl J Med*, **1999**, *340*:1941–1947.

Nightingale JA, Rogers DF, Barnes PJ. Comparison of the effects of salmeterol and formoterol in patients with severe asthma. *Chest*, **2002**, *121*:1401–1406.

O'Byrne PM, Pedersen S, Busse WW, et al. Effects of early intervention with inhaled budesonide on lung function in newly diagnosed asthma. *Chest*, **2006**, *129*:1478–1485.

O'Sullivan S, Akveld M, Burke CM, Poulter LW. Effect of the addition of montelukast to inhaled fluticasone propionate on airway inflammation. *Am J Respir Crit Care Med*, **2003**, *167*:745–750.

Ohta K, Yamashita N. Apoptosis of eosinophils and lymphocytes in allergic inflammation. *J Allergy Clin Immunol*, **1999**, *104*:14–21.

Oliver B, Tomita K, Keller A, et al. Low-dose theophylline does not exert its anti-inflammatory effects in mild asthma through upregulation of interleukin-10 in alveolar macrophages. *Allergy*, **2001**, *56*:1087–1090.

Parameswaran K, Belda J, Rowe BH. Addition of intravenous aminophylline to beta2-agonists in adults with acute asthma. *Cochrane Database Syst Rev*, **2000**, CD002742.

Pavord ID, Chung KF. Management of chronic cough. *Lancet*, **2008**, *371*:1375–1384.

Pedersen S. Do inhaled corticosteroids inhibit growth in children? *Am J Respir Crit Care Med*, **2001**, *164*:521–535.

Pelaia G, Gallelli L, Vatrella A, et al. Potential role of potassium channel openers in the treatment of asthma and chronic obstructive pulmonary disease. *Life Sci*, **2002**, *70*:977–990.

Peters-Golden M, Henderson WR Jr. Leukotrienes. *N Engl J Med*, **2007**, *357*:1841–1854.

Pettipher R, Hansel TT, Armer R. Antagonism of the prostaglandin D2 receptors DP1 and CRTH2 as an approach to treat allergic diseases. *Nat Rev Drug Discov*, **2007**, *6*:313–325.

Poole PJ, Black PN. Oral mucolytic drugs for exacerbations of chronic obstructive pulmonary disease: Systematic review. *BMJ*, **2001**, *322*:1271–1274.

Rabe KF, Atienza T, Magyar P, et al. Reduction in exacerbations with budesonide in combination with formoterol for reliever therapy: A randomised, controlled double-blind study. *Lancet*, **2006**, *368*:707–708.

Rabe KF, Hurd S, Anzueto A, *et al.* Global strategy for the diagnosis, management, and prevention of COPD—2006 update. *Am J Respir Crit Care Med*, **2007**, *176*:532–555.

Ram FS, Jones PW, Castro AA, et al. Oral theophylline for chronic obstructive pulmonary disease. *Cochrane Database Syst Rev*, **2002**, CD003902.

Ray NC, Alcaraz L. Muscarinic antagonist-beta-adrenergic agonist dual pharmacology molecules as bronchodilators: A patent review. *Expert Opin Ther Pat*, **2009**, *19*:1–12.

Rennard SI, Fogarty C, Kelsen S, et al. The safety and efficacy of infliximab in moderate-to-severe chronic obstructive pulmonary disease. *Am J Respir Crit Care Med*, **2007**, *175*:926–934.

Rivington RN, Boulet LP, Cote J, et al. Efficacy of slow-release theophylline, inhaled salbutamol and their combination in asthmatic patients on high-dose inhaled steroids. *Am J Respir Crit Care Med*, **1995**, *151*:325–332.

Robinson DS, Campbell DA, Barnes, PJ. Addition of an anti-leukotriene to therapy in chronic severe asthma in a clinic setting: A double-blind, randomised, placebo-controlled study. *Lancet*, **2001**, *357*:2007–2011.

Rodrigo GJ, Nannini LJ, Rodriguez-Roisin R. Safety of long-acting beta-agonists in stable COPD: A systematic review. *Chest*, **2008**, *133*:1079–1087.

Rogers DF. Pharmacological regulation of the neuronal control of airway mucus secretion. *Curr Opin Pharmacol*, **2002**, *2*:249–255.

Rogers DF, Barnes PJ. Treatment of airway mucus hypersecretion. *Ann Med*, **2006**, *38*:116–125.

Rolland JM, Gardner LM, O'Hehir RE. Allergen-related approaches to immunotherapy. *Pharmacol Ther*, **2009**, *121*:273–284.

Schacke H, Berger M, Rehwinkel H, Asadullah K. Selective glucocorticoid receptor agonists (SEGRAs): Novel ligands with an improved therapeutic index. *Mol Cell Endocrinol*, **2007**, *275*:109–117.

Sears MR, Taylor DR, Print CG, et al. Regular inhaled beta-agonist treatment in bronchial asthma. *Lancet*, **1990**, *336*:1391–1396.

Seddon P, Bara A, Ducharme FM, Lasserson TJ. Oral xanthines as maintenance treatment for asthma in children. *Cochrane Database Syst Rev*, **2006**, CD002885.

Shah L, Wilson AJ, Gibson PG, Coughlan J. Long acting beta-agonists versus theophylline for maintenance treatment of asthma. *Cochrane Database Syst Rev*, **2003**, CD001281.

Sin DD, Tashkin D, Zhang X, *et al.* Budesonide and the risk of pneumonia: A meta-analysis of individual patient data. *Lancet*, **2009**, *374*:712–719.

Singh D, Richards D, Knowles RG, et al. Selective inducible nitric oxide synthase inhibition has no effect on allergen challenge in asthma. *Am J Respir Crit Care Med*, **2007**, *176*:988–993.

Singh S, Amin AV, Loke YK. Long-term use of inhaled corticosteroids and the risk of pneumonia in chronic obstructive pulmonary disease: A meta-analysis. *Arch Intern Med*, **2009**, *169*:219–229.

Skorodin MS, Tenholder MF, Yetter B, et al. Magnesium sulfate in exacerbations of chronic obstructive pulmonary disease. *Arch Intern Med*, **1995**, *155*:496–500.

Spitzer WO, Suissa S, Ernst P, et al. The use of β-agonists and the rate of death and near-death from asthma. *N Engl J Med*, **1992**, *326*:503–506.

Sturton G, Persson C, Barnes PJ. Small airways: An important but neglected target in the treatment of obstructive airway diseases. *Trends Pharmacol Sci*, **2008**, *29*:340–345.

Suissa S, Ernst P, Benayoun S, et al. Low-dose inhaled corticosteroids and the prevention of death from asthma. *N Engl J Med*, **2000**, *343*:332–336.

Suissa S, Ernst P, Vandemheen KL, Aaron SD. Methodological issues in therapeutic trials of COPD. *Eur Respir J*, **2008**, *31*:927–933.

Szczeklik A, Stevenson DD. Aspirin-induced asthma: Advances in pathogenesis, diagnosis, and management. *J Allergy Clin Immuno.*, **2003**, *111*:913–921.

Tantisira KG, Drazen JM. Genetics and pharmacogenetics of the leukotriene pathway. *J Allergy Clin Immunol*, **2009**, *124*:422–427.

Tashkin DP, Celli B, Senn S, et al. A 4-year trial of tiotropium in chronic obstructive pulmonary disease. *N Engl J Med*, **2008**, *359*:1543–1554.

Taylor-Clark TE, Nassenstein C, McAlexander MA, Undem BJ. TRPA1: A potential target for anti-tussive therapy. *Pulm Pharmacol Ther*, **2009**, *22*:71–74.

Ukena D, Harnest U, Sakalauskas R, et al. Comparison of addition of theophylline to inhaled steroid with doubling of the dose of inhaled steroid in asthma. *Eur Respir J*, **1997**, *10*:2754–2760.

Usmani OS, Ito K, Maneechotesuwan K, et al. Glucocorticoid receptor nuclear translocation in airway cells following inhaled combination therapy. *Am J Respir Crit Care Med*, **2005**, *172*:704–712.

van Ganse E, Kaufman L, Derde MP, et al. Effects of antihistamines in adult asthma: A meta-analysis of clinical trials. *Eur Respir J*, **1997**, *10*:2216–2224.

Viola A, Luster AD. Chemokines and their receptors: Drug targets in immunity and inflammation. *Annu Rev Pharmacol Toxicol*, **2008**, *48*:171–197.

Virchow JC, Crompton GK, Dal Negro R, et al. Importance of inhaler devices in the management of airway disease. *Respir Med*, **2008**, *102*:10–19.

Walker S, Monteil M, Phelan K, et al. Anti-IgE for chronic asthma in adults and children. *Cochrane Database Syst Rev*, **2006**, CD003559.

Wenzel SE, Barnes PJ, Bleecker ER, et al. A randomized, double-blind, placebo-controlled study of TNF-α blockade in severe persistent asthma. *Am J Respir Crit Care Med*, **2009**, *179*:549–558.

Wenzel SE, Busse WW. Severe asthma: Lessons from the Severe Asthma Research Program. *J Allergy Clin Immunol*, **2007**, *119*:14–21.

Wessler I, Kirkpatrick CJ. Acetylcholine beyond neurons: The non-neuronal cholinergic system in humans. *Br J Pharmacol*, **2008**, *154*:1558–1571.

Wilson AJ, Gibson PG, Coughlan J. Long acting beta-agonists versus theophylline for maintenance treatment of asthma. *Cochrane Database Syst Rev*, **2000**, CD001281.

Wilson CN. Adenosine receptors and asthma in humans. *Br J Pharmacol*, **2008**, *155*:475–486.

Winkelmann BR, Kullmer TH, Kneissl DG, et al. Low-dose almitrine bismesylate in the treatment of hypoxemia due to chronic obstructive pulmonary disease. *Chest*, **1994**, *105*:1383–1391.

Yang IA, Fong KM, Sim EH, et al. Inhaled corticosteroids for stable chronic obstructive pulmonary disease. *Cochrane Database Syst Rev*, **2007**, CD002991.

Yasui K, Agematsu K, Shinozaki K, et al. Theophylline induces neutrophil apoptosis through adenosine A_{2A} receptor antagonism. *J Leukoc Biol*, **2000**, *67*:529–535.

Zhang ZY, Kaminsky LS. Characterization of human cytochromes P450 involved in theophylline 8-hydroxylation. *Biochem Pharmacol*, **1995**, *50*:205–211.

Zheng JP, Kang J, Huang SG, et al. Effect of carbocisteine on acute exacerbation of chronic obstructive pulmonary disease (PEACE Study): A randomised placebo-controlled study. *Lancet*, **2008**, *371*:2013–2018.

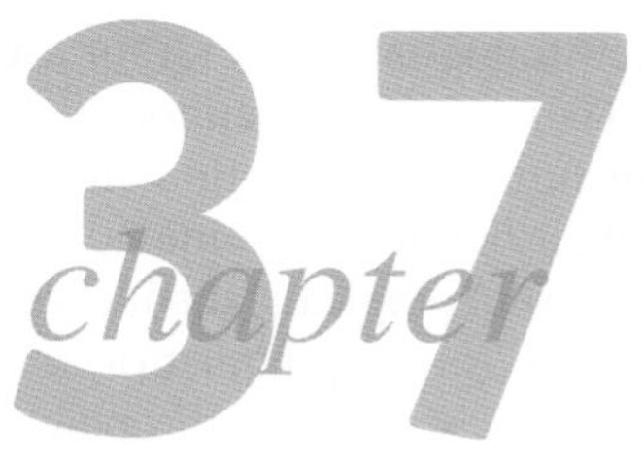

Hematopoietic Agents: Growth Factors, Minerals, and Vitamins

Kenneth Kaushansky
and Thomas J. Kipps

The finite life span of most mature blood cells requires their continuous replacement, a process termed *hematopoiesis.* New cell production must respond to basal needs and states of increased demand. Red blood cell production can increase >20-fold in response to anemia or hypoxemia, white blood cell production increases dramatically in response to a systemic infection, and platelet production can increase 10- to 20-fold when platelet consumption results in thrombocytopenia.

The regulation of blood cell production is complex. Hematopoietic stem cells are rare bone marrow cells that manifest self-renewal and lineage commitment, resulting in cells destined to differentiate into the nine distinct blood-cell lineages. For the most part, this process occurs in the marrow cavities of the skull, vertebral bodies, pelvis, and proximal long bones; it involves interactions among hematopoietic stem and progenitor cells and the cells and complex macromolecules of the marrow stroma, and is influenced by a number of soluble and membrane-bound hematopoietic growth factors. A number of these hormones and cytokines have been identified and cloned, permitting their production in quantities sufficient for therapeutic use. Clinical applications range from the treatment of primary hematologic diseases to use as adjuncts in the treatment of severe infections and in the management of patients who are undergoing cancer chemotherapy or marrow transplantation.

Hematopoiesis also requires an adequate supply of minerals (e.g., iron, cobalt, and copper) and vitamins (e.g., folic acid, vitamin B_{12}, pyridoxine, ascorbic acid, and riboflavin); deficiencies generally result in characteristic anemias, or, less frequently, a general failure of hematopoiesis (Hoffbrand and Herbert, 1999; Wrighting and Andrews, 2008). Therapeutic correction of a specific deficiency state depends on the accurate diagnosis of the anemic state, knowledge about the correct dose, the use of these agents in various combinations, and the expected response. This chapter deals with the growth factors, vitamins, minerals, and drugs that affect the blood and blood-forming organs.

Hematopoietic Growth Factors

History. Modern concepts of hematopoietic cell growth and differentiation arose in the 1950s when cells from the spleen and marrow were shown to play an important role in the restoration of hematopoietic tissue in irradiated animals. In 1961, Till and McCulloch demonstrated that individual hematopoietic cells could form macroscopic hematopoietic colonies in the spleens of irradiated mice. Their work established the concept of discrete hematopoietic stem cells, which can be experimentally identified, albeit in retrospect (i.e., the presence of a multilineage clonal splenic colony appearing 11 days after transplantation implied that a single cell lodged and expanded into several cell lineages). This concept now has been expanded to include normal human marrow cells. Moreover, such cells now can be prospectively identified.

The basis for identifying soluble growth factors was provided by Sachs and independently by Metcalf, who developed clonal, *in vitro* assays for hematopoietic progenitor cells. Initially, such hematopoietic colonies developed only in the presence of conditioned culture medium from leukocytes or tumor cell lines.

Individual growth factors then were isolated based on their activities in clonal *in vitro* assays. Many of these same assays were instrumental in purifying a hierarchy of progenitor cells committed to individual and combinations of mature blood cells (Akashi, 2000; Nakorn, 2003).

The existence of a circulating growth factor that controls red blood cell development was first suggested by the experiments of Paul Carnot in 1906. He observed an increase in the red-cell count in rabbits injected with serum obtained from anemic animals and postulated the existence of a factor that he called hemopoietin. However, it was not until the 1950s that Reissmann, Erslev, and Jacobsen and coworkers defined the origin and actions of the hormone, now called erythropoietin. Subsequently, extensive studies of erythropoietin were carried out in patients with anemia and polycythemia, leading to the purification of erythropoietin from urine and the subsequent cloning of the erythropoietin gene. The high-level expression of erythropoietin in cell lines has allowed for its purification and use in humans with anemia.

Similarly, the existence of specific leukocyte growth factors was suggested by the capacity of different conditioned culture media to induce the *in vitro* growth of colonies containing different combinations of granulocytes and monocytes. An activity that stimulated the production of both granulocytes and monocytes was purified from murine lung-conditioned medium, leading to cloning of granulocyte/macrophage colony-stimulating factor (G-CSF), first from mice (Gough et al., 1984) and subsequently from humans (Wong, 1985). Finding an activity that stimulated the exclusive production of neutrophils permitted the cloning of granulocyte colony-stimulating factor (G-CSF) (Welte et al., 1985). Subsequently, a megakaryocyte colony-stimulating factor termed thrombopoietin was purified and cloned (Kaushansky, 1998).

The growth factors that support lymphocyte growth were not identified using *in vitro* colony-forming assays but rather using assays that measured the capacity of the cytokine to promote lymphocyte proliferation *in vitro*. This permitted the identification of the growth-promoting properties of interleukin (Il)-7, Il-4, or Il-15 for all lymphocytes, B cells, or NK cells, respectively (Goodwin et al., 1989; Grabstein et al., 1994). Again, recombinant expression of these cDNAs permitted production of sufficient quantities of biologically active growth factors for clinical investigations, allowing for the demonstration of the potential clinical utility of such factors.

Growth Factor Physiology. Steady-state hematopoiesis encompasses the production of >400 billion blood cells each day. This production is tightly regulated and can be increased several fold with increased demand. The hematopoietic organ also is unique in adult physiology in that several mature cell types are derived from a much smaller number of multipotent progenitors, which develop from a more limited number of pluripotent hematopoietic stem cells. Such cells are capable of maintaining their own number and differentiating under the influence of cellular and humoral factors to produce the large and diverse number of mature blood cells.

Stem cell differentiation can be described as a series of steps that produce so-called burst-forming units (BFU) and colony-forming units (CFU) for each of the major cell lines. These early progenitors (BFU and CFU) are capable of further proliferation and differentiation, increasing their number by some 30-fold. Subsequently, colonies of morphologically distinct cells form under the control of an overlapping set of additional growth factors (G-CSF, M-CSF, erythropoietin, and thrombopoietin). Proliferation and maturation of the CFU for each cell line can amplify the resulting mature cell product by another 30-fold or more, generating >1000 mature cells from each committed stem cell.

Hematopoietic and lymphopoietic growth factors are glycoproteins produced by a number of marrow cells and peripheral tissues. They are active at very low concentrations and typically affect more than one committed cell lineage. Most interact synergistically with other factors and also stimulate production of additional growth factors, a process called *networking*. Growth factors generally exert actions at several points in the processes of cell proliferation and differentiation and in mature cell function. However, the network of growth factors that contributes to any given cell lineage depends absolutely on a nonredundant, lineage-specific factor, such that absence of factors that stimulate developmentally early progenitors is compensated for by redundant cytokines, but loss of the lineage-specific factor leads to a specific cytopenia. Some of the overlapping and nonredundant effects of the more important hematopoietic growth factors are illustrated in Figure 37–1 and listed in Table 37–1.

ERYTHROPOIESIS STIMULATING AGENTS

Erythropoiesis stimulating agent (ESA) is the term given to a pharmacological substance that stimulates red blood cell production. Although erythropoietin is not the sole growth factor responsible for erythropoiesis, it is the most important regulator of the proliferation of committed erythroid progenitors (CFU-E) and their immediate progeny. In its absence, severe anemia is invariably present, commonly seen in patients with renal failure. Erythropoiesis is controlled by a feedback system in which a sensor in the kidney detects changes in oxygen delivery to modulate the erythropoietin secretion. The sensor mechanism is now understood at the molecular level (Maxwell et al., 2001). Hypoxia-inducible factor (HIF-1) is a heterodimeric (HIF-1α and

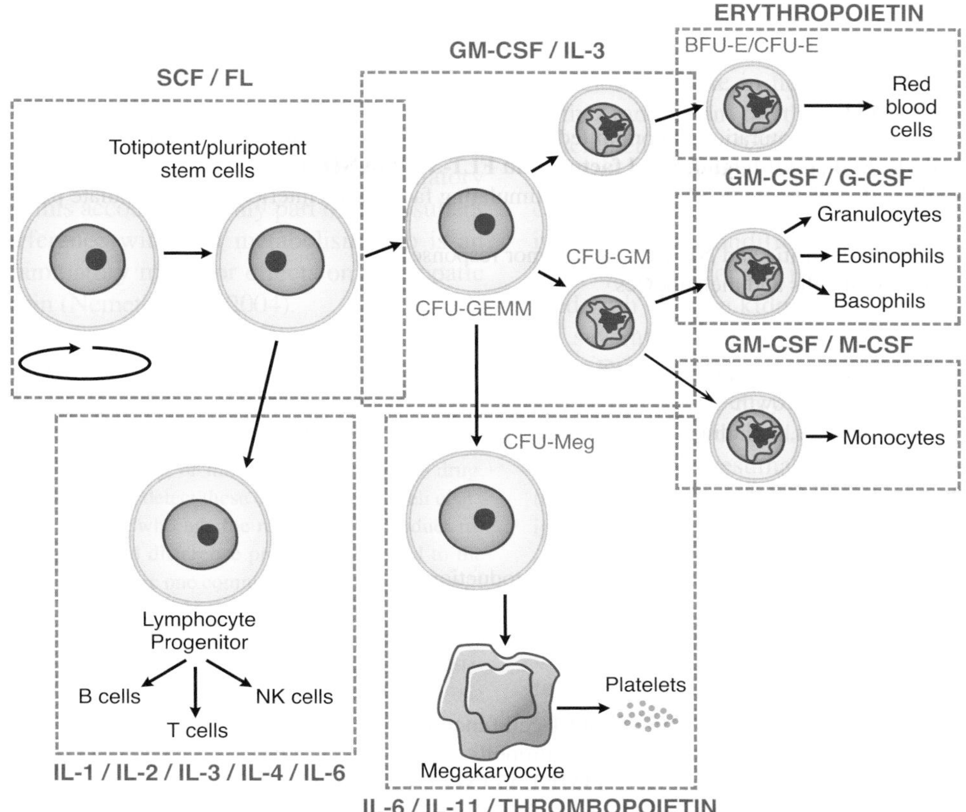

Figure 37–1. *Sites of action of hematopoietic growth factors in the differentiation and maturation of marrow cell lines.* A self-sustaining pool of marrow stem cells differentiates under the influence of specific hematopoietic growth factors to form a variety of hematopoietic and lymphopoietic cells. Stem cell factor (SCF), ligand (FL), interleukin-3 (IL-3), and granulocyte-macrophage colony-stimulating factor (GM-CSF), together with cell–cell interactions in the marrow, stimulate stem cells to form a series of burst-forming units (BFU) and colony-forming units (CFU): CFU-GEMM (granulocyte, erythrocyte, monocyte and megakaryocyte), CFU-GM (granulocyte and macrophage), CFU-Meg (megakaryocyte), BFU-E (erythrocyte), and CFU-E (erythrocyte). After considerable proliferation, further differentiation is stimulated by synergistic interactions with growth factors for each of the major cell lines—granulocyte colony–stimulating factor (G-CSF), monocyte/macrophage-stimulating factor (M-CSF), thrombopoietin, and erythropoietin. Each of these factors also influences the proliferation, maturation, and in some cases the function of the derivative cell line (Table 37–1).

HIF-1β) transcription factor that enhances expression of multiple hypoxia-inducible genes, such as vascular endothelial growth factor and erythropoietin. HIF-1α is labile due to its prolyl hydroxylation and subsequent polyubiquitination and degradation, aided by the von Hippel-Lindau (VHL) protein. During states of hypoxia, the prolyl hydroxylase is inactive, allowing the accumulation of HIF-1α and activating erythropoietin expression, which in turn stimulates a rapid expansion of erythroid progenitors. Specific alteration of VHL leads to an oxygen-sensing defect, characterized by constitutively elevated levels of HIF-1α and erythropoietin, with a resultant polycythemia (Gordeuk et al., 2004). Recently, a potential role for a second isoform of HIF, HIF-2α, was identified in erythropoiesis because genetic gain-of-function mutation of that gene induces erythrocytosis in patients (Percy et al., 2008).

Erythropoietin is encoded by a single copy gene on human chromosome 7 that is expressed primarily in peritubular interstitial cells of the kidney. Erythropoietin contains 193 amino acids, of which the first 27 are cleaved during secretion. The final hormone is heavily glycosylated and has a molecular mass of ~30,000 Da. After secretion, erythropoietin binds to a receptor on the surface of committed erythroid progenitors in the marrow and is internalized. With anemia or hypoxemia, synthesis rapidly increases by 100-fold or more, serum erythropoietin levels rise, and marrow progenitor cell survival, estimated as ~17% based on a meta-analysis of nearly 14,000 cancer patients (Bohlius et al., 2008). The cause(s) of this effect is presently unclear, but some studies suggest that tumor cells bearing the erythropoietin receptor are more likely to be affected by the use of ESAs (Henke et al., 2003). Although epoetin alfa is not associated with direct pressor effects, blood pressure may rise, especially during the early phases of therapy when the hematocrit is increasing. ESAs should not be used in patients with preexisting uncontrolled hypertension. Patients may require initiation of, or increases in, antihypertensive therapy. Hypertensive encephalopathy and seizures have occurred in chronic renal failure patients treated with epoetin alfa. The incidence of seizures appears to be higher during the first 90 days of therapy with epoetin alfa in patients on dialysis (occurring in ~2.5% of patients) when compared with subsequent 90-day periods. Headache, tachycardia, edema, shortness of breath, nausea, vomiting, diarrhea, injection site stinging, and flu-like symptoms (e.g., arthralgias and myalgias) also have been reported in conjunction with epoetin alfa therapy. Pure red-cell aplasia in association with neutralizing antibodies to native erythropoietin has been observed in patients treated with specific epoetin alfa formulations (see earlier discussion). Resistance to therapy can be caused by multiple factors (see following discussion).

Anemia of Chronic Renal Failure. Patients with anemia secondary to chronic kidney disease are ideal candidates for epoetin alfa therapy because the disorder represents a pure erythropoietin deficiency state. The response in predialysis, peritoneal dialysis, and hemodialysis patients depends on the severity of the renal failure, the erythropoietin dose and route of administration, and iron availability (Besarab et al., 1999, Kaufman et al., 1998). The subcutaneous route of administration is preferred over the intravenous route because absorption is slower and the amount of drug required is reduced by 20-40%.

The dose of epoetin alfa should be adjusted to obtain a gradual rise in the hematocrit over a 2- to 4-month period to a final hematocrit of 33-36%. Treatment to hematocrit levels >36% is not recommended because patients treated to a hematocrit >40% showed a higher incidence of myocardial infarction and death (Besarab et al., 1998). The drug should not be used to replace emergency transfusion in patients who need immediate correction of a life-threatening anemia.

Patients are started on doses of 80-120 units/kg of epoetin alfa, given subcutaneously, three times a week. It can be given on a once-weekly schedule, but somewhat more drug is required for an equivalent effect. If the response is poor, the dose should be progressively increased. The final maintenance dose of epoetin alfa can vary from as little as 10 units/kg to >300 units/kg, with an average dose of 75 units/kg, three times a week. Children <5 years of age generally require a higher dose. Resistance to therapy is common in patients who develop an inflammatory illness or become iron deficient, so close monitoring of general health and iron status is essential. Less common causes of resistance include occult blood loss, folic acid deficiency, carnitine deficiency, inadequate dialysis, aluminum toxicity, and osteitis fibrosa cystica secondary to hyperparathyroidism.

The most common side effect of epoetin alfa therapy is aggravation of hypertension, which occurs in 20-30% of patients and most often is associated with a rapid rise in hematocrit. Blood pressure usually can be controlled either by increasing antihypertensive therapy or ultrafiltration in dialysis patients or by reducing the epoetin alfa dose to slow the hematocrit response.

Darbepoetin alfa also is approved for use in patients who are anemic secondary to chronic kidney disease. The recommended starting dose is 0.45 μg/kg administered intravenously or subcutaneously once weekly, with dose adjustments depending on the response. Like epoetin alfa, side effects tend to occur when patients experience a rapid rise in hemoglobin concentration; a rise of <1 g/dL every 2 weeks generally has been considered safe.

Anemia in AIDS Patients. Epoetin alfa therapy has been approved for the treatment of HIV-infected patients, especially those on zidovudine therapy (Fischl et al., 1990). Excellent responses to doses of 100-300 units/kg, given subcutaneously three times a week, generally are seen in patients with zidovudine-induced anemia. In the face of advanced disease, marrow damage, and elevated serum erythropoietin levels (>500 IU/L), therapy is less effective.

Cancer-Related Anemias. Epoetin alfa therapy, 150 units/kg three times a week or 450-600 units/kg once a week, can reduce the transfusion requirement in cancer patients undergoing chemotherapy. Evidence-based guidelines for the therapeutic use of recombinant erythropoietin in patients with cancer have been published (Rizzo et al., 2002). Briefly, the guidelines recommend the use of epoetin alfa in patients with chemotherapy-associated anemia when hemoglobin levels fall below 10 g/dL, basing the decision to treat less severe anemia (Hb, 10-12 g/dL) on clinical circumstances. For anemia associated with hematologic malignancies, the guidelines support the use of recombinant erythropoietin in patients with low-grade myelodysplastic syndrome, although the evidence that the drug is effective in anemic patients with multiple myeloma, non-Hodgkin's lymphoma, or chronic lymphocytic leukemia not receiving chemotherapy is less robust. A baseline serum erythropoietin level may help to predict the response; most patients with blood levels >500 IU/L are unlikely to respond to any dose of the drug. Most patients treated with epoetin alfa experienced an improvement in their anemia, sense of well-being, and quality of life (Littlewood et al., 2001). This improved sense of well-being, particularly in cancer patients, may not be solely due to the rise in the hematocrit. Erythropoietin receptors have been demonstrated in cells of the central nervous system (CNS), and erythropoietin has been found to act as a cytoprotectant in several models of CNS ischemia. Thus high levels of the hormone may directly affect cancer patients' sense of well-being.

Darbepoetin alfa also has been tested in cancer patients undergoing chemotherapy and preliminary studies appear promising. However, recent case reports have suggested a direct effect of both epoetin alfa and darbepoetin alfa in stimulation of tumor cells. For example, patients with cancer of the head and neck randomized to receive recombinant erythropoietin had a statistically significant increase in likelihood of tumor progression during the duration of the study (Henke et al., 2003). A meta-analysis of a large number of patients and clinical trials estimates the risk at ~10% higher than non-treated cancer patients (Bohlius et al., 2008). This finding is being evaluated by the FDA and warrants serious attention.

Surgery and Autologous Blood Donation. Epoetin alfa has been used perioperatively to treat anemia and reduce the need for erythrocyte transfusion. Patients undergoing elective orthopedic and cardiac procedures have been treated with 150-300 units/kg of epoetin alfa once daily for the 10 days preceding surgery, on the day of surgery, and for 4 days after surgery. As an alternative, 600 units/kg can be given on days 21, 14, and 7 before surgery, with an additional dose on the day of surgery. This can correct a moderately severe preoperative anemia (i.e., hematocrit 30-36%) and reduce the need for transfusion. Epoetin alfa also has been used to improve autologous blood donation (Goodnough et al., 1989). However, the potential benefit generally is small, and the expense is considerable. Patients treated for 3-4 weeks with epoetin alfa (300-600 units/kg twice a week) are able to donate only 1 or 2 more units than untreated patients, and most of the time this goes unused. Still, the ability to stimulate erythropoiesis for blood storage can be invaluable in the patient with multiple alloantibodies to red blood cells.

Other Uses. Epoetin alfa has received orphan drug status from the FDA for the treatment of the anemia of prematurity, HIV infection, and myelodysplasia. In the latter case, even very high doses >1000 units/kg two to three times a week have had limited success. The utility of very high-dose therapy in other hematologic disorders, such as sickle cell anemia, is still under study. Highly competitive athletes have used epoetin alfa to increase their hemoglobin levels ("blood doping") and improve performance. Unfortunately, this misuse of the drug has been implicated in the deaths of several athletes and is strongly discouraged.

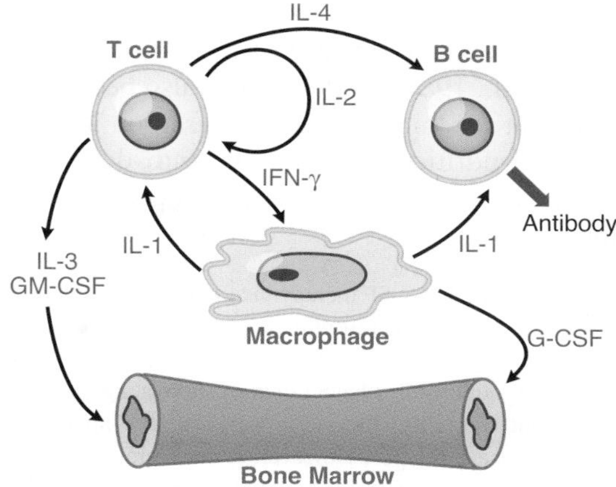

Figure 37–2. *Cytokine–cell interactions.* Macrophages, T cells, B cells, and marrow stem cells interact *via* several cytokines (IL-1, IL-2, IL-3, IL-4, IFN [interferon]-γ, GM-CSF, and G-CSF) in response to a bacterial or a foreign antigen challenge. See Table 37–1 for the functional activities of these various cytokines.

MYELOID GROWTH FACTORS

The myeloid growth factors are glycoproteins that stimulate the proliferation and differentiation of one or more myeloid cell lines. They also enhance the function of mature granulocytes and monocytes. Recombinant forms of several growth factors have been produced, including granulocyte-macrophage colony-stimulating factor (GM-CSF) (Wong et al., 1985), granulocyte colony-stimulating factor (G-CSF) (Welte et al., 1985), IL-3 (Yang et al., 1986), macrophage colony-stimulating g factor (M-CSF) or CSF-1 (Kawasaki et al., 1985), and stem cell factor (SCF) (Huang et al., 1990) (Table 37–1).

The myeloid growth factors are produced naturally by a number of different cells, including fibroblasts, endothelial cells, macrophages, and T cells (Figure 37–2). They are active at extremely low concentrations and act via membrane receptors of the cytokine receptor superfamily to activate the JAK/STAT signal transduction pathway. GM-CSF is capable of stimulating the proliferation, differentiation, and function of a number of the myeloid cell lineages (Figure 37–1). It acts synergistically with other growth factors, including erythropoietin, at the level of the BFU. GM-CSF stimulates the CFU-GEMM, CFU-GM, CFU-M, CFU-E, and CFU-Meg to increase cell production. It also enhances the migration, phagocytosis, superoxide production, and antibody-dependent cell-mediated toxicity of neutrophils, monocytes, and eosinophils (Weisbart et al., 1987).

The activity of G-CSF is restricted to neutrophils and their progenitors, stimulating their proliferation, differentiation, and function. It acts primarily on the CFU-G, although it also can play a synergistic role with IL-3 and GM-CSF in stimulating other cell lines. G-CSF enhances phagocytic and cytotoxic activities of neutrophils. Unlike GM-CSF, G-CSF has little effect on monocytes, macrophages, and eosinophils and reduces inflammation by inhibiting IL-1, tumor necrosis factor, and interferon gamma. G-CSF also mobilizes primitive hematopoietic cells, including hematopoietic stem cells, from the marrow into the peripheral blood (Sheridan et al., 1992). This observation has virtually transformed the practice of stem cell transplantation, such that >90% of all such procedures today use G-CSF–mobilized peripheral blood stem cells as the donor product.

Granulocyte-Macrophage Colony-Stimulating Factor. Recombinant human GM-CSF (sargramostim) is a 127–amino acid glycoprotein produced in yeast. Except for the substitution of a leucine in position 23 and variable levels of glycosylation, it is identical to endogenous human GM-CSF. Although sargramostim, like natural GM-CSF, has a wide range of effects on cells in culture, its primary therapeutic effect is to stimulate myelopoiesis. The initial clinical application of sargramostim was in patients undergoing autologous bone marrow transplantation. By shortening the duration of neutropenia, transplant morbidity was significantly reduced without a change in long-term survival or risk of inducing an early relapse of the malignant process (Brandt et al., 1988). GM-CSF has also been tested as an adjuvant for immunotherapy, based on its stimulation of dendritic cell growth and development. However, its use in that setting is not discussed in this chapter.

The role of GM-CSF therapy in allogeneic transplantation is less clear. Its effect on neutrophil recovery is less pronounced in patients receiving prophylactic treatment for graft-versus-host disease (GVHD), and studies have failed to show a significant effect on transplant mortality, long-term survival, the appearance of GVHD, or disease relapse. However, it may improve survival in transplant patients who exhibit early graft failure (Nemunaitis et al., 1990). It also has been used to mobilize CD34-positive progenitor cells for peripheral blood stem cell collection for transplantation after myeloablative chemotherapy (Haas et al., 1990). Sargramostim has been used to shorten the period of neutropenia and reduce morbidity in patients receiving intensive cancer chemotherapy (Gerhartz et al., 1993). It also stimulates myelopoiesis in some patients with cyclic neutropenia, myelodysplasia, aplastic anemia, or AIDS-associated neutropenia.

Sargramostim (LEUKINE) is administered by subcutaneous injection or slow intravenous infusion at doses of 125-500 μg/m^2 per day. Plasma levels of GM-CSF rise rapidly after subcutaneous injection and then decline with a $t_{1/2}$ of 2-3 hours. When given intravenously, infusions should be maintained over 3-6 hours. With the initiation of therapy, there is a transient decrease in the absolute leukocyte count secondary to margination and sequestration in the lungs. This is followed by a dose-dependent, biphasic increase in leukocyte counts over the next 7-10 days. Once the drug is discontinued, the leukocyte count returns to baseline within 2-10 days. When GM-CSF is given in lower doses, the response is primarily neutrophilic, whereas monocytosis and eosinophilia are observed at larger doses. After hematopoietic stem cell transplantation or intensive chemotherapy, sargramostim is given daily during the period of maximum neutropenia until a sustained rise in the granulocyte count is observed. Frequent blood counts are essential to avoid an excessive rise in the granulocyte count. The dose may be increased if the patient fails to respond after 7-14 days of therapy. However, higher doses are associated with more pronounced side effects, including bone pain, malaise, flu-like symptoms, fever, diarrhea, dyspnea, and rash. An acute reaction to the first dose, characterized by flushing, hypotension, nausea, vomiting, and dyspnea, with a fall in arterial oxygen saturation due to granulocyte sequestration in the pulmonary circulation occurs in sensitive patients. With prolonged administration, a few patients may develop a capillary leak syndrome, with peripheral edema and pleural and pericardial effusions. Other serious side effects include transient supraventricular arrhythmia, dyspnea, and elevation of serum creatinine, bilirubin, and hepatic enzymes.

Granulocyte Colony-Stimulating Factor. Recombinant human G-CSF filgrastim (NEUPOGEN) is a 175–amino acid glycoprotein produced in *Escherichia coli.* Unlike natural G-CSF, it is not glycosylated and carries an extra N-terminal methionine. The principal action of filgrastim is the stimulation of CFU-G to increase neutrophil production (Figure 37–1). It also enhances the phagocytic and cytotoxic functions of neutrophils.

Filgrastim is effective in the treatment of severe neutropenia after autologous hematopoietic stem cell transplantation and high-dose cancer chemotherapy (Lieschke and Burgess, 1992). Like GM-CSF, filgrastim shortens the period of severe neutropenia and reduces morbidity secondary to bacterial and fungal infections. When used as a part of an intensive chemotherapy regimen, it can decrease the frequency of hospitalization for febrile neutropenia and interruptions in the chemotherapy protocol; a positive impact on patient survival has not been demonstrated. G-CSF also is effective in the treatment of severe congenital neutropenias. In patients with cyclic neutropenia, G-CSF therapy will increase the level of neutrophils and shorten the length of the cycle sufficiently to prevent recurrent bacterial infections (Hammond et al., 1989). Filgrastim therapy can improve neutrophil counts in some patients with myelodysplasia or marrow damage (moderately severe aplastic anemia or tumor infiltration of the marrow). The neutropenia of AIDS patients receiving zidovudine also can be partially or completely reversed. Filgrastim is routinely used in patients undergoing peripheral blood stem cell (PBSC) collection for stem cell transplantation. It promotes the release of $CD34^+$ progenitor cells from the marrow, reducing the number of collections necessary for transplant. Moreover, filgrastim-mobilized PBSCs appear more capable of rapid engraftment. PBSC-transplanted patients require fewer days of platelet and red blood cell transfusions and a shorter duration of hospitalization than do patients receiving autologous bone marrow transplants. Finally, G-CSF–induced mobilization of stem cells into the circulation has been promoted as a way to enhance repair of other damaged organs in which PBSC might play a role. For example, many anecdotal reports have claimed improved cardiac function following the treatment of myocardial infarction patients with G-CSF. However, a meta-analysis of these studies have failed to demonstrate an overall benefit (Abdel-Latif et al., 2008).

Filgrastim is administered by subcutaneous injection or intravenous infusion over at least 30 minutes at doses of 1-20 μg/kg per day. The usual starting dose in a patient receiving myelosuppressive chemotherapy is 5 μg/kg per day. The distribution and clearance rate from plasma ($t_{1/2}$ of 3.5 hours) are similar for both routes of administration. As with GM-CSF therapy, filgrastim given daily after hematopoietic stem cell transplantation or intensive cancer chemotherapy will increase granulocyte production and shorten the period of severe neutropenia. Frequent blood counts should be obtained to determine the effectiveness of the treatment and guide dosage adjustment. In patients who received intensive myelosuppressive cancer chemotherapy, daily administration of G-CSF for ≥14-21 days may be necessary to correct the neutropenia. With less intensive chemotherapy, <7 days of treatment may suffice. In AIDS patients on zidovudine or patients with cyclic neutropenia, chronic G-CSF therapy often is required.

One indication for G-CSF presently under investigation is its use to increase the number of peripheral blood neutrophils in leukocyte donors. For many years it had been hoped that, like platelet transfusions for the bleeding associated with severe thrombocytopenia, neutrophil transfusion could diminish the infectious complications of neutropenia. However, given the short circulatory $t_{1/2}$ of neutrophils (~6 hours) and the need for large numbers of cells, the practical collection of sufficient cell numbers has eluded hematologists. With few complications of therapy in >15 years of clinical experience, G-CSF now has been used to increase peripheral neutrophil counts in prospective donors and neutrophil transfusions (Hubel et al., 2002). Although initial results were modest, the therapy is likely to be optimized and greater efficacy is anticipated.

Adverse reactions to filgrastim include mild to moderate bone pain in patients receiving high doses over a protracted period, local skin reactions following subcutaneous injection, and rare cutaneous necrotizing vasculitis. Patients with a history of hypersensitivity to proteins produced by *E. coli* should not receive the drug. Marked granulocytosis, with counts >100,000/μL, can occur in patients receiving filgrastim over a prolonged period of time. However, this is not associated with any reported clinical morbidity or mortality and rapidly resolves once therapy is discontinued. Mild to moderate splenomegaly has been observed in patients on long-term therapy.

Pegylated recombinant human G-CSF pegfilgrastim (NEULASTA) is generated through conjugation of a 20,000-Da polyethylene glycol moiety to the N-terminal methionyl residue of the 175–amino acid G-CSF glycoprotein produced in *E. coli.* The clearance of pegfilgrastim by glomerular filtration is minimized, thus making neutrophil-mediated clearance the primary route of elimination. Consequently the circulating $t_{1/2}$ of pegfilgrastim is longer than that of filgrastim, allowing for more sustained duration of action and less frequent dosing. Clinical studies suggest that neutrophil-mediated clearance of pegfilgrastim may be self-regulating and therefore specific to each patient's hematopoietic recovery (Crawford, 2002). As such, the recommended dose for pegfilgrastim is fixed at 6 mg administered subcutaneously.

The therapeutic roles of other growth factors still need to be defined, although IL-3 and IL-6 have been removed from testing due to poor efficacy and/or significant toxicity. M-CSF may play a role in stimulating monocyte and macrophage production, although with significant side effects, including splenomegaly and thrombocytopenia. Stem cell factor (SCF) has been shown to augment peripheral blood mobilization of primitive hematopoietic progenitor cells (Moskowitz et al., 1997).

Thrombopoietic Growth Factors

Interleukin-11. Interleukin-11 was cloned based on its activity to promote proliferation of an IL-6–dependent myeloma cell line (Du and Williams, 1994). The 23,000-Da cytokine contains 178 amino acids and stimulates hematopoiesis, intestinal epithelial cell growth, and osteoclasto-genesis and inhibits adipogenesis. Interleukin-11 enhances megakaryocyte maturation *in vitro* (Teramura et al., 1992), and its *in vivo* administration to animals modestly increases peripheral blood platelet counts (Neben et al., 1993). Clinical trials in patients who previously demonstrated significant chemotherapy-induced thrombocytopenia demonstrated that administration of the recombinant cytokine was associated with less severe thrombocytopenia and reduced use of platelet transfusions (Tepler et al., 1996), leading to its approval for clinical use by the FDA.

Recombinant human IL-11 oprelvekin (NEUMEGA) is a bacterially derived 19,000-Da polypeptide of 177 amino acids that differs from the native protein only because it lacks the amino terminal proline residue and is not glycosylated. The recombinant protein has a 7-hour $t_{1/2}$ after subcutaneous injection. In normal subjects, daily administration of oprelvekin leads to a thrombopoietic response in 5-9 days.

The drug is available in single-use vials containing 5 mg and is administered to patients at 25-50 μg/kg per day subcutaneously. Oprelvekin is approved for use in patients undergoing chemotherapy for nonmyeloid malignancies that displayed severe thrombocytopenia (platelet count <20,000/μL) on a prior cycle of the same chemotherapy, and it is administered until the platelet count returns to >100,000/μL. The major complications of therapy are fluid retention and associated cardiac symptoms, such as tachycardia, palpitation, edema, and shortness of breath; this is a significant concern in elderly patients and often requires concomitant therapy with diuretics. Fluid retention reverses upon drug discontinuation, but volume status should be carefully monitored in elderly patients, those with a history of heart failure, or those with preexisting fluid collections in the pleura, pericardium, or peritoneal cavity. Also reported are blurred vision, injection-site rash or erythema, and paresthesias.

Thrombopoietin. The cloning and expression of recombinant thrombopoietin, a cytokine that predominantly stimulates megakaryopoiesis, is potentially another milestone in the development of hematopoietic growth factors as therapeutic agents (Lok et al., 1994) (Table 37–1). Thrombopoietin is a 45,000- to 75,000-Da glycoprotein containing 332 amino acids that is produced by the liver, marrow stromal cells, and many other organs. In both humans and mice, genetic elimination of thrombopoietin or its receptor reduces the platelet counts to 10% of normal values. Moreover, blood levels of the hormone are inversely related to the blood platelet count, together indicating that the hormone is the primary regulator of platelet production.

Administration of recombinant thrombopoietin leads to a log-linear increase in the platelet count in mice, rats, dogs, and nonhuman primates (Harker, 1999) that begins on the third day of administration. In a number of human preclinical trials in several models of chemotherapy- and radiation-induced myelosuppression, thrombopoietin accelerated the recovery of platelet counts and other hematologic parameters (Kaushansky et al., 1998). Of note, however, the agent failed to substantially affect hematopoietic recovery when administered after myeloablative therapy and stem cell transplantation, unless given to the stem cell donor (Fibbe et al., 1995).

Two forms of recombinant thrombopoietin have been developed for clinical use. One is a truncated version of the native polypeptide, termed *recombinant human megakaryocyte growth and development factor* (rHuMGDF), which is produced in bacteria and then covalently modified with polyethylene glycol to increase the circulatory $t_{1/2}$. The second is the full-length polypeptide termed *recombinant human thrombopoietin* (rHuTPO), which is produced in mammalian cells. In vitro, both drugs are equally potent in stimulating megakaryocyte growth.

In clinical trials, both drugs are safe in the patient populations selected for study. However, efficacy results using these agents have been mixed. In a small number of patients with gynecological cancers who were receiving carboplatin (Vadhan-Raj et al., 2000), rHuTPO therapy reduced the duration of severe thrombocytopenia and the need for platelet transfusions. In a similar study of patients treated with carboplatin plus cyclophosphamide, patients receiving a cycle of chemotherapy supplemented with G-CSF plus thrombopoietin had higher platelet counts at nadir and a shorter median duration of severe thrombocytopenia than they did after cycles of therapy supplemented only with G-CSF (Basser et al., 2000). When used to augment peripheral blood counts in preparation for platelet donation, a single dose of thrombopoietin in the platelet donors tripled their platelet counts, allowed for a threefold increase in the number of platelets that could be collected in a single apheresis, and led to a fourfold increase in the mean platelet count noted in transfusion recipients (Kuter et al., 2001). However, this particular regimen was associated with several instances of anti-recombinant thrombopoietin antibodies that cross-reacted with the native hormone, resulting in subsequent thrombocytopenia (Li et al., 2001).

In several studies, although the drug was safe, rHuMGDF was not effective. In two studies of patients treated for 7 days with standard aggressive therapy for acute leukemia, the addition of recombinant thrombopoietin failed to accelerate platelet recovery (Archimbaud et al., 1999). A similar lack of efficacy was seen when the drug was used following autologous peripheral blood stem cell transplantation (Bolwell et al., 2000). Failure to improve hematopoiesis in some of these trials may have resulted from the dosing regimen employed; the optimal dose and schedule of administration in various clinical settings need to be established. After a single bolus injection, platelet counts showed a detectable increase by day 4, peaked by 12-14 days, and then returned to normal over the next 4 weeks. The peak platelet response follows a log-linear dose response. Platelet activation and aggregation are not affected, and patients are not at increased risk of thromboembolic disease, unless the platelet count is allowed to rise to very high levels. These kinetics need to be taken into account when planning therapy in cancer chemotherapy patients.

Due to concerns over the immunogenicity of these agents, and to other considerations, efforts now are under way to develop small molecular mimics of recombinant thrombopoietin, discovered either through screening of phage display peptide libraries or of small organic molecules that have been developed for clinical use. Two of these agents are FDA approved for use in patients with immune thrombocytopenic purpura (ITP) who have failed to respond to more conventional treatments. *Romiplostim* (NPLATE) contains four copies of a small peptide that binds with high affinity to the thrombopoietin receptor, grafted onto an immunoglobulin scaffold. Romiplostim was found safe and efficacious in two randomized controlled studies in patients with ITP. Overall, ~84% of patients responded to the drug with substantial increases in platelet levels, of which approximately half were durable (platelets >50,000/μL for 6 of the last 8 weeks of study) (Kuter et al., 2008). The drug is administered weekly by subcutaneous injection, starting with a dose of 1 μg/kg, titrated to a maximum of 10 μg/kg, until platelet count increases above 50,000/μL. Eltrombopag (PROMACTA) is a small organic molecule that binds specifically to the thrombopoietin receptor and is administered orally. The safety and efficacy of eltrombopag were evaluated in two double-blind placebo-controlled clinical studies of >200 adult patients with chronic ITP who had completed at least one prior treatment course and who had severe thrombocytopenia (Bussel et al., 2007). These studies demonstrated that 70-81% of patients with ITP can be expected to respond to a 6-week course of 50-75 mg/day of eltrombopag. The recommended starting dose is 30 g per day, titrated to 75 mg depending on platelet response. Several of these agents are in clinical trials.

Drugs Effective in Iron Deficiency and Other Hypochromic Anemias

IRON AND IRON SALTS

Iron deficiency is the most common nutritional cause of anemia in humans. It can result from inadequate iron intake, malabsorption, blood loss, or an increased requirement, as with pregnancy. When severe, it results in a characteristic microcytic, hypochromic anemia. However, the impact of iron deficiency is not limited to the erythron (Dallman, 1982). Iron also is an essential component of myoglobin; heme enzymes such as the cytochromes, catalase, and peroxidase; and the metalloflavoprotein enzymes, including xanthine oxidase and the mitochondrial enzyme α-glycerophosphate oxidase. Iron deficiency can affect metabolism in muscle independently of the effect of anemia on oxygen delivery. This may reflect a reduction in the activity of iron-dependent mitochondrial enzymes. Iron deficiency also has been associated with behavioral and learning problems in children, abnormalities in catecholamine metabolism, and possibly, impaired heat production. Awareness of the ubiquitous role of iron has stimulated considerable interest in the early and accurate detection of iron deficiency and in its prevention.

History. The modern understanding of iron metabolism began in 1937 with the work of McCance and Widdowson on iron absorption and excretion and Heilmeyer and Plotner's measurement of iron in plasma (Beutler, 2002). In 1947, Laurell described a plasma iron transport protein that he called *transferrin* (Laurell, 1951). Hahn and coworkers first used radioactive isotopes to measure iron absorption and define the role of the intestinal mucosa to regulate this function (Hahn, 1948). In the next decade, Huff and associates initiated isotopic studies of internal iron metabolism. The subsequent development of practical clinical measurements of serum iron, transferrin saturation, plasma ferritin, and red-cell protoporphyrin permitted the definition and detection of the body's iron store status and iron-deficient erythropoiesis. In 1994, Feder and colleagues identified the HFE gene, which is mutated in type 1 hemochromatosis, on the short arm of chromosome 6 at 6p21.3 (Feder et al., 1996). In 2000, Ganz and colleagues discovered a peptide produced by the liver, which was termed *hepcidin* (Park et al., 2001). Soon thereafter hepcidin was found to be the master regulator of iron homeostasis and to play a role in anemia of chronic disease (Ganz, 2003; Ganz and Nemeth, 2009).

Iron and the Environment. Iron exists in the environment largely as ferric oxide or hydroxide or as polymers. In this state, its biological availability is limited unless solubilized by acid or chelating agents. For example, bacteria and some plants produce high-affinity chelating agents that extract iron from the surrounding environment. Most mammals have little difficulty in acquiring iron; this is explained by an ample iron intake and perhaps also by a greater efficiency in absorbing iron. Humans, however, appear to be an exception. Although total dietary intake of elemental iron in humans usually exceeds requirements, the bioavailability of the iron in the diet is limited.

Metabolism of Iron. The body store of iron is divided between essential iron-containing compounds and excess iron, which is held in storage. Quantitatively, hemoglobin dominates the essential fraction (Table 37–2). This protein, with a molecular weight of 64,500 Da, contains four atoms of iron per molecule, amounting to 1.1 mg (20 μmol) of iron per milliliter of red blood cells. Other forms of essential iron include myoglobin and a variety of heme and nonheme iron-dependent enzymes. Ferritin is a protein-iron storage complex that exists as individual molecules or as aggregates. Apoferritin has a molecular weight of ~450,000 and is composed of 24 polypeptide subunits that form an outer shell, within which resides a storage cavity for polynuclear hydrous ferric oxide phosphate. More than 30% of the weight of ferritin may be iron (4000 atoms of iron per ferritin molecule). Ferritin aggregates, referred to as hemosiderin and visible by light microscopy, constitute about one-third of normal stores, a fraction that increases as stores enlarge. The two predominant sites of iron storage are the reticuloendothelial system and the hepatocytes, although some storage also occurs in muscle.

Table 37–2

The Body Content of Iron

	MG/KG OF BODY WEIGHT	
	MALE	FEMALE
Essential iron		
Hemoglobin	31	28
Myoglobin and enzymes	6	5
Storage iron	13	4
Total	50	37

Internal exchange of iron is accomplished by the plasma protein transferrin (Garrick and Garrick, 2009). This 76-kDa β_1-glycoprotein has two binding sites for ferric iron. Iron is delivered from transferrin to intracellular sites by means of specific transferrin receptors in the plasma membrane. The iron-transferrin complex binds to the receptor, and the ternary complex is internalized through clathrin-coated pits by receptor-mediated endocytosis. A proton-pumping ATPase lowers the pH of the intracellular vesicular compartment (the endosomes) to ~5.5. Iron subsequently dissociates and the receptor returns the apotransferrin to the cell surface, where it is released into the extracellular environment.

Cells regulate their expression of transferrin receptors and intracellular ferritin in response to the iron supply (De Domenico et al., 2008). The synthesis of apoferritin and transferrin receptors is regulated post-transcriptionally by two iron-regulatory proteins 1 and 2

(IRP1 and IRP2). Double knockout of the genes encoding these proteins is embryonic lethal, and conditional double knockout of these genes in the intestine results in cellular iron depletion and death of intestinal epithelial cells (Galy et al., 2008). These IRPs are cytosolic RNA-binding proteins that bind to iron regulating elements (IREs) present in the 5′ or 3′ untranslated regions of mRNA encoding apoferritin or the transferrin receptors, respectively. Binding of these IRPs to the 5′ IRE of apoferritin mRNA represses translation, whereas binding to the 3′ IRE of mRNA encoding the transferrin receptors enhances transcript stability, thereby increasing protein production. When iron is abundant, IRP2 undergoes rapid proteolysis and IRP1 is converted from a RNA-binding protein into aconitase, an enzyme that catalyzes the interconversion of citrate and isocitrate. This results in increased production of apoferritin and reduced production of transferrin receptors. Conversely, when iron is in short supply, these IRPs accumulate, thereby repressing translation of apoferritin while enhancing production of transferrin receptors.

The flow of iron through the plasma amounts to a total of 30-40 mg per day in the adult (~0.46 mg/kg of body weight) (Finch and Huebers, 1982). The major internal circulation of iron involves the erythron and reticuloendothelial cells (Figure 37–3). About 80% of the iron in plasma goes to the erythroid marrow to be packaged into new erythrocytes; these normally circulate for ~120 days before being catabolized by the reticuloendothelial system. At that time, a portion of the iron is immediately returned to the plasma bound to transferrin while another portion is incorporated into the ferritin stores of reticuloendothelial cells and returned to the circulation more gradually. Isotopic studies indicate some degree of iron wastage in this process, in which defective cells or unused portions of their iron are transferred to the reticuloendothelial cell during maturation, bypassing the circulating blood. With abnormalities in erythrocyte maturation, the predominant portion of iron assimilated by the erythroid marrow may be rapidly localized in the reticuloendothelial cells as defective red-cell precursors are broken down; this is termed *ineffective erythropoiesis*. The rate of iron turnover in plasma may be reduced by half or more with red-cell aplasia, with all the iron directed to the hepatocytes for storage.

The most remarkable feature of iron metabolism is the degree to which body stores are conserved. Only 10% of the total is lost per year by normal men (i.e., ~1 mg/day). Two-thirds of this iron is excreted from the gastrointestinal (GI) tract as extravasated red cells, iron in bile, and iron in exfoliated mucosal cells. The other third is accounted for by small amounts of iron in desquamated skin and in the urine. Physiological losses of iron in men vary over a narrow range, from 0.5 mg in the iron-deficient individual to 1.5-2 mg per day when excessive iron is consumed. Additional losses of iron occur in women due to menstruation. Although the average loss in menstruating women is ~0.5 mg per day, 10% of menstruating women lose >2 mg per day. Pregnancy and lactation impose an even greater requirement for iron (Table 37–3). Other causes of iron loss include blood donation, the use of anti-inflammatory drugs that cause bleeding from the gastric mucosa, and GI disease with associated bleeding. Two much rarer causes are the hemosiderinuria that follows intravascular hemolysis, and pulmonary siderosis, where iron deposited in the lungs becomes unavailable to the rest of the body.

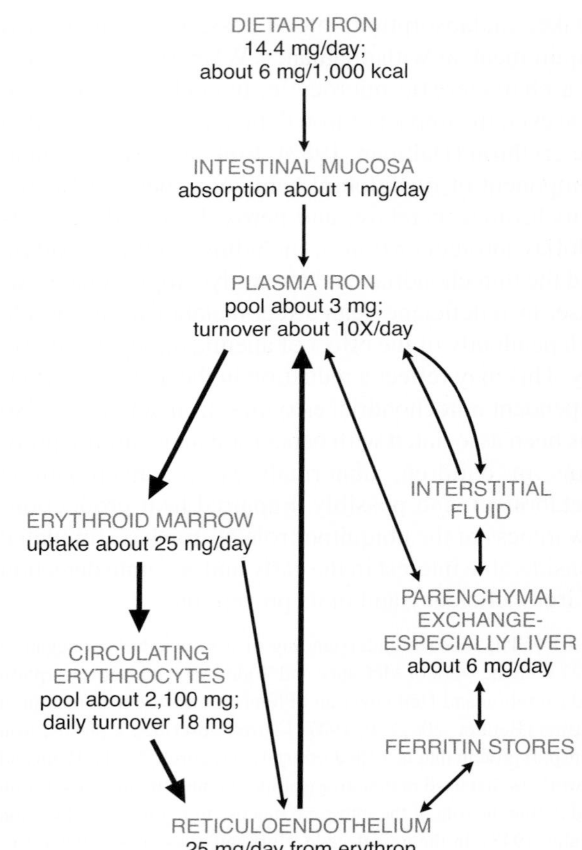

Figure 37–3. *Pathways of iron metabolism in humans (excretion omitted).*

The limited physiological losses of iron point to the primary importance of absorption in determining the body's iron content (Garrick and Garrick, 2009). After acidification and partial digestion of food in the stomach, iron is presented to the intestinal mucosa as either

Table 37–3

Iron Requirements for Pregnancy

	AVERAGE (mg)	RANGE (mg)
External iron loss	170	150–200
Expansion of red cell mass	450	200–600
Fetal iron	270	200–370
Iron in placenta and cord	90	30–170
Blood loss at delivery	150	90–310
Total requirement[a]	980	580–1340
Cost of pregnancy[b]	680	440–1050

[a]Blood loss at delivery not included.
[b]Iron lost by the mother; expansion of red cell mass not included.
Source: Council on Foods and Nutrition. Iron deficiency in the United States. *JAMA* 1968, 203:407–412. Used with permission.

inorganic iron or heme iron. A ferrireductase, duodenal cytochrome B (Dcytb), located on luminal surface of absorptive cells of the duodenum and upper small intestine, reduces the iron to the ferrous state, which is the substrate for the divalent metal (ion) transporter 1 (DMT1). DMT1 transports the iron to basolateral membrane, where it is taken up by another transporter, ferroportin (Fpn; SLC40A1), and subsequently reoxidized to Fe^{3+}, primarily by hephaestin (Hp; HEPH), a transmembrane copper-dependent ferroxidase. Apo-transferrin (Tf) binds the resultant oxidized iron.

Mucosal cell iron transport and the delivery of iron to transferrin from reticuloendothelial stores are both determined by the human hemochromatosis protein, which is a major histocompatibility complex class 1 molecule encoded by the HFE gene (for *H*igh *Fe*) located on the short arm of chromosome 6 at 6p21.3. Regulation is finely tuned to prevent iron overload in times of iron excess while allowing for increased absorption and mobilization of iron stores with iron deficiency. A predominant negative regulator of iron absorption in the small intestine is hepcidin, a 25–amino acid peptide made by hepatocytes (Ganz, 2003). The synthesis of hepcidin is greatly stimulated by inflammation or by iron overload. A deficient hepcidin response to iron loading can contribute to iron overload and one type of hemochromatosis. In anemia of chronic disease, hepcidin production can be increased up to 100-fold, potentially accounting for characteristic features of this condition, namely poor GI uptake and enhanced sequestration of iron in the reticuloendothelial system.

Normal iron absorption is ~1 mg per day in adult men and 1.4 mg per day in adult women; 3-4 mg of dietary iron is the most that normally can be absorbed. Increased iron absorption is seen whenever iron stores are depleted or when erythropoiesis is increased or ineffective. Patients with hereditary hemochromatosis due to HFE mutations demonstrate increased iron absorption and loss of the normal regulation of iron delivery to transferrin by reticuloendothelial cells (Ajioka and Kushner, 2003). The resulting increased saturation of transferrin permits abnormal iron deposition in nonhematopoietic tissues.

Iron Requirements and the Availability of Dietary Iron. Iron requirements are determined by obligatory physiological losses and the needs imposed by growth. Thus adult men require only 13 μg/kg per day (~1 mg), whereas menstruating women require ~21 μg/kg per day (~1.4 mg). In the last two trimesters of pregnancy, requirements increase to ~80 μg/kg per day (5-6 mg), and infants have similar requirements due to their rapid growth. These requirements (Table 37–4) must be considered in the context of the amount of dietary iron available for absorption.

In developed countries, the normal adult diet contains ~6 mg of iron per 1000 calories, providing an average daily intake for adult men of between 12 and 20 mg and for adult women of between 8 and 15 mg. Foods high in iron (>5 mg/100 g) include organ meats such as liver and heart, brewer's yeast, wheat germ, egg yolks, oysters, and certain dried beans and fruits; foods low in iron (<1 mg/100 g) include milk and milk products and most nongreen vegetables. The content of iron in food is affected further by the manner of its preparation because iron may be added from cooking in iron pots.

Although the iron content of the diet obviously is important, of greater nutritional significance is the bioavailability of iron in food. Heme iron, which constitutes only 6% of dietary iron, is far more available and is absorbed independent of the diet composition; it therefore represents 30% of iron absorbed (Conrad and Umbreit, 2002).

The nonheme fraction nonetheless represents far the largest amount of dietary iron ingested by the economically underprivileged. In a vegetarian diet, nonheme iron is absorbed very poorly because of the inhibitory action of a variety of dietary components, particularly phosphates. Ascorbic acid and meat facilitate the absorption of nonheme iron. Ascorbate forms complexes with and/or reduces ferric to ferrous iron. Meat facilitates the absorption of iron by stimulating production of gastric acid; other effects also may be involved. Either of these substances can increase availability several fold. Thus assessment of available dietary iron should include both the amount of iron ingested and an estimate of its availability (Figure 37–4) (Monsen et al., 1978).

A comparison of iron requirements with available dietary iron is seen in Table 37–4. Obviously, pregnancy and infancy represent periods of negative balance. Menstruating women also are at

Table 37–4

Daily Iron Intake and Absorption

SUBJECT	IRON REQUIREMENT (*mg/kg*)	AVAILABLE IRON (*mg/kg*) POOR DIET–GOOD DIET	SAFETY FACTOR *AVAILABLE/REQUIREMENT*
Infant	67	33–66	0.5–1
Child	22	48–96	2–4
Adolescent (male)	21	30–60	1.5–3
Adolescent (female)	20	30–60	1.5–3
Adult (male)	13	26–52	2–4
Adult (female)	21	18–36	1–2
Mid-to-late pregnancy	80	18–36	0.22–0.45

risk, whereas iron balance in adult men and nonmenstruating women is reasonably secure. The difference between dietary supply and requirements is reflected in the size of iron stores, which are low or absent when iron balance is precarious and high when iron balance is favorable (Table 37–2). Thus in infants after the third month of life and in pregnant women after the first trimester, stores of iron are negligible. Menstruating women have approximately one-third the stored iron found in adult men, indicative of the extent to which the additional average daily loss of ~0.5 mg of iron affects iron balance.

Iron Deficiency. Iron deficiency is the most common nutritional disorder (McLean et al., 2009). The prevalence of iron-deficiency anemia in the U.S. is on the order of 1-4% and depends on the economic status of the population. In developing countries, up to 20-40% of infants and pregnant women may be affected. Better iron balance has resulted from the practice of fortifying flour, the use of iron-fortified formulas for infants, and the prescription of medicinal iron supplements during pregnancy.

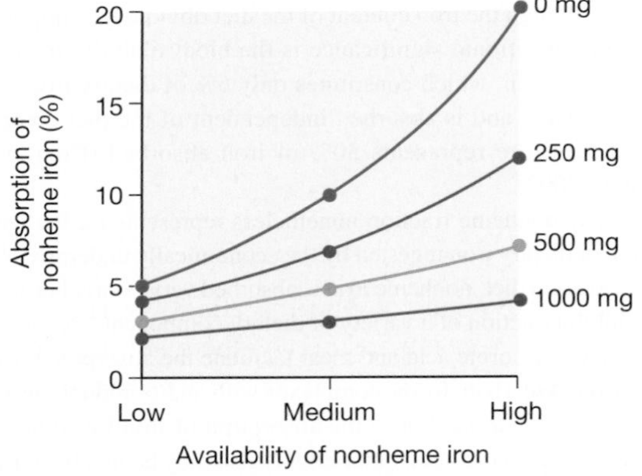

Figure 37–4. *Effect of iron status on the absorption of nonheme iron in food.* The percentages of iron absorbed from diets of low, medium, and high bioavailability in individuals with iron stores of 0, 250, 500, and 1000 mg are portrayed. (After Monsen et al., 1978; reproduced with permission by the American Journal of Clinical Nutrition. © *Am J Clin Nutr*. American Society for Clinical Nutrition.)

Iron-deficiency anemia results from dietary intake of iron that is inadequate to meet normal requirements (nutritional iron deficiency), blood loss, or interference with iron absorption (Clark, 2009). This can have a genetic basis, as in iron-refractory iron deficiency anemia in which patients have iron deficiency that is unresponsive to oral iron, but partially responsive to parenteral iron (Finberg, 2009). Poor oral absorption also can be acquired, as in conditions associated with impaired oral absorption of vitamin B_{12} (Fernandez-Banares et al., 2009), or following partial gastrectomy. More severe iron deficiency is usually the result of blood loss, either from the GI tract, or in women, from the uterus. Finally, treatment of patients with erythropoietin can result in a functional iron deficiency.

Iron deficiency in infants and young children can lead to behavioral disturbances and can impair development, which may not be fully reversible. Iron deficiency in children also can lead to an increased risk of lead toxicity secondary to pica and an increased absorption of heavy metals. Premature and low-birthweight infants are at greatest risk for developing iron deficiency, especially if they are not breast-fed and/or do not receive iron-fortified formula. After the age of 2-3 years, the requirement for iron declines until adolescence when rapid growth combined with irregular dietary habits again increases the risk of iron deficiency. Adolescent girls are at greatest risk; the dietary iron intake of most girls ages 11-18 is insufficient to meet their requirements.

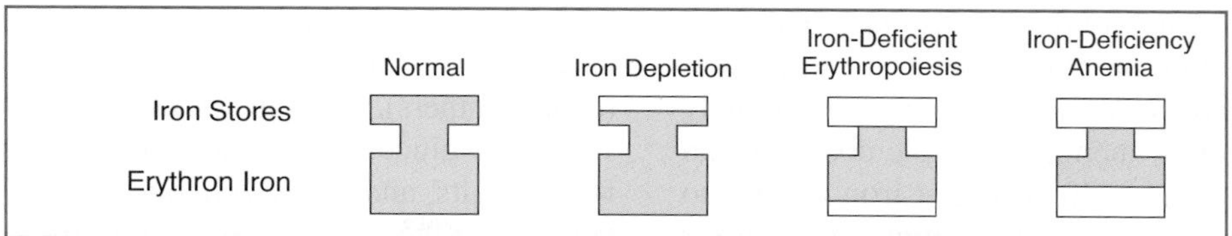

	Normal	Iron Depletion	Iron-Deficient Erythropoiesis	Iron-Deficiency Anemia
Iron Stores / Erythron Iron				
RE marrow Fe	2–3+	0–1+	0	0
Transferrin μg/100 ml (μM)	330 ± 30 (59 ± 5)	360 (64)	390 (70)	410 (73)
Plasma ferritin, μg/l	100 ± 60	20	10	<10
Iron absorption, %	5–10	10–15	10–20	10–20
Plasma iron μg/100 ml (μM)	115 ± 50 (21 ± 9)	115 (21)	<60 (<11)	<40 (<7)
Transferrin saturation, %	35 ± 15	30	<15	<10
Sideroblasts, %	40–60	40–60	<10	<10
RBC protoporphyrin μg/100 ml RBC (μmol per liter RBC)	30 (0.53)	30 (0.53)	100 (1.8)	200 (3.5)
Erythrocytes	Normal	Normal	Normal	Microcytic/ hypochromic

Figure 37–5. *Sequential changes (from left to right) in the development of iron deficiency in the adult.* Red rectangles indicate abnormal test results. RE marrow Fe, reticuloendothelial hemosiderin; RBC, red blood cells. (Adapted from Hillman RS and Finch CA. *Red Cell Manual*, 7th ed. FA Davis Co., Philadelphia, 1997. Used with permission.)

The recognition of iron deficiency rests on an appreciation of the sequence of events that lead to depletion of iron stores. A negative balance first results in a reduction of iron stores and eventually a parallel decrease in red-cell iron and iron-related enzymes (Figure 37–5). In adults, depletion of iron stores may be recognized by a plasma ferritin <12 μg/L and the absence of reticuloendothelial hemosiderin in the marrow aspirate. Iron-deficient erythropoiesis is identified by a decreased saturation of transferrin to <16% and/or by an increase above normal in red-cell protoporphyrin. Iron-deficiency anemia is associated with a recognizable decrease in the concentration of hemoglobin in blood. However, the physiological variation in hemoglobin levels is so great that only about half the individuals with iron-deficient erythropoiesis are identified from their anemia. Moreover, so-called normal hemoglobin and iron values in infancy and childhood are lower because of the more restricted supply of iron in young children (Dallman et al., 1980).

In mild iron deficiency, identifying the underlying cause is more important than any symptoms related to the deficiency state. Because of the frequency of iron deficiency in infants and in menstruating or pregnant women, the need for exhaustive evaluation of such individuals usually is determined by the severity of the anemia. However, iron deficiency in men or postmenopausal women necessitates a search for a site of bleeding.

Although the presence of microcytic anemia is the most common indicator of iron deficiency, laboratory tests—such as measurement of transferrin saturation, red-cell protoporphyrin, and plasma ferritin—are required to distinguish iron deficiency from other causes of microcytosis. Such measurements are particularly useful when circulating red cells are not yet microcytic because of the recent nature of blood loss, but iron supply nonetheless limits erythropoiesis. More difficult is the differentiation of true iron deficiency from iron-deficient erythropoiesis due to inflammation. In the latter condition, iron stores actually are increased, but the release of iron from reticuloendothelial cells is blocked, the concentration of iron in plasma is decreased, and the supply of iron to the erythroid marrow becomes inadequate. The increased stores of iron in this condition may be demonstrated directly by examination of an aspirate of marrow or may be inferred from determination of an elevated plasma concentration of ferritin.

Treatment of Iron Deficiency

General Therapeutic Principles. The response of iron-deficiency anemia to iron therapy is influenced by several factors, including the severity of anemia, the ability of the patient to tolerate and absorb medicinal iron, and the presence of other complicating illnesses. Therapeutic effectiveness is best measured by the resulting increase in the rate of production of red cells. The magnitude of the marrow response to iron therapy is proportional to the severity of the anemia (level of erythropoietin stimulation) and the amount of iron delivered to marrow precursors.

The patient's ability to tolerate and absorb medicinal iron is a key factor in determining the rate of response to therapy. The small intestine regulates absorption, and with increasing doses of oral iron, limits the entry of iron into the bloodstream. This provides a natural ceiling on how much iron can be supplied by oral therapy. In the patient with a moderately severe iron-deficiency anemia, tolerable doses of oral iron will deliver, at most, 40-60 mg of iron per day to the erythroid marrow. This is an amount sufficient for production rates of two to three times normal.

Complicating illness also can interfere with the response of an iron-deficiency anemia to iron therapy. By decreasing the number of red-cell precursors, intrinsic disease of the marrow can blunt the response. Inflammatory illnesses suppress the rate of red-cell production, both by reducing iron absorption and reticuloendothelial release and by direct inhibition of erythropoietin and erythroid precursors. Continued blood loss can mask the response as measured by recovery of the hemoglobin or hematocrit.

Clinically, the effectiveness of iron therapy is best evaluated by tracking the reticulocyte response and the rise in the hemoglobin or the hematocrit. An increase in the reticulocyte count is not observed for at least 4-7 days after beginning therapy. A measurable increase in the hemoglobin level takes even longer. A decision as to the effectiveness of treatment should not be made for 3-4 weeks after the start of treatment. An increase of ≥20 g/L in the concentration of hemoglobin by that time should be considered a positive response, assuming that no other change in the patient's clinical status can account for the improvement and that the patient has not been transfused.

If the response to oral iron is inadequate, the diagnosis must be reconsidered. A full laboratory evaluation should be conducted, and poor compliance by the patient or the presence of a concurrent inflammatory disease must be explored. A source of continued bleeding obviously should be sought. If no other explanation can be found, an evaluation of the patient's ability to absorb oral iron should be considered. There is no justification for merely continuing oral iron therapy beyond 3-4 weeks if a favorable response has not occurred.

Once a response to oral iron is demonstrated, therapy should be continued until the hemoglobin returns to normal. Treatment may be extended if it is desirable to replenish iron stores. This may require a considerable period of time because the rate of absorption of iron by the intestine will decrease markedly as iron stores are reconstituted. The prophylactic use of oral iron should be reserved for patients at high risk, including pregnant women, women with excessive menstrual blood loss, and infants. Iron supplements also may be of value for rapidly growing infants who are consuming substandard diets and for adults with a recognized cause of chronic blood loss. Except for infants, in whom the use of supplemented formulas is routine, the use of over-the-counter mixtures of vitamins and minerals to prevent iron deficiency should be discouraged.

Therapy with Oral Iron. Orally administered ferrous sulfate is the treatment of choice for iron deficiency. Ferrous salts are absorbed about three times as well as ferric salts, and the discrepancy becomes even greater at high dosages. Variations in the particular ferrous salt have relatively little effect on bioavailability; the sulfate (FEOSOL, others), fumarate (HEMOCYTE, FEOSTAT, others), succinate, gluconate (FERGON, others), aspartate, other ferrous salts, and polysaccharide-ferrihydrite complex (NIFEREX, others), are absorbed to approximately the same extent. The effective dose of all of these preparations is based on iron content.

Other iron compounds have utility in fortification of foods. Reduced iron (metallic iron, elemental iron) is as effective as ferrous sulfate, provided that the material employed has a small particle size. Large-particle ferrum reductum and iron phosphate salts have a much lower bioavailability, and their use for the fortification of foods is undoubtedly responsible for some of the confusion concerning effectiveness. Ferric edetate has been shown to have good bioavailability and to have advantages for maintenance of the normal appearance and taste of food.

The amount of iron, rather than the mass of the total salt in iron tablets, is important. It also is essential that the coating of the tablet dissolve rapidly in the stomach. Surprisingly, because iron usually is absorbed in the upper small intestine, certain delayed-release preparations have been reported to be effective and have been said to be even more effective than ferrous sulfate when taken with meals. However, reports of absorption from such preparations vary. Because a number of forms of delayed-release preparations are on the market and information on their bioavailability is limited, the effectiveness of most such preparations must be considered questionable.

A variety of substances designed to enhance the absorption of iron has been marketed, including surface-acting agents, carbohydrates, inorganic salts, amino acids, and vitamins. When present in an amount of ≥200 mg, ascorbic acid increases the absorption of medicinal iron by at least 30%. However, the increased uptake is associated with a significant increase in the incidence of side effects; therefore, the addition of ascorbic acid seems to have little advantage over increasing the amount of iron administered. It is inadvisable to use preparations that contain other compounds with therapeutic actions of their own, such as vitamin B_{12}, folate, or cobalt, because the patient's response to the combination cannot easily be interpreted.

The average dose for the treatment of iron-deficiency anemia is ~200 mg of iron per day (2-3 mg/kg), given in three equal doses of 65 mg. Children weighing 15-30 kg can take half the average adult dose; small children and infants can tolerate relatively large doses of iron, e.g., 5 mg/kg. The dose used is a compromise between the desired therapeutic action and the toxic effects. Prophylaxis and mild nutritional iron deficiency may be managed with modest doses. When the object is the prevention of iron deficiency in pregnant women, e.g., doses of 15 to 30 mg of iron per day are adequate to meet the 3- to 6-mg daily requirement of the last two trimesters. When the purpose is to treat iron-deficiency anemia, but the circumstances do not demand haste, a total dose of ~100 mg (35 mg three times daily) may be used.

The responses expected for different dosage regimens of oral iron are given in Table 37–5. These effects are modified by the severity of the iron-deficiency anemia and by the time of ingestion of iron relative to meals. Bioavailability of iron ingested with food is

Table 37–5

Average Response to Oral Iron

TOTAL DOSE OF IRON (mg/day)	ESTIMATED ABSORPTION %	mg	INCREASE IN BLOOD Hb (g/L/day)
35	40	14	0.7
105	24	25	1.4
195	18	35	1.9
390	12	45	2.2

probably one-half or one-third of that seen in the fasting subject (Grebe et al., 1975). Antacids also reduce iron absorption if given concurrently. It is always preferable to administer iron in the fasting state, even if the dose must be reduced because of GI side effects. For patients who require maximal therapy to encourage a rapid response or to counteract continued bleeding, as much as 120 mg of iron may be administered four times a day. Sustained high rates of red-cell production require an uninterrupted supply of iron, and oral doses should be spaced equally to maintain a continuous high concentration of iron in plasma.

The duration of treatment is governed by the rate of recovery of hemoglobin and the desire to create iron stores. The former depends on the severity of the anemia. With a daily rate of repair of 2 g of hemoglobin per liter of whole blood, the red-cell mass usually is reconstituted within 1-2 months. Thus an individual with a hemoglobin of 50 g per liter may achieve a normal complement of 150 g/L in ~50 days, whereas an individual with a hemoglobin of 100 g/L may take only half that time. The creation of stores of iron requires many months of oral iron administration. The rate of absorption decreases rapidly after recovery from anemia, and after 3-4 months of treatment, stores may increase at a rate of not much more than 100 mg/month. Much of the strategy of continued therapy depends on the estimated future iron balance. Patients with an inadequate diet may require continued therapy with low doses of iron. If the bleeding has stopped, no further therapy is required after the hemoglobin has returned to normal. With continued bleeding, long-term, high-dose therapy clearly is indicated.

Untoward Effects of Oral Preparations of Iron. Intolerance to oral preparations of iron primarily is a function of the amount of soluble iron in the upper GI tract and of psychological factors. Side effects include heartburn, nausea, upper gastric discomfort, and diarrhea or constipation. A good policy is to initiate therapy at a small dosage, to demonstrate freedom from symptoms at that level, and then gradually to increase the dosage to that desired. With a dose of 200 mg of iron per day divided into three equal portions, symptoms occur in ~25% of treated individuals versus 13% among those receiving placebo; this increases to ~40% when the dosage of iron is doubled. Nausea and upper abdominal pain are increasingly common at high dosage. Constipation and diarrhea, perhaps related to iron-induced changes in the intestinal bacterial flora, are not more prevalent at higher dosage, nor is heartburn. If a liquid is given, one can place the iron solution on the back of the tongue with a dropper to prevent transient staining of teeth.

The normal individual apparently is able to control absorption of iron despite high intake, and it is only individuals with underlying disorders that augment the absorption of iron who run the hazard of developing iron overload (hemochromatosis). However, hemochromatosis is a relatively common genetic disorder, present in 0.5% of the population.

Iron Poisoning. Large amounts of ferrous salts are toxic, but fatalities are rare in adults. Most deaths occur in children, particularly between the ages of 12 and 24 months. As little as 1-2 g of iron may cause death, but 2-10 g usually is ingested in fatal cases. The frequency of iron poisoning relates to its availability in the household, particularly the supply that remains after a pregnancy. The colored sugar coating of many of the commercially available tablets gives them the appearance of candy. All iron preparations should be kept in childproof bottles.

Signs and symptoms of severe poisoning may occur within 30 minutes after ingestion or may be delayed for several hours. They include abdominal pain, diarrhea, or vomiting of brown or bloody stomach contents containing pills. Of particular concern are pallor or cyanosis, lassitude, drowsiness, hyperventilation due to acidosis, and cardiovascular collapse. If death does not occur within 6 hours, there may be a transient period of apparent recovery, followed by death in 12-24 hours. The corrosive injury to the stomach may result in pyloric stenosis or gastric scarring. Hemorrhagic gastroenteritis and hepatic damage are prominent findings at autopsy. In the evaluation of a child thought to have ingested iron, a color test for iron in the gastric contents and an emergency determination of the concentration of iron in plasma can be performed. If the latter is <63 μmol (3.5 mg/L), the child is not in immediate danger. However, vomiting should be induced when there is iron in the stomach, and an x-ray should be taken to evaluate the number of pills remaining in the small bowel (iron tablets are radiopaque). Iron in the upper GI tract can be precipitated by lavage with sodium bicarbonate or phosphate solution, although the clinical benefit is questionable. When the plasma concentration of iron is greater than the total iron-binding capacity (63 μmol; 3.5 mg/L), deferoxamine should be administered (Chapter 67). Shock, dehydration, and acid-base abnormalities should be treated in the conventional manner. Most important is the speed of diagnosis and therapy. With early effective treatment, the mortality from iron poisoning can be reduced from as high as 45% to ~1%.

Therapy with Parenteral Iron. When oral iron therapy fails, parenteral iron administration may be an effective alternative (Silverstein and Rodgers, 2004). The rate of response to parenteral therapy is similar to that which follows usual oral doses. Common indications are iron malabsorption (e.g., sprue, short bowel syndrome), severe oral iron intolerance, as a routine supplement to total parenteral nutrition, and in patients who are receiving erythropoietin (Eschbach et al., 1987). In particular, when hemodialysis patients are started on erythropoietin, oral iron therapy alone generally is insufficient to provide an optimal hemoglobin response. It therefore is recommended that sufficient parenteral iron be given to maintain a plasma ferritin level between 100 and 800 μg/L and a transferrin saturation of 20-50% (Goodnough et al., 2000).

Parenteral iron also has been given to iron-deficient patients and pregnant women to create iron stores, something that would take months to achieve by the oral route. The belief that the response to parenteral iron, especially iron dextran, is faster than oral iron is open to debate. In otherwise healthy individuals, the rate of hemoglobin response is determined by the balance between the severity of the anemia (the level of erythropoietin stimulus) and the delivery of iron to the marrow from iron absorption and iron stores. When a large intravenous dose of iron dextran is given to a severely anemic patient, the hematologic response can exceed that seen with oral iron for 1-3 weeks. Subsequently, however, the response is no better than that seen with oral iron.

Parenteral iron therapy should be used only when clearly indicated because acute hypersensitivity, including anaphylactic and anaphylactoid reactions, can occur in 0.2-3% of patients (Faich and Strobos, 1999). Other reactions to intravenous iron include headache, malaise, fever, generalized lymphadenopathy, arthralgias, urticaria, and in some patients with rheumatoid arthritis, exacerbation of the disease.

Four iron formulations are available in the U.S. These are iron dextran (DEXFERRUM or INFED), sodium ferric gluconate (FERRLECIT), ferumoxytol (FERAHEME), and iron sucrose (VENOFER). Ferumoxytol is a semisynthetic carbohydrate-coated superparamagnetic iron oxide nanoparticle that is approved for treatment of iron-deficiency anemia in patients with chronic kidney disease (Balakrishnan et al., 2009). The indications for the iron dextran preparations include treatment of any patient with documented iron deficiency and intolerance or irresponsiveness to oral iron. In contrast, the indications for the ferric gluconate and iron sucrose are limited to patients with chronic kidney disease who have a documented iron deficiency, although broader applications are being advocated (Wish, 2008). Iron dextran is the only preparation that can be given as a total-dose infusion, which is the entire dose of elemental iron required to replace iron stores. However, ferric gluconate and iron sucrose are administered as a fixed dose every week for several weeks until total iron stores are replenished.

Iron Dextran. Iron dextran injection (INFED or DEXFERRUM) is a colloidal solution of ferric oxyhydroxide complexed with polymerized dextran (molecular weight, ~180,000 Da) that contains 50 mg/mL of elemental iron. The use of low-molecular-weight iron dextran has reduced the incidence of toxicity relative to that observed with high molecular weight preparations (IMFERON) (Auerbach and Al Talib, 2008). Iron dextran can be administered by either intravenous (preferred) or intramuscular injection. When given by deep intramuscular injection, it is gradually mobilized via the lymphatics and transported to reticuloendothelial cells; the iron then is released from the dextran complex. Intravenous administration gives a more reliable response. Given intravenously in a dose <500 mg, the iron dextran complex is cleared exponentially with a plasma $t_{1/2}$ of 6 hours. When ≥1 g is administered intravenously as total dose therapy, reticuloendothelial cell clearance is constant at 10-20 mg/hour. This slow rate of clearance results in a brownish discoloration of the plasma for several days and an elevation of the serum iron for 1-2 weeks.

Once the iron is released from the dextran within the reticuloendothelial cells, it is either incorporated into stores or transported via transferrin to the erythroid marrow. Although a portion of the processed iron is rapidly made available to the marrow, a significant fraction is only gradually converted to usable iron stores. All of the iron eventually is released, although many months are required before the process is complete. During this time, the iron dextran stores in reticuloendothelial cells can confuse the clinician who attempts to evaluate the iron status of the patient.

Intramuscular injection of iron dextran should only be initiated after a test dose of 0.5 mL (25 mg of iron). If no adverse reactions are observed, the injections can proceed. The daily dose ordinarily should not exceed 0.5 mL (25 mg of iron) for infants weighing <4.5 kg (10 lb), 1 mL (50 mg of iron) for children weighing <9 kg (20 lb), and 2 mL (100 mg of iron) for other patients. Iron dextran should be injected only into the muscle mass of the upper outer quadrant of the buttock using a z-track technique (displacement of the skin laterally before injection). However, local reactions and the concern about malignant change at the site of injection (Weinbren et al., 1978) make intramuscular administration inappropriate except when the intravenous route is inaccessible.

A test injection of 0.5 mL of undiluted iron dextran or an equivalent amount (25 mg of iron) diluted in saline also should precede intravenous administration of a therapeutic dose of iron dextran. The patient should be observed for signs of immediate anaphylaxis and for an hour after injection for any signs of vascular instability or hypersensitivity, including respiratory distress, hypotension, tachycardia, or back or chest pain. When widely spaced total-dose infusion therapy is given, a test dose injection should be given before each infusion because hypersensitivity can appear at any time. Furthermore, the patient should be monitored closely throughout the infusion for signs of cardiovascular instability. Delayed hypersensitivity reactions also are observed, especially in patients with rheumatoid arthritis or a history of allergies. Fever, malaise, lymphadenopathy, arthralgias, and urticaria can develop days or weeks following injection and last for prolonged periods of time. Therefore, iron dextran should be used with extreme caution in patients with rheumatoid arthritis or other connective tissue diseases, and during the acute phase of an inflammatory illness. Once hypersensitivity is documented, iron dextran therapy must be abandoned.

Before initiating iron dextran therapy, the total dose of iron required to repair the patient's iron-deficient state should be calculated. Relevant factors are the hemoglobin deficit, the need to reconstitute iron stores, and continued excess losses of iron, as seen with hemodialysis and chronic GI bleeding. Iron dextran solution (50 mg/mL of elemental iron) can be administered undiluted in daily doses of 2 mL until the total dose is reached or given off label as a single total-dose infusion. In the latter case, the iron dextran should be diluted in 250-1000 mL of 0.9% saline and infused over an hour or more.

With repeated doses of iron dextran—especially multiple total-dose infusions such as those sometimes used in the treatment of chronic GI blood loss—accumulations of slowly metabolized iron dextran stores in reticuloendothelial cells can be impressive. The plasma ferritin level also can rise to levels associated with iron overload. Although disease-related hemochromatosis has been associated with an increased risk of infections and cardiovascular disease, this has not been shown to be true in hemodialysis patients treated with iron dextran (Owen, 1999). It seems prudent, however, to withhold the drug whenever the plasma ferritin rises above 800 μg/L.

Sodium Ferric Gluconate. Sodium ferric gluconate is an intravenous iron preparation with a molecular size of ~295,000 Da and an osmolality of 990 mOsm/kg^{-1} (Balakrishnan et al., 2009). Administration of ferric gluconate at doses ranging from 62.5-125 mg during hemodialysis is associated with transferrin saturation exceeding 100% (Zanen et al., 1996). Hemodialysis patients who had ferritin levels between 500 and 1200 ng/mL and transferrin saturations of ≤25% while undergoing treatment with erythropoietin had improved hemoglobin values following treatment with ferric gluconate, resulting in reduced requirements for erythropoietin (Kapoian et al., 2008).

Unlike iron dextran, which requires processing by macrophages that may require several weeks, ~80% of sodium ferric gluconate is delivered to transferrin with in 24 hours. Sodium ferric gluconate also has a lower risk of inducing serious anaphylactic reactions than iron dextran (Sengolge et al., 2005). No deaths were reported with 25 million infusions of sodium ferric gluconate, whereas there were 31 infusion-related deaths reported from approximately half the number of patients treated with iron dextran (Faich and Strobos, 1999). Thus, sodium ferric gluconate has become the preferred agent for parenteral iron therapy. Currently iron dextran is reserved for noncompliant patients or for those who are seriously inconvenienced by the multiple infusions that may be required for treatment with sodium ferric gluconate or iron sucrose.

Iron Sucrose. Iron sucrose is complex of polynuclear iron (III)-hydroxide in sucrose with a molecular weight of 252,000 Da and an osmolality of 1316 mOsm/kg^{-1} (Balakrishnan et al., 2009). Following intravenous injection, the complex is taken up by the reticuloendothelial system, where it dissociates into iron and sucrose. Iron sucrose is generally administered in daily amounts of 100-200 mg within a 14-day period to a total cumulative dose of 1000 mg. It can be administered repeatedly to hemodialysis patients as maintenance therapy without inducing hypersensitivity (Aronoff et al., 2004).

Like sodium ferric gluconate, iron sucrose appears to be better tolerated and to cause fewer adverse events than iron dextran (Hayat, 2008). This agent is FDA-approved for the treatment of iron deficiency in patients with chronic kidney disease. However, iron sucrose has been used effectively to treat iron deficiency observed in other clinical settings (al-Momen et al., 1996; Bodemar et al., 2004). However, one study reported that iron sucrose may be most likely of available parenteral iron preparations to induce renal tubular injury because of its high renal uptake (Zager et al., 2004), potentially resulting in tubulointerstitial damage with chronic repeated use (Agarwal, 2006).

Copper

Copper deficiency is extremely rare because the amount present in food is more than adequate to provide the needed body complement of slightly more than 100 mg. There is speculation that marginal deficiency of copper can contribute to development or progression of a number of chronic disorders, such as diabetes or cardiovascular disease (Uriu-Adams and Keen, 2005). However, there is no evidence that copper ever needs to be added to a normal diet, either prophylactically or therapeutically. Even in clinical states associated with hypocupremia (sprue, celiac disease, and nephrotic syndrome), effects of copper deficiency usually are not demonstrable. Anemia due to copper deficiency has been described in individuals who have undergone intestinal bypass surgery (Zidar et al., 1977), in those who are receiving parenteral nutrition (Dunlap et al., 1974), in malnourished infants (Graham and Cordano, 1976), and in patients ingesting excessive amounts of zinc (Hoffman et al., 1988).

Copper has redox properties similar to that of iron, which simultaneously is essential and potentially toxic to the cell (Kim et al., 2008). Cells have virtually no free copper. Instead copper is stored by metallothioneins and distributed by specialized chaperones to sites that make use of its redox properties (Lalioti et al., 2009). Transfer of copper to nascent cuproenzymes is performed by individual or collective activities of P-type ATPases, ATP7A and ATP7B, which are expressed in all tissues (Linz and Lutsenko, 2007). In mammals, the liver is the organ most responsible for the storage, distribution, and excretion of copper. Mutations in ATP7A or ATP7B that interfere with this function have been found responsible for Wilson's disease or Menkes syndrome (steely hair syndrome) (de Bie et al., 2007), respectively, which can result in life-threatening hepatic failure.

Copper deficiency in experimental animals interferes with the absorption of iron and its release from reticuloendothelial cells (Gambling et al., 2008). The associated microcytic anemia is related to a decrease in the availability of iron to the normoblasts, and perhaps even more importantly, to decreased mitochondrial production of heme. It may be that the specific defect in the latter case is a decrease in the activity of cytochrome oxidase. Other pathological effects involving the skeletal, cardiovascular, and nervous systems have been observed in copper-deficient experimental animals. In humans, the prominent findings have been leukopenia, particularly granulocytopenia, and anemia. Concentrations of iron in plasma are variable, and the anemia is not always microcytic. When a low plasma copper concentration is determined in the presence of leukopenia and anemia, a therapeutic trial with copper is appropriate. Daily doses up to 0.1 mg/kg of cupric sulfate have been given by mouth, or 1-2 mg per day may be added to the solution of nutrients for parenteral administration. The daily U.S. Recommended Daily Allowance (RDA) of copper ranges from 1,300 μg for nursing women to 200 μg for infants 0-6 months of age.

Pyridoxine

Harris and associates first described pyridoxine-responsive anemia in 1956. Subsequent reports suggested that the vitamin might improve hematopoiesis in up to 50% of patients with either hereditary or acquired sideroblastic anemia. These patients characteristically have impaired hemoglobin synthesis and accumulate iron in the perinuclear mitochondria of erythroid precursor cells, so-called ringed sideroblasts. Hereditary sideroblastic anemia is an X-linked recessive trait with variable penetrance and expression that results from mutations in the erythrocyte form of δ-aminolevulinate synthase. Affected men typically show a dual population of normal red cells and microcytic, hypochromic cells in the circulation. In contrast, idiopathic acquired sideroblastic anemia and the sideroblastic anemias associated with a number of drugs, inflammatory states, neoplastic disorders, and preleukemic syndromes show a variable morphological picture. Moreover, erythrokinetic studies demonstrate a spectrum of abnormalities, from a hypoproliferative defect with little tendency to accumulate iron to marked ineffective erythropoiesis with iron overload of the tissues (Solomon and Hillman, 1979).

Oral therapy with pyridoxine is of proven benefit in correcting the sideroblastic anemias associated with the antituberculosis drugs isoniazid and pyrazinamide, which act as vitamin B_6 antagonists. A daily dose of 50 mg of pyridoxine completely corrects the defect without interfering with treatment, and routine supplementation of pyridoxine often is recommended (see Chapter 56). In contrast, if pyridoxine is given to counteract the sideroblastic abnormality associated with administration of levodopa, the effectiveness of levodopa in controlling Parkinson's disease is decreased. Pyridoxine therapy does not correct the sideroblastic abnormalities produced by chloramphenicol or lead.

Patients with idiopathic acquired sideroblastic anemia generally fail to respond to oral pyridoxine, and those individuals who appear to have a pyridoxine-responsive anemia require prolonged therapy with large doses of the vitamin, 50-500 mg per day. Unfortunately, the early enthusiasm for treatment with pyridoxine was not reinforced by results of later studies. Moreover, even when a patient with sideroblastic anemia responds, the improvement is only partial because both the ringed sideroblasts and the red-cell defect persist, and the hematocrit rarely returns to normal. Nonetheless, in view of the low toxicity of oral pyridoxine, a therapeutic trial with pyridoxine is appropriate.

As shown in studies of normal subjects, oral pyridoxine in a dosage of 100 mg three times daily produces a maximal increase in red-cell pyridoxine kinase and the major pyridoxal phosphate–dependent enzyme glutamic-aspartic aminotransferase (Solomon and Hillman, 1978). For an adequate therapeutic trial, the drug is administered for at least 3 months while the response is monitored by measuring the reticulocyte index and the hemoglobin concentration. The occasional patient who is refractory to oral pyridoxine may respond to parenteral administration of pyridoxal phosphate. However, oral pyridoxine in doses of 200-300 mg per day produces intracellular concentrations of pyridoxal phosphate equal to or greater than those generated by therapy with the phosphorylated vitamin.

Riboflavin

Pure red-cell aplasia that responded to the administration of riboflavin was reported in patients with protein depletion and complicating infections. Lane and associates induced riboflavin deficiency in humans and demonstrated that a hypoproliferative anemia resulted within a month. The spontaneous appearance in humans of red-cell aplasia due to riboflavin deficiency undoubtedly is rare, if it occurs at all. It has been described in combination with infection and protein deficiency, both of which are capable of producing a hypoproliferative anemia. However, it seems reasonable to include riboflavin in the nutritional management of patients with gross, generalized malnutrition.

B_{12}, Folic Acid, and the Treatment of Megaloblastic Anemias

Vitamin B_{12} and folic acid are dietary essentials (Varela-Moreiras et al., 2009). A deficiency of either vitamin impairs DNA synthesis in any cell in which chromosomal replication and division are taking place. Because tissues with the greatest rate of cell turnover show the most dramatic changes, the hematopoietic system is especially sensitive to deficiencies of these vitamins. An early sign of deficiency is megaloblastic anemia. Abnormal macrocytic red blood cells are produced, and the patient becomes severely anemic. Recognized in the 19th century, this pattern of abnormal hematopoiesis, termed *pernicious anemia,* spurred investigations that ultimately led to the discovery of vitamin B_{12} and folic acid. Even today, the characteristic abnormality in red blood cell morphology is important for diagnosis and as a therapeutic guide following administration of the vitamins.

History. The discovery of vitamin B_{12} and folic acid is a dramatic story that started >180 years ago and includes two discoveries that won the Nobel Prize. The first descriptions of what must have been megaloblastic anemias came from the work of Combe and Addison, who published a series of case reports beginning in 1824. It still is common practice to describe megaloblastic anemia as Addisonian pernicious anemia. Although Combe suggested that the disorder might have some relationship to digestion, it was Austin Flint who in 1860 first described the severe gastric atrophy and called attention to its possible relationship to the anemia.

After the observation by Whipple in 1925 that liver is a source of a potent hematopoietic substance for iron-deficient dogs, Minot and Murphy carried out Nobel Prize–winning experiments that demonstrated the effectiveness of the feeding of liver to reverse pernicious anemia. Soon thereafter, Castle defined the need for both intrinsic factor, a substance secreted by the parietal cells of the gastric mucosa, and extrinsic factor, the vitamin-like material provided by crude liver extracts. Nearly 20 years passed before Rickes and coworkers and Smith and Parker isolated and crystallized vitamin B_{12}; Dorothy Hodgkin received the Nobel Prize for determining its x-ray crystal structure.

As attempts were being made to purify extrinsic factor, Wills and her associates described a macrocytic anemia in women in India that responded to a factor present in crude liver extracts but not in the purified fractions known to be effective in pernicious anemia. This factor, first called Wills' factor and later vitamin M, is now known to be folic acid. The term *folic acid* was coined by Mitchell and coworkers in 1941, after its isolation from leafy vegetables.

More recent work has shown that neither vitamin B_{12} nor folic acid as purified from foodstuffs is the active coenzyme in humans. During extraction, active labile forms are converted to stable congeners of vitamin B_{12} and folic acid, cyanocobalamin and pteroylglutamic acid, respectively. These congeners must then be modified *in vivo* to be effective. Although a great deal has been learned about the intracellular metabolic pathways in which these vitamins function as required cofactors, many questions remain, among them: what is the relationship of vitamin B_{12} deficiency to the neurological abnormalities that occur with this disorder?

Relationships Between Vitamin B_{12} and Folic Acid. The major roles of vitamin B_{12} and folic acid in intracellular metabolism are summarized in Figure 37–6. Intracellular vitamin B_{12} is maintained as two active coenzymes: methylcobalamin and deoxyadenosylcobalamin. Deoxyadenosylcobalamin (deoxyadenosyl B_{12}) is a cofactor for the mitochondrial mutase enzyme that catalyzes the isomerization of l-methylmalonyl CoA to succinyl CoA, an important reaction in carbohydrate and lipid metabolism. This reaction has no direct relationship to the metabolic pathways that involve folate. In contrast, methylcobalamin (CH_3B_{12}) supports the methionine synthetase reaction, which is essential for normal metabolism of folate (Weissbach, 2008). Methyl groups contributed by methyltetrahydrofolate ($CH_3H_4PteGlu_1$) are used to form methylcobalamin, which then acts as a methyl group donor for the conversion of homocysteine to methionine. This folate–cobalamin interaction is pivotal for normal synthesis of purines and pyrimidines, and therefore of DNA. The methionine synthetase reaction is largely responsible for the control of the recycling of folate cofactors; the maintenance of intracellular concentrations of folylpolyglutamates; and, through the synthesis of methionine and its product, S-adenosylmethionine, the maintenance of a number of methylation reactions.

Because methyltetrahydrofolate is the principal folate congener supplied to cells, the transfer of the

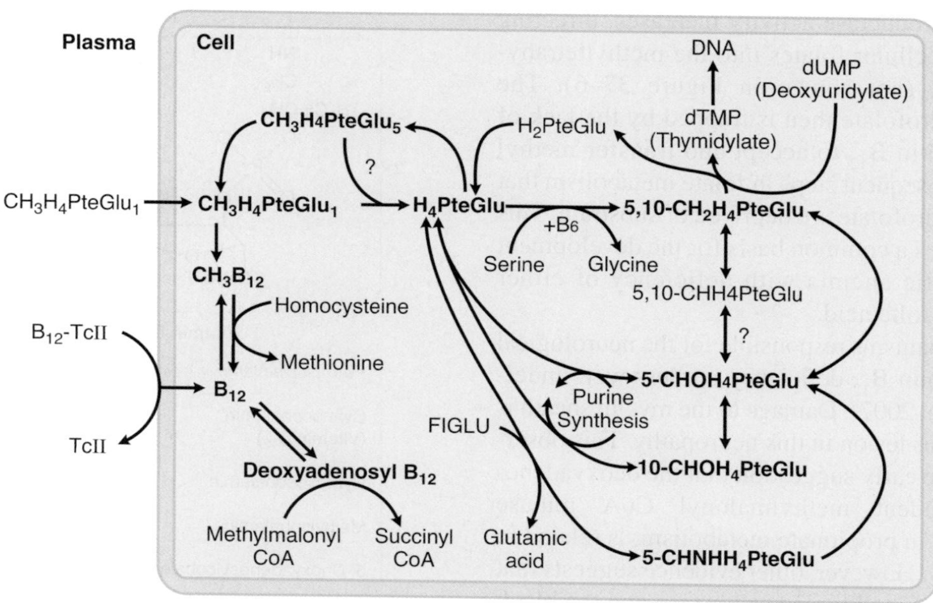

Figure 37–6. *Interrelationships and metabolic roles of vitamin B_{12} and folic acid. See* text for explanation and Figure 37–7 for structures of the various folate coenzymes. FIGLU, formiminoglutamic acid, which arises from the catabolism of histidine; TcII, transcobalamin II; $CH_3H_4PteGlu_1$, methyltetrahydrofolate.

methyl group to cobalamin is essential for the adequate supply of tetrahydrofolate ($H_4PteGlu_1$), the substrate for a number of metabolic steps. Tetrahydrofolate is a precursor for the formation of intracellular folylpolyglutamates; it also acts as the acceptor of a one-carbon unit in the conversion of serine to glycine, with the resultant formation of 5,10-methylenetetrahydrofolate (5,10-CH_2H_4PteGlu). The latter derivative donates the methylene group to deoxyuridylate (dUMP) for the synthesis of thymidylate (dTMP)—an extremely important reaction in DNA synthesis. In the process, the 5,10-CH_2H_4PteGlu is converted to dihydrofolate (H_2PteGlu). The cycle then is completed by the reduction of the H_2PteGlu to H_4PteGlu by dihydrofolate reductase, the step that is blocked by folate antagonists such as methotrexate (Chapter 61). As shown in Figure 37–6, other pathways also lead to the synthesis of 5,10-methylenetetrahydrofolate. These pathways are important in the metabolism of formiminoglutamic acid (FIGLU) and purines and pyrimidines.

In the presence of a deficiency of either vitamin B_{12} or folate, the decreased synthesis of methionine and S-adenosylmethionine interferes with protein biosynthesis, a number of methylation reactions, and the synthesis of polyamines. In addition, the cell responds to the deficiency by redirecting folate metabolic pathways to supply increasing amounts of methyltetrahydrofolate; this tends to preserve essential methylation reactions at the expense of nucleic acid synthesis. With vitamin B_{12} deficiency, methylenetetrahydrofolate reductase activity increases, directing available intracellular folates into the methyltetrahydrofolate pool (not shown in Figure 37–6). The methyltetrahydrofolate then is trapped by the lack of sufficient vitamin B_{12} to accept and transfer methyl groups, and subsequent steps in folate metabolism that require tetrahydrofolate are deprived of substrate. This process provides a common basis for the development of megaloblastic anemia with deficiency of either vitamin B_{12} or folic acid.

The mechanisms responsible for the neurological lesions of vitamin B_{12} deficiency are less well understood (Solomon, 2007). Damage to the myelin sheath is the most obvious lesion in this neuropathy. This observation led to the early suggestion that the deoxyadenosyl B_{12}–dependent methylmalonyl CoA mutase reaction, a step in propionate metabolism, is related to the abnormality. However, other evidence suggests that the deficiency of methionine synthetase and the block of the conversion of methionine to S-adenosylmethionine are more likely to be responsible.

Nitrous oxide (N_2O), used for anesthesia (Chapter 19), can cause megaloblastic changes in the marrow and a neuropathy that resemble those of vitamin B_{12} deficiency. Studies with N_2O have demonstrated a reduction in methionine synthetase and reduced concentrations of methionine and S-adenosylmethionine. The latter is necessary for methylation reactions, including those required for the synthesis of phospholipids and myelin. Significantly, the neuropathy induced with N_2O can be prevented partially by feeding methionine. A neuropathy similar to that occurring with vitamin B_{12} deficiency has been reported in dentists who are exposed to N_2O used as an anesthetic.

Vitamin B_{12}

Chemistry. The structural formula of vitamin B_{12} is shown in Figure 37–7. These are the three major portions of the molecule:

1. A planar group or corrin nucleus—a porphyrin-like ring structure with four reduced pyrrole rings (A-D in Figure 37–7)

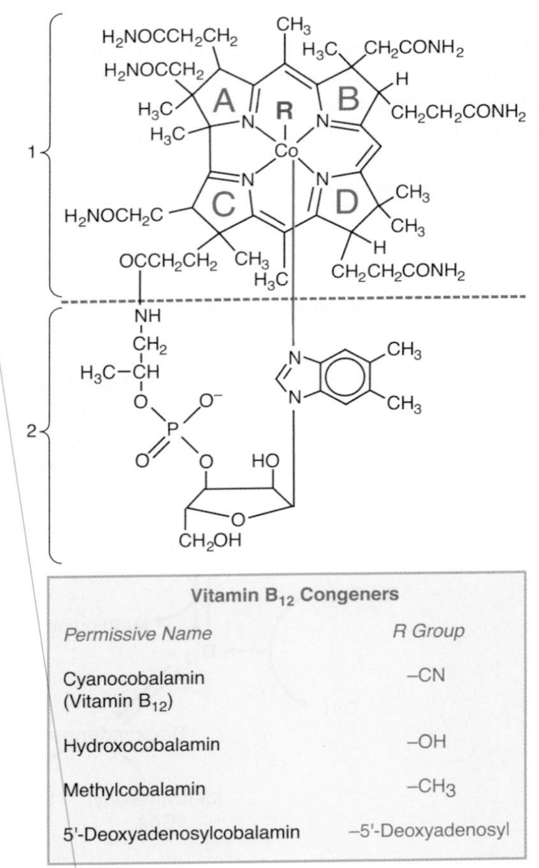

Vitamin B_{12} Congeners

Permissive Name	*R Group*
Cyanocobalamin (Vitamin B_{12})	–CN
Hydroxocobalamin	–OH
Methylcobalamin	$-CH_3$
5'-Deoxyadenosylcobalamin	–5'-Deoxyadenosyl

Figure 37–7. *The structures and nomenclature of vitamin B_{12} congeners.*

linked to a central cobalt atom and extensively substituted with methyl, acetamide, and propionamide residues.

2. A 5,6-dimethylbenzimidazolyl nucleotide, which links almost at right angles to the corrin nucleus with bonds to the cobalt atom and to the propionate side chain of the C pyrrole ring.
3. A variable R group—the most important of which are found in the stable compounds cyanocobalamin and hydroxocobalamin and the active coenzymes methylcobalamin and 5-deoxyadenosylcobalamin.

The terms *vitamin B_{12}* and *cyanocobalamin* are used interchangeably as generic terms for all of the cobamides active in humans. Preparations of vitamin B_{12} for therapeutic use contain either cyanocobalamin or hydroxocobalamin because only these derivatives remain active after storage.

Metabolic Functions. The active coenzymes methylcobalamin and 5-deoxyadenosylcobalamin are essential for cell growth and replication. Methylcobalamin is required for the conversion of homocysteine to methionine and its derivative S-adenosylmethionine. In addition, when concentrations of vitamin B_{12} are inadequate, folate becomes "trapped" as methyltetrahydrofolate to cause a functional deficiency of other required intracellular forms of folic acid (see Figures 37–6 and 37–7 and preceding discussion). The hematologic abnormalities in vitamin B_{12}–deficient patients result from this process. 5-Deoxyadenosylcobalamin is required for the re-arrangement of methylmalonyl CoA to succinyl CoA (Figure 37–6).

Sources in Nature. Humans depend on exogenous sources of vitamin B_{12}. In nature, the primary sources are certain microorganisms that grow in soil, sewage, water, or the intestinal lumen of animals that synthesize the vitamin. Vegetable products are free of vitamin B_{12} unless they are contaminated with such microorganisms, so that animals are dependent on synthesis in their own alimentary tract or the ingestion of animal products containing vitamin B_{12}. The daily nutritional requirement of 3-5 μg must be obtained from animal by-products in the diet. Despite this, strict vegetarians rarely develop vitamin B_{12} deficiency. Some vitamin B_{12} is available from legumes, which are contaminated with bacteria capable of synthesizing vitamin B_{12}, and vegetarians often fortify their diets with a wide range of vitamins and minerals.

Absorption, Distribution, Elimination, and Daily Requirements. In the presence of gastric acid and pancreatic proteases, dietary vitamin B_{12} is released from food and salivary binding protein and bound to gastric intrinsic factor. When the vitamin B_{12}–intrinsic factor complex reaches the ileum, it interacts with a receptor on the mucosal cell surface and is actively transported into circulation. Adequate intrinsic factor, bile, and sodium bicarbonate (to provide a suitable pH) all are required for ileal transport of vitamin B_{12}. Vitamin B_{12} deficiency in adults is rarely the result of a deficient diet per se; rather, it usually reflects a defect in one or another aspect of this complex sequence of absorption (Figure 37–8). Achlorhydria and decreased secretion of intrinsic factor by parietal cells secondary to gastric atrophy or gastric surgery is a common cause of vitamin B_{12} deficiency in adults. Antibodies to parietal cells or intrinsic factor complex also can play a prominent role in producing a deficiency. A number of intestinal diseases can interfere with absorption, including pancreatic disorders (loss of pancreatic protease secretion), bacterial overgrowth, intestinal parasites, sprue, and localized damage to ileal mucosal cells by disease or as a result of surgery.

Once absorbed, vitamin B_{12} binds to transcobalamin II, a plasma β-globulin, for transport to tissues. Two other transcobalamins (I and III) also are present in plasma; their concentrations are related to the rate of turnover of granulocytes. They may represent

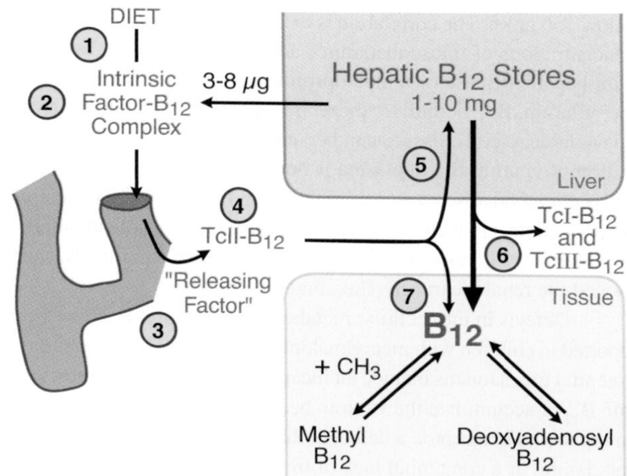

Figure 37–8. *The absorption and distribution of vitamin B_{12}.* Deficiency of vitamin B_{12} can result from a congenital or acquired defect in any one of the following: (1) inadequate dietary supply; (2) inadequate secretion of intrinsic factor (classical pernicious anemia); (3) ileal disease; (4) congenital absence of transcobalamin II (TcII); or (5) rapid depletion of hepatic stores by interference with reabsorption of vitamin B_{12} excreted in bile. The utility of measurements of the concentration of vitamin B_{12} in plasma to estimate supply available to tissues can be compromised by liver disease and (6) the appearance of abnormal amounts of transcobalamins I and III (TcI and III) in plasma. Finally, the formation of methylcobalamin requires (7) normal transport into cells and an adequate supply of folic acid as $CH_3H_4PteGlu_1$.

intracellular storage proteins that are released with cell death. Vitamin B_{12} bound to transcobalamin II is rapidly cleared from plasma and preferentially distributed to hepatic parenchymal cells. The liver is a storage depot for other tissues. In normal adults, as much as 90% of the body's stores of vitamin B_{12}, from 1-10 mg, is in the liver. Vitamin B_{12} is stored as the active coenzyme with a turnover rate of 0.5-8 μg per day, depending on the size of the body stores. The recommended daily intake of the vitamin in adults is 2.4 μg.

Approximately 3 μg of cobalamins are secreted into bile each day, 50-60% of which is not destined for reabsorption. This enterohepatic cycle is important because interference with reabsorption by intestinal disease can progressively deplete hepatic stores of the vitamin. This process may help explain why patients can develop vitamin B_{12} deficiency within 3-4 years of major gastric surgery, even though a daily requirement of 1-2 μg would not be expected to deplete hepatic stores of more than 2 to 3 mg during this time.

The supply of vitamin B_{12} available for tissues is directly related to the size of the hepatic storage pool and the amount of vitamin B_{12} bound to transcobalamin II (Figure 37–8). The plasma concentration of vitamin B_{12} is the best routine measure of B_{12} deficiency, and normally ranges from 150-660 pmol (~200-900 pg/mL). Deficiency should be suspected whenever the concentration falls below 150 pmol. The correlation is excellent except when the plasma concentrations of transcobalamin I and III are increased, as occurs with hepatic disease or a myeloproliferative disorder. Inasmuch as the vitamin B_{12} bound to these transport proteins is relatively unavailable to cells, tissues can become deficient when the concentration of vitamin B_{12} in plasma is normal or even high. In subjects with congenital absence of transcobalamin II, megaloblastic anemia occurs despite relatively normal plasma concentrations of vitamin B_{12}; the anemia will respond to parenteral doses of vitamin B_{12} that exceed the renal clearance (Hakami et al., 1971).

Defects in intracellular metabolism of vitamin B_{12} have been reported in children with methylmalonic aciduria and homocystinuria. Potential mechanisms include an incapacity of cells to transport vitamin B_{12} or accumulate the vitamin because of a failure to synthesize an intracellular acceptor, a defect in the formation of deoxyadenosylcobalamin, or a congenital lack of methylmalonyl CoA isomerase.

Vitamin B_{12} Deficiency. Vitamin B_{12} deficiency is recognized clinically by its impact on the hematopoietic and nervous systems. The sensitivity of the hematopoietic system relates to its high rate of cell turnover. Other tissues with high rates of cell turnover (e.g., mucosa and cervical epithelium) also have high requirements for the vitamin.

As a result of an inadequate supply of vitamin B_{12}, DNA replication becomes highly abnormal. Once a hematopoietic stem cell is committed to enter a programmed series of cell divisions, the defect in chromosomal replication results in an inability of maturing cells to complete nuclear divisions while cytoplasmic maturation continues at a relatively normal rate. This results in the production of morphologically abnormal cells and death of cells during maturation, a phenomenon referred to as *ineffective hematopoiesis.* These abnormalities are readily identified by examination of the marrow and peripheral blood. Maturation of red-cell precursors is highly abnormal (megaloblastic erythropoiesis). Those cells that do leave the marrow also are abnormal, and many cell fragments, poikilocytes, and macrocytes appear in the peripheral blood. The mean red-cell volume increases to values >110 fL. Severe deficiency affects all cell lines, and a pronounced pancytopenia results.

The diagnosis of a vitamin B_{12} deficiency usually can be made using measurements of the serum vitamin B_{12} and/or serum methylmalonic acid. The latter is somewhat more sensitive and has been used to identify metabolic deficiency in patients with normal serum vitamin B_{12} levels. As part of the clinical management of a patient with severe megaloblastic anemia, a therapeutic trial using very small doses of the vitamin can be used to confirm the diagnosis. Serial measurements of the reticulocyte count, serum iron, and hematocrit are performed to define the characteristic recovery of normal red-cell production. The Schilling test can be used to measure the absorption of the vitamin and delineate the mechanism of the disease. By performing the Schilling test with and without added intrinsic factor, it is possible to discriminate between intrinsic factor deficiency by itself and primary ileal cell disease.

Vitamin B_{12} deficiency can irreversibly damage the nervous system. Progressive swelling of myelinated neurons, demyelination, and neuronal cell death are seen in the spinal column and cerebral cortex. This causes a wide range of neurological signs and symptoms, including paresthesias of the hands and feet, decreased vibration and position senses with resultant unsteadiness, decreased deep tendon reflexes, and in the later stages, confusion, moodiness, loss of memory, and even a loss of central vision. The patient may exhibit delusions, hallucinations, or even overt psychosis. Because the neurological damage can be dissociated from the changes in the hematopoietic system, vitamin B_{12} deficiency must be considered in elderly patients with dementia or psychiatric disorders, even if they are not anemic.

Vitamin B_{12} Therapy. Vitamin B_{12} is available for injection or oral administration; combinations with other vitamins and minerals also can be given orally or parenterally. The choice of a preparation always depends on the cause of the deficiency. Although oral preparations may be used to supplement deficient diets, they are of limited value in the treatment of patients with deficiency of intrinsic factor or ileal disease. Even though small amounts of vitamin B_{12} may be absorbed by simple diffusion, the oral administration cannot be relied on for effective therapy in the patient with a marked deficiency of vitamin B_{12} and abnormal hematopoiesis or neurological deficits. Therefore, the preparation of choice for treatment of a vitamin B_{12} deficiency state is cyanocobalamin, and it should be administered by intramuscular or subcutaneous injection.

Cyanocobalamin injection is safe when given by the intramuscular or deep subcutaneous route, but it should never be given intravenously. There have been rare reports of transitory exanthema and anaphylaxis after injection. If a patient reports a previous sensitivity to injections of vitamin B_{12}, an intradermal skin test should be performed before the full dose is administered.

Cyanocobalamin is administered in doses of 1-1000 μg. Tissue uptake, storage, and utilization depend on the availability of transcobalamin II (discussed earlier). Doses >100 μg are cleared rapidly from plasma into the urine, and administration of larger amounts of vitamin B_{12} will not result in greater retention of the vitamin. Administration of 1000 μg is of value in the performance of the Schilling test. After isotopically labeled vitamin B_{12} is administered orally, the compound that is absorbed can be quantitatively recovered in the urine if 1000 μg of cyanocobalamin is administered intramuscularly. This unlabeled material saturates the transport system and tissue binding sites, so >90% of the labeled and unlabeled vitamin is excreted during the next 24 hours.

A number of multivitamin preparations are marketed either as nutritional supplements or for the treatment of anemia. Many of these contain up to 80 μg of cyanocobalamin without or with intrinsic factor concentrate prepared from the stomachs of hogs or other domestic animals. One oral unit of intrinsic factor is defined as that amount of material that will bind and transport 15 μg of cyanocobalamin. Most multivitamin preparations supplemented with intrinsic factor contain 0.5 oral unit per tablet. Although the combination of oral vitamin B_{12} and intrinsic factor would appear to be ideal for patients with an intrinsic factor deficiency, such preparations are not reliable. With prolonged therapy, some patients become refractory to oral intrinsic factor, perhaps related to production of an intraluminal antibody against the hog protein. Patients taking such preparations must be reevaluated at periodic intervals for recurrence of pernicious anemia.

Hydroxocobalamin given in doses of 100 μg intramuscularly has been reported to have a more sustained effect than cyanocobalamin, with a single dose maintaining plasma vitamin B_{12} concentrations in the normal range for up to 3 months. However, some patients show reductions of the concentration of vitamin B_{12} in plasma within 30 days, similar to that seen after cyanocobalamin. Furthermore, the administration of hydroxocobalamin has resulted in the formation of antibodies to the transcobalamin II–vitamin B_{12} complex.

Vitamin B_{12} has an undeserved reputation as a health tonic and has been used for a number of disease states. Effective use of the vitamin depends on accurate diagnosis and an understanding of the following general principles of therapy:

1. Vitamin B_{12} should be given prophylactically only when there is a reasonable probability that a deficiency exists or will exist. Dietary deficiency in the strict vegetarian, the predictable malabsorption of vitamin B_{12} in patients who have had a gastrectomy, and certain diseases of the small intestine constitute such indications. When GI function is normal, an oral prophylactic supplement of vitamins and minerals, including vitamin B_{12}, may be indicated. Otherwise, the patient should receive monthly injections of cyanocobalamin.
2. The relative ease of treatment with vitamin B_{12} should not prevent a full investigation of the etiology of the deficiency. The initial diagnosis usually is suggested by a macrocytic anemia or an unexplained neuropsychiatric disorder. Full understanding of the etiology of vitamin B_{12} deficiency involves studies of dietary supply, GI absorption, and transport.
3. Therapy always should be as specific as possible. Although a large number of multivitamin preparations are available, the use of shotgun vitamin therapy in the treatment of vitamin B_{12} deficiency can be dangerous. With such therapy, there is the danger that sufficient folic acid will be given to result in a hematologic recovery that can mask continued vitamin B_{12} deficiency and permit neurological damage to develop or progress.
4. Although a classical therapeutic trial with small amounts of vitamin B_{12} can help confirm the diagnosis, acutely ill elderly patients may not be able to tolerate the delay in the correction of a severe anemia. Such patients require supplemental blood transfusions and immediate therapy with folic acid and vitamin B_{12} to guarantee rapid recovery.
5. Long-term therapy with vitamin B_{12} must be evaluated at intervals of 6-12 months in patients who are otherwise well. If there is an additional illness or a condition that may increase the requirement for the vitamin (e.g., pregnancy), reassessment should be performed more frequently.

Treatment of the Acutely Ill Patient. The therapeutic approach depends on the severity of the patient's illness. In uncomplicated pernicious anemia, in which the abnormality is restricted to a mild or moderate anemia without leukopenia, thrombocytopenia, or neurological signs or symptoms, the administration of vitamin B_{12} alone will suffice. Moreover, therapy may be delayed until other causes of megaloblastic anemia have been excluded and sufficient studies of GI function have been performed to reveal the underlying cause of the disease. In this situation, a therapeutic trial with small amounts of parenteral vitamin B_{12} (1-10 μg per day) can confirm the presence of an uncomplicated vitamin B_{12} deficiency.

In contrast, patients with neurological changes or severe leukopenia or thrombocytopenia associated with infection or bleeding require emergency treatment. The older individual with a severe anemia (hematocrit <20%) is likely to have tissue hypoxia, cerebrovascular insufficiency, and congestive heart failure. Effective therapy must not wait for detailed diagnostic tests. Once the megaloblastic erythropoiesis has been confirmed and sufficient blood collected for later measurements of vitamin B_{12} and folic acid, the patient should receive intramuscular injections of 100 μg of cyanocobalamin and 1-5 mg of folic acid. For the next 1-2 weeks the patient should receive daily intramuscular injections of 100 μg of cyanocobalamin, together with a daily oral supplement of 1 to 2 mg of folic acid. Because an effective increase in red-cell mass will not occur for 10-20 days, the patient with a markedly depressed hematocrit and tissue hypoxia also should receive a transfusion of 2-3 units of packed red blood cells. If congestive heart failure is present, diuretics can be administered to prevent volume overload.

Patients usually report an increased sense of well-being within the first 24 hours of the initiation of therapy. Objectively, memory and orientation can improve dramatically, although full recovery of mental function may take months, or it may never occur. In addition, even before an obvious hematologic response is apparent, the patient may report an increase in strength, a better appetite, and reduced soreness of the mouth and tongue.

The first objective hematologic change is the disappearance of the megaloblastic morphology of the bone marrow. As the ineffective erythropoiesis is corrected, the concentration of iron in plasma falls dramatically as the metal is used in the formation of hemoglobin. This usually occurs within the first 48 hours. Full correction of precursor maturation in marrow with production of an increased number of reticulocytes begins about the second or third day and peaks 3-5 days later. When the anemia is moderate to severe, the maximal reticulocyte index will be between three and five times the normal value (i.e., a reticulocyte count of 20-40%). The ability of the marrow to sustain a high rate of production determines the rate of recovery of the hematocrit. Patients with complicating iron deficiency, an infection or other inflammatory state, or renal disease may be unable to correct their anemia. Therefore it is important to monitor the reticulocyte index over the first several weeks. If it does not continue at elevated levels while the hematocrit is <35%, plasma concentrations of iron and folic acid should again be determined and the patient reevaluated for an illness that could inhibit the response of the marrow.

The degree and rate of improvement of neurological signs and symptoms depend on the severity and the duration of the abnormalities. Those that have been present for only a few months usually disappear relatively rapidly. When a defect has been present for many months or years, full return to normal function may never occur.

Long-Term Therapy with Vitamin B_{12}. Once begun, vitamin B_{12} therapy must be maintained for life. This fact must be impressed on the patient and family, and a system must be established to guarantee continued monthly injections of cyanocobalamin.

Intramuscular injection of 100 μg of cyanocobalamin every 4 weeks is sufficient to maintain a normal concentration of vitamin B_{12} in plasma and an adequate supply for tissues. Patients with severe neurological symptoms and signs may be treated with larger doses of vitamin B_{12} in the period immediately after the diagnosis. Doses of 100 μg per day or several times per week may be given for several months with the hope of encouraging faster and more complete recovery. It is important to monitor vitamin B_{12} concentrations in plasma and to obtain peripheral blood counts at intervals of 3-6 months to confirm the adequacy of therapy. Because refractoriness to therapy can develop at any time, evaluation must continue throughout the patient's life. Intranasal preparations are available for maintenance following normalization of vitamin B_{12}–deficient patients without nervous system involvement (CALOMIST, NASCOBAL) or as a supplement for vitamin B_{12} deficiencies of various etiologies (NASCOBAL).

Other Therapeutic Uses of Vitamin B_{12}. Vitamin B_{12} has been used in the therapy of a number of conditions, including trigeminal neuralgia, multiple sclerosis and other neuropathies, various psychiatric disorders, poor growth or nutrition, and as a "tonic" for patients complaining of tiredness or easy fatigue. There is no evidence for the validity of such therapy in any of these conditions. Maintenance therapy with vitamin B_{12} has been used with some apparent success in the treatment of children with methylmalonic aciduria.

Folic Acid

Chemistry and Metabolic Functions. The structural formula of pteroylglutamic acid (PteGlu) is shown in Figure 37–9. Major portions of the molecule include a pteridine ring linked by a methylene bridge to para-aminobenzoic acid, which is joined by an amide linkage to glutamic acid. Although pteroylglutamic acid is the common pharmaceutical form of folic acid, it is neither the principal folate congener in food nor the active coenzyme for intracellular metabolism. After absorption, PteGlu is rapidly reduced at the 5, 6, 7, and 8 positions to tetrahydrofolic acid (H_4PteGlu), which then acts as an acceptor of a number of one-carbon units. These are attached at either the 5 or the 10 position of the pteridine ring or may bridge these atoms to form a new five-membered ring. The most important forms of the coenzyme that are synthesized by these reactions are listed in Figure 37–9. Each plays a specific role in intracellular metabolism, summarized as follows (see "Relationships Between Vitamin B_{12} and Folic Acid," as well as Figure 37–6).

Conversion of Homocysteine to Methionine. This reaction requires CH_3H_4PteGlu as a methyl donor and uses vitamin B_{12} as a cofactor.

Conversion of Serine to Glycine. This reaction requires tetrahydrofolate as an acceptor of a methylene group from serine and uses pyridoxal phosphate as a cofactor. It results in the formation of 5,10-CH_2H_4PteGlu, an essential coenzyme for the synthesis of thymidylate.

Synthesis Of thymidylate. 5,10-CH_2H_4PteGlu donates a methylene group and reducing equivalents to deoxyuridylate for the synthesis of thymidylate—a rate-limiting step in DNA synthesis.

Histidine Metabolism. H_4PteGlu also acts as an acceptor of a formimino group in the conversion of formiminoglutamic acid to glutamic acid.

Synthesis of Purines. Two steps in the synthesis of purine nucleotides require the participation of 10-$CHOH_4$PteGlu as a formyl donor in

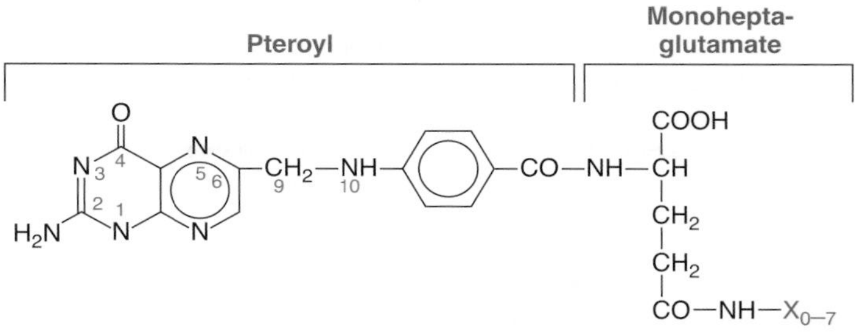

Pteroyl

Monohepta-glutamate

COOH

$-CH_2-NH-$ (C$_6$H$_4$) $-CO-NH-CH$

CH_2

CH_2

$CO-NH-X_{0-7}$

Position	Radical	Congener	
N^5	$-CH_3$	CH_3H_4PteGlu	Methyltetrahydrofolate
N^5	$-CHO$	5-$CHOH_4$PteGlu	Folinic acid (citrovorum factor)
N^{10}	$-CHO$	10-$CHOH_4$PteGlu	10-Formyltetrahydrofolate
$N^{5,10}$	$=CH-$	5,10-CHH_4PteGlu	5,10-Methenyltetrahydrofolate
$N^{5,10}$	$-CH_2-$	5,10-CH_2H_4PteGlu	5,10-Methylenetetrahydrofolate
N^5	$-CHNH$	$CHNHH_4$PteGlu	Formiminotetrahydrofolate
N^{10}	$-CH_2OH$	CH_2OHH_4PteGlu	Hydroxymethyltetrahydrofolate

Figure 37–9. *The structures and nomenclature of pteroylglutamic acid (folic acid) and its congeners.* X represents additional residues of glutamate; polyglutamates are the storage and active forms of the vitamin. The subscript that designates the number of residues of glutamate is frequently omitted because this number is variable.

reactions catalyzed by ribotide transformylases: the formylation of glycinamide ribonucleotide and the formylation of 5-aminoimidazole-4-carboxamide ribonucleotide. By these reactions, carbon atoms at positions 8 and 2, respectively, are incorporated into the growing purine ring.

Utilization or generation of formate. This reversible reaction uses H_4PteGlu and 10-$CHOH_4$PteGlu.

Daily Requirements. Many food sources are rich in folates, especially fresh green vegetables, liver, yeast, and some fruits. However, lengthy cooking can destroy up to 90% of the folate content of such food.

Generally, a standard U.S. diet provides 50-500 μg of absorbable folate per day, although individuals with high intakes of fresh vegetables and meats will ingest as much as 2 mg per day. In the normal adult, the recommended daily intake is 400 μg; pregnant or lactating women and patients with high rates of cell turnover (such as patients with a hemolytic anemia) may require 500-600 μg or more per day. For the prevention of neural tube defects, a daily intake of at least 400 μg of folate in food or in supplements beginning a month before pregnancy and continued for at least the first trimester is recommended. Folate supplementation also is being considered in patients with elevated levels of plasma homocysteine.

Absorption, Distribution, and Elimination. As with vitamin B_{12}, the diagnosis and management of deficiencies of folic acid depend on an understanding of the transport pathways and intracellular metabolism of the vitamin (Figure 37–10). Folates present in food are largely in the form of reduced polyglutamates, and absorption requires transport and the action of a pteroylglutamyl carboxypeptidase associated with mucosal cell membranes. The mucosae of the duodenum and upper part of the jejunum are rich in dihydrofolate reductase and can methylate most or all of the reduced folate that is absorbed. Because most absorption occurs in the proximal portion of the small intestine, it is not unusual for folate deficiency to occur when the jejunum is diseased. Both nontropical and tropical sprue are common causes of folate deficiency and megaloblastic anemia.

Once absorbed, folate is transported rapidly to tissues as CH_3H_4PteGlu. Although certain plasma proteins do bind folate derivatives, they have a greater affinity for nonmethylated analogs. The role of such binding proteins in folate homeostasis is not well understood. An increase in binding capacity is detectable in folate deficiency and in certain disease states, such as uremia, cancer, and alcoholism, but how binding affects transport and tissue supply requires further investigation.

A constant supply of CH_3H_4PteGlu is maintained by food and by an enterohepatic cycle of the vitamin. The liver actively reduces and methylates PteGlu (and H_2 or H_4PteGlu) and then transports the CH_3H_4PteGlu into bile for reabsorption by the gut and subsequent delivery to tissues. This pathway may provide ≥200 μg of folate each day for recirculation to tissues. The importance of the enterohepatic cycle is suggested by animal studies that show a rapid reduction of the plasma folate concentration after either drainage of bile or ingestion of alcohol, which apparently blocks the release of CH_3H_4PteGlu from hepatic parenchymal cells.

Folate Deficiency. Folate deficiency is a common complication of diseases of the small intestine that interferes with the absorption of folate from food and the recirculation of folate through the enterohepatic cycle. In acute

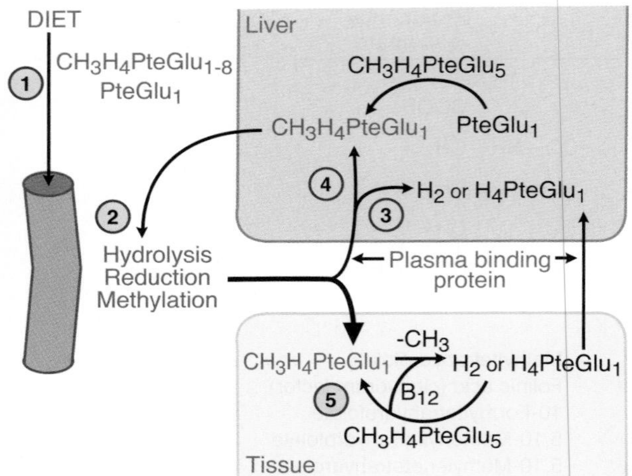

Figure 37–10. *Absorption and distribution of folate derivatives.* Dietary sources of folate polyglutamates are hydrolyzed to the monoglutamate, reduced, and methylated to $CH_3H_4PteGlu_1$ during gastrointestinal transport. Folate deficiency commonly results from (1) inadequate dietary supply and (2) small intestinal disease. In patients with uremia, alcoholism, or hepatic disease there may be defects in (3) the concentration of folate binding proteins in plasma and (4) the flow of $CH_3H_4PteGlu_1$ into bile for reabsorption and transport to tissue (the folate enterohepatic cycle). Finally, vitamin B_{12} deficiency will (5) "trap" folate as $CH_3H_4PteGlu$, thereby reducing the availability of $H_4PteGlu_1$ for its essential roles in purine and pyrimidine synthesis.

or chronic alcoholism, daily intake of folate in food may be severely restricted, and the enterohepatic cycle of the vitamin may be impaired by toxic effects of alcohol on hepatic parenchymal cells; this is the most common cause of folate-deficient megaloblastic erythropoiesis. However, it also is the most amenable to therapy, inasmuch as the reinstitution of a normal diet is sufficient to overcome the effect of alcohol. Disease states characterized by a high rate of cell turnover, such as hemolytic anemias, also may be complicated by folate deficiency. Additionally, drugs that inhibit dihydrofolate reductase (e.g., methotrexate and trimethoprim) or that interfere with the absorption and storage of folate in tissues (e.g., certain anticonvulsants and oral contraceptives) can lower the concentration of folate in plasma and may cause a megaloblastic anemia (Scott and Weir, 1980).

Folate deficiency has been implicated in the incidence of neural tube defects, including spina bifida, encephaloceles, and anencephaly. This is true even in the absence of folate-deficient anemia or alcoholism. A less-than-adequate intake of folate also can result in elevations in plasma homocysteine (Green and Miller, 1999). Because even moderate hyperhomocysteinemia is considered an independent risk factor for coronary artery and peripheral vascular disease and for venous thrombosis, the role of folate as a methyl donor in the homocysteine-to-methionine conversion is getting increased attention. Patients who are heterozygous for one or another enzymatic defect and have high normal to moderate elevations of plasma homocysteine may improve with folic acid therapy.

Folate deficiency is recognized by its impact on the hematopoietic system. As with vitamin B_{12}, this fact reflects the increased requirement associated with high rates of cell turnover. The megaloblastic anemia that results from folate deficiency cannot be distinguished from that caused by vitamin B_{12} deficiency. This finding is to be expected because of the final common pathway of the major intracellular metabolic roles of the two vitamins. At the same time, folate deficiency is rarely if ever associated with neurological abnormalities. Thus the observation of characteristic abnormalities in vibratory and position sense and in motor and sensory pathways is incompatible with an isolated deficiency of folic acid.

After deprivation of folate, megaloblastic anemia develops much more rapidly than it does following interruption of vitamin B_{12} absorption (e.g., gastric surgery). This observation reflects the fact that body stores of folate are limited. Although the rate of induction of megaloblastic erythropoiesis may vary, a folate-deficiency state may appear in 1-4 weeks, depending on the individual's dietary habits and stores of the vitamin.

Folate deficiency is best diagnosed from measurements of folate in plasma and in red cells. However, an empirical trial of folate in cases of suspected deficiency has been proposed as more cost effective (Robinson and Mladenovic, 2001). Indeed, the concentration of folate in plasma is extremely sensitive to changes in dietary intake of the vitamin and the influence of inhibitors of folate metabolism or transport, such as alcohol. Normal folate concentrations in plasma range from 9-45 nmol (4-20 ng/mL); <9 nmol is considered folate deficient. The plasma folate concentration rapidly falls to values indicative of deficiency within 24-48 hours of steady ingestion of alcohol (Eichner and Hillman 1973). The plasma folate concentration will revert quickly to normal once such ingestion is stopped, even while the marrow is still megaloblastic. Such rapid fluctuations detract from the clinical usefulness of the plasma folate concentration. The amount of folate in red cells or the adequacy of stores in lymphocytes (as measured by the deoxyuridine suppression test) may be used to diagnose a longstanding deficiency of folic acid. A positive result on either test shows that the deficiency must have existed for a sufficient time to allow the production of a population of cells with deficient folate stores.

Folic acid is marketed as oral tablets containing pteroylglutamic acid or L-methylfolate, as an aqueous solution for injection (5 mg/mL), and in combination with other vitamins and minerals.

Folinic acid (leucovorin calcium, citrovorum factor) is the 5-formyl derivative of tetrahydrofolic acid. The principal therapeutic uses of folinic acid are to circumvent the inhibition of dihydrofolate reductase as a part of high-dose methotrexate therapy and to potentiate fluorouracil in the treatment of colorectal cancer (Chapter 61). It also has been used as an antidote to counteract the toxicity of folate antagonists such as pyrimethamine or trimethoprim. Although it can be used to treat any folate-deficient state, folinic acid provides no advantage over folic acid, is more expensive, and therefore is not recommended. A single exception is the megaloblastic anemia associated with congenital dihydrofolate reductase deficiency.

Leucovorin should never be used for the treatment of pernicious anemia or other megaloblastic anemias secondary to a deficiency of vitamin B_{12}. Just as is seen with folic acid, its use can result in an apparent response of the hematopoietic system, but neurological damage may occur or progress if already present. Leucovorin is marketed as oral tablets and as products for intravenous infusion.

Untoward Effects. There have been rare reports of reactions to parenteral injections of folic acid and leucovorin. If a patient describes a history of a reaction before the drug is given, caution should be exercised. Oral folic acid usually is not toxic. Even with doses as high as 15 mg/day, there have been no substantiated reports of side effects. Folic acid in large amounts may counteract the antiepileptic effect of phenobarbital, phenytoin, and primidone, and increase the frequency of seizures in susceptible children (Reynolds, 1968). Although some studies have not supported these contentions, the FDA recommends that oral tablets of folic acid be limited to strengths of ≤1 mg.

General Principles of Therapy. The therapeutic use of folic acid is limited to the prevention and treatment of deficiencies of the vitamin. As with vitamin B_{12} therapy, effective use of the vitamin depends on accurate diagnosis and an understanding of the mechanisms that are operative in a specific disease state. The following general principles of therapy should be respected:

1. Prophylactic administration of folic acid should be undertaken for clear indications. Dietary supplementation is necessary when there is a requirement that may not be met by a "normal" diet. The daily ingestion of a multivitamin preparation containing 400-500 μg of folic acid has become standard practice before and during pregnancy to reduce the incidence of neural tube defects and for as long as a woman is breast-feeding. In women with a history of a pregnancy complicated by a neural tube defect, an even larger dose of 4 mg/day has been recommended (MRC Vitamin Study Research Group, 1991). Patients on total parenteral nutrition should receive folic acid supplements as part of their fluid regimen because liver folate stores are limited. Adult patients with a disease state characterized by high cell turnover (e.g., hemolytic anemia) generally require larger doses, 1 mg of folic acid given once or twice a day. The 1-mg dose also has been used in the treatment of patients with elevated levels of homocysteine.
2. As with vitamin B_{12} deficiency, any patient with folate deficiency and a megaloblastic anemia should be evaluated carefully to determine the underlying cause of the deficiency state. This should include evaluation of the effects of medications, the amount of alcohol intake, the patient's history of travel, and the function of the GI tract.
3. Therapy always should be as specific as possible. Multivitamin preparations should be avoided unless there is good reason to suspect deficiency of several vitamins.
4. The potential danger of mistreating a patient who has vitamin B_{12} deficiency with folic acid must be kept in mind. The administration of large doses of folic acid can result in an apparent improvement of the megaloblastic anemia, inasmuch as PteGlu is converted by dihydrofolate reductase to H_4PteGlu; this circumvents the methylfolate "trap." However, folate therapy does not prevent or alleviate the neurological defects of vitamin B_{12} deficiency, and these may progress and become irreversible.

Treatment of the Acutely Ill Patient. As described in detail in the section on vitamin B_{12}, treatment of the patient who is acutely ill with megaloblastic anemia should begin with intramuscular injections of vitamin B_{12} and folic acid. Inasmuch as the patient requires therapy before the exact cause of the disease has been defined, it is important to avoid the potential problem of a combined deficiency of vitamin B_{12} and folic acid. When the patient is deficient in both, therapy with only one vitamin will not provide an optimal response. Longstanding nontropical sprue is one example of a disease in which combined deficiency of B_{12} and folate is common. When indicated, vitamin B_{12} (100 μg) and folic acid (1-5 mg) should be administered intramuscularly, and the patient should then be maintained on daily oral supplements of 1-2 mg of folic acid for the next 1-2 weeks.

Oral administration of folate generally is satisfactory for patients who are not acutely ill, regardless of the cause of the deficiency state. Even the patient with tropical or nontropical sprue and a demonstrable defect in absorption of folic acid will respond adequately to such therapy. Abnormalities in the activity of pteroyl-γ-glutamyl carboxypeptidase and the function of mucosal cells will not prevent passive diffusion of sufficient amounts of PteGlu across the mucosal barrier if the dosage is adequate, and continued ingestion of alcohol or other drugs also will not prevent an adequate therapeutic response. The effects of most inhibitors of folate transport or dihydrofolate reductase are overcome easily by administration of pharmacological doses of the vitamin. Folinic acid is the appropriate form of the vitamin for use in chemotherapeutic protocols, including "rescue" from methotrexate (Chapter 61). Perhaps the only situation in which oral administration of folate will be ineffective is when vitamin C is severely deficient. Patients with scurvy may suffer from a megaloblastic anemia despite increased intake of folate and normal or high concentrations of the vitamin in plasma and cells.

The therapeutic response may be monitored by study of the hematopoietic system in a fashion identical to that described for vitamin B_{12}. Within 48 hours of the initiation of appropriate therapy, megaloblastic erythropoiesis disappears, and as efficient erythropoiesis begins, the concentration of iron in plasma falls to normal or below-normal values. The reticulocyte count begins to rise on the second or third day and reaches a peak by the fifth to seventh days; the reticulocyte index reflects the proliferative state of the marrow. Finally, the hematocrit begins to rise during the second week.

It is possible to use the pattern of recovery as the basis for a therapeutic trial. For this purpose, the patient should receive a daily parenteral injection of 50-100 μg of folic acid. Administration of doses >100 μg/day entails the risk of inducing a hematopoietic response in patients who are deficient in vitamin B_{12}, and oral administration of the vitamin may be unreliable because of intestinal malabsorption. A number of other complications also may interfere with the therapeutic trial. The patient with sprue and deficiencies of other vitamins or iron may fail to respond because of these inadequacies. In cases of alcoholism, the presence of hepatic disease, inflammation, or iron deficiency can blunt the proliferative response of the marrow and prevent the correction of the anemia. For these reasons, the therapeutic trial for the evaluation of the patient with a potential deficiency of folic acid has not gained great popularity.

CLINICAL SUMMARY

Several hematopoietic growth factors are available for clinical use. Recombinant erythropoietin routinely is used for patients with the anemia of renal insufficiency, inflammation, and associated with cancer or the therapy of cancer. Longer-acting growth factors that permit less frequent dosing schedules are coming into increased use. One of the first of these is novel erythropoiesis-stimulating protein (NESP), produced by the insertion of two extra N-linked sialic acid side chains into the erythropoietin molecule. Myeloid growth factors (e.g., GM-CSF and G-CSF) are used to hasten the recovery of granulocytes after myelosuppressive therapy, to help mobilize hematopoietic stem cells into the peripheral blood to allow their harvest for transplantation, and to augment the number of mature leukocytes in the peripheral blood so that they can be used in patients with overwhelming infection. Finally, the development of IL-11 for use in thrombocytopenia and the investigational use of thrombopoietin or mimics of the molecule may provide many of the same therapeutic advances.

BIBLIOGRAPHY

Abdel-Latif A, Bolli R, Zuba-Surma EK, *et al.* Granulocyte colony-stimulating factor therapy for cardiac repair after acute myocardial infarction: A systematic review and meta-analysis of randomized controlled trials. *Am Heart J,* **2008,** *156:* 216–226. e9.

Agarwal R. Proinflammatory effects of iron sucrose in chronic kidney disease. *Kidney Int,* **2006,** *69:*1259–1263.

Ajioka RS, Kushner JP. Clinical consequences of iron overload in hemochromatosis homozygotes. *Blood,* **2003,** *101:*3351–3353; discussion 3354–3358.

Akashi K, Traver D, Miyamoto T, Weissman IL. A clonogenic common myeloid progenitor that gives rise to all myeloid lineages. *Nature,* **2000,** *404:*193–197.

al-Momen, AK, al-Meshari A, al-Nuaim L, *et al.* Intravenous iron sucrose complex in the treatment of iron deficiency anemia during pregnancy. *Eur J Obstet Gynecol Reprod Biol,* **1996,** *69:*21–24.

Archimbaud E, Ottmann OG, Yin JA, *et al.* A randomized, double-blind, placebo-controlled study with pegylated recombinant human megakaryocyte growth and development factor (PEG-rHuMGDF) as an adjunct to chemotherapy for adults with de novo acute myeloid leukemia. *Blood,* **1999,** *94:*3694–3701.

Aronoff GR, Bennett WM, Blumenthal S, *et al.* Iron sucrose in hemodialysis patients: Safety of replacement and maintenance regimens. *Kidney Int,* **2004,** *66:*1193–1198.

Auerbach M, Al Talib K. Low-molecular weight iron dextran and iron sucrose have similar comparative safety profiles in chronic kidney disease. *Kidney Int,* **2008,** *73:*528–530.

Balakrishnan VS, Rao M, Kausz AT, *et al.* Physicochemical properties of ferumoxytol, a new intravenous iron preparation. *Eur J Clin Invest,* **2009,** *39:*489–496.

Basser RL, Underhill C, Davis I, *et al.* Enhancement of platelet recovery after myelosuppressive chemotherapy by recombinant human megakaryocyte growth and development factor in patients with advanced cancer. *J Clin Oncol,* **2000,** *18:*2852–2861.

Bennett CL, Silver SM, Djulbegovic B, *et al.* Venous thromboembolism and mortality associated with recombinant erythropoietin and darbepoetin administration for the treatment of cancer-associated anemia. *JAMA,* **2008,** *299:*914–924.

Besarab A, Bolton WK, Browne JK, *et al.* The effects of normal as compared with low hematocrit values in patients with cardiac disease who are receiving hemodialysis and epoetin. *N Engl J Med,* **1998,** *339:*584–590.

Besarab A, Kaiser JW, Frinak S. A study of parental iron regimens in hemodialysis patients. *Am J Kidney Dis,* **1999,** *34:*21–28.

Beutler E. History of iron in medicine. *Blood Cells Mol Dis,* **2002,** *29:*297–308.

Bodemar G, Kechagias S, Almer S, Danielson BG. Treatment of anaemia in inflammatory bowel disease with iron sucrose. *Scand J Gastroenterol,* **2004,** *39:*454–458.

Bohlius J, Brilliant C, Clarke M, *et al.* Recombinant human erythropoiesis stimulating agents in cancer patients: Individual patient data meta-analysis on behalf of the EPOIPD meta-analysis collaborative group. *Blood,* **2008,** *112:*lba–6.

Bolwell B, Vredenburgh J, Overmoyer B, *et al.* Phase 1 study of pegylated recombinant human megakaryocyte growth and development factor (PEG-rHuMGDF) in breast cancer patients after autologous peripheral blood progenitor cell (PBPC) transplantation. *Bone Marrow Transplant,* **2000,** *26:*141–145.

Brandt SJ, Peters WP, Atwater SK, *et al.* Effect of recombinant human granulocyte-macrophage colony-stimulating factor on hematopoietic reconstitution after high-dose chemotherapy and autologous bone marrow transplantation. *N Engl J Med,* **1988,** *318:*869–876.

Bussel JB, Cheng G, Saleh MN, *et al.* Eltrombopag for the treatment of chronic idiopathic thrombocytopenic purpura. *N Engl J Med,* **2007,** *357:*2237–2247.

Casadevall N. Pure red cell aplasia and anti-erythropoietin antibodies in patients treated with epoetin. *Nephrol Dial Transplant,* **2003,** *18 (suppl 8):*viii37–41.

Clark SF. Iron deficiency anemia: Diagnosis and management. *Curr Opin Gastroenterol,* **2009,** *25:*122–128.

Conrad ME, Umbreit JN. Pathways of iron absorption. *Blood Cells Mol Dis,* **2002,** *29:*336–355.

Crawford J. Neutrophil growth factors. *Curr Hematol Rep,* **2002,** *1:*95–102.

Dallman PR. Manifestations of iron deficiency. *Semin Hematol,* **1982,** *19:*19–30.

Dallman PR, Siimes MA, Stekel A. Iron deficiency in infancy and childhood. *Am J Clin Nutr,* **1980,** *33:*86–118.

de Bie P, Muller P, Wijmenga C, Klomp LW. Molecular pathogenesis of Wilson and Menkes disease: correlation of mutations with molecular defects and disease phenotypes. *J Med Genet,* **2007,** *44:*673–688.

De Domenico I, Nemeth E, Nelson JM, *et al.* The hepcidin-binding site on ferroportin is evolutionarily conserved. *Cell Metab,* **2008,** *8:*146–156.

Du XX, Williams DA. Interleukin-11: A multifunctional growth factor derived from the hematopoietic microenvironment. *Blood,* **1994,** *83:*2023–2030.

Dunlap WM, James GW 3rd, Hume DM. Anemia and neutropenia caused by copper deficiency. *Ann Intern Med,* **1974,** *80:*470–476.

Eichner ER, Hillman RS. Effect of alcohol on serum folate level. *J Clin Invest,* **1973,** *52:*584–591.

Eschbach JW, Egrie JC, Downing MR, *et al.* Correction of the anemia of end-stage renal disease with recombinant human erythropoietin. Results of a combined phase I and II clinical trial. *N Engl J Med,* **1987,** *316:*73–78.

Faich G, Strobos J. Sodium ferric gluconate complex in sucrose: Safer intravenous iron therapy than iron dextrans. *Am J Kidney Dis,* **1999,** *33:*464–470.

Feder JN, Gnirke A, Thomas W, *et al.* A novel MHC class I-like gene is mutated in patients with hereditary haemochromatosis. *Nat Genet,* **1996,** *13:*399–408.

Fernandez-Banares F, Monzon H, Forne M. A short review of malabsorption and anemia. *World J Gastroenterol,* **2009,** *15:*4644–4652.

Fibbe WE, Heemskerk DP, Laterveer L, *et al.* Accelerated reconstitution of platelets and erythrocytes after syngeneic transplantation of bone marrow cells derived from thrombopoietin pretreated donor mice. *Blood,* **1995,** *86:* 3308–3313.

Finberg KE. Iron-refractory iron deficiency anemia. *Semin Hematol,* **2009,** *46:*378–386.

Finch CA, Huebers H. Perspectives in iron metabolism. *N Engl J Med,* **1982,** *306:*1520–1528.

Fischl M, Galpin JE, Levine JD, *et al.* Recombinant human erythropoietin for patients with AIDS treated with zidovudine. *N Engl J Med,* **1990,** *322:*1488–1493.

Galy B, Ferring-Appel D, Kaden S, *et al.* Iron regulatory proteins are essential for intestinal function and control key iron absorption molecules in the duodenum. *Cell Metab,* **2008,** *7:*79–85.

Gambling L, Andersen HS, McArdle HJ. Iron and copper, and their interactions during development. *Biochem Soc Trans,* **2008,** *36:*1258–1261.

Ganz T. Hepcidin, a key regulator of iron metabolism and mediator of anemia of inflammation. Blood, **2003,** *102:*783–788.

Ganz T. Iron homeostasis: Fitting the puzzle pieces together. *Cell Metab,* **2003,** *7:*288–290.

Ganz T, Nemeth E. Iron sequestration and anemia of inflammation. *Semin Hematol,* **2009,** *46:*387–393.

Garrick MD, Garrick LM. Cellular iron transport. *Biochim Biophys Acta,* **2009,** *1790:*309–325.

Gerhartz HH, Engelhard M, Meusers P, *et al.* Randomized, double-blind, placebo-controlled, phase III study of recombinant human granulocyte-macrophage colony-stimulating factor as adjunct to induction treatment of high-grade malignant non-Hodgkin's lymphomas. *Blood,* **1993,** *82:*2329–2339.

Goodnough LT, Rudnick S, Price TH, *et al.* Increased preoperative collection of autologous blood with recombinant human erythropoietin therapy. *N Engl J Med,* **1989,** *321:*1163–1168.

Goodnough LT, Skikne B, Brugnara C. Erythropoietin, iron, and erythropoiesis. *Blood,* **2000,** *96:*823–833.

Goodwin RG, Lupton S, Schmierer A, *et al.* Human interleukin 7: molecular cloning and growth factor activity on human and murine B-lineage cells. *Proc Natl Acad Sci USA*, **1989,** 86:302–306.

Gough NM, Gough J, Metcalf D, *et al.* Molecular cloning of cDNA encoding a murine hematopoietic growth regulator, granulocyte-macrophage colony stimulating factor. *Nature*, **1984,** *309*:763–767.

Gordeuk VR, Sergueeva AI, Miasnikova GY, *et al.* Congenital disorder of oxygen sensing: Association of the homozygous Chuvash polycythemia VHL mutation with thrombosis and vascular abnormalities but not tumors. *Blood,* **2004,** *103:*3924–3932.

Grabstein KH, Eisenman J, Shanebeck K, *et al.* Cloning of a T cell growth factor that interacts with the β chain of the interleukin-2 receptor. *Science*, **1994,** *264*:965–968.

Graham GG, Cordano A. Copper deficiency in human subjects. In: *Trace Elements in Human Health and Diseases, Zinc and Copper*, Academic Press, New York, 1976.

Grebe G, Martinez-Torres C, Layrisse M. Effect of meals and ascorbic acid on the absorption of a therapeutic dose of iron as ferrous and ferric salts. *Curr Ther Res Clin Exp*, **1975,** *17*:382–397.

Green R, Miller JW. Folate deficiency beyond megaloblastic anemia: Hyperhomocysteinemia and other manifestations of dysfunctional folate status. *Semin Hematol*, **1999,** *36*:47–64.

Haas R, Ho AD, Bredthauer U, *et al.* Successful autologous transplantation of blood stem cells mobilized with recombinant human granulocyte-macrophage colony-stimulating factor. *Exp Hematol,* **1990,** *18:*94–98.

Hahn PF. The use of radioactive isotopes in the study of iron and hemoglobin metabolism and the physiology of the erythrocyte. *Adv Biol Med Phys,* **1948,** *1 (1 vol.):*287–319.

Hakami N, Neiman PE, Canellos GP, Lazerson J. Neonatal megaloblastic anemia due to inherited transcobalamin II deficiency in two siblings. *N Engl J Med,* **1971,** *285:*1163–1170.

Hammond WPT, Price TH, Souza LM, Dale DC. Treatment of cyclic neutropenia with granulocyte colony-stimulating factor. *N Engl J Med,* **1989,** *320:*1306–1311.

Harker LA. Physiology and clinical applications of platelet growth factors. *Curr Opin Hematol,* **1999,** *6:*127–134.

Hayat A. Safety issues with intravenous iron products in the management of anemia in chronic kidney disease. *Clin Med Res,* **2008,** *6:*93–102.

Henke M, Laszig R, Rube C, *et al.* Erythropoietin to treat head and neck cancer patients with anaemia undergoing radiotherapy: Randomised, double-blind, placebo-controlled trial. *Lancet,* **2003,** *362:*1255–1260.

Hoffbrand AV, Herbert V. Nutritional anemias. *Semin Hematol,* **1999,** *36:*13–23.

Hoffman HN 2nd, Phyliky RL, Fleming CR. Zinc-induced copper deficiency. *Gastroenterology,* **1988,** *94:*508–512.

Huang E, Nocka K, Beier DR, *et al.* The hematopoietic growth factor KL is encoded by the Sl locus and is the ligand of the c-kit receptor, the gene product of the W locus. *Cell,* **1990,** *63:*225–233.

Hubel K, Carter RA, Liles WC, *et al.* Granulocyte transfusion therapy for infections in candidates and recipients of HPC transplantation: A comparative analysis of feasibility and outcome for community donors versus related donors. *Transfusion,* **2002,** *42:*1414–1421.

Jelkmann W. The enigma of the metabolic fate of circulating erythropoietin (Epo) in view of the pharmacokinetics of the recombinant drugs rhEpo and NESP. *Eur J Haematol,* **2002,** *69:*265–274.

Kapoian T, O'Mara NB, Singh AK, *et al.* Ferric gluconate reduces epoetin requirements in hemodialysis patients with elevated ferritin. *J Am Soc Nephrol,* **2008,** *19:*372–379.

Kaufman JS, Reda DJ, Fye CL, *et al.* Subcutaneous compared with intravenous epoetin in patients receiving hemodialysis. Department of Veterans Affairs Cooperative Study Group on Erythropoietin in Hemodialysis Patients. *N Engl J Med,* **1998,** *339:*578–583.

Kaushansky K. Thrombopoietin. *N Engl J Med,* **1998,** *339:*746–754.

Kawasaki ES, Ladner MB, Wang AM, *et al.* Molecular cloning of a complementary DNA encoding human macrophage-specific colony-stimulating factor (CSF-1). *Science,* **1985,** *230:*291–296.

Kim BE, Nevitt T, Thiele DJ. Mechanisms for copper acquisition, distribution and regulation. *Nat Chem Biol,* **2008,** *4:*176–185.

Kuter DJ, Bussel JB, Lyons RM, *et al.* Efficacy of romiplostim in patients with chronic immune thrombocytopenic purpura: A double-blind randomised controlled trial. *Lancet,* **2008,** *371:*395–403.

Kuter DJ, Goodnough LT, Romo J, *et al.* Thrombopoietin therapy increases platelet yields in healthy platelet donors. *Blood,* **2001,** *98:*1339–1345.

Lalioti V, Muruais G, Tsuchiya Y, *et al.* Molecular mechanisms of copper homeostasis. *Front Biosci,* **2009,** *14:*4878–4903.

Laurell CB. What is the function of transferrin in plasma? *Blood,* **1951,** *6:*183–187.

Li J, Yang C, Xia Y, *et al.* Thrombocytopenia caused by the development of antibodies to thrombopoietin. *Blood,* **2001,** *98:*3241–3248.

Lieschke GJ, Burgess AW. Granulocyte colony-stimulating factor and granulocyte-macrophage colony-stimulating factor (2). *N Engl J Med,* **1992,** *327:*99–106.

Linz R, Lutsenko S. Copper-transporting ATPases ATP7A and ATP7B: cousins, not twins. *J Bioenerg Biomembr,* **2007,** *39:*403–407.

Littlewood TJ, Bajetta E, Nortier JW, *et al.* Effects of epoetin alfa on hematologic parameters and quality of life in cancer patients receiving nonplatinum chemotherapy: Results of a randomized, double-blind, placebo-controlled trial. *J Clin Oncol,* **2001,** *19:*2865–2874.

Lok S, Kaushansky K, Holly RD, *et al.* Cloning and expression of murine thrombopoietin cDNA and stimulation of platelet production in vivo. *Nature,* **1994,** *369:*565–568.

Macdougall IC. Pure red cell aplasia with anti-erythropoietin antibodies occurs more commonly with one formulation of epoetin alfa than another. *Curr Med Res Opin,* **2004,** *20:* 83–86.

Maxwell PH, Pugh CW, Ratcliffe PJ. The pVHL-hIF-1 system. A key mediator of oxygen homeostasis. *Adv Exp Med Biol,* **2001,** *502:*365–376.

McLean E, Cogswell M, Egli I, *et al.* Worldwide prevalence of anaemia, WHO Vitamin and Mineral Nutrition Information System, 1993–2005. *Public Health Nutr,* **2009,** *12:*444–454.

Monsen ER, Hallberg L, Layrisse M, *et al.* Estimation of available dietary iron. *Am J Clin Nutr,* **1978,** *31:*134–141.

Moskowitz CH, Stiff P, Gordon MS, *et al.* Recombinant methionyl human stem cell factor and filgrastim for peripheral blood progenitor cell mobilization and transplantation in non-Hodgkin's lymphoma patients—results of a phase I/II trial. *Blood,* **1997,** *89:*3136–3147.

MRC Vitamin Study Research Group. Prevention of neural tube defects: Results of the Medical Research Council Vitamin Study. *Lancet*, **1991,** *338*:131–137.

Nakorn,TN, Miyamoto T, Weissman IL. Characterization of mouse clonogenic megakaryocyte progenitors. *Proc Natl Acad Sci U S A,* **2003,** *100:*205–210.

Neben TY, Loebelenz J, Hayes L, *et al.* Recombinant human interleukin-11 stimulates megakaryocytopoiesis and increases peripheral platelets in normal and splenectomized mice. *Blood,* **1993,** *81:*901–908.

Nemeth E, Rivera S, Gabayan V, *et al.* IL-6 mediates hypoferremia of inflammation by inducing the synthesis of the iron regulatory hormone hepcidin. *J Clin Invest,* **2004,** *113:* 1271–1276.

Nemunaitis J, Singer JW, Buckner CD, *et al.* Use of recombinant human granulocyte-macrophage colony-stimulating factor in graft failure after bone marrow transplantation. *Blood,* **1990,** *76:*245–253.

Owen WF Jr. Optimizing the use of parenteral iron in end-stage renal disease patients: Focus on issues of infection and cardiovascular disease. Introduction. *Am J Kidney Dis,* **1999,** *34:*S1–2.

Park CH, Valore EV, Waring AJ, Ganz T. Hepcidin, a urinary antimicrobial peptide synthesized in the liver. *J Biol Chem,* **2001,** *276:*7806–7810.

Percy MJ, Beer PA, Campbell G, *et al.* Novel exon 12 mutations in the HIF2A gene associated with erythrocytosis. *Blood,* **2008,** *111:*5400–5402.

Reynolds EH. Mental effects of anticonvulsants and folic acid metabolism. *Brain*, **1968,** *91*:197–214.

Rizzo JD, Lichtin AE, Woolf SH, *et al.* Use of epoetin in patients with cancer: Evidence-based clinical practice guidelines of the American Society of Clinical Oncology and the American Society of Hematology. *Blood,* **2002,** *100:* 2303–2320.

Robinson AR, Mladenovic J. Lack of clinical utility of folate levels in the evaluation of macrocytosis or anemia. *Am J Med,* **2001,** *110:*88–90.

Scott JM, Weir DG. Drug-induced megaloblastic change. *Clin Haematol,* **1980,** *9:*587–606.

Sengolge G, Horl WH, Sunder-Plassmann G. Intravenous iron therapy: Well-tolerated, yet not harmless. *Eur J Clin Invest,* **2005,** *35 (suppl 3):*46–51.

Sheridan WP, Begley CG, Juttner CA, *et al*. Effect of peripheral-blood progenitor cells mobilised by filgrastim (G-CSF) on platelet recovery after high-dose chemotherapy. *Lancet,* **1992,** *339:*640–644.

Silverstein SB, Rodgers GM. Parenteral iron therapy options. *Am J Hematol,* **2004,** *76:*74–78.

Skibeli V, Nissen-Lie G, Torjesen P. Sugar profiling proves that human serum erythropoietin differs from recombinant human erythropoietin. *Blood,* **2001,** *98:*3626–3634.

Solomon LR. Disorders of cobalamin (vitamin B12) metabolism: Emerging concepts in pathophysiology, diagnosis and treatment. *Blood Rev,* **2007,** *21:*113–130.

Solomon LR, Hillman RS. Vitamin B6 metabolism in anaemic and alcoholic man. *Br J Haematol,* **1979,** *41:*343–356.

Solomon LR, Hillman RS. Vitamin B6 metabolism in human red cells. I. Variations in normal subjects. *Enzyme,* **1978,** *23:*262–273.

Solomon LR, Hillman RS. Vitamin B6 metabolism in idiopathic sideroblastic anaemia and related disorders. *Br J Haematol,* **1979,** *42:*239–253.

Tepler I, Elias L, Smith JW 2nd, *et al*. A randomized placebo-controlled trial of recombinant human interleukin-11 in cancer patients with severe thrombocytopenia due to chemotherapy. *Blood,* **1996,** *87:*3607–3614.

Teramura M, Kobayashi S, Hoshino S, *et al.* Interleukin-11 enhances human megakaryocytopoiesis in vitro. *Blood,* **1992,** *79:*327–331.

Uriu-Adams JY, Keen CL. Copper, oxidative stress, and human health. *Mol Aspects Med,* **2005,** *26:*268–298.

Vadhan-Raj S, Verschraegen CF, Bueso-Ramos C, *et al.* Recombinant human thrombopoietin attenuates carboplatin-induced severe thrombocytopenia and the need for platelet transfusions in patients with gynecologic cancer. *Ann Intern Med,* **2000,** *132:*364–368.

Varela-Moreiras G, Murphy MM, Scott JM. Cobalamin, folic acid, and homocysteine. *Nutr Rev,* **2009,** *67 Suppl 1:*S69–72.

Weinbren K, Salm R, Greenberg G. Intramuscular injections of iron compounds and oncogenesis in man. *Br Med J,* **1978,** *1:* 683–685.

Weisbart RH, Kwan L, Golde DW, Gasson JC. Human GM-CSF primes neutrophils for enhanced oxidative metabolism in response to the major physiological chemoattractants. *Blood,* **1987,** *69:*18–21.

Weissbach H. The isolation of the vitamin B12 coenzyme and the role of the vitamin in methionine synthesis. *J Biol Chem,* **2008,** *283:*23497–23504.

Welte K, Platzer E, Lu L, *et al*. Purification and biochemical characterization of human pluripotent hematopoietic colony-stimulating factor. *Proc Natl Acad Sci U S A,* **1985,** *82:* 1526–1530.

Wish JB. Intravenous iron: Not just for hemodialysis patients anymore. *Perit Dial Int,* **2008,** *28:*126–129.

Wong GG, Witek JS, Temple PA, *et al*. Human GM-CSF: Molecular cloning of the complementary DNA and purification of the natural and recombinant proteins. *Science,* **1985,** *228:*810–815.

Wrighting DM, Andrews NC. Iron homeostasis and erythropoiesis. *Curr Top Dev Biol,* **2008,** *82:*141–167.

Yang YC, Ciarletta AB, Temple PA, *et al*. Human IL-3 (multi-CSF): identification by expression cloning of a novel hematopoietic growth factor related to murine IL-3. *Cell,* **1986,** *47:*3–10.

Zager RA, Johnson AC, Hanson SY. Parenteral iron nephrotoxicity: Potential mechanisms and consequences. *Kidney Int,* **2004,** *66:*144–156.

Zanen AL, Adriaansen HJ, van Bommel EF, *et al.* 'Oversaturation' of transferrin after intravenous ferric gluconate (Ferrlecit(R)) in haemodialysis patients. *Nephrol Dial Transplant,* **1996,** *11:*820–824.

Zidar BL, Shadduck RK, Zeigler Z, Winkelstein A. Observations on the anemia and neutropenia of human copper deficiency. *Am J Hematol,* **1977,** *3:*177–185.

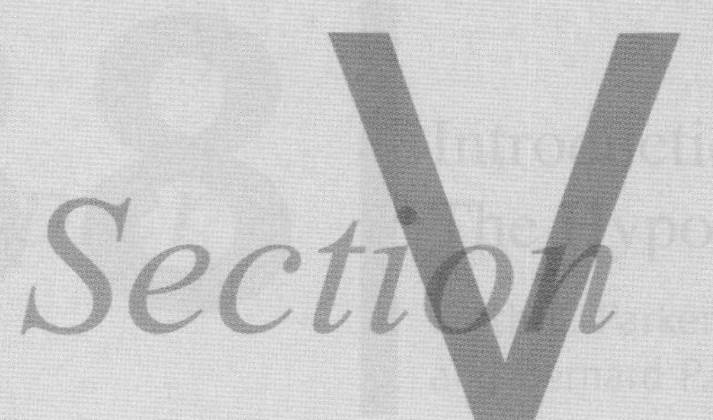

Section V

Hormones and Hormone Antagonists

disorders. Chapters 38 through 44 describe the different endocrine organs and the drugs that are employed to affect their function or to mimic or block their hormonal products.

THE HYPOTHALAMIC-PITUITARY-ENDOCRINE AXIS

Many of the classic endocrine hormones (e.g., cortisol, thyroid hormone, sex steroids, growth hormone) are regulated by complex reciprocal interactions among the hypothalamus, anterior pituitary, and endocrine glands (Table 38–1). These interactions permit precise control over the levels of circulating hormones and also provide a means to alter hormone levels under special physiological or pathological circumstances.

The basic organization of the hypothalamic-pituitary-endocrine axis is summarized in Figure 38–1. Discrete sets of hypothalamic neurons produce different releasing hormones, which are axonally transported to the median eminence. Upon stimulation, these neurons secrete their respective hypothalamic releasing hormones into the hypothalamic-adenohypophyseal plexus, which flows to the anterior pituitary gland. The hypothalamic releasing hormones bind to membrane receptors on specific subsets of pituitary cells and stimulate the secretion of the corresponding pituitary hormones. The pituitary hormones, which can be thought of as the master signals, then circulate to the target endocrine glands, where they again activate specific receptors to stimulate the synthesis and secretion of the target endocrine hormones. These interactions thus represent feed-forward regulation in which the master (signal) hormones stimulate the production of target hormones by the endocrine organs.

Superimposed on this positive feed-forward regulation is negative feedback regulation, which permits precise control of hormone levels. Figures 38–2 and 38–7 show examples of this negative feedback regulation. Typically, the endocrine target hormone circulates to both the hypothalamus and pituitary, where it acts via specific receptors to inhibit the production and secretion of both its hypothalamic releasing hormone and the regulatory pituitary hormone, thereby tightly regulating target hormone levels. In addition, other brain regions have inputs to the hypothalamic releasing neurons, further integrating the regulation of hormone levels in response to diverse stimuli.

An understanding of this regulation facilitates the diagnosis and management of a number of endocrine diseases. Endocrine deficiency states can be divided into those with impaired function at the level of the target endocrine gland (primary disease; as is the case in the autoimmune destruction of the adrenal or thyroid glands) and those with defects at the level of the pituitary gland and/or hypothalamus that impair delivery of the pituitary trophic hormone to its target gland (secondary/tertiary disease). In *primary hypofunction*, the production of the target endocrine hormone will be impaired; however, the hypothalamus and pituitary will sense the diminished feedback inhibition and the anterior pituitary gland will secrete higher than normal levels of the signal hormone. In *secondary hypofunction*, both the signal hormone and the target hormone will be below the normal range.

Table 38–1

Hormones that Integrate the Hypothalamic-Pituitary-Endocrine Axis

HYPOTHALAMIC RELEASING HORMONE	PITUITARY TROPHIC (SIGNAL) HORMONE	TARGET HORMONE(S)
Growth hormone-releasing hormone (GHRH)	Growth hormone (GH)	IGF-1
Somatostatin (SST)[a]	Growth hormone	
Dopamine (DA)[b]	Prolactin	—
Corticotropin-releasing hormone (CRH)	Corticotropin	Cortisol/DHEA
Thyrotropin-releasing hormone (TRH)	Thyroid-stimulating hormone (TSH)	Thyroid hormone
Gonadotropin-releasing hormone (GnRH)	Follicle-stimulating hormone (FSH)	Estrogen
	Luteinizing hormone (LH)	Progesterone/Estrogen (f) Testosterone (m)

[a]Somatostatin inhibits growth hormone release.
[b]Dopamine inhibits prolactin release.
IGF-1, insulin-like growth factor-1; DHEA, dehydroepiandrosterone; f, female; m, male.

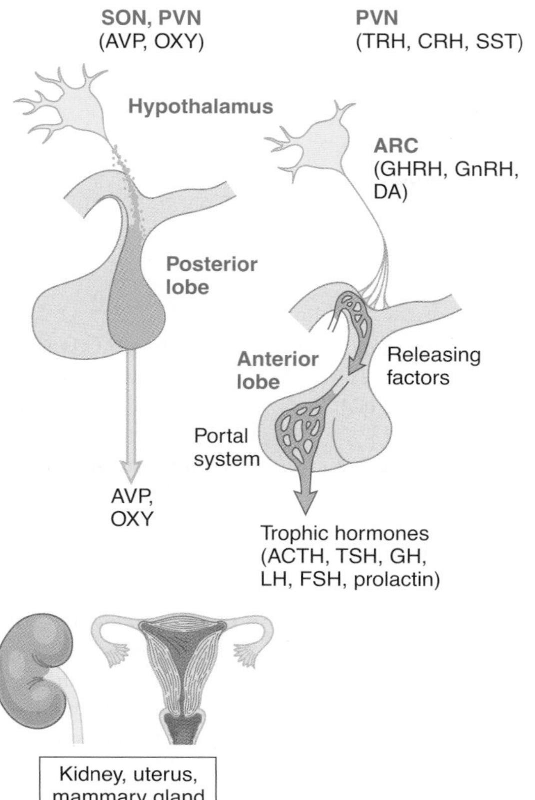

Figure 38–1. *Organization of the anterior and posterior pituitary gland.* Hypothalamic neurons in the supraoptic (SON) and paraventricular (PVN) nuclei synthesize arginine vasopressin (AVP) or oxytocin (OXY). Most of their axons project directly to the posterior pituitary, from which AVP and OXY are secreted into the systemic circulation to regulate their target tissues. Neurons that regulate the anterior lobe cluster in the mediobasal hypothalamus, including the PVH and the arcuate (ARC) nuclei. They secrete hypothalamic releasing hormones, which reach the anterior pituitary via the hypothalamic-adenohypophyseal portal system and stimulate distinct populations of pituitary cells. These cells, in turn, secrete the trophic (signal) hormones, which regulate endocrine organs and other tissues. See Table 38-1 for abbreviations.

Hormone excess similarly can result either from primary disorders at the level of the target endocrine glands (e.g., a hyperfunctioning tumor of the adrenal cortex that oversecretes cortisol) or from secondary disorders at the level of the pituitary gland (e.g., a pituitary corticotrope adenoma that oversecretes corticotropin, the predominant stimulator of adrenal glucocorticoid biosynthesis). Again, knowledge of the levels of the pituitary signal hormone and the target hormone allows the clinician to identify the site of the endocrine disorder.

PITUITARY HORMONES AND THEIR HYPOTHALAMIC RELEASING FACTORS

The peptide hormones of the anterior pituitary are essential for the regulation of growth and development, reproduction, response to stress, and intermediary metabolism. Their synthesis and secretion are controlled by hypothalamic hormones and by hormones from the peripheral endocrine organs. A large number of disease states, as well as a diverse group of drugs, also affect their secretion. The complex interactions among the hypothalamus, pituitary, and target endocrine glands provide elegant examples of the integrated feedback regulation described earlier. Clinically, an improved understanding of the mechanisms that underlie these interactions provides the rationale for diagnosing and treating endocrine disorders and for predicting certain side effects of drugs that affect the endocrine system. Moreover, the elucidation of the structures of the anterior pituitary hormones and hypothalamic releasing hormones and advances in protein chemistry and molecular biology have made it possible to produce synthetic peptide agonists and antagonists that have important diagnostic and therapeutic applications.

The anterior pituitary hormones can be classified into three different groups based on their structural features (Table 38–2). *Corticotropin* (adrenocorticotrophic hormone, ACTH) and *α-melanocyte-stimulating hormone* (α-MSH) are part of a family of peptides derived from *pro-opiomelanocortin* (POMC) by proteolytic processing (Chapters 18 and 42). *Growth hormone* (GH) and *prolactin* belong to the somatotropic family of hormones, which in humans also includes placental lactogen. The glycoprotein hormones—*thyroid-stimulating hormone* (TSH; also called thyrotropin), *luteinizing hormone* (LH; also called lutropin), and *follicle-stimulating hormone* (FSH; also called follitropin)—share a common α-subunit but have different β-subunits that determine their distinct biological activities. In humans, the glycoprotein hormone family also includes *human chorionic gonadotropin* (hCG).

The synthesis and release of anterior pituitary hormones are influenced by the central nervous system (CNS). Their secretion is positively regulated by a group of peptides referred to as *hypothalamic releasing hormones*, which are released from hypothalamic neurons in the region of the median eminence and reach the anterior pituitary through the hypothalamic-adenohypophyseal portal system (Figure 38–1). The hypothalamic- releasing hormones include *corticotropin-releasing hormone* (CRH), *growth hormone–releasing*

Table 38–2

Properties of the Protein Hormones of the Human Adenohypophysis and Placenta

HORMONE	MASS (daltons)	PEPTIDE CHAINS	AMINO ACID RESIDUES	CHROMOSOMAL LOCATION	COMMENTS
Somatotropic hormones					
Growth hormone (GH)	22,000	1	191	17q22-24	
Prolactin (PRL)	23,000	1	199	6p22.2-21.3	
Placental lactogen (PL)	22,125	1	190	17q22-24	
Glycoprotein hormones					
Luteinizing hormone (LH)	29,400	2	α-92 β-121	6q12.q21 19q13.3	Heterodimeric glycoproteins with a common α-subunit and unique β-subunits that determine biological specificity
Follicle-stimulating hormone (FSH)	32,600	2	α-92 β-111	6q12.q21 11p13	
Human chorionic gonadotropin (hCG)	38,600	2	α-92 β-145	6q12.q21 19q13.3	
Thyroid-stimulating hormone (TSH)	28,000	2	α-92 β-118	6q12.q21 1p13	
*POMC-derived hormones**					
Corticotropin (ACTH)	4500	1	39	2p22.3	These peptides are derived by proteolytic hormone processing of the common precursor, pro-opiomelanocortin (POMC)
α-Melanocyte-stimulating (α-MSH)	1650	1	13		

**See* Chapter 42 for further discussion of POMC-derived peptides, including ACTH and α-MSH.

hormone (GHRH), *gonadotropin-releasing hormone* (GnRH), and *thyrotropin-releasing hormone* (TRH). *Somatostatin* (SST), another hypothalamic peptide, negatively regulates secretion of pituitary GH and TSH. The neurotransmitter dopamine inhibits the secretion of prolactin by lactotropes.

The posterior pituitary gland, also known as the neurohypophysis, contains the endings of nerve axons arising from distinct populations of neurons in the supraoptic and paraventicular nuclei of the hypothalamus that synthesize either arginine vasopressin or oxytocin (Figure 38–1). Arginine vasopressin plays an important role in water homeostasis (Chapter 25); oxytocin plays important roles in labor and parturition and in milk letdown, as discussed in the following sections and in Chapter 66.

SOMATOTROPIC HORMONES: GROWTH HORMONE AND PROLACTIN

GH and prolactin are structurally related members of the somatotropic hormone family and share many biological features, thus providing a rationale for discussing them together. The somatotropes and lactotropes, the pituitary cells that produce GH and prolactin, respectively, derive during pituitary development from a common precursor and are eosinophilic in histological sections. Consistent with their common origin, defects in certain transcription factors affect both cell lineages. In addition to their structural similarities, GH and prolactin act via membrane receptors that belong to the cytokine receptor family and modulate target cell function via very similar signal transduction pathways (Chapter 3). The secretion of both hormones is subject to strong inhibitory input from hypothalamic neurons; for prolactin, this negative dopaminergic input clearly is the predominant regulator of secretion. Finally, several drugs that are used to treat excessive secretion of these hormones are effective to varying degrees for both GH and prolactin.

Physiology of the Somatotropic Hormones

Structures of the Somatotropic Hormones. The gene encoding human GH resides on the long arm of chromosome 17 (17q22), which also contains three different variants of placental lactogen and a GH variant, chorionic somatotropin, expressed in the syncytiotrophoblast. GH is secreted by somatotropes as a heterogeneous mixture of peptides; the principal form is a single polypeptide chain of 22 kDa that has two disulfide bonds and is not glycosylated. Alternative splicing deletes residues 32 to 46 of the larger form to produce a smaller form (~20 kDa) with equal bioactivity that makes up 5-10% of circulating GH. Recombinant human GH consists entirely of the 22 kDa form, which provides a way to detect GH abuse for sports performance enhancement.

Additional GH species, differing in size or charge, are found in serum, but their physiological significance is unclear. In the circulation, a 55 kDa protein binds approximately 45% of the 22 kDa and 25% of the 20 kDa forms; this binding protein contains the extracellular domain of the GH receptor and apparently arises from proteolytic cleavage. A second protein unrelated to the GH receptor also binds approximately 5-10% of circulating GH with lower affinity. Bound GH is cleared more slowly and has a biological $t_{1/2}$ ~10 times that of unbound GH, suggesting that the bound hormone may provide a GH reservoir that dampens acute fluctuations in GH levels associated with its pulsatile secretion. Alternatively, the binding protein may decrease GH bioactivity by preventing it from binding to its receptor in target tissues. Obesity increases circulating levels of GH binding proteins and thus may affect the clinical response to exogenous GH.

Human prolactin is a 23 kDa protein with three intramolecular disulfide bonds. It is synthesized by lactotropes, and a portion of the secreted hormone is glycosylated at a single Asn residue. In circulation, dimeric and polymeric forms of prolactin also are found, as are degradation products of 16 kDa and 18 kDa. As with GH, the biological significance of these different forms is not known.

Regulation of Secretion of the Somatotropic Hormones. Daily GH secretion varies throughout life; secretion is high in children, peaks during puberty, and then decreases in an age-related manner in adulthood. GH is secreted in discrete but irregular pulses. Between these pulses, circulating GH falls to levels that are undetectable with most assays. The amplitude of secretory pulses is greatest at night, and the most consistent period of GH secretion is shortly after the onset of deep sleep.

GH secretion, as illustrated in Figure 38–2, incorporates many of the classic features of endocrine regulation. GHRH, produced by hypothalamic neurons found predominantly in the arcuate nucleus, stimulates GH secretion by binding to a specific GPCR on

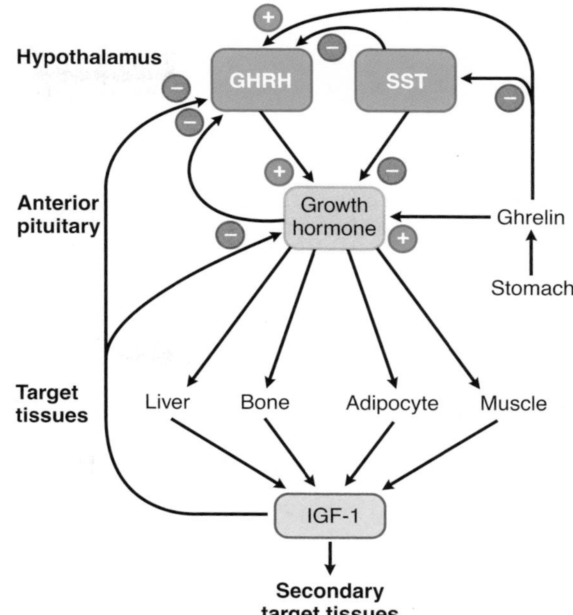

Figure 38–2. *Growth hormone secretion and actions.* Two hypothalamic factors, growth hormone–releasing hormone (GHRH) and somatostatin (SST) stimulate or inhibit the release of growth hormone (GH) from the pituitary, respectively. Insulin-like growth factor-1 (IGF-1), a product of GH action on peripheral tissues, causes negative feedback inhibition of GH release by acting at the hypothalamus and the pituitary. The actions of GH can be direct or indirect (mediated by IGF-1). See text for discussion of the other agents that modulate GH secretion and of the effects of locally produced IGF-1. Inhibition, –; stimulation, +.

somatotropes that resembles most closely the receptors for secretin, vasoactive intestinal polypeptide (VIP), pituitary adenylyl cyclase-activating peptide (PACAP), glucagon, glucagon-like peptide-1 (GLP-1), calcitonin, and parathyroid hormone (PTH). Upon binding GHRH, the GHRH receptor couples to G_s to raise intracellular levels of cyclic AMP and Ca^{2+}, thereby stimulating GH synthesis and secretion. Loss-of-function mutations of the GHRH receptor cause a rare form of short stature in humans, thereby demonstrating its essential role in normal GH secretion (Wajnrajch et al., 1996).

Typical of endocrine systems, GH and its major peripheral effector, insulin-like growth factor 1 (IGF-1), act in negative feedback loops to suppress GH secretion. The negative effect of IGF-1 is predominantly through direct effects on the anterior pituitary gland. In contrast, the negative feedback action of GH is mediated in part by SST, which is synthesized in more widely distributed neurons.

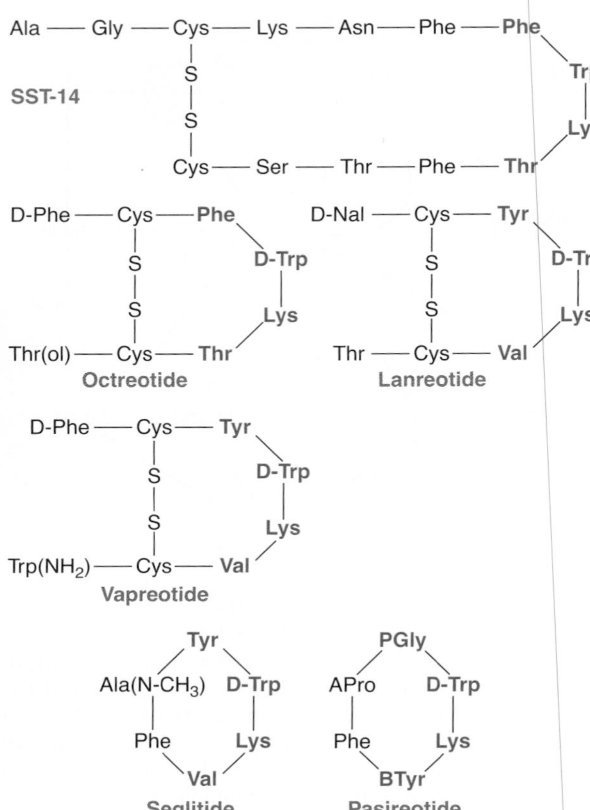

Figure 38–3. *Structures of somatostatin-14 and selected synthetic analogs.* The amino acid sequence of somatostatin (SST)-14 is shown. Residues that play key roles in receptor binding, as discussed in the text, are shown in red. Also shown are the structures of the two clinically available synthetic analogs of somatostatin, octreotide and lanreotide, and three other analogs that have been used in clinical trials, seglitide, vapreotide, and pasireotide. APro, [(2-aminoethyl) aminocarboxyl oxy]-L-proline; D-Nal, (3-(2-napthyl)-D-alanyl; PGly, phenylglycine; BTyr, benzyltyrosine.

Somatostatin is synthesized as a 92–amino acid precursor and processed by proteolytic cleavage to generate two peptides: SST-28 and SST-14. SST-14 consists of the carboxy-terminal 14 amino acids of SST-28, which form an intrapeptide disulfide bond (Figure 38–3). SST exerts its effects by binding to and activating a family of five related GPCRs that signal through G_i to inhibit cyclic AMP accumulation and to activate K^+ channels and protein phosphotyrosine phosphatases.

Each of the SST receptor subtypes (abbreviated SSTRs) binds SST with nanomolar affinity; whereas receptor types 1-4 (SSTR1-4) bind the two SSTs with approximately equal affinity, type 5 (SSTR5) has a 10- to 15-fold greater affinity for SST-28. SSTR2 and SSTR5 are the most important for regulation of GH secretion, and recent studies suggest that these two SSTRs form functional heterodimers with distinctive signaling behavior (Grant et al., 2008). SST exerts direct effects on somatotropes in the pituitary and indirect effects mediated via GHRH neurons in the arcuate nucleus. As discussed later, SST analogs play a key role in the pharmacotherapy of syndromes of GH excess and certain cancers.

Ghrelin, a 28-amino acid peptide that is octanoylated at Ser3, also stimulates GH secretion. Ghrelin is synthesized predominantly in endocrine cells in the fundus of the stomach but also is produced at lower levels at a number of other sites. Both fasting and hypoglycemia stimulate circulating ghrelin levels.

Ghrelin acts primarily through a GPCR called the GH secretagogue receptor. Although the interaction of ghrelin with this receptor directly stimulates GH release by isolated somatotropes, the major action on GH secretion apparently is through actions on the GHRH neurons in the arcuate nucleus. Apart from its effects on GH secretion, ghrelin also stimulates appetite and increases food intake, apparently by central actions on NPY and agouti-related peptide neurons in the hypothalamus. Thus, ghrelin and its receptor act in a complex manner to integrate the functions of the GI tract, the hypothalamus, and the anterior pituitary (Ghigo et al., 2005). Peptide and nonpeptide agonists (termed GH secretagogues) and antagonists of the GH secretagogue receptor are undergoing evaluation as possible modulators of neuroendocrine function.

Several neurotransmitters, drugs, metabolites, and other stimuli modulate the release of GHRH and/or SST and thereby affect GH secretion. DA, 5-HT, and α_2 adrenergic receptor agonists stimulate GH release, as do hypoglycemia, exercise, stress, emotional excitement, and ingestion of protein-rich meals. In contrast, β adrenergic receptor agonists, free fatty acids, IGF-1, and GH itself inhibit release, as does the administration of glucose to normal subjects in an oral glucose-tolerance test.

Many of the physiological factors that influence prolactin secretion also affect GH secretion. Thus sleep, stress, hypoglycemia, exercise, and estrogen increase the secretion of both hormones.

Prolactin is unique among the anterior pituitary hormones in that hypothalamic regulation of its secretion is predominantly inhibitory. The major regulator of prolactin secretion is DA, which is released by tuberoinfundibular neurons and interacts with the D_2 receptor, a GPCR on lactotropes, to inhibit prolactin secretion (Figure 38–4). Recent reports have suggested that the D_2 receptor and the SST_2 receptor can form heterodimers (Baragli et al., 2007), which may have implications for therapy (see following discussion).

A number of putative prolactin-releasing factors have been described, including TRH, VIP, prolactin-releasing peptide, and PACAP, but their physiological roles are unclear. Under certain

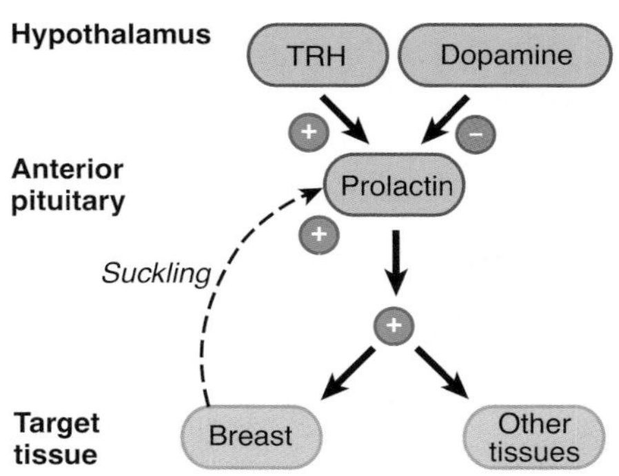

Figure 38–4. *Prolactin secretion and actions.* Prolactin is the only anterior pituitary hormone for which a unique stimulatory releasing factor has not been identified. Thyrotropin-releasing hormone (TRH), however, can stimulate prolactin release and dopamine can inhibit it. Suckling induces prolactin secretion, and prolactin affects lactation and reproductive functions but also has varied effects on many other tissues. Prolactin is not under feedback control by peripheral hormones.

pathological conditions, such as severe primary hypothyroidism, persistently elevated levels of TRH can induce hyperprolactinemia.

Unlike GH, which plays important roles throughout life in both sexes, prolactin acts predominantly in women, both during pregnancy and in the postpartum period in women who breast-feed. Serum prolactin levels remain low in men but are elevated somewhat in normal cycling females. During pregnancy, the maternal serum prolactin level starts to increase at 8 weeks of gestation, increases to peak levels of 250 ng/mL at term, and declines thereafter to prepregnancy levels unless the mother breast-feeds the infant. Suckling or breast manipulation in nursing mothers transmits signals from the breast to the hypothalamus via the spinal cord and the median forebrain bundle, which, in turn, stimulate circulating prolactin levels. Prolactin levels can rise 10- to 100-fold within 30 minutes of stimulation. This response is distinct from milk letdown, which is mediated by oxytocin release from the posterior pituitary gland. The suckling-induced prolactin secretion involves both decreased secretion of dopamine by tuberoinfundibular neurons and possibly increased release of factors that stimulate prolactin secretion. The suckling response becomes less pronounced after several months of breast-feeding, and prolactin concentrations eventually decline to prepregnancy levels.

Prolactin also is synthesized in lactotropes near the end of the luteal phase of the menstrual cycle and by decidual cells early in pregnancy; the latter source is responsible for the very high levels of prolactin in amniotic fluid during the first trimester of human pregnancy. The function of this prolactin and what regulates its expression are not known.

Molecular and Cellular Bases of Somatotropic Hormone Action. All of the effects of GH and prolactin result from their interactions with specific membrane receptors on target tissues (Figure 38–5). Both the GH and prolactin receptors are widely distributed cell surface receptors that belong to the cytokine receptor superfamily and thus share structural similarity with the receptors for leptin, erythropoietin, granulocyte-macrophage colony-stimulating factor, and several of the interleukins. Like other members of the cytokine receptor family, these receptors contain an extracellular hormone-binding domain, a single membrane-spanning region, and an intracellular domain that mediates signal transduction.

The mature human GH receptor contains 620 amino acids, approximately 250 of which are extracellular, 24 of which are transmembrane, and ~350 of which are cytoplasmic. It exists as a preformed homodimer that forms a ternary complex with one molecule of GH. The formation of the GH-GH receptor ternary complex is initiated by high-affinity interaction of GH with one monomer of the GH receptor dimer (mediated by GH site 1), followed by a second, lower affinity interaction of GH with the GH receptor mediated by GH site 2; these interactions induce a conformational change that activates downstream signaling. As discussed later, pegvisomant is a GH analog with amino acid substitutions that disrupt site 2; it binds the receptor and causes its internalization but cannot trigger the conformational change that stimulates downstream events in the signal transduction pathway. Amino acid–substituted versions of human prolactin that act as antagonists at the prolactin receptor are also under development (Goffin et al., 2006).

The ligand-occupied GH receptor dimer lacks inherent tyrosine kinase activity. Rather, it provides docking sites for two molecules of JAK2, a cytoplasmic tyrosine kinase of the Janus kinase family. The juxtaposition of two JAK2 molecules leads to *trans*-phosphorylation and autoactivation of JAK2, with consequent tyrosine phosphorylation of cytoplasmic proteins that mediate downstream signaling events (Lanning and Carter-Su, 2006). These include STAT proteins (*S*ignal *T*ransducers and *A*ctivators of *T*ranscription), Shc (an adapter protein that regulates the Ras/MAPK signaling pathway), and IRS-1 and IRS-2 (insulin-receptor substrate proteins that activate the PI3K pathway). One critical target of STAT5 is the gene encoding IGF-1 (Figure 38–5). The fine control of GH action also involves feedback regulatory events that subsequently turn off the GH signal. As part of its action, GH induces the expression of a family of SOCS (suppressor of cytokine signaling) proteins and a group of protein tyrosine phosphatases that, by different mechanisms, disrupt the communication of the activated GH receptor with JAK2 (Flores-Morales et al., 2006).

Some studies have shown that the GH receptor can translocate to the nucleus and act as a coregulator to activate transcription and cell proliferation (Swanson and Kopchick, 2007). The precise role of this signal transduction pathway in GH physiology and pathophysiology remains to be defined.

The effects of prolactin on target cells also result from interactions with a cytokine receptor that is widely distributed and signals through many of the same pathways as the GH receptor. Alternative splicing of the prolactin receptor gene on chromosome 5 gives rise to multiple forms of the receptor that are identical in the extracellular domain but differ in their cytoplasmic domains. In addition, soluble forms that correspond to the extracellular domain of the receptor are found in circulation. Unlike human GH and placental

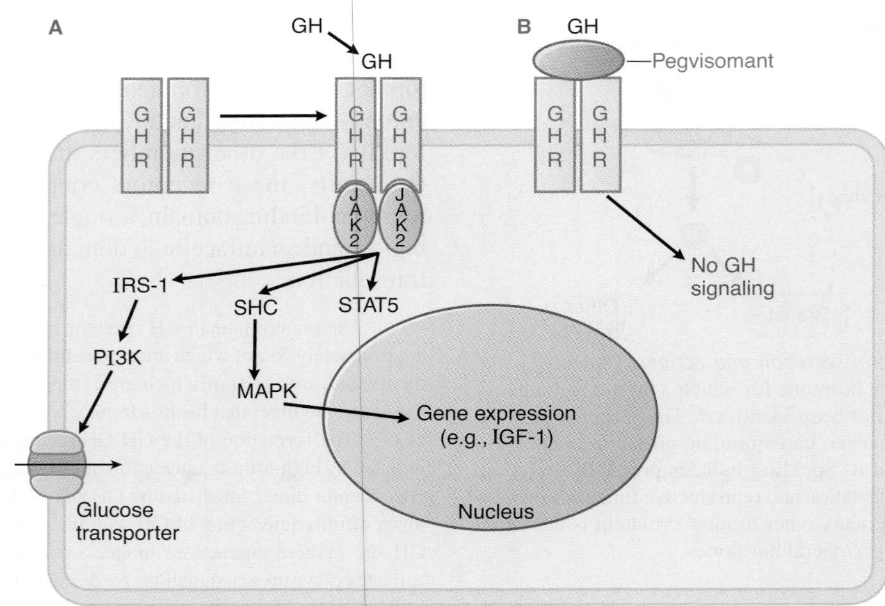

Figure 38–5. *Mechanisms of growth hormone and prolactin action and of GH receptor antagonism.* ***Left (A):*** The binding of GH to a homodimer of the growth hormone receptor (GHR) induces autophosphorylation of JAK2. JAK2 then phosphorylates cytoplasmic proteins that activate downstream signaling pathways, including STAT5 and mediators upstream of MAPK, which ultimately modulate gene expression. The structurally related prolactin receptor also is a ligand activated homodimer that recruits the JAK-STAT signaling pathway (see text for further details). The GHR also activates IRS-1, which may mediate the increased expression of glucose transporters on the plasma membrane. The diagram does not reflect the localization of the intracellular molecules, which presumably exist in multicomponent signaling complexes. JAK2, janus kinase 2; IRS-1, insulin receptor substrate-1; PI3K, phosphatidyl inositol-3 kinase; STAT, signal transducer and activator of transcription; MAPK, mitogen-activated protein kinase; SHC, Src homology containing. ***Right (B):*** Pegvisomant, a recombinant pegylated variant of human GH, contains amino acid substitutions that increase the affinity for one site of the GHR but do not activate its downstream signaling cascade. It thus interferes with GH signaling in target tissues.

lactogen, which also bind to the prolactin receptor and thus are lactogenic, prolactin binds specifically to the prolactin receptor and has no somatotropic (GH-like) activity.

Physiological Effects of the Somatotropic Hormones. The most striking physiological effect of GH—and the basis for its name—is the stimulation of the longitudinal growth of bones (Giustina et al., 2008). GH also increases bone mineral density after the epiphyses have closed and longitudinal growth ceases. These effects of GH involve the differentiation of prechondrocytes to chondrocytes and stimulation of osteoclast and osteoblast proliferation. Other effects of GH include the stimulation of myoblast differentiation (in experimental animals) and increased muscle mass (in human subjects with GH deficiency), increased glomerular filtration rate, and stimulation of preadipocyte differentiation into adipocytes. GH has potent anti-insulin actions in both the liver and peripheral sites (e.g., adipocytes and muscle) that decrease glucose utilization and increase lipolysis. Finally, GH has been implicated in the development and function of the immune system.

Growth hormone acts directly on adipocytes to increase lipolysis and on hepatocytes to stimulate gluconeogenesis, but its anabolic and growth-promoting effects are mediated indirectly through the induction of IGF-1. Although most circulating IGF-1 is made in the liver, IGF-1 produced locally in many tissues is critical for growth, as revealed by normal growth in mice that have a hepatocyte-specific inactivation of IGF-1. Circulating IGF-1 is associated with a family of binding proteins, designated the IGF-binding proteins (IGFBPs), that serve as transport proteins and also may mediate certain aspects of IGF-1 signaling. Most IGF-1 in circulation is bound to IGFBP-3 and another protein called the acid-labile subunit.

The essential role of IGF-1 in growth is evidenced by patients with loss-of-function mutations in both alleles of the *IGF1* gene, whose severe intrauterine and postnatal growth retardation is unresponsive to GH but responsive to recombinant human IGF-1, and by the association of mutations in the IGF-1 receptor with intrauterine growth retardation (Walenkamp and Wit, 2008).

After its synthesis and release, IGF-1 interacts with receptors on the cell surface that mediate its biological activities. The type 1 IGF receptor is closely related to the insulin receptor and consists of a heterotetramer with intrinsic tyrosine kinase activity. This receptor is present in essentially all tissues and binds IGF-1 and the related growth factor, IGF-2, with high affinity; insulin also can activate the type 1 IGF receptor but with an affinity approximately two orders of magnitude less than that of the IGFs. The signal transduction pathway for the insulin receptor is described in detail in Chapter 43.

Unlike GH, prolactin does not induce the synthesis of a second hormone that then mediates many of its effects in an indirect manner. Rather, prolactin effects are limited to tissues that express the prolactin receptor, particularly the mammary gland. A number of hormones—including estrogens, progesterone, placental lactogen, and GH—stimulate development of the breast and prepare it for lactation. Prolactin, acting via prolactin receptors, plays an important role in inducing growth and differentiation of the ductal and lobuloalveolar epithelia and is essential for lactation. Target genes, by which prolactin induces mammary development, include those encoding milk proteins (e.g., caseins), genes important for intracellular structure (e.g., keratins), genes important for cell-cell communication (e.g., amphiregulin and Wnt4), and components of the extracellular matrix (e.g., laminin and collagen).

Prolactin receptors are present in many other sites, including the hypothalamus, liver, adrenal, testes, ovaries, prostate, and immune system, suggesting that prolactin may play multiple roles outside of the breast. The physiological effects of prolactin at these sites remain poorly characterized, and specific defects in their function that result from prolactin deficiency have not been defined.

Pathophysiology of the Somatotropic Hormones

Distinct endocrine disorders result from either excessive or deficient GH production. In contrast, prolactin predominantly impacts endocrine function when produced in excess.

Excess Production of Somatotropic Hormones. Syndromes of excess secretion of GH and prolactin typically are caused by somatotrope or lactotrope adenomas that oversecrete the respective hormones. These adenomas often retain some features of the normal regulation described earlier, thus permitting pharmacological modulation of secretion—an important modality in therapy.

Clinical Manifestations. GH excess causes distinct clinical syndromes depending on the age of the patient. If the epiphyses are unfused, GH excess causes increased longitudinal growth, resulting in gigantism. In adults, GH excess causes acromegaly. The symptoms and signs of acromegaly (e.g., arthropathy, carpal tunnel syndrome, generalized visceromegaly, macroglossia, hypertension, glucose intolerance, headache, lethargy, excess perspiration, and sleep apnea) progress slowly, and diagnosis often is delayed. Mortality is increased at least 2-fold relative to age-matched controls, predominantly due to increased death from cardiovascular disease.

Hyperprolactinemia is a relatively common endocrine abnormality that can result from hypothalamic or pituitary diseases that interfere with the delivery of inhibitory dopaminergic signals, from renal failure, from primary hypothyroidism associated with increased TRH levels, or from treatment with dopamine receptor antagonists. Most often, hyperprolactinemia is caused by prolactin-secreting pituitary adenomas—either microadenomas (≤1 cm in diameter) or macroadenomas (>1 cm in diameter). Manifestations of prolactin excess in women include galactorrhea, amenorrhea, and infertility. In men, hyperprolactinemia causes loss of libido, erectile dysfunction, and infertility.

Diagnosis of Somatotropin Hormone Excess. Although acromegaly should be suspected in patients with the appropriate symptoms and signs, diagnostic confirmation requires the demonstration of increased circulating GH or IGF-1. The "gold standard" diagnostic test for acromegaly is the oral glucose tolerance test. Whereas normal subjects suppress their GH level to <1 ng/mL in response to an oral glucose challenge (the absolute value may vary depending on the sensitivity of the assay), patients with acromegaly either fail to suppress or show a paradoxical increase in GH level.

In patients with hyperprolactinemia, the major question is whether conditions other than a prolactin-producing adenoma are responsible for the elevated prolactin level. A number of medications that inhibit DA signaling can cause moderate elevations in prolactin (e.g., antipsychotics, metoclopramide), as can primary hypothyroidism, pituitary mass lesions that interfere with dopamine delivery to the lactotropes, and pregnancy. Thus thyroid function and pregnancy tests are indicated, as is magnetic resonance imaging (MRI) to look for a pituitary adenoma or other defect that might elevate serum prolactin.

Impaired Production of the Somatotropic Hormones. Prolactin deficiency may result from conditions that damage the pituitary gland, but prolactin is not given as part of endocrine replacement therapy.

Clinical Manifestations of Growth Hormone Deficiency. Clinically, children with GH deficiency present with short stature, delayed bone age, and a low age-adjusted growth velocity. Specific etiologies associated with GH deficiency in children include genetic disorders that affect pituitary development and can cause deficiencies of multiple pituitary hormones, pituitary or hypothalamic tumors, previous CNS irradiation, and infiltrative processes such as histiocytosis. In most patients, however, the deficiency is idiopathic, with normal production of other pituitary hormones and no obvious structural abnormalities.

GH deficiency in adults does not impair linear growth, which ceases with closure of the epiphyses. Rather, GH deficiency in adults is associated with decreased muscle mass and exercise capacity, decreased bone density, impaired psychosocial function, and increased mortality from cardiovascular causes, probably secondary to deleterious changes in fat distribution, increases in circulating lipids, and increased inflammation (Molitch et al., 2006).

Diagnosis of Growth Hormone Deficiency. Because GH secretion is highly pulsatile, random sampling of serum GH is insufficient to diagnose GH deficiency. Whereas tests for substances that provide an estimate of integrated GH levels over time (e.g., IGF-1 and IGFBP-3) are more useful, provocative tests usually are required. After excluding other causes of poor growth, the diagnosis of GH deficiency should be entertained in children with height >2 to 2.5 standard deviations below normal, delayed bone age, a decreased growth velocity, and a predicted adult height substantially below the mean parental height. In this setting, a serum GH level <10 ng/mL following provocative testing (e.g., insulin-induced hypoglycemia, arginine, levodopa, clonidine, or glucagon) indicates GH deficiency; a stimulated value <5 ng/mL reflects severe deficiency.

In adults, overt GH deficiency usually results from pituitary lesions caused by a functioning or nonfunctioning pituitary adenoma, secondary to trauma, or related to surgery or radiotherapy for a pituitary or suprasellar mass (Molitch et al., 2006). Almost all patients with multiple deficits in other pituitary hormones also have deficient GH secretion, and some experts incorporate the number of other pituitary deficiencies into a diagnostic algorithm for diagnosing GH deficiency. Others accept a serum IGF-1 level below the age- and sex-adjusted normal range as indicative of GH deficiency in a patient with known pituitary disease. The converse is not true because an IGF-1 level within the normal range does not exclude adult GH deficiency. Some experts require an inadequate GH response to provocative testing (i.e., a value <5 ng/mL), with either insulin-induced hypoglycemia or a combination of Arg and GHRH as the preferred stimulus for GH secretion. Finally, in patients with known hypothalamic/pituitary disease of recent onset, Arg alone can be used as the stimulus, with the hGH cutoff set at 1.4 ng/mL. The risk of false-positive provocative tests (i.e., a subnormal GH response) is increased in obese subjects.

Pharmacotherapy of Disorders of the Somatotropin Hormones

Pharmacotherapy of Growth Hormone Excess. Treatment options in gigantism/acromegaly include transphenoidal surgery, radiation, and drugs that inhibit GH secretion or action. Pituitary surgery traditionally has been the treatment of choice. In patients with microadenomas, skilled neurosurgeons can achieve cure rates of 65-85%; however, the long-term success rate for patients with macroadenomas typically is <50%. In addition, there is increasing appreciation that acromegalic patients previously considered cured by pituitary surgery actually have persistent GH excess, with its attendant complications. Pituitary irradiation may be associated with significant long-term complications, including visual deterioration and pituitary dysfunction. Thus, increased attention has been given to the pharmacological management of acromegaly, either as primary treatment or for the treatment of persistent GH excess after transphenoidal surgery or irradiation. Another area receiving increased investigation is the potential role of medical therapy before surgery to improve outcome (Carlsen et al., 2008). The favored therapy has been with SST analogs, although the GH receptor antagonist pegvisomant increasingly is used. In patients who refuse these injected treatments, DA agonists may be used, although they are much less effective.

Somatostatin Analogs. The development of synthetic analogs of SST (Figure 38–3) revolutionized the medical treatment of acromegaly. The goal of treatment is to decrease GH levels to <2.5 ng/mL after an oral glucose-tolerance test and to bring IGF-1 levels to within the normal range for age and sex. Some have argued that a basal GH level of <1 ng/mL indicates cure, whereas a basal level of >2 ng/mL is highly suggestive of persistent disease.

Chemistry. Structure-function studies of SST and its derivatives established that the amino acid residues in positions 7-10 of the SST-14 peptide (Phe-Trp-Lys-Thr) are the major determinants of biological activity. Residues Trp^8 and Lys^9 appear to be essential, whereas conservative substitutions at Phe^7 and Thr^{10} are permissible. Active SST analogs retain this core segment constrained in a cyclic structure, formed either by a disulfide bond (octreotide, lanreotide, vapreotide) or an amide linkage (seglitide, pasireotide) that stabilizes the optimal conformation (Pawlikowski and Melen-Mucha, 2004). The endogenous peptides, SST-14 and SST-28, do not show specificity for SST receptor subtypes except for SST_5, which preferentially binds SST-28. Some SST analogs exhibit greater selectivity. For example, the octapeptides octreotide and lanreotide bind to the SST subtypes with the following order of selectivity: SST_2 > SST_5 > SST_3 >> SST_1 and SST_4. The cyclohexapeptide, pasireotide (SOM230), binds with high affinity to all but the SST_4 receptor. Small nonpeptide agonists that exhibit high selectivity for SST receptor subtypes have been isolated from combinatorial chemical libraries; these compounds may lead to a new class of highly selective, orally active SST mimetics (Weckbecker et al., 2003).

A chimeric compound that activates SST receptors and the D_2 receptor (BIM-23A387) is now in clinical trials for therapy of mixed GH- and prolactin-secreting adenomas and for nonfunctioning pituitary adenomas (Pawlikowski and Melen-Mucha, 2004). Based on the apparent formation of heterodimers between the SST_2 and D_2 receptors, such chimeric compounds may have efficacy for certain tumors that do not respond to either classic SST analogs or DA agonists (Florio et al., 2008).

Therapeutic Uses

Currently, the two somatostatin analogs used widely are *octreotide* and *lanreotide*, synthetic derivatives that have longer half-lives and bind preferentially to SST_2 and SST_5 receptors. Octreotide (100 μg) administered subcutaneously three times daily is virtually 100% bioactive, peak effects are seen within 30 min, serum $t_{1/2}$ is ~90 min, and duration of action is ~12 hour. This formulation successfully controls the biochemical parameters of acromegaly in 50-60% of patients.

The need to inject octreotide three times daily poses a significant obstacle to patient compliance. A long-acting, slow-release form (SANDOSTATIN-LAR DEPOT) in which the active species is incorporated into microspheres of a biodegradable polymer greatly reduces the injection frequency. Administered intramuscularly in a dose of 20 or 30 mg once every 4 week, typically to patients who have tolerated and responded to the shorter-acting formulation, octreotide LAR is at least as effective as the regular formulation (Murray and Melmed, 2008). Like the shorter-acting formulation, the longer-acting formulation of octreotide generally is well tolerated with a similar incidence of side effects (see following discussion). A lower dose of 10 mg per injection should be used in patients requiring hemodialysis or with hepatic cirrhosis.

In addition to its effect on GH secretion, octreotide can decrease tumor size, although tumor growth generally resumes after octreotide treatment is stopped.

Lanreotide is another long-acting octapeptide SST analog that causes prolonged suppression of GH secretion when administered in a 30-mg dose intramuscularly. Although its efficacy appears comparable to that of the long-acting formulation of octreotide, its duration of action is shorter; thus, it is administered at 10- or 14-day intervals.

A supersaturated aqueous formulation of lanreotide, *lanreotide autogel* (SOMATULINE DEPOT), has recently been approved for use in the U.S. It is supplied in prefilled syringes containing 60, 90, or 120 mg lanreotide and administered by deep subcutaneous injection. Administered once every 4 weeks, lanreotide autogel provides more uniform drug levels than the depot formulation of octreotide. Results of current clinical trials are at least comparable to those with the slow-release octreotide formulation (Murray and Melmed, 2008).

Adverse Effects. GI side effects—including diarrhea, nausea, and abdominal pain—occur in up to 50% of patients receiving octreotide. In most patients, these symptoms diminish over time and do not require cessation of therapy. Approximately 25% of patients receiving octreotide develop gallbladder sludge or even gallstones, presumably due to decreased gallbladder contraction and bile secretion. In the absence of symptoms, gallstones are not a contraindication to continued use of octreotide. Compared with SST, octreotide reduces insulin secretion to a lesser extent and only infrequently affects glycemic control. Inhibitory effects on TSH secretion may lead to hypothyroidism, and thyroid function tests should be evaluated periodically. The incidence and severity of side effects associated with lanreotide are similar to those of octreotide. Perhaps related to its more global inhibition of SST receptors, pasireotide has exhibited a relatively greater impairment in glycemic control than octreotide or lanreotide. The degree to which this may limit its clinical utility is not yet established.

Other Therapeutic Uses. Somatostatin blocks not only GH secretion but also the secretion of other hormones, growth factors, and cytokines. Thus octreotide and the slow-release formulations of SST analogs have been used to treat symptoms associated with metastatic carcinoid tumors (e.g., flushing and diarrhea) and adenomas secreting vasoactive intestinal peptide (e.g., watery diarrhea). Octreotide also is used for treatment of acute variceal bleeding and for perioperative prophylaxis in pancreatic surgery (see Chapter 46 for discussion of the uses of SST analogs in GI disease). Octreotide also has significant inhibitory effects on TSH secretion, and it is the treatment of choice for patients who have thyrotrope adenomas that oversecrete TSH who are not good candidates for surgery. Finally, modified forms of octreotide labeled with indium or technetium have been used for diagnostic imaging of neuroendocrine tumors such as pituitary adenomas and carcinoids (OCTREOSCAN); modified forms labeled with ß emitters such as ^{90}Y have been used in selective destruction of SST_2 receptor-positive tumors.

Novel uses under evaluation include the treatment of eye diseases associated with excessive proliferation and inflammation (e.g., Graves' orbitopathy and diabetic retinopathy), diabetic nephropathy, and various diseases associated with inflammation (e.g., rheumatoid arthritis, inflammatory bowel disease, pulmonary fibrosis, and psoriasis).

Growth Hormone Antagonists. Pegvisomant (SOMAVERT) is a GH receptor antagonist that is FDA-approved for the treatment of acromegaly. Pegvisomant binds to the GH receptor but does not activate JAK-STAT signaling or stimulate IGF-1 secretion (Figure 38–5).

Pegvisomant is administered subcutaneously as a 40-mg loading dose under physician supervision, followed by self-administration of 10 mg per day. Based on serum IGF-1 levels, the dose is titrated at 4- to 6-week intervals to a maximum of 40 mg per day. Pegvisomant should not be used in patients with an unexplained elevation of hepatic transaminases, and liver function tests should be monitored in all patients. In addition, lipohypertrophy has occurred at injection sites, sometimes requiring cessation of therapy; this is believed to reflect the inhibition of direct actions of GH on adipocytes. Because of concerns that loss of negative feedback by GH and IGF-1 may increase the growth of GH-secreting adenomas, careful follow-up by pituitary MRI is strongly recommended, although this may change as more data become available (Jimenez et al., 2008). Pegvisomant differs structurally from native GH and induces the formation of specific antibodies in ~15% of patients despite the covalent coupling of Lys residues to 4-5 molecules of a polyethylene glycol polymer per modified GH molecule. Nevertheless, the development of tachyphylaxis due to these antibodies has not been reported.

In clinical trials, pegvisomant at higher doses decreased serum IGF-1 to normal age- and sex-adjusted levels in >90% of patients and significantly improved clinical parameters such as ring size, soft-tissue swelling, excessive perspiration, and fatigue. Thus pegvisomant provides a highly effective alternative for use in patients who have not responded to SST analogs, either as sole therapy or as a temporizing measure while waiting for radiation therapy to achieve its full effect; it also is receiving increased scrutiny as first-line therapy.

Therapy of Prolactin Excess. The therapeutic options for patients with prolactinomas include transphenoidal surgery, radiation, and treatment with DA receptor agonists that suppress prolactin production via activation of D_2 receptors. The surgical success rates are 75% for microadenomas and 33% for macroadenomas. Given these results, D_2 receptor agonists are widely recognized as the treatment of choice for most patients (Gillam et al., 2006).

Dopamine Receptor Agonists

These agents generally decrease both prolactin secretion and the size of the adenoma, thereby improving both the endocrine abnormalities and neurological symptoms caused directly by the adenoma (including visual field deficits). Over time, especially with cabergoline, the prolactinoma may decrease in size to the extent that the drug can be discontinued without recurrence of the hyperprolactinemia. Some experts therefore recommend treatment with a dopamine receptor agonist for a minimum of 2 years, followed by a trial of dopamine agonist withdrawal in patients who have responded to dopamine agonist therapy with normalization of prolactin and disappearance of the tumor on MRI scanning (Gillam et al., 2006).

Patients with prolactinomas who wish to become pregnant comprise a special subset of hyperprolactinemic patients because drug safety during pregnancy becomes an important consideration. The dopamine agonists described here relieve the inhibitory effect of prolactin on ovulation and permit most patients with prolactinomas to become pregnant. Clinical experience also indicates that many patients can discontinue the dopaminergic agonist during pregnancy without clinically significant tumor growth. Although drug therapy ideally is discontinued before pregnancy to avoid any fetal exposure, most experts discontinue therapy after pregnancy is confirmed and carefully follow for symptoms or signs of pituitary mass effect throughout gestation. Because of its greater track record, bromocriptine generally is recommended for fertility induction in patients with hyperprolactinemia. Substantial clinical use with cabergoline has not revealed adverse maternal or fetal effects (Colao et al., 2008a), but most endocrinologists still prefer bromocriptine in this setting. Although not definitive, there are data linking quinagolide with fetal abnormalities (reviewed by Gillam et al., 2006), and it should not be used when pregnancy is intended.

Bromocriptine. Bromocriptine (PARLODEL) is the dopamine receptor agonist against which newer agents are compared.

Chemistry. Bromocriptine is a semisynthetic ergot alkaloid (Figure 38–6) that interacts with D_2 receptors to inhibit spontaneous and TRH-induced release of prolactin; to a lesser extent, it also activates D_1 receptors.

Absorption, Distribution, and Elimination. Although a large fraction of the oral dose of bromocriptine is absorbed, only 7% of the dose reaches the systemic circulation because of a high extraction rate and extensive first-pass metabolism in the liver. Bromocriptine has a relatively short elimination $t_{1/2}$ (between 2 and 8 hours) and thus is usually administered in divided doses (see Adverse Effects). To avoid the need for frequent dosing, a slow release oral form is available outside of the U.S. Bromocriptine may be administered vaginally (2.5 mg once daily), reportedly with fewer gastrointestinal side effects.

Therapeutic Uses. Bromocriptine normalizes serum prolactin levels in 70-80% of patients with prolactinomas and decreases tumor size in >50% of patients, including those with macroadenomas. Typically, bromocriptine does not cure the underlying adenoma, and hyperprolactinemia and tumor growth recur upon cessation of therapy.

Adverse Effects. Frequent side effects of bromocriptine include nausea and vomiting, headache, and postural hypotension, particularly on initial use. Less frequently, nasal congestion, digital vasospasm, and CNS effects such as psychosis, hallucinations, nightmares, or insomnia are observed. These adverse effects can be diminished by starting at a low dose (1.25 mg) administered at bedtime with a snack. After 1 week, a morning dose of 1.25 mg can be added. If clinical symptoms persist or serum prolactin levels remain elevated, the dose can be increased gradually, every 3-7 days, to 5 mg two or three times a day as tolerated. Patients often develop tolerance to the adverse effects of bromocriptine. Those who do not respond to bromocriptine or who develop intractable side effects often respond better to cabergoline. At higher concentrations, bromocriptine is used in the management of acromegaly, as noted earlier, and at still higher concentrations is used in the management of Parkinson's disease (Chapter 22).

Cabergoline. Cabergoline (DOSTINEX) is an ergot derivative with a longer $t_{1/2}$ (~65 hours), higher affinity, and greater selectivity for the D_2 receptor (approximately four times more potent) than bromocriptine. It undergoes significant first-pass metabolism in the liver, and the precise oral availability is not known.

Therapeutic Uses. Cabergoline is FDA-approved for the treatment of hyperprolactinemia and has become the preferred drug in most settings for this disorder. Its greater efficacy in decreasing serum prolactin in patients with hyperprolactinemia may reflect

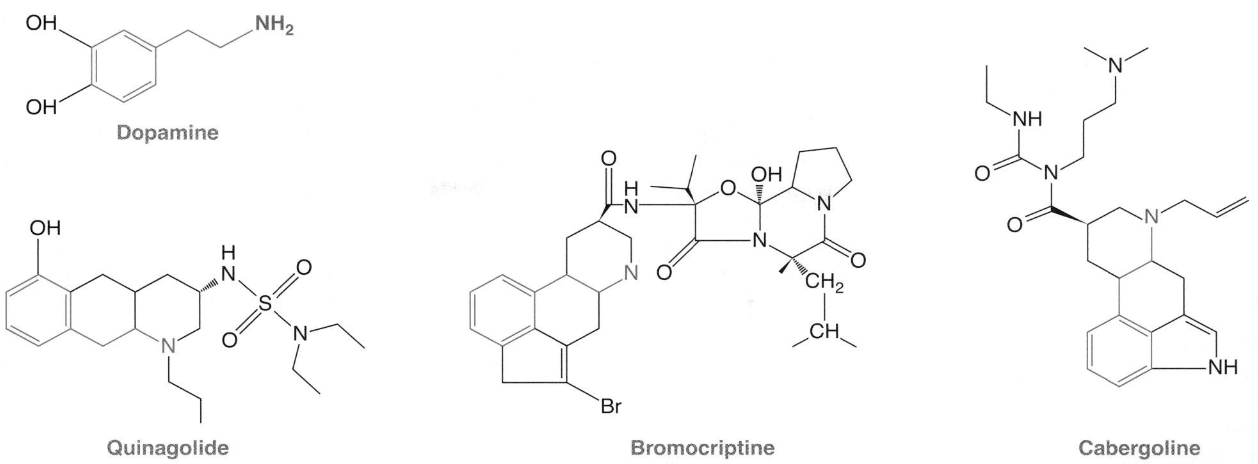

Figure 38–6. *Dopamine receptor agonists used in the treatment of prolactinomas.* The structures of dopamine, the predominant regulator of prolactin secretion, and of dopaminergic agonists that are used to inhibit prolactin secretion are shown. Bromocriptine and cabergoline are ergot derivatives, whereas quinagolide is not. The β-phenylethylamine region of structural similarity between dopamine and the agonists is shown in red.

improved adherence to therapy due to decreased side effects. Therapy is initiated at a dose of 0.25 mg twice a week or 0.5 mg once a week. If the serum prolactin remains elevated, the dose can be increased to a maximum of 1.5-2 mg two or three times a week as tolerated; the dose should not be increased more often than once every 4 weeks.

Cabergoline induces remission in a significant number of patients with prolactinomas, and a trial of drug discontinuation is advocated for the subset of patients with normalization of prolactin and disappearance of a detectable pituitary lesion on MRI scanning.

At higher doses, cabergoline is used in some patients with acromegaly and is now under investigation for patients with Cushing's disease due to corticotrope adenomas (Chapter 42).

Adverse Effects. Compared to bromocriptine, cabergoline has a much lower tendency to induce nausea, although it still may cause hypotension and dizziness. Cabergoline has been linked to valvular heart disease, an effect proposed to reflect agonist activity at the serotonin 5-HT_{2B} receptor. A similar effect has been seen with pergolide (see later). Thus echocardiographic assessment seems appropriate for patients receiving chronic therapy with cabergoline, particularly those on higher doses (Colao et al., 2008b).

Quinagolide. Quinagolide (NORPROLAC) is a non-ergot D_2 agonist (Figure 38–6) with a $t_{1/2}$ (22 hours) between those of bromocriptine and cabergoline. Quinagolide is administered once daily at doses of 0.1-0.5 mg/day. It is not approved by the FDA but has been used extensively in Europe and Canada.

Pergolide. Pergolide (PERMAX), an ergot derivative FDA-approved for treatment of Parkinson disease, also was used off label to treat hyperprolactinemia. In part due to concerns of valvular heart disease, pergolide has been withdrawn from the market.

Therapy of Growth Hormone Deficiency

The pharmacology of somatotropic hormone deficiency is focused on GH because prolactin is not used clinically. Replacement therapy is well established in GH-deficient children and is gaining wider acceptance for GH-deficient adults. Several other indications are also approved, as described later. More recently, recombinant human IGF-1 has been approved for use in patients with mutations in the GH receptor that impair its action, as well as in GH-deficient children who develop antibodies against the recombinant hGH preparation. Although once marketed, a synthetic GHRH analog is no longer available.

Recombinant Human Growth Hormone. Humans do not respond to GH from nonprimate species. In earlier times, GH for therapeutic use was purified from human cadaver pituitaries; it thus was available in very limited quantities and in the mid-1980s was linked to the transmission of Creutzfeldt-Jakob disease. Currently, human GH is produced by recombinant DNA technology, thereby providing virtually unlimited amounts of the hormone while eliminating the risk of disease transmission associated with the pituitary-derived preparations.

Somatropin refers to the many GH preparations whose sequences match that of native GH (ACCRETROPIN, GENOTROPIN, HUMATROPE, NORDITROPIN, NUTROPIN, OMNITROPE, SAIZEN, SEROSTIM, TEV-TROPIN, VALTROPIN, and

ZORBTIVE); *somatrem* refers to a derivative of GH with an additional methionine at the amino terminus that is no longer available in the U.S.

Chemistry. Although the bacterial or yeast systems used to express the recombinant GH subtly affect the structures of these preparations, they all have similar biological actions and potencies (3 IU/mg). An FDA-approved, encapsulated form of somatropin (NUTROPIN DEPOT) injected intramuscularly, either monthly (1.5 mg/kg body weight) or every 2 weeks (0.75 mg/kg body weight), has been discontinued by the manufacturer.

Pharmacokinetics. As a peptide hormone, GH is administered subcutaneously, with a bioavailability of 70%. Although the circulating $t_{1/2}$ of GH is only 20 minutes, its biological $t_{1/2}$ is considerably longer, and once-daily administration is sufficient. To match the usual pattern of secretion, GH typically is administered at bedtime, although this is not essential.

Indications for Growth Hormone Treatment. GH deficiency in children is a well-accepted cause of short stature, and replacement therapy has been used for half a century to treat children with severe GH deficiency. With the advent of essentially unlimited supplies of recombinant GH, therapy has been extended to children with other conditions associated with short stature despite adequate GH production, including Turner's syndrome, Noonan's syndrome, Prader-Willi syndrome, chronic renal insufficiency, children born small for gestational age, and children with idiopathic short stature (i.e., >2.25 standard deviations below mean height for age and sex but with normal laboratory indices of growth hormone levels).

Attention also has shifted to the proper role of GH therapy in GH-deficient adults. The consensus of experts is that at least the most severely affected GH-deficient adults may benefit from GH replacement therapy (Molitch et al., 2006). The FDA also has approved GH therapy for AIDS-associated wasting and for malabsorption associated with the short bowel syndrome. The latter indication is based on the finding that GH stimulates the adaptation of gastrointestinal epithelial cells.

Contraindications. Based on controlled clinical trials showing increased mortality, GH should not be used in patients with acute critical illness due to complications after open heart or abdominal surgery, multiple accidental trauma, or acute respiratory failure. GH also should not be used in patients who have any evidence of neoplasia, and antitumor therapy should be completed before GH therapy is initiated. Other contraindications include proliferative retinopathy or severe nonproliferative diabetic retinopathy. In Prader-Willi syndrome, sudden death has been observed when GH was given to children who were severely obese or who had severe respiratory impairment.

Therapeutic Uses. In GH-deficient children, somatropin typically is administered in a dose of 25-50 μg/kg per day subcutaneously in the evening; higher daily doses (e.g., 50-67 μg/kg) are employed for patients with Noonan's syndrome or Turner's syndrome, who have partial GH resistance. In children with overt GH deficiency, measurement of serum IGF-1 levels sometimes is used to monitor initial response and compliance; long-term response is monitored by close evaluation of height, sometimes in conjunction with measurements of serum IGF-1 levels (Cohen et al., 2007). Although the most pronounced increase in growth velocity occurs during the first 2 years of therapy, GH is continued until the epiphyses are fused and also may be extended into the transition period from childhood to adulthood.

In view of the effects of GH on bone density and visceral adiposity and the manifestations of GH deficiency in adults, many experts now continue therapy into adulthood for children with GH deficiency (Radovick and DiVall, 2007). However, many patients who were GH deficient in childhood based on provocative testing, especially those with idiopathic, isolated GH deficiency, respond normally to provocative tests as adults. Thus, it is essential to confirm GH deficiency after full growth has been achieved, ideally after discontinuation of GH replacement for at least 1 month, to identify patients who will benefit from continuing GH treatment.

For adults, weight-based dosing largely has been supplanted by initiation with relatively low doses irrespective of weight, followed by dose titration as tolerated to raise IGF-1 levels to the mid-normal range adjusted for age and sex. A typical starting dose is 150-300 μg per day, with higher doses used in younger patients transitioning from pediatric therapy; lower doses are used in older patients (e.g., >60 years of age). Either an elevated serum IGF-1 level or persistent side effects mandates a decrease in dose; conversely, the dose can be increased (typically by 100-200 μg per day) if serum IGF-1 has not reached the normal range after 2 months of GH therapy. Because estrogen inhibits GH action, women taking oral—but not transdermal—estrogen may require larger GH doses to achieve the target IGF-1 level. In the setting of AIDS-related wasting, considerably higher doses (e.g., 100 μg/kg) have been used. Studies are also underway to assess the effect of GH therapy on reducing visceral adiposity and increasing lean body mass in HIV-infected patients with the adipose redistribution syndrome (Grunfeld et al., 2007; Lo et al., 2008).

Based on the known age-related decline in GH levels, the use of GH therapy to ameliorate or even reverse the consequences of aging has been widely promoted. Many of the studies supporting this use were not placebo controlled and involved small numbers of subjects. Moreover, one review concluded that there was no significant improvement in strength or aerobic performance with GH therapy in elderly subjects (Liu et al., 2007). Thus, this remains an area of considerable debate. In violation of regulations and standard medical practice, some athletes also use injected GH preparations as anabolic agents to enhance performance (Gibney et al., 2007). In addition to the parenteral GH preparations, oral preparations containing "stacked" amino acids that reputedly stimulate GH release have been marketed as nutritional supplements. Despite the absence of validation in controlled trials, these formulations are part of multibillion dollar anti-aging and performance-enhancing programs (Olshansky and Perls, 2008).

Adverse Effects of Growth Hormone Therapy. In children, GH therapy is associated with remarkably few side effects. Rarely, generally within the first 8 weeks of therapy, patients develop intracranial hypertension, with papilledema, visual changes, headache, nausea, and/or vomiting. Because of this, funduscopic examination is recommended at the initiation of therapy and at periodic intervals thereafter. Leukemia has been reported in some children receiving GH therapy; a causal relationship has not been established, and conditions associated with GH deficiency (e.g., Down's syndrome, cranial irradiation for CNS tumors) probably explain the apparent increased incidence of leukemia. Despite this, the consensus is that GH should not be administered in the first year after treatment of pediatric tumors, including leukemia, or during the first 2 years after therapy for medulloblastomas or ependymomas. Because an increased incidence of type 2 diabetes mellitus has been reported, fasting glucose levels should be followed periodically during therapy. Finally, too-rapid growth may be associated with slipped epiphyses or scoliosis, although a causal link with GH has not been proven.

Side effects associated with the initiation of GH therapy in adults include peripheral edema, carpal tunnel syndrome, arthralgias, and myalgias, which occur most frequently in patients who are older or obese and generally respond to a decrease in dose. These volume-related adverse effects occur less frequently with standard-dose rather than weight-based regimens. Although there are potential concerns about impaired glucose tolerance secondary to anti-insulin actions of GH, this generally has not been a major problem at the recommended doses. In fact, changes in visceral fat composition associated with GH replacement may improve insulin sensitivity in some patients.

Drug Interactions. The effects of estrogen on GH therapy were noted earlier. This effect is much less marked with transdermal estrogen preparations. Recent studies suggest that GH therapy can increase the metabolic inactivation of glucocorticoids in the liver. Thus, GH may precipitate adrenal insufficiency in patients with occult secondary adrenal insufficiency or in patients receiving replacement doses of glucocorticoids. This has been attributed to the inhibition of the type 1 isozyme of steroid 11β-hydroxysteroid dehydrogenase, which normally converts inactive cortisone into the active 11-hydroxy derivative cortisol (Chapter 42).

Insulin-like Growth Factor 1 (IGF-1)

Based on the hypothesis that GH predominantly acts via increases in IGF-1, there has been a longstanding interest in developing IGF-1 preparations for therapeutic use. To this end, recombinant human IGF-1 (mecasermin, INCRELEX) and a combination of recombinant human IGF-1 with its binding protein, IGFBP-3 (mecasermin rinfabate; IPLEX), are FDA-approved. The latter formulation was subsequently discontinued for use in short stature due to patent issues, although it remains available for other conditions such as severe insulin resistance, muscular dystrophy, and HIV-related adipose redistribution syndrome.

Absorption, Distribution, and Elimination. Mecasermin is administered by subcutaneous injection and absorption is virtually complete. As discussed earlier, IGF-1 in circulation is bound by six proteins; a ternary complex that includes IGFBP-3 and the acid labile subunit accounts for >80% of the circulating IGF-1. This protein binding prolongs the $t_{1/2}$ of IGF-1 to ~6 hours. Both the liver and kidney have been shown to metabolize IGF-1.

Therapeutic Uses. Mecasermin is FDA-approved for patients with impaired growth secondary to mutations in the GH receptor or postreceptor signaling pathway, patients with GH deficiency who develop antibodies against GH that interfere with its action, and the very rare patients with IGF-1 gene defects that lead to primary IGF-1 deficiency (Collet-Solberg and Misra, 2008). Typically the starting dose is 40-80 μg/kg per dose twice daily by subcutaneous injection, with a maximum of 120 μg/kg per dose twice daily.

Clinical trials also have examined the efficacy of mecasermin in the much larger cohort of patents with impaired growth secondary to GH deficiency or with idiopathic short stature. In these settings, mecasermin stimulates linear growth but is less effective than conventional therapy using recombinant GH, suggesting direct effects of GH on linear growth independent of IGF-1. Although further study is needed, mecasermin should be reserved for therapy in patients with FDA-approved indications and is unlikely to replace GH as preferred therapy for most patients with GH deficiency or short stature.

Adverse Effects. Side effects of mecasermin include hypoglycemia and lipohypertrophy, both presumably secondary to activation of the insulin receptor. To diminish the frequency of hypoglycemia, mecasermin should be administered shortly before or after a meal or snack. Lymphoid tissue hypertrophy, including enlarged tonsils, also is seen and may require surgical intervention. Other adverse effects are similar to those associated with GH therapy and include intracranial hypertension, slipped epiphyses, and scoliosis.

Contraindications. Mecasermin should not be used for growth promotion in patients with closed epiphyses. It should not be given to patients with active or suspected neoplasia and should be stopped if evidence of neoplasia develops.

Sermorelin. *Sermorelin* (GEREF) is a synthetic form of human GHRH that corresponds in sequence to the first 29 amino acids of human GHRH (a 44–amino acid peptide) and has full biological activity. Although sermorelin is FDA-approved for treatment of GH deficiency and as a diagnostic agent to differentiate between hypothalamic and pituitary disease, the drug was withdrawn from the U.S. market in late 2008.

THE GYCOPROTEIN HORMONES: TSH AND THE GONADOTROPINS

The gonadotropins include LH, FSH, and hCG. They are referred to as the gonadotropins because of their actions on the gonads (Table 38–2). Together with TSH, they constitute the glycoprotein family of pituitary hormones. Each hormone is a glycosylated heterodimer containing a common α-subunit and a distinct β-subunit that confers specificity of action.

LH and FSH were named initially based on their actions on the ovary; appreciation of their roles in male reproductive function came later. LH and FSH are synthesized and secreted by gonadotropes, which make up ~10% of the hormone-secreting cells in the anterior pituitary. hCG, which is produced only in primates and horses, is synthesized by the syncytiotrophoblast of the placenta. Pituitary gonadotropin production is stimulated by GnRH and further

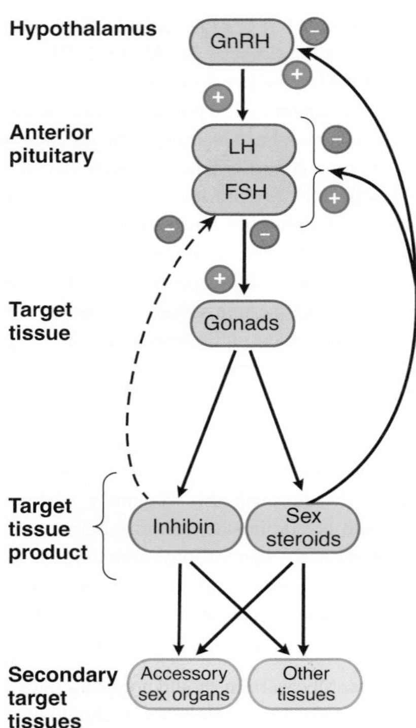

Figure 38–7. *The hypothalamic-pituitary-gonadal axis.* A single hypothalamic releasing factor, gonadotropin-releasing hormone (GnRH), controls the synthesis and release of both gonadotropins (LH and FSH) in males and females. Gonadal steroid hormones (androgens, estrogens, and progesterone) exert feedback inhibition at the level of the pituitary and the hypothalamus. The preovulatory surge of estrogen also can exert a stimulatory effect at the level of the pituitary and the hypothalamus. Inhibins, a family of polypeptide hormones produced by the gonads, specifically inhibit FSH secretion by the pituitary.

regulated by feedback effects of the gonadal hormones (Figures 38–7 and 40-2). Chapters 40 and 41 provide more detailed descriptions of gonadotropin regulation.

TSH is measured in the diagnosis of thyroid disorders, and recombinant TSH is used in the evaluation and treatment of well-differentiated thyroid cancer, as discussed in Chapter 39.

Physiology of the Gonadotropins

Structure-Function Aspects of the Gonadotropins. The carbohydrate residues on the gonadotropins influence their rates of clearance from the circulation, and thus their serum half-lives, and also play a role in activating the gonadotropin receptors. Among the gonadotropin β-subunits, that of hCG is most divergent because it contains a carboxy-terminal extension of 30 amino acids and extra carbohydrate residues that prolong its $t_{1/2}$. The longer $t_{1/2}$ of hCG has some clinical relevance for its use in assisted reproduction technologies (Chapter 66).

Regulation of Gonadotropin Synthesis and Secretion. The predominant regulator of gonadotropin synthesis and secretion is the hypothalamic peptide GnRH. It is a decapeptide with blocked amino and carboxyl termini (Table 38–3) derived by proteolytic cleavage of a 92–amino acid precursor peptide. A separate gene encodes a related GnRH peptide, termed GnRH-II (Millar et al., 2004); its potential functions in reproduction remain to be defined. GnRH release is pulsatile and is governed by a neural pulse generator in the hypothalamus, primarily in the arcuate nucleus, that controls the frequency and amplitude of GnRH release. The GnRH pulse generator is active late in fetal life and for ~1 year after birth but decreases considerably thereafter, presumably secondarily to CNS inhibition. Shortly before puberty, CNS inhibition decreases and the amplitude and frequency of GnRH pulses increase, particularly during sleep. As puberty progresses, the GnRH pulses increase further in amplitude and frequency until the normal adult pattern is established. The intermittent release of GnRH is crucial for the proper synthesis and release of the gonadotropins; the continuous administration of GnRH leads to desensitization and down-regulation of GnRH receptors on pituitary gonadotropes and forms the basis for the clinical use of long-acting GnRH agonists to suppress gonadotropin secretion, as discussed later.

Molecular and Cellular Bases of GnRH Action. GnRH signals through a specific GPCR on gonadotropes that activates $G_{q/11}$ and stimulates the PLC-IP_3-Ca^{2+} pathway (Chapter 3), resulting in increased synthesis and secretion of LH and FSH. Although cyclic AMP is not the major mediator of GnRH action, binding of GnRH to its receptor also increases adenylyl cyclase activity. GnRH receptors also are present in the ovary, testis, and other sites, where their physiological significance remains to be determined. The presence of these receptors on certain tumors has led to investigation of the role of GnRH analogs in cancer therapy (Engel and Schally, 2007).

Other Regulators of Gonadotropin Production. Gonadal steroids regulate gonadotropin production at the level of the pituitary and the hypothalamus, but effects on the hypothalamus predominate. The feedback effects of gonadal steroids are dependent on sex, concentration, and time. In women, low levels of estradiol and progesterone inhibit gonadotropin production, largely through opioid action on the neural pulse generator. Higher and more sustained levels of estradiol have positive feedback effects that ultimately result in the gonadotropin surge that triggers ovulation. In men, testosterone inhibits gonadotropin production, in part through direct actions and in part via its conversion by aromatase to estradiol.

Table 38–3

Structures of Gonadotropin-Releasing Hormone (GnRH) and GnRH Analogs

GnRH CONGENER (TRADE NAME)	AMINO ACID RESIDUE 1	2	3	4	5	6	7	8	9	10	DOSAGE FORMS
Agonists											
GnRH (FACTREL, LUTREPULSE)	PyroGlu	His	Trp	Ser	Tyr	Gly	Leu	Arg	Pro	Gly-NH_2	IV, SC
Goserelin (ZOLADEX)	—	—	—	—	—	D-Ser(tBu)	—	—	—	AzGly-NH_2	SC implant
Nafarelin (SYNAREL)	—	—	—	—	—	D-Nal	—	—	—	—	IN
Triptorelin (TRELSTAR DEPOT, LA)	—	—	—	—	—	D-Trp	—	—	—	—	IM depot
*Buserelin** (SUPREFACT)	—	—	—	—	—	D-Ser(tBu)	—	—	Pro-NHEt		IN, SC
Deslorelin*	—	—	—	—	—	D-Trp	—	—	Pro-NHEt		IM, SC, depot
Histrelin (VANTAS, SUPPRELIN LA)	—	—	—	—	—	D-His(Bzl)	—	—	Pro-NHEt		SC implant
Leuprolide (LUPRON, ELIGARD)	—	—	—	—	—	D-Leu	—	—	Pro-NHEt		IM, SC, depot
Antagonists											
*Abarelix** (PLENAXIS)	Ac-D-Nal	D-Cpa	D-Pal	—	Tyr(N-Me)	D-Asn	—	Lys(iPr)	—	D-Ala-NH_2	SC depot
Cetrorelix (CETROTIDE)	Ac-D-Nal	D-Cpa	D-Pal	—	—	D-Cit	—	—	—	D-Ala-NH_2	SC
Ganirelix (ANTAGON)	Ac-D-Nal	D-Cpa	D-Pal	—	—	D-hArg$(Et)_2$	—	D-hArg$(Et)_2$	—	D-Ala-NH_2	SC

Ac, acetyl; Bzl, benzyl; $EtNH_2$, N-ethylamide; tBu, t butyl; D-Nal, 3-(2-naphthyl)-D-alanyl; Cpa, chlorophenylalanyl; Lys(iPr), isopropyl-lysyl; Pal, 3-pyridylalanyl; AzGly, azaglycyl; hArg$(Et)_2$, ethyl homoarginine; IV, intravenous; SC, subcutaneous; IN, intranasal; IM, intramuscular. A dash (–) denotes amino acid identity with GnRH.

Gonadotropin production also is regulated by the *inhibins*, which are members of the bone morphogenetic protein family of secreted signaling proteins. Inhibin A and B are made by granulosa cells in the ovary and Sertoli cells in the testis in response to the gonadotropins and local growth factors (Bilezikjian et al., 2006). They act directly in the pituitary to inhibit FSH secretion without affecting that of LH. Inhibin A exhibits variation during the menstrual cycle, suggesting that it acts as a dynamic regulator of FSH secretion.

Molecular and Cellular Bases of Gonadotropin Action. The actions of LH and hCG on target tissues are mediated by the LH receptor; those of FSH are mediated by the FSH receptor. Both of these GPCRs have large glycosylated extracellular domains that contribute to their affinity and specificity for their ligands. The FSH and LH receptors couple to $G_{s\alpha}$ to activate the adenylyl cyclase/cyclic AMP pathway. At higher ligand concentrations, the agonist-occupied gonadotropin receptors also activate PKC and Ca^{2+} signaling pathways via G_q-mediated effects on PLCβ. Because most, if not all, actions of the gonadotropins can be mimicked by cyclic AMP analogs, the precise physiological role of Ca^{2+} and PKC in gonadotropin action remains to be determined.

Physiological Effects of Gonadotropins. In men, LH acts on testicular Leydig cells to stimulate the *de novo* synthesis of androgens, primarily testosterone, from cholesterol. Testosterone is required for gametogenesis within the seminiferous tubules and for maintenance of libido and secondary sexual characteristics (Chapter 41). FSH acts on the Sertoli cells to stimulate the production of proteins and nutrients required for sperm maturation.

In women, the actions of FSH and LH are more complicated. FSH stimulates the growth of developing ovarian follicles and induces the expression of LH receptors on theca and granulosa cells. FSH also regulates the expression of aromatase in granulosa cells, thereby stimulating the production of estradiol. LH acts on the theca cells to stimulate the *de novo* synthesis of androstenedione, the major precursor of ovarian estrogens in premenopausal women (Figure 40-1). LH also is required for the rupture of the dominant follicle during ovulation and for the synthesis of progesterone by the corpus luteum.

CLINICAL DISORDERS OF THE HYPOTHALAMIC-PITUITARY-GONADAL AXIS

Clinical disorders of the hypothalamic-pituitary-gonadal axis can manifest either as alterations in levels and effects of sex steroids (hyper- or hypogonadism) or as impaired reproduction. This section focuses on those conditions that specifically affect the hypothalamic-pituitary components of the axis and those for which gonadotropins are used diagnostically or therapeutically.

Deficient sex steroid production resulting from hypothalamic or pituitary defects is termed hypogonadotropic hypogonadism because circulating levels of gonadotropins are either low or undetectable (Layman, 2007). Hypogonadotrophic hypogonadism in some patients results from GnRH receptor mutations; some of these mutations impair targeting of the GnRH receptor to the plasma membrane of gonadotropes, prompting efforts to develop pharmacological strategies to correct receptor trafficking and restore function (Conn et al., 2007). Many other disorders can impair gonadotropin secretion, including pituitary tumors, other genetic disorders such as Kallmann's syndrome, infiltrative processes such as sarcoidosis, and functional disorders such as exercise-induced amenorrhea.

In contrast, reproductive disorders caused by processes that directly impair gonadal function are termed hypergonadotropic because the impaired production of sex steroids leads to a loss of negative feedback inhibition, thereby increasing the synthesis and secretion of gonadotropins.

Precocious Puberty. Puberty normally is a sequential process requiring several years over which the GnRH neurons escape CNS inhibition and initiate pulsatile secretion of GnRH. This stimulates the secretion of gonadotropins and gonadal steroids, thus directing the development of secondary sexual characteristics appropriate for sex. Normally, the initial signs of puberty (breast development in girls and testes enlargement in boys) do not occur before age 8 in girls or age 9 in boys; the initiation of sexual maturation before this time is termed "precocious."

Precocious puberty can be divided into processes that lead to the premature activation of the normal hypothalamic-pituitary-gonadal axis, termed central or GnRH-dependent precocious puberty, and processes that lead to peripheral production of sex steroids in a GnRH-independent manner (Carel and Léger, 2008). Specific etiologies of GnRH-dependent precocious puberty include CNS tumors (including hypothalamic hamartomas), developmental abnormalities of the CNS, and encephalitis or other infectious processes; in most patients and especially in girls, a specific etiology is never defined, and patients are deemed to have an idiopathic process. GnRH-independent precocious puberty results from peripheral production of sex steroids in a manner not driven by pituitary gonadotropins; etiologies include adrenal or gonadal tumors, activating mutations of the LH receptor in boys, and congenital adrenal hyperplasia. As discussed later, synthetic GnRH analogs play important roles in the diagnosis and treatment of GnRH-dependent precocious puberty. In contrast, drugs that interfere with the production of sex steroids, including ketoconazole and aromatase inhibitors, are used in patients with GnRH-independent precocious puberty (Shulman et al., 2008), with varying success.

Sexual Infantilism. The converse of precocious puberty is a failure to initiate the processes of pubertal development at the normal time. This can reflect defects in the GnRH neurons or gonadotropes (secondary hypogonadism) or primary dysfunction in the gonads. In either case, induction of sexual maturation using sex steroids (estrogen followed by estrogen/progesterone in females, testosterone in males) is standard therapy. This suffices to direct sex differentiation in the normal manner. If fertility is the goal, then therapy with either GnRH or gonadotropins is needed to stimulate appropriate germ cell maturation.

Infertility. Infertility, or a failure to conceive after 12 months of unprotected intercourse, is seen in up to 10-15% of couples and is increasing in frequency as women choose to delay childbearing. The rising incidences of obesity, sexually transmitted diseases that disrupt the reproductive tract, and reduced sperm count to due environmental pollution also are contributing factors. When the infertility is due to impaired synthesis or secretion of gonadotropins (hypogonadotropic hypogonadism), various pharmacological approaches are employed. In contrast, when infertility results from intrinsic processes affecting the gonads, pharmacotherapy generally is less effective. Therapeutic approaches to male infertility are described later in this chapter; strategies for female infertility are described in Chapter 66.

Clinical Uses of GnRH and Its Synthetic Analogs

A synthetic peptide comprising the native sequence of GnRH has been used both diagnostically and therapeutically in human reproductive disorders. In addition, as illustrated in Table 38–3, a number of GnRH analogs with structural modifications have been synthesized and brought to market.

Synthetic GnRH. Synthetic GnRH (gonadorelin; FACTREL, LUTREPULSE) is FDA-approved, but ongoing problems with availability have limited its clinical use in the U.S. to a few specialized centers; synthetic analogs have largely supplanted gonadorelin.

Chemistry. The structure of gonadorelin (Table 38–3) corresponds to that of native GnRH; it is a decapeptide with blocked amino and carboxyl termini.

Absorption, Distribution, and Elimination. As a peptide, gonadorelin is administered either subcutaneously or intravenously. It is well-absorbed following subcutaneous injection and has a circulating $t_{1/2}$ of ~2-4 minutes. For therapeutic uses, it must be administered in a pulsatile manner to avoid down-regulation of the GnRH receptor.

Diagnostic and Therapeutic Uses. Because of the limited availability of GnRH, many of its diagnostic and therapeutic uses have been discontinued. For diagnostic purposes, gonadorelin was used in the GnRH stimulation test in patients with hypogonadotropic hypogonadism in an effort to differentiate between hypothalamic and pituitary defects. A blood sample was obtained for a baseline LH value, a single 100-μg dose of GnRH was administered subcutaneously or intravenously, and serum LH levels were measured at various times after injection. A normal LH response to >10 mIU/mL indicated the presence of functional pituitary gonadotropes and prior exposure to GnRH. Inasmuch as the long-term absence of GnRH can impair the responsiveness of otherwise normal gonadotropes, the absence of a response did not always indicate intrinsic pituitary disease. Thus some experts had advocated use of multiple doses of GnRH in an effort to restore gonadotrope responsiveness.

GnRH-stimulation testing also was used to determine whether a child with precocious puberty had a GnRH-dependent (central) or GnRH-independent (peripheral) disorder. A GnRH-induced increase in plasma LH to >10 mIU/mL in boys or >7 mIU/mL in girls indicated true precocious puberty rather than a GnRH-independent process. Currently, some experts in the U.S. and elsewhere have used long-lasting GnRH agonists off label as the stimulating agent for diagnostic assessment (see section on Gonadotropin-Releasing Hormone Agonists).

To treat female infertility secondary to impaired GnRH secretion, gonadorelin was administered by infusion in pulses that promoted a physiological cycle. Advantages over gonadotropin therapy included a lower risk of multifetal pregnancies and a decreased need to monitor plasma estradiol levels or follicle size by ovarian ultrasonography. Side effects usually were minimal; the most common was local irritation due to the infusion device. In women, normal cycling levels of ovarian steroids could be achieved, leading to ovulation and menstruation. The manufacturer has discontinued production for this indication, and gonadorelin is no longer generally available in the U.S.

GnRHA. Synthetic agonists have longer half-lives than native GnRH. After a transient stimulation of gonadotropin secretion, they down-regulate the GnRH receptor and inhibit gonadotropin secretion; this is used

detect the presence of an ectopic pregnancy, hydatidiform mole, or choriocarcinoma. Such assays also are used to follow the therapeutic response of malignancies that secrete hCG, such as germ cell tumors.

Timing of Ovulation. Ovulation occurs ~36 hours after the onset of the LH surge. Therefore urinary concentrations of LH, as measured with an over-the-counter radioimmunoassay kit, can be used to predict the time of ovulation. Urine LH levels are measured every 12- 24 hours, beginning on day 10-12 of the menstrual cycle (assuming a 28-day cycle), to detect the rise in LH and estimate the time of ovulation. This estimate facilitates the timing of sexual intercourse to optimize the chance of achieving pregnancy.

Localization of Endocrine Disease. Measurements of plasma LH and FSH levels with β subunit–specific radioimmunoassays are useful in the diagnosis of several reproductive disorders. Low or undetectable levels of LH and FSH are indicative of hypogonadotropic hypogonadism and suggest hypothalamic or pituitary disease, whereas high levels of gonadotropins suggest primary gonadal diseases. A plasma FSH level of ≥10-12 mIU/mL on day 3 of the menstrual cycle, indicative of decreased ovarian reserve, is associated with reduced fertility, even if a woman is menstruating normally, and predicts a lower likelihood of success in assisted reproduction techniques such as *in vitro* fertilization.

The administration of hCG can be used to stimulate testosterone production and thus to assess Leydig cell function in males suspected of having primary hypogonadism (e.g., in delayed puberty). Serum testosterone levels are assayed after multiple injections of hCG. A diminished testosterone response to hCG indicates Leydig cell failure; a normal testosterone response suggests a hypothalamic-pituitary disorder and normal Leydig cells.

Therapeutic Uses of the Gonadotropins

Male Infertility. In men with impaired fertility secondary to gonadotropin deficiency (hypogonadotropic hypogonadism), gonadotropins can establish or restore fertility. Due to expense and to the occasional development of antibody-mediated resistance to gonadotropins with prolonged use, standard treatment has been to induce sexual development with androgens, reserving gonadotropins until fertility is desired.

Treatment typically is initiated with hCG (1500-2000 IUs intramuscularly or subcutaneously) three times per week until clinical parameters and the plasma testosterone level indicate full induction of steroidogenesis. Thereafter, the dose of hCG is reduced to 2000 IU twice a week or 1000 IU three times a week, and menotropins (FSH + LH) or recombinant FSH is injected three times a week (typical dose of 150 IU) to fully induce spermatogenesis.

Based on the observation that the normal male infant is exposed to high levels of gonadotropins during the first year of life, it has been proposed that therapy with LH and FSH during infancy may be associated with increased spermatogenesis later in life (Grumbach, 2005), and studies addressing this question are in progress.

The most common side effect of gonadotropin therapy in males is gynecomastia, which occurs in up to a third of patients and presumably reflects increased production of estrogens due to the induction of aromatase. Maturation of the prepubertal testes typically requires treatment for >6 months, and optimal spermatogenesis in some patients may require treatment for up to 2 years. Once spermatogenesis has been initiated, either by this combined therapy in patients with prepubertal disease or in patients who developed hypogonadotropic hypogonadism after sexual maturation, ongoing treatment with hCG alone usually is sufficient to support sperm production.

Cryptorchidism. Cryptorchidism, the failure of one or both testes to descend into the scrotum, affects up to 3% of full-term male infants and becomes less prevalent with advancing postnatal age. Cryptorchid testes have defective spermatogenesis and are at increased risk for developing germ cell tumors. Hence the current approach is to reposition the testes as early as possible, typically at 1 year of age but definitely before 2 years of age. The local actions of androgens stimulate descent of the testes; thus hCG has been used by some to induce testicular descent if the cryptorchidism is not secondary to anatomical blockage.

Therapy usually consists of injections of hCG (3000 IU/m^2 body surface area) intramuscularly every other day for six doses. If this does not induce testicular descent, orchiopexy should be performed. Some experts prefer surgery as the initial approach based on the association of hCG treatment with germ cell apoptosis in certain experimental settings (Ritzen, 2008).

POSTERIOR PITUITARY HORMONES: OXYTOCIN AND VASOPRESSIN

The structures of the neurohypophyseal hormones oxytocin and arginine vasopressin (also called antidiuretic hormone, or ADH) and the physiology and pharmacology of vasopressin are presented in Chapter 25. The following discussion emphasizes the physiology of oxytocin. Therapeutic uses of synthetic oxytocin as a uterine-stimulating agent to induce or augment labor in selected pregnant women and to decrease postpartum hemorrhage are described in Chapter 66.

Physiology of Oxytocin

Biosynthesis of Oxytocin. *Oxytocin* is a cyclic nonapeptide that differs from vasopressin by only two amino acids. It is synthesized as a larger precursor in neurons whose cell bodies reside in the paraventricular nucleus and, to a lesser extent, the supraoptic nucleus in the hypothalamus. The precursor peptide is rapidly cleaved to the active hormone and its neurophysin, packaged into secretory granules as an oxytocin-neurophysin complex, and secreted from nerve endings that terminate primarily in the posterior pituitary gland (neurohypophysis). In addition, oxytocinergic neurons that regulate the autonomic nervous system project to regions of the hypothalamus, brainstem, and spinal cord. Other sites of oxytocin synthesis include the luteal cells of the ovary, the endometrium, and the placenta.

Secretion of Oxytocin. Stimuli for oxytocin secretion include sensory stimuli arising from dilation of the cervix and vagina and from suckling at the breast. Increases in circulating oxytocin in women in labor are difficult to detect, partly because of the pulsatile nature of oxytocin secretion and partly because of the activity of circulating oxytocinase. Nevertheless, increased oxytocin in maternal circulation is detected in the second stage of labor, likely triggered by sustained distension of the uterine cervix and vagina.

Estradiol stimulates oxytocin secretion, whereas the ovarian polypeptide relaxin inhibits its release. The inhibitory effect of relaxin appears to be the net result of a direct effect on oxytocin-producing cells and an inhibitory action mediated indirectly by endogenous opiates. Other factors that primarily affect vasopressin secretion also have some impact on oxytocin release; for example, ethanol inhibits release, whereas pain, dehydration, hemorrhage, and hypovolemia stimulate release. Although peripheral actions of oxytocin appear to play no significant role in the response to dehydration, hemorrhage, or hypovolemia, oxytocin may participate in the central regulation of blood pressure.

Pharmacological doses of oxytocin can inhibit free water clearance by the kidney through arginine vasopressin-like activity at vasopressin V_2 receptors, occasionally causing water intoxication if administered with large volumes of hypotonic fluid. Based on the behavior of intravenously administered oxytocin during labor induction, the plasma $t_{1/2}$ of oxytocin is approximately 12-15 minutes.

Mechanism of Action. Oxytocin acts via a specific GPCR (OXT) closely related to the V_{1a} and V_2 vasopressin receptors. In the human myometrium, OXT couples to G_q/G_{11}, activating the PLC_β-IP_3-Ca^{2+} pathway and enhancing activation of voltage-sensitive Ca^{2+} channels. Oxytocin also increases local prostaglandin production, which further stimulates uterine contractions. Figure 66–2 summarizes the interactions of signaling pathways affecting myometrial contractililty.

Effects of Oxytocin

Uterus. The human uterus has a very low level of motor activity during the first two trimesters of pregnancy. During the third trimester, spontaneous motor activity increases progressively until the sharp rise that constitutes the initiation of labor. Oxytocin stimulates the frequency and force of uterine contractions. Uterine responsiveness to oxytocin roughly parallels this increase in spontaneous activity and is highly dependent on estrogen, which increases the expression of the oxytocin receptors. Progesterone antagonizes the stimulatory effect of oxytocin *in vitro,* and refractoriness to progesterone in late pregnancy may contribute to the normal initiation of human parturition.

Because of difficulties associated with the measurement of oxytocin levels and because loss of pituitary oxytocin apparently does not compromise labor and delivery, the physiological role of oxytocin in pregnancy has been highly debated. Exogenous oxytocin can initiate or enhance rhythmic contractions at any time, but a considerably higher dose is required in early pregnancy. An eight-fold increase in uterine sensitivity to oxytocin occurs in the last half of pregnancy, mostly in the last 9 weeks, and is accompanied by a 30-fold increase in oxytocin receptor numbers between week 32 and term. The finding that the oxytocin antagonist atosiban is effective in suppressing preterm labor further supports the physiological importance of oxytocin in this setting.

Breast. Oxytocin plays an important physiological role in milk ejection. Stimulation of the breast through suckling or mechanical manipulation induces oxytocin secretion, causing contraction of the myoepithelium that surrounds alveolar channels in the mammary gland. This action forces milk from the alveolar channels into large collecting sinuses, where it is available to the suckling infant.

Brain. As noted earlier, oxytocin is synthesized by hypothalamic neurons, predominantly located in the paraventricular and supraoptic nuclei. Studies in rodents and humans have implicated oxytocin as an important CNS regulator of trust and of autonomic systems linked to anxiety and fear (Leng et al., 2008).

Brain regions proposed to be critical in the response to fearful stimuli, including the amygdala, midbrain, and striatum, showed decreased activation in response to stressful stimuli following oxytocin treatment (Baumgartner et al., 2008; Huber et al., 2005). The role of perturbations of oxytocin signaling in mental conditions such as social phobia and autism and the possible therapeutic benefit of drugs that manipulate CNS oxytocin effects are exciting areas of ongoing investigation.

Clinical Therapeutics of Oxytocin

Deficiencies of oxytocin associated with disorders of the posterior pituitary impair milk letdown after delivery and may be one of the earliest signs of pituitary insufficiency secondary to postpartum hemorrhage (Sheehan's syndrome); oxytocin is not used clinically in this setting. Rather, oxytocin is used therapeutically to induce or augment labor and to treat or prevent postpartum hemorrhage, as described in Chapter 66.

CLINICAL SUMMARY

Progress continues to be made in the pharmacotherapy of endocrine and reproductive disorders related to the anterior pituitary gland. In children, the indications for therapy with recombinant human GH have been expanded beyond patients with classic, unequivocal GH deficiency, and the drug increasingly is used in conditions such as Turner's syndrome, Noonan's syndrome, chronic renal failure, cystic fibrosis, and other conditions associated with short stature, including idiopathic short stature. Recombinant human GH also is used increasingly to treat adults with GH deficiency, with proposed benefits that include increased muscle mass, decreased adiposity, increased bone mineral density, and improved subjective well-being. Adverse effects occur more commonly in adults, and the dose should be adjusted so that the serum IGF-1 level is in the mid-normal range.

Pharmacotherapy also plays an important role in the treatment of functional tumors that produce GH (gigantism/acromegaly) or prolactin (prolactinomas). For acromegaly, sustained-release preparations of somatostatin analogs (e.g., octreotide and lanreotide) normalize GH and IGF-1 levels in ~65% of patients. Pegvisomant, a GH receptor antagonist, is even more effective, normalizing these parameters in up to 90% of patients. For prolactinomas, dopamine receptor agonists remain the mainstay of treatment. Cabergoline generally is used because of its lower incidence of side effects; when pregnancy is desired, bromocriptine is preferred.

Pituitary hormones also have a role in reproductive medicine. Both GnRH receptor agonists and antagonists are used to down-regulate gonadotropin levels and block endogenous production of sex steroids. Indications include interruption of central precocious puberty, therapy of cancers whose growth is stimulated by sex steroids (e.g., breast and prostate), and suppression of endogenous gonadotropins in assisted reproduction technologies. Gonadotropins are frequently used in assisted reproduction technologies to stimulate follicular maturation and to induce ovulation. Recombinant gonadotropins largely are replacing gonadotropins purified from human urine in clinical use.

BIBLIOGRAPHY

Baragli A, Alturaihi H, Watt HL, et al. Heterooligomerization of human dopamine receptor 2 and somatostatin receptor 2: Co-immunoprecipitation and fluorescence resonance energy transfer analysis. *Cell Signal,* **2007,** *19:*2304–2316.

Baumgartner T, Heinrichs M, Vonlanthen A, et al. Oxytocin shapes the neural circuitry of trust and trust adaptation in humans. *Neuron,* **2008,** *58:*639–650.

Bilezikjian LM, Blount AL, Donaldson CJ, Vale WW. Pituitary actions of ligands of the TGF-beta family: Activins and inhibins. *Reproduction,* **2006,** *132:*207–215.

Brito N, Latronico AC, Arnhold IJ, Mendonca BB. A single luteinizing hormone determination 2 hours after depot leuprolide is useful for therapy monitoring of gonadotropin-dependent precocious puberty in girls. *J Clin Endocrinol Metab,* **2004,** *89:*4338–4342.

Carel JC, Léger J. Precocious puberty. *N Engl J Med,* **2008,** *358:*2366–2377.

Carlsen SM, Lund-Johansen M, Schreiner T, et al. Preoperative octreotide treatment in newly diagnosed acromegalic patients with macroadenomas increases cure short term postoperative rates: a prospective, randomized trial. *J Clin Endocrinol Metab,* **2008,** *93:*2984–2990.

Cohen P, Rogol AD, Howard CP, et al. Insulin-like growth factor-based dosing of growth hormone therapy in children: A randomized, controlled trial. *J Clin Endocrinol Metab,* **2007,** *92:*1480–1486.

Colao A, Abst R, Barcena DG, et al. Pregnancy outcomes following cabergoline treatment: Extended results from a 12-year observational study. *Clin Endocrinol,* **2008a,** *68:*66–71.

Colao A, Galderisi M, Di Sarno A, et al. Increased prevalence of tricuspid regurgitation in patients with prolactinomas chronically treated with cabergoline. *J Clin Endocrinol Metab,* **2008b,** *93:*3777–3784.

Collett-Solberg PF, Misra M. The role of recombinant human insulin-like growth factor-I in treating children with short stature. *J Clin Endocrinol Metab,* **2008,** *93:*10–18.

Conn PM, Ulloa-Aguirre A, Ito J, Janovick JA. G protein-coupled receptor trafficking in health and disease: Lessons learned to prepare for therapeutic mutant rescue in vivo. *Pharmacol Rev,* **2007,** *59:*225–250.

Davis A, Goel S, Picolos M, et al. Pituitary apoplexy after leuprolide. *Pituitary,* **2006,** *9:*263–265.

Elizur SE, Tulandi T. Drugs in infertility and fetal safety. *Fert Steril*, **2008,** *89:*1595–1602.

Engel JB, Schally AV. Drug insight: Clinical use of agonists and antagonists of luteinizing-hormone-releasing hormone. *Nat Clin Pract Endocrinol Metab*, **2007,** *3:*157–167.

Flores-Morales A, Greenhalgh CJ, Norstedt G, Rico-Bautista E. Negative regulation of growth hormone receptor signaling. *Mol. Endocrinol,* **2006,** *20:*241–253.

Florio T, Barbieri F, Spaziante R, et al. Efficacy of a dopamine-somatostatin chimeric molecule, BIM-23A760, in the control of cell growth from primary cultures of human non-functioning pituitary adenomas: A multi-center study. *Endocr Relat Cancer,* **2008,** *15:*583–596.

Ghigo E, Broglio F, Arvat E, et al. Ghrelin: More than a natural GH secretagogue and/or an orexigenic factor. *Clin Endocrinol,* **2005,** *62:*1–17.

Gibney J, Healy M-L, Sonksen PH. The growth hormone/insulin-like growth factor-1 axis in exercise and sport. *Endocr Rev,* **2007,** *28:*603–624.

Giustina A, Mazziotti G, Canalis E. Growth hormone, insulin-like growth factors, and the skeleton. *Endocr Rev,* **2008,** *29:*535–559.

Gillam MP, Molitch ME, Lombardi G, Colao A. Advances in the treatment of prolactinomas. *Endocr Rev*, **2006,** *27:* 485–534.

Goffin V, Touraine P, Culler MD, Kelly PA. Drug insight: Prolactin-receptor antagonists, a novel approach to treatment of unresolved systemic and local hyperprolactinemia? *Nat Clin Pract Endocrinol Metab,* **2006,** *2:*571–581.

Grant M, Alturaihi H, Jaquet P, et al. Cell growth inhibition and functioning of human somatostatin receptor type 2 are modulated by receptor heterodimerization. *Mol Endocrinol,* **2008,** *22:*2278–2292.

Grumbach MM. A window of opportunity: The diagnosis of gonadotropin deficiency in the male infant. *J Clin Endocrinol Metab,* **2005,** *90:*3122–3127.

Grunfeld C, Thompson M, Brown SJ, et al. Recombinant human growth hormone to treat HIV-associated adipose redistribution syndrome: 12-week induction and 24-week maintenance therapy. *J Acquir Immune Defic Syndr,* **2007,** *45:*286–297.

Huber D, Veinante P, Stoop R. Vasopressin and oxytocin excite distinct neuronal populations in the central amygdala. *Science,* **2005,** *308:*245–248.

Jimenez C, Burman P, Abs R, et al. Follow-up of pituitary tumor volume in patients with acromegaly treated with pegvisomant in clinical trials. *Eur J Endocrinol,* **2008,** *159:*517–523.

Lanning NJ, Carter-Su C. Recent advances in growth hormone signaling. *Rev Endocr Metab Disord,* **2006,** *7:*225–235.

Layman LC. Hypogonadotropic hypogonadism. *Endocrinol Metab Clin N Am,* **2007,** *36*:283–296.

Leng G, Meddle SL, Douglas AJ. Oxytocin and the maternal brain. *Curr Opin Pharmacol,* **2008,** *8*:731–734.

Liu H, Bravata DM, Olkin I, et al. Systemic review: The safety and efficacy of growth hormone in the healthy elderly. *Ann Intern Med,* **2007,** *146:*104–115.

Lo J, You SM, Canavan B, et al. Low-dose physiological growth hormone in patients with HIV and abdominal fat redistribution: A randomized controlled trial. *JAMA,* **2008,** *300:* 509–519.

Macklin NS, Stouffer RL, Giudice LC, Fauser BCJM. The science behind 25 years of ovarian stimulation. *Endoc Rev,* **2006,** *27:*170–207.

Millar RP, Lu ZL, Pawson AJ, et al. Gonadotropin-releasing hormone receptors. *Endocr Rev,* **2004,** *25:*235–275.

Molitch ME, Clemmons DR, Malozowski S, et al. Evaluation and treatment of adult growth hormone deficiency: An Endocrine Society Clinical Practice Guideline. *J Clin Endocrinol Metab,* **2006,** *91:*1621–1634.

Murray RD, Melmed S. A critical analysis of clinically available somatostatin analog formulations for therapy of acromegaly. *J Clin Endocrinol Metab,* **2008,** *93*:2957–2968.

Olshansky SJ, Perls TT. New developments in the illegal provision of growth hormone for "anti-aging" and bodybuilding. *JAMA,* **2008,** *299:*2792–2994.

Pawlikowski M, Melen-Mucha G. Somatostatin analogs—from new molecules to new applications. *Curr Opin Pharmacol,* **2004,** *4:*608–613.

Radovick S, DiVall S. Approach to the growth hormone-deficient child during transition to adulthood. *J Clin Endocrinol Metab,* **2007,** *92:*1195–1200.

Reissmann T, Felberbaum R, Diedrich K, et al. Development and applications of luteinizing hormone-releasing hormone antagonists in the treatment of infertility: An overview. *Hum Reprod,* **1995,** *10:*1974–1981.

Ritzen M. Undescended testes: A consensus on management. *Eur J Endocrinol,* **2008,** *159*(suppl 1):S87–S90.

Shulman DI, Francis GL, Palmert MR, Eugster EA. Use of aromatase inhibitors in children and adolescents with disorders of growth and adolescent development. *Pediatrics,* **2008,** *121:*975–983.

Swanson SM, Kopchick JJ. Nuclear localization of growth hormone receptor: Another age of discovery for cytokine action? *Sci STKE,* **2007,** *415*: pe69.

Wajnrajch MP, Gertner JM, Harbison MD, et al. Nonsense mutation in the human growth hormone-releasing hormone receptor causes growth failure analogous to the *little* (*lit*) mouse. *Nat Genet,* **1996,** *12*:88–90.

Walenkamp MJE, Wit JM. Single gene mutations causing SGA. *Best Pract Res Clin Endocrinol Metab,* **2008,** *22:*433–446.

Weckbecker G, Lewis I, Albert R, et al. Opportunities in somatostatin research: Biological, chemical, and therapeutic aspects. *Nat Rev Drug Discov,* **2003,** *2:*999–1017.

Thyroid and Anti-Thyroid Drugs

Gregory A. Brent
and Ronald J. Koenig

Thyroid hormone is essential for normal development, especially of the central nervous system (CNS). In the adult, thyroid hormone maintains metabolic homeostasis and influences the function of virtually all organ systems. Thyroid hormone contains iodine that must be supplied by nutritional intake. The thyroid gland contains large stores of thyroid hormone in the form of thyroglobulin. These stores maintain systemic concentrations of thyroid hormone despite variations in iodine availability and nutritional intake. The thyroidal secretion is predominantly the prohormone thyroxine, which is converted in the liver and other tissues to the active form, triiodothyronine. Local activation of thyroxine also occurs in target tissues (e.g., brain and pituitary) and is increasingly recognized as an important regulatory step in thyroid hormone action. Serum concentrations of thyroid hormones are precisely regulated by the pituitary hormone, thyrotropin (TSH), in a classic negative-feedback system. The predominant actions of thyroid hormone are mediated through binding to nuclear thyroid hormone receptors (TRs) and modulating transcription of specific genes. Thyroid hormones share a common mechanism of action with steroid and steroid-like hormones, such as vitamin D and the retinoids, whose receptors are members of a superfamily of nuclear receptors (Chapter 3). Although the predominant actions of thyroid hormone are nuclear, actions of thyroid hormone outside the nucleus have been reported.

Disorders of the thyroid are common. Thyroid nodules and goiter, thyroid enlargement, are the most common abnormalities and can be either benign or malignant processes. In most of these patients, circulating thyroid hormone levels are normal. Overt hyperthyroidism and hypothyroidism, thyroid hormone excess or deficiency, are usually associated with dramatic clinical manifestations. Milder disease often has a more subtle clinical presentation and is identified based on abnormal biochemical tests of thyroid function. Screening of the newborn population for congenital hypothyroidism occurs in all developed countries, and when followed by the prompt institution of appropriate thyroid hormone replacement therapy, has dramatically decreased the incidence of mental retardation and cretinism. Maternal and neonatal hypothyroidism, due to iodine deficiency, remains the major preventable cause of mental retardation worldwide, although much progress has been made in eradicating iodine deficiency.

Effective treatment of most thyroid disorders is readily available. Treatment of the hypothyroid patient consists of thyroid hormone replacement. Treatment options for the hyperthyroid patient include anti-thyroid drugs to decrease hormone synthesis and secretion, destruction of the gland by the administration of radioactive iodine, or surgical removal. In most patients, disorders of thyroid function can be either cured or have their diseases controlled. Likewise, thyroid malignancies are most often localized and resectable. Metastatic disease often responds to radioiodide treatment but may become highly aggressive and unresponsive to conventional treatment. Newer therapies that target specific genetic mutations in malignancies have shown significant activity in both medullary and papillary thyroid cancers.

THYROID

The thyroid gland is the source of two fundamentally different types of hormones. The thyroid follicle produces the iodothyronine hormones *thyroxine* (T_4) and *3,5,3′-triiodothyronine* (T_3). These hormones are essential for normal growth and development and play an important role in energy metabolism. The thyroid also contains parafollicular cells (C-cells) that produce calcitonin (Chapter 44).

History. The thyroid is named for the Greek word for "shield shaped," from the shape of the nearby tracheal cartilage. It was first recognized as an organ of importance when thyroid enlargement was observed to be associated with changes in the eyes and the heart in the condition we now call *hyperthyroidism.* Parry saw his first patient in 1786 but did not publish his findings until 1825. Graves reported the disorder in 1835 and Basedow in 1840. Hypothyroidism was described later, in 1874, when Gull associated atrophy of the gland with the symptoms characteristic of *hypothyroidism.* The term *myxedema* was applied to the clinical syndrome in 1878 by Ord in the belief that the characteristic thickening of the subcutaneous tissues was due to excessive formation of mucus. In 1891, Murray first treated a case of hypothyroidism by injecting an extract of sheep thyroid gland, later shown to be fully effective when given by mouth. The successful treatment of thyroid deficiency by administering thyroid extract was an important step toward modern endocrinology.

Extirpation experiments to elucidate the function of the thyroid were at first misinterpreted because of the simultaneous removal of the parathyroids. However, Gley's research on the parathyroid glands in the late 19th century allowed the functional differentiation of these two endocrine glands. The structure of parathyroid hormone, however, was not reported until the early 1970s. Calcitonin was discovered in 1961, demonstrating that the thyroid gland produced a hormone in addition to thyroxine.

Chemistry of Thyroid Hormones. The principal hormones of the thyroid gland are the iodine-containing amino acid derivatives of thyronine (T_4 and T_3; Figure 39–1). Following the isolation and the chemical identification of thyroxine, it was generally thought that all the hormonal activity of thyroid tissue could be accounted for by its content of thyroxine. However, careful studies revealed that crude thyroid preparations possessed greater calorigenic activity than could be accounted for by their thyroxine content. The presence of a "second" thyroid hormone was debated, but triiodothyronine was finally detected, isolated, and synthesized by Gross and Pitt-Rivers (1952). Triiodothyronine has a much higher affinity for the nuclear thyroid hormone receptor compared with thyroxine and is much more potent biologically on a molar basis. The subsequent demonstration of T_3 production from T_4 in athyreotic humans led to the practice of effective replacement in hypothyroidism with levothyroxine only (Braverman et al., 1970).

Structure–Activity Relationships. The structural requirements for a significant degree of thyroid hormone activity have been defined (Baxter and Webb, 2009; Yoshihara et al., 2003). The 3′-monosubstituted compounds are more active than the 3′,5′-disubstituted molecules. Thus, triiodothyronine is five times more potent than thyroxine, and 3′-isopropyl-3,5-diiodothyronine has seven times the activity. Substitutions at the 3,5,3′, and 5′ sites influence the conformation of the molecule. In thyronine, the two rings are angulated at ~120° at the ether oxygen and are free to rotate on their axes. As depicted schematically in Figure 39–2, the 3,5 iodines restrict rotation of the two rings, which tend to take up positions perpendicular to one another. In general, the affinity of iodothyronines for the thyroid hormone receptors (TRs) parallels their biological potency (Yen, 2001), but additional factors can affect therapeutic potency, including affinity for plasma proteins, rate of metabolism, and rate of entry into cell nuclei. Specific thyroid hormone transporters, such as MCT8, are likely to be important in specific tissues.

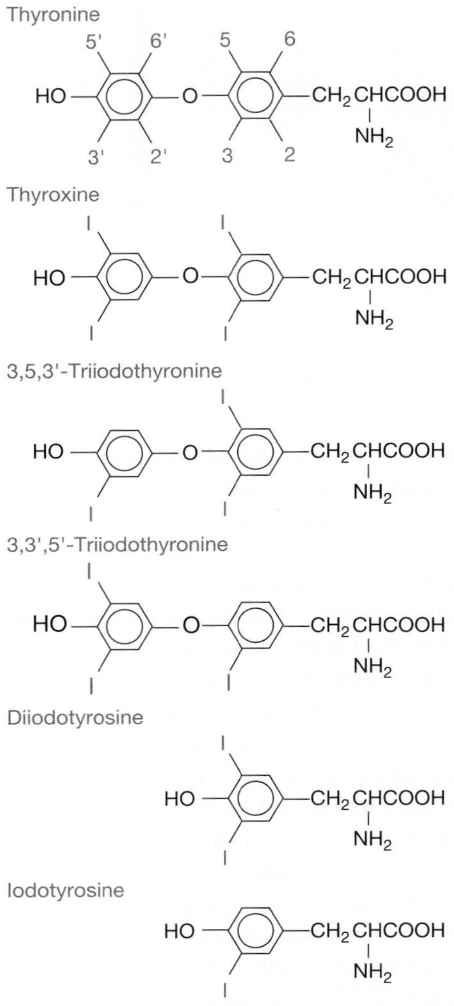

Figure 39–1. *Thyronine, thyroid hormones, and precursors.*

The stereochemical nature of the thyroid hormones plays an important role in defining hormone activity. Many structural analogs of thyroxine have been synthesized to define the structure–activity relationship, to detect antagonists of thyroid hormones, and to find compounds exhibiting a desirable activity while not showing unwanted effects. Introduction of specific arylmethyl groups at the 3′ position of triiodothyronine results in analogs that are liver-selective, cardiac-sparing thyromimetics (Brenta et al., 2007). Solving the x-ray crystallographic structure of the ligand binding domains of the nuclear thyroid hormone receptors α and β has resulted in the rapid development of a range of TR isoform-selective compounds. The difference in the ligand binding domain pocket between TRα and TRβ is only a single amino acid (Ser 277 in TRα

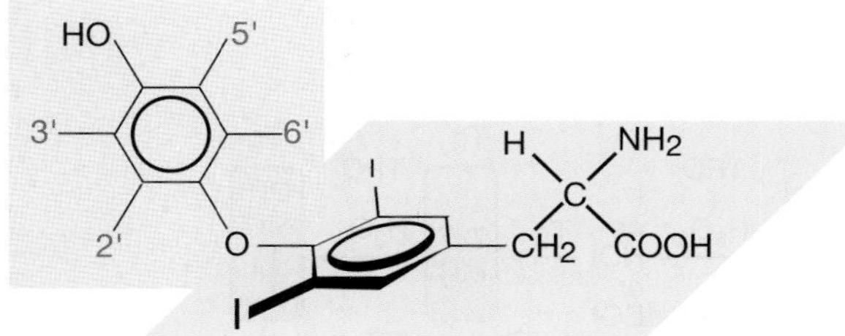

Figure 39–2. *Structural formula of 3,5-diiodothyronine, drawn to show the conformation in which the planes of the aromatic rings are perpendicular to each other.* (Adapted from Jorgensen, 1964.)

and Asn 331 in TRβ). GC-1, a TRβ-specific agonist, stabilizes the ligand binding domain by promoting hydrogen bonding between Asn331 and Arg282. GC-1 has a 10-fold greater affinity for TRβ, the predominant TR isoform in the liver, than TRα, the predominant TR isoform in the heart, and lowers cholesterol without stimulating the heart. Cholesterol lowering with cardiac sparing by GC-1 and other TRβ-selective agonists, however, is also the result of much higher distribution in the liver and less in the heart compared with T_3. Similar compounds, such as KB-141, lower cholesterol in clinical studies (Baxter and Webb, 2009). Interestingly, none of these newer thyroid hormone analogs contains iodine or any halogen.

Biosynthesis of Thyroid Hormones. The synthesis of the thyroid hormones is unique, complex, and seemingly inefficient. The thyroid hormones are synthesized and stored as amino acid residues of thyroglobulin, a protein constituting the vast majority of the thyroid follicular colloid (Rubio and Medeiros-Neto, 2009). The thyroid gland is unique in storing great quantities of potential hormone in this way, and extracellular thyroglobulin can represent a large portion of the thyroid mass. Thyroglobulin is a complex glycoprotein made up of two apparently identical subunits, each of 330,000 Da. Interestingly, molecular cloning has revealed that thyroglobulin belongs to a superfamily of serine hydrolases, including acetylcholinesterase (Chapter 10).

The major steps in the synthesis, storage, release, and interconversion of thyroid hormones are as follows:

1. uptake of iodide ion (I^-) by the gland
2. oxidation of iodide and the iodination of tyrosyl groups of thyroglobulin
3. coupling of iodotyrosine residues by ether linkage to generate the iodothyronines
4. resorption of the thyroglobulin colloid from the lumen into the cell
5. proteolysis of thyroglobulin and the release of thyroxine and triiodothyronine into the blood
6. recycling of the iodine within the thyroid cell via de-iodination of mono- and diiodotyrosines and reuse of the I^-
7. conversion of thyroxine (T_4) to triiodothyronine (T_3) in peripheral tissues as well as in the thyroid

These processes are summarized in Figure 39–3 and described in the correspondingly labeled sections that follow.

1. Uptake of Iodide. Iodine ingested in the diet reaches the circulation in the form of iodide ion (I^-). Under normal circumstances, the I^- concentration in the blood is very low (0.2-0.4 μg/dL; ~15-30 nM), but the thyroid efficiently and actively transports the ion via a specific membrane-bound protein, termed the *sodium-iodide symporter* (NIS) (Dohan et al., 2003). As a result, the ratio of thyroid to plasma iodide concentration is usually between 20 and 50 and can exceed 100 when the gland is stimulated. The iodide transport mechanism is inhibited by a number of ions such as thiocyanate and perchlorate (Figure 39–3). Thyrotropin (thyroid-stimulating hormone [TSH]) stimulates NIS gene expression and promotes insertion of NIS protein into the membrane in a functional configuration. Thus decreased stores of thyroid iodine enhance iodide uptake, and the administration of iodide can reverse this situation by decreasing NIS protein expression (Eng et al., 1999).

NIS has been identified in many other tissues, including the salivary glands, gastric mucosa, midportion of the small intestine, choroid plexus, skin, mammary gland, and perhaps the placenta, all of which maintain a concentration of iodide greater than that of the blood. Iodide accumulation by the placenta and mammary gland may provide adequate supplies for the fetus and infant. Iodine accumulation throughout the body is mediated by a single NIS gene. Individuals with congenital NIS gene mutations have absent or defective iodine concentration in all tissues known to concentrate iodine.

2. Oxidation and Iodination. Consistent with the conditions generally necessary for halogenation of aromatic rings, the iodination of tyrosine residues requires the iodinating species to be in a higher state of oxidation than is the anion. The iodinating species is hypoiodite, either as hypoiodous acid or as an enzyme-linked species (Magnusson et al., 1984).

The oxidation of iodide to its active form is accomplished by thyroid peroxidase, a heme-containing enzyme that uses hydrogen peroxide (H_2O_2) as the oxidant (Dunn and Dunn, 2001). The peroxidase is membrane bound and appears to be concentrated at or near the apical surface of the thyroid cell. The reaction results in the formation of monoiodotyrosyl and diiodotyrosyl residues in

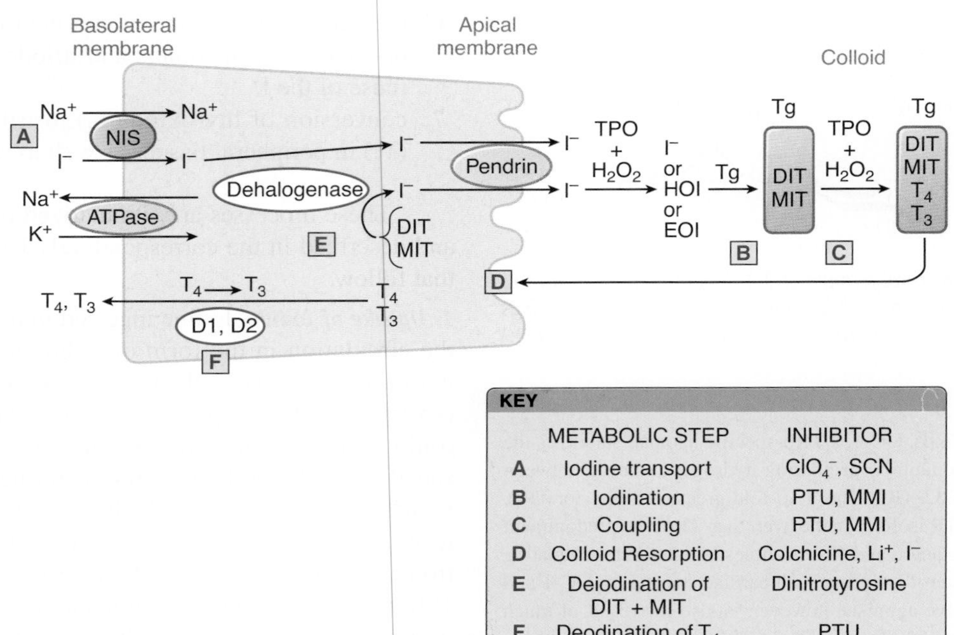

Figure 39–3. *Major pathways of thyroid hormone biosynthesis and release. Abbreviations:* Tg, thyroglobulin; DIT, diiodotyrosine; MIT, monoiodotyrosine; TPO, thyroid peroxidase; HOI, hypoiodous acid; EOI, enzyme-linked species; D1 and D2, deiodinases (see Table 39–1); PTU, propylthiouracil; MMI, methimazole.

thyroglobulin just prior to its extracellular storage in the lumen of the thyroid follicle. The formation of the H_2O_2 that serves as a substrate for the peroxidase probably occurs near its site of utilization and is stimulated by a rise in cytosolic Ca^{2+} (Takasu et al., 1987). The TSH receptor is notably promiscuous in its coupling, stimulating members of four G protein families including G_q, which couples to the PLC-IP_3-Ca^{2+} pathway (Laugwitz et al., 1996); thus, a Ca^{2+}-dependent effect on H_2O_2 production may be a means by which TSH stimulates the organification of iodide in thyroid cells (Figure 39–3).

3. Formation of Thyroxine and Triiodothyronine from Iodotyrosines. The remaining synthetic step is the coupling of two diiodotyrosyl residues to form thyroxine or of monoiodotyrosyl and diiodotyrosyl residues to form triiodothyronine. These oxidative reactions apparently are catalyzed by the same thyroid peroxidase. The mechanism involves the enzymatic transfer of groups, perhaps as iodotyrosyl free radicals or positively charged ions, within thyroglobulin.

Although many other proteins can serve as substrates for the peroxidase, none is as efficient as thyroglobulin in yielding thyroxine. Presumably, conformation of thyroglobulin facilitates this coupling reaction. Thyroxine formation primarily occurs near the amino terminus of the protein, whereas most of the triiodotyrosine is synthesized near the carboxy terminus (Dunn and Dunn, 2001). The relative rates of synthetic activity at the various sites depend on the concentration of TSH and the availability of iodide. Iodine deficiency is associated with an increase in thyroidal T_3 relative to T_4 content (Zimmerman, 2009). Because triiodothyronine is the transcriptionally active iodothyronine and contains only three-fourths as much iodine, a decrease in the quantity of available iodine need have little impact on the effective amount of thyroid hormone elaborated by the gland. Although a decrease in the availability of iodide and the associated increase in the proportion of monoiodotyrosine favor the formation of triiodothyronine over thyroxine, a deficiency in diiodotyrosine ultimately can impair the formation of both compounds. Intrathyroidal and secreted T_3 are also generated by the 5′-deiodination of thyroxine.

4. Resorption; 5. Proteolysis of Colloid; and, 6. Secretion of Thyroid Hormones. Because T_4 and T_3 are synthesized and stored within thyroglobulin, proteolysis is an important part of the secretory process. This process is initiated by endocytosis of colloid from the follicular lumen at the apical surface of the cell, with the participation of a thyroglobulin receptor, megalin. This "ingested" thyroglobulin appears as intracellular colloid droplets, which apparently fuse with lysosomes containing the requisite proteolytic enzymes. It is generally believed that thyroglobulin must be completely broken down into its constituent amino acids for the hormones to be released. The molecular mass of thyroglobulin is 660,000 Da, and the protein is made up of ~300 carbohydrate residues and 5500 amino acid residues, only two to five of which are thyroxine; thus this is an extravagant process.

TSH enhances the degradation of thyroglobulin by increasing the activity of several thiol endopeptidases of the lysosomes. Endopeptidases selectively cleave thyroglobulin, yielding hormone-containing intermediates that subsequently are processed by exopeptidases (Dunn and Dunn, 2001). The liberated hormones then exit the cell, presumably at its basal membrane. When thyroglobulin is hydrolyzed, monoiodotyrosine and diiodotyrosine also are liberated but usually do not leave the thyroid; rather, they are selectively metabolized and the iodine, liberated as I^-, is reincorporated into protein. The iodotyrosine deiodinase enzyme, DHAL1, is essential for conserving iodine and mutations of this gene identified in several kindreds are associated with goitrous hypothyroidism and cognitive deficit (Moreno et al., 2008). Normally, all this iodide is reused; however, when proteolysis is activated intensely by TSH, some of the iodide reaches the circulation, at times accompanied by trace amounts of the iodotyrosines.

7. Thyroid Hormone Metabolism and the Conversion of Thyroxine to Triiodothyronine in Peripheral Tissues. The normal daily production of thyroxine is estimated to range between 80 and 100 μg; that of triiodothyronine is between 30 and 40 μg. Although triiodothyronine is secreted by the thyroid, metabolism of thyroxine by 5′, or outer ring, deiodination in the peripheral tissues accounts for ~80% of circulating triiodothyronine (Figure 39–4). In contrast, removal of the iodine on position 5 of the inner ring produces the metabolically inactive 3,3′,5′-triiodothyronine (reverse T_3, rT_3; Figure 39–1). Under normal conditions, ~40% of T_4 is converted to each of T_3 and rT_3, and ~20% is metabolized *via* other pathways, such as glucuronidation in the liver and excretion in the bile. Normal circulating concentrations of T_4 in plasma range from 4.5-11 μg/dL; those of T_3 are ~1/100 of that (60-180 ng/dL).

Key properties of the three iodothyronine deiodinases are summarized in Table 39–1. The types 1 and 2 deiodinases (D1, D2) convert thyroxine to triiodothyronine (St. Germain et al., 2009). These enzymes contribute approximately equally to the plasma T_3 in rats, but it has not been possible to determine their relative contributions in humans. D1 is expressed primarily in the liver and kidney, and also in the thyroid and pituitary (Figure 39–5). It is upregulated in hyperthyroidism and downregulated in hypothyroidism. A clinically important feature of D1 is its inhibition by the anti-thyroid drug *propylthiouracil*. D1 is localized to the plasma membrane, and the T_3 it produces equilibrates rapidly with the plasma. D2 is expressed primarily in the CNS (including the pituitary and hypothalamus) and brown adipose tissue, also in the thyroid, and at very low levels in other organs such as skeletal muscle. The activity of D2 is unaffected

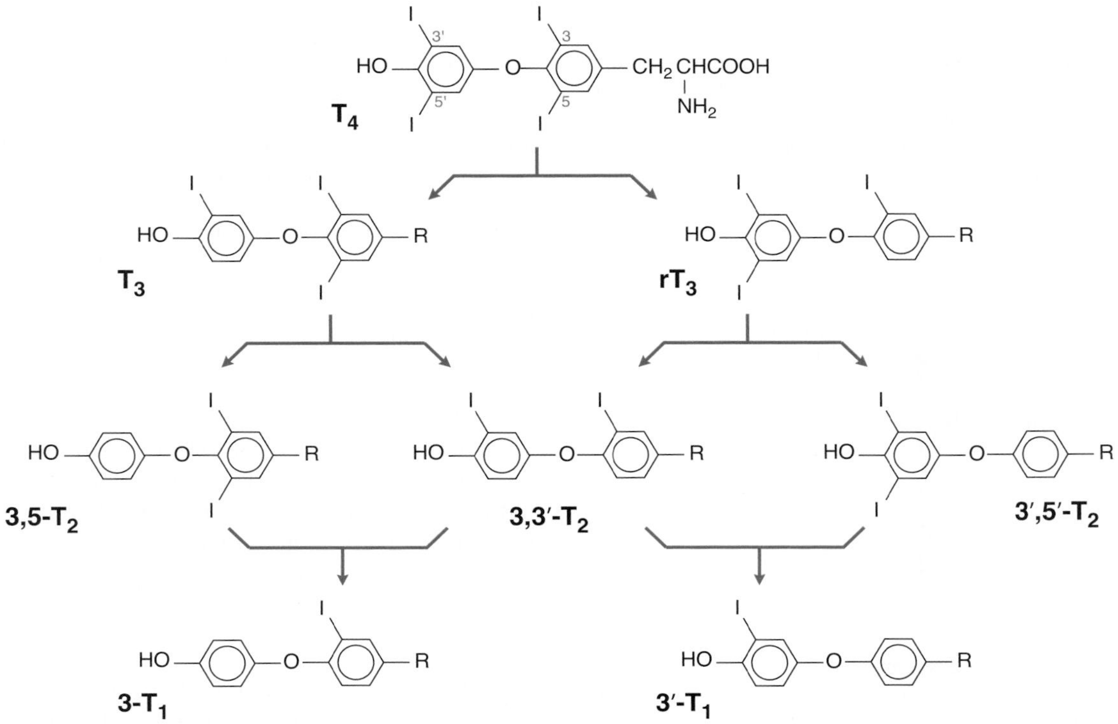

Figure 39–4. *Pathways of iodothyronine deiodination.*

Table 39–1

Properties of Iodothyronine Deiodinases

	TYPE 1 (D1)	TYPE 2 (D2)	TYPE 3 (D3)
Outer ring deiodinase	Yes	Yes	No
Inner ring deiodinase	Yes	No	Yes
Inhibited by PTU	Yes	No	No
Inhibited by amiodarone	Yes	Yes	Unknown
Regulation by thyroid hormone	T_3 induces D1 gene expression	Substrate (T_4) causes D2 protein degradation	T_3 induces D3 gene expression
Location	Liver, kidney, thyroid, pituitary	Brain, pituitary, hypothalamus, thyroid, brown fat, skeletal muscle (very low levels)	Brain, placenta, some sites of inflammation
Selenocysteine in active site	Yes	Yes	Yes

by propylthiouracil. D2 localizes to the endoplasmic reticulum, which facilitates access of D2-generated T_3 to the nucleus. Hence organs that express D2 tend to use the locally generated T_3 to increase the occupancy of nuclear T_3 receptors, and D2-generated T_3 equilibrates slowly with the plasma. D2 is dynamically regulated by its substrate, thyroxine, such that elevated levels of the enzyme are found in hypothyroidism and suppressed levels are found in hyperthyroidism. Thus, D2 autoregulates the intracellular supply of triiodothyronine in organs in which it is expressed.

Inner ring- or 5-deiodination, the main inactivating pathway of T_3 metabolism, is catalyzed mainly by the type 3 deiodinase (D3), and to some extent also by D1. D3 is found at highest levels in the CNS and placenta, and it also is expressed in skin and uterus (St. Germain et al., 2009). It is highly expressed in hemangiomas.

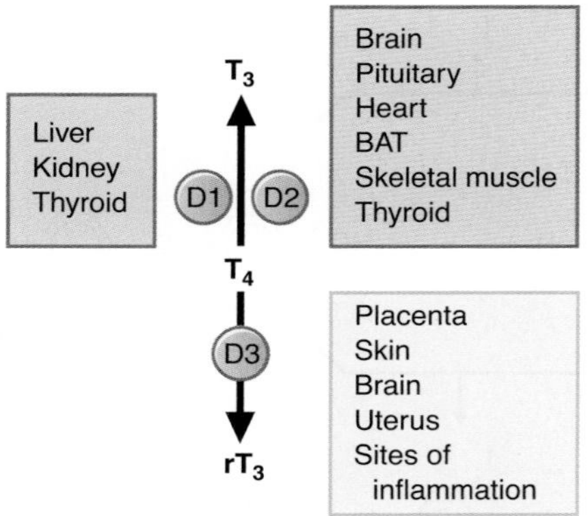

Figure 39–5. *Deiodinase isozymes.*
D1, type I iodothyronine 5′-deiodinase; D2, type II iodothyronine 5′-deiodinase; D3, type III iodothyronine 5-deiodinase; BAT, brown adipose tissue.

D3 can be induced at sites of inflammation, and at least in an animal model this can result in local hypothyroidism (Peeters et al., 2003; Simonides et al., 2008).

D2 and D3 also play important roles in regulating local T3 levels during development, during which thyroid hormone tends to promote differentiation and decrease proliferation. Examples include chondrocyte development and bone differentiation, and auditory (cochlea) development. In the brain, D2 is expressed in glial cells and D3 in neurons. Because T_3 receptors are enriched in neurons, the current model is that glial cells convert T_4 to T_3, which is then exported and taken up by neurons where it activates T_3 receptors, with subsequent degradation by D3 and termination of the T_3 effect. There is a growing recognition of circumstances where D2 and D3 regulate local thyroid hormone levels independent of the plasma T_4 and T_3 concentrations.

The three deiodinases contain the rare amino acid selenocysteine in their active sites. Incorporation of selenocysteine into the growing peptide chain is a complex process involving multiple proteins. Mutations in one such protein, SECIS binding protein 2, are associated with abnormal circulating thyroid hormone levels (Dumitrescu et al., 2005).

Transport of Thyroid Hormones in the Blood. Iodine in the circulation is normally present in several forms, with 95% as organic iodine and ~5% as iodide. Most organic iodine is thyroxine (90-95%); triiodothyronine represents a relatively minor fraction (~5%). The thyroid hormones are transported in the blood in strong but noncovalent association with certain plasma proteins (Schussler, 2000).

Thyroxine-binding globulin (TBG) is the major carrier of thyroid hormones. It is an acidic glycoprotein with a molecular mass of ~63,000 Da that binds one molecule of T_4 per molecule of protein with a very high affinity (the equilibration dissociation constant, K_d, is ~10^{-10} M). T_3 is bound less avidly. Thyroxine, but not triiodothyronine, also is bound by transthyretin (thyroxine-binding prealbumin), a retinol-binding protein. This protein is present in higher concentration than is TBG and primarily binds thyroxine with an equilibrium dissociation constant ~10^{-7} M. Transthyretin has four apparently identical subunits but only a single high-affinity binding site. Albumin also can bind thyroxine when the more avid carriers are saturated, but it is difficult to estimate its quantitative or physiological importance except in *familial dysalbuminemic hyperthyroxinemia.* This syndrome is an autosomal dominant disorder characterized by the increased affinity of albumin for thyroxine due to a point mutation in the albumin gene. There are a number of genetic defects of thyroid-binding globulin (Refetoff, 1989), but these individuals generally have normal circulating free thyroid hormones and serum TSH, and they are euthyroid.

Binding of thyroid hormones to plasma proteins protects the hormones from metabolism and excretion, resulting in their long half-lives in the circulation. The free (unbound) hormone is a small percentage (~0.03% of thyroxine and ~0.3% of triiodothyronine) of the total hormone in plasma. The differential binding affinities for serum proteins also contribute to establishing the 10- to 100-fold differences in circulating hormone concentrations and half-lives of T_4 and T_3.

Essential to understanding the regulation of thyroid function is the "free hormone" concept: Only the unbound hormone has metabolic activity. Thus, because of the high degree of binding of thyroid hormones to plasma proteins, changes in either the concentrations of these proteins or the binding affinity of the hormones for the proteins has major effects on the total serum hormone levels. Certain drugs and a variety of pathological and physiological conditions, such as the changes in circulating concentrations of estrogens during pregnancy or during the administration of oral estrogens, can alter both the binding of thyroid hormones to plasma proteins and the amounts of these proteins (Table 39–2). However, because the pituitary responds to and regulates circulating free hormone levels, minimal changes in free hormone concentrations are seen. Therefore, laboratory tests that measure only total hormone levels can be misleading. Appropriate tests of thyroid function are discussed later in this chapter.

Table 39–2

Factors that Alter Binding of Thyroxine to Thyroxine-Binding Globulin

INCREASE BINDING	DECREASE BINDING
Drugs	
Estrogens	Glucocorticoids
Methadone	Androgens
Clofibrate	L-Asparaginase
5-Fluorouracil	Salicylates
Heroin	Mefenamic acid
Tamoxifen	Antiseizure medications (phenytoin, carbamazepine)
Selective estrogen receptor modulators	Furosemide
Systemic Factors	
Liver disease	Inheritance
Porphyria	Acute and chronic illness
HIV infection	
Inheritance	

Degradation and Excretion (Figure 39–6). Thyroxine is eliminated slowly from the body, with a $t_{1/2}$ of 6-8 days. In hyperthyroidism, the $t_{1/2}$ is shortened to 3-4 days, whereas in hypothyroidism it may be 9-10 days. These changes presumably reflect altered rates of metabolism of the hormone. In conditions associated with increased binding to TBG, such as pregnancy, clearance is retarded. The increase in TBG is due to the estrogen-induced increase in the sialic acid content of the synthesized TBG, resulting in decreased TBG clearance. The opposite effect is observed when there is reduced protein binding of thyroid hormones or when binding to protein is inhibited by certain drugs (Table 39–2). T_3, which is less avidly bound to protein, has a $t_{1/2}$ of ~1 day.

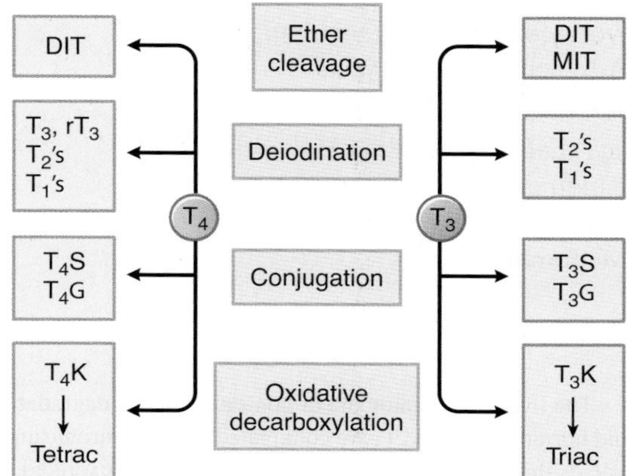

Figure 39–6. *Pathways of metabolism of thyroxine (T_4) and triiodothyronine (T_3).*
DIT, diiodotyrosine; MIT, monoiodotyrosine; T_4S, T_4 sulfate; T_4G, T_4 glucuronide; T_3S, T_3 sulfate; T_3G, T_3 glucuronide; T_4K, T_4 pyruvic acid; T_3K, T_3 pyruvic acid; Tetrac, tetraiodothyroacetic acid; Triac, triiodothyroacetic acid.

Table 39–3

Factors Influencing Oral Levothyroxine Therapy

Drugs and other factors that may increase levothyroxine dosage requirements
Impaired levothyroxine absorption
Aluminum-containing antacids
Bile acid sequestrants (cholestyramine, colestipol, colesevelam)
Calcium carbonate (effect generally small)
Chromium picolinate
Food
Iron salts
Lactose intolerance (single case report)
Phosphate binders (lanthanum carbonate, sevelamer)
Proton pump inhibitors
Raloxifene
Soy products (effect generally very small)
Sucralfate
Increased thyroxine metabolism, CYP3A4 induction of hepatic
Bexarotene
Carbamapzepine
Phenytoin
Rifampin
Sertraline
Impaired $T_4 \rightarrow T_3$ conversion
Amiodarone
Mechanisms uncertain or multifactorial
Estrogen pregnancy
Ethionamide
Tyrosine kinase inhibitors (imatinib, sunitinib)
Lovastatin, simvastatin
Drugs and other factors that may decrease levothyroxine dosage requirements
Advancing age (>65 years)
Androgen therapy in women
Drugs that may decrease TSH without changing free T_4 in levothyroxine-treated patients
Metformin

The liver is the major site of non-deiodinative degradation of thyroid hormones; T_4 and T_3 are conjugated with glucuronic and sulfuric acids through the phenolic hydroxyl group and excreted in the bile. Some thyroid hormone is liberated by hydrolysis of the conjugates in the intestine and reabsorbed. A portion of the conjugated material reaches the colon unchanged, where it is hydrolyzed and eliminated in feces as the free compounds.

As discussed earlier, the major route of metabolism of T_4 is deiodination to either T_3 or reverse T_3. Triiodothyronine and reverse T_3 are deiodinated to three different diiodothyronines, which are further deiodinated to two monoiodothyronines (Figure 39–4), inactive metabolites that are normal constituents of human plasma. Additional metabolites (monoiodotyrosine and diiodotyrosine) in which the diphenyl ether linkage is cleaved have been detected both *in vitro* and *in vivo*.

Regulation of Thyroid Function. Thyrotropin or TSH is a glycoprotein hormone with α and β subunits analogous to those of the gonadotropins. Its structure is discussed with those of the other glycoprotein hormones in Chapter 38. TSH is secreted in a pulsatile manner and circadian pattern; its levels in the circulation are highest during sleep at night. TSH secretion is precisely controlled by the hypothalamic peptide *thyrotropin-releasing hormone* (TRH) and by the concentration of free thyroid hormones in the circulation. Extra thyroid hormone inhibits transcription of both the TRH gene and the genes encoding the α and β subunit of thyrotropin, which suppresses the secretion of TSH and causes the thyroid to become inactive and regress (Chiamolera and Wondisford, 2009). Any decrease in the normal rate of thyroid hormone secretion by the thyroid evokes an enhanced secretion of TSH in the absence of exogenous hormone in an attempt to stimulate the thyroid to secrete more hormone. Additional mechanisms mediating the effect of thyroid hormone on TSH secretion appear to be a reduction in TRH secretion by the hypothalamus and a reduction in the number of TRH receptors on pituitary cells. Figure 39–7 summarizes the regulation of thyroid hormone secretion.

Thyrotropin-Releasing Hormone. TRH stimulates the release of preformed TSH from secretory granules and also stimulates the subsequent synthesis of both α and β subunits of TSH. Somatostatin, dopamine, and pharmacological doses of glucocorticoids inhibit TRH-stimulated TSH secretion.

TRH is a tripeptide with both terminal amino and carboxyl groups blocked (L-pyroglutamyl-L-histidyl-L-proline amide). The mature hormone is derived from a precursor protein that contains six copies of the tripeptide flanked by dibasic residues. TRH is synthesized by the hypothalamus and released into the hypophyseal-portal circulation, where it interacts with TRH receptors on thyrotropes. The binding of TRH to its receptor, a GPCR, stimulates the G_q-PLC-IP_3-Ca^{2+} pathway and activates PKC, ultimately stimulating the synthesis and release of TSH by the thyrotropes (Monga et al., 2008).

TRH also has been localized in the CNS in the cerebral cortex, circumventricular structures, neurohypophysis, pineal gland, and

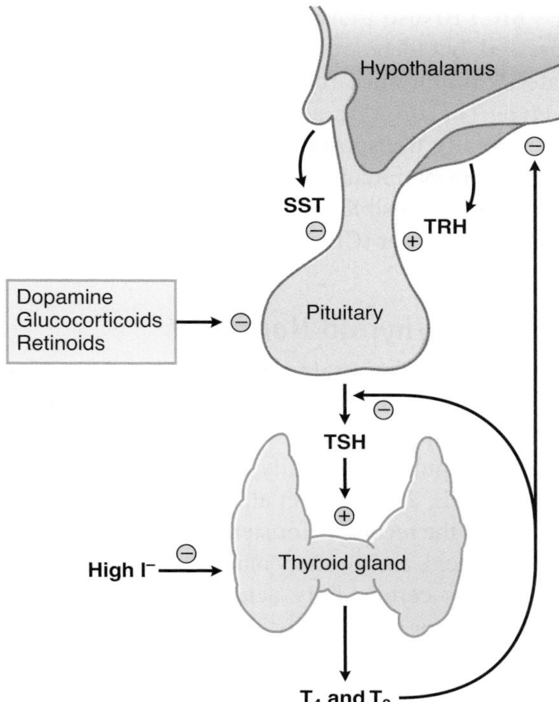

Figure 39–7. *Regulation of thyroid hormone secretion.* Myriad neural inputs influence hypothalamic secretion of thyrotropin-releasing hormone (TRH). TRH stimulates release of thyrotropin (TSH, thyroid-stimulating hormone) from the anterior pituitary; TSH stimulates the synthesis and release of the thyroid hormones T_3 and T_4. T_3 and T_4 feed back to inhibit the synthesis and release of TRH and TSH. Somatostatin (SST) can inhibit TRH action, as can dopamine and high concentrations of glucocorticoids. Low levels of I^- are required for thyroxine synthesis, but high levels inhibit thyroxin synthesis and release.

spinal cord. These findings, as well as its localization in nerve endings, suggest that TRH may act as a neurotransmitter or neuromodulator outside of the hypothalamus. Administration of TRH to animals produces CNS-mediated effects on behavior, thermoregulation, autonomic tone, and cardiovascular function, including increases in blood pressure and heart rate. TRH also has been identified in pancreatic islets, heart, testis, and parts of the gastrointestinal tract. Its physiological role in these sites is not known. Two TRH receptors have now been identified, TRH-R1 and TRH-R2, as well as selective analogs for these receptors (Monga et al., 2008). TRH analogs with CNS activity, but without other hormonal actions, are being developed for therapeutic applications. TRH is no longer available in the U.S.

Actions of Thyroid-Stimulating Hormone on the Thyroid. When TSH is given to experimental animals, the first measurable effect on thyroid hormone metabolism is increased secretion, which is detectable within minutes. All phases of hormone synthesis and release are eventually stimulated: iodide uptake and organification, hormone synthesis, endocytosis, and proteolysis of colloid. There is increased vascularity of the gland and hypertrophy and hyperplasia of thyroid cells.

These effects follow the binding of TSH to its receptor on the plasma membrane of thyroid cells. The TSH receptor is a GPCR that is structurally similar to the receptors for luteinizing hormone and follicle-stimulating hormone (Chapter 38) (Kleinau and Krause, 2009). These receptors share significant amino acid homology and have large extracellular domains that are involved in hormone binding. Binding of TSH to its receptor stimulates the G_s-adenylyl cyclase–cyclic AMP pathway. Higher concentrations of TSH activate the G_q-PLC pathway. Both the adenylyl cyclase and the phospholipase C signaling pathways appear to mediate effects of TSH on thyroid function in humans (Kogai et al., 2006).

Multiple mutations of the TSH receptor result in clinical thyroid dysfunction (Latif et al., 2009). Germline mutations can present as congenital, nonautoimmune hypothyroidism or as autosomal dominant toxic thyroid hyperplasia. Germline mutations of the TSH receptor can cause gestational hyperthyroidism due to a hypersensitivity of the receptor to HCG (Rodien et al., 1998). Somatic mutations that result in constitutive activation of the receptor are associated with hyperfunctioning thyroid adenomas (Krohn and Paschke, 2001). Finally, resistance to TSH has been described, both in families with mutant TSH receptors (Sunthornthepvarakul et al., 1995) and in those with no apparent mutations in either the TSH receptor or in TSH itself (Xie et al., 1997).

Relation of Iodine to Thyroid Function. Normal thyroid function obviously requires an adequate intake of iodine; without it, normal amounts of hormone cannot be made, TSH is secreted in excess, and the thyroid becomes hyperplastic and hypertrophic. The enlarged and stimulated thyroid becomes remarkably efficient at extracting the residual traces of iodide from the blood, developing an iodine gradient that may be 10 times normal; in mild-to-moderate iodine deficiency, the thyroid usually succeeds in producing sufficient hormone and preferentially secreting T_3. In more severe iodine deficiency, adult hypothyroidism and cretinism may occur.

In some areas of the world, simple or nontoxic goiter is prevalent because of insufficient dietary iodine (Zimmerman, 2009). Regions of iodine deficiency exist in Central and South America, Africa, Europe, Southeast Asia, and China. In the U.S., recommended daily allowances for iodine range from 90-120 μg for children, 150 μg for adults, 220 μg for pregnancy, and 290 μg for lactation (Becker et al., 2006). Vegetables, meat, and poultry contain minimal amounts of iodine, whereas dairy products and fish are relatively high in iodine.

Iodine has been used empirically for the treatment of iodine-deficiency goiter for 150 years; however, its modern use evolved from extensive studies using iodine to prevent goiter in school children in Akron, Ohio, where endemic iodine-deficiency goiter was prevalent. The success of these experiments led to the adoption of iodine prophylaxis and therapy in many regions throughout the world where iodine-deficiency goiter was endemic.

The most practical method for providing small supplements of iodine for large segments of the population is the addition of iodide or iodate to table salt; iodate is now preferred. The use of iodized salt is required by law in some countries, but in others such as the U.S., the use is optional. In the U.S., iodized salt provides 100 μg of iodine per gram. Although the U.S. population remains iodine sufficient, iodine intake has steadily decreased over the last 20 years (Hollowell et al., 1998). The most recent data indicate that iodine intake has stabilized, although pregnant women remain a susceptible population for iodine insufficiency (Haddow et al., 2007; Hollowell and Haddow, 2007). Other vehicles for supplying iodine to large populations who are iodine deficient include oral or intramuscular injection of iodized oil (Elnagar et al., 1995), iodized drinking water supplies, iodized irrigation systems, and iodized animal feed.

Thyroid Hormone Transport Into and Out of Cells. Thyroid hormone crosses the cell membrane primarily via specific transporter proteins (Visser et al., 2008). Multiple such transporters likely exist, each expressed in overlapping but different subsets of tissues. To date, the only transporter of proven importance in humans is monocarboxylic acid transporter 8 (MCT8, SLC16A2). Ectopic expression in cultured cells demonstrates that MCT8 transports T_4 and T_3 bidirectionally across the cell membrane. MCT8 is widely expressed, including in liver, heart, and brain. *MCT8* mutations cause Allan-Herndon-Dudley syndrome, characterized by a severe neurological phenotype and abnormal circulating thyroid hormone levels. The serum T_3 typically is about 2-fold elevated, associated with a slight increase in TSH and slight decrease in T_4.

MCT10 also transports T_4 and T_3 and is widely expressed, but there are no mutation studies to demonstrate its importance for thyroid hormone transport *in vivo*. The organic anion transporter OATP1C1 preferentially transports T_4 rather than T_3, is highly expressed in brain capillaries, and has been hypothesized to be responsible for the transport of T_4 across the blood-brain barrier (Chapter 5).

Actions of Thyroid Hormones

Classical Nuclear-Mediated Effects. Thyroid hormone action is mediated largely by the binding of T_3 to thyroid hormone receptors (TRs), which are members of the nuclear receptor superfamily of transcription factors (Bassett et al., 2003; Yen et al., 2006). This superfamily includes the receptors for steroid hormones, vitamin D, retinoic acid, and a variety of small molecule metabolites such as certain fatty acids and bile acids. The nuclear receptor superfamily also includes a number of "orphan receptors" that have no known ligands and may be regulated by posttranslational modifications or other events. The TRs have the classic nuclear receptor structure consisting of an amino terminal domain, a centrally located zinc finger DNA binding domain, and a ligand binding domain that occupies the carboxyl terminal half of the protein (Figure 39–8).

T_3 binds to TRs with ~10-fold greater affinity than does T_4, and T_4 is not thought to be biologically active in normal physiology. TRs bind to specific DNA sequences (thyroid hormone response elements, TREs) in the promoter/regulatory regions of target genes. The transcription of most target genes is repressed by unliganded TRs and induced following the binding of T_3. The mechanisms of these effects have been well studied (Yen, 2001, Yen et al., 2006). In the unliganded state, the TR ligand binding domain interacts with a co-repressor complex that includes

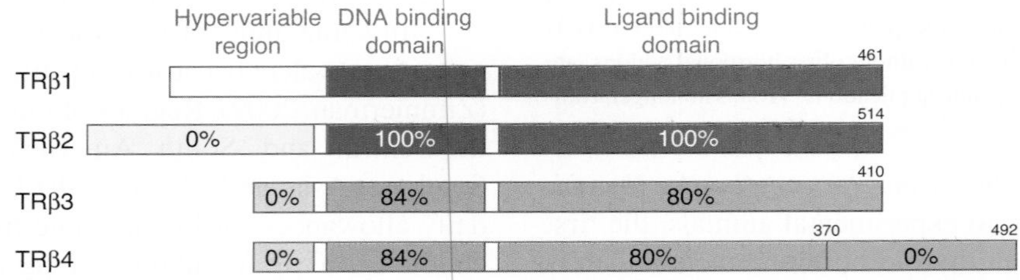

Figure 39–8. *Thyroid hormone receptor isoforms.* The percent amino acid identities of the amino terminal, DNA binding, and ligand binding domains relative to TRβ1 are shown. TRβ1 is 461 amino acids in length. TRα2 does not bind T_3 or any other known ligand.

histone deacetylases and other proteins. The binding of T_3 causes replacement of the co-repressor complex by a co-activator complex that includes histone acetyltransferases, methyltransferases, and other proteins. The actual situation is very complex and probably involves cyclical recruitment of multiple protein complexes to the target gene, leading to cyclical transcription despite the constant presence of T_3 (Liu et al., 2006). Other thyroid hormone target genes, such as those encoding TRH and the TSH subunits, are negatively regulated by T_3. The mechanism is not well defined, but these genes tend to be induced by the unliganded TR in addition to being repressed by T_3.

The TRs are the cellular homologs of the avian retroviral oncoprotein c-*erb*A. There are two genes that encode TRs, *THRA* and *THRB*. *THRA* encodes the receptor TRα1. The biological function of TRα1 is inferred largely through studies of genetically modified mice and cell culture experiments because human mutations in *THRA* have not been described. Although TRα1 is expressed in most cell types, studies in knockout mice demonstrate that the major specific roles for this isoform are in the regulation of heart rate, body temperature, skeletal muscle function, and the development of bone and small intestine (O'Shea and Williams, 2002). Alternative splicing of the TRα primary transcript results in the production of TRα2, which does not bind T_3 because it lacks part of the ligand-binding domain (LBD). TRα2 is expressed ubiquitously and its function is unknown, although there is some evidence that it may inhibit T_3 action. A cryptic promoter within intron 7 of *THRA* drives the production of small proteins that contain only a portion of the TRα LBD. These non-hormone-binding proteins appear to play a role, along with TRα1, in GI development.

The *THRB* gene has two promoters that lead to the production of TRβ1 and TRβ2. These receptors have unique amino terminal domains but otherwise are identical. TRβ1 is ubiquitous, whereas TRβ2 has a highly restricted pattern of expression. Mutations in *THRB* cause the syndrome of resistance to thyroid hormone (Refetoff and Dumitrescu, 2007). Studies in these patients, as well as in genetically modified mice and in cell culture, demonstrate a specific role for TRβ1 in liver metabolism (including the hypocholesterolemic effect of T_3), and for TRβ2 in the negative feedback by T_3 on hypothalamic TRH and pituitary TSH (O'Shea and Williams, 2002). TRβ2 also is important in the development of cones in the retina and in inner ear development.

Non-genomic Effects of Thyroid Hormone. Although nuclear receptors were classically described as being DNA-binding transcription factors, it is now clear that these proteins also can be found outside the nucleus where they can exert biological effects via rapid nongenomic mechanisms (Davis et al., 2008). TRs associate in a T_3-dependent manner with the p85α subunit of phosphatidyl inositol 3-kinase (PI3K), which results in the phosphorylation and activation of PKB/Akt (Hiroi et al., 2006). The PI3K/Akt pathway has broad effects on cellular metabolism. For example, it stimulates NO production by endothelial cells, which leads to vasodilation. Hence, T_3 administration causes rapid vasodilation.

There also is evidence for non-genomic actions of thyroid hormone via a plasma membrane receptor within integrin αVβ3 (Davis et al., 2008). This putative receptor binds extracellular T_4 in preference to T_3, resulting in activation of MAP kinase. However, the importance of non-genomic actions in thyroid hormone physiology and pathophysiology remains uncertain.

Effects of Thyroid Hormone Metabolites. 3-Iodothyronamine and thyronamine, naturally occurring metabolites of T_4, are ligands for the GPCR trace amine-associated receptor 1 (TAAR1) (Scanlan et al., 2004). Administration of 3-iodothyronamine or thyronamine to mice causes hypothermia and bradycardia, presumably through activation of TAAR1 and G_s. 3-Iodothyronamine activation of TAAR1 also induces insulin secretion in the MIN6 cell line (Regard et al., 2007). Interestingly, 3-iodothyronamine also binds to the α_{2A} adrenergic receptor, leading to decreased insulin secretion from mouse islets via a G_i protein-coupled mechanism (Regard et al., 2007). The importance of these effects in human physiology and disease remains to be determined.

MAJOR CLINICAL EFFECTS OF THYROID HORMONES

Growth and Development. Perhaps the most dramatic example of thyroid hormone action is amphibian metamorphosis, in which the tadpole is almost magically transformed into a frog by triiodothyronine. Not only does the animal grow limbs, lungs, and other terrestrial accoutrements, but T_3 also causes the tail to regress.

Thyroid hormone plays a critical role in brain development (Anderson et al., 2003, Bernal, 2007). The absence of thyroid hormone during the period of active neurogenesis (up to 6 months postpartum) leads to irreversible mental retardation (cretinism) and is accompanied by multiple morphological alterations in the brain. These severe morphological alterations result from disturbed neuronal migration, deranged axonal projections, and decreased synaptogenesis. Thyroid hormone supplementation during the first 2 weeks of postnatal life prevents the development of these disturbed morphological changes.

The mechanisms by which thyroid hormone promotes brain development are incompletely understood. Surprisingly, mice with genetic deletions of TRα, TRβ, or both have essentially normal brain development (Gothe et al., 1999). Equally surprisingly, genetic deletion of TRα1 protects mice from the toxic effects of hypothyroidism on brain development (Morte et al., 2002). Perhaps it is the effects of unliganded TRs that result in impaired brain development, such that either T_3 or the absence of TRs is protective. T_3 induces the expression of a number of genes that could plausibly be important in normal brain development, but the exact roles of these specific gene inductions are not known (Anderson et al., 2003). The T_3-dependent expression of many proteins appears to be merely delayed in the hypothyroid animal; normal levels are eventually achieved. Myelin basic protein, a major component of myelin, is induced by T_3 during development. Decreased expression of myelin basic protein in the hypothyroid brain impairs myelinization. RC3/neurogranin, a protein involved in synaptic plasticity, also is induced by T_3. Through its induction of the transcription factor BTEB (basic transcription element binding protein), T3 expands a network of secondary genes in brain development.

The actions of thyroid hormones on protein synthesis and enzymatic activity are not limited to the brain, and in fact most tissues are affected by the administration of thyroid hormone or by its deficiency. The extensive defects in growth and development in cretins vividly illustrate the pervasive effects of thyroid hormones in normal individuals.

Cretinism is usually classified as endemic or sporadic. *Endemic cretinism* occurs in regions of endemic goiter and usually is caused by extreme iodine deficiency. Goiter may or may not be present. *Sporadic cretinism* is a consequence of failure of the thyroid to develop normally or the result of a defect in the synthesis of thyroid hormone. Goiter is present if a synthetic defect is at fault. While detectable at birth, cretinism often is not recognized until 3-5 months of age. When untreated, the condition eventually leads to such gross changes as to be unmistakable: The child is dwarfed, with short extremities, mentally retarded, inactive, uncomplaining, and listless. The face is puffy and expressionless, and the enlarged tongue may protrude through the thickened lips of the half-opened mouth. The skin may have a yellowish hue and feel doughy, dry, and cool to the touch. The heart rate is slow, the body temperature may be low, closure of the fontanels is delayed, and the teeth erupt late. Appetite is poor, feeding is slow and interrupted by choking, constipation is frequent, and there may be an umbilical hernia.

For treatment to be fully effective, the diagnosis must be made long before these changes are obvious. In regions of endemic cretinism due to iodine deficiency, iodine replacement is best instituted before pregnancy. However, iodine replacement given to pregnant women up to the end of the second trimester has been shown to enhance the neurological and psychological development of the children (Cao et al., 1994). Screening of newborn infants for deficient thyroid function is carried out in the U.S. and in most industrialized countries. Concentrations of TSH and thyroxine are measured in blood from the umbilical cord or from a heel stick. The incidence of congenital dysfunction of the thyroid is ~1 per 4000 births.

Thermogenic Effects. Thyroid hormone is necessary for both obligatory thermogenesis (the heat resulting from vital processes) as well as for facultative or adaptive thermogenesis (Silva, 2006). Only a few organs, including the brain, gonads, and spleen, are unresponsive to the thermogenic effects of T_3. Obligatory thermogenesis is the result of T_3 making most biological processes thermodynamically less efficient for the sake of producing heat. Multiple mechanisms underlie the stimulation of obligatory thermogenesis, but the pathways involved and their quantitative contributions have yet to be fully defined. The ability of T_3 to induce the skeletal muscle Ca^{++}-dependent ATPase (SERCA1) contributes to thermogenesis by stimulating the cycling of calcium between cytosol and sarcoplasmic reticulum. Metabolic "futile cycling" (e.g., lipogenesis-lipolysis) has been considered a mechanism to produce heat, but best estimates indicate the contribution is minor. Other than in brown adipose tissue, there is no evidence that a major thermogenic mechanism is uncoupling of phosphorylation, although some groups still believe that T_3 can increase the proton leak through the inner mitochondrial membrane. Regardless of the mechanism, thermogenesis is highly sensitive to thyroid hormone around the physiological range because small changes in L-thyroxine replacement doses may significantly alter resting energy expenditure in the hypothyroid patient. The discovery of type 2 deiodinase in brown fat and its activation by the sympathetic nervous system showed that thyroid hormone also is important for facultative thermogenesis. The ability of T_3 to stimulate thermogenesis has evolved along with ancillary effects to support this thermogenic action, such as the stimulation of appetite and lipogenesis.

Cardiovascular Effects. Changes in the cardiovascular system are prominent in both hyper- and hypothyroidism (Kahaly and Dillmann, 2005). Hyperthyroid patients have tachycardia, increased stroke volume, increased cardiac index, cardiac hypertrophy, decreased peripheral vascular resistance, and increased pulse pressure. Hyperthyroidism is a relatively common cause of atrial fibrillation. Hypothyroid patients have bradycardia, decreased cardiac index, pericardial effusion, increased peripheral vascular resistance, decreased pulse pressure, and elevation of mean arterial pressure.

Triiodothyronine directly regulates myocardial gene expression primarily through TRα1, which is expressed at a higher level in cardiomyocytes than TRβ. T_3 shortens diastolic relaxation (lusitropic effect) by inducing expression of the sarcoplasmic reticulum ATPase SERCa2 and decreasing phospholamban, a SERCa2 inhibitor. T_3 increases the force of myocardial contraction (inotropic effect) in part by inducing expression of the ryanodine channel, the calcium channel of the sarcoplasmic reticulum. T_3 induces the gene encoding the myosin heavy chain (MHC) α isoform and decreases expression of the MHC β gene. Because MHCα endows the myosin holoenzyme with greater ATPase activity, this is one mechanism by which T_3 enhances the velocity of contraction. The chronotropic effect of T_3 is mediated by increases in the pacemaker ion current I_f in the sinoatrial node. Several proteins that comprise the I_f channel are induced by T_3, including HCN2 and HCN4. Interestingly, T_3 also appears to have a direct non-genomic vasodilating effect on vascular smooth muscle (Hiroi et al., 2006), which may contribute to the decreased systemic vascular resistance and increased cardiac output of hyperthyroidism.

Metabolic Effects. Thyroid hormone stimulates the expression of hepatic low-density lipoprotein (LDL) receptors and the metabolism of cholesterol to bile acids, such that hypercholesterolemia is a characteristic feature of hypothyroidism.

Thyroid hormone has complex effects on carbohydrate metabolism (Crunkhorn and Patti, 2008). Thyrotoxicosis is an insulin-resistant state. Post-receptor defects in the liver and peripheral tissues are manifested by depleted glycogen stores and enhanced gluconeogenesis. In addition, the rate of glucose absorption from the gut is increased. Compensatory increases in insulin secretion result in hyperinsulinemia. There may be impaired glucose tolerance or even clinical diabetes, but most hyperthyroid patients are euglycemic. However, diabetic patients already on insulin may have increased insulin requirements in the setting of hyperthyroidism. Conversely, hypothyroidism results in decreased absorption of glucose from the gut, decreased insulin secretion, and a reduced rate of peripheral glucose uptake. Glucose metabolism generally is not affected in a clinically significant manner in nondiabetic patients, although insulin requirements decrease in the hypothyroid patient with diabetes.

Thyroid Hypofunction. Hypothyroidism, known as myxedema when severe, is the most common disorder of thyroid function. Worldwide, hypothyroidism resulting from iodine deficiency remains an all-too-common problem. In non-endemic areas where iodine is sufficient, chronic autoimmune thyroiditis (Hashimoto's thyroiditis) accounts for most cases. This disorder is characterized by high levels of circulating antibodies directed against thyroid peroxidase and, less commonly, against thyroglobulin. In addition, blocking antibodies directed at the TSH receptor may be present, exacerbating the hypothyroidism. The conditions just described are examples of *primary hypothyroidism*, failure of the thyroid gland itself. *Central hypothyroidism* occurs much less often and results from diminished stimulation of the thyroid by TSH because of pituitary failure (*secondary hypothyroidism*) or hypothalamic failure (*tertiary hypothyroidism*). Hypothyroidism present at birth (*congenital hypothyroidism*) is the most common preventable cause of mental retardation in the world. Diagnosis and early intervention with thyroid hormone replacement prevent the development of cretinism, as discussed earlier.

Common symptoms of hypothyroidism include fatigue, lethargy, cold intolerance, mental slowness, depression, dry skin, constipation, mild weight gain, fluid retention, muscle aches and stiffness, irregular menses, and infertility. Common signs include goiter (primary hypothyroidism only), bradycardia, delayed relaxation phase of the deep tendon reflexes, cool and dry skin, hypertension, nonpitting edema, and facial puffiness. Deficiency of thyroid hormone during the first few months of life causes feeding problems, failure to thrive, constipation, and sleepiness. Retardation of mental development is irreversible if not treated promptly. Childhood hypothyroidism impairs linear growth and bone maturation. Because the signs and symptoms of hypothyroidism are nonspecific, diagnosis requires the finding of an elevated serum TSH or, in cases of central hypothyroidism, a decreased serum free T_4. Because physicians maintain a high index of suspicion, the diagnosis usually is made at a relatively early stage. Thus, severe hypothyroidism and myxedema coma are uncommon, except in hypothyroid patients who are noncompliant with their thyroid hormone replacement therapy or individuals without access to medical care.

Thyroid Hyperfunction. Thyrotoxicosis is a condition caused by elevated concentrations of circulating free thyroid hormones. Increased thyroid hormone production is the most common cause, with the common link of TSH receptor stimulation and increased iodine uptake by the thyroid gland as shown by the measurement of the percentage uptake of ^{123}I or ^{131}I in a 24-hour radioactive iodine uptake (RAIU) test. TSH receptor stimulation is either the result of TSH receptor stimulating antibody in Graves' disease or somatic activating TSH receptor mutations in autonomously functioning nodules or a toxic goiter. In contrast, thyroid inflammation or destruction resulting in excess "leak" of thyroid hormones or excess exogenous thyroid hormone intake results in a low 24-hour RAIU. The term *subclinical hyperthyroidism* is defined as those with a subnormal serum TSH and normal concentrations of T_4 and T_3. Atrial arrhythmias, excess cardiac mortality, and excessive bone loss have been associated with this profile of thyroid function tests (Biondi and Cooper, 2008).

Graves' disease is the most common cause of high RAIU thyrotoxicosis (Brent, 2008). It accounts for 60-90% of cases, depending on age and geographic region. Graves' disease is an autoimmune disorder characterized by increased thyroid hormone production, diffuse goiter, and immunoglobulin (Ig)G antibodies that bind to and activate the TSH receptor. This is a relatively common disorder, with an incidence of 0.02-0.4% in the U.S. Endemic areas of iodine deficiency have a lower incidence of autoimmune thyroid disease. As with most types of thyroid dysfunction, women are affected more than men, with a ratio ranging from 5:1-7:1. Graves' disease is more common between the ages of 20 and 50, but it may occur at any age. Major histocompatibility alleles (HLA) B_8 and DR_3 are associated with Graves' disease in whites. Graves' disease is commonly associated with other autoimmune diseases.

The characteristic exophthalmos associated with Graves' disease is an infiltrative ophthalmopathy and is considered an autoimmune-mediated inflammation of the periorbital connective tissue and extraocular muscles. This disorder is clinically evident with various degrees of severity in ~50% of patients with Graves' disease, but it is present on radiological studies, such as ultrasound or CT scan, in almost all patients. The pathogenesis of Graves' ophthalmopathy, including the role of the TSH receptor present in retro-orbital tissues, and the management of this disorder, remain controversial (Khoo and Bahn, 2007).

Toxic uninodular/multinodular goiter accounts for 10-40% of cases of hyperthyroidism and is more common in older patients. Infiltrative ophthalmopathy is absent.

A low RAIU is seen in the destructive thyroiditides and in thyrotoxicosis resulting from exogenous thyroid hormone ingestion. Low RAIU thyrotoxicosis caused by subacute (painful) and silent (painless or lymphocytic) thyroiditis represents ~5-20% of all cases. Silent thyroiditis occurs in 7-10% of postpartum women in the U.S. (Abalovich et al., 2007). Other causes of thyrotoxicosis are much less common.

Most of the signs and symptoms of thyrotoxicosis stem from the excessive production of heat, increased motor activity, and increased sensitivity to catecholamines produced by the sympathetic nervous system. The skin is flushed, warm, and moist; the muscles are weak and tremulous; the heart rate is rapid, the heartbeat is forceful, and the arterial pulses are prominent and bounding. Increased expenditure of energy gives rise to increased appetite and, if intake is insufficient, to loss of weight. There also may be insomnia, difficulty in remaining still, anxiety and apprehension, intolerance to heat, and increased frequency of bowel movements. Angina, arrhythmias, and heart failure may be present in older patients. Older patients may experience less manifestations of sympathetic nervous system stimulation, so called apathetic hyperthyroidism. Some individuals may show extensive muscular wasting as a result of thyroid myopathy. Patients with long-standing undiagnosed or undertreated thyrotoxicosis may develop osteoporosis due to increased bone turnover (Murphy and Williams, 2004).

The most severe form of hyperthyroidism is thyroid storm, which is discussed later in the discussion of therapeutic uses of anti-thyroid drugs.

Thyroid Function Tests. The development of radioimmunoassays and, more recently, chemiluminescent and enzyme-linked immunoassays for T_4, T_3, and TSH have greatly improved the laboratory diagnosis of thyroid disorders (Demers and Spencer, 2003). However, measurement of the total hormone concentration in plasma may not give an accurate picture of the activity of the thyroid gland. The total hormone concentration changes with alterations in either the amount of TBG in plasma or the binding affinity of TBG for hormones. Although equilibrium dialysis of undiluted serum and radioimmunoassay for free thyroxine (FT_4) in the dialysate represent the gold standard for determining FT_4 concentrations, this assay is typically not available in routine clinical laboratories. The FT_4 index is an estimation of the FT_4 concentration and is calculated by multiplying the total thyroxine concentration by the thyroid hormone binding ratio, which estimates the degree of saturation of TBG. The most common assays used for estimating the free T_4 and free T_3 concentrations employ labeled analogs of these iodothyronines in chemiluminescence and enzyme-linked immunoassays. These assays correlate well with free T_4 concentrations measured by the more cumbersome equilibrium dialysis method and are easily adaptable to routine clinical laboratory use. However, the analog assays are affected by extremes of serum binding proteins as well as a wide variety of non-thyroidal disease states, including acute illness, and by certain drugs to a greater degree than are the free T_4 index and free T_4 determined by equilibrium dialysis.

In individuals with normal pituitary function, serum measurement of TSH is the thyroid function test of choice because pituitary secretion of TSH is sensitively regulated in response to circulating concentrations of thyroid hormones.

A major use of the TSH assay is to differentiate between normal and thyrotoxic patients, who should exhibit suppressed TSH values. Indeed, the sensitive TSH assay has replaced evaluation of the response of TSH to injection of synthetic TRH (TRH stimulation test) in the thyrotoxic patient. Although the serum TSH assay is extremely useful in determining the euthyroid state and titrating the replacement dose of thyroid hormone in patients with primary hypothyroidism, abnormal serum TSH concentrations may not always indicate thyroid dysfunction. In such patients, assessment of the circulating thyroid hormone levels will further determine whether or not thyroid dysfunction is truly present. Synthetic preparations of TRH (protirelin) are no longer available in the U.S. for the evaluation of pituitary or hypothalamic failure as a cause of secondary hypothyroidism.

Recombinant human TSH (*thyrotropin alfa*, THYROGEN) is available as an injectable preparation to test the ability of thyroid tissue, both normal and malignant, to take up radioactive iodine and release thyroglobulin (Duntas and Cooper, 2008; Haugen et al., 1999; Pacini and Castangna, 2008).

Therapeutic Uses of Thyroid Hormone

The major indications for the therapeutic use of thyroid hormone are for hormone replacement therapy in patients with hypothyroidism and for TSH suppression therapy in patients with thyroid cancer. Other less common uses also are discussed.

Thyroid Hormone Preparations. Synthetic preparations of the sodium salts of the natural isomers of the thyroid hormones are available and widely used for thyroid hormone therapy.

Levothyroxine. Levothyroxine sodium (L-T_4, LEVOTHROID, LEVOXYL, SYNTHROID, UNITHROID, others) is available in tablets and as a lyophilized powder for injection. Concerns have been raised regarding variations in therapeutic effectiveness among the branded and generic levothyroxine products and the standards used to establish bioequivalence (Hennessey, 2006). More recently, the focus has been on improving uniformity among preparations in tablet content of levothyroxine and stability (Burman et al., 2008). Table 39–3 lists drugs and other factors that may influence levothyroxine dosage requirements.

The potency standards of levothyroxine have been narrowed from the previous standard of 90-110% to 95-105%, and the content must be stable at this level for the designated shelf life. Absorption of thyroxine occurs in the stomach and small intestine and is incomplete (~80% of the dose is absorbed). Absorption is slightly increased when the hormone is taken on an empty stomach, and it is associated with less variability in the TSH when taken this way regularly (Bach-Huynh et al., 2009). The serum T_4 peaks 2-4 hours after oral ingestion, but changes are barely discernable with once-daily dosing due to the 7-day plasma $t_{1/2}$ of the T_4. Given this long $t_{1/2}$, omission of one day's dose does not materially affect the serum TSH or FT_4, but to maintain consistent dosing the patient should be instructed to take a double dose the next day. For any given serum TSH, the serum T_4/T_3 ratio is higher in patients taking levothyroxine than in patients with endogenous thyroid function, due to the fact that ~20% of circulating T_3 normally is supplied by direct thyroidal secretion (Jonklaas et al., 2008). Occasionally this may result in a levothyroxine-treated patient having a marginally elevated free T_4 and a normal TSH, which is acceptable. Follow-up blood tests typically are done ~6 weeks after any dosage change due to the 1-week plasma $t_{1/2}$ of T_4. Dosages are discussed subsequently under specific indications.

In situations where patients cannot take oral medications or where intestinal absorption is in question, levothyroxine may be given intravenously once a day at a dose ~80% of the patient's daily oral requirement.

Liothyronine. Liothyronine sodium (L-T_3) is the salt of triiodothyronine and is available in tablets (CYTOMEL) and in an injectable form (TRIOSTAT, others).

Liothyronine absorption is nearly 100% with peak serum levels 2-4 hours following oral ingestion. Liothyronine may be used occasionally when a more rapid onset of action is desired such as in the rare presentation of myxedema coma or if rapid termination of action is desired such as when preparing a thyroid cancer patient for ^{131}I therapy. Liothyronine is less desirable for chronic replacement therapy due to the requirement for more frequent dosing (plasma $t_{1/2}$ = 0.75 days), higher cost, and transient elevations of serum T_3 concentrations above the normal range. In addition, organs that express the type 2 deiodinase use the locally generated T_3 in addition to plasma T_3, and hence there is theoretical concern that these organs will not maintain physiological intracellular T_3 levels in the absence of plasma T_4. Ten to 15 μg of liothyronine sodium three times per day typically yields a normal serum free T_3 in an athyreotic individual. However, normalization of circulating TSH may require higher levels of free T_3, perhaps because negative feedback normally relies in part on the local generation of T_3 from circulating T_4 (Koutras et al., 1981, Saberi and Utiger, 1974).

Other Preparations. A mixture of thyroxine and triiodothyronine 4:1 by weight is marketed as liotrix (THYROLAR). Desiccated thyroid preparations such as (ARMOUR THYROID, others), with a similar T_4:T_3 ratio, also are available. A 60-mg (1 grain) desiccated thyroid tablet is approximately equivalent in activity to 80 μg of thyroxine. This conversion can be used when changing a patient from replacement therapy with desiccated thyroid to levothyroxine, but typically such patients can be dosed with levothyroxine using dosing guidelines based on age and weight.

Thyroid Hormone Replacement Therapy in Hypothyroidism. Thyroxine (levothyroxine sodium) is the hormone of choice for thyroid hormone replacement therapy due to its consistent potency and prolonged duration of action. With this therapy, one relies on the types 1 and 2 deiodinases to convert T_4 to T_3 to maintain a steady serum level of free T_3.

The average daily adult replacement dose of levothyroxine sodium is 1.7 μg/kg body weight (0.8 μg/lb), although the variation about this average is substantial. Dosing should generally be based on lean body mass (Santini et al., 2005). Although not ideal, once-a-week dosing can be used in situations where compliance is otherwise not possible (Grebe et al., 1997). The goal of therapy is to normalize the serum TSH (in primary hypothyroidism) or free T_4 (in secondary or tertiary hypothyroidism) and to relieve symptoms of hypothyroidism. In primary hypothyroidism, generally it is sufficient to follow TSH without free T_4. A patient with mild primary hypothyroidism will achieve a normal TSH with substantially less than a full replacement dose, but as the endogenous thyroid function declines, the dose will need to be increased. Thus, especially in young healthy patients, it can be simpler to begin with nearly a full replacement dose. In individuals >60 years of age and those with known or suspected cardiac disease or with areas of autonomous thyroid function, institution of therapy at a lower daily dose of levothyroxine sodium (12.5-50 μg per day) is appropriate. The dose can be increased at a rate of 25 μg per day every 6-8 weeks until the TSH is normalized.

Combination therapy with levothyroxine plus liothyronine seems attractive superficially because the thyroid gland secretes T_4 and T_3. However, the T_4:T_3 ratio in human thyroid secretion is ~11:1, compared with 4:1 in the currently available combination pills. Furthermore, the short plasma $t_{1/2}$ of T_3 would necessitate multiple daily dosing to achieve steady circulating T_3 levels. Importantly, randomized blinded controlled trials have failed to uncover evidence of a better therapeutic response to combination therapy with T_4 plus T_3, versus T_4 alone (Grozinsky-Glasberg et al., 2006). Although occasional patients find that they feel better on combination therapy, this is usually short lived. The data indicate that monotherapy with levothyroxine most closely mimics normal physiology and generally is preferred.

Subclinical Hypothyroidism. Subclinical hypothyroidism is the presence of a mildly elevated serum TSH concentration and a normal free T_4 without obvious symptoms. Population screening has shown that subclinical hypothyroidism is very common, with a prevalence of up to 15% in some populations and up to 25% in the elderly. The prevalence is strongly influenced by the definition of the upper limit of normal of serum TSH, which itself is controversial (Surks and Hollowell, 2007). The decision to use levothyroxine therapy in these patients to normalize the serum TSH must be made on an individual basis because treatment may not be appropriate for all patients.

An elevated TSH, especially common among elderly patients and among centenarians, may even be associated with longevity (Atzmon et al., 2009). Patients with subclinical hypothyroidism who may benefit from levothyroxine therapy include those with goiter, autoimmune thyroid disease, hypercholesterolemia, cognitive dysfunction, or pregnancy, and those patients who have nonspecific symptoms that could be due to hypothyroidism (Biondi and Cooper, 2008).

Hypothyroidism During Pregnancy. The dose of levothyroxine in the hypothyroid patient who becomes pregnant usually needs to be increased (Abalovich et al., 2007), perhaps due to the increased serum concentration of TBG induced by estrogen, the expression of type 3 deiodinase by the placenta, and the small amount of transplacental passage of levothyroxine from mother to fetus. In addition, pregnancy may "unmask" hypothyroidism in patients with preexisting autoimmune thyroid disease or in those who reside in a region of iodine deficiency. Overt hypothyroidism during pregnancy is associated with fetal distress and impaired psychoneural development in the progeny. In addition, studies have suggested that subclinical hypothyroidism during pregnancy is associated with mildly impaired psychomotor development in the children and preterm delivery. An increase in miscarriage rate is strongly associated with the presence of anti-thyroid peroxidase antibodies, and early treatment with thyroxine may reduce miscarriages and preterm delivery. These findings strongly suggest that any degree of hypothyroidism, as judged by an elevated serum TSH or perhaps a relatively low T_4, should be treated during pregnancy.

The increased levothyroxine requirement averages 30-50% and can become apparent as early as the fifth week of gestation. The magnitude of thyroxine dose adjustment is greatest for women who are athyreotic from surgical thyroidectomy or radioiodine ablation (Loh et al., 2009). The optimal way to anticipate this increased dosage need and hence to avoid an elevated TSH is not known. Some experts recommend that women increase their levothyroxine dosage by ~30% as soon as pregnancy is confirmed, which can be accomplished by taking two extra pills per week. Most measure a serum TSH in the first trimester and then adjust the thyroxine dose based on this result. Subsequent dosage adjustments would be based on serum TSH, measured 4-6 weeks after each adjustment. For non-pregnant women of reproductive age not using contraception, maintaining the TSH in the lower portion of the reference range (~0.3-2.0 mIU/L) will allow room to move within the reference range during the early part of pregnancy. For similar reasons, dosage adjustments during pregnancy should be made to bring the TSH into the lower portion of the reference range. The increased dosage requirement plateaus at about gestation week 16-20, and dosage needs fall back to prepregnancy levels immediately after delivery.

Myxedema Coma. Myxedema coma is a rare syndrome that represents the extreme expression of severe, long-standing hypothyroidism (Kwaku and Burman, 2007). *It is a medical emergency, and even with early diagnosis and treatment, the mortality rate can be as high as 60%* (Yamamoto et al., 1999). Myxedema coma occurs most often in elderly patients during the winter months. Common precipitating factors include pulmonary infections, cerebrovascular accidents, and congestive heart failure. The clinical course of lethargy proceeding to stupor and then coma is often hastened by drugs, especially sedatives, narcotics, antidepressants, and tranquilizers. Indeed, many cases of myxedema coma have occurred in hypothyroid patients who have been hospitalized for other medical problems.

Cardinal features of myxedema coma are:

- hypothermia, which may be profound
- respiratory depression
- decreased consciousness

Other clinical features include bradycardia, macroglossia, delayed reflexes, and dry, rough skin. Dilutional hyponatremia is common and may be severe. Elevated plasma creatine kinase (CK) and lactate dehydrogenase (LDH) concentrations, acidosis, and anemia are common findings. Lumbar puncture reveals increased opening pressure and high protein content. Hypothyroidism is confirmed by measuring the serum FT_4 and TSH. Ultimately, myxedema coma is a clinical diagnosis.

The mainstay of therapy is supportive care, with ventilatory support, rewarming with blankets, correction of hyponatremia, and treatment of the precipitating cause. Due to a 5-10% incidence of coexisting decreased adrenal reserve in patients with myxedema coma, intravenous steroids are indicated before initiating thyroxine therapy and should be continued until adrenal function has been proven normal (Chapter 42).

There are no randomized controlled clinical trials to evaluate the optimal form of thyroid hormone therapy in myxedema coma. Intravenous administration of thyroid hormone is advised due to uncertain absorption through the gut. Therapy with levothyroxine is commonly begun with a loading dose of 250-500 μg followed by a daily full replacement dose, although some clinicians omit the loading dose. Some clinicians recommend adding liothyronine (10 μg intravenously every 8 hours) with the initial dose of levothyroxine, until the patient is stable and conscious. The limited studies that are available suggest that excessive treatment with either levothyroxine (>500 μg per day) or liothyronine (>75 μg) may be associated with an increased mortality rate.

Congenital Hypothyroidism. Success in the treatment of congenital hypothyroidism depends on the age at which therapy is started. Because of this, newborn screening for congenital hypothyroidism is routine in the U.S., Canada, and many other countries. In cases that do not come to the attention of physicians until retardation of development is clinically obvious, the detrimental effects of thyroid hormone deficiency on mental development will be irreversible. If, however, therapy is instituted within the first 2 weeks of life, normal physical and mental development can be achieved (Rose et al., 2006). Prognosis also depends on the severity of the hypothyroidism at birth and may be worse for infants with thyroid agenesis.

To rapidly normalize the serum thyroxine concentration in the congenitally hypothyroid infant, an initial daily dose of levothyroxine of 10-15 μg/kg is recommended. This dose will increase the serum FT_4 concentration to the upper half of the normal range in most infants within 1-2 weeks. A dose of up to 17 μg/kg has been suggested for the most severely hypothyroid infants, which can normalize the serum T_4 in 3 days (LaFranchi and Austin, 2007). Laboratory evaluations of TSH and FT_4 are performed 2 and 4 weeks after treatment is initiated, every 1-2 months in the first 6 months, every 3-4 months between 6 months and 3 years of age, and every 6-12 months from age 3 years until the end of growth. The goal is to maintain serum FT_4 in the upper half of the reference range and the TSH in the lower normal range during the first 3 years of life. Assessments that are important guides for appropriate hormone replacement include physical growth, motor development, bone maturation, and developmental progress.

Management of premature infants with hypothyroxinemia (~50% of those born at <30 weeks of gestation) remains a therapeutic dilemma. Despite impaired psychomotor development in these patients (Reuss et al., 1996), it is not clear whether levothyroxine therapy may be beneficial, and in some settings it may be detrimental (van Wassenaer et al., 2005).

Thyroid Nodules. Nodular thyroid disease is the most common endocrinopathy. The prevalence of clinically apparent nodules is 4-7% in the U.S., with the frequency increasing throughout adult life. When ultrasound and autopsy data are included, the prevalence of thyroid nodules approaches 50% by age 60. As with other forms of thyroid disease, nodules are more frequent in women. Exposure to ionizing radiation, especially in childhood, increases the rate of nodule development. Approximately 5% of thyroid nodules that come to medical attention are malignant.

The evaluation of the patient with nodular thyroid disease includes a careful physical examination, biochemical analysis of thyroid function, and assessment of the malignant potential of the nodule (Cooper et al., 2006). Thyroid nodules usually are asymptomatic, although they can cause neck discomfort, dysphagia, and a choking sensation. Most patients with thyroid nodules are euthyroid, which should be confirmed by TSH measurement. The most useful diagnostic procedures generally are ultrasound imaging and a fine-needle aspiration biopsy.

TSH suppressive therapy with levothyroxine sometimes is prescribed for the patient with a benign thyroid nodule and a normal serum TSH. The rationale is that a benign nodule will either stop growing or decrease in size after TSH stimulation of the thyroid gland has been suppressed. However, a meta-analysis of randomized trials reveals the shortcomings of this approach (Sdano et al., 2005). Only 22% of nodules decrease in volume by >50% with levothyroxine versus 10% with placebo. Eight patients need to be treated to have one response, and limited data suggest that the nodule will regrow if the levothyroxine is stopped. Furthermore, a 50% decrease in volume represents only about a 20% decrease in linear dimension, a very modest change. The minimum level of TSH suppression needed to achieve this modest response is not known, and long-term exposure to excess thyroid hormone carries risks such as osteoporosis and atrial fibrillation. *Thus the use of levothyroxine to suppress TSH in euthyroid individuals with thyroid nodules cannot be recommended as a general practice. However, if the TSH is elevated, it is appropriate to administer levothyroxine to bring the TSH into the lower portion of the reference range.*

Thyroid Cancer. The mainstays of therapy for well-differentiated thyroid cancer (papillary, follicular) are surgical thyroidectomy, radioiodine, and levothyroxine to suppress TSH (Cooper et al., 2006; Tuttle et al., 2007). The rationale for TSH suppression is that TSH is a growth factor for these cancers. These interventions mainly benefit those patients with stage 2 or higher thyroid cancer (Jonklass et al., 2006).

Given the generally excellent prognosis of well-differentiated thyroid cancer, a prospective randomized controlled trial to assess which patients benefit from suppressive therapy, how low the TSH should be, or how long the suppression should be maintained has not been done. For most low-risk patients with stage 1 or 2 disease, maintaining the TSH just below the reference range for not more than 5 years is one reasonable approach. A greater degree of TSH suppression for a longer duration is recommended for higher risk patients and those with metastatic disease (Cooper et al., 2006).

Non-thyroidal Illness (Sick Euthyroid) Syndrome. Although the circulating free T_3 is low in the non-thyroidal illness syndrome, the current standard of care is not to treat with thyroid hormone because there is no convincing evidence that the low T_3 state contributes to the patient's prognosis or that thyroid hormone therapy would alter the course of the illness. However, there have been very few randomized controlled trials, and these generally involve small numbers of patients and hence have little statistical power. Two trials suggest possible benefit of T_3 therapy in cardiac surgery patients (Klemperer et al., 1995, 1996; Mullis-Jansson et al., 1999).

Depression. Data from several small double-blind placebo-controlled studies suggest potential efficacy of thyroid hormone therapy in euthyroid individuals with major depression, when added to tricyclic antidepressants (Carvalho et al., 2007). It is unclear whether T_3 supplementation of specific serotonin reuptake inhibitor (SSRI) therapy is beneficial (Papakostas et al., 2009). One study suggests that a beneficial effect of T3 added to the SSRI sertraline is seen primarily in subjects with a C785T polymorphism in the type 1 deiodinase gene (Cooper-Kazaz et al., 2009). The mechanism of the T_3 effect (if any) is not known.

Adverse Effects of Thyroid Hormone. Adverse effects of thyroid hormone would generally occur only upon overtreatment and would be similar to the consequences of hyperthyroidism. An excess of thyroid hormone can increase the risk of atrial fibrillation, especially in the elderly, and can increase the risk of osteoporosis, especially in postmenopausal women.

Novel Thyroid Hormone Analogs and Their Potential Therapeutic Applications

The discovery of multiple thyroid hormone receptor isoforms, combined with tissue specific differences in their levels of expression, has led to the development of isoform-specific thyroid hormone analogs with interesting properties (Baxter and Webb, 2009; Brenta et al., 2007). Additional research will be required to determine the therapeutic value of these novel compounds, but their potential merits brief discussion.

TRβ Agonists. Thyroid hormone has long been known to reduce serum cholesterol via effects on hepatic metabolism, but T_4 and T_3 are not useful hypocholesterolemic drugs due to the adverse effects of thyrotoxicosis on the heart and other organs. However, the liver primarily expresses TRβ, whereas the heart primarily expresses TRα. T_3 analogs that have a higher affinity for TRβ than TRα and that accumulate preferentially in the liver have been shown to lower serum cholesterol without causing tachycardia in humans and animals (Erion et al., 2007). These analogs also can induce weight loss in mice with diet-induced obesity. Thyromimetics with preferential action on TRβ also might be useful in the management of thyroid hormone resistance, which in most cases is caused by mutations in TRβ that lower the binding affinity for T_3 (Refetoff and Dumitrescu, 2007).

Thyroid Hormone Receptor α Agonists. Because TRα1 is expressed preferentially in the heart, specific agonists might find use in the management of heart failure or bradycardia. The design of specific agonists for TRα, however, has proven much more difficult than for TRβ (Ocasio and Scanlan, 2008).

Thyromimetics with Altered Entry into Cells. Monocarboxylate transporter 8 (MCT8) transports T_3 into cells and is highly expressed in the brain. Patients with MCT8 mutations have the Allan-Herndon-Dudley syndrome with severe neurological impairment, presumably due to intracellular thyroid hormone deficiency. A thyromimetic that can enter the brain in an MCT8-independent manner could be valuable in treating these patients. The thyroid hormone analog 3,5-diiodothyropropionic acid (DITPA) has this property in mice (Di Cosmo et al., 2009).

Thyroid Hormone Receptor Antagonists. In principle, thyroid hormone receptor antagonists could be useful therapeutics in the medical management of thyrotoxicosis, and possibly even in the management of cardiac arrhythmias. A thyroid hormone analog denoted NH3 antagonizes the cholesterol lowering, TSH lowering, and tachycardic actions of T_3 in rats, but at high doses this drug functions as a T_3 agonist (Grover et al., 2007).

Thyronamines. 3-Iodothyronamine and thyronamine are endogenous thyroid hormone metabolites that functions as agonists for the GRCR Trace Amine Associated Receptor 1 (TAAR1) and the α_{2A} adrenergic receptor. These compounds appear to have broad metabolic effects in experimental animals, such as inducing hypothermia and bradycardia (Scanlan et al., 2004), and conferring protection against brain ischemia (Doyle et al., 2007). The therapeutic potential of these agents or their analogs requires further investigation.

ANTI-THYROID DRUGS AND OTHER THYROID INHIBITORS

A number of compounds are capable of interfering, directly or indirectly, with the synthesis, release, or action of thyroid hormones (Table 39–4). Several are of great clinical value for the temporary or extended control of hyperthyroid states. The major inhibitors may be classified into four categories:

- Anti-thyroid drugs, which interfere directly with the synthesis of thyroid hormones;
- Ionic inhibitors, which block the iodide transport mechanism;
- High concentrations of iodine, which decrease release of thyroid hormones from the gland and also may decrease hormone synthesis;
- Radioactive iodine, which damages the thyroid gland with ionizing radiation.

Adjuvant therapy with drugs that have no specific effects on thyroid hormone synthesis is useful in controlling the peripheral manifestations of thyrotoxicosis. These drugs include inhibitors of the peripheral deiodination of thyroxine to the active hormone, triiodothyronine, β adrenergic receptor antagonists, and Ca^{2+} channel blockers. The anti-thyroid drugs have been reviewed by Cooper (2005). Adrenergic receptor antagonists are discussed more fully in Chapter 12 and Ca^{2+} channel blockers in Chapter 27.

Table 39–4

Anti-thyroid Compounds

PROCESS AFFECTED	EXAMPLES OF INHIBITORS
Active transport of iodide	Complex anions: perchlorate, fluoborate, pertechnetate, thiocyanate
Iodination of thyroglobulin	Thionamides: propylthiouracil, methimazole, carbimazole
	Thiocyanate
	Aniline derivatives; sulfonamides
	Iodide
Coupling reaction	Thionamides
	Sulfonamides
	?All other inhibitors of iodination
Hormone release	Lithium salts
	Iodide
Iodotyrosine deiodination	Nitrotyrosines
Peripheral iodothyronine deiodination	Thiouracil derivatives
	Oral cholecystographic agents
	Amiodarone
Hormone excretion/ inactivation	Inducers of hepatic drug-metabolizing enzymes: phenobarbital, rifampin, carbamazepine, phenytoin
Hormone action	Thyroxine analogs
	Amiodarone
	?Phenytoin
	Binding in gut: cholestyramine

Source: Data adapted from Meier C.A., Burger A.C. Effects of drugs and other substances on thyroid hormone synthesis and metabolism. In: *Werner and Ingbar's The Thyroid*, 9th ed. (Braverman L.E. and Utiger R.D. eds.) Lippincott Williams & Wilkins, Philadelphia, 2005.

Anti-Thyroid Drugs

The anti-thyroid drugs that have clinical utility are the thioureylenes, which belong to the family of thionamides. Propylthiouracil may be considered as the prototype.

History. Studies on the mechanism of the development of goiter began with the observation that rabbits fed a diet composed largely of cabbage often developed goiters. This result was probably due to the presence of precursors of the thiocyanate ion in cabbage leaves. Later, two pure compounds were shown to produce goiter: sulfaguanidine, a sulfanilamide antimicrobial used to treat enteric infections, and phenylthiourea.

Investigation of the effects of thiourea derivatives revealed that rats became hypothyroid despite hyperplastic changes in their thyroid glands that were characteristic of intense thyrotropic stimulation. After treatment was begun, no new hormone was made, and the goitrogen had no visible effect on the thyroid gland following hypophysectomy or the administration of thyroid hormone. This suggested that the goiter was a compensatory change resulting from the induced state of hypothyroidism and that the primary action of the compounds was to inhibit the formation of thyroid hormone. The therapeutic possibilities of such agents in hyperthyroidism were evident, and the substances so used became known as *anti-thyroid drugs* (Astwood, 1945).

Structure–Activity Relationship. The two goitrogens found in the early 1940s proved to be prototypes of two different classes of anti-thyroid drugs. These two, with one later addition, made up three general categories into which most of the agents can be assigned:

- *Thioureylenes* include all the compounds currently used clinically (Figure 39–9);
- *Aniline derivatives,* of which the sulfonamides make up the largest number, embrace a few substances that have been found to inhibit thyroid hormone synthesis;
- *Polyhydric phenols,* such as resorcinol, which have caused goiter in humans when applied to abraded skin.

A few other compounds, mentioned briefly later, do not fit into any of these categories.

Thiourea and its simpler aliphatic derivatives and heterocyclic compounds containing a thioureylene group make up most of the known anti-thyroid agents that are effective in humans. Although most of them incorporate the entire thioureylene group, in some a nitrogen atom is replaced by oxygen or sulfur so that only the thioamide group is common to all. Among the heterocyclic compounds, active representatives are the sulfur derivatives of imidazole, oxazole, hydantoin, thiazole, thiadiazole, uracil, and barbituric acid.

L-5-Vinyl-2-thiooxazolidone (goitrin) is responsible for the goiter that results from consuming turnips or the seeds or green parts of cruciferous plants. These plants are eaten by cows, and the compound is found in cow's milk in areas of endemic goiter in Finland; it is about as active as propylthiouracil in humans.

As the result of industrial exposure, toxicological studies, or clinical trials for various purposes, several other compounds have been noted to possess anti-thyroid activity (Miller et al., 2009). Thiopental and oral hypoglycemic drugs of the sulfonylurea class

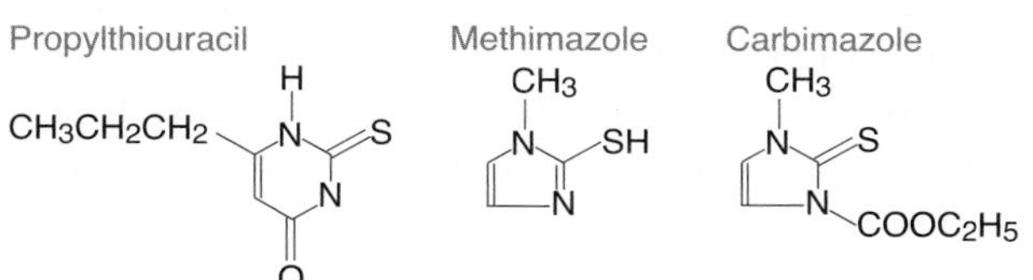

Figure 39–9. *Anti-thyroid drugs of the thiamide type.*

have weak anti-thyroid action in experimental animals. This is not significant at usual doses in humans. However, anti-thyroid effects in humans have been observed from dimercaprol and lithium salts. Polychlorinated biphenyls bear a striking structural resemblance to the thyroid hormones and may function as either agonists or antagonists of thyroid hormone action (Zoeller et al., 2000). Amiodarone, the iodine-rich drug used in the management of cardiac arrhythmias, has complex effects on thyroid function (Basaria and Cooper, 2005). In areas of iodine sufficiency, amiodarone-induced hypothyroidism due to the excess iodine is not uncommon, whereas in iodine-deficient regions, amiodarone-induced thyrotoxicosis predominates, whether because of the excess iodine or the thyroiditis induced by the drug. Amiodarone and its major metabolite, desethylamiodarone, are potent inhibitors of iodothyronine deiodination, resulting in decreased conversion of thyroxine to triiodothyronine. In addition, desethylamiodarone decreases binding of triiodothyronine to its nuclear receptors. Recommendations have been made as to screening methods to identify chemicals that may alter thyroid hormone action or homeostasis (Diamanti-Kandarakis et al., 2009).

Mechanism of Action. The mechanism of action of the thioureylene drugs has been thoroughly reviewed (Cooper, 2005). Anti-thyroid drugs inhibit the formation of thyroid hormones by interfering with the incorporation of iodine into tyrosyl residues of thyroglobulin; they also inhibit the coupling of these iodotyrosyl residues to form iodothyronines. This implies that they interfere with the oxidation of iodide ion and iodotyrosyl groups. The drugs are thought to inhibit the peroxidase enzyme, thereby preventing oxidation of iodide or iodotyrosyl groups to the required active state (Taurog et al., 1996). The anti-thyroid drugs bind to and inactivate the peroxidase only when the heme of the enzyme is in the oxidized state. Over a period of time, the inhibition of hormone synthesis results in the depletion of stores of iodinated thyroglobulin as the protein is hydrolyzed and the hormones are released into the circulation. Only when the preformed hormone is depleted and the concentrations of circulating thyroid hormones begin to decline do clinical effects become noticeable.

There is some evidence that the coupling reaction may be more sensitive to an anti-thyroid drug, such as propylthiouracil, than is the iodination reaction. This may explain why patients with hyperthyroidism respond well to doses of the drug that only partially suppress organification.

When Graves' disease is treated with anti-thyroid drugs, the concentration of thyroid-stimulating immunoglobulins in the circulation often decreases, prompting some to propose that these agents act as immunosuppressants. Perchlorate, which acts by an entirely different mechanism, also decreases thyroid-stimulating immunoglobulins, suggesting that improvement in hyperthyroidism may reduce thyroid antibodies.

In addition to blocking hormone synthesis, propylthiouracil partially inhibits the peripheral deiodination of T_4 to T_3. *Methimazole* does not have this effect; although the quantitative significance of this inhibition has not been established, it provides a rationale for the choice of propylthiouracil over other anti-thyroid drugs in the treatment of severe hyperthyroid states or of thyroid storm, where a decreased rate of $T_4 \rightarrow T_3$ conversion would be beneficial.

Absorption, Metabolism, and Excretion. The anti-thyroid compounds currently used in the U.S. are propylthiouracil (6-*n*-propylthiouracil) and methimazole (1-methyl-2-mercaptoimidazole; TAPAZOLE, others). In Great Britain and Europe, carbimazole (NEO-MERCAZOLE), a carbethoxy derivative of methimazole, is available, and its anti-thyroid action is due to its conversion to methimazole after absorption. Pharmacological properties of propylthiouracil and methimazole are shown in Table 39–5.

Table 39–5

Selected Pharmacokinetic Features of Anti-thyroid Drugs

	PROPYLTHIOURACIL	METHIMAZOLE
Plasma protein binding	~75%	Nil
Plasma $t_{1/2}$	75 minutes	~4-6 hours
Volume of distribution	~20 liters	~40 liters
Concentrated in thyroid	Yes	Yes
Metabolism of drug during illness		
Severe liver disease	Normal	Decreased
Severe kidney disease	Normal	Normal
Dosing frequency	1-4 times daily	Once or twice daily
Transplacental passage	Low	Low
Levels in breast milk	Low	Low

Measurements of the course of organification of radioactive iodine by the thyroid show that absorption of effective amounts of propylthiouracil follows within 20-30 minutes of an oral dose and that the duration of action of the compounds used clinically is brief. The effect of a dose of 100 mg of propylthiouracil begins to wane in 2-3 hours, and even a 500-mg dose is completely inhibitory for only 6-8 hours. As little as 0.5 mg of methimazole similarly decreases the organification of radioactive iodine in the thyroid gland, but a single dose of 10-25 mg is needed to extend the inhibition to 24 hours.

The $t_{1/2}$ of propylthiouracil in plasma is ~75 minutes, whereas that of methimazole is 4-6 hours. The drugs are concentrated in the thyroid, and methimazole, derived from the metabolism of carbimazole, accumulates after carbimazole is administered. Drugs and metabolites appear largely in the urine.

Propylthiouracil and methimazole cross the placenta equally (Mortimer et al., 1997) and also can be found in milk. The use of these drugs during pregnancy is discussed later.

Untoward Reactions. The incidence of side effects from propylthiouracil and methimazole as currently used is relatively low. The overall incidence as compiled from published cases by early investigators was 3% for propylthiouracil and 7% for methimazole, with 0.44% and 0.12% of cases, respectively, developing the most serious reaction, agranulocytosis.

Agranulocytosis usually occurs during the first few weeks or months of therapy but may occur later. Because agranulocytosis can develop rapidly, periodic white cell counts usually are of little help, although a baseline white blood cell count and differential should be obtained before anti-thyroid drug treatment is initiated. Patients should be instructed to immediately report the development of sore throat or fever, which are often signs of the presence of leukopenia. If these signs or symptoms occur, patients should discontinue their anti-thyroid drug and obtain a granuloctye count. Agranulocytosis is reversible upon discontinuation of the offending drug, and the administration of recombinant human granulocyte colony-stimulating factor may hasten recovery (Magner and Snyder, 1994). Mild granulocytopenia, if noted, may be due to thyrotoxicosis or may be the first sign of this dangerous drug reaction. Caution and frequent leukocyte counts are then required.

The most common reaction is a mild, occasionally purpuric, urticarial papular rash. It often subsides spontaneously without interrupting treatment, but it sometimes calls for the administration of an antihistamine, corticosteroids, and changing to another drug (cross-sensitivity between propylthiouracil and methimazole is uncommon). Other less frequent complications are pain and stiffness in the joints, paresthesias, headache, nausea, skin pigmentation, and loss of hair. Drug fever, hepatitis, and nephritis are rare, although abnormal liver function tests are not infrequent with higher doses of propylthiouracil. Although vasculitis was previously thought to be a rare complication, antineutrophilic cytoplasmic antibodies (ANCAs) have been reported to occur in ~50% of patients receiving propylthiouracil and rarely with methimazole (Sato et al., 2000; Sera et al., 2000).

Propylthiouracil-associated hepatic failure has been increasingly recognized, especially in children and pregnant women (Cooper and Rivkees, 2009). There are 47 published reports of propylthiouracil-associated liver failure in adults and children, and 23 liver transplants between 1990 and 2007 due to propylthiouracil-associated liver failure. Methimazole may cause cholestatic dysfunction, but it is not associated with hepatocellular necrosis, and there are no reports of liver transplants due to methimazole-associated liver toxicity. There is increasing concern about using propylthiouracil as a first-line treatment, except in severe thyrotoxicosis when the inhibition of T_4 to T_3 is desired, and possibly in the first trimester of pregnancy. *The FDA has added a "black box" warning to propylthiouracil because of liver failure, recommending close monitoring of liver function during its use. Propylthiouracil should not be used in children except in the case of methimazole allergy.*

Therapeutic Uses. The anti-thyroid drugs are used in the treatment of hyperthyroidism in the following three ways:

- as definitive treatment, to control the disorder in anticipation of a spontaneous remission in Graves' disease
- in conjunction with radioactive iodine, to hasten recovery while awaiting the effects of radiation
- to control the disorder in preparation for surgical treatment (Cooper, 2003)

Methimazole is the drug of choice for Graves' disease; it is effective when given as a single daily dose, has improved adherence, and is less toxic than propylthiouracil. Methimazole has a relatively long plasma and intrathyroidal $t_{1/2}$, as well as a long duration of action. The usual starting dose for methimazole is 15–40 mg per day. The usual starting dose of propylthiouracil is 100 mg every 8 hours. When doses >300 mg daily are needed, further subdivision of the time of administration to every 4-6 hours is occasionally helpful. Failures of response to daily treatment with 300-400 mg of propylthiouracil or 30-40 mg of methimazole are most commonly due to nonadherence but can be seen with very severe disease. Delayed responses also are noted in patients with very large goiters or those in whom iodine in any form has been given beforehand. Once euthyroidism is achieved, usually within 12 weeks, the dose of anti-thyroid drug can be reduced, but not stopped, lest an exacerbation of Graves' disease occur (see later section on remissions).

Response to Treatment. The thyrotoxic state usually improves within 3-6 weeks after the initiation of anti-thyroid drugs. The clinical response is related to the dose of anti-thyroid drug, the size of the goiter, and pretreatment serum T_3 concentrations. The rate of response is determined by the quantity of stored hormone, the rate of turnover of hormone in the thyroid, the $t_{1/2}$ of the hormone in the periphery, and the completeness of the block in synthesis imposed by the dosage given. When large doses are continued, and sometimes with the usual dose, hypothyroidism may develop as a result of overtreatment. The earliest signs of hypothyroidism call for a reduction in dose; if they have advanced to the point of discomfort, thyroid hormone in full replacement doses can be given to hasten recovery;

then the lower maintenance dose of anti-thyroid drug as discussed earlier is instituted for continued therapy. Despite initial suggestions to the contrary, there is no demonstrated benefit of combination levothyroxine and methimazole therapy on either remission rates (Rittmaster et al., 1998) or on changes in serum concentrations of thyroid-stimulating immunoglobulins.

After treatment is initiated, patients should be examined and thyroid function tests (serum FT_4 and total or free triiodothyronine concentrations) measured every 2-4 months. Serum TSH will often remain suppressed for several months after a patient has been hyperthyroid, so the circulating thyroxine and triiodothyronine concentrations are the most reliable assessment of thyroid status (Uy et al., 1995). Once euthyroidism is established, follow-up every 4-6 months is reasonable.

Control of the hyperthyroidism usually is associated with a decrease in goiter size. When this occurs, the dose of the anti-thyroid drug should be significantly decreased and/or levothyroxine can be added once hypothyroidism is confirmed by laboratory testing.

Remissions. There is no highly reliable way of predicting before treatment which patients will eventually achieve a lasting remission and which will relapse. A favorable outcome is unlikely when the disorder is of long standing, the thyroid is quite large, serum T_3 concentration is high relative to serum T_4 concentration, or various forms of treatment have failed. To complicate the issue further, remission and eventual hypothyroidism may represent the natural history of Graves' disease.

During treatment, a positive sign that a remission may have taken place is reduced size of the goiter. The persistence of goiter often indicates failure, unless the patient becomes hypothyroid. Another favorable indication is continued freedom from all signs of hyperthyroidism when the maintenance dose is small. Finally, a decrease in thyroid-stimulating immunoglobulins is associated with remission, although the clinical features and improvement in thyroid function tests are usually sufficient to make this assessment.

The Therapeutic Choice. Because anti-thyroid drug therapy, radioactive iodine, and subtotal thyroidectomy all are effective treatments for Graves' disease, there is no worldwide consensus among endocrinologists about the best therapeutic approach. Prolonged drug therapy of Graves' disease in anticipation of a remission is most successful in patients with small goiters or mild hyperthyroidism. Those with large goiters or severe disease usually require definitive therapy with either surgery or radioactive iodine (^{131}I). Radioactive iodine remains the treatment of choice of many endocrinologists in the U.S.

Many investigators consider coexisting ophthalmopathy to be a relative contraindication for radioactive iodine therapy because worsening of ophthalmopathy has been reported after radioactive iodine (Bartalena et al., 1998a), although this remains controversial. Others suggest that development of hypothyroidism, regardless of the treatment, is the strongest risk factor for progression of ophthalmopathy. Smoking is a risk factor for worsening ophthalmopathy (Bartelena et al., 1998b). In older patients, depleting the thyroid gland of preformed hormone by treatment with anti-thyroid drugs is advisable before therapy with radioactive iodine, thus preventing a severe exacerbation of the hyperthyroid state during the subsequent development of radiation thyroiditis. Subtotal thyroidectomy is advocated for Graves' disease in young patients with large goiters, children who are allergic to anti-thyroid drugs, pregnant women (usually in the second trimester) who are allergic to anti-thyroid drugs, and patients who prefer surgery over anti-thyroid drugs or radioactive iodine. Radioactive iodine or surgery is indicated for definitive therapy in toxic nodular goiter.

Thyrotoxicosis in Pregnancy. Thyrotoxicosis occurs in ~0.2% of pregnancies and is caused most frequently by Graves' disease (Chan and Mandel, 2007). Anti-thyroid drugs are the treatment of choice; radioactive iodine is clearly contraindicated. Historically, propylthiouracil has been preferred over methimazole because transplacental passage was thought to be lower; however, as noted earlier, both propylthiouracil and methimazole cross the placenta equally (Mortimer et al., 1997). Methimazole is also very rarely associated with aplasia cutis and an embryopathy that can include choanal atresia and other anomalies (Diav-Citrin and Ornoy, 2002). Current data suggest that either may be used safely in the pregnant patient (Momotani et al., 1997; Mortimer et al., 1997), although the concern for propylthiouracil-associated liver failure in pregnancy may favor the use of methimazole, especially after organogenesis in the first trimester (Cooper and Rivkees, 2009). Carbimazole is used in the EU during pregnancy and is rarely associated with congenital gut abnormalities (Barwell et al., 2002).

The anti-thyroid drug dosage should be minimized to keep the serum FT_4 index in the upper half of the normal range or slightly elevated. As pregnancy progresses, Graves' disease often improves, and it is not uncommon for patients either to be on very low doses or off anti-thyroid drugs completely by the end of pregnancy. Therefore the anti-thyroid drug dose should be reduced, and maternal thyroid function should be frequently monitored to decrease chances of fetal hypothyroidism. Relapse or worsening of Graves' disease is common after delivery, and patients should be monitored closely. Methimazole up to 20 mg daily in nursing mothers reportedly has no effect on thyroid function in the infant (Azizi et al., 2003), and propylthiouracil is thought to cross into breast milk even less than methimazole.

Adjuvant Therapy. Several drugs that have no intrinsic anti-thyroid activity are useful in the symptomatic treatment of thyrotoxicosis.

β *Adrenergic receptor antagonists* (Chapter 12) are effective in antagonizing the sympathetic/adrenergic effects of thyrotoxicosis, thereby reducing the tachycardia, tremor, and stare, and relieving palpitations, anxiety, and tension. Either propranolol, 20-40 mg four times daily, or atenolol, 50-100 mg daily, is usually given initially. Propranolol or esmolol can be given intravenously if needed. *Ca^{2+} channel blockers* (diltiazem, 60-120 mg four times daily) can be used to control tachycardia and decrease the incidence of supraventricular tachyarrhythmias (Chapters 27 and 29). These drugs, however, should be used as an adjunct to anti-thyroid drug therapy for more rapid improvement of adrenergic-related symptoms and not as the only treatment for hyperthyroidism. Usually only short-term treatment with β adrenergic receptor antagonists or Ca^{2+} channel blockers is required, 2-6 weeks, and it should be discontinued once the patient is euthyroid.

Other drugs that are useful in the rapid treatment of the severely thyrotoxic patient are agents that inhibit the peripheral conversion of thyroxine to triiodothyronine. Dexamethasone (0.5-1 mg, two to four times daily) and the iodinated radiological contrast agents iopanoic acid (500-1000 mg once daily) and sodium ipodate (ORAGRAFIN) (500-1000 mg once daily) are effective in preoperative preparation; neither iopanoic acid nor sodium ipodate is available in the U.S. Cholestyramine has been used in severely toxic patients to bind thyroid hormones in the gut and thus block the enterohepatic circulation of the iodothyronines (Mercado et al., 1996). Immunotherapy has been used for Graves' hyperthyroidism and ophthalmopathy. The B-lymphocyte depleting agent rituximab, when used with methimazole, prolongs remission of Graves' disease (El Fassi et al., 2009). A novel approach that has been successful only *in vitro* uses low-molecular-weight antagonists of the TSH receptor (Neumann et al., 2008). This approach has the potential to provide a rapid and targeted treatment for Graves' disease.

Preoperative Preparation. To reduce operative morbidity and mortality, patients should be rendered euthyroid before subtotal thyroidectomy as definitive treatment for hyperthyroidism. It is possible to bring almost all patients to a euthyroid state with a normal range serum T_4 and T_3 concentration. The serum TSH concentration will be suppressed below normal for several months after serum T_4 and T_3 is normalized, so it is not required that the serum TSH concentration be normal before surgery. The operative mortality in these patients in the hands of an experienced thyroid surgeon is extremely low. Prior treatment with anti-thyroid drugs usually is successful in rendering the patient euthyroid for surgery. Iodide is added to the regimen for 7-10 days before surgery to decrease the vascularity of the gland, making it less friable and decreasing the difficulties for the surgeon. In the patient who is either allergic to anti-thyroid drugs or is noncompliant, a euthyroid state usually can be achieved by treatment with iopanoic acid (not available in the U.S.), dexamethasone, and propranolol for 5-7 days before surgery. All of these drugs should be discontinued after surgery.

Thyroid Storm. Thyroid storm is an uncommon but life-threatening complication of thyrotoxicosis in which a severe form of the disease is usually precipitated by an intercurrent medical problem (Nayak and Burman, 2006). It occurs in untreated or partially treated thyrotoxic patients. Precipitating factors associated with thyrotoxic crisis include infections, stress, trauma, thyroidal or non-thyroidal surgery, diabetic ketoacidosis, labor, heart disease, and, rarely, radioactive iodine treatment.

Clinical features are similar to those of thyrotoxicosis but more exaggerated. Cardinal features include fever (temperature usually >38.5°C) and tachycardia out of proportion to the fever. Nausea, vomiting, diarrhea, agitation, and confusion are frequent presentations. Coma and death may ensue in up to 20% of patients. Thyroid function abnormalities are similar to those found in uncomplicated hyperthyroidism. Therefore thyroid storm is primarily a clinical diagnosis.

Treatment includes supportive measures such as intravenous fluids, antipyretics, cooling blankets, and sedation. Anti-thyroid drugs are given in large doses. Propylthiouracil is preferred over methimazole because it also impairs peripheral conversion of $T_4 \rightarrow T_3$. The recommended initial dose of propylthiouracil is 200-400 mg every 6-8 hours (Nayak and Burman, 2006). Propylthiouracil and methimazole can be administered by nasogastric tube or rectally if necessary. Neither of these preparations is available for parenteral administration in the U.S.

Oral iodides are used after the first dose of an anti-thyroid drug has been administered. The agents mentioned earlier as adjuvant therapies of thyrotoxicosis may be usefully applied. Hydrocortisone (100 mg intravenously every 8 hours) can be used in the setting of hypotension both as an inhibitor of conversion of thyroxine to triiodothyronine and as supportive therapy of possible relative adrenal insufficiency (Nayak and Burman, 2006). Finally, *treatment of the underlying precipitating illness is essential.*

Ionic Inhibitors

The term *ionic inhibitors* designates substances that interfere with the concentration of iodide by the thyroid gland (Diamanti-Kandarakis et al., 2009). The effective agents are anions that resemble iodide: *thiocyanate, perchlorate,* and *fluoroborate*, all monovalent hydrated anions of a size similar to that of iodide.

The most studied example, *thiocyanate,* differs from the others qualitatively; it is not concentrated by the thyroid gland but in large amounts may inhibit the organification of iodine. Thiocyanate is produced following the enzymatic hydrolysis of certain plant glycosides. Thus, certain foods (e.g., cabbage) and cigarette smoking result in an increased concentration of thiocyanate in the blood and urine, as does the administration of sodium nitroprusside. Indeed, cigarette smoking has been reported to worsen both subclinical hypothyroidism (Müller et al., 1995) and Graves' ophthalmopathy (Bartalena et al., 1998b). Dietary precursors of thiocyanate may be a contributing factor in endemic goiter in certain parts of the world, especially in Central Africa, where the intake of iodine is very low.

Among other anions, perchlorate (ClO_4^-) is 10 times as active as thiocyanate (Wolff, 1998). The various NIS inhibitors, perchlorate, thiocyanate, and nitrate, are additive in inhibiting iodine uptake (Tonacchera et al., 2004). Perchlorate blocks the entrance of iodide into the thyroid by competitively inhibiting the NIS. Perchlorate is transported by NIS using a different stoicheiometry, electroneutral, compared with that seen with transport of iodine (Dohan et al., 2007). Although perchlorate can be used to control hyperthyroidism, it has caused fatal aplastic anemia when given in excessive amounts (2-3 g daily). Perchlorate in doses of 750 mg daily has been used in the treatment of Graves' disease and amiodarone-iodine–induced thyrotoxicosis (National Academy of Sciences/National Research Council [NAS/NRC], 2005). Perchlorate can be used to "discharge" inorganic iodide from the thyroid gland in a diagnostic test of iodide organification. Other ions, selected on the basis of their size, also have been found to be active; fluoroborate (BF_4^-) is as effective as perchlorate.

Ammonium perchlorate is an essential oxidizer in the production of rocket fuel, and water supplies have been contaminated with perchlorate derived from the sites of production. A National Academy of Sciences Committee recommended a reference dose of perchlorate exposure of 0.0007 mg/kg per day that would produce no adverse effect. This level of no effect is much higher than that found in most water supplies, indicating a low risk of perchlorate exposure influencing thyroid function (NAS/NRC, 2005). The reference dose was primarily derived from a 2-week study in normal volunteers that determined the daily dose of perchlorate that produced no effect on thyroid function or ^{123}I uptake (Greer et al., 2002). There remain concerns that accumulated perchlorate exposure from multiple sources and combined exposure to other iodine uptake inhibitors may impair thyroid function, especially as it might affect pregnant women and young children (Miller et al., 2009). A study in the U.S. showed a correlation between perchlorate exposure and an increase in serum TSH (still within the normal range), only among women with low iodine intake (Blount et al., 2006). Men and women with adequate iodine intake did not show any influence of perchlorate on thyroid function. Others have argued that the risk of thyroid dysfunction from perchlorate exposure is extremely low and there is little evidence to support this view (Charnley, 2008). A study among pregnant women living in areas of very high natural perchlorate contamination showed no effect on maternal thyroid function or pregnancy outcome for mother or infant (Tellez et al., 2006). Although reassuring, the high iodine content in this region may limit the effects of perchlorate. Because the primary mode of toxicity of perchlorate is inhibition of iodine uptake, the best approach to reduce susceptibility is to maintain adequate iodine intake, especially during pregnancy (Becker et al., 2006).

Lithium has a multitude of effects on thyroid function; its principal effect is decreased secretion of thyroxine and triiodothyronine (Takami, 1994), which can cause overt hypothyroidism in some patients taking Li^+ for the treatment of mania (Chapter 16).

Iodide

Iodide is the oldest remedy for disorders of the thyroid gland. Before the anti-thyroid drugs were used, it was the only substance available for control of the signs and symptoms of hyperthyroidism. Its use in this way is indeed paradoxical, and the explanation for this paradox is still incomplete.

Mechanism of Action. High concentrations of iodide appear to influence almost all important aspects of iodine metabolism by the thyroid gland. The capacity of iodide to limit its own transport was mentioned earlier. Acute inhibition of the synthesis of iodotyrosines and iodothyronines by iodide also is well known (the *Wolff-Chaikoff effect*). This transient 2-day inhibition is observed only above critical concentrations of intracellular rather than extracellular concentrations of iodide. With time, "escape" from this inhibition is associated with an adaptive decrease in iodide transport and a lowered intracellular iodide concentration, associated with a decrease in NIS mRNA and protein (Eng et al., 1999).

An important clinical effect of high $[I^-]_{plasma}$ is inhibition of the release of thyroid hormone. This action is rapid and efficacious in severe thyrotoxicosis. The effect is exerted directly on the thyroid gland and can be demonstrated in the euthyroid subject as well as in the hyperthyroid patient. Studies in a cultured thyroid cell line suggest that some of the inhibitory effects of iodide on thyrocyte proliferation may be mediated by actions of iodide on crucial regulatory points in the cell cycle (Smerdely et al., 1993).

In euthyroid individuals, the administration of doses of iodide from 1.5-150 mg daily results in small decreases in plasma thyroxine and triiodothyronine concentrations and small compensatory increases in serum TSH values, with all values remaining in the normal range. However, euthyroid patients with a history of a wide variety of underlying thyroid disorders may develop iodine-induced hypothyroidism when exposed to large amounts of iodine present in many commonly prescribed drugs (Table 39–6), and these patients do not escape from the acute Wolff-Chaikoff effect (Roti et al., 1997). Among the disorders that predispose patients to iodine-induced hypothyroidism are treated Graves' disease, Hashimoto's thyroiditis, postpartum lymphocytic thyroiditis, subacute painful thyroiditis, and lobectomy for benign nodules. The most commonly prescribed iodine-containing drugs are certain expectorants (e.g., potassium iodide), topical antiseptics (e.g., povidone iodine), and iodinated radiological contrast agents.

Response to Iodide in Hyperthyroidism. The response to iodides in patients with hyperthyroidism is often striking and rapid. The effect usually is discernible within 24 hours, and the basal metabolic rate may fall at a rate comparable to that following thyroidectomy.

Table 39–6

Commonly Used Iodine-Containing Drugs

DRUGS	IODINE CONTENT
Oral or local	
Amiodarone	75 mg/tablet
Calcium iodide syrup	26 mg/mL
Iodoquinol (diiodohydroxyquin)	134-416 mg/ tablet
Echothiophate iodide ophthalmic solution	5-41 μg/drop
Hydriodic acid syrup	13-15 mg/mL
Iodochlorhydroxyquin	104 mg/tablet
Iodine-containing vitamins	0.15 mg/tablet
Idoxuridine ophthalmic solution	18 μg/drop
Kelp/seaweed	0.15 mg/tablet
Lugol's solution	6.3 mg/drop
PONARIS nasal emollient	5 mg/0.8 mL
KI, saturated solution (KISS)	38 mg/drop
Topical antiseptics	
Iodoquinol cream (diiodohydroxyquin)	6 mg/g
Iodine tincture	40 mg/mL
Iodochlorhydroxyquin cream	12 mg/g
Iodoform gauze	4.8 mg/100 mg gauze
Povidone–iodine	10 mg/mL
Radiology contrast agents	
Diatrizoate meglumine sodium	370 mg/mL
Propyliodone	340 mg/mL
Iopanoic acid	333 mg/tablet
Ipodate	308 mg/capsule
Iothalamate	480 mg/mL
Metrizamide (undiluted)	483 mg/mL
Iohexol	463 mg/mL

Source: Adapted from Roti et al., 1997 with permission. Copyright © Lippincott Williams & Wilkins. http://lww.com.

This provides evidence that the release of hormone into the circulation is rapidly blocked. Furthermore, thyroid hormone synthesis also is mildly decreased. In the thyroid gland, vascularity is reduced, the gland becomes much firmer, the cells become smaller, colloid reaccumulates in the follicles, and the quantity of bound iodine increases, as though an excessive stimulus to the gland has been removed or antagonized. The maximal effect is attained after 10-15 days of continuous therapy when the signs and symptoms of hyperthyroidism may have greatly improved.

Unfortunately, iodide therapy usually does not completely control the manifestations of hyperthyroidism, and after a variable period of time, the beneficial effect disappears. With continued treatment, the hyperthyroidism may return in its initial intensity or may become even more severe than it was at first.

Therapeutic Uses. The uses of iodide in the treatment of hyperthyroidism are in the preoperative period in preparation for thyroidectomy, and in conjunction with anti-thyroid drugs and propranolol, in the treatment of thyrotoxic crisis.

Before surgery, iodide is sometimes employed alone, but more frequently it is used after the hyperthyroidism has been controlled by an anti-thyroid drug. It is then given for 7-10 days immediately preceding the operation. Optimal control of hyperthyroidism is achieved if anti-thyroid drugs are first given alone. If iodine also is given from the beginning, variable responses are observed; sometimes the effect of iodide predominates, storage of hormone is promoted, and prolonged anti-thyroid treatment is required before the hyperthyroidism is controlled. These clinical observations may be explained by the capacity of iodide to prevent the inactivation of thyroid peroxidase by anti-thyroid drugs (Taurog et al., 1996).

Another use of iodide is to protect the thyroid from radioactive iodine fallout following a nuclear accident, military exposure, or large scale radioiodination procedures in laboratories. Because the uptake of radioactive iodine is inversely proportional to the serum concentration of stable iodine, the administration of 30-100 mg of iodide daily will markedly decrease the thyroid uptake of radioisotopes of iodine. Following the Chernobyl nuclear reactor accident in 1986, ~10 million children and adults in Poland were given stable iodide to block the thyroid exposure to radioactive iodine from the atmosphere and from dairy products from cows that ate contaminated grass (Nauman and Wolff, 1993).

The dosage or form in which iodide is administered bears little relationship to the response achieved in hyperthyroidism, provided that not less than the minimal effective amount is given; this dosage is 6 mg of iodide per day in most, but not all, patients.

Strong iodine solution (Lugol's solution) is widely used and consists of 5% iodine and 10% potassium iodide, which yields a dose of 8 mg of iodine per drop. The iodine is reduced to iodide in the intestine before absorption. Saturated solution of potassium iodide (SSKI) also is available, containing 50 mg per drop. Typical doses include 16-36 mg (2-6 drops) of Lugol's solution or 50-100 mg (1-2 drops) of SSKI three times a day. A potassium iodide product (THYROSHIELD) is available over the counter in the U.S. to take in the event of a radiation emergency and block the uptake of radioiodide into the thyroid gland. The adult dose is 2 mL (130 mg) every 24 hours, as directed by public health officials, with specific dose recommendations in children and infants based on age and weight.

Untoward Reactions. Occasional individuals show marked sensitivity to iodide or to organic preparations that contain iodine when they are administered intravenously as a supplement (e.g., sodium iodine [IODOPEN]) during total parental nutrition therapy. The onset of an acute reaction may occur immediately or several hours after administration. Angioedema is the outstanding symptom, and laryngeal edema may lead to suffocation. Multiple cutaneous hemorrhages may be present. Also, manifestations of the serum-sickness type of hypersensitivity—such as fever, arthralgia, lymph node enlargement, and eosinophilia—may appear. Thrombotic thrombocytopenic purpura and fatal periarteritis nodosa attributed to hypersensitivity to iodide also have been described.

The severity of symptoms of chronic intoxication with iodide (*iodism*) is related to the dose. The symptoms start with an unpleasant brassy taste and burning in the mouth and throat as well as soreness of the teeth and gums. Increased salivation is noted. Coryza, sneezing, and irritation of the eyes with swelling of the eyelids are commonly observed. Mild iodism simulates a "head cold." The patient often complains of a severe headache that originates in the frontal sinuses. Irritation of the mucous glands of the respiratory tract causes a productive cough. Excess transudation into the bronchial tree may lead to pulmonary edema. In addition, the parotid and submaxillary glands may become enlarged and tender, and the syndrome may be mistaken for mumps parotitis. There also may be inflammation of the pharynx, larynx, and tonsils. Skin lesions are common and vary in type and intensity. They usually are mildly acneform and distributed in the seborrheic areas. Rarely, severe and sometimes fatal eruptions (ioderma) may occur after the prolonged use of iodides. The lesions are bizarre; they resemble those caused by bromism, a rare problem, and as a rule involute quickly when iodide is withdrawn. Symptoms of gastric irritation are common, and diarrhea, which is sometimes bloody, may occur. Fever is occasionally observed, and anorexia and depression may be present.

Fortunately, the symptoms of iodism disappear spontaneously within a few days after stopping the administration of iodide. The renal excretion of I^- can be increased by procedures that promote Cl^- excretion (e.g., osmotic diuresis, chloruretic diuretics, and salt loading). These procedures may be useful when the symptoms of iodism are severe.

Radioactive Iodine

Chemical and Physical Properties. Iodine has several radioactive isotopes, although the primary ones used for the diagnosis and treatment of thyroid disease are ^{123}I and ^{131}I. The short-lived radionuclide of iodine, ^{123}I, is primarily a γ-emitter with a $t_{1/2}$ of only 13 hours and is used in diagnostic studies to measure 24-hour iodine uptake and for thyroid imaging. In contrast, ^{131}I has a $t_{1/2}$ of 8 days and emits both γ rays and β particles. More than 99% of its radiation is expended within 56 days. It is used therapeutically for thyroid destruction of an overactive or enlarged thyroid and in thyroid cancer for thyroid ablation and treatment of metastatic disease.

Effects on the Thyroid Gland. The chemical behavior of the radioactive isotopes of iodine is identical to that of the stable isotope, ^{127}I. ^{131}I is rapidly and efficiently trapped by the thyroid, incorporated into the iodoamino acids, and deposited in the colloid of the follicles, from which it is slowly liberated. Thus the destructive β particles originate within the follicle and act almost exclusively on the parenchymal cells of the thyroid, with little or no damage to surrounding tissue. The γ radiation passes through the tissue and can be quantified by external detection. The effects of the radiation depend on the dosage. When small tracer doses of ^{131}I are administered, thyroid function is not disturbed. However, when large amounts of radioactive iodine gain access to the gland, the characteristic cytotoxic actions of ionizing radiation are observed. Pyknosis and necrosis of the follicular cells are followed by disappearance of colloid and fibrosis of the gland. With properly selected doses of ^{131}I, it is possible to destroy the thyroid gland completely without detectable injury to adjacent tissues. After smaller doses, some of the follicles, usually in the periphery of the gland, retain their function.

Therapeutic Uses. Radioactive iodine finds its widest use in the treatment of hyperthyroidism and in the diagnosis of disorders of thyroid function. Sodium iodide ^{131}I (HICON, others) is available as a solution or in capsules containing essentially carrier-free ^{131}I suitable for oral administration. Sodium iodide ^{123}I is available for scanning procedures. Discussion here is focused on the therapeutic uses of ^{131}I.

Hyperthyroidism. Radioactive iodine is a valuable alternative or adjunctive treatment of hyperthyroidism (Brent, 2008). Stable iodide (non-radioactive) used as treatment for hyperthyroidism, however, may preclude treatment and imaging with radioactive iodine for weeks after the stable iodide has been discontinued. A urinary iodine measurement can be performed to monitor the iodine load. In those patients exposed to stable iodide, a 24-hour radioiodine measurement of a tracer dose of ^{123}I should be performed before ^{131}I administration to ensure there is sufficient uptake to accomplish the desired ablation.

Dosage and Technique. ^{131}I, 7000-10,000 rads per gram of thyroid tissue, is administered orally. The effective dose for a given patient depends primarily on the size of the thyroid, the iodine uptake of the gland, and the rate of release of radioactive iodine from the gland subsequent to the nuclide's deposition in the colloid. Comparison studies have shown little advantage of a standard individualized dose, based on gland weight and radioactive iodine uptake, over a fixed dose (Jarløv et al., 1995). For these reasons, the optimal dose of ^{131}I, expressed in terms of microcuries taken up per gram of thyroid tissue, varies in different laboratories from 80-150 μCi. The usual total dose is 4-15 mCi.

The lower doses produce a lower incidence of hypothyroidism in the early years after treatment; however, many patients with late hypothyroidism may go undetected, and the ultimate incidence of hypothyroidism is probably no less than with the larger doses. In addition, relapse of the hyperthyroid state, or initial failure to alleviate the hyperthyroid state, is increased in patients receiving lower doses of ^{131}I. Thus, many endocrinologists recommend initial treatment with thyroid ablative doses of ^{131}I, with subsequent treatment for hypothyroidism. There also is evidence that pretreatment with an antithyroid drug reduces the therapeutic efficacy of ^{131}I. The medication, therefore, should be discontinued ~1 week before the therapeutic dose of ^{131}I therapy and only resumed 3 days after ^{131}I (Walter et al., 2007). If the anti-thyroid drug cannot be discontinued, the effect can be overcome by adjusting to a higher radioiodine dose.

Course of Disease. The course of hyperthyroidism in a patient who has received an optimal dose of ^{131}I is characterized by progressive recovery. Beginning a few weeks after treatment, the symptoms of hyperthyroidism gradually abate over a period of 2-3 months. If therapy has been inadequate, the necessity for further treatment is apparent within 6-12 months. It is not uncommon, however, for the serum TSH to remain low for several months after ^{131}I therapy, especially if the patient was not rendered euthyroid before receiving the radioactive iodine. Occasionally, this delayed recovery of the hypothalamic-pituitary-thyroid axis results in a picture of central hypothyroidism, with low circulating thyroid hormones. Thus, assessing radioactive iodine failure based on TSH concentrations alone may be misleading and should always be accompanied by determination of free T_4 and usually serum T_3 concentrations. Furthermore, transient hypothyroidism, lasting up to 6 months, may occur in up to 50% of patients receiving a dose of ^{131}I calculated to result in euthyroidism (Aizawa et al., 1997). This is less of a problem if the patient receives a higher, ablative dose of ^{131}I because hypothyroidism occurs far more frequently and persists.

Depending to some extent on the dosage schedule adopted, 80% of patients are cured by a single dose, ~20% require two doses, and a very small fraction require three or more doses before the disorder is controlled. Patients treated with larger doses of ^{131}I almost always develop hypothyroidism within a few months.

β Adrenergic antagonists, anti-thyroid drugs, or both, or stable iodide, can be used to hasten the control of hyperthyroidism while awaiting the full effects of the radioactive iodine.

Advantages. The advantages of radioactive iodine in the treatment of Graves' disease are many. No death as a direct result of the use of the isotope has been reported. There have been reports of increased mortality from cardiovascular and cerebrovascular disease in the first year after radioactive iodine therapy (Franklyn et al., 1998); however, there is no evidence that the increased mortality was related to the radioactive iodine itself, and long-term follow-up of radioactive iodine therapy for Graves' disease has demonstrated no increase in overall cancer mortality in patients treated with ^{131}I (Ron et al., 1998). In the non-pregnant patient, no tissue other than the thyroid is exposed to sufficient ionizing radiation to be detectably altered. Nevertheless, continuing concern about potential effects of radiation on germ cells prompts some endocrinologists to advocate anti-thyroid drugs or surgery in younger patients who are acceptable operative risks. Hypoparathyroidism is a small risk of surgery. With radioactive iodine treatment, the patient is spared the risks and discomfort of surgery. The cost is low, hospitalization is not required in the U.S., and patients can participate in their customary activities during the entire procedure, although there are recommendations to limit exposure to young children.

Disadvantages. The chief consequence of the use of radioactive iodine is the high incidence of delayed hypothyroidism. Even when elaborate procedures are used to estimate iodine uptake and gland size, most patients become hypothyroid.

Several analyses of groups of patients treated ≥10 years previously suggest that the eventual rate may exceed 80%. However, it now appears that the incidence of hypothyroidism also increases progressively after subtotal thyroidectomy or after anti-thyroid drug therapy, and such failure of glandular function is probably part of the natural progression of Graves' disease, no matter what the therapy. Although cancer death rate is not increased after radioiodine therapy, there is a small but significant increase shown in specific types of cancer, including stomach, kidney, and breast (Metso et al., 2007). This finding is especially significant because these tissues all express the iodine transporter NIS and may be especially susceptible to radiation effects.

It is essential that patients treated with radioiodine understand that the resulting hypothyroidism will require lifelong treatment and monitoring. Because there are variations in the interval of time from treatment to the development of hypothyroidism, patients must have regular thyroid function testing after radioiodine. Also, once diagnosed, it is difficult to ensure that patients who need the hormone actually take it. Because the health risks of untreated subclinical hypothyroidism are becoming increasingly evident (Biondi and Cooper, 2008), hypothyroidism, either subclinical or overt, requires long-term follow-up to ensure adequate thyroid hormone status and optimal replacement therapy.

Another disadvantage of radioactive iodine therapy is the long period of time that is sometimes required before the hyperthyroidism is controlled. When a single dose is effective, the response is most satisfactory; however, when multiple doses are needed, it may be many months or a year or more before the patient is well. This disadvantage can be largely overcome if the initial dose is sufficiently large. Other disadvantages include possible worsening of ophthalmopathy after treatment (Bartalena et al., 1998a). Radioactive iodine treatment can induce a radiation thyroiditis, with release of preformed thyroxine and triiodothyronine into the circulation. In most patients, this is asymptomatic, but in some there can be worsening of symptoms of hyperthyroidism and rarely cardiac manifestations, such as atrial fibrillation or ischemic heart disease and very rarely thyroid storm. Pretreatment with anti-thyroid drugs should reduce or eliminate this complication and is indicated especially in those with underlying cardiac disease or the elderly. Finally, salivary gland dysfunction may be seen, especially after the higher doses used for the treatment of thyroid cancer (Mandel and Mandel, 2003). Sialogogic agents to hasten the transit of radioiodine through the salivary glands are used by many clinicians but have unproven efficacy. Salivary gland damage is most strongly linked to the cumulative dose of radioiodine.

Indications. The clearest indication for this form of treatment is hyperthyroidism in older patients and in those with heart disease. Radioactive iodine also is the best form of treatment when Graves' disease has persisted or recurred after subtotal thyroidectomy and when prolonged treatment with anti-thyroid drugs has not led to remission. Finally, radioactive iodine is indicated in patients with toxic nodular goiter because the disease does not go into spontaneous remission.

The risk of inducing hypothyroidism is less in nodular goiter than in Graves' disease, perhaps because of the normal progression of the latter and the preservation of nonautonomous thyroid tissue in the former. Usually, larger doses of radioactive iodine are required in the treatment of toxic nodular goiter than in the treatment of Graves' disease. Radioactive iodine has been used to decrease the size of large nontoxic multinodular goiters that are causing compressive symptoms in patients who are otherwise poor operative risks. Although surgery remains the treatment of choice for patients with compressive multinodular goiters, radioactive iodine therapy may benefit elderly patients, especially those with cardiopulmonary disease. The uptake in multinodular goiters may be low, so some have increased radioiodine uptake by administration of exogenous recombinant human TSH (thyrotropin alfa [THYROGEN]) (Duntas and Cooper, 2008), but caution should be exercised because this treatment may induce transient elevations in serum thyroxine and triiodothyronine that could result in excessive stimulation of the heart.

Contraindications. *The main contraindication for the use of ^{131}I therapy is pregnancy.* After the first trimester, the fetal thyroid will concentrate the isotope and thus suffer damage; even during the first trimester, radioactive iodine is best avoided because there may be adverse effects of radiation on fetal tissues. The risk of causing neoplastic changes in the thyroid gland has been an ongoing concern since radioactive iodine was first introduced, and only small numbers of children have been treated in this way. Indeed, many clinics have declined to treat younger patients for fear of causing cancer and have reserved radioactive iodine for patients older than some arbitrary age, such as 25 or 30 years. Because experience with ^{131}I is now vast, these age limits are lower than they were in the past. The most recent report by the Cooperative Thyrotoxicosis Therapy Follow-up Study Group shows no increase in total cancer mortality following ^{131}I treatment for Graves' disease (Ron et al., 1998). Furthermore, there was no increase in the occurrence of leukemia following large-dose ^{131}I therapy for thyroid cancer, although there was an increase in colorectal cancers in this population (de Vathaire et al., 1997). These data strongly suggest that laxatives be given to all patients receiving ^{131}I therapy for treatment of thyroid cancer to decrease the risk of future digestive tract malignancies. Transient abnormalities in testicular function have been reported following ^{131}I therapy for treatment of thyroid cancer, but no long-term effects on fertility in either men or women have been demonstrated (Dottorini et al., 1995; Pacini et al., 1994). Patients with allergies to iodine contrast agents or to topical iodide-containing products should not have any adverse reaction to ^{131}I. The amount of elemental iodine contained in the treatment is not greater than that contained in iodized salt or flour that is part of regular dietary intake.

Diagnostic Uses. Measurement of the thyroidal accumulation of a tracer dose is helpful in the differential diagnosis of hyperthyroidism and nodular goiter. The response of the thyroid to TSH-suppressive doses of thyroid hormone can be evaluated in this way. Following the administration of a tracer dose, the pattern of localization in the thyroid gland can be depicted by a special scanning apparatus, and this technique is sometimes useful in defining thyroid nodules as functional ("hot") or non-functional ("cold") and in finding ectopic thyroid tissue and occasionally metastatic thyroid tumors.

Thyroid Carcinoma. Because most well-differentiated thyroid carcinomas accumulate very little iodine, stimulation of iodine uptake with TSH is required to treat metastases effectively. Currently, endogenous TSH stimulation is evoked by withdrawal of thyroid hormone replacement therapy in patients previously treated with near-total thyroidectomy with or without radioactive ablation of residual thyroid tissue. Total-body ^{131}I scanning and measurement of serum thyroglobulin when the patient is hypothyroid (TSH >35 mU/L) help to identify metastatic disease or residual thyroid bed tissue. Depending on the residual uptake or the presence of metastatic disease, an ablative dose of ^{131}I ranging from 30 mCi to >150 mCi is administered, and a repeat total body scan is obtained 1 week later. The precise amount of ^{131}I needed to treat residual tissue and metastases is controversial. Thyrotropin alfa (recombinant human TSH) is now available to test the ability of thyroid tissue, both normal and malignant, to take up radioactive iodine and to secrete thyroglobulin (Haugen et al., 1999). Thyrogen allows assessment of the presence of metastatic disease, without the necessity for patients to stop their suppressive levothyroxine therapy and become clinically hypothyroid. Thyrotropin alfa is approved for diagnostic scanning and for thyroid remnant ablation after thyroidectomy in thyroid cancer patients, but not for treatment of metastatic disease. (Duntas and Cooper, 2008; Pacini and Castangna, 2008).

TSH-suppressive therapy with levothyroxine is indicated in all patients after treatment for thyroid cancer. The goal of therapy usually is to keep serum TSH levels in the subnormal range, although relaxing the degree and duration of suppression, especially for stage 1 and 2 cancers, is now recommended (Burmeister et al., 1992; Cooper et al., 2006). Follow-up evaluation every 6 months is reasonable, along with determination of serum thyroglobulin concentrations (Spencer and LoPresti, 2008). Patients with a rise in thyroglobulin but no detectable disease on whole-body scan require additional imaging and consideration of alternative treatments including surgery and external radiation (Kloos, 2008). A rise in serum thyroglobulin concentration is often the first indication of recurrent disease. The prognosis in patients with thyroid cancer depends on the pathology and size of the tumor and is generally worse in older individuals. Overall, the vast majority of patients with thyroid cancer will not die of their disease. Papillary cancer is usually not aggressive; the 10-year survival rate exceeds 80%. Follicular cancer is more aggressive and can metastasize via the bloodstream. Still, prognosis is fair and long-term survival is common. Even in patients with metastatic, differentiated thyroid cancer, ^{131}I therapy is very effective and may be even curative (Cooper et al., 2006). Anaplastic cancer is the exception: It is highly malignant with survival usually <1 year. Medullary thyroid carcinomas do not accumulate I^- and cannot be treated with ^{131}I.

Chemotherapy in Thyroid Cancer

Advanced and metastatic poorly differentiated papillary and follicular thyroid cancer often does not concentrate iodine sufficient for therapy with ^{131}I (Kloos, 2008). There have been significant advances in targeted chemotherapy for thyroid cancer (Sherman, 2009). Recent advances in the molecular genetics of thyroid cancer have resulted in the identification of oncogenic mutations in the *BRAF* and *RAS* genes, known to activate the MAPK signaling pathway. Medullary thyroid carcinoma is associated with mutations in the *RET* gene, which also enhance MAPK signaling. These findings have led to a number of successful clinical trials in poorly differentiated papillary and follicular thyroid cancer and medullary thyroid cancer. Treatment with inhibitors of receptor tyrosine kinases, vascular endothelial growth factor (VEGF), and the VEGF receptor have produced partial response rates in the range of 30%. Agents studied include axitinib, gefitinib, imatinib, motesanib, sorafenib, sunitinib, and vandetanib (Sipos and Shah, 2010). Single agents in poorly differentiated thyroid cancer have most commonly produced disease stabilization, although combining agents to target multiple growth-promoting pathways may improve the disease response.

CLINICAL SUMMARY

Replacement therapy for hypothyroidism typically uses oral L-thyroxine given once daily. The goals of therapy are to restore the serum TSH concentration to the mid-normal or low-normal range, and to relieve the signs and symptoms of hypothyroidism. In patients with central hypothyroidism, the biochemical goal is to restore the serum-free T_4 to the upper half of the normal range. Based on the long $t_{1/2}$ of thyroxine, at least 6-8 weeks are required before a new steady-state level is reached following initiation of therapy or adjustment of dose. Special cases of hypothyroidism include patients following surgical resection of differentiated thyroid carcinoma and pregnancy. In the former setting, the goal is to suppress the TSH level to below normal, thereby removing the potential effect of TSH to stimulate proliferation of the cancer cells. In pregnant patients, the standard replacement dose is usually increased. Realizing the effects of even relatively mild hypothyroidism on neurological development of the fetus and miscarriage, it is especially important to monitor thyroid function tests carefully during pregnancy.

Options available for treating hyperthyroid patients include anti-thyroid drugs (e.g., propylthiouracil and methimazole), radioactive iodine ablation, and surgery. The preferred therapy differs among endocrinologists and geographic regions as well as patient characteristics. Special circumstances, such as the presence of coexisting ophthalmopathy in patients with Graves' disease, also may influence the choice of therapy; radioactive iodine may aggravate the ophthalmopathy. Although younger patients with hyperthyroidism often can be treated effectively with radioactive iodine, medical therapy with anti-thyroid drugs to reduce the levels of thyroid hormone has been the preferred approach. The potential for increased toxicity of anti-thyroid drugs in children and pregnant women may influence this choice. In older patients or those with cardiac disease, radioactive iodine usually is recommended after the patient has been rendered euthyroid with anti-thyroid medication. Surgery remains an option for those who cannot tolerate anti-thyroid drugs or decline radioactive iodine. Surgery is also the most rapid way to treat hyperthyroidism permanently. The initial treatment for thyroid cancer is surgical, usually a total or near-total thyroidectomy. Radioiodine treatment to ablate remnant thyroid tissue or to identify metastatic spread can be done after withdrawal of thyroxine replacement and elevation of endogenous TSH or treatment with recombinant human TSH in patients who are having a total body scan and serum thyroglobulin measurement to determine the presence of residual tissue. Treatment of metastatic disease with radioiodine is performed after thyroxine withdrawal and elevation of endogenous TSH.

BIBLIOGRAPHY

Abalovich M, Amino N, Barbour LA, *et al.* Management of thyroid dysfunction during pregnancy and postpartum: An Endocrine Society Clinical Practice Guideline. *J Clin Endocrinol Metab,* **2007,** *92:*S1–47.

Aizawa Y, Yoshida K, Kaise N, *et al.* The development of transient hypothyroidism after iodine-131 treatment in hyperthyroid patients with Graves' disease: Prevalence, mechanism and prognosis. *Clin Endocrinol (Oxf),* **1997,** *46:*1–5.

Anderson GW, Schoonover CM, Jones SA. Control of thyroid hormone action in the developing rat brain. *Thyroid,* **2003,** *13:*1039–1056

Astwood EB. Chemotherapy of hyperthyroidism. *Harvey Lect,* **1945,** *40:*195–235.

Atzmon G, Barzilai N, Hollowell JG, *et al.* Extreme longevity is associated with increased serum thyrotropin. *J Clin Endocrinol Metab*, **2009,** *94:*1251–1254.

Azizi F, Bahrainian M, Khamseh ME, Khoshniat M. Intellectual development and thyroid function in children who were breast-fed by thyrotoxic mothers taking methimazole. *J Pediatr Endocrinol Metab,* **2003,** *16:*1239–1243.

Bach-Huynh TG, Nayak B, Loh J, *et al.* Timing of levothyroxine administration affects serum thyrotropin concentration. *J Clin Endocrinol Metab,* **2009,** *94:*3905–3912.

Bartalena L, Marcocci C, Bogazzi F, *et al.* Relation between therapy for hyperthyroidism and the course of Graves' ophthalmopathy. *N Engl J Med,* **1998a,** *338:*73–78.

Bartalena L, Marcocci C, Tanda ML, *et al.* Cigarette smoking and treatment outcomes in Graves' ophthalmopathy. *Ann Intern Med,* **1998b,** *129:*632–635.

Barwell J, Fox GF, Round J, Berg, J. Choanal atresia: The result of maternal thyrotoxicosis or fetal carbimazole? *Am J Med Genet,* **2002,** *111:*55–56.

Basaria S, Cooper DS. Amiodarone and the thyroid. *Am J Med,* **2005,** *118:*706–714.

Bassett JH, Harvey CB, Williams GR. Mechanisms of thyroid hormone receptor-specific nuclear and extra nuclear actions. *Mol Cell Endocrinol,* **2003,** *213:*1–11.

Baxter JD, Webb P. Thyroid hormone mimetics: Potential applications in atherosclerosis, obesity and type 2 diabetes. *Nat Rev Drug Discov,* **2009,** *8:*308–320.

Becker DV, Braverman LE, DeLange F, *et al.* Iodine supplementation for pregnancy and lactation—United States and Canada: Recommendations of the American Thyroid Association. *Thyroid,* **2006,** *16:*949–951.

Bernal J. Thyroid hormone receptors in brain development and function. *Nat Clin Pract Endocrinol Metab,* **2007,** *3:*249–259.

Bianco AC, Salvatore D, Gereben B, *et al.* Biochemistry, cellular and molecular biology, and physiological roles of the iodothyronine selenodeiodinases. *Endocr Rev,* **2002,** *23:* 38–89.

Biondi B, Cooper DS. Clinical significance of subclinical thyroid dysfunction. *Endocr Rev,* **2008,** *29:*76–131.

Blount BC, Pirkle JL, Osterloh JD, *et al.* Urinary perchlorate and thyroid hormone levels in adolescent and adult men and women living in the United States. *Environ Health Perspect,* **2006,** *114:*1865–1871.

Braverman LE, Ingbar SH, Sterling K. Conversion of thyroxine (T4) to triiodothyronine (T3) in athyreotic human subjects. *J Clin Invest,* **1970,** *49:*855–864.

Brent GA. Graves' disease. *N Engl J Med,* **2008,** *358:*2594–2605.

Brenta G, Danzi S, Klein I. Potential therapeutic applications of thyroid hormone analogs. *Nat Clin Pract Endocrinol Metab,* **2007,** *3:*632–640.

Burman KD, Hennessey J, McDermott M, *et al.* The FDA revises requirements for levothyroxine products. *Thyroid,* **2008,** *18:*487–490.

Burmeister LA, Goumaz MO, Mariash CN, Oppenheimer JH. Levothyroxine dose requirements for thyrotropin suppression in the treatment of differentiated thyroid cancer. *J Clin Endocrinol Metab,* **1992,** *75:*344–350.

Cao XY, Jiang XM, Dou ZH, *et al.* Timing of vulnerability of the brain to iodine deficiency in endemic cretinism. *N Engl J Med,* **1994,** *331:*1739–1744.

Carvalho AF, Cavalcante JL, Castelo MS, Lima MC. Augmentation strategies for treatment-resistant depression: A literature review. *J Clin Pharm Ther,* **2007,** *32:*415–428.

Chan GW, Mandel SJ. Therapy insights: Management of Graves' disease during pregnancy. *Nat Clin Pract Endocrinol Metab,* **2007,** *3:*470–478.

Charnley G. Perchlorate: Overview of risks and regulations. *Food Chem Toxicol,* **2008,** *46:*2307–2315.

Chiamolera MI, Wondisford FE. Minireview: Thyrotropin-releasing hormone and the thyroid hormone feedback mechanism. *Endocrinology,* **2009,** *150:*1091–1096.

Cooper DS. Antithyroid drugs in the management of patients with Graves' disease: An evidence-based approach to therapeutic controversies. *J Clin Endocrinol Metab,* **2003,** *88:*3474–3481.

Cooper DS. Antithyroid drugs. *N Engl J Med,* **2005,** *352:* 905–917.

Cooper DS, Doherty GM, Haugen BR, *et al.* Management guidelines for patients with thyroid nodules and differentiated thyroid cancer. *Thyroid,* **2006,** *16:*109–142.

Cooper DS, Rivkees S. Putting propylthiouracil in perspective. *J Clin Endocrinol Metab,* **2009,** *94:*1881–1882.

Cooper-Kazaz R, van der Deure WM, Medici M, *et al.* Preliminary evidence that a functional polymorphism in type 1 deiodinase is associated with enhanced potentiation of the antidepressant effect of sertraline by triiodothyronine. *J Affect Disord,* **2009,** *116:*113–116.

Crunkhorn S, Patti ME. Links between thyroid hormone action, oxidative metabolism, and diabetes risk? *Thyroid,* **2008,** *18:*227–237.

Davis PJ, Leonard JL, Davis FB. Mechanisms of nongenomic actions of thyroid hormone. *Front Neuroendocrinol,* **2008,** *29:*211–218.

de Vathaire F, Schlumberger M, Delisle MJ, *et al.* Leukaemias and cancers following iodine-131 administration for thyroid cancer. *Br J Cancer,* **1997,** *75:*734–739.

Demers LM, Spencer CA. Laboratory medicine practice guidelines: Laboratory support for the diagnosis and monitoring of thyroid disease. *Clin Endocrinol (Oxf),* **2003,** *58:*138–140.

Di Cosmo C, Liao X, Dumitrescu AM, *et al.* A thyroid hormone analog with reduced dependence on the monocarboxylate transporter 8 for tissue transport. *Endocrinology,* **2009,** *150:*4450–4458.

Diamanti-Kandarakis E, Boruguignon J-P, Giudice LC, *et al.* Endocrine-disrupting chemicals: An Endocrine Society scientific statement. *Endocr Rev,* **2009,** *30:*293–342.

Diav-Citrin O, Ornoy A. Teratogen update: Antithyroid drugs-methimazole, carbimazole, and propylthiouracil. *Teratology,* **2002,** *65:*38–44.

Dohan O, De la Vieja A, Paroder V, *et al.* The sodium/iodide symporter (NIS): characterization, regulation, and medical significance. *Endocr Rev,* **2003,** *24:*48–77.

Dohan O, Portulano C, Basquin C, *et al.* The Na+/I-symporter (NIS) mediates electroneutral active transport of the environmental pollutant perchlorate. *Proc Natl Acad Sci USA,* **2007,** *104:*20250–20255.

Dottorini ME, Lomuscio G, Mazzucchelli L, e*t al.* Assessment of female fertility and carcinogenesis after iodine-131 therapy for differentiated thyroid carcinoma. *J Nucl Med,* **1995,** *36:*21–27.

Doyle KP, Suchland KL, Ciesielski TM, *et al.* Novel thyroxine derivatives, thyronamine and 3-iodothyronamine, induce transient hypothermia and marked neuroprotection against stroke injury. *Stroke,* **2007,** *38:*2569–2576.

Dumitrescu AM, Liao XH, Abdullah MS, *et al.* Mutations in SECISBP2 result in abnormal thyroid hormone metabolism. *Nat Genet,* **2005,** *37:*1247–1252.

Dunn JT, Dunn AD. Update on intrathyroidal iodine metabolism. *Thyroid,* **2001,** *11:*407–414.

Duntas LH, Cooper DS. Review on the occasion of a decade of recombinant human TSH: Prospects and novel uses. *Thyroid,* **2008,** *18:*509–516.

El Fassi D, Banda JP, Gilbert JA, *et al.* Treatment of Graves' disease with rituximab specifically reduces the production of thyroid stimulating autoantibodies. *Clin Immunol,* **2009,** *130:* 252–258.

Elnagar B, Eltom M, Karlsson FA, *et al.* The effects of different doses of oral iodized oil on goiter size, urinary iodine, and thyroid-related hormones. *J Clin Endocrinol Metab,* **1995,** *80:*891–897.

Eng PH, Cardona GR, Fang SL, *et al*. Escape from the acute Wolff-Chaikoff effect is associated with a decrease in thyroid sodium/iodide symporter messenger ribonucleic acid and protein. *Endocrinology,* **1999,** *140:*3404–3410.

Erion MD, Cable EE, Ito BR, *et al*. Targeting thyroid hormone receptor-beta agonists to the liver reduces cholesterol and triglycerides and improves the therapeutic index. *Proc Natl Acad Sci USA,* **2007,** *104:*15490–15495.

Franklyn JA, Maisonneuve P, Sheppard MC, *et al*. Mortality after the treatment of hyperthyroidism with radioactive iodine. *N Engl J Med,* **1998,** *338:*712–718.

Gothe S, Wang Z, Ng L, *et al*. Mice devoid of all known thyroid hormone receptors are viable but exhibit disorders of the pituitary-thyroid axis, growth, and bone maturation. *Genes Dev,* **1999,** *13:*1329–1341.

Grebe SK, Cooke RR, Ford HC, *et al*. Treatment of hypothyroidism with once weekly thyroxine. *J Clin Endocrinol Metab,* **1997,** *82:*870–875.

Greer MA, Goodman G, Pleus RC, Greer SE. Health effects assessment for environmental perchlorate contamination: The dose response for inhibition of thyroidal radioiodine uptake in humans. *Environ Health Perspect,* **2002,** *110:*927–937.

Gross J, Pitt-Rivers R. The identification of 3:5:3′-l-triiodothyronine in human plasma. *Lancet,* **1952,** *1:*439–441.

Grover GJ, Dunn C, Nguyen NH, *et al*. Pharmacological profile of the thyroid hormone receptor antagonist NH3 in rats. *J Pharmacol Exp Ther,* **2007**, *322:*385–390.

Grozinsky-Glasberg S, Fraser A, Nahshoni E, *et al.* Thyroxine-triiodothyronine combination therapy versus thyroxine monotherapy for clinical hypothyroidism: meta-analysis of randomized controlled trials. *J Clin Endocrinol Metab,* **2006,** *91:*2592–2599.

Haddow JE, McClain MR, Palomaki GE, *et al*. Urine iodine measurements, creatinine adjustment, and thyroid deficiency in an adult United States population. *J Clin Endocrinol Metab,* **2007,** *92:*1019–1022.

Haugen BR, Pacini F, Reiners C, *et al*. A comparison of recombinant human thyrotropin and thyroid hormone withdrawal for the detection of thyroid remnant or cancer. *J Clin Endocrinol Metab,* **1999,** *84:*3877–3885.

Hennessey JV. Levothyroxine dosage and the limitations of current bioequivalence standards. *Nat. Clin Prac Endocrinol Metab*, **2006,** *2:*474–475.

Hiroi Y, Kim HH, Ying H, *et al*. Rapid nongenomic actions of thyroid hormone. *Proc Natl Acad Sci USA*, **2006,** *103:*14104–14109.

Hollowell JG, Haddow JE. The prevalence of iodine deficiency in women of reproductive age in the United States of America. *Public Health Nutr,* **2007,** *10:*1532–1539.

Hollowell JG, Staehling NW, Hannon WH, *et al*. Iodine nutrition in the United States. Trends and public health implications: Iodine excretion data from National Health and Nutrition Examination Surveys I and III (1971–1974 and 1988–1994). *J Clin Endocrinol Metab*, **1998,** *83:*3401–3408.

Jarløv AE, Hegedus L, Kristensen LO, *et al*. Is calculation of the dose in radioiodine therapy of hyperthyroidism worthwhile? *Clin Endocrinol (Oxf),* **1995,** *43:*325–329.

Jonklaas J, Davidson B, Bhagat S, Soldin SJ. Triiodothyronine levels in athyreotic individuals during levothyroxine therapy. *JAMA*, **2008,** *299:*769–777.

Jonklaas J, Sarlis NJ, Litofsky D. Outcomes of patients with differentiated thyroid carcinoma following initial therapy. *Thyroid,* **2006,** *16:*1229–1242.

Jorgensen EC. Stereochemistry of thyroxine and analogues. *Mayo Clin Proc,* **1964,** *39:*560–568.

Kahaly GJ, Dillmann WH. Thyroid hormone action in the heart. *Endocr Rev,* **2005,** *26:*704–728.

Khoo TK, Bahn RS. Pathogenesis of Graves' ophthalmopathy: The role of autoantibodies. *Thyroid,* **2007,** *17:*1013–1018.

Kleinau G, Krause G. Thyrotropin and homologous glycoprotein hormone receptors: Structural and functional aspects of extracellular signaling mechanisms. *Endocr Rev,* **2009,** *30:*133–151.

Klemperer JD, Klein I, Gomez M, et al. Thyroid hormone treatment after coronary-artery bypass surgery. *N Engl J Med,* **1995,** *333:*1522–1527.

Klemperer JD, Klein IL, Ojamaa K, *et al*. Triiodothyronine therapy lowers the incidence of atrial fibrillation after cardiac operations. *Ann Thorac Surg,* **1996,** *61:*1323–1327.

Kloos RT. Approach to the patient with a positive serum thyroglobulin and a negative radioiodine scan after initial therapy for differentiated thyroid cancer. *J Clin Endocrinol Metab,* **2008,** *93:*1519–1525.

Kogai T, Taki K, Brent GA. Enhancement of sodium/iodide symporter expression in thyroid and breast cancer. *Endocr Relat Cancer,* **2006,** *13:*797–826.

Koutras DA, Malamitsi J, Souvatzoglou A, *et al*. Relative ineffectiveness of exogenous triiodothyronine as a thyroid suppressive agent. *J Endocrinol Invest,* **1981,** *4:*343–347.

Krohn K, Paschke R. Progress in understanding the etiology of thyroid autonomy. *J Clin Endocrinol Metab,* **2001,** *86:*3336–3345.

Kwaku MP, Burman KD. Myxedema coma. *J Intensive Care Med,* **2007,** *22:*224–231.

LaFranchi SH, Austin J. How should we be treating children with congenital hypothyroidism? *J Pediatr Endocrinol Metab,* **2007,** *20:*559–578.

Latif R, Morshed SA, Zaidi M, Davies TF. The thyroid-stimulating hormone receptor: Impact of thyroid-stimulating hormone receptor antibodies on multimerization, cleavage, and signaling. *Endocrinol Metab Clin North Am,* **2009,** *38:*319–341.

Laugwitz, K-L, Allgeier A, Offermanns S, *et al*. The human thyrotropin receptor: A heptahelical receptor capable of stimulating members of all four G protein families. *Proc Natl Acad Sci USA,* **1996,** *93:*116–120.

Liu Y, Xia X, Fondell JD, Yen PM. Thyroid hormone-regulated target genes have distinct patterns of coactivator recruitment and histone acetylation. *Mol Endocrinol,* **2006,** *20:*483–490.

Loh JA, Wartofsky L, Jonklaas J, Burman KD. The magnitude of increased levothyroxine requirements in hypothyroid pregnancy women depends upon the etiology of the hypothyroidism. *Thyroid,* **2009,** *19:*269–275.

Magner JA, Snyder DK. Methimazole-induced agranulocytosis treated with recombinant human granulocyte colony-stimulating factor (G-CSF). *Thyroid,* **1994**, *4:*295–296.

Magnusson RP, Taurog A, Dorris ML. Mechanisms of thyroid peroxidase- and lactoperoxidase-catalyzed reactions involving iodide. *J Biol Chem,* **1984,** *259:*13783–13790.

Mandel SJ, Mandel L. Radioactive iodine and the salivary glands. *Thyroid,* **2003,** *13:*265–271.

Mercado M, Mendoza-Zubieta V, Bautista-Osorio R, Espinozade los Monteros AL. Treatment of hyperthyroidism with a combination of methimazole and cholestyramine. *J Clin Endocrinol Metab,* **1996,** *81:*3191–3193.

Metso S, Auvinen A, Huhtala H, *et al.* Increased cancer incidence after radioiodine treatment for hyperthyroidism. *Cancer,* **2007,** *109:*1972–1979.

Miller MD, Crofton KM, Rice DC, Zoeller RT. Thyroid-disrupting chemicals: Interpreting upstream biomarkers of adverse outcomes. *Environ Health Perspect,* **2009,** *117:*1033–1041.

Momotani N, Noh JY, Ishikawa N, Ito K. Effects of propylthiouracil and methimazole on fetal thyroid status in mothers with Graves' hyperthyroidism. *J Clin Endocrinol Metab,* **1997,** *82:*3633–3636.

Monga V, Meena CL, Kaur N, Jain R. Chemistry and biology of thyrotropin-releasing hormone (TRH) and its analogs. *Curr Med Chem,* **2008,** *27:*18–33.

Moreno JC, Klootwijk W, van Toor H, *et al.* Mutations in the iodotyrosine deiodinase gene and hypothyroidism. *N Engl J Med,* **2008,** *358:*1811–1818.

Morte B, Manzano J, Scanlan T, *et al.* Deletion of the thyroid hormone receptor alpha 1 prevents the structural alterations of the cerebellum induced by hypothyroidism. *Proc Natl Acad Sci USA,* **2002,** *99*:3985–3989.

Mortimer RH, Cannell GR, Addison RS, *et al.* Methimazole and propylthiouracil equally cross the perfused human term placental lobule. *J Clin Endocrinol Metab,* **1997,** *82*:3099–3102.

Müller B, Zulewski H, Huber P, *et al.* Impaired action of thyroid hormone associated with smoking in women with hypothyroidism. *N Engl J Med,* **1995,** *333*:964–969.

Mullis-Jansson SL, Argenziano M, Corwin S, *et al.* A randomized double-blind study of the effect of triiodothyronine on cardiac function and morbidity after coronary bypass surgery. *J Thorac Cardiovasc Surg,* **1999,** *117*:1128–1134.

Murphy E, Williams GR. The thyroid and the skeleton. *Clin Endocrinol,* **2004,** *61*: 285–298.

National Academy of Sciences/National Research Council (NAS/NRC). *Health Implications of Perchlorate Ingestion.* National Academy Press, Washington, DC, 2005.

Nauman J, Wolff J. Iodide prophylaxis in Poland after the Chernobyl reactor accident: Benefits and risks. *Am J Med,* **1993,** *94*:524–532.

Nayak B, Burman K. Thyrotoxicosis and thyroid storm. *Endocrinol Metab Clin North Am,* **2006,** *35*:663–686.

Neumann S, Kleinau G, Constanzi S, *et al.* A low-molecular weight antagonist for the human thyrotropin receptor with therapeutic potential for hyperthyroidism. *Endocrinology,* **2008,** *149*:5945–5950.

Ocasio CA, Scanlan TS. Characterization of thyroid hormone receptor alpha (TRalpha)-specific analogs with varying inner- and outer-ring substituents. *Bioorg Med Chem,* **2008,** *16*: 762–770.

O'Shea PJ, Williams GR. Insight into the physiological actions of thyroid hormone receptors from genetically modified mice. *J Endocrinol,* **2002,** *175*:553–570.

Pacini F, Castangna MG. Diagnostic and therapeutic use of recombinant human TSH (rTSH) in differentiated thyroid cancer. *Best Pract Res Clin Endocrinol Metab,* **2008,** *22*: 1009–1021.

Pacini F, Gasperi M, Fugazzola L, *et al.* Testicular function in patients with differentiated thyroid carcinoma treated with radioiodine. *J Nucl Med,* **1994,** *35:*1418–1422.

Papakostas GI, Cooper-Kazaz R, Appelhof BC, *et al.* Simultaneous initiation (coinitiation) of pharmacotherapy with triiodothyronine and a selective serotonin reuptake inhibitor for major depressive disorder: A quantitative synthesis of double-blind studies. *Int Clin Psychopharmacol,* **2009,** *24:*19–25.

Peeters RP, Wouters PJ, Kaptein E, *et al.* Reduced activation and increased inactivation of thyroid hormone in tissues of critically ill patients. *J Clin Endocrinol Metab,* **2003,** *88:*3202–3211.

Refetoff S. Inherited thyroxine-binding globulin abnormalities in man. *Endocr Rev,* **1989,** *10:*275–293.

Refetoff S, Dumitrescu AM. Syndromes of reduced sensitivity to thyroid hormone: Genetic defects in hormone receptors, cell transporters and deiodination. *Best Pract Res Clin Endocrinol Metab,* **2007,** *21:*277–305.

Regard JB, Kataoka H, Cano DA, *et al.* Probing cell type-specific functions of Gi *in vivo* identifies GPCR regulators of insulin secretion. *J Clin Invest,* **2007,** *117:*4034–4043.

Reuss ML, Paneth N, Pinto-Martin JA, *et al.* The relation of transient hypothyroxinemia in preterm infants to neurologic development at two years of age. *N Engl J Med,* **1996,** *334:* 821–827.

Rittmaster RS, Abbott EC, Douglas R, *et al.* Effect of methimazole, with or without L-thyroxine, on remission rates in Graves' disease. *J Clin Endocrinol Metab,* **1998,** *83:* 814–818.

Rodien P, Bremont C, Sanson ML, *et al.* Familial gestational hyperthyroidism caused by a mutant thyrotropin receptor hypersensitive to human chorionic gonadotropin. *N Engl J Med,* **1998,** *339:*1823–1826.

Ron E, Doody MM, Becker DV, *et al.* Cancer mortality following treatment for adult hyperthyroidism. Cooperative Thyrotoxicosis Therapy Follow-up Study Group. *JAMA,* **1998,** *280:*347–355.

Rose SR, Brown RS, Foley T, *et al.* Update of newborn screening and therapy for congenital hypothyroidism. *Pediatrics,* **2006,** *117:*2290–2303.

Roti E, Cozani R, Braverman LE. Adverse effects of iodine on the thyroid. *Endocrinologist,* **1997,** *7:*245–254.

Rubio IG, Medeiros-Neto G. Mutations of the thyroglobulin gene and its relevance to thyroid disorders. *Curr Opin Endocrinol Diabetes Obes,* **2009,** *16:*373–378.

Saberi M, Utiger RD. Serum thyroid hormone and thyrotropin concentrations during thyroxine and triiodothyronine therapy. *J Clin Endocrinol Metab,* **1974,** *39:*923–927.

Santini F, Pinchera A, Marsili A, *et al.* Lean body mass is a major determinant of levothyroxine dosage in the treatment of thyroid disease. *J Clin Endocrinol Metab,* **2005,** *90:*124–127.

Sato H, Hattori M, Fujieda M, *et al.* High prevalence of antineutrophil cytoplasmic antibody positivity in childhood onset Graves' disease treated with propylthiouracil. *J Clin Endocrinol Metab,* **2000,** *85:*4270–4273.

Scanlan TS, Suchland KL, Hart ME, *et al.* 3-Iodothyronamine is an endogenous and rapid-acting derivative of thyroid hormone. *Nat Med,* **2004,** *10:*638–642.

Schussler GC. The thyroxine-binding proteins. *Thyroid,* **2000,** *10:*141–149.

Sdano MT, Falciglia M, Welge JA, Steward DL. Efficacy of thyroid hormone suppression for benign thyroid nodules: Meta-analysis of randomized trials. *Otolaryngol Head Neck Surg,* **2005,** *133:*391–396.

Sera N, Ashizawa K, Ando T, *et al*. Treatment with propylthiouracil is associated with appearance of antineutrophil cytoplasmic antibodies in some patients with Graves' disease. *Thyroid,* **2000,** *10:*595–599.

Silva JE. Thermogenic mechanisms and their hormonal regulation. *Physiol Rev,* **2006,** *86:*435–464.

Simonides WS, Mulcahey MA, Redout EM, *et al*. Hypoxia-inducible factor induces local thyroid hormone inactivation during hypoxic-ischemic disease in rats. *J Clin Invest,* **2008,** *118:*975–983.

Sipos JA, Shah MH. Thyroid cancer: Emerging role for targeted therapies. *Ther Adv Med Oncol,* **2010,** *2:*3–16.

Smerdely P, Pitsiavas V, Boyages SC. Evidence that the inhibitory effects of iodide on thyroid cell proliferation are due to arrest of the cell cycle at G0G1 and G2M phases. *Endocrinology,* **1993,** *133:*2881–2888.

Spencer CA, LoPresti JS. Measuring thyroglobulin and thyroglobulin antibody in patients with differentiated thyroid cancer. *Nat Clin Pract Endocrinol Metab,* **2008,** *4:*223–233.

St. Germain DL, Galton VA, Hernandez A. Minireview: Defining the roles of the iodothyronine deiodinases: Current concepts and challenges. *Endocrinology,* **2009,** *150:*1097–1107.

Sunthornthepvarakul T, Gottschalk ME, Hayashi Y, Refetoff S. Brief report: Resistance to thyrotropin caused by mutations in the thyrotropin-receptor gene. *N Engl J Med,* **1995,** *332:*155–160.

Surks MI, Hollowell JG. Age-specific distribution of serum thyrotropin and antithyroid antibodies in the US population: Implications for the prevalence of subclinical hypothyroidism. *J Clin Endocrinol Metab,* **2007,** *92:*4575–4582.

Takami H. Lithium in the preoperative preparation of Graves' disease. *Int Surg,* **1994,** *79:*89–90.

Takasu N, Yamada T, Shimizu Y. Generation of H_2O_2 is regulated by cytoplasmic free calcium in cultured porcine thyroid cells. *Biochem Biophys Res Commun,* **1987,** *148:*1527–1532.

Taurog A, Dorris ML, Doerge DR. Mechanism of simultaneous iodination and coupling catalyzed by thyroid peroxidase. *Arch Biochem Biophys,* **1996,** *330:*24–32.

Tellez RT, Chacon PM, Abarca CR, *et al.* Long-term environmental exposure to perchlorate through drinking water and thyroid function during pregnancy and the neonatal period. *Thyroid,* **2006,** *15:*963–975.

Tonacchera M, Pinchera A, Dimida A, *et al*. Relative potencies and additivity of perchlorate, thiocyanate, nitrate, and iodide on the inhibition of radioactive iodide uptake by the human sodium iodide symporter. *Thyroid,* **2004,** *14:* 1012–1019.

Tuttle RM, Leboeuf R, Martorella AJ. Papillary thyroid cancer: Monitoring and therapy. *Endocrinol Metab Clin North Am,* **2007,** *36:*753–778.

Uy HL, Reasner CA, Samuels MH. Pattern of recovery of the hypothalamic-pituitary-thyroid axis following radioactive iodine therapy in patients with Graves' disease. *Am J Med,* **1995,** *99:*173–179.

van Wassenaer AG, Westera J, Houtzager BA, Kok JH. Ten-year follow-up of children born at <30 weeks' gestational age supplemented with thyroxine in the neonatal period in a randomized, controlled trial. *Pediatrics,* **2005,** *116:*e613–618.

Visser WE, Friesema EC, Jansen J, Visser TJ. Thyroid hormone transport in and out of cells. *Trends Endocrinol Metab,* **2008,** *19:*50–56.

Walter MA, Briel M, Christ-Crain M, *et al*. Effects of anti-thyroid drugs on radioiodine treatment: Systematic review and meta-analysis of randomised controlled trials. *BMJ,* **2007,** *334:* 514–520.

Wolff J. Perchlorate and the thyroid gland. *Pharmacol Rev,* **1998,** *50:*89–105.

Xie J, Pannain S, Pohlenz J, *et al*. Resistance to thyrotropin (TSH) in three families is not associated with mutations in the TSH receptor or TSH. *J Clin Endocrinol Metab,* **1997,** *82:*3933–3940.

Yamamoto T, Fukuyama J, Fujiyoshi A. Factors associated with mortality of myxedema coma: Report of eight cases and literature survey. *Thyroid,* **1999,** *9:*1167–1174.

Yen PM, Ando S, Feng X, *et al*. Thyroid hormone action at the cellular, genomic and target gene levels. *Mol Cell Endocrinol,* **2006,** *246:*121–127.

Yen PM. Physiological and molecular basis of thyroid hormone action. *Physiol Rev,* **2001,** *81:*1097–1142.

Yoshihara HA, Apriletti JW, Baxter JD, Scanlan TS. Structural determinants of selective thyromimetics. *J Med Chem,* **2003,** *46:*3152–3161.

Zimmerman MB. Iodine deficiency. *Endocr Rev,* **2009,** *30:* 376–408.

Zoeller RT, Dowling AL, Vas AA. Developmental exposure to polychlorinated biphenyls exerts thyroid hormone-like effects on the expression of RC3/neurogranin and myelin basic protein messenger ribonucleic acids in the developing rat brain. *Endocrinology,* **2000,** *141:*181–189.

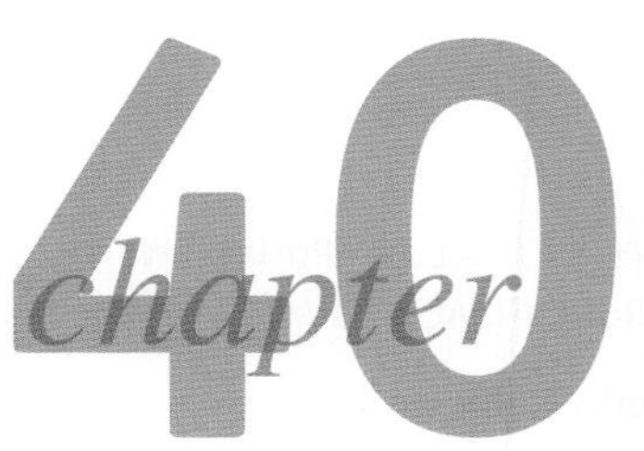

Estrogens and Progestins

Ellis R. Levin
and Stephen R. Hammes

Estrogens and *progestins* are endogenous hormones that produce numerous physiological actions. In women, these include developmental effects, neuroendocrine actions involved in the control of ovulation, the cyclical preparation of the reproductive tract for fertilization and implantation, and major actions on mineral, carbohydrate, protein, and lipid metabolism. Estrogens also have important actions in males, including effects on bone, spermatogenesis, and behavior. The biosynthesis, biotransformation, and disposition of estrogens and progestins are well established. Two well-characterized receptors are present for each hormone, and there is evidence that the receptors mediate biological actions in both the unliganded and steroid hormone-liganded states.

The therapeutic use of estrogens and progestins largely reflects extensions of their physiological activities. The most common uses of these agents are menopausal hormone therapy and contraception in women, but the specific compounds and dosages used in these two settings differ substantially. Estrogen- and progesterone-receptor antagonists also are available. The main uses of anti-estrogens are treatment of hormone-responsive breast cancer and infertility. Selective estrogen receptor modulators (SERMs) that display tissue-selective agonist or antagonist activities are useful to prevent breast cancer and osteoporosis. The main use of anti-progestins has been for medical abortion, but other uses are theoretically possible.

A number of naturally occurring and synthetic environmental chemicals mimic, antagonize, or otherwise affect the actions of estrogens in experimental test systems. The precise effect of these agents on humans is unknown, but this is an area of active investigation. Cancer chemotherapeutic strategies based on blockade of estrogen- and/or progesterone-receptor functions are considered in further detail in Chapter 63. Complementary therapeutic strategies based on suppression of gonadotropin secretion by long-acting gonadotropin-releasing hormone agonists are also discussed in Chapter 63.

History. The hormonal nature of the ovarian control of the female reproductive system was firmly established in 1900 by Knauer when he found that ovarian transplants prevented the symptoms of gonadectomy, and by Halban, who showed that normal sexual development and function occurred when glands were transplanted. In 1923, Allen and Doisy devised a bioassay for ovarian extracts based on the vaginal smear of the rat. Frank and associates in 1925 detected an active sex principle in the blood of sows in estrus, and Loewe and Lange discovered in 1926 that a female sex hormone varied in the urine of women throughout the menstrual cycle. The excretion of estrogen in the urine during pregnancy also was reported by Zondek in 1928 and enabled Butenandt and Doisy in 1929 to crystallize an active substance.

Early investigations indicated that the ovary secretes two substances. Beard had postulated in 1897 that the corpus luteum serves a necessary function during pregnancy, and Fraenkel showed in 1903 that destruction of the corpora lutea in pregnant rabbits caused abortion. Several groups then isolated progesterone from mammalian corpora lutea in the 1930s.

In the early 1960s, pioneering studies by Jensen and colleagues suggested the presence of intracellular receptors for estrogens in target tissues. This was the first demonstration of receptors of the steroid/thyroid superfamily and provided techniques to identify receptors for the other steroid hormones. A second estrogen receptor was identified in 1996 and termed *estrogen receptor* β (ERβ) to distinguish it from the receptor identified by Jensen and others, termed *estrogen receptor* α (ERα). Two protein isoforms, A and B, of the progesterone receptor arise from a single gene by transcription initiation from different promoters. For the primary literature references about the history of this subject, consult the ninth and tenth editions of this text.

ESTROGENS

Chemistry. Many steroidal and nonsteroidal compounds, some of which are shown in Table 40–1 and Figure 40–1, possess estrogenic activity. The most potent naturally occurring estrogen in

Table 40–1

Structural Formulas of Selected Estrogens

STEROIDAL ESTROGENS

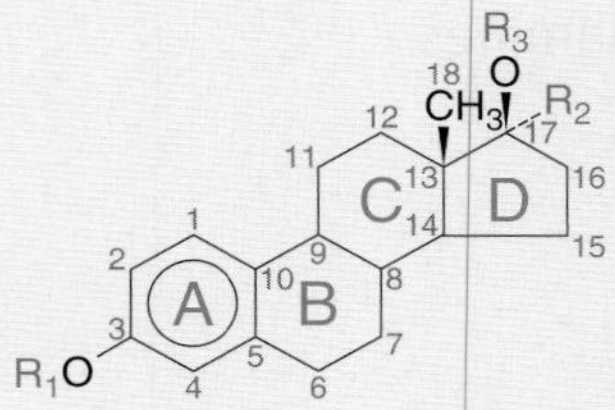

Derivative	R_1	R_2	R_3
Estradiol	—H	—H	—H
Estradiol valerate	—H	—H	$-C(=O)(CH_2)_3CH_3$
Ethinyl estradiol	—H	—C≡CH	—H
Mestranol	$-CH_3$	—C≡CH	—H
Estrone sulfate	$-SO_3H$	—[a]	=O[a]
Equilin[b]	—H	—[a]	=O[a]

[a]Designates C17 Ketone.
[b]Also contains 7, 8 double bond.

NONSTEROIDAL COMPOUNDS WITH ESTROGENIC ACTIVITY

Diethylstilbestrol

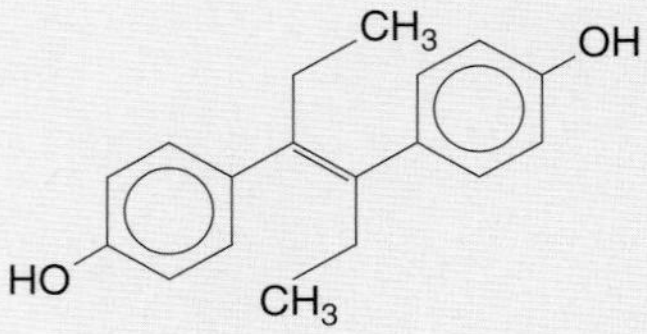

Bisphenol A

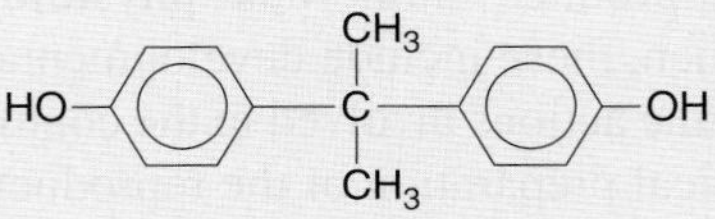

Genistein

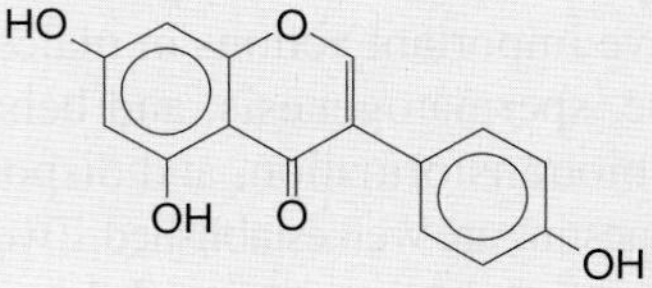

humans, for both ERα- and ERβ-mediated actions, is 17β-estradiol, followed by *estrone* and *estriol*. Each contains a phenolic A ring with a hydroxyl group at carbon 3, and a β-OH or ketone in position 17 of ring D.

The phenolic A ring is the principal structural feature responsible for selective high-affinity binding to both receptors. Most alkyl substitutions on the A ring impair binding, but substitutions on ring C or D may be tolerated. Ethinyl substitutions at the C17 position greatly increase oral potency by inhibiting first-pass hepatic metabolism. Models for the ligand-binding sites of both estrogen receptors have been determined from structure–activity relationships (Harrington et al., 2003) and structural analysis (Pike et al., 2000).

Diethylstilbestrol (DES), which is structurally similar to *estradiol* when viewed in the *trans* conformation, binds with high affinity to both estrogen receptors and it is as potent as estradiol in most assays but has a much longer $t_{1/2}$. DES no longer has widespread use, but it was important historically as an inexpensive orally active estrogen.

Selective ligands for ERα and ERβ are available for experimental studies but are not yet used therapeutically (Harrington et al., 2003).

Nonsteroidal compounds with estrogenic or anti-estrogenic activity—including flavones, isoflavones (e.g., genistein), and coumestan derivatives—occur in plants and fungi. Synthetic agents—including pesticides (e.g., *p,p′*-DDT), plasticizers (e.g., bisphenol A), and a variety of other industrial chemicals (e.g., polychlorinated biphenyls)—also have hormonal or antihormonal activity. Although their affinity is relatively weak, their large number, bioaccumulation, and persistence in the environment have raised concerns about their potential toxicity in humans and wildlife. Over-the-counter and prescription preparations containing naturally occurring estrogenlike compounds from plants (i.e., phytoestrogens) now are available (Fitzpatrick, 2003).

Biosynthesis. Steroidal estrogens arise from androstenedione or testosterone (Figure 40–1) by aromatization of the A ring. The reaction is catalyzed by aromatase (CYP19) that uses nicotinamide adenine dinucleotide phosphate (NADPH) and molecular oxygen as co-substrates. A ubiquitous flavoprotein, NADPH–cytochrome P450 reductase, also is essential. Both proteins are localized in the endoplasmic reticulum of ovarian granulosa cells, testicular Sertoli and Leydig cells, adipose stroma, placental syncytiotrophoblasts, preimplantation blastocysts, bone, various brain regions, and many other tissues (Simpson et al., 2002).

The ovaries are the principal source of circulating estrogen in premenopausal women, with estradiol the main secretory product.

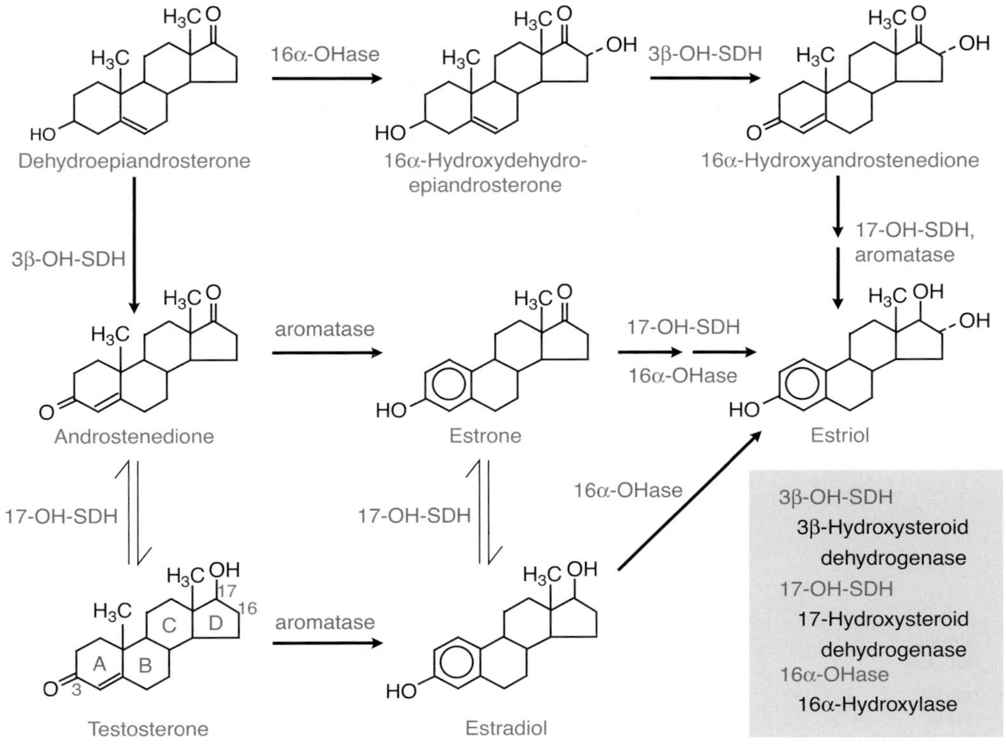

Figure 40–1. *The biosynthetic pathway for the estrogens.*

Gonadotropins, acting via receptors that couple to the G_s-adenylyl cyclase–cyclic AMP pathway, increase the activities of aromatase and the cholesterol side-chain cleavage enzyme and facilitate the transport of cholesterol (the precursor of all steroids) into the mitochondria of cells that synthesize steroids. The ovary contains a form of 17*β*-hydroxysteroid dehydrogenase (type I) that favors the production of testosterone and estradiol from androstenedione and estrone, respectively. However, in the liver, another form of this enzyme (type II) favors oxidation of circulating estradiol to estrone (Peltoketo et al., 1999), and both of these steroids are then converted to estriol (Figure 40–1). All three of these estrogens are excreted in the urine along with their glucuronide and sulfate conjugates.

In postmenopausal women, the principal source of circulating estrogen is adipose tissue stroma, where estrone is synthesized from dehydroepiandrosterone secreted by the adrenals. In men, estrogens are produced by the testes, but extragonadal production by aromatization of circulating C19 steroids (e.g., androstenedione and dehydroepiandrosterone) accounts for most circulating estrogens. Thus, the level of estrogens is regulated in part by the availability of androgenic precursors (Simpson, 2003).

Estrogenic effects most often have been attributed to circulating hormones, but locally produced estrogens also may have important actions (Simpson et al., 2002). For example, estrogens may be produced from androgens by the actions of aromatase or from estrogen conjugates by hydrolysis. Such local production of estrogens could play a causal or promotional role in the development of certain diseases such as breast cancer because mammary tumors contain both aromatase and hydrolytic enzymes. Estrogens also may be produced from androgens via aromatase in the central nervous system (CNS) and other tissues and exert local effects near their production site (e.g., in bone they affect bone mineral density).

The placenta uses fetal dehydroepiandrosterone and its 16*α*-hydroxyl derivative to produce large amounts of estrone and estriol. Human urine during pregnancy is thus an abundant source of natural estrogens, and pregnant mare's urine is the source of *conjugated equine estrogens*, which have been widely used therapeutically for many years.

Physiological and Pharmacological Actions

Developmental Actions. Estrogens are largely responsible for pubertal changes in girls and secondary sexual characteristics. They cause growth and development of the vagina, uterus, and fallopian tubes, and contribute to breast enlargement. They also contribute to molding the body contours, shaping the skeleton, and causing the pubertal growth spurt of the long bones and epiphyseal closure. Growth of axillary and pubic hair, pigmentation of the genital region, and the regional pigmentation of the nipples and areolae that occur after the first trimester of pregnancy are also estrogenic actions. Androgens may also play a secondary role in female sexual development (Chapter 41).

Estrogens appear to play important developmental roles in males. In boys, estrogen deficiency diminishes the pubertal growth spurt and delays skeletal maturation and epiphyseal closure so that linear growth continues into adulthood. Estrogen deficiency in men leads to elevated gonadotropins, macroorchidism, and increased testosterone levels and also may affect carbohydrate and lipid metabolism and fertility in some individuals (Grumbach and Auchus, 1999).

Neuroendocrine Control of the Menstrual Cycle. A neuroendocrine cascade involving the hypothalamus, pituitary, and ovaries controls the menstrual cycle (Figure 40–2). A neuronal oscillator, or "clock," in the hypothalamus fires at intervals that coincide with bursts of gonadotropin-releasing hormone (GnRH) release into the hypothalamic-pituitary portal vasculature (Chapter 38). GnRH interacts with its cognate receptor on pituitary gonadotropes to cause release of luteinizing hormone (LH) and follicle-stimulating hormone (FSH). The frequency of the GnRH pulses, which varies in the different phases of the menstrual cycle, controls the relative synthesis of the unique β subunits of FSH and LH.

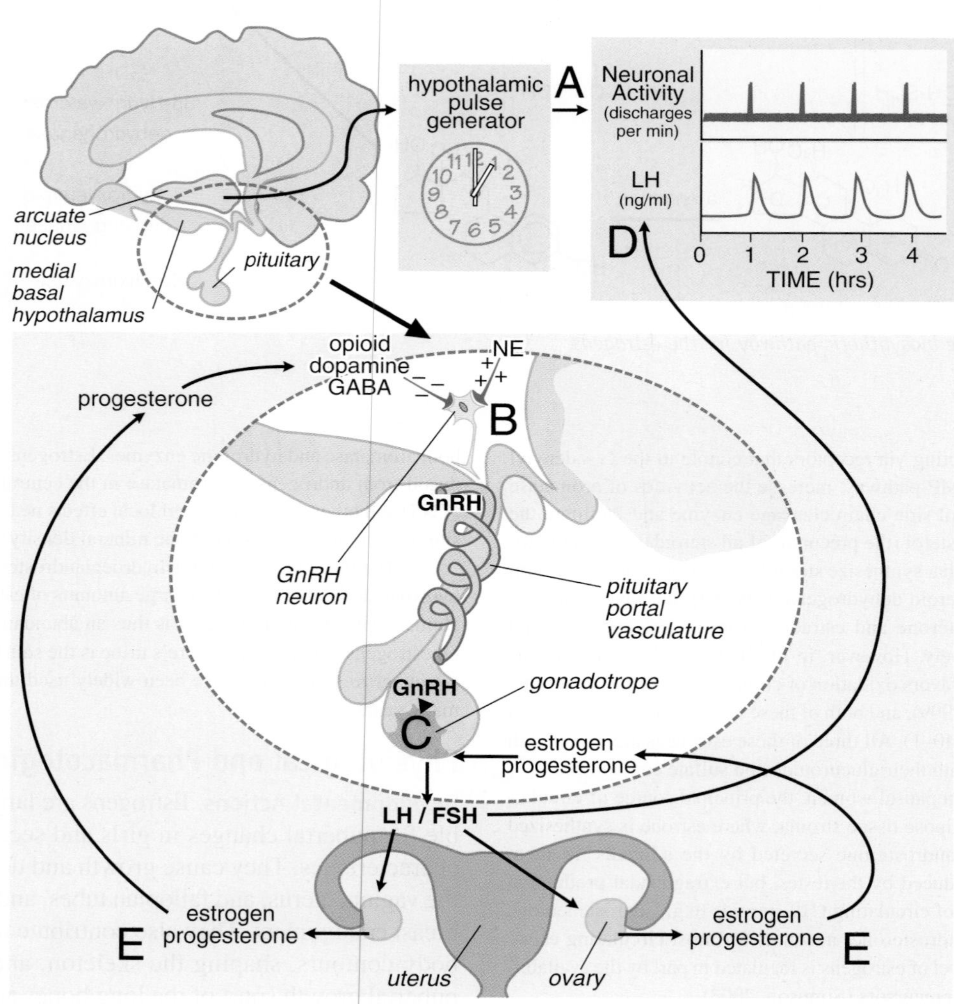

Figure 40–2. *Neuroendocrine control of gonadotropin secretion in females.* The hypothalamic pulse generator located in the arcuate nucleus of the hypothalamus functions as a neuronal "clock" that fires at regular hourly intervals (***A***). This results in the periodic release of gonadotropin-releasing hormone (GnRH) from GnRH-containing neurons into the hypothalamic-pituitary portal vasculature (***B***). GnRH neurons (***B***) receive inhibitory input from opioid, dopamine, and GABA neurons and stimulatory input from noradrenergic neurons (NE, norepinephrine). The pulses of GnRH trigger the intermittent release of luteinizing hormone (LH) and follicle-stimulating hormone (FSH) from pituitary gonadotropes (***C***), resulting in the pulsatile plasma profile (***D***). FSH and LH regulate ovarian production of estrogen and progesterone, which exert feedback controls (***E***). (See text and Figure 40–3 for additional details.)

The gonadotropins (LH and FSH) regulate the growth and maturation of the graafian follicle in the ovary and the ovarian production of estrogen and progesterone, which exert feedback regulation on the pituitary and hypothalamus.

Because the release of GnRH is intermittent, LH and FSH secretion is pulsatile. The pulse *frequency* is determined by the neural "clock" (Figure 40–2), termed the *hypothalamic GnRH pulse generator* (Knobil, 1981), but the amount of gonadotropin released in each pulse (i.e., the pulse *amplitude*) is largely controlled by the actions of estrogens and progesterone on the pituitary. The intermittent, *pulsatile* nature of hormone release is essential for the maintenance of normal ovulatory menstrual cycles because constant infusion of GnRH results in a cessation of gonadotropin release and ovarian steroid production (Chapter 38). The neuropeptide kisspeptin-1, which is released from the hypothalamic anteroventral periventricular nucleus and the arcuate nucleus, may regulate GnRH pulsatility through its G protein-coupled receptor, GPR54, expressed in GnRH neurons. Inactivating mutations in GPR54 have been associated with hypogonadotropic hypogonadism (Seminara, 2006).

Although the precise mechanism that regulates the timing of GnRH release (i.e., pulse frequency) is unclear, hypothalamic cells appear to have an intrinsic ability to release GnRH episodically. The overall pattern of GnRH release likely is regulated by the interplay of intrinsic mechanism(s) and extrinsic synaptic inputs from opioid, catecholamine, and GABAergic neurons (Figure 40–2). Ovarian steroids, primarily progesterone, regulate the frequency of GnRH release, but the cellular and molecular mechanisms of this regulation are not well established. Some GnRH cells have immunoreactive steroid receptors. Some nerve cells that synapse with GnRH neurons also contain steroid receptors, and neighboring glial cells may contain estrogen and progesterone receptors. Steroids may thus directly and indirectly modulate GnRH neuronal function.

At puberty the pulse generator is activated and establishes cyclic profiles of pituitary and ovarian hormones. Although the mechanism of activation is not entirely established, it may involve increases in circulating insulin-like growth factor (IGF)-1 and leptin levels, the latter acting to inhibit neuropeptide Y (NPY) in the arcuate nucleus to relieve an inhibitory effect on GnRH neurons.

Figure 40–3 provides a schematic diagram of the profiles of gonadotropin and gonadal steroid levels in the menstrual cycle. The "average" plasma levels of LH throughout the cycle are shown in panel *A* of Figure 40–3; inserts illustrate the pulsatile patterns of LH during the proliferative and secretory phases in more detail. The average LH levels are similar throughout the early (follicular) and late (luteal) phases of the cycle, but the frequency and amplitude of the LH pulses are quite different in the two phases. This characteristic pattern of hormone secretions results from complex positive and negative feedback mechanisms (Hotchkiss and Knobil, 1994).

In the early follicular phase of the cycle, (1) the pulse generator produces bursts of neuronal activity with a frequency of about one per hour that correspond with pulses of GnRH secretion, (2) these cause a corresponding pulsatile release of LH and FSH from pituitary gonadotropes, and (3) FSH in particular causes the graafian follicle to mature and secrete estrogen. The effects of estrogens on the pituitary are inhibitory at this time and cause the amount of LH and FSH released from the pituitary to decline (i.e., the amplitude of the LH pulse decreases), so gonadotropin levels gradually fall, as seen in Figure 40–3. Inhibin, produced by the ovary, also exerts a negative feedback to selectively decrease serum FSH at this time (Chapter 38). Activin and follistatin, two other peptides released from the ovary, may also regulate FSH production and secretion to a lesser extent, although their levels do not vary appreciably during the menstrual cycle.

At mid-cycle, serum estradiol rises above a threshold level of 150-200 pg/mL for ~36 hours. This sustained elevation of estrogen no longer inhibits gonadotropin release but exerts a brief positive feedback effect on the pituitary to trigger the preovulatory surge of LH and FSH. This effect primarily involves a change in pituitary responsiveness to GnRH. In some species, estrogens may also exert a positive effect on hypothalamic neurons that contributes to a mid-cycle "surge" of GnRH release; this is not yet established in humans. Progesterone may contribute to the mid-cycle LH surge.

The mid-cycle surge in gonadotropins stimulates follicular rupture and ovulation within 1-2 days. The ruptured follicle then develops into the corpus luteum, which produces large amounts of progesterone and lesser amounts of estrogen under the influence of LH during the second half of the cycle. In the absence of pregnancy, the corpus luteum ceases to function, steroid levels drop, and menstruation occurs. When steroid levels drop, the pulse generator reverts to a firing pattern characteristic of the follicular phase, the entire system then resets, and a new ovarian cycle occurs.

Regulation of the frequency and amplitude of gonadotropin secretions by steroids may be summarized as follows: Estrogens act primarily on the pituitary to control the amplitude of gonadotropin pulses, and they may also contribute to the amplitude of GnRH pulses secreted by the hypothalamus.

In the follicular phase of the cycle, estrogens inhibit gonadotropin release but then have a brief mid-cycle stimulatory action that increases the amount released and causes the LH surge. Progesterone, acting on the hypothalamus, exerts the predominant control of the frequency of LH release. It decreases the firing rate of the hypothalamic pulse generator, an action thought to be mediated largely via inhibitory opioid neurons (containing progesterone receptors) that synapse with GnRH neurons. Progesterone also exerts a direct effect on the pituitary to oppose the inhibitory actions of estrogens and thus enhance the amount of LH released (i.e., to increase the amplitude of the LH pulses). These steroid feedback effects, coupled with the intrinsic activity of the hypothalamic GnRH pulse generator, lead to relatively frequent LH pulses of small amplitude in the follicular phase of the cycle, and less frequent pulses of larger amplitude in the luteal phase. Studies in knockout mice indicate that

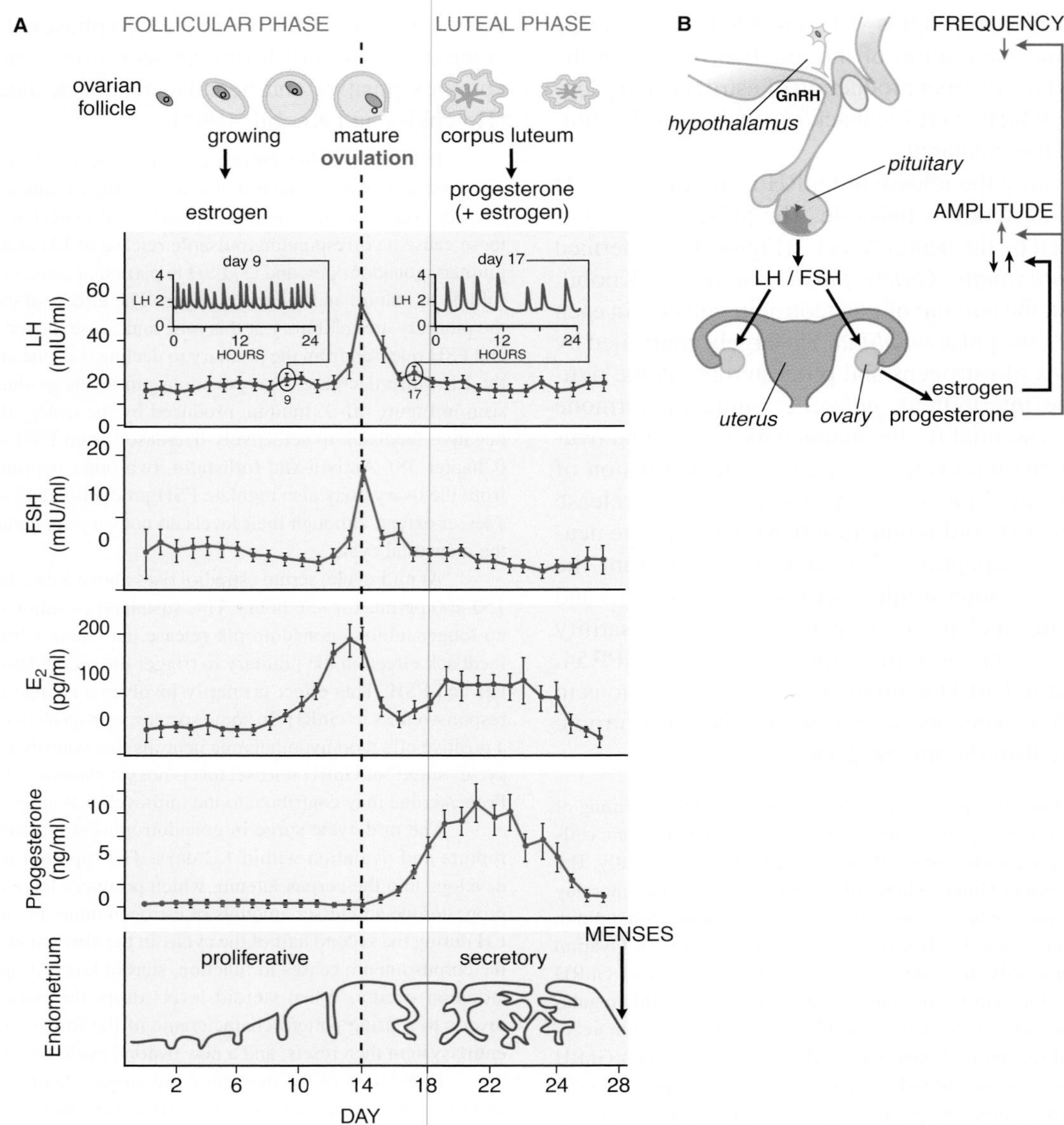

Figure 40–3. *Hormonal relationships of the human menstrual cycle.*

A. Average daily values of LH, FSH, estradiol (E_2), and progesterone in plasma samples from women exhibiting normal 28-day menstrual cycles. Changes in the ovarian follicle (*top*) and endometrium (*bottom*) also are illustrated schematically. Frequent plasma sampling reveals pulsatile patterns of gonadotropin release. Characteristic profiles are illustrated schematically for the follicular phase (day 9, inset on left) and luteal phase (day 17, inset on right). Both the frequency (number of pulses per hour) and amplitude (extent of change of hormone release) of pulses vary throughout the cycle. (Redrawn with permission from Thorneycroft et al., 1971. Copyright © Elsevier).

B. Major regulatory effects of ovarian steroids on hypothalamic-pituitary function. Estrogen decreases the amount of follicle-stimulating hormone (FSH) and luteinizing hormone (LH) released (i.e., gonadotropin pulse amplitude) during most of the cycle and triggers a surge of LH release only at mid-cycle. Progesterone decreases the frequency of GnRH release from the hypothalamus and thus decreases the frequency of plasma gonadotropin pulses. Progesterone also increases the amount of LH released (i.e., the pulse amplitude) during the luteal phase of the cycle.

ERα (Hewitt and Korach, 2003) and the progesterone receptor PR-A (Conneely et al., 2002) mediate the major actions of estrogens and progestins, respectively, on the hypothalamic-pituitary axis.

In males, testosterone regulates the hypothalamic-pituitary-gonadal axis at both the hypothalamic and pituitary levels, and its negative feedback effect is mediated to a substantial degree by estrogen formed via aromatization. Thus, exogenous estrogen administration decreases LH and testosterone levels in men, and anti-estrogens such as *clomiphene* cause an elevation of serum LH, which can be used to evaluate the male reproductive axis.

When the ovaries are removed or cease to function, there is overproduction of FSH and LH, which are excreted in the urine. Measurement of urinary or plasma LH is valuable to assess pituitary function and the effectiveness of therapeutic doses of estrogen. Although FSH levels will also decline upon estrogen administration, they do not return to normal, secondary to production of inhibin by the ovary (Chapter 38). Consequently, the measurement of FSH levels as a means to monitor the effectiveness of hormone therapy is not clinically useful. Additional features of the regulation of gonadotropin secretion and actions are discussed in Chapters 38 and 66.

Effects of Cyclical Gonadal Steroids on the Reproductive Tract. The cyclical changes in estrogen and progesterone production by the ovaries regulate corresponding events in the fallopian tubes, uterus, cervix, and vagina. Physiologically, these changes prepare the uterus for implantation, and the proper timing of events in these tissues is essential for pregnancy. If pregnancy does not occur, the endometrium is shed as the menstrual discharge.

The uterus is composed of an endometrium and a myometrium. The endometrium contains an epithelium lining the uterine cavity and an underlying stroma; the myometrium is the smooth muscle component responsible for uterine contractions. These cell layers, the fallopian tubes, cervix, and vagina display a characteristic set of responses to both estrogens and progestins. The changes typically associated with menstruation occur largely in the endometrium (Figure 40–3).

The luminal surface of the endometrium is a layer of simple columnar epithelial secretory and ciliated cells that is continuous with the openings of numerous glands that extend through the underlying stroma to the myometrial border. Fertilization normally occurs in the fallopian tubes, so ovulation, transport of the fertilized ovum through the fallopian tube, and preparation of the endometrial surface must be temporally coordinated for successful implantation.

The endometrial stroma is a highly cellular connective-tissue layer containing a variety of blood vessels that undergo cyclic changes associated with menstruation. The predominant cells are fibroblasts, but macrophages, lymphocytes, and other resident and migratory cell types also are present.

Menstruation marks the start of the menstrual cycle. During the follicular (or proliferative) phase of the cycle, estrogen begins the rebuilding of the endometrium by stimulating proliferation and differentiation. Numerous mitoses become visible, the thickness of the layer increases, and characteristic changes occur in the glands and blood vessels. In rodent models, ERα mediates the uterotrophic effects of estrogens (Hewitt and Korach, 2003). The overall endometrial response involves estrogen- and progesterone-mediated expression of peptide growth factors and receptors, cell cycle genes, and other regulatory signals. An important response to estrogen in the endometrium and other tissues is induction of the progesterone receptor (PR), which enables cells to respond to this hormone during the second half of the cycle.

In the luteal (or secretory) phase of the cycle, elevated progesterone limits the proliferative effect of estrogens on the endometrium by stimulating differentiation. Major effects include stimulation of epithelial secretions important for implantation of the blastocyst and the characteristic growth of the endometrial blood vessels seen at this time. These effects are mediated by PR-A in animal models (Conneely et al., 2002). Progesterone is thus important in preparation for implantation and for the changes that take place in the uterus at the implantation site (i.e., the decidual response). There is a narrow "window of implantation," spanning days 19-24 of the endometrial cycle, when the epithelial cells of the endometrium are receptive to blastocyst implantation. Because endometrial status is regulated by estrogens and progestins, the efficacy of some contraceptives may be due in part to production of an endometrial surface that is not receptive to implantation. If pregnancy does not occur, the corpus luteum regresses due to lack of continued LH secretion, estrogen and progesterone levels fall, and the endometrium is shed (Figure 40–3).

If implantation occurs, human chorionic gonadotropin (hCG) (Chapter 38), produced initially by the trophoblast and later by the placenta, interacts with the LH receptor of the corpus luteum to maintain steroid hormone synthesis during the early stages of pregnancy. In later stages the placenta itself becomes the major site of estrogen and progesterone synthesis.

Estrogens and progesterone have important effects on the fallopian tube, myometrium, and cervix. In the fallopian tube, estrogens stimulate proliferation and differentiation, whereas progesterone inhibits these processes. Also, estrogens increase and progesterone decreases tubal muscular contractility, which affects transit time of the ovum to the uterus. Estrogens increase the amount of cervical mucus and its water content to facilitate sperm penetration of the cervix, whereas progesterone generally has opposite effects. Estrogens favor rhythmic contractions of the uterine myometrium, and progesterone diminishes contractions. These effects are physiologically important and may also play a role in the action of some contraceptives.

Metabolic Effects. Estrogens affect many tissues and have many metabolic actions in humans and animals. It is not clear in all cases if effects result directly from hormone actions on the tissue in question or secondarily from actions at other sites. Many nonreproductive tissues, including bone, vascular endothelium, liver, CNS, immune system, gastrointestinal (GI) tract, and heart, express low levels of both estrogen receptors, and the ratio of ERα to ERβ varies in a cell-specific manner. Many metabolic effects of estrogens result directly from receptor-mediated events in affected organs. The effects of estrogens on selected aspects of mineral, lipid, carbohydrate, and protein metabolism are particularly important for understanding their pharmacological actions.

Estrogens have positive effects on bone mass (reviewed by Riggs et al., 2002). Bone is continuously remodeled at sites called *bone-remodeling units* by the resorptive action of osteoclasts and the bone-forming action of osteoblasts (Chapter 61). Maintenance of total bone mass requires equal rates of formation and resorption as occurs in early adulthood (ages 18-40 years); thereafter resorption predominates. Osteoclasts and osteoblasts express both ERα and ERβ, with the former apparently playing a greater role. Bone also expresses both androgen and progesterone receptors. Based on animal models, the actions of ERα predominate in bone. Estrogens directly regulate osteoblasts and increase the synthesis of type I collagen, osteocalcin, osteopontin, osteonectin, alkaline phosphatase, and other markers of differentiated osteoblasts. Estrogens also increase osteocyte survival by inhibiting apoptosis. However, the major effect of estrogens is to decrease the number and activity of osteoclasts. Much of the action of estrogens on osteoclasts appears to be mediated by altering cytokine (both paracrine and autocrine) signals from osteoblasts. Estrogens decrease osteoblast and stromal cell production of the osteoclast-stimulating cytokines interleukin (IL)-1, IL-6, and tumor necrosis factor (TNF)-α and increase the production of IGF-1, bone morphogenic protein (BMP)-6, and transforming growth factor (TGF)-β, which are anti-resorptive (reviewed by Spelsberg et al., 1999). Estrogens also increase osteoblast production of the cytokine osteoprotegerin (OPG), a soluble non–membrane-bound member of the TNF superfamily (Chapter 44). OPG acts as a "decoy" receptor that antagonizes the binding of OPG-ligand (OPG-L) to its receptor (termed RANK, or receptor activator of NF-κB) and prevents the differentiation of osteoclast precursors to mature osteoclasts. Estrogens increase osteoclast apoptosis, either directly or by increasing OPG. Estrogens have anti-apoptotic effects on both osteoblasts and osteocytes in animal models, and this action may be mediated by rapid signal transduction mechanisms (Kousteni et al., 2002; Levin, 2008). Estrogens affect bone growth and epiphyseal closure in both sexes. The importance of estrogen in the male skeleton is illustrated by a man with a completely defective ER who had osteoporosis, unfused epiphyses, increased bone turnover, and delayed bone age (Smith et al., 1994), and by the observation that male idiopathic osteoporosis is associated with reduced ERα expression in both osteocytes and osteoblasts (Braidman et al., 2000).

Estrogens have many effects on lipid metabolism; of major interest are their effects on serum lipoprotein and triglyceride levels (Walsh et al., 1994). In general, estrogens slightly elevate serum triglycerides and slightly reduce total serum cholesterol levels. More important, they increase high-density lipoprotein (HDL) levels and decrease the levels of low-density lipoprotein (LDL) and lipoprotein A (LPA) (Chapter 31). This beneficial alteration of the ratio of HDL to LDL is an attractive effect of estrogen therapy in postmenopausal women. The initial conclusions from two large clinical trials—the Heart and Estrogen/Progestin Replacement Study, or HERS (Hulley et al., 1998), and the Women's Health Initiative, or WHI (Anderson et al., 2004; Rossouw et al., 2002)—were that estrogen-progestin or estrogen-only regimens *do not provide any protection from cardiovascular disease*. However, re-examination of the data in women who took hormone replacement within 10 years of the menopause showed a 32% reduction in myocardial infarction (heart attack).

At relatively high concentrations, estrogens have antioxidant activity and may inhibit the oxidation of LDL by affecting superoxide dismutase. Long-term administration of estrogen is associated with decreased plasma renin, angiotensin-converting enzyme, and endothelin-1; expression of the AT_1 receptor for angiotensin II is also decreased. Estrogen actions on the vascular wall include increased production of nitric oxide (NO), which occurs within minutes via a mechanism involving activation of Akt (protein kinase B) (Simoncini et al., 2000), induction of NO synthase, and increased production of prostacyclin. All of these changes promote vasodilation and retard atherogenesis. Estrogens also promote endothelial cell growth while inhibiting the proliferation of vascular smooth muscle cells.

The presence of estrogen receptors in the liver suggests that the beneficial effects of estrogen on lipoprotein metabolism are due partly to direct hepatic actions, but other sites of action cannot be excluded. Estrogens also alter bile composition by increasing cholesterol secretion and decreasing bile acid secretion. This leads to increased saturation of bile with cholesterol and appears to be the basis for increased gallstone formation in some women receiving estrogens. The decline in bile acid biosynthesis may contribute to the decreased incidence of colon cancer in women receiving combined estrogen-progestin treatment. In general, estrogens increase plasma levels of cortisol-binding globulin, thyroxine-binding globulin, and sex hormone-binding globulin (SHBG), which binds both androgens and estrogens. ERα deficiency or aromatase enzyme deficiency in mice is associated with impaired glucose tolerance and other elements of the metabolic syndrome due to increased insulin resistance (Simpson, 2003).

Estrogens alter a number of metabolic pathways that affect the clotting cascade (Mendelsohn and Karas, 1999). Systemic effects include changes in hepatic production of plasma proteins. Estrogens cause a small increase in coagulation factors II, VII, IX, X, and XII, and they decrease the anticoagulation factors protein C, protein S, and antithrombin III (Chapter 30). Fibrinolytic pathways also are affected, and several studies of women treated with estrogen alone or estrogen with a progestin have demonstrated decreased levels of plasminogen-activator inhibitor 1 (PAI-1) protein with a concomitant increase in fibrinolysis (Koh et al., 1997). Thus, estrogens increase both coagulation and fibrinolytic pathways, and imbalance in these two opposing activities may cause adverse effects.

Estrogen Receptors

Estrogens exert their effects by interaction with receptors that are members of the superfamily of nuclear receptors. The two estrogen receptor genes are located on separate chromosomes: ESR1 encodes ERα, and ESR2 encodes ERβ. Both ERs are estrogen-dependent nuclear transcription factors that have different tissue distributions and transcriptional regulatory effects on a wide number of target genes (reviewed by Hanstein et al., 2004). Ligands that discriminate between ERα and ERβ have been developed (Harrington et al., 2003) but are not yet in clinical use. Both ERα and ERβ exist as multiple mRNA isoforms due to differential promoter use and alternative splicing (reviewed by Kos et al., 2001; Lewandowski et al., 2002). The two human ERs are 44% identical in overall amino acid sequence and share the domain structure common to members of this family. The estrogen receptor is divided into six functional domains: The NH_2-terminal A/B domain contains the activation function-1 (AF-1) segment, which can activate transcription independently of ligand; the highly conserved C domain comprises the DNA-binding domain, which contains four cysteines arranged in two zinc fingers; the D domain, frequently called the "hinge region," contains the nuclear localization signal; and the E/F domain has multiple functions, including ligand binding, dimerization, and ligand-dependent transactivation, mediated by the AF-2 domain. There are significant differences between the two receptor isoforms in the ligand-binding domains and in both transactivation domains. Human ERβ does not appear to contain a functional AF-1 domain. The receptors appear to have different biological functions and respond differently to various estrogenic compounds (Kuiper et al., 1997). However, their high homology in the DNA-binding domains suggests that both receptors recognize similar DNA sequences and hence regulate many of the same target genes.

ERα, the first discovered, is expressed most abundantly in the female reproductive tract—especially the uterus, vagina, and ovaries—as well as in the mammary gland, the hypothalamus, endothelial cells, and vascular smooth muscle. ERβ is expressed most highly in the prostate and ovaries, with lower expression in lung, brain, bone, and vasculature. Many cells express both ERα and ERβ, which can form either homo- or heterodimers. Both forms of ER are expressed on breast cancers, although ERα is believed to be the predominant form responsible for growth regulation (Chapter 63). When co-expressed with ERα, ERβ can inhibit ERα-mediated transcriptional activation in many cases (Hall and McDonnell, 1999). Polymorphic variants of ER have been identified, but attempts to correlate specific polymorphisms with the frequency of breast cancer (Han et al., 2003), bone mass (Kurabayashi et al., 2004), endometrial cancer (Weiderpass et al., 2000), or cardiovascular disease (Herrington and Howard, 2003) have led to contradictory results.

A cloned G protein-coupled receptor, GPR30, also appears to interact with estrogens in some cell systems, and its participation in the rapid effects of estrogen is an attractive idea. However, four GPR30 knockout (KO) mice strains show inconsistent data with few stress or developmental phenotypes, and there is no consistent overlap of these models with ERα and ERβ KO phenotypes. There may be interaction/cross-talk between membrane-associated ERα and membrane-localized GPR30 in some cancer cells, but *in vivo* confirmation is lacking (Levin, 2008; Olde et al. 2009).

Mechanism of Action

Both estrogen receptors (ERs) are ligand-activated transcription factors that increase or decrease the transcription of target genes (Figure 40–4). After entering the cell by passive diffusion through the plasma membrane, the hormone binds to an ER in the nucleus. In the nucleus, the ER is present as an inactive monomer bound to heat-shock protein 90 (HSP90), and upon binding estrogen, a change in ER conformation dissociates the heat-shock proteins and causes receptor dimerization, which increases the affinity and the rate of receptor binding to DNA (Cheskis et al., 1997). Homodimers of ERα or ERβ and ER α/ERβ heterodimers can be produced depending on the receptor complement in a given cell. The concept of ligand-mediated changes in ER conformation is central to understanding the mechanism of action of estrogen agonists and antagonists. The ER dimer binds to estrogen response elements (EREs), typically located in the promoter region of target genes with the consensus sequence GGTCANNNTGACC, but several similar sequences can act as estrogen response elements in a promoter-specific context. The type of ERE with which ERs interact also regulates the three-dimensional structure of the activated receptor (Hall et al., 2002).

The ER/DNA complex recruits a cascade of co-activator and other proteins to the promoter region of target genes (Figure 40–4B). Three families of proteins interact with ERs. The first of these has the ability to modify nucleosome structure either in an ATP-dependent manner, like SWI/Snf, or by histone methyltransferase (HMT) activity, as in proteins such as PRMT1. The second family comprises the p160/SRC proteins and includes SRC-1 (steroid-receptor co-activator 1), SRC-2, and SRC-3. The third family includes p300/CBP (cyclic AMP response-element binding protein), co-activators

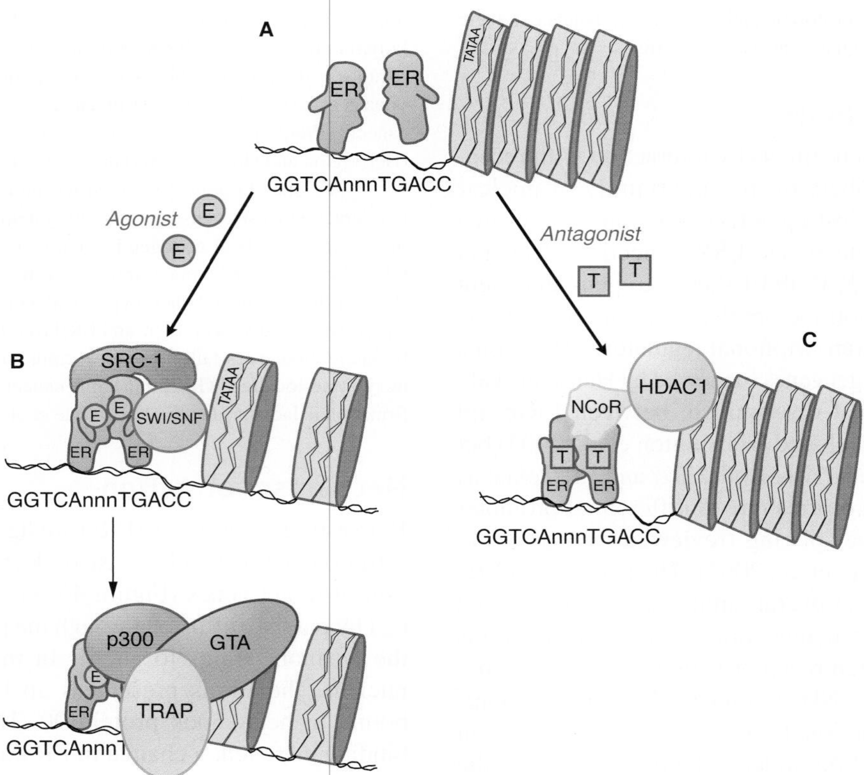

Figure 40–4. *Molecular mechanism of action of nuclear estrogen receptor.* ***A.*** Unliganded estrogen receptor (ER) exists as a monomer within the nucleus. ***B.*** Agonists such as 17β-estradiol ( ) bind to the ER and cause a ligand-directed change in conformation that facilitates dimerization and interaction with specific estrogen response element (ERE) sequences in DNA. The ER-DNA complex recruits co-activators such as SWI/SNF that modify chromatin structure, and co-activators such as steroid-receptor co-activator-1 (SRC-1) that has histone acetyltransferase (HAT) activity that further alters chromatin structure. This remodeling facilitates the exchange of the recruited proteins such that other co-activators (e.g., p300 and the TRAP complex) associate on the target gene promoter and proteins that comprise the general transcription apparatus (GTA) are recruited, with subsequent synthesis of mRNA. ***C.*** Antagonists such as tamoxifen (T) also bind to the ER but produce a different receptor conformation. The antagonist-induced conformation also facilitates dimerization and interaction with DNA, but a different set of proteins called co-repressors, such as nuclear-hormone receptor co-repressor (NcoR), are recruited to the complex. NcoR further recruits proteins such as histone deacetylase I (HDAC1) that act on histone proteins to stabilize nucleosome structure and prevent interaction with the GTA.

that are targets of several signal transduction cascades and may integrate function among diverse pathways and the basal transcriptional apparatus. Agonist-bound ERs appear initially to recruit SWI/Snf and HMT members that modify nucleosome structure and facilitate the subsequent recruitment of p160 members and p300 proteins (Metivier et al., 2003). The co-activators and p300 proteins have histone acetyltransferase (HAT) activity. Acetylation of histones further alters chromatin structure in the promoter region of target genes and allows the proteins that make up the general transcription apparatus to assemble and initiate transcription.

Interaction of ERs with antagonists also promotes dimerization and DNA binding. However, an antagonist produces a conformation of ER that is different from the agonist-occupied receptor (Smith and O'Malley, 2004; Wijayaratne et al., 1999). The antagonist-induced conformation facilitates binding of co-repressors such as NCoR/SMRT (nuclear hormone receptor co-repressor/silencing mediator of retinoid and thyroid receptors) (Figure 40–4C). The co-repressor/ER complex then further recruits other proteins with histone deacetylase activity such as HDAC1. Deacetylation of histones alters chromatin conformation and reduces the ability of the general transcription apparatus to form initiation complexes.

Besides co-activators and co-repressors, both ERα and ERβ can interact physically with other transcription factors such as Sp1 (Saville et al., 2000) or AP-1 (Paech et al., 1997), and these protein-protein interactions provide an alternate mechanism of action. In these circumstances, ER-ligand complexes interact with Sp1 or AP-1 that is already bound to its specific regulatory element, such that the ER complex does not interact directly with an ERE. This may explain how estrogens are able to regulate genes that lack a consensus ERE. Responses to agonists and antagonists mediated by these protein-protein interactions also are ER isoform- and promoter-specific. For example, 17β-estradiol induces transcription of a target gene controlled by an AP-1 site in the presence of an ER α/AP-1 complex but inhibits transcription in the presence of an ERβ/AP-1 complex. Conversely, anti-estrogens are potent activators of ERβ/AP-1 but not of ERα/AP-1 complexes.

Other signaling systems may activate nuclear ER by ligand-independent mechanisms. Phosphorylation of ERα at serine 118 by MAP kinase activates the receptor (Kato et al., 1995). Similarly, PI-3-kinase–activated Akt directly phosphorylates ERα, causing ligand-independent activation of estrogen-target genes (Simoncini et al., 2000). This provides a means of cross-talk between membrane-bound receptor pathways (i.e., EGF/IGF-1) that activate MAPK and the nuclear ER. In a reciprocal fashion ER may interact directly with members of the Src-Shc/Erk signaling pathway. Activation of Erk by an estren that is a novel ER and androgen receptor (AR) agonist is thought to be responsible for the anti-apoptotic action of this drug in bone (reviewed in Manolagas et al., 2002).

Numerous studies indicate that some estrogen receptors are located on the plasma membrane of cells. This cellular pool form of the ER is encoded by the same genes that encode ERα and ERβ (Pedram, 2006) but are transported to the plasma membrane and reside mainly in caveolae. Translocation to the membrane by all sex steroid receptors is mediated by palmitoylation of a nine–amino acid motif in the respective E domains of the receptors (reviewed in Levin, 2008). These membrane-localized ERs mediate the rapid activation of some proteins such as MAPK (phosphorylated in several cell types) and the rapid increase in cyclic AMP caused by the hormone (Aronica and Katzenellenbogen, 1993). The finding that MAPK is activated by estradiol provides an additional level of cross-talk with growth factor receptors for IGF-1 and EGF, which can activate multiple kinase pathways.

Absorption, Fate, and Elimination

Various estrogens are available for oral, parenteral, transdermal, or topical administration. Given the lipophilic nature of estrogens, absorption generally is good with the appropriate preparation. Aqueous or oil-based esters of estradiol are available for intramuscular injection, ranging in frequency from every week to once per month. Conjugated estrogens are available for IV or IM administration. Transdermal patches that are changed once or twice weekly deliver estradiol continuously through the skin. Preparations are available for topical use in the vagina or for application to the skin. For many therapeutic uses, estrogen preparations are available in combination with a progestin. All estrogens are labeled with precautionary statements urging the prescribing of the lowest effective dose and for the shortest duration consistent with the treatment goals and risks for each individual patient.

Oral administration is common and may use estradiol, conjugated estrogens, esters of estrone and other estrogens, and *ethinyl estradiol (in combination with a progestin)*. Estradiol is available in nonmicronized (FEMTRACE) and micronized preparations (ESTRACE, others). The micronized formulations yield a large surface for rapid absorption to partially overcome low absolute oral bioavailability due to first-pass metabolism (Fotherby, 1996). Addition of the ethinyl substituent at C17 (ethinyl estradiol) inhibits first-pass hepatic metabolism. Other common oral preparations contain conjugated equine estrogens (PREMARIN), which are primarily the sulfate esters of estrone, equilin, and other naturally occurring compounds; *esterified esters* (MENEST); or mixtures of synthetic conjugated estrogens prepared from plant-derived sources (CENESTIN; ENJUVIA). These are hydrolyzed by enzymes present in the lower gut that remove the charged sulfate groups and allow absorption of estrogen across the intestinal epithelium. In another oral preparation, *estropipate* (ORTHO-EST, OGEN, others), estrone is solubilized as the sulfate and stabilized with piperazine. Due largely to differences in metabolism, the potencies of various oral preparations differ widely; ethinyl estradiol, e.g., is much more potent than conjugated estrogens.

A number of foodstuffs and plant-derived products, largely from soy, are available as nonprescription items and often are touted as providing benefits similar to those from compounds with established estrogenic activity. These products may contain flavonoids such as genistein (Table 40–1), which display estrogenic activity in laboratory tests, albeit generally much less than that of estradiol. In theory, these preparations could produce appreciable estrogenic effects, but their efficacy at relevant doses has not been established in human trials (Fitzpatrick, 2003).

Administration of estradiol via transdermal patches (ALORA, CLIMARA, ESTRADERM, VIVELLE, others) provides slow, sustained release of the hormone, systemic distribution, and more constant blood levels than oral dosing. Estradiol is also available as a topical emulsion (ESTRASORB), applied to the upper thigh and calf, or as a gel (ESTROGEL), applied once daily to the arm. The transdermal route does not lead to the high level of the drug that occur in the portal circulation after oral administration, and it is thus expected to minimize hepatic effects of estrogens (e.g., effects on hepatic protein synthesis, lipoprotein profiles, and triglyceride levels).

Other preparations are available for intramuscular injection. When dissolved in oil and injected, esters of estradiol are well absorbed. The aryl and alkyl esters of estradiol become less polar as the size of the substituents increases; correspondingly, the rate of absorption of oily preparations is progressively slowed, and the duration of action can be prolonged. A single therapeutic dose of compounds such as *estradiol valerate* (DELESTROGEN, others) or *estradiol cypionate* (DEPO-ESTRADIOL, others) may be absorbed over several weeks following a single intramuscular injection.

Preparations of estradiol (ESTRACE) and conjugated estrogen (PREMARIN) creams are available for topical administration to the vagina. These are effective locally, but systemic effects also are possible due to significant absorption. A 3-month vaginal ring (ESTRING,

FEMRING) may be used for slow release of estradiol, and tablets are also available for vaginal use (VAGIFEM).

Estradiol, ethinyl estradiol, and other estrogens are extensively bound to plasma proteins. Estradiol and other naturally occurring estrogens are bound mainly to SHBG and to a lesser degree to serum albumin. In contrast, ethinyl estradiol is bound extensively to serum albumin but not SHBG. Due to their size and lipophilic nature, unbound estrogens distribute rapidly and extensively.

Variations in estradiol metabolism occur and depend on the stage of the menstrual cycle, menopausal status, and several genetic polymorphisms (Herrington and Klein, 2001). In general, the hormone undergoes rapid hepatic biotransformation, with a plasma $t_{1/2}$ measured in minutes. Estradiol is converted primarily by 17β-hydroxysteroid dehydrogenase to estrone, which undergoes conversion by 16α-hydroxylation and 17-keto reduction to estriol, the major urinary metabolite. A variety of sulfate and glucuronide conjugates also are excreted in the urine. Lesser amounts of estrone or estradiol are oxidized to the 2-hydroxycatechols by CYP3A4 in the liver and by CYP1A in extrahepatic tissues or to 4-hydroxycatechols by CYP1B1 in extrahepatic sites, with the 2-hydroxycatechol being formed to a greater extent. The 2- and 4-hydroxycatechols are largely inactivated by catechol-*O*-methyl transferases (COMTs). However, smaller amounts may be converted by CYP- or peroxidase-catalyzed reactions to yield semiquinones or quinones that are capable of forming DNA adducts or of generating (via redox cycling) reactive oxygen species that could oxidize DNA bases (Yue et al., 2003).

Estrogens also undergo enterohepatic recirculation via (1) sulfate and glucuronide conjugation in the liver, (2) biliary secretion of the conjugates into the intestine, and (3) hydrolysis in the gut (largely by bacterial enzymes) followed by reabsorption.

Many other drugs and environmental agents (e.g., cigarette smoke) act as inducers or inhibitors of the various enzymes that metabolize estrogens, and thus have the potential to alter their clearance. Consideration of the impact of these factors on efficacy and untoward effects is increasingly important with the decreased doses of estrogens currently employed for both menopausal hormone therapy and contraception.

Ethinyl estradiol is cleared much more slowly than estradiol due to decreased hepatic metabolism, and the elimination-phase $t_{1/2}$ in various studies ranges from 13 to 27 hours. Unlike estradiol, the primary route of biotransformation of ethinyl estradiol is via 2-hydroxylation and subsequent formation of the corresponding 2- and 3-methyl ethers. *Mestranol*, another semisynthetic estrogen and a component of some combination oral contraceptives, is the 3-methyl ether of ethinyl estradiol. In the body it undergoes rapid hepatic demethylation to ethinyl estradiol, which is its active form (Fotherby, 1996).

Untoward Responses

Estrogens are highly efficacious, but they do carry a number of risks. Many concerns arose initially from studies of early oral contraceptives, which contained high doses of estrogens. Oral contraceptives now contain much lower amounts of both estrogen and progestins, and this has significantly diminished the risks associated with their use. Nevertheless, major concerns about the use of estrogens remain today, especially regarding cancer, thromboembolic disease, and gallbladder disease.

Concern About Carcinogenic Actions. The risk of developing breast, endometrial, cervical, and vaginal cancer is probably the major concern for the use of estrogens and oral contraceptives. Landmark studies (Greenwald et al., 1971; Herbst et al., 1971) reported an increased incidence of vaginal and cervical adenocarcinoma in female offspring of mothers who had taken diethylstilbestrol (DES) during the first trimester of pregnancy. The incidence of clear cell vaginal and cervical adenocarcinoma in women who were exposed to DES *in utero* was 0.01-0.1% (Food and Drug Administration, 1985); these findings established for the first time that developmental exposure to estrogens was associated with an increase in a human cancer. Estrogen use during pregnancy also can increase the incidence of nonmalignant genital abnormalities in both male and female offspring. Thus, pregnant patients should not be given estrogens because of the possibility of such reproductive tract toxicities.

The use of unopposed estrogen for hormone treatment in postmenopausal women increases the risk of endometrial carcinoma by 5- to 15-fold (Shapiro et al., 1985). This increased risk can be prevented if a progestin is co-administered with the estrogen (Pike et al., 1997), and this is now standard practice.

The association between estrogen and/or estrogen-progestin use and breast cancer is of great concern. The results of two large randomized clinical trials of estrogen/progestin and estrogen-only (i.e., the two arms of WHI) in postmenopausal women clearly established a small but significant increase in the risk of breast cancer, apparently due to the medroxyprogesterone (Anderson et al., 2004; Rossouw et al., 2002). In the WHI study, an estrogen-progestin combination increased the total risk of breast cancer by 25%; the absolute increase in attributable cases of disease was 6 per 1000 women and required 3 or more years of treatment. In women without a uterus who received estrogen alone, the relative risk of breast cancer was actually decreased by 23%, and the decrease only narrowly missed reaching statistical significance. Interestingly, the incidence of colon cancer was reduced by 26% in the WHI trial.

The Million Women Study (MWS) in the U.K. was a cohort study rather than a clinical trial (Beral et al., 2003). It surveyed >1 million women; about half had received some type of hormone treatment and half had never used them. Those receiving an estrogen-progestin combination had an increased relative risk of invasive breast cancer of 2, and those receiving estrogen alone had an increased relative risk of 1.3, but the increase in actual attributable cases of the disease was again small.

Both the WHI and MWS data are thus consistent with earlier studies indicating that the progestin component (e.g., medroxyprogesterone) in combined hormone-replacement therapy plays a major role in this increased risk of breast cancer (Ross et al., 2000; Schairer et al., 2000). Importantly, although long-term data have not accumulated for the WHI trials, the available data suggest that the excess risk of breast cancer associated with menopausal hormone use appears to abate 5 years after discontinuing therapy. Thus, hormone replacement therapy for ≤5 years is often prescribed to mitigate hot flashes and likely has a minimal effect on the risk of breast cancer.

Historically, the carcinogenic actions of estrogens were thought to be related to their trophic effects. An increase in cell proliferation would be expected to cause an increase in spontaneous errors associated with DNA replication, and estrogens would then enhance the growth of clones with mutations introduced by this or other mechanisms (e.g., chemical carcinogens). More recently, another mechanism has been proposed. If catechol estrogens, especially the

4-hydroxycatechols, are converted to semiquinones or quinones prior to "inactivation" by COMT, these products, or reactive oxygen species generated during subsequent biotransformations, may cause direct chemical damage to DNA bases (Yue et al., 2003). In this regard, CYP1B1, which has specific estrogen-4-hydroxylase activity, is present in tissues such as uterus, breast, ovary, and prostate, which often give rise to hormone-responsive cancers (Yue et al., 2003).

Metabolic and Cardiovascular Effects. Although they may slightly elevate plasma triglycerides, estrogens themselves generally have favorable overall effects on plasma lipoprotein profiles. However, as noted in a later section dealing with hormone-replacement regimens, progestins may reduce the favorable actions of estrogens. In contrast, estrogens do increase cholesterol levels in bile and cause a relative 2- to 3-fold increase in gallbladder disease. Currently prescribed doses of estrogens generally do not increase the risk of hypertension, and estrogen engaging the ERβ receptor typically reduces blood pressure.

A number of observational studies, clinical trials using intermediate markers of cardiovascular disease, and numerous animal studies suggested that estrogen therapy in postmenopausal women would reduce the risk of cardiovascular disease by 35-50% (Manson and Martin, 2001). However, two recent randomized clinical trials have not found such protection. HERS (Hulley et al., 1998) followed women with established coronary heart disease (CHD) and found that estrogen plus a progestin increased the relative risk of nonfatal myocardial infarction or CHD death within 1 year of treatment, and found no overall change in 5 years. The HERS II follow-up (Grady et al., 2002) found no overall change in the incidence of CHD after 6.8 years of the treatment. These results indicate no role for hormone replacement in the secondary prevention of atherosclerotic heart disease. In the WHI trials, women *without* existing CHD were treated with an estrogen plus progestin (Rossouw et al., 2002); protective effects were seen but only when hormone replacement was initiated within 10 years of menopause.

It is clear, however, that oral estrogens increase the risk of thromboembolic disease in healthy women and in women with preexisting cardiovascular disease (Grady et al., 2000). The increase in absolute risk is small but significant. In the WHI, e.g., an estrogen-progestin combination led to an increase in eight attributable cases of stroke per 10,000 older women and a similar increase in pulmonary embolism (Rossouw et al., 2002).The latter was seen mainly in women who concomitantly smoked cigarettes.

Effects on Cognition. Several retrospective studies had suggested that estrogens had beneficial effects on cognition and delayed the onset of Alzheimer's disease (Green and Simpkins, 2000). However, the Women's Health Initiative Memory Study (WHIMS) of a group of women ≥65 years of age (Shumaker et al., 2003) found that estrogen-progestin therapy was associated with a doubling in the number of women diagnosed with probable dementia, and no benefit of hormone treatment on global cognitive function was observed (Rapp et al., 2003). Women in the estrogen-only arm also showed a comparable decrease in cognitive function (Espeland et al., 2004), implicating estrogens in these cognitive changes.

Other Potential Untoward Effects. Nausea and vomiting are an initial reaction to estrogen therapy in some women, but these effects may disappear with time and may be minimized by taking estrogens with food or just before sleep. Fullness and tenderness of the breasts and edema may occur but sometimes can be diminished by lowering the dose. A more serious concern is that estrogens may cause severe migraine in some women. Estrogens also may reactivate or exacerbate endometriosis.

Therapeutic Uses

The two major uses of estrogens are for menopausal hormone therapy (MHT) and as components of combination oral contraceptives (see final section of chapter), and the pharmacological considerations for their use and the specific drugs and doses used differ in these settings. Historically, conjugated estrogens have been the most common agents for postmenopausal use (0.625 mg/day most often used). In contrast, most combination oral contraceptives in current use employ 20-35 μg/day of ethinyl estradiol. These preparations differ widely in their oral potencies (e.g., a dose of 0.625 mg of conjugated estrogens generally is considered equivalent to 5-10 μg of ethinyl estradiol). Thus, the "effective" dose of estrogen used for MHT is less than that in oral contraceptives when one considers potency. Furthermore, in the last two decades the doses of estrogens employed in both settings have decreased substantially. The untoward effects of the 20- to 35-μg doses now commonly used thus have a lower incidence and severity than those reported in older studies (e.g., with oral contraceptives that contained 50-150 μg of ethinyl estradiol or mestranol).

Menopausal Hormone Therapy. The established benefits of estrogen therapy in postmenopausal women include amelioration of vasomotor symptoms and the prevention of bone fractures and urogenital atrophy.

Vasomotor Symptoms. The decline in ovarian function at menopause is associated with vasomotor symptoms in most women. The characteristic hot flashes may alternate with chilly sensations, inappropriate sweating, and (less commonly) paresthesias. Treatment with estrogen is specific and is the most efficacious pharmacotherapy for these symptoms (Belchetz, 1994). If estrogen is contraindicated or otherwise undesirable, other options may be considered. Medroxyprogesterone acetate (discussed in the later section on progestins) may provide some relief of vasomotor symptoms for certain patients, and the α_2 adrenergic agonist clonidine diminishes vasomotor symptoms in some women, presumably by blocking the CNS outflow that regulates blood flow to cutaneous vessels. In many women, hot flashes diminish within several years; when prescribed for this purpose the dose and duration of estrogen use should thus be the minimum necessary to provide relief.

Osteoporosis. Osteoporosis is a disorder of the skeleton associated with the loss of bone mass (Chapter 44). The result is thinning and weakening of the bones and an increased incidence of fractures, particularly compression fractures of the vertebrae and minimal-trauma fractures of the hip and wrist. The frequency and severity of these fractures and their associated complications (e.g., death and permanent disability) are a major public health problem, especially as the population continues to age. Osteoporosis is an indication for estrogen therapy, which clearly is efficacious in decreasing the incidence of fractures. However, because of the risks associated with estrogen use, first-line use of other drugs, such as bisphosphonates, should be considered (Chapter 44). Nevertheless, it is important to note that most fractures in the postmenopausal period occur in women without a prior history of osteoporosis, and estrogens are the most efficacious agents available for prevention of fractures at all sites in such women (Anderson et al., 2004; Rossouw et al., 2002).

The primary mechanism by which estrogens act is to decrease bone resorption; consequently, estrogens are more effective at preventing rather than restoring bone loss (Belchetz, 1994; Prince et al., 1991). Estrogens are most effective if treatment is initiated before significant bone loss occurs, and their maximal beneficial effects require continuous use; bone loss resumes when treatment is discontinued. Other options for treatment of osteoporosis are presented in Chapter 44. An appropriate diet with adequate intake of Ca^{2+} and vitamin D and weight-bearing exercise enhance the effects of estrogen treatment. Public health efforts to improve diet and exercise patterns in girls and young women also are rational approaches to increase bone mass.

Vaginal Dryness and Urogenital Atrophy. Loss of tissue lining the vagina or bladder leads to a variety of symptoms in many postmenopausal women (Robinson and Cardozo, 2003). These include dryness and itching of the vagina, dyspareunia, swelling of tissues in the genital region, pain during urination, a need to urinate urgently or often, and sudden or unexpected urinary incontinence. When estrogens are being used solely for relief of vulvar and vaginal atrophy, local administration as a vaginal cream, ring device, or tablets may be considered.

Cardiovascular Disease. The incidence of cardiovascular disease is low in premenopausal women, rising rapidly after menopause, and epidemiological studies consistently showed an association between estrogen use and reduced cardiovascular disease in postmenopausal women. Furthermore, estrogens produce a favorable lipoprotein profile, promote vasodilation, inhibit the response to vascular injury, and reduce atherosclerosis. Studies such as these led to the widespread use of estrogen for prevention of cardiovascular disease in postmenopausal women (Mendelsohn and Karas, 1999). As discussed earlier, estrogens promote coagulation and thromboembolic events. Randomized prospective studies (Grady et al., 2002; Rossouw et al., 2002) unexpectedly have indicated that the incidence of heart disease and stroke in older postmenopausal women treated with conjugated estrogens and a progestin was initially increased, although the trend reversed with time. However, as mentioned, combined estrogen-progestin therapy is associated with a decrease in heart attacks in younger women.

Other Therapeutic Effects. Many other changes occur in postmenopausal women, including a general thinning of the skin; changes in the urethra, vulva, and external genitalia; and a variety of changes including headache, fatigue, and difficulty concentrating. Chronic lack of sleep created by hot flashes and other vasomotor symptoms may be contributing factors. Estrogen replacement may help alleviate or lessen some of these via direct actions (e.g., improvement of vasomotor symptoms) or secondary effects resulting in an improved feeling of well-being (Belchetz, 1994). The WHI demonstrated that a conjugated estrogen in combination with a progestin reduces the risk of colon cancer by roughly one-half in postmenopausal women (Rossouw et al., 2002).

Menopausal Hormone Regimens. In the 1960s and 1970s, there was an increase in *estrogen-replacement therapy*, or ERT (i.e., estrogens alone), in postmenopausal women, primarily to reduce vasomotor symptoms, vaginitis, and osteoporosis. About 1980, epidemiological studies indicated that this treatment increased the incidence of endometrial carcinoma. This led to the use of *hormone-replacement therapy*, or HRT, that includes a progestin to limit estrogen-related endometrial hyperplasia. Although the actions of progesterone on the endometrium are complex, its effects on estrogen-induced hyperplasia may involve a decrease in estrogen-receptor content, increased local conversion of estradiol to the less potent estrone via the induction of 17β hydroxysteroid dehydrogenase in the tissue and/or the conversion of the endometrium from a proliferative to a secretory state. Postmenopausal HRT, when indicated, should include both an estrogen and progestin for women with a uterus (Belchetz, 1994). For women who have undergone a hysterectomy, endometrial carcinoma is not a concern, and estrogen alone avoids the possible deleterious effects of progestins.

Conjugated estrogens and medroxyprogesterone acetate (MPA) historically have been used most commonly in menopausal hormone regimens, although estradiol, estrone, and estriol have been used as estrogens, and *norethindrone, norgestimate, levonorgestrel, norethisterone, and progesterone* also have been widely used (especially in Europe). Various "continuous" or "cyclic" regimens have been used; the latter regimens include drug-free days. An example of a cyclic regimen is as follows: (1) administration of an estrogen for 25 days; (2) the addition of MPA for the last 12-14 days of estrogen treatment; and (3) 5-6 days with no hormone treatment, during which withdrawal bleeding normally occurs due to breakdown and shedding of the endometrium. Continuous administration of combined estrogen plus progestin does not lead to regular, recurrent endometrial shedding but may cause intermittent spotting or bleeding, especially in the first year of use. Other regimens include a progestin intermittently (e.g., every third month), but the long-term endometrial safety of these regimens remains to be firmly established. PREMPRO (conjugated estrogens plus MPA given as a fixed dose daily) and PREMPHASE (conjugated estrogens given for 28 days plus MPA given for 14 of 28 days) are widely used combination formulations. Other combination products available in the U.S. are FEMHRT (ethinyl estradiol plus norethindrone acetate), ACTIVELLA (estradiol plus norethindrone), PREFEST (estradiol and norgestimate), and ANGELIQ (estradiol and drospirenone). Doses and regimens are usually adjusted empirically based on control of symptoms, patient acceptance of bleeding patterns, and/or other untoward effects.

Another pharmacological consideration is the route of estrogen administration. Oral administration exposes the liver to higher concentrations of estrogens than does transdermal administration. Either route effectively relieves vasomotor symptoms and protects against bone loss. Oral but not transdermal estrogen may increase SHBG, other binding globulins, and angiotensinogen; the oral route might be expected to cause greater increases in the cholesterol content of the bile. Transdermal estrogen appears to cause smaller beneficial changes in LDL and HDL profiles (~50% of those seen with the oral route) (Walsh et al., 1994) but may be preferred in women with hypertriglyceridemia.

Tibolone (LIVIAL) is widely used in the E.U. for treatment of vasomotor symptoms and prevention of osteoporosis but is not currently approved in the U.S. The parent compound itself is devoid of activity, but it is metabolized in a tissue-selective manner to three metabolites that have predominantly estrogenic, progestogenic, and androgenic activities. The drug appears to increase bone mineral density and decrease vasomotor symptoms without stimulating the endometrium, but its effects on fractures, breast cancer, and long-term outcomes remain to be established (Modelska and Cummings, 2002).

Regardless of the specific agent or regimen, menopausal hormone therapy with estrogens should use the lowest dose and shortest duration necessary to achieve an appropriate therapeutic goal.

Estrogen Treatment in the Failure of Ovarian Development. In several conditions (e.g., Turner's syndrome), the ovaries do not develop and puberty does not occur. Therapy with estrogen at the appropriate time replicates the events of puberty, and androgens (Chapter 41) and/or growth hormone (Chapter 38) may be used concomitantly to promote normal growth. Although estrogens and androgens promote bone growth, they also accelerate epiphyseal fusion, and their premature use can thus result in a shorter ultimate height.

SELECTIVE ESTROGEN RECEPTOR MODULATORS AND ANTI-ESTROGENS

In the past, estrogen pharmacology was based on a simple model of an agonist binding to a single ER that subsequently affected transcription by the same molecular mechanism in all target tissues and of antagonists that acted by simple competition with agonists for binding. This simple concept is no longer valid. By altering the conformation of the two different ERs and thereby changing interactions with co-activators and co-repressors in a cell-specific and promoter-specific contexts, ligands may have a broad spectrum of activities from purely anti-estrogenic in all tissues, to partially estrogenic in some tissues with anti-estrogenic or no activities in others, to purely estrogenic activities in all tissues. The elucidation of these concepts has been a major breakthrough in estrogen pharmacology and should permit the rational design of drugs with very selective patterns of estrogenic activity (Smith and O'Malley, 2004).

Selective Estrogen Receptor Modulators: Tamoxifen, Raloxifene, and Toremifene. Selective estrogen receptor modulators, or SERMs, are compounds with tissue-selective actions. The pharmacological goal of these drugs is to produce beneficial estrogenic actions in certain tissues (e.g., bone, brain, and liver) during postmenopausal hormone therapy but antagonist activity in tissues such as breast and endometrium, where estrogenic actions (e.g., carcinogenesis) might be deleterious. Currently approved drugs in the U.S. in this class are tamoxifen citrate, raloxifene hydrochloride (EVISTA), and toremifene (FARESTON), which is chemically related and has similar actions to tamoxifen. Tamoxifen and toremifene are used for the treatment of breast cancer, and raloxifene is used primarily for the prevention and treatment of osteoporosis and to reduce the risk of invasive breast cancer in high-risk postmenopausal women. They are considered in detail in Chapter 63.

Anti-Estrogens: Clomiphene and Fulvestrant. These compounds are distinguished from the SERMs in that they are pure antagonists in all tissues studied. Clomiphene (CLOMID, SEROPHENE, others) is approved for the treatment of infertility in anovulatory women, and fulvestrant (FASLODEX) is used for the treatment of breast cancer in women with disease progression after tamoxifen.

Chemistry. The structures of the *trans*-isomer of tamoxifen, and of raloxifene, *trans*-clomiphene (enclomiphene), and fulvestrant are:

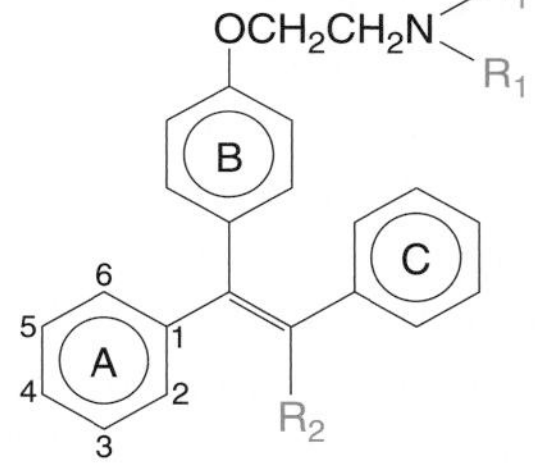

	ENCLOMIPHENE	TAMOXIFEN
R_1:	$-CH_2CH_3$	$-CH_3$
R_2:	$-Cl$	$-CH_2CH_3$

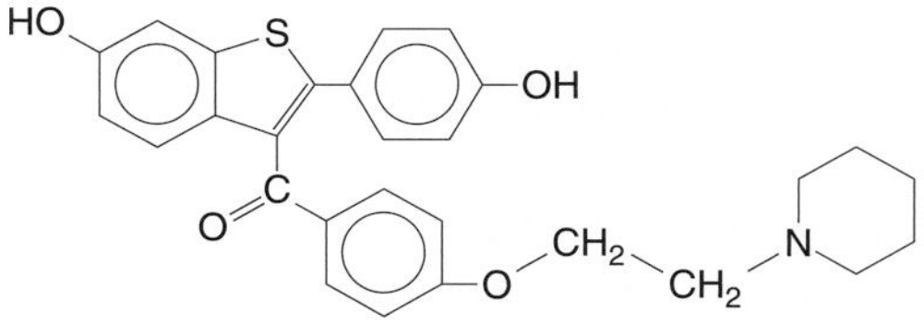

RALOXIFENE

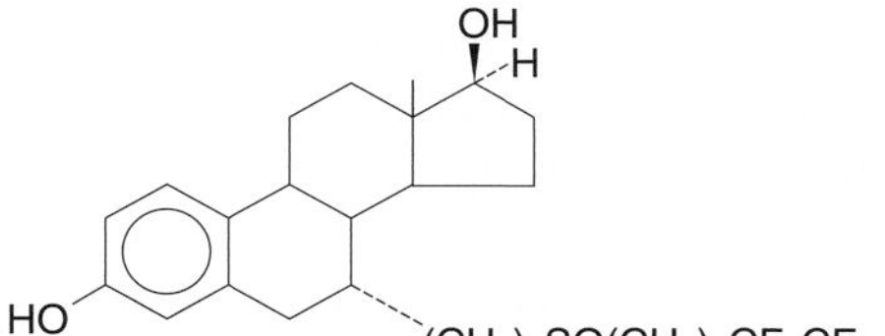

FULVESTRANT (ICI 182, 780)

Tamoxifen is a triphenylethylene with the same stilbene nucleus as DES; compounds of this class display a variety of estrogenic and anti-estrogenic activities. In general, the *trans* conformations have anti-estrogenic activity, whereas the *cis* conformations display estrogenic activity. However, the pharmacological activity of the *trans* compound depends on the species, target tissue, and gene. Hepatic metabolism produces primarily *N*-desmethyltamoxifen, which has affinity for ER comparable to that of tamoxifen, and lesser amounts of the highly active 4-hydroxy metabolite, which has a 25-50 times higher affinity for both ERα and ERβ than does tamoxifen (Kuiper et al., 1997). Tamoxifen is marketed as the pure *trans*-isomer. Toremifene is a triphenylethylene with a chlorine substitution at the R2 position.

Raloxifene is a polyhydroxylated nonsteroidal compound with a benzothiophene core. Raloxifene binds with high affinity for both ERα and ERβ (Kuiper et al., 1997).

Clomiphene citrate is a triphenylethylene; its two isomers, zuclomiphene (*cis*-clomiphene) and enclomiphene (*trans*-clomiphene), are a weak estrogen agonist and a potent antagonist, respectively. Clomiphene binds to both ERα and ERβ, but the individual isomers have not been examined (Kuiper et al., 1997).

Fulvestrant is a 7α-alkylamide derivative of estradiol that interacts with both ERα and ERβ (Van Den Bemd et al., 1999).

Pharmacological Effects

Tamoxifen exhibits anti-estrogenic, estrogenic, or mixed activity depending on the species and target gene measured. In clinical tests or laboratory studies with human cells, the drug's activity depends on the tissue and end point measured. For example, tamoxifen inhibits the proliferation of cultured human breast cancer cells and reduces tumor size and number in women (reviewed in Jaiyesimi et al., 1995), and yet it stimulates proliferation of endometrial cells and causes endometrial thickening (Lahti et al., 1993). The drug has an antiresorptive effect on bone, and in humans it decreases total cholesterol, LDL, and LPA but does not increase HDL and triglycerides (Love et al., 1994). Tamoxifen treatment causes a 2- to 3-fold increase in the relative risk of deep vein thrombosis and pulmonary embolism and a roughly 2-fold increase in endometrial carcinoma (Smith, 2003). Tamoxifen produces hot flashes and other adverse effects, including cataracts and nausea. Due to its agonist activity in bone, it does not increase the incidence of fractures when used in this setting.

Raloxifene is an estrogen agonist in bone, where it exerts an antiresorptive effect. It reduces the number of vertebral fractures by up to 50% in a dose-dependent manner (Delmas et al., 1997; Ettinger et al., 1999). The drug also acts as an estrogen agonist in reducing total cholesterol and LDL, but it does not increase HDL or normalize plasminogen-activator inhibitor 1 in postmenopausal women (Walsh et al., 1998). Raloxifene does not cause proliferation or thickening of the endometrium. Preclinical studies indicate that raloxifene has an antiproliferative effect on ER-positive breast tumors and on proliferation of ER-positive breast cancer cell lines (Hol et al., 1997) and significantly reduces the risk of ER-positive but not ER-negative breast cancer (Cummings et al., 1999). Raloxifene does not alleviate the vasomotor symptoms associated with menopause. Adverse effects include hot flashes and leg cramps and a 3-fold increase in deep vein thrombosis and pulmonary embolism (Cummings et al., 1999).

Initial animal studies with clomiphene showed slight estrogenic activity and moderate anti-estrogenic activity, but the most striking effect was the inhibition of pituitary gonadotropes. In contrast, the most prominent effect in women was enlargement of the ovaries and the drug-induced ovulation in many patients with amenorrhea, polycystic ovarian syndrome, and dysfunctional bleeding with anovulatory cycles. This is the basis for clomiphene's major pharmacological use: to induce ovulation in women with a functional hypothalamic-hypophyseal-ovarian system and adequate endogenous estrogen production. In some cases, clomiphene is used in conjunction with human gonadotropins (Chapter 38) to induce ovulation.

Fulvestrant and its less potent forerunner ICI 164,384 have been purely anti-estrogenic in studies to date. *In vitro*, fulvestrant was more potent than 4-hydroxytamoxifen (DeFriend et al., 1994) in inhibiting proliferation of breast cancer cells, and in clinical trials it is efficacious in treating tamoxifen-resistant breast cancers (Robertson et al., 2003).

All of these agents bind to the ligand-binding pocket of both ERα and ERβ and competitively block estradiol binding. However, the conformation of the ligand-bound ERs is different with different ligands (Smith and O'Malley, 2004), and this has two important mechanistic consequences. The distinct ER-ligand conformations recruit different co-activators and co-repressors onto the promoter of a target gene by differential protein-protein interactions at the receptor surface. The tissue-specific actions of SERMs thus can be explained in part by the distinct conformation of the ER when occupied by different ligands, in combination with different co-activator and co-repressor levels in different cell types that together affect the nature of ER complexes formed in a tissue-selective fashion.

The conformation of ERs, especially in the AF-2 domain, determines whether a co-activator or a co-repressor will be recruited to the ER-DNA complex (Smith and O'Malley, 2004). Whereas 17β-estradiol induces a conformation that recruits co-activators to the receptor, tamoxifen induces a conformation that permits the recruitment of the co-repressor to both ERα and ERβ. The agonist activity of tamoxifen seen in tissues such as the endometrium is mediated by the ligand-independent AF-1 transactivation domain of ER α; because ERβ does not contain a functional AF-1 domain, tamoxifen does not activate ERβ (McInerney et al., 1998).

Raloxifene acts as a partial agonist in bone but does not stimulate endometrial proliferation in postmenopausal women. Presumably this is due to some combination of differential expression of transcription factors in the two tissues and the effects of this SERM on ER conformation. Raloxifene induces a configuration in ERα that is distinct from that of tamoxifen-ERβ (Tamrazi et al., 2003), suggesting that a different set of co-activators/co-repressors may interact with ER-raloxifene compared with ER-tamoxifen.

Clomiphene increases gonadotropin secretion and stimulates ovulation. It increases the amplitude of LH and FSH pulses without changing pulse frequency (Kettel et al., 1993). This suggests that the drug is acting largely at the pituitary level to block inhibitory actions of estrogen on gonadotropin release from the gland and/or is somehow causing the hypothalamus to release larger amounts of GnRH per pulse.

Fulvestrant binds to ERα and ERβ with a high affinity comparable to estradiol but represses transactivation. It also increases dramatically the intracellular proteolytic degradation of ERα while apparently protecting ERβ from degradation (Van Den Bemd et al., 1999). This effect on ERα protein levels may explain fulvestrant's efficacy in tamoxifen-resistant breast cancer.

Absorption, Fate, and Excretion

Tamoxifen is given orally, and peak plasma levels are reached within 4-7 hours after treatment. This drug displays two elimination phases with half-lives of 7-14 hours and 4-11 days. Due to the prolonged $t_{1/2}$, 3-4 weeks of treatment are required to reach steady-state plasma levels. The parent drug is converted largely to metabolites within 4-6 hours after oral administration. Tamoxifen is metabolized in humans by multiple hepatic CYPs, some of which it also induces (Sridar et al., 2002). In humans and other species, 4-hydroxytamoxifen is produced via hepatic metabolism, and this compound is considerably more potent than the parent drug as an anti-estrogen. The major route of elimination from the body involves *N*-demethylation and deamination. The drug undergoes enterohepatic circulation, and excretion is primarily in the feces as conjugates of the deaminated metabolite. Polymorphisms affect the rate of tamoxifen metabolism to its more potent 4-hydroxy metabolite and may impact its therapeutic activity in breast cancer (Chapter 63).

Raloxifene is adsorbed rapidly after oral administration and has an absolute bioavailability of ~2%. The drug has a $t_{1/2}$ of ~28 hours and is eliminated primarily in the feces after hepatic glucuronidation; it does not appear to undergo significant biotransformation by CYPs.

Clomiphene is well absorbed following oral administration, and the drug and its metabolites are eliminated primarily in the feces and to a lesser extent in the urine. The long plasma $t_{1/2}$ (5-7 days) is due largely to plasma-protein binding, enterohepatic circulation, and accumulation in fatty tissues. Other active metabolites with long half-lives also may be produced.

Fulvestrant is administered monthly by intramuscular depot injections. Plasma concentrations reach maximal levels in 7 days and are maintained for a month. Numerous metabolites are formed *in vivo*, possibly by pathways similar to endogenous estrogen metabolism, but the drug is eliminated primarily (90%) via the feces in humans.

Therapeutic Uses

Breast Cancer. Tamoxifen is highly efficacious in the treatment of breast cancer. It is used alone for palliation of advanced breast cancer in women with ER-positive tumors, and it is now indicated as the hormonal treatment of choice for both early and advanced breast cancer in women of all ages (Jaiyesimi et al., 1995). Response rates are ~50% in women with ER-positive tumors. Tamoxifen increases disease-free survival and overall survival; treatment for 5 years reduces cancer recurrence by 50% and death by 27% and is more efficacious than shorter 1- to 2-year treatment periods. Tamoxifen reduces the risk of developing contralateral breast cancer and is approved for primary prevention of breast cancer in women at high risk, in whom it causes a 50% decrease in the development of new tumors. Prophylactic treatment should be limited to 5 years because effectiveness decreases thereafter. The most frequent side effect is hot flashes. Tamoxifen has estrogenic activity in the uterus, increases the risk of endometrial cancer by 2- to 3-fold, and also causes a comparable increase in the risk of thromboembolic disease that leads to serious risks for women receiving anticoagulant therapy (Smith, 2003) and women with a history of deep vein thrombosis or stroke.

Toremifene has therapeutic actions similar to tamoxifen, and fulvestrant may be efficacious in women who become resistant to tamoxifen. Untoward effects of fulvestrant include hot flashes, GI symptoms, headache, back pain, and pharyngitis.

Osteoporosis. Raloxifene reduces the rate of bone loss and may increase bone mass at certain sites. In a large clinical trial, raloxifene increased spinal bone mineral density by >2% and reduced the rate of vertebral fractures by 30-50% but did not significantly reduce nonvertebral fractures (Delmas et al., 2002; Ettinger et al., 1999). Raloxifene does not appear to increase the risk of developing endometrial cancer. The drug has beneficial actions on lipoprotein metabolism, reducing both total cholesterol and LDL; however, HDL is not increased. Adverse effects include hot flashes, deep vein thrombosis, and leg cramps.

Infertility. Clomiphene is used primarily for treatment of female infertility due to anovulation. By increasing gonadotropin levels, primarily FSH, it enhances follicular recruitment. It is relatively inexpensive, orally active, and requires less extensive monitoring than other treatment protocols. However, the drug may exhibit untoward effects, including ovarian hyperstimulation, increased incidence of multiple births, ovarian cysts, hot flashes, and blurred vision. In addition, clomiphene-induced cycles have a relatively high incidence of luteal phase dysfunction due to inadequate progesterone production, and prolonged use (e.g., ≥12 cycles) may increase the risk of ovarian cancer. The drug should not be administered to pregnant women due to reports of teratogenicity in animals, but there is no evidence of this when the drug has been used to induce ovulation. Clomiphene also may be used to evaluate the male reproductive system because testosterone feedback on the hypothalamus and pituitary is mediated to a large degree by estrogens formed from aromatization of the androgen.

Experimental SERM-Estrogen Combinations. There is considerable interest in menopausal hormone therapy using combinations of a pure estrogen agonist (e.g., estradiol) with a SERM that has predominantly antagonist activity in the breast and endometrium but does not distribute to the CNS. The strategy is to obtain the beneficial actions of the agonist (e.g., prevention of hot flashes and bone loss) while the SERM blocks unwanted agonist action at peripheral sites (e.g., proliferative effects in breast and endometrium) but does not enter the brain to cause hot flashes. Animal studies have been encouraging (Labrie et al., 2003), but clinical efficacy and safety of this approach remain to be established.

Estrogen-Synthesis Inhibitors

Several agents can be used to block estrogen biosynthesis. Continual administration of GnRH agonists prevents ovarian synthesis of estrogens but not their peripheral synthesis from adrenal androgens (Chapter 38). *Aminoglutethimide* inhibits aromatase activity, but its use is limited by its lack of selectivity and its side effects (sedation). It was discontinued in the U.S. in 2008.

The recognition that locally produced as well as circulating estrogens may play a significant role in breast cancer has greatly stimulated interest in the use of aromatase inhibitors to selectively block production of estrogens (Chapter 63). Both steroidal (e.g., formestane and exemestane [AROMASIN]) and nonsteroidal agents (e.g., anastrozole [ARIMIDEX], letrozole [FEMARA], and vorozole) are available. Steroidal, or type I, agents are substrate analogs that act as suicide inhibitors to irreversibly inactivate aromatase, whereas the nonsteroidal, or type II, agents interact reversibly with the heme groups of CYPs (Haynes et al., 2003). Exemestane, letrozole, and anastrozole are currently approved in the U.S. for the treatment of breast cancer.

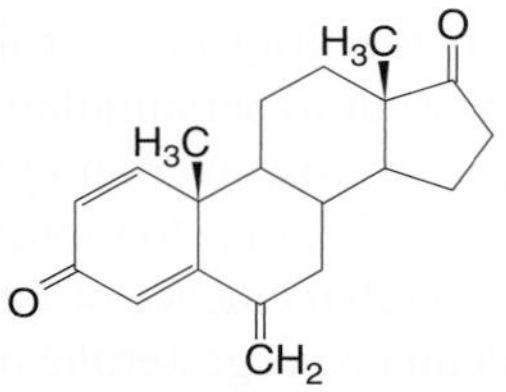

EXEMESTANE

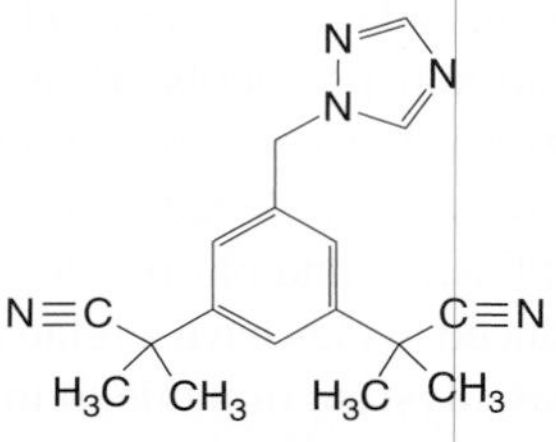

ANASTROZOLE

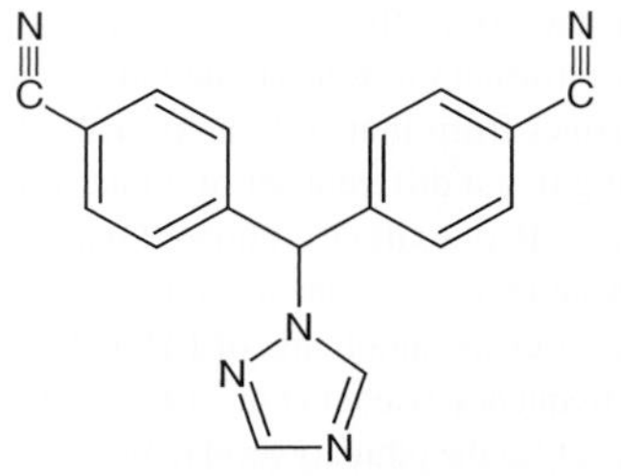

LETROZOLE

As discussed in Chapter 62, these agents may be used as first-line treatment of breast cancer or as second-line drugs after tamoxifen. They are highly efficacious and actually superior to tamoxifen in adjuvant use for postmenopausal women (Coombes et al., 2004), and are indicated either following tamoxifen for 2-5 years or as initial agents. They have the added advantage of not increasing the risk of uterine cancer or venous thromboembolism. Because they dramatically reduce circulating as well as local levels of estrogens, they produce hot flashes. They lack the beneficial effect of tamoxifen to maintain bone density and thus are usually administered with bisphosphonates. Their effects on plasma lipids remain to be established.

PROGESTINS

Compounds with biological activities similar to those of progesterone have been variously referred to in the literature as progestins, progestational agents, progestagens, progestogens, gestagens, or gestogens. The progestins (Figure 40–5) include the naturally occurring hormone progesterone, 17α-acetoxyprogesterone derivatives in the pregnane series, 19-nortestosterone derivatives in the estrane series, and norgestrel and related compounds in the gonane series. Medroxyprogesterone acetate (MPA) and megestrol acetate are C21 steroids in the pregnane family with selective activity very similar to that of progesterone itself. MPA and oral micronized progesterone are widely used with estrogens for MHT and other situations in which a selective progestational effect is desired. Furthermore, depot MPA is used as a long-acting injectable contraceptive. The 19-nortestosterone derivatives (estranes) were developed for use as progestins in oral contraceptives, and although their predominant activity is progestational, they exhibit androgenic and other activities. The gonanes are another family of "19-nor" compounds, containing an ethyl rather than a methyl substituent in the 13-position. They have diminished androgenic activity relative to the estranes. These two classes of 19-nortestosterone derivatives are the progestational components of most oral and some long-acting injectable contraceptives. The remaining oral contraceptives contain a class of progestins derived from

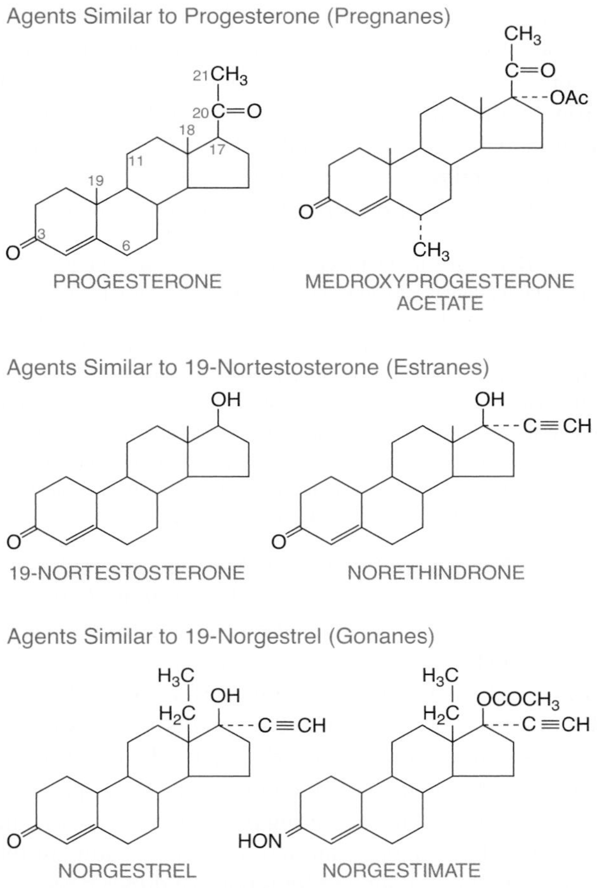

Agents Similar to Progesterone (Pregnanes)

PROGESTERONE

MEDROXYPROGESTERONE ACETATE

Agents Similar to 19-Nortestosterone (Estranes)

19-NORTESTOSTERONE

NORETHINDRONE

Agents Similar to 19-Norgestrel (Gonanes)

NORGESTREL

NORGESTIMATE

Figure 40–5. *Structural features of various progestins.*

spironolactone (e.g., drospirenone) that have anti-mineralocorticoid and anti-androgenic properties.

History. Corner and Allen originally isolated a hormone in 1933 from the corpora lutea of sows and named it "progestin." The next year, several European groups independently isolated the crystalline compound and called it "luteo-sterone," unaware of the previous name. This difference in nomenclature was resolved in 1935 at a garden party in London given by Sir Henry Dale, who helped persuade all parties that the name "progesterone" was a suitable compromise.

Two major advances overcame the early difficulties and expense of obtaining progesterone from animal sources. The first was the synthesis of progesterone by Russel Marker from the plant product diosgenin in the 1940s, which provided a relatively inexpensive and highly pure product. The second was the synthesis of 19-nor compounds, the first orally active progestins, in the early 1950s by Carl Djerassi, who synthesized norethindrone at Syntex, and Frank Colton, who synthesized the isomer *norethynodrel* at Searle. These advances led to the development of effective oral contraceptives.

Chemistry. The structural features of several progestins are shown in Figure 40–5. Unlike the ER, which requires a phenolic A ring for high-affinity binding, the progesterone receptor (PR) favors a Δ^4-3-one A-ring structure in an inverted 1β, 2α-conformation (Duax et al., 1988). Other steroid hormone receptors also bind this nonphenolic A-ring structure, although the optimal conformation differs from that for the PR. Thus, some synthetic progestins (especially the 19-nor compounds) display limited binding to glucocorticoid, androgen, and mineralocorticoid receptors, a property that probably accounts for some of their nonprogestational activities. The spectrum of activities of these compounds is highly dependent on specific substituent groups, especially the nature of the C17 substituent in the D ring, the presence of a C19 methyl group, and the presence of an ethyl group at position C13.

One major class of agents is similar to progesterone and its metabolite 17α-hydroxyprogesterone (Figure 40–5). Compounds such as hydroxyprogesterone caproate have progestational activity but must be used parenterally due to first-pass hepatic metabolism. However, further substitutions at the 6-position of the B ring yield orally active compounds such as medroxyprogesterone acetate and megestrol acetate with selective progestational activity.

The second major class of agents is 19-nor testosterone derivatives. These testosterone derivatives, lacking the C19 methyl group, display primarily progestational rather than androgenic activity. An ethinyl substituent at C17 decreases hepatic metabolism and yields orally active 19-nortestosterone analogs such as norethindrone, norethindrone acetate, norethynodrel, and ethynodiol diacetate. The activity of the latter three compounds is due primarily to their rapid *in vivo* conversion to norethindrone. These compounds are less selective than the 17α-hydroxyprogesterone derivatives just mentioned and have varying degrees of androgenic activity and, to a lesser extent, estrogenic and anti-estrogenic activities.

Replacement of the 13-methyl group of norethindrone with a 13-ethyl substituent yields the gonane norgestrel, which is a more potent progestin than the parent compound but has less androgenic activity. Norgestrel is a racemic mixture of an inactive dextrorotatory isomer and the active levorotatory isomer, levonorgestrel. Preparations containing half as much levonorgestrel as norgestrel thus have equivalent pharmacological activity. Other gonanes—including norgestimate, desogestrel, and gestodene (not available in the U.S.)—have very little if any androgenic activity at therapeutic doses.

Other steroidal progestins include the gonane dienogest; 19-norprogestin derivatives (e.g., nomegestrol, Nestorone, and trimegestone), which have increased selectivity for the progesterone receptor and less androgenic activity than estranes; and the spironolactone derivative drospirenone, which is used in combination with oral contraceptives. Like spironolactone, drospirenone is also a mineralocorticoid and androgen receptor antagonist.

Biosynthesis and Secretion. Progesterone is secreted by the ovary, mainly from the corpus luteum, during the second half of the menstrual cycle (Figure 40–3). LH, acting via its G protein-coupled receptor, stimulates progesterone secretion during the normal cycle.

After fertilization, the trophoblast secretes hCG into the maternal circulation, which then stimulates the LH receptor to sustain the corpus luteum and maintain progesterone production. During the second or third month of pregnancy, the developing placenta begins to secrete estrogen and progesterone in collaboration with the fetal adrenal glands, and thereafter the corpus luteum is not essential to continued gestation. Estrogen and progesterone continue to be secreted in large amounts by the placenta up to the time of delivery.

PHYSIOLOGICAL AND PHARMACOLOGICAL ACTIONS

Neuroendocrine Actions. As discussed earlier in this chapter, progesterone produced in the luteal phase of the cycle has several physiological effects including decreasing the frequency of GnRH pulses. This progesterone-mediated decrease in GnRH pulse frequency is critical for suppressing gonadotropin release and resetting the hypothalamic-pituitary-gonadal axis to transition from the luteal back to the follicular phase. Furthermore, GnRH suppression is the major mechanism of action of progestin-containing contraceptives.

Reproductive Tract. Progesterone decreases estrogen-driven endometrial proliferation and leads to the development of a secretory endometrium (Figure 40–3), and the abrupt decline in progesterone at the end of the cycle is the main determinant of the onset of menstruation. If the duration of the luteal phase is artificially lengthened, either by sustaining luteal function or by treatment with progesterone, decidual changes in the endometrial stroma similar to those seen in early pregnancy can be induced. Under normal circumstances, estrogen antecedes and accompanies progesterone in its action on the endometrium and is essential to the development of the normal menstrual pattern.

Progesterone also influences the endocervical glands, and the abundant watery secretion of the estrogen-stimulated structures is changed to a scant viscid material. As noted previously, these and other effects of progestins decrease penetration of the cervix by sperm.

The estrogen-induced maturation of the human vaginal epithelium is modified toward the condition of pregnancy by the action of progesterone, a change that can be detected in cytological alterations in the vaginal smear. If the quantity of estrogen concurrently acting is known to be adequate, or if it is assured by giving estrogen, the cytological response to a progestin can be used to evaluate its progestational potency.

Progesterone is very important for the maintenance of pregnancy. Progesterone suppresses menstruation and uterine contractility, but other effects also may be important. These effects to maintain pregnancy led to the historical use of progestins to prevent threatened abortion. However, such treatment is of questionable benefit, probably because spontaneous abortion infrequently results from diminished progesterone.

Mammary Gland. Development of the mammary gland requires both estrogen and progesterone. During pregnancy and to a minor degree during the luteal phase of the cycle, progesterone, acting with estrogen, brings about a proliferation of the acini of the mammary gland. Toward the end of pregnancy, the acini fill with secretions and the vasculature of the gland notably increases; however, only after the levels of estrogen and progesterone decrease at parturition does lactation begin.

During the normal menstrual cycle, mitotic activity in the breast epithelium is very low in the follicular phase and then peaks in the luteal phase. This pattern is due to progesterone, which triggers a *single* round of mitotic activity in the mammary epithelium. This effect is transient because continued exposure to the hormone is rapidly followed by arrest of growth of the epithelial cells. Importantly, progesterone may be responsible for the increased risk of breast cancer associated with estrogen-progestin use in postmenopausal women, although controlled studies with only progestin have not been performed (Anderson et al., 2004; Rossouw et al., 2002).

Central Nervous System Effects. During a normal menstrual cycle, an increase in basal body temperature of ~0.6°C (1°F) may be noted at mid-cycle; this correlates with ovulation. This increase is due to progesterone, but the exact mechanism of this effect is unknown. Progesterone also increases the ventilatory response of the respiratory centers to carbon dioxide and leads to reduced arterial and alveolar P_{CO_2} in the luteal phase of the menstrual cycle and during pregnancy. Progesterone also may have depressant and hypnotic actions in the CNS, possibly accounting for reports of drowsiness after hormone administration. This potential untoward effect may be abrogated by giving progesterone preparations at bedtime, which may even help some patients sleep.

Metabolic Effects. Progestins have numerous metabolic actions. Progesterone itself increases basal insulin levels and the rise in insulin after carbohydrate ingestion, but it does not normally alter glucose tolerance. However, long-term administration of more potent progestins, such as norgestrel, may decrease glucose tolerance. Progesterone stimulates lipoprotein lipase activity and seems to enhance fat deposition. Progesterone and analogs such as MPA have been reported to increase LDL and cause either no effects or modest reductions in serum HDL levels. The 19-norprogestins may have more pronounced effects on plasma lipids because of their androgenic activity.

In this regard, a large prospective study has shown that MPA decreases the favorable HDL increase caused by conjugated estrogens during postmenopausal hormone replacement, but it does not significantly affect the beneficial effect of estrogens to lower LDL. In contrast, micronized progesterone does not significantly alter beneficial estrogen effects on either HDL or LDL profiles (Writing

Group for the PEPI Trial, 1995); the spironolactone derivative drospirenone may actually have advantageous effects on the cardiovascular system due to its anti-androgenic and anti-mineralocorticoid activities. Progesterone also may diminish the effects of aldosterone in the renal tubule and cause a decrease in sodium reabsorption that may increase mineralocorticoid secretion from the adrenal cortex.

Mechanism of Action

A single gene that encodes two isoforms of the progesterone receptor, PR-A and PR-B. The first 164 N-terminal amino acids of PR-B are missing from PR-A; this occurs by use of two distinct estrogen-dependent promoters in the PR gene (Giangrande and McDonnell, 1999). The ratios of the individual isoforms vary in reproductive tissues as a consequence of tissue type, developmental status, and hormone levels. Both PR-A and PR-B have AF-1 and AF-2 transactivation domains, but the longer PR-B also contains an additional AF-3 that contributes to its cell- and promoter-specific activity. Because the ligand-binding domains of the two PR isoforms are identical, there is no difference in ligand binding. In the absence of ligand, PR is present primarily in the nucleus in an inactive monomeric state bound to heat-shock proteins (HSP-90, HSP-70, and p59). When receptors bind progesterone, the heat-shock proteins dissociate, and the receptors are phosphorylated and subsequently form dimers (homo- and heterodimers) that bind with high selectivity to PREs (progesterone response elements) located on target genes (Giangrande and McDonnell, 1999). Transcriptional activation by PR occurs primarily via recruitment of co-activators such as SRC-1, NcoA-1, or NcoA-2 (Collingwood et al., 1999). The receptor–co-activator complex then favors further interactions with additional proteins such as CBP and p300, which mediate other processes including histone acetylase activity. Histone acetylation causes a remodeling of chromatin that increases the accessibility of general transcriptional proteins, including RNA polymerase II, to the target promoter. Progesterone antagonists also facilitate receptor dimerization and DNA binding, but, as with ER, the conformation of antagonist-bound PR is different from that of agonist-bound PR. This different conformation favors PR interaction with co-repressors such as NCoR/SMRT, which recruit histone deacetylases. Histone deacetylation increases DNA interaction with nucleosomes and renders a target promoter inaccessible to the general transcription apparatus.

The biological activities of PR-A and PR-B are distinct and depend on the target gene in question. In most cells, PR-B mediates the stimulatory activities of progesterone; PR-A strongly inhibits this action of PR-B and is also a transcriptional inhibitor of other steroid receptors (McDonnell and Goldman, 1994). Current data suggest that co-activators and co-repressors interact differentially with PR-A and PR-B (e.g., the co-repressor SMRT binds much more tightly to PR-A than to PR-B) (Giangrande et al., 2000), and this may account, at least in part, for the differential activities of the two isoforms. Female PR-A knockout mice are infertile, with impaired ovulation and defective decidualization and implantation. Several uterine genes appear to be regulated exclusively by PR-A, including calcitonin and amphiregulin (Mulac-Jericevic et al., 2000), and the antiproliferative effect of progesterone on the estrogen-stimulated endometrium is lost in PR-A knockout mice. In contrast, knockout studies suggest that PR-B is largely responsible for mediating hormone effects in the mammary gland (Mulac-Jericevic et al., 2003).

Certain effects of progesterone, such as increased Ca^{2+} mobilization in sperm, can be seen in as little as 3 minutes (Blackmore, 1999) and are therefore considered transcription independent. Similarly, progesterone can promote oocyte maturation (meiotic resumption) independent of transcription (Hammes, 2004). There is debate regarding the identity of the receptors mediating these progestin-induced processes, as well as their physiological importance in humans.

Absorption, Fate, and Excretion

Progesterone undergoes rapid first-pass metabolism, but high-dose (e.g., 100-200 mg) preparations of micronized progesterone (PROMETRIUM) are available for oral use. Although the absolute bioavailability of these preparations is low (Fotherby, 1996), efficacious plasma levels nevertheless may be obtained. Progesterone also is available in oil solution for injection, as a vaginal gel (CRINONE, PROCHIEVE), as a slow-release intrauterine device (PROGESTASERT) for contraception, and as a vaginal insert (ENDOMETRIN) for assisted reproductive technology.

Esters such as MPA (DEPO-PROVERA) are available for intramuscular administration, and MPA (PROVERA, others) and megestrol acetate (MEGACE, others) may be used orally. The 19-nor steroids have good oral activity because the ethinyl substituent at C17 significantly slows hepatic metabolism. Implants and depot preparations of synthetic progestins are available in many countries for release over very long periods of time (see later section on contraceptives).

In the plasma, progesterone is bound by albumin and corticosteroid-binding globulin but is not appreciably bound to SHBG. 19-Nor compounds, such as norethindrone, norgestrel, and desogestrel, bind to SHBG and albumin, and esters such as MPA bind primarily to albumin. Total binding of all these synthetic compounds to plasma proteins is extensive, ≤90%, but the proteins involved are compound specific.

The elimination $t_{1/2}$ of progesterone is ~5 minutes, and the hormone is metabolized primarily in the liver to hydroxylated metabolites and their sulfate and glucuronide conjugates, which are eliminated in the urine. A major metabolite specific for progesterone is pregnane-3α, 20 α-diol; its measurement in urine and plasma is used as an index of endogenous progesterone secretion. The synthetic progestins have much longer half-lives (e.g., ~7 hours for norethindrone, 16 hours for norgestrel, 12 hours for gestodene, and 24 hours for MPA). The metabolism of synthetic progestins is thought to be primarily hepatic, and elimination is generally via the urine as conjugates and various polar metabolites, although their metabolism is not as clearly defined as that of progesterone.

Therapeutic Uses

The two most frequent uses of progestins are for contraception, either alone or with an estrogen (Chapter 66; see also later in this chapter), and in combination with estrogen for hormone therapy of postmenopausal women.

Progestins also are used diagnostically for secondary amenorrhea. An oral progestin is given to an amenorrheic woman for 5-7 days. If endogenous estrogens are present, withdrawal bleeding will occur. Combinations of estrogens and progestins can also be given to test for endometrial responsiveness in patients with amenorrhea.

In addition, progestins are highly efficacious in decreasing the occurrence of endometrial hyperplasia and carcinoma caused by unopposed estrogens; when used in this setting, there appears to be less irregular uterine bleeding with sequential rather than continuous administration. Local intrauterine application via a hormone-releasing intrauterine device (IUD) containing levonorgestrel can be used to decrease estrogen-induced endometrial hyperplasia while reducing untoward effects (e.g., unfavorable lipid profiles and incidence of breast cancer) of systemically administered progestins.

Finally, levonorgestrel is used as so-called emergency contraception after known or suspected unprotected intercourse. The medication is given orally within 72 hours after intercourse as either a single 1.5-mg dose (PLAN B ONE STEP) or as two 0.75-mg doses (PLAN B) separated by 12 hours. The mechanism of action may involve several factors, including the prevention of ovulation, fertilization, and implantation.

ANTI-PROGESTINS AND PROGESTERONE-RECEPTOR MODULATORS

The first report of an anti-progestin, RU 38486 (often referred to as RU-486) or *mifepristone*, appeared in 1981; this drug is available for the termination of pregnancy (Christin-Maitre et al., 2000). In 2010, the FDA approved ulipristal acetate [ella (U.S.), ellaOne (E.U.)], a partial agonist at the progsterone receptor, for emergency contraception. Anti-progestins also have several other potential applications, including to prevent conception, to induce labor, and to treat uterine leiomyomas, endometriosis, meningiomas, and breast cancer (Spitz and Chwalisz, 2000).

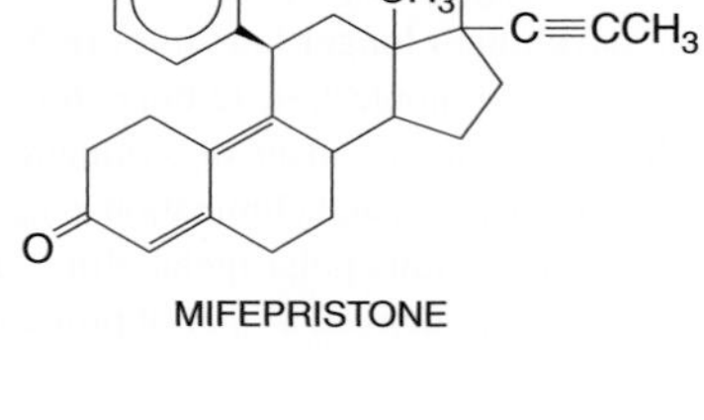

CH_3 OH
$-C{\equiv}CCH_3$

MIFEPRISTONE

CH_3 $CH_2CH_2CH_2OH$
OH

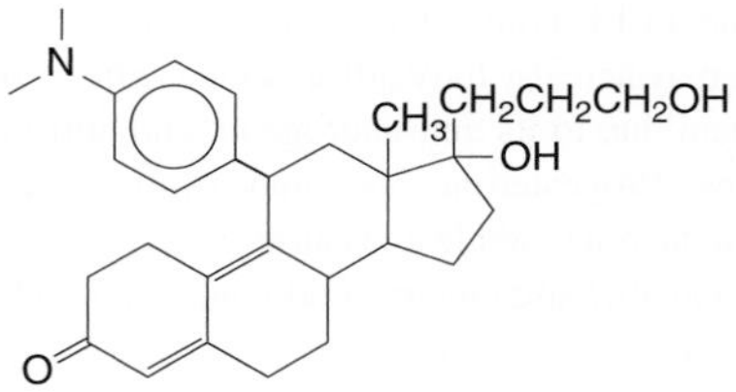

ONAPRISTONE

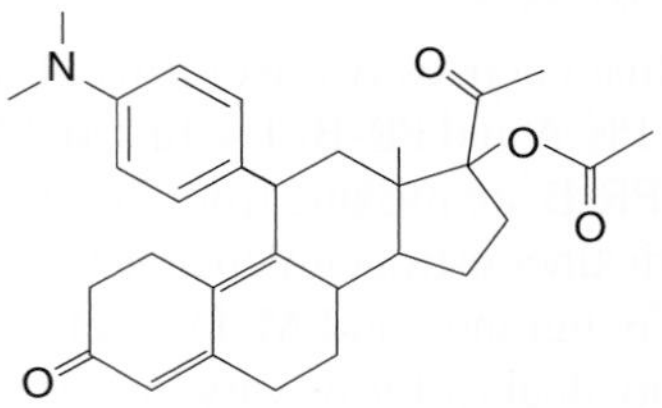

ULIPRISTAL ACETATE

Mifepristone

Chemistry. Mifepristone is a derivative of the 19-norprogestin norethindrone containing a dimethyl-aminophenol substituent at the 11β-position. It effectively competes with both progesterone and glucocorticoids for binding to their respective receptors. Mifepristone was initially thought to be a pure anti-progestin, although it is now considered a progesterone-receptor modulator (PRM) due to its context-dependent activity.

Other PRMs and pure progesterone antagonists now have been synthesized, and most contain an 11β-aromatic group. Another widely studied anti-progestin is onapristone (or ZK 98299), which is similar in structure to mifepristone but contains a methyl substituent in the 13α rather than 13β orientation. More selective progesterone-receptor modulators, such as asoprisnil, are being studied experimentally (DeManno et al., 2003).

Pharmacological Actions. Mifepristone acts primarily as a competitive receptor antagonist for both progesterone receptors, although it may have some agonist activity in certain contexts. In contrast, onapristone appears to be a pure progesterone antagonist. PR complexes of both compounds antagonize the actions of progesterone-PR complexes and also appear to preferentially recruit corepressors (Leonhardt and Edwards, 2002).

When administered in the early stages of pregnancy, mifepristone causes decidual breakdown by blockade of uterine progesterone receptors. This leads to detachment of the blastocyst, which decreases hCG production. This in turn causes a decrease in progesterone secretion from the corpus luteum, which further accentuates decidual breakdown. Decreased endogenous progesterone coupled with blockade of progesterone receptors in the uterus increases uterine prostaglandin levels and sensitizes the myometrium to their contractile actions. Mifepristone also causes cervical softening, which facilitates expulsion of the detached blastocyst.

Mifepristone can delay or prevent ovulation depending on the timing and manner of administration. These effects are due largely to actions on the hypothalamus and pituitary rather than the ovary, although the mechanisms are unclear.

If administered for one or several days in the mid- to late luteal phase, mifepristone impairs the development of a secretory endometrium and produces menses. Progesterone-receptor blockade at this time is the pharmacological equivalent of progesterone withdrawal, and bleeding normally ensues within several days and lasts for 1-2 weeks after anti-progestin treatment.

Mifepristone also binds to glucocorticoid and androgen receptors and exerts anti-glucocorticoid and anti-androgenic actions. A predominant effect in humans is blockade of the feedback inhibition by cortisol of adenocorticotropic hormone secretion from the pituitary, thus increasing both corticotropin and adrenal steroid levels in the plasma.

Absorption, Fate, and Excretion. Mifepristone is orally active with good bioavailability. Peak plasma levels occur within several hours, and the drug is slowly cleared with a plasma $t_{1/2}$ of 20-40 hours. In plasma, it is bound by α_1-acid glycoprotein, which contributes to the drug's long $t_{1/2}$. Metabolites are primarily the mono- and di-demethylated products (thought to have pharmacological activity) formed via CYP3A4-catalyzed reactions and, to a lesser extent, hydroxylated compounds. The drug undergoes hepatic metabolism and enterohepatic circulation; metabolic products are found predominantly in the feces (Jang and Benet, 1997).

Therapeutic Uses and Prospects. Mifepristone (MIFEPREX), in combination with misoprostol or other prostaglandins, is available for the termination of early pregnancy.

When mifepristone is used to produce a medical abortion, a prostaglandin is given 48 hours after the anti-progestin to further increase myometrial contractions and ensure expulsion of the detached blastocyst. Intramuscular *sulprostone*, intravaginal *gemeprost*, and oral misoprostol have been used. The success rate with such regimens is >90% among women with pregnancies of ≤49 days' duration. The most severe untoward effect is vaginal bleeding, which most often lasts 8-17 days but is only rarely (0.1% of patients) severe enough to require blood transfusions. High percentages of women also have experienced abdominal pain and uterine cramps, nausea, vomiting, and diarrhea due to the prostaglandin. Women receiving chronic glucocorticoid therapy should not be given mifepristone because of its anti-glucocorticoid activity. In fact, due to its high affinity for the glucocorticoid receptor, high doses of mifepristone can result in adrenal insufficiency; thus mifepristone is being considered as a chemical treatment for diseases of excess adrenal cortisol secretion.

Ulipristal

Chemistry. Ulipristal, a derivative of 19-norprogesterone, functions as a selective progesterone receptor modulator (SPRM), acting as a partial agonist at progesterone receptors. It has a dimethylaminophenol group at the 11β position, as does mifepristone, with an additional acetoxy group at the C17. Unlike mifepristone, ulipristal appears to be a relatively weak glucocorticoid antagonist.

Pharmacological Actions. In high doses, ulipristal has anti-proliferative effects in the uterus; however, its most relevant actions to date involve its capacity to inhibit ovulation. Ulipristal's anti-ovulatory actions likely occur due to progesterone regulation at many levels, including inhibition of LH release through the hypothalamus and pituitary, and inhibition of LH-induced follicular rupture within the ovary.

A 30-mg dose of ulipristral can inhibit ovulation when taken up to five days after intercourse. Ulipristal can block ovarian rupture at or even just after the time of the LH surge, confirming that at least some of its effects are directly in the ovary. Ulipristal may also block endometrial implantation of the fertilized egg, although whether this contributes to its effects as an emergency contraceptive (see below) is not clear.

Therapeutic Uses. Ulipristal acetate [ella, ellaOne] has recently been licensed in the E.U. and the U.S. as an emergency contraceptive. Studies comparing ulipristal to levonorgestrel (progesterone-only emergency contraception, or POEC) demonstrate that ulipristal is at least as effective when taken up to 72 hours after unprotected sexual intercourse. In addition, ulipristal remains effective up to 120 hours (5 days) after intercourse, making ulipristal a more versatile emergency contraceptive than levonorgestrel, which does not work well beyond 72 hours after unprotected intercourse. The most severe side effect in clinical trials using ulipristal has been a self-limited headache and some abdominal pain.

HORMONAL CONTRACEPTIVES

The incredible growth of the earth's human population stands out as one of the fundamental events of the last two centuries. The Old Testament dictum "Be fruitful and multiply" (Genesis 9:1) has been followed too religiously by readers and nonreaders of the Bible alike. In 1798, Malthus started a great controversy by opposing the prevailing view of unlimited progress for humankind by making two postulates and a conclusion. Malthus postulated "that food is necessary for the existence of man" and that sexual attraction between female and male is necessary and likely to persist, since "toward the extinction of the passion between the sexes, no progress whatever has hitherto been made," barring "individual exceptions." Malthus concluded that "the power of populations is infinitely greater than the power of the earth to produce subsistence for man," producing a "natural inequality" that would someday loom "insurmountable in the way to perfectibility of society."

Malthus was right: The passion between the sexes has persisted, and the power of populations is very great indeed, so much so that our sheer numbers have increased to the point that they are straining the earth's capacity to supply food, energy, and raw materials, and to absorb the detritus of its human burden. Marine fisheries are being depleted, forests and aquifers are disappearing, and the atmosphere is accumulating greenhouse gases from combustion of the fossil fuels that provide the energy needs of almost 7 billion people. Perhaps some of the blame can be laid at the feet of medical science: Advances in public health and medicine have led to a significant decline in mortality and an increased life expectancy. However, medical science has also begun to assume a portion of the responsibility for overpopulation and its adverse effects. To this end, drugs in the form of hormones and their analogs have been developed to control human fertility.

History. Around the beginning of the 20th century, a number of European scientists, including Beard, Prenant, and Loeb, developed the concept that secretions of the corpus luteum suppressed ovulation during pregnancy. The Austrian physiologist Haberlandt then produced temporary sterility in rodents in 1927 by feeding ovarian and placental extracts—a clear example of an oral contraceptive! In 1937, Makepeace and colleagues demonstrated that pure progesterone blocked ovulation in rabbits, and Astwood and Fevold found a similar effect in rats in 1939.

In the 1950s, Pincus, Garcia, and Rock found that progesterone and 19-norprogestins prevented ovulation in women. Ironically, this finding grew out of their attempts to treat infertility with progestins or estrogen-progestin combinations. The initial findings were that either treatment effectively blocked ovulation in most women. However, concern about cancer and other possible side effects of the estrogen they used (i.e., DES) led to the use of a progestin alone in their studies. One of the compounds used was norethynodrel, and early batches of this compound were contaminated with a small amount of mestranol. When mestranol was removed, it was noted that treatment with pure norethynodrel led to increased breakthrough bleeding and less consistent inhibition of ovulation. Mestranol was thus reincorporated into the preparation, and this combination was employed in the first large-scale clinical trial of combination oral contraceptives.

Clinical studies in the 1950s in Puerto Rico and Haiti established the virtually complete contraceptive success of the norethynodrel/mestranol combination. In early 1961, ENOVID (norethynodrel plus mestranol; no longer marketed in the U.S.) was the first "Pill" approved by the FDA for use as a contraceptive agent in the U.S.; this was followed in 1962 by approval for ORTHO-NOVUM (norethindrone plus mestranol). By 1966, numerous preparations using either mestranol or ethinyl estradiol with a 19-norprogestin were available. In the 1960s, the progestin-only minipill and long-acting injectable preparations were developed and introduced.

Millions of women began using oral contraceptives, and frequent reports of untoward effects began appearing in the 1970s. The recognition that these side effects were dose-dependent and the realization that estrogens and progestins synergistically inhibited ovulation led to the reduction of doses and the development of so-called low-dose or second-generation contraceptives. The increasing use of biphasic and triphasic preparations throughout the 1980s further reduced steroid dosages; it may be that currently used doses are the lowest that will provide reliable contraception. In the 1990s, the "third-generation" oral contraceptives, containing progestins with reduced androgenic activity (e.g., norgestimate [ORTHO-CYCLEN, ORTHO TRI-CYCLEN LO, others] and desogestrel [DESOGEN, others]), became available in the U.S. after being used in Europe. A variety of contraceptive formulations are currently available, including pills, injections, skin patches, subdermal implants, vaginal rings, and IUDs that release hormones.

Types of Hormonal Contraceptives

Combination Oral Contraceptives. The most frequently used agents in the U.S. are combination oral contraceptives containing both an estrogen and a progestin. Their theoretical efficacy generally is considered to be 99.9%. Combination oral contraceptives are available in many formulations. Monophasic, biphasic, or triphasic pills are generally provided in 21-day packs. (Virtually all preparations come as 28-day packs, with the pills for the last 7 days containing only inert ingredients.) For the monophasic agents, fixed amounts of the estrogen and progestin are present in each pill, which is taken daily for 21 days, followed by a 7-day "pill-free" period. The biphasic and triphasic preparations provide two or three different pills containing varying amounts of active ingredients, to be taken at different times during the 21-day cycle. This reduces the total amount of steroids administered and more closely approximates the estrogen-to-progestin ratios that occur during the menstrual cycle. With these preparations, predictable menstrual bleeding generally occurs during the 7-day "off" period each month. However, several oral contraceptions are now available whereby progestin withdrawal is only induced every 3 months.

The estrogen content of current preparations ranges from 20 to 50 μg; most contain 30-35 μg. Preparations containing ≤35 μg of an estrogen are generally referred to as "low-dose" or "modern" pills. The dose of progestin is more variable because of differences in potency of the compounds used. For example, monophasic pills currently available in the U.S. contain 0.4-1.5 mg of norethindrone, 0.09-0.15 mg of levonorgestrel, 0.3-0.5 mg of norgestrel, 1 mg of ethynodiol diacetate, 0.25 mg of norgestimate, or 0.15 mg of desogestrel, with slightly different dose ranges in biphasic and triphasic preparations. In contrast, most first-generation preparations (circa 1966) contained 50-100 μg of an estrogen and 2-10 mg of a progestin. These large differences in doses complicate extrapolation of data from early epidemiological studies on the side effects of "high-dose" oral contraceptives to the "low-dose" preparations now used.

A transdermal preparation of norelgestromin and ethinyl estradiol (ORTHO EVRA) is marketed for weekly application to the buttock, abdomen, upper arm, or torso for the first 3 consecutive weeks followed by a patch-free week for each 28-day cycle. A similar 3-week on/1-week off cycle is employed for the intravaginal ring containing ethinyl estradiol and etonogestrel (NUVARING).

Progestin-Only Contraceptives. Several agents are available for progestin-only contraception, with theoretical efficacies of 99%. Specific preparations include the "minipill"; low doses of progestins (e.g., 350 μg of norethindrone [NOR-QD, ORTHO MICRONOR, others]) taken daily without interruption; subdermal implants of 216 mg of norgestrel (NORPLANT II, JADELLE) for long-term contraceptive action (e.g., up to 5 years) or 68 mg of etonogestrel (IMPLANON) for contraception lasting 3 years; and crystalline suspensions of medroxyprogesterone acetate for intramuscular injection of 104 mg (DEPO-SUBQ PROVERA 104) or 150 mg (DEPO-PROVERA, others) of drug; each provides effective contraception for 3 months.

An IUD (PROGESTASERT) that releases low amounts of progesterone locally is available for insertion on a yearly basis. Its effectiveness is considered to be 97-98%, and contraceptive action probably is due to local effects on the endometrium. An intrauterine device (MIRENA) releases levonorgestrel for up to 5 years. It inhibits ovulation in some women but is thought to act primarily by producing local effects.

Mechanism of Action

Combination Oral Contraceptives. Combination oral contraceptives act by preventing ovulation (Lobo and Stanczyk, 1994). Direct measurements of plasma hormone levels indicate that LH and FSH levels are suppressed, a mid-cycle surge of LH is absent, endogenous steroid levels are diminished, and ovulation does not occur. Although either component alone can be shown to exert these effects in certain situations, the combination synergistically decreases plasma gonadotropin levels and suppresses ovulation more consistently than either alone.

Given the multiple actions of estrogens and progestins on the hypothalamic-pituitary-ovarian axis during the menstrual cycle and the extraordinary efficacy of these agents, several effects probably contribute to the blockade of ovulation.

Hypothalamic actions of steroids play a major role in the mechanism of oral contraceptive action. Progesterone diminishes the frequency of GnRH pulses. Because the proper frequency of LH pulses is essential for ovulation, this effect of progesterone likely plays a major role in the contraceptive action of these agents. In monkeys and women with normal menstrual cycles, estrogens do not affect the frequency of the pulse generator. However, in the prolonged absence of a menstrual cycle (e.g., in ovariectomized monkeys and postmenopausal women; Hotchkiss and Knobil, 1994), estrogens markedly diminish pulse-generator frequency, and progesterone enhances this effect. In theory, this hypothalamic effect of estrogens could come into play when oral contraceptives are used for extended time periods.

Multiple pituitary effects of both estrogen and progestin components are thus likely to contribute to oral contraceptive action. Oral contraceptives seem likely to decrease pituitary responsiveness to GnRH. Estrogens also suppress FSH release from the pituitary during the follicular phase of the menstrual cycle, and this effect seems likely to contribute to the lack of follicular development in oral contraceptive users. The progestin component may also inhibit the estrogen-induced LH surge at mid-cycle. Other effects may contribute to a minor extent to the extraordinary efficacy of oral contraceptives. Transit of sperm, the egg, and fertilized ovum are important to establish pregnancy, and steroids are likely to affect transport in the fallopian tube. In the cervix, progestin effects also are likely to produce a thick viscous mucus to reduce sperm penetration and in the endometrium to produce a state that is not receptive to implantation. However, it is difficult to assess quantitatively the contributions of these effects because the drugs block ovulation so effectively.

Progestin-Only Contraceptives. Progestin-only pills and levonorgestrel implants are highly efficacious but block ovulation in only 60-80% of cycles. Their effectiveness is thus thought to be due largely to a thickening of cervical mucus, which decreases sperm penetration, and to endometrial alterations that impair implantation; such local effects account for the efficacy of IUDs that release progestins. Depot injections of MPA are thought to exert similar effects, but they also yield plasma levels of drug high enough to prevent ovulation in virtually all patients, presumably by decreasing the frequency of GnRH pulses.

Untoward Effects

Combination Oral Contraceptives. Shortly after the introduction of oral contraceptives, reports of adverse side effects associated with their use began to appear. Many of the side effects were found to be dose dependent, and this led to the development of current low-dose preparations. Untoward effects of early hormonal contraceptives fell into several major categories: adverse cardiovascular effects, including hypertension, myocardial infarction, hemorrhagic or ischemic stroke, and venous thrombosis and embolism; breast, hepatocellular, and cervical cancers; and a number of endocrine and metabolic effects. The current consensus is that low-dose preparations pose minimal health risks in women who have no predisposing risk factors, and these drugs also provide many beneficial health effects (Burkman et al., 2004).

Cardiovascular Effects. The question of cardiovascular side effects has been reexamined for the newer low-dose oral contraceptives (Burkman et al., 2004; Sherif, 1999). For nonsmokers without other risk factors such as hypertension or diabetes, there is no significant increase in the risk of myocardial infarction or stroke. There is a 28% increase in relative risk for venous thromboembolism, but the estimated absolute increase is very small because the incidence of these events in women without other predisposing factors is low (e.g., roughly half that associated with the risk of venous thromboembolism in pregnancy). Nevertheless, the risk is significantly increased in women who smoke or have other factors that predispose to thrombosis or thromboembolism (Castelli, 1999). Of note, postmarketing epidemiologic studies indicate that women using transdermal contraceptives have a higher than expected exposure to estrogen and are at increased risk for the development of venous thromboembolism. Early high-dose combination oral contraceptives caused hypertension in 4-5% of normotensive women and increased blood pressure in 10-15% of those with preexisting hypertension. This incidence is much lower with newer low-dose preparations, and most reported changes in blood pressure are not significant. The cardiovascular risk associated with oral contraceptive use does not appear to persist after use is discontinued. As noted previously, estrogens increase serum HDL and decrease LDL levels, and progestins tend to have the opposite effect. Recent studies of several low-dose preparations have not found significant changes in total serum cholesterol or lipoprotein profiles, although slight increases in triglycerides have been reported.

Cancer. Given the growth-promoting effects of estrogens, there has been a long-standing concern that oral contraceptives might increase the incidence of endometrial, cervical, ovarian, breast, and other cancers. These concerns were further heightened in the late 1960s by reports of endometrial changes caused by sequential oral contraceptives, which have since been removed from the market in the U.S. However, it is now clear that there is *not* a widespread association between oral contraceptive use and cancer (Burkman et al., 2004; Westhoff, 1999).

Epidemiological evidence suggests that combined oral contraceptive use may increase the risk of cervical cancer by about 2-fold but only in long-term users (>5 years) with persistent human papilloma virus infection (Moodley, 2004).

There have been reports of increases in the incidence of hepatic adenoma and hepatocellular carcinoma in oral contraceptive users. Current estimates indicate there is about a doubling in the risk of liver cancer after 4-8 years of use. However, these are rare cancers, and the absolute increases are small.

The major present concern about the carcinogenic effects of oral contraceptives is focused on breast cancer. Numerous studies have dealt with this issue, and the following general picture has emerged. The risk of breast cancer in women of childbearing age is very low, and current oral contraceptive users in this group have only a very small increase in relative risk of 1.1-1.2, depending on other variables. This small increase is not substantially affected by duration of use, dose or type of component, age at first use, or parity. Importantly, 10 years after discontinuation of oral contraceptive use, there is no difference in breast cancer incidence between past users and never users. In addition, breast cancers diagnosed in women who have ever used oral contraceptives are more likely to be localized to the breast and thus easier to treat (i.e., are less likely to have spread to other sites) (Westhoff, 1999). Thus overall there is no significant difference in the cumulative risk of breast cancer between those who have ever used oral contraceptives and those who have never used them.

Combination oral contraceptives do *not* increase the incidence of endometrial cancer but actually cause a 50% *decrease* in the incidence of this disease, which lasts 15 years after the pills are stopped. This is thought to be due to the inclusion of a progestin, which opposes estrogen-induced proliferation, throughout the entire 21-day cycle of administration. These agents also decrease the incidence of ovarian cancer, and decreased ovarian stimulation by gonadotropins provides a logical basis for this effect. There are accumulating data that oral contraceptive use decreases the risk of colorectal cancer (Fernandez et al., 2001).

Metabolic and Endocrine Effects. The effects of sex steroids on glucose metabolism and insulin sensitivity are complex (Godsland, 1996) and may differ among agents in the same class (e.g., the 19-nor progestins). Early studies with high-dose oral contraceptives generally reported impaired glucose tolerance as demonstrated by increases in fasting glucose and insulin levels and responses to glucose challenge. These effects have decreased as steroid dosages have been lowered, and current low-dose combination contraceptives may even improve insulin sensitivity. Similarly, the high-dose progestins in early oral contraceptives did raise LDL and reduce HDL levels, but modern low-dose preparations do not produce unfavorable lipid profiles (Sherif, 1999). There also have been periodic reports that oral contraceptives increase the incidence of gallbladder disease, but any such effect appears to be weak and limited to current or very long-term users (Burkman et al., 2004).

The estrogenic component of oral contraceptives may increase hepatic synthesis of a number of serum proteins, including those that bind thyroid hormones, glucocorticoids, and sex steroids. Although physiological feedback mechanisms generally adjust hormone synthesis to maintain normal "free" hormone levels, these changes can affect the interpretation of endocrine function tests that measure *total* plasma hormone levels, and may necessitate dose adjustment in patients receiving thyroid-hormone replacement.

The ethinyl estradiol present in oral contraceptives appears to cause a dose-dependent increase in several serum factors known to increase coagulation. However, in healthy women who do not smoke, there also is an increase in fibrinolytic activity, which exerts a counter effect so that overall there is a minimal effect on hemostatic balance. In women who smoke, however, this compensatory effect is diminished, which may shift the hemostatic profile toward a hypercoagulable condition (Fruzzetti, 1999).

Miscellaneous Effects. Nausea, edema, and mild headache occur in some individuals, and more severe migraine headaches may be precipitated by oral contraceptive use in a smaller fraction of women. Some patients may experience breakthrough bleeding during the 21-day cycle when the active pills are being taken. Withdrawal bleeding may fail to occur in a small fraction of women during the 7-day "off" period, thus causing confusion about a possible pregnancy. Acne and hirsutism are thought to be mediated by the androgenic activity of the 19-nor progestins.

Progestin-Only Contraceptives. Episodes of irregular, unpredictable spotting and breakthrough bleeding are the most frequently encountered untoward effect and the major reason women discontinue use of all three types of progestin-only contraceptives. With time, the incidence of these bleeding episodes decreases, especially with the long-acting preparations, and amenorrhea becomes common after a year or more of use.

No evidence indicates that the progestin-only minipill preparations increase thromboembolic events, which are thought to be related to the estrogenic component of combination preparations; blood pressure does not appear to be elevated, and nausea and breast tenderness do not occur. Acne may be a problem, however, because of the androgenic activity of norethindrone-containing preparations. These preparations may be attractive for nursing mothers because they do not decrease lactation as do products containing estrogens.

Aside from bleeding irregularities, headache is the most commonly reported untoward effect of depot MPA. Mood changes and weight gain also have been reported, but controlled clinical studies of these effects are not available. It is of more concern that many studies have found decreases in HDL levels and increases in LDL levels, and there have been several reports of decreased bone density. These effects may be due to reduced endogenous estrogens because depot MPA is particularly effective in lowering gonadotropin levels. Numerous human studies have not found any increases in breast, endometrial, cervical, or ovarian cancer in women receiving MPA (Westhoff, 2003). Because of the time required to completely eliminate the drug, the contraceptive effect of this agent may remain for 6-12 months after the last injection.

Implants of norethindrone may be associated with infection, local irritation, pain at the insertion site, and, rarely, expulsion of the inserts. Headache, weight gain, and mood changes have been reported, and acne is seen in some patients. A number of metabolic studies have been performed in users of norplant (no longer marketed in the U.S.), and in most cases only minimal changes have been observed in lipid, carbohydrate, and protein metabolism. In women desiring pregnancy, ovulation occurs fairly soon after implant removal, reaching 50% in 3 months and almost 90% within 1 year.

Contraindications

Although the use of modern oral contraceptives is considered generally safe in most healthy women, *these agents can contribute to the incidence and severity of cardiovascular, thromboembolic, or malignant disease, particularly if other risk factors are present.* The following conditions are thus considered absolute contraindications for combination oral contraceptive use: the presence or history of thromboembolic disease, cerebrovascular disease, myocardial infarction, coronary artery disease, or congenital hyperlipidemia; known or suspected carcinoma of the breast, carcinoma of the female reproductive tract; abnormal undiagnosed vaginal bleeding; known or suspected pregnancy; and past or present liver tumors or impaired liver function. *The risk of serious cardiovascular side effects is particularly marked in women >35 years of age who smoke heavily* (e.g., >15 cigarettes per day); even low-dose oral contraceptives are contraindicated in such patients.

Several other conditions are relative contraindications and should be considered on an individual basis. These include migraine headaches, hypertension, diabetes mellitus, obstructive jaundice of pregnancy or prior oral contraceptive use, and gallbladder disease. If elective surgery is planned, many physicians recommend discontinuation of oral contraceptives for several weeks to a month to minimize the possibility of thromboembolism after surgery. These agents should be used with care in women with prior gestational diabetes or uterine fibroids, and low-dose pills should generally be used in such cases.

Progestin-only contraceptives are contraindicated in the presence of undiagnosed vaginal bleeding, benign or malignant liver disease, and known or suspected breast cancer. Depot MPA and levonorgestrel inserts are contraindicated in women with a history or predisposition to thrombophlebitis or thromboembolic disorders.

Choice of Contraceptive Preparations

Treatment should generally begin with preparations containing the minimum dose of steroids that provides effective contraceptive coverage. This is typically a pill with 30-35 μg of estrogen, but preparations with 20 μg may be adequate for lighter women or >40 years of age with perimenopausal symptoms; a preparation containing 50 μg of estrogen may be required for heavier women.

In women for whom estrogens are contraindicated or undesirable, progestin-only contraceptives may be an option. The progestin-only minipill may have enhanced effectiveness in several such types of women (e.g., nursing mothers and women >40 years of age, in whom fertility may be decreased).

The choice of a preparation also may be influenced by the specific 19-nor progestin component because this component may have varying degrees of androgenic and other activities. The androgenic activity of this component may contribute to untoward effects such as weight gain, acne due to increased sebaceous gland secretions, and unfavorable lipoprotein profiles. These side effects are greatly reduced in newer low-dose contraceptives that contain progestins with little to no androgenic activity.

In summary, for a given individual, both the efficacy and side effects of hormonal contraceptives may vary considerably among preparations. A number of choices are available to counter the development of side effects and improve patient tolerance, both in terms of specific components and routes of administration, without decreasing contraceptive efficacy. Risks for serious side effects as enumerated earlier should be considered before initiating contraceptives in any individual patient.

Noncontraceptive Health Benefits

It is generally accepted that combination oral contraceptives have substantial health benefits unrelated to their contraceptive use. Oral contraceptives significantly reduce the incidence of ovarian and endometrial cancer within 6 months of use, and the incidence is decreased 50% after 2 years of use. Depot MPA injections also reduce very substantially the incidence of uterine cancer. Furthermore, this protective effect persists for up to 15 years after oral contraceptive use

Grumbach MM, Auchus RJ. Estrogen: Consequences and implications of human mutations in synthesis and action. *J Clin Endocrinol Metab*, **1999,** *84:*4677–4694.

Hall JM, McDonnell DP. The estrogen receptor β-isoform (ER β) of the human estrogen receptor modulates ER β transcriptional activity and is a key regulator of the cellular response to estrogens and antiestrogens. *Endocrinology*, **1999,** *140:* 5566–5578.

Hall JM, McDonnel DP, Korach KS. Allosteric regulation of estrogen receptor structure, function, and coactivator recruiment by different estrogen response elements. *Mol Endocrinol*, **2002,** *16:*469–486.

Hammes SR. Steroids and oocyte maturation—a new look at an old story. *Molecular Endocrinology*, **2004,** *18*:769–775.

Hammes SR, Levin ER. Extra-nuclear steroid receptors: Nature and function. *Endo Rev,* **2007,** *28:*726–741.

Han W, Kang D, Lee KM, *et al*. Full sequencing analysis of estrogen receptor-α gene polymorphism and its association with breast cancer risk. *Anticancer Res*, **2003,** *23:*4703–4707.

Hanstein B, Djahansouzi S, Dall P, *et al*. Insights into the molecular biology of the estrogen receptor define novel therapeutic targets for breast cancer. *Eur J Endocrinol*, **2004,** *150:*243–255.

Harrington WR, Sheng S, Barnett DH, *et al*. Activities of estrogen receptor α- and β-selective ligands at diverse estrogen responsive gene sites mediating transactivation or transrepression. *Mol Cell Endocrinol*, **2003,** *206:*13–22.

Haynes BP, Dowsett M, Miller WR, *et al*. The pharmacology of letrozole. *J Steroid Biochem Mol Biol*, **2003,** *87:*35–45.

Herbst AL, Ulfelder H, Poskanzer DC. Adenocarcinoma of the vagina. Association of maternal stilbestrol therapy with tumor appearance in young women. *N Engl J Med*, **1971,** *284:*878–881.

Herrington DM, Howard TD. ER-α variants and the cardiovascular effects of hormone replacement therapy. *Pharmacogenomics*, **2003,** *4:*269–277.

Herrington DM, Klein, K.P. Pharmacogenetics of estrogen replacement therapy. *J Appl Physiol*, **2001,** *91:*2776–2784.

Hewitt SC, Korach KS. Oestrogen receptor knockout mice: Roles for oestrogen receptors α and β in reproductive tissues. *Reproduction*, **2003,** *125*:143–149.

Hol T, Cox MB, Bryant HU, Draper MW. Selective estrogen receptor modulators and postmenopausal women's health. *J Womens Health*, **1997,** *6:*523–531.

Hotchkiss J, Knobil E. The menstrual cycle and its neuroendocrine control. In: *The Physiology of Reproduction*, 2nd ed. (Knobil E, Neill JD, eds.), Raven Press, New York, **1994,** pp. 711–749.

Hulley S, Grady D, Bush T, *et al*. Randomized trial of estrogen plus progestin for secondary prevention of coronary heart disease in post-menopausal women. Heart and Estrogen/progestin Replacement Study (HERS) Research Group. *JAMA*, **1998,** *280:*605–613.

Jaiyesimi IA, Buzdar AU, Decker DA, Hortobagyi GN. Use of tamoxifen for breast cancer: Twenty-eight years later. *J Clin Oncol*, **1995,** *13:*513–529.

Jang GR, Benet LZ. Antiprogestin pharmacodynamics, pharmacokinetics, and metabolism: Implications for their long-term use. *J Pharmacokinet Biopharm*, **1997,** *25:*647–672.

Jordan VC, Murphy CS. Endocrine pharmacology of antiestrogens as antitumor agents. *Endocr Rev*, **1990,** *11:*578–610.

Kato S, Endoh H, Masuhiro Y, *et al*. Activation of the estrogen receptor through phosphorylation by mitogen-activated protein kinase. *Science*, **1995,** *270:*1491–1494.

Kettel LM, Roseff SJ, Berga SL, *et al*. Hypothalamic-pituitary-ovarian response to clomiphene citrate in women with polycystic ovary syndrome. *Fertil Steril*, **1993,** *59:*532–538.

Knobil E. Patterns of hypophysiotropic signals and gonadotropin secretion in the rhesus monkey. *Biol Reprod*, **1981,** *24:*44–49.

Koh KK, Mincemoyer R, Bui MN, *et al*. Effects of hormone-replacement therapy on fibrinolysis in postmenopausal women. *N Engl J Med*, **1997,** *336:*683–690.

Kos M, Reid G, Denger S, Gannon F. Minireview: Genomic organization of the human ERalpha gene promoter region. *Mol Endocrinol*, **2001,** *15:*2057–2063.

Kousteni S, Chen JR, Bellido T, *et al*. Reversal of bone loss in mice by nongenotropic signaling of sex steroids. *Science*, **2002,** *298:*843–846.

Kuiper GG, Carlsson B, Grandien K, *et al*. Comparison of the ligand binding specificity and transcript tissue distribution of estrogen receptors ER α and β. *Endocrinology*, **1997,** *138:* 863–870.

Kurabayashi T, Matsushita H, Tomita M, *et al*. Association of vitamin D and estrogen receptor gene polymorphism with the effects of long term hormone replacement therapy on bone mineral density. *J Bone Miner Metab*, **2004,** *22:* 241–247.

Labrie F, El-Alfy M, Berger L, *et al*. The combination of a novel selective estrogen receptor modulator with an estrogen protects the mammary gland and uterus in a rodent model: The future of post-menopausal women's health? *Endocrinology*, **2003,** *144:*4700–4706.

Lahti E, Blanco G, Kauppila A, *et al*. Endometrial changes in post-menopausal breast cancer patients receiving tamoxifen. *Obstet Gynecol*, **1993,** *81:*660–664.

Leonhardt SA, Edwards DP. Mechanism of action of progesterone antagonists. *Exp Biol Med*, **2002,** *227:*969–980.

Levin E. G protein-coupled receptor 30: Estrogen receptor or collaborator? *Endocrinol,* **2009,** *150*:1563–1565.

Levin ER. Rapid signaling by steroid receptors. *Am J Physiol,* **2008,** *295*:R1425–R1430.

Lewandowski S, Kalita K, Kaczmarek L. Estrogen receptor β. Potential functional significance of a variety of mRNA isoforms. *FEBS Lett*, **2002,** *524:*1–5.

Lobo RA, Stanczyk FZ. New knowledge in the physiology of hormonal contraceptives. *Am J Obstet Gynecol*, **1994,** *170:* 1499–1507.

Love RR, Wiebe DA, Feyzi JM, *et al*. Effects of tamoxifen on cardiovascular risk factors in postmenopausal women after 5 years of treatment. *J Natl Cancer Inst*, **1994,** *86:*1534–1539.

Manolagas SC, Kousteni S, Jilka RL. Sex steroids and bone. *Recent Prog Horm Res*, **2002,** *57:*385–409.

Manson JE, Martin KA. Clinical practice. Postmenopausal hormone-replacement therapy. *N Engl J Med*, **2001,** *345:*34–40.

McDonnell DP, Goldman ME. RU486 exerts antiestrogenic activities through a novel progesterone receptor A form-mediated mechanism. *J Biol Chem*, **1994,** *269:*11945–11949.

McInerney EM, Weis KE, Sun J, *et al*. Transcription activation by the human estrogen receptor subtype beta (ER beta) studied with ER beta and ER alpha receptor chimeras. *Endocrinology*, **1998,** *139:*4513–4522.

Meis PJ, Klebanoff M, Thom E, *et al.* Prevention of recurrent pre-term delivery by 17 α-hydroxyprogesterone caproate. *N Engl J Med*, **2003,** *348:*2379–2385.

Mendelsohn ME, Karas RH. The protective effects of estrogen on the cardiovascular system. *N Engl J Med*, **1999,** *340:* 1801–1811.

Metivier R, Penot G, Hubner MR, *et al.* Estrogen receptor-α directs ordered, cyclical, and combinatorial recruitment of cofactors on a natural target promoter. *Cell*, **2003,** *115:*751–763.

Modelska K, Cummings S. Tibolone for postmenopausal women: Systematic review of randomized trials. *J Clin Endocrinol Metab*, **2002,** *87:*16–23.

Moodley J. Combined oral contraceptives and cervical cancer. *Curr Opin Obstet Gynecol*, **2004,** *16:*27–29.

Mulac-Jericevic B, Lydon JP, DeMayo FJ, Conneely OM. Defective mammary gland morphogenesis in mice lacking the progesterone receptor B isoform. *Proc Natl Acad Sci USA*, **2003,** *100:*9744–9749.

Mulac-Jericevic B, Mullinax RA, DeMayo FJ, *et al.* Subgroup of reproductive functions of progesterone mediated by progesterone receptor-B isoform. *Science*, **2000,** *289:*1751–1754.

Olde B, Leeb-Lundberg LM. GPR30/GPER1: Searching for a role in estrogen physiology. *Trends Endocrinol Metab*, **2009,** *20*:409–416.

Paech K, Webb P, Kuiper GG, *et al.* Differential ligand activation of estrogen receptors ERα and ERβ at AP1 sites. *Science*, **1997,** *277:*1508–1510.

Pedram A, Razandi M, Levin ER. Nature of functional estrogen receptors at the plasma membrane. *Mol Endocrinol*, **2006,** *20*:1996–2009.

Peltoketo H, Vihko P, Vihko R. Regulation of estrogen action: Role of 17 β-hydroxysteroid dehydrogenases. *Vitam Horm*, **1999,** *55:*353–398.

Pike AC, Brzozowski AM, Hubbard RE. A structural biologist's view of the oestrogen receptor. *J Steroid Biochem Mol Biol*, **2000,** *74:*261–268.

Pike MC, Peters RK, Cozen W, *et al.* Estrogen-progestin replacement therapy and endometrial cancer. *J Natl Cancer Inst*, **1997,** *89:*1110–1116.

Prince RL, Smith M, Dick IM, *et al.* Prevention of postmenopausal osteoporosis. A comparative study of exercise, calcium supplementation, and hormone-replacement therapy. *N Engl J Med*, **1991,** *325:*1189–1195.

Rapp SR, Espeland MA, Shumaker SA, *et al.*, for the WHIMS Investigators. Effect of estrogen plus progestin on global cognitive function in postmenopausal women: The Women's Health Initiative Memory Study: A randomized controlled trial. *JAMA*, **2003,** *289:*2663–2672.

Riggs BL, Khosla S, Melton LJ III. Sex steroids and the construction and conservation of the adult skeleton. *Endocr Rev*, **2002,** *23:*279–302.

Robertson JF, Osborne CK, Howell A, *et al.* Fulvestrant versus anastrozole for the treatment of advanced breast carcinoma in post-menopausal women: A prospective combined analysis of two multi-center trials. *Cancer*, **2003,** *98:*229–238.

Robinson D, Cardozo LD. The role of estrogens in female lower urinary tract dysfunction. *Urology*, **2003,** *62*(suppl 4A):45–51.

Rossouw JE, Anderson GL, Prentice RL, *et al.*, for the Writing Group for the Women's Health Initiative Investigators. Risks and benefits of estrogen plus progestin in healthy postmenopausal women: Principal results from the Women's Health Initiative randomized controlled trial. *JAMA*, **2002,** *288:*321–333.

Saville B, Wormke M, Wang F, *et al.* Ligand-, cell-, and estrogen receptor subtype (α/β)-dependent activation at GC-rich (Sp1) promoter elements. *J Biol Chem*, **2000,** *275:*5379–5387.

Schairer C, Lubin J, Troisi R, *et al.* Menopausal estrogen and estrogen-progestin replacement therapy and breast cancer risk. *JAMA*, **2000,** *283:*485–491.

Seminara SB. Mechanisms of disease: The first kiss-a crucial role for kisspeptin-1 and its receptor G-protein-coupled receptor 54, in puberty and reproduction. *Nat Clin Pract Endocrinol Metab*, **2006,** *2*:328–334.

Shapiro S, Kelly JP, Rosenberg L, *et al.* Risk of localized and widespread endometrial cancer in relation to recent and discontinued use of conjugated estrogens. *N Engl J Med*, **1985,** *313:*969–972.

Sherif K. Benefits and risks of oral contraceptives. *Am J Obstet Gynecol*, **1999,** *180:*S343–S348.

Shumaker SA, Legault C, Rapp SR, *et al.*, for the WHIMS Investigators. Estrogen plus progestin and the incidence of dementia and mild cognitive impairment in postmenopausal women: The Women's Health Initiative Memory Study: A randomized controlled trial. *JAMA*, **2003,** *289:* 2651–2662.

Simoncini T, Hafezi-Moghadam A, Brazil DP, *et al.* Interaction of oestrogen receptor with the regulatory subunit of phosphatidylinositol-3-OH kinase. *Nature*, **2000,** *407:* 538–541.

Simpson ER. Sources of estrogen and their importance. *J Steroid Biochem Mol Biol*, **2003,** *86:*225–230.

Simpson ER, Clyne C, Rubin G, *et al.* Aromatase—a brief overview. *Annu Rev Physiol*, **2002,** *64:*93–127.

Smith CL, O'Malley BW. Coregulator function: A key to understanding tissue specificity of selective receptor modulators. *Endocr Rev*, **2004,** *25:*45–71.

Smith EP, Boyd J, Frank GR, *et al.* Estrogen resistance caused by a mutation in the estrogen-receptor gene in a man. *N Engl J Med*, **1994,** *331:*1056–1061.

Smith RE. A review of selective estrogen receptor modulators and national surgical adjuvant breast and bowel project clinical trials. *Semin Oncol*, **2003,** *30*(5 suppl 16):4–13.

Spelsberg TC, Subramaniam M, Riggs BL, Khosla S. The actions and interactions of sex steroids and growth factors/cytokines on the skeleton. *Mol Endocrinol*, **1999,** *13:*819–828.

Spitz IM, Chwalisz K. Progesterone receptor modulators and progesterone antagonists in women's health. *Steroids*, **2000,** *65:*807–815.

Sridar C, Kent UM, Notley LM, *et al.* Effect of tamoxifen on the enzymatic activity of human cytochrome CYP2B6. *J Pharmacol Exp Ther*, **2002,** *301:*945–952.

Tamrazi A, Carlson KE, Katzenellenbogen JA. Molecular sensors of estrogen receptor conformations and dynamics. *Mol Endocrinol*, **2003,** *17:*2593–2602.

Task Force on Postovulatory Methods of Fertility Regulation. Randomised controlled trial of levonorgestrel versus the Yuzpe regimen of combined oral contraceptives for emergency contraception. *Lancet*, **1998,** *352:*428–433.

Thorneycroft IH, Mishell DR Jr, Stone SC, *et al.* The relation of serum 17-hydroxyprogesterone and estradiol-17β levels during the human menstrual cycle. *Am J Obstet Gynecol*, **1971,** *111:*947–951.

Van Den Bemd GJ, Kuiper GG, Pols HA, Van Leeuwen JP. Distinct effects on the conformation of estrogen receptor α and β by both the antiestrogens ICI 164,384 and ICI 182,780 leading to opposite effects on receptor stability. *Biochem Biophys Res Commun*, **1999,** *261:*1–5.

Walsh BW, Kuller LH, Wild RA, *et al*. Effects of raloxifene on serum lipids and coagulation factors in healthy post-menopausal women. *JAMA*, **1998,** *279:*1445–1451.

Walsh BW, Li H, Sacks FM. Effects of postmenopausal hormone replacement with oral and transdermal estrogen on high density lipoprotein metabolism. *J Lipid Res*, **1994,** *35:*2083–2093.

Weiderpass E, Persson I, Melhus H, *et al*. Estrogen receptor α gene polymorphisms and endometrial cancer risk. *Carcinogenesis*, **2000,** *21:*623–627.

Westhoff C. Depot-medroxyprogesterone acetate injection (Depo-Provera): A highly effective contraceptive option with proven long-term safety. *Contraception*, **2003,** *68:*75–87.

Westhoff CL. Breast cancer risk: Perception versus reality. *Contraception*, **1999,** *59*(suppl):25S–28S.

Wijayaratne AL, Nagel SC, Paige LA, *et al*. Comparative analyses of mechanistic differences among antiestrogens. *Endocrinology*, **1999,** *140:*5828–5840.

Writing Group for the PEPI Trial. Effects of estrogen or estrogen/ progestin regimens on heart disease risk factors in post-menopausal women. The Postmenopausal Estrogen/Progestin Interventions (PEPI) Trial. *JAMA*, **1995,** *273:*199–208.

Yue W, Santen RJ, Wang JP, *et al*. Genotoxic metabolites of estradiol in breast: Potential mechanism of estradiol induced carcinogenesis. *J Steroid Biochem Mol Biol*, **2003,** *86:*477–486.

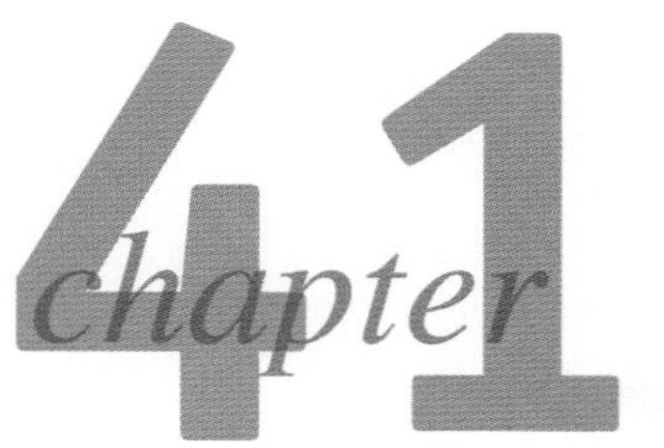

Androgens

Peter J. Snyder

TESTOSTERONE AND OTHER ANDROGENS

In men, testosterone is the principal secreted androgen. The Leydig cells synthesize the majority of testosterone by the pathways shown in Figure 41–1. In women, testosterone also is probably the principal androgen and is synthesized both in the corpus luteum and the adrenal cortex by similar pathways. The testosterone precursors androstenedione and dehydroepiandrosterone are weak androgens that can be converted peripherally to testosterone.

Secretion and Transport of Testosterone. The magnitude of testosterone secretion is greater in men than in women at almost all stages of life, a difference that explains many of the other differences between men and women. In the first trimester *in utero,* the fetal testes begin to secrete testosterone, which is the principal factor in male sexual differentiation, probably stimulated by human chorionic gonadotropin (hCG) from the placenta. By the beginning of the second trimester, the serum testosterone concentration is close to that of mid-puberty, ~250 ng/dL (Figure 41–2) (Dawood and Saxena, 1977; Forest, 1975). Testosterone production then falls by the end of the second trimester, but by birth the value is again ~250 ng/dL, possibly due to stimulation of the fetal Leydig cells by luteinizing hormone (LH) from the fetal pituitary gland. The testosterone value falls again in the first few days after birth, but it rises and peaks again at ~250 ng/dL at 2-3 months after birth and falls to <50 ng/dL by 6 months, where it remains until puberty (Forest, 1975).

During puberty, from ~12 to 17 years of age, the serum testosterone concentration in males increases to a much greater degree than in females, so that by early adulthood the serum testosterone concentration is 500 ng/dL to 700 ng/dL in men, compared to 30 ng/dL to 50 ng/dL in women. The magnitude of the testosterone concentration in the male is responsible for the pubertal changes that further differentiate men from women. As men age, their serum testosterone concentrations gradually decrease, which may contribute to other effects of aging in men.

LH, secreted by the pituitary gonadotropes (Chapter 38), is the principal stimulus of testosterone secretion in men, perhaps potentiated by follicle-stimulating hormone (FSH), also secreted by gonadotropes. The secretion of LH by gonadotropes is positively regulated by hypothalamic gonadotropin-releasing hormone (GnRH), and testosterone directly inhibits LH secretion in a negative feedback loop. LH is secreted in pulses, which occur approximately every 2 hours and are greater in magnitude in the morning. The pulsatility appears to result from pulsatile secretion of GnRH from the hypothalamus. Pulsatile administration of GnRH to men who are hypogonadal due to hypothalamic disease results in normal LH pulses and testosterone secretion, but continuous administration does not (Crowley et al., 1985). Testosterone secretion is likewise pulsatile and diurnal, the highest plasma concentrations occurring at ~8 A.M. and the lowest at ~8 P.M. The morning peaks diminish as men age (Bremner et al., 1983).

In women, LH stimulates the corpus luteum (formed from the follicle after release of the ovum) to secrete testosterone. Under normal circumstances, however, estradiol and progesterone, not testosterone, are the principal inhibitors of LH secretion in women. Sex hormone-binding globulin (SHBG) binds ~40% of circulating testosterone with high affinity, rendering the bound hormone unavailable for biological effects. Albumin binds almost 60% of circulating testosterone with low affinity, leaving ~2% unbound or free. In some testosterone assays, the latter two components are considered as "bioavailable" testosterone.

Metabolism of Testosterone to Active and Inactive Compounds. Testosterone has many different effects in many tissues. One mechanism by which the varied effects are mediated is the metabolism of testosterone to two other active steroids, dihydrotestosterone and estradiol (Figure 41–3). Some effects of testosterone appear

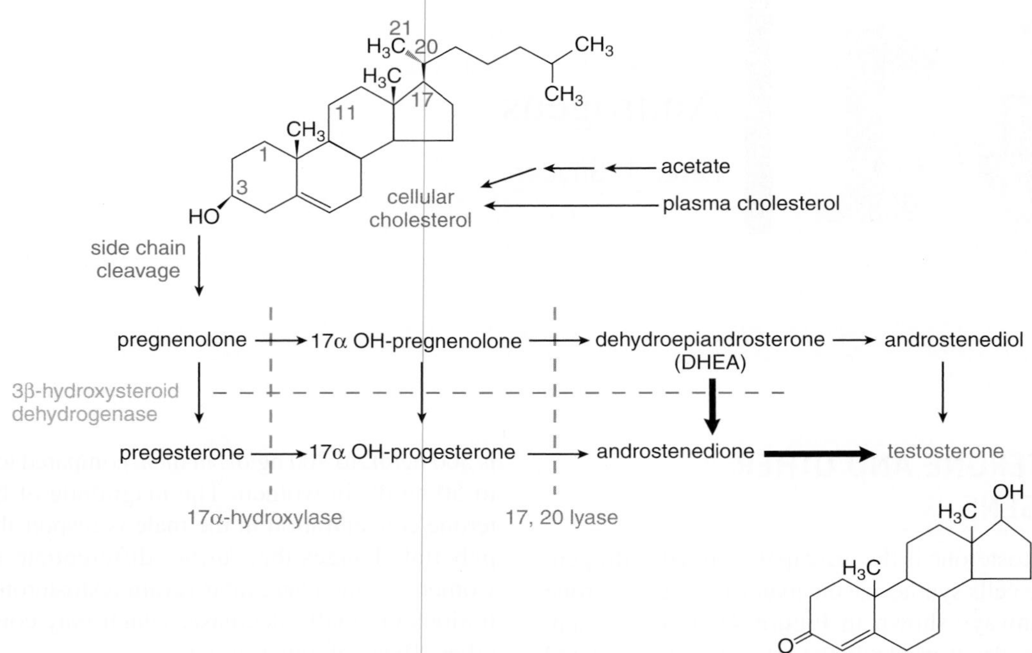

Figure 41–1. *Pathway of synthesis of testosterone in the Leydig cells of the testes.* In Leydig cells, the 11 and 21 hydroxylases (present in adrenal cortex) are absent but CYP17 (17 α-hydroxylase) is present. Thus androgens and estrogens are synthesized; corticosterone and cortisol are not formed. Bold arrows indicate favored pathways.

to be mediated by testosterone itself, some by dihydrotestosterone, and some by estradiol.

The enzyme 5α-reductase catalyzes the conversion of testosterone to dihydrotestosterone. Although both testosterone and dihydrotestosterone act via the androgen receptor, dihydrotestosterone binds with higher affinity (Wilbert et al., 1983) and activates gene expression more efficiently (Deslypere et al., 1992). As a result, acting via dihydrotestosterone and in tissues expressing 5α-reductase, testosterone is able to affect tissues that would otherwise not be affected by circulating levels of testosterone. Two forms of 5α-reductase

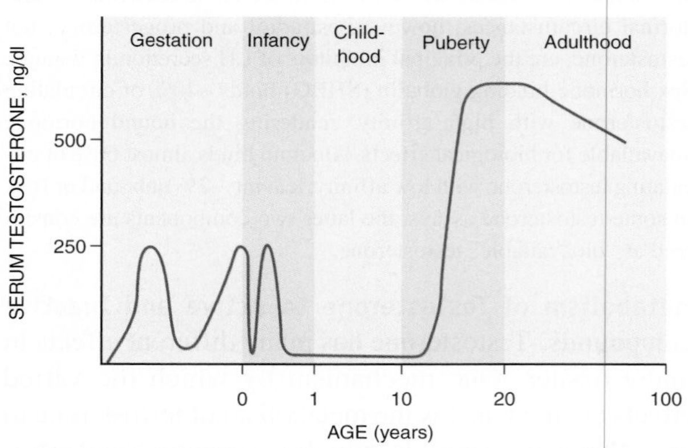

Figure 41–2. *Schematic representation of the serum testosterone concentration from early gestation to old age.*

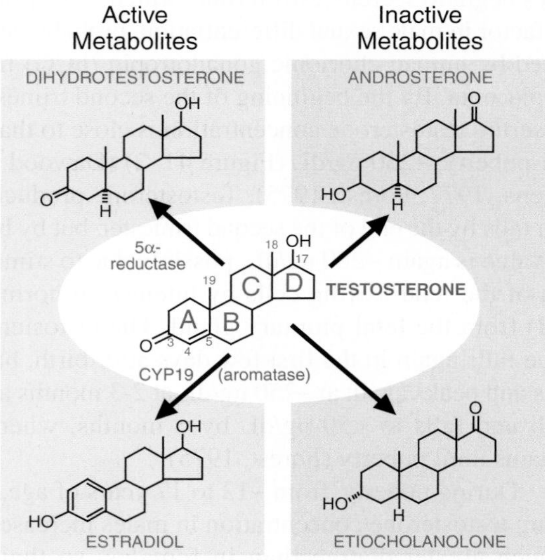

Figure 41–3. *Metabolism of testosterone to its major active and inactive metabolites.*

have been identified: type I, which is found predominantly in nongenital skin, liver and bone, and type II, which is found predominantly in urogenital tissue in men and genital skin in men and women. The effects of dihydrotestosterone in these tissues are described later.

The enzyme complex aromatase, which is present in many tissues, especially the liver and adipose tissue, catalyzes the conversion of testosterone to estradiol. This conversion accounts for ~85% of circulating estradiol in men; the remainder is secreted directly by the testes, probably the Leydig cells (MacDonald et al., 1979). The effects of testosterone thought to be mediated via estradiol are described below.

Testosterone is metabolized in the liver to androsterone and etiocholanolone (Figure 41–3), which are biologically inactive. Dihydrotestosterone is metabolized to androsterone, androstanedione, and androstanediol.

Physiological and Pharmacological Effects of Androgens

The biological effects of testosterone are mediated by the receptor it activates and by the tissues in which the receptor and responses occur at various stages of life. Testosterone can act as an androgen either directly, by binding to the androgen receptor, or indirectly by conversion to dihydrotestosterone, which also binds to the androgen receptor. Testosterone also can act as an estrogen by conversion to estradiol, which binds to the estrogen receptor (Figure 41–4).

Effects That Occur via the Androgen Receptor. Testosterone and dihydrotestosterone act as androgens via a single androgen receptor (Figure 41–5). The androgen receptor—officially designated NR3A—is a member of the nuclear receptor superfamily, which includes steroid hormone receptors, thyroid hormone receptors, and orphan receptors that lack a known ligand (Chapter 3).

The androgen receptor has an amino-terminal domain that contains a polyglutamine repeat of variable length, a DNA-binding domain consisting of two Zn finger motifs, and a carboxyterminal ligand-binding domain. The polyglutamine repeat of variable length is unique to the androgen receptor; a shorter length appears to increase its activity. In the absence of a ligand, the androgen receptor is located in the cytoplasm associated with a heat-shock protein complex. When testosterone or dihydrotestosterone binds to the ligand-binding domain, the androgen receptor dissociates from the heat-shock protein complex, dimerizes, and translocates to the nucleus. The dimer then binds via the DNA-binding domains to androgen response elements on certain responsive genes. The ligand-receptor complex recruits coactivators and acts as a transcription factor complex, stimulating or repressing expression of those genes (Agoulnik and Weigel, 2008; Brinkmann and Trapman, 2000).

The mechanisms by which androgens have different actions in diverse tissues have become clearer in recent years. One mechanism is the higher affinity with which dihydrotestosterone binds to and activates the

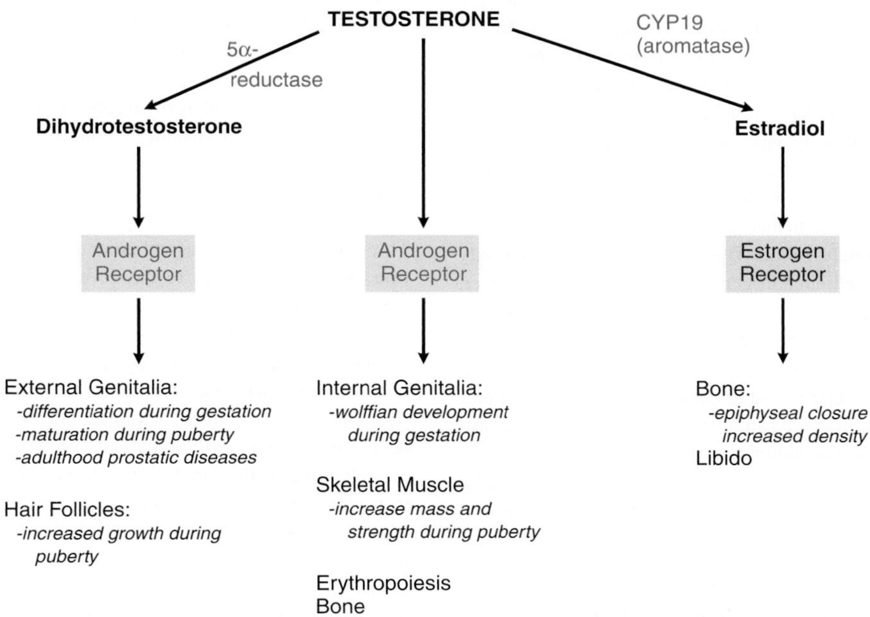

Figure 41–4. *Direct effects of testosterone and effects mediated indirectly via dihydrotestosterone or estradiol.*

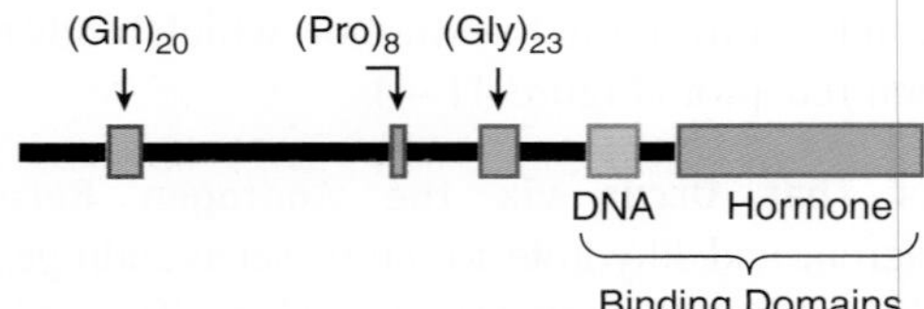

Figure 41–5. *Structure of the androgen receptor.*

androgen receptor compared to testosterone (Deslypere et al., 1992). Another mechanism involves transcription cofactors, both coactivators and corepressors, which are tissue specific. At this time, the roles of cofactors are better described for other nuclear receptors than for the androgen receptor (Smith and O'Malley, 2004).

The importance of the androgen receptor is illustrated by the consequences of its mutations. Predictably, mutations that either alter the primary sequence of the protein or cause a single amino acid substitution in the hormone- or DNA-binding domains result in resistance to the action of testosterone, beginning *in utero* (McPhaul and Griffin, 1999). Male sexual differentiation therefore is incomplete, as is pubertal development.

Another kind of mutation occurs in patients who have spinal and bulbar muscular atrophy, known as Kennedy's disease. These patients have an expansion of the CAG repeat, which codes for glutamine, at the amino terminus of the molecule (Walcott and Merry, 2002). The result is very mild androgen resistance, manifest principally by gynecomastia (Dejager, 2002), and progressively severe motor neuron atrophy. The mechanism by which the neuronal atrophy occurs is unknown but pharmacological induction of autophagy in a model cell system degrades the mutant AR and rescues the cells from damage (Montie et al, 2009). Other trinucleotide repeats are also associated with neurological disorders (Molla et al., 2009).

Other kinds of androgen receptor mutations may explain why prostate cancer that is treated by androgen deprivation eventually becomes androgen-independent. At the time of its clinical presentation, prostate cancer is usually androgen-sensitive, and this sensitivity forms the basis for the initial treatment of metastatic prostate cancer by androgen deprivation. Metastatic prostate cancer often regresses initially in response to this treatment but then becomes unresponsive to continued deprivation. The androgen receptor not only continues to be expressed in androgen-independent prostate cancer, but its signaling remains active, as indicated by expression of the androgen receptor-dependent prostate-specific antigen (PSA). It has been postulated that these observations can be explained by mutations in the androgen receptor gene or changes in androgen receptor co-regulatory proteins. In some patients resistant to standard androgen deprivation therapy, the tumor responds to further depletion of androgens by inhibitors of adrenal androgen synthesis, such as abiraterone, a drug in late stages of clinical development (Chapter 63) (Heinlein and Chang, 2004).

Effects That Occur via the Estrogen Receptor. The effects of testosterone on at least one tissue are mediated by its conversion to estradiol, catalyzed by the aromatase enzyme complex. In the rare cases in which a male does not express aromatase or the estrogen receptor (Smith, 1994), the epiphyses do not fuse and long-bone growth continues indefinitely; moreover, such patients are osteoporotic. Administration of estradiol corrects the bone abnormalities in patients with aromatase deficiency but not in those with an estrogen-receptor defect. Because men have larger bones than women, and bone expresses the androgen receptor (Colvard et al., 1989), testosterone also may have an effect on bone via the androgen receptor. The effect of testosterone on male libido also may be mediated by conversion to estradiol: administration of estradiol to a man with aromatase deficiency increased his libido (Rochira and Carani, 2009).

Effects of Androgens at Different Stages of Life.

In Utero. When the fetal testes, stimulated by hCG, begin to secrete testosterone at about the eighth week of gestation, the high local concentration of testosterone around the testes stimulates the nearby Wolffian ducts to differentiate into the male internal genitalia: the epididymis, vas deferens, and seminal vesicles. Further away, in the anlage of the external genitalia, testosterone is converted to dihydrotestosterone, which causes the development of the male external genitalia: the penis, scrotum, and prostate. The increase in testosterone at the end of gestation may result in further phallic growth.

Infancy. The consequences of the increase in testosterone secretion by the testes during the first few months of life are not yet known.

Puberty. Puberty in the male begins at a mean age of 12 years with an increase in the secretion of FSH and LH from the gonadotropes, stimulated by increased secretion of GnRH from the hypothalamus. The increased secretion of FSH and LH stimulates the testes; not surprisingly, the first sign of puberty is an increase in testicular size. The increase in testosterone production by Leydig cells and the effect of FSH on the Sertoli cells stimulate the development of the seminiferous tubules, which eventually produce mature sperm. Increased secretion of testosterone into the systemic circulation affects many tissues virtually simultaneously, and the changes in most of them occur gradually during the course of several years. The phallus enlarges in length and width, the scrotum becomes rugated, and the prostate begins secreting the fluid it contributes to the semen. The skin becomes coarser and oilier due to increased sebum production, which contributes to the development of acne. Sexual hair begins to grow, initially pubic and axillary hair, then hair on the lower legs, and finally other body hair and facial hair. Full development of the latter two may not occur until 10 years after the start of puberty and marks the completion of puberty. Muscle mass and strength, especially of the shoulder girdle, increase, and subcutaneous fat decreases. Epiphyseal bone growth accelerates, resulting in the pubertal growth spurt, but epiphyseal maturation leads eventually to a slowing and then cessation of growth. Bone also becomes thicker. The increase in muscle mass and bone result in a pronounced increase in weight. Erythropoiesis increases, resulting in higher hematocrit and hemoglobin concentrations in men than boys or women. The larynx thickens, resulting in a lower voice. Libido develops.

Other changes also may result from the increase in testosterone during puberty. Men tend to have a better sense of spatial relations than do women and to exhibit behavior that differs in some ways from that of women, including being more aggressive.

Adulthood. The serum testosterone concentration and the characteristics of the adult man are maintained largely during early adulthood and midlife. One change during this time is the gradual development of male pattern baldness, beginning with recession of hair at the temples and/or at the vertex.

Two changes that can occur in the prostate gland during adulthood are of much greater medical significance. One is the gradual development of benign prostatic hyperplasia, which occurs to a variable degree in almost all men, sometimes obstructing urine outflow by compressing the urethra as it passes through the prostate. This development is mediated by the conversion of testosterone to dihydrotestosterone by 5α-reductase II within prostatic cells (Wilson, 1980).

The other change that can occur in the prostate during adulthood is the development of cancer. Although no direct evidence suggests that testosterone causes the disease, prostate cancer depends on androgen stimulation. This dependency is the basis of treating metastatic prostate cancer by lowering the serum testosterone concentration or by blocking its action at the receptor.

Senescence. As men age, the serum testosterone concentration gradually declines (Figure 41–2), and the SHBG concentration gradually increases, so that by age 80, the total testosterone concentration is ~80% and the free testosterone is ~40% of those at age 20 (Harman et al., 2001). This fall in serum testosterone could contribute to several other changes that occur with increasing age in men, including decreases in energy, libido, muscle mass (Forbes, 1976) and strength (Murray et al., 1980), and bone mineral density. Androgen deprivation also leads to insulin resistance, truncal obesity, and abnormal serum lipids, as observed in patients with metastatic prostate cancer receiving this treatment (see also Chapter 63). A causal role is suggested by the occurrence of similar changes when men develop hypogonadism at a younger age caused by known diseases, as discussed later in this chapter.

Consequences of Androgen Deficiency

The consequences of androgen deficiency depend on the stage of life during which the deficiency first occurs and on the degree of the deficiency.

During Fetal Development. Testosterone deficiency in a male fetus during the first trimester *in utero* causes incomplete sexual differentiation. Testosterone deficiency in the first trimester results only from testicular disease, such as deficiency of 17α-hydroxylase (CYP17); deficiency of LH secretion because of pituitary or hypothalamic disease does not result in testosterone deficiency during the first trimester, presumably because Leydig cell secretion of testosterone at that time is regulated by placental hCG. Complete deficiency of testosterone secretion results in entirely female external genitalia; less severe testosterone deficiency results in incomplete virilization of the external genitalia proportionate to the degree of deficiency. Testosterone deficiency at this stage of development also leads to failure of the wolffian ducts to differentiate into the male internal genitalia, such as the vas deferens and seminal vesicles, but the müllerian ducts do not differentiate into the female internal genitalia as long as testes are present and secrete müllerian inhibitory substance. Similar changes occur if testosterone is secreted normally, but its action is diminished because of an abnormality of the androgen receptor or of the 5α-reductase enzyme. Abnormalities of the androgen receptor can have quite varied effects. The most severe form results in complete absence of androgen action and a female phenotype; moderately severe forms result in partial virilization of the external genitalia; and the mildest forms permit normal virilization *in utero* and result only in impaired spermatogenesis in adulthood (McPhaul and Griffin, 1999). Abnormal 5α-reductase results in incomplete virilization of the external genitalia *in utero* but normal development of the male internal genitalia, which requires only testosterone (Wilson et al., 1993).

Testosterone deficiency during the third trimester, caused either by a testicular disease or a deficiency of fetal LH secretion, has two known consequences. First, the phallus fails to grow as much as it would normally. The result, called microphallus, is a common occurrence in boys later discovered to be unable to secrete LH due to abnormalities of GnRH synthesis. Second, the testes fail to descend into the scrotum; this condition, called cryptorchidism, occurs commonly in boys whose LH secretion is subnormal (Chapter 38).

Before Completion of Puberty. When a boy can secrete testosterone normally in *utero* but loses the ability to do so before the anticipated age of puberty, the result is failure to complete puberty. All of the pubertal changes previously described, including those of the external genitalia, sexual hair, muscle mass, voice, and behavior, are impaired to a degree proportionate to the abnormality of testosterone secretion. In addition, if growth hormone secretion is normal when testosterone secretion is subnormal during the years of expected puberty, the long bones continue to lengthen because the epiphyses do not close. The result is longer arms and legs relative to the trunk; these proportions are referred to as eunuchoid. Another consequence of subnormal testosterone secretion during the age of expected puberty is enlargement of glandular breast tissue, called gynecomastia.

After Completion of Puberty. When testosterone secretion becomes impaired after puberty (e.g., castration or anti-androgen treatment), regression of the pubertal effects of testosterone depends on both the degree and the duration of testosterone deficiency. When the degree of testosterone deficiency is substantial, libido and energy decrease within a week or two, but other testosterone-dependent characteristics decline more slowly. Decreases in muscle mass and strength probably can be detected by testing groups of men within a few months, but a clinically detectable decrease in muscle mass in an individual does not occur for several years. A pronounced decrease in hematocrit and hemoglobin will occur within several months. A decrease in bone mineral density probably can be detected by dual energy absorptiometry within 2 years, but an increase in fracture incidence would not be likely to occur for many years A loss of sexual hair takes many years.

In Women. Loss of androgen secretion in women results in a decrease in sexual hair, but not for many years. Androgens may have other important effects in women, and the loss of androgens (especially with the severe loss of ovarian and adrenal androgens that occurs in panhypopituitarism) may result in the loss of these effects. Testosterone preparations that can yield serum testosterone concentrations in the physiological range in women currently are being developed. The availability of such preparations will allow clinical trials to determine if testosterone replacement in androgen-deficient women improves their libido, energy, muscle mass and strength, and bone mineral density.

Therapeutic Androgen Preparations

The need for a creative approach to pharmacotherapy with androgens arises from the fact that ingestion of testosterone is not an effective means of replacing testosterone deficiency. Even though ingested testosterone is readily absorbed into the hepatic circulation, the rapid hepatic catabolism ensures that hypogonadal men generally cannot ingest it in sufficient amounts and with sufficient frequency to maintain a normal serum testosterone concentration. Most pharmaceutical preparations of androgens, therefore, are designed to bypass hepatic catabolism of testosterone.

Testosterone Esters. Esterifying a fatty acid to the 17α hydroxyl group of testosterone creates a compound that is even more lipophilic than testosterone itself. When an ester, such as testosterone enanthate (heptanoate) or cypionate (cyclopentylpropionate) (Figure 41–6) is dissolved in oil and administered intramuscularly every 2-4 weeks to hypogonadal men, the ester hydrolyzes *in vivo* and results in serum testosterone concentrations that range from higher than normal in the first few days after the injection to low normal just before the next injection (Figure 41–7). Attempts to decrease the frequency of injections by increasing the amount of each injection result in wider fluctuations and poorer therapeutic outcomes. The undecanoate ester of testosterone (Figure 41–6), when dissolved in oil and ingested orally, is absorbed into the lymphatic circulation, thus bypassing initial hepatic catabolism. Testosterone undecanoate in oil also can be injected and produces stable serum testosterone concentrations for 2 months (Schubert et al., 2004). The undecanoate ester of testosterone is not currently marketed in the U.S.

Alkylated Androgens. Several decades ago, chemists found that adding an alkyl group to the 17α position of testosterone (Figure 41–6) retarded its hepatic catabolism. Consequently, 17α-alkylated androgens are androgenic when administered orally; however, they are less androgenic than testosterone itself, and they cause hepatotoxicity (Cabasso, 1994), whereas native testosterone does not.

Transdermal Delivery Systems. Recent attempts to avoid the "first pass" inactivation of testosterone by the liver have employed novel delivery systems; chemicals called excipients are used to facilitate the absorption of native testosterone across the skin in a controlled fashion. These transdermal preparations provide more stable serum testosterone concentrations than do injections of testosterone esters. The first such preparations were patches, one of which (ANDRODERM) is still available. Newer preparations include gels (ANDROGEL, TESTIM) and a buccal tablet (STRIANT). These preparations produce mean serum testosterone concentrations within normal range in hypogonadal men (Figure 41–7).

Attempts to Design Selective Androgens

Alkylated Androgens. Decades ago, investigators attempted to synthesize analogs of testosterone that possessed greater anabolic effects than androgenic effects compared to native testosterone. Several compounds appeared to have such differential effects, based on a greater effect on the levator ani muscle compared to the ventral prostate of the rat. These compounds were called anabolic steroids, and most are 17α-alkylated androgens. None of these compounds, however, has been convincingly demonstrated to have such a differential effect in human beings. Nonetheless, they have

Testosterone
(HISTERONE, others)

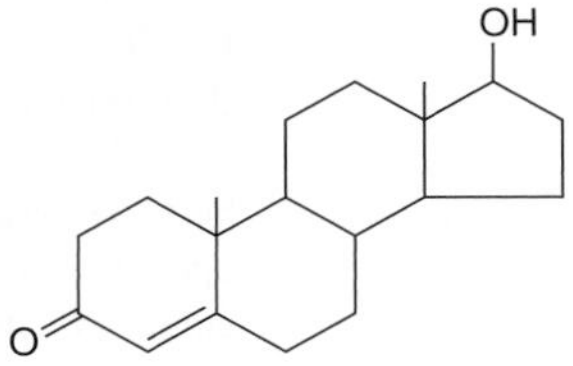

Testosterone Esters

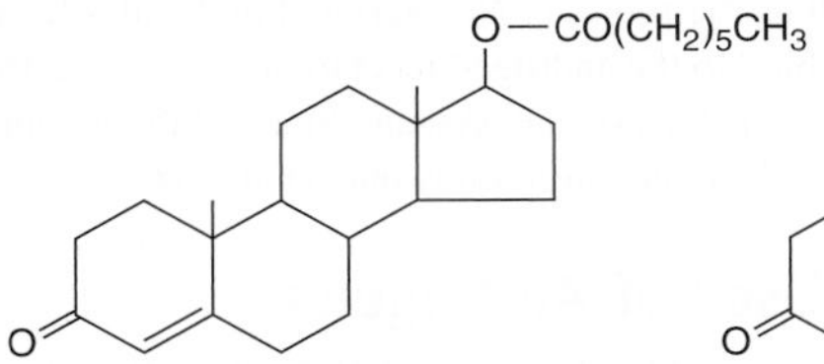

$O-CO(CH_2)_5CH_3$

Testosterone enanthate
(DELATESTRYL, others)

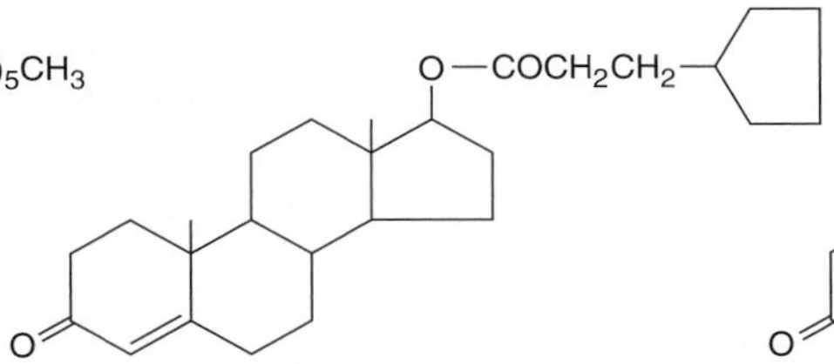

$O-COCH_2CH_2-$

Testosterone cypionate
(DEPO-TESTOSTERONE, others)

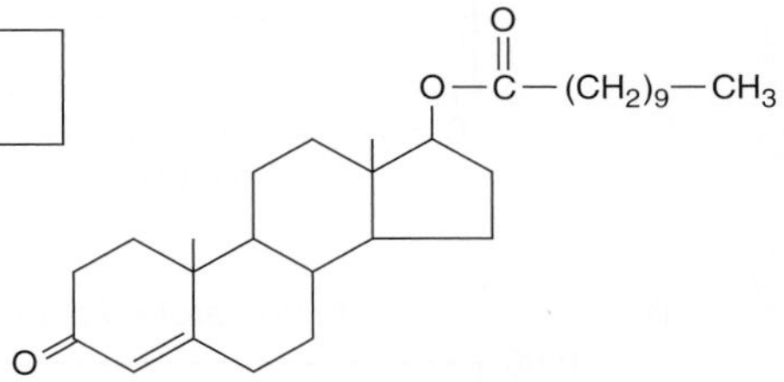

$O-C(=O)-(CH_2)_9-CH_3$

Testosterone undecanoate
(ANDRIOL)

17α-Alkylated Androgens

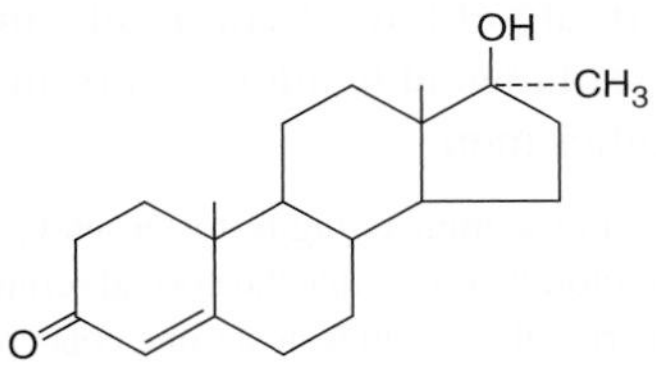

Methyltestosterone
(ORETIN METHYL, others)

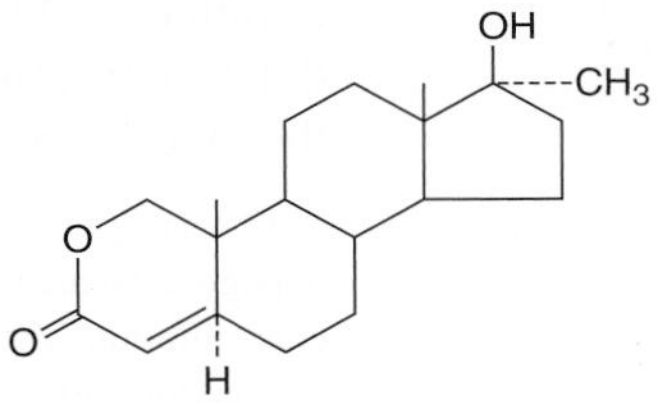

Oxandrolone
(OXANDRIN)

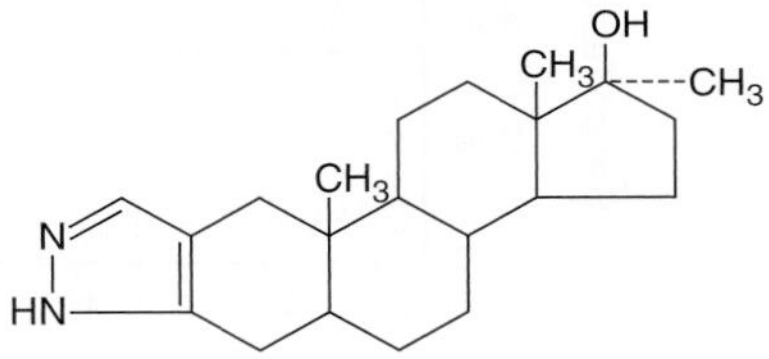

Stanozolol
(WINSTROL)

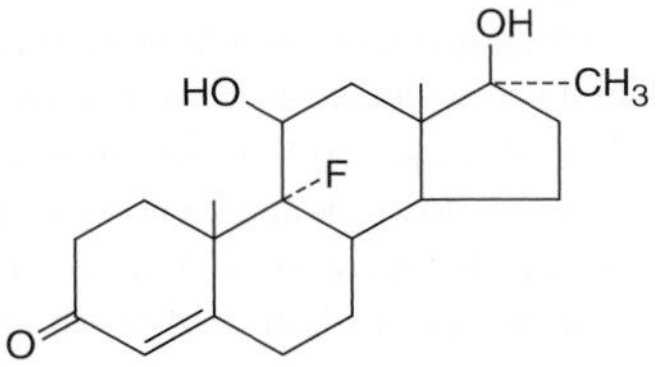

Fluoxymesterone
(HALOTESTIN)

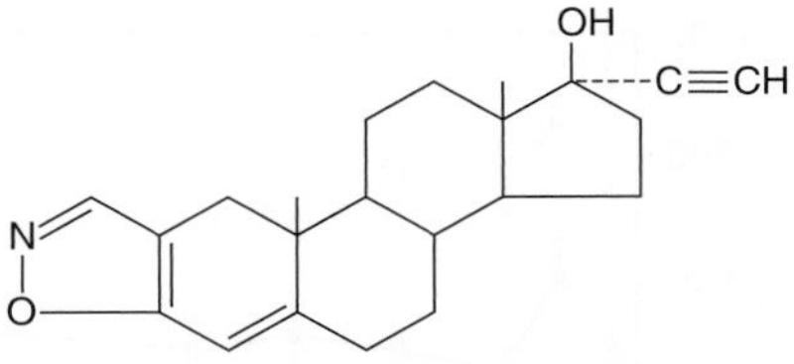

Danazol
(DANOCRINE)

Other

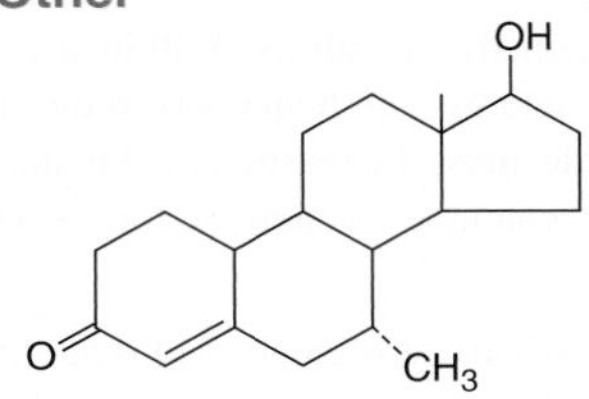

7α-Methyl-19-nortestosterone

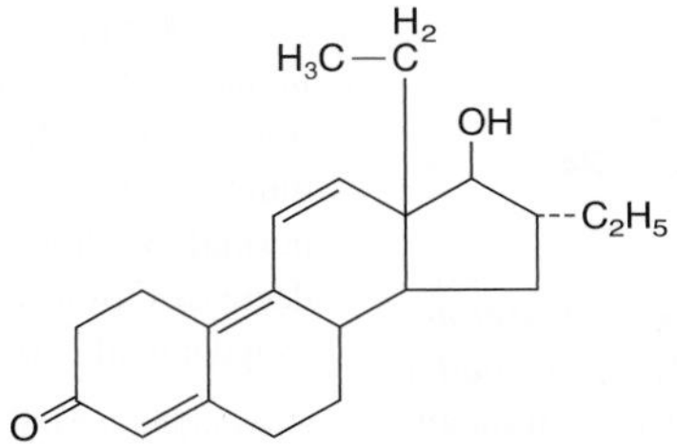

Tetrahydrogestrinone

Figure 41–6. Structures of androgens available for therapeutic use.

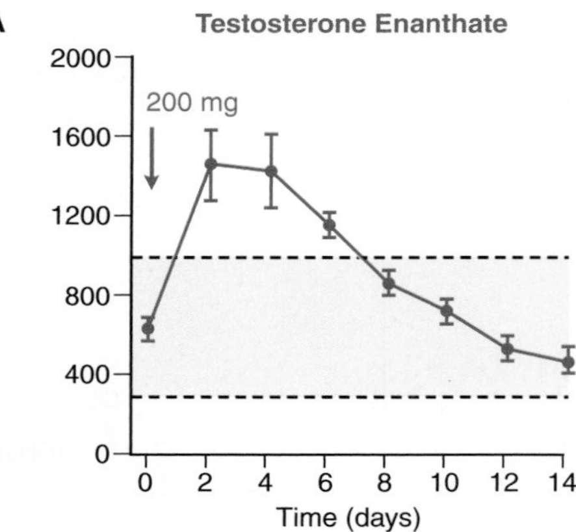

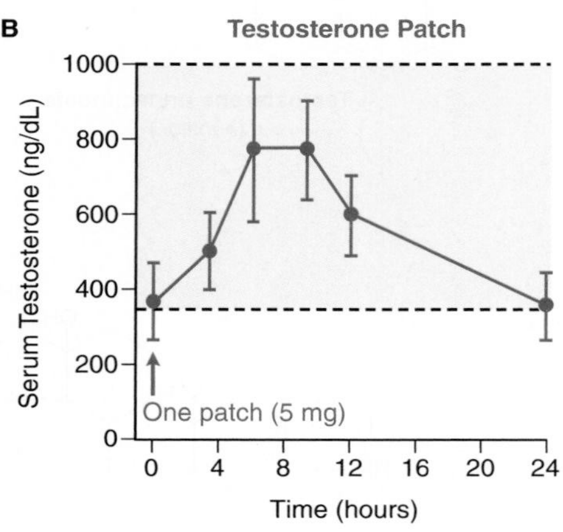

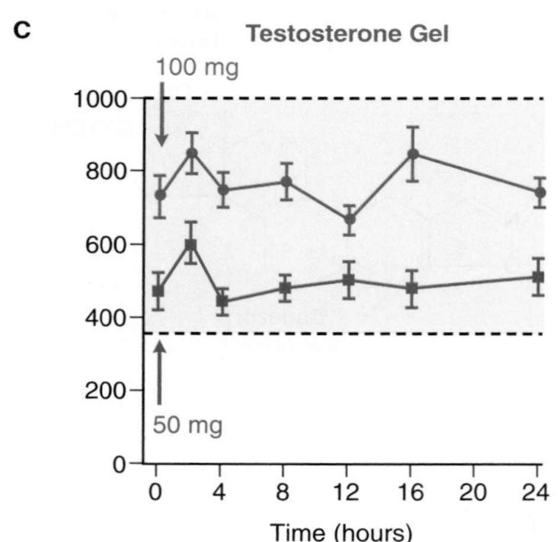

Figure 41–7. *Pharmacokinetic profiles of three testosterone preparations during their chronic administration to hypogonadal men.* Doses of each were given at time 0. Shaded areas indicate range of normal levels. [Data adapted from ***A.*** Snyder and Lawrence (1980); ***B.*** Dobs et al. (1999); **C.** Swerdloff et al. (2000)]

enjoyed popularity among athletes who seek to enhance their performance. Another alkylated androgen, 7α-methyl-19-nortestosterone, is poorly converted to dihydrotestosterone.

Selective Androgen-Receptor Modulators. Stimulated by the development of selective estrogen receptor modulators, which have estrogenic effects in some tissues but not others (Chapter 40), investigators are attempting to develop selective androgen receptor modulators. Another stimulus is the desirable effects of testosterone in some tissues, such as muscle and bone, and the undesirable effects in other tissues, such as the prostate. Nonsteroidal molecules have been developed that bind to the androgen receptor and have greater effect on muscle and bone than on the prostate. Some of these compounds have begun trials in humans (Narayanan et al., 2008).

Therapeutic Uses of Androgens

Male Hypogonadism. The best established indication for administration of androgens is testosterone deficiency in men (i.e., treatment of male hypogonadism). Any of the testosterone preparations or testosterone esters just described can be used to treat testosterone deficiency. Monitoring treatment for beneficial and deleterious effects differs somewhat in adolescents and the elderly from that in other men.

Monitoring for Efficacy. The goal of administering testosterone to a hypogonadal man is to mimic as closely as possible the normal serum concentration. Therefore, measuring the serum testosterone concentration during treatment is the most important aspect of monitoring testosterone treatment for efficacy. When the serum testosterone concentration is measured depends on the testosterone preparation used (Figure 41–7). Occasional random fluctuations can occur, however, so measurements should be repeated for any dose. When the enanthate or cypionate esters of testosterone are administered once every 2 weeks, the serum testosterone concentration measured midway between doses should be normal; if not, the dosage schedule should be adjusted accordingly. If testosterone deficiency results from testicular disease, as indicated by an elevated serum LH concentration, adequacy of testosterone treatment also can be judged indirectly by the normalization of LH within 2 months of treatment initiation (Findlay et al., 1989; Snyder and Lawrence, 1980).

Normalization of the serum testosterone concentration induces normal virilization in prepubertal boys and restores virilization in men who became hypogonadal as adults. Within a few months, and often sooner, libido, energy, and hematocrit return to normal. Within 6 months, muscle mass increases and fat mass decreases. Bone density, however, continues to increase for 2 years (Snyder et al., 2000).

Monitoring for Deleterious Effects. When testosterone itself is administered, as in one of the transdermal preparations or as an ester that is hydrolyzed to testosterone, it has no "side effects" (i.e., no effects that endogenously secreted testosterone does not have), as long as the dose is not excessive. Modified testosterone compounds, such as the 17α-alkylated androgens, do have undesirable effects even when dosages are targeted at physiological replacement. Some of these undesirable effects occur shortly after testosterone administration is initiated, whereas others usually do not occur until administration has been continued for many years. Raising the serum testosterone concentration from prepubertal or mid-pubertal levels to that of an adult male at any age can result in undesirable effects similar to those that occur during puberty, including acne, gynecomastia, and more aggressive sexual behavior. Physiological amounts of testosterone do not appear to affect serum lipids or apolipoproteins. Replacement of physiological levels of testosterone occasionally may have undesirable effects in the presence of concomitant illnesses. For example, stimulation of erythropoiesis would increase the hematocrit from subnormal to normal in a healthy man but would raise the hematocrit above normal in a man with a predisposition to erythrocytosis, such as in chronic pulmonary disease. Similarly, the mild degree of sodium and water retention with testosterone replacement would have no clinical effect in a healthy man but would exacerbate preexisting congestive heart failure. If the testosterone dose is excessive, erythrocytosis and, uncommonly, salt and water retention and peripheral edema occur even in men who have no predisposition to these conditions. When a man's serum testosterone concentration has been in the normal adult male range for many years, whether from endogenous secretion or exogenous administration, and he is >40 years of age, he is subject to certain testosterone-dependent diseases, including benign prostatic hyperplasia and prostate cancer.

The principal adverse effects of the 17α-alkylated androgens are hepatic, including cholestasis and, uncommonly, peliosis hepatis, blood-filled hepatic cysts. Hepatocellular cancer has been reported rarely. Case reports of cancer regression after androgen cessation suggest a possible causal role, but an etiologic link is unproven. The 17α-alkylated androgens, especially in large amounts, may lower serum high-density lipoprotein cholesterol.

Monitoring at the Anticipated Time of Puberty. Administration of testosterone to testosterone-deficient boys at the anticipated time of puberty should be guided by the considerations just described but also by the fact that testosterone accelerates epiphyseal maturation, leading initially to a growth spurt but then to epiphyseal closure and permanent cessation of linear growth. Consequently, the height and growth-hormone status of the boy must be considered. Boys who are short because of growth-hormone deficiency should be treated with growth hormone before their hypogonadism is treated with testosterone.

Male Senescence. Preliminary evidence suggests that increasing the serum testosterone concentration of men whose serum levels are subnormal for no reason other than their age will increase their bone mineral density and lean mass and decrease their fat mass (Amory et al., 2004; Kenny et al., 2001; Snyder et al., 1999a, 1999b). It is entirely uncertain at this time, however, if such treatment will worsen benign prostatic hyperplasia or increase the incidence of clinically detectable prostate cancer.

Female Hypogonadism. Little data exist regarding whether increasing the serum testosterone concentrations of women whose serum testosterone concentrations are below normal will improve their libido, energy, muscle mass and strength, or bone mineral density. In a study of women with low serum testosterone concentrations due to panhypopituitarism, increasing the testosterone concentration to normal was associated with small increases in bone mineral density, fat-free mass, and sexual function compared to placebo (Miller et al., 2006).

Enhancement of Athletic Performance. Some athletes take drugs, including androgens, to attempt to improve their performance. Because androgens for this purpose usually are taken surreptitiously, information about their possible effects is not as complete as that for androgens taken for treatment of male hypogonadism. Citing potentially serious health risks, the FDA has recommended against the use of body-building products that are marketed as containing steroids or steroid-like substances (FDA, 2009).

Kinds of Androgens Used. Virtually all androgens produced for human or veterinary purposes have been taken by athletes. When use by athletes began more than two decades ago, 17α-alkylated androgens and other compounds that were thought to have greater anabolic effects than androgen effects relative to testosterone (so-called anabolic steroids) were used most commonly. Because these compounds can be detected readily by organizations that govern athletic competitions, preparations that increase the serum concentration of testosterone itself, such as the testosterone esters or hCG, have increased in popularity. Testosterone precursors, such as androstenedione and dehydroepiandrosterone (DHEA), also have increased in popularity recently because they are treated as nutritional supplements and thus are not regulated by national governments or athletic organizations.

A new development in use of androgens by athletes is represented by tetrahydrogestrinone (THG), a potent androgen that appears to have been designed and synthesized in order to avoid detection by antidoping laboratories on the basis of its novel structure (Figure 41-6) and rapid catabolism.

Efficacy. There have been few controlled studies of the effects of pharmacological doses of androgens on muscle strength. In one controlled study, 43 normal young men were randomized to one of four groups: strength training ± 600 mg of testosterone enanthate once a week (more than six times the replacement dose); or no exercise ± testosterone. The men who received testosterone experienced an increase in muscle strength compared to those who received placebo, and the men who exercised simultaneously experienced even greater increases (Bhasin et al., 1996). In another study, normal young men were treated with a GnRH analog to reduce endogenous testosterone secretion severely and in a random blinded fashion, weekly doses of testosterone enanthate from 25 mg to 600 mg. There was a dose-dependent effect of testosterone on muscle strength (Bhasin et al., 2001).

In a double-blind study of androstenedione, men who took 100 mg three times a day for 8 weeks did not experience an increase in muscle strength compared to men who took placebo. Failure of this treatment to increase muscle strength is not surprising because it also did not increase the mean serum testosterone concentration (King et al., 1999).

Side Effects. All androgens suppress gonadotropin secretion when taken in high doses and thereby suppress endogenous testicular function. This decreases endogenous testosterone and sperm production, resulting in diminished fertility. If administration continues for many years, testicular size may diminish. Testosterone and sperm production usually return to normal within a few months of discontinuation but may take longer. High doses of androgens also cause erythrocytosis (Drinka et al., 1995).

When administered in high doses, androgens that can be converted to estrogens, such as testosterone itself, cause gynecomastia. Androgens whose A ring has been modified so that it cannot be aromatized, such as dihydrotestosterone, do not cause gynecomastia even in high doses.

The 17α-alkylated androgens are the only androgens that cause hepatotoxicity. These androgens also appear to be much more likely than others, when administered in high doses, to affect serum lipid concentrations, specifically to decrease high-density lipoprotein (HDL) cholesterol and increase low-density lipoprotein (LDL) cholesterol. Other side effects have been suggested by many anecdotes but have not been confirmed, including psychological disorders and sudden death due to cardiac disease, possibly related to changes in lipids or to coagulation activation.

Certain side effects occur specifically in women and children. Both experience virilization, including facial and body hirsutism, temporal hair recession in a male pattern, and acne. Boys experience phallic enlargement, and women experience clitoral enlargement. Boys and girls whose epiphyses have not yet closed experience premature closure and stunting of linear growth.

Detection. An androgen other than testosterone can be detected by gas chromatography and mass spectroscopy if the athlete is still taking it when he is tested. Exogenous testosterone itself can be detected by one of two methods. One is the T/E ratio, the ratio of testosterone glucuronide to its endogenous epimer, epitestosterone glucuronide, in urine. Administration of exogenous testosterone suppresses secretion of both testosterone and epitestosterone and replaces them with only testosterone, so the T/E ratio is higher than normal. This technique is limited, however, by heterozygosity in the UDP-glucuronosyl transferase that converts testosterone to testosterone glucuronide. An athlete who has a deletion of one or both copies of the gene coding for this enzyme and who takes exogenous testosterone will have a much lower T/E ratio than one who have both copies (Schulze, 2008).

A second technique for detecting administration of exogenous testosterone employs gas chromatography-combustion-isotope ratio mass spectrometry to detect the presence of ^{13}C and ^{12}C compounds. Urinary steroids with a low $^{13}C/^{12}C$ ratio are likely to have originated from pharmaceutical sources as opposed to endogenous physiological sources (Aguilera et al., 2001).

Male Contraception. Androgens inhibit LH secretion by the pituitary and thereby decrease endogenous testosterone production. Based on these observations, scientists have tried for more than a decade to use androgens, either alone or in combination with other drugs, as a male contraceptive. Because the concentration of testosterone within the testes, ~100 times that in the peripheral circulation, is necessary for spermatogenesis, suppression of endogenous testosterone production greatly diminishes spermatogenesis. Initial use of testosterone alone, however, required supraphysiologic doses, and addition of GnRH antagonists required daily injections. A more promising approach is the combination of a progestin with a physiological dose of testosterone to suppress LH secretion and spermatogenesis but provide a normal serum testosterone concentration (Bebb et al., 1996). One trial employed injections of testosterone undecanoate with a depot progestin every 2 months (Gu et al., 2004). Another androgen being tested as part of a male contraceptive regimen is 7α-methyl-19-nortestosterone, a synthetic androgen that cannot be metabolized to dihydrotestosterone (Cummings et al., 1998).

Catabolic and Wasting States. Testosterone, because of its anabolic effects, has been used in attempts to ameliorate catabolic and muscle-wasting states, but this has not been generally effective. One exception is in the treatment of muscle wasting associated with acquired immunodeficiency syndrome (AIDS), which often is accompanied by hypogonadism. Treatment of men with AIDS-related muscle wasting and subnormal serum testosterone concentrations increases their muscle mass and strength (Bhasin et al., 2000).

Angioedema. Chronic androgen treatment of patients with angioedema effectively prevents attacks. The disease is caused by hereditary impairment of C1-esterase inhibitor or acquired development of antibodies against it (Cicardi et al., 1998). The 17α-alkylated androgens, such as stanozolol and danazol, stimulate the hepatic synthesis of the esterase inhibitor. In women, virilization is a potential side effect. In children, virilization and premature epiphyseal closure prevent chronic use of androgens for prophylaxis, although they are used occasionally to treat acute episodes. As an alternative to prophylactic androgens, concentrated C1-esterase inhibitor derived from human plasma (CINRYZE) may be used for protection in patients with hereditary angioedema.

Blood Dyscrasias. Androgens once were employed to attempt to stimulate erythropoiesis in patients with anemias of various etiologies, but the availability of erythropoietin has supplanted that use. Androgens, such as danazol, still are used occasionally as adjunctive treatment for hemolytic anemia and idiopathic thrombocytopenic purpura that are refractory to first-line agents.

ANTI-ANDROGENS

Because some effects of androgens are undesirable, at least under certain circumstances, agents have been developed specifically to inhibit androgen synthesis or effects. Other drugs, originally developed for different purposes, have been accidentally found to be antiandrogens and now are used intentionally for this indication. See Chapter 63 for a more detailed discussion of androgen deprivation therapy for prostate cancer.

Inhibitors of Testosterone Secretion. Analogs of GnRH effectively inhibit testosterone secretion by inhibiting LH secretion. GnRH "superactive" analogs, given repeatedly, downregulate the GnRH receptor and are available for treatment of prostate cancer. An extended-release form of the GnRH antagonist, abarelix (PLENAXIS; no longer available in the U.S.) is used for treating prostate cancer (Trachtenberg et al., 2002). Because it does not transiently increase sex steroid production, this preparation may be especially useful in prostate cancer patients in whom any stimulus to tumor growth might have serious adverse consequences, such as patients with metastases impinging on the spinal cord, in whom further tumor growth could cause paralysis.

Some antifungal drugs of the imidazole family, such as ketoconazole (Chapter 57), inhibit CYPs and thereby block the synthesis of steroid hormones, including testosterone and cortisol. Because they may induce adrenal insufficiency and are associated with hepatotoxicity, these drugs generally are not used to inhibit androgen synthesis but sometimes are employed in cases of glucocorticoid excess (Chapter 42).

Inhibitors of Androgen Action

These drugs inhibit the binding of androgens to the androgen receptor or inhibit 5α-reductase.

Androgen Receptor Antagonists.

Flutamide, Bicalutamide, and Nilutamide. These relatively potent androgen receptor antagonists have limited efficacy when used alone because the increased LH secretion stimulates higher serum testosterone concentrations. They are used primarily in conjunction with a GnRH analog in the treatment of metastatic prostate cancer (Chapter 63). In this situation, they block the action of adrenal androgens, which are not inhibited by GnRH analogs. Flutamide also has been used to treat hirsutism in women, and it appears to be as effective as other treatments for this purpose (Venturoli et al., 1999); however, its association with hepatotoxicity warrants caution against its use for this cosmetic purpose.

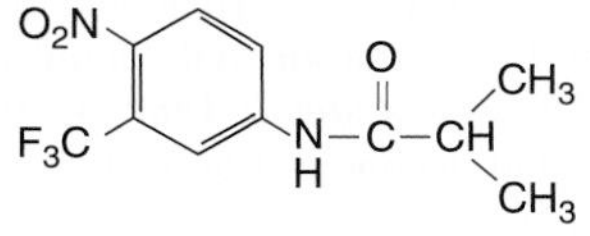

Flutamide

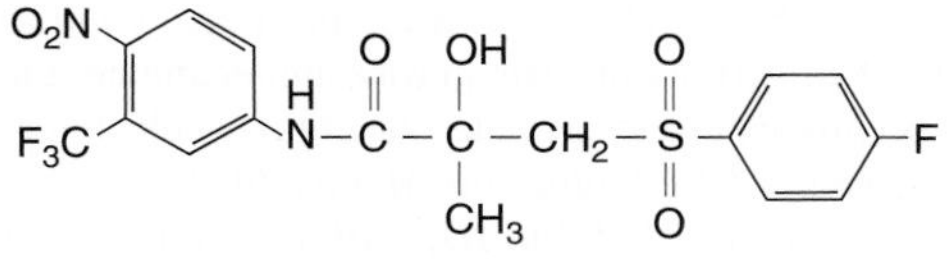

Bicalutamide

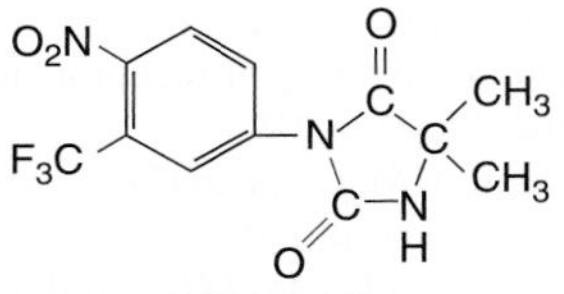

Nilutamide

Spironolactone. *Spironolactone* (ALDACTONE; Chapter 25) is an inhibitor of aldosterone that also is a weak inhibitor of the androgen receptor and a weak inhibitor of testosterone synthesis. When the agent is used to treat fluid retention or hypertension in men, gynecomastia is a common side effect (Caminos-Torres et al., 1977). In part because of this adverse effect, the selective mineralocorticoid receptor antagonist eplerenone (INSPRA) was developed. Spironolactone can be used in women to treat hirsutism; it is moderately effective (Cumming et al., 1982) but may cause irregular menses.

Cyproterone Acetate. Cyproterone acetate is a progestin and a weak antiandrogen by virtue of binding to the androgen receptor. It is moderately effective in reducing hirsutism alone or in combination with an oral contraceptive (Venturoli et al., 1999) but is not approved for use in the U.S.

5α-Reductase Inhibitors. Finasteride (PROSCAR) is an antagonist of 5α-reductase, especially the type II; dutasteride (AVODART) is an antagonist of both type I and type II. Both agents block the conversion of testosterone to dihydrotestosterone, especially in the male external genitalia. These drugs were developed to treat benign prostatic hyperplasia, and they are approved in the U.S. and many other countries for this purpose. When they are administered to men with moderately severe symptoms due to obstruction of urinary tract outflow, serum and prostatic concentrations of dihydrotestosterone decrease, prostatic volume decreases, and urine flow rate increases (McConnell et al., 1998). Impotence is a well-documented, albeit infrequent, side effect of this use, although the mechanism is not understood. Gynecomastia is an even less common side effect (Thompson, 2003).

Finasteride also is approved for use in the treatment of male pattern baldness under the trade name PROPECIA, even though that effect is presumably mediated via the type I enzyme. It appears to be as effective as flutamide and the combination of estrogen and cyproterone in the treatment of hirsutism (Venturoli et al., 1999).

Finasteride

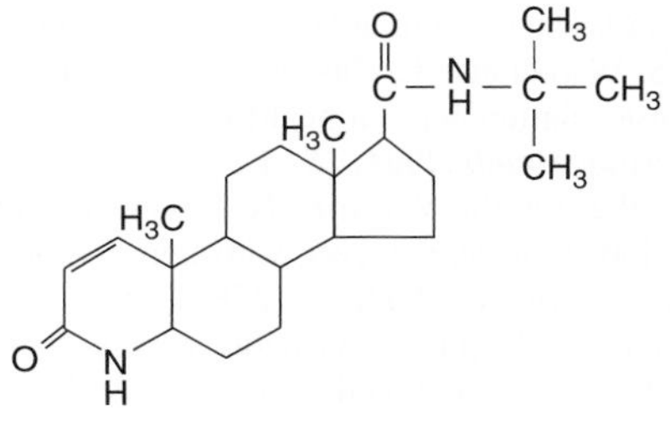

CLINICAL SUMMARY

Testosterone is the principal circulating androgen in men. The varied effects of testosterone are due to its ability to act by at least three mechanisms: by binding to the androgen receptor; by conversion in certain tissues to dihydrotestosterone, which also binds to the androgen receptor; and by conversion to estradiol, which binds to the estrogen receptor. Consequences of testosterone deficiency depend on whether the deficiency occurs in utero, before puberty, or in adulthood.

Testosterone delivery systems are designed to avoid the rapid hepatic catabolism that occurs when native testosterone is ingested orally. Available delivery systems include injectable esters of testosterone, implants, and several transdermal preparations. The major therapeutic indication for testosterone treatment is male hypogonadism. Treatment should be monitored for efficacy by measurement of the serum testosterone concentration and for deleterious effects by evaluating for obstruction to urine flow due to benign prostatic hyperplasia, for prostate cancer, and for erythrocytosis.

BIBLIOGRAPHY

Agoulnik IU, Weigel NL. Androgen receptor coactivators and prostate cancer. *Adv Exp Med Biol*, **2008,** *617*:245–255.

Aguilera R, Chapman TE, Starcevic B, *et al.* Performance characteristics of a carbon isotope ratio method for detecting doping with testosterone based on urine diols: Controls and athletes with elevated testosterone/epitestosterone ratios. *Clin Chem,* **2001,** *47:*292–300.

Amory K, Watts NB, Easley KA, *et al.* Exogenous testosterone or testosterone with finasteride increases bone mineral density in older men with low serum testosterone. *J Clin Endocrinol Metab,* **2004,** *89:*503–510.

Bebb RA, Anawalt B, Christensen RB, *et al.* Combined administration of levonorgestrel and testosterone induces a more rapid and effective suppression of spermatogenesis than testosterone alone: A promising male contraceptive approach. *J Clin Endocrinol Metab,* **1996,** *81:*757–762.

Bhasin S, Storer TW, Berman N, *et al.* The effects of supraphysiologic doses of testosterone on muscle size and strength in normal men. *N Engl J Med,* **1996,** *335:*1–7.

Bhasin S, Storer TW, Javanbakht M, *et al.* Testosterone replacement and resistance exercise in HIV-infected men with weight loss and low testosterone levels. *JAMA,* **2000,** *283*:763–770.

Bhasin S, Woodhouse L, Casaburi R, *et al.* Testosterone dose-response relationships in healthy young men. *Am J Physiol Endocrinol Metab,* **2001,** *281:*E1172–1181.

Bremner WJ, Vitiello V, Prinz PN. Loss of circadian rhythmicity in blood testosterone levels with aging in normal men. *J Clin Endocrinol Metab,* **1983,** *56:*1278–1280.

Brinkmann AO, Trapman J. Genetic analysis of androgen receptors in development and disease. *Adv Pharmacol,* **2000,** *47:*317–341.

Cabasso A. Peliosis hepatis in a young adult bodybuilder. *Med Sci Sports Exerc,* **1994,** *26:*2–4.

Caminos-Torres R, Ma L, Snyder PJ. Gynecomastia and semen abnormalities induced by spironolactone in normal men. *J Clin Endocrinol Metab,* **1977,** *45:*255–260.

Cicardi M, Bergamaschini L, Cugno M, *et al.* Pathogenetic and clinical aspects of C1 esterase inhibitor deficiency. *Immunobiology,* **1998,** *199:*366–376.

Colvard DS, Eriksen EF, Keeting PE, *et al.* Identification of androgen receptors in normal human osteoblast-like cells. *Proc Natl Acad Sci USA,* **1989,** *86:*854–857.

Crowley WF Jr, Filicori M, Spratt DI, Santoro NF. The physiology of gonadotropin-releasing hormone (GnRH) secretion in men and women. *Recent Prog Horm Res,* **1985,** *41:*473–531.

Cumming DC, Yang JC, Rebar RW, *et al.* Treatment of hirsutism with spironolactone. *JAMA,* **1982,** 247*:*1295–1298.

Cummings D, Kumar N, Bardin C, *et al.* Prostate-sparing effects of in primates of the potent androgen 7α-methyl-19-nortestosterone: A potential alternative to testosterone for androgen replacement and male contraception. *J Clin Endocrinol Metab,* **1998,** *84:*4212–4219.

Dawood MY, Saxena BB. Testosterone and dihydrotestosterone in maternal and cord blood and in amniotic fluid. *Am J Obstet Gynecol,* **1977,** *129:*37–42.

Dejager S, Bry-Gauillard H, Bruckert E, *et al.* A comprehensive endocrine description of Kennedy's disease revealing androgen insensitivity linked to CAG repeat length. *J Clin Endocrinol Metab,* **2002,** *87:*3893–3901.

Deslypere J-P, Young M, Wilson JD, *et al.* Testosterone and 5α-dihydrotestosterone interact differently with the androgen receptor to enhance transcription of the MMTV-CAT reporter gene. *Mol Cell Endocrinol,* **1992,** *88:*15–22.

Dobs AS, Meikle AW, Arver S, *et al.* Pharmacokinetics, efficacy, and safety of a permeation-enhanced testosterone transdermal system in comparison with bi-weekly injections of testosterone enanthate for the treatment of hypogonadal men. *J Clin Endocrinol Metab,* **1999,** *84:*3469–3478.

Dole EJ, Holdsworth MT. Nilutamide: An antiandrogen for the treatment of prostate cancer. *Ann Pharmacother,* **1997,** *31:*65–75.

Drinka PJ, Jochen AL, Cuisiner M, *et al.* Polycythemia as a complication of testosterone replacement therapy in nursing home men with low testosterone levels. *J Am Geriat Soc,* **1995,** *43:*899–901.

FDA. Public health advisory: The FDA recommends that consumers should not use body building products marketed as containing steroids or steroid-like substances. Available at: http://www.fda.gov/Drugs/DrugSafety/PublicHealthAdvisories/ucm173935.htm. Accessed May 19,2010.

Findlay JC, Place VA, Snyder PJ. Treatment of primary hypogonadism in men by the transdermal administration of testosterone. *J Clin Endocrinol Metab,* **1989,** *68:*369–373.

Forbes GB. The adult decline in lean body mass. *Human Biol,* **1976,** *48:*161–173.

Forest MG. Differentiation and development of the male. *Clin Endocrinol Metab,* **1975,** *4:*569–596.

Gu YQ, Tong JS, Ma DZ, *et al.* Male hormonal contraception: effects of injections of testosterone undecanoate and depot medroxyprogesterone acetate at eight-week intervals in Chinese men. *J Clin Endocrinol Metab,* **2004,** *89:*2254–2262.

Harman SM, Metter EJ, Tobin JD, *et al.* Longitudinal effects of aging on serum total and free testosterone levels in healthy men. Baltimore Longitudinal Study of Aging. *J Clin Endocrinol Metab,* **2001,** *86:*724–731.

Heinlein CA, Chang C. Androgen receptor in prostate cancer. *Endocr Rev,* **2004,** *25:*276–308.

Kenny AM, Prestwood KM, Gruman CA, *et al.* Effects of transdermal testosterone on bone and muscle in older men with low bioavailable testosterone levels. *J Gerontol A Biol Sci Med Sci,* **2001,** *56:*M266–272.

King DS, Sharp RL, Vukovich MD, et al. Effect of oral androstenedione on serum testosterone and adaptation to resistance training in young men: a randomized controlled trial. *JAMA*. 1999;281:2020–2028.

MacDonald PC, Madden JD, Brenner PF, et al. Origin of estrogen in normal men and in women with testicular feminization. *J Clin Endocrinol Metab*. 1979;49:905–916.

McConnell JD, Bruskewitz R, Walsh P, et al. The effect of finasteride on the risk of acute urinary retention and the need for surgical treatment among men with benign prostatic hyperplasia. Finasteride Long-Term Efficacy and Safety Study Group. *N Engl J Med*. 1998;338:557–563.

McPhaul MJ, Griffin JE. Male pseudohermaphroditism caused by mutations of the human androgen receptor. *J Clin Endocrinol Metab*. 1999;84:3435–3441.

Miller KK, Biller BM, Beauregard C, et al. Effects of testosterone replacement in androgen-deficient women with hypopituitarism: a randomized, double-blind, placebo-controlled study. *J Clin Endocrinol Metab*. 2006;91:1683–1690.

Molla M, Delcher A, Sunyaev S, Cantor C, Kasif S. Triplet repeat length bias and variation in the human transcriptome. *Proc Natl Acad Sci USA*. 2009;106:17095–17100.

Montie HL, Cho M, Holder L, et al. Cytoplasmic retention of polyglutamine-expanded androgen receptor ameliorates disease via autophagy in a mouse model of spinal and bulbar muscular atrophy. *Hum Mol Genet*. 2009;18:1937–1950.

Murray MP, Gardner GM, Mollinger LA, et al. Strength of isometric and isokinetic contractions: Knee muscles of men aged 20 to 86. *Phys Ther*. 1980;60:412–419.

Narayanan R, Mohler ML, Bohl CE, et al. Selective androgen receptor modulators in preclinical and clinical development. *Nucl Recept Signal*. 2008;6:e010.

Rochira V, Carani C. Aromatase deficiency in men: a clinical perspective. *Nat Rev Endocrinol*. 2009;5:559–568.

Schubert M, Minnemann T, Hübler D, et al. Intramuscular testosterone undecanoate: Pharmacokinetic aspects of a novel testosterone formulation during long-term treatment of men with hypogonadism. *J Clin Endocrinol Metab*. 2004;89:5429–5434.

Schulze JJ, Lundmark J, Garle M, Skilving I, Ekström L, Rane A. Substantial advantage of a combined Bayesian and genotyping approach in testosterone doping tests. *Steroids*. 2009;74:365–368.

Schulze JJ, Lorentzon M, Ohlsson C, et al. Genetic aspects of epitestosterone formation and androgen disposition: influence of polymorphisms in CYP17 and UGT2B enzymes. *Pharmacogenet Genomics*. 2008;18:477–485.

Smith CL, O'Malley BW. Coregulator function: A key to understanding tissue specificity of selective receptor modulators. *Endocr Rev*. 2004;25:45–71.

Smith EP, Boyd J, Frank GR. Estrogen resistance caused by a mutation in the estrogen-receptor gene in a man. *N Engl J Med*. 1994;331:1056–1061.

Snyder PJ, Lawrence DA. Treatment of male hypogonadism with testosterone enanthate. *J Clin Endocrinol Metab*. 1980;51:1335–1339.

Snyder PJ, Peachey H, Hannoush P, et al. Effect of testosterone treatment on bone mineral density in men over 65 years of age. *J Clin Endocrinol Metab*. 1999a;84:1966–1972.

Snyder PJ, Peachey H, Hannoush P, et al. Effect of testosterone treatment on body composition and muscle strength in men over 65 years of age. *J Clin Endocrinol Metab*. 1999b;84:2647–2653.

Snyder PJ, Peachey H, Berlin JA, et al. Effects of testosterone replacement in hypogonadal men. *J Clin Endocrinol Metab*. 2000;85:2670–2677.

Swerdloff RS, Wang C, Cunningham G, et al. Long-term pharmacokinetics of transdermal testosterone gel in hypogonadal men. *J Clin Endocrinol Metab*. 2000;85:4500–4510.

Taplin ME, Balk SP. Androgen receptor: A key molecule in the progression of prostate cancer to hormone independence. *J Cell Biochem*. 2004;91:483–490.

Thompson IM, Goodman PJ, Tangen CM, et al. The influence of finasteride on the development of prostate cancer. *N Engl J Med*. 2003;349:215–224.

Tyrrell CJ, Altwein JE, Klippel F, et al. A multicenter randomized trial comparing the luteinizing hormone-releasing hormone analogue goserelin acetate alone and with flutamide in the treatment of advanced prostate cancer. The International Prostate Cancer Study Group. *J Urol*. 1991;146:1321–1326.

Tammela T. Endocrine treatment of prostate cancer. *J Steroid Biochem Mol Biol*. 2004;92:287–295.

Tombal B. The importance of testosterone control in prostate cancer. *Eur Urol Suppl*. 2007;6:834–839.

Tyrrell CJ, Kaisary AV, Iversen P, et al. A randomised comparison of 'Casodex' (bicalutamide) 150 mg monotherapy versus castration in the treatment of metastatic and locally advanced prostate cancer. *Eur Urol*. 1998;33:447–456.

Trachtenberg J, Gittelman M, Steidle C, et al. A phase 3, multicenter, open label, randomized study of abarelix versus leuprolide plus daily antiandrogen in men with prostate cancer. *J Urol*. 2002;167:1670–1674.

Venturoli S, Marescalchi O, Colombo FM, et al. A prospective randomized trial comparing low dose flutamide, finasteride, ketoconazole, and cyproterone acetate-estrogen regimens in the treatment of hirsutism. *J Clin Endocrinol Metab*. 1999;84:1304–1310.

Walcott J, Merry D. Trinucleotide repeat disease. The androgen receptor in spinal and bulbar muscular atrophy. *Vitam Horm*. 2002;65:127–147.

Wilson JD. The pathogenesis of benign prostatic hyperplasia. *Am J Med*. 1980;68:745–756.

Wilson JD, Griffin JE, Russell DW. Steroid 5 alpha-reductase 2 deficiency. *Endocr Rev*. 1993;14:577–593.

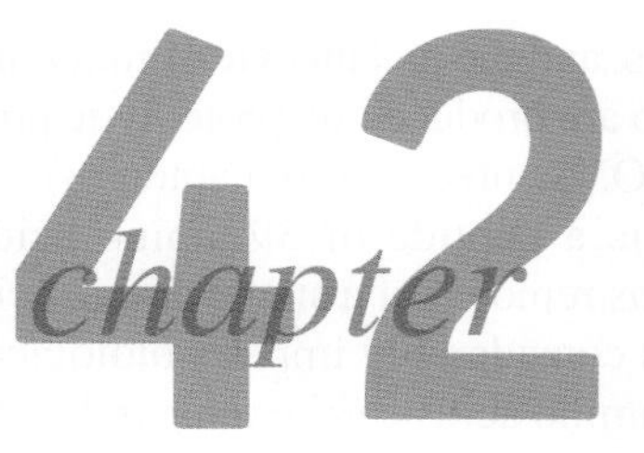

ACTH, Adrenal Steroids, and Pharmacology of the Adrenal Cortex

Bernard P. Schimmer
and John W. Funder

Adrenocorticotropic hormone (ACTH, corticotropin) and the steroid hormone products of the adrenal cortex are considered together because the major physiological and pharmacological effects of ACTH result from its action to increase the circulating levels of adrenocortical steroids. Synthetic derivatives of ACTH are used principally in the diagnostic assessment of adrenocortical function. Because all known therapeutic effects of ACTH can be achieved with corticosteroids, synthetic steroid hormones generally are used therapeutically instead of ACTH.

Corticosteroids and their biologically active synthetic derivatives differ in their metabolic (glucocorticoid) and electrolyte-regulating (mineralocorticoid) activities. These agents are employed at physiological doses for replacement therapy when endogenous production is impaired. In addition, glucocorticoids potently suppress inflammation, and their use in a variety of inflammatory and autoimmune diseases makes them among the most frequently prescribed classes of drugs. Because glucocorticoids exert effects on almost every organ system, the clinical use of and withdrawal from corticosteroids are complicated by a number of serious side effects, some of which are life threatening. Therefore, the decision to institute therapy with systemic corticosteroids always requires careful consideration of the relative risks and benefits in each patient.

Agents that inhibit steps in the steroidogenic pathway and thus alter the biosynthesis of adrenocortical steroids are discussed in this chapter, as are synthetic steroids that inhibit glucocorticoid action. Agents that inhibit the action of aldosterone are presented in Chapter 25; agents used to inhibit growth of steroid-dependent tumors are discussed in Chapters 60-62.

History. Addison described fatal outcomes in patients with adrenal destruction in a presentation to the South London Medical Society in 1849. These studies were soon extended when Brown-Séquard demonstrated that bilateral adrenalectomy was fatal in laboratory animals. It later was shown that the adrenal cortex, rather than the medulla, was essential for survival in these ablation experiments and that the adrenal cortex regulated both carbohydrate metabolism and fluid and electrolyte balance. The isolation and identification of the adrenal steroids by Reichstein and Kendall and the effects of these compounds on carbohydrate metabolism (hence the term *glucocorticoids*) culminated with the synthesis of *cortisone*, the first pharmacologically effective glucocorticoid to become readily available. Subsequently, Tait and colleagues isolated and characterized a distinct corticosteroid, *aldosterone*, which potently affected fluid and electrolyte balance and therefore was termed a *mineralocorticoid*. The isolation of distinct corticosteroids that regulated carbohydrate metabolism or fluid and electrolyte balance led to the concept that the adrenal cortex comprises two largely independent units: an outer zone that produces mineralocorticoids and an inner region that synthesizes glucocorticoids and androgen precursors.

Studies of adrenocortical steroids also played a key part in delineating the role of the anterior pituitary in endocrine function. As early as 1912, Cushing described patients with hypercorticism, and later he recognized that pituitary basophilism caused the adrenal overactivity, thus establishing the link between the anterior pituitary and adrenal function. These studies led to the purification of ACTH and the determination of its chemical structure. ACTH was further shown to be essential for maintaining the structural integrity and steroidogenic capacity of the inner cortical zones. Harris established the role of the hypothalamus in pituitary control and postulated that a soluble factor produced by the hypothalamus activated ACTH release. These investigations culminated with the determination of the structure of corticotropin-releasing hormone (CRH), a hypothalamic peptide that, together with arginine vasopressin, regulates secretion of ACTH from the pituitary.

Shortly after synthetic cortisone became available, Hench and colleagues demonstrated its dramatic effect in the treatment of rheumatoid arthritis. These studies set the stage for the clinical use of corticosteroids in a wide variety of diseases, as discussed in this chapter.

ADRENOCORTICOTROPIC HORMONE (ACTH; CORTICOTROPIN)

As summarized in Figure 42–1, ACTH is synthesized as part of a larger precursor protein, pro-opiomelanocortin (POMC), and is liberated from the precursor through proteolytic cleavage at dibasic residues by the serine endoprotease, prohormone convertase 1 (also known as prohormone convertase 3). The importance of this enzyme in POMC processing is best illustrated in a rare group of patients with prohormone convertase 1 mutations who present with impaired POMC processing, secondary hypocortisolism, childhood obesity, hypogonadotropic hypogonadism, diabetes, and neonatal onset enteropathy (Farooqi et al., 2007). A number of other biologically important peptides, including endorphins, lipotropins, and the melanocyte-stimulating hormones (MSH), also are produced by proteolytic processing of the same POMC precursor (Chapter 18).

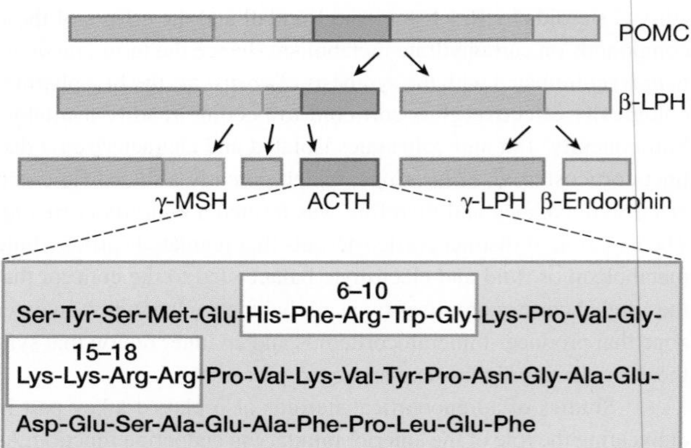

Figure 42–1. *Processing of pro-opiomelanocortin to adrenocorticotropic hormone and the sequence of adrenocorticotropic hormone.* The pathway by which pro-opiomelanocortin (POMC) is converted to adrenocorticotropic hormone (ACTH) and other peptides in the anterior pituitary is depicted. The amino acid sequence of human ACTH is shown. The light blue boxes behind the ACTH structure indicate regions identified as important for steroidogenic activity (residues 6-10) and binding to the ACTH receptor (15-18). α-Melanocyte-stimulating hormone also derives from the POMC precursor and contains the first 13 residues of ACTH. LPH, lipotropin; MSH, melanocyte-stimulating hormone.

Human ACTH is a peptide of 39 amino acids (Figure 42–1). Whereas removal of a single amino acid at the amino terminus considerably impairs biological activity, a number of amino acids can be removed from the carboxyl-terminal end without a marked effect. The structure–activity relationships of ACTH have been studied extensively, and it is believed that a stretch of four basic amino acids at positions 15-18 is an important determinant of high-affinity binding to the ACTH receptor, whereas amino acids 6-10 are important for receptor activation.

The actions of ACTH and the other melanocortins liberated from POMC are mediated by their specific interactions with five melanocortin receptor (MC1-5R) subtypes comprising a distinct subfamily of G protein-coupled receptors. The well-known effects of MSH on pigmentation result from interactions with the MC1R on melanocytes. MC1Rs also are found on cells of the immune system and are thought to mediate the anti-inflammatory effects of α-MSH in experimental models of inflammation. ACTH, which is identical to α-MSH in its first 13 amino acids (Ser-Tyr-Ser-Met-Glu-His-Phe-ArgTrp-Gly-Lys-Pro-Val), exerts its effects on the adrenal cortex through the MC2R. The affinity of ACTH for the MC1R is much lower than for the MC2R; however, under pathological conditions in which ACTH levels are persistently elevated, such as primary adrenal insufficiency, ACTH also can signal through the MC1R and cause hyperpigmentation. Recent studies have defined key roles for β-MSH (Lee et al., 2006) and possibly other melanocortins acting via the MC4R (Farooki et al., 2003) and MC3R (Mencarelli et al., 2008) in the hypothalamic regulation of appetite and body weight, and they therefore are the subject of considerable investigation as possible targets for drugs that affect appetite. The role of MC5R is less well defined, but studies in rodents suggest that MSH triggers aggressive, pheromone-related behavior via the MC5R (Morgan and Cone, 2006).

Actions on the Adrenal Cortex. Acting via MC2R, ACTH stimulates the adrenal cortex to secrete glucocorticoids, mineralocorticoids, and the androgen precursor dehydroepiandrosterone (DHEA) that can be converted peripherally into more potent androgens. The adrenal cortex histologically and functionally can be separated into three zones that produce different steroid products under different regulatory influences. The outer zona glomerulosa secretes the mineralocorticoid aldosterone, the middle zona fasciculata secretes the glucocorticoid cortisol, and the inner zona reticularis secretes DHEA (Figure 42–2) and its sulfated derivative DHEAS, which circulates at concentrations 1000 times greater than DHEA. DHEAS can be converted to DHEA in the periphery by DHEA sulfatase.

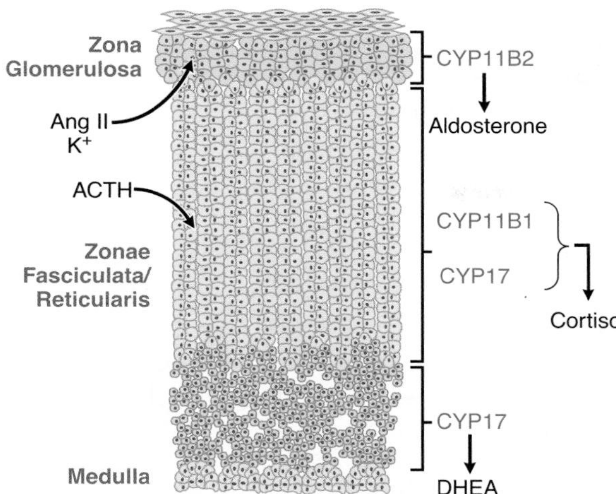

Figure 42–2. *The adrenal cortex contains three anatomically and functionally distinct compartments.* The major functional compartments of the adrenal cortex are shown, along with the steroidogenic enzymes that determine the unique profiles of corticosteroid products. Also shown are the predominant physiological regulators of steroid production: angiotensin II (Ang II) and K^+ for the zona glomerulosa and ACTH for the zona fasciculata. The physiological regulator(s) of dehydroepiandrosterone (DHEA) production by the zona reticularis are not known, although ACTH acutely increases DHEA biosynthesis.

Cells of the outer zone have receptors for angiotensin II and express aldosterone synthase (CYP11B2), an enzyme that catalyzes the terminal reactions in mineralocorticoid biosynthesis. Although ACTH acutely stimulates mineralocorticoid production by the zona glomerulosa, this zone is regulated predominantly by angiotensin II and extracellular K^+ (Chapter 25) and does not undergo atrophy in the absence of ongoing stimulation by the pituitary gland. In the setting of persistently elevated ACTH, mineralocorticoid levels initially increase and then return to normal (a phenomenon termed *ACTH escape*).

In contrast, cells of the zona fasciculata have fewer receptors for angiotensin II and express two enzymes, steroid 17α-hydroxylase (CYP17) and 11β-hydroxylase (CYP11B1), that catalyze the production of glucocorticoids. In the zona reticularis, CYP17 carries out an additional C17-20 lyase reaction that converts C21 corticosteroids to C19 androgen precursors.

In the absence of the anterior pituitary, the inner zones of the cortex atrophy, and the production of glucocorticoids and adrenal androgens is markedly impaired.

Persistently elevated levels of ACTH, due either to repeated administration of large doses of ACTH or to excessive endogenous production, induce hypertrophy and hyperplasia of the inner zones of the adrenal cortex, with overproduction of cortisol and adrenal androgens. Adrenal hyperplasia is most marked in congenital disorders of steroidogenesis, in which ACTH levels are continuously elevated as a secondary response to impaired cortisol biosynthesis. There is some debate regarding the relative roles of ACTH versus other POMC-derived peptides in stimulating adrenal growth, but the essential role of the anterior pituitary in maintaining the integrity of the zona fasciculata is indisputable.

Mechanism of Action. ACTH stimulates the synthesis and release of adrenocortical hormones. Because specific mechanisms for steroid hormone secretion have not been defined and steroids do not accumulate appreciably in the gland, it is believed that the actions of ACTH to increase steroid hormone production are mediated predominantly at the level of *de novo* biosynthesis.

ACTH, binding to MC2R (a GPCR), activates the G_s-adenylyl cyclase-cyclic AMP-PKA pathway. Cyclic AMP is an obligatory second messenger for most, if not all, effects of ACTH on steroidogenesis. Mutations in MC2R account for ~25% of the cases of familial glucocorticoid deficiency, a rare syndrome of familial resistance to ACTH (Clark et al., 2005).

Temporally, the response of adrenocortical cells to ACTH has two phases. The acute phase, which occurs within seconds to minutes, largely reflects increased supply of cholesterol substrate to the steroidogenic enzymes. The chronic phase, which occurs over hours to days, results largely from increased transcription of the steroidogenic enzymes. A summary of the pathways of adrenal steroid biosynthesis and the structures of the major steroid intermediates and products of the human adrenal cortex are shown in Figure 42–3. The rate-limiting step in steroid hormone production is the conversion of cholesterol to pregnenolone, a reaction catalyzed by CYP11A1, the cholesterol side-chain cleavage enzyme. Most of the enzymes required for steroid hormone biosynthesis, including CYP11A1, are members of the cytochrome P450 superfamily of mixed-function oxidases that play important roles in the metabolism of xenobiotics such as drugs and environmental pollutants, as well as in the biosynthesis of such endogenous compounds as steroid hormones, vitamin D, bile acids, fatty acids, prostaglandins, and biogenic amines (Chapter 6). The rate-limiting components in this reaction regulate the mobilization of substrate cholesterol and its delivery to CYP11A1 in the inner mitochondrial matrix.

To ensure an adequate supply of substrate for steroidogenesis, the adrenal cortex uses multiple sources of cholesterol (Kraemer, 2007), including:

- circulating cholesterol and cholesterol esters taken up via the low-density lipoprotein and high-density lipoprotein receptor pathways
- endogenous cholesterol liberated from cholesterol ester stores via activation of cholesterol esterase
- endogenous cholesterol from *de novo* biosynthesis.

The mechanisms by which ACTH stimulates the translocation of cholesterol to the inner mitochondrial matrix are not fully defined. A 37,000-Da phosphoprotein—designated the steroidogenic acute regulatory protein—clearly plays essential roles in cholesterol delivery. Mutations in the gene encoding this phosphoprotein are found in patients with congenital lipoid adrenal hyperplasia, a rare congenital disorder in which adrenal cells become engorged with cholesterol deposits secondary to an inability to synthesize any steroid hormones (Stocco, 2002). An important component of the trophic effect of ACTH is the enhanced transcription of genes that encode the individual steroidogenic enzymes, with associated

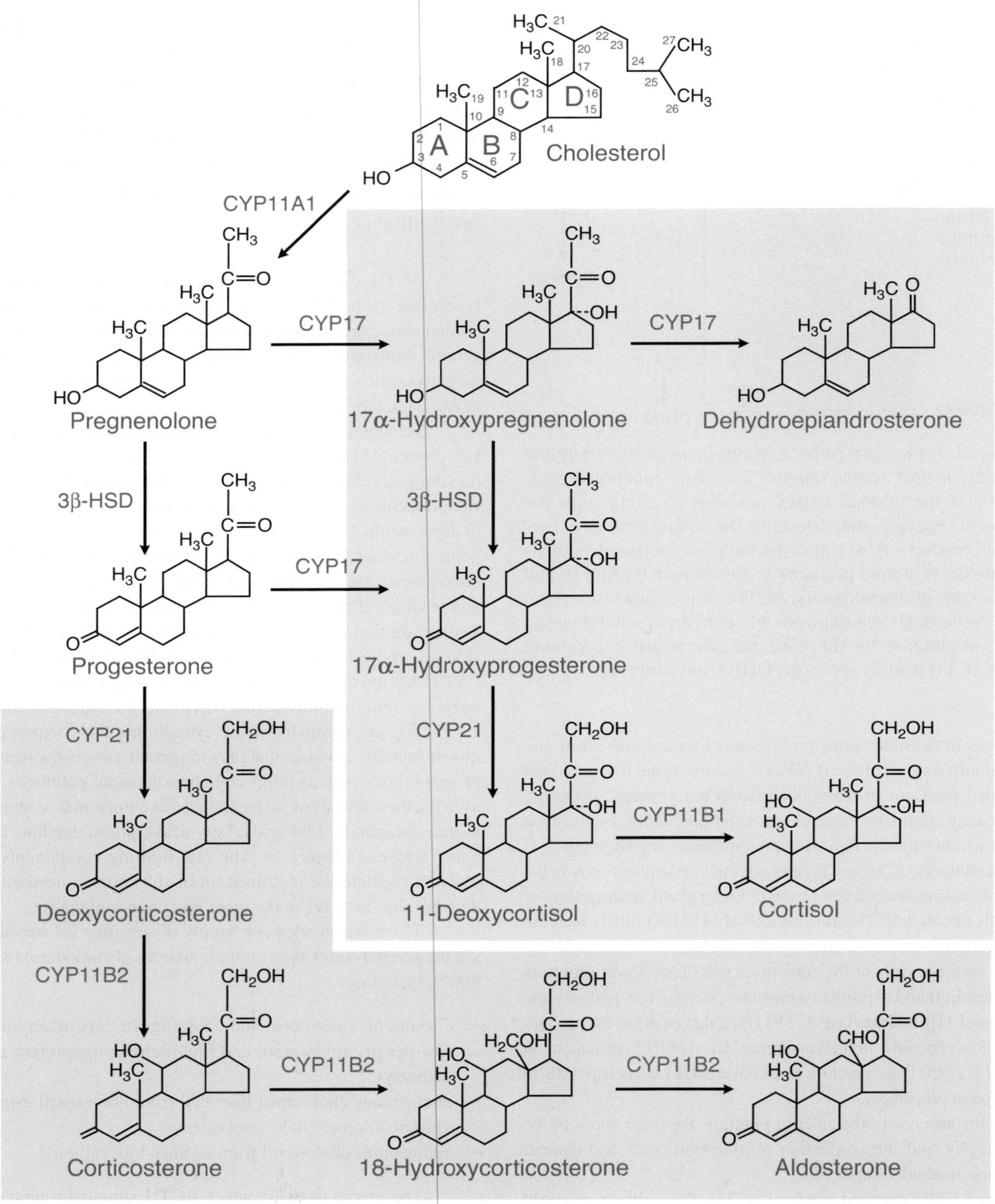

Figure 42–3. *Pathways of corticosteroid biosynthesis.* The steroidogenic pathways used in the biosynthesis of the corticosteroids are shown, along with the structures of the intermediates and products. The pathways unique to the zona glomerulosa are shown in orange box, whereas those that occur in the inner zona fasciculata and zona reticularis are shown in gray box. The zona reticularis does not express 3ß-HSD and thus preferentially synthesizes DHEA. CYP11A1, cholesterol side-chain cleavage enzyme; 3β-HSD, 3β-hydroxysteroid dehydrogenase; CYP17, steroid 17α-hydroxylase; CYP21, steroid 21-hydroxylase; CYP11B2, aldosterone synthase; CYP11B1, steroid 11β-hydroxylase.

increases in the steroidogenic capacity of the gland. Myriad transcriptional regulators participate in the induction of steroid hydroxylases by ACTH. Among these is the nuclear receptor NR5A1 (steroidogenic factor 1), a transcription factor required for the development of the adrenal cortex and for the expression of most of the steroidogenic enzymes (Parker et al., 2002).

Extra-Adrenal Effects of ACTH. In large doses, ACTH causes a number of metabolic changes in adrenalectomized animals, including ketosis, lipolysis, hypoglycemia (immediately after treatment), and resistance to insulin (later after treatment). Given the large doses of ACTH required, the physiological significance of these extra-adrenal effects is questionable. ACTH also reportedly improves learning in experimental animals, an effect postulated to be mediated via distinct receptors in the CNS.

Regulation of ACTH Secretion.

Hypothalamic-Pituitary-Adrenal Axis. The rate of glucocorticoid secretion is determined by fluctuations in the release of ACTH by the pituitary corticotropes. These corticotropes are regulated by corticotropin-releasing hormone (CRH) and arginine vasopressin (AVP), peptide hormones released by specialized neurons of the endocrine hypothalamus, which, in turn, are regulated by several neurotransmitters from the CNS. These three organs collectively are referred to as the hypothalamic-pituitary-adrenal (HPA) axis, an integrated system that maintains appropriate levels of glucocorticoids (Figure 42–4). The three characteristic modes of regulation of the HPA axis are diurnal rhythm in basal steroidogenesis, negative feedback regulation by adrenal corticosteroids, and marked increases in steroidogenesis in response to stress. The diurnal rhythm is entrained by higher neuronal centers in response to sleep-wake cycles, such that levels of ACTH peak in the early morning hours, causing the circulating glucocorticoid levels to peak at ~8 A.M. As discussed later, negative feedback regulation occurs at multiple levels of the HPA axis and is the major mechanism that maintains circulating glucocorticoid levels in the appropriate range. Stress can override the normal negative feedback control mechanisms, leading to marked increases in plasma concentrations of glucocorticoids.

Following release into the hypophyseal plexus, CRH is transported via this portal system to the anterior pituitary, where it binds to specific membrane receptors on corticotropes. Upon CRH binding, the CRH receptor activates the G_s-adenylyl cyclase–cyclic AMP pathway within corticotropes, ultimately stimulating both ACTH biosynthesis and secretion. CRH and CRH-related peptides called urocortins also are produced at other sites, including the amygdala

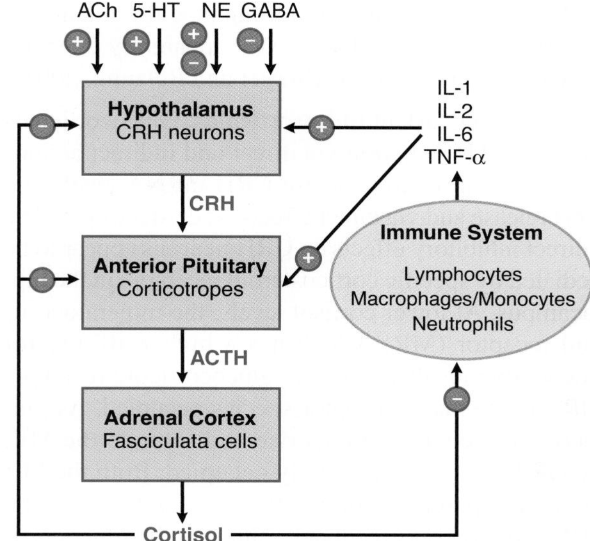

Figure 42–4. *Overview of the hypothalamic-pituitary-adrenal (HPA) axis and the immune inflammatory network.* Also shown are inputs from higher neuronal centers that regulate CRH secretion. + indicates a positive regulator, – indicates a negative regulator, + and – indicates a mixed effect, as for NE (norepinephrine). In addition, arginine vasopressin stimulates release of ACTH from corticotropes.

and hindbrain, gut, skin, adrenal gland, adipose tissue, placenta, and additional sites in the periphery. The classical CRH receptor, now designated CRF_1 receptor, belongs to the class II family of G protein-coupled receptors that includes receptors for calcitonin, parathyroid hormone, growth hormone-releasing hormone, secretin, glucagon, and glucagon-like peptide. A second CRH receptor, designated CRF_2 receptor, shares 70% homology at the amino acid level and is distinguished from the CRF_1 receptor in its binding specificities for CRH and the urocortins. In mice, the CRF_2 receptor opposes those effects mediated by the CRF_1 receptor thereby, providing a highly complex neural network that modulates the adaptive response to stress (Bale and Vale, 2004). The finding that the HPA axis often is altered in patients suffering from major depressive disorders illustrates the complex relationships between stress and mood and has stimulated considerable interest in the possible use of CRH antagonists in disorders such as anxiety and depression (Holsboer and Ising, 2008).

Arginine Vasopressin. Arginine vasopressin (AVP) also acts as a secretagogue for corticotropes, significantly potentiating the effects of CRH. Animal studies suggest that the potentiation of CRH action by AVP probably contributes to the full magnitude of the stress response *in vivo*. Like CRH, AVP is produced in the parvocellular neurons of the paraventricular nucleus and secreted into the pituitary plexus from the median eminence. After binding to V_{1b} receptors, AVP activates the

G_q-PLC-IP_3-Ca^{2+} pathway to enhance the release of ACTH. In contrast to CRH, AVP apparently does not increase ACTH synthesis (Surget and Belzung, 2008).

Negative Feedback of Glucocorticoids. Glucocorticoids inhibit ACTH secretion via direct and indirect actions on CRH neurons to decrease CRH mRNA levels and CRH release and via direct effects on corticotropes. The indirect inhibitory effects on CRH neurons appear to be mediated by specific corticosteroid receptors in the hippocampus. At lower cortisol levels, the mineralocorticoid receptor (MR), which has a higher affinity for glucocorticoids than classical glucocorticoid receptors (GR), is the major receptor species occupied. As glucocorticoid concentrations rise and saturate the MR, the GR becomes increasingly occupied. Both the MR and GR apparently control the basal activity of the HPA axis, whereas feedback inhibition by glucocorticoids predominantly involves the GR.

In the pituitary, glucocorticoids act through the GR to inhibit the release of ACTH from corticotropes and the expression of POMC. These effects are both rapid (occurring within seconds to minutes) and delayed (requiring hours and involving changes in gene transcription mediated through the GR).

The Stress Response. Stress overcomes negative feedback regulation of the HPA axis, leading to a marked rise in corticosteroid production. Examples of stress signals include injury, hemorrhage, severe infection, major surgery, hypoglycemia, cold, pain, and fear. Although the precise mechanisms that underlie this stress response and the essential actions played by corticosteroids are not fully defined, it is clear that their increased secretion is vital to maintain homeostasis in these stressful settings. As discussed later, complex interactions between the HPA axis and the immune system may be a fundamental physiological component of this stress response (Elenkov and Chrousos, 2006).

Assays for ACTH. Initially, ACTH levels were assessed by bioassays that measured induced steroid production or the depletion of adrenal ascorbic acid. Immunochemiluminescent assays that use two separate antibodies directed at distinct epitopes on the ACTH molecule now are widely available. These assays increase considerably the ability to differentiate patients with primary hypoadrenalism due to intrinsic adrenal disease, who have high ACTH levels due to the loss of normal glucocorticoid feedback inhibition, from those with secondary forms of hypoadrenalism, due to low ACTH levels resulting from hypothalamic or pituitary disorders. The immunochemiluminescent ACTH assays also are useful in differentiating between ACTH-dependent and ACTH-independent forms of hypercorticism: High ACTH levels are seen when the hypercorticism results from pituitary adenomas (e.g., Cushing's disease) or nonpituitary tumors that secrete ACTH (e.g., the syndrome of ectopic ACTH), whereas low ACTH levels are seen in patients with excessive glucocorticoid production due to primary adrenal disorders. Despite their considerable utility, one problem with the immunoassays for ACTH is that their specificity for intact ACTH can lead to falsely low values in patients with ectopic ACTH secretion; these tumors can secrete aberrantly processed forms of ACTH that have biological activity but do not react in the antibody assays.

Therapeutic Uses and Diagnostic Applications of ACTH. There are anecdotal reports that selected conditions respond better to ACTH than to corticosteroids (e.g., multiple sclerosis), and some clinicians continue to advocate therapy with ACTH. Despite this, ACTH currently has only limited utility as a therapeutic agent. Therapy with ACTH is less predictable and less convenient than therapy with corticosteroids. In addition, ACTH stimulates mineralocorticoid and adrenal androgen secretion and may therefore cause acute retention of salt and water, as well as virilization. Although ACTH and the corticosteroids are not pharmacologically equivalent, all proven therapeutic effects of ACTH can be achieved with appropriate doses of corticosteroids with a lower risk of side effects.

Testing the Integrity of the HPA Axis. The major clinical use of ACTH is in testing the integrity of the HPA axis. Other tests used to assess the HPA axis include the insulin tolerance test (Chapter 38) and the metyrapone test (discussed later in this chapter). Cosyntropin (CORTROSYN, SYNACTHEN) is a synthetic peptide that corresponds to residues 1-24 of human ACTH. At the considerably supraphysiological dose of 250 μg, cosyntropin maximally stimulates adrenocortical steroidogenesis. In the standard cosyntropin stimulation test, 250 μg of cosyntropin is administered either intramuscularly or intravenously, with cortisol measured just before administration (baseline) and 30-60 minutes after cosyntropin administration. An increase in the circulating cortisol to a level greater than 18-20 μg/dL indicates a normal response. Some accept an increase of 9 μg/dL over the baseline value as a positive response. In patients with pituitary or hypothalamic disease of recent onset or shortly after surgery for pituitary tumors, the standard cosyntropin stimulation test may be misleading because the duration of ACTH deficiency may have been insufficient to cause significant adrenal atrophy with frank loss of steroidogenic capacity. For these patients, some experts advocate a "low-dose" cosyntropin stimulation test, in which 1 μg of cosyntropin is administered intravenously, and cortisol is measured just before and 30 minutes after cosyntropin administration; the cutoff for a normal response is the same as that for the standard test. Care must be taken to avoid adsorption of the cosyntropin to plastic tubing and to measure the plasma cortisol precisely at 30 minutes after the cosyntropin injection. Although some studies indicate that the low-dose test is more sensitive than the standard 250-μg test, others report that this test also may fail to detect secondary adrenal insufficiency.

As already noted, primary adrenocortical insufficiency and secondary adrenocortical insufficiency are reliably distinguished by available sensitive assays for ACTH. More protracted ACTH stimulation tests rarely are used to differentiate between these disorders.

CRH Stimulation Test. Ovine CRH (corticorelin [ACTHREL]) and human CRH are available for diagnostic testing of the HPA axis, with the former used in the U.S. and the latter preferred in Europe. In patients with documented ACTH-dependent hypercorticism, CRH testing may help differentiate between a pituitary source (i.e.,

Cushing's disease) and an ectopic source of ACTH. After two baseline blood samples are obtained 15 minutes apart, CRH (1μg/kg) is administered intravenously over a 30- to 60-second interval, and peripheral blood samples are obtained at 15, 30, and 60 minutes for ACTH measurement. It is important that the blood samples be handled as recommended for the ACTH assay. At the recommended dose, CRH generally is well tolerated, although flushing may occur, particularly if the dose is administered as a bolus. Patients with Cushing's disease respond to CRH with either a normal or an exaggerated increase in ACTH, whereas ACTH levels generally do not increase in patients with ectopic sources of ACTH. This test is not perfect: ACTH levels are induced by CRH in occasional patients with ectopic ACTH, and ~5-10% of patients with Cushing's disease fail to respond.

To improve the diagnostic accuracy of the CRH stimulation test, many authorities advocate sampling of blood from the inferior petrosal sinuses and the peripheral circulation after peripheral administration of CRH. In this test, an inferior petrosal/peripheral ratio of >2.5 supports a pituitary source of ACTH. When performed by a skilled neuroradiologist, this procedure increases diagnostic accuracy with a tolerable risk of complications from the catheterization procedure (Arnaldi et al., 2003).

Absorption and Fate. ACTH is readily absorbed from parenteral sites. The hormone rapidly disappears from the circulation after intravenous administration; in humans, the $t_{1/2}$ in plasma is ~15 minutes, primarily due to rapid enzymatic hydrolysis.

Toxicity of ACTH. Aside from rare hypersensitivity reactions, the toxicity of ACTH is primarily attributable to the increased secretion of corticosteroids. Cosyntropin generally is less antigenic than native ACTH; thus, cosyntropin is the preferred agent for clinical use.

ADRENOCORTICAL STEROIDS

The adrenal cortex synthesizes two classes of steroids: the *corticosteroids* (glucocorticoids and mineralocorticoids), which have 21 carbon atoms, and the *androgens*, which have 19 carbons (Figure 41–3). The actions of corticosteroids historically were described as glucocorticoid (reflecting their carbohydrate metabolism–regulating activity) and mineralocorticoid (reflecting their electrolyte balance–regulating activity). In humans, *cortisol* (*hydrocortisone*) is the main glucocorticoid and aldosterone is the main mineralocorticoid. Table 42–1 shows typical rates of secretion of cortisol and aldosterone, as well as their normal circulating concentrations.

Although the adrenal cortex is an important source of androgen precursors in women, patients with adrenal insufficiency can be restored to normal life expectancy by replacement therapy with glucocorticoids and mineralocorticoids. Adrenal androgens are not essential for survival. The levels of dehydroepiandrosterone (DHEA) and its sulfated derivative DHEA-S peak in the third decade of life and decline progressively thereafter. Moreover, patients with a number of chronic diseases have very low DHEA levels, leading some to propose that DHEA treatment might at least partly alleviate the loss of libido, the decline in cognitive function, the decreased sense of well-being, and other adverse physiological consequences of aging. Whereas some studies have shown that addition of DHEA to the standard replacement regimen in women with adrenal insufficiency improved subjective well-being and sexuality, others have failed to show any benefit of DHEA replacement in either men or women (Chang et al., 2008). Nevertheless, DHEA is widely used as an over-the-counter nutritional supplement for its alleged health benefits, despite the absence of definitive data.

Table 42–1

Normal Daily Production Rates and Circulating Levels of the Predominant Corticosteroids

	CORTISOL	ALDOSTERONE
Rate of secretion under optimal conditions	10 mg/day	0.125 mg/day
Concentration in peripheral plasma:		
8 A.M.	16 μg/100 mL	0.01 μg/100 mL
4 A.M.	4 μg/100 mL	0.01 μg/100 mL

Physiological Functions and Pharmacological Effects

Physiological Actions. Corticosteroids have numerous and widespread effects, which include alterations in carbohydrate, protein, and lipid metabolism; maintenance of fluid and electrolyte balance; and preservation of normal function of the cardiovascular system, the immune system, the kidney, skeletal muscle, the endocrine system, and the nervous system. In addition, corticosteroids endow the organism with the capacity to resist such stressful circumstances as noxious stimuli and environmental changes. In the absence of the adrenal cortex, survival is made possible only by maintaining an optimal environment, including adequate and regular feeding, ingestion of relatively large amounts of sodium chloride, and maintenance of an appropriate environmental temperature; stresses such as infection, trauma, and extremes in temperature in this setting can be life threatening.

Traditionally, the effects of administered corticosteroids have been viewed as physiological (reflecting actions of corticosteroids at doses corresponding to normal daily production levels) or pharmacological (representing effects seen only at doses exceeding the normal daily production of corticosteroids). More recent concepts suggest that the anti-inflammatory and immunosuppressive actions of corticosteroids—one of the major "pharmacological" uses of this class of drugs—also provide a protective mechanism in the physiological setting. Many of the immune mediators associated with the inflammatory response decrease vascular tone and could lead to cardiovascular collapse if unopposed by the adrenal corticosteroids. This hypothesis is supported by the fact that the daily production rate of cortisol can rise at least 10-fold in the setting of severe stress. In addition, the pharmacological actions of corticosteroids in different tissues and the physiological effects are mediated by the same receptor. Thus the various glucocorticoid derivatives used as pharmacological agents generally have side effects on physiological processes that parallel their therapeutic effectiveness.

The actions of corticosteroids are related to those of other hormones. For example, in the absence of lipolytic hormones, cortisol has virtually no effect on the rate of lipolysis by adipocytes. Likewise, in the absence of glucocorticoids, epinephrine and norepinephrine have only minor effects on lipolysis. Administration of a small dose of glucocorticoid, however, markedly potentiates the lipolytic action of these catecholamines. Those effects of corticosteroids that involve concerted actions with other hormonal regulators are termed *permissive* and most likely reflect steroid-induced changes in protein synthesis that, in turn, modify tissue responsiveness to other hormones.

Corticosteroids are grouped according to their relative potencies in Na^+ retention, effects on carbohydrate metabolism (i.e., hepatic deposition of glycogen and gluconeogenesis), and anti-inflammatory effects. In general, potencies of steroids as judged by their ability to sustain life in adrenalectomized animals closely parallel those determined for Na^+ retention, whereas potencies based on effects on glucose metabolism closely parallel those for anti-inflammatory effects. The effects on Na^+ retention and the carbohydrate/anti-inflammatory actions are not closely related and reflect selective actions at distinct receptors.

Based on these differential potencies, the corticosteroids traditionally are divided into mineralocorticoids and glucocorticoids. Estimates of potencies of representative steroids in these actions are listed in Table 42–2. Some steroids that are classified predominantly as glucocorticoids (e.g., cortisol) also possess modest but significant mineralocorticoid activity and thus may affect fluid and electrolyte handling in the clinical setting. At doses used for replacement therapy in patients with primary adrenal insufficiency, the mineralocorticoid effects of these "glucocorticoids" are insufficient to replace that of aldosterone, and concurrent therapy with a more potent mineralocorticoid generally is needed. In contrast, aldosterone is exceedingly potent with respect to Na^+ retention but has only modest potency for effects on carbohydrate metabolism. At normal rates of secretion by the adrenal cortex or in doses that maximally affect electrolyte balance, aldosterone has no significant glucocorticoid activity and thus acts as a pure mineralocorticoid.

General Mechanisms for Corticosteroid Effects. Corticosteroids bind to specific receptor proteins in target tissues to regulate the expression of corticosteroid-responsive genes, thereby changing the levels and array of proteins synthesized by the various target tissues (Figure 42–5). As a consequence of the time required to modulate gene expression and protein synthesis, most effects of corticosteroids are not immediate but become

Table 42–2

Relative Potencies and Equivalent Doses of Representative Corticosteroids

COMPOUND	ANTI-INFLAMMATORY POTENCY	Na^+-RETAINING POTENCY	DURATION OF ACTION[a]	EQUIVALENT DOSE (mg)[b]
Cortisol	1	1	S	20
Cortisone	0.8	0.8	S	25
Fludrocortisone	10	125	I	[c]
Prednisone	4	0.8	I	5
Prednisolone	4	0.8	I	5
6α-Methylprednisolone	5	0.5	I	4
Triamcinolone	5	0	I	4
Betamethasone	25	0	L	0.75
Dexamethasone	25	0	L	0.75

[a]S, short (i.e., 8-12 hour biological $t_{1/2}$); I, intermediate (i.e., 12-36 hour biological $t_{1/2}$); L, long (i.e., 36-72 hour biological $t_{1/2}$).
[b]These dose relationships apply only to oral or intravenous administration, as glucocorticoid potencies may differ greatly following intramuscular or intraarticular administration.
[c]This agent is not used for glucocorticoid effects.

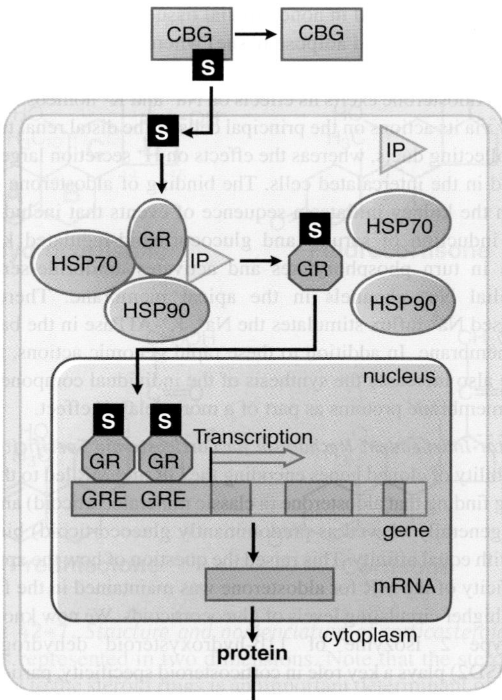

Figure 42–5. *Intracellular mechanism of action of the glucocorticoid receptor.* The figure shows the molecular pathway by which cortisol (labeled S) enters cells and interacts with the glucocorticoid receptor (GR) to change GR conformation (indicated by the change in shape of the GR), induce GR nuclear translocation, and activate transcription of target genes. The example shown is one in which glucocorticoids activate expression of target genes; the expression of certain genes, including pro-opiomelanocortin (POMC) expression by corticotropes, is inhibited by glucocorticoid treatment. CBG, corticosteroid-binding globulin; GR, glucocorticoid receptor; S, steroid hormone; HSP90, the 90-kd heat-shock protein; HSP70, the 70-kd heat-shock protein; IP, the 56-kd immunophilin; GRE, glucocorticoid-response elements in the DNA that are bound by GR, thus providing specificity to induction of gene transcription by glucocorticoids. Within the gene are introns (*gray*) and exons (*red*); transcription and mRNA processing leads to splicing and removal of introns and assembly of exons into mRNA.

apparent after several hours. This fact is of clinical significance because a delay generally is seen before beneficial effects of corticosteroid therapy become manifest. Although corticosteroids predominantly act by increasing gene transcription, there are well-documented examples in which glucocorticoids decrease gene transcription, as discussed later. In addition, corticosteroids may exert some of their immediate effects by nongenomic mechanisms (Stahn and Buttgereit, 2008).

Glucocorticoid Receptors. The receptors for corticosteroids are members of the nuclear receptor family of transcription factors that transduce the effects of a diverse array of small hydrophobic ligands, including the steroid hormones, thyroid hormone, vitamin D, and retinoids. These receptors share two highly conserved domains: a region of ~70 amino acids forming two zinc-binding domains, called *zinc fingers*, that are essential for the interaction of the receptor with specific DNA sequences, and a region at the carboxyl terminus that interacts with ligand (the ligand-binding domain). The GR resides predominantly in the cytoplasm in an inactive form until it binds glucocorticoids (Figure 42–5). Steroid binding results in receptor activation and translocation to the nucleus. The inactive GR is complexed with other proteins, including heat-shock protein (HSP) 90, a member of the heat-shock family of stress-induced proteins; HSP70; and a 56,000-Da immunophilin, one of the group of intracellular proteins that bind the immunosuppressive agents cyclosporine and tacrolimus (see Chapter 35). HSP90, through interactions with the steroid-binding domain, may facilitate folding of the GR into an appropriate conformation that permits ligand binding.

The gene encoding the GR is located on human chromosome 5 and gives rise to several receptor isoforms as the result of alternative RNA splicing. Of these, GRα is the prototypical glucocorticoid-responsive isoform already discussed and is the best studied. A second major GR isoform, GRβ, is a truncated dominant negative variant that lacks 35 amino acids at the C-terminus and is unable to bind glucocorticoids or activate gene expression. GRβ expression is enhanced by tumor necrosis factor α and other pro-inflammatory cytokines and its relative abundance is thought to contribute to glucocorticoid resistance in some patients. Other splice variants have been identified that retain their ligand-binding activity but have amino acid insertions or deletions of the DNA-binding domain that reduce their transcriptional activity (Gross and Cidlowski, 2008). Finally, polymorphisms have been identified in the human GR that are associated with differences in GR function and have been linked to glucocorticoid insensitivity (Derijk et al., 2008).

Although complete loss of GR function apparently is lethal, mutations leading to partial loss of GR function occur in rare patients with generalized glucocorticoid resistance (Charmandari et al., 2008). These patients harbor mutations in the GR, most of which impair glucocorticoid binding and decrease transcriptional activation. As a consequence of these mutations, cortisol levels that normally mediate feedback inhibition fail to suppress the HPA axis completely. In this setting of partial loss of GR function, the HPA axis resets to a higher level to provide compensatory increases in ACTH and cortisol secretion. Because the GR defect is partial, adequate compensation for the end-organ insensitivity can result from the elevated cortisol level, but the excess ACTH secretion also stimulates the production of mineralocorticoids and adrenal androgens. Because the mineralocorticoid receptor (MR) and the androgen receptor are intact, these subjects present with manifestations of mineralocorticoid excess (hypertension and hypokalemic alkalosis) and/or of increased androgen levels (acne, hirsutism, male pattern baldness, menstrual irregularities, anovulation, and infertility). In children, the excess adrenal androgens can cause precocious sexual development.

Regulation of Gene Expression by Glucocorticoids. After ligand binding, the GR dissociates from its associated proteins and translocates

effect of other agents, such as growth hormone and β adrenergic receptor agonists, resulting in an increase in free fatty acids after glucocorticoid administration.

One hypothesis for the redistribution of body fat is that peripheral and truncal adipocytes differ in their relative sensitivities to insulin and to glucocorticoid-facilitated lipolytic effects. Truncal adipocytes respond predominantly to elevated levels of insulin resulting from glucocorticoid-induced hyperglycemia, whereas peripheral adipocytes are less sensitive to insulin and respond mostly to the glucocorticoid-facilitated effects of other lipolytic hormones. This differential sensitivity may reflect differences in the expression of 11βHSD1 that converts inactive cortisone into active cortisol in target tissues (Figure 42–6). Consistent with this idea, overexpression of 11βHSD1 in adipocytes causes obesity in a transgenic mouse model. The potential role of this enzyme in adipocyte function has prompted speculation that 11βHSD1 inhibitors may have a role in the treatment of obesity.

Electrolyte and Water Balance. Aldosterone is by far the most potent endogenous corticosteroid with respect to fluid and electrolyte balance. Thus, electrolyte balance is relatively normal in patients with adrenal insufficiency due to pituitary disease, despite the loss of glucocorticoid production by the inner cortical zones. Mineralocorticoids act on the distal tubules and collecting ducts of the kidney to enhance reabsorption of Na^+ from the tubular fluid; they also increase the urinary excretion of K^+ and H^+. Conceptually, it is useful to think of aldosterone as stimulating a renal exchange between Na^+ and K^+ or H^+, although this does not involve a simple 1:1 exchange of cations in the renal tubule.

These actions on electrolyte transport, in the kidney and in other tissues (e.g., colon, salivary glands, and sweat glands), appear to account for the physiological and pharmacological activities that are characteristic of mineralocorticoids. Thus, the primary features of hyperaldosteronism are positive Na^+ balance with consequent expansion of extracellular fluid volume, normal or slight increases in plasma Na^+ concentration, normal or low plasma K^+, and alkalosis. Mineralocorticoid deficiency, in contrast, leads to Na^+ wasting and contraction of the extracellular fluid volume, hyponatremia, hyperkalemia, and acidosis. Indeed, mineralocorticoid-deficient patients are especially predisposed to Na^+ loss and volume depletion through excessive sweating in hot environments. Chronically, hyperaldosteronism causes hypertension, whereas aldosterone deficiency can lead to hypotension and vascular collapse.

Further insights into the roles of aldosterone target genes in fluid and electrolyte balance have emerged from analyses of patients with rare genetic disorders of mineralocorticoid action, such as *pseudohypoaldosteronism* and *pseudoaldosteronism.* Despite elevated levels of mineralocorticoids, patients with classical pseudohypoaldosteronism (i.e., type 1 disease) present with clinical manifestations suggestive of deficient mineralocorticoid action (i.e., volume depletion, hypotension, hyperkalemia, and metabolic acidosis). Molecular analyses have defined discrete subpopulations of patients with this disorder. One form of the disease is caused by autosomal dominant mutations in the MR that impair its activity. A second, autosomal recessive form results from loss-of-function mutations in genes encoding subunits of the amiloride-sensitive epithelial Na^+ channel. A nonclassical pseudohypoaldosteronism (type 2, also known as Gordon's syndrome) presents with hyperkalemia, mild metabolic acidosis, and familial hypertension. In some of these patients, the disease is caused by autosomal dominant mutations in the protein kinase genes *WNK1* and *WNK4* that inhibit the sodium chloride cotransporter. Pseudoaldosteronism, also termed Liddle's syndrome, is an autosomal dominant disease that results from mutations in subunits of the amiloride-sensitive Na^+ channel that interfere with its downregulation. The constitutive activity of this channel leads to hypertension, hypokalemia, and metabolic alkalosis, despite low levels of plasma renin and aldosterone.

Glucocorticoids also exert effects on fluid and electrolyte balance, largely due to permissive effects on tubular function and actions that maintain glomerular filtration rate. Glucocorticoids play a permissive role in the renal excretion of free water. In part, the inability of patients with glucocorticoid deficiency to excrete free water results from the increased secretion of AVP, which stimulates water reabsorption in the kidney.

In addition to their effects on monovalent cations and water, glucocorticoids also exert multiple effects on Ca^{2+} metabolism. Steroids lower Ca^{2+} uptake from the gut and increase Ca^{2+} excretion by the kidney. These effects collectively lead to decreased total body Ca^{2+} stores.

Cardiovascular System. The most striking effects of corticosteroids on the cardiovascular system result from mineralocorticoid-induced changes in renal Na^+, as is evident in primary aldosteronism. Studies have shown direct effects of MR activation on the heart and vessel wall; aldosterone induces hypertension and interstitial cardiac fibrosis in animal models. The increased cardiac fibrosis is proposed to result from direct mineralocorticoid actions in the heart rather than from the effect of hypertension because treatment with spironolactone, a MR antagonist, blocks the development of fibrosis without altering blood pressure. Indeed, in age-, sex-, and blood pressure-matched hypertensive patients, those with primary aldosteronism have a higher prevalence of atrial fibrillation, stroke, and myocardial infarction, indicating direct effects of increased aldosterone on the cardiovascular system. Similar cardiac effects of MR activation in human beings may explain the beneficial effects of spironolactone in patients with congestive heart failure (Chapter 28).

The second major action of corticosteroids on the cardiovascular system is to enhance vascular reactivity to other vasoactive substances. Hypoadrenalism is associated with reduced responsiveness to vasoconstrictors such as norepinephrine and angiotensin II, perhaps due to decreased expression of adrenergic receptors in the vascular wall. Conversely, hypertension is seen in patients with excessive glucocorticoid secretion, occurring in most patients with Cushing's syndrome and in a subset of patients treated with synthetic glucocorticoids (even those lacking any significant mineralocorticoid action).

The underlying mechanisms in glucocorticoid-induced hypertension also are unknown; the hypertension related to the endogenous secretion of cortisol, as seen in patients with Cushing's syndrome, likely results from multiple effects mediated by the GR and MR. Unlike hypertension caused by high aldosterone levels, the hypertension secondary to excess glucocorticoids is generally resistant to Na^+ restriction (Magiakou et al., 2006).

Skeletal Muscle. Permissive concentrations of corticosteroids are required for the normal function of skeletal muscle, and diminished work capacity is a prominent sign of adrenocortical insufficiency. In patients with Addison's disease, weakness and fatigue are frequent symptoms. Excessive amounts of either glucocorticoids or mineralocorticoids also impair muscle function. In primary aldosteronism, muscle weakness results primarily from hypokalemia rather than from direct effects of mineralocorticoids on skeletal muscle. In contrast, glucocorticoid excess over prolonged periods, either secondary to glucocorticoid therapy or endogenous hypercorticism, causes skeletal muscle wasting. This effect, termed *steroid myopathy*, accounts in part for weakness and fatigue in patients with glucocorticoid excess and is discussed in more detail later.

Central Nervous System. Corticosteroids exert a number of indirect effects on the CNS, through maintenance of blood pressure, plasma glucose concentrations, and electrolyte concentrations. Increasingly, direct effects of corticosteroids on the CNS have been recognized, including effects on mood, behavior, and brain excitability.

Patients with adrenal insufficiency exhibit a diverse array of neurological manifestations, including apathy, depression, and irritability; some patients are frankly psychotic. Appropriate replacement therapy corrects these abnormalities. Conversely, glucocorticoid administration can induce multiple CNS reactions. Most patients respond with mood elevation, which may impart a sense of well-being despite the persistence of underlying disease. Some patients exhibit more pronounced behavioral changes, such as mania, insomnia, restlessness, and increased motor activity. A smaller but significant percentage of patients treated with glucocorticoids become anxious, depressed, or overtly psychotic. A high incidence of neuroses and psychoses is seen in patients with Cushing's syndrome. These abnormalities usually disappear after cessation of glucocorticoid therapy or treatment of the Cushing's syndrome.

The mechanisms whereby corticosteroids affect neuronal activity are unknown, but it has been proposed that steroids produced locally in the brain (termed *neurosteroids*) may regulate neuronal excitability. In rodent models, very high doses of glucocorticoids decrease survival and function of hippocampal neurons; in association with these changes, memory also is diminished. In one study in human subjects, basal cortisol levels correlated directly with hippocampal atrophy and memory deficits. To the extent that these results are confirmed, they may have important prognostic implications for age-related memory decline, and for therapeutic approaches directed at diminishing the negative effects of glucocorticoids on hippocampal neurons with aging.

Formed Elements of Blood. Glucocorticoids exert minor effects on hemoglobin and erythrocyte content of blood, as evidenced by the frequent occurrence of polycythemia in Cushing's syndrome and of normochromic, normocytic anemia in adrenal insufficiency. More profound effects are seen in the setting of autoimmune hemolytic anemia, in which the immunosuppressive effects of glucocorticoids can diminish the self-destruction of erythrocytes.

Corticosteroids also affect circulating white blood cells. Addison's disease is associated with an increased mass of lymphoid tissue and lymphocytosis. In contrast, Cushing's syndrome is characterized by lymphocytopenia and decreased mass of lymphoid tissue. The administration of glucocorticoids leads to a decreased number of circulating lymphocytes, eosinophils, monocytes, and basophils. A single dose of hydrocortisone leads to a decline of these circulating cells within 4-6 hours; this effect persists for 24 hours and results from the redistribution of cells away from the periphery rather than from increased destruction. In contrast, glucocorticoids increase circulating polymorphonuclear leukocytes as a result of increased release from the marrow, diminished rate of removal from the circulation, and decreased adherence to vascular walls. Finally, certain lymphoid malignancies are destroyed by glucocorticoid treatment, an effect that may relate to the ability of glucocorticoids to activate programmed cell death.

Anti-inflammatory and Immunosuppressive Actions. In addition to their effects on lymphocyte number, corticosteroids profoundly alter the immune responses of lymphocytes. These effects are an important facet of the anti-inflammatory and immunosuppressive actions of the glucocorticoids. Glucocorticoids can prevent or suppress inflammation in response to multiple inciting events, including radiant, mechanical, chemical, infectious, and immunological stimuli. Although the use of glucocorticoids as anti-inflammatory agents does not address the underlying cause of the disease, the suppression of inflammation is of enormous clinical utility and has made these drugs among the most frequently prescribed agents. Similarly, glucocorticoids are of immense value in treating diseases that result from undesirable immune reactions. These diseases range from conditions that predominantly result from humoral immunity, such as urticaria (Chapter 65), to those that are mediated by cellular immune mechanisms, such as transplantation rejection (Chapter 35). The immunosuppressive and anti-inflammatory actions of glucocorticoids are inextricably linked, perhaps because they both involve inhibition of leukocyte functions.

Multiple mechanisms are involved in the suppression of inflammation by glucocorticoids. Glucocorticoids inhibit the production by multiple cells of factors that are critical in generating the inflammatory response. As a result, there is decreased release of vasoactive and chemoattractive factors, diminished secretion of lipolytic and proteolytic enzymes, decreased extravasation of leukocytes to areas of injury, and ultimately, decreased fibrosis. Glucocorticoids can also reduce expression of pro-inflammatory cytokines, as well as COX-2 and NOS2. Some of the cell types and mediators that are inhibited by glucocorticoids are summarized in Table 42–3. The net effect of these actions on various cell types is to diminish markedly the inflammatory response.

The influence of stressful conditions on immune defense mechanisms is well documented, as is the contribution of the HPA axis to the stress response (Elenkov and Chrousos, 2006). This has led to a growing appreciation of the importance of glucocorticoids as physiological modulators of the immune system, where glucocorticoids appear to protect the organism against life-threatening consequences of a full-blown inflammatory response (Chrousos, 1995).

Stresses such as injury, infection, and disease result in the increased production of cytokines, a network of signaling molecules that integrate actions of macrophages/monocytes, T lymphocytes, and B lymphocytes in mounting immune responses. Among these cytokines, interleukin (IL)-1, IL-6, and tumor necrosis factor α (TNF-α) stimulate the HPA axis, with IL-1 having the broadest range of actions. IL-1 stimulates the release of CRH by hypothalamic neurons, interacts directly with the pituitary to increase the release of ACTH, and may directly stimulate the adrenal gland to produce glucocorticoids. As detailed earlier, the increased production of glucocorticoids, in turn, profoundly inhibits the immune system at multiple sites. Factors that are inhibited include components of the cytokine network, including interferon γ (IFN-γ), granulocyte-macrophage colony-stimulating factor (GM-CSF), interleukins (IL-1, IL-2, IL-3, IL-6, IL-8, and IL-12), and TNF-α. Thus, the HPA axis and the immune system are capable of bidirectional interactions in response to stress, and these interactions appear to be important for homeostasis (Chrousos, 1995).

Absorption, Transport, Metabolism, and Excretion

Absorption. Hydrocortisone and numerous congeners, including the synthetic analogs, are orally effective. Certain water-soluble esters of hydrocortisone and its

Table 42–3

Effects of Glucocorticoids on Components of Inflammatory/Immune Responses

CELL TYPE	FACTOR	COMMENTS
Macrophages and monocytes	Arachidonic acid and its metabolites (prostaglandins and leukotrienes)	Mediated by glucocorticoid inhibition of COX-2 and PLA_2.
	Cytokines, including: interleukin (IL)-1, IL-6, and tumor necrosis factor-α (TNF-α)	Production and release are blocked. The cytokines exert multiple effects on inflammation (e.g., activation of T cells, stimulation of fibroblast proliferation).
	Acute phase reactants	These include the third component of complement.
Endothelial cells	ELAM-1 and ICAM-1	ELAM-1 and ICAM-1: critical for leukocyte localization.
	Acute phase reactants Cytokines (e.g., IL-1) Arachidonic acid derivatives	Same as above, for macrophages and monocytes.
Basophils	Histamine, LTC_4	IgE-dependent release inhibited by glucocorticoids.
Fibroblasts	Arachidonic acid metabolites	Same as above for macrophages and monocytes. Glucocorticoids also suppress growth factor–induced DNA synthesis and fibroblast proliferation.
Lymphocytes	Cytokines (IL-1, IL-2, IL-3, IL-6, TNF-α, GM-CSF, interferon-γ)	Same as above for macrophages and monocytes.

ELAM-1, endothelial-leukocyte adhesion molecule-1; ICAM-1, intercellular adhesion molecule-1.

synthetic congeners are administered intravenously to achieve high concentrations of drug rapidly in body fluids. More prolonged effects are obtained by intramuscular injection of suspensions of hydrocortisone, its esters, and congeners. Minor changes in chemical structure may markedly alter the rate of absorption, time of onset of effect, and duration of action.

Glucocorticoids also are absorbed systemically from sites of local administration, such as synovial spaces, the conjunctival sac, skin, and respiratory tract. When administration is prolonged, when the site of application is covered with an occlusive dressing, or when large areas of skin are involved, absorption may be sufficient to cause systemic effects, including suppression of the HPA axis.

Transport, Metabolism, and Excretion. After absorption, ≥90% of cortisol in plasma is reversibly bound to protein under normal circumstances. Only the fraction of corticosteroid that is unbound is active and can enter cells. Two plasma proteins account for almost all of the steroid-binding capacity: corticosteroid-binding globulin (CBG; also called transcortin), and albumin. CBG is an α-globulin secreted by the liver that has high affinity for steroids (estimated dissociation constant of ~1.3×10^{-9} M) but relatively low total binding capacity, whereas albumin, also produced by the liver, has a relatively large binding capacity but low affinity (estimated dissociation constant of 1×10^{-3} M). Because of its higher dissociation constant, albumin-bound corticosteroid makes a greater contribution to the active corticosteroid fraction in tissues that have a slow capillary transit time (e.g., liver and spleen) than in tissues with rapid capillary transit times (e.g., kidney). At normal or low concentrations of corticosteroids, most of the hormone is protein bound. At higher steroid concentrations, the capacity of protein binding is exceeded, and a greater fraction of the steroid exists in the free state. Corticosteroids compete with each other for binding sites on CBG. CBG has relatively high affinity for cortisol and some of its synthetic congeners and low affinity for aldosterone and glucuronide-conjugated steroid metabolites; thus, greater percentages of these latter steroids are found in the free form.

A special state of physiological hypercorticism occurs during pregnancy. The elevated circulating estrogen levels induce CBG production, and CBG and total plasma cortisol increase severalfold. The physiological significance of these changes remains to be established.

All of the biologically active adrenocortical steroids and their synthetic congeners have a double bond in the 4,5 position and a ketone group at C3 (Figure 42–7). As a general rule, the metabolism of steroid hormones involves sequential additions of oxygen or hydrogen atoms, followed by conjugation to form water-soluble derivatives. Reduction of the 4,5 double bond occurs at both hepatic and extrahepatic sites, yielding inactive compounds. Subsequent reduction of the 3-ketone substituent to the 3-hydroxyl derivative, forming tetrahydrocortisol, occurs only in the liver. Most of these A ring–reduced steroids are conjugated through the 3-hydroxyl group with sulfate or glucuronide by enzymatic reactions that take place in the liver and, to a lesser extent, in the kidney. The resultant sulfate esters and glucuronides are water soluble and the predominant forms excreted in urine. Neither biliary nor fecal excretion is of quantitative importance in humans.

Synthetic steroids with an 11-keto group, such as cortisone and prednisone, must be enzymatically reduced to the corresponding 11β-hydroxy derivative before they are biologically active. The type 1 isozyme of 11β-hydroxysteroid dehydrogenase (11βHSD1) catalyzes this reduction, predominantly in the liver, but also in specialized sites such as adipocytes, bone, eye, and skin. In settings in which this enzymatic activity is impaired, it is prudent to use steroids that do not require enzymatic activation (e.g., hydrocortisone or prednisolone rather than cortisone or prednisone). Such settings include severe hepatic failure and patients with the rare condition of cortisone reductase deficiency, who are unable to activate the 11-keto steroids because of a defect in the enzyme hexose-6-phosphate dehydrogenase, which regulates the activity of 11β-hydroxysteroid dehydrogenase by supplying required reducing equivalents (Lavery et al., 2008).

Structure–Activity Relationships

Chemical modifications to the cortisol molecule have generated derivatives with greater separations of glucocorticoid and mineralocorticoid activity; for a number of synthetic glucocorticoids, the effects on electrolytes are minimal even at the highest doses used (Table 42–2). In addition, these modifications have led to derivatives with greater potencies and with longer durations of action. A vast array of steroid preparations is available for oral, parenteral, and topical use. Some of these agents are summarized in Table 42–4. None of these currently available derivatives effectively separates anti-inflammatory effects from effects on carbohydrate, protein, and fat metabolism, or from suppressive effects on the HPA axis.

The structures of hydrocortisone (cortisol) and some of its major derivatives are shown in Figure 42–7. Changes in chemical structure may alter the specificity and/or potency due to changes in affinity and intrinsic activity at corticosteroid receptors, and alterations in absorption, protein binding, rate of metabolic transformation, rate of excretion, or membrane permeability. The effects of various substitutions on glucocorticoid and mineralocorticoid activity and on duration of action are summarized in Table 42–2. The 4,5 double bond and the 3-keto group on ring A are essential for glucocorticoid and mineralocorticoid activity; an 11β-hydroxyl group on ring C is required for glucocorticoid activity but not mineralocorticoid activity; a hydroxyl group at C21 on ring D is present on all natural corticosteroids and on most of the active synthetic analogs, and seems to be an absolute requirement for mineralocorticoid but not glucocorticoid activity. The 17α-hydroxyl group on ring D is a substituent on cortisol and on all of the currently used synthetic glucocorticoids. Although steroids without the 17α -hydroxyl group (e.g., corticosterone) have appreciable glucocorticoid activity, the 17α-hydroxyl group gives optimal potency.

Introduction of an additional double bond in the 1,2 position of ring A, as in prednisolone or prednisone, selectively increases glucocorticoid activity, and results in an enhanced glucocorticoid/mineralocorticoid potency ratio. This modification also results in compounds that are metabolized more slowly than hydrocortisone.

Fluorination at the 9α position on ring B enhances both glucocorticoid and mineralocorticoid activity, possibly related to an electron-withdrawing effect on the nearby 11β-hydroxyl group. Fludrocortisone (9α-fluorocortisol) has enhanced activity at the GR (10 times relative to cortisol) but even greater activity at the MR (125 times relative to cortisol). It is used in mineralocorticoid replacement therapy and has no appreciable glucocorticoid effect at usual daily doses of 0.05-0.2 mg. When combined with the 1,2 double bond in ring A plus other substitutions at C16 on ring D (Figure 42–7), the 9α-fluoro derivatives formed (e.g., triamcinolone, dexamethasone, and betamethasone) have marked glucocorticoid activity—the substitutions at C16 virtually eliminate mineralocorticoid activity.

Other Substitutions. 6α Substitution on ring B has somewhat unpredictable effects. 6α-Methylcortisol has increased glucocorticoid and mineralocorticoid activity, whereas 6α-methylprednisolone has somewhat greater glucocorticoid activity and somewhat less mineralocorticoid activity than prednisolone. A number of modifications convert the glucocorticoids to more lipophilic molecules with enhanced topical/systemic potency ratios. Examples include the introduction of an acetonide between hydroxyl groups at C16 and C17, esterification of the hydroxyl group with valerate at C17, esterification of hydroxyl groups with propionate at C17 and C21, and substitution of the hydroxyl group at C21 with chlorine. Other approaches to achieve local glucocorticoid activity while minimizing systemic effects involve the formation of analogs that are rapidly inactivated after absorption (e.g., C21 carboxylate or carbothioate glucocorticoid esters, which are rapidly metabolized to inactive 21-carboxylic acids) or the formation of inactive analogs that are selectively activated at their site of action (e.g., glucocorticoid C21 isobutyryl or propionyl esters that are hydrolyzed to active C21 alcohols by airway-specific esterases).

Toxicity of Adrenocortical Steroids

Two categories of toxic effects result from the therapeutic use of corticosteroids: those resulting from withdrawal of steroid therapy and those resulting from continued use at supraphysiological doses. The side effects from both categories are potentially life threatening and require a careful assessment of the risks and benefits in each patient.

Withdrawal of Therapy. The most frequent problem in steroid withdrawal is flare-up of the underlying disease for which steroids were prescribed. Several other complications are associated with steroid withdrawal. The most severe complication of steroid cessation, acute adrenal insufficiency, results from overly rapid withdrawal of corticosteroids after prolonged therapy has suppressed the HPA axis. The therapeutic approach to acute adrenal insufficiency is detailed later. There is significant variation among patients with respect to the degree and duration of adrenal suppression after glucocorticoid therapy, making it difficult to establish the relative risk in any given patient. Many patients recover from glucocorticoid-induced HPA suppression within several weeks to months; however, in some individuals the time to recovery can be a year or longer.

In an effort to diminish the risk of iatrogenic acute adrenal insufficiency, protocols for discontinuing corticosteroid therapy in patients receiving long-term treatment with corticosteroids have been proposed, generally without rigorous documentation of their efficacy. Patients who have received supraphysiological doses of glucocorticoids for a period of 2-4 weeks within the preceding year should be considered to have some degree of HPA impairment in settings of acute stress and should be treated accordingly.

In addition to this most severe form of withdrawal, a characteristic glucocorticoid withdrawal syndrome consists of fever, myalgia, arthralgia, and malaise, which may be difficult to differentiate from some of the underlying diseases for which steroid therapy was instituted (Hochberg et al., 2003). Finally, *pseudotumor cerebri*, a clinical syndrome that includes increased intracranial pressure with papilledema, is a rare condition that sometimes is associated with reduction or withdrawal of corticosteroid therapy.

Continued Use of Supraphysiological Glucocorticoid Doses. Besides the consequences that result from the suppression of the HPA axis, a number of other complications result from prolonged therapy with corticosteroids. These include fluid and electrolyte abnormalities, hypertension, hyperglycemia, increased susceptibility to infection, osteoporosis, myopathy, behavioral disturbances, cataracts, growth arrest, and the characteristic habitus of steroid overdose, including fat redistribution, striae, and ecchymoses.

Fluid and Electrolyte Handling. Alterations in fluid and electrolyte handling can cause hypokalemic alkalosis and hypertension, particularly in patients with primary hyperaldosteronism secondary to an adrenal adenoma or in patients treated with potent mineralocorticoids. Similarly, hypertension is a relatively common manifestation of glucocorticoid excess, even in patients treated with glucocorticoids lacking appreciable mineralocorticoid activity.

Metabolic Changes. The effects of glucocorticoids on intermediary metabolism have already been described. Hyperglycemia with glycosuria usually can be managed with diet and/or insulin, and its occurrence should not be a major factor in the decision to continue corticosteroid therapy or to initiate therapy in diabetic patients.

Immune Responses. Because of their multiple effects to inhibit the immune system and the inflammatory response, glucocorticoid use is associated with an increased susceptibility to infection and a risk for reactivation of latent tuberculosis. In the presence of known infections of some consequence, glucocorticoids should be administered only if absolutely necessary and concomitantly with appropriate and effective antimicrobial or antifungal therapy.

Table 42–4

Available Preparations of Adrenocortical Steroids and Their Synthetic Analogs

NONPROPRIETARY NAME	TRADE NAME	TYPE OF PREPARATION
Alclometasone dipropionate	ACLOVATE	Topical
Amcinonide		Topical
Betamethasone acetate and sodium phosphate	CELESTONE SOLUSPAN	Injectable
Beclomethasone dipropionate	BECONASE AQ, QVAR40, QVAR80	Inhaled
	DIPROLENE, DIPROLINE AF	Topical
Betamethasone sodium phosphate	CELESTONE	Oral
Betamethasone valerate	BETA-VAL, DERMABET, LUXIQ	Topical
Budesonide	ENTOCORT EC	Oral
	PULMICORT	Inhaled
	RHINOCORT	Nasal
Ciclesonide	ALVESCO, OMNARIS	Inhaled
Clobetasol propionate	CLOBEX, CORMAX EMBELINE, OLUX, TEMOVATE	Topical
Clocortolone pivalate	CLODERM	Topical
Desonide	DESONATE, DESOWEN, VERDESO	Topical
Desoximetasone	TOPICORT	Topical
Dexamethasone		Oral
Dexamethasone sodium phosphate	MAXIDEX	Ophthalmic
Diflorasone diacetate	PSORCON	Topical
Fludrocortisone acetate*		Oral
Flunisolide	AEROBID, AEROSPAN HFA	Inhaled
	NASAREL	Nasal
Fluocinolone acetonide	DERMA-SMOOTHE/FS, FS, SYNALAR	Topical
	RETISERT	Intravitreal implant
Fluocinonide	LIDEX, LIDEX-E, VANOS	Topical
Fluorometholone	FML, FML FORTE	Ophthalmic
Fluorometholone acetate	FLAREX	Ophthalmic
Flurandrenolide	CORDRAN CORDRAN SP	Topical
Halcinonide	HALOG	Topical
Hydrocortisone	ALA-CORT, HYTONE, NUTRACORT, STIE-CORT, SYNACORT, TEXACORT	Topical
	CORTEF	Oral
Hydroxycortisone acetate	MICORT-HC	Topical
	CORTIFOAM	Rectal
Hydroxycortisone butyrate	LOCOID	Topical

(Continued)

Table 42–4

Available Preparations of Adrenocortical Steroids and Their Synthetic Analogs (Continued)

NONPROPRIETARY NAME	TRADE NAME	TYPE OF PREPARATION
Hydrocortisone cypionate	CORTEF	Oral
Hydrocortisone sodium succinate	A-HYDROCORT, SOLU-CORTEF	Injectable
Hydrocortisone valerate	WESTCORT	Topical
Methylprednisolone acetate	MEDROL	Oral
	DEPO-MEDROL	Injectable
Methylprednisolone sodium succinate	A-METHAPRED, SOLU-MEDROL	Injectable
Mometasone furoate	ASMANEX	Inhaled
	NASONEX	Nasal
	ELOCON	Topical
Prednisolone		Oral
Prednisolone acetate	FLO-PRED	Oral
	OMNIPRED, PRED FORT, PRED MILD	Ophthalmic
Prednisolone sodium phosphate	ORAPRED, ORAPRED ODT, PEDIAPRED	Oral
Prednisone		Oral
Triamcinolone acetonide	AZMACORT	Inhaled
	NASACORT AQ	Nasal
	KENOLOG	Topical
	KENOLOG-10, KENALOG-40, TRIESENCE, TRIVARIS	Injectable
Triamcinolone hexacetonide	ARISTOSPAN	Injectable
	AZMACORT	Inhaled

*Fludrocortisone acetate is intended for use as a mineralocorticoid.
Note: *Topical* preparations include agents for application to skin or mucous membranes in creams, solutions, ointments, gels, pastes (for oral lesions), and aerosols; *ophthalmic* preparations include solutions, suspensions, and ointments; *inhalation* preparations include agents for nasal or oral inhalation.

Possible Risk of Peptic Ulcers. There is considerable debate about the association between peptic ulcers and glucocorticoid therapy. The possible onset of hemorrhage and perforation in these ulcers and their insidious onset make peptic ulcers a serious therapeutic problem (Chapter 45); estimating the degree of risk from corticosteroids has received much study. Most patients who develop gastrointestinal bleeding while receiving corticosteroids also receive nonsteroidal anti-inflammatory agents, which are known to promote ulceration, such that the pathogenic role of corticosteroids remains open to debate. Nonetheless, it is prudent to be especially vigilant for peptic ulcer formation in patients receiving therapy with corticosteroids, especially if administered concomitantly with nonsteroidal anti-inflammatory drugs.

Myopathy. Myopathy, characterized by weakness of proximal limb muscles, can occur in patients taking large doses of corticosteroids and also is part of the clinical picture in patients with endogenous Cushing's syndrome. It can be of sufficient severity to impair ambulation and is an indication for withdrawal of therapy. Attention also has focused on steroid myopathy of the respiratory muscles in patients with asthma or chronic obstructive pulmonary disease (Chapter 36); this complication can diminish respiratory function. Recovery from the steroid myopathies may be slow and incomplete.

Behavioral Changes. Behavioral disturbances are common after administration of corticosteroids and in patients who have Cushing's syndrome secondary to endogenous hypercorticism; these disturbances may take many forms, including nervousness, insomnia, changes in mood or psyche, and overt psychosis. Suicidal tendencies are not uncommon. A history of previous psychiatric illness does not preclude the use of steroids in patients for whom they are otherwise indicated. Conversely, the absence of a history of previous psychiatric illness does not guarantee that a given patient will not develop psychiatric disorders while on steroids.

Cataracts. Cataracts are a well-established complication of glucocorticoid therapy and related to dosage and duration of therapy. Children appear to be particularly at risk. Cessation of therapy may not lead to complete resolution of opacities, and the cataracts may progress despite reduction or cessation of therapy. Patients on long-term glucocorticoid therapy at doses of prednisone of ≥10-15 mg/day should receive periodic slit-lamp examinations to detect glucocorticoid-induced posterior subcapsular cataracts.

Osteoporosis. Osteoporosis, a frequent serious complication of glucocorticoid therapy, occurs in patients of all ages and is related to dosage and duration of therapy (Woolf, 2007). A reasonable estimate is that 30-50% of all patients who receive chronic glucocorticoid therapy ultimately will develop osteoporotic fractures. Glucocorticoids preferentially affect trabecular bone and the cortical rim of the vertebral bodies; the ribs and vertebrae are the most frequent sites of fracture. Glucocorticoids decrease bone density by multiple mechanisms, including inhibition of gonadal steroid hormones, diminished gastrointestinal absorption of Ca^{2+}, and inhibition of bone formation due to suppressive effects on osteoblasts and stimulation of resorption by osteoclasts via changes in the production of osteoprotegerin and RANK ligand. In addition, glucocorticoid inhibition of intestinal Ca^{2+} uptake may lead to secondary increases in parathyroid hormone, thereby increasing bone resorption.

The considerable morbidity of glucocorticoid-related osteoporosis has led to efforts to identify patients at risk for fractures and to prevent or reverse bone loss in patients requiring chronic glucocorticoid therapy. The initiation of glucocorticoid therapy—that is, ≥5 mg/day prednisone (or its equivalent) for ≥3 months—is considered an indication for bone densitometry to detect abnormalities in trabecular bone. Because bone loss associated with glucocorticoids predominantly occurs within the first 6 months of therapy, densitometric evaluation, preferably with techniques such as dual-energy x-ray absorptiometry of the lumbar spine and hip, along with prophylactic measures should be initiated with therapy or shortly thereafter. Most authorities advocate maintaining a Ca^{2+} intake of 1500 mg/day by diet plus Ca^{2+} supplementation and vitamin D intake of 800 IU/day, assuming that these measures do not increase urinary calcium excretion above the normal range. Although gonadal hormone replacement therapy has been widely used in specific groups of patients receiving chronic glucocorticoid therapy, this is the subject of considerable debate based on recently published results from randomized placebo-controlled trials (Chapter 40). Recombinant parathyroid hormone 1-34 (teriparatide, FORTEO) also has received considerable attention as a potential therapy of glucocorticoid-induced osteoporosis.

The most important advance to date in the prevention of glucocorticoid-related osteoporosis is the successful use of bisphosphonates, which have been shown to decrease the decline in bone density and the incidence of fractures in patients receiving glucocorticoid therapy. Additional discussion of these issues is found in Chapters 40 and 44.

Osteonecrosis. Osteonecrosis (also known as avascular or aseptic necrosis) is a relatively common complication of glucocorticoid therapy. The femoral head is affected most frequently, but this process also may affect the humeral head and distal femur. Joint pain and stiffness usually are the earliest symptoms, and this diagnosis should be considered in patients receiving glucocorticoids who abruptly develop hip, shoulder, or knee pain. Although the risk increases with the duration and dose of glucocorticoid therapy, osteonecrosis also can occur when high doses of glucocorticoids are given for short periods of time. Osteonecrosis generally progresses, and most affected patients ultimately require joint replacement.

Regulation of Growth and Development. Growth retardation in children can result from administration of relatively small doses of glucocorticoids. Although the precise mechanism is unknown, there are reports that collagen synthesis and linear growth in these children can be restored by treatment with growth hormone; further studies are needed to define the role of concurrent treatment with growth hormone in this setting. Further studies also are needed to explore the possible effects of exposure to corticosteroids *in utero*. In experimental animals, antenatal exposure to glucocorticoids is clearly linked to cleft palate and altered neuronal development, ultimately resulting in complex behavioral abnormalities. Thus, although the actions of glucocorticoids to promote cellular differentiation play important physiological roles in human development in late gestation and in the neonatal period (e.g., production of pulmonary surfactant and induction of hepatic gluconeogenic enzymes), the possibility remains that antenatal steroids can lead to subtle abnormalities in fetal development.

Therapeutic Uses

With the exception of replacement therapy in deficiency states, the use of glucocorticoids largely is empirical. Based on extensive clinical experience, a number of therapeutic principles can be proposed. Given the number and severity of potential side effects, the decision to institute therapy with glucocorticoids always requires a careful consideration of the relative risks and benefits in each patient. For any disease and in any patient, the appropriate dose to achieve a given therapeutic effect must be determined by trial and error and must be reevaluated periodically as the activity of the underlying disease changes or as complications of therapy arise. *A single dose of glucocorticoid, even a large one, is virtually without harmful effects, and a short course of therapy (up to 1 week), in the absence of specific contraindications, is unlikely to be harmful. As the duration of glucocorticoid therapy is increased beyond 1 week, there are time- and dose-related increases in the incidence of disabling and potentially lethal effects.* Except in patients receiving replacement therapy, glucocorticoids are neither specific nor curative; rather, they are palliative by virtue of their anti-inflammatory and immunosuppressive actions. Finally, *abrupt cessation of glucocorticoids after prolonged therapy is associated with the risk of adrenal insufficiency, which may be fatal.*

These principles have several implications for clinical practice. When glucocorticoids are to be given over long periods, the dose must be determined by trial and error and must be the lowest that will achieve the desired effect. When the therapeutic goal is relief of painful or distressing symptoms not associated with an immediately life-threatening disease, complete relief is not sought, and the steroid dose is reduced gradually until worsening symptoms indicate that the minimal acceptable dose has been found. Where possible, the substitution of other medications, such as nonsteroidal anti-inflammatory drugs, may facilitate tapering the glucocorticoid dose once the initial benefit of therapy has been achieved. When therapy is directed at a life-threatening disease (e.g., pemphigus or lupus cerebritis), the initial dose should be a large one aimed at achieving rapid control of the crisis. If some benefit is not observed quickly, then the dose should be doubled or tripled. After initial control in a potentially lethal disease, dose reduction should be carried out under conditions that permit frequent accurate observations of the patient. It is always essential to weigh carefully the relative dangers of therapy and of the disease being treated.

The lack of demonstrated deleterious effects of a single dose of glucocorticoids within the conventional therapeutic range justifies their administration to critically ill patients who may have adrenal insufficiency. If the underlying condition does result from deficiency of glucocorticoids, then a single intravenous injection of a soluble glucocorticoid may prevent immediate death and allow time for a definitive diagnosis to be made. If the underlying disease is not adrenal insufficiency, the single dose will not harm the patient.

In the absence of specific contraindications, short courses of high-dose systemic glucocorticoids also may be given for diseases that are not life threatening, but the general rule is that long courses of therapy at high doses should be reserved for life-threatening disease. In selected settings, as when a patient is threatened with permanent disability, this rule is justifiably violated.

In an attempt to dissociate therapeutic effects from undesirable side effects, various regimens of steroid administration have been used. To diminish HPA axis suppression, the intermediate-acting steroid preparations (e.g., prednisone or prednisolone) should be given in the morning as a single dose. Alternate-day therapy with the same glucocorticoids also has been employed because certain patients obtain adequate therapeutic responses on this regimen. Alternatively, pulse therapy with higher glucocorticoid doses (e.g., doses as high as 1 to 1.5 g/day of methylprednisolone for 3 days) frequently is used to initiate therapy in patients with fulminant, immunologically related disorders such as acute transplantation rejection, necrotizing glomerulonephritis, and lupus nephritis. The benefit of such pulse therapy in long-term maintenance regimens remains to be defined.

Replacement Therapy. Adrenal insufficiency can result from structural or functional lesions of the adrenal cortex (primary adrenal insufficiency or Addison's disease) or from structural or functional lesions of the anterior pituitary or hypothalamus (secondary adrenal insufficiency). In developed countries, primary adrenal insufficiency most frequently is secondary to autoimmune adrenal disease, whereas tuberculous adrenalitis is the most frequent etiology in developing countries. Other causes include adrenalectomy, bilateral adrenal hemorrhage, neoplastic infiltration of the adrenal glands, acquired immunodeficiency syndrome, inherited disorders of the steroidogenic enzymes, and X-linked adrenoleukodystrophy (Carey, 1997). Secondary adrenal insufficiency resulting from pituitary or hypothalamic dysfunction generally presents in a more insidious manner than does the primary disorder, probably because mineralocorticoid biosynthesis is preserved.

Acute Adrenal Insufficiency. This life-threatening disease is characterized by GI symptoms (nausea, vomiting, and abdominal pain), dehydration, hyponatremia, hyperkalemia, weakness, lethargy, and hypotension. It usually is associated with disorders of the adrenal rather than the pituitary or hypothalamus, and it sometimes follows abrupt withdrawal of glucocorticoids used at high doses or for prolonged periods.

The immediate management of patients with acute adrenal insufficiency includes intravenous therapy with isotonic sodium chloride solution supplemented with 5% glucose and corticosteroids and appropriate therapy for precipitating causes such as infection, trauma, or hemorrhage. Because cardiac function often is reduced in the setting of adrenocortical insufficiency, the patient should be monitored for evidence of volume overload such as rising central venous pressure or pulmonary edema. After an initial intravenous bolus of 100 mg, hydrocortisone (cortisol) should be given by continuous infusion at a rate of 50-100 mg every 8 hours. At this dose, which approximates the maximum daily rate of cortisol secretion in response to stress, hydrocortisone alone has sufficient mineralocorticoid activity to meet all requirements. As the patient stabilizes, the hydrocortisone dose may be decreased to 25 mg every 6-8 hours. Thereafter, patients are treated in the same fashion as those with chronic adrenal insufficiency.

For the treatment of suspected but unconfirmed acute adrenal insufficiency, 4 mg of dexamethasone sodium phosphate can be substituted for hydrocortisone because dexamethasone does not cross-react in the cortisol assay and will not interfere with the measurement of cortisol (either basally or in response to the cosyntropin stimulation test). A failure to respond to cosyntropin in this setting is diagnostic of adrenal insufficiency. Often, a sample for the measurement of plasma ACTH also is obtained because it will provide information about the underlying etiology if the diagnosis of adrenocortical insufficiency is established.

Chronic Adrenal Insufficiency. Patients with chronic adrenal insufficiency present with many of the same manifestations seen in adrenal crisis but with lesser severity. These patients require daily treatment with corticosteroids (Coursin and Wood, 2002).

Studies with other forms of renal disease, such as membranous and membranoproliferative glomerulonephritis and focal sclerosis, have provided conflicting data on the role of glucocorticoids. In clinical practice, patients with these disorders often are given a therapeutic trial of glucocorticoids with careful monitoring of laboratory indices of response. In the case of membranous glomerulonephritis, many nephrologists recommend a trial of alternate-day glucocorticoids for 8-10 weeks (e.g., prednisone, 120 mg every other day), followed by a 1- to 2-month period of tapering.

Allergic Disease. The onset of action of glucocorticoids in allergic diseases is delayed, and patients with severe allergic reactions such as anaphylaxis require immediate therapy with epinephrine. The manifestations of allergic diseases of limited duration—such as hay fever, serum sickness, urticaria, contact dermatitis, drug reactions, bee stings, and angioneurotic edema—can be suppressed by adequate doses of glucocorticoids given as supplements to the primary therapy. In severe disease, intravenous glucocorticoids (methylprednisolone, 125 mg intravenously every 6 hours, or equivalent) are appropriate. In less severe disease, antihistamines are the drugs of first choice. In allergic rhinitis, intranasal steroids are now viewed as the drug of choice by many experts.

Bronchial Asthma and Other Pulmonary Conditions. Corticosteroids frequently are used in bronchial asthma (Chapter 36). Although they sometimes are employed in chronic obstructive pulmonary disease (COPD), particularly when there is some evidence of reversible obstructive disease, data supporting the efficacy of corticosteroids are much less convincing than for bronchial asthma. The increased use of corticosteroids in asthma reflects an increased appreciation of the role of inflammation in the immunopathogenesis of this disorder. In severe asthma attacks requiring hospitalization, treatment with high-dose parenteral glucocorticoids is essential. Symptomatic relief sometimes is very rapid; however, the onset of a maintained response may take up to 6-12 hours. Intravenous administration of 60-120 mg methylprednisolone (or equivalent) every 6 hours is used initially, followed by daily oral doses of prednisone (30-60 mg) as the acute attack resolves. The dose then is tapered gradually, with withdrawal planned for 10 days to 2 weeks after initiation of steroid therapy. In general, patients subsequently can be managed on their prior medical regimen.

Less severe acute exacerbations of asthma (as well as acute flares of COPD) often are treated with brief courses of oral glucocorticoids. In adult patients, 30-60 mg prednisone is administered daily for 5 days; an additional week of therapy at lower doses also may be required. Upon resolution of the acute exacerbation, the glucocorticoids generally can be rapidly tapered without significant deleterious effects. Any suppression of adrenal function usually dissipates within 1-2 weeks. In the treatment of severe chronic bronchial asthma (or, less frequently, COPD) that is not controlled by other measures, the long-term administration of glucocorticoids may be necessary. As with other long-term uses of these agents, the lowest effective dose is used, and care must be exercised when withdrawal is attempted. Given the risks of long-term treatment with glucocorticoids, it is especially important to document objective evidence of a response (e.g., an improvement in pulmonary function tests). In addition, these risks dictate that long-term glucocorticoid therapy be reserved for those patients who have failed to respond to adequate regimens of other medications (Chapter 36).

In many patients, inhaled steroids (see Table 42–4) can either reduce the need for oral corticosteroids or replace them entirely. Many physicians prefer inhaled glucocorticoids over previously recommended oral theophylline in the treatment of children with moderately severe asthma, in part because of the behavioral toxicity associated with chronic theophylline administration. The oral bioavailability of inhaled corticosteroids varies considerably; however, when used as recommended, inhaled glucocorticoids are effective in reducing bronchial hyperreactivity and are less likely to suppress adrenal function than are the oral glucocorticoids. Dysphonia or oropharyngeal candidiasis may develop, but the incidence of such side effects can be reduced substantially by maneuvers that reduce drug deposition in the oral cavity, such as spacers and mouth rinsing or by using corticosteroids with low oral bioavailability. For example, ciclesonide (ALVESCO, OMNARIS) and beclomethasone dipropionate (BECONASE AQ, QVAR), are inactive compounds that are activated on site by lung esterases; therefore they are less likely to adversely affect the oral cavity (Derendorf et al., 2006). The status of glucocorticoids in asthma therapy is discussed in Chapter 36.

Antenatal glucocorticoids are used frequently in the setting of premature labor, decreasing the incidence of respiratory distress syndrome, intraventricular hemorrhage, and death in infants delivered prematurely. Betamethasone (12 mg intramuscularly every 24 hours for two doses) or dexamethasone (6 mg intramuscularly every 12 hours for four doses) is administered to women with definitive signs of premature labor between 26 and 34 weeks of gestation (Roberts and Dalziel, 2006). Due to evidence of decreased birthweight and adrenal suppression in infants whose mothers were given repeated courses of glucocorticoids, only a single course of glucocorticoids should be administered.

Infectious Diseases. Although the use of immunosuppressive glucocorticoids in infectious diseases may seem paradoxical, there are a limited number of settings in which they are indicated in the therapy of specific infectious pathogens. One dramatic example of such beneficial effects is seen in AIDS patients with *Pneumocystis carinii* pneumonia and moderate to severe hypoxia; addition of glucocorticoids to the antibiotic regimen increases oxygenation and lowers the incidence of respiratory failure and mortality. Similarly, glucocorticoids clearly decrease the incidence of long-term neurological impairment associated with *Haemophilus influenzae* type b meningitis in infants and children ≥2 months of age.

A long-standing controversy in medicine is the use of glucocorticoids in septic shock (Sprung et al., 2008). Supraphysiological doses of glucocorticoids had been used routinely as adjunctive therapy in subjects with septic shock associated with gram-negative bacteremia until it was recognized that glucocorticoid therapy in supraphysiologic doses actually increased mortality. Subsequent studies then examined the benefit of somewhat lower doses of glucocorticoids (e.g., 100 mg hydrocortisone every 8 hours) administered to patients early in the course of their disease. In one multicenter randomized placebo-controlled trial, beneficial effects of hydrocortisone plus fludrocortisone were seen only in subjects with adrenal insufficiency as determined by the rapid cosyntropin stimulation test. Although a second large study using hydrocortisone alone failed to demonstrate a beneficial effect regardless of adrenal status, current guidelines suggest that hydrocortisone be used in adult patients with septic shock whose blood pressure fails to respond adequately to fluids and vasopressors (Dellinger et al., 2008).

Ocular Diseases. Ocular pharmacology, including some consideration of the use of glucocorticoids, is discussed in Chapter 64. Glucocorticoids frequently are used to suppress inflammation in the eye and can preserve sight when used properly. They are administered topically for diseases of the outer eye and anterior segment and attain therapeutic concentrations in the aqueous humor after instillation into the conjunctival sac. For diseases of the posterior segment, intraocular injection or systemic administration is required. Generally, ocular use of glucocorticoids should be supervised by an ophthalmologist.

A typical prescription is 0.1% dexamethasone sodium phosphate solution (ophthalmic), 2 drops in the conjunctival sac every 4 hours while awake, and 0.05% dexamethasone sodium phosphate ointment (ophthalmic) at bedtime. For inflammation of the posterior segment, typical doses are 30 mg of prednisone or equivalent per day, administered orally in divided doses.

Topical glucocorticoid therapy frequently increases intraocular pressure in normal eyes and exacerbates intraocular hypertension in patients with antecedent glaucoma. The glaucoma is not always reversible on cessation of glucocorticoid therapy. Intraocular pressure should be monitored when glucocorticoids are applied to the eye for >2 weeks.

Topical administration of glucocorticoids to patients with bacterial, viral, or fungal conjunctivitis can mask evidence of progression of the infection until sight is irreversibly lost. Glucocorticoids are contraindicated in herpes simplex keratitis because progression of the disease may lead to irreversible clouding of the cornea. Topical steroids should not be used in treating mechanical lacerations and abrasions of the eye because they delay healing and promote the development and spread of infection.

Skin Diseases. Glucocorticoids are remarkably efficacious in the treatment of a wide variety of inflammatory dermatoses. As a result, a large number of different preparations and concentrations of topical glucocorticoids of varying potencies are available. A typical regimen for an eczematous eruption is 1% hydrocortisone ointment applied locally twice daily. Effectiveness is enhanced by application of the topical steroid under an occlusive film, such as plastic wrap; unfortunately, the risk of systemic absorption also is increased by occlusive dressings, and this can be a significant problem when the more potent glucocorticoids are applied to inflamed skin. Glucocorticoids are administered systemically for severe episodes of acute dermatological disorders and for exacerbations of chronic disorders. The dose in these settings is usually 40 mg/day of prednisone. Systemic steroid administration can be lifesaving in pemphigus, which may require daily doses of up to 120 mg of prednisone. Further discussion of the treatment of skin diseases is presented in Chapter 65.

Gastrointestinal Diseases. Glucocorticoid therapy is indicated in selected patients with inflammatory bowel disease (chronic ulcerative colitis and Crohn's disease; Chapter 47). Patients who fail to respond to more conservative management (i.e., rest, diet, and sulfasalazine) may benefit from glucocorticoids; steroids are most useful for acute exacerbations. In mild ulcerative colitis, hydrocortisone (100 mg) can be administered as a retention enema with beneficial effects. In more severe acute exacerbations, oral prednisone (10-30 mg/day) frequently is employed. For severely ill patients—with fever, anorexia, anemia, and impaired nutritional status—larger doses should be used (40-60 mg prednisone per day). Major complications of ulcerative colitis or Crohn's disease may occur despite glucocorticoid therapy, and glucocorticoids may mask signs and symptoms of complications such as intestinal perforation and peritonitis.

Budesonide, a highly potent synthetic glucocorticoid that is inactivated by first-pass hepatic metabolism, reportedly exhibits diminished systemic side effects commonly associated with glucocorticoids. Oral administration of budesonide in delayed-release capsules (ENTOCORT, 9 mg/day) facilitates drug delivery to the ileum and ascending colon; the drug also has been used as a retention enema in the treatment of ulcerative colitis.

Hepatic Diseases. The use of corticosteroids in hepatic disease has been highly controversial. Glucocorticoids clearly are of benefit in autoimmune hepatitis, where as many as 80% of patients show histological remission when treated with prednisone (40-60 mg daily initially, with tapering to a maintenance dose of 7.5-10 mg daily after serum transaminase levels fall). The role of corticosteroids in alcoholic liver disease is not fully defined; the most recent meta-analysis of previously published reports failed to establish a beneficial role of corticosteroids, even in patients with severe disease (Rambaldi et al., 2008). Further studies are needed to confirm or refute the role of steroids in this setting. In the setting of severe hepatic disease, prednisolone should be used instead of prednisone, which requires hepatic conversion to be active.

Malignancies. Glucocorticoids are used in the chemotherapy of acute lymphocytic leukemia and lymphomas because of their antilymphocytic effects. Most commonly, glucocorticoids are one component of combination chemotherapy administered under scheduled protocols. Glucocorticoids once were frequently employed in the setting of hypercalcemia of malignancy, but more effective agents, such as the bisphosphonates, now are the preferred therapy.

Cerebral Edema. Corticosteroids are of value in the reduction or prevention of cerebral edema associated with parasites and neoplasms, especially those that are metastatic. Although corticosteroids are frequently used for the treatment of cerebral edema caused by trauma or cerebrovascular accidents, controlled clinical trials do not support their use in these settings.

Miscellaneous Diseases and Conditions. Sarcoidosis. Corticosteroids are indicated therapy for patients with debilitating symptoms or life-threatening forms of sarcoidosis. Patients with severe pulmonary involvement are treated with 10-20 mg per day of prednisone, or an equivalent dose of alternative steroids, to induce remission. Higher doses may be required for other forms of this disease. Maintenance doses, which often are required for long periods of time, may be as low as 5 mg/day of prednisone. These patients, like all patients who require chronic glucocorticoid therapy at doses exceeding the normal daily production rate, are at increased risk of secondary tuberculosis; therefore, patients with a positive tuberculin reaction or other evidence of tuberculosis should receive prophylactic antituberculosis therapy.

Thrombocytopenia. In thrombocytopenia, prednisone (0.5 mg/kg) is used to decrease the bleeding tendency. In more severe cases, and for initiation of treatment of idiopathic thrombocytopenia, daily doses of prednisone (1-1.5 mg/kg) are employed. Patients with refractory idiopathic thrombocytopenia may respond to pulsed high-dose glucocorticoid therapy.

Autoimmune Destruction of Erythrocytes. Patients with autoimmune destruction of erythrocytes (i.e., hemolytic anemia with a positive

Coombs test) are treated with prednisone (1 mg/kg per day). In the setting of severe hemolysis, higher doses may be used, with tapering as the anemia improves. Small maintenance doses may be required for several months in patients who respond.

Organ Transplantation. In organ transplantation, high doses of prednisone (50-100 mg) are given at the time of transplant surgery, in conjunction with other immunosuppressive agents, and most patients are kept on a maintenance regimen that includes lower doses of glucocorticoids (Chapter 35). For some solid organ transplants (e.g., pancreas), protocols that either withdraw corticosteroids early after transplantation or that avoid them completely are becoming more common (Meier-Kriesche et al., 2006).

Spinal Cord Injury. A meta-analysis of several randomized, controlled trials (Bracken, 2002) demonstrated significant decreases in neurological defects in patients with acute spinal cord injury treated within 8 hours of injury with large doses of methylprednisolone sodium succinate (30 mg/kg initially followed by an infusion of 5.4 mg/kg per hour for 23 hours). One trial showed further improvement with an additional 24 hours of treatment. The ability of corticosteroids at these high doses to decrease neurological injury may reflect inhibition of free radical–mediated cellular injury, as occurs following ischemia and reperfusion. Potential side effects include increased susceptibility to infection and other wound complications.

Diagnostic Applications of Adrenocortical Steroids

In addition to its therapeutic uses, dexamethasone is used as a first-line agent to diagnose hypercortisolism and to differentiate among the different causes of Cushing's syndrome (Arnaldi et al., 2003).

To determine if patients with clinical manifestations suggestive of hypercortisolism have biochemical evidence of increased cortisol biosynthesis, an overnight dexamethasone suppression test has been devised. Patients are given 1 mg of dexamethasone orally at 11 P.M., and cortisol is measured at 8 A.M. the following morning. Suppression of plasma cortisol to <1.8 μg/dL suggests strongly that the patient does not have Cushing's syndrome. Drugs such as barbiturates that enhance dexamethasone metabolism or drugs (estrogens) or conditions (pregnancy) that increase the concentrations of corticosteroid binding globulin can interfere with suppression and compromise the test. The formal dexamethasone suppression test is used in the differential diagnosis of biochemically documented Cushing's syndrome. Following determination of baseline cortisol levels for 48 hours, dexamethasone (0.5 mg every 6 hours) is administered orally for 48 hours. This dose markedly suppresses cortisol levels in normal subjects, including those who have nonspecific elevations of cortisol due to obesity or stress, but it does not suppress levels in patients with Cushing's syndrome. In the high-dose phase of the test, dexamethasone is administered orally at 2 mg every 6 hours for 48 hours. Patients with pituitary-dependent Cushing's syndrome (i.e., Cushing's disease) generally respond with decreased cortisol levels. In contrast, patients with ectopic production of ACTH or with adrenocortical tumors generally do not exhibit decreased cortisol levels. Despite these generalities, dexamethasone may suppress cortisol levels in some patients with ectopic ACTH production, particularly with tumors such as bronchial carcinoids, and many experts prefer to use inferior petrosal sinus sampling after CRH administration to make this distinction.

INHIBITORS OF THE BIOSYNTHESIS AND ACTION OF ADRENOCORTICAL STEROIDS

Hypercortisolism with its attendant morbidity and mortality is most frequently caused by corticotroph adenomas that overproduce ACTH (Cushing's disease) or by adrenocortical tumors or bilateral hyperplasias that overproduce cortisol (Cushing's syndrome). Less frequently, hypercortisolism may result from adrenocortical carcinomas or ectopic ACTH- or CRH-producing tumors. Although surgery is the treatment of choice, it is not always effective, and adjuvant therapy with inhibitors of steroidogenesis becomes necessary (Biller et al., 2008). In these settings, ketoconazole, metyrapone, etomidate, and mitotane are clinically useful. Ketoconazole, etomidate, and mitotane are discussed in more detail in other chapters. All of these agents pose the common risk of precipitating acute adrenal insufficiency; thus, they must be used in appropriate doses, and the status of the patient's HPA axis must be carefully monitored. Agents that act as glucocorticoid receptor antagonists (antiglucocorticoids) are discussed later in this chapter; mineralocorticoid antagonists are discussed in Chapter 25.

Ketoconazole. Ketoconazole (NIZORAL) is an antifungal agent, and this remains its most important clinical role (Chapter 57). In doses higher than those employed in antifungal therapy, it is an effective inhibitor of adrenal and gonadal steroidogenesis, primarily because of its inhibition of the activity of CYP17 (17α-hydroxylase). At even higher doses, ketoconazole also inhibits CYP11A1, effectively blocking steroidogenesis in all primary steroidogenic tissues. Ketoconazole is the best tolerated and most effective inhibitor of steroid hormone biosynthesis in patients with hypercortisolism. In most cases, a dosage regimen of 600-800 mg/day (in two divided doses) is required, and some patients may require up to 1200 mg/day given in two to three doses. Side effects include hepatic dysfunction, which ranges from asymptomatic elevations of transaminase levels to severe hepatic injury. The potential of ketoconazole to interact with CYP isoforms can lead to drug interactions of serious consequence (Chapter 6). Further studies are needed to define the precise role of ketoconazole in the medical management of patients with excessive steroid hormonal production, and the FDA has not approved this indication for ketoconazole use.

Metyrapone. Metyrapone (METOPIRONE) is a relatively selective inhibitor of CYP11B1 (11β-hydroxylase), which converts 11-deoxycortisol to cortisol in the terminal reaction of the glucocorticoid biosynthetic pathway. Because of this inhibition, the biosynthesis of cortisol is markedly impaired, and the levels of steroid precursors (e.g., 11-deoxycortisol) are markedly increased. Although the biosynthesis of aldosterone also is impaired, the elevated levels of 11-deoxycortisol sustain mineralocorticoid-dependent functions. In a diagnostic test of the entire HPA axis, metyrapone (30 mg/kg, maximum dose of 3 g) is administered orally with a snack at midnight, and plasma cortisol and 11-deoxycortisol are measured at 8 A.M. the next morning. A plasma cortisol <8 μg/dL validates adequate inhibition of CYP11B1; in this setting, an 11-deoxycortisol level <7 μg/dL is highly suggestive of impaired hypothalamic-pituitary-adrenal function. An abnormal response does not identify the site of the defect; hypothalamic CRH release, ACTH production, or adrenal biosynthetic capacity could be impaired. Some authorities avoid overnight metyrapone testing in outpatients thought to have a reasonable probability of impaired HPA function because there is some risk of precipitating acute adrenal insufficiency. Others believe that the ability to assess the entire HPA axis with a relatively easy test justifies the use of metyrapone testing in outpatients.

Metyrapone also is used to diagnose patients with Cushing's syndrome who respond equivocally to the formal dexamethasone suppression test. Those with pituitary-dependent Cushing's syndrome exhibit a normal response, whereas those patients with ectopic secretion of ACTH exhibit no changes in ACTH or 11-deoxycortisol levels.

Therapeutically, metyrapone has been used to treat the hypercorticism resulting from either adrenal neoplasms or tumors producing ACTH ectopically. Maximal suppression of steroidogenesis requires doses of 4 g/day. More frequently, metyrapone is used as adjunctive therapy in patients who have received pituitary irradiation or in combination with other agents that inhibit steroidogenesis. In this setting, a dose of 500-750 mg three or four times daily is employed. The use of metyrapone in the treatment of Cushing's syndrome secondary to pituitary hypersecretion of ACTH is more controversial. Chronic administration of metyrapone can cause hirsutism, which results from increased synthesis of adrenal androgens upstream from the enzymatic block, and hypertension, which results from elevated levels of 11-deoxycortisol. Other side effects include nausea, headache, sedation, and rash.

Etomidate. Etomidate (AMIDATE), a substituted imidazole used primarily as an anaesthetic agent and sedative, inhibits cortisol secretion at subhypnotic doses primarily by inhibiting CYP11B1 activity. It is administered intravenously and has been used off-label to treat hypercortisolism when rapid control is required in a patient who cannot take medication by the oral route. An international consensus panel recommends that etomidate be administered as a bolus of 0.03 mg/kg intravenously, followed by an infusion of 0.1 mg/kg per hour to a maximum of 0.3 mg/kg per hour (Biller et al., 2008).

Mitotane. Mitotane (o,p'-DDD; LYSODREN) is an adrenocorticolytic agent used to treat inoperable adrenocortical carcinoma. Its cytolytic action is due to its metabolic conversion to a reactive acyl chloride by adrenal mitochondrial CYPs and subsequent reactivity with cellular proteins. In a few centers, it has been used for long-term control of hypercortisolism. Doses range from 0.5-3 g administered three times daily. Its onset of action takes weeks to months, and GI disturbances and ataxia are its major toxicities.

Aminoglutethimide. Aminoglutethimide (α-ethyl-*p*-aminophenylglutarimide; CYTADREN) primarily inhibits CYP11A1, which catalyzes the initial and rate-limiting step in the biosynthesis of all physiological steroids and also inhibits CYP11B1 and CYP19 (aromatase). As a result, the production of all classes of steroid hormones is impaired. Although used at one time to treat hypercortisolism and advanced cancer of the breast and prostate, aminoglutethimide recently has been withdrawn from the market by the manufacturer and is no longer available.

Trilostane. Trilostane (4α,5α,17β)-4-5-epoxy-3,17-dihydroxyandrost-2-ene-2-carbonitrile), a competitive inhibitor of the type II 3β-hydroxysteroid dehydrogenase (Figure 42–3), also interferes with the synthesis of both adrenal and gonadal hormones, but it is more effective in dogs than in humans. For this reason, trilostane is not used in humans but still has a place in veterinary medicine.

ANTIGLUCOCORTICOIDS

The progesterone receptor antagonist *mifepristone* (MIFEPREX; RU-486; 11β-[*p*-(dimethylamino)phenyl]-17β-hydroxy-17-(1-propynyl)estra-4,9-dien-3-one) has received considerable attention because of its use as an antiprogestogen that can terminate early pregnancy (Chapter 66). At higher doses, mifepristone also inhibits the GR, blocking feedback regulation of the HPA axis and secondarily increasing endogenous ACTH and cortisol levels. Because of its ability to inhibit glucocorticoid action, mifepristone also has been studied as a potential therapeutic agent in a small number of patients with hypercortisolism (Johanssen and Allolio, 2007). Currently, its use for this purpose is considered investigational and is restricted to patients with inoperable causes of cortisol excess that have not responded to other agents.

CLINICAL SUMMARY

Glucocorticoids are administered in multiple formulations (e.g., oral, parenteral, and topical) for disorders that share an inflammatory or immunological basis. Except in patients receiving replacement therapy for adrenal insufficiency, glucocorticoids are neither specific nor curative, but rather are palliative because of their anti-inflammatory and immunosuppressive actions. Given the number and severity of potential side effects, the decision to institute therapy with glucocorticoids always requires a careful consideration of the relative risks and benefits in each patient. After therapy is initiated, the minimal dose needed to achieve a given therapeutic effect must be determined by trial and error and must be reevaluated periodically as the activity of the underlying disease changes or as complications of therapy arise. A single dose of glucocorticoid, even a large one, is virtually without harmful effects, and a short course of therapy (up to 1 week) is unlikely to cause harm in the absence of specific contraindications. As the duration of glucocorticoid therapy increases beyond 1 week, adverse effects increase in a time- and dose-related manner. Abrupt cessation of glucocorticoids after prolonged therapy is associated with the risk of adrenal insufficiency due to suppression of the HPA axis, and it may be fatal.

BIBLIOGRAPHY

Allolio B, Arlt W. DHEA treatment: Myth or reality? *Trends Endocrinol Metab*, **2002,** *341:*288–294.

Arnaldi G, Angeli A, Atkinson AB, *et al.* Diagnosis and complications of Cushing's syndrome: A consensus statement. *J Clin Endocrinol Metab*, **2003,** *88:*5593–5602.

Axelrod L. Perioperative management of patients treated with glucocorticoids. *Endocrinol Metab Clin North Am*, **2003,** *32:*367–383.

Bale TL, Vale W. CRF and CRF receptors: role in stress responsivity and other behaviors. *Annu Rev Pharmacol Toxicol*, **2004,** *44:*525–557.

Bray PJ, Cotton RG. Variations of the human glucocorticoid receptor gene (NR3C1): pathological and in vitro mutations and polymorphisms. *Hum Mutat*, **2003,** *21:*557–568.

Biller BM, Grossman AB, Stewart PM, *et al.* Treatment of adrenocorticotropin-dependent Cushing's syndrome: A consensus statement. *J Clin Endocrinol Metab*, **2008,** *93:*2454-2462.

Bracken MB. Steroids for acute spinal cord injury. *Cochrane Database Syst Rev*, **2002,** CD001046.DOI: 10.1002/14651858.CD001046.

Carey RM. The changing clinical spectrum of adrenal insufficiency. *Ann Intern Med*, **1997,** *127:*1103–1105.

Chang AY, Ghayee HK, Auchus RJ. Dehydroepiandrosterone replacement therapy—panacea, snake oil, or a bit of both? *Nat Clin Pract Endocrinol Metab*, **2008,** *4:*442–443.

Charmandari E, Kino T, Ichijo T, Chrousos GP. Generalized glucocorticoid resistance: Clinical aspects, molecular mechanisms, and implications of a rare genetic disorder. *J Clin Endocrinol Metab*, **2008,** *93:*1563–1572.

Chrousos GP. The hypothalamic-pituitary-adrenal axis and immune-mediated inflammation. *N Engl J Med*, **1995,** *332:* 1351–1362.

Clark AJ, Metherell LA, Cheetham ME, Huebner A. Inherited ACTH insensitivity illuminates the mechanisms of ACTH action. *Trends Endocrinol Metab*, **2005,** *16:*451–457.

Coursin DB, Wood KE. Corticosteroid supplementation for adrenal insufficiency. *JAMA*, **2002,** *287:*236–240.

De Bosscher K, Vanden Berghe W, Haegeman G. The interplay between the glucocorticoid receptor and nuclear factor-kB or activator protein-1: Molecular mechanisms for gene repression. *Endocr Rev*, **2003,** *24:*488–522.

Dellinger RP, Levy MM, Carlet JM, et al. Surviving Sepsis Campaign: International guidelines for management of severe sepsis and septic shock: 2008. *Crit Care Med*, **2008,** *36:*296–327.

Derendorf H, Nave R, Drollmann A, *et al.* Relevance of pharmacokinetics and pharmacodynamics of inhaled corticosteroids to asthma. *Eur Respir J*, **2006,** *28:*1042–1050.

Derijk RH, van Leeuwen N, Klok MD, Zitman FG. Corticosteroid receptor-gene variants: Modulators of the stress-response and implications for mental health. *Eur J Pharmacol*, **2008,** *585:*492–501.

Elenkov IJ, Chrousos GP. Stress system—organization, physiology and immunoregulation. *Neuroimmunomodulation*, **2006,** *13:*257–267.

Farooki IS, Keogh JM, Yeo GSH, *et al.* Clinical spectrum of obesity and mutations in the melanocortin 4 receptor gene. *N Engl J Med*, **2003,** *348:*1085–1095.

Farooqi IS, Volders K, Stanhope R, *et al.* Hyperphagia and early-onset obesity due to a novel homozygous missense mutation in prohormone convertase 1/3. *J Clin Endocrinol Metab*, **2007,** *92:*3369–3373.

Gross KL, Cidlowski JA. Tissue-specific glucocorticoid action: A family affair. *Trends Endocrinol Metab*, **2008,** *19:*331–339.

Hammer F, Stewart PM. Cortisol metabolism in hypertension. *Best Pract Res Clin Endocrinol Metab*, **2006,** *20*:337–353.

Hochberg Z, Pacak K, Chrousos GP. Endocrine withdrawal syndromes. *Endocr Rev*, **2003,** *24:*523–538.

Holsboer F, Ising M. Central CRH system in depression and anxiety—evidence from clinical studies with CRH1 receptor antagonists. *Eur J Pharmacol*, **2008,** *583:*350–357.

Johanssen S, Allolio B. Mifepristone (RU 486) in Cushing's syndrome. *Eur J Endocrinol*, **2007,** *157:*561–569.

Kraemer FB. Adrenal cholesterol utilization. *Mol Cell Endocrinol*, **2007,** *265–266:*42–45.

Lavery GG, Walker EA, Tiganescu A, *et al.* Steroid biomarkers and genetic studies reveal inactivating mutations in hexose-6-phosphate dehydrogenase in patients with cortisone reductase deficiency. *J Clin Endocrinol Metab*, **2008,** *93:*3827–3832.

Lee YS, Challis BG, Thompson DA, *et al.* A POMC variant implicates [beta]-melanocyte-stimulating hormone in the control of human energy balance. *Cell Metabolism*, **2006,** *3:*135–140.

Magiakou MA, Smyrnaki P, Chrousos GP. Hypertension in Cushing's syndrome. *Best Pract Res Clin Endocrinol Metab*, **2006,** *20:*467–482.

McMaster A, Ray DW. Drug insight: Selective agonists and antagonists of the glucocorticoid receptor. *Nat Clin Pract Endocrinol Metab*, **2008,** *4*:91–101.

Meier-Kriesche HU, Li S, Gruessner RW, et al. Immunosuppression: Evolution in practice and trends, 1994–2004. *Am J Transplant*, **2006,** *6:*1111–1131.

Mencarrelli M, Walker GE, Maestrini S, et al. Sporadic mutations in melanocortin receptor 3 in morbid obese individuals. *Eur J Hum Genet*, **2008,** *16*:581–586.

Morgan C, Cone RD. Melanocortin-5 receptor deficiency in mice blocks a novel pathway influencing pheromone-induced aggression. *Behav Genet*, **2006,** *36:*291–300.

Norman AW, Mizwicki MT, Norman DP. Steroid-hormone rapid actions, membrane receptors, and a conformational ensemble model. *Nat Rev Drug Discov*, **2004,** *3:*27–41.

Parker KL, Rice DA, Lala DS, et al. Steroidogenic factor 1: An essential mediator of endocrine development. *Rec Prog Hormone Res*, **2002,** *57:*19–36.

Rambaldi A, Saconato HH, Christensen E, *et al.* Systematic review: Glucocorticosteroids for alcoholic hepatitis—a Cochrane Hepato-Biliary Group systematic review with meta-analyses and trial sequential analyses of randomized clinical trials. *Aliment Pharmacol Ther*, **2008,** *27:*1167–1178.

Roberts D, Dalziel S. Antenatal corticosteroids for accelerating fetal lung maturation for women at risk of preterm birth. *Cochrane Database Syst Rev*, **2006,** *3:*CD004454.

Sprung CL, Annane D, Keh D, et al. Hydrocortisone therapy for patients with septic shock. *N Engl J Med*, **2008,** *358*: 111–124.

Stahn C, Buttgereit F. Genomic and nongenomic effects of glucocorticoids. *Nat Clin Pract Rheumatol*, **2008,** *4:*525–533.

Stocco DM. Clinical disorders associated with abnormal cholesterol transport: Mutations in the steroidogenic acute regulatory protein. *Mol Cell Endocrinol*, **2002,** *191:*19–25.

Surget A, Belzung C. Involvement of vasopressin in affective disorders. *Eur J Pharmacol*, **2008,** *583:*340–349.

Woolf AD. An update on glucocorticoid-induced osteoporosis. *Curr Opin Rheumatol*, **2007,** *19*:370–375.

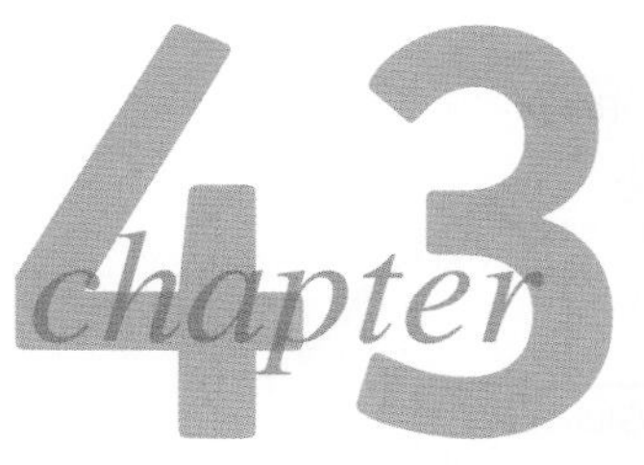

Endocrine Pancreas and Pharmacotherapy of Diabetes Mellitus and Hypoglycemia

Alvin C. Powers
and David D'Alessio

Diabetes mellitus is a spectrum of common metabolic disorders, arising from a variety of pathogenic mechanisms, all resulting in hyperglycemia. The number of individuals with diabetes is rising rapidly throughout the world. Both genetic and environmental factors contribute to its pathogenesis, which involves insufficient insulin secretion, reduced responsiveness to endogenous or exogenous insulin, increased glucose production, and/or abnormalities in fat and protein metabolism. The resulting hyperglycemia may lead to both acute symptoms and metabolic abnormalities. However, the major sources of the morbidity of diabetes are the chronic complications that arise from prolonged hyperglycemia, including retinopathy, neuropathy, nephropathy, and cardiovascular disease. Fortunately, these chronic complications can be mitigated in many patients by sustained control of the blood glucose. There are now a wide variety of treatment options for hyperglycemia that target different processes involved in glucose regulation or dysregulation.

Following a brief review of glucose homeostasis and the pathogenesis of diabetes, this chapter discusses the general approaches and specific agents used in the therapy of diabetes. The last section describes agents used for hypoglycemia.

PHYSIOLOGY OF GLUCOSE HOMEOSTASIS

Regulation of Blood Glucose. In healthy humans, blood glucose is tightly maintained despite wide fluctuations in glucose consumption, utilization, and production. The maintenance of glucose homeostasis, generally termed *glucose tolerance,* is a highly developed systemic process involving the integration of several major organs through multilayered communication (Figure 43–1). Although endocrine control of blood glucose, primarily through the actions of insulin, is of central importance, myriad levels of inter-organ communication, via other hormones, nerves, local factors and substrates, also play a vital role. The pancreatic β cell is central in this homeostatic process, adjusting the amount of insulin secreted very precisely to promote glucose uptake after meals and to regulate glucose output from the liver during fasting.

In the fasting state (Figure 43–1A), most of the fuel demands of the body are met by the oxidation of fatty acids. Importantly, the brain does not effectively utilize fatty acids to meet energy needs and in the fasting state requires glucose for normal function; glucose requirements are ~2 mg/kg per minute in adult humans, largely to supply the central nervous system (CNS) with an energy source. Fasting glucose requirements are primarily provided by the liver, with a minor contribution from the kidney. Liver glycogen stores provide some of this glucose; conversion of gluconeogenic precursors, primarily lactate, alanine and glycerol, into glucose accounts for the remainder. The dominant regulation of hepatic glycogenolysis and gluconeogenesis are the pancreatic islet hormones insulin and glucagon. Insulin inhibits hepatic glucose production at several levels, and the decline of circulating insulin concentrations in the postabsorptive state (fasting) is permissive for higher rates of glucose output. Glucagon maintains blood glucose concentrations at physiological levels in the absence of exogenous carbohydrate (overnight and in between meals) by stimulating gluconeogenesis and glycogenolysis by the liver.

Ingestion of a meal provides a substantial challenge to glucose homeostasis (Figure 43–1B). Adults

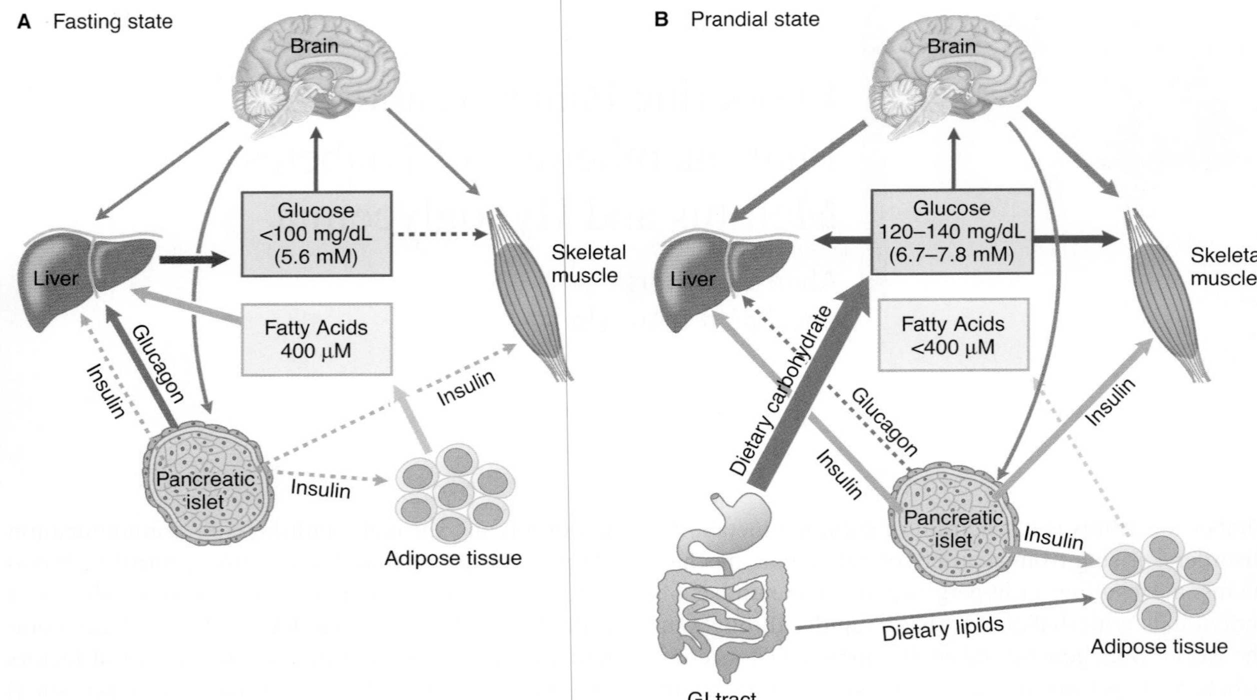

Figure 43–1. *Insulin, glucagon, and glucose homeostasis.* **A.** Fasting State–In healthy humans plasma glucose is maintained in a range from 4.4-5 mM, and fatty acids near 400 μM. In the absence of nutrient absorption from the GI tract, glucose is supplied primarily from the liver and fatty acids from adipose tissue. With fasting, plasma insulin levels are low, and plasma glucagon is elevated, contributing to increased hepatic glycogenolysis and gluconeogenesis; low insulin also releases adipocytes from inhibition, permitting increased lipogenesis. Most tissues oxidize primarily fatty acids during fasting, sparing glucose for use by the CNS. **B.** Prandial State–During feeding, nutrient absorption causes an increases in plasma glucose, resulting in release of incretins from the gut and neural stimuli that promote insulin secretion. Under the control of insulin, the liver, sekletal muscle and adipose tissue actively take up glucose. Hepatic glucose production and lipolysis are inhibited, and total body glucose oxidation increases. The brain senses plasma glucose concentrations and provides regulatory inputs contributing to fuel homeostasis. The boldness of the arrows reflects relative intensity of action; a dashed line indicates little or no activity.

typically consume 30-90 g of carbohydrate in a single meal, considerably more than the extracellular glucose pool, which typically contains 15-20 g of glucose. Therefore, uptake and disposition of meal-derived glucose requires effective coordination of a range of processes, from digestion and absorption to intracellular glycolysis and glycogen synthesis, to prevent major shifts in plasma glucose concentrations. Regulation of nutrient disposition after meals is under the primary control of insulin. Insulin secretion is stimulated by food ingestion, nutrient absorption, and increases in blood glucose, and insulin promotes glucose, lipid, and protein anabolism. The centrality of insulin in glucose metabolism is emphasized by the fact that all the forms of human diabetes have as a root cause some abnormality of insulin secretion or action.

In healthy humans, β cell function is primarily controlled by plasma glucose concentrations. Elevations of blood glucose are necessary for insulin release above basal levels, and other stimuli are relatively ineffective when plasma glucose is in the fasting range (4.4-5.5 mM or 80-100 mg %). These other stimuli include nutrient substrates, insulinotropic hormones released from the gastrointestinal (GI) tract, and autonomic neural pathways. As a result, the pancreatic β cell is stimulated from the time of food presentation, through nutrient absorption, and until blood glucose returns to fasting levels. Neural stimuli cause some increase of insulin secretion prior to food consumption. In addition to these cephalic responses, neural stimulation of insulin secretion occurs throughout the meal and contributes significantly to glucose tolerance. Arrival of nutrient chyme to the intestine leads to the release of insulinotropic peptides from specialized endocrine cells in the intestinal mucosa. Glucose-dependent insulinotropic polypeptide (GIP) and glucagon-like peptide 1 (GLP-1), together termed *incretins,* are the essential gut hormones contributing to glucose tolerance. They are secreted in proportion to the nutrient load ingested and relay this information to the islet as part of a feed-forward mechanism that allows an insulin response appropriate to meal size. Insulin secretion rates in healthy humans are highest in the early digestive phase of meals, preceding and limiting the peak in blood glucose. This pattern of premonitory insulin secretion is an essential feature of normal glucose tolerance. How to mimic this pattern is one of the key challenges for successful insulin therapy in diabetic patients.

Elevated circulating insulin concentrations lower glucose in blood by inhibiting hepatic glucose production and stimulating the uptake and metabolism of glucose by muscle and adipose tissue. These two important effects occur at different concentrations of insulin. Production of glucose is inhibited half-maximally by an insulin concentration of ~120 pmol/L, whereas glucose utilization is stimulated half-maximally at ~300 pmol/L. Some of the effects of insulin on the liver occur rapidly, within the first 20 minutes of meal ingestion, whereas stimulation of peripheral glucose uptake may require up to an hour to reach significant rates. This is probably due to the quick access of insulin to hepatocytes, via the hepatic-portal circulation and the liver sinusoids, and the slower passage of insulin to its receptors on muscle and adipose cells. Insulin has potent effects to reduce lipolysis from adipocytes, primarily through the inhibition of hormone-sensitive lipase, and increases lipid storage by promoting lipoprotein lipase synthesis and adipocyte glucose uptake. Finally, insulin stimulates amino acid uptake and protein synthesis and inhibits protein degradation in muscle and other tissues; it thus causes a decrease in the circulating concentrations of most amino acids.

The demand for glucose as an energy source for skeletal muscle increases dramatically during exercise. Glycogen stored in skeletal muscle is mobilized for some of these needs, but there are limited supplies that are used, mostly at the onset of activity. Most of the glucose support of exercise comes from hepatic gluconeogenesis. The dominant regulation of hepatic glucose production during exercise comes from epinephrine and norepinephrine. The catecholamines stimulate glycogenolysis and gluconeogenesis, inhibit insulin secretion, and enhance release of glucagon, all contributing to increased hepatic glucose output. In addition, catecholamines promote lipolysis, freeing fatty acids for oxidation in exercising muscle and glycerol for hepatic gluconeogenesis.

Pancreatic Islet Physiology and Insulin Secretion. The pancreatic islets comprise 1-2% of the pancreatic volume and are scattered throughout the exocrine pancreas. The pancreatic islet is a highly vascularized, highly innervated mini-organ containing five endocrine cell types: α cells that secrete glucagon, β cells that secrete glucose, δ cells that secrete somatostatin, cells that secrete pancreatic polypeptide, and ε cells that secrete ghrelin. The endocrine, exocrine, and ductal cells of the pancreas share a common embryologic heritage but in the adult are functionally distinct. Insulin and glucagon are important pharmacological agents in the treatment of diabetes, and an understanding of their synthesis, secretion, and action are important in the therapeutic efforts related to diabetes.

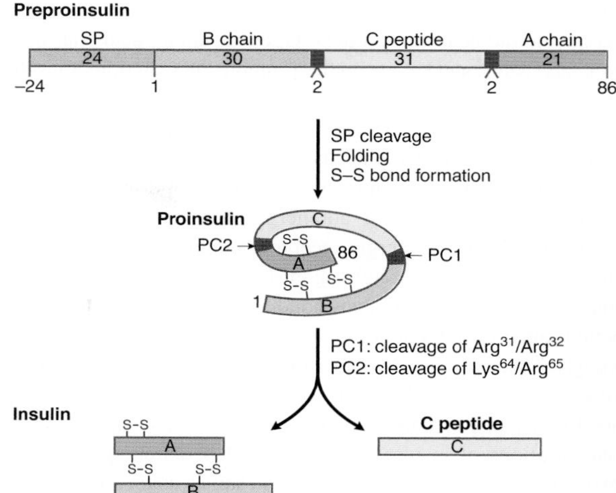

Figure 43–2. *Synthesis and processing of insulin.* The initial peptide, preproinsulin (110 amino acids) consists of a signal peptide (SP), B chain, C peptide, and A chain. The SP is cleaved and S-S bonds form as the proinsulin folds. Two prohormone convertases, PC1 and PC2, cleave proinsulin into insulin, C peptide, and two dipeptides. Insulin and C peptide are stored in granules and co-secreted in equimolar quantities.

Insulin is initially synthesized as a single polypeptide chain, preproinsulin (110 amino acid), which is processed first to proinsulin and then to insulin and C-peptide (Figure 43–2). This complex and highly regulated process involves the Golgi complex, the endoplasmic reticulum, and importantly the distinctive secretory granules of the β cell. Secretory granules are critical not only in bringing insulin to the cell surface for exocytosis, but also in the cleavage and processing of the prohormone to the final secretion products, insulin and C-peptide. The structure of insulin is discussed in the section describing its therapeutic use. Equimolar quantities of insulin and C-peptide (31 amino acids) are co-secreted. Insulin has a $t_{1/2}$ of 5-6 minutes due to extensive hepatic clearance. C-peptide, in contrast, with no known physiological function or receptor, has a $t_{1/2}$ of ~30 minutes. Because almost all of the C-peptide released into the portal vein reaches the peripheral circulation where it can be measured, this peptide is useful in assessment of β-cell secretion, and to distinguish endogenous and exogenous hyperinsulinemia (for example in the evaluation of insulin-induced hypoglycemia). Importantly, the β cell also synthesizes and secretes islet amyloid polypeptide (IAPP) or amylin, a 37–amino acid peptide. IAPP is not essential for life but influences GI motility and the speed of glucose absorption. Pramlintide is an agent used in the treatment of diabetes that mimics the action of IAPP. As reflected by its name, IAPP forms amyloid fibrils in the islets of individuals with type 2 diabetes; whether this is a cause or a consequence of the islet dysfunction of type 2 diabetes is not yet clear.

Insulin secretion is a tightly regulated process designed to provide stable concentrations of glucose in blood during both fasting and feeding. This regulation is achieved by the coordinated interplay of various nutrients, GI hormones, pancreatic hormones, and autonomic neurotransmitters. Glucose, amino acids (arginine, etc.), fatty acids, and ketone bodies promote the secretion of insulin. Glucose is the primary insulin secretagogue, and insulin secretion is tightly coupled to the extracellular glucose concentration. Insulin secretion is much greater when the same amount of glucose is delivered orally compared to intravenously (incretin effect). Islets are richly innervated by both adrenergic and cholinergic nerves. Stimulation of α_2 adrenergic receptors inhibits insulin secretion, whereas β_2 adrenergic receptor agonists and vagal nerve stimulation enhance release. In general, any condition that activates the sympathetic branch of the autonomic nervous system (such as hypoxia, hypoglycemia, exercise, hypothermia, surgery, or severe burns) suppresses the secretion of insulin by stimulation of α_2 adrenergic receptors. Predictably, α_2 adrenergic receptor antagonists increase basal concentrations of insulin in plasma, and β_2 adrenergic receptor antagonists decrease them. Glucagon and somatostatin inhibit insulin secretion.

The pancreatic β cell is a highly specialized cell that has considerable structural and functional similarities to a sensory neuron: Both cell types quickly sense and respond to external stimuli. The molecular events controlling glucose-stimulated insulin secretion begin with the transport of glucose into the β cell via a facilitative glucose transporter (Figure 43–3). In rodents, this is the GLUT2, which has a distinctive, low affinity for glucose and is also the primary glucose transporter in hepatocytes. Human β cells express primarily GLUT1 but little GLUT2. Upon entry into the β cell, glucose is quickly phosphorylated by glucokinase (GK; hexokinase IV); this phosphorylation is the rate-limiting step in glucose metabolism in the β cell. GK's distinctive affinity for glucose leads to a marked increase in glucose metabolism over the range of 5-10 mM glucose, where glucose-stimulated insulin secretion is most pronounced. The glucose-6-phosphate produced by GK activity enters the glycolytic pathway, producing changes in NADPH and the ratio of ADP/ATP. Elevated ATP inhibits an ATP-sensitive K^+ channel (K_{ATP} channel), leading to cell membrane depolarization. This K_{ATP} channel is a heteromeric protein that consists of an inward rectifying K^+ channel (Kir6.2) and a closely associated protein known as the sulfonylurea receptor (SUR), which was identified originally because of its interaction with this class of drugs. Mutations in the K_{ATP} channel are responsible for some types of neonatal diabetes or hypoglycemia. Membrane depolarization then leads to opening of a voltage-dependent Ca^{2+} channel and increased intracellular Ca^{2+}, resulting in exocytotic release of insulin from storage vesicles. These intracellular events are modulated by a number of processes, such as changes in cAMP production, amino acid metabolism, and the level of transcription factors. GPCRs for glucagon, GIP, and GLP-1 couple to G_s to stimulate adenylyl cyclase and insulin secretion; receptors for somatostatin and α_2 adrenergic agonists couple to G_i to reduce cellular cAMP production and secretion.

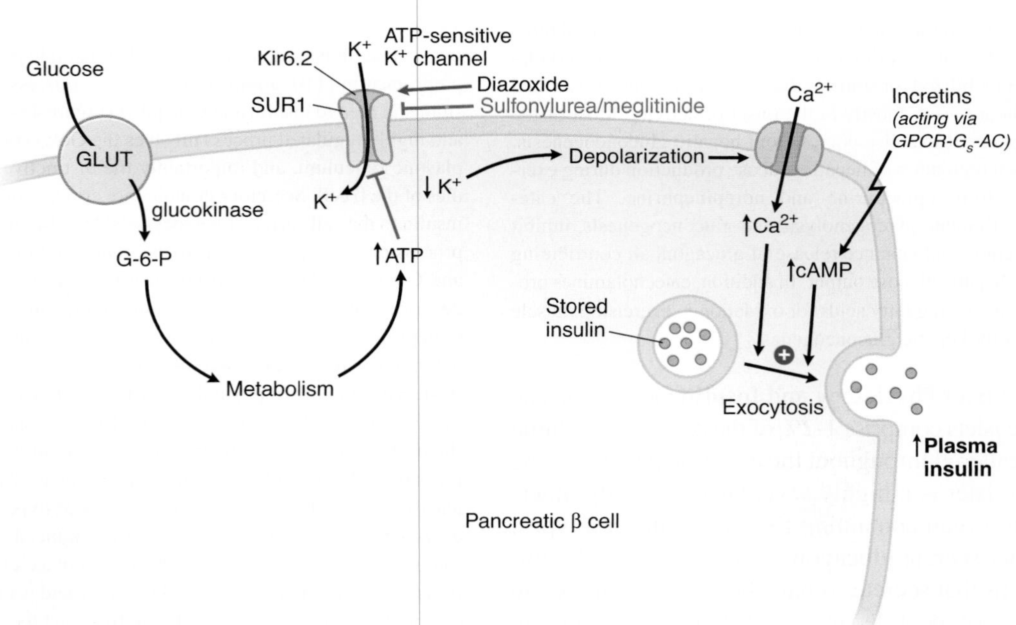

Figure 43–3. *Regulation of insulin secretion from a pancreatic β cell.* The pancreatic β cell in a resting state (fasting blood glucose) is hyperpolarized. Glucose, entering via GLUT transporters (primarily GLUT1 in humans, GLUT2 in rodents), is metabolized and elevates cellular ATP, which inhibits. K^+ entry through the K_{ATP} channel; the decreased K^+ conductance results in depolarization, leading to Ca^{2+}- dependent exocytosis of stored insulin. The K_{ATP} channel, actually a hetero-octamer composed of SUR1 and Kir 6.2 subunits, is the site of action of several classes of drugs: ATP binds to and inhibits Kir 6.2; sulfonylureas and meglitinides bind to and inhibit SUR1; all 3 agents thereby promote insulin secretion. Diazoxide and ADP-Mg^{2+} (low ATP) bind to and activate SUR1, thereby inhibiting insulin secretion. Incretins enhance insulin secretion.

The pancreatic α cell, which has considerable similarity to the β cell, secretes glucagon, primarily in response to hypoglycemia. Glucagon biosynthesis begins with preproglucagon, which is processed in a cell-specific fashion to several biologically active peptides such as glucagon, GLP-1, and glucagon-like peptide-2 (GLP-2) (Figure 43-9). The molecular mechanisms that control glucagon secretion are unclear but may involve paracrine regulation by the β cell and neural input. *In general, glucagon and insulin secretion are regulated in a reciprocal fashion; that is, the agents or processes that stimulate insulin secretion inhibit glucagon secretion. Notable exceptions are arginine and somatostatin: arginine stimulates and somatostatin inhibits the secretion of both hormones.*

Insulin Action. The insulin receptor is expressed on virtually all mammalian cell types, explaining the broad array of biological responses to insulin. The tissues that are considered critical for regulation of blood glucose are liver, skeletal muscle, and fat (Figure 43–1). However, recent evidence suggests that specific regions of the brain and the pancreatic islet are also important targets for insulin. Systemically, the actions of insulin are anabolic, and insulin signaling is critical for promoting the uptake, use, and storage of the major nutrients: glucose, lipids, and amino acids. Importantly, while insulin action stimulates glycogenesis, lipogenesis, and protein synthesis, it also inhibits the catabolism of these compounds. On a cellular level, insulin stimulates transport of substrates and ions into cells, promotes translocation of proteins between cellular compartments, regulates the action of specific enzymes, and controls gene transcription and mRNA translation. Some effects of insulin occur within seconds or minutes, such as activation of glucose and ion transport systems and phosphorylation or dephosphorylation of specific enzymes. Other effects, such as those promoting protein synthesis and regulating gene transcription, manifest over minutes to hours. The effects of insulin on cell proliferation and differentiation occur over days. Metabolic effects such as inhibition of lipolysis or hepatic glucose production occur rapidly, within minutes of increasing concentrations of plasma insulin; detectable increases in glucose clearance from the blood may take nearly an hour. The variability in the kinetics of insulin action probably relate to variable access to insulin receptors in different tissues, distinct intracellular signaling pathways, and the inherent kinetics of the various processes controlled by insulin.

The Insulin Receptor. Insulin action is transmitted through a receptor tyrosine kinase that bears functional similarity to the insulin-like growth factor 1 (IGF-1) receptor (Taniguchi et al., 2006). The insulin receptor is composed of linked (α/β subunit dimers that are products of a single gene; dimers linked by disulfide bonds form a transmembrane heterotetramer glycoprotein composed of two extracellular α-subunits and two membrane-spanning β-subunits (Figure 43–4). The number of receptors varies from as few as 40 per cell on the relatively insulin-insensitive erythrocytes, to 300,000 per cell on adipocytes and hepatocytes, cell types that are highly responsive to insulin.

The α-subunits inhibit the inherent tyrosine kinase activity of the β-subunits. Insulin binding to the α-subunits releases this inhibition and allows transphosphorylation of one β-subunit by the other, and autophosphorylation at specific sites from the juxtamembrane region to the intracellular tail of the receptor. There are two splice variants of the α-subunits, which lead to insulin receptors with differential expression and ligand binding. In addition, insulin receptor dimers can form complexes with IGF-1 receptor α/β dimers, creating another distinct receptor isoform. Activation of the insulin receptor initiates signaling by phosphorylating a set of intracellular proteins such as the insulin receptor substrates (IRS) and Src-homology-2-containing protein (Shc). These insulin receptor substrates interact with effectors that amplify and extend the signaling cascade. As an example, binding of Shc to IRS1 leads to activation of the GTPase Ras and initiation of the protein kinase cascade involving MAPK and ERK that are involved in insulin-mediated gene transcription and cell growth .

Insulin action, at least for glucose transport, is critically dependent on the activation of phosphatidylinositol-3-kinase (PI3K). PI3K is activated by interaction with IRS proteins and generates phosphatidylinositol 3,4,5-trisphosphate (PIP3), which regulates the localization and activity of several downstream kinases, including Akt, atypical isoforms of protein kinase C (PKC ζ and λ/τ), and mammalian target of rapamycin (mTOR) (Huang and Czech, 2007). The isoform Akt2 appears to control the downstream steps that are important for glucose uptake in skeletal muscle and adipose tissue, and to regulate glucose production in the liver. Substrates of Akt2 coordinate the translocation of the glucose transporter 4 (GLUT4) to the plasma membrane through processes involving actin remodeling and other membrane trafficking systems (Zaid et al., 2008). Despite the centrality of PI3K/Akt2 in mediating insulin signaling in key target tissues, it seems likely that there are additional effects mediated by the insulin receptor that do not directly involve these enzymes. Actions of small G-proteins, such as Rac and TC10, have been implicated in the actin remodeling necessary for GLUT4 translocation.

GLUT4 is expressed in insulin-responsive tissues such as skeletal muscle and adipose tissue that constitute important sites of glucose disposal after meal ingestion. GLUT4 is one of a family of 13 glucose transporters in humans that share 12 membrane-spanning domains. GLUT4 is noteworthy among these transporters as the most dependent on discrete stimuli by insulin or other effectors; in the basal state, most GLUT4 resides in the intracellular space; following activation of insulin receptors, GLUT4 is shifted rapidly and

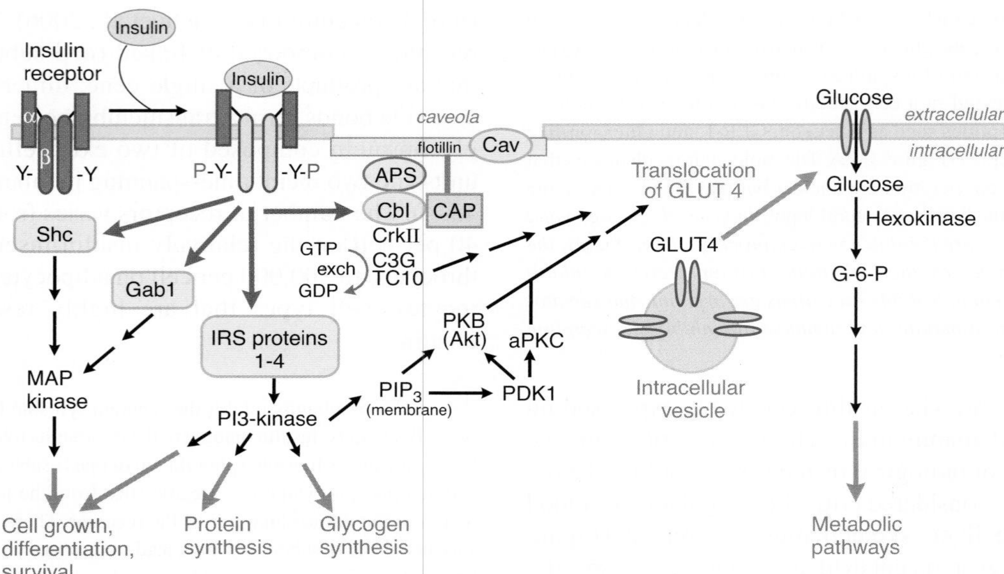

Figure 43–4. *Pathways of insulin signaling.* The binding of insulin to its plasma membrane receptor activates a cascade of downstream signaling events. Insulin binding activates the intrinsic tyrosine kinase activity of the receptor dimer, resulting in the tyrosine phosphorylation (Y-P) of the receptor's β subunits and a small number of specific substrates (yellow shapes): the Insulin Receptor Substrate (IRS) proteins, Gab-1 and SHC; within the membrane, a caveolar pool of insulin receptor phosphorylates caveolin (Cav), APS, and Cbl. These tyrosine-phosphorylated proteins interact with signaling cascades via SH2 and SH3 domains to mediate the effects of insulin, with specific effects resulting from each pathway. In target tissues such as skeletal muscle and adipocytes, a key event is the translocation of the Glut4 glucose transporter from intracellular vesicles to the plasma membrane; this translocation is stimulated by both the caveolar and non-caveolar pathways. In the non-caveolar pathway, the activation of PI3K is crucial, and PKB/Akt (anchored at the membrane by PIP3) and/or an atypical form of PKC is involved. In the caveolar pathway, caveolar protein flotillin localizes the signaling complex to the caveola; the signaling pathway involves series of SH2 domain interactions that add the adaptor protein CrkII, the guanine nucleotide exchange protein C3G, and small GTP-binding protein, TC10. The pathways are inactivated by specific phosphoprotein phosphatases (eg, PTB1B). In addition to the actions shown, insulin also stimulates the plasma membrane Na^+,K^+-ATPase by a mechanism that is still being elucidated; the result is an increase in pump activity and a net accumulation of K^+ in the cell. Abbreviations: APS, adaptor protein with PH and SH2 domains; CAP, Cbl associated protein; CrkII, chicken tumor virus regulator of kinase II; GLUT4, glucose transporter 4; Gab-1, Grb-2 associated binder; MAP kinase, mitogen-activated protein kinase; PDK, phosphoinositide-dependent kinase; PI3 kinase, phosphatidylinositol-3-kinase; PIP3, phosphatidylinositol trisphosphate; PKB, protein kinase B (also called Akt); aPKC, atypical isoform of protein kinase C; Y, tyrosine residue; Y-P, phosphorylated tyrosine residue.

in abundance to the plasma membrane, where it facilitates inward transport of glucose from the circulation. Insulin signaling also reduces GLUT4 endocytosis, increasing the residence time of the protein in the plasma membrane.

Following the facilitated diffusion into cells along a concentration gradient, glucose is phosphorylated to glucose-6-phosphate (G-6-P) by a family of hexokinases. Hexokinase II is found in association with GLUT4 in skeletal and cardiac muscle and in adipose tissue. Like GLUT4, hexokinase II is regulated transcriptionally by insulin. G-6-P is a branch-point substrate that can enter several pathways. G-6-P can be isomerized to G-1-P by phosphoglucomutase, and then the G-1-P can be stored as glycogen (insulin enhances the activity of glycogen synthase); G-6-P can enter the glycolytic pathway (leading to ATP production); G-6-P can also enter the pentose phosphate pathway.

PATHOPHYSIOLOGY AND DIAGNOSIS OF DIABETES MELLITUS

Glucose Homeostasis and the Diagnosis of Diabetes

Broad categories of glucose homeostasis as defined by the fasting blood glucose or the glucose level following an oral glucose challenge include:

- Normal glucose homeostasis: Fasting plasma glucose <5.6 mmol/L (100 mg/dL)
- Impaired fasting glucose (IFG): 5.6-6.9 mmol/L (100-125 mg/dL)

- Impaired glucose tolerance (IGT): Glucose level between 7.8 and 11.1 mmol/L (140-199 mg/dL) 120 minutes after ingestion of 75 g liquid glucose solution
- Diabetes mellitus (see Table 43–1)

The diagnosis of diabetes mellitus is currently based on the correlation of a diabetes-specific complication with a particular level of glycemia, that is, the level of glycemia at which a diabetes-specific complication like retinopathy begins to appear. The boundaries between normal glucose homeostasis, abnormal glucose homeostasis, and diabetes are described as abrupt transitions, but the data are best viewed as a spectrum.

Organizations such as the American Diabetes Association (ADA) and the World Health Organization (WHO) have adopted criteria for the diagnosis of diabetes, based on the fasting blood glucose, the glucose value following an oral glucose challenge, or the level of hemoglobin A_{1c} (HbA_{1c}; exposure of proteins to elevated [glucose] produces nonenzymatic glycation of proteins including Hb. Thus the level of HbA_{1c} represents a measure of the average glucose concentration to which the Hb has been exposed) (Table 43–1). Fasting plasma glucose is most widely used because of its convenience and low cost. The diagnostic criteria have recently (2009) been changed to also include a hemoglobin A_{1c} (A1C) value ≥6.5%. Impaired fasting glucose (IFG) and impaired glucose tolerance (IGT), previously termed prediabetes, or an A1C of 5.7-6.4% portend a markedly increased risk of progressing to type 2 diabetes. An A1C of 5.7-6.4%, IFG, and IGT do not identify the same group of individuals, but all are associated with increased risk of cardiovascular disease.

Table 43–1

Criteria for the Diagnosis of Diabetes

- Symptoms of diabetes plus random blood glucose concentration ≥11.1 mM (200 mg/dL)[a] or
- Fasting plasma glucose ≥7.0 mM (126 mg/dL)[b] or
- Two-hour plasma glucose ≥11.1 mM (200 mg/dL) during an oral glucose tolerance test[c]
- HbA_{1c} ≥6.5%

[a]Random is defined as without regard to time since the last meal.
[b]Fasting is defined as no caloric intake for at least 8 h.
[c]The test should be performed using a glucose load containing the equivalent of 75 g anhydrous glucose dissolved in water; this test is not recommended for routine clinical use.
Note: In the absence of unequivocal hyperglycemia and acute metabolic decompensation, these criteria should be confirmed by repeat testing on a different day.
Adapted from Diabetes Care, **2010**; 33:S62-S69.

The four broad categories of diabetes include type 1 diabetes, type 2 diabetes, other forms of diabetes, and gestational diabetes (Table 43–2). Although hyperglycemia is common to all forms of diabetes, the pathogenic mechanisms leading to diabetes are quite distinct. As our current understanding of the molecular pathogenesis of the hyperglycemia improves, these categories will likely be subdivided into a number of other types of diabetes.

Screening for Diabetes and Categories of Increased Risk Of Diabetes. Many individuals with type 2 diabetes are asymptomatic at the time of diagnosis, and diabetes is often found on routine blood testing as an outpatient or upon admission to the hospital for nonglucose-related reasons. A long, asymptomatic phase in type 2 diabetes (up to a decade) is likely responsible for the observation that up to 50% of individuals with diabetes may have a diabetes-related complication at the time of diagnosis. For these reasons, the ADA recommends widespread screening for type 2 diabetes of these individuals with the following features:

- >45 years of age or
- Body mass index >25 kg/m^2 with one of these additional risk factors: hypertension, low high-density lipoprotein, family history of type 2 diabetes, high-risk ethnic group (African American, Latino, Native American, Asian American, and Pacific Islander), abnormal glucose testing (IFG, IGT, A1C of 5.7-6.4%), cardiovascular disease, and women with polycystic ovary syndrome or who have previously delivered a large infant.

Earlier diagnosis and treatment of type 2 diabetes should delay diabetes-related complications and reduce the burden of the disease. Many also feel that earlier treatment may alter the natural history of the disease, but conclusive proof of this hypothesis is lacking. Likewise, informing individuals who are at increased risk for developing diabetes provides impetus to take steps to slow the progression to diabetes. A number of interventions including pharmacological agents and lifestyle modification are effective. Screening for type 1 diabetes is not currently recommended.

Pathogenesis of Type 1 Diabetes. Type 1 diabetes accounts for 5-10% of diabetes and results from autoimmune-mediated destruction of the β cells of the islet leading to total or near total insulin deficiency (von Herrath et al., 2007). Prior terminology included juvenile-onset diabetes mellitus or insulin-dependent diabetes mellitus. Although traditionally considered a disease of children and adolescents, type 1 diabetes resulting from autoimmune β cell destruction can occur at any age. In fact, in some reports, more than one-third of individuals developed type 1 diabetes after adolescence. Individuals with type 1 diabetes and their families have an increased prevalence of autoimmune diseases such

Table 43–2

Different Forms of Diabetes Mellitus

I. Type 1 diabetes β-cell destruction, usually leading to absolute insulin deficiency)
   A. Immune-mediated
   B. Idiopathic
II. Type 2 diabetes (may range from predominantly insulin resistance with relative insulin deficiency to a predominantly insulin secretory defect with insulin resistance)
III. Other specific types of diabetes
   A. Genetic defects of β cell function characterized by mutations in:
      1. Hepatocyte nuclear transcription factor (HNF) 4α (MODY 1)
      2. Glucokinase (MODY 2)
      3. HNF-1α (MODY 3)
      4. Insulin promoter factor-1 (IPF-1; MODY 4)
      5. HNF-1β (MODY 5)
      6. NeuroD1 (MODY 6)
      7. Mitochondrial DNA
      8. Subunits of ATP-sensitive K^+ channel
      9. Proinsulin or insulin sequence conversion
   B. Genetic defects in insulin action
      1. Type A insulin resistance
      2. Leprechaunism
      3. Rabson-Mendenhall syndrome
      4. Lipodystrophy syndromes
   C. Diseases of the exocrine pancreas—pancreatitis, pancreatectomy, neoplasia, cystic fibrosis, hemochromatosis, fibrocalculous pancreatopathy, mutations in carboxyl ester lipase
   D. Endocrinopathies—acromegaly, Cushing's syndrome, glucagonoma, pheochromocytoma, hyperthyroidism, somatostatinoma, aldosteronoma
   E. Drug- or chemical-induced—Vacor (a rodenticide); see Table 43-3
   F. Infections—congenital rubella, cytomegalovirus
   G. Uncommon forms of immune-mediated diabetes—"stiff-person" syndrome, anti-insulin receptor antibodies
   H. Other genetic syndromes sometimes associated with diabetes—Wolfram's syndrome, Down's syndrome, Klinefelter's syndrome, Turner's syndrome, Friedreich's ataxia, Huntington's chorea, Laurence-Moon-Biedl syndrome, myotonic dystrophy, porphyria, Prader-Willi syndrome
IV. Gestational diabetes mellitus (GDM)

MODY- maturity onset of diabetes of the young. Copyright 2010 American Diabetes Association. From *Diabetes Care*, Vol. 33 (Suppl 1), **2010**; S62. Reprinted with permission from the American Diabetes Association.

as autoimmune adrenal insufficiency (Addison's disease), autoimmune thyroid disease (Graves' and Hashimoto's disease), pernicious anemia, vitiligo, and celiac sprue.

The concordance of type 1 diabetes in genetically identical twins is 40-60%, indicating a significant genetic component. The major genetic risk (40-50%) is conferred by HLA class II genes encoding HLA-DR and HLA-DQ (and possibly other genes with the HLA locus). Candidate gene association studies and recently genome-wide association studies have identified >20 additional loci that confer genetic susceptibility to type 1 diabetes (INS, PTPN22, CTLA4, and IL2RA, among others) (Concannon et al., 2009). However, there clearly is a critical interaction of genetics and an environmental or infectious agent. Most individuals with type 1 diabetes (~75%) do not have a family member with type 1 diabetes, and the genes conferring genetic susceptibility are found in a significant fraction of the nondiabetic population.

Genetically susceptible individuals are thought to have a normal β cell number or mass until β cell–directed autoimmunity develops and β cell loss begins. The first physiological abnormality that is detectable in affected subjects is loss of the first phase of glucose-stimulated insulin secretion. Prior to this, islet cell autoantibodies can be detected in the serum (known autoantigens include insulin, glutamate decarboxylase, protein tyrosine phosphatase IA-2[ICA-512], and zinc transporter 8 [SLC30A8]). The initiating or triggering stimulus for the autoimmune process is not known, but most favor exposure to viruses (enterovirus, etc.) or other ubiquitous environmental agents. Histological examinations of human pancreata during the prediabetic period and at presentation are quite limited, but animal models of type 1 diabetes show a T cell infiltrate with a predominance of CD8+ cells (insulitis). The β cell destruction is cell mediated, and there is also evidence that infiltrating cells produce local inflammatory agents such as TNF-α, IFN-γ, and IL-1, all of which can lead to β cell death. The β cell destruction occurs over a period of months to years and when >80% of the β cells are destroyed, hyperglycemia ensues and the clinical diagnosis of type 1 diabetes is made. Sometimes the clinical presentation of type 1 diabetes is with a concurrent illness (viral syndrome) and this may result in diabetic ketoacidosis; at other times, the typical symptoms of diabetes lead to the diagnosis. Most patients report several weeks of polyuria and polydipsia, fatigue, and often abrupt and significant weight loss. Some adults with the phenotypic appearance of type 2 diabetes (obese, not insulin-requiring initially) have islet cell autoantibodies suggesting autoimmune-mediated β cell destruction and are diagnosed as expressing latent-autoimmune diabetes of adults (LADA).

Pathogenesis of Type 2 Diabetes. The pathogenesis of type 2 diabetes mellitus is complex, and the condition is best thought of as a heterogeneous syndrome of dysregulated glucose homeostasis associated with impaired insulin secretion and insulin action (Das and Elbein, 2006; Doria et al., 2008; Taylor, 2008). Overweight or obesity is a common correlate of type 2 diabetes that occurs in ~ 80% of affected individuals. Increased lipid accumulation in depots in the abdomen, skeletal muscle cells, and hepatocytes has been linked to some of the common impairments. For the vast majority of persons developing type 2 diabetes, there is no clear inciting incident, but rather the condition is thought to develop gradually over years with progression through identifiable prediabetic stages.

In fundamental terms, type 2 diabetes results when there is insufficient insulin action to maintain plasma glucose levels in the normal range. Insulin action is the composite effect of plasma insulin concentrations (determined by islet β cell function) and insulin sensitivity of key target tissues (liver, skeletal muscle, and adipose tissue). These sites of regulation are all impaired to variable extents in patients with type 2 diabetes (Figure 43–5).

The etiology of type 2 diabetes has a strong genetic component (Das and Elbein, 2006; Grant et al., 2009). It is a heritable condition with a relative 4-fold increased risk of disease for persons having a diabetic parent or sibling, increasing to 6-fold if both parents have type 2 diabetes. Consistent with this, the concordance rates of diabetes in monozygotic twins are 2- to 3-fold those in dizygotic twins. Based on linkage analysis, candidate gene searches, and genome-wide association studies, type 2 diabetes appears to be a complex multigenic condition, with many loci of susceptibility contributing to the ultimate phenotype. Although more than 20 genetic loci with clear associations to type 2 diabetes have been identified through recent genome-wide association studies, the contribution of each is relatively small. The genetic locus with the largest relative risk is the transcription factor TCF7L2. Of note, most of the genes currently associated with type 2 diabetes have a relevant connection to β cell function, with fewer linked to the action of insulin in target cells.

Impaired β Cell Function. In persons with type 2 diabetes, the sensitivity of the β cell to glucose is impaired, and there is also a loss of responsiveness to other stimuli such as insulinotropic GI hormones and neural signaling. This results in delayed secretion of insufficient amounts of insulin, allowing the blood glucose to rise dramatically after meals, and failure to restrain liver glucose release during

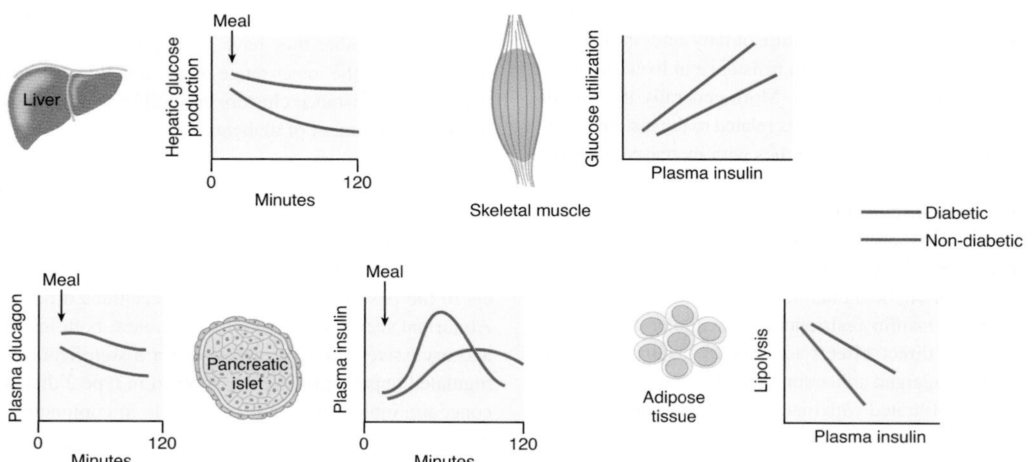

Figure 43–5. *Pathophysiology of type 2 diabetes mellitus.* Graphs show data from diabetic (———) and non-diabetic (———) patients, comparing postprandial insulin and glucagon secretion and hepatic glucose production, and the sensitivities of muscle glucose use and adipocyte lipolysis to insulin.

fasting. Beyond the defect in functional properties of the β cell, the absolute mass of β cells is reduced in type 2 diabetes patients. It is estimated that persons with early type 2 diabetes have ~50% of the normal complement of β cells (Butler et al., 2003). This deficit is compounded by a gradual loss of β cell mass over time, potentially related to toxic effects of hyperglycemia. Progressive reduction of β cell mass and function explains the natural history of type 2 diabetes in most patients who require steadily increasing therapy to maintain glucose control.

Type 2 diabetic patients frequently have elevated levels of fasting insulin. This is not a reflection of accentuated β cell function but a result of their higher fasting glucose levels and insulin resistance. Another factor contributing to apparently high insulin levels early in the course of the disease is the presence of increased amounts of proinsulin. Proinsulin, the precursor to insulin, is inefficiently processed in the diabetic islet. Whereas healthy subjects have only 2-4% of total circulating insulin as proinsulin, type 2 diabetic patients can have 10-20% of the measurable plasma insulin in this form. Proinsulin has a considerably attenuated effect for lowering blood glucose compared to insulin.

Insulin Resistance. Insulin sensitivity is a quantifiable parameter that is measured as the amount of glucose cleared from the blood in response to a dose of insulin. The failure of normal amounts of insulin to elicit the expected response is referred to as *insulin resistance.* This is a relative term because there is inherent variability of insulin sensitivity among cells, tissues, and individuals. Insulin sensitivity is affected by many factors including age, body weight, physical activity levels, illness, and medications. Furthermore, insulin sensitivity varies within individuals over time and across groups or populations of subjects, even among healthy adults. Thus, insulin resistance is a relative designation but has considerable pathological significance because persons with type 2 diabetes or glucose intolerance have reduced responses to insulin and can easily be distinguished from groups with normal glucose tolerance.

The major insulin-responsive tissues are skeletal muscle, adipose tissue, and liver. Insulin resistance in muscle and fat is generally marked by a decrease in transport of glucose from the circulation. Hepatic insulin resistance generally refers to a blunted ability of insulin to suppress glucose production. Insulin resistance in adipocytes causes increased rates of lipolysis and release of fatty acids into the circulation, which can contribute to insulin resistance in liver and muscle, hepatic steatosis, and dyslipidemia. More generally the role of obesity in the etiology of type 2 diabetes is related to the insulin resistance in skeletal muscle and liver that comes with increased amounts of lipid storage, particularly in specific fat depots. The sensitivity of humans to the effects of insulin administration is inversely related to the amount of fat stored in the abdominal cavity; more visceral adiposity leads to more insulin resistance (Kahn, 2003). Similarly, intrahepatocyte or intramuscular fat, both commonly associated with obesity, are strongly linked to insulin resistance. Intracellular lipid or its byproducts may have direct effects to impede insulin signaling (Savage et al., 2007). Enlarged collections of adipose tissue, visceral or otherwise, is often infiltrated with macrophages and can become a site of chronic inflammation. Adipocytokines, secreted from adipocytes and immune cells, including TNF-α, IL-6, resistin, and retinol-binding protein 4, can also cause systemic insulin resistance. Insulin resistance is even more severe in obese persons with type 2 diabetes who have further reductions of insulin-stimulated glucose uptake into skeletal muscle and relatively low rates of nonoxidative glucose metabolism (glycogen synthesis), and impaired suppression of hepatic glucose production and adipocyte lipolysis, despite insulin concentrations that are often elevated.

Another important variable in determining insulin sensitivity is activity level. Sedentary persons are more insulin resistant than active ones, and physical training can improve insulin sensitivity. Physical activity can decrease the risk of developing diabetes and improve glycemic control in persons who have diabetes (Crandall et al., 2008). Insulin resistance is more common in the elderly; within populations, insulin sensitivity decreases linearly with age. Older individuals tend to be less physically active, which can contribute to insulin resistance. In addition, over the normal course of aging there is a decrease in muscle mass and an increase in fat mass, with an increased percentage of fat stored in the abdominal cavity.

At the cellular level, insulin resistance involves blunted steps in the cascade from the insulin receptor tyrosine kinase to translocation of GLUT4 transporters, but the molecular mechanisms are incompletely defined. There have been >75 different mutations in the insulin receptor discovered, most of which cause significant impairment of insulin action. These mutations affect insulin receptor number, movement to and from the plasma membrane, binding, and phosphorylation. Mutations involving the insulin binding domains of the extracellular α-chain cause the most severe syndromes, but specific variants in the intracellular portions of the receptor also cause severe insulin resistance. However, most insulin resistance associated with obesity and type 2 diabetes is not due to abnormalities of the insulin receptor. A central feature of the more common forms of insulin resistance is increased phosphorylation of serine, rather than tyrosine, in the insulin receptor and IRS proteins, inhibiting their activation and signaling. This process is mediated by protein serine/threonine kinases, which respond to an increased intracellular flux of fatty acids, specific lipid products, particularly diacylglycerol and ceramide, inflammatory mediators such as TNFα, and endoplasmic reticulum stress. In addition, chronic hyperinsulinemia, the typical correlate of insulin resistance, seems to increase IRS protein catabolism. It is known that insulin sensitivity is under genetic control, but it is unclear whether insulin-resistant individuals have mutations in specific components of the insulin signaling cascade or whether they have a complement of signaling effectors that operate at the lower range of normal. Regardless, it is apparent that insulin resistance clusters in families and is a major risk factor for the development of diabetes.

Dysregulated Hepatic Glucose Metabolism. In type 2 diabetes, hepatic glucose output is excessive in the fasting state and inadequately suppressed after meals. These are key components to the abnormal glycemic profile in diabetic patients, who have elevated glucose levels in the postabsorptive state and accentuated postprandial rises. Abnormal secretion of the islet hormones, both insufficient insulin and excessive glucagon, accounts for a significant portion of dysregulated hepatic glucose metabolism in type 2 diabetes. Increased concentrations of glucagon, especially in conjunction with hepatic insulin resistance, can lead to excessive hepatic gluconeogenesis and glycogenolysis and abnormally high fasting glucose concentrations.

The liver is also resistant to insulin action in type 2 diabetes. This contributes to the reduced potency of insulin to suppress hepatic glucose production and promote hepatic glucose uptake and glycogen synthesis after meals. Despite ineffective insulin effects on hepatic glucose metabolism, the lipogenic effects of insulin in the liver are maintained and even accentuated by fasting hyperinsulinemia. This contributes to hepatic steatosis and further worsening of insulin resistance.

Pathogenesis of Other Forms of Diabetes. Mutations in key genes involved in glucose homeostasis cause monogenic diabetes, which is inherited in an autosomal dominant fashion. These fall in two broad categories: diabetes onset in the immediate neonatal period (<6 months of age) and diabetes in children or adults (Murphy et al., 2008; Vaxillaire and Froguel, 2008). Some forms of neonatal diabetes are caused by mutations in the sulfonylurea receptor or its accompanying inward rectifying K^+ channel and mutations in the insulin gene. Monogenic diabetes beyond the first year of life may appear clinically similar to type 1 or type 2 diabetes. In other instances, young individuals (adolescence to young adulthood) may have monogenic forms of diabetes known as maturity onset diabetes of the young (MODY). Phenotypically, these individuals are not obese and are not insulin resistant, or they may initially have modest hyperglycemia. The most common causes are mutations in key islet-enriched transcription factors or glucokinase (see discussion about molecular mechanisms of insulin secretion; Table 43–2 and Figure 43–3). Most individual with MODY are treated similarly to those with type 2 diabetes. Importantly, sulfonylureas may be a particularly effective treatment of individuals with MODY-3 or neonatal diabetes caused by a mutation in the K_{ATP} channel complex.

Diabetes may also be the result of other pathological processes such as acromegaly and Cushing's disease (Table 43–2). A number of medications promote hyperglycemia or lead to diabetes by either impairing insulin secretion or insulin action (Table 43–3). Most notable are asparaginase, glucocorticoids, pentamidine, nicotinic acid, α-interferon, protease inhibitors, and in particular, atypical antipsychotics (Chapter 16).

Table 43–3

Some Drugs that may Promote Hyperglycemia or Hypoglycemia

HYPERGLYCEMIA	HYPOGLYCEMIA
Glucocorticoids	β Adrenergic antagonists
Antipsychotics (atypical, others)	Ethanol
Protease inhibitors	Salicylates
β Adrenergic agonists	Non-steroidal anti-inflammatory drugs
Diuretics (thiazide, loop)	Pentamidine
Hydantoins (phenytoin, others)	ACE inhibitors
Opioids (fentanyl, morphine, others)	Lithium chloride
Diazoxide	Theophylline
Nicotinic Acid	Bromocriptine
Pentamidine	Mebendazole
Epinephrine	
Interferons	
Amphotericin B	
Asparaginase	
Acamprosate	
Basiliximab	
Thyroid hormones	

For additional details, see Murad et al., 2009.

Epidemiology of Diabetes. The number of individuals with diabetes is increasing worldwide. Although the annual rate of type 1 diabetes has increased modestly over the past decade, the increased frequency of type 2 diabetes has been dramatic. In the U.S., 7-10% of adults are affected, with up to three times that many at risk. There is clear ethnic variability in the prevalence of type 2 diabetes. Among adults living in the U.S., there is a spectrum of prevalence with Native Americans (15%), Hispanics (12%), and African Americans (12%) having greater rates than persons of European ancestry (8%). While the upward trends in the industrialized world have been similar in many countries, there are now alarming increases in rates of type 2 diabetes worldwide. Most notable are China, India, and other countries in the Far East where the disease was previously uncommon (Chan et al., 2009). The largest increase in the number of people with diabetes is predicted to take place in the regions or countries with developing economies. Parallel increases in obesity rates and changes in diet and activity appear to be the major factors in this marked increase in diabetes.

Diabetes-Related Complications. Diabetes can cause metabolic derangements or acute complications, such as the life-threatening metabolic disorders of diabetic ketoacidosis and hyperglycemic hyperosmolar state. These require hospitalization for insulin administration, rehydration with intravenous fluids, and careful monitoring of electrolytes and metabolic parameters. Chronic complications of diabetes have been described in all forms of the disease and are commonly divided into microvascular and macrovascular complications. Microvascular complications occur only in individuals with diabetes, whereas macrovascular complications occur more frequently in individuals with diabetes but are not diabetes specific. The common microvascular complications include retinopathy, nephropathy and neuropathy. Macrovascular complications refer to increased atherosclerosis-related events such as myocardial infarction and stroke. The pharmacological management of diabetes-related complications is discussed elsewhere (e.g., Chapters 25, 28, 31, 64).

In the U.S., diabetes is the leading cause of blindness in adults, the leading reason for renal failure requiring dialysis or renal transplantation, and the leading cause of nontraumatic lower extremity amputations. Fortunately, most of these diabetes-related complications can be prevented, delayed, or reduced by near normalization of the blood glucose on a consistent basis. How chronic hyperglycemia causes these complications is unclear. For microvascular complications, current hypothesis are that hyperglycemia leads to advanced glycosylation end products (AGEs), increased glucose metabolism via the sorbitol pathway, increased formation of diacylglycerol leading to PKC activation, and increased flux through the hexosamine pathway. Growth factors such as vascular endothelial growth factor α may be involved in diabetic retinopathy and TGF-β in diabetic nephropathy.

Therapy of Diabetes

Goals of Therapy. The goals of therapy for diabetes are to alleviate the symptoms related to hyperglycemia (fatigue, polyuria, etc.) and to prevent or reduce the acute and chronic complications of diabetes. Accomplishment of these goals requires a multidisciplinary team (physicians, nurse educators, pharmacists) with expertise in pharmacology, nutrition, and patient education. Central to the treatment plan is the patient who must actively participate in the care of his or her diabetes.

Glycemic control is assessed using both short-term (blood glucose self-monitoring) and long-term metrics (A1C, fructosamine). Using capillary blood glucose measurements, the patient assesses capillary blood glucose on a regular basis (fasting, before meals, or postprandially) and reports these values to the diabetes management team. A1C reflects glycemic control over the prior 3 months; glycosylated albumin (fructosamine) is a measure of glycemic control over the preceding 2 weeks.

Approaches to diabetes care are sometimes termed intensive insulin therapy, intensive glycemic control, and tight control. This chapter use the term *comprehensive diabetes care* to describe optimal therapy, which involves more than glucose management and includes aggressive treatment of abnormalities in blood pressure and lipids and detection and management of diabetes-related complications (Figure 43–6). Table 43–4 shows the ADA-recommended treatment goals for comprehensive diabetes care, for glucose, blood pressure, and lipids (Brunzell et al., 2008). Improved glycemic control reduces the complications when started relatively early in the course of both type 1 and type 2 diabetes, but very intensive glucose lowering (with A_{1c} near 6.0) has not shown benefit in individuals with type 2 diabetes and atherosclerotic disease (Duckworth et al., 2009; Holman et al., 2008; Skyler et al., 2009). A summary of available pharmacologic agents for the treatment of diabetes is at the end of this chapter (Table 43–9).

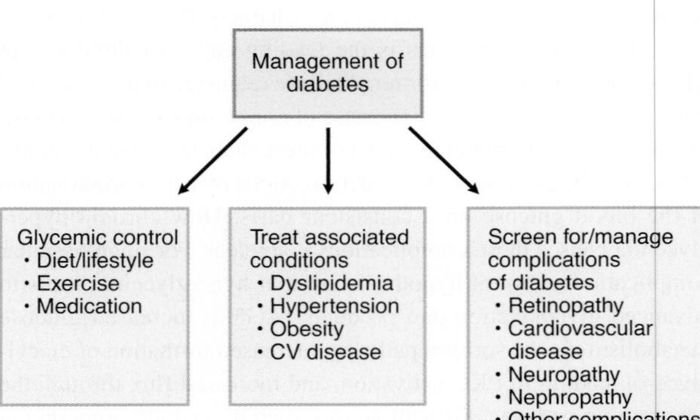

Figure 43–6. *Components of comprehensive diabetes care.*

Nonpharmacologic Aspects of Diabetes Therapy. The patient with diabetes should be educated about nutrition, exercise, and medications aimed at lowering the plasma glucose. The role of the certified diabetes educator, a healthcare professional (nurse, dietician, or pharmacist) with specialized patient education skills, is critical. In terms of diet, the ADA uses the term *medical nutrition therapy* to describe the diet that coordinates calorie intake and other aspects of diabetes therapy such as pharmacological agents and exercise. In type 1 diabetes, matching caloric intake and insulin dosing is very important. In type 2 diabetes, the diet is directed at weight loss and reducing blood pressure and atherosclerotic risk. Exercise provides multiple benefits for patients with diabetes, but dosing of the glucose-lowering therapy may require adjustment to avoid exercise-related hypoglycemia.

In addition to lifestyle modification, the other major nonpharmacological means to reduce the progression of abnormal glucose metabolism is bariatric surgery (Sjostrom et al., 2004). A number of procedures, including gastric banding, gastric bypass, and biliopancreatic diversion, improve glucose tolerance and prevent or reverse type 2 diabetes.

Insulin Therapy

Insulin is the mainstay for treatment of virtually all type 1 and many type 2 diabetes patients. Insulin may be administered intravenously, intramuscularly, or subcutaneously. Long-term treatment relies predominantly on subcutaneous injection. Subcutaneous administration of insulin differs from physiological secretion of insulin in two major ways:

- The absorption kinetics do not reproduce the rapid rise and decline of endogenous insulin in response to glucose following intravenous or oral administration.
- Injected insulin is delivered into the peripheral circulation instead of being released into the portal circulation. Thus the portal/peripheral insulin concentration is not physiological, and this may alter the influence of insulin on hepatic metabolic processes.

Nonetheless, insulin delivered into the peripheral circulation can lead to normal or near-normal glycemia.

History. The discovery of insulin is a dramatic story. The discovery is attributed to Frederick Banting, Charles Best, J.J.R. Macleod, and J.B. Collip at the University of Toronto, but others provided important observations and techniques that made it possible (Bliss, 2005). In 1869, a German medical student, Paul Langerhans, noted that the pancreas contains two distinct groups of cells—the acinar cells, which secrete digestive enzymes, and cells that are clustered in islands, or islets, which he suggested served a second function. Direct evidence for this function came in 1889, when Minkowski and von Mering showed that pancreatectomized dogs exhibit a syndrome similar to human diabetes mellitus. Thereafter, there were numerous attempts to extract the pancreatic substance responsible for regulating blood glucose. Between 1903 and 1909, the Romanian

Table 43–4

Goals of Therapy in Diabetes

INDEX	GOAL[a]
Glycemic control[b]	
A1C	<7.0%[c]
Preprandial capillary plasma glucose	3.9-7.2 mmol/L (70-130 mg/dL)
Peak Postprandial capillary plasma glucose	10.0 mmol/L (<180 mg/dL)[d]
Blood pressure	<130/80
Lipids[e]	
Low-density lipoprotein	<2.6 mmol/L (<100 mg/dL)[f]
High-density lipoprotein	>1.1 mmol/L (>40 mg/dL)[g]
Triglycerides	<1.7 mmol/L (<150 mg/dL)

[a]As recommended by the ADA goals should be individualized for each patient. Goals may be different for certain patient populations.
[b]A1C is primary goal.
[c]While the ADA recommends an A1C <7.0% in general, in the individual patient it recommends that an approprpate goal for the individual patient based on age, duration of diabetes, life expectancy, other medical conditions, cardiovascular disease).
[d]One to two hours after beginning of a meal.
[e]In decreasing order of priority
[f]In individuals with conronary artery disease, an LDL <1.8 mmol (70 mg/dL) is the goal.
[g]For women, some suggest a goal that is 0.25 mmol/L (10 mg/dL) higher.
Adapted from *Diabetes Care* 33:S11, **2010**.

physiologist Nicolas Paulesco found that injections of pancreatic extracts reduced urinary sugar and ketones in diabetic dogs and published results clearly indicating isolation of a glucose-lowering compound. The significance of these findings was recognized only years later.

Unaware of much of this work, Frederick Banting, a young Canadian surgeon, convinced J.J.R. Macleod, a professor of physiology in Toronto, to allow him access to a laboratory to search for the antidiabetic principle of the pancreas. Banting began work on the assumption that the islets secreted a glucose-lowering hormone that was destroyed by proteolytic digestion prior to or during extraction. Together with Charles Best, a fourth-year medical student, he attempted to overcome the problem by ligating the pancreatic ducts so that the acinar tissue degenerated, leaving the islets undisturbed. Using an ethanol and acid extraction procedure, Banting and Best obtained a pancreatic isolate that decreased the concentration of blood glucose in diabetic dogs. Under the guidance of Macleod, Banting and Best received help from J.B. Collip, a chemist with expertise in extraction and purification of epinephrine. The first patient to receive the active extracts was Leonard Thompson, age 14. He presented at the Toronto General Hospital with a blood glucose level of 500 mg/dL (28 mM). Despite rigid control of his diet (450 kcal/day), he continued to excrete large quantities of glucose, and, without insulin, would likely have died within a few months. The administration of the pancreatic extracts reduced the plasma concentration and urinary excretion of glucose, and the patient demonstrated marked clinical improvement. Replacement therapy with the newly discovered hormone, insulin, had interrupted what was clearly an otherwise fatal metabolic disorder. Stable extracts eventually were obtained, and patients in many parts of North America soon were being treated with insulin from porcine and bovine sources. The first of several Nobel Prizes associated with insulin was awarded to Banting and Macleod in 1923. A furor over credit followed immediately, and Banting announced that he would share his prize with Best; Macleod did the same with Collip (Bliss, 2005). Frederick Sanger established the amino acid sequence of insulin and received the Nobel Prize in 1958. Dorothy Hodgkin (Nobel prize for chemistry, 1964) and coworkers elucidated insulin's three-dimensional structure. Insulin was the hormone for which Yalow and Berson first developed the radioimmunoassay, which was recognized with the Nobel Prize in 1977.

Insulin Preparation and Chemistry. Human insulin, produced by recombinant DNA technology, is soluble in aqueous solution. Most preparations are supplied at neutral pH, which improves stability and permits short-term storage at room temperature. Beginning shortly after its discovery in 1921, patients were treated with insulin preparations prepared from porcine or bovine pancreatic extracts for >70 years. With the advent of human insulin, beef and pork insulin are no longer produced. A number of other insulin preparations that once were widely used such as lente, ultralente, and protamine zinc insulin are no longer available.

Doses and concentration of clinically used insulin preparations are expressed in international units. This tradition dates to a time when preparations of hormones were impure and the concentration of the hormone was standardized by bioassay. One unit of insulin is defined as the amount required to reduce the blood glucose concentration in a fasting rabbit to 45 mg/dL (2.5 mM).

Commercial preparations of insulin are supplied in solution or suspension at a concentration of 100 units/mL, which is ~3.6 mg insulin per milliliter (0.6 mM) and termed U-100. Insulin also is available in a more concentrated solution (500 units/mL or U-500) for patients who are resistant to the hormone. In the past, other concentrations of insulin such as U-40 were available. Other insulin formulations such as inhaled insulin and injected human proinsulin were tested but either were not clinically useful or were used for only a brief period of time. Work is ongoing to develop delivery approaches that do not involve injection.

Insulin Formulations. Preparations of insulin are classified according to their duration of action into short-acting and long-acting (Table 43–5). Within the short-acting acting category, some distinguish the very rapid-acting insulins (aspart, glulisine, lispro) from regular insulin. Likewise, some distinguish formulations with a longer duration of action (detemir, glargine) from NPH insulin. Two approaches are used to modify the absorption and pharmacokinetic profile of insulin. The first approach, which has been used for >70 years to alter the absorption profile of native insulin, is based on formulations that slow the absorption following subcutaneous injection. The other approach is to alter the amino acid sequence or protein structure of human insulin so that it retains its ability to bind the insulin receptor, but its behavior in solution or following injection is either accelerated or prolonged in comparison to native or regular insulin (Figure 43–7).

The wide variability in the kinetics of insulin action between and even within individuals must be emphasized. The time to peak hypoglycemic effect and insulin levels can vary by 50%. This variability is caused, at least in part, by large variations in the rate of subcutaneous absorption.

Short-Acting Regular Insulin. Native or regular insulin molecules associate as hexamers in aqueous solution at a neutral pH and this aggregation slows absorption following subcutaneous injection. Regular insulin should be injected 30-45 minutes before a meal. Regular insulin also may be given intravenously or intramuscularly.

Short-Acting Insulin Analogs. The development of short-acting insulin analogs that retain a monomeric or dimeric configuration is a major advance in insulin therapy (Figures 43–7 and 43–8; Table 43–5). These analogs are absorbed more rapidly from subcutaneous sites than regular insulin. Consequently, there is a more rapid increase in plasma insulin concentration and an earlier response. Insulin analogs should be injected ≤15 minutes before a meal.

Insulin lispro (HUMALOG) is identical to human insulin except at positions B28 and B29, where the sequence of the two residues has been reversed to match the sequence in IGF-1 (which does not self-associate). Like regular insulin, lispro exists as a hexamer in commercially available formulations. Unlike regular insulin, lispro

Table 43–5

Properties of Insulin Preparations

PREPARATION	TIME OF ACTION: ONSET, h	PEAK, h	EFFECTIVE DURATION, h
Short-acting			
Aspart	<0.25	0.5-1.5	3-4
Glulisine	<0.25	0.5-1.5	3-4
Lispro	<0.25	0.5-1.5	3-4
Regular	0.5-1.0	2-3	4-6
Long-acting			
Detemir	1-4	—[a]	20-24
Glargine	1-4	—[a]	20-24
NPH	1-4	6-10	10-16
Insulin combinations			
75/25-75% protamine lispro, 25% lispro	<0.25	1.5 h	Up to 10-16
70/30-70% protamine aspart, 30% aspart	<0.25	1.5 h	Up to 10-16
50/50-50% protamine lispro, 50% lispro	<0.25	1.5 h	Up to 10-16
70/30-70% NPH, 30% regular	0.5-1	Dual[b]	10-16

[a]Glargine and detemir have minimal peak activity.
[b]Dual: two peaks - one at 2-3 h; the second one several hours later.
Copyright 2004 American Diabetes Association. Adapted with permission from Skyler JS. Insulin treatment. In HE Lebovitz, ed., *Therapy for Diabetes Mellitus*. American Diabetes Association, Alexandria, VA, **2004**.

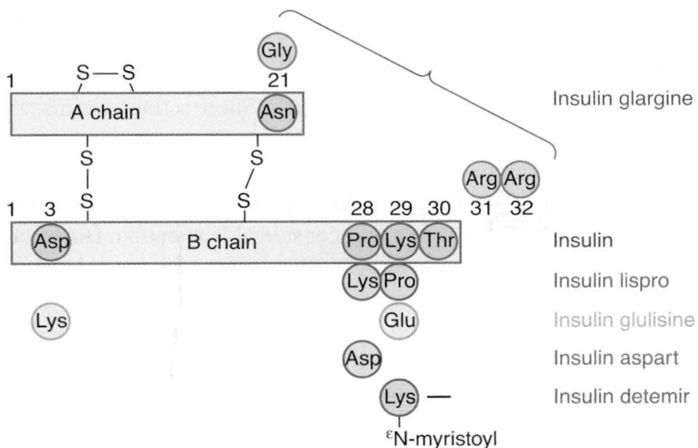

Figure 43–7. *Insulin analogs.* Modifications of native insulin can alter its pharmacokinetic profile. Reversing amino acids 28 and 29 in the B chain (lispro) or substituting Asp for Pro^{28B} (aspart) gives analogs with reduced tendencies for molecular self-association that are faster acting. Altering Asp^{3B} to Lys and Lys^{29B} to Glu produces an insulin (glulisine) with a more rapid onset and a shorter duration of action. Substituting Gly for Asn^{21A} and lengthening the B chain by adding Arg^{31} and Arg^{32} produces a derivative (glargine) with reduced solubility at pH 7.4 that is, consequently, absorbed more slowly and acts over a longer period of time. Deleting Thr^{30B} and adding a myristoyl group to the ε-amino group of Lys^{29B} (detemir) enhances reversible binding to albumin, thereby slowing transport across vascular endothelium to tissues and providing prolonged action.

dissociates into monomers almost instantaneously following injection. This property results in the characteristic rapid absorption and shorter duration of action compared with regular insulin. Two therapeutic advantages have emerged with lispro as compared with regular insulin. First, the prevalence of hypoglycemia is reduced with lispro; second, glucose control, as assessed by A1C, is modestly but significantly improved (0.3-0.5%).

Insulin aspart (NOVOLOG) is formed by the replacement of proline at B28 with aspartic acid. This reduces self-association to a degree similar to lispro. Like lispro, insulin aspart dissociates rapidly into monomers following injection. Comparison of a single subcutaneous dose of aspart and lispro in a group of type 1 diabetes patients revealed similar plasma insulin profiles. In clinical trials, insulin aspart and insulin lispro have had similar effects on glucose control and hypoglycemia frequency, with lower rates of nocturnal hypoglycemia as compared with regular insulin.

Insulin glulisine (APIDRA) is formed when glutamic acid replaces lysine at B29, and lysine replaces asparagine at B23; these substitutions result in a reduction in self-association and rapid dissociation into active monomers. The time–action profile of insulin glulisine is similar to that of insulin aspart and insulin lispro. Similar to insulin aspart, insulin glulisine has been approved in the U.S. for continuous subcutaneous insulin infusion (CSII) pump use.

Long-Acting Insulins. Neutral protamine hagedorn (NPH; insulin isophane) is a suspension of native insulin complexed with zinc and protamine in a phosphate buffer. This produces a cloudy or whitish solution in contrast to the clear appearance of other insulin solutions. Because of this formulation, the insulin dissolves more gradually when injected subcutaneously and thus its duration of action is prolonged. NPH insulin is usually given either once a day (at bedtime) or twice a day in combination with short-acting insulin. In patients with type 2 diabetes, long-acting insulin is often given at bedtime to help normalize fasting blood glucose. It should be noted that the use of long-acting basal insulin alone will not control postprandial glucose elevation in insulin-deficient type 1 or type 2 diabetes.

Insulin glargine (LANTUS) is a long-acting analog of human insulin that is produced following two alterations of human insulin. Two arginine residues are added to the C terminus of the B chain, and an asparagine molecule in position 21 on the A chain is replaced with glycine. Insulin glargine is a clear solution with a pH of 4.0,

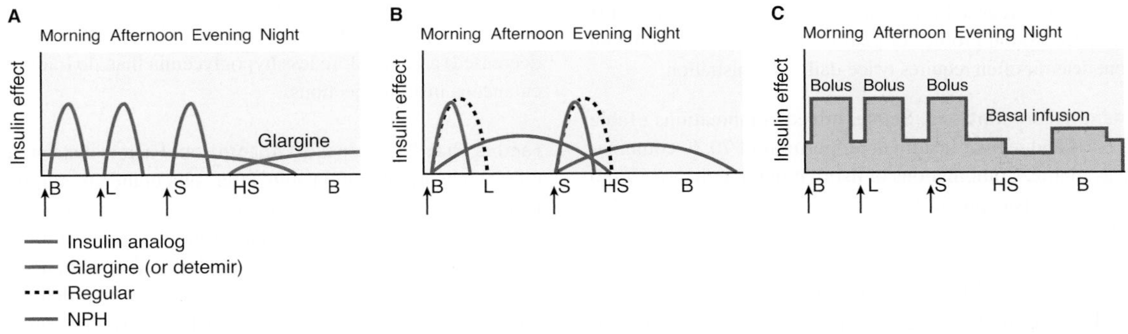

Figure 43–8. *Commonly used insulin regimens.* Panel A shows administration of a long-acting insulin like glargine (detemir could also be used but often requires twice-daily administration) to provide basal insulin and a pre-meal short-acting insulin analog (Table 43–5). Panel B shows a less intensive insulin regimen with BID injection of NPH insulin providing basal insulin and regular insulin or an insulin analog providing meal-time insulin coverage. Only one type of shorting-acting insulin would be used. Panel C shows the insulin level attained following subcutaneous insulin (short-acting insulin analog) by an insulin pump programmed to deliver different basal rates. At each meal, an insulin bolus is delivered. B=breakfast; L=lunch; S=supper; HS=bedtime. Upward arrow shows insulin administration at mealtime. (Copyright 2008 American Diabetes Association. From Kaufman FR (ed), *Medical Management of Type 1 Diabetes*, Fifth Edition. Modified with permission from the American Diabetes Association.)

which stabilizes the insulin hexamer. When injected into the neutral pH of the subcutaneous space, aggregations occurs, resulting in prolonged, but predictable, absorption from the injection site. Owing to insulin glargine's acidic pH, it cannot be mixed with short-acting insulin preparations (i.e., regular insulin, aspart, or lispro) that are formulated at a neutral pH.

In clinical studies glargine has a sustained peakless absorption profile, and provides a better once-daily 24-hour insulin coverage than NPH insulin. Evidence from clinical trials also suggests that glargine has a lower risk of hypoglycemia, particularly overnight compared to NPH insulin. Glargine may be administered at any time during the day with equivalent efficacy and does not accumulate after several injections. Glargine has been shown in clinical studies to normalize fasting (postabsorptive) glucose levels following once-daily administration in patients with type 2 diabetes. Sometimes, splitting the dose of glargine may be needed in very insulin-sensitive type 1 diabetes patients to achieve fasting (basal) glucose levels in the target range and avoid hypoglycemia. Unlike traditional insulin preparations that are absorbed more rapidly from the abdomen than from the arm or leg, the site of administration does not influence the time–action profile of glargine. Similarly, exercise does not influence glargine's unique absorption kinetics, even when the insulin is injected into a working limb.

Glargine binds with a slightly greater affinity to IGF-1 receptors as compared with human insulin. However, this slightly increased binding is still approximately two log scales lower than that of IGF-1. Controversy currently exists whether glargine insulin is associated with an increased chance of malignancy or an acceleration of underlying malignancy, but most feel that the available evidence is circumstantial and not sufficiently convincing to change prescribing patterns (Pocock and Smeeth, 2009; Smith and Gale, 2009; Weinstein et al., 2009).

Insulin determir (LEVEMIR) is an insulin analog modified by the addition of a saturated fatty acid to the ε amino group of LysB29, yielding a myristoylated insulin. When insulin detemir is injected subcutaneously, it binds to albumin via its fatty acid chain. Clinical studies in patients with type 1 diabetes have demonstrated that when insulin detemir is administered twice a day, it has a smoother time–action profile and produces a reduced prevalence of hypoglycemia than NPH insulin. The absorption profiles of glargine and determir insulin are similar, but detemir often requires twice-daily administration.

Other Insulin Formulations. Stable, mixed combinations (Table 43–5) of NPH and regular insulin in proportions of 70:30 combinations are available. Combinations of lispro protamine/lispro (50/50 and 75/25) and aspart protamine/aspart (70/30) are also available in the U.S.

Insulin Delivery. Most insulin is injected subcutaneously. Pen devices containing prefilled regular, lispro, NPH, glargine, premixed lispro protamine-lispro, or premixed aspart protamine-aspart have proven to be popular with many diabetic patients. Jet injector systems that enable patients to receive subcutaneous insulin injections without a needle are available. Intravenous infusions of insulin are useful in patients with ketoacidosis or when requirements for insulin may change rapidly, such as during the perioperative period, during labor and delivery, and in intensive care situations.

Continuous Subcutaneous Insulin Infusion. Short-acting insulins are the only form of the hormone used in subcutaneous infusion pumps. A number of pumps are available for continuous subcutaneous insulin infusion (CSII) therapy. CSII, or pump, therapy is not suitable for all patients because it demands considerable attention. However, for patients interested in intensive insulin therapy, a pump may be an attractive alternative to several daily injections. Insulin pumps provide a constant basal infusion of insulin and have the option of different infusion rates during the day and night to help avoid the dawn phenomenon (rise in blood glucose that occurs just prior to awakening from sleep) and bolus injections that are programmed according to the size and nature of a meal.

Glucose sensors that measure the interstitial glucose are now available and may be helpful in patients with labile blood glucose and frequent hypoglycemia (Juvenile Diabetes Research Foundation Continuous Glucose Monitoring Study Group, 2008). Although patients can use both a pump and a sensor, these devices are not yet integrated into a closed-loop system. Similar to the collected evidence with CSII, the benefits of continuous glucose monitoring have not been conclusively demonstrated, nor have clear selection criteria for appropriate patient groups been developed. However, the results from recent studies suggest that real-time glucose monitoring may lead to modest improvements in glycemic control and improved patient/family quality of life.

Pump therapy presents some unique problems. Because all the insulin used is short acting and there is a minimal amount of insulin in the subcutaneous pool at any given time, insulin deficiency and ketoacidosis may develop rapidly if therapy is interrupted accidentally. Although modern pumps have warning devices that detect changes in line pressure, mechanical problems such as pump failure, dislodgement of the needle, aggregation of insulin in the infusion line, or accidental kinking of the infusion catheter may occur. There also is a possibility of subcutaneous abscesses and cellulitis. Selection of the most appropriate patients is extremely important for success with pump therapy. Offsetting these potential problems, pump therapy is capable of producing a more physiological profile of insulin replacement during exercise (where insulin production is decreased) and therefore less hypoglycemia than do traditional subcutaneous insulin injections.

Factors That Affect Insulin Absorption. Factors that determine the rate of absorption of insulin after subcutaneous administration include the site of injection, the type of insulin, subcutaneous blood flow, smoking, regional muscular activity at the site of the injection, the volume and concentration of the injected insulin, and depth of injection (insulin has a more rapid onset of action if delivered intramuscularly rather than subcutaneously). Increased subcutaneous blood flow (brought about by massage, hot baths, or exercise) increases the rate of absorption.

Insulin usually is injected into the subcutaneous tissues of the abdomen, buttock, anterior thigh, or dorsal arm. Absorption is usually most rapid from the abdominal wall, followed by the arm, buttock, and thigh. If a patient is willing to inject into the abdomen, injections can be rotated throughout the entire area, thereby eliminating the injection site as a cause of variability in the rate of absorption. The abdomen currently is the preferred site of injection in the morning because insulin is absorbed 20-30% faster from that site than from the arm. If the patient refuses to inject into the abdominal area, it is preferable to select a consistent injection site for each component of insulin treatment (e.g., before-breakfast dose into the thigh, evening dose into the arm). Rotation of insulin injection sites traditionally has been advocated to avoid lipohypertrophy or lipoatrophy, although these conditions are infrequent with current preparations of insulin. In a small group of patients, subcutaneous degradation of insulin has been observed, and this has necessitated the injection of large amounts of insulin for adequate metabolic control.

Insulin Dosing and Regimens. In most patients, insulin-replacement therapy includes long-acting insulin (basal) and a short-acting insulin to provide postprandial needs. In a mixed population of type 1 diabetes patients, the average dose of insulin is usually 0.6-0.7 units/kg body weight per day, with a range of 0.2-1 units/kg per day. Obese patients generally and pubertal adolescents require more (~1-2 units/kg per day) because of resistance of peripheral tissues to insulin. Patients who require less insulin than 0.5 units/kg per day may have some endogenous production of insulin or may be more sensitive to the hormone because of good physical conditioning. The basal dose suppresses lipolysis, proteolysis, and hepatic glucose production; it is usually 40-50% of the total daily dose with the remainder as prandial or pre-meal insulin. The insulin dose at meal time should reflect the anticipated carbohydrate intake (many patients with type 1 diabetes calculate a ratio of the insulin dose to the number of grams of carbohydrate). A supplemental scale of short-acting insulin is added to the prandial insulin dose to allow correction of the BG. With all insulin dosing, the provider should consider the insulin sensitivity of the patient and adjust the insulin dosing accordingly. *Insulin administered as a single daily dose of long-acting insulin, alone or in combination with short-acting insulin, is rarely sufficient to achieve euglycemia. More complex regimens that include multiple injections of long-acting or short-acting insulin are needed to reach this goal. In all patients, careful monitoring of therapeutic end points directs the insulin dose used. This approach is facilitated by self-glucose monitoring and measurements of A1C.*

A number of commonly used dosage regimens that include mixtures of insulin given in two or more daily injections are depicted in Figure 43–8. An effective regimen involving multiple daily injections consisting of basal administration of long-acting insulin (e.g., insulin glargine or determir) either before breakfast or at bedtime and preprandial injections of a short-acting insulin (Weng et al., 2008). This method is called *basal/bolus* and is very similar to the pattern of insulin administration achieved with a subcutaneous infusion pump. Another regimen used is the *split-mixed regimen* involving the pre-breakfast and pre-supper injection of a mixture of short- and long-acting insulins. When the pre-supper NPH insulin is not sufficient to control hyperglycemia throughout the night, the evening dose may be divided into a pre-supper dose of regular insulin followed by NPH insulin at bedtime.

Individuals with diabetes may sometimes consume smaller amounts of food than originally planned. This, in the presence of a previously injected dose of insulin that was based on anticipation of a larger meal, could result in postprandial hypoglycemia. Thus, in patients who have gastroparesis or loss of appetite, injection of a short-acting analog postprandially, based on the amount of food actually consumed, may provide smoother glycemic control.

Adverse Events. The most common adverse reaction during insulin therapy is hypoglycemia. Hypoglycemia is the major risk that must be weighed against benefits of efforts to normalize glucose control. Additional information about hypoglycemia and its treatment is provided later in this chapter. Insulin is an anabolic hormone, and insulin treatment of both type 1 and type 2 diabetes is associated with modest weight gain. Paradoxically, improved glycemic control may initially lead to the deterioration of retinopathy in rare patients, but this is followed by a long-term reduction in diabetes-related complications. There has been a dramatic decrease in the incidence of allergic reactions to insulin with the transition to recombinant human insulin; these may still occur as a result of reaction to the small amounts of aggregated or denatured insulin in preparations, to minor contaminants, or because of sensitivity to one of the components added to insulin in its formulation (protamine, Zn^{2+}, etc.). Human insulin, as delivered to patients with diabetes, is immunogenic as reflected by the observation that many patients have circulating anti-insulin antibodies, but these do not alter insulin pharmacokinetics or action. Atrophy of subcutaneous fat at the site of insulin injection (lipoatrophy) was a rare side effect of older insulin preparations. Lipohypertrophy (enlargement of subcutaneous fat depots) has been ascribed to the lipogenic action of high local concentrations of insulin.

Insulin Treatment of Ketoacidosis and Other Special Situations. Acutely ill diabetic patients may have metabolic disturbances that are sufficiently severe or labile to justify intravenous administration of insulin (Kitabchi et al., 2009). Such treatment is most appropriate in patients with ketoacidosis or severe hyperglycemia with a hyperosmolar state. Insulin infusion inhibits lipolysis and gluconeogenesis completely and produces near-maximal stimulation of glucose uptake. In most patients with diabetic ketoacidosis, blood glucose concentrations will fall by ~10% per hour; the acidosis is corrected more slowly. As treatment proceeds, it often is necessary to administer glucose along with the insulin to prevent hypoglycemia but to allow clearance of all ketones. Some physicians prefer to initiate therapy with a loading dose of insulin, but this tactic appears unnecessary because steady-state concentrations of the hormone are achieved within 30 minutes with a constant infusion. Patients with nonketotic hyperglycemic hyperosmolar state may be more sensitive to insulin than are those with ketoacidosis. Appropriate replacement of fluid and electrolytes is an integral part of the therapy in both situations because there is always a major deficit. *Regardless of the insulin regimen, the key to effective therapy is careful and frequent monitoring of the patient's clinical status, glucose, and electrolytes.* A frequent error in the management of such patients is the failure to administer long-acting insulin subcutaneously before the insulin infusion is discontinued.

Treatment of Diabetes in Children or Adolescents. Diabetes is one of the most common chronic diseases of childhood, and rates of type 1 diabetes in American youth are estimated at 1 in 300, with an increasing incidence over the past 20 years. One of the unfortunate corollaries of the growing rates of obesity over the past three decades is an increase in the numbers of children and adolescents with nonautoimmune, or type 2, diabetes. Current estimates are that 15-20% of new cases of pediatric diabetes may in fact be type 2 diabetes; rates vary by ethnicity, with disproportionately high rates in Native Americans, African Americans, and Latinos. Because of a paucity of clinical trials performed in children, there is only limited information on which to base decisions for appropriate therapy. Thus the results in the Diabetes Control and Complications Trial with young and middle-aged adults have been extrapolated to the pediatric population such that current practice is for more intensive, physiologically based insulin replacement with a goal of tight glucose control (Diabetes Control Complications Trial Research Group, 1993). This is achieved with combinations of basal and prandial insulin replacement. The primary limiting factor of more aggressive insulin therapy is hypoglycemia, a problem with special concerns in young children. Diabetic patients <5 years old are at greater risk for hypoglycemia, have increased rates of severe hypoglycemia with seizures and coma, and may suffer permanent cognitive dysfunction as a result of repeated episodes of low blood glucose. Older children and adolescents do not seem to have demonstrable cognitive impairment related to hypoglycemia; good glycemic control is associated with better mental function (Kodl and Seaquist, 2008).

The treatment of type 1 diabetes in children and adolescents has changed with the availability of newer technologies. The standard for insulin treatment now includes multiple dose regimens with three to five injections per day or CSII. Split/mixed regimens using NPH and regular insulin have been increasingly supplanted by regimens using insulin analogs because they offer more flexibility in dosing and meal patterns. Similarly, CSII is used with increasing frequency in the pediatric diabetic population. Moreover, recent studies show that this approach is applicable to young children as well as older children and adolescents.

Because of the nearly uniform association of type 2 diabetes with obesity in the pediatric age group, lifestyle management is the recommended first step in therapy. Goals of reducing body weight while maintaining normal linear growth, and increasing physical activity, are broadly recommended and can be effective when patients are compliant. There have been few clinical trials of glucose lowering therapy in pediatric type 2 diabetes. The only medication currently approved by the FDA specifically for medical treatment of type 2 diabetes is *metformin*. Metformin is approved for children as young as 10 years of age and is available in a liquid formulation (100 mg/mL). Results from clinical trials have shown that both metformin and glimepiride effectively lower blood glucose in affected patients. Insulin is the typical second line of therapy after metformin; basal insulin can be added to oral agent therapy or multiple daily injections can be used when simpler regimens are not successful. Weight gain is a more significant problem than hypoglycemia with insulin treatment in pediatric type 2 diabetes. Other diabetes medications, such as thiazolidinediones, α-glucosidase inhibitors, DPP-4 inhibitors, and exenatide, have been tried empirically in type 2 diabetic adolescents, but there is no systematically collected data on efficacy or safety of these agents in the pediatric population.

Management of Diabetes in Hospitalized Patients. Hyperglycemia is common in hospitalized patients. Depending on how hyperglycemia is defined, prevalence estimates of elevated blood glucose among inpatients with and without a prior diagnosis of diabetes range between 20% and 100% for patients treated in intensive care units (ICUs) and 30% and 83% outside the ICU. Although most of these individuals will have known diabetes, ~30% of hospitalized patients will have elevated blood glucose levels without a prior diagnosis of diabetes (Falciglia, 2007). Patients admitted to the hospital often have a number of challenges to glucose regulation in addition to those faced by diabetic outpatients (Donner and Flammer, 2008). Stress of illness has been associated with insulin resistance, possibly the result of counterregulatory hormone secretion, cytokines, and other inflammatory mediators. Food intake is often variable due to concurrent illness or preparation for diagnostic testing. Medications used in the hospital, such as glucocorticoids or dextrose-containing intravenous solutions, can exacerbate tendencies toward hyperglycemia. Finally fluid balance and tissue perfusion can affect the absorbance of subcutaneous insulin and the clearance of glucose. Therapy of hyperglycemia in hospitalized patients needs to be adjusted for these variables.

There is an emerging body of information indicating that hyperglycemia portends poor outcomes in hospitalized patients, most notably in the critically ill, and that this effect is independent of severity of illness (Finfer et al., 2009; van den Berghe et al., 2001). The mechanisms for this association have not been fully explained, and controversy persists about the optimal level of glycemia in hospitalized patients. The ADA currently suggests these blood glucose targets: 140-180 m/dL (7.8-10.0 mM) in critically ill patients and random glucose of 180 mg/dL (10 mM) or pre-meal glucose of 140 mg/dL (7.8 mM) in noncritically ill patients. Great emphasis should be placed on steps taken to minimize hypoglycemia in both settings.

Insulin is the cornerstone of treatment of hyperglycemia in hospitalized patients (Moghissi et al., 2009). For critically ill patients and those with variable blood pressure, edema, and tissue perfusion, intravenous insulin is the treatment of choice. This method of insulin administration has been firmly established in the care of critically ill patients with elevated blood glucose and provides the most flexible and precise means of treatment. A number of algorithms have been adapted to allow rapid titration with adjustments to maintain blood glucose in a target range. For patients who are more stable, subcutaneous insulin regimens using combinations of basal and prandial insulin is the standard. There is considerable evidence that reactive treatment, using sliding scale regimens, is inferior and associated with wider fluctuations in blood glucose and greater rates of both hyper- and hypoglycemia. Oral agents have a limited place in treatment of hyperglycemic patients in the hospital because of slow onset of action, insufficient potency, need for intact GI function, and side effects. In general, oral glucose-lowering medications should be discontinued on hospital admission and can be restarted at discharge.

Intravenous administration of insulin also is well suited to the treatment of diabetic patients during the perioperative period and during childbirth. There is debate, however, about the optimal route of insulin administration during surgery. Although some clinicians advocate subcutaneous insulin administration, most recommend intravenous insulin infusion. Some physicians give patients half their normal daily dose of insulin as long-acting insulin subcutaneously on the morning of an operation and then administer 5% dextrose infusions during surgery to maintain glucose concentrations. This approach provides less minute-to-minute control than is possible with intravenous regimens and also may increase the likelihood of hypoglycemia. For patients with type 1 diabetes, failure to provide some basal insulin at all times can precipitate diabetic ketoacidosis.

INSULIN SECRETAGOGUES AND ORAL HYPOGLYCEMIC AGENTS

A variety of sufonylureas, meglitinides, GLP-1 agonists, and inhibitors of dipeptidyl peptidase-4 (DPP-4) are used as secretagogues to stimulate insulin release (Table 43–6).

K_{ATP} Channel Modulators:Sulfonylureas

Chemistry. All members of this class of drugs are substituted arylsulfonylureas. They differ by substitutions at the para position on the benzene ring and at one nitrogen residue of the urea moiety. The sulfonylureas are divided into two groups or generations of agents. The first generation sulfonylureas (tolbutamide, tolazamide, and chlorpropamide) are rarely used now in the treatment of type 2 diabetes and are not discussed (information is available in prior editions of this book). The second, more potent generation of hypoglycemic sulfonylureas includes glyburide (glibenclamide; DIABETA, others), glipizide (GLUCOTROL, others), and glimepiride (AMARYL, others) (Table 43–7). Some are available in an extended-release (glipizide) or a micronized (glyburide) formulation.

Mechanism of Action. Sulfonylureas stimulate insulin release by binding to a specific site on the β cell K_{ATP} channel complex (the sulfonylurea receptor, SUR) and inhibiting its activity. K_{ATP} channel inhibition causes cell membrane depolarization and the cascade of events leading to insulin secretion (Figure 43–3). The acute administration of sulfonylureas to type 2 diabetes patients increases insulin release from the pancreas. Sulfonylureas may also reduce hepatic clearance of insulin, further increasing plasma insulin levels. In the initial months of sulfonylurea treatment, fasting plasma insulin levels and insulin responses to oral glucose challenges are increased. With chronic administration, circulating insulin levels decline to those that existed before treatment, but despite this reduction in insulin levels, reduced plasma glucose levels are maintained. The explanation for this is not clear, but it may relate to the fact that chronic hyperglycemia *per se* impairs insulin secretion (glucose toxicity), and with the initial

Table 43–6

Properties of Insulin Secretagogues

CLASS/GENERIC NAME	DAILY DOSAGE[a], mg	DURATION OF ACTION, h
Sulfonylureas - first generation		
Chlorpropamide	100-500	>48
Tolazamide	100-1000	12-24
Tolbutamide	1000-3000	6-12
Sulfonylureas - second generation		
Glimepiride	1-8	24
Glipizide	5-40	12-18
Glipizide (extended release)	5-20	24
Glyburide	1.25-20	12-24
Glyburide (micronized)	0.75-12	12-24
Nonsulfonylureas (Meglitinides)		
Repaglinide	0.5-16	2-6
Nateglinide	180-360	2-4
GLP-1 agonist		
Exenatide	0.01-0.02	4-6
Dipeptidyl Peptidase-4 Inhibitors		
Saxagliptin	2.5-5	
Sitagliptin	100	12-16
Vildagliptin	50-100	12-24

[a]Dose may be lower in some patients

Table 43–7

Structural Formulas of the Sulfonylureas

General structure: R_1–(benzene ring)–$SO_2NHC(=O)NH$–R_2

SECOND-GENERATION AGENTS	R_1	R_2
Glyburide (Glibenclamide, MICRONASE, DIABETA, others)	Cl, OCH_3 (substituted benzene ring)–$CONH(CH_2)_2$–	cyclohexyl
Glipizide (GLUCOTROL, others)	H_3C–(pyrazine ring, N, N)–$CONH(CH_2)_2$–	cyclohexyl
Gliclazide (DIAMICRON, others; unavailable in the U.S.)	H_3C–	–N (bicyclic ring)
Glimepiride (AMARYL)	H_3C, H_5C_2, O (pyrrolinone ring) N–C(=O)–$NH-CH_2-CH_2$–	cyclohexyl–CH_3

correction of plasma glucose circulating insulin has improved effects on its target tissues. The absence of acute stimulatory effects of sulfonylureas on insulin secretion during chronic treatment is attributed to downregulation of cell surface receptors for sulfonylureas on the pancreatic β cell. If chronic sulfonylurea therapy is discontinued, pancreatic β cell response to acute administration of the drug is restored.

Absorption, Distribution, and Elimination. Although the rates of absorption of the different sulfonylureas vary, all are effectively absorbed from the GI tract. However, food and hyperglycemia can reduce absorption. Sulfonylureas in plasma are largely (90-99%) bound to protein, especially albumin; plasma protein binding is greatest for glyburide. The volumes of distribution of most of the sulfonylureas are ~0.2 L/kg. Although their half-lives are short (3-5 hours), their hypoglycemic effects are evident for 12-24 hours, and they often can be administered once daily. The reason for the discrepancies between their half-lives and duration of action is not clear. The liver metabolizes all sulfonylureas, and the metabolites are excreted in the urine. Thus, sulfonylureas should be administered with caution to patients with either renal or hepatic insufficiency.

Adverse Effects and Drug Interactions. Not unexpectedly, sulfonylureas may cause hypoglycemic reactions, including coma. This is a particular concern in elderly patients with impaired hepatic or renal function who are taking longer-acting sulfonylureas (a major reason first-generation agents are rarely used). Because of the long $t_{1/2}$ of some sulfonylureas, it may be necessary to monitor or treat elderly hypoglycemic patients for 24-48 hours with an intravenous glucose infusion in the in-patient setting. Weight gain of 1-3 kg is a common side effect of improving glycemic control with sulfonylurea treatment.

Less frequent side effects of sulfonylureas include nausea and vomiting, cholestatic jaundice, agranulocytosis, aplastic and hemolytic anemias, generalized hypersensitivity reactions, and dermatological reactions. Rarely, patients treated with these drugs develop an alcohol-induced flush similar to that caused by disulfiram or hyponatremia. A long-running debate has centered on whether treatment with sulfonylureas is associated with increased cardiovascular mortality (Bell, 2006). This likely reflects the expression of the sulfonylurea receptor on vascular smooth muscle cells and cardiac myocytes, where activation of the sulfonylurea prevents the beneficial effects of ischemic preconditioning. Glyburide, but not glimepiride, interacts with the sulfonylurea receptor in these non-islet sites and may be associated with increased cardiovascular risk. However, a recent randomized trial of glyburide, metformin, and rosiglitazone found a slightly lower cardiovascular mortality in individuals treated with glyburide (Kahn et al., 2006).

The hypoglycemic effect of sulfonylureas may be enhanced by various mechanisms (decreased hepatic metabolism or renal excretion, displacement from protein-binding sites). For example, some drugs (sulfonamides, clofibrate, and salicylates) displace the sulfonylureas from binding proteins, thereby transiently increasing the concentration of free drug. Ethanol may enhance the action of sulfonylureas and cause hypoglycemia. In addition, hypoglycemia may be more frequent in patients taking a sulfonylurea and one of these agents: androgens, anticoagulants, azole antifungals, chloramphenicol, fenfluramine, fluconazole, gemfibrozil, histamine H_2 antagonists, magnesium salts, methyldopa, monoamine oxidase inhibitors (MAOIs), probenecid, sulfinpyrazone, sulfonamides, tricyclic antidepressants, and urinary acidifiers. Other drugs may decrease the glucose-lowering effect of sulfonylureas by increased hepatic metabolism, increased renal excretion, or inhibiting insulin secretion (β-blockers, Ca^{2+} channel blockers, cholestyramine, diazoxide, estrogens, hydantoins, isoniazid, nicotinic acid, phenothiazines, rifampin, sympathomimetics, thiazide diuretics, and urinary alkalinizers).

Dosage Forms Available. Treatment is initiated at lower end of the dose range and titrated upward based on the patient's glycemic response. Some have a longer duration of action and can be prescribed in a single daily dose (glimepiride), whereas others are formulated as extended-release or micronized formulations to extend their duration of action (Table 43–7). The dose for the extended-release glipizide or micronized glyburide is lower. Glyburide is not recommended when the creatinine clearance is < 50 mL/minute or in elderly individuals because reduced drug and metabolite clearance greatly increases the risk of hypoglycemia. Other sulfonylureas such as glipizide or glimepiride appear safer in elderly individuals with type 2 diabetes.

Therapeutic Uses. Sulfonylureas are used to treat hyperglycemia in type 2 diabetes. Between 50% and 80% of properly selected patients respond to this class of agents. All members of the class appear be equally efficacious. A significant number of patients who respond initially later cease to respond to the sulfonylurea and develop unacceptable hyperglycemia (secondary failure). This may occur as a result of a change in drug metabolism or more likely from a progression of β-cell failure. A recent randomized trial found that the initial improvement in glycemic control was less durable with glyburide monotherapy (compared to metformin or rosiglitazone monotherapy), suggesting that the secondary failure rate is higher with this class of drugs (Kahn et al., 2006). Some individuals with neonatal diabetes or MODY-3 respond to these agents (this is an off-label use). Combinations of insulin and sulfonylureas and other oral agents are discussed later. Contraindications to the use of these drugs include type 1 diabetes, pregnancy, lactation, and, for the older preparations, significant hepatic or renal insufficiency.

K_{ATP} Channel Modulators: Non-Sulfonylureas

Repaglinide. Repaglinide (PRANDIN) is an oral insulin secretagogue of the meglitinide class (Table 43–6). It is a benzoic acid derivative structurally unrelated to the sulfonylureas, but like sulfonylureas, it stimulates insulin release by closing K_{ATP} channels in pancreatic β cells. The drug is absorbed rapidly from the GI tract, and peak blood levels are obtained within 1 hour. The $t_{1/2}$ is ~1 hour. These features allow for multiple preprandial use as compared with the classical once- or twice-daily dosing of sulfonylureas.

Repaglinide is metabolized primarily by the liver (CYP3A4) to inactive derivatives. Repaglinide should be used cautiously in patients with hepatic insufficiency. Because a small proportion (~10%) is metabolized by the kidney, dosing of the drug in patients with renal insufficiency also should be performed cautiously. As with sulfonylureas, the major side effect of repaglinide is hypoglycemia. Like sulfonylureas, repaglinide is associated with a decline in efficacy (secondary failure) after initially improving glycemic control. Certain drugs may potentiate the action of repaglinide by displacing it from plasma protein binding sites (β-blockers, chloramphenicol, coumarins, MAOIs, nonsteroidal anti-inflammatory drugs [NSAIDs], probenecid, salicylates, and sulfonamide) or altering its metabolism (gemfibrozil, itraconazole, trimethoprim, cyclosporine, simvastatin, clarithromycin).

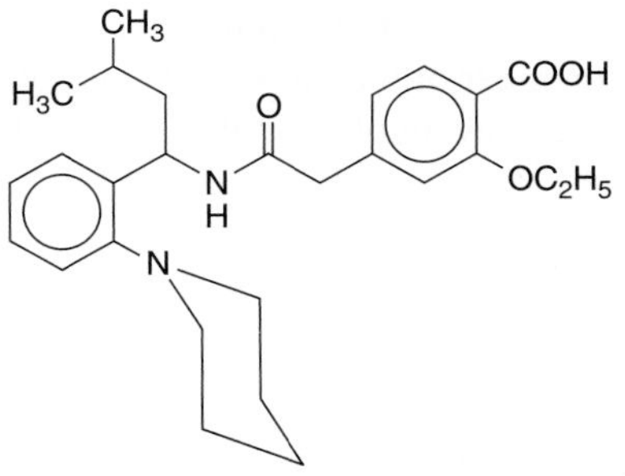

REPAGLINIDE

Nateglinide. Nateglinide (STARLIX) is an orally effective insulin secretagogue derived from d-phenylalanine. Like sulfonylureas and repaglinide, nateglinide stimulates insulin secretion by blocking K_{ATP} channels in pancreatic β cells (Rosenstock et al., 2004). Nateglinide promotes a more rapid but less sustained secretion of insulin than other available oral antidiabetic agents. The drug's major therapeutic effect is reducing postprandial glycemic elevations in type 2 diabetes patients. Nateglinide is approved by the FDA for use in type 2 diabetes. It is most effective when administered in a dose of 120 mg, 1-10 minutes before a meal.

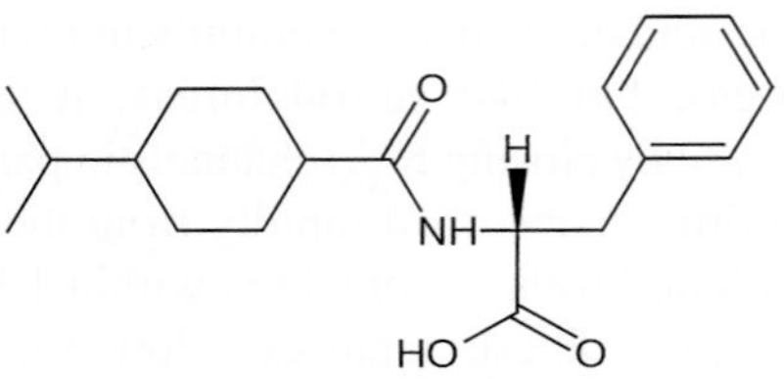

NATEGLINIDE

Nateglinide is metabolized primarily by hepatic CYPs [2C9, 70%; 3A4, 30%] and thus should be used cautiously in patients with hepatic insufficiency. About 16% of an administered dose is excreted by the kidney as unchanged drug. Dosage adjustment is unnecessary in renal failure. Some drugs reduce the glucose-lowering effect of nateglinide (corticosteroids, rifamycins, sympathomimetics, thiazide diuretics, thyroid products); others (alcohol, NSAIDs, salicylates, MAOIs, and nonselective β blockers) may increase the risk of hypoglycemia with nateglinide. Nateglinide therapy may produce fewer episodes of hypoglycemia than other currently available oral insulin secretagogues including repaglinide. As with sulfonylureas and repaglinide, secondary failure occurs.

A$_{MPK}$ and PPAR γ activators

Metformin

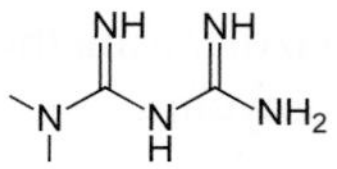

METFORMIN

Mechanism of Action. Metformin (GLUCOPHAGE, others) is the only member of the biguanide class of oral hypoglycemic drugs available for use today (Bailey and Turner, 1996). Metformin increases the activity of the AMP-dependent protein kinase (AMPK) (Zhou et al., 2001). AMPK is activated by phosphorylation when cellular energy stores are reduced (i.e., lower concentrations of ATP and phosphocreatine). Activated AMPK stimulates fatty acid oxidation, glucose uptake, and nonoxidative metabolism, and it reduces lipogenesis and gluconeogenesis. The net result of these actions is increased glycogen storage in skeletal muscle, lower rates of hepatic glucose production, increased insulin sensitivity, and lower blood glucose levels.

Metformin causes a similar profile of effects and is dependent on AMPK activation (Shaw et al., 2005). Although the molecular mechanism by which metformin activates AMPK is not known, it is thought to be indirect, possibly by reducing intracellular energy stores. Consistent with this, metformin has been shown to inhibit cellular respiration by specific actions on mitochondrial complex I. Metformin has little effect on blood glucose in normoglycemic states and does not affect the release of insulin or other islet hormones and rarely causes hypoglycemia. However, even in persons with only mild hyperglycemia, metformin lowers blood glucose by reducing hepatic glucose production and increasing peripheral glucose uptake. This effect is at least partially mediated by reducing insulin resistance at key target tissues. The hepatic effect is probably the dominant mode of action and involves primarily suppression of gluconeogenesis. Table 43–8 compares metformin and thiazolidinediones (glitazones).

Table 43–8

Comparison of Metformin and Thiazolidinediones

PARAMETER	METFORMIN	THIAZOLIDINEDIONES
Molecular target	AMPK	PPARγ
Pharmacologic action	Suppression of HGP	Enhanced insulin sensitivity
Reduction of HbA_{1c} [a]	1.0-1.25	0.5-1.4
Reduction of FFA	Minimal	Moderate
Stimulation of adiponectin	Minimal	Significant
Effect on body weight	Minimal	Increased
Peripheral edema	Minimal	Moderate
Fracture risk	None	Increased
Lactic Acidosis	Rare[b]	None

[a]Magnitude of absolute reduction dependent on starting A1C value
[b]In renal insufficiency
HGP = hepatic glucose production

Absorption, Distribution, and Elimination. Metformin is absorbed primarily from the small intestine. The drug is stable, does not bind to plasma proteins, and is excreted unchanged in the urine. It has a $t_{1/2}$ in the circulation of ~2 hours. The transport of metformin into cells is mediated in part by organic cation transporters (see Chapter 5). Organic cation transporter 1 (OCT 1) is believed to carry the drug into cells such as hepatocytes and myocytes where it is pharmacologically active. Organic cation transporter 2 (OCT 2) is thought to transport metformin into renal tubules for excretion. There is recent evidence suggesting that genetic variation in OCT 1 among humans may affect the response to metformin.

Therapeutic Uses and Dosage. Metformin is currently the most commonly used oral agent to treat type 2 diabetes and is generally accepted as the first-line treatment for this condition. Metformin is effective as monotherapy and in combination with nearly every other therapy for type 2 diabetes, and its utility is supported by data from a large number of clinical trials. Fixed-dose combinations of metformin in conjunction with glipizide, glyburide, pioglitazone, repaglinide, rosiglitazone, and sitagliptin are available. Metformin is available as an immediate-release form, and treatment is best started with low doses and titrated over days to weeks to minimize side effects. The currently recommended dosing is 0.5-1.0 g twice daily, with a maximum dose of 2550 mg; there is no advantage of thrice-daily administration. A sustained-release preparation is available that is effective for once-daily dosing; the maximum dose for this compound is 2 g.

Metformin has superior or equivalent efficacy of glucose lowering compared to other oral agents used to treat diabetes, and reduces diabetes-related complications in patients with type 2 diabetes. Unlike many of the other oral agents, metformin does not typically cause weight gain and in some cases causes weight reduction. Metformin is not effective in the treatment of type 1 diabetes. Several observational studies suggest that diabetic patients treated with metformin may have lower rates of cardiovascular disease and mortality, compared to individuals treated with alternative therapies (Evans et al., 2006; Johnson et al., 2005). The results of the Diabetes Prevention Program indicate that in persons with impaired glucose tolerance, treatment with metformin delays the progression to diabetes. Metformin has been used as a treatment for infertility in women with the polycystic ovarian syndrome. Although not formally approved for this purpose, metformin has demonstrable effects to improve ovulation and menstrual cyclicity and reduce circulating androgens and hirsutism.

Adverse Effects and Drug Interactions. The most common side effects of metformin are gastrointestinal. Approximately 10-25% of patients starting this medication report nausea, indigestion, abdominal cramps or bloating, diarrhea, or some combination of these. Metformin has direct effects on GI function including glucose and bile salt absorption. Use of metformin is associated with 20-30% lower blood levels of vitamin B_{12} (DeFronzo et al., 1995), probably due to malabsorption, but neurological or hematological consequences of this have not been reported. Most GI adverse effects of metformin abate over time with continued use of the drug, and can be minimized by starting at low doses and gradually titrating to a target dose over several weeks, and by having patients take it with meals.

Like phenformin, metformin has been associated with lactic acidosis. The most concrete evidence of this is from cases of metformin overdose where very high circulating levels of the drug were associated with high plasma lactate and acidemia. However, the estimated incidence of lactic acidosis attributable to metformin use is 3-6 per 100,000 patient-years of treatment (Lalau and Race, 2001; Scarpello and Howlett, 2008), which is comparable to rates in type 2 diabetic patients not using metformin. Moreover, several recent analyses of this association have raised doubts as to whether the association of lactic acidosis with metformin is causal (Kamber et al., 2008). Many cases of lactic acidosis associated with the use of metformin have been reported in patients with concurrent conditions that can cause poor tissue perfusion such as sepsis, myocardial infarction, and congestive heart failure. Renal failure is another common comorbidity reported in patients having lactic acidosis associated with metformin use, and decreased glomerular filtration rates are thought to increase plasma metformin levels by reducing clearance of drug from the circulation. There are no consensus guidelines for renal contraindications for metformin use; because clearance of the drug is not altered significantly until the creatinine clearance drops below 50 mL/minute, metformin is probably safe in patients with this level of renal function (Herrington and Levy, 2008). It is important to assess renal function before starting metformin and to monitor function at least annually. Metformin should be discontinued preemptively in situations where renal function could decline precipitously, such as before radiographic procedures that use contrast dyes and during admission to hospital for severe illness. Metformin should not be used in severe pulmonary disease, decompensated heart failure, severe liver disease, or chronic alcohol abuse.

Cationic drugs that are eliminated by renal tubular secretion have the potential for interaction with metformin by competing for common renal tubular transport systems. Careful patient monitoring and dose adjustment of metformin is recommended in patients who are taking cationic medications such as cimetidine, furosemide, and nifedipine, excreted via the proximal renal tubular secretory system.

Thiazolidinediones

Chemistry and Mechanism of Action. Thiazolidinediones are ligands for the peroxisome proliferation activating receptor γ (PPARγ) receptors, a group of nuclear hormone receptors that are involved in the regulation of genes related to glucose and lipid metabolism (Yki-Jarvinen, 2004). Two thiazolidinediones are currently available to treat patients with type 2 diabetes, rosiglitazone (AVANDIA) and pioglitazone (ACTOS). These compounds are generally similar but have several important differences. Although much is understood about the molecular mechanisms of action of the thiazolidinediones, they have complex effects on a wide variety of tissues, and much remains to be learned about their overall clinical impact and their specific role in therapeutics. Table 43–8 compares metformin and thiazolidinediones.

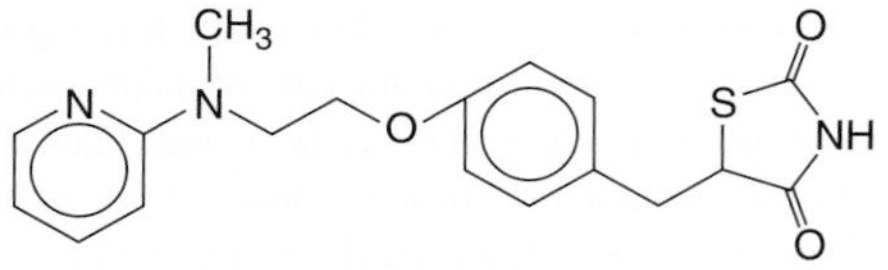

ROSIGLITAZONE

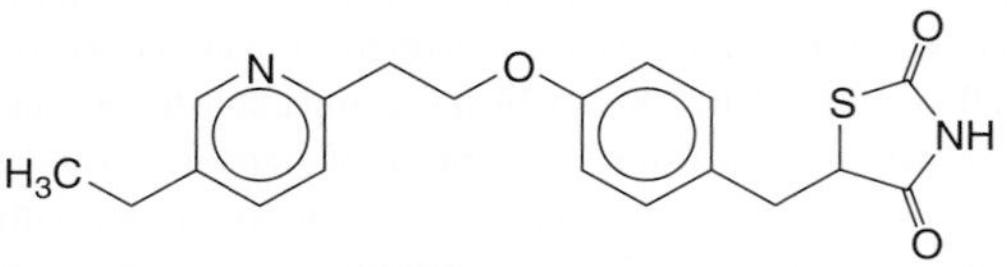

PIOGLITAZONE

PPARγ is expressed primarily in adipose tissue with lesser expression in cardiac, skeletal, and smooth muscle cells, islet β cells, macrophages, and vascular endothelial cells. The endogenous ligands for PPARγ include small lipophilic molecules such as oxidized linoleic acid, arachidonic acid and the prostaglandin metabolite 15d-PGJ2; rosiglitazone and pioglitazone are synthetic ligands for PPARγ. Ligand binding to PPARγ causes heterodimer formation with the retinoid X receptor and interaction with PPAR response elements on specific genes, an interaction that is modulated by complex interactions with co-repressors and co-activators. The principal response to PPARγ activation is adipocyte differentiation. Preclinical gain-of-function models show increased numbers of adipocytes and expansion of fat mass; loss-of-function models demonstrate lipodystrophy. Along with adipocyte differentiation, PPARγ activity promotes uptake of circulating fatty acids into fat cells and shifts of lipid stores from extra-adipose to adipose tissue. One consequence of the concerted cellular responses to PPARγ activation is increased tissue sensitivity to insulin, and this is the basis for the pharmacological application of thiazolidinediones to clinical medicine.

Pioglitazone and rosiglitazone are insulin sensitizers and increase insulin-mediated glucose uptake by 30-50% in patients with type 2 diabetes. Although adipose tissue seems to be the primary target for PPARγ agonists, both clinical and preclinical models support a role for skeletal muscle, the major site for insulin-mediated glucose disposal, in the response to thiazolidinediones. It is still not clear whether thiazolidinedione-induced improvement of insulin resistance is due to direct effects on key target tissues (skeletal muscle and liver), indirect effects mediated by secreted products of adipocytes (e.g., adiponectin), or some combination of these. In addition to promoting glucose uptake into muscle and adipose tissue, the thiazolidinediones reduce hepatic glucose production and increase hepatic glucose uptake.

Beyond effects on insulin sensitivity and blood glucose, thiazolidinediones also affect lipid metabolism. Treatment with rosiglitazone or pioglitazone reduces plasma levels of fatty acids by increasing clearance and reducing lipolysis. These drugs also cause a shift of triglyceride stores from nonadipose to adipose tissues, and from visceral to subcutaneous fat depots. In clinical trials, pioglitazone reduces plasma triglycerides by 10-15%, and raises HDL-cholesterol levels. This has been attributed to a dual effect on PPARα as well as PPARγ; rosiglitazone does not interact with PPARα and has minimal effects on plasma triglycerides and cholesterol. Because of these actions on plasma lipids, and beneficial effects on inflammatory markers, coagulation, and endothelial function, thiazolidinediones were predicted to reduce macrovascular complications of diabetes and insulin resistance. However, recently completed randomized clinical trials demonstrated a questionable benefit of pioglitazone (Dormandy et al., 2005), and no effect of rosiglitazone on major events related to atherosclerosis (Home et al., 2009). Because thiazolidinediones reduce hepatic triglyceride, they have been applied to the treatment of nonalcoholic fatty liver disease. Although results of these studies have been encouraging (Kashi et al., 2008), the thiazolidinediones are not yet approved for this use.

Absorption, Distribution, and Elimination. Both agents are absorbed within 2-3 hours, and bioavailability does not seem to be affected by food. The thiazolidinediones are metabolized by the liver and may be administered to patients with renal insufficiency, but should not be used if there is active hepatic disease or significant elevations of serum liver transaminases. The thiazolidinediones are metabolized by hepatic CYPs. CYPs 2C8 and 3A4 metabolize pioglitazone; rosiglitazone is metabolized by CYPs 2C9 and 2C8. Rifampin induces these enzymes and causes a significant decrease in plasma concentrations of rosiglitazone and pioglitazone; gemfibrozil impedes metabolism of the thiazolidinediones and can increase plasma levels by ~2-fold. It may be prudent to reduce the doses of the thiazolidinediones when they are used in conjunction with gemfibrozil. Rosiglitazone and pioglitazone do not seem to significantly affect the pharmacokinetics of other drugs.

Therapeutic Uses and Dosage. Rosiglitazone and pioglitazone are dosed once daily. The starting dose of rosiglitazone is 4 mg and should not exceed 8 mg daily. The starting dose of pioglitazone is 15-30 mg, up to a maximum of 45 mg daily. Thiazolidinediones have proven effects to enhance insulin action on liver, adipose tissue, and skeletal muscle. These composite effects on glucose metabolism confer improvements in glycemic control in persons with type 2 diabetes and cause average reductions in A1C of 0.5-1.4%. Thiazolidinediones require the presence of insulin for pharmacological activity and are not indicated to treat type 1 diabetes. Both pioglitazone and rosiglitazone are effective as monotherapy and as additive therapy to metformin, sulfonylureas, or insulin. The onset of action of thiazolidinediones is relatively slow; maximal effects on glucose homeostasis develop gradually over the course of 1-3 months.

There is evidence in drug-naive diabetic subjects that the glucose-lowering effect of primary treatment with rosiglitazone is more durable than that of metformin or glyburide (Kahn et al., 2006). Treatment with rosiglitazone also reduced progression from prediabetes to type 2 diabetes (Gerstein et al., 2006).

Adverse Effects and Drug Interactions. The most common adverse effects of the thiazolidinediones are weight gain and edema. Edema attributable to thiazolidinedione treatment occurs in up to 10% of patients in clinical trials and has been reported equally with pioglitazone and rosiglitazone. Beyond the effects of edema, treatment with thiazolidinediones causes an increase in body adiposity and an average weight gain of 2-4 kg over the first year of treatment. Importantly, in both preclinical models and in human studies the gain of body weight occurs peripherally, in subcutaneous adipose tissue, and visceral fat changes little or is reduced. The use of insulin with thiazolidinedione treatment roughly doubles the incidence of edema and amount of weight gain, compared with either drug alone.

Macular edema has been reported in patients using both rosiglitazone and pioglitazone (Ryan et al., 2006), usually in association with more general fluid retention. Beyond regular annual retinal exams, diabetic patients taking thiazolidinediones should be observed for visual changes.

Of greatest concern among the adverse effects of thiazolidinediones is the increased incidence of congestive heart failure. This has generally been attributed to the effect of the drugs to cause plasma volume expansion in type 2 diabetic patients who have significantly increased risk for heart failure. There does not appear to be an acute effect of pioglitazone or rosiglitazone to reduce myocardial contractility or ejection fraction. Yet exposure to these drugs over several years in clinical trials has been associated with an increased incidence of heart failure of up to 2-fold (Home et al., 2009). The use of thiazolidinediones in diabetic patients without a history of heart failure, or with compensated heart failure, can be initiated, but monitoring for signs and symptoms of congestive heart failure is important, especially when insulin is also used. Thiazolidinediones should not be used in patients with moderate to severe heart failure, and they should be discontinued in those who develop clinically apparent heart failure while being treated (Nesto et al., 2003).

Recent evidence suggests that rosiglitazone, but not pioglitazone, increases the risk of cardiovascular events (myocardial infarction, stroke). While the degree of the risk remains controversial, an expert panel reviewing this question for the FDA recommended caution in the use of rosiglitazone, but did not recommend its removal from the market (Rosen, 2010). Rather, as of September, 2010, the FDA requires that new prescriptions for rosiglitazone be issued under a risk evaluation and mitigation strategy and be limited to patients whose diabetes could not be adequately controlled by other medications (including pioglitazone). The European Medicines Agency has suspended marketing of rosiglitazone-containing formulations and recommended removal of rosiglitazone and rosiglitazone-containing formulations from the European market.

Evidence from clinical trials indicates that treatment with thiazolidinediones can increase the risk of bone fracture in women (Home et al., 2009; Kahn et al., 2006; Meier et al., 2008). This effect has been proposed to result from increased shunting of mesenchymal stem cells into the adipocyte lineage, and away from osteogenesis, as a result of increased PPARγ activity. Treatment with thiazolidinediones has also been associated with a small but consistent reduction in the hematocrit. This has generally been attributed to hemodilution due to plasma volume expansion, but thiazolidinediones may conceivably shunt erythroid precursors into adipose tissue development.

The first thiazolidinedione released for treatment of diabetic patients, troglitazone, was removed from the market because of rare but severe, and sometimes fatal, hepatic failure. There have been few cases of severe hepatocellular damage attributable to the newer thiazolidinediones, and these have not caused death or required transplantation. In general, pioglitazone and rosiglitazone have been associated with a lowering of transaminases, probably reflective of reductions in hepatic steatosis. It is recommended that thiazolidinediones be withheld from patients with clinically apparent liver disease and that liver function be monitored intermittently during treatment.

GLP-1-Based Agents

Incretins are GI hormones that are released after meals and stimulate insulin secretion. The two best known incretins are GLP-1 and GIP. Although these peptides share many similarities, they differ in that GIP is not effective for stimulating insulin release and lowering blood glucose in persons with type 2 diabetes, whereas GLP-1 is effective. Consequently, the GLP-1 signaling system has been a successful drug target.

Both GLP-1 and glucagon are products derived from preproglucagon, a 180–amino acid precursor with five separately processed domains (Figure 43–9) (Drucker, 2006). An amino-terminal signal peptide is followed by glicentin-related pancreatic peptide, glucagon, GLP-1, and glucagon-like peptide 2 (GLP-2). Processing of the protein is sequential and occurs in a tissue-specific fashion. Pancreatic α-cells cleave proglucagon into glucagon and a large C-terminal peptide that includes both of the GLPs. Intestinal L-cells and specific hindbrain neurons process proglucagon into a large N-terminal peptide that includes glucagon or GLP-1 and GLP-2. GLP-2 impacts the proliferation of epithelial cells lining the GI tract. Teduglutide, a GLP-2 analog, is under development as a treatment for short bowel syndrome and has received orphan drug designation for the treatment of short bowel syndrome from the U.S. FDA and the European Medicines Agency.

Given intravenously to diabetic subjects in supraphysiologic amounts, GLP-1 stimulates insulin secretion, inhibits glucagon release, delays gastric emptying, reduces food intake, and normalizes fasting and postprandial insulin secretion. The insulinotropic effect of GLP-1 is glucose dependent in that insulin secretion at fasting glucose concentrations, even with high levels of circulating GLP-1, is minimal. The effects of GLP-1 to promote glucose homeostasis and the glucose dependence of these effects are beneficial aspects of this signaling system for treating type 2 diabetes. GLP-1 is rapidly inactivated by the enzyme dipeptidyl peptidase IV (DPP-4), with a plasma $t_{1/2}$ of 1-2 minutes; thus, the natural peptide, itself, is not a useful therapeutic agent.

Two broad strategies have been taken to applying GLP-1 to therapeutics, the development of injectable, DPP-4 resistant peptide agonists of the GLP-1 receptor, and the creation of small molecule inhibitors of DPP-4 (Figure 43–10; Table 43–6).

GLP-1 Receptor Agonists. There are currently two GLP-1 receptor agonists that have been approved for

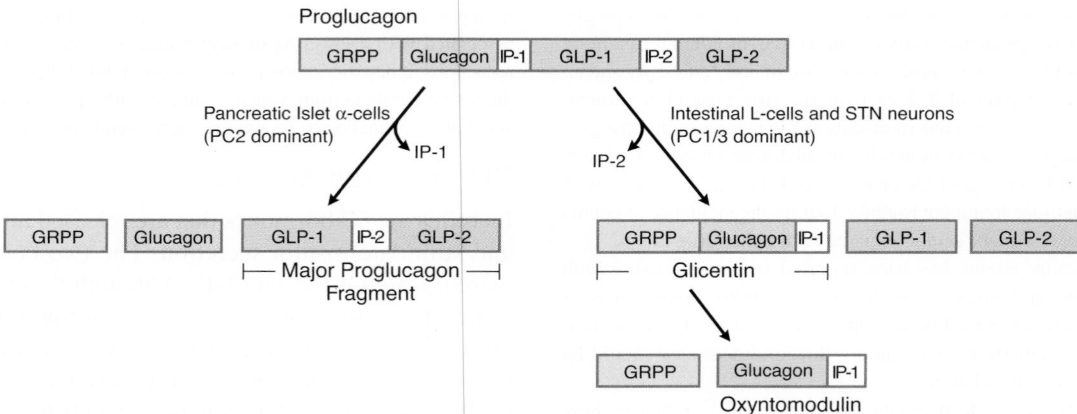

Figure 43–9. *Processing of proglucagon to glucagon, GLP1. GLP-2, and GRPP.* Proglucagon is synthesized in islet α cells, intestinal enteroendocrine cells (L cells) and a subset of neurons in the hindbrain. In α cells, prohormone processing is primarily by proconvertase 2, releasing glucagon, glicentin-related pancreatic polypeptide (GRPP), and a major proglucagon fragment, containing the two glucagon-like peptides (GLPs). In L cells and neurons, proglucagon cleavage is mostly through proconvertase 1/3, giving the larger C-terminal peptides, glicentin and oxyntomodulin, and the smaller GLP-1 and GLP-2. STN, solitary tract nucleus.

treatment diabetic patients in the U.S. and several others in advanced phases of development. Exendin-4 is a naturally occurring reptilian peptide of 39 amino acids with considerable homology to GLP-1. It is a potent GLP-1 receptor agonist that shares many of the physiological and pharmacological effects of GLP-1. It is not metabolized by DPP-4 and so has a plasma $t_{1/2}$ of 2-3 hours following subcutaneous injection. Importantly,

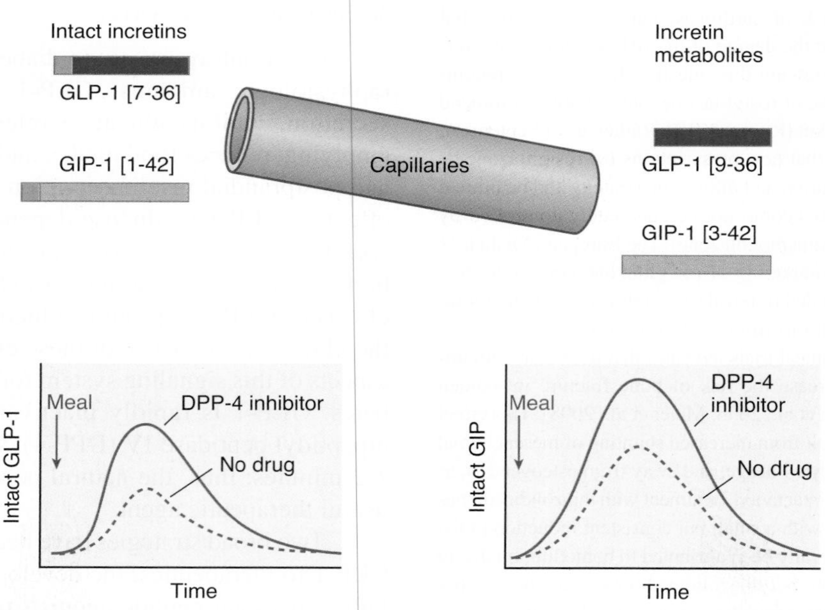

Figure 43–10. *Pharmacological effects of DDP-4 inhibition.* DPP-4, an ectoenzyme located on the luminal side of capillary endothelial cells metabolizes the incretins, glucagon-like peptide 1 (GLP-1). and glucose-dependent insulinotropic polypeptide (GIP), by removing the two N-terminal amino acids. The target for DPP-4 cleavage is a proline or alanine residue in the second position of the primary peptide sequence. The truncated metabolites GLP-1[9-36] and GIP[3-42] are the major forms of the incretins in plasma and are inactive as insulin secretagogues. Treatment with a DPP-4 inhibitor increases the concentrations of intact GLP-1 and GIP.

exendin-4 causes glucose-dependent insulin secretion, delayed gastric emptying, lower glucagon levels, and reduced food intake.

Exenatide (BYETTA), synthetic exendin-4, is approved for use as monotherapy and as adjunctive therapy for type 2 diabetes patients not achieving glycemic targets with metformin, sulfonylurea, the combination of metformin and sulfonylurea, or thiazolidinedione. In clinical trials, exenatide, alone or in combination with metformin, sulfonylurea, or thiazolidinedione, was associated with improved glycemic control, as reflected in an ~1% decrease in HbA1C, and weight loss that averaged 2.5-4 kg (Amori et al., 2007).

Liraglutide is a second GLP-1 receptor agonist. Structurally, liraglutide is nearly identical to native GLP-1, with Lys^{34} to Arg substitution and addition of a α-glutamic acid spacer coupled to a C16 fatty acyl group. The fatty acid side chain permits binding to albumin and other plasma proteins and accounts for an extended $t_{1/2}$ permitting once a day administration. The pharmacodynamic profile of liraglutide mimics GLP-1 and exenatide, and in clinical trials liraglutide caused both improvement in glycemic control and weight loss. In a single comparative trial, liraglutide reduced A1C~30% more than exenatide (Buse et al., 2009). Liraglutide is indicated for adjunctive therapy in patients not achieving glycemic control with metformin, sulfonylurea, or the combination of metformin/sulfonylurea or metformin/thiazolidinedione.

There are a number of other GLP-1 receptor agonists in development. A sustained-release form of exenatide, exenatide LAR, is being tested as a once-weekly injection. This compound is composed of exenatide in microspheres with the biodegradable polymer D,L lactic-co-glycolic acid. In phase 3 studies, exenatide LAR shares the pharmacodynamic properties of exenatide but may be more potent (Kim et al., 2007). Other long-acting GLP-1 receptor agonists in advanced stages of development include albiglutide, a recombinant protein fusion of GLP-1 and albumin; taspoglutide, a modified GLP-1; lixisenatide, a modified exendin-4 based molecule; and CJC-1134, an exendin-4/albumin conjugate. These agonists all have extended half-lives relative to exenatide and liraglutide and may be suitable for once-weekly injection. The distinguishing feature among the drugs currently available or under investigation is their pharmacokinetics and the exposure time to the GLP-1 receptor.

Mechanism of Action. All GLP-1 receptor agonists share a common mechanism, activation of the GLP-1 receptor. GLP-1 receptors are expressed by β cells, cells in the peripheral and central nervous system, the heart and vasculature, kidney, lung, and GI mucosa. Binding of agonists to the GLP-1 receptor activates the cAMP-PKA pathway and several GEFs (guanine nucleotide exchange factors) (Drucker, 2006). GLP-1 receptor activation also initiates signals through PKC and PI3K, and it alters the activity of several ion channels. In β cells, the end result of these actions is increased insulin biosynthesis and exocytosis in a glucose-dependent manner (Figure 43-3).

Absorption, Distribution, Metabolism, Excretion, and Dosing. Exenatide is given as a subcutaneous injection twice daily, typically before meals. Exenatide is rapidly absorbed, reaches peak concentrations in ~2 hours, undergoes little metabolism in the circulation, and has a volume of distribution of nearly 30 L. Clearance of the drug occurs primarily by glomerular filtration, with tubular proteolysis and minimal reabsorption. Exenatide is marketed as a pen that delivers 5 or 10 μg; dosing is typically started at the lower amount and increased as the response to therapy warrants.

Liraglutide is given as a subcutaneous injection once daily. Peak levels occur in 8-12 hours and the elimination $t_{1/2}$ is 12-14 hours. There is little renal or intestinal excretion of liraglutide, and clearance is primarily through the metabolic pathways of large plasma proteins. Liraglutide is supplied in a pen injector that delivers 0.6, 1.2, or 1.8 mg of drug; the low dose is for treatment initiation and generally advanced to the two higher doses based on clinical response.

Adverse Effects and Drug Interactions. The side effects of GLP-1 receptor agonists mimic the pharmacology of native GLP-1. Intravenous or subcutaneous administration of GLP-1 causes nausea and vomiting in a dose-dependent manner; the doses above which GLP-1 causes GI side effects are higher than those needed to regulate blood glucose. Despite this therapeutic window that minimizes adverse effects, nausea, vomiting, and other problems related to GI function are common with these drugs. Based on data from clinical trials, up to 40-50% of subjects given a GLP-1 receptor agonist report nausea at the initiation of therapy. Because the GI side effects of these drugs wane over time, most affected patients are able to continue a course of therapy. The activation of the GLP-1 receptor can delay gastric emptying; thus exenatide and other drugs of this class should be used with caution with other compounds that affect gastric emptying. Moreover, GLP-1 agonists may alter the pharmacokinetics of drugs that require rapid GI absorption, such as oral contraceptives and antibiotics.

In the absence of other diabetes drugs that cause low blood glucose, hypoglycemia associated with GLP-1 agonist treatment is rare. The combination of exenatide or liraglutide with sulfonylurea drugs causes an increased rate of hypoglycemia compared to sulfonylurea treatment alone. Because of the high degree of renal clearance, exenatide should not be given to persons with moderate to severe renal failure (creatinine clearance <30 mL/minute). There is no current recommendation for dose adjustments of other GLP-1 receptor agonists for decreased renal function. Exenatide has also been rarely associated with acute renal failure. Based on surveillance data, there is a possible association of exenatide treatment with pancreatitis, including fatal and nonfatal hemorrhagic or necrotizing pancreatitis. There is currently no mechanism to explain this association, and cases linking exenatide to pancreatitis are rare.

Mechanism of Action. DPP-4 is a serine protease that is widely distributed throughout the body, expressed as an ectoenzyme on endothelial cells, on the surface of T-lymphocytes, and in a circulating form. DPP-4 cleaves the two N-terminal amino acids from peptides with a proline or alanine in the second position. Although there are many potential substrates for this enzyme, it seems to be especially critical for the inactivation of GLP-1 and GIP (*glucose-dependent insulinotropic polypeptide; gastric inhibitory peptide*) (Drucker, 2007). DPP-4 inhibitors increase the AUC of GLP-1 and GIP when their secretion is by a meal (Figure 43-10).

Dosage Forms. Several agents provide nearly complete and long-lasting inhibition of DPP-4, thereby increasing the proportion of active GLP-1 from 10-20% of total circulating GLP-1 immunoreactivity to nearly 100%. Two of these, sitagliptin (JANUVIA) and saxagliptin (ONGLYZA), are now available in the U.S.; a third, vildagliptin, is available in the E.U.; a fourth compound, alogliptin, is in advanced stages of clinical trials. Sitagliptin and alogliptin are competitive inhibitors of DPP-4, whereas vildagliptin and saxagliptin bind the enzyme covalently. Despite these differences, all four drugs can be given in doses that lower measurable activity of DPP-4 by >95% for 12 hours. This causes a greater than 2-fold elevation of plasma concentrations of active GIP and GLP-1 and is associated with increased insulin secretion, reduced glucagon levels, and improvements in both fasting and postprandial hyperglycemia. Inhibition of DPP-4 does not appear to have direct effects on insulin sensitivity, gastric motility, or satiety, nor does chronic treatment with DPP-4 inhibitors affect body weight. DPP-4 inhibitors, used as monotherapy in type 2 diabetic patients, reduced HbA_{1c} levels by an average ~0.8%. These compounds are also effective for chronic glucose control when added to the treatment of diabetic patients receiving metformin, thiazolidinediones, sulfonylureas, and insulin. The effects of DPP-4 inhibitors in combination regimens appear to be additive. The recommended dose of sitagliptin is 100 mg once daily. The recommended dose of saxagliptin is 5 mg once daily.

Absorption, Distribution, Metabolism, and Excretion. DPP-4 inhibitors are absorbed effectively from the small intestine. They circulate in primarily in unbound form and are excreted mostly unchanged in the urine. DPP-4 inhibitors do not bind to albumin, nor do they affect the hepatic cytochrome oxidase system. Both sitagliptin and saxagliptin are excreted renally, and lower doses should be used in patients with reduced renal function. Sitagliptin has minimal metabolism by hepatic microsomal enzymes. Saxagliptin is metabolized by CYP 3A4/5 to an active metabolite. The dose saxagliptin should be lowered to 2.5 mg daily when co-administered with strong CYP3A4 inhibitors (e.g., ketoconazole, atazanavir, clarithromycin, indinavir, itraconazole, nefazodone, nelfinavir, ritonavir, saquinavir, and telithromycin).

Adverse Effects and Drug Interactions. There are no consistent adverse effects that have been noted in clinical trials with any of the DPP-4 inhibitors. With few exceptions the incidence of adverse effects in drug-treated and placebo-treated patients has been similar. DPP-4 is expressed on lymphocytes; in the immunology literature, the enzyme is referred to as CD26. Although there is some evidence of minor effects on *in vitro* lymphocyte function with DPP-4 inhibitors, there is no evidence from clinical studies of major adverse effects in humans. This area bears scrutiny as more patients are treated with these compounds.

OTHER HYPOGLYCEMIC AGENTS

Alpha Glucosidase Inhibitors

Mechanism of Action. α-Glucosidase inhibitors reduce intestinal absorption of starch, dextrin, and disaccharides by inhibiting the action of α-glucosidase in the intestinal brush border. Inhibition of this enzyme slows the absorption of carbohydrates from the GI tract and blunts the rate of rise of postprandial plasma glucose. These drugs also increase the release of the glucoregulatory hormone GLP-1 into the circulation, which may contribute to their glucose-lowering effects.

Dosage Forms. The drugs in this class are acarbose (PRECOSE, others), miglitol (GLYSET), and voglibose; only acarbose and miglitol are available in the U.S. Dosing of acarbose and miglitol are similar. Both are provided as 25, 50, or 100 mg tablets that are taken before meals. It is recommended that treatment start with lower doses and be titrated as indicated by balancing postprandial glucose, A1C, and GI symptoms. Acarbose and miglitol are most effective when given with a starchy, high-fiber diet with restricted amounts of glucose and sucrose.

Absorption, Distribution, Metabolism, Excretion, and Dosing. Acarbose is minimally absorbed and the small amount of drug reaching the systemic circulation is cleared by the kidney. Miglitol absorption is saturable, with 50-100% of any dose taken into the circulation. Miglitol is cleared almost entirely by the kidney, and dose reductions are recommended for patients with creatinine clearance <30 mL/minute.

Adverse Effects and Drug Interactions. The most prominent adverse effects related to α-glucosidase inhibitors are malabsorption, flatulence, diarrhea, and abdominal bloating. These side effects are dose dependent and related to the mechanism of action of the drugs, with greater amounts of carbohydrate available in the lower intestinal tract for metabolism by bacteria. Mild to moderate elevations of hepatic transaminases have been reported with acarbose, but symptomatic liver disease is very rare. Cutaneous hypersensitivity has been described but is also rare. α-Glucosidase inhibitors do not stimulate insulin release and therefore do not result in hypoglycemia when given alone. Hypoglycemia has been described when α-glucosidase inhibitors are added to insulin or an insulin secretagogue. For hypoglycemia in the setting of α-glucosidase use, glucose rather than sucrose or more complex carbohydrates should be used for treatment. Acarbose can decrease the absorption of digoxin and miglitol can decrease the absorption of propranolol and ranitidine. Alpha glucosidase inhibitors are contraindicated in patients with stage 4 renal failure.

Parenteral						
Insulin	↑ Glucose utilization, ↓ Hepatic glucose production, and other anabolic actions	See text and Table 43-5	Not limited	Known safety profile	Injection, weight gain, hypoglycemia	
GLP-1 agonists[c]	↑ Insulin, ↓ Glucagon, slow gastric emptying, satiety	Exenatide, liraglutide	0.5-1.0	Weight loss	Injection, nausea, ↑ risk of hypoglycemia with insulin secretagogues, pancreatitis	Renal disease, agents that also slow GI motility, pancreatitis
Amylin agonists[b,c]	Slow gastric emptying, ↓ Glucagon	Pramlintide	0.25-0.5	Reduce postprandial glycemia; weight loss	Injection, nausea, ↑ risk of hypoglycemia with insulin	Agents that also slow GI motility
Medical nutrition therapy and physical activity[c]	↓ Insulin, resistance, ↑ insulin secretion	Low-calorie, low-fat diet, exercise	1-3	Other health benefits	Compliance difficult, long-term success low	

[a]A1C reduction (absolute) depends partly on starting A1C value.
[b]Used in conjunction with insulin for treatment of type 1 diabetes
[c]Used for treatment of type 2 diabetes
Adapted with permission from *Harrison's Principles of Internal Medicine*, 17e (Fauci AS, Braunwald E, Kasper DL, Hauser SL, Longo DL, Jameson JL, Loscalzo J, eds.) New York: McGraw-Hill, 2008.

system that prevents acute hypoglycemia, a hazardous and potentially lethal situation. The two major clinical scenarios for hypoglycemia are:

- treatment of diabetes
- inappropriate production of endogenous insulin or an insulin-like substance by a pancreatic islet tumor (insulinoma) or a non-islet tumor

Hypoglycemia in the first scenario can occur either in the fasting or fed state, whereas in the second scenario, hypoglycemia occurs almost exclusively in the fasting or postabsorptive state. Some drugs not used for the treatment of diabetes promote hypoglycemia (Table 43–3; Murad et al., 2009). After a brief discussion of the physiological responses to hypoglycemia, agents used to treat hypoglycemia are discussed.

The most common and serious adverse event related to diabetes therapy is hypoglycemia. Although an adverse reaction to a number of oral therapies, it is most pronounced and serious with insulin therapy. Hypoglycemia may result from an inappropriately large dose, from a mismatch between the time of peak delivery of insulin and food intake, or from superimposition of additional factors that increase sensitivity to insulin (e.g., adrenal or pituitary insufficiency) or that increase insulin-independent glucose uptake (e.g., exercise). The more vigorous the attempt to achieve euglycemia, the more frequent are the episodes of hypoglycemia (Cryer, 2008; Heller, 2008). In the Diabetes Control and Complications Trial, the incidence of severe hypoglycemic reactions was three times higher in the intensive insulin therapy group than in the conventional therapy group. Milder but significant hypoglycemic episodes were much more common than were severe reactions, and their frequency also increased with intensive therapy. Hypoglycemia is the major risk that always must be weighed against benefits of efforts to normalize glucose control.

There is a hierarchy of physiological responses to hypoglycemia. The first response is a reduction of endogenous insulin secretion, which occurs at a plasma glucose level of ~70 mg/dL (3.9 mM); thereafter, the counter-regulatory hormones—epinephrine, glucagon, growth hormone, cortisol, and norepinephrine—are released. Symptoms of hypoglycemia are first discerned at a plasma glucose level of 60-80 mg/dL (3.3-4.4 mM). Sweating, hunger, paresthesias, palpitations, tremor, and anxiety, principally of autonomic origin, usually are seen first. Difficulty in concentrating, confusion, weakness, drowsiness, a feeling of warmth, dizziness, blurred vision, and loss of consciousness (i.e., most importantneuroglycopenic symptoms) usually occur at lower plasma glucose levels than do autonomic symptoms.

Glucagon and epinephrine are the most important counter-regulatory hormones in acute hypoglycemia in newly diagnosed diabetes patients and normal subjects. In patients with type 1 and type 2 diabetes of longer duration, the glucagon secretory response to hypoglycemia becomes deficient, but effective glucose counter-regulation still occurs because epinephrine plays a compensatory role. Diabetic patients thus become dependent on epinephrine for counter-regulation, and if this mechanism becomes deficient, the incidence of severe hypoglycemia increases. This occurs in patients with diabetes of long duration who may also have autonomic neuropathy. The absence of both glucagon and epinephrine can lead to prolonged hypoglycemia, particularly during the night, when some individuals can have extremely low plasma glucose levels for several hours. Severe hypoglycemia can lead to convulsions and coma. In addition to autonomic neuropathy, several related syndromes of defective counter-regulation contribute to the increased incidence of severe hypoglycemia in intensively treated type 1 diabetes patients. These include hypoglycemic unawareness, altered thresholds for release of counter-regulatory hormones, and deficient secretion of counter-regulatory hormones. With the ready availability of home glucose monitoring, hypoglycemia can be documented in most patients who experience suggestive symptoms. Hypoglycemia that occurs during sleep may be difficult to detect but should be suspected from a history of morning headaches, night sweats, or symptoms of hypothermia.

All diabetic patients who receive insulin or oral agents that can cause hypoglycemia should be aware of the symptoms of hypoglycemia, carry some form of easily ingested glucose, and carry an identification card or bracelet containing pertinent medical information. When possible, patients who suspect that they are experiencing hypoglycemia should document the glucose concentration with a measurement. Mild-to-moderate hypoglycemia may be treated simply by ingestion of glucose (15 g of carbohydrate). When hypoglycemia is severe, it should be treated with intravenous glucose or an injection of glucagon (Figure 43–10).

Agents Used to Treat Hypoglycemia

Glucagon is a single-chain polypeptide of 29 amino acids and is produced by recombinant DNA technology. Glucagon interacts with a GPCR on the plasma membrane of target cells that signals through G_s. The primary effects of glucagon on the liver are mediated by cAMP. Glucagon is used to treat severe hypoglycemia, particularly in diabetic patients when the patient cannot safely consume oral glucose and intravenous glucose is not available (Figure 43–12). For hypoglycemic reactions, 1 mg is administered intravenously, intramuscularly, or subcutaneously, usually by the patient's family member, who must be trained to administer this.

The intramuscular route is preferred in such an emergency. The hyperglycemic action of glucagon is transient and may be inadequate if hepatic stores of glycogen are depleted. After the initial response to glucagon, patients should be given glucose or urged to eat to prevent recurrent hypoglycemia. Glucagon also is sometimes used to relax the intestinal tract to facilitate radiographic examination of the upper and lower gastrointestinal tract with barium and retrograde ileography and in magnetic resonance imaging of the gastrointestinal tract. Nausea and vomiting are the most frequent adverse effects.

Diazoxide (PROGLYCEM) is an antihypertensive, antidiuretic benzothiadiazine derivative with potent hyperglycemic actions when given orally. Hyperglycemia

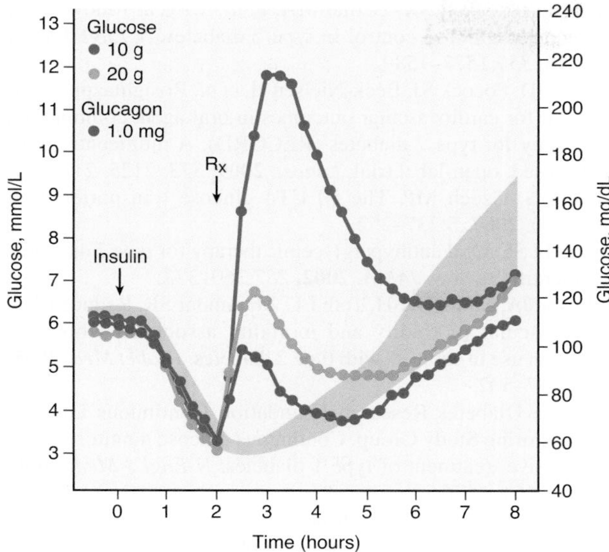

Figure 43–12. *Treatment of hypoglycemia with glucose or glucagon.* The blood glucose falls following administration of insulin (at time = 0). Following administration of oral glucose (10 or 20 g) or subcutaneous glucagon (at arrow marked "R_x"), the blood glucose rises. The blue band shows the recovery when glucose or glucagon was not administered. (Copyright 1993 American Diabetes Association. From Wiethop and Cryer. *Diabetes Care*, Vol. 16, 1993; 1131–1136. Reprinted with permission from The American Diabetes Association.)

results primarily from inhibition of insulin secretion. Diazoxide interacts with the K_{ATP} channel on the β cell membrane and either prevents its closing or prolongs the open time; this effect is opposite to that of the sulfonylureas (Figure 43–3). Diazoxide has been used to treat patients with various forms of chronic or recurring hypoglycemia.

The usual oral dose is 3-8 mg/kg per day in adults and children and 8 to 15 mg/kg per day in infants and neonates. The drug can cause nausea and vomiting and thus usually is given in divided doses with meals. Diazoxide circulates largely bound to plasma proteins and has a $t_{1/2}$ of ~48 hours. Thus the patient should be maintained at the chosen dosage for several days before evaluating the therapeutic result. Diazoxide has a number of adverse effects, including retention of Na^+ and fluid, hyperuricemia, hypertrichosis (especially in children), thrombocytopenia, and leucopenia, which sometimes limit its use. Despite these side effects, the drug may be useful in patients with inoperable insulinomas and in children with neonatal hyperinsulinism (leucine sensitivity, islet cell hyperplasia, nesidioblastosis, extrapancreatic malignancy, or islet cell adenoma).

OTHER PANCREATIC ISLET HORMONES

Somatostatin was identified as an inhibitor of GH secretion from the pituitary. Somatostatin (SST) is produced by δ cells of the pancreatic islet, cells of the GI tract, and in the CNS. Somatostatin, produced as a 14–amino acid or a 28–aminoacid peptide molecule, acts through a family of five GPCRs, $SSTR_{1-5.}$ SST inhibits a wide variety of endocrine and exocrine secretions, including TSH and GH from the pituitary, gastrin, motilin, VIP, glicentin, and insulin, glucagon, and pancreatic polypeptide from the pancreatic islet. The physiological role of somatostatin has not been defined precisely, but its short $t_{1/2}$ (3-6 minutes) prevents its use therapeutically. Longer-acting analogs such as octreotide (SANDOSTATIN) and lanreotide (SOMATULINE) are useful for treatment of carcinoid tumors, glucagonomas, VIPomas, and acromegaly (Chapter 38).

A depot form of octreotide or lanreotide can be administered intramuscularly every 4 weeks. Octreotide or lanreotide successfully controls excess secretion of growth hormone in most patients, and both have been reported to reduce the size of pituitary tumors in about one-third of cases. Octreotide has been used to treat severe hypoglycemia related to sulfonylurea ingestion (Cryer et al., 2009). Because octreotide also can decrease blood flow to the GI tract, it has been used to treat bleeding esophageal varices, peptic ulcers, and postprandial orthostatic hypotension. Gallbladder abnormalities (stones and biliary sludge) occur frequently with chronic use of the somatostatin analogs, as do GI symptoms. Hypoglycemia, hyperglycemia, hypothyroidism, and goiter have been reported in patients being treated with somatostatin analogs for acromegaly.

BIBLIOGRAPHY

Amori RE, Lau J, Pittas AG. Efficacy and safety of incretin therapy in type 2 diabetes: systematic review and meta-analysis. *JAMA,* **2007,** *298*:194–206.

Bailey CJ, Turner RC. Metformin. *N Engl J Med,* **1996,** *334*: 574–579.

Bell DSH. Do sulfonylurea drugs increase the risk of cardiac events? *CMAJ,* **2006,** *174*:185–186.

Bliss M. Resurrections in Toronto: the emergence of insulin. *Horm Res,* **2005,** *64*(suppl 2):98–102.

Bretzel RG, Nuber U, Landgraf W, *et al.* Once-daily basal insulin glargine versus thrice-daily prandial insulin lispro in people with type 2 diabetes on oral hypoglycaemic agents (APOLLO): an open randomised controlled trial. *Lancet,* **2008,** *371*: 1073–1084.

Brunzell JD, Davidson M, Furberg CD, *et al.* Lipoprotein management in patients with cardiometabolic risk. *Diabetes Care,* **2008,** *31*:811–822.

Buse JB, Rosenstock J, Sesti G, *et al.* Liraglutide once a day versus exenatide twice a day for type 2 diabetes: A 26-week randomised, parallel-group, multinational, open-label trial (LEAD-6). *Lancet,* **2009,** *374*:39–47.

Butler AE, Janson J, Bonner-Weir S, *et al.* Beta-cell deficit and increased beta-cell apoptosis in humans with type 2 diabetes. *Diabetes,* **2003,** 52:102–110.

Chan JC, Malik V, Jia W, *et al.* Diabetes in Asia: Epidemiology, risk factors, and pathophysiology. *JAMA,* **2009,** 301: 2129–2140.

Concannon P, Rich SS, Nepom GT. Genetics of type 1A diabetes. *N Engl J Med,* **2009,** *360*:1646–1654.

Crandall JP, Knowler WC, Kahn SE, *et al.* The prevention of type 2 diabetes. *Nat Clin Pract Endocrinol Metab,* **2008,** *4*:382–393.

Cryer PE. Glucose hoemostasis and hypoglycemia. In: *Williams Textbook of Endocrinology* (Kronenberg HM, Melmed S, Polonsky KS, Larsen PR, eds.), Philadelphia, Saunders Elsevier, **2008.**

Cryer PE, Axelrod L, Grossman AB, *et al.* Evaluation and management of adult hypoglycemic disorders: An Endocrine Society Clinical Practice Guideline. *J Clin Endocrinol Metab,* **2009,** *94*:709–728.

Das SK, Elbein SC. The genetic basis of type 2 diabetes. *Cellscience,* **2006,** *2*:100–131.

DeFronzo RA, Goodman AM. The Multicenter Metformin Study Group. Efficacy of metformin in patients with non-insulin-dependent diabetes mellitus. *N Engl J Med,* **1995,** *333*: 541–549.

Diabetes Control Complications Trial Research Group. The effect of intensive treatment of diabetes on the development and progression of long-term complications in insulin-dependent diabetes mellitus. *N Engl J Med,* **1993,** *329*:977–986.

Donner TW, Flammer KM. Diabetes management in the hospital. *Med Clin North Am,* **2008,** *92*:407–425, ix–x.

Doria A, Patti ME, Kahn CR. The emerging genetic architecture of type 2 diabetes. *Cell Metab,* **2008,** *8*:186–200.

Dormandy JA, Charbonnel B, Eckland DJ, *et al.* Secondary prevention of macrovascular events in patients with type 2 diabetes in the Proactive Study (Prospective Pioglitazone Clinical Trial in Macrovascular Events): A randomised controlled trial. *Lancet,* **2005,** *366*:1279–1289.

Drucker DJ. The biology of incretin hormones. *Cell Metab,* **2006,** *3*:153–165.

Drucker DJ. Dipeptidyl peptidase-4 inhibition and the treatment of type 2 diabetes: Preclinical biology and mechanisms of action. *Diabetes Care,* **2007,** *30*:1335–1343.

Duckworth W, Abraira C, Moritz T, *et al.* Glucose control and vascular complications in veterans with type 2 diabetes. *N Engl J Med,* **2009,** *360*:129–139.

Evans JM, Ogston SA, Emslie-Smith A, Morris AD. Risk of mortality and adverse cardiovascular outcomes in type 2 diabetes: A comparison of patients treated with sulfonylureas and metformin. *Diabetologia,* **2006,** *49*:930–936.

Falciglia M. Causes and consequences of hyperglycemia in critical illness. *Curr Opin Clin Nutr Metab Care,* **2007,** *10*:498–503.

Finfer S, Chittock DR, Su SY, *et al.* Intensive versus conventional glucose control in critically ill patients. *N Engl J Med,* **2009,** *360*:1283–1297.

Gerstein HC, Yusuf S, Bosch J, *et al.* Effect of rosiglitazone on the frequency of diabetes in patients with impaired glucose tolerance or impaired fasting glucose: A randomised controlled trial. *Lancet,* **2006,** *368*:1096–10105.

Grant RW, Moore AF, Florez JC. Genetic architecture of type 2 diabetes: Recent progress and clinical implications. *Diabetes Care,* **2009,** *32*:1107–1114.

Heller SR. Minimizing hypoglycemia while maintaining glycemic control in diabetes. *Diabetes,* **2008,** *57*: 3177–3183.

Herrington WG, Levy JB. Metformin: Effective and safe in renal disease? *Int Urol Nephrol,* **2008,** *40*:411–417.

Holman RR, Paul SK, Bethel MA, *et al.* 10-year follow-up of intensive glucose control in type 2 diabetes. *N Engl J Med,* **2008,** *359*:1577–1589.

Home PD, Pocock SJ, Beck-Nielsen H, *et al.* Rosiglitazone evaluated for cardiovascular outcomes in oral agent combination therapy for type 2 diabetes (RECORD): A multicentre, randomised, open-label trial. *Lancet,* **2009,** *373*: 2125–2135.

Huang S, Czech MP. The GLUT4 glucose transporter. *Cell Metab,* **2007,** 5:237–252.

Inzucchi SE. Oral antihyperglycemic therapy for type 2 diabetes: Scientific review. *JAMA,* **2002,** *287*:360–372.

Johnson JA, Simpson SH, Toth EL, Majumdar SR. Reduced cardiovascular morbidity and mortality associated with metformin use in subjects with type 2 diabetes. *Diabet Med,* **2005,** *22*:497–502.

Juvenile Diabetes Research Foundation Continuous Glucose Monitoring Study Group. Continuous glucose monitoring and intensive treatment of type 1 diabetes. *N Engl J Med,* **2008,** *359*:1464–1476.

Kahn SE. The relative contributions of insulin resistance and beta-cell dysfunction to the pathophysiology of type 2 diabetes. *Diabetologia,* **2003,** *46*:3–19.

Kahn SE, Haffner SM, Heise MA, *et al.* Glycemic durability of rosiglitazone, metformin, or glyburide monotherapy. *N Engl J Med,* **2006,** *355*:2427–2443.

Kamber N, Davis WA, Bruce DG, Davis TM. Metformin and lactic acidosis in an Australian community setting: The Fremantle Diabetes Study. *Med J Aust,* **2008,** *188*:446–449.

Kashi MR, Torres DM, Harrison SA. Current and emerging therapies in nonalcoholic fatty liver disease. *Semin Liver Dis,* **2008,** *28*:396–406.

Kim D, MacConell L, Zhuang D, *et al.* Effects of once-weekly dosing of a long-acting release formulation of exenatide on glucose control and body weight in subjects with type 2 diabetes. *Diabetes Care,* **2007,** *30*:1487–1493.

Kitabchi AE, Umpierrez GE, Miles, JM, Fisher JN. Hyperglycemic crises in adult patients with diabetes. *Diabetes Care,* **2009,** *32*:1335–1343.

Kodl CT, Seaquist ER. Cognitive dysfunction and diabetes mellitus. *Endocr Rev,* **2008,** *29*:494–511.

Lalau JD, Race JM. Lactic acidosis in metformin therapy: Searching for a link with metformin in reports of 'metformin-associated lactic acidosis.' *Diabetes Obes Metab,* **2001,** *3*:195–201.

Lasserson DS, Glasziou P, Perera R, *et al.* Optimal insulin regimens in type 2 diabetes mellitus: Systematic review and meta-analyses. *Diabetologia,* **2009,** *52*:1990–2000.

Meier C, Kraenzlin ME, Bodmer M, *et al.* Use of thiazolidinediones and fracture risk. *Arch Intern Med,* **2008,** *168*: 820–825.

Moghissi ES, Korytkowski MT, DiNardo M, *et al.* American Association of Clinical Endocrinologists and American Diabetes Association Consensus Statement on Inpatient Glycemic Control. *Diabetes Care,* **2009,** *32*:1119–1131.

Monami M, Lamanna C, Marchionni N, Mannucci E. Comparison of different drugs as add-on treatments to metformin in type 2 diabetes: A meta-analysis. *Diabetes Res Clin Pract,* **2008,** *79*:196–203.

Murad MH, Coto-Yglesias F, Wang AT, *et al.* Clinical review: Drug-induced hypoglycemia; a systematic review. *J Clin Endocrinol Metab,* **2009,** *94*:741–745.

Murphy R, Ellard S, Hattersley AT. Clinical implications of a molecular genetic classification of monogenic beta-cell diabetes. *Nat Clin Pract Endocrinol Metab,* **2008,** *4*:200–213.

Nathan DM, Buse JB, Davidson MB, *et al.* Medical management of hyperglycemia in type 2 diabetes: A consensus algorithm for the initiation and adjustment of therapy; a consensus statement of the American Diabetes Association and the European Association for the Study of Diabetes. *Diabetes Care,* **2009,** *32*:193–203.

Nesto RW, Bell D, Bonow RO, *et al.* Thiazolidinedione use, fluid retention, and congestive heart failure: A consensus statement from the American Heart Association and American Diabetes Association. *Circulation,* **2003,** *108*: 2941–2948.

Pocock SJ, Smeeth L. Insulin glargine and malignancy: an unwarranted alarm. *Lancet,* **2009,** *374*:511–513.

Rosen CJ, Revisiting the Rosiglitazone story—Lessons Learned. *N Engl J Med,* **2010**, *363*:803-806.

Rosenstock J, Hassman DR, Madder RD, *et al.* Repaglinide versus nateglinide monotherapy. *Diabetes Care,* **2004,** *27*:1265–1270.

Ryan EH Jr, Han DP, Ramsay RC, *et al.* Diabetic macular edema associated with glitazone use. *Retina,* **2006,** *26*:562–570.

Savage DB, Petersen KF, Shulman GI. Disordered lipid metabolism and the pathogenesis of insulin resistance. *Physiol Rev,* **2007,** *87*:507–520.

Scarpello JH, Howlett HC. Metformin therapy and clinical uses. *Diab Vasc Dis Res,* **2008,** *5*:157–167.

Shaw RJ, Lamia KA, Vasquez D, *et al.* The kinase LKB1 mediates glucose homeostasis in liver and therapeutic effects of metformin. *Science,* **2005,** *310*:1642–1646.

Sjostrom L, Lindroos A-K, Peltonen M, *et al.* Lifestyle, diabetes, and cardiovascular risk factors 10 years after bariatric surgery. *N Engl J Med,* **2004,** *351*:2683–2693.

JS Skyler, Therapy for Diabetes Mellitus and Related Disorders., Alexandria, VA: American Diabetes Association, **2004**.

Skyler JS, Bergenstal R, Bonow RO, *et al.* Intensive glycemic control and the prevention of cardiovascular events: Implications of the ACCORD, ADVANCE, and VA Diabetes Trials; a position statement of the American Diabetes Association and a Scientific Statement of the American College of Cardiology Foundation and the American Heart Association. *J Am Coll Cardiol,* **2009,** *53*:298–304.

Smith U, Gale EA. Does diabetes therapy influence the risk of cancer? *Diabetologia,* **2009,** *52*:1699–1708.

Sonnett TE, Levien TL, Neumiller, JJ, *et al.* Colesevelam hydrochloride for the treatment of type 2 diabetes mellitus. *Clin Ther,* **2009,** *31*:245–259.

Taniguchi CM, Emanuelli B, Kahn CR. Critical nodes in signalling pathways: insights into insulin action. *Nat Rev Mol Cell Biol,* **2006,** *7*:85–96.

Taylor R. Pathogenesis of type 2 diabetes: Tracing the reverse route from cure to cause. *Diabetologia,* **2008,** *51*:1781–1789.

van den Berghe G, Wouters P, Weekers F, *et al.* Intensive insulin therapy in the critically ill patients. *N Engl J Med,* **2001,** *345*:1359–1367.

Vaxillaire M, Froguel P. Monogenic diabetes in the young, pharmacogenetics and relevance to multifactorial forms of type 2 diabetes. *Endocr Rev,* **2008,** *29*:254–264.

von Herrath M, Sanda S, Herold K. Type 1 diabetes as a relapsing-remitting disease? *Nat Rev Immunol,* **2007,** *7*:988–994.

Weinstein D, Simon M, Yehezkel E, *et al.* Insulin analogues display IGF-I-like mitogenic and anti-apoptotic activities in cultured cancer cells. *Diabetes Metab Res Rev,* **2009,** *25*:41–49.

Weithop BV, Cryer PE. Glycemic actions of alanine and terbutaline in IDDM. *Diabetes Care,* **1993,** *16*:1124–1130.

Weng J, Li Y, Xu W, *et al.* Effect of intensive insulin therapy on beta-cell function and glycaemic control in patients with newly diagnosed type 2 diabetes: A multicentre randomised parallel-group trial. *Lancet,* **2008,** *371*:1753–1760.

Yki-Jarvinen H. Thiazolidinediones. *N Engl J Med,* **2004,** *351*:1106–1118.

Zaid H, Antonescu CN, Randhawa VK, Klip A. Insulin action on glucose transporters through molecular switches, tracks and tethers. *Biochem J,* **2008,** *413*:201–215.

Zhou G, Myers R, Li Y, *et al.* Role of AMP-activated protein kinase in mechanism of metformin action. *J Clin Invest,* **2001,** *108*:1167–1174.

Murray P, Chune GW, Raghavan VA. Clinical implications of a molecular structural classification of monogenic forms of diabetes. *Nat Clin Pract Endocrinol Metab.* 2008;4:200–213.
Nathan DM, Buse JB, Davidson MB, et al. Medical management of hyperglycemia in type 2 diabetes: a consensus algorithm for the initiation and adjustment of therapy: a consensus statement of the American Diabetes Association and the European Association for the Study of Diabetes. *Diabetes Care.* 2009; 32(1):193–203.
Nesto RW, Bell D, Bonow RO, et al. Thiazolidinedione use, fluid retention, and congestive heart failure: A consensus statement from the American Heart Association and American Diabetes Association. *Circulation.* 2003;108:2941–2948.
Pocock SJ, Smeeth L. Insulin glargine and malignancy: an unwarranted alarm. *Lancet.* 2009;374:511–513.
Rosen CJ. Revisiting the Rosiglitazone story—Lessons Learned. *N Engl J Med.* 2010;363:803–806.
Rosenstock J, Hassman DR, Madder RD, et al. Repaglinide versus nateglinide monotherapy. *Diabetes Care.* 2004; 27:1265–1270.
Ryan KB Jr, Han DP, Ramsay RC, et al. Diabetic macular edema associated with glitazone use. *Retina.* 2006;26:562–570.
Savage DB, Petersen KF, Shulman GI. Disordered lipid metabolism and the pathogenesis of insulin resistance. *Physiol Rev.* 2007;87:507–520.
Scarpello JH, Howlett HC. Metformin therapy and clinical uses. *Diab Vasc Dis Res.* 2008;5:157–167.
Shaw RJ, Lamia KA, Vasquez D, et al. The kinase LKB1 mediates glucose homeostasis in liver and therapeutic effects of metformin. *Science.* 2005;310:1642–1646.
Sjöström L, Lindroos A-K, Peltonen M, et al. Lifestyle, diabetes and cardiovascular risk factors 10 years after bariatric surgery. *N Engl J Med.* 2004;351:2683–2693.
JS Skyler. *Therapy for Diabetes Mellitus and Related Disorders.* Alexandria, VA: American Diabetes Association; 2004.
Skyler JS, Bergenstal R, Bonow RO, et al. Intensive glycemic control and the prevention of cardiovascular events: implications of the ACCORD, ADVANCE, and VA Diabetes Trials: a position statement of the American Diabetes Association and a Scientific Statement of the American College of Cardiology Foundation and the American Heart Association. *J Am Coll Cardiol.* 2009;53:298–304.
Smith U, Gale EA. Does diabetes therapy influence the risk of cancer? *Diabetologia.* 2009;52:1699–1708.
Sorensen TB, Lewis CP, Vermillion N, et al. Cadaveric donor islet transplantation for people with type 1 diabetes mellitus. *Curr Diab Rep.* 2009;9:...
Tamborlane CM, Kamath...S, Kahn CR. Critical nodes in signalling pathways: insights into insulin action. *Nat Rev Mol Cell Biol.* 2006;7:85–96.
Taylor SI. Pathogenesis of type 2 diabetes: Tracing the reverse route from cure to cause. *Diabetologia.* 2008;51:1781–1789.
van den Berghe G, Wouters P, Weekers F, et al. Intensive insulin therapy in the critically ill patients. *N Engl J Med.* 2001; 345:1359–1367.
Vasilakou V, Fraser F. Monogenic diabetes in the young: ... consequences and ... in maturity-onset forms of type ... diabetes. *Endocr Rev.* 2008;29:254–264.
von Herrath M, Sanda S, Herold K. Type 1 diabetes as a relapsing-remitting disease? *Nat Rev Immunol.* 2007;7:988–994.
Weinstein D, Simon M, Yehezkel E, et al. Insulin analogues display IGF-I-like mitogenic and anti-apoptotic activities in cultured cancer cells. *Diabetes Metab Res Rev.* 2009;25:41–49.
Weiner RV, Lyon PR. Metabolic actions of amylin and leptin in (IDDM). *Diabetes Care.* 1993;16:1234–1238.
Weng J, Li Y, Xu W, et al. Effect of intensive insulin therapy on beta-cell function and glycaemic control in patients with newly diagnosed type 2 diabetes: A multicentre randomised parallel-group trial. *Lancet.* 2008;371:1753–1760.
Von Herrath M. Immunomodulation. *N Engl J Med.* 2004; 350:1084–1086.
Zaid H, Antonescu CN, Randhawa VK, Klip A. Insulin action on glucose transporters through molecular switches, tracks and tethers. *Biochem J.* 2008;413:201–215.
Zhou G, Myers R, Li Y, et al. Role of AMP-activated protein kinase in mechanism of metformin action. *J Clin Invest.* 2001; 108:1167–1174.

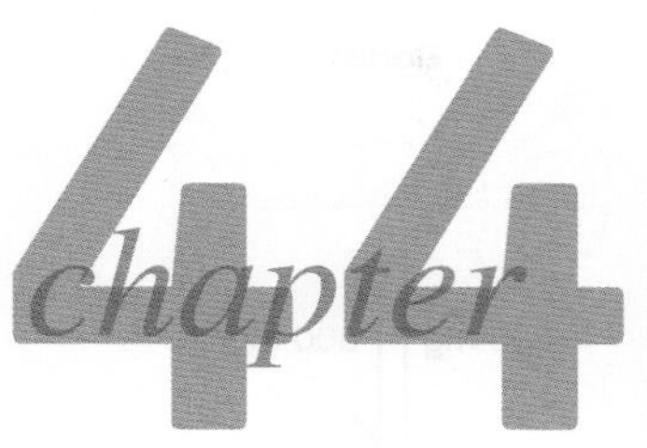

Agents Affecting Mineral Ion Homeostasis and Bone Turnover

Peter A. Friedman

To understand why, when, and how to employ pharmacological agents that affect mineral ion homeostasis, one must first understand some basic physiology and pathophysiology of the subject. This chapter presents a primer on mineral ion homeostasis and the endocrinology of Ca^{2+} and phosphate metabolism, then some relevant pathophysiology, and, finally, pharmacotherapeutic options in treating disorders of mineral ion homeostasis.

PHYSIOLOGY OF MINERAL ION HOMEOSTASIS

Calcium

Elemental calcium is essential for a variety of micromolecular and macroscopic biological functions. Its ionized form, Ca^{2+}, is an important component of current flow across excitable membranes. Ca^{2+} is vital for muscle contraction, fusion, and release of storage vesicles. In the submicromolar range, intracellular Ca^{2+} acts as a critical second messenger (Chapter 3). In extracellular fluid, millimolar concentrations of calcium promote blood coagulation and support the formation and continuous remodeling of the skeleton.

Ca^{2+} has an adaptable coordination sphere that facilitates binding to the irregular geometry of proteins. The capacity of an ion to cross-link two proteins requires a high coordination number, which dictates the number of electron pairs that can be formed and generally is six to eight for Ca^{2+}. Unlike disulfide or sugar–peptide cross-links, Ca^{2+} linking is readily reversible. Cross-linking of structural proteins in bone matrix is enhanced by the relatively high extracellular concentration of calcium.

In the face of millimolar extracellular Ca^{2+}, intracellular free Ca^{2+} is maintained at a low level, ~100 nM in cells in their basal state, by active extrusion by Ca^{2+}–ATPases and by Na^+/Ca^{2+} exchange. As a consequence, changes in cytosolic Ca^{2+} (whether released from intracellular stores or entering via membrane Ca^{2+} channels) can modulate effector targets, often by interacting with the Ca^{2+}-binding protein calmodulin. The rapid association–dissociation kinetics of Ca^{2+} and the relatively high affinity and selectivity of Ca^{2+}-binding domains permit effective regulation of Ca^{2+} over the 100 nM to 1 μM range.

The body content of calcium in healthy adult men and women, respectively, is ~1300 and 1000 g, of which >99% is in bone and teeth. Ca^{2+} is the major extracellular divalent cation. Although the portion of calcium in extracellular fluids is small, this fraction is stringently regulated within narrow limits. In adult humans, the normal serum calcium concentration ranges from 8.5-10.4 mg/dL (4.25-5.2 mEq/L, 2.1-2.6 mM) and includes three distinct chemical forms of Ca^{2+}: ionized (50%), protein-bound (40%), and complexed (10%). Thus, whereas total plasma calcium concentration is ~2.54 mM, the concentration of ionized Ca^{2+} in human plasma is ~1.2 mM.

The various pools of calcium are illustrated schematically in Figure 44–1. Only diffusible calcium (i.e., ionized plus complexed) can cross cell membranes. Albumin accounts for some 90% of the serum calcium bound to plasma proteins. Smaller percentages are bound, albeit with greater affinity, to β-globulin, α_2-globulin, α_1-globulin, and γ-globulin. The remaining 10% of the serum calcium is complexed in ion pairs with small polyvalent anions, primarily phosphate and citrate. The degree of complex formation depends on the ambient pH and the concentrations of ionized calcium and complexing anions. Ionized Ca^{2+} is the physiologically relevant component, mediates calcium's biological effects, and, when perturbed, produces the characteristic signs and symptoms of hypo- or hypercalcemia.

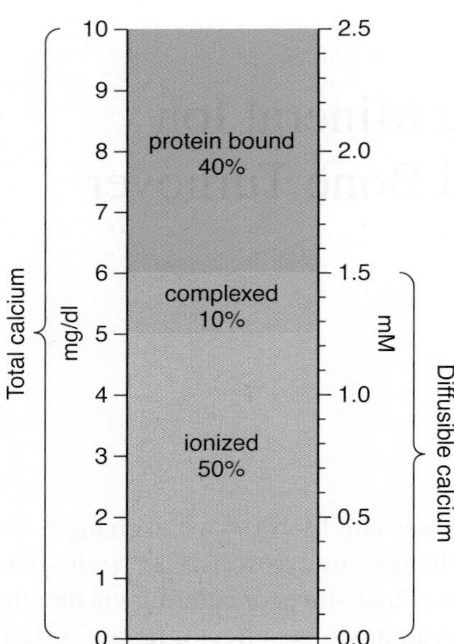

Figure 44–1. *Pools of calcium in serum.* Concentrations are expressed as mg/dL on the left-hand axis and as mM on the right. The total serum calcium concentration is 10 mg/dL or 2.5 mM, divided into three pools: protein-bound (40%), complexed with small anions (10%), and ionized calcium (50%). The complexed and ionized pools represent the diffusable forms of calcium.

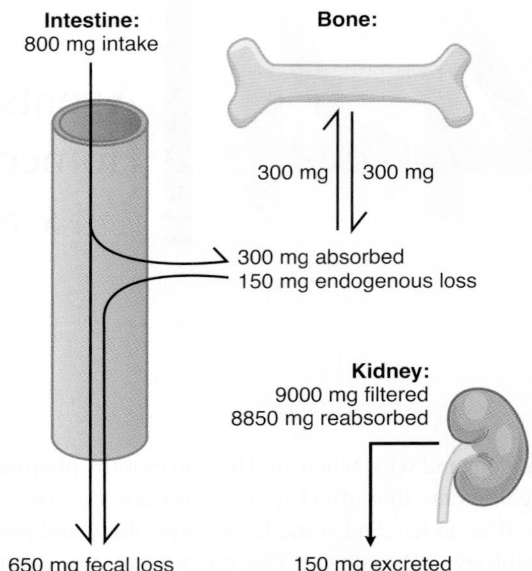

Figure 44–2. *Schematic representation of the whole body daily turnover of calcium.* (Adapted with permission from Yanagawa N, Lee DBN. Renal handling of calcium and phosphorus. In: *Disorders of Bone and Mineral Metabolism* (Coe FL, Favus MJ, eds.), Raven Press, New York, 1992, pp. 3–40.)

The total plasma calcium concentration can be interpreted only by correcting for the concentration of plasma proteins. A change of plasma albumin concentration of 1.0 g/dL from the normal value of 4.0 g/dL can be expected to alter total calcium concentration by ~0.8 mg/dL.

The extracellular Ca^{2+} concentration is tightly controlled by hormones that affect calcium entry at the intestine and its exit at the kidney; when needed, these same hormones regulate withdrawal from the large skeletal reservoir.

Calcium Stores. The skeleton contains 99% of total body calcium in a crystalline form resembling the mineral hydroxyapatite [$Ca_{10}(PO_4)_6(OH)_2$]; other ions, including Na^+, K^+, Mg^{2+}, and F^-, also are present in the crystal lattice. The steady-state content of calcium in bone reflects the net effect of bone resorption and bone formation, coupled with aspects of bone remodeling. In addition, a labile pool of bone Ca^{2+} exchanges readily with interstitial fluid. This exchange is modulated by hormones, vitamins, drugs, and other factors that directly alter bone turnover or that influence the Ca^{2+} level in interstitial fluid.

Calcium Absorption and Excretion. In the U.S., ~75% of dietary calcium is obtained from milk and dairy products. The adequate intake value for calcium is 1300 mg/day in adolescents and 1000 mg/day in adults. After age 50, the adequate intake is 1200 mg/day. This contrasts with median intakes of calcium for boys and girls ≥9 years of age of 865 and 625 mg, respectively, and a median daily calcium intake of 517 mg for women >50 years of age.

Figure 44–2 illustrates the components of whole-body daily calcium turnover. Ca^{2+} enters the body only through the intestine. *Active vitamin D–dependent transport* occurs in the proximal duodenum, whereas *facilitated diffusion* throughout the small intestine accounts for most total Ca^{2+} uptake. This uptake is counterbalanced by an obligatory daily intestinal calcium loss of ~150 mg/day that reflects the calcium content of mucosal and biliary secretions and in sloughed intestinal cells.

The efficiency of intestinal Ca^{2+} absorption is inversely related to calcium intake. Thus, a diet low in calcium leads to a compensatory increase in fractional absorption owing partly to activation of vitamin D. In older persons, this response is considerably less robust. Disease states associated with steatorrhea, diarrhea, or chronic malabsorption promote fecal loss of calcium, whereas drugs such as glucocorticoids and phenytoin depress intestinal Ca^{2+} transport.

Urinary Ca^{2+} excretion is the net difference between the quantity filtered at the glomerulus and the amount reabsorbed. About 9 g of Ca^{2+} are filtered each day. Tubular reabsorption is very efficient, with >98% of filtered Ca^{2+} returned to the circulation. The efficiency of reabsorption is highly regulated by parathyroid hormone (PTH) but also is influenced by filtered Na^+, the presence of nonreabsorbed anions, and diuretic agents (Chapter 25). Sodium intake, and therefore sodium excretion, is directly related to urinary calcium excretion. Diuretics that act on the ascending limb of the loop of Henle (e.g., furosemide) increase calcium excretion. By contrast, thiazide diuretics uncouple the relationship between Na^+ and Ca^{2+} excretion, increasing sodium excretion but diminishing calcium excretion (Friedman and Bushinsky, 1999). Urine Ca^{2+} excretion is a direct function of dietary protein intake, presumably owing to the effect of sulfur-containing amino acids on renal tubular function.

Phosphate

Phosphate is an essential component of all body tissues, present in plasma, extracellular fluid, cell membrane phospholipids, intracellular fluid, collagen, and bone tissue. More than 80% of total body phosphorus is found in bone, and ~15% is in soft tissue. Additionally, phosphate subserves roles as a dynamic constituent of intermediary and energy metabolism and as a key regulator of enzyme activity when transferred by protein kinases from ATP to phosphorylatable serine, threonine, and tyrosine residues.

Biologically, phosphorus (P) exists in both organic and inorganic (P_i) forms. Organic forms include phospholipids and various organic esters. In extracellular fluid, the bulk of phosphorus is present as inorganic phosphate in the form of NaH_2PO_4 and Na_2HPO_4; at pH 7.4, the ratio of disodium to monosodium phosphate is 4:1, so plasma phosphate has an intermediate valence of 1.8. Owing to its relatively low concentration in extracellular fluid, phosphate contributes little to buffering capacity. The aggregate level of inorganic phosphate (P_i) modifies tissue concentrations of Ca^{2+} and plays a major role in renal H^+ excretion. Within bone, phosphate is complexed with calcium as hydroxyapatites having the general formula $Ca_{10}(PO_4)_6(OH)_2$ and as calcium phosphate.

Absorption, Distribution, and Excretion. Phosphate is absorbed from and, to a limited extent, secreted into the GI tract. Phosphate is a ubiquitous component of ordinary foods; thus even an inadequate diet rarely causes phosphate depletion. Transport of phosphate from the intestinal lumen is an active, energy-dependent process that is regulated by several factors, primarily vitamin D, which stimulates absorption. In adults, about two-thirds of ingested phosphate is absorbed and is excreted almost entirely into the urine. In growing children, phosphate balance is positive, and plasma concentrations of phosphate are higher than in adults.

Phosphate excretion in the urine represents the difference between the amount filtered and that reabsorbed. More than 90% of plasma phosphate is freely filtered at the glomerulus, and 80% is actively reabsorbed, predominantly in the initial segment of the proximal convoluted tubule but also in the proximal straight tubule (pars recta). Renal phosphate absorption is regulated by a variety of hormones and other factors; the most important are PTH and dietary phosphate, with extracellular volume and acid–base status playing lesser roles. Dietary phosphate deficiency upregulates renal phosphate transporters and decreases excretion, whereas a high-phosphate diet increases phosphate excretion; these changes are independent of any effect on plasma P_i, Ca^{2+}, or PTH. PTH increases urinary phosphate excretion by blocking phosphate absorption. Expansion of plasma volume increases urinary phosphate excretion. Effects of vitamin D and its metabolites on proximal tubular phosphate are modest at best.

Role of Phosphate in Urine Acidification. Despite the fact that the concentration and buffering capacity of phosphate in extracellular fluid are low, phosphate is concentrated progressively in the renal tubule and becomes the most abundant buffer system in the distal tubule and terminal nephron. The exchange of H^+ and Na^+ in the tubular urine converts disodium hydrogen phosphate (Na_2HPO_4) to sodium dihydrogen phosphate (NaH_2PO_4), permitting the excretion of large amounts of acid without lowering the urine pH to a degree that would block H^+ transport.

Actions of Phosphate. If large amounts of phosphate are introduced into the GI tract by oral administration or enema, a cathartic action will result. Thus, phosphate salts are employed as mild laxatives (Chapter 46). If excessive phosphate salts are introduced either intravenously or orally, they may reduce the concentration of Ca^{2+} in the circulation and induce precipitation of calcium phosphate in soft tissues.

HORMONAL REGULATION OF CALCIUM AND PHOSPHATE HOMEOSTASIS

A number of hormones interact to regulate extracellular calcium and phosphate balance. The most important are parathyroid hormone (PTH) and 1,25-dihydroxyvitamin D (calcitriol), which regulate mineral homeostasis by effects on the kidney, intestine, and bone (Figure 44–3).

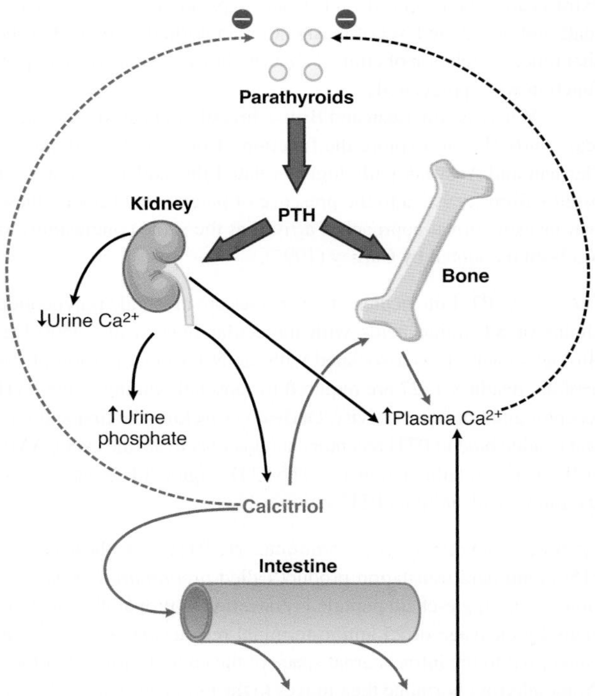

Figure 44–3. *Calcium homeostasis and its regulation by parathyroid hormone (PTH) and 1,25-dihydroxyvitamin D.* PTH has stimulatory effects on bone and kidney, including the stimulation of 1α-hydroxylase activity in kidney mitochondria leading to the increased production of 1,25-dihydroxyvitamin D (calcitriol) from 25-hydroxycholecalciferol, the monohydroxylated vitamin D metabolite (Figure 44–6). Calcitriol is the biologically active metabolite of vitamin D.

Parathyroid Hormone

Parathyroid hormone (PTH) is a polypeptide hormone that helps to regulate plasma Ca^{2+} by affecting bone resorption/formation, renal Ca^{2+} excretion/reabsorption, and calcitriol synthesis (thus GI Ca^{2+} absorption).

History. Sir Richard Owen, the curator of the British Museum of Natural History, discovered the parathyroid glands in 1852 while dissecting a rhinoceros that had died in the London Zoo. Credit for discovery of the human parathyroid glands usually is given to Sandstrom, a Swedish medical student who published an anatomical report in 1890. In 1891, von Recklinghausen reported a new bone disease, which he termed "osteitis fibrosa cystica," which Askanazy subsequently described in a patient with a parathyroid tumor in 1904. The glands were rediscovered a decade later by Gley, who determined the effects of their extirpation with the thyroid. Vassale and Generali then successfully removed only the parathyroids and noted that tetany, convulsions, and death quickly followed unless calcium was given postoperatively.

MacCallum and Voegtlin first noted the effect of parathyroidectomy on plasma Ca^{2+}. The relation of low plasma Ca^{2+} concentration to symptoms was quickly appreciated, and a comprehensive picture of parathyroid function began to form. Active glandular extracts alleviated hypocalcemic tetany in parathyroidectomized animals and raised the level of plasma Ca^{2+} in normal animals. For the first time, the relation of clinical abnormalities to parathyroid hyperfunction was appreciated.

Whereas American and British investigators used physiological approaches to explore the function of the parathyroid glands, German and Austrian pathologists related the skeletal changes of osteitis fibrosa cystica to the presence of parathyroid tumors; these two investigational approaches arrived at the same conclusions, as has been recounted by Carney (1997).

Chemistry. PTH molecules of all species are all single polypeptide chains of 84 amino acids with molecular masses of ~9500 Da. Biological activity is associated with the N-terminal portion of the peptide; residues 1–27 are required for optimal binding to the PTH receptor and hormone activity. Derivatives lacking the first and second residue bind to PTH receptors but do not activate the cyclic AMP or IP_3–Ca^{2+} signaling pathways. The PTH fragment lacking the first six amino acids inhibits PTH action.

Synthesis, Secretion, and Immunoassay. PTH is synthesized as a 115-amino-acid translation product called *preproparathyroid hormone.* This single-chain peptide is converted to proparathyroid hormone by cleavage of 25 amino-terminal residues as the peptide is transferred to the intracisternal space of the endoplasmic reticulum. Proparathyroid hormone then moves to the Golgi complex, where it is converted to PTH by cleavage of six amino acids. PTH(1-84) resides within secretory granules until it is discharged into the circulation. Neither preproparathyroid hormone nor proparathyroid hormone appears in plasma. The synthesis and processing of PTH have been reviewed (Jüppner et al., 2001).

A major proteolytic product of PTH is PTH(7–84). PTH(7–84) and other amino-truncated PTH fragments accumulate significantly during renal failure in part because they are normally cleared from the circulation predominantly by the kidneys, whereas intact PTH is also removed by extrarenal mechanisms. Rather than competing with PTH(1–84) binding at the receptor, PTH(7–84) may cause the PTH receptor to internalize from the plasma membrane in a cell-specific manner (Sneddon et al., 2003).

During periods of hypocalcemia, more PTH is secreted and less is hydrolyzed. In this setting, PTH(7–84) release is augmented. In prolonged hypocalcemia, PTH synthesis also increases, and the gland hypertrophies.

PTH(1–84) has a $t_{1/2}$ in plasma of ~4 minutes; removal by the liver and kidney accounts for ~90% of its clearance. Proteolysis of PTH (in the storage granule and in plasma) generates smaller fragments (e.g., a 33–36 amino acid N-terminal fragment that is fully active, a larger C-terminal peptide, and PTH[7–84]). Much of what circulates in the blood and is measured by older RIAs is the inactive C-terminal fragment that has a longer $t_{1/2}$ than the active N-terminal fragment or the intact PTH(1–84). Second-generation enzyme-linked immunosorbent assays for PTH, by contrast, can distinguish among these forms, but the clinical value of such information and whether it should affect therapeutic intervention remains controversial (D'Amour, 2008; Herberth et al., 2009).

Physiological Functions. The primary function of PTH is to maintain a constant concentration of Ca^{2+} and P_i in the extracellular fluid. The principal processes regulated are renal Ca^{2+} and P_i absorption, and mobilization of bone Ca^{2+} (Figure 44–3). PTH also affects a variety of tissues not involved in mineral ion homeostasis that include cartilage, vascular smooth muscle, placenta, liver, pancreatic islets, brain, dermal fibroblasts, and lymphocytes. The actions of PTH on its target tissues are mediated by at least two receptors. The PTH_1 receptor (PTH1R or PTH/PTHrP receptor) also binds PTH-related protein (PTHrP); the PTH_2 receptor, found in vascular tissues, brain, pancreas, and placenta, binds only PTH. Both of these are GPCRs that can couple with G_s and G_q in cell-type specific manners; thus cells may show one, the other, or both types of responses. There is also evidence that PTH can activate phospholipase D through a $G_{12/13}$–RhoA pathway (Singh et al., 2005). A third receptor, designated the CPTH receptor, interacts with forms of PTH that are truncated in the amino-terminal region, contain most of the carboxy terminus, and are inactive at the PTH_1 receptor; these CPTH receptors reportedly are expressed on osteocytes (Selim et al., 2006).

Regulation of Secretion. Plasma Ca^{2+} is the major factor regulating PTH secretion. As the concentration of Ca^{2+} diminishes, PTH secretion increases. Sustained hypocalcemia induces parathyroid hypertrophy and hyperplasia. Conversely, if the concentration of Ca^{2+} is high, PTH secretion decreases. Studies of parathyroid cells in culture show that amino acid transport, nucleic acid and protein synthesis, cytoplasmic growth, and PTH secretion are all stimulated by low concentrations of Ca^{2+} and suppressed by high concentrations. Thus, Ca^{2+} itself appears to regulate parathyroid gland growth as well as hormone synthesis and secretion.

Changes in plasma Ca^{2+} regulate PTH secretion by the plasma membrane–associated calcium-sensing receptor (CaSR) on parathyroid cells. The CaSR is a GPCR that couples with G_q and G_i. Occupancy of the CaSR by Ca^{2+} thus stimulates the G_q-PLC-IP_3-Ca^{2+} pathway leading to activation of PKC; this results in inhibition of PTH secretion, an unusual case in which elevation of cellular Ca^{2+} inhibits secretion (another being the granular cells in the juxtaglomerular complex of the kidney, where elevation of cellular Ca^{2+}

inhibits renin secretion). Simultaneous activation of the G_i pathway by Ca^{2+} reduces cAMP synthesis and lowers the activity of PKA, also a negative signal for PTH secretion. Conversely, reduced occupancy of CaSR by Ca^{2+} reduces signaling through G_i and G_q, lessening inhibition of adenylyl cyclase and lowering activation of the G_q pathway, thereby promoting PTH secretion. Thus, the extracellular concentration of Ca^{2+} is controlled by a classical negative-feedback system, the afferent limb of which is sensitive to the ambient activity of Ca^{2+} and the efferent limb of which releases PTH. Acting via the CaSR, hypercalcemia reduces intracellular cyclic AMP content and activates PKC, whereas hypocalcemia does the reverse. The precise links between these changes and alterations in PTH secretion remain to be defined. Other agents that increase parathyroid cell cyclic AMP levels, such as β adrenergic receptor agonists and *dopamine,* also increase PTH secretion, but the magnitude of response is far less than that seen with hypocalcemia. The active vitamin D metabolite, 1,25-dihydroxyvitamin D (*calcitriol*), directly suppresses PTH gene expression. There appears to be no relation between physiological concentrations of extracellular phosphate and PTH secretion, except insofar as changes in phosphate concentration alter circulating Ca^{2+}. Severe hypermagnesemia or hypomagnesemia can inhibit PTH secretion.

Effects on Bone. PTH exerts both catabolic and anabolic effects on bone. Normally, these processes are tightly coupled. Chronically elevated PTH enhances bone resorption and thereby increases Ca^{2+} delivery to the extracellular fluid, whereas intermittent exposure to PTH promotes anabolic actions. The primary skeletal target cell for PTH is the osteoblast, although evidence points to the presence of functional PTH receptors on osteocytes (O'Brien et al., 2008). PTH also recruits osteoclast precursor cells to form new bone remodeling units. Sustained increases in circulating PTH cause characteristic histological changes in bone that include an increase in the prevalence of osteoclastic resorption sites and in the proportion of bone surface that is covered with unmineralized matrix (Martin and Ng, 1994).

Direct effects of PTH on osteoblasts *in vitro* generally are inhibitory and include reduced formation of type I collagen, alkaline phosphatase, and osteocalcin. However, the response to PTH *in vivo* reflects not only hormone action on individual cells but also the increased total number of active osteoblasts, owing to initiation of new remodeling units. Thus, plasma levels of osteocalcin and alkaline phosphatase activity actually may be increased. No simple model can fully explain the molecular basis of PTH effects on bone. PTH stimulates cyclic AMP production in osteoblasts, but there also is evidence that intracellular Ca^{2+} mediates some PTH actions.

Effects on Kidney. In the kidney, PTH enhances the efficiency of Ca^{2+} reabsorption, inhibits tubular reabsorption of phosphate, and stimulates conversion of vitamin D to its biologically active form, calcitriol (Figure 44–3). As a result, filtered Ca^{2+} is avidly retained, and its concentration increases in plasma, whereas phosphate is excreted, and its plasma concentration falls. Newly synthesized calcitriol interacts with specific high-affinity receptors in the intestine to increase the efficiency of intestinal Ca^{2+} absorption, thereby contributing to the increase in plasma (Ca^{2+}).

Calcium. PTH increases tubular reabsorption of Ca^{2+} with concomitant decreases in urinary Ca^{2+} excretion. The effect occurs at distal nephron sites. This action, along with mobilization of calcium from bone and increased absorption from the intestine, increases the concentration of Ca^{2+} in plasma. Eventually, the increased glomerular filtration of Ca^{2+} overwhelms the stimulatory effect of PTH on tubular reabsorption, and hypercalciuria ensues. Conversely, reduction of serum PTH depresses tubular reabsorption of Ca^{2+} and thereby increases urinary Ca^{2+} excretion. When the plasma Ca^{2+} concentration falls below 7 mg/dL (1.75 mM), Ca^{2+} excretion decreases as the filtered load of Ca^{2+} reaches the point where the cation is almost completely reabsorbed despite reduced tubular capacity.

Phosphate. PTH increases renal excretion of inorganic phosphate by decreasing its reabsorption by proximal tubules. This action is mediated by retrieval of the luminal membrane Na–P_i cotransport protein, NPT2a, rather than an effect on its activity. Patients with primary hyperparathyroidism therefore typically have low tubular phosphate reabsorption.

Cyclic AMP apparently mediates the renal effects of PTH on proximal tubular phosphate reabsorption. PTH-sensitive adenylyl cyclase is located in the renal cortex, and cyclic AMP synthesized in response to the hormone affects tubular transport mechanisms. A portion of the cyclic AMP synthesized at this site, so-called nephrogenous cyclic AMP, escapes into the urine. Measurement of urinary cyclic AMP is used as a surrogate for parathyroid activity and renal responsiveness.

Other Ions. PTH reduces renal Mg^{2+} excretion. This effect reflects the net result of enhanced renal Mg^{2+} reabsorption and increased mobilization of the ion from bone (Quamme, 2010). PTH increases excretion of water, amino acids, citrate, K^+, bicarbonate, Na^+, Cl^-, and SO_4^{2-}, whereas it decreases the excretion of H^+. These effects are minor and generally can be seen only under tightly controlled circumstances.

Calcitriol Synthesis. The final step in the activation of vitamin D to calcitriol occurs in kidney proximal tubule cells. Three primary regulators govern the enzymatic activity of the 25-hydroxyvitamin D_3-1α-hydroxylase that catalyzes this step: P_i, PTH, and Ca^{2+} (see later for further discussion). Reduced circulating or tissue phosphate content rapidly increases calcitriol production, whereas hyperphosphatemia or hypercalcemia suppresses it. PTH powerfully stimulates calcitriol synthesis. Thus, when hypocalcemia causes a rise in PTH concentration, both the PTH-dependent lowering of circulating P_i and a more direct effect of the hormone on the 1α-hydroxylase lead to increased circulating concentrations of calcitriol.

Integrated Regulation of Extracellular Ca^{2+} Concentration by PTH. Even modest reductions of serum Ca^{2+} stimulate PTH secretion. For minute-to-minute regulation of Ca^{2+}, adjustments in renal Ca^{2+} handling more than suffice to maintain plasma calcium homeostasis. With more prolonged hypocalcemia, the renal 1α-hydroxylase is induced, enhancing the synthesis and release of calcitriol that directly stimulates intestinal calcium absorption (Figure 44–3). In addition, delivery of calcium from bone into the extracellular fluid is augmented. In the face of prolonged and severe hypocalcemia, new bone remodeling units are activated to restore circulating Ca^{2+} concentrations, albeit at the expense of skeletal integrity.

When plasma Ca^{2+} activity rises, PTH secretion is suppressed, and tubular Ca^{2+} reabsorption decreases. The reduction in circulating PTH promotes renal phosphate conservation, and both the decreased PTH and the increased phosphate depress calcitriol production and thereby decrease intestinal Ca^{2+} absorption. Finally, bone remodeling is suppressed. These integrated physiological events ensure a coherent response to positive or negative excursions of plasma Ca^{2+} concentrations. In humans, the importance of other hormones, such as FGF23 and calcitonin, to this scheme remains unsettled. They may modulate the Ca^{2+}–parathyroid–vitamin D axis or, in the case of FGF23, serve as primary regulators (Razzaque, 2009).

Vitamin D

Vitamin D traditionally was viewed as a permissive factor in calcium metabolism because it was thought to permit efficient absorption of dietary calcium and to allow full expression of the actions of PTH. We know now that vitamin D exerts a more active role in calcium homeostasis. Vitamin D is actually a hormone rather than a vitamin; it is synthesized in mammals and, under ideal conditions, probably is not required in the diet. Receptors for the activated form of vitamin D are expressed in many cells that are not involved in calcium homeostasis, including hematopoietic cells, lymphocytes, epidermal cells, hair follicles, adipose tissue, pancreatic islets, muscle, and neurons.

History. Vitamin D is the name applied to two related fat-soluble substances, *cholecalciferol* (vitamin D_3) and *ergocalciferol* (vitamin D_2) (Figure 44–4), that share the capacity to prevent or cure rickets. Prior to the discovery of vitamin D, a high percentage of urban children living in temperate zones developed rickets. Some researchers believed that the disease was due to lack of fresh air and sunshine; others claimed a dietary factor was responsible. Mellanby and Huldschinsky showed both notions to be correct; addition of cod liver oil to the diet or exposure to sunlight prevented or cured the disease. In 1924, it was found that ultraviolet irradiation of animal rations was as efficacious at curing rickets as was irradiation of the animal itself. These observations led to the elucidation of the structures of chole- and ergocalciferol and eventually to the discovery that these compounds require further processing in the body to become active. The discovery of metabolic activation is attributable primarily to studies conducted in the laboratories of DeLuca and Kodicek (DeLuca, 1988). The biological actions of vitamin D are mediated by the vitamin D receptor (VDR), a nuclear receptor, that was cloned in 1987 (McDonnell et al., 1987).

Chemistry and Occurrence. Ultraviolet irradiation of several animal and plant sterols results in their conversion to compounds possessing vitamin D activity. The principal provitamin found in animal tissues is 7-dehydrocholesterol, which is synthesized in the skin. Exposure of the skin to sunlight converts 7-dehydrocholesterol to cholecalciferol (vitamin D_3) (Figure 44–4). Ergosterol, which is present only in plants and fungi, is the provitamin for vitamin D_2 (ergocalciferol). Ergosterol and vitamin D_2 differ from 7-dehydrocholesterol and vitamin D_3, respectively, by the presence of a double bond between C22 and C23 and a methyl group at C24. Vitamin D_2 is the active constituent of a number of commercial vitamin preparations and is in irradiated bread and irradiated milk. In humans there is no practical difference between the antirachitic potencies of vitamin D_2 and vitamin D_3. Therefore, "vitamin D" is used here as a collective term for vitamins D_2 and D_3.

Human Requirements and Units. Although sunlight provides adequate vitamin D supplies in the equatorial belt, in temperate climates insufficient cutaneous solar radiation especially in winter may necessitate dietary vitamin D supplementation. It was assumed that vitamin D deficiency had been eliminated as a significant medical problem in the U.S. However, upward adjustment of estimates of normal vitamin D levels, improved analytical methodology, and more comprehensive data collection have led to an appreciation of the common finding of low circulating levels of vitamin D and a re-emergence of vitamin D–dependent rickets. Potential factors contributing to the rise of vitamin D deficiency include diminished consumption of vitamin D–fortified foods owing to concerns about fat intake; reduced intake of calcium-rich foods, including milk, in adolescents and young women of reproductive age; increased use of sunscreens and decreased exposure to sunlight to reduce the risk of skin cancer and prevent premature aging from exposure to ultraviolet radiation; and an increased prevalence and duration of exclusive breast-feeding (the combination of human milk, a poor source of vitamin D, and the high prevalence of low circulating vitamin D levels in U.S. women, particularly African-American mothers) (Bodnar et al., 2007).

There is no consensus regarding optimal vitamin D intake, and determination of vitamin D requirements is remarkably unsupported by clinical measurements. The recommended dietary allowance of vitamin D for infants and children is 400 IU, or 10 μg, daily. The basis for this dose was that it approximates that in a teaspoon (5 mL) of cod liver oil, which had long been considered safe and effective in preventing rickets (Vieth, 1999). Because adults require less vitamin D than infants, the adult dose was set arbitrarily at 200 IU.

The Food and Nutrition Board of the Institute of Medicine has developed Dietary Reference Intakes (DRI) for vitamins (Institute of Medicine, 2003). In both premature and normal infants, intake of 200 units per day of vitamin D from any source is considered adequate for optimal growth. Recently, the American Academy of Pediatrics recommended an intake of 400 IU of vitamin D per day from infants through adolescence (Wagner and Greer, 2008). Beyond adolescence, this amount probably may be sufficient, although nutritionists now recommend high daily intake, up to 4000 IU/day (Bischoff-Ferrari et al., 2009). There is some evidence that vitamin D requirements increase during pregnancy and lactation (Hollis and Wagner, 2004), where vitamin D doses of <1000 IU/day may be inadequate to maintain normal circulating 25-hydroxyvitamin D concentrations. Doses of $\leq 10{,}000$ IU/day of vitamin D for up to 5 months do not elevate circulating 25-hydroxyvitamin D to concentrations >90 ng/mL.

Absorption, Fate, and Excretion. Vitamins D_2 and D_3 are absorbed from the small intestine, although vitamin D_3 may be absorbed more efficiently. Most of the vitamin appears first within chylomicrons in lymph. Bile is essential for adequate absorption of vitamin D; deoxycholic acid is the major constituent of bile in this regard (Chapter 46). The primary route of vitamin D_3 excretion is the bile; with a smaller percentage found in the urine. Patients who have intestinal bypass surgery or otherwise have severe shortening or inflammation of the small intestine may fail to absorb vitamin D sufficiently to maintain normal levels; hepatic or biliary dysfunction also may seriously impair vitamin D absorption.

Absorbed vitamin D circulates in the blood in association with vitamin D–binding protein, a specific α-globulin. The vitamin

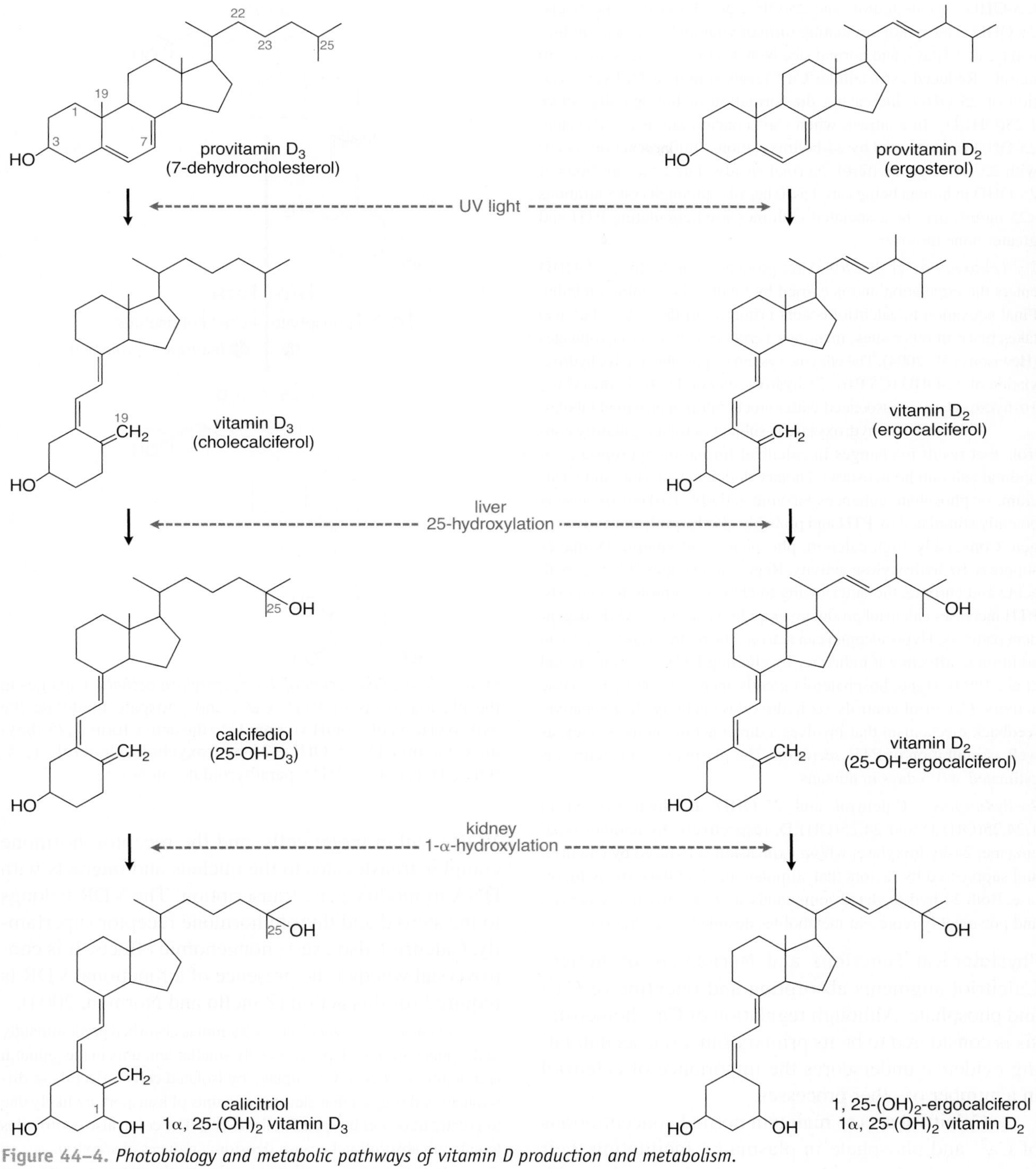

provitamin D_3 (7-dehydrocholesterol)

provitamin D_2 (ergosterol)

UV light

vitamin D_3 (cholecalciferol)

vitamin D_2 (ergocalciferol)

liver 25-hydroxylation

calcifediol (25-OH-D_3)

vitamin D_2 (25-OH-ergocalciferol)

kidney 1-α-hydroxylation

calicitriol 1α, 25-$(OH)_2$ vitamin D_3

1, 25-$(OH)_2$-ergocalciferol 1α, 25-$(OH)_2$ vitamin D_2

Figure 44–4. *Photobiology and metabolic pathways of vitamin D production and metabolism.*

disappears from plasma with a $t_{1/2}$ of 20–30 hours but is stored in fat depots for prolonged periods.

Metabolic Activation. Whether derived from diet or endogenously synthesized, vitamin D requires modification to become biologically active. The primary active metabolite of the vitamin is calcitriol [1α,25-dihydroxyvitamin D, 1,25$(OH)_2$D], the product of two successive hydroxylations of vitamin D (Figure 44–4).

25-Hydroxylation of Vitamin D. The initial step in vitamin D activation occurs in the liver, where cholecalciferol and ergocalciferol are hydroxylated in the 25-position to generate 25-OH-cholecalciferol

(25-OHD, or calcifediol) and 25-OH-ergocalciferol, respectively. 25-OHD is the major circulating form of vitamin D_3; it has a biological $t_{1/2}$ of 19 days, and normal steady-state concentrations are 15-50 ng/mL. Reduced extracellular Ca^{2+} levels stimulate 1α-hydroxylation of 25-OHD, increasing the formation of biologically active $1,25(OH)_2D_3$. In contrast, when Ca^{2+} concentrations are elevated, 25-OHD is inactivated by 24-hydroxylation. Similar reactions occur with 25-OH-ergocalciferol. Normal steady-state concentrations of 25-OHD in human beings are 15-50 ng/mL, although concentrations <25 ng/mL may be associated with increased circulating PTH and greater bone turnover.

1α-Hydroxylation of 25-OHD. After production in the liver, 25-OHD enters the circulation and is carried by vitamin D–binding globulin. Final activation to calcitriol occurs primarily in the kidney but also takes place in other sites, including keratinocytes and macrophages (Hewison et al., 2004). The enzyme system responsible for 1α-hydroxylation of 25-OHD (CYP1α, 25-hydroxyvitamin D_3-1α-hydroxylase, 1α-hydroxylase) is associated with mitochondria in proximal tubules.

Vitamin D 1α-hydroxylase is subject to tight regulatory controls that result in changes in calcitriol formation appropriate for optimal calcium homeostasis. Dietary deficiency of vitamin D, calcium, or phosphate enhances enzyme activity. 1α-Hydroxylase is potently stimulated by PTH and probably also by prolactin and estrogen. Conversely, high calcium, phosphate, and vitamin D intakes suppress 1α-hydroxylase activity. Regulation (Figure 44–5) is both acute and chronic, the latter owing to changes in protein synthesis. PTH increases calcitriol production rapidly via a cyclic AMP–dependent pathway. Hypocalcemia can activate the hydroxylase directly in addition to affecting it indirectly by eliciting PTH secretion (Bland et al., 1999). Hypophosphatemia greatly increases 1α-hydroxylase activity. Calcitriol controls 1α-hydroxylase activity by a negative-feedback mechanism that involves a direct action on the kidney, as well as inhibition of PTH secretion. The plasma $t_{1/2}$ of calcitriol is estimated at 3-5 days in humans.

24-Hydroxylase. Calcitriol and 25-OHD are hydroxylated to $1,24,25(OH)_2D$ and $24,25(OH)_2D$, respectively, by another renal enzyme, 24-hydroxylase, whose expression is induced by calcitriol and suppressed by factors that stimulate the 25-OHD-1α-hydroxylase. Both 24-hydroxylated compounds are less active than calcitriol and presumably represent metabolites destined for excretion.

Physiological Functions and Mechanism of Action. Calcitriol augments absorption and retention of Ca^{2+} and phosphate. Although regulation of Ca^{2+} homeostasis is considered to be its primary function, accumulating evidence underscores the importance of calcitriol in a number of other processes.

Calcitriol acts to maintain normal concentrations of Ca^{2+} and phosphate in plasma by facilitating their absorption in the small intestine, by interacting with PTH to enhance their mobilization from bone, and by decreasing their renal excretion. It also exerts direct physiological and pharmacological effects on bone mineralization (Suda et al., 2003).

The mechanism of action of calcitriol is mediated by its interaction with VDR. Calcitriol binds to cytosolic

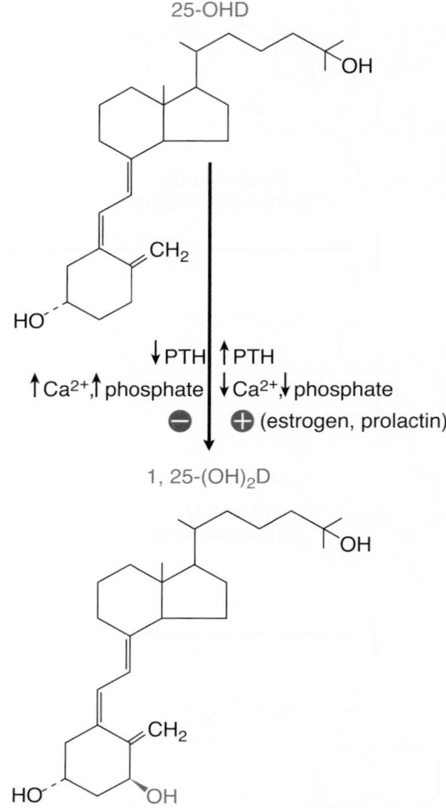

Figure 44–5. *Regulation of 1α-hydroxylase activity.* Changes in the plasma levels of PTH, Ca^{2+}, and phospate modulate the hydroxylation of 25-OH vitamin D to the active form, 1,25-dihydroxyvitamin D. 25-OHD, 25-hydroxycholecalciferol; 1,25-$(OH)_2$-D, calcitriol; PTH, parathyroid hormone.

VDRs within target cells, and the receptor–hormone complex translocates to the nucleus and interacts with DNA to modify gene transcription. The VDR belongs to the steroid and thyroid hormone receptor superfamily. Calcitriol also exerts nongenomic effects. It is controversial whether the presence of a functional VDR is required for this action (Zanello and Norman, 2004).

Intestinal Absorption of Calcium. Calcium is absorbed predominantly in the duodenum, with progressively smaller amounts in the jejunum and ileum. Studies of Ca^{2+} uptake by isolated cells reflect these differences and suggest that elevated amounts of transport are likely due to greater transport by each duodenal cell. The colon also contributes to calcium absorption because ileostomy reduces absorption.

In the absence of calcitriol, calcium absorption is inefficient and proceeds in a thermodynamically passive manner through the lateral intercellular spaces (paracellular pathway). Calcitriol increases the transcellular movement of Ca^{2+} from the mucosal to the serosal surface of the duodenum. Transcellular Ca^{2+} movement involves three processes: Ca^{2+} entry across the mucosal surface, diffusion through the cell, and energy-dependent extrusion across the serosal cell membrane. Calcium is also secreted from serosal to mucosal compartments. Thus, net calcium absorption is the difference between the two oppositely oriented vectorial processes. The complex mechanisms and the proteins mediating calcium absorption are still incompletely understood (Perez et al., 2008). Evidence implicates TRPV6 Ca^{2+} channels in mediating mucosal calcium entry in the intestine (Bianco et al., 2007). In humans, TRPV6 is expressed in the duodenum and proximal jejunum. A calcium-poor diet upregulates intestinal TRPV6 expression in mice (Van Cromphaut et al., 2001). This effect is greatly reduced in VDR knockout mice, suggesting that TRPV6 mediates calcium entry and is vitamin D dependent.

Ca^{2+} absorption is potently augmented by calcitriol. It is likely that calcitriol enhances all three steps involved in intestinal Ca^{2+} absorption: entry across mucosal brush border membranes, diffusion through the enterocytes, and active extrusion across serosal plasma membranes. Calcitriol upregulates the synthesis of calbindin-D_{9K} and calbindin-D_{28K} and the serosal plasma membrane Ca–ATPase. Calbindin-D_{9K} enhances the extrusion of Ca^{2+} by the Ca–ATPase, whereas the precise function of calbindin-D_{28K} is unsettled.

Mobilization of Bone Mineral. Although vitamin D–deficient animals show obvious deficits in bone mineral, there is little evidence that calcitriol directly promotes mineralization. Thus, even though VDR knockout mice exhibit severely impaired bone formation and mineralization, these deficiencies can be entirely corrected by a high-calcium diet. These results support the view that the primary role of calcitriol is to stimulate intestinal absorption of calcium, which, in turn, indirectly promotes bone mineralization. Indeed, children with rickets caused by mutations of the VDR have been treated successfully with intravenous infusions of Ca^{2+} and phosphate. In contrast, physiological doses of vitamin D promote mobilization of Ca^{2+} from bone, and large doses cause excessive bone turnover. Although calcitriol-induced bone resorption may be reduced in parathyroidectomized animals, the response is restored when hyperphosphatemia is corrected. Thus, PTH and calcitriol act independently to enhance bone resorption.

Calcitriol increases bone turnover by multiple mechanisms (Suda et al., 2003). Mature osteoclasts apparently lack the VDR. Acting by a non-VDR mechanism, calcitriol promotes the recruitment of osteoclast precursor cells to resorption sites, as well as the development of differentiated functions that characterize mature osteoclasts.

Osteoblasts, the cells responsible for bone formation, express the VDR, and calcitriol induces their production of several proteins, including osteocalcin, a vitamin K–dependent protein that contains γ-carboxyglutamic acid residues, and interleukin-1 (IL-1), a lymphokine that promotes bone resorption (Spear et al., 1988). Thus the current view is that calcitriol is a bone-mobilizing hormone but not a bone-forming hormone. Osteoporosis is a disease in which osteoclast responsiveness to calcitriol or other bone-resorbing agents is profoundly impaired, leading to deficient bone resorption.

Renal Retention of Calcium and Phosphate. The effects of calcitriol on the renal handling of Ca^{2+} and phosphate are of uncertain importance. Calcitriol increases retention of Ca^{2+} independently of phosphate. The effect on Ca^{2+} is thought to proceed in distal tubules, whereas enhanced phosphate absorption occurs in proximal tubules.

Other Effects of Calcitriol. It now is evident that the effects of calcitriol extend well beyond calcium homeostasis. Receptors for calcitriol are distributed widely throughout the body (Pike and Shevde, 2005). Calcitriol affects maturation and differentiation of mononuclear cells and influences cytokine production and immune function (Nagpal et al., 2005). One focus of research is the potential use of calcitriol to inhibit proliferation and to induce differentiation of malignant cells (van den Bemd et al., 2000). The possibility of dissociating the hypercalcemic effect of calcitriol from its actions on cell differentiation has encouraged the search for analogs that might be useful in cancer therapy. Calcitriol inhibits epidermal proliferation and promotes epidermal differentiation and therefore is a potential treatment for psoriasis vulgaris (Kragballe and Iversen, 1993) (Chapter 65). Calcitriol also affects the function of skeletal muscle, brain (Carswell, 1997), and blood pressure (Nagpal et al., 2005).

Calcitonin

Calcitonin is a hypocalcemic hormone whose actions generally oppose those of PTH.

History and Source. Copp observed in 1962 that perfusion of canine parathyroid and thyroid glands with hypercalcemic blood caused a transient hypocalcemia that occurred significantly earlier than that caused by total parathyroidectomy. He concluded that the parathyroid glands secreted a calcium-lowering hormone (calcitonin) in response to hypercalcemia and in this way normalized plasma Ca^{2+} concentrations. The physiological relevance of calcitonin has been challenged vigorously: calcitonin normally circulates at remarkably low levels; surgical removal of the thyroids has no appreciable effect on calcium metabolism; and conditions associated with profound elevations of serum calcitonin concentration are not accompanied by hypocalcemia (Hirsch and Baruch, 2003). The primary interest in calcitonin arises from its pharmacological use in treating Paget's disease and hypercalcemia and in its diagnostic use as a tumor marker for medullary carcinoma of the thyroid.

The thyroid parafollicular C cells are the site of production and secretion of calcitonin. Human C cells, which are derived from neural crest ectoderm, are distributed widely in the thyroid, parathyroid, and thymus. In non-mammalian vertebrates, calcitonin is found in ultimobranchial bodies, which are separate organs from the thyroid gland.

The calcitonin gene is localized on human chromosome 11p and contains six exons (Figure 44–6). The primary transcript is alternatively spliced in a tissue-specific manner. In thyroid C cells, the calcitonin/calcitonin gene-related peptide (CGRP) pre-mRNA is processed primarily with common exons 2 and 3 to include exon 4. This leads to production of the 32-amino-acid peptide calcitonin, along with a flanking 21-amino-acid peptide called katacalcin, whose physiological significance is unknown. In neuronal cells, in contrast, most of the calcitonin/CGRP pre-mRNA, is processed to exclude exon 4, resulting in inclusion of exons 5 and 6 with common exons 2 and 3, which ultimately gives rise to CGRP. This results in the production of the 37-amino-acid CGRP. Calcitonin is the most potent peptide inhibitor of osteoclast-mediated bone resorption and helps to protect the skeleton during periods of "calcium stress," such as growth, pregnancy, and lactation. CGRP and the closely related peptide adrenomedullin are potent endogenous vasodilators.

Chemistry and Immunoreactivity. Calcitonin is a single-chain peptide of 32 amino acids with a disulfide bridge linking the cysteine residues in positions 1 and 7 (Figure 44–7). In all species, 8 of the

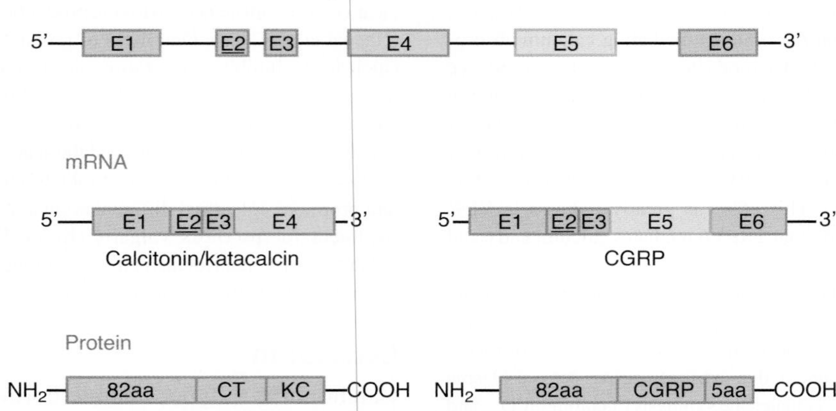

Figure 44–6. *Alternative splicing of calcitonin/calcitonin gene–related peptide (CGRP).*

32 residues are invariant, including the disulfide bridge and a carboxyl-terminal proline amide; both structural features are essential for biological activity. The residues in the middle portion of the molecule (positions 10–27) are more variable and apparently influence potency and/or duration of action. Calcitonins derived from salmon and eel differ from the human hormone by 13 and 16 amino acid residues, respectively, and are more potent than mammalian calcitonin. Salmon calcitonin is used therapeutically in part because it is cleared more slowly from the circulation.

Regulation of Secretion. The biosynthesis and secretion of calcitonin are regulated by the plasma Ca^{2+} concentration. Calcitonin secretion increases when plasma Ca^{2+} is high and decreases when plasma Ca^{2+} is low. Multiple forms of calcitonin are found in plasma, including high-molecular-weight aggregates or cross-linked products. Assays for the intact monomeric peptide are now available. The circulating concentrations of calcitonin are low, normally <15 and 10 pg/mL for males and females, respectively. The circulating $t_{1/2}$ of calcitonin is ~10 minutes. Abnormally elevated levels of calcitonin are characteristic of thyroid C-cell hyperplasia and medullary thyroid carcinoma.

Calcitonin secretion is stimulated by a number of agents, including catecholamines, glucagon, gastrin, and cholecystokinin, but there is little evidence for a physiological role for secretion in response to these stimuli.

Mechanism of Action. Calcitonin actions are mediated by the calcitonin receptor (CTR), which is a member of the PTH/secretin subfamily of GPCRs (Lin et al., 1991). Six human CTR subtypes occur through alternative splicing of coding and noncoding exons (Purdue et al., 2002). These isoforms exhibit distinct ligand-binding specificity and/or signal-transduction pathways and are distributed in a tissue-specific pattern. Of the more abundant isoforms, hCTRI1$^-$, which lacks a 16-amino acid insert in the first intracellular loop, preferentially couples with the G_s–adenylyl cyclase pathway (Gorn et al., 1995). The hCTRI1$^+$ isoform, which includes this casette, does not couple with PLC (Naro et al., 1998) and therefore does not activate PKC or trigger an increase in Ca^{2+}. Calcitonin receptors can dimerize with RAMPs (receptor-activity modifying proteins) to create receptors with high affinity for amylin (Hay et al., 2005) (Chapter 43).

The hypocalcemic and hypophosphatemic effects of calcitonin are caused predominantly by direct inhibition of osteoclastic bone resorption. Although calcitonin inhibits the effects of PTH on osteolysis, it inhibits neither PTH activation of bone cell adenylyl cyclase nor PTH-induced uptake of Ca^{2+} into bone. Calcitonin interacts directly with receptors on osteoclasts to produce a rapid and profound decrease in ruffled border surface area, thereby diminishing resorptive activity.

Depressed bone resorption reduces urinary excretion of Ca^{2+}, Mg^{2+}, and hydroxyproline. Plasma phosphate concentrations are lowered owing also to increased urinary phosphate excretion. Direct renal effects of calcitonin vary with species. Acute administration of pharmacological doses of calcitonin increases urinary calcium excretion, whereas calcitonin inhibits renal calcium excretion at physiological concentrations. In humans, calcitonin increases fractional urinary calcium excretion in a dose-dependent manner in subjects given a modest calcium load (Carney, 1997).

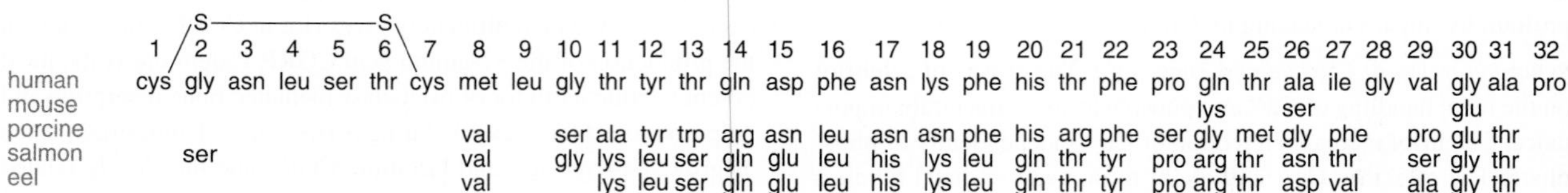

	1	2	3	4	5	6	7	8	9	10	11	12	13	14	15	16
human	cys	gly	asn	leu	ser	thr	cys	met	leu	gly	thr	tyr	thr	gln	asp	phe
mouse																
porcine								val		ser	ala	tyr	trp	arg	asn	leu
salmon		ser						val		gly	lys	leu	ser	gln	glu	leu
eel								val			lys	leu	ser	gln	glu	leu

	17	18	19	20	21	22	23	24	25	26	27	28	29	30	31	32
human	asn	lys	phe	his	thr	phe	pro	gln	thr	ala	ile	gly	val	gly	ala	pro
mouse								lys		ser				glu		
porcine	asn	asn	phe	his	arg	phe	ser	gly	met	gly	phe		pro	glu	thr	
salmon	his	lys	leu	gln	thr	tyr	pro	arg	thr	asn	thr		ser	gly	thr	
eel	his	lys	leu	gln	thr	tyr	pro	arg	thr	asp	val		ala	gly	thr	

Figure 44–7. *Comparison of calcitonins from several species.* Calcitonin is a 32-amino-acid polypeptide with a disulfide bond between residues 1 and 7 and a proline-amide at the C-terminus. The figure highlights the differences in amino acid sequence between human calcitonin and calcitonins of other species; lack of an entry indicates identity with human calcitonin. Salmon calcitonin is ~20 times more potent in humans than is human calcitonin.

The amount of vitamin D necessary to cause hypervitaminosis varies widely. As a rough approximation, continued daily ingestion of ≥50,000 units by a person with normal parathyroid function and sensitivity to vitamin D may result in poisoning. Hypervitaminosis D is particularly dangerous in patients who are receiving digoxin because the toxic effects of the cardiac glycosides are enhanced by hypercalcemia (Chapter 28).

The initial signs and symptoms of vitamin D toxicity are those associated with hypercalcemia. Because hypercalcemia in vitamin D intoxication generally is due to very high circulating levels of 25-OHD, the plasma concentrations of PTH and calcitriol typically (but not uniformly) are suppressed. In children, a single episode of moderately severe hypercalcemia may arrest growth completely for ≥6 months, and the deficit in height may never be fully corrected. Vitamin D toxicity in the fetus is associated with excess maternal vitamin D intake or extreme sensitivity and may result in congenital supravalvular aortic stenosis. In infants, this anomaly frequently is associated with other stigmata of hypercalcemia.

Vitamin D Deficiency. Vitamin D deficiency results in inadequate absorption of Ca^{2+} and phosphate. The consequent decrease of plasma Ca^{2+} concentration stimulates PTH secretion, which acts to restore plasma Ca^{2+} at the expense of bone. Plasma concentrations of phosphate remain subnormal because of the phosphaturic effect of increased circulating PTH. In children, the result is a failure to mineralize newly formed bone and cartilage matrix, causing the defect in growth known as *rickets*. As a consequence of inadequate calcification, bones of individuals with rickets are soft, and the stress of weight bearing gives rise to bowing of the long bones.

In adults, vitamin D deficiency results in osteomalacia, a disease characterized by generalized accumulation of undermineralized bone matrix. Severe osteomalacia may be associated with extreme bone pain and tenderness. Muscle weakness, particularly of large proximal muscles, is typical and may reflect both hypophosphatemia and inadequate vitamin D action on muscle. Gross deformity of bone occurs only in advanced stages of the disease. Circulating 25-OHD concentrations <8 ng/mL are highly predictive of osteomalacia.

Metabolic Rickets and Osteomalacia. These disorders are characterized by abnormalities in calcitriol synthesis or response.

Hypophosphatemic vitamin D–resistant rickets, in its most common form, is an X-linked disorder (XLH) of calcium and phosphate metabolism. Calcitriol levels are inappropriately normal for the observed degree of hypophosphatemia. Patients experience clinical improvement when treated with large doses of vitamin D, usually in combination with inorganic phosphate. Even with vitamin D treatment, calcitriol concentrations may remain lower than expected. The genetic basis for XLH has been defined. The affected protein, a phosphate-regulating gene with homologies to endopeptidases on the X chromosome (PHEX), is a neutral endoprotease. The substrate for this enzyme likely is involved in renal phosphate transport. Syndromes closely related to XLH, in which phosphate levels are altered without significant net changes in serum concentrations of calcium, PTH, or $1,25(OH)_2D_3$, include *hereditary hypophosphatemic rickets with hypercalciuria* (HHRH) and *autosomal dominant hypophosphatemic rickets.* The latter disorder maps to chromosome 12p13.3 and is associated with mutations in the gene encoding fibroblast growth factor 23 (White et al., 2001; Bergwitz and Jüppner, 2010).

Vitamin D–dependent rickets (also called *vitamin D–dependent rickets type I, VDDR-1* or *pseudovitamin D-deficiency rickets* (PDDR) is an autosomal recessive disease caused by an inborn error of vitamin D metabolism involving defective conversion of 25-OHD to calcitriol owing to mutations in CYP1α (1α-hydroxylase). The condition responds to physiological doses of calcitriol. An initial dose of 1-3 μg/day is used to heal rickets, after which a maintenance dose of 0.25-1 μg/day can be used. 1αOHD is also effective as slightly higher dosages (2-5 μg/day and 1-2 μg/day, respectively). Other vitamin D analogs upstream of the 1α-hydroxylase have little activity.

Hereditary 1,25-dihydroxyvitamin D resistance (HVDDR, also called *vitamin D–dependent rickets type II*) is an autosomal recessive disorder that is characterized by hypocalcemia, osteomalacia, rickets, and total alopecia. Multiple heterogenous mutations of the vitamin D receptor cause vitamin D–dependent rickets type II (Malloy et al., 2005). Absolute hormone resistance results from premature stop mutations, missense mutations in the zinc finger DNA-binding domain, mutations of the receptor ligand-binding domain, or mutations that affect heterodimerization of the VDR with the retinoid X receptor (RXR).

Serum abnormalities include low serum concentrations of calcium and phosphate and elevated serum alkaline phosphatase activity. The hypocalcemia leads to secondary hyperparathyroidism with elevated PTH levels and hypophosphatemia. The 25(OH)-vitamin D values are normal, whereas $1,25(OH)_2$-vitamin D levels are elevated in type II vitamin D–dependent rickets. This clinical feature distinguishes hereditary vitamin D–dependent rickets type II from CYP1α deficiency (vitamin D–dependent rickets type I), where serum 1,25(OH)2-vitamin D values are depressed. Children affected by vitamin D–dependent rickets type II are refractory even to massive doses of vitamin D and calcitriol, and they may require prolonged treatment with parenteral Ca^{2+}. Some remission of symptoms has been observed during adolescence, but the basis of remission is unknown. Notably, missense mutations in the ligand-binding domain have been described that result only in partial hormone resistance. Thus, the use of calcitriol analogs that bind to the VDR at different amino acids may provide therapeutic opportunities not otherwise available. This represents a prime application of pharmacogenetics, where "personalized" treatment based on the specific VDR mutations can be envisioned.

Renal osteodystrophy (renal rickets) refers to the disordered bone morphology that attends chronic kidney disease. It is characterized by abnormalities of bone turnover, mineralization, volume, linear growth, or strength, as well as underlying defects in mineral ion, PTH, or vitamin D metabolism. In the early phase of chronic renal failure, physiological concentrations of 1,25(OH)2D in circulation may become insufficient to regulate parathyroid cell function normally. As a result, the set point of PTH secretion to plasma Ca^{2+} concentration shifts to the right, PTH synthesis becomes enhanced at the transcriptional level, and parathyroid cells begin to proliferate. This resistance of the parathyroid cells to the physiological concentration of 1,25(OH)2D may be partially due to decreased conversion of 25-OHD to calcitriol. Phosphate retention and diminished serum calcium also increase PTH mRNA levels but at the post-transcriptional level. In addition, calcitriol deficiency impairs intestinal Ca^{2+} absorption and mobilization from bone. Hypocalcemia commonly results (although in some patients, prolonged and severe hyperparathyroidism eventually may lead to hypercalcemia). Aluminum deposition in bone, once a cause of renal osteodystrophy, is no longer an issue since aluminum was removed from dialysis solutions.

Osteoporosis

Osteoporosis is a condition of low bone mass and microarchitectural disruption that results in fractures with minimal trauma. Osteoporosis is a major and growing public health problem in developed nations. Many women (30-50%) and men (15-30%) suffer a fracture related to osteoporosis. Characteristic sites of fracture include vertebral bodies, the distal radius, and the proximal femur, but osteoporotic individuals have generalized skeletal fragility, and fractures at sites such as ribs and long bones also are common. Fracture risk increases exponentially with age, and spine and hip fractures are associated with reduced survival. Fractures of distal forearm, foot, or ankle are not associated with increased mortality (Teng et al., 2008).

Osteoporosis can be categorized as *primary* or *secondary*. In 1948, Albright and Reifenstein concluded that primary osteoporosis included two separate entities: one related to menopausal estrogen loss and the other to aging. This concept was extended by the recognition that primary osteoporosis represents two fundamentally different conditions: *type I osteoporosis,* characterized by loss of trabecular bone owing to estrogen lack at menopause, and *type II osteoporosis,* characterized by loss of cortical and trabecular bone in men and women due to long-term remodeling inefficiency, dietary inadequacy, and activation of the parathyroid axis with age. It is not clear, however, that these two entities are truly distinct. Although many osteoporotic women undoubtedly have experienced excessive menopausal bone loss, it may be more appropriate to consider osteoporosis as the result of multiple physical, hormonal, and nutritional factors acting alone or in concert.

Secondary osteoporosis is due to systemic illness or medications such as glucocorticoids or phenytoin. The most successful approach to secondary osteoporosis is prompt resolution of the underlying cause or drug discontinuation. Whether primary or secondary, osteoporosis is associated with characteristic disordered bone remodeling, so the same therapies can be used.

Paget's Disease. Paget's disease is characterized by single or multiple sites of disordered bone remodeling. The etiology of the disease is uncertain but is thought to be the result of infection with the measles virus of the paramyxovirus family (Roodman and Windle, 2005). It affects up to 2-3% of the population >60 years of age. The primary pathologic abnormality is increased bone resorption followed by exuberant bone formation. However, the newly formed bone is disorganized and of poor quality, resulting in characteristic bowing, stress fractures, and arthritis of joints adjoining the involved bone. Pagetic lesions contain many abnormal multinucleated osteoclasts associated with a disordered mosaic pattern of bone formation. Pagetic bone is thickened and has abnormal microarchitecture. The altered bone structure can produce secondary problems, such as deafness, spinal cord compression, high-output cardiac failure, and pain. Malignant degeneration to osteogenic sarcoma is a rare but lethal complication of Paget's disease.

Renal Osteodystrophy. Bone disease is a frequent consequence of chronic renal failure and dialysis. Pathologically, lesions are typical of hyperparathyroidism (osteitis fibrosa), vitamin D deficiency (osteomalacia), or a mixture of both. The underlying pathophysiology reflects increased serum phosphate and decreased calcium, leading to secondary events that strive to preserve circulating levels of mineral ions at the expense of bone.

PHARMACOLOGICAL TREATMENT OF DISORDERS OF MINERAL ION HOMEOSTASIS AND BONE METABOLISM

Hypercalcemia

Hypercalcemia can be life threatening. Such patients frequently are severely dehydrated because hypercalcemia compromises renal concentrating mechanisms. Thus, fluid resuscitation with large volumes of isotonic saline must be early and aggressive (6-8 L/day). Agents that augment Ca^{2+} excretion, such as loop diuretics (Chapter 25), may help to counteract the effect of plasma volume expansion by saline but are contraindicated until volume is repleted because they otherwise will aggravate volume depletion and hypercalcemia.

Corticosteroids administered at high doses (e.g., 40-80 mg/day of prednisone) may be useful when hypercalcemia results from sarcoidosis, lymphoma, or hypervitaminosis D (Chapter 42). The response to steroid therapy is slow; from 1-2 weeks may be required before plasma Ca^{2+} concentration falls.

Calcitonin (CALCIMAR, MIACALCIN) may be useful in managing hypercalcemia. Reduction in Ca^{2+} can be rapid, although "escape" from the hormone commonly occurs within several days. The recommended starting dose is 4 units/kg of body weight administered subcutaneously every 12 hours; if there is no response within 1-2 days, the dose may be increased to a maximum of 8 units/kg every 12 hours. If the response after 2 more days still is unsatisfactory, the dose may be increased to a maximum of 8 units/kg every 6 hours. Calcitonin can lower serum calcium by 1-2 mg/dL.

Intravenous *bisphosphonates* (*pamidronate, zoledronate*) have proven very effective in the management of hypercalcemia (see further discussion of bisphosphonates later in the chapter). These agents potently inhibit osteoclastic bone resorption. Oral bisphosphonates are less effective for treating hypercalcemia. Therefore, pamidronate (AREDIA) is given as an intravenous infusion of 60-90 mg over 4-24 hours; the more prolonged infusion (>4 hours) is reserved primarily for patients with renal dysfunction. With pamidronate, resolution of hypercalcemia occurs over several days, and the effect usually persists for several weeks. Zoledronate (ZOMETA) has superseded pamidronate because of its more rapid normalization of serum calcium and longer duration of action.

Plicamycin (mithramycin, MITHRACIN) is a cytotoxic antibiotic that also decreases plasma Ca^{2+} concentrations by inhibiting bone resorption. Reduction in plasma Ca^{2+} concentrations occurs within 24-48 hours when a relatively low dose of this agent is given

(15-25 μg/kg of body weight) to minimize the high systemic toxicity of the drug; indeed, its toxicity generally precludes its use.

Oral sodium phosphate lowers plasma Ca^{2+} concentrations and may offer short-term calcemic control of some patients with primary hyperparathyroidism who are awaiting surgery. However, the risk of precipitating calcium phosphate salts in soft tissues throughout the body is of concern. In light of satisfactory responses to other agents, administration of intravenous sodium phosphate is not recommended as a treatment for hypercalcemia.

Once the hypercalcemic crisis has resolved or in patients with milder calcium elevations, therapy turns to more durable resolution of the hypercalcemic state. Parathyroidectomy remains the only definitive treatment for primary hyperparathyroidism. Specific indications for surgery have been proposed (Bilezikian et al., 2002). In the hands of a skilled parathyroid surgeon, resection of a single adenoma (~80% of cases) or of the hyperplastic glands (~15% of cases) cures hyperparathyroidism. Complications include transient postoperative hypocalcemia, which may reflect temporary disruption of blood supply to the remaining parathyroid tissue or skeletal avidity for calcium, and permanent hypoparathyroidism. As described later, a calcium mimetic that stimulates the calcium-sensing receptor is a promising new therapy for hyperparathyroidism that may be used increasingly in the future.

Therapy of hypercalcemia of malignancy ideally is directed at the underlying cancer. When this is not possible, parenteral bisphosphonates often will maintain calcium levels within an acceptable range.

Hypocalcemia and Other Therapeutic Uses of Calcium. Hypoparathyroidism is treated primarily with vitamin D. Dietary supplementation with Ca^{2+} also may be necessary.

Calcium is used in the treatment of calcium deficiency states and as a dietary supplement. Ca^{2+} salts are specific in the immediate treatment of hypocalcemic tetany regardless of etiology. In severe tetany, symptoms are best brought under control by intravenous medication. *Calcium chloride* ($CaCl_2 \cdot 2H_2O$) contains 27% Ca^{2+}; it is valuable in the treatment of hypocalcemic tetany and laryngospasm. The salt is given intravenously and *must never be injected into tissues.* Injections of calcium chloride are accompanied by peripheral vasodilation and a cutaneous burning sensation. The salt usually is given intravenously in a concentration of 10% (equivalent to 1.36 mEq Ca^{2+}/mL). The rate of injection should be slow (not >1 mL/minute) to prevent cardiac arrhythmias from a high concentration of Ca^{2+}. The injection may induce a moderate fall in blood pressure owing to vasodilation. Because calcium chloride is an acidifying salt, it is usually undesirable in the treatment of the hypocalcemia caused by renal insufficiency. *Calcium gluceptate* injection (a 22% solution; 18 mg or 0.9 mEq of Ca^{2+}/mL) is administered intravenously at a dose of 5-20 mL for the treatment of severe hypocalcemic tetany; the injection produces a transient tingling sensation when given too rapidly. When the intravenous route is not possible, injections may be given intramuscularly in the gluteal region at a dose of up to 5 mL. A mild local reaction may result. *Calcium gluconate* injection (a 10% solution; 9.3 mg of Ca^{2+}/mL) given intravenously is the treatment of choice for severe hypocalcemic tetany. Patients with moderate-to-severe hypocalcemia may be treated by intravenous infusion of calcium gluconate at a dose of 10-15 mg of Ca^{2+}/kg of body weight over 4-6 hours. Because the usual 10-mL vial of a 10% solution contains only 93 mg Ca^{2+}, many vials are needed. The intramuscular route should not be employed because abscess formation at the injection site may result.

For control of milder hypocalcemic symptoms, oral medication suffices, frequently in combination with vitamin D or one of its active metabolites. Calcium salts are acidifying, and different forms can be interchanged to avoid gastric irritation. Available Ca^{2+} salts include calcium carbonate, lactate, gluconate, phosphate, citrate, and hydroxyapatite. Calcium carbonate is prescribed most frequently, whereas calcium citrate may be absorbed more efficiently than other salts. However, absorption efficiency for most commonly prescribed calcium products is reasonable, and for many patients, cost and palatability outweigh modest differences in efficacy. Average doses for hypocalcemic patients are calcium gluconate, 15 g/day in divided doses; calcium lactate, 7.7 g plus 8 g lactose with each meal; and calcium carbonate or calcium phosphate, 1-2 g with meals.

Calcium carbonate and calcium acetate are used to restrict phosphate absorption in patients with chronic renal failure and oxalate absorption in patients with inflammatory bowel disease. Acute administration of calcium may be lifesaving in patients with extreme hyperkalemia (serum K^+>7 mEq/L). Calcium gluconate (10-30 mL of a 10% solution) can reverse some of the cardiotoxic effects of hyperkalemia, providing time while other efforts are taken to lower the plasma K^+ concentration.

Additional FDA-approved uses of calcium include intravenous treatment for black widow spider envenomation and management of magnesium toxicity. Use of supplemental calcium in the prevention and treatment of osteoporosis is discussed later.

THERAPEUTIC USES OF VITAMIN D

Clinical Forms of Vitamin D. Calcitriol (1,25-dihydroxycholecalciferol; CALCIJEX, ROCALTROL) is available for oral administration or injection. Intravenous treatment regimens with high doses of calcitriol or one of its derivatives have become predominant for managing patients with chronic kidney disease and end-stage kidney disease. Its specific therapeutic uses are discussed later. Several derivatives of vitamin D (Figure 44–10) are of considerable therapeutic and experimental interest.

Doxercalciferol (1α-hydroxyvitamin D_2, HECTOROL) is a prodrug that first must be activated by hepatic 25-hydroxylation to generate the biologically active compound, 1α,25-$(OH)_2D_2$ (Figure 44–10). The FDA has approved oral and intravenous preparations of 1α-hydroxyvitamin D_2 for use in treating secondary hyperparathyroidism, starting at 10 mg three times per week.

Dihydrotachysterol (DHT, ROXANE) is a reduced form of vitamin D_2. In the liver DHT is converted to its active form, 25-hydroxydihydrotachysterol. DHT is <1% as active as calcitriol in antirachitic assays but is much more effective in mobilizing bone mineral at high doses; it therefore can be used to maintain plasma Ca^{2+} in hypoparathyroidism. DHT is well absorbed from the GI tract and maximally increases serum calcium concentration after 2 weeks of daily

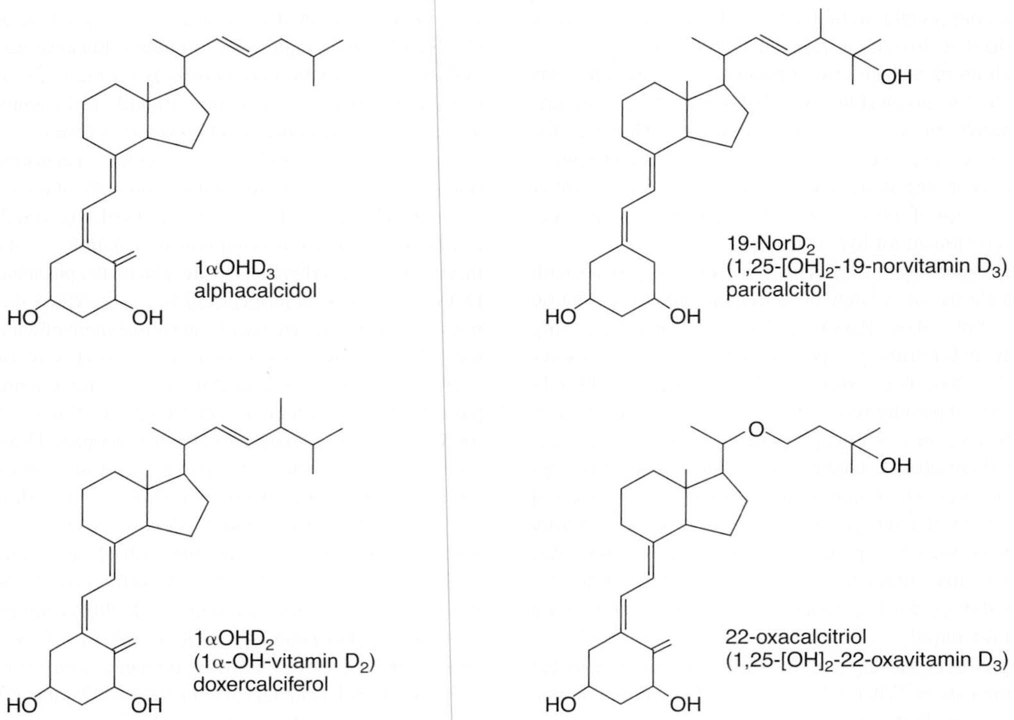

Figure 44–10. *Vitamin D analogs.*

administration. The hypercalcemic effects typically persist for 2 weeks but can last for up to 1 month. DHT is available for oral administration in doses ranging from 0.2-1 mg/day (average 0.6 mg/day).

1α-Hydroxycholecalciferol (1-OHD$_3$, alphacalcidol; ONE-ALPHA) was introduced as a substitute for 1,25(OH)$_2$D$_3$; alphacalcidol is a synthetic vitamin D$_3$ derivative that is already hydroxylated in the 1α position and is rapidly hydroxylated by 25-hydroxylase to form 1,25-(OH)$_2$D$_3$. It is equal to calcitriol in assays for stimulation of intestinal absorption of Ca^{2+} and bone mineralization and does not require renal activation. It therefore has been used to treat renal osteodystrophy and is available in the U.S. for experimental purposes.

Ergocalciferol (calciferol, DRISDOL) is pure vitamin D$_2$. It is available for oral, intramuscular, or intravenous administration. Ergocalciferol is indicated for the prevention of vitamin D deficiency and the treatment of familial hypophosphatemia, hypoparathyroidism, and vitamin D–resistant rickets type II, typically in doses of 50,000-200,000 units/day in conjunction with calcium supplements.

Analogs of Calcitriol. Several vitamin D analogs (Figure 44–10) suppress PTH secretion by the parathyroid glands but have less or negligible hypercalcemic activity. They therefore offer a safer and more effective means of controlling secondary hyperparathyroidism.

Calcipotriol (calcipotriene) is a synthetic derivative of calcitriol with a modified side chain that contains a 22–23 double bond, a 24(*S*)-hydroxy functional group, and carbons 25-27 incorporated into a cyclopropane ring. Calcipotriol has comparable affinity with calcitriol for the vitamin D receptor, but it is <1% as active as calcitriol in regulating calcium metabolism. This reduced calcemic activity largely reflects the pharmacokinetics of calcipotriol (Kissmeyer and Binderup, 1991). Calcipotriol has been studied extensively as a treatment for psoriasis (Chapter 65), although its mode of action is not known; a topical preparation (DOVONEX) is available for that purpose. In clinical trials, topical calcipotriol has been found to be slightly more effective than glucocorticoids with a good safety profile.

Paricalcitol (1,25-dihydroxy-19-norvitamin D$_2$, ZEMPLAR) is a synthetic calcitriol derivative that lacks the exocyclic C19 and has a vitamin D$_2$ rather than vitamin D$_3$ side chain (Figure 44–10). It reduces serum PTH levels without producing hypercalcemia or altering serum phosphorus (Martin et al., 1998). In an animal model, paricalcitol prevented or reversed PTH-induced high-turnover bone disease (Slatopolsky et al., 2003). Paricalcitol administered intravenously is FDA-approved for treating secondary hyperparathyroidism in patients with chronic renal failure.

22-Oxacalcitriol (1,25-dihydroxy-22-oxavitamin D$_3$, OCT, maxacalcitol, OXAROL) differs from calcitriol only in the substitution of C-22 with an oxygen atom. Oxacalcitriol has a low affinity for vitamin D–binding protein; as a result, more of the drug circulates in the free (unbound) form, allowing it to be metabolized more rapidly than calcitriol with a consequent shorter $t_{1/2}$. Oxacalcitriol is a potent suppressor of PTH gene expression and shows very limited activity on intestine and bone. It is a useful compound in patients with overproduction of PTH in chronic renal failure. It should be borne in mind that persuasive evidence supports the use of cinacalcet for treatment of secondary hyperparathyroidism (Drueke and Ritz, 2009). Indeed, emerging findings show the clinical efficacy of cinacalcet for managing primary hyperparathyroidism (Peacock et al., 2009).

Therapeutic Indications for Vitamin D

The major therapeutic uses of vitamin D may be divided into four categories:

- prophylaxis and cure of nutritional rickets
- treatment of metabolic rickets and osteomalacia, particularly in the setting of chronic renal failure
- treatment of hypoparathyroidism
- prevention and treatment of osteoporosis (discussed in the section on osteoporosis)

Vitamin D supplementation may help prevent fractures, but the relationship between blood vitamin D concentrations and fracture risk is unclear (Cauley et al., 2008).

Nutritional Rickets. Nutritional rickets results from inadequate exposure to sunlight or deficiency of dietary vitamin D. The condition, once extremely rare in the U.S. and other countries where food fortification with the vitamin is practiced, is now increasing. Infants and children receiving adequate amounts of vitamin D–fortified food do not require additional vitamin D; however, breast-fed infants or those fed unfortified formula should receive 400 units of vitamin D daily as a supplement (Wagner and Greer, 2008). The usual practice is to administer vitamin A in combination with vitamin D. A number of balanced vitamin A and D preparations are available for this purpose. *Because the fetus acquires >85% of its calcium stores during the third trimester, premature infants are especially susceptible to rickets and may require supplemental vitamin D.*

Treatment of fully developed rickets requires a larger dose of vitamin D than that used prophylactically. One thousand units daily will normalize plasma Ca^{2+} and phosphate concentrations in ~10 days, with radiographic evidence of healing within ~3 weeks. However, a larger dose of 3000–4000 units daily often is prescribed for more rapid healing, particularly when respiration is compromised by severe thoracic rickets.

Vitamin D may be given prophylactically in conditions that impair its absorption (e.g., diarrhea, steatorrhea, and biliary obstruction). Parenteral administration also may be used in such cases.

Treatment of Osteomalacia and Renal Osteodystrophy. Osteomalacia, distinguished by undermineralization of bone matrix, occurs commonly during sustained phosphate depletion. Patients with chronic renal disease are at risk for developing osteomalacia but also may develop a complex bone disease called *renal osteodystrophy*. In this setting, bone metabolism is stimulated by an increase in PTH and by a delay in bone mineralization that is due to decreased renal synthesis of calcitriol. In renal osteodystrophy, low bone mineral density may be accompanied by high-turnover bone lesions typically seen in patients with uncontrolled hyperparathyroidism or by low bone remodeling activity seen in patients with adynamic bone disease. The therapeutic approach to the patient with renal osteodystrophy depends on its specific type. In high-turnover (hyperparathyroid) or mixed high-turnover disease with deficient mineralization, dietary phosphate restriction, generally in combination with a phosphate binder, is recommended because phosphate restriction is limited by the need to provide adequate protein intake to maintain nitrogen balance. Although highly effective, *aluminum* is no longer used as a phosphate binder because it promotes adynamic bone disease, anemia, myopathy, and occasionally dementia. Calcium-containing phosphate binders along with calcitriol administration may contribute to oversuppression of PTH secretion and likewise result in adynamic bone disease and an increased incidence of vascular calcification. Highly effective non-calcium-containing phosphate binders have been developed. Sevelamer hydrochloride (RENAGEL), a nonabsorbable phosphate-binding polymer, effectively lowers serum phosphate concentration in hemodialysis patients, with a corresponding reduction in the calcium × phosphate product. Sevelamer hydrochloride consists of cross-linked poly[allylamine hydrochloride] that is resistant to digestive degradation. Its partially protonated amines spaced one carbon from the polymer backbone chelate phosphate ions. Sevelamer is modestly water soluble and only trace amounts are absorbed from the GI tract. However, with continued use, progressive accumulation has been reported in experimental animals. Side effects of sevelamer include vomiting, nausea, diarrhea, and dyspepsia. Sevelamer does not affect the bioavailability of digoxin, warfarin, enalapril, or metoprolol. Lanthanum carbonate (FOSRENOL) is a poorly permeable trivalent cation that is useful in treating the hyperphosphatemia associated with renal osteodystrophy.

Renal osteodystrophy associated with low bone turnover (adynamic bone disease) is increasingly common and may be due to oversuppression of PTH with aggressive use of either calcitriol or other vitamin D analogs. Although PTH levels generally are low (<100 pg/mL), a high PTH level does not exclude the presence of adynamic bone disease, especially with PTH assays that do not distinguish between biologically active and inactive PTH fragments (Monier-Faugere et al., 2001). Current guidelines suggest that treatment with an active vitamin D preparation is indicated if serum 25-OHD levels are <30 ng/mL and serum calcium is <9.5 mg/dL (2.37 mM). However, if 25-OHD and serum calcium levels are elevated, vitamin D supplementation should be discontinued. If the serum calcium level is <9.5 mg/dL, treatment with a vitamin D analog is warranted irrespective of the 25-OHD level (Eknoyan et al., 2003).

Hypoparathyroidism. Vitamin D and its analogs are a mainstay of the therapy of hypoparathyroidism. Dihydrotachysterol (DHT) has a faster onset, shorter duration of action, and a greater effect on bone mobilization than does vitamin D and traditionally has been a preferred agent. Calcitriol also is effective in the management of hypoparathyroidism and certain forms of pseudohypoparathyroidism in which endogenous levels of calcitriol are abnormally low. However, most hypoparathyroid patients respond to any form of vitamin D. Calcitriol may be preferred for temporary treatment of hypocalcemia while awaiting effects of a slower-acting form of vitamin D.

Miscellaneous Uses of Vitamin D. Vitamin D is used to treat hypophosphatemia associated with Fanconi's syndrome. Large doses of vitamin D (>10,000 units/day) are not useful in patients with osteoporosis and even can be dangerous. However, administration of 400-800 units/day of vitamin D to frail elderly men and women has been shown to suppress bone remodeling, protect bone mass, and reduce fracture incidence (see later section on osteoporosis). Clinical trials suggest that calcitriol may become an important agent for the treatment of psoriasis (Kowalzick, 2001). As such nontraditional uses of vitamin D are discovered, it will become important to develop noncalcemic analogs of calcitriol that achieve effects on cellular differentiation without the risk of hypercalcemia.

Adverse Effects of Vitamin D Therapy

The primary toxicity associated with calcitriol reflects its potent effect to increase intestinal calcium and phosphate absorption, along with the potential to mobilize osseous calcium and phosphate. Hypercalcemia, with or without hyperphosphatemia, commonly complicates calcitriol therapy and may limit its use at doses that effectively suppress PTH secretion. As described earlier, noncalcemic vitamin D analogs provide alternative interventions, although they do not obviate the need to monitor serum calcium and phosphorus concentrations.

Hypervitaminosis D is treated by immediate withdrawal of the vitamin, a low-calcium diet, administration of glucocorticoids, and vigorous fluid support. As noted earlier under hypercalcemia, forced saline diuresis with loop diuretics is also useful. With this regimen, the plasma Ca^{2+} concentration falls to normal, and Ca^{2+} in soft tissue tends to be mobilized. Conspicuous improvement in renal function occurs unless renal damage has been severe.

CALCITONIN

Diagnostic Uses of Calcitonin. Calcitonin is a sensitive and specific marker for the presence of medullary thyroid carcinoma (MTC), a neuroendocrine malignancy originating in thyroid parafollicular C cells. MTC can be hereditary (25%) or sporadic (75%) and is present in all patients with the multiple endocrine neoplasia type 2 (MEN2) syndromes. Because one form of MEN2 is inherited as a dominant trait, relatives of patients should be examined repeatedly by calcitonin measurements from early childhood. Because calcitonin levels may be low in early tumor stages or in premalignant C-cell hyperplasia, pentagastrin-induced calcitonin provides greater sensitivity and increased MTC detection. The identification of discrete mutations in the *RET* protooncogene in subjects with MEN2 offers hope that genetic screening will supplant reliance on testing serum calcitonin, which can give spurious results.

Therapeutic Uses. Calcitonin lowers plasma Ca^{2+} and phosphate concentrations in patients with hypercalcemia; this effect results from decreased bone resorption and is greater in patients in whom bone turnover rates are high. Although calcitonin is effective for up to 6 hours in the initial treatment of hypercalcemia, patients become refractory after a few days. This is likely due to receptor downregulation (Takahashi et al., 1995). Use of calcitonin does not substitute for aggressive fluid resuscitation, and the bisphosphonates are the preferred agents.

Calcitonin is effective in disorders of increased skeletal remodeling, such as Paget's disease, and in some patients with osteoporosis. In Paget's disease, chronic use of calcitonin produces long-term reductions of serum alkaline phosphatase activity and symptoms. Development of antibodies to calcitonin occurs with prolonged therapy, but this is not necessarily associated with clinical resistance. Side effects of calcitonin include nausea, hand swelling, urticaria, and, rarely, intestinal cramping. Side effects appear to occur with equal frequency with human and salmon calcitonin. *Salmon calcitonin* is approved for clinical use. The latter product also is available as a nasal spray, introduced for once-daily treatment of postmenopausal osteoporosis. For Paget's disease, calcitonin generally is administered by subcutaneous injection because intranasal delivery is relatively ineffective owing to limited bioavailability. After initial therapy at 100 units/day, the dose typically is reduced to 50 units three times a week.

BISPHOSPHONATES

Bisphosphonates are analogs of pyrophosphate (Figure 44–11) that contain two phosphonate groups attached to a geminal (central) carbon that replaces the oxygen in pyrophosphate. Because they form a three-dimensional structure capable of chelating divalent cations such as Ca^{2+}, the bisphosphonates have a strong affinity for bone, targeting especially bone surfaces undergoing remodeling. Accordingly, they are used extensively in conditions characterized by osteoclast-mediated bone resorption, including osteoporosis, steroid-induced osteoporosis, Paget's disease, tumor-associated osteolysis, breast and prostate cancer, and hypercalcemia. Calcium supplements, antacids, food or medications containing divalent cations, such as iron, may interfere with intestinal absorption of bisphosphonates. Recent evidence suggests that second- and third-generation bisphosphonates also may be effective anticancer drugs. For a review of the basic and clinical pharmacology of bisphosphonates, see Russell, 2007.

The clinical utility of bisphosphonates resides in their direct inhibition of bone resorption. First-generation bisphosphonates contain minimally modified side chains (R_1 and R_2 in Figure 44-11) (medronate, clodronate, and etidronate) or posses a chlorophenol group (tiludronate) (Figure 44-11). They are the least potent and in some instances cause bone demineralization. Second-generation aminobisphosphonates (e.g., alendronate and pamidronate) contain a nitrogen group in the side chain. They are 10-100 times more potent than first-generation compounds. Third-generation bisphosphonates (e.g., risedronate and zoledronate) contain a nitrogen atom within a heterocyclic ring and are up to 10,000 times more potent than first-generation agents.

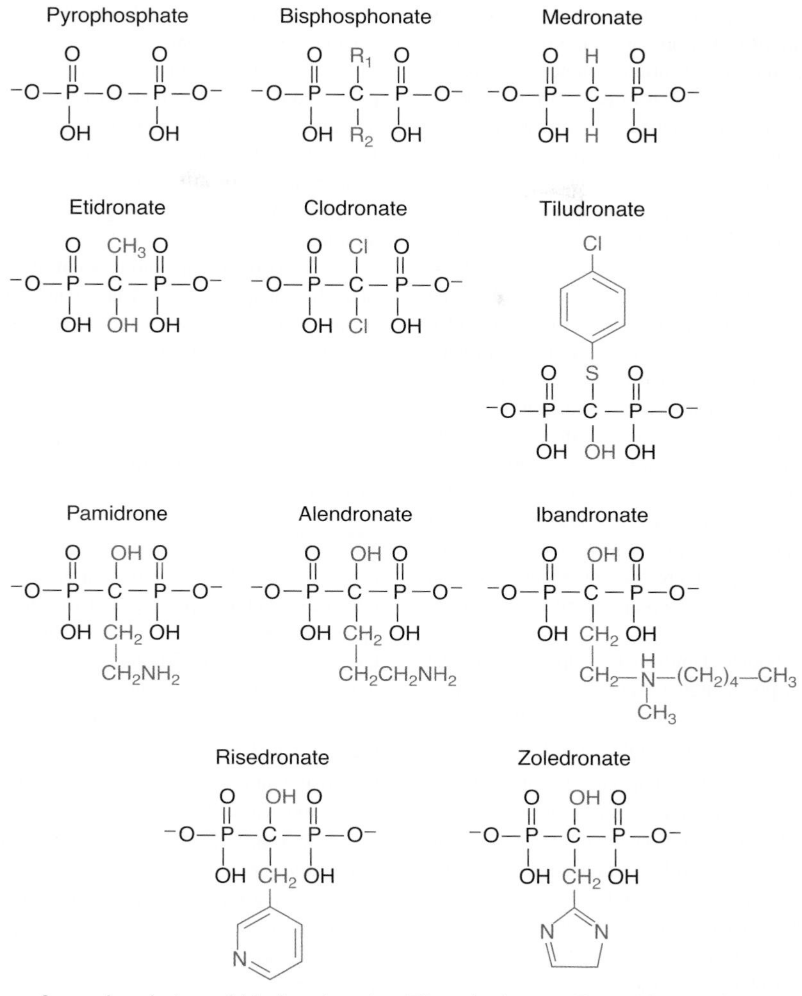

Figure 44–11. *Structures of pyrophosphate and bisphosphonates.* The substituents (R_1 and R_2) on the central carbon of the bisphosphonate parent structure are shown in blue.

Bisphosphonates concentrate at sites of active remodeling. Because they are highly negatively charged, bisphosphonates are membrane impermeable but are incorporated into the bone matrix by fluid-phase endocytosis (Stenbeck and Horton, 2000). Bisphosphonates remain in the matrix until the bone is remodeled and then are released in the acid environment of the resorption lacunae beneath the osteoclast as the overlying mineral matrix is dissolved. The importance of this process for the antiresorptive effect of bisphosphonates is evidenced by the fact that calcitonin blocks the antiresorptive action.

Although bisphosphonates prevent hydroxyapatite dissolution, their antiresorptive action is due to direct inhibitory effects on osteoclasts rather than strictly physiochemical effects. The antiresorptive activity apparently involves two primary mechanisms: osteoclast apoptosis and inhibition of components of the cholesterol biosynthetic pathway.

The current model is that apoptosis accounts for the antiresorptive effect of first-generation bisphosphonates, whereas the inhibitory action of aminobisphosphonates proceeds through the latter mechanism. Consistent with this view, the antiresorptive effect of aminobisphosphonates such as alendronate and risedronate, but not of clodronate or etidronate, persists when apoptosis is suppressed (Halasy-Nagy et al., 2001). First-generation bisphosphonates are metabolized into a nonhydrolyzable ATP analog (AppCCl_2p) that accumulates within osteoclasts and induces apoptosis (Rogers, 2003). In contrast, the aminobisphosphonates such as *alendronate* and *ibandronate* directly inhibit multiple steps in the pathway from mevalonate to cholesterol and isoprenoid lipids, such as geranylgeranyl diphosphate, that are required for the prenylation of proteins that are important for osteoclast function. The potency of aminobisphosphonates for inhibiting farnesyl synthase correlates directly with their antiresorptive activity (Dunford et al., 2001).

Available Bisphosphonates

Several bisphosphonates are available in the U.S. (Figure 44–11). Etidronate sodium (DIDRONEL) is used for treatment of Paget's disease and may be used parenterally to treat hypercalcemia. Because etidronate is the only bisphosphonate that inhibits mineralization, it has been supplanted largely by pamidronate and zoledronate for treating hypercalcemia. Pamidronate (AREDIA) is approved for management of hypercalcemia and for prevention of bone loss in breast cancer and multiple myeloma, but it also is effective in other skeletal disorders. Pamidronate is available in the U.S. only for parenteral administration. For treatment of hypercalcemia, pamidronate may be given as an intravenous infusion of 60-90 mg over 4-24 hours.

Several newer bisphosphonates have been approved for treatment of Paget's disease. These include tiludronate (SKELID), alendronate (FOSAMAX), and risedronate (ACTONEL). Tiludronate is approved for treatment of Paget's disease of bone. Standard dosing is 400 mg/day orally for 3 months. Tiludronate in recommended doses does not interfere with bone mineralization, unlike etidronate. Zoledronate (ZOMETA) is approved for treating Paget's disease and administered as a single 5-mg infusion decreased bone turnover markers for 6 months with no loss of therapeutic effect (Reid et al., 2005). Zometa is widely used for prevention of osteoporosis in prostate and breast cancer patients receiving hormonal therapy. It is also approved for treating hypercalcemia of malignancies and for preventing fractures and skeletal complications in cancer patients with bone metastases. It is widely used to prevent osteoporosis and fractures in breast and prostate cancer patients receiving hormone-antagonist treatment.

The potent bisphosphonate ibandronate is approved for the prevention and treatment of postmenopausal osteoporosis. The recommended oral dose is 2.5 mg daily or 150 mg once monthly, which appears to be as effective as daily treatment and is well tolerated.

Absorption, Fate, and Excretion. All oral bisphosphonates are very poorly absorbed from the intestine and have remarkably limited bioavailability (<1% [alendronate, risedronate] to 6% [etidronate, tiludronate]). Hence these drugs should be administered with a full glass of water following an overnight fast and at least 30 minutes before breakfast. Oral bisphosphonates have not been used widely in children or adolescents because of uncertainty of long-term effects of bisphosphonates on the growing skeleton.

Bisphosphonates are excreted primarily by the kidneys. Adjusted doses for patients with diminished renal function have not been determined; bisphosphonates currently are not recommended for patients with a creatinine clearance of <30 mL/minute.

Adverse Effects. Oral bisphosphonates, including alendronate, ibandronate, and risedronate, can cause heartburn, esophageal irritation, or esophagitis. Other GI side effects include abdominal pain and diarrhea. Symptoms often abate when patients take the medication after an overnight fast, with tap or filtered water (not mineral water), and remain upright. Esophageal complications are infrequent when the drug is taken as described. If symptoms persist despite these precautions, use of a nonsteroidal anti-inflammatory drug or acetaminophen can diminish these symptoms; a proton pump inhibitor at bedtime may be helpful (Chapter 45). Both drugs may be better tolerated on a once-weekly regimen with no reduction of efficacy. Patients with active upper GI disease should not be given oral bisphosphonates.

Serious osteonecrosis of the jaw is associated with use of bisphosphonates (Edwards et al., 2008). In 2008 the FDA issued an alert on the use of bisphosphonates (http://www.fda.gov/Drugs/DrugSafety/PostmarketDrugSafetyInformationforPatientsandProviders/ucm124165.htm) and product labeling was modified to highlight the severe musculoskeletal pain that may occur and its relation to osteonecrosis of the jaw.

Owing to cytokine release, initial parenteral infusion of pamidronate, may cause skin flushing, flu-like symptoms, muscle and joint aches and pains, nausea and vomiting, abdominal discomfort and diarrhea (or constipation) but mainly when given in higher concentrations or at faster rates than those recommended. These symptoms are short lived and generally do not recur with subsequent administration.

Zoledronate has more potent effects on calcium than some other bisphosphonates and is capable of causing severe hypocalcemia. It has been associated with renal toxicity, deterioration of renal function, and potential renal failure. Thus, the infusion should be given over at least 15 minutes, and the dose should be 4 mg. Patients who receive zoledronate should have standard laboratory and clinical parameters of renal function assessed prior to treatment and periodically after treatment to monitor for deterioration in renal function.

Other Therapeutic Uses

Hypercalcemia. The use of pamidronate in the management of malignancy-associated hypercalcemia was described earlier. Zoledronate appears to be more effective than pamidronate and at least as safe, can be infused over 15 minutes rather than 2-4 hours, and is FDA-approved for this indication.

Postmenopausal Osteoporosis. Much interest is focused on the role of bisphosphonates in the treatment of osteoporosis. Clinical trials show that treatment is associated with increased bone mineral density and protection against fracture.

Cancer. Bisphosphonates may also have direct antitumor action by inhibiting oncogene activation and through their anti-angiogenic effects. Randomized clinical trials of bisphosphonates in patients with breast cancer suggest that they delay or prevent development of metastases as a component of endocrine adjuvant therapy (Gnant et al., 2009).

PARATHYROID HORMONE

Continuous administration of parathyroid hormone (PTH) or high-circulating PTH levels achieved in primary hyperparathyroidism causes bone demineralization and osteopenia. However, *intermittent* PTH administration promotes bone growth. Selye first described the anabolic action of PTH some 80 years ago, but this observation was largely ignored and generally forgotten. Beginning in the 1970s, studies focused on the anabolic action of PTH, culminating with FDA approval of synthetic human 34-amino-acid amino-terminal PTH fragment [hPTH(1-34), teriparatide (FORTEO)] for use in treating severe osteoporosis (Hodsman et al., 2005).

Full-length human recombinant PTH(1-84) is in phase III trials for hypoparathyroidism, for which teriparatide is not approved. Intermittent PTH(1-84) may soon be approved for use in osteoporosis, but its benefits over PTH(1-34) remain to be established.

Absorption, Fate, and Excretion. Pharmacokinetics and systemic actions of teriparatide on mineral metabolism are the same as for PTH. Teriparatide is administered by once-daily subcutaneous injection of 20 μg into the thigh or abdomen. With this regimen, serum PTH concentrations peak at 30 minutes after the injection and decline to undetectable concentrations within 3 hours, whereas the serum calcium concentration peaks at 4-6 hours after administration. Based on aggregate data from different dosing regimens, teriparatide bioavailability averages 95%. Teriparatide clearance averages 62 L/hour in women and 94 L/hour in men, which exceeds normal liver plasma flow, consistent with both hepatic and extrahepatic PTH removal. The serum $t_{1/2}$ of teriparatide is ~1 hour when administered subcutaneously versus 5 minutes when administered intravenously. The longer $t_{1/2}$ following subcutaneous administration reflects the time required for absorption from the injection site. The elimination of PTH(1-34) and full-length PTH proceeds by nonspecific enzymatic mechanisms in the liver, followed by renal excretion.

Clinical Effects. In postmenopausal women with osteoporosis, teriparatide increases BMD and reduces the risk of vertebral and nonvertebral fractures. Several laboratories have examined the effects of intermittent PTH on BMD in patients with osteoporosis. In these studies, teriparatide increased axial bone mineral, although initial reports of effects on cortical bone were disappointing. Co-administration of hPTH(1-34) with estrogen or synthetic androgen led to impressive gains in vertebral bone mass or trabecular bone. However, in some early studies there was only maintenance or even loss of cortical bone. Vitamin D insufficiency in patients at baseline or pharmacokinetic differences involving bioavailability or circulating half-life may have contributed to observed differences on cortical bone. The most comprehensive studies to date established the value of daily hPTH(1–34) administration on total BMD, with significant elevations of BMD in lumbar spine and femoral neck and with significant reductions of vertebral and nonvertebral fracture risk in osteoporotic women (Neer et al., 2001) and men (Finkelstein et al., 2003).

Candidates for teriparatide treatment include women who have a history of osteoporotic fracture, who have multiple risk factors for fracture, or who failed or are intolerant of previous osteoporosis therapy. Men with primary or hypogonadal osteoporosis are also candidates for treatment with teriparatide. However, the effect on fracture incidence in this group has not been established.

Adverse Effects. In rats, teriparatide increased the incidence of osteosarcoma (Vahle et al., 2004). Because of these findings, a black box warning appears on the FORTEO package insert. The clinical relevance of this finding is unclear, especially because patients with primary hyperparathyroidism have marked elevation of serum PTH without a greater incidence of osteosarcoma. Nonetheless, teriparatide should not be used in patients who are at increased baseline risk for osteosarcoma (including those with Paget's disease of bone, unexplained elevations of alkaline phosphatase, open epiphyses, or prior radiation therapy involving the skeleton). The safety and efficacy of FORTEO have not been evaluated for extended use beyond 2 years of treatment and therapy should be limited to no more than 2 years. A tumor registry-based analysis of the occurrence of osteosarcoma in teriparatide-treated patients is ongoing; cases of osteosarcoma associated with the drug should be reported to the FDA. Increases in bone density acquired during therapy with teriparatide can maintained or extended with subsequent use of bisphosphonates (Black et al., 2005).

Full-length PTH(1-84) has been associated with osteosarcomas in rats (Jolette et al., 2006) although not in humans. The significance and interpretation of the toxicological findings has been questioned (Tashjian and Goltzman, 2008). However, adverse effects include exacerbation of nephrolithiasis and elevation of serum uric acid levels.

CALCIUM SENSOR MIMETICS: CINACALCET

Calcimimetics are drugs that mimic the stimulatory effect of calcium on the calcium-sensing receptor (CaSR) to inhibit PTH secretion by the parathyroid glands. By enhancing the sensitivity of the CaSR to extracellular Ca^{2+}, calcimimetics lower the concentration of Ca^{2+} at which PTH secretion is suppressed. Inorganic di- and trivalent cations, along with polycations such as spermine, aminoglycosides (e.g., streptomycin, gentamicin, and neomycin) and polybasic amino acids (e.g., polylysine) are full agonists and are referred to a type I calcimimetics. Phenylalkylamine derivatives that are allosteric CaSR modulators that require the presence of Ca^{2+} or other full agonists to enhance the sensitivity of activation without altering the maximal response are designated type II calcimimetics. Cinacalcet (SENSIPAR) (Figure 44–12) is approved for the treatment of secondary hyperparathyroidism owing to chronic renal disease and for patients with hypercalcemia associated with parathyroid carcinoma. Cinacalcet lowers serum PTH levels in patients with normal or reduced renal function (Padhi and Harris, 2009).

In clinical trials, cinacalcet at 20- to 100-mg doses lowered PTH levels in a concentration-dependent manner by 15–50% and the serum calcium × phosphate product by 7% compared with placebo (Franceschini et al., 2003). Cinacalcet also effectively reduced PTH levels in patients with primary hyperparathyroidism and provided sustained normalization of serum calcium without altering bone mineral density (Shoback et al., 2003). Long-term control of PTH levels was achieved during a 3-year study of cinacalcet, suggesting that resistance does not develop. There currently is insufficient information to know whether reducing serum PTH levels with

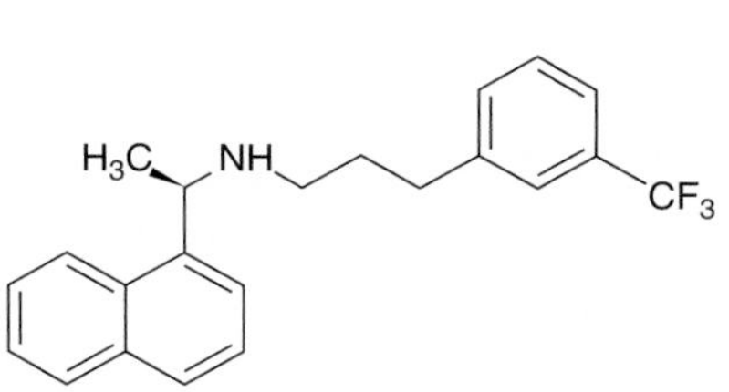

Figure 44–12. *Structure of cinacalcet.* Cinacalcet exists as optical isomers. The *R*-enantiomer, which is more active, is shown.

cinacalcet improves outcomes such as risk of cardiovascular events, bone disease, or mortality (Evenepoel, 2008).

Absorption, Fate, and Excretion. Cinacalcet (αR)-(–)α-methyl-*N*-[3-[3-[trifluoromethylphenyl]propyl]-1-napthalenemethanamine hydro-chloride) exhibits first-order absorption, with maximal serum concentrations achieved 2-6 hours after oral administration. Maximal effects, as defined by the nadir of serum PTH, occur 2–4 hours after administration. After absorption, plasma concentrations of cinacalcet decrease with a $t_{1/2}$ of 30-40 hours. Cinacalcet is eliminated primarily by renal excretion, with some 85% recovered in the urine after oral administration; the drug is also metabolized by multiple hepatic cytochromes, including CYPs 3A4, 2D6, and 1A2.

Cinacalcet is available in 30-, 60-, and 90-mg tablets. Optimal doses have not been defined. The recommended starting dose for treatment of secondary hyperparathyroidism in patients with chronic kidney disease on dialysis is 30 mg once daily, with a maximum of 180 mg/day. For treatment of parathyroid carcinoma, a starting dose of 30 mg twice daily is recommended, with a maximum of 90 mg four times daily. The starting dose is titrated upward every 2-4 weeks to maintain the PTH level between 150 and 300 pg/mL (secondary hyperparathyroidism) or to normalize serum calcium (parathyroid carcinoma).

Adverse Reactions. The principal adverse event with cinacalcet is hypocalcemia. Thus, the drug should not be used if the initial serum [Ca^{2+}] is <8.4 mg/dL; serum calcium and phosphorus concentrations should be measured within 1 week, and PTH should be measured within 4 weeks after initiating therapy or after changing dosage.

Hypocalcemia can be diminished by initiating therapy with a low dose and gradually titrating it as necessary or adjusting the dose when vitamin D and/or phosphate binders are administered concomitantly. Patients on hemodialysis with low-calcium dialysate need to be monitored closely for hypocalcemia. Seizure threshold is lowered by significant reductions in serum Ca^{2+}, so patients with a history of seizure disorders should be monitored especially closely. Finally, adynamic bone disease may develop if the PTH level is <100 pg/mL, and the drug should be discontinued or the dose decreased if the PTH level falls below 150 pg/mL.

Drug Interactions. Potential drug interactions can be anticipated with drugs that interfere with calcium homeostasis or that hinder cinacalcet absorption. Based on these considerations, potentially interfering drugs may include vitamin D analogs, phosphate binders, bisphosphonates, calcitonin, glucocorticoids, gallium, and cisplatin. The other category of drug interactions is for compounds metabolized by CYPs. Caution is recommended when cinacalcet is coadministered with inhibitors of CYP3A4 (e.g., ketoconazole, erythromycin, or itraconazole), CYP2D6 (many β adrenergic receptor blockers, flecainide, vinblastine, and most tricyclic antidepressants), and many other drugs.

INTEGRATED APPROACH TO PREVENTION AND TREATMENT OF OSTEOPOROSIS

Osteoporosis is a major and growing public health problem in developed nations. Ten million Americans are afflicted with osteoporosis, and an estimated 44 million individuals >50 years of age have low bone mass placing them at risk for osteoporosis. Osteoporosis is associated with a significant risk for bone fracture, especially of the hip, spine, and wrist. Approximately 50% women and 25% of men >50 years of age will experience an osteoporosis-related fracture. However, important reductions in fracture risk can be achieved with appropriate lifelong attention to prevention. Regular weight-bearing and muscle-strengthening exercise of reasonable intensity is endorsed at all ages. For children and adolescents, adequate dietary calcium and vitamin D are important if peak bone mass is to reach the level appropriate for genetic endowment. Attention to nutritional status (i.e., increased dietary calcium or calcium and/or vitamin D supplements) also may be required, particularly in elderly patients and those at risk of vitamin D deficiency. Smoking and excessive alcohol are significant risk factors and should be avoided. Although the administration of estrogen to women at menopause is a powerful intervention to preserve bone and protect against fracture, the detrimental effects of hormone-replacement therapy (HRT) have mandated a major reexamination on treatment options (see later and Chapter 40).

Pharmacological agents used to manage osteoporosis act by decreasing the rate of bone resorption and thereby slowing the rate of bone loss (antiresorptive therapy) or by promoting bone formation (anabolic therapy). Because bone remodeling is a coupled process, antiresorptive drugs ultimately decrease the rate of bone formation and therefore do not promote substantial gains in BMD. They nonetheless reduce fracture risk, particularly in the spine but also in the hip (for alendronate and risedronate). Increases in BMD during the first years of antiresorptive therapy represent a constriction of the remodeling space to a new steady-state level, after which BMD reaches a plateau (Figure 44–13). One consequence of this phenomenon is that therapeutic trials in osteoporosis must be of sufficient duration (i.e., at least 2 years) to determine whether an increase in BMD represents anything more than a simple reduction in remodeling space.

Pharmacological treatment of osteoporosis is aimed at restoring bone strength and preventing fractures. The long-standing centerpiece of this approach has been antiresorptive drugs such as the bisphosphonates, estrogen, or the selective estrogen receptor modulator (SERM) raloxifene, and, to some extent, calcitonin. These drugs inhibit osteoclast-mediated bone loss, thereby reducing bone turnover.

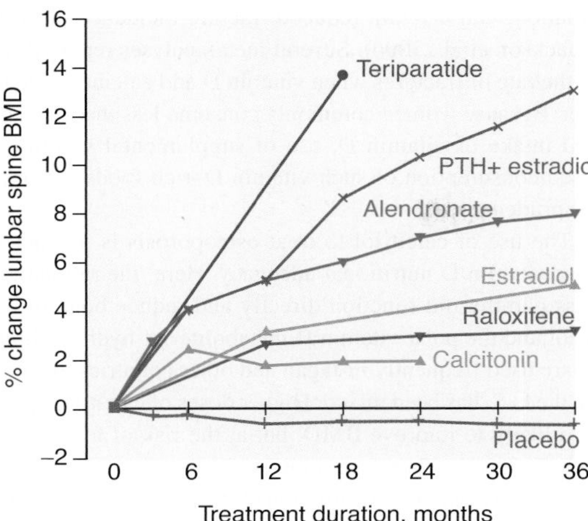

Figure 44–13. *Relative efficacy of different therapeutic interventions on bone mineral density of the lumbar spine.* Teriparatide (40 μg) (Neer et al., 2001), PTH (25 μg) + estradiol, alendronate (10 mg), estradiol (0.625 mg/day), raloxifene (120 mg), calcitonin (200 IU). Typical results with placebo treatment underscore the inexorable bone loss without intervention. Some of the indicated treatment interventions involved combination therapy, and absolute comparisons should not be made. For additional references, see legend to Figure 61-13 in the 11th edition of this text.

Until recently, antiresorptive drugs were the only agents approved in the U.S. for treating osteoporosis. The increase in bone density that they produce is variable and depends on the site and the particular drug; generally, the increase is <10% after 3 years (Figure 44–12). This situation changed in 2002 when the FDA approved the biologically active PTH fragment PTH(1–34) (teriparatide, FORTEO) for use in treating postmenopausal women with osteoporosis and to increase bone mass in men with primary or hypogonadal osteoporosis. For a review and proposed guidelines for teriparatide/PTH use, see Hodsman et al. (2005). This agent should be used only after consideration of the risks (potential cause of osteosarcoma) and benefits in patients refractory to bisphosphonates or at serious risk of fracture. Therapeutic approaches likely will evolve considerably as newer treatment paradigms are developed and combinations of antiresorptive agents and PTH are introduced, and as the molecular physiology of osteoblast and osteoclast function is elucidated (Grey et al., 2005).

Antiresorptive Agents. Bisphosphonates. Bisphosphonates are the most frequently used drugs for the prevention and treatment of osteoporosis. Second- and third-generation oral bisphosphonates alendronate and risedronate have sufficient potency to suppress bone resorption at doses that do not inhibit mineralization.

Alendronate (FOSAMAX), risedronate (ACTONEL), and ibandronate (BONIVA) are approved for prevention and treatment of osteoporosis and for the treatment of glucocorticoid-associated osteoporosis. Multiple appropriate formulations are available. Studies of daily treatment with alendronate established its efficacy to increase bone mineral density, decrease bone turnover, and reduce the risk of vertebral fracture among women with osteoporosis (Bone et al., 2004; Liberman et al., 1995; Tonino et al., 2000; Tucci et al., 1996). Similar results were obtained with risedronate (Delmas et al., 2008). The results of 10-year daily treatment with 10 mg of alendronate (with 500 mg of supplemental calcium) reported a 14% increase of lumbar spine BMD, with smaller increments at the trochanter, total hip, and femoral neck (Bone et al., 2004). On reduction and discontinuation of treatment, BMD at the lumbar spine was maintained. Although significant decreases of BMD occurred at the total hip, femoral neck, and forearm, BMD at the lumbar spine, trochanter, total hip, and total body remained significantly above baseline values at year 10.

For patients in whom oral bisphosphonates cause severe esophageal distress despite countermeasures, intravenous zoledronate (RECLAST) or ibandronate offer skeletal protection without causing adverse GI effects. For treatment of osteoporosis, ibandronate (3 mg) is given intravenously every 3 months; zoledronate is administered as 5 mg once yearly. Zoledronate is the first bisphosphonate to be approved from once-yearly intravenous treatment of osteoporosis. Intravenous ibandronate significantly increased BMD of the lumbar spine. No fracture prevention data for intravenous ibandronate are available. Zoledronate reduces both vertebral and nonvertebral fractures (Black et al., 2007). Optimal duration of treatment and long-term safety remain to be established. A 4-mg formulation (ZOMETA) is available for intravenous treatment of hypercalcemia of malignancy, multiple myeloma, or bone metastasis resulting from solid tumors.

Denosumab. As described earlier, RANKL binds to its cognate receptor RANK on the surface of precursor and mature osteoclasts, and stimulates these cells to mature and resorb bone. OPG, which competes with RANK for binding to RANKL, is the physiological inhibitor of RANKL. Denosumab is an investigational human monoclonal antibody that binds with high affinity to RANKL, mimicking the effect of OPG, and thereby reducing the binding of RANKL to RANK. Denosumab blocks osteoclast formation and activation. It increases BMD and decreases bone turnover markers when given subcutaneously once every 6 months. Denosumab, administered subcutaneously at 60 mg doses every 6 months, resulted in 68%, 41%, and 20% reductions in vertebral, hip and nonvertebral fractures, respectively, in a phase III clinical trial (Cummings et al., 2008). In the 3-year Fracture Reduction Evaluation with Denosumab and Osteoporosis Every Six Months (FREEDOM) Trial, denosumab significantly reduced morphometric vertebral fractures, and decreased hip and nonvertebral fractures and changes in BMD and bone turnover markers (Cummings et al., 2008). This novel therapy may soon gain FDA approval.

Selective Estradiol Receptor Modulators (SERMs). Considerable work has been undertaken to develop estrogenic compounds with tissue-selective activities. One of these, raloxifene (EVISTA), acts as an estrogen agonist on bone and liver, is inactive on the uterus, and acts as an anti-estrogen on the breast (Chapter 40). In postmenopausal women, raloxifene stabilizes and modestly increases BMD and has been shown to reduce the risk of vertebral compression fracture (Ettinger et al., 1999). Raloxifene is approved for both the prevention and treatment of osteoporosis. With the decreased use of estrogen for treating osteoporosis, the SERM raloxifene would seem to be an ideal alternative to HRT because raloxifene reduces the risk of vertebral fractures (albeit without a positive effect on nonvertebral fractures), breast cancer, and coronary events (coronary death, nonfatal myocardial infarction, and hospitalized acute coronary syndromes other than myocardial infarction) (Clemett and Spencer, 2000). The major drawback of raloxifene is that it can worsen vasomotor symptoms.

Estrogen. There is an unambiguous relationship between estrogen deficiency and osteoporosis. Postmenopausal status or estrogen deficiency at any age significantly increases a patient's risk for osteoporosis and fractures. Likewise, overwhelming evidence supports the positive impact of estrogen replacement on the conservation of bone and protection against osteoporotic fracture after menopause (Chapter 40). The outcome of the Women's Health Initiative (WHI) studies, however, strikingly altered the view of the therapeutic use of HRT for long-term prevention or treatment of osteoporosis. Significantly increased risks of heart disease and breast cancer were found (Anderson et al., 2004; Cauley et al., 2003). The consensus among experts now is to reserve HRT only for the short-term relief of vasomotor symptoms associated with menopause. HRT should be limited to osteoporosis prevention in women with significant ongoing vasomotor symptoms who are not at an increased risk for cardiovascular disease. An annual individualized risk-benefit reassessment should be performed on these patients.

Calcium. The physiological roles of Ca^{2+} and its use in the treatment of hypocalcemic disorders were discussed earlier. The rationale for using supplemental calcium to protect bone varies with time of life.

For preteens and adolescents, adequate substrate calcium is required for bone accretion. Controlled trials indicate that supplemental calcium promotes adolescent bone acquisition (Johnston et al., 1992), but its impact on peak bone mass is not known. Higher calcium intake during the third decade of life is positively related to the final phase of bone acquisition (Recker et al., 1992). There is controversy about the role of calcium during the early years after menopause, when the primary basis for bone loss is estrogen withdrawal. Although little effect of calcium on trabecular bone has been reported, reduction in cortical bone loss with calcium supplementation has been observed (Elders et al., 1994), even in populations with high dietary calcium intake. In elderly subjects, supplemental calcium suppresses bone turnover, improves BMD. Although some studies found a concomitant decreases in the incidence of fracture (Dawson-Hughes et al., 1997), three randomized trials found that it did not reduce fracture rate in older women (Jackson et al., 2006).

Patients who are unable or unwilling to increase calcium by dietary means alone may choose from many palatable, low-cost calcium preparations. As noted previously, numerous oral calcium preparations are available. The most frequently prescribed is carbonate, which should be taken with meals to facilitate dissolution and absorption. Traditional dosing of calcium is ~1000 mg/day, nearly the amount present in a quart of milk. Adults >50 years of age need 1200 mg of calcium daily. More may be necessary to overcome endogenous intestinal calcium losses, but daily intakes of ≥2000 mg frequently are reported to be constipating.

Vitamin D and Its Analogs. Modest supplementation with vitamin D (400-800 IU/day) may improve intestinal Ca^{2+} absorption, suppress bone remodeling, and improve BMD in individuals with marginal or deficient vitamin D status. A prospective study found that neither dietary calcium nor vitamin D intake was of major importance for the primary prevention of osteoporotic fractures in women (Michaelsson et al., 2003). However, supplemental vitamin D in combination with calcium reduced fracture incidence in multiple trials (Jackson et al., 2006). Several meta-analyses reported reduction in the rate of fractures when vitamin D and calcium were taken together. Because women commonly consume less than the recommended intake of vitamin D, use of supplemental vitamin D or increased consumption of such vitamin D–rich foods as dark fish may be prudent.

The use of calcitriol to treat osteoporosis is distinct from ensuring vitamin D nutritional adequacy. Here, the rationale is to suppress parathyroid function directly and reduce bone turnover. Calcitriol and the polar vitamin D metabolite 1α-hydroxycholecalciferol are used frequently in Japan and other countries, but experience in the U.S. has been mixed. Higher doses of calcitriol appear to be more likely to improve BMD, but at the risk of hypercalciuria and hypercalcemia; therefore, close scrutiny of patients and dose modification are required. Restriction of dietary calcium may reduce toxicity during calcitriol therapy (Gallagher and Goldgar, 1990). A low incidence of hypercalciuric and hypercalcemic complications of therapy in Japan may reflect relatively poor calcium intakes in that country.

Calcitonin. Calcitonin inhibits osteoclastic bone resorption and modestly increases bone mass in patients with osteoporosis; the largest increases occurred in patients with high intrinsic rates of bone turnover. One study showed that calcitonin nasal spray (200 units/day) reduced the incidence of vertebral compression fractures by ~40% in osteoporotic women (Chesnut et al., 2000).

Thiazide Diuretics. Although not strictly antiresorptive, *thiazides* reduce urinary Ca^{2+} excretion and constrain bone loss in patients with hypercalciuria. Whether they will prove to be useful in patients who are not hypercalciuric is not clear, but data suggest that they reduce hip fracture risk. No sustained effect is observed (Schoofs et al., 2003). Hydrochlorothiazide, 25 mg once or twice daily, may reduce urinary Ca^{2+} excretion substantially. Effective doses of thiazides for reducing urinary Ca^{2+} excretion generally are lower than those necessary for blood pressure control. For a more detailed discussion of thiazide diuretics, see Chapter 25.

Anabolic Agents. Teriparatide. Teriparatide (FORTEO) is the only agent currently available that increases new bone formation. It is FDA-approved for treatment of osteoporosis for up to 2 years in both men and postmenopausal women at high risk for fractures. Teriparatide significantly decreased the incidence of vertebral (4-5% vs. 14%) and nonvertebral fractures (3% vs. 6%) compared to placebo in a prospective, randomized control study (FPT) (Neer et al., 2001). Teriparatide increases predominantly trabecular bone at the lumbar spine and femoral neck; it has less significant effects at cortical sites. Although initial studies showed dose-dependent actions, and side effects, because of concern (and black box label warning), teriparatide is approved at the 20 μg dose, administered once daily by subcutaneous injection in the thigh or abdominal wall. The most common adverse effects associated with teriparatide include injection-site pain, nausea, headaches, leg cramps, and dizziness.

Combination Therapies

Osteoporosis. Because teriparatide stimulates bone formation, whereas bisphosphonates reduce bone resorption, it was predicted that therapy combining the two would enhance the effect on BMD more than treatment with either one alone. However, addition of alendronate to PTH treatment provided no additional benefit for BMD and reduced the anabolic effect of PTH in both women and men (Cosman, 2008). Sequential treatment with PTH(1-84) followed by alendronate increased vertebral BMD to a greater degree than alendronate or estrogen alone (Rittmaster et al., 2000). Recent work underscores the beneficial action of alendronate in consolidating the gains in lumbar spine BMD achieved by antecedent teriparatide treatment in men.

The fracture outcome 30 months after cessation of teriparatide therapy was studied in a cohort of patients included in the FPT. Approximately 50% of each group (teriparatide or control) were treated with a bisphosphonate for some period of time during the 30-month period. Patients treated with bisphosphonates after discontinuation of teriparatide showed continued increments in BMD, whereas those who received no treatment had declines (Prince et al., 2005).

Paget's Disease. Although most patients with Paget's disease require no treatment, factors such as severe pain, neural compression, progressive deformity, hypercalcemia, high-output congestive heart failure, and repeated fracture risk are considered indications for treatment. Bisphosphonates and calcitonin decrease the elevated biochemical markers of bone turnover, such as plasma alkaline phosphatase activity and urinary excretion of hydroxyproline. An initial course of bisphosphonate typically is given once daily or once weekly for 6 months. With treatment, most patients experience a decrease in bone pain over several weeks. Such treatment may induce long-lasting remission. If symptoms recur, additional courses of therapy can be effective. When etidronate is given at higher doses (10-20 mg/kg per day) or continuously for >6 months, there is a substantial risk for osteomalacia. At lower doses (5-7.5 mg/kg per day), focal osteomalacia has been observed occasionally. Defective mineralization has not been observed with other bisphosphonates or with calcitonin.

Choice of optimal therapy for Paget's disease varies among patients. Bisphosphonates are the standard therapy. Intravenous pamidronate induces long-term remission following a single infusion. Zoledronate seems to exhibit greater response rates and a longer median duration of complete response (Major et al., 2001). Compared with calcitonin, bisphosphonates have the advantage of oral administration, lower cost, lack of antigenicity, and generally fewer side effects. Resistance to calcitonin develops in most patients. However, calcitonin is highly reliable and may have a distinct skeletal analgesic property. Mithramycin (plicamycin) has been used in difficult cases of Paget's disease that do not respond to bisphosphonates or calcitonin. Therapeutic utility of this agent is limited by a high potential for hemorrhagic and other toxicities, and it is not generally recommended.

FLUORIDE

Fluoride is discussed because of its toxic properties and its effect on dentition and bone.

Absorption, Distribution, and Excretion. Human beings obtain fluoride predominantly from the ingestion of plants and water, with most absorption taking place in the intestine. The degree of fluoride absorption correlates with its water solubility. Relatively soluble compounds, such as sodium fluoride, are absorbed almost completely, whereas relatively insoluble compounds, such as cryolite (Na_3AlF_6) and the fluoride found in bone meal (fluoroapatite) are absorbed poorly. A second route of absorption is through the lungs, and inhalation of fluoride present in dusts and gases constitutes the major route of industrial exposure.

Fluoride is distributed widely in organs and tissues but is concentrated in bone and teeth, and the skeletal burden is related to intake and age. Bone deposition reflects skeletal turnover; growing bone shows greater deposition than mature bone.

The kidneys are the major site of fluoride excretion. Small amounts of fluoride also appear in sweat, milk, and intestinal secretions; in a very hot environment, sweat can account for nearly 50% of total fluoride excretion.

Pharmacological Actions and Uses. Because it is concentrated in the bone, the radionuclide ^{18}F has been used in skeletal imaging. Sodium fluoride enhances osteoblast activity and increases bone volume. These effects may be bimodal, with low doses stimulating and higher doses suppressing osteoblasts; if true, this may account for the poorly mineralized and mechanically defective bone seen in some studies. In doses of 30-60 mg/day, fluoride increases trabecular bone mineral density in many, but not all, patients. In one controlled trial, fluoride increased lumbar spine density (cancellous bone) but decreased cortical bone mineral density; these changes were associated with a significant increase in peripheral fractures and stress fractures (Riggs et al., 1990). In one study, sustained-release fluoride, which provided lower blood fluoride levels, increased bone mineral density and decreased fractures (Pak et al., 1994). Intermittent courses of slow-release fluoride also have been evaluated. When the total fluoride dose was kept constant (Balena et al., 1998), there was no difference in outcome between continuous and intermittent fluoride treatment; notably, both regimens increased cancellous and trabecular thickness to the same extent. *Unfortunately, increased bone mass is not synonymous with increased bone strength* (Riggs et al., 1990). Thus, the apparent effects of fluoride in osteoporosis are slight compared with those achieved with PTH or other agents.

Other pharmacological actions of fluoride can be classified as toxic. Fluoride inhibits several enzyme systems and diminishes tissue respiration and anaerobic glycolysis.

Acute Poisoning. Acute fluoride poisoning usually results from accidental ingestion of fluoride-containing insecticides or rodenticides. Initial symptoms (salivation, nausea, abdominal pain, vomiting, and diarrhea) are secondary to the local action of fluoride on the intestinal mucosa. Systemic symptoms are varied and severe: increased irritability of the central nervous system consistent with the Ca^{2+}-binding effect of fluoride and the resulting hypocalcemia; hypotension, presumably owing to central vasomotor depression as well as direct cardiotoxicity; and stimulation and then depression of respiration. Death can result from respiratory paralysis or cardiac failure. The lethal dose of sodium fluoride for humans is ~5 g, although there is considerable variation. Treatment includes the intravenous administration of glucose in saline and gastric lavage with lime water (0.15% calcium hydroxide solution) or other Ca^{2+} salts to precipitate the fluoride. Calcium gluconate is given intravenously for tetany; urine volume is kept high with vigorous fluid resuscitation.

Chronic Poisoning. In humans, the major manifestations of chronic ingestion of excessive fluoride are osteosclerosis and mottled enamel. Osteosclerosis is characterized by increased bone density secondary both to elevated osteoblastic activity and to the replacement of hydroxyapatite by the denser fluoroapatite. The degree of skeletal involvement varies from changes that are barely detectable radiologically to marked cortical thickening of long bones, numerous exostoses scattered throughout the skeleton, and calcification of ligaments, tendons, and muscle attachments. In its severest form, it is a disabling and crippling disease.

Mottled enamel, or dental fluorosis, was first described >60 years ago. In very mild mottling, small, opaque, paper-white areas are scattered irregularly over the tooth surface. In severe cases, discrete or confluent, deep brown- to black-stained pits give the tooth a corroded appearance. Mottled enamel results from a partial failure of the enamel-forming ameloblasts to elaborate and lay down enamel. Because mottled enamel is a developmental injury, fluoride ingestion following the eruption of teeth has no effect. Mottling is one of the first visible signs of excess fluoride intake during childhood. Continuous use of water containing ~1 ppm of fluoride may result in very mild mottling in 10% of children; at 4-6 ppm the incidence approaches 100%, with a marked increase in severity.

Severe dental fluorosis formerly occurred in regions where local water supplies had a very high fluoride content (e.g., Pompeii, Italy, and Pike's Peak, Colorado). Current regulations in the U.S. require lowering the fluoride content of the water supply or providing an alternative source of acceptable drinking water for affected communities. Sustained consumption of water with a fluoride content of 4 mg/L (4 ppm) is associated with deficits in cortical bone mass and increased rates of bone loss over time (Sowers et al., 1991).

Fluoride and Dental Caries. After a new water supply was established, children in Bauxite, Arkansas, had a much higher incidence of caries than those who had been exposed to the former fluoride-containing water. Subsequent studies established definitely that supplementation of water fluoride content to 1.0 ppm is a safe and practical intervention that substantially reduces the incidence of caries in permanent teeth.

There are partial benefits for children who begin drinking fluoridated water at any age; however, optimal benefits are obtained at ages before permanent teeth erupt. Topical application of fluoride solutions by dental personnel appears to be particularly effective on newly erupted teeth and can reduce the incidence of caries by 30-40%. Dietary fluoride supplements should be considered for children <12 years of age whose drinking water contains <0.7 ppm fluoride. Conflicting results have been reported from studies of fluoride-containing toothpastes.

Adequate incorporation of fluoride into teeth hardens the outer layers of enamel and increases resistance to demineralization. Fluoride deposition apparently involves exchange with hydroxyl or citrate anions in the enamel apatite crystal surface. The mechanism by which fluoride prevents caries is not completely understood. There is no convincing evidence that fluoride from any source reduces the development of caries after the permanent teeth are completely formed (usually ~14 years of age).

The fluoride salts usually employed in dentifrices are sodium fluoride and stannous fluoride. Sodium fluoride also is available in a variety of preparations for oral and topical use, including tablets, drops, rinses, and gels.

Since its inception, regulation of the fluoride concentration of community water supplies periodically has encountered vocal opposition, including allegations of putative adverse health consequences of fluoridated water. Careful examination of these issues indicates that cancer and all-cause mortalities do not differ significantly between communities with fluoridated and nonfluoridated water (Richmond, 1985).

CLINICAL SUMMARY

Increasing evidence supports the concept that regular physical activity, adequate calcium intake, and lifestyle changes have a positive impact on bone remodeling, constrain bone loss, and reduce fracture risk. Antiresorptive agents such as bisphosphonates, estrogen, selective estrogen response modulators (SERMs), and calcium slow bone resorption. Recombinant human PTH is available for the treatment of osteoporosis and provides significant intervention for restoring normal bone mass.

Cinacalcet, a drug that acts directly on the parathyroid calcium-sensing receptor, provides a novel approach to decreasing PTH secretion in secondary hyperparathyroidism and parathyroid carcinoma. Improved assays for measuring biologically active and inactive forms of PTH may facilitate the diagnosis and treatment of diseases associated with PTH resistance.

Estrogen-replacement therapy, once a mainstay treatment for osteoporosis in women, has been curtailed by the findings of the Women's Health Initiative: Despite estrogen's beneficial effects on bone and fracture risk, alone or in combination with *progestin,* estrogen promotes an array of serious adverse cardiovascular consequences. The FDA now recommends that estrogen be reserved for women at significant risk of osteoporosis who cannot take other medications.

BIBLIOGRAPHY

Alon US, Levy-Olomucki R, Moore WV, et al. Calcimimetics as an adjuvant treatment for familial hypophosphatemic rickets. *Clin J Am Soc Nephrol,* **2008,** *3*:658–664.

Anderson GL, Limacher M, Assaf AR, et al. Effects of conjugated equine estrogen in postmenopausal women with hysterectomy: The Women's Health Initiative randomized controlled trial. *JAMA,* **2004,** *291*:1701–1712.

Anonymous. Drugs for postmenopausal osteoporosis. *Treat Guidel Med Lett,* **2008,** *6*:67–74.

Anonymous. Drugs for prevention and treatment of postmenopausal osteoporosis. *Treat Guidel Med Lett,* **2005,** *3*:69–74.

Balena R, Kleerekoper M, Foldes JA, et al. Effects of different regimens of sodium fluoride treatment for osteoporosis on the structure, remodeling and mineralization of bone. *Osteoporos Int,* **1998,** *8*:428–435.

Ballock RT, O'Keefe RJ. The biology of the growth plate. *J Bone Joint Surg,* **2003,** *85-A*:715–726.

Bergwitz C, Jüppner H. Regulation of phosphate homeostasis by PTN, vitamin D, and FGF 23. *Annu Rev Med*, **2010,** *61*: 91–104.

Bianco SD, Peng JB, Takanaga H, et al. Marked disturbance of calcium homeostasis in mice with targeted disruption of the Trpv6 calcium channel gene. *J Bone Miner Res,* **2007,** *22*: 274–285.

Bilezikian JP, Potts JT Jr, Fuleihan Gel H, et al. Summary statement from a workshop on asymptomatic primary hyperparathyroidism: A perspective for the 21st century. *J Bone Miner Res,* **2002,** *17 suppl 2*:N2–N11.

Bischoff-Ferrari HA, Shao A, Dawson-Hughes B, et al. Benefit-risk assessment of vitamin D supplementation. *Osteoporos Int,* **2009** December 3 (Epub ahead of print).

Black DM, Bilezikian JP, Ensrud KE, et al. One year of alendronate after one year of parathyroid hormone (1-84) for osteoporosis. *N Engl J Med,* **2005,** *353*:555–565.

Black DM, Delmas PD, Eastell R, et al. Once-yearly zoledronic acid for treatment of postmenopausal osteoporosis. *N Engl J Med,* **2007,** *356*:1809–1822.

Bland R, Walker EA, Hughes SV, et al. Constitutive expression of 25-hydroxyvitamin D_3-1a-hydroxylase in a transformed human proximal tubule cell line: Evidence for direct regulation of vitamin D metabolism by calcium. *Endocrinology,* **1999,** *140*:2027–2034.

Bodnar LM, Simhan HN, Powers RW, et al. High prevalence of vitamin D insufficiency in black and white pregnant women residing in the northern United States and their neonates. *J Nutr,* **2007,** *137*:447–452.

Bone HG, Hosking D, Devogelaer JP, et al. Ten years' experience with alendronate for osteoporosis in postmenopausal women. *N Engl J Med,* **2004,** *350*:1189–1199.

Carney SL. Calcitonin and human renal calcium and electrolyte transport. *Miner Electrolyte Metab,* **1997,** *23*:43–47.

Carswell S. Vitamin D in the nervous system: Action and therapeutic potential. In: *Vitamin D.* (Feldman D, Glorieux FH, Pike JW, eds.), Academic Press, San Diego, **1997,** pp. 1197–1212.

Cauley JA, Lacroix AZ, Wu L, et al. Serum 25-hydroxyvitamin D concentrations and risk for hip fractures. *Ann Intern Med,* **2008,** *149*:242–250.

Cauley JA, Robbins J, Chen Z, et al. Effects of estrogen plus progestin on risk of fracture and bone mineral density: The Women's Health Initiative randomized trial. *JAMA,* **2003,** *290*: 1729–1738.

Chesnut CH 3rd, Silverman S, Andriano K, et al. A randomized trial of nasal spray salmon calcitonin in postmenopausal women with established osteoporosis: The prevent recurrence of osteoporotic fractures study. PROOF Study Group. *Am J Med,* **2000,** *109*:267–276.

Clemett D, Spencer CM. Raloxifene: A review of its use in postmenopausal osteoporosis. *Drugs,* **2000,** *60*:379–411.

Cosman F. Parathyroid hormone treatment for osteoporosis. *Curr Opin Endocrinol, Diabetes Obes,* **2008,** *15*:495–501.

Costante G, Meringolo D, Durante C, *et al.* Predictive value of serum calcitonin levels for preoperative diagnosis of medullary thyroid carcinoma in a cohort of 5817 consecutive patients with thyroid nodules. *J Clin Endocrinol Metab,* **2007,** *92*:450–455.

Cummings SR, McClung MR, Christiansen C, et al. A phase III study of the effects of denosumab on vertebral, nonvertebral, and hip fracture in women with osteoporosis: results from the FREEDOM trail. *J Bone Miner Res,* **2008,** *12*:S80.

D'Amour P. Lessons from a second- and third-generation parathyroid hormone assays in renal failure patients. *J Endocrinol Invest,* **2008,** *31*:459–462.

Dawson-Hughes B, Harris SS, Krall EA, et al. Effect of calcium and vitamin D supplementation on bone density in men and women 65 years of age or older. *N Engl J Med,* **1997,** *337*:670–676.

Delmas PD, Benhamou CL, Man Z, et al. Monthly dosing of 75 mg risedronate on 2 consecutive days a month: Efficacy and safety results. *Osteoporos Int,* **2008,** *19*:1039–1045.

DeLuca HF. The vitamin D story: A collaborative effort of basic science and clinical medicine. *FASEB J,* **1988,** *2*:224–236.

Drueke TB, Ritz E. Treatment of secondary hyperparathyroidism in CKD patients with cinacalcet and/or vitamin D derivatives. *Clin J Am Soc Nephrol,* **2009,** *4*:234–241.

Dunford JE, Thompson K, Coxon FP, et al. Structure-activity relationships for inhibition of farnesyl diphosphate synthase in vitro and inhibition of bone resorption in vivo by nitrogen-containing bisphosphonates. *J Pharmacol Exp Ther,* **2001,** *296*:235–242.

Edwards BJ, Gounder M, McKoy JM, et al. Pharmacovigilance and reporting oversight in US FDA fast-track process: Bisphosphonates and osteonecrosis of the jaw. *Lancet Oncol,* **2008,** *9*:1166–1172.

Eknoyan G, Levin A, Levin NW. Bone metabolism and disease in chronic kidney disease. *Am J Kidney Dis,* **2003,** *42*:1–201.

Elders PJ, Lips P, Netelenbos JC, et al. Long-term effect of calcium supplementation on bone loss in perimenopausal women. *J Bone Miner Res,* **1994,** *9*:963–970.

Ettinger B, Black DM, Mitlak BH, et al. Reduction of vertebral fracture risk in postmenopausal women with osteoporosis treated with raloxifene: results from a 3-year randomized clinical trial. Multiple Outcomes of Raloxifene Evaluation (MORE) Investigators. *JAMA,* **1999,** *282*:637–645.

Evenepoel P. Calcimimetics in chronic kidney disease: Evidence, opportunities and challenges. *Kidney Int,* **2008,** *74*:265–275.

Finkelstein JS, Hayes A, Hunzelman JL, et al. The effects of parathyroid hormone, alendronate, or both in men with osteoporosis. *N Engl J Med,* **2003,** *349*:1216–1226.

Franceschini N, Joy MS, Kshirsagar A. Cinacalcet HCl: A calcimimetic agent for the management of primary and secondary hyperparathyroidism. *Expert Opin Investig Drugs,* **2003,** *12*:1413–1421.

Friedman PA, Bushinsky DA. Diuretic effects on calcium metabolism. *Semin Nephrol,* **1999,** *19*:551–556.

Gallagher JC, Goldgar D. Treatment of postmenopausal osteoporosis with high doses of synthetic calcitriol. A randomized controlled study. *Ann Intern Med,* **1990,** *113*:649–655.

Gnant M, Mlineritsch B, Schippinger W, et al. Endocrine therapy plus zoledronic acid in premenopausal breast cancer. *N Engl J Med,* **2009,** *360*:679–691.

Gorn AH, Rudolph SM, Flannery MR, et al. Expression of two human skeletal calcitonin receptor isoforms cloned from a giant cell tumor of bone. The first intracellular domain modulates ligand binding and signal transduction. *J Clin Invest,* **1995,** *95*:2680–2691.

Greenspan SL, Bone HG, Ettinger MP, et al. Effect of recombinant human parathyroid hormone (1-84) on vertebral fracture and bone mineral density in postmenopausal women with osteoporosis: A randomized trial. *Ann Intern Med,* **2007,** *146*: 326–339.

Grey A, Lucas J, Horne A, et al. Vitamin D repletion in patients with primary hyperparathyroidism and coexistent vitamin D insufficiency. *J Clin Endocrinol Metab,* **2005,** *90*:2122–2126.

Grill V, Rankin W, Martin TJ. Parathyroid hormone related protein (PTHrP) and hypercalcaemia. *Eur J Cancer [A],* **1998,** *34*:222–229.

Halasy-Nagy JM, Rodan GA, Reszka AA. Inhibition of bone resorption by alendronate and risedronate does not require osteoclast apoptosis. *Bone,* **2001,** *29*:553–559.

Hay DL, Christopoulos G, Christopoulos A, et al. Pharmacological discrimination of calcitonin receptor: receptor activity-modifying protein complexes. *Mol Pharmacol,* **2005,** *67*: 1655–1665.

Herberth J, Monier-Faugere MC, Mawad HW, et al. The five most commonly used intact parathyroid hormone assays are useful for screening but not for diagnosing bone turnover abnormalities in CKD-5 patients. *Clin Nephrol,* **2009,** *72*: 5–14.

Hewison M, Zehnder D, Chakraverty R, et al. Vitamin D and barrier function: A novel role for extra-renal 1α-hydroxylase. *Mol Cell Endocrinol,* **2004,** *215*:31–38.

Hirsch PF, Baruch H. Is calcitonin an important physiological substance? *Endocrine,* **2003,** *21*:201–208.

Hodsman AB, Bauer DC, Dempster DW, et al. Parathyroid hormone and teriparatide for the treatment of osteoporosis: A review of the evidence and suggested guidelines for its use. *Endocrine Rev,* **2005,** *26*:688–703.

Hollis BW, Wagner CL. Assessment of dietary vitamin D requirements during pregnancy and lactation. *Am J Clin Nutr,* **2004,** *79*:717–726.

Institute of Medicine (U.S.). *Dietary Reference Intakes: Applications in Dietary Planning*. National Academy Press, Washington, **2003,** pp 969–998.

Jackson RD, LaCroix AZ, Gass M, et al. Calcium plus vitamin D supplementation and the risk of fractures. *N Engl J Med,* **2006,** *354*:669–683.

Johnston CC Jr, Miller JZ, Slemenda CW, et al. Calcium supplementation and increases in bone mineral density in children. *N Engl J Med,* **1992,** *327*:82–87.

Jolette J, Wilker CE, Smith SY, et al. Defining a noncarcinogenic dose of recombinant human parathyroid hormone 1-84 in a 2-year study in Fischer 344 rats. *Toxicol Pathol,* **2006,** *34*: 929–940.

Jüppner H, Potts JT Jr. Immunoassays for the detection of parathyroid hormone. *J Bone Miner Res,* **2002,** *17 suppl 2*:N81–N86.

Jüppner HW, Gardella TJ, Brown EM, et al. Parathyroid hormone and parathyroid hormone-related peptide in the regulation of calcium homeostasis and bone development. In: *Endocrinology*. (DeGroot LJ, Jameson JL, eds.), W.B. Saunders Company, Philadelphia, **2001,** pp. 969–998.

Khosla S. Minireview: The OPG/RANKL/RANK system. *Endocrinology,* **2001,** *142*:5050–5055.

Kissmeyer AM, Binderup L. Calcipotriol (MC 903): Pharmacokinetics in rats and biological activities of metabolites. A comparative study with $1,25(OH)_2D_3$. *Biochem Pharmacol,* **1991,** *41*:1601–1606.

Kowalzick L. Clinical experience with topical calcitriol (1,25-dihydroxyvitamin D_3) in psoriasis. *Br J Dermatol,* **2001,** *144 Suppl 58*:21–25.

Kragballe K, Iversen L. Calcipotriol. A new topical antipsoriatic. *Dermatol Clin,* **1993,** *11*:137–141.

Levine MA, Germain-Lee E, Jan de Beur S. Genetic basis for resistance to parathyroid hormone. *Horm Res,* **2003,** *60 suppl 3*:87–95.

Liberman UA, Weiss SR, Broll J, et al. Effect of oral alendronate on bone mineral density and the incidence of fractures in postmenopausal osteoporosis. The Alendronate Phase III Osteoporosis Treatment Study Group. *N Engl J Med,* **1995,** *333*:1437–1443.

Lin HY, Harris TL, Flannery MS, et al. Expression cloning of an adenylate cyclase-coupled calcitonin receptor. *Science,* **1991,** *254*:1022–1024.

Major P, Lortholary A, Hon J, et al. Zoledronic acid is superior to pamidronate in the treatment of hypercalcemia of malignancy: A pooled analysis of two randomized, controlled clinical trials. *J Clin Oncol,* **2001,** *19*:558–567.

Malloy PJ, Pike JW, Feldman D. Hereditary 1,25-dihydroxyvitamin D-resistant rickets. In: *Vitamin D* (Feldman D, Pike JW, Glorieux FH, eds.), Elsevier, Burlington, MA, **2005,** pp. 1207–1237.

Manolagas SC, Kousteni S, Jilka RL. Sex steroids and bone. *Recent Prog Horm Res,* **2002,** *57*:385–409.

Martin KJ, Gonzalez EA, Gellens M, et al. 19-Nor-1-α-25-dihydroxyvitamin D_2 (Paricalcitol) safely and effectively reduces the levels of intact parathyroid hormone in patients on hemodialysis. *J Am Soc Nephrol,* **1998,** *9*:1427–1432.

Martin TJ, Ng KW. Mechanisms by which cells of the osteoblast lineage control osteoclast formation and activity. *J Cell Biochem,* **1994,** *56*:357–366.

McDonnell DP, Mangelsdorf DJ, Pike JW, et al. Molecular cloning of complementary DNA encoding the avian receptor for vitamin D. *Science,* **1987,** *235*:1214–1217.

Michaelsson K, Melhus H, Bellocco R, et al. Dietary calcium and vitamin D intake in relation to osteoporotic fracture risk. *Bone,* **2003,** *32*:694–703.

Monier-Faugere MC, Geng Z, Mawad H, et al. Improved assessment of bone turnover by the PTH-(1-84)/large C-PTH fragments ratio in ESRD patients. *Kidney Int,* **2001,** *60*:1460–1468.

Morony S, Warmington K, Adamu S, et al. The inhibition of RANKL causes greater suppression of bone resorption and hypercalcemia compared with bisphosphonates in two models of humoral hypercalcemia of malignancy. *Endocrinology,* **2005,** *146*:3235–3243.

Nagpal S, Na S, Rathnachalam R. Noncalcemic actions of vitamin D receptor ligands. *Endocrine Rev,* **2005,** *26*:662–687.

Naro F, Perez M, Migliaccio S, et al. Phospholipase D- and PKC isoenzyme-dependent signal transduction pathways activated by the calcitonin receptor. *Endocrinology,* **1998,** *139*: 3241–3248.

Neer RM, Arnaud CD, Zanchetta JR, et al. Effect of parathyroid hormone (1-34) on fractures and bone mineral density in postmenopausal women with osteoporosis. *N Engl J Med,* **2001,** *344*:1434–1441.

O'Brien CA, Plotkin LI, Galli C, et al. Control of bone mass and remodeling by PTH receptor signaling in osteocytes. *PLoS ONE,* **2008,** *3*:e2942.

Okazaki M, Ferrandon S, Vilardaga JP, et al. Prolonged signaling at the parathyroid hormone receptor by peptide ligands targeted to a specific receptor conformation. *Proc Natl Acad Sci USA,* **2008,** *105*:16525–16530.

Padhi D, Harris R. Clinical pharmacokinetic and pharmacodynamic profile of cinacalcet hydrochloride. *Clin Pharmacokinet,* **2009,** *48*:303–311.

Pak CY, Sakhaee K, Piziak V, et al. Slow-release sodium fluoride in the management of postmenopausal osteoporosis. A randomized controlled trial. *Ann Intern Med,* **1994,** *120*: 625–632.

Peacock M, Bolognese MA, Borofsky M, et al. Cinacalcet treatment of primary hyperparathyroidism: Biochemical and bone densitometric outcomes in a five-year study. *J Clin Endocrinol Metab,* **2009,** *94*:4860–4867.

Perez AV, Picotto G, Carpentieri AR, et al. Minireview on regulation of intestinal calcium absorption. Emphasis on molecular mechanisms of transcellular pathway. *Digestion,* **2008,** *77*:22–34.

Pike JW, Shevde NK. The vitamin D receptor. In: *Vitamin D.* (Feldman D, Pike JW, Glorieux FH, eds.), Elsevier, Burlington, MA, **2005,** pp. 167–191.

Plotkin H, Gundberg C, Mitnick M, et al. Dissociation of bone formation from resorption during 2-week treatment with human parathyroid hormone-related peptide-(1-36) in humans: Potential as an anabolic therapy for osteoporosis. *J Clin Endocrinol Metab,* **1998,** *83*:2786–2791.

Pollak MR, Seidman CE, Brown EM. Three inherited disorders of calcium sensing. *Medicine,* **1996,** *75*:115–123.

Prince R, Sipos A, Hossain A, et al. Sustained nonvertebral fragility fracture risk reduction after discontinuation of teriparatide treatment. *J Bone Miner Res,* **2005,** *20*:1507–1513.

Purdue BW, Tilakaratne N, Sexton PM. Molecular pharmacology of the calcitonin receptor. *Receptors Channels,* **2002,** *8*: 243–255.

Quamme GA. Molecular identification of ancient and modern mammalian magnesium transporters. *Am J Physiol Cell Physiol,* **2010,** *298*:C407–429.

Razzaque MS. FGF23-mediated regulation of systemic phosphate homeostasis: Is Klotho an essential player? *Am J Physiol,* **2009,** *296*:F470–476.

Recker RR, Davies KM, Hinders SM, *et al.* Bone gain in young adult women. *JAMA,* **1992,** *268*:2403–2408.

Reid IR, Miller P, Lyles K, et al. Comparison of a single infusion of zoledronic acid with risedronate for Paget's disease. *N Engl J Med,* **2005,** *353*:898–908.

Richmond VL. Thirty years of fluoridation: A review. *Am J Clin Nutr,* **1985,** *41*:129–138.

Riggs BL, Hodgson SF, O'Fallon WM, et al. Effect of fluoride treatment on the fracture rate in postmenopausal women with osteoporosis. *N Engl J Med,* **1990,** *322*:802–809.

Rittmaster RS, Bolognese M, Ettinger MP, et al. Enhancement of bone mass in osteoporotic women with parathyroid hormone followed by alendronate. *J Clin Endocrinol Metab,* **2000,** *85*:2129–2134.

Rogers MJ. New insights into the molecular mechanisms of action of bisphosphonates. *Curr Pharm Des,* **2003,** *9*:2643–2658.

Roodman GD, Windle JJ. Paget disease of bone. *J Clin Invest* **2005,** *115*:200–208.

Russell RG. Bisphosphonates: Mode of action and pharmacology. *Pediatrics,* **2007,** *119 Suppl 2*:S150–162.

Schoofs MW, van der Klift M, Hofman A, et al. Thiazide diuretics and the risk for hip fracture. *Ann Intern Med,* **2003,** *139*: 476–482.

Shoback DM, Bilezikian JP, Turner SA, et al. The calcimimetic cinacalcet normalizes serum calcium in subjects with primary hyperparathyroidism. *J Clin Endocrinol Metab,* **2003,** *88*: 5644–5649.

Selim AA, Mahon M, Juppner H, Bringhurst FR, Divieti P. Role of calcium channels in carboxyl-terminal parathyroid hormone receptor signaling. *Am J Physiol Cell Physiol,* **2006,** *291*: C114–C121.

Singh AT, Gilchrist A, Voyno-Yasenetskaya T, et al. $G\alpha_{12}/G\alpha_{13}$ subunits of heterotrimeric G proteins mediate parathyroid hormone activation of phospholipase D in UMR-106 osteoblastic cells. *Endocrinology,* **2005,** *146*:2171–2175.

Slatopolsky E, Cozzolino M, Lu Y, *et al.* Efficacy of 19-nor-1,25-$(OH)_2D_2$ in the prevention and treatment of hyperparathyroid bone disease in experimental uremia. *Kidney Int,* **2003,** *63*:2020–2027.

Sneddon WB, Syme CA, Bisello A, et al. Activation-independent parathyroid hormone receptor internalization is regulated by NHERF1 (EBP50). *J Biol Chem,* **2003,** *278*:43787–43796.

Sowers MF, Clark MK, Jannausch ML, et al. A prospective study of bone mineral content and fracture in communities with differential fluoride exposure. *Am J Epidemiol,* **1991,** *133*: 649–660.

Spear GT, Paulnock DM, Helgeson DO, et al. Requirement of differentiative signals of both interferon-gamma and 1,25-dihydroxyvitamin D_3 for induction and secretion of interleukin-1 by HL-60 cells. *Cancer Res,* **1988,** *48*:1740–1744.

Stenbeck G, Horton MA. A new specialized cell-matrix interaction in actively resorbing osteoclasts. *J Cell Sci,* **2000,** *113*: 1577–1587.

Suda T, Takahashi N, Udagawa N, *et al.* Modulation of osteoclast differentiation and function by the new members of the tumor necrosis factor receptor and ligand families. *Endocrine Rev,* **1999,** *20*:345–357.

Suda T, Ueno Y, Fujii, K, et al. Vitamin D and bone. *J Cell Biochem,* **2003,** *88*:259–266.

Takahashi S, Goldring S, Katz M, et al. Downregulation of calcitonin receptor mRNA expression by calcitonin during human osteoclast-like cell differentiation. *J Clin Invest,* **1995,** *95*:167–171.

Tashjian AH Jr, Goltzman D. On the interpretation of rat carcinogenicity studies for human PTH(1-34) and human PTH(1-84). *J Bone Miner Res,* **2008,** *23*:803–811.

Teng GG, Curtis JR, Saag KG. Mortality and osteoporotic fractures: Is the link causal, and is it modifiable? *Clin Exp Rheumatol,* **2008,** *26*:S125–S137.

Tonino RP, Meunier PJ, Emkey R, et al. Skeletal benefits of alendronate: 7-year treatment of postmenopausal osteoporotic women. Phase III Osteoporosis Treatment Study Group. *J Clin Endocrinol Metab,* **2000,** *85*:3109–3115.

Tucci JR, Tonino RP, Emkey RD, et al. Effect of three years of oral alendronate treatment in postmenopausal women with osteoporosis. *Am J Med,* **1996,** *101*:488–501.

Vahle JL, Long GG, Sandusky G, *et al.* Bone neoplasms in F344 rats given teriparatide [rhPTH(1-34)] are dependent on duration of treatment and dose. *Toxicol Pathol,* **2004,** *32*: 426–438.

Van Cromphaut SJ, Dewerchin M, Hoenderop JG, *et al.* Duodenal calcium absorption in vitamin D receptor-knockout mice: Functional and molecular aspects. *Proc Natl Acad Sci USA,* **2001,** *98*:13324–13329.

van den Bemd GJ, Pols HA, van Leeuwen JP. Anti-tumor effects of 1,25-dihydroxyvitamin D_3 and vitamin D analogs. *Curr Pharm Des,* **2000,** *6*:717–732.

Vieth R. Vitamin D supplementation,25-hydroxyvitamin D concentrations, and safety. *Am J Clin Nutr*, **1999,** 69:842-856.

Wagner CL, Greer FR. Prevention of rickets and vitamin D deficiency in infants, children, and adolescents. *Pediatrics,* **2008,** *122*:1142–1152.

White KE, Jonsson KB, Carn G, et al. The autosomal dominant hypophosphatemic rickets (ADHR) gene is a secreted polypeptide overexpressed by tumors that cause phosphate wasting. *J Clin Endocrinol Metab,* **2001,** *86*:497–500.

Yu DW, Yu SH, Schuster V, *et al.* Identification of two novel deletion mutations within the $G_s\alpha$ gene (*GNAS1*) in Albright hereditary osteodystrophy. *J Clin Endocrinol Metab,* **1999,** *84*:3254–3259.

Zanello LP, Norman AW. Rapid modulation of osteoblast ion channel responses by 1α,25(OH)$_2$-vitamin D_3 requires the presence of a functional vitamin D nuclear receptor. *Proc Natl Acad Sci USA,* **2004,** *101*:1589–1594.

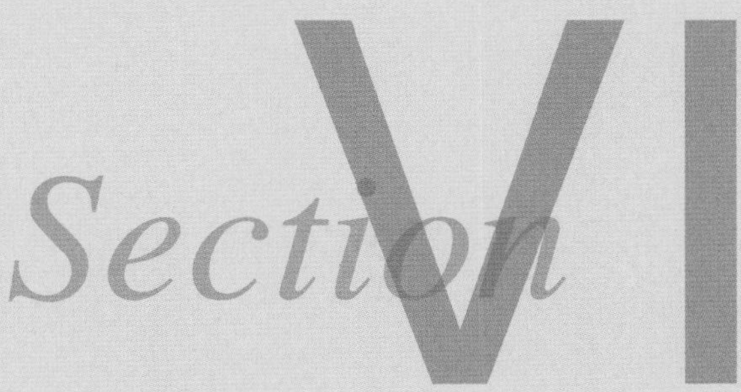

Drugs Affecting Gastrointestinal Function

Pharmacotherapy of Gastric Acidity, Peptic Ulcers, and Gastroesophageal Reflux Disease

John L. Wallace and
Keith A. Sharkey

The acid-peptic diseases are those disorders in which gastric acid and pepsin are necessary, but usually not sufficient, pathogenic factors. Although inherently caustic, acid and pepsin in the stomach normally do not produce damage or symptoms because of intrinsic defense mechanisms. Barriers to the reflux of gastric contents into the esophagus comprise the primary esophageal defense. If these protective barriers fail and reflux occurs, dyspepsia and/or erosive esophagitis may result. Therapies are directed at decreasing gastric acidity, enhancing the lower esophageal sphincter, or stimulating esophageal motility (Chapter 46). The stomach is protected by a number of factors, collectively referred to as "mucosal defense," many of which are stimulated by the local generation of prostaglandins and NO (Wallace, 2008). If these defenses are disrupted, a gastric or duodenal ulcer may form. The treatment and prevention of these acid-related disorders are accomplished by decreasing gastric acidity and enhancing mucosal defense. The appreciation that an infectious agent, *Helicobacter pylori*, plays a key role in the pathogenesis of acid-peptic diseases has stimulated new approaches to prevention and therapy.

PHYSIOLOGY OF GASTRIC SECRETION

Gastric acid secretion is a complex, continuous process in which multiple central and peripheral factors contribute to a common end point: the secretion of H^+ by parietal cells. Neuronal (acetylcholine, ACh), paracrine (histamine), and endocrine (gastrin) factors all regulate acid secretion (Figure 45–1). Their specific receptors (M_3, H_2, and CCK_2, respectively) are on the basolateral membrane of parietal cells in the body and fundus of the stomach. Some of these receptors are also present on enterochromaffin-like cells (ECL), where they regulate the release of histamine. The H_2 receptor is a GPCR (Chapters 3 and 32) that activates the G_s–adenylyl cyclase–cyclic AMP–PKA pathway. ACh and gastrin signal through GPCRs that couple to the G_q–PLC-IP_3–Ca^{2+} pathway in parietal cells. In parietal cells, the cyclic AMP and the Ca^{2+}-dependent pathways activate H^+, K^+-ATPase (the proton pump), which exchanges hydrogen and potassium ions across the parietal cell membrane. This pump generates the largest ion gradient known in vertebrates, with an intracellular pH of ~7.3 and an intracanalicular pH of ~0.8.

The most important structures for CNS stimulation of gastric acid secretion are the dorsal motor nucleus of the vagal nerve, the hypothalamus, and the solitary tract nucleus. Efferent fibers originating in the dorsal motor nuclei descend to the stomach via the vagus nerve and synapse with ganglion cells of the enteric nervous system. ACh release from postganglionic vagal fibers directly stimulates gastric acid secretion through muscarinic M_3 receptors on the basolateral membrane of parietal cells. The CNS predominantly modulates the activity of the enteric nervous system via ACh, stimulating gastric acid secretion in response to the sight, smell, taste, or anticipation of food (the "cephalic" phase of acid secretion). ACh also indirectly affects parietal cells by increasing the release of histamine from the ECL cells in the fundus of the stomach and of gastrin from G cells in the gastric antrum.

ECL cells, the source of gastric histamine, usually are in close proximity to parietal cells. Histamine acts as a paracrine mediator, diffusing from its site of release to nearby parietal cells, where it activates H_2 receptors. The critical role of histamine in gastric acid secretion is dramatically demonstrated by the efficacy of H_2 receptor antagonists in decreasing gastric acid secretion.

Gastrin, which is produced by antral G cells, is the most potent inducer of acid secretion. Multiple pathways stimulate gastrin release, including CNS activation, local distention, and chemical

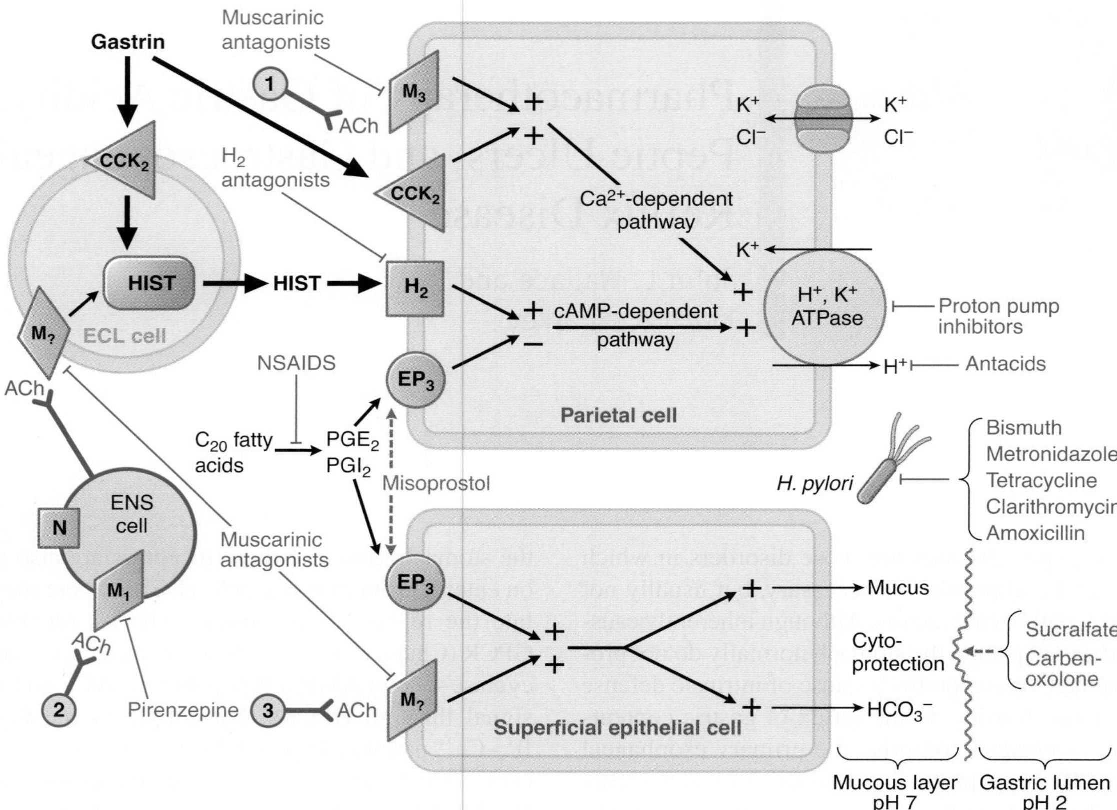

Figure 45–1. *Physiological and pharmacological regulation of gastric secretion: the basis for therapy of acid-peptic disorders.* Shown are the interactions among an enterochromaffin-like (ECL) cell that secretes histamine, a ganglion cell of the enteric nervous system (ENS), a parietal cell that secretes acid, and a superficial epithelial cell that secretes mucus and bicarbonate. Physiological pathways, shown in solid black, may be stimulatory (+) or inhibitory (–). ***1*** and ***3*** indicate possible inputs from postganglionic cholinergic fibers; ***2*** shows neural input from the vagus nerve. Physiological agonists and their respective membrane receptors include acetylcholine (ACh), muscarinic (M), and nicotinic (N) receptors; gastrin, cholecystokinin receptor 2 (CCK_2); histamine (HIST), H_2 receptor; and prostaglandin E_2 (PGE_2), EP_3 receptor. A red ——┤ indicates targets of pharmacological antagonism. A light blue dashed arrow indicates a drug action that mimics or enhances a physiological pathway. Shown in red are drugs used to treat acid-peptic disorders. NSAIDs are nonsteroidal anti-inflammatory drugs, which can induce ulcers via inhibition of cyclooxygenase.

components of the gastric contents. Gastrin stimulates acid secretion indirectly by inducing the release of histamine by ECL cells; a direct effect on parietal cells also plays a lesser role.

Somatostatin (SST), which is produced by antral D cells, inhibits gastric acid secretion. Acidification of the gastric luminal pH to <3 stimulates SST release, which in turn suppresses gastrin release in a negative feedback loop. SST-producing cells are decreased in patients with *H. pylori* infection, and the consequent reduction of SST's inhibitory effect may contribute to excess gastrin production.

Gastric Defenses Against Acid. The extremely high concentration of H^+ in the gastric lumen requires robust defense mechanisms to protect the esophagus and the stomach. The primary esophageal defense is the lower esophageal sphincter, which prevents reflux of acidic gastric contents into the esophagus. The stomach protects itself from acid damage by a number of mechanisms that require adequate mucosal blood flow, perhaps because of the high metabolic activity and oxygen requirements of the gastric mucosa. One key defense is the secretion of a mucus layer that helps to protect gastric epithelial cells by trapping secreted bicarbonate at the cell surface. Gastric mucus is soluble when secreted but quickly forms an insoluble gel that coats the mucosal surface of the stomach, slows ion diffusion, and prevents mucosal damage by macromolecules such as pepsin. Mucus production is stimulated by prostaglandins E_2 and I_2, which also directly inhibit gastric acid secretion by parietal cells. Thus, drugs that inhibit prostaglandin formation (e.g., NSAIDs, ethanol) decrease mucus secretion and predispose to the development of acid-peptic disease.

Figure 45–1 outlines the rationale and pharmacological basis for the therapy of acid-peptic diseases. The proton pump inhibitors are used most commonly, followed by the histamine H_2 receptor antagonists.

PROTON PUMP INHIBITORS

Chemistry; Mechanism of Action; Pharmacology. The most potent suppressors of gastric acid secretion are inhibitors of the gastric H^+, K^+-ATPase (proton pump) (Figure 45–2). In typical doses, these drugs diminish the daily production of acid (basal and stimulated) by 80-95%. Six proton pump inhibitors are available for clinical use: omeprazole (PRILOSEC, others) and its S-isomer, esomeprazole (NEXIUM), lansoprazole (PREVACID) and its R-enantiomer, dexlansoprazole (KAPIDEX), rabeprazole (ACIPHEX), and pantoprazole (PROTONIX, others). These drugs have different substitutions on their pyridine and/or benzimidazole groups but are remarkably similar in their pharmacological properties (Appendix II). Omeprazole is a racemic mixture of R- and S-isomers; the S-isomer, esomeprazole (S-omeprazole), is eliminated less rapidly than R-omeprazole, which theoretically provides a therapeutic advantage because of the increased $t_{1/2}$. Despite claims to the contrary, all proton pump inhibitors have equivalent efficacy at comparable doses.

Proton pump inhibitors (PPIs) are prodrugs that require activation in an acid environment. After absorption into the systemic circulation, the prodrug diffuses into the parietal cells of the stomach and accumulates in the acidic secretory canaliculi. Here, it is activated by proton-catalyzed formation of a tetracyclic sulfenamide (Figure 45–2), trapping the drug so that it cannot diffuse back across the canalicular membrane. The activated form then binds covalently with sulfhydryl groups of cysteines in the H^+, K^+-ATPase, irreversibly inactivating the pump molecule. Acid secretion resumes only after new pump molecules are synthesized and inserted into the luminal membrane, providing a prolonged (up to 24- to 48-hour) suppression of acid secretion, despite the much shorter plasma half-lives (0.5-2 hours) of the parent compounds. Because they block the final step in acid production, the proton pump inhibitors are effective in acid suppression regardless of other stimulating factors.

To prevent degradation of proton pump inhibitors by acid in the gastric lumen, oral dosage forms are supplied in different formulations:

- enteric-coated drugs contained inside gelatin capsules (omeprazole, dexlansoprazole, esomeprazole, and lansoprazole)

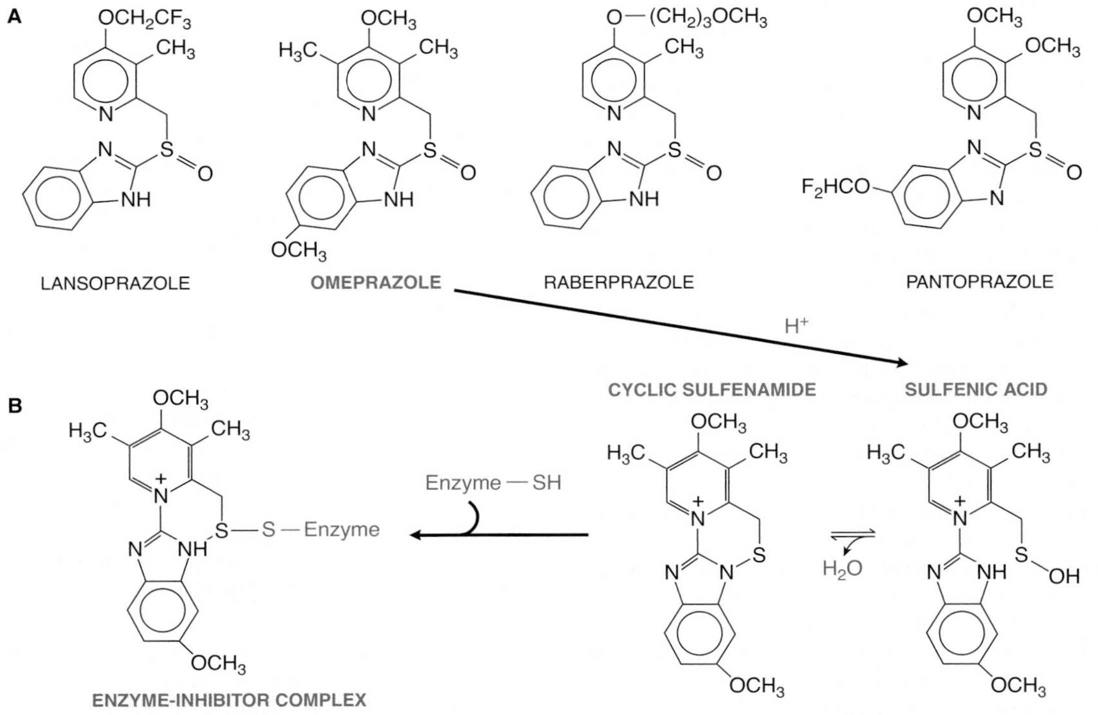

A

LANSOPRAZOLE

OMEPRAZOLE

RABERPRAZOLE

PANTOPRAZOLE

H^+

B

CYCLIC SULFENAMIDE

SULFENIC ACID

Enzyme — SH

S — S — Enzyme

H_2O

ENZYME-INHIBITOR COMPLEX

Figure 45–2. *Proton pump inhibitors.* ***A.*** Inhibitors of gastric H^+, K^+-ATPase (proton pump). ***B.*** Conversion of omeprazole to a sulfenamide in the acidic secretory canaliculi of the parietal cell. The sulfenamide interacts covalently with sulfhydryl groups in the proton pump, thereby irreversibly inhibiting its activity. The other three proton pump inhibitors undergo analogous conversions.

- enteric-coated granules supplied as a powder for suspension (lansoprazole)
- enteric-coated tablets (pantoprazole, rabeprazole, and omeprazole)
- powdered omeprazole combined with *sodium bicarbonate* (ZEGERID) contained in capsules and formulated for oral suspension

The delayed-release and enteric-coated tablets dissolve only at alkaline pH, whereas admixture of omeprazole with sodium bicarbonate simply neutralizes stomach acid; both strategies substantially improve the oral bioavailability of these acid-labile drugs. Until recently, the requirement for enteric coating posed a challenge to the administration of proton pump inhibitors in patients for whom the oral route of administration is not available (Freston et al., 2003). These patients and those requiring immediate acid suppression now can be treated parenterally with esomeprazole, pantoprazole, or lansoprazole, which are approved for intravenous administration in the U.S. A single intravenous bolus of 80 mg of pantoprazole inhibits acid production by 80-90% within an hour, and this inhibition persists for up to 21 hours, permitting once-daily dosing to achieve the desired degree of hypochlorhydria. The FDA-approved dose of intravenous pantoprazole for gastroesophageal reflux disease is 40 mg daily for up to 10 days. Higher doses (e.g., 160-240 mg in divided doses) are used to manage hypersecretory conditions such as the Zollinger-Ellison syndrome.

Pharmacokinetics. Because an acidic pH in the parietal cell acid canaliculi is required for drug activation and food stimulates acid production, these drugs ideally should be given ~30 minutes before meals. Concurrent administration of food may reduce somewhat the rate of absorption of proton pump inhibitors, but this effect is not thought to be clinically significant. Concomitant use of other drugs that inhibit acid secretion, such as H_2 receptor antagonists, might be predicted to lessen the effectiveness of the proton pump inhibitors, but the clinical relevance of this potential interaction is unknown.

Once in the small bowel, proton pump inhibitors are rapidly absorbed, highly protein bound, and extensively metabolized by hepatic CYPs, particularly CYP2C19 and CYP3A4. Several variants of CYP2C19 have been identified. Asians are more likely than whites or African Americans to have the CYP2C19 genotype that correlates with slow metabolism of proton pump inhibitors (23% vs. 3%, respectively), which has been suggested to contribute to heightened efficacy and/or toxicity in this ethnic group (Dickson and Stuart, 2003). Although the CYP2C19 genotype is correlated with the magnitude of gastric acid suppression by proton pump inhibitors in patients with gastroesophageal reflux disease, there is no evidence that the CYP2C19 genotype predicts clinical efficacy of these drugs (Chong and Ensom, 2003).

Because not all pumps or all parietal cells are active simultaneously, maximal suppression of acid secretion requires several doses of the proton pump inhibitors. For example, it may take 2-5 days of therapy with once-daily dosing to achieve the 70% inhibition of proton pumps that is seen at steady state (Wang and Hunt, 2008). More frequent initial dosing (e.g., twice daily) will reduce the time to achieve full inhibition but is not proven to improve patient outcome. Because the proton pump inhibition is irreversible, acid secretion will be suppressed for 24-48 hours, or more, until new proton pumps are synthesized and incorporated into the luminal membrane of parietal cells.

Chronic renal failure does not lead to drug accumulation with once-a-day dosing of the proton pump inhibitors. Hepatic disease substantially reduces the clearance of esomeprazole and lansoprazole. Thus, in patients with severe hepatic disease, dose reduction is recommended for esomeprazole and should be considered for lansoprazole.

Adverse Effects and Drug Interactions. Proton pump inhibitors generally cause remarkably few adverse effects. The most common side effects are nausea, abdominal pain, constipation, flatulence, and diarrhea. Subacute myopathy, arthralgias, headaches, and skin rashes also have been reported. As noted earlier, proton pump inhibitors are metabolized by hepatic CYPs and therefore may interfere with the elimination of other drugs cleared by this route. Proton pump inhibitors have been observed to interact with warfarin (esomeprazole, lansoprazole, omeprazole, and rabeprazole), diazepam (esomeprazole and omeprazole), and cyclosporine (omeprazole and rabeprazole). Among the proton pump inhibitors, only omeprazole inhibits CYP2C19 (thereby decreasing the clearance of disulfiram, phenytoin, and other drugs) and induces the expression of CYP1A2 (thereby increasing the clearance of imipramine, several antipsychotic drugs, tacrine, and theophylline). There is emerging evidence that omeprazole can interact adversely with the anticlotting agent, clopidogrel, at the level of CYP2C19, for which both are substrates; thus, omeprazole can inhibit conversion of clopidogrel to the active anticoagulating form. Pantoprazole is less likely to result in this interaction (Ferreiro and Angiolillo, 2009; Norgard et al., 2009); concurrent use of clopidogrellarry and PPIs (mainly pantoprazole) significantly reduced GI bleeding without increasing adverse cardiac events (Ray et al., 2010). For the pharmacological issues involved in the concurrent use of dual antiplatelet therapy and proton pump inhibitors, see Chapter 30, "Regulation of Blood Coagulation."

Chronic treatment with omeprazole decreases the absorption of vitamin B_{12}, but the clinical relevance of this effect is not clear. Loss of gastric acidity also may affect the bioavailability of such drugs as ketoconazole, ampicillin esters, and iron salts. Chronic use of proton pump inhibitors has been reported to be associated with an increased risk of bone fracture and with increased susceptibility to certain infections (e.g., hospital-acquired pneumonia, community-acquired *Clostridium difficile*) (Coté and Howden, 2008). Hypergastrinemia is more frequent and more severe with proton pump inhibitors than with H_2 receptor antagonists, and gastrin levels of >500 ng/L occur in ~5-10% of users with chronic omeprazole administration. This hypergastrinemia may predispose to rebound hypersecretion of gastric acid upon discontinuation of therapy and also may promote the growth of gastrointestinal (GI) tumors. In rats, long-term administration of proton pump inhibitors causes hyperplasia of enterochromaffin-like cells and the development of gastric carcinoid tumors. Although the gastrin levels observed in rats are ~10-fold higher than those seen in human beings, this finding has raised concerns about the possibility of similar complications of proton pump inhibitors in humans, for which there is no unequivocal evidence.

Therapeutic Uses. Prescription proton pump inhibitors are used to promote healing of gastric and duodenal ulcers and to treat *g*astro*e*sophageal *r*eflux *d*isease (GERD), including erosive esophagitis, which is either complicated or unresponsive to treatment with H_2 receptor antagonists. Over-the-counter omeprazole is approved for the self-treatment of heartburn. Proton pump inhibitors also are the mainstay in the treatment of pathological hypersecretory conditions, including the Zollinger-Ellison syndrome. Lansoprazole and esomeprazole are FDA approved for treatment and prevention of recurrence of nonsteroidal anti-inflammatory drug (NSAID)-associated gastric ulcers in patients who continue NSAID use. It is not clear if proton pump inhibitors affect the susceptibility to NSAID-induced damage and bleeding in the small and large intestine. In addition, all proton pump inhibitors are approved for reducing the risk of duodenal ulcer recurrence associated with *H. pylori* infections. Therapeutic applications of proton pump inhibitors are further discussed later under "Specific Acid-Peptic Disorders and Therapeutic Strategies."

Use in Children. In children, omeprazole is safe and effective for treatment of erosive esophagitis and GERD. Younger patients generally have increased metabolic capacity, which may explain the need for higher dosages of omeprazole per kilogram in children compared with adults.

H_2 RECEPTOR ANTAGONISTS

The description of selective histamine H_2 receptor blockade was a landmark in the treatment of acid-peptic disease (Black, 1993). Before the availability of the H_2 receptor antagonists, the standard of care was simply acid neutralization in the stomach lumen, generally with inadequate results. The long history of safety and efficacy with the H_2 receptor antagonists eventually led to their availability without a prescription. Increasingly, however, proton pump inhibitors are replacing the H_2 receptor antagonists in clinical practice.

Chemistry; Mechanism of Action; Pharmacology. The H_2 receptor antagonists inhibit acid production by reversibly competing with histamine for binding to H_2 receptors on the basolateral membrane of parietal cells. Four different H_2 receptor antagonists, which differ mainly in their pharmacokinetics (Appendix II) and propensity to cause drug interactions, are available in the U.S. (Figure 45–3): cimetidine (TAGAMET, others), ranitidine (ZANTAC, others), famotidine (PEPCID, others), and nizatidine (AXID, others). These drugs are less potent than proton pump inhibitors but still suppress 24-hour gastric acid secretion by ~70%. The H_2 receptor antagonists predominantly inhibit basal acid secretion, which accounts for their efficacy in suppressing nocturnal acid secretion. Because the most important determinant of duodenal ulcer healing is the level of nocturnal acidity, evening dosing of H_2 -receptor antagonists is adequate therapy in most instances. Ranitidine and nizatidine also may stimulate GI motility, but the clinical importance of this effect is unknown.

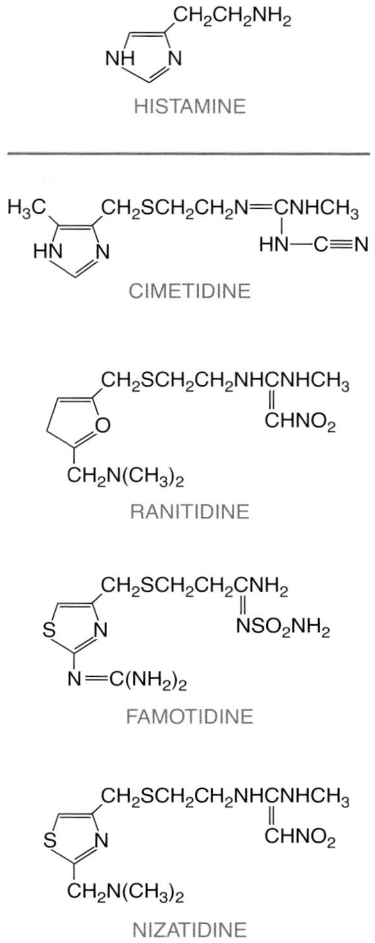

HISTAMINE

CIMETIDINE

RANITIDINE

FAMOTIDINE

NIZATIDINE

Figure 45–3. *Histamine and H_2 receptor antagonists.*

All four H_2 receptor antagonists are available as prescription and over-the-counter formulations for oral administration. Intravenous and intramuscular preparations of cimetidine, ranitidine, and famotidine also are available. When the oral or nasogastric routes are not an option, these drugs can be given in intermittent intravenous boluses or by continuous intravenous infusion (Table 45–1). The latter provides better control of gastric pH but is not proven to be more effective in preventing significant bleeding in critically ill patients.

Pharmacokinetics. The H_2 receptor antagonists are rapidly absorbed after oral administration, with peak serum concentrations

Table 45–1

Intravenous Doses of H_2 Receptor Antagonists

	CIMETIDINE	RANITIDINE	FAMOTIDINE
Intermittent bolus	300 mg every 6-8 hours	50 mg every 6-8 hours	20 mg every 12 hours
Continuous infusion	37.5-100 mg/hour	6.25-12.5 mg/hour	1.7-2.1 mg/hour

within 1-3 hours. Absorption may be enhanced by food or decreased by antacids, but these effects probably are unimportant clinically. Therapeutic levels are achieved rapidly after intravenous dosing and are maintained for 4-5 hours (cimetidine), 6-8 hours (ranitidine), or 10-12 hours (famotidine). Unlike proton pump inhibitors, only a small percentage of H_2 receptor antagonists are protein bound. Small amounts (from <10% to ~35%) of these drugs undergo metabolism in the liver, but liver disease *per se* is not an indication for dose adjustment. The kidneys excrete these drugs and their metabolites by filtration and renal tubular secretion, and it is important to reduce doses of H_2 receptor antagonists in patients with decreased creatinine clearance. Neither hemodialysis nor peritoneal dialysis clears significant amounts of the drugs.

Adverse Reactions and Drug Interactions. Like the proton pump inhibitors, the H_2 receptor antagonists generally are well tolerated, with a low (<3%) incidence of adverse effects. Side effects usually are minor and include diarrhea, headache, drowsiness, fatigue, muscular pain, and constipation. Less common side effects include those affecting the CNS (confusion, delirium, hallucinations, slurred speech, and headaches), which occur primarily with intravenous administration of the drugs or in elderly subjects. Long-term use of cimetidine at high doses—seldom used clinically today—decreases testosterone binding to the androgen receptor and inhibits a CYP that hydroxylates estradiol. Clinically, these effects can cause galactorrhea in women and gynecomastia, reduced sperm count, and impotence in men. Several reports have associated H_2 receptor antagonists with various blood dyscrasias, including thrombocytopenia. H_2 receptor antagonists cross the placenta and are excreted in breast milk. Although no major teratogenic risk has been associated with these agents, caution nevertheless is warranted when they are used in pregnancy.

All agents that inhibit gastric acid secretion may alter the rate of absorption and subsequent bioavailability of the H_2 receptor antagonists (see "Antacids" section). Drug interactions with H_2 receptor antagonists occur mainly with cimetidine, and its use has decreased markedly. Cimetidine inhibits CYPs (e.g., CYP1A2, CYP2C9, and CYP2D6), and thereby can increase the levels of a variety of drugs that are substrates for these enzymes. Ranitidine also interacts with hepatic CYPs, but with an affinity of only 10% of that of cimetidine; thus, ranitidine interferes only minimally with hepatic metabolism of other drugs. Famotidine and nizatidine are even safer in this regard, with no significant drug interactions mediated by inhibiting hepatic CYPs. Slight increases in blood-alcohol concentration may result from concomitant use of H_2 receptor antagonists, but this is unlikely to be clinically significant.

Therapeutic Uses. The major therapeutic indications for H_2-receptor antagonists are to promote healing of gastric and duodenal ulcers, to treat uncomplicated GERD, and to prevent the occurrence of stress ulcers. More information about the therapeutic applications of H_2 receptor antagonists is provided in the section "Specific Acid-Peptic Disorders and Therapeutic Strategies."

TOLERANCE AND REBOUND WITH ACID-SUPPRESSING MEDICATIONS

Tolerance to the acid-suppressing effects of H_2 receptor antagonists is well described and may account for a diminished therapeutic effect with continued drug administration (Sandevik et al., 1997). Tolerance can develop within 3 days of starting treatment and may be resistant to increased doses of the medications. Diminished sensitivity to these drugs may result from the effect of the secondary hypergastrinemia to stimulate histamine release from ECL cells. Proton pump inhibitors, despite even greater elevations of endogenous gastrin, do not cause this phenomenon, probably because their site of action is distal to the action of histamine on acid release. However, rebound increases in gastric acidity can occur when either of these drug classes is discontinued, possibly reflecting changes in function and justifying a gradual drug taper or the substitution of alternatives (e.g., antacids) in at-risk patients.

AGENTS THAT ENHANCE MUCOSAL DEFENSE

Prostaglandin Analogs: Misoprostol

Chemistry; Mechanism of Action; Pharmacology. Prostaglandin E_2 (PGE_2) and prostacyclin (PGI_2) are the major prostaglandins synthesized by the gastric mucosa. Contrary to their cyclic AMP-elevating effects on many cells via EP_2 and EP_4 receptors, these prostanoids bind to the EP_3 receptor on parietal cells (Chapters 33 and 34) and stimulate the G_i pathway, thereby decreasing intracellular cyclic AMP and gastric acid secretion. PGE_2 also can prevent gastric injury by cytoprotective effects that include stimulation of mucin and bicarbonate secretion and increased mucosal blood flow. Although smaller doses than those required for acid suppression can protect the gastric mucosa in laboratory animals, this has not been convincingly demonstrated in humans; acid suppression appears to be the most important effect clinically (Wolfe and Sachs, 2000).

Because NSAIDs diminish prostaglandin formation by inhibiting cyclooxygenase, synthetic prostaglandin analogs offer a logical approach to reducing NSAID-induced mucosal damage. Misoprostol (15-deoxy-16-hydroxy-16-methyl-PGE_1; CYTOTEC, others) is a synthetic analog of PGE_1. Structural modifications include an additional methyl ester group at C1 that increases potency and duration of antisecretory effect, and transfer of a hydroxyl group from C15 to C16 and addition of a methyl group that increases oral bioactivity, duration of antisecretory action, and safety. The degree of inhibition of gastric acid secretion by misoprostol is directly related to dose; oral doses of 100-200 μg significantly inhibit basal acid secretion (up to 85-95% inhibition) or food-stimulated acid secretion (up to 75-85% inhibition). The usual recommended dose for ulcer prophylaxis is 200 μg four times a day.

Pharmacokinetics. Misoprostol is rapidly absorbed after oral administration and then is rapidly and extensively de-esterified to form misoprostol acid, the principal and active metabolite of the drug. Some of this conversion may occur in the parietal cells. A single dose inhibits acid production within 30 minutes; the therapeutic effect peaks at 60-90 minutes and lasts for up to 3 hours. Food and antacids decrease the rate of misoprostol absorption, resulting in delayed and decreased peak plasma concentrations of the active metabolite. The free acid is excreted mainly in the urine, with an elimination $t_{1/2}$ of 20-40 minutes.

Adverse Effects. Diarrhea, with or without abdominal pain and cramps, occurs in up to 30% of patients who take misoprostol. Apparently dose related, it typically begins within the first 2 weeks after therapy is initiated and often resolves spontaneously within a week; more severe or protracted cases may necessitate drug discontinuation. *Misoprostol can cause clinical exacerbations of inflammatory bowel disease* (Chapter 47) and should be avoided in patients with this disorder. *Misoprostol is contraindicated during pregnancy* because it can increase uterine contractility.

Therapeutic Use. Misoprostol is FDA-approved to prevent NSAID-induced mucosal injury. However, it rarely is used because of its adverse effects and the inconvenience of four-times-daily dosing.

SUCRALFATE

Chemistry; Mechanism of Action; Pharmacology. In the presence of acid-induced damage, pepsin-mediated hydrolysis of mucosal proteins contributes to mucosal erosion and ulcerations. This process can be inhibited by sulfated polysaccharides. Sucralfate (CARAFATE, others) consists of the octasulfate of sucrose to which $Al(OH)_3$ has been added. In an acid environment (pH <4), sucralfate undergoes extensive cross-linking to produce a viscous, sticky polymer that adheres to epithelial cells and ulcer craters for up to 6 hours after a single dose. In addition to inhibiting hydrolysis of mucosal proteins by pepsin, sucralfate may have additional cytoprotective effects, including stimulation of local production of prostaglandins and epidermal growth factor. Sucralfate also binds bile salts; thus some clinicians use sucralfate to treat individuals with the syndromes of biliary esophagitis or gastritis (the existence of which is controversial).

Therapeutic Uses. The use of sucralfate to treat peptic acid disease has diminished in recent years. Nevertheless, because increased gastric pH may be a factor in the development of nosocomial pneumonia in critically ill patients, sucralfate may offer an advantage over proton pump inhibitors and H_2 receptor antagonists for the prophylaxis of stress ulcers. Due to its unique mechanism of action, sucralfate also has been used in several other conditions associated with mucosal inflammation/ulceration that may not respond to acid suppression, including oral mucositis (radiation and aphthous ulcers) and bile reflux gastropathy. Administered by rectal enema, sucralfate also has been used for radiation proctitis and solitary rectal ulcers.

Because it is activated by acid, sucralfate should be taken on an empty stomach 1 hour before meals. The use of antacids within 30 minutes of a dose of sucralfate should be avoided. The usual dose of sucralfate is 1 g four times daily (for active duodenal ulcer) or 1 g twice daily (for maintenance therapy).

Adverse Effects. The most common side effect of sucralfate is constipation (~2%). Because some aluminum can be absorbed, sucralfate should be avoided in patients with renal failure who are at risk for aluminum overload. Likewise, aluminum-containing antacids should not be combined with sucralfate in these patients. Sucralfate forms a viscous layer in the stomach that may inhibit absorption of other drugs, including phenytoin, digoxin, cimetidine, ketoconazole, and fluoroquinolone antibiotics. Sucralfate therefore should be taken at least 2 hours after the administration of other drugs. The "sticky" nature of the viscous gel produced by sucralfate in the stomach also may be responsible for the development of bezoars in some patients, particularly in those with underlying gastroparesis.

ANTACIDS

Although hallowed by tradition, the antacids largely have been replaced by more effective and convenient drugs. Nevertheless, they continue to be used by patients for a variety of indications, and some knowledge of their pharmacology is important for the medical professional (Table 45–2 compares some commonly used antacid preparations).

Many factors, including palatability, determine the effectiveness and choice of antacid. Although sodium bicarbonate effectively neutralizes acid, it is very water soluble and rapidly absorbed from the stomach, and the alkali and sodium loads may pose a risk for patients with cardiac or renal failure. Depending on particle size and crystal structure, $CaCO_3$ rapidly and effectively neutralizes gastric H^+, but the release of CO_2 from bicarbonate- and carbonate-containing antacids can cause belching, nausea, abdominal distention, and flatulence. Calcium also may induce rebound acid secretion, necessitating more frequent administration.

Combinations of Mg^{2+} (rapidly reacting) and Al^{3+} (slowly reacting) hydroxides provide a relatively balanced and sustained neutralizing capacity and are preferred by most experts. Magaldrate is a hydroxymagnesium aluminate complex that is converted rapidly in gastric acid to $Mg(OH)_2$ and $Al(OH)_3$, which are absorbed poorly and thus provide a sustained antacid effect. Although fixed combinations of magnesium and aluminum theoretically counteract the adverse effects of each other on the bowel (Al^{3+} can relax gastric smooth muscle, producing delayed gastric emptying and constipation; Mg^{2+} exerts the opposite effects), such balance is not always achieved in practice.

Simethicone, a surfactant that may decrease foaming and hence esophageal reflux, is included in many antacid preparations. However, other fixed combinations, particularly those with aspirin, that are marketed for "acid indigestion" are irrational choices, are potentially unsafe in patients predisposed to gastroduodenal ulcers, and should not be used.

Table 45–2

Composition and Acid Neutralizing Capacities of Popular Antacid Preparations

PRODUCT	$Al(OH)_3$[a]	$Mg(OH)_2$[a]	$CaCO_3$[a]	SIMETHICONE[a]	ACID NEUTRALIZING CAPACITY[b]
Tablets					
Gelusil	200	200	0	25	10.5
Maalox Quick Dissolve	0	0	600	0	12
Mylanta Double Strength	400	400	0	40	23
Riopan Plus Double Strength	Magaldrate, 1080			20	30
Calcium Rich Rolaids		80	412	0	11
Tums EX	0	0	750	0	15
Liquids					
Maalox TC	600	300	0	0	28
Milk of Magnesia	0	400	0	0	14
Mylanta Maximum Strength	400	400	0	40	25
Riopan	Magaldrate, 540			0	15

[a]Contents, milligrams per tablet or per 5 ml.
[b]Acid neutralizing capacity, milliequivalents per tablet or per 5 ml.
The U.S. marketplace for antacids is fluid. The current trend of "reusing" well-known brand names to introduce new products that contain an active ingredient different from expected is a source of confusion that can present a danger to patients. Medication safety experts encourage clinical practitioners to refer to the active ingredient(s) in conjunction with the proprietary (brand) name when selecting OTC products.

The relative effectiveness of antacid preparations is expressed as milliequivalents of acid-neutralizing capacity (defined as the quantity of 1N HCl, expressed in milliequivalents, that can be brought to pH 3.5 within 15 minutes); according to FDA requirements, antacids must have a neutralizing capacity of at least 5 mEq per dose. Due to discrepancies between *in vitro* and *in vivo* neutralizing capacities, antacid doses in practice are titrated simply to relieve symptoms. For uncomplicated ulcers, antacids are given orally 1 and 3 hours after meals and at bedtime. This regimen, providing ~120 mEq of a Mg-Al combination per dose, may be almost as effective as conventional dosing with an H_2 receptor antagonist. For severe symptoms or uncontrolled reflux, antacids can be given as often as every 30-60 minutes. In general, antacids should be administered in suspension form because this probably has a greater neutralizing capacity than powder or tablet dosage forms. If tablets are used, they should be thoroughly chewed for maximum effect.

Antacids are cleared from the empty stomach in ~30 minutes. However, the presence of food is sufficient to elevate gastric pH to ~5 for ~1 hour and to prolong the neutralizing effects of antacids for ~2-3 hours.

Antacids vary in the extent to which they are absorbed, and hence in their systemic effects. In general, most antacids can elevate urinary pH by ~1 pH unit. Antacids that contain Al^{3+}, Ca^{2+}, or Mg^{2+} are absorbed less completely than are those that contain $NaHCO_3$. With normal renal function, the modest accumulations of Al^{3+} and Mg^{2+} do not pose a problem; with renal insufficiency, however, absorbed Al^{3+} can contribute to osteoporosis, encephalopathy, and proximal myopathy. About 15% of orally administered Ca^{2+} is absorbed, causing a transient hypercalcemia. Although this is not a problem in normal patients, the hypercalcemia from as little as 3-4 g of $CaCO_3$ per day can be problematic in patients with uremia. In the past, when large doses of $NaHCO_3$ and $CaCO_3$ were administered commonly with milk or cream for the management of peptic ulcer, the *milk-alkali syndrome* (alkalosis, hypercalcemia, and renal insufficiency) occurred frequently. Today, this syndrome is rare and generally results from the chronic ingestion of large quantities of Ca^{2+} (five to forty 500-mg tablets per day of calcium carbonate) taken with milk. Patients may be asymptomatic or may present with the insidious onset of hypercalcemia, reduced secretion of parathyroid hormone, retention of phosphate, precipitation of Ca^{2+} salts in the kidney, and renal insufficiency.

By altering gastric and urinary pH, antacids may affect a number of drugs (e.g., thyroid hormones, allopurinol, and imidazole antifungals, by altering rates of dissolution and absorption, bioavailability, and renal elimination). Al^{3+} and Mg^{2+} antacids also are notable for their propensity to chelate other drugs present in the GI tract, forming insoluble complexes that pass through the GI tract without absorption. Thus it generally is prudent to avoid concurrent administration of antacids and drugs intended for systemic absorption. Most interactions can be avoided by taking antacids 2 hours before or after ingestion of other drugs.

Other Acid Suppressants and Cytoprotectants

The M_1 muscarinic receptor antagonists pirenzepine and telenzepine (Chapter 9) can reduce basal acid production by 40-50% and long have been used to treat patients with peptic ulcer disease in countries other than the U.S. The ACh receptor on the parietal cell itself is of the M_3 subtype, and these drugs are believed to suppress neural stimulation of acid production via actions on M_1 receptors of intramural ganglia (Figure 45–1). Because of their relatively poor efficacy, significant and undesirable anticholinergic side effects, and risk of blood disorders (pirenzepine), they rarely are used today.

In the hope of providing more rapid onset of action and sustained acid suppression, reversible inhibitors of the gastric H^+, K^+-ATPase (e.g., the pyrrolopyridazine derivative AKU517) are being developed for clinical use. Antagonists of the CCK2 gastrin receptor on parietal cells also are under study. The precise role that these agents will play in the therapy of acid-peptic disorders in the future is yet to be determined.

Rebamipide (2-(4-chlorobenzoylamino)-3-[2(1H)-quinolinon-4-yl]-propionic acid) is used for ulcer therapy in parts of Asia. It appears to exert a cytoprotective effect both by increasing prostaglandin generation in gastric mucosa and by scavenging reactive oxygen species. Ecabet (GASTROM; 12-sulfodehydroabietic acid monosodium), which appears to increase the formation of PGE_2 and PGI_2, also is used for ulcer therapy, mostly in Japan. Carbenoxolone, a derivative of glycyrrhizic acid found in licorice root, has been used with modest success for ulcer therapy in Europe. Its exact mechanism of action is not clear, but it may alter the composition and quantity of mucin. Unfortunately, carbenoxolone inhibits the type I isozyme of 11β-hydroxysteroid dehydrogenase, which protects the mineralocorticoid receptor from activation by cortisol in the distal nephron; it therefore causes hypokalemia and hypertension due to excessive mineralocorticoid receptor activation (Chapter 42). Bismuth compounds (Chapter 46) may be as effective as cimetidine in patients with peptic ulcers and are frequently prescribed in combination with antibiotics to eradicate *H. pylori* and prevent ulcer recurrence. Bismuth compounds bind to the base of the ulcer, promote mucin and bicarbonate production, and have significant antibacterial effects. Bismuth compounds are an important component of many anti-*Helicobacter* regimens; however, given the availability of more effective drugs, bismuth compounds seldom are used alone as cytoprotective agents.

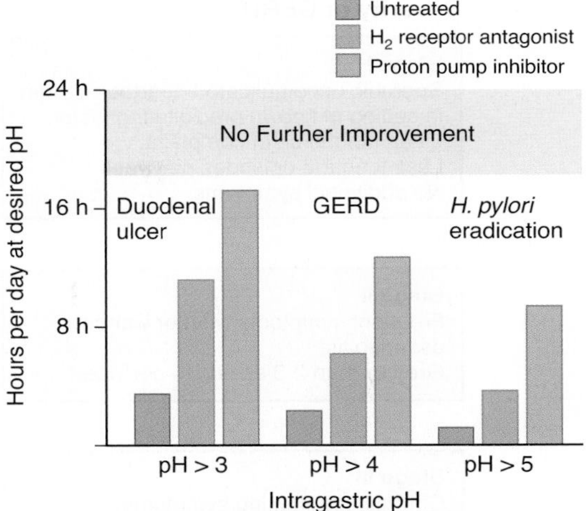

Figure 45–4. *Comparative success of therapy with proton pump inhibitors and H_2 receptor antagonists.* Data show the effects of a proton pump inhibitor (given once daily) and an H_2 receptor antagonist (given twice daily) in elevating gastric pH to the target ranges (i.e., pH 3 for duodenal ulcer, pH 4 for GERD, and pH 5 for antibiotic eradication of *H. pylori*).

SPECIFIC ACID-PEPTIC DISORDERS AND THERAPEUTIC STRATEGIES

The success of acid-suppressing agents in a variety of conditions is critically dependent on their ability to keep intragastric pH above a certain target, generally pH 3-5; this target varies to some extent with the disease being treated (Figure 45–4).

Gastroesophageal Reflux Disease

In the U.S., it is estimated that one in five adults has symptoms of heartburn or gastroesophageal regurgitation at least once a week. Although most cases follow a relatively benign course, these symptoms, often referred to as "gastroesophageal reflux disease" (GERD), can be associated with severe erosive esophagitis; stricture formation and Barrett's metaplasia (replacement of squamous by intestinal columnar epithelium), in turn, is associated with a small but significant risk of adenocarcinoma. Most of the symptoms of GERD reflect injurious effects of the refluxed acid-peptic content on the esophageal epithelium, providing the rationale for suppression of gastric acid. The goals of GERD therapy are complete resolution of symptoms and healing of esophagitis. Proton pump inhibitors clearly are more effective than H_2 receptor antagonists in achieving these goals. Healing rates after 4 weeks and 8 weeks of therapy with protein pump inhibitors are ~80% and 90%, respectively; the corresponding healing rates with H_2 receptor antagonists are 50% and 75%, respectively. Indeed, proton pump inhibitors are so effective that their empirical use is advocated as a therapeutic trial in patients in whom GERD is suspected to play a role in the pathogenesis of symptoms.

Because of the wide clinical spectrum associated with GERD, the therapeutic approach is best tailored to the level of severity in the individual patient (Figure 45–5). In general, the optimal dose for each patient is determined based on symptom control, and routine measurement of esophageal pH to guide dosing is not recommended. Strictures associated with GERD also respond better to proton pump inhibitors than to H_2 receptor antagonists; indeed, the use of proton pump inhibitors reduces the requirement for esophageal dilation. Unfortunately, one of the other complications of GERD, Barrett's esophagus, appears to be more refractory to therapy because neither acid suppression nor antireflux surgery has been shown convincingly to produce regression of metaplasia or to decrease the incidence of tumors.

Regimens for the treatment of GERD with proton pump inhibitors and histamine H_2 receptor antagonists are listed in Table 45–3. Although some patients with mild GERD symptoms may be managed by nocturnal doses of H_2 receptor antagonists,

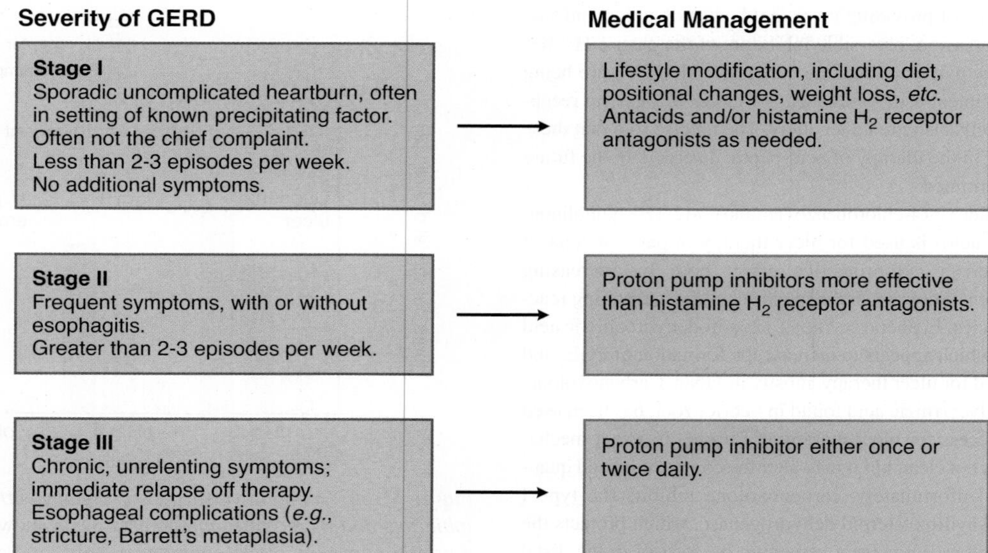

Severity of GERD
Medical Management
Stage I
Sporadic uncomplicated heartburn, often in setting of known precipitating factor.
Often not the chief complaint.
Less than 2-3 episodes per week.
No additional symptoms.
Lifestyle modification, including diet, positional changes, weight loss, etc.
Antacids and/or histamine H2 receptor antagonists as needed.
Stage II
Frequent symptoms, with or without esophagitis.
Greater than 2-3 episodes per week.
Proton pump inhibitors more effective than histamine H2 receptor antagonists.
Stage III
Chronic, unrelenting symptoms; immediate relapse off therapy.
Esophageal complications (e.g., stricture, Barrett's metaplasia).
Proton pump inhibitor either once or twice daily.

Figure 45–5. *General guidelines for the medical management of gastroesophageal reflux disease (GERD).* Only medications that suppress acid production or that neutralize acid are shown. (Adapted from Wolfe and Sachs, 2000, with permission from Elsevier. Copyright © Elsevier.)

twice-daily dosing usually is required. Antacids are recommended only for the patient with mild, infrequent episodes of heartburn. In general, prokinetic agents (Chapter 46) are not particularly useful for GERD, either alone or in combination with acid-suppressant medications.

GERD is a chronic disorder that requires long-term therapy. Some experts advocate "stepdown" approaches that attempt to maintain symptomatic remission by either decreasing the dose of the proton pump inhibitor or switching to an H_2 receptor antagonist. Other experts have advocated intermittent, "on-demand" therapy with proton pump inhibitors for symptomatic relief in patients who have responded initially but continue to have symptoms. However, many patients will maintain their requirement for proton pump inhibitors, and several studies suggest that these drugs are better than H_2 receptor antagonists for maintaining remission in GERD.

Table 45–3

Antisecretory Drug Regimens for Treatment and Maintenance of GERD

DRUG	DOSAGE
H_2 Receptor Antagonists	
Cimetidine	400*/800* mg *bid*
Famotidine	20/40 mg *bid*
Nizatidine	150*/300* mg *bid*
Ranitidine	150/300 mg *bid*
Proton Pump Inhibitors	
Esomeprazole	20/40 mg daily/40* mg *bid*
Lansoprazole	30*/60* mg daily/30* mg *bid*
Omeprazole	20/40* mg daily/20* mg *bid*
Pantoprazole	40/80* mg daily/40* mg *bid*
Rabeprazole	20/40* mg daily/20* mg *bid*

bid, twice daily.
*Indicates unlabeled use.

Severe Symptoms and Nocturnal Acid Breakthrough. In patients with severe symptoms or extraintestinal manifestations of GERD, twice-daily dosing with a proton pump inhibitor may be needed. However, it is difficult if not impossible to render patients achlorhydric—even on twice-daily doses of proton pump inhibitors—and two-thirds or more of subjects will continue to make acid, particularly at night. This phenomenon, called *nocturnal acid breakthrough*, has been invoked as a cause of refractory symptoms in some patients with GERD. However, decreases in gastric pH at night while on therapy generally are not associated with acid reflux into the esophagus, and the rationale for suppressing nocturnal acid secretion (even if feasible) remains to be established. Nevertheless, patients with continuing symptoms on twice-daily proton pump inhibitors are often treated by adding an H_2 receptor antagonist at night. Although this can further suppress acid production, the effect is short lived, probably due to the development of tolerance, as described earlier (Fackler et al., 2002).

Therapy for Extraintestinal Manifestations of GERD. With varying levels of evidence, acid reflux has been implicated in a variety of atypical symptoms, including noncardiac chest pain, asthma, laryngitis, chronic cough, and other ear, nose, and throat conditions. Proton pump inhibitors have been used with some success in certain patients with these disorders, generally in higher doses and for longer periods of time than those used for patients with more classic symptoms of GERD.

GERD and Pregnancy. Heartburn is estimated to occur in 30-50% of pregnancies, with an incidence approaching 80% in some populations (Richter, 2003). In the vast majority of cases, GERD ends soon after delivery and thus does not represent an exacerbation of a preexisting condition. Nevertheless, because of its high prevalence and the fact that it can contribute to the nausea of pregnancy, treatment often is required. Treatment choice in this setting is complicated by the paucity of data for the most commonly used drugs. In general, most drugs used to treat GERD fall in FDA Category B, with the exception of omeprazole (FDA Category C).

Mild cases of GERD during pregnancy should be treated conservatively; antacids or sucralfate are considered the first-line drugs. If symptoms persist, H_2 receptor antagonists can be used, with ranitidine having the most established track record in this setting. PPIs are reserved for women with intractable symptoms or complicated reflux disease. In these situations, lansoprazole is considered the preferred choice among the proton pump inhibitors, based on animal data and available experience in pregnant women.

PEPTIC ULCER DISEASE

The pathophysiology of peptic ulcer disease is best viewed as an imbalance between mucosal defense factors (bicarbonate, mucin, prostaglandin, NO, and other peptides and growth factors) and injurious factors (acid and pepsin). On average, patients with duodenal ulcers produce more acid than do control subjects, particularly at night (basal secretion). Although patients with gastric ulcers have normal or even diminished acid production, ulcers rarely if ever occur in the complete absence of acid. Presumably, a weakened mucosal defense and reduced bicarbonate production contribute to the injury from the relatively lower levels of acid in these patients. *H. pylori* and exogenous agents such as NSAIDs interact in complex ways to cause an ulcer. Up to 60% of peptic ulcers are associated with *H. pylori* infection of the stomach. This infection may lead to impaired production of somatostatin by D cells and, in time, decreased inhibition of gastrin production, resulting in increased acid production and reduced duodenal bicarbonate production.

NSAIDs also are very frequently associated with peptic ulcers and bleeding. Topical injury by the luminal presence of the drug appears to play a minor role in the pathogenesis of these ulcers, as evidenced by the fact that ulcers can occur with very low doses of aspirin (10 mg) or with parenteral administration of NSAIDs (Wallace, 2008). The effects of these drugs are instead mediated systemically; the critical element is suppression of mucosal prostaglandin synthesis (particularly PGE_2 and PGI_2). Most of the mucosal prostaglandin synthesis occurs via the constitutively expressed cyclooxygenase-1 (COX-1), but COX-2, which can be very rapidly induced, also contributes significantly to the generation of mucosal-protective prostaglandins. Thus suppression of COX-1 and COX-2 by NSAIDs contributes to the induction of mucosal injury. COX-2-derived prostaglandins are particularly important in repair of mucosal injury (Wallace, 2008).

Table 45–4 summarizes current recommendations for drug therapy of gastroduodenal ulcers. Proton pump inhibitors relieve symptoms of duodenal ulcers and promote healing more rapidly than do H_2 receptor antagonists, although both classes of drugs are very effective in this setting. Peptic ulcer represents a chronic disease, and recurrence within 1 year is expected in the majority of patients who do not receive prophylactic acid suppression. With the appreciation

Table 45–4

Recommendations for Treatment of Gastroduodenal Ulcers

DRUG	ACTIVE ULCER	MAINTENANCE THERAPY
H_2 Receptor Antagonists		
Cimetidine	800 mg at bedtime/400 mg twice daily	400 mg at bedtime
Famotidine	40 mg at bedtime	20 mg at bedtime
Nizatidine/ranitidine	300 mg after evening meal or at bedtime/150 mg twice daily	150 mg at bedtime
Proton Pump Inhibitors		
Lansoprazole	15 mg (DU; NSAID risk reduction) daily 30 mg (GU including NSAID-associated) daily	
Omeprazole	20 mg daily	
Rabeprazole	20 mg daily	
Prostaglandin Analog		
Misoprostol	200 μg four times daily (NSAID-associated ulcer prevention)*	

DU, duodenal ulcer; GU, gastric ulcer.
*Only misoprostol 800 μg/day has been directly shown to reduce the risk of ulcer complications such as perforation, hemorrhage, or obstruction (Rostom et al., 2009).

that *H. pylori* plays a major etiopathogenic role in the majority of peptic ulcers, prevention of relapse is focused on eliminating this organism from the stomach. Chronic acid suppression, once the mainstay of ulcer prevention, now is used mainly in patients who are *H. pylori*–negative or, in some cases, for maximum prevention of recurrence in patients who have had life-threatening complications.

Intravenous pantoprazole or lansoprazole clearly is the preferred therapy in patients with acute bleeding ulcers. The theoretical benefit of maximal acid suppression in this setting is to accelerate healing of the underlying ulcer. In addition, a higher gastric pH enhances clot formation and retards clot dissolution.

Treatment of *Helicobacter pylori* Infection. *H. pylori*, a gram-negative rod, has been associated with gastritis and the subsequent development of gastric and duodenal ulcers, gastric adenocarcinoma, and gastric B-cell lymphoma (Suerbaum and Michetti, 2002). Because of the critical role of *H. pylori* in the pathogenesis of peptic ulcers, to eradicate this infection is standard care in patients with gastric or duodenal ulcers. Provided that patients are not taking NSAIDs, this strategy almost completely eliminates the risk of ulcer recurrence. Eradication of *H. pylori* also is indicated in the treatment of mucosa-associated lymphoid tissue lymphomas of the stomach, which can regress significantly after such treatment.

Many regimens for *H. pylori* eradication have been proposed. Evidence-based literature review suggests that the ideal regimen in this setting should achieve a cure rate of at least 80%. Five important considerations influence the selection of an eradication regimen (Chey and Wong, 2007; Graham, 2000) (Table 45–5). First, single-antibiotic regimens are ineffective in eradicating *H. pylori* infection and lead to microbial resistance. Combination therapy with two or three antibiotics (plus acid-suppressive therapy) is associated with the highest rate of *H. pylori* eradication. Second, a proton pump inhibitor or H_2 receptor antagonist significantly enhances the effectiveness of *H. pylo*ri antibiotic regimens containing amoxicillin or clarithromycin. Third, a regimen of 10-14 days of treatment appears to be better than shorter treatment regimens; in the U.S., a 14-day course of therapy generally is preferred. Fourth, poor patient compliance is linked to the medication-related side effects experienced by as many as half of patients taking triple-agent regimens, and to the inconvenience of three- or four-drug regimens administered several times per day. Packaging that combines the daily doses into one convenient unit is available and may improve patient compliance (Table 45–5). Finally, the emergence of resistance to clarithromycin and metronidazole increasingly is recognized as an important factor in the failure to eradicate *H. pylori*. Clarithromycin resistance is related to mutations that prevent binding of the antibiotic to the ribosomes of the pathogen and is an all-or-none phenomenon. In contrast, metronidazole resistance is relative rather than absolute and may involve several adaptations by the bacteria. In the presence of *in vitro* evidence of resistance to metronidazole, amoxicillin should be used instead. In areas with a high frequency of resistance to clarithromycin and metronidazole, a 14-day quadruple-drug regimen (three antibiotics combined with a proton pump inhibitor) generally is effective therapy.

Table 45–5

Therapy of *Helicobacter pylori* Infection

Triple therapy × 14 days: Proton pump inhibitor + clarithromycin 500 mg plus metronidazole 500 mg or amoxicillin 1 g twice a day (tetracycline 500 mg can be substituted for amoxicillin or metronidazole)

Quadruple therapy × 14 days: Proton pump inhibitor twice a day + metronidazole 500 mg three times daily plus bismuth subsalicylate 525 mg + tetracycline 500 mg four times daily

or

H_2 receptor antagonist twice a day plus bismuth subsalicylate 525 mg + metronidazole 250 mg + tetracycline 500 mg four times daily

Dosages:

Proton pump inhibitors:	H_2 receptor antagonists:
Omeprazole: 20 mg	Cimetidine: 400 mg
Lansoprazole: 30 mg	Famotidine: 20 mg
Rabeprazole: 20 mg	Nizatidine: 150 mg
Pantoprazole: 40 mg	Ranitidine: 150 mg
Esomeprazole: 40 mg	

See Chey and Wong, 2007.

NSAID-Related Ulcers. Chronic NSAID users have a 2-4% risk of developing a symptomatic ulcer, GI bleeding, or perforation. Ideally, NSAIDs should be discontinued in patients with an ulcer if at all possible. If continued therapy is needed, selective COX-2 inhibitors may be considered, although this does not eliminate the risk of subsequent ulcer formation and the possible association of these drugs with adverse cardiovascular events mandates caution (Chapter 34). Moreover, any GI benefit of selective COX-2 inhibitors is lost if the patient is also taking low-dose aspirin. Healing of ulcers despite continued NSAID use is possible with the use of acid-suppressant agents, usually at higher doses and for a considerably longer duration than standard regimens (e.g., ≥8 weeks). Again, proton pump inhibitors are superior to H_2 receptor antagonists and misoprostol in promoting the healing of active ulcers (healing rates of 80-90% for proton pump inhibitors vs. 60-75% for the H_2 receptor antagonists), and in preventing recurrence of gastric and duodenal ulcers in the setting of continued NSAID administration (Lanas and Hunt, 2006; Rostom et al., 2009).

Stress-Related Ulcers. Stress ulcers are ulcers of the stomach or duodenum that occur in the context of a profound illness or trauma requiring intensive care. The etiology of stress-related ulcers differs somewhat from that of other peptic ulcers, involving acid and mucosal ischemia. Because of limitations on the oral administration of drugs in many patients with stress-related ulcers, intravenous H_2 receptor antagonists have been used extensively to reduce the incidence of GI hemorrhage due to stress ulcers. Now that intravenous preparations of proton pump inhibitors are available, it is likely that they will prove to be equally beneficial. *However, there is some concern over the risk of pneumonia secondary to gastric colonization by bacteria in an alkaline milieu.* In this setting, sucralfate appears to provide reasonable prophylaxis against bleeding without increasing the risk of aspiration pneumonia. This approach also appears to provide reasonable prophylaxis against bleeding, but it is less convenient (Cook et al., 1998).

Zollinger-Ellison Syndrome. Patients with this syndrome develop pancreatic or duodenal gastrinomas that stimulate the secretion of very large amounts of acid, sometimes in the setting of multiple endocrine neoplasia, type I. This can lead to severe gastroduodenal ulceration and other consequences of uncontrolled hyperchlorhydria. Proton pump inhibitors clearly are the drugs of choice, usually given at twice the routine dosage for peptic ulcers with the therapeutic goal of reducing acid secretion to 1-10 mmol/hour.

Nonulcer Dyspepsia. This term refers to ulcer-like symptoms in patients who lack overt gastroduodenal ulceration. It may be associated with gastritis (with or without *H. pylori*) or with NSAID use, but the pathogenesis of this syndrome remains controversial. Although empirical treatment with acid-suppressive agents is used routinely in patients with nonulcer dyspepsia, there is no convincing evidence of their benefit in controlled trials.

CLINICAL SUMMARY

The control of acid-peptic disease represents a major triumph for modern pharmacology. Proton pump inhibitors are considered superior for acid suppression in most clinically significant acid-peptic diseases, including gastroesophageal reflux disease, peptic ulcers, and NSAID-induced ulcers. Proton pump inhibitors also are employed in combination with antibiotics to eradicate infection with *H. pylori* and thereby play a role in preventing recurrent peptic ulcers. These agents largely have replaced the use of misoprostol and sucralfate, although the latter still is a low-cost alternative for prophylaxis against stress ulcers. The delay in maximal inhibition of acid secretion with the proton pump inhibitors (3-5 days) makes them less suited for use on an as-needed basis for symptom relief. In this setting, H_2 receptor antagonists, although less effective than proton pump inhibitors in suppressing acid secretion, have a more rapid onset of action that makes them useful for patient-directed management of mild or infrequent symptoms.

BIBLIOGRAPHY

Black J. Reflections on the analytical pharmacology of histamine H_2-receptor antagonists. *Gastroenterology*, **1993,** *105:*963–968.

Chey WD, Wong BCY. American College of Gastroenterology Guideline on the Management of Helicobacter pylori Infection. *Am J Gastroenterol,* **2007,** *102:*1808–1825.

Chong E, Ensom MH. Pharmacogenetics of the proton pump inhibitors: A systematic review. *Pharmacotherapy*, **2003,** *23:*460–471.

Cook D, Guyatt G, Marshall J, et al. Comparison of sucralfate and ranitidine for the prevention of upper gastrointestinal bleeding in patients requiring mechanical ventilation. Canadian Critical Care Trials Group. *N Engl J Med*, **1998,** *338:*791–797.

Coté GA, Howden CW. Potential adverse effects of proton pump inhibitors. *Curr Gastroenterol Rep,* **2008,** *10:*208–214.

Dickson EJ, Stuart RC. Genetics of response to proton pump inhibitor therapy: Clinical implications. *Am J Pharmacogenomics*, **2003,** *3:*303–315.

Fackler WK, Ours TM, Vaezi MF, Richter JE. Long-term effect of H2RA therapy on nocturnal gastric acid breakthrough. *Gastroenterology*, **2002,** *122:*625–632.

Ferreiro JL, Angiolillo DJ. Antiplatelet therapy: Clopidogrel plus PPIs—a dangerous combination? *Nature Rev Cardiol,* **2009,** *6:*392–394.

Freston J, Chiu YL, Pan WJ, Lukasik N, Taubel J. Oral bioavailability of pantoprazole suspended in sodium bicarbonate solution. *Am J Health Syst Pharm*, **2003,** *60:*1324–1329.

Graham DY. Therapy of *Helicobacter pylori*: Current status and issues. *Gastroenterology*, **2000,** *118:*S2–S8.

Lanas A, Hunt RH. Prevention of anti-inflammatory drug-induced gastrointestinal damage: Benefits and risks of therapeutic strategies. *Ann Med*, **2006,** *38:*415–428.

Norgard NB, Mathews KD, Wall GC. Drug-drug interaction between clopidogrel and the proton pump inhibitors. *Ann Pharmacother,* **2009,** *43:*1266–1274.

Ray WA, Murray KT, Griffin MR, et al. Outcomes with concurrent use of clopidogrel and proton-pump inhibitors: a cohort study. *Ann Intern Med,* **2010,** *152:*337–345.

Richter JE. Gastroesophageal reflux disease during pregnancy. *Gastroenterol Clin North Am,* **2003,** *32:*235–261.

Rostom A, Moayyedi P, Hunt R. Canadian Association of Gastroenterology Consensus Group. Canadian consensus guidelines on long-term nonsteroidal anti-inflammatory drug therapy and the need for gastroprotection: Benefits versus risks. *Aliment Pharmacol Ther,* **2009,** *29:*481–496.

Sandevik AK, Brenna E, Waldum HL. Review article: The pharmacological inhibition of gastric acid secretion-tolerance and rebound. *Aliment Pharmacol Ther,* **1997,** *11:*1013–1018.

Suerbaum S, Michetti P. *Helicobacter pylori* infection. *N Engl J Med,* **2002,** *347:*1175–1186.

Wallace JL. Prostaglandins, NSAIDs and mucosal defence. Why doesn't the stomach digest itself? *Physiol Rev,* **2008,** *88:* 1547–1565.

Wang C, Hunt RH. Medical management of gastroesophageal reflux disease. *Gastroenterol Clin North Am,* **2008,** *37:* 879–899.

Wolfe MM, Sachs G. Acid suppression: Optimizing therapy for gastroduodenal ulcer healing, gastroesophageal reflux disease, and stress-related erosive syndrome. *Gastroenterology,* **2000,** *118:*S9–S31.

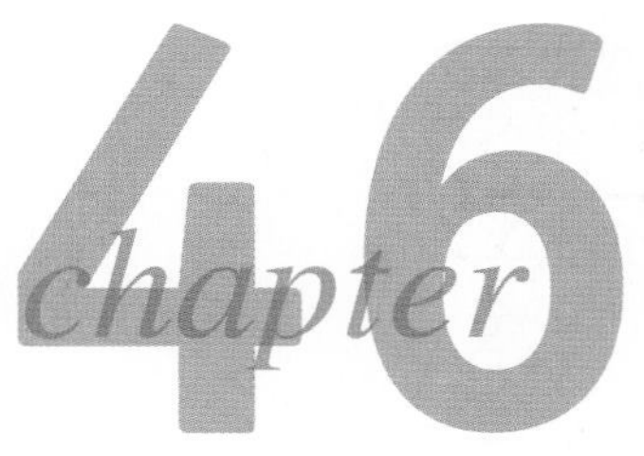

Treatment of Disorders of Bowel Motility and Water Flux; Anti-Emetics; Agents Used in Biliary and Pancreatic Disease

Keith A. Sharkey and
John L. Wallace

The longer I live, the more I am convinced that half the unhappiness in the world proceeds from little stoppages, from a duct choked up, from food pressing in the wrong place, from a vexed duodenum or an agitated pylorus.

—Sydney Smith (1771–1845)

INTRODUCTION TO GASTROINTESTINAL MOTILITY

The gastrointestinal (GI) tract is in a continuous contractile, absorptive, and secretory state. The control of this state is complex, with contributions by the muscle and epithelium themselves, as well as local nerves of the enteric nervous system (ENS), the autonomic nervous system (ANS), and circulating hormones (De Giorgio et al., 2007; Furness, 2006; Grundy et al., 2006; Wood, 2008). Of these, perhaps the most important regulator of physiological gut function is the ENS (Figure 46–1). The ENS is an extensive collection of nerves that constitutes the third division of the ANS. It is the only part of the ANS truly capable of autonomous function if separated from the central nervous system (CNS). The ENS lies within the wall of the GI tract organized into two connected networks of neurons and nerve fibers: the *myenteric (Auerbach's) plexus*, found between the circular and longitudinal muscle layers, and the *submucosal (Meissner's) plexus*, located in the submucosa. The former is largely responsible for motor control, whereas the latter regulates secretion, fluid transport, and blood flow. The ENS and the ANS are also involved in host defense and innervate organs and cells of the immune system (Rhee et al., 2009).

Generation and Regulation of GI Activity

The ENS is responsible for the largely autonomous nature of most GI activity. This activity is organized into relatively distinct programs that respond to input from the local environment of the gut, as well as the ANS-CNS. Each program consists of a series of complex, but coordinated, patterns of secretion and movement that show regional and temporal variation. The fasting program of the gut is called the MMC (*migrating myoelectric complex* when referring to electrical activity and *migrating motor complex* when referring to the accompanying contractions) and consists of a series of four phasic activities. The most characteristic, phase III, consists of clusters of rhythmic contractions that occupy short segments of the intestine for a period of 6-10 minutes before proceeding caudally (toward the anus). Phase II of the MMC is associated with the release of the peptide hormone motilin. Agonists of motilin stimulate motility in the proximal gut and are used clinically (Sanger, 2008). One whole MMC cycle (i.e., all four phases) takes ~80-110 minutes. The migrating motor complex occurs in the fasting state, during which it helps sweep debris caudad in the gut and serves to limit the overgrowth of luminal bacteria. The migrating motor complex cycles continually in animals that feed constantly but is interrupted by another pattern of contractions—the fed program—in intermittently feeding animals such as humans. The fed program consists of high-frequency (12-15 per minute) contractions that are either propagated for short segments (*propulsive*) or are irregular and not propagated (*mixing*).

Reflex circuits within the ENS underlie the stereotyped behaviors of the gut, such as peristalsis. Physiologically, peristalsis is a series of reflex responses to a bolus in the lumen of a given segment of the intestine; the ascending excitatory reflex results in contraction of the circular muscle on the oral side of the bolus, whereas the descending inhibitory reflex results in relaxation on the anal side. The net pressure gradient moves the bolus caudad. Three neural elements, responsible for sensory, relay, and effector functions, are required to produce these reflexes. Luminal factors stimulate sensory elements in the mucosa, leading to a coordinated pattern of

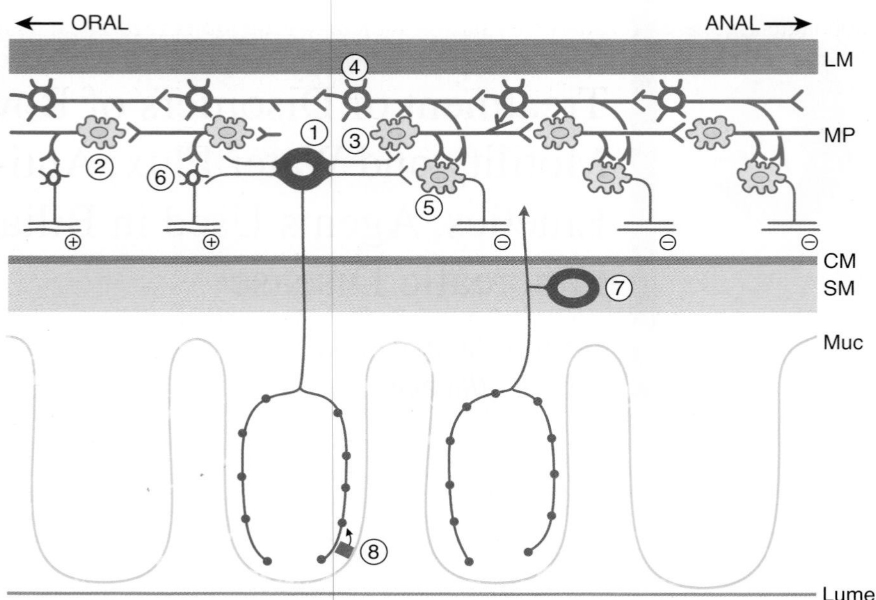

Figure 46–1. *The neuronal network that initiates and generates the peristaltic response.* Mucosal stimulation leads to release of serotonin by enterochromaffin cells (8), which excites the intrinsic primary afferent neurons (1), which then communicate with ascending (2) and descending (3) interneurons in the local reflex pathways. The reflex results in contraction at the oral end via the excitatory motor neuron (6) and aboral relaxation via the inhibitory motor neuron (5). The migratory myoelectric complex (see text) is shown here as being conducted by a different chain of interneurons (4). Another intrinsic primary afferent neuron with its cell body in the submucosa also is shown (7). MP, myenteric plexus; CM, circular muscle; LM, longitudinal muscle; SM, submucosa; Muc, mucosa. (Adapted from Kunze and Furness, 1999, with permission from Annual Reviews. www.annualreviews.org.)

muscle activity that is directly controlled by the motor neurons of the myenteric plexus to provide the effector component of the peristaltic reflex. Motor neurons receive input from ascending and descending interneurons (which constitute the relay and programming systems) that are of two broad types, excitatory and inhibitory. The primary neurotransmitter of the excitatory motor neurons is acetylcholine (ACh), although tachykinins, co-released by these neurons, also play a role. The principal neurotransmitter in the inhibitory motor neurons appears to be NO, although important contributions may also be made by ATP, vasoactive intestinal peptide, and pituitary adenylyl cyclase–activating peptide (PACAP), all of which are variably coexpressed with NO synthase. Substantial progress has been made in elucidating the mucosal sensor for initiating peristalsis and other reflexes. Enterochromaffin cells, scattered throughout the epithelium of the intestine, release serotonin (5-HT) to initiate many gut reflexes (Gershon and Tack, 2007) by acting locally on enteric neurons. Excessive release of 5-HT from the gut wall (e.g., by chemotherapeutic agents) leads to vomiting by actions of 5-HT on vagal nerve endings in the proximal small intestine. Compounds targeting the 5-HT system are important modulators of motility, secretion, and emesis.

This view of nerve–muscle interaction within the GI tract is in many ways oversimplified, and other cell types are important. One of these is the interstitial cell of Cajal, distributed within the gut wall and responsible for setting the electrical rhythm, and hence the pace of contractions, in various regions of the gut. These cells also translate or modulate excitatory and inhibitory neuronal communication to the smooth muscle (Ward et al., 2004).

Excitation-Contraction Coupling in GI Smooth Muscle

Control of tension in GI smooth muscle is in large part dependent on the intracellular Ca^{2+} concentration. In general, there are two types of excitation-contraction coupling. Ionotropic receptors can mediate changes in membrane potential, which in turn activate voltage-dependent Ca^{2+} channels to trigger an influx of Ca^{2+} (electromechanical coupling); metabotropic receptors activate various signal transduction pathways to release Ca^{2+} from intracellular stores (pharmaco-mechanical coupling). Inhibitory receptors also exist on smooth muscle and generally act via PKA and PKG, whose kinase activities can lead to hyperpolarization, decreased cytosolic $[Ca^{2+}]$, and reduced interaction of actin and myosin. As an example, NO may induce relaxation via activation of guanylyl cyclase-cyclic GMP pathway, and the opening of several types of K^+ channels.

OVERVIEW OF FUNCTIONAL AND MOTILITY DISORDERS OF THE BOWEL

GI motility disorders are a complex and heterogeneous group of syndromes whose pathophysiology is not completely understood. Typical motility disorders include achalasia of the esophagus (impaired relaxation of the lower esophageal sphincter associated with defective esophageal peristalsis that results in dysphagia and regurgitation), gastroparesis (delayed gastric emptying), myopathic and neuropathic forms of intestinal dysmotility, and others. These disorders can be congenital, idiopathic, or secondary to systemic diseases (e.g., diabetes mellitus or scleroderma). This term also has traditionally (and perhaps inaccurately) included disorders—such as irritable bowel syndrome (IBS) and noncardiac chest pain—in which disturbances in pain processing or sensory function may be more important than any associated motor patterns. For most of these disorders, treatment remains empirical and symptom based, reflecting our ignorance of the specific derangements in pathophysiology involved.

PROKINETIC AGENTS AND OTHER STIMULANTS OF GI CONTRACTILITY

Activation of muscarinic receptors with the older cholinomimetic agents (Chapter 9) or AChE inhibitors (Chapter 10), is not a very effective strategy for treating GI motility disorders because these agents enhance contractions in a relatively uncoordinated fashion that produces little or no net propulsive activity. The use of cholinergic agents is discussed in the previous edition of this book.

By contrast, *prokinetic* agents are medications that enhance coordinated GI motility and transit of material in the GI tract. Although ACh, when released from primary motor neurons in the myenteric plexus, is the principal immediate mediator of muscle contractility, most of the clinically useful prokinetic agents act "upstream" of ACh, at receptor sites on the motor neuron itself, or even more indirectly, on neurons or non-neuronal cells one or two orders removed from it. Although pharmacologically and chemically diverse, these agents appear to enhance the release of excitatory neurotransmitter at the nerve-muscle junction without interfering with the normal physiological pattern and rhythm of motility. Coordination of activity among the segments of the gut, necessary for propulsion of luminal contents, therefore is maintained.

Agents useful clinically in altering GI motility are considered next.

Dopamine Receptor Antagonists

Dopamine (DA) is present in significant amounts in the GI tract and has several inhibitory effects on motility, including reduction of lower esophageal sphincter and intragastric pressures. These effects, which apparently result from suppression of ACh release from myenteric motor neurons, are mediated by D_2 dopaminergic receptors. By antagonizing the inhibitory effect of dopamine on myenteric motor neurons, DA receptor antagonists are effective as prokinetic agents; they have the additional advantage of relieving nausea and vomiting by antagonism of DA receptors in the chemoreceptor trigger zone. Examples of such agents are metoclopramide and domperidone.

Metoclopramide. Chemistry, Mechanism of Action, and Pharmacological Properties. Metoclopramide (REGLAN, others) and other substituted benzamides are derivatives of *para*-aminobenzoic acid and are structurally related to procainamide.

Cl, $CONHCH_2CH_2N(C_2H_5)_2$, H_2N, OCH_3

METOCLOPRAMIDE

The mechanisms of action of metoclopramide are complex and involve 5-HT_4 receptor agonism, vagal and central 5-HT_3 antagonism, and possible sensitization of muscarinic receptors on smooth muscle, in addition to DA receptor antagonism. Metoclopramide is one of the oldest true prokinetic agents; its administration results in coordinated contractions that enhance transit. Its effects are confined largely to the upper digestive tract, where it increases lower esophageal sphincter tone and stimulates antral and small intestinal contractions. Despite having *in vitro* effects on the contractility of colonic smooth muscle, metoclopramide has no clinically significant effects on large-bowel motility.

Pharmacokinetics. Metoclopramide is absorbed rapidly after oral ingestion, undergoes sulfation and glucuronide conjugation by the liver, and is excreted principally in the urine, with a $t_{1/2}$ of 4-6 hours. Peak concentrations occur within 1 hour after a single oral dose; the duration of action is 1-2 hours.

Therapeutic Use. Metoclopramide has been used in patients with gastroesophageal reflux disease to produce symptomatic relief of, but not healing of, associated esophagitis. It clearly is less effective than modern acid-suppressive medications, such as proton pump inhibitors or histamine H_2 receptor antagonists, and now rarely is used in this setting. Metoclopramide is indicated more often in symptomatic patients with gastroparesis, in whom it may cause mild to modest improvements of gastric emptying (Tonini et al., 2004). Metoclopramide injection is used as an adjunctive measure in medical or diagnostic procedures such as intestinal intubation or contrast radiography of the GI tract. Although it has been used in patients with postoperative ileus, its ability to improve transit in disorders of small-bowel motility appears to be limited. *In general, its greatest utility lies in its ability to ameliorate the nausea and vomiting that often accompany GI dysmotility syndromes.* Metoclopramide has also been used in the treatment of persistent hiccups, but its efficacy in this condition is equivocal at best.

Metoclopramide is available in oral dosage forms (tablets and solution) and as a parenteral preparation for intravenous or intramuscular use. The usual initial oral dose range is 10 mg, 30 minutes before each meal and at bedtime. The onset of action is within 30-60 minutes after an oral dose. In patients with severe nausea, an initial dose of 10 mg can be given intramuscularly (onset of action 10-15 minutes) or intravenously (onset of action 1-3 minutes). For prevention of chemotherapy-induced emesis, metoclopramide can be given as an infusion of 1-2 mg/kg administered over at least 15 minutes, beginning 30 minutes before the chemotherapy is begun and repeated as needed every 2 hours for two doses, then every 3 hours for three doses.

Adverse Effects. The major side effects of metoclopramide include extrapyramidal effects, such as those seen with the phenothiazines (Chapter 16). Dystonias, usually occurring acutely after intravenous administration, and parkinsonian-like symptoms that may occur several weeks after initiation of therapy generally respond to treatment with anticholinergic or antihistaminic drugs and are reversible upon discontinuation of metoclopramide. Tardive dyskinesia also can occur with chronic treatment (months to years) and may be irreversible. Extrapyramidal effects appear to occur more commonly in children and young adults and at higher doses. Like other DA antagonists, metoclopramide also can cause galactorrhea by blocking the inhibitory effect of dopamine on prolactin release, but this adverse effect is relatively infrequent in clinical practice. Methemoglobinemia has been reported occasionally in premature and full-term neonates receiving metoclopramide.

Domperidone; D_2 Receptor Antagonists

In contrast to metoclopramide, domperidone predominantly antagonizes the D_2 receptor without major involvement of other receptors. It is not available for use in the U.S. but has been used elsewhere (MOTILIUM, others) and has modest prokinetic activity in doses of 10-20 mg three times a day. Although it does not readily cross the blood-brain barrier to cause extrapyramidal side effects, domperidone exerts effects in the parts of the CNS that lack this barrier, such as those regulating emesis, temperature, and prolactin release. As is the case with metoclopramide, domperidone does not appear to have any significant effects on lower GI motility. Other D_2 receptor antagonists being explored as prokinetic agents include levosulpiride, the levo-enantiomer of sulpiride.

Serotonin Receptor Agonists

5-HT plays an important role in the normal motor and secretory function of the gut (Gershon and Tack, 2007) (Chapter 13). Indeed, >90% of the total 5-HT in the body exists in the GI tract. The enterochromaffin cell, a specialized cell found in the epithelium lining the mucosa of the gut, produces most of this 5-HT and rapidly releases 5-HT in response to chemical and mechanical stimulation (e.g., food boluses; noxious agents such as cisplatin; certain microbial toxins; adrenergic, cholinergic, and purinergic receptor agonists). 5-HT triggers the peristaltic reflex (Figure 46–1) by stimulating intrinsic sensory neurons in the myenteric plexus (via 5-HT_{1p} and 5-HT_4 receptors), as well as extrinsic vagal and spinal sensory neurons (via 5-HT_3 receptors). Additionally, stimulation of submucosal intrinsic afferent neurons activates secretomotor reflexes resulting in epithelial secretion. 5-HT receptors also are found on other neurons in the enteric nervous system, where they can be either stimulatory (5-HT_3 and 5-HT_4) or inhibitory (5-HT_{1a}). In addition, serotonin also stimulates the release of other neurotransmitters, depending on the receptor subtype. Thus, 5-HT_1 stimulation of the gastric fundus results in release of NO and reduces smooth muscle tone. 5-HT_4 stimulation of excitatory motor neurons enhances ACh release at the neuromuscular junction, and both 5-HT_3 and 5-HT_4 receptors facilitate interneuronal signaling. Developmentally, 5-HT acts as a neurotrophic factor for enteric neurons via the 5-HT_{2B} and 5-HT_4 receptors.

Reuptake of serotonin by enteric neurons and epithelium is mediated by the same transporter (SERT; Chapters 5 and 13) as 5-HT reuptake by serotonergic neurons in the CNS. This reuptake therefore also is blocked by selective serotonin reuptake inhibitors (SSRIs, Chapter 15), which explains the common side effect of diarrhea that accompanies the use of these agents. Modulation of the multiple, complex, and sometimes opposing effects of 5-HT on gut motor function has become a major target for drug development.

The availability of serotonergic prokinetic drugs has in recent years been restricted because of serious adverse cardiac events. Tegaserod maleate (ZELNORM) was discontinued in 2007 and cisapride is available only via a restricted investigational drug protocol. A novel 5-HT_4 agonist, prucalopride (RESOLOR), is approved for use in Europe for symptomatic treatment of chronic constipation in women in whom laxatives fail to provide adequate relief.

Cisapride. Cisapride (PROPULSID) is a substituted piperidinyl benzamide (Figure 46–2) that appears to stimulate 5-HT_4 receptors and increase adenylyl cyclase activity within neurons. It also has weak 5-HT_3 antagonistic properties and may directly stimulate smooth muscle. Cisapride was a commonly used prokinetic agent, particularly for gastroesophageal reflux disease and gastroparesis. However, it no longer is generally available in the U.S. because of its potential to induce serious and occasionally fatal cardiac arrhythmias, including ventricular tachycardia, ventricular fibrillation, and torsades de pointes. These arrhythmias result from a prolonged QT interval through an interaction with pore-forming subunits of the HERG K^+ channel. HERG K^+ channels conduct the rapid delayed rectifier K^+ current that is important for normal repolarization of the ventricle (Chapter 29). Cisapride-induced ventricular arrhythmias occur most

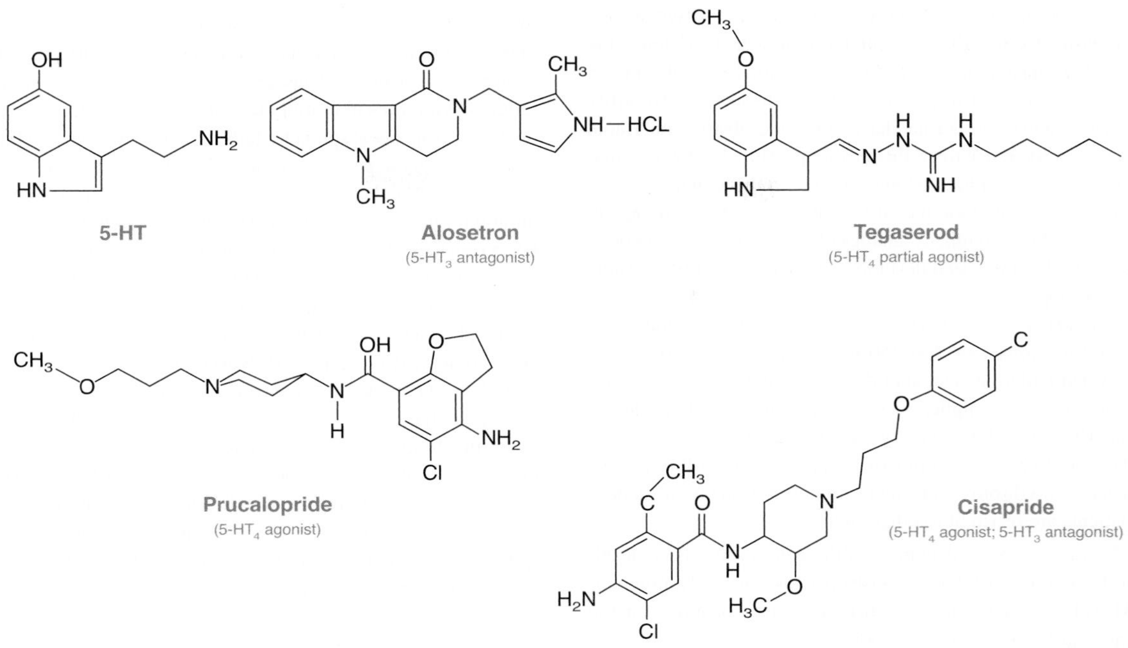

Figure 46–2. *Ligands of 5-HT$_3$ and 5-HT$_4$ receptors modulating GI motility.*

often when the drug is combined with other drugs that inhibit CYP3A4 (Chapter 6); such combinations inhibit the metabolism of cisapride and lead to high plasma concentrations of the drug. Due to its association with ventricular arrhythmias, cisapride is contraindicated in patients with a history of prolonged QT interval, renal failure, ventricular arrhythmias, ischemic heart disease, congestive heart failure, respiratory failure, uncorrected electrolyte abnormalities (e.g., hypokalemia and hypomagnesemia), or concomitant medications known to prolong the QT interval. At this time, cisapride is available only through an investigational, limited-access program for patients with GERD, gastroparesis, pseudo-obstruction, refractory severe chronic constipation, and neonatal enteral feeding intolerance who have failed all standard therapeutic modalities and who have undergone a thorough diagnostic evaluation, including an ECG.

Prucalopride (RESELOR; Figure 46–2) is a benzofuran derivative and a specific 5-HT$_4$-receptor agonist that facilitates cholinergic neurotransmission. It acts throughout the length of the intestine, increasing oral-cecal transit and colonic transit without affecting gastric emptying in healthy volunteers. In patients with chronic idiopathic constipation, prucalopride was able to improve colonic transit and stool frequency. Given in doses of 2 and 4 mg orally, once daily, there were significant normalization of bowel habits including increased stool frequency and consistency (Gale, 2009). This drug recently gained approval in Europe for use in women with chronic constipation in whom laxatives fail to provide adequate relief.

Motilides

Macrolides and Erythromycin. Motilin, a 22–amino acid peptide hormone found in the GI M cells and in some enterochromaffin cells of the upper small bowel, is a potent contractile agent of the upper GI tract. Motilin levels fluctuate in association with the migrating motor complex and appear to be responsible for the amplification, if not the actual induction, of phase III activity. In addition, motilin receptors are found on smooth muscle cells and enteric neurons.

The effects of motilin can be mimicked by erythromycin, a discovery that arose from the frequent occurrence of GI side effects with the use of this antibiotic. This property is shared to varying extents by other macrolide antibiotics (Chapter 55), including oleandomycin, azithromycin, and clarithromycin. In addition to its motilin-like effects, which are most pronounced at higher doses (250-500 mg), erythromycin at lower doses (e.g., 40-80 mg) also may act by other poorly defined mechanisms that may involve cholinergic facilitation.

Erythromycin induces phase III migrating motor complex activity in dogs and increases smooth muscle contractility. It has multiple effects on upper GI motility, increasing lower esophageal pressure and stimulating gastric and small-bowel contractility. By contrast, it has little or no effect on colonic motility. At doses higher than 3 mg/kg, it can produce a spastic type of contraction in the small bowel, resulting in cramps, impairment of transit, and vomiting.

Therapeutic Use. The best established use of erythromycin as a prokinetic agent is in patients with diabetic gastroparesis, where it can improve gastric emptying in the short term. Erythromycin-stimulated gastric contractions can be intense and result in "dumping" of relatively undigested food into the small bowel. This potential disadvantage can be exploited clinically to clear the stomach of undigestible residue such as plastic tubes or bezoars. Anecdotally, erythromycin also has been of benefit in patients with small-bowel dysmotility such as that seen in scleroderma, ileus, or pseudo-obstruction. Rapid development of tolerance to erythromycin, possibly by downregulation of the motilin receptor, and undesirable (in this context) antibiotic effects have limited the use of this drug as a prokinetic agent. Several non-antibiotic synthetic analogs of erythromycin and peptide analogs of motilin have been developed; to date, the clinical results have been disappointing.

A standard dose of erythromycin for gastric stimulation is 3 mg/kg intravenously or 200-250 mg orally every 8 hours. For small-bowel stimulation, a smaller dose (e.g., 40 mg intravenously) may be more useful, as higher doses may actually retard motility of this organ. Concerns about toxicity, pseudomembranous colitis, and the induction of resistant strains of bacteria, among other things, limit the use of erythromycin to acute situations or in circumstances where patients are resistant to other medications.

Motilin Receptor Agonists. A number of these drugs have been developed for the treatment of diabetic gastroparesis. Currently, mitemcinal (GM-611), a macrolide nonantibiotic, shows promise for the treatment of gastroparesis (Gale, 2009).

Miscellaneous Agents for Stimulating Motility

The GI hormone cholecystokinin (CCK) is released from the intestine in response to meals and delays gastric emptying, causes contraction of the gallbladder, stimulates pancreatic enzyme secretion, increases intestinal motility, promotes satiety, and has a host of other actions. The C-terminal octapeptide of CCK, sincalide (KINEVAC), is useful for stimulating the gallbladder and/or pancreas and may also be used for accelerating barium transit through the small bowel for diagnostic testing of these organs. This drug is administered intravenously 0.02-0.04 μg/kg over 30-60 seconds or up to 30-45 minutes depending on the test. Administration of this agent is frequently accompanied by nausea and abdominal pain, and much less frequently dizziness. Concerns that should be noted using this agent are related to the expulsion of small gallstones into the common bile duct or cystic duct. *Dexloxiglumide* is a CCK_1 (or CCK-A)–receptor antagonist that can improve gastric emptying and was investigated as a treatment for gastroparesis and for constipation-dominant IBS, but may also have uses in feeding intolerance in critically ill individuals. Clonidine also has been reported to be of benefit in patients with gastroparesis. Octreotide acetate (SANDOSTATIN, others), a somatostatin analogue, also is used in some patients with intestinal dysmotility.

In some disorders of motility, effective treatment does not necessarily require a "neuroenteric" approach. One such example is gastroesophageal reflux disease. Acid reflux is associated with transient lower esophageal sphincter relaxations that occur in the absence of a swallow. Because the damage to the esophagus ultimately is inflicted by acid, the most effective therapy for gastroesophageal reflux disease still is the suppression of acid production by the stomach (Chapter 45). Neither metoclopramide nor cisapride by itself is particularly effective in gastroesophageal reflux disease. However, a new approach under investigation relies on suppression of the transient lower esophageal sphincter relaxations, as achieved by CCK_1-receptor antagonists (such as dexloxiglumide), GABA agonists (such as baclofen), and inhibitors of NO synthesis.

Agents that Suppress Motility

Smooth muscle relaxants such as organic nitrates and Ca^{2+} channel antagonists (Chapters 27 and 28) often produce temporary, if partial, relief of symptoms in motility disorders such as achalasia, in which the lower esophageal sphincter fails to relax, resulting in a functional obstruction to the passage of food and severe difficulty in swallowing. A more recent approach relies on the use of preparations of botulinum toxin (BOTOX, DYSPORT, MYOBLOC), injected directly into the lower esophageal sphincter via an endoscope, in doses of 80-100 units (Zhao and Pasricha, 2003). This potent agent inhibits ACh release from nerve endings (Chapter 11) and can produce partial paralysis of the sphincter muscle, with significant improvements in symptoms and esophageal clearance. However, its effects dissipate over a period of several months, requiring repeated injections; there is also some potential for post-administration "spread" of the toxin that can result in life-threatening consequences. Botulinum toxin preparations likely will be more widely used especially in the elderly and in those with other risks for pneumatic dilation. Other GI conditions in which botulinum toxin A has been used include gastroparesis, sphincter of Oddi dysfunction, and anal fissures, although currently there are not strong trial data to support its efficacy.

LAXATIVES, CATHARTICS, AND THERAPY FOR CONSTIPATION

Overview of GI Water and Electrolyte Flux. Fluid content is the principal determinant of stool volume and consistency; water normally accounts for 70-85% of total stool weight. Net stool fluid content reflects a balance between luminal input (ingestion and secretion of water and electrolytes) and output (absorption) along the length of the GI tract. The daily challenge for the gut is to extract water, minerals, and nutrients from the luminal contents, leaving behind a manageable pool of fluid for proper expulsion of waste material via the process of defecation. Normally ~8-9 L of fluid enter the small intestine daily from exogenous and endogenous sources (Figure 46–3). Net absorption of the water occurs in the small intestine in response to osmotic gradients that result from the uptake and secretion of ions and the absorption of nutrients (mainly sugars and amino acids), with only ~1-1.5 L crossing the ileocecal valve. The colon then extracts most of the remaining fluid, leaving ~100 mL of fecal water daily.

Under normal circumstances, these quantities are well within the range of the total absorptive capacity of the small bowel (~16 L) and colon (4-5 L). Neurohumoral mechanisms, pathogens, and drugs can alter these processes, resulting in changes in either secretion or absorption of fluid by the intestinal epithelium. Altered motility also contributes in a general way to this process, as the extent of absorption parallels transit time. With decreased motility and excess fluid removal,

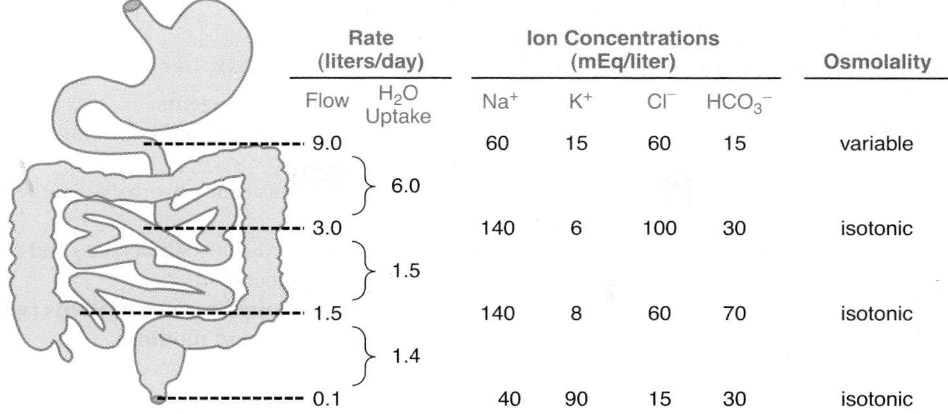

Rate
(liters/day)
Flow
H_2O Uptake
Ion Concentrations
(mEq/liter)
Na^+
K^+
Cl^-
HCO_3^-
Osmolality
9.0
60 15 60 15
variable
6.0
3.0
140 6 100 30
isotonic
1.5
1.5
140 8 60 70
isotonic
1.4
0.1
40 90 15 30
isotonic

Figure 46–3. *The approximate volume and composition of fluid that traverses the small and large intestines daily.* Of the 9 L of fluid typically presented to the small intestine each day, 2 L are from the diet and 7 L are from secretions (salivary, gastric, pancreatic, and biliary). The absorptive capacity of the colon is 4-5 L per day.

feces can become inspissated and impacted, leading to constipation. When the capacity of the colon to absorb fluid is exceeded, diarrhea occurs.

Constipation: General Principles of Pathophysiology and Treatment. Scientific definitions rely mostly on stool number; most surveys have found the normal stool frequency on a Western diet to be at least three times a week. However, patients use the term *constipation* not only for decreased frequency, but also for difficulty in initiation or passage, passage of firm or small-volume feces, or a feeling of incomplete evacuation. By questionnaire, 25% of the population of the U.S., more commonly women and elderly people, complain of constipation. A survey of bowel habits of adults in the U.S. showed that 18% of respondents used laxatives at least once a month, but nearly one-third of users did not have constipation. Approximately 2.5 million physician visits per year are attributed to constipation.

Constipation has many reversible or secondary causes, including lack of dietary fiber, drugs, hormonal disturbances, neurogenic disorders, and systemic illnesses. In most cases of chronic constipation, no specific cause is found. Up to 60% of patients presenting with constipation have normal colonic transit. These patients either have IBS or define constipation in terms other than stool frequency (e.g., changes in consistency, excessive straining, or a feeling of incomplete evacuation). In the rest, attempts usually are made to categorize the underlying pathophysiology either as a disorder of delayed colonic transit because of an underlying defect in colonic motility or, less commonly, as an isolated disorder of defecation or evacuation (outlet disorder) due to dysfunction of the neuromuscular apparatus of the rectoanal region. Colonic motility is responsible for mixing luminal contents to promote absorption of water and moving them from proximal to distal segments by means of propulsive contractions. Mixing in the colon is accomplished in a way similar to that in the small bowel: by short- or long-duration, stationary (nonpropulsive) contractions. Propulsive contractions in the colon include giant migrating contractions, also known as colonic mass actions or mass movements, which propagate caudally over extended lengths in the colon and evoke mass transfer of feces from the right to the left colon once or twice a day. Disturbances in motility therefore may have complex effects on bowel movements. "Decreased motility" of the mass action type and "increased motility" of the nonpropulsive type may lead to constipation. In any given patient, the predominant factor often is not obvious. Consequently, the pharmacological approach to constipation remains empirical and is based, in most cases, on nonspecific principles.

In many cases, constipation can be corrected by adherence to a fiber-rich (20-35 g daily) diet, adequate fluid intake, appropriate bowel habits and training, and avoidance of constipating drugs. However, the association between constipation and either fluid intake or exercise has not withstood scientific scrutiny. Constipation related to medications can be corrected by use of alternative drugs where possible, or adjustment of dosage. If non-pharmacological measures alone are inadequate or unrealistic (e.g., because of elderly age or infirmity), they may be supplemented with bulk-forming agents or osmotic laxatives. When stimulant laxatives are used, they should be administered at the lowest effective dosage and for the shortest period of time to avoid abuse. In addition to perpetuating dependence on drugs, the laxative habit may lead to excessive loss of water and electrolytes; secondary aldosteronism may occur if volume depletion is prominent. Steatorrhea, protein-losing enteropathy with hypoalbuminemia, and osteomalacia due to excessive loss of calcium in the stool have been reported.

In addition to treating constipation, laxatives frequently are employed before surgical, radiological, and endoscopic procedures where an empty colon is desirable.

The terms *laxatives, cathartics, purgatives, aperients*, and *evacuants* often are used interchangeably. There is a distinction, however, between *laxation* (the evacuation of formed fecal material from the rectum) and *catharsis* (the evacuation of unformed, usually watery fecal material from the entire colon). Most of the commonly used agents promote laxation, but some are actually cathartics that act as laxatives at low doses.

Laxatives generally act in one of the following ways: (1) enhancing retention of intraluminal fluid by hydrophilic or osmotic mechanisms; (2) decreasing net absorption of fluid by effects on small- and large-bowel fluid and electrolyte transport; or (3) altering motility by either inhibiting segmenting (nonpropulsive) contractions or stimulating propulsive contractions. Based on their actions, laxatives can be classified as shown in Table 46–1; their known effects on motility and secretion are listed in Table 46–2. However, studies indicate considerable overlap among these traditional categories. A variety of laxatives, both osmotic agents and stimulants, increase the activity of NO synthase and the biosynthesis of platelet-activating factor in the gut. Platelet-activating factor is a phospholipid proinflammatory mediator that stimulates colonic secretion and GI motility (Izzo et al., 1998). NO also may stimulate intestinal secretion and inhibit segmenting contractions in the colon, thereby promoting laxation. Agents that reduce the expression of NO synthase or its activity can prevent the laxative effects of castor oil, cascara, and bisacodyl (but not senna), as well as magnesium sulfate.

Table 46–1

Classification of Laxatives

1. **Luminally active agents**
   Hydrophilic colloids; bulk-forming agents (bran, psyllium, etc.)
   Osmotic agents (non-absorbable inorganic salts or sugars)
   Stool-wetting agents (surfactants) and emollients (docusate, mineral oil)
2. **Nonspecific stimulants or irritants (with effects on fluid secretion and motility)**
   Diphenylmethanes (bisacodyl)
   Anthraquinones (senna and cascara)
   Castor oil
3. **Prokinetic agents (acting primarily on motility)**
   5-HT_4 receptor agonists
   Dopamine receptor antagonists
   Motilides (erythromycin)

An alternate way to classify laxatives is by the pattern of effects produced by the usual clinical dosage (Table 46–3).

Dietary Fiber and Supplements

Under normal circumstances, the bulk, softness, and hydration of feces depend on the fiber content of the diet. Fiber is defined as that part of food that resists enzymatic digestion and reaches the colon largely unchanged. Colonic bacteria ferment fiber to varying

Table 46–2

Summary of Effects of Some Laxatives on Bowel Function

	SMALL BOWEL		COLON		
AGENT	TRANSIT TIME	MIXING CONTRACTIONS	PROPULSIVE CONTRACTIONS	MASS ACTIONS	STOOL WATER
Dietary fiber	↓	?	↑	?	↑
Magnesium	↓	—	↑	↑	↑↑
Lactulose	↓	?	?	?	↑↑
Metoclopramide	↓	?	↑	?	—
Cisapride	↓	?	↑	?	↑
Erythromycin	↓	?	?	?	?
Naloxone	↓	↓	—	—	↑
Anthraquinones	↓	↓	↑	↑	↑↑
Diphenylmethanes	↓	↓	↑	↑	↑↑
Docusates	—	?	?	?	—

↑, increased; ↓, decreased; ?, no data available; —, no effect on this parameter. Modified from Kreek, 1994, with permission. http://lww.com.

Table 46–3

Classification and Comparison of Representative Laxatives

LAXATIVE EFFECT AND LATENCY IN USUAL CLINICAL DOSAGE		
SOFTENING OF FECES, 1-3 DAYS	SOFT OR SEMIFLUID STOOL, 6-8 HOURS	WATERY EVACUATION, 1-3 HOURS
Bulk-forming laxatives	***Stimulant laxatives***	***Osmotic laxatives***[a]
Bran	Diphenylmethane derivatives	Sodium phosphates
Psyllium preparations	Bisacodyl	Magnesium sulfate
Methylcellulose		Milk of magnesia
Calcium polycarbophil		Magnesium citrate
Surfactant laxatives	***Anthraquinone derivatives***	***Castor oil***
Docusates	Senna	
Poloxamers	Cascara sagrada	
Lactulose		

[a]Employed in high dosage for rapid cathartic effect and in lower dosage for laxative effect.

degrees, depending on its chemical nature and water solubility. Fermentation of fiber has two important effects:

- it produces short-chain fatty acids that are trophic for colonic epithelium
- it increases bacterial mass

Although fermentation of fiber generally decreases stool water, short-chain fatty acids also may have a prokinetic effect, and increased bacterial mass may contribute to increased stool volume. However, fiber that is not fermented can attract water and increase stool bulk. The net effect on bowel movement therefore varies with different compositions of dietary fiber (Table 46–4). In general, insoluble, poorly fermentable fibers, such as lignin, are most effective in increasing stool bulk and transit.

Bran, the residue left when flour is made from cereal grains, contains >40% dietary fiber. Wheat bran, with its high lignin content, is most effective at increasing stool weight. Fruits and vegetables contain more *pectins* and *hemicelluloses*, which are more readily fermentable and produce less effect on stool transit. *Psyllium husk*, derived from the seed of the plantago herb (*Plantago ovata*; known as ispaghula or isabgol in many parts of the world), is a component of many commercial products for constipation (METAMUCIL, others). Psyllium husk contains a hydrophilic mucilloid that undergoes significant fermentation in the colon, leading to an increase in colonic bacterial mass. The usual dose is 2.5-4 g (1-3 teaspoonfuls in 250 mL of fruit juice), titrated upward until the desired goal is reached. A variety of semisynthetic celluloses—e.g., methylcellulose (CITRUCEL, others) and the hydrophilic resin calcium polycarbophil (FIBERCON, FIBERALL, others), a polymer of acrylic acid resin—also are available. These poorly fermentable compounds absorb water and increase fecal bulk. Malt soup extract (MALSTSUPEX, others), an extract of malt from barley grains that contains small amounts of polymeric carbohydrates, proteins, electrolytes, and vitamins, is another orally administered bulk-forming agent.

Fiber is contraindicated in patients with obstructive symptoms and in those with megacolon or megarectum. Fecal impaction should be treated before initiating fiber supplementation. Bloating is the most common side effect of soluble fiber products (perhaps due to colonic fermentation), but it usually decreases with time. Calcium polycarbophil preparations release Ca^{2+} in the GI tract and thus should be avoided by patients who must restrict their intake of calcium or who are taking tetracycline. Sugar-free bulk laxatives may contain aspartame and are contraindicated in patients with phenylketonuria. Allergic reactions to psyllium have been reported.

Osmotically Active Agents

Saline Laxatives. Laxatives containing magnesium cations or phosphate anions commonly are called *saline laxatives*: magnesium sulfate, magnesium hydroxide, magnesium citrate, sodium phosphate. Their cathartic action is believed to result from osmotically mediated water retention, which then stimulates peristalsis. Other mechanisms may contribute to their effects, including the production of inflammatory mediators. Magnesium-containing laxatives may stimulate the release of cholecystokinin, which leads to intraluminal fluid and electrolyte accumulation and to increased intestinal motility. It is estimated that for every additional mEq of Mg^{2+} in the intestinal lumen, fecal weight increases by ~7 g. The usual dose of magnesium salts contains 40-120 mEq of Mg^{2+} and produces 300-600 mL of stool within 6 hours. The intensely bitter taste of some

Table 46–4

Properties of Different Dietary Fibers

TYPE OF FIBER	WATER SOLUBILITY	% FERMENTED
Nonpolysaccharides		
Lignin	Poor	0
Cellulose	Poor	15
Noncellulose polysaccharides		
Hemicellulose	Good	56-87
Mucilages and gums	Good	85-95
Pectins	Good	90-95

preparations may induce nausea and can be masked with citrus juices.

Phosphate salts are better absorbed than magnesium-based agents and therefore need to be given in larger doses to induce catharsis. The most frequently employed preparations of sodium phosphate are an oral solution (FLEET PHOSPHO-SODA) and tablets (VISICOL, OSMOPREP). Over-the-counter oral sodium phosphate products for bowel cleansing were withdrawn from the market in 2008 following the determination by the FDA that only prescription medications should be available for this purpose. To reduce the likelihood of acute phosphate nephropathy, oral phosphates should be avoided in patients at risk (the elderly, patients with known bowel pathology or renal dysfunction, and patients on angiotensin-converting enzyme [ACE] inhibitors, angiotensin receptor blockers [ARBs], and nonsteroidal anti-inflammatory drugs [NSAIDs]) and the two-dose regimens should be split evenly with the first dose taken the evening before the exam and the second starting 3-5 hours before the exam. Adequate fluid intake (1-3 L) is essential for any oral sodium phosphate regimen used for colonic preparation.

Magnesium- and phosphate-containing preparations must be used with caution or avoided in patients with renal insufficiency, cardiac disease, or preexisting electrolyte abnormalities, and in patients on diuretic therapy. Patients taking >45 mL of oral sodium phosphate as a prescribed bowel preparation may experience electrolyte shifts that pose a risk for the development of symptomatic dehydration, renal failure, metabolic acidosis, tetany from hypocalcemia, and even death in vulnerable populations.

Nondigestible Sugars and Alcohols. *Lactulose* (CEPHULAC, CHRONULAC, others) is a synthetic disaccharide of galactose and fructose that resists intestinal disaccharidase activity. This and other non-absorbable sugars such as sorbitol and mannitol are hydrolyzed in the colon to short-chain fatty acids, which stimulate colonic propulsive motility by osmotically drawing water into the lumen. Sorbitol and lactulose are equally efficacious in the treatment of constipation caused by opioids and vincristine, of constipation in the elderly, and of idiopathic chronic constipation.

They are available as 70% solutions, which are given in doses of 15-30 mL at night, with increases as needed up to 60 mL per day in divided doses. Effects may not be seen for 24-48 hours after dosing is begun. Abdominal discomfort or distention and flatulence are relatively common in the first few days of treatment but usually subside with continued administration. A few patients dislike the sweet taste of the preparations; dilution with water or administering the preparation with fruit juice can mask the taste.

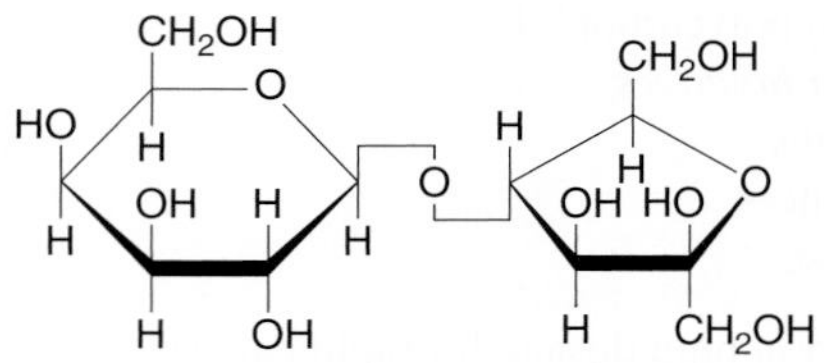

LACTULOSE

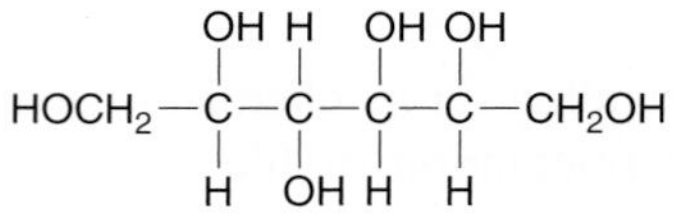

SORBITOL

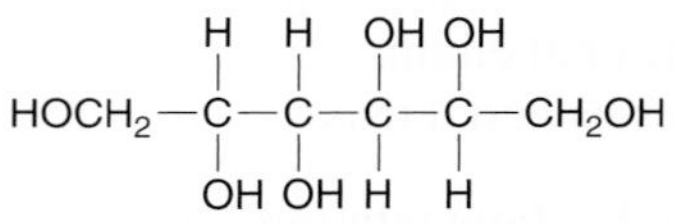

MANNITOL

Lactulose also is used to treat hepatic encephalopathy. Patients with severe liver disease have an impaired capacity to detoxify ammonia coming from the colon, where it is produced by bacterial metabolism of fecal urea. The drop in luminal pH that accompanies hydrolysis to short-chain fatty acids in the colon results in "trapping" of the ammonia by its conversion to the polar ammonium ion. Combined with the increases in colonic transit, this therapy significantly lowers circulating ammonia levels. The therapeutic goal in this condition is to give sufficient amounts of lactulose (usually 20-30 g, three to four times per day) to produce two to three soft stools a day with a pH of 5-5.5.

Polyethylene Glycol–Electrolyte Solutions. Long-chain polyethylene glycols (PEGs; molecular weight ~3350 Da) are poorly absorbed, and PEG solutions are retained in the lumen by virtue of their high osmotic nature. When used in high volume, aqueous solutions of PEGs with electrolytes (COLYTE, GOLYTELY, others) produce an effective catharsis and have replaced oral sodium phosphates as the most widely used preparations for colonic cleansing prior to radiological, surgical, and endoscopic procedures. Usually 240 mL of this solution is taken every 10 minutes until 4 L is consumed or the rectal effluent is clear. To avoid net transfer of ions across the intestinal wall, these preparations contain an isotonic mixture of sodium sulfate, sodium bicarbonate, sodium chloride, and potassium chloride. The osmotic activity of the PEG molecules retains the added water and the electrolyte concentration assures little or no net ionic shifts.

PEGs (without electrolytes) are also increasingly being used in smaller doses (250-500 mL daily) for the treatment of constipation in difficult cases. A powder form of polyethylene glycol 3350 (MIRALAX, others) is now available for the short-term treatment (≤2 weeks) of occasional constipation, although the agent has been prescribed safely for longer periods in clinical practice. The usual dose is 17 g of powder per day in 8 ounces of water. This preparation does not contain electrolytes, so larger volumes may represent a risk for ionic shifts. As with other laxatives, prolonged, frequent, or excessive use may result in dependence or electrolyte imbalance.

Stool-Wetting Agents and Emollients

Docusate salts are anionic surfactants that lower the surface tension of the stool to allow mixing of aqueous and fatty substances, softening the stool and permitting easier defecation. However, these agents also stimulate intestinal fluid and electrolyte secretion (possibly by increasing mucosal cyclic AMP) and alter intestinal mucosal permeability. Docusate sodium (diocytl sodium sulfosuccinate; COLACE, DOXINATE, others) and docusate calcium (dioctyl calcium sulfosuccinate; SURFAK, others), are available in several dosage forms. Despite their widespread use, these agents have marginal, if any, efficacy in most cases of constipation.

Mineral oil is a mixture of aliphatic hydrocarbons obtained from petrolatum. The oil is indigestible and absorbed only to a limited extent. When mineral oil is taken orally for 2-3 days, it penetrates and softens the stool and may interfere with resorption of water. The side effects of mineral oil preclude its regular use and include interference with absorption of fat-soluble substances (such as vitamins), elicitation of foreign-body reactions in the intestinal mucosa and other tissues, and leakage of oil past the anal sphincter. Rare complications such as lipid pneumonitis due to aspiration also can occur, so "heavy" mineral oil should not be taken at bedtime and "light" (topical) mineral oil should never be administered orally.

Stimulant (Irritant) Laxatives

Stimulant laxatives have direct effects on enterocytes, enteric neurons, and GI smooth muscle. These agents probably induce a limited low-grade inflammation in the small and large bowel to promote accumulation of water and electrolytes and stimulate intestinal motility. Proposed mechanisms include activation of prostaglandin–cyclic AMP and NO–cyclic GMP pathways, platelet-activating factor production (see earlier), and inhibition of Na^+, K^+-ATPase. Included in this group are diphenylmethane derivatives, anthraquinones, and ricinoleic acid.

Diphenylmethane Derivatives. Bisacodyl (DULCOLAX, CORRECTOL, others) is the only diphenylmethane derivative available in the U.S. It is marketed as enteric-coated and regular tablets and as a suppository for rectal administration.

The usual oral daily dose of bisacodyl is 10-15 mg for adults and 5-10 mg for children ages 6-12 years old. The drug requires hydrolysis by endogenous esterases in the bowel for activation, and so the laxative effects after an oral dose usually are not produced in <6 hours; taken at bedtime, it will produce its effect the next morning. Suppositories work much more rapidly, within 30-60 minutes. Due to the possibility of developing an atonic nonfunctioning colon, bisacodyl should not be used for >10 consecutive days.

Bisacodyl is mainly excreted in the stool; ~5% is absorbed and excreted in the urine as a glucuronide. Overdosage can lead to catharsis and fluid and electrolyte deficits. The diphenylmethanes can damage the mucosa and initiate an inflammatory response in the small bowel and colon. To avoid drug activation in the stomach with consequent gastric irritation and cramping, patients should swallow tablets without chewing or crushing and avoid milk or antacid medications within 1 hour of the ingestion of bisacodyl.

Phenolphthalein, once among the most popular components of laxatives, has been withdrawn from the market in the U.S. because of potential carcinogenicity. Oxyphenisatin, another older drug, was withdrawn due to hepatotoxicity. Sodium picosulfate (LUBRILAX, SUR-LAX) is a diphenylmethane derivative widely available outside of the U.S. It is hydrolyzed by colonic bacteria to its active form, and hence acts locally only in the colon. Effective doses of the diphenylmethane derivatives vary as much as 4- to 8-fold in individual patients. Consequently, recommended doses may be ineffective in some patients but may produce cramps and excessive fluid secretion in others.

Anthraquinone Laxatives. These derivatives of plants such as aloe, cascara, and senna share a tricyclic anthracene nucleus modified with hydroxyl, methyl, or carboxyl groups to form monoanthrones, such as rhein and frangula. Monoanthrones are irritating to the oral mucosa; however, the process of aging or drying converts them to more innocuous dimeric (dianthrones) or glycoside forms. This process is reversed by bacterial action in the colon to generate the active forms.

Senna (SENOKOT, EX-LAX, others) is obtained from the dried leaflets on pods of *Cassia acutifolia* or *Cassia angustifolia* and contains the rhein dianthrone glycosides sennoside A and B. *Cascara sagrada* is obtained from the bark of the buckthorn tree and contains the glycosides barbaloin and chrysaloin. Barbaloin is also found in aloe. The rhubarb plant also produces anthraquinone compounds that have been used as laxatives. Anthraquinones can also be synthesized; however, the synthetic monoanthrone danthron was withdrawn from the U.S. market because of concerns over possible carcinogenicity. In addition, all aloe and cascara sagrada products sold as laxatives have been categorized by FDA as not generally recognized as safe and effective for over-the-counter use because of a lack of scientific information about potential carcinogenicity.

Although these ingredients may still be sold over-the-counter in the U.S., legally they cannot be labeled for use as laxatives. This judgment is medically prudent but may provoke a longing for times past in Joyceans, who recall that cascara sagrada, the *sacred bark*, worked well for Leopold Bloom, in Dublin, on June 16, 1904:

> *Midway, his last resistance yielding, he allowed his bowels to ease themselves quietly as he read, reading still patiently that slight constipation of yesterday quite gone. Hope its not too big to bring on piles again. No, just right. So. Ah! Costive one tabloid of cascara sagrada. Life might be so. (Joyce, 1922)*

Anthraquinone laxatives can produce giant migrating colonic contractions and induce water and electrolyte secretion. They are poorly absorbed in the small bowel, but because they require activation in the colon, the laxative effect is not noted until 6-12 hours after ingestion. Active compounds are absorbed to a variable degree from the colon and excreted in the bile, saliva, milk, and urine.

The adverse consequences of long-term use of these agents have limited their use. A melanotic pigmentation of the colonic mucosa (*melanosis coli*) has been observed in patients using anthraquinone laxatives for long periods (at least 4-9 months). Histologically, this is caused by the presence of pigment-laden macrophages within the lamina propria. The condition is benign and reversible on discontinuation of the laxative. These agents also have been associated with the development of "cathartic colon," which can be seen in patients (typically women) who have a long-standing history (typically years) of laxative abuse. Regardless of whether a definitive causal relationship can be demonstrated between the use of these agents and colonic pathology, it is clear that they should not be recommended for chronic or long-term use.

Castor Oil. A bane of childhood since the time of the ancient Egyptians, castor oil (PURGE, NEOLOID, others) is derived from the bean of the castor plant, *Ricinus communis*. The castor bean is the source of an extremely toxic protein, ricin, as well as the oil (chiefly of the triglyceride of ricinoleic acid). The triglyceride is hydrolyzed in the small bowel by the action of lipases into glycerol and the active agent, ricinoleic acid, which acts primarily in the small intestine to stimulate secretion of fluid and electrolytes and speed intestinal transit. When taken on an empty stomach, as little as 4 mL of castor oil may produce a laxative effect within 1-3 hours; however, the usual dose for a cathartic effect is 15-60 mL for adults. Because of its unpleasant taste and its potential toxic effects on intestinal epithelium and enteric neurons, castor oil is seldom recommended now.

Prokinetic and Other Agents for Constipation

Although several of the agents already described stimulate motility, they do so in nonspecific or indirect ways. By contrast, the term *prokinetic* generally is reserved for agents that enhance GI transit via interaction with specific receptors involved in the regulation of motility.

Newer agents, such as the potent 5-HT$_4$-receptor agonist prucalopride, may be useful for the treatment of chronic constipation. Another potentially useful agent is misoprostol, a synthetic prostaglandin analog primarily used for protection against gastric ulcers resulting from the use of NSAIDs (Chapters 34 and 45). Prostaglandins can stimulate colonic contractions, particularly in the descending colon, and this may account for the diarrhea that limits the usefulness of misoprostol as a gastroprotectant. However, this property may be utilized for therapeutic gain in patients with intractable constipation. Colchicine, a microtubule formation inhibitor used for gout (Chapter 34), also has been shown to be effective in constipation (mechanism unknown), but its toxicity has limited widespread use. A novel biological agent, neurotrophin-3 (NT-3), recently was shown to be effective in improving frequency and stool consistency and decreasing straining, again by an unknown mechanism of action.

A new development in the treatment of constipation is the introduction of drugs that enhance fluid secretion by acting locally on ion channels in the colonic epithelium, to promote secretion. Lubiprostone (AMITIZA) is a prostanoid activator of Cl^- channels. The drug appears to bind to EP$_4$ receptors linked to activation of adenylyl cyclase, leading to enhanced apical Cl^- conductance; the identity of the Cl^- channel(s) involved is not certain, possibly CFTR and ClC-2. Lubiprostone was recently introduced for treatment of chronic constipation in adults and irritable bowel syndrome with constipation (IBS-C) in adult women. The drug promotes the secretion of a chloride-rich fluid and so improves stool consistency and promotes increased frequency by reflexly activating motility. A dose of 8 μg twice daily was found to be effective in IBS-C, though higher doses (24 μg twice daily) is given for chronic constipation. The drug is poorly bioavailable, acting only in the lumen of the bowel. Side effects of lubiprostone include nausea, headache, diarrhea, allergic reactions, and dyspnea.

Another class of secretory agent is represented by linaclotide, a 14–amino acid peptide agonist of guanylate cyclase C that stimulates secretion and motility. This compound shows promise in the treatment of IBS-C and chronic constipation, and it appears to have few serious side effects (Gale, 2009). Recent work in rodents suggests it may also be antinociceptive, reducing visceral pain (Eutamene et al., 2009), a major factor in IBS-C.

Opioid-Induced Constipation

Opioids are the main class of analgesics in the treatment and palliation of cancer, as well as other chronic pain states. Opioids cause severe constipation, which significantly limits their acceptability and reduces quality of life considerably. Laxatives and dietary strategies are frequently ineffective in the management of opioid-induced constipation. A promising strategy is the prevention of opioid-induced constipation with peripherally acting μ opioid receptor antagonists that specifically target the underlying reason for this condition, without limiting centrally produced analgesia. Methylnaltrexone (RELISTOR) was approved for the treatment of opioid-induced constipation by the FDA in 2008. Approval was based on multicenter trials demonstrating good efficacy in initiating bowel movements after injection of the drug in end-stage cancer patients in a hospice setting. When methylnaltrexone (0.15-0.3 mg/kg) was administered repeatedly every other day for 2 weeks, bowel movements occurred in 50% of the patients, compared with 8–15% of patients receiving placebo (Holzer, 2009). Another μ opioid antagonist, alvimopan (ENTEREG, 0.5-1 mg twice daily for 6 weeks) has also been tested in this setting where it increased spontaneous bowel movements and improved other symptoms of opioid-induced constipation without compromising analgesia (Holzer, 2009). Opioid-induced constipation represents an off-label use for alvimopan.

Post-operative Ileus

Post-operative ileus refers to the intolerance to oral intake and non-mechanical obstruction of the bowel that occurs after abdominal and non-abdominal surgery. It generally lasts 1-3 days after surgery with some variation along the length of the bowel. The pathogenesis is complex and is a combination of activation of neural inhibitory reflexes involving enteric μ opioid receptors and the activation of local inflammatory mechanisms that reduce smooth muscle contractility. The condition is exacerbated by opioids, which are the mainstay of post-operative analgesia. The extent to which endogenous opioids are involved in post-operative ileus remains to be determined. Prolonged post-operative ileus is hard to treat, and therefore considerable efforts are made to prevent its occurrence, including use of epidural anesthetics, minimally invasive surgeries, and reduced narcotic administration. Prokinetic agents typically do not have much effect in this condition, but recently, two new therapeutic agents have been introduced that have benefit in reducing GI recovery time after surgery.

Alvimopan (ENTEREG) is an orally active peripherally restricted μ opioid receptor antagonist that is FDA approved for limited indications following surgery (12 mg prior to surgery and then once daily for up to 7 days or until discharge; not to exceed 15 doses total). Methylnaltrexone (RELISTOR) is another peripherally restricted μ opioid receptor antagonist that lacks anti-analgesic actions. Methylnaltrexone reportedly enhanced GI transit but did not reduce time to discharge compared to standard approaches (Holzer, 2009). It is FDA approved for the treatment of opioid-induced constipation in patients receiving palliative care when laxative therapy is insufficient.

Dexpanthenol (ILOPAN, others) is the alcohol of pantothenic acid (vitamin B_5). The drug is a congener of pantothenic acid, a precursor of coenzyme A, which serves as a cofactor in the synthesis of ACh by choline acetyl transferase. It is proposed to act by enhancing ACh synthesis. ACh is the major excitatory transmitter of the gut. Dexpanthenol is used as an injection immediately postoperatively after major abdominal surgery to minimize the occurrence of paralytic ileus. It is given by intramuscular injection (200-500 mg) immediately and then 2 hours later and every 6 hours after that until the situation has resolved. It may cause mild hypotension and shortness of breath as well as local irritation.

Enemas and Suppositories

Enemas commonly are employed, either by themselves or as adjuncts to bowel preparation regimens, to empty the distal colon or rectum of retained solid material. Bowel distention by any means will produce an evacuation reflex in most people, and almost any form of enema, including normal saline solution, can achieve this. Specialized enemas contain additional substances that are either osmotically active or irritant; however, their safety and efficacy have not been studied in a rigorous manner. Repeated enemas with tap water or other hypotonic solutions can cause hyponatremia; repeated enemas with sodium phosphate–containing solution can cause hypocalcemia. Phosphate-containing enemas also are known to alter the appearance of rectal mucosa and contribute to acute phosphate nephropathy in susceptible patients.

Glycerin is a trihydroxy alcohol that is absorbed orally but acts as a hygroscopic agent and lubricant when given rectally. The resultant water retention stimulates peristalsis and usually produces a bowel movement in less than an hour. Glycerin is for rectal use only and is given in a single daily dose as a 2- or 3-g rectal suppository or as 5-15 mL of an 80% solution in enema form. Rectal glycerin may cause local discomfort, burning, or hyperemia and (minimal) bleeding. Some glycerin suppositories contain sodium stearate, which can cause local irritation.

Another agent for occasional constipation makes use of rectal distension to initiate laxation. CEO-TWO suppositories contain sodium bicarbonate and potassium bitartrate. When administered rectally, the suppository produces CO_2, which initiates a bowel movement in 5-30 minutes.

ANTI-DIARRHEAL AGENTS

Diarrhea: General Principles and Approach to Treatment. Diarrhea (Greek and Latin: *dia*, through, and *rheein*, to flow or run) does not require any definition to people who suffer from "the too rapid evacuation of too fluid stools." Scientists usually define diarrhea as excessive fluid weight, with 200 g per day representing the upper limit of normal stool water weight for healthy adults in the Western world. Because stool weight is largely determined by stool water, most cases of diarrhea result from disorders of intestinal water and electrolyte transport.

An appreciation and knowledge of the underlying causative processes in diarrhea facilitates effective treatment. From a mechanistic perspective, diarrhea can be caused by an increased osmotic load within the intestine (resulting in retention of water within the lumen); excessive secretion of electrolytes and water into the intestinal lumen; exudation of protein and fluid from the mucosa; and altered intestinal motility resulting in rapid transit (and decreased fluid absorption). In most instances, multiple processes are affected simultaneously, leading to a net increase in stool volume and weight accompanied by increases in fractional water content.

Many patients with sudden onset of diarrhea have a benign, self-limited illness requiring no treatment or evaluation. In severe cases, dehydration and electrolyte imbalances are the principal risk, particularly in infants, children, and frail elderly patients. *Oral rehydration therapy* therefore is a cornerstone for patients with acute illnesses resulting in significant diarrhea. This is of particular importance in developing countries, where the use of such therapy saves many thousands of lives every year. This therapy exploits the fact that nutrient-linked cotransport of water and electrolytes remains intact in the small bowel in most cases of acute diarrhea. Sodium and chloride absorption is linked to glucose uptake by the enterocyte; this is followed by movement of water in the same direction. A balanced mixture of glucose and electrolytes in volumes matched to losses therefore can prevent dehydration. This can be provided by many commercial premixed formulas using glucose-electrolyte or rice-based physiological solutions.

Pharmacotherapy of diarrhea in adults should be reserved for patients with significant or persistent symptoms. Nonspecific anti-diarrheal agents typically do not address the underlying pathophysiology responsible for the diarrhea; their principal utility is to provide symptomatic relief in mild cases of acute diarrhea. Many of these agents act by decreasing intestinal motility and should be avoided as much as possible in acute diarrheal illnesses caused by invasive organisms. In such cases, these agents may mask the clinical picture, delay clearance of organisms, and increase the risk of systemic invasion by the infectious organisms; they also may induce local complications such as toxic megacolon.

Bulk-Forming and Hydroscopic Agents. Hydrophilic and poorly fermentable colloids or polymers such as *carboxymethylcellulose* and calcium polycarbophil absorb water and increase stool bulk (calcium polycarbophil absorbs 60 times its weight in water). They usually are used for constipation but are sometimes useful in acute episodic diarrhea and in mild chronic diarrheas in patients suffering with IBS. The mechanism of this effect is not clear, but they may work as gels to modify stool texture and viscosity and to produce a perception of decreased stool fluidity. Some of these agents also may bind bacterial toxins and bile salts. Clays such as kaolin (a hydrated aluminum silicate) and other silicates such as attapulgite (magnesium aluminum disilicate; DIASORB, others) bind water avidly (attapulgite absorbs eight times its weight in water) and also may bind enterotoxins. However, binding is not selective and may involve other drugs and nutrients; hence these agents are best avoided within 2-3 hours of taking other medications. A mixture of kaolin and pectin (a plant polysaccharide) is a popular over-the-counter remedy (KAOPECTOLIN, others) and may provide useful symptomatic relief of mild diarrhea.

Bile Acid Sequestrants. Cholestyramine, colestipol, and colesevalam effectively bind bile acids and some bacterial toxins. Cholestyramine is useful in the treatment of bile salt–induced diarrhea, as in patients with resection of the distal ileum. In these patients, there is partial interruption of the normal enterohepatic circulation of bile salts, resulting in excessive concentrations reaching the colon and stimulating water and electrolyte secretion. Patients with extensive ileal resection (usually >100 cm) eventually develop net bile salt depletion, which can produce steatorrhea because of inadequate micellar formation required for fat absorption. In such patients, the use of cholestyramine aggravates the diarrhea. The drug also has had an historic role in treating mild antibiotic-associated diarrhea and mild colitis due to *Clostridium difficile*. However, its use in infectious diarrheas generally is discouraged because it may decrease clearance of the pathogen from the bowel.

In patients suspected of having bile salt–induced diarrhea, a trial of cholestyramine (QUESTRAN, QUESTRAN LIGHT, others) can be given at a dose of 4 g of the dried resin (four times a day). If successful, the dose may be titrated down to achieve the desired stool frequency.

Cholestyramine resin also is helpful for the relief of pruritus associated with partial biliary obstruction and in conditions such as primary biliary cirrhosis. In such conditions, excessive bile acids are thought to be deposited in the skin and cause irritation. Cholestyramine increases fecal excretion of bile acids and reduces circulating and eventually systemic levels with relief of pruritus in ~1-3 weeks.

Bismuth. Bismuth compounds have been used to treat a variety of GI diseases and symptoms for centuries, although their mechanism of action remains poorly understood. PEPTO-BISMOL (or generic formulations of bismuth subsalicylate) is an over-the-counter preparation estimated to be used by 60% of American households. It is a crystal complex consisting of trivalent bismuth and salicylate suspended in a mixture of magnesium aluminum silicate clay. In the low pH of the stomach, the bismuth subsalicylate reacts with hydrochloric acid to form bismuth oxychloride and salicylic acid. Although 99% of the bismuth passes unaltered and unabsorbed into the feces, the salicylate is absorbed in the stomach and small intestine. Thus, the product carries the same labeled warning regarding Reye's syndrome as other salicylates, and patients taking other forms of salicylates should be made aware of the overlap in adverse effect.

Bismuth is thought to have anti-secretory, anti-inflammatory, and antimicrobial effects. Nausea and abdominal cramps also are relieved by bismuth. The clay in PEPTO-BISMOL and generic formulations also may have some additional benefits in diarrhea, but this is not clear. Bismuth subsalicylate has been used extensively for the prevention and treatment of traveler's diarrhea, but it also is effective in other forms of episodic diarrhea and in acute gastroenteritis. Today, the most common antibacterial use of this agent is in the treatment of *Helicobacter pylori* (Chapter 45). A recommended dose of the bismuth subsalicylate (30 mL of regular strength liquid or two tablets) contains approximately equal amounts of bismuth and salicylate (262 mg each). For control of indigestion, nausea, or diarrhea, the dose is repeated every 30-60 minutes, as needed, up to eight times a day. Bismuth products have a long track record of safety at recommended doses, although impaction may occur in infants and debilitated patients. Dark stools (sometimes mistaken for melena) and black staining of the tongue in association with bismuth compounds are caused by bismuth sulfide formed in a reaction between the drug and bacterial sulfides in the GI tract.

Probiotics. The GI tract contains a vast commensal microflora that is necessary for health. Alterations in the balance or composition of the microflora are responsible for antibiotic-associated diarrhea, and possibly other disease conditions. The administration of nonpathogenic bacteria to recolonize the gut is an area of intense investigation (Sartor, 2005). Probiotic preparations containing a variety of bacterial strains have shown some degree of benefit in acute diarrheal conditions, antibiotic-associated diarrhea, and infectious diarrhea, but most clinical studies have been small and conclusions are therefore limited. Because these agents are generally safe, their use continues despite mainly anecdotal evidence of efficacy.

Anti-Motility and Anti-Secretory Agents

Opioids. Opioids continue to be widely used in the treatment of diarrhea. They act by several different mechanisms, mediated principally through either μ- or δ-opioid receptors on enteric nerves, epithelial cells, and muscle (Chapter 18). These mechanisms include effects on intestinal motility (μ receptors), intestinal secretion (δ receptors), or absorption (μ and δ receptors). Commonly used anti-diarrheals such as diphenoxylate, difenoxin, and loperamide act principally via peripheral μ opioid receptors and are preferred over opioids that penetrate the CNS.

Loperamide. Loperamide (IMODIUM, IMODIUM A-D, others), a piperidine butyramide derivative with μ receptor activity, is an orally active anti-diarrheal agent. The drug is 40-50 times more potent than morphine as an anti-diarrheal agent and penetrates the CNS poorly. It increases small intestinal and mouth-to-cecum transit times. Loperamide also increases anal sphincter tone, an effect that may be of therapeutic value in some patients who suffer from anal incontinence. In addition, loperamide has anti-secretory activity against cholera toxin and some forms of *Escherichia coli* toxin, presumably by acting on G_i-linked receptors and countering the increase in cellular cyclic AMP generated in response to the toxins.

Because of its effectiveness and safety, loperamide is marketed for over-the-counter distribution and is available in capsule, solution, and chewable tablet forms. It acts quickly after an oral dose, with peak plasma levels achieved within 3-5 hours. It has a $t_{1/2}$ of ~11 hours and undergoes extensive hepatic metabolism. The usual adult dose is 4 mg initially followed by 2 mg after each subsequent loose stool, up to 16 mg per day. If clinical improvement in acute diarrhea does not occur within 48 hours, loperamide should be discontinued. Recommended maximum daily doses for children are 3 mg for ages 2-5 years, 4 mg for ages 6-8 years, and 6 mg for ages 8-12 years. Loperamide is not recommended for use in children <2 years of age.

Loperamide has been shown to be effective against traveler's diarrhea, used either alone or in combination with antimicrobial agents (trimethoprim, trimethoprim-sulfamethoxazole, or a fluoroquinolone). Loperamide also has been used as adjunct treatment in almost all forms of chronic diarrheal disease, with few adverse effects. Loperamide lacks significant abuse potential and is more effective in treating diarrhea than diphenoxylate. Overdosage, however, can result in CNS depression (especially in children) and paralytic ileus. In patients with active inflammatory bowel disease involving the colon (Chapter 47), loperamide should be used with great caution, if at all, to prevent development of toxic megacolon.

Loperamide N-*oxide*, an investigational agent, is a site-specific prodrug; it is chemically designed for controlled release of loperamide in the intestinal lumen, thereby reducing systemic absorption.

Diphenoxylate and Difenoxin. Diphenoxylate and its active metabolite difenoxin (diphenoxylic acid) are piperidine derivatives that are related structurally to meperidine. As anti-diarrheal agents, diphenoxylate and difenoxin are somewhat more potent than morphine.

Both compounds are extensively absorbed after oral administration, with peak levels achieved within 1-2 hours. Diphenoxylate is rapidly deesterified to difenoxin, which is eliminated with a $t_{1/2}$ of ~12 hours. Both drugs can produce CNS effects when used in higher doses (40-60 mg per day) and thus have a potential for abuse and/or addiction. They are available in preparations containing small doses of atropine (considered subtherapeutic) to discourage abuse and deliberate overdosage: 25 μg of atropine sulfate per tablet with either 2.5 mg diphenoxylate hydrochloride (LOMOTIL) or 1 mg of difenoxin hydrochloride (MOTOFEN). The usual dosage is two tablets initially, then one tablet every 3-4 hours, not to exceed eight tablets per day. With excessive use or overdose, constipation and (in inflammatory conditions of the colon) toxic megacolon may develop. In high doses, these drugs cause CNS effects as well as anticholinergic effects from the atropine (dry mouth, blurred vision, etc.) (Chapter 9).

Other opioids used for diarrhea include codeine (in doses of 30 mg given three or four times daily) and opium-containing compounds. Paregoric (camphorated opium tincture) contains the equivalent of 2 mg of morphine per 5 mL (0.4 mg/mL); deodorized tincture of opium, which is 25 times stronger, contains the equivalent of 50 mg of morphine per 5 mL (10 mg/mL). The two tinctures sometimes are confused in prescribing and dispensing, resulting in dangerous overdoses. The anti-diarrheal dose of opium tincture for adults is 0.6 mL (equivalent to 6 mg morphine) four times daily; the adult dose of paregoric is 5-10 mL (equivalent to 2-4 mg morphine) one to four times daily. Paregoric is used in children at a dose of 0.25-0.5 mL/kg (equivalent to 0.1-0.2 mg morphine/kg) one to four times daily.

Enkephalins are endogenous opioids that are important enteric neurotransmitters. Enkephalins inhibit intestinal secretion without affecting motility. Racecadotril (acetorphan), a dipeptide inhibitor of enkephalinase, reinforces the effects of endogenous enkephalins on the δ-opioid receptor to produce an anti-diarrheal effect.

α_2 Adrenergic Receptor Agonists. α_2 Adrenergic receptor agonists such as clonidine can interact with specific receptors on enteric neurons and enterocytes, thereby stimulating absorption and inhibiting secretion of fluid and electrolytes and increasing intestinal transit time. These agents may have a special role in diabetics with chronic diarrhea, in whom autonomic neuropathy can lead to loss of noradrenergic innervation. Oral clonidine (beginning at 0.1 mg twice a day) has been used in these patients; the use of a topical preparation (e.g., CATAPRES TTS, two patches a week) may result in more steady plasma levels of the drug. Clonidine also may be useful in patients with diarrhea caused by opiate withdrawal. Side effects such as hypotension, depression, and perceived fatigue may be dose limiting in susceptible patients.

Octreotide and Somatostatin. Octreotide (SANDOSTATIN, others) (Chapter 43) is an octapeptide analog of somatostatin (SST) that is effective in inhibiting the severe secretory diarrhea brought about by hormone-secreting tumors of the pancreas and the GI tract. Its mechanism of action appears to involve inhibition of hormone secretion, including 5-HT and various other GI peptides (e.g., gastrin, vasoactive intestinal polypeptide (VIP), insulin, secretin, etc.). Octreotide has been used off label, with varying success, in other forms of secretory diarrhea such as chemotherapy-induced diarrhea, diarrhea associated with human immunodeficiency virus (HIV), and diabetes-associated diarrhea. Its greatest utility, however, may be in the "dumping syndrome" seen in some patients after gastric surgery and pyloroplasty. In this condition, octreotide inhibits the release of hormones (triggered by rapid passage of food into the small intestine) that are responsible for distressing local and systemic effects.

Octreotide has a $t_{1/2}$ of 1-2 hours and is administered either subcutaneously or intravenously as a bolus dose. Standard initial therapy with octreotide is 50-100 μg, given subcutaneously two or three times a day, with titration to a maximum dose of 500 μg three times a day based on clinical and biochemical responses. A long-acting preparation of octreotide acetate enclosed in biodegradable microspheres (SANDOSTATIN LAR DEPOT) is available for use in the treatment of diarrheas associated with carcinoid tumors and VIP–secreting tumors, as well as in the treatment of acromegaly (Chapter 44). This preparation is injected intramuscularly once per month in a dose of 20 or 30 mg. Side effects of octreotide depend on the duration of therapy. Short-term therapy leads to transient nausea, bloating, or pain at sites of injection. Long-term therapy can lead to gallstone formation and hypo- or hyperglycemia. Another long-acting SST analog, lanreotide (SOMATULIN, others), is available in Europe but not in the U.S.; another, vapreotide, is under development. SST (STILAMIN) also is available in Europe.

Variceal Bleeding. Vasoactive agents have been used to control variceal bleeding. Traditionally, vasopressin has been used (Chapter 26), but its significant side effects—such as myocardial ischemia, peripheral vascular disease, and the release of plasminogen activator and factor VIII—have led to its decline. SST and octreotide are effective in reducing hepatic blood flow, hepatic venous wedge pressure, and azygos blood flow. These agents constrict the splanchnic arterioles by a direct action on vascular smooth muscle and by inhibiting the release of peptides contributing to the hyperdynamic circulatory syndrome of portal hypertension. Octreotide also may act through the autonomic nervous system. These agents can control bleeding acutely and decrease bleeding-related mortality, with an efficacy comparable to endoscopic therapy or balloon tamponade. The major advantage of somatostatin and octreotide over vasopressin is their safety. Because of its short $t_{1/2}$ (1-2 minutes), SST can be given only by intravenous infusion (a 250 μg bolus dose followed by 250 μg hourly for 5 days). Higher doses (up to 500 μg/hour) are more efficacious and can be used for patients who continue to bleed on the lower dose (Moitinho et al., 2001). For patients with variceal bleeding, therapy with octreotide usually is initiated while the patient is awaiting endoscopy.

Intestinal Dysmotility. Octreotide has complex and apparently conflicting effects on GI motility, including inhibition of antral motor activity and colonic tone. However, octreotide also can rapidly induce phase III activity of the migrating motor complex in the small bowel to produce longer and faster contractions than those occurring spontaneously. Its use has been shown to result in improvement in selected patients with scleroderma and small-bowel dysfunction.

Pancreatitis. Both SST and octreotide inhibit pancreatic secretion and have been used for the prophylaxis and treatment of acute pancreatitis. The rationale for their use is to "put the pancreas to rest" so as to not aggravate inflammation by the continuing production of proteolytic enzymes, to reduce intraductal pressures, and to ameliorate pain. Octreotide probably is less effective than SST in this regard because it may cause an increase in sphincter of Oddi pressure and perhaps also have a deleterious effect on pancreatic blood flow. Although some studies have suggested that these agents improve mortality in patients with acute pancreatitis, definitive data are lacking.

Other Agents

Calcium channel blockers such as verapamil and nifedipine (Chapters 25 and 27) reduce motility and may promote intestinal electrolyte and water absorption. Constipation, in fact, is a significant side effect of these drugs. However, because of their systemic effects and the availability of other agents, they seldom if ever are used for diarrheal illnesses.

Berberine is a plant alkaloid that has been used for millennia in traditional Indian and Chinese medicine. It is produced by several genera of the families Ranuculaceae and Berberidaceae (e.g., *Berberis*, *Mahonia*, and *Coptis*) and has complex pharmacological actions that include antimicrobial actions, stimulation of bile flow, inhibition of ventricular tachyarrhythmias, and possible antineoplastic activity. It is used most commonly in bacterial diarrhea and cholera, but is also apparently effective against intestinal parasites. The anti-diarrheal effects in part may be related to its antimicrobial activity, as well as its ability to inhibit smooth muscle contraction and delay intestinal transit by antagonizing the effects of ACh (by competitive and noncompetitive mechanisms) and blocking the entry of Ca^{2+} into cells. In addition, it inhibits intestinal secretion.

Chloride channel blockers are effective anti-secretory agents *in vitro* but are too toxic for human use and have not proven to be effective anti-diarrheal agents *in vivo*. Calmodulin inhibitors, which include chlorpromazine, also are anti-secretory. Zaldaride maleate, an investigational drug in this class, may be effective in traveler's diarrhea by reducing secretion without affecting intestinal motility.

IRRITABLE BOWEL SYNDROME (IBS)

IBS, a condition that affects up to 15% of the population in the U.S., is perhaps one of the more challenging nonfatal illnesses seen by gastroenterologists (Mertz, 2003). Patients may complain of a variety of symptoms, the most characteristic of which is recurrent abdominal pain associated with altered bowel movements. The pathophysiology of this condition is not clear; it appears to result from a varying combination of disturbances in visceral motor and sensory function, often associated with significant affective disorders. The disturbances in bowel function, which can be either constipation or diarrhea or both at different times, have led to the classical interpretation of IBS as being a "motility disorder," but motor disturbances cannot explain the entire clinical picture. Recently, more emphasis has been devoted to the pathogenesis of pain in these patients, and there now is considerable evidence to suggest a specific enhancement of visceral (as opposed to somatic) sensitivity to noxious, as well as physiological stimuli in this syndrome. The etiopathogenesis of this visceral hypersensitivity probably is multifactorial; a popular hypothesis is that transient visceral injury in genetically predisposed individuals leads to long-lasting sensitization of the neural pain circuit despite complete resolution of the initiating event. Increasingly, this concept is being extended to other so-called functional disorders of the gut characterized by unexplained pain, including noncardiac chest pain and nonulcer dyspepsia. These disorders, also considered for many years to arise from motor disturbances, may in fact represent part of a spectrum of a new syndrome of "visceral hyperalgesia."

Many patients can be managed satisfactorily with a strong patient-physician relationship, simple counseling, and adjunctive measures, including dietary restrictions and fiber supplementation; overt psychological abnormalities should be treated appropriately. Despite these measures, a significant proportion of patients remain plagued by severe symptoms, and drug therapy is attempted almost invariably. However, there are very few effective pharmacological options for these patients, a situation that in part reflects our limited understanding of the pathogenesis of this syndrome.

The pharmacological approach to IBS reflects its multifaceted nature. Treatment of bowel symptoms (either diarrhea or constipation) is predominantly symptomatic and nonspecific. Patients with mild symptoms often are started on fiber supplements; this approach may work for constipation and diarrhea (by binding water). Patients with episodic, discrete pain episodes often are treated with agents that may reduce smooth muscle contractility in the gut. These so-called antispasmodics include anticholinergic agents, Ca^{2+} channel antagonists, and peripheral opioid receptor antagonists. The use of most such drugs is hallowed by years of tradition but seldom has been subjected to critical assessment; however, these drugs may be modestly effective in a subset of patients and are useful adjuncts.

In recent years, an increasing emphasis is being placed on the pharmacological treatment of visceral sensitivity. Although the biological basis of visceral hyperalgesia in IBS patients is not known, a possible role for serotonin has been suggested based on its known involvement in sensitization of nociceptor neurons in inflammatory conditions. This has led to the development of specific receptor modulators, such as the 5-HT_3 antagonist alosetron (Figure 46–2). Buspirone and sumatriptan are 5-HT_1 receptor agonists (Chapter 13) that can reduce gastric and colonic sensitivity to distention and are being evaluated in clinical trials.

The most effective class of agents in this regard has been the tricyclic anti-depressants (Chapter 15), which can have neuromodulatory and analgesic properties independent of their anti-depressant effect. Tricyclic anti-depressants have a proven track record in the management of chronic "functional" visceral pain. Effective analgesic doses of these drugs (e.g., 25-75 mg per day of nortryptiline) are significantly lower than those required to treat depression. Although changes in mood usually do not occur at these doses, there may be some diminution of anxiety and restoration of sleep patterns, which can be considered desirable effects in this group of patients. Selective serotonin reuptake inhibitors have fewer side effects and have been advocated particularly for patients with functional constipation because they can increase bowel movements and even cause diarrhea. However, they probably are not as effective as tricyclic anti-depressants in the management of visceral pain.

a_2 Adrenergic agonists, such as clonidine (Chapter 12), also can increase visceral compliance and reduce distention-induced pain. The SST analog octreotide has selective inhibitory effects on peripheral afferent nerves projecting from the gut to the spinal cord in healthy human beings and has been shown to blunt the perception of rectal distention in patients with IBS. Fedotozine, an investigational opioid that appears to be a peripherally active, selective κ receptor antagonist, produces marginal improvement in symptoms in patients with IBS and functional dyspepsia. The lack of CNS effects is an advantage in such patients in whom chronic medication use is anticipated. Other agents of unproven value include leuprolide, a gonadotropin-releasing hormone analog (Chapter 42).

Alosetron and Other 5-HT_3 Antagonists

The 5-HT_3 receptor participates in several important processes in the gut, including sensitization of spinal sensory neurons, vagal signaling of nausea, and peristaltic reflexes. Some of these effects in experimental models are potentially conflicting, with release of excitatory and inhibitory neurotransmitters. However, the clinical effect of 5-HT_3 antagonism is a general reduction in GI contractility with decreased colonic transit, along with an increase in fluid absorption. In general, therefore, these antagonists produce the opposite effects seen with 5-HT_4 agonists. Although they also may blunt visceral sensation, a direct effect on spinal afferents has not been fully established. Alosetron (LOTRONEX) was the first agent in this class specifically approved for the treatment of diarrhea-predominant IBS in women. Alosetron is a much more potent antagonist of the 5-HT_3 receptor than ondansetron and causes significant (although modest) improvements in abdominal pain as well as stool frequency, consistency, and urgency in these patients. Shortly after its initial release, alosetron was withdrawn from the U.S. market because of an unusually high incidence of ischemic colitis (up to 3 per 1000 patients), leading to surgery and even death in a small number of cases. The mechanism of this effect is not fully established but may result from the drug's ability to suppress intestinal relaxation, thereby causing severe spasm in segments of the colon in susceptible individuals. It is not clear whether this is a nonspecific effect or involves serotoninergic mechanisms. Nevertheless, the FDA has reapproved this drug for diarrhea-predominant IBS under a limited distribution system. However, concerns about the consequences of prescribing this drug are important, and the manufacturer requires a prescription program that includes physician certification and an elaborate patient education and consent protocol before dispensing.

Alosetron is rapidly absorbed from the GI tract; its duration of action (~10 hours) is longer than expected from its $t_{1/2}$ of 1.5 hours. It is metabolized by hepatic CYPs. The drug should be started at 1 mg per day for the first 4 weeks and advanced to a maximum of 1 mg twice daily if an adequate response is not achieved.

Other 5-HT_3 antagonists currently available in the U.S. are approved for nausea and vomiting (see later in this chapter and Chapter 13).

ANTI-SPASMODICS AND OTHER AGENTS

Anticholinergic agents ("spasmolytics" or "anti-spasmodics") often are used in patients with IBS. The most common agents of this class available in the U.S. are nonspecific antagonists of the muscarinic receptor (Chapter 9) and include the tertiary amines dicyclomine (BENTYL, others) and hyoscyamine (LEVSIN, others) and the quaternary ammonium compounds glycopyrrolate (ROBINUL, others) and methscopolamine (PAMINE, others). The advantage of the latter two compounds is that they have a limited propensity to cross the blood-brain barrier and hence a lower risk for neurological side effects such as lightheadedness, drowsiness, or nervousness. These agents typically are given either on an as-needed basis (with the onset of pain) or before meals to prevent the pain and fecal urgency that predictably occur in some patients with IBS (with presumed exaggerated gastrocolic reflex).

Dicyclomine is given in doses of 20 mg orally every 6 hours initially and increased to 40 mg every 6 hours unless limited by side effects. Doses <160 mg/day are not usually effective and should be discontinued after a 2-week trial period. Hyoscyamine is available as immediate-release oral capsules, tablets, elixir, drops, and a nonaerosol spray (all administered as 0.125-0.25 mg every 4 hours as needed), and extended-release forms for oral use (0.25-0.375 mg every 12 hours as needed). An injectable is available for subcutaneous, intravenous, or intramuscular administration. Regardless of the formulation, the adult dose of hyoscyamine usually should not exceed 1.5 mg in 24 hours. Glycopyrrolate is available as immediate-release tablets; the dose is 1-2 mg two or three times daily, not to exceed 8 mg/day. Methscopolamine is provided as 2.5-mg and 5-mg tablets; the dose is 2.5 mg a half hour before meals and 2.5-5 mg at bedtime.

Other Drugs. Cimetropium, an antimuscarinic compound that reportedly is effective in patients with IBS, is not available in the U.S. Otilonium bromide is a quaternary ammonium salt with antimuscarinic effects that also appears to block Ca^{2+} channels and neurokinin

NK_2 receptors; it is not available in the U.S. but has been used extensively for patients with IBS in other parts of the world. Mebeverine hydrochloride is a derivative of hydroxybenzamide that appears to have a direct effect on the smooth muscle cell, blocking K^+, Na^+, and Ca^{2+} channels. It is widely used outside of the U.S. as an anti-spasmodic agent for patients with IBS.

ANTI-NAUSEANTS AND ANTI-EMETIC AGENTS

Nausea and Vomiting

The act of emesis and the sensation of nausea that accompanies it generally are viewed as protective reflexes that serve to rid the stomach and intestine of toxic substances and prevent their further ingestion. Vomiting is a complex process that consists of a pre-ejection phase (gastric relaxation and retroperistalsis), retching (rhythmic action of respiratory muscles preceding vomiting and consisting of contraction of abdominal and intercostal muscles and diaphragm against a closed glottis), and ejection (intense contraction of the abdominal muscles and relaxation of the upper esophageal sphincter). This is accompanied by multiple autonomic phenomena including salivation, shivering, and vasomotor changes. During prolonged episodes, marked behavioral changes including lethargy, depression, and withdrawal may occur. The process appears to be coordinated by a central emesis center in the lateral reticular formation of the mid-brainstem adjacent to both the chemoreceptor trigger zone (CTZ) in the area postrema (AP) at the bottom of the fourth ventricle and the solitary tract nucleus (STN). The lack of a blood-brain barrier allows the CTZ to monitor blood and cerebrospinal fluid constantly for toxic substances and to relay information to the emesis center to trigger nausea and vomiting. The emesis center also receives information from the gut, principally by the vagus nerve (via the STN) but also by splanchnic afferents via the spinal cord. Two other important inputs to the emesis center come from the cerebral cortex (particularly in anticipatory nausea or vomiting) and the vestibular apparatus (in motion sickness). In turn, the center sends out efferents to the nuclei responsible for respiratory, salivary, and vasomotor activity, as well as to striated and smooth muscle involved in the act. The CTZ has high concentrations of receptors for serotonin ($5\text{-}HT_3$), dopamine (D_2), and opioids; the STN is rich in receptors for enkephalin, histamine, and ACh, and also contains $5\text{-}HT_3$ receptors. A variety of these neurotransmitters are involved in nausea and vomiting (Figure 46–4), and an understanding of their nature has allowed a rational approach to the pharmacological treatment of nausea and vomiting (Hornby, 2001; Scuderi, 2003).

Anti-emetics generally are classified according to the predominant receptor on which they are proposed to act (Table 46–5). However, considerable overlap among these mechanisms exists, particularly for the older agents (Table 46–6). For treatment and prevention of the nausea and emesis associated with cancer chemotherapy, several anti-emetic agents from different pharmacological classes may be used in combination (Table 46–7). The individual classes of agents are presented next.

$5\text{-}HT_3$ Receptor Antagonists

Chemistry, Pharmacological Effects, and Mechanism of Action. Ondansetron (ZOFRAN, others) is the prototypical drug in this class. Since their introduction in the early 1990s, the $5\text{-}HT_3$ receptor antagonists have become the most widely used drugs for chemotherapy-induced emesis. Other agents in this class include granisetron (KYTRIL, others), dolasetron (ANZEMET), palonosetron (ALOXI), and tropisetron (available in some countries but not in the U.S.). The differences among these agents are related mainly to their chemical structures, $5\text{-}HT_3$ receptor affinities, and pharmacokinetic profiles (Table 46–8). Alosetron was discussed separately earlier.

There is evidence that effects at peripheral and central sites contribute to the efficacy of these agents. $5\text{-}HT_3$ receptors are present in several critical sites involved in emesis, including vagal afferents, the STN (which receives signals from vagal afferents), and the area postrema itself (Figure 46–4). Serotonin is released by the enterochromaffin cells of the small intestine in response to chemotherapeutic agents and may stimulate vagal afferents (via $5\text{-}HT_3$ receptors) to initiate the vomiting reflex. Experimentally, vagotomy has been shown to prevent cisplatin-induced emesis. However, the highest concentrations of $5\text{-}HT_3$ receptors in the CNS are found in the STN and CTZ, and antagonists of $5\text{-}HT_3$ receptors also may suppress nausea and vomiting by acting at these sites.

Pharmacokinetics. The anti-emetic effects of these drugs persist long after they disappear from the circulation, suggesting their continuing interaction at the receptor level. In fact, all of these drugs can be administered effectively just once a day.

These agents are absorbed well from the GI tract. Ondansetron is extensively metabolized in the liver by CYP1A2, CYP2D6, and CYP3A4, followed by glucuronide or sulfate conjugation. Patients with hepatic dysfunction have reduced plasma clearance, and some adjustment in the dosage is advisable. Although ondansetron clearance also is reduced in elderly patients, no adjustment in dosage for age is recommended. Granisetron also is metabolized predominantly by the liver, a process that appears to involve

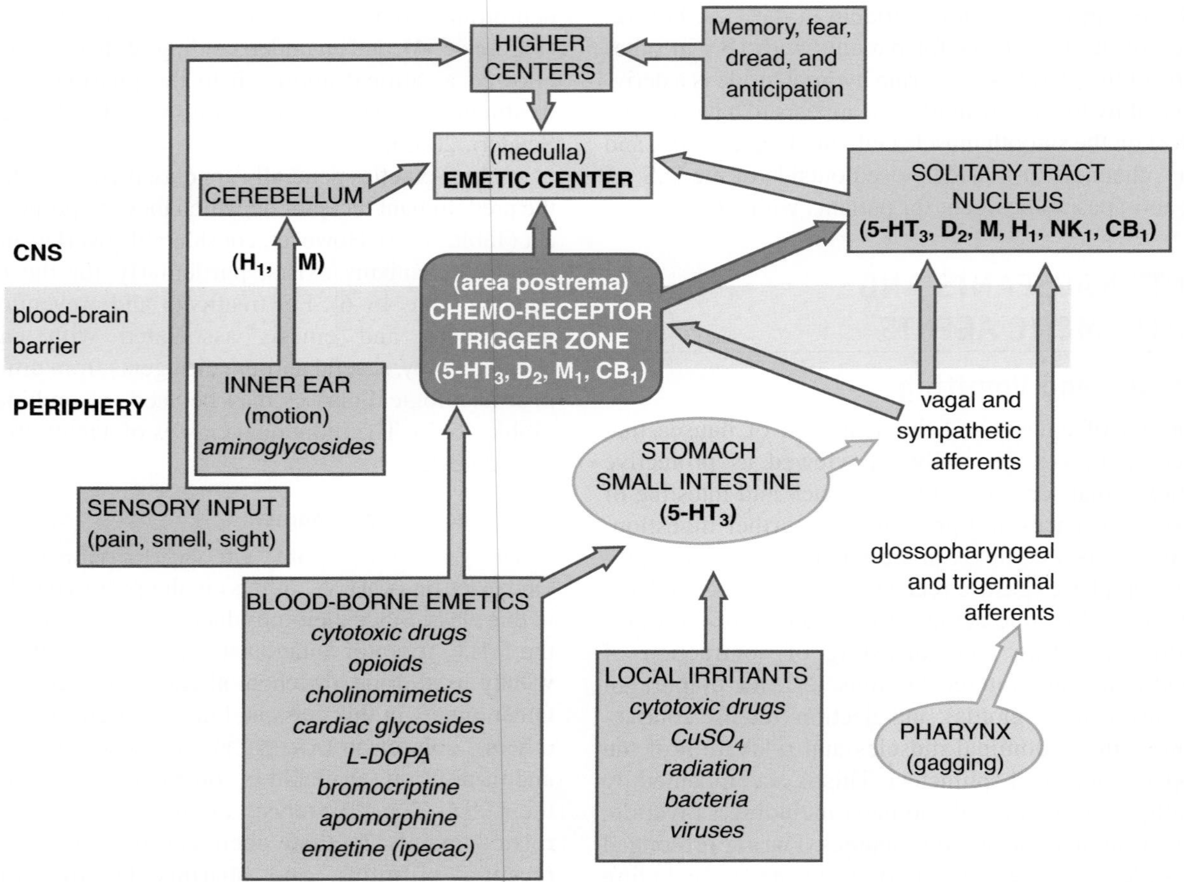

Figure 46–4. *Pharmacologist's view of emetic stimuli.* Myriad signaling pathways lead from the periphery to the emetic center. Stimulants of these pathways are noted in *italics*. These pathways involve specific neurotransmitters and their receptors (**bold** type). Receptors are shown for dopamine (D_2), acetylcholine (muscarinic, M), histamine (H_1), cannabinoids (CB_1), substance P (NK_1), and 5-hydroxytryptamine ($5\text{-}HT_3$). Some of these receptors also may mediate signaling in the emetic center.

Table 46–5

General Classification of Anti-emetic Agents

ANTI-EMETIC CLASS	EXAMPLES	TYPE OF VOMITING MOST EFFECTIVE AGAINST
$5\text{-}HT_3$ receptor antagonists[a]	Ondansetron	Cytotoxic drug induced emesis
Centrally acting dopamine receptor antagonists	Metoclopramide[b]	Cytotoxic drug induced emesis
	Promethazine[c]	
Histamine H_1 receptor antagonists	Cyclizine	Vestibular (motion sickness)
Muscarinic receptor antagonists	Hyoscine (scopolamine)	Motion sickness
Neurokinin receptor antagonists	Aprepitant	Cytotoxic drug induced emesis (delayed vomiting)
Cannabinoid receptor agonists	Dronabinol	Cytotoxic drug induced emesis

[a]The most effective agents for chemotherapy-induced nausea and vomiting are the $5\text{-}HT_3$ antagonists and metoclopramide. In addition to their use as single agents, they are often combined with other drugs to improve efficacy as well as reduce the incidence of side effects.
[b]Also has some peripheral activity at $5\text{-}HT_3$ receptors.
[c]Also has some antihistaminic and anticholinergic activity.

Table 46–6

Receptor Specificity of Anti-emetic Agents

PHARMACOLOGIC CLASS Drugs in Class	DOPAMINE (D_2)	ACETYLCHOLINE (MUSCARINIC)	HISTAMINE	SEROTONIN
Anticholinergics				
Scopolamine	+	++++	+	–
Antihistamines				
Cyclizine	+	+++	++++	–
Dimenhydrinate, diphenhydramine, hydroxyzine	+	++	++++	–
Promethazine	++	++	++++	–
Anti-serotonins				
Dolasetron, granisetron, ondansetron, palonosetron, ramosetron	–	–	–	++++
Benzamides				
Domperidone	++++	–	–	+
Metoclopramide	+++	–	–	++
Butyrophenones				
Droperidol	++++	–	+	+
Haloperidol	++++	–	+	–
Phenothiazines				
Chlorpromazine	++++	++	++++	+
Fluphenazine	++++	+	++	–
Perphenazine	++++	+	++	+
Prochlorperazine	++++	++	++	+
Steroids				
Betamethasone, dexamethasone	–	–	–	–

For details, see Scuderi, 2003. Plus signs indicate some (+) to considerable (++++) interaction. (–) indicates no effect.

the CYP3A family, as it is inhibited by ketoconazole. Dolasetron is converted rapidly by plasma carbonyl reductase to its active metabolite, hydrodolasetron. A portion of this compound then undergoes subsequent biotransformation by CYP2D6 and CYP3A4 in the liver while about one-third of it is excreted unchanged in the urine. Palonosetron is metabolized principally by CYP2D6 and excreted in the urine as the metabolized and the unchanged forms in about equal proportions.

Therapeutic Use. These agents are most effective in treating chemotherapy-induced nausea and in treating nausea secondary to upper abdominal irradiation, where all three agents appear to be equally efficacious. They also are effective against hyperemesis of pregnancy, and to a lesser degree, postoperative nausea, but not against motion sickness. Unlike other agents in this class, palonosetron also may be helpful in delayed emesis, perhaps a reflection of its long $t_{1/2}$.

These agents are available as tablets, oral solution, and intravenous preparations for injection. For patients on cancer chemotherapy, these drugs can be given in a single intravenous dose (Table 46–8) infused over 15 minutes, beginning 30 minutes before chemotherapy, or in 2-3 divided doses, with the first usually given 30 minutes before and subsequent doses at various intervals after chemotherapy. The drugs also can be used intramuscularly (ondansetron only) or orally. Granisetron is available as a transdermal formulation that is applied 24-48 hours before chemotherapy and worn for up to 7 days.

Adverse Effects. In general, these drugs are very well tolerated, with the most common adverse effects being constipation or diarrhea, headache, and lightheadedness. As a class, these agents have been shown experimentally to induce minor electrocardiographic changes, but these are not expected to be clinically significant in most cases.

Dopamine-Receptor Antagonists

Phenothiazines such as prochlorperazine, thiethylperazine (discontinued in the U.S.), and chlorpromazine (Chapter 16) are among the most commonly used "general-purpose" anti-nauseants and anti-emetics. Their effects in this regard are complex, but their principal mechanism of action is D_2 receptor antagonism at the CTZ. Compared with metoclopramide or ondansetron, these drugs do not appear to be as uniformly effective in cancer chemotherapy–induced emesis. But they also possess antihistaminic and anticholinergic activities, which are of value in other forms of nausea, such as motion sickness.

Table 46–7

A. Some Anti-emetic Regimens Used in Cancer Chemotherapy

ANTI-EMETIC AGENT	INITIAL DOSE
For Severe Chemotherapy-Induced Emesis	
(Several Anti-emetic Agents Used in Combination)	
Dexamethasone	20 mg IV
Metoclopramide	3 mg/kg body weight IV every 2 h × 2
Diphenhydramine	25-50 mg IV every 2 h × 2
Lorazepam	1-2 mg IV
Dexamethasone	20 mg IV
Ondansetron	32 mg IV daily, in divided doses
For Moderate Chemotherapy-Induced Emesis	
(Anti-emetic Agents Used Singly)	
Prochlorperazine	5-10 mg orally or IV, or 25 mg by rectal suppository
Thiethylperazine	10 mg orally, IM, or by rectal suppository
Dexamethasone	10-20 mg IV
Ondansetron	8 mg orally or 10 mg IV
Dronabinol	10 mg orally

B. Useful Combinations of Anti-emetic Agents for Improved Anti-emetic Effect

PRIMARY AGENT	SUPPLEMENTAL AGENT
5-HT_3 receptor antagonist	Corticosteroid, phenothiazine, butyrophenone, NK_1 antagonist
Substituted benzamide	Corticosteroid ± muscarinic receptor antagonist
Phenothiazine/ butyrophenone	Corticosteroid
Corticosteroid	Benzodiazepine
Cannabinoid	Corticosteroid

C. Useful Combinations of Anti-emetic Agents Providing Decreased Toxicity of the Primary Agent

PRIMARY AGENT	SUPPLEMENTAL AGENT
Substituted benzamide	H_1 receptor antagonist, corticosteroid, benzodiazepine
Phenothiazine/ butyrophenone	H_1 receptor antagonist
Cannabinoid	Phenothiazine

H, histamine, 5-HT, serotonin; IV, intravenous; IM, intramuscular.
Source: All combination regimens are from Grunberg and Hesketh, 1993, with permission.

Antihistamines

Histamine H_1 antagonists are primarily useful for motion sickness and postoperative emesis. They act on vestibular afferents and within the brainstem. Cyclizine, hydroxyzine, promethazine, and diphenhydramine are examples of this class of agents. Cyclizine has additional anticholinergic effects that may be useful for patients with abdominal cancer. For a detailed discussion of these drugs, see Chapter 32.

Anticholinergic Agents

The most commonly used muscarinic receptor antagonist is scopolamine (hyoscine), which can be injected as the hydrobromide, but usually is administered as the free base in the form of a transdermal patch (TRANSDERM-SCOP). Its principal utility is in the prevention and treatment of motion sickness, although it has been shown to have some activity in postoperative nausea and vomiting tool. In general, anticholinergic agents have no role in chemotherapy-induced nausea. For a detailed discussion of these drugs, see Chapter 9.

Substance P Receptor Antagonists

The nausea and vomiting associated with cisplatin (Chapter 61) have two components: an acute phase that universally is experienced (within 24 hours after chemotherapy) and a delayed phase that affects only some patients (on days 2-5). 5-HT_3 receptor antagonists are not very effective against delayed emesis. Antagonists of the NK_1 receptors for substance P, such as aprepitant (and its parenteral formulation, fosaprepitant; EMEND), have anti-emetic effects in delayed nausea and improve the efficacy of standard anti-emetic regimens in patients receiving multiple cycles of chemotherapy.

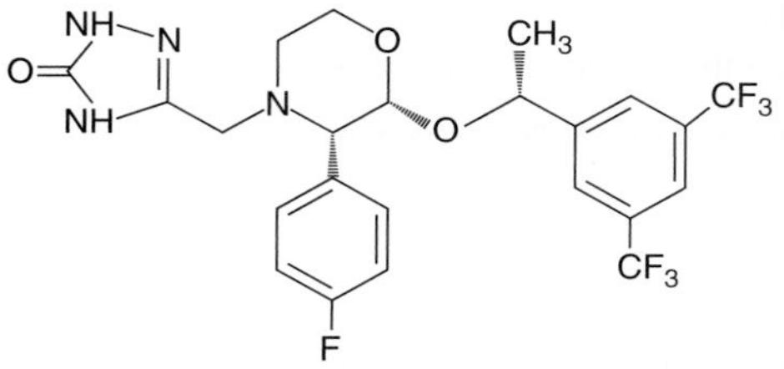

APREPITANT

After absorption, aprepitant is bound extensively to plasma proteins (>95%); it is metabolized avidly, primarily by hepatic CYP3A4, and is excreted in the stools; its $t_{1/2}$ is 9-13 hours. Aprepitant has the potential to interact with other substrates of CYP3A4, requiring adjustment of other drugs, including dexamethasone, methylprednisolone (whose dose may need to be reduced by 50%), and warfarin. Aprepitant is contraindicated in patients on cisapride or pimozide, in whom life-threatening QT prolongation has been reported.

Aprepitant is supplied in 40-, 80- and 125-mg capsules and is administered for 3 days in conjunction with highly emetogenic chemotherapy, along with a 5-HT_3 antagonist and a corticosteroid. The recommended adult dosage of aprepitant is 125 mg administered 1 hour before chemotherapy on day 1, followed by 80 mg once daily in the morning on days 2 and 3 of the treatment regimen.

Cannabinoids

Dronabinol (Δ-9-tetrahydrocannabinol; marinol) is a naturally occurring cannabinoid that can be synthesized chemically or

Table 46–8

5-HT_3 Antagonists in Chemotherapy-Induced Nausea/Emesis

DRUG	CHEMICAL NATURE	RECEPTOR INTERACTIONS	$t_{1/2}$	DOSE (IV)
Ondansetron	Carbazole derivative	5-HT_3 antagonist and weak 5-HT_4 antagonist	3.9 h	0.15 mg/kg
Granisetron	Indazole	5-HT_3 antagonist	9-11.6 h	10 μg/kg
Dolasetron	Indole moiety	5-HT_3 antagonist	7-9 h	1.8 mg/kg
Palonosetron	Isoquinoline	5-HT_3 antagonist; highest affinity for 5-HT_3 receptor in this class	40 h	0.25 mg

IV, intravenous.

extracted from the marijuana plant, *Cannabis sativa*. The exact mechanism of the anti-emetic action of dronabinol is not known but probably relates to stimulation of the CB_1 subtype of cannabinoid receptors on neurons in and around the vomiting center in the brainstem (Van Sickle et al., 2001).

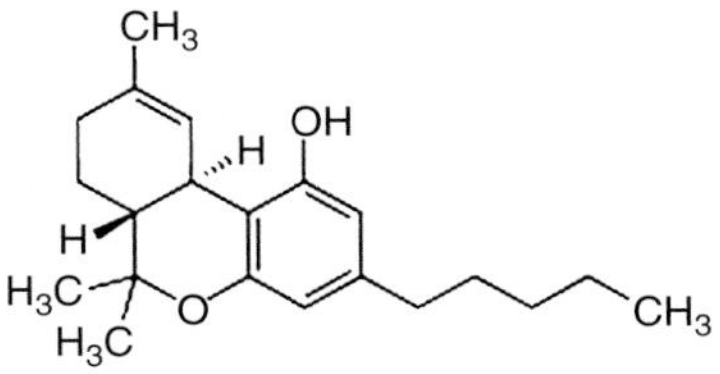

CH_3 OH H H H_3C H_3C O CH_3

DRONABINOL

Pharmacokinetics. Dronabinol is a highly lipid-soluble compound that is absorbed readily after oral administration; its onset of action occurs within an hour, and peak levels are achieved within 2-4 hours. It undergoes extensive first-pass metabolism with limited systemic bioavailability after single doses (only 10-20%). Active and inactive metabolites are formed in the liver; the principal active metabolite is 11-OH-delta-9-tetrahydrocannabinol.

These metabolites are excreted primarily via the biliary-fecal route, with only 10-15% excreted in the urine. Both dronabinol and its metabolites are highly bound (>95%) to plasma proteins. Because of its large volume of distribution, a single dose of dronabinol can result in detectable levels of metabolites for several weeks.

Therapeutic Use. Dronabinol is a useful prophylactic agent in patients receiving cancer chemotherapy when other anti-emetic medications are not effective. It also can stimulate appetite and has been used in patients with acquired immunodeficiency syndrome (AIDS) and anorexia. As an anti-emetic agent, it is administered at an initial dose of 5 mg/m^2 given 1-3 hours before chemotherapy and then every 2-4 hours afterward for a total of four to six doses. If this is not adequate, incremental increases can be made up to a maximum of 15 mg/m^2 per dose. For other indications, the usual starting dose is 2.5 mg twice a day; this can be titrated up to a maximum of 20 mg per day.

Adverse Effects. Dronabinol has complex effects on the CNS, including a prominent central sympathomimetic activity. This can lead to palpitations, tachycardia, vasodilation, hypotension, and conjunctival injection (bloodshot eyes). Patient supervision is necessary because marijuana-like "highs" (e.g., euphoria, somnolence, detachment, dizziness, anxiety, nervousness, panic, etc.) can occur, as can more disturbing effects such as paranoid reactions and thinking abnormalities. After abrupt withdrawal of dronabinol, an abstinence syndrome (irritability, insomnia, and restlessness) can occur. Because of its high affinity for plasma proteins, dronabinol can displace other plasma protein-bound drugs, whose doses may have to be adjusted as a consequence. Dronabinol should be prescribed with great caution to persons with a history of substance abuse (alcohol, drugs) because it also may be abused by these patients.

Nabilone (CESAMET) is a synthetic cannabinoid with a mode of action similar to that of dronabinol.

Pharmacokinetics. Nabilone, like dronabinol, is a highly lipid-soluble compound that is rapidly absorbed after oral administration; its onset of action occurs within an hour, and peak levels are achieved within 2 hours. The $t_{1/2}$ is ~2 hours for the parent compound and 35 hours for metabolites. The metabolites are excreted primarily via the biliary-fecal route (60%), with only ~25% excreted in the urine.

Therapeutic Use. Nabilone is a useful prophylactic agent in patients receiving cancer chemotherapy when other anti-emetic medications are not effective. A dose (1-2 mg) can be given the night before chemotherapy; usual dosing starts 1-3 hours before treatment and then every 8-12 hours during the course of chemotherapy and for 2 days following its cessation.

Adverse Effects. The adverse effects are largely the same as for dronabinol, with significant CNS actions in >10% of patients. Cardiovascular, GI, and other side effects are also common and together with the CNS actions limit the usefulness of this agent.

Glucocorticoids and Anti-Inflammatory Agents

Glucocorticoids such as dexamethasone can be useful adjuncts (Table 46–7) in the treatment of nausea in patients with widespread cancer, possibly by suppressing peritumoral inflammation and prostaglandin production. A similar mechanism has been invoked to explain beneficial effects of NSAIDs in the nausea and vomiting induced by systemic irradiation. For a detailed discussion of these drugs, see Chapters 34 and 42.

Benzodiazepines

Benzodiazepines, such as lorazepam and alprazolam, by themselves are not very effective anti-emetics, but their sedative, amnesic, and anti-anxiety effects can be helpful in reducing the anticipatory component of nausea and vomiting in patients. For a detailed discussion of these drugs, see Chapter 17.

Phosphorated Carbohydrate Solutions

Aqueous solutions of glucose, fructose, and phosphoric acid (EMETROL, NAUSETROL) are available over the counter to relieve nausea. Their mechanism of action is not well established. They may be safely taken for a short period (1 hour with a dose every 15 minutes).

AGENTS USED FOR MISCELLANEOUS GI DISORDERS

Chronic Pancreatitis and Steatorrhea

Pancreatic Enzymes. Chronic pancreatitis is a debilitating syndrome that results in symptoms from loss of glandular function (exocrine and endocrine) and inflammation (pain). Because there is no cure for chronic pancreatitis, the goals of pharmacological therapy are prevention of malabsorption and palliation of pain. The cornerstone of therapy for malabsorption is the use of pancreatic enzymes. Although also used for pain, these agents are much less effective for this symptom.

Enzyme Formulations. In the past, two preparations (and many brands thereof) of pancreatic enzymes were available for replacement therapy, pancreatin and pancrelipase. As of 2009, only pancrelipase (CREON, ZENPEP) is licensed for sale in the U.S. Pancreatic enzymes are typically prescribed on the basis of the lipase content. Pancrelipase products contain various amounts of lipase, protease, and amylase and thus may not be interchangeable. Excess lipase administration has been implicated in the development of fibrosing colonopathy and adherence to published dosing guidelines is thought to minimize this risk (Borowitz et al., 2002).

Replacement Therapy for Malabsorption. Fat malabsorption (steatorrhea) and protein maldigestion occur when the pancreas loses >90% of its ability to produce digestive enzymes. The resultant diarrhea and malabsorption can be managed reasonably well if 30,000 USP units of pancreatic lipase are delivered to the duodenum during a 4-hour period with and after meals; this represents ~10% of the normal pancreatic output. Alternatively, one can titrate the dosage to the fat content of the diet, with ~8000 USP units of lipase activity required for each 17 g of dietary fat. Available preparations of pancreatic enzymes contain up to 20,000 units of lipase and 76,000 units of protease, and the typical dose of pancrelipase is one to three capsules or tablets with or just before meals and snacks, adjusted until a satisfactory symptomatic response is obtained. The loss of pancreatic amylase does not present a problem because of other sources of this enzyme (e.g., salivary glands). The commercially available products are formulated as delayed-release capsules to overcome the need to control gastric acid pharmacologically.

Enzymes for Pain. Pain is the other cardinal symptom of chronic pancreatitis. The rationale for its treatment with pancreatic enzymes is based on the principle of negative feedback inhibition of the pancreas by the presence of duodenal proteases. The release of cholecystokinin (CCK), the principal secretagogue for pancreatic enzymes, is triggered by CCK-releasing monitor peptide in the duodenum, which normally is denatured by pancreatic trypsin. In chronic pancreatitis, trypsin insufficiency leads to persistent activation of this peptide and an increased release of CCK, which is thought to cause pancreatic pain because of continuous stimulation of pancreatic enzyme output and increased intraductal pressure. Delivery of active proteases to the duodenum (which can be done reliably only with uncoated preparations) therefore is important for the interruption of this loop. Although enzymatic therapy has become firmly entrenched for the treatment of painful pancreatitis, the evidence supporting this practice is equivocal at best.

In general, pancreatic enzyme preparations are tolerated extremely well by patients. Hyperuricosuria in patients with cystic fibrosis can occur, and malabsorption of folate and iron has been reported.

Medium-chain triglycerides. Medium-chain triglycerides (MCTs) may provide an additional source of calories in patients with weight loss and a poor response to diet and pancreatic enzyme therapy. MCTs are readily degraded by gastric and pancreatic lipase, and they do not require bile for digestion. In addition, they can be directly absorbed in the intestine. Oral administration of an enteral formula such as PEPTAMEN, which is enriched in MCTs and hydrolyzed peptides, may be of benefit.

Octreotide. Octreotide (Chapter 38) also has been used, with questionable efficacy, to decrease refractory abdominal pain in patients with chronic pancreatitis.

Enzyme Deficiencies

Congenital or acquired deficiencies in digestive enzymes may lead to malabsorption and diarrhea as well as other GI symptoms. Most commonly seen are lactose intolerance, which occurs in the West (10-20%) but in some Asian populations may exceed 90%. Clinically, diarrhea, pain and flatulence occur. Treatment consists of reducing dietary intake of lactose, primarily by reducing consumption of milk and dairy products. Enzyme replacements are over the counter and can be added to meals. They are bacterial or yeast-derived β-galactosidases, with varying efficacy (LACTAID, LACTRASE, DAIRYEASE, others). Because of considerable individual variation and the uncertain degree of efficacy of these preparations, patients must establish an effective dosing regime empirically. Because of the essential requirements to maintain protein, calcium, and vitamin D intake, these must be supplemented or alternative sources provided in the diet if dairy products are limited.

Congenital sucrase-isomaltase deficiency is less common. The symptoms include diarrhea, abdominal pain, and weight loss. This is a congenital disease and may be diagnosed in children who are failing to thrive and are susceptible to repeated infections. Treatment with enzyme replacement therapy is effective. Sacrosidase (SUCRAID) taken with meals reduces or attenuates symptoms in most cases. Elimination of sugars and carbohydrates from the diet is not practical.

BILE ACIDS

Bile acids and their conjugates are essential components of bile that are synthesized from cholesterol in the liver. The major bile acids in human adults are depicted in Figure 46–5. Bile acids induce bile flow,

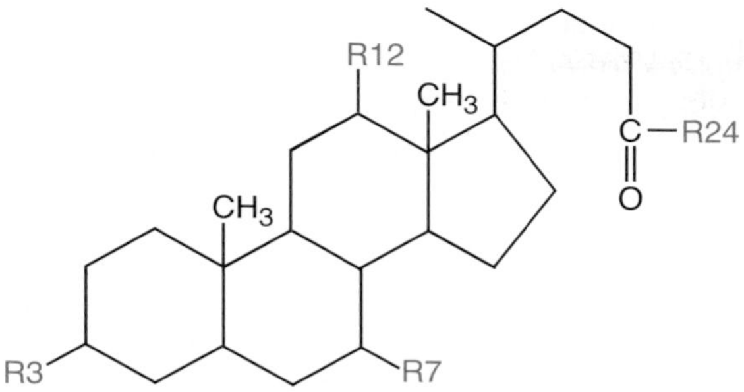

Bile Acid	R3	R7	R12	R24
Cholic acid	–OH	–OH	–OH	glycine (75%) taurine (24%) –OH (<1%)
Chenodeoxycholic acid	–OH	–OH	–H	
Deoxycholic acid	–OH	–H	–OH	
Lithocholic acid	$-SO_2^-$ / –OH	–H	–H	
Ursodeoxycholic acid	–OH	◄OH	–H	

Figure 46–5. *Major bile acids in adults.*

feedback-inhibit cholesterol synthesis, promote intestinal excretion of cholesterol, and facilitate the dispersion and absorption of lipids and fat-soluble vitamins. After secretion into the biliary tract, bile acids are largely (95%) reabsorbed in the intestine (mainly in the terminal ileum), returned to the liver, and then again secreted in bile (enterohepatic circulation). Cholic acid, chenodeoxycholic acid, and deoxycholic acid constitute 95% of bile acids; lithocholic acid and ursodeoxycholic acid are minor constituents. The bile acids exist largely as glycine and taurine conjugates, the salts of which are called bile salts. Colonic bacteria convert primary bile acids (cholic and chenodeoxycholic acid) to secondary acids (mainly deoxycholic and lithocholic acid) by sequential deconjugation and dehydroxylation. These secondary bile acids also are absorbed in the colon and join the primary acids in the enterohepatic pool.

Dried bile from the Himalayan bear (Yutan) has been used for centuries in China to treat liver disease. Ursodeoxycholic acid (UDCA; ursodiol, ACTIGALL, others) (Figure 46–5) is a hydrophilic, dehydroxylated bile acid that is formed by epimerization of the bile acid chenodeoxycholic acid (CDCA; chenodiol) in the gut by intestinal bacteria; it comprises ~1-3% of the total bile acid pool in human beings but is present at much higher concentrations in bears. When administered orally, litholytic bile acids such as chenodiol and ursodiol can alter relative concentrations of bile acids, decrease biliary lipid secretion, and reduce the cholesterol content of the bile so that it is less lithogenic. Ursodiol also may have cytoprotective effects on hepatocytes and effects on the immune system that account for some of its beneficial effects in cholestatic liver diseases.

Bile acids were first used therapeutically for gallstone dissolution; use for this indication requires a functional gallbladder because the modified bile must enter the gallbladder to interact with gallstones. To be amenable to dissolution, the gallstones must be composed of cholesterol monohydrate crystals and generally must be <15 mm in diameter to provide a favorable ratio of surface to size. For these reasons, the overall efficacy of litholytic bile acids in the treatment of gallstones has been disappointing (partial dissolution occurs in 40-60% of patients completing therapy and is complete in only 33-50% of these). Although a combination of chenodiol and ursodiol probably is better than either agent alone, ursodiol is preferred as a single agent because of its greater efficacy and less-frequent side effects (e.g., hepatotoxicity).

Primary biliary cirrhosis is a chronic, progressive, cholestatic liver disease of unknown etiology that typically affects middle-aged to elderly women. Ursodiol (administered at 13-15 mg/kg per day in two divided doses) reduces the concentration of primary bile acids and improves biochemical and histological features of primary biliary cirrhosis, especially in early disease. Patients with advanced primary biliary cirrhosis and complications such as ascites do not benefit from this treatment. Ursodiol also has been used in a variety of other cholestatic liver diseases, including primary sclerosing cholangitis, and in cystic fibrosis; in general, it is less effective in these conditions than in primary biliary cirrhosis.

ANTI-FLATULENCE AGENTS

"Gas" is a common but relatively vague GI complaint, used in reference not only to flatulence and eructation but also bloating or fullness. Although few symptoms can be directly attributable to excessive intestinal gas, over-the-counter and herbal preparations that are touted as anti-flatulent are very popular. One of these is simethicone (MYLICON, GAS-X, others), a mixture of siloxane polymers stabilized with silicon dioxide.

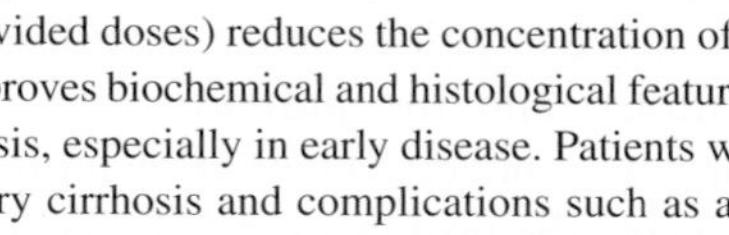

$$(H_3C)_3Si{-}[OSi(CH_3)_2]_n{-}CH_3 \quad + \quad SiO_2$$

Simethicone is an inert, non-toxic insoluble liquid. Because of its ability to collapse bubbles by forming a thin layer on their surface, it is an effective anti-foaming agent. Although it may be effective in diminishing gas volumes in the GI tract, it is not clear whether this accomplishes a therapeutic effect. Simethicone is available in chewable tablets, liquid-filled capsules, suspensions, and orally disintegrating strips, either by itself or in combination with other over-the-counter medications including antacids and other digestants. The usual dosage in adults is 40-25 mg four times daily. Activated charcoal may also be used alone or in combination with simethicone, but has not been shown conclusively to have much benefit.

An alpha-galactosidase preparation (BEANO) is available over-the-counter to reduce gas from baked beans.

CLINICAL SUMMARY

GI Motility Disorders. As a group, these are difficult disorders to treat because of a lack of effective therapeutic options. For patients with gastroparesis, first-line therapy consists of metoclopramide, which accelerates gastric emptying and also has anti-emetic effects. Erythromycin, a motilin agonist, also has been employed, but is most effective for short-term use. For patients with small-bowel dysmotility, the choices are even more limited: Metoclopramide and erythromycin generally do not work; therapy with octreotide may benefit a subset of patients.

Constipation. Although many choices exist for this condition, most therapies are empirical and non-specific. Constipation often can be addressed by simple measures such as increasing fiber intake, avoiding constipating medications, and the judicious use of osmotic laxatives on an as-needed basis. For more persistent symptoms, a specific prokinetic 5-HT_4 receptor agonist or Cl^- channel agonist may be effective in some patients. Stimulant laxatives, although effective, should be avoided for long-term use. Patients with chronic constipation who do not respond to simple measures should undergo further testing to discover uncommon but specific disorders of colonic or anorectal motility.

Diarrhea. In most cases, an attempt should be made to find the underlying cause and to target it specifically. If no such cause is found, chronic diarrhea can be treated empirically, with the simplest approach being bulk-forming and hygroscopic agents, followed by opioids such as loperamide for diarrhea associated with inflammatory bowel disease or diphenoxylate/difenoxin can be used to manage acute exacerbations of chronic functional diarrhea.

Irritable Bowel Syndrome. IBS consists of abdominal pain and discomfort associated with diarrhea, constipation, or alternating bouts of diarrhea and constipation. This common syndrome requires a combination of pharmacological and behavioral approaches that include dietary modifications and psychological counseling. No one therapy will work for all patients and currently there are no therapies focused on IBS that treat both the pain and GI symptoms. Anti-spasmodics are useful by themselves in mild cases and as adjuncts in a regimen that includes tricyclic anti-depressants for more persistent pain.

Nausea and Vomiting. The development of the 5-HT_3 receptor antagonists has led to a major advances in the treatment of nausea and vomiting, especially in the post-chemotherapy and post-operative settings. Anticholinergics are most effective in motion sickness. Antihistamines and related drugs still are useful for empirical treatment of nausea from a variety of causes. Dronabinol or nabilone may be an effective agent for some refractory cases. The clinical utility of newer agents such as aprepitant in situations other than post-chemotherapy nausea will be tested in coming years.

BIBLIOGRAPHY

Borowitz D, Baker RD, Stallings V. Consensus report on nutrition for pediatric patients with cystic fibrosis. *J Pediatr Gastroenterol Nutr,* **2002,** *35:*246–259.

De Giorgio R, Barbara G, Furness JB, Tonini M. Novel therapeutic targets for enteric nervous system disorders. *Trends Pharmacol Sci,* **2007,** *28:*473–481.

Eutamene H, Bradesi S, Larauche M, *et al.* Guanylate cyclase C-mediated antinociceptive effects of linaclotide in rodent models of visceral pain. *Neurogastroenterol Motil,* **2009** August 25 (Epub ahead of print).

Furness JB. *The Enteric Nervous System.* Wiley-Blackwell, Oxford, **2006**, pp 286.

Gale JD. The use of novel promotility and prosecretory agents for the treatment of chronic idiopathic constipation and irritable bowel syndrome with constipation. *Adv Ther,* **2009,** *26:*519–530.

Gershon MD, Tack J. The serotonin signalling system: From basic understanding to drug development for functional GI disorders. *Gastroenterology,* **2007,** *132:*397–414.

Grunberg SM, Hesketh PJ. Control of chemotherapy-induced emesis. *N Engl J Med*, **1993,** *329:*1790–1796.

Grundy D, Al-Chaer ED, Aziz Q, *et al.* Fundamentals of neurogastroenterology: Basic science. *Gastroenterology,* **2006,** *130:*1391–1411.

Hornby PJ. Central neurocircuitry associated with emesis. *Am J Med*, **2001,** *111(suppl 8A):*106S–112S.

Holzer P. Opioid receptors in the gastrointestinal tract. *Reg Peptides,* **2009,** *155:*11–17.

Izzo AA, Gaginella TS, Mascolo N, Capasso F. Recent findings on the mode of action of laxatives: The role of platelet activating factor and nitric oxide. *Trends Pharmacol Sci*, **1998,** *19:*403–405.

Joyce J. *Ulysses* (1922). The Gabler edition, Random House, NY, 1986, p. 56.

Kreek MJ. Constipation syndromes. In: *A Pharmacological Approach to Gastrointestinal Disorders*. (Lewis JH, ed.), Williams & Wilkins, Baltimore, **1994,** pp. 179–208.

Kunze WA, Furness JB. The enteric nervous system and regulation of intestinal motility. *Annu Rev Physiol*, **1999,** *61:* 117–142.

Mertz HR. Drug therapy: Irritable bowel syndrome. *N Engl J Med*, **2003,** *349:*2136–2146.

Moitinho E, Planas R, Banares R, *et al.* Multicenter randomized controlled trial comparing different schedules of somatostatin in the treatment of acute variceal bleeding. *J Hepatol*, **2001,** *35:*712–718.

Rhee SH, Pothoulakis C, Mayer EA. Principles and clinical implications of the brain-gut-enteric microbiota axis. *Nat Rev Gastroenterol Hepatol,* **2009,** *6:*306–314.

Sanger GJ. Motilin, ghrelin and related neuropeptides as targets for the treatment of GI diseases. *Drug Disc Today,* **2008,** *13:*234–239.

Sartor RB. Probiotic therapy of intestinal inflammation and infections. *Curr Opin Gastroenterol,* **2005,** *21:*44–50.

Scuderi PE. Pharmacology of anti-emetics. *Int Anesthesiol Clin,* **2003,** *41:*41–66.

Tonini M, Cipollina L, Poluzzi E, *et al*. Review article: Clinical implications of enteric and central D_2 receptor blockade by anti-dopaminergic gastrointestinal prokinetics. *Aliment Pharmacol Ther*, **2004,** *19:*379–390.

Van Sickle MD, Oland LD, Ho W, *et al.* Cannabinoids inhibit emesis through CB1 receptors in the brainstem of the ferret. *Gastroenterology,* **2001,** *121:*767–774.

Ward SM, Sanders KM, Hirst GD. Role of interstitial cells of Cajal in neural control of gastrointestinal smooth muscles. *Neurogastroenterol Motil,* **2004,** *16(suppl 1):*112–117.

Wood JD. Enteric nervous system: Reflexes, pattern generators and motility. *Curr Opin Gastroenterol,* **2008,** *24:*149–158.

Zhao X, Pasricha PJ. Botulinum toxin for spastic GI disorders: A systematic review. *Gastrointest Endosc*, **2003,** *57:* 219–235.

Pharmacotherapy of Inflammatory Bowel Disease

John L. Wallace and
Keith A. Sharkey

Inflammatory bowel disease (IBD) is a spectrum of chronic, idiopathic, inflammatory intestinal conditions. IBD causes significant gastrointestinal (GI) symptoms that include diarrhea, abdominal pain, bleeding, anemia, and weight loss. IBD also is associated with a variety of extraintestinal manifestations, including arthritis, ankylosing spondylitis, sclerosing cholangitis, uveitis, iritis, pyoderma gangrenosum, and erythema nodosum.

IBD conventionally is divided into two major subtypes: ulcerative colitis and Crohn's disease. Ulcerative colitis is characterized by confluent mucosal inflammation of the colon starting at the anal verge and extending proximally for a variable extent (e.g., proctitis, left-sided colitis, or pancolitis). Crohn's disease, by contrast, is characterized by transmural inflammation of any part of the GI tract but most commonly the area adjacent to the ileocecal valve. The inflammation in Crohn's disease is not necessarily confluent, frequently leaving "skip areas" of relatively normal mucosa. The transmural nature of the inflammation may lead to fibrosis and strictures or, alternatively, fistula formation.

Medical therapy for IBD is problematic. Because no unique abnormality has been identified, current therapy for IBD seeks to dampen the generalized inflammatory response; however, no agent can reliably accomplish this, and the response of an individual patient to a given medicine may be limited and unpredictable. Based on this variable response, clinical trials generally employ standardized quantitative assessments of efficacy that take into account both clinical and laboratory parameters (e.g., the Crohn's Disease Activity Index). The disease also exhibits marked fluctuations in activity—even in the absence of therapy—leading to a significant "placebo effect" in therapeutic trials.

Specific goals of pharmacotherapy in IBD include controlling acute exacerbations of the disease, maintaining remission, and treating specific complications such as fistulas. Specific drugs may be better suited for one or the other of these aims (Table 47–1). For example, glucocorticoids remain the treatment of choice for moderate to severe flares but are inappropriate for long-term use because of side effects and their inability to maintain remission. Other immunosuppressive agents, such as azathioprine, that require several weeks to achieve their therapeutic effect, have a limited role in the acute setting but are preferred for long-term management.

For many years glucocorticoids, sulfasalazine and 5-aminosalicylic acid were the mainstays of pharmacotherapy for IBD. More recently, agents used in other immune/inflammatory conditions, such as azathioprine and cyclosporine, have been adapted for IBD therapy. Advances in the understanding of the inflammatory response and improved biotechnology have led to the development of biological agents that can target single steps in the immune cascade, a successful and widely accepted strategy. Drug delivery to the appropriate site(s) along the GI tract also has been a major challenge, and second-generation agents have improved drug delivery, increased efficacy, and decreased side effects.

PATHOGENESIS OF INFLAMMATORY BOWEL DISEASE

Crohn's disease and ulcerative colitis are chronic idiopathic inflammatory disorders of the GI tract; a summary of proposed pathogenic events and potential sites of therapeutic intervention is shown in Figure 47–1.

Table 47–1

Medications Commonly Used to Treat Inflammatory Bowel Disease

	CROHN'S DISEASE					ULCERATIVE COLITIS			
	ACTIVE DISEASE			MAINTENANCE		ACTIVE DISEASE			
CLASS/Drug	Mild-Moderate	Moderate-Severe	Fistula	Medical Remission	Surgical Remission	Distal Colitis	Mild-Moderate	Moderate-Severe	Maintenance
Mesalamine									
Enema	+[a]	–	–	–	–	+	+[a,b]	–	+
Oral	+	–	–	+/–	+[c]	+	+	–	+
Antibiotics									
(metronidazole ciprofloxacin, others)	+	+	+	?	+[c]	–	–	–	+[c]
Corticosteroids									
Enema, foam, suppository	+[a]	–	–	–	+	+[b]	–	–	–
Oral	+	+	–	–	–	+	+	+	–
Intravenous	–	+	–	–	–	+[d]	–	+	–
Immunomodulators									
6-MP/AZA	–	+	+	+	+[c]	+[d]	–	+[d]	+[d]
Methotrexate	–	?	?	?	?	–	–	–	–
Cyclosporine	–	+[d]	+[d]	–	–	+[d]	–	+[d]	–
Biological response modifiers									
Infliximab	+[d]	+	+	+[c]	?	+	–	+	?
Adalimumab	+	+	+	+	?	?	?	?	?
Certolizumab pegol	+	+	?	+	?	?	?	+	?
Natalizumab	–	+	?	+	?	?	?	?	?

[a]Distal colonic disease only.
[b]For adjunctive therapy.
[c]Some data to support use; remains controversial.
[d]Selected patients.
ABBREVIATIONS: 6-MP, 6-mercaptopurine; AZA, azathioprine. (From Sands BE. Therapy of inflammatory bowel disease. *Gastroenterology*. **2000**;118(2 Suppl 1): S68-S82. Table 1, Pg S71. With permission from Elsevier. Copyright © Elsevier.)

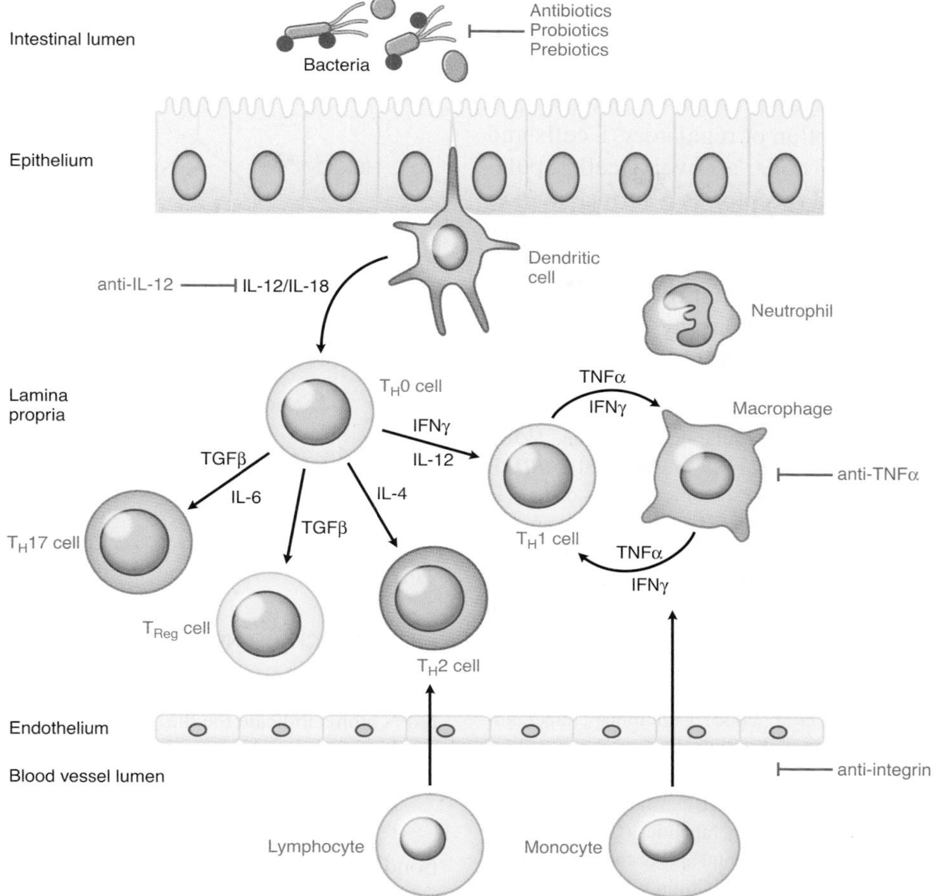

Figure 47–1. *Proposed pathogenesis of inflammatory bowel disease and target sites for pharmacological intervention.* Shown are the interactions among bacterial antigens in the intestinal lumen and immune cells in the intestinal wall. If the epithelial barrier is impaired, bacterial antigens can gain access to antigen-presenting cells (APC) such as dendritic cells in the lamina propria. These cells then present the antigen(s) to $CD4^+$ lymphocytes and also secrete cytokines such interleukin (IL)-12 and IL-18, thereby inducing the differentiation of T_H1 cells in Crohn's disease (or, under the control of IL-4, type 2 helper T cells [T_H2] in ulcerative colitis). The balance of pro-inflammatory and anti-inflammatory events is also governed by regulatory T_H17 and T_{Reg} cells, both of which serve to limit immune and inflammatory responses in the GI tract. Transforming growth factor (TGF)β and IL-6 are important cytokines that drive the expansion of the regulatory T cell subsets. The T_H1 cells produce a characteristic array of cytokines, including interferon (IFN)γ and TNFα, which in turn activate macrophages. Macrophages positively regulate T_H1 cells by secreting additional cytokines, including IFNγ and TNFα. Recruitment of a variety of leukocytes is mediated by activation of resident immune cells including neutrophils. Cell adhesion molecules such as integrins are important in the infiltration of leukocytes and novel biological therapeutic strategies aimed at blocking leukocyte recruitment are effective at reducing inflammation. General immunosuppressants (e.g., glucocorticoids, thioguanine derivatives, methotrexate, and cyclosporine) affect multiple sites of inflammation. More site-specific intervention involve intestinal bacteria (antibiotics, prebiotics, and probiotics) and therapy directed at TNFα or IL-12 (see text for further details).

Although Crohn's disease and ulcerative colitis share a number of GI and extraintestinal manifestations and can respond to a similar array of drugs, emerging evidence suggests that they result from fundamentally distinct pathogenetic mechanisms (Xavier and Podolsky, 2007). Histologically, the transmural lesions in Crohn's disease exhibit marked infiltration of lymphocytes and macrophages, granuloma formation, and submucosal fibrosis, whereas the superficial lesions in ulcerative colitis have lymphocytic and neutrophilic infiltrates. Within the diseased bowel in Crohn's disease, the cytokine profile includes increased levels of interleukin (IL)-12, IL-23, interferon-γ, and tumor necrosis factor-α (TNFα), findings characteristic of T-helper 1 (T_H1)–

mediated inflammatory processes. In contrast, the inflammatory response in ulcerative colitis resembles aspects of that mediated by the T_H2 pathway. Recently, this relatively simplistic classification has been revised in the light of the description of regulatory T cells and pro-inflammatory T_H17 cells, a novel T-cell population that expresses IL-23 receptor as a surface marker and produces, among others, the pro-inflammatory cytokines IL-17, IL-21, IL-22, and IL-26. Several studies have demonstrated an important role of T_H17 cells in intestinal inflammation, particularly in Crohn's disease (Cho, 2008; Strober et al., 2007).

Important insights into pathogenesis have emerged from genetic analyses of Crohn's disease. Mutations in the gene *NOD2* (*nucleotide-binding oligomerization domain-2*; also called *CARD15*) are associated with both familial and sporadic Crohn's disease in whites (Hugot et al., 2001; Ogura et al., 2001). *NOD2* is expressed in monocytes, granulocytes, dendritic cells, Paneth cells, and epithelial cells. It is proposed to function as an intracellular sensor for bacterial infection by recognizing peptidoglycans, thereby playing an important role in the natural immunity to bacterial pathogens. Consistent with this model, other studies have identified bacterial antigens, including pseudomonal protein I2 (Dalwadi et al., 2001) and a flagellin protein (Lodes et al., 2004), as dominant superantigens that induce the T_H1 response in Crohn's disease (shown as bacterial products in Figure 47–1). More recently, genome-wide studies have revealed other genes associated with IBD, whose identification may lead to the development of novel therapeutics (Cho, 2008).

Thus, these converging experimental approaches are generating novel insights into the pathogenesis of Crohn's disease that soon may translate into novel therapeutic approaches to IBD. The major therapeutic agents available for IBD are described next.

MESALAMINE (5-ASA)-BASED THERAPY

Chemistry, Mechanism of Action, and Pharmacological Properties. First-line therapy for mild to moderate ulcerative colitis generally involves mesalamine (5-aminosalicylic acid, or 5-ASA). The archetype for this class of medications is sulfasalazine (AZULFIDINE), which consists of 5-ASA linked to sulfapyridine by an azo bond (Figure 47–2). Although this drug was developed originally as therapy for rheumatoid arthritis, clinical trials serendipitously demonstrated a beneficial effect on the GI symptoms of subjects with concomitant ulcerative colitis. Sulfasalazine is a prime example of an oral drug that is delivered effectively to the distal GI tract. Given individually, either 5-ASA or sulfapyridine is absorbed in the upper GI tract; the azo linkage in sulfasalazine prevents absorption in the stomach and small intestine, and the individual components are not liberated for absorption until colonic bacteria cleave the bond. 5-ASA is now regarded as the therapeutic moiety, with little, if any, contribution by sulfapyridine.

Sulfasalazine

5-ASA Mesalamine

Sulfapyridine

Olsalazine

Balsalazide

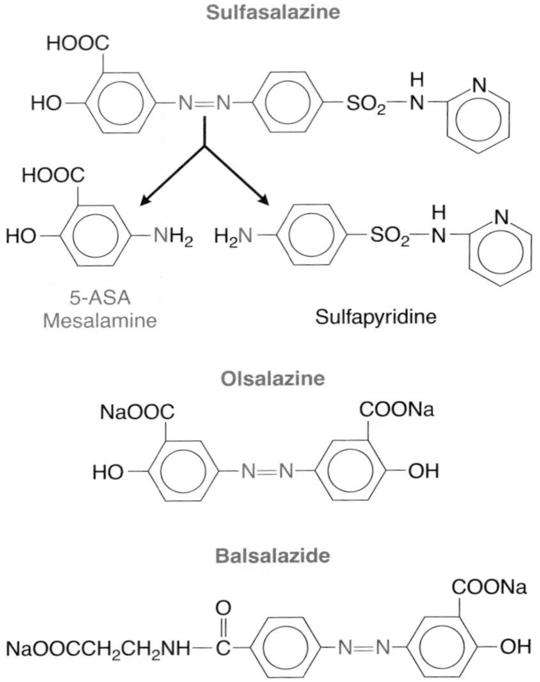

Figure 47–2. *Structures of sulfasalazine and related agents.* The red N atoms indicate the diazo linkage that is cleaved to generate the active moiety.

Mesalamine is a salicylate, but its therapeutic effect does not appear to relate to cyclooxygenase inhibition; indeed, traditional nonsteroidal anti-inflammatory drugs and selective inhibitors of cyclooxygenase-2 ("coxibs") may exacerbate IBD. Many potential sites of action have been demonstrated *in vitro* for either sulfasalazine or mesalamine: inhibition of the production of IL-1 and TNFα, inhibition of the lipoxygenase pathway, scavenging of free radicals and oxidants, and inhibition of NF-κB, a transcription factor pivotal to production of inflammatory mediators. Specific mechanisms of action of these drugs have not been identified.

Although not active therapeutically, sulfapyridine causes many of the adverse effects observed in patients taking sulfasalazine. To preserve the therapeutic effect of 5-ASA without the adverse effects of sulfapyridine, several second-generation 5-ASA compounds have been developed (Figures 47–2, 47–3, and 47–4). They are divided into two groups: prodrugs and coated drugs. Prodrugs contain the same azo bond as sulfasalazine but replace the linked sulfapyridine with either another 5-ASA (olsalazine, DIPENTUM) or an inert compound

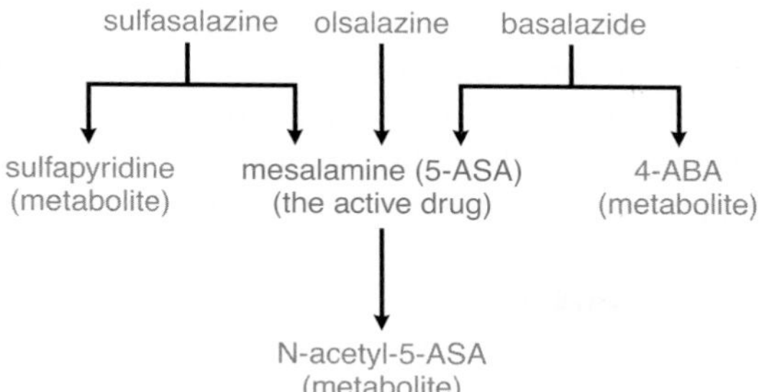

Figure 47–3. *Metabolic fates of the different oral formulations of mesalamine (5-ASA).* Chemical structures are in Figure 47–2.

(balsalazide, COLAZIDE). Thus, these compounds act at sites along the GI tract similar to those of sulfasalazine. The alternative approaches employ either a delayed-release formulation (PENTASA) or a pH-sensitive coating (ASACOL; LIALDA/MEZAVANT). Delayed-release mesalamine is released throughout the small intestine and colon, whereas pH-sensitive mesalamine is released in the terminal ileum and colon. These different distributions of drug delivery have potential therapeutic implications.

Oral sulfasalazine is effective in patients with mild or moderately active ulcerative colitis, with response rates in the range of 60-80% (Prantera et al., 1999). The usual dose is 4 g/day in four divided doses with food; to avoid adverse effects, the dose is increased gradually from an initial dose of 500 mg twice a day. Doses as high as 6 g/day can be used but cause an increased incidence of side effects. For patients with severe colitis, sulfasalazine is of less certain value, even though it is often added as an adjunct to systemic glucocorticoids. Regardless of disease severity, the drug plays a useful role in preventing relapses once remission has been achieved. In general, newer 5-ASA preparations have similar therapeutic efficacy in ulcerative colitis with fewer side effects. Because they lack the dose-related side effects of sulfapyridine, the newer formulations can be used to provide higher doses of mesalamine with some improvement in disease control. The usual doses to treat active disease are 800 mg three times a day for ASACOL and 1 g four times a day for PENTASA. Lower doses are used for maintenance (e.g., ASACOL, 800 mg twice a day). Although some studies have suggested that a given preparation may be superior in treating colonic disease, there is no consensus on this issue.

The efficacy of 5-ASA preparations (e.g., sulfasalazine) in Crohn's disease is less striking, with modest benefit at best in controlled trials. Sulfasalazine has not been shown to be effective in maintaining remission and has been replaced by newer 5-ASA preparations. Some studies have reported that both ASACOL and PENTASA are more effective than placebo in inducing remission in patients with Crohn's disease (particularly colitis), although higher doses than those typically used in ulcerative colitis are required. The role of mesalamine in maintenance therapy for Crohn's disease is controversial, and there is no clear benefit of continued 5-ASA therapy in patients who achieve medical remission (Camma et al., 1997). Because they largely bypass the small intestine, the second-generation 5-ASA prodrugs such as olsalazine and balsalazide do not have a significant effect in small-bowel Crohn's disease.

Topical preparations of mesalamine suspended in a wax matrix suppository (ROWASA) or in a suspension enema (CANASA) are effective in active proctitis and distal ulcerative colitis, respectively. They appear to be superior to topical hydrocortisone in this setting, with response rates of 75-90%. Mesalamine enemas (4 g/60 mL) should be used at bedtime and retained for at least 8 hours; the suppository (500 mg) should be used two to three times a day with the objective of retaining it for at least 3 hours. Response to local therapy with mesalamine may occur within 3-21 days; however, the usual course of therapy is from 3-6 weeks. Once remission has occurred, lower doses are used for maintenance.

Pharmacokinetics. Approximately 20-30% of orally administered sulfasalazine is absorbed in the small intestine. Much of this is taken up by the liver and excreted unmetabolized in the bile; the rest (~10%) is excreted unchanged in the urine. The remaining 70% reaches the colon, where, if cleaved completely by bacterial enzymes, it generates 400 mg mesalamine for every gram of the parent compound. Thereafter, the individual components of sulfasalazine follow different metabolic pathways. Sulfapyridine, which is highly lipid soluble, is absorbed rapidly from the colon. It undergoes extensive hepatic metabolism, including acetylation and hydroxylation, conjugation with glucuronic acid, and excretion in the urine. The acetylation phenotype of the patient determines plasma levels of sulfapyridine and the probability of side effects;

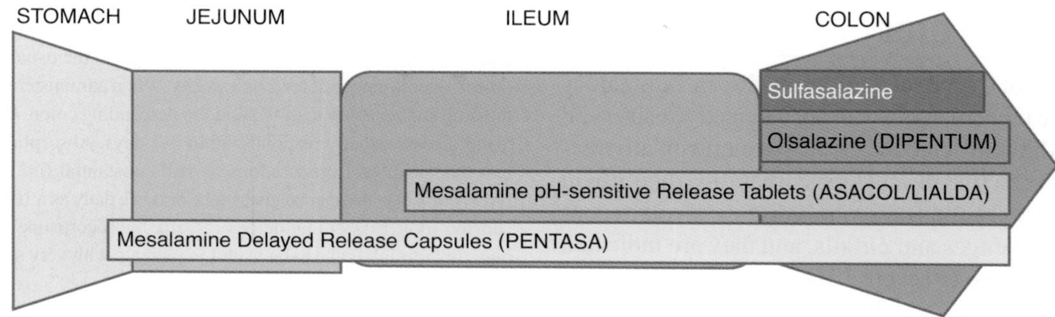

Figure 47–4. *Sites of release of mesalamine (5-ASA) in the GI tract from different oral formulations.*

rapid acetylators have lower systemic levels of the drug and fewer adverse effects. By contrast, only 25% of mesalamine is absorbed from the colon, and most of the drug is excreted in the stool. The small amount that is absorbed is acetylated in the intestinal mucosal wall and the liver and then excreted in the urine. Intraluminal concentrations of mesalamine therefore are very high (~1500 μg/mL or 10 mM in patients taking a typical dose of 3 g/day).

The pH-sensitive coatings (methyl-methacrylate methacrylic acid copolymer) of ASACOL (EUDAGRIT) and LIALDA/MEZAVANT limit gastric and small intestinal absorption of 5-ASA, as assessed by urinary, ileostomal, and fecal measurements of the various metabolites. The pharmacokinetics of PENTASA differ somewhat. The ethylcellulose-coated micro-granules are released in the upper GI tract as discrete prolonged-release units of mesalamine. Acetylated mesalamine can be detected in the circulation within an hour after ingestion, indicating some rapid absorption, but some intact micro-granules also can be detected in the colon. Because it is released in the small bowel, a greater fraction of PENTASA is absorbed systemically compared with the other 5-ASA preparations.

Adverse Effects. Side effects of sulfasalazine occur in 10-45% of patients with ulcerative colitis and are related primarily to the sulfa moiety. Some are dose related, including headache, nausea, and fatigue. These reactions can be minimized by giving the medication with meals or by decreasing the dose. Allergic reactions include rash, fever, Stevens-Johnson syndrome, hepatitis, pneumonitis, hemolytic anemia, and bone marrow suppression. Sulfasalazine reversibly decreases the number and motility of sperm but does not impair female fertility. Sulfasalazine inhibits intestinal folate absorption and is usually administered with folate.

The newer mesalamine formulations generally are well tolerated, and side effects are relatively infrequent and minor. Headache, dyspepsia, and skin rash are the most common. Diarrhea appears to be particularly common with olsalazine (occurring in 10-20% of patients); this may be related to its ability to stimulate chloride and fluid secretion in the small bowel. Nephrotoxicity, although rare, is a more serious concern. Mesalamine has been associated with interstitial nephritis; although its pathogenic role is controversial, renal function should be monitored in all patients receiving these drugs. Both sulfasalazine and its metabolites cross the placenta but have not been shown to harm the fetus. Although less well studied, the newer formulations appear to be safe in pregnancy. The risks to the fetus from the consequences of uncontrolled IBD in pregnant women are believed to outweigh the risks associated with the therapeutic use of these agents.

GLUCOCORTICOIDS

The effects of glucocorticoids on the inflammatory response are numerous and well documented (Chapters 38 and 42). Although glucocorticoids are universally recognized as effective in acute exacerbations, their use in either ulcerative colitis or Crohn's disease involves considerable challenges and pitfalls, and they are indicated only for moderate to severe IBD.

The response to glucocorticoids in individual patients with IBD divides them into three general classes: responsive, dependent, and unresponsive. Glucocorticoid-responsive patients improve clinically, generally within 1-2 weeks and remain in remission as the steroids are tapered and then discontinued. Glucocorticoid-dependent patients also respond to glucocorticoids but then experience a relapse of symptoms as the steroid dose is tapered. Glucocorticoid-unresponsive patients do not improve even with prolonged high-dose steroids. Approximately 40% of patients are glucocorticoid responsive, 30-40% have only a partial response or become glucocorticoid dependent, and 15-20% of patients do not respond to glucocorticoid therapy.

Glucocorticoids sometimes are used for prolonged periods to control symptoms in corticosteroid-dependent patients. However, the failure to respond to steroids with prolonged remission (i.e., a disease relapse) should prompt consideration of alternative therapies, including immunosuppressive agents and anti-TNFα therapies. Glucocorticoid are not effective in maintaining remission in either ulcerative colitis or Crohn's disease (Steinhart et al., 2003); their significant side effects have led to increased emphasis on limiting the duration and cumulative dose of corticosteroids in IBD.

The approach to glucocorticoid therapy in IBD differs somewhat from that in diseases such as asthma or rheumatoid arthritis. Initial doses are 40-60 mg of prednisone or equivalent per day; higher doses generally are no more effective. The glucocorticoid dose in IBD is tapered over weeks to months. Even with these slow tapers, however, efforts should be made to minimize the duration of therapy. Glucocorticoids induce remission in most patients with either ulcerative colitis or Crohn's disease (Faubion et al., 2001). Oral prednisone is the preferred agent for moderate to severe disease, and the typical dose is 40-60 mg once a day. Most patients improve substantially within 5 days of initiating treatment; others require treatment for several weeks before remission occurs. For more severe cases, glucocorticoids are given intravenously. Generally, *methylprednisolone* or *hydrocortisone* is used for intravenous therapy, although some experts believe that corticotropin (ACTH) is more effective in patients who have not previously received any steroids.

Topically acting agents (i.e., given by enema) have fewer adverse effects than systemic steroids but are also less effective in reducing remission. Glucocorticoid enemas are useful mainly in patients whose disease is limited to the rectum and left colon. Hydrocortisone is available as a retention enema (100 mg/60 mL), and the usual dose is one 60-mL enema per night for 2 or 3 weeks. When administered optimally, the drug can reach up to or beyond the descending colon. Patients with distal disease usually respond within 3-7 days. Absorption, although less than with oral preparations, is still substantial (up to 50-75%). Hydrocortisone also can be given once or twice daily as a 10% foam suspension (CORTIFOAM) that delivers 80 mg hydrocortisone per application; this formulation can be useful in patients with very short areas of distal proctitis and difficulty retaining fluid.

Budesonide (ENTOCORT ER) is an enteric-release form of a synthetic steroid that is used for ileocecal Crohn's disease

(Greenberg et al., 1994; McKeage and Goa, 2002). It is proposed to deliver adequate steroid therapy to a specific portion of inflamed gut while minimizing systemic side effects owing to extensive first-pass hepatic metabolism to inactive derivatives. Topical therapy (e.g., enemas and suppositories) also is effective in treating colitis limited to the left side of the colon. Although the topical potency of budesonide is 200 times higher than that of hydrocortisone, its oral systemic bioavailability is only 10%. In some studies, budesonide was associated with a lower incidence of systemic side effects than prednisone, although data also indicate that systemic steroids are more effective in patients with higher Crohn's Disease Activity Index scores. Budesonide (9 mg/day for up to 8 weeks followed by 6 mg/day for maintenance of remission for up to 3 months) is effective in the acute management of mild-to-moderate exacerbations of Crohn's disease, but its role in maintaining remission has not been fully delineated (Hofer, 2003).

A significant number of patients with IBD fails to respond adequately to glucocorticoids and are either steroid-resistant or steroid-dependent. The reasons for this failure are poorly understood but may involve complications such as fibrosis or strictures in Crohn's disease, which will not respond to anti-inflammatory measures alone; local complications such as abscesses, in which case the use of glucocorticoids may lead to uncontrolled sepsis; and intercurrent infections with organisms such as cytomegalovirus and *Clostridium difficile*. Steroid failures also may be related to specific pharmacogenomic factors such as upregulation of the multidrug resistance (*mdr*) gene (Farrell et al., 2000) or altered levels of corticosteroid-binding globulin.

IMMUNOSUPPRESSIVE AGENTS

Several drugs developed initially for cancer chemotherapy or as immunosuppressive agents in organ transplants have been adapted for treatment of IBD. Although their initial use in IBD was based on their immunosuppressive effects, their specific mechanisms of action are unknown. Increasing clinical experience has defined specific roles for each of these agents as mainstays in the pharmacotherapy of IBD. However, their potential for serious adverse effects mandates a careful assessment of risks and benefits in each patient.

Thiopurine Derivatives

The cytotoxic thiopurine derivatives *mercaptopurine* (6-MP, PURINETHOL) and azathioprine (IMMURAN) (Chapters 51 and 52) are used to treat patients with severe IBD or those who are steroid resistant or steroid dependent (Prefontaine et al., 2009). These thiopurine antimetabolites impair purine biosynthesis and inhibit cell proliferation. Both are prodrugs: azathioprine is converted to mercaptopurine, which is subsequently metabolized to 6-thioguanine nucleotides that are the presumed active moiety (Figure 47–5).

These drugs generally are used interchangeably with appropriate dose adjustments, typically azathioprine (2-2.5 mg/ kg) or mercaptopurine (1.5 mg/kg). As discussed later, the pathways by which they are metabolized are clinically relevant, and specific assays can be used to assess clinical response and to avoid side effects. Because of concerns about side effects, these drugs were used initially only in Crohn's disease, which lacks a surgical curative option. They now are considered equally effective in Crohn's disease and ulcerative colitis. These drugs effectively maintain remission in both diseases; they also may prevent (or, more typically, delay) recurrence of Crohn's disease after surgical resection. Finally, they are used successfully to treat fistulas in Crohn's disease. The clinical response to azathioprine or mercaptopurine may take weeks to months, such that other drugs with a more rapid onset of action (e.g., mesalamine, glucocorticoids, or infliximab) are preferred in the acute setting.

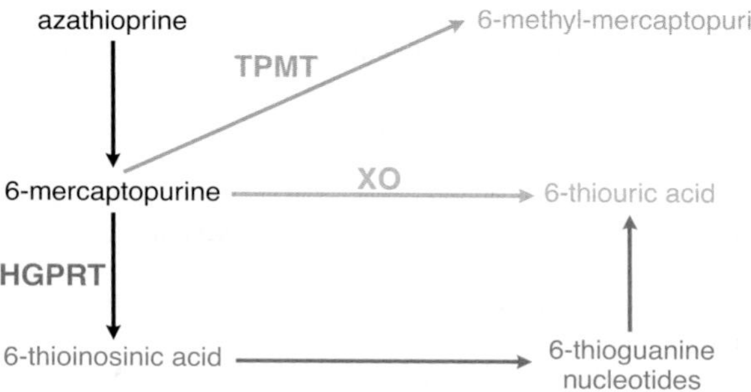

Figure 47–5. *Metabolism of azathioprine and 6-mercaptopurine.* HGPRT, hypoxanthine–guanine phosphoribosyl transferase; TPMT, thiopurine methyltransferase; XO, xanthine oxidase. The activities of these enzymes vary among humans because genetic polymorphisms are expressed differentially, explaining responses and side effects when azathioprine–mercaptopurine therapy is employed (see text for details).

The decision to initiate immunosuppressive therapy depends on an accurate assessment of the risk/benefit ratio. In general, physicians who treat IBD believe that the long-term risks of azathioprine–mercaptopurine are lower than those of steroids. Thus these purines are used in glucocorticoid-unresponsive or glucocorticoid-dependent disease and in patients who have had recurrent flares of disease requiring repeated courses of steroids. Additionally, patients who have not responded adequately to mesalamine but are not acutely ill may benefit by conversion from glucocorticoids to immunosuppressive drugs. Immunosuppressives therefore may be viewed as steroid-sparing agents.

Adverse effects of azathioprine–mercaptopurine can be divided into three general categories: idiosyncratic, dose related, and possible. Although the therapeutic effects of azathioprine–mercaptopurine often are delayed, their adverse effects occur at any time after initiation of treatment and can affect up to 10% of patients. The most serious idiosyncratic reaction is pancreatitis, which affects ~5% of patients treated with these drugs. Fever, rash, and arthralgias are seen occasionally, whereas nausea and vomiting are somewhat more frequent. The major dose-related adverse effect is bone marrow suppression, and circulating blood counts should be monitored closely when therapy is initiated and at less frequent intervals during maintenance therapy (e.g., every 3 months). Elevations in liver function tests also may be dose related. Although keeping drug levels in the appropriate range diminishes these adverse effects, they can occur even with therapeutic serum levels of 6-thioguanine nucleotides. The serious adverse effect of cholestatic hepatitis is relatively rare. Although the increased risk of infection is a significant concern with immunosuppressives, especially if pancytopenia occurs, infections are linked more closely to concomitant glucocorticoid therapy than to the immunosuppressives (Aberra et al., 2003).

Immunosuppressive regimens given in the setting of cancer chemotherapy or organ transplants have been associated with an increased incidence of malignancy, particularly non-Hodgkin's lymphoma. Definitive conclusions about the causative roles of azathioprine–mercaptopurine in lymphomas are complicated by the possible increased incidence of lymphomas in IBD per se and by the relative rarity of these cancers. The increased risk, if any, must be relatively small.

Metabolism and Pharmacogenetics. Favorable responses to azathioprine–mercaptopurine are seen in up to two-thirds of patients. Recent insights into the metabolism of the thiopurine agents and appreciation of genetic polymorphisms in these pathways have provided new insights into variability in response rates and adverse effects. As shown in Figure 47–4, mercaptopurine has three metabolic fates:

- conversion by xanthine oxidase to 6-thiouric acid
- metabolism by thiopurine methyltransferase (TPMT) to 6-methyl-mercaptopurine (6-MMP)
- conversion by hypoxanthine–guanine phosphoribosyl transferase (HGPRT) to 6-thioguanine nucleotides and other metabolites

The relative activities of these different pathways may explain, in part, individual variations in efficacy and adverse effects of these immunosuppressives.

The plasma $t_{1/2}$ of mercaptopurine is limited by its relatively rapid (i.e., within 1-2 hours) uptake into erythrocytes and other tissues. Following this uptake, differences in TPMT activity determine the drug's fate. Approximately 80% of the U.S. population has what is considered "normal" metabolism, whereas 1 in 300 individuals has minimal TPMT activity. In the latter setting, mercaptopurine metabolism is shifted away from 6-methyl-mercaptopurine and driven toward 6-thioguanine nucleotides, which can severely suppress the bone marrow. About 10% of people have intermediate TPMT activity; given a similar dose, these individuals will tend to have higher 6-thioguanine levels than the normal metabolizers. Finally, ~10% of the population is considered rapid metabolizers. In these individuals, mercaptopurine is shunted away from 6-thioguanine nucleotides toward 6-MMP, which has been associated with abnormal liver function tests. In addition, relative to normal metabolizers, the 6-thioguanine levels of these rapid metabolizers are lower for an equivalent oral dose, possibly reducing therapeutic response. Given this variability, some experts evaluate an individual's TPMT activity status prior to initiating treatment with thiopurines and also measure 6-thioguanine/6-MMP levels in individuals not responding to therapy. To avoid these complexities, treatment with 6-thioguanine was explored; unfortunately, 6-thioguanine is associated with a high incidence of an uncommon liver abnormality, hepatic nodular regeneration, and associated portal hypertension; 6-thioguanine therapy of IBD therefore has been abandoned.

Xanthine oxidase in the small intestine and liver converts mercaptopurine to thiouric acid, which is inactive as an immunosuppressant. Inhibition of xanthine oxidase by allopurinol diverts mercaptopurine to more active metabolites such as 6-thioguanine and increases both immunosuppressant and potential toxic effects. Thus, patients on mercaptopurine should be warned about potentially serious interactions with medications used to treat gout or hyperuricemia, and the dose should be decreased to 25% of the standard dose in subjects who are already taking allopurinol.

Methotrexate

Methotrexate was engineered to inhibit dihydrofolate reductase, thereby blocking DNA synthesis and causing cell death. First used in cancer treatment, methotrexate subsequently was recognized to have beneficial effects in autoimmune diseases such as rheumatoid arthritis and psoriasis (Chapter 62 discusses the use of methotrexate in dermatological disorders). The anti-inflammatory effects of methotrexate may involve mechanisms in addition to inhibition of dihydrofolate reductase.

As with azathioprine–mercaptopurine, methotrexate generally is reserved for patients whose IBD is either steroid-resistant or steroid-dependent. In Crohn's disease, it both induces and maintains remission, generally with a more rapid response than that seen with mercaptopurine or azathioprine (Feagan et al., 1995). Its use in ulcerative colitis has not been thoroughly investigated.

Therapy of IBD with methotrexate differs somewhat from its use in other autoimmune diseases. Most important, higher doses (e.g., 15-25 mg/week) are given parenterally. The increased efficacy with parenteral administration may reflect the unpredictable intestinal absorption at higher doses of methotrexate. For unknown reasons, the incidence of methotrexate-induced hepatic fibrosis in patients with IBD is lower than that seen in patients with psoriasis. Use of methotrexate for treatment of IBD has largely been supplanted by biological therapies (such as anti-TNFα antibodies).

Cyclosporine

The calcineurin inhibitor cyclosporine is a potent immunomodulator used most frequently after organ transplantation (Chapter 35). It is effective in specific clinical settings in IBD, but the high frequency of significant adverse effects limits its use as a first-line medication.

Cyclosporine is effective in patients with severe ulcerative colitis who have failed to respond adequately to glucocorticoid therapy. Between 50% and 80% of these severely ill patients improve significantly (generally within 7 days) in response to intravenous cyclosporine (2-4 mg/kg per day), sometimes avoiding emergent colectomy. Careful monitoring of cyclosporine levels is necessary to maintain a therapeutic level in whole blood between 300 and 400 ng/mL.

Oral cyclosporine is less effective as maintenance therapy in Crohn's disease, perhaps because of its limited intestinal absorption. In this setting, long-term therapy with NEORAL or GENGRAF (formulations of cyclosporine with increased oral bioavailability) may be more effective, but this has not been studied fully. The calcineurin inhibitors can be used to treat fistulous complications of Crohn's disease. A significant rapid response to intravenous cyclosporine has been observed; however, frequent relapses accompany oral cyclosporine therapy, and other medical strategies are required to maintain fistula closure. Thus, the calcineurin inhibitors generally are used to treat specific problems over a short term while providing a bridge to longer-term therapy (Sandborn, 1995).

Other immunomodulators that are being evaluated in IBD include the calcineurin inhibitor tacrolimus (FK 506, PROGRAF), mycophenolate mofetil and mycophenolate (CELLCEPT, MYFORTIC), inhibitors of inosine monophosphate dehydrogenase to which lymphocytes are especially susceptible (Chapter 35).

BIOLOGICAL THERAPIES

Infliximab (REMICADE, cA2) is a chimeric immunoglobulin (25% mouse, 75% human) that binds to and neutralizes TNFα. Although many, both pro- and anti-inflammatory cytokines, are generated in the inflamed gut in IBD (Figure 47–1), there is some rationale for targeting TNF-α because it is one of the principal cytokines mediating the T_H1 immune response characteristic of Crohn's disease (Targan et al., 1997).

Although infliximab was designed specifically to target TNFα, it may have more complex actions. Infliximab binds membrane-bound TNFα and may cause lysis of these cells by antibody-dependent or cell-mediated cytotoxicity. Thus, infliximab may deplete specific populations of subepithelial inflammatory cells. These effects, together with its mean terminal plasma $t_{1/2}$ of 8-10 days, may explain the prolonged clinical effects of infliximab.

Infliximab (5 mg/kg infused intravenously at intervals of several weeks to months) decreases the frequency of acute flares in approximately two-thirds of patients with moderate to severe Crohn's disease and also facilitates the closing of enterocutaneous fistulas associated with Crohn's disease (Present et al., 1999). Its longer-term role in Crohn's disease is evolving, but emerging evidence supports its efficacy in maintaining remission (Rutgeerts et al., 2004) and in preventing recurrence of fistulas (Sands et al., 2004). The combination of infliximab and azathioprine is more effective than infliximab alone in induction of remission and mucosal healing in steroid-resistant patients (Rutgeerts et al., 2009). In contrast, there appears to be no synergistic benefit of the combination of methotrexate and infliximab. Infliximab has also proven to be an effective treatment for refractory ulcerative colitis (Rutgeerts et al., 2009).

The use of infliximab as a biological response modifier raises several important considerations. Both acute (fever, chills, urticaria, or even anaphylaxis) and subacute (serum sickness–like) reactions may develop after infliximab infusion, but a frank lupus-like syndrome occurs only rarely. Antibodies to infliximab can decrease its clinical efficacy. Each year, at least 10% of patients on infliximab have to stop therapy because of loss of response or intolerance (Rutgeerts et al., 2009). Strategies to minimize the development of these antibodies (e.g., treatment with glucocorticoids or other immunosuppressives) may be critical to preserving infliximab efficacy for either recurrent or chronic therapy (Farrell et al., 2003). Other proposed strategies to overcome the problem of "antibody resistance" include increasing the dose of infliximab or decreasing the interval between infusions.

Infliximab therapy is associated with increased incidence of respiratory infections; of particular concern is potential reactivation of tuberculosis or other granulomatous infections with subsequent dissemination. The FDA recommends that candidates for infliximab therapy be tested for latent tuberculosis with purified protein derivative, and patients who test positive should be treated prophylactically with isoniazid. However, anergy with a false-negative skin test has been noted in some patients with Crohn's disease, and some experts routinely perform chest radiographs to look for active or latent pulmonary disease. Infliximab also is contraindicated in patients with severe congestive heart failure (New York Heart Association classes III and IV) and should be used cautiously in class I or II patients. As with the immunosuppressives, there is concern about the possible increased incidence of non-Hodgkin's lymphoma, but a causal role has not been established. Finally, the significant cost of biological therapies such as infliximab is an important consideration.

Adalimumab (HUMIRA) is a humanized recombinant human IgG_1 monoclonal antibody against TNFα. It is effective in inducing remission in mild to moderate, severe, and fistulizing Crohn's disease (Rutgeerts et al., 2009). Unfortunately, adalimumab cannot be used to rescue patients who have lost responsiveness to another anti-TNFα antibody, such as infliximab. Certolizumab pegol (CIMZIA) is a pegylated humanized fragment antigen binding (Fab) that binds TNFα. It is approved in the U.S. for the treatment of Crohn's disease. It appears to have comparable efficacy to that of adalimumab and infliximab for the treatment of Crohn's disease, although direct comparative studies have not been performed (Rutgeerts et al., 2009). With both adalimumab and certolizumab pegol, immunogenicity appears to be less of a problem than that associated with infliximab.

Another anti-TNFα agent, Etanercept (ENBREL), is a fusion protein of the ligand-binding portion of the TNFα receptor and the Fc portion of human IgG_1. This construct binds to TNFα and blocks its biologic effects but is ineffective in Crohn's disease.

Natalizumab (TYSABRI) is a humanized monoclonal antibody against α4-integrin (also known as VLA-4). Binding of the antibody to this adhesion molecule will reduce extravasation of certain leukocytes (e.g., lymphocytes), preventing them from migrating to sites of inflammation where they may exacerbate tissue injury. In 2008, natalizumab was approved in the U.S. for induction and maintenance of remission of moderate to severe Crohn's disease. Natalizumab had previously been withdrawn from the market and carries a black box warning because it appears to interact with other immune-modulating drugs to increase the risk of progressive multifocal leukoencephalopathy (PML). Thus, natalizumab is contraindicated for use with other immunomodulators. Because of the capacity of corticosteroids to produce immunosuppression, patients taking natalizumab for the treatment of Crohn's disease should have their doses reduced before starting natalizumab treatment.

The role of anti-TNF therapies for steroid-refractory or steroid-dependent ulcerative colitis is less clear. The rationale for their use is based on finding elevated levels of TNFα in the mucosa of patients. Large controlled clinical trials have demonstrated that anti-TNF agents significantly reduce the severity of the inflammation. The rates of clinical remission range from 26-34%, with endoscopic healing in about half the treated patients. Unlike Crohn's disease, ulcerative colitis is cured with surgery; thus the cost and serious adverse events associated with anti-TNF therapy need to be balanced with the effectiveness of the drug at preventing the need for colectomy. Currently, it is not known how effective anti-TNF therapies are for prevention, as opposed to delay, of colectomy.

ANTIBIOTICS AND PROBIOTICS

An emerging concept is that a balance in the GI tract normally exists among the mucosal epithelium, the normal gut flora, and the immune response (Preidis & Versalovic, 2009). Moreover, there are experimental and clinical data that colonic bacteria may either initiate or perpetuate the inflammation of IBD (Salzmann and Bevins, 2008), and, as mentioned earlier ("Pathogenesis of Inflammatory Bowel Disease"), recent studies have implicated specific bacterial antigens in the pathogenesis of Crohn's disease. Thus, certain bacterial strains may be either pro- (e.g., *Bacteroides*) or anti-inflammatory (e.g., *Lactobacillus*), prompting attempts to manipulate the colonic flora in patients with IBD. Traditionally, antibiotics have been used to this end, most prominently in Crohn's disease. More recently, probiotics have been used to treat specific clinical situations in IBD.

Antibiotics can be used as:

- adjunctive treatment along with other medications for active IBD
- treatment for a specific complication of Crohn's disease
- prophylaxis for recurrence in postoperative Crohn's disease

Metronidazole (Sutherland et al., 1991), ciprofloxacin (Arnold et al., 2002), and clarithromycin are the antibiotics used most frequently. They are more beneficial in Crohn's disease involving the colon than in disease restricted to the ileum. Specific Crohn's disease-related complications that may benefit from antibiotic therapy include intra-abdominal abscess and inflammatory masses, perianal disease (including fistulas and perirectal abscesses), small-bowel bacterial overgrowth secondary to partial small-bowel obstruction, secondary infections with organisms such as *C. difficile*, and post-operative complications. Metronidazole may be particularly effective for the treatment of perianal disease. Post-operatively, metronidazole and related compounds have been shown to delay the recurrence of Crohn's disease. In one study, a 3-month course of metronidazole (20 mg/kg per day) prolonged the time to both endoscopic and clinical recurrence (Rutgeerts et al., 1995). The significant side effects of prolonged systemic antibiotic use must be balanced against their potential benefits, and definitive data to support their routine use are lacking.

Probiotics are mixtures of putatively beneficial lyophilized bacteria given orally. Several studies have provided evidence for beneficial effects of probiotics in ulcerative colitis and pouchitis (Hedin et al., 2007). However, the studies have involved relatively small numbers of patients and the various studies had different end points. Thus, the utility of probiotics as a primary therapy for IBD remains unclear.

SUPPORTIVE THERAPY IN INFLAMMATORY BOWEL DISEASE

Analgesic, anticholinergic, and antidiarrheal agents play supportive roles in reducing symptoms and improving quality of life. These drugs should be individualized based on a patient's symptoms and are supplementary to anti-inflammatory medications. Oral iron, folate, and vitamin B_{12} should be administered as indicated. Loperamide or diphenoxylate (Chapter 46) can be used to reduce the frequency of bowel movements and relieve rectal urgency in patients with mild disease; these agents are contraindicated in patients with severe disease because they may predispose to the development of toxic megacolon. Cholestyramine can be used to prevent bile salt–induced colonic secretion in patients who have undergone limited ileocolic resections. Anticholinergic agents (dicyclomine hydrochloride, etc.; Chapter 9) are used to reduce abdominal cramps, pain, and rectal urgency. As with the antidiarrheal agents, they are contraindicated in severe disease or when obstruction is suspected. Care should be taken to differentiate exacerbation of IBD from symptoms that may be related to coexistent functional bowel disease (Chapter 46).

THERAPY OF INFLAMMATORY BOWEL DISEASE DURING PREGNANCY

IBD is a chronic disease that affects women in their reproductive years; thus, the issue of pregnancy often has a significant impact on medical management. The effects of IBD on pregnancy and the effects of pregnancy on IBD are beyond the scope of this chapter. In general, decreased disease activity increases fertility and improves pregnancy outcomes. At the same time, limiting medication during pregnancy is always desired but sometimes conflicts with the goal of controlling the disease.

Mesalamine and glucocorticoids are FDA Category B drugs that are used frequently in pregnancy and generally are considered safe, whereas methotrexate is clearly contraindicated in pregnant patients. The use of thiopurine immunosuppressives is more controversial. Because these medications are given long term, both their initiation and discontinuation are major management decisions. Although there are no controlled trials of these medications in pregnancy, considerable experience has emerged over the last several years. There does not appear to be an increase in adverse outcomes in pregnant patients maintained on thiopurine-based immunosuppressives (Francella et al., 2003). Nonetheless, decisions regarding the use of these medications in patients contemplating pregnancy are complex and necessarily must involve consideration of the risks and benefits involved.

CLINICAL SUMMARY

The treatment of IBD in any given patient may have several different goals, such as relief of symptoms, induction of remission in patients with active disease, prevention of relapse (i.e., maintenance therapy), healing of fistulas, and avoidance of emergent surgery. Further, therapy may be tailored to some extent to the severity and location of disease. Acute exacerbations of ulcerative colitis are treated with colonic-release preparations of 5-ASA and, in most patients with significant inflammation, with glucocorticoids. For milder cases involving only the rectum, these drugs may be given topically (by enema). Maintenance therapy for patients with ulcerative colitis is principally in the form of 5-ASA compounds, which generally are effective and safe. In patients who relapse on these preparations, purine metabolites (e.g., azathioprine–mercaptopurine) may be used. Other approaches being tested in this setting include the use of probiotic bacteria.

Drugs used in mild to moderately active Crohn's disease include sulfasalazine, budesonide, and oral corticosteroids. In contrast to their use in ulcerative colitis, the role of 5-ASA preparations in maintenance therapy of Crohn's disease is limited. Patients who relapse frequently may be treated with immunosuppressive agents (azathioprine–mercaptopurine or methotrexate). Glucocorticoid-dependent patients may be treated with long-term budesonide. Infliximab is particularly useful in closing fistulas associated with Crohn's disease; increasingly, along with other biological agents, it is used in acute flares of this condition. The efficacy of the biological agents in maintaining patients in remission must be balanced against the risk of adverse effects. Antibiotics, particularly metronidazole, may be useful adjuncts for the acute treatment of complications associated with Crohn's disease (including perianal disease) but are not established as a routine therapy in this disorder.

BIBLIOGRAPHY

Aberra FN, Lewis JD, Hass D, *et al*. Corticosteroids and immuno-modulators: postoperative infectious complication risk in inflammatory bowel disease. *Gastroenterology*, **2003,** *125*:320–327.

Arnold GL, Beaves MR, Pryjdun VO, Mook WJ. Preliminary study of ciprofloxacin in active Crohn's disease. *Inflamm Bowel Dis,* **2002,** *8*:10–15.

Camma C, Giunta M, Rosselli M, Cotton M. Mesalamine in the maintenance treatment of Crohn's disease: A meta-analysis adjusted for confounding variables. *Gastroenterology*, **1997,** *113*:1465–1473.

Cho JH. The genetics and immunopathogenesis of inflammatory bowel disease. *Nature Rev Immunol,* **2008,** *8*:458-466.

Dalwadi H, Wei B, Kronenberg M, *et al.* The Crohn's disease–associated bacterial protein I2 is a novel enteric T-cell superantigen. *Immunity,* **2001,** *15*:149–158.

Farrell RJ, Alsahli M, Jeen YT, *et al.* Intravenous hydrocortisone premedication reduces antibodies to infliximab in Crohn's disease: A randomized, controlled trial. *Gastroenterology,* **2003,** *124*:917–924.

Farrell RJ, Murphy A, Long A, *et al.* High multidrug resistance (P-glycoprotein 170) expression in inflammatory bowel disease patients who fail medical therapy. *Gastroenterology,* **2000,** *118*:279–288.

Faubion WA Jr, Loftus EV, Harmsen WS, *et al.* The natural history of corticosteroid therapy for inflammatory bowel disease: A population-based study. *Gastroenterology,* **2001,** *121*:255–260.

Feagan BG, Rochon J, Fedorak RN, *et al.* Methotrexate for the treatment of Crohn's disease. *N Engl J Med,* **1995,** *332*:292–297.

Francella A, Dyan A, Bodian C, *et al.* The safety of 6-mercaptopurine for childbearing patients with inflammatory bowel disease: A retrospective cohort study. *Gastroenterology,* **2003,** *124*:9–17.

Greenberg GR, Feagan BR, Martin, F, *et al.* Oral budesonide for active Crohn's disease. *N Engl J Med,* **1994,** *331*:836–841.

Hedin C, Whelan K, Lindsay JO. Evidence for the use of probiotics and prebiotics in inflammatory bowel disease: A review of clinical trials. *Proc Nutr Soc,* **2007,** *66*:307–315.

Hofer KN. Oral budesonide in management of Crohn's disease. *Ann Pharmacother,* **2003,** *37*:1457–1464.

Hugot JP, Chamaillard M, Zouali H, *et al.* Association of NOD2 leucine-rich repeat variants with susceptibility to Crohn's disease. *Nature,* **2001,** *411*:599–603.

Lodes MJ, Cong Y, Elson CO, *et al.* Bacterial flagellin is a dominant antigen in Crohn's disease. *J Clin Invest,* **2004,** *113*:1296–1306.

McKeage K, Goa KL. Budesonide (ENTOCORT EC capsules). *Drugs,* **2002,** *62*:2263–2282.

Ogura Y, Bonen DK, Inohara N, *et al.* A frameshift mutation in *NOD2* associated with susceptibility to Crohn's disease. *Nature,* **2001,** *411*:603–606.

Prantera C, Cottone M, Pallone F, *et al*. Mesalamine in the treatment of mild to moderate active Crohn's ileitis: Results of a randomized, multicenter trial. *Gastroenterology,* **1999,** *116*:521–526.

Prefontaine E, Macdonald JK, Sutherland LR. Azathioprine or 6-mercaptopurine for induction of remission in Crohn's disease. *Cochrane Database Syst Rev,* **2009,** CD000545.

Preidis GA, Versalovic J. Targeting the human microbiome with antibiotics, probiotics, and prebiotics: Gastroenterology enters the metagenomics era. *Gastroenterology,* **2009,** *136*: 2015–2031.

Present DH, Rutgeerts P, Targan S, *et al*. Infliximab for the treatment of fistulas in patients with Crohn's disease. *N Engl J Med,* **1999,** *340*:1398–1405.

Rutgeerts P, Vermeire S, Van Assche G. Biological therapies for inflammatory bowel disease. *Gastroenterology,* **2009,** *136*: 1182–1197.

Rutgeerts P, Feagan BF, Lichtenstein GR, *et al*. Comparison of scheduled and episodic treatment strategies of infliximab in Crohn's disease. *Gastroenterology,* **2004,** *126*:402–413.

Rutgeerts P, Hiele M, Geboes K, *et al*. Controlled trial of metronidazole treatment for prevention of Crohn's recurrence after ileal resection. *Gastroenterology,* **1995,** *108*:1617–1621.

Salzmann NH, Bevins CL. Negative interactions with the microbiota: IBD. *Adv Exp Biol Med,* **2008,** *635*:67–78.

Sandborn WJ. A critical review of cyclosporine therapy in inflammatory bowel disease. *Inflamm Bowel Dis,* **1995,** *1*: 48–63.

Sands BE, Anderson, FH, Bernstein CN, *et al*. Infliximab maintenance therapy for fistulizing Crohn's disease. *N Engl J Med,* **2004,** *350*:876–885.

Steinhart AH, Ewe K, Griffiths AM, *et al.* Corticosteroids for maintenance of remission in Crohn's disease. *Cochrane Database Syst Rev,* **2003,** CD000301.

Strober W, Fuss I, Mannon P. The fundamental basis of inflammatory bowel disease. *J Clin Invest*, **2007,** *117*:514–521.

Sutherland L, Singleton J, Sessions J, *et al*. Double blind, placebo-controlled trial of metronidazole in Crohn's disease. *Gut,* **1991,** *32*:1071–1075.

Targan SR, Hanauer SB, van Deventer SJ, *et al*. A short-term study of chimeric monoclonal antibody cA2 to tumor necrosis factor alpha for Crohn's disease. *N Engl J Med,* **1997,** *337*: 1029–1035.

Xavier RJ, Podolsky DK. Unravelling the pathogenesis of inflammatory bowel disease. *Nature,* **2007,** *448*: 427–434.

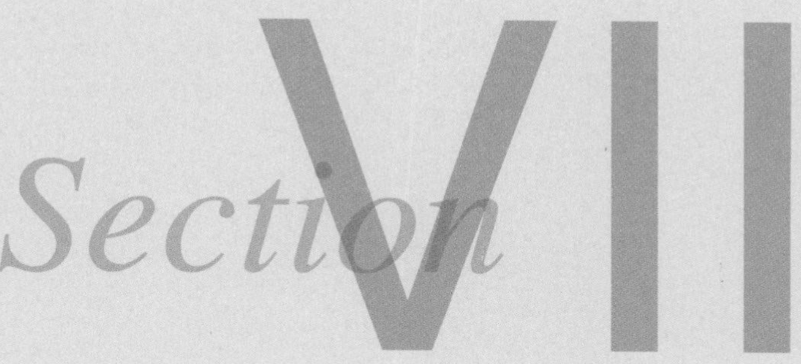

Chemotherapy of Microbial Diseases

General Principles of Antimicrobial Therapy

Tawanda Gumbo

SCIENTIFIC BASIS OF ANTIMICROBIAL CHEMOTHERAPY

An important revolution in human understanding of nature was the germ theory of disease based on the work of Louis Pasteur and Robert Koch, which linked specific microorganisms to specific diseases (Koch, 1876; Pasteur, 1861). Modern chemotherapy is predicated on this idea, radical in its time. The germ theory developed considerably in the 20th century, with identification and characterization of many microbial pathogens and their pathogenic mechanisms and the introduction of antimicrobial drugs. With the use of these drugs came issues of appropriate regimens, drug resistance, drug interactions, and toxicity.

Although the antimicrobials are a large group of diverse structures with myriad mechanisms of actions against bacteria, viruses, fungi, and parasites, we can, nonetheless, develop generalizations about important issues surrounding the use of antimicrobial agents. This chapter reviews the general classes of antimicrobial drugs, their mechanisms of action, mechanisms of resistance, and patterns of kill by different classes of the drugs. It also discusses principles for the selection of an appropriate antibiotic, dose, dose schedule, and type of antibiotic therapy. The pharmacological properties and uses of individual classes of antimicrobials are discussed in Chapters 49 through 59.

Classes and Actions of Antimicrobial Agents. Microorganisms of medical importance fall into four categories: bacteria, viruses, fungi, and parasites. The first broad classification of antibiotics follows this classification closely, so that we have (1) antibacterial, (2) antiviral, (3) antifungal, and (4) antiparasitic agents. Within each of these major categories, drugs are further categorized by their biochemical properties. Antimicrobial molecules should be viewed as ligands whose receptors are microbial proteins. The term *pharmacophore,* first introduced by Ehrlich, defines that active chemical moiety of the drug that binds to the microbial receptor. The microbial proteins targeted by the antibiotic are essential components of biochemical reactions in the microbes, and interference with these physiological pathways kills the microorganisms. To the extent that an antimicrobial agent targets a protein that is not widely expressed in other bacteria, the drug will be relatively selective in its antimicrobial effect. The biochemical processes commonly inhibited include cell wall synthesis in bacteria and fungi, cell membrane synthesis, synthesis of 30s and 50s ribosomal subunits, nucleic acid metabolism, function of topoisomerases, viral proteases, viral integrases, viral envelope fusion proteins, folate synthesis in parasites, and parasitic chemical detoxification processes. Classification of an antibiotic is based on:

- the class and spectrum of microorganisms it kills
- the biochemical pathway it interferes with
- the chemical structure of its pharmacophore

Because antimicrobial agents are ligands that bind to their targets to produce effects, the relationship between drug concentration and effect on a population of organisms is still modeled using the standard Hill-type curve for receptor and agonist (Chapters 2 and 3), characterized by three parameters: the inhibitory concentration 50, or IC_{50} (also termed EC_{50}), a measure of the antimicrobial agent's potency; the maximal effect, E_{max}; and H, the slope of the curve, or Hill factor. In antimicrobial therapy, the relationship is often expressed as an inhibitory sigmoid E_{max} model, to take into account the control bacterial population without treatment (E_{con}) as a fourth parameter (Equation 48–1 and

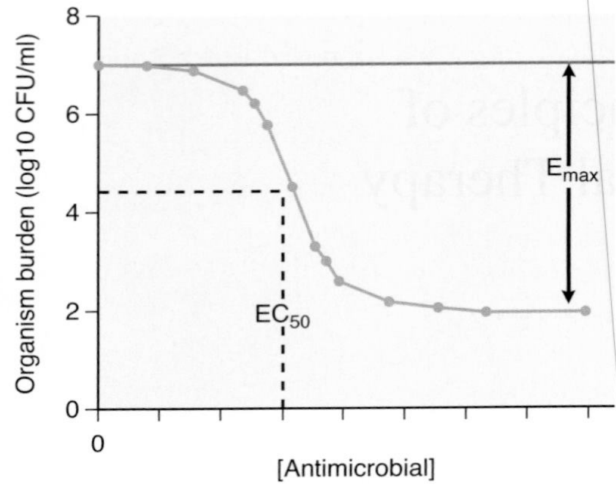

Figure 48–1. *Inhibitory sigmoid E_{max} curve.* CFU, colony-forming units.

Figure 48–1), where E is effect as measured by microbial burden.

$$E = E_{con} - E_{max} \times [IC]^H / ([IC]^H + [IC_{50}]^H)$$

(Equation 48–1)

THE PHARMACOKINETIC BASIS OF ANTIMICROBIAL THERAPY

Penetration of Antimicrobial Agents into Anatomic Compartments. In many infections, the pathogen causes disease not in the whole body, but in specific organs. Moreover, only specific pathological compartments may be infected within these organs. Antibiotics are often administered far away from these sites of infection. To be effective, each antibiotic has to get to where the pathogen is, to penetrate into the infected compartment. Therefore, in choosing an antimicrobial agent for therapy, a crucial consideration is whether the drug can penetrate to the site of infection.

For example, the antibiotic levofloxacin achieves skin tissue/plasma peak concentration ratio of 1.4, epithelial lining fluid to plasma ratio of 2.8, and urine to plasma ratios of 67 (Chow et al., 2002; Conte et al., 2006; Wagenlehner et al., 2006). In a clinical trial on patients treated with levofloxacin, the two most important factors in predicting successful clinical and microbiological outcomes in the patients were a sufficient maximal plasma concentration of the drug (C_{Pmax}), which needed to achieve a level of 12 times the minimum inhibitory concentration (MIC) (C_{Pmax}/MIC ≥12), and the site of infection. The failure rate of therapy was 0% in patients with urinary tract infections, 3% in patients with pulmonary infections, and 16% in patients with skin and soft tissue infections (Preston et al., 1998). Clearly, the poorer the penetration into the anatomical compartment, the higher the likelihood of failure.

The penetration of a drug into an anatomical compartment depends on the physical barriers that the molecule must traverse, the chemical properties of the drug, and the presence of multidrug transporters. The physical barriers are usually due to layers of epithelial and endothelial cells, and the type of junctions formed between these cells. Penetration across this physical barrier generally correlates with the octanol-water partition coefficient of the antimicrobial agent, a measure of the hydrophilicity or hydrophobicity of a chemical. Hydrophobic molecules get concentrated in the bi-lipid cell membrane bi-layer, whereas hydrophilic molecules tend to concentrate in the blood, the cytosol, and other aqueous compartments. Thus, the higher the octanol-water partition coefficient (P), the greater the likelihood that an antimicrobial agent will cross physical barriers erected by layers of cells. Conversely, the more charged a molecule is, and the larger it is, the poorer its penetration across membranes and other physical barriers (see Figure 2–3).

Another barrier is due to membrane transporters, which actively export drugs from the cellular or tissue compartment back into the blood (Chapter 5). A well-known example is the P-glycoprotein. Although the octanol-water partition coefficient would favor lipophilic molecules to transverse across cell barriers, P-glycoprotein exports structurally unrelated amphiphilic and lipophilic molecules of 3-4 kDa, reducing their effective penetration. Examples of antimicrobial agents that are P-glycoprotein substrates include HIV protease inhibitors, the antiparasitic agent ivermectin, the antibacterial agent telithromycin, and the antifungal agent itraconazole.

The central nervous system (CNS) is guarded by the blood-brain barrier. The movement of antibiotics across the blood-brain barrier is restricted by tight junctions that connect endothelial cells of cerebral microvessels to one another in the brain parenchyma, as well as by protein transporters (Miller et al., 2008). Antimicrobial agents that are polar at physiological pH generally penetrate poorly; some, such as *penicillin G*, are actively transported out of the cerebrospinal fluid (CSF) and achieve CSF concentrations of only 0.5-5% of that achieved in plasma. However, the integrity of the blood-brain barrier is diminished during active bacterial infection; tight junctions in cerebral capillaries open, leading to a marked increase in the penetration of even polar drugs (Quagliarello and Scheld, 1997). As the infection is eradicated and the inflammatory reaction subsides, penetration diminishes to normal. Because this may occur while viable microorganisms persist in the CSF, drug dosage should not be reduced as the patient improves.

Drug penetration into the eye is especially pertinent in the treatment of endophthalmitis (infection and inflammation of ocular cavity and surrounding tissue) and infections of the retina. There is generally poor penetration of drug from plasma to this compartment, so that the standard therapy is direct instillation of antibiotics into the ocular cavity. In fungal endophthalmitis, however, systemic administration of amphotericin B and triazole is recommended (Pappas et al., 2009) because these agents, especially the triazoles, have sufficient penetration ratios into the vitreous space.

In patients with pulmonary infections such as pneumonia, drugs must penetrate into the epithelial lining fluid, where the pathogens are found. Among antibacterial agents, many β-lactam antibiotics have poor epithelial lining fluid-to-plasma ratios (0.1-0.4:1); macrolides have ratios of 2-40:1, fluoroquinolones have ratios ≥1:1; pyrazinamide has ratios of ~20:1; isoniazid, >1:1; and linezolid, 2.4-4.2:1 (Kiem and Schentag, 2008).

Other important compartments requiring special drug penetration are endocardial vegetations and the biofilm formed by bacteria and fungi on prosthetic devices such as artificial heart valves, long-dwelling intravascular catheters, artificial hips, and devices for internal fixation of bone fractures. Bacterial and fungal biofilms are colonies of slowly growing cells that are enclosed within an exopolymer matrix. The exopolysaccharide is negatively charged, which restricts positively charged antibiotics from reaching their target. This physical barrier restricts the diffusion of antimicrobial molecules and sometimes binds them (Lewis, 2001). To be effective against infections in these compartments, antibiotics have to be able to penetrate the biofilm and endothelial barriers.

Pharmacokinetic Compartments. Once an antibiotic has penetrated to the site of infection, it may be subjected to processes of elimination and distribution that differ from those in the blood. These sites where the concentration-time profiles differ from each other are considered separate pharmacokinetic compartments, thus, the human body is viewed as multicompartmental. The concentration of antibiotic within each compartment is assumed to be homogeneous. If two compartments have similar concentration profiles, then they may be considered a single compartment. Antibiotic concentrations can be analyzed using any number of such compartments, with the best number of compartments chosen based on the least number of compartments that can adequately explain the findings. The model is also defined as *open* or *not open;* an open model is one in which the drug is eliminated out of the body from the compartment (e.g., kidneys). The order of the process must also be specified (Chapter 2): a first-order process is directly correlated to concentration of drug D, or $[D]^1$, as opposed to zero order, which is independent of [D] and reflects a process that is saturated at ambient levels of D (such as the elimination of ethanol; Chapter 23).

Suppose a patient has pneumonia with the pathogen in the lung epithelial lining fluid (ELF). The patient ingests an antibiotic that is absorbed via the GI tract (*g*) into blood or central compartment (compartment 1), as a first-order input. In this process, the transfer constant from the GI tract to central compartment is termed the *absorption constant* and is designated k_a. The antibiotic in the central compartment is then delivered to the lungs where it penetrates into the ELF (compartment 2). However, it also penetrates into other tissues of the body peripheral to the site of infection, termed the *peripheral compartment* (compartment 3). Thus, we have four compartments (including *g*), each with its own concentration-time profile, as shown in Figure 48–2. The penetration of drug from compartment 1 to 2 is based on the penetration factors discussed earlier and is defined by the transfer constant k_{12}. However, the drug also redistributes from compartment 2 back to 1, defined by transfer constant k_{21}. A similar process between the blood and peripheral tissues leads to transfer constants k_{13} and k_{31}. The drug may also be lost from the body (i.e., open system) via the lungs and other peripheral tissues (e.g., kidneys or liver) at a rate proportional to the concentration.

Antibiotic concentrations within each compartment change with time. The changes in the amount of antibiotic in each compartment with time are described using standard differential equations (Gibaldi and Perrier, 1975). If X is the amount of antibiotic in a compartment, SCL the drug clearance, and V_c the volume of central compartment, then equations for absorption compartment (Equation 48–2), central compartment (Equation 48–3), site of infection or compartment 2 (Equation 48–4), and peripheral compartment (Equation 48–5) are as follows:

$$dX_g/dt = -K_a \cdot X_g \qquad \text{(Equation 48–2)}$$

$$dX_1/dt = K_a \cdot X_g - [(SCL/V_c) + K_{12} + K_{13}] \cdot X_1 + K_{21} \cdot X_2 + K_{31} \cdot X_3 \qquad \text{(Equation 48–3)}$$

$$dX_2/dt = K_{12} \cdot X_1 - K_{21} \cdot X_2 \qquad \text{(Equation 48–4)}$$

$$dX_3/dt = K_{13} \cdot X_3 - K_{31} \cdot X_3 \qquad \text{(Equation 48–5)}$$

Such models have been used in conjunction with population pharmacokinetics to describe and model a plethora of antimicrobials used to treat bacteria, fungi, viruses, and parasites (Hope et al., 2007; Tarning et al., 2008; Wilkins et al., 2008; Zhou et al., 1999).

In recent years, semi-mechanistic models have related pathogen response to drug concentrations within these pharmacokinetic compartments in preclinical disease models and in patients (Gumbo et al., 2006; Jumbe et al., 2003; Neumann et al., 1998; Pukrittayakamee et al., 2003; Talal et al., 2006). Pathogens within one or more of these compartments are exposed to dynamic drug concentrations within the compartments, as described by Equations 48–2 to 48–5. A pathogen population (N) may be described as consisting of at least two subpopulations, drug-susceptible (N_S) and drug-resistant (N_R) organisms. The organisms are either killed,

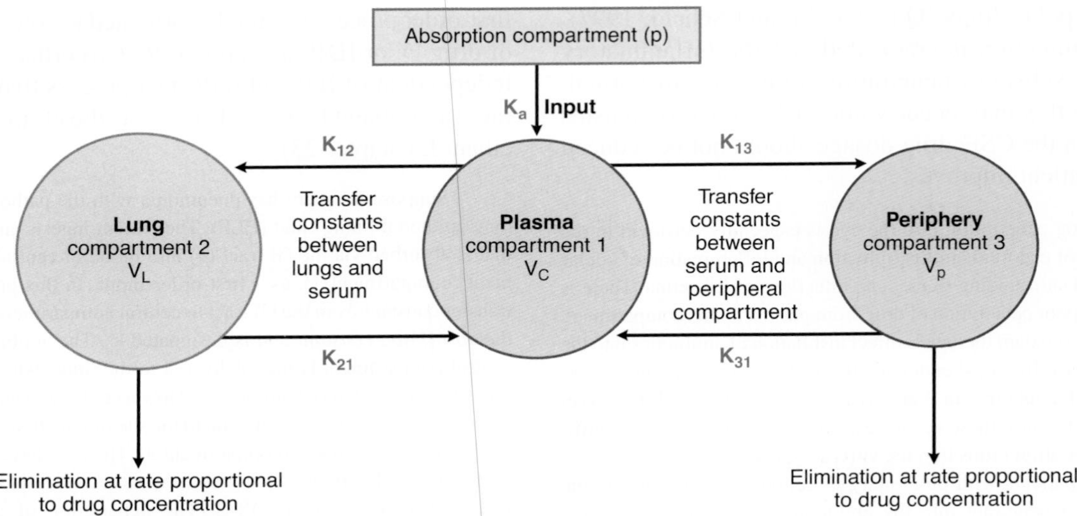

Figure 48–2. *Diagrammatic depiction of a multi-compartment model.*

inhibited, or continued to grow in response to the antibiotic concentration. For some pathogens such as fungi and bacteria, it is assumed they are in logarithmic growth phase in the absence of drug, exhibiting an exponential density-limited growth rate so that they will reach a stationary phase at a maximal pathogen density, POPMAX. E is a logistic carrying function, so that

$$E = 1 - (N/POPMAX) \quad \text{(Equation 48–6)}$$

where N is the pathogen burden in a particular compartment. For replications rates of parasites and viruses, unique models may be specified. The drug will affect the growth rate either independent of kill or via killing the pathogen. The drug effect that is independent of kill is through a saturable Michaelis-Menten-type kinetic event (L).

$$L = (X_1/V_c)^H/[(X_1/V_c)^H + IC_{50}{}^H], \text{ where } H = H_{g\text{-}s} \text{ or } H_{g\text{-}r} \quad \text{(Equation 48–7)}$$

where H and IC_{50} are as described in Equation 48–1. Microbial kill is based on the concentrations within the compartment, and is modeled as a sigmoid E_{max} effect model M:

$$M = K_{kmax} *(X_1/V_c)^H/[(X_1/V_c)^H + IC_{50}{}^H], \text{ where } H = H_{k\text{-}s} \text{ or } H_{k\text{-}r} \quad \text{(Equation 48–8)}$$

where K_{kmax} is the maximal kill rate. Because the microbial density (N) is in fact a balance between growth (maximal growth rate = K_{gmax}) and microbial kill, the change in pathogen density as a function of time is described by Equation 48–9:

$$dN/dt = K_{gmax} \cdot N \cdot E - K_{kmax} \cdot M \cdot N \quad \text{(Equation 48–9)}$$

The changes in drug-susceptible subpopulation of pathogen with time and the drug-resistant subpopulation are described by:

$$dN_S/dt = K_{gmax\text{-}S} \cdot (1 - Ls) \cdot N_S \cdot E - K_{kmax\text{-}S} \cdot Ms \cdot N_S \quad \text{(Equation 48–10)}$$

$$dN_R/dt = K_{gmax\text{-}R} \cdot (1 - L_R) \cdot N_R \cdot E - K_{kmax\text{-}R} \cdot M_R \cdot NR \quad \text{(Equation 48–11)}$$

This can be made more complex and predictive adding parameters describing the effect of inoculum, delay in microbial effect, or splitting the drug-resistant population to smaller subpopulations based on molecular mechanism of resistance (Bulitta et al., 2009).

Population Pharmacokinetics and Variability in Drug Response. The framework for the models central to population pharmacokinetics evolved from a series of publications by Lewis Sheiner (Sheiner et al., 1977). What are population pharmacokinetics? Consider a simple example. When multiple patients are treated with the same dose of a drug, each patient will achieve pharmacokinetic parameters that differ from others. This is termed *between-patient variability*. Even when the same dose is administered to the same patient on two separate occasions, the patient may achieve a different concentration-time profile of the drug between the two occasions. This is termed *inter-occasion or within-patient variability*. The variability is reflected at the level of the compartmental pharmacokinetic parameters such as k_a, k_{12}, k_{21}, SCL, V_c, and so on. Even when a recommended dose is administered, the drug may fail to reach a therapeutic concentration in some patients. In other patients, the drug may reach high and toxic concentrations. Such variability could be due to factors that can be explained, such as genetic variability. In addition, anthropometric measures such as weight, height, and age also lead to variability. Furthermore, patients may have comorbid conditions such as renal and liver dysfunction, which may lead to variability. Drug interactions are an important source of variability with potentially dangerous consequences. These interactions usually occur when one drug inhibits or induces uptake or clearance mechanisms affecting another drug (i.e., modulation of the activities of xenobiotic metabolic enzymes, drug transporters, and excretion mechanisms; Chapters 5 and 6).

Even when such factors are accounted for, there remains residual variability due to computational noise, assay variability, and unexplainable factors. The common practice of using an "average" value of data or "naive pooling," has implications of smoothing out data and failing to recognize subgroups of patients at risk for therapeutic failure or increased toxicity of antibiotic. Thus the variability itself, the extent of such variability, and any factors that may explain part of the variability of drug response are more important to understand than measures of central tendency and dispersion for a hypothetical average patient. Such variability reflects the fact that pathogens within patients given the same dose of antibiotic will be exposed to different antibiotic concentrations from patient to patient, leading to effective kill in some and resistance emergence in others. Knowledge of covariates associated with pharmacokinetic variability leads to better dose adjustments, or switching therapy from one antibiotic to another, or changing concomitant medications.

IMPACT OF SUSCEPTIBILITY TESTING ON SUCCESS OF ANTIMICROBIAL AGENTS

The microbiology laboratory plays a central role in the decision to choose a particular antimicrobial agent over others. First, identification and isolation of the culprit organism takes place when the patients' specimens are sent to the microbiology laboratory. Once the microbial species causing the disease has been identified, a rational choice of the class of antibiotics likely to work in the patient can be made. The microbiology laboratory then plays a second role, which is to perform susceptibility testing. This step is crucial in narrowing down the list of possible antimicrobials that could be used.

Millions of individuals across the globe get infected by many different isolates of the same species of pathogen. Evolutionary processes cause each isolate to be slightly different from the next, so that each will have a unique susceptibility to antimicrobial agents. As the microorganisms divide within the patient, they may undergo further evolution between the time of infection and when the disease is diagnosed. As an example, a relatively narrow range of variants are transmitted when patients become infected with HIV. However, HIV replication has poor fidelity and has replication rates that result in up to 10^{10} viral particles each day. Moreover, viral recombination occurs commonly. Over many months, under immune pressure, numerous variants arise. The emergence of a quasi species that harbors a mutation associated with drug resistance to at least one drug is high, based on probability factors in the context of high replication rates and the massive numbers of viral particles. Therefore, we expect that there will be a wide distribution of concentrations of antimicrobial agents that can kill pathogens. Often, this distribution is Gaussian, with a skew that depends on where the patient lives. These factors will affect the shape of the inhibitory sigmoid E_{max} model curve described by Equation 48–1.

With changes in susceptibility, the sigmoid E_{max} curve shifts in one of two basic ways. The first is a shift to the right, an increase in IC_{50}, as shown in Figure 48–3A. This means that much higher concentrations than before are now needed to show specific effect. Susceptibility tests for bacteria, fungi, parasites, and viruses have been developed to determine whether these shifts have occurred at a sufficient magnitude to warrant higher doses of drug to achieve particular effect. The change in IC_{50} may become so large that it is not possible to overcome the concentration deficit by increasing the antimicrobial dose without causing toxicity to the patient. At that stage, the organism is now "resistant" to the particular antibiotic. A second possible change in the curve is decrease in E_{max} (Figure 48–3B), such that increasing the dose of the antimicrobial agent beyond a certain point will achieve no further effect; i.e., changes in the microbe are such that eradication of the microbe by the particular drug can never be achieved. This occurs because the available target proteins have been reduced or the microbe has developed an alternative pathway to overcome the biochemical inhibition. As an example, maraviroc is an allosteric, noncompetitive antagonist that binds to the CCR5 receptor of patient's CD4 cells to deny HIV entry into the cell. Viral resistance occurs by a mechanism that involves HIV adapting to use of the maraviroc-bound CCR5, which results in decrease of E_{max} in phenotypic susceptibility assays (Hirsch et al., 2008).

Bacteria. For bacteria, dilution tests employ antibiotics in serially diluted concentrations on solid agar or in

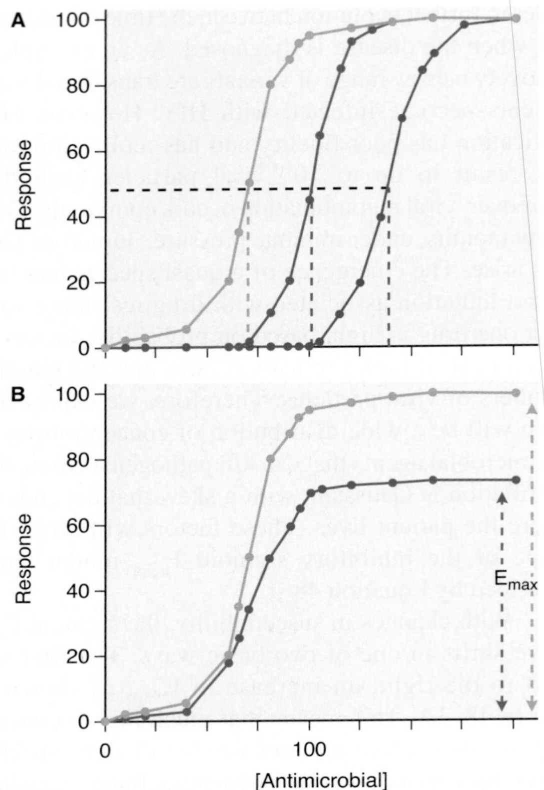

Figure 48–3. *Changes in sigmoid E_{max} model with increases in drug resistance.* Increase in resistance may show changes in IC_{50} (**panel A:** the IC_{50} increases from 70 (orange line) to 100 (green line), to 140 (blue line)) or decrease in E_{max} (**panel B**: efficacy decreases from full response (orange line) to 70% (green line))

broth medium that contains a culture of the test microorganism. The lowest concentration of the agent that prevents visible growth after 18-24 hours of incubation is known as the *minimum inhibitory concentration* (MIC).

Automated systems also use a broth-dilution method. The optical density of a broth culture of the clinical isolate incubated in the presence of drug is determined. If the density of the culture exceeds a threshold optical density, then growth has occurred at that concentration of drug. The MIC is the concentration at which the optical density remains below the threshold.

The disk-diffusion technique provides only qualitative or semi-quantitative information on antimicrobial susceptibility. The test is performed by applying commercially available filter-paper disks impregnated with a specific amount of the drug onto an agar surface, over which a culture of the microorganism has been streaked. After 18-24 hours of incubation, the size of the clear zone of inhibition around the disk is measured. The diameter of the zone depends on the activity of the drug against the test strain. Standardized values for zone sizes for each bacterial species and antibiotic permit classification of the clinical isolate as either resistant or susceptible. A variant of the disk diffusion tests is the Epsilometer test, or E-test. A rectangular test strip impregnated with changing concentrations of antimicrobial agent, usually across 15 dilutions, is placed on an agar plate that has a heavy inoculum of test organism. The drug concentrations are printed along this long test strip. The cultures are then incubated under favorable conditions for 24 hours, 48 hours, or 5 days, depending on the test organism. There is no growth with higher concentrations and heavy microbial growth where there is lower drug concentration, so that a clear elliptical zone is formed that bisects the test strip at the MIC. This test has the virtue of determining an actual MIC value, rather than the dichotomous categorization of "susceptible" or "resistant." There are test strips for hundreds of antibacterial agents as well as for some antifungal agents active against Candida species.

Sometimes, a biochemical or immunological reaction that leads to a color change is used to detect susceptibility. As an example, methicillin resistance in *Staphylococcus aureus* (methicillin-resistant *S. aureus,* or MRSA) occurs because of acquisition of a low-affinity penicillin-binding protein 2' (2a), or PBP2' (PBP2a). The PBP2' is extracted from isolates of the MRSA, and supernatant mixed with a latex reagent with monoclonal antibody against PBP2'. Visible clumping within 3 minutes indicates presence of PBP2', indicating MRSA.

Fungi. For fungi that are yeasts (i.e., Candida), susceptibility testing methods are similar to those used for bacteria. However, the definitions of MIC differ based on drug and the type of yeast, so there are cutoff points of 50% decrease in turbidity compared to controls at 24 hours, or 80% at 48 hours, or total clearance of the turbidity. Susceptibility tests and MICs for triazoles have been extensively shown to correlate with clinical outcomes.

Standardized tests for echinocandin antifungals and amphotericin B-based compounds are available. However, the correlation of these tests with clinical outcomes is still weak. Susceptibility tests for molds have also been developed, but the clinical correlations are still being examined. Different terminology from MICs has been adopted when evaluating echinocandins against molds because the fungal burden can not be measured by counting discrete cells in molds, given that hyphae will break up into unpredictable numbers of discrete fungi when under antifungal pressure. Furthermore, echinocandins often do not completely inhibit mold growth, but instead cause damage reflected by morphological changes in hyphae. Thus, the minimum effective concentration (MEC) for echinocandins is the lowest drug concentration at which short, stubby, and highly branched hyphae are observed on microscopic examination.

Viruses. In HIV phenotypic assays, the patient's HIV-RNA is extracted from plasma, and genes for targets of antiretroviral drugs such as reverse transcriptase and protease are amplified. The genes are then inserted into a standard HIV vector that lacks analogous gene sequences to produce a recombinant virus, which is co-incubated with drug of interest in a mammalian cell

enzyme (Harshey and Ramakrishnan, 1976; Wehrli et al., 1968). The PAE of the rifampin is long and concentration dependent (Gumbo et al., 2007a). This means that administering combined doses on a more intermittent basis (i.e., once a day) will maximize effect for these drugs. Toxicity generated by intermittent dosing may preclude such use for some drugs such as rifampin, whereas for others (i.e., aminoglycosides) such infrequent dosing may actually decrease toxicity.

There is a third group of drugs for which dosing schedule has no effect on efficacy, but where it is the cumulative dose that matters. Thus, it is more the total concentration (AUC) to MIC ratio that matters and not the time that concentration persists above a certain threshold. Antibacterial agents such as daptomycin fall into this class (Louie et al., 2001). These agents also have a good PAE. The AUC/IC_{50} explains why the nucleoside analogue reverse transcriptase inhibitors tenofovir and emtricitabine have been combined into one pill, administered once a day for the treatment of AIDS.

The shape of concentration-time curve that optimizes resistance suppression is often different from that which optimizes microbial kill. In many instances, the drug exposure associated with resistance suppression is much higher than for optimal kill. It should actually be this higher exposure that should be achieved by each dose in patients for optimal effect, rather than the EC_{80} as discussed earlier. However, this is often precluded by increased drug toxicity when doses are increased. Second, although the relationship between kill and exposure is based on the inhibitory sigmoid E_{max} model, experimental work with preclinical models demonstrates that this model does not apply to resistance suppression (Gumbo, 2007b; Tam et al., 2007).

The optimal dose should be designed to achieve a high probability of exceeding the EC_{80} microbial PK/PD index, or index associated with suppression of resistance, given the population pharmacokinetic variability and the MIC distribution of clinical microbe isolates. The population pharmacokinetic variability enables integration of pharmacogenetics, anthropometric measures, and residual variability into the decision to choose optimal dose (Gumbo, 2008). Once that has been achieved, the dose schedule is chosen according to whether efficacy is driven by AUC/MIC (or AUC/EC_{95}), C_{Pmax}/MIC, or T > MIC. Duration of therapy is then chosen, based on best available evidence.

TYPES AND GOALS OF ANTIMICROBIAL THERAPY

When an infection occurs, the numbers of microorganisms are often small in the beginning. Pathogen burden eventually increases with replication of the organism. Sometimes, the immune system manages to eliminate the infection before it causes any further damage. In other instances, the organism is not entirely eliminated but hides inside the patient's own cells and become dormant, only to reactivate when immune function is compromised in the future. In some patients, the organism may overcome immune defenses and then cause disease. In a subset of such patients, the disease is self-limited. For example, many viral upper respiratory infections are self-limited and should not be treated with antimicrobial agents. Other diseases, however, require antimicrobial therapy. In these patients, therapy should be discontinued after resolution of disease. In special cases where the immune or anatomical defect that led to the infection is still present, suppressive or "maintenance" therapy may be required. A useful way to organize the types and goals of antimicrobial therapy is to consider where along the disease progression timetable therapy is initiated (Figure 48–5); therapy can be prophylactic, preemptive, empirical, definitive, or suppressive.

Prophylactic Therapy. Prophylaxis involves treating patients who are not yet infected or have not yet developed disease. The goal of prophylaxis is to prevent infection in some patients or to prevent development of a potentially dangerous disease in those who already have evidence of infection. Ideally, a single, effective, nontoxic drug is successful in preventing infection by a specific microorganism or eradicating an early infection. The main principle behind prophylaxis is targeted therapy. However, prophylaxis to prevent

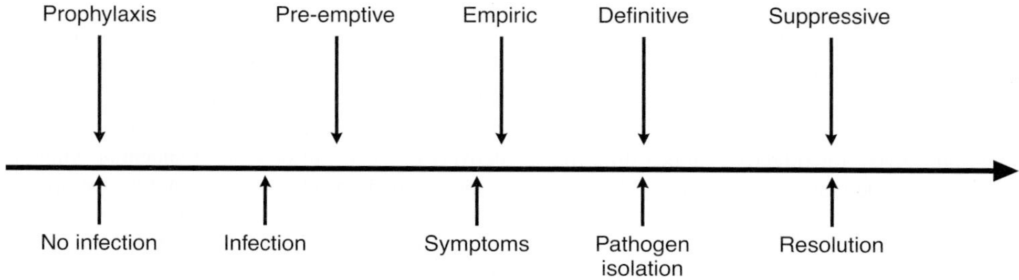

Figure 48–5. *Aantimicrobial therapy-disease progression timeline.* Stages of disease progression are below the horizontal arrow; categories of antimicrobial therapy are above the arrow.

colonization or infection by any or all microorganisms present in the environment of a patient often fails.

Prophylaxis is used in immunosuppressed patients such as those with HIV-AIDS or are post-transplantation and on anti-rejection medications. The efficacy of prophylaxis in these patients is based on excellent evidence (Anonymous, 2000; DHHS Panel on Guidelines for the Prevention and Treatment of Opportunistic Infections in HIV-Infected Adults and Adolescents, 2008). In these groups of patients, specific antiparasitic, antibacterial, antiviral, and antifungal therapy is administered based on the well-defined pattern of pathogens that are major causes of morbidity during immunosuppression. A risk-benefit analysis is used to determine choice and duration of prophylaxis. Prophylaxis of opportunistic infections in patients with AIDS is started when the CD4 count falls below 200 cells per mm^3. In post-transplant patients, prophylaxis depends on time since the transplant procedure, which is related to intensity of use and type of immunosuppressive therapy. Prophylaxis should be discontinued in patients who are doing well at certain time points, such as 1 year post-transplant. In AIDS patients, prophylaxis is discontinued when the CD4 count climbs above 200 cells/mm^3. Infections for which prophylaxis is given include *Pneumocystis jiroveci, Mycobacterium avium-intracellulare, Toxoplasma gondii, Candida* species, *Aspergillus* species, *Cytomegalovirus,* and other Herpesviridae. In general, lower doses of prophylactic agent are given compared to when the same drug is used for treatment.

Chemoprophylaxis is also used to prevent wound infections after various surgical procedures. Wound infection results when a critical number of bacteria are present in the wound at the time of closure. Antimicrobial agents directed against the invading microorganisms may reduce the number of viable bacteria below the critical level and thus prevent infection. Several factors are important for the effective and judicious use of antibiotics for surgical prophylaxis. First, antimicrobial activity must be present at the wound site at the time of its closure. Thus, infusion of the first antimicrobial dose should begin within 60 minutes before surgical incision and should be discontinued within 24 hours of the end of surgery (Bratzler and Houck, 2004). Second, the antibiotic must be active against the most likely contaminating microorganisms for that type of surgery. A number of studies indicate that chemoprophylaxis can be justified in dirty or contaminated surgical procedures (e.g., resection of the colon), where the incidence of wound infections is high. These include <10% of all surgical procedures. In clean surgical procedures, which account for ~75% of the total, the expected incidence of wound infection is <5%, and antibiotics should not be used routinely. When the surgery involves insertion of a prosthetic implant (e.g., prosthetic valve, vascular graft, prosthetic joint), cardiac surgery, or neurosurgical procedures, the complications of infection are so drastic that most authorities currently agree to chemoprophylaxis for these indications.

Patients at the highest risk for infective endocarditis for which prophylaxis is recommended fall into four groups (Wilson et al., 2007):

- those with a prosthetic material used for heart valve repair or replacement
- previous infective endocarditis
- congenital heart disease such as unrepaired cyanotic heart disease, or within 6 months of repair of the heart disease with prosthetic material, or those with residual defects adjacent to prosthetic material
- postcardiac transplant patients with heart valve defects

Chemoprophylaxis is reasonable in these patients when undergoing dental procedures if there is manipulation of gingival tissue or periapical region of teeth, or perforation of oral mucosa, but not for other dental procedures. Recommended therapy is a single dose of oral amoxicillin 30 minutes to 1 hour before the procedure or intravenous ampicillin or ceftriaxone in those unable to take oral medication. A macrolide or clindamycin may be administered for patients who are allergic to β-lactam agents. Therapy may be administered no more than 2 hours after the procedure for patients who failed to receive the prophylaxis prior to the procedure (Wilson et al., 2007). Prophylaxis is also reasonable for procedures that will involve infected skin and soft tissues as well as infected respiratory tract, but not in routine genitourinary and GI tract procedures. If the organism causing the infection is known, then the prophylactic antibiotic for patients undergoing these procedures should be tailored toward that particular organism.

Prophylaxis may be used to protect healthy persons from acquisition of or invasion by specific microorganisms to which they are exposed. This is termed *post-exposure prophylaxis.* Successful examples of this practice include rifampin administration to prevent meningococcal meningitis in people who are in close contact with a case, prevention of gonorrhea or syphilis after contact with an infected person, and macrolides after contact with confirmed cases of pertussis. Post-exposure prophylaxis is recommended in those patients inadvertently exposed to HIV infection. Currently, combination therapy from one of the classes of antiretrovirals, nucleoside reverse transcriptase inhibitors, nucleotide reverse transcriptase inhibitors, non-nucleoside reverse transcriptase inhibitors, protease inhibitors, and fusion inhibitors is administered for 4 weeks (Panlilio et al., 2005). For influenza, the neuraminidase inhibitor oseltamivir has been recommended for prevention of influenza A and B in healthy adults and children with close contact of laboratory-confirmed cases (Hayden and Pavia, 2006).

Mother-to-child transmission of HIV and syphilis are important public health problems for which specific chemotherapeutic regimens have been devised, based on locality. Anti-retroviral therapy is administered for HIV prophylaxis during the pregnancy and peripartum periods. Prophylactic therapy for syphilis during pregnancy is effective in reducing neonatal death and infant neurological, auditory, and bone malformations.

Pre-emptive therapy. Pre-emptive therapy is used as a substitute for universal prophylaxis and as early targeted therapy in high-risk patients who already have a laboratory or other test indicating that an asymptomatic patient has become infected. The principle is that delivery of therapy prior to development of symptoms (presymptomatic) aborts impending disease, and the therapy is for a short and defined duration (Singh, 2001). This has been applied in the clinic to therapy for cytomegalovirus (CMV) after both hematopoietic stem cell transplants and after solid organ transplantation. It is unclear whether this method is superior to keeping all at-risk patients on ganciclovir. Recent evidence in liver transplant patients suggest this approach may be as efficacious as universal prophylaxis while using far less antiviral medications (Gerna et al., 2008; Singh et al., 2008).

Empirical Therapy in the Symptomatic Patient. Once a patient is symptomatic, should the patient be treated immediately? The first consideration in selecting an antimicrobial is to determine if the drug is indicated. *The reflex action to associate fever with treatable infections and prescribe antimicrobial therapy without further evaluation is irrational and potentially dangerous.*

The diagnosis may be masked if therapy is started and appropriate cultures are not obtained. Antimicrobial agents are potentially toxic and may promote selection of resistant microorganisms. For some diseases, the cost of waiting a few days is low. These patients can wait for microbiological evidence of infection without empirical treatment. In a second group of patients, the risks of waiting are high, based either on the patient's immune status or other known risk factors for poor outcome with therapy delay. Initiation of optimal empirical antimicrobial therapy should rely on the clinical presentation, which may suggest the specific microorganism, and knowledge of the microorganisms most likely to cause specific infections in a given host. In addition, simple and rapid laboratory techniques are available for the examination of infected tissues.

The most valuable and time-tested method for immediate identification of bacteria is examination of the infected secretion or body fluid with Gram stain. In malaria-endemic areas, or in travelers returning from such an area, a simple thick and thin blood smear may mean the difference between a patient's receiving appropriate therapy and surviving or death while on wrong therapy for presumed bacterial infection. Such tests help to narrow the list of potential pathogens and permit more rational selection of initial antibiotic therapy. Similarly, neutropenic patients with fever have high risks of mortality, and, when febrile, they are presumed to have either a bacterial or fungal infection; thus a broad-spectrum combination of antibacterial and antifungal agents that cover common infections encountered in granulocytopenic patients are given. Performance of cultures is still mandatory with a view to modify antimicrobial therapy with culture results.

Definitive Therapy with Known Pathogen. Once a pathogen has been isolated and susceptibilities results are available, therapy should be streamlined to a narrow targeted antibiotic. Monotherapy is preferred to decrease the risk of antimicrobial toxicity and selection of antimicrobial-resistant pathogens. Proper antimicrobial doses and dose schedules are crucial to maximizing efficacy and minimizing toxicity. In addition, the duration of therapy should be as short as is necessary. The practice of keeping a patient indefinitely on antimicrobial therapy without a particular reason is discouraged. In fact, both experimental and clinical evidence have shown that unnecessarily prolonged therapies lead to the emergence of resistance.

Combination therapy is an exception, rather than a rule. Once a pathogen has been isolated, there should be no reason to use multiple antibiotics, except when evidence overwhelmingly suggests otherwise. Using two antimicrobial agents where one is required leads to increased toxicity and unnecessary damage to the patient's otherwise protective fungal and bacterial flora. This is true, even when intuition suggests use of two agents. As an example, Cosgrove and colleagues recently demonstrated increased nephrotoxicity of low-dose gentamicin administered only for 4 days as "synergistic therapy" with vancomycin or an antistaphylococcal penicillin for *S. aureus* bacteremia and endocarditis, without improving efficacy (Cosgrove et al., 2009).

However, there are special circumstances where evidence is unequivocal in favor of combination therapy. The principles behind such antimicrobial use include:

- preventing resistance to monotherapy
- accelerating the rapidity of microbial kill
- enhancing therapeutic efficacy by use of synergistic interactions or enhancing kill by a drug based on a mutation generated by resistance to another drug
- paradoxically, reducing toxicity (i.e., when full efficacy of a standard antibacterial agent can only be achieved at doses that are toxic to the patient, and a second drug is co-administered to exert additive effects)

Clinical situations for which combination therapy is advised are discussed in the relevant chapters but include antiretroviral therapy for AIDS, antiviral therapy for hepatitis B and C, the treatment of tuberculosis, *Mycobacterium avium-intracellulare* and leprosy, fixed-dose combinations of antimalarial drugs, the treatment of *Cryptococcus neoformans* with flucytosine and amphotericin B, during empirical therapy for patients with febrile neutropenia, and advanced AIDS with fever. The combination of a sulfonamide and an inhibitor of dihydrofolate reductase, such as trimethoprim, is synergistic owing to the blocking of sequential steps in microbial folate synthesis. A fixed combination of sulfamethoxazole and trimethoprim is active against organisms that may be resistant to sulfonamides alone, is effective for many infections, and is rarely given as its separate components.

Post-treatment suppressive therapy. In some patients, after the initial disease is controlled by the antimicrobial agent, therapy is continued at a lower dose. This is because in these patients the infection is not completely eradicated and the immunological or anatomical defect that led to the original infection is still present. This is common in AIDS patients and post-transplant patients, for example. The goal is more as secondary prophylaxis. Nevertheless, risks of toxicity from long durations of the therapy are still real. In this group of patients, the suppressive therapy is eventually discontinued if the patient's immune system improves.

MECHANISMS OF RESISTANCE TO ANTIMICROBIAL AGENTS

Antimicrobial agents were viewed as miracle cures when first introduced into clinical practice. However, it became evident rather soon after the discovery of penicillin that resistance developed quickly, terminating the miracle. This serious development is ever present with each new antimicrobial agent and threatens the end of the antimicrobial era. Today, every major class of antibiotic is associated with the emergence of significant resistance. *Two major factors are associated with emergence of antibiotic resistance: evolution and clinical/environmental practices*. A species that is subjected to pressure, chemical or otherwise, that threatens its extinction often evolves mechanisms to survive under that stress. Pathogens will evolve to develop resistance to the chemical warfare to which we subject them. This evolution is mostly aided by poor therapeutic practices by healthcare workers, as well as indiscriminant use of antibiotics for agricultural and animal husbandry purposes. Poor clinical practices that fail to incorporate the pharmacological properties of antimicrobials amplify the speed of development of drug resistance.

Antimicrobial resistance can develop at any one or more of steps in the processes by which a drug reaches and combines with its target. Thus, resistance development may develop due to:

- reduced entry of antibiotic into pathogen
- enhanced export of antibiotic by efflux pumps
- release of microbial enzymes that destroy the antibiotic
- alteration of microbial proteins that transform pro-drugs to the effective moieties
- alteration of target proteins
- development of alternative pathways to those inhibited by the antibiotic

Mechanisms by which such resistance develops can include acquisition of genetic elements that code for the resistant mechanism, mutations that develop under antibiotic pressure, or constitutive induction.

Resistance Due to Reduced Entry of Drug into Pathogen. The outer membrane of gram-negative bacteria is a permeable barrier that excludes large polar molecules from entering the cell. Small polar molecules, including many antibiotics, enter the cell through protein channels called *porins*. Absence of, mutation in, or loss of a favored porin channel can slow the rate of drug entry into a cell or prevent entry altogether, effectively reducing drug concentration at the target site. If the target is intracellular and the drug requires active transport across the cell membrane, a mutation or phenotypic change that slows or abolishes this transport mechanism can confer resistance. As an example, *Trypanosoma brucei* is treated with suramin and pentamidine during early stages, but with melarsoprol and eflornithine when CNS disease (sleeping sickness) is present. Melarsoprol is actively taken up by trypanosome P2 protein transporter. When the parasite either lacks the P2 transporter, or has a mutant form, resistance to melarsoprol and cross resistance to pentamidine occur due to reduced uptake (Ouellette, 2001).

Resistance Due to Drug Efflux. Microorganisms can overexpress efflux pumps and then expel antibiotics to which the microbes would otherwise be susceptible. There are five major systems of efflux pumps that are relevant to antimicrobial agents:

- the multidrug and toxic compound extruder (MATE)
- the major facilitator superfamily (MFS) transporters
- the small multidrug resistance (SMR) system
- the resistance nodulation division (RND) exporters
- ATP binding cassette (ABC) transporters

Efflux pumps are a prominent mechanism of resistance for parasites, bacteria, and fungi. One of the tragic consequences of resistance emergence has been the development of drug resistance by *Plasmodium falciparum*. Drug resistance to most antimalarial drugs, specifically chloroquine, quinine, mefloquine, halofantrine, lumefantrine, and the artemether-lumefantrine combination is mediated by an ABC transporter encoded by *Plasmodium falciparum* multidrug resistance gene 1 (Pf*mdr1*) (Happi et al., 2009). Point mutations in the Pf*mdr1* gene lead to drug resistance and failure of chemotherapy. Drug efflux sometimes works in tandem with chromosomal resistance, as is seen in *Streptococcus pneumoniae,* and perhaps, *Myobacterium tuberculosis*. In these situations, induction of efflux pumps occurs early, which increases the MIC only modestly. However, this MIC increase is enough to allow further microbial replication and an increased mutation frequency, which enable the development of resistance via more robust chromosomal mutations (Gumbo et al., 2007b; Jumbe et al., 2006).

Resistance Due to Destruction of Antibiotic. Drug inactivation is a common mechanism of drug resistance. Bacterial resistance to aminoglycosides and to β-lactam antibiotics usually is due to production of an aminoglycoside-modifying enzyme or β-lactamase, respectively.

Resistance Due to Reduced Affinity of Drug to Altered Target Structure. A common consequence of either single point or multiple point mutations is change in amino acid composition and conformation of target protein. This change leads to a reduced affinity of drug for its target, or of a prodrug for the enzyme that converts the prodrug to active drug. Such alterations may be due to mutation of the natural target (e.g., fluoroquinolone resistance), target modification (e.g., ribosomal protection type of resistance to macrolides and tetracyclines), or acquisition of a resistant form of the native, susceptible target (e.g., staphylococcal methicillin resistance caused by production of a low-affinity penicillin-binding protein) (Hooper, 2002; Lim and Strynadka, 2002; Nakajima, 1999). Similarly, in HIV resistance mutations associated with reduced affinity are encountered in protease inhibitors, integrase inhibitors, fusion inhibitors, and nonnucleoside reverse transcriptase inhibitors (Nijhuis et al., 2009). Similarly, benzimidazoles are used against myriad worms and protozoa and work by binding to the parasite's tubulin; point mutations in the β-tubulin gene lead to modification of the tubulin and drug resistance (Ouellette, 2001).

Incorporation of Drug. An uncommon situation occurs when an organism not only becomes resistant to an antimicrobial agent but subsequently starts requiring it for growth. Enterococcus, which easily develops vancomycin resistance, can, after prolonged exposure to the antibiotic, develop vancomycin-requiring strains.

Resistance Due to Enhanced Excision of Incorporated Drug. Nucleoside reverse transcriptase inhibitors such as zidovudine are 2′-deoxyribonucleoside analogs that are converted to their 5′-triphosphate form and compete with natural nucleotides. These drugs are incorporated into the viral DNA chain and cause chain termination. When resistance emerges via mutations at a variety of points in the reverse transcriptase gene, phosphorolytic excision of the incorporated chain-terminating nucleoside analog is enhanced (Arion et al., 1998).

Hetero-resistance and Viral Quasi Species. Hetero-resistance is said to be present when a subset of the total microbial population is resistant, despite the total population being considered susceptible on testing (Falagas et al., 2008; Rinder, 2001). In a way, this should not be a surprise given that chromosomal mutations are a stochastic process and there is a baseline mutation rate for each gene. Therefore, a subclone that has alterations in genes associated with drug resistance is expected to reflect the normal mutation rates and occur at between 10^{-6} and 10^{-5} colonies. In bacteria, hetero-resistance has been described especially for vancomycin in *S. aureus*, vancomycin in *Enterococcus faecium*, colistin in *Acinetobacter baumannii-calcoaceticus*, rifampin, isoniazid, and streptomycin in *M. tuberculosis,* and penicillin in *S. pneumoniae* (Falagas et al., 2008; Rinder, 2001). Increased therapeutic failures and mortality have been reported in patients with hetero-resistant staphylococci and *M. tuberculosis* (Falagas et al., 2008; Hofmann-Thiel et al., 2009). For fungi, hetero-resistance leading to clinical failure has been described for fluconazole in *Cryptococcus neoformans* and *Candida albicans* (Marr et al., 2001; Mondon et al., 1999).

Viral replication is more error prone than replication in bacteria and fungi. Viral evolution under drug and immune pressure occurs relatively easily, commonly resulting in variants or quasi species that may contain drug-resistant subpopulations. This is not often termed hetero-resistance, but the principle is the same as described for bacteria and fungi: A virus may be considered susceptible to a drug because either phenotypic or genotypic tests reveal "lack" of resistance, when there is a resistant subpopulation just below the limit of assay detection. These minority quasi species that are resistant to antiretroviral agents have been associated with failure of antiretroviral therapy (Metzner et al., 2009).

EVOLUTIONARY BASIS OF RESISTANCE EMERGENCE

Development of Resistance via Mutation Selection. Mutation and antibiotic selection of the resistant mutant are the molecular basis for resistance for many bacteria, viruses, and fungi. Mutations may occur in the gene encoding (1) the target protein, altering its structure so that it no longer binds the drug; (2) a protein involved in drug transport; (3) a protein important for drug activation or inactivation; or (4) in a regulatory gene or promoter affecting expression of the target, a transport protein, or an inactivating enzyme. Mutations are not caused by drug exposure per se. They are random events that confer a survival advantage when drug is present. Any large population of drug susceptible bacteria is likely to contain rare mutants that are only slightly less susceptible than the parent. However, suboptimal dosing strategies lead to selective kill of the more susceptible population, which leaves the resistant isolates to flourish.

In some instances, a single-step mutation results in a high degree of resistance. Examples include *M. tuberculosis katG* Ser315 mutations that cause resistance to isoniazid; the M814V mutation in the reverse transcriptase gene of HIV-1, causing resistance to lamivudine; a cytochrome-b gene mutation causing resistance to the antimalaria drug atovaquone; and *Candida albicans fks1* Ser645 mutations causing resistance to echinocandins.

In other circumstances, however, it is the sequential acquisition of more than one mutation that leads to clinically significant resistance. As an example, the combination of pyrimethamine and sulfadoxine inhibits *Plasmodium falciparum*'s folate biosynthetic pathway via inhibition of dihydrofolate reductase (DHFR) by the pyrimethamine and inhibition of dihydropteroate synthetase (DHPS) by sulfadoxine. Clinically meaningful resistance occurs when there is a single point mutation in the *DHPS* gene accompanied by at least a double mutation in the *DHFR* gene.

Hypermutable Phenotypes. The ability to protect genetic information from disintegrating and also to be flexible enough to allow genetic changes that lead to adaptation to the environment is essential to all living things. This is accomplished principally by the insertion of the correct base pair by DNA polymerase III, proofreading by the polymerase, and postreplicative repair. The development of a defect in one of these repair mechanisms leads to a high degree of mutations in many genes; such isolates are termed *mutator (Mut) phenotypes* and may include mutations in genes causing antibiotic resistance (Giraud et al., 2002). This second-order selection of hypermutable (mutator) alleles based on alterations in DNA repair genes has been implicated in the emergence of multidrug resistant strains of *M. tuberculosis* Beijing genotype (Rad et al., 2003).

Resistance by External Acquisition of Genetic Elements. Drug resistance may be acquired by mutation and selection, with passage of the trait *vertically* to daughter cells. For mutation and selection to be successful in generating resistance, the mutation cannot be lethal and should not appreciably alter virulence. For the trait to be passed on, the original mutant or its progeny also must disseminate and replicate; otherwise, the mutation will be lost until it is "rediscovered" by some other mutant arising from within a wild-type population.

Drug resistance more commonly is acquired by *horizontal transfer* of resistance determinants from a donor cell, often of another bacterial species, by transduction, transformation, or conjugation. Resistance acquired by horizontal transfer can disseminate rapidly and widely either by clonal spread of the resistant strain or by subsequent transfers to other susceptible recipient strains. Horizontal transfer of resistance offers several advantages over mutation selection. Lethal mutation of an essential gene is avoided; the level of resistance often is higher than that produced by mutation, which tends to yield incremental changes; the gene, which still can be transmitted vertically, can be mobilized and rapidly amplified within a population by transfer to susceptible cells; and the resistance gene can be eliminated when it no longer offers a selective advantage.

Horizontal Gene Transfer. Horizontal transfer of resistance genes is greatly facilitated by and is largely dependent on mobile genetic elements. Mobile genetic elements include plasmids and transducing phages. Other mobile elements—transposable elements, integrons, and gene cassettes—also participate in the process. *Transposable elements* are of three general types: insertion sequences, transposons, and transposable phages. Only insertion sequences and transposons are important for resistance.

Insertion sequences (Mahillon and Chandler, 1998) are short segments of DNA encoding enzymatic functions (e.g., transposase and resolvase) for site-specific recombination with inverted repeat sequences at either end. They can copy themselves and insert themselves into a chromosome or a plasmid. Insertion sequences do not encode resistance, but they function as sites for integration of other resistance-encoding elements (e.g., plasmids or transposons). *Transposons* are insertion sequences that also code for other functions, one of which can be drug resistance. Because transposons move between chromosome and plasmid, the resistance gene can "hitchhike" with a transferable element out of the host and into a recipient. Transposons are mobile elements that excise and integrate in the bacterial genomic or plasmid DNA (i.e., from plasmid to plasmid, from plasmid to chromosome, or from chromosome to plasmid). *Integrons* (Fluit and Schmitz, 2004) are not formally mobile and do not copy themselves, but they encode an integrase and provide a specific site into which mobile gene cassettes integrate. *Gene cassettes* encode resistance determinants, usually lacking a promoter, with a downstream repeat sequence. The integrase recognizes this repeat sequence and directs insertion of the cassette into position behind a strong promoter that is present on the integron. Integrons may be located within transposons or in plasmids, and therefore may be mobilizable, or located on the chromosome.

Transduction is acquisition of bacterial DNA from a phage (a virus that propagates in bacteria) that has incorporated DNA from a previous host bacterium within its outer protein coat. If the DNA includes a gene for drug resistance, the newly infected bacterial cell may acquire resistance. Transduction is particularly important in the transfer of antibiotic resistance among strains of *S. aureus*. *Transformation* is the uptake and incorporation into the host genome by homologous recombination of free DNA released into the environment by other bacterial cells. Transformation is the molecular basis of penicillin resistance in pneumococci and *Neisseria* (Spratt, 1994). *Conjugation*, as the name implies, is gene transfer by direct cell-to-cell contact through a sex pilus or bridge. This complex and fascinating mechanism for the spread of antibiotic resistance is extremely important because multiple resistance genes can be transferred in a single event. The transferable genetic material consists of two different sets of plasmid-encoded genes that may be on the same or different plasmids. One set encodes the actual resistance; the second encodes genes necessary for the bacterial conjugation process. Conjugation with genetic exchange between nonpathogenic and pathogenic microorganisms probably occurs in the GI tracts of humans and animals. The efficiency of transfer is low; however, antibiotics can exert a powerful selective pressure to allow emergence of the resistant strain. Genetic transfer by conjugation is common among gram-negative bacilli, and resistance is conferred on a susceptible cell as a single event. Enterococci also contain a broad range of host-range conjugative plasmids that are involved in the transfer and spread of resistance genes among gram-positive organisms.

CLINICAL SUMMARY

Antimicrobial agents work by targeting specific biochemical properties of pathogens, and therefore have a narrow spectrum of organisms that they can kill. Infection is usually in a particular anatomical compartment. Important determinants of success of antimicrobial therapy include proper selection of antimicrobial therapy based on microbiology results and susceptibility testing, knowledge of drug penetration into the infected compartment, and knowledge of compartmental pharmacokinetics. The proper dose and dosing schedule are chosen by integrating microbial pharmacokinetic-pharmacodynamic information, expected pharmacokinetic variability, and the minimum inhibitory concentration of the pathogen. The goals of therapy should be clear. Prophylaxis, pre-emptive therapy, empirical therapy, and definitive therapy should have treatment goals and duration of therapy clearly spelled out in the beginning, based on proper evidence. The general rule is monotherapy, except in select situations where combination therapy has been shown to be superior. Poor dosing strategies lead to catastrophic outcomes such as drug-resistant pathogens and untoward toxicity to the patients.

BIBLIOGRAPHY

Ambrose PG, Bhavnani SM, Rubino CM, *et al.* Pharmacokinetics-pharmacodynamics of antimicrobial therapy: It's not just for mice anymore. *Clin Infect Dis,* **2007,** *44:*79–86.

Andes D, van Ogtrop M. In vivo characterization of the pharmacodynamics of flucytosine in a neutropenic murine disseminated candidiasis model. *Antimicrob Agents Chemother,* **2000,** *44:*938–942.

Anonymous. Guidelines for preventing opportunistic infections among hematopoietic stem cell transplant recipients. *MMWR Recomm Rep,* **2000,** *49:*1–7.

Arion D, Kaushik N, McCormick S, *et al.* Phenotypic mechanism of HIV-1 resistance to 3′-azido-3′-deoxythymidine (AZT): Increased polymerization processivity and enhanced sensitivity to pyrophosphate of the mutant viral reverse transcriptase. *Biochemistry,* **1998,** *37:*15908–15917.

Bratzler DW, Houck PM. Antimicrobial prophylaxis for surgery: An advisory statement from the National Surgical Infection Prevention Project. *Clin Infect Dis*, **2004,** *38:* 1706–1715.

Bulitta JB, Ly NS, Yang JC, *et al.* Development and qualification of a pharmacodynamic model for the pronounced inoculum effect of ceftazidime against *Pseudomonas aeruginosa. Antimicrob Agents Chemother*, **2009,** *53:* 46–56.

Chow AT, Chen A, Lattime H, *et al.* Penetration of levofloxacin into skin tissue after oral administration of multiple 750 mg once-daily doses. *J Clin Pharm Ther,* **2002,** *27:*143–150.

Conte JE Jr, Golden JA, McIver M, Zurlinden E. Intrapulmonary pharmacokinetics and pharmacodynamics of high-dose levofloxacin in healthy volunteer subjects. *Int J Antimicrob Agents*, **2006,** *28:*114–121.

Cosgrove SE, Vigliani GA, Fowler VG Jr, *et al.* Initial low-dose gentamicin for *Staphylococcus aureus* bacteremia and endocarditis is nephrotoxic. *Clin Infect Dis,* **2009,** *48:*713–721.

Craig WA. Pharmacokinetic/pharmacodynamic parameters: Rationale for antibacterial dosing of mice and men. *Clin Infect Dis,* **1998,** *26:*1–10.

Craig WA. Pharmacodynamics of antimicrobials: General concepts and applications. In: *Antimicrobial Pharmacodynamics in Theory and Practice,* 2nd ed. (Nightangle CH, Ambrose PG, Drusano G.L, Murakawa T, eds.), Informa Healthcare USA, New York, **2007,** pp. 1–19.

Craig WA, Kunin CM. Significance of serum protein and tissue binding of antimicrobial agents. *Annu Rev Med,* **1976,** *27:* 287–300.

DHHS Panel on Guidelines for the Prevention and Treatment of Opportunistic Infections in HIV-Infected Adults and Adolescents. Guidelines for Prevention and Treatment of Opportunistic Infections in HIV-Infected Adults and Adolescents. Available at: http://aidsinfo.nih.gov/contentfiles/Adult_OI.pdf. Accessed February 15, 2009.

Eagle H, Fleishman R, Musselman AD. Effect of schedule of administration on the therapeutic efficacy of penicillin; importance of the aggregate time penicillin remains at effectively bactericidal levels. *Am J Med,* **1950,** *9:*280–299.

Falagas ME, Makris GC, Dimopoulos G, Matthaiou DK. Heteroresistance: A concern of increasing clinical significance? *Clin Microbiol Infect,* **2008,** *14:*101–104.

Fluit AC, Schmitz FJ. Resistance integrons and super-integrons. *Clin Microbiol Infect,* **2004,** *10:*272–288.

Gerna G, Lilleri D, Callegaro A, et al. Prophylaxis followed by preemptive therapy versus preemptive therapy for prevention of human cytomegalovirus disease in pediatric patients undergoing liver transplantation. *Transplantation,* **2008,** *86:*163–166.

Gibaldi M, Perrier D. *Pharmacokinetics,* Marcel Dekker, New York, **1975.**

Giraud A, Matic I, Radman M, *et al.* Mutator bacteria as a risk factor in treatment of infectious diseases. *Antimicrob Agents Chemother,* **2002,** *46:*863–865.

Gumbo T. Integrating pharmacokinetics, pharmacodynamics and pharmacogenomics to predict outcomes in antibacterial therapy. *Curr Opin Drug Discov Devel,* **2008,** *11:*32–42.

Gumbo T, Drusano GL, Liu W, et al. Anidulafungin pharmacokinetics and microbial response in neutropenic mice with disseminated candidiasis. *Antimicrob Agents Chemother,* **2006,** *50:*3695–3700.

Gumbo T, Louie A, Deziel MR, et al. Concentration-dependent *Mycobacterium tuberculosis* killing and prevention of resistance by rifampin. *Antimicrob Agents Chemother*, **2007a,** *51:* 3781–3788.

Gumbo T, Louie A, Liu W, et al. Isoniazid bactericidal activity and resistance emergence: Integrating pharmacodynamics and pharmacogenomics to predict efficacy in different ethnic populations. *Antimicrob Agents Chemother,* **2007b,** *51:* 2329–2336.

Hanna GJ, D'Aquila RT. Clinical use of genotypic and phenotypic drug resistance testing to monitor antiretroviral chemotherapy. *Clin Infect Dis,* **2001,** *32:*774–782.

Happi CT, Gbotosho GO, Folarin OA, et al. Selection of *Plasmodium falciparum* multidrug resistance gene 1 alleles in asexual stages and gametocytes by artemether-lumefantrine in Nigerian children with uncomplicated falciparum malaria. *Antimicrob Agents Chemother,* **2009,** *53:*888–895.

Harshey RM, Ramakrishnan T. Purification and properties of DNA-dependent RNA polymerase from *Mycobacterium tuberculosis* H37RV. *Biochim Biophys Acta,* **1976,** *432:*49–59.

Hayden FG, Pavia AT. Antiviral management of seasonal and pandemic influenza. *J Infect Dis*, **2006,** *194* (suppl 2)*:* S119–S126.

Hertogs K, de Bethune MP, Miller V, et al. A rapid method for simultaneous detection of phenotypic resistance to inhibitors of protease and reverse transcriptase in recombinant human immunodeficiency virus type 1 isolates from patients treated with antiretroviral drugs. *Antimicrob Agents Chemother,* **1998,** *42:*269–276.

Hirsch MS, Gunthard HF, Schapiro JM, et al. Antiretroviral drug resistance testing in adult HIV-1 infection: 2008 recommendations of an International AIDS Society-USA panel. *Clin Infect Dis,* **2008,** *47:*266–285.

Hofmann-Thiel S, van Ingen J, Feldmann K, et al. Mechanisms of heteroresistance to isoniazid and rifampin of *Mycobacterium tuberculosis* in Tashkent, Uzbekistan. *Eur Respir J*, **2009,** *33:*368–374.

Hooper DC. Fluoroquinolone resistance among Gram-positive cocci. *Lancet Infect Dis,* **2002,** *2:*530–538.

Hope WW, Seibel NL, Schwartz CL, et al. Population pharmacokinetics of micafungin in pediatric patients and implications for antifungal dosing. *Antimicrob Agents Chemother,* **2007,** *51:*3714–3719.

Jumbe N, Louie A, Leary R, *et al.* Application of a mathematical model to prevent in vivo amplification of antibiotic-resistant bacterial populations during therapy. *J Clin Invest*, **2003,** *112:*275–285.

Jumbe NL, Louie A, Miller MH, *et al.* Quinolone efflux pumps play a central role in emergence of fluoroquinolone resistance in *Streptococcus pneumoniae*. *Antimicrob Agents Chemother*, **2006,** *50:*310–317.

Kiem S, Schentag JJ. Interpretation of antibiotic concentration ratios measured in epithelial lining fluid. *Antimicrob Agents Chemother*, **2008,** *52:*24–36.

Koch R. Die aetiologie der Milzbrand-Krankheit, begründet auf die Entwicklungsgeschichte des *Bacillus Anthracis*. *Beiträge zur Biologie der Pflanzen,* **1876,** *2:*277–310.

Lewis K. Riddle of biofilm resistance. *Antimicrob Agents Chemother,* **2001,** *45:*999–1007.

Lim D, Strynadka NC. Structural basis for the beta lactam resistance of PBP2a from methicillin-resistant *Staphylococcus aureus*. *Nat Struct Biol,* **2002,** *9:*870–876.

Louie A, Kaw P, Liu W, *et al.* Pharmacodynamics of daptomycin in a murine thigh model of *Staphylococcus aureus* infection. *Antimicrob Agents Chemother*, **2001,** *45:*845–851.

Mahillon J, Chandler M. Insertion sequences. *Microbiol Mol Biol Rev,* **1998,** *62:*725–774.

Marr KA, Lyons CN, Ha K, *et al.* Inducible azole resistance associated with a heterogeneous phenotype in *Candida albicans*. *Antimicrob Agents Chemother*, **2001,** *45:*52–59.

Metzner KJ, Giulieri SG, Knoepfel SA, *et al.* Minority quasispecies of drug-resistant HIV-1 that lead to early therapy failure in treatment-naive and -adherent patients. *Clin Infect Dis*, **2009,** *48:*239–247.

Miller DS, Bauer B, Hartz AM. Modulation of P-glycoprotein at the blood-brain barrier: Opportunities to improve central nervous system pharmacotherapy. *Pharmacol Rev,* **2008,** *60:*196–209.

Moise-Broder PA, Sakoulas G, Eliopoulos GM, *et al.* Accessory gene regulator group II polymorphism in methicillin-resistant *Staphylococcus aureus* is predictive of failure of vancomycin therapy. *Clin Infect Dis*, **2004,** *38:*1700–1705.

Mondon P, Petter R, Amalfitano G, *et al.* Heteroresistance to fluconazole and voriconazole in *Cryptococcus neoformans*. *Antimicrob Agents Chemother*, **1999,** *43:* 1856–1861.

Nakajima Y. Mechanisms of bacterial resistance to macrolide antibiotics. *J Infect Chemother,* **1999,** *5:*61–74.

Neumann AU, Lam NP, Dahari H, *et al.* Hepatitis C viral dynamics in vivo and the antiviral efficacy of interferon-alpha therapy. *Science*, **1998,** *282:*103–107.

Nijhuis M, van Maarseveen NM, Boucher CA. Antiviral resistance and impact on viral replication capacity: Evolution of viruses under antiviral pressure occurs in three phases. *Handb Exp Pharmacol*, **2009,** *189:*299–320.

Ouellette M. Biochemical and molecular mechanisms of drug resistance in parasites. *Trop Med Int Health*, **2001,** *6:* 874–882.

Panlilio AL, Cardo DM, Grohskopf LA, *et al.* Updated U.S. Public Health Service guidelines for the management of occupational exposures to HIV and recommendations for postexposure prophylaxis. *MMWR Recomm Rep,* **2005,** *54:*1–17.

Pappas PG, Kauffman CA, Andes D, *et al.* Clinical practice guidelines for the management of candidiasis: 2009 update by the Infectious Diseases Society of America. *Clin Infect Dis*, **2009,** *48:*503–535.

Pasteur L. Mémoire sur les corpuscles organisés qui existent dans l'atmosphère. Examen de la doctrine des générations spontanées. *Annales des sciences naturelles,* **1861,** *16:* 5–98.

Petropoulos CJ, Parkin NT, Limoli KL, *et al.* A novel phenotypic drug susceptibility assay for human immunodeficiency virus type 1. *Antimicrob Agents Chemother,* **2000,** *44:* 920–928.

Preston SL, Drusano GL, Berman AL, et al. Pharmacodynamics of levofloxacin: A new paradigm for early clinical trials. *JAMA,* **1998,** *279:*125–129.

Pukrittayakamee S, Wanwimolruk S, Stepniewska K, *et al.* Quinine pharmacokinetic-pharmacodynamic relationships in uncomplicated falciparum malaria. *Antimicrob Agents Chemother*, **2003,** *47:*3458–3463.

Quagliarello VJ, Scheld WM. Treatment of bacterial meningitis. *N Engl J Med,* **1997,** *336:*708–716.

Rad ME, Bifani P, Martin C, *et al.* Mutations in putative mutator genes of *Mycobacterium tuberculosis* strains of the W-Beijing family. *Emerg Infect Dis,* **2003,** *9:*838–845.

Rinder H. Hetero-resistance: An under-recognised confounder in diagnosis and therapy? *J Med Microbiol*, **2001,** *50:* 1018–1020.

Sheiner LB, Rosenberg B, Marathe VV. Estimation of population characteristics of pharmacokinetic parameters from routine clinical data. *J Pharmacokinet Biopharm,* **1977,** *5:*445–479.

Singh N. Preemptive therapy versus universal prophylaxis with ganciclovir for cytomegalovirus in solid organ transplant recipients. *Clin Infect Dis,* **2001,** *32:*742–751.

Singh N, Wannstedt C, Keyes L, et al. Valganciclovir as preemptive therapy for cytomegalovirus in cytomegalovirus-seronegative liver transplant recipients of cytomegalovirus-seropositive donor allografts. *Liver Transpl*, **2008,** *14:*240–244.

Spratt BG. Resistance to antibiotics mediated by target alterations. *Science,* **1994,** *264:*388–393.

Stepniewska K, Chotivanich K, Brockman A, *et al.* Overestimating resistance in field testing of malaria parasites: Simple methods for estimating high EC50 values using a Bayesian approach. *Malar J*, **2007,** *6:*4.

Talal AH, Ribeiro RM, Powers KA, *et al.* Pharmacodynamics of PEG-IFN alpha differentiate HIV/HCV coinfected sustained virological responders from nonresponders. *Hepatology*, **2006,** *43:*943–953.

Tam VH, Louie A, Deziel MR, *et al.* The relationship between quinolone exposures and resistance amplification is characterized by an inverted U: A new paradigm for optimizing pharmacodynamics to counterselect resistance. *Antimicrob Agents Chemother,* **2007,** *51:*744–747.

Tarning J, Ashley EA, Lindegardh N, *et al.* Population pharmacokinetics of piperaquine after two different treatment regimens with dihydroartemisinin-piperaquine in patients with *Plasmodium falciparum* malaria in Thailand. *Antimicrob Agents Chemother,* **2008,** *52:*1052–1061.

Vogelman B, Gudmundsson S, Leggett J, *et al.* Correlation of antimicrobial pharmacokinetic parameters with therapeutic efficacy in an animal model. *J Infect Dis,* **1988,** *158:* 831–847.

Wagenlehner FM, Kinzig-Schippers M, Sorgel F, *et al.* Concentrations in plasma, urinary excretion and bactericidal activity of levofloxacin (500 mg) versus ciprofloxacin (500 mg) in healthy volunteers receiving a single oral dose. *Int J Antimicrob Agents,* **2006,** *28:*551–519.

Wehrli W, Knusel F, Schmid K, Staehelin M. Interaction of rifamycin with bacterial RNA polymerase. *Proc Natl Acad Sci U S A*, **1968,** *61:*667–673.

Wilkins JJ, Savic RM, Karlsson MO, *et al.* Population pharmacokinetics of rifampin in pulmonary tuberculosis patients, including a semimechanistic model to describe variable absorption. *Antimicrob Agents Chemother*, **2008,** *52:* 2138–2148.

Wilson W, Taubert KA, Gewitz M, *et al.* Prevention of infective endocarditis: Guidelines from the American Heart Association; a guideline from the American Heart Association Rheumatic Fever, Endocarditis, and Kawasaki Disease Committee, Council on Cardiovascular Disease in the Young, and the Council on Clinical Cardiology, Council on Cardiovascular Surgery and Anesthesia, and the Quality of Care and Outcomes Research Interdisciplinary Working Group. *Circulation*, **2007,** *116:*1736–1754.

Zhou XJ, Sheiner LB, D'Aquila RT, *et al.* Population pharmacokinetics of nevirapine, zidovudine, and didanosine in human immunodeficiency virus-infected patients. The National Institute of Allergy and Infectious Diseases AIDS Clinical Trials Group Protocol 241 Investigators. *Antimicrob Agents Chemother,* **1999,** *43:*121–128.

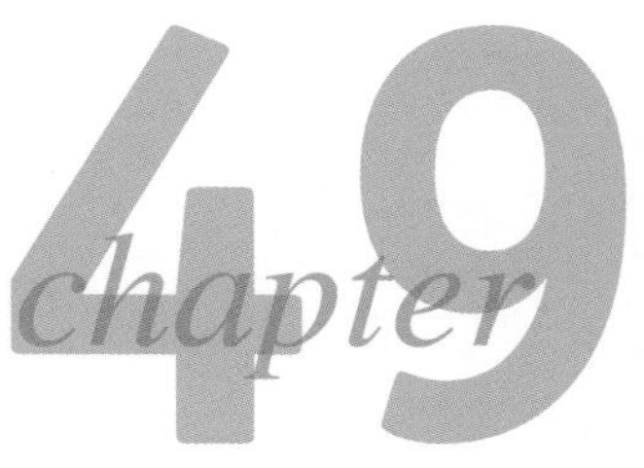

Chemotherapy of Malaria

Joseph M. Vinetz, Jérôme Clain, Viengngeun Bounkeua, Richard T. Eastman, and David Fidock

Malaria affects about a quarter of a billion people and leads to almost 900,000 deaths annually (World Health Organization, 2009). This disease is caused by infection with single-celled protozoan parasites of the genus *Plasmodium.* Five *Plasmodium* spp. are known to infect humans: *P. falciparum, P. vivax, P. ovale, P. malariae,* and *P. knowlesi. P. falciparum* and *P. vivax* cause most of the malarial infections worldwide. Of these, *P. falciparum* accounts for the majority of the burden of malaria in sub-Saharan Africa and is associated with the most severe disease. *P. vivax* accounts for half of the malaria burden in South and East Asia and >80% of the malarial infections in the America. Malaria due to *P. ovale* and *P. malariae* is relatively uncommon but requires identification both for treatment (*P. ovale*, like *P. vivax*, forms hypnozoites with the potential for relapse) and for epidemiological purposes (malarial infection, due mostly to *P. malariae,* can arise from blood transfusion). *P. knowlesi,* previously thought to infect only nonhuman primates, has emerged as a zoonotic malarial parasite and now is an important, sometimes lethal, cause of human malaria in parts of Southeast Asia (including Malaysia, Indonesia, Thailand, Singapore, and the Philippines; Cox-Singh et al., 2008). *P. knowlesi* should therefore be considered as a potential cause of malaria among travelers returning from this region. The vast majority of malaria cases occur via infection from *Anopheles* mosquitoes in endemic regions. Infections acquired congenitally or via transfusions or contaminated needles are known to occur but are rare. Screening of blood donors has reduced the risk of transfusion-transmitted malaria to 1:4,000,000 in the U.S.

Research on malaria has entered the genomic era; the complete genome sequence has been determined for multiple *Plasmodium* species, including *P. falciparum, P. vivax, P. knowlesi,* and other species infecting rodents and non-human primates. The availability of a robust culture system for *P. falciparum* erythrocytic stages, combined with methods to experimentally infect mosquitoes and generate sporozoite and liver stage parasites, has generated key platforms for drug discovery. These platforms include genetic modifications by gene knockout, heterologous expression and complementation, allelic replacement, high throughput screening of the pathogenic asexual blood stage parasites, and lower throughput assays against other stages of the parasite life cycle (Hayton and Su, 2008; Winzeler, 2008). Similar laboratory approaches have not yet been successful for *P. vivax.* Methods for sustained *in vitro* culture of blood stage forms of *P. vivax* are not yet available but are being developed for *P. knowlesi* and *P. cynomolgi*, which share important biological similarities with *P. vivax.*

BIOLOGY OF MALARIAL INFECTION

Plasmodium sporozoites, which initiate infection in humans, are inoculated into the dermis and enter the bloodstream following the bite of a *Plasmodium*-infected female anopheline mosquito. Within minutes, sporozoites travel to the liver, where they infect hepatocytes via cell surface receptor-mediated events. This process initiates the *asymptomatic prepatent period*, or *exoerythrocytic stage* of infection, which typically lasts ~1 week. During this period, the parasite undergoes asexual replication within hepatocytes, resulting in production of liver stage schizonts. Upon rupture of the infected hepatocytes, tens of thousands of merozoites are released into the bloodstream and infect red blood cells. After the initial exoerythrocytic stage, *P. falciparum* and *P. malariae* are no longer found in the liver. *P. vivax* and *P. ovale*, however, can maintain a quiescent hepatocyte infection as a dormant form of the parasite known as the hypnozoite. Consequently, *P. vivax* and *P. ovale* can reinitiate symptomatic disease long after the initial symptoms of malaria are recognized and treated. Erythrocytic forms cannot reestablish infection of hepatocytes.

Transmission of human-infecting malarial parasites is maintained in human populations both by the extended persistence of hypnozoites (lasting from months to no more than a few years for *P. vivax* and *P. ovale*), by antigenic variation in *P. falciparum* (probably months), and presumably by antigen variation in *P. malariae* (for as long as several decades) (Vinetz et al., 1998).

The *asexual erythrocytic stages* of malarial parasites are responsible for the clinical manifestations of malaria. This part of the *Plasmodium* life cycle is initiated by merozoite recognition of red blood cells, mediated by cell surface receptors, followed by red blood cell invasion. Once inside a red blood cell, the merozoite develops into a ring form, which becomes a trophozoite that matures into an asexually dividing blood stage schizont. Upon rupture of the infected erythrocyte, these schizonts release 8-32 merozoites that can establish new infections in nearby red blood cells. The erythrocytic replication cycle lasts for 24 hours (for *P. knowlesi*), 48 hours (for *P. falciparum, P. vivax, and P. ovale*), and 72 hours (for *P. malariae*). As such, infections due to *P. vivax* and *P. ovale* can produce tertian fever patterns (48 hours), whereas those due to *P. malariae* can result in quartan fever (72 hours, as classically described in Hippocrates' *Epidemics*). Although most invading merozoites develop into schizonts, a small proportion become gametocytes, the form of the parasite that is infective to mosquitoes. Gametocytes are ingested into the mosquito midgut during an infectious blood meal and then transform into gametes that can fertilize to become zygotes. Zygotes mature into ookinetes, which penetrate the mosquito midgut wall and develop into oocysts. Numerous rounds of asexual replication occur in the oocyst to generate sporozoites over 10-14 days. Fully developed sporozoites rupture from oocysts and invade the mosquito salivary glands, from which they can initiate a new infection during subsequent mosquito blood meals (Figure 49–1). Understanding the subtleties of the life cycles of *Plasmodium* parasites is important for tailoring drug therapies to the various species and geographic contexts.

Mechanisms of erythrocyte invasion include initial binding by merozoites to specific red blood cell surface ligands. *P. falciparum* has a family of binding proteins that can recognize a variety of host cell molecules. *P. falciparum* invades all stages of erythrocytes and therefore can achieve high parasitemias. *P. vivax* selectively binds to the Duffy chemokine receptor protein as well as reticulocyte-specific proteins. Thus, *P. vivax* does not establish infection in Duffy-negative individuals and only invades reticulocytes. (However, *P. vivax* has reportedly mutated in Madagascar to enable infection of Duffy-negative individuals [Ménard et al., 2010].) Because of this restricted subpopulation of suitable erythrocytes, *P. vivax* rarely exceeds 1% parasitemia in the bloodstream. *P. ovale* is similar to *P. vivax* in its predilection for young red blood cells, but the mechanism of its erythrocyte recognition is unknown. *P. malariae* parasitizes senescent red blood cells, maintains a very low parasitemia, and typically causes an indolent infection.

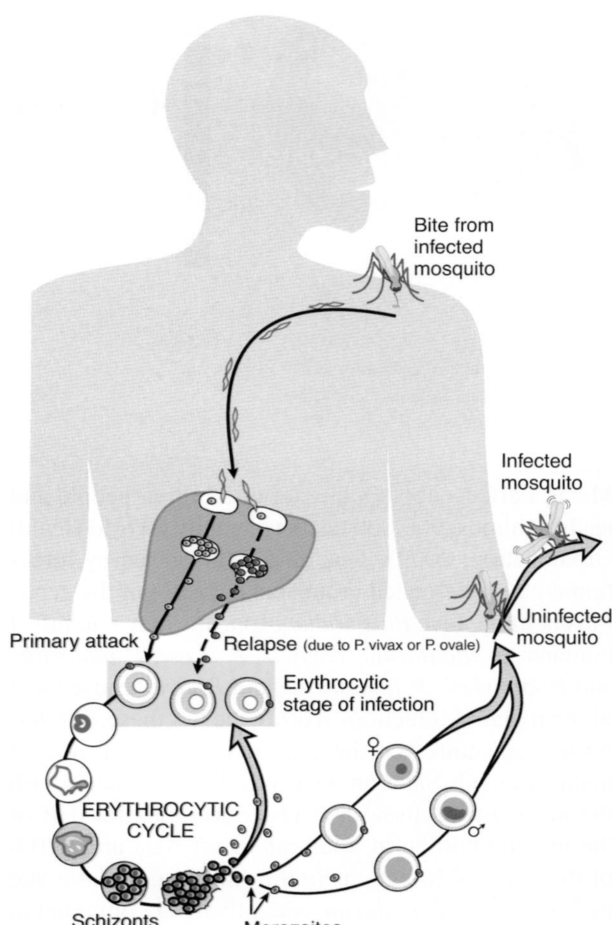

Figure 49–1. *Life cycle of malaria parasites.*

P. falciparum assembles cytoadherence proteins (PfEMP1s, encoded by a highly variable family of *var* genes) into structures called knobs that are presented on the erythrocyte surface. Knobs allow the *P. falciparum*-parasitized erythrocyte to bind to postcapillary vascular endothelium, so as to avoid spleen-mediated clearance and allow the parasite to grow in a low oxygen, high carbon dioxide microenvironment. For the patient, the consequences are microvascular blockage in the brain and organ beds, and local release of cytokines and direct vascular intermediates such as nitric oxide. These lead to severe complications such as cerebral malaria, pulmonary edema, acute renal failure, and placental malaria. These can result in low birthweight and translocation of bacteria from the gastrointestinal (GI) tract to the blood (septic complications, so-called algid malaria).

Attention is increasingly being focused on measures to prevent parasite transmission from a human host to a mosquito vector. Bed nets and residual indoor insecticide treatment are the mainstay of malaria prevention in endemic areas. Drugs are being used to prevent transmission, but this strategy presents special problems related to toxicity. Whereas some antimalarials, such as 4-aminoquinolines and sulfadoxine-pyrimethamine, promote increased gametocytemia, others, including 8-aminoquinolines and artemisinins, can reduce gametocyte levels and thus reduce transmission. Although the gametocytocidal activity of primaquine and tafenoquine is potentially important, these agents cannot be used for mass treatment without first assessing glucose-6-phosphate dehydrogenase (G6PD) levels, because of the potential for hemolytic anemia in G6PD-deficient individuals.

Clinical Manifestations of Malaria

The cardinal signs and symptoms of malaria are high, spiking fevers (with or without periodicity), chills, headaches, myalgias, malaise, and GI symptoms. Severe headache, a characteristic early symptom in malaria caused by all *Plasmodium* spp., often heralds the onset of infection, before fever and chills. *P. falciparum* causes the most severe disease and may lead to organ failure and death. Placental malaria, of particular danger for primigravidae, is due to *P. falciparum* adherence to chondroitin sulfate A (CSA) in the placenta. This often leads to severe complications, including miscarriage. When treated early, symptoms of malarial infection usually improve within 24-48 hours.

Acute illness due to *P. vivax* infection may appear severe due to high fever and prostration. Indeed, the pyrogenic threshold of this parasite (i.e., parasite burden associated with fever) is lower than that of *P. falciparum*. Nonetheless, *P. vivax* malaria generally has a low mortality rate. *P. vivax* malaria is characterized by relapses caused by the reactivation of latent tissue forms. Clinical manifestations of relapse are the same as those of primary infection. In recent years, severe *P. vivax* malaria from Oceania (Papua New Guinea, Indonesia) and India possess important similarities to severe malaria caused by *P. falciparum*. These include neurological symptoms (diminished consciousness, seizure) and pulmonary edema. Rare but life-threatening complications can occur, including splenic rupture, acute lung injury, and profound anemia.

P. ovale causes a clinical syndrome similar to that of *P. vivax* but may be milder with lower levels of parasitemia. It shares with *P. vivax* the ability to form the hypnozoite (dormant liver stage) that may relapse after months to 2 years later. *P. ovale* is more common in sub-Saharan Africa and some islands in Oceania.

P. malariae causes a generally indolent infection with very low levels of parasitemia and often does not produce clinical symptoms. This parasite can be found in all malaria-endemic areas but is most common in sub-Saharan Africa and the southwest Pacific. Interestingly, *P. malariae* prevalence increases during the dry season and can be found as a co-infection with *P. falciparum*. Although uncommon, a potentially fatal complication of *P. malariae* is a glomerulonephritis syndrome that does not respond to antimalarial treatment.

P. knowlesi infection is often misdiagnosed as *P. malariae* by light microscopy. This infection is distinguished by a shorter erythrocytic cycle (24 hours compared with 72 hours for *P. malariae*) and higher levels of parasitemia. Like *P. malariae, P. knowlesi* is generally sensitive to chloroquine, but patients presenting with advanced disease nonetheless may progress to death despite adequate drug dosing.

Asymptomatic *P. falciparum* and *P. vivax* infections are common in endemic regions, and they represent important potential reservoirs for malaria transmission. Although different studies are not entirely consistent in the definition of "asymptomatic," generally this state implies a lack of fever, headache, and other systemic complaints, within a defined time period prior to a positive test for malaria parasitemia. Migration of asymptomatic individuals, to areas where malaria is not present but vector mosquitoes are (i.e., anophelism without malaria), is an important mechanism for the introduction or reintroduction of malaria, in addition to facilitating the spread of drug-resistant isolates. Novel approaches to preventing transmission from asymptomatic reservoirs—whether through new drugs or vaccines—will be essential for future malaria control, elimination, and eradication strategies.

CLASSIFICATION OF ANTIMALARIAL AGENTS

The various stages of the malarial parasite life cycle that occur in humans differ from one another in their morphology, metabolism, and drug sensitivity. Thus, antimalarial drugs can be classified based on their activities during this life cycle as well as by their intended use for either chemoprophylaxis or treatment.

The spectrum of antimalarial drug activity (Table 49–1) leads to several generalizations. The first relates to chemoprophylaxis: *Because no antimalarial drug kills sporozoites, it is not truly possible to prevent infection; drugs can only prevent the development of symptomatic malaria caused by the asexual erythrocytic forms.*

The second relates to the treatment of an established infection: *No single antimalarial is effective against all liver and intra-erythrocytic stages of the life cycle that may co-exist in the same patient. Complete elimination of the parasite infection, therefore, may require more than one drug.*

The patterns of clinically useful activity fall into three general categories (Table 49–1). The first group

Table 49–1

Malarial Parasite Developmental Stages Targeted by Antimalarial Drugs

		EFFECT OF DRUG ON PARASITE VIABILITY				
			LIVER STAGES		BLOOD STAGES	
GROUP	DRUGS	SPOROZOITE	PRIMARY	HYPNOZOITE	ASEXUAL	GAMETOCYTE
1	Artemisinins	–	–	–	+	+
	Chloroquine	–	–	–	+	+/–
	Mefloquine	–	–	–	+	–
	Quinine/Quinidine	–	–	–	+	+/–
	Pyrimethamine	–	–	–	+	–
	Sulfadoxine	–	–	–	+	–
	Tetracycline	–	–	–	+	–
2	Atovaquone/ Proguanil	–	+	–	+	+/–
3	Primaquine	–	+	+	–	+

–, no activity; +/–, low to moderate activity; +, important activity.

of agents (artemisinins, chloroquine, mefloquine, quinine and quinidine, pyrimethamine, sulfadoxine, and tetracycline) are not reliably effective against primary or latent liver stages. Instead, their action is directed against the asexual blood stages responsible for disease. These drugs will treat, or prevent, clinically symptomatic malaria. When used as chemoprophylaxis, these drugs must continue to be taken for several weeks after exposure, until parasites complete their intrahepatic stage of development and become susceptible to therapy.

The spectrum is somewhat expanded for a second category of drugs (typified by atovaquone and proguanil), which target not only the asexual erythrocytic forms but also the primary liver stages of *P. falciparum*. This additional activity shortens to several days the required period for postexposure chemoprophylaxis.

The third category, currently comprised solely of primaquine, is effective against primary and latent liver stages as well as gametocytes. Primaquine has no place in the treatment of symptomatic malaria but rather is used most commonly to eradicate the intrahepatic hypnozoites of *P. vivax* and *P. ovale* that are responsible for relapsing infections. Primaquine also has anti-gametocytic activity.

Aside from their antiparasitic activity, the utility of antimalarials for chemoprophylaxis or therapy depends on their pharmacokinetics and their safety. Thus quinine and primaquine, which have significant toxicity and relatively short half-lives, generally are reserved for the treatment of established infection and are not used for chemoprophylaxis in a healthy traveler. In contrast, chloroquine is relatively free from toxicity and has a long $t_{1/2}$ that is convenient for chemoprophylactic dosing (in those few areas still reporting chloroquine-sensitive malaria).

Regimens currently recommended for chemoprophylaxis in travelers are given in Table 49–2, whereas regimens for the treatment and presumptive self-treatment (based on symptom presentation) of malaria in travelers are provided in Table 49–3 and Table 49–4, respectively. Individual agents are discussed in greater detail later in this chapter, listed alphabetically.

ARTEMISININ AND DERIVATIVES

History. Artemisinin is a sesquiterpene lactone endoperoxide derived from *qing hao* (*Artemisia annua*), also called *sweet wormwood* or *annual wormwood*. The Chinese have ascribed medicinal value to this plant for >2000 years (White, 2008). As early as 340 A.D., Ge Hong prescribed tea made from *qing hao* as a remedy for fevers, and in 1596, Li Shizhen recommended it to relieve malarial symptoms. By 1972, Chinese scientists had identified the major antimalarial ingredient, *qinghaosu*, now known as *artemisinin*.

Chemistry. The structures of artemisinin and its three major semisynthetic derivatives in clinical use, dihydroartemisinin, artemether, and artesunate, are as follows:

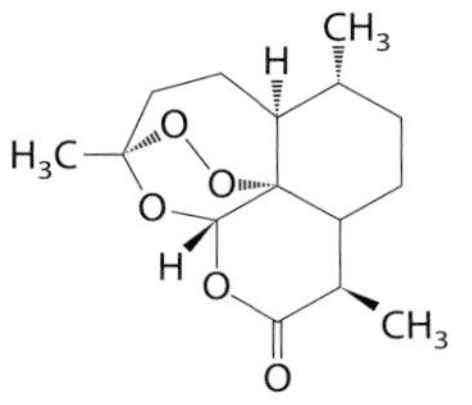

ARTEMISININ

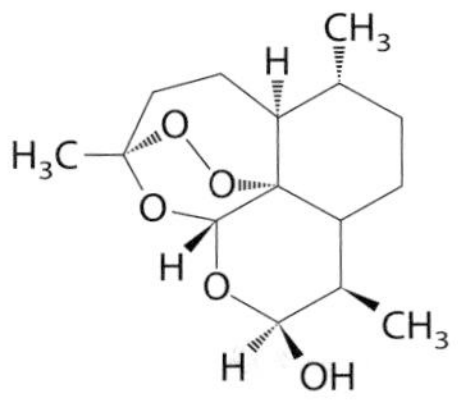

DIHYDROARTEMISININ

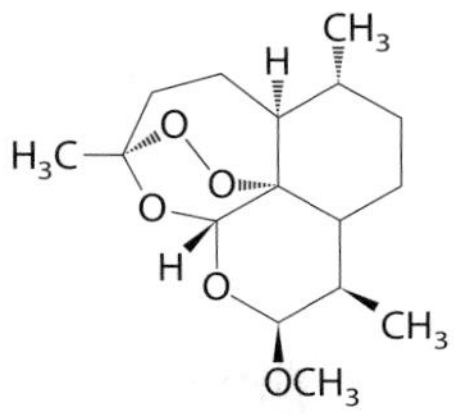

ARTEMETHER

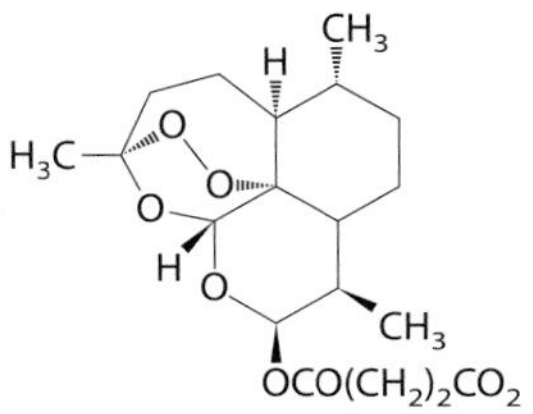

ARTESUNATE

Table 49–2

Regimens for the Prevention of Malaria in Non-immune Individuals

DRUG	USAGE	ADULT DOSE	PEDIATRIC DOSE	COMMENTS
Atovaquone/ proguanil (MALARONE)	Prophylaxis in all areas	Adult tablets contain 250 mg atovaquone and 100 mg proguanil hydrochloride. 1 adult tablet orally, daily	Pediatric tablets (62.5 mg atovaquone/25 mg proguanil HCl). 5-8 kg: 1/2 ped tab/day >8-10 kg: 3/4 ped tab/day >10-20 kg: 1 ped tab/day >20-30 kg: 2 ped tab/day >30-40 kg: 3 ped tab/day >40 kg: 1 adult tablet daily	Begin 1-2 days before travel to malarious areas. Take daily at the same time each day while in the malarious area and for 7 days after leaving such areas. Contraindicated in persons with severe renal impairment (creatinine clearance <30 mL/minute). Atovaquone/proguanil should be taken with food or a milky drink. Not recommended for prophylaxis for children <5 kg, pregnant women, and women breast-feeding infants weighing <5 kg.
Chloroquine phosphate (ARALEN and generic)	Prophylaxis only in areas with chloroquine-sensitive malaria	300 mg base (500 mg salt) orally, once/week	5 mg/kg base (8.3 mg/kg salt) orally, once/week, up to max adult dose (300 mg base)	Begin 1-2 weeks before travel to malarious areas. Take weekly on the same day of the week while in the malarious area and for 4 weeks after leaving such areas. May exacerbate psoriasis.
Doxycycline	Prophylaxis in all areas	100 mg orally, daily	≥8 years of age: 2 mg/kg up to adult dose of 100 mg/day	Begin 1-2 days before travel to malarious areas. Take daily at the same time each day while in the malarious area and for 4 weeks after leaving such areas. Contraindicated in children <8 years of age and pregnant women.
Hydroxy-chloroquine sulfate (PLAQUENIL)	An alternative to chloroquine for prophylaxis only in areas with chloroquine-sensitive malaria	310 mg base (400 mg salt) orally, once/week	5 mg/kg base (6.5 mg/kg salt) orally, once/week, up to max adult dose (310 mg base)	Begin 1-2 weeks before travel to malarious areas. Take weekly on the same day of the week while in the malarious area and for 4 weeks after leaving such areas.

(*Continued*)

Table 49–2

Regimens for the Prevention of Malaria in Non-immune Individuals (*Continued*)

DRUG	USAGE	ADULT DOSE	PEDIATRIC DOSE	COMMENTS
Mefloquine (LARIAM and generic)	Prophylaxis in areas with mefloquine-sensitive malaria	228 mg base (250 mg salt) orally, once/week	≤9 kg: 4.6 mg/kg base (5 mg/kg salt) orally, once/week; >9-19 kg: 1/4 tablet once/week; >19-30 kg: 1/2 tablet once/week; >31-45 kg: 3/4 tablet once/week; ≥45 kg: 1 tablet once/week	Begin 1-2 weeks before travel to malarious areas. Take weekly on same day of the week while in malarious area and for 4 weeks after leaving such areas. Contraindicated in persons allergic to mefloquine or related compounds (e.g., quinine, quinidine) and in persons with active depression, a recent history of depression, generalized anxiety disorder, psychosis, schizophrenia, other major psychiatric disorders, or seizures. Use with caution in persons with psychiatric disturbances or a previous history of depression. Not recommended for persons with cardiac conduction abnormalities.
Primaquine	Prophylaxis for short-duration travel to areas with principally *P. vivax*	30 mg base (52.6 mg salt) orally, daily	0.5 mg/kg base (0.8 mg/kg salt) up to adult dose orally, daily	Begin 1-2 days before travel to malarious areas. Take daily at same time each day while in malarious area and for 7 days after leaving such areas. Contraindicated in persons with G6PD[a] deficiency, and during pregnancy and lactation unless the infant being breastfed has documented normal G6PD level.
Primaquine	For presumptive anti-relapse therapy (terminal prophylaxis) to decrease the risk of relapses (*P. vivax*, *P. ovale*)	30 mg base (52.6 mg salt) orally, once/day for 14 days after departure from the malarious area.	0.5 mg/kg base (0.8 mg/kg salt) up to adult dose orally, once/day for 14 days after departure from the malarious area	Indicated for persons who have had prolonged exposure to *P. vivax* and *P. ovale* or both. Contraindicated in persons with G6PD[a] deficiency. Also contraindicated during pregnancy and lactation unless the infant being breastfed has a documented normal G6PD level.

[a]Glucose-6-phosphate dehydrogenase. All persons who take primaquine should have a documented normal G6PD level before starting the medication. These regimens are based on published recommendations of the United States Centers for Disease Control and Prevention (CDC). These recommendations may change over time. Up-to-date information should be obtained from www.cdc.gov/travel. Recommendations and available treatment differ among countries in the industrialized world, developing world, and malaria-endemic regions; in the latter, some antimalarial treatments may be available without prescription, but the most effective drugs usually are controlled by governmental agencies.

Source: From the United States Centers for Disease Control and Prevention, Health Information for International Travel 2010 (Yellow Book). Available at: (http://wwwnc.cdc.gov/travel/content/yellowbook/home-2010.aspx. Accessed January 12, 2010.

Table 49–3

Regimens for the Treatment of Malaria

DRUG	INDICATION	ADULT DOSAGE	PEDIATRIC DOSAGE[a]	POTENTIAL ADVERSE EFFECTS	COMMENTS
Artemether-lumefantrine (COARTEM)	P. *falciparum* from chloroquine resistant or unknown areas	Tablet: 20 mg artemether, limefantrine. Dose: 4 tablets Day 1: 2 doses separated by 8 hours; thereafter bid × 2d	Wt. (kg) — Tablets (per dose) 5-15 — 1 15-25 — 2 25-<35 — 3 >35 — 4 Use same 3-day schedule as adluts	Adults; headache anorexia, dizziness, asthenia, arthralgia myalgia Children: fever, cough, vomiting, loss of appetite, headache	Take with food or whole milk. If patient vomits within 30 minutes, repeat dose. Contraindicated in pregnancy
Artesunate (IV; available from U.S. Center for Disease Control and Prevention)	Severe malaria (see CDC guidelines)	U.S. treatment IND (CDC): 4 equal doses of artesunate (2.4 mg/kg each) over a 3-day period followed by oral treatment with atovaquone-proguanil, doxycycline, clindamycin, or mefloquine (to avoid emergence of resistance)		See Artemether	See Artemether and CDC guidelines
Atovaquone-proguanil MALARONE (oral)	*Plasmodium falciparum* from chloroquine-resistant areas; can be used for *P. vivax*	Adult tablet 250 mg atovaquone/100 mg, proguanil 4 Adult tablets orally per day × 3 d	Pediatric tablet = 62.5 mg atovaquone/25 mg proguanil 5-8 kg: 2 ped tab orally per day × 3 d >8-10 kg: 3 ped tab orally daily × 3 d >10-20 kg: 1 adult tab orally daily × 3 d >20-30 kg: 2 adult tab orally daily × 3 d >30-40 kg: 3 adult tab orally daily × 3 d >40 kg: 4 adult tab orally daily × 3 d	Abdominal pain, nausea, vomiting, diarrhea, headache, rash, mild reversible elevations in liver aminotransferase levels	Not indicated for use in pregnant women due to limited data Contraindicated if hypersensitivity to atovaquone or proguanil; severe renal impairment (creatinine clearance <30 mL/min) Should be taken with food to increase absorption of atovaquone

(*Continued*)

Table 49–3

Regimens for the Treatment of Malaria (*Continued*)

DRUG	INDICATION	ADULT DOSAGE	PEDIATRIC DOSAGE[a]	POTENTIAL ADVERSE EFFECTS	COMMENTS
Chloroquine phosphate	*P. falciparum* from chloroquine sensitive areas *P vivax* from chloroquine sensitive areas All *P. ovale* All *P malariae* All *P. knowlesi*	600 mg base (1000 mg salt) orally immediately, followed by 300 mg base (500 mg salt) orally at 6, 24, and 48 h Total dose: 1500 mg base (2500 mg salt)	10 mg base/kg orally immediately, followed by 5 mg base/kg orally at 6, 24, and 48 h Total dose: 25 mg base/kg	Nausea, vomiting, rash, headache, dizziness, urticaria, abdominal pain, pruritus	Safe in children and pregnant women Give for chemoprophylaxis (500 mg salt orally every week) in pregnant women with chloroquine-sensitive *P. vivax* Contraindicated if retinal or visual field change; hypersensitivity to 4-aminoquinolines Use with caution in those with impaired liver function since the drug is concentrated in the liver
Clindamycin (oral or IV)	*P. falciparum* from chloroquine-resistant areas *P vivax* from chloroquine-resistant areas	Oral: 20 mg base/kg/d orally divided 3 times daily × 7 d IV: 10 mg base/kg loading dose IV followed by 5 mg base/kg IV every 8 h; switch to oral clindamycin (as above) as soon as patient can take oral meds; duration = 7 d	Oral: 20 mg base/kg/d orally divided 3 times daily × 7 d IV: 10 mg base/kg loading dose IV followed by 5 mg base/kg IV every 8 h; switch to oral clindamycin (oral dose as above) as soon as patient can take oral medication; treatment course = 7 d	Diarrhea, nausea, rash	Always use in combination with quinine-quinidine Safe in children and pregnant women

Doxycycline (oral or IV)	*P falciparum* from chloroquine-resistant areas *P vivax* from chloroquine-resistant areas	Oral: 100 mg orally twice daily × 7 d IV: 100 mg IV every 12 h and then switch to oral doxycycline (as above) as soon as patient can take oral medication; treatment course = 7 d	Oral: 2.2 mg/kg orally every12 h × 7 d IV: IV only if patient is not able to take oral medication; for children <45 kg, give 2.2 mg/kg IV every 12 h and then switch to oral doxycycline (dose as above) as soon as patient can take oral medication; for children >45 kg, use same dosing as for adults; duration = 7 d	Nausea, vomiting, diarrhea, abdominal pain, dizziness, photosensitivity, headache, esophagitis, odynophagia Rarely hepatotoxicity, pancreatitis, and benign intracranial hypertension seen with tetracycline class of drugs	Always use in combination with quinine or quinidine Contraindicated in children < 8 y, pregnant women, and persons with known hypersensitivity to tetracyclines Food and milk decrease absorption of doxycycline, will decrease GI disturbances To prevent esophagitis, take tetracyclines with large amounts of fluids, (patients should not lie down for 1 h after taking the drugs) Barbiturates, carbamazepine, or phenytoin may cause reduction in C_p of doxycycline
Hydroxychloroquine (oral)	Second-line alternative for treatment of: *P. falciparum* and *P. vivax* from chloroquine-sensitive areas All *P. ovale* All *P. malariae*	620-mg base (= 800 mg salt) orally immediately, followed by 310 mg base (= 400 mg salt) orally at 6, 24, and 48 h Total dose: 1550-mg base (= 2000 mg salt)	10-mg base/kg orally immediately, followed by 5-mg base/kg orally at 6, 24, and 48 h Total dose: 25-mg base/kg	Nausea, vomiting, rash, headache, dizziness, urticaria, abdominal pain, pruritus[b]	Safe in children and pregnant women Contraindicated if retinal or visual field change; hypersensitivity to 4-aminoquinolines Use with caution in those with impaired liver function

(*Continued*)

Table 49–3

Regimens for the Treatment of Malaria (*Continued*)

DRUG	INDICATION	ADULT DOSAGE	PEDIATRIC DOSAGE[a]	POTENTIAL ADVERSE EFFECTS	COMMENTS
Mefloquine[c]	*P. falciparum* from chloroquine-resistant areas, except Thailand-Burmese and Thailand-Cambodian border regions *P. vivax* from chloroquine-resistant areas	684 mg base (= 750 mg salt) orally as initial dose, followed by 456 mg base (= 500 mg salt) orally given 6-12 h after initial dose Total dose = 1250 mg salt	13.7 mg base/kg (= 15 mg salt/kg) orally as initial dose, followed by 9.1 mg base/kg (= 10 mg salt/kg) orally given 6-12 h after initial dose Total dose = 25 mg salt/kg	GI complaints (nausea, vomiting, diarrhea, abdominal pain), mild CNS complaints (dizziness, headache, somnolence, sleep disorders), myalgia, mild skin rash, and fatigue; moderate to severe neuropsychiatric reactions, ECG changes, including sinus arrhythmia, sinus bradycardia, first degree A-V block, QTc prolongation, and abnormal T waves	Contraindicated if hypersensitive to the drug or to related compounds; cardiac conduction abnormalities; psychiatric disorders; and seizure disorders Do not administer if patient has received related drugs (chloroquine, quinine, quinidine) less than 12 h ago
Primaquine phosphate	Radical cure of *P. vivax* and *P. ovale* (to eliminate hypnozoites)	30 mg base orally per day × 14 d	0.5 mg base/kg orally per day × 14 d	GI disturbances, methemoglobinemia (self-limited), hemolysis in persons with G6PD deficiency	Must screen for G6PD deficiency prior to use Contraindicated in persons with G6PD deficiency; pregnant women Should be taken with food to minimize GI adverse effects

Quinine sulfate (oral)	*P. falciparum* from chloroquine-resistant areas *P. vivax* from chloroquine-resistant areas	542 mg base (650 mg salt)[d] orally 3 times daily × 3 d (infections acquired outside Southeast Asia) to 7 d (infections acquired in SE Asia)	8.3 mg base/kg (10 mg salt/kg) orally 3 times daily × 3 d (infections acquired outside Southeast Asia) to 7 d (infections acquired in SE Asia)	Cinchonism[e], sinus arrhythmia, junctional rhythms, atrioventricular block, prolonged QT interval, ventricular tachycardia, ventricular fibrillation (these are rare and more commonly seen with quinidine), hypoglycemia	Combine with tetracycline, doxycycline, or clindamycin, except for *P. vivax* infections in children <8 y or pregnant women Contraindicated in hypersensitivity including history of blackwater fever, thrombocytopenic purpura, or thrombocytopenia associated with quinine or quinidine use; many cardiac conduction defects and arrhythmias[f]; myasthenia gravis; optic neuritis
Quinidine gluconate (IV)	Severe malaria (all species, independently of chloroquine resistance) Patient unable to take oral medication Parasitemia >10%	6.25 mg base/kg (= 10 mg salt/kg) loading dose IV over 1-2 h, then 0.0125 mg base/kg/min (0.02 mg salt/kg/min) continuous infusion for at least 24 h Alternative regimen:[g]	Same as adult	Cinchonism, tachycardia, prolongation of QRS and QTc intervals, flattening of T-wave (effects are often transient) Ventricular arrhythmias, hypotension, hypoglycemia	Combine with tetracycline, doxycycline, or clindamycin Contraindicated in hypersensitivity; history of blackwater fever including history of blackwater fever, thrombocytopenic purpura or thrombocytopenia associated with quinine or quinidine use; many cardiac conduction defects and arrhythmias[h]; myasthenia gravis; optic neuritis

(Continued)

Table 49–3

Regimens for the Treatment of Malaria (*Continued*)

DRUG	INDICATION	ADULT DOSAGE	PEDIATRIC DOSAGE[a]	POTENTIAL ADVERSE EFFECTS	COMMENTS
Tetracycline (oral or IV)	*P. falciparum* (chloroquine-resistant areas) *P. vivax* from chloroquine-resistant areas (with quinine/quinidine)	Oral: 250 mg 4 times daily × 7 d IV: dosage same as for oral	25 mg/kg/d orally divided 4 times daily × 7 d IV: dosage same as for oral	See doxycycline	See doxycycline

G6PD, glucose-6-phosphate dehydrogenase; IV, intravenous.

[a]Pediatric dosage should never exceed adult dosage.

[b]Extrapolated from chloroquine literature.

[c]Mefloquine should not be used to treat *P. falciparum* infections acquired in the following areas: borders of Thailand with Burma (Myanmar) and Cambodia, western provinces of Cambodia, eastern states of Burma (Myanmar), border between Burma and China, Laos along borders of Laos and Burma (and adjacent parts of Thailand-Cambodia border), and southern Vietnam due to resistant strains.

[d]Quinine sulfate capsule manufactured in the U.S. is in a 324-mg dose; therefore, two capsules should be sufficient for adult dosing.

[e]Nausea, vomiting, headache, tinnitus, deafness, dizziness, and visual disturbances.

[f]Refer to quinine sulfate, package insert (Mutual Pharmaceutical Inc, Philadelphia, PA, Rev 08, November 2009).

[g]Alternative dosing hypoglycemia optic neuritis regimen for quinidine gluconate (IV): 15 mg base/kg (24 mg salt/kg) loading dose IV infused over 4 h, followed by 7.5 mg base/kg (= 12 mg salt/kg) infused over 4 h every 8 h, starting 8 h after the loading dose (see package insert); once parasite density <1% and patient can take oral medication, complete treatment with oral quinine, dose as above Quinidine or quinine course = 7 d in SE Asia (3 d in Africa or South America)

[h]Refer to quinidine gluconate, package insert (Eli Lilly Co, Indianapolis, IN, February 2002).

These regimens are based on published recommendations of the U.S. Centers for Disease Control and Prevention (CDC). Although current at the time of writing, these recommendations may change over time. Up-to-date information should be obtained from the CDC website at www.cdc.gov/travel. Recommendations and available treatment differ among countries in the industrialized world, developing world, and malaria-endemic regions; in the latter, some anti-malarial treatments may be available without prescription, but the most effective drugs usually are controlled by governmental agencies.

From http://wwwnc.cdc.gov/travel/content/yellowbook/home-2010.aspx; accessed January 12, 2010.

Table 49–4

Regimen for Presumptive Self-Treatment of Malaria

DRUG	ADULT DOSE	PEDIATRIC DOSE	COMMENTS
Atovaquone/proguanil (MALARONE) Self-treatment drug to be used if professional medical care is not available within 24 hours. Medical care should be sought immediately after treatment.	4 tablets (each dose contains 1000 mg atovaquone and 400 mg proguanil) orally as a single daily dose for 3 consecutive days.	Daily dose to be taken for 3 consecutive days: 5-8 kg: 2 pediatric tablets; 9-10 kg: 3 pediatric tablets; 11-20 kg: 1 adult tablet; 21-30 kg: 2 adult tablets; 31-40 kg: 3 adult tablets; >41 kg: 4 adult tablets	Contraindicated in persons with severe renal impairment (creatinine clearance <30 mL/min). Not recommended for self-treatment in persons on atovaquone/ proguanil prophylaxis. Not currently recommended for children <5 kg, pregnant women, and women breast-feeding infants weighing <5 kg

These regimens are based on published recommendations of the United States Centers for Disease Control and Prevention (CDC). These recommendations may change over time. Up-to-date information should be obtained from www.cdc.gov/travel. Recommendations and available treatment differ among countries in the industrialized world, developing world, and malaria-endemic regions; in the latter, some antimalarial treatments may be available without prescription but the most effective drugs usually will be controlled by governmental agencies.
Source: From http://wwwnc.cdc.gov/travel/content/yellowbook/home-2010.aspx. Accessed January 12, 2010.

The derivatives display improved potency and bioavailability and have largely replaced the use of artemisinin. *Dihydroartemisinin* is a reduced product, *artesunate* is the water-soluble hemisuccinate ester of dihydroartemisinin, and *artemether* is a lipophilic methyl ether. Extensive structure-activity studies have confirmed the requirement for an endoperoxide moiety for antimalarial activity.

Mechanisms of Antimalarial Action and Resistance. As a class, the artemisinins are very potent and fast-acting antimalarials, inducing more rapid parasite clearance and fever resolution than any other currently licensed antimalarial drug. They are particularly well suited for the treatment of severe *P. falciparum* malaria and are also effective against the asexual erythrocytic stages of *P. vivax*. Increasingly, the standard treatment of malaria employs artemisinin-based combination therapies (ACTs) to increase treatment efficacy and reduce selection pressure for the emergence of drug resistance. Artemisinins cause a significant reduction of the parasite burden, with a four-$\log_{10}$ reduction in the parasite population for each 48-hour cycle of intraerythrocytic invasion, replication, and egress. As such, only three to four cycles (6-8 days) of treatment are required to remove all the parasites from the blood (White, 2008). Additionally, artemisinins possess some gametocytocidal activity, leading to a decrease in malarial parasite transmission. ACTs have low toxicity and are considered safe for use in nonpregnant adults and children. Of concern, however, is the widespread distribution of counterfeit or clinically substandard drugs that contain small quantities of the artemisinin derivative, a practice that threatens the effective administration of ACTs.

The mechanisms by which ACTs exert their antimalarial activity remain contentious (Golenser et al., 2006). Nevertheless, most studies concur that the activity of artemisinin and its potent derivatives results from reductive scission of the peroxide bridge by reduced heme-iron, which is produced inside the highly acidic digestive vacuole (DV) of the parasite as it digests hemoglobin. In addition to the formation of potentially toxic heme-adducts, activated artemisinin (for which the site of action remains unclear) might in turn generate free radicals that alkylate and oxidize proteins and possibly lipids in parasitized erythrocytes (Eastman and Fidock, 2009).

Artemisinins do not display significant clinical cross-resistance with other drugs. Indeed, sensitivity to artemisinins may even be increased in at least some strains of chloroquine-resistant parasites. Recent evidence has nonetheless suggested the emergence of *P. falciparum* isolates with an increased tolerance to artemisinins, manifesting as longer parasite clearance times (Dondorp et al., 2009). This has triggered significant efforts to elucidate the mechanistic basis of resistance and implement means to limit its spread. The World Health Organization (WHO) and most authorities strenuously recommend using artemisinins only in combination therapy, both to increase treatment efficacy and prevent the emergence of drug resistance.

Absorption, Fate, and Excretion. The semisynthetic artemisinins have been formulated for oral (dihydroartemisinin, artesunate, and artemether), intramuscular (artesunate and artemether), intravenous (artesunate), and rectal (artesunate) routes. Bioavailability after oral dosing typically is ≤30%. Although artemisinins rapidly achieve peak serum levels; intramuscular administration of the lipid-soluble artemether peaks in 2-6 hours, due to a depot effect at the injection site. Both artesunate and artemether have modest levels of plasma protein binding, ranging from 43% to 82%. These derivatives are extensively metabolized and converted to dihydroartemisinin, which has a plasma $t_{1/2}$ of 1-2 hours (German and Aweeka, 2008). Rectal administration of artesunate has emerged as an important administration route, especially in tropical countries where it can be lifesaving. However, drug bioavailability via rectal administration is highly variable among individual patients (Medhi et al., 2009).

With repeated dosing, artemisinin and artesunate induce their own CYP-mediated metabolism, primarily via CYPs 2B6 and 3A4. This may enhance clearance by up to 5-fold. Recent studies have found no clinically significant pharmacokinetic or toxic interactions between artemisinins and its partner drugs.

Therapeutic Uses. Given their rapid and potent activity against even multidrug-resistant parasites, the artemisinins are valuable for the treatment of severe *P. falciparum* malaria. Intravenous artesunate is more than comparable to a standard quinine regimen, likely possessing higher efficacy and a better safety profile in many patient populations (Rosenthal, 2008). The artemisinins generally are not used alone because of their limited ability to eradicate infection completely. In numerous studies in Africa, South America, and Asia, artemisinins have proven highly effective, when combined with other antimalarials, for the first-line treatment of malaria (Sinclair et al., 2009). Artemisinins should not be used for chemoprophylaxis because of their short $t_{1/2}$, which translates into high recrudescence rates. In the U.S., the Food and Drug Administration (FDA) has approved the use of artemether-lumefantrine for oral treatment of uncomplicated *P. falciparum* malaria. Although useful in treating presumptively chloroquine-resistant *P. vivax*, artemether-lumefantrine does not have a formal FDA-approved indication for this infection. Under an investigational new drug (IND) application, intravenous artesunate is now indicated for the treatment of severe malaria; this drug currently can be obtained through the Centers for Disease Control and Prevention (CDC) Drug Service or CDC Quarantine Stations.

Toxicity and Contraindications. The increasing usage of ACTs has focused attention on the safety profile of artemisinins, especially with regard to potential toxic effects in infants and during the first trimester of pregnancy. In pregnant rats and rabbits, artemisinins can cause increased embryo lethality or malformations early postconception. Preclinical toxicity studies have identified the brain (and brainstem), liver, bone marrow, and fetus as the principal target organs. In patients, the many neurological changes that accompany severe malaria confound the evaluation of drug neurotoxicity; however, no systematic neurological changes were attributable to treatment in patients >5 years of age. As in small animals, patients may develop dose-related and reversible decreases in reticulocyte and neutrophil counts and increases in transaminase levels in patients. About 1 in 3000 patients develops an allergic reaction. Studies of artemisinin treatment during the first trimester have found no evidence of adverse effects on fetal development (Eastman and Fidock, 2009). Nonetheless, out of general concern, it is recommended that ACTs not be used for the treatment of children ≤5 kg or during the first trimester of pregnancy.

ACT Partner Drugs. The short plasma $t_{1/2}$ of artemisinin and its derivatives translates into substantial treatment failure rates when artemisinins are used as monotherapy. Combining an artemisinin derivative with a longer-lasting partner drug assures sustained antimalarial activity. Current ACT regimens that are well tolerated in adults and children ≥5 kg include artemether-lumefantrine, artesunate-mefloquine, artesunate-amodiaquine, artesunate-sulfoxadine-pyrimethamine, and dihydroartemisinin-piperaquine. Artesunate-pyronaridine has also recently completed phase III clinical trials. Combination with mefloquine or sulfadoxine-pyrimethamine is discussed in a separate section. Properties of other partner drugs are discussed later.

Lumefantrine shares structural similarities with the arylaminoalcohol drugs mefloquine and halofantrine (Figure 49–2) and is formulated with artemether (COARTEM).

This combination has proven to be highly effective for the treatment of uncomplicated malaria and is the most widely used first-line antimalarial across Africa. The pharmacokinetic properties of lumefantrine include a large apparent volume of distribution and a terminal elimination $t_{1/2}$ of 4-5 days. Human pharmacokinetic and pharmacodynamic studies correlate the risk of clinical failure (the likelihood to recrudesce) with plasma lumefantrine concentrations falling below 280 ng/mL. These findings, combined with a report of up to 15-fold variability in lumefantrine plasma concentrations in clinical trial volunteers, highlight the importance of appropriate dosing with lumefantrine-containing combinations (Checchi et al., 2006). Administration with a high-fat meal is recommended because it significantly increases absorption. Recently a sweetened dispersible formulation of artemether-lumefantrine (COARTEM *Dispersible*) has been approved for treatment of children. This formulation has comparable pharmacokinetics to crushed tablets and provides substantially improved ease of administration.

Amodiaquine is a congener of chloroquine (Figure 49–2) that is no longer recommended in the U.S. for chemoprophylaxis of *P. falciparum* malaria because of its toxicity (hepatic and agranulocytosis). These adverse events, however, were generally associated with its prophylactic use. A meta-analysis of clinical studies found that therapeutic amodiaquine regimes, with a total dose of up to 35 mg/kg body weight administered over 3 days, were as well tolerated as chloroquine for the treatment of uncomplicated *P. falciparum* malaria (Olliaro and Mussano, 2003). One

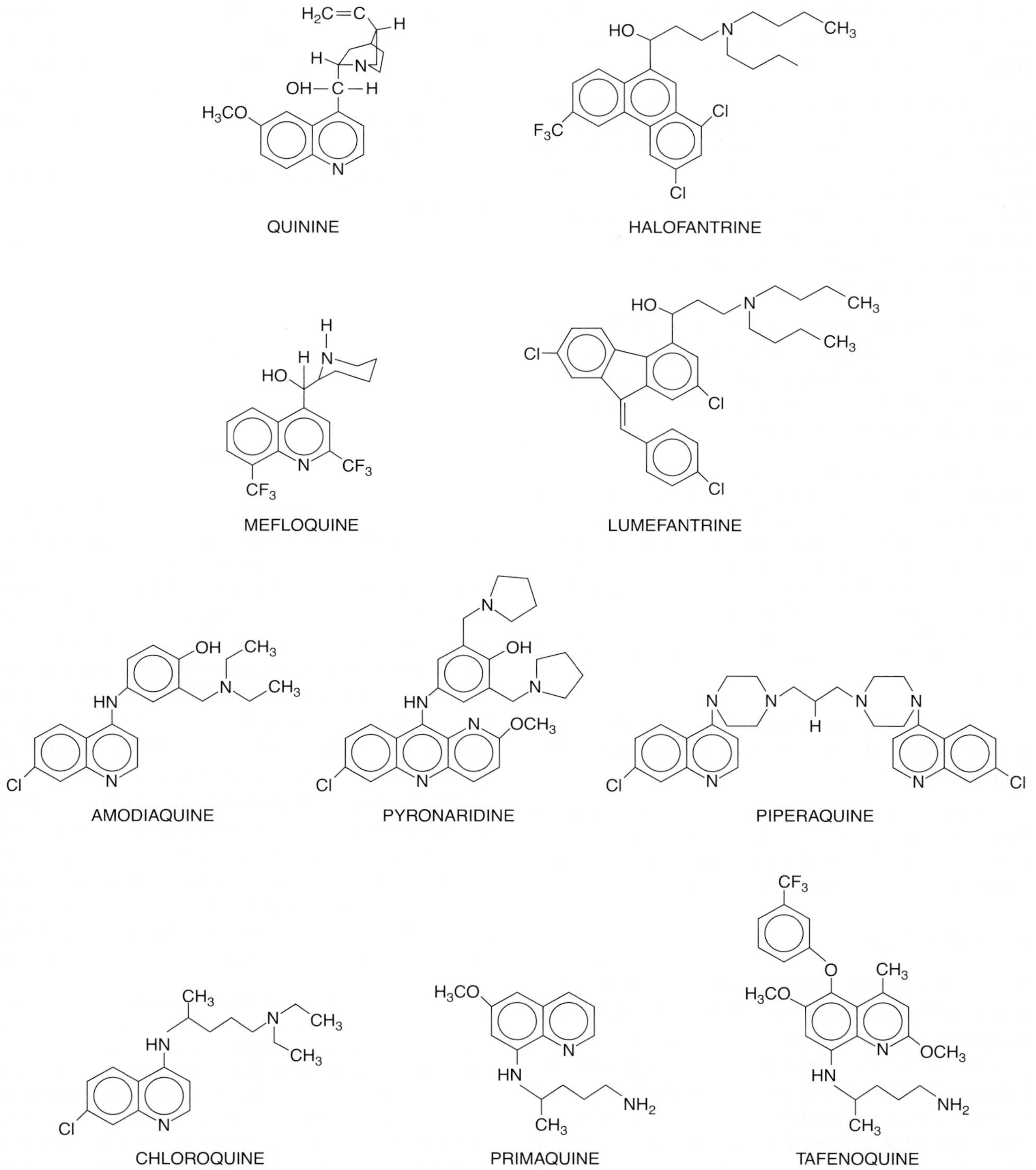

QUININE

HALOFANTRINE

MEFLOQUINE

LUMEFANTRINE

AMODIAQUINE

PYRONARIDINE

PIPERAQUINE

CHLOROQUINE

PRIMAQUINE

TAFENOQUINE

Figure 49–2. *Chemical structure of antimalarial quinolines and related compounds.*

recent study reported an increased risk of neutropenia with amodiaquine therapy in HIV patients receiving antiretroviral therapy (Gasasira et al., 2008).

In vivo, amodiaquine is rapidly converted by hepatic CYPs into monodesethyl-amodiaquine. This metabolite, which retains substantial antimalarial activity, has a plasma $t_{1/2}$ of 9-18 days and reaches a peak concentration of ~500 nM 2 hours after oral administration. By contrast, amodiaquine has a $t_{1/2}$ of ~3 hours, attaining a peak concentration of ~25 nM within 30 minutes of oral administration (Eastman and Fidock, 2009). *In vivo* clearance rates of amodiaquine, however, display a variation between individuals that ranges from 78 to 943 mL/min/kg.

Piperaquine, a potent and well-tolerated bisquinoline compound (Figure 49–2) structurally related to chloroquine, became the primary antimalarial in China during the 1970s and 1980s in response to increasing rates of chloroquine resistance.

Piperaquine has a large volume of distribution and reduced rates of excretion after multiple doses. This lipophilic drug is rapidly absorbed, with a T_{max} (time to reach the highest concentration) of 2 hours after a single dose. In clinical trials, the combination of piperaquine and dihydroartemisinin produced cure rates and cleared fever and parasites in a time frame similar to artesunate-mefloquine (Wells et al., 2009). Piperaquine has the longest plasma $t_{1/2}$ (5 weeks) of all ACT partner drugs, suggesting that piperaquine-dihydroartemisinin might also be effective in reducing rates of reinfection following treatment.

Pyronaridine, an antimalarial structurally related to amodiaquine (Figure 49–2), was developed by the Chinese in the 1970s.

Pyronaridine is well tolerated and highly potent against both *P. falciparum* and *P. vivax*, causing fever to subside in 1-2 days and parasite clearance in 2-3 days. Clinical data from trials of artesunate-pyronaridine should soon be available (Wells et al., 2009).

ATOVAQUONE

History. Based on the antiprotozoal activity of hydroxynaphthoquinones, atovaquone (MEPRON) was developed as a promising synthetic derivative with potent activity against *Plasmodium* species and the opportunistic pathogens *Pneumocystis jiroveci* (previously called *Pneumocystis carinii*) and *Toxoplasma gondii* (Schlitzer, 2007). The FDA approved this compound in 1992 for treatment of mild-to-moderate *P. jiroveci* pneumonia in patients intolerant of trimethoprim-sulfamethoxazole. Subsequent clinical studies in patients with uncomplicated *P. falciparum* malaria revealed that atovaquone produced good initial responses, but parasites recrudesced and were highly atovaquone resistant. In contrast, the combination of atovaquone and proguanil produced high cure rates with minimal toxicity. A fixed combination of atovaquone with proguanil hydrochloride (MALARONE) is available in the U.S. for malaria chemoprophylaxis and for the treatment of uncomplicated *P. falciparum* malaria in adults and children (Boggild et al., 2007).

Chemistry. Atovaquone is a highly lipophilic analog of ubiquinone.

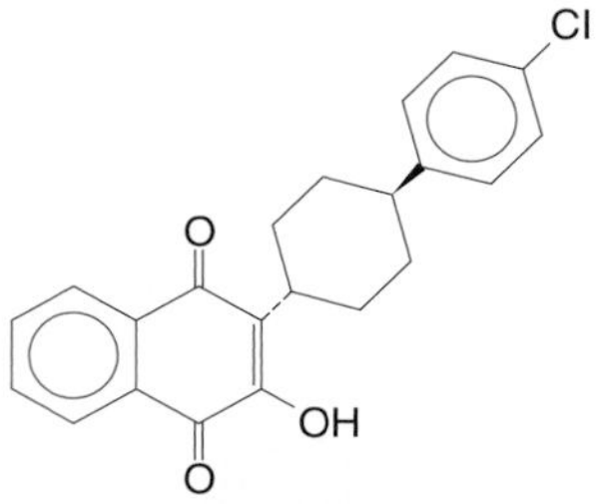

ATOVAQUONE

Mechanisms of Antimalarial Action and Resistance. Atovaquone is highly active against *P. falciparum* asexual blood stage parasites *in vitro* (with low nanomolar activity) and *in vivo* in humans and the *Aotus* primate model. This drug is effective against liver stages of *P. falciparum* but not against *P. vivax* liver stage hypnozoites. Atovaquone acts selectively on the mitochondrial cytochrome bc_1 complex to inhibit electron transport and collapse the mitochondrial membrane potential (Vaidya and Mather, 2009). The primary function of mitochondrial electron transport in *P. falciparum* is to regenerate ubiquinone, which is the electron acceptor for parasite dihydroorotate dehydrogenase, an enzyme essential for pyrimidine biosynthesis in the parasite (Painter et al., 2007). Synergy between proguanil and atovaquone results from the ability of nonmetabolized proguanil to enhance the mitochondrial toxicity of atovaquone (Fivelman et al., 2004; Srivastava et al., 1999).

Resistance to atovaquone alone in *P. falciparum* develops easily *in vitro* and *in vivo*, and it is conferred by single non-synonymous nucleotide polymorphisms in the cytochrome b gene located in the mitochondrial genome (Kessl et al., 2007). In the *Saccharomyces cerevisiae* cytochrome bc_1 complex, atovaquone binding is inhibited by the introduction of resistance mutations found in *P. falciparum*. Similar mutations have been reported in resistant isolates of rodent malarial species, as well as in *T. gondii* and perhaps *P. jiroveci*. Addition of proguanil markedly reduces the frequency of appearance of atovaquone resistance, as based on *in vivo* treatment cure rate. However, once atovaquone resistance is present, the synergy of the partner drug proguanil diminishes. In the key mutation associated with clinical atovaquone-proguanil resistance, tyrosine is replaced by serine, cysteine, or asparagine at codon 268 (Y268S/C/N) of the cytochrome b gene. Reports of atovaquone-proguanil treatment failures are rare. However, when atovaquone-proguanil treatment fails because of parasite resistance, the recurrent malarial attack commonly occurs ~20-30 days after treatment initiation. Treatment with different drugs should then be started. Earlier treatment failures (during the first 2 weeks after treatment initiation) are more likely related to lack of compliance or inadequate drug levels (Musset et al., 2006; Rose et al., 2008).

Absorption, Fate, and Excretion. Atovaquone absorption after a single oral dose is slow, erratic, and variable due to its highly lipophilic nature and low aqueous solubility. Absorption improves when the drug is taken with a fatty meal (Boggild et al., 2007). More than 99% of the drug is bound to plasma protein, and cerebrospinal fluid levels are <1% of those in plasma. Profiles of drug concentration versus time often show a double peak, albeit with considerable variability. The first peak appears in 1-8 hours, whereas the second occurs 1-4 days after a single dose. This pattern suggests an enterohepatic circulation. In the absence of a CYP-inducing second medication, humans do not metabolize atovaquone significantly. The drug is excreted in bile, and >94% of the drug is recovered unchanged in feces; only traces appear in the urine. Atovaquone has a reported elimination $t_{1/2}$ from plasma of 2-3 days in adults and 1-2 days in children. Clearance is unaffected by dose or co-administration of proguanil (Boggild et al., 2007).

Therapeutic Uses. Atovaquone-proguanil is used for malaria chemoprophylaxis in adults and children ≥11 kg and for treatment of uncomplicated *P. falciparum* malaria in adults and children ≥5 kg.

A tablet containing a fixed dose of 250 mg atovaquone and 100 mg proguanil hydrochloride, taken orally, is highly effective and safe in a 3-day regimen for treating mild-to-moderate attacks of chloroquine- or sulfadoxine-pyrimethamine-resistant *P. falciparum* malaria (Looareesuwan et al., 1999). Although the same regimen followed by a primaquine course is effective in treatment of *P. vivax* malaria (Lacy et al., 2002), evidence for atovaquone-proguanil efficacy as treatment of non–*P. falciparum* malaria is limited (Boggild et al., 2007). The CDC does not recommend the combination for non-*P. falciparum* treatment, except for malaria caused by chloroquine-resistant *P. vivax*. Atovaquone-proguanil is a standard agent for malaria chemoprophylaxis. It can be discontinued 1 week after leaving the endemic area because both components are active against liver stage parasites. Experience in prevention of non–*P. falciparum* malaria is also limited (Ling et al., 2002). *P. vivax* infection may occur after drug discontinuation, indicating imperfect activity against exo-erythrocytic stages of this parasite.

Toxicity. Atovaquone may cause side effects (abdominal pain, nausea, vomiting, diarrhea, headache, rash) that require cessation of therapy. Vomiting and diarrhea may decrease drug absorption, resulting in therapeutic failure. However, readministration of this drug within an hour of vomiting may still be effective in patients with *P. falciparum* malaria. Atovaquone occasionally causes transient elevations of serum transaminase or amylase.

Precautions and Contraindications. Although atovaquone is generally considered to be safe, it needs further evaluation in children <11 kg, pregnant women, and lactating mothers. Accordingly, although the drug is not formally recommended for these individuals, the risks and benefits of its use (both as chemoprophylaxis and treatment) should be considered carefully for individual patients, taking known toxicities into account. Preclinical evaluations for carcinogenicity, mutagenicity, and teratogenicity have been negative. Atovaquone may compete with certain drugs for binding to plasma proteins, and therapy with rifampin, a potent inducer of CYP-mediated drug metabolism, can reduce plasma levels of atovaquone substantially, whereas atovaquone may raise plasma levels of rifampin. Co-administration with tetracycline is associated with a 40% reduction in plasma concentration of atovaquone.

DIAMINOPYRIMIDINES

History. Based on their structural analogy with the antimalarial proguanil (see section on proguanil), large numbers of 2,4-diaminopyrimidines were tested for inhibitory activity against malarial parasites, leading to the identification of the potent antimalarial agent pyrimethamine. Studies also observed marked antimalarial synergy between sulfonamides and proguanil. Accordingly, pyrimethamine was formulated and marketed as a fixed combination with sulfadoxine, a sulfonamide with pharmacokinetics that match those of pyrimethamine. For several decades sulfadoxine-pyrimethamine (FANSIDAR) has been a primary treatment for uncomplicated *P. falciparum* malaria, especially against chloroquine-resistant strains, but widespread resistance now seriously compromises its efficacy and it is no longer recommended for the treatment of uncomplicated malaria.

CH_3CH_2 N NH_2 N NH_2 Cl

PYRIMETHAMINE

Mechanisms of Antimalarial Action and Resistance. Pyrimethamine is a slow-acting blood schizontocide with antimalarial effects *in vivo* similar to those of proguanil, resulting from inhibition of folate biosynthesis in *Plasmodium*. However, pyrimethamine has greater antimalarial potency, and its $t_{1/2}$ is much longer than that of cycloguanil, the active metabolite of proguanil. The efficacy of pyrimethamine against hepatic forms of *P. falciparum* is less than that of proguanil, and at therapeutic doses pyrimethamine fails to eradicate *P. vivax* hypnozoites or gametocytes of any *Plasmodium* species. It increases the number of circulating *P. falciparum* mature infecting gametocytes, likely leading to increased transmission to mosquitoes during the period of treatment.

The 2,4-diaminopyrimidines more potently inhibit the *Plasmodium* dihydrofolate reductase compared to the mammalian enzyme. Unlike its counterpart in human cells, the malarial dihydrofolate reductase resides on the same polypeptide chain as thymidylate synthase and, importantly, protein production is not increased in response to inhibition. The latter property favors the selective anti-plasmodial toxicity of pyrimethamine (Zhang and Rathod, 2002).

Synergy of pyrimethamine and the sulfonamides or sulfones results from inhibition of two key metabolic steps in folate biosynthesis in the parasite:

- the utilization of *p*-aminobenzoic acid for the synthesis of dihydropteroic acid, which is catalyzed by dihydropteroate synthase and inhibited by sulfonamides
- the reduction of dihydrofolate to tetrahydrofolate, which is catalyzed by dihydrofolate reductase and inhibited by pyrimethamine (Figure 52–2).

Dietary *p*-aminobenzoic acid or folate may affect the therapeutic response to antifolates. Both of these metabolites can be imported by the malarial parasite and can reduce drug efficacy substantially (Hyde, 2007). Resistance to pyrimethamine has developed in regions of prolonged or extensive drug use and can be attributed to mutations in dihydrofolate reductase that decrease the binding affinity of pyrimethamine (Gregson and Plowe, 2005). Interestingly, the pattern of amino acid substitutions is different in parasites resistant to cycloguanil, even though cross-resistance can occur between these structurally related inhibitors of plasmodial dihydrofolate reductase. The key mutation associated with pyrimethamine resistance is the substitution of asparagine for serine at codon 108 (S108N). The stepwise accumulation of additional single-amino-acid changes at codons 51, 59, and 164 is associated with progressively increasing resistance, as determined with *P. falciparum* isolates and with recombinant proteins. The triple mutant N51I/C59R/S108N (predominant in Africa) and the quadruple mutant N51I/C59R/S108N/I164L (predominant in Southeast Asia) exhibit high levels of pyrimethamine resistance and contribute to pyrimethamine-sulfadoxine therapeutic failure. Remarkably, studies exploring the mutational trajectories leading to the most resistant quadruple mutant N51I/C59R/S108N/I164L suggest a specific ordering of mutational events that balance the acquisition of resistance with the maintenance of pathogen fitness (Lozovsky et al., 2009). These studies also suggest that this quadruple mutant is substantially less fit in the absence of drugs when compared to its wild-type counterpart. Compensatory mechanisms might therefore be necessary to alleviate this fitness cost. An increase in the number of copy of the GTP cyclohydrolase I gene, which encodes the first enzyme in the *Plasmodium* folate biosynthesis pathway, is closely associated with the dihydrofolate reductase I164L mutation, suggesting a potential compensatory function (Nair et al., 2008).

Absorption, Fate, and Distribution. After oral administration, pyrimethamine is slowly but completely absorbed, reaching peak plasma levels in 2-6 hours. The compound is significantly distributed in the tissues and is ~90% bound to plasma proteins (German and Aweeka, 2008). Pyrimethamine is slowly eliminated from plasma with a $t_{1/2}$ of 85-100 hours. Concentrations that are suppressive for responsive *Plasmodium* strains remain in the blood for ~2 weeks, but levels are lower in patients with active infection. Several metabolites of pyrimethamine appear in the urine; however, their identities and antimalarial properties have not been fully characterized. Pyrimethamine also enters the milk of nursing mothers.

Therapeutic Uses. Pyrimethamine-sulfadoxine is no longer recommended for the treatment of uncomplicated malaria or for chemoprophylaxis due to increasing drug resistance. However, for those living in malaria-endemic areas, some still recommend it for the intermittent preventive treatment of malaria in pregnancy, and it is being evaluated for intermittent preventive treatment in infants (Aponte et al., 2009). Pyrimethamine is typically administered with either a sulfonamide or sulfone to enhance its antifolate activity. Most malaria-endemic areas currently have a high prevalence of pyrimethamine-resistant parasites.

Toxicity, Precautions, and Contraindications. Antimalarial doses of pyrimethamine alone cause minimal toxicity except for occasional skin rashes and reduced hematopoiesis. Excessive doses can produce a megaloblastic anemia, resembling that of folate deficiency, which responds readily to drug withdrawal or treatment with folinic acid. At high doses, pyrimethamine is teratogenic in animals, and in humans the related combination, trimethoprim-sulfamethoxazole, may cause birth defects (Hernandez-Diaz et al., 2000).

Sulfonamides or sulfones, rather than pyrimethamine, usually account for the toxicity associated with coadministration of these antifolate drugs. The combination of pyrimethamine and sulfadoxine is no longer recommended for malaria chemoprophylaxis because in ~1 in 5000 to 1 in 8000 individuals, this combination causes severe and even fatal cutaneous reactions, such as erythema multiforme, Stevens-Johnson syndrome, or toxic epidermal necrolysis. It has also been associated with serum sickness–type reactions, urticaria, exfoliative dermatitis, and hepatitis. Pyrimethamine-sulfadoxine is contraindicated for individuals with previous reactions to sulfonamides, for lactating mothers, and for infants <2 months of age. Administration of pyrimethamine with dapsone (MALOPRIM), a drug combination unavailable in the U.S., has occasionally been associated with agranulocytosis.

PROGUANIL

History. Proguanil is the common name for chloroguanide, a biguanide derivative that emerged in 1945 as a product of British antimalarial research. The antimalarial activity of proguanil eventually was ascribed to cycloguanil, a cyclic triazine metabolite and selective inhibitor of the bifunctional plasmodial dihydrofolate reductase-thymidylate synthetase that is crucial for parasite *de novo* purine and pyrimidine synthesis. Indeed, investigation of compounds bearing a structural resemblance to cycloguanil resulted in the development of antimalarial dihydrofolate reductase inhibitors such as pyrimethamine. Accrued evidence also indicates that proguanil itself has intrinsic antimalarial activity independent of its metabolite's effect on parasite dihydrofolate reductase-thymidylate synthetase (Fidock and Wellems, 1997).

Chemistry. Proguanil and its triazine metabolite cycloguanil have the following chemical structures:

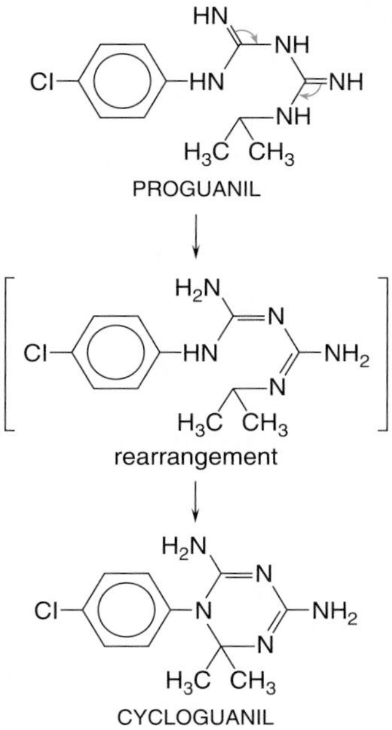

PROGUANIL

rearrangement

CYCLOGUANIL

Proguanil has the widest margin of safety of a large series of antimalarial biguanide analogs examined. Dihalogen substitution in positions 3 and 4 of the benzene ring yields chlorproguanil, a more potent prodrug than proguanil. Cycloguanil, the metabolite, is structurally related to pyrimethamine.

Mechanisms of Antimalarial Action and Resistance. In drug-sensitive *P. falciparum* malaria, proguanil exerts activity against both the primary liver stages and the asexual red blood cell stages, thus adequately controlling the acute attack and usually eradicating the infection. Proguanil is also active against acute *P. vivax* malaria, but because the latent tissue stages of *P. vivax* are unaffected, relapses may occur after the drug is withdrawn. Proguanil treatment does not destroy gametocytes, but oocytes in the gut of the mosquito can fail to develop normally.

Cycloguanil selectively inhibits the bifunctional dihydrofolate reductase–thymidylate synthetase of sensitive plasmodia, causing inhibition of DNA synthesis and depletion of folate cofactors (Kamchonwongpaisan et al., 2004). As referred to earlier, a series of amino acid changes near the dihydrofolate reductase–binding site have been identified that cause resistance to cycloguanil, pyrimethamine, or both (Gregson and Plowe, 2005). Specifically, resistance to cycloguanil (and chlorcycloguanil) can be linked to mutations leading to paired A16V/S108T substitutions in *Plasmodium* dihydrofolate reductase. In addition, cross-resistance between cycloguanil and pyrimethamine has been observed *in vitro* for both the triple (N51I/C59R/S108N) and quadruple (N51I/C59R/S108N/I164L) dihydrofolate reductase–thymidylate synthetase mutants, prevalent in Africa and South America, respectively (Peterson et al., 1990). Malarial isolates demonstrate varying degrees of cross-resistance to cycloguanil and pyrimethamine, indicating that the evolution of mutation patterns in individual organisms during treatment may be quite complex.

The presence of *Plasmodium* dihydrofolate reductase is not required for the intrinsic antimalarial activity of proguanil or chlorproguanil (Fidock and Wellems, 1997); however, the molecular basis for this alternative activity remains enigmatic. Proguanil as the biguanide accentuates the mitochondrial membrane-potential-collapsing action of atovaquone against *P. falciparum* but displays no such activity by itself (Vaidya and Mather, 2009) (see section on atovaquone). In contrast to cycloguanil, resistance to the parent drug, proguanil, either alone or in combination with atovaquone, is not well documented.

Absorption, Fate, and Excretion. Proguanil is slowly but adequately absorbed from the GI tract. After a single oral dose, peak plasma concentrations usually are attained within 5 hours. The mean plasma elimination $t_{1/2}$ is ~180-200 hours or longer (German and Aweeka, 2008).

The metabolism of proguanil in mammals cosegregates with mephenytoin oxidation polymorphisms, controlled by isoforms in the CYP2C subfamily. Only ~3% of whites are deficient in this oxidation phenotype, contrasted with ~20% of Asians and Kenyans. Proguanil is oxidized to two major metabolites, cycloguanil and an inactive 4-chlorophenylbiguanide. On a 200 mg daily dosage regimen, plasma levels of cycloguanil in extensive metabolizers exceed the therapeutic range, whereas cycloguanil levels in poor metabolizers fail to reach a therapeutic level. Proguanil itself does not accumulate appreciably in tissues during long-term administration, except in red blood cells where its concentration is about three times that in plasma. The inactive metabolite 4-chlorophenyl-biguanide is not readily detected in plasma but appears in increased quantities in the urine of poor proguanil metabolizers. In humans, 40-60% of the absorbed proguanil is excreted in urine, either as the parent drug or as the active metabolite.

Therapeutic Uses. Proguanil as a single agent is not available in the U.S. but has been prescribed as chemoprophylaxis in England and Europe for individuals traveling to malarious areas in Africa. Strains of *P. falciparum* resistant to proguanil emerge rapidly in areas where the drug is used exclusively, but breakthrough infections may also result from deficient conversion of proguanil to its active antimalarial metabolite. Proguanil has been reported to be ineffective against multidrug-resistant strains of *P. falciparum* in Thailand and New Guinea. This drug can protect against chloroquine and pyrimethamine-sulfadoxine resistant strains of *P. falciparum* found in sub-Saharan Africa.

Proguanil is effective and tolerated well in combination with atovaquone, once daily for 3 days, to treat drug-resistant strains of *P. falciparum* or *P. vivax* (see section on atovaquone). Indeed, this drug combination has been successful in Southeast Asia, where highly drug-resistant strains of *P. falciparum* prevail. *P. falciparum* readily develops clinical resistance to monotherapy with either proguanil or atovaquone; however resistance to the combination is uncommon unless the strain is initially resistant to atovaquone. In contrast, some strains resistant to proguanil do respond to proguanil plus atovaquone.

Toxicity and Side Effects. In chemoprophylactic doses of 200-300 mg daily, proguanil causes relatively few adverse effects, except occasional nausea and diarrhea. Large doses (≥1 g daily) may cause vomiting, abdominal pain, diarrhea, hematuria, and the transient appearance of epithelial cells and casts in the urine. Gross accidental or deliberate overdose (as much as 15 g) has failed to produce lasting sequelae. Doses as high as 700 mg twice daily have been taken for >2 weeks without serious toxicity. Proguanil is considered safe for use during pregnancy. It is remarkably safe when used in conjunction with other antimalarial drugs such as chloroquine, atovaquone, tetracyclines, and other antifolates.

QUINOLINES AND RELATED COMPOUNDS

Quinolines have been the mainstay of antimalarial chemotherapy starting with quinine nearly 400 years ago. In the last century, legions of related compounds were synthesized and tested for antimalarial activity. These efforts produced several drugs for the chemoprophylaxis and treatment of malaria. The most important of these are shown in Figure 49–2.

Chloroquine and Hydroxychloroquine

History. Chloroquine (ARALEN) is one of a large series of 4-aminoquinolines synthesized as part of the extensive cooperative program of antimalarial research in the U.S. during World War II. Chloroquine proved most promising and was released for field trial. When hostilities ceased, it was discovered that the compound had been synthesized and studied as early as 1934 under the name of Resochin at the Bayer laboratories in Germany but had been rejected because of toxicity in avian models.

Chemistry. The d-, l-, and dl- forms of chloroquine (see structure in Figure 49–2) have equal potency against *P. lophurae* malaria (a duck parasite), but the d-isomer is somewhat less toxic than the l-isomer in mammals. A chlorine atom attached to position 7 of the quinoline ring confers the most potent antimalarial activity in both avian and human malarias. Research on the structure-activity relationships of chloroquine and related alkaloid compounds continues in an effort to find new effective antimalarials with improved safety profiles that can be used successfully against chloroquine- and multidrug-resistant strains of *P. falciparum*. One example is the synthesis of short-chain derivatives that can demonstrate full efficacy against chloroquine-resistant strains of *P. falciparum*. Another important example is piperaquine, a bisquinoline that was extensively used in China to treat chloroquine-resistant malaria. It is highly efficacious in combination with dihydroartemisinin (Davis et al., 2005); see earlier section on artemisinin-based combination therapies.

Hydroxychloroquine, in which one of the *N*-ethyl substituents of chloroquine is *β*-hydroxylated, is essentially equivalent to chloroquine against *P. falciparum* malaria. This analog is preferred over chloroquine for treatment of mild rheumatoid arthritis and lupus erythematosus because, in the high doses required, it may cause less ocular toxicity. Care should be taken when these compounds are administered to patients with known G6PD deficiency.

Mechanisms of Action and Resistance. Asexual malarial parasites flourish in host erythrocytes by digesting hemoglobin in their acidic digestive vacuoles, a process that generates free radicals and iron-bound heme (ferriprotoporphyrin IX) as highly reactive by-products (Goldberg, 2005). Perhaps aided by histidine-rich proteins and lipids, heme is sequestered as an insoluble, chemically inert malarial pigment termed *hemozoin*. Many theories for the mechanism of action of chloroquine have been advanced (Valderramos and Fidock, 2006). Current evidence suggests that quinolines interfere with heme detoxification. Chloroquine, a weak base, concentrates in the highly acidic digestive vacuoles of susceptible *Plasmodium*, where it binds to heme and disrupts its sequestration. Failure to inactivate heme or even enhanced toxicity of drug-heme complexes is thought to kill the parasites via oxidative damage to membranes, digestive proteases, or other critical biomolecules. Other quinolines such as quinine, amodiaquine, and mefloquine, as well as other amino alcohol analogs (lumefantrine, halofantrine) and mannich base analogs (pyronaridine), may act by a similar mechanism, although differences in their actions have been proposed (Bray et al., 2005; Eastman and Fidock, 2009).

Resistance of erythrocytic asexual forms of *P. falciparum* to antimalarial quinolines, especially chloroquine, now is common in most parts of the world (Figure 49–3). Reports of chloroquine failures in the treatment of *P. vivax* are fairly common in Indonesia, East Timor, and Papua New Guinea, in which case alternative treatments (mefloquine, or quinine plus doxycycline or tetracycline, or atovaquone-proguanil) should be considered (Price et al., 2009). Chloroquine-resistant *P. vivax* has also been recently detected in Ethiopia, where *P. vivax* is an important cause of morbidity (Yeshiwondim et al., 2010). Chloroquine-resistant *P. vivax* isolates do not appear to have significant alterations in their *pfcrt* ortholog and may have a different resistance mechanism.

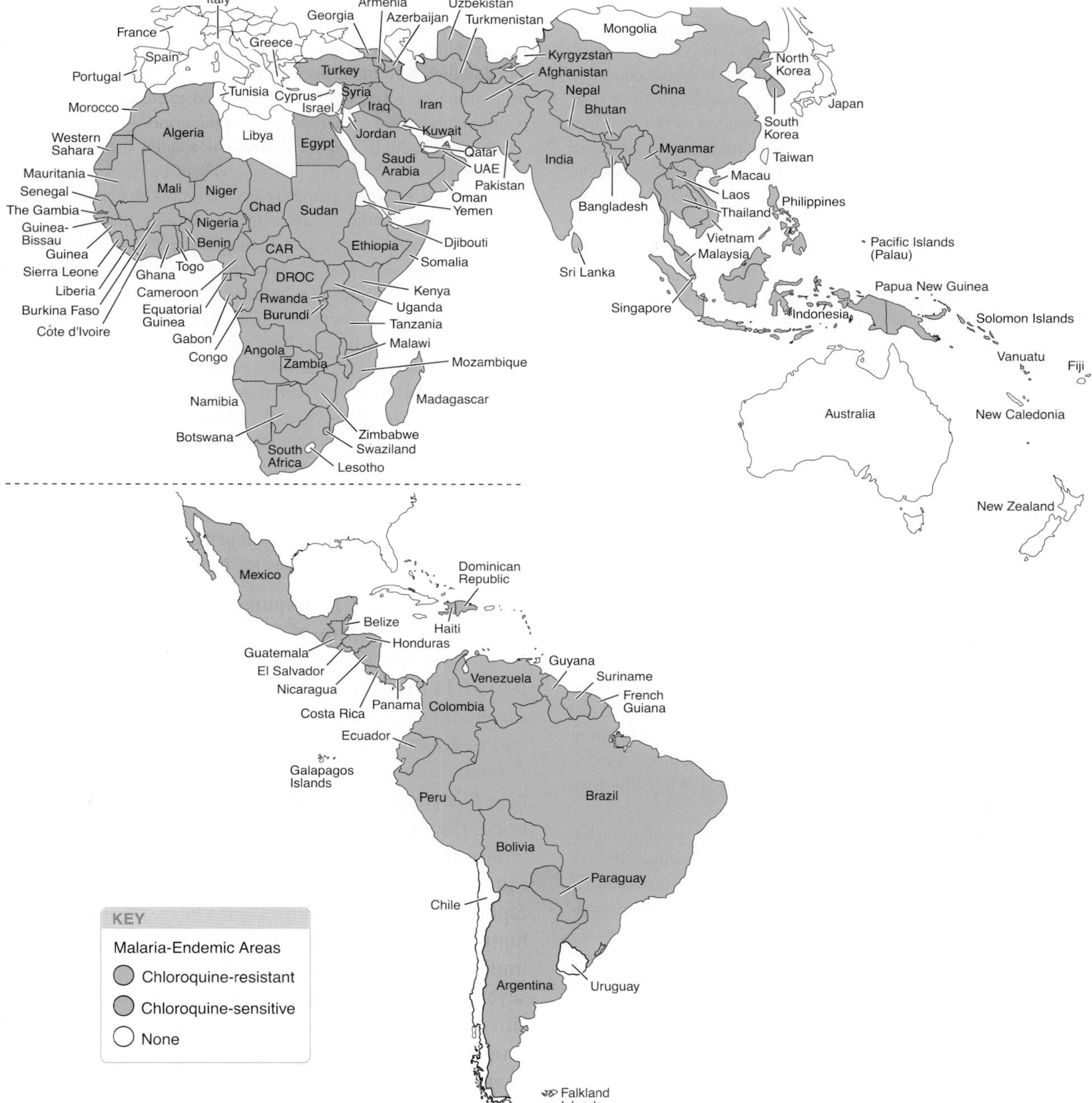

Figure 49–3. *Malaria-endemic countries in the Americas (bottom) and in Africa, the Middle East, Asia, and the South Pacific (top), 2007.* CAR, Central African Republic; DCOR, Democratic Republic of the Congo; UAE, United Arab Emirates. (Reproduced with permission from Anthony S. Fauci, Eugene Braunwald, Dennis L Kasper, Stephen L Hauser, Dan L Longo, J Larry Jameson, and Joseph Loscalzo, Eds. *Harrison's Principles of Internal Medicine, 17 ed.* McGraw-Hill, Inc., New York, 2008. Figure 203-2, p. 1282.)

Forty years ago, Fitch and coworkers noted that chloroquine-sensitive *P. falciparum* parasites concentrated the drug to higher levels than did chloroquine-resistant organisms (Fitch et al., 1969). A parasite-encoded efflux mechanism may account for the reduced levels of chloroquine in the digestive vacuoles of chloroquine-resistant parasites (Martin et al., 2009; Valderramos and Fidock, 2006).

By studying the progeny of a genetic cross between a chloroquine-sensitive clone and a chloroquine-resistant clone, Wellems, Fidock, and colleagues identified a polymorphic gene (*pfcrt*, for *P. falciparum* chloroquine resistance transporter) that segregates with chloroquine resistance. Geographically distinct *pfcrt* alleles, possessing 4-8 point mutations compared to the invariant chloroquine-sensitive allele, were found to be highly associated with chloroquine resistance in clinical field isolates from across the malaria-endemic areas of the globe (Fidock et al., 2000). Multiple mutations are needed to confer resistance, including the K76T mutation that is ubiquitous to chloroquine-resistant strains. The *pfcrt* gene encodes a putative transporter that resides in the membrane of the acidic digestive vacuole, the site of hemoglobin degradation and chloroquine action. Its physiological function, however, remains unknown. Chloroquine binding and accumulation studies, with genetically modified isogenic lines differing in their *pfcrt* allele, suggest that mutant *pfcrt* confers chloroquine resistance by actively effluxing chloroquine away from its heme target in the digestive vacuole, seemingly via an energy-dependent process (Sanchez et al., 2007). Heterologous expression of codon-adjusted *pfcrt* alleles in *Xenopus laevis* oocytes has recently provided compelling evidence that mutant PfCRT can efflux chloroquine, and has found that this property was not solely dependent on the K76T mutation (Martin et al., 2009). Genomic studies suggest that *pfcrt* has been under intense selection pressure in recent decades, consistent with its role as the primary resistance determinant and the prevalence of chloroquine use in populations exposed to parasites (Mu et al, 2010). Studies from Malawi have found that mutant *pfcrt* alleles essentially disappear upon prolonged cessation of chloroquine use. This implies that mutant *pfcrt* alleles can impart a significant fitness cost to the organism. This cost of fitness results in attrition of mutant forms in areas where polyclonal infections are common and subjects are sufficiently immune such that a substantial proportion of infections are not subject to the pressure of drug selection.

In addition to chloroquine, variant *pfcrt* alleles may impact parasite susceptibility to other antimalarials. As an example, the 7G8 allele, representative of *pfcrt* sequences from South America and the Pacific region, imparts low-level cross resistance to monodesethylamodiaquine, the active metabolite of amodiaquine (Sidhu et al., 2002). Cross-resistance to quinine has also been observed with some *pfcrt* alleles in certain genetic backgrounds. In contrast, mutant *pfcrt* increases parasite susceptibility to lumefantrine and artemisinin derivatives, which bodes well for the use of artemether-lumefantrine in areas where the prevalence of mutant *pfcrt* is high (Sisowath et al., 2009). In addition to PfCRT, the P-glycoprotein transporter encoded by *pfmdr1*, and other transporters including PfMRP, may play a modulatory role in chloroquine resistance (Duraisingh and Cowman, 2005, Raj et al., 2009), and the glutathione system also could contribute (Ginsburg and Golenser, 2003).

Absorption, Fate, and Excretion. Chloroquine is well absorbed from the GI tract and rapidly from intramuscular and subcutaneous sites. This drug extensively sequesters in tissues, particularly liver, spleen, kidney, lung, melanin-containing tissues, and, to a lesser extent, brain and spinal cord. Chloroquine binds moderately (60%) to plasma proteins and undergoes appreciable biotransformation via hepatic CYPs to two active metabolites, desethylchloroquine and bisdesethylchloroquine (Ducharme and Farinotti, 1996). These metabolites may reach plasma concentrations of 40% and 10% of that of chloroquine, respectively. The renal clearance of chloroquine is about half of its total systemic clearance. Unchanged chloroquine and desethylchloroquine account for >50% and 25% of the urinary drug products, respectively, and the renal excretion of both compounds is increased by acidification of the urine.

Both in adults and in children, chloroquine exhibits complex pharmacokinetics such that plasma levels of the drug shortly after dosing are determined primarily by the rate of distribution rather than the rate of elimination (Krishna and White, 1996). Because of extensive tissue binding, a loading dose is required to achieve effective concentrations in plasma. After parenteral administration, rapid entry into the bloodstream together with slow exit from this compartment can result in transiently high and potentially lethal concentrations of the drug in plasma. Hence, parenteral chloroquine is given either slowly by constant intravenous infusion or in small divided doses by the subcutaneous or intramuscular route. Chloroquine is safer when given orally because the rates of absorption and distribution are more closely matched. Peak plasma levels are achieved in ~3-5 hours after dosing by this route. The $t_{1/2}$ of chloroquine increases from a few days to weeks as plasma levels decline, reflecting release of drug from extensive tissue stores. The terminal $t_{1/2}$ ranges from 30 to 60 days, and traces of the drug can be found in the urine for years after a therapeutic regimen.

Therapeutic Uses. Chloroquine is highly effective against the erythrocytic forms of *P. vivax, P. ovale, P. malariae, P. knowlesi*, and chloroquine-sensitive strains of *P. falciparum*. For infections caused by *P. ovale* and *P. malariae,* it remains the agent of choice for chemoprophylaxis and treatment. Chloroquine is also widely used to treat *P. vivax;* however, as mentioned earlier, resistant strains have been detected, mostly in Asia and the Pacific region. For *P. falciparum* this drug has been largely replaced by artemisinin-based combination therapies (Eastman and Fidock, 2009). Gametocytocidal activity has been reported for the four main *Plasmodium* species infecting humans, with activity against *P. falciparum* restricted to immature gametocytes exposed to concentrations that are several fold higher than those effective against drug-sensitive asexual blood stage *P. falciparum* parasites. The drug has no activity against latent hypnozoite forms of *P. vivax* or *P. ovale*.

Chloroquine is inexpensive and safe, but its usefulness has declined across most malaria-endemic regions of the world because of the spread of chloroquine-resistant *P. falciparum*. Except in areas where resistant strains of *P. vivax* are reported, chloroquine is very effective in chemoprophylaxis or treatment of acute attacks of malaria caused by *P. vivax, P. ovale*, and *P. malariae* (Table 49–3). Chloroquine has no activity against primary or latent liver stages of the parasite. To prevent relapses in *P. vivax* and *P. ovale* infections, primaquine can be given either with chloroquine or used after a patient leaves an endemic area. Chloroquine rapidly controls the clinical symptoms and parasitemia of acute malarial attacks. Most patients become completely afebrile within 24-48 hours after receiving therapeutic doses, and thick smears of peripheral blood generally are negative by 48-72 hours. If patients fail to respond during the second day of chloroquine therapy, resistant strains should be suspected and therapy instituted with quinine plus tetracycline or doxycycline, or atovaquone-proguanil, or artemether-lumefantrine, or mefloquine if the others are not available. Although chloroquine can be given safely by parenteral routes to comatose or vomiting patients, quinidine gluconate usually is given in the U.S. In comatose children, chloroquine is well absorbed and effective when given through a nasogastric tube. Tables 49–2 and 49–3 provide information about recommended chemoprophylactic and therapeutic dosage regimens involving the use of chloroquine. These regimens are subject to modification according to clinical judgment, geographic patterns of chloroquine resistance, and regional usage.

Chloroquine and its analogs are also used to treat certain nonmalarial conditions, including hepatic amebiasis. Chloroquine and hydroxychloroquine have also been used as secondary drugs to treat a variety of chronic diseases because both alkaloids concentrate in lysosomes and have anti-inflammatory properties. Thus, these compounds, often together with other agents, have clinical efficacy in rheumatoid arthritis, systemic lupus erythematosus, discoid lupus, sarcoidosis, and photosensitivity diseases such as porphyria cutanea tarda and severe polymorphous light eruption.

Toxicity and Side Effects. Taken in proper doses and for recommended total durations, chloroquine is very safe. However, its safety margin is narrow, and a single dose of 30 mg/kg may be fatal (Taylor and White, 2004).

Acute chloroquine toxicity is encountered most frequently when therapeutic or high doses are administered too rapidly by parenteral routes. Toxic manifestations relate primarily to the cardiovascular system and the CNS. Cardiovascular effects include hypotension, vasodilation, suppressed myocardial function, cardiac arrhythmias, and eventual cardiac arrest. Confusion, convulsions, and coma may also result from overdose. Chloroquine doses of >5 g given parenterally usually are fatal. Prompt treatment with mechanical ventilation, epinephrine, and diazepam may be lifesaving.

Doses of chloroquine used for oral therapy of the acute malarial attack may cause GI upset, headache, visual disturbances, and urticaria. Pruritus also occurs, most commonly among dark-skinned persons. Prolonged treatment with suppressive doses occasionally causes side effects such as headache, blurring of vision, diplopia, confusion, convulsions, lichenoid skin eruptions, bleaching of hair, widening of the QRS interval, and T-wave abnormalities. These complications usually disappear soon after the drug is withheld. Rare instances of hemolysis and blood dyscrasias have been reported. Chloroquine may cause discoloration of nail beds and mucous membranes. This drug has also been reported to interfere with the immunogenicity of certain vaccines (Pappaioanou et al, 1986).

High daily doses of chloroquine or hydroxychloroquine (>250 mg) leading to cumulative total doses of >1 g/kg, such as those used for treatment of diseases other than malaria, can result in irreversible retinopathy and ototoxicity. Retinopathy presumably is related to drug accumulation in melanin containing tissues and can be avoided if the daily dose is ≤250 mg (Rennie, 1993). Prolonged therapy with high doses of chloroquine or hydroxychloroquine also can cause toxic myopathy, cardiopathy, and peripheral neuropathy. These reactions improve if the drug is withdrawn promptly (Estes et al., 1987). Rarely, neuropsychiatric disturbances, including suicide, may be related to overdose.

Precautions and Contraindications. Chloroquine is not recommended for treating individuals who have epilepsy or myasthenia gravis. This drug should be used cautiously if at all in the presence of advanced liver disease or severe GI, neurological, or blood disorders. In individuals with decreased renal function, dosage should be adjusted to avoid elevated plasma concentrations. In rare cases, chloroquine can cause hemolysis in patients with G6PD deficiency (see later section on primaquine). Concomitant use of gold or phenylbutazone (no longer available in the U.S.) with chloroquine, in the treatment of rheumatoid arthritis, should be avoided because of the tendency of all three agents to produce dermatitis. Chloroquine should not be prescribed for patients with psoriasis or other exfoliative skin conditions because it can cause severe reactions. Because of the danger of cutaneous reactions, it should also not be used to treat malaria in patients with porphyria cutanea tarda; however it can be used in lower doses for treatment of manifestations of this form of porphyria. Chloroquine inhibits CYP2D6 and interacts with a variety of different drugs. It attenuates the efficacy of the yellow fever vaccine when administered at the same time. It should not be given with mefloquine because of increased risk of seizures and lack of added benefit. Most important, chloroquine opposes the action of anticonvulsants and increases the risk of ventricular arrhythmias when co-administered with amiodarone or halofantrine. By increasing plasma levels of digoxin and cyclosporine, chloroquine also can increase the risk of toxicity from these agents. Patients receiving long-term, high-dose therapy should undergo ophthalmological and neurological evaluations every 3-6 months.

Quinine and Quinidine

History. The medicinal use of quinine dates back >350 years (Rocco, 2003). Quinine is the chief alkaloid of cinchona, the powdered bark of the South American cinchona tree, otherwise known as Peruvian, Jesuit's, or Cardinal's bark. It had been used by indigenous Peruvians to treat shivering. In 1633, an Augustinian monk named Calancha, of Lima, Peru, first wrote that a powder of cinchona "given as a beverage, cures the fevers and tertians." By 1640, cinchona was used to treat fevers in Europe. The Jesuit fathers were the main importers and distributors of cinchona in Europe.

For almost two centuries the bark was employed for medicine as a powder, extract, or infusion. In 1820, Pelletier and Caventou isolated quinine from cinchona. Quinine still is a mainstay for treating attacks of chloroquine- and multidrug-resistant *P. falciparum* malaria (Table 49–3). However, combination therapy (now standard artemisinin-derivative combinations) with other antimalarials is supplanting quinine regimens because of increasing resistance of *P. falciparum* to quinine in Southeast Asia and parts of the Amazon basin. Quinine toxicity, usually seen in overdose, can include pulmonary edema, immune thrombocytopenic purpura, irreversible deafness, or arrhythmias.

Oral quinine is FDA approved for the treatment of uncomplicated *P. falciparum* malaria and is currently available from one manufacturer in the U.S. Intravenous quinine is not available in the U.S. The more potent enantiomer, quinidine, is the preferred intravenous form.

Chemistry. Cinchona contains a mixture of >20 structurally related alkaloids, the most important of which are quinine and quinidine. Both compounds contain a quinoline group attached through a secondary alcohol linkage to a quinuclidine ring (Figure 49–2). A methoxy side chain is attached to the quinoline ring and a vinyl to the quinuclidine. They differ only in the steric configuration at two of the three asymmetrical centers: the carbon bearing the secondary alcohol group and at the quinuclidine junction. Although quinine and quinidine have been synthesized, the procedures are complex; hence they still are obtained from natural sources. Quinidine is both somewhat more potent as an antimalarial and more toxic than quinine (Griffith et al., 2007). Structure-activity analysis of the cinchona alkaloids provided the basis for the discovery of more recent antimalarials such as mefloquine.

Mechanisms of Action and Parasite Resistance. Quinine acts against asexual erythrocytic forms and has no significant effect on hepatic forms of malarial parasites. This drug is more toxic and less effective than chloroquine against malarial parasites susceptible to both drugs. However, quinine, along with its stereoisomer quinidine, is especially valuable for the parenteral treatment of severe illness owing to drug-resistant strains of *P. falciparum*. Of note, however, some strains from Southeast Asia and South America have become more resistant to both agents. Because of its toxicity and short $t_{1/2}$, quinine is generally not used for chemoprophylaxis.

The antimalarial mechanism of quinine is thought to share similarities to chloroquine in being able to bind heme and prevent its detoxification. The basis of *P. falciparum* resistance to quinine, nonetheless, is complex. Patterns of *P. falciparum* resistance to quinine correlate in some strains with resistance to chloroquine yet in others correlate more closely with resistance to mefloquine and halofantrine. Gene amplification of *pfmdr1* in *P. falciparum*, implicated in resistance to mefloquine and halofantrine, can contribute to reduced quinine susceptibility *in vitro*. Similarly, *pfmdr1* point mutations can also contribute to quinine resistance, in particular the N1042D mutation (Duraisingh and Cowman, 2005; Sidhu et al., 2005). Despite their close chemical similarity, quinine and quinidine sensitivity can also diverge in some strains harboring novel PfCRT haplotypes (Cooper et al., 2002). Recent evidence suggests that other transporter genes participate in conferring resistance to quinine, potentially including the sodium-hydrogen exchanger PfNHE (Hayton and Su, 2008; Nkrumah et al., 2009).

Action on Skeletal Muscle. Quinine and related cinchona alkaloids exert effects on skeletal muscle that can have clinical implications. Quinine increases the tension response to a single maximal stimulus delivered to muscle directly or through nerves, but it also increases the refractory period of muscle so that the response to tetanic stimulation is diminished. The excitability of the motor end-plate region decreases so that responses to repetitive nerve stimulation and to acetylcholine are reduced. Thus, quinine can antagonize the actions of physostigmine on skeletal muscle as effectively as curare. Quinine may also produce alarming respiratory distress and dysphagia in patients with myasthenia gravis. The effect on skeletal muscle can be augmented by concurrent administration of gentamicin. Quinine may also cause symptomatic relief of myotonia congenita. This disease is the pharmacological antithesis of myasthenia gravis, such that drugs effective in one syndrome aggravate the other.

Absorption, Fate, and Excretion. Quinine is readily absorbed when given orally or intramuscularly. In the former case, absorption occurs mainly from the upper small intestine and is >80% complete, even in patients with marked diarrhea. After an oral dose, plasma levels reach a maximum in 3-8 hours and, after distributing into an apparent volume of ~1.5 L/kg in healthy individuals, decline with a $t_{1/2}$ of ~11 hours. The pharmacokinetics of quinine may change according to the severity of malarial infection (Krishna and White, 1996). Values for both the apparent volume of distribution and the systemic clearance of quinine decrease, the latter more than the former, such that the average elimination $t_{1/2}$ increases to 18 hours. In patients with severe infection, standard therapeutic doses may produce peak plasma levels of quinine as high as 15-20 mg/L without causing major toxicity. In contrast, levels >10 mg/L can produce severe drug reactions. The high levels of plasma α_1-acid glycoprotein produced in severe malaria may prevent toxicity by binding quinine and thereby reducing the free fraction of drug. Concentrations of quinine are lower in erythrocytes (33-40%) and CSF (2-5%) than in plasma, and the drug readily reaches fetal tissues.

The cinchona alkaloids are metabolized extensively, especially by hepatic CYP3A4; thus only ~20% of an administered dose is excreted in an unaltered form in the urine. These drugs do not accumulate in the body upon continued administration. However, the major metabolite of quinine, 3-hydroxyquinine, retains some antimalarial activity and can accumulate and possibly cause toxicity in patients with renal failure. Renal excretion of quinine itself is more rapid when the urine is acidic.

Therapeutic Uses. Quinine and quinidine have historically been treatments of choice for drug-resistant and severe *P. falciparum* malaria. However, the advent of artemisinin therapy is changing this situation because both oral and intravenous artemisinins have entered clinical practice (Table 49–3). In severe illness, the prompt use of loading doses of intravenous quinine (or quinidine, where intravenous quinine is not available, as is the case in the U.S.) is imperative and can be lifesaving. Oral medication to maintain therapeutic concentrations is then given as soon as tolerated and is continued for 5-7 days. Especially for treatment of infections with multidrug-resistant strains of *P. falciparum*, slower-acting blood schizonticides such as tetracyclines or clindamycin are given concurrently to enhance quinine efficacy. Formulations of quinine and quinidine and specific regimens for their use in the treatment of *P. falciparum* malaria are shown in Table 49–3.

In a series of studies over the past two decades, White and associates designed rational regimens, including the institution of loading doses, for the use of quinine and quinidine in the treatment of *P. falciparum* malaria in Southeast Asia (Krishna and White, 1996). Between 0.2 and 2.0 mg/L has been estimated as the therapeutic range for "free" quinine. Regimens needed to achieve this target may vary based on patient age, severity of illness, and the responsiveness of *P. falciparum* to the drug. For example, lower doses are more effective in treating children in Africa than adults in Southeast Asia because the pharmacokinetics of quinine differ in the two populations, as does the susceptibility of *P. falciparum* to the drug (Krishna and White, 1996). Dosage regimens for quinidine are similar to those for quinine, although quinidine binds less to plasma proteins and has a larger apparent volume of distribution, greater systemic clearance, and shorter terminal elimination $t_{1/2}$ than quinine (Griffith et al., 2007; Miller et al., 1989). Thompson et al. (2003) suggest that the dose of quinidine currently recommended by the CDC (10 mg salt/kg initially, followed by 0.02 mg salt/kg per minute) may be too low and should be 10 mg salt/kg and 0.02 mg/kg of base/minute (60% of the salt is base). Clinical data on which to base a firm recommendation are lacking.

Treatment of Nocturnal Leg Cramps. It is commonly believed that night cramps might be relieved by quinine taken at bedtime at a dose of 200-300 mg (available until 1995 in products that did not require a prescription). Some consider this condition severe. The degree of symptomatic relief appears to vary substantially between individuals. In 1995, the FDA issued a ruling that required drug manufacturers to stop marketing over-the-counter quinine products for nocturnal leg cramps, stating that data supporting safety and efficacy of quinine for this indication were inadequate and that risks outweighed the potential benefits.

Toxicity and Side Effects. The fatal oral dose of quinine for adults is ~2-8 g. Quinine is associated with a triad of dose-related toxicities when given at full therapeutic or excessive doses. These are cinchonism, hypoglycemia, and hypotension. Mild forms of cinchonism—consisting of tinnitus, high-tone deafness, visual disturbances, headache, dysphoria, nausea, vomiting, and postural hypotension—occur frequently and disappear soon after the drug is withdrawn. Hypoglycemia is also common, mostly in the treatment of severe malaria, and can be life threatening if not treated promptly with intravenous glucose. Hypotension is rarer but also serious and most often is associated with excessively rapid intravenous infusions of quinine or quinidine. Prolonged medication or high single doses also may produce GI, cardiovascular, and skin manifestations, as discussed next.

Hearing and vision are particularly affected. Functional impairment of the eighth nerve results in tinnitus, decreased auditory acuity, and vertigo. Visual signs consist of blurred vision, disturbed color perception, photophobia, diplopia, night blindness, constricted visual fields, scotomata, mydriasis, and even blindness (Bateman and Dyson, 1986). These visual and auditory effects probably result from direct neurotoxicity, although secondary vascular changes may have a role. Marked spastic constriction of the retinal vessels leads to retinal ischemia, pale optic discs, and retinal edema, with the potential for severe optic atrophy.

GI symptoms are also prominent in cinchonism. Nausea, vomiting, abdominal pain, and diarrhea result from the local irritant action of quinine, but the nausea and emesis also have a central basis. Cutaneous manifestations may include flushing, sweating, rash, and angioedema, especially of the face. Quinine and quinidine, even at therapeutic doses, may cause hyperinsulinemia and severe hypoglycemia through their powerful stimulatory effect on pancreatic beta cells. Despite treatment with glucose infusions, this complication can be serious and possibly life threatening, especially in pregnancy and prolonged severe infection. Hypoglycemia is seen occasionally in uninfected patients who take quinine.

Quinine rarely causes cardiac complications unless therapeutic plasma concentrations are exceeded (Krishna and White, 1996). QTc prolongation is mild and does not appear to be affected by concurrent mefloquine treatment. Acute overdosage also may cause serious and even fatal cardiac dysrhythmias such as sinus arrest, junctional rhythms, AV block, and ventricular tachycardia and fibrillation (Bateman and Dyson, 1986). Quinidine is even more cardiotoxic than quinine. Cardiac monitoring of patients on intravenous quinidine is advisable where possible.

Severe hemolysis can result from hypersensitivity to these cinchona alkaloids. Hemoglobinuria and asthma from quinine may occur more rarely. "Blackwater fever"—the triad of massive hemolysis, hemoglobinemia, and hemoglobinuria leading to anuria, renal failure, and in some instances death—is a rare type of hypersensitivity reaction to quinine therapy that can occur during treatment of malaria. Quinine may cause milder hemolysis upon occasion, especially in people with G6PD deficiency. Thrombotic thrombocytopenic purpura is a rare but clinically significant adverse effect. This reaction can occur even in response to ingestion of tonic water, which has ~4% the therapeutic oral dose per 12 oz ("cocktail purpura"). Other rare adverse effects include hypoprothrombinemia, leukopenia, and agranulocytosis.

Precautions, Contraindications, and Interactions. Quinine must be used with considerable caution, if at all, in patients who manifest hypersensitivity (balanced against risks primarily of not urgently treating severe malaria in the absence of other effective antimalarial drugs). Quinine should be discontinued immediately if evidence of hemolysis appears.

This drug should be avoided in patients with tinnitus or optic neuritis. In patients with cardiac dysrhythmias, the administration of quinine requires the same precautions as for quinidine. Quinine appears to be safe in pregnancy and is used commonly for the treatment of pregnancy-associated malaria. However, glucose levels must be monitored because of the increased risk of hypoglycemia.

Because parenteral solutions of quinine and quinidine are highly irritating, the drug should not be given subcutaneously. Concentrated solutions may cause abscesses when injected intramuscularly, or thrombophlebitis when infused intravenously. Antacids that contain aluminum can delay absorption of quinine from the GI tract. Quinine and quinidine can delay the absorption and elevate plasma levels of digoxin and related cardiac glycosides. Likewise, these alkaloids may raise plasma levels of warfarin and related anticoagulants. The action of quinine at neuromuscular junctions enhances the effect of neuromuscular blocking agents and opposes the action of acetylcholinesterase inhibitors. Prochlorperazine can amplify quinine's cardiotoxicity, as can halofantrine. The renal clearance of quinine can be decreased by cimetidine and increased by urine acidification and by rifampin.

Mefloquine

History. Mefloquine (LARIAM) is a product of the Malaria Research Program established by the Walter Reed Institute for Medical Research in 1963 to develop promising new compounds to address the alarming growth of drug-resistant malaria. Of the many 4-quinoline methanols tested based on their structural similarity to quinine, mefloquine displayed high antimalarial activity in animal models, and emerged from clinical trials as safe and effective against drug-resistant strains of *P. falciparum*. Mefloquine was first used to treat chloroquine-resistant *P. falciparum* malaria in Thailand. However, the slow elimination of mefloquine fostered the emergence of drug-resistant parasites.

Chemistry. The structure of the mefloquine raceme is illustrated in Figure 49–2. Recent work has demonstrated that the (−)-enantiomer is associated with adverse CNS effects, whereas the (+)-enantiomer retains antimalarial activity with fewer side effects. Mefloquine can be paired with artesunate, thereby reducing the selection pressure for resistance. This combination has proved efficacious for the treatment of *P. falciparum* malaria, even in regions with high prevalence of mefloquine-resistant parasites.

Mechanisms of Action and Parasite Resistance. Mefloquine is a highly effective blood schizonticide. However, it possesses no activity against hepatic stages or mature gametocytes of *P. falciparum* or latent tissue forms of *P. vivax*.

Earlier work showed that mefloquine associates with intraerythrocytic hemozoin, suggesting similarities to the mode of action of chloroquine (Sullivan et al., 1998). However, evidence that this association might be secondary to a primarily cytosolic mode of action comes from studies with transgenic *P. falciparum* lines expressing different *pfmdr1* copy numbers. Increased *pfmdr1* copy numbers are associated with both reduced parasite susceptibility to mefloquine (and artemisinin) and increased PfMDR1-mediated solute import into the digestive vacuole of intraerythrocytic parasites (Rohrbach et al., 2006). Therefore, if the drug's target resides outside of this vacuolar compartment, increased import of mefloquine into the digestive vacuole, potentially driven by PfMDR1 activity, would be beneficial for the parasite and reduce its susceptibility to the drug.

A comprehensive clinical and molecular epidemiological study conducted with parasites from Thailand identified *pfmdr1* gene amplification as a major determinant of mefloquine treatment failure and *in vitro* mefloquine resistance (Price et al., 2004). Some individuals in that study nonetheless failed mefloquine treatment despite not having parasites with multiple *pfmdr1* copies, implying secondary mechanisms of resistance. Mefloquine susceptibility *in vitro* can also be affected by the presence of point mutations in *pfmdr1* or *pfcrt* (Valderramos and Fidock, 2006).

Absorption, Fate, and Excretion. Mefloquine is taken orally because parenteral preparations cause severe local reactions. The drug is rapidly absorbed, with marked variability between individuals. Probably owing to extensive enterogastric and enterohepatic circulation, plasma levels of mefloquine rise in a biphasic manner to their peak in ~17 hours. Mefloquine has a variable and long $t_{1/2}$, 13-24 days, reflecting its high lipophilicity, extensive tissue distribution, and extensive binding (~98%) to plasma proteins. Mefloquine is extensively metabolized in the liver. CYP3A4 has been implicated in the metabolism of mefloquine; this CYP can be inhibited by ketoconazole and induced by rifampicin (German and Aweeka, 2008). Excretion of mefloquine is mainly by the fecal route; only ~10% of mefloquine appears unchanged in the urine. The stereoisomers of mefloquine exhibit quite different pharmacokinetic characteristics that relate to their biodisposition (Hellgren et al., 1997).

Therapeutic Uses. Mefloquine should be reserved for the prevention and treatment of malaria caused by drug-resistant *P. falciparum* and *P. vivax,* but it is no longer considered first-line treatment of malaria in most clinical contexts. The drug is especially useful as a chemoprophylactic agent for travelers spending weeks, months, or years in areas where these infections are endemic (Table 49–2). In areas where malaria is due to multiply drug-resistant strains of *P. falciparum* (particularly in Southeast Asia), mefloquine is more effective when used in combination with an artemisinin compound.

Toxicity and Side Effects. The use of mefloquine for the chemoprophylaxis or treatment of malaria must balance concerns about clinically significant risks and benefits. The major adverse effects of mefloquine have been reviewed in detail (Chen et al., 2006). Mefloquine given orally is generally well tolerated at chemoprophylactic dosages, although vivid dreams are common. Significant neuropsychiatric signs and symptoms can occur in 10% (or more) of people receiving treatment doses, although serious adverse events (psychosis, seizures) are rare. Short-term adverse effects of treatment include nausea, vomiting, and dizziness. Dividing the dose improves tolerance. The full dose should be repeated if vomiting occurs within the first hour.

Estimates for frequency of severe CNS toxicity after mefloquine treatment can be as high as 0.5%. Adverse reactions include seizures, confusion or decreased sensorium, acute psychosis, and disabling vertigo. Such symptoms generally are reversible upon drug discontinuation. At chemoprophylactic dosages, the risk of serious neuropsychiatric effects is estimated to be ~0.01% (about the same as for chloroquine). Mild-to-moderate toxicities (e.g., disturbed sleep, dysphoria, headache, GI disturbances, and dizziness) occur even at chemoprophylactic dosages. Whether these symptoms are more common than with other antimalarial regimens is debated. Adverse effects usually manifest after the first to third doses and often abate even with continued treatment. Reports of cardiac abnormalities, hemolysis, and agranulocytosis are rare.

Contraindications and Interactions. At very high doses, mefloquine is teratogenic in rodents. Studies have suggested an increased rate of stillbirths with mefloquine use, especially during the first trimester (Taylor and White, 2004). The significance of these data has been debated, but it is fair to say that the evidence for mefloquine's safety in pregnancy is not convincing, and mefloquine may be used if it is the only available treatment option. Pregnancy should be avoided for 3 months after mefloquine use because of the prolonged $t_{1/2}$ of this agent.

This drug is contraindicated for patients with a history of seizures, depression, bipolar disorder and other severe neuropsychiatric conditions, or adverse reactions to quinoline antimalarials such as quinine, quinidine, halofantrine, mefloquine, and chloroquine. Mefloquine may counteract seizures in epileptic patients. Although this drug can be taken safely 12 hours after a last dose of quinine, taking quinine shortly after mefloquine can be very hazardous because the latter is eliminated so slowly. Treatment with or after halofantrine or within 2 months of prior mefloquine administration is contraindicated.

Recent studies do not indicate that mefloquine compromises the performance of tasks that require good motor coordination, e.g., driving or operating machinery. Although some advise against the use of mefloquine for patients in occupations that require focused concentration, dexterity and cognitive function in safety-sensitive settings, such as pilots, controlled studies suggest that mefloquine does not impair performance in persons who tolerate the drug.

Primaquine

History. The weak anti-*Plasmodium* activity of methylene blue, first discovered by Ehrlich in 1891, led to the development of the 8-aminoquinoline antimalarials, of which pamaquine was the first introduced into medicine. During World War II the search for more potent and less toxic 8-aminoquinoline antimalarials resulted in the discovery of primaquine (Figure 49–2).

Primaquine, in contrast to other antimalarials, acts on exoerythrocytic tissue stages of plasmodia in the liver to prevent and cure relapsing malaria. The striking hemolysis that may follow primaquine therapy led directly to the landmark discovery of G6PD deficiency, the first genetic disorder associated with an enzyme. Hemolysis remains notoriously identified with primaquine. Patients should be screened for G6PD deficiency prior to therapy with this drug. The pressing need for alternatives to this important drug has resulted in the evaluation of multiple 8-aminoquinoline analogs (Vale et al., 2009). These include tafenoquine, a compound under clinical evaluation that is active against relapsing liver stage forms of *P. vivax,* and multidrug resistant asexual blood stage forms of *P. falciparum* (Wells et al., 2009).

Mechanisms of Action and Parasite Resistance. Primaquine acts against primary and latent hepatic stages of *Plasmodium spp*. and prevents relapses in *P. vivax* and *P. ovale* infections. This drug and other 8-aminoquinolines also display gametocytocidal activity against *P. falciparum* and other *Plasmodium* species. However, primaquine is inactive against asexual blood stage parasites.

The mechanism of action of the 8-aminoquinolines has not been elucidated. Primaquine may be converted to electrophilic intermediates that act as oxidation-reduction mediators. Such activity could contribute to antimalarial effects by generating reactive oxygen species or by interfering with mitochondrial electron transport in the parasite (Vale et al., 2009). Some strains of *P. vivax* can exhibit partial resistance to primaquine (Baird, 2009).

Absorption, Fate, and Excretion. Absorption of primaquine from the GI tract approaches 100%. After a single dose, the plasma concentration reaches a maximum within 3 hours and then falls with a variable elimination $t_{1/2}$ averaging 7 hours.

The apparent volume of distribution is several times that of total-body water, due to extensive tissue distribution. Primaquine binds preferentially to the acute-phase reactant protein α1-glycoprotein, which may alter the distribution of free drug depending on its concentration in the blood. Primaquine is metabolized rapidly, and only a small fraction of an administered dose is excreted as the parent drug. Importantly, primaquine induces CYP1A2. Thus, caution should be taken in administering primaquine with drugs metabolized by CYP1A2 (including warfarin) (Hill et al., 2006). The major metabolite, carboxyprimaquine, is inactive.

Therapeutic Uses. Primaquine is used primarily for terminal chemoprophylaxis and radical cure of *P. vivax* and *P. ovale* (relapsing) infections because of its high activity against the latent tissue forms (hypnozoites) of these *Plasmodium* species. The compound is given together with a blood schizonticide, usually chloroquine, to eradicate erythrocytic stages of these plasmodia and reduce the possibility of emerging drug resistance.

For terminal chemoprophylaxis, primaquine regimens should be initiated shortly before or immediately after a subject leaves an endemic area (Table 49–2). Radical cure of *P. vivax* or *P. ovale* malaria can be achieved if the drug is given either during an asymptomatic latent period of presumed infection (based on travel to or residence within an endemic region) or during an acute attack. Simultaneous administration of a schizonticidal drug plus primaquine is more effective in radical cure than sequential treatment. Limited studies have shown efficacy in prevention of *P. falciparum* and *P. vivax* malaria when primaquine is taken as chemoprophylaxis (Taylor and White, 2004). Gametocytocidal activity of primaquine should also reduce the transmission potential during drug treatment of *P. falciparum*. However, this approach to prophylaxis is not routine clinical practice. Primaquine is generally well tolerated when taken for up to 1 year.

Toxicity and Side Effects. Primaquine has few side effects when given to most whites in the usual therapeutic doses. Primaquine can cause mild to moderate abdominal distress in some individuals. Taking the drug at mealtime often alleviates these symptoms. Mild anemia, cyanosis (methemoglobinemia), and leukocytosis are less common. High doses (60-240 mg daily) worsen the abdominal symptoms and cause some degree of methemoglobinemia in most subjects. Methemoglobinemia can occur even with usual doses of primaquine and can be severe in individuals with congenital deficiency of NADH methemoglobin reductase (Coleman and Coleman, 1996). Chloroquine and dapsone may synergize with primaquine to produce methemoglobinemia in these patients. Granulocytopenia and agranulocytosis are rare complications of therapy and usually are associated with overdosage. Other rare adverse reactions are hypertension, arrhythmias, and symptoms referable to the CNS.

Therapeutic or higher doses of primaquine may cause acute hemolysis and hemolytic anemia in humans with G6PD deficiency (Vale et al., 2009). This X-linked condition, primarily owing to amino acid substitutions in the G6PD enzyme, affects >200 million people worldwide. More than 400 genetic variants of G6PD produce variable responses to oxidative stress. About 11% of African Americans have the A variant of G6PD, and are therefore vulnerable to hemolysis caused by pro-oxidant drugs such as primaquine. G6PD deficiency is uncommon in Latin America but may be present in those residents of African descent. Primaquine-induced hemolysis can be even more severe in white ethnic groups, including Sardinians, Sephardic Jews, Greeks, and Iranians; these populations have a G6PD variant in which two amino acid substitutions impair both enzyme stability and activity. Because primaquine sensitivity is inherited through an X-linked gene, hemolysis is often of intermediate severity in heterozygous females who have two populations of red blood cells, one normal and the other deficient in G6PD. Owing to "variable penetrance," these females may be affected less frequently than predicted. Primaquine is the prototype of >50 drugs, including antimalarial sulfonamides, that cause hemolysis in G6PD-deficient individuals.

Precautions and Contraindications. G6PD deficiency should be ruled out prior to administration of primaquine. Primaquine has been used cautiously in subjects with the A form of G6PD deficiency, although benefits of treatment may not necessarily outweigh the risks. The drug should not be used in patients with more severe deficiency. If a daily dose of >30 mg primaquine base (>15 mg in potentially sensitive patients) is given, then blood counts should be followed carefully. Patients should be counseled to look for dark or blood-colored urine, which would indicate hemolysis. Primaquine should not be given to pregnant women, and, in treating lactating mothers, it should be prescribed only after ascertaining that the breast-feeding infant has a normal G6PD level (which can be difficult to assess soon after birth).

Primaquine is contraindicated for acutely ill patients suffering from systemic disease characterized by a tendency to granulocytopenia (e.g., active forms of rheumatoid arthritis and lupus erythematosus). Primaquine should not be given to patients receiving other drugs capable of causing hemolysis or depressing the myeloid elements of the bone marrow.

SULFONAMIDES AND SULFONES

History. Shortly after their introduction into clinical practice, the sulfonamides were found to have antimalarial activity, a property investigated extensively during World War II. The efficacy of sulfones was demonstrated in the first trial of dapsone against *P. falciparum* in 1943. The sulfonamides combined with pyrimethamine have been used to treat chloroquine-resistant *P. falciparum* malaria, particularly in parts of Africa. The sulfonamides and sulfones are slow-acting blood schizonticides and more active against *P. falciparum* than *P. vivax*.

Mechanism of Action. Sulfonamides are *p*-aminobenzoic acid analogs that competitively inhibit *Plasmodium* dihydropteroate synthase. These agents are combined with an inhibitor of parasite dihydrofolate reductase to enhance their antimalarial action. The synergistic "antifolate" combination of sulfadoxine, a long-acting sulfonamide, with pyrimethamine has been extensively used to treat malaria. As observed for pyrimethamine, sulfadoxine resistance appeared quickly *in vivo* after the introduction of this treatment as monotherapy.

Drug Resistance. Sulfadoxine resistance is conferred by several point mutations in the dihydropteroate synthase gene; the more widespread is the substitution Ala437Gly. These sulfadoxine-resistance mutations, when combined with mutations of dihydrofolate reductase and conferring pyrimethamine resistance, greatly increase the likelihood of sulfadoxine-pyrimethamine treatment failure. Sulfadoxine-pyrimethamine, given intermittently during the second and third trimesters of pregnancy, is a routine component of antenatal care throughout Africa. Intermittent preventive treatment strategies might also benefit infants (Aponte et al., 2009). However, there are substantial concerns about these strategies in the face of the expanding profile of resistance to pyrimethamine-sulfadoxine. A recent report found that intermittent preventive treatment in pregnancy exacerbated placental inflammation and caused increased levels of parasitemia and increased selective pressure for drug-resistant infections (Harrington et al., 2009). Thus, there is a clear need to identify alternative intermittent preventive treatment regimens. Generally, one can anticipate that, in the absence of novel antifolates effective against existing drug-resistant strains, the use of these antimalarials for either prevention or treatment will continue to decline.

TETRACYCLINES AND OTHER ANTIBIOTIC AGENTS

Tetracyclines are a group of antibiotic agents initially derived from *Streptomyces.* The pharmacological properties of tetracyclines are presented in Chapter 55. Two members of this group, tetracycline and doxycycline, are useful in malaria treatment. In addition, clindamycin, a lincosamide antibiotic (Chapter 55), is also recommended. These agents are slow-acting blood schizonticides that can be used alone for short-term chemoprophylaxis in areas with chloroquine- and mefloquine-resistant malaria (only doxycycline is recommended for malaria chemoprophylaxis). All of these antibiotics act via a delayed death mechanism resulting from their inhibition of protein translation in the parasite plastid. This effect on malarial parasites manifests as death of the progeny of drug-treated parasites, resulting in slow onset of antimalarial activity (Dahl and Rosenthal, 2008). Their relatively slow mode of action makes these drugs ineffective as single agents for malaria treatment. However, their efficacy as treatment is increased when they are used as an adjunct to quinine, quinidine, or artesunate, and in this context, they can be used to treat uncomplicated or severe *P. falciparum* malaria. These antibiotics are not clinically used to eliminate liver stage infection.

Dosage regimens for tetracyclines and clindamycin are listed in Tables 49–2 and 49–3. Because of their adverse effects on bones and teeth, tetracyclines should not be given to pregnant women or to children <8 years of age. In these subjects, clindamycin is a reasonable alternative. Photosensitivity reactions or drug-induced superinfections may mandate discontinuation of therapy or chemoprophylaxis with tetracyclines. As an alternative antibiotic, the macrolide azithromycin also displays antimalarial activity through a similar delayed-death mechanism and is undergoing further evaluation. As with clindamycin, azithromycin is safe for use in young children and pregnant women.

PRINCIPLES AND GUIDELINES FOR CHEMOPROPHYLAXIS AND CHEMOTHERAPY OF MALARIA

Pharmacological prevention of malaria poses a difficult challenge because *P. falciparum*, which causes nearly all the deaths from human malaria, has become progressively more resistant to available antimalarial drugs. Chloroquine had been the drug of choice to prevent all forms of malaria until resistance became widespread in the past decades. Chloroquine remains effective against malaria caused by *P. ovale*, *P. malariae*, *P. knowlesi*, most strains of *P. vivax*, and chloroquine-sensitive strains of *P. falciparum* found in some geographic areas. However, chloroquine-resistant strains of *P. falciparum* are now the rule, not the exception, in most malaria-endemic regions except Mexico, Central America west of the Panama Canal Zone, the Caribbean, and parts of the Middle East (Figure 49–3). Except for parts of Africa, extensive geographic overlap also exists between chloroquine resistance and resistance to pyrimethamine-sulfadoxine. Multidrug-resistant *P. falciparum* malaria is especially prevalent and severe in Southeast Asia and Oceania. These infections may not respond adequately even to mefloquine or quinine.

Genetic studies indicate that isolates of *P. falciparum* from patients in highly endemic areas contain many parasite clones with different drug resistance phenotypes (Druilhe et al., 1998). A patient with severe malaria may have up to 10^{12} parasites. Because single point mutations occur with an estimated frequency of 10^{-9}, based on *in vitro* studies (Cooper et al., 2002), single point mutations that confer resistance could potentially arise in virtually every patient and double point mutations would arise occasionally. Most of these new mutant strains will not survive because of immunity, decreased fitness, and additional factors; nonetheless, successful drugs or drug combinations must ideally not be susceptible to resistance resulting from single point mutations. Mutations by gene amplification are expected to be even more frequent than single point mutations (Nair et al., 2008). Looking back in time, one notes that decades of intense chloroquine use preceded development of resistance to this agent. This delay was likely due to the requirement for at least four point mutations in the *pfcrt* gene to confer resistance (Valderramos and Fidock, 2006). Pharmacokinetics can also be a determinant in the generation of resistance. Drugs with a long $t_{1/2}$ are thought to generally be more likely to select for resistance (White, 2004).

On a population level, the fitness of resistant parasites is another important parameter: If mutation causes a reduced ability to survive or grow, the parasites are less likely to spread. However, in the case of antifolates, treatment actually induces gametocytogenesis, which promotes transmission; this effect, together with other forces (intense selection pressure from preventive drug use; parasite migrations driven by humans), may explain the spread of particular resistance alleles across Southeast Asia and Africa. These considerations strongly argue for regimens that combine two or more antimalarial agents with different mechanisms of action (and therefore, hopefully, with different mechanisms of resistance) to treat drug-resistant *P. falciparum* malaria (White, 2004). ACTs are the most important combination treatment currently available.

The following section presents an overview of the chemoprophylaxis and chemotherapy of malaria. For more current details about individual drugs, their clinical and chemoprophylactic applications, and about malaria risk areas, consult the latest information available from the CDC (www.cdc.gov/travel/travel). Consultation and emergency advice about treatment are available 24 hours a day from the duty officer, Division of Parasitic Diseases, CDC.

Current CDC recommendations for drugs and dosing regimens for the chemoprophylaxis and treatment of malaria in nonimmune individuals are shown in Tables 49–2 and 49–3. These will change and should serve only as general guidelines to be modified appropriately according to the status and habitat of the patient; the geographic origin, species, and drug-resistance profile of infecting parasites; and the agents used for malaria prevention.

Importantly, *drugs should not replace simple, inexpensive measures for malaria prevention*. Individuals visiting malarious areas should take appropriate steps to prevent mosquito bites. One such measure is to avoid exposure to mosquitoes at dusk and dawn, usually the times of maximal feeding. Others include using insect repellents containing at least 30% *N,N′*-diethylmetatoluamide (DEET) and sleeping in well-screened rooms or under bed nets impregnated with a pyrethrin insecticide such as permethrin (Kain and Jong, 2003).

Malaria Chemoprophylaxis. Regimens for malaria chemoprophylaxis include primarily three drugs: atovaquone-proguanil and doxycycline that can both be used in all areas, and mefloquine that can be used in areas with mefloquine-sensitive malaria. Other available options are chloroquine or hydroxychloroquine (but their use is restricted to the few areas with chloroquine-sensitive malaria), and primaquine (for short duration travel to areas with principally *P. vivax*).

In general, dosing should be started before exposure, ideally before the traveler leaves home, to establish therapeutic blood levels and to detect early signs or symptoms of intolerance so the regimen can be modified before departure. As described earlier, the duration of post-exposure dosing is dictated by the spectrum of drug action (Table 49–1).

In those few areas where chloroquine-sensitive strains of *P. falciparum* are found, chloroquine is still suitable for chemoprophylaxis. It also remains the drug of choice for chemoprophylaxis and control of infections due to *P. vivax*, *P. ovale*, *P. malariae*, and *P. knowlesi*. In areas where chloroquine-resistant malaria is endemic, mefloquine and atovaquone-proguanil are the regimens of choice for chemoprophylaxis. There is more experience with mefloquine and more evidence for its efficacy against *P. vivax*, an important consideration in areas where this species co-exists with *P. falciparum*. However, there are more contraindications to the use of mefloquine and perhaps greater toxicity than for alternative regimens. Doxycycline is an alternative chemoprophylactic agent. In cases where mefloquine, atovaquone-proguanil, and doxycycline all are contraindicated, primaquine is a possibility for chemoprophylaxis. Primaquine, like atovaquone-proguanil, is active against liver stages and can be discontinued shortly after leaving the endemic area. Attempts at radical cure of *P. vivax* malaria with primaquine should be delayed until the patient leaves an endemic area.

For chemoprophylaxis in long-term travelers, chloroquine is safe at the doses used, but some recommend yearly retinal examinations, and there is a finite dose limit for which chemoprophylaxis with chloroquine is recommended because of ocular toxicity (Tehrani et al., 2008). Mefloquine and doxycycline are well tolerated. Mefloquine is the best documented drug for long-term travelers and, if well tolerated, can be used for prolonged periods. Atovaquone-proguanil has been studied for up to 20 weeks but probably is acceptable for years based on experience with the individual components.

The diagnosis of malaria must be considered for patients presenting with acute febrile illness after returning from a malaria-endemic region (Table 49–5). *If proven to be malaria, such an illness should be considered a medical emergency, especially for vulnerable populations such as nonimmune travelers, pregnant women, and young children. Severe* P. falciparum *malaria is as acute as any other life-threatening illness and demands close attention and aggressive treatment. An organized, rational approach to diagnosis, parasite identification, and appropriate treatment is crucial* (see Figure 49–4). Treatment with a rapidly acting blood schizonticide must be instituted promptly if *P. falciparum* malaria is suspected from a travel history and clinical findings. One should not wait for a definitive parasitological diagnosis to initiate therapy in such patients because their clinical status may deteriorate rapidly. Moreover, the clinical presentation may be atypical, and thick blood smears may fail to reveal malarial parasites in early stages of this infection.

Table 49–5

Criteria for the Diagnosis of Malaria

Signs and symptoms consistent with malaria, including fever, chills, headache, ± severe malaria criteria (below), *plus*	
Demonstration of the presence of malaria parasite:	
Light microscope examination of stained thin or thick smear	
Rapid diagnostic test	
Molecular or biophysical-based testing	
Criteria for the Diagnosis of Severe Malaria[a]	
Prostration	Jaundice
Impaired consciousness/coma	Severe anemia
Respiratory distress (acidotic breathing)	Acute renal failure
Multiple convulsions	Disseminated intravascular coagulation
Circulatory shock	Acidosis
Pulmonary edema	Hemoglobinuria
Acute respiratory distress syndrome	Parasitemia >5%
Abnormal bleeding	

[a]Adapted from: WHO Management of Severe Malaria (2000), http://malaria.who.int/docs/hbsm_toc.htm, accessed January 12, 2010; and WHO Guidelines for the Treatment of Malaria (2006), www.who.int/malaria/docs/TreatmentGuidelines2006.pdf, accessed January 12, 2010.

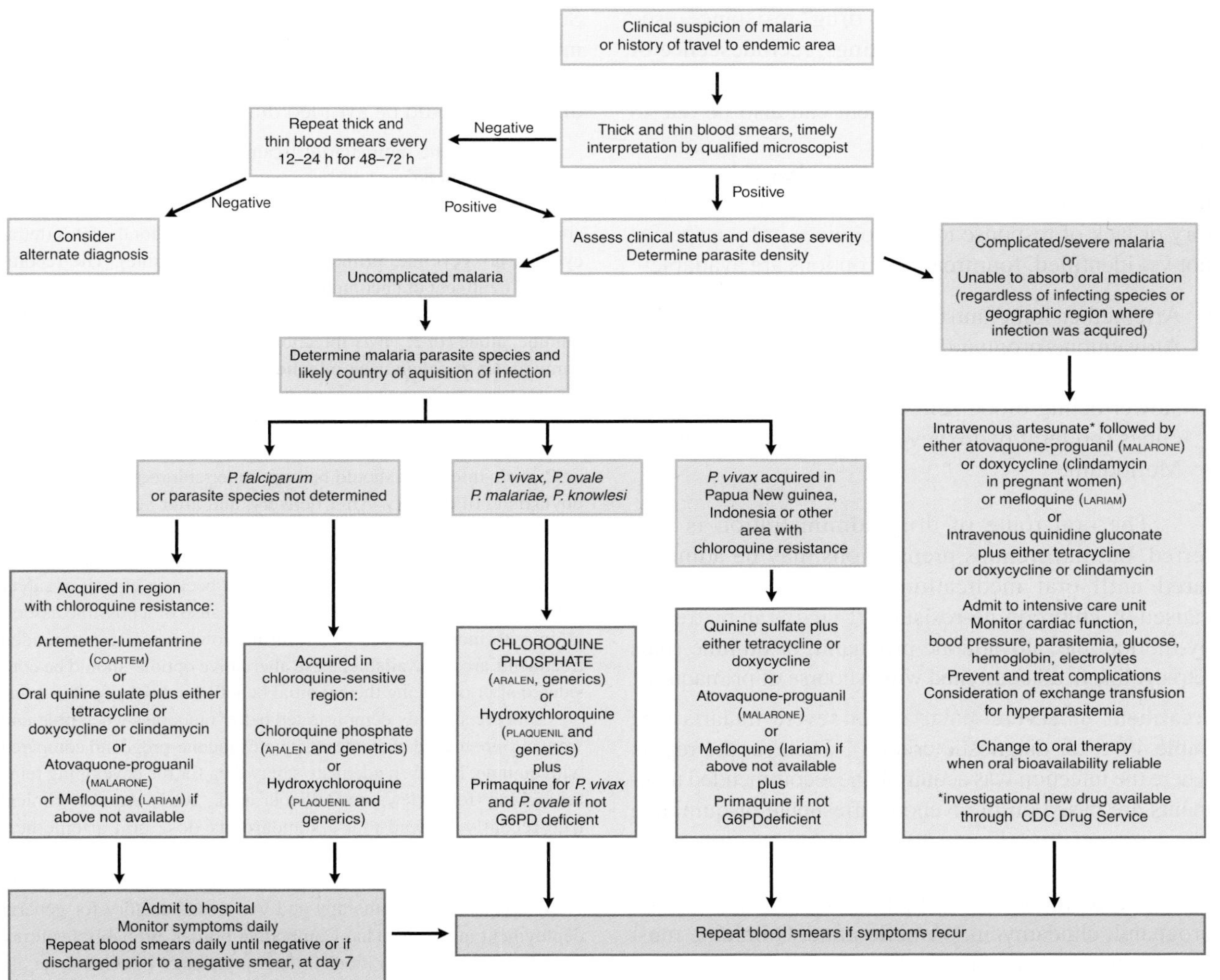

Figure 49–4. *Approach to the treatment of malaria.* Atovaquone-proguanil, mefloquine, artemether-lumefantrine, tetracycline, and doxycycline are not indicated during pregnancy. Tetracycline and doxycycline are not indicated in children <8 years of age. G6PD, glucose- 6-phosphate dehydrogenase. (Adapted from Griffith KS, Lewis LS, Mali S, Parise ME. Treatment of malaria in the United States: A systematic review. *JAMA,* 297(20):2264–77, 2007, with permission of the American Medical Association © 2007. All rights reserved.)

Guidelines for treatment of malaria in the U.S. are provided by the CDC and are shown in Table 49–3. Updates should be checked on the CDC website. Figure 49–4 presents an overview of the general strategy for treatment of malaria in the U.S.

Treatment of Uncomplicated Malaria. Chloroquine is the drug of choice for *P. ovale*, *P. malariae*, *P. knowlesi*, and chloroquine-sensitive strains of *P. vivax* and *P. falciparum*. For *P. vivax* and *P. ovale* infections, a 2-week course of primaquine should be added to eradicate hypnozoites that may remain dormant in the liver, and thus prevent relapse. Some patients with *P. vivax* infection may require more than one course of primaquine to obtain radical cure. Primaquine must not be given to patients with G6PD deficiency or to pregnant women. The oral route of administration should be used if feasible. Within 48-72 hours of initiating therapy, patients should show marked clinical improvement (especially clearance of fever) and a substantial decrease in parasitemia as monitored by daily thin and thick blood smears. Under controlled administration of treatment, lack of such a response or failure to clear asexual forms of the parasite from the blood by 7 days suggests the presence of drug resistance (except for atovaquone-proguanil).

For clinical classification of drug resistance, see Bloland (2001). In endemic settings, recrudescence of *P. falciparum* clinical episodes or asymptomatic parasitemia after appropriate treatment can also be due to reinfection.

For uncomplicated malaria caused by chloroquine-resistant *P. falciparum* (suspected either from travel history or lack of response to chloroquine) or by a species not yet identified, four treatment options are available:

- Artemether-lumefantrine
- Atovaquone-proguanil
- Oral quinine given along with other effective but slower-acting blood schizonticides such as tetracyclines (preferably doxycycline) or clindamycin
- Mefloquine

The oral route of drug administration is preferred, but intravenous preparations may be administered until oral medication can be taken. Malaria caused by chloroquine-resistant *P. vivax* can be treated by mefloquine, atovaquone-proguanil, or quinine (plus tetracyclines), all combined with a course of primaquine.

Treatment of Severe Malaria. For severe malaria (see Table 49–5 for diagnostic criteria), whatever the region where the infection was acquired, the recommended treatments are based on intravenous artesunate or quinidine plus a second drug (Figure 49–4). Artesunate, now available in the U.S. from the CDC under an investigational new drug protocol, should be followed by atovaquone-proguanil, clindamycin, or mefloquine. Quinidine must be substituted for quinine (no longer available) and combined with doxycycline, tetracycline, or clindamycin (reviewed in Griffith et al., 2007). Exchange transfusion may be of additional value in severe *P. falciparum* malaria with high levels of parasitemia (Griffith et al., 2007; Miller et al., 1989).

Children and pregnant women are the most susceptible to severe malaria. With appropriate dosage adjustments and safety precautions, the treatment of children generally is the same as for adults (pediatric dose should never exceed adult dose). However, tetracyclines should not be given to children <8 years of age except in an emergency, and atovaquone-proguanil as treatment has been approved only for children weighing >5 kg (for current information, see the CDC website and Boggild et al., 2007).

Chemoprophylaxis and Treatment During Pregnancy. Pregnant women should be urged not to travel to endemic areas if possible (Freedman, 2008). Chemoprophylaxis during pregnancy is complex, and women should evaluate with expert medical staff the benefits and risks of different strategies with regard to their particular situation. Severe malaria during pregnancy should be treated with intravenous antimalarial treatment according to the general guidelines for severe malaria, taking into account the drugs that should be avoided during pregnancy.

Among the antimalarial treatments available in the U.S., many should not be used during pregnancy because of lack of sufficient formal safety data (antifolates, atovaquone-proguanil, and artemether-lumefantrine) or known potential risks for the fetus (tetracycline, doxycycline, primaquine, and mefloquine). The recommended treatment of uncomplicated malaria during pregnancy relies on chloroquine in areas with chloroquine-sensitive parasites, and quinine, alone (in *P. vivax* infections) or in combination with clindamycin (in *P. falciparum* infections), in areas with chloroquine-resistant parasites. Appropriate caution should be exercised when administering quinine, given the frequency of hypoglycemia as an adverse reaction in pregnant women. Pregnant patients with *P. vivax* or *P. ovale* infections should be kept under chloroquine chemoprophylaxis until delivery. After delivery, and after verifying that the patient is not G6PD deficient, treatment with primaquine should be initiated to eradicate hypnozoites. Atovaquone-proguanil and artemether-lumefantrine are not indicated because of lack of safety data. Mefloquine is also not indicated because of a possible association with increased risk of stillbirth. However, if recommended treatments are not available, these alternative options should be considered after balancing the potential benefits and risks for the fetus.

A recent study demonstrated better outcomes when pregnant women were treated with artesunate-atovaquone-proguanil compared with quinine; however, adequate safety data for the developing fetus are lacking (for review, see Dellicour et al., 2007). Another clinical trial recently showed that a standard six-dose oral artemether-lumefantrine regimen was well tolerated and safe in pregnant women with uncomplicated *falciparum* malaria, but efficacy was inferior to 7-day artesunate monotherapy and was unsatisfactory for general deployment along the Thai Cambodian border, probably resulting from low drug concentrations in later pregnancy (McGready et al., 2008). The use of antimalarial drugs in pregnancy has been well reviewed (Ward et al., 2007).

In lactating mothers, treatment with most compounds is acceptable, although chloroquine and hydroxychloroquine are the preferred agents. The use of atovaquone-proguanil is not recommended unless breast-feeding infants weigh >5 kg. Also, the breast-feeding infant should be shown to have a normal G6PD level before receiving primaquine (Schlagenhauf and Petersen, 2008).

New Targets, New Drugs

In the face of evolving drug resistance and the necessity to increase the useful life span of antimalarial drugs through combination therapies, novel and potent antimalarial drugs are urgently needed. The malaria research pipeline includes either compounds derived from known antimalarials through modification of their chemical structure (likely to retain activity against the original targets), drugs previously developed for other infectious organisms or diseases (and likely act on the same target in *Plasmodium*), or inhibitors of novel targets (exploiting differences in the biology of host and parasite). This latter strategy of drug discovery benefits from the genome sequencing projects of the different *Plasmodium* species and the human host. Perspectives in malaria chemotherapy (including new drug targets and antimalarial drugs in discovery, preclinical and clinical phases) have recently been extensively discussed (Biot and Chibale, 2006; de Beer et al., 2009; Gardiner et al., 2009; Olliaro and Wells, 2009; Wells et al., 2009).

Among the novel antimalarial drugs undergoing clinical development, two notable examples act on new metabolic pathways:

1. *TE3*, a prodrug of a bis-ammonium compound that acts on phospholipid metabolism through the inhibition of *de novo* phosphatidylcholine synthesis, combined with a putative activity on heme detoxification. This new class of compounds has shown potent *in vivo* antimalarial activity in the primate model *Aotus* and is not cross resistance *in vitro* with known antimalarials.
2. *Fosmidomycin*, which inhibits the 1-desoxy-D-xylulose-5-phosphate reductoisomerase in the mevalonate-independent pathway of isoprenoid synthesis in the apicoplast (Wiesner and Jomaa, 2007). The apicoplast, a specialized parasite organelle of algal origin, appears to be important for lipid and heme biosynthesis, and is a major focus of current drug development efforts (Wiesner et al., 2008). Fosmidomycin was initially developed as an antibacterial drug, but has shown efficacy in combination with clindamycin or azithromycin against *P. falciparum* malaria.

A nonexhaustive list of the molecular targets under current experimental or clinical investigation includes two clinically validated antimalarial drug targets (dihydrofolate reductase and cytochrome bc1 complex), for which inhibitors are being developed to overcome existing resistance (this strategy is also being explored to derive new 4-aminoquinolines and amino-alcohols) and a series of novel, experimental antimalarial drug targets: dihydro-orotate dehydrogenase (involved in pyrimidine synthesis), purine nucleoside phosphorylase (nucleotide synthesis), adenosine deaminase (regulation of intracellular nucleoside pools), subtilisin-like proteases (egress from erythrocytes), falcipains (hemoglobin proteolysis), histone deacetylase (DNA replication), protein kinases (signal transduction), and fatty acid biosynthesis (apicoplast lipid synthesis). The rationale focusing on these targets for antimalarial drug development can be found in the reviews cited.

CLINICAL SUMMARY

Agents available for the treatment of acute malaria due to *Plasmodium falciparum* in the U.S. have been expanded beyond previously used quinolines (chloroquine, quinine/quinidine, mefloquine) with or without adjunctive doxycycline and clindamycin, to include atovaquone-proguanil and artemisinin derivatives: artemether plus lumefantrine approved for oral use, and intravenous artesunate (available from the CDC under an IND protocol). Mefloquine is no longer considered first-line therapy for the treatment of any form of malaria in the U.S. because of adverse effects in the higher treatment doses and the availability of better tolerated alternatives. Sulfadoxine-pyrimethamine is no longer reliable due to widespread resistance and diminished efficacy. Chloroquine resistance must be assumed for *P. falciparum* originating anywhere other than Mexico, Central America, and the Caribbean. Mefloquine resistance is likely for *P. falciparum* arising from border areas along Thailand and infections of similar geographic origin.

Chloroquine is the preferred drug in *P. vivax* infections originating in most geographic regions, with the exception of Papua New Guinea and Indonesia where resistance is prevalent. Radical therapy with primaquine is recommended to eradicate latent infection for both *P. vivax* and *P. ovale*, after normal erythrocyte levels of G6PD are confirmed. Primaquine is most effective if administered concurrently with the indicated therapy for acute malaria, although *P. vivax* in some regions seems to require higher or prolonged dosing to minimize the risk of relapse.

For malaria chemoprophylaxis, long-acting quinolines (chloroquine and mefloquine) are used, although they are of limited utility in specific geographic areas due to drug resistance. Because of a better side-effect profile, atovaquone-proguanil is often preferred. Doxycycline remains a viable option for malaria chemoprophylaxis, particularly in long-term travelers living in malaria-endemic regions where mefloquine resistance is present. Pregnant women should avoid travel to malaria endemic regions. If travel cannot be avoided and the risk of contracting malaria is considered to exceed the risk of adverse effects on fetus, chloroquine and mefloquine are the drugs of choice.

Atovaquone-proguanil is now the only recommended drug for the presumptive self-treatment of malaria.

BIBLIOGRAPHY

Aponte JJ, Schellenberg D, Egan A, *et al.* Efficacy and safety of intermittent preventive treatment with sulfadoxine-pyrimethamine for malaria in African infants: A pooled analysis of six randomised, placebo-controlled trials. *Lancet,* **2009,** *374:*1533–1542.

Baird JK. Resistance to therapies for infection by *Plasmodium vivax. Clin Microbiol Rev,* **2009,** *22:*508–534.

Bateman DN, Dyson EH. Quinine toxicity. *Adverse Drug React Acute Poisoning Rev,* **1986,** *5:*215–233.

Biot C, Chibale K. Novel approaches to antimalarial drug discovery. *Infect Disord Drug Targets,* **2006,** *6:*173–204.

Bloland PB. Drug resistance in malaria, WHO/CSR, 2001. Available at: http://www.who.int/csr/resources/publications/drugresist/malaria.pdf. Accessed January 12, 2010.

Boggild AK, Parise ME, Lewis LS, Kain KC. Atovaquone-proguanil: Report from the CDC expert meeting on malaria chemoprophylaxis (II). *Am J Trop Med Hyg,* **2007,** *76:*208–223.

Bray PG, Ward SA, O'Neill PM. Quinolines and artemisinin: Chemistry, biology and history. *Curr Top Microbiol Immunol,* **2005,** *295:*3–38.

Checchi F, Piola P, Fogg C, *et al.* Supervised versus unsupervised antimalarial treatment with six-dose artemether-lumefantrine: Pharmacokinetic and dosage-related findings from a clinical trial in Uganda. *Malar J,* **2006,** *5:*59.

Chen LH, Wilson ME, Schlagenhauf P. Prevention of malaria in long-term travelers. *JAMA,* **2006,** *296:*2234–2244.

Coleman MD, Coleman NA. Drug-induced methaemoglobinaemia. Treatment issues. *Drug Saf,* **1996,** *14:*394–405.

Cooper RA, Ferdig MT, Su XZ, *et al.* Alternative mutations at position 76 of the vacuolar transmembrane protein PfCRT are associated with chloroquine resistance and unique stereospecific quinine and quinidine responses in *Plasmodium falciparum. Mol Pharmacol,* **2002,** *61:*35–42.

Cox-Singh J, Davis TM, Lee KS, *et al. Plasmodium knowlesi* malaria in humans is widely distributed and potentially life threatening. *Clin Infect Dis,* **2008,** *46:*165–171.

Dahl EL, Rosenthal PJ. Apicoplast translation, transcription and genome replication: Targets for antimalarial antibiotics. *Trends Parasitol,* **2008,** *24:*279–284.

Davis TM, Karunajeewa HA, Ilett KF. Artemisinin-based combination therapies for uncomplicated malaria. *Med J Aust,* **2005,** *182:*181–185.

de Beer TA, Wells GA, Burger PB, *et al.* Antimalarial drug discovery: In silico structural biology and rational drug design. *Infect Disord Drug Targets,* **2009,** *9:*304–318.

Dellicour S, Hall S, Chandramohan D, Greenwood B. The safety of artemisinins during pregnancy: A pressing question. *Malar J,* **2007,** *6:*15.

Dondorp AM, Nosten F, Yi P, *et al.* Artemisinin resistance in *Plasmodium falciparum* malaria. N *Engl J Med,* **2009,** *361:*455–467.

Druilhe P, Daubersies P, Patarapotikul J, *et al.* A primary malarial infection is composed of a very wide range of genetically diverse but related parasites. *J Clin Invest,* **1998,** *101:* 2008–2016.

Ducharme J, Farinotti R. Clinical pharmacokinetics and metabolism of chloroquine. Focus on recent advancements. *Clin Pharmacokinet,* **1996,** *31:*257–274.

Duraisingh MT, Cowman AF. Contribution of the *pfmdr1* gene to antimalarial drug-resistance. *Acta Trop,* **2005,** *94:*181–190.

Eastman RT, Fidock DA. Artemisinin-based combination therapies: A vital tool in efforts to eliminate malaria. *Nat Rev Microbiol,* **2009,** *7:*864–874.

Estes ML, Ewing-Wilson D, Chou SM, *et al.* Chloroquine neuromyotoxicity. Clinical and pathologic perspective. *Am J Med,* **1987,** *82:*447–455.

Fidock DA, Nomura T, Talley AK, *et al.* Mutations in the *P. falciparum* digestive vacuole transmembrane protein PfCRT and evidence for their role in chloroquine resistance. *Mol Cell,* **2000,** *6:*861–871.

Fidock DA, Wellems TE. Transformation with human dihydrofolate reductase renders malaria parasites insensitive to WR99210 but does not affect the intrinsic activity of proguanil. *Proc Natl Acad Sci USA,* **1997,** *94:*10931–10936.

Fitch, CD. Choloroquine resistance in malaria: A deficiency of chloroquine binding. *Proc Natl Acad Sci USA*, **1969,** *64*:1181–1187.

Fivelman QL, Adagu IS, Warhurst DC. Modified fixed-ratio isobologram method for studying *in vitro* interactions between atovaquone and proguanil or dihydroartemisinin against drug-resistant strains of *Plasmodium falciparum. Antimicrob Agents Chemother,* **2004,** *48:*4097–4102.

Freedman DO. Clinical practice. Malaria prevention in short-term travelers. *N Engl J Med,* **2008,** *359:*603–612.

Gardiner DL, Skinner-Adams TS, Brown CL, *et al. Plasmodium falciparum*: New molecular targets with potential for antimalarial drug development. *Expert Rev Anti Infect Ther,* **2009,** *7:*1087–1098.

Gasasira AF, Kamya MR, Achan J, *et al.* High risk of neutropenia in HIV-infected children following treatment with artesunate plus amodiaquine for uncomplicated malaria in Uganda. *Clin Infect Dis,* **2008,** *46:*985–991.

German PI, Aweeka FT. Clinical pharmacology of artemisinin-based combination therapies. *Clin Pharmacokinet,* **2008,** *47:*91–102.

Ginsburg H, Golenser J. Glutathione is involved in the antimalarial action of chloroquine and its modulation affects drug sensitivity of human and murine species of *Plasmodium. Redox Rep,* **2003,** *8:*276–279.

Goldberg DE. Hemoglobin degradation. *Curr Top Microbiol Immunol,* **2005,** *295:*275–291.

Golenser J, Waknine JH, Krugliak M, *et al.* Current perspectives on the mechanism of action of artemisinins. *Int J Parasitol,* **2006,** *36:*1427–1441.

Gregson A, Plowe CV. Mechanisms of resistance of malaria parasites to antifolates. *Pharmacol Rev,* **2005,** *57:*117–145.

Griffith KS, Lewis LS, Mali S, Parise ME. Treatment of malaria in the United States: A systematic review. *JAMA,* **2007,** *297:* 2264–2277.

Harrington WE, Mutabingwa TK, Muehlenbachs A, *et al.* Competitive facilitation of drug-resistant *Plasmodium falciparum* malaria parasites in pregnant women who receive preventive treatment. *Proc Natl Acad Sci USA,* **2009,** *106:* 9027–9032.

Hayton K, Su XZ. Drug resistance and genetic mapping in *Plasmodium falciparum. Curr Genet,* **2008,** *54:*223–239.

Hellgren U, Berggren-Palme I, Bergqvist Y, Jerling M. Enantioselective pharmacokinetics of mefloquine during long-term intake of the prophylactic dose. *Br J Clin Pharmacol,* **1997,** *44:*119–124.

Hernandez-Diaz S, Werler MM, Walker AM, Mitchell AA. Folic acid antagonists during pregnancy and the risk of birth defects. *N Engl J Med,* **2000,** *343:*1608–1614.

Hill DR, Baird JK, Parise ME, *et al.* Primaquine: Report from CDC expert meeting on malaria chemoprophylaxis I. *Am J Trop Med Hyg,* **2006,** *75:*402–415.

Hyde JE. Targeting purine and pyrimidine metabolism in human apicomplexan parasites. *Curr Drug Targets,* **2007,** *8:*31–47.

Kain KC, Jong EC. Malaria prevention. In: *Malaria Prevention* (Jong E.C., McMullen R., eds.), Saunders, Philadelphia, **2003,** 52–74.

Kamchonwongpaisan S, Quarrell R, Charoensetakul N, *et al.* Inhibitors of multiple mutants of *Plasmodium falciparum* dihydrofolate reductase and their antimalarial activities. *J Med Chem,* **2004,** *47:*673–680.

Kessl JJ, Meshnick SR, Trumpower BL. Modeling the molecular basis of atovaquone resistance in parasites and pathogenic fungi. *Trends Parasitol,* **2007,** *23:*494–501.

Krishna S, White, NJ. Pharmacokinetics of quinine, chloroquine and amodiaquine. Clinical implications. *Clin Pharmacokinet,* **1996,** *30:*263–299.

Lacy MD, Maguire JD, Barcus MJ, *et al.* Atovaquone/proguanil therapy for *Plasmodium falciparum* and *Plasmodium vivax* malaria in Indonesians who lack clinical immunity. *Clin Infect Dis,* **2002,** *35:*e92–95.

Ling J, Baird JK, Fryauff DJ, *et al.* Randomized, placebo-controlled trial of atovaquone/proguanil for the prevention of *Plasmodium falciparum* or *Plasmodium vivax* malaria among migrants to Papua, Indonesia. *Clin Infect Dis,* **2002,** *35:*825–833.

Looareesuwan S, Chulay JD, Canfield CJ, Hutchinson DB. Malarone (atovaquone and proguanil hydrochloride): A review of its clinical development for treatment of malaria. Malarone Clinical Trials Study Group. *Am J Trop Med Hyg,* **1999,** *60:*533–541.

Lozovsky ER, Chookajorn T, Brown KM, *et al.* Stepwise acquisition of pyrimethamine resistance in the malaria parasite. *Proc Natl Acad Sci USA,* **2009,** *106:*12025–12030.

Martin RE, Marchetti RV, Cowan AI, *et al.* Chloroquine transport via the malaria parasite's chloroquine resistance transporter. *Science,* **2009,** *325:*1680–1682.

McGready R, Tan SO, Ashley EA, *et al.* A randomised controlled trial of artemether-lumefantrine versus artesunate for uncomplicated plasmodium falciparum treatment in pregnancy. *PLoS Med,* **2008,** *5:*e253.

Medhi B, Patyar S, Rao RS, *et al.* Pharmacokinetic and toxicological profile of artemisinin compounds: An update. *Pharmacology,* **2009,** *84:*323–332.

Ménard D, Barnadas C, Bouchier C, et al. *Plasmodium vivax* clinical malaria is commonly observed in Duffy-negative Malagasy people. *Proc Natl Acad Sci,* **2010,** *107:*5967–5971.

Miller KD, Greenberg AE, Campbell CC. Treatment of severe malaria in the United States with a continuous infusion of quinidine gluconate and exchange transfusion. *N Engl J Med,* **1989,** *321:*65–70.

Musset L, Bouchaud O, Matheron S, *et al.* Clinical atovaquone-proguanil resistance of *Plasmodium falciparum* associated with cytochrome b codon 268 mutations. *Microbes Infect,* **2006,** *8:*2599–2604.

Nair S, Miller B, Barends M, *et al.* Adaptive copy number evolution in malaria parasites. *PLoS Genet,* **2008,** *4:*e1000243.

Nkrumah LJ, Riegelhaupt PM, Moura P, *et al.* Probing the multifactorial basis of *Plasmodium falciparum* quinine resistance: Evidence for a strain-specific contribution of the sodium-proton exchanger PfNHE. *Mol Biochem Parasitol,* **2009,** *165:* 122–131.

Olliaro P, Mussano P. Amodiaquine for treating malaria. *Cochrane Database Syst Rev,* **2003,** CD000016.

Olliaro P, Wells TN. The global portfolio of new antimalarial medicines under development. *Clin Pharmacol Ther,* **2009,** *85:*584–595.

Painter HJ, Morrisey JM, Mather MW, Vaidya AB. Specific role of mitochondrial electron transport in blood-stage *Plasmodium falciparum. Nature,* **2007,** *446:*88–91.

Peterson DS, Milhous WK, Wellems TE. Molecular basis of differential resistance to cycloguanil and pyrimethamine in *Plasmodium falciparum* malaria. *Proc Natl Acad Sci USA,* **1990,** *87:*3018–3022.

Price RN, Douglas NM, Anstey NM. New developments in *Plasmodium vivax* malaria: Severe disease and the rise of chloroquine resistance. *Curr Opin Infect Dis,* **2009,** *22:*430–435.

Price RN, Uhlemann A-C, Brockman A, *et al.* Mefloquine resistance in *Plasmodium falciparum* and increased *pfmdr1* gene copy number. *Lancet,* **2004,** *364:*438–447.

Raj DK, Mu J, Jiang H, *et al.* Disruption of a *Plasmodium falciparum* multidrug resistance-associated protein (PfMRP) alters its fitness and transport of antimalarial drugs and glutathione. *J Biol Chem,* **2009,** *284:*7687–7696.

Rennie IG. Clinically important ocular reactions to systemic drug therapy. *Drug Saf,* **1993,** *9:*196–211.

Rocco F. *The Miraculous Fever-Tree: Malaria and the Quest for a Cure That Changed the World.* HarperCollins, New York, **2003.**

Rohrbach P, Sanchez CP, Hayton K, *et al.* Genetic linkage of *pfmdr1* with food vacuolar solute import in *Plasmodium falciparum. EMBO J,* **2006,** *25:*3000–3011.

Rose GW, Suh KN, Kain KC, *et al.* Atovaquone-proguanil resistance in imported *falciparum* malaria in a young child. *Pediatr Infect Dis J,* **2008,** *27:*567–569.

Rosenthal PJ. Artesunate for the treatment of severe falciparum malaria. *N Engl J Med,* **2008,** *358:*1829–1836.

Sanchez CP, Rohrbach P, McLean JE, *et al.* Differences in trans-stimulated chloroquine efflux kinetics are linked to PfCRT in *Plasmodium falciparum. Mol Microbiol,* **2007,** *64:*407–420.

Schlagenhauf P, Petersen E. Malaria chemoprophylaxis: Strategies for risk groups. *Clin Microbiol Rev,* **2008,** *21:*466–472.

Schlitzer M. Malaria chemotherapeutics part I: History of antimalarial drug development, currently used therapeutics, and drugs in clinical development. *Chem Med Chem,* **2007,** *2:*944–986.

Sidhu AB, Verdier-Pinard D, Fidock DA. Chloroquine resistance in *Plasmodium falciparum* malaria parasites conferred by *pfcrt* mutations. *Science,* **2002,** *298:*210–213.

Sidhu ABS, Valderramos SG, Fidock DA. *pfmdr1* mutations contribute to quinine resistance and enhance mefloquine and artemisinin sensitivity in *Plasmodium falciparum. Mol Microbiol,* **2005,** *57:*913–926.

Sinclair D, Zani B, Donegan S, *et al.* Artemisinin-based combination therapy for treating uncomplicated malaria. *Cochrane Database Syst Rev,* **2009,** CD007483.

Sisowath C, Petersen I, Veiga MI, *et al. In vivo* selection of *Plasmodium falciparum* parasites carrying the chloroquine-susceptible *pfcrt* K76 allele after treatment with artemether-lumefantrine in Africa. *J Infect Dis,* **2009,** *199:*750–757.

Srivastava IK, Morrisey JM, Darrouzet E, *et al.* Resistance mutations reveal the atovaquone-binding domain of cytochrome b in malaria parasites. *Mol Microbiol,* **1999,** *33:*704–711.

Sullivan DJ Jr, Matile H, Ridley RG, Goldberg DE. A common mechanism for blockade of heme polymerization by antimalarial quinolines. *J Biol Chem,* **1998,** *273:*31103–31107.

Taylor WR, White NJ. Antimalarial drug toxicity: A review. *Drug Saf,* **2004,** *27:*25–61.

Tehrani R, Ostrowski RA, Hariman R, Jay WM. Ocular toxicity of hydroxychloroquine. *Semin Ophthalmol,* **2008,** *23:*201–209.

Thompson MJ, White N, Jong EC. Malaria diagnosis and treatment. In: *Malaria Diagnosis and Treatment* (Jong EC, McMullen R, eds.), Saunders, Philadelphia, **2003,** 269–288.

Vaidya AB, Mather MW. Mitochondrial evolution and functions in malaria parasites. *Annu Rev Microbiol,* **2009,** *63:*249–267.

Valderramos SG, Fidock DA. Transporters involved in resistance to antimalarial drugs. *Trends Pharmacol Sci,* **2006,** *27:* 594–601.

Vale N, Moreira R, Gomes P. Primaquine revisited six decades after its discovery. *Eur J Med Chem,* **2009,** *44:*937–953.

Vinetz JM, Li J, McCutchan TF, Kaslow DC. *Plasmodium malariae* infection in an asymptomatic 74-year-old Greek woman with splenomegaly. *N Engl J Med,* **1998,** *338:* 367–371.

Ward SA, Sevene EJ, Hastings IM, Nosten F, McGready R. Antimalarial drugs and pregnancy: safety, pharmacokinetics, and pharmacovigilance. *Lancet Infect Dis*, **2007,** *7*:136–144.

Wells TN, Alonso PL, Gutteridge WE. New medicines to improve control and contribute to the eradication of malaria. *Nat Rev Drug Discov,* **2009,** *8:*879–891.

World Health Organization. World Malaria Report, 2009. Available at: http://www.who.int/malaria/world_malaria_report_2009/en/index.html. Accessed January 12, 2010.

White NJ. Antimalarial drug resistance. *J Clin Invest,* **2004,** *113:*1084–1092.

White NJ. Qinghaosu (artemisinin): The price of success. *Science,* **2008,** *320:*330–334.

Wiesner J, Jomaa H. Isoprenoid biosynthesis of the apicoplast as drug target. *Curr Drug Targets,* **2007,** *8:*3–13.

Wiesner J, Reichenberg A, Heinrich S, *et al.* The plastid-like organelle of apicomplexan parasites as drug target. *Curr Pharm Des,* **2008,** *14:*855–871.

Winzeler EA. Malaria research in the post-genomic era. *Nature,* **2008,** *455:*751–756.

Yeshiwondim AK, Tekle AH, Dengela DO, *et al.* Therapeutic efficacy of chloroquine and chloroquine plus primaquine for the treatment of *Plasmodium vivax* in Ethiopia. *Acta Trop,* **2010,** *113:*105–113.

Zhang K, Rathod PK. Divergent regulation of dihydrofolate reductase between malaria parasite and human host. *Science,* **2002,** *296:*545–547.

Chemotherapy of Protozoal Infections: Amebiasis, Giardiasis, Trichomoniasis, Trypanosomiasis, Leishmaniasis, and Other Protozoal Infections

Margaret A. Phillips
and Samuel L. Stanley, Jr.

Humans host a wide variety of protozoal parasites that can be transmitted by insect vectors, directly from other mammalian reservoirs or from one person to another. Because protozoa multiply rapidly in their hosts and effective vaccines are unavailable, chemotherapy has been the only practical way to both treat infected individuals and reduce transmission. The immune system plays a crucial role in protecting against the pathological consequences of protozoal infections. Thus, opportunistic infections with protozoa are prominent in infants, individuals with cancer, transplant recipients, those receiving immunosuppressive drugs or extensive antibiotic therapy, and persons with advanced human immunodeficiency virus (HIV) infection. Treatment of protozoal infections in immunocompromised individuals is especially difficult, and the outcome is often unsatisfactory.

Most antiprotozoal drugs have been in use for years despite major advances in bioscience relevant to parasite biology, host defenses, and mechanisms of disease. Satisfactory agents for treating important protozoal infections such as African trypanosomiasis (sleeping sickness) and chronic Chagas' disease still are lacking. Many effective antiprotozoal drugs are toxic at therapeutic doses, a problem exacerbated by increasing drug resistance. Development of drug resistance also poses a serious threat to better tolerated antiprotozoal agents in current use. Unfortunately, many of these diseases afflict the poor in developing countries, and there is little economic incentive for pharmaceutical companies to develop new antiparasitic drugs. Scientists and physicians working in this field must be creative and have turned to drugs developed originally for other indications (e.g., amphotericin and miltefosine for leishmaniasis), to investigational drugs made available directly from the Centers for Disease Control and Prevention (CDC), or to agents developed for veterinary use to discover new antiparasitic therapies.

This chapter describes important human protozoal infections other than malaria and the drugs used to treat them.

INTRODUCTION TO PROTOZOAL INFECTIONS OF HUMANS

Amebiasis. Amebiasis affects ~10% of the world's population, causing invasive disease in ~50 million people and death in ~100,000 of these annually (Stanley, 2003). In the U.S., amebiasis is seen most commonly in the states that border Mexico and among individuals living in poverty, crowded conditions, and areas with poor sanitation. Three morphologically identical but genetically distinct species of *Entamoeba* (i.e., *E. histolytica, E. dispar, and E. moshkovskii*) have been isolated from infected persons. Although the proportions vary worldwide, *E. dispar* and *E. moshkovskii* account for ~90% of human infections, with *E. histolytica* responsible for only 10%. However, only *E. histolytica* is capable of causing disease and thus requires treatment.

The organisms can be differentiated by antigen-detection enzyme-linked immunosorbent assays or by polymerase chain reaction (PCR)–based diagnostics. Humans are the only known hosts for these protozoa, which are transmitted almost exclusively by the fecal-oral route. Ingested *E. histolytica* cysts from contaminated food or water survive acid gastric contents and transform into *trophozoites* that reside in the large intestine. The outcome of *E. histolytica* infection is variable. Many individuals remain asymptomatic but excrete the infectious cyst form, making them a source for further infections. In other individuals, *E. histolytica* trophozoites invade into the colonic mucosa with resulting colitis and bloody diarrhea (amebic dysentery). In a smaller proportion of patients, *E. histolytica* trophozoites invade through the colonic mucosa, reach the portal circulation, and travel to the liver, where they establish an amebic liver abscess.

The cornerstone of therapy for amebiasis is the nitroimidazole compound metronidazole or its analogs tinidazole and ornidazole. Metronidazole and tinidazole are the only nitroimidazoles available in the U.S. and are the drugs of choice for the treatment of amebic colitis, amebic liver abscess, and any other extraintestinal form of amebiasis. Because metronidazole is so well absorbed in the gut, levels may not be therapeutic in the colonic lumen, and the drug is less effective against cysts. Hence patients with amebiasis (amebic colitis or amebic liver abscess) also should receive a luminal agent to eradicate any *E. histolytica* trophozoites residing within the gut lumen. Luminal agents are also used to treat asymptomatic individuals found to be infected with *E. histolytica*. The nonabsorbed aminoglycoside paromomycin and the 8-hydroxyquinoline compound iodoquinol are two effective luminal agents. Diloxanide furoate, previously considered the luminal agent of choice for amebiasis, is no longer available in the U.S. Nitazoxanide (ALINIA), a drug approved in the U.S. for the treatment of cryptosporidiosis and giardiasis, is also active against *E. histolytica*.

Giardiasis. Giardiasis, caused by the flagellated protozoan *Giardia intestinalis*, is prevalent worldwide and is the most commonly reported intestinal protozoal infection in the U.S. (Hlavsa et al., 2005). Infection results from ingestion of the cyst form of the parasite, which is found in fecally contaminated water or food. *Giardia* is a zoonosis, and cysts shed from animals or from infected humans can contaminate recreational and drinking water supplies. Human-to-human transmission via the fecal-oral route is especially common among children in day-care centers and nurseries, as well as among institutionalized individuals and male homosexuals.

Infection with *Giardia* results in one of three syndromes: an asymptomatic carrier state, acute self-limited diarrhea, or chronic diarrhea. Asymptomatic infection is most common; these individuals excrete *Giardia* cysts and serve as a source for new infections. Most adults with symptomatic infection develop an acute self-limited illness with watery, foul-smelling stools, abdominal distension, and flatus. However, a significant proportion of these individuals go on to develop a chronic diarrhea syndrome (>2 weeks of illness) with signs of malabsorption (steatorrhea) and weight loss.

The diagnosis of giardiasis is made by identification of cysts or trophozoites in fecal specimens or of trophozoites in duodenal contents. Chemotherapy with a 5-day course of metronidazole usually is successful, although therapy may have to be repeated or prolonged in some instances. A single dose of tinidazole (TINDAMAX, others) probably is superior to metronidazole for the treatment of giardiasis. Paromomycin (HUMATIN, others) has been used to treat pregnant women to avoid any possible mutagenic effects of the other drugs. Nitazoxanide (ALINIA), N-(nitrothiazolyl) salicylamide, and tinidazole were approved recently for the treatment of giardiasis in immune-competent children <12 years of age. Furazolidone, previously used for the treatment of giardiasis, has been discontinued in the U.S.

Trichomoniasis. Trichomoniasis is caused by the flagellated protozoan *Trichomonas vaginalis*. This organism inhabits the genitourinary tract of the human host, where it causes vaginitis in women and, uncommonly, urethritis in men. Trichomoniasis is a sexually transmitted disease, with >200 million people infected worldwide and at least 3 million women infected in the U.S. annually. Infection with *Trichomonas* has been associated with an increased risk of acquiring HIV infection. Only *trophozoite* forms of *T. vaginalis* have been identified in infected secretions.

Metronidazole remains the drug of choice for the treatment of trichomoniasis. However, treatment failures owing to metronidazole-resistant organisms are becoming more frequent (Dunne et al., 2003). Tinidazole, another nitroimidazole that was approved recently by the FDA, appears to be better tolerated than metronidazole and has been used successfully at higher doses to treat metronidazole-resistant *T. vaginalis* (Sobel et al., 2001). Nitazoxanide shows activity against *T. vaginalis in vitro* but has not undergone clinical trials and is not licensed for the treatment of trichomoniasis.

Toxoplasmosis. Toxoplasmosis is a cosmopolitan zoonotic infection caused by the obligate intracellular protozoan *Toxoplasma gondii* (Montoya and Liesenfeld, 2004). Although cats and other feline species are the natural hosts, tissue cysts (*bradyzoites*) have been recovered from all mammalian species examined. The four most common routes of infection in humans are:

- ingestion of undercooked meat containing tissue cysts
- ingestion of vegetable matter contaminated with soil containing infective *oocysts*
- direct oral contact with feces of cats shedding oocysts
- transplacental fetal infection with *tachyzoites* from acutely infected mothers

Primary infection with *T. gondii* produces clinical symptoms in ~10% of immunocompetent individuals. The acute illness is usually self-limiting, and treatment rarely is required. Individuals who are immunocompromised, however, are at risk of developing toxoplasmic encephalitis from reactivation of tissue cysts deposited in the brain. The vast majority of cases of toxoplasmic encephalitis are seen in patients with AIDS, in whom the disease is fatal if it is not recognized and treated appropriately. Clinical manifestations of congenital toxoplasmosis vary widely, but chorioretinitis, which may present decades after perinatal exposure, is the most commonly recognized finding.

The primary treatment for toxoplasmic encephalitis consists of the antifolates pyrimethamine (DARAPRIM) and sulfadiazine along with folinic acid (leucovorin). However, therapy must be discontinued in ~40% of cases because of toxicity owing primarily to the sulfa compound. In this instance, clindamycin can be substituted for sulfadiazine without loss of efficacy. Alternative regimens combining azithromycin, clarithromycin, atovaquone, or dapsone with either trimethoprim-sulfamethoxazole or pyrimethamine and folinic acid are less toxic but also less effective than the combination of pyrimethamine and sulfadiazine.

Spiramycin, which concentrates in placental tissue, is used for the treatment of acute acquired toxoplasmosis in pregnancy to prevent transmission to the fetus. If fetal infection is detected, the combination of pyrimethamine, sulfadiazine, and folinic acid is administered to the mother (only after the first 12-14 weeks of pregnancy) and to the newborn in the postnatal period. Spiramycin is not available in the U.S.

Cryptosporidiosis. Cryptosporidia are coccidian protozoan parasites that can cause diarrhea in a number of animal species, including humans (Ramirez et al., 2004). Their taxonomy is evolving, but *Cryptosporidium parvum* and the newly named *C. hominis* appear to account for almost all infections in humans.

Infectious *oocysts* in feces may be spread either by direct human-to-human contact or by contaminated water supplies, the latter being recognized as an established route of epidemic infection. Groups at risk include travelers, children in day-care facilities, male homosexuals, animal handlers, veterinarians, and other healthcare personnel. Immunocompromised individuals are especially vulnerable. After ingestion, the mature oocyte is digested, releasing *sporozoites* that invade host epithelial cells, penetrating the cell membrane but not actually entering the cytoplasm. In most individuals, infection is self-limited. However, in AIDS patients and other immunocompromised individuals, the severity of voluminous, secretory diarrhea may require hospitalization and supportive therapy to prevent severe electrolyte imbalance and dehydration.

The most effective therapy for cryptosporidiosis in AIDS patients is restoration of their immune function through highly active antiretroviral therapy (HAART) (Chapter 59). Nitazoxanide has shown activity in treating cryptosporidiosis in immunocompetent children and is possibly effective in immunocompetent adults (Rossignol et al., 2001). Its efficacy in children and adults with HIV infection and AIDS is not clearly established, although some studies showed a modest benefit in a subset of adult men with AIDS and chronic cryptosporidiosis (Rossignol, 2006; Sears and Kirkpatrick, 2007). Nevertheless, nitazoxanide is currently the only drug approved for the treatment of cryptosporidiosis in the U.S.

Trypanosomiasis. African trypanosomiasis, or "sleeping sickness," is caused by subspecies of the hemoflagellate *Trypanosoma brucei* that are transmitted by bloodsucking tsetse flies of the genus *Glossinia* (Barrett et al., 2007; Kennedy, 2008; Stuart et al., 2008). Largely restricted to sub-Saharan Africa, the infection causes serious human illness and also threatens livestock (*nagana*), leading to protein malnutrition. In humans, the infection is fatal unless treated. Owing to strict surveillance, vector control, and early therapy, the prevalence of African sleeping sickness declined to its nadir in the early 1960s. However, relaxation of these measures, together with massive population displacement and breakdowns in societal infrastructure owing to armed conflict, led to a resurgence of this disease in the 1990s. An estimated 500,000 Africans carry the infection, and >50 million people are at risk for the disease. It is extremely rare in travelers returning to the U.S. and can be difficult to diagnose in its more chronic form (Lejon et al., 2003).

The parasite is entirely extracellular, and early human infection is characterized by the finding of replicating parasites in the bloodstream or lymph without CNS involvement (stage 1); stage 2 disease is characterized by CNS involvement (Blum et al., 2006). Symptoms of early-stage disease include febrile illness, lymphadenopathy, splenomegaly, and occasional myocarditis that result from systemic dissemination of the parasites. There are two types of African trypanosomiasis, the East African (Rhodesian) and West

African (Gambian), caused by *T. brucei rhodesiense* and *T. brucei gambiense*, respectively. *T. brucei rhodesiense* produces a progressive and rapidly fatal form of disease marked by early involvement of the CNS and frequent terminal cardiac failure; *T. brucei gambiense* causes illness that is characterized by later involvement of the CNS and a more long-term course that progresses to the classical symptoms of sleeping sickness over months to years. Neurological symptoms include confusion, poor coordination, sensory deficits, an array of psychiatric signs, disruption of the sleep cycle, and eventual progression into coma and death.

Four drugs are used for the treatment of sleeping sickness, and only one, eflornithine, has been developed since the 1950s (Barrett et al., 2007; Croft, 2008; Fries and Fairlamb, 2003; Kennedy, 2008; Stuart et al., 2008). Standard therapy for early-stage disease is pentamidine for *T. brucei gambiense* and suramin for *T. brucei rhodesiense*. Both compounds must be given parenterally over long periods and are not effective against late-stage disease. The CNS phase has traditionally been treated with melarsoprol (available from the CDC), which is a highly toxic agent that causes a fatal reactive encephalopathy in 2-10% of treated patients. Moreover, lack of response to this agent is leading to increasing numbers of treatment failures (Pepin and Mpia, 2005, Robays et al., 2008b). Eflornithine, which was developed originally as an anticancer agent and approved as an orphan drug, offers the only alternative for the treatment of late-stage disease. This compound is an inhibitor of ornithine decarboxylase, a key enzyme in polyamine metabolism. It has shown marked efficacy against both early and late stages of human *T. brucei gambiense* infection; however, it is ineffective as monotherapy for infections of *T. brucei rhodesiense*. Notably, eflornithine has significantly fewer side effects than melarsoprol and is more effective than melarsoprol for treatment of late-stage Gambian trypanosomiasis, suggesting that eflornithine is the best available first-line treatment for this form of the disease (Chappuis, 2007). Although eflornithine is expensive and difficult to administer, nifurtimox-eflornithine combination therapy (NECT) allows a shorter exposure to eflornithine with good efficacy and a reduction in adverse events (Priotto et al., 2009).

Recent efforts by not-for-profit agencies have fostered significant new efforts to develop new therapies for the neglected tropical diseases including African sleeping sickness, Chagas' disease, and Leishmaniasis (Croft, 2007; Frearson et al., 2007; Nwaka and Hudson, 2006; Pink et al., 2005; Stuart et al., 2008). These efforts involve partnerships with academic and industrial groups. The recent increase in high throughput screening centers within academic groups with interest in developing drugs for these applications is also helping to fuel discovery of lead compounds. The genome data is being exploited to develop publicly accessible databases that organize data relevant to drug discovery projects (Aguero et al., 2008). From these efforts an orally available novel diamidine, pafuramidine maleate (DB289), was recently advanced to phase IV trials for the treatment of early-stage (stage 1) sleeping sickness, representing the only new clinical candidate since the discovery of eflornithine (Mdachi et al., 2009). Although the trials were stopped due to toxicity issues (Kennedy, 2008), the discovery of pafuramidine provides hope that the current approaches and increased effort will yield new clinical entities for these diseases in the near future.

American trypanosomiasis, or *Chagas' disease*, a zoonotic infection caused by *Trypanosoma cruzi*, affects ~15 million people from Mexico to Argentina and Chile, with 50,000-200,000 new infections added each year (Bern et al., 2007; Stuart et al., 2008; Tarleton et al., 2007). The chronic form of the disease in adults is a major cause of cardiomyopathy, megaesophagus, megacolon, and death. Blood-sucking triatomid bugs infesting poor rural dwellings most commonly transmit this infection to young children; transplacental transmission also may occur in endemic areas.

Reactivation of disease also may occur in patients who are immunosuppressed after organ transplantation or because of infection (e.g., AIDS, leukemia, and other neoplasias). Occurrences of *T. cruzi* infection in transplant patients or through blood transfusions have been reported in the U.S., and as a consequence the FDA-approved diagnostic blood screening for the parasite (Bern et al., 2008). Reports of autochthonous Chagas cases are also on the rise in the U.S. Acute infection is evidenced by a raised tender skin nodule (*chagoma*) at the site of inoculation; other signs may be absent or range from fever, adenitis, skin rash, and hepatosplenomegaly to, albeit rarely, acute myocarditis, and death. Invading metacyclic *trypomastigotes* penetrate host cells, especially macrophages, where they proliferate as *amastigotes*. These then differentiate into trypomastigotes that enter the bloodstream. Circulating trypomastigotes do not multiply until they invade other cells or are ingested by an insect vector during a blood meal. After recovery from the acute infection that lasts a few weeks to months, individuals usually remain asymptomatic for years despite sporadic parasitemia. During this period, their blood can transmit the parasites to transfusion recipients and accidentally to laboratory workers. Approximately 20-30% of infected individuals eventually progress to clinically evident disease that is characterized by chronic disease of the heart and GI tract as they age. Progressive destruction of myocardial cells and neurons of the myenteric plexus results from the special tropism of *T. cruzi* for muscle cells. Recent studies with improved techniques indicate the presence of *T. cruzi* at sites of cardiac lesions, and it is now well recognized that parasite persistence is linked directly to pathology and disease outcome (Tarleton, 2003). Whether an undefined autoimmune response also contributes to the pathogenesis of Chagas' disease is unknown; however, the data indicate that immunological defenses, especially cell-mediated immunity, do modulate the course of disease.

Two nitroheterocyclic drugs, nifurtimox (available from the CDC) and benznidazole are used to treat this infection (Bern et al., 2007; Croft, 2008; Tarleton et al., 2007). Both agents suppress parasitemia and can cure the acute phase of Chagas' disease in 60-80% of cases; however, both drugs are toxic and must be taken for long periods. A long-term clinical trial with results expected in 2011 (BENEFIT) is currently underway to provide clarification of the role of treatment in modulating disease progression and preventing death (http://clinicaltrials.gov/show/NCT00123916; Marin-Neto et al., 2008). Field isolates vary with respect to their susceptibility to nifurtimox and benznidazole. Moreover, cross-resistance to both compounds can be induced in the laboratory (Wilkinson et al., 2008).

Clearly, new drugs with better potency against parasites in the chronic phase and with reduced toxicities are needed. A key factor in new drug development for Chagas' disease is the need for better methods to assess parasitological cure. Several important reports documenting significant advances in this area have recently been published (Bustamante et al., 2008; Cooley et al., 2008). Additionally, some promising strides toward the development of new agents have been made. Inhibitors of an essential protease, cruzipain, have anti-parasite activity, and one (K777) is in preclinical development for the treatment of Chagas' disease (Doyle et al., 2007). In the absence of new drugs, however, alternative measures such as improved vector control and housing accommodations have been used to reduce the transmission of Chagas' disease substantially in Brazil, Chile, and Venezuela (World Health Organization, 1999).

Leishmaniasis. Leishmaniasis is a complex vector-borne zoonosis caused by ~20 different species of obligate intramacrophage protozoa of the genus *Leishmania* (Chappuis et al., 2007; Croft 2008; Stuart et al., 2008). Small mammals and canines generally serve as reservoirs for these pathogens, which can be transmitted to humans by the bites of some 30 different species of female phlebotomine sandflies.

Various forms of leishmaniasis affect people in southern Europe and many tropical and subtropical regions throughout the world. Flagellated extracellular free *promastigotes*, regurgitated by feeding flies, enter the host, where they attach to and become phagocytized by tissue macrophages. These transform into *amastigotes*, which reside and multiply within phagolysosomes until the cell bursts. Released amastigotes then propagate the infection by invading more macrophages. Amastigotes taken up by feeding sandflies transform back into promastigotes, thereby completing the transformation cycle. The particular localized or systemic disease syndrome caused by *Leishmania* depends on the species or subspecies of infecting parasite, the distribution of infected macrophages, and especially the host's immune response. In increasing order of systemic involvement and potential clinical severity, major syndromes of human leishmaniasis have been classified into *cutaneous, mucocutaneous, diffuse cutaneous*, and *visceral* (*kala azar*) forms. Leishmaniasis increasingly is becoming recognized as an AIDS-associated opportunistic infection.

The classification, clinical features, course, and chemotherapy of human leishmaniasis syndromes as well as the biochemistry and immunology of the parasite and host germane to chemotherapy have been recently reviewed (Chappuis et al., 2007; Croft and Coombs, 2003; Stuart et al., 2008). Cutaneous forms of leishmaniasis generally are self-limiting, with cures occurring in 3-18 months after infection. However, this form of the disease can leave disfiguring scars. The mucocutaneous, diffuse cutaneous, and visceral forms of the disease do not resolve without therapy. Visceral leishmaniasis caused by *L. donovani* is fatal unless treated.

The list of current drugs useful for the treatment of all forms of leishmaniasis has been described (Alvar et al., 2006; Croft, 2008; Olliaro et al., 2005). The classic therapy for all species of *Leishmania* is pentavalent antimony (sodium antimony gluconate; sodium stibogluconate; PENTOSTAM); resistance to this compound has led to widespread failure of this drug in India, although it remains useful in other parts of the world. As an alternative, liposomal amphotericin B is a highly effective agent for visceral leishmaniasis, and it is currently the drug of choice for antimony-resistant disease (Chappuis et al., 2007) (Chapter 57). Importantly, treatment of leishmania has undergone major changes owing to the success of the first orally active agent, miltefosine, in clinical trials (Berman, 2008; Bhattacharya et al., 2007). Miltefosine was approved in India for the treatment of visceral leishmaniasis in 2002. The drug also appears to have promise for the treatment of the cutaneous disease and for the treatment of dogs, which serve as an important animal reservoir of the disease (Berman, 2008). Paromomycin has been used with success as a parenteral agent for visceral disease (Sundar et al., 2007), and topical formulations of paromomycin have efficacy against cutaneous disease. Pentamidine may also be used for cutaneous disease (Croft, 2008).

Other Protozoal Infections. Just a few of the many less common protozoal infections of humans are highlighted here.

Babesiosis, caused by either *Babesia microcoti* or *B. divergens*, is a tick-borne zoonosis that superficially resembles malaria in that the parasites invade erythrocytes, producing a febrile illness, hemolysis, and hemoglobinuria. This infection usually is mild and self-limiting but can be severe or even fatal in asplenic or severely immunocompromised individuals. Currently recommended therapy is with a combination of clindamycin and quinine for severe disease, and the combination of azithromycin and atovaquone for mild or moderate infections.

Balantidiasis, caused by the ciliated protozoan *Balantidium coli*, is an infection of the large intestine that may be confused with amebiasis. Unlike amebiasis, however, this infection usually responds to tetracycline therapy.

Isospora belli, a coccidian parasite, causes diarrhea in AIDS patients and responds to treatment with trimethoprim-sulfamethoxazole. *Cyclospora cayetanensis*, another coccidian parasite, causes self-limited diarrhea in normal hosts and can cause prolonged diarrhea in individuals with AIDS. It is susceptible to trimethoprim-sulfamethoxazole.

Microsporidia are spore-forming unicellular eukaryotic fungal parasites that can cause a number of disease syndromes, including diarrhea in immunocompromised individuals. Infections with microsporidia of the *Encephalitozoon* genus, including *E. hellum*, *E. intestinalis*, and *E. cuniculi*, have been treated successfully with albendazole, a benzimidazole derivative and inhibitor of β-tubulin polymerization (Gross, 2003) (Chapter 51). Immunocompromised individuals with intestinal microsporidiosis due to *E. bieneusi* (which does not respond as well to albendazole) have been treated successfully with the antibiotic fumagillin (Molina et al., 2002).

ANTI-PROTOZOAL DRUGS

The myriad agents used to treat nonmalarial protozoal diseases are presented alphabetically.

Amphotericin B

The pharmacology, formulation, and toxicology of amphotericin B are presented in Chapter 57. Only those features of the drug pertinent to its use in leishmaniasis are described here.

Antiprotozoal Effects. In 1997, the FDA approved liposomal amphotericin B (AMBISOME) for the treatment of visceral leishmaniasis. Amphotericin B is a highly effective antileishmanial agent that cures >90% of the cases of visceral leishmaniasis in clinical studies, and it has become the drug of choice for antimonial-resistant cases (Bern et al., 2006; Croft, 2008, Olliaro et al., 2005). It is considered a second-line drug for cutaneous or mucosal leishmaniasis, where it has been shown effective for the treatment of immunocompromised patients (Alvar et al., 2006). However, because cutaneous leishmaniasis is typically self-limiting, the drug has not been evaluated for treatment of a broader range of patient populations. The lipid preparations of the drug have reduced toxicity, but the cost of the drug and the difficulty of administration remain a problem in endemic regions.

The mechanism of action of amphotericin B against leishmania is similar to the basis for the drug's antifungal activities (Chapter 57). Amphotericin complexes with ergosterol precursors in the cell membrane, forming pores that allow ions to enter the cell. Leishmania has similar sterol composition to fungal pathogens, and the drug binds to these sterols preferentially over the host cholesterol. No significant resistance to the drug has been encountered after nearly 30 years of use as an antifungal agent.

Therapeutic Uses. Numerous dosing schedules have been reported for the treatment of visceral leishmaniasis, with most achieving high cure rates and good safety (Alvar et al., 2006, Bern et al., 2006; Olliaro et al., 2005). Typical schemes of 10-20 mg/kg total dose given in divided doses over 10-20 days by intravenous infusion have yielded >95% cure rates. In the U.S., the FDA recommends 3 mg/kg intravenously on days 1-5, 14, and 21 for a total dose of 21 mg/kg (Meyerhoff, 1999). Shorter courses of the drug have been tested with good efficacy and provide a potential alternative with lower cost, although only a limited number of patients have been tested: Cure rates of 89-91% were observed for single doses of 3.75, 5, and 7.5 mg/kg. Recent data suggest that a single dose of 5 mg/kg followed by 7-14 days treatment with oral miltefosine was effective at curing visceral leishmaniasis, and this dosing scheme warrants additional study (Sundar et al., 2008).

Chloroquine

The pharmacology and toxicology of chloroquine are presented in Chapter 49 (anti-malarials). Chloroquine does have an FDA-approved use for *extra-intestinal amebiasis* at a dose of 1 g (600 mg base) daily for 2 days, followed by 500 mg daily for at least 2-3 weeks. Treatment is usually combined with an effective intestinal amebicide. The interested reader should consult the 11th edition of this book for further details.

Diloxanide Furoate

Diloxanide furoate (FURAMIDE, others) is the furoate ester of diloxanide, a derivative of dichloroacetamide. Diloxanide furoate is a very effective luminal agent for the treatment of *E. histolytica* infection but is no longer available in the U.S. The interested reader should consult the 10th edition of this book for further details on this agent.

Eflornithine

Eflornithine (α-D,L difluoromethylornithine, DFMO, ORNIDYL) is an irreversible catalytic (suicide) inhibitor of ornithine decarboxylase, the enzyme that catalyzes the first and rate-limiting step in the biosynthesis of polyamines (Casero and Marton, 2007). The polyamines—putrescine, spermidine, and in mammals, spermine—are required for cell division and for normal cell differentiation. In trypanosomes, spermidine additionally is required for the synthesis of trypanothione, which is a conjugate of spermidine and glutathione that replaces many of the functions of glutathione in the parasite cell (Fries and Fairlamb, 2003).

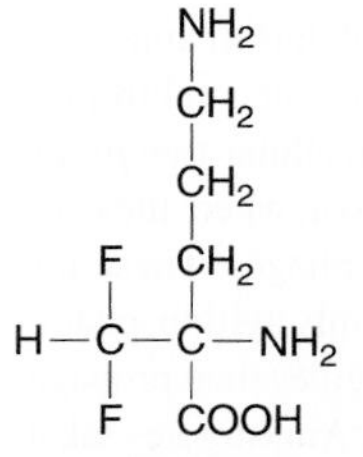

$$H{-}CF_2{-}C(NH_2)(COOH){-}CH_2{-}CH_2{-}CH_2{-}NH_2$$

EFLORNITHINE

Both in animal models and *in vitro*, eflornithine arrests the growth of several types of tumor cells, providing the basis for its clinical evaluation as an antitumor agent. The discovery that eflornithine cured rodent infections with *T. brucei* first focused attention on protozoal polyamine biosynthesis as a potential target for chemotherapeutic attack (Bacchi et al., 1980). Eflornithine currently is used to treat West African (Gambian) trypanosomiasis caused by *T. brucei gambiense* (Balasegaram et al., 2006a, 2009; Chappuis,

2007, Chappuis et al., 2005; Priotto et al., 2006, 2008; Robays et al., 2008a). In contrast, the drug is largely ineffective for East African trypanosomiasis. Eflornithine's difficult treatment regimen is the primary limitation to its use in the field. However, the negotiation of the World Health Organization (WHO) of a stable supply of eflornithine through 2011 has led to the widespread availability of the drug and to its use in control and research programs run by world health agencies.

Eflornithine is both safer and more efficacious than melarsoprol for late-stage Gambiense sleeping sickness, and it is now the recommended first-line treatment for this disease when adequate care can be provided for its administration. Eflornithine is no longer available for systemic use in the U.S. but is available for treatment of Gambian trypanosomiasis by special request from the CDC.

Antitrypanosomal Effects. The effects of eflornithine have been evaluated both on drug-susceptible and drug-resistant *T. brucei in vitro* and in infections with these parasites in rodent models (reviewed in: Barrett et al., 2007). Eflornithine is a cytostatic agent that has multiple biochemical effects on trypanosomes, all of which are a consequence of polyamine depletion. The polyamine putrescine is depleted to undetectable levels, intracellular levels of spermidine and trypanothine are reduced by 25-50%, and methionine metabolism is altered. Depletion of the polyamines, or of trypanothione, would be expected to be lethal to the cells based on genetic studies that have disrupted the biosynthetic genes in the pathway. As a consequence, macromolecular biosynthesis is depressed, and the parasites transform from the long, slender dividing forms into the short, stumpy nonreplicating forms. These latter parasites are unable to synthesize variable cell surface glycoprotein and eventually are cleared by the immune system.

The molecular mechanism of eflornithine action clearly is inhibition of ornithine decarboxylase. Eflornithine irreversibly inhibits both mammalian and trypanosomal ornithine decarboxylases, thereby preventing the synthesis of putrescine, a precursor of polyamines needed for cell division. Eflornithine inactivates the enzyme through covalent labeling of an active-site cysteine residue, and an X-ray structure of the *T. brucei* enzyme bound to the drug has been reported (Grishin et al., 1999). A number of studies demonstrate conclusively that ornithine decarboxylase is the target of eflornithine action that leads to cell death. Mutant bloodstream trypanosomes lacking ornithine decarboxylase or wild-type trypanosomes treated with eflornithine cannot replicate, and mice inoculated with these null parasites become resistant to infection by wild-type parasites (Mutomba et al., 1999). The product of the ornithine decarboxylase reaction, putrescine, rescues the growth deficit in both the mutant parasites and eflornithine-treated cells. The null mutant parasites grown with putrescine are not affected by eflornithine, demonstrating the selectivity of the drug for the target enzyme.

The mechanisms of selective toxicity between the host and parasite, or between the different species of *T. brucei*, are less clear (Barrett et al., 2007). The parasite and human enzymes are equally susceptible to inhibition by eflornithine; however, the mammalian enzyme is turned over rapidly, whereas the parasite enzyme is stable, and this difference likely plays a role in the selective toxicity. In addition, mammalian cells may be able to replenish polyamine pools through uptake of extracellular polyamines, whereas the slender bloodstream forms of human trypanosomes divide within human blood, which contains only very low levels of these essential compounds. Further, the parasites lack efficient transport mechanisms.

T. brucei rhodesiense cells are less sensitive to eflornithine inhibition than *T. brucei gambiense* cells, and studies *in vitro* suggest that the effective doses are increased by 10-20 times in the refractory cells. The molecular basis for the higher dose requirement in *T. brucei rhodesiense* is still poorly understood; however, it has been postulated to involve differences both in enzyme stability and in the metabolism of *S*-adenosylmethionine compared with the sensitive *T. brucei gambiense* cell lines.

Absorption, Fate, and Excretion. Eflornithine is given by intravenous infusion. The drug does not bind to plasma proteins but is well distributed and penetrates into the CSF, where it is estimated that concentrations of at least 50 μM must be reached to clear parasites (Burri and Brun, 2003). Despite the ability of the drug to penetrate the blood-brain barrier, studies in mice suggest that eflornithine crosses the healthy blood-CNS interface poorly, and that it is the breakdown of this barrier caused by *T. brucei* infection that allows greater penetration to occur (Sanderson et al., 2008). In these studies, suramin enhanced eflornithine uptake into the CNS, suggesting that this combination might lead to lower dose requirements for eflornithine. Renal clearance after intravenous administration is rapid (2 mL/minute per kilogram), with >80% of the drug cleared by the kidney largely in unchanged form (Burri and Brun, 2003). There is some evidence that eflornithine displays dose-dependent pharmacokinetics at the highest doses used clinically.

Therapeutic Uses. Eflornithine is used for the treatment of late-stage West African trypanosomiasis caused by *T. brucei gambiense* (Balasegaram et al., 2006a, 2008; Chappuis, 2007; Chappuis et al., 2005; Priotto et al., 2006, 2008; Robays et al., 2008a). Most patients in the reported studies had advanced disease with CNS complications. The preferred regimen for adult patients was found to be 100 mg/kg given intravenously every 6 hours as a 2-hour infusion for 14 days. Virtually all patients improved on this regimen unless they were extremely ill, and the WHO and Médecins Sans Frontières report improved rates >90%. The probability of disease-free survival 2 years after treatment was calculated to be 0.88 in one study (Priotto et al., 2008) and the case-fatality rate of 1% for eflornithine was the lowest reported for second-stage sleeping sickness in any study (Chappuis et al., 2005). Children (<12 years of age) received higher doses of eflornithine (150 mg/kg given intravenously every 6 hours for 14 days) based on prior findings that eflornithine trough concentrations in both the CSF and blood were significantly lower among children than in adults (Milord et al., 1993). Patients who failed therapy in this study tended to have trough CSF concentrations <50 μM. Equal doses of eflornithine were less effective when given by the oral route probably because of limited bioavailability. The problem cannot be overcome simply by increasing the oral dose because of ensuing osmotic diarrhea.

Eflornithine has proven to be less successful for treating AIDS patients with West African trypanosomiasis, presumably because host defenses play a critical role in clearing drug-treated *T. brucei gambiense* from the bloodstream.

The standard course eflornithine treatment regime is very challenging to administer in rural settings in Africa. A randomized phase III trial testing nifurtimox-eflornithine combination therapy for second-stage *T. brucel gambiense* suggested that the treatment course for eflornithine could be reduced to 7 days in combination with nifurtimox. A recently concluded clinical trial confirms the efficacy of nifurtimox used in combination with eflornithine (NECT) (Priotto, 2009). This new protocol uses a shortened course of eflornithine in combination with oral nifurtimox, with dosing as follows: 400 mg/kg per day given intravenously every 12 h by 2 h infusion for 7 days plus nifurtimox (orally at 15 mg/kg per day in 3 divided doses [every 8 h]) for 10 days. This combination is logistically easier to administer and it requires less eflornithine, which is expensive to synthesize. Importantly, compared to eflornithine alone, NECT achieves a higher cure rate (96.5% vs. 91.5%). NECT has been added to the WHO essentials medicines list and is likely to become the front line treatment for the indication. Drug combination may also reduce the potential for eflornithine resistance to develop in the field. Given the paucity of drugs available for the treatment of late stage disease, the development of eflornithine resistance would represent a very serious problem.

Toxicity and Side Effects. Eflornithine is reported to cause adverse reactions in most of the treated patients (Balasegaram et al., 2008; Burri and Brun, 2003; Chappuis, 2007; Chappuis et al., 2005; Priotto et al., 2006, 2008); however, they are generally reversible on withdrawal of the drug. Abdominal pain, both mild and moderate, and headache were the predominant complaints followed by reactions at the injection sites. Tissue infections and pneumonia were also observed. The most severe reactions reported for one study, with numbers given for events classified as major, included fever peaks (6%), seizures (4%), and diarrhea (2%) (Priotto et al., 2008). The case fatality rate for eflornithine (~1.2%) is significantly lower than for melarsoprol (4.9%), and overall eflornithine is superior to melarsoprol with respect to both safety and efficacy. Reversible hearing loss can occur after prolonged therapy with oral doses. Although this has been a problem in the use of eflornithine for cancer chemotherapy, hearing loss has not been observed during the treatment of sleeping sickness.

Therapeutic doses of eflornithine are large and require coadministration of substantial volumes of intravenous fluid. This poses significant practical limitations in remote settings and can cause fluid overload in susceptible patients. For NECT, the severe adverse events were reduced compared to eflornithine alone (14% vs. 29%), and treatment related deaths were also fewer (0.7% vs. 2%) (Priotto, 2009). Both NECT and eflornithine alone showed significantly fewer treatment-related deaths than what has been reported for melarsoprol. With eflornithine alone, most reported deaths were due to septic shock. The typical side effects of eflornithine (diarrhea, fever, infection, hypertension, and skin rash) were reduced in the NECT arm of the study, however more patients experienced tremors, nausea and vomiting.

Emetine and Dehydroemetine

The use of emetine, an alkaloid derived from *ipecac* ("Brazil root"), as a direct-acting systemic amebicide dates from the early part of the 20th century. Dehydroemetine (MEBADIN) has similar pharmacological properties but is considered to be less toxic. Although both drugs were once used widely to treat severe invasive intestinal amebiasis and extraintestinal amebiasis, they have been replaced by metronidazole, which is as effective and far safer. Thus, emetine and dehydroemetine should not be used unless metronidazole is contraindicated. In the U.S., dehydroemetine is available under an investigational new drug protocol from the CDC drug service. Details of the pharmacology and toxicology of emetine and dehydroemetine are presented in the fifth and earlier editions of this book.

Fumagillin

Fumagillin (FUMIDIL B, others) is an acyclic polyene macrolide produced by the fungus *Aspergillus fumigatus*.

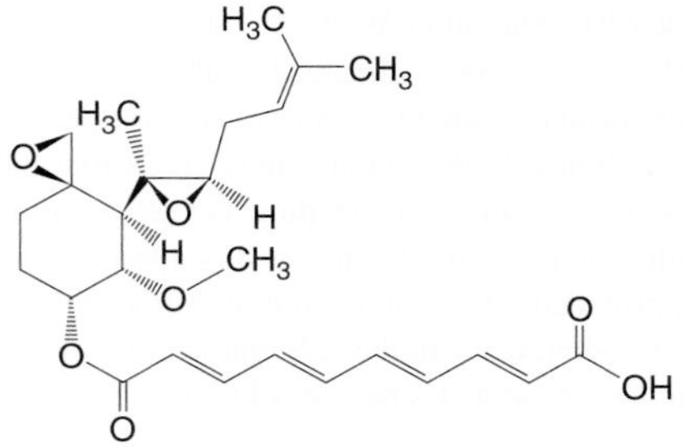

FUMAGILLIN

Both fumagillin and its synthetic analog TNP-470 are toxic to microsporidia, and fumagillin is used widely to treat the microsporidian *Nosema apis*, a pathogen of honey bees. Fumagillin and TNP-470 also inhibit angiogenesis and suppress tumor growth, and TNP-470 is undergoing clinical trials as an anticancer agent (Chapter 61). Human methionine-aminopeptidase-2 (MetAP2) has been identified as the target for the drugs' antitumor activity, and a gene encoding MetAP2 has been identified in the genome of the microsporidian parasite *E. cuniculi.*

Fumagillin is used topically to treat keratoconjunctivitis caused by *E. hellem* at a dose of 3-10 mg/mL in a balanced salt suspension. For the treatment of intestinal microsporidiosis caused by *E. bieneusi*, fumagillin was used at a dose of 20 mg orally three times daily for 2 weeks (Molina et al., 2002). Adverse effects of fumagillin may include abdominal cramps, nausea, vomiting, and diarrhea. Reversible thrombocytopenia and neutropenia also have been reported (Molina et al., 2002). Fumagillin has not been approved for the systemic treatment of microsporidia infection in the U.S.

8-Hydroxyquinolines

The halogenated 8-hydroxyquinolines iodoquinol (diiodohydroxyquin) and clioquinol (iodochlorhydroxyquin) have been used as luminal agents to eliminate intestinal colonization with *E. histolytica*. Iodoquinol (YODOXIN) is the safer of the two agents and is the only one available for use as an oral agent in the U.S. When used at appropriate doses (never to exceed 2 g/day and duration of therapy not greater than 20 days in adults), adverse effects are unusual. However, the use of these drugs, especially at doses exceeding 2 g/day, for long periods is associated with significant risk. The most important toxic reaction, which has been ascribed primarily to clioquinol, is subacute myelo-optic neuropathy. This disease is a myelitis-like illness that was first described in epidemic form (thousands of afflicted patients) in Japan; only sporadic cases have been reported elsewhere, but the actual prevalence is undoubtedly higher. Peripheral neuropathy is a less severe manifestation of neurotoxicity owing to these drugs. Administration of iodoquinol in high doses to children with chronic diarrhea has been associated with optic atrophy and permanent loss of vision.

Because of its superior adverse-event profile, paromomycin is preferred by many authorities as the luminal agent used to treat amebiasis; however, iodoquinol is a reasonable alternative. Iodoquinol is used in combination with metronidazole to treat individuals with amebic colitis or amebic liver abscess but may be used as a single agent for asymptomatic individuals found to be infected with *E. histolytica*. For adults, the recommended dose of iodoquinol is 650 mg orally three times daily for 20 days, whereas children receive 10 mg/kg of body weight orally three times a day (not to exceed 1.95 g/day) for 20 days.

The pharmacology and toxicology of the 8-hydroxyquinolines are described in greater detail in the fifth and earlier editions of this book.

Melarsoprol

In 1949, Friedheim demonstrated that melarsoprol, the dimercaptopropanol derivative of melarsen oxide, was effective in the treatment of late-stage trypanosomiasis. It was considerably safer than other trypanocides available at the time. Despite the fact that it causes an often fatal encephalopathy in 2-10% of the patients, melarsoprol has remained the only drug for the treatment of late (CNS) stages of East African trypanosomiasis caused by *T. brucei rhodesiense* (Barrett et al., 2007; Croft, 2008; Kennedy, 2008). Although melarsoprol is also effective against late-stage West African trypanosomiasis caused by *T. brucei gambiense*, eflornithine has become the first-line treatment for this disease. The continued use of melarsoprol in the field is indicative of the paucity of alternative therapies for late-stage sleeping sickness.

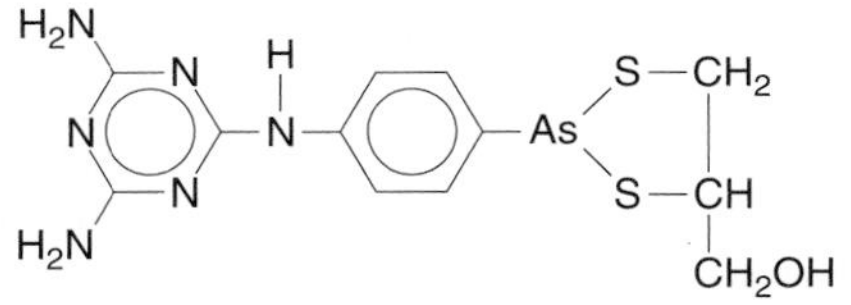

H_2N, N, H, N, N, N, H_2N, As, S—CH_2, S—CH, CH_2OH

MELARSOPROL

Melarsoprol (MEL B; ARSOBAL), consisting of two arsenic-containing stereoisomers in a 3:1 ratio, is insoluble in water and is supplied as a 3.6% (w/v) solution in propylene glycol for intravenous administration. It is available in the U.S. only from the CDC.

Antiprotozoal Effects. Melarsoprol has many wide-ranging nonspecific effects on both the trypanosome and host cells (Fries and Fairlamb, 2003). Melarsoprol is a prodrug and is metabolized rapidly ($t_{1/2}$ = 30 minutes) to melarsen oxide, the active form of the drug. Arsen-oxides react avidly and reversibly with vicinal sulfhydryl groups, including those of proteins, and thereby inactivate a great number and variety of enzymes. The same nonspecific mechanisms by which melarsoprol is lethal to parasites are probably responsible for its toxicity to host tissues. The basis for the trypanocidal action of melarsoprol is not understood, probably owing to its high reactivity with many biomolecules. Disruption of energy metabolism by inhibition of glycolytic enzyme was long thought to explain its trypanocidal activity. Other evidence suggests, however, that this is not a primary effect. Melarsoprol reacts with trypanothione, the spermidine-glutathione adduct that substitutes for glutathione in these parasites. Binding of melarsoprol to trypanothione results in formation of melarsen oxide-trypanothione adduct (Mel T), a compound that is a potent competitive inhibitor of trypanothione reductase, the enzyme responsible for maintaining trypanothione in its reduced form. Both the sequestering of trypanothione and the inhibition of trypanothione reductase would be expected to have lethal consequences to the cell. However, critical evidence directly linking melarsoprol's action on the trypanothione system to parasite death is still lacking.

The number of treatment failures owing to increasing resistance of trypanosomes to melarsoprol has risen sharply in recent years. Failure rates of 20-27% in Uganda, Angola, and the Congo have been reported (Burri and Keiser, 2001; Pepin and Mpia, 2005; Robays et al., 2008b). *In vitro* analysis of field isolates indicates that resistant strains are an order of magnitude less sensitive to the drug than sensitive strains (Brun et al., 2001). However, not all treatment failures can be linked to drug resistance, suggesting that additional factors contribute to lack of efficacy (Maina et al., 2007).

Resistance to melarsoprol is likely to involve transport defects, although the situation is complicated by evidence for multiple transport mechanisms of the drug (de Koning, 2008). The best characterized transporter is an unusual adenine-adenosine transporter termed the *P2 transporter* that has activity on melarsoprol as well as pentamidine and berenil. Cross-resistance between these compounds is observed frequently. Point mutations in this transporter are found in melarsoprol-resistant field isolates. However, null mutant cell lines that lack this transporter were resistant to berenil but had only two-fold resistance to melarsoprol and pentamidine. Another transporter, HAPT1, has been identified, and the concomitant loss of both the P2 and HAPT transporters led to high-level cross-resistance to both melarsen and pentamidine (de Koning, 2008).

Absorption, Fate, and Excretion. Melarsoprol is always administered intravenously. A small but therapeutically significant amount of the drug enters the CSF and has a lethal effect on trypanosomes infecting the CNS. The compound is excreted rapidly, with 70-80% of the arsenic appearing in the feces.

Therapeutic Uses. Melarsoprol is the only effective drug available for treatment of the late meningoencephalitic stage of East African (Rhodesian) trypanosomiasis, which is 100% fatal if untreated. The drug is also effective in the early hemolymphatic stage of these infections, but because of its toxicity, it is reserved for therapy of late-stage infections. Patients infected with *T. brucei rhodesiense* who relapse after a course of melarsoprol usually respond to a second course of the drug. In contrast, patients infected with *T. brucei gambiense* who are not cured with melarsoprol rarely benefit from repeated treatment with this drug. Such patients often respond well to eflornithine.

The original treatment schedules for melarsoprol were derived empirically >40 years ago; new clinical trials have been undertaken with dosage schemes based on a better knowledge of melarsoprol pharmacokinetics, and these have yielded new recommendations for treatment protocols (Pepin and Mpia, 2006; Schmid et al., 2005). Melarsoprol is administered by slow intravenous injection, with care to avoid leakage into the surrounding tissues because the drug is intensely irritating. For *T. brucei gambiense* a continuous 10-day course of 2.2 mg/kg per day is equivalent to the longer course treatment and is now recommended (Pepin and Mpia, 2006; Schmid et al., 2005). The 10-day therapy has not reduced the incidence of encephalopathy (the treatment-related death rate was still 5.9% for this protocol), but it has the advantage of easier administration, and in an area where hospitalization is difficult, this is particularly important. These studies further demonstrated that historically used graded dosing schemes led to increased incidence of convulsions and reduced efficacy; thus these schedules should not be used for the treatment of *T. brucei gambiense* (Pepin and Mpia, 2006).

The 10-day therapy is currently undergoing clinical testing for *T. brucei rhodesiense*. However, until clinical data are available to support a dosing change, patients with Rhodesian sleeping sickness should instead receive one of several older schedules developed for this disease. A number of dosing schemes are in use or recommended by various agencies, including the WHO (1998) and Médecins Sans Frontières (2007). In the U.S., the CDC recommends the following treatment schedule: three series of three daily doses with a 7-day rest period between series. The first series gives 1.8, 2.7, and 3.6 mg/kg on days 1, 2, and 3, respectively. The subsequent series are 3.6 mg/kg daily. Encephalopathy develops more frequently in patients with *T. brucei rhodesiense* compared to *T. brucei gambiense*, possibly related to this graded dosing regimen. Concurrent administration of prednisolone is frequently employed throughout the treatment course; prednisolone it is not proven to reduce the frequency of reactive encephalopathy (Schmid et al., 2005) but it does help to control hypersensitivity reactions that occur most often during the second or subsequent courses of melarsoprol therapy.

Toxicity and Side Effects. Treatment with melarsoprol is associated with significant toxicity and morbidity (Balasegaram et al., 2006b; Burri and Brun, 2003; Kennedy, 2008; Schmid et al., 2005). A febrile reaction often occurs soon after drug injection, especially if parasitemia is high. The most serious complications involve the nervous system. A reactive encephalopathy occurs in ~5-10% of patients, leading to death in about half of these. The cause is unknown, but encephalopathy, when it occurs, typically develops 9-11 days after treatment starts (Schmid et al., 2005). Peripheral neuropathy, noted in ~10% of patients receiving melarsoprol, probably is due to a direct toxic effect of the drug. Hypertension and myocardial damage are not uncommon, although shock is rare. Albuminuria occurs frequently, and occasionally the appearance of numerous casts in the urine or evidence of hepatic disturbances may necessitate modification of treatment. Vomiting and abdominal colic also are common, but their incidence can be reduced by injecting melarsoprol slowly into the supine, fasting patient. The patient should remain in bed and not eat for several hours after the injection is given.

Precautions and Contraindications. Melarsoprol should be given only to patients under hospital supervision so that the dosage regimen may be modified if necessary. Initiation of therapy during a febrile episode has been associated with an increased incidence of reactive encephalopathy. Administration of melarsoprol to leprous patients may precipitate erythema nodosum. Use of the drug is contraindicated during epidemics of influenza. Severe hemolytic reactions have been reported in patients with deficiency of glucose-6-phosphate dehydrogenase. Pregnancy is not a contraindication for treatment with melarsoprol.

Metronidazole

Isolation of the antibiotic azomycin (2-nitro-imidazole) from a streptomycete by Maeda and collaborators in 1953 and demonstration of its trichomonacidal properties by Horie in 1956 led to the chemical synthesis and biological testing of many nitroimidazoles. One compound, 1-(β-hydroxyethyl)-2-methyl-5-nitroimidazole, or metronidazole (FLAGYL, others), had especially high activity *in vitro* and *in vivo* against the anaerobic protozoa *T. vaginalis* and *E. histolytica*. In 1960, Durel and associates reported that oral doses of the drug imparted trichomonacidal activity to semen and urine and that high cure rates could be obtained in both male and female patients with trichomoniasis. Later studies revealed that metronidazole had extremely useful clinical activity against a variety of anaerobic pathogens that included both gram-negative and gram-positive bacteria and the protozoan *G. lamblia* (Freeman et al., 1997). Other clinically effective 5-nitroimidazoles closely related in structure and activity to metronidazole include tinidazole (TINDAMAX, FASIGYN, others), secnidazole (SECZOL-DS, others), and ornidazole (TIBERAL, others). Among these, only tinidazole is available in the U.S. Benznidazole (ROCHAGAN), another 5-nitroimidazole derivative, is unusual in that it is effective in acute Chagas' disease.

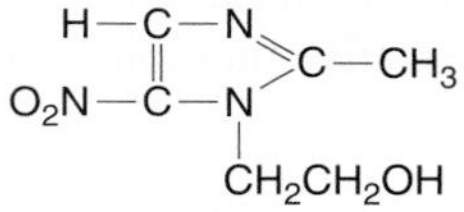

H—C—N
O_2N—C—N —C—CH_3
CH_2CH_2OH

METRONIDAZOLE

Antiparasitic and Antimicrobial Effects. Metronidazole and related nitroimidazoles are active *in vitro* against a wide variety of anaerobic protozoal parasites and anaerobic bacteria (Freeman et al., 1997). The compound is directly trichomonacidal. Sensitive isolates of *T. vaginalis* are killed by <0.05 μg/mL of the drug under anaerobic conditions; higher concentrations are required when 1% oxygen is present or to affect isolates from patients who display poor therapeutic responses to metronidazole. The drug also has potent amebicidal activity against *E. histolytica*. Trophozoites of *G. lamblia* are affected by metronidazole at concentrations of 1-50 μg/mL *in vitro*. *In vitro* studies on drug-sensitive and drug-resistant protozoan parasites indicate that the nitro group on C5 of metronidazole is essential for activity and that substitutions at the 2 position of the imidazole ring that enhance the resonance conjugation of the chemical structure increase antiprotozoal activity. In contrast, substitution of an acyl group at the 2 position ablates such conjugation and reduces antiprotozoal activity (Upcroft et al., 1999).

Metronidazole manifests antibacterial activity against all anaerobic cocci and both anaerobic gram-negative bacilli, including *Bacteroides* spp., and anaerobic spore-forming gram-positive bacilli. Nonsporulating gram-positive bacilli often are resistant, as are aerobic and facultatively anaerobic bacteria.

Metronidazole is clinically effective in trichomoniasis, amebiasis, and giardiasis, as well as in a variety of infections caused by obligate anaerobic bacteria, including *Bacteroides, Clostridium*, and microaerophilic bacteria such as *Helicobacter* and *Campylobacter* spp. Metronidazole may facilitate extraction of adult guinea worms in dracunculiasis even though it has no direct effect on the parasite (Chapter 51).

Mechanism of Action and Resistance. Metronidazole is a prodrug; it requires reductive activation of the nitro group by susceptible organisms. Its selective toxicity toward anaerobic and microaerophilic pathogens such as the amitochondriate protozoa *T. vaginalis, E. histolytica*, and *G. lamblia* and various anaerobic bacteria derives from their energy metabolism, which differs from that of aerobic cells (Land and Johnson, 1997; Samuelson, 1999; Upcroft and Upcroft, 1999). These organisms, unlike their aerobic counterparts, contain electron transport components such as ferredoxins, small Fe–S proteins that have a sufficiently negative redox potential to donate electrons to metronidazole. The single electron transfer forms a highly reactive nitro radical anion that kills susceptible organisms by radical-mediated mechanisms that target DNA and possibly other vital biomolecules. Metronidazole is catalytically recycled; loss of the active metabolite's electron regenerates the parent compound. Increasing levels of O_2 inhibit metronidazole-induced cytotoxicity because O_2 competes with metronidazole for electrons generated by energy metabolism. Thus, O_2 can both decrease reductive activation of metronidazole and increase recycling of the activated drug. Anaerobic or microaerophilic organisms susceptible to metronidazole derive energy from the oxidative fermentation of ketoacids such as pyruvate. Pyruvate decarboxylation, catalyzed by pyruvate:ferredoxin oxidoreductase (PFOR), produces electrons that reduce ferredoxin, which, in turn, catalytically donates its electrons to biological electron acceptors or to metronidazole.

Clinical resistance to metronidazole is well documented for *T. vaginalis, G. lamblia*, and a variety of anaerobic and microaerophilic bacteria but has yet to be shown for *E. histolytica*. Resistant strains of *T. vaginalis* derived from nonresponsive patients have shown two major types of abnormalities when tested under aerobic conditions. The first correlates with impaired oxygen-scavenging capabilities, leading to higher local O_2 concentrations, decreased activation of metronidazole, and futile recycling of the activated drug. The second type is associated with lowered levels of PFOR and ferredoxin, the latter owing to reduced transcription of the ferredoxin gene. That PFOR and ferredoxin are not completely absent may explain why infections with such strains usually respond to higher doses of metronidazole or more prolonged therapy. Studies on metronidazole-resistant isolates of *G. intestinalis* indicate that similar mechanisms may be operating, with PFOR levels reduced 5-fold compared with susceptible strains (Upcroft and Upcroft, 2001). Metronidazole resistance has not been found in clinical isolates of *E. histolytica* but has been induced *in vitro* by culturing trophozoites in gradually increasing concentrations of the drug. Interestingly, although some decrease in PFOR levels was reported, metronidazole resistance was mediated primarily by increased expression of superoxide dismutase and peroxiredoxin in amebic trophozoites (Wassmann et al., 1999). Resistance of anaerobic bacteria to metronidazole is being recognized increasingly and has important clinical consequences. In the case of *Bacteroides* spp., metronidazole resistance has been linked to a family of nitroimidazole (*nim*) resistance genes, *nimA, -B, -C, -D, -E*, and *-F*, that can be encoded chromosomally or episomally (Gal and Brazier, 2004). The exact mechanisms underlying resistance are not known, but *nim* genes appear to encode a nitroimidazole reductase capable of converting a 5-nitroimidazole to a 5-aminoimidazole, thus stopping the formation of the reactive nitroso group responsible for microbial killing. Metronidazole has been used widely for the treatment of the microaerophilic organism *Helicobacter pylori*, the major cause of ulcer disease and gastritis worldwide. However, *Helicobacter* can develop resistance to metronidazole rapidly. Multiple mechanisms probably are operating, but there are data associating loss-of-function mutations in an oxygen-independent NADPH nitroreductase (*rdxA* gene) with resistance to metronidazole (Mendz and Mégraud, 2002).

Absorption, Fate, and Excretion. The pharmacokinetic properties of metronidazole and its two major metabolites have been investigated intensively (Lamp et al., 1999). Preparations of metronidazole are available for oral, intravenous, intravaginal, and topical administration. The drug usually is absorbed completely and promptly after oral intake, reaching concentrations in plasma of 8-13 μg/mL within 0.25-4 hours after a single 500-mg dose. (Mean effective concentrations of the compound are ≤8 μg/mL for most susceptible protozoa and bacteria.) A linear relationship between dose and plasma concentration pertains for doses of 200-2000 mg. Repeated doses every 6-8 hours result in some accumulation of the drug; systemic clearance exhibits dose dependence. The $t_{1/2}$ of metronidazole in plasma is ~8 hours; its volume of distribution approximates total body water. Less than 20% of the drug is bound to plasma proteins. With the exception of the placenta, metronidazole penetrates well into body tissues and fluids, including vaginal secretions, seminal fluid, saliva, breast milk, and CSF.

After an oral dose, >75% of labeled metronidazole is eliminated in the urine largely as metabolites; ~10% is recovered as unchanged drug. The liver is the main site of metabolism, and this accounts for >50% of the systemic clearance of metronidazole. The two principal metabolites result from oxidation of side chains, a hydroxy derivative and an acid. The hydroxy metabolite has a longer $t_{1/2}$ (~12 hours) and has ~50% of the antitrichomonal activity of metronidazole. Formation of glucuronides also is observed. Small quantities of reduced metabolites, including ring-cleavage products, are formed by the gut flora. The urine of some patients may be reddish brown owing to the presence of unidentified pigments derived from the drug. Oxidative metabolism of metronidazole is induced by phenobarbital, prednisone, rifampin, and possibly ethanol. Cimetidine appears to inhibit hepatic metabolism of the drug.

Therapeutic Uses. The uses of metronidazole for anti-protozoal therapy have been reviewed extensively (Freeman et al., 1997; Nash, 2001; Stanley, 2003). Metronidazole cures genital infections with *T. vaginalis* in both females and males in >90% of cases. The preferred treatment regimen is 2 g metronidazole as a single oral dose for both males and females. Tinidazole, which has a longer $t_{1/2}$ than metronidazole, is also used at a 2-g single dose and appears to provide equivalent or better responses than metronidazole. For patients who cannot tolerate a single 2-g dose of metronidazole (or 1 g twice daily in the same day), an alternative regimen is a 250-mg dose given three times daily or a 375-mg dose given twice daily for 7 days. When repeated courses or higher doses of the drug are required for uncured or recurrent infections, it is recommended that intervals of 4-6 weeks elapse between courses. In such cases, leukocyte counts should be carried out before, during, and after each course of treatment.

Treatment failures owing to the presence of metronidazole-resistant strains of *T. vaginalis* are becoming increasingly common. Most of these cases can be treated successfully by giving a second 2-g dose to both patient and sexual partner. In addition to oral therapy, the use of a topical gel containing 0.75% metronidazole or a 500- to 1000-mg vaginal suppository will increase the local concentration of drug and may be beneficial in refractory cases. Metronidazole is an effective amebicide and is the agent of choice for the treatment of all symptomatic forms of amebiasis, including amebic colitis and amebic liver abscess. The recommended dose is 500-750 mg metronidazole taken orally three times daily for 7-10 days, or for children, 35-50 mg/kg/day given in three divided doses for 7-10 days.

Although standard recommendations are for 7-10 days' duration of therapy, amebic liver abscess has been treated successfully by short courses (2.4 g daily as a single oral dose for 2 days) of metronidazole or tinidazole (Stanley, 2003). *E. histolytica* persist in most patients who recover from acute amebiasis after metronidazole therapy, so it is recommended that all such individuals also be treated with a luminal amebicide.

Although effective for the therapy of giardiasis, metronidazole has yet to be approved for treatment of this infection in the U.S. However, tinidazole is approved for the treatment of giardiasis as a single 2-g dose and is appropriate first-line therapy. Metronidazole is a relatively inexpensive, highly versatile drug with clinical efficacy against a broad spectrum of anaerobic and microaerophilic bacteria. It is used for the treatment of serious infections owing to susceptible anaerobic bacteria, including *Bacteroides*, *Clostridium*, *Fusobacterium*, *Peptococcus*, *Peptostreptococcus*, *Eubacterium*, and *Helicobacter*. The drug is also given in combination with other antimicrobial agents to treat polymicrobial infections with aerobic and anaerobic bacteria. Metronidazole achieves clinically effective levels in bones, joints, and the CNS. Metronidazole can be given intravenously when oral administration is not possible. A loading dose of 15 mg/kg is followed 6 hours later by a maintenance dose of 7.5 mg/kg every 6 hours, usually for 7-10 days. Metronidazole is used as a component of prophylaxis for colorectal surgery and is employed as a single agent to treat bacterial vaginosis. It is used in combination with other antibiotics and a proton pump inhibitor in regimens to treat infection with *H. pylori* (Chapter 45).

Metronidazole is used as primary therapy for *Clostridium difficile* infection, the major cause of pseudomembranous colitis. Given at doses of 250-500 mg orally three times daily for 7-14 days (or even longer), metronidazole is an effective and cost-saving alternative to oral vancomycin therapy. However, a reported increase in treatment failures and higher rates of disease recurrence with metronidazole (as compared to oral vancomycin) are raising questions about the role of metronidazole as first-line therapy (McFarland, 2008). Finally, metronidazole is also used in the treatment of patients with Crohn's disease who have perianal fistulas, and it can help control colonic (but not small bowel) Crohn's disease. However, high doses (750 mg three times daily) for prolonged periods may be necessary, and neurotoxicity may be limiting (Podolsky, 2002). Metronidazole and other nitroimidazoles can sensitize hypoxic tumor cells to the effects of ionizing radiation, but these drugs are not used clinically for this purpose.

Toxicity, Contraindications, and Drug Interactions. The toxicity of metronidazole has been reviewed (Raether and Hanel, 2003). Side effects only rarely are severe enough to discontinue therapy. The most common are headache, nausea, dry mouth, and a metallic taste. Vomiting, diarrhea, and abdominal distress are experienced occasionally. Furry tongue, glossitis, and stomatitis occurring during therapy may be associated with an exacerbation of candidiasis. Dizziness, vertigo, and very rarely, encephalopathy, convulsions, incoordination, and ataxia are neurotoxic effects that warrant discontinuation of metronidazole. The drug also should be withdrawn if numbness or paresthesias of the extremities occur. Reversal of serious sensory neuropathies may be slow or incomplete. Urticaria, flushing, and pruritus are indicative of drug sensitivity that can require withdrawal of metronidazole. Metronidazole is a rare cause of Stevens-Johnson syndrome (toxic epidermal necrolysis); one report described a high rate of this syndrome among individuals receiving high doses of metronidazole and concurrent therapy with the antihelminthic mebendazole (Chen et al., 2003).

Dysuria, cystitis, and a sense of pelvic pressure have been reported. Metronidazole has a well-documented disulfiram-like effect, and some patients experience abdominal distress, vomiting, flushing, or headache if they drink alcoholic beverages during or within 3 days of therapy with this drug. Patients should be cautioned to avoid consuming alcohol during metronidazole treatment even though the risk of a severe reaction is low. By the same token, metronidazole and disulfiram or any disulfiram-like drug should not be taken together because confusional and psychotic states may occur. Although related chemicals have caused blood dyscrasias, only a temporary neutropenia, reversible after discontinuation of therapy, occurs with metronidazole.

Metronidazole should be used with caution in patients with active disease of the CNS because of its potential neurotoxicity. The drug also may precipitate CNS signs of lithium toxicity in patients receiving high doses of lithium. Plasma levels of metronidazole can be elevated by drugs such as cimetidine that inhibit hepatic microsomal metabolism. Moreover, metronidazole can prolong the prothrombin time of patients receiving therapy with coumadin anticoagulants. The dosage of metronidazole should be reduced in patients with severe hepatic disease.

Given in high doses for prolonged periods, metronidazole is carcinogenic in rodents; it also is mutagenic in bacteria (Raether and Hanel, 2003). Mutagenic activity is associated with metronidazole and several of its metabolites found in the urine of patients treated with therapeutic doses of the drug. However, there is no evidence that therapeutic doses of metronidazole pose any significant increased risk of cancer to human patients. There is conflicting evidence about the teratogenicity of metronidazole in animals. Although metronidazole has been taken during all stages of pregnancy with no apparent adverse effects, its use during the first trimester generally is not advised.

Miltefosine

Miltefosine (IMPAVIDO) is an alkylphosphocholine (APC) analog that was developed originally as an anticancer agent. Its antiprotozoal activity was discovered in the 1980s during the time that it was being evaluated for cancer chemotherapy. In 2002, it was approved in India as the first orally active treatment available for visceral leishmaniasis. Miltefosine is the first orally available therapy for leishmaniasis. It is highly curative against visceral leishmaniasis in the trials conducted to date and also appears to be effective against the cutaneous forms of the disease (Berman, 2008; Bhattacharya et al., 2007). Its main drawback is its teratogenicity; consequently, it must not be used in pregnant woman.

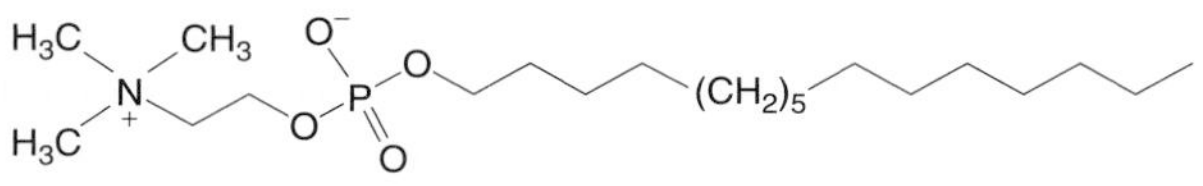

MILTEFOSINE

Antiprotozoal Effects. *In vitro* analysis of a large number of alkylglycerophosphoethanolamines (AGPEs), alkylglycerophosphocholines (AGPCs), and APCs, originally developed as anticancer agents, demonstrated that a number of these compounds had potent antileishmanial activity against cultured promastigote or amastigote parasites (Croft et al., 2003). Of the APCs, miltefosine demonstrated the best activity against both stages of parasites. The potency of miltefosine varies for different *Leishmania* spp., with *L. donovani* being the most sensitive ($1.2<ED_{50}<5$ μM against amastigotes) and *L. major* being the least sensitive ($8<ED_{50}<40$ μM against amastigotes). Several phospholipid analogs also had good potency against cultured *T. cruzi* parasites, whereas they were relatively inactive against *T. brucei*. *In vivo*, miltefosine had the best activities of the tested APCs, and by 5 days of treatment with 20 mg/kg orally, it gave >95% suppression of *L. donovani* and *L. infantum* amastigotes in the affected organs of mice. It also had good activity when administered as a 6% ointment to skin lesions of *L. mexicana* or *L. major* on *BALB/c* mice.

Against visceral leishmaniasis, 95-98% cure rates were observed with a 100 mg/day oral dose for 28-42 days (Croft et al., 2003) and 95% with a 28-day regimen of 100 mg/day orally for adults and 2.5 mg/kg daily for children (Bhattacharya et al., 2007). Thus, oral miltefosine appears to be a safe and effective treatment for visceral leishmaniasis (Berman, 2008). Recent studies of oral miltefosine also have shown >90% efficacy against some species of cutaneous leishmaniasis (registered in Colombia for this use in 2005). However, significant strain variation has been observed in the clinical trials (Soto and Berman, 2006; Soto et al., 2007): For *L. panamensis* in Colombia, cure rates were from 84-91% (versus the placebo cure rate of 37%), and it was considerably less effective for *L. brasiliensis* in Guatemala.

The mechanism of action of miltefosine is not yet understood. Potential targets in mammalian cells include PKC; CTP:phosphocholine-cytidylyltransferase inhibition, which disrupts phosphatidylcholine biosynthesis; and altered sphingomyelin biosynthesis, where increased levels of cellular ceramide may trigger apoptosis (Croft et al., 2003). Studies in *Leishmania* suggest that the drug may alter ether-lipid metabolism, cell signaling, or glycosylphosphatidylinositol anchor biosynthesis. A transporter for miltefosine has been cloned recently by functional rescue of a laboratory-generated resistant strain of *L. donovani*. The transporter is a P-type ATPase that belongs to the aminophospholipid translocase subfamily, and the basis for the drug resistance appears to be point mutation in the transporter leading to decreased drug uptake. Mutations in this transporter lead to miltefosine resistance in laboratory models (Croft et al., 2006; Seifert et al., 2007).

Absorption, Fate, and Excretion. Miltefosine is well absorbed orally and distributed throughout the human body. Detailed pharmacokinetic data are lacking, with the exception that miltefosine has a long $t_{1/2}$ in humans (Berman, 2008). Plasma concentrations are proportional to the dose, and maximum serum concentrations for dosing of 50-150 mg per day were 20-70 μg/mL with a $t_{1/2}$ of 1 week and a terminal $t_{1/2}$ of ~4 weeks. The C_{max} in children was ~30% less than in adults.

Therapeutic Uses. Oral miltefosine is registered for use in India for the treatment of visceral leishmaniasis with clinical trial study patients receiving the following oral doses (Bhattacharya, 2007): for adults >25 kg, 100 mg daily divided into two parts, and for adults <25 kg, 50 mg daily in 1 dose for 28 days; for children, 2.5 mg/kg/day in two divided doses. For cutaneous disease, the dose in clinical testing is 2.5 mg/kg per day orally (maximum, 150 mg/day) for 28 days. In the U.S., the recommended dose for both visceral and cutaneous disease is 2.5 mg/kg per day (maximum dose of 150 mg/day) for 28 days, given in two divided doses (Medical Letter, 2007). Miltefosine is also available in Afghanistan, Pakistan, and South America. Because of its teratogenic potential, miltefosine is contraindicated in pregnant women. Women should receive a negative pregnancy test prior to treatment, and birth control is required during and for at least 2 months after treatment. The compound cannot be given intravenously because it has hemolytic activity.

Toxicity and Side Effects. Vomiting and diarrhea have been reported as frequent side effects in up to 60% of the patients. Elevations in hepatic transaminases and serum creatinine also have been reported. These effects are typically mild and reversible, and they resolve quickly once the drug is withdrawn.

Nifurtimox and Benznidazole

A variety of nitrofurans and nitroimidazole analogs are effective in experimental infections with American trypanosomiasis caused by *T. cruzi* (Bern et al., 2007; Tarleton et al., 2007). Of these, nifurtimox and benznidazole are currently used clinically to treat the disease. Nifurtimox (Bayer 2502, LAMPIT), a nitrofuran analog, and benznidazole (Roche 7-1051, ROCHAGAN), a nitroimidazole analog, can be obtained in the U.S. from the CDC.

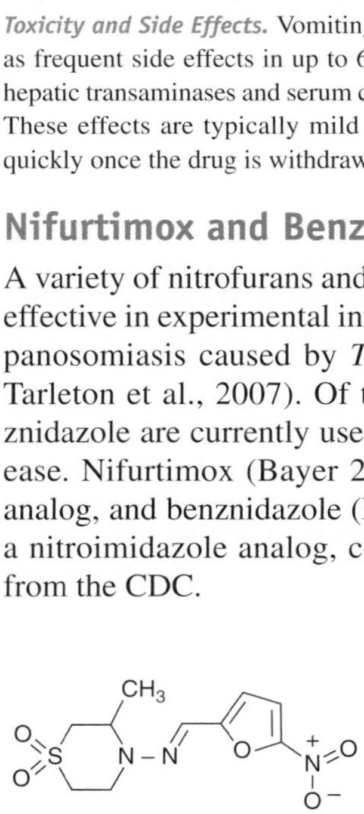

NIFURTIMOX

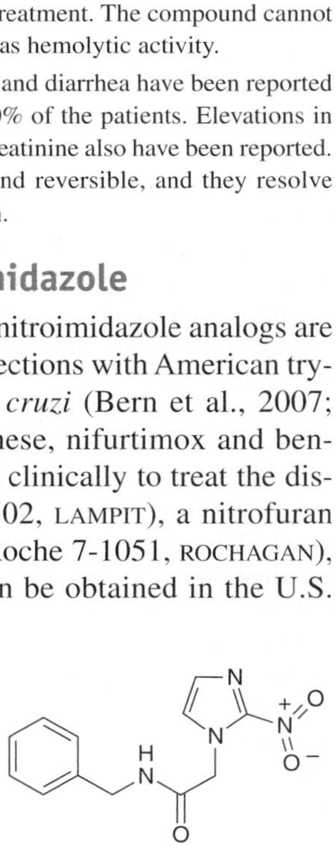

BENZNIDAZOLE

Antiprotozoal Effects and Mechanisms of Action. Nifurtimox and benznidazole are trypanocidal against both the trypomastigote and amastigote forms of *T. cruzi*. Nifurtimox also has activity against

T. brucei and can be curative against both early- and late-stage disease (see earlier discussion on nifurtimox-eflornithine combination therapy.

Both nifurtimox and benznidazole are activated by a NADH-dependent mitochondrial nitroreductase, leading to the intracellular generation of nitro radical anions that are thought to account for the trypanocidal effects. The generated nitro anion radicals form covalent attachments to macromolecules leading to cellular damage that kills the parasites. Transfer of electrons from the activated drug regenerates the native nitrofuran and forms superoxide radical anions and other reactive oxygen species such as hydrogen peroxide and hydroxyl radical. Reaction of free radicals with cellular macromolecules results in cellular damage that includes lipid peroxidation and membrane injury, enzyme inactivation, and damage to DNA. Reduced nitroreductase expression through single allele gene knockout experiments or through drug selection leads to drug resistance (Wilkinson et al., 2008).

Absorption, Fate, and Excretion. Nifurtimox is well absorbed after oral administration, with peak plasma levels observed after ~3.5 hours (Paulos et al., 1989). Despite this, only low concentrations of the drug (10-20 μM) are present in plasma, and <0.5% of the dose is excreted in urine. The elimination $t_{1/2}$ is ~3 hours. High concentrations of several unidentified metabolites are found, however, and nifurtimox clearly undergoes rapid biotransformation, probably via a presystemic first-pass effect. Whether the metabolites have any trypanocidal activity is unknown.

Therapeutic Uses. Nifurtimox and benznidazole are employed in the treatment of American trypanosomiasis (Chagas' disease) caused by *T. cruzi* (Bern et al., 2007; Tarleton et al., 2007). However, because of toxicity issues, benznidazole is the preferred treatment. Both drugs markedly reduce the parasitemia, morbidity, and mortality of acute Chagas' disease, with parasitological cures obtained in 80% of these cases. Parasitological cure is defined by a negative result in PCR and serological tests for the parasite. In the chronic form of the disease, parasitological cures are still possible in up to 50% of the patients, although the drug is less effective than in the acute stage. Treatment with nifurtimox or benznidazole has no effect on irreversible organ lesions. Although a component of tissue destruction may be autoimmune in nature, the continued presence of parasites in the infected organs of patients with chronic disease argues that Chagas' disease should be treated as a parasitic disease.

The clinical response of the acute illness to drug therapy varies with geographic region; parasite strains present in Argentina, southern Brazil, Chile, and Venezuela appear to be more susceptible than those in central Brazil. A large-scale clinical trial (BENEFIT) is currently underway to test the efficacy of benznidazole in the treatment of both acute and chronic Chagas' disease (http://clinicaltrials.gov/show/NCT00123916); (Marin-Neto et al., 2008); until the trial's results are available, the current recommendations are that patients <50 years of age with either acute- or recent chronic-phase disease, without advanced cardiomyopathy, should be treated (Bern et al., 2007); in patients >50 years of age, treatment is optional because of lowered drug tolerability in this group; dosing is 5 mg/kg per day for 60 days. Therapy is strongly encouraged for patients that will receive immunosuppressive therapy or who are HIV positive. For patients with late chronic-phase disease (>10 years) with advanced cardiomyopathy, parasitological cure is less likely, and the general consensus is not to treat these patients. However, the decision to treat should be made on an individual basis. Therapy with nifurtimox or benznidazole should start promptly after exposure for persons at risk of *T. cruzi* infection from laboratory accidents or from blood transfusions.

Both drugs are given orally. The treatment schedules recommended by the CDC in the U.S. are as follows: for nifurtimox, adults (>17 years of age) with acute infection should receive 8-10 mg/kg per day in three to four divided doses for 90 days; children 1-10 years of age should receive 15-20 mg/kg per day in three to four divided doses for 90 days; for individuals 11-16 years old, the daily dose is 12.5-15 mg/kg given according to the same schedule. For benznidazole, the recommended treatment for adults (>13 years) is 5-7 mg/kg per day in two divided doses for 60 days, with children up to 12 years receiving 10 mg/kg per day (Bern et al., 2007). Gastric upset and weight loss can occur during treatment. If the latter occurs, dosage should be reduced. The ingestion of alcohol should be avoided during treatment because the incidence of side effects may increase.

Nifurtimox is used in combination with eflornithine in treating late stage *T.b. gambiense* sleeping sickness (see "Eflornithine" earlier in this chapter).

Toxicity and Side Effects. Children tolerate nifurtimox and benznidazole better than adults. Nonetheless, drug-related side effects are common. They range from hypersensitivity reactions (e.g., dermatitis, fever, icterus, pulmonary infiltrates, and anaphylaxis) to dose- and age-dependent complications primarily referable to the GI tract and both the peripheral and central nervous systems. Nausea and vomiting are common, as are myalgia and weakness. Peripheral neuropathy and GI symptoms are especially common after prolonged treatment; the latter complication may lead to weight loss and preclude further therapy. Headache, psychic disturbances, paresthesias, polyneuritis, and CNS excitability are less frequent. Leukopenia and decreased sperm counts also have been reported. Because of the seriousness of Chagas' disease and the lack of superior drugs, there are few absolute contraindications to the use of these drugs.

Nitazoxanide

Nitazoxanide (*N*-[nitrothiazolyl] salicylamide, ALINA) is an oral synthetic broad-spectrum antiparasitic agent that was synthesized originally in the 1980s based on the structure of the antihelminthic niclosamide (Chapter 51). It was found initially to have activity against tapeworms (Rossignol and Maisonneuve, 1984); subsequent *in vitro* studies suggested that it was effective against a number of intestinal helminths and protozoans. Nitazoxanide is FDA-approved for the treatment of cryptosporidiosis and giardiasis in children.

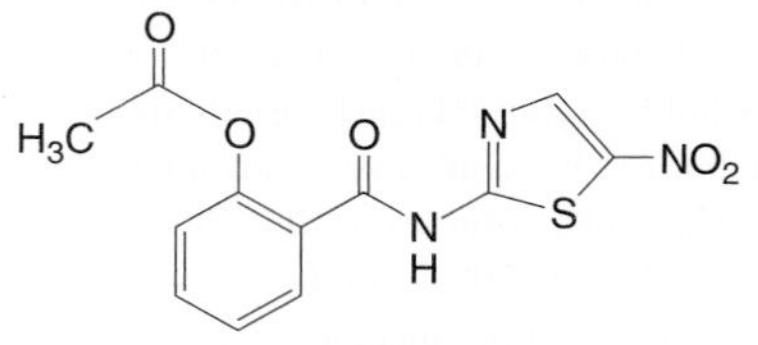

O
H_3C O O N NO_2
N S
H

NITAZOXANIDE

Antimicrobial Effects. Nitazoxanide and its active metabolite, tizoxanide (desacetyl-nitazoxanide), inhibit the growth of sporozoites and oocytes of *C. parvum* and inhibit the growth of the trophozoites of *G. intestinalis*, *E. histolytica*, and *T. vaginalis in vitro* (Adagu et al., 2002). Activity against other protozoans, including *Blastocystis hominis*, *Isospora belli*, and *Cyclospora cayetanensis* also has been reported. Nitazoxanide also demonstrated activity against the intestinal helminths: *Hymenolepis nana, Trichuris trichiura, Ascaris lumbricoides, Enterobius vermicularis, Ancylostoma duodenale, Strongyloides stercoralis*, and the liver fluke *Fasciolahepatica*. Effects against some anaerobic or microaerophilic bacteria, including *Clostridium* spp. and *H. pylori*, also have been reported. Nitazoxanide reportedly displays antiviral activity and is now undergoing clinical trials for the treatment of hepatitis C (Rossignol and Keeffe, 2008).

Mechanism of Action and Resistance. Nitazoxanide interferes with the PFOR enzyme-dependent electron-transfer reaction, which is essential to anaerobic metabolism in protozoan and bacterial species. One proposed mechanism of nitazoxanide is blockade of the first step in the PFOR chain by inhibiting the binding of pyruvate to the thiamine pyrophosphate cofactor (Hoffman et al., 2007). Resistance to nitazoxanide has been induced in Giardia *in vitro*, but clinically resistant clinical isolates have not yet been reported.

Absorption, Fate, and Excretion. Following oral administration, nitazoxanide is hydrolyzed rapidly to its active metabolite, tizoxanide, which undergoes conjugation primarily to tizoxanide glucuronide. Bioavailability after an oral dose is excellent, and maximum plasma concentrations of the metabolites are detected within 1-4 hours following administration of the parent compound. Tizoxanide is >99.9% bound to plasma proteins. Tizoxanide is excreted in the urine, bile, and feces; tizoxanide glucuronide is excreted in the urine and bile. The pharmacokinetics of nitazoxanide in individuals with impaired hepatic or renal function have not been reported.

Therapeutic Uses. In the U.S., nitazoxanide is approved for the treatment of *G. intestinalis* infection (therapeutic efficacy of 85-90% for clinical response) and for the treatment of diarrhea caused by cryptosporidia (therapeutic efficacy, 56-88% for clinical response) in adults and children >1 year of age (Amadi et al., 2002; Rossignol et al., 2001). The efficacy of nitazoxanide in children (or adults) with cryptosporidia infection and AIDS has not been clearly established. For children ages 12-47 months, the recommended dose is 100 mg nitazoxanide every 12 hours for 3 days; for children ages 4-11 years, the dose is 200 mg nitazoxanide every 12 hours for 3 days. A 500-mg tablet, suitable for adult dosing (every 12 hours), is available.

Nitazoxanide has been used as a single agent to treat mixed infections with intestinal parasites (protozoa and helminths) in several trials. Effective parasite clearance (based on negative follow-up fecal samples) after nitazoxanide treatment was shown for *G. intestinalis, E. histolytica/E. dispar, B. hominis, C. parvum, C. cayetanensis, I. belli, H. nana, T. trichiura, A. lumbricoides*, and *E. vermicularis* (Romero-Cabello et al., 1997), although more than one course of therapy was required in some cases. Nitazoxanide may have some efficacy against *Fasciola hepatica* infections (Favennec et al., 2003) and has been used to treat infections with *G. intestinalis* that are resistant to metronidazole and albendazole (Abboud et al., 2001).

Toxicity and Side Effects. To date, adverse effects appear to be rare with nitazoxanide. Abdominal pain, diarrhea, vomiting, and headache have been reported, but rates were no different from those in patients receiving placebo. A greenish tint to the urine is seen in most individuals taking nitazoxanide. Nitazoxanide is a pregnancy Category B agent, based on animal teratogenicity and fertility studies, but there is no clinical experience with its use in pregnant women or nursing mothers.

Paromomycin

Paromomycin (aminosidine, HUMATIN) is an aminoglycoside of the neomycin/kanamycin family (Chapter 54) that is used as an oral agent to treat *E. histolytica* infection. The drug is not absorbed from the GI tract and thus the actions of an oral dose are confined to the GI tract. Paromomycin also has been used orally to treat cryptosporidiosis and giardiasis. A topical formulation has been used to treat trichomoniasis, and parenteral administration has been used for visceral leishmaniasis.

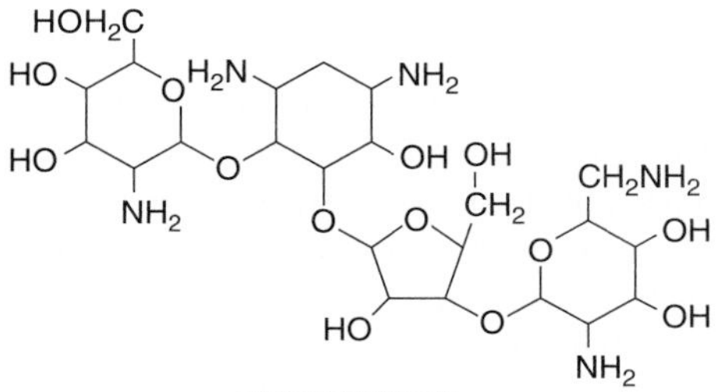

PAROMOMYCIN

Mechanism of Action. Paromomycin shares the same mechanism of action as neomycin and kanamycin (binding to the 30S ribosomal subunit) and has the same spectrum of antibacterial activity. Paromomycin is available only for oral use in the U.S. Following oral administration, 100% of the drug is recovered in the feces, and even in cases of compromised gut integrity, there is little evidence for clinically significant absorption of paromomycin. *Parenteral administration carries the same risks of nephrotoxicity and ototoxicity seen with other aminoglycosides.*

Antimicrobial Effects; Therapeutics Uses. Paromomycin is the drug of choice for treating intestinal colonization with *E. histolytica*. It is used in combination with metronidazole to treat amebic colitis and amebic liver abscess and can be used as a single agent for asymptomatic individuals found to have *E. histolytica* intestinal colonization. Recommended dosing for adults and children is 25-35 mg/kg per day orally in three divided doses. Adverse effects are rare with oral usage but include abdominal pain and cramping, epigastric pain, nausea and vomiting, steatorrhea, and diarrhea. Rarely, rash and headache have been reported. Paromomycin has been used to treat cryptosporidiosis in AIDS patients both as a single agent and in combination with azithromycin, but in a randomized controlled trial, paromomycin was no more effective than placebo for this indication (Hewitt et al., 2000). Paromomycin has been advocated as a treatment for giardiasis in pregnant women, especially during the first trimester, when metronidazole is contraindicated and as an alternative agent for metronidazole-resistant isolates of *G. intestinalis*. Although there is limited clinical experience, response rates of 55-90% have been reported (Gardner and Hill, 2001). Dosing in adults is 500 mg orally three times daily for 10 days, whereas children have been treated with 25-30 mg/kg per day in three divided oral doses. Paromomycin formulated as a 6.25% cream has been used to treat vaginal trichomoniasis in patients who had failed metronidazole therapy or could not receive metronidazole. Some cures have been reported, but vulvovaginal ulcerations and pain have complicated treatment and absorption via this route (and the possibility of aminoglycoside-related toxicities) must be anticipated.

Paromomycin is also efficacious as a topical formulation containing 15% paromomycin in combination with 12% methylbenzonium chloride for the treatment of cutaneous leishmaniasis (Alvar et al., 2006). The drug has been administered parenterally alone or in combination with antimony to treat visceral leishmaniasis. Paromomycin (intramuscular injection, 11 mg/kg per day for 21 days) produced a cure rate for visceral leishmaniasis (94.6%) that was statistically equivalent to liposomal amphotericin B (Sundar et al., 2007). However, adverse events were more common with paromomycin than with liposomal amphotericin B.

Pentamidine

Pentamidine is a positively charged aromatic diamine that was discovered in 1937 as a fortuitous consequence of the search for hypoglycemic compounds that might compromise parasite energy metabolism. Of the compounds tested, three were found to possess outstanding activity: stilbamidine, pentamidine, and propamidine. Pentamidine was the most useful clinically because of its relative stability, lower toxicity, and ease of administration. Pentamidine is a broad-spectrum agent with activity against several species of pathogenic protozoa and some fungi.

$$(HN{=})(H_2N)C\text{–}C_6H_4\text{–}OCH_2(CH_2)_3CH_2O\text{–}C_6H_4\text{–}C(=NH)(NH_2)$$

PENTAMIDINE

Pentamidine as the di-isethionate salt is marketed for injection (PENTAM 300, others) or for use as an aerosol (NEBUPENT). One milligram of pentamidine base is equivalent to 1.74 mg of the pentamidine isethionate. The di-isethionate salt is highly water soluble; however, solutions should be used promptly after preparation because pentamidine is unstable in solution.

Antiprotozoal and Antifungal Effects. The positively charged aromatic diamidines are toxic to a number of different protozoa yet show rather marked selectivity of action. Pentamidine is used for the treatment of early-stage *T. brucei gambiense* infection (Barrett et al., 2007; Kennedy, 2008) but is ineffective in the treatment of late-stage disease and has reduced efficacy against *T. brucei rhodesiense*. Its use is therefore limited to treatment of first-stage *T. brucei gambiense* sleeping sickness. Pentamidine is an alternative agent for the treatment of cutaneous leishmaniasis (Alvar et al., 2006; Croft, 2008). It has been used for the treatment of visceral disease but less toxic agents are preferred. Pentamidine is an alternative agent for the treatment and prophylaxis of Pneumocystis pneumonia caused by the ascomycetous fungus *Pneumocystis jiroveci* (formerly known as *Pneumocystis carinii*) (Thomas and Limper, 2004).

Diminazene (BERENIL) is a related diamidine that is used as an inexpensive alternative to pentamidine for the treatment of early African trypanosomiasis and has been used outside the U.S. for the treatment of early-stage *T. b. gambiense* in periods of pentamidine shortage.

Mechanism of Action and Resistance. The mechanism of action of the diamidines is unknown. The dicationic compounds appear to display multiple effects on any given parasite and act by disparate mechanisms in different parasites (Barrett et al., 2007). In *T. brucei*, for example, the diamidines are concentrated via an energy-dependent high-affinity uptake system to millimolar concentrations in cells; this selective uptake is essential to their efficacy. The best-characterized diamidine transporter is the P2 purine transporter used by the melamine-based arsenicals, which explains the cross-resistance to diamidines exhibited by certain arsenical-resistant strains of *T. brucei in vitro* (de Koning, 2008). It is increasingly clear that multiple transporters are responsible for pentamidine uptake, and this may account for the fact that little resistance to this drug is observed in field isolates despite its years of use as a prophylactic agent. Although failure to concentrate diamidines is the usual cause of pentamidine resistance *in vitro*, other mechanisms also may be involved.

The positively charged hydrophobic diamidines may exert their trypanocidal effects by reacting with a variety of negatively charged intracellular targets. Indeed, ribosomal aggregation, inhibition of DNA and protein synthesis, inhibition of several enzymes, and loss of trypanosomal kinetoplast DNA have been reported. The loss of kinetoplast DNA may be mediated through inhibition of topoisomerase II. It is doubtful that an effect on topoisomerase accounts for the drug's broad antimicrobial activity or fully explains its mechanism of action. Inhibition of S-adenosyl-L-methionine decarboxylase *in vitro* (but no change in polyamine levels in vivo) and inhibition of a plasma Ca^{2+}, Mg^{2+}-ATPase also have been reported.

Absorption, Fate, and Excretion. The pharmacokinetics and biodisposition of pentamidine isethionate have been studied most extensively in AIDS patients with *P. jiroveci* infections (Vöhringer and Arastéh, 1993); information from patients with Gambian trypanosomiasis is more limited (Bronner et al., 1995). Pentamidine isethionate is fairly well absorbed from parenteral sites of administration. Following a single intravenous dose, the drug disappears from plasma with an apparent $t_{1/2}$ of several minutes to a few hours and maximum plasma concentrations after intramuscular injection occurring at 1 hour. The $t_{1/2}$ of elimination is very slow, lasting from weeks to months, and the drug is 70% bound to plasma proteins. This highly charged compound is poorly absorbed orally and does not cross the blood-brain barrier, explaining why it is ineffective against late-stage trypanosomiasis.

After multiple parenteral doses, the liver, kidney, adrenal, and spleen contain the highest concentrations of drug, whereas only traces are found in the brain (Donnelly et al., 1988). The lungs contain intermediate but therapeutic concentrations after five daily doses of 4 mg/kg. Inhalation of pentamidine aerosols is used for prophylaxis of *Pneumocystis* pneumonia; delivery of drug by this route results in little systemic absorption and decreased toxicity compared with intravenous administration in both adults and children (Hand et al., 1994; Leoung et al., 1990). The actual dose delivered to the lungs depends on both the size of particles generated by the nebulizer and the patient's ventilatory patterns.

Therapeutic Uses. Pentamidine isethionate is used for the treatment of early-stage *T. brucei gambiense* and is given by intramuscular injection in single doses of 4 mg/kg per day for 7 days. Pentamidine has been used successfully in courses of 15-20 intramuscular doses of 4 mg/kg every other day to treat visceral leishmaniasis (Alvar et al., 2006). This compound provides an alternative to antimonials, lipid formulations of amphotericin B, or miltefosine but it is overall the least well tolerated of the available therapies and is not used routinely for this disease. Pentamidine isethionate given as 4-7 intramuscular doses of 4 mg/kg every other day has enjoyed some success in the treatment of cutaneous leishmaniasis (Oriental sore caused by *L. tropica*) but is not used routinely to treat this infection (Alvar et al., 2006).

Pentamidine is one of several drugs or drug combinations used to treat or prevent *Pneumocystis* infection. *Pneumocystis* pneumonia (PCP) is a major cause of mortality in individuals with HIV infection and AIDS and can occur in patients who are immunosuppressed by other mechanisms (e.g., high-dose corticosteroids or underlying malignancy). The availability of highly active antiretroviral therapy (HAART) has reduced the number of cases of PCP significantly within the U.S. and E.U. and greatly reduced the number of individuals requiring prophylaxis for PCP. Trimethoprim-sulfamethoxazole is the drug of choice for the treatment and prevention of PCP (Chapter 52). Pentamidine is reserved for two indications. Pentamidine given intravenously as a 4 mg/kg single daily dose for 21 days is used to treat severe PCP in individuals who cannot tolerate trimethoprim-sulfamethoxazole and are not candidates for alternative agents such as atovaquone or the combination of clindamycin and primaquine. Pentamidine has been recommended as a "salvage" agent for individuals with PCP who failed to respond to initial therapy (usually trimethoprim-sulfamethoxazole), but a meta-analysis suggested that pentamidine is less effective than other therapies (specifically the combination of clindamycin and primaquine or atovaquone) for this indication (Smego et al., 2001). Pentamidine administered as an aerosol preparation is used for the prevention of PCP in at-risk individuals who cannot tolerate trimethoprim-sulfamethoxazole and are not deemed candidates for either dapsone (alone or in combination with pyrimethamine) or atovaquone. Candidates for PCP prophylaxis are individuals with HIV infection and a CD4 count of <200/mm^3 and individuals with HIV infection and persistent unexplained fever or oropharyngeal candidiasis. Secondary prophylaxis is recommended for everyone with a documented PCP episode. For prophylaxis, pentamidine isethionate is given monthly as a 300-mg dose in a 5-10% nebulized solution over 30-45 minutes. Although the monthly dosage regimen is convenient, aerosolized pentamidine has several disadvantages, including its failure to treat any extrapulmonary sites of *Pneumocystis*, the lack of efficacy against any other potential opportunistic pathogens (compared with trimethoprim-sulfamethoxazole), and a slightly increased risk for pneumothorax. Long-term aerosolized pentamidine prophylaxis (≥5 years) has not been associated with the development of any pulmonary disease (Obaji et al., 2003). For individuals who receive HAART and develop CD4 counts persistently above 200/mm^3 for 3 months, primary or secondary PCP prophylaxis can be stopped.

Toxicity and Side Effects. Pentamidine is a toxic agent, and ~50% of individuals receiving the drug at recommended doses (4 mg/kg per day) show some adverse effect. Intravenous administration of pentamidine may be associated with hypotension, tachycardia, and headache. These effects are probably secondary to the ability of pentamidine to bind imidazoline receptors (Chapter 14) and can be ameliorated by slowing the rate of the intravenous infusion (Wood et al., 1998). As noted earlier, the diamidines were designed originally for use as hypoglycemics, and pentamidine retains that property. Hypoglycemia, which can be life threatening, may occur at any time during pentamidine treatment, even weeks into therapy. Careful monitoring of blood sugar is key. Paradoxically, pancreatitis, hyperglycemia, and the development of insulin-dependent diabetes have been seen in some patients. Pentamidine is nephrotoxic (~25% of treated patients show signs of renal dysfunction), and if the serum creatinine concentration rises >1.0-2.0 mg/dL, it may be necessary to withhold the drug temporarily or change to an alternative agent. Individuals developing pentamidine-induced renal dysfunction are at higher risk for hypoglycemia. Other adverse effects include skin rashes, thrombophlebitis, anemia, neutropenia, and elevation of hepatic enzymes. Intramuscular administration of pentamidine, while effective, is associated with the development of sterile abscesses at the injection site, which can become infected secondarily. For this reason, most authorities recommend intravenous administration. Aerosolized pentamidine is associated with few adverse events.

Quinacrine

Quinacrine is an acridine derivative used widely during World War II as an antimalarial agent. *Quinacrine hydrochloride* is very effective against *G. lamblia*, producing cure rates of at least 90%. However, quinacrine is no longer available in the U.S. For a description of the pharmacology and toxicology of quinacrine, consult the fifth and earlier editions of this book.

Sodium Stibogluconate

Antimonials were introduced in 1945 and have been used for therapy of leishmaniasis and other protozoal infections (Alvar et al., 2006; Croft, 2008; Olliaro et al., 2005). The first trivalent antimonial compound used to treat cutaneous leishmaniasis and kala azar was antimony potassium tartrate (tartar emetic), which was both toxic and difficult to administer. Tartar emetic and other trivalent arsenicals eventually were replaced by pentavalent antimonial derivatives of phenylstibonic acid. An early member of this family of compounds was sodium stibogluconate (sodium antimony gluconate, PENTOSTAM). This drug is used widely today and, together with meglumine antimonate (GLUCANTIME), a pentavalent antimonial compound preferred in French-speaking countries, has been the mainstay of the treatment of leishmaniasis. However, increasing resistance to antimonials has reduced their efficacy and they are no longer useful in India (Croft, 2008; Croft et al.,

2006), where lipid-based amphotericin B and miltefosine are now recommended instead.

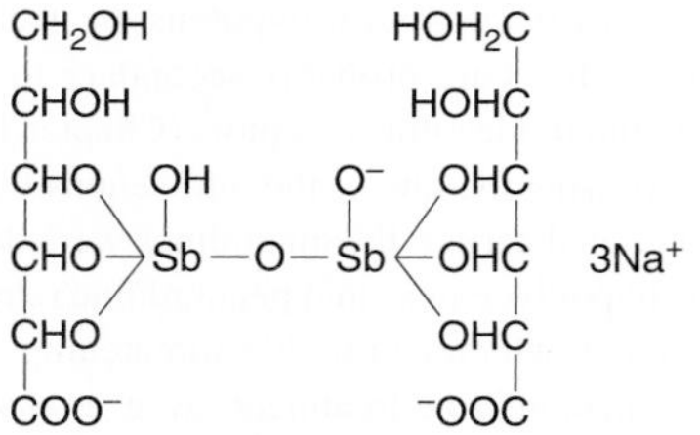

```
CH2OH                  HOH2C
|                          |
CHOH                    HOHC
|                          |
CHO   OH         O-     OHC
|      \    |         |    /     |
CHO — Sb — O — Sb — OHC     3Na+
|                          |
CHO                     OHC
|                          |
COO-                    -OOC
```

SODIUM STIBOGLUCONATE

Clinical formulations of sodium stibogluconate consist of multiple uncharacterized molecular forms, some of which have higher molecular masses than the compound shown. Typical preparations contain 30-34% pentavalent antimony by weight and *m*-chlorocresol (as a preservative). In the U.S., sodium stibogluconate can be obtained from the CDC.

Antiprotozoal Effects and Drug Resistance. The mechanism of the antileishmanial action of sodium stibogluconate remains an active area of research, and recent studies have provided interesting new insights (Croft et al., 2006). These studies support the old hypothesis that relatively nontoxic pentavalent antimonials act as prodrugs. These compounds are reduced to the more toxic Sb^{3+} species that kill amastigotes within the phagolysosomes of macrophages. This reduction preferentially occurs in the intracellular amastigote stage, and recently an enzyme, As^{5+} reductase, was characterized that is able to reduce Sb^{5+} to the active Sb^{3+} form. Furthermore, the overexpression of this enzyme in promastigotes increased their sensitivity to the drugs. Classically, it was thought that the antiparasitic effects of antimonials occurred through inhibition of glucose catabolism and fatty acid oxidation; however, recent studies suggest that the drugs operate by interfering with the trypanothione redox system. In drug-sensitive cell lines, Sb^{3+} induces a rapid efflux of trypanothione and glutathione from the cells, and also inhibits trypanothione reductase, thereby causing a significant loss of thiol reduction potential in the cells. This hypothesis is further supported by the observation that laboratory-generated resistance to antimonials leads to overexpression of glutathione and polyamine biosynthetic enzymes, resulting in increased trypanothione levels, which conjugate to the drug. Elevated levels of ABC efflux transporters (see Chapter 5) were observed, though these transporters seem to play only a minor role in drug resistance.

Absorption, Fate, and Excretion. The pentavalent antimonials attain much higher concentrations in plasma than do the trivalent compounds. Consequently, most of a single dose of sodium stibogluconate is excreted in the urine within 24 hours. Its pharmacokinetic behavior is similar whether the drug is given intravenously or intramuscularly; it is not active orally (Chulay et al., 1988). The agent is absorbed rapidly, distributed in an apparent volume of ~0.22 L/kg, and eliminated in two phases. The first has a $t_{1/2}$ of ~2 hours, and the second is much slower ($t_{1/2}$ = 33-76 hours). The prolonged terminal elimination phase may reflect conversion of the Sb^{5+} to the more toxic Sb^{3+} that is concentrated and slowly released from tissues. Indeed, ~20% of the plasma antimony is present in the trivalent form after pentavalent antimonial administration. Sequestration of antimony in macrophages also may contribute to the prolonged antileishmanial effect after plasma antimony levels have dropped below the minimal inhibitory concentration observed *in vitro*.

Therapeutic Uses. The changing use of sodium stibogluconate, meglumine antimonate, and other agents for the chemotherapy of leishmaniasis has been reviewed extensively (Alvar et al., 2006; Croft, 2008; Olliaro et al., 2005). Sodium stibogluconate is given parenterally, with the dosage regimen individualized depending on the local responsiveness of a particular form of leishmaniasis to this compound. The standard course is 20 mg/kg per day for 21 days for cutaneous disease and for 28 days for visceral disease. In some regions of the world prolonged dosage schedules with maximally tolerated doses are now needed for successful therapy of visceral, mucosal, and some cutaneous forms of leishmaniasis, in part to overcome increasing clinical resistance to antimonial drugs. Even high-dose regimens may no longer produce satisfactory results. Increased resistance has greatly compromised the effectiveness of these drugs, and the drug is now obsolete in India. This is in contrast to previous cure rates of >85% for both visceral and cutaneous disease. Liposomal amphotericin B is the recommended alternative for treatment of either visceral leishmaniasis (kala azar) in India or mucosal leishmaniasis in general; the orally effective compound miltefosine is likely to see much wider use in the coming years. Intralesional treatment has also been advocated as a safer, alternative method for treating cutaneous disease (Munir et al., 2008).

Children usually tolerate the drug well, and the dose per kilogram is the same as that given to adults. Patients who respond favorably show clinical improvement within 1-2 weeks of initiation of therapy. The drug may be given on alternate days or for longer intervals if unfavorable reactions occur in especially debilitated individuals. Patients infected with HIV present a challenge because they usually relapse after successful initial therapy with either pentavalent antimonials or amphotericin B.

Toxicity and Side Effects. The toxicity of the pentavalent antimonials is best evaluated in patients without systemic disease (i.e., visceral leishmaniasis). In general, high-dose regimens of sodium stibogluconate are fairly well tolerated; toxic reactions usually are reversible, and most subside despite continued therapy. Effects noted most commonly include pain at the injection site after intramuscular administration; chemical pancreatitis in nearly all patients; elevation of serum hepatic transaminase levels; bone marrow suppression manifested by decreased red cell, white cell, and platelet counts in the blood; muscle and joint pain; weakness and malaise; headache; nausea and abdominal pain; and skin rashes. Changes in the electrocardiogram that include T-wave flattening and inversion and prolongation of the QT interval found in patients with systemic disease are uncommon in other forms of leishmaniasis (Navin et al., 1992). Reversible polyneuropathy has been reported. Hemolytic anemia and renal damage are rare manifestations of antimonial toxicity, as are shock and sudden death.

Suramin

Based on the trypanocidal activity of the dyes *trypan red*, *trypan blue*, and *afridol violet*, research in Germany resulted in the introduction of suramin into therapy in 1920. Today, the drug is used primarily for treatment of African trypanosomiasis; it has no clinical utility against American trypanosomiasis. Although suramin is effective in clearing adult filariae in *onchocerciasis*, ivermectin has supplanted suramin for the treatment of this condition (Chapter 51). Suramin is a potent inhibitor of retroviral reverse transcriptase *in vitro*, but it is ineffective in HIV infection. The antiproliferative activity of suramin led to its experimental use, alone and with other compounds, for the therapy of a variety of tumors, particularly in androgen-independent prostate cancer. However, only modest palliative effects were observed and treatment for this indication was complicated by high toxicity. The antiparasitic and antineoplastic properties of suramin, along with its clinical uses and limitations, have been the topic of numerous reviews (Kennedy, 2008; McGeary et al., 2008).

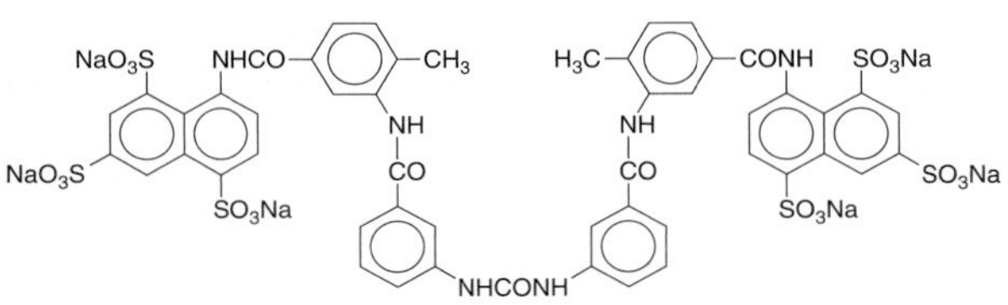

NaO_3S NHCO– –CH_3 H_3C– –CONH SO_3Na
NH NH
NaO_3S CO CO SO_3Na
SO_3Na SO_3Na
NHCONH
SURAMIN SODIUM

Suramin sodium (BAYER 205, formerly GERMANIN, others) is soluble in water, but solutions deteriorate quickly in air; only freshly prepared solutions should be used. In the U.S., suramin is available only from the CDC.

Antiparasitic Effects. Suramin is a relatively slowly acting trypanocide (>6 hours *in vitro*) with high clinical activity against both *T. b. gambiense* and *T. b. rhodesiense*. Its mechanism of action is unknown (Barrett et al., 2007). Selective toxicity is likely to result from the ability of the parasite to take up the drug by receptor-mediated endocytosis of the protein-bound drug, with low-density lipoproteins the most important interacting proteins for this event. Suramin reacts reversibly with a variety of biomolecules *in vitro*, inhibiting many trypanosomal and mammalian enzymes and receptors unrelated to its antiparasitic effects. Compartmentation protects many vital molecules, such as the glycolytic enzymes inside trypanosomal glycosomes, from suramin because this compound does not cross membrane barriers by passive diffusion. Suramin-treated trypanosomes exhibit damage to intracellular membrane structures other than lysosomes, but whether or not this relates to the drug's primary action is unknown. Inhibition of a trypanosomal cytosolic serine oligopeptidase may account for part of the activity of suramin, but the drug is also an inhibitor of dihydrofolate reductase, thymidine kinase, and several glycolytic enzymes. No clear consensus for the mechanism of action has emerged, and the lack of any significant field resistance points to multiple potential targets.

Absorption, Fate, and Excretion. The clinical pharmacology of suramin was determined during clinical trials for its application as an antitumor agent. Because it is not absorbed after oral intake, suramin is given intravenously to avoid local inflammation and necrosis associated with subcutaneous or intramuscular injections. After its administration, the drug displays complex pharmacokinetics with marked interindividual variability. The drug is 99.7% serum protein bound and has a terminal elimination $t_{1/2}$ of 41-78 days. Suramin is not appreciably metabolized, and renal clearance accounts for elimination of ~80% of the compound from the body. This large polar anion does not enter cells readily, and tissue concentrations are uniformly lower than those in plasma. In experimental animals the kidneys contain considerably more suramin than do other organs. Such retention may account for the fairly frequent occurrence of albuminuria following injection of the drug in humans. Very little suramin penetrates the CSF, consistent with its lack of efficacy once the CNS has been invaded by trypanosomes.

Therapeutic Uses. Suramin is the first-line therapy for early-stage *T. brucei rhodesiense* infection (Barrett et al., 2007; Kennedy, 2008). Although it shows activity against *T. brucei gambiense,* it is not used for this application because other drugs are available for the treatment of this disease that are not complicated by the high activity of suramin against Onchocerca and Brugia, and possible immunological reactions resulting from killing of these parasitic worms. Because only small amounts of the drug enter the brain, suramin is used only for the treatment of early-stage African trypanosomiasis (before CNS involvement). Suramin will clear the hemolymphatic system of trypanosomes even in late-stage disease, so it is often administered before initiating melarsoprol to reduce the risk of reactive encephalopathy associated with the administration of that arsenical. Suramin is given by slow intravenous injection as a 10% aqueous solution. Treatment of active African trypanosomiasis should not be started until 24 hours after diagnostic lumbar puncture to ensure no CNS involvement, and caution is required if the patient has onchocerciasis (river blindness) because of the potential for eliciting a Mazzotti reaction (i.e., pruritic rash, fever, malaise, lymph node swelling, eosinophilia, arthralgias, tachycardia, hypotension, and possibly permanent blindness). The normal single dose for adults with *T. brucei rhodesiense* infection is 1 g. It is advisable to employ a test dose of 200 mg initially to detect sensitivity, after which the normal dose is given intravenously on days 1, 3, 7, 14, and 21, although a wide range of schedules are in use. The pediatric dose is 20 mg/kg, given according to the same schedule. Patients in poor condition should be treated with lower doses during the first week. Patients who relapse after suramin therapy should be treated with melarsoprol.

Toxicity and Side Effects. Suramin can cause a variety of untoward reactions that vary in intensity and frequency and tend to be more severe in debilitated patients. Fortunately, the most serious immediate reaction consisting of nausea, vomiting, shock, and loss of consciousness is rare (~1 in 2000 patients). Malaise, nausea, and fatigue are also common immediate reactions. Parasite destruction may cause febrile episodes and skin hypersensitivity rashes that are reduced by pretreatment with glucocorticoids; concomitant onchocerciasis optimally should be treated first with ivermectin to minimize these reactions (Chapter 51). The most common problem encountered after several doses of suramin is renal toxicity, manifested by albuminuria, and delayed neurological complications, including headache, metallic taste, paresthesias, and peripheral neuropathy. These complications usually disappear spontaneously despite continued therapy. Other, less prevalent reactions include vomiting, diarrhea, stomatitis, chills, abdominal pain, and edema. Laboratory abnormalities noted in 12-26% of patients with AIDS include leukopenia and occasional agranulocytosis, thrombocytopenia, proteinuria, and elevations of plasma creatinine, transaminases, and bilirubin, which are reversible. Unexpected findings in patients with AIDS include adrenal insufficiency and vortex keratopathy.

Precautions and Contraindications. Patients receiving suramin should be followed closely. Therapy should not be continued in patients who show intolerance to initial doses, and the drug should be employed with great caution in individuals with renal insufficiency. Moderate albuminuria is common during control of the acute phase, but persisting, heavy albuminuria calls for caution as well as modification of the treatment schedule. If casts appear, treatment with suramin should be discontinued. The occurrence of palmar-plantar hyperesthesia may presage peripheral neuritis.

BIBLIOGRAPHY

Abboud P, Lemee V, Gargala G, *et al.* Successful treatment of metronidazole- and albendazole-resistant giardiasis with nitazoxanide in a patient with acquired immunodeficiency syndrome. *Clin Infect Dis*, **2001,** *32:*1792–1794.

Adagu IS, Nolder D, Warhurst DC, Rossignol JF. *In vitro* activity of nitazoxanide and related compounds against isolates of *Giardia intestinalis*, *Entamoeba histolytica*, and *Trichomonas vaginalis*. *J Antimicrob Chemother*, **2002,** *49:*103–111.

Aguero F, Al-Lazikani B, Aslett M, *et al.* Genomic-scale prioritization of drug targets: The TDR Targets database. *Nat Rev Drug Discov,* **2008,** *7:*900–907.

Alvar J, Croft S, Olliaro P. Chemotherapy in the treatment and control of leishmaniasis. *Adv Parasitol,* **2006,** *61:*223–274.

Amadi B, Mwiya M, Musuku J, *et al.* Effect of nitazoxanide on morbidity and mortality in Zambian children with cryptosporidiosis: A randomized, controlled trial. *Lancet*, **2002,** *360:*1375–1380.

Bacchi CJ, Nathan HC, Hunter SH, *et al.* Polyamine metabolism: A potential therapeutic target in trypanosomes. *Science*, **1980,** *210:*332–334.

Balasegaram M, Harris S, Checchi F, *et al.* Melarsoprol versus eflornithine for treating late-stage Gambian trypanosomiasis in the Republic of the Congo. *Bull World Health Organ,* **2006a,** *84:*783–791.

Balasegaram M, Harris S, Checchi F, *et al.* Treatment outcomes and risk factors for relapse in patients with early-stage human African trypanosomiasis (HAT) in the Republic of the Congo. *Bull World Health Organ,* **2006b,** *84:*777–782.

Balasegaram M, Young H, Chappuis F, *et al.* Effectiveness of melarsoprol and eflornithine as first-line regimens for gambiense sleeping sickness in nine Médecins Sans Frontières programmes. *Trans R Soc Trop Med Hyg,* **2009,** *103:*280–290.

Barrett MP, Boykin DW, Brun R, Tidwell RR. Human African trypanosomiasis: Pharmacological re-engagement with a neglected disease. *Br J Pharmacol,* **2007,** *152:*1155–1171.

Berman JJ. Treatment of leishmaniasis with miltefosine: 2008 status. *Expert Opin Drug Metab Toxicol,* **2008,** *4:* 1209–1216.

Bern C, Montgomery SP, Herwaldt BL, *et al.* Evaluation and treatment of Chagas disease in the United States: A systematic review. *JAMA,* **2007,** *298:*2171–2181.

Bern C, Montgomery SP, Katz L, *et al.* Chagas disease and the US blood supply. *Curr Opin Infect Dis,* **2008,** *21:*476–482.

Bhattacharya SK, Sinha PK, Sundar S, *et al.* Phase 4 trial of miltefosine for the treatment of Indian visceral leishmaniasis. *J Infect Dis,* **2007,** *196:*591–598.

Blum J, Schmid C, Burri C. Clinical aspects of 2541 patients with second stage human African trypanosomiasis. *Acta Trop,* **2006,** *97:*55–64.

Bronner U, Gustafsson LL, Doua F, *et al.* Pharmacokinetics and adverse reactions after a single dose of pentamidine in patients with *Trypanosoma gambiense* sleeping sickness. *Br J Clin Pharmacol*, **1995,** *39:*289–295.

Brun R, Schumacher R, Schmid C, *et al.* The phenomenon of treatment failures in human African trypanosomiasis. *Trop Med Int Health*, **2001,** *6:*906–914.

Burri C, Brun R. Eflornithine for the treatment of human African trypanosomiasis. *Parasitol Res*, **2003,** *90*(suppl):49–52.

Burri C, Keiser J. Pharmacokinetic investigations in patients from northern Angola refractory to melarsoprol treatment. *Trop Med Int Health*, **2001,** *6:*412–420.

Bustamante JM, Bixby LM, Tarleton RL. Drug-induced cure drives conversion to a stable and protective CD8+ T central memory response in chronic Chagas disease. *Nat Med,* **2008,** *14:*542–550.

Casero RA Jr, Marton LJ. Targeting polyamine metabolism and function in cancer and other hyperproliferative diseases. *Nat Rev Drug Discov,* **2007,** *6:*373–390.

Chappuis F. Melarsoprol-free drug combinations for second-stage Gambian sleeping sickness: The way to go. *Clin Infect Dis,* **2007,** *45:*1443–1445.

Chappuis F, Sundar S, Hailu A, *et al.* Visceral leishmaniasis: What are the needs for diagnosis, treatment and control? *Nat Rev Microbiol,* **2007,** *5:*873–882.

Chappuis F, Udayraj N, Stietenroth K, *et al.* Eflornithine is safer than melarsoprol for the treatment of second-stage Trypanosoma brucei gambiense human African trypanosomiasis. *Clin Infect Dis,* **2005,** *41:*748–751.

Chen KT, Twu SJ, Chang HJ, Lin RS. Outbreak of Stevens-Johnson syndrome/toxic epidermal necrolysis associated with mebendazole and metronidazole use among Filipino laborers in Taiwan. *Am J Public Health,* **2003,** *93:*489–492.

Chulay JD, Fleckenstein L, Smith DH. Pharmacokinetics of antimony during treatment of visceral leishmaniasis with sodium stibogluconate or meglumine antimonate. *Trans R Soc Trop Med Hyg*, **1988,** *82:*69–72.

Cooley G, Etheridge RD, Boehlke C, *et al.* High throughput selection of effective serodiagnostics for *Trypanosoma cruzi* infection. *PLoS Negl Trop Dis,* **2008,** *2:*e316.

Croft SL. Neglected diseases: Progress in drug development. *Curr Opin Invest Drugs,* **2007,** *8:*103–104.

Croft SL. Kinetoplastida: New therapeutic strategies. *Parasite,* **2008,** *15:*522–527.

Croft SL, Coombs GH. Leishmaniasis: Current chemotherapy and recent advances in the search for novel drugs. *Trends Parasitol*, **2003,** *19:*502–508.

Croft SL, Sundar S, Fairlamb AH. Drug resistance in leishmaniasis. *Clin Microbiol Rev,* **2006,** *19:*111–126.

de Koning HP. Ever-increasing complexities of diamidine and arsenical cross resistance in African trypanosomes. *Trends Parasitol,* **2008,** *24:*345–349.

Donnelly H, Bernard EM, Rothkotter H, *et al.* Distribution of pentamidine in patients with AIDS. *J Infect Dis*, **1988,** *157:*985–989.

Doyle PS, Zhou YM, Engel JC, McKerrow JH. A cysteine protease inhibitor cures Chagas' disease in an immunodeficient-mouse model of infection. *Antimicrob Agents Chemother,* **2007,** *51:*3932–3939.

Dunne RL, Dunn LA, Upcroft P, *et al.* Drug resistance in the sexually transmitted protozoan *Trichomonas vaginalis. Cell Res*, **2003,** *13:*239–249.

Favennec L, Jave-Ortiz J, Gargala G, *et al.* Double-blind, randomized, placebo-controlled study of nitazoxanide in the treatment of fascioliasis in adults and children from northern Peru. *Aliment Pharmacol Therm*, **2003,** *17:*265–270.

Frearson JA, Wyatt PG, Gilbert IH, Fairlamb AH. Target assessment for antiparasitic drug discovery. *Trends Parasitol,* **2007,** *23:*589–595.

Freeman CD, Klutman NE, Lamp KC. Metronidazole: A therapeutic review and update. *Drugs*, **1997,** *54:*679–708.

Gal M, Brazier JS. Metronidazole resistance in *Bacteroides* spp. carrying *nim* genes and the selection of slow-growing metronidazole-resistant mutants. *J Antimicrob Chemother*, **2004,** *54:*109–116.

Gardner TB, Hill DR. Treatment of giardiasis. *Clin Microbiol Rev*, **2001,** *14:*114–128.

Grishin NV, Osterman AL, Brooks HB, *et al.* The X-ray structure of ornithine decarboxylase from *Trypanosoma brucei:* The native structure and the structure in complex with α-difluoromethylornithine. *Biochemistry*, **1999,** *38:*15174–15184.

Gross U. Treatment of microsporidiosis including albendazole. *Parasitol Res*, **2003,** *90*(suppl):14–18.

Hand IL, Wiznia AA, Porricolo M, *et al.* Aerosolized pentamidine for prophylaxis of *Pneumocystis carinii* pneumonia in infants with human immunodeficiency virus infection. *Pediatr Infect Dis J*, **1994,** *13:*100–104.

Hewitt RG, Yiannoutsos CT, Higgs ES, *et al.* Paromomycin: No more effective than placebo for treatment of cryptosporidiosis in patients with advanced human immunodeficiency virus infection. AIDS Clinical Trial Group. *Clin Infect Dis*, **2000,** *31:*1084–1092.

Hlavsa MC, Watson JC, Beach MJ. Giardiasis surveillance—United States, 1998–2002. *MMWR* **2005,** *54:*9–16.

Hoffman PS, Sisson G, Croven MA, *et al.* Antiparasitc drug nitazoxanide inhibits the pyruvate oxidoreductases of *Helicobacter pylori,* selected anaerobic bacteria and parasites and *Campylobacter jejuni. Antimicrob Agents Chemother*, **2007,** *51:*868–876.

Kennedy PG. The continuing problem of human African trypanosomiasis (sleeping sickness). *Ann Neurol,* **2008,** *64:*116–126.

Lamp KC, Freeman CD, Klutman NE, Lacy MK. Pharmacokinetics and pharmacodynamics of the nitroimidazole antimicrobials. *Clin Pharmacokinet*, **1999,** *36:*353–373.

Land KM, Johnson PJ. Molecular mechanisms underlying metronidazole resistance in trichomonads. *Exp Parasitol*, **1997,** *87:*305–308.

Lejon V, Boelaert M, Jannin J, *et al.* The challenge of *Trypanosoma brucei gambiense* sleeping sickness diagnosis outside of Africa. *Lancet Infect Dis*, **2003,** *3:*804–808.

Leoung SG, Feigal DW Jr, Montgomery AB, *et al.* Aerosolized pentamidine for prophylaxis against *Pneumocystis carinii* pneumonia: The San Francisco community prophylaxis trial. *N Engl J Med*, **1990,** *323:*769–775.

Maina N, Maina KJ, Maser P, Brun R. Genotypic and phenotypic characterization of Trypanosoma brucei gambiense isolates from Ibba, South Sudan, an area of high melarsoprol treatment failure rate. *Acta Trop,* **2007,** *104:*84–90.

Marin-Neto JA, Rassi A Jr, Morillo CA, *et al.* Rationale and design of a randomized placebo-controlled trial assessing the effects of etiologic treatment in Chagas' cardiomyopathy: the BENznidazole Evaluation For Interrupting Trypanosomiasis (BENEFIT). *Am Heart J,* **2008,** *156:*37–43.

McFarland LV. Renewed interest in a difficult disease: *Clostridium difficile* infections—epidemiology and current treatment strategies. *Curr Opin Gastroenterol,* **2008,** *25:*24–35.

McGeary RP, Bennett AJ, Tran QB, *et al.* Suramin: Clinical uses and structure-activity relationships. *Mini Rev Med Chem,* **2008,** *8:*1384–1394.

Mdachi RE, Thuita JK, Kagira JM, *et al.* Efficacy of the novel diamidine compound 2, 5-bis (4-amidinophenyl)-furan-bis-O-methylamidoxime (pafuramidine, DB289) against T. b. rhodesiense infection in vervet monkeys after oral administration. *Antimicrob Agents Chemother,* **2009,** *53:*953–957.

Medecins Sans Frontieres. Clinical guidelines, **2007**; available at: www.refbooks.msf.org/msf_docs/en/clinical_guide/CG_en.pdf; accessed June 2, 2010.

Medical Letter. Drugs for parasitic infections. *Met Lett Drugs Ther,* **2007,** *5:*e1–e15.

Mendz GL, Mégraud F. Is the molecular basis of metronidazole resistance in microaerophilic organisms understood? *Trends Microbiol*, **2002,** *10:*370–375.

Meyerhoff A. U.S. Food and Drug Administration approval of AmBicome (liposomal amphotericin B) for the treatment of visceral leishmaniasis. *Clin Infect Dis*, **1999,** *28:*42–48.

Milord F, Loko L, Éthier L, *et al.* Eflornithine concentrations in serum and cerebrospinal fluid of 63 patients treated for *Trypanosoma brucei gambiense* sleeping sickness. *Trans R Soc Trop Med Hyg*, **1993,** *87:*473–477.

Molina JM, Tourneur M, Sarfati C, *et al.* Fumagillin treatment of intestinal microsporidiosis. *N Engl J Med*, **2002,** *346:*1963–1969.

Montoya JG, Liesenfield O. Toxoplasmosis. *Lancet*, **2004,** *363:*1965–1976.

Munir A, Janjua SA, Hussain I. Clinical efficacy of intramuscular meglumine antimoniate alone and in combination with intralesional meglumine antimoniate in the treatment of old world cutaneous leishmaniasis. *Acta Dermatovenerol Croat,* **2008,** *16:*60–64.

Mutomba MC, Li F, Gottesdiener KM, Wang CC. A *Trypanosoma brucei* bloodstream form mutant deficient in ornithine decarboxylase can protect against wild-type infection in mice. *Exp Parasitol*, **1999,** *91:*176–184.

Nash TE. Treatment of *giardia lamblia* infections. *Pediatr Infect Dis J*, **2001**, *20*:193–195.

Navin TR, Arana BA, Arana FE, *et al.* Placebo-controlled clinical trial of sodium stibogluconate (Pentostam) versus ketoconazole for treating cutaneous leishmaniasis in Guatemala. *J Infect Dis*, **1992,** *165:*528–534.

Nwaka S, Hudson A. Innovative lead discovery strategies for tropical diseases. *Nat Rev Drug Discov,* **2006,** *5:*941–955.

Obaji J, Lee-Pack LR, Gutierrez C, Chan CK. The pulmonary effects of long-term exposure to aerosol pentamidine: A 5-year surveillance study in HIV-infected patients. *Chest*, **2003,** *123:*1983–1987.

Olliaro PL, Guerin PJ, Gerstl S, *et al.* Treatment options for visceral leishmaniasis: A systematic review of clinical studies done in India, 1980–2004. *Lancet Infect Dis,* **2005,** *5:*763–774.

Paulos C, Paredes J, Vasquez I, *et al.* Pharmacokinetics of a nitrofuran compound, nifurtimox, in healthy volunteers. *Int J Clin Pharmacol Ther Toxicol*, **1989,** *27:*454–457.

Pepin J, Mpia B. Trypanosomiasis relapse after melarsoprol therapy, Democratic Republic of Congo, 1982–2001. *Emerg Infect Dis,* **2005,** *11:*921–927.

Pepin J, Mpia B. Randomized controlled trial of three regimens of melarsoprol in the treatment of *Trypanosoma brucei gambiense* trypanosomiasis. *Trans R Soc Trop Med Hyg,* **2006,** *100:*437–441.

Pink R, Hudson A, Mouries MA, Bendig M. Opportunities and challenges in antiparasitic drug discovery. *Nat Rev Drug Discov,* **2005,** *4:*727–740.

Podolsky DK. Inflammatory bowel disease. *N Engl J Med*, **2002,** *347:*417–429.

Priotto G, Fogg C, Balasegaram M, *et al.* Three drug combinations for late-stage *Trypanosoma brucei gambiense* sleeping sickness: A randomized clinical trial in Uganda. *PLoS Clin Trials,* **2006,** *1:*e39.

Priotto G, Kasparian S, Mutombo W, et al. Nifurtimox-eflornithine combination therapy for seond-stage African *Trypanosoma brucei gambiense* trypanosomiasis: a multi-centre, randomized, phase III, non-inferiority trial. *Lancet*, **2009**, *374*:56–64.

Priotto G, Pinoges L, Fursa IB, *et al.* Safety and effectiveness of first line eflornithine for *Trypanosoma brucei gambiense* sleeping sickness in Sudan: Cohort study. *BMJ,* **2008,** *336:*705–708.

Raether W, Hänel H. Nitroheterocyclic drugs with broad-spectrum activity. *Parasitol Res*, **2003,** *90*(suppl):19–39.

Ramirez NE, Ward LA, Sreevatsan, S. A review of the biology and epidemiology of cryptosporidiosis in humans and animals. *Microbes Infect*, **2004,** *6:*773–785.

Robays J, Nyamowala G, Sese C, *et al.* High failure rates of melarsoprol for sleeping sickness, Democratic Republic of Congo. *Emerg Infect Dis,* **2008b,** *14:*966–967.

Robays J, Raguenaud ME, Josenando T, Boelaert M. Eflornithine is a cost-effective alternative to melarsoprol for the treatment of second-stage human West African trypanosomiasis in Caxito, Angola. *Trop Med Int Health,* **2008a,** *13:*265–271.

Romero-Cabello R, Guerrero LR, Munoz-Garcia MR, Geyne-Cruz A. Nitazoxanide for the treatment of intestinal protozoan and helminthic infections in Mexico. *Trans R Soc Trop Med Hyg*, **1997,** *91:*701–703.

Rossignol J. Nitazoxanide in the treatment of acquired immune deficiency syndrome-related cryptosporidiosis: results of the United States compassionate use program in 365 patients. *Aliment Pharmacol Ther,* **2006,** *24:*887–894.

Rossignol JF, Ayoub A, Ayers MS. Treatment of diarrhea caused by *Cryptosporidium parvum:* A prospective, randomized, double-blind, placebo-controlled study of nitazoxanide. *J Infect Dis*, **2001,** *184:*103–106.

Rossignol JF, Keeffe EB. Thiazolides: A new class of drugs for the treatment of chronic hepatitis B and C. *Future Microbiol,* **2008,** *3:*539–545.

Rossignol JF, Maisonneuve H. Nitazoxanide in the treatment of *Taenia saginata* and *Hymenolepis nana* infections. *Am J Trop Med Hyg*, **1984,** *33:*511–512.

Sanderson L, Dogruel M, Rodgers J, *et al.* The blood-brain barrier significantly limits eflornithine entry into *Trypanosoma brucei brucei* infected mouse brain. *J Neurochem,* **2008,** *107:*1136–1146.

Schmid C, Richer M, Bilenge CM, *et al.* Effectiveness of a 10-day melarsoprol schedule for the treatment of late-stage human African trypanosomiasis: Confirmation from a multinational study (IMPAMEL II). *J Infect Dis,* **2005,** *191:* 1922–1931.

Sears CL, Kirkpatrick BD. Is nitazoxanide an effective treatment for patients with acquired immune deficiency syndrome-related cryptosporidiosis? *Nature Clin Pract,* **2007,** *4:* 136–137.

Seifert K, Perez-Victoria FJ, Stettler M, *et al.* Inactivation of the miltefosine transporter, LdMT, causes miltefosine resistance that is conferred to the amastigote stage of Leishmania donovani and persists in vivo. *Int J Antimicrob Agents,* **2007,** *30:*229–235.

Smego RA Jr, Nagar S, Maloba B, Popara M. A meta-analysis of salvage therapy for *Pneumocystis carinii* pneumonia. *Arch Intern Med*, **2001,** *161:*1529–1533.

Sobel JD, Nyirjesy P, Brown W. Tinidazole therapy for metronidazole-resistant vaginal trichomoniasis. *Clin Infect Dis*, **2001,** *33:*1341–1346.

Soto J, Berman J. Treatment of New World cutaneous leishmaniasis with miltefosine. *Trans R Soc Trop Med Hyg,* **2006,** *100*(suppl 1)*:*S34–40.

Soto J, Toledo J, Valda L, *et al.* Treatment of Bolivian mucosal leishmaniasis with miltefosine. *Clin Infect Dis,* **2007,** *44:*350–356.

Stanley SL Jr. Amoebiasis. *Lancet*, **2003,** *361:*1025–1034.

Stuart K, Brun R, Croft S, *et al.* Kinetoplastids: Related protozoan pathogens, different diseases. *J Clin Invest,* **2008,** *118:* 1301–1310.

Sundar S, Jha TK, Thakur CP, *et al.* Injectable paromomycin for visceral leishmaniasis in India. *N Engl J Med,* **2007,** *356:*2571–2581.

Sundar S, Rai M, Chakravarty J, *et al.* New treatment approach in Indian visceral leishmaniasis: Single-dose liposomal amphotericin B followed by short-course oral miltefosine. *Clin Infect Dis,* **2008,** *47:*1000–1006.

Tarleton RL. Chagas disease: A role for autoimmunity? *Trends Parasitol,* **2003,** *19:*447–451.

Tarleton RL, Reithinger R, Urbina JA, *et al.* The challenges of Chagas Disease—grim outlook or glimmer of hope. *PLoS Med,* **2007,** *4:*e332.

Thomas CF Jr, Limper AH. *Pneumocystis* pneumonia. *N Engl J Med*, **2004,** *350:*2487–2498.

Upcroft JA, Campbell RW, Benakli K, *et al.* Efficacy of new 5-nitroimidazoles against metronidazole-susceptible and -resistant *Giardia, Trichomonas*, and *Entamoeba* spp. *Antimicrob Agents Chemother*, **1999,** *43:*73–76.

Upcroft JA, Upcroft P. Keto-acid oxidoreductases in the anaerobic protozoa. *J Eukaryot Microbiol*, **1999,** *46:*447–449.

Upcroft P, Upcroft JA. Drug targets and mechanisms of resistance in the anaerobic protozoa. *Clin Microbiol Rev*, **2001,** *14:*150–164.

Vöhringer HF, Arastéh K. Pharmacokinetic optimisation in the treatment of *Pneumocystis carinii* pneumonia. *Clin Pharmacokinet*, **1993,** *24:*388–412.

Wassmann C, Hellberg A, Tannich E, Bruchhaus I. Metronidazole resistance in the protozoan parasite *Entamoeba histolytica* is associated with increased expression of iron-containing superoxide dismutase and peroxiredoxin and decreased expression of ferredoxin 1 and flavin reductase. *J Biol Chem*, **1999,** *274:*26051–26056.

Wilkinson SR, Taylor MC, Horn D, *et al.* A mechanism for cross-resistance to nifurtimox and benznidazole in trypanosomes. *Proc Natl Acad Sci USA,* **2008,** *105:*5022–5027.

Wood DH, Hall JE, Rose BG, Tidwell RR. 1,5-Bis(4amidinophenoxy)pentane (pentamidine) is a potent inhibitor of [^{3}H]idazoxan binding to imidazoline I_2 binding sites. *Eur J Pharmacol*, **1998,** *353:*97–103.

World Health Organization. Control and surveillance of African trypanosomiasis. *World Health Organization, Technical Report Series,* **1998,** 881.

World Health Organization. Chile and Brazil to be certified free of transmission of Chagas' disease. *TDR News*, **1999,** *59:*10.

Chemotherapy of Helminth Infections

James McCarthy, Alex Loukas, and Peter J. Hotez

Infections with helminths, or parasitic worms, affect more than two billion people worldwide. In regions of rural poverty in the tropics, where prevalence is greatest, simultaneous infection with more than one type of helminth is common. The relative incidence of common helminthic infections in humans worldwide is illustrated in Figure 51–1.

Worms pathogenic for humans are Metazoa and can be classified into roundworms (nematodes) and two types of flatworms, flukes (trematodes) and tapeworms (cestodes). These biologically diverse eukaryotes vary with respect to life cycle, bodily structure, development, physiology, localization within the host, and susceptibility to chemotherapy. Immature forms invade humans via the skin or GI tract and evolve into well-differentiated adult worms with characteristic tissue distributions. With few exceptions, such as *Strongyloides* and *Echinococcus*, these organisms cannot complete their life cycle and replicate within the human host to produce mature offspring. Therefore, the extent of exposure to these parasites dictates the number of parasites infecting the host, a characteristic recognized as infection intensity, which itself determines the morbidity caused by infection. Secondly, any reduction in the number of adult organisms by chemotherapy is sustained unless reinfection occurs. The burden of parasitic helminths within an infected population is not uniformly distributed, and it typically displays a negative binomial distribution whereby relatively few persons carry the heaviest parasite burden, resulting in increased morbidity in these individuals who also contribute disproportionately to transmission.

Anthelmintics are drugs that act either locally within the gut lumen to cause expulsion of worms from the GI tract, or systemically against helminths residing outside the GI tract. Safe and effective broad-spectrum anthelmintics, initially developed for veterinary use, are currently available for use in humans. However, therapy for many tissue-dwelling helminths, such as filarial parasites, is not fully effective. For many reasons, including their long-lived and relatively complex life cycles, acquired resistance to anthelmintics in humans has yet to become a major clinical problem. However, with the increasing deployment of mass drug therapy, and considering the veterinary experience with resistance, the potential for drug resistance among helminths in humans requires monitoring.

Primarily as a result of stepped-up advocacy by the World Health Organization (WHO), the World Bank, the Global Network for Neglected Tropical Diseases, and smaller nongovernmental organizations such as the London-based Partnership for Child Development (PCD), there is increasing appreciation for the impact of helminth infections on the health and education of school-aged children. These organizations have promoted the periodic and frequent use of anthelmintic drugs in schools as a means to control morbidity caused by soil-transmitted helminths and schistosomes in developing countries. In addition, interest has grown in eliminating arthropod-borne helminth infections by interrupting their transmission through the widespread use of anthelmintics. Today, control programs employing anthelmintics rank among the world's largest health efforts, and hundreds of millions of people receive treatment annually (Hotez et al., 2009).

This chapter is divided into two main parts:

- clinical presentation and recommended chemotherapy for common helminth infections in humans
- pharmacological properties of specific anthelmintics

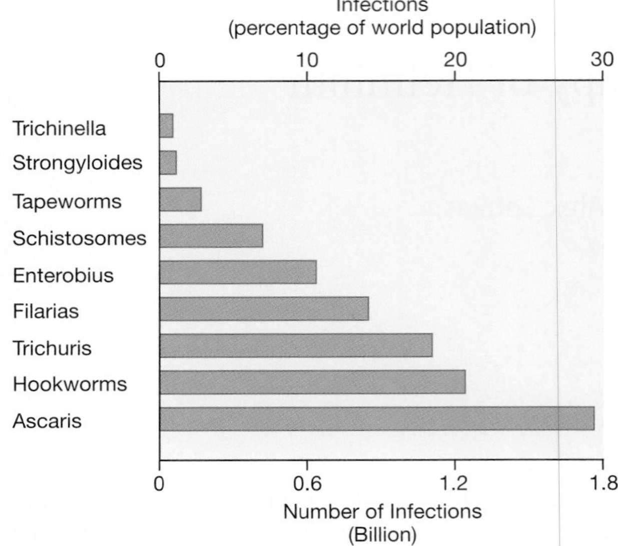

Figure 51–1. *Relative incidence of helminth infections worldwide.*

HELMINTH INFECTIONS AND THEIR TREATMENT

Nematodes (Roundworms)

The major nematode parasites of humans include the soil-transmitted helminths (STHs; sometimes referred to as "geohelminths") and the filarial nematodes.

The major STH infections (ascariasis [roundworm], trichuriasis [whipworm], and hookworm infection) are among the most prevalent infections in developing countries. Because STH worm burdens are higher in school-aged children than in any other single group, the WHO and the PCD advocate school-based administration of broad-spectrum anthelmintics on a periodic and frequent basis. The agents most widely employed for reducing morbidity are the benzimidazole anthelmintics (BZ), either albendazole (ALBENZA and ZENTEL) or mebendazole (VERMOX, others) (Table 51–1, p. 1450).

Single dose therapy with a BZ reduces worm burden to a varying degree, with greatest efficacy for ascariasis, followed by whipworm and hookworm (Keiser and Utzinger, 2008) and subsequently reduces morbidity attributable to the parasite. Treatment improves host iron stores and hemoglobin levels, physical growth, cognition, educational achievement, and school absenteeism, as well as having a positive influence on the entire community by reducing transmission (Bethony et al., 2006). In 2001, the World Health Assembly adopted a resolution urging that by 2010 member states should regularly administer anthelmintics to at least 75% of all school-age children at risk for morbidity (WHO, 2002). Concerns with this recommendation have included:

- The scope of the undertaking
- The high rate of post-treatment reinfection that occur in areas of high transmission
- Documented drug failures against hookworm with mebendazole
- The possibility that widespread treatment will lead to the emergence of BZ drug resistance
- The possibility that by focusing exclusively on school-aged children, other groups and vulnerable populations, such as preschool children and women of reproductive age, will be omitted

In addition to targeting STH infections among school-aged children, there are ongoing programs to eliminate lymphatic filariasis (LF) and onchocerciasis (river blindness) over the next 10-20 years (Molyneux and Zagaria, 2002; Molyneux et al., 2003). The term *elimination,* as opposed to *eradication,* refers to the reduction of disease incidence to zero or close to zero, with a requirement for ongoing control efforts (Hotez et al., 2004). The major goals for the LF elimination program (and to some extent, the onchocerciasis elimination programs) are to interrupt arthropod-borne transmission by administering combination therapy with either diethylcarbamazine (DEC; HETRAZAN; available from CDC in the U.S.) and albendazole (in LF-endemic regions such as India and Egypt), or ivermectin (STROMECTOL) and albendazole (in LF regions where onchocerciasis and/or loiasis are co-endemic). For onchocerciasis, ivermectin also reduces the microfilarial load in the skin, leading to reductions in so-called troublesome itching and ultimately, in preventing river blindness. DEC and ivermectin target the microfilarial stages of the parasite, which circulate in blood and are taken up by arthropod vectors where further parasite development takes place. Both control programs rely heavily on the generosity of major drug companies that donate ivermectin and albendazole, respectively (Burnham and Mebrahtu, 2004; Molyneux et al., 2003).

Ascaris lumbricoides and Toxocara canis. *Ascaris lumbricoides*, known as the "roundworm," parasitizes a billion or more people worldwide (de Silva et al., 2003; Hotez et al, 2009). Ascariasis may affect from 70-90% of persons in some tropical regions; it is also seen in temperate climates. People become infected by ingesting food or soil contaminated with embryonated *A. lumbricoides* eggs. The highest ascaris worm burdens occur in school-aged children in whom the parasite can cause intestinal obstruction or hepatobiliary ascariasis (Crompton, 2001).

Effective and safe anthelmintics have replaced the older ascaricides. The preferred agents are the benzimidazoles (BZ), mebendazole and albendazole, and the broad spectrum drug pyrantel pamoate. Cure with any of these drugs can be achieved in nearly 100% of cases. Mebendazole and albendazole are preferred for therapy of asymptomatic to moderate ascariasis, as well as for mass drug administration campaigns because those agents have a broad spectrum of activity against GI nematodes. Both compounds should be used with caution to treat heavy *Ascaris* infections, alone or with hookworms. In rare instances, following chemotherapy hyperactive ascarids may migrate to unusual loci and cause serious complications such as appendicitis, occlusion of the common bile duct, and intestinal obstruction and perforation with peritonitis. For this reason, some clinicians recommend the use of pyrantel for heavy *Ascaris* infections because this agent paralyzes the worms prior to their expulsion. Surgery may be required to alleviate obstructive complications. Pyrantel is considered safe for use during pregnancy, whereas BZ should be avoided during the first trimester. Albendazole is available off-label for treatment of ascariasis in the U.S.

Toxocariasis, a zoonotic infection caused by the canine ascarid *Toxocara canis*, is a common helminthiasis in North America and Europe. Although precise information is not available, toxocariasis may have displaced pinworm as the most common helminth infection in the U.S. (Hotez and Wilkins, 2009). In the U.S., the highest rates of infection are found within African American and Hispanic American populations, with some evidence to suggest that toxocariasis is the most common neglected infection associated with poverty (Hotez, 2008; Hotez and Wilkins, 2009).

Three major syndromes are caused by *T. canis* infection: visceral larva migrans (VLM), ocular larva migrans (OLM), and covert toxocariasis (CTox). CTox may represent an under-appreciated cause of asthma and seizures (Sharghi et al., 2001). Specific treatment of VLM is reserved for patients with severe, persistent, or progressive symptoms (Bethany et al., 2006). Albendazole is the drug of choice. In contrast, anthelmintic therapy for treatment of OLM and CT is controversial. In the case of OLM, surgical management often is indicated, sometimes accompanied by systemic or topical steroids (Sabrosa and de Souza, 2001).

Hookworm

Necator americanus, Ancylostoma duodenale. These closely related hookworm species infect ~1 billion people in developing countries (Figure 51–1).

N. americanus is the predominant hookworm worldwide, especially in the Americas, sub-Saharan Africa, South China, and Southeast Asia, whereas *A. duodenale* is focally endemic in Egypt and in parts of northern India and China. Infection also occurs farther north in unusual but relatively warm settings such as mines and large mountain tunnels, hence the terms *miner's disease* and *tunnel disease*. Hookworm larvae live in the soils and penetrate exposed skin. After reaching the lungs, the larvae migrate to the oral cavity and are swallowed. After attaching to the small intestinal mucosa, the derived adult worms feed on host blood. There is a general relationship between the number of hookworms (hookworm burden) as determined by quantitative fecal egg counts and fecal blood loss. In individuals with low iron reserves, the correlation extends to hookworm burden and degree of iron-deficiency anemia. Unlike heavy *Ascaris* and *Trichuris* infections, which occur predominantly in children, heavy hookworm infections also occur in adults, including women of reproductive age. In some endemic areas, the heaviest hookworm burdens occur exclusively in adult populations.

Although iron supplementation (and transfusion in severe cases) often is helpful in individuals with severe iron-deficiency anemia, the major goal of treatment is to remove blood-feeding adult hookworms from the intestines. Albendazole is the agent of first choice against both *A. duodenale* and *N. americanus*. This drug has the advantage of activity against other GI nematodes (Hotez, 2009). Mebendazole is also commonly used; however, especially when used in a single dose, albendazole is considered far superior to mebendazole at removing adult hookworms from the GI tract (Keiser and Utzinger, 2008). Oral albendazole is the drug of choice for treating *cutaneous larva migrans,* or "creeping eruption," which is due most commonly to skin migration by larvae of the dog hookworm, *A. braziliense*. Oral ivermectin or topical *thiabendazole* also can be used.

Trichuris trichiura. *Trichuris* (whipworm) infection occurs in ~1 billion people in developing countries (Bethony et al., 2006; de Silva et al., 2003; Hotez et al, 2009). The infection is acquired by ingestion of embryonated eggs. In children, heavy *Trichuris* worm burdens can lead to colitis, *Trichuris* dysentery syndrome, and rectal prolapse (Bundy and Cooper, 1989).

Mebendazole and albendazole are the most effective agents for treatment of whipworm, either as a single agent or together with *Ascaris* and hookworm infections. Both drugs provide significant reductions in host worm burdens even when used in a single dose, such as what might be used in mass drug administration campaigns (Hotez, 2009). However, single-dose therapy with either drug is often ineffective for achieving "cure" (i.e., total worm burden removal), so that a 3-day course of therapy is typically required (Keiser and Utzinger, 2008).

Strongyloides stercoralis. *S. stercoralis*, sometimes called the threadworm or dwarf threadworm, is almost unique among helminths in being able to complete its life cycle within the human host. The organism infects 30-100 million people worldwide, most frequently in the tropics and other hot, humid locales. In the U.S., strongyloidiasis is still endemic in the Appalachian region and in parts of the American South (Hotez, 2008). It also is found in institutionalized individuals living in unsanitary conditions and in immigrants, travelers, and military personnel who lived in endemic areas.

Infective larvae in fecally contaminated soil penetrate the skin or mucous membranes, travel to the lungs, and ultimately mature into adult worms in the small intestine, where they reside. Many infected individuals are asymptomatic, but some experience skin rashes, nonspecific GI symptoms, and cough. Life-threatening disseminated disease, known as the hyperinfection syndrome, can occur in immunosuppressed persons, even decades after the initial infection when parasite replication in the small intestine is unchecked by a competent immune response. Most deaths caused by parasites in the U.S. probably are due to *Strongyloides* hyperinfection. Ivermectin is the drug of choice for treatment of strongyloidiasis. Hyperinfection may require prolonged or repeated therapy. Although the BZ drugs show some efficacy, they are less effective than ivermectin.

Enterobius vermicularis. *Enterobius*, the pinworm, is one of the most common helminth infections in temperate climates, including the U.S. Although this parasite rarely causes serious complications, pruritus in the perianal and perineal region can be severe, and scratching may cause secondary infection. In female patients, worms may wander into the genital tract and penetrate into the peritoneal cavity. Salpingitis or even peritonitis may ensue. Because the infection easily spreads throughout members of a family, a school, or an institution, the physician must decide whether to treat all individuals in close contact with an infected person. More than one course of therapy may be required.

Pyrantel pamoate, mebendazole, and albendazole are highly effective. Single oral doses of each should be repeated after 2 weeks. When their use is combined with rigid standards of personal hygiene, a very high proportion of cures can be obtained. Treatment is simple and almost devoid of side effects.

Trichinella spiralis. *T. spiralis* is an ubiquitous zoonotic nematode parasite. Trichinosis in the U.S. and the developing world is usually caused by eating under- or uncooked venison and wild pigs. When released by acid stomach contents, encysted larvae mature into adult worms in the intestine. Adults then produce infectious larvae that invade tissues, especially skeletal muscle and heart.

Severe infection can be fatal, but more typically causes marked muscle pain and cardiac complications. Fortunately, infection is readily preventable. All pork, including pork sausages, should be thoroughly cooked before being eaten. The encysted larvae are killed by exposure to heat of 60°C for 5 minutes.

Albendazole and mebendazole are effective against the intestinal forms of *T. spiralis* that are present early in infection. The efficacy of these agents or any anthelmintic agent on larvae that have migrated to muscle is questionable. Glucocorticoids may be of considerable value in controlling the acute and dangerous manifestations of established infection, although steroids can alter the metabolism of albendazole.

Lymphatic Filariasis: Wuchereria bancrofti, Brugia malayi, and B. timori. Adult worms that cause human lymphatic filariasis (LF) dwell in the lymphatic vessels. Transmission occurs through the bite of infected mosquitoes; ~90% of cases are due to *W. bancrofti,* most of the rest are due to *B. malayi.* The major endemic regions are sub-Saharan Africa, the Indian subcontinent, Southeast Asia and the Pacific region, and in four tropical countries of the Americas (Haiti, Dominican Republic, Guyana, and Brazil).

In LF, host reaction to the adult worms initially cause lymphatic inflammation manifested by fevers, lymphangitis, and lymphadenitis. This can progress to lymphatic obstruction and is often exacerbated by secondary attacks of bacterial cellulitis, leading to lymphedema manifested by hydrocele and elephantiasis. An accentuated immune reaction to microfilariae, termed *tropical pulmonary eosinophilia*, also occurs in some persons.

The Global Program for the Elimination of LF recommends that all at-risk individuals be treated once yearly with an oral two-drug combination (Molyneux and Zagaria, 2002). Today, >500 million people are treated annually (Hotez, 2009). For most countries, the WHO recommends diethylcarbamate (DEC) for its micro- and macrofilaricidal effect in combination with albendazole to enhance macrofilaricidal activity. The exceptions are in many parts of sub-Saharan Africa and Yemen, where either loiasis or onchocerciasis are co-endemic. In these regions, ivermectin is substituted for DEC (Molyneux et al., 2003). DEC and ivermectin clear circulating microfilariae from infected subjects (Molyneux and Zagaria, 2002), thereby reducing the likelihood that mosquitoes will transmit LF to other individuals. The number of serious adverse events from LF-control chemotherapy programs has been remarkably low, 1 out of 4.5 million subjects treated (Molyneux et al., 2003).

DEC is the drug of choice for specific therapy directed against adult worms. However, the anthelmintic effect on the adult worms is variable. Although chemotherapy decreases the incidence of filarial lymphangitis, it is unclear whether it reverses lymphatic damage or other chronic manifestations of LF. In longstanding elephantiasis, surgical measures may be required to improve lymph drainage and remove redundant tissue.

Loa loa (loiasis). *L. loa* is a tissue-migrating filarial parasite found in large river regions of Central and West Africa; the parasite is transmitted by deerflies. Adult worms reside in subcutaneous tissues, and infection may be recognized when these migrating worms cause episodic and transient subcutaneous "Calabar" swellings. Adult worms may also pass across the sclera, causing "eyeworm." Rarely, encephalopathy, cardiopathy, or nephropathy occurs in association with heavy infection, particularly following chemotherapy.

DEC currently is the best single drug for the treatment of loiasis, but it is advisable to start with a small initial dose to diminish host reactions that result from destruction of microfilariae. Glucocorticoids may be administered to ameliorate post-treatment acute reactions. In rare instances, life-threatening encephalopathy follows the treatment of loiasis, probably due to the inflammatory reaction to dead or dying microfilariae lodged in the cerebral microvasculature. Guidelines have been developed aimed at screening out populations with heavy infection so that they are not administered ivermectin, which has also been associated with fatal encephalopathy. The potential complications of unmonitored DEC treatment of loiasis are a major reason why this agent is not recommended for mass chemoprophylaxis of LF in regions of sub-Saharan Africa where *L. loa* is co-endemic.

Onchocerca volvulus (Onchocerciasis or River Blindness). Transmitted by blackflies near fast-flowing streams and rivers, *O. volvulus* infects 17-37 million people in 22 countries in sub-Saharan Africa (Hotez et al., 2009; Molyneux et al., 2003), and <100,000 people in six Latin American countries (Mexico, Guatemala, Ecuador, Colombia, Venezuela, and Brazil). Cases also occur in Yemen. Inflammatory reactions, primarily to microfilariae rather than adult worms, affect the subcutaneous tissues, lymph nodes, and eyes. Onchocerciasis is a leading cause of infectious blindness worldwide and results from the cumulative destruction of microfilariae in the eyes, a process that evolves over decades.

Ivermectin is the drug of choice for control and treatment of onchocerciasis. DEC is no longer recommended because ivermectin produces far milder systemic reactions and few if any ocular complications. Ivermectin treatment clears microfilariae in the tissues, prevents the development of blindness, and interrupts transmission. It also results in delayed resumption of production of microfilariae in the uterus of female worms. The African Programme for Onchocerciasis Control coordinates treatment of river blindness in Central and West Africa (www.who.int/pbd/blindness/onchocerciasis). Although suramin (Chapter 50) kills adult *O. volvulus* worms, treatment with this relatively toxic agent is generally not advised.

Dracunculus medinensis. Known as the guinea, dragon, or Medina worm, this parasite causes dracunculiasis, an infection in decline with <5000 cases as of 2009, most of which occurred in rural Sudan, Ghana, and Mali. People become infected by drinking water containing copepods that carry infective larvae. After ~1 year, the adult female worms migrate and emerge through the skin, usually of the lower legs or feet. Through the advocacy and work of the Carter Center in partnership with WHO, strategies such as filtering drinking water and reducing contact of infected individuals with water have markedly reduced the transmission and prevalence of dracunculiasis in most endemic regions.

There is no effective anthelmintic for treatment of *D. medinensis* infection. Traditional treatment for this disabling condition is to draw the live adult female worm out day by day by rolling it onto a small piece of wood. This procedure risks significant secondary bacterial infection. *Metronidazole*, 250 mg given three times a day for 10 days, may provide symptomatic and functional relief by facilitating removal of the worm through indirect suppression of host inflammatory responses.

Cestodes (Flatworms)

Taenia saginata. Humans are the definitive hosts for *Taenia saginata*, known as the beef tapeworm. This most common form of tapeworm usually is detected after passage of proglottids from the intestine. It is cosmopolitan, occurring most commonly in sub-Saharan Africa and the Middle East, where undercooked or raw beef is consumed. Preventable by cooking beef to 60°C for >5 minutes, this infection rarely produces serious clinical disease, but it must be distinguished from that produced by *Taenia solium*.

Praziquantel (BILTRICIDE) is the drug of choice for treatment of infection by *T. saginata*, although niclosamide can also be used. Both drugs are very effective, simple to administer, and comparatively free from side effects. Assessment of cure can be difficult because the worm (segments as well as scolex) usually is passed in a partially digested state. If the parasitological diagnosis is uncertain, niclosamide (not available in the U.S.) is the preferred drug because of the danger of an inadvertent secondary inflammatory response to occult cysticercosis.

Taenia solium. *Taenia solium*, or pork tapeworm, also has a cosmopolitan distribution; immigrant populations are a common source of infection in the U.S. This cestode causes two types of infection. The intestinal form with adult tapeworms is caused by eating undercooked meat containing cysticerci, or more commonly by fecal-oral transmission of infective *T. solium* eggs from another infected human host. *Cysticercosis*, the far more dangerous systemic form that usually coexists with the intestinal form, is caused by invasive larval forms of the parasite (Garcia and Del Brutto, 2000). Systemic infection results either from ingestion of fecally contaminated infectious material, or from eggs liberated from a gravid segment passing upward into the duodenum, where the outer layers are digested. In either case, larvae gain access to the circulation and tissues, exactly as in their cycle in the intermediate host, usually the pig. The seriousness of the resulting disease depends on the particular tissue involved. Invasion of the brain (neurocysticercosis) is common and dangerous. Epilepsy, meningitis, and increased intracranial pressure can develop, depending on the inflammatory reactions to the cysticerci and/or their size and location.

Niclosamide is preferred for treatment of intestinal infections with *T. solium* because it will have no effect on occult neurocysticercosis. Albendazole is the drug of choice for treating cysticercosis. The advisability of chemotherapy for neurocysticercosis is controversial (Salinas and Prasad, 2000), being appropriate only when it is directed at live cysticerci and not against dead or dying cysticerci (as evidenced by neuroimaging using contrast agents) or in settings where cerebral imaging reveals a large burden of parasites. Pretreatment with glucocorticoids is strongly advised in this situation to minimize inflammatory reactions to dying parasites (Evans et al., 1997). Anthelmintic treatment can shrink brain cysts but also can have adverse consequences leading to seizures and hydrocephalus especially if corticosteroids are not administered beforehand. Some experts advocate use of albendazole therapy for patients with multiple cysts or viable cysts (as determined by absence of ring enhancement on contrast neuroimaging studies).

Diphyllobothrium latum. *Diphyllobothrium latum*, the fish tapeworm, is found most commonly in rivers and lakes of the Northern Hemisphere. In North America, the pike is the most common second intermediate host. The eating of inadequately cooked infested fish introduces the larvae into the human intestine; the larvae can develop into adult worms up to 25 m long. Most infected individuals are asymptomatic. The most frequent manifestations include abdominal symptoms and weight loss; megaloblastic anemia develops due to a deficiency of vitamin B_{12}, which is taken up by the parasite.

Therapy with praziquantel readily eliminates the worm and ensures hematological remission.

Hymenolepis nana. *Hymenolepis nana*, the dwarf tapeworm, is the smallest and most common tapeworm parasitizing humans. Infection with this cestode is cosmopolitan, more prevalent in tropical than temperate climates, and most common among institutionalized children, including those in the southern U.S. *H. nana* is the only cestode that can develop from ovum to mature adult in humans without an intermediate host. Cysticerci develop in the villi of the intestine and then regain access to the intestinal lumen where larvae mature into adults. Treatment therefore must be adapted to this cycle of autoinfection.

Praziquantel is effective against *H. nana* infections, but higher doses than used for other tapeworm infections usually are required. In addition, therapy may have to be repeated. Treatment failure or reinfection is indicated by the appearance of eggs in the stool ~4 weeks after the last dose. Albendazole is partially efficacious against *H. nana*; in 277 cases from 11 studies, 69.5% of patients were cured by albendazole (400 mg daily for 3 days) (Horton, 2000).

Echinococcus Species. Humans serve as one of several intermediate hosts for larval forms of *Echinococcus* species that cause "cystic" (*E. granulosus*) and "alveolar" (*E. multilocularis* and *E. vogeli*) hydatid disease. Dogs and related canids are definitive hosts for these tapeworms. Parasite eggs from canine stools are a major worldwide cause of disease in associated livestock (e.g., sheep and goats). *E. granulosus* produces unilocular, slowly growing cysts, most often in liver and lung, whereas *E. multilocularis* creates multilocular invasive cysts, predominantly in the same organs. Removal of the cysts by surgery is the preferred treatment, but leakage from ruptured cysts may spread disease to other organs.

Prolonged regimens of albendazole, either alone or as an adjunct to surgery, are reportedly of some benefit. However, some patients are not cured despite multiple courses of therapy, especially in alveolar echinococcosis where lifelong therapy with albendazole may be required. Treatment of infected dogs with praziquantel eradicates adult worms and interrupts transmission of these infections. New treatment methods, such as percutaneous puncture, aspiration, injection of scolicidal agents, and re-aspiration–based techniques, have received much attention, and they yield rates of cure and relapse equivalent to those following surgery. Benzimidazole treatment should be administered in the perioperative period (Kern, 2003).

Trematodes (Flukes)

Schistosoma haematobium, Schistosoma mansoni, Schistosoma japonicum. These are the main species of blood flukes that cause human schistosomiasis; less common species are *Schistosoma intercalatum* and *Schistosoma mekongi*. The infection affects >200 million people (Figure 51–1), and >700 million are at risk (Steinmann et al., 2006). In the Americas, schistosomiasis occurs in Brazil, Suriname, Venezuela and certain Caribbean islands (*S. mansoni*), much of Africa and the Arabian Peninsula (*S. mansoni* and *S. haematobium*), and China, the Philippines, and Indonesia (*S. japonicum*). More than 90% of the cases of schistosomiasis occur in sub-Saharan Africa, with approximately two-thirds of the cases caused by *S. haematobium* and one-third caused by *S. mansoni*. Infected freshwater snails act as intermediate hosts for transmission of the infection, which continues to spread as agriculture and water resources increase. Like most helminth infections, the clinical manifestations of schistosomiasis generally correlate with the intensity of infection, with pathology primarily involving the liver, spleen, and GI tract (for *S. mansoni* and *S. japonicum*) or the urinary and genital tracts (*S. haematobium*). Heavy infection with *S. haematobium* predisposes to squamous cell carcinoma of the bladder. Chronic infections can cause porto-systemic shunting due to hepatic granuloma formation and periportal fibrosis in the liver.

Praziquantel is the drug of choice for treatment of schistosomiasis. The drug is safe and effective when given in single or divided oral doses on the same day. These properties make praziquantel especially suitable for population-based chemotherapy. Moreover, repeated chemotherapy with praziquantel is thought to accelerate protective immune responses by increasing exposure to antigens released from dying worms that induce a T_H2 response (Mutapi et al., 1998). In sub-Saharan Africa, praziquantel is typically administered in mass drug administration campaigns for populations infected with schistosomiasis, with the use of a height pole as a guide to drug dosage. Sadly, even the modest cost of US $0.08 per tablet is beyond the health budgets of many sub-Saharan African countries (Hotez, 2009). Although not effective clinically against *S. haematobium* and *S. japonicum*, oxamniquine is effective for treatment of *S. mansoni* infections, particularly in South America, where the sensitivity of most strains may permit single-dose therapy. However, resistance has

Anthelmintic Action. After rapid and reversible uptake, praziquantel has two major effects on adult schistosomes. At the lowest effective concentrations, it causes increased muscular activity, followed by contraction and spastic paralysis. Affected worms detach from blood vessel walls and migrate from the mesenteric veins to the liver. At slightly higher concentrations, praziquantel causes tegumental damage and exposes a number of tegumental antigens (Redman et al., 1996). The clinical efficacy of this drug correlates better with tegumental action (Xiao et al., 1985). The drug is ineffective against juvenile schistosomes and therefore is relatively ineffective in early infection. An intact immune response is believed to be important for the clinical efficacy of the drug.

The primary site of action of praziquantel is uncertain (Aragon et al., 2009). The drug may act through generation of reactive oxygen species. It also promotes an influx of Ca^{2+}, and possibly interacts with the variant Ca^{2+} channel Ca-varβ (Jeziorski and Greenberg, 2006), which is found in schistosomes and other praziquantel-sensitive parasites. However, Ca^{2+} influx does not correlate with sensitivity to the drug an all settings (Pica-Mattoccia et al., 2008). Prazifuantel inhibits adenosine flux (Angelucci et al., 2007), but definitive evidence that this action contributes to the anthelmintic effect is lacking.

Absorption, Fate, and Excretion. Praziquantel is readily absorbed after oral administration, the drug reaching maximal levels in human plasma in 1-2 hours. The pharmacokinetics of praziquantel are dose related. Extensive first-pass metabolism to many inactive hydroxylated and conjugated products limits the bioavailability of this drug and results in plasma concentrations of metabolites at least 100-fold higher than that of praziquantel. The drug is ~80% bound to plasma proteins. Its plasma $t_{1/2}$ is 0.8-3 hours, depending on the dose, compared with 4-6 hours for its metabolites; this may be prolonged in patients with severe liver disease, including those with hepatosplenic schistosomiasis. About 70% of an oral dose of praziquantel is recovered as metabolites in the urine within 24 hours; most of the remainder is metabolized in the liver and eliminated in the bile.

Therapeutic Uses. Praziquantel is approved in the U.S. for therapy of schistosomiasis and liver fluke infections. However, the drug has activity against many other trematodes and cestodes. Praziquantel should be stored at temperatures <30°C and swallowed with water without chewing because of its bitter taste.

Praziquantel is the drug of choice for treating schistosomiasis caused by all *Schistosoma* species that infect humans. Although dosage regimens vary, a single oral dose of 40 mg/kg or three doses of 20 mg/kg each, given 4-6 hours apart, generally produce cure rates of 70-95% and consistently high reductions (>85%) in egg counts. Tablets of 600 mg currently are available from generic manufacturers; on average, treatment of a school-aged child in Africa requires 2.5 tablets (WHO, 2002).

The absence of weighing scales in Africa and elsewhere in developing countries led to the development dosing in proportion to height (WHO 2006; www.who.int/wormcontrol).

Strains of *S. mansoni* and *S. japonicum* resistant to praziquantel have been selected in laboratory studies (Fallon et al., 1996). Moreover, decreased clinical efficacy of praziquantel against infections with *S. mansoni* has been reported in two human populations (Ismail et al., 1999). However, praziquantel-tolerant or -resistant schistosome strains are not currently of clinical importance (Fallon et al., 1996).

Three doses of 25 mg/kg taken 4-8 hours apart on the same day result in high rates of cure for infections with either the liver flukes *Clonorchis sinensis* and *Opisthorchis viverrini*, or the intestinal flukes *Fasciolopsis buski, Heterophyes heterophyes*, and *Metagonimus yokogawai*. The same three-dose regimen, used over 2 days, is highly effective against infections with the lung fluke, *Paragonimus westermani*. Of note, the liver fluke *Fasciola hepatica* is resistant to praziquantel and should be treated with the BZ drug triclabendazole.

Low doses of praziquantel can be used successfully to treat intestinal infections with adult cestodes, for example, a single oral dose of 25 mg/kg for *Hymenolepis nana* and 10 to 20 mg/kg for *Diphyllobothrium latum, Taenia saginata*, or *T. solium*. Retreatment after 7-10 days is advisable for individuals heavily infected with *H. nana*. Although albendazole is preferred for therapy of human cysticercosis, praziquantel represents an alternative agent, but its use for this indication is hampered by the important pharmacokinetic interaction with dexamethasone and other corticosteroids that should be co-administered in this condition (Evans et al., 1997). Neither the "cystic" nor "alveolar" hydatid disease caused by larval stages of *Echinococcus* tapeworms responds to praziquantel, but the drug may have a role in the uncommon setting of perioperative cyst spillage (Horton, 1997; Schantz, 1999).

Toxicity, Precautions, and Interactions. Abdominal discomfort, particularly pain and nausea, diarrhea, headache, dizziness, and drowsiness may occur shortly after taking praziquantel; these direct effects are transient and dose related. Indirect effects such as fever, pruritus, urticaria, rashes, arthralgia, and myalgia are noted occasionally. Such side effects and increases in eosinophilia often relate to parasite burden and are therefore believed to be a consequence of parasite killing and antigen release. In neurocysticercosis, inflammatory reactions to praziquantel may produce meningismus, seizures, mental changes, and cerebrospinal fluid pleocytosis. These effects usually are delayed in onset, last 2-3 days, and respond to appropriate symptomatic therapy such as analgesics and anticonvulsants.

Praziquantel is considered safe in children >4 years of age (or >94 cm in height), who probably tolerate the drug better than adults. Low levels of the drug appear in the breast milk, but there is no evidence that this compound is mutagenic or carcinogenic. High doses of praziquantel increase abortion rates in rats, but a retrospective study showed that treatment of pregnant women in Sudan resulted in no significant differences between treated and untreated women in the rates of abortion or preterm deliveries. Moreover, no congenital abnormalities were noted by clinical examination in any of the infants born to either group (Adam et al., 2004).

The bioavailability of praziquantel is reduced by inducers of hepatic CYPs such as carbamazepine and phenobarbital; predictably, co-administration of the CYP inhibitor, cimetidine, has the opposite effect (Dachman et al., 1994). Dexamethasone reduces the bioavailability of praziquantel. Under certain conditions, praziquantel may increase the bioavailability of albendazole (Homeida et al., 1994).

Praziquantel is contraindicated in ocular cysticercosis because the host response can irreversibly damage the eye. Shortly after taking the drug, driving, operating machinery, and other tasks requiring mental alertness should be avoided. Severe hepatic disease can prolong the $t_{1/2}$ of praziquantel, requiring dosage adjustment in such patients (Mandour et al., 1990).

Metrifonate

Metrifonate (trichlorfon; BILARCIL) is an organophosphorus compound used first as an insecticide and later as an anthelmintic, especially for treatment of *Schistosoma haematobium*.

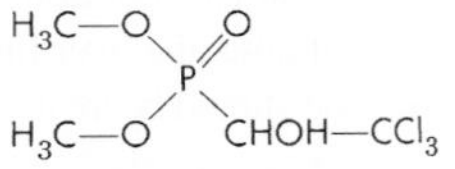

H_3C—O, H_3C—O, P(=O), CHOH—CCl_3

METRIFONATE

Metrifonate is a prodrug; at physiological pH, it is converted nonenzymatically to *dichlorvos* (2,2-dichlorovinyl dimethyl phosphate, DDVP), a potent cholinesterase inhibitor (Chapter 10) However, inhibition of cholinesterase alone is unlikely to explain the antischistosomal properties of metrifonate (Bloom, 1981). *In vitro*, dichlorvos is about equally potent as an inhibitor of both *S. mansoni* and *S. haematobium* acetylcholinesterases, yet metrifonate is effective clinically only against infections with *S. haematobium*. The molecular basis for this species-selective effect is not understood. Trichlorfon is the formulation of metrifonate approved for veterinary purposes in the U.S. More complete information on the pharmacology and therapeutic uses of metrifonate can be found in the tenth edition of this book.

Oxamniquine

Oxamniquine is a 2-aminomethyltetrahydroquinoline derivative that is used as a second-line drug after praziquantel for the treatment of *Schistosoma mansoni* infection. *S. haematobium* and *S. japonicum* are refractory to this drug. Although it has largely been replaced by praziquantel and is not commercially available in the U.S., it continues to be used in *S. mansoni* control programs, especially in South America. More details on the pharmacology and therapeutic uses of oxamniquine can be found in the ninth edition of this book.

Niclosamide

Niclosamide, a halogenated salicylanilide derivative, was introduced in the 1960s for human use as a taeniacide. This compound was considered as a second-choice drug to praziquantel for treating human intestinal infections with *Taenia saginata, Diphyllobothrium latum, Hymenolepis nana*, and most other cestodes because it was cheap, effective, and readily available in many parts of the world. However, therapy with niclosamide poses a risk to people infected with *T. solium* because ova released from drug-damaged gravid worms develop into larvae that can cause cysticercosis, a dangerous infection that responds poorly to chemotherapy. Niclosamide is no longer approved for use in the U.S. More complete information on the pharmacology and therapeutic uses of niclosamide can be found in the ninth edition of this book.

Piperazine

Piperazine, a cyclic secondary amine, has been superseded as a first-line anthelmintic by the better tolerated and more easily administered benzimidazole anthelmintics (BZs). Piperazine is highly effective against *Ascaris lumbricoides* and *Enterobius vermicularis*. The predominant effect of piperazine on *Ascaris* is a flaccid paralysis that results in expulsion of the worm by peristalsis. Affected worms recover if incubated in drug-free medium. Piperazine acts as a GABA-receptor agonist. By increasing chloride ion conductance of *Ascaris* muscle membrane, the drug produces hyperpolarization and reduced excitability that leads to muscle relaxation and flaccid paralysis (Martin, 1985). Piperazine and dipiperazine are licensed as veterinary medications in the U.S. More complete information on the pharmacology and therapeutic uses of piperazine may be found in the tenth edition of this book.

Pyrantel Pamoate

Pyrantel pamoate first was introduced into veterinary practice as a broad-spectrum anthelmintic directed against pinworm, roundworm, and hookworm infections. Its effectiveness and lack of toxicity led to its trial against related intestinal helminths in humans. *Oxantel pamoate*, an *m*-oxyphenol analog of pyrantel, is effective for single-dose treatment of trichuriasis.

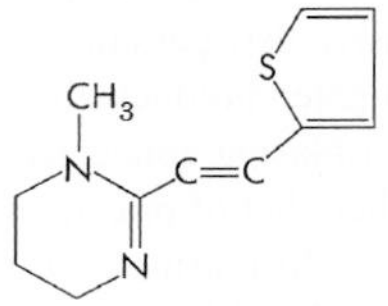

CH_3, N, C=C, S, N

PYRANTEL

Antihelmintic Action. Pyrantel and its analogs are depolarizing neuromuscular blocking agents. They open nonselective cation channels and induce persistent activation of nicotinic acetylcholine receptors and spastic paralysis of the worm (Robertson et al., 1994).

Pyrantel also inhibits cholinesterases. It causes a slowly developing contracture of isolated preparations of *Ascaris* at 1% of the concentration of acetylcholine required to produce the same effect. Pyrantel exposure leads to depolarization and increased spike-discharge frequency, accompanied by increases in tension, in isolated helminth muscle preparations. Pyrantel is effective against hookworm, pinworm, and roundworm but is ineffective against *Trichuris trichiura,* which responds paradoxically to the analog oxantel.

Absorption, Fate, and Excretion. Pyrantel pamoate is poorly absorbed from the GI tract, a property that confines its action to intralumenal GI nematodes. Less than 15% is excreted in the urine as parent drug and metabolites. The major proportion of an administered dose is recovered in the feces.

Therapeutic Uses. Pyrantel pamoate is an alternative to mebendazole or albendazole in the treatment of ascariasis and enterobiasis. High cure rates have been achieved after a single oral dose of 11 mg/kg, to a maximum of 1 g. Pyrantel also is effective against hookworm infections caused by *Ancylostoma duodenale* and *Necator americanus*, although repeated doses are needed to cure heavy infections by *N. americanus*. The drug should be used in combination with oxantel for mixed infections with *T. trichiura*. In the case of pinworm, it is wise to repeat the treatment after an interval of 2 weeks. In the U.S., pyrantel is sold as an over-the-counter pinworm treatment (PIN-X, others).

Precautions. When given parenterally to experimental animals, pyrantel can produce complete neuromuscular blockade; only very large oral doses produce toxic effects. Transient and mild GI symptoms occasionally are observed in humans, as are headache, dizziness, rash, and fever. Pyrantel pamoate has not been studied in pregnant women. Thus its use in pregnant patients and children <2 years of age is not recommended. Because pyrantel pamoate and piperazine are mutually antagonistic with respect to their neuromuscular effects on parasites, they should not be used together.

BIBLIOGRAPHY

Adam I, el Elwasila T, Homeida M. Is praziquantel therapy safe during pregnancy? *Trans R Soc Trop Med Hyg,* **2004,** *98:* 540–543.

Addiss D, Critchley J, Ejere H, *et al.* International Filariasis Review Group. *Cochrane Database Syst Rev,* **2004,** CD003753.

Addiss DG, Dreyer G. Treatment of lymphatic filariasis. In: *Lymphatic Filariasis* (Nutman TB, ed.), Imperial College Press, London, **2000,** pp. 151–191.

Andrews P. Praziquantel: Mechanisms of anti-schistosomal activity. *Pharmacol Ther,* **1985,** *29:*129–156.

Angelucci T, Basso A, Bellelli A, et al. The anti-schistosomal drug praziquantel is an adenosine antagonist. *Parasitology*, **2007,** *134*:1215–1221.

Aragon AD, Imani RA, Blackburn VP, et al. Towards an understanding of the mechanism of action of praziquantel. *Mol Biochem Parasitol*, **2009**, *164*:57–65.

Arena JP, Liu KK, Paress PS, *et al.* The mechanism of action of avermectins in *Caenorhabditis elegans:* Correlation between activation of glutamate-sensitive chloride current, membrane binding, and biological activity. *J Parasitol,* **1995,** *81:*286–294.

Awadzi K, Adjepon-Yamoah KK, Edwards G, *et al.* The effect of moderate urine alkalinisation on low dose diethylcarbamazine therapy in patients with onchocerciasis. *Br J Clin Pharmacol,* **1986,** *21:*669–676.

Bagheri H, Simiand E, Montastruc JL, Magnaval JF. Adverse drug reactions to anthelmintics. *Ann Pharmacother,* **2004,** *38:*383–388.

Bethony J, Brooker S, Albonico M, *et al.* Soil-transmitted helminth infections: ascariasis, trichuriasis, and hookworm. *Lancet*, **2006,** *367:*1521–1532.

Bloom A. Studies of the mode of action of metrifonate and DDVP in schistosomes—cholinesterase activity and the hepatic shift. *Acta Pharmacol Toxicol (Copenh),* **1981,** *49*(suppl 5):109–113.

Boatin BA, Hougard JM, Alley ES, *et al.* The impact of Mectizan on the transmission of onchocerciasis. *Ann Trop Med Parasitol,* **1998,** *92*(suppl 1):S46–S60.

Brooker S, Hotez PJ, Bundy DA. Hookworm-related anaemia among pregnant women: A systematic review. *PLoS Negl Trop Dis*, **2008,** *2:*e291.

Brown KR. Changes in the use profile of Mectizan: 1987–1997. *Ann Trop Med Parasitol,* **1998,** *92*(suppl 1):S61–S64.

Bundy DA, Cooper ES. *Trichuris* and trichuriasis in humans. *Adv Parasitol,* **1989,** *28:*107–173.

Burnham G, Mebrahtu T. The delivery of ivermectin (Mectizan). *Trop Med Int Health,* **2004,** *9:*A26–A44.

Campbell WC. Ivermectin, an antiparasitic agent. *Med Res Rev,* **1993,** *13:*61–79.

Campbell WC, ed. *Ivermectin and Abamectin.* Springer-Verlag, New York, **1989.**

Chiodini PL, Reid AJ, Wiselka MJ, *et al.* Parenteral ivermectin in Strongyloides hyperinfection. *Lancet,* **2000,** *355:*43–44.

Court JP, Bianco AE, Townson S, *et al.* Study on the activity of antiparasitic agents against *Onchocerca lienalis* third stage larvae *in vitro. Trop Med Parasitol,* **1985,** *36:*117–119.

Crompton DW. *Ascaris* and ascariasis. *Adv Parasitol,* **2001,** *48:*285–375.

Cully DF, Wilkinson H, Vassilatis DK, *et al.* Molecular biology and electrophysiology of glutamate-gated chloride channels of invertebrates. *Parasitology,* **1996,** *113*(suppl)*:*S191–S200.

Cupp EW, Onchoa AO, Collins RC, *et al.* The effect of multiple ivermectin treatments on infection of *Simulium ochraceum* with *Onchocerca volvulus. Am J Trop Med Hyg,* **1989,** *40:* 501–506.

Dachman WD, Adubofour KO, Bikin DS, *et al.* Cimetidine-induced rise in praziquantel levels in a patient with neurocysticercosis being treated with anticonvulsants. *J Infect Dis,* **1994,** *169:*689–691.

Davies HD, Sakuls P, Keystone JS. Creeping eruption. A review of clinical presentation and management of 60 cases presenting to a tropical disease unit. *Arch Dermatol,* **1993,** *129:* 588–591.

Davis A, Dixon H, Pawlowski ZS. Multicentre clinical trials of benzimidazole-carbamates in human cystic echinococcosis (phase 2). *Bull World Health Organ,* **1989,** *67:*503–508.

Dayan AD. Albendazole, mebendazole and praziquantel. Review of non-clinical toxicity and pharmacokinetics. *Acta Trop,* **2003,** *86:*141–159.

de Silva NR, Brooker S, Hotez PJ, *et al.* Soil-transmitted helminth infections: updating the global picture. *Trends Parasitol,* **2003,** *19:*547–551.

Diawara A, Drake LJ, Suswillo RR, *et al*. Assays to detect beta-tubulin codon 200 polymorphism in *Trichuris trichiura* and *Ascaris lumbricoides*. *PLoS Negl Trop Dis,* **2009,** *3:*e397.

Dominguez-Vazquez A, Taylor HR, Greene BM, *et al.* Comparison of flubendazole and diethylcarbamazine in treatment of onchocerciasis. *Lancet,* **1983,** *1:*139–143.

Drake LJ, Jukes MCH, Sternberg RJ, Bundy DAP. Geohelminth infections (ascariasis, trichuriasis, and hookworm): Cognitive and developmental impacts. *Semin Pediatr Infect Dis,* **2000,** *11:*245–251.

Driscoll M, Dean E, Reilly E, *et al.* Genetic and molecular analysis of *Caenorhabditis elegans* β-tubulin that conveys benzimidazole sensitivity. *J Cell Biol,* **1989,** *109:*2993–3003.

Dull HB, Meredith SE. The Mectizan Donation Programme—a 10-year report. *Ann Trop Med Parasitol,* **1998,** *92*(suppl 1): S69–S71.

Evans C, Garcia HH, Gilman RH, Friedland JS. Controversies in the management of cysticercosis. *Emerg Infect Dis,* **1997,** *3:*403–405.

Fallon PG, Tao LF, Ismail MM, Bennett JL. Schistosome resistance to praziquantel: Fact or artifact? *Parasitol Today,* **1996,** *12:*316–320.

Flohr C, Tuyen LN, Lewis S, *et al.* Low efficacy of mebendazole against hookworm in Vietnam: Two randomized controlled trials. *Am J Trop Med Hyg,* **2007,** *76:*732–736.

Gao J, Liu Y, Wang X, Hu P. Triclabendazde in the treatment of *Paragonimiasis skrjabini. Chin Med J (Engl),* **2003,** *116:* 1683–1686.

Garcia HH, Del Brutto OH. *Taenia solium* cysticercosis. *Infect Dis Clin North Am,* **2000,** *14:*97–119.

Gardon J, Gardon-Wendel N, Demanga-Ngangue, *et al.* Serious reactions after mass treatment of onchocerciasis with ivermectin in an area endemic for *Loa loa* infection. *Lancet,* **1997,** *350:*18–22.

Gelband H. Diethylcarbamazine salt in the control of lymphatic filariasis. *Am J Trop Med Hyg,* **1994,** *50:*655–662.

Gleizes C, Eeckhoutte C, Pineau T, *et al.* Inducing effect of oxfendazole on cytochrome P450IA2 in rabbit liver. Consequences on cytochrome P450-dependent monooxygenases. *Biochem Pharmacol,* **1991,** *41:*1813–1820.

Goa KL, McTavish D, Clissold SP. Ivermectin. A review of its antifilarial activity, pharmacokinetic properties and clinical efficacy in onchocerciasis. *Drugs,* **1991,** *42:*640–658.

Gottschall DW, Theodorides VJ, Wang R. The metabolism of benzimidazole anthelmintics. *Parasitol Today,* **1990,** *6:* 115–124.

Hejmadi MV, Jagannathan S, Delany NS, *et al.* L-glutamate binding sites of parasitic nematodes: Association with ivermectin resistance? *Parasitology,* **2000,** *120:*535–545.

Hoerauf A, Volkmann L, Hamelmann C, *et al.* Endosymbiotic bacteria in worms as targets for a novel chemotherapy in filariasis. *Lancet,* **2000,** *355:*1242–1243.

Homeida M, Leahy W, Copeland S, *et al.* Pharmacokinetic interaction between praziquantel and albendazole in Sudanese men. *Ann Trop Med Parasitol,* **1994,** *88:*551–559.

Horton J. Albendazole: A review of anthelmintic efficacy and safety in humans. *Parasitology,* **2000,** *121:*S113–S132.

Horton RJ. Albendazole in treatment of human cystic echinococcosis: 12 years of experience. *Acta Trop,* **1997,** *64:*79–93.

Hotez P. Mass drug administration and integrated control of the world's high-prevalence neglected tropical diseases. *Clin Pharmacol Ther,* **2009,** *85:*659–664.

Hotez PJ. Neglected infections of poverty in the United States of America. *PLoS Negl Trop Dis,* **2008,** *2:*e256.

Hotez PJ, Fenwick A, Savioli L, Molyneux DH. Rescuing the bottom billion through control of neglected tropical diseases. *Lancet,* **2009,** *373:*1570–1575.

Hotez PJ, Remme JHF, Buss P, *et al.* Combating tropical infectious diseases: Report of the disease control priorities in developing countries project. *Clin Infect Dis,* **2004,** *38:* 871–878.

Hotez PJ, Wilkins PP. Toxocariasis: America's most common neglected infection of poverty and a helminthiasis of global importance. *PLoS Negl Trop Dis,* **2009,** *3:*e400.

Ismail M, Botros S, Metwally A, *et al.* Resistance to praziquantel: Direct evidence from *Schistosoma mansoni* isolated from Egyptian villagers. *Am J Trop Med Hyg,* **1999,** *60:*932–935.

James CE, Davey MW. Increased expression of ABC transport proteins is associated with ivermectin resistance in the model nematode *C. elegans. Int J Parasitol,* **2009,** *39:*213–220.

Jeziorski MC, Greenberg RM. Voltage-gated calcium channel subunits from platyhelminths: Potential role in praziquantel action. *Int J Parasitol,* **2006,** *36:*625–632.

Katiyar SK, Edlind TD. *In vitro* susceptibilities of the AIDS-associated microsporidian *Encephalitozoon intestinalis* to albendazole, its sulfoxide metabolite, and 12 additional benzimidazole derivatives. *Antimicrob Agents Chemother,* **1997,** *41:*2729–2732.

Keiser J, Utzinger J. Efficacy of current drugs against soil-transmitted helminth infections: Systematic review and meta-analysis. *JAMA,* **2008,** *299:*1937–1948.

Kern P. *Echinococcus granulosus* infection: Clinical presentation, medical treatment and outcome. *Langenbecks Arch Surg,* **2003,** *388:*413–420.

Klion AD, Horton J, Nutman TB. Albendazole therapy for loiasis refractory to diethylcarbamazine treatment. *Clin Infect Dis,* **1999,** *29:*680–682.

Krishna DR, Klotz U. Determination of ivermectin in human plasma by high-performance liquid chromatography. *Arzneimittelforshung,* **1993,** *43:*609–611.

Kwa MS, Veenstra JG, Van Dijk M, Roos MH. Beta-tubulin genes from the parasitic nematode *Haemonchus contortus* modulate drug resistance in *Caenorhabditis elegans. J Mol Biol,* **1995,** *246:*500–510.

Liu LX, Weller PF. Strongyloidiasis and other intestinal nematode infections. *Infect Dis Clin North Am,* **1993,** *7:*655–682.

Mandour ME, el Turabi H, Homeida MM, *et al.* Pharmacokinetics of praziquantel in healthy volunteers and patients with schistosomiasis. *Trans R Soc Trop Med Hyg,* **1990,** *84:*389–393.

Marques MP, Takayanagui OM, Bonato PS, *et al.* Enantioselective kinetic disposition of albendazole sulfoxide in patients with neurocysticercosis. *Chirality,* **1999,** *11:* 218–223.

Marti H, Haji HJ, Savioli L, *et al.* A comparative trial of a single-dose ivermectin versus three days of albendazole for treatment of *Strongyloides stercoralis* and other soil-transmitted helminth infections in children. *Am J Trop Med Hyg,* **1996,** *55:*477–481.

Martin RJ. γ-Aminobutyric acid- and piperazine-activated single-channel currents from *Ascaris suum* body muscle. *Br J Pharmacol,* **1985,** *84:*445–461.

Martin RJ, Robertson A, Bjorn H. Target sites of anthelmintics. *Parasitology,* **1997,** *114*(suppl):S111–S124.

Molyneux DH, Zagaria N. Lymphatic filariasis elimination: progress in global programme development. *Ann Trop Med Parasitol,* **2002,** *96*(suppl. 2):S15–S40.

Molyneux DH, Bradley M, Hoerauf A, *et al.* Mass drug treatment for lymphatic filariasis and onchocerciasis. *Trends Parasitol,* **2003,** *19:*516–522.

Morris DL, Chinnery JB, Georgiou G, *et al.* Penetration of albendazole sulfoxide into hydatid cysts. *Gut,* **1987,** *28:*75–80.

Mutapi F, Ndhlovu PD, Hagan P, *et al.* Chemotherapy accelerates the development of acquired immune responses to *Schistosoma haematobium* infection. *J Infect Dis,* **1998,** *178:*289–293.

Newland HS, White AT, Greene BM, *et al.* Effect of single-dose ivermectin therapy on human *Onchocerca volvulus* infection with onchocercal ocular involvement. *Br J Ophthalmol,* **1988,** *72:*561–569.

Osei-Atweneboana MY, Eng JK, Boakye DA, *et al.* Prevalence and intensity of Onchocerca volvulus infection and efficacy of ivermectin in endemic communities in Ghana: A two-phase epidemiological study. *Lancet,* **2007,** *369:*2021–2029.

Ottesen EA, Ramachandran CP. Lymphatic filariasis infection and disease: Control strategies. *Parasitol Today,* **1995,** *11:*129–131.

Ottesen EA, Ismail MM, Horton J. The role of albendazole in programmes to eliminate lymphatic filariasis. *Parasitol Today,* **1999,** *15:*382–386.

Peixoto CA, Rocha A, Aguiar-Santos A, Florencio MS. The effects of diethylcarbamazine on the ultrastructure of *Wuchereria bancrofti in vivo* and *in vitro*. *Parasitol Res,* **2004,** *92:*513–517.

Pica-Mattocia L, Orcini T, Basso A, et al. *Schistosoma mansoni*: lack of correlation between praziquantel-induced intraworm calcium influx and parasitic death. *Exp Parasitol,* **2008,** *119:*332–335.

Prichard R. Anthelmintic resistance. *Vet Parasitol,* **1994,** *54:* 259–268.

Redman CA, Robertson A, Fallon PG, *et al.* Praziquantel: An urgent and exciting challenge. *Parasitol Today,* **1996,** *12:*14–20.

Redondo PA, Alvarez AI, Garcia JL, *et al.* Presystemic metabolism of albendazole: Experimental evidence of an efflux process of albendazole sulfoxide to intestinal lumen. *Drug Metab Dispos,* **1999,** *27:*736–740.

Roberts LJ, Huffam SE, Walton SF, Currie BJ. Crusted scabies: Clinical and immunological findings in seventy-eight patients and a review of the literature. *J Infect,* **2005,** *50:*375–381.

Robertson SJ, Pennington AJ, Evans AM, Martin RJ. The action of pyrantel as an agonist and an open-channel blocker at acetylcholine receptors in isolated *Ascaris suum* muscle vesicles. *Eur J Pharmacol,* **1994,** *271:*273–282.

Roos MH. The role of drugs in the control of parasitic nematode infections: Must we do without? *Parasitology,* **1997,** *114*(suppl): S137–S144.

Saba R, Korkmaz M, Inan D, *et al.* Human fascioliasis. *Clin Microbiol Infect,* **2004,** *10:*385–387.

Sabrosa NA, de Souza EC. Nematode infections of the eye: Toxocariasis and diffuse unilateral subacute neuroretinitis. *Curr Opin Ophthalmol,* **2001,** *12:*450–454.

Salinas R, Prasad K. Drugs for treating neurocysticercosis (tapeworm infection of the brain). *Cochrane Database Syst Rev,* **2000,** *2:*CD000215.

Sangster NC, Gill J. Pharmacology of anthelmintic resistance. *Parasitol Today,* **1999,** *15:*141–146.

Schaeffer JM, Haines HW. Avermectin binding in *Caenorhabditis elegans*. A two-state model for the avermectin binding site. *Biochem Pharmacol,* **1989,** *38:*2329–2338.

Schantz PM. Editorial response: Treatment of cystic echinococcosis—improving but still limited. *Clin Infect Dis,* **1999,** *29:*310–311.

Schinkel AH, Smit JJ, van Tellingen O, *et al.* Disruption of the mouse *mdr1a* P-glycoprotein gene leads to a deficiency in the blood-brain barrier and to increased sensitivity to drugs. *Cell,* **1994,** *77:*491–502.

Schwab AE, Boakye DA, Kyelem D, Prichard RK. Detection of benzimidazole resistance-associated mutations in the filarial nematode *Wuchereria bancrofti* and evidence for selection by albendazole and ivermectin combination treatment. *Am J Trop Med Hyg,* **2005**, *73:*234–238.

Sharghi N, Schantz PM, Caramico L, *et al.* Environmental exposure to *Toxocara* as a possible risk factor for asthma: A clinic-based case-control study. *Clin Infect Dis,* **2001,** *32:* E111–E116.

Shoop WL, Ostlind DA, Roher SP, *et al.* Avermectins and milbemycins against *Fasciola hepatica: In vivo* drug efficacy and *in vitro* receptor binding. *Int J Parasitol,* **1995,** *25:*923–927.

Spiro RC, Parsons WG, Perry SK, *et al.* Inhibition of post-translational modification and surface expression of a melanoma-associated chondroitin sulfate proteoglycan by diethylcarbamazine or ammonium chloride. *J Biol Chem,* **1986,** *261:*5121–5129.

Steinmann P, Keiser J, Bos R, *et al.* Schistosomiasis and water resources development: Systematic review, meta-analysis, and estimates of people at risk. *Lancet Infect Dis,* **2006,** *6:*411–425.

Symposium. (Various authors.) Biltricide symposium on African schistosomiasis. (Classen HG, Schramm V, eds.) *Arzneimittelforschung,* **1981,** *31:*535–618.

Taylor MJ, Hoerauf A. A new approach to the treatment of filariasis. *Curr Opin Infect Dis,* **2001,** *14:*727–731.

Urbani C, Albonico M. Anthelminthic drug safety and drug administration in the control of soil-transmitted helminthiasis in community campaigns. *Acta Trop,* **2003,** *86:*215–223.

Venkatesan P. Albendazole. *J Antimicrob Chemother,* **1998,** *41:* 145–147.

World Health Organization. *Prevention and Control of Schistosomiasis and Soil-Transmitted Helminthiasis*, Report of a WHO Expert Committee. WHO Technical Report Series 912, **2002,** Geneva.

World Health Organization. Preventive Chemotherapy in Human Helminthiasis. Coordinated use of anthelminthic drugs in control interventions: A manual for health professionals and programmatic managers. WHO, **2006**.

Wilmshurst JM, Robb SA. Can mebendazole cause lateralized occipital seizures? *Eur J Paediatr Neurol,* **1998,** *2:*323–324.

Xiao SH, Catto BA, Webster LT Jr. Effects of praziquantel on different developmental stages of *Schistosoma mansoni in vitro* and *in vivo*. *J Infect Dis,* **1985,** *151:*1130–1137.

Xu M, Molento M, Blackhall W, *et al.* Ivermectin resistance in nematodes may be caused by alteration of P-glycoprotein homolog. *Mol Biochem Parasitol,* **1998,** *91:*327–335.

Zeng Z, Andrew NW, Arison BH, *et al.* Identification of cytochrome P4503A4 as the major enzyme responsible for the metabolism of ivermectin by human liver microsomes. *Xenobiotica,* **1998,** *28:*313–321.

Zufall F, Franke C, Hatt H. The insecticide avermectin B_{1a} activates a chloride channel in crayfish muscle membrane. *J Exp Biol,* **1989,** *142:*191–205.

Sulfonamides, Trimethoprim-Sulfamethoxazole, Quinolones, and Agents for Urinary Tract Infections

William A. Petri, Jr.

SULFONAMIDES

The sulfonamide drugs were the first effective chemotherapeutic agents to be employed systemically for the prevention and cure of bacterial infections in humans. The considerable medical and public health importance of their discovery and their subsequent widespread use was quickly reflected in the sharp decline in morbidity and mortality figures for treatable infectious diseases. The advent of penicillin and subsequently of other antibiotics has diminished the usefulness of the sulfonamides, and they presently occupy a relatively small place in the therapeutic armamentarium of the physician. However, the introduction in the mid-1970s of the combination of trimethoprim and sulfamethoxazole has increased the use of sulfonamides for the prophylaxis and treatment of specific microbial infections.

History. Investigations in 1932 at the I. G. Farbenindustrie resulted in the patenting of PRONTOSIL and several other azo dyes containing a sulfonamide group. Prompted by the knowledge that synthetic azo dyes had been studied for their action against streptococci, Domagk tested the new compounds and observed that mice with streptococcal and other infections could be protected by PRONTOSIL. In 1933, Foerster reported giving PRONTOSIL to a 10-month-old infant with staphylococcal septicemia and achieving a dramatic cure. Favorable clinical results with PRONTOSIL and its active metabolite, sulfanilamide, in puerperal sepsis and meningococcal infections awakened the medical profession to the new field of antibacterial chemotherapy, and experimental and clinical articles soon appeared in profusion. The development of the carbonic anhydrase inhibitor–type diuretics and the sulfonylurea hypoglycemic agents followed from observations made with the sulfonamide antibiotics. For discovering the chemotherapeutic value of PRONTOSIL, Domagk was awarded the Nobel Prize in Medicine for 1938 (Lesch, 2007).

Chemistry. The term *sulfonamide* is employed herein as a generic name for derivatives of *para*-aminobenzenesulfonamide (sulfanilamide); the structural formulas of selected members of this class are shown in Figure 52–1. Most of them are relatively insoluble in water, but their sodium salts are readily soluble. The minimal structural prerequisites for antibacterial action are all embodied in sulfanilamide itself. The SO_2NH_2 group is not essential as such, but the important feature is that the sulfur is linked directly to the benzene ring. The *para*-NH_2 group (the N of which has been designated as N4) is essential and can be replaced only by moieties that can be converted *in vivo* to a free amino group. Substitutions made in the amide NH_2 group (position N1) have variable effects on antibacterial activity of the molecule. However, substitution of heterocyclic aromatic nuclei at N1 yields highly potent compounds.

Effects on Microbes

Sulfonamides have a wide range of antimicrobial activity against both gram-positive and gram-negative bacteria. However, resistant strains have become common, and the usefulness of these agents has diminished correspondingly. In general, the sulfonamides exert only a bacteriostatic effect, and cellular and humoral defense mechanisms of the host are essential for final eradication of the infection.

Antibacterial Spectrum. Resistance to sulfonamides is increasingly a problem. Microorganisms that may be susceptible *in vitro* to sulfonamides include *Streptococcus pyogenes*, *Streptococcus pneumoniae, Haemophilus influenzae, Haemophilus ducreyi, Nocardia, Actinomyces, Calymmato-bacterium granulomatis*, and *Chlamydia trachomatis*. Minimal inhibitory concentrations (MICs) range from 0.1 μg/mL for *C. trachomatis* to 4-64 μg/mL for *Escherichia coli*. Peak plasma drug concentrations achievable *in vivo* are ~100-200 μg/mL.

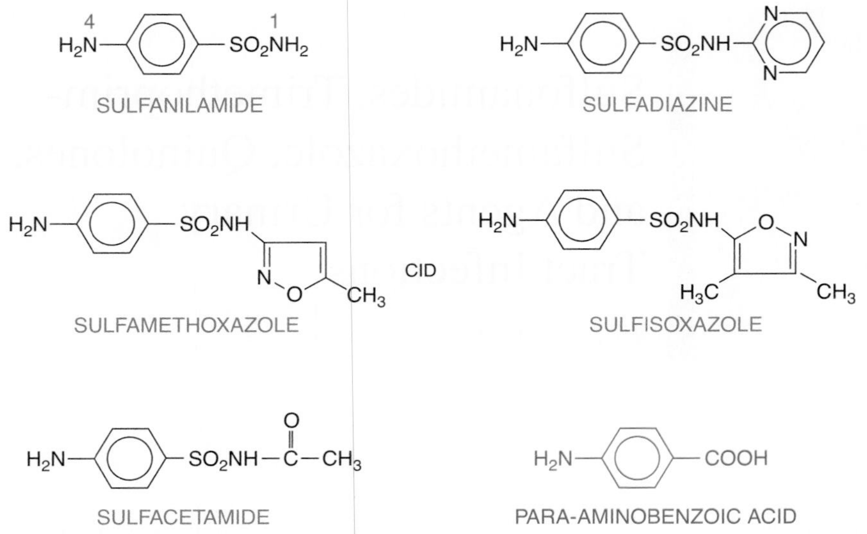

SULFANILAMIDE

SULFADIAZINE

SULFAMETHOXAZOLE

SULFISOXAZOLE

SULFACETAMIDE

PARA-AMINOBENZOIC ACID

Figure 52–1. *Structural formulas of selected sulfonamides and para-aminobenzoic acid.* The N of the *para*-NH_2 group is designated as N4; that of the amide NH_2, as N1.

Although sulfonamides were used successfully for the management of meningococcal infections for many years, most isolates of *Neisseria meningitidis* of serogroups B and C in the U.S. and group A isolates from other countries are now resistant. A similar situation prevails with respect to *Shigella*. Strains of *E. coli* isolated from patients with urinary tract infections (community acquired) often are resistant to sulfonamides, which are no longer the therapy of choice for such infections.

Mechanism of Action. Sulfonamides are competitive inhibitors of dihydropteroate synthase, the bacterial enzyme responsible for the incorporation of PABA into dihydropteroic acid, the immediate precursor of folic acid (Figure 52–2). Thus, these structural analogs of *para*-aminobenzoic acid (PABA) prevent normal bacterial use of PABA for the synthesis of folic acid (pteroylglutamic acid). Sensitive microorganisms are those that must synthesize their own folic acid; bacteria that can use preformed folate are not affected. Bacteriostasis induced by sulfonamides is counteracted by PABA competitively. Mammalian cells require preformed folic acid, cannot synthesize it, and are insensitive to drugs acting by this mechanism. Thus, mammalian cells are comparable to sulfonamide-insensitive bacteria that use preformed folate.

Synergists of Sulfonamides. One of the most active agents that exerts a synergistic effect when used with a sulfonamide is trimethoprim (Bushby and Hitchings, 1968). This compound is a potent and selective competitive inhibitor of microbial dihydrofolate reductase, the enzyme that reduces dihydrofolate to tetrahydrofolate. It is this reduced form of folic acid that is required for one-carbon transfer reactions. The simultaneous administration of a sulfonamide and trimethoprim thus introduces sequential blocks in the pathway by which microorganisms synthesize tetrahydrofolate from precursor molecules (Figure 52–2). The expectation that

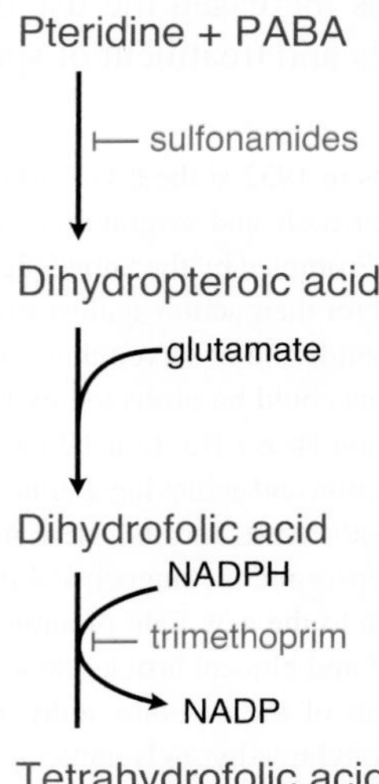

Figure 52–2. *Steps in folate metabolism blocked by sulfonamides and trimethoprim.*

such a combination would yield synergistic antimicrobial effects has been realized both *in vitro* and *in vivo*.

Acquired Bacterial Resistance to Sulfonamides. Bacterial resistance to sulfonamides presumably originates by random mutation and selection or by transfer of resistance by plasmids (Chapter 48). Such resistance, once it is maximally developed, usually is persistent and irreversible, particularly when produced *in vivo*. Acquired resistance to sulfonamide usually does not involve cross-resistance to antimicrobial agents of other classes. The *in vivo* acquisition of resistance has little or no effect on either virulence or antigenic characteristics of microorganisms.

Resistance to sulfonamide probably is the consequence of an altered enzymatic constitution of the bacterial cell; the alteration may be characterized by (1) a lower affinity of dihydropteroate synthase for sulfonamides, (2) decreased bacterial permeability or active efflux of the drug, (3) an alternative metabolic pathway for synthesis of an essential metabolite, or (4) an increased production of an essential metabolite or drug antagonist. For example, some resistant staphylococci may synthesize 70 times as much PABA as do the susceptible parent strains. Nevertheless, an increased production of PABA is not a constant finding in sulfonamide-resistant bacteria, and resistant mutants may possess enzymes for folate biosynthesis that are less readily inhibited by sulfonamides. Plasmid-mediated resistance is due to plasmid-encoded drug-resistant dihydropteroate synthetase.

Absorption, Fate, and Excretion

Except for sulfonamides especially designed for their local effects in the bowel (Chapter 47), this class of drugs is absorbed rapidly from the GI tract. Approximately 70-100% of an oral dose is absorbed, and sulfonamide can be found in the urine within 30 minutes of ingestion. Peak plasma levels are achieved in 2-6 hours, depending on the drug. The small intestine is the major site of absorption, but some of the drug is absorbed from the stomach. Absorption from other sites, such as the vagina, respiratory tract, or abraded skin, is variable and unreliable, but a sufficient amount may enter the body to cause toxic reactions in susceptible persons or to produce sensitization.

All sulfonamides are bound in varying degree to plasma proteins, particularly to albumin. The extent to which this occurs is determined by the hydrophobicity of a particular drug and its pK_a; at physiological pH, drugs with a high pK_a exhibit a low degree of protein binding, and *vice versa*.

Sulfonamides are distributed throughout all tissues of the body. The diffusible fraction of sulfadiazine is distributed uniformly throughout the total-body water, whereas sulfisoxazole is confined largely to the extracellular space. The sulfonamides readily enter pleural, peritoneal, synovial, ocular, and similar body fluids and may reach concentrations therein that are 50-80% of the simultaneously determined concentration in blood. Because the protein content of such fluids usually is low, the drug is present in the unbound active form.

After systemic administration of adequate doses, sulfadiazine and sulfisoxazole attain concentrations in cerebrospinal fluid that may be effective in meningeal infections. At steady state, the concentration ranges between 10% and 80% of that in the blood. However, because of the emergence of sulfonamide-resistant microorganisms, these drugs are used rarely for the treatment of meningitis.

Sulfonamides pass readily through the placenta and reach the fetal circulation. The concentrations attained in the fetal tissues are sufficient to cause both antibacterial and toxic effects.

The sulfonamides undergo metabolic alterations *in vivo*, especially in the liver. The major metabolic derivative is the N4-acetylated sulfonamide. Acetylation, which occurs to a different extent with each agent, is disadvantageous because the resulting products have no antibacterial activity and yet retain the toxic potential of the parent substance.

Sulfonamides are eliminated from the body partly as the unchanged drug and partly as metabolic products. The largest fraction is excreted in the urine, and the $t_{1/2}$ of sulfonamides in the body thus depends on renal function. In acid urine, the older sulfonamides are insoluble and may precipitate, forming crystalline deposits that can cause urinary obstruction. Small amounts are eliminated in the feces, bile, milk, and other secretions.

Pharmacological Properties of Individual Sulfonamides

The sulfonamides may be classified on the basis of the rapidity with which they are absorbed and excreted (Table 52–1):

- agents that are absorbed and excreted rapidly, such as sulfisoxazole and sulfadiazine
- agents that are absorbed very poorly when administered orally and hence are active in the bowel lumen, such as sulfasalazine
- agents that are used mainly topically, such as sulfacetamide, mafenide, and silver sulfadiazine
- long-acting sulfonamides, such as sulfadoxine, that are absorbed rapidly but excreted slowly

Rapidly Absorbed and Eliminated Sulfonamides

Sulfisoxazole. Sulfisoxazole is a rapidly absorbed and excreted sulfonamide with excellent antibacterial activity. Because its high solubility eliminates much of the renal toxicity inherent in the use of older sulfonamides, it has essentially replaced the less soluble agents.

Sulfisoxazole is bound extensively to plasma proteins. Following an oral dose of 2-4 g, peak concentrations in plasma of 110-250 μg/mL are found in 2-4 hours. From 28-35% of sulfisoxazole in the blood and ~30% in the urine is in the acetylated form. The kidney excretes ~95% of a single dose in 24 hours. Concentrations of the drug in urine thus greatly exceed those in blood and may be bactericidal. The concentration in cerebrospinal fluid averages about a third of that in the blood.

Table 52–1

Classes of Sulfonamides

CLASS	SULFONAMIDE	SERUM $t_{1/2}$ (hours)
Absorbed and excreted rapidly	Sulfisoxazole	5-6
	Sulfamethoxazole	11
	Sulfadiazine	10
Poorly absorbed–active in bowel lumen	Sulfasalazine	—
Topically used	Sulfacetamide	—
	Silver sulfadiazine	—
Long-acting	Sulfadoxine	100-230

Sulfisoxazole acetyl is tasteless and hence preferred for oral use in children. Sulfisoxazole acetyl is marketed in combination with erythromycin ethylsuccinate for use in children with otitis media.

Fewer than 0.1% of patients receiving sulfisoxazole suffer serious toxic reactions. The untoward effects produced by this agent are similar to those which follow the administration of other sulfonamides, as discussed later. Because of its relatively high solubility in the urine as compared with sulfadiazine, sulfisoxazole only infrequently produces hematuria or crystalluria (0.2-0.3%). Despite this, patients taking this drug should ingest an adequate quantity of water. Sulfisoxazole and all sulfonamides that are absorbed must be used with caution in patients with impaired renal function. Like all sulfonamides, sulfisoxazole may produce hypersensitivity reactions, some of which are potentially lethal. Sulfisoxazole currently is preferred over other sulfonamides by most clinicians when a rapidly absorbed and rapidly excreted sulfonamide is indicated.

Sulfamethoxazole. Sulfamethoxazole is a close congener of sulfisoxazole, but its rates of enteric absorption and urinary excretion are slower. It is administered orally and employed for both systemic and urinary tract infections. Precautions must be observed to avoid sulfamethoxazole crystalluria because of the high percentage of the acetylated, relatively insoluble form of the drug in the urine. The clinical uses of sulfamethoxazole are the same as those for sulfisoxazole. In the U.S., it is marketed only in fixed-dose combinations with trimethoprim.

Sulfadiazine. Sulfadiazine given orally is absorbed rapidly from the GI tract, and peak blood concentrations are reached within 3-6 hours after a single dose. Following an oral dose of 3 g, peak concentrations in plasma are 50 μg/mL. About 55% of the drug is bound to plasma protein at a concentration of 100 μg/mL when plasma protein levels are normal. Therapeutic concentrations are attained in cerebrospinal fluid within 4 hours of a single oral dose of 60 mg/kg.

Sulfadiazine is excreted quite readily by the kidney in both the free and acetylated forms, rapidly at first and then more slowly over a period of 2-3 days. It can be detected in the urine within 30 minutes of oral ingestion. About 15-40% of the excreted sulfadiazine is in acetylated form. This form of the drug is excreted more readily than the free fraction, and the administration of alkali accelerates the renal clearance of both forms by further diminishing their tubular reabsorption.

In adults and children who are being treated with sulfadiazine, every precaution must be taken to ensure fluid intake adequate to produce a urine output of at least 1200 mL in adults and a corresponding quantity in children. If this cannot be accomplished, sodium bicarbonate may be given to reduce the risk of crystalluria.

Poorly Absorbed Sulfonamides

Sulfasalazine. Sulfasalazine (AZULFIDINE, others) is very poorly absorbed from the GI tract. It is used in the therapy of ulcerative colitis and regional enteritis (Chapter 47). Intestinal bacteria break sulfasalazine down to sulfapyridine, an active sulfonamide that is absorbed and eventually excreted in the urine, and 5-aminosalicylate (5-ASA, mesalamine; Figures 47–2 through 47–4), which reaches high levels in the feces. Whereas sulfapyridine is responsible for most of the toxicity 5-ASA is the effective agent in inflammatory bowel disease. Toxic reactions include Heinz-body anemia, acute hemolysis in patients with glucose-6-phosphate dehydrogenase deficiency, and agranulocytosis. Nausea, fever, arthralgias, and rashes occur in up to 20% of patients treated with the drug; desensitization has been an effective treatment. Sulfasalazine can cause a reversible infertility in males owing to changes in sperm number and morphology.

Sulfonamides for Topical Use

Sulfacetamide. Sulfacetamide is the N1-acetyl-substituted derivative of sulfanilamide. Its aqueous solubility (1:140) is ~90 times that of sulfadiazine. Solutions of the sodium salt of the drug are employed extensively in the management of ophthalmic infections. Although topical sulfonamide for most purposes is discouraged because of lack of efficacy and a high risk of sensitization, sulfacetamide has certain advantages. Very high aqueous concentrations are not irritating to the eye and are effective against susceptible microorganisms. A 30% solution of the sodium salt has a pH of 7.4, whereas the solutions of sodium salts of other sulfonamides are highly alkaline. The drug penetrates into ocular fluids and tissues in high concentration. Sensitivity reactions to sulfacetamide are rare, but the drug should not be used in patients with known hypersensitivity to sulfonamides. See Chapters 64 and 65 for ocular and dermatogical uses.

Silver Sulfadiazine. Silver sulfadiazine (SILVADENE, others) inhibits the growth *in vitro* of nearly all pathogenic bacteria and fungi, including some species resistant to sulfonamides. The compound is used topically to reduce microbial colonization and the incidence of infections from burns. It should not be used to treat an established deep infection. Silver is released slowly from the preparation in concentrations that are selectively toxic to the microorganisms. However, bacteria may develop resistance to silver sulfadiazine. Although little silver is absorbed, the plasma concentration of sulfadiazine may approach therapeutic levels if a large surface area is involved. Adverse reactions—burning, rash, and itching—are infrequent. Silver sulfadiazine is considered by most authorities to be an agent of choice for the prevention of burn infections.

Mafenide. This sulfonamide (α-amino-*p*-toluene-sulfonamide) is marketed as mafenide acetate (SULFAMYLON). When applied topically, it effectively prevents colonization of burns by a large variety of gram-negative and gram-positive bacteria. It should not be used in treatment of an established deep infection. Superinfection with *Candida* occasionally may be a problem. The cream is applied once or twice daily to a thickness of 1-2 mm over the burned skin. Cleansing of the wound and removal of debris should be carried out before each application of the drug. Therapy is continued until skin grafting is possible. Mafenide is rapidly absorbed systemically and converted to *para*-carboxybenzenesulfonamide. Studies of absorption from the burn surface indicate that peak plasma concentrations are reached in 2-4 hours. Adverse effects include intense pain at sites of application, allergic reactions, and loss of fluid by evaporation from the burn surface because occlusive dressings are not used. The drug and its primary metabolite inhibit carbonic anhydrase, and the urine becomes alkaline. Metabolic acidosis with compensatory tachypnea and hyperventilation may ensue; these effects limit the usefulness of mafenide.

Long-Acting Sulfonamides

Sulfadoxine. This agent, N1-[5,6-dimethoxy-4-pyrimidiny] sulfanilamide, has a particularly long plasma $t_{1/2}$ (7-9 days). It is used in combination with pyrimethamine (500 mg sulfadoxine plus 25 mg pyrimethamine as FANSIDAR) for the prophylaxis and treatment of malaria caused by mefloquine-resistant strains of *Plasmodium falciparum* (Chapter 49). However, because of severe and sometimes fatal reactions, including the Stevens-Johnson syndrome, and the emergence of resistant strains, the drug has limited usefulness for the treatment of malaria.

Sulfonamide Therapy

The number of conditions for which the sulfonamides are therapeutically useful and constitute drugs of first choice has been reduced sharply by the development of more effective antimicrobial agents and by the gradual increase in the resistance of a number of bacterial species to this class of drugs. However, the combination of sulfamethoxazole and trimethoprim is widely employed.

Urinary Tract Infections. Because a significant percentage of urinary tract infections in many parts of the world are caused by sulfonamide-resistant microorganisms, sulfonamides are no longer a therapy of first choice. Trimethoprim-sulfamethoxazole, a quinolone, trimethoprim, fosfomycin, or ampicillin are the preferred agents. However, sulfisoxazole may be used effectively in areas where the prevalence of resistance is not high or when the organism is known to be sensitive. The usual dosage is 2-4 g initially followed by 1-2 g, orally four times a day for 5-10 days. Patients with acute pyelonephritis with high fever and other severe constitutional manifestations are at risk of bacteremia and shock and should not be treated with a sulfonamide.

Nocardiosis. Sulfonamides are of value in the treatment of infections due to *Nocardia* spp. A number of instances of complete recovery from the disease after adequate treatment with a sulfonamide have been recorded. Sulfisoxazole or sulfadiazine may be given in dosages of 6-8 g daily. Concentrations of sulfonamide in plasma should be 80-160 μg/mL. This schedule is continued for several months after all manifestations have been controlled. The administration of sulfonamide together with a second antibiotic has been recommended, especially for advanced cases, and ampicillin, erythromycin, and streptomycin have been suggested for this purpose. The clinical response and the results of sensitivity testing may be helpful in choosing a companion drug. Notably, there are no clinical data to show that combination therapy is better than therapy with a sulfonamide alone. Trimethoprim-sulfamethoxazole also has been effective, and some authorities consider it to be the drug of choice.

Toxoplasmosis. The combination of pyrimethamine and sulfadiazine is the treatment of choice for toxoplasmosis (Montoya et al., 2005) (Chapter 50). Pyrimethamine is given as a loading dose of 75 mg followed by 25 mg orally per day, with sulfadiazine 1 g orally every 6 hours, plus folinic acid (leucovorin) 10 mg orally each day for at least 3-6 weeks. Patients should receive at least 2 L of fluid intake daily to prevent crystalluria during therapy.

Use of Sulfonamides for Prophylaxis. The sulfonamides are as efficacious as oral penicillin in preventing streptococcal infections and recurrences of rheumatic fever among susceptible subjects. Despite the efficacy of sulfonamides for long-term prophylaxis of rheumatic fever, their toxicity and the possibility of infection by drug-resistant streptococci make sulfonamides less desirable than penicillin for this purpose. They should be used, however, without hesitation in patients who are hypersensitive to penicillin. If untoward responses occur, they usually do so during the first 8 weeks of therapy; serious reactions after this time are rare. White blood cell counts should be carried out once weekly during the first 8 weeks.

Untoward Reactions to Sulfonamides

The untoward effects that follow the administration of sulfonamides are numerous and varied; the overall incidence of reactions is ~5%.

Disturbances of the Urinary Tract. Although the risk of crystalluria was relatively high with the older, less soluble sulfonamides, the incidence of this problem is very low with more soluble agents such as sulfisoxazole. Crystalluria has occurred in dehydrated patients with acquired immune deficiency syndrome (AIDS) who were receiving sulfadiazine for *Toxoplasma* encephalitis. Fluid intake should be sufficient to ensure a daily urine volume of at least 1200 mL (in adults). Alkalinization of the urine may be desirable if urine volume or pH is unusually low because the solubility of sulfisoxazole increases greatly with slight elevations of pH.

Disorders of the Hematopoietic System.

Acute Hemolytic Anemia. The mechanism of the acute hemolytic anemia produced by sulfonamides is not always readily apparent. In some cases, it may be a sensitization phenomenon; in other instances, the hemolysis is related to an erythrocytic deficiency of glucose-6-phosphate dehydrogenase activity. Hemolytic anemia is rare after treatment with sulfadiazine (0.05%); its exact incidence following therapy with sulfisoxazole is unknown.

Agranulocytosis. Agranulocytosis occurs in ~0.1% of patients who receive sulfadiazine; it also can follow the use of other sulfonamides. Although return of granulocytes to normal levels may be delayed for weeks or months after sulfonamide is withdrawn, most patients recover spontaneously with supportive care.

Aplastic Anemia. Complete suppression of bone marrow activity with profound anemia, granulocytopenia, and thrombocytopenia is an extremely rare occurrence with sulfonamide therapy. It probably results from a direct myelotoxic effect and may be fatal. However, reversible suppression of the bone marrow is quite common in patients with limited bone marrow reserve (e.g., patients with AIDS or those receiving myelosuppressive chemotherapy).

Hypersensitivity Reactions. The incidence of other hypersensitivity reactions to sulfonamides is quite variable. Among the skin and mucous membrane manifestations attributed to sensitization to sulfonamide are morbilliform, scarlatinal, urticarial, erysipeloid, pemphigoid, purpuric, and petechial rashes, as well as erythema nodosum, erythema multiforme of the Stevens-Johnson type, Behçet's syndrome, exfoliative dermatitis, and photosensitivity. These hypersensitivity reactions occur most often after the first week of therapy but may appear earlier in previously sensitized individuals. Fever, malaise, and pruritus frequently are present simultaneously. The incidence of untoward dermal effects is ~2% with sulfisoxazole, although patients with AIDS manifest a higher frequency of rashes with sulfonamide treatment than do other individuals. A syndrome similar to serum sickness may appear after several days of sulfonamide therapy. Drug fever is a common untoward manifestation of sulfonamide treatment; the incidence approximates 3% with sulfisoxazole.

Focal or diffuse necrosis of the liver owing to direct drug toxicity or sensitization occurs in <0.1% of patients. Headache, nausea, vomiting, fever, hepatomegaly, jaundice, and laboratory evidence of hepatocellular dysfunction usually appear 3-5 days after sulfonamide administration is started, and the syndrome may progress to acute yellow atrophy and death.

Miscellaneous Reactions. Anorexia, nausea, and vomiting occur in 1-2% of persons receiving sulfonamides, and these manifestations probably are central in origin. The administration of sulfonamides to newborn infants, especially if premature, may lead to the displacement of bilirubin from plasma albumin. In newborn infants, free bilirubin can become deposited in the basal ganglia and subthalamic nuclei of the brain, causing an encephalopathy called *kernicterus*. Sulfonamides should not be given to pregnant women near term because these drugs pass through the placenta and are secreted in milk.

Drug Interactions. The most important interactions of the sulfonamides involve those with the oral anticoagulants, the sulfonylurea hypoglycemic agents, and the hydantoin anticonvulsants. In each case, sulfonamides can potentiate the effects of the other drug by mechanisms that appear to involve primarily inhibition of metabolism and, possibly, displacement from albumin. Dosage adjustment may be necessary when a sulfonamide is given concurrently.

TRIMETHOPRIM-SULFAMETHOXAZOLE

The introduction of trimethoprim in combination with sulfamethoxazole constitutes an important advance in the development of clinically effective antimicrobial agents and represents the practical application of a theoretical consideration; that is, if two drugs act on sequential steps in the pathway of an obligate enzymatic reaction in bacteria (Figure 52–2), the result of their combination will be synergistic (Hitchings, 1961). In much of the world the combination of trimethoprim with sulfamethoxazole is known as cotrimoxazole. In addition to its combination with sulfamethoxazole (BACTRIM, SEPTRA, others), trimethoprim also is available as a single-entity preparation.

Chemistry. Sulfamethoxazole was discussed earlier in this chapter, and its structural formula is shown in Figure 52–1. Trimethoprim, a diaminopyrimidine, inhibits bacterial dihydrofolate reductase. The drug's properties are reviewed in Chapter 49.

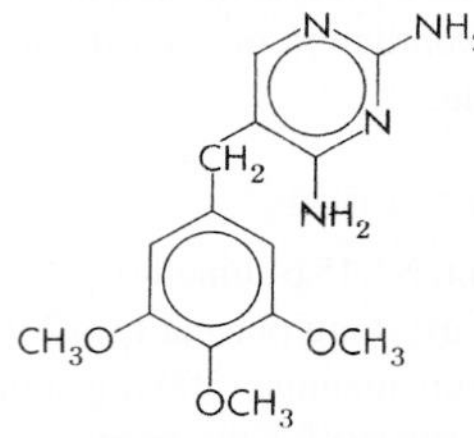

TRIMETHOPRIM

Antibacterial Spectrum. The antibacterial spectrum of trimethoprim is similar to that of sulfamethoxazole, although the former drug usually is 20-100 times more potent than the latter. Most gram-negative and gram-positive microorganisms are sensitive to trimethoprim, but resistance can develop when the drug is used alone. *Pseudomonas aeruginosa, Bacteroides fragilis*, and enterococci usually are resistant. There is significant variation in the susceptibility of Enterobacteriaceae to trimethoprim in different geographic locations because of the spread of resistance mediated by plasmids and transposons (see Chapter 48).

Efficacy of Trimethoprim-Sulfamethoxazole in Combination. *Chlamydia diphtheriae* and *N. meningitidis* are susceptible to trimethoprim-sulfamethoxazole. Although most *S. pneumoniae* are susceptible, there has been a disturbing increase in resistance. From 50-95% of strains of *Staphylococcus aureus, Staphylococcus epidermidis, S. pyogenes*, the *viridans* group of streptococci, *E. coli, Proteus mirabilis, Proteus morganii, Proteus rettgeri, Enterobacter* spp., *Salmonella, Shigella, Pseudomonas pseudomallei, Serratia*, and *Alcaligenes* spp. are inhibited. Also sensitive are *Klebsiella* spp., *Brucella abortus, Pasteurella haemolytica, Yersinia pseudotuberculosis, Yersinia enterocolitica*, and *Nocardia asteroides*.

Mechanism of Action. The antimicrobial activity of the combination of trimethoprim and sulfamethoxazole results from its actions on two steps of the enzymatic pathway for the synthesis of tetrahydrofolic acid. Sulfonamide inhibits the incorporation of PABA into folic acid, and trimethoprim prevents the reduction of dihydrofolate to tetrahydrofolate (Figure 52–2). Tetrahydrofolate is essential for one-carbon transfer reactions (e.g., the synthesis of thymidylate from deoxyuridylate). Selective toxicity for microorganisms is achieved in two ways. Mammalian cells use preformed folates from the diet and do not synthesize the compound. Furthermore, trimethoprim is a highly selective inhibitor of dihydrofolate reductase of lower organisms: ~100,000 times more drug is required to inhibit human reductase than the bacterial enzyme. This relative selectivity is vital because this enzymatic function is essential to all species.

The synergistic interaction between sulfonamide and trimethoprim is predictable from their respective mechanisms. There is an optimal ratio of the concentrations of the two agents for synergism that equals the ratio of the minimal inhibitory concentrations of the drugs acting independently. Although this ratio varies for different bacteria, the most effective ratio for the greatest number of microorganisms is 20 parts sulfamethoxazole to 1 part trimethoprim. The combination is thus formulated to achieve a sulfamethoxazole concentration *in vivo* that is 20 times greater than that of trimethoprim. The pharmacokinetic properties of the sulfonamide chosen to be in combination with trimethoprim are critical because relative constancy of the concentrations of the two compounds in the body is desired.

Bacterial Resistance. Bacterial resistance to trimethoprim-sulfamethoxazole is a rapidly increasing problem, although resistance is lower than it is to either of the agents alone. Resistance often is due to the acquisition of a plasmid that codes for an altered dihydrofolate reductase. Resistance to trimethoprim-sulfamethoxazole is reportedly formed in almost 30% of urinary isolates of *E. coli* (Olson, et al., 2009).

Absorption, Distribution, and Excretion. The pharmacokinetic profiles of sulfamethoxazole and trimethoprim are closely but not perfectly matched to achieve a constant ratio of 20:1 in their concentrations in blood and tissues. The ratio in blood is often >20:1, and that in tissues is frequently less. After a single oral dose of the combined preparation, trimethoprim is absorbed more rapidly than sulfamethoxazole. The concurrent administration of the drugs appears to slow the absorption of sulfamethoxazole. Peak blood concentrations of trimethoprim usually occur by 2 hours in most patients, whereas peak concentrations of sulfamethoxazole occur by 4 hours after a single oral dose. The half-lives of trimethoprim and sulfamethoxazole are ~11 and 10 hours, respectively.

When 800 mg sulfamethoxazole is given with 160 mg trimethoprim (the conventional 5:1 ratio) twice daily, the peak concentrations of the drugs in plasma are ~40 and 2 μg/mL, the optimal ratio. Peak concentrations are similar (46 and 3.4 μg/mL) after intravenous infusion of 800 mg sulfamethoxazole and 160 mg trimethoprim over a period of 1 hour.

Trimethoprim is distributed and concentrated rapidly in tissues, and ~40% is bound to plasma protein in the presence of sulfamethoxazole. The volume of distribution of trimethoprim is almost nine times that of sulfamethoxazole. The drug readily enters cerebrospinal fluid and sputum. High concentrations of each component of the mixture also are found in bile. About 65% of sulfamethoxazole is bound to plasma protein.

About 60% of administered trimethoprim and from 25% to 50% of administered sulfamethoxazole are excreted in the urine in 24 hours. Two-thirds of the sulfonamide is unconjugated. Metabolites of trimethoprim also are excreted. The rates of excretion and the concentrations of both compounds in the urine are reduced significantly in patients with uremia.

Therapeutic Uses.

Urinary Tract Infections. Treatment of uncomplicated lower urinary tract infection (UTI) with trimethoprim-sulfamethoxazole often is highly effective for sensitive bacteria. The preparation has been shown to produce a better therapeutic effect than does either of its components given separately when the infecting microorganisms are of the family Enterobacteriaceae. Single-dose therapy (320 mg trimethoprim plus 1600 mg sulfamethoxazole in adults) has been effective in some cases for the treatment of acute uncomplicated UTI, but a minimum of 3 days of therapy is more likely to be effective (Fihn, 2003; Zinner and Mayer, 2005).

The combination appears to have special efficacy in chronic and recurrent infections of the urinary tract. Small doses (200 mg sulfamethoxazole plus 40 mg trimethoprim per day and postcoitally or 2-4 times these amounts once or twice per week) effectively reduce the number of recurrent urinary tract infections in women. This effect may be related to the presence of therapeutic concentrations of trimethoprim in vaginal secretions. Enterobacteriaceae surrounding the urethral orifice may be eliminated or markedly reduced in number, thus diminishing the chance of an ascending reinfection. Trimethoprim also is found in therapeutic concentrations in prostatic secretions, and trimethoprim-sulfamethoxazole is often effective for the treatment of bacterial prostatitis.

Bacterial Respiratory Tract Infections. Trimethoprim-sulfamethoxazole is effective for acute exacerbations of chronic bronchitis. Administration of 800-1200 mg sulfamethoxazole plus 160-240 mg trimethoprim twice a day appears to be effective in decreasing fever, purulence and volume of sputum, and sputum bacterial count. Trimethoprim-sulfamethoxazole should *not* be used to treat streptococcal pharyngitis because it does not eradicate the microorganism. It is effective for acute otitis media in children and acute maxillary sinusitis in adults caused by susceptible strains of *H. influenzae* and *S. pneumoniae*.

GI Infections. The combination is an alternative to a fluoroquinolone for treatment of shigellosis because many strains of the causative agent now are resistant to ampicillin; however, resistance to trimethoprim-sulfamethoxazole is increasingly common. It also is a second-line drug (ceftriaxone or a fluoroquinolone is the preferred treatment) for typhoid fever, but resistance is an increasing problem. In adults, trimethoprim-sulfamethoxazole appears to be effective when the dose is 800 mg sulfamethoxazole plus 160 mg trimethoprim every 12 hours for 15 days. The same regimen has been used for 5 days for Travelers' diarrhea.

Trimethoprim-sulfamethoxazole appears to be effective in the management of carriers of sensitive strains of *Salmonella typhi* and other *Salmonella* spp. One proposed schedule is the administration of 800 mg sulfamethoxazole plus 160 mg trimethoprim twice a day for 3 months; however, failures have occurred. The presence of chronic disease of the gallbladder may be associated with a high incidence of failure to clear the carrier state. Acute diarrhea owing to sensitive strains of enteropathogenic *E. coli* can be treated or prevented with either trimethoprim or trimethoprim plus sulfamethoxazole (Hill et al., 2006). However, antibiotic treatment (either trimethoprim-sulfamethoxazole or cephalosporin) of diarrheal illness owing to enterohemorrhagic *E. coli* O157:H7 may increase the risk of hemolytic-uremic syndrome, perhaps by increasing the release of Shiga toxin by the bacteria (Wong et al., 2000).

Infection by Pneumocystis jiroveci. High-dose therapy (trimethoprim 15-20 mg/kg per day plus sulfamethoxazole 75-100 mg/kg per day in three or four divided doses) is effective for this severe infection in patients with AIDS (Thomas and Limper, 2004). This combination compares favorably with pentamidine for treatment of this disease. Adjunctive corticosteroids should be given at the onset of anti-*Pneumocystis* therapy in patients with a Po_2 <70 mm Hg or an alveolar-arterial gradient >35 mm Hg (Centers for Disease Control and Prevention, 2009). However, the incidence of side effects is high for both regimens. Prophylaxis with 800 mg sulfamethoxazole and 160 mg trimethoprim once daily or three times a week is effective in preventing pneumonia caused by this organism in patients with AIDS (Centers for Disease Control and Prevention, 2009). Adverse reactions are less frequent with the lower prophylactic doses of trimethoprim-sulfamethoxazole. The most common problems are rash, fever, leukopenia, and hepatitis.

Prophylaxis in Neutropenic Patients. Several studies have demonstrated the effectiveness of low-dose therapy (150 mg/m^2 of body surface area of trimethoprim and 750 mg/m^2 of body surface area of sulfamethoxazole) for the prophylaxis of infection by *P. jiroveci*. In addition, significant protection against sepsis caused by gram-negative bacteria was noted when 800 mg sulfamethoxazole and 160 mg trimethoprim were given twice daily to severely neutropenic patients. The emergence of resistant bacteria may limit the usefulness of trimethoprim-sulfamethoxazole for prophylaxis (Hughes et al., 2002).

Miscellaneous Infections. *Nocardia* infections have been treated successfully with the combination, but failures also have been reported. Although a combination of doxycycline and streptomycin or gentamicin now is considered to be the treatment of choice for brucellosis, trimethoprim-sulfamethoxazole may be an effective substitute for the doxycycline combination. Trimethoprim-sulfamethoxazole also has been used successfully in the treatment of Whipple's disease, infection by *Stenotrophomonas maltophilia*, and infection by the intestinal parasites *Cyclospora* and *Isospora*. Wegener's granulomatosis may respond, depending on the stage of the disease.

Untoward Effects. There is no evidence that trimethoprim-sulfamethoxazole, when given in the recommended doses, induces folate deficiency in normal persons. However, the margin between toxicity for bacteria and that for humans may be relatively narrow when the cells of the patient are deficient in folate. In such cases, trimethoprim-sulfamethoxazole may cause or precipitate megaloblastosis, leukopenia, or thrombocytopenia. In routine use, the combination appears to exert little toxicity. About 75% of the untoward effects involve the skin. However, trimethoprim-sulfamethoxazole has been reported to cause up to three times as many dermatological reactions as does sulfisoxazole alone (5.9% versus 1.7%).

Exfoliative dermatitis, Stevens-Johnson syndrome, and toxic epidermal necrolysis (Lyell's syndrome) are rare, occurring primarily in older individuals. Nausea and vomiting constitute the bulk of GI reactions; diarrhea is rare. Glossitis and stomatitis are relatively common. Mild and transient jaundice has been noted and appears to have the histological features of allergic cholestatic hepatitis. Central nervous system reactions consist of headache, depression, and hallucinations, manifestations known to be produced by sulfonamides. Hematological reactions, in addition to those just mentioned, are various anemias (including aplastic, hemolytic, and macrocytic), coagulation disorders, granulocytopenia, agranulocytosis, purpura, Henoch-Schönlein purpura, and sulfhemoglobinemia. Permanent impairment of renal function may follow the use of trimethoprim-sulfamethoxazole in patients with renal disease, and a reversible decrease in creatinine clearance has been noted in patients with normal renal function.

Patients with AIDS frequently have hypersensitivity reactions to trimethoprim-sulfamethoxazole (rash, neutropenia, Stevens-Johnson syndrome, Sweet's syndrome, and pulmonary infiltrates). It may be possible to continue therapy in such patients following rapid oral desensitization (Gluckstein and Ruskin, 1995).

THE QUINOLONES

The first quinolone, *nalidixic acid*, was isolated as a by-product of the synthesis of *chloroquine* and made available for the treatment of urinary tract infections. The introduction of fluorinated 4-quinolones, such as ciprofloxacin (CIPRO, others), and moxifloxacin (AVELOX), represents a particularly important therapeutic advance: These agents have broad antimicrobial activity and are effective after oral administration for the treatment of a wide variety of infectious diseases (Table 52–2) (Hooper, 2005a). Rare and potentially fatal side effects, however, have resulted in the withdrawal from the U.S. market of lomefloxacin sparfloxacin (phototoxicity, QTc prolongation), gatifloxacin (hypoglycemia), temafloxacin (immune hemolytic anemia), trovafloxacin (hepatotoxicity), grepafloxacin (cardiotoxicity), and clinafloxacin (phototoxicity). In all these cases, the side effects were detected by postmarketing surveillance (Sheehan and Chew, 2003).

Chemistry. The compounds that are currently available for clinical use in the U.S. are quinolones containing a carboxylic acid moiety at position 3 of the primary ring structure. Many of the newer fluoroquinolones also contain a fluorine substituent at position 6 and a piperazine moiety at position 7 (Table 52–2).

Mechanism of Action. The quinolone antibiotics target bacterial DNA gyrase and topoisomerase IV (Hooper, 2005a). For many gram-positive bacteria (such as *S. aureus*), topoisomerase IV is the primary activity inhibited by the quinolones. In contrast, DNA gyrase is the primary quinolone target in many gram-negative microbes (such as *E. coli*) (Alovero et al., 2000; Hooper, 2005a). Individual strands of double-helical DNA must be separated to permit DNA replication or transcription. However, anything that separates the strands results in "overwinding" or excessive positive supercoiling of the DNA in front of the point of separation. To combat this mechanical obstacle, the bacterial enzyme DNA gyrase is responsible for the continuous introduction of negative supercoils into

Table 52–2

Structural Formulas of Selected Quinolones and Fluoroquinolones

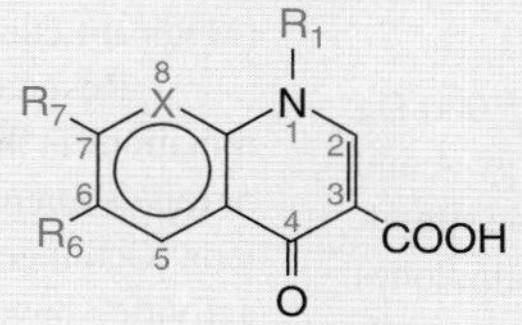

(General structure: quinolone nucleus with R_1 on N-1, COOH at C-3, O at C-4, R_6 at C-6, R_7 at C-7, X at position 8)

CONGENER	R_1	R_6	R_7	X
Nalidixic acid	$-C_2H_5$	$-H$	$-CH_3$	$-N-$
Cinoxacin (*N replaces C2*)	$-C_2H_5$	(Fused dioxolo ring)*		$-CH-$
Norfloxacin	$-C_2H_5$	$-F$	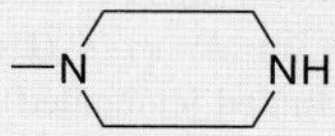 piperazinyl (–N ring NH)	$-CH-$
Ciprofloxacin	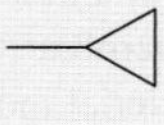 cyclopropyl	$-F$	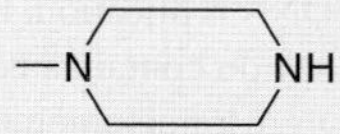 piperazinyl (–N ring NH)	$-CH-$
Ofloxacin	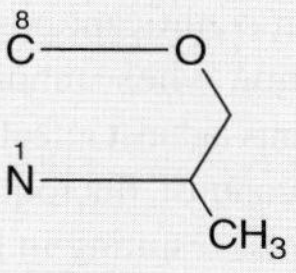 C8–O–CH2–CH(CH3)–N1 bridge	$-F$	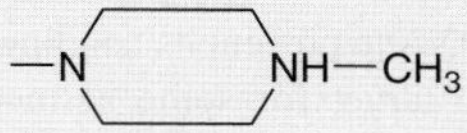 4-methylpiperazinyl (–N ring NH–CH_3)	$-CH-$
Sparfloxacin (*—NH_2 on C5*)	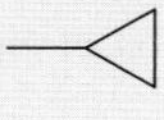 cyclopropyl	$-F$	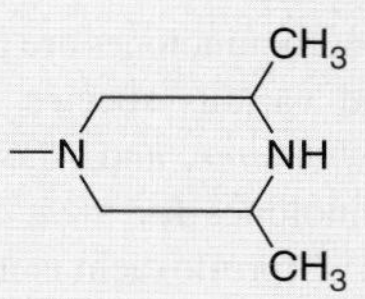 3,5-dimethylpiperazinyl (–N ring NH, two CH_3)	$-\overset{F}{C}-$
Fleroxacin	$-CH_2-CH_2-F$	$-F$	4-methylpiperazinyl (–N ring NH–CH_3)	$-\overset{F}{C}-$
Pefloxacin	$-C_2H_5$	$-F$	4-methylpiperazinyl (–N ring NH–CH_3)	$-CH-$
Levofloxacin	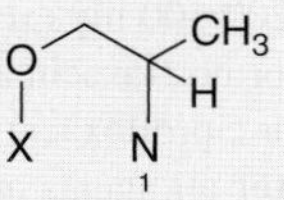 X–O–CH2–CH(CH3)(H)–N1 bridge	$-F$	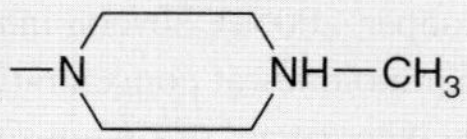 4-methylpiperazinyl (–N ring NH–CH_3)	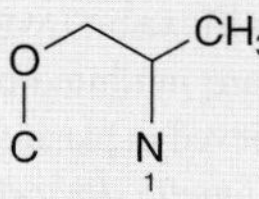 O–CH2–CH(CH_3)–N1 bridge to C
Garenoxacin	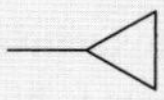 cyclopropyl	$-H$	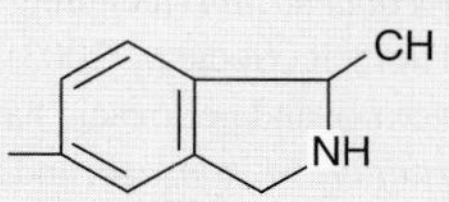 isoindolinyl (CH, NH)	$OCHF_2$ on $-C-$
Gemifloxacin	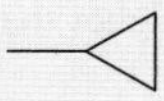 cyclopropyl	$-F$	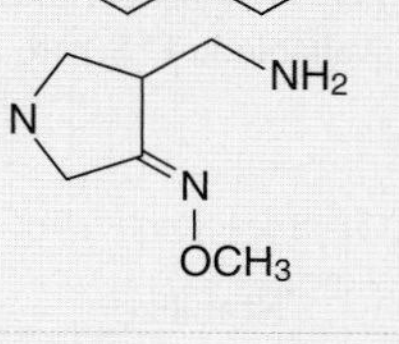 3-(aminomethyl)-4-(methoxyimino)pyrrolidinyl (NH_2, N–OCH_3)	$-N-$

*[C with –O– and –O– (dioxolo)]

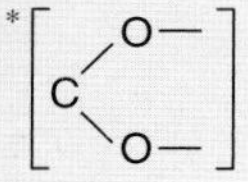

DNA via an ATP-dependent reaction requiring that both strands of the DNA be cut to permit passage of a segment of DNA through the break; the break then is resealed.

The DNA gyrase of *E. coli* is composed of two 105,000 Da A subunits and two 95,000 Da B subunits encoded by the *gyrA* and *gyrB* genes, respectively. The A subunits, which carry out the strand-cutting function of the gyrase, are the site of action of the quinolones (Figure 52–3). The drugs inhibit gyrase-mediated DNA supercoiling at concentrations that correlate well with those required to inhibit bacterial growth (0.1-10 μg/mL). Mutations of the gene that encodes the A subunit polypeptide can confer resistance to these drugs (Hooper, 2005a).

Topoisomerase IV is also composed of four subunits encoded by the *parC* and *parE* genes in *E. coli* (Hooper, 2005a). Topoisomerase IV separates interlinked (catenated) daughter DNA molecules that are the product of DNA replication. Eukaryotic cells do not contain DNA gyrase, but they do contain a conceptually and mechanistically similar type II DNA topoisomerase that removes positive supercoils from DNA to prevent its tangling during replication. This enzyme is the target for some antineoplastic agents (Chapters 60 and 61). Quinolones inhibit eukaryotic type II topoisomerase only concentrations (100-1000 μg/mL) much higher than those that inhibit bacterial DNA gyrase (Mitscher and Ma, 2003).

Antibacterial Spectrum. The fluoroquinolones are potent bactericidal agents against *E. coli* and various species of *Salmonella, Shigella, Enterobacter, Campylobacter*, and *Neisseria* (Hooper, 2005a). MICs of the fluoroquinolones for 90% of these strains (MIC_{90}) usually are <0.2 μg/mL. Ciprofloxacin is more active than norfloxacin (NOROXIN) against *P. aeruginosa*; values of MIC_{90} range from 0.5-6 μg/mL. Fluoroquinolones also have good activity against staphylococci, but not against methicillin-resistant strains (MIC_{90} = 0.1-2 μg/mL).

Activity against streptococci is limited to a subset of the quinolones, including levofloxacin (LEVAQUIN), gatifloxacin, and moxifloxacin (AVELOX) (Hooper, 2005a). Several intracellular bacteria are inhibited by fluoroquinolones at concentrations that can be achieved in plasma; these include species of *Chlamydia, Mycoplasma, Legionella, Brucella*, and *Mycobacterium* (including *Mycobacterium tuberculosis)* (American Thoracic Society, 2003). Ciprofloxacin (CIPRO, others), ofloxacin (FLOXIN), and pefloxacin have MIC_{90} values from 0.5-3 μg/mL for *M. fortuitum, M. kansasii*, and *M. tuberculosis*; ofloxacin and pefloxacin (not available in U.S.) are active in animal models of leprosy (Hooper, 2005a). However, clinical experience with these pathogens remains limited.

Several fluoroquinolones, including garenoxacin (not available in U.S.) and gemifloxacin, have activity against anaerobic bacteria (Medical Letter, 2000, 2004).

Resistance to quinolones may develop during therapy via mutations in the bacterial chromosomal genes encoding DNA gyrase or topoisomerase IV or by active transport of the drug out of the bacteria (Oethinger et al., 2000). No quinolone-modifying or -inactivating activities have been identified in bacteria (Gold and Moellering, 1996). Resistance has increased after the introduction of fluoroquinolones, especially in *Pseudomonas* and staphylococci. Increasing fluoroquinolone resistance also is being observed in *C. jejuni, Salmonella, N. gonorrhoeae*, and *S. pneumoniae*.

As mentioned in Chapter 48, the pharmacokinetic and pharmacodynamic parameters of antimicrobial agents are important in preventing the selection and spread of resistant strains and have led to description of the mutation-prevention concentration, which is the lowest concentration of antimicrobial that prevents selection of resistant bacteria from high bacterial inocula. β-Lactams are time-dependent agents without significant post-antibiotic effects, resulting in bacterial eradication when unbound serum concentrations exceed MICs of these agents against infecting pathogens for >40-50% of the dosing interval. By contrast, fluoroquinolones are concentration- and time-dependent agents, resulting in bacterial eradication when unbound serum area under the curve-to-MIC ratios exceed 25-30. An extended release formulation of ciprofloxacin (PROQUIN XR) exemplifies this principle.

Absorption, Fate, and Excretion. The quinolones are well absorbed after oral administration and are distributed widely in body tissues. Peak serum levels of the fluoroquinolones are obtained within 1-3 hours of an oral dose of 400 mg, with peak levels ranging from 1.1 μg/mL for sparfloxacin to 6.4 μg/mL for levofloxacin. Relatively low serum levels are reached with norfloxacin and limit its usefulness to the treatment of urinary tract infections. Food does not impair oral absorption but may delay the time to peak serum concentrations. Oral doses in adults are 200-400 mg every 12 hours for ofloxacin, 400 mg every 12 hours for norfloxacin and pefloxacin, and 250 to 750 mg every 12 hours for ciprofloxacin. Bioavailability of the fluoroquinolones is >50% for all agents and >95% for several. The serum $t_{1/2}$ is 3-5 hours for norfloxacin and ciprofloxacin. The volume of distribution of quinolones is high, with concentrations of quinolones in urine, kidney, lung and prostate tissue, stool, bile, and macrophages and neutrophils higher than serum levels. Quinolone

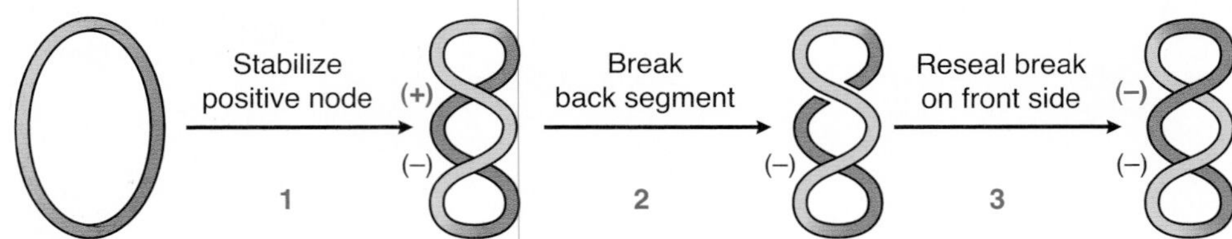

Figure 52–3. *Model of the formation of negative DNA supercoils by DNA gyrase.* The enzyme binds to two segments of DNA (1), creating a node of positive (+) superhelix. The enzyme then introduces a double-strand break in the DNA and passes the front segment through the break (2). The break is then resealed (3), creating a negative (–) supercoil. Quinolones inhibit the nicking and closing activity of the gyrase and, at higher concentrations, block the decatenating activity of topoisomerase IV. From Cozzarelli NR. DNA gyrase and the supercoiling of DNA. *Science*, 1980, 207:953–960. Reprinted with permission from AAAS.

concentrations in cerebrospinal fluid, bone, and prostatic fluid are lower than in serum. Pefloxacin and ofloxacin levels in ascites fluid are close to serum levels, and ciprofloxacin, ofloxacin, and pefloxacin have been detected in human breast milk.

Most quinolones are cleared predominantly by the kidney, and dosages must be adjusted for renal failure. Exceptions are pefloxacin and moxifloxacin, which are metabolized predominantly by the liver and should not be used in patients with hepatic failure. None of the agents is removed efficiently by peritoneal dialysis or hemodialysis.

Therapeutic Uses

Urinary Tract Infections. Nalidixic acid is useful only for UTI caused by susceptible microorganisms. The fluoroquinolones are significantly more potent and have a much broader spectrum of antimicrobial activity. Norfloxacin is approved for use in the U.S. only for urinary tract infections. Comparative clinical trials indicate that the fluoroquinolones are more efficacious than trimethoprim-sulfamethoxazole for the treatment of UTI (Hooper, 2005b). Ciprofloxacin XR is FDA-approved only for UTI.

Prostatitis. Norfloxacin, ciprofloxacin, and ofloxacin all have been effective in uncontrolled trials for the treatment of prostatitis caused by sensitive bacteria. Fluoroquinolones administered for 4-6 weeks appear to be effective in patients not responding to trimethoprim-sulfamethoxazole.

Sexually Transmitted Diseases. The quinolones are contraindicated in pregnancy. Fluoroquinolones lack activity for *Treponema pallidum* but have activity *in vitro* against *C. trachomatis* and *H. ducreyi*. For chlamydial urethritis/cervicitis, a 7-day course of ofloxacin is an alternative to a 7-day treatment with doxycycline or a single dose of azithromycin; other available quinolones have not been reliably effective. A single oral dose of a fluoroquinolone such as ofloxacin or ciprofloxacin had been effective treatment for sensitive strains of *N. gonorrhoeae*, but increasing resistance to fluoroquinolones has led to ceftriaxone being the first-line agent for this infection (Newman et al., 2004). Chancroid (infection by *H. ducreyi*) can be treated with 3 days of ciprofloxacin.

GI and Abdominal Infections. For traveler's diarrhea (frequently caused by enterotoxigenic *E. coli*), the quinolones are equal to trimethoprim-sulfamethoxazole in effectiveness, reducing the duration of loose stools by 1-3 days (Hill et al., 2006). Norfloxacin, ciprofloxacin, and ofloxacin given for 5 days all have been effective in the treatment of patients with shigellosis, with even shorter courses effective in many cases. Ciprofloxacin and ofloxacin treatment cures most patients with enteric fever caused by *S. typhi*, as well as bacteremic nontyphoidal infections in AIDS patients, and it clears chronic fecal carriage. Shigellosis is treated effectively with either ciprofloxacin or azithromycin. The *in vitro* ability of the quinolones to induce the Shiga toxin *stx2* gene (the cause of the hemolytic-uremic syndrome) in *E. coli* suggests that the quinolones should not be used for Shiga toxin–producing *E. coli* (Miedouge et al., 2000). Ciprofloxacin and ofloxacin have been less effective in treating episodes of peritonitis occurring in patients on chronic ambulatory peritoneal dialysis likely owing to the higher MICs for these drugs for the coagulase-negative staphylococci that are a common cause of peritonitis in this setting.

Respiratory Tract Infections. The major limitation to the use of quinolones for the treatment of community-acquired pneumonia and bronchitis had been the poor *in vitro* activity of ciprofloxacin, ofloxacin, and norfloxacin against *S. pneumoniae* and anaerobic bacteria. However, newer fluoroquinolones, including gatifloxacin (available only for ophthalmic use in U.S.) and moxifloxacin, have excellent activity against *S. pneumoniae*. The fluoroquinolones have *in vitro* activity against the rest of the commonly recognized respiratory pathogens, including *H. influenzae, Moraxella catarrhalis, S. aureus, M. pneumoniae, Chlamydia pneumoniae*, and *Legionella pneumophila*. Either a fluoroquinolone (ciprofloxacin or levofloxacin) or azithromycin is the antibiotic of choice for *L. pneumophila* (Edelstein & Cianciotto, 2005). Fluoroquinolones have been very effective at eradicating both *H. influenzae* and *M. catarrhalis* from sputum. Mild to moderate respiratory exacerbations owing to *P. aeruginosa* in patients with cystic fibrosis have responded to oral fluoroquinolone therapy. Emerging clinical data are demonstrating a clear role for the newer fluoroquinolones as single agents for treatment of community-acquired pneumonia (Hooper, 2005b). However, on the horizon is a decreasing susceptibility of *S. pneumoniae* to fluoroquinolones (Chen et al., 1999; Wortmann and Bennett, 1999).

Bone, Joint, and Soft Tissue Infections. The treatment of chronic osteomyelitis requires prolonged (weeks to months) antimicrobial therapy with agents active against *S. aureus* and gram-negative rods. The fluoroquinolones, by virtue of their oral administration and appropriate antibacterial spectrum for these infections, may be used appropriately in some cases; recommended doses are 500 mg every 12 hours or, if severe, 750 mg twice daily. Bone and joint infections may require treatment for 4-6 weeks or more. Dosage should be reduced for patients with severely impaired renal function. Clinical cures have been as high as 75% in chronic osteomyelitis in which gram-negative rods predominated (Hooper, 2005b). Failures have been associated with the development of resistance in *S. aureus, P. aeruginosa*, and *Serratia marcescens*. In diabetic foot infections, which are commonly caused by a mixture of bacteria including gram-negative rods, anaerobes, streptococci, and staphylococci, the fluoroquinolones in combination with an agent with antianaerobic activity are a reasonable choice.

Other Infections. Ciprofloxacin received wide usage for the prophylaxis of anthrax and has been shown to be effective for the treatment of tularemia (Chocarro et al., 2000; Swartz, 2001). The quinolones may be used as part of multiple-drug regimens for the treatment of multidrug-resistant tuberculosis and for the treatment of atypical mycobacterial infections as well as *Myobacterium avium* complex infections in AIDS (Chapter 56). Quinolones, when used as prophylaxis in neutropenic patients, have decreased the incidence of gram-negative rod bacteremias (Hughes et al., 2002).

Adverse Effects. Quinolones and fluoroquinolones generally are well tolerated (Mandell, 2003). The most common adverse reactions involve the GI tract, with 3-17% of patients reporting mostly mild nausea, vomiting, and/or abdominal discomfort. Ciprofloxacin is the most common cause of *C. difficile* colitis. Gatifloxacin is associated with both hypo- and hyperglycemia in older adults (Park-Wyllie et al., 2006). CNS side effects, predominantly mild headache and dizziness, have been seen in 0.9-11% of patients. Rarely, hallucinations, delirium, and seizures have occurred, predominantly in patients who were also receiving theophylline or a nonsteroidal anti-inflammatory drug. Ciprofloxacin and pefloxacin inhibit the metabolism of theophylline, and toxicity from elevated concentrations of the methylxanthine may occur (Schwartz et al., 1988). Nonsteroidal anti-inflammatory drugs may augment displacement of γ-aminobutyric acid (GABA) from its receptors by the quinolones (Halliwell et al., 1993). Rashes, including photosensitivity reactions, also can occur. Achilles tendon rupture or tendinitis is a recognized adverse effect, especially in those >60 years old, patients taking corticosteroids, and in solid organ transplant recipients (Mandell, 2003). All these agents can produce arthropathy in several species of immature animals. Traditionally, the use of quinolones in children has been contraindicated for this reason. However, children with cystic fibrosis given ciprofloxacin, norfloxacin, and nalidixic acid have had few, and reversible, joint symptoms (Burkhardt et al., 1997; Sabharwal & Marchant, 2006). Therefore, in some cases the benefits may outweigh the risks of quinolone therapy in children. Ciprofloxacin should not be given to pregnant women.

Leukopenia, eosinophilia, and mild elevations in serum transaminases occur rarely. QT_c interval (QT interval corrected for heart rate) prolongation has been observed with sparfloxacin and to a lesser extent with gatifloxacin and moxifloxacin. Quinolones probably should be used only with caution in patients on class III (amiodarone) and class IA (quinidine, procainamide) antiarrhythmics (Chapter 29).

ANTISEPTIC AND ANALGESIC AGENTS FOR URINARY TRACT INFECTIONS

Urinary tract antiseptics are concentrated in the renal tubules where they inhibit the growth of many species of bacteria. These agents cannot be used to treat systemic infections because effective concentrations are not achieved in plasma with safe doses; however, they can be administered orally to treat infections of the urinary tract. Furthermore, effective antibacterial concentrations reach the renal pelves and the bladder. Treatment with such drugs can be thought of as local therapy: Only in the kidney and bladder, with the rare exceptions mentioned below, are adequate therapeutic levels achieved (Hooper, 2005b).

Methenamine. Methenamine is a urinary tract antiseptic and pro-drug that owes its activity to its capacity to generate formaldehyde.

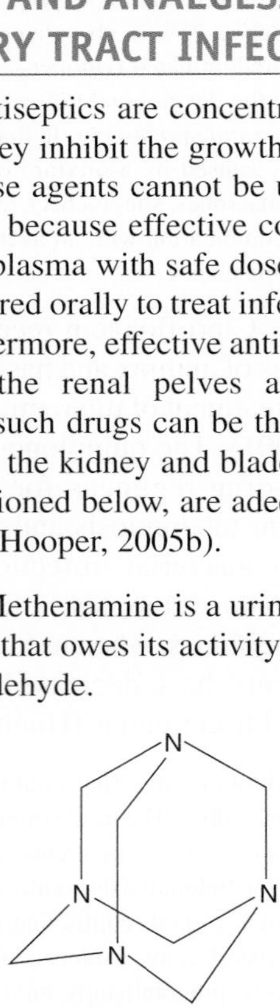

METHENAMINE

Chemistry. Methenamine is hexamethylenetetramine (hexamethylenamine). The compound decomposes in water to generate formaldehyde, according to the following reaction:

$$NH_4(CH_2)_6 + 6H_2O + 4H^+ \rightarrow 4NH_4^+ + 6HCHO$$

At pH 7.4, almost no decomposition occurs; the yield of formaldehyde is 6% of the theoretical amount at pH 6 and 20% at pH 5. Thus, acidification of the urine promotes formaldehyde formation and the formaldehyde-dependent antibacterial action. The decomposition reaction is fairly slow, and 3 hours are required to reach 90% completion.

Antimicrobial Activity. Nearly all bacteria are sensitive to free formaldehyde at concentrations of ~20 μg/mL. Urea-splitting microorganisms (e.g., *Proteus* spp.) tend to raise the pH of the urine and thus inhibit the release of formaldehyde. Microorganisms do not develop resistance to formaldehyde.

Pharmacology and Toxicology. Methenamine is absorbed orally, but 10-30% decomposes in the gastric juice unless the drug is protected by an enteric coating. Because of the ammonia produced, methenamine is contraindicated in hepatic insufficiency. Excretion in the urine is nearly quantitative. When the urine pH is 6 and the daily urine volume is 1000-1500 mL, a daily dose of 2 g will yield a urine concentration of 18-60 μg/mL of formaldehyde; this is more than the MIC for most urinary tract pathogens. Various poorly metabolized acids can be used to acidify the urine. Low pH alone is bacteriostatic, so acidification serves a double function. The acids commonly used are mandelic acid and hippuric acid (UREX, HIPREX).

GI distress frequently is caused by doses >500 mg four times a day, even with enteric-coated tablets. Painful and frequent micturition, albuminuria, hematuria, and rashes may result from doses of 4 to 8 g/day given for longer than 3-4 weeks. Once the urine is sterile, a high dose should be reduced. Because systemic methenamine has low toxicity at the typically used doses, renal insufficiency does not constitute a contraindication to the use of methenamine alone, but the acids given concurrently may be detrimental; methenamine mandelate is contraindicated in renal insufficiency. Crystalluria from the mandelate moiety can occur. Methenamine combines with sulfamethizole and perhaps other sulfonamides in the urine, which results in mutual antagonism; therefore, these drugs should not be used in combination.

Therapeutic Uses and Status. Methenamine is not a primary drug for the treatment of acute urinary tract infections, but it is of value for chronic suppressive treatment (Fihn, 2003). The agent is most useful when the causative organism is *E. coli*, but it usually can suppress the common gram-negative offenders and often *S. aureus* and *S. epidermidis* as well. *Enterobacter aerogenes* and *Proteus vulgaris* are usually resistant. Urea-splitting bacteria (mostly *Proteus*) make it difficult to control the urine pH. The physician should strive to keep the pH <5.5.

Nitrofurantoin. Nitrofurantoin (FURADANTIN, MACROBID, others) is a synthetic nitrofuran that is used for the prevention and treatment of infections of the urinary tract.

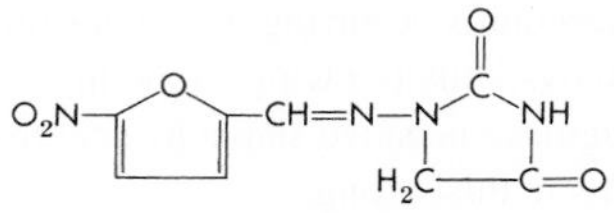

NITROFURANTOIN

Antimicrobial Activity. Enzymes capable of reducing nitrofurantoin appear to be crucial for its activation. Highly reactive intermediates are formed, and these seem to be responsible for the observed capacity of the drug to damage DNA. Bacteria reduce nitrofurantoin more rapidly than do mammalian cells, and this is thought to account for the selective antimicrobial activity of the compound. Bacteria that are susceptible to the drug rarely become resistant during therapy. Nitrofurantoin is active against many strains of *E. coli* and enterococci. However, most species of *Proteus* and *Pseudomonas* and many species of *Enterobacter* and *Klebsiella* are resistant. Nitrofurantoin is bacteriostatic for most susceptible microorganisms at concentrations of ≤32 μg/mL or less and is bactericidal at concentrations of ≥100 μg/mL. The antibacterial activity is higher in an acidic urine.

Pharmacology and Toxicity. Nitrofurantoin is absorbed rapidly and completely from the GI tract. The macrocrystalline form of the drug is absorbed and excreted more slowly. Antibacterial concentrations are not achieved in plasma following ingestion of recommended doses because the drug is eliminated rapidly. The plasma $t_{1/2}$ is 0.3-1 hour; ~40% is excreted unchanged into the urine. The average dose of nitrofurantoin yields a concentration in urine of ~200 μg/mL. This concentration is soluble at pH >5, but the urine should not be alkalinized because this reduces antimicrobial activity. The rate of excretion is linearly related to the creatinine clearance, so in patients with impaired glomerular function, the efficacy of the drug may be decreased and the systemic toxicity increased. Nitrofurantoin colors the urine brown.

The most common untoward effects are nausea, vomiting, and diarrhea; the macrocrystalline preparation is better tolerated than traditional formulations. Various hypersensitivity reactions occur occasionally. These include chills, fever, leukopenia, granulocytopenia, hemolytic anemia (associated with G6PD deficiency), cholestatic jaundice, and hepatocellular damage. Chronic active hepatitis is an uncommon but serious side effect. Acute pneumonitis with fever, chills, cough, dyspnea, chest pain, pulmonary infiltration, and eosinophilia may occur within hours to days of the initiation of therapy; these symptoms usually resolve quickly after discontinuation of the drug. More insidious subacute reactions also may be noted, and interstitial pulmonary fibrosis can occur in patients taking the drug chronically. This appears to be due to generation of oxygen radicals as a result of redox cycling of the drug in the lung. Elderly patients are especially susceptible to the pulmonary toxicity of nitrofurantoin. Megaloblastic anemia is rare. Various neurological disorders are observed occasionally. Headache, vertigo, drowsiness, muscular aches, and nystagmus are readily reversible, but severe polyneuropathies with demyelination and degeneration of both sensory and motor nerves have been reported; signs of denervation and muscle atrophy result. Neuropathies are most likely to occur in patients with impaired renal function and in persons on long-continued treatment.

The oral dosage of nitrofurantoin for adults is 50-100 mg four times a day with meals and at bedtime, less for the macrocrystalline formulation (100 mg every 12 hours for 7 days). Alternatively, the daily dosage is better expressed as 5-7 mg/kg in four divided doses (not to exceed 400 mg). A single 50-100-mg dose at bedtime may be sufficient to prevent recurrences. The daily dose for children is 5 to 7 mg/kg but may be as low as 1 mg/kg for long-term therapy. A course of therapy should not exceed 14 days, and repeated courses should be separated by rest periods. Pregnant women, individuals with impaired renal function (creatinine clearance <40 mL/minute), and children <1 month of age should not receive nitrofurantoin.

Nitrofurantoin is approved only for the treatment of urinary tract infections caused by microorganisms known to be susceptible to the drug. Currently, bacterial resistance to nitrofurantoin is more frequent than resistance to fluoroquinolones or trimethoprim-sulfamethoxazole, making nitrofurantoin a second-line agent for treatment of urinary tract infections (Fihn, 2003). Nitrofurantoin is not recommended for treatment of pyelonephritis or prostatitis.

Phenazopyridine. Phenazopyridine hydrochloride (PYRIDIUM, others) is *not* a urinary antiseptic. However, it does have an analgesic action on the urinary tract and alleviates symptoms of dysuria, frequency, burning, and urgency.

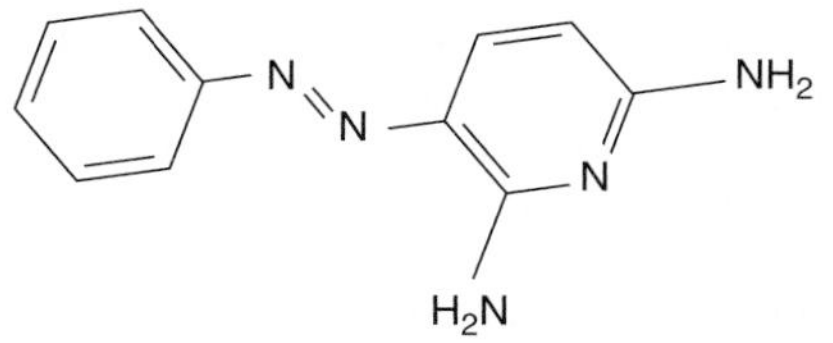

N N NH₂ N H₂N

PHENAZOPYRIDINE

The usual dose is 200 mg three times daily. The compound is an azo dye, which colors urine orange or red; the patient should be so informed. GI upset is seen in up to 10% of patients and can be reduced by administering the drug with food; overdosage may result in methemoglobinemia. Phenazopyridine has been marketed since 1925 and has had dual prescription/over-the-counter (OTC) marketing status since 1951. As part of their ongoing review of OTC drug products, the Food and Drug Administration (FDA) is currently in the process of evaluating products containing <200 mg phenazopyridine to determine whether these products generally are recognized as safe and effective as urinary analgesics. The outcome of this evaluation will determine the continued availability of OTC phenazopyridine products in the U.S. Products containing 200 mg phenazopyridine are sold by prescription, but their long-term availability in the marketplace also may be affected by the FDA's final OTC ruling. Phenazopyridine is no longer available in Canada.

BIBLIOGRAPHY

Alovero FL, Pan XS, Morris JE, *et al.* Engineering the specificity of antibacterial fluoroquinolones: benzenesulfonamide modifications at C-7 of ciprofloxacin change its primary target in *Streptococcus pneumoniae* from topoisomerase IV to gyrase. *Antimicrob Agents Chemother*, **2000,** *44:*320–325.

American Thoracic Society, CDC and Infectious Diseases Society of America. Practice guidelines for the treatment of tuberculosis. *MMWR*, **2003,** *52* (No. RR-11).

Burkhardt JE, Walterspeil JN, Schaad UB. Quinolone arthropathy in animals versus children. *Clin Infect Dis*, **1997,** *25:* 1196–1204.

Bushby SR, Hitchings GH. Trimethoprim, a sulphonamide potentiator. *Br J Pharmacol*, **1968,** *33:*72–90.

Centers for Disease Control and Prevention. Guidelines for prevention and treatment of opportunistic infections in HIV-infected adults and adolescents *MMWR*, **2009,** *58* (No. RR-4):1–207. Available at: http://aidsinfo.nih.gov/contentfiles/Adult_OI.pdf. Accessed December 16, 2009.

Chen DK, McGeer A, de Azavedo JC, Low DE. Decreased susceptibility of *Streptococcus pneumoniae* to fluoroquinolones in Canada. Canadian Bacterial Surveillance Network. *N Engl J Med*, **1999,** *341:*233–239.

Chocarro A, Gonzalez A, Garcia I. Treatment of tularemia with ciprofloxacin. *Clin Infect Dis*, **2000,** *31:*623.

Cozzarelli NR. DNA gyrase and the supercoiling of DNA. *Science*, **1980,** *207*:953–960.

Edelstein PH, Cianciotto NP. *Legionella*. In: *Mandell, Douglas, and Bennett's Principles and Practice of Infectious Diseases*, 6th ed. (Mandell GL, Bennett JE, Dolin R, eds.), Churchill Livingstone, New York, **2005**, pp. 2711–2727.

Fihn SD. Acute uncomplicated urinary tract infection in women. *N Engl J Med*, **2003,** *349:*259–266.

Gluckstein D, Ruskin J. Rapid oral desensitization to trimethoprim-sulfamethoxazole (TMP-SMZ): Use in prophylaxis for *Pneumocystis carinii* pneumonia in patients with AIDS who were previously tolerant to TMP-SMZ. *Clin Infect Dis*, **1995,** *20:*849–853.

Gold HS, Moellering RC Jr. Antimicrobial-drug resistance. *N Engl J Med*, **1996,** *335:*1445–1453.

Halliwell RF, Davey PG, Lambert JJ. Antagonism of $GABA_A$ receptors by 4-quinolones. *J Antimicrob Chemother*, **1993,** *31:*457–462.

Hill DR, Ericsson CD, Pearson RD, *et al.* The practice of travel medicine: Guidelines by the Infectious Diseases Society of America. *Clin Infect Dis,* **2006,** *43:*1499–1539.

Hitchings GH. A biochemical approach to chemotherapy. *Ann NY Acad Sci*, **1961,** *23:*700–708.

Hooper DC. Quinolones. In: *Mandell, Douglas, and Bennett's Principles and Practice of Infectious Diseases*, 6th ed. (Mandell GL, Bennett JE, Dolin R, eds.), Churchill Livingstone, New York, **2005a,** pp. 451–467.

Hooper DC. Urinary tract agents: Nitrofurantoin and methenamine. In: *Mandell, Douglas, and Bennett's Principles and Practice of Infectious Diseases*, 6th ed. (Mandell GL, Bennett JE, Dolin R, eds.), Churchill Livingstone, New York, **2005b,** pp. 473–476.

Hughes WT, Armstrong D, Bodey GP, *et al.* 2002 guidelines for the use of antimicrobial agents in neutropenic patients with cancer. *Clin Infect Dis,* **2002,** *34:*730–751.

Lesch JE. *The First Miracle Drugs: How the Sulfa Drugs Transformed Medicine*. Oxford University Press, New York, **2007.**

Mandell LA. Improved safety profile of newer fluoroquinolone. In: *Fluoroquinolone Antibiotics* (Ronald AR, Low DE, eds.), Birkhauser, Basel, **2003,** pp. 73–86.

Medical Letter. Gatifloxacin and moxifloxacin: Two new fluoroquinolones. *Med Lett Drugs Ther*, **2000,** *42:*15–17.

Medical Letter. Gemifloxacin. *Med Lett Drugs Ther*, **2004,** *46:* 78–80.

Miedouge M, Hacini J, Grimont F, Watine J. Shiga toxin–producing *Escherichia coli* urinary tract infection associated with hemolytic-uremic syndrome in an adult and possible adverse effect of ofloxacin therapy. *Clin Infect Dis*, **2000,** *30:*395–396.

Mitscher LA, Ma Z. Structure-activity relationships of quinolones. In: *Fluoroquinolone Antibiotics* (Ronald AR, Low DE, eds.), Birkhauser, Basel, **2003,** pp. 11–48.

Montoya JG, Kovacs JA, Remington JS. *Toxoplasma gondii*. In: *Mandell, Douglas, and Bennett's Principles and Practice of Infectious Diseases*, 6th ed. (Mandell GL, Bennett JE, Dolin R, eds.), Churchill Livingstone, New York, **2005,** 3170–3193.

Newman LM, Wang SA, Ohye RG, *et al*. The epidemiology of fluoroquinolone-resistant *Neisseria gonorrhoeae* in Hawaii, 2001. *Clin Infect Dis*, **2004,** *38:*649–654.

Oethinger M, Kern WV, Jellen-Ritter AS, *et al.* Ineffectiveness of topoisomerase mutations in mediating clinically significant fluoroquinolone resistance in *Escherichia coli* in the absence of the AcrAB efflux pump. *Antimicrob Agents Chemother*, **2000,** *44:*10–13.

Olson RP, Harrell LJ, Kaye KS, Antibiotic Resistance in Urinary Isolates of E. coli from College Women with Urinary Tract Infections. *Antimicrob Agents Chemother*, **2009,** *53*: 1285–1286.

Park-Wyllie LY, Juurlink DN, Kopp A, *et al.* Outpatient gatifloxacin therapy and dysglycemia in older adults. *N Engl J Med*, **2006,** *354:*1352–1361.

Sabharwal V, Marchant CD. Fluoroquinolone use in children. *Pediatr Infect Dis J,* **2006,** *25:*257–258.

Schwartz J, Jauregui L, Lettieri J, Bachmann K. Impact of ciprofloxacin on theophylline clearance and steady-state concentrations in serum. *Antimicrob Agents Chemother*, **1988,** *32:*75–77.

Sheehan G, Chew NSY. The history of quinolones. In: *Fluoroquinolone Antibiotics* (Ronald AR, Low DE, eds.), Birkhauser, Basel, **2003,** pp. 1–10.

Swartz MN. Recognition and management of anthrax: An update. *N Engl J Med*, **2001,** *345:*1621–1626.

Thomas CF, Limper AH. *Pneumocystis* pneumonia. *N Engl J Med*, **2004,** *350:*2487–2498.

Wong CS, Jelacic S, Habeeb RL, *et al.* The risk of the hemolytic-uremic syndrome after antibiotic treatment of *Escherichia coli* O157:H7. *N Engl J Med*, **2000,** *342:*1930–1936.

Wortmann GW, Bennett SP. Fatal meningitis due to levofloxacin-resistant *Streptococcus pneumoniae. Clin Infect Dis*, **1999,** *29:*1599–1600.

Zinner SH, Mayer KH. Sulfonamides and trimethoprim. In: *Mandell, Douglas, and Bennett's Principles and Practice of Infectious Diseases*, 6th ed. (Mandell GL, Bennett JE, Dolin R, eds.), Churchill Livingstone, New York, **2005,** pp. 440–443.

Gonococcal Infections. Gonococci gradually have become more resistant to penicillin G, and penicillins are no longer the therapy of choice, unless it is known that gonococcal strains in a particular geographic area are susceptible. Uncomplicated gonococcal urethritis is the most common infection, and a single intramuscular injection of 250 mg ceftriaxone is the recommended treatment (Handsfield and Sparling, 2005).

Gonococcal arthritis, disseminated gonococcal infections with skin lesions, and gonococcemia should be treated with ceftriaxone 1 g daily given either intramuscularly or intravenously for 7-10 days. Ophthalmia neonatorum also should be treated with ceftriaxone for 7-10 days (25-50 mg/kg per day intramuscularly or intravenously).

Syphilis. Therapy of syphilis with penicillin G is highly effective. Primary, secondary, and latent syphilis of <1-year duration may be treated with penicillin G procaine (2.4 million units per day intramuscularly) plus probenecid (1.0 g/day orally) for 10 days or with 1-3 weekly intramuscular doses of 2.4 million units of penicillin G benzathine (three doses in patients with HIV infection). Patients with late latent syphilis, neurosyphilis, or cardiovascular syphilis may be treated with a variety of regimens. Because the latter two conditions are potentially lethal and their progression can be halted (but not reversed), intensive therapy with 20 million units of penicillin G daily for 10 days is recommended. There are no proven alternatives for treating syphilis in pregnant women, so penicillin-allergic individuals must be acutely desensitized to prevent anaphylaxis (Centers for Disease Control and Prevention, 2006).

Infants with congenital syphilis discovered at birth or during the postnatal period should be treated for at least 10 days with 50,000 units/kg daily of aqueous penicillin G in two divided doses or 50,000 units/kg of procaine penicillin G in a single daily dose (Tramont, 2005).

Most patients (70-90%) with secondary syphilis develop the Jarisch-Herxheimer reaction. This also may be seen in patients with other forms of syphilis. Several hours after the first injection of penicillin, chills, fever, headache, myalgias, and arthralgias may develop. The syphilitic cutaneous lesions may become more prominent, edematous, and brilliant in color. Manifestations usually persist for a few hours, and the rash begins to fade within 48 hours. It does not recur with the second or subsequent injections of penicillin. This reaction is thought to be due to release of spirochetal antigens with subsequent host reactions to the products. Aspirin gives symptomatic relief, and therapy with penicillin should not be discontinued.

Actinomycosis. Penicillin G is the agent of choice for the treatment of all forms of actinomycosis. The dose should be 10-20 million units of penicillin G intravenously per day for 6 weeks. Some physicians continue therapy for 2-3 months with oral penicillin V (500 mg four times daily). Surgical drainage or excision of the lesion may be necessary before cure is accomplished.

Diphtheria. There is no evidence that penicillin or any other antibiotic alters the incidence of complications or the outcome of diphtheria; specific antitoxin is the only effective treatment. However, penicillin G eliminates the carrier state. The parenteral administration of 2-3 million units per day in divided doses for 10-12 days eliminates the diphtheria bacilli from the pharynx and other sites in practically 100% of patients. A single daily injection of penicillin G procaine for the same period produces comparable results.

Anthrax. Strains of *Bacillus anthracis* resistant to penicillin have been recovered from human infections. When penicillin G is used, the dose should be 12-20 million units per day.

Clostridial Infections. Penicillin G is the agent of choice for gas gangrene; the dose is in the range of 12-20 million units per day given parenterally as an adjunct to the antitoxin. Adequate debridement of the infected areas is essential. Antimicrobial drugs probably have no effect on the ultimate outcome of tetanus. Débridement and administration of human tetanus immune globulin may be indicated. Penicillin is administered, however, to eradicate the vegetative forms of the bacteria that may persist.

Fusospirochetal Infections. Gingivostomatitis, produced by the synergistic action of *Leptotrichia buccalis* and spirochetes that are present in the mouth, is readily treatable with penicillin. For simple "trench mouth," 500 mg penicillin V given every 6 hours for several days is usually sufficient to clear the disease.

Rat-Bite Fever. The two microorganisms responsible for this infection, *Spirillum minor* in the Far East and *Streptobacillus moniliformis* in America and Europe, are sensitive to penicillin G, the therapeutic agent of choice. Because most cases due to *Streptobacillus* are complicated by bacteremia and, in many instances, by metastatic infections, especially of the synovia and endocardium, the dose should be large; a daily dose of 12-15 million units given parenterally for 3-4 weeks has been recommended.

Listeria Infections. Ampicillin (with gentamicin for immunosuppressed patients with meningitis) and penicillin G are the drugs of choice in the management of infections owing to *L. monocytogenes*. The recommended dose of ampicillin is 1-2 g intravenously every 4 hours. The recommended dose of penicillin G is 15-20 million units parenterally per day for at least 2 weeks. When endocarditis is the problem, the dose is the same, but the duration of treatment should be no less than 4 weeks.

Lyme Disease. Although a tetracycline is the usual drug of choice for early disease, amoxicillin is effective; the dose is 500 mg three times daily for 21 days. Severe disease is treated with a third-generation cephalosporin or up to 20 million units of intravenous penicillin G daily for 10-14 days.

Erysipeloid. The causative agent of this disease, *Erysipelothrix rhusiopathiae*, is sensitive to penicillin. The uncomplicated infection responds well to a single injection of 1.2 million units of penicillin G benzathine. When endocarditis is present, penicillin G, 12-20 million units per day, has been found to be effective; therapy should be continued for 4-6 weeks.

Pasteurella multocida. Pasteurella multocida is the cause of wound infections after a cat or dog bite. It is uniformly susceptible to penicillin G and ampicillin and resistant to penicillinase-resistant penicillins and first-generation cephalosporins (Goldstein et al., 1988). When the infection causes meningitis, a third-generation cephalosporin is preferred because the MICs are slightly lower than for penicillin.

Prophylactic Uses of the Penicillins. The demonstrated effectiveness of penicillin in eradicating microorganisms was followed quickly and quite naturally by attempts to prove that it also was effective in preventing infection in susceptible hosts. As a result, the antibiotic has been administered in almost every situation in which a risk of bacterial invasion has been present. As prophylaxis has been investigated under controlled conditions, it has become clear that penicillin is highly effective in some situations, useless and potentially dangerous in others, and of questionable value in still others (Chapter 48).

Streptococcal Infections. The administration of penicillin to individuals exposed to *S. pyogenes* affords protection from infection. The oral ingestion of 200,000 units of penicillin G or penicillin V twice a day or a single injection of 1.2 million units of penicillin G benzathine is effective. Indications for this type of prophylaxis include outbreaks of streptococcal disease in closed populations, such as boarding schools or military bases. Patients with extensive deep burns are at high risk of severe wound infections with *S. pyogenes;* "low-dose" prophylaxis for several days appears to be effective in reducing the incidence of this complication.

Recurrences of Rheumatic Fever. The oral administration of 200,000 units of penicillin G or penicillin V every 12 hours produces a striking decrease in the incidence of recurrences of rheumatic fever in susceptible individuals. Because of the difficulties of compliance, parenteral administration is preferable, especially in children. The intramuscular injection of 1.2 million units of penicillin G benzathine once a month yields excellent results. In cases of hypersensitivity to penicillin, sulfisoxazole or sulfadiazine, 1 g twice a day for adults, also is effective; for children weighing <27 kg, the dose is halved. Prophylaxis must be continued throughout the year. The duration of such treatment is an unsettled question. It has been suggested that prophylaxis should be continued for life because instances of acute rheumatic fever have been observed in the fifth and sixth decades. However, the necessity for such prolonged prophylaxis has not been established and may be unnecessary for young adults judged to be at low risk for recurrence (Berrios et al., 1993).

Syphilis. Prophylaxis for a contact with syphilis consists of a course of therapy as described for primary syphilis. A serological test for syphilis should be performed at monthly intervals for at least 4 months thereafter.

Surgical Procedures in Patients with Valvular Heart Disease. About 25% of cases of subacute bacterial endocarditis follow dental extractions. This observation, together with the fact that up to 80% of persons who have teeth removed experience a transient bacteremia, emphasizes the potential importance of chemoprophylaxis for those who have congenital or acquired valvular heart disease of any type and need to undergo dental procedures. Since transient bacterial invasion of the bloodstream occurs occasionally after surgical procedures (e.g., tonsillectomy and genitourinary and GI procedures) and during childbirth, these, too, are indications for prophylaxis in patients with valvular heart disease. Whether the incidence of bacterial endocarditis actually is altered by this type of chemoprophylaxis remains to be determined.

Detailed recommendations for adults and children with valvular heart disease have been formulated (Wilson et al., 2007).

The Penicillinase-Resistant Penicillins

The penicillins described in this section are resistant to hydrolysis by staphylococcal penicillinase. Their appropriate use should be restricted to the treatment of infections that are known or suspected to be caused by staphylococci that elaborate the enzyme, which now includes the vast majority of strains of this bacterium that are encountered clinically. These drugs are much less active than penicillin G against other penicillin-sensitive microorganisms, including non-penicillinase-producing staphylococci.

The role of the penicillinase-resistant penicillins as the agents of choice for most staphylococcal disease is changing with the increasing incidence of isolates of so-called *methicillin-resistant microorganisms.* As commonly used, this term denotes resistance of these bacteria to all the penicillinase-resistant penicillins and cephalosporins. Hospital-acquired strains usually are resistant to the aminoglycosides, tetracyclines, erythromycin, and clindamycin as well. Vancomycin is considered the drug of choice for such infections, although intermediate-level resistance is emerging (Centers for Disease Control and Prevention, 2004). Some physicians use a combination of vancomycin and rifampin, especially for life-threatening infections and those involving foreign bodies. Community-acquired methicillin-resistant strains are less likely to be resistant to other classes of antibiotics with the exception of macrolides (Okuma et al., 2002). MRSA contains an additional high-molecular-weight PBP with a very low affinity for β-lactam antibiotics (Spratt, 1994). From 40-60% of strains of *S. epidermidis* also are resistant to the penicillinase-resistant penicillins by the same mechanism. As with MRSA, these strains may appear to be susceptible to cephalosporins on disk-sensitivity testing, but there usually is a significant population of microbes that is resistant to cephalosporins and emerges during such therapy. Vancomycin also is the drug of choice for serious infection caused by methicillin-resistant *S. epidermidis;* rifampin is given concurrently when a foreign body is involved.

The Isoxazolyl Penicillins: Oxacillin, Cloxacillin, and Dicloxacillin. These three congeneric semisynthetic penicillins are similar pharmacologically and thus conveniently are considered together. Their structural formulas are shown in Table 53–1. All are relatively stable in an acidic medium and absorbed adequately after oral administration. All are markedly resistant to cleavage by penicillinase. These drugs are not substitutes for penicillin G in the treatment of diseases amenable to it, and they are not active against enterococci or *Listeria.* Furthermore, because of variability in intestinal absorption, oral administration is not a substitute for the parenteral route in the treatment of serious staphylococcal infections that require a penicillin unaffected by penicillinase.

Pharmacological Properties. The isoxazolyl penicillins are potent inhibitors of the growth of most penicillinase-producing staphylococci.

This is their valid clinical use. Dicloxacillin is the most active, and many strains of *S. aureus* are inhibited by concentrations of 0.05-0.8 μg/mL. Comparable values for cloxacillin (not currently marketed in the U.S.) and oxacillin are 0.1-3 and 0.4-6 μg/mL, respectively. These differences may have little practical significance, however, because dosages are adjusted accordingly. These agents are, in general, less effective against microorganisms susceptible to penicillin G, and they are not useful against gram-negative bacteria.

These agents are absorbed rapidly but incompletely (30-80%) from the GI tract. Absorption of the drugs is more efficient when they are taken on an empty stomach; preferably they are administered 1 hour before or 2 hours after meals to ensure better absorption. Peak concentrations in plasma are attained by 1 hour and ~5-10 μg/mL after the ingestion of 1 g oxacillin. Slightly higher concentrations are achieved after the administration of 1 g cloxacillin, whereas the same oral dose of dicloxacillin yields peak plasma concentrations of 15 μg/mL. There is little evidence that these differences are of clinical significance. All these congeners are bound to plasma albumin to a great extent (~90-95%); none is removed from the circulation to a significant degree by hemodialysis.

The isoxazolyl penicillins are excreted rapidly by the kidney. Normally, ~50% of a dose of these drugs is excreted in the urine in the first 6 hours after oral administration. There also is significant hepatic elimination of these agents in the bile. The half-lives for all are between 30 and 60 minutes. Intervals between doses of oxacillin, cloxacillin, and dicloxacillin do not have to be altered for patients with renal failure. The differences just noted in plasma concentrations produced by the isoxazolyl penicillins are related mainly to differences in rate of urinary excretion and degree of resistance to degradation in the liver.

Nafcillin. This semisynthetic penicillin is highly resistant to penicillinase and has proven effective against infections caused by penicillinase-producing strains of *S. aureus*. Its structural formula is shown in Table 53–1.

Pharmacological Properties. Nafcillin is slightly more active than oxacillin against penicillin G–resistant *S. aureus* (most strains are inhibited by 0.06–2 μg/mL). Although it is the most active of the penicillinase-resistant penicillins against other microorganisms, it is not as potent as penicillin G. The peak plasma concentration is ~8 μg/mL 60 minutes after a 1-g intramuscular dose. Nafcillin is ~90% bound to plasma protein. Peak concentrations of nafcillin in bile are well above those found in plasma. Concentrations of the drug in CSF appear to be adequate for therapy of staphylococcal meningitis.

The Aminopenicillins: Ampicillin, Amoxicillin, and Their Congeners

These agents have similar antibacterial activity and a spectrum that is broader than the antibiotics already discussed. They all are destroyed by β-lactamase (from both gram-positive and gram-negative bacteria).

Antimicrobial Activity. Ampicillin and the related aminopenicillins are bactericidal for both gram-positive and gram-negative bacteria. The meningococci and *L. monocytogenes* are sensitive to this class of drugs. Many pneumococcal isolates have varying levels of resistance to ampicillin. Penicillin-resistant strains should be considered ampicillin/amoxicillin-resistant. *H. influenzae* and the *viridans* group of streptococci exhibit varying degrees of resistance. Enterococci are about twice as sensitive to ampicillin on a weight basis as they are to penicillin G (MIC for ampicillin averages 1.5 μg/mL). Although most strains of *N. gonorrhoeae, E. coli, P. mirabilis*, *Salmonella,* and *Shigella* were highly susceptible when ampicillin was first used in the early 1960s, an increasing percentage of these species now is resistant. From 30% to 50% of *E. coli*, a significant number of *P. mirabilis*, and practically all species of *Enterobacter* presently are insensitive. Resistant strains of *Salmonella* (plasmid mediated) have been recovered with increasing frequency in various parts of the world. Most strains of *Shigella* now are resistant. Most strains of *Pseudomonas, Klebsiella*, *Serratia*, *Acinetobacter,* and indole-positive *Proteus* also are resistant to this group of penicillins; these antibiotics are less active against *B. fragilis* than penicillin G. However, concurrent administration of a β-lactamase inhibitor such as clavulanate or *sulbactam* markedly expands the spectrum of activity of these drugs.

Ampicillin. This drug is the prototype of the group. Its structural formula is shown in Table 53–1.

Pharmacological Properties. Ampicillin (PRINCIPEN, others) is stable in acid and is well absorbed after oral administration. An oral dose of 0.5 g produces peak concentrations in plasma of ~3 μg/mL at 2 hours. Intake of food prior to ingestion of ampicillin diminishes absorption. Intramuscular injection of 0.5 or 1 g sodium ampicillin yields peak plasma concentrations of ~7 or 10 μg/mL, respectively, at 1 hour; these decline exponentially, with a $t_{1/2}$ of ~80 minutes. Severe renal impairment markedly prolongs the persistence of ampicillin in the plasma. Peritoneal dialysis is ineffective in removing the drug from the blood, but hemodialysis removes ~40% of the body store in ~7 hours. Adjustment of the dose of ampicillin is required in the presence of renal dysfunction. Ampicillin appears in the bile, undergoes enterohepatic circulation, and is excreted in appreciable quantities in the feces.

Amoxicillin. This drug, a penicillinase-susceptible semi-synthetic penicillin, is a close chemical and pharmacological relative of ampicillin (Table 53–1). The drug is stable in acid and designed for oral use. It is absorbed more rapidly and completely from the GI tract than ampicillin, which is the major difference between the two. The antimicrobial spectrum of amoxicillin is essentially identical to that of ampicillin, with the important exception that amoxicillin appears to be less effective than ampicillin for shigellosis.

Peak plasma concentrations of amoxicillin (AMOXIL, others) are 2-2.5 times greater for amoxicillin than for ampicillin after oral

Table 53–1

Chemical Structures and Major Properties of Various Penicillins

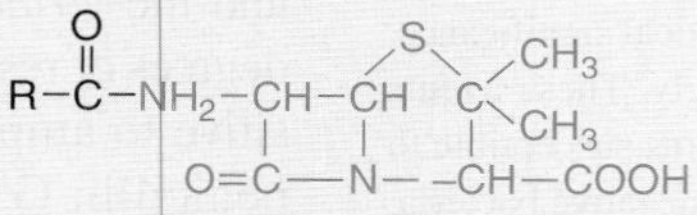

$$R{-}\overset{O}{\overset{\|}{C}}{-}NH_2{-}CH{-}CH\ \ C(CH_3)_2 \quad (\text{S ring}); \quad O{=}C{-}N{-}CH{-}COOH$$

Penicillins are substituted 6-aminopenicillanic acids

R	NONPROPRIETARY NAME	MAJOR PROPERTIES: *Absorption after Oral Administration*	MAJOR PROPERTIES: *Resistance to Penicillinase*	MAJOR PROPERTIES: *Useful Antimicrobial Spectrum*
$C_6H_5{-}CH_2{-}$	Penicillin G	Variable (poor)	No	*Streptococcus* species,[a] Enterococci,[a] *Listeria, Neisseria meningitidis*, many anaerobes (not *Bacteroides fragilis*),[b] spirochetes, *Actinomyces, Erysipelothrix* spp., *Pasteurella multocida*[b]
$C_6H_5{-}OCH_2{-}$	Penicillin V	Good	No	
2,6-(OCH_3)$_2$$C_6H_3{-}$	Methicillin	Poor (not given orally)	Yes	
Phenyl (R_1, R_2)–isoxazolyl (CH_3)	Oxacillin ($R_1 = R_2 = H$) Cloxacillin (R_1 = Cl; R_2 = H) Dicloxacillin ($R_1 = R_2$ = Cl)	Good	Yes	Indicated only for non-methicillin-resistant strains of *Staphylococcus aureus* and *Staphylococcus epidermidis*. Compared to other penicillins, these penicillinase-resistant penicillins lack activity against *Listeria monocytogenes* and *Enterococcus* spp.
2-OC_2H_5-naphthyl	Nafcillin	Variable	Yes	
$R_1{-}C_6H_4{-}CH(NH_2){-}$	Ampicillin[c] (R_1 = H)	Good	No	
	Amoxicillin (R_1 = OH)	Excellent		Extends spectrum of penicillin to include sensitive strains of Enterobacteriaceae,[b] *Escherichia coli, Proteus mirabilis, Salmonella, Shigella, Haemophilus influenzae*,[b] and *Helicobacter pylori*. Superior to penicillin for treatment of *Listeria monocytogenes* and sensitive enterococci. Amoxicillin most active of all oral β-lactams against penicillin-resistant *Streptococcus pneumoniae*

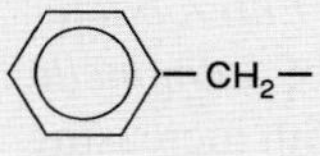

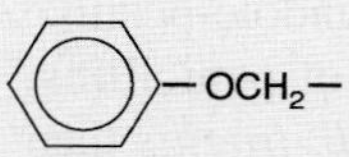

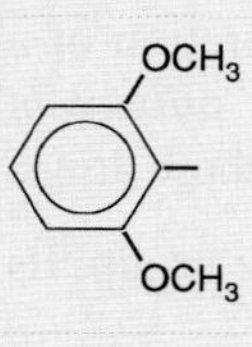

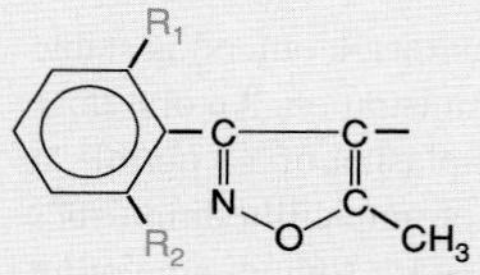

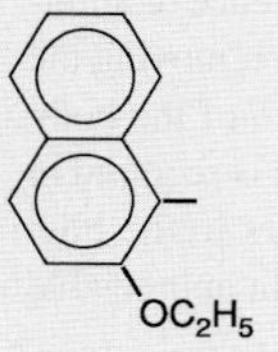

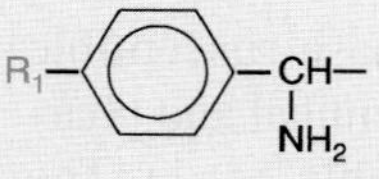

(*Continued*)

Table 53–1

Chemical Structures and Major Properties of Various Penicillins (*Continued*)

R	NONPROPRIETARY NAME	MAJOR PROPERTIES: *Absorption after Oral Administration*	*Resistance to Penicillinase*	*Useful Antimicrobial Spectrum*
Phenyl–CH(COOR$_1$)–	Carbenicillin (R_1 = H)	Poor (not given orally)		
	Carbenicillin indanyl (R_1 = 5-indanol)	Good	No	Less active than ampicillin against Streptococcus species, *Enterococcus faecalis, Klebsiella*, and *Listeria monocytogenes*. Activity against *Pseudomonas aeruginosa* is inferior to that of mezlocillin and piperacillin
Thienyl–CH(COOH)–	Ticarcillin	Poor (not given orally)	No	
Phenyl–CH(NHCO–N-imidazolidinone–N–SO_2CH_3)–	Mezlocillin	Poor (not given orally)	No	
Phenyl–CH(NHCO–N-dioxopiperazine–N–C_2H_5)–	Piperacillin	Poor (not given orally)	No	Extends spectrum of ampicillin to include *Psuedomonas aeruginosa*,[d] Enterobacteriaceae,[b] Bacteroides species[b]

[a]Many strains are resistant due to altered penicillin-binding proteins. [b]Many strains are resistant due to production of β-lactamases. [c]There are other congeners of ampicillin; *see* the text. [d]Some strains are resistant due to decreased entry or active efflux.

administration of the same dose; they are reached at 2 hours and average ~4 μg/mL when 250 mg is administered. Food does not interfere with absorption. Perhaps because of more complete absorption of this congener, the incidence of diarrhea with amoxicillin is less than that following administration of ampicillin. The incidence of other adverse effects appears to be similar. Although the $t_{1/2}$ of amoxicillin is similar to that for ampicillin, effective concentrations of orally administered amoxicillin are detectable in the plasma for twice as long as with ampicillin, again because of the more complete absorption. About 20% of amoxicillin is protein bound in plasma, a value similar to that for ampicillin. Most of a dose of the antibiotic is excreted in an active form in the urine. Probenecid delays excretion of the drug.

Therapeutic Indications for the Aminopenicillins

Upper Respiratory Infections. Ampicillin and amoxicillin are active against *S. pyogenes* and many strains of *S. pneumoniae* and *H. influenzae*, which are major upper respiratory bacterial pathogens. The drugs constitute effective therapy for sinusitis, otitis media, acute exacerbations of chronic bronchitis, and epiglottitis caused by sensitive strains of these organisms. Amoxicillin is the most active of all the oral β-lactam antibiotics against both penicillin-sensitive and penicillin-resistant *S. pneumoniae*. Based on the increasing prevalence of pneumococcal resistance to penicillin, an increase in dose of oral amoxicillin (from 40-45 up to 80-90 mg/kg per day) for empirical treatment of acute otitis media in children is recommended (Dowell et al., 1999). Ampicillin-resistant *H. influenzae* may be a problem in many areas. The addition of a β-lactamase inhibitor (amoxicillin-clavulanate or ampicillin-sulbactam) extends the spectrum to β-lactamase-producing *H. influenzae* and Enterobacteriaceae. Bacterial pharyngitis should be treated with penicillin G or penicillin V because *S. pyogenes* is the major pathogen.

Urinary Tract Infections. Most uncomplicated urinary tract infections are caused by Enterobacteriaceae, and *E. coli* is the most common species; ampicillin often is an effective agent, although resistance is increasingly common. Enterococcal urinary tract infections are treated effectively with ampicillin alone.

Meningitis. Acute bacterial meningitis in children is most frequently due to *S. pneumoniae* or *N. meningitidis*. Because 20-30% of strains of *S. pneumoniae* now may be resistant to this antibiotic, ampicillin is not indicated for single-agent treatment of meningitis. Ampicillin has excellent activity against *L. monocytogenes*, a cause of meningitis in immunocompromised persons. Thus, the combination of ampicillin and vancomycin plus a third-generation cephalosporin is a rational regimen for empirical treatment of suspected bacterial meningitis.

Salmonella Infections. Disease associated with bacteremia, disease with metastatic foci, and the enteric fever syndrome (including typhoid fever) respond favorably to antibiotics. A fluoroquinolone or ceftriaxone is considered by some to be the drug of choice, but the administration of trimethoprim-sulfamethoxazole or high doses of ampicillin (12 g/day for adults) also is effective. In some geographic areas, resistance to ampicillin is common. The typhoid carrier state has been eliminated successfully in patients without gallbladder disease with ampicillin, trimethoprim-sulfamethoxazole, or ciprofloxacin.

Anti-Pseudomonal Penicillins: The Carboxypenicillins and the Ureidopenicillins

The carboxypenicillins, carbenicillin (discontinued in the U.S.) and ticarcillin (marketed in combination with clavulanate in the U.S.) and their close relatives, are active against some isolates of *P. aeruginosa* and certain indole-positive *Proteus* spp. that are resistant to ampicillin and its congeners. They are ineffective against most strains of *S. aureus, Enterococcus faecalis, Klebsiella,* and *L. monocytogenes. B. fragilis* is susceptible to high concentrations of these drugs, but penicillin G is actually more active on the basis of weight. The ureidopenicillins, mezlocillin (discontinued in the U.S.) and piperacillin, have superior activity against *P. aeruginosa* compared with carbenicillin and ticarcillin. In addition, mezlocillin and piperacillin are useful for treatment of infections with *Klebsiella.* The carboxypenicillins and the ureidopenicillins are sensitive to destruction by β-lactamases.

Carbenicillin. This drug is a penicillinase-susceptible derivative of 6-aminopenicillanic acid. Its structural formula is shown in Table 53–1. Carbenicillin was the first penicillin with activity against *P. aeruginosa* and some *Proteus* strains that are resistant to ampicillin. Because carbenicillin is supplied as a disodium salt, it contains ~5 mEq Na^+ per gram of drug, and this results in the administration of >100 mEq Na^+ to patients treated for *P. aeruginosa* infections. In the U.S., carbenicillin has been superseded by piperacillin.

Preparations of carbenicillin may cause adverse effects in addition to those that follow the use of other penicillins. Congestive heart failure may result from the administration of excessive Na^+. Hypokalemia may occur because of obligatory excretion of cation with the large amount of nonreabsorbable anion (carbenicillin) presented to the distal renal tubule. The drug interferes with platelet function, and bleeding may occur because of abnormal aggregation of platelets.

Carbenicillin Indanyl Sodium. This congener is the indanyl ester of carbenicillin; it is acid stable and is suitable for oral administration. After absorption, the ester is converted rapidly to carbenicillin by hydrolysis of the ester linkage. The antimicrobial spectrum of the drug is therefore that of carbenicillin. Although the concentration of carbenicillin reached in the serum is not high enough to treat a systemic *Pseudomonas* infection, the active moiety is excreted rapidly in the urine, where it achieves effective concentrations. Thus, the only use of this drug is for the management of urinary tract infections caused by *Proteus* spp. other than *P. mirabilis* and by *P. aeruginosa.*

Piperacillin. Piperacillin extends the spectrum of ampicillin to include most strains of *P. aeruginosa*, Enterobacteriaceae (non-β-lactamase-producing), many *Bacteroides* spp., and *E. faecalis*. In combination with a β-lactamase inhibitor (piperacillin-tazobactam, ZOSYN) it has the broadest antibacterial spectrum of the penicillins. Pharmacokinetic properties are reminiscent of the other ureidopenicillins. High biliary concentrations are achieved.

Therapeutic Indications. Piperacillin and related agents are important agents for the treatment of patients with serious infections caused by gram-negative bacteria. Such patients frequently have impaired immunological defenses, and their infections often are acquired in the hospital. Therefore, these penicillins find their greatest use in treating bacteremias, pneumonias, infections following burns, and urinary tract infections owing to microorganisms resistant to penicillin G and ampicillin; the bacteria especially responsible include *P. aeruginosa,* indole-positive strains of *Proteus,* and *Enterobacter* spp. Because *Pseudomonas* infections are common in neutropenic patients, therapy for severe bacterial infections in such individuals should include a β-lactam antibiotic such as piperacillin with good activity against these microorganisms.

Ticarcillin. This semisynthetic penicillin (Table 53–1) is very similar to carbenicillin, but it is two to four times more active against *P. aeruginosa*. Ticarcillin is inferior to piperacillin for the treatment of serious infections caused by *Pseudomonas*. Ticarcillin is only marketed in combination with clavulanate (TIMENTIN) in the U.S.

Mezlocillin. This ureidopenicillin is more active against *Klebsiella* than is carbenicillin; its activity against *Pseudomonas in vitro* is similar to that of ticarcillin. It is more active than ticarcillin against *E. faecalis. Mezlocillin sodium* has been discontinued in the U.S.

Untoward Reactions to Penicillins

Hypersensitivity Reactions. Hypersensitivity reactions are by far the most common adverse effects noted with the penicillins, and these agents probably are the most common cause of drug allergy. Allergic reactions complicate 0.7-4% of all treatment courses. There is no convincing evidence that any single penicillin differs from the group in its potential for causing true allergic reactions. In approximate order of decreasing frequency, manifestations of allergy to penicillins include maculopapular rash, urticarial rash, fever, bronchospasm, vasculitis, serum sickness, exfoliative dermatitis, Stevens-Johnson syndrome, and anaphylaxis (Weiss and Adkinson, 2005). The reported overall incidence of such reactions to the penicillins is 0.7-10%. Hypersensitivity to penicillins generally extends to the other β-lactams (e.g., cephalosporins, some carbapenems).

Hypersensitivity reactions may occur with any dosage form of penicillin; allergy to one penicillin exposes the patient to a greater risk of reaction if another is given. But the occurrence of an untoward effect does not necessarily imply repetition on subsequent exposures. Hypersensitivity reactions may appear in the absence of a previous known exposure to the drug. This may be caused by unrecognized prior exposure to penicillin in the environment (e.g., in foods of animal origin or from the fungus-producing penicillin). Although elimination of the antibiotic usually results in rapid clearing of the allergic manifestations, they may persist for 1-2 weeks or longer after therapy has been stopped. In some cases, the reaction is mild and disappears even when the penicillin is continued; in others, immediate cessation of penicillin treatment is required. In a few instances, it is necessary to interdict the future use of penicillin because of the risk of death, and the patient should be so warned. It must be stressed that fatal episodes of anaphylaxis have followed the ingestion of very small doses of this antibiotic or skin testing with minute quantities of the drug.

Penicillins and their breakdown products act as haptens after covalent reaction with proteins. The most abundant breakdown product is the penicilloyl moiety (major determinant moiety [MDM]), which is formed when the β-lactam ring is opened. A large percentage of immunoglobulin (Ig)E-mediated reactions are to the MDM, but at least 25% of reactions are to other breakdown products, and the severities of the reactions to the various components are comparable. These products are formed *in vivo* and can be found in solutions of penicillin prepared for administration. The terms *major* and *minor determinants* refer to the frequency with which antibodies to these haptens appear to be formed. They do not describe the severity of the reaction that may result. In fact, anaphylactic reactions to penicillin usually are mediated by IgE antibodies against the minor determinants.

Antipenicillin antibodies are detectable in virtually all patients who have received the drug and in many who have never knowingly been exposed to it. Recent treatment with the antibiotic induces an increase in major-determinant-specific antibodies that are skin sensitizing. The incidence of positive skin reactors is three to four times higher in atopic than in nonatopic individuals. Clinical and immunological studies suggest that immediate allergic reactions are mediated by skin-sensitizing or IgE antibodies, usually of minor-determinant specificities. Accelerated and late urticarial reactions usually are mediated by major-determinant–specific skin-sensitizing antibodies. The recurrent-arthralgia syndrome appears to be related to the presence of skin-sensitizing antibodies of minor-determinant specificities. Some maculopapular and erythematous reactions may be due to toxic antigen-antibody complexes of major-determinant-specific IgM antibodies. Accelerated and late urticarial reactions to penicillin may terminate spontaneously because of the development of blocking antibodies.

Skin rashes of all types may be caused by allergy to penicillin. Scarlatiniform, morbilliform, urticarial, vesicular, and bullous eruptions may develop. Purpuric lesions are uncommon and usually are the result of a vasculitis; thrombocytopenic purpura may occur very rarely. Henoch-Schönlein purpura with renal involvement has been a rare complication. Contact dermatitis is observed occasionally in pharmacists, nurses, and physicians who prepare penicillin solutions. Fixed-drug reactions also have occurred. More severe reactions involving the skin are exfoliative dermatitis and exudative erythema multiforme of either the erythematopapular or vesiculobullous type; these lesions may be very severe and atypical in distribution and constitute the characteristic Stevens-Johnson syndrome. The incidence of skin rashes appears to be highest following the use of ampicillin, at ~9%; rashes follow the administration of ampicillin in nearly all patients with infectious mononucleosis. When allopurinol and ampicillin are administered concurrently, the incidence of rash also increases. Ampicillin-induced skin eruptions in such patients may represent a "toxic" rather than a truly allergic reaction. Positive skin reactions to the major and minor determinants of penicillin sensitization may be absent. The rash may clear even while administration of the drug is continued.

The most serious hypersensitivity reactions produced by the penicillins are angioedema and anaphylaxis. Angioedema, with marked swelling of the lips, tongue, face, and periorbital tissues, frequently accompanied by asthmatic breathing and "giant hives," has been observed after topical, oral, or systemic administration of penicillins of various types.

Acute anaphylactic or anaphylactoid reactions induced by various preparations of penicillin constitute the most important immediate danger connected with their use. Among all drugs, the penicillins are most often responsible for this type of untoward effect. Anaphylactoid reactions may occur at any age. Their incidence is thought to be 0.004-0.04% in persons treated with penicillins (Kucers and Bennett, 1987). About 0.001% of patients treated with these agents die from anaphylaxis. It has been estimated that at least 300 deaths per year are due to this complication of therapy. About 70% have had penicillin previously, and one-third of these reacted to it on a prior occasion. Anaphylaxis most often has followed the injection of penicillin, although it also has been observed after oral ingestion of the drug and even has resulted from the intradermal instillation of a very small quantity for the purpose of testing for the presence of hypersensitivity. The clinical pictures that develop vary in severity. The most dramatic is sudden, severe hypotension and rapid death. In other instances, bronchoconstriction with severe asthma; abdominal pain, nausea, and vomiting; extreme weakness and a fall in blood pressure; or diarrhea and purpuric skin eruptions have characterized the anaphylactic episodes.

Serum sickness varies from mild fever, rash, and leukopenia to severe arthralgia or arthritis, purpura, lymphadenopathy, splenomegaly, mental changes, electrocardiographic abnormalities suggestive of myocarditis, generalized edema, albuminuria, and hematuria. It is mediated by IgG antibodies. This reaction is rare, but when it occurs, it appears after penicillin treatment has been continued for 1 week or more; it may be delayed, however, until 1 or 2 weeks after the drug has been stopped. Serum sickness caused by penicillin may persist for a week or longer.

Vasculitis of the skin or other organs may be related to penicillin hypersensitivity. The Coombs reaction frequently becomes positive during prolonged therapy with a penicillin or cephalosporin, but hemolytic anemia is rare. Reversible neutropenia may occur. It is not known if this is truly a hypersensitivity reaction; it has been noted with all the penicillins and has been seen in up to 30% of patients treated with 8-12 g nafcillin for >21 days. The bone marrow shows an arrest of maturation.

Fever may be the only evidence of a hypersensitivity reaction to the penicillins. It may reach high levels and be maintained, remittent, or intermittent; chills occur occasionally. The febrile reaction usually disappears within 24-36 hours after administration of the drug is stopped but may persist for days.

Eosinophilia is an occasional accompaniment of other allergic reactions to penicillin. At times, it may be the sole abnormality, and eosinophils may reach levels of ≥10-20% of the total number of circulating white blood cells.

Penicillins rarely cause interstitial nephritis; methicillin has been implicated most frequently. Hematuria, albuminuria, pyuria, renal cell and other casts in the urine, elevation of serum creatinine, and even oliguria have been noted. Biopsy shows a mononuclear infiltrate with eosinophilia and tubular damage. IgG is present in the interstitium. This reaction usually is reversible.

Management of the Patient Potentially Allergic to Penicillin. Evaluation of the patient's history is the most practical way to avoid the use of penicillin in patients who are at the greatest risk of adverse reaction. Most patients who give a history of allergy to penicillin should be treated with a different type of antibiotic. Unfortunately, there is no totally reliable means to confirm a history of penicillin allergy (Romano et al., 2003). Skin testing for IgE-mediated immediate-type responses is compromised by the lack of a commercially available minor-determinant mixture. A National Institute of Allergy and Infectious Diseases (NIAID) multicenter study used major and minor determinants for skin testing. Of 726 patients with a history of penicillin allergy, 566 had negative skin tests. Of those, only 7 of 566 (1.2%) had possibly IgE-mediated immediate or accelerated penicillin allergy when given penicillin (Sogn et al., 1992). Radioallergosorbent tests (RASTs) for IgE antipenicilloyl determinants suffer from the same limitations as skin tests (Weiss and Adkinson, 2005).

Occasionally, *desensitization* is recommended for penicillin-allergic patients who must receive the drug. This procedure consists of administering gradually increasing doses of penicillin in the hope of avoiding a severe reaction and should be performed only in an intensive care setting. This may result in a subclinical anaphylactic discharge and the binding of all IgE before full doses are administered. Penicillin may be given in doses of 1, 5, 10, 100, and 1000 units intradermally in the lower arm, with 60-minute intervals between doses. If this is well tolerated, then 10,000 and 50,000 units may be given subcutaneously. Desensitization also may be accomplished by the oral administration of penicillin. When full doses are reached, penicillin should not be discontinued and then restarted because immediate reactions may recur (see Weiss and Adkinson, 2005, for details). The patient should be observed constantly during the desensitizing procedure, an intravenous line must be in place, and epinephrine and equipment and expertise for artificial ventilation must be on hand. It must be emphasized that this procedure may be dangerous, and its efficacy is unproven.

Patients with life-threatening infections (e.g., endocarditis or meningitis) may be continued on penicillin despite the development of a maculopapular rash, although alternative antimicrobial agents should be used whenever possible. The rash often resolves as therapy is continued, perhaps owing to the development of blocking antibodies of the IgG class. The rash may be treated with antihistamines or glucocorticoids, although there is no evidence that this therapy is efficacious. Rarely, exfoliative dermatitis with or without vasculitis develops in these patients if therapy with penicillin is continued.

Other Adverse Reactions. The penicillins have minimal direct toxicity. Apparent toxic effects that have been reported include bone marrow depression, granulocytopenia, and hepatitis. The last-named effect is rare but is seen most commonly following the administration of oxacillin and nafcillin. The administration of penicillin G, carbenicillin, piperacillin, or ticarcillin has been associated with a potentially significant defect of hemostasis that appears to be due to an impairment of platelet aggregation; this may be caused by interference with the binding of aggregating agents to platelet receptors (Fass et al., 1987).

Most common among the irritative responses to penicillin are pain and sterile inflammatory reactions at the sites of intramuscular injections—reactions that are related to concentration. Serum transaminases and lactic dehydrogenase may be elevated as a result of local damage to muscle. In some individuals who receive penicillin intravenously, phlebitis or thrombophlebitis develops. Many persons who take various penicillin preparations by mouth experience nausea, with or without vomiting, and some have mild to severe diarrhea. These manifestations often are related to the dose of the drug.

When penicillin is injected accidentally into the sciatic nerve, severe pain occurs and dysfunction in the area of distribution of this nerve develops and persists for weeks. Intrathecal injection of penicillin G may produce arachnoiditis or severe and fatal encephalopathy. Because of this, intrathecal or intraventricular administration of penicillins should be avoided. The parenteral administration of large doses of penicillin G (>20 million units per day, or less with renal insufficiency) may produce lethargy, confusion, twitching, multifocal myoclonus, or localized or generalized epileptiform seizures. These are most apt to occur in the presence of renal insufficiency, localized lesions of the central nervous system (CNS), or hyponatremia. When the concentration of penicillin G in CSF exceeds 10 μg/mL, significant dysfunction of the CNS is frequent. The rapid intravenous administration of 20 million units of penicillin G potassium, which contains 34 mEq of K^+, may lead to severe or even fatal hyperkalemia in persons with renal dysfunction.

Injection of penicillin G procaine may result in an immediate reaction, characterized by dizziness, tinnitus, headache, hallucinations, and sometimes seizures. This is due to the rapid liberation of toxic concentrations of procaine. It has been reported to occur in 1 of 200 patients receiving 4.8 million units of penicillin G procaine to treat venereal disease.

Reactions Unrelated to Hypersensitivity or Toxicity. Regardless of the route by which the drug is administered, but most strikingly when it is given by mouth, penicillin changes the composition of the microflora in the GI tract by eliminating sensitive microorganisms. This phenomenon is usually of no clinical significance, and normal microflora are typically reestablished shortly after therapy is stopped. In some persons, however, superinfection results from pathological changes to the flora. Pseudomembranous colitis, related to overgrowth and production of a toxin by *Clostridium difficile,* has followed oral and, less commonly, parenteral administration of penicillins.

THE CEPHALOSPORINS

Cephalosporium acremonium, the first source of the cephalosporins, was isolated in 1948 by Brotzu from the sea near a sewer outlet off the Sardinian coast. Crude filtrates from cultures of this fungus were found to inhibit the *in vitro* growth of *S. aureus* and to cure staphylococcal infections and typhoid fever in humans. Culture fluids in which the Sardinian fungus was cultivated were found to contain three distinct antibiotics, which were named *cephalosporin P, N,* and *C*. With isolation of the active nucleus of cephalosporin C, 7-aminocephalosporanic acid, and with the addition of side chains, it became possible to produce semisynthetic compounds with antibacterial activity very much greater than that of the parent substance.

Chemistry. Cephalosporin C contains a side chain derived from D-α-aminoadipic acid, which is condensed with a dihydrothiazine β-lactam ring system (7-aminocephalosporanic acid). Compounds containing 7-aminocephalosporanic acid are relatively stable in dilute acid and highly resistant to penicillinase regardless of the nature of their side chains and their affinity for the enzyme.

Cephalosporin C can be hydrolyzed by acid to 7-aminocephalosporanic acid. This compound subsequently has been modified by the addition of different side chains to create a whole family of cephalosporin antibiotics. It appears that modifications at position 7 of the β-lactam ring are associated with alteration in antibacterial activity and that substitutions at position 3 of the dihydrothiazine ring are associated with changes in the metabolism and pharmacokinetic properties of the drugs.

The cephamycins are similar to the cephalosporins but have a methoxy group at position 7 of the β-lactam ring of the 7-aminocephalosporanic acid nucleus. The structural formulas of representative cephalosporins and cephamycins are shown in Table 53–2, along with dosages schedules and half-lives.

Mechanism of Action. Cephalosporins and cephamycins inhibit bacterial cell wall synthesis in a manner similar to that of penicillin.

Classification. The large number of cephalosporins makes a system of classification most desirable. Although cephalosporins may be classified by their chemical structure, clinical pharmacology, resistance to β-lactamase, or antimicrobial spectrum, the well-accepted system of classification by "generations" is very useful, although admittedly somewhat arbitrary (Table 53–3). It is important to remember that none of the cephalosporins has activity against MRSA, listeria, or enterococci.

Classification by generations is based on general features of antimicrobial activity (Andes and Craig, 2005). The *first-generation* cephalosporins, epitomized by cephalothin (discontinued in the U.S.) and cefazolin, have good activity against gram-positive bacteria and relatively modest activity against gram-negative microorganisms. Most gram-positive cocci (with the exception of enterococci, methicillin-resistant *S. aureus*, and *S. epidermidis*) are susceptible. Most oral cavity anaerobes are sensitive, but the *B. fragilis* group is resistant. Activity against *Moraxella catarrhalis, E. coli, K. pneumoniae*, and *P. mirabilis* is good. The *second-generation* cephalosporins have somewhat increased activity against gram-negative microorganisms but are much less active than the third-generation agents. A subset of second-generation agents (cefoxitin, cefotetan, and cefmetazole, which have been discontinued in the U.S.) also is active against the *B. fragilis* group. *Third-generation* cephalosporins generally are less active than first-generation agents against gram-positive cocci; these agents are much more active against the Enterobacteriaceae, although resistance is dramatically increasing due to β-lactamase-producing strains. A subset of third-generation agents (ceftazidime and cefoperazone, which are discontinued in the U.S.) also is active against *P. aeruginosa* but less active than other third-generation agents against gram-positive cocci. *Fourth-generation* cephalosporins, such as cefepime, have an extended spectrum of activity compared with the third generation and have increased stability from hydrolysis by plasmid and chromosomally mediated β-lactamases (but not the KPC class A β-lactamases). Fourth-generation agents are useful in the empirical treatment of serious infections in hospitalized patients when gram-positive microorganisms, Enterobacteriaceae, and *Pseudomonas* all are potential etiologies. It is important to remember that none of the cephalosporins has reliable activity against the following bacteria: penicillin-resistant *S. pneumoniae*, MRSA, methicillin-resistant *S. epidermidis* and other coagulase-negative staphylococci, *Enterococcus, L. monocytogenes, Legionella pneumophila, L. micdadei, C. difficile, Xanthomonas maltophilia, Campylobacter jejuni,* KPC-producing *Enterobacteriaceae,* and *Acinetobacter* spp.

Mechanisms of Bacterial Resistance to the Cephalosporins. Resistance to the cephalosporins may be related to the inability of the antibiotic to reach its sites of action or to alterations in the penicillin-binding proteins (PBPs) that are targets of the cephalosporins such that the antibiotics bind to bacterial enzymes (β-lactamases) that can hydrolyze the β-lactam ring and inactivate the cephalosporin. Alterations in two PBPs (1A and 2X) that decrease their affinity for cephalosporins render pneumococci resistant to third-generation cephalosporins because the other three high-molecular-weight PBPs have inherently low affinity (Spratt, 1994).

The most prevalent mechanism of resistance to cephalosporins is destruction of the cephalosporins by hydrolysis of the β-lactam ring.

Table 53–2

Names, Structural Formulas, Dosage, and Dosage Forms of Selected Cephalosporins and Related Compounds

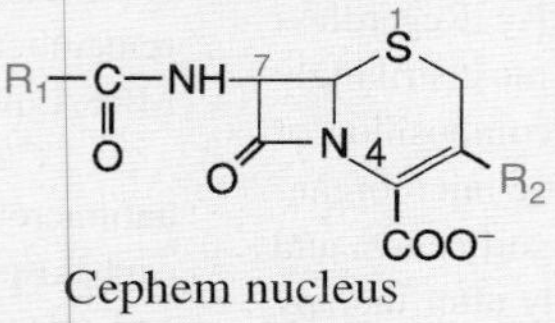

Cephem nucleus

COMPOUND (TRADE NAMES)	R_1	R_2	DOSAGE FORMS,[a] ADULT DOSAGE FOR SEVERE INFECTION, AND $t_{\frac{1}{2}}$
First generation			
Cefadroxil (DURICEF)	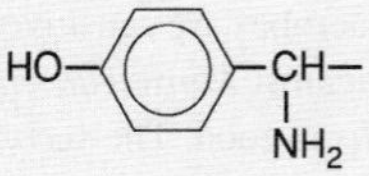 HO–(phenyl)–CH(NH_2)–	$-CH_3$	O: 1 g every 12 hours $t_{\frac{1}{2}}$ = 1.1 hours
Cefazolin (ANCEF, KEFZOL, others)	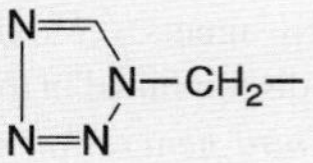 (tetrazol-1-yl)–CH_2–	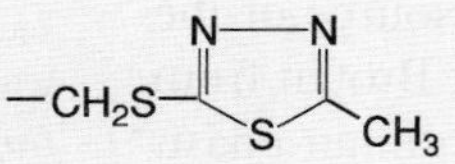 $-CH_2S$–(5-methyl-1,3,4-thiadiazol-2-yl)	I: 1-1.5 g every 6 hours $t_{\frac{1}{2}}$ = about 2 hours
Cephalexin (KEFLEX, others)	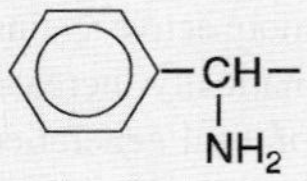 (phenyl)–CH(NH_2)–	$-CH_3$	O: 1 g every 6 hours $t_{\frac{1}{2}}$ = 0.9 hour
Second generation			
Cefaclor (CECLOR)	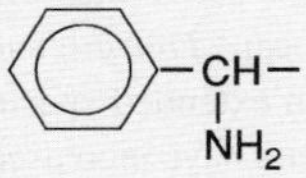 (phenyl)–CH(NH_2)–	–Cl	O: 1 g every 8 hours $t_{\frac{1}{2}}$ = 0.7 hours
Ceforanide (PRECEF)	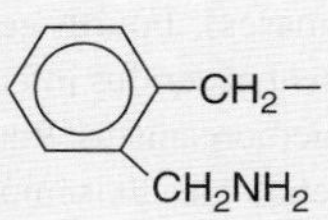 (2-(CH_2NH_2)phenyl)–CH_2–	$-CH_2S$–(1-carboxymethyl-tetrazol-5-yl)	I: 1 g every 12 hours $t_{\frac{1}{2}}$ = 2.6 hours
Cefotetan (CEFOTAN)	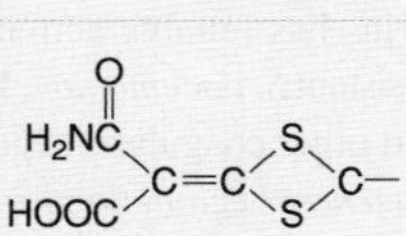 $H_2NC(=O)(HOOC)C$=C(1,3-dithietane)–C–	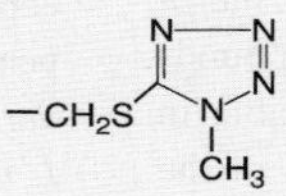 $-CH_2S$–(1-methyl-tetrazol-5-yl)	I: 2-3 g every 12 hours $t_{\frac{1}{2}}$ = 3.3 hours
Cefoxitin[b] (MEFOXIN)	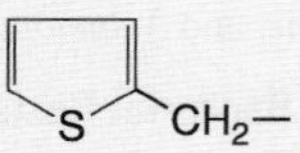 (2-thienyl)–CH_2–	$-CH_2OC(=O)NH_2$	I: 2 g every 4 hours or 3 g every 6 hours $t_{\frac{1}{2}}$ = 0.7 hours
Cefprozil (CEFZIL)	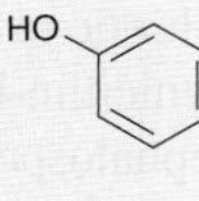 HO–(phenyl)–CH(NH_2)–	CH=CH–CH_3	O: 500 mg every 12 hours $t_{\frac{1}{2}}$ = 1.3 hours
Cefuroxime acetil[c] (CEFTIN) Cefuroxime (ZINACEF)	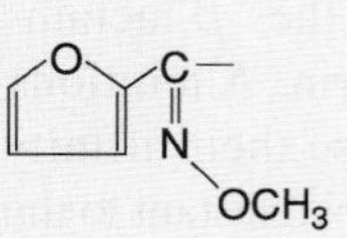 (2-furyl)–C(=N–OCH_3)–	$-CH_2OC(=O)NH_2$	I: up to 3 g every 8 hours $t_{\frac{1}{2}}$ = 1.7 hours T: 500 mg every 12 hours

(Continued)

Table 53–2

Names, Structural Formulas, Dosage, and Dosage Forms of Selected Cephalosporins and Related Compounds (*Continued*)

COMPOUND (TRADE NAMES)	R_1	R_2	DOSAGE FORMS,[a] ADULT DOSAGE FOR SEVERE INFECTION, AND $t_{\frac{1}{2}}$
Third generation			
Cefdinir (OMNICEF)	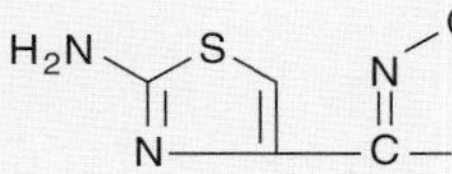 H_2N, S, N, N–OH, C (aminothiazole oxime)	$-CH=CH_2$	O: 300 mg every 12 hours or 600 mg every 24 hours $t_{\frac{1}{2}}$ = 1.7 hours
Cefditoren pivoxil (SPECTRACEF)	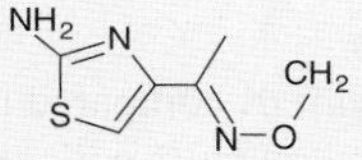 NH_2, N, S, CH_2, N–O	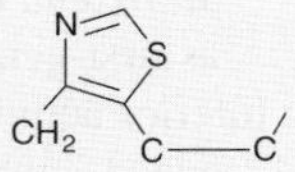 N, S, CH_2, C–C (methylthiazolyl vinyl)	O: 400 mg every 12 hours $t_{\frac{1}{2}}$ = 1.6 hours
Cefibuten (CEDAX)	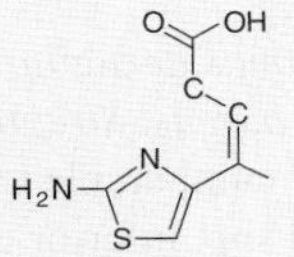 O, OH, C, C, H_2N, N, S	$-H$	O: 400 mg every 24 hours $t_{\frac{1}{2}}$ = 2.4 hours
Cefixime	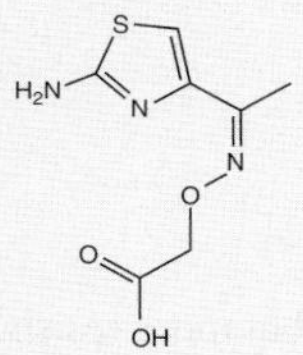 S, H_2N, N, N, O, O, OH	$-CH=CH_2$	O: 400 mg/day or 200 mg every 12 hours $t_{\frac{1}{2}}$ = 3.5 hours
Cefotaxime (CLAFORAN)	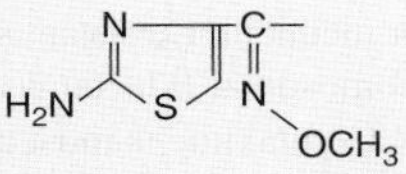 N, C–, H_2N, S, N, OCH_3	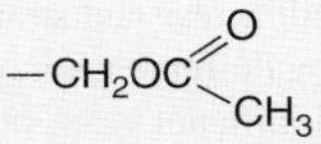 $-CH_2OC(=O)CH_3$	I: 2 g every 4-8 hours $t_{\frac{1}{2}}$ = 1.1 hours
Cefpodoxime proxetil[d] (VANTIN)	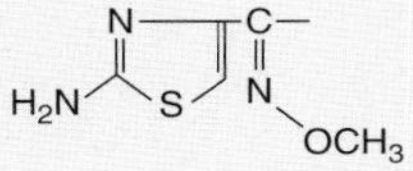 N, C–, H_2N, S, N, OCH_3	$-CH_2OCH_3$	O: 200-400 mg every 12 hours $t_{\frac{1}{2}}$ = 2.2 hours
Ceftizoxime (CEFIZOX)	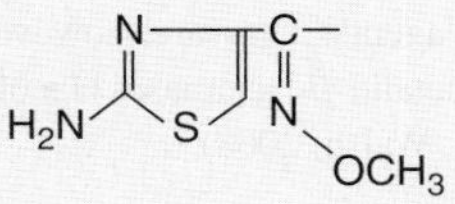 N, C–, H_2N, S, N, OCH_3	$-H$	I: 3-4 g every 8 hours $t_{\frac{1}{2}}$ = 1.8 hours
Ceftazidime (HORTAZ, others)	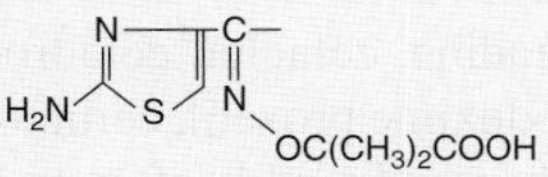 N, C–, H_2N, S, N, $OC(CH_3)_2COOH$	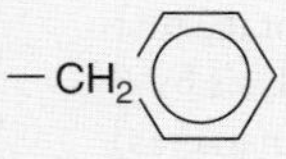 $-CH_2$–(pyridinium)	I: 2 g every 8 hours $t_{\frac{1}{2}}$ = 1.8 hours
Ceftriaxone (ROCHEPHIN)	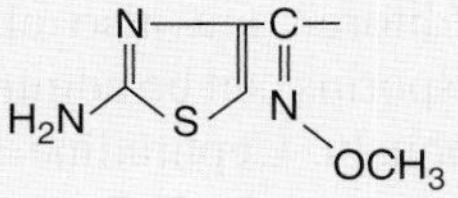 N, C–, H_2N, S, N, OCH_3	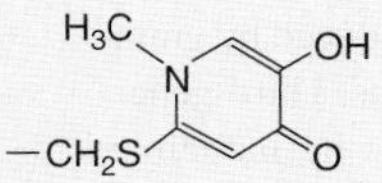 H_3C, N, OH, O, $-CH_2S$– (triazinedione)	I: 2 g every 12-24 hours $t_{\frac{1}{2}}$ = 8 hours
Fourth generation			
Cefepime (MAXIPIME)	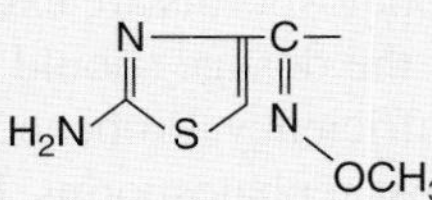 N, C–, H_2N, S, N, OCH_3	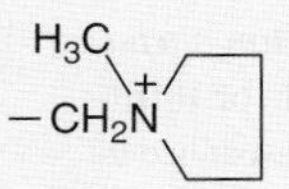 H_3C, $-CH_2N^+$ (pyrrolidinium)	I: 2 g every 8 hours $t_{\frac{1}{2}}$ = 2 hours

[a]T, tablet; C, capsule; O, oral suspension; I, injection [b]Cefoxitin, a cophamycin, has a $-OCH_3$ group at position 7 of cephem nucleus. [c]Cefuroxime axctil is the acetyloxyethyl ester of cefuroxime. [d]Cefpodoxime proxetil has a $-COOCH(CH_3)OCOOCH(CH_3)_2$ group at position 4 of cephem nucleus.

Table 53–3

Cephalosporin Generations

EXAMPLES	USEFUL SPECTRUM[a]
First Generation	
Cefazolin (ANCEF, ZOLICEF, others)	Streptococci[b]; *Staphylococcus aureus.*[c]
Cephalexin monohydrate (KEFTAB)	
Cefadroxil (DURACEF)	
Cephradine (VELOSEF)	
Second Generation	
Cefuroxime (ZINACEF)	*Escherichia coli, Klebsiella, Proteus, Haemophilus influenzae, Moraxella catarrhalis*. Not as active against gram-positive organisms as first-generation agents.
Cefuroxime axetil (CEFTIN)	
Cefprozil (CEFZIL)	
Cefmetazole (ZEFAZONE)	Inferior activity against *S. aureus* compared to cefuroxime but with added activity against *Bacteroides fragilis* and other *Bacteroides spp.*
Loracarbef (LORABID)	
Third Generation	
Cefotaxime (CLAFORAN)	Enterobacteriaceae[d]; *Pseudomonas aeruginosa*[e]; *Serratia; Neisseria gonorrhoeae*; activity for *S. aureus, Streptococcus pneumoniae*, and *Streptococcus pyogenes*[f] comparable to first-generation agents. Activity against *Bacteroides* spp. inferior to that of cefoxitin and cefotetan.
Ceftriaxone (ROCEPHIN)	
Cefdinir (OMNICEF)	
Cefditoren pivoxil (SPECTRACEF)	
Ceftibuten (CEDAX)	
Cefpodoxime proxetil (VANTIN)	
Ceftizoxime (CEFIZOX)	
Cefoperazone (CEFOBID)	Active against *Pseudomonas*
Ceftazidime (FORTAZ, others)	
Fourth Generation	
Cefepime (MAXIPINE)	Comparable to third generation but more resistant to some β-lactamases.

[a]All cephalosporins lack activity against enterococci, *Listeria monocytogenes, Legionella* spp., methicillin-resistant *S. aureus, Xanthomonas maltophilia*, and *Acinetobacter* species. [b]Except for penicillin-resistant strains. [c]Except for methicillin-resistant strains. [d]Resistance to cephalosporins may be induced rapidly during therapy by de-repression of bacterial chromosomal β-lactamases, which destroy the cephalosporins. [e]Ceftazidime only. [f]Ceftazidime lacks significant gram-positive activity. Cefotaxime is most active in class against *S. aureus* and *S. pyogenes*.

Many gram-positive microorganisms release relatively large amounts of β-lactamase into the surrounding medium. Although gram-negative bacteria seem to produce less β-lactamase, the location of their enzyme in the periplasmic space may make it more effective in destroying cephalosporins because they diffuse to their targets on the inner membrane, as is the case for the penicillins. The cephalosporins have variable susceptibility to β-lactamase. For example, of the first-generation agents, cefazolin is more susceptible to hydrolysis by β-lactamase from *S. aureus* than is cephalothin (no longer marketed). Cefoxitin, cefuroxime, and the third-generation cephalosporins are more resistant to hydrolysis by the β-lactamases produced by gram-negative bacteria than first-generation cephalosporins. Third-generation cephalosporins are susceptible to hydrolysis by inducible, chromosomally encoded (type I) β-lactamases. Induction of type I β-lactamases by treatment of infections owing to aerobic gram-negative bacilli (especially *Enterobacter* spp., *Citrobacter freundii, Morganella, Serratia, Providencia,* and *P. aeruginosa*) with second- or third-generation cephalosporins and/or imipenem may result in resistance to all third-generation cephalosporins. The fourth-generation cephalosporins, such as cefepime, are poor inducers of type I β-lactamases and are less susceptible to hydrolysis by type I β-lactamases than are the third-generation agents. They are, however, susceptible to degradation by KPC and metallo-β-lactamases (Jacoby and Munoz-Price, 2005; Jones et al., 2008; Walsh, 2008).

General Features of the Cephalosporins. Cephalexin, cephradine, cefaclor, cefadroxil, loracarbef, cefprozil, cefpodoxime proxetil, ceftibuten, and cefuroxime axetil are absorbed readily after oral administration. Cefdinir and cefditoren are also effective orally. The other cephalosporins can be administered intramuscularly or intravenously. Cephradine and loracarbef have been discontinued in the U.S.

Cephalosporins are excreted primarily by the kidney; thus the dosage should be altered in patients with renal insufficiency. Probenecid slows the tubular secretion of most cephalosporins. Exceptions are cefpiramide and cefoperazone, which are excreted predominantly in the bile (neither is available in the U.S.). Cefotaxime is deacetylated *in vivo*. The metabolite has less antimicrobial activity than the parent compound and is excreted by the kidneys. None of the other cephalosporins appears to undergo appreciable metabolism.

Several cephalosporins penetrate into the CSF in sufficient concentration to be useful for the treatment of meningitis. These include cefotaxime, ceftriaxone, and cefepime (see "Therapeutic Uses" section). Cephalosporins also cross the placenta, and they are found in high concentrations in synovial and pericardial fluids. Penetration into the aqueous humor of the eye is relatively good after systemic administration of third-generation agents, but penetration into the vitreous humor is poor. Some evidence indicates that concentrations sufficient for therapy of ocular infections owing to gram-positive and certain gram-negative microorganisms can be achieved after systemic administration. Concentrations in bile usually are high, with those achieved after administration of cefoperazone and cefpiramide the highest.

Specific Agents

First-Generation Cephalosporins. Cefazolin has an antibacterial spectrum that is typical of other first-generation cephalosporins except that it also has activity against some *Enterobacter* spp. Cefazolin is relatively well tolerated after either intramuscular or intravenous administration, and concentrations of the drug in plasma after a 1-g intramuscular injection reach 64 μg/mL. Cefazolin is excreted by glomerular filtration and is bound to plasma proteins to a great extent (~85%). Cefazolin usually is preferred among the first-generation cephalosporins because it can be administered less frequently owing to its longer $t_{1/2}$.

Cephalexin is available for oral administration, and it has the same antibacterial spectrum as the other first-generation cephalosporins. However, it is somewhat less active against penicillinase-producing staphylococci. Oral therapy with cephalexin results in peak concentrations in plasma of 16 μg/mL after a dose of 0.5 g; this is adequate for the inhibition of many gram-positive and gram-negative pathogens. The drug is not metabolized, and 70-100% is excreted in the urine.

Cephradine is similar in structure to cephalexin, and its activity *in vitro* is almost identical. Cephradine is not metabolized and, after rapid absorption from the GI tract, is excreted unchanged in the urine. Cephradine can be administered orally, intramuscularly, or intravenously. When administered orally, it is difficult to distinguish cephradine from cephalexin; some authorities believe these two drugs can be used interchangeably. Because cephradine is so well absorbed, the concentrations in plasma are nearly equivalent after oral or intramuscular administration.

Cefadroxil is the *para*-hydroxy analog of cephalexin. Concentrations of cefadroxil in plasma and urine are at somewhat higher levels than are those of cephalexin. The drug may be administered orally once or twice a day for the treatment of urinary tract infections. Its activity *in vitro* is similar to that of cephalexin.

Second-Generation Cephalosporins. Second-generation cephalosporins have a broader spectrum than do the first-generation agents and are active against sensitive strains of *Enterobacter* spp., indole-positive *Proteus* spp., and *Klebsiella* spp.

Cefoxitin is a cephamycin produced by *Streptomyces lactam durans*. It is resistant to some β-lactamases produced by gram-negative rods. This antibiotic is less active than the first-generation cephalosporins against gram-positive bacteria. Cefoxitin is more active than other first- or second-generation agents (except cefotetan) against anaerobes, especially *B. fragilis*. After an intramuscular dose of 1 g, concentrations in plasma are ~22 μg/mL. The $t_{1/2}$ is ~40 minutes. Cefoxitin's special role seems to be for treatment of certain anaerobic and mixed aerobic-anaerobic infections, such as pelvic inflammatory disease and lung abscess.

Cefaclor is used orally. The concentration in plasma after oral administration is ~50% of that achieved after an equivalent oral dose of cephalexin. However, cefaclor is more active against *H. influenzae* and *Moraxella catarrhalis*, although some β-lactamase-producing strains of these organisms may be resistant.

Loracarbef is an orally administered carbacephem, similar in activity to cefaclor, that is more stable against some β-lactamases. The serum $t_{1/2}$ is 1.1 hours.

Cefuroxime is similar to loracarbef with broader gram-negative activity against some *Citrobacter* and *Enterobacter* spp. Unlike cefoxitin, cefmetazole (discontinued in the U.S.), and cefotetan, cefuroxime lacks activity against *B. fragilis*. The $t_{1/2}$ is 1.7 hours, and the drug can be given every 8 hours. Concentrations in CSF are ~10% of those in plasma, and the drug is effective (but inferior to ceftriaxone) for treatment of meningitis owing to *H. influenzae* (including strains resistant to ampicillin), *N. meningitidis*, and *S. pneumoniae* (Schaad et al., 1990).

Cefuroxime axetil is the 1-acetyloxyethyl ester of cefuroxime. Between 30% and 50% of an oral dose is absorbed, and the drug then is hydrolyzed to cefuroxime; resulting concentrations in plasma are variable.

Cefprozil is an orally administered agent that is more active than first-generation cephalosporins against penicillin-sensitive streptococci, *E. coli, P. mirabilis, Klebsiella* spp., and *Citrobacter* spp. It has a serum $t_{1/2}$ of ~1.3 hours.

Third-Generation Cephalosporins. Cefotaxime is highly resistant to many (but not the extended-spectrum product) of the bacterial β-lactamases and has good activity against many gram-positive and gram-negative aerobic bacteria. However, activity against *B. fragilis* is poor compared with agents such as clindamycin and metronidazole. Cefotaxime has a $t_{1/2}$ in plasma of ~1 hour and should be administered every 4–8 hours for serious infections. The drug is metabolized *in vivo* to desacetylcefotaxime, which is less active against most microorganisms than is the parent compound. However, the metabolite acts synergistically with the parent compound against certain microbes. Cefotaxime has been used effectively for meningitis caused by *H. influenzae,* penicillin-sensitive *S. pneumoniae*, and *N. meningitides*.

Ceftizoxime has a spectrum of activity *in vitro* that is very similar to that of cefotaxime, except that it is less active against *S. pneumoniae* and more active against *B. fragilis* (Haas et al., 1995). The $t_{1/2}$ is somewhat longer, 1.8 hours, and the drug thus can be administered every 8-12 hours for serious infections. Ceftizoxime is not metabolized, and 90% is recovered in urine.

Ceftriaxone has activity *in vitro* very similar to that of ceftizoxime and cefotaxime. A $t_{1/2}$ of ~8 hours is the outstanding feature. Administration of the drug once or twice daily has been effective for patients with meningitis, whereas dosage once a day has been effective for other infections. About half the drug can be recovered from the urine; the remainder appears to be eliminated by biliary secretion. A single dose of ceftriaxone (125-250 mg) is effective in the treatment of urethral, cervical, rectal, or pharyngeal gonorrhea, including disease caused by penicillinase-producing microorganisms.

Cefpodoxime proxetil is an orally administered third-generation agent that is very similar in activity to the fourth-generation agent cefepime except that it is not more active against *Enterobacter* or *Pseudomonas* spp. It has a serum $t_{1/2}$ of 2.2 hours.

Cefditoren pivoxil is a prodrug that is hydrolyzed by esterases during absorption to the active drug, cefditoren. Cefditoren has a $t_{1/2}$ of ~1.6 hours and is eliminated unchanged in the urine. The drug is active against methicillin-susceptible strains *of S. aureus*, penicillin-susceptible strains *of S. pneumoniae, S. pyogenes, H. influenzae, H. parainfluenzae,* and *Moraxella catarrhalis*. Cefditoren pivoxil is only indicated for the treatment of mild-to-moderate pharyngitis, tonsillitis, uncomplicated skin and skin structure infections, and acute exacerbations of chronic bronchitis.

Cefixime is an oral third-generation cephalosporin with clinical efficacy against urinary tract infections caused by *E. coli* and *P. mirabilis*, otitis media caused by *H. influenza* and *S. pyogenes*, pharyngitis due to *S. pyogenes*, and uncomplicated gonorrhea. It is available as an oral suspension (SUPREX, others). Cefixime has a plasma $t_{1/2}$ of 3–4 hours and is both excreted in the urine and eliminated in the bile. The standard dose for adults is 400 mg/day for 5-7 days, and for a longer interval in patients with *S. pyogenes*. Doses must be reduced in patients with renal impairment (300 mg/day for creatinine clearance between 20 and 60 mL/minute, and 200 mg day for <20 mL/minute). Pediatric dosing varies with patient weight.

Ceftibuten is an orally effective cephalosporin with a $t_{1/2}$ of 2.4 hours. It is less active against gram-positive and gram-negative organisms than cefixime, with activity limited to *S. pneumonia* and *S. pyogenes*, *H. influenzae*, and *M. catarrhalis*. Ceftibuten is only indicated for acute bacterial exacerbations of chronic bronchitis, acute bacterial otitis media, pharyngitis, and tonsillitis. It lacks useful activity against *S. aureus*.

Cefdinir is effective orally, with a $t_{1/2}$ of ~1.7 hours; it is eliminated primarily unchanged in the urine. Cefdinir has greater activity than the second-generation agents for facultative gram-negative bacteria but lacks anaerobic activity. It is also inactive against *Pseudomonas* and *Enterobacter* spp.

Third-Generation Cephalosporins with Good Activity Against Pseudomonas

Ceftazidime is one-quarter to one-half as active by weight against gram-positive microorganisms as is cefotaxime. Its activity against the Enterobacteriaceae is very similar, but its major distinguishing feature is excellent activity against *Pseudomonas* and other gram-negative bacteria. Ceftazidime has poor activity against *B. fragilis*. Its $t_{1/2}$ in plasma is ~1.5 hours, and the drug is not metabolized. Ceftazidime is more active *in vitro* against *Pseudomonas* than piperacillin is (Edmond et al., 1999).

Fourth-Generation Cephalosporins. Cefepime and cefpirome are fourth-generation cephalosporins. Only cefepime is available for use in the U.S. Cefepime is stable to hydrolysis by many of the previously identified plasmid-encoded β-lactamases (called TEM-1, TEM-2, and SHV-1). It is a poor inducer of, and is relatively resistant to, the type I chromosomally encoded and some extended-spectrum β-lactamases. Thus, it is active against many Enterobacteriaceae that are resistant to other cephalosporins via induction of type I β-lactamases but remains susceptible to many bacteria expressing extended-spectrum plasmid-mediated β-lactamases (such as KPC, TEM-3, and TEM-10).

Against the fastidious gram-negative bacteria (*H. influenzae, N. gonorrhoeae,* and *N. meningitidis*), cefepime has comparable or greater *in vitro* activity than cefotaxime. For *P. aeruginosa*, cefepime has comparable activity to ceftazidime, although it is less active than ceftazidime for other *Pseudomonas* spp. and *X. maltophilia*. Cefepime has higher activity than ceftazidime and comparable activity to cefotaxime for streptococci and methicillin-sensitive *S. aureus*. It is not active against methicillin-resistant *S. aureus*, penicillin-resistant pneumococci, enterococci, *B. fragilis, L. monocytogenes, Mycobacterium avium* complex, or *M. tuberculosis*. Cefepime is excreted almost 100% renally, and doses should be adjusted for renal failure. Cefepime has excellent penetration into the CSF in animal models of meningitis. When given at the recommended dosage for adults of 2 g intravenously every 12 hours, peak serum concentrations in humans range from 126 to 193 μg/mL. The serum $t_{1/2}$ is 2 hours.

Adverse Reactions. Hypersensitivity reactions to the cephalosporins are the most common side effects, and there is no evidence that any single cephalosporin is more or less likely to cause such sensitization. The reactions appear to be identical to those caused by the penicillins, perhaps related to the shared β-lactam structure of both groups of antibiotics. Immediate reactions such as anaphylaxis, bronchospasm, and urticaria are observed. More commonly, maculopapular rash develops, usually after several days of therapy; this may or may not be accompanied by fever and eosinophilia.

Because of the similar structures of the penicillins and cephalosporins, patients who are allergic to one class of agents may manifest cross-reactivity to a member of the other class. Immunological studies have demonstrated cross-reactivity in as many as 20% of patients who are allergic to penicillin, but clinical studies indicate a much lower frequency (~1%) of such reactions. There are no skin tests that can reliably predict whether a patient will manifest an allergic reaction to the cephalosporins.

Patients with a history of a mild or a temporally distant reaction to penicillin appear to be at low risk of rash or other allergic reaction following the administration of a cephalosporin. However, patients who have had a recent severe, immediate reaction to a penicillin should be given a cephalosporin with great caution, if at all. A positive Coombs reaction appears frequently in patients who receive large doses of a cephalosporin. Hemolysis usually is not associated with this phenomenon, although it has been reported and has been associated with fatalities. Cephalosporins have produced rare instances of bone marrow depression, characterized by granulocytopenia.

The cephalosporins have been implicated as potentially nephrotoxic agents, although they are not nearly as toxic to the kidney as the aminoglycosides or the polymyxins. Renal tubular necrosis has followed the administration of cephaloridine in doses >4 g/day; this agent is no longer available in the U.S. Other cephalosporins are much less toxic and, when used by themselves in recommended doses, rarely produce significant renal toxicity. High doses of cephalothin (no longer available in the U.S.) have produced acute tubular necrosis in certain instances, and usual doses (8-12 g/day) have caused nephrotoxicity in patients with preexisting renal disease. There is good evidence that the concurrent administration of cephalothin and gentamicin or tobramycin act synergistically to cause nephrotoxicity, especially in patients >60 years of age. Diarrhea can result from the administration of cephalosporins and may be more frequent with cefoperazone, perhaps because of its greater biliary excretion. Intolerance to alcohol (a disulfiram-like reaction) has been noted with cephalosporins that contain the methylthiotetrazole (MTT) group, including cefotetan, cefamandole, moxalactam, and cefoperazone (the latter three are no longer available in the U.S.). Serious bleeding related either to hypoprothrombinemia owing to the MTT group, thrombocytopenia, and/or platelet dysfunction has been reported with several β-lactam antibiotics.

Therapeutic Uses. The cephalosporins are used widely and are therapeutically important antibiotics. Clinical studies have shown cephalosporins to be effective as both therapeutic and prophylactic agents. Unfortunately, a wide array of bacteria is resistant to their activity.

The first-generation cephalosporins are excellent agents for skin and soft tissue infections owing to *S. pyogenes* and methicillin-susceptible *S. aureus*. A single dose of cefazolin just before surgery is the preferred prophylaxis for procedures in which skin flora are the likely pathogens (Medical Letter, 2006). For colorectal surgery, where prophylaxis for intestinal anaerobes is desired, the second-generation agent cefoxitin is preferred.

The second-generation cephalosporins generally have been displaced by third-generation agents. They have inferior activity against penicillin-resistant *S. pneumoniae* compared with either the third-generation agents or ampicillin and therefore should not be used for empirical treatment of meningitis or pneumonia. The oral second-generation cephalosporins can be used to treat respiratory tract infections, although they are suboptimal (compared with oral amoxicillin) for treatment of penicillin-resistant *S. pneumoniae* pneumonia and otitis media. In situations where facultative gram-negative bacteria and anaerobes are involved, such as intra-abdominal infections, pelvic inflammatory disease, and diabetic foot infection, cefoxitin and cefotetan both are effective.

The third-generation cephalosporins, with or without aminoglycosides, have been considered to be the drugs of choice for serious infections caused by *Klebsiella, Enterobacter, Proteus, Providencia, Serratia*, and *Haemophilus* spp. Ceftriaxone is the therapy of choice for all forms of gonorrhea and for severe forms of Lyme disease. The third-generation cephalosporins cefotaxime or ceftriaxone are used for the initial treatment of meningitis in nonimmunocompromised adults and children >3 months of age (in combination with vancomycin and ampicillin pending identification of the causative agent) because of their antimicrobial activity, good penetration into CSF, and record of clinical success. They are the drugs of choice for the treatment of meningitis caused by *H. influenzae*, sensitive *S. pneumoniae*, *N. meningitidis*, and gram-negative enteric bacteria. Cefotaxime has failed in the treatment of meningitis owing to resistant *S. pneumoniae;* thus vancomycin should be added (Quagliarello and Scheld, 1997). Ceftazidime plus an aminoglycoside is the treatment of choice for *Pseudomonas* meningitis. Third-generation cephalosporins, however, lack activity against *L. monocytogenes* and penicillin-resistant pneumococci, which may cause meningitis. The antimicrobial spectra of cefotaxime and ceftriaxone are excellent for the treatment of community-acquired pneumonia, i.e., pneumonia caused by some pneumococci (achievable serum concentrations exceed MICs for many or most penicillin-resistant isolates), *H. influenzae*, or *S. aureus*.

The fourth-generation cephalosporins are indicated for the empirical treatment of nosocomial infections where antibiotic resistance owing to extended-spectrum β-lactamases or chromosomally induced β-lactamases are anticipated. For example, cefepime has superior activity against nosocomial isolates of *Enterobacter, Citrobacter*, and *Serratia* spp. compared with ceftazidime and piperacillin. However KPC- or metallo-β-lactamase expressing strains are resistant to cefepime.

OTHER β-LACTAM ANTIBIOTICS

Important therapeutic agents with a β-lactam structure that are neither penicillins nor cephalosporins have been developed.

Carbapenems

Carbapenems are β-lactams that contain a fused β-lactam ring and a five-member ring system that differs from the penicillins because it is unsaturated and contains a carbon atom instead of the sulfur atom. This class of antibiotics has a broader spectrum of activity than most other β-lactam antibiotics.

Imipenem. Imipenem is marketed in combination with cilastatin, a drug that inhibits the degradation of imipenem by a renal tubular dipeptidase.

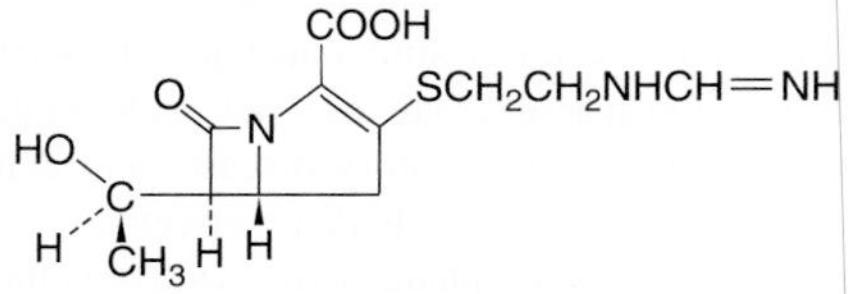

IMIPENEM

Imipenem is derived from a compound produced by *Streptomyces cattleya*. The compound thienamycin is unstable, but imipenem, the *N*-formimidoyl derivative, is stable.

Antimicrobial Activity. Imipenem, like other β-lactam antibiotics, binds to penicillin-binding proteins, disrupts bacterial cell wall synthesis, and causes death of susceptible microorganisms. It is very resistant to hydrolysis by most β-lactamases.

The activity of imipenem is excellent *in vitro* for a wide variety of aerobic and anaerobic microorganisms. Streptococci (including penicillin-resistant *S. pneumoniae*), enterococci (excluding *E. faecium* and non-β-lactamase-producing penicillin-resistant strains), staphylococci (including penicillinase-producing strains), and *Listeria* all are susceptible. Although some strains of methicillin-resistant staphylococci are susceptible, many strains are not. Activity was excellent against the Enterobacteriaceae until the emergence of KPC carbapenemase-producing strains (Jones et al., 2008; Walsh, 2008). Most strains of *Pseudomonas* and *Acinetobacter* are inhibited. *S. maltophilia* is resistant. Anaerobes, including *B. fragilis*, are highly susceptible.

Pharmacokinetics and Adverse Reactions. Imipenem is not absorbed orally. The drug is hydrolyzed rapidly by a dipeptidase found in the brush border of the proximal renal tubule. Because concentrations of active drug in urine were low, cilastatin, an inhibitor of the dehydropeptidase, was synthesized. A preparation has been developed that contains equal amounts of imipenem and cilastatin (PRIMAXIN).

After the intravenous administration of 500 mg imipenem and cilastatin, peak concentrations in plasma average 33 μg/mL. Both imipenem and cilastatin have a $t_{1/2}$ of ~1 hour. When administered concurrently with cilastatin, ~70% of administered imipenem is recovered in the urine as the active drug. Dosage should be modified for patients with renal insufficiency.

Nausea and vomiting are the most common adverse reactions (1-20%). Seizures also have been noted in up to 1.5% of patients, especially when high doses are given to patients with CNS lesions and to those with renal insufficiency. Patients who are allergic to other β-lactam antibiotics may have hypersensitivity reactions when given imipenem.

Therapeutic Uses. Imipenem–cilastatin is effective for a wide variety of infections, including urinary tract and lower respiratory infections; intra-abdominal and gynecological infections; and skin, soft tissue, bone, and joint infections. The drug combination appears to be especially useful for the treatment of infections caused by cephalosporin-resistant nosocomial bacteria, such as *Citrobacter freundii* and *Enterobacter* spp. (with the exception of the increasingly common KPC-producing strains). It would be prudent to use imipenem for empirical treatment of serious infections in hospitalized patients who have recently received other β-lactam antibiotics because of the increased risk of infection with cephalosporin- and/or penicillin-resistant bacteria. Imipenem should not be used as monotherapy for infections owing to *P. aeruginosa* because of the risk of resistance developing during therapy.

Meropenem. Meropenem (MERREM iv) is a dimethylcarbamoyl pyrolidinyl derivative of thienamycin. It does not require co-administration with cilastatin because it is not sensitive to renal dipeptidase. Its toxicity is similar to that of imipenem except that it may be less likely to cause seizures (0.5% for meropenem; 1.5% for imipenem). Its *in vitro* activity is similar to that of imipenem, with activity against some imipenem-resistant *P. aeruginosa* but less activity against gram-positive cocci. Clinical experience with meropenem demonstrates therapeutic equivalence with imipenem.

Doripenem. Doripenem (DORIBAX) has a spectrum of activity that is similar to that of imipenem and meropenem, with greater activity against some resistant isolates of Pseudomonas (Medical Letter, 2008).

Ertapenem. Ertapenem (INVANZ) differs from imipenem and meropenem by having a longer $t_{1/2}$ that allows once-daily dosing and by having inferior activity against *P. aeruginosa* and *Acinetobacter* spp. Its spectrum of activity against gram-positive organisms, Enterobacteriaceae, and anaerobes makes it attractive for use in intra-abdominal and pelvic infections (Solomkin et al., 2003).

Aztreonam. Aztreonam (AZACTAM) is a monocyclic β-lactam compound (a monobactam) isolated from *Chromobacterium violaceum* (Sykes et al., 1981).

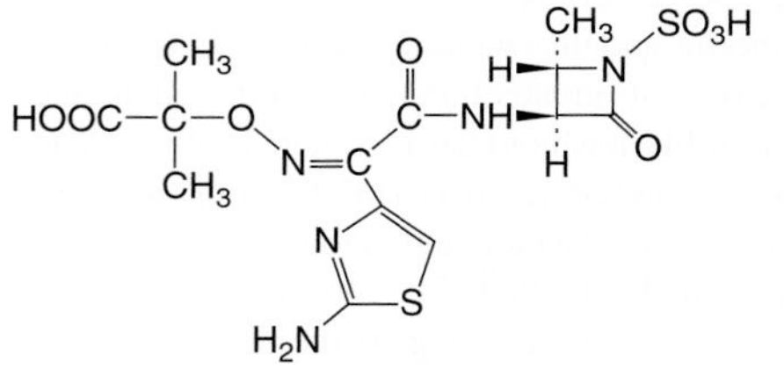

AZTREONAM

Aztreonam interacts with penicillin-binding proteins of susceptible microorganisms and induces the formation of long filamentous bacterial structures. The compound is resistant to many of the β-lactamases that are elaborated by most gram-negative bacteria, including the metallo-β-lactamases but not the KPC β-lactamases (Jones et al., 2008; Walsh, 2008).

The antimicrobial activity of aztreonam differs from those of other β-lactam antibiotics and more closely resembles that of an aminoglycoside. Aztreonam has activity only against gram-negative bacteria; it has no activity against gram-positive bacteria and anaerobic organisms. However, activity against Enterobacteriaceae is excellent, as is that against *P. aeruginosa*. It is also highly active *in vitro* against *H. influenzae* and gonococci.

Aztreonam is administered either intramuscularly or intravenously. Peak concentrations of aztreonam in plasma average nearly 50 μg/mL after a 1-g intramuscular dose. The $t_{1/2}$ for elimination is 1.7 hours, and most of the drug is recovered unaltered in the urine. The $t_{1/2}$ is prolonged to ~6 hours in anephric patients.

Aztreonam generally is well tolerated. Interestingly, patients who are allergic to penicillins or cephalosporins appear not to react to aztreonam, with the exception of ceftazidime.

The usual dose of aztreonam for severe infections is 2 g every 6-8 hours. This should be reduced in patients with renal insufficiency. Aztreonam has been used successfully for the therapy of a variety of infections. One of its notable features is little allergic cross-reactivity with β-lactam antibiotics, with the possible exception of ceftazidime (Perez Pimiento et al., 1998), with which it has considerable structural similarity. Aztreonam is therefore quite useful for treating gram-negative infections that normally would be treated with a β-lactam antibiotic were it not for the history of a prior allergic reaction.

β-LACTAMASE INHIBITORS

Certain molecules can inactivate β-lactamases, thereby preventing the destruction of β-lactam antibiotics that are substrates for these enzymes. β-Lactamase inhibitors are most active against plasmid-encoded β-lactamases (including the enzymes that hydrolyze ceftazidime and cefotaxime), but they are inactive at clinically achievable concentrations against the type I chromosomal β-lactamases induced in gram-negative bacilli (such as *Enterobacter, Acinetobacter,* and *Citrobacter*) by treatment with second- and third-generation cephalosporins.

Clavulanic acid is produced by *Streptomyces clavuligerus;* its structural formula is:

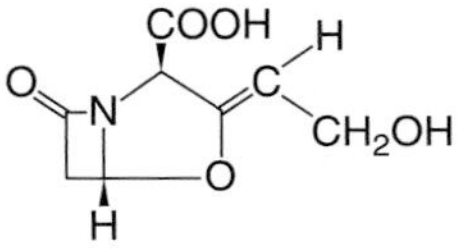

CLAVULANIC ACID

It has poor intrinsic antimicrobial activity, but it is a "suicide" inhibitor that irreversibly binds β-lactamases produced by a wide range of gram-positive and gram-negative microorganisms. Clavulanic acid is well absorbed by mouth and also can be given parenterally. It has been combined with amoxicillin as an oral preparation (AUGMENTIN, others) and with ticarcillin as a parenteral preparation (TIMENTIN).

Amoxicillin plus clavulanate is effective *in vitro* and *in vivo* for β-lactamase-producing strains of staphylococci, *H. influenzae,* gonococci, and *E. coli*. Amoxicillin-clavulanate plus ciprofloxacin has been shown to be an effective oral treatment for low-risk febrile patients with neutropenia from cancer chemotherapy (Freifeld et al., 1999; Kern et al., 1999). It also is effective in the treatment of acute otitis media in children, sinusitis, animal or human bite wounds, cellulitis, and diabetic foot infections. The addition of clavulanate to ticarcillin (timentin) extends its spectrum such that it resembles imipenem to include aerobic gram-negative bacilli, *S. aureus*, and *Bacteroides* spp. There is no increased activity against *Pseudomonas* spp. The dosage should be adjusted for patients with renal insufficiency. The combination is especially useful for mixed nosocomial infections and is used often with an aminoglycoside.

Sulbactam is another β-lactamase inhibitor similar in structure to clavulanic acid. It may be given orally or parenterally along with a β-lactam antibiotic. It is available for intravenous or intramuscular use combined with ampicillin (UNASYN, others). Dosage must be adjusted for patients with impaired renal function. The combination has good activity against gram-positive cocci, including β-lactamase-producing strains of *S. aureus*, gram-negative aerobes (but not resistant strains of *E. coli* or *Pseudomonas*), and anaerobes; it also has been used effectively for the treatment of mixed intra-abdominal and pelvic infections.

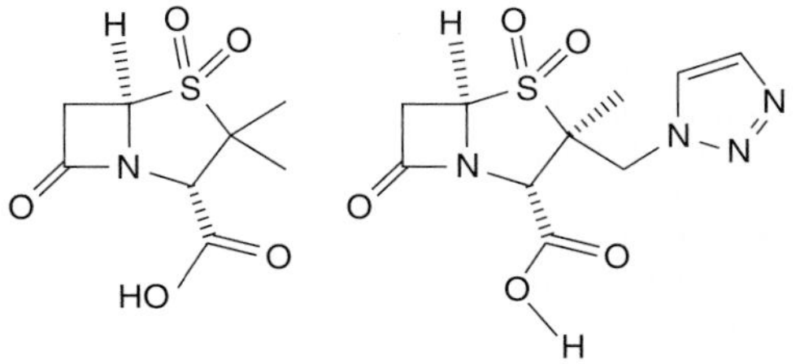

SULBACTAM

TAZOBACTAM

Tazobactam is a penicillanic acid sulfone β-lactamase inhibitor. In comparison with the other available inhibitors, it has poor activity against the inducible chromosomal β-lactamases of Enterobacteriaceae but has good activity against many of the plasmid β-lactamases, including some of the extended-spectrum class. It has been combined with piperacillin as a parenteral preparation (ZOSYN).

The combination of piperacillin and tazobactam does not increase the activity of piperacillin against *P. aeruginosa* because resistance is due to either chromosomal β-lactamases or decreased permeability of piperacillin into the periplasmic space. Because the currently recommended dose (3 g piperacillin per 375 mg tazobactam every 4-8 hours) is less than the recommended dose of piperacillin when used alone for serious infections (3-4 g every 4-6 hours), concern has been raised that piperacillin-tazobactam may prove ineffective in the treatment of some *P. aeruginosa* infections that would have responded to piperacillin. The combination of piperacillin plus tazobactam should be equivalent in antimicrobial spectrum to ticarcillin plus clavulanate.

BIBLIOGRAPHY

Andes DR, Craig WA. Cephalosporins. In: *Mandell, Douglas, and Bennett's Principles and Practice of Infectious Diseases,* 6th ed. (Mandell GL, Bennett JE, Dolin R, eds.), Churchill Livingstone, Philadelphia, **2005,** pp. 294–307.

Bayles KW. The bactericidal action of penicillin: New clues to an unsolved mystery. *Trends Microbiol,* **2000,** *8:*81274–81278.

Berrios X, del Campo E, Guzman B, Bisno AL. Discontinuing rheumatic fever prophylaxis in selected adolescents and young adults: A prospective study. *Ann Intern Med,* **1993,** *118:*401–406.

Bisno AL, Stevens DL. Streptococcal infections of skin and soft tissues. *N Engl J Med*, **1996,** *334:*240–245.

Brown EJ. The molecular basis of streptococcal toxic shock syndrome. *N Engl J Med,* **2004,** *350:*2093–2094.

Bush K. New *β*-lactamases in gram-negative bacteria: Diversity and impact on the selection of antimicrobial therapy. *Clin Infect Dis,* **2001,** *32:*1085–1089.

Carratalá J, Alcaide F, Fernandez-Sevilla A, et al. Bacteremia due to *viridans* streptococci that are highly resistant to penicillin: Increase among neutropenic patients with cancer. *Clin Infect Dis,* **1995,** *20:*1169–1173.

Catalan MJ, Fernandez JM, Vazquez A, et al. Failure of cefotaxime in the treatment of meningitis due to relatively resistant *Streptococcus pneumoniae. Clin Infect Dis,* **1994,** *18:* 766–769.

Centers for Disease Control and Prevention. Vancomycin-intermediate/resistant *Staphylococcus aureus. MMWR,* **2004,** *53:*322–323. Available at: http://www.cdc.gov/ncidod/dhqp/ar_visavrsa.html.

Centers for Disease Control and Prevention. Sexually transmitted diseases guidelines. 2006. Available at: http://www.cdc.gov/std/treatment/. Accessed December 22, 2009.

Chambers HF. Penicillins. In: *Mandell, Douglas, and Bennett's Principles and Practice of Infectious Diseases,* 6th ed. (Mandell GL, Bennett JE, Dolin R, eds.), Churchill Livingstone, Philadelphia, **2005.**

de Gans J, van de Beek D. Dexamethasone in adults with bacterial meningitis. *N Engl J Med,* **2002,** *347:*1549–1556.

Donlan RM. Biofilm formation: A clinically relevant microbiologic process. *Clin Infect Dis,* **2001,** *33:*1387–1392.

Dowell SF, Butler JC, Giebink GS, et al. Acute otitis media: Management and surveillance in an era of pneumococcal resistance—a report from the Drug-resistant *Streptococcus pneumoniae* Therapeutic Working Group. *Pediatr Infect Dis J,* **1999,** *18:*1–9.

Edmond MB, Wallace SE, McClish DK, et al. Nosocomial bloodstream infections in United States hospitals: A three-year analysis. *Clin Infect Dis,* **1999,** *29:*239–244.

Fass RJ, Copelan EA, Brandt JT, *et al.* Platelet-mediated bleeding caused by broad-spectrum penicillins. *J Infect Dis,* **1987,** *155:*1242–1248.

Fiore AE, Moroney JF, Farley MM, et al. Clinical outcomes of meningitis caused by *Streptococcus pneumoniae* in the era of antibiotic resistance. *Clin Infect Dis,* **2000,** *30:*71–77.

Freifeld A, Marchigiani D, Walsh T, et al. A double-blind comparison of empirical oral and intravenous antibiotic therapy for low-risk febrile patients with neutropenia during cancer chemotherapy. *N Engl J Med,* **1999,** *341:*305–311.

Ghuysen JM. Serine *β*-lactamases and penicillin-binding proteins. *Annu Rev Microbiol,* **1991,** *45:*37–67.

Goldstein EJ, Citron DM, Richwald GA. Lack of *in vitro* efficacy of oral forms of certain cephalosporins, erythromycin, and oxacillin against *Pasteurella multocida. Antimicrob Agents Chemother,* **1988,** *32:*213–215.

Haas DW, Stratton CW, Griffin JP, et al. Diminished activity of ceftizoxime in comparison to cefotaxime and ceftriaxone against *Streptococcus pneumoniae. Clin Infect Dis,* **1995,** *20:* 671–676.

Handsfield HH, Sparling PF. *Neisseria gonorrhoeae.* In: *Mandell, Douglas, and Bennett's Principles and Practice of Infectious Diseases,* 6th ed. (Mandell GL, Bennett JE, Dolin R, eds.), Churchill Livingstone, Philadelphia, **2005,** pp. 2514–2527.

Jacoby GA, Munoz-Price L. The new beta-lactamases. *N Engl J Med,* **2005,** *352:*380–391.

John CC. Treatment failure with use of a third-generation cephalosporin for penicillin-resistant pneumococcal meningitis: Case report and review. *Clin Infect Dis,* **1994,** *18:*188–193.

Jones RN, Kirby JT, Rhomberg PR. Comparative activity of meropenem in US medical centers (2007): Initiating the 2nd decade of MYSTIC program surveillance. *Diagn Microbiol Infect Dis,* **2008,** *61:*203–213.

Kern WV, Cometta A, De Bock R, et al. Oral versus intravenous empirical antimicrobial therapy for fever in patients with granulocytopenia who are receiving cancer chemotherapy. International Antimicrobial Therapy Cooperative Group of the European Organization for Research and Treatment of Cancer. *N Engl J Med,* **1999,** *341:*312–318.

Kucers A, Bennett NM. *The Use of Antibiotics: A Comprehensive Review with Clinical Emphasis.* Lippincott, Philadelphia, **1987.**

Levison ME, Mangura CT, Lorber B, et al. Clindamycin compared with penicillin for the treatment of anaerobic lung abscess. *Ann Intern Med,* **1983,** *98:*466–471.

Lovering AL, de Castro LH, Lim D, Strynadka NCJ. Structural insight into the transglyosylation step of bacterial cell-wall biosynthesis. *Science,* **2007,** *315:*1402–1405.

Medical Letter. Antimicrobial prophylaxis for surgery: Treatment guidelines. *Med Lett Drugs Ther,* **2006,** *4:*83–88.

Medical Letter. Choice of antibacterial drugs: Treatment guidelines. *Med Lett Drugs Ther,* **2007,** *5:*33–50.

Medical Letter. Doripenem (Doribax)—a new parenteral carbapenem. *Med Lett Drugs Ther,* **2008,** *50:*5–6.

Moran GL, Krishnadasan A, Gorwitz, et al. Methicillin-resistant *S. aureus* infection among patients in the emergency department. *N Engl J Med,* **2006,** *355:*666.

Nakae T. Outer-membrane permeability of bacteria. *Crit Rev Microbiol,* **1986,** *13:*1–62.

Nikaido H. Antibiotic resistance caused by gram-negative multidrug efflux pumps. *Clin Infect Dis,* **1998,** *27*(suppl I):S32–S41.

Nikaido H. Prevention of drug access to bacterial targets: Permeability barriers and active efflux. *Science,* **1994,** *264:*382–388.

Okuma K, Iwakawa K, Turnidge JD. Dissemination of new methicillin-resistant *Staphylococcus aureus* clones in the community. *J Clin Microbiol,* **2002,** *40:*4289–4294.

Perez Pimiento A, Gomez Martinez M, Minguez Mena A, et al. Aztreonam and ceftazidime: Evidence of *in vivo* cross allergenicity. *Allergy,* **1998,** *53:*624–625.

Quagliarello V, Scheld WM. Drug therapy: Treatment of bacterial meningitis. *N Engl J Med,* **1997,** *336:*708–716.

Romano A, Mondino C, Viola M, Montuschi P. Immediate allergic reactions to *β*-lactams: Diagnosis and therapy. *Int J Immunopathol Pharmacol,* **2003,** *16:*19–23.

Schaad UB, Suter S, Gianella-Borradori A, et al. A comparison of ceftriaxone and cefuroxime for the treatment of bacterial meningitis in children. *N Engl J Med,* **1990,** *322:*141–147.

Sogn DD, Evans R, Shepherd GM, et al. Results of the NIAID collaborative clinical trial to test the predictive value of skin testing with major and minor penicillin derivatives in hospitalized adults. *Arch Intern Med,* **1992,** *152:*1025–1032.

Solomkin JS, Yellin AE, Rutstein OD, et al. Ertapenem vs. piperacillin/tazobactam in the treatment of complicated intra-abdominal infections: Results of a double-blind, randomized comparative phase III trial. *Ann Surg,* **2003,** *237:*235–242.

Spratt BG. Resistance to antibiotics mediated by target alterations. *Science,* **1994,** *264:*388–393.

Swartz MN. Cellulitis. *N Engl J Med*, **2004,** *350:*904–912.

Sykes RB, Cimarusti CM, Bonner DP, et al. Monocyclic β-lactam antibiotics produced by bacteria. *Nature,* **1981,** *291:*489–491.

Tramont EC. *Treponema pallidum* (syphilis). In: *Mandell, Douglas, and Bennett's Principles and Practice of Infectious Diseases,* 6th ed. (Mandell GL, Bennett JE, Dolin R, eds.), Churchill Livingstone, Philadelphia, **2005,** pp. 2768–2783.

Walsh TR. Clinically significant carbapenemases: An update. *Curr Opin Infect Dis,* **2008,** *21:*367–371.

Weiss ME, Adkinson NF Jr. β-Lactam allergy. In: *Mandell, Douglas, and Bennett's Principles and Practice of Infectious Diseases,* 6th ed. (Mandell GL, Bennett JE, Dolin R, eds.), Churchill Livingstone, Philadelphia, **2005.**

Wilson W, Taubert K, Gewitz M, et al. Prevention of infective endocarditis. *Circulation,* **2007,** *116:*1736.

Wilson WR, Wilkowske CJ, Wright AJ, et al. Treatment of streptomycin-susceptible and streptomycin-resistant enterococcal endocarditis. *Ann Intern Med,* **1984,** *100:*816–823.

Aminoglycosides

Conan MacDougall
and Henry F. Chambers

The aminoglycoside group includes gentamicin, tobramycin, amikacin, netilmicin (not available in the U.S.), kanamycin, streptomycin, paromomycin, and neomycin. These drugs are used primarily to treat infections caused by aerobic gram-negative bacteria; streptomycin is an important agent for the treatment of tuberculosis, and paromomycin is used orally for intestinal amebiasis and in the management of hepatic coma. In contrast to most inhibitors of microbial protein synthesis, which are bacteriostatic, the aminoglycosides are bactericidal inhibitors of protein synthesis. Mutations affecting proteins in the bacterial ribosome, the target for these drugs, can confer marked resistance to their action. However, most commonly resistance is due to acquisition of plasmids or transposon-encoding genes for aminoglycoside-metabolizing enzymes or from impaired transport of drug into the cell. Thus, there can be cross-resistance between members of the class.

These agents contain amino sugars linked to an aminocyclitol ring by glycosidic bonds (Figure 54–1). They are polycations, and their polarity is responsible in part for pharmacokinetic properties shared by all members of the group. For example, none is absorbed adequately after oral administration, inadequate concentrations are found in cerebrospinal fluid (CSF), and all are excreted relatively rapidly by the normal kidney. Although aminoglycosides are widely used and important agents, serious toxicity limits their utility. All members of the group share the same spectrum of toxicity, most notably nephrotoxicity and ototoxicity, which can involve the auditory and vestibular functions of the eighth cranial nerve.

History and Source. Aminoglycosides are natural products or semisynthetic derivatives of compounds produced by a variety of soil actinomycetes. Streptomycin was first isolated from a strain of *Streptomyces griseus*. Gentamicin and netilmicin are derived from species of the actinomycete *Micromonospora*. The difference in spelling (*-micin*) compared with the other aminoglycoside antibiotics (*-mycin*) reflects this difference in origin. Tobramycin is one of several components of an aminoglycoside complex (nebramycin) that is produced by *S. tenebrarius*. It is most similar in antimicrobial activity and toxicity to gentamicin. In contrast to the other aminoglycosides, amikacin, a derivative of kanamycin, and netilmicin, a derivative of sisomicin, are semisynthetic products. Other aminoglycoside antibiotics have been developed (e.g., arbekacin, isepamicin, and sisomicin), but they have not been introduced into clinical practice in the U.S. because numerous potent, less toxic alternatives (e.g., broad-spectrum β-lactam antibiotics and quinolones) are available.

Chemistry. The aminoglycosides consist of two or more amino sugars joined in glycosidic linkage to a hexose nucleus, which usually is in a central position (Figure 54–1). This hexose, or aminocyclitol, is either streptidine (found in streptomycin) or 2-deoxystreptamine (found in all other available aminoglycosides). These compounds thus are aminoglycosidic aminocyclitols, although the simpler term *aminoglycoside* is used commonly. A related compound, *spectinomycin*, is an aminocyclitol that does not contain amino sugars (Chapter 55).

The aminoglycoside families are distinguished by the amino sugars attached to the aminocyclitol. In the neomycin family, which includes neomycin B and paromomycin, three amino sugars are attached to the central 2-deoxystreptamine. The kanamycin and gentamicin families have only two such amino sugars.

In the kanamycin family, which includes kanamycins A and B, amikacin, and tobramycin, two amino sugars are linked to a centrally located 2-deoxystreptamine moiety; one of these is a 3-aminohexose (Figure 54–1).

Amikacin is a semisynthetic derivative prepared from kanamycin A by acylation of the 1-amino group of the 2-deoxystreptamine moiety with 2-hydroxy-4-aminobutyric acid.

The gentamicin family, which includes gentamicins C_1, C_{1a}, and C_2, sisomicin, and netilmicin (the 1-N-ethyl derivative of sisomicin), contains a different 3-amino sugar (garosamine). Variations in methylation of the other amino sugar result in the different components of gentamicin (Figure 54–1). These modifications appear to have little effect on biological activity.

Streptomycin differs from the other aminoglycoside antibiotics in that it contains streptidine rather than 2-deoxystreptamine, and the aminocyclitol is not in a central position, as shown here.

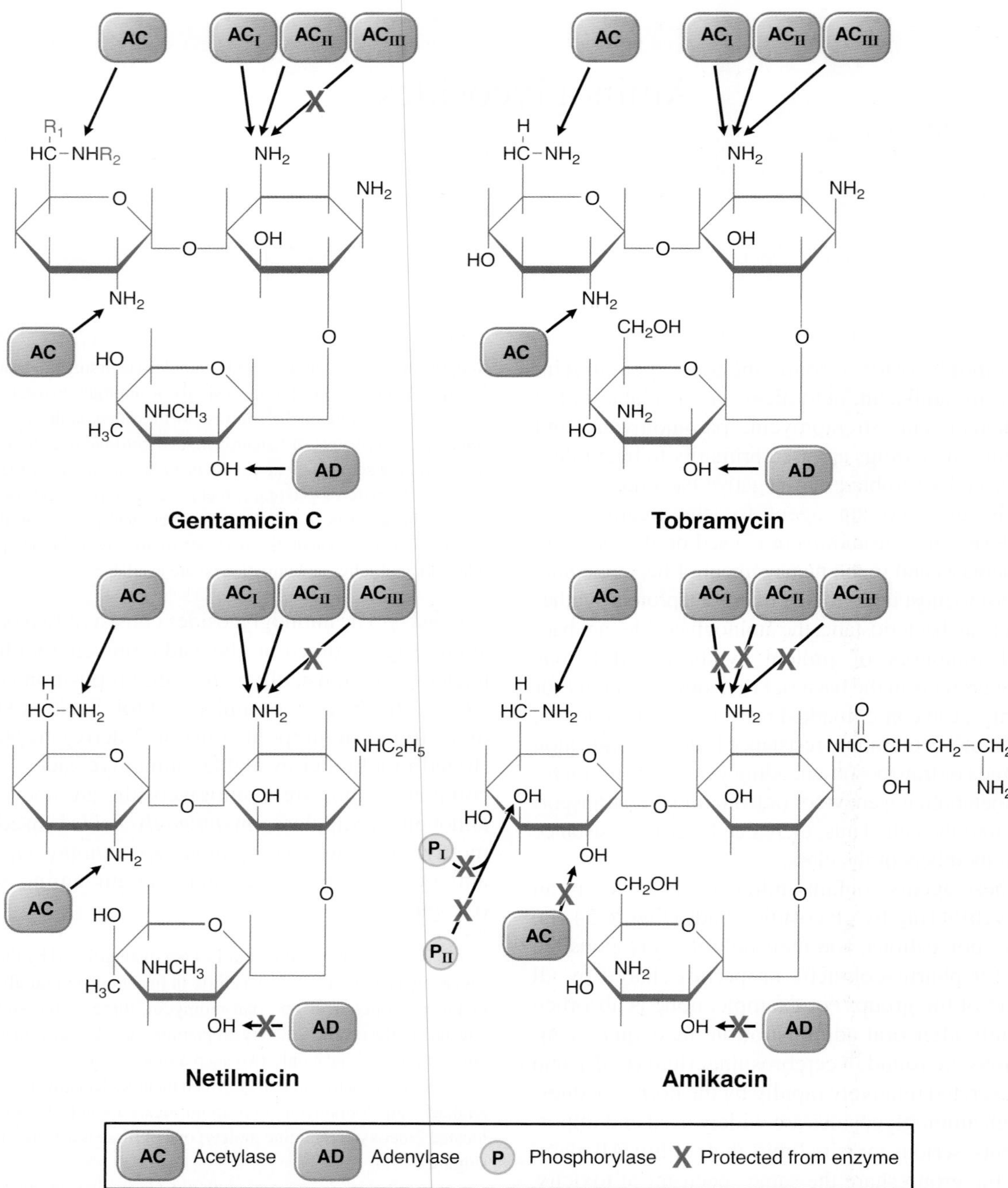

Figure 54–1. *Sites of activity of various plasmid-mediated enzymes capable of inactivating aminoglycosides.* The red **X** indicates regions of the molecules that are protected from the designated enzyme. In gentamicin C_1, R_1=R_2=CH_3; in gentamicin C_2, R_1=CH_3, R_2=H; in gentamicin C_{1a}, R_1=R_2=H. (Reproduced with permission from Moellering RC Jr. Microbiological considerations in the use of tobramycin and related aninoglycosidic aminocyclitol antibiotics. *MJA* 1977;2S:4–8. Copyright 1977. The Medical Journal of Australia.)

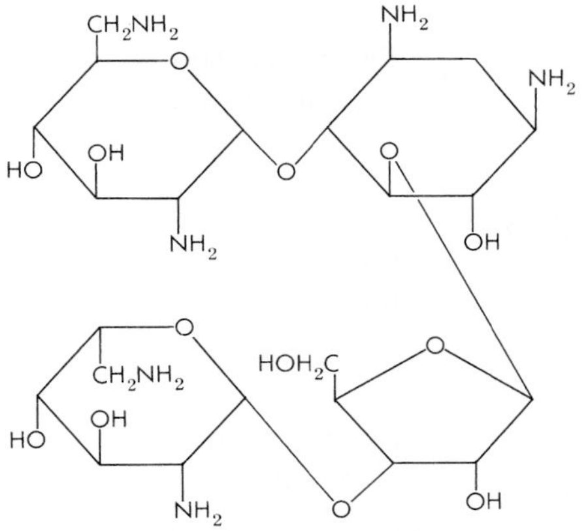

NEOMYCIN B

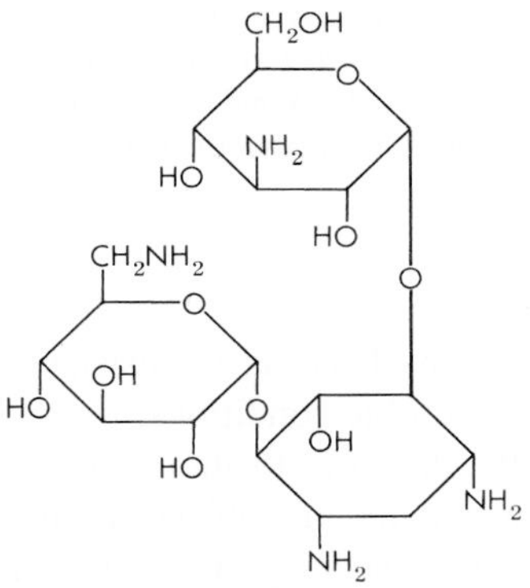

KANAMYCIN A

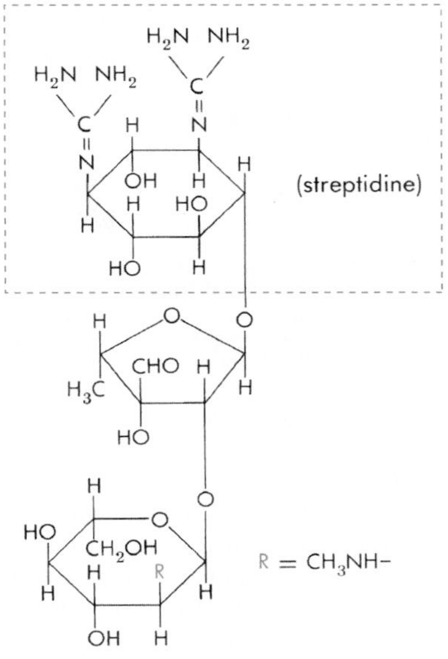

(streptidine)

R = CH_3NH–

STREPTOMYCIN

Mechanism of Action. The aminoglycoside antibiotics are rapidly bactericidal. Bacterial killing is concentration dependent: The higher the concentration, the greater is the rate at which bacteria are killed. A post-antibiotic effect, that is, residual bactericidal activity persisting after the serum concentration has fallen below the minimum inhibitory concentration (MIC), also is characteristic of aminoglycoside antibiotics; the duration of this effect also is concentration dependent. These properties probably account for the efficacy of high-dose, extended-interval dosing regimens of aminoglycosides.

Aminoglycosides diffuse through aqueous channels formed by porin proteins in the outer membrane of gram-negative bacteria to enter the periplasmic space. Transport of aminoglycosides across the cytoplasmic (inner) membrane depends on electron transport, in part because of a requirement for a membrane electrical potential (interior negative) to drive permeation of these antibiotics. This phase of transport has been termed *energy-dependent phase I* (EDP_1). It is rate limiting and can be blocked or inhibited by divalent cations (e.g., Ca^{2+} and Mg^{2+}), hyperosmolarity, a reduction in pH, and anaerobic conditions. The last two conditions impair the ability of the bacteria to maintain the membrane potential, which is the driving force for transport. Thus, the antimicrobial activity of aminoglycosides is reduced markedly in the anaerobic environment of an abscess, in hyperosmolar acidic urine, and in other conditions that limit EDP_1 (Mingeot-Leclercq et al., 1999).

Once inside the cell, aminoglycosides bind to polysomes and interfere with protein synthesis by causing misreading and premature termination of mRNA translation (Figure 54–2).

The primary intracellular site of action of the aminoglycosides is the 30S ribosomal subunit, which consists of 21 proteins and a single 16S molecule of RNA. At least three of these ribosomal proteins, and perhaps the 16S ribosomal RNA as well, contribute to the streptomycin-binding site, and alterations of these molecules markedly affect the binding and subsequent action of streptomycin. For example, a single amino acid substitution of asparagine for lysine at position 42 of the S_{12} ribosomal protein prevents binding of the drug; the resulting mutant is totally resistant to streptomycin. Substitution of glutamine for lysine creates a mutant that actually requires streptomycin for survival. The other aminoglycosides also bind to the 30S ribosomal subunit; however, they also appear to bind to several sites on the 50S ribosomal subunit (Davis, 1988).

Aminoglycosides disrupt the normal cycle of ribosomal function by interfering, at least in part, with the initiation of protein synthesis, leading to the accumulation of abnormal initiation complexes, or *streptomycin monosomes*, shown schematically in Figure 54–2B (Luzzatto et al., 1969). Aminoglycosides also cause misreading of the mRNA template and incorporation of incorrect amino acids into the growing polypeptide chains. Aminoglycosides vary in their

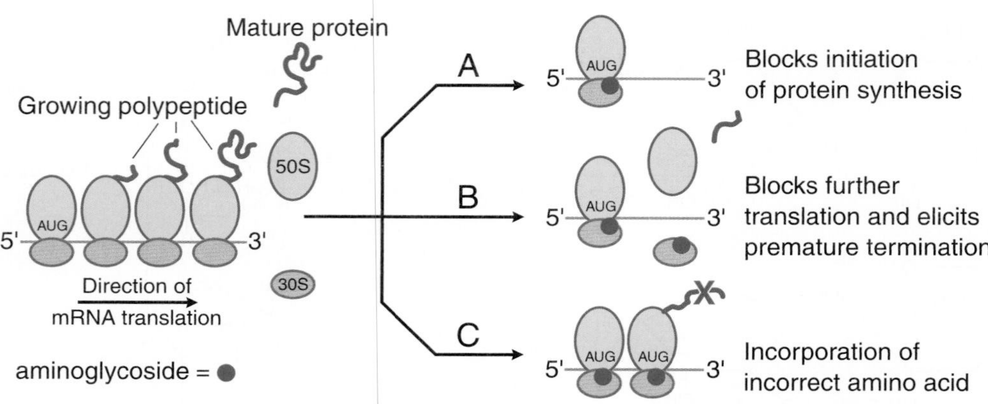

Figure 54–2. *Effects of aminoglycosides on protein synthesis.* **A.** Aminoglycoside (represented by red circles) binds to the 30S ribosomal subunit and interferes with initiation of protein synthesis by fixing the 30S–50S ribosomal complex at the start codon (AUG) of mRNA. As 30S–50S complexes downstream complete translation of mRNA and detach, the abnormal initiation complexes, so-called streptomycin monosomes, accumulate, blocking further translation of the message. Aminoglycoside binding to the 30S subunit also causes misreading of mRNA, leading to ***B,*** premature termination of translation with detachment of the ribosomal complex and incompletely synthesized protein or ***C,*** incorporation of incorrect amino acids (indicated by the red X), resulting in the production of abnormal or nonfunctional proteins.

capacity to cause misreading, presumably owing to differences in their affinities for specific ribosomal proteins. Although there appears to be a strong correlation between bactericidal activity and the ability to induce misreading (Hummel and Böck, 1989), it is not clear whether misreading is the primary mechanism of aminoglycoside-induced cell death.

The resulting aberrant proteins may be inserted into the cell membrane, leading to altered permeability and further stimulation of aminoglycoside transport (Busse et al., 1992). This phase of aminoglycoside transport, termed *energy-dependent phase II* (EDP_2), is poorly understood; however, EDP_2 may link to disruption of the structure of the cytoplasmic membrane, perhaps by the aberrant proteins. This concept is consistent with the observed progression of the leakage of small ions, followed by larger molecules and, eventually, by proteins from the bacterial cell prior to aminoglycoside-induced death. This progressive disruption of the cell envelope, as well as other vital cell processes, may help to explain the lethal action of aminoglycosides (Bryan, 1989).

Microbial Resistance to the Aminoglycosides. Bacteria may be resistant to aminoglycosides because of failure of the antibiotic to penetrate intracellularly, inactivation of the drug by microbial enzymes, or low affinity of the drug for the bacterial ribosome. Intrinsic resistance to aminoglycosides may be caused by failure of the drug to penetrate the cytoplasmic (inner) membrane. Penetration of drug across the outer membrane of gram-negative microorganisms into the periplasmic space can be slow, but resistance on this basis is unimportant clinically. Transport of aminoglycosides across the cytoplasmic membrane is an oxygen-dependent active process. Strictly anaerobic bacteria thus are resistant to these drugs because they lack the necessary transport system. Similarly, facultative bacteria are resistant when they are grown under anaerobic conditions.

Clinically, drug inactivation is the most common mechanism for acquired microbial resistance to aminoglycosides. The genes encoding aminoglycoside-modifying enzymes are acquired primarily by conjugation and transfer of resistance plasmids (Davies, 1994) (Chapter 48). These enzymes phosphorylate, adenylate, or acetylate specific hydroxyl or amino groups (Figure 54–1). Amikacin is a suitable substrate for only a few of these inactivating enzymes (Figure 54–1); thus, strains that are resistant to multiple other aminoglycosides tend to be susceptible to amikacin. The metabolites of the aminoglycosides may compete with the unaltered drug for transport across the inner membrane, but they are incapable of binding effectively to ribosomes and interfering with protein synthesis. A significant percentage of clinical isolates of *Enterococcus faecalis* and *E. faecium* are highly resistant to all aminoglycosides. Infections caused by aminoglycoside-resistant strains of enterococci can be especially difficult to treat because of the loss of the synergistic bactericidal activity between a penicillin or vancomycin and an aminoglycoside (Spera and Farber, 1992; Vemuri and Zervos, 1993). Resistance to gentamicin indicates cross-resistance to tobramycin, amikacin, kanamycin, and netilmicin because the inactivating enzyme is bifunctional and can modify all these aminoglycosides. Owing to differences in the chemical structures of streptomycin and other aminoglycosides, this enzyme does not modify streptomycin, which is inactivated by another enzyme;

consequently, gentamicin-resistant strains of enterococci may be susceptible to streptomycin.

Resistance owing to mutations that alter ribosomal structure and reduce aminoglycoside binding is relatively uncommon. Missense mutations in *Escherichia coli* that substitute a single amino acid in a crucial ribosomal protein may prevent binding of streptomycin. Although highly resistant to streptomycin, these strains are not widespread in nature. Similarly, only 5% of strains of *Pseudomonas aeruginosa* exhibit such ribosomal resistance to streptomycin. Resistance in ~50% of streptomycin-resistant strains of enterococci is attributable to ribosomal mutations (Eliopoulos et al., 1984). Because ribosomal resistance usually is specific for streptomycin, these strains of enterococci remain sensitive to a combination of penicillin and gentamicin *in vitro*.

Antibacterial Spectrum of the Aminoglycosides. The antibacterial activity of gentamicin, tobramycin, kanamycin, netilmicin, and amikacin is directed primarily against aerobic gram-negative bacilli. Kanamycin, like streptomycin, has a more limited spectrum compared with other aminoglycosides; in particular, it should not be used to treat infections caused by *Serratia* or *P. aeruginosa*. The aerobic gram-negative bacilli vary in their susceptibility to the aminoglycosides (Table 54–1). Tobramycin and gentamicin exhibit similar activity against most gram-negative bacilli, although tobramycin usually is more active against *P. aeruginosa* and some *Proteus* spp., whereas gentamicin is usually more active against *Serratia*. Many gram-negative bacilli that are resistant to gentamicin because of plasmid-mediated inactivating enzymes also are resistant to tobramycin. Amikacin and, in some instances, netilmicin retain their activity against gentamicin-resistant strains because they are a poor substrate for many of the aminoglycoside-inactivating enzymes.

Aminoglycosides have little activity against anaerobic microorganisms or facultative bacteria under anaerobic conditions. Their action against most gram-positive bacteria is limited, and they should not be used as single agents to treat infections caused by gram-positive bacteria. In combination with a cell wall–active agent, such as a penicillin or vancomycin, an aminoglycoside produces a synergistic bactericidal effect *in vitro*. Clinically, the superiority of aminoglycoside combination regimens over β-lactams alone is not proven except in relatively few infections (discussed later).

Absorption, Distribution, Dosing, and Elimination of the Aminoglycosides

Absorption. The aminoglycosides are highly polar cations and therefore are very poorly absorbed from the GI tract. Less than 1% of a dose is absorbed after either oral or rectal administration. The drugs are not inactivated in the intestine and are eliminated quantitatively in the feces. Long-term oral or rectal administration of aminoglycosides may result in accumulation to toxic concentrations in patients with renal impairment. Absorption of gentamicin from the GI tract may be increased by GI disease (e.g., ulcers or inflammatory bowel disease). Instillation of these drugs into body cavities with serosal surfaces also may result in rapid absorption and unexpected toxicity (i.e., neuromuscular blockade). Similarly, intoxication may occur when aminoglycosides are applied topically for long periods to large

Table 54–1

Typical Minimal Inhibitory Concentrations of Aminoglycosides That Will Inhibit 90% (MIC_{90}) of Clinical Isolates for Several Species

	MIC_{90} µg/ml				
SPECIES	KANAMYCIN	GENTAMICIN	NETILMICIN	TOBRAMYCIN	AMIKACIN
Citrobacter freundii	8	0.5	0.25	0.5	1
Enterobacter spp.	4	0.5	0.25	0.5	1
Escherichia coli	16	0.5	0.25	0.5	1
Klebsiella pneumoniae	32	0.5	0.25	1	1
Proteus mirabilis	8	4	4	0.5	2
Providencia stuartii	128	8	16	4	2
Pseudomonas aeruginosa	>128	8	32	4	2
Serratia spp.	>64	4	16	16	8
Enterococcus faecalis	—	32	2	32	≥64
Staphylococcus aureus	2	0.5	0.25	0.25	16

Adapted with permission from Wiedemann B, Atkinson BA. Susceptibility to antibiotics: Species incidence and trends. In: *Antibiotics in Laboratory Medicine*, 3rd ed. (Lorian V, ed.), Lippincott Williams & Wilkins, Baltimore, 1991, pp. 962–1208.)

wounds, burns, or cutaneous ulcers, particularly if there is renal insufficiency.

All the aminoglycosides are absorbed rapidly from intramuscular sites of injection. Peak concentrations in plasma occur after 30-90 minutes and are similar to those observed 30 minutes after completion of an intravenous infusion of an equal dose over a 30-minute period. These concentrations typically range from 4-12 μg/mL following a 1.5-2 mg/kg dose of gentamicin, tobramycin, or netilmicin and from 20 to 35 μg/mL following a 7.5 mg/kg dose of amikacin or kanamycin. In critically ill patients, especially those in shock, absorption of drug may be reduced from intramuscular sites because of poor perfusion.

There is increasing use of aminoglycosides administered via inhalation, primarily for the management of patients with cystic fibrosis who have chronic *Pseudomonas aeruginosa* pulmonary infections. Amikacin and tobramycin solutions for injection have been used, as well as a commercial formulation of tobramycin designed for inhalation (TOBI, others). Studies of this formulation indicate that high sputum concentrations are obtained (mean of 1200 μg/g), but serum concentrations remain low (mean peak concentration of 0.95 μg/mL) (Geller et al., 2002).

Distribution. Because of their polar nature, the aminoglycosides do not penetrate into most cells, the CNS, or the eye. Except for streptomycin, there is negligible binding of aminoglycosides to plasma albumin. The apparent volume of distribution of these drugs is 25% of lean body weight and approximates the volume of extracellular fluid. The aminoglycosides distribute poorly into adipose tissue, which must be considered when using weight-based dosing regimens in obese patients. Approaches using ideal or adjusted body weight are recommended in conjunction with drug-level monitoring to avoid excessive serum concentrations.

Concentrations of aminoglycosides in secretions and tissues are low. High concentrations are found only in the renal cortex and the endolymph and perilymph of the inner ear; the high concentration in these sites likely contribute to the nephrotoxicity and ototoxicity caused by these drugs. As a result of active hepatic secretion, concentrations in bile approach 30% of those found in plasma, but this represents a very minor excretory route for the aminoglycosides. Penetration into respiratory secretions is poor (Panidis et al., 2005). Diffusion into pleural and synovial fluid is relatively slow, but concentrations that approximate those in the plasma may be achieved after repeated administration. Inflammation increases the penetration of aminoglycosides into peritoneal and pericardial cavities.

Concentrations of aminoglycosides achieved in CSF with parenteral administration usually are subtherapeutic. In patients, concentrations in CSF in the absence of inflammation are <10% of those in plasma; this value may approach 25% when there is meningitis (Kearney and Aweeka, 1999). Given the limit on dosage escalation due to the toxicity of aminoglycosides, treatment of meningitis with intravenous administration is generally suboptimal. Intrathecal or intraventricular administration of aminoglycosides has been used to achieve therapeutic levels, but the availability of third- and fourth-generation cephalosporins has made this unnecessary in most cases. Penetration of aminoglycosides into ocular fluids is so poor that effective therapy of bacterial endophthalmitis requires periocular and intraocular injections of the drugs.

Administration of aminoglycosides to women late in pregnancy may result in accumulation of drug in fetal plasma and amniotic fluid. Streptomycin and tobramycin can cause hearing loss in children born to women who receive the drug during pregnancy. Insufficient data are available regarding the other aminoglycosides; it is therefore recommended that they be used with caution during pregnancy and only for strong clinical indications in the absence of suitable alternatives.

Elimination. The aminoglycosides are excreted almost entirely by glomerular filtration, and urine concentrations of 50-200 μg/mL are achieved. A large fraction of a parenterally administered dose is excreted unchanged during the first 24 hours, with most of this appearing in the first 12 hours. The half-lives of the aminoglycosides in plasma are similar, 2-3 hours in patients with normal renal function. Renal clearance of aminoglycosides is approximately two-thirds of the simultaneous creatinine clearance; this observation suggests some tubular reabsorption of these drugs.

After a single dose of an aminoglycoside, disappearance from the plasma exceeds renal excretion by 10-20%; however, after 1-2 days of therapy, nearly 100% of subsequent doses eventually is recovered in the urine. This lag period probably represents saturation of binding sites in tissues. The rate of elimination of drug from these sites is considerably longer than from plasma; the $t_{1/2}$ for tissue-bound aminoglycoside has been estimated to range from 30 to 700 hours. For this reason, small amounts of aminoglycosides can be detected in the urine for 10-20 days after drug administration is discontinued. Aminoglycoside bound to renal tissue exhibits antibacterial activity and protects experimental animals against bacterial infections of the kidney even when the drug no longer can be detected in serum (Bergeron et al., 1982).

The concentration of aminoglycoside in plasma produced by the initial dose depends only on the volume of distribution of the drug. Because the elimination of aminoglycosides depends almost entirely on the kidney, a linear relationship exists between the concentration of creatinine in plasma and the $t_{1/2}$ of all aminoglycosides in patients with moderately compromised renal function. In anephric patients, the $t_{1/2}$ varies from 20-40 times that is determined in normal individuals. *Because the incidence of nephrotoxicity and ototoxicity is likely related to the overall drug exposure to aminoglycosides, it is critical to reduce the maintenance dosage of these drugs in patients with impaired renal function.*

Aminoglycosides can be removed from the body by either hemodialysis or peritoneal dialysis. Approximately 50% of the administered dose is removed in 12 hours by hemodialysis, which has been used for the treatment of overdosage. As a general rule, a dose equal to half the loading dose administered after each hemodialysis should maintain the plasma concentration in the desired range; however, a number of variables make this a rough approximation at best. Continuous arteriovenous hemofiltration (CAVH) and continuous venovenous hemofiltration (CVVH) will result in aminoglycoside clearances approximately equivalent to 15 and 15-30 mL/min of creatinine clearance, respectively, depending on the flow rate. The amount of aminoglycoside removed can be replaced by administering ~15-30% of the maximum daily dose (Table 54–2) each day. Frequent monitoring of plasma drug concentrations is again crucial.

Peritoneal dialysis is less effective than hemodialysis in removing aminoglycosides. Clearance rates are ~5-10 mL/min for the various drugs but are highly variable. If a patient who requires

Table 54–2

Algorithm for Dose Reduction of Aminoglycosides Based on Calculated Creatinine Clearance

CREATININE CLEARANCE (mL/min)	% OF MAXIMUM DAILY DOSE*	FREQUENCY OF DOSING
100	100	Every 24 hours
75	75	
50	50	
25	25	
20	80	Every 48 hours
10	60	
<10	40	

*The maximum adult daily dose for amikacin, kanamycin, and streptomycin is 15 mg/kg; for gentamicin and tobramycin, 5.5 mg/kg; and for netilmicin, 6.5 mg/kg.

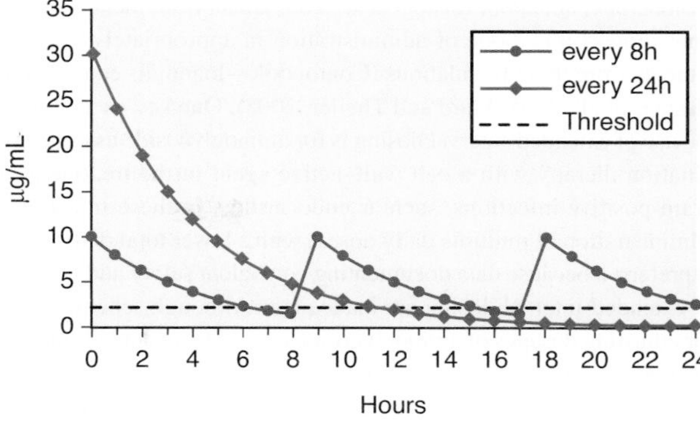

Figure 54–3. *Plasma concentrations (μg/mL) after administration of 5.1 mg/kg of gentamicin intravenously to a hypothetical patient either as a single dose (every 24h) or as three divided doses (every 8h).* The threshold for toxicity has been chosen to correspond to a plasma concentration of 2 μg/mL, the maximum recommended. The high-dose, extended-interval (once-daily) regimen produces a 3-fold higher plasma concentration, which enhances efficacy that otherwise might be compromised due to prolonged sub-MIC concentrations later in the dosing interval compared with the every-8-hours regimen. The once-daily regimen provides a 12-hour period during which plasma concentrations are below the threshold for toxicity, thereby minimizing the toxicity that otherwise might result from the high plasma concentrations early on. The every-8-hours regimen, in contrast, provides only a brief period during which plasma concentrations are below the threshold for toxicity.

dialysis has bacterial peritonitis, a therapeutic concentration of the aminoglycoside probably will not be achieved in the peritoneal fluid because the ratio of the concentration in plasma to that in peritoneal fluid may be 10:1 (Smithivas et al., 1971). Thus, it is recommended that antibiotic be added to the dialysate to achieve concentrations equal to those desired in plasma.

Aminoglycosides can be inactivated by various penicillins *in vitro* and thus should not be admixed in solution. Some reports indicate that this inactivation may occur *in vivo* in patients with end-stage renal failure (Blair et al., 1982), thus making monitoring of aminoglycoside plasma concentrations even more necessary in such patients. Amikacin appears to be the aminoglycoside least affected by this interaction, and penicillins with more nonrenal elimination (such as piperacillin) may be less prone to cause this interaction.

Although excretion of aminoglycosides is similar in adults and children >6 months of age, half-lives of the drugs may be prolonged significantly in the newborn: 8-11 hours in the first week of life in newborns weighing <2 kg and ~5 hours in those weighing >2 kg (Yow, 1977). Thus, it is critically important to monitor plasma concentrations of aminoglycosides during treatment of neonates (Philips et al., 1982). For unknown reasons, aminoglycoside clearances are increased and half-lives are reduced in patients with cystic fibrosis compared to subjects without cystic fibrosis, after controlling for age and weight (Mann et al., 1985). Larger doses of aminoglycosides may likewise be required in burn patients because of more rapid drug clearance, possibly because of drug loss through burn tissue.

Dosing. Recommended doses of individual aminoglycosides in the treatment of specific infections are given in later sections of this chapter. Historically, aminoglycosides have been administered as two or three equally divided doses, based on the short $t_{1/2}$ of the drugs. However, studies of the pharmacokinetic/pharmacodynamic properties of aminoglycosides demonstrate that administering higher doses at extended intervals (typically once daily in patients with normal renal function) is likely to be at least equally efficacious and potentially less toxic than administration of divided doses. A comparison of this high-dose, extended-interval dosing method to traditional divided-dose methods is illustrated in Figure 54–3. Because of the post-antibiotic effect of aminoglycosides, good therapeutic response can be attained even when concentrations of aminoglycosides fall below inhibitory concentrations for a substantial fraction of the dosing interval. High-dose, extended-interval dosing schemes for aminoglycosides may also reduce the characteristic oto- and nephrotoxicity of these drugs. This diminished toxicity is probably due to a threshold effect from accumulation of drug in the inner ear or in the kidney. More drug accumulates with higher plasma concentrations, particularly at trough, and with prolonged periods of exposure. Net elimination of aminoglycoside from these organs occurs more slowly when plasma concentrations are relatively high. High-dose, extended-interval regimens, despite the higher peak concentration, provide a longer period when concentrations fall below the threshold for toxicity than does a multiple-dose regimen (12 hours versus <3 hours total in the example shown in Figure 54–3), potentially accounting for the lower toxicity of this approach.

Numerous studies and meta-analyses demonstrate that administration of the total dose once daily is associated with less nephrotoxicity and is just as effective as multiple-dose regimens (Bailey et al., 1997; Buijk et al., 2002). Extended-interval dosing also costs less and is administered more easily. For these reasons, high-dose, extended-interval administration of aminoglycosides is the preferred means of administering aminoglycosides for most indications and patient populations. Although the use of extended-interval dosing has been controversial in pregnancy, neonatal, and pediatric infections

(Knoderer et al., 2003; Rastogi et al., 2002), data from meta-analyses now support this mode of administration in appropriately selected patients from these populations (Contopoulos-Ioannidis et al., 2004; Nestaas et al., 2005; Ward and Theiler, 2008). One key exception to the use of extended-interval dosing is for aminoglycoside use as combination therapy with a cell wall–active agent in the treatment of gram-positive infections, such as endocarditis. In these infections, administration of multiple daily doses (with a lower total daily dose) is preferred because data documenting equivalent safety and efficacy of extended-interval dosing are inadequate. Although schemes exist for adjusting dosages of aminoglycosides dosed by extended-interval methods in patients with significant renal dysfunction (i.e., creatinine clearance <25 mL/minute), some clinicians prefer to use the traditional multiple-dose regimen in such patients.

Nomograms may be helpful in selecting initial doses, but variability in aminoglycoside clearance among patients is too great for these to be relied on for more than a few days (Bartal et al., 2003). If it is anticipated that the patient will be treated with an aminoglycoside for >3-4 days, then plasma concentrations should be monitored to avoid drug accumulation. Whether extended-interval or multiple-daily dosing is chosen, the dose must be adjusted for patients with creatinine clearances of <80-100 mL/minute (Table 54–2), and plasma concentrations must be monitored. Determination of the concentration of drug in plasma is an essential guide to the proper administration of aminoglycosides. In patients with life-threatening systemic infections, aminoglycoside concentrations should be determined several times per week (more frequently if renal function is changing) and should be determined within 24-48 hours of a change in dosage. The size of the individual dose, the interval between doses, or both can be altered based on the results of monitoring of drug levels in plasma. Methods for calculation of dosage are described in Appendix II. There are obvious difficulties in using any of these approaches for ill patients with rapidly changing renal function. In addition, even when known factors are taken into consideration, concentrations of aminoglycosides achieved in plasma after a given dose vary widely among patients. If the extracellular volume is expanded, the volume of distribution is increased, and concentrations will be reduced.

For twice- or thrice-daily dosing regimens, both peak and trough plasma concentrations are determined. The trough sample is obtained just before a dose, and the peak sample is obtained 60 minutes after intramuscular injection or 30 minutes after an intravenous infusion given over 30 minutes. The peak concentration documents that the dose produces therapeutic concentrations, generally accepted to be 4-10 μg/mL for gentamicin, netilmicin, and tobramycin and 15-30 μg/mL for amikacin and streptomycin. The trough concentration is used to avoid toxicity by monitoring for accumulation of drug. Trough concentrations should be <1-2 μg/mL for gentamicin, netilmicin, and tobramycin and <10 μg/mL for amikacin and streptomycin.

Monitoring of aminoglycoside plasma concentrations also is important when using an extended-interval dosing regimen, although peak concentrations are not determined routinely (these will be three to four times higher than the peak achieved with a multiple-daily-dosing regimen). Several approaches may be used to determine that drug is being cleared and not accumulating.

The most accurate method for monitoring plasma levels for dose adjustment is to measure the concentration in two plasma samples drawn several hours apart (e.g., at 2 and 12 hours after a dose). The clearance then can be calculated and the dose adjusted to achieve the desired target range.

Another approach relies on nomograms to target a range of concentrations in a sample obtained earlier in the dosing interval. For example, if the plasma concentration from a sample obtained 8 hours after a dose of gentamicin is between 1.5 and 6 μg/mL, then the concentration at 18 hours will be <1 μg/mL (Chambers et al., 1998). Target ranges of 1-1.5 μg/mL for gentamicin at 18 hours for patients with creatinine clearances >50 mL/min and 1-2.5 μg/mL for those with clearances <50 mL/min also have been used. This method also tends to be inaccurate, particularly when conditions that alter aminoglycoside clearance are present (Bartal et al., 2003; Toschlog et al., 2003).

The simplest method is to obtain a trough sample 24 hours after dosing and adjust the dose to achieve the recommended plasma concentration, (e.g., <1-2 μg/mL in the case of gentamicin or tobramycin). This approach probably is the least desirable. An undetectable trough concentration could reflect grossly inadequate dosing in patients who clear the drug rapidly with prolonged periods (perhaps well over half the dosing interval) during which concentrations are subtherapeutic. In contrast, a 24-hour trough concentration target of 1-2 μg/mL actually would increase aminoglycoside exposure compared with a multiple-daily-dosing regimen (Barclay et al., 1999), which defeats the goal of providing a washout with concentrations of 0-1 μg/mL between 18 and 24 hours after a dose.

Untoward Effects

All aminoglycosides have the potential to produce reversible and irreversible vestibular, cochlear, and renal toxicity. These side effects complicate the use of these compounds and make their proper administration difficult.

Ototoxicity. Vestibular and auditory dysfunction can follow the administration of any of the aminoglycosides, and ototoxicity may become a dose-limiting adverse effect. Aminoglycoside induced ototoxicity results in irreversible, bilateral high-frequency hearing loss and temporary vestibular hypofunction. Degeneration of hair cells and neurons in the cochlea correlates with the loss of hearing. With increasing dosage and prolonged exposure, damage progresses from the base of the cochlea, where high-frequency sounds are processed, to the apex, which is necessary for the perception of low frequencies. Although these histological changes correlate with the ability of the cochlea to generate an action potential in response to sound, the biochemical mechanism for ototoxicity is poorly understood. Early changes induced by aminoglycosides in experimental ototoxicity are reversible by Ca^{2+}. Once sensory cells are lost, however, regeneration does not occur; retrograde degeneration of the auditory nerve follows, resulting in irreversible hearing loss.

Aminoglycosides may interfere with the active transport system essential for the maintenance of the ionic balance of the endolymph (Neu and Bendush, 1976). Ototoxicity is largely irreversible and results from progressive destruction of vestibular or cochlear sensory cells, which are highly sensitive to damage by aminoglycosides. The degree of permanent dysfunction correlates with the number of destroyed or altered sensory hair cells and is related to sustained exposure to the drug. An iron-aminoglycoside complex is postulated to potentiate reactive oxygen species–induced cellular degeneration in the cochlea (Guthrie, 2008).

Accumulation within the perilymph and endolymph occurs predominantly when aminoglycoside concentrations in plasma are high. Diffusion back into the bloodstream is slow; the half-lives of the aminoglycosides are five to six times longer in the otic fluids than in plasma. Back diffusion is concentration dependent and facilitated at the trough concentration of drug in plasma Thus, it is generally thought that ototoxicity is more likely to occur in patients with persistently elevated concentrations of drug in plasma. However, studies have not consistently shown an association between ototoxicity and putative risk factors such as aminoglycoside serum levels, total dose and duration of aminoglycoside exposure, and renal dysfunction (including aminoglycoside-induced nephrotoxicity) (de Jager and van Altena, 2002; Peloquin et al., 2004). Drugs such as ethacrynic acid and furosemide potentiate the ototoxic effects of the aminoglycosides in animals, but data from humans implicating furosemide are less convincing (Moore et al., 1984). Hearing loss following exposure to these agents also is more likely to develop in patients with pre-existing auditory impairment.

The description of families where several members experienced profound deafness from as little as a single dose of aminoglycoside led to the investigation of a potential genetic predisposition for this toxicity. Subsequent studies have identified several predisposing mutations in mitochondrial ribosomal RNA genes (Fischel-Ghodsian, 2005). The contribution of genetic susceptibility to the overall incidence of aminoglycoside-induced ototoxicity is unclear, but surveys of subjects of European origin put the prevalence of one of these mutations at 1 in 500 (Vandebona et al., 2009).

Although all aminoglycosides can affect cochlear and vestibular function, there is some preferential toxicity. Streptomycin and gentamicin produce predominantly vestibular effects, whereas amikacin, kanamycin, and neomycin primarily affect auditory function; tobramycin affects both equally. The incidence of ototoxicity is difficult to determine. Audiometric data suggest that the incidence may be as high as 25% (de Jager and van Altena, 2002); however, these data need to be interpreted in the context of the limitations of audiometric testing in acutely ill patients and day-to-day variability of audiometric testing (Brummett and Morrison, 1990). The relative incidence appears to be equal for tobramycin, gentamicin, and amikacin. Initial studies suggested that netilmicin is less ototoxic than other aminoglycosides (Lerner et al., 1983); however, the incidence of ototoxicity from netilmicin is not negligible—such complications developed in 10% of patients in one clinical trial of netilmicin. The incidence of vestibular toxicity is particularly high in patients receiving streptomycin; nearly 20% of individuals who received 500 mg twice daily for 4 weeks for enterococcal endocarditis developed clinically detectable irreversible vestibular damage (Wilson et al., 1984). In addition, up to 75% of patients who received 2 g streptomycin for >60 days showed evidence of nystagmus or postural imbalance.

Because the initial symptoms may be reversible, patients receiving high doses and/or prolonged courses of aminoglycosides should be monitored carefully for ototoxicity; however, deafness may occur several weeks after therapy is discontinued. Screening patients for a family history of aminoglycoside-induced deafness seems reasonable, but the cost effectiveness of genetic screening for mutations predisposing to aminoglycoside ototoxicity is not yet clear.

Clinical Symptoms of Cochlear Toxicity. A high-pitched tinnitus often is the first symptom of toxicity. If the drug is not discontinued, auditory impairment may develop after a few days. The tinnitus may persist for several days to 2 weeks after therapy is stopped. Because perception of sound in the high-frequency range (outside the conversational range) is lost first, the affected individual is not always aware of the difficulty, and it will not be detected except by careful audiometric examination. If the hearing loss progresses, the lower sound ranges are affected, and conversation becomes difficult.

Clinical Symptoms of Vestibular Toxicity. Moderately intense headache lasting 1-2 days may precede the onset of labyrinthine dysfunction. This is followed immediately by an acute stage in which nausea, vomiting, and difficulty with equilibrium develop and persist for 1-2 weeks. Prominent symptoms include vertigo in the upright position, inability to perceive termination of movement ("mental past-pointing"), and difficulty in sitting or standing without visual cues. Drifting of the eyes at the end of a movement so that both focusing and reading are difficult, a positive Romberg test, and rarely, pendular trunk movement and spontaneous nystagmus, are prominent signs. The acute stage ends suddenly and is followed by the appearance of manifestations of chronic labyrinthitis, in which, although symptomless while in bed, the patient has difficulty when attempting to walk or make sudden movements; ataxia is the most prominent feature. The chronic phase persists for ~2 months; it is gradually superseded by a compensatory stage in which symptoms are latent and appear only when the eyes are closed. Adaptation to the impairment of labyrinthine function is accomplished by the use of visual cues and deep proprioceptive sensation for determining movement and position. It is more adequate in the young than in the old but may not be sufficient to permit the high degree of coordination required in many special trades. Recovery from this phase may require 12-18 months, and most patients have some permanent residual damage. Although there is no specific treatment for the vestibular deficiency, early discontinuation of the drug may permit recovery before irreversible damage of the hair cells.

Nephrotoxicity. Approximately 8-26% of patients who receive an aminoglycoside for several days develop mild renal impairment that is almost always reversible. The toxicity results from accumulation and retention of aminoglycoside in the proximal tubular cells (Lietman and Smith, 1983). The initial manifestation of damage at this site is excretion of enzymes of the renal tubular brush border (Banday et al., 2008). After several days, there is a defect in renal concentrating ability, mild proteinuria, and the appearance of hyaline and granular casts. The glomerular filtration rate is reduced after several additional days (Schentag et al., 1979). The non-oliguric phase of renal insufficiency is thought to be due to the effects of aminoglycosides on the distal portion of the nephron with a reduced sensitivity of the collecting-duct epithelium to endogenous antidiuretic hormone (Appel, 1982). Although severe acute tubular necrosis may occur rarely, the most common significant finding is a mild rise in plasma creatinine (5-20 μg/mL; 40-175 μM). Hypokalemia, hypocalcemia, and hypophosphatemia are seen very infrequently. The impairment in renal function is almost always reversible because the proximal tubular cells have the capacity to regenerate.

The biochemical events leading to tubular cell damage and glomerular dysfunction are poorly understood but may involve perturbations of the structure of cellular membranes. Aminoglycosides inhibit various phospholipases, sphingomyelinases, and ATPases, and they alter the function of mitochondria and ribosomes (Humes et al., 1984; Queener et al., 1983). Because of the ability of cationic aminoglycosides to interact with anionic phospholipids, these drugs may impair the synthesis of membrane-derived autacoids and intracellular second messengers such as prostaglandins, inositol phosphates, and diacylglycerol.

Several variables appear to influence nephrotoxicity from aminoglycosides. Toxicity correlates with the total amount of drug administered. Consequently, toxicity is more likely to be encountered with longer courses of therapy. Continuous infusion is more nephrotoxic in animals than intermittent dosing (Powell et al., 1983). High-dose, extended-interval dosing approaches lead to less nephrotoxicity at the same level of total drug exposure (as measured by area under the curve) than divided-dose approaches (Figure 54-3). Advanced age, liver disease, diabetes mellitus, and septic shock have been suggested as risk factors for the development of nephrotoxicity from aminoglycosides, but data are not convincing. Note, however, that renal function in the elderly patient is overestimated by measurement of creatinine concentration in plasma, and overdosing will occur if this value is used as the only guide in this patient population (Baciewicz et al., 2003).

The nephrotoxic potential varies among individual aminoglycosides. The relative toxicity correlates with the concentration of drug found in the renal cortex in experimental animals. Neomycin, which concentrates to the greatest degree, is highly nephrotoxic in human beings and should not be administered systemically. Streptomycin does not concentrate in the renal cortex and is the least nephrotoxic. Most of the controversy has concerned the relative toxicities of gentamicin and tobramycin. If differences between the renal toxicity of these two aminoglycosides do exist in human beings, they appear to be slight. Comparative studies with amikacin, sisomicin, and netilmicin are not conclusive. Other drugs, such as amphotericin B, vancomycin, angiotensin-converting enzyme inhibitors, cisplatin, and cyclosporine, may potentiate aminoglycoside-induced nephrotoxicity (Wood et al., 1986). Clinical studies have not proven conclusively that furosemide potentiates aminoglycoside nephrotoxicity (Smith and Lietman, 1983), but volume depletion and wasting of K^+ that accompany the use of furosemide may predispose to aminoglycoside toxicity.

Neuromuscular Blockade. An unusual toxic reaction of acute neuromuscular blockade and apnea has been attributed to the aminoglycosides. The order of decreasing potency for blockade is neomycin, kanamycin, amikacin, gentamicin, and tobramycin. In humans, neuromuscular blockade generally has occurred after intrapleural or intraperitoneal instillation of large doses of an aminoglycoside; however, the reaction can follow intravenous, intramuscular, and even oral administration of these agents. Most episodes have occurred in association with anesthesia or the administration of other neuromuscular blocking agents. Patients with myasthenia gravis are particularly susceptible to neuromuscular blockade by aminoglycosides (Chapter 11).

Aminoglycosides may inhibit prejunctional release of acetylcholine while also reducing postsynaptic sensitivity to the transmitter, but Ca^{2+} can overcome this effect, and the intravenous administration of a calcium salt is the preferred treatment for this toxicity (Sarkar et al., 1992). Inhibitors of acetylcholinesterase (e.g., edrophonium and neostigmine) also have been used with varying degrees of success.

Other Untoward Effects. In general, the aminoglycosides have little allergenic potential; anaphylaxis and rash are unusual. Rare hypersensitivity reactions—including skin rashes, eosinophilia, fever, blood dyscrasias, angioedema, exfoliative dermatitis, stomatitis, and anaphylactic shock—have been reported as cross-hypersensitivity among drugs in this class. Parenterally administered aminoglycosides are not associated with pseudomembranous colitis, probably because they do not disrupt the normal anaerobic flora. Other reactions that have been attributed to individual drugs are discussed next.

Therapeutic Uses of Gentamicin and Other Aminoglycosides

Gentamicin is an important agent for the treatment of many serious gram-negative bacillary infections. It is the aminoglycoside of first choice because of its lower cost and reliable activity against all but the most resistant gram-negative aerobes. Gentamicin preparations are available for parenteral, ophthalmic, and topical administration.

Gentamicin, tobramycin, amikacin, and netilmicin can be used interchangeably for the treatment of most of the following infections and therefore are discussed together. For most indications, gentamicin is the preferred agent because of long experience with its use and its lower cost. Many different types of infections can be treated successfully with these aminoglycosides; however, owing to their toxicities, prolonged use should be restricted to the therapy of life-threatening infections and those for which a less toxic agent is contraindicated or less effective.

Aminoglycosides frequently are used in combination with a cell wall–active agent (β-lactam or glycopeptide) for the therapy of serious proven or suspected bacterial infections. Three rationales exist for this approach:

- To expand the empiric spectrum of activity of the antimicrobial regimen to ensure the presence of at least one drug active against a suspected pathogen.

- To provide synergistic bacterial killing.
- To prevent the emergence of resistance to the individual agents.

The first rationale is the most common justification for the use of combination therapy in infections such as healthcare-associated pneumonia or sepsis, where multidrug-resistant gram-negative organisms such as *P. aeruginosa, Enterobacter, Klebsiella,* and *Serratia* may be causative and the consequences of failing to provide initially active therapy are dire (Dupont et al., 2001). This approach leverages the high levels of coverage that aminoglycosides continue to provide against this organism. The use of aminoglycosides to achieve synergistic bacterial killing and improve microbiological eradication and clinical response is most well established for the treatment of endocarditis due to gram-positive organisms, most importantly *Enterococcus*. Clinical data do not support the use of combination therapy for synergistic killing of gram-negative organisms, with the possible exceptions of serious *P. aeruginosa* infections (Paul et al., 2003, 2004; Safdar et al., 2004). With the exception of mycobacterial infections, the use of aminoglycosides to prevent the emergence of resistance is not supported by clinical data, despite establishment as an *in vitro* phenomenon (Bliziotis et al., 2005).

Gentamicin

The typical recommended intramuscular or intravenous dose of gentamicin sulfate when used for the treatment of known or suspected gram-negative organisms as a single agent or in combination therapy for adults with normal renal function is 5-7 mg/kg daily given over 30-60 minutes. For patients with renal dysfunction, the interval may be extended. For patients who are not candidates for extended-interval dosing, a typical dosing regimen for gram-negative coverage is a loading dose of 2 mg/kg and then 3-5 mg/kg per day, one-third given every 8 hours when administered as a multiple-daily-dosing regimen. Dosages at the upper end of this range may be required to achieve therapeutic levels for trauma or burn patients, those with septic shock, patients with cystic fibrosis, and others in whom drug clearance is more rapid or volume of distribution is larger than normal. Several dosage schedules have been suggested for newborns and infants: 3 mg/kg once daily for preterm newborns <35 weeks of gestation (Hansen et al., 2003; Rastogi et al., 2002); 4 mg/kg once daily for newborns >35 weeks of gestation; 5 mg/kg daily in two divided doses for neonates with severe infections; and 2-2.5 mg/kg every 8 hours for children up to 2 years of age. Peak plasma concentrations range from 4-10 mg/mL (dosing: 1.7 mg/kg every 8 hours) and 16-24 mg/ mL (dosing: 5.1 mg/kg once daily). It should be emphasized that the recommended doses of gentamicin do not always yield desired concentrations. Periodic determinations of the plasma concentration of aminoglycosides are recommended strongly, especially in seriously ill patients, to confirm that drug concentrations are in the desired range (see earlier sections on dosing for more details).

Urinary Tract Infections. Aminoglycosides usually are not indicated for the treatment of uncomplicated urinary tract infections, although a single intramuscular dose of gentamicin (5 mg/kg) has been effective in uncomplicated infections of the lower urinary tract. However, as strains of *E. coli* have acquired resistance to β-lactams, trimethoprim-sulfamethoxazole, and fluoroquinolones, use of aminoglycosides may increase. In the seriously ill patient with pyelonephritis, an aminoglycoside alone or in combination with a β-lactam antibiotic offers broad and effective initial coverage. Once the microorganism is isolated and its sensitivities to antibiotics are determined, the aminoglycoside should be discontinued if the infecting microorganism is sensitive to less toxic antibiotics.

Pneumonia. The organisms that cause community-acquired pneumonia are susceptible to broad-spectrum β-lactam antibiotics, macrolides, or a fluoroquinolone, and usually it is not necessary to add an aminoglycoside. Therapy with an aminoglycoside alone is likely to be ineffective; therapeutic concentrations are difficult to achieve owing to relatively poor penetration of drug into inflamed tissues and the associated conditions of low O_2 tension and low pH—both of which interfere with aminoglycoside antibacterial activity. Aminoglycosides are ineffective for the treatment of pneumonia due to anaerobes or *S. pneumoniae*, which are common causes of community-acquired pneumonia. They should not be considered as effective single-drug therapy for any aerobic gram-positive cocci (including *S. aureus* or streptococci), the microorganisms commonly responsible for suppurative pneumonia or lung abscess. An aminoglycoside in combination with a β-lactam antibiotic is recommended as standard therapy for hospital-acquired pneumonia in which a multiple-drug-resistant gram-negative aerobe is a likely causative agent (American Thoracic Society, 2005). Once it is established that the β-lactam is active against the causative agent, there is generally no benefit from continuing the aminoglycoside. Patients presenting with pulmonary exacerbations of cystic fibrosis often receive aminoglycosides as a component of therapy. Due to the altered pharmacokinetics of aminoglycosides in cystic fibrosis patients, higher daily doses (up to 10 mg/kg/day) may be necessary.

Meningitis. Availability of third-generation cephalosporins, especially cefotaxime and ceftriaxone, has reduced the need for treatment with aminoglycosides in most cases of meningitis, except for infections caused by gram-negative organisms resistant to β-lactam antibiotics (e.g., species of *Pseudomonas* and *Acinetobacter*). If therapy with an aminoglycoside is necessary, in adults, 5 mg of a preservative-free formulation of gentamicin (or equivalent dose of another aminoglycoside) is administered directly intrathecally or intraventricularly once daily (Barnes et al., 2003).

Peritonitis Associated with Peritoneal Dialysis. Patients who develop peritonitis as a result of peritoneal dialysis may be treated with aminoglycoside diluted into the dialysis fluid to a concentration of 4-8 mg/L for gentamicin, netilmicin, or tobramycin or 6-12 mg/L for amikacin. Intravenous or intramuscular administration of drug is unnecessary because serum and peritoneal fluid will equilibrate rapidly.

Bacterial Endocarditis. "Synergistic" or low-dose gentamicin (3 mg/kg per day in three divided doses) in combination with a penicillin or vancomycin has been recommended in certain circumstances for treatment of infections due to gram-positive organisms, primarily bacterial endocarditis. Penicillin and gentamicin in combination are effective as a short-course (i.e., 2-week) regimen for uncomplicated native-valve streptococcal endocarditis. In cases of enterococcal endocarditis, concomitant administration of penicillin and gentamicin for 4-6 weeks has been recommended because of an unacceptably high relapse rate with penicillin alone. A large case series from Sweden, however, found that cure rates were not substantially affected by shortening the duration of aminoglycoside therapy to a median of 15 days (Olaison and Schadewitz, 2002). A 2-week regimen of gentamicin or tobramycin in combination with nafcillin is effective for the treatment of selected cases of staphylococcal tricuspid native-valve endocarditis in intravenous drug users (Chambers et al., 1988), although the need to include the aminoglycoside is not established (Le and Bayer, 2003). For patients with native mitral or aortic valve staphylococcal endocarditis, the risks of aminoglycoside administration likely outweigh the benefits (Cosgrove et al., 2009). Administration of an aminoglycoside in combination with a cell wall–active agent and rifampin is recommended for treatment of staphylococcal prosthetic valve endocarditis, but clinical studies supporting this practice are limited.

Sepsis. Inclusion of an aminoglycoside in an empirical regimen is commonly recommended for the febrile patient with granulocytopenia and for sepsis when *P. aeruginosa* is a potential pathogen. Most studies that demonstrate a benefit for combination aminoglycoside therapy in these infections compared weak β-lactams (e.g., carbenicillin, no longer marketed in the U.S.) alone versus these agents plus an aminoglycoside (Paul et al., 2003, 2004). More recent studies using potent broad-spectrum β-lactams (e.g., carbapenems and antipseudomonal cephalosporins) have demonstrated no benefit from adding an aminoglycoside to the regimen. If there is concern that an infection may be caused by a multiple-drug-resistant organism that may be susceptible only to an aminoglycoside, then adding this antibiotic to the regimen is reasonable. Evidence that aminoglycosides are beneficial for other gram-negative infections is weak if the isolate is susceptible to other antibiotics. *To avoid toxicity, aminoglycosides should be used briefly and sparingly as long as other alternatives are available.*

Topical Applications. Gentamicin is absorbed slowly when it is applied topically in an ointment and somewhat more rapidly when it is applied as a cream. When the antibiotic is applied to large areas of denuded body surface, as may be the case in burned patients, plasma concentrations can reach 4 μg/mL, and 2-5% of the drug used may appear in the urine.

Untoward Effects. Like other aminoglycosides, the most important and serious side effects of the use of gentamicin are nephrotoxicity and irreversible ototoxicity. Intrathecal or intraventricular administration is used rarely because it may cause local inflammation and can result in radiculitis and other complications.

Tobramycin

The antimicrobial activity, pharmacokinetic properties, and toxicity profile of tobramycin are very similar to those of gentamicin. Tobramycin may be given either intramuscularly, intravenously, or by inhalation. Tobramycin (TOBREX, others) also is available in ophthalmic ointments and solutions.

Therapeutic Uses. Indications for the use of tobramycin are the same as those for gentamicin. The superior activity of tobramycin against *P. aeruginosa* makes it the preferred aminoglycoside for treatment of serious infections known or suspected to be caused by this organism; the drug has been usefully administered by inhalation to combat *P. aeruginosa* infections (LoBue, 2005). Tobramycin usually is used with an anti-pseudomonal β-lactam antibiotic. In contrast to gentamicin, tobramycin shows poor activity in combination with penicillin against many strains of enterococci. Most strains of *E. faecium* are highly resistant. Tobramycin is ineffective against mycobacteria. Dosages and serum concentrations are identical with those for gentamicin.

Untoward Effects. Tobramycin, like other aminoglycosides, causes nephrotoxicity and ototoxicity. Studies in experimental animals suggest that tobramycin may be less toxic to hair cells in the cochlear and vestibular end organs and cause less renal tubular damage than gentamicin. However, clinical data are less convincing.

Amikacin

The spectrum of antimicrobial activity of amikacin is the broadest of the group. Because of its resistance to many of the aminoglycoside-inactivating enzymes, it has a special role in hospitals where gentamicin- and tobramycin-resistant microorganisms are prevalent.

Therapeutic Uses. Amikacin is the preferred agent for the initial treatment of serious nosocomial gram-negative bacillary infections in hospitals where resistance to gentamicin and tobramycin has become a significant problem. Amikacin is active against the vast majority of aerobic gram-negative bacilli in the community and the hospital. This includes most strains of *Serratia, Proteus*, and *P. aeruginosa*. It is active against nearly all strains of *Klebsiella, Enterobacter*, and *E. coli* that are resistant to gentamicin and tobramycin. Most resistance to amikacin is found among strains of *Acinetobacter, Providencia*, and *Flavobacter* and strains of *Pseudomonas* other than *P. aeruginosa*; these all are unusual pathogens. Like tobramycin, amikacin is less active than gentamicin against enterococci and should not be used for this organism. Amikacin is not active against the majority of gram-positive anaerobic bacteria. It is active against *M. tuberculosis* (99% of strains inhibited by 4 μg/mL), including streptomycin-resistant strains and atypical mycobacteria. It has been used in the treatment of disseminated atypical mycobacterial infections in patients with acquired immunodeficiency syndrome (AIDS).

The recommended dose of amikacin is 15 mg/kg per day as a single daily dose or divided into two or three equal portions, which must be reduced for patients with renal failure. The drug is absorbed rapidly after intramuscular injection, and peak concentrations in plasma approximate 20 μg/mL after injection of 7.5 mg/kg. An intravenous infusion of the same dose over a 30-minute period produces a peak concentration in plasma of nearly 40 μg/mL at the end of the infusion, which falls to ~20 μg/mL 30 minutes later. The concentration 12 hours after a 7.5 mg/kg dose typically is 5-10 μg/mL. A 15 mg/kg once-daily dose produces peak concentrations 50-60 μg/mL and a trough of <1 μg/mL. For treatment of mycobacterial infections, thrice-weekly dosing schedules of amikacin are often used, with doses up to 25 mg/kg.

Untoward Effects. As with the other aminoglycosides, amikacin causes ototoxicity, hearing loss, and nephrotoxicity.

Netilmicin

Netilmicin is the latest of the aminoglycosides to be marketed. It is similar to gentamicin and tobramycin in its pharmacokinetic properties and dosage. Its antibacterial activity is broad against aerobic gram-negative bacilli. Like amikacin, it is not metabolized by most of the aminoglycoside-inactivating enzymes, and it therefore may be active against certain bacteria that are resistant to gentamicin.

Therapeutic Uses. Netilmicin is useful for the treatment of serious infections owing to susceptible Enterobacteriaceae and other aerobic gram-negative bacilli. It is effective against certain gentamicin-resistant pathogens, with the exception of enterococci (Panwalker et al., 1978).

The recommended dose of netilmicin for complicated urinary tract infections in adults is 1.5-2 mg/kg every 12 hours. For other serious systemic infections, a total daily dose of 4-7 mg/kg is administered as a single dose or two to three divided doses. Children should receive 3-7 mg/kg per day in two to three divided doses; neonates receive 3.5-5 mg/kg per day as a single daily dose (Gosden et al., 2001). The distribution and elimination of netilmicin, gentamicin, and tobramycin are very similar. The $t_{1/2}$ for elimination is usually 2–2.5 hours in adults and increases with renal insufficiency.

Untoward Effects. As with other aminoglycosides, netilmicin also may produce ototoxicity and nephrotoxicity. Animal models suggest that netilmicin may be less toxic than other aminoglycosides, but this remains to be proven in humans (Tange et al., 1995).

Streptomycin

Streptomycin is used for the treatment of certain unusual infections generally in combination with other antimicrobial agents. Because it generally is less active than other members of the class against aerobic gram-negative rods, it is rarely used.

Therapeutic Uses. ***Bacterial Endocarditis.*** Streptomycin and penicillin in combination are synergistically bactericidal *in vitro* and in animal models of infection against strains of enterococci, group D streptococci, and the various oral streptococci of the *viridans* group. The combination of penicillin G, which by itself is only bacteriostatic against enterococci, and streptomycin is effective as bactericidal therapy for enterococcal endocarditis. Gentamicin is generally preferred for its lesser toxicity; also, gentamicin should be used when the strain of enterococcus is resistant to streptomycin (MIC >2 mg/mL). Streptomycin should be used instead of gentamicin when the strain is resistant to the latter and susceptibility has been demonstrated to streptomycin, which may occur because the enzymes that inactivate these two aminoglycosides are different.

Streptomycin may be administered by deep intramuscular injection or intravenously. Intramuscular injection may be painful, with a hot tender mass developing at the site of injection. The dose of streptomycin is 15 mg/kg per day for patients with creatinine clearances >80 mL/minute. It typically is administered as a 1000-mg single daily dose for tuberculosis or 500 mg twice daily, resulting in peak serum concentrations of ~50-60 and 15-30 μg/mL and trough concentrations of <1 and 5-10 μg/mL, respectively. The total daily dose should be reduced in direct proportion to the reduction in creatinine clearance for creatinine clearances >30 mL/minute (Table 54–2).

Tularemia. Streptomycin (or gentamicin) is the drug of choice for the treatment of tularemia. Most cases respond to the administration of 1-2 g (15-25 mg/kg) streptomycin per day (in divided doses) for 10-14 days. Fluoroquinolones and tetracyclines also are effective, although the failure rate may be higher with tetracyclines.

Plague. Streptomycin is effective agent for the treatment of all forms of plague. The recommended dose is 2 g/day in two divided doses for 10 days. Gentamicin is probably as efficacious (Boulanger et al., 2004).

Tuberculosis. Streptomycin is a second-line agent for the treatment of active tuberculosis, and streptomycin always should be used in combination with at least one or two other drugs to which the causative strain is susceptible. The dose for patients with normal renal function is 15 mg/kg per day as a single intramuscular injection for 2-3 months and then two or three times a week thereafter.

Untoward Effects. Streptomycin has been replaced by gentamicin for most indications because the toxicity of gentamicin is primarily renal and reversible, whereas that of streptomycin is vestibular and irreversible. The administration of streptomycin may produce dysfunction of the optic nerve, including scotomas, presenting as enlargement of the blind spot. Among the less common toxic reactions to streptomycin is peripheral neuritis. This may be due either to accidental injection of a nerve during the course of parenteral therapy or to toxicity involving nerves remote from the site of antibiotic administration.

Kanamycin

The use of kanamycin has declined markedly because its spectrum of activity is limited compared with other aminoglycosides, and it is among the most toxic aminoglycosides. Kanamycin sulfate is available for injection and oral use. The parenteral dose for adults is 15 mg/kg per day (2-4 equally divided and spaced doses), with a maximum of 1.5 g/day. Children may be given up to 15 mg/kg per day.

Therapeutic Uses. Kanamycin is all but obsolete, and there are few indications for its use. Kanamycin has been employed to treat tuberculosis in combination with other effective drugs. It has no therapeutic advantage over streptomycin or amikacin and probably is more toxic; either should be used instead, depending on susceptibility of the isolate.

Prophylactic Uses. Kanamycin can be administered orally as adjunctive therapy in cases of hepatic encephalopathy. The dose is 4-6 g/day for 36-72 hours; quantities as large as 12 g/day (in divided doses) have been given.

Untoward Effects. Kanamycin is ototoxic and nephrotoxic. Like neomycin, its oral administration can cause malabsorption and superinfection. The untoward effects of the oral administration of aminoglycosides are considered in the section on neomycin.

Neomycin

Neomycin is a broad-spectrum antibiotic. Susceptible microorganisms usually are inhibited by concentrations of ≤10 μg/mL. Gram-negative species that are highly sensitive are *E. coli, Enterobacter aerogenes, Klebsiella pneumoniae*, and *Proteus vulgaris*. Gram-positive microorganisms that are inhibited include *S. aureus* and *E. faecalis. M. tuberculosis* also is sensitive to neomycin. Strains of *P. aeruginosa* are resistant to neomycin. Neomycin sulfate is available for topical and oral administration. Neomycin currently is available in many brands of creams, ointments, and other products alone and in combination with polymyxin, bacitracin, other antibiotics, and a variety of corticosteroids. There is no evidence that these topical preparations shorten the time required for healing of wounds or that those containing a steroid are more effective.

Therapeutic Uses. Neomycin has been used widely for topical application in a variety of infections of the skin and mucous membranes caused by microorganisms susceptible to the drug. These include infections associated with burns, wounds, ulcers, and infected dermatoses. However, such treatment does not eradicate bacteria from the lesions.

The oral administration of neomycin (usually in combination with erythromycin base) has been employed primarily for "preparation" of the bowel for surgery. For therapy of hepatic encephalopathy, an oral daily dose of 4-12 g (in divided doses) is given, provided that renal function is normal. Because renal insufficiency is a complication of hepatic failure and neomycin is nephrotoxic, it is used rarely for this indication.

Neomycin and polymyxin B have been used for irrigation of the bladder. For this purpose, 1 mL of a preparation (NEOSPORIN G.U. IRRIGANT) containing 40 mg neomycin and 200,000 units polymyxin B per milliliter is diluted in 1 L of 0.9% sodium chloride solution and is used for continuous irrigation of the urinary bladder through appropriate catheter systems. The goal is to prevent bacteriuria and bacteremia associated with indwelling catheters. The bladder is irrigated at the rate of 1 L every 24 hours.

Absorption and Excretion. Neomycin is poorly absorbed from the GI tract and is excreted by the kidney, as are the other aminoglycosides. An oral dose of 3 g produces a peak plasma concentration of 1-4 μg/mL; a total daily intake of 10 g for 3 days yields a blood concentration below that associated with systemic toxicity if renal function is normal. Patients with renal insufficiency may accumulate the drug. About 97% of an oral dose of neomycin is not absorbed and is eliminated unchanged in the feces.

Untoward Effects. Hypersensitivity reactions, primarily skin rashes, occur in 6-8% of patients when neomycin is applied topically. Individuals sensitive to this agent may develop cross-reactions when exposed to other aminoglycosides. The most important toxic effects of neomycin are renal damage and nerve deafness; as a consequence, the drug is no longer available for parenteral administration. Toxicity has been reported in patients with normal renal function after topical application or irrigation of wounds with 0.5% neomycin solution. Neuromuscular blockade with respiratory paralysis also has occurred after irrigation of wounds or serosal cavities. Individuals treated with 4-6 g/day of the drug by mouth sometimes develop a sprue-like syndrome with diarrhea, steatorrhea, and azotorrhea. Overgrowth of yeasts in the intestine also may occur; this is not associated with diarrhea or other symptoms in most cases.

CLINICAL SUMMARY

The role of aminoglycosides in the treatment of bacterial infections has diminished steadily as alternative drugs have become available. The aminoglycosides are narrow-spectrum agents, with their activity limited mainly to gram-negative aerobes. Compared with other antibacterials, aminoglycosides are among the most toxic, particularly if used for prolonged periods of time; serum concentrations must be monitored to avoid drug accumulation. These agents are first-line therapy for only a limited number of very specific, often historically prominent infections, such as plague, tularemia, and tuberculosis. Gentamicin or amikacin may have a role as a backup agent in the treatment of nosocomial infections caused by multidrug-resistant gram-negative pathogens such as *Pseudomonas* or *Acinetobacter*. Gentamicin also may be useful for the treatment of serious urinary tract infections caused by enteric organisms that have acquired resistance to sulfa drugs, penicillins, cephalosporins, and fluoroquinolones. Although gentamicin has been recommended for use in combination with vancomycin or a β-lactam to enhance bactericidal effect (i.e., synergism), the clinical benefit of such combinations is unproven for most infections. Because more effective and less toxic alternatives usually are available, aminoglycosides should be used sparingly and reserved for specific indications. If an aminoglycoside must be used, the duration of therapy should be kept to a minimum to avoid toxicity, and serum concentrations should be monitored.

BIBLIOGRAPHY

American Thoracic Society. Guidelines for the management of adults with hospital-acquired, ventilator-associated, and healthcare-associated pneumonia. *Am J Resp Crit Care Med*, **2005,** *171:*388–416.

Appel GB. Aminoglycoside nephrotoxicity: Physiologic studies of the sites of nephron damage. In: *The Aminoglycosides: Microbiology, Clinical Use, and Toxicity* (Whelton A, Neu HC, eds.), Marcel Dekker, New York, **1982,** pp. 269–282.

Baciewicz AM, Sokos DR, Cowan RI. Aminoglycoside-associated nephrotoxicity in the elderly. *Ann Pharmacother*, **2003,** *37:*182–186.

Bailey TC, Little JR, Littenberg B, et al. A meta-analysis of extended-interval dosing versus multiple daily dosing of aminoglycosides. *Clin Infect Dis*, **1997,** *24:*786–795.

Banday AA, Farooq N, Priyamvada S, et al. Time dependent effects of gentamicin on the enzymes of carbohydrate metabolism, brush border membrane and oxidative stress in rat kidney tissues. *Life Sciences*, **2008,** *82:*450–459.

Barclay ML, Kirkpatrick CM, Begg EJ. Once-daily aminoglycoside therapy: Is it less toxic than multiple daily doses and how should it be monitored? *Clin Pharmacokinet*, **1999,** *36:*89–98.

Barnes BJ, Wiederhold NP, Micek ST, et al. *Enterobacter cloacae* ventriculitis successfully treated with cefepime and gentamicin: Case report and review of the literature. *Pharmacotherapy*, **2003,** *23:*537–542.

Bartal C, Danon A, Schlaeffer F, et al. Pharmacokinetic dosing of aminoglycosides: A controlled trial. *Am J Med*, **2003,** *114:* 194–198.

Bergeron MG, Bastille A, Lessard C, Gagnon PM. Significance of intrarenal concentrations of gentamicin for the outcome of experimental pyelonephritis in rats. *J Infect Dis*, **1982,** *146:* 91–96.

Blair DC, Duggan DO, Schroeder ET. Inactivation of amikacin and gentamicin by carbenicillin in patients with end-stage renal failure. *Antimicrob Agents Chemother*, **1982,** *22:*376–379.

Bliziotis IA, Samonis, G, Vardakas KZ, et al. Effect of aminoglycoside and beta-lactam combination therapy versus beta-lactam monotherapy on the emergence of antimicrobial resistance: a meta-analysis of randomized, controlled trials. *Clin Infect Dis*, **2005,** *41:*149–158.

Boulanger LL, Ettestad P, Fogarty JD, et al. Gentamicin and tetracyclines for the treatment of human plague: Review of 75 cases in New Mexico, 1985–1999. *Clin Infect Dis*, **2004,** *38:* 663–669.

Brummett RE, Morrison RB. The incidence of aminoglycoside antibiotic-induced hearing loss. *Arch Otolaryngol Head Neck Surg*, **1990,** *116:*406–410.

Bryan LE. Cytoplasmic membrane transport and antimicrobial resistance. In: *Microbial Resistance to Drugs: Handbook of Experimental Pharmacology*, Vol. 91 (Bryan LE, ed.), Springer-Verlag, Berlin, **1989,** pp. 35–57.

Buijk SE, Mouton JW, Gyssens IC, et al. Experience with a once-daily dosing program of aminoglycosides in critically ill patients. *Intensive Care Med*, **2002,** *28:*936–942.

Busse HJ, Wöstmann C, Bakker EP. The bactericidal action of streptomycin: Membrane permeabilization caused by the insertion of mistranslated proteins into the cytoplasmic membrane of *Escherichia coli* and subsequent caging of the antibiotic inside the cells due to degradation of these proteins. *J Gen Microbiol*, **1992,** *138:*551–561.

Chambers HF, Hadley WK, Jawetz E. Aminoglycosides and spectinomycin. In: *Basic and Clinical Pharmacology*, 7th ed. (Katzung BG, ed.), Appleton & Lange, Stamford, CT, **1998,** pp. 752–760.

Chambers HF, Miller RT, Newman MD. Right-sided *Staphylococcus aureus* endocarditis in intravenous drug abusers: Two-week combination study. *Ann Intern Med*, **1988,** *109:*619–624.

Contopoulos-Ioannidis DG, Giotis ND, Baliatsa DV, et al. Extended-interval aminoglycoside administration for children: A meta-analysis. *Pediatrics*, **2004,** *114:*e111–118.

Cosgrove SE, Vigliani GA, Fowler VG Jr, et al. Initial low-dose gentamicin for *Staphylococcus aureus* bacteremia and endocarditis is nephrotoxic. *Clin Infect Dis*, **2009,** *48:*713–721.

Davies J. Inactivation of antibiotics and the dissemination of resistance genes. *Science*, **1994,** *264:*375–382.

Davis BB. The lethal action of aminoglycosides. *J Antimicrob Chemother*, **1988,** *22:*1–3.

de Jager P, van Altena R. Hearing loss and nephrotoxicity in long-term aminoglycoside treatment in patients with tuberculosis. *Int J Tuberc Lung Dis*, **2002,** *6:*622–627.

Dupont H, Menlec H, Sollet JP, Bleichner G. Impact of appropriateness of initial antibiotic therapy on the outcome of ventilator-associated pneumonia. *Intensive Care Med*, **2001,** *27:* 355–362.

Eliopoulos GM, Farber BF, Murray BE, et al. Ribosomal resistance of clinical enterococcal to streptomycin isolates. *Antimicrob Agents Chemother*, **1984,** *25:*398–399.

Fischel-Ghodsian N. Genetic factors in aminoglycoside toxicity. *Pharmacogenomics*, **2005,** *6:*27–36.

Geller DE, Pitlick WH, Nardella PA, et al. Pharmacokinetics and bioavailability of aerosolized tobramycin in cystic fibrosis. *Chest*, **2002,** *122:*219–226.

Gosden PE, Bedford KA, Dixon JJ, et al. Pharmacokinetics of once-a-day netilmicin (4.5 mg/kg) in neonates. *J Chemother*, **2001,** *13:*270–276.

Guthrie OW. Aminoglycoside-induced ototoxicity. *Toxicology,* **2008,** *249:*91–96.

Hansen A, Forbes P, Arnold A, O'Rourke E. Once-daily gentamicin dosing for the preterm and term newborn: Proposal for a simple regimen that achieves target levels. *J Perinatol*, **2003,** *23:*635–639.

Humes HD, Sastrasinh M, Weinberg JM. Calcium is a competitive inhibitor of gentamicin-renal membrane binding interactions, and dietary calcium supplementation protects against gentamicin nephrotoxicity. *J Clin Invest*, **1984,** *73:* 134–147.

Hummel H, Böck A. Ribosomal changes resulting in antimicrobial resistance. In: *Microbial Resistance to Drugs. Handbook of Experimental Pharmacology*. Vol. 91. (Bryan LE, ed.), Springer-Verlag, Berlin, **1989,** pp. 193–226.

Kearney BP, Aweeka FT. The penetration of anti-infectives into the central nervous system. *Neurol Clin*, **1999,** *17:* 883–900.

Knoderer CA, Everett JA, Buss WF. Clinical issues surrounding once-daily aminoglycoside dosing in children. *Pharmacotherapy*, **2003,** *23:*44–56.

Le T, Bayer AS. Combination antibiotic therapy for infective endocarditis. *Clin Infect Dis*, **2003,** *36:*615–621.

Lerner AM, Reyes MP, Cone LA, et al. Randomised, controlled trial of the comparative efficacy, auditory toxicity, and nephrotoxicity of tobramycin and netilmicin. *Lancet*, **1983,** *1:* 1123–1126.

Lietman PS, Smith CR. Aminoglycoside nephrotoxicity in humans. *J Infect Dis*, **1983,** *5*(suppl. 2):S284–S292.

LoBue PA. Inhaled tobramycin. *Chest,* **2005,** *127:*1098–1101.

Luzzatto L, Apirion D, Schlessinger D. Polyribosome depletion and blockage of the ribosome cycle by streptomycin in *Escherichia coli. J Mol Biol*, **1969,** *42:*315–335.

Mann HJ, Canafax DM, Cipolle RJ, et. al. Increased dosage requirements of tobramycin and gentamicin for treating *Pseudomonas* pneumonia in patients with cystic fibrosis. *Pediatr Pulmonol*, **1985,** *1:*238–243.

Mingeot-Leclercq MP, Glupczynski Y, Tulkens PM. Aminoglycosides: Activity and resistance. *Antimicrob Agents Chemother*, **1999,** *43:*727–737.

Moore RD, Smith CR, Lietman PS. Risk factors for the development of auditory toxicity in patients receiving aminoglycosides. *J Infect Dis*, **1984,** *149:*23–30.

Nestaas E, Bangstad HJ, Sandvik L, Wathne KO. Aminoglycoside extended interval dosing in neonates is safe and effective: A meta-analysis. *Arch Dis Child Fetal Neonatal Ed*, **2005,** *90:*F294–300.

Neu HC, Bendush CL. Ototoxicity of tobramycin: A clinical overview. *J Infect Dis*, **1976,** *134:*S206–S218.

Olaison L, Schadewitz K. Swedish Society of Infectious Diseases Quality Assurance Study Group for Endocarditis. Enterococcal endocarditis in Sweden, 1995–1999: Can shorter therapy with aminoglycosides be used? *Clin Infect Dis*, **2002,** *34:*159–166.

Panidis D, Markantonis SL, Boutzouka E, et al. Penetration of gentamicin into the alveolar lining fluid of critically ill patients with ventilator-associated pneumonia. *Chest*, **2005,** *128:* 545–552.

Panwalker AP, Malow JB, Zimelis VM, Jackson GG. Netilmicin: Clinical efficacy, tolerance, and toxicity. *Antimicrob Agents Chemother*, **1978,** *13:*170–176.

Paul M, Benuri-Silbiger I, Soards-Weiser K, Leibovici L. Beta lactam monotherapy versus beta lactam-aminoglycoside combination therapy for sepsis in immunocompetent patients: Systematic review and meta-analysis of randomised trials. *BMJ*, **2004,** *328:*668.

Paul M, Soares-Weiser K, Leibovici L. Beta lactam monotherapy versus beta lactam-aminoglycoside combination therapy for fever with neutropenia: Systematic review and meta-analysis. *BMJ*, **2003,** *326:*1111.

Peloquin CA, Berning SE, Nitta AT, et al. Aminoglycoside toxicity: Daily versus thrice-weekly dosing for treatment of mycobacterial diseases. *Clin Infect Dis,* **2004,** *38:*1538–1544.

Philips JB III, Satterwhite C, Dworsky ME, Cassady G. Recommended amikacin doses in newborns often produce excessive serum levels. *Pediatr Pharmacol (New York)*, **1982,** *2:*121–125.

Powell SH, Thompson WL, Luthe MA, et al. Once-daily vs. continuous aminoglycoside dosing: Efficacy and toxicity in animal and clinical studies of gentamicin, netilmicin, and tobramycin. *J Infect Dis*, **1983,** *147:*918–932.

Queener SF, Luft FC, Hamel FG. Effect of gentamicin treatment on adenylate cyclase and Na^+,K^+-ATPase activities in renal tissues of rats. *Antimicrob Agents Chemother*, **1983,** *24:*815–818.

Rastogi A, Agarwal G, Pyati S, Pildes RS. Comparison of two gentamicin dosing schedules in very low birth weight infants. *Pediatr Infect Dis J*, **2002,** *21:*234–240.

Safdar N, Handelsman J, Maki DG. Does combination antimicrobial therapy reduce mortality in gram-negative bacteraemia? A meta-analysis. *Lancet Infect Dis*, **2004,** *4:*519–527.

Sarkar A, Koley BN, Koley J, Sarkar R. Calcium as a counteractive agent to streptomycin induced respiratory depression: an in vivo electrophysiological observation. *Acta Physiol Hungar*, **1992,** *79:*305–321.

Schentag JJ, Gengo FM, Plaut ME, et al. Urinary casts as an indicator of renal tubular damage in patients receiving aminoglycosides. *Antimicrob Agents Chemother*, **1979,** *16:*468–474.

Smith CR, Lietman PS. Effect of furosemide on aminoglycoside-induced nephrotoxicity and auditory toxicity in humans. *Antimicrob Agents Chemother*, **1983,** *23:*133–137.

Smithivas T, Hyams PJ, Matalon R, et al. The use of gentamicin in peritoneal dialysis: I. Pharmacologic results. *J Infect Dis*, **1971,** *124*(suppl):77–83.

Spera RV Jr, Farber BF. Multiply-resistant *Enterococcus faecium:* The nosocomial pathogen of the 1990s. *JAMA*, **1992,** *268:*2563–2564.

Tange RA, Dreschler WA, Prins JM, et al. Ototoxicity and nephrotoxicity of gentamicin vs. netilmicin in patients with serious infections: A randomized clinical trial. *Clin Otolaryngol*, **1995,** *20:*1118–1123.

Toschlog EA, Blount KP, Rotondo MF, et al. Clinical predictors of subtherapeutic aminoglycoside levels in trauma patients undergoing once-daily dosing. *J Trauma*, **2003,** *55:*255–260; discussion 260–262.

Vandebona H, Mitchell P, Manwaring N, et al. Prevalence of mitochondrial 1555A->G mutation in adults of European descent. *N Engl J Med*, **2009,** *360:*642–644.

Vemuri RK, Zervos MJ. Enterococcal infections: The increasing threat of nosocomial spread and drug resistance. *Postgrad Med J*, **1993,** *93:*121–124, 127–128.

Ward K, Theiler RN. Once-daily dosing of gentamicin in obstetrics and gynecology. *Clin Obstet Gynecol*, **2008,** *51:*498–506.

Wilson WR, Wilkowske CJ, Wright AJ, et al. Treatment of streptomycin-susceptible and streptomycin-resistant enterococcal endocarditis. *Ann Intern Med*, **1984,** *100:*816–823.

Wood CA, Kohlhepp SJ, Kohnen PW, et al. Vancomycin enhancement of experimental tobramycin nephrotoxicity. *Antimicrob Agents Chemother*, **1986,** *30:*20–24.

Yow MD. An overview of pediatric experience with amikacin. *Am J Med*, **1977,** *62:*954–958.

Protein Synthesis Inhibitors and Miscellaneous Antibacterial Agents

Conan MacDougall and Henry F. Chambers

The antimicrobial agents discussed in this chapter may be assigned to three groups:

- Bacteriostatic, protein-synthesis inhibitors that target the ribosome, such as tetracyclines and glycylcyclines, chloramphenicol, macrolides and ketolides, lincosamides (clindamycin), streptogramins (quinupristin/dalfopristin), oxazolidinones (linezolid), and aminocyclitols (spectinomycin).
- Agents acting on the cell wall or cell membrane such as polymyxins, glycopeptides (vancomycin and teicoplanin), and lipopeptides (daptomycin).
- Miscellaneous compounds acting by diverse mechanisms with limited indications: bacitracin and mupirocin.

TETRACYCLINES AND GLYCYLCYCLINES

Sources and Chemistry. The tetracyclines are close congeners of polycyclic naphthacenecarboxamide. Structural formulas of the tetracyclines are shown in Table 55–1.

Chlortetracycline, the prototype of this class, was introduced in 1948 but is no longer marketed in the U.S. Oxytetracycline is a natural product elaborated by *Streptomyces rimosus*. Tetracycline is a semisynthetic derivative of chlortetracycline. Demeclocycline is the product of a mutant strain of *S. aureofaciens,* and methacycline (not available in the U.S.), doxycycline, and minocycline all are semisynthetic derivatives.

Because of their activity against *Rickettsia*, aerobic and anaerobic gram-positive and gram-negative bacteria, and *Chlamydia*, tetracyclines became known as "broad-spectrum" antibiotics. The spread of antimicrobial resistance has eroded the activity of tetracyclines against many gram-positive and gram-negative organisms. A new group of tetracycline derivatives, the glycyclines, have regained much of this activity. The glycylcyclines are synthetic analogs of the tetracyclines; the glycycline currently approved is tigecycline, the *9-tert*-butyl-glycylamido derivative of minocycline.

Antimicrobial Activity. Tetracyclines are bacteriostatic antibiotics with activity against a wide range of aerobic and anaerobic gram-positive and gram-negative bacteria.

They also are effective against some microorganisms, such as *Rickettsia, Coxiella burnetii, Mycoplasma pneumoniae, Chlamydia* spp., *Legionella* spp., *Ureaplasma*, some atypical mycobacteria, and *Plasmodium* spp., that are resistant to cell-wall-active antimicrobial agents. The tetracyclines are active against many spirochetes, including *Borrelia recurrentis, Borrelia burgdorferi* (Lyme disease), *Treponema pallidum* (syphilis), and *Treponema pertenue.* Tetracyclines are active against *Chlamydia* and *Mycoplasma*. Some nontuberculosis strains of mycobacteria (e.g., *M. marinum*) also are susceptible. They are not active against fungi. Demeclocycline, tetracycline, minocycline, and doxycycline are available in the U.S. for systemic use. Other derivatives are available in other countries. The more lipophilic drugs, minocycline and doxycycline, usually are the most active by weight, followed by tetracycline. Resistance of a bacterial strain to any one member of the class may or may not result in cross-resistance to other tetracyclines. Tigecycline is generally, although not universally, active against organisms that are susceptible to tetracyclines as well as those with acquired resistance to tetracyclines (Gales et al., 2008).

Bacterial strains with tetracycline minimum inhibitory concentrations (MICs) ≤4 μg/mL are considered susceptible except for *Haemophilus influenzae* and *Streptococcus pneumoniae*, whose susceptibility breakpoints (defined as the upper limit of the concentration at which bacteria are still considered susceptible to a given drug) are ≤2 μg/mL, and *Neisseria gonorrhoeae*, with a breakpoint of ≤0.25 μg/mL. The MIC breakpoint for susceptible anaerobic bacteria is 8 μg/mL. Tetracyclines intrinsically are more active against gram-positive than gram-negative microorganisms, but acquired resistance is common. Recent data from the U.S. on the activity of tetracycline and other agents discussed in this chapter against selected gram-positive aerobes are displayed in Table 55–2. However, prevalence of resistant strains varies in different regions. For example, ~10% of *S. pneumoniae* isolates in the U.S. are resistant

Table 55–1

Structural Formulas of the Tetracyclines

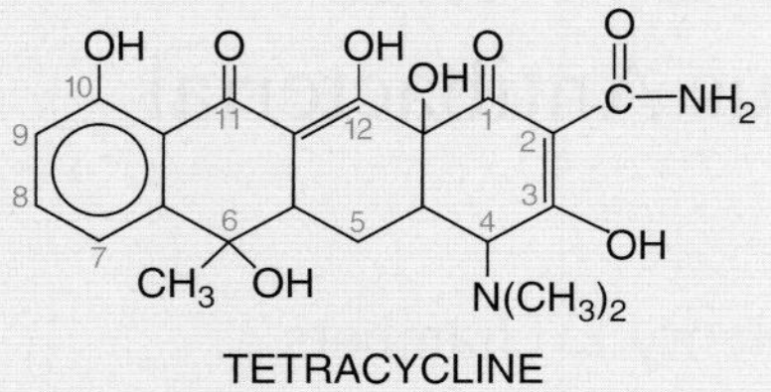

TETRACYCLINE

CONGENER	SUBSTITUENT(S)	POSITION(S)
Chlortetracycline	–Cl	7
Oxytetracycline	–OH,–H	5
Demeclocycline	–OH,–H; –Cl	6; 7
Methacycline	–OH,–H; CH_2	5; 6
Doxycycline	–OH,–H; $–CH_3$, –H	5; 6
Minocycline	–H,–H; $–N(CH_3)_2$	6; 7

to tetracycline versus 40% in the Asia-Pacific region (Hoban et al., 2001). *Bacillus anthracis* and *Listeria monocytogenes* are susceptible. Of note, the tetracyclines, doxycycline and minocycline in particular, have generally retained excellent levels of activity against staphylococci, including methicillin-resistant *Staphylococcus aureus* (MRSA). Doxycycline and minocycline can be active against some tetracycline-resistant isolates.

H. influenzae is generally susceptible, but many Enterobacteriaceae have acquired resistance. Although all strains of *Pseudomonas aeruginosa* are resistant, 90% of strains of *Burkholderia pseudomallei* (the cause of melioidosis) are sensitive. Most strains of *Brucella* also are susceptible. Tetracyclines remain useful for infections caused by *Haemophilus ducreyi* (chancroid), *Vibrio cholerae* and *V. vulnificus*, and inhibit the growth of *Legionella pneumophila, Campylobacter jejuni, Helicobacter pylori, Yersinia pestis, Yersinia enterocolitica, Francisella tularensis*, and *Pasteurella multocida*. Strains of *Neisseria gonorrhoeae* no longer are predictably susceptible to tetracycline, which is not recommended for treatment of gonococcal infections. The tetracyclines are active against many anaerobic and facultative microorganisms. A variable number of anaerobes (e.g.,

Table 55–2

Activity of Selected Antimicrobials Against Key Gram-positive Pathogens

	CONCENTRATION OF ANTIMICROBIAL AGENT REQUIRED TO INHIBIT GROWTH OF 90% OF ISOLATES, µg/mL (% SUSCEPTIBLE AT CLINICALLY ACHIEVABLE CONCENTRATIONS OF DRUG)						
		Streptococcus Pneumoniae		*Staphylococcus Aureus*			
	Streptococcus Pyogenes	PCN-S	PCN-R	MSSA	MRSA	*Enterococcus Faecalis*	*Enterococcus Faecium*
Tetracycline	4 (89.7)	≤2 (94.6)	>8 (36.7)	≤2 (95.7)	≤2 (93.4)	>8 (24.6)	>8 (58.7)
Tigecycline	≤0.03 (100)	≤0.03 (NR)	≤0.03 (NR)	0.25 (100)	0.25 (99.9)	0.25 (99.9)	0.12 (NR)
Erythromycin	1 (89.7)	>2 (87.3)	>2 (17.2)	>2 (70.8)	>2 (6.1)	>2 (9.1)	>2 (3.0)
Clindamycin	≤0.25 (97.7)	≤0.25 (97.1)	>2 (44.4)	≤0.25 (94.6)	>2 (57.9)	NA	NA
Quinupristin/ dalfopristin	≤0.12 (100)	0.5 (99)	0.5 (100)	0.25 (100)	0.5 (100)	8 (3.9)	2 (92.6)
Linezolid	1 (100)	1 (100)	1 (100)	2 (99.9)	2 (99.9)	2 (99.9)	2 (98.0)
Vancomycin	0.25 (100)	≤1 (100)	≤1 (100)	1 (99.9)	1 (99.9)	2 (94.5)	>16 (26.6)
Daptomycin	0.06 (100)	0.12 (NA)	0.12 (NA)	0.25 (100)	0.5 (100)	2 (100)	4 (100)

Entries are drug concentrations, in µg/mL, required to inhibit growth of 90% of isolates of that organism. In parentheses below each drug concentration is the percentage of isolates inhibited at clinically useful drug concentrations. PCN-S = penicillin-susceptible; PCN-R = penicillin-resistant; MSSA = methicillin-susceptible *Staphylococcus aureus*; MRSA = methicillin-resistant *Staphylococcus aureus*; NR = not reported; NA = not applicable.
Sources: Gales *et al*., 2008; Critchley *et al*., 2003.

Bacteroides spp., *Propionibacterium, Peptococcus*) are sensitive to doxycycline, but other antibiotics (e.g., chloramphenicol, clindamycin, metronidazole, and certain β-lactam antibiotics) have better activity. Tetracycline is active against *Actinomyces* and is a drug of choice for treating actinomycosis.

Currently established breakpoints for tigecycline susceptibility vary by organism: for *S. aureus* ≤0.5 μg/mL; for *Streptococcus, Haemophilus,* and *Enterococcus* species, ≤0.25 μg/mL; for *S. pneumoniae*, ≤0.06 μg/mL; for Enterobacteriaceae ≤2 μg/mL; and for anaerobic organisms ≤4 μg/mL. In general, tigecycline is equally or more active *in vitro* against bacteria than the tetracyclines (Table 55–1), including activity against tetracycline-resistant organisms, especially gram-negative organisms. There are a few exceptions where other tetracyclines may be more active against certain organisms, such as *Stenotrophomonas* and *Ureaplasma*. There is currently a lack of clinical experience with tigecycline for infections caused by organisms such as *Burkholderia, Brucella, Yersinia, Francisella,* and *Pasteurella*. Notable holes in the spectrum of activity of tigecycline (as with the tetracyclines) include *Pseudomonas, Proteus, and Providencia* spp.

Mechanism of Action. Tetracyclines and glycylcyclines inhibit bacterial protein synthesis by binding to the 30S bacterial ribosome and preventing access of aminoacyl tRNA to the acceptor (A) site on the mRNA-ribosome complex (Figure 55–1). These drugs enter gram-negative bacteria by passive diffusion through the hydrophilic channels formed by the porin proteins of the outer cell membrane and by active transport via an energy-dependent system that pumps all tetracyclines across the cytoplasmic membrane. Entry of these drugs into gram-positive bacteria requires metabolic energy, but the process is not as well understood.

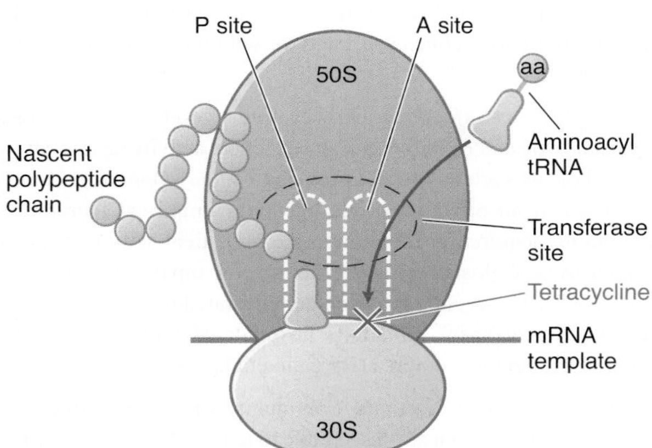

Figure 55–1. *Inhibition of bacterial protein synthesis by tetracyclines.* Messenger RNA (mRNA) attaches to the 30S subunit of bacterial ribosomal RNA. The P (peptidyl) site of the 50S ribosomal RNA subunit contains the nascent polypeptide chain; normally, the aminoacyl tRNA charged with the next amino acid (aa) to be added to the chain moves into the A (acceptor) site, with complementary base pairing between the anticodon sequence of tRNA and the codon sequence of mRNA. *Tetracyclines* inhibit bacterial protein synthesis by binding to the 30S subunit and blocking tRNA binding to the A site.

Resistance to Tetracyclines and Glycylcyclines. Resistance is primarily plasmid mediated and often inducible. The three main resistance mechanisms are (1) decreased accumulation of tetracycline as a result of either decreased antibiotic influx or acquisition of an energy-dependent efflux pathway; (2) production of a ribosomal protection protein that displaces tetracycline from its target, a "protection" that also may occur by mutation; and (3) enzymatic inactivation of tetracyclines. Cross-resistance, or lack thereof, among tetracyclines depends on which mechanism is operative. For example, *S. aureus* strains that are tetracycline resistant on the basis of efflux mediated by *tetK* still may be susceptible to minocycline. Tetracycline resistance due to a ribosomal protection mechanism (*tetM*) produces cross-resistance to doxycycline and minocycline because the target site protected is the same for all tetracyclines.

The glycylamido moiety characteristic of tigecycline reduces its affinity for most efflux pumps, restoring activity against many organisms displaying tetracycline resistance due to this mechanism. Binding of glycyclines to ribosomes is also enhanced, improving activity against organisms that harbor ribosomal protection proteins that confer resistance to other tetracyclines (Petersen et al., 1999).

Absorption, Distribution, and Excretion

Absorption. Oral absorption of most tetracyclines is incomplete. The percentage of an oral dose that is absorbed with an empty stomach is modest for demeclocycline and tetracycline (60-80%) and high for doxycycline (95%) and minocycline (100%). The percentage of unabsorbed drug rises as the dose increases. Tigecycline is not appreciably absorbed from the gastrointestinal (GI) tract and is only available for parenteral administration. Absorption of orally administered tetracyclines mostly takes place in the stomach and upper small intestine and is greater in the fasting state. Absorption may be impaired by the concurrent ingestion of divalent and trivalent cations (e.g., Ca^{2+}, Mg^{2+}, Al^{3+}, $Fe^{2+/3+}$, and Zn^{2+}). Thus, dairy products, antacids, aluminum hydroxide gels; calcium, magnesium, and iron or zinc salts; bismuth subsalicylate (e.g., PEPTO-BISMOL), and dietary Fe and Zn supplements can interfere with absorption of tetracyclines. The decreased absorption apparently results from chelation with these cations and formation of complexes with poor solubility. Doxycycline and minocycline are less affected than tetracyclines and administration with milk or calcium-containing foods is unlikely to impair absorption substantially, but co-administration of antacids or mineral supplements should be avoided.

Variable absorption of orally administered tetracyclines leads to a wide range of plasma concentrations in different individuals. Tetracycline is incompletely absorbed. After a single oral dose, the peak plasma concentration is attained in 2-4 hours. These drugs have half-lives in the range of 6-12 hours and frequently are administered two to four times daily. The administration of 250 mg tetracycline every 6 hours produces peak plasma concentrations of 2-2.5 μg/mL. Increasing the dosage above 1 g every 6 hours does not further increase plasma concentrations. Demeclocycline, which also is incompletely absorbed, can be administered in lower daily dosages than the congeners just mentioned because its $t_{1/2}$ of 16 hours provides effective plasma concentrations for 24-48 hours.

Oral doses of doxycycline and minocycline are well absorbed (90-100%) and have half-lives of 16-18 hours; they therefore can be administered less frequently and at lower doses than tetracycline or demeclocycline. After an oral dose of 200 mg of doxycycline, a maximum plasma concentration of 3 μg/mL is achieved at 2 hours, and the plasma concentration remains above 1 μg/mL for 8-12 hours. Plasma concentrations are equivalent whether doxycycline is given orally or parenterally.

Distribution. Tetracyclines distribute widely throughout the body and into tissues and secretions, including urine and prostate. They accumulate in reticuloendothelial cells of the liver, spleen, and bone marrow, and in bone, dentine, and enamel of unerupted teeth. Tigecycline distributes rapidly and extensively into tissues, with an estimated apparent volume of 7-10 L/kg. Because of this extensive distribution, peak serum levels of tigecycline are relatively low (~1 μg/mL).

Inflammation of the meninges is not required for the passage of tetracyclines into the cerebrospinal fluid (CSF). Penetration of these drugs into most other fluids and tissues is excellent. Concentrations in synovial fluid and the mucosa of the maxillary sinus approach that in plasma. Tetracyclines cross the placenta and enter the fetal circulation and amniotic fluid. Relative to the maternal circulation, tetracycline concentrations in umbilical cord plasma and amniotic fluid are 60% and 20%, respectively. Relatively high concentrations of these drugs also are found in breast milk.

Excretion. The primary route of elimination of most older tetracyclines (e.g., demeclocycline, tetracycline) is the kidney, although they also are concentrated in the liver and excreted in bile. After biliary excretion, they are partially reabsorbed via enterohepatic recirculation. Elimination via the intestinal tract occurs even when the drugs are given parenterally. Comparable amounts of tetracycline (i.e., 20-60%) are excreted in the urine within 24 hours following oral or intravenous administration.

Doxycycline is largely excreted unchanged both in the bile and urine, tigecycline is mostly excreted unchanged along with a small amount of glucuronidated metabolites, and minocycline is extensively metabolized by the liver before excretion. Doses of these agents do not require adjustment in patients with renal dysfunction. Decreased hepatic function or obstruction of the common bile duct reduces the biliary excretion of these agents, resulting in longer half-lives and higher plasma concentrations. Specific dosage adjustment recommendations in hepatic disease are available only for tigecycline. Because of their enterohepatic circulation, these drugs may remain in the body for a long time after cessation of therapy. There is some evidence for drug interactions between doxycycline and hepatic enzyme-inducing agents such as phenytoin and rifampin, but not for minocycline or tigecycline.

Therapeutic Uses and Dosage. The tetracyclines have been used extensively to treat infectious diseases and as an additive to animal feeds to facilitate growth. These uses have increased resistance to tetracyclines among gram-positive and gram-negative organisms, limiting their use for a number of common bacterial infections. However, the drugs remain useful as first-line therapy for infections caused by rickettsiae, mycoplasmas, and chlamydiae. The glycylcyclines have restored much of the antibacterial activity lost to the tetracyclines due to resistance and can be used for a number of infections due to gram-positive and gram-negative organisms.

Children >8 years of age should receive 25-50 mg/kg daily in four divided doses. The total daily dose of intravenous tetracycline (no longer available in the U.S.) for most acute infections is 1 g (or 2 g for severe infection), divided into equal doses and administered at 6- or 12-hour intervals. The low pH of tetracycline, but not doxycycline or minocycline, invariably causes phlebitis if infused into a peripheral vein. The recommended dose of demeclocycline is 150 mg every 6 hours or 300 mg every 12 hours for adults and 6.6-13.2 mg/kg in two to four divided doses for children >8 years of age. Demeclocycline is used rarely as an antimicrobial agent because of its higher risks of photosensitivity reactions and nephrogenic diabetes insipidus. The oral or intravenous dose of doxycycline for adults is 100 mg every 12 hours on the first day and then 50 mg every 12 hours, 100 mg once a day, or 100 mg twice daily when severe infection is present; for children >8 years of age, the dose is 4-5 mg/kg per day in two divided doses the first day, then 2-2.5 mg/kg given once or twice daily. The dose of minocycline for adults is 200 mg orally or intravenously initially, followed by 100 mg every 12 hours; for children, it is 4 mg/kg initially followed by 2 mg/kg every 12 hours. Tigecycline is administered intravenously to adults as a 100-mg loading dose, followed by 50 mg every 12 hours. For patients with severe hepatic impairment, the loading dose should be followed by a reduced maintenance dose of 25 mg every 12 hours. Dosage data are not available for tigecycline in pediatrics.

Tetracyclines should not be administered intramuscularly because of local irritation and poor absorption. GI distress, nausea, and vomiting can be minimized by administration of tetracyclines with food. Generally, oral administration of tetracyclines should occur 2 hours before or 2 hours after co-administration with any of the agents listed. Cholestyramine and colestipol also bind orally administered tetracyclines and interfere with the absorption of the antibiotic.

Respiratory Tract Infections. Doxycycline's good activity against *S. pneumoniae* and *H. influenzae* and excellent activity against atypical pathogens such as *Mycoplasma* and *Chlamydophilia pneumoniae* make it an effective single agent for empirical therapy of community-acquired pneumonia in the outpatient setting or as an adjunct to cephalosporin-based therapy for inpatients (Mandell et al., 2007). Tigecycline has been demonstrated to be effective for use as a single agent for adults hospitalized with community-acquired bacterial pneumonia (Bergallo et al., 2009).

Skin and Soft-Tissue Infections. Community strains of methicillin-resistant *S. aureus* often are susceptible to tetracycline, doxycycline, or minocycline, which appear to be effective for uncomplicated skin and soft-tissue infections, although published data are limited (Cenizal et al., 2007). Tigecycline is approved by the Food and Drug Administration (FDA) for the treatment of complicated skin and soft-tissue infections.

Tetracyclines have been used to treat acne. They may act by inhibiting propionibacteria, which reside in sebaceous follicles and metabolize lipids into irritating free fatty acids. The relatively low doses of tetracycline used for acne (e.g., 250 mg orally twice a day) are associated with few side effects.

Intra-abdominal Infections. Increasing resistance among Enterobacteriaceae and gram-negative anaerobes limit the utility of the tetracyclines for intra-abdominal infections. However, tigecycline possesses excellent activity against these pathogens as well as *Enterococcus* and has demonstrated effectiveness in clinical trials for complicated intra-abdominal infections (Oliva et al., 2005).

GI Infections. Therapy with the tetracyclines is often ineffective in infections caused by *Shigella, Salmonella*, or other Enterobacteriaceae because of a high prevalence of drug-resistant strains in many areas. Resistance limits the usefulness of tetracyclines for travelers' diarrhea. Doxycycline (300 mg as a single dose) is effective in reducing stool volume and eradicating *Vibrio cholerae* from the stool within 48 hours. Antimicrobial agents, however, are not substitutes for fluid and electrolyte replacement in this disease. In addition, some strains of *V. cholerae* are resistant to tetracyclines.

Urinary Tract Infections. Tetracyclines are no longer recommended for routine treatment of urinary tract infections because many enteric organisms that cause these infections, including *E. coli*, are resistant. There is little experience in using tigecycline for urinary tract infections; based on its *in vitro* activity, it should be adequate.

Sexually Transmitted Diseases. Because of resistance, doxycycline no longer is recommended for gonococcal infections. If coinfection with *C. trachomatis* has not been excluded, then either doxycycline or azithromycin should be administered in addition to an agent effective for gonococcal urethritis (Workowski and Berman, 2006).

C. trachomatis often is a coexistent pathogen in acute pelvic inflammatory disease, including endometritis, salpingitis, parametritis, and/or peritonitis. Doxycycline, 100 mg intravenously twice daily, is recommended for at least 48 hours after substantial clinical improvement, followed by oral therapy at the same dosage to complete a 14-day course. Doxycycline usually is combined with cefoxitin or cefotetan (Chapter 53) to cover anaerobes and facultative aerobes.

Acute epididymitis is caused by infection with *C. trachomatis* or *N. gonorrhoeae* in men <35 years of age. Effective regimens include a single injection of ceftriaxone (250 mg) plus doxycycline, 100 mg orally twice daily for 10 days. Sexual partners of patients with any of these conditions also should be treated.

Nonspecific urethritis is often due to *Chlamydia trachomatis*. Doxycycline, 100 mg every 12 hours for 7 days, is effective; however, azithromycin is usually preferred because it can be given as a single 1-g dose. Doxycycline (100 mg twice daily for 21 days) is first-line therapy for treatment of lymphogranuloma venereum. The size of buboes decreases within 4 days, and inclusion and elementary bodies entirely disappear from the lymph nodes within 1 week. Rectal pain, discharge, and bleeding of lymphogranulomatous proctitis are decreased markedly. When relapses occur, treatment is resumed with full doses and is continued for longer periods.

Nonpregnant penicillin-allergic patients who have primary, secondary, or latent syphilis can be treated with a tetracycline regimen such as doxycycline, 100 mg orally twice daily for 2 weeks. Tetracyclines should not be used for treatment of neurosyphilis.

Rickettsial Infections. Tetracyclines are effective and may be lifesaving in rickettsial infections, including Rocky Mountain spotted fever, recrudescent epidemic typhus (Brill's disease), murine typhus, scrub typhus, rickettsialpox, and Q fever. Clinical improvement often is evident within 24 hours after initiation of therapy. Doxycycline is the drug of choice for treatment of suspected or proven Rocky Mountain spotted fever in adults and in children, including those <9 years of age, in whom the risk of staining of permanent teeth is outweighed by the seriousness of this potentially fatal infection (Masters et al., 2003).

Anthrax. Doxycycline, 100 mg every 12 hours (2.2 mg/kg every 12 hours for children weighing <45 kg), is indicated for prevention or treatment of anthrax. It should be used in combination with another agent when treating inhalational or GI infection. The recommended duration of therapy is 60 days for exposures occurring as an act of bioterrorism.

Local Application. Except for local use in the eye, topical use of the tetracyclines is not recommended. Their use in ophthalmic therapy is discussed in previous versions of this text. Minocycline sustained-release microspheres for subgingival administration are used in dentistry as an adjunct to scaling and root planing procedures to reduce pocket depth in patients with adult periodontitis.

Other Infections. Tetracyclines in combination with rifampin or streptomycin are effective for acute and chronic infections caused by *Brucella melitensis, Brucella suis*, and *Brucella abortus*. Effective regimens are doxycycline, 200 mg per day, plus rifampin, 600-900 mg daily for 6 weeks, or the usual dose of doxycycline plus streptomycin 1 g daily, intramuscularly. Relapses usually respond to a second course of therapy. Although streptomycin is preferable, tetracyclines also are effective in tularemia (Ellis et al., 2002). Both the ulceroglandular and typhoidal types of the disease respond well. Actinomycosis, although most responsive to penicillin G, may be successfully treated with a tetracycline. Minocycline is an alternative for the treatment of nocardiosis, but a sulfonamide should be used concurrently. Yaws and relapsing fever respond favorably to the tetracyclines. Tetracyclines are useful in the acute treatment and for prophylaxis of leptospirosis (*Leptospira* spp.). *Borrelia* spp., including *B. recurrentis* (relapsing fever) and *B. burgdorferi* (Lyme disease), respond to therapy with a tetracycline. The tetracyclines have been used to treat susceptible atypical mycobacterial pathogens, including *M. marinum*.

Untoward Effects

Gastrointestinal. All tetracyclines can produce GI irritation, most commonly after oral administration. GI distress is also characteristic of tigecycline administration. Epigastric burning and distress, abdominal discomfort, nausea, vomiting, and diarrhea may occur. Tolerability can be improved by administering these drugs with food, but tetracyclines should not be taken with dairy products or antacids. Tetracycline has been associated with esophagitis, esophageal ulcers, and pancreatitis.

Many of the tetracyclines are incompletely absorbed from the GI tract, and high concentrations in the bowel can markedly alter enteric flora. Sensitive aerobic and anaerobic coliform microorganisms and gram-positive spore-forming bacteria are suppressed markedly during long-term tetracycline regimens. As the fecal coliform count declines, overgrowth of tetracycline-resistant microorganisms occurs, particularly of yeasts (*Candida* spp.), enterococci, *Proteus*, and *Pseudomonas*. Moniliasis, thrush, or *Candida*-associated esophagitis may arise during therapy with tetracyclines. Tetracyclines and glycylcyclines may occasionally produce pseudomembranous colitis caused by *Clostridium difficile; pseudomembranous colitis caused by overgrowth of* C. difficile *is a potentially life-threatening complication.*

Photosensitivity. Demeclocycline, doxycycline, and other tetracyclines and glycylcyclines to a lesser extent may produce mild-to-severe photosensitivity reactions in the skin of treated individuals exposed to sunlight. Onycholysis and pigmentation of the nails may develop with or without accompanying photosensitivity.

Hepatic Toxicity. Hepatic toxicity has developed in patients with renal failure receiving ≥2 g of drug per day parenterally, but this effect also may occur when large quantities are administered orally. Cases of hepatotoxicity have been reported rarely with doxycycline, minocycline, and tigecycline administration. Pregnant women are particularly susceptible to tetracycline-induced hepatic damage.

Renal Toxicity. Tetracyclines may aggravate azotemia in patients with renal disease because of their catabolic effects. Doxycycline, minocycline, and tigecycline have fewer renal side effects than other tetracyclines. Nephrogenic diabetes insipidus has been observed in some patients receiving demeclocycline, and this phenomenon has been exploited for the treatment of the syndrome of inappropriate secretion of antidiuretic hormone (Chapter 25).

Fanconi syndrome, characterized by nausea, vomiting, polyuria, polydipsia, proteinuria, acidosis, glycosuria, and aminoaciduria, has been observed in patients ingesting outdated and degraded tetracycline. These symptoms presumably result from a toxic effect of the degradation products on proximal renal tubules. Under no circumstances should outdated tetracyclines be administered.

Effects on Teeth. Children receiving long- or short-term therapy with a tetracycline or glycylcycline may develop permanent brown discoloration of the teeth. The larger the drug dose relative to body weight, the more intense the enamel discoloration. The duration of therapy appears to be less important than the total quantity of antibiotic administered. The risk of this untoward effect is highest when a tetracycline is given to neonates and infants before the first dentition. However, pigmentation of the permanent teeth may develop if the drug is given between the ages of 2 months and 5 years when these teeth are being calcified. The deposition of the drug in the teeth and bones probably is due to its chelating property and the formation of a tetracycline–calcium orthophosphate complex.

Treatment of pregnant patients with tetracyclines may produce discoloration of the teeth in their children. The period of greatest danger to the teeth is from midpregnancy to ~4-6 months of the postnatal period for the deciduous anterior teeth, and from a few months to 5 years of age for the permanent anterior teeth when the crowns are being formed. However, children up to 8 years old may be susceptible to this complication of tetracycline therapy.

Other Toxic and Irritative Effects. Tetracyclines are deposited in the skeleton during gestation and throughout childhood and may depress bone growth in premature infants. This is readily reversible if the period of exposure to the drug is short.

Thrombophlebitis frequently follows intravenous administration. This irritative effect of tetracyclines has been used therapeutically in patients with malignant pleural effusions, where drug is instilled into the pleural space in a procedure called pleurodesis.

Long-term tetracycline therapy may produce leukocytosis, atypical lymphocytes, toxic granulation of granulocytes, and thrombocytopenic purpura.

The tetracyclines may cause increased intracranial pressure (pseudotumor cerebri) in young infants, even when given in the usual therapeutic doses. Except for the elevated pressure, the spinal fluid is normal. The pressure promptly returns to normal when therapy is discontinued, and this complication rarely occurs in older individuals.

Patients receiving minocycline may experience vestibular toxicity, manifested by dizziness, ataxia, nausea, and vomiting. The symptoms occur soon after the initial dose and generally disappear within 24-48 hours after drug administration is stopped. Long-term use of minocycline can pigment the skin, producing a brownish discoloration. Various skin reactions, including morbilliform rashes, urticaria, fixed drug eruptions, and generalized exfoliative dermatitis, rarely may follow the use of any of the tetracyclines. Among the more severe allergic responses are angioedema and anaphylaxis; anaphylactoid reactions can occur even after the oral use of these agents. Other hypersensitivity reactions are burning of the eyes, cheilosis, atrophic or hypertrophic glossitis, pruritus ani or vulvae, and vaginitis. Although the exact cause of these reactions is unknown, they can persist for weeks or months after cessation of tetracycline therapy. Fever of varying degrees and eosinophilia may occur when these agents are administered. Asthma also has been observed. Cross-sensitization among the various tetracyclines is common.

Tetracyclines have a variety of effects on mammalian cells unrelated to their capacity to inhibit bacterial protein synthesis. Doxycycline is being studied as an inhibitor of matrix metalloproteinases (Villareal et al., 2003).

CHLORAMPHENICOL

Chloramphenicol, an antibiotic produced by *Streptomyces venezuelae*, was introduced into clinical practice in 1948. With the drug's wide use, it became evident that chloramphenicol could cause serious and fatal blood dyscrasias. For this reason, chloramphenicol is now reserved for treatment of life-threatening infections (e.g., meningitis, rickettsial infections) in patients who cannot take safer alternatives because of resistance or allergies (Wareham and Wilson, 2002).

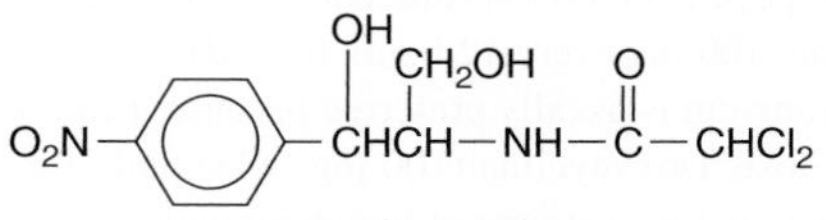

$$O_2N-C_6H_4-CH(OH)-CH(CH_2OH)-NH-C(=O)-CHCl_2$$

CHLORAMPHENICOL

The antibiotic is unique among natural compounds in that it contains a nitrobenzene moiety and is a derivative of dichloroacetic acid. The biologically active form is levorotatory.

Antimicrobial Activity. Chloramphenicol possesses a broad spectrum of antimicrobial activity. Strains are considered sensitive if they are inhibited by concentrations of ≤8 μg/mL, except *S. pneumoniae where the breakpoint is* 4 μg/mL, and *H. influenzae*, which has a breakpoint of 2 μg/mL. Chloramphenicol is bacteriostatic against most species, although it may be bactericidal against *H. influenzae*, *Neisseria meningitidis*, and *S. pneumoniae*. More than 95% of strains of the following gram-negative bacteria are inhibited *in vitro* by 8 μg/mL or less of chloramphenicol: *H. influenzae*, *N. meningitidis*, *N. gonorrhoeae*, *Brucella* spp., and *Bordetella pertussis*. Likewise, most anaerobic bacteria, including gram-positive cocci and *Clostridium* spp., and gram-negative rods including *B. fragilis*, are inhibited by this concentration of the drug. Strains of *S. aureus* tend to be less susceptible, with MICs >8 μg/mL. Chloramphenicol is active against *Mycoplasma*, *Chlamydia*, and *Rickettsia*.

The Enterobacteriaceae are variably sensitive to chloramphenicol. Most strains of *Escherichia coli* (≥75%) and *Klebsiella pneumoniae* are susceptible. *Proteus mirabilis* and indole-positive *Proteus* spp. are susceptible. *P. aeruginosa* is resistant to even very high concentrations of chloramphenicol. Strains of *V. cholerae* have remained largely susceptible to chloramphenicol. Strains of *Shigella* and *Salmonella* resistant to multiple drugs, including chloramphenicol, are prevalent. Of special concern is the increasing prevalence of multiple-drug-resistant strains of *Salmonella* serotype typhi, particularly for strains acquired outside the U.S.

Mechanism of Action. Chloramphenicol inhibits protein synthesis in bacteria, and to a lesser extent, in eukaryotic cells. The drug readily penetrates bacterial cells, probably by facilitated diffusion. Chloramphenicol acts primarily by binding reversibly to the 50S ribosomal subunit (near the binding site for the macrolide antibiotics and clindamycin, which chloramphenicol inhibits competitively). Although binding of tRNA at the codon recognition site on the 30S ribosomal subunit is undisturbed, the drug apparently prevents the binding of the amino acid–containing end of the aminoacyl tRNA to the acceptor site on the 50S ribosomal subunit. The interaction between peptidyltransferase and its amino acid substrate cannot occur, and peptide bond formation is inhibited (Figure 55–2).

Chloramphenicol also can inhibit mitochondrial protein synthesis in mammalian cells, perhaps because mitochondrial ribosomes resemble bacterial ribosomes (both are 70S) more than they do the 80S cytoplasmic ribosomes of mammalian cells. The peptidyltransferase of mitochondrial ribosomes, but not of cytoplasmic ribosomes, is inhibited by chloramphenicol. Mammalian erythropoietic cells are particularly sensitive to the drug.

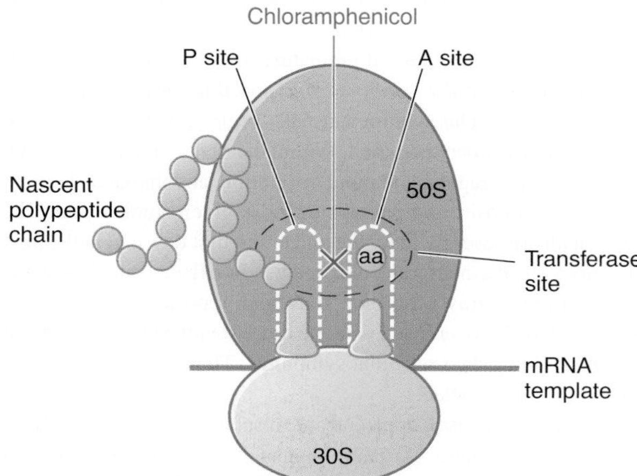

Figure 55–2. *Inhibition of bacterial protein synthesis by chloramphenicol.* Chloramphenicol binds to the 50S ribosomal subunit at the peptidyltransferase site and inhibits the transpeptidation reaction. Chloramphenicol binds to the 50S ribosomal subunit near the site of action of clindamycin and the macrolide antibiotics. These agents interfere with the binding of chloramphenicol and thus may interfere with each other's actions if given concurrently. See Figure 55–1 and its legend for additional information.

Resistance to Chloramphenicol. Resistance to chloramphenicol usually is caused by a plasmid-encoded acetyltransferase that inactivates the drug. Resistance also can result from decreased permeability and from ribosomal mutation. Acetylated derivatives of chloramphenicol fail to bind to bacterial ribosomes.

Absorption, Distribution, Fate, and Excretion. Chloramphenicol is absorbed rapidly from the GI tract, and peak concentrations of 10-13 μg/mL occur within 2-3 hours after the administration of a 1-g dose. The product for oral administration is no longer available in the U.S. The preparation of chloramphenicol for parenteral use is the water-soluble, inactive prodrug sodium succinate. Similar concentrations of chloramphenicol succinate in plasma are achieved after intravenous and intramuscular administration. Hydrolysis of chloramphenicol succinate by esterases occurs *in vivo*. Chloramphenicol succinate is rapidly cleared from plasma by the kidneys; this may reduce overall bioavailability of the drug because as much as 30% of the dose may be excreted before hydrolysis. Poor renal function in the neonate and other states of renal insufficiency result in increased plasma concentrations of chloramphenicol succinate. Decreased esterase activity has been observed in the plasma of neonates and infants, prolonging time to peak concentrations of active chloramphenicol (up to 4 hours) and extending the period over which renal clearance of chloramphenicol succinate can occur.

Chloramphenicol is widely distributed in body fluids and readily reaches therapeutic concentrations in CSF, where values are ~60% of those in plasma (range, 45-99%) in the presence or absence of meningitis. The drug actually may accumulate in the brain. Chloramphenicol is present in bile, milk, and placental fluid. It also is found in the aqueous humor after subconjunctival injection.

Hepatic metabolism to the inactive glucuronide is the major route of elimination. This metabolite and chloramphenicol itself are excreted in the urine following filtration and secretion. Patients with cirrhosis or otherwise impaired hepatic function have decreased metabolic clearance, and dosage should be adjusted in these individuals. The $t_{1/2}$ of chloramphenicol correlates with plasma bilirubin concentrations. About 50% of chloramphenicol is bound to plasma proteins; such binding is reduced in cirrhotic patients and in neonates. Half-life is not altered significantly by renal insufficiency or hemodialysis, and dosage adjustment usually is not required. However, if the dose of chloramphenicol has been reduced because of cirrhosis, clearance by hemodialysis may be significant. This effect can be minimized by administering the drug at the end of hemodialysis. Significant variability in the metabolism and pharmacokinetics of chloramphenicol in neonates, infants, and children necessitates monitoring of drug concentrations in plasma.

Therapeutic Uses and Dosage. Therapy with chloramphenicol must be limited to infections for which the benefits of the drug outweigh the risks of the potential toxicities. When other antimicrobial drugs that are equally effective and potentially less toxic are available, they should be used instead of chloramphenicol (Wareham and Wilson, 2002).

Typhoid Fever. Third-generation cephalosporins and quinolones are drugs of choice for the treatment of typhoid fever because they are less toxic and because strains of *Salmonella typhi* often are resistant to chloramphenicol (Parry, 2003).

The adult dose of chloramphenicol for typhoid fever is 1 g every 6 hours for 4 weeks. Although intravenous and oral routes have been used, the response is more rapid with oral administration. Provided that the primary isolate is sensitive, relapses respond satisfactorily to retreatment.

Bacterial Meningitis. Third-generation cephalosporins have replaced chloramphenicol in the therapy of bacterial meningitis (Quagliarello and Scheld, 1997). Chloramphenicol remains an alternative drug for the treatment of meningitis caused by *H. influenzae*, *N. meningitidis*, and *S. pneumoniae* in patients who have severe allergy to β-lactams and in developing countries (Fuller et al., 2003). The total daily dose for children should be 50 mg/kg of body weight, divided into four equal doses given intravenously every 6 hours. Results with chloramphenicol used for pneumococcal meningitis may be unsatisfactory because some strains are inhibited but not killed. Moreover, penicillin-resistant strains frequently also are resistant to chloramphenicol (Hoban et al., 2001). In the rare situation in which chloramphenicol must be used to treat pneumococcal meningitis, lumbar puncture should be repeated 2-3 days after treatment is initiated to ensure that an adequate response has occurred.

Rickettsial Diseases. The tetracyclines usually are the preferred agents for the treatment of rickettsial diseases. However, in patients allergic to these drugs, in those with reduced renal function, in pregnant women, and in children <8 years of age who require prolonged or repeated courses of therapy, chloramphenicol may be the drug of choice. Rocky Mountain spotted fever, epidemic, murine, scrub, and recrudescent typhus, and Q fever respond well to chloramphenicol. For adults and children with these diseases, a dosage of 50 mg/kg/day divided into 6-hour intervals is recommended. For severe or resistant infections, doses up to 100 mg/kg/day may be used for short intervals, but the dose be reduced to 50 mg/kg/day as soon as possible. Therapy should be continued until the general condition has improved and the patient is afebrile for 24-48 hours.

Untoward Effects. Chloramphenicol inhibits the synthesis of proteins of the inner mitochondrial membrane, probably by inhibiting the ribosomal peptidyltransferase. These include subunits of cytochrome *c* oxidase, ubiquinone-cytochrome *c* reductase, and the proton-translocating ATPase critical for aerobic metabolism. Much of the toxicity observed with this drug can be attributed to these effects.

Hypersensitivity Reactions. Although relatively uncommon, macular or vesicular skin rashes result from hypersensitivity to chloramphenicol. Fever may appear simultaneously or be the sole manifestation. Angioedema is a rare complication. Jarisch-Herxheimer reactions may occur after institution of chloramphenicol therapy for syphilis, brucellosis, and typhoid fever.

Hematological Toxicity. The most important adverse effect of chloramphenicol is on the bone marrow. Chloramphenicol affects the hematopoietic system in two ways: a dose-related toxicity that presents as anemia, leukopenia, or thrombocytopenia, and an idiosyncratic response manifested by aplastic anemia, leading in many cases to fatal pancytopenia. Pancytopenia seems to occur more commonly in individuals who undergo prolonged therapy and especially in those who are exposed to the drug on more than one occasion. A genetic predisposition is suggested by the occurrence of pancytopenia in identical twins. Although the incidence of the reaction is low, ~1 in ≥30,000 courses of therapy, the fatality rate is high when bone marrow aplasia is complete, and there is an increased incidence of acute leukemia in those who recover. Aplastic anemia accounts for ~70% of cases of blood dyscrasias due to chloramphenicol; hypoplastic anemia, agranulocytosis, and thrombocytopenia make up the remainder. The exact biochemical mechanism has not yet been elucidated but is hypothesized to involve conversion of the nitro group to a toxic intermediate by intestinal bacteria.

The risk of aplastic anemia does not contraindicate the use of chloramphenicol in situations in which it may be lifesaving. The drug should never be used, however, in undefined situations or in diseases readily, safely, and effectively treatable with other antimicrobial agents.

Dose-related, reversible erythroid suppression probably reflects an inhibitory action of chloramphenicol on mitochondrial protein synthesis in erythroid precursors, which in turn impairs iron incorporation into heme. Leukopenia and thrombocytopenia also may occur. Bone marrow suppression occurs regularly when plasma concentrations are ≥25 μg/mL and is observed with the use of large doses of chloramphenicol, prolonged treatment, or both. Dose-related suppression of the bone marrow may progress to fatal aplasia if treatment is continued, but most cases of bone marrow aplasia develop suddenly, without prior dose-related marrow suppression. Some patients who developed chronic bone marrow hypoplasia after chloramphenicol treatment subsequently developed acute myeloblastic leukemia. The administration of chloramphenicol in the presence of hepatic disease frequently depresses erythropoiesis. About one-third of patients with severe renal insufficiency exhibit the same reaction.

Other Toxic and Irritative Effects. Nausea and vomiting, unpleasant taste, diarrhea, and perineal irritation may follow the oral administration of chloramphenicol. Blurring of vision and digital paresthesias may rarely occur. Tissues that have a high rate of oxygen consumption may be particularly susceptible to chloramphenicol effects on mitochondrial enzyme systems; encephalopathy and cardiomyopathy have been reported.

Neonates, especially if premature, may develop a serious illness termed *gray baby syndrome* if exposed to excessive doses of chloramphenicol. This syndrome usually begins 2-9 days (average of 4 days) after treatment is started. Within the first 24 hours, vomiting, refusal to suck, irregular and rapid respiration, abdominal distention, periods of cyanosis, and passage of loose green stools occur. The children all are severely ill by the end of the first day, and in the next 24 hours turn an ashen-gray color and become flaccid and hypothermic. A similar "gray syndrome" has been reported in adults who were accidentally overdosed with the drug. Death occurs in ~40% of patients within 2 days of initial symptoms. Those who recover usually exhibit no sequelae.

Two mechanisms apparently are responsible for chloramphenicol toxicity in neonates: (1) a developmental deficiency of glucuronyl transferase, the hepatic enzyme that metabolizes chloramphenicol, in the first 3-4 weeks of life; and (2) inadequate renal excretion of unconjugated drug. At the onset of the clinical syndrome, chloramphenicol concentrations in plasma usually exceed 100 μg/mL, although they may be as low as 75 μg/mL. Children ≤2 weeks of age should receive chloramphenicol in a daily dose no larger than 25 mg/kg of body weight; after this age, full-term infants may be given daily quantities up to 50 mg/kg. Toxic effects have not been observed in the newborns when as much as 1 g of the antibiotic has been given every 2 hours to the mothers during labor.

Drug Interactions. Chloramphenicol inhibits hepatic CYPs and thereby prolongs the half-lives of drugs that are metabolized by this system, including warfarin, dicumarol, phenytoin, chlorpropamide, antiretroviral protease inhibitors, rifabutin, and tolbutamide. Severe toxicity and death have occurred because of failure to recognize such effects. Conversely, other drugs may alter the elimination of chloramphenicol. Concurrent administration of phenobarbital or rifampin, which potently induce CYPs, shortens the $t_{1/2}$ of the antibiotic and may result in subtherapeutic drug concentrations.

MACROLIDES AND KETOLIDES

Erythromycin was discovered in 1952 by McGuire and coworkers in the metabolic products of a strain of *Streptomyces erythreus*. Clarithromycin (BIAXIN, others) and azithromycin (ZITHROMAX, others) are semisynthetic derivatives of erythromycin. Ketolides are semisynthetic derivatives of erythromycin with activity against some macrolide-resistant strains. Telithromycin (KETEK) is the only ketolide currently approved in the U.S. Although the ketolides are promising agents against drug-resistant organisms, substantial hepatotoxicity seen with telithromycin has limited their use.

Macrolide antibiotics contain a many-membered lactone ring (14-membered rings for erythromycin and clarithromycin and a 15-membered ring for azithromycin) to which are attached one or more deoxy sugars. Clarithromycin differs from erythromycin only by methylation of the hydroxyl group at the 6 position, and azithromycin differs by the addition of a methyl-substituted nitrogen atom into the lactone ring. These structural modifications improve acid stability and tissue penetration and broaden the spectrum of activity.

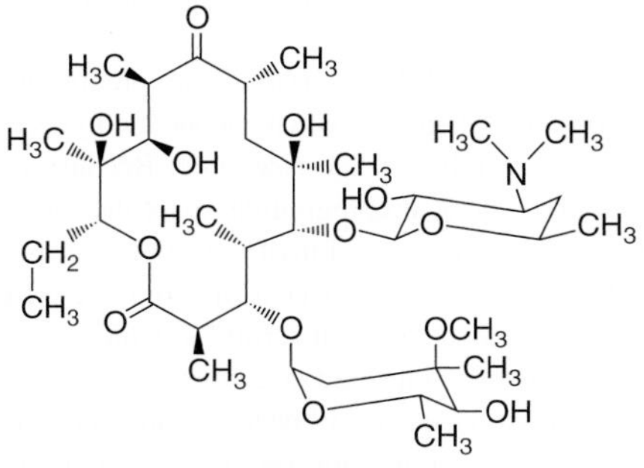

ERYTHROMYCIN

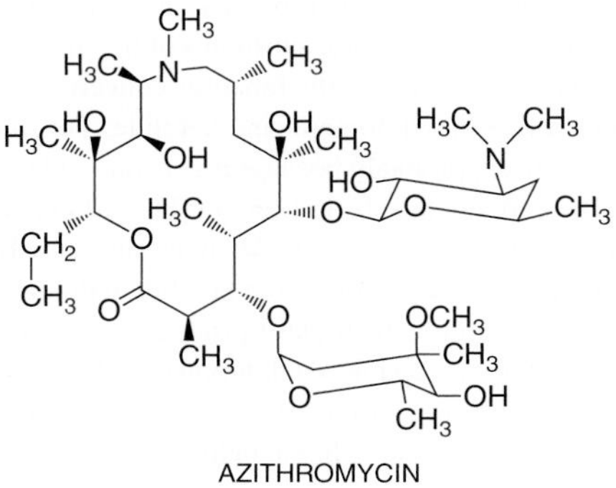

AZITHROMYCIN

Telithromycin differs from erythromycin in that a 3-keto group replaces the α-L-cladinose of the 14-member macrolide ring, and there is a substituted carbamate at C11-C12. These modifications render ketolides less susceptible to methylase-mediated (*erm*) and efflux-mediated (*mef* or *msr*) mechanisms of resistance. Ketolides therefore are active against many macrolide-resistant gram-positive strains. The structural formula of telithromycin is:

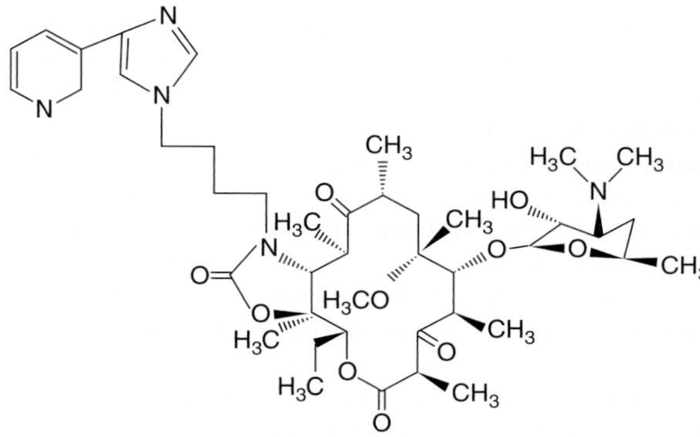

TELITHROMYCIN

Antimicrobial Activity. Erythromycin usually is bacteriostatic but may be bactericidal in high concentrations against susceptible organisms. The antibiotic is most active *in vitro* against aerobic gram-positive cocci and bacilli (Table 55–2). Staphylococci are considered susceptible at ≤0.5 μg/mL and streptococci at ≤0.25 μg/mL. Macrolide resistance among *S. pneumoniae* often co-exists with penicillin resistance Staphylococci are not reliably sensitive to erythromycin, especially methicillin-resistant strains. Macrolide-resistant strains of *S. aureus* are potentially cross-resistant to clindamycin and streptogramin B (quinupristin). Gram-positive bacilli also are sensitive to erythromycin; typical MICs are 1 μg/mL for *Clostridium perfringens*, from 0.2 to 3 μg/mL for *Corynebacterium diphtheriae*, and from 0.25 to 4 μg/mL for *Listeria monocytogenes*.

Erythromycin is inactive against most aerobic enteric gram-negative bacilli. It has modest activity *in vitro* against other gram-negative organisms, including *H. influenzae* (MIC, 1-32 μg/mL) and *N. meningitidis* (MIC, 0.4-1.6 μg/mL), and good activity against most strains of *N. gonorrhoeae* (MIC, 0.12-2 μg/mL). Useful antibacterial activity also is observed against *Pasteurella multocida*, *Borrelia* spp., and *Bordetella pertussis*. Resistance is common for *B. fragilis* (the MIC ranging from 2-32 μg/mL). Macrolides are usually active against *Campylobacter jejuni* (MIC, 0.5-4 μg/mL). Erythromycin is active against *M. pneumoniae* (MIC, 0.004-0.02 μg/mL) and *Legionella pneumophila* (MIC, 0.01-2 μg/mL). Most strains of *C. trachomatis* are inhibited by 0.06-2 μg/mL of erythromycin. Some of the atypical mycobacteria, including *M. scrofulaceum*, are sensitive to erythromycin *in vitro*; *M. kansasii* and *M. avium-intracellulare* vary in sensitivity. *M. fortuitum* is resistant. Macrolides have no effect on viruses, yeasts, or fungi.

In general, organisms are considered susceptible to clarithromycin and azithromycin at MICs ≤2 μg/mL.

Clarithromycin and azithromycin have some activity against *H. influenzae*, with MIC breakpoints of ≤8 μg/mL and ≤4 μg/mL, respectively. However, these agents are not drugs of choice for documented *H. influenzae* infections because of their lesser activity compared to β-lactams or fluoroquinolones. Clarithromycin is slightly more potent than erythromycin against sensitive strains of streptococci and staphylococci, and has modest activity against *H. influenzae* and *N. gonorrhoeae*. Azithromycin generally is less active than erythromycin against gram-positive organisms and slightly more active than either erythromycin or clarithromycin against *H. influenzae* and *Campylobacter* spp. Clarithromycin and azithromycin have good activity against *M. catarrhalis*, *Chlamydia* spp., *L. pneumophila*, *B. burgdorferi*, *Mycoplasma pneumoniae*, and *H. pylori*. Azithromycin and clarithromycin have enhanced activity against *M. avium-intracellulare*, as well as against some protozoa (e.g., *Toxoplasma gondii*, *Cryptosporidium*, and *Plasmodium* spp.). Clarithromycin has good activity against *Mycobacterium leprae*.

Telithromycin's spectrum of activity is similar to clarithromycin and azithromycin. MIC breakpoints for telithromycin are ≤0.25 μg/mL for *S. aureus*, ≤1 μg/mL for *S. pneumoniae*, and ≤4 μg/mL for *H. influenzae*. Telithromycin's ability to withstand many macrolide resistance mechanisms increases its activity against macrolide-resistant *S. pneumoniae* and *S. aureus*.

Mechanism of Action. Macrolide antibiotics are bacteriostatic agents that inhibit protein synthesis by binding reversibly to 50S ribosomal subunits of sensitive microorganisms (Figure 55–3), at or very near the site that binds chloramphenicol (Figure 55–2). Erythromycin does not inhibit peptide bond formation per se but rather inhibits the translocation step wherein a newly synthesized peptidyl tRNA molecule moves from the acceptor site on the ribosome to the peptidyl donor site. Gram-positive bacteria accumulate ~100 times more erythromycin than do gram-negative bacteria. Cells are considerably more permeable to the unionized form of the drug, which probably explains the increased antimicrobial activity at alkaline pH. Ketolides and macrolides have the same ribosomal target site. The principal difference between the two is that structural modifications within ketolides neutralize the common resistance mechanisms that make macrolides ineffective (Nilius and Ma, 2002).

Resistance to Macrolides and Ketolides. Resistance to macrolides usually results from one of four mechanisms:

- drug efflux by an active pump mechanism (encoded by *mrsA*, *mefA*, or *mefE* in staphylococci, group A streptococci, or *S. pneumoniae*, respectively)
- ribosomal protection by inducible or constitutive production of methylase enzymes, mediated by expression of *ermA*, *ermB*, and *ermC*, which modify the ribosomal target and decrease drug binding
- macrolide hydrolysis by esterases produced by Enterobacteriaceae (Lina et al., 1999; Nakajima, 1999)
- chromosomal mutations that alter a 50S ribosomal protein (found in *B. subtilis*, *Campylobacter* spp., mycobacteria, and gram-positive cocci)

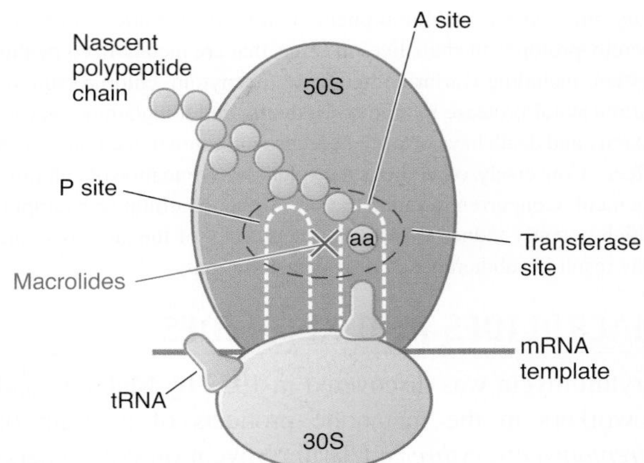

Figure 55–3. *Inhibition of bacterial protein synthesis by the macrolide antibiotics erythromycin, clarithromycin, and azithromycin.* Macrolide antibiotics are bacteriostatic agents that inhibit protein synthesis by binding reversibly to the 50S ribosomal subunits of sensitive organisms. Erythromycin appears to inhibit the translocation step such that the nascent peptide chain temporarily residing at the A site of the transferase reaction fails to move to the P, or donor, site. Alternatively, macrolides may bind and cause a conformational change that terminates protein synthesis by indirectly interfering with transpeptidation and translocation. See Figure 55–1 and its legend for additional information.

The MLS_B (macrolide-lincosamide-streptogramin B) phenotype is conferred by *erm* genes, which encode methylases that modify the macrolide binding of the ribosome. Because macrolides, lincosamides, and type B streptogramins share the same ribosomal binding site, constitutive expression of *erm* confers cross-resistance to all three drug classes. If resistance is due to inducible expression of *erm*, there is resistance to the macrolides, which are inducers of *erm*, but not to lincosamides and streptogramin B, which are not inducers. Cross-resistance can still occur if constitutive mutants are selected by exposure to lincosamides or streptogramin B. Efflux-mediated resistance to macrolides may not result in cross-resistance to lincosamides or streptogramin B because they are structurally dissimilar to macrolides and are not substrates of the macrolide pump.

Introduction of the 3-keto function converts a methylase-inducing macrolide into a noninducing ketolide. This moiety also prevents drug efflux, probably because it generates a less-desirable substrate. The carbamate substitution at C11-C12 enhances binding to the ribosomal target site, even when the site is methylated, by introducing an extra interaction of the ketolide with the ribosome. Inducible and constitutive methylase-producing strains of *S. pneumoniae* are therefore susceptible to telithromycin. However, constitutive methylase-producing strains of *S. aureus* and *S. pyogenes* are telithromycin resistant because the strength of the ketolide interaction with the fully methylated ribosomal binding site is insufficient to overcome resistance. Constitutive methylase producers can be selected from strains with the inducible *erm* phenotype.

Absorption, Distribution, and Excretion.

Absorption. Erythromycin base is incompletely but adequately absorbed from the upper small intestine. Because it is inactivated by gastric acid, the drug is administered as enteric-coated tablets, as capsules containing enteric-coated pellets that dissolve in the duodenum, or as an ester. Food, which increases gastric acidity, may delay absorption.

Peak serum concentrations are 0.3-0.5 μg/mL, 4 hours after oral administration of 250 mg of the base, and 0.3-1.9 μg/mL after a single dose of 500 mg. Esters of erythromycin base (e.g., stearate, estolate, and ethylsuccinate) have improved acid stability, and their absorption is less altered by food. A single oral 250-mg dose of erythromycin estolate produces peak serum concentrations of ~1.5 μg/mL after 2 hours, and a 500-mg dose produces peak concentrations of 4 μg/mL. Peak serum concentrations of erythromycin ethylsuccinate are 1.5 μg/mL (0.5 μg/mL of base) 1-2 hours after administration of a 500-mg dose. These peak values include the inactive ester and the free base, the latter of which comprises 20-35% of the total. The concentration of microbiologically active erythromycin base in serum therefore is similar for the various preparations. Higher concentrations of erythromycin can be achieved by intravenous administration. Values are ~10 μg/mL 1 hour after intravenous administration of 500-1000 mg of erythromycin lactobionate.

Clarithromycin is absorbed rapidly from the GI tract after oral administration, but first-pass metabolism reduces its bioavailability to 50-55%. Peak concentrations occur ~2 hours after drug administration. Clarithromycin may be given with or without food, but the extended-release form, typically given once daily as a 1-g dose, should be administered with food to improve bioavailability. Steady-state peak concentrations in plasma of 2-3 μg/mL are achieved after 2 hours with a regimen of 500 mg every 12 hours, or after 2-4 hours with two 500-mg extended-release tablets given once daily.

Azithromycin administered orally is absorbed rapidly and distributes widely throughout the body, except to the brain and CSF. Concomitant administration of aluminum and magnesium hydroxide antacids decreases the peak serum drug concentrations but not overall bioavailability. Azithromycin should not be administered with food. A 500-mg loading dose will produce a peak plasma drug concentration of ~0.4 μg/mL. When this loading dose is followed by 250 mg once daily for 4 days, the steady-state peak drug concentration is 0.24 μg/mL. Azithromycin also can be administered intravenously, producing plasma concentrations of 3-4 μg/mL after a 1-hour infusion of 500 mg.

Telithromycin is formulated as a 400-mg tablet for oral administration. There is no parenteral form. It is well absorbed with ~60% bioavailability. Peak serum concentrations, averaging 2 μg/mL following a single 800-mg oral dose, are achieved within 30 minutes to 4 hours.

Distribution. Erythromycin diffuses readily into intracellular fluids, achieving antibacterial activity in essentially all sites except the brain and CSF. Erythromycin penetrates into prostatic fluid, achieving concentrations ~40% of those in plasma. Concentrations in middle ear exudate reach only 50% of serum concentrations and thus may be inadequate for the treatment of otitis media caused by *H. influenzae.* Protein binding is ~70-80% for erythromycin base and even higher, 96%, for the estolate. Erythromycin traverses the placenta, and drug concentrations in fetal plasma are ~5-20% of those in the maternal circulation. Concentrations in breast milk are 50% of those in serum.

Clarithromycin and its active metabolite, 14-hydroxyclarithromycin, distribute widely and achieve high intracellular concentrations throughout the body. Tissue concentrations generally exceed serum concentrations. Concentrations in middle-ear fluid are 50% higher than simultaneous serum concentrations for clarithromycin and the active metabolite. Protein binding of clarithromycin ranges from 40% to 70% and is concentration dependent.

Azithromycin's unique pharmacokinetic properties include extensive tissue distribution and high drug concentrations within cells (including phagocytes), resulting in much greater concentrations of drugs in tissue or secretions compared to simultaneous serum concentrations. Tissue fibroblasts act as the natural reservoir for the drug *in vivo*. Protein binding is 50% at very low plasma concentrations and less at higher concentrations.

Telithromycin is 60-70% bound by serum protein, principally albumin. It penetrates well into most tissues, exceeding plasma concentrations by ~2-fold to ≥10-fold. Telithromycin is concentrated into macrophages and white blood cells, where concentrations of 40 μg/mL (500 times the simultaneous plasma concentration) are maintained 24 hours after dosing.

Elimination. Only 2-5% of orally administered erythromycin is excreted in active form in the urine; this value is from 12-15% after intravenous infusion. The antibiotic is concentrated in the liver and excreted in the bile, which may contain as much as 250 μg/mL when serum concentrations are very high. The serum elimination $t_{1/2}$ of erythromycin is ~1.6 hours. Although the $t_{1/2}$ may be prolonged in patients with anuria, dosage reduction is not routinely recommended in renal failure patients. The drug is not removed significantly by either peritoneal dialysis or hemodialysis.

Clarithromycin is eliminated by renal and nonrenal mechanisms. It is metabolized in the liver to several metabolites; the active 14-hydroxy metabolite is the most significant. Primary metabolic pathways are oxidative *N*-demethylation and hydroxylation at the 14 position. The elimination half-lives are 3-7 hours for clarithromycin and 5-9 hours for 14-hydroxyclarithromycin. Metabolism is saturable, resulting in nonlinear pharmacokinetics with higher dosages; longer half-lives are observed after larger doses. The amount of clarithromycin excreted unchanged in the urine ranges from 20% to 40%, depending on the dose administered and the formulation (tablet versus oral suspension). An additional 10-15% of a dose is excreted in the urine as 14-hydroxyclarithromycin. Although the pharmacokinetics of clarithromycin are altered in patients with either hepatic or renal dysfunction, dose adjustment is not necessary unless the creatinine clearance is <30 mL/minute.

Azithromycin undergoes some hepatic metabolism to inactive metabolites, but biliary excretion is the major route of elimination. Only 12% of drug is excreted unchanged in the urine. The elimination $t_{1/2}$, 40-68 hours, is prolonged because of extensive tissue sequestration and binding.

With a $t_{1/2}$ of 9.8 hours, telithromycin can be given once daily. The drug is cleared primarily by hepatic metabolism, 50% by CYP3A4 and 50% by CYP-independent metabolism. No adjustment of the dose is required for hepatic failure or mild-to-moderate renal failure. No dose has been established for patients in whom creatinine clearance is <30 mL/minute, although a reduction in dosage probably is advisable (Shi et al., 2004).

Therapeutic Uses and Dosage. Depending on the nature and severity of the infection, the usual oral dose of erythromycin (erythromycin base) for adults ranges from 1-2 g per day, in equally divided and spaced amounts, usually given every 6 hours. Erythromycin base is available as immediate release (film-coated) and delayed-release (enteric-coated) tablets. Daily doses of erythromycin as large as 8 g orally, given for 3 months, have been well tolerated. Food should not be taken concurrently, if possible, with erythromycin base or the stearate formulations, but this is not necessary with erythromycin estolate. The oral dose of erythromycin for children is 30-50 mg/kg per day, divided into four portions; this dose may be doubled for severe infections. Intramuscular administration of erythromycin is not recommended because of pain upon injection. Intravenous administration is generally reserved for the therapy of severe infections, such as legionellosis. The usual dose is 0.5-1 g every 6 hours; 1 g of erythromycin gluceptate (not available in the U.S.) has been given intravenously every 6 hours for as long as 4 weeks with no adverse effects except for thrombophlebitis at the site of injection. Erythromycin lactobionate is available for intravenous injection. The combination of erythromycin and sulfisoxazole appears to have synergistic antibacterial activity; it is available as a suspension used primarily for treatment of otitis media in children.

Clarithromycin (BIAXIN, others) usually is given twice daily at a dose of 250 mg for children >12 years and adults with mild to moderate infection. Larger doses (e.g., 500 mg twice daily) are indicated for more severe infection such as pneumonia or when infection is caused by more resistant organisms such as *H. influenzae*. Children <12 years old have received 7.5 mg/kg twice daily in clinical studies. The 500-mg extended-release formulation is given as two tablets once daily. Clarithromycin (500 mg) is also packaged with lansoprazole (30 mg) and amoxicillin (1 g) as a combination regimen (PREVPAC) that is administered twice daily for 10 or 14 days to eradicate *H. pylori* and to reduce the associated risk of duodenal ulcer recurrence (Chapter 45).

Azithromycin (ZITHROMAX, other) should be given 1 hour before or 2 hours after meals when administered orally. For outpatient therapy of community-acquired pneumonia, pharyngitis, or skin and skin-structure infections, a loading dose of 500 mg is given on the first day, and then 250 mg per day is given for days 2 through 5. A single 2-g dose of extended-release microspheres is an alternative regimen for treatment of community-acquired pneumonia or acute exacerbations of chronic bronchitis. Treatment or prophylaxis of *M. avium-intracellulare* infection in AIDS patients requires higher doses: 600 mg daily in combination with one or more other agents for treatment, or 1200 mg once weekly for primary prevention (Kovacs and Masur, 2000). Azithromycin is useful in treatment of sexually transmitted diseases, especially during pregnancy when tetracyclines are contraindicated. The treatment of uncomplicated nongonococcal urethritis presumed to be caused by *C. trachomatis* consists of a single 1-g dose of azithromycin. This dose also is effective for chancroid. Azithromycin (1 g per week for 3 weeks) is an alternative regimen for treatment of granuloma inguinale or lymphogranuloma venereum.

In children, the recommended dose of azithromycin oral suspension for acute otitis media and pneumonia is 10 mg/kg on the first day (maximum: 500 mg) and 5 mg/kg (maximum: 250 mg per day) on days 2 through 5. A single 30 mg/kg dose is approved as an alternative for otitis media. The dose for tonsillitis or pharyngitis is 12 mg/kg per day, up to 500 mg total, for 5 days.

Respiratory Tract Infections. Macrolides and ketolides are suitable drugs for the treatment of a number of respiratory tract infections due to their activity against *Streptococcus pneumoniae*, *Haemophilus influenzae*, and atypical pathogens (*Mycoplasma*, *Chlamydophilia*, *Legionella*). Azithromycin and clarithromycin are suitable choices for treatment of mild to moderate community-acquired pneumonia among ambulatory patients. In hospitalized patients, a macrolide is commonly added to a cephalosporin for coverage of atypical respiratory pathogens. Macrolides, fluoroquinolones, and tetracyclines are drugs of choice for treatment of pneumonia caused by *Chlamydia pneumoniae* or *Mycoplasma pneumoniae*. Erythromycin has been considered as the drug of choice for treatment of pneumonia caused by *L. pneumophila*, *L. micdadei*, or other *Legionella* spp. Because of excellent *in vitro* activity, superior tissue concentration, the ease of administration as a single daily dose, and better tolerability compared to erythromycin, azithromycin (or a fluoroquinolone) has supplanted erythromycin as the first-line agent for treatment of legionellosis (Garey and Amsden, 1999). The recommended dose is 500 mg daily, intravenously or orally, for a total of 10-14 days.

Macrolides are also appropriate alternative agents for the treatment of acute exacerbations of chronic bronchitis, acute otitis media, acute streptococcal pharyngitis, and acute bacterial sinusitis. Azithromycin or clarithromycin are generally preferred to erythromycin for these indications due to their broader spectrum and superior tolerability.

Telithromycin has shown to be effective in the treatment of community-acquired pneumonia, acute exacerbations of chronic bronchitis, and acute bacterial sinusitis, and has a potential advantage over macrolides in regions where macrolide-resistant strains are common. However, due to a number of cases of severe hepatotoxicity due to telithromycin, telithromycin's U.S. FDA approval for treatment of acute exacerbations of chronic bronchitis and sinusitis have been rescinded, leaving only its indication for community-acquired pneumonia. *Because of the substantial risk of serious hepatotoxicity, telithromycin should be used only in circumstances where it provides a substantial advantage over less toxic therapies.*

Skin and Soft-Tissue Infections. Macrolides are alternatives for treatment of erysipelas and cellulitis among patients who have a serious allergy to penicillin. Unfortunately, macrolide-resistant strains of staphylococci and streptococci are increasingly encountered. Erythromycin has been an alternative agent for the treatment of relatively minor skin and soft-tissue infections caused by either penicillin-sensitive or penicillin-resistant *S. aureus*. However, many strains of *S. aureus* are resistant to macrolides, and they no longer can be relied on unless *in vitro* susceptibility has been documented.

Chlamydial Infections. Chlamydial infections can be treated effectively with any of the macrolides. A single 1-g dose of azithromycin is recommended for patients with uncomplicated urethral, endocervical, rectal, or epididymal infections because of the ease of compliance. During pregnancy, erythromycin base, 500 mg four times daily for 7 days, is recommended as first-line therapy for chlamydial urogenital infections. Azithromycin, 1 g orally as a single dose, is a suitable alternative. Erythromycin base is preferred for chlamydial pneumonia of infancy and ophthalmia neonatorum (50 mg/kg per day in four divided doses for 10-14 days). Azithromycin, 1 g/week for 3 weeks, may be effective for lymphogranuloma venereum.

Diphtheria. Erythromycin, 250 mg four times daily for 7 days, is very effective for acute infections or for eradicating the carrier state. The other macrolides also are likely to be effective; because clinical experience with them is lacking, they are not FDA-approved for this indication. The presence of an antibiotic does not alter the course of an acute infection with the diphtheria bacillus or the risk of complications. Antitoxin is indicated in the treatment of acute infection.

Pertussis. Erythromycin is the drug of choice for treating persons with *B. pertussis* disease and for postexposure prophylaxis of household members and close contacts. A 7-day regimen of erythromycin estolate (40 mg/kg per day; maximum: 1 g/day; not available in U.S) is as effective as the 14-day regimens traditionally recommended (Halperin et al., 1997). Clarithromycin and azithromycin also are effective (Bace et al., 1999). If administered early in the course of whooping cough, erythromycin may shorten the duration of illness; it has little influence on the disease once the paroxysmal stage is reached, although it may eliminate the microorganisms from the nasopharynx. Nasopharyngeal cultures should be obtained from people with pertussis who do not improve with erythromycin therapy because resistance has been reported.

Campylobacter Infections. The treatment of gastroenteritis caused by *C. jejuni* with erythromycin (250-500 mg orally four times a day for 7 days) hastens eradication of the microorganism from the stools and reduces the duration of symptoms. Availability of fluoroquinolones, which are highly active against *Campylobacter* species and other enteric pathogens, largely has replaced the use of erythromycin for this disease in adults. Erythromycin remains useful for treatment of *Campylobacter* gastroenteritis in children.

Helicobacter pylori Infection. Clarithromycin, 500 mg, in combination with omeprazole, 20 mg, and amoxicillin, 1 g (PREVPAC), each administered twice daily for 10-14 days, is effective for treatment of peptic ulcer disease caused by *H. pylori* (Peterson et al., 2000). Numerous other regimens, some effective as 7-day treatments, have been studied and also are effective. The more effective regimens generally include three agents, one of which usually is clarithromycin (Chapter 45).

Mycobacterial Infections. Clarithromycin or azithromycin is recommended as first-line therapy for prophylaxis and treatment of disseminated infection caused by *M. avium-intracellulare* in AIDS patients and for treatment of pulmonary disease in patients not infected with HIV (Kovacs and Masur, 2000). Azithromycin (1.2 g once weekly) or clarithromycin (500 mg twice daily) is recommended for primary prevention for AIDS patients with <50 CD4 cells/mm^3. Single-agent therapy should not be used for treatment of active disease or for secondary prevention in AIDS patients. Clarithromycin (500 mg twice daily) plus ethambutol (15 mg/kg once daily) with or without rifabutin is an effective combination regimen. Azithromycin (500 mg once daily) may be used instead of clarithromycin, but clarithromycin appears to be slightly more efficacious (Ward et al., 1998). Clarithromycin also has been used with minocycline for the treatment of *Mycobacterium leprae* in lepromatous leprosy.

Prophylactic Uses. Penicillin is the drug of choice for the prophylaxis of recurrences of rheumatic fever. Erythromycin is an effective alternative for individuals who are allergic to penicillin. Clarithromycin or azithromycin (or clindamycin) are recommended alternatives for the prevention of bacterial endocarditis in patients undergoing dental procedures who are at high risk for endocarditis (Wilson et al., 2007).

Untoward Effects.

Hepatotoxicity. Cholestatic hepatitis is the most striking side effect. It is caused primarily by erythromycin estolate and rarely by the ethylsuccinate or the stearate. The illness starts after 10-20 days of treatment and is characterized initially by nausea, vomiting, and abdominal cramps. The pain often mimics that of acute cholecystitis. These symptoms are followed shortly thereafter by jaundice, which may be accompanied by fever, leukocytosis, eosinophilia, and elevated transaminases in plasma. Biopsy of the liver reveals cholestasis, periportal infiltration by neutrophils, lymphocytes, and eosinophils, and occasionally, necrosis of neighboring parenchymal cells. Findings usually resolve within a few days after cessation of drug therapy and rarely are prolonged. The syndrome may represent a hypersensitivity reaction to the estolate ester.

Hepatotoxicity has also been observed with clarithromycin and azithromycin, although at a lower rate than with erythromycin. After its regulatory approval and widespread use, a number of post-marketing reports of severe telithromycin-induced hepatotoxicity emerged. These cases tended to have a short latency between drug initiation and manifestation of hepatotoxicity, with some leading to death or liver transplantation (Brinker et al., 2009). Because of this toxicity, telithromycin should only be used in circumstances where it represents a clear advantage over alternative agents.

GI Toxicity. Oral administration of erythromycin, especially of large doses, frequently is accompanied by epigastric distress, which may be quite severe. Intravenous administration of erythromycin may cause similar symptoms, with abdominal cramps, nausea, vomiting, and diarrhea. Erythromycin stimulates GI motility by acting on motilin receptors. Because of this property, erythromycin is used postoperatively to promote peristalsis; it has been exploited to speed gastric emptying in patients with gastroparesis (Chapter 46). The GI symptoms are dose related and occur more commonly in children and young adults; they may be reduced by prolonging the infusion time to 1 hour or by pretreatment with glycopyrrolate (Bowler et al., 1992). Intravenous infusion of 1-g doses, even when dissolved in a large volume, often is followed by thrombophlebitis. This can be minimized by slow rates of infusion. Clarithromycin, azithromycin, and telithromycin also may cause GI distress, but typically to a lesser degree than that seen with erythromycin.

Cardiac toxicity. Erythromycin, clarithromycin, and telithromycin have been reported to cause cardiac arrhythmias, including QT prolongation with ventricular tachycardia. Most patients have had underlying risk factors, such as prolonged QT syndrome, uncorrected hypokalemia or hypomagnesemia, profound bradycardia, or in patients receiving certain antiarrhythmics (e.g., quinidine, procainamide, amiodarone) or other agents that prolong QTc (e.g., cisapride, pimozide).

Other Toxic and Irritative Effects. Among the allergic reactions observed are fever, eosinophilia, and skin eruptions, which may occur alone or in combination; each disappears shortly after therapy is stopped. Transient auditory impairment is a potential complication of treatment with erythromycin; it has been observed to follow intravenous administration of large doses of the gluceptate or lactobionate (4 g per day) or oral ingestion of large doses of the estolate. Visual disturbances due to slowed accommodation have been reported to occur in ~1% of treatment courses with telithromycin, and they include blurred vision, difficulty focusing, and diplopia. Telithromycin is contraindicated in patients with myasthenia gravis due to reports of exacerbation of neurological symptoms by the antibiotic in these patients. Loss of consciousness and visual disturbances are associated with telithromycin.

Drug Interactions. Erythromycin, clarithromycin, and telithromycin inhibit CYP3A4 and are associated with clinically significant drug interactions (Periti et al., 1992). Erythromycin potentiates the effects of carbamazepine, corticosteroids, cyclosporine, digoxin, ergot alkaloids, theophylline, triazolam, valproate, and warfarin, probably by interfering with CYP-mediated metabolism of these drugs (Chapter 6). Clarithromycin, which is structurally related to erythromycin, has a similar drug interaction profile. Telithromycin is both a substrate and a strong inhibitor of CYP3A4. Co-administration of rifampin, a potent inducer of CYP, decreases the serum concentrations of telithromycin by 80%. CYP3A4 inhibitors (e.g., itraconazole) increase peak serum concentrations of telithromycin. Azithromycin, which differs from erythromycin and clarithromycin because of its 15-membered lactone ring structure, and dirithromycin, which is a longer-acting 14-membered lactone ring analog of erythromycin, appear to be free of these drug interactions. Caution is advised, nevertheless, when using azithromycin in conjunction with drugs known to interact with erythromycin.

LINCOSAMIDES (CLINDAMYCIN)

Clindamycin is a lincosamide, a derivative of the amino acid *trans*-L-4-*n*-propylhygrinic acid, attached to a sulfur-containing derivative of an octose. It is a congener of lincomycin:

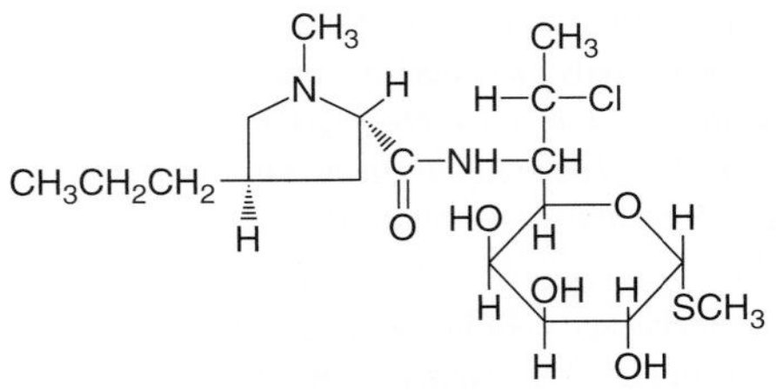

CLINDAMYCIN

Antimicrobial Activity. Bacterial strains are susceptible to clindamycin at MICs of ≤0.5 μg/mL. Clindamycin generally is similar to erythromycin in its *in vitro* activity against susceptible strains of pneumococci, *S. pyogenes*, and viridans streptococci (Table 55–2). Methicillin-susceptible strains of *S. aureus* usually are susceptible to clindamycin, but methicillin-resistant strains of *S. aureus* and coagulase-negative staphylococci frequently are resistant.

Clindamycin is more active than erythromycin or clarithromycin against anaerobic bacteria, especially *B. fragilis*; some strains are inhibited by <0.1 μg/mL, and most are inhibited by 2 μg/mL. The MICs for other anaerobes are as follows: *Bacteroides melaninogenicus*, 0.1 to 1 μg/mL; *Fusobacterium*, <0.5 μg/mL (although most strains of *Fusobacterium varium* are resistant); *Peptostreptococcus*, <0.1-0.5 μg/mL; *Peptococcus*, 1-100 μg/mL (with 10% of strains resistant); and *C. perfringens*, <0.1-8 μg/mL. From 10-20% of clostridial species other than *C. perfringens* are resistant. Resistance to clindamycin in *Bacteroides* spp. increasingly is encountered (Hedberg and Nord, 2003). Strains of *Actinomyces israelii* and *Nocardia asteroides* are sensitive. Essentially all aerobic gram-negative bacilli are resistant.

With regard to atypical organisms and parasites, *M. pneumoniae* is resistant. *Chlamydia* spp. are variably sensitive, although the clinical relevance is not established. Clindamycin plus primaquine and clindamycin plus pyrimethamine are second-line regimens for *Pneumocystis jiroveci* pneumonia and *T. gondii* encephalitis, respectively. Clindamycin has been used for treatment of babesiosis.

Mechanism of Action. Clindamycin binds exclusively to the 50S subunit of bacterial ribosomes and suppresses protein synthesis. Although clindamycin, erythromycin, and chloramphenicol are not structurally related, they act at sites in close proximity (Figures 55–2 and 55–3), and binding by one of these antibiotics to the ribosome may inhibit the interaction of the others. There are no clinical indications for the concurrent use of these antibiotics.

Resistance to Clindamycin. Macrolide resistance due to ribosomal methylation by *erm*-encoded enzymes also may produce resistance to clindamycin. Because clindamycin does not induce the methylase, there is cross-resistance only if the enzyme is produced constitutively. However, strains with inducible resistance may develop constitutive production of the methylase during therapy. Thus, many clinicians avoid use of clindamycin in the treatment of deep-seated infections due to organisms displaying an inducible resistance phenotype. Detection of this phenotype can be accomplished by approximating erythromycin and clindamycin on an agar plate with a lawn of the organism; a blunting of the zone of inhibition between clindamycin and erythromycin suggests inducible resistance (this is known as the "D-test") (Lewis & Jorgensen, 2005). Clindamycin is not a substrate for macrolide efflux pumps; thus strains that are resistant to macrolides by this mechanism are susceptible to clindamycin.

These strains would not display a blunting of inhibition on a D-test, and clindamycin use would be appropriate. Altered metabolism occasionally causes clindamycin resistance (Bozdogan et al., 1999).

Absorption, Distribution, and Excretion

Absorption. Clindamycin is nearly completely absorbed following oral administration. Peak plasma concentrations of 2-3 μg/mL are attained within 1 hour after the ingestion of 150 mg. The presence of food in the stomach does not reduce absorption significantly. The $t_{1/2}$ of the antibiotic is ~2.9 hours, and modest accumulation of drug is thus expected if it is given every 6 hours.

Clindamycin palmitate, an oral preparation for pediatric use, is an inactive prodrug that is hydrolyzed rapidly *in vivo*. Its rate and extent of absorption are similar to those of clindamycin. After several oral doses at 6-hour intervals, children attain plasma concentrations of 2-4 μg/mL with the administration of 8-16 μg/kg.

The phosphate ester of clindamycin, which is given parenterally, also is rapidly hydrolyzed *in vivo* to the active parent compound. After intramuscular injection, peak concentrations in plasma are not attained until 3 hours in adults and 1 hour in children; these values approximate 6 μg/mL after a 300-mg dose and 9 μg/mL after a 600-mg dose in adults.

Distribution. Clindamycin is widely distributed in many fluids and tissues, including bone. Significant concentrations are not attained in CSF, even when the meninges are inflamed. Concentrations sufficient to treat cerebral toxoplasmosis are achievable (Gatti et al., 1998). The drug readily crosses the placental barrier. Ninety percent or more of clindamycin is bound to plasma proteins. Clindamycin accumulates in polymorphonuclear leukocytes, alveolar macrophages, and in abscesses.

Excretion. Only ~10% of the clindamycin administered is excreted unaltered in the urine, and small quantities are found in the feces. However, antimicrobial activity persists in feces for ≥5 days after parenteral therapy with clindamycin is stopped; growth of clindamycin-sensitive microorganisms in colonic contents may be suppressed for up to 2 weeks.

Clindamycin is inactivated by metabolism to *N*-demethylclindamycin and clindamycin sulfoxide, which are excreted in the urine and bile. Accumulation of clindamycin can occur in patients with severe hepatic failure, and dosage adjustments thus may be required.

Therapeutic Uses and Dosage. The oral dose of clindamycin (clindamycin hydrochloride; CLEOCIN, others) for adults is 150-300 mg every 6 hours; for severe infections, it is 300-600 mg every 6 hours. Children should receive 8-12 mg/kg per day of clindamycin palmitate hydrochloride (CLEOCIN PEDIATRIC) in three or four divided doses (some physicians recommend 10-30 mg/kg per day in six divided doses) or for severe infections, 13-25 mg/kg per day. However, children weighing ≤10 kg should receive $^1/_2$ teaspoonful of clindamycin palmitate hydrochloride (37.5 mg) every 8 hours as a minimal dose. Clindamycin phosphate (CLEOCIN PHOSPHATE, others) is available for intramuscular or intravenous use. For serious infections, intravenous or intramuscular administration is recommended in dosages of 1200-2400 mg per day, divided into three or four equal doses for adults. Daily doses as high as 4.8 g have been given intravenously to adults. Children should receive 15-40 mg/kg per day in three or four divided doses; in severe infections, a minimal daily dose of 300 mg is recommended, regardless of body weight.

Skin and Soft-Tissue Infections. Because of clindamycin's good activity against aerobic and anaerobic gram-positive cocci and good oral bioavailability, it is an alternative agent for the treatment of skin and soft-tissue infections, especially in patients with β-lactam allergies. However, *the high incidence of diarrhea and the occurrence of pseudomembranous colitis should limit its use to infections where it represents a clear therapeutic advantage.* Clindamycin has been employed in the treatment of necrotizing skin and soft-tissue infections based on its potential to reduce toxin expression.

Respiratory Tract Infections. On the basis of one clinical trial which found that clindamycin (600 mg intravenously every 8 hours) was superior to penicillin (1 million units intravenously every 4 hours; Levison et al., 1983), clindamycin has replaced penicillin as the drug of choice for treatment of lung abscess and anaerobic lung and pleural space infections. Clindamycin (600 mg intravenously every 8 hours, or 300-450 mg orally every 6 hours for less severe disease) in combination with primaquine (15 mg of base once daily) is useful for the treatment of mild to moderate cases of *P. jiroveci* pneumonia in AIDS patients.

Other Infections. Clindamycin (600-1200 mg given intravenously every 6 hours) in combination with pyrimethamine (a 200-mg loading dose followed by 75 mg orally each day) and *leucovorin* (folinic acid, 10 mg/day) is effective for acute treatment of encephalitis caused by *T. gondii* in patients with AIDS. Clindamycin also is available as a topical solution, gel, or lotion (CLEOCIN T, others) and as a vaginal cream (CLEOCIN, others). It is effective topically (or orally) for acne vulgaris and bacterial vaginosis. Clindamycin is not predictably useful for the treatment of bacterial brain abscesses because penetration into the CSF is poor; metronidazole, in combination with penicillin or a third-generation cephalosporin, is preferred.

Untoward Effects.

Gastrointestinal Effects. The reported incidence of diarrhea associated with the administration of clindamycin ranges from 2% to 20%. A number of patients (variously reported as 0.01-10%) have developed pseudomembranous colitis caused by the toxin from the organism *C. difficile*. This colitis is characterized by watery diarrhea, fever, and elevated peripheral white blood cell counts. Proctoscopic examination reveals white to yellow plaques on the mucosa of the colon. *This syndrome may be lethal.* Discontinuation of the drug, combined with administration of metronidazole or oral vancomycin usually is curative, but relapses occur in up to 20% of cases. Agents that inhibit peristalsis, such as opioids, may prolong and worsen the condition.

Other Toxic and Irritative Effects. Skin rashes occur in ~10% of patients treated with clindamycin and may be more common in patients with HIV infection. Other reactions, which are uncommon, include exudative erythema multiforme (Stevens-Johnson syndrome), reversible elevation of aspartate aminotransferase and alanine aminotransferase, granulocytopenia, thrombocytopenia, and anaphylactic reactions. Local thrombophlebitis may follow intravenous administration of the drug. Clindamycin can inhibit neuromuscular transmission and may potentiate the effect of a neuromuscular blocking agent administered concurrently.

STREPTOGRAMINS (QUINUPRISTIN/ DALFOPRISTIN)

Quinupristin/dalfopristin (SYNERCID) is a combination of quinupristin, a streptogramin B, with dalfopristin, a streptogramin A, in a 30:70 ratio. These compounds are semisynthetic derivatives of naturally occurring pristinamycins, produced by *Streptomyces pristinaespiralis*. Pristinamycin has been available in France for >30 years for oral treatment of staphylococcal infections. Quinupristin and dalfopristin are more soluble derivatives of pristinamycin IA and pristinamycin IIA, respectively, and therefore are suitable for intravenous administration.

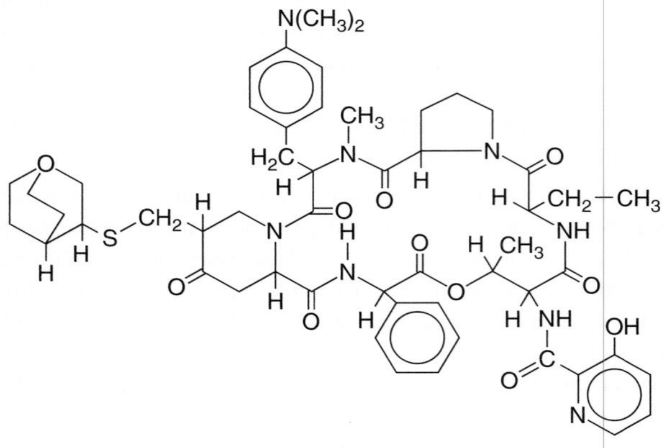

QUINUPRISTIN

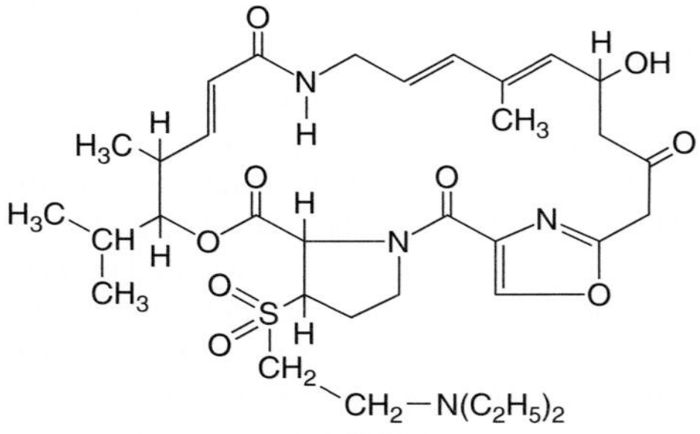

DALFOPRISTIN

Antimicrobial Activity. Quinupristin/dalfopristin is active against gram-positive cocci, including *S. pneumoniae*, beta- and alpha-hemolytic strains of streptococci, *E. faecium* (but not *E. faecalis*), and coagulase-positive and coagulase-negative strains of staphylococci (Table 55–2). Strains are considered sensitive if they are inhibited by concentrations of ≤1 μg/mL. The combination is largely inactive against gram-negative organisms, although *Moraxella catarrhalis* and *Neisseria* spp. are susceptible. It also is active against organisms responsible for atypical pneumonia, *M. pneumoniae, Legionella* spp., and *Chlamydia pneumoniae*. The combination is bactericidal against streptococci and many strains of staphylococci but bacteriostatic against *E. faecium.*

Mechanism of Action. Quinupristin and dalfopristin are protein synthesis inhibitors that bind the 50S ribosomal subunit. Quinupristin binds at the same site as macrolides and has a similar effect, with inhibition of polypeptide elongation and early termination of protein synthesis. Dalfopristin binds at a site nearby, resulting in a conformational change in the 50S ribosome, synergistically enhancing the binding of quinupristin at its target site. Dalfopristin directly interferes with polypeptide-chain formation. In many bacterial species, the net result of the cooperative and synergistic binding of these two molecules to the ribosome is bactericidal activity.

Resistance to Streptogramins. Resistance to quinupristin is mediated by MLS type B resistance determinants (e.g., *ermA* and *ermC* in staphylococci and *ermB* in enterococci), encoding a ribosomal methylase that prevents binding of drug to its target; or *vgb* or *vgbB*, which encode lactonases that inactivate type B streptogramins (Allignet et al., 1998; Bozdogan and Leclercq, 1999). Resistance to dalfopristin is mediated by *vat, vatB, vatC, vatD*, and *satA*, which encode acetyltransferases that inactivate type A streptogramins (Soltani et al., 2000); or staphylococcal genes *vga* and *vgaB*, which encode ATP-binding efflux proteins that pump type A streptogramins out of the cell (Bozdogan and Leclercq, 1999). These resistance determinants are located on plasmids that may be transferable by conjugative mobilization. Resistance to quinupristin/dalfopristin always is associated with a resistance gene for type A streptogramins. Genes encoding resistance to type B streptogramins also may be present but are not sufficient by themselves to produce resistance. Methylase-encoding *erm* genes, however, can render the combination bacteriostatic instead of bactericidal, making it ineffective in certain infections in which bactericidal activity is necessary for cure, such as endocarditis.

Absorption, Distribution, and Excretion. The combination of quinupristin/dalfopristin is administered only by intravenous infusion over at least 1 hour. It is incompatible with saline and heparin and should be dissolved in 5% dextrose in water. Steady-state peak serum concentrations in healthy male volunteers are ~3 μg/mL of quinupristin and 7 μg/mL of dalfopristin with a 7.5-mg/kg dose administered every 8 hours. The $t_{1/2}$ is 0.85 hour for quinupristin and 0.7 hour for dalfopristin. The volume of distribution is 0.87 L/kg for quinupristin and 0.71 L/kg for dalfopristin. Hepatic metabolism by conjugation is the principal means of clearance for both compounds, with 80% of an administered dose eliminated by biliary excretion. Renal elimination of active compound accounts for most of the remainder. No dosage adjustment is necessary for renal insufficiency. Pharmacokinetics are not significantly altered by peritoneal dialysis or hemodialysis. The area under the plasma concentration curve of active component and its metabolites is increased by 180% for quinupristin and 50% for dalfopristin by hepatic insufficiency. No adjustment is recommended unless the patient is unable to tolerate the drug, in which case the dosing frequency should be reduced from 8 to 12 hours.

Therapeutic Uses and Dosage. Quinupristin/dalfopristin is approved in the U.S. for treatment of infections caused by vancomycin-resistant strains of *E. faecium* and complicated skin and skin-structure infections caused by methicillin-susceptible strains of *S. aureus* or *S. pyogenes* (Nichols et al., 1999). In Europe it also is approved for treatment of nosocomial pneumonia and infections caused by methicillin-resistant strains of *S. aureus* (Fagon et al., 2000). In open-label, nonrandomized studies, clinical and microbiological cure rates for a variety of infections caused by vancomycin-resistant *E. faecium* were ~70% with quinupristin/dalfopristin at a dose of 7.5 mg/kg every 8-12 hours (Moellering et al., 1999). Quinupristin/dalfopristin should be reserved for treatment of serious infections caused by multiple-drug-resistant gram-positive organisms such as vancomycin-resistant *E. faecium.*

Untoward Effects. The most common side effects are infusion-related events, such as pain and phlebitis at the infusion site and arthralgias and myalgias. Phlebitis and pain can be minimized by infusion of drug through a central venous catheter. Arthralgias and myalgias, which are more likely to be a problem in patients with hepatic insufficiency and may be due to accumulation of metabolites, are managed by reducing the infusion frequency to every 12 hours.

Drug Interactions. Quinupristin/dalfopristin inhibits CYP3A4. The concomitant administration of other CYP3A4 substrates (Chapter 6) with quinupristin/dalfopristin may raise blood pressure and/or result in significant toxicity. Examples include antihistamines (e.g., azelastine and clemastine); some anticonvulsants (e.g., fosphenytoin and felbamate), macrolide antibiotics; some fluoroquinolones (e.g., moxifloxacin) and ketoconazole; some antimalarials (e.g., chloroquine, mefloquine, and quinine); some antidepressants (e.g., fluoxetine, imipramine, venlafaxine); some antipsychotics (e.g., haloperidol, risperidone, and quetiapine); tacrolimus; and doxepin. Appropriate caution and monitoring are recommended for drugs in which the toxic therapeutic window is narrow or for drugs that prolong the QTc interval.

OXAZOLIDINONES (LINEZOLID)

Linezolid (ZYVOX) is a synthetic antimicrobial agent of the oxazolidinone class (Clemett and Markham, 2000; Diekema and Jones, 2000; Hamel et al., 2000). Several other oxazolidinones are in clinical development.

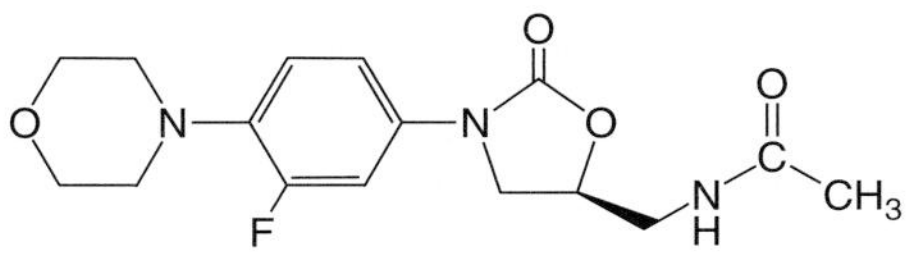

LINEZOLID

Antimicrobial Activity. Linezolid is active against gram-positive organisms including staphylococci, streptococci, enterococci, gram-positive anaerobic cocci, and gram-positive rods such as *Corynebacterium* spp. and *Listeria monocytogenes* (Table 55–2). It has poor activity against most gram-negative aerobic or anaerobic bacteria. It is bacteriostatic against enterococci and staphylococci and bactericidal against streptococci. Breakpoints for susceptibility are ≤4 μg/mL for staphylococci and ≤2 μg/mL for enterococci and streptococci. *Mycobacterium tuberculosis* is moderately susceptible, with MICs of 2 μg/mL.

Mechanism of Action and Resistance to Oxazolidinones. Linezolid inhibits protein synthesis by binding to the P site of the 50S ribosomal subunit and preventing formation of the larger ribosomal-fMet-tRNA complex that initiates protein synthesis. Because of its unique mechanism of action, linezolid is active against strains that are resistant to multiple other agents, including penicillin-resistant strains of *S. pneumoniae;* methicillin-resistant, vancomycin-intermediate, and vancomycin-resistant strains of staphylococci; and vancomycin-resistant strains of enterococci. Resistance in enterococci and staphylococci is due to point mutations of the 23S rRNA (Wilson et al., 2003). Because multiple copies of 23S rRNA genes are present in bacteria, resistance generally requires mutations in two or more copies.

Absorption, Distribution, and Excretion. Linezolid is well absorbed after oral administration and may be administered without regard to food. With oral bioavailability approaching 100%, dosing for oral and intravenous preparations is the same. Peak serum concentrations average 13 μg/mL 1-2 hours after a single 600-mg dose in adults and ~20 μg/mL at steady state with dosing every 12 hours. The $t_{1/2}$ is ~4-6 hours. Linezolid is 30% protein-bound and distributes widely to well-perfused tissues, with a 0.6-0.7 L/kg volume of distribution.

Linezolid is broken down by nonenzymatic oxidation to aminoethoxyacetic acid and hydroxyethyl glycine derivatives. Approximately 80% of the dose of linezolid appears in the urine, 30% as active compound and 50% as the two primary oxidation products. Ten percent of the administered dose appears as oxidation products in feces. Although serum concentrations and $t_{1/2}$ of the parent compound are not appreciably altered by renal insufficiency, oxidation products accumulate in renal insufficiency, with half-lives increasing by ~50-100%. The clinical significance of this is unknown, and no dose adjustment in renal insufficiency is currently recommended. Linezolid and its breakdown products are eliminated by dialysis; therefore the drug should be administered after hemodialysis. One case report noted sustained therapeutic concentrations of linezolid in peritoneal dialysis fluid with oral administration of 600 mg of linezolid twice daily (DePestel et al., 2003).

Therapeutic Uses and Dosage. Linezolid is FDA approved for treatment of infections caused by vancomycin-resistant *E. faecium;* nosocomial pneumonia caused by methicillin-susceptible and resistant strains of *S. aureus;* community-acquired pneumonia caused by penicillin-susceptible strains of *S. pneumoniae;* complicated skin and skin structure infections caused by streptococci and methicillin-susceptible and -resistant strains of *S. aureus;* and uncomplicated skin and skin-structure infections (Clemett and Markham, 2000). Linezolid is bacteriostatic for staphylococci and enterococci; it should not be first-line therapy for treatment of suspected endocarditis, although there are reports of cure of endocarditis with linezolid in salvage situations (Falagas et al., 2006).

Infections Due to Vancomycin-resistant E. faecium. In noncomparative studies, linezolid (600 mg twice daily) has had clinical and microbiological cure rates in the range of 85-90% in treatment of a variety of infections (soft tissue, urinary tract, and bacteremia) caused by vancomycin-resistant *E. faecium.*

Skin and Soft-Tissue Infections. Efficacy of linezolid was similar to that of either oxacillin or vancomycin for complicated and uncomplicated skin and skin-structure infections, most microbiologically documented cases are caused by *S. aureus.* Linezolid, 600 mg twice daily (with or without aztreonam), was as effective as ampicillin/sulbactam (with or without vancomycin or aztreonam) for the management of diabetic foot infections. A 400-mg twice-daily dosage regimen is recommended only for treatment of uncomplicated skin and skin-structure infections.

Respiratory Tract Infections. In randomized, comparative studies, cure rates with linezolid (~60%) were similar to those with vancomycin for nosocomial pneumonia caused by methicillin-resistant or methicillin-susceptible *S. aureus* (Rubinstein et al., 2001; Wunderink et al., 2003a). A post hoc analysis suggested that linezolid may be superior to vancomycin for nosocomial pneumonia caused by methicillin-resistant *S. aureus*, but this needs to be confirmed in a prospective randomized trial (Wunderink et al., 2003b). Linezolid also may be an effective alternative for patients with MRSA infections who are failing vancomycin therapy or whose isolates have reduced susceptibility to vancomycin (Howden et al., 2004).

Linezolid should be reserved as an alternative agent for treatment of infections caused by multiple-drug-resistant strains. It should not be used when other agents are likely to be effective (e.g., community-acquired pneumonia, even though it has the indication).

Indiscriminant use and overuse will hasten selection of resistant strains and the eventual loss of this valuable newer agent.

Untoward Effects

Hematological Toxicity. Myelosuppression, including anemia, leukopenia, pancytopenia, and thrombocytopenia, has been reported in patients receiving linezolid. Thrombocytopenia or a significant reduction in platelet count has been associated with linezolid in 2.4% of treated patients, and its occurrence is related to duration of therapy. Platelet counts should be monitored in patients with risk of bleeding, preexisting thrombocytopenia, or intrinsic or acquired disorders of platelet function (including those potentially caused by concomitant medication) and in patients receiving courses of therapy lasting beyond 2 weeks.

Other Toxic and Irritative Effects. The drug seems to be well tolerated, with generally minor side effects (e.g., GI complaints, headache, rash). Patients receiving long-term (e.g., >8 weeks) treatment with linezolid have developed peripheral neuropathy, optic neuritis, and lactic acidosis (Narita et al., 2007). It is believed that these toxicities may originate from effects of linezolid on the mitochondria. Because these effects have not always been reversible, linezolid should be generally not be used for long-term therapy if there are alternative agents.

Drug Interactions. Linezolid is a weak nonspecific inhibitor of monoamine oxidase. Patients receiving concomitant therapy with an adrenergic or serotonergic agent (including selective serotonin reuptake inhibitors [SSRIs]) or consuming >100 mg of tyramine a day may experience serotonin syndrome, characterized by palpitations, headache, or hypertensive crisis. Co-administration of these agents is best avoided if possible. However, in patients receiving SSRIs who acutely require linezolid therapy for short-term (10-14 days) treatment, co-administration with careful monitoring is reasonable because SSRIs generally require tapering to avoid discontinuation syndrome. Linezolid is neither a substrate nor an inhibitor of CYPs.

AMINOCYCLITOLS (SPECTINOMYCIN)

Spectinomycin is an antibiotic produced by *Streptomyces spectabilis.* The drug is an aminocyclitol:

SPECTINOMYCIN

Antimicrobial Activity, Mechanism of Action, and Resistance to Spectinomycin. Spectinomycin is active against a number of gram-negative bacterial species, but it is inferior to other drugs to which such microorganisms are susceptible. *Its only therapeutic use is in the treatment of gonorrhea caused by strains resistant to first-line drugs or if there are contraindications to the use of these drugs.* Spectinomycin selectively inhibits protein synthesis in gram-negative bacteria. The antibiotic binds to and acts on the 30S ribosomal subunit. Its action is similar to that of the aminoglycosides, but spectinomycin is not bactericidal and does not cause misreading of messenger RNA. Bacterial resistance may be mediated by mutations in the 16S ribosomal RNA or by modification of the drug by adenylyltransferase (Clark et al., 1999).

Absorption, Distribution, and Excretion. Spectinomycin is rapidly absorbed after intramuscular injection. A single dose of 2 g produces peak serum concentrations of 100 μg/mL at 1 hour. Eight hours after injection, the concentration is ~15 μg/mL. The drug is not significantly bound to plasma protein, and all of an administered dose is recovered in the urine within 48 hours.

Therapeutic Uses and Dosage. The Centers for Disease Control and Prevention recommends ceftriaxone or cefixime for the treatment of uncomplicated gonococcal infection (Workowski and Berman, 2006). Fluoroquinolones are no longer recommended because of increasing resistance. Spectinomycin is recommended as an alternative regimen in patients who are intolerant or allergic to β-lactam antibiotics; however, the drug is not currently available in the U.S. Spectinomycin also is useful in pregnancy when patients are intolerant to β-lactams. The recommended dose for men and women is a single deep intramuscular injection of 2 g. One of the disadvantages of this regimen is that spectinomycin has no effect on incubating or established syphilis, and it is not active against *Chlamydia* spp. It also is less effective for pharyngeal infections, and follow-up cultures to document cure should be obtained.

Untoward Effects. Spectinomycin, when given as a single intramuscular injection, produces few significant untoward effects. Urticaria, chills, and fever have been noted after single doses, as have dizziness, nausea, and insomnia. The injection may be painful.

POLYMYXINS

The polymyxins, discovered in 1947, are a group of closely related antibiotics elaborated by various strains of *Bacillus polymyxa.* Colistin (polymyxin E) is produced by *Bacillus (Aerobacillus) colistinus.* These drugs, which are cationic detergents, are relatively simple basic peptides with molecular masses of ~1000 Da. Polymyxin B is a mixture of polymyxins B_1 and B_2:

R—L-DAB—L-Thr—L-DAB—L-DAB (—L-DAB—D-Phe—L-Leu; —L-Thr—L-DAB—L-DAB)

Polymyxin B_1: R = (+)-methyloctanoyl
Polymyxin B_2: R = 6-methylheptanoyl
DAB = α,γ-diaminobutyric acid

Colistin has a similar structure.

Antimicrobial Activity, Mechanism of Action, and Resistance to Polymyxins. The antimicrobial activities of polymyxin B and colistin are similar and restricted to gram-negative bacteria, including *Enterobacter, E. coli, Klebsiella, Salmonella, Pasteurella, Bordetella,* and *Shigella,* which usually are sensitive to concentrations of 0.05-2 μg/mL. Most strains of *P. aeruginosa* and *Acinetobacter* are inhibited by <8 μg/mL *in vitro. Proteus* and *Serratia* spp. are intrinsically resistant.

Polymyxins are surface-active amphipathic agents. They interact strongly with phospholipids and disrupt the structure of cell membranes. The permeability of the bacterial membrane changes immediately on contact with the drug. Sensitivity to polymyxin B apparently is related to the phospholipid content of the cell wall–membrane complex. The cell walls of certain resistant bacteria may prevent access of the drug to the cell membrane. Polymyxin B binds to the lipid A portion of endotoxin (the lipopolysaccharide of the outer membrane of gram-negative bacteria) and inactivates this molecule. Polymyxin B attenuates pathophysiological consequences of the release of endotoxin in several experimental systems, but the clinical utility of polymyxin B for this indication has not yet been established.

Although resistance to polymyxins among normally susceptible species is rare (likely owing to the minimal systemic use of this agent for many years), emergence of resistance while on treatment has been documented. Dosing regimens, including combination therapies, able to suppress the emergence of resistance are currently being studied.

Absorption, Distribution, and Excretion. Polymyxin B and colistin are not absorbed when given orally and are poorly absorbed from mucous membranes and the surfaces of large burns. They are cleared renally, and modification of the dose is required in patients with impaired renal function.

Therapeutic Uses and Dosage

Topical Uses. Polymyxin B sulfate is available for ophthalmic, otic, and topical use in combination with a variety of other compounds. Colistin is available as otic drops. Infections of the skin, mucous membranes, eye, and ear due to polymyxin B–sensitive microorganisms respond to local application of the antibiotic in solution or ointment. External otitis, frequently due to *Pseudomonas*, may be cured by the topical use of the drug. *P. aeruginosa* is a common cause of infection of corneal ulcers; local application or subconjunctival injection of polymyxin B often is curative. Polymyxin B, in combination with neomycin (NEOSPORIN G.U. IRRIGANT), is administered as a urinary bladder irrigant in conjunction with the use of indwelling catheters.

Systemic Uses. Colistin is available as colistin sulfate for oral use and as colistimethate sodium for parenteral administration. Due to the emergence of multidrug-resistant gram-negative organisms (especially *Stenotrophomonas maltophilia*, *Acinetobacter* spp., *P. aeruginosa*, and *Klebsiella* spp), there has been a resurgence in the systemic use of polymyxins, despite their toxicity when administered via this route. There are no prospective clinical trials of polymyxin use for systemic infections; however, a number of studies have described their use as salvage therapy for treatment of infections caused by multidrug-resistant organisms (Linden et al., 2003; San Gabriel et al., 2004). Because dosing of these agents varies by drug (polymyxin B or colistin), by the particular commercial preparation, and by the patient's degree of renal dysfunction, expert consultation is recommended before using these agents.

Untoward Effects. Polymyxin B applied to intact or denuded skin or mucous membranes produces no systemic reactions because of its almost complete lack of absorption from these sites. Hypersensitization is uncommon with topical application. Polymyxins are nephrotoxic, and administration with aminoglycosides or other nephrotoxins should be avoided if possible. Polymyxins interfere with neurotransmission at the neuromuscular junction, resulting in muscle weakness and apnea. Other neurological reactions include paresthesias, vertigo, and slurred speech.

GLYCOPEPTIDES (VANCOMYCIN AND TEICOPLANIN)

Vancomycin. Vancomycin is a tricyclic glycopeptide antibiotic produced by *Streptococcus orientalis*. Teicoplanin, a glycopeptide antibiotic produced by *Actinoplanes teichomyetius*, is available in Europe (Biavasco et al., 1997). A number of derivatives, the lipoglycopeptides (including telavancin, oritavancin, and dalbavancin), are in late-stage development.

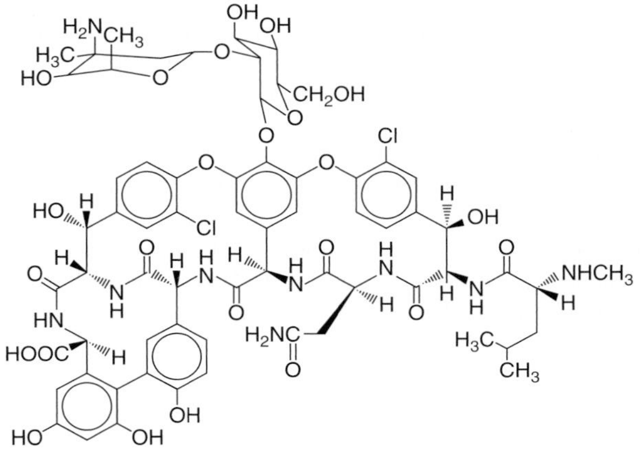

VANCOMYCIN

Teicoplanin. This agent is a mixture of six closely related compounds: One compound has a terminal hydrogen at the oxygen indicated by an asterisk; five compounds have an R substituent of either a decanoic acid [*n*-, 8-methyl-, 9-methyl, (Z)-4-] or of a nonanoic acid [8-methyl]. Although not FDA approved for use in the U.S., it is available in Europe. It is similar to vancomycin in chemical structure, mechanism of action, spectrum of activity, and route of elimination (i.e., primarily renal).

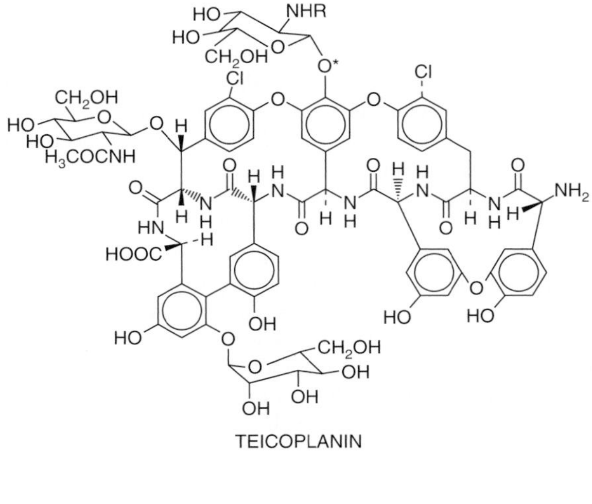

TEICOPLANIN

Antimicrobial Activity. Vancomycin possesses activity against a broad spectrum of gram-positive bacteria (Table 55–2). Strains are considered susceptible at MICs of ≤2 μg/mL for *S. aureus,* ≤4 μg/mL for *S. epidermidis,* and ≤1 μg/mL for streptococci. *Bacillus* spp., including *B. anthracis*, are inhibited by ≤2 μg/mL. *Corynebacterium* spp. (diphtheroids) are inhibited by <0.04-3.1 μg/mL of vancomycin; most species of *Actinomyces*, by 5-10 μg/mL; and *Clostridium* spp., by 0.39-6 μg/mL. Essentially all species of gram-negative bacilli and mycobacteria are resistant to vancomycin.

Teicoplanin is active against methicillin-susceptible and methicillin-resistant staphylococci, which typically have MICs of <4 μg/mL. The MICs for *Listeria monocytogenes, Corynebacterium* spp., *Clostridium* spp., and anaerobic gram-positive cocci range from 0.25-2 μg/mL. Nonviridans and viridans streptococci, *S. pneumoniae*, and enterococci are inhibited by concentrations ranging from 0.01-1 μg/mL. Some strains of staphylococci, coagulase positive and coagulase negative, as well as enterococci and other organisms that are intrinsically resistant to vancomycin (i.e., *Lactobacillus* spp. and *Leuconostoc* spp.), are resistant to teicoplanin.

Mechanism of Action. Vancomycin and teicoplanin inhibit the synthesis of the cell wall in sensitive bacteria by binding with high affinity to the D-alanyl-D-alanine terminus of cell wall precursor units (Figure 55–4). Because of their large molecular size, they are unable to penetrate the outer membrane of gram-negative bacteria.

Glycopeptides are generally bactericidal against susceptible strains, except for enterococci. The activity of glycopeptides is best predicted by the ratio of the total drug exposure (area under the curve [AUC]) of glycopeptide to minimum inhibitory concentration (MIC) of the infecting organism. This AUC-to-MIC ratio is established as being predictive of organism killing and cure in *in vitro* and animal models, and in some limited clinical data (Rybak, 2006). An AUC-to-MIC ratio of 400 was predictive of efficacy in patients with MRSA pneumonia (Moise-Broder et al., 2004). One implication of the potential importance of this parameter is that increases in organism MIC, even below the cutoff for susceptibility, can make achieving this target ratio difficult without substantial dosage increases. Thus, although an isolate of *S. aureus* with an MIC of 2 μg/mL would be considered susceptible, it would be difficult to achieve an AUC-to-MIC ratio of 400 at standard doses. The validity and target value of this parameter requires confirmation in further clinical studies with a variety of organisms and infections. The potential contribution to toxicity of using higher doses to achieve these target values also requires consideration (see later in the chapter).

Resistance to Glycopeptides. Strains of enterococci once were uniformly susceptible to glycopeptides. Glycopeptide-resistant strains

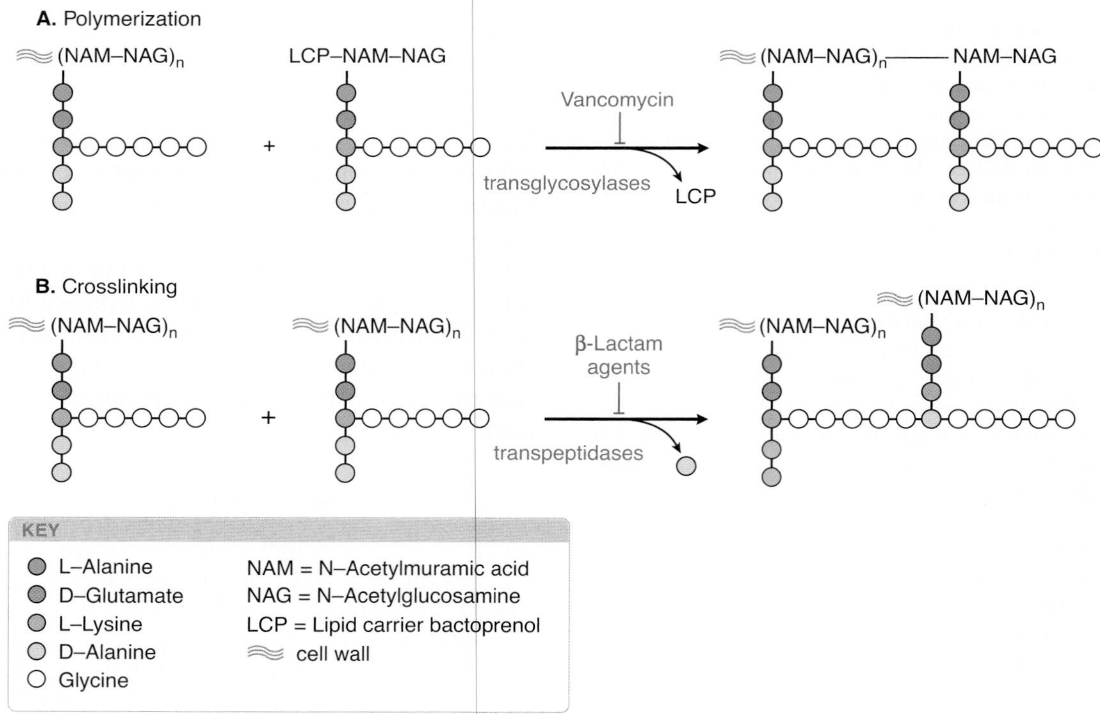

Figure 55–4. *Inhibition of bacterial cell wall synthesis: vancomycin and β-lactam agents.* Vancomycin inhibits the polymerization or transglycosylase reaction (A) by binding to the D-alanyl-D-alanine terminus of the cell wall precursor unit attached to its lipid carrier and blocks linkage to the glycopeptide polymer (indicated by the subscript n). These $(NAM–NAG)_n$ peptidoglycan polymers are located within the cell wall. Van A-type resistance is due to expression of enzymes that modify cell wall precursor by substituting a terminal D-lactate for D-alanine, reducing vancomycin binding affinity by 1000 times. β-Lactam antibiotics inhibit the cross-linking or transpeptidase reaction (B) that links glycopeptide polymer chains by formation of a cross-bridge with the stem peptide (the five glycines in this example) of one chain, displacing the terminal D-alanine of an adjacent chain. See also Figure 53–3.

of enterococci, primarily *Enterococcus faecium*, have emerged as major nosocomial pathogens in hospitals in the U.S. Vancomycin resistance determinants in *E. faecium* and *E. faecalis* are located on a transposon that is part of a conjugative plasmid, rendering it readily transferable among enterococci and, potentially, other gram-positive bacteria. These strains typically are resistant to multiple antibiotics, including streptomycin, gentamicin, and ampicillin, effectively eliminating these as alternative therapeutic agents. Resistance to streptomycin and gentamicin is of special concern because the combination of an aminoglycoside with a cell-wall-synthesis inhibitor is the only reliably bactericidal regimen for treatment of enterococcal endocarditis.

Enterococcal resistance to glycopeptides is the result of alteration of the D-alanyl-D-alanine target to D-alanyl-D-lactate or D-alanyl-D-serine (Arias et al., 2000), which bind glycopeptides poorly, due to the lack of a critical site for hydrogen bonding. Several enzymes within the *van* gene cluster are required for this target alteration to occur. Several phenotypes of resistance to glycopeptides have been described. The *Van A* phenotype confers inducible resistance to teicoplanin and vancomycin in *E. faecium* and *E. faecalis*. The *Van B* phenotype, which tends to be a lower level of resistance, also has been identified in *E. faecium* and *E. faecalis*. The trait is inducible by vancomycin but not teicoplanin, and consequently, many strains remain susceptible to teicoplanin. The *Van C* phenotype, the least important clinically and least well characterized, confers resistance only to vancomycin, is constitutive, and is present in no species of enterococci other than *E. faecalis* and *E. faecium*. *Van D* and *Van E* gene clusters also have been identified, and presumably others will follow.

S. aureus and coagulase-negative staphylococci may express reduced or "intermediate" susceptibility to vancomycin (MIC, 4-8 μg/mL) (Garrett et al., 1999; Hiramatsu et al., 1997; Smith et al., 1999) or high-level resistance (MIC ≥16 μg/mL). Intermediate resistance is associated with (and may be preceded by) a heterogeneous phenotype in which a small proportion of cells within the population (1 in 10^5 to 1 in 10^6) will grow in the presence of vancomycin concentrations >4 μg/mL. The genetic and biochemical basis of the intermediate phenotype is unknown. Intermediate strains produce an abnormally thick cell wall, and resistance may be due to false targets for vancomycin. Several genetic elements and multiple mutations are involved, and many of the genes that have been implicated encode enzymes of the cell-wall biosynthetic pathway (Sieradzki and Tomasz, 1999; Sieradzki et al., 1999). Infections caused by vancomycin-intermediate strains have failed to respond to vancomycin clinically and in animal models (Climo et al., 1999; Moore et al., 2003). Prior treatment courses and low vancomycin levels may predispose patients to infection and treatment failure with vancomycin-intermediate strains. These strains typically are resistant to methicillin and multiple other antibiotics; their emergence is a major concern because until recently vancomycin has been the only antibiotic to which staphylococci were reliably susceptible.

The first high-level vancomycin-resistant *S. aureus* strain (MIC ≥32 μg/mL) was isolated in June 2002 (Weigel et al., 2003). This strain, like others that have subsequently been isolated, harbored a conjugative plasmid into which the *Van A* transposon, Tn1546, was integrated as a consequence of an interspecies horizontal gene transfer from *E. faecalis* to a methicillin-resistant strain of *S. aureus*. These isolates have been variably susceptible to teicoplanin and the investigational lipoglycopeptides.

Absorption, Distribution, and Excretion

Absorption. Vancomycin is poorly absorbed after oral administration. For parenteral therapy, the drug should be administered intravenously, never intramuscularly. Teicoplanin can be administered safely by intramuscular injection as well as intravenous administration.

Distribution. A single intravenous dose of 1 g in adults produces plasma concentrations of 15-30 μg/mL 1 hour after a 1- to 2-hour infusion. Approximately 30% of vancomycin is bound to plasma protein. Vancomycin appears in various body fluids, including the CSF when the meninges are inflamed (7-30%); bile; and pleural, pericardial, synovial, and ascitic fluids. Teicoplanin is highly bound by plasma proteins (90-95%).

Elimination. About 90% of an injected dose of vancomycin is excreted by glomerular filtration. The drug has a serum elimination $t_{1/2}$ of ~6 hours. The drug accumulates if renal function is impaired, and dosage adjustments must be made under these circumstances. The drug can be cleared rapidly from plasma with high-flux methods of hemodialysis. In contrast to vancomycin, teicoplanin has an extremely long serum elimination $t_{1/2}$ (up to 100 hours in patients with normal renal function).

Therapeutic Uses and Dosage. Vancomycin and teicoplanin have been used to treat a wide variety of infections, including osteomyelitis and endocarditis, caused by methicillin-resistant and methicillin-susceptible staphylococci, streptococci, and enterococci. Teicoplanin has been found to be comparable to vancomycin in efficacy, except for treatment failures from low doses used for such serious infections as endocarditis. In general, recommendations for teicoplanin follow those of vancomycin, except where noted later. Although extensively studied for >10 years, teicoplanin has not yet been licensed for use in the U.S.

Vancomycin hydrochloride (VANCOCIN, others) is marketed for *intravenous* use as a sterile powder for solution. It should be diluted and infused over at least a 60-minute period to avoid infusion-related adverse reactions. The recommended dose of vancomycin for adults is 30-45 mg/kg per day in 2-3 divided doses. The "therapeutic range" for this agent is somewhat controversial. Current recommendations call for monitoring serum trough concentrations (within 30 minutes prior to a dose) at steady state, typically before the fourth dose of a given dosage regimen. A minimum target trough serum concentration of 10 μg/mL is recommended in the most recent consensus guidelines (Rybak et al., 2009). For patients with more serious infections (including endocarditis, osteomyelitis, meningitis, and MRSA pneumonia), trough levels of 15-20 μg/mL are recommended. General pediatric dosage ranges for vancomycin are as follows: for newborns during the first week of life, 15 mg/kg initially, followed by 10 mg/kg every 12 hours; for infants 8-30 days old, 15 mg/kg followed by 10 mg/kg every 8 hours; for older infants (>30 days) and children, 10-15 mg/kg every 6 hours (Frymoyer et al, 2009).

Alteration of dosage is required for patients with impaired renal function. Serum drug concentrations may help guide dose adjustment, but caution should be used in interpreting concentrations in patients with rapidly changing renal function. In functionally anephric patients and patients receiving dialysis with non-high-flux membranes, administration of 1 g (~15 mg/kg) every 5-7 days typically achieves adequate serum levels. In patients receiving intermittent high-efficiency or high-flux dialysis, maintenance doses administered after each dialysis session are typically required because these modalities clear vancomycin efficiently. Because there is so much variation in how well vancomycin is dialyzed with different membranes, it is recommended that blood levels be monitored to decide how frequently the drug needs to be administered to maintain therapeutic concentrations.

Skin/Soft-Tissue and Bone/Joint Infections. Vancomycin is frequently used in the empirical and definitive treatment of skin/soft-tissue and bone/joint infections, where gram-positive organisms including MRSA are the leading pathogens.

Respiratory Tract Infections. Vancomycin is employed for the treatment of pneumonia when MRSA is suspected, either because of healthcare-associated acquisition or in patients with community-acquired pneumonia with risk factors for staphylococcal infection (e.g., influenza). Because vancomycin penetration into lung tissue is relatively low, aggressive dosing (targeting trough levels of 15-20 μg/mL) is generally recommended.

CNS Infections. Because of vancomycin's excellent activity against *Streptococcus pneumoniae*, it is a key component in the initial empirical treatment of community-acquired bacterial meningitis in locations where penicillin-resistant *Streptococcus pneumoniae* is common (Tunkel et al., 2004). Penetration of vancomycin across inflamed meningitis is modest to poor; thus aggressive dosing is typically warranted. Vancomycin is also used to treat nosocomial meningitis, usually associated with neurosurgical procedures and often caused by staphylococci. Intraventricular administration of vancomycin (via a shunt or reservoir) has been necessary in a few cases of CNS infections due to susceptible microorganisms that did not respond to intravenous therapy alone.

Endocarditis and Vascular Catheter Infections. Vancomycin is standard therapy for staphylococcal endocarditis when the isolate is methicillin resistant or patients have a severe penicillin allergy (Baddour et al., 2005). Administration of an adjunctive aminoglycoside is no longer recommended unless there is a prosthetic valve. Vancomycin is an effective alternative for the treatment of endocarditis caused by viridans streptococci in patients who are allergic to penicillin. In combination with an aminoglycoside, it may be used for enterococcal endocarditis in patients with serious penicillin allergy or for isolates that are not susceptible to penicillins.

Vancomycin is commonly used for the treatment of vascular catheter infections due to gram-positive organisms, such as staphylococci, viridans streptococci, *Corynebacterium* spp, and *Bacillus* spp. In situations when removal of the catheter is not desired, adjunctive treatment with vancomycin as an "antibiotic lock" may aid in salvaging the catheter. In this procedure, a concentrated solution of vancomycin is instilled into the catheter hub and allowed to dwell for variable amounts of time when the catheter is not in use (Carratala, 2002).

Other Infections. Vancomycin can be administered orally to patients with pseudomembranous colitis due to *C. difficile*, and it may be more efficacious than metronidazole in patients with severe disease. The dose for adults is 125-250 mg every 6 hours; the total daily dose for children is 40 mg/kg, given in three to four divided doses. Commercially available capsules can be used for this purpose, or the intravenous formulation can be administered orally with or without compounding into a more palatable oral solution.

The standard dose of teicoplanin in adults is 3-6 mg/kg per day, with higher dosages possible for treatment of serious staphylococcal infections. Once-daily dosing is possible for the treatment of most infections because of the prolonged serum elimination half-life. As with vancomycin, teicoplanin doses must be adjusted in patients with renal insufficiency. For functionally anephric patients, administration once weekly has been appropriate, but serum drug concentrations should be monitored to determine that the therapeutic range has been maintained (e.g., trough concentration of 15-20 μg/mL). Oral teicoplanin has also been studied for the treatment of *C. difficile* disease, at a dose of 100 mg twice daily.

Untoward Effects. Among the hypersensitivity reactions produced by vancomycin and teicoplanin are macular skin rashes and anaphylaxis. Phlebitis and pain at the site of intravenous injection are relatively uncommon. Chills, rash, and fever may occur. Rapid intravenous infusion of vancomycin may cause erythematous or urticarial reactions, flushing, tachycardia, and hypotension. The extreme flushing that can occur is sometimes called "red-neck" or "red-man" syndrome. This is not an allergic reaction but a direct toxic effect of vancomycin on mast cells, causing them to release histamine. This reaction is generally not observed with teicoplanin.

Auditory impairment, sometimes permanent, may follow the use of vancomycin or teicoplanin. Ototoxicity is associated with excessively high concentrations of these drugs in plasma (60-100 μg/mL of vancomycin). Nephrotoxicity, formerly very problematic due to the impurities in earlier formulations of vancomycin, has become less common with modern formulations at standard dosages. However, the more aggressive dosing regimens recently advocated have been demonstrated to increase nephrotoxicity risk. In a recent observational study, nephrotoxicity occurred in 33% of patients with initial vancomycin trough concentrations of >20 μg/mL, compared to 5% among patients with trough concentrations of <10 μg/mL (Lodise et al., 2009). Thus, careful dosing and monitoring of vancomycin is necessary to balance the risks and benefits. Additionally, caution should be exercised when ototoxic or nephrotoxic drugs, such as aminoglycosides, are administered concurrently with vancomycin.

LIPOPEPTIDES (DAPTOMYCIN)

Daptomycin (CUBICIN) is a cyclic lipopeptide antibiotic derived from *Streptomyces roseosporus*. Discovered >25 years ago, its clinical development has been resumed in response to increasing need for bactericidal antibiotics effective against vancomycin-resistant gram-positive bacteria (Carpenter and Chambers, 2004; Eisenstein and Tally, 2006).

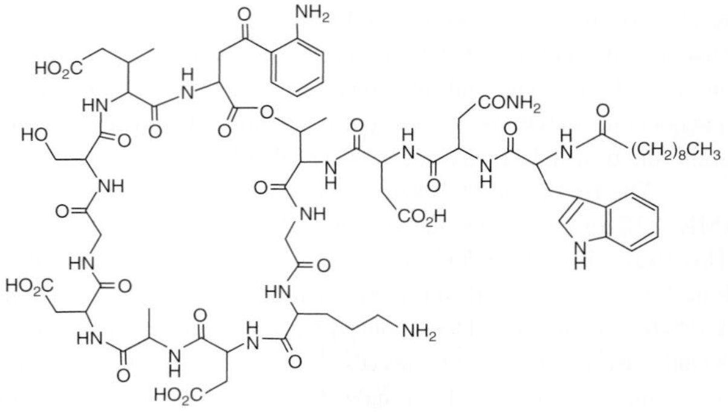

DAPTOMYCIN

Antimicrobial Activity. Daptomycin is a bactericidal antibiotic selectively active against aerobic, facultative, and anaerobic gram-positive bacteria (Table 55–2) (Jevitt et al., 2003; Streit et al., 2004). The MIC susceptibility breakpoint for staphylococci and streptococci is ≤1 μg/mL; for enterococci it is ≤4 μg/mL. Daptomycin may be active against vancomycin-resistant strains, although MICs tend to be higher for these organisms than for their vancomycin-susceptible counterparts. MICs of *Corynebacterium* spp., *Peptostreptococcus*, propionibacteria, and *Clostridium perfringens* are generally inhibited by ≤0.5-1 μg/mL (Goldstein et al., 2004). *Actinomyces* spp. are inhibited over the concentration range of 4-32 μg/mL. *In vitro* activity of daptomycin is Ca^{2+} dependent, and MIC tests should be performed in medium containing 50 mg/L calcium.

Mechanisms of Action and Resistance to Daptomycin. Daptomycin binds to bacterial membranes resulting in depolarization, loss of membrane potential, and cell death. It has concentration-dependent bactericidal activity. During initial clinical trials for treatment of skin and soft-tissue infections, resistance was rarely observed. Subsequently, during clinical use, daptomycin resistance has been reported to emerge while on therapy, typically during treatment of deep-seated infections (e.g., osteomyelitis, endocarditis, infections of prosthetic material). In a trial of vancomycin for staphylococcal bacteremia and right-sided endocarditis, increases in daptomycin MIC associated with microbiological treatment failure were seen in 6 of 120 patients (5%) (Fowler et al., 2006). The mechanisms of resistance to daptomycin have not been fully characterized, although genetic changes in the *mprF* gene (regulating cell membrane charge) correlating to daptomycin resistance have been described (Yang et al., 2009). Staphylococci with decreased susceptibility to vancomycin have higher daptomycin MICs than fully susceptible strains (Jevitt et al., 2003).

Absorption, Fate, and Excretion. Daptomycin is poorly absorbed orally and should only be administered intravenously. Direct toxicity to muscle precludes intramuscular injection. The steady-state peak serum concentration following intravenous administration of 4 mg/kg in healthy volunteers is ~58 μg/mL. Daptomycin displays linear pharmacokinetics at doses up to 8 mg/kg. It is reversibly bound to albumin; protein binding is 92%. The serum $t_{1/2}$ is 8-9 hours in normal subjects, permitting once-daily dosing. Although the drug penetrates adequately into the lung, the drug is inactivated by pulmonary surfactant (Silverman et al., 2005). Approximately 80% of the administered dose is recovered in urine; a small amount is excreted in feces. Dosage adjustment is required for creatinine clearance <30 mL/minute; this is accomplished by administering the recommended dose every 48 hours. For hemodialysis patients the dose should be administered immediately after dialysis.

Therapeutic Uses and Dosage. Daptomycin is indicated for treatment of complicated skin and soft tissue infections (at 4 mg/kg per day) and complicated bacteremia and right-sided endocarditis (at 6 mg/kg per day) (Carpenter and Chambers, 2004). Its efficacy was comparable to that of vancomycin or semisynthetic penicillins. Higher doses (up to 10-12 mg/kg per day) appear to be well tolerated and may be incorporated into future recommendations (Figueroa et al., 2009). Daptomycin was inferior to comparators for treatment of community-acquired pneumonia, likely due to its inactivation in pulmonary surfactant, and it should not be used for this indication (Pertel et al., 2008).

Untoward Effects. The primary toxicity of daptomycin is damage to the musculoskeletal system. In humans, elevations of creatine kinase may occur; this does not require discontinuation of the drug unless there are findings of an otherwise unexplained myopathy. Rhabdomyolysis has been reported to occur rarely. In phase 1 and 2 clinical trials, a few patients had evidence of possible neuropathy, although this was not observed in phase 3 studies.

Drug Interactions. Daptomycin neither inhibits nor induces CYPs, and there are no important drug–drug interactions. However, caution is recommended when administering daptomycin in conjunction with aminoglycosides or statins because of potential risks of nephrotoxicity and myopathy, respectively.

BACITRACIN

Bacitracin is an antibiotic produced by the Tracy-I strain of *Bacillus subtilis*. The bacitracins are a group of polypeptide antibiotics; multiple components have been demonstrated in the commercial products. The major constituent is bacitracin A; its probable structural formula is:

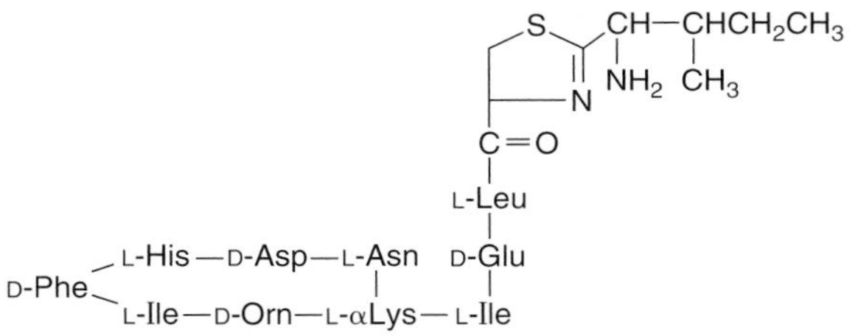

S
CH—CHCH₂CH₃
NH₂ CH₃
N
C=O
L-Leu
L-His—D-Asp—L-Asn D-Glu
D-Phe
L-Ile—D-Orn—L-αLys—L-Ile

BACITRACIN

A unit of the antibiotic is equivalent to 26 μg of the USP standard.

Antimicrobial Activity, Mechanism of Action, and Resistance to Bacitracin. Bacitracin inhibits the synthesis of the bacterial cell wall. A variety of gram-positive cocci and bacilli, *Neisseria, H. influenzae,* and *Treponema pallidum,* are sensitive to ≤0.1 unit of bacitracin per milliliter. *Actinomyces* and *Fusobacterium* are inhibited by concentrations of 0.5-5 units/mL. Enterobacteriaceae, *Pseudomonas, Candida* spp., and *Nocardia* are resistant to the drug.

Therapeutic Uses and Dosage. Although bacitracin previously has been employed parenterally, current use is restricted to topical application because of the toxicity of intravenous administration. Bacitracin is available in ophthalmic and dermatologic ointments; the antibiotic also is available as a powder (BACI-RX) for the extemporaneous compounding of topical solutions. The ointments are applied directly to the involved surface one or more times daily. A number of topical preparations of bacitracin, to which neomycin or polymyxin or both have been added, are available, and some contain the three antibiotics plus hydrocortisone.

Topical bacitracin alone or in combination with other antimicrobial agents has no established value in the treatment of furunculosis, pyoderma, carbuncle, impetigo, and superficial and deep abscesses. For open infections such as infected eczema and infected dermal ulcers, the local application of the antibiotic may be of some help in eradicating sensitive bacteria. Unlike several other antibiotics used topically, bacitracin rarely produces hypersensitivity. Suppurative conjunctivitis and infected corneal ulcer respond well to the topical use of bacitracin when caused by susceptible bacteria. Bacitracin has been used with limited success for eradication of nasal carriage of staphylococci. Oral bacitracin has been used with some success for the treatment of antibiotic-associated diarrhea caused by *C. difficile*. Bacitracin is used by neurosurgeons to irrigate the meninges intraoperatively as an alternative to vancomycin. It has no direct toxicity on neurons.

Untoward Effects. Serious nephrotoxicity results from the parenteral use of this antibiotic. Hypersensitivity reactions rarely result from topical application.

MUPIROCIN

Mupirocin (BACTROBAN) is derived from a fermentation product of *Pseudomonas fluorescens*. It is for topical use only.

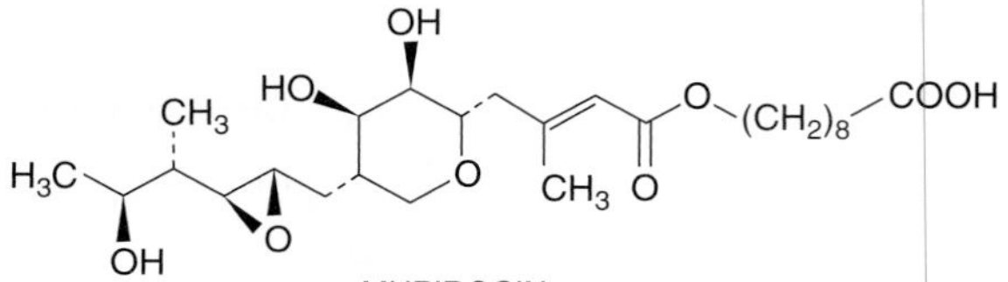

MUPIROCIN

Antimicrobial Activity. Mupirocin is active against many gram-positive and selected gram-negative bacteria. It has good activity with MICs ≤1 μg/mL against *Streptococcus pyogenes* and methicillin-susceptible and methicillin-resistant strains of *S. aureus*. It is bactericidal at concentrations achieved with topical application.

Mechanism of Action and Mupirocin Resistance. Mupirocin inhibits bacterial protein synthesis by reversible binding and inhibition of isoleucyl transfer-RNA synthetase. There is no cross-resistance with other classes of antibiotics. Low-level resistance, which is not clinically significant, is due to mutations of the host gene encoding isoleucyl transfer-RNA synthetase or an extra chromosomal copy of a gene encoding a modified isoleucyl transfer-RNA synthetase (Ramsey et al., 1996; Udo et al., 2001). High-level resistance (MIC >1 mg/mL) is mediated by a plasmid or chromosomal copy of *mupA*, which encodes a "bypass" synthetase that binds mupirocin poorly (Udo et al., 2001).

Absorption, Fate, and Excretion. Systemic absorption through intact skin or skin lesions is minimal. Any mupirocin that is absorbed is rapidly metabolized to inactive monic acid.

Therapeutic Uses and Dosage. Mupirocin is available as a 2% cream and a 2% ointment for dermatologic use and as a 2% ointment for intranasal use. The dermatologic preparations are indicated for treatment of traumatic skin lesions and impetigo secondarily infected with *S. aureus* or *S. pyogenes*.

The nasal ointment is approved for eradication of *S. aureus* nasal carriage. Mupirocin is highly effective in eradicating *S. aureus* carriage (Laupland and Conly, 2003). Because *S. aureus* colonization often precedes infection, eradication of carriage by intranasal application of mupirocin might reduce the risk of later infection. However, two clinical trials failed to demonstrate that mupirocin prophylaxis reduces nosocomial *S. aureus* infections (Kalmeijer et al., 2002; Wertheim et al., 2004). A third large study found that *S. aureus* nasal carriers had fewer *S. aureus* nosocomial infections of any site, but it failed to show a reduction in *S. aureus* surgical site infections, the primary end point of the study (Perl et al., 2002). The accumulated evidence indicates that patients who stand to benefit from mupirocin prophylaxis are those with proven *S. aureus* nasal colonization plus risk factors for distant infection or a history of skin or soft-tissue infections. General inpatient populations and individuals lacking specific risk factors for *S. aureus* infection are not likely to benefit from mupirocin prophylaxis.

Untoward Effects. Mupirocin may cause irritation and sensitization at the site of application. Contact with the eyes should be avoided because mupirocin causes tearing, burning, and irritation that may take several days to resolve. Systemic reactions to mupirocin occur rarely, if at all. Polyethylene glycol present in the ointment can be absorbed from damaged skin. Application of the ointment to large surface areas should be avoided in patients with moderate to severe renal failure to avoid accumulation of polyethylene glycol.

CLINICAL SUMMARY

Doxycycline, the most important member of the tetracyclines, is a drug of choice for sexually transmitted diseases, rickettsial infections, plague, brucellosis, tularemia, and spirochetal infections. It is also an important agent for treatment of respiratory tract infections, given its activity against *S. pneumoniae*, *Haemophilus* spp., and atypical pneumonia pathogens; and for skin and soft-tissue infections caused by community strains of methicillin-resistant *S. aureus*, for which minocycline also is particularly active. Glycylcyclines, beginning with tigecycline, have restored much of the activity of the tetracyclines against bacteria that have become refractory to first- and second-generation tetracyclines, including aerobic and anaerobic gram-negative organisms as well as refractory gram-positive organisms.

Macrolides and ketolides are effective for treatment of respiratory tract infections caused by the common pathogens of community-acquired pneumonia, including *S. pneumoniae*, *Haemophilus* spp., *Chlamydia*, mycoplasma, and *Legionella*. They generally are well-tolerated, orally bioavailable, and except for erythromycin, effective in once or twice-daily dosing. All except azithromycin have important drug interactions because they inhibit hepatic CYPs.

Chloramphenicol is rarely indicated in the U.S. and Europe because it can cause irreversible bone marrow toxicity and because less toxic drugs are readily available. However, it continues to be an important antibiotic in developing nations because it is inexpensive and highly effective for a broad range of infections.

Spectinomycin is indicated only for the treatment of gonococcal infection when a β-lactam or fluoroquinolone cannot be given. Clindamycin has excellent activity against gram-positive cocci but principally is used to treat anaerobic infections. Vancomycin, daptomycin, quinupristin/dalfopristin, and linezolid are indicated for the treatment of gram-positive infections caused by drug-resistant organisms such as penicillin-resistant pneumococci and methicillin-resistant staphylococci. Quinupristin/dalfopristin and linezolid are indicated for the treatment of vancomycin-resistant *E. faecium* infections. These drugs, along with daptomycin, also are active against vancomycin-insensitive strains of *S. aureus*, although clinical trials have not established their clear clinical efficacy to date.

Polymyxins, bacitracin, and mupirocin are effective for the topical treatment of minor skin infections. Colistin (polymyxin E) can be administered systemically and is active against drug-resistant gram-negative bacteria, including *Pseudomonas*, *Stenotrophomonas*, and *Acinetobacter*; its significant toxicity makes it an agent of last resort. Mupirocin is effective for eradication of *S. aureus* nasal colonization.

BIBLIOGRAPHY

Arias CA, Courvalin P, Reynolds PE. vanC cluster of vancomycin-resistant *Enterococcus gallinarum* BM4174. *Antimicrob Agents Chemother*, **2000,** *44:*1660–1666.

Bace A, Zrnic T, Begovac J, et al. Short-term treatment of pertussis with azithromycin in infants and young children. *Eur J Clin Microbiol Infect Dis*, **1999,** *18:*296–298.

Baddour LM, Wilson WR, Bayer AS, et al. Infective endocarditis: Diagnosis, antimicrobial therapy, and management of complications: a statement for healthcare professionals from the Committee on Rheumatic Fever, Endocarditis, and Kawasaki Disease, Council on Cardiovascular Disease in the Young, and the Councils on Clinical Cardiology, Stroke, and Cardiovascular Surgery and Anesthesia, American Heart Association: endorsed by the Infectious Diseases Society of America. *Circulation*, **2005,** *111:* e394–434.

Bergallo C, Jasovich A, Teglia O, et al. Safety and efficacy of intravenous tigecycline in treatment of community-acquired pneumonia: Results from a double-blind randomized phase 3 comparison study with levofloxacin. *Diagn Microbiol Infect Disease*, **2009,** *63:*52–61.

Biavasco F, Vignaroli C, Lupidi R, *et al*. In vitro antibacterial activity of LY333328, a new semisynthetic glycopeptide. *Antimicrob Agents Chemother*, **1997,** *41:*2165–2172.

Bowler WA, Hostettler C, Samuelson D, et al. Gastrointestinal side effects of intravenous erythromycin: Incidence and reduction with prolonged infusion time and glycopyrrolate pretreatment. *Am J Med*, **1992,** *92:*249–253.

Bozdogan B, Berrezouga L, Kuo MS, et al. A new resistance gene, linB, conferring resistance to lincosamides by nucleotidylation in *Enterococcus faecium* HM1025. *Antimicrob Agents Chemother*, **1999,** *43:*925–929.

Bozdogan B, Leclercq R. Effects of genes encoding resistance to streptogramins A and B on the activity of quinupristin-dalfopristin against *Enterococcus faecium*. *Antimicrob Agents Chemother*, **1999,** *43:*2720–2725.

Brinker AD, Wassel RT, Lyndly J, et al. Telithromycin-associated hepatotoxicity: Clinical spectrum and causality assessment of 42 cases. *Hepatology*, **2009,** *49:* 250–257.

Carpenter CF, Chambers HF. Daptomycin: Another novel agent for treating infections due to drug-resistant gram-positive pathogens. *Clin Infect Dis*, **2004,** *38:*994–1000.

Carratala J. The antibiotic-lock technique for therapy of 'highly needed' infected catheters. *Clin Microbiol Infect*, **2002,** *8:*282–289.

Cenizal MJ, Skiest D, Luber S, et al. Prospective randomized trial of empiric therapy with trimethoprim-sulfamethoxazole or doxycycline for outpatient skin and soft tissue infections in an area of high prevalence of methicillin-resistant *Staphylococcus aureus*. *Antimicrob Agents Chemother*, **2007,** *51:*2628–2630.

Centers for Disease Control and Prevention. Vancomycin-resistant *Staphylococcus aureus*—New York. *MMWR Morb Mortal Wkly Rep*, **2004,** *53:*322–323.

Clark NC, Olsvik O, Swenson JM, et al. Detection of a streptomycin/spectinomycin adenylyltransferase gene (aadA) in *Enterococcus faecalis*. *Antimicrob Agents Chemother*, **1999,** *43:*157–160.

Clemett D, Markham A. Linezolid. *Drugs*, **2000,** *59:*815–827; discussion 828.

Climo MW, Patron RL, Archer GL. Combinations of vancomycin and β-lactams are synergistic against staphylococci with reduced susceptibilities to vancomycin. *Antimicrob Agents Chemother*, **1999,** *43:*1747–1753.

Critchley IA, Blosser-Middleton RS, Jones ME, et al. Baseline study to determine in vitro activities of daptomycin against gram-positive pathogens isolated in the United States in 2000–2001. *Antimicrob Agents Chemother*, **2003,** *47:*1689–1693.

DePestel DD, Peloquin CA, Carver PL. Peritoneal dialysis fluid concentrations of linezolid in the treatment of vancomycin-resistant *Enterococcus faecium* peritonitis. *Pharmacotherapy*, **2003,** *23:*1322–1326.

Diekema DI, Jones RN. Oxazolidinones: A review. *Drugs*, **2000,** *59:*7–16.

Eisenstein BI, Tally FP. The new and continuing epidemics of drug-resistant *Staphylococcus aureus*: Daptomycin as a case study in antibiotic development. Goodman & Gilman Online. December 2006. http://www.accessmedicine.com/updates.aspx?resourceID=58. Accessed December 19, 2009.

Ellis J, Oyston PC, Green M, Titball RW. Tularemia. *Clin Microbiol Rev*, **2002,** *15:*631–646.

Fagon J, Patrick H, Haas DW, et al. Treatment of gram-positive nosocomial pneumonia. Prospective randomized comparison of quinupristin/dalfopristin versus vancomycin. Nosocomial Pneumonia Group. *Am J Respir Crit Care Med*, **2000,** *161:* 753–762.

Falagas ME, Manta KG, Ntziora F, Vardakas KZ. Linezolid for the treatment of patients with endocarditis: A systematic review of the published evidence. *J Antimicrob Chemother*, **2006,** *58:*273–280.

Figueroa DA, Mangini E, Amodio-Groton M, et al. Safety of high-dose intravenous daptomycin treatment: Three-year cumulative experience in a clinical program. *Clin Infect Dis*, **2009,** *49:*177–180.

Fowler VG Jr, Boucher HW, Corey GR, et al. Daptomycin versus standard therapy for bacteremia and endocarditis caused by *Staphylococcus aureus. N Engl J Med,* **2006,** *355:*653–665.

Frymoyer A, Hersh AL, Benet LZ, Guglielmo BJ. Current recommended dosing of vancomycin for children with invasive methicillin-resistant *staphylococcus aureus* infections is inadequate. *Pediatr Infect Dis*, **2009,** *28:*398–402.

Fuller DG, Duke T, Shann R, Curtis N. Antibiotic treatment for bacterial meningitis in children in developing countries. *Ann Trop Paediatr*, **2003,** *23:*233–253.

Gales AC, Sader HS, Fritsche TR. Tigecycline activity tested against 11808 bacterial pathogens recently collected from US medical centers. *Diagn Microbiol Infect Dis*, **2008,** *60:*421–427.

Garey KW, Amsden GW. Intravenous azithromycin. *Ann Pharmacother*, **1999,** *33:*218–228.

Garrett DO, Jochimsen E, Murfitt K, et al. The emergence of decreased susceptibility to vancomycin in *Staphylococcus epidermidis. Infect Control Hosp Epidemiol*, **1999,** *20:*167–170.

Gatti G, Malena M, Casazza R, et al. Penetration of clindamycin and its metabolite *N*-demethylclindamycin into cerebrospinal fluid following intravenous infusion of clindamycin phosphate in patients with AIDS. *Antimicrob Agents Chemother*, **1998,** *42:*3014–3017.

Goldstein EJ, Citron DM, Merriam CV, et al. In vitro activities of the new semisynthetic glycopeptide telavancin (TD-6424), vancomycin, daptomycin, linezolid, and four comparator agents against anaerobic gram-positive species and *Corynebacterium* spp. *Antimicrob Agents Chemother*, **2004,** *48:*2149–2152.

Halperin SA, Bortolussi R, Langley JM, et al. Seven days of erythromycin estolate is as effective as fourteen days for the treatment of *Bordetella pertussis* infections. *Pediatrics*, **1997,** *100:*65–71.

Hamel JC, Stapert D, Moerman JK, Ford CW. Linezolid, critical characteristics. *Infection*, **2000,** *28:*60–64.

Hedberg M, Nord CE. Antimicrobial susceptibility of *Bacteroides fragilis* group isolates in Europe. *Clin Microbiol Infect*, **2003,** *9:*475–488.

Hiramatsu K, Aritaka N, Hanaki H, et al. Dissemination in Japanese hospitals of strains of *Staphylococcus aureus* heterogeneously resistant to vancomycin. *Lancet*, **1997,** *350:*1670–1673.

Hoban DJ, Doern GV, Fluit AC, et al. Worldwide prevalence of antimicrobial resistance in *Streptococcus pneumoniae*, *Haemophilus influenzae*, and *Moraxella catarrhalis* in the SENTRY Antimicrobial Surveillance Program, 1997–1999. *Clin Infect Dis*, **2001,** *32:*S81–S93.

Howden BP, Ward PB, Charles PG, et al. Treatment outcomes for serious infections caused by methicillin-resistant *Staphylococcus aureus* with reduced vancomycin susceptibility. *Clin Infect Dis*, **2004,** *38:*521–528.

Jevitt LA, Smith AJ, Williams PP, et al. In vitro activities of Daptomycin, Linezolid, and Quinupristin-Dalfopristin against a challenge panel of Staphylococci and Enterococci, including vancomycin-intermediate *Staphylococcus aureus* and vancomycin-resistant *Enterococcus faecium. Microb Drug Resist*, **2003,** *9:*389–393.

Kalmeijer MD, Coertjens H, van Nieuwland-Bollen PM, et al. Surgical site infections in orthopedic surgery: The effect of mupirocin nasal ointment in a double-blind, randomized, placebo-controlled study. *Clin Infect Dis*, **2002,** *35:*353–358.

Kovacs JA, Masur H. Prophylaxis against opportunistic infections in patients with human immunodeficiency virus infection. *N Engl J Med*, **2000,** *342:*1416–1429.

Laupland KB, Conly JM. Treatment of *Staphylococcus aureus* colonization and prophylaxis for infection with topical intranasal mupirocin: An evidence-based review. *Clin Infect Dis*, **2003,** *37:*933–938.

Levison ME, Mangura CT, Lorber B, et al. Clindamycin compared with penicillin for the treatment of anaerobic lung abscess. *Ann Intern Med*, **1983,** *98:*466–471.

Lewis JS, Jorgensen JH. Inducible clindamycin resistance in Staphylococci: Should clinicians and microbiologists be concerned? *Clin Infect Dis*, **2005,** *40:*280–285.

Lina G, Quaglia A, Reverdy ME, et al. Distribution of genes encoding resistance to macrolides, lincosamides, and streptogramins among staphylococci. *Antimicrob Agents Chemother*, **1999,** *43:*1062–1066.

Linden PK, Kusne S, Coley K, et al. Use of parenteral colistin for the treatment of serious infection due to antimicrobial-resistant *Pseudomonas aeruginosa. Clin Infect Dis*, **2003,** *37:*154–160.

Lodise TP, Patel N, Lomaestro BM, et al. Relationship between initial vancomycin concentration-time profile and nephrotoxicity in hospitalized patients. *Clin Infect Dis*, **2009,** *49:*507–514.

Mandell LA, Wunderink RG, Anzueto A, et al. Infectious Diseases Society of America/American Thoracic Society consensus guidelines on the management of community-acquired pneumonia in adults. *Clin Infect Dis*, **2007,** *44*(suppl): S27–S72.

Masters EJ, Olson GS, Weiner SJ, et al. Rocky Mountain spotted fever: A clinician's dilemma. *Arch Intern Med*, **2003,** *163:*769–774.

Moellering RC, Linden PK, Reinhardt J, et al. The efficacy and safety of quinupristin/dalfopristin for the treatment of infections caused by vancomycin-resistant *Enterococcus faecium. J Antimicrob Chemother*, **1999,** *44:*251–261.

Moise-Broder PA, Forrest A, Birmingham MC, Schentag JJ. Pharmacodynamics of vancomycin and other antimicrobials in patients with *Staphylococcus aureus* lower respiratory tract infections. *Clin Pharmacokinet*, **2004,** *43:*925–942.

Moore MR, Perdreau-Remington F, Chambers HF, et al. Vancomycin treatment failure associated with heterogeneous vancomycin-intermediate *Staphylococcus aureus* in a patient with endocarditis and in the rabbit model of endocarditis. *Antimicrob Agents Chemother*, **2003**, *47:*1262–1266.

Nakajima Y. Mechanisms of bacterial resistance to macrolide antibiotics. *J Infect Chemother*, **1999,** *5:*61–74.

Narita M, Tsuji BT, Yu VL. Linezolid-associated peripheral and optic neuropathy, lactic acidosis, and serotonin syndrome. *Pharmacotherapy*, **2007,** *27:*1189–1197.

Nichols RL, Graham DR, Barriere SL, et al. Treatment of hospitalized patients with complicated gram-positive skin and skin structure infections: Two randomized, multicentre studies of quinupristin/dalfopristin versus cefazolin, oxacillin or vancomycin. Synercid Skin and Skin Structure Infection Group. *J Antimicrob Chemother*, **1999,** *44:*263–273.

Nilius AM, Ma Z. Ketolides: The future of the macrolides? *Curr Opin Pharmacol*, **2002,** *2:*493–500.

Oliva ME, Rekha A, Yellin A, et al. A multicenter trial of the efficacy and safety of tigecycline versus imipenem/cilastatin in patients with complicated intra-abdominal infections. *BMC Infect Dis*, **2005,** *5:*88.

Parry CM. Antimicrobial drug resistance in *Salmonella enterica*. *Curr Opin Infect Dis*, **2003,** *16:*467–472.

Periti P, Mazzei T, Mini E, Novelli A. Pharmacokinetic drug interactions of macrolides. *Clin Pharmacokinet*, **1992,** *23:*106–131.

Perl TM, Cullen JJ, Wenzel RP, et al. Intranasal mupirocin to prevent postoperative *Staphylococcus aureus* infections. *N Engl J Med*, **2002,** *346:*1871–1877.

Pertel PE, Bernardo P, Fogarty C, et al. Effects of prior effective therapy on the efficacy of daptomycin and ceftriaxone for the treatment of community-acquired pneumonia. *Clin Infect Dis*, **2008,** *46:*1142–1151.

Petersen PJ, Jacobus NV, Weiss WJ, et al. In vitro and in vivo antibacterial activities of a novel glycylcycline, the 9-t-butylglycylamido derivative of minocycline (GAR-936). *Antimicrob Agents Chemother*, **1999,** *43:*738–744.

Peterson WL, Fendrick AM, Cave DR, et al. *Helicobacter pylori*–related disease: Guidelines for testing and treatment. *Arch Intern Med*, **2000**, *160:*1285–1291.

Quagliarello VJ, Scheld WM. Treatment of bacterial meningitis. *N Engl J Med*, **1997,** *336:*708–716.

Ramsey MA, Bradley SF, Kauffman CA, Morton TM. Identification of chromosomal location of mupA gene, encoding low-level mupirocin resistance in staphylococcal isolates. *Antimicrob Agents Chemother*, **1996,** *40:*2820–2823.

Rubinstein E, Cammarata S, Oliphant T, et al. Linezolid (PNU-100766) versus vancomycin in the treatment of hospitalized patients with nosocomial pneumonia: a randomized, double-blind, multicenter study. *Clin Infect Dis*, **2001,** *32:*402–412.

Rybak MJ. The pharmacokinetic and pharmacodynamic properties of vancomycin. *Clin Infect Dis,* **2006,** *42*(suppl):S35–S39.

Rybak MJ, Lomaestro BM, Rotschfer JC, et al. Vancomycin therapeutic guidelines: a summary of consensus recommendations from the Infectious Diseases Society of America, the American Society of Health-System Pharmacists, and the Society of Infectious Diseases Pharmacists. *Clin Infect Dis*, **2009,** *49:*325–327.

San Gabriel P, Zhou J, Tabibi S, et al. Antimicrobial susceptibility and synergy studies of *Stenotrophomonas maltophilia* isolates from patients with cystic fibrosis. *Antimicrob Agents Chemother*, **2004,** *48:*168–171.

Shi J, Montay G, Chapel S, et al. Pharmacokinetics and safety of the ketolide telithromycin in patients with renal impairment. *J Clin Pharmacol*, **2004,** *44:*234–244.

Sieradzki K, Tomasz A. Gradual alterations in cell wall structure and metabolism in vancomycin-resistant mutants of *Staphylococcus aureus*. *J Bacteriol*, **1999,** *181:*7566–7570.

Sieradzki K, Wu SW, Tomasz A. Inactivation of the methicillin resistance gene mecA in vancomycin-resistant *Staphylococcus aureus*. *Microb Drug Resist*, **1999,** *5:*253–237.

Silverman JA, Mortin LI, Vanpraagh AD, et al. Inhibition of daptomycin by pulmonary surfactant: In vitro modeling and clinical impact. *J Infect Dis*, **2005,** *191:*2149–2152.

Smith TL, Pearson ML, Wilcox KR, et al. Emergence of vancomycin resistance in *Staphylococcus aureus.* Glycopeptide-Intermediate *Staphylococcus aureus* Working Group. *N Engl J Med*, **1999,** *340:*493–501.

Soltani M, Beighton D, Philpott-Howard J, Woodford N. Mechanisms of resistance to quinupristin-dalfopristin among isolates of *Enterococcus faecium* from animals, raw meat, and hospital patients in Western Europe. *Antimicrob Agents Chemother*, **2000,** *44:*433–436.

Streit JM, Jones RN, Sader HS. Daptomycin activity and spectrum: a worldwide sample of 6737 clinical gram-positive organisms. *J Antimicrob Chemother,* **2004,** *53:*669–674.

Tunkel AR, Hartman BJ, Kaplan SL, et al. Practice guidelines for the management of bacterial meningitis. *Clin Infect Dis,* **2004,** *39:*1267–1284.

Udo EE, Jacob LE, Mathew B. Genetic analysis of methicillin-resistant *Staphylococcus aureus* expressing high and low-level mupirocin resistance. *J Med Microbiol*, **2001,** *50:* 909–915.

Villareal FJ, Griffin M, Owens J, et al. Early short-term treatment with doxycycline modulates post-infarction left ventricular remodeling. *Circulation*, **2003,** *108:*1487–1492.

Ward TT, Rimland D, Kauffman C, et al. Randomized, open-label trial of azithromycin plus ethambutol vs. clarithromycin plus ethambutol as therapy for *Mycobacterium avium* complex bacteremia in patients with human immunodeficiency virus infection. Veterans Affairs HIV Research Consortium. *Clin Infect Dis*, **1998,** *27:*1278–1285.

Wareham DW, Wilson P. Chloramphenicol in the 21st century. *Hosp Med*, **2002,** *63:*157–161.

Weigel LM, Clewell DB, Gill SR, et al. Genetic analysis of a high-level vancomycin-resistant isolate of *Staphylococcus aureus*. *Science*, **2003,** *302:*1569–1571.

Wertheim HF, Vos MC, Ott A, et al. Mupirocin prophylaxis against nosocomial *Staphylococcus aureus* infections in non-surgical patients: a randomized study. *Ann Intern Med*, **2004,** *140:*419–425.

Wilson P, Andrews JA, Charlesworth R, et al. Linezolid resistance in clinical isolates of *Staphylococcus aureus*. *J Antimicrob Chemother*, **2003,** *51:*186–188.

Wilson W, Taubert KA, Gewitz M, *et al.* Prevention of infective endocarditis: Guidelines from the American Heart Association: A guideline from the American Heart Association Rheumatic Fever, Endocarditis and Kawasaki Disease Committee, Council on Cardiovascular Disease in the Young, and the Council on Clinical Cardiology, Council on Cardiovascular Surgery and Anesthesia, and the Quality of Care and Outcomes Research Interdisciplinary Working Group. *J Am Dent Assoc,* **2007,** *138:*739–745, 747–760.

Workowski KA, Berman SM. Sexually transmitted diseases treatment guidelines, 2006. *MMWR*, **2006**; *55*(RR-11):1–94. Available at: www.cdc.gov/mmwr/preview/ mmwrhtml/ rr5511a1.htm. Accessed December 16, 2009.

Wunderink RG, Cammarata SK, Olliphant TH, et al. Continuation of a randomized, double-blind, multicenter study of linezolid versus vancomycin in the treatment of patients with nosocomial pneumonia. *Clin Ther*, **2003a,** *25:*980–992.

Wunderink RG, Rello J, Cammarata SK, et al. Linezolid vs. vancomycin: analysis of two double-blind studies of patients with methicillin-resistant *Staphylococcus aureus* nosocomial pneumonia. *Chest*, **2003b,** *124:*1789–1797.

Yang S-J, Xiong YQ, Schrenzel J, et al. Regulation of mprF in daptomycin-nonsusceptible *Staphylococcus aureus* strains. *Antimicrob Agents Chemother*, **2009,** *53:*2636–2637.

Chemotherapy of Tuberculosis, *Mycobacterium Avium* Complex Disease, and Leprosy

Tawanda Gumbo

Mycobacteria have caused epic diseases: Tuberculosis (TB) and leprosy have terrorized humankind since antiquity. Although the burden of leprosy has decreased, TB is still the most important infectious killer of humans. *Mycobacterium avium-intracellulare* (or *Mycobacterium avium* complex; MAC) infection continues to be difficult to treat.

Mycobacterium, from the Greek "mycos," refers to Mycobacteria's waxy appearance, which is due to the composition of their cell walls. More than 60% of the cell wall is lipid, mainly mycolic acids composed of 2-branched, 3-hydroxy fatty acids with chains made of 76-90 carbon atoms! This extraordinary shield prevents many pharmacological compounds from getting to the bacterial cell membrane or inside the cytosol.

A second layer of defense comes from an abundance of efflux pumps in the cell membrane. These transport proteins pump out potentially harmful chemicals from the bacterial cytoplasm back into the extracellular space and are responsible for the native resistance of mycobacteria to many standard antibiotics (Morris et al., 2005). As an example, ATP binding cassette (ABC) permeases comprise a full 2.5% of the genome of *Mycobacterium tuberculosis*.

A third barrier is the propensity of some of the bacilli to hide inside the patient's cells, thereby surrounding themselves with an extra physicochemical barrier that antimicrobial agents must cross to be effective.

Mycobacteria are separated into two groups, defined by their rate of growth on agar. A list of pathogenic *rapid* and *slow* growers is shown in Table 56–1. Rapid growers are visible to the naked eye within 7 days; slow growers are visible later. Slow growers tend to be susceptible to antibiotics specifically developed for Mycobacteria, whereas rapid growers tend to be also susceptible to antibiotics used against many other bacteria. The pharmacology of drugs developed against slow growers is discussed in this chapter.

The mechanisms of action of the anti-mycobacterial drugs are summarized in Figure 56–1. The mycobacterial mechanisms of resistance to these drugs are summarized in Figure 56–2. Pharmacokinetic parameters are presented in terms of Figure 48–1 and Equation 48–1.

History. The first successful drug for treating TB was para-amino salicylic acid (PAS), developed by Lehman in 1943. A more dramatic success came when Waksman and Schatz developed streptomycin. Further efforts led to development of thiacetazone by Domagk in 1946, isoniazid at Squibb, Hoffman La Roche, and Bayer in 1952, pyrazinamide by Kushner and colleagues in 1952, and rifamycins by Sensi and Margalith in 1957. Ethambutol was discovered at Lederle Laboratories in 1961. As might be anticipated, the use all of these drugs presents problems of drug resistance, adverse events, and drug interactions. Therefore, newer classes of agents are being developed. Moxifloxacin, PA-824, and TMC-207 have reached advanced clinical testing.

ANTI-MYCOBACTERIAL DRUGS

Rifamycins: Rifampin, Rifapentine, and Rifabutin

Rifampin or rifampicin (RIFADIN; RIMACTANE, others), rifapentine (PRIFTIN), and rifabutin (MYCOBUTIN) are important in treatment of mycobacterial diseases.

Chemistry. Rifamycins are macrocyclic antibiotics characterized by a chromophoric naphthohydroquinone group that is spanned by a

Table 56–1

Pathogenic Mycobacterial Rapid and Slow Growers (Runyon Classification)

SLOW GROWERS
Runyon I: Photochromogens
Mycobacterium kansasii
Mycobacterium marinum
Runyon II: Scotochromogens
Mycobacterium scrofulaceum
Mycobacterium szulgai
Mycobacterium gordonae
Runyon III: Non-chromogens
Mycobacterium avium complex
Mycobacterium haemophilum
Mycobacterium xenopi
RAPID GROWERS
Runyon IV:
Mycobacterium fortuitum complex
Mycobacterium smegmatis group

Slow growers tend to be susceptible to antibiotics specifically developed for Mycobacteria; rapid growers tend to be susceptible to antibiotics also used against many other bacteria.

long aliphatic bridge, with an acetyl group at C25. Rifapentine and rifabutin are derivatives of rifampin, whose structure is:

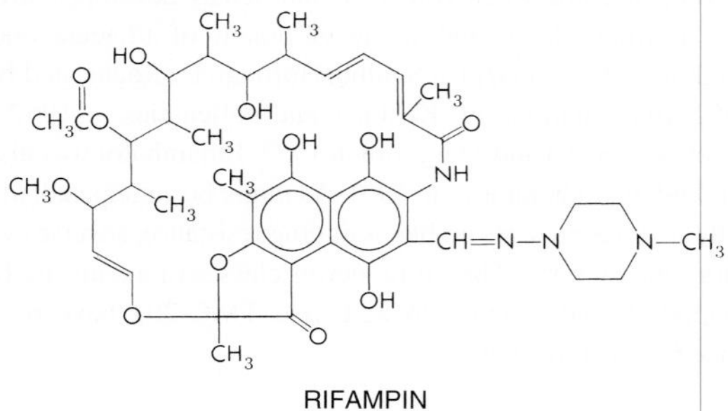

RIFAMPIN

Mechanism of Action. The mechanism of action for rifamycins is typified by rifampin's action against *M. tuberculosis.* Rifampin enters bacilli in a concentration dependent manner, achieving steady-state concentrations within 15 minutes (Gumbo et al., 2007a). Rifampin binds to the β subunit of DNA-dependent RNA polymerase (*rpoB*) to form a stable drug–enzyme complex. Drug binding suppresses chain formation in RNA synthesis.

Antibacterial Activity. Rifampin inhibits the growth of most gram-positive bacteria as well as many gram-negative microorganisms such as *Escherichia coli, Pseudomonas*, indole-positive and indole-negative *Proteus*, and *Klebsiella*. Rifampin is very active against *Staphylococcus aureus* and coagulase-negative staphylococci. The drug also is highly active against *Neisseria meningitidis* and *Haemophilus influenzae*. Rifampin inhibits the growth of *Legionella* species in cell culture and in animal models.

Rifampin inhibits the growth of many *M. tuberculosis* clinical isolates *in vitro* at concentrations of 0.06-0.25 mg/L (Heifets, 1991). Rifampin is also bactericidal against *M. leprae*. *M. kansasii* is inhibited by 0.25-1 mg/L. Most strains of *Mycobacterium scrofulaceum, Mycobacterium intracellulare*, and *M. avium* are suppressed by concentrations of 4 mg/L. *Mycobacterium fortuitum* is highly resistant to the drug. Rifapentine minimum inhibitory concentrations (MICs) are similar to those of rifampin. Rifabutin inhibits the growth of most MAC isolates at concentrations ranging from 0.25-1 mg/L. Rifabutin also inhibits the growth of many strains of *M. tuberculosis* at concentrations of ≤0.125 mg/L and *in vitro* has better MICs than rifampin.

Bacterial Resistance. The prevalence of rifampin-resistant isolates are 1 in every 10^7 to 10^8 bacilli. Microbial resistance to rifampin is due to an alteration of the target of this drug, *rpoB,* with resistance in 86% of cases due to mutations at codons 526 and 531 of the *rpoB* gene (Somoskovi et al., 2001). Rifamycin monoresistance occurs at higher rates when patients with AIDS and multi-cavitary TB are treated with either rifapentine or rifabutin (Burman et al., 2006a).

Mutations in genes involved in DNA repair mechanisms will impair the repair of multiple genes, which may lead to hyper-mutable strains (Chapter 48). *M. tuberculosis* Beijing genotype clinical isolates have been associated with higher rates of simultaneous rifampin and isoniazid resistance associated with mutations in the repair genes *mut* and *ogt* (Nouvel et al., 2006; Rad et al., 2003). Inducible or environment-dependent mutators may be a more common phenomenon than these stable mutator phenotypes (Warner and Mizrahi, 2006). Antibiotics, endogenous oxidative and metabolic stressors lead to DNA damage, which induces *dnaE2*. The induction is associated with error-prone DNA repair. This leads to higher rates of rifampin resistance (Boshoff et al., 2003).

Absorption, Distribution, and Excretion. After oral administration, the rifamycins are absorbed to variable extents (Table 56–2) (Burman et al., 2001). Food decreases the rifampin C_{Pmax} by one third; a high-fat meal increases the area under the curve (AUC) of rifapentine by 50%. Food has no effect on rifabutin absorption. Thus rifampin should be taken on an empty stomach, whereas rifapentine should be taken with food, if possible.

Rifamycins are metabolized by microsomal B-esterases and cholinesterases that remove the acetyl group at position 25, resulting in 25-*O*-desacetyl rifamycins. Rifampin is also metabolized by hydrolysis to 3-formyl rifampin, whereas rifapentine is metabolized to 3-formyl rifapentine and 3-formyl-25-*O*-desacetyl-rifapentine. A major pathway for rifabutin elimination is CYP3A. Due to autoinduction, all three rifamycins reduce their own area

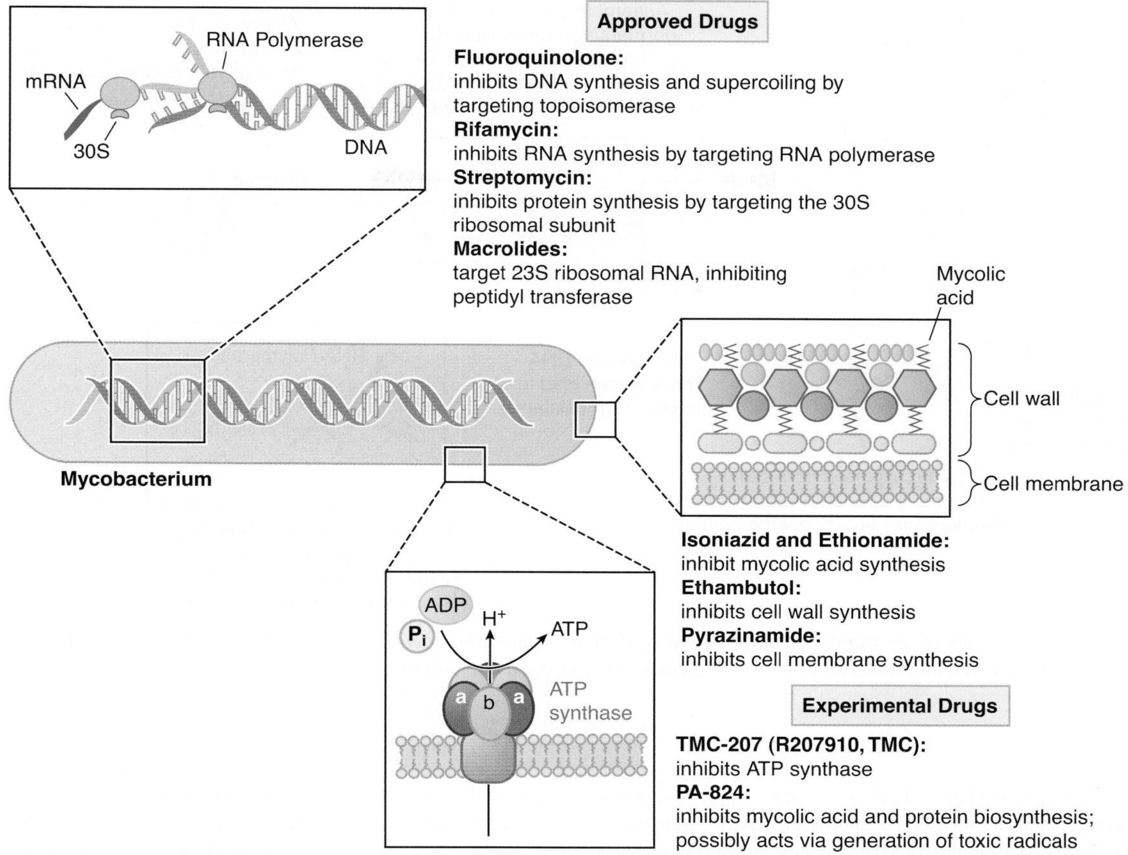
RNA Polymerase
mRNA
30S
DNA
Approved Drugs
Fluoroquinolone:
inhibits DNA synthesis and supercoiling by targeting topoisomerase
Rifamycin:
inhibits RNA synthesis by targeting RNA polymerase
Streptomycin:
inhibits protein synthesis by targeting the 30S ribosomal subunit
Macrolides:
target 23S ribosomal RNA, inhibiting peptidyl transferase
Mycolic acid
Cell wall
Cell membrane
Mycobacterium
Isoniazid and Ethionamide:
inhibit mycolic acid synthesis
Ethambutol:
inhibits cell wall synthesis
Pyrazinamide:
inhibits cell membrane synthesis
ADP
Pi
H+
ATP
a
b
a
ATP synthase
Experimental Drugs
TMC-207 (R207910, TMC):
inhibits ATP synthase
PA-824:
inhibits mycolic acid and protein biosynthesis; possibly acts via generation of toxic radicals

Figure 56–1. *Mechanisms of action of established and experimental drugs used for the chemotherapy of mycobacterial infections.* Shown at the top are the sites of action of approved drugs for the chemotherapy of mycobacterial diseases. Rifamycin is used as a generic term for several drugs, of which rifampin is used most frequently. Also included are two experimental drugs now under investigation: TMC-207 and PA-824. Clofazimine, whose mode of action is not understood, is omitted.

under the concentration-time curves (AUC) with repeated administration (Table 56–3). They have good penetration into many tissues, but levels in the CNS reach only ~5% of those in plasma, likely due to the activity of P-glycoprotein. The drugs and metabolites are excreted by bile and eliminated via feces, with urine elimination accounting for only one-third and less of metabolites.

The population pharmacokinetics (PK) of rifampin are best described using a one-compartment model with transit compartment absorption (Wilkins et al., 2008), using the PK parameters in Table 56–2. Single-drug formulations increase mean transit time during absorption by ~100% and systemic clearance (SCL) by 24% in comparison to fixed-dose combinations of rifampin and other anti-TB drugs. Thus the absorption of rifampin will be slower, and the peak concentration (C_{Pmax}) of rifampin lower, with some formulations compared to others (Wilkins et al., 2008).

Rifapentine pharmacokinetics are likewise best described using a one-compartment open model with first-order absorption and elimination (Langdon et al., 2005). The PK parameters are summarized in Table 56–2. However, for each 1-kg weight increase above 50 kg, SCL increases by 0.05 L/hour and V_d by 0.69 L. Thus, C_{Pmax} and AUC decrease with increasing patient weight above 50 kg.

Rifabutin pharmacokinetics are best described by a two-compartment open model with first-order absorption and elimination. Rifabutin disposition is biexponential. Rifabutin concentrations are substantially higher in tissue than in plasma due to its lipophilic properties, leading to the very high apparent volumes of distribution (Table 56–2). The consequence is that C_{Pmax} values for rifabutin are lower than one would predict by comparison with other rifamycins. The volume of peripheral compartment decreases by 27% with concomitant azithromycin administration; tobacco smoking increases the volume by 39%.

Pharmacokinetics-Pharmacodynamics. Rifampin's bactericidal activity is best optimized by a high AUC/MIC ratio (Gumbo et al., 2007a). However, resistance suppression and rifampin's enduring post-antibiotic effect are best optimized by high C_{max}/MIC. Therefore, the duration of time that the rifampin concentration persists above the MIC is of less importance.

These results predict that the $t_{1/2}$ of a rifamycin is less of an issue in optimizing therapy, and that if patients could tolerate it, higher doses

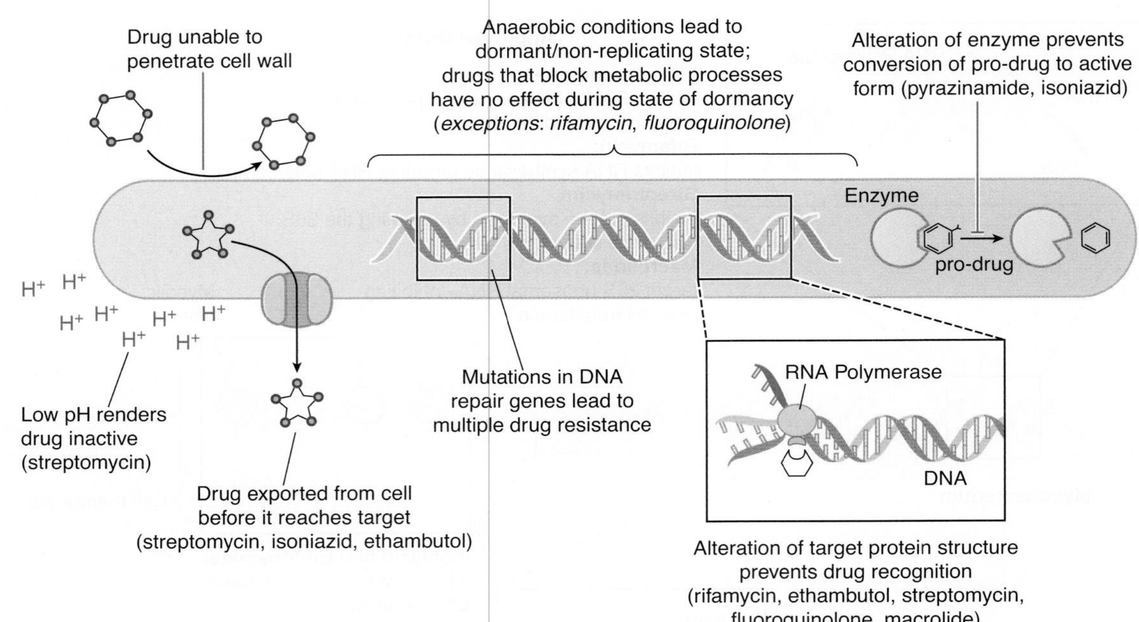

Figure 56–2. *Mechanisms of resistance of Mycobacteria to different chemotherapeutic drugs.* Shown are the various mechanisms by which mycobacteria resist antibacterial effects of the currently approved chemotherapeutic agents.

would lead to higher bactericidal activities while suppressing resistance. In a recent clinical study, TB patients in South Africa were treated with 20 mg/kg/day of rifampin for 5 days, and the rate of sputum bacillary decline compared to that for doses of 3 mg/kg/day, 6 mg/kg/day, and 12 mg/kg/day (Diacon et al., 2007). There was a linear increase in the rate of kill, with a 2-fold increase between the 600 mg dose and the 1200 mg dose. Currently, efficacy of higher doses of rifapentine and rifampin is being examined in clinical studies.

Therapeutic Uses. Rifampin for oral administration is available alone and as a fixed-dose combination with isoniazid (150 mg of isoniazid, 300 mg of rifampin; rifamate, others) or with isoniazid and pyrazinamide (50 mg of isoniazid, 120 mg of rifampin, and 300 mg pyrazinamide; RIFATER). A parenteral form of rifampin is also available. The dose of rifampin for treatment of tuberculosis in adults is 600 mg, given once daily, either 1 hour before or 2 hours after a meal. Children should receive 10-20 mg/kg given in the same way. Rifabutin is administered at 5 mg/kg/day and rifapentine at 10 mg/kg once a week.

Rifampin is also useful for the prophylaxis of meningococcal disease and *H. influenzae* meningitis. To prevent meningococcal disease, adults may be treated with 600 mg twice daily for 2 days or 600 mg once daily for 4 days; children >1 month of age should receive 10-15 mg/kg, to a maximum of 600 mg. Combined with a β-lactam antibiotic or vancomycin, rifampin may be useful for therapy in selected cases of staphylococcal endocarditis or osteomyelitis, especially those caused by staphylococci "tolerant" to penicillin. Rifampin may also be indicated for the eradication of the staphylococcal nasal carrier state in patients with chronic furunculosis.

Untoward Effects. Rifampin is generally well tolerated in patients. Usual doses result in <4% of patients with TB developing significant adverse reactions; the most common are rash (0.8%), fever (0.5%), and nausea and vomiting (1.5%). Rarely, hepatitis and deaths due to liver failure have been observed in patients who received other hepatotoxic agents in addition to rifampin or who had preexisting liver disease. Chronic liver disease, alcoholism, and old age appear to increase the incidence of severe hepatic problems. GI disturbances have occasionally required discontinuation of the drug. Various nonspecific symptoms related to the nervous system also have been noted.

Hypersensitivity reactions may be encountered. Hemolysis, hemoglobinuria, hematuria, renal insufficiency, and acute renal failure have been observed rarely; these also are thought to be hypersensitivity reactions. High-dose rifampin should not be administered on a dosing schedule of less than twice weekly because this is associated with a flu-like syndrome of fever, chills, and myalgias in 20% of patients so treated. The syndrome also may include eosinophilia, interstitial nephritis, acute tubular necrosis, thrombocytopenia, hemolytic anemia, and shock. Light chain proteinuria has also been documented with rifampin use. Thrombocytopenia, transient leukopenia, and anemia have occurred during therapy. Because the potential teratogenicity of rifampin is unknown and the drug is known to cross the placenta, it is best to avoid the use of this agent during pregnancy.

Rifabutin is generally well tolerated; primary reasons for discontinuation of therapy include rash (4%), GI intolerance (3%), and neutropenia (2%) (Nightingale et al., 1993). Neutropenia occurred in

Table 56–2

Population Pharmacokinetic Parameter Estimates for Antimycobacterial Drugs in Adult Patients

	PARAMETER ESTIMATE		
	k_a (h^{-1})	SCL (L/h)	V_d (L)
First-line Drugs			
Rifampin	1.15	19	53
Rifapentine	0.6	2.03	37.8
Rifabutin	0.2	61	231/1,050[a]
Pyrazinamide	3.56	3.4	29.2
Isoniazid	2.3	22.1	35.2
Ethambutol	0.7	1.3[b]	6.0[b]
Clofazimine	0.7	0.6/76.7	1470
Dapsone	1.04	1.83	69.6
Second-line Agents			
Ethionamide	0.25	1.9[b]	3.2[b]
Para-aminosalicylic acid	0.4	0.3[b]	0.9[b]
Cycloserine	1.9	0.04[b]	0.5[b]

[a]Volume of central compartment/volume of peripheral compartment. [b]Expressed per kilogram of body weight. k_a, absorption constant (see Chapter 48); SCL, systemic clearance; V_d, volume of distribution.

Table 56–3

Pharmacokinetic Parameters of Rifampin, Rifabutin, and Rifapentine

	RIFABUTIN	RIFAMPIN	RIFAPENTINE
Protein binding (%)	71	85	97
Oral bioavailability (%)	20	68	—
t_{max} (hours)	2.5-4.0	1.5-2.0	5.0-6.0
C_{max} total (μg/mL)	0.2-0.6	8-20	8-30
C_{max} free drug (μg/mL)	0.1	1.5	0.5
Half-life (hours)	32-67	2-5	14-18
Intracellular/extracellular penetration	9	5	24-60
Autoinduction (AUC decrease)	40%	38%	20%
CYP3A induction	Weak	Pronounced	Moderate
CYP3A substrate	Yes	No	No

AUC, area under the curve.

25% of patients with severe HIV infection who received rifabutin. Uveitis and arthralgias have occurred in patients receiving rifabutin doses >450 mg daily in combination with clarithromycin or fluconazole. Patients should be cautioned to discontinue the drug if visual symptoms (pain or blurred vision) occur. Rifabutin causes an orange-tan discoloration of skin, urine, feces, saliva, tears, and contact lenses, like rifampin. Rarely, thrombocytopenia, a flu-like syndrome, hemolysis, myositis, chest pain, and hepatitis develop in patients treated with rifabutin. Unique side effects include polymyalgia, pseudojaundice, and anterior uveitis.

Rifamycin Overdose. Rifampin overdose is uncommon and has been poorly studied. Doses of up to 12 g have produced serum rifampin concentrations of 400 mg/L with no change in the serum elimination rate. The most prominent symptoms are the orange discoloration of skin, fluids, and mucosal surfaces, leading to the term *red-man syndrome*. Overdose can be life-threatening; treatment consists of supportive measures; there is no antidote.

Drug Interactions. Because rifampin potently induces CYPs 1A2, 2C9, 2C19, and 3A4, its administration results in a decreased $t_{1/2}$ for a number of compounds, including HIV protease and non-nucleoside reverse transcriptase inhibitors, digitoxin, digoxin, quinidine, disopyramide, mexiletine, tocainide, ketoconazole, propranolol, metoprolol, clofibrate, verapamil, methadone, cyclosporine, corticosteroids, coumarin anticoagulants, theophylline, barbiturates, oral contraceptives, halothane, fluconazole, and the sulfonylureas. It leads to therapeutic failure of these agents, with potentially catastrophic consequences. Prior to putting a patient on rifampin, therefore, all the patient's medications should be examined for potential interactions. Rifabutin is a less potent inducer of CYPs than rifampin, both in terms of potency and number of CYP enzymes involved; however, rifabutin does induce hepatic microsomal enzymes and decreases the $t_{1/2}$ of zidovudine, prednisone, digitoxin, quinidine, ketoconazole, propranolol, phenytoin, sulfonylureas, and warfarin. It has less effect than rifampin on serum levels of indinavir and nelfinavir. Compared to rifabutin and rifampin, the CYP-inducing effects of rifapentine are intermediate.

Pyrazinamide

Pyrazinamide is the synthetic pyrazine analog of nicotinamide. Pyrazinamide is also known as pyrazinoic acid amide, pyrazine carboxylamide, and pyrazinecarboxamide.

PYRAZINAMIDE

Mechanism of Action. Pyrazinamide is "activated" by acidic conditions. Initially it was assumed that the acidic conditions under which pyrazinamide works were inside macrophage phagosomes. However, pyrazinamide may not be very effective within macrophages; rather, the acidic conditions for activation may be at the edges of necrotic TB cavities where inflammatory cells produce lactic acid (Blumberg et al., 2003).

Mycobacterium tuberculosis nicotinamidase, or pyrazinaminidase deaminates pyrazinamide to pyrazinoic acid (POA^-), which is then transported to the extracellular milieu by an efflux pump (Zhang et al., 1999). In an acidic extracellular milieu, a fraction of POA^- is protonated to POAH, a more lipid-soluble form that enters the bacillus. The Henderson-Hasselbalch equilibrium (Chapter 2) progressively favors the formation of POAH and its equilibration across membrances as the pH of the extracellular medium declines toward the pK_a of pyrazinoic acid, 2.9, a condition that also enhances microbial killing (Zhang et al., 2002). Although the actual mechanism of microbial kill is still unclear, three mechanisms have been proposed (Zhang et al., 2003; Zimhony et al., 2000):

- inhibition of fatty acid synthase type I leading to interference with mycolic acid synthesis
- reduction of intracellular pH
- disruption of membrane transport by HPOA

Antibacterial Activity. Pyrazinamide exhibits antimicrobial activity *in vitro* only at acidic pH. At pH of 5.8-5.95, 80-90% of clinical isolates have an MIC of ≤100 mg/L (Salfinger and Heifets, 1988).

Mechanisms of Resistance. Pyrazinamide-resistant *M. tuberculosis* have pyrazinamidase with reduced affinity for pyrazinamide. This reduced affinity decreases the conversion of pyrazinamide to POA. Single point mutations in the *pncA* gene are encountered in up to 70% of resistant clinical isolates. The mechanisms contributing to resistance in 30% of resistant clinical isolates is unclear.

Absorption, Distribution, and Excretion. Pyrazinamide oral bioavailability is >90%. Pharmacokinetics are best described by a one-compartment model. GI absorption segregates patients into two groups: fast absorbers (56%) with an absorption rate constant of 3.56/hour and slow absorbers (44%) with an absorption rate of 1.25/hour (Wilkins et al., 2006). The drug is concentrated 20-fold in lung epithelial lining fluid (Conte et al., 2000). Pyrazinamide is metabolized by microsomal deamidase to POA and subsequently hydroxylated to 5-hydroxy-POA, which is then excreted by the kidneys. CL (clearance) and V_d (volume of distribution) increase with patient mass (0.5 L/hour and 4.3 L for every 10 kg above 50 kg), and V_d is larger in males (by 4.5 L) (see Table 56–2) This has several implications: The $t_{1/2}$ of pyrazinamide will vary considerably based on weight and gender, and the AUC_{0-24} will decrease with increase in weight for the same dose (same mg drug/kg body weight). Pyrazinamide clearance is reduced in renal failure; therefore, the dosing frequency is reduced to three times a week at low glomerular filtration rates. Hemodialysis removes pyrazinamide; therefore, the drug needs to be re-dosed after each session of hemodialysis (Malone et al., 1999b).

Microbial Pharmacokinetics-Pharmacodynamics. Pyrazinamide's sterilizing effect is closely linked to AUC_{0-24}/MIC (Gumbo et al., 2008). However, resistance suppression is linked to the fraction of time that C_P persists above MIC (T > MIC). Because patient weight impacts both SCL and volume, both AUC and $t_{1/2}$ will be impacted by high weight. Clinical trial simulations that account for patient weight reveal that optimal AUC_{0-24}/MIC and T > MIC are likely to be achieved only by doses much higher than the currently recommended 15-30 mg/kg/day (Gumbo et al., 2008). The safety of such higher doses in actual patients is unclear.

Therapeutic Uses. The co-administration of pyrazinamide with isoniazid or rifampin has led to a one-third reduction in the duration of anti-TB therapy, and a two-thirds reduction in TB relapse. This led to reduction in length of therapy to 6 months, producing the current "short course" chemotherapy. Pyrazinamide is administered at an oral dose of 15-30 mg/kg/day.

Untoward Effects. Injury to the liver is the most serious side effect of pyrazinamide. When a dose of 40-50 mg/kg is administered orally, signs and symptoms of hepatic disease appear in ~15% of patients, with jaundice in 2-3% and death due to hepatic necrosis in rare instances. However, these rates were determined in an era when pyrazinamide was administered for durations much longer than the current 2 months. Elevations of plasma alanine/aspartate aminotransferases are the earliest abnormalities produced by the drug. Regimens employed currently (15-30 mg/kg/day) are much safer. Prior to pyrazinamide administration, all patients should undergo studies of hepatic function, and these studies should be repeated at frequent intervals during the entire period of treatment. If evidence of significant hepatic damage becomes apparent, therapy must be stopped. Pyrazinamide should not be given to individuals with hepatic dysfunction unless this is absolutely unavoidable.

Pyrazinamide inhibits excretion of urate, resulting in hyperuricemia in nearly all patients, and may cause acute episodes of gout. Other untoward effects observed with pyrazinamide include arthralgias, anorexia, nausea and vomiting, dysuria, malaise, and fever. In the U.S., the use of pyrazinamide is not approved during pregnancy because of inadequate data on teratogenicity.

There are minimal data on pyrazinamide overdose, and no antidote has been studied.

Isoniazid

Isoniazid (NYDRAZID, others) is a primary drug for the chemotherapy of tuberculosis. All patients infected with isoniazid-sensitive strains of the tubercle bacillus should receive the drug if they can tolerate it. The use of combination therapy (isoniazid + pyrazinamide + rifampin) provides the basis for "short-course" therapy and improved remission rates.

Chemistry. Isoniazid (*Isoni*cotinic acid hydr*azide*), also called INH, is a small water-soluble molecule (MW = 137) that is structurally related to pyrazinamide (see Figure 56–3).

Mechanism of Action. Isoniazid enters bacilli by passive diffusion. The drug is not directly toxic to the bacillus but must be activated to its toxic form within the bacillus by KatG, a multifunctional catalase-peroxidase. KatG catalyzes the production from isoniazid of an isonicotinoyl radical that subsequently interacts with mycobacterial NAD and NAPD to produce a dozen adducts (Argyrou et al., 2007). One of these, a nicotinoyl-NAD isomer, inhibits the activities of enoyl acyl carrier protein reductase (InhA) and β-ketoacyl acyl carrier protein synthase (KasA). Inhibition of these enzymes inhibits synthesis of mycolic acid, an essential component of the mycobacterial cell wall, leading to bacterial cell death. Another adduct, a nicotinoyl-NADP isomer, potently inhibits (K_i<1nM) mycobacterial dihydrofolate reductase, thereby interfering with nucleic acid synthesis (Argyrou et al., 2006). See Figure 56–3.

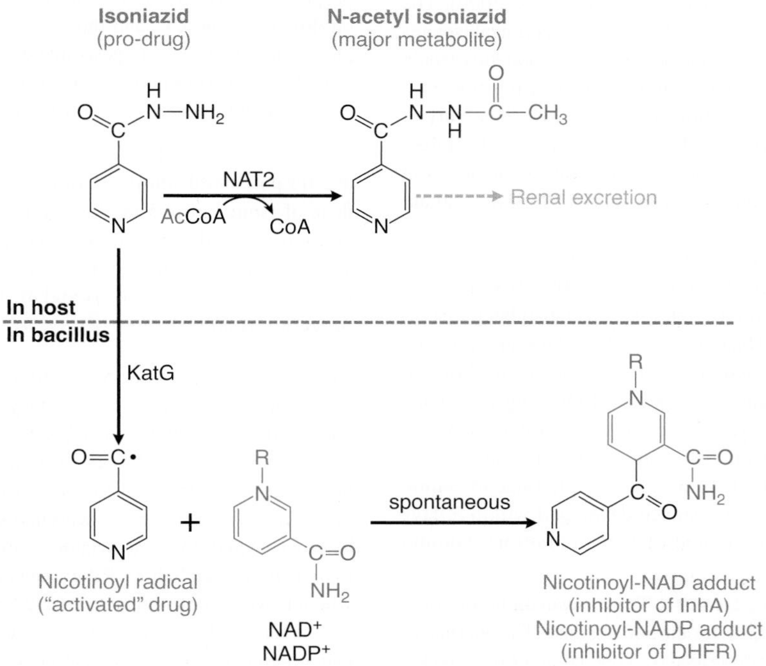

Isoniazid (pro-drug)
N-acetyl isoniazid (major metabolite)
NAT2
AcCoA
CoA
Renal excretion
In host
In bacillus
KatG
spontaneous
Nicotinoyl radical ("activated" drug)
NAD^+
$NADP^+$
Nicotinoyl-NAD adduct (inhibitor of InhA)
Nicotinoyl-NADP adduct (inhibitor of DHFR)

Figure 56–3. *Metabolism and activation of isoniazid.* The pro-drug isoniazid is metabolized in humans by NAT2 isoforms to its principal metabolite, N-acetyl isoniazid, which is excreted by the kidney. Isoniazid diffuses into mycoplasma where it is "activated" by KatG (oxidase/peroxidase) to the nicotinoyl radical, which reacts spontaneously with NAD^+ or $NADP^+$ to produce adducts that inhibit important enzymes in cell-wall and nucleic acid synthesis. DHFR, dihydrofolate reductase.

Other products of KatG activation of INH include superoxide, H_2O_2, alkyl hydroperoxides, and the NO radical, which may also contribute to the mycobactericidal effects of INH (Timmins and Deretic, 2006). *M. tuberculosis* could be especially sensitive to damage from these radicals because the bacilli have a defect in the central regulator of the oxidative stress response, *oxyR*. Backup defense against radicals is provided by alkyl hydroperoxide reductase (encoded by *ahpC*), which detoxifies organic peroxides. Increased expression of *ahpC* reduces isoniazid effectiveness.

Antibacterial Activity. The isoniazid MICs with clinical *M. tuberculosis* strains vary from country to country. In the U.S., e.g., the MICs are 0.025-0.05 mg/L (Heifets, 1991). Activity against *M. bovis* and *M. kansasii* is moderate. Isoniazid has poor activity against MAC. It has no activity against any other microbial genus.

Mechanisms of Resistance. The prevalence of drug-resistant mutants is ~1 in 10^6 bacilli. Because TB cavities may contain as many as 10^7 to 10^9 microorganisms, preexistent resistance can be expected in pulmonary TB cavities of untreated patients. These spontaneous mutants can be selected by monotherapy; indeed, strains resistant to isoniazid will be selected and amplified by isoniazid monotherapy. Thus two or more agents are usually used. Because the mutations resulting in drug resistance are independent events, the probability of resistance to two antimycobacterial agents is small, ~1 in 10^{12} ($1 \times 10^6 \times 10^6$), a low probability considering the number of bacilli involved.

Resistance to INH is associated with mutation or deletion of katG, overexpression of the genes for inhA (confers low-level resistance to INH and some cross-resistance to ethionamide), and ahpC and mutations in the *kasA* and *katG* genes. KatG mutants exhibit a high level of resistance to isoniazid (Zhang and Yew, 2009). The most common mechanism of isoniazid resistance in clinical isolates is due to single point mutations in the heme binding catalytic domain of KatG, especially a serine to asparagine change at position 315. Although isolates with this mutation completely lose the ability to form nicotinoyl-NAD^+/$NADP^+$ adducts, they retain good catalase activity and maintain good biofitness. Compensatory mutations in the *ahpC* promoter occur and increase survival of *katG* mutant strains under oxidative stress.

KatG 315 mutants have a high probability of co-occurrence with ethambutol resistance (Hazbón et al., 2006; Parsons et al., 2005). Mutations in *katG*, *ahpC*, and *inhA* have also been associated with *rpoB* mutations (Hazbón et al., 2006). This suggests that mutations at different loci associated with resistance to different drugs may somehow interact to make multiple drug resistance more likely. In the laboratory, efflux pump induction by isoniazid has been demonstrated, and it also confers resistance to ethambutol (Colangeli et al., 2005). In an *in vitro* pharmacodynamic model, efflux pump-induced resistance developed within 3 days and was followed by development of *katG* mutations (Gumbo et al., 2007b).

Absorption, Distribution, and Excretion. The bioavailability of orally administered isoniazid is ~100% for the 300 mg dose. The pharmacokinetics of isoniazid are best described by a one-compartment model, with the pharmacokinetic parameters in Table 56–2 (Kinzig-Schippers et al., 2005). The ratio of isoniazid in the epithelial lining fluid to that in plasma is 1-2 and for CSF is 0.9 (Conte et al., 2002). Approximately 10% of drug is bound to protein. From 75-95% of a dose of isoniazid is excreted in the urine within 24 hours, mostly as acetylisoniazid and isonicotinic acid.

Isoniazid is metabolized by hepatic arylamine *N*-acetyltransferase type 2 (NAT2), encoded by a variety of NAT2* alleles (Figure 56–3). The drug is N-acetylated to N-acetylisoniazid in a reaction that uses acetyl-coA. Isoniazid clearance in patients has been traditionally classified as one of two phenotypic groups: "slow" and "fast" acetylators, as seen in Figure 56–4. Recently, the phenotypic groups have been expanded to fast, intermediate, and slow acetylators, and population pharmacokinetic parameters of isoniazid have been estimated and related to *NAT2* genotype; the number of NAT2*4 alleles account for 88% of the variability of INH clearance (Kinzig-Schippers et al., 2005).

The frequency of each acetylation phenotype depends on race but is not influenced by sex or age. Fast acetylation is found in Inuit and Japanese. Slow acetylation is the predominant phenotype in most Scandinavians, Jews, and North African whites. The incidence of "slow acetylators" among various racial types in the U.S. is ~50%. Because high acetyltransferase activity (fast acetylation) is inherited as an autosomal dominant trait, "fast acetylators" of isoniazid are either heterozygous or homozygous. Although it has been useful to categorize different "racial" groups dominated by one or the other of these phenotypes, the more precise approach will be to determine the NAT2*4 alleles for each patient to guide therapy for that patient in the future.

Microbial Pharmacokinetics-Pharmacodynamics. Isoniazid's microbial kill is best explained by the AUC_{0-24}-to-MIC ratio (Gumbo et al., 2007c). Resistance emergence is closely related to both AUC/MIC and C_{max}/MIC (Gumbo et al., 2007c). Because AUC is proportional to dose/CL, this means that efficacy is most dependent on drug dose and CL, and thus on the activity of *NAT-2* polymorphic forms. This also suggests that dividing the isoniazid dose into more frequent doses may be detrimental in terms of resistance emergence, and more intermittent dosing would be better (Chapter 48).

Therapeutic Uses. Isoniazid is available as a pill, as an elixir, and for parenteral administration. The commonly used total daily dose of isoniazid is 5 mg/kg, with a maximum of 300 mg; oral and intramuscular doses are identical. Children should receive 10-15 mg/kg/day (300 mg maximum). Dosing information in the treatment of *M. tuberculosis* and *M. kansasii* infections is given in section II and VI.

Untoward Effects. After NAT2 converts isoniazid to acetylisoniazid, which is excreted by the kidney; acetylisoniazid can also be converted to acetylhydrazine (Roy et al., 2008), and then to hepatotoxic metabolites by CYP2E1. Alternatively, acetylhydrazine may be further acetylated by NAT-2 to diacetylhydrazine, which is nontoxic. In this scenario, rapid acetylators will rapidly remove acetylhydrazine while slower acetylators or induction of CYP2E1 will lead to more toxic metabolites. Rifampin is a potent inducer of CYP2E1, which is why it potentiates isoniazid hepatotoxicity.

Elevated serum aspartate and alanine transaminases are encountered commonly in patients on isoniazid. However, the enzyme levels often normalize even when isoniazid therapy is continued (Blumberg et al., 2003). Severe hepatic injury occurs in ~0.1% of all patients taking the drug. Hepatic damage is rare in patients <20 years old but the incidence increases with age to 1.2%

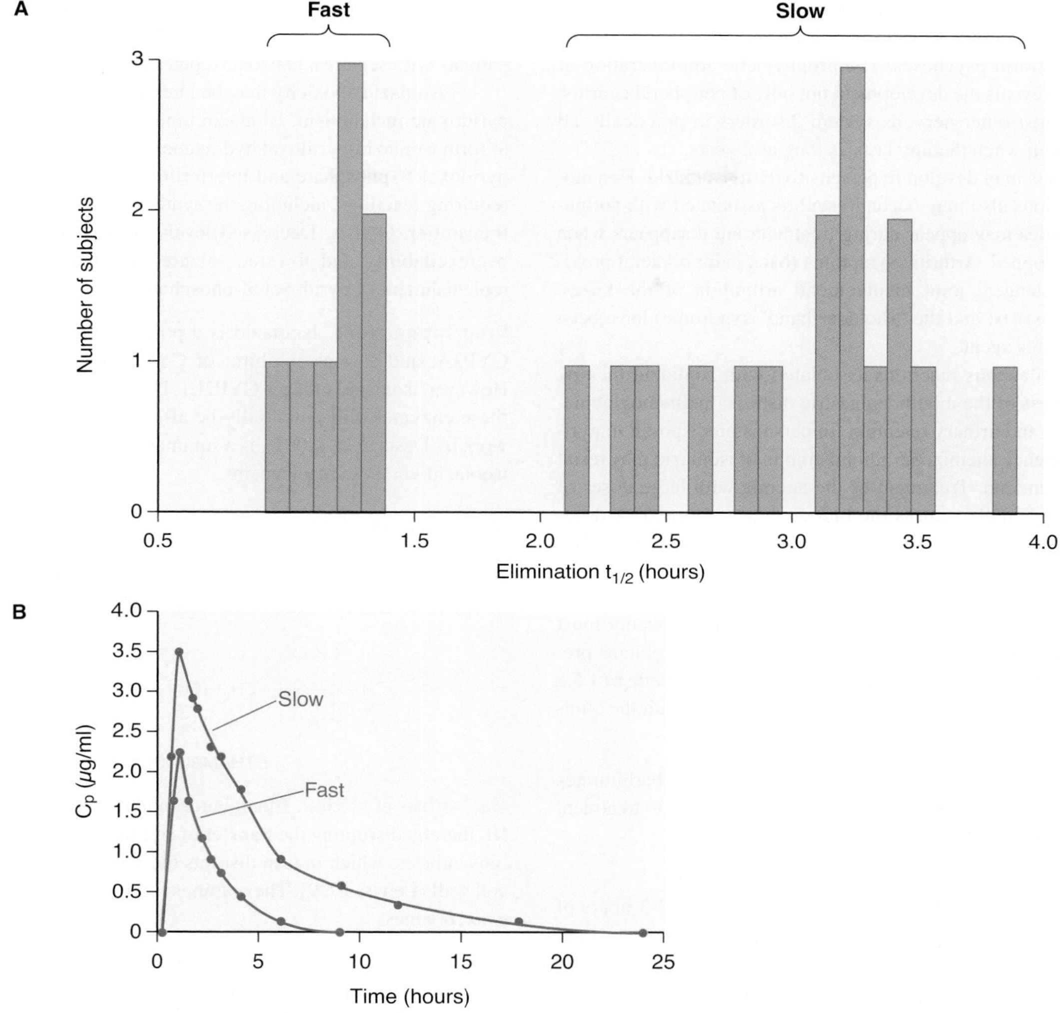

Figure 56–4. *Multi-modal distribution of INH clearance due to NAT2 polymorphisms.* Twenty-four male volunteers were given INH (250 mg orally [3.3 ± 0.5 mg/kg; all subjects within 10% of estimated lean body mass]) and the time courses of plasma levels (C_p) were assessed. (Modified with permission from Peloquin CA et al. Population pharmacokinetic modeling of isoniazid, rifampin, and pyrazinamide. *Antimicrob Agents Chemother*; 1997, 41:2670. With permission from American Society for Microbiology.) **A.** *Frequency distribution of elimination half-times*. Plotting elimination half-times ($t_{1/2}$) as a frequency distribution demonstrates a group of 8 subjects with $t_{1/2}$ values < 1.5 hours (mean = 1.2 hours), the *fast acetylators*, and a group of 16 with $t_{1/2}$ values > 2 hours (mean = 3.3 hours), the *slow acetylators.* **B.** *Time course of plasma levels*. The mean data (C_p vs time after administration) fall into two major groups (see panel A). Both groups reached C_{Pmax} at 1 hour. One group (red line) achieved a higher C_p (3.6 μg/mL) with a mean elimination $t_{1/2}$ = 3.3 hours (*slow acetylators*); the other group (green line) reached a lower maximal C_p (2.3 μg/mL) with a mean elimination $t_{1/2}$ = 1.2 hours (*fast acetylators*).
Variation in expression of active and defective polymorphic forms of NAT2 characterize the fast and slow acetylators. Slow acetylators may be a greater risk for adverse effects from INH, sulfonamides, and procainamide, whereas fast acetylators may have diminished responses to standard doses of these agents but greater risk from bioactivation by NAT2 of arylamine/hydrazine carcinogens. Recently, researchers have identified three elimination subgroups for INH metabolism, *fast*, *slow*, and *intermediate* (codominant fast and slow alleles).

between 35 and 49 years and to 2.3% over 50 years of age. Overall risk is increased by co-administration with rifampin to ~3%. Fatal hepatitis is even rarer (0.02%). Most cases of hepatitis occur 4-8 weeks after the start of therapy.

If pyridoxine is not given concurrently, peripheral neuritis (most commonly paresthesias of feet and hands) is encountered in ~2% of patients receiving isoniazid 5 mg/kg of the drug daily. Neuropathy is more frequent in "slow" acetylators and in individuals with diabetes mellitus, poor nutrition, or anemia. Other neurological toxicities include convulsions in patients with seizure disorders, optic neuritis and atrophy, muscle twitching, dizziness, ataxia, paresthesias, stupor, and toxic encephalopathy. Mental abnormalities may appear during the use of this drug, including euphoria, transient impairment of memory, separation of ideas and reality, loss of self-control, and florid psychoses. The prophylactic administration of pyridoxine prevents the development not only of peripheral neuritis, as well as most other nervous system disorders in practically all instances, even when therapy lasts as long as 2 years.

Patients may develop hypersensitivity to isoniazid. Hematological reactions also may occur. Vasculitis associated with antinuclear antibodies may appear during treatment but disappears when the drug is stopped. Arthritic symptoms (back pain; bilateral proximal interphalangeal joint involvement; arthralgia of the knees, elbows, and wrists; and the "shoulder-hand" syndrome) have been attributed to this agent.

Miscellaneous reactions associated with isoniazid therapy include dryness of the mouth, epigastric distress, methemoglobinemia, tinnitus, and urinary retention. In persons predisposed to pyridoxine-deficiency anemia, the administration of isoniazid may result in dramatic anemia. Treatment of the anemia with large doses of vitamin B_6 gradually returns the blood count to normal. A drug-induced syndrome resembling systemic lupus erythematosus has also been reported.

Isoniazid Overdose. Intentional isoniazid overdose occurs most often in young women with concomitant psychiatric problems prescribed isoniazid for latent TB (Sullivan et al., 1998). As little as 1.5 g can be toxic. Isoniazid overdose has been associated with the clinical triad of:

- seizures refractory to treatment with phenytoin and barbiturates
- metabolic acidosis with an anion gap that is resistant to treatment with sodium bicarbonate
- coma

The common early symptoms appear within 0.5-3 hours of ingestion and include ataxia, peripheral neuropathy, dizziness, and slurred speech. The most dangerous are grand mal seizures and coma, encountered when patients ingests ≥30 mg/kg of the drug. Mortality in these circumstances is as high as 20%. Intravenous pyridoxine is administered over 5-15 minutes on a gram-to-gram basis with the ingested isoniazid. If the dose of ingested isoniazid is unknown, then a pyridoxine dose of 70 mg/kg should be used. In patients with seizures, benzodiazepines are utilized.

Isoniazid's toxicity may be interpreted in terms of effects on pyridoxine metabolism. Isoniazid binds to pyridoxal 5′-phosphate to form isoniazid-pyridoxal hydrazones, thereby depleting neuronal pyridoxal 5′-phosphate and interfering with pyridoxal phosphate-requiring reactions, including the synthesis of the inhibitory neurotransmitter, GABA. Decreased levels of GABA lead to cerebral overexcitability and lowered seizure threshold. The antidote is replenishment of pyridoxal 5′-phosphate.

Drug Interactions. Isoniazid is a potent inhibitor of CYP2C19, CYP3A, and a weak inhibitor of CYP2D6 (Desta et al., 2001). However, isoniazid induces CYP2E1. Drugs that are metabolized by these enzymes will potentially be affected. Table 56–4, based on work by Desta et al. (2001), is a summary of drugs that interact with isoniazid via these mechanisms.

Ethambutol

Ethambutol hydrochloride (MYAMBUTOL) is a water-soluble and heat-stable compound:

$$\mathrm{H{-}\underset{C_2H_5}{\overset{CH_2OH}{C}}{-}NH{-}CH_2{-}CH_2{-}HN{-}\underset{CH_2OH}{\overset{C_2H_5}{C}}{-}H}$$

ETHAMBUTOL

Mechanism of Action. Ethambutol inhibits arabinosyl transferase III, thereby disrupting the transfer of arabinose into arabinogalactan biosynthesis, which in turn disrupts the assembly of mycobacterial cell wall (Lewis, 1999). The arabinosyl transferases are encoded by *embAB* genes.

Antibacterial Activity. Ethambutol has activity against a wide range of mycobacteria but has no activity against any other genus. Ethambutol MICs are 0.5-2 mg/L in clinical isolates of *M. tuberculosis*, ~0.8 mg/L for *M. kansasii,* and 2-7.5 mg/L for *M. avium* (Heifets, 1991;

Table 56–4

Isoniazid-Drug Interactions via Inhibition and Induction of CYPs

CO-ADMINISTERED DRUG	CYP ISOFORM	ADVERSE EFFECTS
Acetaminophen	CYP2E1 inhibition-induction	Hepatotoxicity
Carbamazepine	CYP3A inhibition	Neurological toxicity
Diazepam	CYP3A and CYP2C19 inhibition	Sedation and respiratory depression
Ethosuximide	CYP3A inhibition	Psychotic behavior
Isoflurane and enflurane	CYP2E1 induction	Decreased effectiveness
Phenytoin	CYP2C19 inhibition	Neurological toxicity
Theophylline	CYP3A inhibition	Seizures, palpitation, nausea
Vincristine	CYP3A inhibition	Limb weakness and tingling
Warfarin	CYP2C9 inhibition	Possibility of increased bleeding (single case reported)

Lewis, 1999). The following species are also susceptible: *M. gordonae, M. marinum, M. scrofulaceum, M. szulgai*. However, the majority of *M. xenopi, M. fortuitum*, and *M. chelonae* have been reported as resistant (Lewis, 1999).

Mechanisms of Resistance. *In vitro*, mycobacterial resistance to the drug develops via mutations in the *embB* gene. In 30-70% of clinical isolates that are resistant to ethambutol, mutations are encountered at codon 306 of the *embB* gene. However, mutations in this codon are also encountered in ethambutol-susceptible mycobacteria, as though this mutation is necessary, but not sufficient, to confer ethambutol resistance (Safi et al., 2008). In addition, enhanced efflux pump activity may induce resistance to both isoniazid and ethambutol in the laboratory.

Absorption, Distribution, Metabolism, and Excretion. The oral bioavailability of ethambutol is ~80%. Approximately 10-40% of the drug is bound to plasma protein. Ethambutol drug concentrations have been modeled using a two-compartment open model, with first-order absorption and elimination (Peloquin et al., 1999; Zhu et al., 2004). The decline in ethambutol is biexponential, with a $t_{1/2}$ of 3 hours in the first 12 hours, and a $t_{1/2}$ of 9 hours between 12 and 24 hours, due to redistribution of drug. Clearance and V_d are greater in children than in adults on a per kilogram basis. Slow and incomplete absorption is common in children, so that good peak concentrations of drug are often not achieved with standard dosing (Zhu et al., 2004). In addition, these C_{max} values are not very impressive given the typical MIC values for most clinical isolates of mycobacteria. See Table 56–2 for PK data on this drug.

Alcohol dehydrogenase oxidizes ethambutol to an aldehyde, which is then oxidized by aldehyde dehydrogenase to dicarboxylic acid. However, 80% of the drug is not metabolized at all and is renally excreted. Therefore, in renal failure ethambutol should be dosed at 15-25 mg/kg, three times a week instead of daily, even in patients receiving hemodialysis.

Microbial pharmacokinetics-pharmacodynamics. Ethambutol's microbial kill of *M. tuberculosis* is optimized by AUC/MIC, while that against disseminated MAC is optimized by C_{max}/MIC (Srivastava et al., 2010; Deshpande et al., 2010). Thus, to optimize microbial kill, high intermittent doses such as 25 mg/kg every other day to 50 mg/kg twice a week may be superior to daily doses of 15 mg/kg.

Therapeutic Uses. Ethambutol is available for oral administration in tablets containing the D-isomer. It is used for the treatment of TB, disseminated MAC, and in *M. kansasii* infection. Ethambutol is administered at 15-25 mg/kg per day for both adults and children.

Untoward Effects. Ethambutol produces very few serious untoward reactions. Fewer than 2% of patients who receive daily doses of 15 mg/kg of ethambutol have adverse reactions: ~1% experience diminished visual acuity, 0.5% a rash, and 0.3% drug fever. Other side effects that have been observed are pruritus, joint pain, GI upset, abdominal pain, malaise, headache, dizziness, mental confusion, disorientation, and possible hallucinations. Numbness and tingling of the fingers owing to peripheral neuritis are infrequent. Anaphylaxis and leukopenia are rare. Therapy with ethambutol results in an increased concentration of urate in the blood in ~50% of patients, owing to decreased renal excretion of uric acid.

The most important side effect is optic neuritis, resulting in decreased visual acuity and loss of ability to differentiate red from green. The incidence of this reaction is proportional to the dose of ethambutol and is observed in 15% of patients receiving 50 mg/kg/day, in 5% of patients receiving 25 mg/kg/day, and in <1% of patients receiving daily doses of 15 mg/kg. The intensity of the visual difficulty is related to the duration of therapy after the decreased visual acuity first becomes apparent and may be unilateral or bilateral. Tests of visual acuity and red-green discrimination prior to the start of therapy and periodically thereafter are thus recommended. Recovery usually occurs when ethambutol is withdrawn; the time required is a function of the degree of visual impairment.

Cases of ethambutol overdose are rare; drug interactions involving ethambutol are not significant.

Aminoglycosides: Streptomycin, Amikacin, and Kanamycin

The aminoglycosides streptomycin, amikacin, and kanamycin are used for the treatment of mycobacterial diseases. The MICs for *M. tuberculosis* in Middlebrook broth are 0.25-3.0 mg/L for all three aminoglycosides (Heifets, 1991). For *M. avium* streptomycin and amikacin, MICs are 1-8 mg/L; those of kanamycin are 3-12 mg/L. *M. kansasii* is frequently susceptible to these agents, but other nontuberculous mycobacteria are only occasionally susceptible. The pharmacological properties and therapeutic uses of aminoglycosides are discussed in full in Chapter 54.

Bacterial Resistance. Primary resistance to streptomycin is found in 2-3% of *M. tuberculosis* clinical isolates. Streptomycin and the two other aminoglycosides inhibit protein synthesis by binding to the 30S ribosomal subunit and causing misreading of the genetic code during translation. The 30s ribosomal unit is made of the 16S mRNA (encoded by *rpsL*), which binds to the ribosomal protein S12 (encoded by *rrs*) to optimize tRNA binding and mRNA decoding. Mutations in *rpsL* and *rrs* are associated with high-level aminoglycoside resistance in mycobacteria. However, mutations in these genes are only encountered in half of clinical isolates with aminoglycoside resistance. GidB is an rRNA methyltransferase for 16S rRNA, and mutations in *gidB* gene are associated with low-level streptomycin resistance (Okamoto et al., 2007). The *gidB* mutations lead to high-level streptomycin resistant mutants at a rate 2000 times that in wild type. Mutations in *gidB* are encountered in 33% of streptomycin-resistant clinical isolates of *M. tuberculosis*. Finally, efflux pump–mediated resistance was recently demonstrated in clinical isolates with low-level streptomycin-resistant *M. tuberculosis* and interacted with chromosomal mutations in *gidB* (Spies et al., 2008). Thus resistance to aminoglycosides involves several genetic loci, as well as efflux pumps.

Therapeutic Uses. Therapeutic uses of aminoglycosides in treatment of mycobacterial infections are discussed later.

Clofazimine

Clofazimine (LAMPRENE) is a fat-soluble riminophenazine dye. It was discontinued in 2005 but remains licensed as an orphan drug.

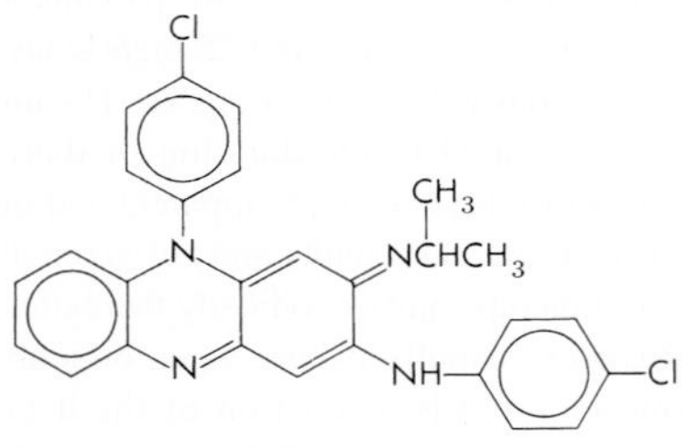

CLOFAZIMINE

Mechanism of Action. The biochemical basis for the antimicrobial actions of clofazimine remains to be established (Anonymous, 2008a). Possible mechanisms of action include:

- membrane disruption
- inhibition of mycobacterial phospholipase A_2
- inhibition of microbial K^+ transport
- generation of hydrogen peroxide
- interference with the bacterial electron transport chain

However, it is known that clofazimine has both antibacterial activity as well as anti-inflammatory effects via inhibition of macrophages, T cells, neutrophils, and complement.

Antibacterial Activity. The MICs for *M. avium* clinical isolates are 1-5 mg/L. The MICs for *M. tuberculosis* are ~1.0 mg/L. The compound also is useful for treatment of chronic skin ulcers (Buruli ulcer) produced by *Mycobacterium ulcerans*. It has activity against many gram-positive bacteria with an MIC ≤1.0 mg/L against *S. aureus*, coagulase-negative Staphylococci, *Streptococcus pyogenes*, and *Listeria monocytogenes*. Gram-negative bacteria have MICs >32 mg/L.

Bacterial Resistance. Mechanisms of resistance are unknown.

Absorption, Distribution, and Excretion. Clofazimine's oral bioavailability is highly variable, 45-60%; bioavailability is increased 2-fold by high-fat meals and decreased 30% by antacids (Nix et al., 2004). After a single dose, clofazimine is best modeled using a one-compartment model and has a prolonged absorption phase; after 200 mg of clofazimine, the t_{max} is 5.3-7.8 hours. After prolonged repeated dosing , the $t_{1/2}$ is ~70 days. For PK data, see Table 56–2 and Nix et al. (2004). As a result of the good penetration into many tissues, a reddish black discoloration of skin and body secretions may occur and take a long time to resolve. Crystalline deposits of the drug have been encountered in many tissues at autopsy (Anonymous, 2008a). Clofazimine is metabolized in the liver in four steps: hydrolytic dehalogenation, hydrolytic deamination, glucuronidation, and hydroxylation.

Dosing. Clofazimine is administered orally at doses up to 300 mg a day.

Untoward Effects. GI problems are encountered in 40-50% of patients and include abdominal pain, diarrhea, nausea, and vomiting. In patients who have died following the abdominal pain, crystal deposition in intestinal mucosa, liver, spleen, and abdominal lymph nodes has been demonstrated (Anonymous, 2008a). Body secretion discoloration, eye discoloration, and skin discoloration occur in most patients and can lead to depression in some patients.

Drug interactions. Anti-inflammatory effects may be inhibited by dapsone.

Fluoroquinolones

Fluoroquinolones are DNA gyrase inhibitors. Their chemistry, spectrum of activity, pharmacology, and adverse events are discussed in greater detail in Chapter 52. Drugs such as ofloxacin and ciprofloxacin have been second-line anti-TB agents for many years, but they are limited by the rapid development of resistance. Adding C8 halogen and C8 methoxy groups markedly reduces the propensity for drug resistance. Of the C8 methoxy quinolones, moxifloxacin (approved by the Food and Drug Administration for nontubercular infections) is furthest along in clinical testing as an anti-TB agent. Moxifloxacin is being studied to replace either isoniazid or ethambutol.

Microbial Pharmacokinetics-Pharmacodynamics Relevant to TB. Fluoroquinolone microbial kill is best explained by AUC_{0-24}/MIC ratio. In preclinical models, moxifloxacin AUC_{0-24}/MIC exposures equivalent to those from the standard 400-mg dose were associated with good microbial kill but amplified the drug-resistant subpopulation, so that resistance emerged in 7-13 days with monotherapy (Gumbo et al., 2004). This time to emergence of resistance harmonizes well with speed of resistance emergence in patients (Ginsburg et al., 2003). Moxifloxacin exposure best associated with minimizing emergence of resistance was an AUC_{0-24}/MIC of 53. Clinical trial simulations revealed that doses >400 mg a day might better achieve this AUC/MIC, which experiments in mice substantiate (Almeida et al., 2007). Given that rifamycins reduce moxifloxacin AUC, these results point to a potential concern of quinolone resistance. Unfortunately, the safety of moxifloxacin doses >400 mg has not been established.

Therapeutic Uses in Treatment of TB. In TB patients, moxifloxacin (400 mg/day) has bactericidal effects similar to that of standard doses of isoniazid (Johnson et al., 2006). When replacing ethambutol in the standard multi-drug regimen, 400 mg/day of moxifloxacin produces faster sputum conversion at 4 weeks than ethambutol (Burman et al., 2006b). In a comparison study of moxifloxacin, gatifloxacin, ofloxacin, and ethambutol as the fourth drug administered concurrently with isoniazid, rifampin, and pyrazinamide (Rustomjee et al., 2008b), moxifloxacin led to faster rates of bacterial kill during the early phases, gatifloxacin was equivalent by the eighth week, and ofloxacin was no better than ethambutol. Moxifloxacin is currently being studied in a phase 3 trial that may eventually lead to 4-month duration of anti-TB therapy compared to the current 6 months.

Drug Interactions Relevant to TB. In a study of volunteers treated with rifampin, moxifloxacin, or both drugs, rifampin reduced the moxifloxacin AUC_{0-24} by 27% via induction of sulfate conjugation (Weiner et al., 2007). In another study, rifapentine reduced moxifloxacin AUC_{0-24} by 17% (Dooley et al., 2008). These studies suggest that the most important cause of pharmacokinetic variability for moxifloxacin is concomitantly administered drugs for tuberculosis.

TMC-207 (R207910)

TMC-207 is a diarylquinone discovered by Andries et al. in 2005.

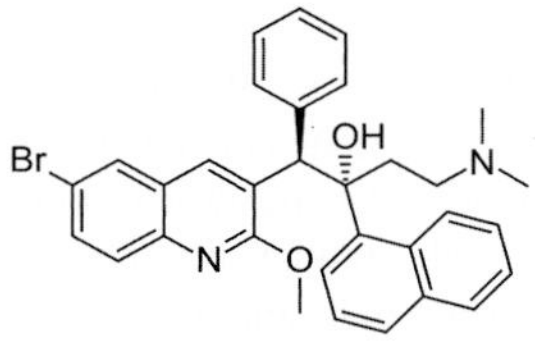

TMC207

Mechanism of Action. TMC-207 acts by targeting subunit c of the ATP synthase of *M. tuberculosis*, leading to inhibition of the proton pump activity of the ATP synthase (Andries et al., 2005; Koul et al., 2007). Thus, the compound targets bacillary energy metabolism.

Antibacterial Activity. The TMC-207 MIC for *M. tuberculosis* is 0.03-0.12 mg/L. It has good activity against *MAC, M. leprae, M. bovis, M. marinum, M. kansasii, M. ulcerans, M. fortuitum, M. szulgai,* and *M. abscessus* (Andries et al., 2005; Huitric et al., 2007).

Bacterial Resistance. The proportion of *M. tuberculosis* mutants resistant to four times the MIC is 5×10^{-7} to 2×10^{-8}. Resistance is associated with two point mutations: D32V and A63P. This region of the gene encodes the membrane-spanning domain of the ATP synthase *c* subunit.

Absorption, Distribution, and Excretion. After oral ingestion of 400 mg of TMC-207, the t_{max} was 4 hours, the C_{max} was 5.5 mg/L after 400 mg/day, and the $AUC_{0\text{-}24}$ was 65 mg·h/L. Based on these data, the CL is ~6.2 L/h, although systemic clearance reportedly is "triexponential." Population pharmacokinetic studies have not been published.

Pharmacokinetics, Efficacy, and Therapeutic Use. The anti-TB activity of TMC-207 is correlated with time above MIC. In murine TB, TMC-207 had superior bactericidal activity compared to isoniazid and rifampin, and accelerated sterilization when combined with rifampin, isoniazid, and pyrazinamide (Andries et al., 2005). In patients with drug-susceptible TB, the rate of sputum bacillary decline was similar to rifampin and isoniazid (Rustomjee et al., 2008a). A regimen of TMC207 400 mg daily for 2 weeks followed by 200 mg three times day thereafter was added to a background second-line regimen of either kanamycin or amikacin, ofloxacin with or without ethambutol in patients with TB resistant to both isoniazid and rifampin (MDR-TB), and led to an 8-week sputum conversion of ~50% with TMC207 compared to 9% without (Diacon et al., 2009).

Untoward Effects. The adverse events encountered with TMC207 are mild and include nausea in 26% of patients and diarrhea in 13% of patients, with others such as arthralgia, pain in extremities, and hyperuricemia in a small proportion of patients (Diacon et al., 2009). However, only a limited number of patients have been exposed to this drug, so that the full side-effect profile is unclear.

PA-824

PA-824 is a nitroimidazopyran discovered by Stover et al. in 2000.

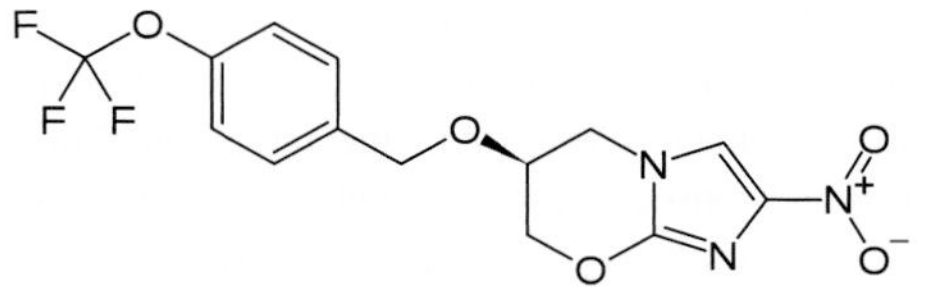

PA-824

Mechanism of Action. PA-824 inhibits *M. tuberculosis* mycolic acid and protein synthesis at the step between hydroxymycolate and keto-mycolate (Stover et al., 2000). Similar to the structurally related metronidazole, PA-824 is a pro-drug that requires activation by the bacteria via a nitro-reduction step that requires, among other factors, a specific glucose-6-phosphate dehydrogenase, FGD1, and the reduced deazaflavin co-factor F_{420} (Bashiri et al., 2008). Another mechanism involves generation of reactive nitrogen species such as NO by PA-824's des-nitro metabolite, which then augment the kill of intracellular nonreplicating persistent bacilli by the innate immune system (Singh et al., 2008).

Antibacterial Activity. *In vitro*, the drug kills both nonreplicating *M. tuberculosis* that are under anaerobic conditions as well as replicating bacteria in ambient air. The MICs of PA-824 against *M. tuberculosis* range from 0.015–0.25 mg/L, but the drug lacks activity against other mycobacteria.

Bacterial Resistance. The proportion of mutants resistant to 5 mg/L of PA-824 is 10^{-6}. Resistance arises due to changes in structure of FGD, which is due to a variety of point mutations in *fgd* gene. However, resistant isolates have also been identified that lack *fgd* mutations, so that resistance may also be due to other mechanisms (Stover et al., 2000).

Pharmacokinetics and Efficacy. In murine and guinea pig TB, PA-824 was equivalent to standard doses of isoniazid (Stover et al., 2000). In a recent murine TB study, 100 mg/kg/day of PA-824 with pyrazinamide and rifampin showed total sterilization at 2 months and no relapse, versus 15% relapse with the standard isoniazid, rifampin, and pyrazinamide regimen (Tasneen et al., 2008). Phase 1 studies have been performed, but the pharmacokinetic data have not been published. Phase 2 studies are in progress.

Ethionamide

Ethionamide (TRECATOR) is a congener of thioisonicotinamide.

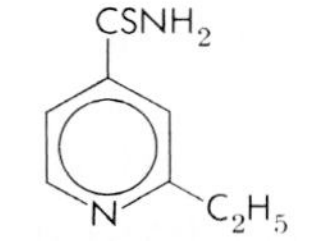

ETHIONAMIDE

Mechanism of Action. Mycobacterial EthaA, an NADPH-specific, FAD-containing monooxygenase, converts ethionamide to a sulfoxide, and then to 2-ethyl-4-aminopyridine (Vannelli et al., 2002). Although these products are not toxic to mycobacteria, it is believed that a closely related and transient intermediate is the active antibiotic. Ethionamide inhibits mycobacterial growth by inhibiting the activity of the *inhA* gene product, the enoyl-ACP reductase of fatty acid synthase II (Larsen et al., 2002). This is the same enzyme that activated isoniazid inhibits. Although the exact mechanisms of inhibition may differ, the results are the same: inhibition of mycolic acid biosynthesis and consequent impairment of cell-wall synthesis.

Antibacterial Activity. The multiplication of *M. tuberculosis* is suppressed by concentrations of ethionamide ranging from 0.6-2.5 mg/L. A concentration of ≤10 mg/L will inhibit ~75% of photochromogenic mycobacteria; the scotochromogens are more resistant.

Bacterial Resistance. Resistance occurs mainly via changes in the enzyme that activates ethionamide, and mutations are encountered in a transcriptional repressor gene that controls its expression, *etaR*. Mutations in *inhA* gene lead to resistance to both ethionamide and isoniazid.

Absorption, Distribution, and Excretion. The oral bioavailability of ethionamide approaches 100%. The pharmacokinetics are adequately explained by a one-compartment model with first-order absorption and elimination (Zhu et al., 2002); see PK values in Table 56–2. After oral administration of 500 mg of ethionamide, a C_{max} of 1.4 mg/L is achieved in 2 hours. The $t_{1/2}$ is ~2 hours. The concentrations in the blood and various organs are approximately equal. Ethionamide is cleared by hepatic metabolism; six metabolites have been identified. Metabolites are eliminated in the urine, with <1% of ethionamide excreted in an active form.

Therapeutic Uses. Ethionamide is administered only orally. The initial dosage for adults is 250 mg twice daily; it is increased by 125 mg/day every 5 days until a dose of 15-20 mg/kg/day is achieved. The maximal dose is 1 g daily. The drug is best taken with meals in divided doses to minimize gastric irritation. Children should receive 10-20 mg/kg/day in two divided doses, not to exceed 1 g/day.

Untoward effects. Approximately 50% of patients are unable to tolerate a single dose larger than 500 mg because of GI upset. The most common reactions are anorexia, nausea and vomiting, gastric irritation, and a variety of neurologic symptoms. Severe postural hypotension, mental depression, drowsiness, and asthenia are common. Convulsions and peripheral neuropathy are rare. Other reactions referable to the nervous system include olfactory disturbances, blurred vision, diplopia, dizziness, paresthesias, headache, restlessness, and tremors. Pyridoxine (vitamin B_6) relieves the neurologic symptoms, and its concomitant administration is recommended. Severe allergic skin rashes, purpura, stomatitis, gynecomastia, impotence, menorrhagia, acne, and alopecia have also been observed. A metallic taste also may be noted. Hepatitis has been associated with the use of the ethionamide in ~5% of cases. Hepatic function should be assessed at regular intervals in patients receiving the drug.

Para-Aminosalicylic Acid

Para-aminosalicylic acid (PAS), discovered by Lehman in 1943, was the first effective treatment for TB.

COOH, OH, NH_2

AMINOSALICYLIC ACID

Mechanism of Action. PAS is a structural analog of *para*-aminobenzoic acid, the substrate of dihydropteroate synthase (*fol*P1/P2). As a result, PAS is thought to be a competitive inhibitor *fol*P1. However, *in vitro* the inhibitory activity against *fol*P1 is very poor. However, mutation of the thymidylate synthase gene (thyA) results in resistance to PAS, but only 37% of the PAS-resistant clinical isolates or spontaneous mutants encode a mutation in *thyA* gene, or in any genes encoding enzymes in the folate pathway or biosynthesis of thymine nucleotides (Mathys et al., 2009). Unidentified actions of PAS likely play more important roles in its anti-TB effects.

Antibacterial Activity. PAS is bacteriostatic. *In vitro*, most strains of *M. tuberculosis* are sensitive to a concentration of 1 mg/L. It has no activity against other bacteria.

Bacterial Resistance. Mutations in *thyA* gene lead to drug resistance in a minority of drug-resistant isolates.

Absorption, Distribution, and Excretion. PAS oral bioavailability is >90%. PAS pharmacokinetics are described by a one-compartment model (Peloquin et al., 2001); see the PK values in Table 56–2. The C_{max} increases 1.5-fold and AUC 1.7-fold with food compared to fasting (Peloquin et al., 2001). These results mean that PAS should be administered with food, which also greatly reduces gastric irritation. Protein binding is 50-60%. PAS is N-acetylated in the liver to N-acetyl PAS, a potential hepatotoxin. Over 80% of the drug is excreted in the urine; >50% is in the form of the acetylated compound. Excretion of PAS acid is reduced by renal dysfunction; thus the dose must be reduced in renal dysfunction.

Therapeutic Uses. PAS is administered orally in a daily dose of 12 g. The drug is best administered after meals, with the daily dose divided into three equal portions. Children should receive 150-300 mg/kg/day in 3-4 divided doses.

Untoward Effects. The incidence of untoward effects associated with the use of PAS is ~10-30%. GI problems predominate and often limit patient adherence. Hypersensitivity reactions to PAS are seen in 5-10% of patients and manifest as skin eruptions, fever, eosinophilia, and other hematological abnormalities.

Cycloserine

Cycloserine (SEROMYCIN) is D-4-amino-3-isoxazolidone. It is a broad-spectrum antibiotic produced by *Streptococcus orchidaceous.*

O, NH, H_2N, O

CYCLOSERINE

Mechanism of Action. Cycloserine and d-alanine are structural analogs; thus cycloserine inhibits alanine racemase which converts L-alanine to d-alanine and d-alanine: d-alanine ligase, stopping reactions in which d-alanine is incorporated into bacterial cell-wall synthesis (Anonymous, 2008b).

Antibacterial Activity. Cycloserine is a broad-spectrum antibiotic. It inhibits *M. tuberculosis* at concentrations of 5-20 mg/L. It has good activity against MAC, enterococci, *E. coli, S. aureus, Nocardia* species, and *Chlamydia*.

Mechanisms of Resistance. Mutations involved in cycloserine resistance to pathogenic *Mycobacteria* are currently unknown. However, resistance in clinical isolates of M. tuberculosis has been detected in 10-82% of isolates (Anonymous, 2008b).

Absorption, Distribution, and Excretion. Oral cycloserine is almost completely absorbed. The population pharmacokinetics are best described using a one-compartment model with first-order absorption and elimination (Zhu et al., 2001). The drug's $t_{1/2}$ is 9 hours. C_{max} in plasma is reached in 45 minutes in fasting subjects, but is delayed for up to 3.5 hours with a high-fat meal. See Table 56–2 for PK values. Cycloserine is well distributed throughout body. There is no appreciable barrier to CNS entry for cycloserine, and cerebrospinal fluid (CSF) concentrations are approximately the same as those in plasma. About 50% of cycloserine is excreted unchanged in the urine in the first 12 hours; a total of 70% is recoverable in the active form over a period of 24 hours. The drug may accumulate to toxic concentrations in patients with renal failure. About 60% of it is removed by hemodialysis, and the drug must be re-dosed after each hemodialysis session (Malone et al., 1999a).

Therapeutic Uses. Cycloserine is available for oral administration. The usual dose for adults is 250-500 mg twice daily.

Untoward Effects. Neuropsychiatric symptoms are common and occur in 50% of patients on 1 g/day, so much so that the drug has earned the nickname "psych-serine." Symptoms range from headache and somnolence to severe psychosis, seizures, and suicidal ideas. Large doses of cycloserine or the concomitant ingestion of alcohol increases the risk of seizures. Cycloserine is contraindicated in individuals with a history of epilepsy and should be used with caution in individuals with a history of depression.

Capreomycin

Capreomycin (CAPASTAT) is an antimycobacterial cyclic peptide. It consists of four active components: capreomycins IA, IB, IIA, and IIB. The agent used clinically contains primarily IA and IB. Antimycobacterial activity is similar to that of aminoglycosides as are adverse effects, and capreomycin should not be administered with other drugs that damage cranial nerve VIII.

Bacterial resistance to capreomycin develops when it is given alone; such microorganisms show cross-resistance with kanamycin and neomycin. The adverse reactions associated with the use of capreomycin are hearing loss, tinnitus, transient proteinuria, cylindruria, and nitrogen retention. Severe renal failure is rare. Eosinophilia is common. Leukocytosis, leukopenia, rashes, and fever have also been observed. Injections of the drug may be painful. Capreomycin is a second-line antituberculosis agent. The recommended daily dose is 1g (no more than 20 mg/kg) per day for 60-120 days, followed by 1 g two to three times a week.

Macrolides

The pharmacology, bacterial activity, resistance mechanisms of macrolides are discussed in Chapter 55. Azithromycin and clarithromycin are used for the treatment of MAC.

Dapsone

Dapsone (DDS, diamino-diphenylsulfone) or 4′-diaminodiphenylsulfone, was synthesized by Fromm and Wittman in 1908, and its similarity to sulphonamides led to the establishment of anti-streptococcal effects by Buttle et al. and Forneau et al. in 1937.

H_2N — NH_2

DAPSONE

Mechanism of Action. Dapsone is a structural analog of *para*-aminobenzoic acid (PABA) and a competitive inhibitor of dihydropteroate synthase (*fol*P1/P2) in the folate pathway, shown in Figure 56–5. The effect on this evolutionarily conserved pathway also explains why dapsone is a broad-spectrum agent with antibacterial, anti-protozoal, and antifungal effects.

The anti-inflammatory effects of dapsone occur via inhibition of tissue damage by neutrophils (summarized by Wolf et al., 2002). First, dapsone inhibits neutrophil myeloperoxidase activity and respiratory burst. Second, it inhibits activity of neutrophil lysosomal enzymes. Third, it may also act as a free radical scavenger, counteracting the effect of free radicals generated by neutrophils. Fourth, dapsone may also inhibit migration of neutrophils to inflammatory lesions (Wolf et al., 2002). Dapsone is extensively used for acne, but this therapy is not recommended.

Antimicrobial Effects. *Antibacterial.* Dapsone is bacteriostatic against *M. leprae* at concentrations of 1-10 mg/L. More than 90% of clinical isolates of MAC and *M. kansasii* have an MIC of ≤8 mg/L, but the MICs for *M. tuberculosis* isolates are high. It has little activity against other bacteria.

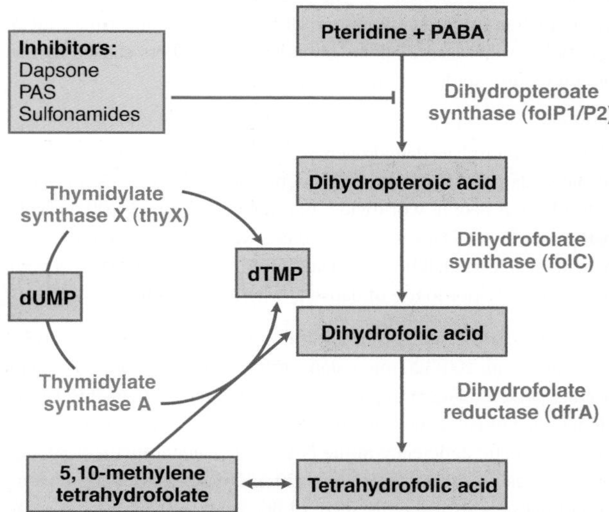

Figure 56–5. *Effects of antimicrobials on folate metabolism and deoxynucleotide synthesis.*

Anti-parasitic. Dapsone is also highly effective against *Plasmodium falciparum* with IC_{50} of 0.006-0.013 mg/mL (0.6-1.3 mg/L) even in sulfadoxine-pyrimethamine–resistant strains. Dapsone has an IC_{50} of 0.55 mg/L against *Toxoplasma gondii* tachyzoites.

Antifungal. Dapsone is effective at concentrations of 0.1/mg/L against the fungus *Pneumocystic jiroveci*.

Drug Resistance. Resistance to dapsone in *P. falciparum*, *P. jiroveci*, and *M. leprae* results primarily from mutations in genes encoding dihydropteroate synthase (Figure 56–5). In *P. falciparum* mutations occur at several positions such as 436, 437, 540, 58, and 613. In *P. jiroveci* isolates, mutations are often amino acid substitutions at positions 55 and 57. In *M. leprae*, mutations are encountered at codons 53 and 55.

Absorption, Distribution, and Excretion. After oral administration, absorption is complete; the elimination $t_{1/2}$ is 20-30 hours. The population pharmacokinetics of dapsone are shown in Table 56–2 (Simpson et al., 2006). CL increases 0.03 L/hour and V_d 0.7 L increases for each 1-kg increase in body weight above 62.3 kg. Dapsone undergoes N-acetylation by NAT2. N-oxidation to dapsone hydroxylamine is via CYP2E1, and to a lesser extent by CYP2C. Dapsone hydroxylamine enters red blood cells, leading to methemoglobin formation. Sulfones tend to be retained for up to 3 weeks in skin and muscle and especially in liver and kidney. Intestinal reabsorption of sulfones excreted in the bile contributes to long-term retention in the bloodstream; periodic interruption of treatment is advisable for this reason. Epithelial lining fluid to plasma ratio is between 0.76 and 2.91; CSF-to-plasma ratio is 0.21-2.01 (Gatti et al., 1997). Approximately 70-80% of a dose of dapsone is excreted in the urine as an acid-labile mono-*N*-glucuronide and mono-*N*-sulfamate.

Therapeutic Uses. Dapsone is administered as an oral agent. Therapeutic uses of dapsone in the treatment of leprosy are described later. Dapsone is combined with chlorproguanil for the treatment of malaria. Dapsone is also used for *P. jiroveci* infection and prophylaxis, and for the prophylaxis for *T. gondii,* as discussed in chapters devoted to these infections. The anti-inflammatory effects are the basis for therapy for pemphigoid, dermatitis herpetiformis, linear IgA bullous disease, relapsing chondritis, and ulcers caused by the brown recluse spider (Wolf et al., 2002).

Dapsone and Glucose-6-Phosphate Dehydrogenase Deficiency. Glucose-6-phosphate dehydrogenase (G6PD) protects red cells against oxidative damage. However, G6PD deficiency is encountered in nearly half a billion people worldwide, the most common of 100 variants being G6PD-A$^-$. Dapsone, an oxidant, causes severe hemolysis in patients with G6PD deficiency. Thus, G6PD deficiency testing should be performed prior to use of dapsone wherever possible.

Other Untoward Effects. Hemolysis develops in almost every individual treated with 200-300 mg of dapsone per day. Doses of ≤100 mg in healthy persons and ≤50 mg in healthy individuals with a G6PD deficiency do not cause hemolysis. Methemoglobinemia also is common. A genetic deficiency in the NADH-dependent methemoglobin reductase can result in severe methemoglobinemia after administration of dapsone. Isolated instances of headache, nervousness, insomnia, blurred vision, paresthesias, reversible peripheral neuropathy (thought to be due to axonal degeneration), drug fever, hematuria, pruritus, psychosis, and a variety of skin rashes have been reported. An infectious mononucleosis-like syndrome, which may be fatal, occurs occasionally.

PRINCIPLES OF ANTITUBERCULOSIS CHEMOTHERAPY

Evolution and Pharmacology. *Mycobacterium tuberculosis* is not a single species, but a complex of species with 99.9% similarity at nucleotide level. The complex includes *M. tuberculosis (typus humanus)*, *M. canettii, M. africanum, M. bovis,* and *M. microti*. They all cause tuberculosis (TB), with *M. microti* responsible for only a handful of human cases.

Antituberculosis Therapy. Isoniazid, pyrazinamide, rifampin, ethambutol, and streptomycin are currently considered first-line anti-TB agents. Moxifloxacin is being studied as a first-line agent. First-line agents are more efficacious and better tolerated, relative to second-line agents. Second-line agents are used in case of poor tolerance or resistance to first-line agents. Second-line drugs include ethionamide, PAS, cycloserine, amikacin, kanamycin, and capreomycin.

When anti-TB drug monotherapy was administered to TB patients, resistance emergence terminated the effectiveness of these drugs. The mutation rates to first-line anti-TB drugs are between 10^{-7} and 10^{-10}, so that the likelihood of resistance is high to any single anti-TB drugs in patients with cavitary TB who have ~10^9 CFU of bacilli in a 3-cm pulmonary lesion. However, the likelihood that bacilli would develop mutations to two or more different drugs is the product of two mutation rates (between 1 in 10^{14} and 1 in 10^{20}), which makes the probability of resistance emergence to more than two drugs acceptably small. Thus, only combination therapy anti-TB therapy is currently recommended for treatment of TB. Multidrug therapy has led to a reduction in length of therapy.

Types of Antituberculosis Therapy

Prophylaxis. After infection with *M. tuberculosis*, ~10% of people will develop active disease over a lifetime. The highest risk of reactivation TB is in patients with Mantoux tuberculin skin test reaction ≥5 mm who also fall into one of the following categories: recently exposed to TB, have HIV co-infection, have fibrotic changes on chest radiograms, or are immunosuppressed due to HIV infection, post-transplantation, or are taking immunosuppressive medications for any reason. If the tuberculin skin test is ≥10 mm, high risk of TB is encountered in recent (≤5 years) immigrants from areas of high TB prevalence, children <4 years of age, children exposed to adults with TB, intravenous drug users, as well as residents and employees of high-risk congregate settings. Any person with a skin test >15 mm is also at high risk of disease. In these patients at high risk of active TB, prophylaxis is recommended to prevent active disease. Prophylaxis consists of oral isoniazid, 300 mg daily or twice weekly, for 6 months in adults. Those who cannot take isoniazid should be given rifampin, 10 mg/kg daily, for 4 months. In children, isoniazid 10-15 mg/kg daily (maximum 300 mg) is administered, or 20-30 mg/kg two times a week directly observed, for 9 months. In children who cannot tolerate isoniazid, rifampin 10-20 mg/kg daily for 6 months is recommended.

Definitive Therapy. All active TB cases should be confirmed by culture and have antimicrobial susceptibilities determined. The current standard regimen for drug-susceptible TB consists of isoniazid (5 mg/kg, maximum 300 mg/day), rifampin (10 mg/kg, maximum 600 mg/day), and pyrazinamide (15-30 mg/kg, maximum of 2 g/day) for 2 months, followed by intermittent 10 mg/kg rifampin and 15 mg/kg isoniazid two or three times a week for 4 months. Children should receive 10-20 mg/kg isoniazid per day (300 mg maximum). Rifabutin 5 mg/kg/day can be used for the entire 6 months of therapy in adult HIV-infected patients because rifampin can adversely interact with some antiretroviral agents to reduce their effectiveness. In case there is resistance to isoniazid, initial therapy also may include ethambutol (15-20 mg/kg/day) or streptomycin (1 g/day) until isoniazid susceptibility is documented. Ethambutol doses in children are 15-20 mg/kg/day (maximum 1 g) or 50 mg/kg twice weekly (2.5 g). Because monitoring of visual acuity is difficult in children <5 years old, caution should be exercised in using ethambutol in these children.

The first 2 months of the four-drug regimen is termed the initial phase of therapy, and the last 4 months the continuation phase of therapy. Rifapentine (10 mg/kg once a week) may be substituted for rifampin in the continuation phase in patients with no evidence of HIV infection or cavitary TB. Pyridoxine, vitamin B_6, (10-50 mg/day) should be administered with isoniazid to minimize the risks of neurological toxicity in patients predisposed to neuropathy (e.g., the malnourished, elderly, pregnant women, HIV-infected individuals, diabetic patients, alcoholic patients, and uremic patients). To ensure compliance, therapy is administered as directly observed therapy (DOT). Although DOT is the standard of care, an analysis of a series of 11 randomized clinical trials found no difference in outcome between DOT and self-administered therapy (Volmink and Garner, 2007).

The duration of therapy for drug-susceptible pulmonary TB is 6 months. A 9-month duration should be used for patients with cavitary disease who are still sputum culture positive at 2 months. HIV-infected patients with CD4+ lymphocyte cell counts <100/mm^3 are at increased risk of developing rifamycin resistance. Therefore, daily therapy is recommended during the continuation phase. Most cases of extrapulmonary TB are treated for 6 months. TB meningitis is an exception that requires a 9- to 12-month duration. In addition, corticosteroids are recommended for TB pericarditis, and results of a meta-analysis suggest they should also be used in TB meningitis (Prasad and Singh, 2008).

Drug-Resistant TB. According to the fourth global report of the World Health Organization (WHO), from 2002 to 2006, the proportion of new TB cases resistant to at least one anti-TB drug was 17%; isoniazid resistance was 10%, and MDR (multidrug resistant) was 3%. MDR-TB is said to be present if an isolate is resistant simultaneously to isoniazid and rifampin. According to the CDC, in the U.S., resistance to isoniazid was 8% and MDR was 1%. In previously treated patients, resistance to at least one drug was 35%, isoniazid resistance was 28%, and MDR was 15%; resistance to isoniazid in previously treated cases was 13%, and MDR was 4%; of the MDR, only 3% was extensively drug resistant TB [XDR]. XDR-TB is MDR-TB that is also resistant to fluoroquinolones and at least one of three injectable second-line drugs (i.e., amikacin, kanamycin, or capreomycin).

In documented drug resistance, therapy should be based on evidence of susceptibility and should include:

- at least three drugs to which the pathogen is susceptible, with at least one of the injectable anti-TB agents
- in the case of MDR-TB, use of four to six medications for better outcomes
- at least 18 months of therapy (Blumberg et al., 2003; Orenstein et al., 2009)

The addition to the regimen of a fluoroquinolone and surgical resection of the main lesions have been associated with improved outcome (Chan et al., 2004). There are currently no data to support intermittent therapy.

PRINCIPLES OF THERAPY AGAINST *MYCOBACTERIUM AVIUM* COMPLEX

The *Mycobacterium avium* complex (MAC) is made up of at least two species: *M. intracellulare* and *M. avium*. *M. intracellulare* causes pulmonary disease often in immunocompetent individuals. *M. avium* is further divided into a number of subspecies: *M. avium* subsp. *hominissuis* causes disseminated disease in immunocompromised patients, *M. avium* subsp. *paratuberculosis* has been implicated in the etiology of Crohn's disease, and *M. avium* subsp. *avium* causes TB of birds. These bacteria are ubiquitous in the environment and can be encountered in water, food, and soil. Therefore, when MAC bacteria are isolated from a nonsterile site in patient's body, one cannot assume they are causing an infection.

Therapy of MAC Pulmonary Infection

M. intracellulare often infects immunocompetent patients. The first decision after isolating MAC from pulmonary specimens is to determine whether disease is actually present or if the organism is merely part of environmental contamination. Criteria in favor of therapy includes bacteriological evidence, which consists of positive cultures from at least two sputums, or one positive culture from bronchoalveolar lavage or pulmonary biopsy with a positive culture or histopathological features, *and* clinical evidence of infection, *and* radiological evidence of infection such as pulmonary cavitation, nodular lesions, and/or bronchiectasis (Griffith et al., 2007).

In newly diagnosed patients with MAC pneumonia, triple drug therapy is recommended. These include a rifamycin, ethambutol, and a macrolide (Griffith et al., 2007; Kasperbauer and Daley, 2008). For the macrolides, either oral clarithromycin or azithromycin may be used. Rifampin is often the rifamycin of choice. Clarithromycin, 1000 mg, or azithromycin, 500 mg, are combined with ethambutol, 25 mg/kg, and rifampin, 600 mg, and administered three times a week for nodular and bronchiectatic disease. Therapy is continued for 12 months after the last negative culture. The same drugs are administered for patients with cavitary disease, but the dosing regimens are azithromycin 250 mg, ethambutol 15 mg/kg, and rifampin 600 mg. Parenteral streptomycin or amikacin at 15 mg/kg are recommended as a fourth drug. The effect of the aminoglycosides on clinical outcomes is unclear. Duration of therapy is as for nodular disease. In advanced pulmonary disease or during re-treatment, rifabutin 300 mg daily may replace rifampin. Because clarithromycin susceptibility correlates with outcome, risk of failure is high when high clarithromycin MICs are documented. Patients at risk for failure also include those with cavitary disease, presumably due to higher bacillary load. Even with these therapies, long-term success is still fairly limited. Only half of patients have successful outcomes as defined by both culture conversion and clinical outcomes.

Therapy for Disseminated *M. Avium* Complex

Disseminated MAC disease is caused by *M. avium* in 95% of patients. This is a disease of the immunocompromised patient, especially with reduced cell-mediated immunity. MAC usually occurs in patients whose CD4 cell count is <50/mm^3. Patients at risk for infection are those who have had other opportunistic infections, are colonized with MAC, or have an HIV RNA burden >5 log copies/mm^3.

The symptoms and laboratory findings of disseminated disease are nonspecific and include fever, night sweats, weight loss, elevated serum alkaline phosphates, and anemia at the time of diagnosis. However, when disease occurs in patients already on antiretroviral therapy, it may manifest as a focal disease of the lymph nodes, osteomyelitis, pneumonitis, pericarditis, skin or soft-tissue abscesses, genital ulcers, or CNS infection (DHHS Panel, 2008). In addition to a compatible clinical picture, isolation of MAC from cultures of blood, lymph node, bone marrow, or other normally sterile tissue or body fluids is required for diagnosis.

Prophylactic Therapy. The goals of prophylactic therapy are to prevent the development of disease during the time when a patient's CD4 count is low. Monotherapy with either oral azithromycin 1200 mg once a week or clarithromycin 500 mg twice a day is started when patients present with a CD4 count <50/mm^3 (DHHS Panel, 2008). For patients intolerant to macrolides, rifabutin 300 mg a day is administered. Once the CD4 count is >100 per mm^3 for ≥3 months, MAC prophylaxis should be discontinued.

Definitive and Suppressive Therapy. In patients with disease due to MAC, the goals of therapy include suppression of symptoms and conversion to negative blood cultures. The infection itself is not completely eradicated until immune reconstitution. Therapy is divided into initial therapy and chronic suppressive therapy. Recommended therapy consists of a combination of clarithromycin 500 mg twice a day with ethambutol 15 mg/kg daily, administered orally (DHHS Panel, 2008). Azithromycin 500-600 mg daily is an acceptable alternative to clarithromycin, especially in those patients in whom clarithromycin would adversely interact with other drugs. The addition of rifabutin 300 mg a day may improve outcomes. Mortality in disseminated MAC is high in patients with either a CD4 cell count <50/mm^3 or a MAC burden of >2 $\log_{10}$ CFU/mm^3 of blood, or in the absence of effective antiretroviral therapy. In these patients, a fourth drug may be added, based on susceptibility testing. Potential fourth agents include amikacin, 10-15 mg/kg intravenously daily; streptomycin, 1 g intravenously or intramuscularly daily; ciprofloxacin, 500-750 mg orally twice daily; levofloxacin, 500 mg orally daily; or moxifloxacin, 400g orally daily. Patients should be continued on suppressive therapy until all three of the following criteria are met:

- therapy duration of at least 12 months
- CD4 count >100/mm^3 for at least 6 months
- asymptomatic for MAC infection

PRINCIPLES OF ANTI-LEPROSY THERAPY

The global prevalence of leprosy has markedly declined, largely due to the global initiative of the WHO to eliminate leprosy (Hansen's disease) as a public health problem by providing multidrug therapy (rifampin, clofazimine, and dapsone) free of charge. Prevalence of the disease has dropped by ~90% since 1985. Nevertheless, there are pockets of disease around the world, especially in Africa, Asia, and South America. In the U.S., <200 new cases were reported in 2005, mainly among immigrants.

Four major clinical types of leprosy impact therapy. At one end of the spectrum is *tuberculoid leprosy,* also termed paucibacillary leprosy because the bacterial burden is low and *M. leprae* is rarely found in smears. On the other end of the spectrum is the *lepromatous* form of the disease (Levis and Ernst, 2005). This is characterized by a disseminated infection and a high bacillary burden. Two major intermediate forms of the disease are recognized: borderline (dimorphous) tuberculoid disease, which has features of both tuberculoid and lepromatous leprosy, and indeterminate disease, which has early hypopigmented lesions without features of the lepromatous and tuberculoid leprosy.

Mycobacterium leprae was discovered by Armauer Hansen in 1873. The *M. leprae* genome has undergone reductive evolution and has radically downsized its genome (Cole et al., 2001). As a result, *M. leprae* cannot produce ATP from NADH or utilize acetate or galactose as carbon sources; moreover, it has lost the anaerobic electron transfer system and cannot survive under hypoxic conditions. It has a long doubling time (14 days) and is an obligate intracellular pathogen. As a result, *M. leprae* is difficult to culture on synthetic media, an impediment to basic research on the disease.

Types of Anti-Leprosy Therapy

Therapy for leprosy is based on multi-drug regimens using rifampin, clofazimine, and dapsone. The reasons for using combinations of agents include reduction in the development of resistance, the need for adequate therapy when primary resistance already exists, and reduction in the duration of therapy. The most bactericidal drug in current regimens is rifampin. Because of high kill rates and massive release of bacterial antigens, rifampin is not often given during a "reversal" reaction (see below) or in patients with erythema nodosum leprosum. Clofazimine is only bacteriostatic against *M. leprae*. However, it also has anti-inflammatory effects and can treat reversal reactions and erythema nodosum leprosum. The third major agent in the regimen is dapsone. The objective of administering these drugs is total cure.

Definitive Therapy; Standard Therapy

Pauci-Bacillary Leprosy. The WHO regimen consists of a single dose of oral rifampin, 600 mg, combined with dapsone, 100 mg, administered under direct supervision once every month for 6 months, and dapsone, 100 mg a day, in between for 6 months. In the U.S., the regimen consists of dapsone, 100 mg, and rifampin, 600 mg, daily for 6 months, followed by dapsone monotherapy for 3-5 years.

Multibacillary Therapy. The WHO recommends the same regimen as for paucibacillary leprosy, with two major changes. First, clofazimine, 300 mg a day, is added for the entirety of therapy. Second, the regimen lasts 1 year instead of 6 months. In the U.S., the regimen is also the same as for paucibacillary, but dual therapy continues for 3 years, followed by dapsone monotherapy for 10 years. Clofazimine (an orphan drug) is added when there is dapsone resistance or chronically reactional patients.

The duration of therapy for multi-bacillary leprosy is a drawback. Studies in murine leprosy, and in patients, have demonstrated that viable bacilli are killed within 3 months of therapy (Ji et al., 1996) suggesting that the length of current therapy for multibacillary leprosy may be unnecessarily long. Recently, the WHO proposed that all forms of leprosy be treated with the same dose as for paucibacillary leprosy; a clinical trial was promising (Kroger et al., 2008). This new shorter regimen promises to reduce duration of therapy radically.

Treatment of Reactions in Leprosy. Patients with tuberculoid leprosy may develop "reversal reactions," manifestations of delayed

Table 56–5

Drugs Used in the Treatment of Mycobacteria Other Than for Tuberculosis, Leprosy, or MAC

MYCOBACTERIAL SPECIES	FIRST-LINE THERAPY	ALTERNATIVE AGENTS
M. kansasii	Isoniazid + rifampin[a] + ethambutol	Trimethoprim-sulfamethoxazole; ethionamide; cycloserine; clarithromycin; amikacin; streptomycin; moxifloxacin or gatifloxacin
M. fortuitum complex	Amikacin + doxycycline	Cefoxitin; rifampin; a sulfonamide; moxifloxacin or gatifloxacin; clarithromycin; trimethoprim-sulfamethoxazole; imipenem
M. marinum	Rifampin + ethambutol	Trimethoprim-sulfamethoxazole; clarithromycin; minocycline; doxycycline
Mycobacterium ulcerans	Rifampin + streptomycin[c]	Clarithromycin[b]; rifapentine[b]
M. malmoense	Rifampin + ethambutol ± clarithromycin	Fluoroquinolone
M. haemophilum	Clarithromycin + rifampin + quinolone	-

[a]In HIV-infected patients, the substitution of rifabutin for rifampin minimizes drug interactions with the HIV protease inhibitors and non-nucleoside reverse transcriptase inhibitors. [b]Based on animal models. [c]For *Mycobacterium ulcerans*, surgery is the primary therapy.

hypersensitivity to antigens of *M. leprae*. Cutaneous ulcerations and deficits of peripheral nerve function may occur. Early therapy with corticosteroids or clofazimine is effective. Reactions in the lepromatous form of the disease (erythema nodosum leprosum) are characterized by the appearance of raised, tender, intracutaneous nodules, severe constitutional symptoms, and high fever. This reaction may be triggered by several conditions but is often associated with therapy. It is thought to be an Arthus-type reaction related to release of microbial antigens in patients harboring large numbers of bacilli. Treatment with clofazimine or thalidomide is effective.

Therapy for Other Nontuberculous Mycobacteria

Mycobacteria other than those already discussed can be recovered from a variety of lesions in humans. Because they frequently are resistant to many of the commonly used agents, they must be examined for sensitivity *in vitro* and drug therapy selected on this basis. Therapy for infections from these organisms is summarized in Table 56–5. In some instances, surgical removal of the infected tissue followed by long-term treatment with effective agents is necessary. *M. kansasii* causes disease similar to that caused by *M. tuberculosis*, but it may be milder. The microorganisms may be resistant to isoniazid. Therapy with isoniazid, rifampin, and ethambutol has been successful.

CLINICAL SUMMARY

Combination therapy is almost always the desirable approach for mycobacterial disease, to ensure effective eradication and to prevent the emergence of resistance. Isoniazid, rifampin, ethambutol, streptomycin, and pyrazinamide are first-line agents for the treatment of tuberculosis. Moxifloxacin promises to replace either isoniazid or ethambutol and shorten therapy. Antimicrobial agents with excellent activity against *Mycobacterium avium* complex include rifabutin, clarithromycin, azithromycin, and fluoroquinolones. Clinical monitoring of patients with mycobacterial infections is important because drug interactions and adverse drug reactions are common with the multiple-drug regimens used. Considerable progress has been achieved in eliminating leprosy through the use of multiple-drug chemotherapy including dapsone, rifampin, and clofazimine.

BIBLIOGRAPHY

Almeida D, Nuermberger E, Tyagi S, et al. In vivo validation of the mutant selection window hypothesis with moxifloxacin in a murine model of tuberculosis. *Antimicrob Agents Chemother*, **2007,** *51*:4261–4266.

Andries K, Verhasselt P, Guillemont J, et al. A diarylquinoline drug active on the ATP synthase of Mycobacterium tuberculosis. *Science,* **2005,** *307*:223–227.

Anonymous. Clofazimine. *Tuberculosis (Edinb),* **2008a,** *88*:96–99.

Anonymous. Cycloserine. *Tuberculosis (Edinb),* **2008b,** *88*: 100–101.

Argyrou A, Vetting MW, Aladegbami B, Blanchard JS. Mycobacterium tuberculosis dihydrofolate reductase is a target for isoniazid. *Nat Struct Mol Biol,* **2006,** *13*:408–413.

Argyrou A, Vetting MW, Blanchard JS. New insight into the mechanism of action of and resistance to isoniazid: Interaction of *Mycobacterium tuberculosis* enoyl-ACP reductase with INH-NADP. *J Am Chem Soc,* **2007,** *129*:9582–9583.

Bashiri G, Squire CJ, Moreland NJ, Baker EN. Crystal structures of F_{420}-dependent glucose-6-phosphate dehydrogenase FGD1 involved in the activation of the anti-tuberculosis drug candidate PA-824 reveal the basis of coenzyme and substrate binding. *J Biol Chem,* **2008,** *283*:17531–17541.

Blumberg HM, Burman WJ, Chaisson RE, et al; American Thoracic Society/Centers for Disease Control and Prevention/Infectious Diseases Society of America. Treatment of tuberculosis. *Am J Respir Crit Care Med,* **2003,** *167*:603–662.

Boshoff HI, Reed MB, Barry CE III, Mizrahi V. DnaE2 polymerase contributes to in vivo survival and the emergence of drug resistance in *Mycobacterium tuberculosis*. *Cell,* **2003,** *113*:183–193.

Burman W, Benator D, Vernon A, *et al*. Acquired rifamycin resistance with twice-weekly treatment of HIV-related tuberculosis. *Am J Respir Crit Care Med,* **2006a,** *173*:350–356.

Burman WJ, Gallicano K, Peloquin C. Comparative pharmacokinetics and pharmacodynamics of the rifamycin antibacterials. *Clin Pharmacokinet,* **2001,** *40*:327–341.

Burman WJ, Goldberg S, Johnson JL, et al. Moxifloxacin versus ethambutol in the first 2 months of treatment for pulmonary tuberculosis. *Am J Respir Crit Care Med,* **2006b,** *174*:331–338.

Chan ED, Laurel V, Strand MJ, et al. Treatment and outcome analysis of 205 patients with multidrug-resistant tuberculosis. *Am J Respir Crit Care Med,* **2004,** *169*:1103–1109.

Colangeli R, Helb D, Sridharan S, et al. The *Mycobacterium tuberculosis* iniA gene is essential for activity of an efflux pump that confers drug tolerance to both isoniazid and ethambutol. *Mol Microbiol,* **2005,** *55*:1829–1840.

Cole ST, Eiglmeier K, Parkhill J, et al. Massive gene decay in the leprosy bacillus. *Nature,* **2001,** *409*:1007–1011.

Conte JE Jr, Golden JA, McQuitty M, et al. Effects of gender, AIDS, and acetylator status on intrapulmonary concentrations of isoniazid. *Antimicrob Agents Chemother,* **2002,** *46*:2358–2364.

Conte JE Jr, Lin E, Zurlinden E. High-performance liquid chromatographic determination of pyrazinamide in human plasma, bronchoalveolar lavage fluid, and alveolar cells. *J Chromatogr Sci,* **2000,** *38*:33–37.

Desta Z, Soukhova NV, Flockhart DA. Inhibition of cytochrome P450 (CYP450) isoforms by isoniazid: potent inhibition of CYP2C19 and CYP3A. *Antimicrob Agents Chemother,* **2001,** *45*:382–392.

DHHS Panel. Guidelines for Prevention and Treatment of Opportunistic Infections in HIV-Infected Adults and Adolescents. **2008.** Available at: http://aidsinfo.nih.gov/contentfiles/Adult_OI.pdf. Accessed March 16, 2008.

Diacon AH, Patientia RF, Venter A, et al. Early bactericidal activity of high-dose rifampin in patients with pulmonary tuberculosis evidenced by positive sputum smears. *Antimicrob Agents Chemother,* **2007,** *51*:2994–2996.

Diacon AH, Pym A, Grobusch M, et al. The diarylquinoline TMC207 for multidrug-resistant tuberculosis. *N Engl J Med,* **2009,** *360*:2397–2405.

Dooley K, Flexner C, Hackman J, et al. Repeated administration of high-dose intermittent rifapentine reduces rifapentine and moxifloxacin plasma concentrations. *Antimicrob Agents Chemother,* **2008,** *52*:4037–4042.

Gatti G, Hossein J, Malena M, Cruciani M, Bassetti M. Penetration of dapsone into cerebrospinal fluid of patients with AIDS. *J Antimicrob Chemother*, **1997,** *40*:113–115.

Ginsburg AS, Woolwine SC, Hooper N, et al. The rapid development of fluoroquinolone resistance in *M. tuberculosis*. *N Engl J Med,* **2003,** *349*:1977–1978.

Griffith DE, Aksamit T, Brown-Elliott BA, et al. An official ATS/IDSA statement: Diagnosis, treatment, and prevention of nontuberculous mycobacterial diseases. *Am J Respir Crit Care Med,* **2007,** *175*:367–416.

Gumbo T, Louie A, Deziel MR, et al. Concentration-dependent *Mycobacterium tuberculosis* killing and prevention of resistance by rifampin. *Antimicrob Agents Chemother,* **2007a,** *51*:3781–3788.

Gumbo T, Louie A, Deziel MR, et al. Selection of a moxifloxacin dose that suppresses drug resistance in *Mycobacterium tuberculosis*, by use of an in vitro pharmacodynamic infection model and mathematical modeling. *J Infect Dis,* **2004,** *190*:1642–1651.

Gumbo T, Louie A, Liu W, et al. Isoniazid bactericidal activity and resistance emergence: integrating pharmacodynamics and pharmacogenomics to predict efficacy in different ethnic populations. *Antimicrob Agents Chemother,* **2007b,** *51*: 2329–2336.

Gumbo T, Louie A, Liu W, *et al.* Isoniazid's bactericidal activity ceases because of the emergence of resistance, not depletion of *Mycobacterium tuberculosis* in the log phase of growth. *J Infect Dis,* **2007c,** *195*:194–201.

Gumbo T, Siyambalapitiyage Dona CS, Meek C, Leff R. Pharmacokinetics-pharmacodynamics of pyrazinamide in a novel *in vitro* model of tuberculosis for sterilizing effect: a paradigm for faster assessment of a new antituberculosis drugs. *Antimicrob Agents Chemother*, **2009,** *53*:3197–3204.

Hazbón MH, Brimacombe M, Bobadilla del Valle M, et al. Population genetics study of isoniazid resistance mutations and evolution of multidrug-resistant *Mycobacterium tuberculosis*. *Antimicrob Agents Chemother*, **2006,** *50*:2640–2649.

Heifets LB. Antituberculosis drugs: Antimicrobial activity *in vitro*. In: *Drug Susceptibility in the Chemotherapy of Mycobacterial Infections* (Heifets LB, ed.), CRC Press, Boca Raton, FL, **1991,** pp.13–57.

Huitric E, Verhasselt P, Andries K, Hoffner SE. In vitro antimycobacterial spectrum of a diarylquinoline ATP synthase inhibitor. *Antimicrob Agents Chemother,* **2007,** *51*:4202–4204.

Jayaram R, Shandil RK, Gaonkar S, et al. Isoniazid pharmacokinetics-pharmacodynamics in an aerosol infection model of tuberculosis. *Antimicrob Agents Chemother,* **2004,** *48*:2951–2957.

Ji B, Perani EG, Petinom C, Grosset JH. Bactericidal activities of combinations of new drugs against *Mycobacterium leprae* in nude mice. *Antimicrob Agents Chemother,* **1996,** *40*:393–399.

Johnson JL, Hadad DJ, Boom WH, et al. Early and extended early bactericidal activity of levofloxacin, gatifloxacin and moxifloxacin in pulmonary tuberculosis. *Int J Tuberc Lung Dis,* **2006,** *10*:605–612.

Kasperbauer SH, Daley CL. Diagnosis and treatment of infections due to *Mycobacterium avium* complex. *Semin Respir Crit Care Med,* **2008,** *29*:569–576.

Kinzig-Schippers M, Tomalik-Scharte D, Jetter A, *et al.* Should we use N-acetyltransferase type 2 genotyping to personalize isoniazid doses? *Antimicrob Agents Chemother,* **2005,** *49*:1733–1738.

Koul A, Dendouga N, Vergauwen K, et al. Diarylquinolines target subunit c of mycobacterial ATP synthase. *Nat Chem Biol,* **2007,** *3*:323–324.

Kroger A, Pannikar V, Htoon MT, et al. International open trial of uniform multi-drug therapy regimen for 6 months for all types of leprosy patients: Rationale, design and preliminary results. *Trop Med Int Health,* **2008,** *13*:594–602.

Langdon G, Wilkins J, McFadyen L, et al. U. S. Population pharmacokinetics of rifapentine and its primary desacetyl metabolite in South African tuberculosis patients. *Antimicrob Agents Chemother,* **2005,** *49*:4429–4436.

Larsen MH, Vilcheze C, Kremer L, et al. Overexpression of inhA, but not kasA, confers resistance to isoniazid and ethionamide in *Mycobacterium smegmatis, M. bovis* BCG and *M. tuberculosis*. *Mol Microbiol,* **2002,** *46*:453–466.

Levis WR, Ernst JD. *Mycobacterium leprae* (Leprosy, Hansen's disease). In: *Mandell, Douglas, and Bennett's Principles and Practices of Infectious Diseases* (Mandell GL, Bennett JE, Dolin R, eds.), Elsevier Churchill Livingstone, Philadelphia, **2005,** pp. 2886–2896.

Lewis M. Antimycobacterial agents: Ethambutol. In: *Antimicrobial Therapy and Vaccines* (Yu LV, Merigan TC, Barriere SL, eds.), Williams & Wilkins, Baltimore, **1999,** pp. 643–650.

Lounis N, Veziris N, Chauffour A, et al. Combinations of R207910 with drugs used to treat multidrug-resistant tuberculosis have the potential to shorten treatment duration. *Antimicrob Agents Chemother,* **2006,** *50*:3543–3547.

Malone RS, Fish DN, Spiegel DM, et al. The effect of hemodialysis on cycloserine, ethionamide, para-aminosalicylate, and clofazimine. *Chest,* **1999a,** *116*:984–990.

Malone RS, Fish DN, Spiegel DM, et al. The effect of hemodialysis on isoniazid, rifampin, pyrazinamide, and ethambutol. *Am J Respir Crit Care Med,* **1999b,** *159*:1580–1584.

Mathys V, Wintjens R, Lefevre P, et al. Molecular genetics of para-aminosalicylic acid (PAS) resistance in clinical isolates and spontaneous mutants of *Mycobacterium tuberculosis*. *Antimicrob Agents Chemother,* **2009,** *53*:2100–2109.

Morris RP, Nguyen L, Gatfield J, et al. Ancestral antibiotic resistance in *Mycobacterium tuberculosis*. *Proc Natl Acad Sci USA,* **2005,** *102*:12200–12205.

Nightingale SD, Cameron DW, Gordin FM, et al. Two controlled trials of rifabutin prophylaxis against *Mycobacterium avium* complex infection in AIDS. *N Engl J Med,* **1993,** *329*:828–833.

Nix DE, Adam RD, Auclair B, et al. Pharmacokinetics and relative bioavailability of clofazimine in relation to food, orange juice and antacid. *Tuberculosis (Edinb),* **2004,** *84*:365–373.

Nouvel LX, Kassa-Kelembho E, Dos Vultos T, et al. Multidrug-resistant *Mycobacterium tuberculosis*, Bangui, Central African Republic. *Emerg Infect Dis,* **2006,** *12*:1454–1456.

Okamoto S, Tamaru A, Nakajima C, et al. Loss of a conserved 7-methylguanosine modification in 16S rRNA confers low-level streptomycin resistance in bacteria. *Mol Microbiol,* **2007,** *63*:1096–1106.

Orenstein EW, Basu S, Shah NS, et al. Treatment outcomes among patients with multidrug-resistant tuberculosis: systematic review and meta-analysis. *Lancet Infect Dis,* **2009,** *9*:153–161.

Parsons LM, Salfinger M, Clobridge A, et al. Phenotypic and molecular characterization of *Mycobacterium tuberculosis* isolates resistant to both isoniazid and ethambutol. *Antimicrob Agents Chemother,* **2005,** *49*:2218–2225.

Peloquin CA, Bulpitt AE, Jaresko GS, et al. Pharmacokinetics of ethambutol under fasting conditions, with food, and with antacids. *Antimicrob Agents Chemother,* **1999,** *43*:568–572.

Peloquin CA, Zhu M, Adam RD, et al. Pharmacokinetics of para-aminosalicylic acid granules under four dosing conditions. *Ann Pharmacother,* **2001,** *35*:1332–1338.

Prasad K, Singh MB. Corticosteroids for managing tuberculous meningitis. *Cochrane Database Syst Rev*, **2008,** CD002244.

Rad ME, Bifani P, Martin C, et al. Mutations in putative mutator genes of *Mycobacterium tuberculosis* strains of the W-Beijing family. *Emerg Infect Dis,* **2003,** *9*:838–845.

Roy PD, Majumder M, Roy B. Pharmacogenomics of anti-TB drugs-related hepatotoxicity. *Pharmacogenomics,* **2008,** *9*:311–321.

Rustomjee R, Diacon AH, Allen J, et al. Early bactericidal activity and pharmacokinetics of the diarylquinoline TMC207 in treatment of pulmonary tuberculosis. *Antimicrob Agents Chemother,* **2008a,** *52*:2831–2835.

Rustomjee R, Lienhardt C, Kanyok T, et al. A Phase II study of the sterilising activities of ofloxacin, gatifloxacin and moxifloxacin in pulmonary tuberculosis. *Int J Tuberc Lung Dis,* **2008b,** *12*:128–138.

Safi H, Sayers B, Hazbón MH, Alland D. Transfer of embB codon 306 mutations into clinical *Mycobacterium tuberculosi*s strains alters susceptibility to ethambutol, isoniazid, and rifampin. *Antimicrob Agents Chemother,* **2008,** *52*: 2027–2034.

Salfinger M, Heifets LB. Determination of pyrazinamide MICs for *Mycobacterium tuberculosis* at different pHs by the radiometric method. *Antimicrob Agents Chemother,* **1988,** *32*:1002–1004.

Simpson JA, Hughes D, Manyando C, et al. Population pharmacokinetic and pharmacodynamic modeling of the antimalarial chemotherapy chloproguanil/dapsone. *Br j Clin Pharmacol,* **2006,** *61*:289–300.

Singh R, Manjunatha U, Boshoff HI, et al. PA-824 kills nonreplicating *Mycobacterium tuberculosis* by intracellular NO release. Science, **2008,** *322*:1392–1395.

Somoskovi A, Parsons LM, Salfinger M. The molecular basis of resistance to isoniazid, rifampin, and pyrazinamide in *Mycobacterium tuberculosis. Respir Res,* **2001,** *2*:164–168.

Spies FS, da Silva PE, Ribeiro MO, et al. Identification of mutations related to streptomycin resistance in clinical isolates of *Mycobacterium tuberculosis* and possible involvement of efflux mechanism. *Antimicrob Agents Chemother,* **2008,** *52*:2947–2949.

Stover CK, Warrener P, VanDevanter DR, et al. A small-molecule nitroimidazopyran drug candidate for the treatment of tuberculosis. *Nature,* **2000,** *405*:962–966.

Sullivan EA, Geoffroy P, Weisman R, et al. Isoniazid poisonings in New York City. *J Emerg Med,* **1998,** *16*:57–59.

Tasneen R, Tyagi S, Williams K, et al. Enhanced bactericidal activity of rifampin and/or pyrazinamide when combined with PA-824 in a murine model of tuberculosis. *Antimicrob Agents Chemother,* **2008,** *52*:3664–3668.

Timmins GS, Deretic V. Mechanisms of action of isoniazid. *Mol Microbiol,* **2006,** *62*:1220–1227.

Vannelli TA, Dykman A, Ortiz de Montellano PR. The antituberculosis drug ethionamide is activated by a flavoprotein monooxygenase. *J Biol Chem,* **2002,** *277*:12824–12829.

Volmink J, Garner P. Directly observed therapy for treating tuberculosis. *Cochrane Database Syst Rev*, **2007,** CD003343.

Warner DF, Mizrahi V. Tuberculosis chemotherapy: The influence of bacillary stress and damage response pathways on drug efficacy. *Clin Microbiol Rev,* **2006,** *19*:558–570.

Weiner M, Burman W, Luo CC, et al. Effects of rifampin and multidrug resistance gene polymorphism on concentrations of moxifloxacin. *Antimicrob Agents Chemother,* **2007,** *51*:2861–2866.

Wilkins JJ, Langdon G, McIlleron H, et al. Variability in the population pharmacokinetics of pyrazinamide in South African tuberculosis patients. *Eur J Clin Pharmacol,* **2006,** *62*:727–735.

Wilkins JJ, Savic RM, Karlsson MO, et al. Population pharmacokinetics of rifampin in pulmonary tuberculosis patients, including a semimechanistic model to describe variable absorption. *Antimicrob Agents Chemother,* **2008,** *52*:2138–2148.

Wolf R, Matz H, Orion E, Tuzun B, Tuzun Y. Dapsone. *Dermatol Online J*, **2002**, *8*:2.

Zhang Y, Permar S, Sun Z. Conditions that may affect the results of susceptibility testing of *Mycobacterium tuberculosis* to pyrazinamide. *J Med Microbiol,* **2002,** *51*:42–49.

Zhang Y, Scorpio A, Nikaido H, Sun Z. Role of acid pH and deficient efflux of pyrazinoic acid in unique susceptibility of *Mycobacterium tuberculosis* to pyrazinamide. *J Bacteriol,* **1999,** *181*:2044–2049.

Zhang Y, Wade MM, Scorpio A, et al. Mode of action of pyrazinamide: Disruption of *Mycobacterium tuberculosis* membrane transport and energetics by pyrazinoic acid. *J Antimicrob Chemother,* **2003,** *52*:790–795.

Zhu M, Burman WJ, Starke JR, et al. Pharmacokinetics of ethambutol in children and adults with tuberculosis. *Int J Tuberc Lung Dis,* **2004,** *8*:1360–1367.

Zhu M, Namdar R, Stambaugh JJ, et al. Population pharmacokinetics of ethionamide in patients with tuberculosis. *Tuberculosis (Edinb),* **2002,** *82*:91–96.

Zhu M, Nix DE, Adam RD, et al. Pharmacokinetics of cycloserine under fasting conditions and with high-fat meal, orange juice, and antacids. *Pharmacotherapy,* **2001,** *21*:891–897.

Zimhony O, Cox JS, Welch JT, et al. Pyrazinamide inhibits the eukaryotic-like fatty acid synthetase I (FASI) of *Mycobacterium tuberculosis. Nat Med,* **2000,** *6*:1043–1047.

Antifungal Agents

John E. Bennett

There are 200,000 known species of fungi, and estimates of the total size of Kingdom Fungi range to well over a million. Residents of the kingdom are quite diverse and include yeasts, molds, mushrooms, smuts, the pathogens *Aspergillus fumigatus* and *Candida albicans,* and the source of penicillin, *Penicillium chrysogenum*. Fortunately, only ~400 fungi cause disease in animals, and even fewer cause significant human disease. However, fungal infections are becoming more common: Patients with AIDS and patients whose immune systems are compromised by drug therapy are especially susceptible to mycotic infections. Fungi are eukaryotes with unique cell walls containing glucans and chitin, and their eradication requires different strategies than those for treatment of bacterial infections. Available agents have effects on the synthesis of membrane and cell-wall components, on membrane permeability, on the synthesis of nucleic acids, and on microtubule/mitotic spindle function (Figure 57–1).

Antifungal agents described in this chapter are discussed under two major headings, systemic and topical, although this distinction is somewhat arbitrary. The imidazole, triazole, and polyene antifungal agents may be used either systemically or topically, and many superficial mycoses can be treated either systemically or topically.

Although *Pneumocystis jirovecii,* responsible for life-threatening pneumonia in immunocompromised patients, is a fungus and not a protozoan, its treatment is discussed elsewhere because the drugs used are primarily antibacterial or antiprotozoal rather than antifungal.

Major pharmaceutical companies have closed their antifungal development programs, although a few small firms continue to sponsor research in this field. Thus, the near future in this area is likely to be limited to expansion of experience with existing compounds (Table 57–1). The most recent systemic antifungals to reach clinical development, posaconazole (NOXAFIL) and isavuconazole (in phase III trials in the U.S.), are both triazoles.

SYSTEMIC ANTIFUNGAL AGENTS: SYSTEMIC DRUGS FOR DEEPLY INVASIVE FUNGAL INFECTIONS

Amphotericin B

Chemistry. Amphotericin B is one of a family of some 200 polyene macrolide compounds with antifungal activity. Those studied to date share the characteristics of four to seven conjugated double bonds, an internal cyclic ester, poor aqueous solubility, substantial toxicity on parenteral administration, and a common mechanism of antifungal action. Amphotericin B (see following structure) is a heptaene macrolide containing seven conjugated double bonds in the *trans* position and 3-amino-3,6-dideoxymannose (mycosamine) connected to the main ring by a glycosidic bond. The amphoteric behavior for which the drug is named derives from the presence of a carboxyl group on the main ring and a primary amino group on mycosamine; these groups confer aqueous solubility at extremes of pH. X-ray crystallography has shown the molecule to be rigid and rod-shaped, with the hydrophilic hydroxyl groups of the macrolide ring forming an opposing face to the lipophilic polyenic portion.

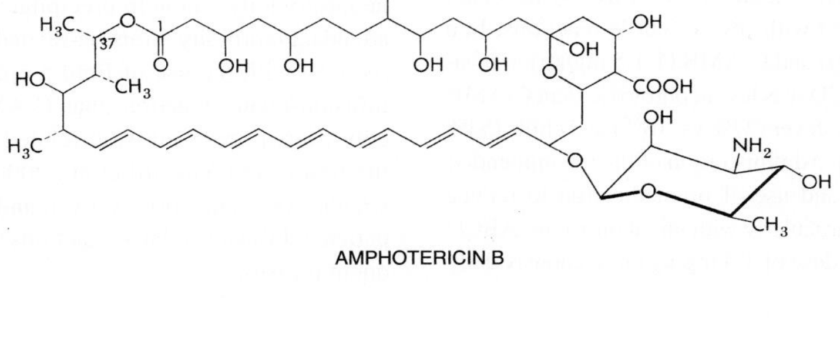

AMPHOTERICIN B

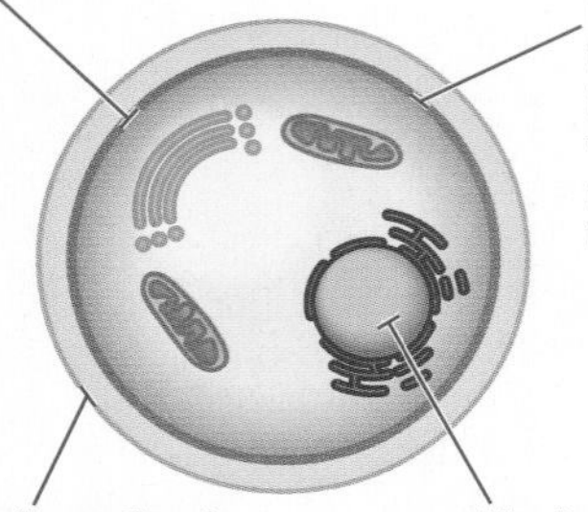

Figure 57–1. *Sites of action of antifungal drugs.* Amphotericin B and other polyenes, such as nystatin, bind to ergosterol in fungal cell membranes and increase membrane permeability. The imidazoles and triazoles, such as itraconazole and fluconazole, inhibit 14-α-sterol demethylase, prevent ergosterol synthesis, and lead to the accumulation of 14-α-methylsterols. The allylamines, such as naftifine and terbinafine, inhibit squalene epoxidase and prevent ergosterol synthesis. The echinocandins, such as caspofungin, inhibit the formation of glucans in the fungal cell wall.

Drug Formulations. There are currently four formulations of amphotericin B commercially available: conventional amphotericin B (C-AMB), liposomal amphotericin B (L-AMB), amphotericin B lipid complex (ABLC), and amphotericin B colloidal dispersion (ABCD). Table 57–2 summarizes the pharmacokinetic properties of these preparations.

C-AMB (Conventional amphotericin B, FUNGIZONE). Amphotericin B is insoluble in water but is formulated for intravenous infusion by complexing it with the bile salt deoxycholate. The complex is marketed as a lyophilized powder for injection. C-AMB forms a colloid in water, with particles largely <0.4 μm in diameter. Filters in intravenous infusion lines that trap particles >0.22 μm in diameter will remove significant amounts of drug. Addition of electrolytes to infusion solutions causes the colloid to aggregate.

ABCD. Amphotericin B colloidal dispersion (AMPHOTEC, AMPHOCIL) contains roughly equimolar amounts of amphotericin B and cholesteryl sulfate formulated for injection. Like C-AMB, ABCD forms a colloidal solution when dispersed in aqueous solution. ABCD provides much lower blood levels than C-AMB in mice and humans. In a study in patients with neutropenic fever comparing daily ABCD (4 mg/kg) with C-AMB (0.8 mg/kg), chills and hypoxia were significantly more common with ABCD than with C-AMB (White et al., 1998). Hypoxia was associated with severe febrile reactions. In a comparison of ABCD (6 mg/kg) and C-AMB (1-1.5 mg/kg) in invasive aspergillosis patients, ABCD was less nephrotoxic than C-AMB (49% vs. 15%) but caused more fever (27% vs. 16%) and chills (53% vs. 30%) (Bowden et al., 2002). Administration of the recommended ABCD dose over 3-4 hours and use of premedication to reduce febrile reactions are advised, particularly with initial infusions. ABCD is approved at a recommended dose of 3-4 mg/kg intravenously daily for patients with invasive aspergillosis who are not responding to or are unable to tolerate C-AMB.

L-AMB. Liposomal amphotericin B is a small, unilamellar vesicle formulation of amphotericin B (AMBISOME). The drug is supplied as a lyophilized powder, which is reconstituted with sterile water for injection. Blood levels following intravenous infusion are almost equivalent to those obtained with C-AMB, and because L-AMB can be given at higher doses, blood levels have been achieved that exceed those obtained with C-AMB (Boswell et al., 1998) (Table 57–2). Amphotericin B accumulation in the liver and spleen is higher with L-AMB than with C-AMB. Adverse effects include nephrotoxicity, hypokalemia, and infusion-related reactions, such as fever, chills, hypoxia, hypotension, and hypertension, but these do not commonly lead to drug discontinuation. Infusion-related pain in the back, abdomen, or chest occurs in occasional patients, usually with the first few doses. Anaphylaxis also has been reported. As empirical therapy or prophylaxis in febrile neutropenic patients, CAMB and L-AMB are equivalent. As induction therapy of disseminated histoplasmosis in AIDS patients, L-AMB 3 mg/kg was superior to C-AMB 0.7 mg/kg (Johnson, 2002). L-AMB is approved for initial therapy of cryptococcal meningitis of AIDS patients and is listed as an alternative to C-AMB for induction therapy of both disseminated histoplasmosis and cryptococcal meningoencephalitis in AIDS patients (Kaplan et al., 2009). L-AMB is approved for empirical therapy of fever in the neutropenic host not responding to appropriate antibacterial agents, as well as for salvage therapy of aspergillosis and candidiasis. The recommended daily intravenous dose for empirical therapy is 3 mg/kg; for treatment of mycoses, the dosage is 3-5 mg/kg. L-AMB also is effective in visceral leishmaniasis at doses of 3-4 mg/kg daily. The drug is administered in 5% dextrose in water, with initial doses infused over 2 hours. If well tolerated, infusion duration can be shortened to 1 hour. Doses up to 10 mg/kg have been used but are associated with higher toxicity and, in one randomized trial of aspergillosis, no improvement in efficacy (Cornely, 2007a).

ABLC (ABELCET). Amphotericin B lipid complex is a complex of amphotericin B with lipids (dimyristoylphosphatidylcholine and dimyristoylphosphatidylglycerol). ABLC is given in a dose of 5 mg/kg in 5% dextrose in water, infused intravenously once daily over 2 hours. Blood levels of amphotericin B are much lower with ABLC than with the same dose of C-AMB. ABLC is effective in a variety of mycoses, with the possible exception of cryptococcal meningitis. The drug is approved for salvage therapy of deep mycoses.

The three lipid formulations collectively appear to reduce the risk of the patient's serum creatinine doubling during therapy by 58% (Barrett et al., 2003). In patients at high risk for nephrotoxicity, ABLC is more nephrotoxic than L-AMB (Wingard et al., 2000). In some patients, the additive burden of amphotericin B nephrotoxicity can help precipitate advanced renal failure, with attendant morbidity. Infusion-related reactions are not consistently reduced with the use of lipid preparations. ABCD causes more infusion-related reactions than C-AMB. Although L-AMB reportedly causes fewer infusion-related reactions than ABLC during the first dose (Wingard et al., 2000), the difference depends on whether premedication is given and varies considerably between patients. Infusion-related reactions typically decrease with subsequent infusions.

Table 57–1

Pharmacotherapy of Mycoses

DEEP MYCOSES	DRUGS	SUPERFICIAL MYCOSES	DRUGS
Invasive aspergillosis		***Candidiasis***	
Immunosuppressed	Voriconazole, amphotericin B	Vulvovaginal	*Topical*
Non-immunosuppressed	Voriconazole, amphotericin B, itraconazole		Butoconazole, clotrimazole, miconazole, nystatin, terconazole, tioconazole
Blastomycosis			*Oral*
Rapidly progressive or CNS	Amphotericin B		Fluconazole
Indolent and non-CNS	Itraconazole	Oropharyngeal	*Topical*
Candidiasis			Clotrimazole, nystatin
Deeply invasive	Amphotericin B, fluconazole, voriconazole, caspofungin, micafungin, anidulafungin		*Oral (systemic)* Fluconazole, itraconazole Posaconazole
Coccidioidomycosis		Cutaneous	*Topical*
Rapidly progressing	Amphotericin B		Amphotericin B, clotrimazole,
Indolent	Itraconazole, fluconazole		ciclopirox, econazole, ketoconazole, miconazole, nystatin
Meningeal	Fluconazole, intrathecal amphotericin B	***Ringworm***	*Topical* Butenafine, ciclopirox, clotrimazole,
Cryptococcosis			econazole, haloprogin, ketoconazole,
Non-AIDS and initial AIDS	Amphotericin B, flucytosine		miconazole, naftifine, oxiconazole,
Maintenance AIDS	Fluconazole		sertaconazole, sulconazole,
Histoplasmosis			terbinafine, tolnaftate, undecylenate
Chronic pulmonary	Itraconazole		*Systemic*
Disseminated			Griseofulvin, itraconazole, terbinafine
Rapidly progressing or CNS	Amphotericin B		
Indolent non-CNS	Itraconazole		
Maintenance AIDS	Itraconazole		
Mucormycosis	Amphotericin B		
Pseudallescheriasis	Voriconazole, itraconazole		
Sporotrichosis			
Cutaneous	Itraconazole		
Extracutaneous	Amphotericin B, itraconazole		
Prophylaxis in the immunocompromised host	Fluconazole Posaconazole Micafungin		
Empirical therapy in the immunocompromised host (*category not recognized by FDA*)	Amphotericin B Caspofungin Fluconazole		

The cost of the lipid formulations of amphotericin B greatly exceeds that of C-AMB, making them unavailable in many countries.

Mechanism of Action. The antifungal activity of amphotericin B depends principally on its binding to a sterol moiety, primarily ergosterol in the membrane of sensitive fungi. By virtue of their interaction with these sterols, polyenes appear to form pores or channels that increase the permeability of the membrane, allowing leakage of a variety of small molecules (Figure 57–1).

Absorption, Distribution, and Excretion. Gastrointestinal (GI) absorption of all amphotericin B formulations is negligible. Pharmacokinetic properties differ markedly between preparations with L-AMB having the highest plasma concentrations at therapeutic doses

Table 57-2

Pharmocokinetic Parameters for Amphotericin B Formulations after Multiple Administrations in Humans

PRODUCT	DOSE (MG/KG)	C_{MAX} (μg/mL)	$AUC_{(1\text{-}24hr)}$ (μg.hr/mL)	V (L/kg)	Cl (mL/hr/kg)
AmBisome (L-AMB)	5	83±35.2	555±311	0.11±0.08	11±6
Amphotec (ABCD)	5	3.1	43	4.3	117
Ablecet (ABLC)	5	1.7±0.8	14±7	131±7.7	426±188.5
Fungizone (C-AMB)	0.6	1.1±0.2	17.1±5	5±2.8	38±15

For details, see Boswell et al. (1998). From Boswell GW, Buell D, Bekersky I. AmBisome (liposomal amphotericin B): A comparative review. *J Clin Pharmacol*, **1998**, 38:583–592.

(Table 57–2). C-AMB is released from its complex with deoxycholate in the bloodstream, and the amphotericin B that remains in plasma is more than 90% bound to proteins, largely β-lipoprotein. Excretion into the urine is negligible with all the formulations. Azotemia, liver failure, or hemodialysis does not have a measurable impact on plasma concentrations. Concentrations of amphotericin B (via C-AMB) in fluids from inflamed pleura, peritoneum, synovium, and aqueous humor are approximately two-thirds of trough concentrations in plasma. Little amphotericin B from any formulation penetrates into cerebrospinal fluid (CSF), vitreous humor, or normal amniotic fluid.

Antifungal Activity. Amphotericin B has useful clinical activity against *Candida* spp., *Cryptococcus neoformans, Blastomyces dermatitidis, Histoplasma capsulatum, Sporothrix schenckii, Coccidioides* spp., *Paracoccidioides braziliensis, Aspergillus* spp., *Penicillium marneffei*, and the agents of mucormycosis. Amphotericin B has limited activity against the protozoa *Leishmania* spp. and *Naegleria fowleri*. The drug has no antibacterial activity.

Fungal Resistance. Some isolates of *Candida lusitaniae* have been relatively resistant to amphotericin B. *Aspergillus terreus* and perhaps *Aspergillus nidulans* may be more resistant to amphotericin B than other *Aspergillus* species (Steinbach et al., 2004). Mutants selected *in vitro* for resistance to nystatin (a polyene antifungal discussed later) or amphotericin B replace ergosterol with certain precursor sterols. The rarity of significant amphotericin B resistance arising during therapy has left it unclear whether ergosterol-deficient mutants retain sufficient pathogenicity to survive in deep tissue.

Therapeutic Uses. The recommended doses were given earlier for each formulation. Candida esophagitis responds to much lower doses than deeply invasive mycoses. Intrathecal infusion of C-AMB is useful in patients with meningitis caused by *Coccidioides.* Too little is known about intrathecal administration of lipid formulations to recommend them. C-AMB can be injected into the CSF of the lumbar spine, cisterna magna, or lateral cerebral ventricle. Fever and headache are common reactions that may be decreased by intrathecal administration of 10-15 mg of hydrocortisone. Local injections of amphotericin B into a joint or peritoneal dialysate fluid commonly produce irritation and pain. Intraocular injection following pars plana vitrectomy has been used successfully for fungal endophthalmitis.

Intravenous administration of amphotericin B is the treatment of choice for mucormycosis and is used for initial treatment of cryptococcal meningitis, severe or rapidly progressing histoplasmosis, blastomycosis, coccidioidomycosis, and penicilliosis marneffei, as well as in patients not responding to azole therapy of invasive aspergillosis, extracutaneous sporotrichosis, fusariosis, alternariosis, and trichosporonosis. Amphotericin B (C-AMB or L-AMB) is often given to selected patients with profound neutropenia who have fever that does not respond to broad-spectrum antibacterial agents over 5-7 days.

Untoward Effects. The major acute reactions to intravenous amphotericin B formulations are fever and chills. Infusion-related reactions are worst with ABCD, slightly less with C-C-AMB, even less with ABLC, and least with L-AMB. Tachypnea and respiratory stridor or modest hypotension also may occur, but true bronchospasm or anaphylaxis is rare. Patients with pre-existing cardiac or pulmonary disease may tolerate the metabolic demands of the reaction poorly and develop hypoxia or hypotension. The reaction ends spontaneously in 30-45 minutes; meperidine may shorten it. Pretreatment with oral acetaminophen or use of intravenous hydrocortisone hemisuccinate, 0.7 mg/kg, at the start of the infusion decreases reactions. Febrile reactions abate with subsequent infusions. Infants, children, and patients receiving therapeutic doses of glucocorticoids are less prone to reactions.

Azotemia occurs in 80% of patients who receive C-AMB for deep mycoses (Carlson and Condon, 1994). Lipid formulations are less nephrotoxic, being much less with ABLC, even less with L-AMB, and minimal with ABCD. Toxicity is dose-dependent and usually transient and increased by concurrent therapy with other nephrotoxic agents, such as aminoglycosides or cyclosporine. Although permanent histological changes in renal tubules occur even during short courses of C-AMB, permanent functional impairment is uncommon in adults with normal renal function prior to treatment unless the cumulative dose exceeds 3-4 g. Renal tubular acidosis and renal wasting of K^+ and Mg^{2+} also may be seen during and for several weeks after therapy. Supplemental K^+ is required in one-third of patients on prolonged therapy. Saline loading has decreased nephrotoxicity, even in the absence of water or salt deprivation. Administration of 1 L of normal saline intravenously on the day that C-AMB is to be given has been recommended for adults who are able to tolerate the Na^+ load and who are not already receiving that amount in intravenous fluids.

Hypochromic, normocytic anemia commonly occurs during treatment with C-AMB. Anemia is less with lipid formulations and usually not seen over the first 2 weeks. The anemia is most likely due to decreased production of erythropoietin. Patients with low plasma erythropoietin may respond to administration of recombinant erythropoietin. Anemia reverses slowly following cessation of therapy. Headache, nausea, vomiting, malaise, weight loss, and phlebitis at peripheral infusion sites are common. Thrombocytopenia or mild leukopenia is observed rarely. Hepatotoxicity is not firmly established with any amphotericin B formulation. Arachnoiditis has been observed as a complication of injecting C-AMB into the CSF.

Flucytosine

Chemistry. Flucytosine is 5-fluorocytosine, a fluorinated pyrimidine related to fluorouracil and floxuridine.

FLUCYTOSINE

Mechanism of Action. All susceptible fungi are capable of deaminating flucytosine to 5-fluorouracil (Figure 57–2), a potent antimetabolite that is used in cancer chemotherapy (Chapter 61). Fluorouracil is metabolized first to 5-fluorouracil-ribose monophosphate (5-FUMP) by the enzyme uracil phosphoribosyl transferase (UPRTase; also called uridine monophosphate pyrophosphorylase). As in mammalian cells, 5-FUMP then is either incorporated into RNA (via synthesis of 5-fluorouridine triphosphate) or metabolized to 5-fluoro-2′-deoxyuridine-5′-monophosphate (5-FdUMP), a potent inhibitor of thymidylate synthetase. DNA synthesis is impaired as the ultimate result of this latter reaction. The selective action of flucytosine is due to the lack of cytosine deaminase in mammalian cells, which prevents metabolism to fluorouracil.

Antifungal Activity. Flucytosine has clinically useful activity against *Cryptococcus neoformans, Candida* spp., and the agents of chromoblastomycosis. Within these species, determination of susceptibility *in vitro* has been extremely dependent on the method employed, and susceptibility testing performed on isolates obtained prior to treatment has not correlated with clinical outcome.

Fungal Resistance. Drug resistance arising during therapy (secondary resistance) is an important cause of therapeutic failure when flucytosine is used alone for cryptococcosis and candidiasis. In chromoblastomycosis, resurgence of lesions after an initial response has led to the presumption of secondary drug resistance. In isolates of *Cryptococcus* and *Candida* species, secondary drug resistance has been accompanied by a change in the minimal inhibitory concentration from <2.5 μg/mL to >360 μg/mL. The mechanism for this resistance can be loss of the permease necessary for cytosine transport or decreased activity of either UPRTase or cytosine deaminase (Figure 57–2). In *Candida albicans,* substitution of thymidine for cytosine at nucleotide 301 in the gene encoding UPRTase (*FURl*) causes a cysteine to become an arginine, modestly increasing flucytosine resistance (Dodgson et al., 2004). Flucytosine resistance is further increased if both *FURl* alleles in the diploid fungus are mutated.

Absorption, Distribution, and Excretion. Flucytosine is absorbed rapidly and well from the GI tract. It is widely distributed in the body,

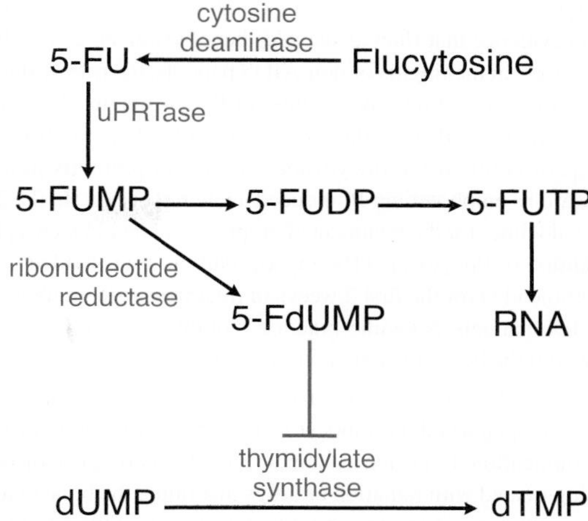

Figure 57–2. *Action of flucytosine in fungi.* Flucytosine is transported by cytosine permease into the fungal cell, where it is deaminated to 5-fluorouracil (5-FU). The 5-FU is then converted to 5-fluorouracil-ribose monophosphate (5-FUMP) and then is either converted to 5-fluorouridine triphosphate (5-FUTP) and incorporated into RNA or converted by ribonucleotide reductase to 5-fluoro-2′-deoxyuridine-5′-monophosphate (5-FdUMP), which is a potent inhibitor of thymidylate synthase. 5-FUDP, 5-fluorouridine-5′-diphosphate; dUMP, deoxyuridine-5′-monophosphate; dTMP, deoxythymidine-5′-monophosphate.

with a volume of distribution that approximates total body water, and is minimally bound to plasma proteins. The peak plasma concentration in patients with normal renal function is ~70-80 μg/mL, achieved 1-2 hours after a dose of 37.5 mg/kg. Approximately 80% of a given dose is excreted unchanged in the urine; concentrations in the urine range from 200-500 μg/mL. The $t_{1/2}$ of the drug is 3-6 hours in normal individuals. In renal failure, the $t_{1/2}$ may be as long as 200 hours. The clearance of flucytosine is approximately equivalent to that of creatinine. Reduction of dosage is necessary in patients with decreased renal function, and concentrations of drug in plasma should be measured periodically. Peak concentrations should range between 50 and 100 μg/mL. Flucytosine is cleared by hemodialysis, and patients undergoing such treatment should receive a single dose of 37.5 mg/kg after dialysis; the drug also is removed by peritoneal dialysis.

Flucytosine concentration in CSF is ~65-90% of that found simultaneously in the plasma. The drug also appears to penetrate into the aqueous humor.

Therapeutic Uses. Flucytosine (ANCOBON) is given orally at 50-150 mg/kg per day, in four divided doses at 6-hour intervals. Dosage must be adjusted for decreased renal function. Flucytosine is used predominantly in combination with amphotericin B. Flucytosine caused no added toxicity when added to 0.7 mg/kg of amphotericin B for the initial 2 weeks of therapy of cryptococcal meningitis in AIDS patients. Although the CSF colony count diminished more rapidly with combination therapy, there was no apparent impact on mortality or morbidity (van der Horst et al., 1997). An all-oral regimen of flucytosine plus fluconazole also has been advocated for therapy of AIDS patients with cryptococcosis, but the combination has substantial GI toxicity with no evidence that flucytosine adds benefit (Larsen et al., 1994). In cryptococcal meningitis of non-AIDS patients, the role of flucytosine is more conjectural. The addition of flucytosine to ≥6 weeks of therapy with C-AMB runs the risk of substantial bone marrow suppression or colitis if the flucytosine dose is not promptly adjusted downward as amphotericin B–induced azotemia occurs. In the 2008 IDSA guidelines for the treatment of cryptococcal meningoencephalitis, addition of flucytosine (100 mg/kg orally in four divided doses) is recommended for the first 2 weeks of treatment with amphotericin B in AIDS patients. A similar practice is often used in HIV-negative patients but the benefit is unknown (Pappas et al., 2001).

Untoward Effects. Flucytosine may depress the bone marrow and lead to leukopenia and thrombocytopenia; patients are more prone to this complication if they have an underlying hematological disorder, are being treated with radiation or drugs that injure the bone marrow, or have a history of treatment with such agents. Other untoward effects—including rash, nausea, vomiting, diarrhea, and severe enterocolitis—have been noted. In ~5% of patients, plasma levels of hepatic enzymes are elevated, but this effect reverses when therapy is stopped. Toxicity is more frequent in patients with AIDS or azotemia (including those who are receiving amphotericin B concurrently) and when plasma drug concentrations exceed 100 μg/mL. Toxicity may result from conversion of flucytosine to 5-fluorouracil by the microbial flora in the intestinal tract of the host.

Imidazoles and Triazoles

The azole antifungals include two broad classes, imidazoles and triazoles, which share the same antifungal spectrum and mechanism of action. The systemic triazoles are metabolized more slowly and have less effect on human sterol synthesis than the imidazoles. Because of these advantages, new congeners under development are mostly triazoles. Of the drugs now on the market in the U.S., clotrimazole, miconazole, ketoconazole, econazole, butoconazole, oxiconazole, sertaconazole, and sulconazole are imidazoles; terconazole, itraconazole, fluconazole, voriconazole, posaconazole, and isavuconazole (an experimental drug) are triazoles. The topical use of azole antifungals is described in the second section of this chapter. The basic triazole structure is:

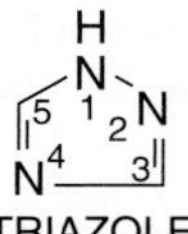

Mechanism of Action. At concentrations achieved following systemic administration, the major effect of imidazoles and triazoles on fungi is inhibition of 14-α-sterol demethylase, a microsomal CYP (Figure 57–1). Imidazoles and triazoles thus impair the biosynthesis of ergosterol for the cytoplasmic membrane and lead to the accumulation of 14-α-methylsterols. These methylsterols may disrupt the close packing of acyl chains of phospholipids, impairing the functions of certain membrane-bound enzyme systems, thus inhibiting growth of the fungi. Some azoles directly increase permeability of the fungal cytoplasmic membrane, but the concentrations required are likely only obtained with topical use.

Antifungal Activity. Azoles as a group have clinically useful activity against *Candida albicans, Candida tropicalis, Candida parapsilosis, Candida glabrata, Cryptococcus neoformans, Blastomyces dermatitidis, Histoplasma capsulatum, Coccidioides* spp., *Paracoccidioides brasiliensis,* and ringworm fungi (dermatophytes). *Aspergillus* spp., *Scedosporium apiospermum (Pseudallescheria boydii), Fusarium*, and *Sporothrix schenckii* are intermediate in susceptibility. *Candida krusei* and the agents of mucormycosis are more resistant. Thus, these drugs do not have any useful antibacterial or antiparasitic activity, with the possible exception of antiprotozoal effects against *Leishmania major.* Posaconazole has slightly improved activity *in vitro* against the agents of mucormycosis.

Resistance. Azole resistance emerges gradually during prolonged azole therapy, causing clinical failure in patients with far-advanced HIV infection and oropharyngeal or esophageal candidiasis. The primary mechanism of resistance in *C. albicans* is accumulation of mutations in *ERG11*, the gene coding for the 14-α-sterol demethylase. These mutations protect heme in the enzyme pocket from binding to the azole but allow access of the natural substrate for the enzyme lanosterol. Cross-resistance is conferred to all azoles. Increased azole efflux by both ATP-binding cassette (ABC) and major facilitator superfamily transporters can add to fluconazole resistance in *C. albicans* and *C. glabrata.* Increased production of C14-α-sterol demethylase is another potential cause of resistance. Mutation of the C5,6 sterol reductase gene *ERG3* also can increase azole resistance in some species.

Primary azole resistance has been described in some isolates of *Aspergillus fumigatus* with increased azole transport and decreased ergosterol content, but the clinical significance is unknown. Decreased fluconazole susceptibility has been described in *Cryptococcus neoformans* isolated from AIDS patients failing prolonged therapy.

Interaction of Azole Anti-Fungals with Other Drugs. The azoles interact with hepatic CYPs as substrates and inhibitors (Table 57–3), providing myriad possibilities for the interaction of azoles with many other medications. Thus, azoles can elevate plasma levels of some co-administered drugs (Table 57–4). Other co-administered drugs can decrease plasma concentrations of azole antifungal agents (Table 57–5). As a consequence of myriad interactions, combinations of certain drugs with azole antifungal medications may be contraindicated (Table 57–6).

Ketoconazole

Ketoconazole, administered orally, has been replaced by itraconazole for the treatment of all mycoses except when the lower cost of ketoconazole outweighs the advantage of itraconazole. Itraconazole lacks ketoconazole's corticosteroid suppression while retaining most of ketoconazole's pharmacological properties and expanding the antifungal spectrum. Ketoconazole sometimes is used to inhibit excessive production of glucocorticoids in patients with Cushing's syndrome (Chapter 42) and is available for topical use, as described later.

Itraconazole

This synthetic triazole is an equimolar racemic mixture of four diastereoisomers (two enantiomeric pairs), each

Table 57-3

Interaction of Azole Antifungal Agents with Hepatic CYPs

FLUCONAZOLE	VORICONAZOLE	ITRACONAZOLE	POSACONAZOLE
CYP3A4 inhibitor CYP2C9 inhibitor CYP2C19 inhibitor	CYP2C9 inhibitor and substrate CYP3A4 inhibitor CYP2C19 inhibitor	CYP3A4 inhibitor	CYP3A4 inhibitor

Table 57-4

Drugs Exhibiting Elevated Plasma Concentrations When Co-Administered with Azole Anti-Fungal Agents

Alfentanil
Alprazolam
Astemizole
Buspirone
Busulfan
Carbamazepine
Cisapride
Cyclosporine
Digoxin
Docetaxel
Dofetilide
Efavirenz
Eletriptan
Eplerenone
Ergot alkaloids
Erlotinib
Eszopiclone
Felodipine
Fexofenadine
Gefitinib
Glimepiride
Glipizide
Halofantrine
Haloperidol
Imatinib
Irinotecan
Losartan
Lovastatin
Methadone
Methylprednisolone
Midazolam
Nevirapine
Omeprazole
Phenytoin
Pimozide
Quinidine
Ramelteon
Ranolazine
Risperidone
Saquinavir
Sildenafil
Sirolimus
Solifenacin
Sunitinib
Tacrolimus
Triazolam
Vardenafil
Vinca alkaloids
Warfarin
Zidovudine
Zolpidem

Mechanism of interaction presumably occurs largely at the level of hepatic CYPs, especially CYPs 3A4, 2C9, and 2D6, but can also involve P-glycoprotein and other mechanisms. Not all drugs listed interact equally with all azoles. For details, see Chapter 6 and Zonios (2008).

Table 57-5

Some Drugs that Decrease Azole Concentration When Co-Administered

DRUG	FLUCONAZOLE	VORICONAZOLE	ITRACONAZOLE	POSACONAZOLE
Antacids (simultaneous)	–		+	–
Barbiturates		+	+[a]	
Carbamazepine	+	+	+	+
H_2 antagonists			+	+
Didanosine			+	
Efavirenz		+	+	
Nevirapine		+	+	
Proton pump inhibitors	–	–[b]	+	+
Phenytoin	–	+	+	+
Rifampin	+	+	+	+
Rifabutin		+	+	+
Ritonavir		+		

[a]Phenobarbital only. [b]Omeprazole and voriconazole increase each other's concentrations in plasma; reduce omeprazole dose by 50% when initiating voriconazole therapy. For additional information, see Zonios, 2008.

Table 57-6

Some Additional Contraindicated Azole Drug Combinations

DRUG	FLUCONAZOLE	VORICONAZOLE	ITRACONAZOLE	POSACONAZOLE
Alfuzosin		x	x	x
Artemether	x	x		
Bepridil	x			
Clopidogrel	x			
Conivaptan	x	x	x	x
Dabigatran			x	
Darunavir		x		
Dronedarone	x	x	x	x
Everolimus	x	x	x	x
Lopinavir		x		
Lumefantrine	x	x		
Mesoridazine	x			
Nilotinib	x	x	x	x
Nisoldipine	use with caution	x	x	x
Quinine	x	x		
Rifapentine		x	use with caution	use with caution
Ritonavir		x	use with caution	
Rivaroxaban		x	x	
Salmeterol		x	x	x
Silodosin		x	x	x
Simvastatin	use with caution		x	
St. John's wort		x		
Tetrabenazine	x	x		
Thioridazine	x	x		
Tolvaptan	x	x		x
Tolvaptan	x		x	
Topotecan			x	
Ziprasidone	x	x		

possessing three chiral centers. The structure is similar to that of the imidazole ketoconazole.

Absorption, Distribution, and Excretion. Itraconazole (SPORANOX, others) is available as a capsule and a solution in hydroxypropyl-β-cyclodextrin for oral use. The capsule form of the drug is best absorbed in the fed state, but the oral solution is better absorbed in the fasting state, providing peak plasma concentrations >150% of those obtained with the capsule. Itraconazole is metabolized in the liver. It is both a substrate for and a potent inhibitor of CYP3A4. Itraconazole is present in plasma with an approximately equal concentration of a biologically active metabolite, hydroxy-itraconazole. Bioassays may report up to 3.3 times as much itraconazole in plasma as do physical methods such as high-performance liquid chromatography, depending on the susceptibility of the bioassay organism to hydroxy-itraconazole. The native drug and metabolite are >99%

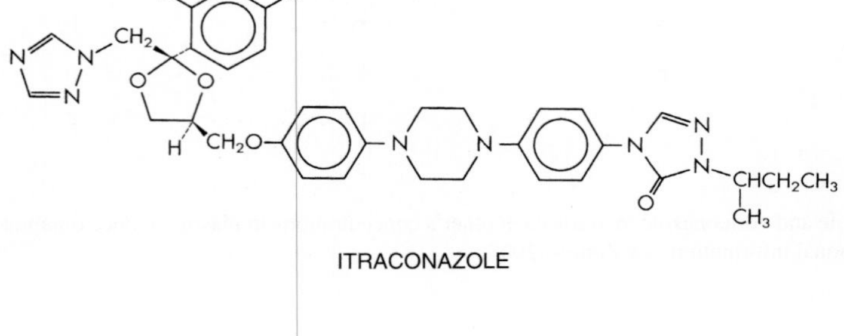

ITRACONAZOLE

bound to plasma proteins. Neither appears in urine or CSF. The $t_{1/2}$ of itraconazole at steady state is ~30-40 hours. Steady-state levels of itraconazole are not reached for 4 days and those of hydroxy-itraconazole for 7 days; thus, loading doses are recommended when treating deep mycoses. Severe liver disease will increase itraconazole plasma concentrations, but azotemia and hemodialysis have no effect. Itraconazole is not carcinogenic but is teratogenic in rats and contraindicated for the treatment of onychomycosis during pregnancy or for women contemplating pregnancy (Category C).

Drug Interactions. Tables 57–4, 57–5, and 57–6 list select interactions of azoles with other drugs. Many of the interactions can result in serious toxicity from the companion drug, such as inducing potentially fatal cardiac arrhythmias when used with quinidine, halofantrine (an orphan drug used for malaria), levomethadyl (an orphan drug used for heroin addiction), pimozide (ORAP) or cisapride (only available under an investigational limited access program in the U.S.). Other drugs may decrease itraconazole serum levels below therapeutic concentrations (Table 57–5).

Therapeutic Uses. Itraconazole is the drug of choice for patients with indolent, nonmeningeal infections due to *B. dermatitidis, H. capsulatum, P. brasiliensis,* and *C. immitis*. The drug also is useful in the therapy of indolent invasive aspergillosis outside the CNS, particularly after the infection has been stabilized with amphotericin B. Approximately half the patients with distal subungual onychomycosis respond to itraconazole (Evans and Sigurgeirsson, 1999). Although not an approved use, itraconazole is a reasonable choice for the treatment of pseudallescheriasis, an infection not responding to amphotericin B therapy, as well as cutaneous and extracutaneous sporotrichosis, tinea corporis, and extensive tinea versicolor. HIV-infected patients with disseminated histoplasmosis or *Penicillium marneffei* infections have a decreased incidence of relapse if given prolonged itraconazole "maintenance" therapy. According to the 2008 CDC/IDSA guidelines, discontinuation of itraconazole may be considered in AIDS patients with disseminated histoplasmosis who have completed 1 year of itraconazole, have responded to highly active antiretroviral therapy (HAART) with a CD4 >150/mm^3 for 6 months, have a urine histoplasma antigen <2 units and a negative blood culture for histoplasma (Kaplan et al., 2009) (Chapter 59). Itraconazole is not recommended for maintenance therapy of cryptococcal meningitis in HIV-infected patients because of a high incidence of relapse. Long-term therapy has been used in non-HIV–infected patients with allergic bronchopulmonary aspergillosis to decrease the dose of glucocorticoids and reduce attacks of acute bronchospasm (Salez et al., 1999).

Itraconazole solution is effective and approved for use in oropharyngeal and esophageal candidiasis. Because the solution has more GI side effects than fluconazole tablets, itraconazole solution usually is reserved for patients not responding to fluconazole.

Untoward Effects. Adverse effects of itraconazole therapy can occur as a result of interactions with many other drugs (Tables 57–3 and 57–4). Serious hepatotoxicity has rarely led to hepatic failure and death. If symptoms of hepatotoxicity occur, the drug should be discontinued and liver function assessed. Intravenous itraconazole causes a dose-dependent inotropic effect that can lead to congestive heart failure in patients with impaired ventricular function. In the absence of interacting drugs, itraconazole capsules and suspension are well tolerated at 200 mg daily. Some patients complain of the taste of the solution, and GI side effects are common, although adherence is generally unimpaired. Diarrhea, abdominal cramps, anorexia, and nausea are more common than with the capsules. In one series of patients receiving 50-400 mg of the capsules per day, nausea and vomiting were recorded in 10%, hypertriglyceridemia in 9%, hypokalemia in 6%, increased serum aminotransferase in 5%, rash in 2%, and at least one side effect in 39%. Occasionally, rash necessitates drug discontinuation, but most adverse effects can be handled with dose reduction. Profound hypokalemia has been seen in patients receiving ≥600 mg daily and in those who recently have received prolonged amphotericin B therapy. Doses of 300 mg twice daily have led to other side effects, including adrenal insufficiency, lower limb edema, hypertension, and in at least one case, rhabdomyolysis. Doses >400 mg per day are not recommended for long-term use. Anaphylaxis has been observed rarely, as well as severe rash, including Stevens-Johnson syndrome.

Dosage. In treating deep (life-threatening) mycoses, a loading dose of 200 mg of itraconazole is administered three times daily for the first 3 days. After the loading doses, two 100-mg capsules are given twice daily with food. The divided doses are alleged to increase the area under the plasma concentration versus time curve (AUC), even though the $t_{1/2}$ is ~30 hours. For maintenance therapy of HIV-infected patients with disseminated histoplasmosis, 200 mg once daily is used. Onychomycosis can be treated with either 200 mg once daily for 12 weeks or for infections isolated to fingernails, two monthly cycles consisting of 200 mg twice daily for 1 week followed by a 3-week period of no therapy—so-called pulse therapy (Evans and Sigurgeirsson, 1999). Retention of active drug in the nail keratin permits intermittent treatment. Daily therapy is preferred by some authorities for infections likely to be more refractory, but it costs twice as much as pulse therapy. Once-daily terbinafine (250 mg), however, is superior to pulse therapy with itraconazole. For oropharyngeal candidiasis, itraconazole oral solution should be taken fasting in a dose of 100 mg (10 mL) once daily and swished vigorously in the mouth before swallowing to optimize any topical effect. Patients with esophageal thrush unresponsive or refractory to treatment with fluconazole tablets are given 100 mg of the solution twice a day for 2-4 weeks.

Fluconazole

Fluconazole is a fluorinated bistriazole.

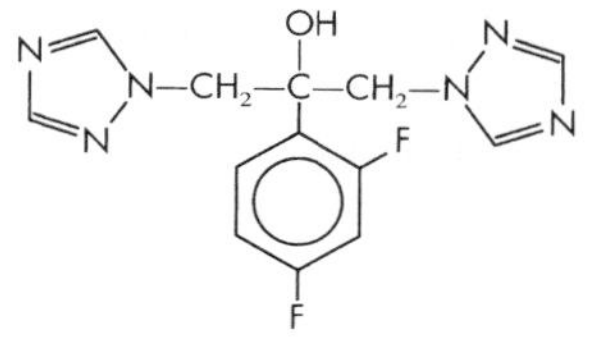

FLUCONAZOLE

Absorption, Distribution, and Excretion. Fluconazole is almost completely absorbed from the GI tract. Plasma concentrations are essentially the same whether the drug is given orally or intravenously, and its bioavailability is unaltered by food or gastric acidity. Peak plasma concentrations are 4-8 μg/mL after repetitive doses of 100 mg. Renal excretion accounts for >90% of elimination, and the elimination $t_{1/2}$ is 25-30 hours. Fluconazole diffuses readily into body fluids, including breast milk, sputum, and saliva; concentrations in CSF can reach 50-90% of the simultaneous values in plasma. The dosage interval should be increased from 24-48 hours with a creatinine clearance of 21-40 mL/minute and to 72 hours at 10-20 mL/minute. A dose of 100-200 mg should be given after each hemodialysis. About 11-12% of drug in the plasma is protein bound.

Drug Interactions. Fluconazole is an inhibitor of CYP3A4 and CYP2C9. Fluconazole's drug–drug interactions are shown in Tables 57–3 and 57–4. Patients who receive >400 mg daily or azotemic patients who have elevated fluconazole blood levels may experience drug interactions not otherwise seen.

Therapeutic Uses. ***Candidiasis.*** Fluconazole, 200 mg on the first day and then 100 mg daily for at least 2 weeks, is effective in oropharyngeal candidiasis. Doses of 100-200 mg daily have been used to decrease candiduria in high-risk patients. A single dose of 150 mg is effective in uncomplicated vaginal candidiasis. A dose of 400 mg daily decreases the incidence of deep candidiasis in allogeneic bone marrow transplant recipients and is useful in treating candidemia of nonimmunosuppressed patients. In patients who have not been receiving fluconazole prophylaxis, the drug has been used successfully as empirical treatment of febrile neutropenia in patients not responding to antibacterial agents and who are not judged to be at high risk of mould infections. Although response to *C. glabrata* bloodstream infections in randomized trials using fluconazole has been comparable to that with *C. albicans*, *C. glabrata* becomes resistant upon prolonged exposure to fluconazole. Empirical use of fluconazole for suspected candidemia may not be advisable in patients who have been receiving long-term fluconazole prophylaxis and may be colonized with azole-resistant *C. glabrata*. Based on resistance *in vitro, Candida krusei* would not be expected to respond to fluconazole or other azoles.

Cryptococcosis. Following IDSA guidelines (Perfect et al., 2010), fluconazole, 400 mg daily, is used for the initial 8 weeks in the treatment of cryptococcal meningitis in patients with AIDS after the patient's clinical condition has been stabilized with at least 2 weeks of intravenous amphotericin B. After 8 weeks in patients no longer symptomatic, the dose is decreased to 200 mg daily and continued indefinitely. If the patient has completed 12 months of treatment for cryptococcosis, responds to HAART, has a CD4 count maintained >200/mm^3 for at least 6 months, and is asymptomatic from cryptococcal meningitis, it is reasonable to discontinue maintenance fluconazole as long as the CD4 response is maintained. Some would add that an undetectable viral load for 3 months is required. Fluconazole, 400 mg daily, has been recommended as continuation therapy in non-AIDS patients with cryptococcal meningitis who have responded to an initial course of C-AMB or L-AMB and for patients with pulmonary cryptococcosis.

Other Mycoses. Fluconazole is the drug of choice for treatment of coccidioidal meningitis because of good penetration into the CSF and much less morbidity than with intrathecal amphotericin B. In other forms of coccidioidomycosis, fluconazole is comparable to itraconazole. Fluconazole has no useful activity against histoplasmosis, blastomycosis, or sporotrichosis. Fluconazole is not effective in the prevention or treatment of aspergillosis. Fluconazole has some activity in ringworm but is not approved for that indication. As with other azoles, with the possible exception of posaconazole, there is no activity in mucormycosis.

Untoward Effects. Side effects in patients receiving >7 days of drug, regardless of dose, include the following: nausea 3.7%, headache 1.9%, skin rash 1.8%, vomiting 1.7%, abdominal pain 1.7%, and diarrhea 1.5%. Use of high doses may be limited by nausea. Reversible alopecia may occur with prolonged therapy at 400 mg daily. Rare cases of deaths due to hepatic failure or Stevens-Johnson syndrome have been reported. Fluconazole is teratogenic in rodents and has been associated with skeletal and cardiac deformities in at least three infants born to two women taking high doses during pregnancy. Fluconazole is a Category C agent that should be avoided during pregnancy unless the potential benefit justifies the possible risk to the fetus.

Dosage. Fluconazole (DIFLUCAN, others) is marketed in the U.S. as tablets of 50, 100, 150, and 200 mg for oral administration, powder for oral suspension providing 10 and 40 mg/mL, and intravenous solutions containing 2 mg/mL in saline and in dextrose solution. The daily dose of fluconazole should be based on the infecting organism and the patient's response to therapy. Generally recommended dosages are 50-400 mg once daily for either oral or intravenous administration. A loading dose of twice the daily maintenance dose is generally administered on the first day of therapy. Prolonged maintenance therapy may be required to prevent relapse. Children are treated with 3-12 mg/kg once daily (maximum: 600 mg/day).

Voriconazole

Voriconazole (VFEND) is a triazole with a structure similar to fluconazole but with increased activity *in vitro*, an expanded spectrum, and poor aqueous solubility.

VORICONAZOLE

Absorption, Distribution, and Excretion. Oral bioavailability is 96% and protein binding 56% (Jeu et al., 2003). Volume of distribution is high (4.6 L/kg), with extensive drug distribution in tissues. Metabolism occurs through CYP2C19 and to a lesser extent CYP2C9; CYP3A4 plays a limited role. Less than 2% of parent drug is recovered from urine, although 80% of the inactive metabolites are excreted in the urine. The oral dose does not have to be adjusted for azotemia or hemodialysis. Peak plasma concentrations after oral doses of 200 mg orally twice daily are ~3 μg/mL. CSF concentrations of 1-3 μg/mL have been reported in a patient with fungal meningitis.

Plasma elimination $t_{1/2}$ is 6 hours. Voriconazole exhibits nonlinear metabolism so that higher doses cause greater-than-linear increases in systemic drug exposure. Genetic polymorphisms in CYP2C19 can cause up to 4-fold differences in drug exposure; 15-20% of Asians are homozygous poor metabolizers, compared with 2% of whites and African Americans. Patients >65 years and patients with mild or moderate hepatic insufficiency have elevated areas under the curve (AUCs). Patients with mild-to-moderate cirrhosis should receive the same loading dose of voriconazole but half the maintenance dose. There are no data to guide dosing in patients with severe hepatic insufficiency.

The intravenous formulation of voriconazole contains sulfobutyl ether β-cyclodextrin (SBECD). When voriconazole is given intravenously, SBECD is excreted completely by the kidney. Significant accumulation of SBECD occurs with a creatinine clearance <50 mL/minute. Because toxicity of SBECD at high plasma concentrations is unclear, oral voriconazole is preferred in azotemic patients.

Drug Interactions. Voriconazole is metabolized by, and inhibits, CYPs 2C19, 2C9, and CYP3A4 (in that order of decreasing potency) The major metabolite of voriconazole, the voriconazole N-oxide, also inhibits these CYPs. Inhibitors or inducers of these CYPs may increase or decrease voriconazole plasma concentrations, respectively. In addition, there is potential for voriconazole and its major metabolite to increase the plasma concentrations of other drugs metabolized by these enzymes (Tables 57–3, 57–4, and 57–5). Because the sirolimus AUC increases 11-fold when voriconazole is given, co-administration is contraindicated. *When starting voriconazole in a patient receiving ≥40 mg/day of omeprazole, the dose of omeprazole should be reduced by half.*

Therapeutic Uses. In an open randomized trial, voriconazole provided superior efficiency to C-AMB in the primary therapy of invasive aspergillosis (Herbrecht et al., 2002). In a secondary analysis, survival also was superior in the voriconazole arm. Voriconazole was compared to L-AMB in an open randomized trial in the empirical therapy of neutropenic patients whose fever did not respond to >96 hours of antibacterial therapy. Because the 95% confidence interval in this noninferiority trial permitted the possibility that voriconazole might be >10% worse than L-AMB, the Food and Drug Administration did not approve voriconazole for this use (Walsh et al., 2002). However, in a secondary analysis, there were fewer breakthrough infections with voriconazole (1.9%) than with L-AMB (5%). Voriconazole is approved for use in esophageal candidiasis on the basis of a double-blind randomized comparison with fluconazole (Ally et al., 2001). In non-neutropenic patients with candidemia, voriconazole was comparable in efficacy and less toxic than initial C-AMB followed by fluconazole (Kullberg, 2005). Voriconazole is approved for initial treatment of candidemia and invasive aspergillosis, as well as for salvage therapy in patients with *Pseudallescheria boydii (Scedosporium apiospermum)* and *Fusarium* infections. Positive response of patients with cerebral fungal suggest that the drug penetrates infected brain.

Untoward Effects. Voriconazole is teratogenic in animals and generally contraindicated in pregnancy (Category D). Women of child-bearing potential should use effective contraception during treatment. Although voriconazole is generally well tolerated, occasional cases of hepatotoxicity have been reported, and liver function should be monitored. Voriconazole, like some other azoles, causes a prolongation of the QTc interval, which can become significant in patients with other risk factors for torsades de pointes. Patients must be warned about possible visual effects. Transient visual or auditory hallucinations are frequent after the first dose, usually at night and particularly with intravenous administration. Symptoms diminish with time (Zonios et al., 2008). Patients receiving their first intravenous infusion have had anaphylactoid reactions, with faintness, nausea, flushing, feverishness, and rash. In such patients, the infusion should be stopped. Rash has been reported in 5.8% of patients.

Dosage. Voriconazole for intravenous infusion is packaged as 200 mg with 3.2 g SBECD. Treatment is usually initiated with an intravenous infusion of 6 mg/kg every 12 hours for two doses, followed by 3-4 mg/kg every 12 hours. It should be administered no faster than 3 mg/kg/hr (e.g., over 1-2 hours, not as an intravenous bolus). As the patient improves, oral administration is continued as 200 mg every 12 hours. Patients failing to respond may be given 300 mg every 12 hours. Voriconazole is available as 50- or 200-mg tablets or a suspension of 40 mg/mL when hydrated. The tablets, but not the suspension, contain lactose. Because high-fat meals reduce voriconazole bioavailability, oral drug should be given either 1 hour before or 1 hour after meals. Children metabolize voriconazole more rapidly that adults (Walsh, 2004a).

Posaconazole

Posaconazole (NOXAFIL) is a synthetic structural analog of itraconazole with the same broad antifungal spectrum but with up to 4-fold greater activity *in vitro* against yeasts and filamentous fungi, including the agents of mucormycosis (Guinea et al., 2008; Frampton, 2008). Activity against yeasts *in vitro* is similar to voriconazole. The mechanism of action is the same as other imidazoles, inhibition of sterol 14-α demethylase.

Absorption, Distribution, and Excretion. Posaconazole is available as a cherry-flavored suspension containing 40 mg/mL. Bioavailability is significantly enhanced by the presence of food (Courtney et al., 2003; Krieter, 2004). The drug has a long terminal phase $t_{1/2}$ (25-31 hours), a large volume of distribution (331-1341 L), and extensive binding (>98%) to protein, predominantly albumin. Systemic exposure is four times higher in homozygous CYP2C19 slow metabolizers than in homozygous wild-type metabolizers. Steady-state concentrations are reached in 7-10 days when dosed four times daily. Saturation of absorption occurs at 800 mg/day (Ezzet et al., 2005; Ullmann et al., 2006). Renal impairment does not alter plasma concentrations; hepatic impairment causes a modest increase (Moton, 2008). With radiolabeled drug given to volunteers, 77% was excreted in the stool, with 66% of the administered dose appearing as unchanged drug. The major metabolic pathway is hepatic UDP glucuronidation (Krieter, 2004). Hemodialysis does not remove detectable amounts of this highly protein-bound drug from the circulation. Gastric acid improves absorption in that an acidic beverage, ginger ale, increased the AUC by 70% in the fasting state (Krishna et al., 2009b). Drugs that reduce gastric acid (e.g., cimetidine and esomeprazole) decreased posaconazole exposure by 32-50% (Frampton and Scott, 2008). Diarrhea reduced the average plasma concentration by 37% (Smith et al., 2009). Plasma concentrations in allogeneic stem cell transplant recipients were 52% lower than in patients not receiving a stem cell transplant (Ullmann et al., 2006). Although monitoring plasma concentrations has been advocated (Smith et al., 2009), the lower limit of therapeutic effect for any indication is unknown.

Therapeutic Use. Posaconazole is not inferior to fluconazole for treatment of oropharyngeal candidiasis, although fluconazole is the preferred drug because of safety, cost, and extensive experience. The dose is 100 mg twice daily the first day and once daily thereafter for

13 days. Posaconazole is approved for prophylaxis against candidiasis and aspergillosis in patients >13 years of age who have prolonged neutropenia or severe graft-vs-host disease (GVHD) (Ullmann et al., 2007). Posaconazole and other "azoles" have recently been compared for prophylaxis effect in patients with neutropenia (Cornely et al., 2007b). The broad applicability of posaconazole for prophylaxis of patients with prolonged neutropenia or GVHD remains unsettled, although the drug clearly remains an option for those indications (De Pauw, 2007).

Posaconazole is approved in the E.U. as salvage therapy for aspergillosis and several other infections, as are itraconazole and voriconazole. A number of clinical reports of favorable response to posaconazole as salvage therapy in mucormycosis have appeared in the literature, leaving the issue unresolved (Dannaoui et al., 2003; Greenberg et al., 2006). Lack of an intravenous formulation continues to limit studies of critically ill patients.

Drug Interactions. Posaconazole inhibits CYP3A4. Co-administration with rifabutin or phenytoin increases the plasma concentration of these drugs and decreases posaconazole exposure by 2-fold. The mechanism of induced posaconazole clearance is unknown but may involve hepatic phase 2 glucuronidation, rather than phase 1 oxidative enzymes. Oxidative products have not been recovered in the serum of treated patients. Posaconazole increases the AUC of cyclosporine, tacrolimus (121%), sirolimus (790%), midazolam (83%) and other CYP3A4 substrates (Table 57–4) (Frampton and Scott, 2008; Krishna et al., 2009a; Moton et al., 2009). Posaconazole is not known to prolong cardiac repolarization, as other azoles may, but posaconazole should not be co-administered with drugs that are CYP3A4 substrates and prolong the QTc interval, such as methadone, haloperidol, pimozide, quinidine, risperidone, sunitinib, tacrolimus, and halofantrine (Table 57–6).

Untoward Effects. The safety profile of posaconazole is good, with nausea, vomiting, diarrhea, abdominal pain, and headache the most commonly reported adverse effects (Smith et al., 2009). Although adverse effects occur in at least a third of patients, discontinuation due to adverse effects in long-term studies has been only 8%, Posaconazole causes fetal bone malformation in pregnant rats and is pregnancy Category C. Safety in children <8 years of age has not been established.

Dosage. Dosage for adults and children >8 years of age is 200 mg (5 mL suspension) three times daily for prophylaxis. Treatment of active infection is begun at 200 mg four times daily and changed to 400 mg twice daily once infection has improved. All doses should be taken with a full meal.

Isavuconazole

Isavuconazole (BAL8557) is an investigational water-soluble pro-drug of the synthetic triazole, BAL4815.

The pro-drug is readily cleaved by esterases in the human body to release the active triazole. *In vitro* activity is comparable to voriconazole (Guinea et al., 2008; Perkhofer et al., 2009).

Absorption, Distribution, and Excretion. Oral administration of once-daily doses equivalent to 100 mg BAL4815 for loading followed by 50 mg daily and 200 mg loading followed by 100 mg resulted in peak plasma concentrations at 21 days of 1.37 μg/mL and 3.5 μg/mL at 2.25 and 3.5 hours, respectively. The $AUCs_{0\text{-}24h}$ were 21.6 and 40.3 μg·h/mL, respectively (Schmitt-Hoffman et al., 2006). With intravenous administration there was close to a linear dose response, with a 5-fold accumulation over 14 days, a $t_{1/2}$ of 84.5-117 hours, and a volume of distribution at steady state of 308-542 L. Excretion is by the liver with most drug appearing in feces.

Therapeutic Use. Isavuconazole has been found comparable to fluconazole in *Candida* esophagitis with all three isavuconazole regimens tested: loading dose of 200 followed by 50 mg daily, loading dose of 400 mg followed by 100 mg daily, or 400 mg once weekly for 14 days (Odds, 2006). The drug was well tolerated. Phase III trials are enrolling patients with deeply invasive candidiasis and aspergillosis.

Echinocandins

Screening natural products of fungal fermentation in the 1970s led to the discovery that *echinocandins* had activity against *Candida* and that the biological activity was directed against formation of 1,3-β-D-glucans in the fungal cell wall (Wiederhold and Lewis, 2003). The inhibition of glucan synthesis reduces structural integrity of the fungal cell wall (Figure 57–3), resulting in osmotic instability and cell death. Three echinocandins are approved for clinical use: caspofungin, anidulafungin, and micafungin. All are cyclic lipopeptides with a hexapeptide nucleus. All have the same mechanism of action but differ in pharmacological properties. Susceptible fungi include *Candida* species and *Aspergillus* species (Bennett, 2006).

General Pharmacological Characteristics. Echinocandins differ somewhat pharmacokinetically (Table 57–7) but all share lack of oral bioavailability, extensive protein binding (>97%), inability to penetrate into CSF, lack of renal clearance, and only a slight to modest effect of hepatic insufficiency on plasma drug concentration (Kim et al., 2007; Wagner et al., 2006). Adverse effects are minimal and rarely lead to drug discontinuation (Kim et al., 2007). All three agents are pregnancy Category C. For a review of the basic and clinical pharmacology of the echinocandins, see Wiederhold and Lewis (2007).

The minimum inhibitory concentration (MIC) of *Candida albicans* and several other Candida species are in the range of 0.015-0.5 μg/mL, higher for caspofungin than micafungin or anidulafungin. In *Candida* spp., echinocandins cause cell death at concentrations only 2- to 4-fold higher than that needed to inhibit growth. Azole-resistant Candida species remain susceptible to echinocandins. MIC of *Candida parapsilosis* and *C. guilliermondii* are consistently higher than other *Candida* spp., usually 2 μg/mL with all three echinocandins. In none of the clinical trials of the three echinocandins has the higher MIC of *C. parapsilosis* been reflected in lower response rates. An unexplained and paradoxical effect of increased growth at concentrations above the MIC has been seen more often in *C. parapsilosis* than with other *Candida* spp. and more commonly with caspofungin than micafungin or anidulafungin (Chamilos et al., 2007). In *Aspergillus,* echinocandins are not cidal but change the shape of hyphae; thus, *in vitro* susceptibility testing is done with a "morphological" end point (change in hyphal shape). Animal models do not suggest activity against dimorphic fungi such

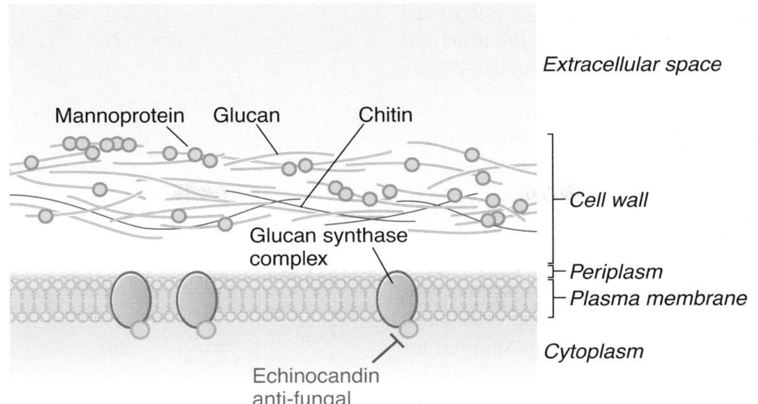

Figure 57–3. *The fungal cell wall and membrane and the action of echinocandins.* The strength of the fungal cell wall is maintained by fibrillar polysaccharides, largely β-1,3-glucan and chitin, which bind covalently to each other and to proteins. A glucan synthase complex in the plasma membrane catalyzes the synthesis of beta-1,3-glucan; the glucan is extruded into the periplasm and incorporated into the cell wall. Echinocandins inhibit the activity of the glucan synthase complex, resulting in loss of the structural integrity of the cell wall. A subunit of glucan synthase designated Fks1p is thought to be the target of the echinocandin. Mutations in Fks1p, coded for by *FSK1,* cause resistance to echinocandins.

as *Histoplasma capsulatum.* Echinocandins have no activity against *Cryptococcus neoformans*, *Trichosporon* spp., or agents of mucormycosis. *In vitro* studies have consistently failed to show synergism or antagonism between echinocandins and amphotericin B. There is no antagonism between echinocandins and azoles; an additive effect has been reported with Aspergillus in some *in vitro* systems and animals models. Echinocandin resistance can be selected in *Candida albicans* under drug pressure both *in vitro* and clinically during prolonged echinocandin therapy. Resistance is from mutations in a conserved region of the *FKS1* gene, coding for amino acids Phe ^{641}-Asp ^{658} (Park et al., 2005). FKS1p is an essential component of the 1,3-β-D-glucan synthase complex (Figure 57–3).

Caspofungin

Caspofungin acetate (CANCIDAS) is a water-soluble, semisynthetic lipopeptide synthesized from the fermentation product of *Glarea lozoyensis* (Johnson and Perfect, 2003; Keating and Figgit, 2003).

CASPOFUNGIN

Table 57-7

Pharmacokinetics of Echinocandins in Humans

DRUG	DOSE (mg)	C_{max} (μg/mL)	$AUC_{0\text{-}24h}$ (mg•h/L)	$t_{1/2}$ (h)	Cl (mL/min/kg)	V_d (L)
Caspofungin	70	12	93.5	10	0.15	9.5
Micafungin	75	7.1	59.9	13	0.16	14
Anidulafungin	200	7.5	104.5	25.6	0.16	33.4

For details, see Wagner et al. (2006).

Metabolism and Excretion. Catabolism is largely by hydrolysis and *N*-acetylation, with excretion of the metabolites in the urine and feces. Mild and moderate hepatic insufficiency increases the AUC by 55% and 76%, respectively.

Drug Interactions. Caspofungin increase tacrolimus levels by 16%, which should be managed by standard monitoring. Cyclosporine slightly increases caspofungin levels. Rifampin and other drugs activating CYP3A4 can cause a slight reduction in caspofungin levels.

Therapeutic Use. Caspofungin is approved for initial therapy of deeply invasive candidiasis and as salvage therapy for patients with invasive aspergillosis who are failing or intolerant of approved drugs, such as amphotericin B formulations or voriconazole. Approval for salvage therapy of aspergillosis was based on a study of 63 patients in a noncomparative salvage trial. Caspofungin is also approved for esophageal candidiasis, based on randomized trials that found noninferiority to fluconazole and C-AMB (Villanueva et al., 2001). A blinded randomized clinical trial of caspofungin in deeply invasive candidiasis found noninferiority to C-AMB, leading to approval for that indication (Mora-Duarte et al., 2002). Most patients in that multicenter study were not neutropenic and had catheter-acquired candidemia. Efficacy was comparable to that of fluconazole in other studies of the same general patient population. Caspofungin is also approved for the treatment of persistently febrile neutropenic patients with suspected fungal infections, based on noninferiority to L-AMB in a randomized trial (Walsh et al., 2004b).

Untoward Effects. Caspofungin has been remarkably well tolerated, with the exception of phlebitis at the infusion site. Histamine-like effects have been reported with rapid infusions. Other symptoms have been equivalent to those observed in patients receiving fluconazole in the comparator arm.

Dosage. Caspofungin is administered intravenously once daily over 1 hour. In candidemia and salvage therapy of aspergillosis, the initial dose is 70 mg, followed by 50 mg daily. The dose should be increased to 70 mg daily in patients receiving rifampin as well as in those failing to respond to 50 mg. Esophageal candidiasis is treated with 50 mg daily. In moderate hepatic failure, the dose should be reduced to 35 mg daily.

Micafungin

Micafungin (MYCAMINE) is a water-soluble semisynthetic echinocandin derived from the fungus *Coleophoma empedri*.

Absorption, Distribution, and Excretion. Micafungin has linear pharmacokinetics over a large range of doses (1-3 mg/kg) and ages (premature infants to elderly). Feces contain 71% of intravenously administered radiolabeled drug, including both native drug and metabolites (Wiederhold and Lewis, 2007). Small amounts of drug are metabolized in the liver by arylsulfatase and catechol *O*-methyltransferase. Hydroxylation by CYP3A4 is barely detectable. Reduction of dose in moderate hepatic failure is not required. Clearance is more rapid in premature infants and intermediate in children 2-8 years of age, compared to older children and adults.

Drug Interactions. In normal volunteers, micafungin appears to be a mild inhibitor of CYP3A4, increasing AUC of nifedipine by 18%

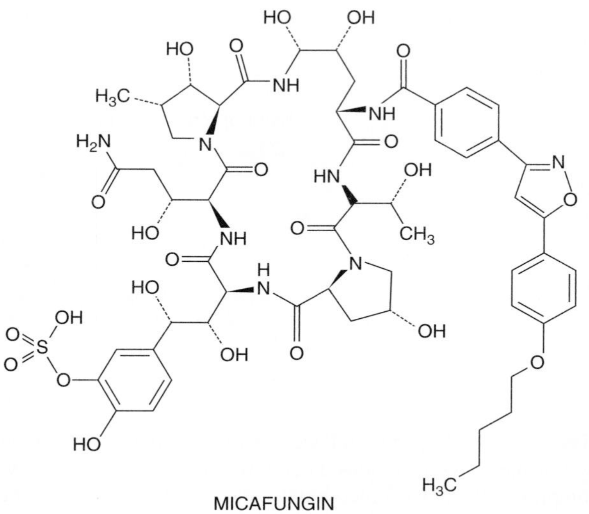

MICAFUNGIN

and sirolimus by 21%. Micafungin has no effect on tacrolimus clearance.

Therapeutic Use. Micafungin is approved for the treatment of deeply invasive candidiasis (Fritz et al., 2008). Doses of 100 mg and 150 mg daily of micafungin were equivalent to caspofungin (Pappas et al., 2007). Micafungin, 100 mg/day, was also not inferior to L-AMB, 3 mg/kg (Kuse et al., 2007). Micafungin is also approved for treatment of esophageal candidiasis and prophylaxis of deeply invasive candidiasis in hematopoietic stem cell transplant recipients.

Doses. Micafungin is given intravenously as 100 mg daily over 1 hour for adults, with 50 mg recommended for prophylaxis and 150 mg for esophageal candidiasis. No loading dose is needed.

Anidulafungin

Anidulafungin (ERAXIS) is a water-insoluble semisynthetic compound extracted from the fungus *Aspergillus nidulans*, from which the drug's name derives.

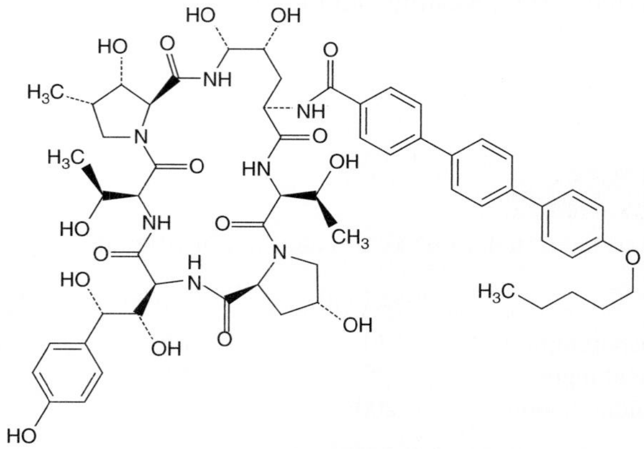

ANIDULAFUNGIN

Absorption, Distribution and Excretion. Anidulafungin is cleared from the body by slow chemical degradation, first by opening the hexapeptide ring and then proteolysis of peptide bonds (Vazquez and Sobel, 2006). No metabolism by the liver or renal excretion of active drug occurs. No dose adjustment for hepatic or renal failure is needed. The drug diluent for intravenous infusion contains 3 mg ethanol for every 50 mg anidulafungin, an amount of ethanol insufficient to have a pharmacological effect.

Drug interactions. None are known.

Therapeutic Use. In a randomized double-blinded clinical trial, anidulafungin was noninferior to fluconazole in candidemia of non-neutropenic patients (Reboli et al., 2007). Anidulafungin is also approved for the treatment of esophageal candidiasis.

Dose. Drug dissolved in the supplied diluent is infused once daily in saline or 5% dextrose in water at a rate not exceeding 1.1 mg/minute. For deeply invasive candidiasis, anidulafungin is given daily as a loading dose of 200 mg followed by 100 mg daily. For esophageal candidiasis, a loading dose of 100 mg is followed by 50 mg daily.

Griseofulvin

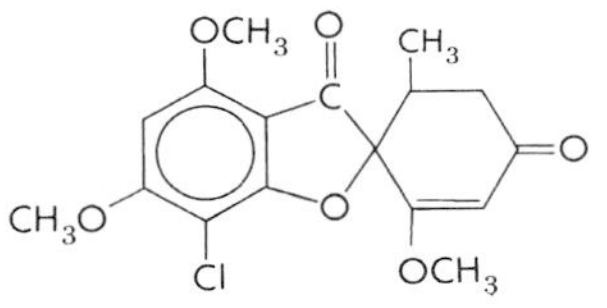

OCH_3 CH_3 CH_3O Cl OCH_3

GRISEOFULVIN

The drug is practically insoluble in water.

Mechanism of Action. Griseofulvin inhibits microtubule function and thereby disrupts assembly of the mitotic spindle. Thus, a prominent morphological manifestation of the action of griseofulvin is the production of multinucleate cells as the drug inhibits fungal mitosis. Although the effects of the drug are similar to those of *colchicine* and the vinca alkaloids, griseofulvin's binding sites on the microtubular protein are distinct. In addition to its binding to tubulin, griseofulvin interacts with microtubule-associated protein.

Absorption, Distribution, and Excretion. The oral administration of a 0.5 g dose of griseofulvin produces peak plasma concentrations of ~1 μg/mL in ~4 hours. Blood levels are quite variable, however. Some studies have shown improved absorption when the drug is taken with a fatty meal. Because the rates of dissolution and disaggregation limit the bioavailability of griseofulvin, micro-sized and ultra-micro-sized powders are now used in preparations (GRIFULVIN V and GRIS-PEG, respectively). Although the bioavailability of the ultra-microcrystalline preparation is said to be 50% greater than that of the conventional micro-sized powder, this may not always be true. Griseofulvin has a plasma $t_{1/2}$ of ~1 day, and ~50% of the oral dose can be detected in the urine within 5 days, mostly in the form of metabolites. The primary metabolite is 6-methylgriseofulvin. Barbiturates decrease griseofulvin absorption from the GI tract.

Griseofulvin is deposited in keratin precursor cells; when these cells differentiate, the drug is tightly bound to, and persists in, keratin, providing prolonged resistance to fungal invasion. For this reason, the new growth of hair or nails is the first to become free of disease. As the fungus-containing keratin is shed, it is replaced by normal tissue. Griseofulvin is detectable in the stratum corneum of the skin within 4-8 hours of oral administration. Sweat and transepidermal fluid loss play an important role in the transfer of the drug in the stratum corneum. Only a very small fraction of a dose of the drug is present in body fluids and tissues.

Antifungal Activity. Griseofulvin is fungistatic *in vitro* for various species of the dermatophytes *Microsporum, Epidermophyton,* and *Trichophyton.* The drug has no effect on bacteria or on other fungi. Although failure of ringworm lesions to improve is not rare, isolates from these patients usually are still susceptible to griseofulvin *in vitro.*

Therapeutic Uses. Mycotic disease of the skin, hair, and nails due to *Microsporum, Trichophyton,* or *Epidermophyton* responds to griseofulvin therapy. For tinea capitis in children, griseofulvin remains the drug of choice for efficacy, safety, and availability as an oral suspension; efficacy is best for tinea capitis caused by *Microsporum canis, Microsporum audouinii, Trichophyton schoenleinii,* and *Trichophyton verrucosum.* Griseofulvin is also effective for ringworm of the glabrous skin; tinea cruris and tinea corporis caused by *M. canis, Trichophyton rubrum, T. verrucosum,* and *Epidermophyton floccosum;* and tinea of the hands (*T. rubrum* and *T. mentagrophytes*) and beard (*Trichophyton* species). Griseofulvin also is highly effective in tinea pedis, the vesicular form of which is most commonly due to *T. mentagrophytes* and the hyperkeratotic type to *T. rubrum.* Topical therapy is sufficient for most cases of tinea pedis. *T. rubrum* and *T. mentagrophytes* infections may require higher-than-conventional doses of griseofulvin.

Dosage. The recommended daily dose of griseofulvin is 2.3 mg/ kg (up to 500 mg) for children and 500 mg to 1 g for adults. Doses of 1.5-2 g daily may be used for short periods in severe or extensive infections. Best results are obtained when the daily dose is divided and given at 6-hour intervals, although the drug often is given once or twice per day. Treatment must be continued until infected tissue is replaced by normal hair, skin, or nails, which requires 1 month for scalp and hair ringworm, 6-9 months for fingernails, and at least a year for toenails. Itraconazole or terbinafine is much more effective for onychomycosis.

Untoward Effects. The incidence of serious reactions due to griseofulvin is very low. One of the minor effects is headache (incidence as high as 15%), which is sometimes severe and usually disappears as therapy is continued. Other nervous system manifestations include peripheral neuritis, lethargy, mental confusion, impairment of performance of routine tasks, fatigue, syncope, vertigo, blurred vision, transient macular edema, and augmentation of the effects of alcohol. Among the side effects involving the alimentary tract are nausea, vomiting, diarrhea, heartburn, flatulence, dry mouth, and angular stomatitis. Hepatotoxicity also has been observed. Hematological effects include leukopenia, neutropenia, punctate basophilia, and monocytosis; these often disappear despite continued therapy. Blood studies should be carried out at least once a week during the first month of treatment or longer. Common renal effects include albuminuria and cylindruria without evidence of renal insufficiency. Reactions involving the skin are cold and warm urticaria, photosensitivity, lichen planus, erythema, erythema multiforme–like rashes, and vesicular and morbilliform eruptions. Serum sickness syndromes and severe angioedema develop rarely during treatment with griseofulvin. Estrogen-like effects have been observed in children. A moderate but inconsistent increase of fecal protoporphyrins has been noted with chronic use.

Griseofulvin induces hepatic CYPs, thereby increasing the rate of metabolism of warfarin; adjustment of the dosage of the latter agent may be necessary in some patients. The drug may reduce the efficacy of low-estrogen oral contraceptive agents, probably by a similar mechanism.

Terbinafine

Terbinafine is a synthetic allylamine, structurally similar to the topical agent naftifine.

TERBINAFINE

Terbinafine is well absorbed, but bioavailability is decreased to ~40% because of first-pass metabolism in the liver. Proteins bind >99% of the drug in plasma. Drug accumulates in skin, nails, and fat. The initial $t_{1/2}$ is ~12 hours but extends to 200-400 hours at steady state. Terbinafine is not recommended in patients with marked azotemia or hepatic failure because in the latter condition, terbinafine plasma levels are increased by unpredictable amounts. Rifampin decreases and cimetidine increases plasma terbinafine concentrations. The drug is well tolerated, with a low incidence of GI distress, headache, or rash. Very rarely, fatal hepatotoxicity, severe neutropenia, Stevens-Johnson syndrome, or toxic epidermal necrolysis may occur. The drug is pregnancy Category B and it is recommended that systemic terbinafine therapy for onychomycosis be postponed until after pregnancy is complete. Its mechanism of action is inhibition of fungal squalene epoxidase, blocking ergosterol biosynthesis. Increased intracellular squalene also impairs cell growth.

Terbinafine (LAMISIL, others), given as one 250-mg tablet daily for adults, is somewhat more effective for nail onychomycosis than 200 mg daily of itraconazole, and definitely more effective than pulse itraconazole therapy (Fernandez-Obregon et al., 2007). Duration of treatment varies with the site being treated but typically is 6-12 weeks. Efficacy in onychomycosis can be improved by the simultaneous use of amorolfine 5% nail lacquer (Baran et al., 2007). Terbinafine (250 mg daily) also is effective in tinea capitis and is used off-label for ringworm elsewhere on the body. Oral granules are available for use against tinea capitis, usually a disease of children. The recommended dose is 125-250 mg (depending on weight) daily for 6 weeks. The topical use of terbinafine is discussed later.

Topical Antifungal Agents

Topical treatment is useful in many superficial fungal infections, i.e., those confined to the stratum corneum, squamous mucosa, or cornea. Such diseases include dermatophytosis (ringworm), candidiasis, tinea versicolor, piedra, tinea nigra, and fungal keratitis. Topical administration of antifungal agents usually is not successful for mycoses of the nails (onychomycosis) and hair (tinea capitis) and has no place in the treatment of subcutaneous mycoses, such as sporotrichosis and chromoblastomycosis. The efficacy of topical agents in the treatment of superficial mycoses depends not only on the type of lesion and the mechanism of action of the drug but also on the viscosity, hydrophobicity, and acidity of the formulation. Regardless of formulation, penetration of topical drugs into hyperkeratotic lesions often is poor. Removal of thick, infected keratin is sometimes a useful adjunct to therapy and is the principal mode of action of Whitfield's ointment. Similarly, 40% urea paste can be applied under occlusion to soften infected nails.

Among the topical agents, the preferred formulation for cutaneous application usually is a cream or solution. Ointments are messy and are too occlusive for macerated or fissured intertriginous lesions. The use of powders, whether applied by shake containers or aerosols, is largely confined to the feet and moist lesions of the groin and other intertriginous areas.

The systemic agents used for the treatment of superficial mycoses were discussed earlier. Some of these agents also are administered topically; their uses are described here and also in Chapter 65.

Imidazoles and Triazoles for Topical Use

These closely related classes of drugs are synthetic antifungal agents that are used both topically and systemically. Indications for their topical use include ringworm, tinea versicolor, and mucocutaneous candidiasis. Resistance to imidazoles or triazoles is very rare among the fungi that cause ringworm. Selection of one of these agents for topical use should be based on cost and availability because testing *in vitro* for fungal susceptibility to these drugs does not predict clinical responses.

Cutaneous Application. The preparations for cutaneous use described below are effective for tinea corporis, tinea pedis, tinea cruris, tinea versicolor, and cutaneous candidiasis. They should be applied twice a day for 3-6 weeks. Despite some activity *in vitro* against bacteria, this effect is not clinically useful. The cutaneous formulations are not suitable for oral, vaginal, or ocular use.

Vaginal Application. Vaginal creams, suppositories, and tablets for vaginal candidiasis are all used once a day for 1-7 days, preferably at bedtime to facilitate retention. None is useful in trichomoniasis, despite some activity *in vitro*. Most vaginal creams are administered in 5-g amounts. Three vaginal formulations—clotrimazole tablets, miconazole suppositories, and terconazole cream—come in both low- and high-dose preparations. A shorter duration of therapy is recommended for the higher dose of each. These preparations are administered for 3-7 days. Approximately 3-10% of the vaginal dose is absorbed. Although some imidazoles are teratogenic in rodents, no adverse effects on the human fetus have been attributed to the vaginal use of imidazoles or triazoles. The most common side effect is vaginal burning or itching. A male sexual partner may experience mild penile irritation. Cross-allergenicity among these compounds is assumed to exist, based on their structural similarities.

Oral Use. Use of the oral troche of clotrimazole is properly considered as topical therapy. The only indication for this 10-mg troche is oropharyngeal candidiasis. Antifungal activity is due entirely to the local concentration of the drug; there is no systemic effect.

Clotrimazole

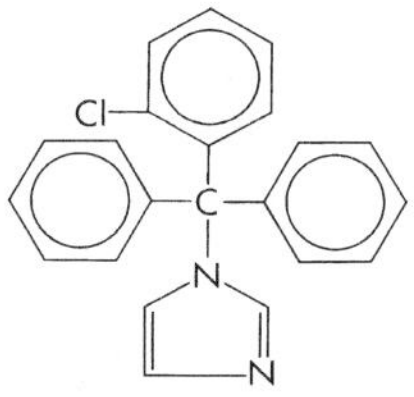

CLOTRIMAZOLE

Absorption of clotrimazole is <0.5% after application to the intact skin; from the vagina, it is 3-10%. Fungicidal concentrations remain in the vagina for as long as 3 days after application of the drug. The small amount absorbed is metabolized in the liver and excreted in bile. In adults, an oral dose of 200 mg/day will give rise initially to plasma concentrations of 0.2-0.35 μg/mL, followed by a progressive decline.

In a small fraction of recipients, clotrimazole on the skin may cause stinging, erythema, edema, vesication, desquamation, pruritus, and urticaria. When it is applied to the vagina, ~1.6% of recipients complain of a mild burning sensation, and rarely of lower abdominal cramps, a slight increase in urinary frequency, or skin rash. Occasionally, the sexual partner may experience penile or urethral irritation. By the oral route, clotrimazole can cause GI irritation. In patients using troches, the incidence of this side effect is ~5%.

Therapeutic Uses. Clotrimazole is available as a 1% cream, lotion, powder, aerosol solution, and solution (LOTRIMIN AF, MYCELEX, others), 1% or 2% vaginal cream, or vaginal tablets of 100, 200, or 500 mg (GYNE-LOTRIMIN, others), and 10-mg troches (MYCELEX, others). On the skin, applications are made twice a day. For the vagina, the standard regimens are one 100-mg tablet once a day at bedtime for 7 days, one 200-mg tablet daily for 3 days, one 500-mg tablet inserted only once, or 5 g of cream once a day for 3 days (2% cream) or 7 days (1% cream). For oropharyngeal candidiasis, troches are to be dissolved slowly in the mouth five times a day for 14 days.

Topical clotrimazole cures dermatophyte infections in 60-100% of cases. The cure rates in cutaneous candidiasis are 80-100%. In vulvovaginal candidiasis, the cure rate is usually >80% when the 7-day regimen is used. A 3-day regimen of 200 mg once a day appears to be similarly effective, as does single-dose treatment (500 mg). Recurrences are common after all regimens. The cure rate with oral troches for oral and pharyngeal candidiasis may be as high as 100% in the immunocompetent host.

Econazole

Econazole is the deschloro derivative of miconazole. Econazole readily penetrates the stratum corneum and is found in effective concentrations down to the mid-dermis. However, <1% of an applied dose appears to be absorbed into the blood. Approximately 3% of recipients have local erythema, burning, stinging, or itching. Econazole nitrate (SPECTAZOLE, ECOSTATIN, others) is available as a water-miscible cream (1%) to be applied twice a day.

Miconazole

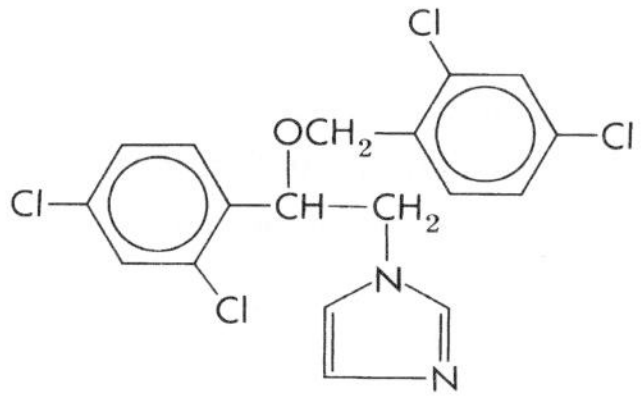

MICONAZOLE

Miconazole readily penetrates the stratum corneum of the skin and persists there for >4 days after application. Less than 1% is absorbed into the blood. Absorption is no more than 1.3% from the vagina.

Adverse effects from topical application to the vagina include burning, itching, or irritation in ~7% of recipients, and infrequently, pelvic cramps (0.2%), headache, hives, or skin rash. Irritation, burning, and maceration are rare after cutaneous application. Miconazole is considered safe for use during pregnancy, although some authors avoid its vaginal use during the first trimester.

Therapeutic Uses. Miconazole nitrate is available as a 2% cream, ointment, lotion, powder, gel, aerosol powder, and aerosol solution (MICATIN, ZEASORB-AF, others). To avoid maceration, only the lotion should be applied to intertriginous areas. Miconazole is available as a 2% and 4% vaginal cream, and as 100-mg, 200-mg, or 1200-mg vaginal suppositories (MONISTAT 7, MONISTAT 3, MONISTAT 1, others), to be applied high in the vagina at bedtime for 7, 3, or 1 day(s), respectively.

In the treatment of tinea pedis, tinea cruris, and tinea versicolor, the cure rate may be >90%. In the treatment of vulvovaginal candidiasis, the mycologic cure rate at the end of 1 month is ~80-95%. Pruritus sometimes is relieved after a single application. Some vaginal infections caused by *Candida glabrata* also respond.

Terconazole and Butoconazole

Terconazole (TERAZOL, others) is a ketal triazole. The mechanism of action of terconazole is similar to that of the imidazoles. The 80-mg vaginal suppository is inserted at bedtime for 3 days; the 0.4% vaginal cream is used for 7 days and the 0.8% cream for 3 days. Clinical efficacy and patient acceptance of both preparations are at least as good as for clotrimazole in patients with vaginal candidiasis.

Butoconazole is an imidazole that is pharmacologically quite comparable to clotrimazole. Butoconazole nitrate (FEMSTAT 3, others) is available as a 2% vaginal cream; it is used at bedtime in nonpregnant females. Because of the slower response during pregnancy, a 6-day course is recommended (during the second and third trimester).

Tioconazole

Tioconazole (VAGISTAT 1, others) is an imidazole marketed for treatment of *Candida* vulvovaginitis. A single 4.6-g dose of ointment (300 mg) is given at bedtime.

Oxiconazole, Sulconazole, and Sertaconazole

These imidazole derivatives are used for the topical treatment of infections caused by the common pathogenic dermatophytes. Oxiconazole nitrate (OXISTAT) is available as a 1% cream and lotion; sulconazole nitrate (EXELDERM, SULCOSYN) is supplied as a 1% solution and/or cream. Sertaconazole (ERTACZO) is a 2% cream marketed for tinea pedis.

Ketoconazole

This imidazole is available as a 0.5% cream, foam, gel, and shampoo (NIZORAL, others) for common skin dermatophytes infections, for tinea versicolor, and seborrheic dermatitis.

Ciclopirox Olamine

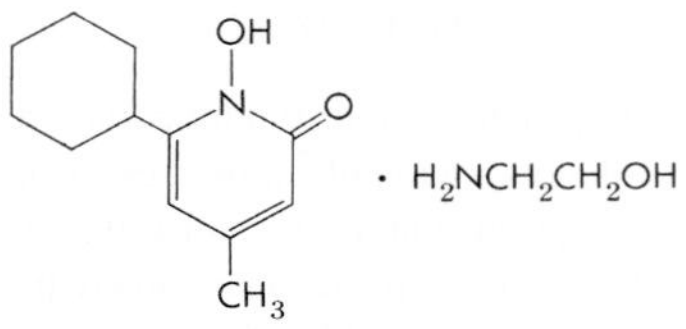

CICLOPIROX OLAMINE

Ciclopirox olamine (LOPROX, others) has broad-spectrum antifungal activity. It is fungicidal to *C. albicans, E. floccosum, M. canis, T. mentagrophytes,* and *T. rubrum.* It also inhibits the growth of *Malassezia furfur.* After application to the skin, it penetrates through the epidermis into the dermis, but even under occlusion, <1.5% is absorbed into the systemic circulation. Because the $t_{1/2}$ is 1.7 hours, no systemic accumulation occurs. The drug penetrates into hair follicles and sebaceous glands. It can sometimes cause hypersensitivity. It is available as a 0.77% cream, gel, suspension, and lotion for the treatment of cutaneous candidiasis and for tinea corporis, cruris, pedis, and versicolor. An 8% nail lacquer is available for onychomycosis. Cure rates in the dermatomycoses and candidal infections are 81-94%. No topical toxicity has been noted.

Ciclopirox 0.77% gel and 1% shampoo are also used for the treatment of seborrheic dermatitis of the scalp. An 8% topical solution (PENLAC NAIL LACQUER, others) is an effective treatment for mild to moderate superficial white onychomycosis. An oral agent would be preferred for distal or lateral onychomycosis.

Haloprogin

Haloprogin is a halogenated phenolic ether:

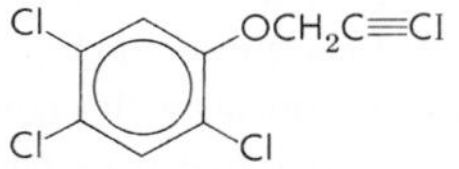

HALOPROGIN

It is fungicidal to various species of *Epidermophyton, Pityrosporum, Microsporum, Trichophyton,* and *Candida.* During treatment with this drug, irritation, pruritus, burning sensations, vesiculation, increased maceration, and "sensitization" (or exacerbation of the lesion) occasionally occur, especially on the foot if occlusive footgear is worn. Haloprogin is poorly absorbed through the skin; it is converted to trichlorophenol in the body. The systemic toxicity from topical application appears to be low.

Haloprogin (HALOTEX) cream or solution is applied twice a day for 2-4 weeks. Its principal use is against tinea pedis, for which the cure rate is ~80%; it is thus approximately equal in efficacy to tolnaftate. It also is used against tinea cruris, tinea corporis, tinea manuum, and tinea versicolor. Haloprogin is no longer available in the U.S.

Tolnaftate

Tolnaftate is a thiocarbamate with the following structure:

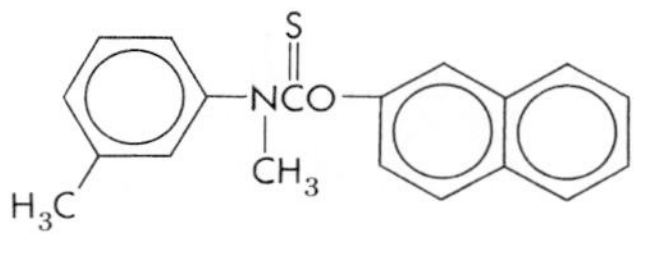

TOLNAFTATE

Tolnaftate is effective in the treatment of most cutaneous mycoses caused by *T. rubrum, T. mentagrophytes, T. tonsurans, E. floccosum, M. canis, M. audouinii, Microsporum gypseum,* and *M. furfur,* but it is ineffective against *Candida.* In tinea pedis, the cure rate is ~80%, compared with ~95% for miconazole. Toxic or allergic reactions to tolnaftate have not been reported.

Tolnaftate (AFTATE, TINACTIN, others) is available in a 1% concentration as a cream, gel, powder, aerosol powder, and topical solution, or as a topical aerosol liquid. The preparations are applied locally twice a day. Pruritus is usually relieved in 24-72 hours. Involution of interdigital lesions caused by susceptible fungi is very often complete in 7-21 days.

Naftifine

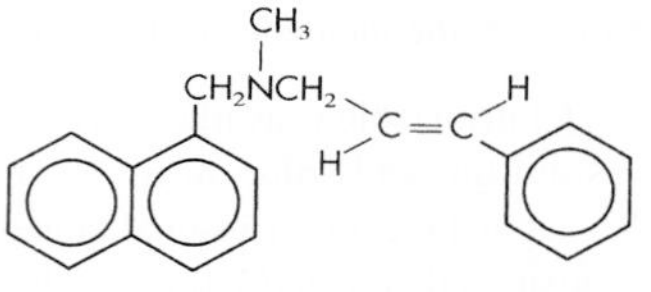

NAFTIFINE

Naftifine is representative of the allylamine class of synthetic agents that inhibit squalene-2,3-epoxidase and thus inhibit fungal biosynthesis of ergosterol. The drug has broad-spectrum fungicidal activity *in vitro.* Naftifine hydrochloride (NAFTIN) is available as a 1% cream or gel. It is effective for the topical treatment of tinea cruris and tinea corporis; twice-daily application is recommended. The drug is well tolerated, although local irritation has been observed in 3% of treated patients. Allergic contact dermatitis also has been reported. Naftifine also may be efficacious for cutaneous candidiasis and tinea versicolor, although the drug is not approved for these uses.

Terbinafine

Terbinafine 1% cream or spray is applied twice daily and is effective in tinea corporis, tinea cruris, and tinea pedis. Terbinafine is less active against *Candida* species and *Malassezia furfur,* but the cream also can be used in cutaneous candidiasis and tinea versicolor. The systemic use of terbinafine was discussed earlier.

Butenafine

Butenafine hydrochloride (MENTAX, LOTRIMIN ULTRA) is a benzylamine derivative with a mechanism of action similar to that of terbinafine and naftifine. Its spectrum of antifungal activity and use also are similar to those of the allylamines.

Polyene Antifungal Antibiotics

Nystatin. Nystatin was discovered in the New York State Health Laboratory and was named accordingly; it is a tetraene macrolide produced by *Streptomyces noursei*, is structurally similar to amphotericin B, and has the same mechanism of action. The drug is not absorbed from the GI tract, skin, or vagina. A liposomal formulation (NYOTRAN) is in clinical trials for candidemia.

Nystatin (MYCOSTATIN, NILSTAT, others) is useful only for candidiasis and is supplied in preparations intended for cutaneous, vaginal, or oral administration for this purpose. Infections of the nails and hyperkeratinized or crusted skin lesions do not respond. Powders are preferred for moist lesions and are applied two to three times daily. Creams or ointments are used twice daily. Combinations of nystatin with antibacterial agents or corticosteroids also are available. Allergic reactions to nystatin are very uncommon. Although vaginal tablets of nystatin are well tolerated, imidazoles or triazoles are more effective agents than nystatin for vaginal candidiasis.

Nystatin suspension is usually effective for oral candidiasis of the immunocompetent host. Patients should be instructed to swish the drug around in the mouth and then swallow; otherwise, the patient may expectorate the bitter liquid and fail to treat the infected mucosa in the posterior pharynx or esophagus. Other than the bitter taste and occasional complaints of nausea, adverse effects are uncommon.

Miscellaneous Antifungal Agents

Undecylenic Acid. Undecylenic acid is 10-undecenoic acid, an 11-carbon unsaturated compound. It is a yellow liquid with a characteristic rancid odor. It is primarily fungistatic, although fungicidal activity may be observed with long exposure to high concentrations of the agent. The drug is active against a variety of fungi, including those that cause ringworm. Undecylenic acid (DESENEX, others) is available in a cream, powder, spray powder, soap, and liquid. Zinc undecylenate is marketed in combination with other ingredients. The zinc provides an astringent action that aids in the suppression of inflammation. Compound undecylenic acid ointment contains both undecylenic acid (~5%) and zinc undecylenate (~20%). Calcium undecylenate (CALDESENE, CRUEX) is available as a powder.

Undecylenic acid preparations are used in the treatment of various dermatomycoses, especially tinea pedis. Concentrations of the acid as high as 10%, as well as those of the acid and salt in the compound ointment, may be applied to the skin. The preparations as formulated are usually not irritating to tissue, and sensitization to them is uncommon. It is of undoubted benefit in retarding fungal growth in tinea pedis, but the infection frequently persists despite intensive treatment with preparations of the acid and the zinc salt. At best, the clinical "cure" rate is ~50%, which is much lower than that obtained with the imidazoles, haloprogin, or tolnaftate. Efficacy in the treatment of tinea capitis is marginal, and the drug is no longer used for that purpose. Undecylenic acid preparations also are approved for use in the treatment of diaper rash, tinea cruris, and other minor dermatologic conditions.

Benzoic Acid and Salicylic Acid. An ointment containing benzoic and salicylic acids is known as Whitfield's ointment. It combines the fungistatic action of benzoate with the keratolytic action of salicylate. It contains benzoic acid and salicylic acid in a ratio of 2:1 (usually 6-3%) and is used mainly in the treatment of tinea pedis. Because benzoic acid is only fungistatic, eradication of the infection occurs only after the infected stratum corneum is shed, and continuous medication is required for several weeks to months. The salicylic acid accelerates the desquamation. The ointment also is sometimes used to treat tinea capitis. Mild irritation may occur at the site of application.

BIBLIOGRAPHY

Ally R, Schürmann D, Kreisel W, et al., for the Esophageal Candidiasis Study Group. A randomized, double-blind, double-dummy, multicenter trial of voriconazole and fluconazole in the treatment of esophageal candidiasis in immunocompromised patients. *Clin Infect Dis,* **2001**, *33:*1447–1454.

Baran R, Sigurgeirsson B, de Berker D, et al. A multicentre, randomized, controlled study of the efficacy, safety and cost-effectiveness of a combination therapy with amorolfine nail lacquer and oral terbinafine compared with oral terbinafine alone for the treatment of onychomycosis with matrix involvement. *Br J Dermatol,* **2007**, *157:*149–157.

Barrett JP, Vardulaki KA, Conlon C, et al., for the Amphotericin B Systematic Review Study Group. A systematic review of the antifungal effectiveness and tolerability of amphotericin B formulations. *Clin Ther,* **2003**, *25:*1295–1320.

Bennett JE. Echinocandins for candidemia in adults without neutropenia. *N Engl J Med,* **2006**, *355:*1154–1159.

Boswell GW, Buell D, Bekersky I. AmBisome (liposomal amphotericin B): A comparative review. *J Clin Pharmacol,* **1998**, *38:*583–592.

Bowden R, Chandrasekar P, White MH, et al. A double-blind, randomized, controlled trial of amphotericin B colloidal dispersion versus amphotericin B for treatment of invasive aspergillosis in immunocompromised patients. *Clin Infect Dis,* **2002**, *35:*359–366.

Carlson MA, Condon RE. Nephrotoxicity of amphotericin B. *J Am Coll Surg,* **1994**, *179:*361–381.

Chamilos G, Lewis, RE, Albert N, Kontoyiannis DP. Paradoxical effect of echinocandins across *Candida* species in vitro: Evidence for echinocandin-specific and *Candida* species-related differences. *Antimicrob Agents Chemother,* **2007**, *51:*2257–2259.

Cornely OA, Maertens J, Bresnik M, et al. Liposomal amphotericin B as initial therapy for invasive mold infection: A randomized trial comparing a high-loading dose regimen with standard dosing (AmBiLoad trial). *Clin Infect Dis,* **2007a**, *44:*1289–1297.

Cornely OA, Maertens J, Winston DJ. Posaconazole vs fluconazole or itraconazole prophylaxis in patients with neutropenia. *N Engl J Med,* **2007b**, *356:*348–359.

Courtney R, Wexler D, Radwanski E, et al. Effect of food on the relative bioavailability of posaconazole in healthy adults. *Br J Clin Pharmacol,* **2003**, *57:*218–222.

Dannaoui R, Meis JGM, Loebenberg D, Verweij P. Activity of posaconazole in treatment of disseminated zygomycosis. *Antimicrob Agents Chemother,* **2003**, *47:*3647–3650.

De Pauw BE, Donnelly JP. Prophylaxis and aspergillosis—has the principle been proven? *N Engl J Med,* **2007**, *356:*409–411.

Dodgson AR, Dodgson KJ, Pujol C, et al. Clade-specific flucytosine resistance is due to a single nucleotide change in the *FURl* gene of *Candida albicans. Antimicrob Agents Chemother,* **2004**, *48:*2223–2227.

Evans EG, Sigurgeirsson B. Double blind, randomised study of continuous terbinafine compared with intermittent itraconazole in treatment of toenail onychomycosis. The LION Study Group. *BMJ,* **1999**, *318:*1031–1035.

Ezzet F, Wexler D, Courtney R, et al. Oral bioavailability of posaconazole in fasted healthy subjects. *Clin Pharmacokinet,* **2005**, *44:*211–220.

Fernandez-Obregon AC, Rohrback J, Reichel MA, et al. Current use of anti-infectives in dermatology. *Expert Rev Anti Infect Ther,* **2005**, *3:*557–591.

Frampton JE, Scott LJ. Posaconazole. A review of its use in the prophylaxis of invasive fungal infections. *Drugs,* **2008**, *68:*99–1016.

Fritz JM, Brielmaier BD, Dubberke ER. Micafungin for the prophylaxis and treatment of Candida infections. *Expert Rev Anti-Infect Ther,* **2008**, *6:*153–162.

Greenberg RN, Mullane K, van Burik J-AH, et al. Posaconazole as salvage therapy for zygomycosis. *Antimicrob Agents Chemother,* **2006**, *50*:126–133.

Guinea J, Peláez T, Recio S, *et al.* In vitro antifungal activities of isavuconazole (BAL4815), voriconazole, and fluconazole against 1,007 isolates of Zygomycete, *Candida, Aspergillus, Fusarium* and *Scedosporium* species. *Antimicrob Agents Chemother*, **2008**, *52:*1396–1400.

Herbrecht R, Denning DW, Patterson TF, *et al.* Voriconazole versus amphotericin B for primary therapy of invasive aspergillosis. *N Engl J Med,* **2002**, *347:*408–415.

Jeu L, Piacenti FJ, Lyakhovetskiy AG, Fung HB. Voriconazole. *Clin Ther,* **2003**, *25:*1321–1381.

Johnson MD, Perfect JR. Caspofungin: First approved agent in a new class of antifungals. *Expert Opin Pharmacother,* **2003**, *4:*807–823.

Johnson PC, Wheat LJ, Cloud GA, et al. Safety and efficacy of liposomal amphotericin B compared with conventional amphotericin B for induction therapy of histoplasmosis in patients with AIDS. *Ann Intern Med,* **2002**, *137*:105–109.

Kaplan JE, Benson C, Holmes KH, et al. Guidelines for prevention and treatment of opportunistic infections in adults and adolescents. Recommendations from CDC, the National Institutes of Health, the HIV Medicine Association of the Infectious Diseases Society of America. *MMWR Recomm Rep,* **2009**, *58:*1–207.

Keating G, Figgitt D. Caspofungin: A review of its use in oesophageal candidiasis, invasive candidiasis and invasive aspergillosis. *Drugs,* **2003**, *63:*2235–2263.

Kim R, Khachikian D, Reboli AC. A comparative evaluation of properties and clinical efficacy of the echinocandins. *Expert Opin Pharmacother,* **2007**, *8:*1479–1492.

Krieter P, Flannery B, Musick T, et al. Disposition of posaconazole following single-dose oral administration in healthy subjects. *Antimicrob Agents Chemother,* **2004**, *48*:3543–3551.

Krishna G, Moton A, Ma L, et al. Effects of oral posaconazole on the pharmacokinetics properties of oral and intravenous midazolam: A phase 1, randomized, open-label, crossover study in healthy volunteers. *Clin Ther,* **2009a**, *31:* 286–298.

Krishna G, Moton A, Ma L, et al. Pharmacokinetics and absorption of posaconazole oral suspension under various gastric conditions in healthy volunteers. *Antimicrob Agents Chemother*, **2009b**, *53:*948–966.

Kullberg BJ, Sobel JD, Ruhnke M, et al. Voriconazole versus a regimen of amphotericin B followed by fluconazole for candidaemia in non-neutropenic patients: A randomized non-inferiority trial. *Lancet,* **2005**, *366:*1435–1442.

Kuse E-R, Chetchotisakd P, daCunha CA, et al. Micafungin versus liposomal amphotericin B for candidaemia and invasive candidosis: A phase III randomized double blind trial. *Lancet,* **2007**, *369:*1519–1527.

Larsen RA, Bozzette SA, Jones BE, et al. Fluconazole combined with flucytosine for treatment of cryptococcal meningitis in patients with AIDS. *Clin Infect Dis*, **1994**, *19*:741–745.

Mora-Duarte J, Betts R, Rotstein C, et al. Comparison of caspofungin and amphotericin B for invasive candidiasis. *N Engl J Med,* **2002**, *347:*2020–2029.

Moton A, Ma L, Krishna G, *et al.* Effects of oral posaconazole on the pharmacokinetics of serolimus. *Curr Med Res Opin*, **2009**, *25*:701–707.

Odds FC. Drug evaluation: BAL-8577—a novel broad-spectrum triazole antifungal. *Curr Opin Investig Drugs,* **2006**, *7:*766–772.

Pappas PG, Perfect JR, Cloud GA, et al. Cryptococcosis in human immunodeficiency virus-negative patients in the era of effective azole therapy. *Clin Infect Dis,* **2001**, *33:*690–699.

Pappas PG, Rotstein CM, Betts RF, et al. Micafungin versus caspofungin for treatment of candidemia and other forms of invasive candidiasis. *Clin Infect Dis,* **2007**, *45*:883–893.

Park S, Kelly R, Nielsen Kahn J, et al. Specific substitutions in the echinocandin target Fks1p account for reduced susceptibility of rare laboratory and clinical *Candida* sp isolates. *Antimicrob Agents Chemother*, **2005**, *49:*3264–3273.

Perfect JR, Dismukes WE, Dromer F, et al. Clinical practice guidelines for the management of cryptococcal disease: 2010 update by the Infectious Diseases Society of America. *Clin Infect Dis*, **2010**, *50*:291–322.

Perkhofer S, Lechner V, Lass-Flörl C. *In vitro* activity of isavuconazole against Aspergillus species and Zygomycetes according to the methodology of the European Committee on Antimicrobial Susceptibility Testing. *Antimicrob Agents Chemother,* **2009**, *53:*1645–1647.

Reboli AC, Rotstein C, Pappas PG, et al. Anidulafungin versus fluconazole for invasive candidiasis. *N Engl J Med*, **2007**, *356:*2472–2482.

Salez F, Brichet A, Desurmont S, et al. Effects of itraconazole therapy in allergic bronchopulmonary aspergillosis. *Chest,* **1999**, *116:*1665–1668.

Schmitt-Hoffman A, Roos B, Marres J, et al. Multiple dose pharmacokinetics and safety of the new antifungal triazole BAL4815 after intravenous infusion and oral administration of its prodrug, BAL8557, in healthy volunteers. *Antimicrob Agents Chemother,* **2006**, *50:*286–293.

Smith WJ, Drew RH, Perfect JR. Posaconazole's impact on prophylaxis and treatment of invasive fungal infections: An update. *Expert Rev Anti Infective Ther,* **2009**, *7:*165–181.

Steinbach WJ, Perfect JR, Schell WA, et al. *In vitro* analyses, animal models, and 60 clinical cases of invasive *Aspergillus terreus* infection. *Antimicrob Agents Chemother,* **2004**, *48:* 3217–3225.

Ullmann AJ, Cornely OA, Burchardt A, et al. Pharmacokinetics, safety and efficacy of posaconazole in patients with persistent febrile neutropenia or refractory invasive fungal infections. *Antimicrob Agents Chemother*, **2006**, *50:*658–666.

Ullmann AJ, Lipton JH, Vesole DH, et al. Posaconazole or fluconazole for prophylaxis in severe graft-versus-host disease. *N Engl J Med,* **2007**, *356:*335–347.

van der Horst CM, Saag MS, Cloud GA, et al. Treatment of cryptococcal meningitis associated with the acquired immunodeficiency syndrome. National Institute of Allergy and Infectious Diseases Mycoses Study Group and AIDS Clinical Trials Group. *N Engl J Med,* **1997**, *337:*15–21.

Vazquez JA, Sobel JD. Anidulafungin: A novel echinocandin. *Clin Infect Dis,* **2006**, *43:*215–222.

Villanueva A, Arathoon EG, Gotuzzo E, et al. A randomized double-blind study of caspofungin versus amphotericin for the treatment of candidal esophagitis. *Clin Infect Dis,* **2001**, *33:*1529–1535.

Wagner C, Graninger W, Presterl E, Joukhadar C. The echinocandins: Comparison of their pharmacokinetics, pharmacodynamics and clinical applications. *Pharmacology,* **2006**, *78:*161–177.

Walsh TJ, Karlsson MO, Driscoll T, et al. Pharmacokinetics and safety of intravenous voriconazole in children after single- or multiple-dose administration. *Antimicrob Agents Chemother,* **2004a**, *48:*2166–2172.

Walsh TJ, Pappas P, Winston DJ, et al., for the National Institute of Allergy and Infectious Diseases Mycoses Study Group. Voriconazole compared with liposomal amphotericin B for empirical antifungal therapy in patients with neutropenia and persistent fever. *N Engl J Med,* **2002**, *346:*225–234.

Walsh TJ, Teppler H, Donowitz GR, et al. Caspofungin versus liposomal amphotericin B for empirical antifungal therapy in patients with persistent fever and neutropenia. *N Engl J Med,* **2004**, *351:*1391–1402.

White MH, Bowden RA, Sandler ES, et al. Randomized, double-blind clinical trial of amphotericin B colloidal dispersion vs. amphotericin B in the empirical treatment of fever and neutropenia. *Clin Infect Dis,* **1998**, *27:*296–302.

Wiederhold NP, Lewis JS 2nd. The echinocandin micafungin: A review of the pharmacology, spectrum of activity, clinical efficacy and safety. *Expert Opin Pharmacother,* **2007**, *8:*1155–1166.

Wiederhold NP, Lewis RE. The echinocandin antifungals: An overview of the pharmacology, spectrum and clinical efficacy. *Expert Opin Invest Drugs*, **2003**, *12:*1313–1333.

Wingard JR, White MH, Anaissie E, et al. A randomized, double-blind comparative trial evaluating the safety of liposomal amphotericin B versus amphotericin B lipid complex in the empirical treatment of febrile neutropenia. *Clin Infect Dis,* **2000**, *31:*1155–1163.

Zonios DI, Bennett JE. Update on azole antifungals. *Semin Respir Crit Care Med,* **2008**, *29:*198–210.

Zonios DI, Gea-Banacloche J, Childs R, Bennett JE. Hallucinations during voriconazole use. *Clin Infect Dis*, **2008**, *47:*e7–10.

Antiviral Agents (Nonretroviral)

Edward P. Acosta
and Charles Flexner

Most antivirals currently available in the U.S. have been developed and approved in the last two decades. This flurry of activity was driven by successes in rational drug design and approval that began with the anti-herpesvirus nucleoside analog acyclovir, whose discovery and development resulted in the awarding of a Nobel Prize to Gertrude Elion and George Hitchings in 1988. Because viruses are obligatory intracellular microorganisms and rely on host biosynthetic machinery to reproduce, there were doubts about the possibility of developing antiviral drugs with selective toxicity, but those doubts have long been erased. Viruses are now obvious targets for effective antimicrobial chemotherapy, and it is certain that the number of available agents in this category will continue to increase.

Viruses are simple microorganisms that consist of either double- or single-stranded DNA or RNA enclosed in a protein coat called a *capsid.* Some viruses also possess a lipid envelope derived from the infected host cell, which, like the capsid, may contain antigenic glycoproteins. There are distinct stages of viral replication and the classes of antiviral agents that can act at each stage (Table 58–1). Effective antiviral agents inhibit virus-specific replicative events or preferentially inhibit *virus-directed rather than host cell–directed* nucleic acid or protein synthesis. Host cell molecules that are essential to viral replication also offer targets for intervention. Some effective antiviral agents (e.g., interferons; see Chapter 35) have multiple mechanisms of action that include modulation of host immune responses. Figure 58–1 gives a schematic diagram of the replicative cycle of typical DNA and RNA viruses. DNA viruses (and the diseases they cause) include poxviruses (smallpox), herpesviruses (chickenpox, shingles, oral and genital herpes), adenoviruses (conjunctivitis, sore throat), hepadnaviruses (hepatitis B [HBV]), and papillomaviruses (warts). Most DNA viruses enter the host cell nucleus, where the viral DNA is transcribed into mRNA by host cell polymerase; mRNA is translated in the usual host cell fashion into virus-specific proteins. An exception to this strategy are poxviruses, which carry their own RNA polymerase and replicate in the host cell cytoplasm.

For RNA viruses, the replication strategy relies either on enzymes in the virion to synthesize mRNA or has the viral RNA serving as its own mRNA. The mRNA is translated into various viral proteins, including RNA polymerase, which directs the synthesis of more viral mRNA and genomic RNA (Figure 58–1B). Most RNA viruses complete their replication in the cytoplasm, but some, such as influenza, are transcribed in the host cell nucleus. Examples of RNA viruses (and the diseases they cause) include rubella virus (German measles), rhabdoviruses (rabies), picornaviruses (poliomyelitis, meningitis, colds, hepatitis A), arenaviruses (meningitis, Lassa fever), flaviviruses (West Nile meningoencephalitis, yellow fever, hepatitis C), orthomyxoviruses (influenza), paramyxoviruses (measles, mumps), and coronaviruses (colds, severe acute respiratory syndrome [SARS]). Retroviruses are a special group of RNA viruses that include human immunodeficiency virus (HIV); chemotherapy for retroviruses is described in Chapter 59.

Table 58–2 summarizes currently approved drugs for nonretroviral infections. Their pharmacological properties are presented below, class by class, as listed in the table.

ANTI-HERPESVIRUS AGENTS

Infection with herpes simplex virus type 1 (HSV-1) typically causes diseases of the mouth, face, skin, esophagus, or brain. Herpes simplex virus type 2 (HSV-2) usually causes infections of the genitals, rectum, skin,

Table 58–1

Stages of Virus Replication and Possible Targets of Action of Antiviral Agents

STAGE OF REPLICATION	CLASSES OF SELECTIVE INHIBITORS
Cell entry	
Attachment	Soluble receptor decoys, antireceptor antibodies, fusion protein inhibitors
Penetration	
Uncoating	Ion channel blockers, capsid stabilizers
Release of viral genome	
Transcription of viral genome[a]	Inhibitors of viral DNA polymerase, RNA polymerase, reverse transcriptase, helicase, primase, or integrase
Transcription of viral messenger RNA	
Replication of viral genome	
Translation of viral proteins	Interferons, antisense oligonucleotides, ribozymes
Regulatory proteins (early)	Inhibitors of regulatory proteins
Structural proteins (late)	
Post-translational modifications	
Proteolytic cleavage	Protease inhibitors
Myristoylation, glycosylation	
Assembly of virion components	Interferons, assembly protein inhibitors
Release	Neuraminidase inhibitors, antiviral antibodies, cytotoxic lymphocytes
Budding, cell lysis	

[a]Depends on specific replication strategy of virus, but virus-specified enzyme required for part of process.

hands, or meninges. Both cause serious infections in neonates. HSV infection may be a primary one in a naive host, a nonprimary initial one in a host previously infected by other viruses, or the consequence of activation of a latent infection.

The first systemically administered anti-herpesvirus agent, vidarabine (no longer marketed in the U.S.), was approved by the FDA in 1977. However, toxicities restricted its use to life- or vision-threatening infections of HSV and varicella-zoster virus (VZV). The discovery and development of acyclovir, approved in 1982, provided the first effective treatment for less severe HSV and VZV infections in ambulatory patients. Intravenous acyclovir is superior to vidarabine in terms of efficacy and toxicity in HSV encephalitis and in VZV infections of immunocompromised patients. Acyclovir is the prototype of a group of antiviral agents that are phosphorylated intracellularly by a viral kinase and subsequently by host cell enzymes to become inhibitors of viral DNA synthesis. Other agents employing this strategy include penciclovir and ganciclovir.

Acyclovir and Valacyclovir

Chemistry and Antiviral Activity. Acyclovir is an acyclic guanine nucleoside analog that lacks a 3′-hydroxyl on the side chain. Valacyclovir is the L-valyl ester prodrug of acyclovir. Acyclovir and valacyclovir chemical structures are depicted in Figure 58–2.

Acyclovir's clinically useful antiviral spectrum is limited to herpesviruses. *In vitro,* acyclovir is most active against HSV-1 (0.02-0.9 μg/mL), approximately half as active against HSV-2 (0.03-2.2 μg/mL), a tenth as potent against VZV (0.8-4.0 μg/mL) and Epstein-Barr virus (EBV), and least active against cytomegalovirus (CMV) (generally >20 μg/mL) and human herpesvirus 6 (HHV-6). Uninfected mammalian cell growth generally is unaffected by high acyclovir concentrations (>50 μg/mL).

Mechanisms of Action and Resistance. Acyclovir inhibits viral DNA synthesis via a mechanism outlined in Figure 58–3 (Elion, 1986). Its selectivity of action depends on interaction with two distinct viral proteins: HSV thymidine kinase and DNA polymerase. Cellular uptake and initial phosphorylation are facilitated by HSV thymidine kinase. The affinity of acyclovir for HSV thymidine kinase is ~200 times greater than for the mammalian enzyme. Cellular enzymes convert the monophosphate to acyclovir triphosphate, which is present in 40-100-fold higher concentrations in HSV-infected than in uninfected cells and competes for endogenous deoxyguanosine triphosphate (dGTP).

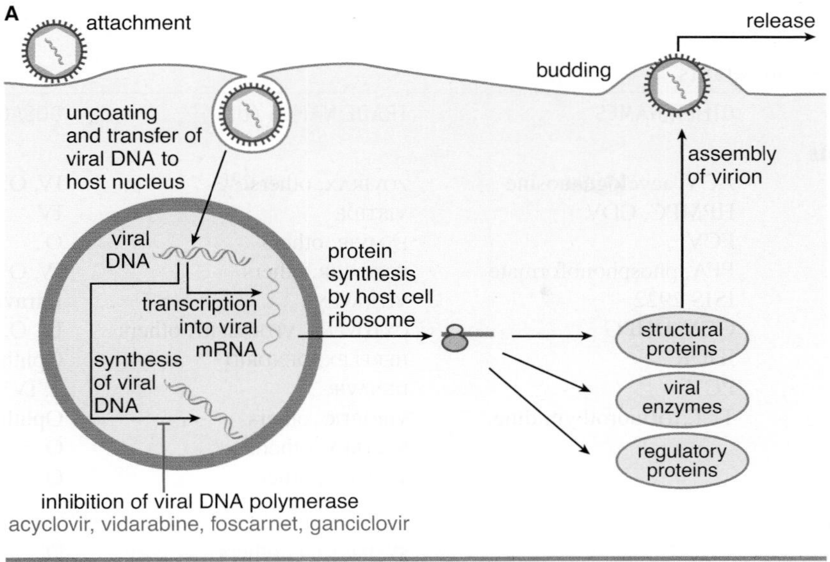

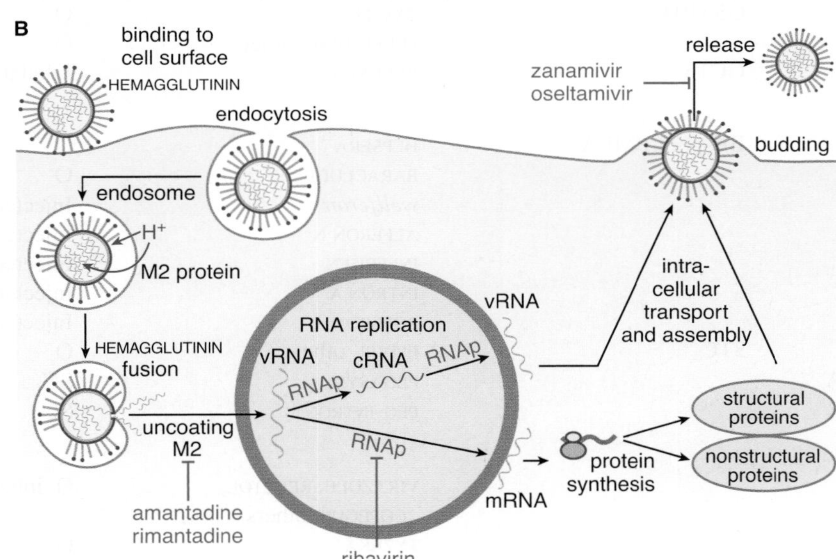

Figure 58–1. *Replicative cycles of DNA (A) and RNA (B) viruses.* The replicative cycles of herpesvirus (A) and influenza (B) are examples of DNA-encoded and RNA-encoded viruses, respectively. Sites of action of antiviral agents also are shown. Key: mRNA = messenger RNA; cDNA = complementary DNA; vRNA = viral RNA; DNAp = DNA polymerase; RNAp = RNA polymerase; cRNA = complementary RNA. The symbol ——┤ indicates a block to virus growth.

A. Replicative cycles of herpes simplex virus, a DNA virus, and the probable sites of action of antiviral agents. Herpesvirus replication is a regulated multistep process. After infection, a small number of immediate-early genes are transcribed; these genes encode proteins that regulate their own synthesis and are responsible for synthesis of early genes involved in genome replication, such as thymidine kinases, DNA polymerases, etc. After DNA replication, the bulk of the herpesvirus genes (called late genes) are expressed and encode proteins that either are incorporated into or aid in the assembly of progeny virions.

B. Replicative cycles of influenza, an RNA virus, and the loci for effects of antiviral agents. The mammalian cell shown is an airway epithelial cell. The M2 protein of influenza virus allows an influx of hydrogen ions into the virion interior, which in turn promotes dissociation of the RNP (ribonuclear protein) segments and release into the cytoplasm (uncoating). Influenza virus mRNA synthesis requires a primer cleared from cellular mRNA and used by the viral RNAp complex. The neuraminidase inhibitors zanamivir and oseltamivir specifically inhibit release of progeny virus. Small capitals indicate virus proteins.

Table 58–2

Nomenclature of Antiviral Agents

GENERIC NAME	OTHER NAMES	TRADE NAMES (U.S.)	DOSAGE FORMS AVAILABLE
Antiherpesvirus agents			
Acyclovir	ACV, acycloguanosine	ZOVIRAX, others	IV, O, T, ophth[a]
Cidofovir	HPMPC, CDV	VISTIDE	IV
Famciclovir	FCV	FAMVIR, others	O
Foscarnet	PFA, phosphonoformate	FOSCAVIR, others	IV, O[a]
Fomivirsena	ISIS 2922	VITRAVENE	Intravitreal
Ganciclovir	GCV, DHPG	CYTOVENE, VITRASERT, others	IV, O, intravitreal
Idoxuridine	IDUR	HERPLEX, DENDRID	Ophth
Penciclovir	PCV	DENAVIR	T, IV[a]
Trifluridine	TFT, trifluorothymidine	VIROPTIC, others	Ophth
Valacyclovir		VALTREX, others	O
Valganciclovir		VALCYTE, others	O
Anti-influenza agents			
Amantadine		SYMMETREL, others	O
Oseltamivir	GS4104	TAMIFLU	O
Rimantadine		FLUMADINE, others	O
Zanamivir	GC167	RELENZA	Inhalation
Antihepatitis agents			
Adefovir dipivoxil	Bis-pom-PMEA	HEPSERA	O
Entecavir		BARACLUDE	O
Interferon alfa-N1		*wellferon*[a]	Injected
Interferon alfa-N3		ALFERON N	Injected
Interferon alfacon-1		INFERGEN	Injected
Interferon alfa-2B		INTRON A	Injected
Interferon alfa-2A		ROFERON A	Injected
Lamivudine	3TC	EPIVIR, others	O
Peginterferon alfa 2A		PEGASYS	SC
Peginterferon alfa 2B		PEG-INTRON	SC
Other antiviral agents			
Ribavirin		VIRAZOLE, REBETOL, COPEGUS, others	O, inhalation, IV
Telbivudine		TYZEKA	O
Tenofovir disoproxil fumarate	TDF	VIREAD, others	O
Imiquimod		ALDARA	Topical

[a]Not currently approved for use in U.S. ABBREVIATIONS: IV, intravenous; O, oral; T, topical; ophth, ophthalmic.

The immunosuppressive agent mycophenolate mofetil (Chapter 35) potentiates the anti-herpes activity of acyclovir and related agents by depleting intracellular dGTP pools. Acyclovir triphosphate competitively inhibits viral DNA polymerases and, to a much lesser extent, cellular DNA polymerases. Acyclovir triphosphate also is incorporated into viral DNA, where it acts as a chain terminator because of the lack of a 3′- hydroxyl group. By a mechanism termed *suicide inactivation,* the terminated DNA template containing acyclovir binds the viral DNA polymerase and leads to its irreversible inactivation.

Acyclovir resistance in HSV has been linked to one of three mechanisms: impaired production of viral thymidine kinase, altered thymidine kinase substrate specificity (e.g., phosphorylation of thymidine but not acyclovir), or altered viral DNA polymerase. Alterations in viral enzymes are caused by point mutations and base insertions or deletions in the corresponding genes. Resistant variants are present in native virus populations and in isolates from treated patients. The most common resistance mechanism in clinical HSV isolates is absent or deficient viral thymidine kinase activity; viral DNA polymerase mutants are rare. Phenotypic resistance

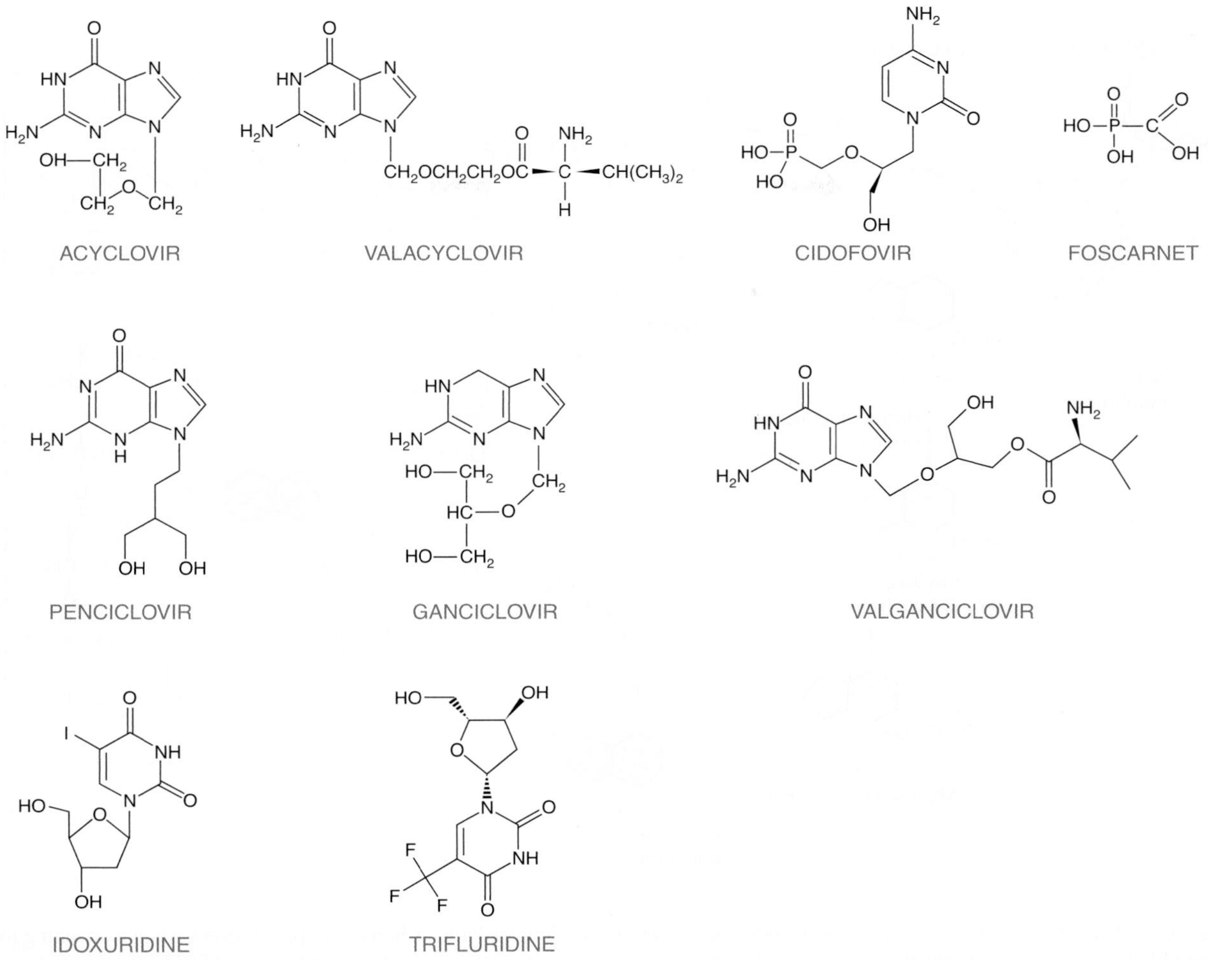

Figure 58–2. *Chemical Structures of Anti-Herpes Drugs.*

typically is defined by *in vitro* inhibitory concentrations of >2-3 μg/mL, which predict failure of therapy in immunocompromised patients.

Acyclovir resistance in VZV isolates is caused by mutations in VZV thymidine kinase and less often by mutations in viral DNA polymerase.

Absorption, Distribution, and Elimination. The oral bioavailability of acyclovir ranges from 10-30% and decreases with increasing dose (Wagstaff et al., 1994). Peak plasma concentrations average 0.4-0.8 μg/mL after 200-mg doses and 1.6 μg/mL after 800-mg doses. Following intravenous dosing, peak and trough plasma concentrations average 9.8 and 0.7 μg/mL after 5 mg/kg every 8 hours and 20.7 and 2.3 μg/mL after 10 mg/kg every 8 hours, respectively.

Valacyclovir is converted rapidly and virtually completely to acyclovir after oral administration in healthy adults. This conversion is thought to result from first-pass intestinal and hepatic metabolism through enzymatic hydrolysis. Unlike acyclovir, valacyclovir is a substrate for intestinal and renal peptide transporters. The relative oral bioavailability of acyclovir increases 3-5 fold to ~70% following valacyclovir administration (Steingrimsdottir et al., 2000). Peak acyclovir concentrations average 5-6 μg/mL following single 1000-mg doses of oral valacyclovir and occur ~2 hours after dosing. Peak plasma concentrations of valacyclovir are only 4% of acyclovir levels. Less than 1% of an administered dose of valacyclovir is recovered in the urine; most is eliminated as acyclovir.

Acyclovir distributes widely in body fluids, including vesicular fluid, aqueous humor, and cerebrospinal fluid (CSF). Compared with plasma, salivary concentrations are low, and vaginal secretion concentrations vary widely. Acyclovir is concentrated in breast milk, amniotic fluid, and placenta. Newborn plasma levels are similar to maternal ones. Percutaneous absorption of acyclovir after topical administration is low.

The mean plasma elimination $t_{1/2}$ of acyclovir is ~2.5 hours (range: 1.5-6 hours in adults with normal renal function). The elimination $t_{1/2}$ of acyclovir is ~4 hours in neonates and increases to 20 hours in anuric patients (Wagstaff et al., 1994). Renal excretion of unmetabolized acyclovir by glomerular filtration and tubular

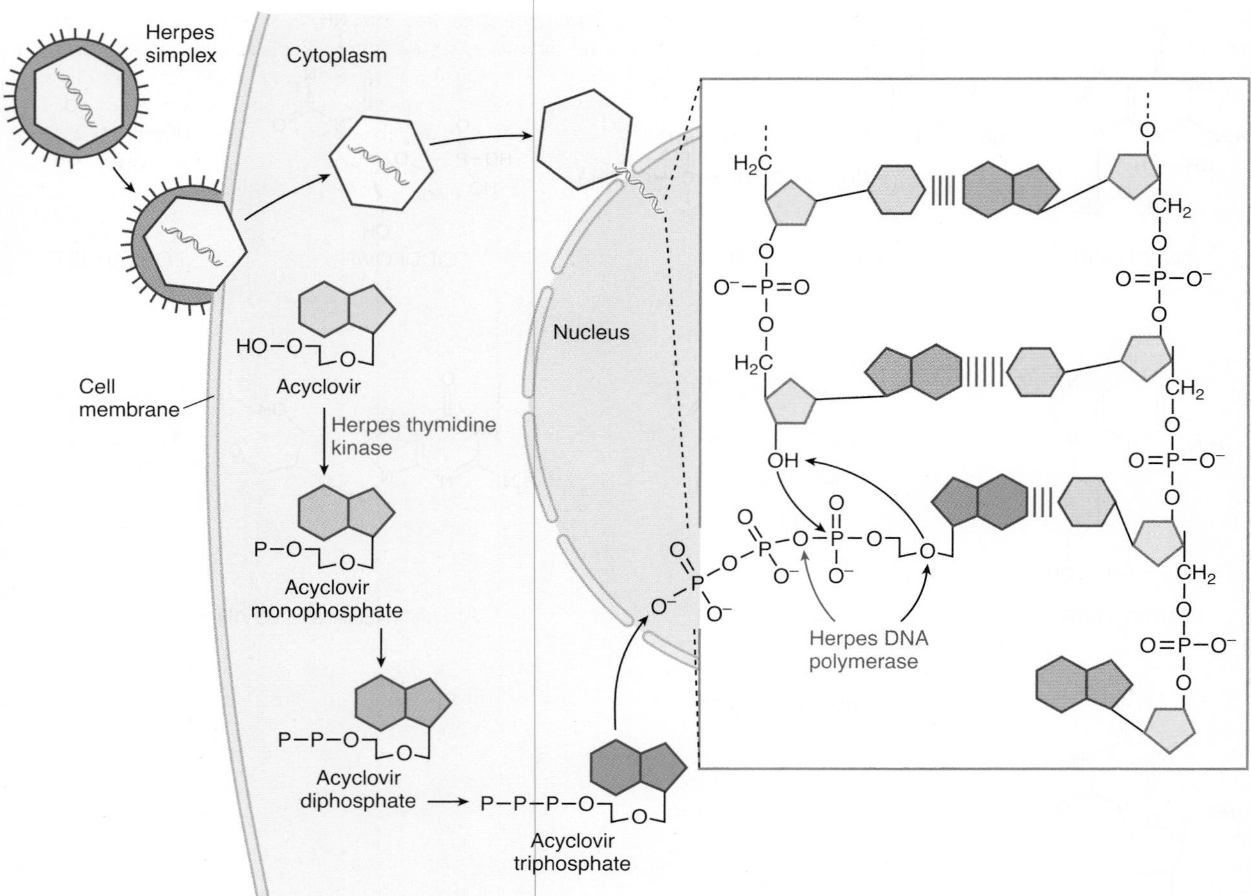

Figure 58–3. *Mechanism of Action of Acyclovir in Cells Infected by Herpes Simplex Virus.* A herpes simplex virion is shown attaching to a susceptible host cell, fusing its envelope with the cell membrane, and releasing naked capsids that deliver viral DNA into the nucleus, where it initiates synthesis of viral DNA. Acyclovir molecules entering the cell are converted to acyclovir monophosphate by virus-induced thymidine kinase. Host-cell enzymes add two more phosphates to form acyclovir triphosphate, which is transported into the nucleus. After the herpes DNA polymerase cleaves pyrophosphate from acyclovir triphosphate (indicated by the red arrow in the inset), viral DNA polymerase inserts acyclovir monophosphate rather than 2′-deoxyguanosine monophosphate into the viral DNA (indicated by black arrows in the inset). Further elongation of the chain is impossible because acyclovir monophosphate lacks the 3′ hydroxyl group necessary for the insertion of an additional nucleotide, and the exonuclease associated with the viral DNA polymerase cannot remove the acyclovir moiety. In contrast, ganciclovir and penciclovir have a 3′ hydroxyl group; therefore, further synthesis of viral DNA is possible in the presence of these drugs. Foscarnet acts at the pyrophosphate-binding site of viral DNA polymerase and prevents cleavage of the pyrophosphate from nucleoside triphosphates, thus stalling further primer template extension. The red bands between the viral DNA strands in the inset indicate hydrogen bonding of the base pairs. (Adapted with permission from Balfour HH. Antiviral drugs. *N Engl J Med*, **1999,** *340:*1255–1268. Copyright © 1999. Massachusetts Medical Society. All rights reserved.)

secretion is the principal route of elimination. Less than 15% is excreted as 9-carboxymethoxymethylguanine or minor metabolites. The pharmacokinetics of oral acyclovir and valacyclovir appear to be similar in pregnant and nonpregnant women (Kimberlin et al., 1998).

Untoward Effects. Acyclovir generally is well tolerated. Topical acyclovir in a polyethylene glycol base may cause mucosal irritation and transient burning when applied to genital lesions.

Oral acyclovir has been associated infrequently with nausea, diarrhea, rash, or headache and very rarely with renal insufficiency or neurotoxicity. Valacyclovir also may be associated with headache, nausea, diarrhea, nephrotoxicity, and central nervous system (CNS) symptoms. High doses of valacyclovir have been associated with confusion and hallucinations, nephrotoxicity, and uncommonly, severe thrombocytopenic syndromes, sometimes fatal, in immunocompromised patients. Acyclovir has been associated with neutropenia in neonates. Chronic acyclovir suppression of genital herpes has been used safely for up to 10 years. No excess frequency of congenital abnormalities has been recognized in infants born to women exposed to acyclovir during pregnancy (Ratanajamit et al., 2003).

The principal dose-limiting toxicities of intravenous acyclovir are renal insufficiency and CNS side effects. Preexisting renal insufficiency, high doses, and high acyclovir plasma levels (>25 μg/mL) are risk factors for both. Reversible renal dysfunction occurs in ~5% of patients, probably related to high urine levels causing crystalline nephropathy. Manifestations include nausea, emesis, flank pain, and increasing azotemia. Rapid infusion, dehydration, and inadequate urine flow increase the risk. Infusions should be given at a constant rate over at least an hour. Nephrotoxicity usually resolves with drug cessation and volume expansion. Neurotoxicity occurs in 1-4% of patients and may be manifested by altered sensorium, tremor, myoclonus, delirium, seizures, or extrapyramidal signs. Phlebitis following extravasation, rash, diaphoresis, nausea, hypotension, and interstitial nephritis also have been described. Hemodialysis may be useful in severe cases.

Severe somnolence and lethargy may occur with combinations of zidovudine and acyclovir. Concomitant cyclosporine and probably other nephrotoxic agents enhance the risk of nephrotoxicity. Probenecid decreases the acyclovir renal clearance and prolongs the elimination $t_{1/2}$. Acyclovir may decrease the renal clearance of other drugs eliminated by active renal secretion, such as methotrexate.

Therapeutic Uses. In immunocompetent persons, the clinical benefits of acyclovir and valacyclovir are greater in initial HSV infections than in recurrent ones, which typically are milder in severity. These drugs are particularly useful in immunocompromised patients because these individuals experience both more frequent and more severe HSV and VZV infections. Because VZV is less susceptible than HSV to acyclovir, higher doses must be used for treating varicella-zoster infections than for HSV infections. Oral valacyclovir is as effective as oral acyclovir in HSV infections and more effective for treating herpes zoster.

Herpes Simplex Virus Infections. In initial genital HSV infections, oral acyclovir (200 mg five times daily or 400 mg three times daily for 7-10 days) and valacyclovir (1000 mg twice daily for 7-10 days) are associated with significant reductions in virus shedding, symptoms, and time to healing (Kimberlin and Rouse, 2004). Intravenous acyclovir (5 mg/kg every 8 hours) has similar effects in patients hospitalized with severe primary genital HSV infections. Topical acyclovir is much less effective than systemic administration. None of these regimens reproducibly reduces the risk of recurrent genital lesions. Acyclovir (200 mg five times daily or 400 mg three times daily for 5 days or 800 mg three times daily for 2 days) or valacyclovir (500 mg twice daily for 3 or 5 days) shortens the manifestations of recurrent genital HSV episodes by 1-2 days. Frequently recurring genital herpes can be suppressed effectively with chronic oral acyclovir (400 mg twice daily or 200 mg three times daily) or with valacyclovir (500 mg or, for very frequent recurrences, 1000 mg once daily). During use, the rate of clinical recurrences decreases by ~90%, and subclinical shedding is markedly reduced, although not eliminated. Valacyclovir suppression of genital herpes reduces the risk of transmitting infection to a susceptible partner by ~50% over an 8-month period (Corey et al., 2004). Chronic suppression may be useful in those with disabling recurrences of herpetic whitlow or HSV-related erythema multiforme.

Oral acyclovir is effective in primary herpetic gingivostomatitis (600 mg/m^2 four times daily for 10 days in children) but provides only modest clinical benefit in recurrent orolabial herpes. Short-term, high-dose valacyclovir (2 g twice over 1 day) shortens the duration of recurrent orolabial herpes by ~1 day (Elish et al., 2004). The FDA has approved an acyclovir/hydrocortisone combination (LIPSOVIR) for early treatment of recurrent herpes cold sores. Topical acyclovir cream is modestly effective in recurrent labial (Spruance et al., 2002) and genital herpes simplex virus infections. Preexposure acyclovir prophylaxis (400 mg twice daily for 1 week) reduces the overall risk of recurrence by 73% in those with sun-induced recurrences of HSV infections. Acyclovir during the last month of pregnancy reduces the likelihood of viral shedding and the frequency of cesarean delivery in women with primary or recurrent genital herpes (Corey and Wald, 2009).

In immunocompromised patients with mucocutaneous HSV infection, intravenous acyclovir (250 mg/m^2 every 8 hours for 7 days) shortens healing time, duration of pain, and the period of virus shedding. Oral acyclovir (800 mg five times per day) and valacyclovir (1000 mg twice daily) for 5-10 days are also effective. Recurrences are common after cessation of therapy and may require long-term suppression. In those with very localized labial or facial HSV infections, topical acyclovir may provide some benefit. Intravenous acyclovir may be beneficial in viscerally disseminating HSV in immunocompromised patients and in patients with HSV-infected burn wounds.

Systemic acyclovir prophylaxis is highly effective in preventing mucocutaneous HSV infections in seropositive patients undergoing immunosuppression. Intravenous acyclovir (250 mg/m2 every 8-12 hours) begun prior to transplantation and continuing for several weeks prevents HSV disease in bone marrow transplant recipients. For patients who can tolerate oral medications, oral acyclovir (400 mg five times daily) is effective, and long-term oral acyclovir (200-400 mg three times daily for 6 months) also reduces the risk of VZV infection (Steer et al., 2000). In HSV encephalitis, acyclovir (10 mg/kg every 8 hours for a minimum of 10 days) reduces mortality by >50% and improves overall neurologic outcome compared with vidarabine. Higher doses (15-20 mg/kg every 8 hours) and prolonged treatment (up to 21 days) are recommended by many experts. Intravenous acyclovir (20 mg/kg every 8 hours for 21 days) is more effective than lower doses in viscerally invasive neonatal HSV infections (Kimberlin et al., 2001). In neonates and immunosuppressed patients and, rarely, in previously healthy persons, relapses of encephalitis following acyclovir may occur. The value of continuing long-term suppression with valacyclovir after completing intravenous acyclovir is under study.

An ophthalmic formulation of acyclovir (not available in the U.S.) is at least as effective as topical vidarabine or trifluridine in herpetic keratoconjunctivitis.

Infection owing to resistant HSV is rare in immunocompetent persons; however, in immunocompromised hosts, acyclovir-resistant HSV isolates can cause extensive mucocutaneous disease and, rarely, meningoencephalitis, pneumonitis, or visceral disease. Resistant HSV can be recovered from 6-17% of immunocompromised patients receiving acyclovir treatment (Bacon et al., 2003). Recurrences after cessation of acyclovir usually are due to sensitive virus but may be due to acyclovir-resistant virus in AIDS patients. In patients with progressive disease, intravenous foscarnet therapy is effective, but vidarabine is not (Chilukuri and Rosen, 2003).

Varicella-Zoster Virus Infections. If begun within 24 hours of rash onset, oral acyclovir has therapeutic effects in varicella of children and adults. In children weighing up to 40 kg, acyclovir (20 mg/kg, up to 800 mg per dose, four times daily for 5 days) reduces fever and new lesion formation by ~1 day. Routine use in uncomplicated pediatric varicella is not recommended but should be considered in those at risk of moderate-to-severe illness (persons >12 years of age, secondary household cases, those with chronic cutaneous or pulmonary disorders, or those receiving corticosteroids or long-term salicylates) (Committee on Infectious Diseases, American Academy of Pediatrics, 2003). In adults treated within 24 hours, oral acyclovir (800 mg five times daily for 7 days) reduces the time to crusting of lesions by ~2 days, the maximum number of lesions by one-half, and the duration of fever. Intravenous acyclovir appears to be effective in varicella pneumonia or encephalitis of previously healthy adults. Oral acyclovir (10 mg/kg four times daily) given between 7 and 14 days after exposure may reduce the risk of varicella.

In older adults with localized herpes zoster, oral acyclovir (800 mg five times daily for 7 days) reduces pain and healing times if treatment can be initiated within 72 hours of rash onset. A reduction in ocular complications, particularly keratitis and anterior uveitis, occurs with treatment of zoster ophthalmicus. Prolonged acyclovir and concurrent prednisone for 21 days speed zoster healing and improve quality-of-life measures compared with each therapy alone. Valacyclovir (1000 mg three times daily for 7 days) provides more prompt relief of zoster-associated pain than acyclovir in older adults (≥50 years) with zoster.

In immunocompromised patients with herpes zoster, intravenous acyclovir (500 mg/m^2 every 8 hours for 7 days) reduces viral shedding, healing time, and the risks of cutaneous dissemination and visceral complications, as well as the length of hospitalization, in disseminating zoster. In immunosuppressed children with varicella, intravenous acyclovir decreases healing time and the risk of visceral complications.

Acyclovir-resistant VZV isolates uncommonly have been recovered from HIV-infected children and adults who may manifest chronic hyperkeratotic or verrucous lesions and sometimes meningoradiculitis. Intravenous foscarnet also appears to be effective for acyclovir-resistant VZV infections.

Other Viruses. Acyclovir is ineffective therapeutically in established cytomegalovirus (CMV) infections but ganciclovir is effective for CMV prophylaxis in immunocompromised patients. High-dose intravenous acyclovir (500 mg/m^2 every 8 hours for 1 month) in CMV-seropositive bone marrow transplant recipients is associated with ~50% lower risk of CMV disease and, when combined with prolonged oral acyclovir (800 mg four times daily through 6 months), improves survival. Following engraftment, valacyclovir (2000 mg four times daily to day 100) appears as effective as intravenous ganciclovir prophylaxis in such patients (Winston et al., 2003). High-dose oral acyclovir or valacyclovir (2000 mg four times daily) suppression for 3 months may reduce the risk of CMV disease and its sequelae in certain solid-organ transplant recipients (Lowance et al., 1999), but oral valganciclovir is the preferred agent for mismatched graft recipients (Pereyra and Rubin, 2004). Compared with acyclovir, high-dose valacyclovir reduces CMV disease in advanced HIV infection but is associated with greater toxicity and possibly shorter survival.

In infectious mononucleosis, acyclovir is associated with transient antiviral effects but no clinical benefits. EBV-related oral hairy leukoplakia may improve with acyclovir. Oral acyclovir in conjunction with systemic corticosteroids appears beneficial in treating Bell's palsy, but valacyclovir is ineffective in acute vestibular neuritis.

Cidofovir

Chemistry and Antiviral Activity. Cidofovir is a cytidine nucleotide analog with inhibitory activity against human herpes, papilloma, polyoma, pox, and adenoviruses (Hitchcock et al., 1996). It structure is shown in Figure 58–2.

In vitro inhibitory concentrations range from >0.2 to 0.7 μg/mL for CMV, 0.4 to 33 μg/mL for HSV, and 0.02-17 μg/mL for adenoviruses. Because cidofovir is a phosphonate that is phosphorylated by cellular but not virus enzymes, it inhibits acyclovir-resistant thymidine kinase (TK)–deficient or TK-altered HSV or VZV strains, ganciclovir-resistant CMV strains with UL97 mutations but not those with DNA polymerase mutations, and some foscarnet-resistant CMV strains. Cidofovir synergistically inhibits CMV replication in combination with ganciclovir or foscarnet.

Mechanisms of Action and Resistance. Cidofovir inhibits viral DNA synthesis by slowing and eventually terminating chain elongation. Cidofovir is metabolized to its active diphosphate form by cellular enzymes; the levels of phosphorylated metabolites are similar in infected and uninfected cells. The diphosphate acts as both a competitive inhibitor with respect to dCTP and as an alternative substrate for viral DNA polymerase. The diphosphate has a prolonged intracellular $t_{1/2}$ and competitively inhibits CMV and HSV DNA polymerases at concentrations one-eighth to one six-hundredth of those required to inhibit human DNA polymerases (Hitchcock et al., 1996). A phosphocholine metabolite also has a long intracellular $t_{1/2}$ (~87 hours) and may serve as an intracellular reservoir of drug. The prolonged intracellular $t_{1/2}$ of cidofovir diphosphate allows infrequent dosing regimens, and single doses are effective in experimental HSV, varicella, and poxvirus infections.

Cidofovir resistance in CMV is due to mutations in viral DNA polymerase. Low-level resistance to cidofovir develops in up to ~30% of retinitis patients by 3 months of therapy. Highly ganciclovir-resistant CMV isolates that possess DNA polymerase and UL97 kinase mutations are resistant to cidofovir, and prior ganciclovir therapy may select for cidofovir resistance. Some foscarnet-resistant CMV isolates show cross-resistance to cidofovir, and triple-drug-resistant variants with DNA polymerase mutations occur.

Absorption, Distribution, and Elimination. Cidofovir is dianionic at physiological pH and has very low oral bioavailability (Cundy, 1999). The plasma levels after intravenous dosing decline in a biphasic pattern with a terminal $t_{1/2}$ that averages 2.6 hours. The volume of distribution approximates total-body water. Penetration into the

CNS or eye has not been well characterized, but CSF levels are low. Extemporaneously compounded topical cidofovir gel may result in low plasma concentrations (<0.5 μg/mL) in patients with large mucocutaneous lesions.

Cidofovir is cleared by the kidney via glomerular filtration and tubular secretion. Over 90% of the dose is recovered unchanged in the urine without significant metabolism in humans. The probenecid-sensitive organic anion transporter 1 mediates uptake of cidofovir into proximal renal tubular epithelial cells (Ho et al., 2000). High-dose probenecid (2 g three hours before and 1 g two and eight hours after each infusion) blocks tubular transport of cidofovir and reduces renal clearance and associated nephrotoxicity. At cidofovir doses of 5 mg/kg, peak plasma concentrations increase from 11.5-19.6 μg/mL with probenecid, and renal clearance is reduced to the level of glomerular filtration. Elimination relates linearly to creatinine clearance, and the $t_{1/2}$ increases to 32.5 hours in patients on chronic ambulatory peritoneal dialysis (CAPD). Hemodialysis removes >50% of the administered dose (Cundy, 1999).

Untoward Effects. Nephrotoxicity is the principal dose-limiting side effect of intravenous cidofovir. Proximal tubular dysfunction includes proteinuria, azotemia, glycosuria, metabolic acidosis, and uncommonly, Fanconi's syndrome. Concomitant oral probenecid and saline prehydration reduce the risk of renal toxicity. On maintenance doses of 5 mg/kg every 2 weeks, up to 50% of patients develop proteinuria, 10-15% show an elevated serum creatinine concentration, and 15-20% develop neutropenia. Anterior uveitis that is responsive to topical corticosteroids and cycloplegia occurs commonly and low intraocular pressure occurs infrequently with intravenous cidofovir. Concurrent probenecid administration is associated with gastrointestinal (GI) upset, constitutional symptoms, and hypersensitivity reactions, including fever, rash, and uncommonly, anaphylactoid manifestations. Administration with food and pretreatment with antiemetics, antihistamines, and/or acetaminophen may improve tolerance.

Probenecid, but not cidofovir, alters zidovudine pharmacokinetics such that zidovudine doses should be reduced when probenecid is present, as should the doses of other drugs whose renal secretion probenecid inhibits (e.g., β-lactam antibiotics, nonsteroidal anti-inflammatory drugs [NSAIDs], acyclovir, lorazepam, furosemide, methotrexate, theophylline, and rifampin). Concurrent nephrotoxic agents are contraindicated, and at least 7 days should elapse between the end of aminoglycoside therapy and initiation of cidofovir. The same interval should separate intravenous pentamidine, amphotericin B, foscarnet, NSAID, or contrast dye and cidofovir. Cidofovir and oral ganciclovir are poorly tolerated in combination at full doses.

Topical application of cidofovir is associated with dose-related application-site reactions (e.g., burning, pain, and pruritus) in up to one-third of patients and occasionally ulceration. Intravitreal cidofovir may cause vitreitis, hypotony, and visual loss and is contraindicated.

Preclinical studies indicate that cidofovir has mutagenic, gonadotoxic, embryotoxic, and teratogenic effects. Because cidofovir is carcinogenic in rats, it is considered a potential human carcinogen. It may cause infertility and is classified as pregnancy Category C.

Therapeutic Uses. Intravenous cidofovir is approved for the treatment of CMV retinitis in HIV-infected patients.

Intravenous cidofovir (5 mg/kg once a week for 2 weeks followed by dosing every 2 weeks) increases the time to progression of CMV retinitis in previously untreated patients and in those failing or intolerant of ganciclovir and foscarnet therapy. CMV viremia may persist during cidofovir administration. Maintenance doses of 5 mg/kg are more effective but less well tolerated than 3 mg/kg doses. Intravenous cidofovir has been used for treating acyclovir-resistant mucocutaneous HSV infection, adenovirus disease in transplant recipients (Ljungman et al., 2003), and extensive molluscum contagiosum in HIV patients. Reduced doses (0.25-1 mg/kg every 2-3 weeks) without probenecid may be beneficial in BK virus nephropathy in renal transplant patients (Vats et al., 2003).

Extemporaneously compounded topical cidofovir gel eliminates virus shedding and lesions in some HIV-infected patients with acyclovir-resistant mucocutaneous HSV infections and has been used in treating anogenital warts and molluscum contagiosum in immunocompromised patients and cervical intraepithelial neoplasia in women. Intralesional cidofovir induces remissions in adults and children with respiratory papillomatosis.

Famciclovir and Penciclovir

Chemistry and Antiviral Activity. Famciclovir is the diacetyl ester prodrug of 6-deoxy penciclovir and lacks intrinsic antiviral activity. Penciclovir is an acyclic guanine nucleoside analog. The side chain differs structurally in that the oxygen has been replaced by a carbon, and an additional hydroxymethyl group is present Figure 58–2.

Penciclovir is similar to acyclovir in its spectrum of activity and potency against HSV and VZV. The inhibitory concentrations of penciclovir depend on cell type but are usually within 2-fold of those of acyclovir for HSV and VZV. It also is inhibitory for HBV.

Mechanisms of Action and Resistance. Penciclovir is an inhibitor of viral DNA synthesis. In HSV- or VZV-infected cells, penciclovir is phosphorylated initially by viral thymidine kinase. Penciclovir triphosphate serves as a competitive inhibitor of viral DNA polymerase (Figure 58–3). Although penciclovir triphosphate is approximately one one-hundredth as potent as acyclovir triphosphate in inhibiting viral DNA polymerase, it is present in much higher concentrations and for more prolonged periods in infected cells than acyclovir triphosphate. The prolonged intracellular $t_{1/2}$ of penciclovir triphosphate, 7-20 hours, is associated with prolonged antiviral effects. Because penciclovir has a 3′-hydroxyl group, it is not an obligate chain terminator but does inhibit DNA elongation.

Resistant variants owing to thymidine kinase or DNA polymerase mutations can be selected by passage *in vitro,* but the occurrence of resistance during clinical use is currently low (Bacon et al., 2003). Thymidine kinase–deficient, acyclovir-resistant herpes viruses are cross-resistant to penciclovir.

Absorption, Distribution, and Elimination. Oral penciclovir has low (<5%) bioavailability. In contrast, famciclovir is well absorbed orally (bioavailability ~75%) and is converted rapidly to penciclovir by deacetylation of the side chain and oxidation of the purine ring during and following absorption from the intestine (Gill and Wood, 1996). Thus, the bioavailability of penciclovir is ~75% following oral administration of famciclovir.

Food slows absorption but does not reduce overall bioavailability. After single 250- or 500-mg doses of famciclovir, the peak plasma concentration of penciclovir averages 1.6 and 3.3 μg/mL, respectively. A small quantity of the 6-deoxy precursor but no famciclovir is detectable in plasma. After intravenous infusion of penciclovir at 10 mg/kg, peak plasma levels average 12 μg/mL. The volume of distribution is about twice the volume of total-body water. The plasma elimination $t_{1/2}$ of penciclovir averages ~2 hours, and >90% is excreted unchanged in the urine, probably by both filtration and active tubular secretion. Following oral famciclovir administration, nonrenal clearance accounts for ~10% of each dose, primarily through fecal excretion, but penciclovir (60% of dose) and its 6-deoxy precursor (<10% of dose) are eliminated primarily in the urine. The plasma $t_{1/2}$ averages 9.9 hours in renal insufficiency (Cl_{cr} <30 mL/minute); hemodialysis efficiently removes penciclovir. Lower peak plasma concentrations of penciclovir, but no reduction in overall bioavailability of famciclovir, occur in compensated chronic hepatic insufficiency (Boike et al., 1994).

Untoward Effects. Oral famciclovir is well tolerated but may be associated with headache, diarrhea, and nausea. Urticaria, rash, and hallucinations or confusional states (predominantly in the elderly) have been reported. Topical penciclovir, which is formulated in 40% propylene glycol and a cetomacrogol base, is associated infrequently with application-site reactions (~1%). The short-term tolerance of famciclovir is comparable with that of acyclovir.

Penciclovir is mutagenic at high concentrations *in vitro*. Although studies in laboratory animals indicate that chronic famciclovir administration is tumorigenic and decreases spermatogenesis and fertility in rodents and dogs, long-term administration (1 year) does not affect spermatogenesis in men. No teratogenic effects have been observed in animals, but safety during pregnancy has not been established. No clinically important drug interactions have been identified to date with famciclovir or penciclovir (Gill and Wood, 1996).

Therapeutic Uses. Oral famciclovir, topical penciclovir, and intravenous penciclovir are approved for managing HSV and VZV infections (Sacks and Wilson, 1999).

Oral famciclovir (250 mg three times a day for 7-10 days) is as effective as acyclovir in treating first-episode genital herpes (Kimberlin and Rouse, 2004). In patients with recurrent genital HSV, patient-initiated famciclovir treatment (125 or 250 mg twice a day for 5 days) reduces healing time and symptoms by ~1 day. Famciclovir (250 mg twice a day for up to 1 year) is effective for suppression of recurrent genital HSV, but single daily doses are less effective. Higher doses (500 mg twice a day) reduce HSV recurrences in HIV-infected persons. Intravenous penciclovir (5 mg/kg every 8 or 12 hours for 7 days) (not available in the U.S.) is comparable to intravenous acyclovir for treating mucocutaneous HSV infections in immunocompromised hosts. In immunocompetent persons with recurrent orolabial HSV, topical 1% penciclovir cream (applied every 2 hours while awake for 4 days) shortens healing time and symptoms by ~1 day (Raborn et al., 2002).

In immunocompetent adults with herpes zoster of ≤3 days' duration, famciclovir (500 mg three times a day for 10 days) is at least as effective as acyclovir (800 mg five times daily) in reducing healing time and zoster-associated pain, particularly in those ≥50 years of age. Famciclovir is comparable with valacyclovir in treating zoster and reducing associated pain in older adults (Tyring et al., 2000). Famciclovir (500 mg three times a day for 7-10 days) also is comparable with high-dose oral acyclovir in treating zoster in immunocompromised patients and in those with ophthalmic zoster (Tyring et al., 2001).

Famciclovir is associated with dose-related reductions in HBV DNA and transaminase levels in patients with chronic HBV hepatitis but is less effective than lamivudine (Lai et al., 2002). Famciclovir is also ineffective in treating lamivudine-resistant HBV infections owing to emergence of multiply resistant variants.

Fomivirsen

Fomivirsen, a 21-base phosphorothioate oligionucleotide, was the first FDA-approved antisense therapy for viral infections. It is complementary to the messenger RNA sequence for the major immediate-early transcriptional region of CMV and inhibits CMV replication through sequence-specific and nonspecific mechanisms, including inhibition of virus binding to cells. Fomivirsen is active against CMV strains resistant to ganciclovir, foscarnet, and cidofovir. CMV variants with 10-fold reduced susceptibility to fomivirsen have been selected by *in vitro* passage.

Fomivirsen is given by intravitreal injection in the treatment of CMV retinitis for patients intolerant of or unresponsive to other therapies. Following injection, it is cleared slowly from the vitreous ($t_{1/2}$ ~55 hours) through distribution to the retina and probable exonuclease digestion (Geary et al., 2002). Local metabolism by exonucleases accounts for elimination. In HIV-infected patients with refractory, sight-threatening CMV retinitis, fomivirsen injections (330 μg weekly for 3 weeks and then every 2 weeks or on days 1 and 15 followed by monthly) significantly delay time to retinitis progression (Vitravene Study Group, 2002). Ocular side effects include iritis in up to one-quarter of patients, which can be managed with topical corticosteroids; vitritis; cataracts; and increases in intraocular pressure in 15-20% of patients. Recent cidofovir use may increase the risk of inflammatory reactions. The drug is no longer available in the U.S.

Foscarnet

Chemistry and Antiviral Activity. Foscarnet (trisodium phosphonoformate; Figure 58–2) is an inorganic pyrophosphate analog that is inhibitory for all herpesviruses and HIV.

In vitro inhibitory concentrations are generally 100-300 μM for CMV and 80-200 μM for other herpesviruses, including most ganciclovir-resistant CMV and acyclovir-resistant HSV and VZV strains. Combinations of foscarnet and ganciclovir synergistically inhibit CMV replication *in vitro*. Concentrations of 500-1000 μM reversibly inhibit the proliferation and DNA synthesis of uninfected cells.

Mechanisms of Action and Resistance. Foscarnet inhibits viral nucleic acid synthesis by interacting directly with herpesvirus DNA polymerase or HIV reverse transcriptase (Figure 58–3). It is taken up slowly by cells and does not undergo significant intracellular metabolism. Foscarnet reversibly blocks the pyrophosphate binding site of the viral polymerase in a noncompetitive manner and inhibits cleavage of pyrophosphate from deoxynucleotide triphosphates. Foscarnet has ~100-fold greater inhibitory effects against herpesvirus DNA polymerases than against cellular DNA polymerase-α. Herpesviruses resistant to foscarnet have point mutations in the viral DNA polymerase and are associated with 3- to 7-fold reductions in foscarnet activity *in vitro*.

Absorption, Distribution, and Elimination. Oral bioavailability of foscarnet is low. Following an intravenous infusion of 60 mg/kg every 8 hours, peak and trough plasma concentrations are ~450-575 and 80-150 μM, respectively. Vitreous levels approximate those in plasma, and CSF levels average 66% of those in plasma at steady state.

Over 80% of foscarnet is excreted unchanged in the urine by glomerular filtration and probably tubular secretion. Plasma clearance decreases proportionately with creatinine clearance, and dose adjustments are indicated for small decreases in renal function. Plasma elimination is complex, with initial bimodal half-lives totaling 4-8 hours and a prolonged terminal elimination $t_{1/2}$ averaging 3-4 days. Sequestration in bone with gradual release accounts for the fate of an estimated 10-20% of a given dose. Foscarnet is cleared efficiently by hemodialysis (~50% of a dose).

Untoward Effects. Foscarnet's major dose-limiting toxicities are nephrotoxicity and symptomatic hypocalcemia. Increases in serum creatinine occur in up to one-half of patients but are reversible after cessation in most patients. High doses, rapid infusion, dehydration, prior renal insufficiency, and concurrent nephrotoxic drugs are risk factors. Acute tubular necrosis, crystalline glomerulopathy, nephrogenic diabetes insipidus, and interstitial nephritis have been described. Saline loading may reduce the risk of nephrotoxicity.

Foscarnet is highly ionized at physiological pH, and metabolic abnormalities are very common. These include increases or decreases in Ca^{2+} and phosphate, hypomagnesemia, and hypokalemia. Decreased serum ionized Ca^{2+} may cause paresthesia, arrhythmias, tetany, seizures, and other CNS disturbances. Concomitant intravenous pentamidine administration increases the risk of symptomatic hypocalcemia. Parenteral magnesium sulfate does not alter foscarnet-induced hypocalcemia or symptoms (Huycke et al., 2000).

CNS side effects include headache in ~25% of patients, tremor, irritability, seizures, and hallucinosis. Other reported side effects are generalized rash, fever, nausea or emesis, anemia, leukopenia, abnormal liver function tests, electrocardiographic changes, infusion-related thrombophlebitis, and painful genital ulcerations. Topical foscarnet may cause local irritation and ulceration, and oral foscarnet may cause GI disturbance. Preclinical studies indicate that high foscarnet concentrations are mutagenic and may cause tooth and skeletal abnormalities in developing laboratory animals. Safety in pregnancy or childhood is uncertain.

Therapeutic Uses. Intravenous foscarnet is effective for treatment of CMV retinitis, including ganciclovir-resistant infections, other types of CMV infection, and acyclovir-resistant HSV and VZV infections. Foscarnet is poorly soluble in aqueous solutions and requires large volumes for administration.

In CMV retinitis in AIDS patients, foscarnet (60 mg/kg every 8 hours or 90 mg/kg every 12 hours for 14-21 days followed by chronic maintenance at 90 to 120 mg/kg every day in one dose) is associated with clinical stabilization in ~90% of patients. A comparative trial of foscarnet with ganciclovir found comparable control of CMV retinitis in AIDS patients but improved overall survival in the foscarnet-treated group (Studies of Ocular Complications of AIDS, 1992). This improved survival with foscarnet may be related to the drug's intrinsic anti-HIV activity, but patients stop taking foscarnet over three times as often as ganciclovir because of side effects. A combination of foscarnet and ganciclovir is more effective than either drug alone in refractory retinitis; combinations may be useful in treating ganciclovir-resistant CMV infections in solid-organ transplant patients. Foscarnet benefits other CMV syndromes in AIDS or transplant patients but is ineffective as monotherapy in treating CMV pneumonia in bone marrow transplant patients (possibly effective if started early). When used for preemptive therapy of CMV viremia in bone marrow transplant recipients, foscarnet (60 mg/kg every 12 hours for 2 weeks followed by 90 mg/kg daily for 2 weeks) is as effective as intravenous ganciclovir and causes less neutropenia (Reusser et al., 2002). When used for CMV infections, foscarnet may reduce the risk of Kaposi's sarcoma in HIV-infected patients. Intravitreal injections of foscarnet also have been used.

In acyclovir-resistant mucocutaneous HSV infections, lower doses of foscarnet (40 mg/kg every 8 hours for ≥7 days) are associated with cessation of viral shedding and with complete healing of lesions in about three-quarters of patients. Foscarnet also appears to be effective in acyclovir-resistant VZV infections. Topical foscarnet cream is ineffective in treating recurrent genital HSV in immunocompetent persons but appears to be useful in chronic acyclovir-resistant infections in immunocompromised patients.

Resistant clinical isolates of herpesviruses have emerged during therapeutic use and may be associated with poor clinical response to foscarnet treatment.

Ganciclovir and Valganciclovir

Chemistry and Antiviral Activity. Ganciclovir is an acyclic guanine nucleoside analog that is similar in structure to acyclovir except in having an additional hydroxymethyl group on the acyclic side chain. Valganciclovir is the L-valyl ester prodrug of ganciclovir. Their structures are shown in Figure 58–2.

Ganciclovir has inhibitory activity against all herpesviruses but is especially active against CMV (Noble and Faulds, 1998). Inhibitory concentrations are similar to those of acyclovir for HSV and VZV but 10-100 times lower for human CMV strains (0.2-2.8 μg/mL).

Inhibitory concentrations for human bone marrow progenitor cells are similar to those inhibitory for CMV replication, a finding predictive of ganciclovir's myelotoxicity during clinical use. Inhibition of human lymphocyte blastogenic responses also occurs at clinically achievable concentrations of 1-10 μg/mL.

Mechanisms of Action and Resistance. Ganciclovir inhibits viral DNA synthesis. It is monophosphorylated intracellularly by viral thymidine kinase during HSV infection and by a viral phosphotransferase encoded by the UL97 gene during CMV infection. Ganciclovir diphosphate and ganciclovir triphosphate are formed by cellular enzymes. At least 10-fold higher concentrations of ganciclovir triphosphate are present in CMV-infected than in uninfected cells. The triphosphate is a competitive inhibitor of deoxyguanosine triphosphate incorporation into DNA and preferentially inhibits viral rather than host cellular DNA polymerases. Ganciclovir is incorporated into both viral and cellular DNA. Incorporation into viral DNA causes eventual cessation of DNA chain elongation (Figures 58–1B and 58–3).

Intracellular ganciclovir triphosphate concentrations are 10-fold higher than those of acyclovir triphosphate and decline much more slowly with an intracellular elimination $t_{1/2}$ >24 hours. These differences may account in part for ganciclovir's greater anti-CMV activity and provide the rationale for single daily doses in suppressing human CMV infections.

CMV can become resistant to ganciclovir by one of two mechanisms: reduced intracellular ganciclovir phosphorylation owing to mutations in the viral phosphotransferase encoded by the UL97 gene and mutations in viral DNA polymerase (Schreiber et al., 2009). Resistant CMV clinical isolates have from 4- to >20-fold increases in inhibitory concentrations. Resistance has been associated primarily with impaired phosphorylation but sometimes only with DNA polymerase mutations. Highly resistant variants with dual UL97 and polymerase mutations are cross-resistant to cidofovir and variably to foscarnet. Ganciclovir also is much less active against acyclovir-resistant thymidine kinase–deficient HSV strains.

Absorption, Distribution, and Elimination. The oral bioavailability of ganciclovir averages 6-9% following ingestion with food. Peak and trough plasma levels are ~0.5-1.2 and 0.2-0.5 μg/mL, respectively, after 1000-mg doses every 8 hours. Oral valganciclovir is well absorbed and hydrolyzed rapidly to ganciclovir; the bioavailability of ganciclovir averages 61% following valganciclovir (Curran and Noble, 2001). Food increases the bioavailability of valganciclovir by ~25%, and peak ganciclovir concentrations average 6.1 μg/mL after 875-mg doses. High oral valganciclovir doses in the fed state provide ganciclovir exposures comparable with intravenous dosing (Brown et al., 1999). Following intravenous administration of 5 mg/kg doses of ganciclovir, peak and trough plasma concentrations average 8-11 and 0.6-1.2 μg/mL, respectively. Following intravenous dosing, vitreous fluid levels are similar to or higher than those in plasma and average ~1 μg/mL. Vitreous levels decline with a $t_{1/2}$ of 23-26 hours. Intraocular sustained-release ganciclovir implants provide vitreous levels of ~4.1 μg/mL.

The plasma elimination $t_{1/2}$ is ~2-4 hours in patients with normal renal function. Over 90% of ganciclovir is eliminated unchanged by renal excretion through glomerular filtration and tubular secretion. Consequently, the plasma $t_{1/2}$ increases almost linearly as creatinine clearance declines and may reach 28-40 hours in patients with severe renal insufficiency.

Untoward Effects. Myelosuppression is the principal dose-limiting toxicity of ganciclovir. Neutropenia occurs in ~15-40% of patients and thrombocytopenia in 5-20%. Neutropenia is observed most commonly during the second week of treatment and usually is reversible within 1 week of drug cessation. Persistent fatal neutropenia has occurred. Oral valganciclovir is associated with headache and GI disturbance (i.e., nausea, pain, and diarrhea) in addition to the toxicities associated with intravenous ganciclovir, including neutropenia. Recombinant granulocyte colony-stimulating factor (G-CSF; filgrastim, lenograstim) may be useful in treating ganciclovir-induced neutropenia (Chapter 37).

CNS side effects occur in 5-15% of patients and range in severity from headache to behavioral changes to convulsions and coma. About one-third of patients must interrupt or prematurely stop intravenous ganciclovir therapy because of bone marrow or CNS toxicity. Infusion-related phlebitis, azotemia, anemia, rash, fever, liver function test abnormalities, nausea or vomiting, and eosinophilia also have been described.

Teratogenicity, embryotoxicity, irreversible reproductive toxicity, and myelotoxicity have been observed in animals at ganciclovir dosages comparable with those used in humans. Ganciclovir is classified as pregnancy Category C.

Zidovudine and probably other cytotoxic agents increase the risk of myelosuppression, as do nephrotoxic agents that impair ganciclovir excretion. Probenecid and possibly acyclovir reduce renal clearance of ganciclovir. Oral ganciclovir increases the absorption and peak plasma concentrations of didanosine by approximately 2-fold and that of zidovudine by ~20%.

Therapeutic Uses. Ganciclovir is effective for treatment and chronic suppression of CMV retinitis in immunocompromised patients and for prevention of CMV disease in transplant patients.

In CMV retinitis, initial induction treatment (5 mg/kg intravenously every 12 hours for 10-21 days) is associated with improvement or stabilization in ~85% of patients (Faulds and Heel, 1990). Reduced viral excretion is usually evident by 1 week, and funduscopic improvement is seen by 2 weeks. Because of the high risk of relapse, AIDS patients with retinitis require suppressive therapy with high doses of ganciclovir (5 mg/kg/day). Oral ganciclovir (1000 mg three times daily) is effective for suppression of retinitis after initial intravenous treatment but has been replaced in practice by oral valganciclovir. Oral valganciclovir (900 mg twice daily for 21 days initial treatment) is comparable with intravenous dosing for initial control and sustained suppression (900 mg daily) of CMV retinitis (Schreiber et al., 2009). Intravitreal ganciclovir injections have been used in some patients, and an intraocular sustained-release ganciclovir implant (VITRASERT) is more effective than systemic dosing in suppressing retinitis progression.

Ganciclovir therapy (5 mg/kg every 12 hours for 14-21 days) may benefit other CMV syndromes in AIDS patients or solid-organ transplant recipients (Infectious Disease Community of Practice et al., 2004). Response rates of ≥67% have been found in combination with a decrease in immunosuppressive therapy. The duration of therapy depends on demonstrating clearance of viremia; early switch from intravenous ganciclovir to oral valganciclovir is feasible. Recurrent CMV disease occurs commonly after initial treatment. In bone marrow transplant recipients with CMV pneumonia, ganciclovir alone appears ineffective. However, ganciclovir combined with intravenous immunoglobulin or CMV immunoglobulin reduces the mortality of CMV pneumonia by about one-half. Ganciclovir treatment improved hearing outcomes in neonates with symptomatic congenital CMV infections involving the CNS (Kimberlin et al, 2003).

Ganciclovir has been used for both prophylaxis and preemptive therapy of CMV infections in transplant recipients (Schreiber et al., 2009). In bone marrow transplant recipients, preemptive ganciclovir treatment (5 mg/kg every 12 hours for 7-14 days followed by 5 mg/kg every day to days 100-120 after transplant) starting when CMV is isolated from bronchoalveolar lavage or from other sites is highly effective in preventing CMV pneumonia and appears to reduce mortality in these patients. Initiation of ganciclovir at the time of engraftment also reduces CMV disease rates but does not improve survival in part because of infections owing to ganciclovir-related neutropenia.

Intravenous ganciclovir, oral ganciclovir, and oral valganciclovir reduce the risk of CMV disease in solid-organ transplant recipients (Infectious Disease Community of Practice et al., 2004). Oral ganciclovir (1000 mg three times daily for 3 months) reduces CMV disease risk in liver transplant recipients, including high-risk patients with primary infection or those receiving antilymphocyte antibodies. Oral valganciclovir prophylaxis generally is more effective than high-dose oral acyclovir. Oral valganciclovir (900 mg once daily) provides somewhat greater antiviral effects and similar reductions in CMV disease as oral ganciclovir in mismatched solid-organ transplant recipients (Schreiber et al., 2009). Valganciclovir has recently been approved for prevention of CMV in pediatric transplant patients.

In advanced HIV disease, oral ganciclovir (1000 mg three times daily) may reduce the risk of CMV disease and possibly mortality in those not receiving didanosine (Brosgart et al., 1998) but has been replaced for prophylaxis by oral valganciclovir. The addition of oral high-dose ganciclovir (1500 mg three times daily) to the intraocular ganciclovir implant further delays the time to retinitis progression and reduces the risk of new CMV disease and possibly the risk of Kaposi's sarcoma.

Ganciclovir resistance emerges in a minority of transplant patients, especially mismatched solid-organ recipients (Limaye et al., 2000), and is associated with poorer prognosis. The use of antithymocyte globulin and prolonged ganciclovir exposure are risk factors. Recovery of ganciclovir-resistant CMV isolates has been associated with progressive CMV disease in AIDS and other immunocompromised patients. Over one-quarter of retinitis patients have resistant isolates by 9 months of therapy, and resistant CMV has been recovered from CSF, vitreous fluid, and visceral sites.

A ganciclovir ophthalmic gel formulation (ZIRGAN) is effective in treating HSV keratitis (Colin et al., 1997). Oral ganciclovir also reduces HBV DNA levels and aminotransferase levels in chronic hepatitis B virus infection (Hadziyannis et al., 1999), but the drug is not approved for this indication.

Docosanol

Docosanol is a long-chain saturated alcohol that is FDA-approved as an over-the-counter 10% cream for the treatment of recurrent orolabial herpes. Docosanol inhibits the in vitro replication of many lipid-enveloped viruses, including HSV, at millimolar concentrations. It does not inactivate HSV directly but appears to block fusion between the cellular and viral envelope membranes and inhibits viral entry into the cell. Topical treatment beginning within 12 hours of prodromal symptoms or lesion onset reduces healing time by ~1 day and appears to be well tolerated (Elish et al., 2004). Treatment initiation at papular or later stages provides no benefit.

Idoxuridine

Idoxuridine (5-iodo-2′-deoxyuridine) is an iodinated thymidine analog that inhibits the in vitro replication of various DNA viruses, including herpesviruses and poxviruses (Prusoff, 1988).

Inhibitory concentrations of idoxuridine for HSV-1 are 2-10 μg/mL, at least 10-fold higher than those of acyclovir. Idoxuridine lacks selectivity, in that low concentrations inhibit the growth of uninfected cells. The triphosphate inhibits viral DNA synthesis and is incorporated into both viral and cellular DNA. Such altered DNA is more susceptible to breakage and also leads to faulty transcription. Resistance to idoxuridine develops readily in vitro and occurs in viral isolates recovered from idoxuridine-treated patients with HSV keratitis.

In the U.S., idoxuridine is approved only for topical (ophthalmic) treatment of HSV keratitis. Idoxuridine formulated in dimethylsulfoxide is available outside the U.S. for topical treatment of herpes labialis, genitalis, and zoster. In ocular HSV infections, topical idoxuridine is more effective in epithelial infections, especially initial episodes, than in stromal infections. Adverse reactions include pain, pruritus, inflammation, and edema involving the eye or lids; rarely do allergic reactions occur.

Trifluridine

Trifluridine (5-trifluoromethyl-2′-deoxyuridine) is a fluorinated pyrimidine nucleoside that has in vitro inhibitory activity against HSV types 1 and 2, CMV, vaccinia, and to a lesser extent, certain adenoviruses.

Concentrations of trifluridine of 0.2-10 μg/mL inhibit replication of herpesviruses, including acyclovir-resistant strains. Trifluridine also inhibits cellular DNA synthesis at relatively low concentrations.

Trifluridine monophosphate irreversibly inhibits thymidylate synthase, and trifluridine triphosphate is a competitive inhibitor of thymidine triphosphate incorporation into DNA;

trifluridine is incorporated into viral and cellular DNA. Trifluridine-resistant HSV with altered thymidine kinase substrate specificity can be selected in vitro, and resistance in clinical isolates has been described.

Trifluridine currently is approved in the U.S. for treatment of primary keratoconjunctivitis and recurrent epithelial keratitis owing to HSV types 1 and 2. Topical trifluridine is more active than idoxuridine and comparable with vidarabine in HSV ocular infections. Adverse reactions include discomfort on instillation and palpebral edema. Hypersensitivity reactions, irritation, and superficial punctate or epithelial keratopathy are uncommon. Topical trifluridine also appears to be effective in some patients with acyclovir-resistant HSV cutaneous infections.

ANTI-INFLUENZA AGENTS

Four drugs are currently approved for the treatment and prevention of influenza virus infection. Over the past several years, there has been increasing concern about the possibility of new influenza pandemics, stemming from small but severe outbreaks of H5N1 avian influenza and the novel 2009 influenza A H1N1, thought to be of swine origin. This has prompted stockpiling of existing agents and motivated new drug discovery. Regulatory responses include Emergency Use Authorization (EUA) granted by the FDA, Centers for Disease Control and Prevention, and the World Health Organization to allow for treatment and prophylaxis of H1N1 in pediatric patients ≤1 year of age even though the four available agents were never granted conventional approval for this age group. In addition, peramivir, an investigational neuraminidase inhibitor, was made available for intravenous use via EUA authorization.

In the 2008–2009 influenza season, virtually all strains of influenza A H1N1 were resistant to the neuraminidase inhibitor oseltamivir (Moscona, 2009). This has arisen as a consequence of overuse of these drugs, including in veterinary applications. Fortunately the majority of 2009 H1N1 "swine" viruses were susceptible to oseltamivir; however, sporadic cases of oseltamivir resistance have been detected even with this strain. All such viruses tested to date were resistant to the adamantine antivirals, amantadine and rimantadine. Development of resistance to these drugs, and the spread of resistant viruses, is a major challenge in the chemotherapy and chemoprophylaxis of influenza and is likely to drive future recommendations for use of these drugs in global populations.

Amantadine and Rimantadine

Chemistry and Antiviral Activity. Amantadine (1-adamantanamine hydrochloride) and its α-methyl derivative rimantadine (α-methyl-1-adamantane methylamine hydrochloride) are uniquely configured tricyclic amines. Their structures are depicted in Figure 58–4.

Low concentrations of either agent specifically inhibit the replication of influenza A viruses (Schmidt, 2004). Depending on the assay method and strain, inhibitory concentrations of the drugs range from ~0.03-1.0 μg/mL for influenza A viruses. Rimantadine generally is 4-10 times more active than amantadine. Concentrations of ≥10 μg/mL inhibit other enveloped viruses but are not achievable in humans and may be cytotoxic. Rimantadine is inhibitory *in vitro* for *Trypanosoma brucei,* a cause of African sleeping sickness, at concentrations of 1-2.5 μg/mL. These agents do not inhibit hepatitis C virus (HCV) enzymes or internal ribosomal entry site–mediated translation but block the ion channel activity of the HCV p7 protein *in vitro* (Griffin et al., 2003).

Mechanisms of Action and Resistance. Amantadine and rimantadine share two mechanisms of antiviral action. They inhibit an early step in viral replication, probably viral uncoating; for some strains, they also have an effect on a late step in viral assembly probably mediated through altering hemagglutinin processing. The primary locus of action is the influenza A virus M2 protein, an integral membrane protein that functions as an ion channel. By interfering with this function of the M2 protein, the drugs inhibit the acid-mediated dissociation of the ribonucleoprotein complex early in replication and potentiate acidic pH–induced conformational changes in the hemagglutinin during its intracellular transport later in replication.

Absorption, Distribution, and Elimination. Amantadine and rimantadine are well absorbed after oral administration (Schmidt, 2004) (Table 58–3). Peak plasma concentrations of amantadine average 0.5-0.8 μg/mL on a 100-mg twice-daily regimen in healthy young adults. Comparable doses of rimantadine give peak and trough plasma concentrations of ~0.4-0.5 and 0.2-0.4 μg/mL, respectively. The elderly require only one-half the weight-adjusted dose of amantadine needed for young adults to achieve equivalent trough plasma levels of 0.3 μg/mL. Both drugs have very large volumes of distribution. Nasal secretion and salivary levels of amantadine approximate those found in the serum. Amantadine is excreted in breast milk. Rimantadine concentrations in nasal mucus average 50% higher than those in plasma.

Amantadine is excreted largely unmetabolized in the urine through glomerular filtration and probably tubular secretion. The plasma $t_{1/2}$ of elimination is ~12-18 hours in young adults. Because amantadine's elimination is highly dependent on renal function, the elimination $t_{1/2}$ increases up to 2-fold in the elderly and even more in those with renal impairment. Dose adjustments are advisable in those with mild decrements in renal function. In contrast,

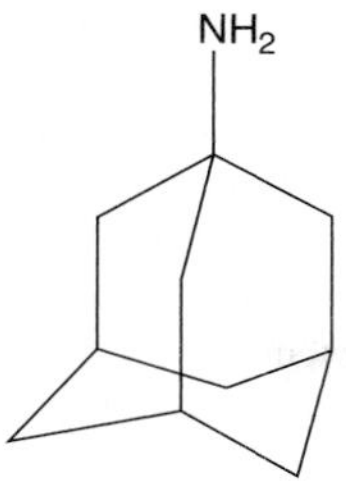

AMANTADINE

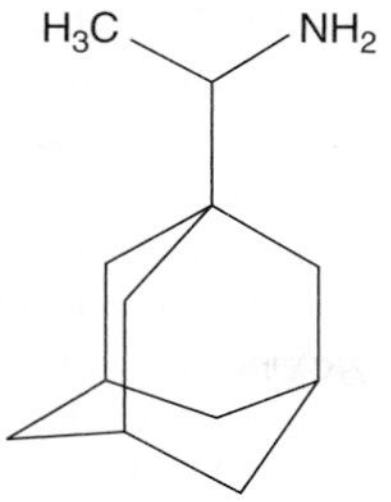

RIMANTADINE

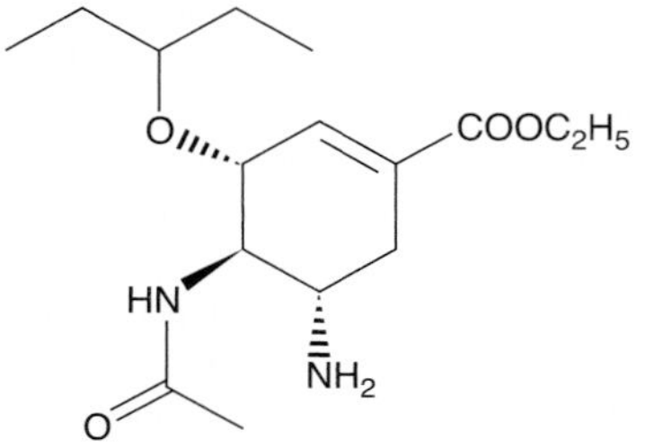

OSELTAMIVIR

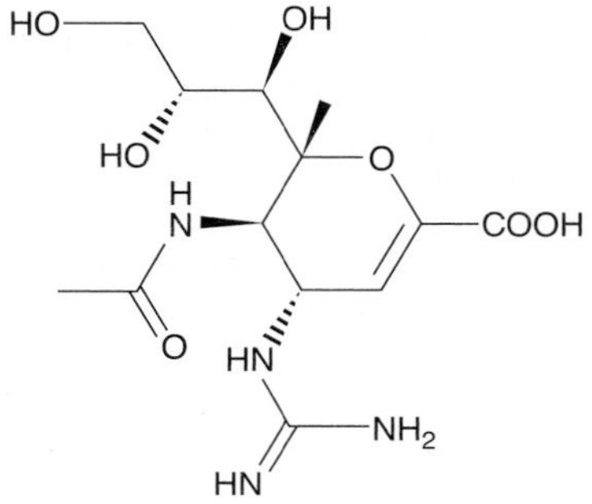

ZANAMIVIR

Figure 58–4. *Chemical Structures of the Anti-Influenza Drugs.*

rimantadine is metabolized extensively by hydroxylation, conjugation, and glucuronidation prior to renal excretion. Following oral administration, the elimination $t_{1/2}$ of rimantadine averages 24-36 hours, and 60-90% is excreted in the urine as metabolites. Renal clearance of unchanged rimantadine is similar to creatinine clearance.

Untoward Effects. The most common side effects related to amantadine and rimantadine are minor dose-related CNS and gastrointestinal (Schmidt, 2004). These include nervousness, light-headedness, difficulty concentrating, insomnia, and loss of appetite or nausea. CNS side effects occur in 5-33% of patients treated with amantadine at doses of 200 mg/day but are significantly less frequent with rimantadine. The neurotoxic effects of amantadine appear to be increased by concomitant ingestion of antihistamines and psychotropic or anticholinergic drugs, especially in the elderly. Amantadine dose reductions are required in older adults (100 mg/day) because of decreased renal function, but 20-40% of infirm elderly will experience side effects even at this lower dose. At comparable doses of 100 mg/day, rimantadine is significantly better tolerated in nursing home residents than amantadine (Keyser et al., 2000).

High amantadine plasma concentrations (1.0-5.0 μg/mL) have been associated with serious neurotoxic reactions, including delirium, hallucinosis, seizures, and coma, and cardiac arrhythmias. Exacerbations of preexisting seizure disorders and psychiatric symptoms may occur with amantadine and possibly with rimantadine. Amantadine is teratogenic in animals. Both drugs are considered pregnancy Category C because safety has not been established in pregnancy.

Therapeutic Uses. Seasonal prophylaxis with either amantadine or rimantadine (a total of 200 mg/day in one or two divided doses in young adults) is ~70-90% protective against influenza A illness.

Efficacy has been shown during pandemic influenza, in preventing nosocomial influenza, and in curtailing nosocomial outbreaks. Doses of 100 mg/day are better tolerated and still appear to be protective against influenzal illness. Postexposure prophylaxis with either drug provides protection of exposed family contacts if ill young children are not concurrently treated (Schmidt, 2004).

Seasonal prophylaxis is an alternative in high-risk patients if the influenza vaccine cannot be administered or may be ineffective (i.e., in immunocompromised patients). Prophylaxis should be started as soon as influenza is identified in a community or region and should be continued throughout the period of risk (usually 4-8 weeks) because any protective effects are lost several days after cessation of therapy. Alternatively, the drugs can be started in conjunction with immunization and continued for 2 weeks until protective immune responses develop.

The amantadines are effective against influenza A H1N1 in adults and children if treatment is initiated within 2 days of the onset of symptoms (Schmidt, 2004). Therapy reduces duration of viral excretion, fever, and other systemic complaints, but resistance has become more widespread with use. Duration of illness is shortened by ~1 day. In uncomplicated influenza A illness of adults, early amantadine or rimantadine treatment (200 mg/day for 5 days) reduces the duration of fever and systemic complaints by 1-2 days, speeds functional recovery, and sometimes decreases the duration of virus shedding (Schmidt, 2004). In children, rimantadine treatment may be associated with less illness and lower viral titers during the first 2 days of treatment, but rimantadine-treated children have more prolonged shedding of virus. The usual regimen in children (≥1 year of age) is 5 mg/kg/day, up to 150 mg, administered once or twice daily.

Resistant variants have been recovered from ~30% of treated children or outpatient adults by the fifth day of therapy (Schmidt, 2004). Resistant variants also arise commonly in immunocompromised patients (Englund et al., 1998). Illnesses owing to apparent transmission of resistant virus associated with failure of drug prophylaxis have been documented in contacts of drug-treated ill persons in households and in nursing homes (Schmidt, 2004). Resistant variants appear to be pathogenic and can cause typical disabling influenza.

Although both drugs are useful for the prevention and treatment of infections caused by influenza A virus, vaccination against influenza is a more cost-effective means of reducing disease burden. The utility of the amantadines has been limited by the development of resistance. Amantadine and rimantadine are active only against susceptible influenza A viruses (not influenza B); rimantadine is 4- to 10-fold more active than amantadine. Currently, virtually all H3N2 strains of influenza circulating worldwide are resistant to these drugs. Resistance to these drugs results from a mutation in the RNA sequence encoding for the M2 protein transmembrane domain (Schmidt, 2004), and resistant isolates typically appears in the treated patient within 2-3 days of starting therapy.

Oseltamivir

Chemistry and Antiviral Activity. Oseltamivir carboxylate (Figure 58–4) is a transition-state analog of sialic acid that is a potent selective inhibitor of influenza A and B virus neuraminidases. Oseltamivir phosphate is an ethyl ester prodrug that lacks antiviral activity.

Oseltamivir carboxylate has an antiviral spectrum and potency similar to that of zanamivir. It inhibits amantadine and rimantadine-resistant influenza A viruses and some zanamivir-resistant variants.

Mechanisms of Action and Resistance. Influenza neuraminidase cleaves terminal sialic acid residues and destroys the receptors recognized by viral hemagglutinin, which are present on the cell surface, in progeny virions, and in respiratory secretions (Schirmer and Holodniy, 2009). This enzymatic action is essential for release of virus from infected cells. Interaction of oseltamivir carboxylate with the neuraminidase causes a conformational change within the enzyme's active site and inhibits its activity. Inhibition of neuraminidase activity leads to viral aggregation at the cell surface and reduced virus spread within the respiratory tract.

Influenza variants selected *in vitro* for resistance to oseltamivir carboxylate contain hemagglutinin and/or neuraminidase mutations. The most commonly recognized variants (mutations at positions 292 in N2 and 274 in N1 neuraminidases) have reduced infectivity and virulence in animal models. Outpatient oseltamivir therapy has been associated with recovery of resistant variants in ~0.5% of adults and 5.5% of children; a higher frequency (~18%) occurs in hospitalized children. Seasonal influenza A (H1N1) has become virtually 100% resistant to oseltamivir worldwide (Moscona, 2009; Schirmer and Holodniy, 2009). Importantly, novel H1N1 (nH1N1 or swine influenza) remains susceptible to oseltamivir.

Absorption, Distribution, and Elimination. Oral oseltamivir phosphate is absorbed rapidly (Table 58–3) and cleaved by esterases in the GI tract and liver to the active carboxylate. Low blood levels of the phosphate are detectable, but exposure is only 3-5% of that of the metabolite. The bioavailability of the carboxylate is estimated to be ~80%. The time to maximum plasma concentrations of the carboxylate is ~2.5-5 hours. Food does not decrease bioavailability but reduces the risk of GI intolerance. After 75-mg doses, peak plasma concentrations average 0.07 μg/mL for oseltamivir phosphate and 0.35 μg/mL for the carboxylate. The carboxylate has a volume of distribution similar to extracellular water. Bronchoalveolar lavage levels in animals and middle ear fluid and sinus concentrations in humans are comparable with plasma levels. Following oral administration, the plasma $t_{1/2}$ of oseltamivir phosphate is 1-3 hours; that of the carboxylate is 6-10 hours. Both the prodrug and active metabolite are eliminated primarily unchanged through the kidney. Probenecid doubles the plasma $t_{1/2}$ of the carboxylate, which indicates tubular secretion by the anionic pathway. Children <2 years of age exhibit age-related changes in oseltamivir carboxylate clearance and total drug exposure (Kimberlin et al., 2009).

Untoward Effects. Oral oseltamivir is associated with nausea, abdominal discomfort, and, less often, emesis, probably owing to local irritation. GI complaints usually are mild to moderate in intensity, typically resolve in 1-2 days despite continued dosing, and are preventable by administration with food. The frequency of such complaints is ~10-15% when oseltamivir is used for the treatment of influenza illness and <5% when used for prophylaxis. An increased frequency of headache was reported in one prophylaxis study in elderly adults.

Oseltamivir phosphate and the carboxylate do not interact with CYPs *in vitro*. Their binding to protein is low. No clinically significant drug interactions have been recognized to date. Oseltamivir does not appear to impair fertility or to be teratogenic in animal studies, but safety in pregnancy is uncertain (pregnancy Category C). Very high doses have been associated with increased mortality, perhaps related to increased brain concentrations, in unweaned rats.

Therapeutic Uses. Oral oseltamivir is effective in the treatment and prevention of influenza A and B virus infections.

Treatment of previously healthy adults (75 mg twice daily for 5 days) or children 1-12 years of age (weight-adjusted dosing) with acute influenza reduces illness duration by ~1-2 days, speeds functional recovery, and reduces the risk of complications leading to antibiotic use by 40-50% (Whitley et al., 2001). Treatment is associated with approximate halving of the risk of subsequent hospitalization in adults (Kaiser et al., 2003). When used for prophylaxis during the typical influenza season, oseltamivir (75 mg once daily) is effective (~70-90%) in reducing the likelihood of influenza illness in both unimmunized working adults and in immunized nursing

Table 58–3

Pharmacological Characteristics of Antivirals for Influenza

	AMANTADINE	RIMANTADINE	ZANAMIVIR	OSELTAMIVIR
Spectrum (types of influenza)	A	A	A, B	A, B
Route/formulations	Oral (tablet/ capsule/syrup)	Oral (tablet/syrup)	Inhaled (powder) Intravenous[a]	Oral (capsule/ syrup) Intravenous[a]
Oral bioavailability	> 90%	> 90%	< 5%[b]	80%[c]
Effect of meals on AUC	Negligible	Negligible	Not applicable	Negligible
Elimination $t_{1/2}$, h	12-18	24-36	2.5-5	6-10[c]
Protein binding, %	67%	40%	< 10%	3%[c]
Metabolism, %	< 10%	~75%	Negligible	Negligible
Renal excretion, % (parent drug)	>90%	~25%	100%	95%[c]
Dose adjustments	$Cl_{cr} \leq 50$ Age ≥ 65 yrs	$Cl_{cr} \leq 10$ Age ≥ 65 years	None[d]	$Cl_{cr} \leq 30$

A fifth agent, permavir, is investigational in the U.S. and approved in Japan at a dose of 600 mg intravenously once daily in adults. Its elimination is primarily renal, with dosage adjustment required for renal insufficiency.
[a]Investigational at present. [b]Systemic absorption 4-17% after inhalation. [c]For antivirally active oseltamivir carboxylate. [d]Inhaled formulation only. Cl_{cr}, creatinine clearance

home residents; short-term use (7-10 days) protects against influenza in household contacts (Schirmer and Holodniy, 2009).

Because of the global development of resistance of H1N1 seasonal influenza, treatment recommendations issued by the CDC for the 2008–2009 influenza season required the co-administration of an adamantine and a neuraminidase inhibitor. An intravenous formulation of oseltamivir is being evaluated in adults and children under the 2009 EUA. Until recently, oseltamivir was only licensed for patients >2 years of age; however, with the introduction of 2009 nH1N1, an EUA allows for therapy for all ages (Centers for Disease Control and Prevention, 2009).

Zanamivir

Chemistry and Antiviral Activity. Zanamivir (Figure 58–4) is a sialic acid analog that potently and specifically inhibits the neuraminidases of influenza A and B viruses.

Depending on the strain, zanamivir competitively inhibits influenza neuraminidase activity at concentrations of ~0.2-3 ng/mL but affects neuraminidases from other pathogens and mammalian sources only at 106-fold higher concentrations. Zanamivir inhibits *in vitro* replication of influenza A and B viruses, including amantadine- and rimantadine-resistant strains and several oseltamivir-resistant variants. It is active after topical administration in animal influenza models.

Mechanisms of Action and Resistance. Like oseltamivir, zanamivir inhibits viral neuraminidase and thus causes viral aggregation at the cell surface and reduced spread of virus within the respiratory tract (Eiland and Eiland, 2007).

In vitro selection of viruses resistant to zanamivir is associated with mutations in the viral hemagglutinin and/or neuraminidase. Hemagglutinin variants generally have mutations in or near the receptor binding site that make them less dependent on neuraminidase action for release from cells *in vitro,* although they typically retain susceptibility *in vivo*. Hemagglutinin variants are cross-resistant to other neuraminidase inhibitors. Neuraminidase variants contain mutations in the enzyme active site that diminish binding of zanamivir, but the altered enzymes show reduced activity or stability. Zanamivir-resistant variants usually have decreased infectivity in animals. Resistance has not been documented in immunocompetent hosts to date but has been seen rarely in highly immunocompromised patients (Eiland and Eiland, 2007).

Absorption, Distribution, and Elimination. The oral bioavailability of zanamivir is low (<5%) (Table 58–3), and the commercial form is delivered by oral inhalation of dry powder in a lactose carrier. The proprietary inhaler device is breath-actuated and requires a cooperative patient. Following inhalation of the dry powder, ~15% is deposited in the lower respiratory tract and ~80% in the oropharynx. Overall bioavailability is 4-17%, and plasma levels after 10-mg inhaled doses average ~35-100 ng/mL in adults and children. Median zanamivir concentrations in induced sputum samples are 1336 ng/mL at 6 hours and 47 ng/mL at 24 hours after a single 10-mg dose in healthy volunteers. The plasma $t_{1/2}$ of zanamivir averages 2.5-5 hours after oral inhalation but only 1.7 hours following intravenous dosing. Over 90% is eliminated in the urine as the parent compound (Eiland and Eiland, 2007).

Untoward Effects. Orally inhaled zanamivir generally is well tolerated in ambulatory adults and children with influenza. Wheezing and bronchospasm have been reported in some influenza-infected patients without known airway disease, and acute deteriorations in lung function, including fatal outcomes, have occurred in those with underlying asthma or chronic obstructive airway disease. Tolerability in more serious bronchopulmonary disorders or in intubated patients is uncertain. Zanamivir is not generally recommended for treatment of patients with underlying airway disease (e.g., asthma or chronic obstructive pulmonary disease) because of the risk of serious adverse events.

Preclinical studies of zanamivir revealed no evidence of mutagenic, teratogenic, or oncogenic effects (pregnancy Category C). No clinically significant drug interactions have been recognized to date. Zanamivir does not diminish the immune response to injected influenza vaccine.

Therapeutic Uses. Inhaled zanamivir is effective for the prevention and treatment of influenza A and B virus infections.

Early zanamivir treatment (10 mg [two inhalations] twice daily for 5 days) of febrile influenza in ambulatory adults and children ≥5 years of age shortens the time to illness resolution by 1-3 days (Eiland and Eiland, 2007) and in adults reduces by 40% the risk of lower respiratory tract complications leading to antibiotic use (Kaiser et al., 2000). Once-daily inhaled, but not intranasal, zanamivir is highly protective against community-acquired influenza illness, and when given for 10 days, it protects against household transmission (Eiland and Eiland, 2007). Intravenous zanamivir is protective against experimental human influenza and is being evaluated for the 2009 nH1N1 EUA.

ANTI-HEPATITIS VIRUS AGENTS

A number of agents are available for treatment of hepatitis B virus (HBV) and hepatitis C virus (HCV) infections. Several agents (e.g., interferons, ribavirin, and the nucleoside/nucleotide analogs lamivudine, telbivudine, and tenofovir) have other uses as well (Chapters 59 and 65). Therapeutic strategies for these two chronic viral infections, hepatitis B and C, are very different and are described separately.

Drugs Used Mainly for Hepatitis C Virus Infection

Hepatitis C is one of the most common chronic virus infections in the developed world and is associated with significant morbidity and mortality. Untreated, this virus can cause progressive hepatocellular injury with fibrosis and eventual cirrhosis. Chronic HCV is also a major risk factor for hepatocellular carcinoma.

Although the virus is quite prolific, producing several billion new particles every few days in an infected individual, this RNA virus does not integrate into chromosomal DNA, and it does not establish latency per se. Therefore the infection is, in theory, curable in all affected individuals. The current standard of care for treatment is a combination of peginterferon alfa and ribavirin, which produces a high cure rate in selected virus genotypes only (McHutchison et al., 2009). Recent advent of highly effective oral agents that are pharmacologically selective for this pathogen, including HCV protease inhibitors and polymerase inhibitors, bring hope for curative combinations of oral agents. It is likely that treatment recommendations for this infection will change radically in the coming decade.

Interferons

Classification and Antiviral Activity. Interferons (IFNs) are potent cytokines that possess antiviral, immunomodulatory, and antiproliferative activities (Biron, 2001; Samuel, 2001) (Chapter 35). These proteins are synthesized by host cells in response to various inducers and, in turn, cause biochemical changes leading to an antiviral state in cells. Three major classes of human interferons with significant antiviral activity currently are recognized: α (>18 individual species), β, and γ. Clinically used recombinant α-IFNs (Table 58–2) are non-glycosylated proteins of ~19,500 Da, the pegylated forms predominating in the U.S. market.

IFN-α and IFN-β may be produced by nearly all cells in response to viral infection and a variety of other stimuli, including double-stranded RNA and certain cytokines (e.g., interleukin 1, interleukin 2, and tumor necrosis factor). IFN-γ production is restricted to T-lymphocytes and natural killer cells responding to antigenic stimuli, mitogens, and specific cytokines. IFN-α and IFN-β exhibit antiviral and antiproliferative actions; stimulate the cytotoxic activity of lymphocytes, natural killer cells, and macrophages; and upregulate class I major histocompatibility (MHC) antigens and other surface markers. IFN-γ has less antiviral activity but more potent immunoregulatory effects, particularly macrophage activation, expression of class II MHC antigens, and mediation of local inflammatory responses. In addition, interferons downregulate production of a number of cellular proteins, which may be an equally important mediator of the pharmacological benefit of these agents.

Most animal viruses are inhibited by IFNs, although many DNA viruses are relatively insensitive. Considerable differences in sensitivity to the effects of IFNs exist among different viruses and assay systems. The biological activity of IFN usually is measured in terms of antiviral effects in cell culture and generally is expressed as international units (IU) relative to reference standards.

Mechanisms of Action. Following binding to specific cellular receptors, IFNs activate the JAK-STAT signal-transduction pathway and lead to the nuclear translocation of a cellular protein complex that binds to genes

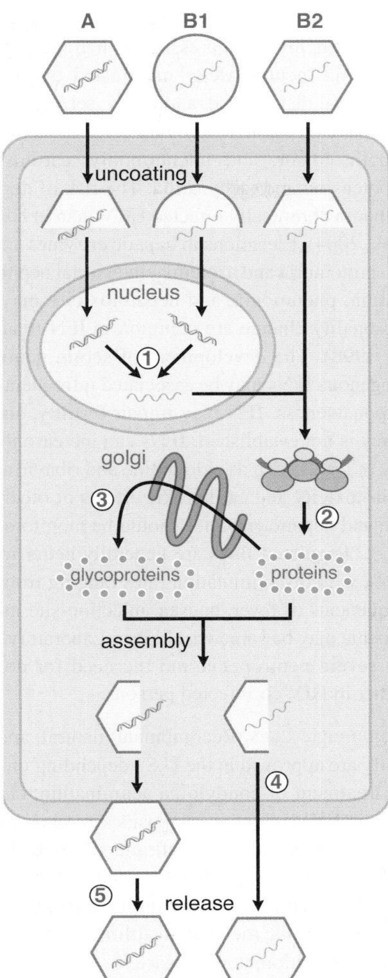

Viruses

A. DNA
B. RNA
1. orthomyxoviruses and retroviruses
2. picornaviruses and most RNA viruses

IFN Effects

① **inhibition of transcription**
activates Mx protein
blocks mRNA synthesis

② **inhibition of translation**
activates methylase, thereby reducing mRNA cap methylation

activates 2′5′ oligoadenylate synthetase ⟶ 2′5′A ⟶ inhibits mRNA splicing and activates RNaseL ⟶ cleaves viral RNA

activates protein kinase P1 ⟶ blocks eIL-2a function ⟶ inhibits initiation of mRNA translation

activates phosphodiesterase ⟶ blocks tRNA function

③ **inhibition of post-translational processing**
inhibits glycosyltransferase, thereby reducing protein glycosylation

④ **inhibition of virus maturation**
inhibits glycosyltransferase, thereby reducing glycoprotein maturation

⑤ **inhibition of virus release**
causes membrane changes ⟶ blocks budding

Figure 58–5. *Interferon-Mediated Antiviral Activity Occurs via Multiple Mechanisms.* The binding of IFN to specific cell surface receptor molecules signals the cell to produce a series of antiviral proteins. The stages of viral replication that are inhibited by various IFN-induced antiviral proteins are shown. Most of these act to inhibit the translation of viral proteins (mechanism 2), but other steps in viral replication also are affected (mechanisms 1, 3, and 4). The roles of these mechanisms in the other actions of IFNs are under study. Key: IFN = interferon; mRNA = messenger RNA; Mx = IFN-induced cellular protein with anti-viral activity; tRNA = transfer RNA; RNase L = latent cellular endoribonuclease; 2′5′A = 2′-5′-oligoadenylates; eIF-2α = protein synthesis initiation factor. (Modified from Baron et al., 1992, with permission.)

containing an IFN-specific response element. This, in turn, leads to synthesis of over two dozen proteins that contribute to viral resistance mediated at different stages of viral penetration (Samuel, 2001) (Figure 58–5).

Inhibition of protein synthesis is the major inhibitory effect for many viruses. IFN-induced proteins include 2′-5′-oligoadenylate [2-5(A)] synthetase and a protein kinase, either of which can inhibit protein synthesis in the presence of double-stranded RNA. The 2-5(A) synthetase produces adenylate oligomers that activate a latent cellular endoribonuclease (RNase L) to cleave both cellular and viral single-stranded RNAs. The protein kinase selectively phosphorylates and inactivates a protein involved in protein synthesis, eukaryotic initiation factor 2 (eIF-2). IFN-induced protein kinase also may be an important effector of apoptosis. In addition, IFN induces a phosphodiesterase that cleaves a portion of transfer RNA and thus prevents peptide elongation. A given virus may be inhibited at several steps, and the principal inhibitory effect differs among virus families. Certain viruses are able to counter IFN effects by blocking production or activity of selected IFN-inducible proteins. For example, IFN resistance in hepatitis C virus is attributable to inhibition of the IFN-induced protein kinase, among other mechanisms.

Complex interactions exist between IFNs and other parts of the immune system, so IFNs may ameliorate viral infections by exerting direct antiviral effects and/or by modifying the immune response to infection (Biron, 2001). For example, IFN-induced expression of MHC antigens may contribute to the antiviral actions of IFN by enhancing the lytic effects of cytotoxic T-lymphocytes. Conversely, IFNs may mediate some of the systemic symptoms associated with viral infections and contribute to immunologically mediated tissue damage in certain viral diseases.

Absorption, Distribution, and Elimination. Oral administration does not result in detectable IFN levels in serum or increases in 2-5(A) synthetase activity in peripheral blood mononuclear cells (used as a marker of IFN's biologic activity). After intramuscular or subcutaneous injection of IFN-α, absorption exceeds 80%. Plasma levels are dose related, peaking at 4-8 hours and returning to baseline by 18-36 hours. Levels of 2-5(A) synthetase in peripheral blood mononuclear cells show increases beginning at 6 hours and lasting through 4 days after a single injection. An antiviral state in peripheral blood mononuclear cells peaks at 24 hours and decreases slowly to baseline by 6 days after injection. Intramuscular or subcutaneous injections of IFN-β result in negligible plasma levels, although increases in 2-5(A) synthetase levels may occur. After systemic administration, low levels of IFN are detected in respiratory secretions, CSF, eye, and brain.

Because IFNs induce long-lasting cellular effects, their activities are not easily predictable from usual pharmacokinetic measures. After intravenous dosing, clearance of IFN from plasma occurs in a complex manner (Bocci, 1992). With subcutaneous or intramuscular dosing, the plasma $t_{1/2}$ of IFN-α ranges is variable, 3-8 hours. Elimination from the blood relates to distribution to the tissues, cellular uptake, and catabolism primarily in the kidney and liver. Negligible amounts are excreted in the urine. Clearance of IFN-α2B is reduced by ~80% in hemodialysis patients (Uchiharaa et al., 1998).

Attachment of IFN proteins to large inert polyethylene glycol (PEG) molecules (pegylation) slows absorption, decreases clearance, and provides higher and more prolonged serum concentrations that enable once-weekly dosing (Bruno et al., 2004). Two pegylated IFNs are available commercially: peginterferon alfa-2a (PEGASYS) and peginterferon alfa-2B (PEGINTRON). PegIFN alfa-2B has a straight-chain 12,000-Da type of PEG that increases the plasma $t_{1/2}$ from ~2-3 hours to ~30-54 hours (Glue et al., 2000). PegIFN alfa-2a consists of an ester derivative of a branched-chain 40,000-Da PEG bonded to IFN-α2A and has a plasma $t_{1/2}$ averaging ~80-90 hours. PegIFN alfa-2A is more stable and dispensed in solution, whereas pegIFN alfa-2B requires reconstitution prior to use. For pegIFN alfa-2A, peak serum concentrations occur up to 120 hours after dosing and remain detectable throughout the weekly dosing interval (Bruno et al., 2004); steady-state levels occur 5-8 weeks after initiation of weekly dosing (Keating and Curran, 2003). For pegIFN alfa-2A, dose-related maximum plasma concentrations occur at 15-44 hours after dosing and decline by 96-168 hours. These differences in pharmacokinetics may be associated with differences in antiviral effects (Bruno et al., 2004). Increasing PEG size is associated with longer $t_{1/2}$ and less renal clearance. About 30% of pegIFN alfa-2B is cleared by the kidneys; pegIFN alfa-2A also is cleared primarily by the liver. Dose reductions in both pegylated IFNs are indicated in end-stage renal disease.

Untoward Effects. Injection of recombinant IFN doses of ≥1 to 2 million units (MU) usually is associated with an acute influenza-like syndrome beginning several hours after injection. Symptoms include fever, chills, headache, myalgia, arthralgia, nausea, vomiting, and diarrhea. Fever usually resolves within 12 hours. Tolerance develops gradually in most patients. Febrile responses can be moderated by pretreatment with antipyretics. Up to one-half of patients receiving intralesional therapy for genital warts experience the influenzal illness initially, as well as discomfort at the injection site, and leukopenia.

The principal dose-limiting toxicities of systemic IFN are depression, myelosuppression with granulocytopenia and thrombocytopenia; neurotoxicity manifested by somnolence, confusion, behavioral disturbance, and rarely, seizures; debilitating neurasthenia and depression; autoimmune disorders including thyroiditis and hypothroidism; and uncommonly, cardiovascular effects with hypotension and tachycardia. The risk of depression appears to be higher in chronically infected HCV than in HBV patients (Marcellin et al., 2004). Elevations in hepatic enzymes and triglycerides, alopecia, proteinuria and azotemia, interstitial nephritis, autoantibody formation, pneumonia, and hepatotoxicity may occur. Alopecia and personality change are common in IFN-treated children (Sokal et al., 1998). The development of serum neutralizing antibodies to exogenous IFNs may be associated infrequently with loss of clinical responsiveness. IFN may impair fertility, and safety during pregnancy is not established. IFNs can increase the hematological toxicity of drugs such as zidovudine and ribavirin and may increase the neurotoxicity and cardiotoxic effects of other drugs. Thyroid function and hepatic enzymes should be monitored during IFN therapy.

Pegylated IFNs are generally better tolerated than standard IFNs, with discontinuation rates ranging from 2-11%, although the frequencies of fever, nausea, injection-site inflammation, and neutropenia may be somewhat higher. Laboratory abnormalities, including severe neutropenia and the need for dose modifications, are higher in HIV-co-infected persons.

Therapeutic Uses. Recombinant, natural, and pegylated IFNs currently are approved in the U.S., depending on the specific IFN type, for treatment of condyloma acuminatum, chronic HCV infection, chronic HBV infection, Kaposi's sarcoma in HIV-infected patients, other malignancies, and multiple sclerosis. In addition, interferons have been granted orphan drug status for a variety of rare disease states including idiopathic pulmonary fibrosis, laryngeal papillomatosis, juvenile rheumatoid arthritis, and infections associated with chronic granulomatous disease.

Hepatitis B Virus. In patients with chronic HBV infection, parenteral administration of various IFNs is associated with loss of HBV DNA, loss of HBeAg and development of anti-HBe antibody, and biochemical and histological improvement in ~25-50% of the patients.

Lasting responses require moderately high IFN doses and prolonged administration (typically 5 MU/day or 10 MU in adults and 6 MU/m^2 in children three times per week of IFNα-2B for 4 to 6 weeks) (Sokal et al., 1998). Plasma HBV DNA and polymerase activity decline promptly in most patients, but complete disappearance is sustained in only about one-third of patients or less. Low pretherapy serum HBV DNA levels and high aminotransferase levels are predictors of response. Sustained responses are infrequent in those with vertically acquired infection, anti-HBe positivity, or concurrent immunosuppression owing to HIV. PegIFN alfa-2A appears superior to conventional IFN alfa-2A in HbeAg-positive patients (Cooksley et al., 2003), and treatment (180 μg once weekly for 24-48 weeks) is associated with normalization of aminotransferases in ~60% and sustained viral suppression in ~20% of HBeAg-negative patients (Marcellin et al., 2004). Responses with seroconversion to anti-HBe usually are associated with aminotransferase elevations and often a hepatitis-like illness during the second or third month of therapy, likely related to immune clearance of infected hepatocytes. High-dose

IFN can cause myelosuppression and clinical deterioration in those with decompensated liver disease.

Remissions in chronic hepatitis B induced by IFN are sustained in >80% of patients treated and frequently are followed by loss of HBV surface antigen (HbsAg), histological improvement or stabilization, and reduced risk of liver-related complications and mortality (Lau et al., 1997). IFN may benefit some patients with nephrotic syndrome and glomerulonephritis owing to chronic HBV infection. Antiviral effects and improvements occur in about one-half of chronic hepatitis D virus (HDV) infections, but relapse is common unless HbsAg disappears. IFN does not appear to be beneficial in acute HBV or HDV infections.

Hepatitis C Virus. In chronic HCV infection, IFN alfa-2B monotherapy (3 MU three times a week) is associated with an approximate 50-70% rate of aminotransferase normalization and loss of plasma viral RNA, but relapse rates are high, and sustained virologic remission (absence of detectable HCV RNA) is observed in only 10-25% of patients.

Sustained viral responses are associated with long-term histological improvement and probably reduced risk of hepatocellular carcinoma and hepatic failure (Coverdale et al., 2004). Viral genotype and pretreatment RNA level influence response to treatment, but early viral clearance is the best predictor of sustained response. Failure to achieve an early viral response (nondetectable HCV RNA or reduction ≥2 $\log_{10}$ units compared with baseline at 12 weeks) predicts lack of sustained viral response with continued treatment (Seeff and Hoofnagle, 2002). Nonresponders generally do not benefit from IFN monotherapy retreatment, but they and patients relapsing after monotherapy often respond to combined pegylated IFN and ribavirin treatment. IFN treatment may benefit HCV-associated cryoglobulinemia and glomerulonephritis. IFN administration during acute HCV infection appears to reduce the risk of chronicity (Alberti et al., 2002).

Pegylated IFNs are superior to conventional thrice-weekly IFN monotherapy in inducing sustained remissions in treatment-naive patients. Monotherapy with pegIFN alfa-2A (180 μg subcutaneously weekly for 48 weeks) or pegIFN alfa-2B (weight-adjusted doses of 1.5 μg/kg/week for 1 year) is associated with sustained response in 30-39%, including stable cirrhotic patients (Heathcote et al., 2000), and it is a treatment option in patients unable to take ribavirin. Studies of prolonged (4 years) maintenance monotherapy with pegylated IFNs are in progress for those not responding to IFN-ribavirin combinations. A large randomized comparison of pegIFN alfa-2A versus alfa-2B combined with ribavirin found no difference in response rates (McHutchison et al., 2009).

The efficacy of conventional and pegylated IFNs is enhanced by the addition of ribavirin to the treatment regimens, particularly for genotype 1 infections. Combined therapy with pegIFN alfa-2A (180 μg once weekly for 48 weeks) and ribavirin (1000-1200 mg/day in divided doses) gives higher sustained viral response rates than IFN-ribavirin combinations in previously untreated patients (Fried et al., 2002). A shorter duration of therapy (24 weeks) and lower ribavirin dose (800 mg/day) are effective in genotype 2 and 3 infections, but prolonged therapy and higher ribavirin doses are needed for genotype 1 and 4 infections (Hadziyannis et al., 2004). Approximately 15-20% of those failing to respond to combined IFN-ribavirin will have sustained responses to combined pegIFN-ribavirin. Histological improvement may occur in patients who do not achieve sustained viral responses. In patients with compensated cirrhosis, treatment may reverse cirrhotic changes and possibly reduce the risk of hepatocellular carcinoma (Poynard et al., 2002).

Papillomavirus. In refractory condylomata acuminata (genital warts), intralesional injection of various natural and recombinant IFNs is associated with complete clearance of injected warts in 36-62% of patients, but other treatments are preferred (Wiley et al., 2002). Relapse occurs in 20-30% of patients. Verruca vulgaris may respond to intralesional IFN-α. Intramuscular or subcutaneous administration is associated with some regression in wart size but greater toxicity. Systemic IFN may provide adjunctive benefit in recurrent juvenile laryngeal papillomatosis and in treating laryngeal disease in older patients.

Other Viruses. IFNs have been shown to have virological and clinical effects in various herpesvirus infections including genital HSV infections, localized herpes-zoster infection of cancer patients or of older adults, and CMV infections of renal transplant patients. However, IFN generally is associated with more side effects and inferior clinical benefits compared with conventional antiviral therapies. Topically applied IFN and trifluridine combinations appear active in acyclovir-resistant mucocutaneous HSV infections.

In HIV-infected persons, IFNs have been associated with antiretroviral effects. In advanced infection, however, the combination of zidovudine and IFN is associated with only transient benefit and excessive hematological toxicity. IFN-α (3 MU three times weekly) is effective for treatment of HIV-related thrombocytopenia resistant to zidovudine therapy.

Except for adenovirus, IFN has broad-spectrum antiviral activity against respiratory viruses *in vitro*. However, prophylactic intranasal IFN-α is protective only against rhinovirus colds, and chronic use is limited by the occurrence of nasal side effects. Intranasal IFN is therapeutically ineffective in established rhinovirus colds. Systemically administered IFN-α may be beneficial in early treatment of SARS (Loutfy et al., 2003).

Ribavirin

Chemistry and Antiviral Activity. Ribavirin is a purine nucleoside analog with a modified base and D-ribose sugar (Figure 58–6).

Ribavirin inhibits the replication of a wide range of RNA and DNA viruses, including orthomyxo-, paramyxo-, arena-, bunya-, and flaviviruses *in vitro*. *In vitro* inhibitory concentrations range from 3 to 10 μg/mL for influenza viruses, parainfluenza viruses, and respiratory syncytial viruses (RSV). Similar concentrations may reversibly inhibit macromolecular synthesis and proliferation of uninfected cells, suppress lymphocyte responses, and alter cytokine profiles *in vitro*.

Mechanisms of Action and Resistance. The antiviral mechanism of ribavirin is incompletely understood but relates to alteration of cellular nucleotide pools and inhibition of viral messenger RNA synthesis (Tam et al., 2002).

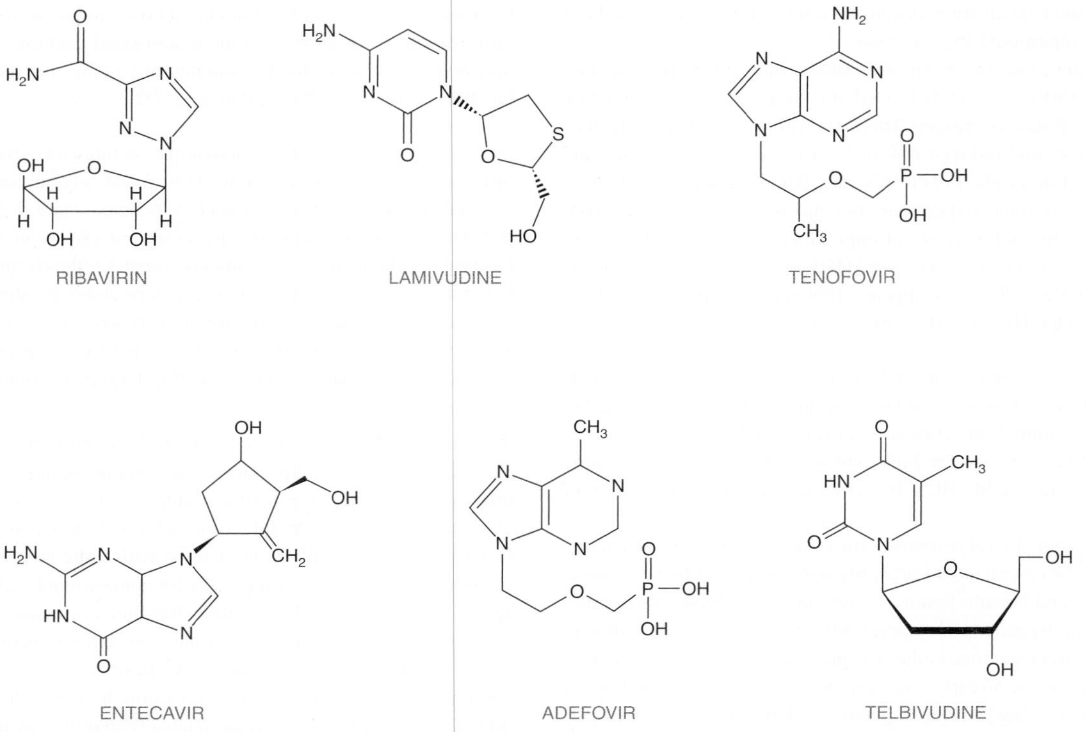

RIBAVIRIN

LAMIVUDINE

TENOFOVIR

ENTECAVIR

ADEFOVIR

TELBIVUDINE

Figure 58–6. *Chemical Structures of the Anti-Hepatitis Drugs.*

Intracellular phosphorylation to the mono-, di-, and triphosphate derivatives is mediated by host cell enzymes. In both uninfected and RSV-infected cells, the predominant derivative (>80%) is the triphosphate, which has an intracellular $t_{1/2}$ <2 hours.

Ribavirin monophosphate competitively inhibits cellular inosine-5′-phosphate dehydrogenase and interferes with the synthesis of GTP and thus nucleic acid synthesis in general. Ribavirin triphosphate also competitively inhibits the GTP-dependent 5′ capping of viral messenger RNA and specifically influenza virus transcriptase activity. Ribavirin appears to have multiple sites of action, and some of these (e.g., inhibition of GTP synthesis) may potentiate others (e.g., inhibition of GTP-dependent enzymes). Ribavirin also may enhance viral mutagenesis to an extent that some viruses may be inhibited from effective replication, so-called lethal mutagenesis (Hong and Cameron, 2002).

Emergence of viral resistance to ribavirin has not been documented in most viruses but has been reported in Sindbis and HCV (Young et al., 2003); it has been possible to select cells that do not phosphorylate ribavirin to its active forms.

Absorption, Distribution, and Elimination. Ribavirin is actively taken up by nucleoside transporters in the proximal small bowel; oral bioavailability averages ~50% (Glue, 1999). Extensive accumulation occurs in plasma, and steady state is reached by ~4 weeks. Food increases plasma levels substantially (Glue, 1999). Following single or multiple oral doses of 600 mg, peak plasma concentrations average ~0.8 and 3.7 μg/mL, respectively. After intravenous doses of 1000 and 500 mg, plasma concentrations average ~24 and 17 μg/mL, respectively. With aerosol administration, plasma levels increase with the duration of exposure and range from 0.2 to 1.0 μg/mL after 5 days (Englund et al., 1990). Levels in respiratory secretions are much higher but vary up to 1000-fold.

The apparent volume of distribution for ribavirin is large (~10 L/kg) owing to its cellular uptake. Plasma protein binding is negligible. The elimination of ribavirin is complex. The plasma $t_{1/2}$ increases to ~200-300 hours at steady state. Erythrocytes concentrate ribavirin triphosphate; the drug exits red cells gradually, with a $t_{1/2}$ of ~40 days. Hepatic metabolism and renal excretion of ribavirin and its metabolites are the principal routes of elimination. Hepatic metabolism involves deribosylation and hydrolysis to yield a triazole carboxamide. Ribavirin clearance decreases by two-thirds in those with advanced renal insufficiency (Cl_{cr} = 10-30 mL/minute); the drug should be used cautiously in patients with creatinine clearances of <50 mL/minute (Glue, 1999).

Untoward Effects. Aerosolized ribavirin may cause conjunctival irritation, rash, transient wheezing, and occasional reversible deterioration in pulmonary function. When used in conjunction with mechanical ventilation, equipment modifications and frequent monitoring are required to prevent plugging of ventilator valves and tubing with ribavirin. Techniques to reduce environmental exposure of healthcare workers are recommended.

Systemic ribavirin causes dose-related reversible anemia owing to extravascular hemolysis and suppression of bone marrow. Associated increases occur in reticulocyte counts and in serum bilirubin, iron, and uric acid concentrations. High ribavirin triphosphate levels may cause oxidative damage to membranes, leading to erythrophagocytosis by the reticuloendothelial system. About 20% of chronic HCV infection patients receiving combination IFN-ribavirin therapy discontinue treatment early because of side effects. In addition to IFN toxicities, oral ribavirin increases the risk of fatigue, cough, rash, pruritus, nausea, insomnia, dyspnea, depression, and particularly, anemia. Preclinical studies indicate that ribavirin is teratogenic, embryotoxic, oncogenic, and possibly gonadotoxic. To prevent possible teratogenic effects, up to 6 months is required for washout following cessation of long-term treatment (Glue, 1999). Bolus intravenous infusion may cause rigors.

Pregnant women should not directly care for patients receiving ribavirin aerosol (FDA pregnancy Category X).

Ribavirin inhibits the phosphorylation and antiviral activity of pyrimidine nucleoside HIV reverse-transcriptase inhibitors such as zidovudine and stavudine but increases the activity of purine nucleoside reverse-transcriptase inhibitors (e.g., didanosine) *in vitro*. It appears to increase the risk of mitochondrial toxicity from didanosine (Chapter 59).

Therapeutic Uses. Oral ribavirin in combination with injected pegIFN alfa-2A or -2B has become standard treatment for chronic HCV infection (Reddy et al., 2009; Seeff and Hoofnagle, 2002).

Ribavirin monotherapy for 6-12 months reversibly decreases aminotransferase elevations to normal in ~30% of patients but does not affect HCV RNA levels. Combination therapy with pegIFN alfa-2A and oral ribavirin (500 mg, or 600 mg if weight is >75 kg, twice daily for 24-48 weeks) increases the likelihood of sustained biochemical and virologic responses to ~56% depending on genotype (Fried et al., 2002). The combination is superior to IFN or pegIFN monotherapy and combinations of pegIFN alfa-2 and ribavirin in both treatment-naive patients and those not responding to, or relapsing after, IFN monotherapy. A longer duration of therapy (48 weeks) appears necessary in those with genotype 1 infections, whereas 24 weeks' therapy is adequate in genotype 2 and 3 infections (Hadziyannis et al., 2004). Combined ribavirin and pegIFN alfa-2A or -2B is effective in achieving sustained viral responses in a minority of HCV/HIV co-infected patients (Reddy et al., 2009). Combined therapy has been used in the management of recurrent HCV infection after liver transplantation.

Ribavirin aerosol is approved in the U.S. for treatment of RSV bronchiolitis and pneumonia in hospitalized children. Aerosolized ribavirin (usual dose of 20 mg/mL as the starting solution in the drug reservoir of the small particle aerosol generator unit for 18 hours' exposure per day for 3-7 days) may reduce some illness measures, but its use generally is not recommended (Committee on Infectious Diseases, American Academy of Pediatrics, 2003). No consistent beneficial effects on duration of hospitalization, ventilatory support, mortality, or long-term pulmonary function have been found. High-dose, reduced-duration therapy (60 mg/mL in the drug reservoir of the small particle aerosol generator unit for 2 hours three times daily) has been used. Aerosol ribavirin combined with intravenous immunoglobulin appears to reduce mortality of RSV infection in bone marrow transplant and other highly immunocompromised patients (Ghosh et al., 2000).

Intravenous and/or aerosol ribavirin has been used occasionally in treating severe influenza virus infection and in the treatment of immunosuppressed patients with adenovirus, vaccinia, parainfluenza, or measles virus infections. Aerosolized ribavirin is associated with reduced duration of fever but no other clinical or antiviral effects in influenza infections in hospitalized children. Intravenous ribavirin decreases mortality in Lassa fever and has been used in treating other arenavirus-related hemorrhagic fevers. Intravenous ribavirin is beneficial in hemorrhagic fever with renal syndrome owing to Hantavirus infection but appears ineffective in hantavirus-associated cardiopulmonary syndrome or SARS. Oral ribavirin has been used for the treatment and prevention of Crimean-Congo hemorrhagic fever and treatment of Nipah virus infections (Mardani et al., 2003). Intravenous ribavirin is investigational in the U.S.

Drugs for Hepatitis B Virus Infection

Unlike hepatitis C virus, hepatitis B virus is transcribed into DNA that can be integrated into host chromosomal DNA and is capable of establishing lifelong chronic infection in ~10% of patients. Those with chronic HBV may develop active hepatitis that can lead to fibrosis and cirrhosis, but all such individuals have a greatly increased incidence of hepatocellular carcinoma.

Interferon, or a combination of interferon and ribavirin, can cure patients with chronic infection but is associated with a high rate of side effects, often leading to premature treatment discontinuation. Several antiretroviral nucleoside or nucleotide analog polymerase inhibitors, including lamivudine, telbivudine, and tenofovir, have potent anti-HBV activity and have provided a popular alternative therapy: chronic suppressive oral single agent or combination treatment. These regimens are much better tolerated than IFN-containing regimens but are not usually curative.

Adefovir

Chemistry and Antiviral Activity. Adefovir dipivoxil (9-[2-[bis[(pivaloyloxy)methoxy]phosphinyl]methoxyl]ethyl]adenine, bis-POM PMEA) is a diester prodrug of adefovir, an acyclic phosphonate nucleotide analog of adenosine monophosphate (Figure 58–6).

It is inhibitory *in vitro* against a range of DNA and RNA viruses, but its clinical use is limited to HBV infections (De Clercq, 2003). Inhibitory concentrations for HBV range from 0.2 to 1.2 μM in cell culture, and it is active against lamivudine-resistant HBV strains. Oral adefovir dipivoxil shows dose-dependent inhibition of hepadnavirus replication in animal models. *In vitro* combinations of adefovir and lamivudine or other anti-HBV nucleosides show enhanced antihepadnavirus activity *in vitro* (Delaney et al., 2004), and trials of dual therapy are in progress.

Mechanisms of Action and Resistance. Adefovir dipivoxil enters cells and is deesterified to adefovir. Adefovir is converted by cellular enzymes to the diphosphate, which acts as a competitive inhibitor of viral DNA polymerases and reverse transcriptases with respect to deoxyadenosine triphosphate and also serves as a chain terminator of viral DNA synthesis (Cundy, 1999). Its selectivity relates to a higher affinity for HBV DNA polymerase compared with cellular polymerases.

The intracellular $t_{1/2}$ of the diphosphate is prolonged, ranging from 5 to 18 hours, so once-daily dosing is feasible. Adefovir resistance has been detected in a small proportion (~4%) of chronically infected HBV patients during 3 years of treatment. Such variants have unique point mutations in the HBV polymerase but retain susceptibility to lamivudine. The consequences of the emergence of resistance remain to be determined.

Absorption, Distribution, and Elimination. The parent compound has low oral bioavailability (<12%), whereas the dipivoxil prodrug is absorbed rapidly and hydrolyzed by esterases in the intestine and blood to adefovir with liberation of pivalic acid, providing a bioavailability ~30-60%. After 10-mg doses of the pro-drug, peak serum concentrations of adefovir average 0.02 μg/mL, and the pro-drug is not detectable. Food does not affect bioavailability. Adefovir is scantily protein bound (<5%) and has a volume of distribution similar to body water (~0.4 L/kg).

Adefovir is eliminated unchanged by renal excretion through a combination of glomerular filtration and tubular secretion. After oral administration of adefovir dipivoxil, ~30-45% of the dose is recovered within 24 hours; the serum $t_{1/2}$ of elimination is 5-7.5 hours. Dose reductions are recommended for Cl_{Cr} values <50 mL/minute. Adefovir is removed by hemodialysis, but the effects of peritoneal dialysis or severe hepatic insufficiency on pharmacokinetics are unknown.

Pivalic acid is a product of adefovir dipivoxil metabolism that can cause reduced free carnitine levels. Although L-carnitine has been given in some investigational HIV studies of adefovir, supplementation generally is not recommended at the doses used in chronic HBV infection.

Untoward Effects. Adefovir dipivoxil causes dose-related nephrotoxicity and tubular dysfunction, manifested by azotemia and hypophosphatemia, acidosis, glycosuria, and proteinuria that usually are reversible months after discontinuation. The lower dose (10 mg/day) used in chronic HBV infection patients has been associated with few adverse events (*e.g.*, headache, abdominal discomfort, diarrhea, and asthenia) and negligible renal toxicity compared with a 3-fold higher dose (Hadziyannis et al., 2003; Marcellin et al., 2003). Adverse events lead to premature discontinuation in ~2% of patients. After 2 years of dosing, the risk of serum creatinine levels rising above 0.5 mg/dL is ~2% but is higher in those with preexisting renal insufficiency. Acute, sometimes severe exacerbations of hepatitis can occur in patients stopping adefovir or other anti-HBV therapies. Close monitoring is necessary, and resumption of antiviral therapy may be required in some patients.

No clinically important drug interactions have been recognized to date, although drugs that reduce renal function or compete for active tubular secretion could decrease adefovir clearance. Ibuprofen increases adefovir exposure modestly. An increased risk of lactic acidosis and steatosis may exist when adefovir is used in conjunction with nucleoside analogs or other antiretroviral agents. Adefovir is transported efficiently into tubular epithelium by a probenecid-sensitive organic anion transporter (hOAT1).

Adefovir is genotoxic, and high doses cause hepatotoxicity, lymphoid toxicity, and renal tubular nephropathy in animals. The diphosphate's inhibitory effects on renal adenylyl cyclase may contribute to nephrotoxicity. Adefovir dipivoxil is not associated with reproductive toxicity, although high intravenous doses of adefovir cause maternal and embryotoxicity with fetal malformations in rats (pregnancy Category C).

Therapeutic Uses. Adefovir dipivoxil is approved for treatment of chronic HBV infections.

In patients with HBV e-antigen (HbeAg)–positive chronic hepatitis B, adefovir dipivoxil (10 mg/day) reduces serum HBV DNA levels by 99% and, in about one-half of patients, improves hepatic histology and normalization of aminotransferase levels by 48 weeks (Marcellin et al., 2003). Continued therapy is associated with increasing frequencies of aminotransferase normalization and HbeAg seroconversion (De Clercq, 2003). In patients with HbeAg-negative chronic HBV, adefovir is associated with similar biochemical and histological benefits (Hadziyannis et al., 2003). Regression of cirrhosis may occur in some patients.

In patients with lamivudine-resistant HBV infections, adefovir dipivoxil monotherapy results in sustained reductions in serum HBV DNA levels, but lamivudine alone or added to adefovir is not beneficial (Peters et al., 2004). In patients with dual HIV and lamivudine-resistant HBV infections, adefovir dipivoxil (10 mg/day) causes significant HBV DNA level reductions (Benhamou et al., 2001), and it also has been used successfully in patients with lamivudine-resistant HBV infections both before and following liver transplantation. The optimal duration of treatment in different populations, possible long-term effects on HBV complications, and combined use with other anti-HBV agents are under study.

Entecavir

Chemistry and Antiviral Activity. Entecavir is a guanosine nucleoside analog with selective activity against HBV polymerase (Figure 58–6).

Mechanisms of Action and Resistance. Entecavir requires intracellular phosphorylation. Entecavir triphosphate competes with endogenous deoxyguanosine triphosphate and inhibits all three activities of the HBV polymerase (reverse transcriptase):

- base priming
- reverse transcription of the negative strand from the pregenomic messenger RNA
- synthesis of the positive strand of HBV DNA

Entecavir triphosphate is a weak inhibitor of cellular DNA polymerases α, β, and δ and mitochondrial DNA polymerase γ. The inhibitory concentration against HBV is 0.004 μM in transfected cells and ranges from 0.01 to 0.059 μM against lamivudine-resistant (L180M, M204V) HBV. Eight- to 30-fold reductions in entecavir susceptibility were observed for lamivudine-resistant strains in cell-based assays (Scott and Keating, 2009).

Entecavir selected for an M184I substitution in HIV reverse transcriptase at μM concentrations in cell culture, and HIV variants containing the M184V substitution showed loss of susceptibility to entecavir. In patients, entecavir decreased HIV-1 RNA in three persons with HIV-1 and HBV co-infection and led to HIV-1 variants with the M184V lamivudine-resistant mutation in one subject (McMahon et al., 2007). Lamivudine and telbivudine resistance confers decreased susceptibility to entecavir. In patients with preexisting lamivudine resistance, entecavir resistance emerged in 7% and 43% after 1 and 4 years, respectively (Dienstag, 2009).

Absorption, Distribution, and Elimination. Following multiple daily doses ranging from 0.1 to 1.0 mg, C_{max} and area under the concentration-time curve (AUC) at steady-state increased in proportion to dose. Time to peak occurs in 0.5-1.5 hours. Steady-state is reached after 6-10 days of once daily dosing. The tablet and oral solution can be used interchangeably. Administration with food decreases C_{max} by 44-46% and AUC by 18-20%; thus entecavir should be administered on an empty stomach.

Entecavir is extensively distributed in tissues and is 13% bound to serum proteins. It is primarily eliminated unchanged in the kidney. Renal clearance is independent of dose and ranges from 360 to 471 mL/minute, suggesting that entecavir undergoes both glomerular filtration and net tubular secretion. Entecavir exhibits biphasic elimination, with a terminal $t_{1/2}$ of 128-149 hours; the active triphosphate has an elimination $t_{1/2}$ of 15 hours. Dose reductions are needed for patients with Cl_{Cr} <50 mL/minute, typically by extension of the dosing interval (Scott and Keating, 2009).

Untoward Effects. Severe acute exacerbations of hepatitis B have been reported in patients who have discontinued anti-HBV therapy, including entecavir. Hepatic function should be monitored closely with both clinical and laboratory follow-up for at least several months in patients who discontinue anti-HBV therapy. There is a potential for development of resistance to nucleoside reverse transcriptase inhibitors in HBV/HIV co-infection especially if HIV is not being treated. Lactic acidosis and severe hepatomegaly with steatosis, including fatal cases, have been reported, mostly in women with some antiretroviral nucleoside analogs (Chapter 59), but not with entecavir. Other common adverse reactions include headache, fatigue, dizziness, and nausea (Scott and Keating, 2009).

Therapeutic Uses. Entecavir is indicated for the treatment of chronic HBV infection in adults with active viral replication and either evidence of persistent elevations in serum aminotransferases or histologically active disease.

The recommended dose for nucleoside-treatment-naive adults (>16 years of age) is 0.5 mg once daily. For patients with lamivudine or telbivudine resistance, the dose is 1 mg once daily. Entecavir is superior to lamivudine in the degree of suppression and associated with a more frequent fall of HBV DNA to undetectable levels (Dienstag, 2009). Durability of HBeAg responses is comparable to other oral agents. Entecavir had negligible resistance (≤1%) for up to 4 years and is active against adefovir-resistant HBV.

Lamivudine

Chemistry and Antiviral Activity. Lamivudine, the (–)-enantiomer of 2′,3′-dideoxy-3′-thiacytidine, is a nucleoside analog that inhibits HIV reverse transcriptase and HBV DNA polymerase (Figure 58–6). Its use as an antiretroviral agent is discussed in Chapter 59.

It inhibits HBV replication *in vitro* by 50% at concentrations of 4-7 ng/mL with negligible cellular cytotoxicity. Cellular enzymes convert lamivudine to the triphosphate, which competitively inhibits HBV DNA polymerase and causes chain termination.

Mechanisms of Action and Resistance. Lamivudine triphosphate is a potent inhibitor of the DNA polymerase/reverse transcriptase of HBV; the intracellular $t_{1/2}$ of the triphosphate averages 17-19 hours in HBV-infected cells, so once-daily dosing is possible.

Oral lamivudine is active in animal models of hepadnavirus infection. Lamivudine shows enhanced antiviral activity in combination with adefovir or penciclovir against hepadnaviruses. Point mutations in the *YMDD* motif of HBV DNA polymerase result in a 40- to 104-fold reduction in *in vitro* susceptibility (Ono et al., 2001). Lamivudine resistance confers cross-resistance to related agents such as emtricitabine and the investigational agent, clevudine, and is often associated with an additional non-*YMDD* mutation that confers cross-resistance to famciclovir. Lamivudine-resistant HBV retains susceptibility to adefovir, tenofovir, and partially to entecavir (Ono et al., 2001). Viruses bearing *YMDD* mutations are less replication competent *in vitro* than wild-type HBV. However, lamivudine resistance is associated with elevated HBV DNA levels, decreased likelihood of HbeAg loss or seroconversion, hepatitis exacerbations, and progressive fibrosis and graft loss in transplant recipients (Dienstag et al., 2003; Lai et al., 2002).

Absorption, Distribution, and Elimination. The pharmacokinetic properties of lamivudine are described in detail in Chapter 59. In HBV-infected children, doses of 3 mg/kg/day provide plasma exposure and trough plasma levels comparable with those in adults receiving 100 mg daily (Sokal et al., 2000). Dose reductions are indicated for moderate renal insufficiency (creatinine clearance <50 mL/minute). Trimethoprim decreases the renal clearance of lamivudine.

Untoward Effects. At the doses used for chronic HBV infection, lamivudine generally has been well tolerated. Aminotransferase rises after therapy occur more often in lamivudine recipients, and flares in post-treatment aminotransferase elevations (>500 IU/mL) occur in ~15% of patients after cessation.

Therapeutic Uses. Lamivudine is approved for the treatment of chronic HBV hepatitis in adults and children.

In adults, doses of 100 mg/day for 1 year cause suppression of HBV DNA levels, normalization of aminotransferase levels in

≥41% of patients, and reductions in hepatic inflammation in >50% of patients (Dienstag et al., 1999; Lai et al., 2002). Seroconversion with antibody to HbeAg occurs in <20% of recipients at 1 year. In children 2-17 years of age, lamivudine (3 mg/kg/day to a maximum of 100 mg/day for 1 year) is associated with normalization of aminotransferase levels in about one-half and seroconversion to anti-Hbe in about one-fifth of cases (Jonas et al., 2002). In those without emergence of resistant variants, prolonged therapy is associated with sustained suppression of HBV DNA, continued histological improvement, and an increased proportion of patients experiencing a virological response (loss of HbeAg and undetectable HBV DNA). Prolonged therapy is associated with an approximate halving of the risk of clinical progression and development of hepatocellular carcinoma in those with advanced fibrosis or cirrhosis (Liaw et al., 2004). However, the frequency of lamivudine-resistant variants increases progressively with continued drug administration, reaching 67% after 4 years of treatment (Liaw et al., 2004). The risk of resistance development is higher after transplantation and in HIV/HBV co-infected patients.

Combined use of IFN or pegIFN alfa-2A with lamivudine has not improved responses in HBeAg-positive patients consistently. The addition of lamivudine to pegINF alfa-2A for 1 year of therapy does not improve post-treatment response rates in HBeAg-negative patients (Marcellin et al., 2004). In HIV and HBV co-infections, higher lamivudine doses are associated with antiviral effects and uncommonly anti-HBe seroconversion. Administration of lamivudine before and after liver transplantation may suppress recurrent HBV infection.

Telbivudine

Chemistry and Antiviral Activity. Telbivudine (Figure 58–6) is a synthetic thymidine nucleoside analog with activity against HBV DNA polymerase.

Mechanisms of Action and Resistance. Telbivudine is phosphorylated by cellular kinases to the active triphosphate form, which has a $t_{1/2}$ of 14 hours. Telbivudine 5′-triphosphate inhibits HBV DNA polymerase (reverse transcriptase) by competing with the natural substrate, thymidine 5′-triphosphate. Incorporation of telbivudine 5′-triphosphate into viral DNA causes chain termination. Telbivudine 5′-triphosphate at concentrations up to 100 μM did not inhibit human cellular DNA polymerases α, β, or γ.

In cell-based assays, lamivudine-resistant HBV strains expressing either the M204I substitution or the L180M/M204V double substitution had ≥1000-fold reduced susceptibility. Telbivudine retained wild-type phenotypic activity against the lamivudine resistance–associated substitution M204V alone. HBV encoding the adefovir mutation A181V showed 3- to 5-fold reduced susceptibility, but N236T remained susceptible. The A181S and A181T substitutions conferred 2.7- and 3.5-fold reductions in susceptibility to telbivudine, respectively. The A181T substitution is associated with decreased clinical response in patients with HBV treated with adefovir and entecavir (Hadziyannis and Vassilopoulos, 2008).

In a cell culture model, the EC_{50} for inhibition of viral DNA synthesis by telbivudine was 0.2 μM. The anti-HBV activity of telbivudine is additive with that of adefovir in cell culture, and it is not antagonized by the HIV-1 nucleoside analogs didanosine and stavudine (Hadziyannis and Vassilopoulos, 2008).

Absorption, Distribution, and Elimination. At 600 mg once daily, steady-state peak concentrations are ~3.7 μg/mL at a median of 2 hours post-dose. Steady state is achieved after ~5-7 days of once-daily administration with ~1.5-fold accumulation. *In vitro* protein binding is low (3.3%) and telbivudine is widely distributed into tissues. Telbivudine concentrations decline biexponentially with an elimination $t_{1/2}$ of 40-49 hours. The drug is eliminated unchanged in the urine.. Patients with moderate-to-severe renal dysfunction and those undergoing hemodialysis require dose adjustments.

Untoward Effects. Telbivudine is generally well tolerated and safe. The most common adverse events resulting in telbivudine discontinuation included increased creatine kinase, nausea, diarrhea, fatigue, myalgia, and myopathy. Elevations of creatine kinase activity, mostly asymptomatic grade 3-4, were more common in telbivudine-treated patients after 2 years of therapy than with lamivudine.

Therapeutic Uses. Similar to other oral HBV agents, telbivudine is indicated for the treatment of chronic HBV in adult patients with evidence of viral replication and either evidence of persistent elevations in serum aminotransferases (ALT or AST) or histologically active disease.

The recommended dose is 600 mg orally once daily without regard to food. An oral solution is also available. This dose is based on pharmacodynamic analyses showing a relationship between telbivudine dose and changes in HBV DNA from baseline to week 4 (Lai et al., 2004). The dose producing the maximum effect was between 400 and 800 mg/day. The drug has not been studied in patients with HBV/HIV co-infection. Telbivudine resistance is substantial (25%) after 2 years of treatment and higher than observed with other oral anti-HBV agents (Dienstag, 2009; Hadziyannis and Vassilopoulos, 2008). Cross-resistance and treatment-emergent resistance have limited the use of telbivudine for patients with chronic HBV, compared to alternative agents.

Tenofovir

Tenofovir is a nucleotide analog with activity against both HIV-1 and HBV (Figure 58–6). It is administered orally as the disoproxil prodrug. *Chemistry, pharmacokinetic properties, untoward effects, precautions, and interactions* for this drug are covered in more detail in Chapter 59.

In *in vitro* cell cultures, the EC_{50} for tenofovir against HBV ranged from 0.14 to 1.5 μM, with cytotoxicity concentrations >100 μM. No antagonistic activity was observed when combined with other oral anti-HBV agents. In cell-based assays, mutant HBV (V173L, L180M, and M204I/V) associated with resistance to lamivudine and telbivudine showed a susceptibility to tenofovir of 0.7-3.4 times that of wild-type virus. Overall, tenofovir has a favorable resistance profile and has been effective in treating lamivudine-resistant HBV (Dienstag, 2009).

Therapeutic Uses. Tenofovir is approved for treatment of HBV infection in adults at a dose of 300 mg once daily without regard to food. In HBeAg-negative patients, tenofovir suppressed HBV DNA to <400 copies/mL in 93% of subjects at 48 weeks, compared to 63% for adefovir. Tenofovir resistance was not evident over 48 weeks of treatment. Due to the safety, efficacy, and resistance profile of tenofovir, it will likely supersede most adefovir use for the treatment of chronic HBV infection.

The tenofovir dose should be adjusted for impaired renal function: For Cl_{cr} of 30-49 mL/minute, 300 mg every 48 hours; 10-29 mL/minute, 300 mg every 72-96 hours. During hemodialysis the dose is 300 mg every 7 days or after 12 hours of dialysis.

Clevudine

Clevudine is a nucleoside analog with potent activity against HBV. The oral drug is approved for use in South Korea and the Philippines. However the drug caused myopathy in large Phase 3 clinical trials, casting doubt on its future approval in the U.S.

OTHER AGENTS

Imiquimod

Imiquimod [1-(2-methylpropyl)-1*H*-imidazo[4,5-*c*]quinolin-4 amine] is a novel immunomodulatory agent that is effective for topical treatment of condylomata acuminata, molluscum contagiosum, and certain other dermatologic conditions associated with DNA virus infections (Skinner, 2003). It lacks direct antiviral or antiproliferative effects *in vitro* but rather induces cytokines and chemokines with antiviral and immunomodulating effects.

Imiquimod shows antiviral activity in animal models after systemic or topical administration. When applied topically as a 5% cream to genital warts in humans, it induces local IFN-α, -β, and -γ and TNFα responses and causes reductions in viral load and wart size. When applied topically (three times weekly for up to 16 weeks), imiquimod cream is associated with complete clearance of treated genital and perianal warts in ~50% of patients, with response rates higher in women than in men (Skinner, 2003; Wiley et al., 2002). The median time to clearance is 8-10 weeks; relapses are not uncommon. Application is associated with local erythema in ~20% of patients, excoriation/flaking in 18-26%, itching in 10-20%, burning in 5-12%, and less often, erosions or ulcerations.

BIBLIOGRAPHY

Alberti A, Boccato S, Vario A, Benvegnu L. Therapy of acute hepatitis C. *Hepatology,* **2002**, *36:*S195–S200.

Bacon TH, Levin MJ, Leary JJ, *et al.* Herpes simplex virus resistance to acyclovir and penciclovir after two decades of antiviral therapy. *Clin Microbiol Rev,* **2003**, *16:*114–128.

Baron S, Coppenhaver DH, Dianzani F, *et al.* Introduction to the interferon system. In: *Interferons: Principles and Medical Applications.* (Baron S, Dianzani F, Stanton GJ, *et al.,* eds.), University of Texas Medical Branch Dept. of Microbiology, Galveston, TX, **1992**, pp. 1–15.

Benhamou Y, Bochet M, Thibault V, et al. Safety and efficacy of adefovir dipivoxil in patients co-infected with HIV-1 and lamivudine-resistant hepatitis B virus: An open-label pilot study. *Lancet,* **2001**, *358:*718–723.

Biron C. Interferons alpha and beta as immune regulators: A new look. *Immunity,* **2001**, *14:*661–664.

Bocci, V. Physiochemical and biologic properties of interferons and their potential uses in drug delivery systems. *Crit Rev Ther Drug Carrier Syst,* **1992,** *9:*91–133.

Boike S, Pue M, Audet P, *et al.* Pharmacokinetics of famciclovir in subjects with chronic hepatic disease. *J Clin Pharmacol,* **1994**, *34:*1199–1207.

Brosgart C, Louis T, Hillman D, *et al.* A randomized, placebo-controlled trial of the safety and efficacy of oral ganciclovir for prophylaxis of cytomegalovirus disease in HIV-infected individuals. Terry Beirn Community Programs for Clinical Research on AIDS. *AIDS,* **1998**, *12:*269–277.

Brown F, Banken L, Saywell K, Arum I. Pharmacokinetics of valganciclovir and ganciclovir following multiple oral dosages of valganciclovir in HIVand CMV-seropositive volunteers. *Clin Pharmacokinet,* **1999**, *37:*167–176.

Bruno R, Sacchi P, Ciappina V, et al. Viral dynamics and pharmacokinetics of peginterferon alpha-2a and peginterferon alpha-2b in naïve patients with chronic hepatitis C: A randomized, controlled study. *Antiviral Ther,* **2004**, *9:*491–497.

Centers for Disease Control and Prevention. Emergency use authorization of Tamiflu. Available from: http://www.cdc.gov/h1n1flu/eua/tamiflu.htm. Accessed January 4, **2010**.

Chilukuri S, Rosen T. Management of acyclovir-resistant herpes simplex virus. *Dermatol Clin,* **2003**, *21:*311–320.

Chrisp P, Clissold SP. Foscarnet: A review of its antiviral activity, pharmacokinetic properties and therapeutic use in immunocompromised patients with cytomegalovirus retinitis. *Drugs,* **1991**, *41:*104–129.

Colin J, Hoh H, Easty D, et al. Ganciclovir ophthalmic gel (Virgan: 0.15%) in the treatment of herpes simplex keratitis. *Cornea,* **1997**, *16:*393–399.

Committee on Infectious Diseases, American Academy of Pediatrics, *Red Book: 2003 Report of the Committee on Infectious Diseases.* American Academy of Pediatrics, Elk Grove Village, IL, **2003**.

Cooksley W, Piratvisuth T, Lee S, et al. Peginterferon alpha-2a (40 kDa): An advance in the treatment of hepatitis B e antigen–positive chronic hepatitis B. *J Viral Hepat,* **2003**, *10:*298–305.

Corey L, Wald A. Maternal and neonatal herpes simplex virus infections. *N Engl J Med,* **2009**, *361:*1376–1385.

Corey L, Wald A, Patel R, *et al.* Once-daily valacyclovir to reduce the risk of transmission of genital herpes. *N Engl J Med,* **2004**, *350:*11–20.

Coverdale S, Khan M, Byth K, et al. Effects of interferon treatment response on liver complications of chronic hepatitis C: 9-year followup study. *Am J Gastroenterol,* **2004**, *99:*636–644.

Cundy K. Clinical pharmacokinetics of the antiviral nucleotide analogues cidofovir and adefovir. *Clin Pharmacokinet,* **1999**, *36:*127–143.

Curran M, Noble S. Valganciclovir. *Drugs,* **2001**, *61:*1145–1150.

De Clercq E. Clinical potential of the acyclic nucleoside phosphonates cidofovir, adefovir, and tenofovir in treatment of DNA virus and retrovirus infections. *Clin Microbiol Rev*, **2003**, *16:*569–596.

Delaney W, Yang H, Miller M, et al. Combinations of adefovir with nucleoside analogs produce additive antiviral effects against hepatitis B virus *in vitro*. *Antimicrob Agents Chemother,* **2004**, *48:*3702–3710.

Dienstag JL. Benefits and risks of nucleoside analog therapy for hepatitis B. *Hepatology,* **2009**, *49:*S112–S121.

Dienstag J, Goldin R, Heathcote E, et al. Histological outcome during long-term lamivudine therapy. *Gastroenterology*, **2003**, *124:*105–117.

Dienstag J, Schiff E, Wright T, et al. Lamivudine as initial treatment for chronic hepatitis B in the United States. *N Engl J Med,* **1999**, *341:*1256–1263.

Eiland LS, Eiland EH. Zanamivir for the prevention of influenza in adults and children age 5 years and older. *Ther Clin Risk Manag,* **2007**, *3:*461–465.

Elion GB. History, mechanism of action, spectrum and selectivity of nucleoside analogs. In: *Antiviral Chemotherapy: New Directions for Clinical Application and Research* (Mills J, Corey L, eds.), Elsevier, New York, **1986**, pp. 118–137.

Elish D, Singh F, Weinberg JM. Therapeutic options for herpes labialis. II: Topical agents. *Cutis,* **2004**, *74:*35–40.

Fried M, Shiffman M, Reddy K, et al. Peginterferon alfa-2a plus ribavirin for chronic hepatitis C virus infection. *N Engl J Med,* **2002**, *347*:975–982.

Geary R, Henry S, Grillone L. Fomivirsen: Clinical pharmacology and potential drug interactions. *Clin Pharmacokinet*, **2002**, *41:*255–260.

Ghosh S, Champlin RI, Englund J, et al. Respiratory syncytial virus upper respiratory tract illnesses in adult blood and marrow transplant recipients: Combination therapy with aerosolized ribavirin and intravenous immunoglobulin. *Bone Marrow Transplant,* **2000**, *25:*751–755.

Gill KS, Wood MJ. The clinical pharmacokinetics of famciclovir. *Clin Pharmacokinet,* 1**996**, *31*:1–8.

Glue P. The clinical pharmacology of ribavirin. *Semin Liver Dis,* **1999**, *19*(suppl 1):17–24.

Glue P, Fang J, Rouzier-Panis R, et al. Pegylated interferon-alpha2b: Pharmacokinetics, pharmacodynamics, safety, and preliminary efficacy data. Hepatitis C Intervention Therapy Group. *Clin Pharmacol Ther,* **2000**, *68*:556–567.

Griffin S, Beales L, Clarke D, et al. The P7 protein of hepatitis C virus forms an ion channel that is blocked by the antiviral drug, amantadine. *FEBS Lett,* **2003**, *535:*34–38.

Hadziyannis SJ, Manesis EK, Papakonstantinou A. Oral ganciclovir treatment in chronic hepatitis B virus infection: A pilot study. *J Hepatol,* **1999**, *31*:210–214.

Hadziyannis S, Sette H, Morgan T, et al. Peginterferon-alpha2a and ribavirin combination therapy in chronic hepatitis C: A randomized study of treatment duration and ribavirin dose. *Ann Intern Med,* **2004**, *140:*346–355.

Hadziyannis S, Tassopoulos N, Heathcote E, et al. Adefovir dipivoxil for the treatment of hepatitis B e antigen–negative chronic hepatitis B. *N Engl J Med,* **2003**, *348:*800–807.

Hadziyannis SJ, Vassilopoulos D. Telbivudine in the treatment of chronic hepatitis B. *Expert Rev Gastroenterol Hepatol*, **2008**, *2:*13–22.

Hayden F. Perspectives on antiviral use during pandemic influenza. *Phil Trans Soc Lond,* **2001**, *356:*1877–1884.

Hayden F, Belshe R, Villanueva C, et al. Management of influenza in households: A prospective, randomized comparison of oseltamivir treatment with or without post-exposure prophylaxis. *J Infect Dis,* **2004**, *189:*440–449.

Heathcote J, Shiffman M, Cooksley G, et al. Peginterferon alfa-2a in patients with chronic hepatitis C and cirrhosis. *N Engl J Med,* **2000**, *343:*1673–1680.

Hitchcock M, Jaffe H, Martin J, Stagg R. Cidofovir, a new agent with potent anti-herpesvirus activity. *Antiviral Chem Chemother,* **1996**, *7:*115–127.

Ho E, Lin D, Mendel D, Cihlar T. Cytotoxicity of antiviral nucleotides adefovir and cidofovir is induced by the expression of human renal organic anion transporter 1. *J Am Soc Nephrol,* **2000**, *11:*383–393.

Hong Z, Cameron C. Pleiotropic mechanisms of ribavirin antiviral activities. *Prog Drug Res,* **2002**, *59*:41–69.

Infectious Disease Community of Practice, American Society of Transplantation, Guidelines for the prevention and management of infectious complications of solid organ transplantation: Cytomegalovirus. *Am J Transplant,* **2004**, *4*(suppl 10): 51–58.

Jonas M, Kelly D, Mizerski J, et al. Clinical trial of lamivudine in children with chronic hepatitis B. *N Engl J Med,* **2002**, *346*:1706–1713.

Kaiser L, Keene O, Hammond J, et al. Impact of zanamivir on antibiotics use for respiratory events following acute influenza in adolescents and adults. *Arch Intern Med,* **2000**, *160*: 3234–3240.

Kaiser L, Wat C, Mills T, et al. Impact of oseltamivir treatment on influenza-related lower respiratory tract complications and hospitalizations**.** *Arch Intern Med,* **2003**, *163:*1667–1672.

Keating G, Curran M. Peginterferon-alpha-2a (40 kDa) plus ribavirin: A review of its use in the management of chronic hepatitis C. *Drugs,* **2003**, *63*:701–730.

Keyser L, Karl M, Nafziger A, Bertino J Jr. Comparison of central nervous system adverse effects of amantadine and rimantadine used as sequential prophylaxis of influenza A in elderly nursing home patients. *Arch Intern Med*, **2000**, *160:* 1485–1488.

Kimberlin D, Weller S, Whitley R, *et al.* Pharmacokinetics of oral valacyclovir and acyclovir in late pregnancy. *Am J Obstet Gynecol,* **1998**, *179*:846–851.

Kimberlin DW, Lin CY, Jacobs RF, et al,. Safety and efficacy of high-dose intravenous acyclovir in the management of neonatal herpes simplex virus infections. *Pediatrics,* **2001**, *108:* 230–238.

Kimberlin DW, Lin CY, Sanchez PJ, et al. Effect of ganciclovir therapy on hearing in symptomatic congenital cytomegalovirus disease involving the central nervous system: A randomized, controlled trial. *J Pediat*, **2003**, *143:*16–25.

Kimberlin D, Rouse D. Clinical practice: Genital herpes. *N Engl J Med,* **2004**, *350:*1970–1977.

Kimberlin D, Acosta E, Sanchez P, *et al.* Oseltamivir pharmacokinetics (PK) in infants: Interim results from multicenter trial. Paper presented at: 47th Annual Meeting of the Infectious Diseases Society of America (IDSA); Philadelphia, PA; **2009**.

Lai C, Yuen M, Hui C, et al. Comparison of the efficacy of lamivudine and famciclovir in Asian patients with chronic hepatitis B: Results of 24 weeks of therapy. *J Med Virol,* **2002**, *67:*334–338.

Lai CL, Lim SG, Brown NA, et al. A dose-finding study of once-daily oral telbivudine in HBeAg-positive patients with chronic hepatitis B virus infection. *Hepatology,* **2004**, *40:*719–726.

Lau D, Everhart J, Kleiner D, et al. Long-term follow-up of patients with chronic hepatitis B treated with interferon alfa. *Gastroenterology,* **1997**, *113*:1660–1667.

Liaw Y, Sung J, Chow W, et al. Lamivudine for patients with chronic hepatitis B and advanced liver disease. *N Engl J Med,* **2004**, *351:*1521–1531.

Limaye A, Corey L, Koelle D, et al. Emergence of ganciclovir-resistant cytomegalovirus disease among recipients of solid-organ transplants. *Lancet,* **2000**, *356:*645–649.

Ljungman P, Ribaud P, Eyrich M, *et al.* Cidofovir for adenovirus infections after allogeneic hematopoietic stem cell transplantation: A survey by the Infectious Diseases Working Party of the European Group for Blood and Marrow Transplantation. *Bone Marrow Transplant,* **2003**, *31*:481–486.

Loutfy MR, Blatt LM, Siminovitch KA, et al. Interferon alfacon-1 plus corticosteroids in severe acute respiratory syndrome: A preliminary study. *JAMA,* **2003,** *290*:3222–3228.

Lowance D, Neumayer H, Legendre CM, et al. Valacyclovir for the prevention of cytomegalovirus disease after renal transplantation. *N Engl J Med,* **1999**, *340:*1462–1470.

Marcellin P, Chang TT, Lim SG, et al. Adefovir dipivoxil for the treatment of hepatitis B e antigen–positive chronic hepatitis B. *N Engl J Med,* **2003**, *348:*808–816.

Marcellin P, Lau GK, Bonino F. Peginterferon alfa-2a alone, lamivudine alone, and the two in combination in patients with HBeAg-negative chronic hepatitis B. *N Engl J Med,* **2004**, *351*:1206–1217.

Mardani M, Jahromi MK, Naieni KH, Zeinali M. The efficacy of oral ribavirin in the treatment of Crimean-Congo hemorrhagic fever in Iran. *Clin Infect Dis,* **2003**, *36:*1613–1618.

McHutchison JG, Everson GT, Gordon SC, et al. Telaprevir with peginterferon and ribavirin for chronic HCV genotype 1 infection. *N Engl J Med,* **2009**, *360:*1827–1838.

McHutchison JG, Lawitz EJ, Shiffman ML, et al. Peginterferon alfa-2b or alfa-2a with ribavirin for treatment of hepatitis C infection. *N Engl J Med,* **2009**, *361:*580–593.

McMahon MA, Jilek BL, Brennan TP, et al. The HBV drug entecavir—effects on HIV-1 replication and resistance. *N Engl J Med,* **2007**, *356:*2614–2621.

Moscona A. Global transmission of oseltamivir-resistant influenza. *N Engl J Med,* **2009**, *360:*953–956.

Noble S, Faulds D. Ganciclovir: An update of its use in the prevention of cytomegalovirus infection and disease in transplant recipients. *Drugs,* **1998**, *56:*115–146.

Ono SK, Kato N, Shiratori Y, et al. The polymerase L528M mutation cooperates with nucleotide binding-site mutations, increasing hepatitis B virus replication and drug resistance. *J Clin Invest,* **2001**, *107*:449–455.

Peters MG, Hann H, Martin P, et al. Adefovir dipivoxil alone or in combination with lamivudine in patients with lamivudine-resistant chronic hepatitis B. *Gastroenterology,* **2004**, *126:* 91–101.

Poynard T, McHutchison J, Manns M, et al. Impact of pegylated interferon alfa-2b and ribavirin on liver fibrosis in patients with chronic hepatitis C. *Gastroenterology,* **2002**, *122:*1303–1313.

Prusoff WH. Idoxuridine or how it all began. In: *Clinical Use of Antiviral Drugs.* (DeClercq, E, ed.), Martinus Nijhoff, Boston, **1988**, pp. 15–24.

Raborn GW, Martel AY, Lassonde M, et al. Effective treatment of herpes simplex labialis with penciclovir cream: Combined results of two trials. *J Am Dent Assoc,* **2002**, *133:*303–309.

Ratanajamit C, Vinther S, Jepsen P, et al. Adverse pregnancy outcome in women exposed to acyclovir during pregnancy: A population-based observational study. *Scand J Infect Dis,* **2003**, *35:*255–259.

Reddy KR, Nelson DR, Zeuzem S. Ribavirin: Current role in the optimal clinical management of chronic hepatitis C. *J Hepatol,* **2009**, *50:*402–411.

Reusser P, Einsele H, Lee J, et al. Randomized multicenter trial of foscarnet versus ganciclovir for preemptive therapy of cytomegalovirus infection after allogeneic stem cell transplantation. *Blood,* **2002**, *99:*1159–1164.

Sacks SL, Wilson B. Famciclovir/penciclovir. *Adv Exp Med Biol,* **1999**, *458*:135–147.

Samuel CE. Antiviral actions of interferons. *Clin Microbiol Rev,* **2001**, *14:*778–809.

Schirmer P, Holodniy M. Oseltamivir for treatment and prophylaxis of influenza infection. *Expert Opin Drug Saf,* **2009**, *8:*357–371.

Schmidt AC. Antiviral therapy for influenza: A clinical and economic comparative review. *Drugs,* **2004**, *64:*2031–2046.

Schreiber A, Härter G, Schubert A, et al. Antiviral treatment of cytomegalovirus infection and resistant strains. *Expert Opin Pharmacother,* **2009**, *10:*191–209.

Scott LJ, Keating GM. Entecavir: A review of its use in chronic hepatitis B. *Drugs,* **2009**, *69:*1003–1033.

Seeff LB, Hoofnagle JH. National Institutes of Health Consensus Development Conference statement: Management of hepatitis C. *Hepatology,* **2002**, *36*(5 suppl 1):S1–S2.

Skinner RB Jr. Imiquimod. *Dermatol Clin,* **2003**, *21:*291–300.

Sokal EM, Conjeevaram HS, Roberts EA, et al. Interferon alfa therapy for chronic hepatitis B in children: A multinational randomized, controlled trial. *Gastroenterology,* **1998**, *114:* 988–995.

Sokal EM, Roberts EA, Mieli-Vergani G, et al. Dose ranging study of the pharmacokinetics, safety, and preliminary efficacy of lamivudine in children and adolescents with chronic hepatitis B. *Antimicrob Agents Chemother,* **2000**, *44:* 590–597.

Spruance SL, Nett R, Marbury T, et al. Acyclovir cream for treatment of herpes simplex labialis: Results of two randomized, doubleblind, vehicle-controlled, multicenter clinical trials. *Antimicrob Agents Chemother,* **2002**, *46:*2238–2243.

Steer CB, Szer J, Sasadeusz J, et al. Varicella-zoster infection after allogeneic bone marrow transplantation: Incidence, risk factors and prevention with low-dose aciclovir and ganciclovir. *Bone Marrow Transplant,* **2000**, *25:*657–664.

Steingrimsdottir H, Gruber A, Palm C, et al. Bioavailability of aciclovir after oral administration of acyclovir and its prodrug valaciclovir to patients with leukopenia after chemotherapy. *Antimicrob Agents Chemother,* **2000**, *44:*207–209.

Studies of Ocular Complications of AIDS (SOCA) Research Group, in Collaboration with the AIDS Clinical Trials Group. Mortality in patients with the acquired immunodeficiency syndrome treated with either foscarnet or ganciclovir for cytomegalovirus retinitis (published erratum appears in *N Engl J Med,* **1992**, *326:*1172). *N Engl J Med,* **1996**, *326:* 213–220.

Tam RC, Lau JY, Hong Z. Mechanisms of action of ribavirin in antiviral therapies. *Antiviral Chem Chemother,* **2002**, *12:* 261–272.

Tyring S, Engst R, Corriveau C. Famciclovir for ophthalmic zoster: A randomised acyclovir controlled study. *Br J Ophthalmol,* **2001**, *85:*576–581.

Tyring SK, Beutner K, Tucker BA, et al. Antiviral therapy for herpes zoster. *Arch Fam Med,* **2000**, *9*:863–869.

Vats A, Shapiro R, Singh R, et al. Quantitative viral load monitoring and cidofovir therapy for the management of BK virus–associated nephropathy in children and adults. *Transplantation,* **2003**, *75*:105–112.

Vitravene Study Group. Randomized dose-comparison studies of intravitreous fomivirsen for treatment of cytomegalovirus retinitis that has reactivated or is persistently active despite other therapies in patients with aids. *Am J Ophthalmol,* **2002**, *133:*475–483.

Wagstaff AJ, Faulds D, Goa KL. Acyclovir: A reappraisal of its antiviral activity, pharmacokinetic properties and therapeutic efficacy. *Drugs,* **1994**, *47*:153–205.

Whitley RJ, Hayden FG, Reisinger K, et al. Oral oseltamivir treatment of influenza in children. *Pediatr Infect Dis J,* **2001**, *20*:127–133.

Wiley DJ, Douglas J, Beutner K, et al. External genital warts: Diagnosis, treatment, and prevention. *Clin Infect Dis,* **2002**, *35*:S210–S224.

Winston DJ, Yeager AM, Chandrasekar PH, et al. Randomized comparison of oral valacyclovir and intravenous ganciclovir for prevention of cytomegalovirus disease after allogeneic bone marrow transplantation. *Clin Infect Dis,* **2003**, *36:*749–758.

Young KC, Lindsay KL, Lee KJ. Identification of a ribavirin resistant NS5B mutation of hepatitis C virus during ribavirin monotherapy. *Hepatology,* **2003,** *38*:869–878.

Antiretroviral Agents and Treatment of HIV Infection

Charles Flexner

I. Overview of HIV Infection and its Treatment

There are currently several million people taking chronic combination antiretroviral therapy to suppress human immunodeficiency virus (HIV) infection, including >3 million in sub-Saharan Africa alone. This is an amazing achievement for a disease that was uniformly fatal and with few treatment options just two decades ago. Combination antiretroviral therapy prolongs life and prevents progression of disease caused by HIV. The pharmacotherapy of HIV infection is a rapidly moving field. In 2009, 24 antiretroviral drugs were available in the U.S. Three-drug combinations are the minimum standard of care for this infection, so current agents constitute several thousand possible regimens. The long-term management of a patient on antiretroviral therapy can be daunting, even for experienced healthcare providers. Knowing the essential features of the pathophysiology of this disease and how chemotherapeutic agents affect the virus and the host is critical in developing a rational approach to therapy. *Unique features of this drug class include the need for lifelong administration to control virus replication and the possibility of rapid emergence of permanent drug resistance if these agents are not used properly.*

Increasingly, the public health impact of this epidemic has shifted to those regions least able to afford treatment. Because combination antiretroviral therapy has the capacity to improve the quality of human health and to produce near-normal life expectancies (Lee et al., 2001), there is a strong impetus to provide these drugs to as many infected individuals as possible. Through a combination of increased foreign aid, access to generic antiretrovirals, and willingness on the part of legacy pharmaceutical companies to allow violation of intellectual property law for this class of drugs, HIV treatment is now a possibility for much of the world. Because the number of effective treatment options is large, emphasis is shifting from efficacy to long-term convenience, tolerability, and safety. One outcome has been the development of single tablet fixed-dose combinations of drugs that can be taken orally once or twice a day. Because treatment is taken for years if not decades, the potential adverse effects of each drug take on increasing importance.

PATHOGENESIS OF HIV-RELATED DISEASE

Human immunodeficiency viruses (HIV) are lentiviruses, a family of mammalian retroviruses evolved to establish chronic persistent infection with gradual onset of clinical symptoms. Unlike herpesviruses, replication is constant following infection, and although some infected cells may harbor nonreplicating virus for years, in the absence of treatment there generally is no true period of viral latency following infection (Greene and Peterlin, 2002). Humans and nonhuman primates are the only natural hosts for these viruses.

There are two major families of HIV. Most of the epidemic involves HIV-1; HIV-2 is more closely related to simian immunodeficiency virus (SIV) and is concentrated in western Africa. HIV-1 is genetically diverse, with at least five distinct subfamilies or clades. HIV-1 and HIV-2 have similar *in vitro* sensitivity to most antiretroviral drugs, although the non-nucleoside reverse transcriptase inhibitors (NNRTIs) are HIV-1-specific and have no activity against HIV-2. Within HIV-1 isolates, clade *per se* does not seem to have a major effect on drug sensitivity.

Virus Structure. HIV is a typical retrovirus with a small RNA genome of 9300 base pairs. Two copies of the genome are contained in a nucleocapsid core surrounded by a lipid bilayer, or envelope, that is derived from the host cell plasma membrane (Figure 59–1). The viral genome encodes three major open reading frames: *gag* encodes a polyprotein that is processed to release the major structural proteins of the virus; *pol* overlaps *gag* and encodes three important enzyme activities—an RNA-dependent DNA polymerase or reverse transcriptase with RNAase activity, protease, and the viral integrase; and *env* encodes the large transmembrane envelope protein responsible for cell binding and entry. Several small genes encode regulatory proteins that enhance virion production or combat host defenses. These include *tat, rev, nef*, and *vpr* (Greene and Peterlin, 2002).

Virus Life Cycle. HIV tropism is controlled by the envelope protein gp160 (env) (Figure 59–1). The major target for env binding is the CD4 receptor present on lymphocytes and macrophages, although cell entry also requires binding to a coreceptor, generally the chemokine receptor CCR5 or CXCR4 (Greene and Peterlin, 2002). CCR5 is present on macrophage lineage cells. Most infected individuals harbor predominantly the CCR5-tropic virus; HIV with this tropism is responsible for nearly all naturally acquired infections. A shift from CCR5 to CXCR4 utilization is associated with advancing disease, and the increased affinity of HIV-1 for CXCR4 allows infection of T-lymphocyte lines (Berger et al., 1999). A phenotypic switch from CCR5 to CXCR4 heralds accelerated loss of CD4+ helper T cells and increased risk of immunosuppression. Whether coreceptor switch is a cause or a consequence of advancing disease is still unknown, but it is possible to develop clinical AIDS without this switch.

The gp41 domain of env controls the fusion of the virus lipid bilayer with that of the host cell. Following fusion, full-length viral RNA enters the cytoplasm, where it undergoes replication to a short-lived RNA-DNA duplex; the original RNA is degraded by RNase H to allow creation of a full-length double-stranded DNA copy of the virus (Figure 59–1). Because the HIV reverse transcriptase is error prone and lacks a proofreading function, mutation is quite frequent and estimated

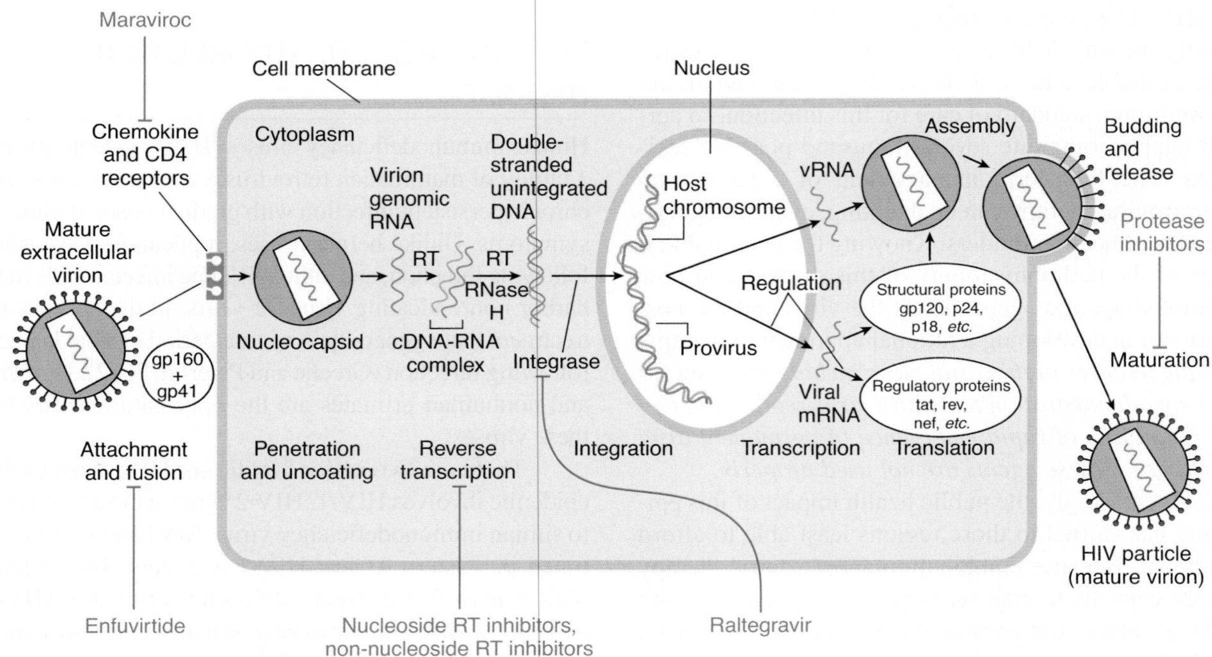

Figure 59–1. *Replicative cycle of HIV-1 showing the sites of action of available antiretroviral agents.* Available antiretroviral agents are shown in blue. Key: RT, reverse transcriptase; cDNA, complementary DNA; mRNA, messenger RNA; RNase H, ribonuclease H; gp120 + gp41, extracellular and intracellular domains, respectively, of envelope glycoprotein. (Adapted from Hirsch and D'Aquila, 1993.)

to occur at approximately three bases out of every full-length (9300-base-pair) replication (Coffin, 1995). Virus DNA is transported into the nucleus, where it is integrated into a host chromosome by the viral integrase in a random or quasi-random location (Greene and Peterlin, 2002).

Following integration, the virus may remain in a quiescent state, not producing RNA or protein but replicating as the cell divides. When a cell that harbors the virus is activated, viral RNA and proteins are produced. Structural proteins assemble around full-length genomic RNA to form a nucleocapsid (Figure 59–1). The envelope and structural proteins assemble at the cell surface, concentrated in cholesterol-rich lipid rafts. The nucleocapsid cores are directed to these sites and bud through the cell membrane, creating new enveloped HIV particles containing two complete single-stranded RNA genomes. Reverse transcriptase is incorporated into virus particles so replication can begin immediately after the virus enters a new cell (Greene and Peterlin, 2002).

How the Virus Causes Disease. Sexual acquisition of HIV infection is thought to be mediated by one or, at most, a handful of infectious virus particles. Soon after infection, there is a rapid burst of replication peaking at 2-4 weeks, with $\geq 10^9$ cells becoming infected. This peak is associated with a transient dip in the number of peripheral CD4+ (helper) T-lymphocytes. As a result of new host immune responses and target cell depletion, the number of infectious virions as reflected by the plasma HIV RNA concentration (also known as *viral load*) declines to a quasi-steady state. This level of virus activity has been termed the *set point* and reflects the interplay between host immunity and the pathogenicity of the infecting virus (Coffin, 1995). Most viruses are derived from CD4+ cells that turn over with a $t_{1/2}$ of 2.2 days (Perelson et al., 1996). Thus, in the average infected individual, several billion infectious virus particles are produced every few days.

Eventually, the host CD4+ T-lymphocyte count begins a steady decline, accompanied by a rise in the plasma HIV RNA concentration. Once the peripheral CD4 cell count falls below 200 cells/mm^3, there is an increasing risk of opportunistic diseases and ultimately death. Sexual acquisition of CCR5-tropic HIV-1 is associated with a median time to clinical AIDS of 8-10 years. Some patients, termed *long-term nonprogressors*, can harbor HIV for more than two decades without significant decline in peripheral CD4 cell count or clinical immunosuppression; this may reflect a combination of favorable host immunogenetics and immune responses (Fauci, 1996).

An important question relevant to treatment is whether HIV disease is a consequence of CD4+ lymphocyte depletion alone. Most natural history data suggest that this is true, although both the amount of virus measurable in the patient's circulation and the CD4 cell count are independent predictors of disease progression (Mellors et al., 1996, 1997). Regardless, successful therapy is based on inhibition of HIV replication; interventions designed specifically to boost the host immune response without exerting a direct antiviral effect have had no reliable clinical benefit.

History of Antiretroviral Therapy. The first effective antiretroviral agent, zidovudine, was synthesized by Horwitz in 1964 as a false nucleoside with disappointing anticancer activity. The drug was shown by Osterag in 1972 to inhibit the *in vitro* replication of a murine type D retrovirus (McLeod and Hammer, 1992). Mitsuya and Broder, working in Bethesda in 1985, reported that this drug had potent *in vitro* anti-HIV activity (Mitsuya et al., 1985). Clinical studies of zidovudine began that same year, and by 1987 this drug was approved and marketed for the control of HIV infection based on the results of a small but definitive randomized clinical trial (Fischl et al., 1987). Large numbers of nucleoside analogs already had been synthesized as potential anticancer and immunomodulatory drugs, and this made it possible for similar nucleoside reverse transcriptase inhibitors (NRTIs) to be tested efficiently and approved.

Selective non-nucleoside reverse transcriptase inhibitors (NNRTIs) were identified by iterative screening using purified viral enzyme (Pauwels et al., 1990). The clinical development of these drugs was hindered by the rapid emergence of drug resistance (Wei et al., 1995). However, three drugs in this category were approved by 1998 (Table 59–1). HIV protease inhibitors (PIs) were the products of rational drug design, relying on technology developed to identify transition-state peptidomimetic antagonists of proteases in the renin-angiotensin cascade (Flexner, 1998). Highly selective antagonists of the HIV protease were reported as early as 1987. Phase 1 trials of the first of these drugs, saquinavir, began in 1989, and this drug was approved for prescription use in 1995. Two additional protease inhibitors, ritonavir and indinavir, were approved within the next 4 months.

Innovation in drug approval and regulation facilitated the availability of multiple agents capable of fighting this infection. In 1989, the FDA agreed to make promising agents available to patients with advanced disease through an expanded access program. The capacity to measure plasma HIV RNA concentrations and CD4 cell counts, and proof of the predictive value of these surrogate end points (Mellors et al., 1996) made it possible to collapse the time frame for clinical drug development. The most promising drug combinations were identified by their effect on these end points in clinical trials as short as 6 months.

A detailed understanding of the molecular basis of drug resistance guides the search for new agents and informs the selection of combination strategies for existing drugs. The large number of possible drug combinations has given patients more chances at virus

Table 59–1

Antiretroviral Agents Approved for Use in the U.S.

GENERIC NAME [U.S. TRADE NAME]	ABBREVIATION; CHEMICAL NAMES
Nucleoside Reverse Transcriptase Inhibitors	
Zidovudine [RETROVIR, others][a]	ZDV; azidothymidine (AZT)
Didanosine [VIDEX; VIDEX EC, others]	ddI; dideoxyinosine
Stavudine [ZERIT]	d4T; didehydrodeoxythymidine
Zalcitabine [HIVID][c]	DDC; dideoxycytidine
Lamivudine [EPIVIR][a]	3TC; dideoxythiacytidine
Abacavir [ZIAGEN][a]	ABC; cyclopropylaminopurinylcyclopentene
Tenofovir disoproxil [VIREAD][a]	TDF; phosphinylmethoxypropyladenine (PMPA)
Emtricitabine [EMTRIVA][a]	FTC; fluorooxathiolanyl cytosine
Non-nucleoside Reverse Transcriptase Inhibitors	
Nevirapine [VIRAMUNE]	NVP
Efavirenz [SUSTIVA; STOCRIN][a]	EFV
Delavirdine [RESCRIPTOR]	DLV
Etravirine [INTELENCE]	ETV
Protease Inhibitors	
Saquinavir [INVIRASE]	SQV
Indinavir [CRIXIVAN]	IDV
Ritonavir [NORVIR]	RTV
Nelfinavir [VIRACEPT]	NFV
Amprenavir [AGENERASE; PROZEI][c]	APV
Lopinavir [KALETRA; ALUVIA][b]	LPV/r
Atazanavir [REYATAZ; ZRIVADA]	ATV
Fosamprenavir [LEXIVA; TELZIR]	FPV
Tipranavir [APTIVUS]	TPV
Darunavir [PREZISTA]	DRV
Entry Inhibitors	
Enfuvirtide [FUZEON]	T-20
Maraviroc [SELZENTRY; CELSENTRI]	MVC
Integrase Inhibitor	
Raltegravir [ISENTRESS]	RAL

[a]A number of fixed-dose co-formulations are available: zidovudine + lamivudine (COMBIVIR); zidovidine + lamivudine + abacavir (TRIZIVIR); abacavir + lamivudine (EPZICOM); tenofovir + emtricitabine (TRUVADA); tenofivir + efavirenz + emtricitabine (ATRIPLA). [b]Lopinavir is available only as part of a fixed-dose co-formulation with ritonavir (KALETRA/ALUVIA). [c]No longer marketed worldwide.

control but also complicates the practice of HIV medicine. Current challenges include access to effective long-term treatment in resource-poor countries and the continuing need for identification of new drugs for treatment-experienced patients with resistance to approved drugs (Flexner, 2007).

PRINCIPLES OF HIV CHEMOTHERAPY

Current treatment assumes that all aspects of disease derive from the direct toxic effects of HIV on host cells, mainly CD4+ T-lymphocytes. All treatment regimens associated with long-term suppression of HIV replication (as measured by decreased plasma HIV RNA) and repletion of peripheral CD4 cells are clinically beneficial (Lee et al., 2001). The goal of therapy is to suppress virus replication as much as possible for as long as possible.

Deciding when to start antiretroviral therapy has been a shifting target during the epidemic. Current guidelines in the U.S. recommend starting therapy in all those with a CD4 count of ≤350 cells/mm^3 (Department of Health and Human Services, 2010). Treatment is also recommended for HIV-infected pregnant women, those with HIV nephropathy, and those with concurrent hepatitis B virus infection requiring treatment regardless of CD4 count. Increasing evidence supports the clinical benefit and cost effectiveness of starting treatment at higher CD4 counts. With more active drug combinations, large systematic reviews of observational studies and a few randomized clinical trials suggest measurable clinical benefit the earlier treatment is initiated, beginning at CD4 counts ≤500 (Kitahata et al., 2009; When to Start Consortium, 2009). In the foreseeable future, treatment may be recommended for all infected adults and children (Flexner, 2007).

Increasing evidence supports the value of antiretroviral therapy in preventing transmission of the virus from person to person. Although most antiretroviral therapy is used in chronic treatment of established infection, these medications are also used in short courses to prevent infection in post-exposure settings and to prevent mother-to-child transmission (Department of Health and Human Services, 2010). Epidemiological modeling suggests that overall transmission rates are likely to fall in endemic areas where antiretroviral therapy is widely used (Granich et al., 2009). The possible value of targeted antiretroviral therapy to reduce new infections, or even to reduce or eliminate epidemic transmission, has not been adequately explored (Dieffenbach and Fauci, 2009).

A number of studies have confirmed the low likelihood that HIV can be eradicated with drug therapy.

A reservoir of long-lived quiescent T cells harboring infectious HIV DNA integrated into the host chromosome was identified independently by several groups of investigators (Chun et al., 1998; Finzi et al., 1997). Infectious HIV can be produced by these quiescent cells after chemical activation *ex vivo* (and presumably if the cells are activated by immune stimuli *in vivo*), but the nonreplicating form of the viral genome is not susceptible to antiretroviral drugs. Most estimates suggest that at least some of these cells will survive for decades and probably for the life of the patient (Siliciano et al., 2003) regardless of the type of anti-HIV treatment. Fortunately, in the presence of suppressive combination antiretroviral therapy it appears that residual viremia is the consequence of release of virus from pre-formed latent reservoirs, and the risk of developing drug resistance in such treated patients is negligible (Nettles et al., 2005). Episodic detection of low level plasma HIV RNA in otherwise suppressed individuals (also known as *blips*) almost certainly represents release of previously formed virus from resting cells; intermittent detection of HIV RNA at a concentrations <500 copies/mL is not associated with increased risk of treatment failure or drug resistance, unless this is accompanied by nonadherence (Kieffer et al., 2004).

Drug resistance is a key problem that must be prevented and circumvented through a combination of regimen selection and patient education. There is a high likelihood that all untreated infected individuals harbor viruses with single-amino-acid mutations conferring some degree of resistance to every known antiretroviral drug because of the high mutation rate of HIV and the tremendous number of infectious virions (Coffin, 1995). Starting treatment with only a single antiretroviral drug inevitably provokes the emergence of drug-resistant virus, in some cases within a few weeks (Wei et al., 1995). Drug therapy does not cause mutation but rather provides the necessary selective pressure to promote growth of drug-resistant viruses that arise naturally (Coffin, 1995). A combination of active agents therefore is required to prevent drug resistance, analogous to strategies employed in the treatment of tuberculosis (Chapter 56). Intentional drug holidays, also known as *structured treatment interruptions*, allow the virus to replicate anew and increase the risk of drug resistance and disease progression (Lawrence et al., 2003). Recrudescent replication of HIV after stopping therapy is associated with an acute increase in the risk of death, mainly from cardiovascular events (El-Sadr et al., 2006). This may be the consequence of increased immune activation that accompanies replication of the virus; HIV infection is associated with endothelial cell dysfunction, although the absolute increase in cardiovascular risk after controlling for other risk factors is small (Aberg, 2009).

The current standard of care is to use at least three drugs simultaneously for the entire duration of treatment. The expected outcome of initial therapy in a previously untreated patient is an undetectable *viral load* (plasma HIV RNA <50 copies/mL) within 24 weeks of starting treatment (Department of Health and Human Services, 2010). In prospective comparative trials, two-drug regimens were more effective than single-drug regimens (Fischl et al., 1995; Hammer et al., 1996; Saag et al., 1998), and three-drug regimens are more effective still (Collier et al., 1996; Gulick et al., 1997; Hammer et al., 1997). Mathematical models of HIV replication suggested that three is the minimum number of agents required to guarantee effective long-term suppression of HIV replication without resistance (Muller and Bonhoeffer, 2003). However, earlier models may not adequately predict the effects of newer and more potent antiretrovirals.

Randomized controlled trials found that a combination of two potent drugs (e.g., an NNRTI plus a PI) had equivalent virologic efficacy to either agent plus two NRTIs (Riddler et al., 2008). In treatment-naive patients, a regimen containing a non-nucleoside plus two nucleoside reverse transcriptase inhibitors was as effective as a regimen containing an additional nucleoside (Shafer et al., 2003), indicating the equivalence of these three-drug and four-drug regimens. Four or more drugs may be used simultaneously in pretreated patients harboring drug-resistant virus, but the number of agents a patient can take is limited by toxicity and inconvenience. Even for heavily treatment-experienced patients, a three-drug regimen containing at least two potent active agents is often as effective as regimens containing additional active agents (Steigbigel et al., 2008).

Several small studies have now shown that patients who are fully suppressed (HIV plasma RNA <50 copies/mL) for months on a triple drug combination may be switched to a single "boosted" protease inhibitor (e.g., lopinavir/ritonavir or atazanavir/ritonavir) and maintain full suppression of viral replication for years on antiretroviral monotherapy. Such simplification strategies are investigational and should only be used in patients who are known to be highly adherent and are closely monitored, because randomized trials have found higher failure rates in patients maintained on only a single active agent (Wilkin et al., 2009).

Pharmacodynamic synergy is probably not an important consideration in regimen selection, although most prescribers prefer to use drugs that attack at least two different molecular sites. This could include NRTIs that target the active site of the enzyme combined with an NNRTI that binds to a different site on the same enzyme, or an inhibitor of a different enzyme, such as HIV protease or integrase. Regimens containing an NNRTI or PI plus two NRTIs have similar long-term efficacy.

Failure of an antiretroviral regimen is defined as a persistent increase in plasma HIV RNA concentrations in a patient with previously undetectable virus, despite continued treatment with that regimen (Department of Health and Human Services, 2010). This indicates resistance to one or more drugs in the regimen and necessitates a change in treatment. Once resistance occurs, resistant strains remain in cells (mainly T-lymphocytes) indefinitely, even though the resistant virus may not be detectable in the plasma. For example, women who received a single dose of nevirapine to prevent mother-to-child transmission of HIV (and thus were more likely to harbor nevirapine-resistant virus) had a higher treatment failure rate if initiating therapy with nevirapine within 6 months, compared to treated women who had never received nevirapine (Lockman et al., 2007). The selection of new agents is therefore informed by the patient's treatment history, as well as viral resistance testing, preferably obtained while the patient is still taking a failing regimen to facilitate proper recovery and characterization of the patient's virus (Kuritzkes, 2004). Treatment failure generally requires implementation of a completely new combination of drugs. Adding a single active agent to a failing regimen is functional monotherapy if the patient is resistant to all drugs in the regimen and is likely to produce resistance to the new agent.

Treatment failure is usually the consequence of non-adherence. The risk of failing a regimen depends on the percentage of prescribed doses taken during any given period of treatment, but it also depends on the drugs in the regimen. Efavirenz-based regimens may be more forgiving of occasional skipped doses, and thus more useful because of the long $t_{1/2}$ of that drug; ritonavir-boosted PI regimens may be relatively more forgiving because of their higher genetic barrier to resistance (Gardner et al., 2009).

As antiretroviral therapy becomes more effective and easier to take, long-term toxicity of these drugs is of greater concern. An important consequence of long-term therapy is the development of a metabolic syndrome characterized by insulin resistance, fat redistribution, and hyperlipidemia and known as the *HIV lipodystrophy syndrome*. Lipodystrophy occurs in 10-40% of treated patients and has been seen with most drug combinations used in clinical trials. Symptomatic manifestations have been most strongly linked to the older generation of NRTIs, especially stavudine, which had more substantial mitochondrial toxicities; these drugs are now less commonly used in the developed world. The pathogenesis is still somewhat mysterious but involves phenotypic and metabolic changes similar to those seen with other human lipodystrophy syndromes (Garg, 2004). Clinical features include peripheral fat wasting (lipoatrophy), central fat accumulation including enlarged breasts and buffalo hump, insulin resistance and hyperglycemia, and elevations in serum cholesterol and triglycerides. Switching from one drug regimen to another may not reverse the symptoms, emphasizing its ubiquitous nature and possible role of HIV infection *per se*. Treatment is symptom directed and should include management of hyperlipidemias as recommended by the American Heart Association (Chapter 31). Lipodystrophy has been associated with an increased risk of myocardial infarction in virologically controlled patients, emphasizing the importance of cardiovascular risk factor reduction.

There is evidence that chronic HIV infection *per se* increases long-term cardiovascular risks, but the quantitative contribution of drug therapy to this risk is not well defined. Metabolic abnormalities associated with chronic HIV infection and possibly exacerbated by some drugs include insulin resistance, hyperglycemia, and increased risk of diabetes mellitus, as well as osteopenia and its attendant complications (Calmy et al., 2009).

A potential concern that applies to all protease inhibitors and NNRTIs is clinically significant pharmacokinetic drug interactions (Piscitelli and Gallicano, 2001). All agents in these two drug classes can act as inhibitors and/or inducers of hepatic CYPs and other drug metabolizing enzymes, as well as drug transport proteins. Prescribing practices should be guided by up-to-date knowledge of these potential effects. Internet-based educational resources are updated frequently (see, e.g., Flexner and Pham, 2009) and are an excellent way to track evolving knowledge about the undesired effects of drugs used in combination with antiretrovirals.

An increasingly recognized complication of initiating antiretroviral therapy is accelerated inflammatory reaction to overt or subclinical opportunistic infections or malignancies. This is thought to reflect reversal of immunodeficiency, resulting in new antimicrobial host defenses. This *immune reconstitution inflammatory syndrome (IRIS)* is most commonly seen when initiating therapy in individuals with low CD4 counts and/or advanced HIV disease, and it is associated with a better virologic response to therapy (Manabe et al., 2007). Not surprisingly, this is now most prevalent in resource-poor countries, where it may occur in >10% of newly treated patients. Infections most commonly associated with IRIS include tuberculosis and other mycobacterial diseases, cryptococcosis, hepatitis virus infections, and Pneumocystis pneumonia. Duration of symptoms ranges from a few days to more than a year. Symptomatic relief can be obtained with anti-inflammatory drugs, but systemic corticosteroids do not appear to shorten the course of symptoms (Manabe et al., 2007).

II. Drugs Used to Treat HIV Infection

NUCLEOSIDE AND NUCLEOTIDE REVERSE TRANSCRIPTASE INHIBITORS

The HIV-encoded, RNA-dependent DNA polymerase, also called *reverse transcriptase*, converts viral RNA into proviral DNA that is then incorporated into a host cell chromosome. Available inhibitors of this enzyme are either nucleoside/nucleotide analogs or non-nucleoside inhibitors (Figure 59–2 and Table 59–2).

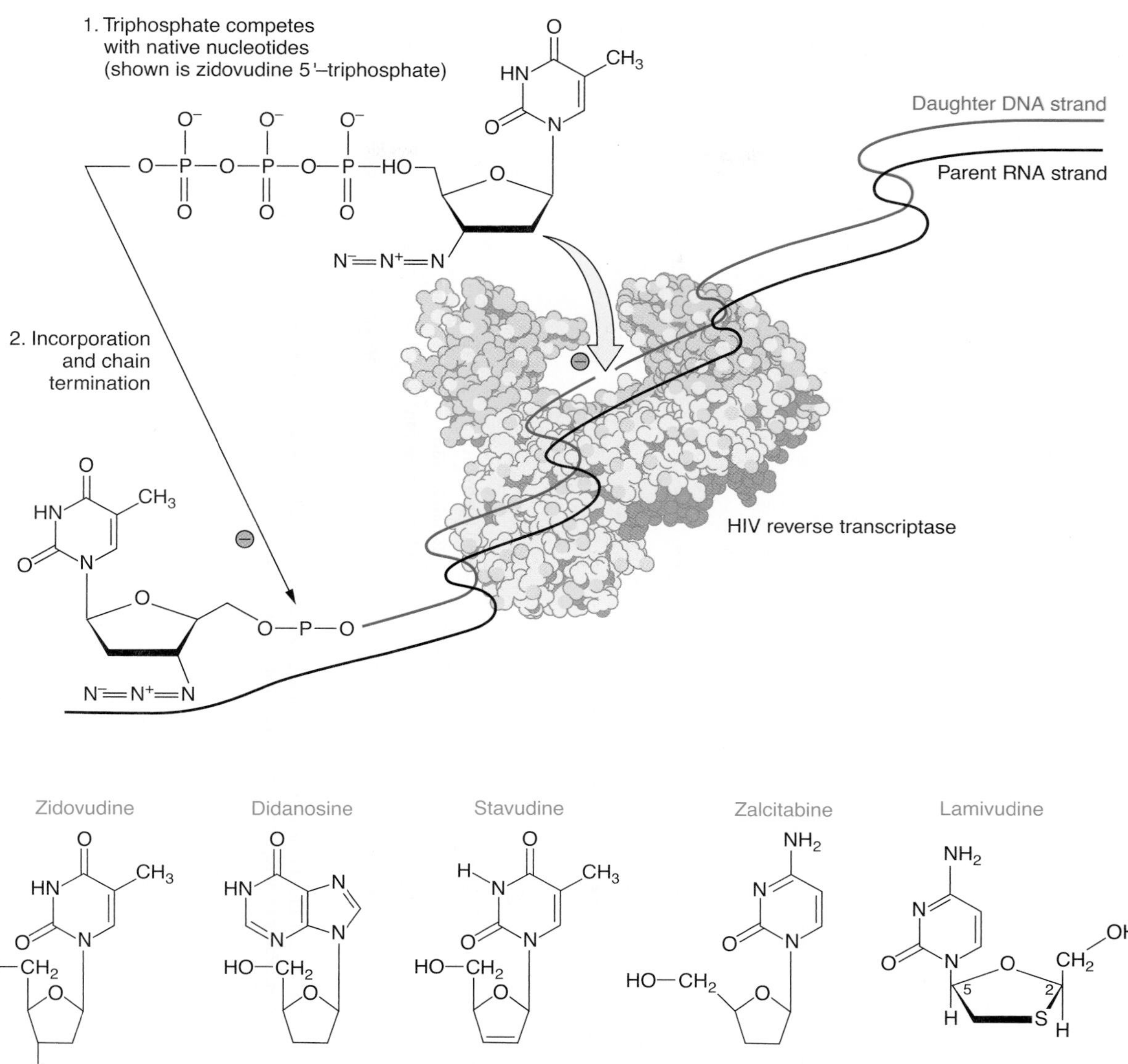

Figure 59–2. *Structures and mechanism of nucleoside and nucleotide reverse transcriptase inhibitors.*

Table 59–2

Pharmacokinetic Properties of Nucleoside Reverse Transcriptase Inhibitors[a]

PARAMETER	ZIDOVUDINE	LAMIVUDINE	STAVUDINE[b]	DIDANOSINE[c]	ABACAVIR	TENOFOVIR	EMTRICITABINE
Oral bioavailability, %	64	86-87	86	42	83	25	93
Effect of meals on AUC	↓24% (high fat)	↔	↔	↓55% (acidity)	↔	↑40% (high fat)	↔
Plasma $t_{1/2}$, elim, h	1.0	5-7	1.1-1.4	1.5	0.8-1.5	14-17	10
Intracellular $t_{1/2}$, elim of triphosphate, h	3-4	12-18	3.5	25-40	21	10-50	39
Plasma protein binding, %	20-38	<35	<5	<5	50	<8	<4
Metabolism, %	60-80 (glucuronidation)	<36	ND	50 (purine metabolism)	>80 (dehydrogenation and glucuronidation)	ND	13
Renal excretion of parent drug, %	14	71	39	18-36	<5	70-80	86

ABBREVIATIONS: AUC, area under plasma concentration time curve; $t_{1/2}$, elim, half-life of elimination; ↑, increase; ↓, decrease; ↔, no effect; ND, not determined.
[a]Reported mean values in adults with normal renal and hepatic function. [b]Parameters reported for the stavudine capsule formulation. [c]Parameters reported for the didanosine chewable tablet formulation.

Like all available antiretroviral drugs, nucleoside and nucleotide reverse transcriptase inhibitors prevent infection of susceptible cells but do not eradicate the virus from cells that already harbor integrated proviral DNA. Nucleoside and nucleotide analogs must enter cells and undergo phosphorylation to generate synthetic substrates for the enzyme (Table 59–2). The fully phosphorylated analogs block replication of the viral genome both by competitively inhibiting incorporation of native nucleotides and by terminating elongation of nascent proviral DNA because they lack a 3′-hydroxyl group (Dudley, 1995).

All but one of the drugs in this class are nucleosides that must be triphosphorylated at the 5′-hydroxyl to exert activity. The sole exception, tenofovir, is a nucleotide monophosphate analog that requires two additional phosphates to acquire full activity. These compounds inhibit both HIV-1 and HIV-2, and several have broad-spectrum activity against other human and animal retroviruses; emtricitabine, lamivudine, and tenofovir are active against hepatitis B virus (HBV), and tenofovir also has activity against herpesviruses (Chapter 58; De Clercq, 2003).

The selective toxicity of these drugs depends on their ability to inhibit the HIV reverse transcriptase without inhibiting host cell DNA polymerases. Although the intracellular triphosphates for all these drugs have low affinity for human DNA polymerase-α and -β, some are capable of inhibiting human DNA polymerase-γ, which is the mitochondrial enzyme. As a result, the important toxicities common to this class of drugs result in part from the inhibition of mitochondrial DNA synthesis (Lee et al., 2003). These toxicities include anemia, granulocytopenia, myopathy, peripheral neuropathy, and pancreatitis. Lactic acidosis with or without hepatomegaly and hepatic steatosis is a rare but potentially fatal complication seen with stavudine, zidovudine, and didanosine; it is probably not associated independently with the other drugs (Tripuraneni et al., 2004). Phosphorylated emtricitabine, lamivudine, and tenofovir have low affinity for DNA polymerase-γ and are largely devoid of mitochondrial toxicity.

The chemical structures of nucleoside and nucleotide reverse transcriptase inhibitors approved for treating HIV infection are shown in Figure 59–2; their pharmacokinetic properties are summarized in Table 59–2. Phosphorylation pathways for these eight drugs are summarized in Figure 59–3. Most nucleoside and nucleotide reverse transcriptase inhibitors are

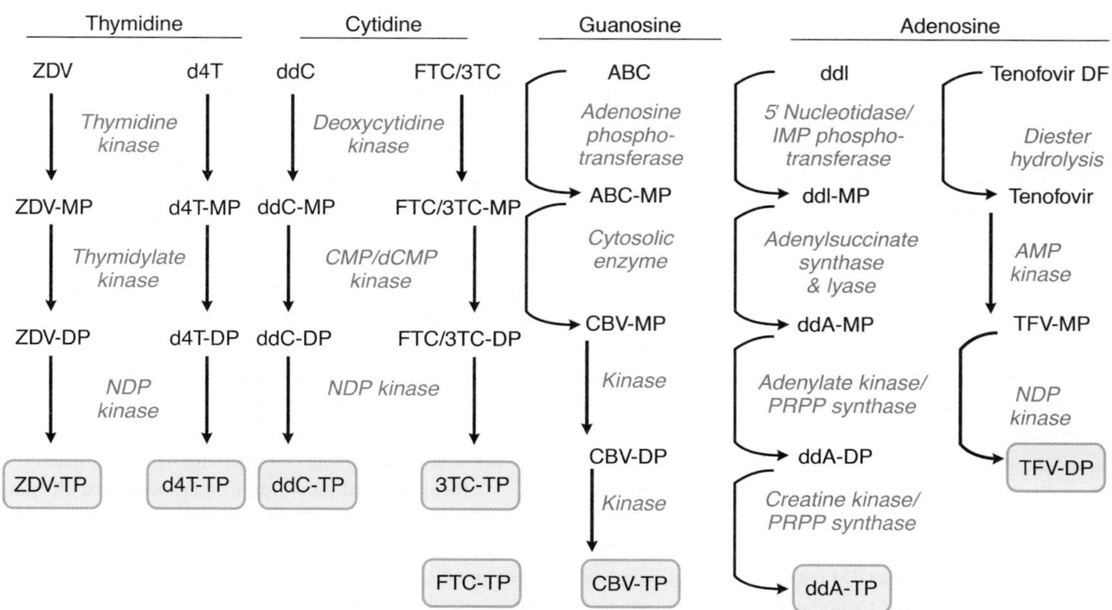

Figure 59–3. *Intracellular activation of nucleoside analog reverse transcriptase inhibitors.* Drugs and phosphorylated anabolites are abbreviated; the enzymes responsible for each conversion are spelled out. The active antiretroviral anabolite for each drug is shown in the blue box. Key: ZDV, zidovudine; d4T, stavudine; ddC, dideoxycytidine; FTC, emtricitabine; 3TC, lamivudine; ABC, abacavir; ddI, didanosine; DF, disoproxil fumarate; MP, monophosphate; DP, diphosphate; TP, triphosphate; AMP, adenosine mono phosphate; CMP, cytidine monophosphate; dCMP, deoxycytidine monophosphate; IMP, inosine 5′-monophosphate; PRPP, phosphoribosyl pyrophosphate; NDP, nucleoside diphosphate. (Adapted with permission from Khoo *et al.,* 2002. Copyright © Elsevier.)

eliminated from the body primarily by renal excretion. Zidovudine and abacavir, however, are cleared mainly by hepatic glucuronidation. Most of the parent compounds are eliminated rapidly from the plasma, with elimination half-lives of 1-10 hours, with the exception of tenofovir ($t_{1/2}$ ~14-17 hours) (Table 59–2). Despite rapid clearance from the plasma, the critical pharmacological pathway for these agents is production and elimination of the intracellular nucleoside triphosphate or nucleotide diphosphate, which is the active anabolite. In general, the phosphorylated anabolites are eliminated from cells much more gradually than the parent drug is eliminated from the plasma. Estimated elimination half-lives for intracellular triphosphates range from 2 to 50 hours (Table 59–2). This allows for less frequent dosing than would be predicted from plasma half-lives of the parent compounds. All available nucleoside and nucleotide reverse transcriptase inhibitors are dosed once or twice daily.

These drugs generally are not involved in clinically significant pharmacokinetic drug interactions because they are not major substrates for hepatic CYPs. Pharmacokinetic drug interactions involving tenofovir and protease inhibitors are likely to be explained by inhibition of OATP drug transporters (Chapman et al., 2003; see Chapter 5).

High-level resistance to nucleoside/nucleotide reverse transcriptase inhibitors, especially thymidine analogs, occurs slowly by comparison to NNRTIs and first-generation protease inhibitors. For example, zidovudine resistance was noted in only one-third of treated subjects after 1 year of monotherapy (Fischl et al., 1995). High-level resistance can occur rapidly with lamivudine and emtricitabine. In most cases, high-level resistance requires accumulation of a minimum of three to four codon substitutions, although a two-amino-acid insertion is associated with resistance to all drugs in this class (Gallant et al., 2003). Cross-resistance is common but often confined to drugs having similar chemical structures; zidovudine is a thymidine analog, and a zidovudine-resistant isolate is much more likely to be cross-resistant to the thymidine analog stavudine than to the cytidine analog lamivudine.

Nucleoside/nucleotide analogs are generally less active as single agents than other antiretroviral drugs. When used investigationally as monotherapy, most of these drugs produced only a 30-90% mean peak decrease in plasma concentrations of HIV RNA; abacavir monotherapy, however, produced up to a 99% decrease (Hervey and Perry, 2000). CD4 lymphocyte count increases were also modest with nucleoside monotherapy (mean increases of 50-100 cells/mm^3, depending on disease stage). Nonetheless, these drugs remain a critical component of therapy, and nearly all patients starting antiretroviral treatment do so with at least one agent from this class. Although modest in their own antiviral potency, several nucleoside analogs have favorable safety and tolerability profiles and are useful in suppressing the emergence of HIV isolates resistant to the more potent drugs in combination regimens.

Zidovudine

Chemistry and Antiviral Activity. Zidovudine (3′-azido-3′-deoxythymidine; AZT) is a synthetic thymidine analog with potent *in vitro* activity against a broad spectrum of retroviruses including HIV-1, HIV-2, and human T-cell lymphotrophic viruses (HTLV) I and II (McLeod and Hammer, 1992). Its IC_{50} against laboratory and clinical isolates of HIV-1 ranges from 10 to 48 nM.

Zidovudine is active in lymphoblastic and monocytic cell lines but is substantially less active in chronically infected cells (Geleziunas et al., 1993), probably because it has no impact on cells already infected with HIV. Zidovudine appears to be more active in lymphocytes than in monocyte-macrophage cells because of enhanced phosphorylation in the former. For the same reason, the drug is more potent in activated than in resting lymphocytes because the phosphorylating enzyme, thymidine kinase, is S-phase-specific (Gao et al., 1994).

Mechanisms of Action and Resistance. Like other nucleoside analogs, intracellular zidovudine is phosphorylated by thymidine kinase to zidovudine 5′-monophosphate, which is then phosphorylated by thymidylate kinase to the diphosphate and by nucleoside diphosphate kinase to zidovudine 5′-triphosphate (Figure 59–3). Zidovudine 5′-triphosphate terminates the elongation of proviral DNA because it is incorporated by reverse transcriptase into nascent DNA but lacks a 3′-hydroxyl group. The monophosphate competitively inhibits cellular thymidylate kinase, and this may reduce the amount of intracellular thymidine triphosphate. Zidovudine 5′-triphosphate only weakly inhibits cellular DNA polymerase-α but is a more potent inhibitor of mitochondrial polymerase-γ.

Because the conversion of zidovudine 5′-monophosphate to diphosphate is very inefficient, high concentrations of the monophosphate accumulate inside cells (Dudley, 1995) and may serve as a precursor depot for formation of triphosphate. As a consequence, there is little correlation between extracellular concentrations of parent drug and intracellular concentrations of triphosphate, and higher plasma concentrations of zidovudine do not increase intracellular triphosphate concentrations proportionately.

Resistance to zidovudine is associated with mutations at reverse transcriptase codons 41, 44, 67, 70, 210, 215, and 219 (Gallant et al., 2003). These mutations are referred to as *thymidine analog mutations* (TAMs) because of their ability to confer cross-resistance to other thymidine analogs such as stavudine. Two clusters of resistance mutations occur commonly. The pattern of 41L, 210W, and 215Y is associated with high-level resistance to zidovudine, as well as cross-resistance to other drugs in this class, including tenofovir and abacavir. The pattern 67N, 70R, 215F, and 219Q is less common and also associated with lower levels of resistance and cross-resistance. TAMs associated with resistance to zidovudine and stavudine promote excision of the incorporated nucleotide anabolites through pyrophosphorolysis (Naeger et al., 2002). Mutations accumulated gradually when zidovudine was used as the sole antiretroviral agent, and clinical resistance developed in only 31% of patients after 1 year of zidovudine monotherapy (Fischl et al., 1995). Cross-resistance to multiple nucleoside analogs has been reported following prolonged therapy and has been associated with a mutation cluster involving codons 62, 75, 77, 116, and 151. A mutation at codon 69 (typically T69S) followed by a two-amino-acid insertion produces cross-resistance to all available nucleoside and nucleotide analogs (Gallant et al., 2003).

The M184V substitution in the reverse transcriptase gene associated with the use of lamivudine or emtricitabine greatly restores sensitivity to zidovudine (Gallant et al., 2003). The combination of zidovudine and lamivudine produces greater long-term suppression of plasma HIV RNA than does zidovudine alone (Eron et al., 1995). As a result, this agent is usually combined with lamivudine in clinical practice.

Absorption, Distribution, and Elimination. Zidovudine is absorbed rapidly and reaches peak plasma concentrations within 1 hour (Dudley, 1995). Like other nucleoside analogs, the elimination $t_{1/2}$ of the parent compound (~1 hour) is considerably shorter than that of the intracellular triphosphate, which is 3-4 hours (Table 59–2). Failure to recognize this led to serious overdosing of the drug when it was first approved; the recommended dose was 250 mg every 4 hours in 1987, compared with 300 mg twice a day presently.

Zidovudine undergoes rapid first-pass hepatic metabolism by conversion to 5-glucuronyl zidovudine, which limits systemic bioavailability to ~64%. Food may slow absorption but does not alter the *AUC* (area under the plasma concentration-time curve) (Table 59–2), and the drug can be administered regardless of food intake (Dudley, 1995). The pharmacokinetic profile of zidovudine is not altered significantly during pregnancy, and drug concentrations in the newborn approach those of the mother. Parent drug crosses the blood-brain barrier relatively well and achieves a cerebrospinal fluid (CSF)-to-plasma ratio of ~0.6. Zidovudine also is detectable in breast milk, semen, and fetal tissue. Zidovudine concentrations are higher in the male genital tract than in the peripheral circulation, suggesting active transport or trapping.

Untoward Effects. Patients initiating zidovudine treatment often complain of fatigue, malaise, myalgia, nausea, anorexia, headache, and insomnia. These symptoms usually resolve within the first few weeks of treatment. Bone marrow suppression, mainly anemia and granulocytopenia, occurs most often in individuals with advanced HIV disease and very low CD4 counts and also was more common with the higher doses used when the drug was first approved. Erythrocytic macrocytosis is seen in ~90% of all patients but usually is not associated with anemia.

Chronic zidovudine administration has been associated with nail hyperpigmentation. Skeletal muscle myopathy can occur and is associated with depletion of mitochondrial DNA, most likely as a consequence of inhibition of DNA polymerase-γ. Serious hepatic toxicity, with or without steatosis and lactic acidosis, is rare but can be fatal. Risk factors for the lactic acidosis-steatosis syndrome include female sex, obesity, and prolonged exposure to the drug (Tripuraneni et al., 2004).

Precautions and Interactions. Zidovudine is not a substrate or inhibitor of CYPs. However, probenecid, fluconazole, atovaquone, and valproic acid may increase plasma concentrations of zidovudine probably through inhibition of glucuronosyl transferase (Dudley, 1995). The clinical significance of these interactions is unknown because intracellular triphosphate levels may be unchanged despite higher plasma concentrations. Zidovudine can cause bone marrow suppression and should be used cautiously in patients with preexisting anemia or granulocytopenia and in those taking other marrow-suppressive drugs. Stavudine and zidovudine compete for intracellular phosphorylation and should not be used concomitantly. Three clinical trials found a significantly worse virologic outcome in patients taking these two drugs together as compared with either agent used alone (Havlir et al., 2000).

Therapeutic Use. Zidovudine is FDA-approved for the treatment of adults and children with HIV infection and for preventing mother-to-child transmission of HIV infection; it is still recommended for post-exposure prophylaxis in HIV-exposed healthcare workers because of the large amount of data supporting its effectiveness in this setting (Centers for Disease Control and Prevention, 2005).

Despite being the oldest antiretroviral drug, zidovudine is still in widespread use, especially in resource-poor settings. This is a consequence of broad experience with the drug and its well-known tolerability, toxicity, and efficacy profiles. Zidovudine (RETROVIR, others) is marketed in oral tablets, capsules, and solution as well as a solution for intravenous injection. Zidovudine is available in coformulated tablets with lamivudine (COMBIVIR) or with lamivudine and abacavir (TRIZIVIR). Zidovudine monotherapy reduced the risk of perinatal transmission of HIV by 67% (Connor et al., 1994), and combining zidovudine with other antiretroviral drugs is even more efficacious in this setting.

Stavudine

Chemistry and Antiviral Activity. Stavudine (2′,3′-didehydro-2′,3′-dideoxythymidine; d4T) is a synthetic thymidine analog reverse transcriptase inhibitor that is active *in vitro* against HIV-1 and HIV-2. Its IC_{50} in lymphoblastoid and monocytic cell lines and in primary mononuclear cells ranges from 0.009 to 4 μM (Hurst and Noble, 1999).

Mechanisms of Action and Resistance. Intracellular stavudine is phosphorylated by thymidine kinase to stavudine 5′-monophosphate, which is then phosphorylated by thymidylate kinase to the diphosphate and by nucleoside diphosphate kinase to stavudine 5′-triphosphate (Hurst and Noble, 1999) (Figure 59–3). Unlike zidovudine monophosphate, stavudine monophosphate does not accumulate in the cell, and the rate-limiting step in activation appears to be generation of the monophosphate. Like zidovudine, stavudine is most potent in activated cells, probably because thymidine kinase is an S-phase-specific enzyme (Gao et al., 1994). Stavudine and zidovudine are antagonistic *in vitro*, and thymidine kinase has a higher affinity for zidovudine than for stavudine.

Stavudine resistance is seen most frequently with mutations at reverse transcriptase codons 41, 44, 67, 70, 210, 215, and 219 (Gallant et al., 2003), which are the same mutations associated with zidovudine resistance. Clusters of resistance mutations that include M41L, K70R, and T215Y are associated with a lower level of *in vitro* resistance than seen with zidovudine but are found in up to 38% of patients who fail to respond to stavudine. TAMs associated with resistance to zidovudine and stavudine promote excision of the incorporated triphosphate anabolites through pyrophosphorolysis (Naeger et al., 2002). As with zidovudine, resistance mutations for stavudine appear to accumulate slowly. Cross-resistance to multiple nucleoside analogs has been reported following prolonged therapy and has been associated with a mutation cluster involving codons 62, 75, 77, 116, and 151. In addition, a mutation at codon 69 (typically T69S) followed by a 2-amino acid insertion produces cross-resistance to all current nucleoside and nucleotide analogs (Gallant et al., 2003).

Absorption, Distribution, and Elimination. Stavudine is well absorbed and reaches peak plasma concentrations within 1 hour (Hurst and Noble, 1999). Bioavailability is not affected by food. The drug undergoes active tubular secretion, and renal elimination accounts for ~40% of parent drug.

Stavudine concentrations are higher in patients with low body weight, and the dose should be decreased from 40 to 30 mg twice daily in patients weighing <60 kg, although WHO recommends 30 mg twice daily in all patients. Dose also should be adjusted in patients with renal insufficiency (Jayasekara et al., 1999).

Plasma protein binding is <5%. The drug penetrates well into the CSF, achieving concentrations that are ~40% of those in plasma. Placental concentrations of stavudine are about half those of zidovudine, possibly reflecting stavudine's lower lipid solubility.

Untoward Effects. The most common serious toxicity of stavudine is peripheral neuropathy.

Neuropathy occurred in up to 71% of patients in initial monotherapy trials with a dose of 4 mg/kg per day. With the current recommended dose of 40 mg twice daily, the neuropathy incidence is ~12% (Hurst and Noble, 1999). Although this is thought to reflect mitochondrial toxicity, stavudine is a less potent inhibitor of DNA polymerase-γ than either didanosine or zalcitabine, suggesting that other mechanisms may be involved. Peripheral neuropathy is more common with higher doses or concentrations of stavudine and is more prevalent in patients with underlying HIV-related neuropathy or in those receiving other neurotoxic drugs. Stavudine is also associated with a progressive motor neuropathy characterized by weakness and in some cases respiratory failure, similar to Guillain-Barré syndrome (HIV Neuromuscular Syndrome Study Group, 2004).

Lactic acidosis and hepatic steatosis have been associated with stavudine use. This may be more common when stavudine and didanosine are combined. Elevated serum lactate is more common with stavudine than with zidovudine or abacavir (Tripuraneni et al., 2004), but the comparative risk of hepatic steatosis is unknown. Acute pancreatitis is not highly associated with stavudine but is more common when stavudine is combined with didanosine than when didanosine is given alone (Havlir et al., 2001).

Of all nucleoside analogs, stavudine use is associated most strongly with fat wasting, or *lipoatrophy* (Calmy et al., 2009). Whether this is a consequence of the extensive use of this agent combined with its mitochondrial toxicity or reflects a pathogenetic mechanism that has yet to be discovered remains to be determined. Stavudine has fallen out of favor in the developed world largely because of this toxicity. Other reported adverse effects include elevated hepatic transaminases, headache, nausea, and rash; however, these side effects are almost never severe enough to cause discontinuation of the drug.

Precautions and Interactions. Stavudine is mainly renally cleared and is not subject to metabolic drug interactions. The incidence and severity of peripheral neuropathy may be increased when stavudine is combined with other neuropathic medications, and therefore drugs such as ethambutol, isoniazid, phenytoin, and vincristine should be avoided.

Combining stavudine with didanosine leads to increased risk and severity of peripheral neuropathy and potentially fatal pancreatitis; therefore, *these two drugs should not be used together* (Havlir et al., 2001). Stavudine and zidovudine compete for intracellular phosphorylation and should not be used concomitantly. Three clinical trials found a significantly worse virologic outcome in patients taking these two drugs together as compared with either agent used alone (Havlir et al., 2000).

Therapeutic Use. Stavudine (ZERIT, others) is approved for use in HIV-infected adults and children, including neonates.

In early monotherapy trials, stavudine reduced plasma HIV RNA by 70-90% and delayed disease progression compared with continued zidovudine therapy. Lamivudine improves the long-term virologic response to stavudine, possibly reflecting the benefits of the M184V mutation (Kuritzkes et al., 1999). Many large prospective clinical trials have demonstrated potent and durable suppression of viremia and sustained increases in CD4+ cell counts when stavudine is combined with other nucleoside analogs plus NNRTIs or protease inhibitors (Hurst and Noble, 1999). Stavudine is no longer a popular drug in the developed world because of toxicity. However, it continues to be widely used in resource-poor settings because of its availability as an inexpensive generic version, often co-formulated with nevirapine and lamivudine.

Lamivudine

Chemistry and Antiviral Activity. Lamivudine [(–)2′, 3′-dideoxy, 3′-thiacytidine; 3TC] is a cytidine analog reverse transcriptase inhibitor that is active against HIV-1, HIV-2, and HBV.

The molecule has two chiral centers and is manufactured as the pure 2*R*, *cis*(–)-enantiomer (Figure 59–2). The racemic mixture from which lamivudine originates has antiretroviral activity but is less potent and substantially more toxic than the pure (−)-enantiomer. Compared with the (+)-enantiomer, the phosphorylated (−)-enantiomer is more resistant to cleavage from nascent RNA/DNA duplexes by cellular 3′-5′ exonucleases, which may contribute to its greater potency. The IC_{50} of lamivudine against laboratory strains of HIV-1 ranges from 2 to 670 nM, although the IC_{50} in primary human peripheral blood mononuclear cells is as high as 15 μM (Perry and Faulds, 1997).

Mechanisms of Action and Resistance. Lamivudine enters cells by passive diffusion, is converted to the monophosphate by deoxycytidine kinase, and undergoes further phosphorylation by deoxycytidine monophosphate kinase and nucleoside diphosphate kinase to yield lamivudine 5′-triphosphate, which is the active anabolite (Perry and Faulds, 1997) (Figure 59–3). Lamivudine is phosphorylated more efficiently in resting cells, which may explain its reduced potency in primary peripheral blood mononuclear cells as compared with cell lines (Gao et al., 1994). Lamivudine has low affinity for human DNA polymerases, explaining its low toxicity to the host.

High-level resistance to lamivudine occurs with single-amino-acid substitutions, M184V or M184I. These mutations can reduce *in vitro* sensitivity to lamivudine by up to 1000-fold (Perry and Faulds, 1997). The same mutations confer high-level cross-resistance to emtricitabine and a lesser degree of resistance to abacavir (Gallant et al., 2003). The M184V mutation restores zidovudine susceptibility in zidovudine-resistant HIV (Larder et al., 1995) and also partially restores tenofovir susceptibility in tenofovir-resistant HIV harboring the K65R mutation (Wainberg et al., 1999). The same K65R mutation confers resistance to lamivudine, emtricitabine, didanosine, stavudine, and abacavir.

HIV-1 isolates harboring the M184V mutation have increased transcriptional fidelity *in vitro* (Wainberg et al., 1996) and decreased replication capacity (Miller et al., 1999). Variants with the M184I mutation are even more impaired with regard to *in vitro* replication (Larder et al., 1995) and usually are replaced in lamivudine-treated patients by the M184V mutation. The reduced fitness of lamivudine-resistant viruses harboring these mutations, and their ability to prevent or partially reverse the effect of thymidine analog mutations, may contribute to the sustained virologic benefits of zidovudine and lamivudine combination therapy (Eron et al., 1995).

Lamivudine is used to treat HBV infection (Chapter 58), and some parallels in drug resistance are worth noting. High-level resistance to lamivudine occurs with a single mutation in the HBV DNA polymerase gene; as with HIV, this consists of a methionine-to-valine substitution (M2041V) in the enzyme active site. Resistance to lamivudine occurs in up to 90% of HIV/HBV co-infected patients after 4 years of treatment. However, virologic benefits persist in some treated patients harboring lamivudine-resistant HBV possibly because the mutated virus has substantially reduced replicative capacity (Leung et al., 2001).

Absorption, Distribution, and Elimination. The oral bioavailability of lamivudine is >80% and is not affected by food. Although lamivudine was marketed originally with a recommended dose of 150 mg twice daily based on the short plasma $t_{1/2}$ of the parent compound, the intracellular $t_{1/2}$ of lamivudine 5′-triphosphate is 12-18 hours, and the drug is now approved for use once daily at 300 mg (Moore et al., 1999).

Lamivudine is excreted primarily unchanged in the urine, and dose adjustment is recommended for patients with a creatinine clearance <50 mL/minute (Jayasekara et al., 1999). Lamivudine does not bind significantly to plasma proteins and freely crosses the placenta into the fetal circulation. Like zidovudine, lamivudine concentrations are higher in the male genital tract than in the peripheral circulation, suggesting active transport or trapping. Penetration to the CNS appears to be moderate, with a CSF-to-plasma concentration ratio of ≤0.15 (Perry and Faulds, 1997). The clinical significance of the low CSF penetration is unknown.

Untoward Effects. Lamivudine is one of the least toxic antiretroviral drugs and has few significant adverse effects.

Neutropenia, headache, and nausea have been reported at higher than recommended doses. Pancreatitis has been reported in pediatric patients, but this has not been confirmed in controlled trials of adults or children. Because lamivudine also has activity against HBV and substantially lowers plasma HBV DNA concentrations, caution is warranted in using this drug in patients co-infected with HBV or in HBV-endemic areas; discontinuation of lamivudine may be associated with a rebound of HBV replication and exacerbation of hepatitis.

Precautions and Interactions. Because lamivudine and emtricitabine have nearly identical resistance and activity patterns, there is no rationale for their combined use. Lamivudine is synergistic with most other nucleoside analogs *in vitro* (Perry and Faulds, 1997).

Therapeutic Use. Lamivudine (EPIVIR) is approved for HIV in adults and children ≥3 months of age.

In early monotherapy studies, initial declines in plasma HIV-1 RNA concentrations of up to 90% occurred within 14 days but rebounded rapidly with emergence of lamivudine-resistant HIV (Perry and Faulds, 1997). Patients randomized to the combination of lamivudine plus zidovudine had substantially better mean decreases in plasma HIV-1 RNA at 52 weeks (97% vs. 70% decrease in copies/mL) and increases in CD4+ lymphocyte counts (+61 versus −53 cells/mm^3) compared with those receiving zidovudine alone (Eron et al., 1995). In a large randomized double-blind trial, combining lamivudine with zidovudine or stavudine caused ~12-fold further decline in viral load at 24 weeks compared with zidovudine or stavudine monotherapy (Kuritzkes et al., 1999); in the same trial, combining lamivudine with didanosine conferred no additional benefits. Lamivudine has been effective in combination with other antiretroviral drugs in both treatment-naive and experienced patients (Perry and Faulds, 1997) and is a common component of therapy, given its safety, convenience, and efficacy.

Lamivudine (EPIVIR-HBV) also is approved for treatment of chronic hepatitis B.

Abacavir

Chemistry and Antiviral Activity. Abacavir is a synthetic carbocyclic purine analog (Figure 59–2).

Carbovir, a related guanine analog, was withdrawn from clinical development owing to poor oral bioavailability (Hervey and Perry, 2000). The IC_{50} of abacavir for primary clinical HIV-1 isolates is 0.26 μM, and its IC_{50} for laboratory strains ranges from 0.07 to 5.8 μM.

Mechanisms of Action and Resistance. Abacavir is the only approved antiretroviral that is active as a guanosine analog. It is initially monophosphorylated by adenosine phosphotransferase. The monophosphate is then converted to (−)-carbovir 3′-monophosphate, which is then phosphorylated to the di- and triphosphates by cellular kinases (Figure 59–3). Carbovir 5′-triphosphate terminates the elongation of proviral DNA because it is incorporated by reverse transcriptase into nascent DNA but lacks a 3′-hydroxyl group.

Clinical resistance to abacavir is associated with four specific codon substitutions: K65R, L74V, Y115F, and M184V (Gallant et al., 2003). Individually, these substitutions produce only modest (2- to 4-fold) resistance to abacavir, but in combination can reduce susceptibility by up to 10-fold. The Y115F mutation is seen uniquely with abacavir and causes low-level resistance. The L74V mutation is associated with cross-resistance to the purine analog didanosine. K65R confers cross-resistance to all nucleosides except zidovudine. An alternate pathway for abacavir resistance involves mutations at codons 41, 210, and 215, which have been associated with a reduced likelihood of virologic response. Abacavir sensitivity is greatly reduced by the multinucleoside resistance clusters, including that associated with the Q151M, as well as the 2-amino acid insertion following codon 69 (Gallant et al., 2003).

Absorption, Distribution, and Elimination. Abacavir's oral bioavailability is >80% regardless of food intake (Table 59–2). Abacavir is eliminated by metabolism to the 5′-carboxylic acid derivative catalyzed by alcohol dehydrogenase, and by glucuronidation to the 5′-glucuronide (Figure 59–3). These metabolites account for 30% and 36% of elimination, respectively (Hervey and Perry, 2000). Abacavir is not a substrate or inhibitor of CYPs. Abacavir is 50% bound to plasma proteins, and the CSF/plasma AUC ratio is ~0.3. Although the introduced dose of abacavir was 300 mg twice daily, carbovir triphosphate accumulates inside the cell and has a reported elimination $t_{1/2}$ of up to 21 hours (Hervey and Perry, 2000); thus a regimen of 600 mg once daily is approved now.

Untoward Effects. The most important adverse effect of abacavir is a unique and potentially fatal hypersensitivity syndrome. This syndrome is characterized by fever, abdominal pain, and other gastrointestinal (GI) complaints; a mild maculopapular rash; and malaise or fatigue. Respiratory complaints (cough, pharyngitis, dyspnea), musculoskeletal complaints, headache, and paresthesias are reported less commonly. Median time to onset of symptoms is 11 days, and 93% of cases occur within 6 weeks of initiating therapy (Hetherington et al., 2002). The presence of concurrent fever, abdominal pain, and rash within 6 weeks of starting abacavir is diagnostic and necessitates immediate discontinuation of the drug. Patients having only one of these symptoms may be observed to see if additional symptoms appear. Unlike many hypersensitivity syndromes, this condition worsens with continued treatment. *Abacavir can never be restarted once discontinued for hypersensitivity because reintroduction of the drug leads to rapid recurrence of severe symptoms, accompanied by hypotension, a shocklike state, and possibly death.* The reported mortality rate of restarting abacavir in sensitive individuals is 4% (Hervey and Perry, 2000).

Abacavir hypersensitivity occurs in 2-9% of patients depending on the population studied. The cause is a genetically mediated immune response linked to both the *HLA-B*5701* locus and the M493T allele in the heat-shock locus *Hsp70-Hom* (Mallal et al., 2008). The latter gene is implicated in antigen presentation, and this haplotype is associated with aberrant tumor necrosis factor-α release after exposure of human lymphocytes to abacavir *ex vivo*. This is one of the strongest pharmacogenetic associations ever described. In one white population, the combination of these two markers occurred in 94.4% of cases and <0.5% of controls for a positive predictive value of 93.8% and a negative predictive value of 99.5% (Mallal et al., 2008). *Abacavir should not be given to those with the HLA-B*5701 genotype*; in all others, the risk of true hypersensitivity is essentially zero (Mallal et al., 2008). Aside from hypersensitivity, abacavir is a well-tolerated drug. Carbovir 5′-triphosphate is a weak inhibitor of human DNA polymerases, including DNA polymerase-γ (Hervey and Perry, 2000). Abacavir therefore has not been associated with adverse events thought to be due to mitochondrial toxicity. Epidemiological associations link abacavir use and increased risk of myocardial infarction (D:A:D Study Group et al., 2008).

Precautions and Interactions. Abacavir is not associated with any clinically significant pharmacokinetic drug interactions. However, a large dose of ethanol (0.7 g/kg) increased the abacavir plasma AUC by 41% and prolonged the elimination $t_{1/2}$ by 26% (McDowell et al., 2000) possibly owing to competition for alcohol dehydrogenase.

Therapeutic Use. Abacavir (ZIAGEN) is approved for the treatment of HIV-1 infection, in combination with other antiretroviral agents. In initial monotherapy studies, abacavir reduced HIV plasma RNA concentrations up to 300 times more than that seen with other antiretroviral nucleosides, and it increased CD4+ lymphocyte counts by 80-200 cells/mm^3 (Hervey and Perry, 2000). Abacavir is not a more potent inhibitor of HIV replication than other nucleosides *in vitro*, and the mechanism for its more potent *in vivo* monotherapy activity is unexplained.

Abacavir is effective in combination with other nucleoside analogs, NNRTIs, and protease inhibitors. Adding abacavir to zidovudine and lamivudine resulted in a substantially greater decrease in plasma HIV-1 RNA than seen with the two-drug regimen of zidovudine plus lamivudine in adults or children (Hervey and Perry, 2000). Abacavir is available in a co-formulation with zidovudine and lamivudine (TRIZIVIR) for twice-daily dosing. However, the combination of abacavir, zidovudine, and lamivudine was less effective in a randomized, double-blind, placebo-controlled trial in treatment-naive patients than was the combination of zidovudine, lamivudine, and efavirenz or the four-drug regimen of zidovudine, lamivudine, abacavir, and efavirenz; 79% of patients in the abacavir, zidovudine, lamivudine group had undetectable plasma HIV RNA at 32 weeks as compared with 89% with the other regimens (Gulick et al., 2004).

Abacavir is available in a co-formulation with lamivudine (EPZICOM) for once-daily dosing, which is how it is most commonly used. Abacavir is approved for use in adult and pediatric patients ≥3 months of age, with dosing in the latter based on body weight.

Tenofovir

Chemistry and Antiviral Activity. Tenofovir disoproxil is a derivative of adenosine 5′-monophosphate lacking a complete ribose ring, and it is the only nucleotide analog currently marketed for the treatment of HIV infection (Figure 59–2).

Because the parent compound had very poor oral bioavailability, tenofovir is available only as the disoproxil prodrug, which substantially improves oral absorption and cellular penetration. Like lamivudine and emtricitabine, tenofovir is active against HIV-1, HIV-2, and HBV. The IC_{50} of tenofovir disoproxil against laboratory strains of HIV-1 ranges from 2 to 7 nM, making the prodrug ~100-fold more active *in vitro* than the parent compound (Chapman et al., 2003).

Mechanisms of Action and Resistance. Tenofovir disoproxil is hydrolyzed rapidly to tenofovir and then is phosphorylated by cellular kinases to its active metabolite, tenofovir diphosphate (which is actually a triphosphate: the parent drug is a monophosphate) (Figure 59–3). Tenofovir diphosphate is a competitive inhibitor of viral reverse transcriptases and is incorporated into HIV DNA to cause chain termination because it has an incomplete ribose ring. Although tenofovir diphosphate has broad-spectrum activity against viral DNA polymerases, it has low affinity for human DNA polymerases-α, -β, and -γ, which is the basis for its selective toxicity.

Specific resistance occurs with a single substitution at codon 65 of reverse transcriptase (K65R). This mutation reduces *in vitro* sensitivity by only 3- to 4-fold but has been associated with clinical failure of tenofovir-containing regimens (Chapman et al., 2003). Tenofovir sensitivity and virologic efficacy also are reduced in patients harboring HIV isolates with high-level resistance to zidovudine or stavudine, specifically those having three or more TAMs, including M41L or L120W. However, HIV variants that are resistant to zidovudine show only partial resistance to tenofovir, possibly reflecting less efficient excision of tenofovir diphosphate by pyrophosphorolysis (Naeger et al., 2002). The M184V mutation associated with lamivudine or emtricitabine resistance partially restores susceptibility in tenofovir-resistant HIV harboring the K65R mutation (Wainberg et al., 1999).

The K65R mutation was reported in only 2-3% of tenofovir-treated patients in initial clinical studies, and this mutation usually was not associated with treatment failure. Patients failing most tenofovir-containing regimens are more likely to harbor genotypic resistance to the other drugs in the regimen. Notable exceptions are once-daily combination regimens of three nucleosides, specifically tenofovir plus didanosine and lamivudine and tenofovir plus abacavir and lamivudine. Both of these regimens were associated with very high early rates of virologic failure or nonresponse, and at the time of failure, the K65R mutation was present in 36-64% of virus isolated from patients (Department of Health and Human Services, 2010); these combinations should be avoided.

Absorption, Distribution, and Elimination. Tenofovir disoproxil has an oral bioavailability of 25%. A high-fat meal increases the bioavailability to 39%, but the drug can be taken without regard to food (Chapman et al., 2003). Tenofovir is not bound significantly to plasma proteins. The plasma elimination $t_{1/2}$ ranges from 14 to 17 hours. The reported $t_{1/2}$ of intracellular tenofovir diphosphate is 11 hours in activated peripheral blood mononuclear cells and ≥49 hours in resting cells (Chapman et al., 2003). The drug therefore can be dosed once daily. Tenofovir undergoes both glomerular filtration and active tubular secretion. Following an intravenous dose, 70-80% of the drug is recovered unchanged in the urine. Doses should be decreased in those with renal insufficiency (Chapman et al., 2003).

Untoward Effects. Tenofovir generally is well tolerated, with few significant adverse effects reported except for flatulence.

In placebo-controlled double-blinded trials, the drug had no other adverse effects reported more frequently than with placebo after treatment for up to 24 weeks. Unlike the antiviral nucleotides adefovir and cidofovir (Chapter 58), tenofovir is not toxic to human renal tubular cells *in vitro* (Chapman et al., 2003). However, rare episodes of acute renal failure and Fanconi's syndrome have been reported with tenofovir, and this drug should be used with caution in patients with preexisting renal disease. Tenofovir use is associated with small declines in estimated creatinine clearance after months of treatment in some patients (Gallant and Moore, 2009), and because the dose needs to be reduced if renal insufficiency is present, renal function (creatinine and phosphorus) should be monitored regularly in patient taking this drug. Because tenofovir also has activity against HBV and may lower plasma HBV DNA concentrations, caution is warranted in using this drug in patients co-infected with HBV and in regions with high HBV seroprevalence because discontinuation of tenofovir may be associated with a rebound of HBV replication and exacerbation of hepatitis.

Precautions and Interactions. Tenofovir is not metabolized to a significant extent by CYPs and is not known to inhibit or induce these enzymes. However, tenofovir has been associated with a few potentially important pharmacokinetic drug interactions.

A 300-mg dose of tenofovir increased the didanosine AUC by 44-60%, probably as a consequence of inhibition of purine nucleoside phosphorylase by both tenofovir and tenofovir monophosphate (Robbins et al., 2003). These two drugs probably should not be used together; if the combination is essential, the dose of didanosine should be reduced from 400 to 250 mg/day (Chapman et al., 2003). Although tenofovir is not known to induce CYPs, it has been reported to reduce the atazanavir AUC by ~26%. In addition, low-dose ritonavir (100 mg twice daily) increases the mean tenofovir AUC by 34%, lopinavir/ritonavir increases the AUC by 32%, and atazanavir increases the tenofovir AUC by 25%. These interactions are most likely mediated by tenofovir's interaction with drug transport proteins.

Therapeutic Use. Tenofovir (VIREAD) is FDA approved for treating HIV infection in adults in combination with other antiretroviral agents.

The use of tenofovir in antiretroviral-experienced patients resulted in a further sustained decrease in HIV plasma RNA concentrations of 4.5-7.4-fold relative to placebo after 48 weeks of treatment (Chapman et al., 2003). Several large trials have confirmed the antiretroviral activity of tenofovir in three-drug regimens with other agents, including other nucleoside analogs, protease inhibitors, and/or NNRTIs. In a randomized double-blind comparison trial in which treatment-naive patients also received lamivudine and efavirenz, tenofovir 300 mg once daily was as effective and less toxic than stavudine 40 mg twice daily (Gallant et al., 2004). Tenofovir is also being investigated as a component of prophylactic regimens, including in the prevention of mother-to-child transmission, and it may have advantages over zidovudine in these settings (Foster et al., 2009).

Tenofovir is also approved for the treatment of chronic hepatitis B in adults.

Emtricitabine

Chemistry and Antiviral Activity. Emtricitabine is a cytidine analog chemically related to lamivudine and shares many of that drug's pharmacodynamic properties.

Like lamivudine, it has two chiral centers and is manufactured as the enantiomerically pure (2*R*,5*S*)-5-fluoro-1-[2-(hydroxymethyl)-1,3-oxathiolan-5-yl]cytosine (FTC) (Figure 59–2). Emtricitabine is active against HIV-1, HIV-2, and HBV. The IC_{50} of emtricitabine against laboratory strains of HIV-1 ranges from 2 to 530 nM, although, on average, the drug is ~10 times more active *in vitro* than lamivudine (Saag, 2006).

Mechanisms of Action and Resistance. Emtricitabine enters cells by passive diffusion and is phosphorylated by deoxycytidine kinase and cellular kinases to its active metabolite, emtricitabine 5′-triphosphate (Figure 59–3). Like lamivudine, emtricitabine has low affinity for human DNA polymerases, explaining its low toxicity to the host.

High-level resistance to emtricitabine occurs with the same mutations affecting lamivudine (mainly the methionine-to-valine substitution at codon 184), although these appear to occur less frequently with emtricitabine. In three studies, M184V/I occurred about half as frequently with emtricitabine-containing regimens as with lamivudine, and patients presenting with virologic failure were two to three times as likely to have wild-type virus at the time of failure as compared with lamivudine (Saag, 2006). The M184V mutation restores zidovudine susceptibility to zidovudine-resistant HIV and also partially restores tenofovir susceptibility to tenofovir-resistant HIV harboring the K65R mutation (Wainberg et al., 1999). The same K65R mutation confers resistance to emtricitabine and the other cytidine analog lamivudine, as well as didanosine, stavudine, and abacavir.

Absorption, Distribution, and Elimination. Emtricitabine is absorbed rapidly and has an oral bioavailability of 93%. Food reduces the C_{max} but does not affect the AUC, and the drug can be taken without regard to meals. Emtricitabine is not bound significantly to plasma proteins. Compared with other nucleoside analogs, the drug has a slow systemic clearance and long elimination $t_{1/2}$ of 8-10 hours (Saag, 2006). In addition, the estimated $t_{1/2}$ of the intracellular triphosphate is long, possibly up to 39 hours, providing the pharmacokinetic rationale for once-daily dosing. Emtricitabine is excreted primarily unchanged in the urine, undergoing glomerular filtration and active tubular secretion. The dose should be reduced in those with estimated creatinine clearances of <50 mL/minute.

Untoward Effects. Emtricitabine is one of the least toxic antiretroviral drugs and, like its chemical relative lamivudine, has few significant adverse effects and no effect on mitochondrial DNA *in vitro* (Saag, 2006).

Prolonged exposure has been associated with hyperpigmentation of the skin, especially in sun-exposed areas. Elevated hepatic transaminases, hepatitis, and pancreatitis have been reported, but these have occurred in association with other drugs known to cause these toxicities. Because emtricitabine also has *in vitro* activity against HBV, caution is warranted in using this drug in patients co-infected with HBV and in regions with high HBV seroprevalence; discontinuation of lamivudine, which is closely related to emtricitabine, has been associated with a rebound of HBV replication and exacerbation of hepatitis.

Precautions and Interactions. Emtricitabine is not metabolized to a significant extent by CYPs, and it is not susceptible to any known metabolic drug interactions. The possibility of a pharmacokinetic interaction involving renal tubular secretion, such as that between trimethoprim and lamivudine, has not been investigated for emtricitabine; the drug does not alter the pharmacokinetics of tenofovir.

Therapeutic Use. Emtricitabine (EMTRIVA) is FDA-approved for treating HIV infection in adults in combination with other antiretroviral agents. Emtricitabine is available co-formulated with tenofovir ± efavirenz.

Two small monotherapy trials showed that the maximal antiviral effect of emtricitabine (mean 1.9 log unit decrease in plasma HIV RNA concentration) was achieved with a dose of 200 mg/day. Several large trials have confirmed the antiretroviral activity of emtricitabine in three-drug regimens with other agents, including nucleoside or nucleotide analogs, protease inhibitors, and/or NNRTIs. In two randomized comparison studies, emtricitabine- and lamivudine-based triple-combination regimens had similar efficacy (Saag, 2006).

Didanosine

Chemistry and Antiviral Activity. Didanosine (2′,3′-dideoxyinosine; ddI) is a purine nucleoside analog active against HIV-1, HIV-2, and other retroviruses including HTLV-1 (Perry and Noble, 1999). Its IC_{50} against HIV-1 ranges from 10 nM in monocytes-macrophage cells, to 10 μM in lymphoblast cell lines. Didanosine has been supplanted by less toxic drugs.

Mechanisms of Action and Resistance. Didanosine is transported into cells by a nucleobase carrier and undergoes initial phosphorylation by 5′-nucleotidase and inosine 5′-monophosphate phosphotransferase (Dudley, 1995; Khoo et al., 2002). Didanosine 5′-monophosphate is then converted to dideoxyadenosine 5′-monophosphate by adenylosuccinate synthetase and adenylosuccinate lyase (Figure 59–3). Adenylate kinase and phosphoribosyl pyrophosphate synthetase produce dideoxyadenosine 5′-diphosphate, which is converted to the triphosphate by creatine kinase and phosphoribosyl pyrophosphate synthetase. Dideoxyadenosine 5′-triphosphate is the active anabolite of didanosine, which therefore functions as an antiviral adenosine analog. Dideoxyadenosine 5′-triphosphate terminates the elongation of proviral DNA because it is incorporated by reverse transcriptase into nascent HIV DNA but lacks a 3′-hydroxyl group.

Resistance to didanosine is associated with mutations at reverse transcriptase codons 65 and 74. The L74V substitution, which reduces susceptibility 5- to 26-fold *in vitro*, is seen most commonly in patients failing to respond to didanosine. Other nucleoside analog mutations, including thymidine analog mutations, can contribute to didanosine resistance even though the drug does not appear to select for these mutations *de novo*. The reverse transcriptase insertion mutations at codon 69 produce cross-resistance to all current nucleoside analogs, including didanosine (Gallant et al., 2003). The M184V mutation seen in response to emtricitabine and lamivudine reduces didanosine susceptibility *in vitro* but probably plays no role in clinical resistance to this drug.

Absorption, Distribution, and Elimination. Didanosine is acid labile and is degraded at low gastric pH (Dudley, 1995). An antacid buffer is used in some formulations to improve bioavailability. Chewable tablets contain calcium carbonate and magnesium hydroxide, whereas the powder form contains citrate–phosphate buffer. The pediatric powder formulation lacks buffer and is reconstituted with purified water and mixed with a liquid antacid preparation. Food decreases didanosine bioavailability (AUC) by ~55%, so all formulations of didanosine must be administered at least 30 minutes before or 2 hours after eating (Moreno et al., 2007). This complicates dosing of didanosine in combination with antiretroviral drugs that must be given with food, as is the case for most HIV protease inhibitors. The enzyme purine nucleoside phosphorylase (PNP) probably contributes to the presystemic clearance of didanosine because tenofovir, which inhibits PNP, greatly increases concentrations of orally administered didanosine (Robbins et al., 2003). PNP converts didanosine to hypoxanthine, which is ultimately converted to uric acid.

Peak plasma concentrations of didanosine are seen ~1 hour after oral administration of the chewable tablets or powder formulations and 2 hours after delayed-release capsules. The plasma elimination $t_{1/2}$ of parent drug is ~1.5 hours, but the estimated intracellular $t_{1/2}$ of dideoxyadenosine 5′-triphosphate is substantially longer, 25-40 hours (Moreno et al., 2007). As a result, didanosine can be administered once daily. Didanosine is excreted both by glomerular filtration and by tubular secretion and does not undergo metabolism to a significant degree. Drug doses therefore must be adjusted in patients with renal insufficiency or renal failure (Jayasekara et al., 1999). Didanosine is not protein bound to a significant degree. The cerebrospinal penetration of didanosine is less than that of zidovudine, with a CSF-to-plasma ratio of 0.2, but the clinical significance of this is unclear.

Untoward Effects. The most serious toxicities associated with didanosine include peripheral neuropathy and pancreatitis, both of which are thought to be a consequence of mitochondrial toxicity. Up to 20% of patients reported peripheral neuropathy in early clinical trials (Moreno et al., 2007). As with other dideoxynucleosides, peripheral neuropathy is more common with higher doses or concentrations of didanosine and is more prevalent in patients with underlying HIV-related neuropathy, low CD4 count, or in those receiving other neurotoxic drugs. Typically, this is a symmetrical distal sensory neuropathy that begins in the feet and lower extremities but may involve the hands as it progresses (stocking/glove distribution). Patients complain of pain, numbness, and tingling in the affected extremities. If the drug is stopped as soon as symptoms appear, the neuropathy will stabilize and should improve or resolve. However, irreversible neuropathy can occur with continued use. Retinal changes and optic neuritis also have been reported with didanosine, and patients should undergo periodic retinal examinations.

Acute pancreatitis is a rare but potentially fatal complication of didanosine. Acute pancreatitis is associated with higher doses and concentrations of didanosine but has occurred in up to 7% of patients using the recommended dose of 200 mg twice daily (Moreno et al., 2007). Pancreatitis is more common with advanced HIV disease, and other risk factors include a previous history of pancreatitis, alcohol or illicit drug use, and hypertriglyceridemia. Combining didanosine with stavudine, which is also associated with peripheral neuropathy and pancreatitis, increases the risk and severity of both toxicities (Havlir et al., 2001).

As with other dideoxynucleosides and zidovudine, serious hepatic toxicity—with or without steatosis, hepatomegaly, and lactic acidosis—occurs very rarely but can be fatal. Risk factors for the lactic acidosis-steatosis syndrome include female sex, obesity, and prolonged exposure to the drug (Tripuraneni et al., 2004).

Other reported adverse effects include elevated hepatic transaminases, headache, and asymptomatic hyperuricemia and portal hypertension. The impact of didanosine on heart attack risk is under review. Diarrhea is reported more frequently with didanosine than with other nucleoside analogs and has been attributed to the antacid in the buffered oral preparations (Moreno et al., 2007). Didanosine chewable tablets contain 36.5 mg phenylalanine and should be avoided in those with phenylketonuria. Buffered powder for oral solution contains 1.4 g sodium per packet and should be used cautiously in those on sodium-restricted diets.

Precautions and Interactions. Buffering agents included in didanosine formulations can interfere with the bioavailability of some co-administered drugs because of altered pH or chelation with cations in the buffer. For example, the ciprofloxacin AUC is decreased by up to 98% when given with didanosine, and concentrations of ketoconazole and itraconazole, whose absorption is pH dependent, also are diminished (Piscitelli and Gallicano, 2001). A 200-mg dose of buffered didanosine reduced the indinavir AUC by 84%. These interactions generally can be avoided by separating administration of didanosine from that of other agents by at least 2 hours after or 6 hours before the interacting drug. The enteric-coated formulation of didanosine does not alter ciprofloxacin or indinavir absorption.

Didanosine is excreted renally, and shared renal excretory mechanisms provide a basis for drug interactions. Oral ganciclovir can increase plasma didanosine concentrations approximately 2-fold and may be associated with an increase in didanosine toxicity. Allopurinol can increase the didanosine AUC more than 4-fold and is contraindicated. Tenofovir increases the didanosine AUC by 44-60% and also may increase the risk of didanosine toxicity. If these two drugs must be given together, it is recommended to decrease the didanosine dose from 400 to 250 mg once daily for patients >60 kg (Chapman et al., 2003). Methadone decreases the didanosine AUC by 57-63% (Rainey et al., 2000) possibly as a consequence of altered GI motility and delayed absorption, although this has not been associated with a higher risk of failing didanosine treatment.

Didanosine should be avoided in patients with a history of pancreatitis or neuropathy because the risk and severity of both complications increase. Co-administration of other drugs that cause pancreatitis or neuropathy also will increase the risk and severity of these symptoms. Ethambutol, isoniazid, vincristine, cisplatin, and pentamidine also should be avoided.

The combination of didanosine and hydroxyurea was used to exploit a beneficial interaction that creates a favorable intracellular ratio of concentrations of dideoxyadenosine 5′-triphosphate to deoxythymidine 5′-triphosphate (Frank et al., 2004). Although this combination may boost didanosine antiviral activity modestly, it also increases toxicity, producing peripheral neuropathy and fatal pancreatitis, and should be avoided (Havlir et al., 2001).

Therapeutic Use. Didanosine (VIDEX, VIDEX EC) is FDA-approved for adults and children with HIV infection in combination with other antiretroviral agents. Didanosine has long-term efficacy when combined with other nucleoside analogs and HIV protease inhibitors or NNRTIs. Didanosine as a component of combination therapy also has beneficial effects in infants and children (Moreno et al., 2007). However, this drug is no longer widely prescribed in the developed world because of the availability of other agents with less toxicity.

Zalcitabine

Zalcitabine (2′,3′-dideoxycytidine; ddC) is a synthetic cytidine analog reverse transcriptase inhibitor that is designated as an orphan drug for the treatment of advanced HIV infection. It is no longer marketed because of toxicity (mainly peripheral neuropathy) and the need for thrice daily dosing. It is active against HIV-1, HIV-2, and hepatitis B virus (HBV). For additional information on this drug, see the 11th edition of this book.

NON-NUCLEOSIDE REVERSE TRANSCRIPTASE INHIBITORS

Non-nucleoside reverse transcriptase inhibitors (NNRTIs) include a variety of chemical substrates that bind to a hydrophobic pocket in the p66 subunit of the HIV-1 reverse transcriptase. The NNRTI-binding pocket is not essential for the function of the enzyme and is distant from the active site. These compounds induce a conformational change in the three-dimensional structure of the enzyme that greatly reduces its activity, and thus they act as noncompetitive inhibitors. Unlike nucleoside and nucleotide reverse transcriptase inhibitors, these compounds do not require intracellular phosphorylation to attain activity. Because the binding site for NNRTIs is virus-strain-specific, the approved agents are active against HIV-1 but not HIV-2 or other retroviruses and should not be used to treat HIV-2 infection (Harris and Montaner, 2000). These compounds also have no activity against host cell DNA polymerases. The two most commonly used agents in this category, efavirenz and nevirapine, are quite potent and transiently decrease plasma HIV RNA concentrations by two orders of magnitude or more when used as sole agents (Havlir et al., 1995; Wei et al., 1995). The chemical structures of the four approved NNRTIs are shown in Figure 59–4, and their pharmacokinetic properties are summarized in Table 59–3.

All approved NNRTIs are eliminated from the body by hepatic metabolism. Nevirapine and delavirdine are primarily substrates for CYP3A4, whereas efavirenz is a substrate for CYPs 2B6 and 3A4, and etravirine is subject to mixed metabolism. The steady-state elimination half-lives of efavirenz and nevirapine range from 24 to 72 hours, allowing daily dosing. Efavirenz, etravirine, and nevirapine are moderately potent inducers of hepatic drug-metabolizing enzymes including CYP3A4, whereas delavirdine is mainly a CYP3A4 inhibitor. Pharmacokinetic drug interactions are thus an important consideration with this class of compounds and represent a potential toxicity.

All NNRTIs except etravirine are susceptible to high-level drug resistance caused by single-amino-acid changes in the NNRTI-binding pocket (usually in codons 103 or 181). Unlike nucleoside analogs or protease inhibitors, efavirenz or nevirapine can induce resistance and virologic relapse within a few days or weeks if given as monotherapy (Wei et al., 1995). Exposure to even a single dose of nevirapine in the absence of other antiretroviral drugs is associated with resistance mutations in up to one-third of patients (Eshleman et al., 2004). *These agents are potent and highly effective but must be combined with at least two other active agents to avoid resistance.*

The use of efavirenz or nevirapine in combination with other antiretroviral drugs is associated with favorable long-term suppression of viremia and elevation of CD4+ lymphocyte counts (Sheran, 2005). Efavirenz in particular is a common component of first regimens

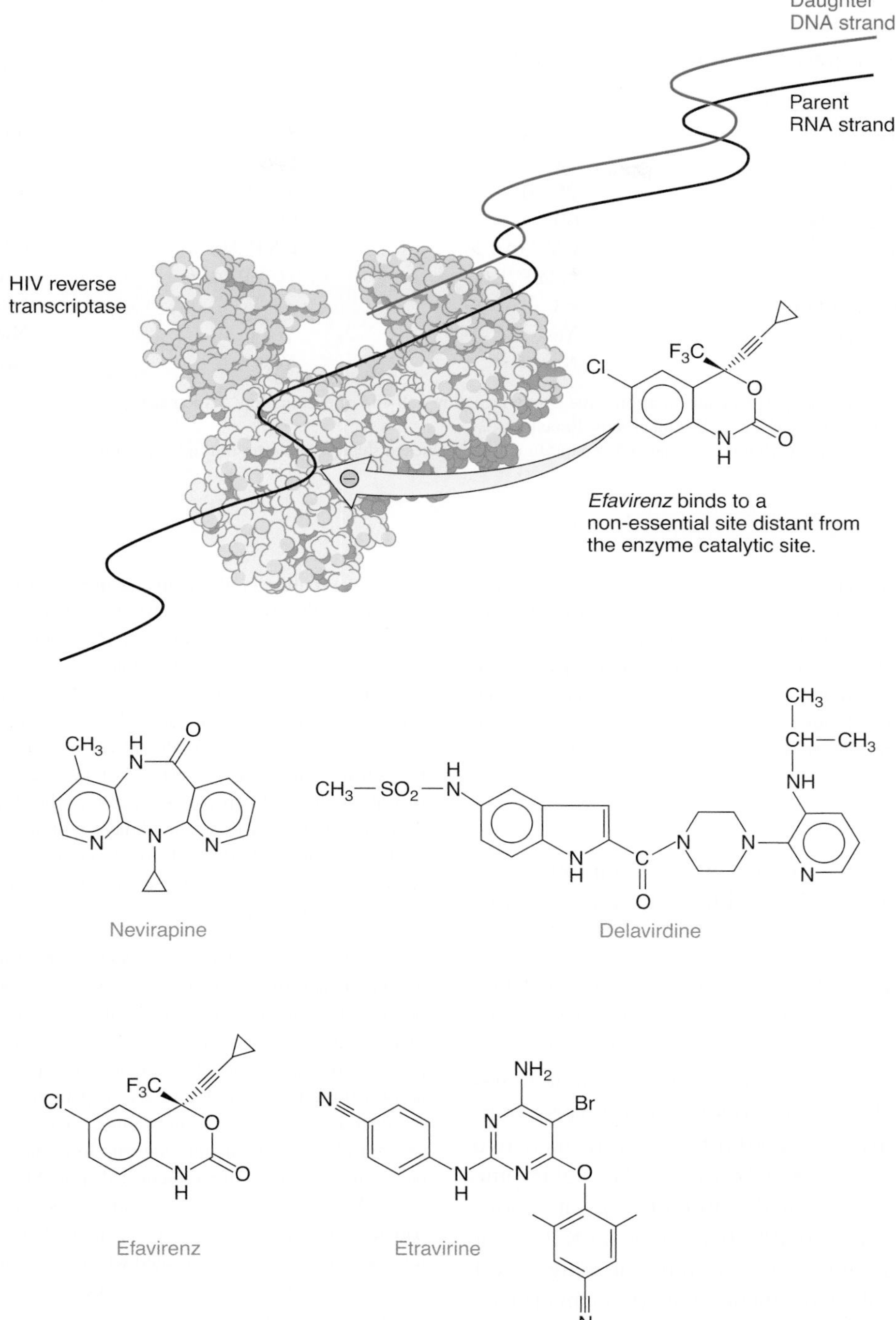

Figure 59–4. *Structures and mechanism of non-nucleoside reverse transcriptase inhibitors.*

Table 59–3

Pharmacokinetic Properties of Non-nucleoside Reverse Transcriptase Inhibitors[a]

PARAMETER	NEVIRAPINE[b]	EFAVIRENZ[b]	ETRAVIRINE
Oral bioavailability, %	90-93	50	NR
Effect of meals on *AUC*	↔	↑17-28%	↑33-102%
Plasma $t_{1/2}$, elim, h	25-30	40-55	41
Plasma protein binding, %	60	99	99.9
Metabolism	CYP3A4 > CYP2B6	CYP2B6 > CYP3A4	CYP3A4, 2C9, 2C19, UGT
Renal excretion of parent drug, %	<3	<3	1%
Autoinduction of metabolism	Yes	Yes	NR
Inhibition of CYP3A	No	Yes	No

ABBREVIATIONS: *AUC*, area under plasma concentration–time curve; $t_{1/2}$, elim, half-life of elimination; ↑, increase; ↓, decrease; ↔, no effect; NR, not reported; CYP, cytochrome P450; UGT, UDP-glucuronosyltransferase.
[a]Reported mean values in adults with normal renal and hepatic function. [b]Values at steady state after multiple oral doses.

for treatment-naive patients in recognition of its convenience, tolerability, and potency. Rashes occur frequently with all NNRTIs, usually during the first 4 weeks of therapy. These generally are mild and self-limited, although rare cases of potentially fatal Stevens-Johnson syndrome have been reported with nevirapine, efavirenz, and etravirine. Fat accumulation can be seen after long-term use of NNRTIs (Calmy et al., 2009), and fatal hepatitis has been associated with nevirapine use.

Nevirapine

Chemistry and Antiviral Activity. Nevirapine is a dipyridodiazepinone NNRTI with potent activity against HIV-1 (Figure 59–4).

The *in vitro* IC_{50} of this drug ranges from 10 to 100 nM. Like other compounds in this class, nevirapine does not have significant activity against HIV-2 or other retroviruses (Sheran, 2005).

Mechanisms of Action and Resistance. A single mutation at either codon 103 or codon 181 of reverse transcriptase decreases susceptibility by more than two orders of magnitude (Kuritzkes, 2004). Nevirapine resistance is also associated with mutations at codons 100, 106, 108, 188, and 190, but either the K103N or the Y181C mutation is sufficient to produce high-level resistance and clinical treatment failure (Eshleman et al., 2004). *Cross-resistance extends to efavirenz and delavirdine, and any patient who fails treatment with this NNRTI should not be treated with those drugs.*

Absorption, Distribution, and Elimination. Nevirapine is well absorbed, and its bioavailability is not altered by food or antacids. The drug readily crosses the placenta and has been found in breast milk, a feature that has encouraged use of nevirapine for prevention of mother-to-child transmission of HIV (Mirochnick et al., 1998).

Nevirapine is eliminated mainly by oxidative metabolism involving CYP3A4 and CYP2B6. Less than 3% of the parent drug is eliminated unchanged in the urine. Nevirapine has a long elimination $t_{1/2}$ of 25-30 hours at steady state, but $t_{1/2}$ may be longer in some individuals, especially those of African descent (Sheran, 2005). The drug is a moderate inducer of CYPs, including CYP3A4; thus the drug induces its own metabolism, which decreases the $t_{1/2}$ from 45 hours following the first dose to 25-30 hours after 2 weeks. To compensate for this, it is recommended that the drug be initiated at a dose of 200 mg once daily for 14 days, with the dose then increased to 200 mg twice daily if no adverse reactions have occurred. Clinical studies of nevirapine have investigated once-daily use, but this dosing regimen is not approved.

Untoward Effects. The most frequent adverse event associated with nevirapine is rash, which occurs in ~16% of patients. Mild macular or papular eruptions commonly involve the trunk, face, and extremities and generally occur within the first 6 weeks of therapy. Pruritus is also common. In most patients the rash resolves with continued administration of drug. Up to 7% of patients discontinue therapy owing to rash; administration of glucocorticoids may cause a more severe rash. Life-threatening Stevens-Johnson syndrome is rare but occurs in up to 0.3% of recipients (Sheran, 2005).

Elevated hepatic transaminases occur in up to 14% of patients. Clinical hepatitis occurs in up to 1% of patients. Severe and fatal hepatitis has been associated with nevirapine use, and this may be more common in women with CD4 counts >250 cells/mm^3, especially during pregnancy (Sheran, 2005). Other reported side effects include fever, fatigue, headache, somnolence, and nausea.

Precautions and Interactions. Because nevirapine induces CYP3A4, this drug may lower plasma concentrations of co-administered CYP3A4 substrates. Methadone withdrawal has been reported in patients receiving nevirapine, presumably as a consequence of enhanced methadone clearance. Plasma ethinyl estradiol and norethindrone concentrations decrease by 20% with nevirapine, and alternative methods of birth control are advised.

Therapeutic Use. Nevirapine (VIRAMUNE) is FDA approved for the treatment of HIV-1 infection in adults and children in combination with other antiretroviral agents.

In original monotherapy studies, a rapid fall in plasma HIV RNA concentrations of ≥99% was followed by a return toward baseline within 8 weeks because of rapid emergence of resistance (Havlir et al., 1995; Wei et al., 1995). *Nevirapine should never be used as a single agent or as the sole addition to a failing regimen.* Nevirapine is approved for use in infants and children ≥15 days old, with dosing based on body surface area.

Single-dose nevirapine has been used commonly in pregnant HIV-infected women to prevent mother-to-child transmission. A single oral intrapartum dose of 200 mg nevirapine followed by a single dose given to the newborn reduced neonatal HIV infection to 13% compared with 21.5% infection with a more complicated zidovudine regimen (Sheran, 2005). Although this regimen is very inexpensive and generally well tolerated, the high prevalence of nevirapine resistance following the single oral dose (Eshleman et al., 2004), coupled with the recent recognition of fatal nevirapine hepatitis, has prompted a reexamination of the role this regimen should play in the prevention of vertical transmission (Department of Health and Human Services, 2010).

Efavirenz

Chemistry and Antiviral Activity. Efavirenz is a 1,4-dihydro-2H-3,1-benzoxazin-2-one NNRTI (Figure 59–4) with potent activity against HIV-1. The *in vitro* IC_{50} of this drug ranges from 3 to 9 nM (Sheran, 2005). Like other compounds in this class, efavirenz does not have significant activity against HIV-2 or other retroviruses.

Mechanisms of Resistance. The most common efavirenz resistance mutation seen clinically is at codon 103 of reverse transcriptase (K103N), and this decreases susceptibility up to ≥100-fold (Kuritzkes, 2004). Additional resistance mutations have been seen at codons 100, 106, 108, 181, 188, 190, and 225, but either the K103N or Y181C mutation is sufficient to produce clinical treatment failure. Cross-resistance extends to nevirapine and delavirdine.

Absorption, Distribution, and Elimination. Efavirenz is well absorbed from the GI tract and reaches peak plasma concentrations within 5 hours. There is diminished absorption of the drug with increasing doses. Bioavailability (AUC) is increased by 22% with a high-fat meal.

Efavirenz is >99% bound to plasma proteins and, as a consequence, has a low CSF-to-plasma ratio of 0.01. The clinical significance of this low CNS penetration is unclear, especially because the major toxicities of efavirenz involve the CNS. The drug should be taken initially on an empty stomach at bedtime to reduce side effects (Sheran, 2005).

Efavirenz is cleared *via* oxidative metabolism, mainly by CYP2B6 and to a lesser extent by CYP3A4. The parent drug is not excreted renally to a significant degree. Efavirenz is cleared slowly, with an elimination $t_{1/2}$ of 40-55 hours at steady state. This safely allows once-daily dosing. Clearance is even slower in recipients with the 516G→T and 983C→T CYP 2B6 genotype (Haas et al., 2009), a common polymorphism in those of Japanese and African ancestry.

Untoward Effects. The most important adverse effects of efavirenz involve the CNS. Up to 53% of patients report some CNS or psychiatric side effects, but <5% discontinue the drug for this reason. CNS symptoms may occur with the first dose and last for hours; more severe symptoms may require weeks to resolve. Patients commonly report dizziness, impaired concentration, dysphoria, vivid or disturbing dreams, and insomnia. Episodes of frank psychosis (depression, hallucinations, and/or mania) have been associated with initiating efavirenz. Fortunately, CNS side effects generally become more tolerable and resolve within the first 4 weeks of therapy.

Rash occurs frequently with efavirenz, in up to 27% of adult patients (Sheran, 2005). Rash usually occurs within the first few weeks of treatment but resolves spontaneously and rarely requires drug discontinuation. Life-threatening skin eruptions such as Stevens-Johnson syndrome have been reported during postmarketing experience with efavirenz but are rare.

Other side effects reported with efavirenz include headache, increased hepatic transaminases, and elevated serum cholesterol. False-positive urine screening tests for marijuana metabolites also can occur depending on the assay used (Sheran, 2005).

Efavirenz is the only antiretroviral drug that is unequivocally teratogenic in primates. When efavirenz was administered to pregnant cynomolgus monkeys, 25% of fetuses developed malformations. In 13 known cases where women were exposed to efavirenz during the first trimester of pregnancy, fetuses or infants had significant malformations, mainly of the brain and spinal cord. *Women of childbearing potential therefore should use two methods of birth control and avoid pregnancy while taking efavirenz.*

Precautions and Interactions. Efavirenz is a moderate inducer of hepatic enzymes, especially CYP3A4, but also a weak to moderate CYP inhibitor; because of the drug's long $t_{1/2}$, there is no need to alter drug dose during the first few weeks of treatment.

Efavirenz decreases concentrations of phenobarbital, phenytoin, and carbamazepine; the methadone AUC is reduced by 33-66% at steady state. Rifampin concentrations are unchanged by concurrent efavirenz, but rifampin may reduce efavirenz concentrations slightly. Efavirenz reduces the rifabutin AUC by 38% on average. Efavirenz has a variable effect on HIV protease inhibitors. Indinavir, saquinavir, and amprenavir concentrations are reduced, but ritonavir and nelfinavir concentrations are increased. Drugs that induce CYPs 2B6 or 3A4 (e.g., phenobarbital, phenytoin, and carbamazepine) would be expected to increase the clearance of efavirenz and should be avoided (Sheran, 2005).

Therapeutic Use. Efavirenz (SUSTIVA) was the first antiretroviral agent approved by the FDA for once-daily administration. Initial short-term monotherapy studies showed substantial decreases in plasma HIV RNA, but the drug should only be used in combination with other effective agents and should not be added as the sole new agent to a failing regimen. Efavirenz has also been effective in patients who have failed previous antiretroviral therapy not containing an NNRTI (Sheran, 2005).

Efavirenz is used widely in the developed world because of its convenience, effectiveness, and long-term tolerability. Especially popular is the once-daily single pill co-formulation of efavirenz, tenofovir, and emtrictabine (ATRIPLA). To date, no antiretroviral regimen has produced better long-term treatment responses than efavirenz-containing regimens in randomized prospective clinical trials. As a result, efavirenz plus two nucleoside reverse transcriptase inhibitors remains a preferred regimen for treatment-naive patients. Generic versions of efavirenz are increasingly used in treatment regimens in resource-poor countries because of this drug's better toxicity profile compared to nevirapine. Efavirenz can be safely combined with rifampin and is useful in patients also being treated for tuberculosis.

Efavirenz is approved for adult and pediatric patients ≥3 years of age and weighing at least 10 kg. Efavirenz is only available as tablets and capsules; pediatric dosing is based on weight range.

Etravirine

Chemistry and Antiviral Activity. Etravirine is a diarylpyrimidine NNRTI that is active against HIV-1 (Figure 59–4). The IC_{50} for HIV-1 in various *in vitro* assays ranges from 1 to 5 nM, but like other NNRTIs, etravirine has no activity against HIV-2 (Deeks and Keating, 2008).

Mechanisms of Action and Resistance. Etravirine is unique in its ability to inhibit reverse transcriptase that is resistant to other available NNRTIs. Specifically, activity of the drug is not affected by the K103N, Y181C, or Y188L mutations or the K103N/Y181C double mutations that confer high-level resistance to efavirenz, nevirapine, and delavirdine.

Etravirine appears to have conformational and positional flexibility in the NNRTI binding pocket that allow it to inhibit the function of the HIV-1 reverse transcriptase in the presence of common NNRTI resistance mutations (Deeks and Keating, 2008). Clinically significant drug resistance and treatment failure require the presence of multiple mutations, including V90I, A98G, L100I, K101E/P, V106I, V179D/F, Y181C/I/V, and G190A/S. Best response to an etravirine-containing regimen is seen in patients harboring three or fewer resistance mutations, although likelihood of virologic benefit decreases with each additional mutation. One limitation of etravirine resistance data is that most information comes from patients also receiving darunavir, and few resistance and response data are available for other regimens (Fulco and McNicholl, 2009).

Absorption, Distribution, and Elimination. Etravirine is absorbed rapidly after oral administration with peak concentrations occurring 2.5-4 hours after dosing. Food increases the etravirine AUC by 50% (Deeks and Keating, 2008), and it is therefore recommended that the drug be administered with food. Methyl- and dimethyl-hydroxylated metabolites are produced in the liver primarily by CYPs 3A4, 2C9, and 2C19, accounting for most of the elimination of this drug. No unchanged drug is detected in the urine. The terminal elimination $t_{1/2}$ is ~41 hours; twice-daily dosing of this drug is the historical consequence of enormous pill burdens from older formulations that are no longer in use, and it is likely that the drug could be given once daily (Deeks and Keating, 2008). Etravirine is 99% bound to plasma proteins, mainly to albumin and α_1-acid glycoprotein.

Untoward Effects. In randomized placebo-controlled trials combining etravirine with darunavir in treatment-experienced patients, the only side effect occurring more commonly with etravirine than with placebo was rash (17% versus 9%), usually occurring within a few weeks of starting therapy and resolving within 1-3 weeks. Overall, 2% of patients in these trials discontinued etravirine because of rash. Severe rash including Stevens-Johnson syndrome and toxic epidermal necrolysis have been reported. Etravirine was not associated with more neuropsychiatric or hepatic adverse effects than placebo (Deeks and Keating, 2008).

Precautions and Interactions. Etravirine is an inducer of CYP3A4 and glucuronosyl transferases, and an inhibitor of CYPs 2C9 and 2C19, and can therefore be involved in a number of clinically significant pharmacokinetic drug interactions.

Etravirine can be combined with darunavir/ritonavir, lopinavir/ritonavir, and saquinavir/ritonavir without the need for dose adjustments. The dose of maraviroc should be doubled to 600 mg twice daily when these two drugs are combined. Etravirine should not be administered with tipranavir/ritonavir, fosamprenavir/ritonavir, or atazanavir/ritonavir in the absence of better data to guide dosing. Etravirine should not be combined with efavirenz, nevirapine, or delavirdine. Unlike other NNRTIs, etravirine does not appear to alter the clearance of methadone (Fulco and McNicholl, 2009).

Therapeutic Use. Etravirine (INTELENCE) is approved for use only in treatment-experienced HIV-infected adults. NNRTI-experienced patients should not receive etravirine plus NRTIs alone. Etravirine has not yet been approved for pediatric use.

In a pooled analysis of >1200 treatment-experienced patients taking darunavir/ritonavir, 61% of patients randomized to etravirine achieved a plasma HIV RNA <50 copies/mL at 48 weeks compared to 40% on placebo ($p < 0.0001$). Etravirine-treated patients also had a moderately better mean CD4 cell count increase at week 48 (98 vs. 73 cells/mm^3). Week 48 virologic responses were dependent on the number of baseline etravirine-resistance mutations, with a differential versus placebo of 75% versus 44% if no mutations were present, falling to 25% versus 17% if four or more were present (Fulco and McNicholl, 2009). In small studies, virologic response with etravirine was poor unless the regimen contained at least one other active antiretroviral.

Delavirdine

Delavirdine is a bisheteroarylpiperazine NNRTI that selectively inhibits HIV-1 (Figure 59–4). The *in vitro* IC_{50} ranges from 6 to 30 nM for laboratory HIV-1 isolates to 1 to 700 nM for clinical isolates (Scott and Perry, 2000). Delavirdine (RESCRIPTOR) is no longer used widely because of its short $t_{1/2}$ and requirement for thrice-daily dosing.

Delavirdine does not have significant activity against HIV-2 or other retroviruses. Delavirdine shares resistance mutations with efavirenz and nevirapine, and any patient who fails treatment with this NNRTI should not be treated with those drugs.

Delavirdine is well absorbed, especially at pH<2. Antacids, histamine H_2-receptor antagonists, proton pump inhibitors, and achlorhydria may decrease its absorption. Standard meals do not alter the delavirdine AUC, and the drug can be administered irrespective of food. The drug may have nonlinear pharmacokinetics because the plasma $t_{1/2}$ increases with increasing doses (Scott and Perry, 2000). Delavirdine clearance is primarily through oxidative metabolism by CYP3A4, with <5% of a dose recovered unchanged in the urine. At the recommended dose of 400 mg three times daily, the mean elimination $t_{1/2}$ is 5.8 hours (range: 2-11 hours because of the considerable interpatient variability in clearance).

As with all drugs in this class, the most common side effect of delavirdine is rash, which occurs in 18-36% of subjects. Rash usually is seen in the first few weeks of treatment and often resolves despite continued therapy. Severe dermatitis, including erythema multiforme and Stevens-Johnson syndrome, has been reported but is rare. Elevated hepatic transaminases and hepatic failure also have been reported. Neutropenia also may occur rarely (Scott and Perry, 2000).

Delavirdine is both a substrate for and an inhibitor of CYP3A4 and can alter the metabolism of other CYP3A4 substrates. Potent inducers of CYP3A4, such as carbamazepine, phenobarbital, phenytoin, rifabutin, and rifampin, may decrease delavirdine concentrations and should be avoided. Delavirdine increases the plasma concentrations of most HIV protease inhibitors (Scott and Perry, 2000).

Initial monotherapy studies with delavirdine produced only transient decreases in plasma HIV RNA concentrations owing to rapid emergence of resistance. Later studies of delavirdine in combination with nucleoside analogs showed sustained decreases in HIV-1 RNA.

HIV PROTEASE INHIBITORS

HIV protease inhibitors are peptide-like chemicals that competitively inhibit the action of the virus aspartyl protease (Figure 59–5). This protease is a homodimer consisting of two 99-amino acid monomers; each monomer contributes an aspartic acid residue that is essential for catalysis (Flexner, 1998). The preferred cleavage site for this enzyme is the N-terminal side of proline residues, especially between phenylalanine and proline. Human aspartyl proteases (i.e., renin, pepsin, gastricsin, and cathepsins D and E) contain only one polypeptide chain and are not significantly inhibited by HIV protease inhibitors.

These drugs prevent proteolytic cleavage of HIV gag and pol precursor polypeptides that include essential structural (p17, p24, p9, and p7) and enzymatic (reverse transcriptase, protease, and integrase) components of the virus. This prevents the metamorphosis of HIV virus particles into their mature infectious form (Flexner, 1998). Infected patients treated with HIV protease inhibitors as sole agents experienced a 100- to 1000-fold mean decrease in plasma HIV RNA concentrations within 12 weeks, an effect similar in magnitude to that produced by NNRTIs (Ho et al., 1995).

The pharmacokinetic properties of HIV protease inhibitors are characterized by high interindividual variability, which may reflect differential activity of intestinal and hepatic CYPs (Flexner, 1998). Clearance is mainly through hepatic oxidative metabolism. All except nelfinavir are metabolized predominantly by CYP3A4 (and nelfinavir's major metabolite is cleared by CYP3A4). Elimination half-lives of the HIV protease inhibitors range from 1.8 to 10 hours (Table 59–4), and most of these drugs can be dosed once or twice daily. Most HIV protease inhibitors are highly protein bound in plasma, and adding plasma proteins will increase their *in vitro* IC_{50} (Molla et al., 1998). Fractional penetration into the CSF is also low for most of these agents, although the clinical significance is unknown.

An important toxicity common to all approved HIV protease inhibitors is the potential for metabolic drug interactions. Most of these drugs inhibit CYP3A4 at clinically achieved concentrations, although the magnitude of inhibition varies greatly, with ritonavir by far the most potent (Piscitelli and Gallicano, 2001). It is now a common practice to combine HIV protease inhibitors with a low dose of ritonavir to take advantage of that drug's remarkable capacity to inhibit CYP3A4 metabolism (Flexner, 2000).

Although the approved dose of ritonavir for antiretroviral treatment is 600 mg twice daily, doses of 100 or 200 mg once or twice daily are sufficient to inhibit CYP3A4 and increase ("boost") the concentrations of most concurrently administered CYP3A4 substrates. Lower doses of ritonavir are much better tolerated. The enhanced pharmacokinetic profile of HIV protease inhibitors administered with ritonavir reflects inhibition of both first-pass and systemic clearance, resulting in improved oral bioavailability and a longer elimination $t_{1/2}$ of the co-administered drug. This allows a reduction in both drug dose and dosing frequency while increasing systemic concentrations (Flexner, 2000). Combinations of darunavir, lopinavir, fosamprenavir, and atazanavir with ritonavir are approved for once-daily administration.

Most HIV protease inhibitors are substrates for the P-glycoprotein efflux pump (P-gp) (Chapter 5).

P-gp in capillary endothelial cells of the blood-brain barrier limits the penetration of HIV protease inhibitors into the brain (Kim et al., 1998), although the low CSF-to-plasma drug concentration ratio characteristic of these drugs also may reflect extensive binding to plasma proteins. Most HIV protease inhibitors penetrate less well into semen than do nucleoside reverse transcriptase inhibitors and NNRTIs. Virologic responses in plasma, CSF, and semen usually are concordant (Taylor et al., 1999), and the clinical significance of P-gp and protein-binding effects is unclear.

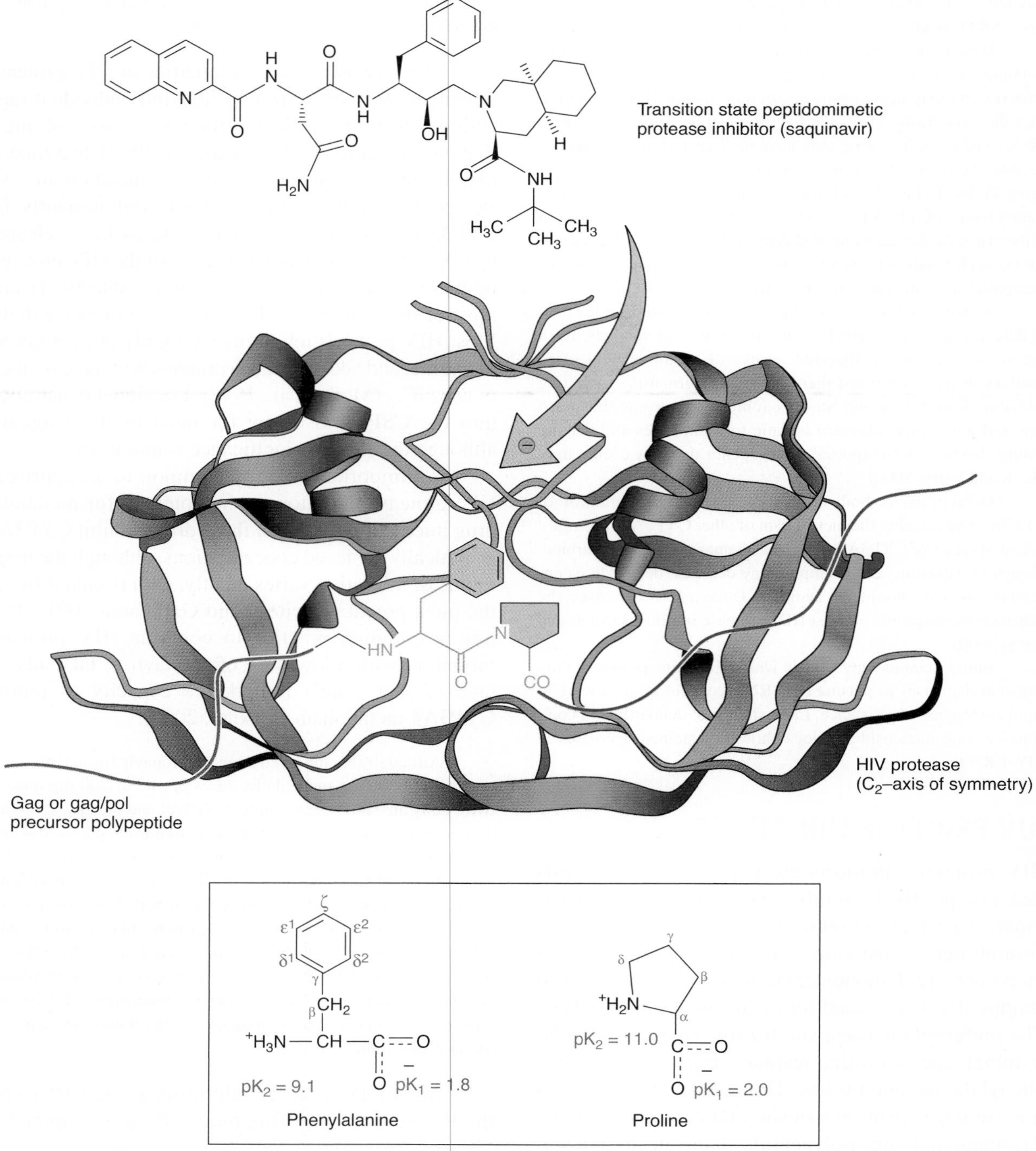

Figure 59–5. *Mechanism of action of an HIV protease inhibitor.* Shown here is a phenylalanine-proline target peptide sequence (in blue) for the protease enzyme (in golden brown) with chemical structures of the native amino acids (in lower box) to emphasize homology of their structures to that of saquinavir (at top).

Table 59–4

Pharmacokinetic Properties of HIV-1 Protease Inhibitors[a]

PARAMETER	SAQUINAVIR[b]	INDINAVIR	RITONAVIR	NELFINAVIR	FOSAMPRENAVIR	LOPINAVIR[c]	ATAZANAVIR	TIPRANAVIR	DARUNAVIR
Oral bioavailability, %	13	60-65	>60	20-80 (formulation- and food-dependent)	ND	ND	ND	ND	82
Effect of meals on *AUC*	↑570% (high fat)	↓77% (high fat)	↑13% (capsule)	↑100–200%	↔	↑27% (moderate fat)	↑70% (light meal)	↔	↑30%
Plasma $t_{1/2}$, h	1-2	1.8	3-5	3.5-5	7.7	5-6	6.5-7.9	4.8-6.0	15
Plasma protein binding, %	98	60	98-99	>98	90	98-99	86	99.9	95
Metabolism	CYP3A4	CYP3A4	CYP3A4 > CYP2D6	CYP2C19 > CYP3A4	CYP3A4	CYP3A4	CYP3A4	CYP3A4	CYP3A4
Autoinduction of metabolism	No	No	Yes	Yes	No	Yes	No	Yes	ND
Renal excretion of parent drug, %	<3	9-12	3.5	1-2	1	<3	7	0.5	8
Inhibition of CYP3A4	+	++	+++	++	++	+++	++	+++	+++

ABBREVIATIONS: *AUC* area under plasma concentration–time curve; $t_{1/2}$ half-life of elimination; ↑, increase; ↓, decrease; ↔, no effect; CYP, cytochrome P450; ND, not determined; +, weak; ++, moderate; +++, substantial. [a]Reported mean values in adults with normal renal and hepatic function. [b]Parameters reported for the saquinavir soft-gel capsule formulation. [c]Values for lopinavir, tipranavir, and darunavir reflect coadministration with ritonavir.

GI side effects including nausea, vomiting, and diarrhea are common, although symptoms generally resolve within 4 weeks of starting treatment.

The speed with which HIV develops resistance to unboosted protease inhibitors is intermediate between that of nucleoside analogs and NNRTIs. In initial monotherapy studies, the median time to rebound in HIV plasma RNA concentrations of one log or greater was 3-4 months (Flexner, 1998). In contrast to NNRTIs, high-level resistance to these drugs generally requires accumulation of a minimum of four to five codon substitutions, which may take many months.

Initial (primary) resistance mutations in the enzymatic active site confer only a 3- to 5-fold drop in sensitivity to most drugs; these are followed by secondary mutations often distant from the active site that compensate for the reduction in proteolytic efficiency. Accumulation of secondary resistance mutations increases the likelihood of cross-resistance to other PIs (Flexner, 1998; Kuritzkes, 2004). Patients failing boosted PI-based combination regimens are more likely to have resistance mutations to the other drugs in the regimen, especially NRTIs (Kuritzkes, 2004), suggesting a high genetic barrier to resistance.

With potent activity and favorable resistance profiles, these drugs are a common component of regimens for treatment-experienced patients. However, the virologic benefits of these drugs must be balanced against short- and long-term toxicities, including the risk of insulin resistance and lipodystrophy (Garg, 2004). Improvements in pill burden, convenience, and tolerability have greatly improved adherence to drugs in this class (Gardner et al., 2009).

Saquinavir

Chemistry and Antiviral Activity. Saquinavir, the first approved HIV protease inhibitor, is a peptidomimetic hydroxyethylamine (Figure 59–6). It is a transition-state analog of a phenylalanine-proline cleavage site in one of the native substrate sequences for the HIV aspartyl protease and was the product of a rational drug-design program (Roberts et al., 1990). Saquinavir inhibits both HIV-1 and HIV-2 replication and has an *in vitro* IC_{50} in peripheral blood lymphocytes that ranges from 3.5 to 10 nM (Noble and Faulds, 1996).

Mechanisms of Resistance. As is typical of HIV protease inhibitors, high-level resistance requires accumulation of multiple resistance mutations.

The primary saquinavir resistance mutation occurs at HIV protease codon 90 (a leucine-to-methionine substitution), although primary resistance also has been reported with a glycine-to-valine substitution at codon 48. Secondary resistance mutations occur at codons 36, 46, 82, 84, and others, and these are associated with clinical saquinavir resistance as well as cross-resistance to most other HIV protease inhibitors (Noble and Faulds, 1996).

Absorption, Distribution, and Elimination. Fractional oral bioavailability is low (~4%) owing mainly to extensive first-pass metabolism (Flexner, 1998), and so this drug should always be given in combination with ritonavir. Low doses of ritonavir increase the saquinavir steady-state AUC by 20- to 30-fold (Flexner, 2000), allowing administration once or twice daily.

Substances that inhibit intestinal but not hepatic CYP3A4, such as grapefruit juice, increase the saquinavir AUC by 3-fold at most (Flexner, 2000). Saquinavir is metabolized primarily by intestinal and hepatic CYP3A4 (Fitzsimmons and Collins, 1997); its metabolites are not known to be active against HIV-1. The parent drug and its metabolites are eliminated through the biliary system and feces (>95% of drug), with minimal urinary excretion (<3%).

Untoward Effects. The most frequent side effects of saquinavir are GI: nausea, vomiting, diarrhea, and abdominal discomfort. Most side effects of saquinavir are mild and short lived, although long-term use is associated with lipodystrophy.

Precautions and Interactions. Saquinavir clearance is increased with CYP3A4 induction; thus, co-administration of inducers of CYP3A4 such as rifampin, phenytoin, or carbamazepine lowers saquinavir concentrations and should be avoided (Flexner, 1998). The effect of nevirapine or efavirenz on saquinavir may be partially or completely reversed with ritonavir. Most drug interactions seen with saquinavir/ritonavir reflect the effect of the boosting agent.

Therapeutic Use. Saquinavir is available as a hard-gelatin capsule (INVIRASE). In initial clinical trials, unboosted saquinavir at the approved dose (600 mg three times daily) produced only modest virologic benefit because of its poor oral bioavailability. When combined with ritonavir and nucleoside analogs, saquinavir produces viral load reductions comparable with those of other HIV protease inhibitor regimens (Flexner, 2000). Saquinavir is no longer widely prescribed in the developed world because of its relatively high pill burden, but the drug remains popular as a generic combined with ritonavir in resource-limited settings because of its favorable toxicity and efficacy profile.

Ritonavir

Chemistry and Antiviral Activity. Ritonavir is a peptidomimetic HIV protease inhibitor designed to complement the C_2 axis of symmetry of the enzyme active site (Flexner, 1998) (Figure 59–5). Ritonavir is active against both HIV-1 and HIV-2, although it may be slightly less active against the latter. Its IC_{50} for wild-type HIV-1 variants in the absence of human serum ranges from 4 to 150 nM.

Mechanisms of Resistance. Ritonavir is mostly used as a pharmacokinetic enhancer (CYP 3A4 inhibitor), and

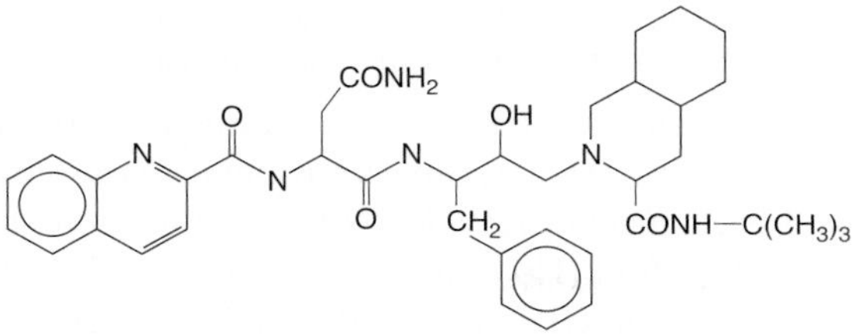

SAQUINAVIR

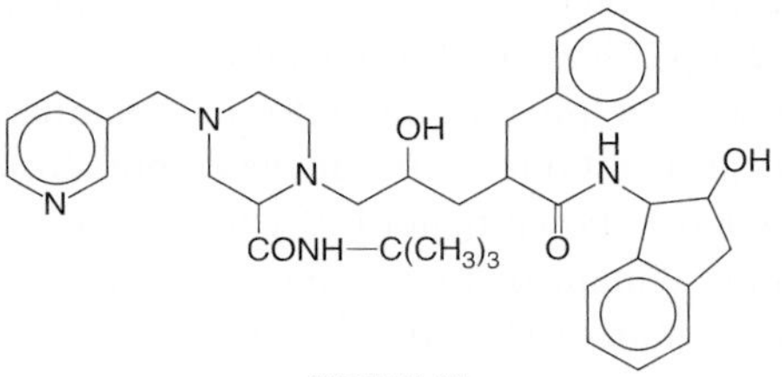

INDINAVIR

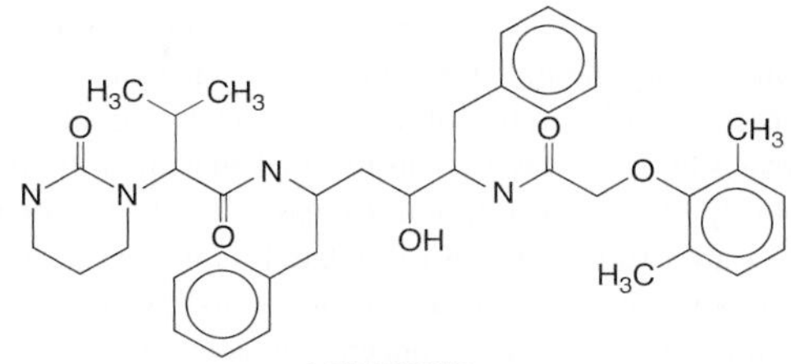

LOPINAVIR

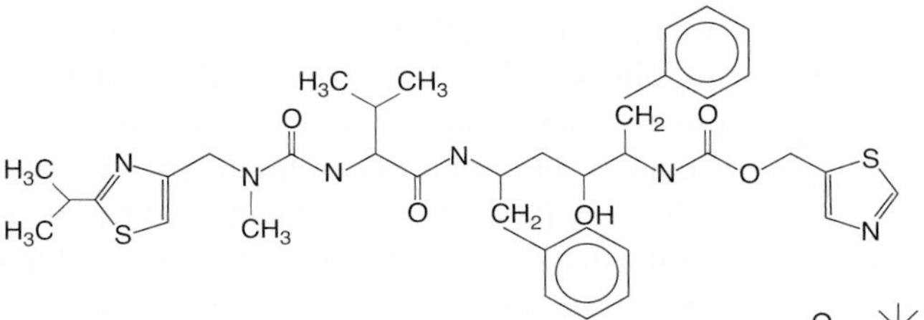

RITONAVIR

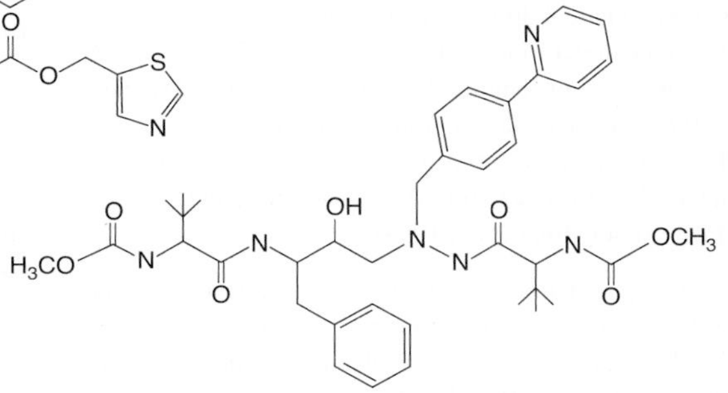

ATAZANAVIR

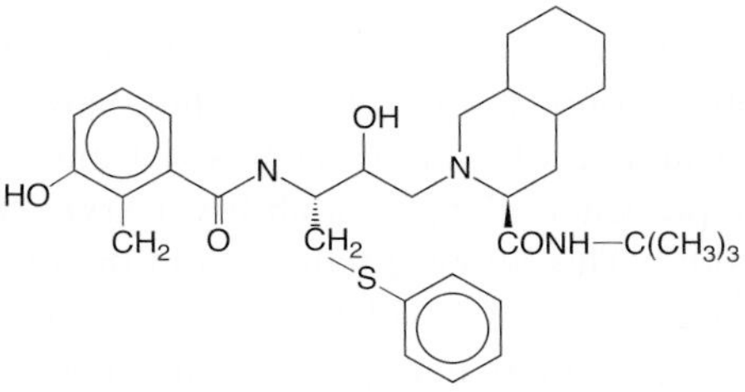

NELFINAVIR

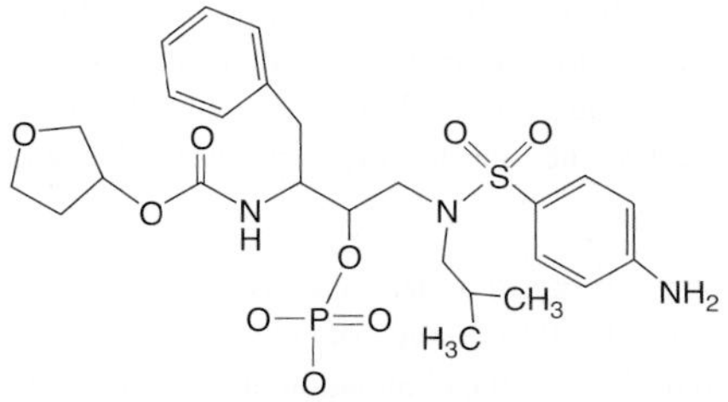

FOSAMPRENAVIR

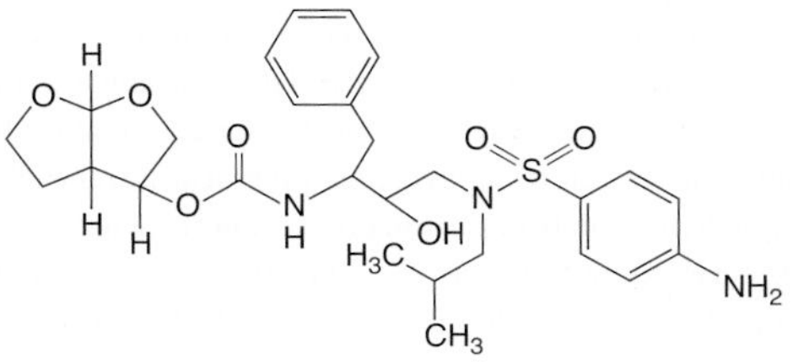

DARUNAVIR

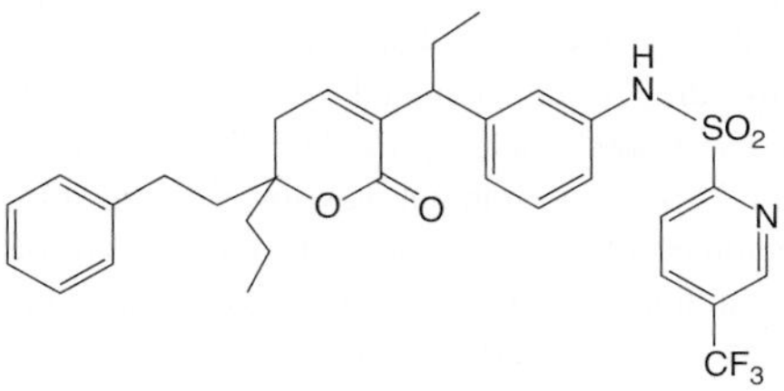

TIPRANAVIR

Figure 59–6. *Structure of available HIV protease inhibitors.*

the low doses used for this purpose are not known to induce ritonavir resistance mutations.

The primary ritonavir resistance mutation is usually at protease codon 82 (several possible substitutions for valine) or codon 84 (isoleucine-to-valine substitution). Additional mutations associated with increasing resistance occur at codons 20, 32, 46, 54, 63, 71, 84, and 90. High-level resistance requires accumulation of multiple mutations.

Absorption, Distribution, and Elimination. Absorption of ritonavir is rapid and is only slightly affected by food, depending on the formulation. The overall absorption of ritonavir from the capsule formulation increases by 13% when the capsule is taken with meals, but the bioavailability of the oral solution decreases by 7% (Flexner, 1998). A heat-stable 100-mg tablet formulation is now available. Interindividual variability in pharmacokinetics is high, with a variability exceeding 6-fold in trough concentrations among patients given 600 mg ritonavir every 12 hours as capsules (Hsu et al., 1998).

Ritonavir is metabolized primarily by CYP3A4 and to a lesser extent by CYP2D6. Ritonavir and its metabolites are mainly eliminated in feces (86% of parent drug and metabolites), with only 3% of drug eliminated unchanged in the urine. Ritonavir induces its own metabolism; steady-state concentrations are reached within 2 weeks. Ritonavir is 98-99% bound to plasma proteins, mainly to α_1-acid glycoprotein. Physiological concentrations of α_1-acid glycoprotein increase the *in vitro* IC_{50} by a factor of 10, whereas albumin increases the IC_{50} by a factor of 4 (Molla et al., 1998).

Untoward Effects. The major side effects of ritonavir are GI and include dose-dependent nausea, vomiting, diarrhea, anorexia, abdominal pain, and taste perversion. GI toxicity may be reduced if the drug is taken with meals. Peripheral and perioral paresthesias can occur at the therapeutic dose of 600 mg twice daily. These side effects generally abate within a few weeks of starting therapy. Ritonavir also causes dose-dependent elevations in serum total cholesterol and triglycerides, as well as other signs of lipodystrophy, and it could increase the long-term risk of atherosclerosis in some patients.

Precautions and Interactions. Ritonavir is one of the most potent known inhibitors of CYP3A4, markedly increasing the plasma concentrations and prolonging the elimination of many drugs. Ritonavir should be used with caution in combination with any CYP3A4 substrate and should not be combined with drugs that have a narrow therapeutic index such as midazolam, triazolam, fentanyl, and ergot derivatives (Flexner, 1998). Ritonavir is a mixed competitive and irreversible inhibitor of CYP 3A4 and its effects can persist for 2-3 days after the drug is discontinued (Washington et al., 2003). Ritonavir is also a weak inhibitor of CYP2D6. Potent inducers of CYP3A4 activity such as rifampin may lower ritonavir concentrations and should be avoided or dosage adjustments considered. The capsule and solution formulations of ritonavir contain alcohol and should not be administered with disulfiram or metronidazole (Chapter 23).

Ritonavir is also a moderate inducer of CYP3A4, glucuronosyl *S*-transferase, and possibly other hepatic enzymes and drug transport proteins. The concentrations of some drugs therefore will be decreased in the presence of ritonavir. Ritonavir reduces the ethinyl estradiol AUC by 40%, and alternative forms of contraception should be used (Piscitelli and Gallicano, 2001).

Therapeutic Use. Among patients with susceptible strains of HIV-1, ritonavir (NORVIR) as a sole agent lowered plasma HIV-1 RNA concentrations by 100- to 1000-fold (Ho et al., 1995). In a trial in patients with advanced HIV disease, the addition of ritonavir to current therapy reduced HIV-related mortality and disease progression by ~50% over a median of 6 months of follow-up (Flexner, 1998). Ritonavir is used infrequently as the sole protease inhibitor in combination regimens because of GI toxicity. However, numerous clinical trials have shown benefit of ritonavir as a pharmacokinetic enhancer in various dual protease inhibitor combinations (Flexner, 2000).

Use of Ritonavir as a CYP3A4 Inhibitor. Ritonavir inhibits the metabolism of all current HIV protease inhibitors and is frequently used in combination with most of these drugs, with the exception of nelfinavir, to enhance their pharmacokinetic profile and allow a reduction in dose and dosing frequency of the co-administered drug (Flexner, 2000). Ritonavir also overcomes the deleterious effect of food on indinavir bioavailability. Under most circumstances, low doses of ritonavir (100 or 200 mg once or twice daily) are just as effective at inhibiting CYP3A4 and are much better tolerated than the 600 mg twice-daily treatment dose.

Fosamprenavir

Chemistry and Antiviral Activity. Fosamprenavir is a phosphonooxy prodrug of amprenavir that has the advantage of greatly increased water solubility and improved oral bioavailability (Arvieux and Tribut, 2005). This allowed reduction in the pill burden from 16 capsules to 4 tablets per day. Fosamprenavir is as effective, more convenient, and generally better tolerated than amprenavir, and as a result, amprenavir is no longer marketed.

Amprenavir is an *N,N*-disubstituted (hydroxyethyl) amino sulfonamide nonpeptide HIV protease inhibitor. Although developed using a sophisticated structure-based drug-design program, the same compound was identified previously using a more traditional high-throughput screen of an available chemical library (Werth, 1994). Amprenavir contains a sulfonamide moiety, which may play a role in its dermatologic side effects. The drug is active against both HIV-1 and HIV-2, with an IC_{90} for wild-type HIV-1 of ~80 nM.

Mechanisms of Resistance. Amprenavir's primary resistance mutation occurs at HIV protease codon 50; this isoleucine-to-valine substitution confers only 2-fold decreased susceptibility *in vitro*. Primary resistance occurs less frequently at codon 84. Secondary resistance mutations occur at codons 10, 32, 46, 47, 54, 73, and 90, which greatly increase resistance and cross-resistance (Arvieux and Tribut, 2005).

Absorption, Distribution, and Elimination. Fosamprenavir is dephosphorylated rapidly to amprenavir in the intestinal mucosa. The phosphorylated prodrug is ~2000 times more water soluble than amprenavir. Meals have no significant effect on fosamprenavir pharmacokinetics (Arvieux and Tribut, 2005). Amprenavir is 90% bound to plasma proteins, mostly α_1-acid glycoprotein. This binding is relatively weak, and physiological concentrations of α_1-acid glycoprotein increase the *in vitro* IC_{50} only 3- to 5-fold. Amprenavir clearance is mainly by hepatic CYP3A4, and excretion is by the biliary route. Amprenavir is a moderate inhibitor and inducer of CYP3A4. Ritonavir increases amprenavir concentrations by inhibiting CYP3A4, allowing lower fosamprenavir doses. The daily fosamprenavir dose may be reduced from 1400 mg twice daily to 1400 mg plus 200 mg ritonavir when given once daily, or 700 mg (one tablet) plus 100 mg ritonavir twice daily.

Untoward Effects. The most common adverse effects associated with fosamprenavir are GI and include diarrhea, nausea, and vomiting. Hyperglycemia, fatigue, paresthesias, and headache also have been reported. Fosamprenavir can produce skin eruptions; moderate to severe rash is reported in up to 8% of recipients, and onset is usually within 2 weeks of starting therapy (Arvieux and Tribut, 2005). Fosamprenavir has fewer effects on plasma lipid profiles than lopinavir-based regimens.

Precautions and Interactions. Inducers of hepatic CYP3A4 activity (e.g., rifampin and efavirenz) may lower plasma amprenavir concentrations. Because amprenavir is both a CYP3A4 inhibitor and inducer, pharmacokinetic drug interactions can occur and may be unpredictable. For example, atorvastatin, ketoconazole, and rifabutin concentrations increase significantly when fosamprenavir is given without ritonavir, whereas methadone concentrations decrease.

Therapeutic Use. Clinical trials have demonstrated long-term virologic benefit in treatment-naive and treatment-experienced patients receiving fosamprenavir (LEXIVA) with or without ritonavir, in combination with nucleoside analogs (Arvieux and Tribut, 2005).

Twice-daily fosamprenavir/ritonavir produces virologic outcomes equivalent to lopinavir/ritonavir in both treatment-naive and treatment-experienced patients (Arvieux and Tribut, 2005). However, once-daily fosamprenavir/ritonavir is inferior to lopinavir/ritonavir in protease-inhibitor experienced patients, and the drug should only be given twice daily in this patient population. Fosamprenavir is approved for use in treatment-naive pediatric patients ≥2 years of age and treatment-experienced patients ≥6 years of age, at a dose of 30 mg/kg twice daily or 18 mg/kg plus ritonavir 3 mg/kg twice daily.

Lopinavir

Chemistry and Antiviral Activity. Lopinavir is a peptidomimetic HIV protease inhibitor that is structurally similar to ritonavir (Figure 59–6) but is 3- to 10-fold more potent against HIV-1 *in vitro*. Lopinavir is active against both HIV-1 and HIV-2; its IC_{50} for wild-type HIV variants in the presence of 50% human serum ranges from 65 to 290 nM. Lopinavir is available only in co-formulation with low doses of ritonavir (KALETRA), which is used to inhibit CYP3A4 metabolism and increase concentrations of lopinavir (Oldfield and Plosker, 2006).

Mechanisms of Action and Resistance. Treatment-naive patients who fail a first regimen containing lopinavir generally do not have HIV protease mutations but may have genetic resistance to the other drugs in the regimen (Oldfield and Plosker, 2006). For treatment-experienced patients, accumulation of four or more HIV protease inhibitor resistance mutations is associated with a reduced likelihood of virus suppression after starting lopinavir (Kuritzkes, 2004).

Mutations most likely to be associated with resistance include I47A/V, V32I, and L76V. Additional mutations associated with lopinavir failure in treatment-experienced patients include those at HIV protease codons 10, 20, 24, 33, 46, 50, 53, 54, 63, 71, 73, 82, 84, and 90 (Oldfield and Plosker, 2006). There is no evidence that exposure to the low doses of ritonavir in the lopinavir/ritonavir co-formulation selects for ritonavir-specific resistance mutations.

Absorption, Distribution, and Elimination. Lopinavir is absorbed rapidly after oral administration. Food has a minimal effect on bioavailability of lopinavir/ritonavir tablets, and the drug can be taken with or without food. Although the tablets contain lopinavir/ritonavir in a fixed 4:1 ratio, the observed plasma concentration ratio for these two drugs following oral administration is nearly 20:1, reflecting the sensitivity of lopinavir to the inhibitory effect of ritonavir on CYP3A4. Lopinavir undergoes extensive hepatic oxidative metabolism by CYP3A4. Approximately 90% of total drug in plasma is the parent compound, and <3% of a dose is eliminated unchanged in the urine. Both lopinavir and ritonavir are highly bound to plasma proteins, mainly to α_1-acid glycoprotein, and have a low fractional penetration into CSF and semen.

When administered orally without ritonavir, lopinavir plasma concentrations were exceedingly low mainly owing to first-pass metabolism. Both the first-pass metabolism and systemic clearance of lopinavir are very sensitive to inhibition by ritonavir.

A single 50-mg dose of ritonavir increased the lopinavir AUC by 77-fold compared with 400 mg lopinavir alone; 100 mg ritonavir increased the lopinavir AUC by 155-fold. Lopinavir trough concentrations were increased 50- to 100-fold by co-administration of low doses of ritonavir (Oldfield and Plosker, 2006). Multiple-dose pharmacokinetic studies have not been conducted with lopinavir in the absence of ritonavir. Adding 100 mg ritonavir twice daily to the lopinavir/ritonavir co-formulation (a total of 200 mg twice daily of ritonavir) has only a modest further effect on lopinavir concentrations, increasing the mean steady-state AUC by 46%.

Untoward Effects. The most common adverse events reported with the lopinavir/ritonavir co-formulation have been GI: loose stools, diarrhea, nausea, and vomiting. These are less frequent and less severe than those reported with the 600 mg twice-daily standard dose of ritonavir but more common compared to those of boosted atazanavir and darunavir. The most common laboratory abnormalities include elevated total cholesterol and triglycerides. Because the same adverse effects occur with ritonavir, it is unclear whether these side effects are due to ritonavir, lopinavir, or both.

Precautions and Interactions. Because lopinavir metabolism is highly dependent on CYP3A4, concomitant administration of agents that induce CYP3A4, such as rifampin, may lower plasma lopinavir concentrations considerably. St. John's wort is a known inducer of CYP3A4, leading to lower concentrations of lopinavir and possible loss of antiviral effectiveness. Co-administration of other antiretrovirals that can induce CYP3A4, including amprenavir, nevirapine or efavirenz, may require increasing the dose of lopinavir (Oldfield and Plosker, 2006).

Although lopinavir is a weak inhibitor of CYP3A4 *in vitro*, the ritonavir in the co-formulated capsule strongly inhibits CYP3A4 activity and probably dwarfs any lopinavir effect. The liquid formulation of lopinavir contains 42% ethanol and should not be administered with disulfiram or metronidazole (Chapter 23). Ritonavir is also a moderate CYP inducer at the dose employed in the co-formulation and can adversely decrease concentrations of some co-administered drugs (e.g., oral contraceptives). There is no direct proof that lopinavir is a CYP inducer *in vivo*; however, concentrations of some co-administered drugs (e.g., amprenavir and phenytoin) are lower with the lopinavir/ritonavir co-formulation than would have been expected with low-dose ritonavir alone (Oldfield and Plosker, 2006).

Therapeutic Use. In comparative clinical trials, lopinavir has antiretroviral activity at least comparable with that of other potent HIV protease inhibitors and better than that of nelfinavir. Lopinavir also has considerable and sustained antiretroviral activity in patients who failed previous HIV protease inhibitor–containing regimens.

In one study, 70 subjects who had failed therapy with one previous HIV protease inhibitor were treated for 2 weeks with lopinavir, followed by the addition of nevirapine. At 48 weeks, 60% of subjects had plasma HIV-1 RNA levels of <50 copies/mL despite substantial phenotypic resistance to other HIV protease inhibitors (Oldfield and Plosker, 2006). Because plasma concentrations of lopinavir generally are much higher than those required to suppress HIV replication *in vitro*, the drug may be capable of suppressing HIV isolates with low-level protease inhibitor resistance.

The adult lopinavir/ritonavir dose is 400/100 mg (two tablets) twice daily, or 800/200 mg (four tablets) once daily, with or without food. Lopinavir/ritonavir should not be dosed once daily in treatment-experienced patients. Lopinavir/ritonavir is approved for use in pediatric patients ≥14 days, with dosing based on either weight or body surface area. A pediatric tablet formulation is available for use in children >6 months of age.

Atazanavir

Chemistry and Antiviral Activity. Atazanavir is an azapeptide protease inhibitor with a C_2-symmetrical chemical structure that is active against both HIV-1 and HIV-2 (Croom et al., 2009) (Figure 59–6). The IC_{50} for HIV-1 in various *in vitro* assays ranges from 2 to 15 nM. In the presence of 40% human serum, the *in vitro* IC_{50} is increased 3- to 4-fold (Croom et al., 2009).

Mechanisms of Resistance. The primary atazanavir resistance mutation occurs at HIV protease codon 50 and confers abut a 9-fold decreased susceptibility. This isoleucine-to-leucine substitution (I50L) is distinct from the isoleucine-to-valine substitution selected by fosamprenavir and darunavir.

This mutation was present in 100% of viruses isolated from patients failing therapy in one clinical trial (Croom et al., 2009). Isolates with only this mutation are still susceptible to inhibition by other protease inhibitors. Sensitivity to atazanavir is affected by various primary and secondary mutations that accumulate in patients who have failed other HIV protease inhibitors, with high-level resistance more likely if five or more additional mutations are present (Croom et al., 2009).

Absorption, Distribution, and Elimination. Atazanavir is absorbed rapidly after oral administration, with peak concentrations occurring ~2 hours after dosing. Atazanavir absorption is sensitive to food: a light meal increases the AUC by 70%, whereas a high-fat meal increases the AUC by 35% (Croom et al., 2009). It is therefore recommended that the drug be administered with food, which also decreases the interindividual variability in pharmacokinetics, unless given with ritonavir. Absorption is pH dependent, and proton pump inhibitors or other acid-reducing agents substantially reduce atazanavir concentrations after oral dosing; this effect is only partially reversed by concomitant ritonavir.

Atazanavir undergoes oxidative metabolism in the liver primarily by CYP3A4, which accounts for most of the elimination of this drug. Only 7% of the parent drug is excreted unchanged in the urine. The mean elimination $t_{1/2}$ of atazanavir at the standard 400-mg once-daily dose is ~7 hours; however, the drug has nonlinear pharmacokinetics, and the $t_{1/2}$ increases to nearly 10 hours at a dose of 600 mg (Croom et al., 2009). Atazanavir is 86% bound to plasma proteins, both to albumin and α_1-acid glycoprotein. It is present in CSF at <3% of plasma concentrations but has excellent penetration into seminal fluid (Croom et al., 2009).

Untoward Effects. Like indinavir, atazanavir frequently causes unconjugated hyperbilirubinemia, although this is mainly a cosmetic side effect and not associated with hepatotoxicity.

Approximately 40% of subjects receiving 400 mg atazanavir once daily in initial clinical trials developed a significant increase in total bilirubin (Croom et al., 2009), although only 5% developed jaundice. This is a consequence of inhibition of UDP-glucuronosyl transferase by atazanavir, and the side effect occurs more prominently in those who are genetically deficient in this enzyme, e.g., patients with Gilbert's syndrome (Rotger et al., 2005). Postmarketing reports include hepatic adverse reactions of cholecystitis, cholelithiasis, cholestasis, and other hepatic function abnormalities.

Other side effects reported with atazanavir include diarrhea and nausea, mainly during the first few weeks of therapy. Overall,

6% of patients discontinued atazanavir because of side effects during 48 weeks of treatment. Patients treated with atazanavir in randomized clinical trials had significantly lower fasting triglyceride and cholesterol concentrations than patients treated with nelfinavir, lopinavir, or efavirenz (Croom et al., 2009), suggesting a reduced propensity to cause these side effects. In addition, atazanavir is not known to cause glucose intolerance or changes in insulin sensitivity.

Precautions and Interactions. Because atazanavir is metabolized by CYP3A4, concomitant administration of agents that induce this enzyme (e.g., rifampin) is contraindicated. Efavirenz 600 mg once daily reduced the unboosted atazanavir AUC by 74%. Atazanavir is a moderate inhibitor of CYP3A4 and may alter plasma concentrations of other CYP3A4 substrates. Atazanavir inhibits CYP3A4 less than ritonavir and does not appear to inhibit other CYP isoforms. Atazanavir is a moderate UGT 1A1 inhibitor, and when given with or without ritonavir increases the raltegravir AUC 41-72% and increases the raltegravir C_{12h} approximately 2-fold. Atazanavir is not known to induce hepatic drug-metabolizing enzymes.

Ritonavir significantly increases the atazanavir AUC and reduces atazanavir systemic clearance. Ritonavir 100 mg once daily increases the atazanavir 300 mg once-daily steady-state AUC by 2.5-fold and increases the C_{min} 6.5-fold (Croom et al., 2009). Low-dose ritonavir also counters the effect of some inducers, for example efavirenz, on the atazanavir AUC.

Proton pump inhibitors reduce atazanavir concentrations substantially with concomitant administration. These drugs and H_2 blockers should be avoided in patients receiving atazanavir without ritonavir.

Therapeutic Use. In treatment-experienced patients, atazanavir (REYATAZ) 400 mg once daily without ritonavir was inferior to the lopinavir/ritonavir co-formulation given twice daily; 81% of lopinavir/ritonavir-treated patients had plasma HIV RNA concentrations <400 copies/mL at week 24 compared with 61% of atazanavir-treated patients. The combination of atazanavir and low-dose ritonavir had a similar viral-load effect as the lopinavir/ritonavir co-formulation in one study (Croom et al., 2009), suggesting that this drug should be combined with ritonavir in treatment-experienced patients—and perhaps in treatment-naive patients with high baseline viral load—in order to take advantage of the enhanced pharmacokinetic profile.

In addition to its use for treatment-naive and experienced adults, atazanavir, in combination with ritonavir, is approved for treatment of pediatric patients >6 years of age, with dosing based on weight.

Darunavir

Chemistry and Antiviral Activity. Darunavir is a non-peptidic protease inhibitor that is active against both HIV-1 and HIV-2 (Figure 59–6). The IC_{50} for HIV-1 in various *in vitro* assays ranges from 1 to 5 nM, although human serum and α_1-acid glycoprotein increase the IC_{50} by 20-fold (McKeage et al., 2009).

Mechanisms of Action and Resistance. Darunavir binds tightly but reversibly to the active site of HIV protease but has also been shown to prevent protease dimerization.

Clinically significant drug resistance requires accumulation of multiple primary mutations. At least three darunavir-associated resistance mutations are required to confer resistance, and the most commonly seen are V32I, L33F, I47V, I54L and L89V (McKeage et al., 2009). Pretreatment resistance to darunavir is highly unlikely in treatment-naive patients and occurs in <10% of protease inhibitor-experienced patients.

Absorption, Distribution, and Elimination. Darunavir is absorbed rapidly after oral administration with ritonavir, with peak concentrations occurring 2-4 hours after dosing. Ritonavir increases darunavir bioavailability and increases the darunavir AUC by up to 14-fold. The drug should be taken with food because food increases the darunavir AUC by 30% (McKeage et al., 2009).

Darunavir undergoes oxidative metabolism in the liver primarily by CYP3A4, accounting for most of the elimination of this drug. About 8% of the parent drug is excreted unchanged in the urine. When combined with ritonavir, the mean elimination $t_{1/2}$ of darunavir is ~15 hours. In the presence of ritonavir 100 mg twice daily, the AUC after a 600-mg dose administered twice daily was increased 14-fold (McKeage et al., 2009). Darunavir is 95% bound to plasma proteins, mainly to α_1-acid glycoprotein.

Untoward Effects. Because darunavir must be combined with a low dose of ritonavir, drug administration can be accompanied by all of the side effects caused by ritonavir, including GI complaints in up to 20% of patients. Darunavir, like fosamprenavir, contains a sulfa moiety, and rash has been reported in up to 10% of recipients.

Overall, 3% of patients in randomized clinical trials discontinued darunavir because of side effects during 48 weeks of treatment, compared to 7% of patients treated with lopinavir/ritonavir. Darunavir/ritonavir is associated with increases in plasma triglycerides and cholesterol, although the magnitude of increase is lower than that seen with lopinavir/ritonavir (McKeage et al., 2009). Although causality is not firmly established, darunavir has been associated with episodes of hepatotoxicity.

Precautions and Interactions. Because darunavir is metabolized by CYP3A4, concomitant administration of agents that induce this enzyme (e.g., rifampin) is contraindicated. The drug interaction profile of darunavir/ritonavir is dominated by those expected with ritonavir.

Efavirenz 600 mg once daily reduced the darunavir AUC by 13% when combined with darunavir/ritonavir 300/100 mg twice daily. Darunavir/ritonavir 600/100 twice daily increased the maraviroc AUC by 344%, and the maraviroc dose should be reduced to 150 mg twice daily when combined with darunavir.

Therapeutic Use. Darunavir (PREZISTA) in combination with ritonavir is approved for use in HIV-infected adults.

In treatment-naive patients receiving tenofovir plus emtricitabine randomized to darunavir/ritonavir 800/100 mg once daily, virologic outcomes after 48 weeks were comparable to those seen with lopinavir/ritonavir 800/200 mg once daily (84% vs. 78%, respectively, achieved plasma HIV RNA <50 copies/mL). In protease inhibitor–experienced patients receiving an optimized background regimen and randomized to darunavir/ritonavir 600/100 mg twice daily, virologic outcomes after 48 weeks were better than those seen with lopinavir/ritonavir 400/100 mg twice daily (71% vs. 60%, respectively, achieving plasma HIV RNA <50 copies/mL) (McKeage et al., 2009).

Darunavir/ritonavir can be used as a once-daily (800/100 mg) or twice-daily (600/100 mg) regimen with nucleosides in treatment-naive adults and as a twice-daily regimen in treatment-experienced adults, taken with food. Darunavir/ritonavir twice daily is approved for use in pediatric patients >6 years of age, with dosing based on weight.

Indinavir

Chemistry and Antiviral Activity. Indinavir is a peptidomimetic hydroxyethylene HIV protease inhibitor (Figure 59–6) whose structure was based on a renin inhibitor with some similarity to the phenylalanine-proline cleavage site in the HIV gag polyprotein (Plosker and Noble, 1999), although indinavir is not itself a renin inhibitor. Indinavir is 10-fold more potent against the HIV-1 protease than that of HIV-2, and its 95% inhibitory concentration (IC_{95}) for wild-type HIV-1 ranges from 25 to 100 nM.

Mechanisms of Resistance. The primary indinavir resistance mutations occur at HIV protease codons 46 (a methionine-to-isoleucine or leucine), 82, and 84. However, secondary resistance mutations can accumulate at codons 10, 20, 24, 46, 54, 63, 71, 82, 84, and 90, and these are associated with clinical indinavir resistance as well as cross-resistance to other HIV protease inhibitors (Plosker and Noble, 1999).

Absorption, Distribution, and Elimination. Indinavir is absorbed rapidly after oral administration, with peak concentrations achieved in ~1 hour. Unlike other drugs in this class, food can adversely affect indinavir bioavailability; a high-calorie, high-fat meal reduces plasma concentrations by 75% (Plosker and Noble, 1999). Therefore, indinavir must be taken with ritonavir or while fasting or with a light low-fat meal.

Indinavir has the lowest protein binding of the HIV protease inhibitors, with only 60% of drug bound to plasma proteins (Plosker and Noble, 1999). As a consequence, indinavir has higher fractional CSF penetration than other drugs in this class, although the clinical significance of this is unknown.

The short $t_{1/2}$ of indinavir makes thrice-daily (every 8 hours) dosing necessary unless the drug is combined with ritonavir. Indinavir clearance is greatly reduced by low doses of ritonavir, which also overcome the deleterious effects of food on bioavailability (Flexner, 2000). This allows indinavir to be dosed twice daily regardless of meals.

Untoward Effects. A unique and common adverse effect of indinavir is crystalluria and nephrolithiasis. This stems from the poor solubility of the drug, which is lower at pH 7.4 than at pH 3.5 (Plosker and Noble, 1999). Precipitation of indinavir and its metabolites in urine can cause renal colic, and nephrolithiasis occurs in ~3% of patients. Patients must drink sufficient fluids to maintain dilute urine and prevent renal complications. Risk of nephrolithiasis is related to higher plasma drug concentrations, which presumably produce higher urine concentrations, regardless of whether or not the drug is combined with ritonavir (Dieleman et al., 1999).

Like atazanavir, indinavir frequently causes unconjugated hyperbilirubinemia, and 10% of patients develop an indirect serum bilirubin concentration >2.5 mg/dL (Plosker and Noble, 1999). This is generally asymptomatic and not associated with serious long-term sequelae. As with other HIV protease inhibitors, prolonged administration of indinavir is associated with the HIV lipodystrophy syndrome, especially fat accumulation. Indinavir has been associated with hyperglycemia and can induce a relative state of insulin resistance in healthy HIV-seronegative volunteers following a single 800-mg dose (Noor et al., 2002). Dermatologic complications have been reported, including hair loss, dry skin, dry and cracked lips, and ingrown toenails (Plosker and Noble, 1999).

Precautions and Interactions. Patients taking indinavir should drink at least 2 L of water daily to prevent renal complications. *This is especially problematic for those who live in warm climates.* Because indinavir solubility decreases at higher pH, antacids or other buffering agents *should not* be taken at the same time. Didanosine formulations containing an antacid buffer should not be taken within 2 hours before or 1 hour after indinavir. Like most other HIV protease inhibitors, indinavir is metabolized by CYP3A4 and is a moderately potent CYP3A4 inhibitor. Indinavir should not be co-administered with other CYP3A4 substrates that have a narrow therapeutic index. Drugs that induce CYP3A4 may lower indinavir concentrations and should be avoided.

Therapeutic Use. Indinavir (CRIXIVAN) is no longer widely prescribed because of problems with nephrolithiasis and other nephrotoxicities, and it lacks significant advantages over other available HIV protease inhibitors. When combined with ritonavir and nucleoside analogs, twice-daily indinavir produces viral load reductions comparable with those of other HIV protease inhibitor regimens (Flexner, 2000).

Nelfinavir

Chemistry and Antiviral Activity. Nelfinavir is a nonpeptidic protease inhibitor that is active against both HIV-1 and HIV-2 (Bardsley-Elliot and Plosker, 2000) (Figure 59–6). The mean IC_{95} for HIV-1 in various *in vitro* assays is 59 nM.

Mechanisms of Action and Resistance. The primary nelfinavir resistance mutation is unique to this drug and occurs at HIV protease codon 30 (aspartic acid-to-asparagine substitution); this mutation results in a 7-fold decrease in susceptibility. Isolates with only this mutation retain full sensitivity to other HIV protease inhibitors (Bardsley-Elliot and Plosker, 2000). Less commonly, a primary resistance mutation occurs at position 90, which can confer cross-resistance. In addition, secondary resistance mutations can accumulate at codons 35, 36, 46, 71, 77, 88, and 90, and these are associated with further resistance to nelfinavir, as well as cross-resistance to other HIV protease inhibitors.

Absorption, Distribution, and Elimination. Nelfinavir absorption is very sensitive to food effects; a moderate-fat meal increases the AUC 2- to 3-fold, and higher concentrations are achieved with high-fat meals (Bardsley-Elliot and Plosker, 2000). Intraindividual and interindividual variabilities in plasma nelfinavir concentrations are large as a consequence of variable absorption. Originally approved at a dose of 750 mg three times daily, nelfinavir is now administered at a dose of 1250 mg twice daily using a reduced-volume 625-mg tablet. Nelfinavir's high dependence on fatty foods for optimal absorption, combined with the fact that nelfinavir is the only HIV protease inhibitor whose pharmacokinetics are not substantially improved with ritonavir, have reduced its popularity.

Nelfinavir undergoes oxidative metabolism primarily by CYP2C19 but also by CYP3A4 and CYP2D6. Its major hydroxy-*t*-butylamide metabolite, M8, is formed by CYP2C19 and has *in vitro* antiretroviral activity similar to that of the parent drug. This is the only known active metabolite of any HIV protease inhibitor. Nelfinavir induces its own metabolism, and average trough concentrations after 1 week of therapy are approximately one-half those at day 2 of therapy (Bardsley-Elliot and Plosker, 2000).

Untoward Effects. The most important side effect of nelfinavir is diarrhea or loose stools, which resolve in most patients within the first 4 weeks of therapy. Up to 20% of patients report chronic occasional diarrhea lasting >3 months, although <2% of patients discontinue the drug because of diarrhea. Nelfinavir augments intestinal calcium-dependent chloride channel secretory responses *in vitro*, and electrolyte analysis of stool is most consistent with a secretory diarrhea (Rufo et al., 2004). Otherwise, nelfinavir is generally well tolerated but has been associated with glucose intolerance, elevated cholesterol levels, and elevated triglycerides, like other drugs in this class.

Precautions and Interactions. Because nelfinavir is metabolized by CYPs 2C19 and 3A4, concomitant administration of agents that induce these enzymes may be contraindicated (as with rifampin) or may necessitate an increased nelfinavir dose (as with rifabutin). Nelfinavir is a moderate inhibitor of CYP3A4 and may alter plasma concentrations of other CYP3A4 substrates. Nelfinavir inhibits CYP3A4 much less than does ritonavir and does not appear to inhibit other CYP isoforms. Nelfinavir also induces hepatic drug-metabolizing enzymes, reducing the AUC of ethinyl estradiol by 47% and norethindrone by 18% (Flexner, 1998). Combination oral contraceptives therefore should not be used as the sole form of contraception in patients taking nelfinavir. Nelfinavir reduces the zidovudine AUC by 35%, suggesting induction of glucuronosyl *S*- transferase.

Therapeutic Use. Nelfinavir (VIRACEPT) is approved for the treatment of HIV infection in adults and children in combination with other antiretroviral drugs. In large randomized comparative trials, long-term virologic suppression with nelfinavir-based combination regimens is statistically significantly inferior to lopinavir/ritonavir, atazanavir, or efavirenz-based regimens. This possibly reflects the unpredictable nature of nelfinavir absorption but contributes to the decreasing popularity of this drug. Nelfinavir is well tolerated in pregnant HIV-infected women and shows no evidence of teratogenesis (Bardsley-Elliot and Plosker, 2000) but detection of a potentially carcinogenic containant in 2007 led to a recommendation that the drug not be used pregnant women.

Tipranavir

Chemistry and Antiviral Activity. Tipranavir is a non-peptidic, dihydropyrone protease inhibitor that is active against both HIV-1 and HIV-2 (Figure 59–6). The IC_{50} for HIV-1 *in vitro* ranges from 30 to 70 nM, although human plasma increases the IC_{50} by 4-fold (Orman and Perry, 2008).

Mechanisms of Action and Resistance. Tipranavir binding to the active site of the HIV protease depends less on water-mediated hydrogen bonding than other molecules in this class, which may explain, in part, its unique resistance profile.

Clinically significant drug resistance requires accumulation of multiple mutations. The three mutations most commonly associated with treatment failure were L33F/I/V, V82T/L and I84V, although 21 mutations in 16 amino acids have been associated with reduced susceptibility to this drug. In general, tipranavir-resistant HIV retains sensitivity only to saquinavir and darunavir (Orman and Perry, 2008). Fewer than 3% of patients who have failed other protease inhibitors harbor virus with >10-fold resistance tipranavir. Because most HIV strains sensitive to tipranavir are also sensitive to darunavir, the latter drug is preferred for most treatment-experienced patients because of its better tolerability and toxicity profile.

Absorption, Distribution, and Elimination. Tipranavir must be administered with ritonavir because of poor oral bioavailability. The recommended regimen of tipranavir/ritonavir 500/200 mg twice daily includes a ritonavir dose higher than that of other boosted HIV protease inhibitors; lower doses of ritonavir should not be used. Food does not alter pharmacokinetics in the presence of ritonavir but may reduce GI side effects. Tipranavir is 99.9% bound in the presence of plasma proteins (Orman and Perry, 2008). Metabolism is mainly via CYP3A4; mean elimination $t_{1/2}$ is 5-6 hours in the presence of ritonavir.

Untoward Effects. Tipranavir use has been associated with rare fatal hepatotoxicity. Through 48 weeks of treatment, grade 3 or 4 elevation of hepatic transaminases occurred in 20% of treatment-naive and 10% of treatment-experienced patients. Tipranavir use has been associated with rare intracranial hemorrhage (including fatalities) and bleeding episodes in patients with hemophilia. The drug has anticoagulant properties *in vitro* and in animal models, and these effects are potentiated by vitamin E (Flexner et al., 2005). Tipranavir is more likely to cause elevation in lipids and triglycerides than other boosted PIs, possibly due to the higher dose of ritonavir. Tipranavir contains a sulfa moiety, and ~10% of treated patients report a transient rash. The current formulation contains a high amount of vitamin E, and patients should not take supplements containing this fat-soluble vitamin while taking tipranavir (Orman and Perry, 2008).

Precautions and Interactions. Like ritonavir, tipranavir is a substrate, inhibitor, and inducer of CYP enzymes. In combination, these two agents produce a broad array of clinically significant pharmacokinetic drug interactions. Tipranvir/ritonavir reduces the concentrations (AUC) of all co-administered protease inhibitors by 44-76% and should not be administered with any of these agents (Orman and Perry, 2008). This reflects the combined effect of the increased ritonavir dose, as well as tipranavir's unique capacity among PIs to induce expression of the P-glycoprotein drug transporter.

Therapeutic Use. Tipranavir (APTIVUS) is approved for use only in treatment-experienced adult and pediatric patients whose HIV is resistant to one or more protease inhibitors. In nearly 1500 patients with at least one major PI resistance mutation randomized to tipranavir/ritonavir or a comparator PI regimen, 34% had at least a one log sustained drop in plasma HIV RNA by week 48 compared to 15% of controls. However, 5.4% of tipranavir recipients discontinued treatment because of adverse events, compared to 1.6% of controls (Orman and Perry, 2008). Combining tipranavir with at least one other active antiretroviral drug, usually enfuvirtide, greatly improved virologic responses in these studies. Tipranavir/ritonavir is approved for use in adults and pediatric patients >2 years of age, with pediatric dosing based on weight or body surface area.

ENTRY INHIBITORS

There are two drugs available in this class, enfuvirtide and maraviroc, that have different mechanisms of action (Figure 59–1). Enfuvirtide inhibits fusion of the viral and cell membranes mediated by gp41 and CD4 interactions. Maraviroc is a chemokine receptor antagonist and binds to the host cell CCR5 receptor to block binding of viral gp120. As such, maraviroc is the only approved antiretroviral drug that targets a host protein. One other CCR5 receptor antagonist, vicriviroc, is in advanced clinical development.

CXCR4, the co-receptor for T-lymphocyte tropic HIV, would seem to be an equally good target for antiretroviral drug development. However, two investigational CXCR4 antagonists produced no substantial drop in plasma HIV RNA in most treated patients, even though they efficiently eliminated CXCR4-tropic virus from the circulation (Stone et al., 2007), suggesting that these drugs cause rapid selection for HIV that is CCR5-tropic. Although these compounds are no longer in development for HIV infection, they do cause an increase in circulating leukocytes, presumably as a direct consequence of CXCR4 blockade. One of these compounds, plerixafor, is now approved as an adjunct to stem cell mobilization after cancer chemotherapy (Chapter 37).

Maraviroc

Chemistry and Mechanisms of Action and Resistance. Maraviroc blocks the binding of the HIV outer envelope protein gp120 to the CCR5 chemokine receptor (Figure 59–7). Maraviroc is active only against CCR5-tropic strains of HIV and has no activity against viruses that are CXCR4-tropic or dual-tropic. The reported *in vitro* IC_{50} for CCR5-tropic HIV-1 ranges from 0.1 to 4.5 nM depending on the virus strain and testing method employed (MacArthur and Novak, 2008). Maraviroc retains activity against viruses that have become resistant to antiretroviral agents of other classes because of its unique mechanism of action.

HIV can develop resistance to this drug through two distinct pathways. A patient starting maraviroc therapy with HIV that is predominantly CCR5-tropic may experience a shift in tropism to CXCR4- or dual/mixed-tropism predominance. This is especially likely in patients harboring low-level but undetected CXCR4- or dual/mixed-tropic virus prior to initiation of maraviroc. Alternatively, HIV can retain its CCR5-tropism but gain resistance to the drug through specific mutations in the V3 loop of gp 120 that allow virus binding in the presence of inhibitor (MacArthur and Novak, 2008). This results in both an increase in IC_{50} and a decrease in maximum percent inhibition of virus replication for such viruses *in vitro*.

Absorption, Distribution, and Elimination. The oral bioavailability of maraviroc, 23-33%, is dose dependent. Food decreases bioavailability (AUC) as much as 50%, but there are no food requirements for drug administration because clinical efficacy trials were conducted without food restrictions. Maraviroc is 76% protein bound in human plasma, with a volume of distribution of 194 L. Elimination is mainly via CYP3A4 with an elimination $t_{1/2}$ of 10.6 hours (MacArthur and Novak, 2008).

Untoward Effects. Maraviroc is generally well tolerated, with little significant toxicity.

One case of serious hepatotoxicity with allergic features has been reported, but in controlled trials significant (grade 3 or 4) hepatotoxicity was no more frequent with maraviroc than with placebo. There is a theoretical concern that CCR5 inhibition might interfere with immune function; for example, humans with the Δ-32 genetic deletion in CCR5 that prevents HIV-1 entry are also more likely to develop severe West Nile virus encephalopathy (MacArthur and Novak, 2008). However, to date there has been no obvious increase in serious infections or malignancies with maraviroc treatment.

Precautions and Interactions. Maraviroc is a CYP3A4 substrate and susceptible to pharmacokinetic drug interactions involving CYP3A4 inhibitors or inducers. Recommended dosing of this drug depends on concomitant medications. Maraviroc is not itself a CYP inhibitor or inducer *in vivo*, although high-dose maraviroc (600 mg daily) increased concentrations of the CYP2D6 substrate debrisoquine.

Therapeutic Uses. Maraviroc (SELZENTRY) is approved for use in HIV-infected adults who have baseline evidence of predominantly CCR5-tropic virus. Maraviroc is the only antiretroviral drug approved at three different starting doses, depending on concomitant medications. When combined with most CYP3A inhibitors, the starting dose is 150 mg twice daily; when combined with most CYP3A inducers, the starting dose is 600 mg twice daily; for other concomitant medications, the starting dose is 300 mg twice daily.

In phase 3 clinical trials involving heavily pretreated patients with documented multidrug-resistant HIV-1, the addition of maraviroc to optimized background therapy (OBT) resulted in an undetectable (<50 copies/mL) plasma HIV-1 RNA in 44% of patients after 24 weeks, compared to 17% with OBT alone; maraviroc-treated patients also had higher mean CD4 lymphocyte count increases (120 versus 61 cells/mL). A maraviroc-based regimen was inferior to an efavirenz-based regimen in one clinical trial in treatment-naive patients (MacArthur and Novak, 2008). Maraviroc has little to no efficacy in patients harboring CXCR4- or dual/mixed-tropic virus at

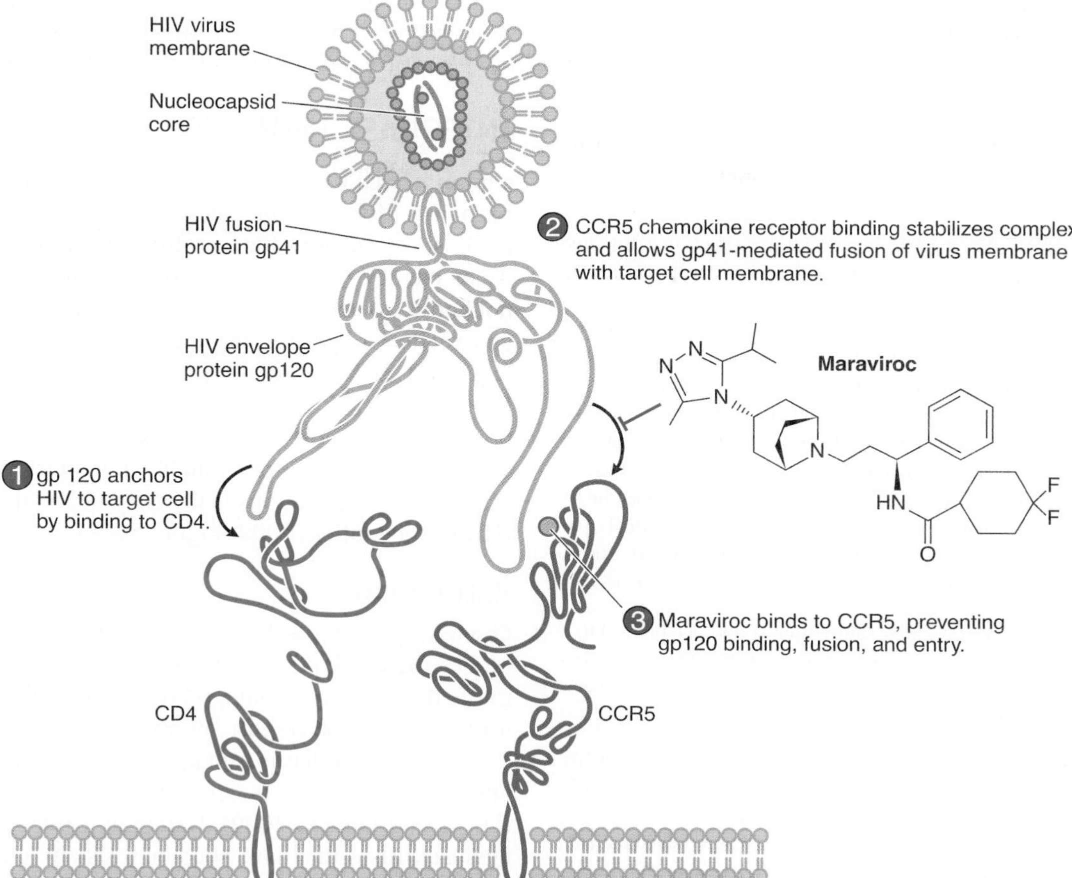

Figure 59–7. *Mechanism of action of the HIV entry inhibitor maraviroc.*

baseline. In addition, the requirement for an expensive baseline phenotype test limits its cost effectiveness.

Enfuvirtide

Chemistry and Antiviral Activity. Enfuvirtide is a 36-amino-acid synthetic peptide whose sequence is derived from a part of the transmembrane gp41 region of HIV-1 that is involved in fusion of the virus membrane lipid bilayer with that of the host cell membrane. Enfuvirtide is not active against HIV-2 but has a broad range of potencies against HIV-1 laboratory and clinical isolates. The reported *in vitro* IC_{50} ranges from 0.1 nM to 1.7 μM depending on the HIV-1 strain and testing method employed (Dando and Perry, 2003).

Enfuvirtide was investigated originally as a possible vaccine component, in part because of a high degree of sequence conservation among HIV-1 strains. This peptide turned out to have potent anti-HIV activity *in vitro*, a property eventually attributed to selective inhibition of HIV-mediated membrane fusion (Jiang et al., 1993; Wild et al., 1994). Enfuvirtide is expensive to manufacture and must be administered by subcutaneous injection twice daily. Thus cost and route of administration limit its use to those with no other treatment options.

Mechanisms of Action and Resistance. Enfuvirtide has a unique mechanism of antiretroviral action. The peptide blocks the interaction between the N36 and C34 sequences of the gp41 glycoprotein by binding to a hydrophobic groove in the N36 coil. This prevents formation of a six-helix bundle critical for membrane fusion and viral entry into the host cell. Enfuvirtide inhibits infection of CD4+ cells by free virus particles, as well as cell-to-cell transmission of HIV *in vitro*. Enfuvirtide retains activity against viruses that have become resistant to antiretroviral agents of other classes because of its unique mechanism of action.

HIV can develop resistance to this drug through specific mutations in the enfuvirtide-binding domain of gp41. Of the patients experiencing virologic failure during enfuvirtide treatment, 94% had virus with mutations in the gp41 region associated with enfuvirtide resistance *in vitro*. The most common mutations involve a V38A or N43D substitution. Single-amino-acid substitutions can confer up to 450-fold resistance *in vitro*, although high-level clinical resistance is usually associated with two or more amino acid changes (Dando and Perry, 2003).

Absorption, Distribution, and Elimination. Enfuvirtide is the only approved antiretroviral drug that must be administered parenterally. The bioavailability of subcutaneous enfuvirtide is 84% compared with an intravenous dose (Dando and Perry, 2003). Pharmacokinetics of the subcutaneous drug are not affected by site of injection.

The major route of elimination for enfuvirtide has not been determined; only a deamidated metabolite at the C-terminal phenylalanine has been detected (Dando and Perry, 2003). The mean elimination $t_{1/2}$ of parenteral drug is 3.8 hours, necessitating twice-daily administration. Enfuvirtide is 98% bound to plasma proteins, mainly albumin.

Untoward Effects. The most prominent adverse effects of enfuvirtide are injection-site reactions. About 98% of patients develop local side effects including pain, erythema, and induration at the site of injection; 80% of patients develop nodules or cysts (Dando and Perry, 2003). Between 4% and 5% of patients discontinue treatment because of local reactions. Use of enfuvirtide has been associated with a higher incidence of lymphadenopathy and pneumonia in at least one study. Whether these are direct drug effects, a secondary consequence of drug-related immune dysfunction, or effects from another mechanism is the subject of investigation. Enfuvirtide suppresses interleukin-12 production *in vitro* by >90% at concentrations equal to or less than those required to inhibit HIV replication (Braun et al., 2001); the role this might play in clinical immunosuppression is unclear.

Precautions and Interactions. Enfuvirtide is not metabolized to a significant extent and not known to alter the concentrations of any co-administered drugs. Ritonavir, rifampin, or ritonavir plus saquinavir did not alter enfuvirtide concentrations (Dando and Perry, 2003).

Therapeutic Use. Enfuvirtide (FUZEON) is FDA-approved for use only in treatment-experienced adults who have evidence of HIV replication despite ongoing antiretroviral therapy.

In phase 3 clinical trials involving heavily pretreated patients with documented multidrug-resistant HIV-1, inclusion of enfuvirtide (90 mg subcutaneously twice daily) in combination with an optimized background regimen enhanced the fraction of patients with undetectable (<50 copies/mL) plasma HIV-1 RNA concentrations after 24 weeks of treatment (~16% on enfuvirtide versus ~6% without) (Dando and Perry, 2003). Treatment response is more likely in patients with at least two other active drugs in the regimen, based on history and HIV genotype. *Given the cost, inconvenience, and cutaneous toxicity of this drug, enfuvirtide generally is reserved for patients who have failed all other feasible antiretroviral regimens.*

INTEGRASE INHIBITORS

Chromosomal integration is a defining characteristic of retrovirus life cycles and allows viral DNA to remain in the host cell nucleus for a prolonged period of inactivity or latency (Figure 59–1). Because human DNA is not known to undergo excision and reintegration, this is an excellent target for antiviral intervention. The first approved HIV integrase inhibitor, raltegravir, was licensed in 2007. It prevents the formation of covalent bonds between host and viral DNA—a process known as *strand transfer*—presumably by interfering with essential divalent cations in the enzyme's catalytic core (Hicks and Gulick, 2009; Figure 59–8).

Raltegravir

Chemistry and Mechanism of Action. Raltegravir blocks the catalytic activity of the HIV-encoded integrase, thus preventing integration of virus DNA into the host chromosome (Figure 59–8).

Raltegravir has potent activity against both HIV-1 and HIV-2, with an *in vitro* IC_{95} range of 6-30 nM (Hicks and Gulick, 2009). Raltegravir retains activity against viruses that have become resistant to antiretroviral agents of other classes because of its unique mechanism of action.

The two major raltegravir resistance pathways involve primary mutations Q184R/H/K, or N155H in the integrase gene. Either mutation can confer 25- to 50-fold changes in drug sensitivity *in*

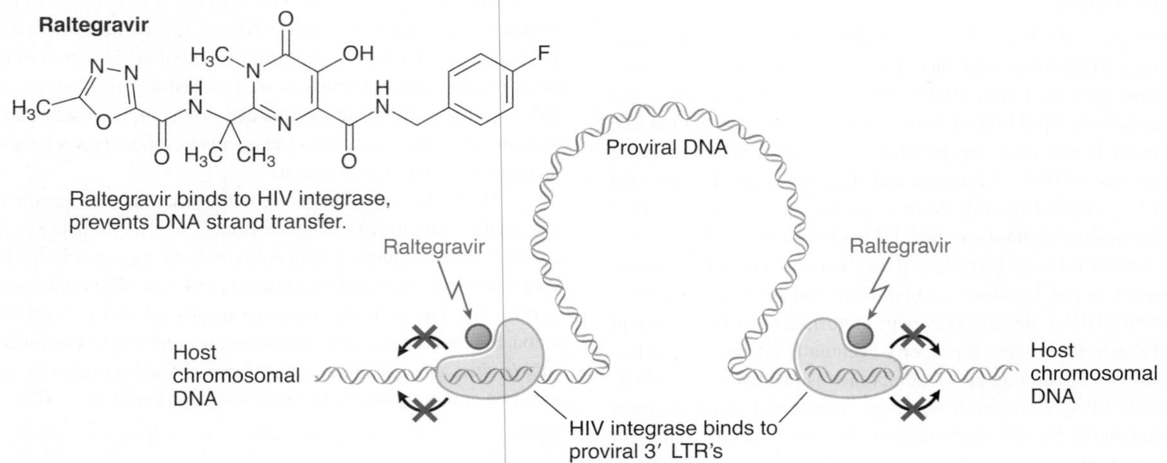

Figure 59–8. *Mechanism of action of the HIV integrase inhibitor raltegravir.*

vitro. The Y143C/H/R mutation has also been observed. In one phase 3 clinical trial, 64% of patients failing raltegravir combination therapy harbored at least one of these primary resistance mutations (Hicks and Gulick, 2009). Additional secondary mutations can accumulate and cause high-level resistance, including cross-resistance to investigational integrase inhibitors.

Absorption, Distribution, and Elimination. Peak concentrations of raltegravir occur ~1-3 hours after oral dosing. Elimination is biphasic, with a β-phase $t_{1/2}$ of ~1 hour and a terminal β-phase $t_{1/2}$ of 9 hours. The pharmacokinetics of raltegravir are highly variable. Moderate- and high-fat meals increased raltegravir apparent bioavailability (AUC) by as much as 2-fold; a low-fat meal decreased AUC modestly (46%). There are no food requirements for raltegravir administration because clinical efficacy trials were conducted without food restrictions and because initial antiviral effects were maximal at all concentrations produced with the 400 mg twice-daily dose in clinical studies. Raltegravir is 83% protein bound in human plasma. Raltegravir is eliminated mainly via glucuronidation by UGT1A1.

Untoward Effects. Raltegravir is generally well tolerated, with remarkably little clinical toxicity. In clinical trials, the most common complaints occurring at a frequency higher than in placebo recipients were headache, nausea, asthenia, and fatigue. Creatine kinase elevations, myopathy, and rhabdomyolysis have been reported, although a causal relationship to drug exposure is unproven. Exacerbation of depression has also been reported (Hicks and Gulick, 2009).

Precautions and Interactions. As a UGT1A1 substrate, raltegravir is susceptible to pharmacokinetic drug interactions involving inhibitors or inducers of this enzyme. Atazanavir, a moderate UGT1A1 inhibitor, increases the raltegravir AUC 41-72%. Tenofovir increased the raltegravir AUC by 49%, but the mechanism for this interaction is unknown. When raltegravir is combined with the CYP inducer rifampin, the raltegravir dose should be doubled to 800 mg twice daily, although no clinical data on this combination have been published. Raltegravir is not a significant enzyme inhibitor or inducer *in vitro* and has little effect on the pharmacokinetics of co-administered drugs.

Therapeutic Uses. Raltegravir (ISENTRESS) is approved for use in HIV-infected adults.

In phase 3 clinical trials involving heavily pretreated patients with documented multidrug-resistant HIV-1, the addition of raltegravir to optimized background therapy (OBT) resulted in an undetectable (<50 copies/mL) plasma HIV-1 RNA in 62% of patients after 48 weeks, compared to 33% with placebo (Hicks and Gulick, 2009). Response rates in this study ranged from 45-77%, depending on the number of additional active drugs in the regimen (0, 1, or 2). Raltegravir-treated patients also had higher mean CD4 lymphocyte count increases (109 versus 45 cells/mL).

Raltegravir has also been studied in treatment-naive patients and was recently approved for use in patients who have not taken prior antiretroviral therapy. In 10-day monotherapy studies, raltegravir decreased mean HIV-1 RNA by 1.7 log at a dose of 400 mg twice daily. In a prospective randomized comparison, raltegravir was as efficacious as efavirenz when combined with two nucleosides, with 83% and 84% of subjects, respectively, having undetectable HIV-1 RNA (<50 copies/mL) after 96 weeks of treatment. Raltegravir-treated subjects achieve an undetectable plasma HIV RNA faster than efavirenz-treated subjects, although the clinical significance of this effect is unknown (Hicks and Gulick, 2009).

CLINICAL SUMMARY

Although there has been great progress in the management of HIV and its complications, enormous challenges remain. Whereas a decade ago most treatment took place in developed countries, today most treated patients reside in resource-poor settings. In these locations, decision making is driven by availability of low-cost generic drugs. In addition, concurrent infections such as tuberculosis and hepatitis B virus are common and alter the choice of antiretroviral drugs. Potentially detrimental drug interactions and effects of traditional and herbal medicines are of increasing concern (Dooley et al., 2008). Although co-formulation of antiretroviral agents is a current trend intended to improve convenience and adherence, this can complicate management of those who require dose individualization, e.g., young children or those with hepatic or renal insufficiency.

Several expert panels issue periodic recommendations for use of antiretroviral drugs for treatment-naive and treatment-experienced adults and children. In the U.S., the Panel on Clinical Practices for Treatment of HIV Infection issues updated guidelines approximately every 6 months; their most recent guidelines can be accessed at http://www.aidsinfo.nih.gov/Guidelines (Department of Health and Human Services). These recommendations are based on a consensus assessment of the results of published clinical studies. Practitioners need to be aware that such documents are intended to provide general guidance rather than absolute recommendations and may need to be modified based on intercurrent disease, concurrent medications, and other circumstances. U.S. guidelines sometimes are contradicted by guidelines designed for use in other countries or specific patient populations; these differences may reflect different priorities assigned to drug costs, as well as the relative importance of long-term and short-term toxicities.

Current treatment recommendations center around making two important clinical decisions:

- When to start therapy in treatment-naive individuals
- When to change therapy in individuals who are failing their current regimen

In each of these settings, there is a complex algorithm of possible drug choices depending on patient and viral characteristics. The specific drugs recommended may change from year to year as new choices become available and clinical research data accumulate. Selection of drugs in the developed world will be driven by genotypic and phenotypic resistance testing. However, it is likely that future treatment guidelines will continue to be driven by three principles:

- Use of combination therapy to prevent the emergence of resistant virus;
- Emphasis on regimen convenience, tolerability, and adherence to chronically suppress HIV replication;
- Realization of the need for lifelong treatment under most circumstances.

Treatment guidelines are not sufficient to dictate all aspects of patient management. Prescribers of antiretroviral therapy must maintain a comprehensive and current fund of knowledge regarding this disease and its pharmacotherapy. Because the treatment of HIV infection is a long-lived and complex affair, and because mistakes can have dire and irreversible consequences for the patient, the prescribing of these drugs should be limited to those with specialized training.

BIBLIOGRAPHY

Aberg JA. Cardiovascular complications in HIV management: Past, present, and future. *J Acquir Immune Defic Syndr*, **2009,** *50:*54–64.

Arvieux C, Tribut O. Amprenavir or fosamprenavir plus ritonavir in HIV infection: pharmacology, efficacy and tolerability profile. *Drugs*, **2005,** *65:*633–659.

Bardsley-Elliot A, Plosker GL. Nelfinavir: An update on its use in HIV infection. *Drugs*, **2000,** *59:*581–620.

Berger EA, Murphy PM, Farber JM. Chemokine receptors as HIV-1 coreceptors: Roles in viral entry, tropism, and disease. *Annu Rev Immunol*, **1999,** *17:*657–700.

Braun MC, Wang JM, Lahey E, et al. Activation of the formyl peptide receptor by the HIV-derived peptide T-20 suppresses interleukin-12 p70 production by human monocytes. *Blood*, **2001,** *97:*3531–3536.

Calmy A, Hirschel B, Cooper DA, Carr A. A new era of antiretroviral drug toxicity. *Antivir Ther*, **2009,** *14:*165–179.

Centers for Disease Control and Prevention. Updated U.S. Public Health Service guidelines for the management of occupational exposures to HIV and recommendations for postexposure prophylaxis. *MMWR*, **2005,** *54*(RR-9):1–17.

Chapman T, McGavin J, Noble S. Tenofovir disoproxil fumarate. *Drugs*, **2003,** *63:*1597–1608.

Chun TW, Engel D, Berrey MM, et al. Early establishment of a pool of latently infected, resting CD4(+) T cells during primary HIV-1 infection. *Proc Natl Acad Sci USA*, **1998,** *95:* 8869–8873.

Coffin JM. HIV population dynamics *in vivo*: Implications for genetic variation, pathogenesis, and therapy. *Science*, **1995,** *267:*483–489.

Collier AC, Coombs RW, Schoenfeld DA, et al. Treatment of human immunodeficiency virus infection with saquinavir, zidovudine, and zalcitabine, *N Eng J Med*, **1996,** *334*: 1011–1017.

Connor EM, Sperling RS, Gelber R, et al. Reduction of maternal-infant transmission of human immunodeficiency virus type 1 with zidovudine treatment. Pediatric AIDS Clinical Trials Group Protocol 076 Study Group. *N Engl J Med*, **1994,** *331:* 1173–1180.

Croom KF, Dhillon S, Keam SJ. Atazanavir: A review of its use in the management of HIV-1 infection. *Drugs*, **2009,** *69*: 1107–1140.

D:A:D Study Group, Sabin CA, Worm SW, Weber R, et al. Use of nucleoside reverse transcriptase inhibitors and risk of myocardial infarction in HIV-infected patients enrolled in the D:A:D study: A multi-cohort collaboration. *Lancet*, **2008,** *371:*1417–1426.

Dando TM, Perry CM. Enfuvirtide. *Drugs*, **2003,** *63:*2755–2766.

De Clercq E. Clinical potential of the acyclic nucleoside phosphonates cidofovir, adefovir, and tenofovir in treatment of DNA virus and retrovirus infections. *Clin Microbiol Rev*, **2003,** *16:*569–596.

Deeks ED, Keating GM. Etravirine. *Drugs*, **2008,** *68:* 2357–2372.

Department of Health and Human Services (DHHS). AIDS Info: Clinical Guidelines portal. Available at: http://www.aidsinfo.nih.gov/Guidelines/. Accessed January 10, 2010.

Dieffenbach CW, Fauci AS. Universal voluntary testing and treatment for prevention of HIV transmission. *JAMA*, **2009,** *301:*2380–2382.

Dieleman JP, Gyssens IC, van der Ende ME, et al. Urological complaints in relation to indinavir plasma concentrations in HIV-infected patients. *AIDS*, **1999,** *13:*473–478.

Dooley K, Flexner C, Andrade ASA. Drug interactions involving combination antiretroviral therapy and other anti-infective agents: Repercussions for resource-limited countries. *J Infect Dis*, **2008,** *198:*948–961.

Dudley MN. Clinical pharmacokinetics of nucleoside antiretroviral agents. *J Infect Dis*, **1995,** *171:*S99–112.

El-Sadr WM, Lundgren JD, Neaton JD, et al. CD4+ count-guided interruption of antiretroviral treatment. *N Engl J Med*, **2006,** *355:*2283–2296.

Eron JJ, Benoit SL, Jemsek J, et al. Treatment with lamivudine, zidovudine, or both in HIV-positive patients with 200 to 500 CD4+ cells per cubic millimeter. North American HIV Working Party. *N Engl J Med*, **1995,** *333:*1662–1669.

Eshleman SH, Guay LA, Mwatha A, et al. Comparison of nevirapine (NVP) resistance in Ugandan women 7 days vs. 6–8 weeks after single-dose NVP prophylaxis: HIVNET 012. *AIDS Res Hum Retroviruses*, **2004,** *20*:595–599.

Fauci AS. Host factors and the pathogenesis of HIV-induced disease. *Nature*, **1996,** *384:*529–534.

Finzi D, Hermankova M, Pierson T, et al. Identification of a reservoir for HIV-1 in patients on highly active antiretroviral therapy. *Science*, **1997,** *278:*1295–1300.

Fischl MA, Richman DD, Grieco MH, et al. The efficacy of azidothymidine (AZT) in the treatment of patients with AIDS and AIDS-related complex: A double-blind, placebo-controlled trial. *N Engl J Med*, **1987,** *317:*185–191.

Fischl MA, Stanley K, Collier AC, et al. Combination and monotherapy with zidovudine and zalcitabine in patients with advanced HIV disease. The NIAID AIDS Clinical Trials Group. *Ann Intern Med*, **1995,** *122:*24–32.

Fitzsimmons ME, Collins JM. Selective biotransformation of the human immunodeficiency virus protease inhibitor saquinavir by human small-intestinal cytochrome P4503A4: Potential contribution to high first-pass metabolism. *Drug Metab Dispos*, **1997,** *25:*256–266.

Flexner C. HIV-protease inhibitors. *N Engl J Med*, **1998,** *338:* 1281–1292.

Flexner C. Dual protease inhibitor therapy in HIV-infected patients: Pharmacologic rationale and clinical benefits. *Annu Rev Pharmacol Toxicol*, **2000,** *40:*649–674.

Flexner C. HIV drug development: The next 25 years. *Nature Rev Drug Disc,* **2007,** *6:*959–966.

Flexner C, Bate G, Kirkpatrick P. Tipranavir. *Nature Rev Drug Disc*, **2005,** *4:*955–956.

Flexner C, Pham P. Drug-drug interactions in HIV-infected patients: An interactive decision support tool. Clinical Care Options, LLC, Washington, DC. First published August 14, 2006; last updated May 30, 2009. Available at http://clinicaloptions.com/HIV/Treatment%20Updates/Drug-Drug.

Foster C, Lyall H, Olmscheid B, et al. Tenofovir disoproxil fumarate in pregnancy and prevention of mother-to-child transmission of HIV-1: Is it time to move on from zidovudine? *HIV Med*, **2009,** *10:*397–406.

Frank I, Bosch RJ, Fiscus S, et al., for the ACTG 307 Protocol Team. Activity, safety, and immunologic effects of hydroxyurea added to didanosine in antiretroviral naïve and experienced HIV-1 infected subjects: A randomized, placebo-controlled trial, ACTG 307. *AIDS Res Hum Retroviruses*, **2004,** *20:*916–926.

Fulco PP, McNicholl IR. Etravirine and rilpivirine: Nonnucleoside reverse transcriptase inhibitors with activity against human immunodeficiency virus type 1 strains resistant to previous nonnucleoside agents. *Pharmacotherapy*, **2009,** *29:*281–294.

Gallant JE, Gerondelis PZ, Wainberg MA, et al. Nucleoside and nucleotide analogue reverse transcriptase inhibitors: A clinical review of antiretroviral resistance. *Antivir Ther*, **2003,** *8:*489–506.

Gallant JE, Moore RD. Renal function with use of a tenofovir-containing initial antiretroviral regimen. *AIDS*, **2009,** *23:* 1971–1975.

Gallant JE, Staszewski S, Pozniak AL, et al., for the 903 Study Group. Efficacy and safety of tenofovir DF vs stavudine in combination therapy in antiretroviral-naive patients: A 3-year randomized trial. *JAMA*, **2004,** *292:*191–201.

Gao WY, Agbaria R, Driscoll JS, Mitsuya H. Divergent anti-human immunodeficiency virus activity and anabolic phosphorylation of 2′,3′-dideoxynucleoside analogs in resting and activated human cells. *J Biol Chem*, **1994,** *269:*12633–12638.

Gardner EM, Burman WJ, Steiner JF, et al. Antiretroviral medication adherence and the development of class-specific antiretroviral resistance. *AIDS*, **2009,** *23:*1035–1046.

Garg A. Acquired and inherited lipodystrophies. *N Engl J Med*, **2004,** *350:*1220–1234.

Geleziunas R, Arts EJ, Boulerice F, et al. Effect of 3′-azido-3′-deoxythymidine on human immunodeficiency virus type 1 replication in human fetal brain macrophages. *Antimicrob Agents Chemother*, **1993,** *37:*1305–1312.

Granich RM, Gilks CF, Dye C, et al. Universal voluntary HIV testing with immediate antiretroviral therapy as a strategy for elimination of HIV transmission: a mathematical model. *Lancet*, **2009,** *373:*48–57.

Greene WC, Peterlin BM. Charting HIV's remarkable voyage through the cell: Basic science as a passport to future therapy. *Nature Med*, **2002,** *8:*673–680.

Gulick RM, Mellors JW, Havlir D, et al. Treatment with indinavir, zidovudine and lamivudine in adults with human immunodeficiency virus infection and prior antiretroviral therapy. *N Eng Med*, **1997**, *337*:734–739.

Gulick RM Ribaudo HJ, Shikuma CM et al. Triple nucleoside regimens versus efavirenz-containing regimens for the initial treatment of HIV-1 infection. *N Eng J Med*, **2004**, *350*:1850–1861.

Haas DW, Gebretsadik T, Mayo G, et al. Associations between CYP2B6 polymorphisms and pharmacokinetics after a single dose of nevirapine or efavirenz in African Americans. *J Infect Dis*, **2009,** *199:*872–880.

Hammer SM, Katzenstein DA, Hughes MD, et al. A trial comparing nucleoside monotherapy with combination therapy in HIV-infected adults with CD4 cell counts from 200 to 500 per cubic millimeter. AIDS Clinical Trials Group Study 175 Study Team. *N Engl J Med*, **1996,** *335:*1081–1090.

Hammer SM, Squires KE, Hughes MD, et al. A controlled trial of two nucleoside analogues plus indinavir in persons with human immunodeficiency virus infection and CD4 cells counts of 200 per cubic millimeter or less. *N Eng J Med*, **1997**, *337*: 725–733.

Harris M, Montaner JS. Clinical uses of non-nucleoside reverse transcriptase inhibitors. *Rev Med Virol*, **2000,** *10:*217–229.

Havlir DV, Gilbert PB, Bennett K, et al., for the ACTG 5025 Study Group. Effects of treatment intensification with hydroxyurea in HIV-infected patients with virologic suppression. *AIDS*, **2001,** *15:*1379–1388.

Havlir D, McLaughlin MM, Richman DD. A pilot study to evaluate the development of resistance to nevirapine in asymptomatic human immunodeficiency virus-infected patients with CD4 cell counts of >500/mm^3: AIDS Clinical Trials Group Protocol 208. *J Infect Dis*, **1995,** *172:*1379–1383.

Havlir DV, Tierney C, Friedland GH, et al. *In vivo* antagonism with zidovudine plus stavudine combination therapy. *J Infect Dis*, **2000,** *182:*321–325.

Hervey PS, Perry CM. Abacavir: A review of its clinical potential in patients with HIV infection. *Drugs*, **2000,** *60:*447–479.

Hetherington S, Hughes AR, Mosteller M, et al. Genetic variations in HLA-B region and hypersensitivity reactions to abacavir. *Lancet*, **2002,** *359:*1121–1122.

Hicks C, Gulick RM. Raltegravir: The first HIV type 1 integrase inhibitor. *Clin Infect Dis,* **2009,** *48:*931–939.

Hirsch MS, D'Aquila RT. Therapy for human immunodeficiency virus infection. *N Engl J Med*, **1993,** *328:*1686–1695.

HIV Neuromuscular Syndrome Study Group. HIV-associated neuromuscular weakness syndrome. *AIDS*, **2004,** *18:*1403–1412.

Ho DD, Neumann AU, Perelson AS, et al. Rapid turnover of plasma virions and CD4 lymphocytes in HIV-1 infection. *Nature*, **1995,** *373:*123–126.

Hsu A, Granneman GR, Bertz RJ. Ritonavir: Clinical pharmacokinetics and interactions with other anti-HIV agents. *Clin Pharmacokinet*, **1998,** *35:*275–291.

Hurst M, Noble S. Stavudine: An update of its use in the treatment of HIV infection. *Drugs*, **1999,** *58:*919–949.

Jayasekara D, Aweeka FT, Rodriguez R, et al. Antiviral therapy for HIV patients with renal insufficiency. *J Acquir Immune Defic Syndr*, **1999,** *21:*384–395.

Jiang S, Lin K, Strick N, Neurath AR. HIV-1 inhibition by a peptide. *Nature*, **1993,** *365:*113.

Khoo SH, Back DJ, Merry C. Pharmacology. In: *Practical Guidelines in Antiviral Therapy* (Boucher CAB, Galasso GAJ, eds.), Elsevier, Amsterdam, **2002,** pp. 13–35.

Kieffer TL, Finucane MM, Nettles RE, et al. Genotypic analysis of HIV-1 drug resistance at the limit of detection: Virus production without evolution in treated adults with undetectable HIV loads. *J Infect Dis*, **2004,** *189:*1452–1465.

Kim RB, Fromm MF, Wandel C, et al. The drug transporter P-glycoprotein limits oral absorption and brain entry of HIV-1 protease inhibitors. *J Clin Invest*, **1998,** *101:*289–294.

Kitahata MM, Gange SJ, Abraham AG, *et al.* Effect of early versus deferred antiretroviral therapy for HIV on survival. *N Engl J Med*, **2009,** *360:*1815–1826.

Kuritzkes DR. Preventing and managing antiretroviral drug resistance. *AIDS Patient Care STDs*, **2004,** *18*:259–273.

Kuritzkes DR, Marschner I, Johnson VA, et al. Lamivudine in combination with zidovudine, stavudine, or didanosine in patients with HIV-1 infection: A randomized, double-blind, placebo-controlled trial. National Institute of Allergy and Infectious Disease AIDS Clinical Trials Group Protocol 306 Investigators. *AIDS*, **1999,** *13:*685–694.

Larder BA, Kemp SD, Harrigan PR. Potential mechanism for sustained antiretroviral efficacy of AZT-3TC combination therapy. *Science*, **1995,** *269:*696–699.

Lawrence J, Mayers DL, Hullsiek KH, et al., for the 064 Study Team of the Terry Beirn Community Programs for Clinical Research on AIDS. Structured treatment interruption in patients with multi-drug-resistant human immunodeficiency virus. *N Engl J Med*, **2003,** *349:*837–846.

Lee H, Hanes J, Johnson KA. Toxicity of nucleoside analogues used to treat AIDS and the selectivity of the mitochondrial DNA polymerase. *Biochemistry*, **2003,** *42:*14711–14719.

Lee LM, Karon JM, Selik R, et al. Survival after AIDS diagnosis in adolescents and adults during the treatment era, United States, 1984–1997. *JAMA*, **2001,** *285:*1308–1315.

Leung NW, Lai CL, Chang TT, et al., on behalf of the Asia Hepatitis Lamivudine Study Group. Extended lamivudine treatment in patients with chronic hepatitis B enhances hepatitis B e antigen sero-conversion rates: Results after 3 years of therapy. *Hepatology*, **2001,** *33*:1527–1532.

Lockman S, Shapiro RL, Smeaton LM, et al. Response to antiretroviral therapy after a single, peripartum dose of nevirapine. *N Engl J Med*, **2007,** *356:*135–147.

MacArthur RD, Novak RM. Maraviroc: The first of a new class of antiretroviral agents. *Clin Infect Dis*, **2008,** *47:*236–241.

Mallal S, Phillips E, Carosi G, et al. HLA-B*5701 screening for hypersensitivity to abacavir. *N Engl J Med*, **2008,** *358:*568–579.

Manabe YC, Campbell JD, Sydnor E, Moore RD. Immune reconstitution inflammatory syndrome: Risk factors and treatment implications. *J Acquir Immune Defic Syndr*, **2007,** *46:*456–462.

McDowell JA, Chittick GE, Stevens CP, et al. Pharmacokinetic interaction of abacavir (1592U89) and ethanol in human immunodeficiency virus–infected adults. *Antimicrob Agents Chemother*, **2000,** 44*:*1686–1690.

McKeage K, Perry CM, Keam SJ. Darunavir: A review of its use in the management of HIV infection in adults. *Drugs*, **2009,** *69:*477–503.

McLeod GX, Hammer SM. Zidovudine: Five years later. *Ann Intern Med,* **1992,** *117:*487–501.

Mellors JW, Munoz A, Giorgi JV, et al. Plasma viral load and CD4+ lymphocytes as prognostic markers of HIV-1 infection. *Ann Intern Med*, **1997,** *126:*946–954.

Mellors JW, Rinaldo CR Jr, Gupta P, et al. Prognosis in HIV-1 infection predicted by the quantity of virus in plasma. *Science*, **1996,** *272:*1167–1170.

Miller MD, Anton KE, Mulato AS, et al. Human immunodeficiency virus type 1 expressing the lamivudine-associated M184V mutation in reverse transcriptase shows increased susceptibility to adefovir and decreased replication capability *in vitro. J Infect Dis*, **1999,** *179:*92–100.

Mirochnick M, Fenton T, Gagnier P, et al. Pharmacokinetics of nevirapine in human immunodeficiency virus type 1–infected pregnant women and their neonates. Pediatric AIDS Clinical Trials Group Protocol 250 Team. *J Infect Dis*, **1998,** *178:* 368–374.

Mitsuya H, Weinhold KJ, Furman PA, et al. 3′-Azido-3′-deoxythymidine (BW A509U): An antiviral agent that inhibits the infectivity and cytopathic effect of human T-lymphotropic virus type III/lymphadenopathy-associated virus *in vitro. Proc Natl Acad Sci USA*, **1985,** *82:*7096–7100.

Molla A, Vasavanonda S, Kumar G, et al. Human serum attenuates the activity of protease inhibitors toward wild-type and mutant human immunodeficiency virus. *Virology*, **1998,** *250:*255–262.

Moore KH, Barrett JE, Shaw S, *et al.* The pharmacokinetics of lamivudine phosphorylation in peripheral blood mononuclear cells from patients infected with HIV-1. *AIDS*, **1999,** *13:*2239–2250.

Moreno S, Hernández B, Dronda F. Didanosine enteric-coated capsule: Current role in patients with HIV-1 infection. *Drugs*, **2007,** *67:*1441–1462.

Muller V, Bonhoeffer S. Mathematical approaches in the study of viral kinetics and drug resistance in HIV-1 infection. *Curr Drug Targets Infect Disord,* **2003,** *3:*329–344.

Naeger LK, Margot NA, Miller MD. ATP-dependent removal of nucleoside reverse transcriptase inhibitors by human immunodeficiency virus type 1 reverse transcriptase. *Antimicrob Agents Chemother*, **2002,** *46:*2179–2184.

Nettles RE, Kieffer TL, Kwon P, et al. Intermittent HIV-1 viremia (blips) and drug resistance in patients receiving HAART. *JAMA*, **2005,** *293:*817–829.

Noble S, Faulds D. Saquinavir: A review of its pharmacology and clinical potential in the management of HIV infection. *Drugs,* **1996,** *52:*93–112.

Noor MA, Seneviratne T, Aweeka FT, et al. Indinavir acutely inhibits insulin-stimulated glucose disposal in humans: A randomized, placebo-controlled study. *AIDS*, **2002,** *16:*F1–F8.

Oldfield V, Plosker GL. Lopinavir/ritonavir: A review of its use in the management of HIV infection. *Drugs*, **2006,** *66:* 1275–1299.

Orman JS, Perry CM. Tipranavir: A review of its use in the management of HIV infection. *Drugs*, **2008,** *68:*1435–1463.

Pauwels R, Andries K, Desmyter J, et al. Potent and selective inhibition of HIV-1 replication *in vitro* by a novel series of TIBO derivatives. *Nature*, **1990,** *343:*470–474.

Perelson AS, Neumann AU, Markowitz M, et al. HIV-1 dynamics *in vivo*: Virion clearance rate, infected cell life-span, and viral generation time. *Science*, **1996,** *271:*1582–1586.

Perry CM, Faulds D. Lamivudine: A review of its antiviral activity, pharmacokinetic properties and therapeutic efficacy in the management of HIV infection. *Drugs*, **1997,** *53:*657–680.

Perry CM, Noble S. Saquinavir soft-gel capsule formulation: A review of its use in patients with HIV infection. *Drugs*, **1998,** *55:*461–486.

Piscitelli SC, Gallicano KD. Interactions among drugs for HIV and opportunistic infections. *N Engl J Med*, **2001,** *344:*984–996.

Plosker GL, Noble S. Indinavir: A review of its use in the management of HIV infection. *Drugs*, **1999,** *58:*1165–1203.

Rainey PM, Friedland G, McCance-Katz EF, et al. Interaction of methadone with didanosine and stavudine. *J Acquir Immune Defic Syndr*, **2000,** 24:241–248.

Riddler SA, Haubrich R, DiRienzo, et al. Class-sparing regimens for initial treatment of HIV-1 infection. *N Engl J Med*, **2008,** *358:*2095–2106.

Robbins BL, Wilcox CK, Fridland A, Rodman JH. Metabolism of tenofovir and didanosine in quiescent or stimulated human peripheral blood mononuclear cells. *Pharmacotherapy*, **2003,** *23:*695–701.

Roberts NA, Martin JA, Kinchington D, et al. Rational design of peptide-based HIV proteinase inhibitors. *Science*, **1990,** *248:*358–361.

Rotger M, Taffe P, Bleiber G, et al. Gilbert syndrome and the development of antiretroviral therapy-associated hyperbilirubinemia. *J Infect Dis*, **2005,** *192*:1381–1386.

Rufo P, Lin PW, Andrade A, et al. Diarrhea-associated HIV-1 aspartyl protease-inhibitors potentiate muscarinic activation of Cl^-secretion by T84 cells *via* prolongation of cytosolic Ca^{2+} signaling. *Am J Physiol Cell Physiol*, **2004,** *286*: 998–1008.

Saag MS. Emtricitabine, a new antiretroviral agent with activity against HIV and hepatitis B virus. *Clin Infect Dis*, **2006,** *42:*126–131.

Saag MS, Sonnerborg A, Torres RA, et al. Antiretroviral effect and safety of abacavir alone and in combination with zidovudine in HIV-infected adults. Abacavir Phase 2 Clinical Team. *AIDS*, **1998,** *12:*F203–F209.

Scott LJ, Perry CM. Delavirdine: A review of its use in HIV infection. *Drugs*, **2000,** *60:*1411–1444.

Shafer RW, Smeaton LM, Robbins GK, et al., for the AIDS Clinical Trials Group 384 Team. Comparison of four-drug regimens and pairs of sequential three-drug regimens as initial therapy for HIV-1 infection. *N Engl J Med*, **2003,** *349:* 2304–2315.

Sheran M. The nonnucleoside reverse transcriptase inhibitors efavirenz and nevirapine in the treatment of HIV. *HIV Clin Trials*, **2005,** *6:*158–168.

Siliciano JD, Kajdas J, Finzi D, et al. Long-term follow-up studies confirm the stability of the latent reservoir for HIV-1 in resting CD4+ T cells. *Nature Med*, **2003,** *9:*727–728.

Steigbigel RT, Cooper DA, Kumar PN, et al. Raltegravir with optimized background therapy for resistant HIV-1 infection. *N Engl J Med*, **2008,** *359:*339–354.

Stone ND, Dunaway SB, Flexner C, et al. Multiple dose escalation study of the safety, pharmacokinetics, and biologic activity of oral AMD070, a selective CXCR4 receptor inhibitor, in human subjects (ACTG A5191). *Antimicrob Agents Chemother,* **2007,** *51:*2351–2358.

Taylor S, Back DJ, Workman J, et al. Poor penetration of the male genital tract by HIV-1 protease inhibitors. *AIDS*, **1999,** *13:*859–860.

Tripuraneni NS, Smith PR, Weedon J, et al. Prognostic factors in lactic acidosis syndrome caused by nucleoside reverse transcriptase inhibitors: Report of eight cases and review of the literature. *AIDS Patient Care STDs*, **2004,** *18:*379–384.

Wainberg MA, Drosopoulos WC, Salomon H, et al. Enhanced fidelity of 3TC-selected mutant HIV-1 reverse transcriptase. *Science*, **1996,** *271:*1282–1285.

Wainberg MA, Miller MD, Quan Y, et al. *In vitro* selection and characterization of HIV-1 with reduced susceptibility to PMPA. *Antivir Ther*, **1999,** *4:*87–94.

Washington CB, Flexner C, Sheiner LB, et al. Effect of simultaneous versus staggered dosing on pharmacokinetic interactions of protease inhibitors. *Clin Pharmacol Ther,* **2003,** *73:* 406–416.

Wei X, Ghosh SK, Taylor ME, et al. Viral dynamics in human immunodeficiency virus type 1 infection. *Nature*, **1995,** *373:* 117–122.

Werth B. *The Billion Dollar Molecule: One Company's Quest for the Perfect Drug.* Simon & Schuster, New York, **1994.**

When to Start Consortium. Timing of initiation of antiretroviral therapy in AIDS-free HIV-1-infected patients: A collaborative analysis of 18 HIV cohort studies. *Lancet,* **2009,** *373:*1352–1363.

Wild CT, Shugars DC, Greenwell TK, et al. Peptides corresponding to a predictive alpha-helical domain of human immunodeficiency virus type 1 gp41 are potent inhibitors of virus infection. *Proc Natl Acad Sci USA*, **1994,** *91:*9770–9774.

Wilkin TJ, McKinnon JE, DiRienzo AG, et al. Regimen simplification to atazanavir-ritonavir alone as maintenance antiretroviral therapy: Final 48-week clinical and virologic outcomes. *J Infect Dis*, **2009,** *199:*866–871.

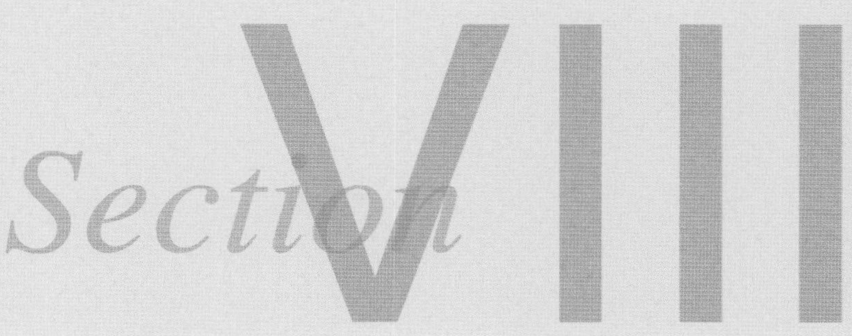

Chemotherapy of Neoplastic Diseases

General Principles of Cancer Chemotherapy

Bruce A. Chabner

Introduction. The practice of cancer medicine has changed dramatically as curative treatments have been identified for many previously fatal malignancies such as testicular cancer, lymphomas, and leukemia. Adjuvant chemotherapy and hormonal therapy can extend life and prevent disease recurrence following surgical resection of localized breast, colorectal, and lung cancers. Chemotherapy is also employed as part of the multimodal treatment of locally advanced head and neck, breast, lung, and esophageal cancers, soft-tissue sarcomas, and pediatric solid tumors, thereby allowing for more limited surgery and even cure in these formerly incurable cases. Colony-stimulating factors restore bone marrow function and expand the utility of high-dose chemotherapy. Chemotherapeutic drugs are increasingly used in nonmalignant diseases: cytotoxic antitumor agents have become standard in treating autoimmune diseases, including rheumatoid arthritis (methotrexate and cyclophosphamide), Crohn's disease (6-mercaptopurine), organ transplantation (methotrexate and azathioprine), sickle cell anemia (hydroxyurea), and psoriasis (methotrexate). Despite these therapeutic successes, few categories of medication have a narrower therapeutic index and greater potential for causing harmful effects than the cytotoxic antineoplastic drugs. A thorough understanding of their pharmacology, including drug interactions and clinical pharmacokinetics, is essential for their safe and effective use in humans.

The compounds used in the chemotherapy of neoplastic disease are quite varied in structure and mechanism of action, including alkylating agents; antimetabolite analogs of folic acid, pyrimidine, and purine; natural products; hormones and hormone antagonists; and a variety of agents directed at specific molecular targets. Tables 60-1 through 60-5 summarize of the main classes and examples of these drugs. Figure 60–1 depicts the cellular targets of chemotherapeutic agents.

The strategy for the discovery of anticancer drugs has undergone a dramatic transformation in the past 15 years, based largely on advances in understanding the molecular basis of malignant transformation. In prior years, cancer drugs were discovered through the large-scale testing of synthetic chemicals and natural products against rapidly proliferating animal tumor systems, primarily murine leukemias (Chabner and Roberts, 2005). Most of the agents discovered in these screens interacted with DNA or its precursors, inhibiting the synthesis of new genetic material and causing broad-based damage to DNA in both normal and malignant cells. The rapidly expanding knowledge of cancer biology has led to the discovery of entirely new and more cancer-specific targets (e.g., growth factor receptors, intracellular signaling pathways, epigenetic processes, tumor vascularity, DNA repair defects, and cell death pathways). For example, in many tumors, proliferation and survival depends on the constitutive activity of a single growth factor pathway, or so-called oncogene addiction (i.e., the "Achilles heel"), and inhibition of that pathway leads to cell death (Weinstein and Joe, 2006). Thus, imatinib (GLEEVEC) attacks the unique and specific *bcr-abl* translocation in chronic myelocytic leukemia. Imatinib also inhibits c-kit and produces extended control of gastrointestinal stromal tumors that express a mutated and constitutively activated form of c-kit. Monoclonal antibodies effectively inhibit tumor-associated antigens such as the amplified her-2/neu receptor in breast cancer cells. These examples emphasize that entirely new strategies for drug discovery and development, and advances in patient care, will result from new knowledge of cancer biology. Figure 60–1 outlines the common targets of cancer

Table 60–1

Alkylating Agents

TYPE OF AGENT	NONPROPRIETARY NAMES	DISEASE
Nitrogen mustards	Mechlorethamine	Hodgkin's disease
	Cyclophosphamide Ifosfamide	Acute and chronic lymphocytic leukemia; Hodgkin's disease; non-Hodgkin's lymphoma; multiple myeloma; neuroblastoma; breast, ovary, lung cancer; Wilms' tumor; cervix, testis cancer; soft-tissue sarcoma
	Melphalan	Multiple myeloma
	Chlorambucil	Chronic lymphocytic leukemia; macroglobulinemia
Methylhydrazine derivative	Procarbazine (*N*-methylhydrazine, MIH)	Hodgkin's disease
Alkyl sulfonate	Busulfan	Chronic myelogenous leukemia, bone marrow transplantation
Nitrosoureas	Carmustine (BCNU)	Hodgkin's disease; non-Hodgkin's lymphoma; glioblastoma
	Streptozocin (streptozotocin)	Malignant pancreatic insulinoma; malignant carcinoid
	Bendamustine	Non-Hodgkin's lymphoma
Triazenes	Dacarbazine (DTIC; dimethyltriazenoimidazole carboxamide),	Malignant melanoma; Hodgkin's disease; soft-tissue sarcomas; melanoma
	Temozolomide	Malignant gliomas
Platinum coordination complexes	Cisplatin, carboplatin, oxaliplatin	Testicular, ovarian, bladder, esophageal, lung, head and neck, colon, breast cancer

Table 60–2

Antimetabolites

TYPE OF AGENT	NONPROPRIETARY NAMES	DISEASE
Folic acid analogs	Methotrexate (amethopterin)	Acute lymphocytic leukemia; choriocarcinoma; breast, head, neck and lung cancers; osteogenic sarcoma; bladder cancer
	Pemetrexed	Mesothelioma, lung cancer
Pyrimidine analogs	Fluorouracil (5-fluorouracil; 5-FU), capecitabine	Breast, colon, esophageal, stomach, pancreas, head and neck; premalignant skin lesion (topical)
	Cytarabine (cytosine arabinoside)	Acute myelogenous and acute lymphocytic leukemia; non-Hodgkin's lymphoma
	Gemcitabine	Pancreatic, ovarian, lung cancer
	5-aza-cytidine	Myelodysplasia
	Deoxy-5-aza-cytidine	"
Purine analogs and related inhibitors	Mercaptopurine (6-mercaptopurine; 6-MP)	Acute lymphocytic and myelogenous leukemia; small cell non-Hodgkin's lymphoma
	Pentostatin (2′-deoxycoformycin)	Hairy cell leukemia; chronic lymphocytic leukemia; small cell non-Hodgkin's lymphoma
	Fludarabine	Chronic lymphocytic leukemia
	Clofarabine	Acute myelogenous leukemia
	Nelarabine	T-cell leukemia, lymphoma

Table 60–3

Natural Products

TYPE OF AGENT	NONPROPRIETARY NAMES	DISEASE
Vinca alkaloids	Vinblastine	Hodgkin's disease; non-Hodgkin's lymphoma; testis cancer.
	Vinorelbine	Breast and lung cancer
	Vincristine	Acute lymphocytic leukemia; neuroblastoma; Wilms' tumor; rhabdomyosarcoma; Hodgkin's disease; non-Hodgkin's lymphoma
Taxanes	Paclitaxel, docetaxel	Ovarian, breast, lung, prostate, bladder, head and neck cancer
Epipodophyllotoxins	Etoposide	Testis, small cell lung and other lung cancer; breast cancer; Hodgkin's disease; non-Hodgkin's lymphomas; acute myelogenous leukemia; Kaposi's sarcoma
	Teniposide	Acute lymphoblastic leukemia in children
Camptothecins	Topotecan	Ovarian cancer; small cell lung cancer
	irinotecan	Colon cancer
Antibiotics	Dactinomycin (actinomycin D)	Choriocarcinoma; Wilms' tumor; rhabdomyosarcoma; testis; Kaposi's sarcoma
	Daunorubicin (daunomycin, rubidomycin)	Acute myelogenous and acute lymphocytic leukemia
	Doxorubicin	Soft-tissue, osteogenic, and other sarcoma; Hodgkin's disease; non-Hodgkin's lymphoma; acute leukemia; breast, genitourinary, thyroid, lung, and stomach cancer; neuroblastoma and other childhood and adult sarcomas
Echinocandins	Yondelis	Soft-tissue sarcomas, ovarian cancer
Anthracenedione	Mitoxantrone	Acute myelogenous leukemia; breast and prostate cancer
	Bleomycin	Testis and cervical cancer; Hodgkin's disease; non-Hodgkin's lymphoma
	Mitomycin C	Stomach, anal, and lung cancer
Enzymes	L-Asparaginase	Acute lymphocytic leukemia

chemotherapeutic agents. New clinical trial designs, aimed at determining effects of new drugs at the molecular level, increasingly employ biomarkers derived from samples of biological fluids or tumors to assess the effects of these new agents on signaling pathways, tumor proliferation and cell death, and angiogenesis (Maheswaran et al., 2008). Imaging of molecular, metabolic, and physiological effects of drugs will become increasingly important in establishing that drugs effectively engage their targets.

Although molecularly targeted drugs have had outstanding successes in selected types of cancer, new therapies are not likely to replace cytotoxics in the foreseeable future. Rather, the targeted drugs and cytotoxics will continue to be used in combination. For instance, monoclonal antibodies or small targeted molecules, used as single agents against solid tumors, produce low response rates and modest benefits; however, in combination with cytotoxics and in early stages of disease, monoclonal antibodies such as trastuzumab (HERCEPTIN) and bevacizumab (AVASTIN) are dramatically effective (Romond et al., 2005; Slamon et al., 2001). At the same time, the toxicities of cytotoxic drugs have become more manageable with the development of better anti-nausea medications (Chapters 13 and 46) and with granulocyte colony-stimulating factor and erythropoietin to restore bone marrow function (Chapters 37 and 62). Finally, targeted drugs are helping to overcome resistance to chemotherapeutic agents by normalizing blood flow, promoting apoptosis, and inhibiting prosurvival signals from growth factor pathways. Tumor angiogenesis leads to increased interstitial pressure and diminishes delivery of drugs to tumor cells; inhibitors of angiogenesis (e.g., bevacizumab) normalize blood flow and interstitial pressure (Batchelor et al., 2007), improve drug delivery, and are thus synergistic with cytotoxic drugs in the treatment of lung, breast, and other cancers.

Table 60–4

Hormones and Antagonists

TYPE OF AGENT	NONPROPRIETARY NAMES	DISEASE
Adrenocortical suppressants	Mitotane (*o,p′*-DDD)	Adrenal cortex cancer
Adrenocortico-steroids	Prednisone (other equivalent preparations available)	Acute and chronic lymphocytic leukemia; non-Hodgkin's lymphoma; Hodgkin's disease; breast cancer, multiple myeloma
Progestins	Hydroxyprogesterone caproate, medroxyprogesterone acetate, megestrol acetate	Endometrial, breast cancer
Estrogens	Diethylstilbestrol, ethinyl estradiol (other preparations available)	Breast, prostate cancer
Anti-estrogens	Tamoxifen, toremifene	Breast cancer
Aromatase inhibitors	Anastrozole, letrozole, exemestane	Breast cancer
Androgens	Testosterone propionate, fluoxymesterone (other preparations available)	Breast cancer
Anti-androgen	Flutamide, casodex	Prostate cancer
GnRH analog	Leuprolide	Prostate cancer

Table 60–5

Miscellaneous Agents

TYPE OF AGENT	NONPROPRIETARY NAMES	DISEASE
Substituted urea	Hydroxyurea	Chronic myelogenous leukemia; polycythemia vera; essential thrombocytosis
Differentiating agents	Tretinoin, arsenic trioxide	Acute promyelocytic leukemia
	Histone deacetylase inhibitor (vorinostat)	Cutaneous T-cell lymphoma
Protein tyrosine kinase inhibitors	Imatinib	Chronic myelogenous leukemia; GI stromal tumors (GIST); hypereosinophilia syndrome
	Dasatinib, nilotinib	Chronic myelogenous leukemia
	Gefitinib, erlotinib	EGFR inhibitors: Non–small cell lung cancer
	Sorafenib	Hepatocellular cancer, renal cancer
	Sunitinib	GIST, renal cancer
	Lapatinib	Breast cancer
Proteasome inhibitor	Bortezomib	Multiple myeloma
Biological response modifiers	Interferon-alfa, interleukin-2	Hairy cell leukemia; Kaposi's sarcoma; melanoma; carcinoid; renal cell; non-Hodgkin's lymphoma; mycosis fungoides; chronic myelogenous leukemia
Immunomodulators	Thalidomide	Multiple myeloma
	Lenalidomide	Myelodysplasia ($5q^-$ syndrome); multiple myeloma
mTOR Inhibitors	Temsirolimus, everolimus	Renal cancer
Monoclonal antibodies		(*see* Tables 62–1 and 62–2)

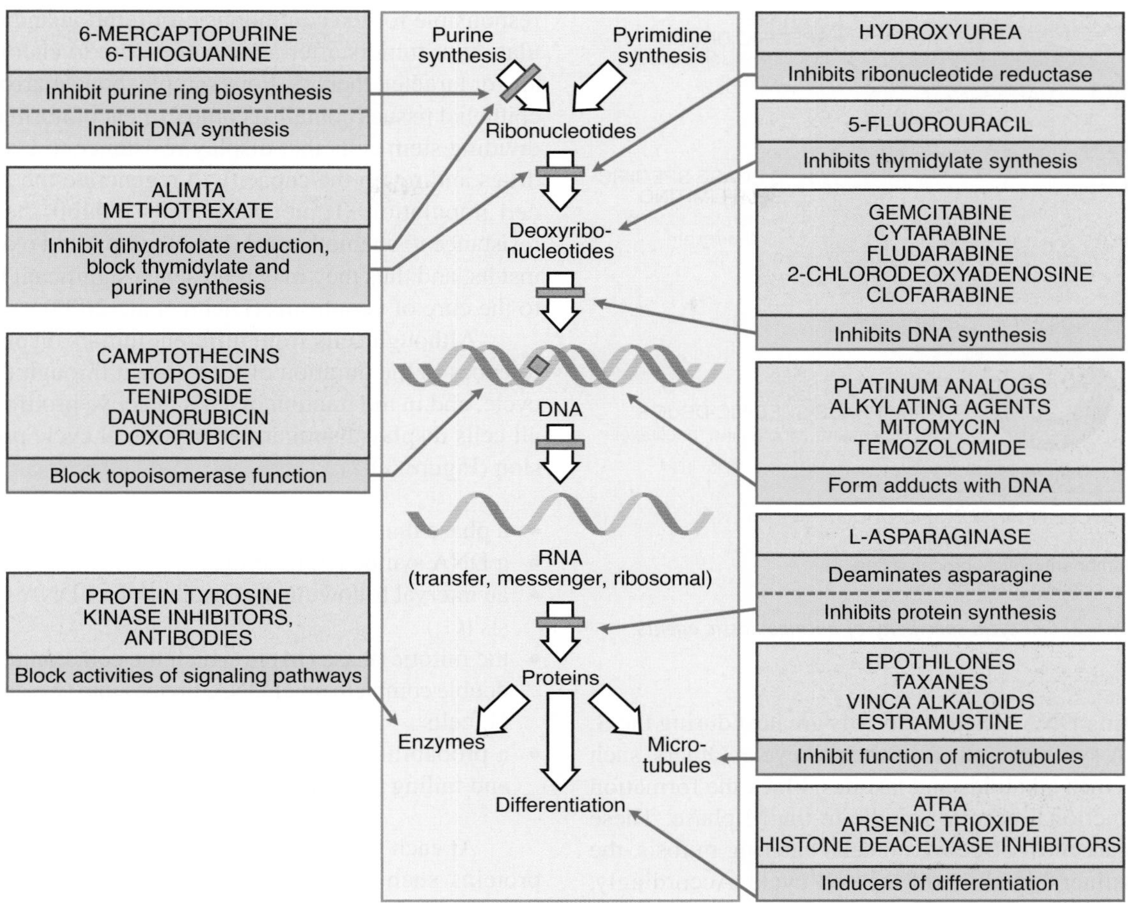

Figure 60–1. *Summary of the mechanisms and sites of action of some chemotherapeutic agents useful in neoplastic disease.*

Drug resistance remains a major obstacle to successful cancer treatment. Resistance results from a variety of pharmacokinetic and molecular changes that can defeat the best designed treatments, including poor drug absorption and delivery; genetically determined variability in drug transport, activation, and clearance; and mutations, amplifications, or deletions in drug targets. The resistance process is best understood for targeted agents. Tumors developing resistance to bcr-abl inhibitors and to inhibitors of the epidermal growth factor receptor (EGFR) express mutations in the target enzyme. Cells exhibiting drug-resistant mutations exist in the patient prior to drug treatment and are selected by drug exposure. Resistance to inhibitors of the EGFR may develop through expression of an alternative receptor, c-met, which bypasses EGFR blockade and stimulates proliferation (Engelman et al., 2008). Defects in recognition of DNA breaks and overexpression of specific repair enzymes may also contribute to resistance to cytotoxic drugs (Holleman et al., 2006), and a loss of apoptotic pathways can lead to resistance to both cytotoxic and targeted agents.

In designing specific clinical regimens, a number of factors must be considered. Drugs in combination can negate the effects of a resistance mechanism specific for a single agent, and they may be synergistic because of their biochemical interactions. Ideally, drug combinations should not overlap in their major toxicities. In general, cytotoxic drugs are used as close as possible to their maximally tolerated individual doses and should be given as frequently as tolerated to discourage tumor regrowth. Because the tumor cell population in patients with clinically detectable disease exceeds 1 g, or 10^9 cells, and each cycle of therapy kills <99% of the cells, it is necessary to repeat treatments in multiple, carefully timed cycles to achieve cure.

The Cell Cycle. An understanding of the life cycle of tumors is essential for the rational use of antineoplastic agents (Figure 60–2). Many cytotoxic agents act by

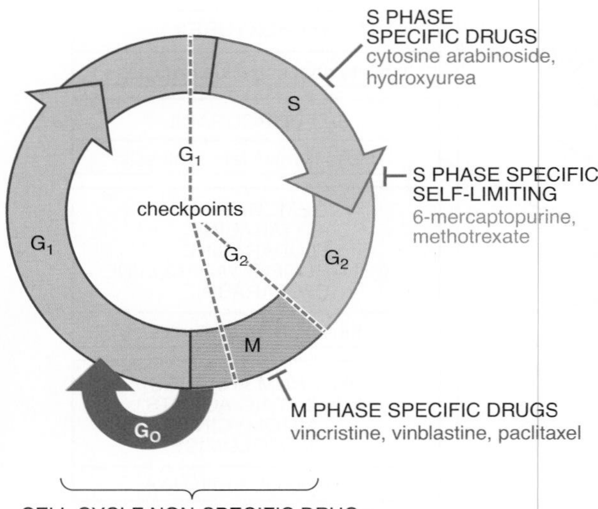

Figure 60–2. *Cell cycle specificity of antineoplastic agents.*

damaging DNA. Their toxicity is greatest during the S, or DNA synthetic, phase of the cell cycle. Others, such as the vinca alkaloids and taxanes, block the formation of a functional mitotic spindle in the M phase. These agents are most effective on cells entering mitosis, the most vulnerable phase of the cell cycle. Accordingly, human neoplasms most susceptible to chemotherapeutic measures, including leukemias and lymphomas, are those having a high percentage of proliferating cells. Normal tissues that proliferate rapidly (bone marrow, hair follicles, and intestinal epithelium) are thus highly susceptible to damage from cytotoxic drugs.

Slowly growing tumors with a small growth fraction (e.g., carcinomas of the colon or non–small cell lung cancer) are less responsive to cycle-specific drugs. More effective are agents that inflict high levels of DNA damage (e.g., alkylating agents) or those that remain at high concentrations inside the cell for extended periods of time (e.g., fluoropyrimidines). The results of comparative clinical trials provide evidence for the most effective regimens for specific tumors. The clinical benefit of cytotoxic drugs has primarily been measured by radiological assessment of drug effects on tumor size; newer "targeted" agents, however, may simply slow or halt tumor growth so their effects may best be measured in the assessment of time to disease progression. More recently, there is growing interest in designing drugs that selectively kill the stem cell component of tumors because these cells are believed to be responsible for the continuous proliferation and repopulation of tumors after a toxic exposure to chemotherapy or targeted therapy. For example, bone marrow and epithelial tissues contain a compartment of normal nondividing stem cells that display resistance to cytotoxic drugs and retain the capacity to regenerate the normal cell population. Tumor stem cells exhibit the same resistance to chemotherapy, radiotherapy, and oxidative insults, and thus they may represent a significant barrier to the cure of neoplasms (Diehn et al., 2009).

Although cells from different tumors display differences in the duration of their transit through the cell cycle, and in the fraction of cells in active proliferation, all cells display a similar pattern of cell cycle progression (Figure 60-2):

- a phase that precedes DNA synthesis (G_1)
- a DNA synthetic phase (S)
- an interval following the termination of DNA synthesis (G_2)
- the mitotic phase (M) in which the cell, containing a double complement of DNA, divides into two daughter G_1 cells
- a probability of moving into a quiescent state (G_0) and failing to move forward for long periods of time

At each transition point in the cell cycle, specific proteins such as p53 and chk-1 and 2, monitor the integrity of DNA and, upon detection of DNA damage, may initiate DNA repair processes or, in the presence of massive damage, direct cells down a cell death (apoptosis) pathway. Some cancer chemotherapeutic drugs act at specific phases, in the cell cycle, mainly at the S phase and M phase; other agents are cytoxic at any point in the cell cycle and are termed cell cycle phase nonspecific agents.

Each transition point in the cell cycle requires the activation of specific cyclin-dependent kinases (CDKs), which, in their active forms, couple with corresponding regulatory proteins called cyclins. The proliferative impact of CDKs is in turn dampened by inhibitory proteins such as p16. Tumor cells often exhibit changes in cell-cycle regulation that lead to relentless proliferation (e.g., mutations or loss of p16 or other inhibitory components of the so-called retinoblastoma pathway, enhanced cyclin or CDK activity). Consequently, CDKs and their effector proteins have become attractive targets for discovery of anti-neoplastic agents.

Because of the central importance of DNA to the identity and functionality of a cell, elaborate mechanisms ("checkpoints") have evolved to monitor DNA integrity. If a cell possesses normal checkpoint function, drug-induced DNA damage will activate apoptosis when the cell reaches the G_1/S or G_2/M boundary. If the p53 gene product or other checkpoint proteins are mutated or absent and the checkpoint function fails, damaged cells will not divert to the apoptotic pathway but will proceed through the S phase and mitosis. The cell progeny will emerge as a mutated and potentially drug-resistant population. Thus, alterations in the regulation of cell-cycle kinetics and checkpoint controls are critical factors in determining sensitivity to cytotoxic drugs and understanding the success or failure of new agents.

Achieving Therapeutic Integration and Efficacy. The treatment of cancer patients requires a skillful interdigitation of pharmacotherapy with other modalities of treatment (e.g., surgery and irradiation). Each treatment modality carries its own risks and benefits, with the potential for both antagonistic and synergistic interactions between modalities, particularly between drugs and irradiation. Furthermore, individual patient characteristics determine the choice of modalities. Not all patients can tolerate drugs, and not all drug regimens are appropriate for a given patient. Renal and hepatic function, bone marrow reserve, general performance status, and concurrent medical problems all come into consideration in making a therapeutic plan. Other less quantifiable considerations, such as the natural history of the tumor, the patient's willingness to undergo difficult and potentially dangerous treatments, and the patient's physical and emotional tolerance for side effects, enter the equation, with the goal of balancing the likely long-term gains and risks in the individual patient.

One of the great challenges of therapeutics is to adjust drug regimens to achieve a therapeutic but nontoxic outcome. Although it is customary to base dose on body surface area for individual patients, this practice is not necessarily supported by evidence in the literature (Sawyer and Ratain, 2001). Orally administered drugs are now frequently prescribed using uniform dosing for all adult patients. Dose adjustment based on renal function, on hepatic function, or on pharmacokinetic monitoring does facilitate meeting specific targets such as desired drug concentration in plasma or area under the concentration-time curve (AUC), a measure of the pattern of systemic exposure to the agent in question. Unfortunately, there are few good guidelines for adjusting dose on the basis of obesity or age. Elderly patients, particularly those >70 years of age, exhibit less tolerance for chemotherapy because of decreased renal and hepatic drug clearance, lower protein binding, and less bone marrow reserve, but individuals vary widely. Drug clearance decreases in morbidly obese patients, and dosage should probably be capped for these patients at no more than 150% of the dosage for patients of average body surface area (1.73 m^2) (Rodvold et al., 1988), with adjustment upward for tolerance after each subsequent dose.

Even patients with normal renal and hepatic function exhibit significant variability in pharmacokinetics of anticancer drugs that can reduce efficacy or cause excess toxicity. The following examples illustrate the potential of using pharmacokinetic targeting to improve therapy:

1. The thrombocytopenia caused by carboplatin is a direct function of AUC, which in turn is determined by renal clearance of the parent drug. Calvert and Egorin (2002) have devised a formula for targeting a desired AUC based on creatinine clearance.
2. Monitoring of 5-fluorouracil levels in plasma allows dose adjustment to improve response rates in patients with rapid drug clearance, and to avoid toxicity in those with slow drug clearance (Gamelin et al., 2008).
3. High-dose methotrexate therapy requires drug-level monitoring to detect patients at high risk for renal failure and severe myelosuppression. Patients with inappropriately high concentrations of methotrexate at specific time points can be rescued from toxicity by the administration of leucovorin, and in extreme cases, by dialysis or administration of a methotrexate-cleaving enzyme and orphan drug, glucarpidase (VORAXAZE; recombinant carboxypeptidase G2).

Molecular Testing to Select Patients for Chemotherapy. Molecular tests are increasingly employed to identify patients likely to benefit from treatment and those at highest risk of toxicity (Roberts and Chabner, 2004). Pretreatment testing has become standard practice to select patients for hormonal therapy of breast cancer and for treatment with antibodies such as trastuzumab (her-2/neu receptor) and rituximab (CD20). The presence of a mutated k-ras gene indicates that a colorectal cancer patient's tumor will not respond to anti-EGFR antibodies (Tol et al., 2009); mutations of EGFR signal a 70% likelihood of response to erlotinib (TARCEVA) and gefitinib (IRESSA), both inhibitors of this receptor (Sequist and Lynch, 2008). Although *not* yet routinely employed in traditional cytotoxic therapy, molecular testing of tumors could improve outcomes by pairing patients with drugs likely to be effective against mutations that drive tumor proliferation or survival. Mutations of the *b-Raf, HER 2/neu,* and *Alk*, which are found in subsets of solid tumors in human subjects, represent examples of promising targets for solid tumor chemotherapy.

Inherited differences in protein sequence polymorphisms or levels of RNA expression influence toxicity and anti-tumor response. For example, tandem repeats in the promoter region of the gene encoding thymidylate synthase, the target of 5-fluorouracil, determine the level of expression of the enzyme. Increased numbers of repeats are associated with increased gene expression, a lower incidence of toxicity, and a decreased rate of response in patients with colorectal cancer (Pullarkat et al., 2001). Polymorphisms of the dihydropyrimidine dehydrogenase gene, the product of which is responsible for degradation of 5-fluorouracil, are associated with decreased enzyme activity and a significant risk of overwhelming drug toxicity, particularly in the rare individual homozygous for the polymorphic genes (Van Kuilenburg et al., 2002). Other polymorphisms appear to affect the clearance and therapeutic activity of cancer drugs, including tamoxifen (Schroth et al., 2007), methotrexate, irinotecan, and 6-mercaptopurine (Cheok and Evans, 2006).

Other aspects of molecular biology are entering into clinical decision making in oncology. Gene expression profiling, in which the levels of messenger RNA from thousands of genes are randomly surveyed using gene arrays, has revealed tumor profiles that are highly associated with metastasis (Ramaswamy et al., 2003). The expression of the transcription factor HOX B13 correlates with disease recurrence in patients receiving adjuvant hormonal therapy in breast cancer (Ma et al., 2004). Gene expression profiles also predict the benefit of adjuvant chemotherapy for breast cancer patients (Sotiriou and Pusztai, 2009) and the response of ovarian cancer patients to platinum-based therapy (Dressman et al., 2007).

New molecular tests and their more widespread use likely will shorten the time for drug development and approval, realize savings by avoiding the cost and toxicity of ineffective drugs, and ultimately improve patient outcome (Chabner and Roberts, 2005; Roberts and Chabner, 2004). Undoubtedly, molecular testing to select patients for specific treatments will be a cornerstone of cancer chemotherapy for years to come.

A Cautionary Note. Although advances in drug discovery and molecular profiling of tumors offer great promise for improving the outcomes of cancer treatment, a final word of caution regarding all treatment regimen deserves emphasis. *The pharmacokinetics and toxicities of cancer drugs vary among individual patients.* It is imperative to *recognize toxicities early*, to *alter doses or discontinue offending medication* to relieve symptoms and reduce risk, and to *provide vigorous supportive care* (platelet transfusions, antibiotics, and hematopoietic growth factors). Toxicities affecting the heart, lungs, or kidneys may be irreversible if recognized late in their course, leading to permanent organ damage or death. Fortunately, such toxicities can be minimized by early recognition and by adherence to standardized protocols and to the guidelines for drug use.

BIBLIOGRAPHY

Batchelor TA, Sorensen AG, di Tomaso E, et al. AZD2171, a pan-VEGF receptor tyrosine kinase inhibitor, normalizes tumor vasculature and alleviates edema in glioblastoma patients. *Cancer Cell*, **2007,** *11:*83–95.

Calvert AH, Egorin MJ. Carboplatin dosing formulae: Gender bias and the use of creatinine-based methodologies. *Eur J Cancer*, **2002,** *38:*11–16.

Chabner BA, Roberts TG. Timeline: Chemotherapy and the war on cancer. *Nat Rev Cancer*, **2005,** *5:*65–72.

Cheok MH, Evans WE. Acute lymphoblastic leukaemia: A model for the pharmacogenomics of cancer therapy. *Nat Rev Cancer*, **2006,** *6:*117–129. Erratum in: *Nat Rev Cancer*, **2006,** *6:*249.

Diehn M, Cho RW, Lobo NA, et al. Association of reactive oxygen species levels and radioresistance in cancer stem cells. *Nature*, **2009,** *458:*780–783.

Dressman HK, Berchuck A, Chan G, et al. An integrated genomic-based approach to individualized treatment of patients with advanced-stage ovarian cancer. *J Clin Oncol*, **2007,** *25:*517–525.

Engelman JA, Chen L, Tan X, et al. Effective use of PI3K and MEK inhibitors to treat mutant Kras G12D and PIK3CA H1047R murine lung cancers. *Nat Med*, **2008,** *14:* 1351–1356.

Gamelin E, Delva R, Jacob J, et al. Individual fluorouracil dose adjustment based on pharmacokinetic follow-up compared with conventional dosage: Results of a multicenter randomized trial of patients with metastatic colorectal cancer. *J Clin Oncol*, **2008,** *26:*2099–2105.

Holleman A, den Boer ML, de Menezes RX, et al. The expression of 70 apoptosis genes in relation to lineage, genetic subtype, cellular drug resistance, and outcome in childhood acute lymphoblastic leukemia. *Blood*, **2006,** *107:*769–776.

Ma XJ, Wang Z, Ryan, PD, et al. A two-gene expression ratio predicts clinical outcome in breast cancer patients treated with tamoxifen. *Cancer Cell*, **2004,** *5:*607–616.

Maheswaran S, Sequist LV, Nagrath S, et al. Detection of mutations in EGFR in circulating lung-cancer cells. *N Engl J Med*, **2008,** *359:*366–377.

Pullarkat ST, Stoehlmacher J, Ghaderi V, et al. Thymidylate synthase gene polymorphism determines response and toxicity of 5-FU chemotherapy. *Pharmacogenomics J*, **2001,** *1:*65–70.

Ramaswamy S, Ross KN, Lander, ES, Golub TR. A molecular signature of metastasis in primary solid tumors. *Nat Genet*, **2003,** *33:*49–54.

Roberts TG Jr, Chabner BA. Beyond fast track for drug approvals. *N Engl J Med, **2004,** 351:*501–505.

Rodvold KA, Rushing DA, Tewksbury DA. Doxorubicin clearance in the obese. *J Clin Oncol*, **1988,** *6:*1321–1327.

Romond EH, Perez EA, Bryant J, et al. Trastuzumab plus adjuvant chemotherapy for operable HER2-positive breast cancer. *N Engl J Med*, **2005,** *353:*1673–1684.

Sawyer M, Ratain MJ. Body surface area as a determinant of pharmacokinetics and drug dosing. *Invest New Drugs*, **2001,** *19:*171–177.

Schroth W, Antoniadou L, Fritz P, et al. Breast cancer treatment outcome with adjuvant tamoxifen relative to patient CYP2D6 and CYP2C19 genotypes. *J Clin Oncol*, **2007,** *25:*5187–5193.

Sequist LV, Lynch TJ. EGFR tyrosine kinase inhibitors in lung cancer: An evolving story. *Annu Rev Med*, **2008,** *59:*429–442.

Sotiriou C, Pusztai L. Gene-expression signatures in breast cancer. *N Engl J Med*, **2009,** *360:*790–800.

Slamon DJ, Leyland-Jones B, Shak S, et al. Use of chemotherapy plus a monoclonal antibody against HER2 for metastatic breast cancer that overexpresses HER2. *N Engl J Med*, **2001,** *344:*783–792.

Tol J, Koopman M, Cats A, et al. Chemotherapy, bevacizumab, and cetuximab in metastatic colorectal cancer. *N Engl J Med*, **2009,** *360:*563–572.

Van Kuilenburg AB, Meinsma R, Zoetekouw L, Van Gennip AH. High prevalence of the IVS14 + 1G>A mutation in the dihydropyrimidine dehydrogenase gene of patients with severe 5-fluorouracil-associated toxicity. *Pharmacogenetics,* **2002,** *12:*555–558.

Weinstein IB, Joe AK. Mechanisms of disease: Oncogene addiction—a rationale for molecular targeting in cancer therapy. *Nat Clin Pract Oncol*, **2006,** *8:*448–457.

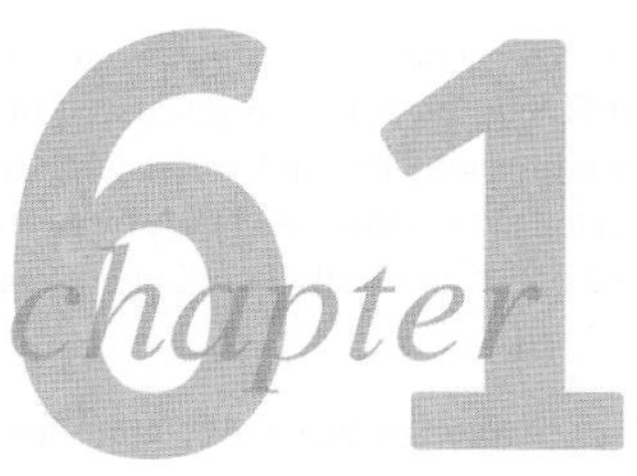

Cytotoxic Agents

Bruce A. Chabner, Joseph Bertino, James Cleary, Taylor Ortiz, Andrew Lane, Jeffrey G. Supko, and David Ryan

I. Alkylating Agents and Platinum Coordination Complexes

The pervasive toxic effects of sulfur mustard gas were noted as the result of its use in World War I. A potent vesicant, the gas caused a topical burn to skin, eyes, lungs, and mucosa and, after massive exposure, aplasia of the bone marrow and lymphoid tissue and ulceration of the GI tract. Early clinical experiments with topically applied sulfur mustard led to regression of penile tumors. Thereafter, Goodman, Gilman, the originators of this text, working with colleagues at Yale in a consortium organized by the U.S. Department of Defense, confirmed the antineoplastic action of the nitrogen mustards against a murine lymphoma. In 1942, they began clinical studies of intravenous nitrogen mustards in patients with lymphoma, launching the modern era of cancer chemotherapy (Gilman and Philips, 1946).

At present, six major types of alkylating agents are used in the chemotherapy of neoplastic diseases:

- nitrogen mustards
- ethyleneimines
- alkyl sulfonates
- nitrosoureas
- the triazenes
- DNA-methylating drugs, including procarbazine, temozolomide, and dacarbazine

In addition, because of similarities in their mechanisms of action and resistance, platinum complexes are discussed with classical alkylating agents, even though they do not alkylate DNA but instead form covalent metal adducts with DNA. The mechanism of action of alkylating agents is shown in Figure 61–1.

Chemistry. The chemotherapeutic alkylating agents have in common the property of forming highly reactive carbonium ion intermediates. These reactive intermediates covalently link to sites of high electron density, such as phosphates, amines, sulfhydryl, and hydroxyl groups. Their chemotherapeutic and cytotoxic effects are directly related to the alkylation of reactive amines, oxygens, or phosphates on DNA. The N7 atom of guanine is particularly susceptible to the formation of a covalent bond with bifunctional alkylating agents and may represent the key target that determines their biological effects. Other atoms in the purine and pyrimidine bases of DNA, including N1 and N3 of the adenine ring, N3 of cytosine, and O6 of guanine, react with these agents, as do the amino and sulfhydryl groups of proteins and the sulfhydryls of glutathione.

The possible actions of alkylating agents on DNA are illustrated in Figure 61–1 with mechlorethamine (nitrogen mustard). First, one 2-chloroethyl side chain undergoes a first-order (S_N1) intramolecular cyclization, with release of Cl^- and formation of a highly reactive ethyleneimine intermediate (Figure 61–1). The unstable quaternary amine then reacts with a variety of electron-dense sites. This latter reaction proceeds as a second-order (S_N2) nucleophilic substitution. Alkylation of the N7 of guanine in DNA, a highly favored reaction, exerts several biologically important effects. Guanine residues in DNA exist predominantly as the keto tautomer and readily make Watson-Crick base pairs by hydrogen bonding with cytosine residues. However, when the N7 of guanine is alkylated (to become a quaternary ammonium nitrogen) the guanine residue is more acidic and the enol tautomer is favored. The modified guanine can mispair with thymine residues during DNA synthesis, leading to the substitution of thymine for cytosine. Second, alkylation of the N7 creates lability in the imidazole ring, leading to opening of the ring and excision of the damaged guanine residue. Mispairing and imidazole ring opening can lead to attempts to repair the damaged stretch of DNA, causing strand breakage. Third, with bifunctional alkylating agents such as nitrogen mustard, the second 2-chloroethyl side chain can undergo a similar cyclization

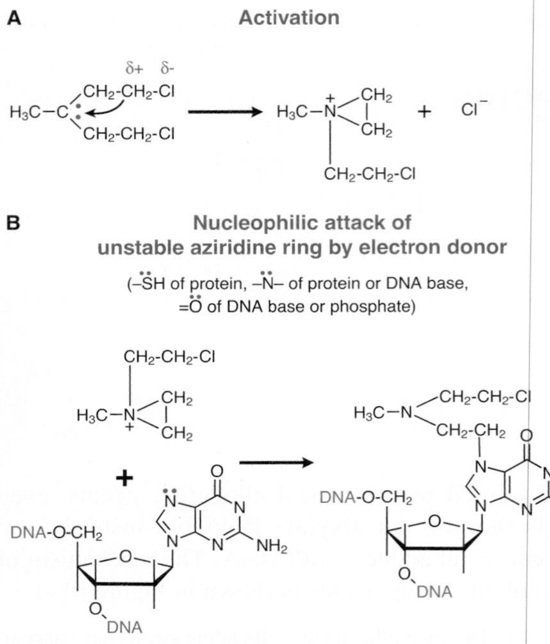

Figure 61–1. *Mechanism of action of alkylating agents.* **A.** Activation reaction. **B.** Alkylation of N7 of guanine.

reaction and alkylate a second guanine residue or another nucleophilic moiety, resulting in the cross-linking of two nucleic acid chains or the linking of a nucleic acid to a protein, alterations that would cause a major disruption in nucleic acid function. Any of these effects could contribute to both the mutagenic and cytotoxic effects of alkylating agents. The extreme cytotoxicity of bifunctional alkylators correlates very closely with interstrand cross-linkage of DNA (Garcia et al., 1988).

The ultimate cause of cell death related to DNA damage is not known. Specific cellular responses include cell-cycle arrest and attempts to repair DNA. The specific repair enzyme complex utilized will depend on two factors: the chemistry of the adduct formed and the repair capacity of the cell involved. The process of recognizing and repairing DNA generally requires an intact nucleotide excision repair (NER) complex, but, as discussed in the rest of this section, may differ with each drug and with each tumor. Alternatively, recognition of extensively damaged DNA by p53 can trigger apoptosis. Mutations of p53 lead to alkylating agent resistance (Kastan, 1999).

Structure-Activity Relationships. Although these alkylating agents share the capacity to alkylate biologically important molecules, modification of the basic chloroethylamino structure changes reactivity, lipophilicity, active transport across biological membranes, sites of macromolecular attack, and mechanisms of DNA repair, all of which properties determine drug activity *in vivo.* With several of the most valuable agents (e.g., cyclophosphamide, ifosfamide), the active alkylating moieties are generated *in vivo* through hepatic metabolism.

The biological activity of alkylators of the nitrogen mustard type is based on the presence of the *bis*-(2-chloroethyl) group. Although mechlorethamine has been widely used in the past, linkage of the *bis*-(2-chloroethyl) group to election-rich substitutions such as unsaturated ring systems has yielded more stable drugs with better pharmacodynamic properties and with greater selective killing of tumor cells. *Bis*-(2-chloroethyl) groups linked to amino acids (phenylalanine) and substituted phenyl groups (aminophenol butyric acid, as in chlorambucil) create a more stable and orally available form. The structures of important nitrogen mustards are shown in Figure 61–2.

A classical example of the role of host metabolism in the activation and degradation of an alkylating agent is seen with cyclophosphamide, now the most widely used agent of this class. The drug undergoes metabolic activation (hydroxylation) by CYP2B (Figure 61–3), with subsequent transport of the activated intermediate to sites of action. The selectivity of cyclophosphamide against certain malignant tissues may result in part from the capacity of normal tissues to degrade the activated intermediates via aldehyde dehydrogenase, glutathione transferase, and other pathways.

Ifosfamide is an oxazaphosphorine, similar to cyclophosphamide. Cyclophosphamide has two chloroethyl groups on the exocyclic nitrogen atom, whereas one of the 2-chloroethyl groups of

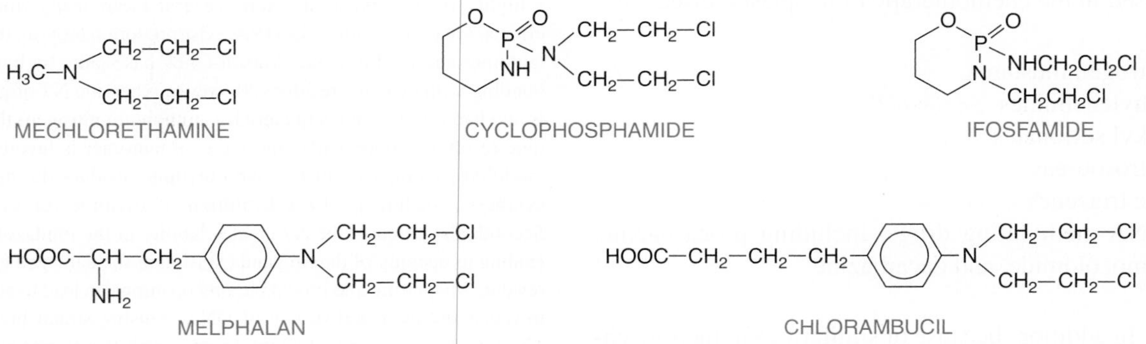

Figure 61–2. *Nitrogen mustards employed in therapy.*

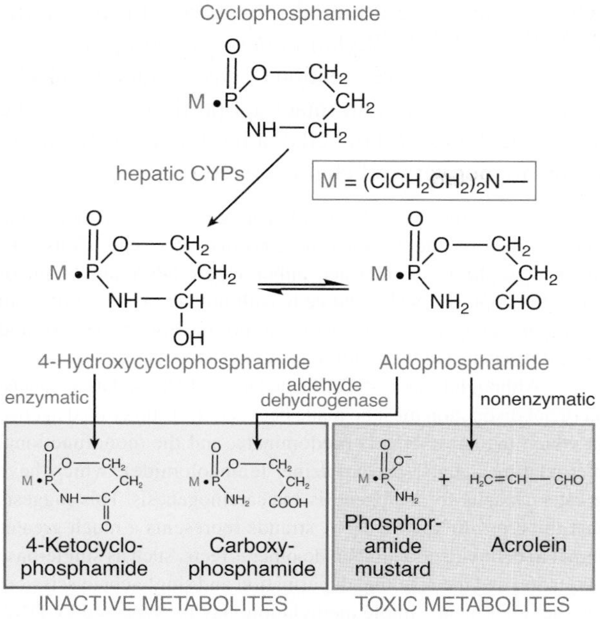

Cyclophosphamide

hepatic CYPs

M = $(ClCH_2CH_2)_2N$—

4-Hydroxycyclophosphamide

Aldophosphamide

enzymatic

aldehyde dehydrogenase

nonenzymatic

4-Ketocyclophosphamide

Carboxyphosphamide

Phosphoramide mustard

Acrolein

INACTIVE METABOLITES

TOXIC METABOLITES

Figure 61–3. *Metabolism of cyclophosphamide.*

ifosfamide is on the cyclic phosphoramide nitrogen of the oxazaphosphorine ring. Ifosfamide is activated in the liver by CYP3A4. The activation of ifosfamide proceeds more slowly, with greater production of dechlorinated metabolites and chloroacetaldehyde. These differences in metabolism likely account for the higher doses of ifosfamide required for equitoxic effects, the greater neurotoxicity of ifosfamide, and the possible differences in antitumor spectrum of the two agents.

The newest approved alkylating agent, bendamustine, has the typical chloroethyl reactive groups attached to a benzimidazole backbone.

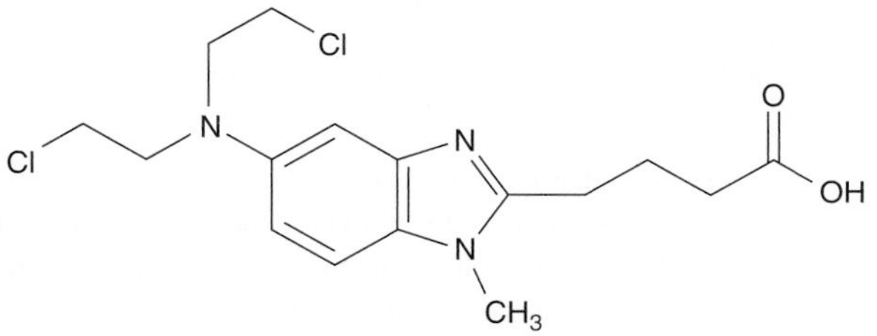

BENDAMUSTINE

The unique properties and activity of this drug may derive from this purine-like structure; the agent produces slowly repaired DNA cross-links, lacks cross-resistance with other classical alkylators (Leoni et al., 2008), and has significant activity in chronic lymphocytic leukemia (CLL) and large-cell lymphomas refractory to standard alkylators.

A unique class of alkylating agents transfers methyl rather than ethyl groups to DNA. The triazene derivative 5-(3,3-dimethyl-1-triazeno)-imidazole-4-carboxamide, usually referred to as dacarbazine or DTIC, is prototypical of methylating agents.

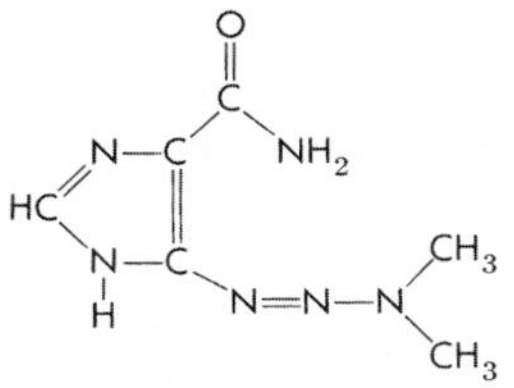

DACARBAZINE

Dacarbazine requires initial activation by hepatic CYPs through an *N*-demethylation reaction. In the target cell, spontaneous cleavage of the metabolite, methyl-triazeno-imidazole-carboxamide (MTIC), yields an alkylating moiety, a methyl diazonium ion. A related triazene, temozolomide, undergoes spontaneous, nonenzymatic activation to MTIC and has significant activity against gliomas.

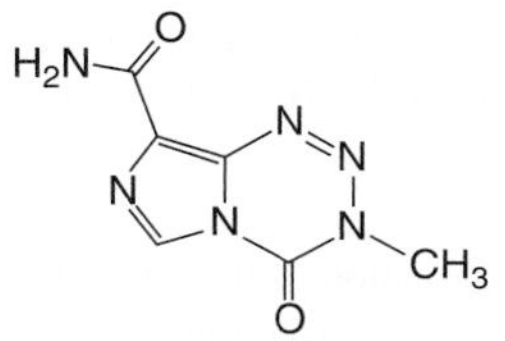

TEMOZOLOMIDE

The nitrosoureas, which include compounds such as 1,3-*bis*-(2-chloroethyl)-1-nitrosourea (carmustine; BCNU), 1-(2-chloroethyl)-3-cyclohexyl-1-nitrosourea (lomustine; CCNU), and its methyl derivative (semustine; methyl-CCNU), as well as the antibiotic streptozocin (streptozotocin), exert their cytotoxicity through the spontaneous breakdown to an alkylating intermediate, the 2-chloroethyl diazonium ion.

$ClCH_2CH_2$—N(N=O)—C(=O)—$NHCH_2CH_2Cl$

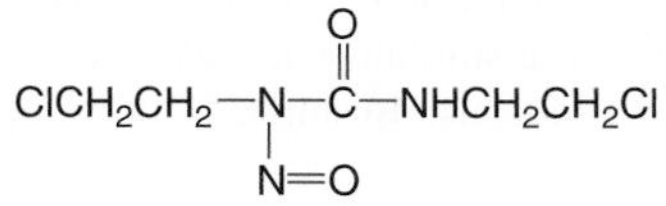

CARMUSTINE (BCNU)

The 2-chloroethyl diazonium ion, a strong electrophile, can alkylate guanine, cytidine, and adenine bases (Ludlum, 1990). Displacement of the halogen atom can then lead to interstrand or intrastrand cross-linking of DNA. The formation of cross-links after the initial alkylation reaction proceeds relatively slowly and can be reversed by the DNA repair enzyme O^6-alkyl, methyl guanine methyltransferase (MGMT), which displaces the chloroethyl adduct from its binding to guanine in a suicide reaction. The same enzyme, when expressed in human gliomas, produces resistance to nitrosoureas and to other methylating agents, including DTIC, temozolomide, and procarbazine. As with the nitrogen mustards, interstrand cross-linking appears to be the primary lesion responsible for the cytotoxicity of nitrosoureas (Ludlum, 1990). The reactions of the nitrosoureas with macromolecules are shown in Figure 61–4.

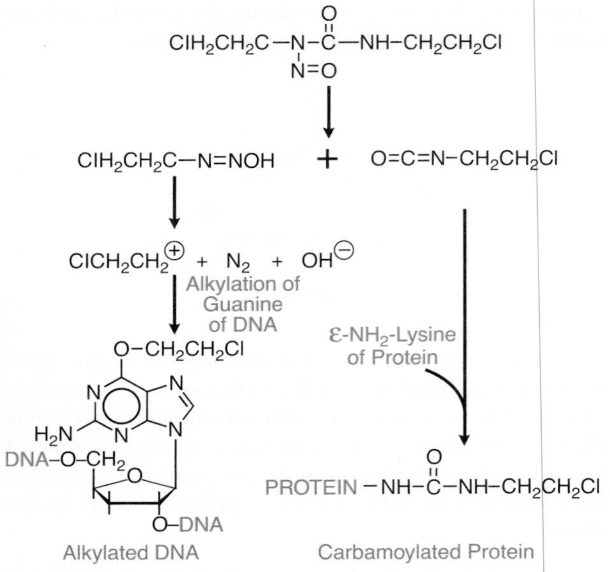

$ClH_2CH_2C-N(N{=}O)-C(=O)-NH-CH_2CH_2Cl$

$\downarrow$

$ClH_2CH_2C-N{=}NOH \quad + \quad O{=}C{=}N-CH_2CH_2Cl$

$\downarrow$

$ClCH_2CH_2^{\oplus} + N_2 + OH^{\ominus}$

Alkylation of Guanine of DNA

ε-NH_2-Lysine of Protein

$O-CH_2CH_2Cl$ (guanine) ... $DNA-O-CH_2$ ... $O-DNA$

$PROTEIN-NH-C(=O)-NH-CH_2CH_2Cl$

Alkylated DNA   Carbamoylated Protein

Figure 61–4. Degradation of carmustine (BCNU) with generation of alkylating and carbamylating intermediates.

Because the formation of the ethyleneimine ion constitutes the initial reaction of the nitrogen mustards, it is not surprising that stable ethyleneimine derivatives have antitumor activity. Several compounds of this type, including triethylenemelamine (TEM) and triethylenethiophosphoramide (thiotepa), have been used clinically. In standard doses, thiotepa produces little toxicity other than myelosuppression; it also is used for high-dose chemotherapy regimens, in which it causes both mucosal and central nervous system toxicity. Altretamine (hexamethylmelamine; HMM) is mentioned here because of its chemical similarity to TEM. The methylmelamines are *N*-demethylated by hepatic microsomes with the release of formaldehyde, and there is a direct relationship between the degree of the demethylation and their activity against murine tumors.

Esters of alkane sulfonic acids alkylate DNA through the release of methyl radicals. Busulfan is of value in high-dose chemotherapy.

$H_3C-S(=O)_2-O-CH_2-CH_2-CH_2-CH_2-O-S(=O)_2-CH_3$

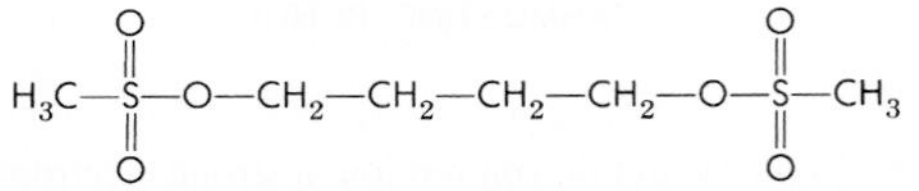

BUSULFAN

Pharmacological Actions

Cytotoxic Actions. The capacity of alkylating agents to interfere with DNA integrity and function and to induce cell death in rapidly proliferating tissues provides the basis for their therapeutic and toxic properties. Acute effects manifest primarily against rapidly proliferating tissues; however, certain alkylating agents may have damaging effects on tissues with normally low mitotic indices (e.g., liver, kidney, and mature lymphocytes), which usually are affected in a delayed time frame. Lethality of DNA alkylation depends on the recognition of the adduct, the creation of DNA strand breaks by repair enzymes, and an intact apoptotic response. The actual mechanism(s) of cell death related to DNA alkylation are not yet well characterized.

In non-dividing cells, DNA damage activates a checkpoint that depends on the presence of a normal p53 gene. Cells thus blocked in the G_1/S interface either repair DNA alkylation or undergo apoptosis. Malignant cells with mutant or absent p53 fail to suspend cell-cycle progression, do not undergo apoptosis, and exhibit resistance to these drugs.

Although DNA is the ultimate target of all alkylating agents, a crucial distinction must be made between the bifunctional agents, in which cytotoxic effects predominate, and the monofunctional methylating agents (procarbazine, temozolomide), which have greater capacity for mutagenesis and carcinogenesis. This suggests that the cross-linking of DNA strands represents a much greater threat to cellular survival than do other effects, such as single-base alkylation and the resulting depurination and single-chain scission. On the other hand, simple methylation may be bypassed by DNA polymerases, leading to mispairing reactions that permanently modify DNA sequence. These new sequences are transmitted to subsequent generations and may result in mutagenesis or carcinogenesis. Some methylating agents, such as procarbazine, are highly carcinogenic.

DNA repair systems play an important role in removing adducts, and thereby determine the selectivity of action against particular cell types, and acquired resistance to alkylating agents. Alkylation of a single strand of DNA (mono-adducts) is repaired by the nucleotide excision repair pathway, while the less frequent cross-links require participation of nonhomologous end joining, an error-prone pathway, or the error-free homologous recombination pathway. After drug infusion in humans, mono-adducts appear rapidly and peak within 2 hours of drug exposure, while cross-links peak at 8 hours. The $t_{1/2}$ for repair of adducts varies among normal tissues and tumors; in peripheral blood mononuclear cells, both mono-adducts and cross-links disappear with a $t_{1/2}$ of 12-16 hours (Souliotis et al., 1990).

The homologous end-joining pathway has multiple components (Wang et al., 2001):

- sensors of DNA integrity (such as p53)
- activation signals such as the ataxia-telangiectasia-mutated (ATM) and ataxia-telangiectasia and rad-related (ATR) proteins
- the activated repair complex composed of Fanconi anemia proteins and BRCA2, all of which localize at the site of DNA damage and initiate removal of the cross-linked segment of DNA
- homologous recombination, which allows resynthesis of the damaged DNA sequence followed by re-ligation of the repaired sequences

The process depends on the presence and accurate functioning of multiple proteins. Their absence or mutation, as in Fanconi anemia or ataxia telangiectasia, leads to extreme sensitivity to DNA cross-linking agents such as mitomycin, cisplatin, or classical alkylators.

Other repair enzymes are specific for removing methyl and ethyl adducts from the O-6 of guanine (MGMT) and for repair of alkylation of the N-3 of adenine and N-7 of guanine (3-methyladenine-DNA glycosylase) (Matijasevic et al., 1993). High expression of MGMT protects cells from cytotoxic effects of nitrosoureas and methylating agents and confers drug resistance, while methylation and silencing of the gene in brain tumors are associated with clinical response to BCNU and temozolomide (Hegi et al., 2008).

Bendamustine differs from classical chloroethyl alkylators in activating base excision repair, rather than the more complex double-strand break repair or MGMT. It impairs physiological arrest of adduct-containing cells at mitotic checkpoints and leads to mitotic catastrophe rather than apoptosis, and does not require an intact p53 to cause cytotoxicity.

Finally, recognition of DNA adducts is an essential step in promoting attempts at repair and ultimately leading to apoptosis. The Fanconi pathway, consisting of 12 proteins, recognizes adducts and signals the need for repair of a broad array of DNA-damaging drugs and irradiation (Chen et al., 2007). Absence or inactivation of components of this pathway leads to increased sensitivity to DNA damage. Conversely, for the methylating drugs, nitrosoureas, cisplatin and carboplatin, and thiopurine analogs, the mismatch repair (MMR) pathway is essential for cytotoxicity, causing strand breaks at sites of adduct formation, creating mispairing of thymine residues, and triggering apoptosis.

Mechanisms of Resistance to Alkylating Agents. Resistance to an alkylating agent develops rapidly when it is used as a single agent. Specific biochemical changes implicated in the development of resistance include:

- Decreased permeation of actively transported drugs (mechlorethamine and melphalan).
- Increased intracellular concentrations of nucleophilic substances, principally thiols such as glutathione, which can conjugate with and detoxify electrophilic intermediates.
- Increased activity of DNA repair pathways, which may differ for the various alkylating agents.

Increased activity of the complex NER pathway correlates with resistance to most chloroethyl and platinum adducts. MGMT activity determines response to BCNU and to methylating drugs such as the triazenes, procarbazine, temozolomide, and busulfan. Methylation of the MGMT gene found that pretreatment in 20% of brain tumor patients decreases MGMT expression and strongly correlates with response and survival after BCNU or temozolomide for malignant gliomas. MGMT activity increases with each round of alkylator treatment and with disease progression (Wiewrodt et al., 2008).

- Increased rates of metabolic degradation of the activated forms of cyclophosphamide and ifosfamide to their inactive keto and carboxy metabolites by aldehyde dehydrogenase (Figure 61–3), and detoxification of most alkylating intermediates by glutathione transferases.
- Loss of ability to recognize adducts formed by nitrosoureas and methylating agents, as the result of defective MMR capability, confers resistance, as does defective checkpoint function for virtually all alkylating drugs.

The MSH6 component of the MMR system seems particularly susceptible to mutation by exposure to alkylating agents; in studies of brain tumor resistance to therapy, loss of MSH6 conferred resistance to temozolomide and related drugs (Cahill et al., 2008).

- Impaired apoptotic pathways, with overexpression of bcl-2 as an example, confer resistance.

To reverse cellular changes that lead to resistance, strategies that are effective in selected experimental tumors have been devised. These include the use of compounds that deplete glutathione, such as l-buthionine-sulfoximine; sulfhydryl compounds such as amifostine (WR-2721) that selectively detoxify alkylating species in normal cells and thereby prevent toxicity; O^6-benzylguanine, which inactivates MGMT; and compounds such as ethacrynic acid, which inhibits glutathione transferases. Although each of these modalities has experimental evidence to support its use, their clinical efficacy has not yet been proven.

TOXICITIES OF ALKYLATING AGENTS

Bone Marrow Toxicity

The alkylating agents differ in their patterns of antitumor activity and in the sites and severity of their side effects. Most cause dose-limiting toxicity to bone marrow elements and, to a lesser extent, intestinal mucosa. Most alkylating agents (i.e., melphalan, chlorambucil, cyclophosphamide, and ifosfamide) cause acute myelosuppression, with a nadir of the peripheral blood granulocyte count at 6-10 days and recovery in 14-21 days.

Cyclophosphamide has lesser effects on peripheral blood platelet counts than do the other agents. Busulfan suppresses all blood elements, particularly stem cells, and may produce a prolonged and cumulative myelosuppression lasting months or even years. For this reason, it is used as a preparative regimen in allogenic bone marrow transplantation. Carmustine and other chloroethylnitrosoureas cause delayed and prolonged suppression of both platelets and granulocytes, reaching a nadir 4-6 weeks after drug administration and reversing slowly thereafter.

Both cellular and humoral immunity are suppressed by alkylating agents, which have been used to treat various auto-immune diseases. Immunosuppression is reversible at usual doses, but opportunistic infections such as *Pneumocystis jiroveci* pneumonia, or fungal infections, may occur with extended treatment, and reactivation of hepatitis B has been described, prompting some authors to advocate antiviral prophylaxis in hepatitis B carriers undergoing intensive alkylating agent chemotherapy (Grewal et al., 2007).

Mucosal Toxicity

Alkylating agents are highly toxic to dividing mucosal cells and to hair follicles, leading to oral mucosal ulceration, intestinal denudation, and alopecia.

The mucosal effects are particularly damaging in high-dose chemotherapy protocols associated with bone marrow reconstitution, as they predispose to bacterial sepsis arising from the GI tract. In these protocols, cyclophosphamide, melphalan, and thiotepa have the advantage of causing less mucosal damage than the other agents. In high-dose protocols, however, other toxicities become limiting, as delineated in Table 61–1.

Neurotoxicity

Nausea and vomiting commonly follow agent administration of nitrogen mustard or BCNU. Ifosfamide is the most neurotoxic agent of this class and may produce altered mental status, coma, generalized seizures, and cerebellar ataxia. These side effects result from the release of chloroacetaldehyde from the phosphate-linked chloroethyl side chain of ifosfamide. High-dose busulfan can cause seizures; in addition, it accelerates the clearance of phenytoin, an anti-seizure medication.

Other Organ Toxicities. Although mucosal and bone marrow toxicities occur predictably and acutely with conventional doses of these drugs, other organ toxicities may supervene after prolonged or high-dose use; these effects can appear after months or years and may be irreversible and even lethal. All alkylating agents, including temozolomide, have caused pulmonary fibrosis, usually several months after treatment. In high-dose regimens, particularly those employing busulfan or BCNU, vascular endothelial damage may precipitate veno-occlusive disease (VOD) of the liver, an often fatal side effect that is successfully reversed by the investigational drug defibrotide (Richardson et al., 2003). The nitrosoureas and ifosfamide, after multiple cycles of therapy, may lead to renal failure. Cyclophosphamide and ifosfamide release a nephrotoxic and urotoxic metabolite, acrolein, which causes a severe hemorrhagic cystitis in high-dose regimens. This adverse effect can be prevented by co-administration of 2-mercaptoethanesulfonate (mesna; MESNEX), which conjugates acrolein in urine. Ifosfamide in high doses for transplant causes a chronic, and often irreversible, renal toxicity. Proximal and, less commonly, distal tubules may be affected, leading to defective Ca^{2+} and Mg^{2+} reabsorption, glycosuria, and renal tubular acidosis. Nephrotoxicity correlates with the total dose of drug received and increases in frequency in children <5 years of age. The syndrome may be due to chloroacetaldehyde and/or acrolein excreted in the urine.

The more unstable alkylating agents (particularly mechlorethamine and the nitrosoureas) have strong vesicant properties, damage veins with repeated use and, if extravasated, produce ulceration.

Finally, all alkylating agents have toxic effects on the male and female reproductive systems, causing an often permanent amenorrhea, particularly in perimenopausal women, and an irreversible azoospermia in men.

Leukemogenesis. As a class of drugs, the alkylating agents are highly leukemogenic. Acute nonlymphocytic leukemia, often associated with partial or total deletions of chromosome 5 or 7, peaks in incidence ~4 years after therapy and may affect up to 5% of patients treated on regimens containing alkylating drugs. Leukemia often is preceded by a period of neutropenia or anemia and by bone marrow morphology consistent with myelodysplasia. Melphalan, the nitrosoureas, and the methylating agent procarbazine have the greatest propensity to cause leukemia, while it is less common after cyclophosphamide.

Table 61–1

Dose-Limiting Extramedullary Toxicities of Single Alkylating Agents

DRUG	MTD,[a] mg/m²	FOLD INCREASE OVER STANDARD DOSE	MAJOR ORGAN TOXICITIES
Cyclophosphamide	7000	7	Cardiac, hepatic VOD
Ifosfamide	16,000	2.7	Renal, CNS, hepatic VOD
Thiotepa	1000	18	GI, CNS, hepatic VOD
Melphalan	180	5.6	GI, hepatic VOD
Busulfan	640	9	GI, hepatic VOD
Carmustine (BCNU)	1050	5.3	Lung, hepatic VOD
Cisplatin	200	2	PN, renal
Carboplatin	2000	5	Renal, PN, hepatic VOD

[a]Maximum tolerated dose (MTD; cumulative) in treatment protocols.
CNS, central nervous system; GI, gastrointestinal; PN, peripheral neuropathy; VOD, veno-occlusive disease.

CLINICAL PHARMACOLOGY

Nitrogen Mustards

The chemistry and the pharmacological actions of the alkylating agents as a group, and of the nitrogen mustards, have been presented in the preceding sections. Only the unique pharmacological characteristics of the individual agents are considered in this section.

Mechlorethamine. Mechlorethamine was the first clinically used nitrogen mustard and is the most reactive of the drugs in this class. It rarely is used in current practice.

Absorption and Fate. Severe local reactions of exposed tissues necessitate rapid intravenous injection of mechlorethamine for most clinical uses. In either water or body fluids, at rates affected markedly by pH, mechlorethamine rapidly undergoes chemical degradation as it combines with either water or cellular nucleophiles, and the parent compound disappears from the bloodstream within minutes.

Therapeutic Uses. Mechlorethamine HCl (MUSTARGEN) formerly was used in the combination chemotherapy regimen MOPP (mechlorethamine, vincristine, procarbazine, and prednisone) in patients with Hodgkin's disease. It is given by intravenous bolus administration in doses of 6 mg/m^2 on days 1 and 8 of the 28-day cycles of each course of treatment. It has been largely replaced by cyclophosphamide, melphalan, and other, more stable alkylating agents.

It also is used topically for treatment of cutaneous T-cell lymphoma (CTCL) as a solution that is rapidly mixed and applied to affected areas of the skin.

Clinical Toxicity. The major acute toxic manifestations of mechlorethamine are nausea and vomiting, lacrimation, and myelosuppression. Leukopenia and thrombocytopenia limit the amount of drug that can be given in a single course.

Cyclophosphamide

Absorption, Fate, and Excretion. Cyclophosphamide is well absorbed orally and is activated to the 4-hydroxy intermediate (Xie et al., 2003) (Figure 61–3). 4-Hydroxycyclophosphamide exists in equilibrium with the acyclic tautomer aldophosphamide. The rate of metabolic activation of cyclophosphamide exhibits significant interpatient variability and increases with successive doses in high-dose regimens but appears to be saturable at infusion rates of >4 g/90 min and concentrations of the parent compound >150 μM (Chen et al., 1995). 4-Hydroxycyclophosphamide may be oxidized further by aldehyde oxidase, either in liver or in tumor tissue, to inactive metabolites. The hydroxyl metabolite of ifosfamide similarly is inactivated by aldehyde dehydrogenase. 4-Hydroxycyclophosphamide and its tautomer, aldophosphamide, travel in the circulation to tumor cells where aldophosphamide cleaves spontaneously, generating stoichiometric amounts of phosphoramide mustard and acrolein. Phosphoramide mustard is responsible for antitumor effects, while acrolein causes hemorrhagic cystitis often seen during therapy with cyclophosphamide. Cystitis can be reduced in intensity or prevented by the parenteral co-administration of mesna. Mesna does not negate the systemic antitumor activity of the drug.

Patients should receive vigorous intravenous hydration during high-dose treatment. Brisk hematuria in a patient receiving daily oral therapy should lead to immediate drug discontinuation. Refractory bladder hemorrhage can become life-threatening, and cystectomy may be necessary for control of bleeding.

Inappropriate secretion of antidiuretic hormone has been observed in patients receiving cyclophosphamide, usually at doses >50 mg/kg (see Chapter 25). It is important to be aware of the possibility of water intoxication, because these patients usually are vigorously hydrated to prevent bladder toxicity.

Pretreatment with CYP inducers such as phenobarbital enhances the rate of activation of the azoxyphosphorenes but does not alter total exposure to active metabolites over time and does not affect toxicity or therapeutic activity in humans. Cyclophosphamide can be used in full doses in patients with renal dysfunction, because it is eliminated by hepatic metabolism. Patients with mild hepatic dysfunction (bilirubin <3 mg/dL) can be treated with full doses of this drug, but those with more significant hepatic dysfunction should receive reduced doses.

Urinary and fecal excretion of unchanged cyclophosphamide is minimal after intravenous administration. Maximal concentrations in plasma are achieved 1 hour after oral administration, and the $t_{1/2}$ of parent drug in plasma is ~7 hours.

Therapeutic Uses. Cyclophosphamide (LYOPHILIZED CYTOXAN, others) is administered orally or intravenously. Recommended doses vary widely, and standard protocols for determining the schedule and dose of cyclophosphamide in combination with other chemotherapeutic agents should be consulted.

As a single agent, a daily oral dose of 100 mg/m^2 for 14 days has been recommended for patients with lymphomas and CLL. Higher doses of 500 mg/m^2 intravenously every 2-4 weeks are used in combination with other drugs in the treatment of breast cancer and lymphomas. The neutrophil nadir of 500-1000 cells/mm^3 generally serves as a lower limit for dosage adjustments in prolonged therapy. In regimens associated with bone marrow or peripheral stem cell rescue, cyclophosphamide may be given in total doses of 5-7 g/m^2 over a 3- to 5-day period. GI ulceration, cystitis (counteracted by mesna and diuresis), and, less commonly, pulmonary, renal, hepatic, and cardiac toxicities (a hemorrhagic myocardial necrosis) may occur after high-dose therapy with total doses >200 mg/kg.

The clinical spectrum of activity for cyclophosphamide is very broad. It is an essential component of many effective drug combinations for non-Hodgkin's lymphomas, other lymphoid malignancies, breast and ovarian cancers, and solid tumors in children. Complete remissions and presumed cures have been reported when cyclophosphamide was given as a single agent for Burkitt's lymphoma. It frequently is used in combination with doxorubicin and a taxane as adjuvant therapy after surgery for carcinoma of the breast.

Because of its potent immunosuppressive properties, cyclophosphamide has been used to treat auto-immune disorders, including Wegener's granulomatosis, rheumatoid arthritis, and the nephrotic syndrome. Caution is advised when the drug is considered for non-neoplastic conditions, not only because of its acute toxic effects but also because of its potential for inducing sterility, teratogenic effects, and leukemia.

Ifosfamide. Ifosfamide (IFEX, others) is an analog of cyclophosphamide. Severe urinary tract and central nervous system (CNS) toxicity limited the use of ifosfamide when it first was introduced in the early 1970s.

However, adequate hydration and co-administration of mesna have reduced its bladder toxicity.

Therapeutic Uses. Ifosfamide is approved for treatment of relapsed germ cell testicular cancer and is frequently used for first-time treatment of pediatric and adult sarcomas. It is a common component of high-dose chemotherapy regimens with bone marrow or stem cell rescue; in these regimens, in total doses of 12-14 g/m^2, it may cause severe neurological toxicity, including hallucinations, coma, and death, with symptoms appearing 12 hours to 7 days after beginning the ifosfamide infusion. This toxicity is thought to result from a metabolite, chloroacetaldehyde. In addition, ifosfamide causes nausea, vomiting, anorexia, leukopenia, nephrotoxicity, and VOD of the liver.

In nonmyeloablative regimens, ifosfamide is infused intravenously over at least 30 minutes at a dose of ≤1.2 g/m^2/day for 5 days. Intravenous mesna is given as bolus injections in a dose equal to 20% of the ifosfamide dose concomitantly and an additional 20% again 4 and 8 hours later, for a total mesna dose of 60% of the ifosfamide dose. For ifosfamide doses ≤2 g/m^2, oral mesna, at a dose equal to 40% of the ifosfamide dose, can be substituted for the second and third IV mesna doses, given at 2 and 6 hours after each dose of ifosfamide, for a total mesna dose equal to the ifosfamide dose. Alternatively, mesna may be given concomitantly in a single dose equal to the ifosfamide dose. Patients also should receive at least 2 L of oral or intravenous fluid daily. Treatment cycles are repeated every 3-4 weeks after hematological recovery.

Pharmacokinetics. The parent compound, ifosfamide, has an elimination $t_{1/2}$ in plasma of ~1.5 hours after doses of 3.8-5 g/m^2 and a somewhat shorter $t_{1/2}$ at lower doses, although its pharmacokinetics are highly variable from patient to patient due to variable rates of hepatic metabolism. Hydroxylation by CYPs generates an active phosphoramide mustard.

Toxicity. Ifosfamide has virtually the same toxicity profile as cyclophosphamide, although it causes greater platelet suppression, neurotoxicity, nephrotoxicity, and in the absence of mesna, urothelial damage.

Melphalan. This alkylating agent primarily is used to treat multiple myeloma and, less commonly, in high-dose chemotherapy with marrow transplantation.

Pharmacological and Cytotoxic Actions. The general pharmacological and cytotoxic actions of melphalan are similar to those of other bifunctional alkylators. The drug is not a vesicant.

Absorption, Fate, and Excretion. Oral melphalan is absorbed in an inconsistent manner and, for most indications, is given as an intravenous infusion. The drug has a $t_{1/2}$ in plasma of ~45-90 minutes, and 10-15% of an administered dose is excreted unchanged in the urine. Patients with decreased renal function may develop unexpectedly severe myelosuppression.

Therapeutic Uses. Melphalan (ALKERAN) for multiple myeloma is given in doses of 4-10 mg orally for 4-7 days every 28 days, with dexamethasone or thalidomide. Treatment is repeated at 4-week intervals based on response and tolerance. Dosage adjustments should be based on blood cell counts. Melphalan also may be used in myeloablative regimens followed by bone marrow or peripheral blood stem cell reconstitution. For this use, the dose is 180-200 mg/m^2.

Clinical Toxicity. The clinical toxicity of melphalan is mostly hematological and is similar to that of other alkylating agents. Nausea and vomiting are less frequent. The drug causes less alopecia and, rarely, renal or hepatic dysfunction.

Chlorambucil. This agent is almost exclusively used in treating CLL, and in this disease has largely been replaced by fludarabine and cyclophosphamide.

Pharmacological and Cytotoxic Actions. The cytotoxic effects of chlorambucil on the bone marrow, lymphoid organs, and epithelial tissues are similar to those observed with other nitrogen mustards. As an orally administered agent, chlorambucil is well tolerated in small daily doses and provides flexible titration of blood counts. Nausea and vomiting may result from single oral doses of ≥20 mg.

Absorption, Fate, and Excretion. Oral absorption of chlorambucil is adequate and reliable. The drug has a $t_{1/2}$ in plasma of ~1.5 hours, and is hydrolyzed to inactive products.

Therapeutic Uses. In treating CLL, the standard initial daily dose of chlorambucil (LEUKERAN) is 0.1-0.2 mg/kg, given once daily and continued for 3-6 weeks. With a fall in the peripheral total leukocyte count or clinical improvement, the dosage is titrated to maintain neutrophils and platelets at acceptable levels. Maintenance therapy (usually 2 mg daily) often is required to maintain clinical response.

Clinical Toxicity. In CLL, chlorambucil treatment may continue for months or years, achieving its effects gradually and often without significant toxicity to a compromised bone marrow.

Although it is possible to induce marked hypoplasia of the bone marrow with excessive doses, its myelosuppressive effects are moderate, gradual, and rapidly reversible. GI discomfort, azoospermia, amenorrhea, pulmonary fibrosis, seizures, dermatitis, and hepatotoxicity rarely may be encountered. A marked increase in the incidence of acute myelocytic leukemia (AML) and other tumors was noted in the treatment of polycythemia vera and in patients with breast cancer receiving chlorambucil as adjuvant chemotherapy (Lerner, 1978).

Bendamustine. This drug is approved for treatment of CLL and non-Hodgkin's lymphoma.

Bendamustine is given as a 30-minute intravenous infusion in dosages of 100 mg/m^2/day on days 1 and 2 of a 28-day cycle. Lower doses may be indicated in heavily pretreated patients. It is rapidly degraded through sulfhydryl interaction and adduct formation with macromolecules, and <5% of the parent drug is excreted in the urine intact. *N*-demethylation and oxidation produces metabolites that have antitumor activity, but less than that of the parent molecule. The parent drug has a $t_{1/2}$ in plasma of ~30 minutes (Teichert et al., 2007).

The clinical toxicity pattern of bendamustine is typical of classical alkylators, with a rapidly reversible myelosuppression and mucositis, both generally tolerable in the 28-day regimen.

MISCELLANEOUS ALKYLATING DRUGS

Although nitrogen mustards containing chloroethyl groups constitute the most widely used class of alkylating agents, alternative alkylators with greater chemical stability and well-defined activity in specific types of cancer have value in clinical practice.

Ethyleneimines and Methylmelamines

Altretamine

Pharmacology and Cytotoxic Effects. Altretamine (HEXALEN), formerly known as hexamethylmelamine, is structurally similar to triethylenemelamine (tretamine). However, *in vitro* tests for alkylating activity of altretamine and its metabolites have been negative, and the precise mechanism of the cytotoxic action of altretamine is unknown. It is a palliative treatment for persistent or recurrent ovarian cancer following cisplatin-based combination therapy.

The usual dosage of altretamine as a single agent in ovarian cancer is 260 mg/m^2/day in four divided doses, for 14 or 21 consecutive days out of a 28-day cycle, for up to 12 cycles.

Absorption, Fate, and Excretion. Following oral administration, altretamine is well absorbed from the GI tract and undergoes rapid demethylation in the liver. The principal metabolites are pentamethylmelamine and tetramethyl melamine, and the elimination $t_{1/2}$ is 4-10 hours.

Clinical Toxicities. The main toxicities of altretamine are myelosuppression and neurotoxicity. Altretamine causes both peripheral and central neurotoxicity (ataxia, depression, confusion, drowsiness, hallucinations, dizziness, and vertigo). Neurological symptoms abate upon discontinuation of therapy. Peripheral blood counts and a neurological examination should be performed prior to the initiation of each course of therapy. Therapy should be interrupted for at least 14 days and subsequently restarted at a lower dosage of 200 mg/m^2/day if the white cell count falls to <2000 cells/mm^3 or the platelet count falls to <75,000 cells/mm^3 or if neurotoxic or intolerable GI symptoms occur. If neurological symptoms fail to stabilize on the reduced-dose schedule, altretamine should be discontinued. Nausea and vomiting also are common side effects and may be dose limiting. Renal dysfunction may necessitate discontinuing the drug. Other rare adverse effects include rashes, alopecia, and hepatic toxicity. Severe, life-threatening orthostatic hypotension may develop in patients who receive monoamine oxidase (MAO) inhibitors, amitriptyline, imipramine, or phenelzine concurrently with altretamine.

Thiotepa

Pharmacological and Cytotoxic Effects. Thiotepa (THIOPLEX, others) consists of three ethyleneimine groups stabilized by attachment to the nucleophilic thiophosphoryl base. Its current use primarily is for high-dose chemotherapy regimens.

Both thiotepa and its desulfurated primary metabolite, triethylenephosphoramide (TEPA), to which it is rapidly converted by hepatic CYPs, form DNA cross-links. The aziridine rings open after protonation of the ring-nitrogen, leading to a reactive molecule.

Absorption, Fate, and Excretion. TEPA becomes the predominant form of the drug present in plasma within hours of thiotepa administration. The parent compound has a plasma $t_{1/2}$ of 1.2-2 hours, as compared to a longer $t_{1/2}$ of 3-24 hours for TEPA. Thiotepa pharmacokinetics essentially are the same in children as in adults at conventional doses (≤80 mg/m^2), and drug and metabolite $t_{1/2}$ are unchanged in children receiving high-dose therapy of 300 mg/m^2/day for 3 days. Less than 10% of the administered drug appears in urine as the parent drug or the primary metabolite. Multiple secondary metabolites and chemical degradation products account for the remainder of the administered dose.

Clinical Toxicities. The toxicities of thiotepa essentially are the same as those of the other alkylating agents, namely myelosuppression, and to a lesser extent mucositis. Myelosuppression tends to develop somewhat later than with cyclophosphamide, with leukopenic nadirs at 2 weeks and platelet nadirs at 3 weeks. In high-dose regimens, thiotepa may cause neurotoxic symptoms, including coma and seizures.

Alkyl Sulfonates

Busulfan. Busulfan exerts few pharmacological actions other than myelosuppression at conventional doses and, prior to the advent of imatinib mesylate (GLEEVEC), was a standard agent for patients in the chronic phase of myelocytic leukemia and caused a severe and prolonged pancytopenia in some patients. Busulfan now is primarily used in high-dose regimens, in which pulmonary fibrosis, GI mucosal damage, and hepatic veno-occlusive disease (VOD) are important toxicities.

Absorption, Fate, and Excretion. Busulfan is well absorbed after oral administration in dosages of 2-6 mg/day and has a plasma $t_{1/2}$ of 2-3 hours. The drug is conjugated to GSH by glutathione S-transferase A1A and further metabolized by CYP-dependent pathways; its major urinary metabolite is methane sulfonic acid. In high doses, children <18 years of age clear the drug two to four times faster than adults and tolerate higher doses (Vassal et al., 1993). An intravenous preparation is available for high-dose regimens. With doses of 1 mg/kg every 6 hours for 4 days, peak drug concentrations reach 10 μM in adults but only 1-5 μM in children 1-3 years of age, because of faster clearance. Busulfan clearance varies considerably among patients. VOD is associated with high area under the curve (AUC) (AUC >1500 μM × min) peak drug levels and slow clearance, leading to recommendations for dose adjustment based on drug level monitoring (Grochow, 1993). A target steady-state concentration of 600-900 ng/mL in plasma in adults or AUC <1000 μM × min in children achieves an appropriate balance between toxicity and therapeutic benefit (Witherspoon et al., 2001).

Therapeutic Uses. In treating chronic myelogenous leukemia (CML), the initial oral dose of busulfan (MYLERAN, BUSULFEX) varies with the total leukocyte count and the severity of the disease; daily doses of 2-8 mg for adults (~60 μg/kg or 1.8 mg/m^2 for children) are used to initiate therapy and are adjusted appropriately to subsequent hematological and clinical responses, with the aim of reducing the total leukocyte count to ≤10,000 cells/mm^3. A decrease in the leukocyte count usually is not seen during the first 10-15 days of treatment, and the leukocyte count may actually increase; during this period, an increase in leukocyte count should not be interpreted as drug resistance nor should the dose be increased. Because the leukocyte count may fall for >1 month after discontinuing the drug, it is recommended that busulfan be withdrawn when the total leukocyte count has declined to ~15,000 cells/mm^3. A normal leukocyte count usually is achieved within 12-20 weeks. During remission, daily treatment resumes when the total leukocyte count reaches ~50,000 cells/mm^3. Daily maintenance doses are 1-3 mg. In high-dose therapy, doses of 1 mg/kg are given every 6 hours for 4 days, with adjustment based on pharmacokinetics.

In high-dose regimens, busulfan is given at 0.8 mg/kg every 6 hours for 4 days. Anticonvulsants must be used concomitantly to protect against acute CNS toxicities, including tonic-clonic seizures, which may occur several hours after each dose. Busulfan induces the metabolism of phenytoin. In patients requiring anti-seizure medication, non-enzyme-inducing drugs such as lorazepam are recommended as an alternative to phenytoin. When phenytoin is used concurrently, plasma busulfan levels should be monitored and the busulfan dose adjusted accordingly.

Clinical Toxicity. The major toxic effects of busulfan are related to its myelosuppressive properties, and prolonged thrombocytopenia may be a hazard. Occasionally, patients experience nausea, vomiting, and diarrhea. Long-term use leads to impotence, sterility, amenorrhea, and fetal malformation. Rarely, patients develop asthenia and hypotension, a syndrome resembling Addison's disease, but without abnormalities of corticosteroid production.

High-dose busulfan causes VOD of the liver in ≤10% of patients, as well as seizures, hemorrhagic cystitis, permanent alopecia, and cataracts. The coincidence of VOD and hepatotoxicity is increased by its co-administration with drugs that inhibit CYPs, including imidazoles and metronidazole, possibly through inhibition of the clearance of busulfan and/or its toxic metabolites (Nilsson et al., 2003).

Nitrosoureas

The nitrosoureas have an important role in the treatment of brain tumors and find occasional use in treating lymphomas and in high-dose regimens with bone marrow reconstitution. They function as bifunctional alkylating agents but differ from conventional nitrogen mustards in both pharmacological and toxicological properties.

Carmustine (BCNU) and lomustine (CCNU) are highly lipophilic and thus readily cross the blood-brain barrier, an important property in the treatment of brain tumors. Unfortunately, with the exception of streptozocin, nitrosoureas cause profound and delayed myelosuppression with recovery 4-6 weeks after a single dose. Long-term treatment with the nitrosoureas, especially semustine (methyl-CCNU), has resulted in renal failure. As with other alkylating agents, the nitrosoureas are highly carcinogenic and mutagenic. They generate both alkylating and carbamylating moieties as illustrated in Figure 61–4.

Carmustine (BCNU). Carmustine's major action is its alkylation of DNA at the O^6-guanine position, an adduct repaired by MGMT. Methylation of the MGMT promoter inhibits its expression in ~30% of primary gliomas and is associated with sensitivity to nitrosoureas. In high doses with bone marrow rescue, it produces hepatic VOD, pulmonary fibrosis, renal failure, and secondary leukemia (Tew et al., 2001).

Absorption, Fate, and Excretion. Carmustine is unstable in aqueous solution and in body fluids. After intravenous infusion, it disappears from the plasma with a highly variable $t_{1/2}$ of ≥15-90 minutes. Approximately 30-80% of the drug appears in the urine within 24 hours as degradation products. The alkylating metabolites enter rapidly into the cerebrospinal fluid (CSF), and their concentrations in the CSF reach 15-30% of the concurrent plasma values.

Therapeutic Uses. When used alone, carmustine (BICNU) is administered intravenously at doses of 150-200 mg/m^2, given by infusion over 1-2 hours and repeated every 6 weeks.

Because of its ability to cross the blood-brain barrier, carmustine has been used in the treatment of malignant gliomas but has been increasingly replaced by temozolomide. An implantable carmustine wafer (GLIADEL) is available for use as an adjunct to surgery and radiation in newly diagnosed high-grade malignant glioma patients and as an adjunct to surgery for recurrent glioblastoma multiforme.

Streptozocin. This antibiotic has a methylnitrosourea (MNU) moiety attached to the 2-carbon of glucose. It has a high affinity for cells of the islets of Langerhans and causes diabetes in experimental animals.

Absorption, Fate, and Excretion. Streptozocin is rapidly degraded following intravenous administration. The $t_{1/2}$ of the drug is ~15 minutes. Only 10-20% of a dose is recovered intact in the urine.

Therapeutic Uses. Streptozocin (ZANOSAR) is used exclusively in the treatment of human pancreatic islet cell carcinoma and malignant carcinoid tumors. It is administered intravenously, 500 mg/m^2 once daily for 5 days; this course is repeated every 6 weeks. Alternatively, 1000 mg/m^2 can be given weekly for 2 weeks, and the weekly dose then can be increased to a maximum of 1500 mg/m^2, depending on tolerance and response.

Clinical Toxicity. Nausea is frequent. Mild, reversible renal or hepatic toxicity occurs in approximately two-thirds of cases; in <10% of patients, renal toxicity may be cumulative with each dose and may lead to irreversible renal failure. Proteinuria is an early sign of tubular damage and impending renal failure. Streptozocin should not be given with other nephrotoxic drugs. Hematological toxicity—anemia, leukopenia, or thrombocytopenia—occurs in 20% of patients.

Triazenes

Dacarbazine (DTIC). Dacarbazine functions as a methylating agent after metabolic activation to the monomethyl triazeno metabolite, MTIC. It kills cells in all phases of the cell cycle. Resistance has been ascribed to the removal of methyl groups from the O^6-guanine bases in DNA by MGMT.

Absorption, Fate, and Excretion. Dacarbazine is administered intravenously. After an initial rapid phase of disappearance ($t_{1/2}$ of ~20 minutes), dacarbazine is cleared from plasma with a terminal $t_{1/2}$ of ~5 hours. The $t_{1/2}$ is prolonged in the presence of hepatic or renal disease. Almost 50% of the compound is excreted intact in the urine by tubular secretion. Elevated urinary concentrations of 5-aminoimidazole-4-carboxamide reflect from the catabolism of dacarbazine, rather than inhibition of *de novo* purine biosynthesis.

Therapeutic Uses. Dacarbazine (DTIC-DOME) for malignant melanoma is given intravenously in dosages of 2-4.5 mg/kg/day for a 10-day period, repeated every 28 days. Alternatively, 250 mg/m^2 can be given daily for 5 days and repeated every 3 weeks. Extravasation of the drug may cause tissue damage and severe pain. In combination with other drugs for Hodgkin's disease, dacarbazine is given in dosages of 150 mg/m^2/day for 5 days, repeated every 4 weeks, or a single dose of 375 mg/m^2 is given and repeated every 15 days.

At present, the primary clinical indication for dacarbazine is in the combination chemotherapy of Hodgkin's disease. It is modestly effective against malignant melanoma and adult sarcomas.

Clinical Toxicity. DTIC induces nausea and vomiting in >90% of patients; vomiting usually develops 1-3 hours after treatment and may last up to 12 hours. Myelosuppression, with both leukopenia and thrombocytopenia, is mild and readily reversible within 1-2 weeks. A flulike syndrome consisting of chills, fever, malaise, and myalgias may occur during treatment with DTIC. Hepatotoxicity, alopecia, facial flushing, neurotoxicity, and dermatological reactions are less common adverse effects.

Temozolomide. Temozolomide (TEMODAR) is the standard agent in combination with radiation therapy for patients with malignant glioma and for astrocytoma. Temozolomide, like dacarbazine, forms the methylating metabolite MTIC and kills cells in all phases of the cell cycle. Resistance arises by any of the common mechanisms attributed to other alkylating agents, but particularly the *loss* of MLH6, a component of MMR.

Absorption, Fate, and Excretion. Temozolomide is administered orally in dosages of ~200 mg/day; it has a bioavailability approaching 100%. Maximum drug concentration reaches 5 μg/mL, or ~10 μM in plasma, ~1 hour after administration of a dose of 200 mg and declines with an elimination $t_{1/2}$ of 1-2 hours. The primary active metabolite MTIC reaches a maximum plasma concentration of 150 ng/mL 90 minutes after a dose and declines with a $t_{1/2}$ of 2 hours. Little intact drug is recovered in the urine, the primary urinary metabolite being the inactive imidazole carboxamide (Baker et al., 1999).

Clinical Toxicity. Temozolomide is available for oral and intravenous administration. It is administered cyclically, and hematological monitoring is necessary to guide dosing adjustments. The toxicities of temozolomide mirror those of DTIC.

Methylhydrazines

Procarbazine. The methylhydrazine derivatives were synthesized in a search for inhibitors of monoamine neurotransmitters. Several compounds in this series had anticancer activity, but only procarbazine (*N*-isopropyl-α-(2-methylhydrazino)-*p*-toluamide), an agent formerly useful in Hodgkin's disease and currently employed for second-line therapy in malignant brain tumors, has a role in clinical chemotherapy.

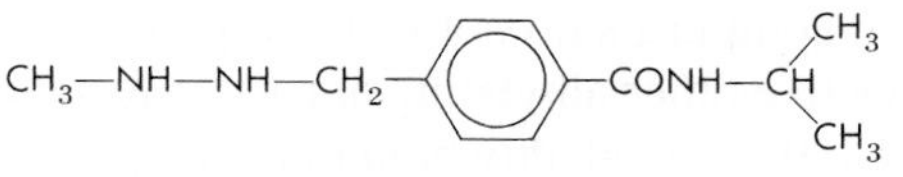

CH_3—NH—NH—CH_2—C_6H_4—CONH—CH(CH_3)$_2$

PROCARBAZINE

Cytotoxic Action. The antineoplastic activity of procarbazine results from its conversion by CYP-mediated hepatic oxidative metabolism to highly reactive alkylating species, which methylate DNA. The activation pathways are complex and not fully understood; free-radical intermediates may be cytotoxic. Activated procarbazine can produce chromosomal damage, including chromatid breaks and translocations, consistent with its mutagenic and carcinogenic actions. Resistance to procarbazine develops rapidly when it is used as a single agent. One mechanism results from the increased expression of MGMT, which repairs methylation of guanine.

Absorption, Fate, and Excretion. The pharmacokinetic behavior of procarbazine has not yet been thoroughly defined. The drug is extensively metabolized by CYP isoenzymes to azo, methylazoxy, and benzylazoxy intermediates, which are found in the plasma and yield the alkylating metabolites in tumor cells. In brain cancer patients, it is surprising that the concurrent use of anti-seizure drugs that induce hepatic CYPs does not significantly alter the pharmacokinetics of the parent drug (He et al., 2004).

Therapeutic Uses. The recommended dosage of procarbazine (MATULANE) for adults is 100 mg/m^2/day for 10-14 days in combination regimens such as MOPP (nitrogen mustard, oncovin, procarbazine, and prednisone) for Hodgkin's disease. The drug rarely is used in current practice, the MOPP combination having been replaced by alternative drugs.

Clinical Toxicity. The most common toxic effects include leukopenia and thrombocytopenia, which begin during the second week of therapy and reverse within 2 weeks off treatment. GI symptoms such as mild nausea and vomiting occur in most patients; diarrhea and rash are noted in 5-10% of cases. Behavioral disturbances also have been reported. Because procarbazine augments sedative effects, the concomitant use of CNS depressants should be avoided. The drug is a weak MAO inhibitor; it blocks the metabolism of catecholamines, sympathomimetics, and dietary tyramine and may provoke hypertension in patients concurrently exposed to these. Procarbazine has disulfiram-like actions, and therefore the ingestion of alcohol should be avoided. The drug is highly carcinogenic, mutagenic, and teratogenic and is associated with a 5-10% risk of acute leukemia in patients treated with MOPP. The highest risk is for patients who also receive radiation therapy. In addition, procarbazine is a potent immunosuppressive agent. It causes infertility, particularly in males.

PLATINUM COORDINATION COMPLEXES

The platinum coordination complexes have broad antineoplastic activity and have become the foundation for treatment of ovarian, head and neck, bladder, esophagus, lung, and colon cancers. The analogs differ in their pharmacological properties, and oxaliplatin has mechanistic differences that may explain its unique activity in colorectal cancer (see "Mechanism of Action") (Dolan and Fitch, 2007). Although cisplatin and other platinum complexes do not form carbonium ion intermediates like other alkylating agents or formally alkylate DNA, they covalently bind to nucleophilic sites on DNA and share many pharmacological attributes with alkylators.

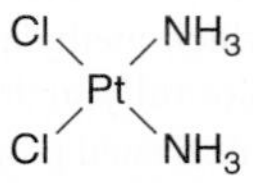

CISPLATIN 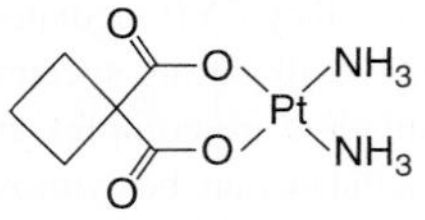 CARBOPLATIN

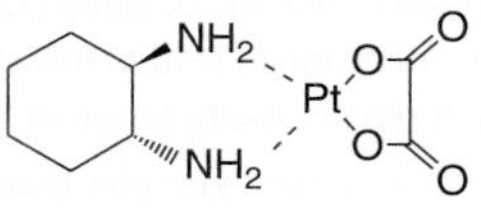

OXALIPLATIN

Chemistry. Cisplatin and carboplatin are divalent, inorganic, water-soluble, platinum-containing complexes. Oxaliplatin, a tetravalent complex, does not display cross-resistance to the divalent compounds in some experimental tumors. The coordination of di- or tetravalent platinum with various organic adducts reduces its renal toxicity and stabilizes the metal ion, as compared to the inorganic divalent platinum ion.

Mechanism of Action. Cisplatin, carboplatin, and oxaliplatin enter cells by an active Cu^{2+} transporter, CTR1, and in doing so rapidly degrade the transporter (Kruh, 2003). The compounds are actively extruded from cells by ATP7A and ATP7B copper transporters and by multidrug resistance protein 1 (MRP 1); variable expression of these transporters may contribute to clinical resistance (Dolan and Fitch, 2007). Inside the cell, the chloride, cyclohexane, or oxalate ligands of the three analogs are displaced by water molecules, yielding a positively charged and highly reactive molecule. In the primary cytotoxic reaction, the aquated species of the drug then reacts with nucleophilic sites on DNA and proteins.

Aquation of cisplatin is favored at the low concentrations of chloride inside the cell and in the urine. High concentrations of chloride stabilize the drug, explaining the effectiveness of chloride diuresis in preventing nephrotoxicity (see "Clinical Toxicities"). The activated platinum complexes can react with electron-rich molecules, such as sulfhydryls, and with various sites on DNA, forming both intrastrand and interstrand cross-links. The N-7 of guanine is a particularly reactive site, leading to platinum cross-links between adjacent guanines (GG intrastrand cross-links) on the same DNA strand; guanine–adenine cross-links also form and may contribute to cytotoxicity. Interstrand cross-links form less frequently. DNA-platinum adducts inhibit replication and transcription, lead to single- and double-stranded breaks and miscoding, and if recognized by p53 and other checkpoint proteins, cause induction of apoptosis. Although no quantitative relationship between platinum-DNA adduct formation and efficacy has been documented, the ability of patients to form and sustain platinum adducts appears to be an important predictor of clinical response (Reed et al., 1988). The analogs differ in the conformation of their adducts and the effects of adduct on DNA structure and function. Oxaliplatin and carboplatin are slower to form adducts. The oxaliplatin adducts are bulkier and less readily repaired, create a different pattern of distortion of the DNA helix, and differ from cisplatin adducts in the pattern of hydrogen bonding to adjacent segments of DNA (Sharma et al., 2007).

Unlike the other platinum analogs, oxaliplatin exhibits a cytotoxicity that does not depend on an active MMR system, which may explain its greater activity in colorectal cancer. It also seems less dependent on the presence of high mobility group (HMG) proteins that are required by the other platinum derivatives. Testicular cancers have a high concentration of HMG proteins and are quite sensitive to cisplatin. Basal-type breast cancers, such as those with BRCA1 and BRCA2 mutations, lack Her 2 amplification and hormone-receptor expression and appear to be uniquely susceptible to cisplatin through their upregulation of apoptotic pathways governed by p63 and p73 (Deyoung and Ellisen, 2007). The specificity of cisplatin with regard to phase of the cell cycle differs among cell types, although the effects of cross-linking are most pronounced during the S phase.

The platinum analogs are mutagenic, teratogenic, and carcinogenic. Cisplatin- or carboplatin-based chemotherapy for ovarian cancer is associated with a 4-fold increased risk of developing secondary leukemia.

Resistance to Platinum Analogs. Resistance to the platinum analogs likely is multifactorial, and the compounds differ in their degree of cross-resistance. Carboplatin shares cross-resistance with cisplatin in most experimental tumors, while oxaliplatin does not. A number of factors influence sensitivity to platinum analogs in experimental cells, including intracellular drug accumulation, as determined by the uptake and efflux transporters; intracellular levels of glutathione and other sulfhydryls such as metallothionein that bind to and inactivate the drug (Meijer et al., 1990); and rates of repair of DNA adducts. Repair of platinum-DNA adducts requires participation of the NER pathway. Inhibition or loss of NER increases sensitivity to cisplatin in ovarian cancer patients, while overexpression of NER components is associated with poor response to cisplatin or oxaliplatin-based therapy in lung, colon, and gastric cancer (Paré et al., 2008). Higher levels of expression of the NER component, ERCC1, in tumor cells and peripheral white blood cells are associated with a lower response rate in patients with solid tumors (Dolan and Fitch, 2007).

Resistance to cisplatin, but not oxaliplatin, appears to be partly mediated through loss of function in the MMR proteins (hMLH1, hMLH2, or hMSH6), which recognize platinum-DNA adducts and initiate apoptosis.

In the absence of effective repair of DNA-platinum adducts, sensitive cells cannot replicate or transcribe affected portions of the DNA strand. However, it is clear that some DNA polymerases can bypass adducts, especially those created by cisplatin. Oxaliplatin adducts are less easily bypassed. It remains unproven whether these polymerases contribute to resistance. Cisplatin resistance related to loss of active uptake has been demonstrated in yeast; overexpression of copper efflux transporters, ATP7A and ATP7B, correlates with poor survival after cisplatin-based therapy for ovarian cancer (Kruh, 2003).

Cisplatin

Absorption, Fate, and Excretion. After intravenous administration, cisplatin has an initial plasma elimination $t_{1/2}$ of 25-50 minutes; concentrations of total (bound and unbound) drug fall thereafter, with a $t_{1/2}$ of ≥24 hours. More than 90% of the platinum in the blood is covalently bound to plasma proteins. The unbound fraction, composed predominantly of parent drug, diminishes within minutes. High concentrations of cisplatin are found in the tissues of the kidney, liver, intestine, and testes but poorly penetrate into the CNS. Only a small portion of the drug is excreted by the kidney during the first 6 hours; by 24 hours, up to 25% is excreted, and by 5 days, up to 43% of the administered dose is recovered in the urine, mostly covalently bound to protein and peptides. Biliary or intestinal excretion of cisplatin is minimal.

Therapeutic Uses. Cisplatin (PLATINOL, others) is given only by the intravenous route. The usual dosage is 20 mg/m²/day for 5 days, 20-30 mg weekly for 3-4 weeks, or 100 mg/m² given once every 4 weeks. *To prevent renal toxicity, it is important to establish a chloride diuresis by the infusion of 1-2 L of normal saline prior to treatment.* The appropriate amount of cisplatin then is diluted in a solution containing dextrose, saline, and mannitol and administered intravenously over 4-6 hours. Because aluminum reacts with and inactivates cisplatin, the drug should not come in contact with needles or other infusion equipment that contain aluminum during its preparation or administration.

Cisplatin, in combination with bleomycin, etoposide, ifosfamide, or vinblastine, cures 90% of patients with testicular cancer. Used with paclitaxel, cisplatin or carboplatin induces complete response in the majority of patients with carcinoma of the ovary. Cisplatin produces responses in cancers of the bladder, head and neck, cervix, and endometrium; all forms of carcinoma of the lung; anal and rectal carcinomas; and neoplasms of childhood. Interestingly, the drug also sensitizes cells to radiation therapy and enhances control of locally advanced lung, esophageal, and head and neck tumors when given with irradiation.

Clinical Toxicities. Cisplatin-induced nephrotoxicity has been largely abrogated by adequate pretreatment hydration and chloride diuresis. Amifostine (ETHYOL, others) is a thiophosphate cytoprotective agent that reduces renal toxicity associated with repeated administration of cisplatin, but is not commonly used. Ototoxicity caused by cisplatin is unaffected by diuresis and is manifested by tinnitus and high-frequency hearing loss. The ototoxicity can be unilateral or bilateral, tends to be more frequent and severe with repeated doses, and may be more pronounced in children. Marked nausea and vomiting occur in almost all patients and usually can be controlled with 5-HT_3 antagonists, NK1-receptor antagonists, and high-dose corticosteroids (see Chapter 46).

At higher doses, or after multiple cycles of treatment, cisplatin causes a progressive peripheral motor and sensory neuropathy, which may worsen after discontinuation of the drug and may be aggravated by subsequent or simultaneous treatment with taxanes or other neurotoxic drugs. Cisplatin causes mild to moderate myelosuppression, with transient leukopenia and thrombocytopenia. Anemia may become prominent after multiple cycles of treatment. Electrolyte disturbances, including hypomagnesemia, hypocalcemia, hypokalemia, and hypophosphatemia, are common. Hypocalcemia and hypomagnesemia secondary to tubular damage and renal electrolyte wasting may produce tetany if untreated. Routine measurement of Mg^{2+} concentrations in plasma is recommended. Hyperuricemia, hemolytic anemia, and cardiac abnormalities are rare side effects. Anaphylactic-like reactions, characterized by facial edema, bronchoconstriction, tachycardia, and hypotension, may occur within minutes after administration and should be treated by intravenous injection of epinephrine and with corticosteroids or antihistamines. Like other DNA adduct–forming drugs, cisplatin has been associated with the development of AML, usually ≥4 years after treatment.

Carboplatin

The mechanisms of action and resistance and the spectrum of clinical activity of carboplatin (CBDCA, JM-8) are similar to cisplatin (see "Cisplatin"). However, the two drugs differ significantly in their chemical, pharmacokinetic, and toxicological properties.

Because carboplatin is much less reactive than cisplatin, the majority of drug in plasma remains in its parent form, unbound to proteins. Most drug is eliminated via renal excretion, with a $t_{1/2}$ in plasma of ~2 hours. A small fraction of platinum binds irreversibly to plasma proteins and disappears slowly, with a $t_{1/2}$ of ≥5 days.

Carboplatin is relatively well tolerated clinically, causing less nausea, neurotoxicity, ototoxicity, and nephrotoxicity than cisplatin. Instead, the dose-limiting toxicity is myelosuppression, primarily thrombocytopenia. It is more likely to cause a hypersensitivity reaction; in patients with a mild reaction, premedication, graded doses of drug, and more prolonged infusion lead to desensitization.

Carboplatin and cisplatin are equally effective in the treatment of suboptimally debulked ovarian cancer, non–small cell lung cancer, and extensive-stage small cell lung cancer; however, carboplatin may be less effective than cisplatin in germ cell, head and neck, and esophageal cancers (Go and Adjei, 1999). Carboplatin is an effective alternative for responsive tumors in patients unable to tolerate cisplatin because of impaired renal function, refractory nausea, significant hearing impairment, or neuropathy, but doses must be adjusted for renal function. In addition, it may be used in high-dose therapy with bone marrow or peripheral stem cell rescue. The dose of carboplatin should be adjusted in proportion to the reduction in creatinine clearance (CrCl) for patients with a CrCl <60 mL/min. The following formula is useful for calculation of dose:

$$\text{Dose (mg)} = \text{AUC} \times (\text{GFR} + 25)$$

where the target AUC (area under the plasma concentration–time curve) is ~5-7 min/mg/mL for acceptable toxicity in patients receiving single-agent carboplatin (GFR = glomerular filtration rate).

Carboplatin (PARAPLATIN) is administered as an intravenous infusion over at least 15 minutes, using the above-mentioned formula for dose calculation, and is given once every 21-28 days.

Oxaliplatin

Absorption, Fate, and Excretion. Oxaliplatin, like cisplatin, has a very brief $t_{1/2}$ in plasma, probably as a result of its rapid uptake by tissues and its reactivity. Maximum concentrations in plasma range from 1-1.5 μg platinum/mL for patients receiving 80-130 mg/m² intravenously and decline thereafter, with an initial $t_{1/2}$ of 0.28 hour. Although the ultrafiltrable component has a slow terminal clearance from plasma, most of the low-molecular-weight platinum species represent inactive degradation products. These metabolites undergo renal excretion at a rate dependent on the CrCl. No dose adjustment is required for patients with a CrCl ≥20 mL/min; decreased renal function does not affect the rapid chemical inactivation of the drug in the systemic circulation and tissues (Takimoto et al., 2007). Dose adjustment is not required for hepatic dysfunction (Synold et al., 2007).

Therapeutic Uses. Oxaliplatin exhibits a range of antitumor activity (colorectal and gastric cancer) that differs from other platinum agents. Oxaliplatin's effectiveness in colorectal cancer is perhaps due to its MMR- and HMG-independent effects (see "Mechanism of Action" under "Platinum Coordination Complexes"). It also suppresses expression of thymidylate synthase (TS), the target enzyme of 5-fluorouracil (5-FU) action, which may promote synergy of these two drugs (Fischel et al., 2002). In combination with 5-FU, it is approved for treatment of patients with colorectal cancer.

Clinical Toxicity. The dose-limiting toxicity of oxaliplatin is a peripheral neuropathy. An acute form, often triggered by exposure to cold liquids, manifests as paresthesias and/or dysesthesias in the upper and lower extremities, mouth, and throat. It may be caused by rapid release of oxalate, with depletion of calcium and magnesium, and responds to infusion of these electrolytes. A second type of peripheral neuropathy is more closely related to cumulative dose and has features similar to cisplatin neuropathy; 75% of patients receiving a cumulative dose of 1560 mg/m^2 experience some progressive sensory neurotoxicity, with dysesthesias, ataxia, and numbness of the extremities. Hematological toxicity is mild to moderate, except for rare immune-mediated cytopenias, and nausea is well controlled with 5-HT_3-receptor antagonists. Like other platinum analogs, oxaliplatin causes leukemia and pulmonary fibrosis months to years after administration. Oxaliplatin may cause an acute allergic response with urticaria, hypotension, and bronchoconstriction.

II. Antimetabolites

FOLIC ACID ANALOGS

Folic acid is an essential dietary factor that is converted by enzymatic reduction to a series of tetrahydrofolate (FH_4) cofactors that provide methyl groups for the synthesis of precursors of DNA (thymidylate and purines) and RNA (purines). Interference with FH_4 metabolism reduces the cellular capacity for one-carbon transfer and the necessary methylation reactions in the synthesis of purine ribonucleotides and thymidine monophosphate (TMP), thereby inhibiting DNA replication.

History. Antifolate chemotherapy occupies a special place in the history of cancer treatment: This class of drugs produced the first striking, although temporary, remissions in leukemia (Farber et al., 1948) and the first cure of a solid tumor, choriocarcinoma (Berlin et al., 1963). Interest in folate antagonists further increased with the development of curative combination therapy for childhood acute lymphocytic leukemia; in this therapy, methotrexate played a critical role in both systemic treatment and intrathecal therapy. Introduction of high-dose regimens with "rescue" of host toxicity by the reduced folate, leucovorin (folinic acid, citrovorum factor, 5-formyl tetrahydrofolate, N^5-formyl FH_4), further extended the effectiveness of this drug to both systemic and CNS lymphomas, osteogenic sarcoma, and leukemias. Most recently, pemetrexed, an analog that differs from methotrexate in its transport properties and sites of action, has proven useful in treating mesothelioma and lung cancer.

Recognition that methotrexate, an inhibitor of dihydrofolate reductase (DHFR), also directly inhibits the folate-dependent enzymes of *de novo* purine and thymidylate synthesis led to development of antifolate analogs that specifically target these other folate-dependent enzymes (Figure 61–5). New inhibitors have resulted from synthetic modifications of the basic folate molecule (replacement of the N5 and/or N8 nitrogens of the pteridine ring and the N10 nitrogen of the bridge between the pteridine and benzoate rings of folate, as well as various side-chain substitutions). These

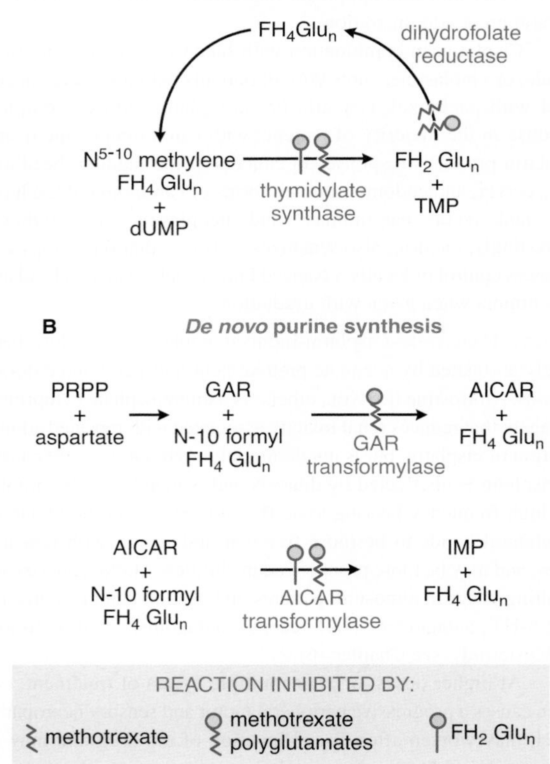

Figure 61–5. *Sites of action of methotrexate and its polyglutamates.* AICAR, aminoimidazole carboxamide; TMP, thymidine monophosphate; dUMP, deoxyuridine monophosphate; FH_2Glu_n, dihydrofolate polyglutamate; FH_4Glu_n, tetrahydrofolate polyglutamate; GAR, glycinamide ribonucleotide; IMP, inosine monophosphate; PRPP, 5-phosphoribosyl-1-pyrophosphate.

new agents have greater capacity for transport into tumor cells (pralatrexate) and exert their primary inhibitory effect on TS (raltitrexed, TOMUDEX), early steps in purine biosynthesis (lometrexol), or both (the multitargeted antifolate, pemetrexed, ALIMTA) (Vogelzang et al., 2003; O'Connor et al., 2007).

Aside from its antineoplastic activity, methotrexate also has been used with benefit in the therapy of psoriasis (see Chapter 65). Additionally, methotrexate inhibits cell-mediated immune reactions and is employed to suppress graft-versus-host disease in allogenic bone marrow and organ transplantation and for the treatment of dermatomyositis, rheumatoid arthritis, Wegener's granulomatosis, and Crohn's disease (see Chapters 35 and 47).

Structure-Activity Relationship. The primary target of methotrexate is the enzyme DHFR (Figure 61–5). Inhibition of DHFR leads to partial depletion of the FH_4 cofactors (5-10 methylene tetrahydrofolic acid and N-10 formyl tetrahydrofolic acid) required for the respective synthesis of thymidylate and purines. In addition, methotrexate, like its physiological counterparts (the folates), undergoes conversion to a series of polyglutamates (MTX-PGs) in both normal and tumor cells. These MTX-PGs constitute an intracellular storage form of folates and folate analogs and dramatically increase inhibitory potency of the analog for additional sites, including TS and two early enzymes in the purine biosynthetic pathway (Figure 61–5). Finally, the dihydrofolic acid polyglutamates that accumulate in cells behind the blocked DHFR reaction also act as inhibitors of TS and other enzymes (Figure 61–5) (Allegra et al., 1987b).

Because folic acid and many of its analogs are polar, they cross the blood-brain barrier poorly and require specific transport mechanisms to enter mammalian cells. Three inward folate transport systems are found on mammalian cells: 1) a folate receptor, which has high affinity for folic acid but much reduced ability to transport methotrexate and other analogs; 2) the reduced folate transporter, the major transit protein for methotrexate, raltitrexed, pemetrexed, and most analogs (Westerhof et al., 1995); and 3) a transporter that is active at low pH. The importance of transport in determining drug sensitivity is illustrated by the finding that the reduced folate transporter is highly expressed in the hyperdiploid subtype of acute lymphoblastic leukemia, due to the presence of multiple copies of chromosome 21, on which its gene resides; these cells have extreme sensitivity to methotrexate (Pui et al., 2004). Once in the cell, additional glutamyl residues are added to the molecule by the enzyme folylpolyglutamate synthetase. Intracellular methotrexate polyglutamates have been identified with up to six glutamyl residues. Because these higher polyglutamates are strongly charged and cross cellular membranes poorly, if at all, polyglutamation serves as a mechanism of entrapment and may account for the prolonged retention of methotrexate in chorionic epithelium (where it is a potent abortifacient); in tumors derived from this tissue, such as choriocarcinoma cells; and in normal tissues subject to cumulative drug toxicity, such as liver. Polyglutamylated folates and analogs have substantially greater affinity than the monoglutamate form for folate-dependent enzymes that are required for purine and thymidylate synthesis and have at least equal affinity for DHFR.

New folate antagonists that are better substrates for the reduced folate carrier have been identified. In efforts to bypass the obligatory membrane transport system and to facilitate penetration of the blood-brain barrier, lipid-soluble folate antagonists also have been synthesized. Trimetrexate (NEUTREXIN), a lipid-soluble analog that lacks a terminal glutamate, was one of the first to be tested for clinical activity. The analog has modest antitumor activity, primarily in combination with leucovorin rescue. However, it is beneficial in the treatment of *P. jiroveci* (*Pneumocystis carinii*) pneumonia (Allegra et al., 1987a), where leucovorin provides differential rescue of the host but not the parasite.

The most important new folate analog, MTA or pemetrexed (ALIMTA) (Figure 61–6), is a pyrrole–pyrimidine structure. It is avidly transported into cells via the reduced folate carrier. It readily is converted to polyglutamates that inhibit TS and glycine amide ribonucleotide transformylase, as well as DHFR. It has shown activity against ovarian cancer, mesothelioma, and non–small cell adenocarcinomas of the lung (Vogelzang et al., 2003).

Inhibitors of DHFR differ in their relative potency for blocking enzymes from different species. Agents have been identified that have little effect on the human enzyme but have strong activity against bacterial and parasitic infections (see discussions of trimethoprim, Chapter 52, and pyrimethamine, Chapter 49). By contrast, methotrexate effectively inhibits DHFR in all species investigated. Crystallographic studies have revealed the structural basis for the high affinity of methotrexate for DHFR (Blakley and Sorrentino, 1998) and the species specificity of the various DHFR inhibitors.

Mechanism of Action. To function as a cofactor in one-carbon transfer reactions, folate must first be reduced by DHFR to FH_4. Single-carbon fragments are added enzymatically to FH_4 in various configurations and then may be transferred in specific synthetic reactions. In a key metabolic event catalyzed by TS (Figure 61–5), deoxyuridine monophosphate (dUMP) is converted to thymidine monophosphate (TMP), an essential component of DNA. In this reaction, a one-carbon group is transferred to dUMP from 5,10-methylene FH_4, and the reduced folate cofactor is oxidized to dihydrofolate (FH_2). To function again as a cofactor, FH_2 must be reduced to FH_4 by DHFR. Inhibitors such as methotrexate, with a high affinity for DHFR (K_i ~0.01-0.2 nM), prevent the formation of FH_4 and allow an accumulation of the toxic inhibitory substrate, FH_2 polyglutamate, behind the blocked reaction. The absence of reduced folates shuts down the one-carbon transfer reactions crucial for the *de novo* synthesis of purine nucleotides and thymidylate and interrupts the synthesis of DNA and RNA. The toxic effects of methotrexate may be terminated by administering leucovorin, a fully reduced folate coenzyme, which repletes the intracellular pool of FH_4 cofactors.

As with most antimetabolites, methotrexate is only partially selective for tumor cells and kills rapidly

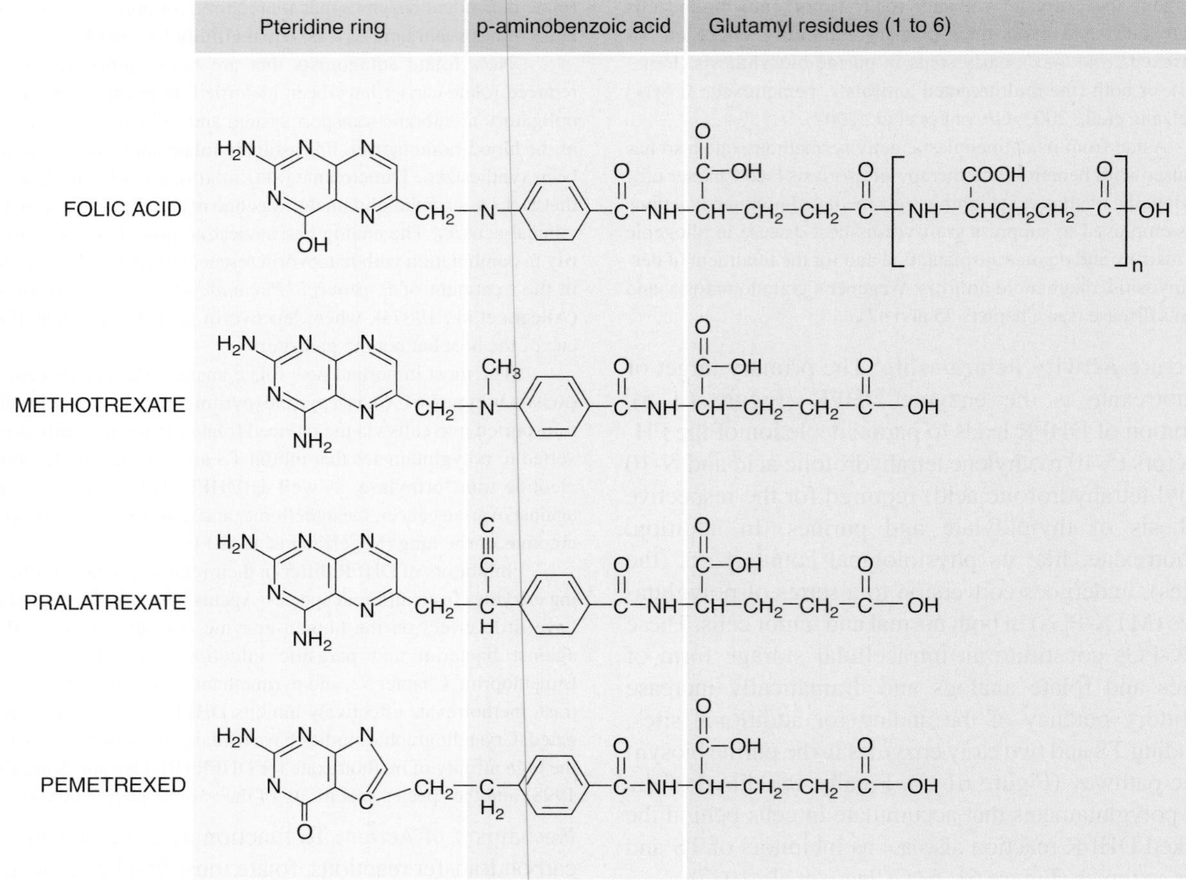

Figure 61–6. *Structures of folic acid and anti-folates.* The shading identifies common structural features and areas of modification.

dividing normal cells, such as those of the intestinal epithelium and bone marrow. Folate antagonists kill cells during the S phase of the cell cycle and are most effective when cells are proliferating rapidly.

Pemetrexed and its polyglutamates have a somewhat different spectrum of biochemical actions. Like methotrexate, pemetrexed inhibits DHFR, but as a polyglutamate, it even more potently inhibits glycinamide ribonucleotide formyltransferase (GART) and thymidylate synthase (TS). Unlike methotrexate, it produces little change in the pool of reduced folates, indicating that the distal sites of inhibition (TS and GART) predominate. Its pattern of deoxynucleotide depletion, as studied in cell lines, also differs from methotrexate, as it causes a greater fall in thymidine triphosphate (TTP) than in other triphosphates (Chen et al., 1998). Like methotrexate, it induces p53 and cell-cycle arrest, but this effect does not seem to depend on downstream induction of p21. Pralatrexate is more effectively taken up and polyglutamated than methotrexate. Pralatrexate is approved for treatment of cutanous T-cell lymphoma (O'Connor et al, 2007).

Mechanisms of Resistance to Antifolates. In experimental and clinical chemotherapy, acquired resistance to methotrexate affects each known step in methotrexate action, including:

- Impaired transport of methotrexate into cells
- Production of altered forms of DHFR that have decreased affinity for the inhibitor
- Increased concentrations of intracellular DHFR through gene amplification or altered gene regulation
- Decreased ability to synthesize methotrexate polyglutamates
- Increased expression of a drug efflux transporter of the MRP class (see Chapter 5)

DHFR levels in leukemic cells increase within 24 hours after treatment of patients with methotrexate; this likely reflects induction of new enzyme synthesis. The unbound DHFR protein may bind to its own message and inhibit translational efficiency of its own synthesis, while the DHFR-MTX complex is ineffective in blocking the DHFR translation. With longer periods of drug exposure, tumor cell populations that contain markedly increased levels of DHFR emerge. These cells contain multiple gene copies of DHFR either in mitotically unstable double-minute chromosomes (extrachromosomal elements formed by amplification of DHFR genes in response to methotrexate treatment) or in stably integrated, homogeneously staining chromosomal regions or amplicons. First identified as an explanation for resistance to methotrexate (Schimke et al., 1978), gene amplification of a target protein has since been implicated in the resistance to many antitumor agents, including 5-FU and pentostatin (2′-deoxycoformycin) and has been observed in patients with lung cancer (Curt et al., 1985) and leukemia. Impaired transport and polyglutamation have been implicated as mechanisms of resistance in childhood leukemia.

To overcome resistance, high doses of methotrexate may permit entry of the drug into transport-defective cells and may permit the intracellular accumulation of methotrexate in concentrations that inactivate high levels of DHFR.

The understanding of resistance to pemetrexed is incomplete. In various cell lines, resistance to this agent seems to arise from loss of influx transport, TS amplification, changes in purine biosynthetic pathways, or loss of polyglutamation.

Absorption, Fate, and Excretion. Methotrexate is readily absorbed from the GI tract at doses of <25 mg/m^2, but larger doses are absorbed incompletely and are routinely administered intravenously. Peak concentrations of 1-10 μM in the plasma are obtained after doses of 25-100 mg/m^2, and concentrations of 0.1-1 mM are achieved after high-dose infusions of 1.5-20 g/m^2. After intravenous administration, the drug disappears from plasma in a triphasic fashion (Sonneveld et al., 1986). The rapid distribution phase is followed by a second phase, which reflects renal clearance ($t_{1/2}$ of ~2-3 hours). A third phase has a $t_{1/2}$ of ~8-10 hours. This terminal phase of disappearance, if unduly prolonged by renal failure, may be responsible for major toxic effects of the drug on the marrow, GI epithelium, and skin. Distribution of methotrexate into body spaces, such as the pleural or peritoneal cavity, occurs slowly. However, if such spaces are expanded (e.g., by ascites or pleural effusion), they may act as a site of storage and slow release of the drug, resulting in prolonged elevation of plasma concentrations and more severe bone marrow toxicity.

Approximately 50% of methotrexate binds to plasma proteins and may be displaced from plasma albumin by a number of drugs, including sulfonamides, salicylates, tetracycline, chloramphenicol, and phenytoin; caution should be used if these drugs are given concomitantly. Up to 90% of a given dose is excreted unchanged in the urine within 48 hours, mostly within the first 8-12 hours. Metabolism of methotrexate in humans usually is minimal. After high doses, however, metabolites are readily detectable; these include 7-hydroxy-methotrexate, which is potentially nephrotoxic. Renal excretion of methotrexate occurs through a combination of glomerular filtration and active tubular secretion. Therefore, the concurrent use of drugs that reduce renal blood flow (e.g., nonsteroidal anti-inflammatory agents), that are nephrotoxic (e.g., cisplatin), or that are weak organic acids (e.g., aspirin, piperacillin) can delay drug excretion and lead to severe myelosuppression. Particular caution must be exercised in treating patients with renal insufficiency. In such patients, the dose should be adjusted in proportion to decreases in renal function, and high-dose regimens should be avoided.

Methotrexate is retained in the form of polyglutamates for long periods—for example, for weeks in the kidneys and for several months in the liver.

It is important to emphasize that concentrations of methotrexate in CSF are only 3% of those in the systemic circulation at steady state; hence, neoplastic cells in the CNS probably are not killed by standard dosage regimens. When high doses of methotrexate are given (>1.5 g/m^2; see "Therapeutic Uses"), cytotoxic concentrations of methotrexate reach the CNS.

Pharmacogenetics may influence the response to antifolates and their toxicity. The C677T substitution in methylenetetrahydrofolate reductase reduces the activity of the enzyme that generates methylenetetrahydrofolate, the cofactor for TS, and thereby increases methotrexate toxicity (Pullarkat et al., 2001). The presence of this polymorphism in leukemic cells confers increased sensitivity to methotrexate and might also modulate the toxicity and therapeutic effect of pemetrexed, a predominant TS inhibitor. Likewise, polymorphisms in the promoter region of TS govern the translation efficiency of this message and, by governing the intracellular levels of TS, modulate the response and toxicity of both antifolates (Pui et al., 2004) and fluoropyrimidines.

Therapeutic Uses. Methotrexate (Amethopterin; RHEUMATREX, TREXALL, others) has been used in the treatment of severe, disabling psoriasis in doses of 2.5 mg orally for 5 days, followed by a rest period of at least 2 days, or 10-25 mg intravenously weekly. It also is used at low dosage to induce remission in refractory rheumatoid arthritis (Hoffmeister, 1983). Awareness of the pharmacology, toxic potential, and drug interactions associated with methotrexate is a prerequisite for its use in these non-neoplastic disorders.

Methotrexate is a critical drug in the management of acute lymphoblastic leukemia (ALL) in children. High-dose methotrexate is of great value in remission induction and consolidation and in the maintenance of remissions in this highly curable disease. A 6- to 24-hour infusion of relatively large doses of methotrexate may be employed every 2-4 weeks (≥1-7.5 g/m^2) but only when leucovorin rescue follows within 24 hours of the methotrexate infusion. Such regimens produce cytotoxic concentrations of drug in the CSF and protect against leukemic meningitis. For maintenance therapy, it is administered weekly in doses of 20 mg/m^2 orally. Outcome of treatment in children correlates inversely with the rate of drug clearance. During methotrexate infusion, high steady-state levels are associated with a lower leukemia relapse rate (Pui et al., 2004). Methotrexate is of limited value in adults with AML, except for treatment and prevention of leukemic meningitis. The intrathecal administration of methotrexate has been employed for treatment or prophylaxis of meningeal leukemia or lymphoma and for treatment of meningeal carcinomatosis. This route of administration achieves high concentrations of methotrexate in the CSF and also is effective in patients whose systemic disease has become resistant to methotrexate. The recommended intrathecal dose in all patients >3 years of age is 12 mg (Bleyer, 1978). The dose is repeated every 4 days until malignant cells no longer are evident in the CSF. Leucovorin may be administered to counteract the potential toxicity of methotrexate that escapes into the systemic circulation, although this generally is not necessary. Because methotrexate administered into the lumbar space distributes poorly over the cerebral convexities, the drug may be given via an intraventricular Ommaya reservoir in the treatment of active intrathecal disease. Methotrexate is of established value in choriocarcinoma and related trophoblastic tumors of women; cure is achieved in ~75% of advanced cases treated sequentially with methotrexate and dactinomycin and in >90% when early diagnosis is made. In the treatment of choriocarcinoma, 1 mg/kg of methotrexate is administered intramuscularly every other day for four doses, alternating with leucovorin (0.1 mg/kg every other day). Courses are repeated at 3-week intervals, toxicity permitting, and urinary β-human chorionic gonadotropin titers are used as a guide for persistence of disease.

Beneficial effects also are observed in the combination therapy of Burkitt's and other non-Hodgkin's lymphomas. Methotrexate is a component of regimens for carcinomas of the breast, head and neck, ovary, and bladder. High-dose methotrexate with leucovorin rescue (HDM-L) is a standard agent for adjuvant therapy of osteosarcoma and produces a high complete response rate in CNS lymphomas. The administration of HDM-L has the potential for renal toxicity, probably related to the precipitation of the drug, a weak acid, in the acidic tubular fluid. Thus, vigorous hydration and alkalinization of urine pH are required prior to drug administration. HDM-L should be performed only by experienced clinicians who are familiar with hydration regimens and who have access to laboratories that monitor concentrations of methotrexate in plasma. If methotrexate values measured 48 hours after drug administration are 1 μM or higher, higher doses (100 mg/m^2) of leucovorin must be given until the plasma concentration of methotrexate falls to <50 nM (Stoller et al., 1977). With appropriate hydration and urine alkalinization, and in patients with normal renal function, the incidence of nephrotoxicity following HDM-L is <2%. In patients who become oliguric, intermittent hemodialysis is ineffective in reducing methotrexate levels. Continuous-flow hemodialysis can eliminate methotrexate at ~50% of the clearance rate in patients with intact renal function (Wall et al., 1996). Alternatively, a methotrexate-cleaving enzyme, carboxypeptidase G2, can be obtained from the Cancer Therapy Evaluation Program at the National Cancer Institute. When administered intravenously, it rapidly clears the drug (DeAngelis et al., 1996). Methotrexate concentrations in plasma fall by ≥99% within 5-15 minutes following enzyme administration, with insignificant rebound. Systemically administered carboxypeptidase G2 has little effect on methotrexate levels in the CSF.

Clinical Toxicities. As previously stated, the primary toxicities of antifolates affect the bone marrow and the intestinal epithelium and correct within 10-14 days. Myelosuppressed patients may be at risk for spontaneous hemorrhage or life-threatening infection, and they may require prophylactic transfusion of platelets and broad-spectrum antibiotics if febrile. Side effects usually reverse completely within 2 weeks, but prolonged myelosuppression may occur in patients with compromised renal function who have delayed excretion of the drug. The dosage of methotrexate (and likely pemetrexed) must be reduced in proportion to any reduction in CrCl.

Additional toxicities of methotrexate include alopecia, dermatitis, an allergic interstitial pneumonitis, nephrotoxicity (after high-dose therapy), defective oogenesis or spermatogenesis, abortion, and teratogenesis. Low-dose methotrexate may lead to cirrhosis after long-term continuous treatment, as in patients with psoriasis. Intrathecal administration of methotrexate often causes meningismus and an inflammatory response in the CSF. Seizures, coma, and death may occur rarely. Leucovorin does not reverse neurotoxicity.

A toxicity of particular significance in chronic administration to patients with psoriasis or rheumatoid arthritis is hepatic fibrosis and cirrhosis. Increased hepatic portal fibrosis is detected with higher frequency than in control patients after ≥6 months of continuous oral methotrexate treatment of psoriasis. Its presence mandates discontinuation of methotrexate. High-dose administration regularly causes acute elevation of hepatic transaminases, but these changes rapidly reverse and are not associated with permanent liver damage.

Folic acid antagonists are toxic to developing embryos. Methotrexate is highly effective when used with the prostaglandin analog misoprostol in inducing abortion in first-trimester pregnancy (Hausknecht, 1995).

Pemetrexed toxicity mirrors that of methotrexate, with the additional feature of a prominent erythematous and pruritic rash in 40% of patients. Dexamethasone, 4 mg twice daily on days −1, 0, and +1, markedly diminishes this toxicity. Unpredictably severe myelosuppression with pemetrexed, seen especially in patients with preexisting homocystinemia and possibly reflecting folate deficiency, largely is eliminated by concurrent administration of low dosages of folic acid, 350-1000 mg/day, beginning 1-2 weeks prior to pemetrexed and continuing while the drug is administered. Patients should receive intramuscular vitamin B_{12} (1 mg) with the first dose of pemetrexed to correct possible B_{12} deficiency. These small doses of folate and B_{12} do not compromise the therapeutic effect.

PYRIMIDINE ANALOGS

The antimetabolites as a class encompass a diverse group of drugs that inhibit RNA and DNA function. The fluoropyrimidines and certain purine analogs (6-mercaptopurine and 6-thioguanine) inhibit the synthesis of essential precursors of DNA. Others, such as the cytidine and adenosine nucleoside analogs, become incorporated into DNA and block its further elongation and function. Other inhibitory effects of these analogs may contribute to their cytotoxicity and even their ability to induce differentiation.

To understand the role of these drugs, it is useful to review the nomenclature of the DNA bases and their metabolic intermediates. Four bases, shown in Figure 61–7, form DNA; these are two pyrimidines, thymine and cytosine, and two purines, guanine and adenine. Some bases (guanine) are found in mammalian cells as free bases, while others (the pyrimidines) are present in their active form only as nucleosides (a base attached to a ribose or deoxyribose). These precursor forms then are converted to a nucleoside triphosphate (base, sugar, and 5′-phosphate, also known as a nucleotide). Mammalian cells lack the ability to utilize cytosine, thymine, and adenine as bases, and so these bases are found in the bloodstream as nucleosides and in cells as nucleosides or nucleotides. The various purine and pyrimidine triphosphates form the intracellular pool of precursors for both RNA (with ribose sugars) and DNA (with deoxyribose sugars). The composition of RNA also differs from DNA in that RNA incorporates uracil instead of thymine as one of its bases.

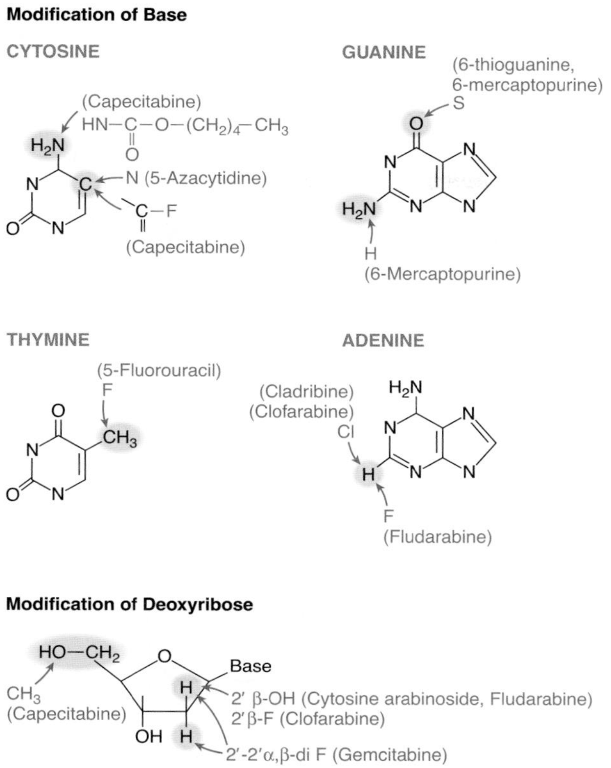

Modification of Base

Modification of Deoxyribose

Figure 61–7. *Structural modification of base and deoxyribonucleoside analogs.* The yellow ellipses indicate sites modified to create antimetabolites. The specific substitutions are indicated in red for each drug. Modifications occur in the base ring systems, in their amino or hydroxyl side groups, and in the deoxyribose sugar found in deoxyribonucleosides.

Strategies for inhibiting DNA synthesis are based on the ability to create analogs of these precursors that readily enter tumor cells and become activated by intracellular enzyme. As an example, the first successful pyrimidine analog, 5-FU, is converted to a deoxynucleotide, fluorodeoxyuridine monophosphate (FdUMP), which in turn blocks the enzyme; TS, required for the physiological conversion of dUMP to dTMP, a component of DNA. Other analogs incorporate into DNA itself and thereby block its function.

Cells can make the purine and pyrimidine bases *de novo* and convert them to their active triphosphates (dNTPs). The dNTPs then act as substrates for DNA polymerase and become linked in 3′-5′ phosphate ester bonds to form DNA strands; their base sequence provides the code for subsequent RNA and protein sequences.

As an alternative to synthesis of new precursor molecules, cells can salvage either free bases or their deoxynucleosides (Figure 61–7) from the bloodstream, presumably the products of degradation of DNA. Certain bases, such as uracil, guanine, and their analogs, can be taken up by cells and converted intracellularly to (deoxy) nucleotides by the addition of deoxyribose and phosphate groups. Antitumor analogs of these bases (5-FU, 6-thioguanine) can be formulated as simple substituted bases. Other bases, including cytosine, thymine, and adenine, and their analogs can only be utilized as deoxynucleosides, which are readily transported into cells and activated to deoxynucleotides by intracellular kinases. Thus, cytarabine (cytosine arabinoside; Ara-C), gemcitabine, 5-azacytidine, and adenosine analogs (cladribine), are nucleosides readily taken up by cells, converted to nucleotides, and incorporated into DNA (Figure 61–8).

Fludarabine phosphate, a nucleotide, is dephosphorylated rapidly in plasma, releasing the nucleoside that is readily taken up by cells. Analogs may differ from the physiological bases in a variety of ways: by altering in the purine or pyrimidine ring; by altering the sugar attached to the base, as in the arabinoside, Ara-C; or by altering both the base and sugar, as in fludarabine phosphate (Figure 61–7). These alterations produce inhibitory effects on vital enzymatic pathways and prevent DNA synthesis.

Fluorouracil, Capecitabine, and Floxuridine (Fluorodeoxyuridine)

5-fluorouracil (5-FU)

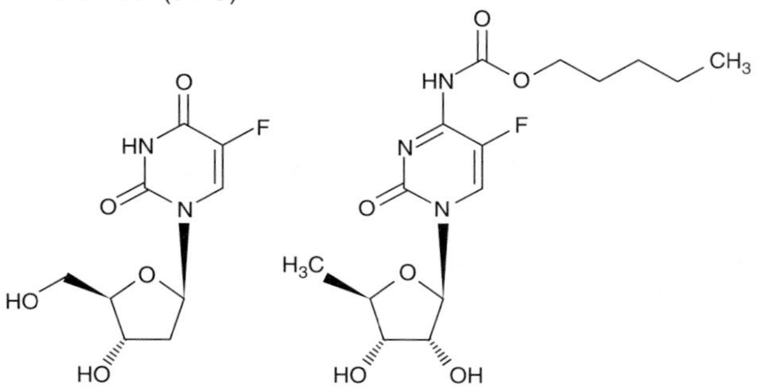

Mechanism of Action. 5-FU requires enzymatic conversion to the nucleotide status (ribosylation and phosphorylation) in order to exert its cytotoxic activity (Figure 61–9). Several routes are available for the formation of floxuridine monophosphate (FUMP). 5-FU may be converted to fluorouridine by uridine phosphorylase and then to FUMP by uridine kinase, or it may react directly with 5-phosphoribosyl-1-pyrophosphate (PRPP), as catalyzed by orotate phosphoribosyl transferase, to form FUMP. Further metabolic pathways are available to FUMP. As the triphosphate FUTP, it is incorporated into RNA. In an alternative reaction sequence crucial for antineoplastic activity, it is reduced to FUDP by ribonucleotide reductase (RNR) to the deoxynucleotide level and forming of FdUMP. 5-FU also may be converted by thymidine phosphorylase to the deoxyriboside fluorodeoxyuridine (FUdR) and then by thymidine kinase to FdUMP, a potent inhibitor of thymidylate synthesis. This complex metabolic pathway for the generation of FdUMP may be bypassed through administration of floxuridine (fluorodeoxyuridine; FUdR), which is converted directly to FdUMP by thymidine kinase. FUdR rarely is used in clinical practice.

FdUMP inhibits TS and blocks the synthesis of TTP, a necessary constituent of DNA (Figure 61–10). The folate cofactor, 5,10-methylenetetrahydrofolate, and FdUMP form a covalently bound ternary complex with TS. This inhibited complex resembles the transition state formed during the enzymatic conversion of dUMP to

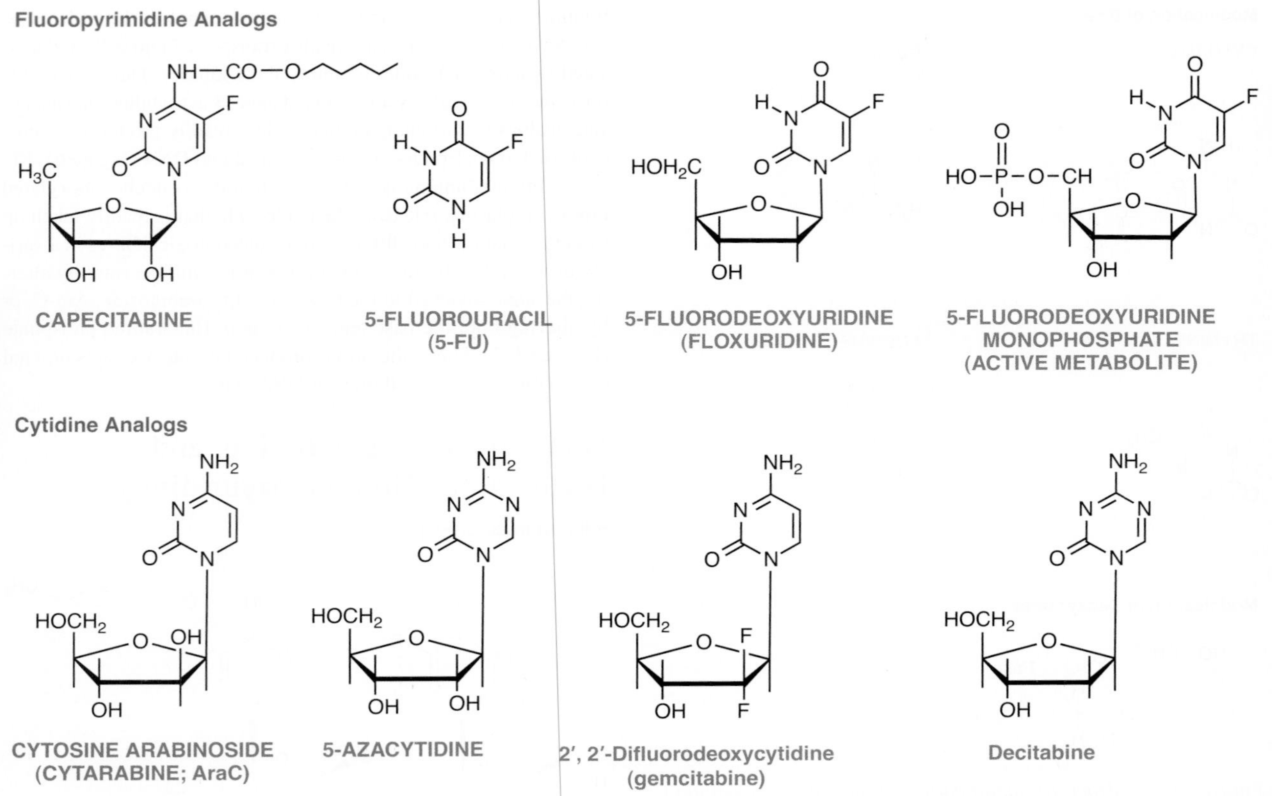

CAPECITABINE

5-FLUOROURACIL (5-FU)

5-FLUORODEOXYURIDINE (FLOXURIDINE)

5-FLUORODEOXYURIDINE MONOPHOSPHATE (ACTIVE METABOLITE)

Cytidine Analogs

CYTOSINE ARABINOSIDE (CYTARABINE; AraC)

5-AZACYTIDINE

2′, 2′-Difluorodeoxycytidine (gemcitabine)

Decitabine

Figure 61–8. *Structures of available pyrimidine analogs.*

thymidylate. The physiological complex of TS-folate-dUMP progresses to the synthesis of thymidylate by transfer of the methylene group and two hydrogen atoms from folate to dUMP, but this reaction is blocked in the inhibited complex of TS-FdUMP-folate by the stability of the fluorine carbon bond on FdUMP; sustained inhibition of the enzyme results.

5-FU is incorporated into both RNA and DNA. In 5-FU-treated cells, both fluorodeoxyuridine triphosphate (FdUTP) and deoxyuridine triphosphate (dUTP) (the substrate that accumulates behind the blocked TS reaction) incorporate into DNA in place of the depleted physiological TTP. The significance of the incorporation of FdUTP and dUTP into DNA is unclear. Presumably, the incorporation of

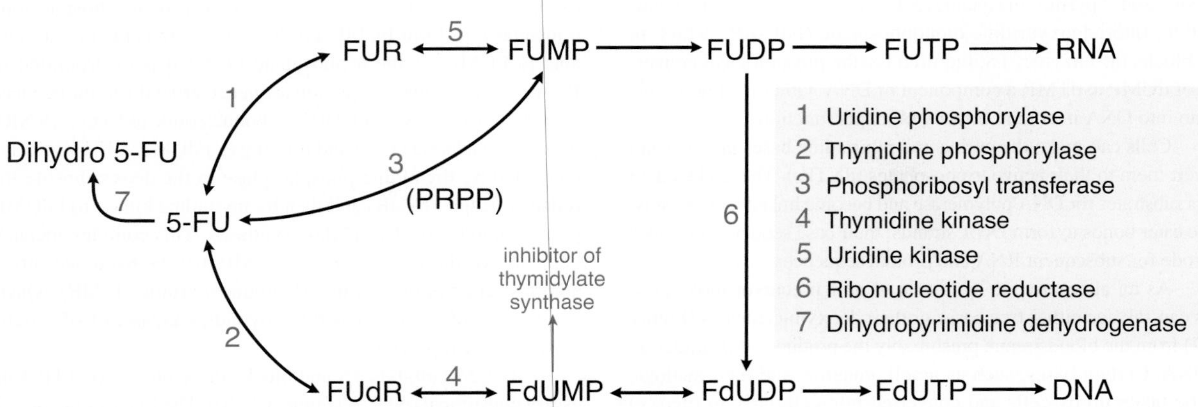

Figure 61–9. *Activation pathways for 5-fluorouracil (5-FU) and 5-floxuridine (FUR).* FUDP, floxuridine diphosphate; FUMP, floxuridine monophosphate; FUTP, floxuridine triphosphate; FUdR, fluorodeoxyuridine; FdUDP, fluorodeoxyuridine diphosphate; FdUMP, fluorodeoxyuridine monophosphate; FdUTP, fluorodeoxyuridine triphosphate; PRPP, 5-phosphoribosyl-1-pyrophosphate.

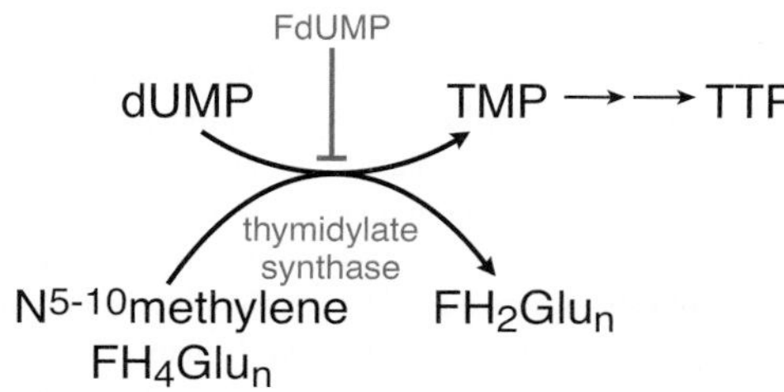

Other actions of 5-FU nucleotides:
· Inhibition of RNA processing
· Incorporation into DNA

Figure 61–10. *Site of action of 5-fluoro-2′-deoxyuridine-5′-phosphate (5-FdUMP).* 5-FU, 5-fluorouracil; dUMP, deoxyuridine monophosphate; TMP, thymidine monophosphate; TTP, thymidine triphosphate; FdUMP, fluorodeoxyuridine monophosphate; FH_2Glu_n, dihydrofolate polyglutamate; FH_4Glu_n, tetrahydrofolate polyglutamate.

deoxyuridylate and/or fluorodeoxyuridylate into DNA would call into action the excision-repair process. This process may result in DNA strand breakage because DNA repair requires TTP, but this substrate is lacking as a result of TS inhibition. 5-FU incorporation into RNA also causes toxicity as the result of major effects on both the processing and functions of RNA.

Resistance to the cytotoxic effects of 5-FU or FUdR has been ascribed to loss or decreased activity of the enzymes necessary for activation of 5-FU, amplification of TS (Washtein, 1982), mutation of TS to a form that is not inhibited by FdUMP (Barbour et al., 1990), and high levels of the degradative enzymes dihydrouracil dehydrogenase and thymidine phosphorylase (Van Triest et al., 2000). TS levels are finely controlled by an autoregulatory feedback mechanism wherein the unbound enzyme interacts with and inhibits the translational efficiency of its own mRNA, which provides for the rapid TS modulation needed for cellular division. When TS is bound to FdUMP, inhibition of translation is relieved, and levels of free TS rise, restoring thymidylate synthesis. Thus, TS autoregulation may be an important mechanism by which malignant cells become insensitive to the effects of 5-FU (Chu et al., 1991).

Some malignant cells appear to have insufficient concentrations of 5,10-methylenetetrahydrofolate, and thus cannot form maximal levels of the inhibited ternary complex with TS. Addition of exogenous folate in the form of N^5-formyl FH_4 (leucovorin) increases formation of the complex and enhances responses to 5-FU in clinical trials (Grogan et al., 1993).

In addition to leucovorin, a number of other agents have been combined with 5-FU in attempts to enhance the cytotoxic activity through biochemical modulation. Methotrexate, by inhibiting purine synthesis and increasing cellular pools of PRPP, enhances the activation of 5-FU and increases antitumor activity of 5-FU when given prior to but not following 5-FU. In clinical trials, the combination of cisplatin and 5-FU has yielded impressive responses in tumors of the upper aerodigestive tract, but the molecular basis of their interaction is not well understood. Oxaliplatin, which downregulates TS expression, is commonly used with 5-FU and leucovorin for treating metastatic colorectal cancer. Perhaps the most important interaction is the enhancement of irradiation by fluoropyrimidines, the basis for which is unclear. 5-FU with simultaneous irradiation cures anal cancer and enhances local tumor control in head and neck, cervical, rectal, gastroesophageal, and pancreatic cancer.

Absorption, Fate, and Excretion. 5-FU is administered parenterally, because absorption after oral ingestion of the drug is unpredictable and incomplete. Metabolic degradation occurs in many tissues, particularly the liver. 5-FU is inactivated by reduction of the pyrimidine ring in a reaction carried out by dihydropyrimidine dehydrogenase (DPD), which is found in liver, intestinal mucosa, tumor cells, and other tissues. Inherited deficiency of this enzyme leads to greatly increased sensitivity to the drug (Milano et al., 1999). The rare individual who totally lacks this enzyme may experience profound drug toxicity following conventional doses of the drug. DPD deficiency can be detected either by enzymatic or molecular assays using peripheral white blood cells or by determining the plasma ratio of 5-FU to its metabolite, 5-fluoro-5,6-dihydrouracil.

Intravenous administration of 5-FU produces peak plasma concentrations of 0.1-0.5 mM; plasma clearance is rapid (with a $t_{1/2}$ of 10-20 minutes). Only 5-10% of a single intravenous dose of 5-FU is excreted intact in the urine. Although the liver contains high concentrations of DPD, the dose does not have to be modified in patients with hepatic dysfunction, presumably because of degradation of the drug at extrahepatic sites. Given by continuous intravenous infusion for 24-120 hours, 5-FU achieves steady-state plasma concentrations in the range of 0.5-0.8 μM. 5-FU enters the CSF in minimal amounts.

Therapeutic Uses

5-Fluorouracil. 5-FU produces partial responses in 10-20% of patients with metastatic colon carcinomas, upper GI tract carcinomas, and breast carcinomas but rarely is used as a single agent. 5-FU in combination with leucovorin and oxaliplatin or irinotecan in the adjuvant setting is associated with a survival advantage for patients with colorectal cancers.

For average-risk patients in good nutritional status with adequate hematopoietic function, the weekly dosage regimen employs 500-600 mg/m^2 with leucovorin once each week for 6 of 8 weeks. Other regimens use daily doses of 500 mg/m^2 for 5 days, repeated in monthly cycles. When used with leucovorin, doses of daily 5-FU for 5 days must be reduced to 375-425 mg/m^2 because of mucositis and diarrhea. 5-FU increasingly is used as a biweekly infusion, in which a loading dose is followed by a 48-hour continuous infusion, a schedule that has less overall toxicity as well as superior response rates and progression-free survival for patients with metastatic colon cancer (De Gramont et al., 1998).

Floxuridine (FUdR). FUdR (fluorodeoxyuridine; FUDR, others) is used primarily by continuous infusion into the hepatic artery for treatment of metastatic carcinoma of the colon or following resection of hepatic metastases (Kemeny et al., 1999); the response rate to such infusion is 40-50%, or double that observed with intravenous administration.

Intrahepatic arterial infusion for 14-21 days causes minimal systemic toxicity; however, there is a significant risk of biliary sclerosis if this route is used for multiple cycles of therapy. Treatment should be discontinued at the earliest manifestation of toxicity (usually stomatitis or diarrhea) because the maximal effects of bone marrow suppression and gut toxicity will not be evident until days 7-14.

Capecitabine **(XELODA).** Capecitabine, an orally administered prodrug of 5-FU, is approved for the treatment of 1) metastatic breast cancer in patients who have not responded to a regimen of paclitaxel and an anthracycline antibiotic; 2) metastatic breast cancer when used in combination with docetaxel in patients who have had a prior anthracycline-containing regimen; and 3) metastatic colorectal cancer.

The recommended dosage is 2500 mg/m^2/day, given in two divided doses with food, for 2 weeks, followed by a rest period of 1 week. Capecitabine is well absorbed orally. It is rapidly de-esterified and deaminated, yielding high plasma concentrations of an inactive prodrug 5′-deoxyfluorodeoxyuridine (5′-dFdU), which disappears with a $t_{1/2}$ of ~1 hour. The conversion of 5′-dFdU to 5-FU by thymidine phosphorylase occurs in liver tissues, peripheral tissues, and tumors. 5-FU levels are <10% of those of 5′-dFdU, reaching a maximum of 0.3 mg/L or 1 μM at 2 hours. Liver dysfunction delays the conversion of the parent compound to 5′-dFdU and 5-FU, but there is no consistent effect on toxicity (Twelves et al., 1999).

Combination Therapy. Higher response rates are seen when 5-FU or capecitabine is used in combination with other agents (e.g., with cisplatin in head and neck cancer, with oxaliplatin or irinotecan in colon cancer).

The combination of 5-FU and oxaliplatin or irinotecan has become the standard first-line treatment for patients with metastatic colorectal cancer, although equivalent results are reported for capecitabine and oxaliplatin. 5-FU in combination regimens has improved survival in the adjuvant treatment for breast cancer and, with oxaliplatin and leucovorin, for colorectal cancer. 5-FU also is a potent radiation sensitizer. Beneficial effects also have been reported when combined with irradiation as primary treatment for locally advanced cancers of the esophagus, stomach, pancreas, cervix, anus, and head and neck. 5-FU produces very favorable results for the topical treatment of premalignant keratoses of the skin and multiple superficial basal cell carcinomas.

Clinical Toxicities. The clinical manifestations of toxicity caused by 5-FU and floxuridine are similar. The earliest untoward symptoms during a course of therapy are anorexia and nausea, followed by stomatitis and diarrhea, which constitute reliable warning signs that a sufficient dose has been administered. Mucosal ulcerations occur throughout the GI tract and may lead to fulminant diarrhea, shock, and death, particularly in patients who are DPD deficient. The major toxic effects of bolus-dose regimens result from the myelosuppressive action of 5-FU. The nadir of leukopenia usually is between days 9 and 14 after the first injection of drug. Thrombocytopenia and anemia also may occur. Loss of hair, occasionally progressing to total alopecia, nail changes, dermatitis, and increased pigmentation and atrophy of the skin may be encountered. Hand-foot syndrome, a particularly prominent adverse effect of capecitabine, consists of erythema, desquamation, pain, and sensitivity to touch of the palms and soles. Acute chest pain with evidence of ischemia in the electrocardiogram may result from coronary artery vasospasms during or shortly after 5-FU infusion. In general, myelosuppression, mucositis, and diarrhea occur less often with infusional regimens than with bolus regimens, while hand-foot syndrome occurs more often with infusional regimens than with bolus regimens. The significant risk of toxicity with fluoropyrimidines emphasizes the need for very skillful supervision by physicians familiar with the action and possible hazards.

Capecitabine causes much the same spectrum of toxicities as 5-FU (diarrhea, myelosuppression), but the hand-foot syndrome occurs more frequently and may require dose reduction or cessation of therapy.

CYTIDINE ANALOGS

Cytarabine (Cytosine Arabinoside; Ara-C)

Cytarabine (1-β-D-arabinofuranosylcytosine; Ara-C) is the most important antimetabolite used in the therapy of AML. It is the single most effective agent for induction of remission in this disease.

Mechanism of Action. Ara-C is an analog of 2′-deoxycytidine with the 2′-hydroxyl in a position *trans* to the 3′-hydroxyl of the sugar (Figure 61–7). The 2′-hydroxyl hinders rotation of the pyrimidine base around the nucleoside bond and interferes with base pairing. The drug enters cells via a nucleoside transporter and is converted to its active form, the 5′-monophosphate ribonucleotide, by deoxycytidine kinase (CdK), an enzyme that shows polymorphic expression among patients, as detailed in the following paragraphs.

Ara-C penetrates cells by a carrier-mediated process shared by physiological nucleosides. Several candidate carriers bring nucleosides into cells, but the hENT1 transporter appears to be the primary mediator of Ara-C influx. In infants and adults with ALL and t(4;11) mixed-lineage leukemia (MLL) translocation, high-dose Ara-C is particularly effective; in these patients, the nucleoside transporter, hENT1, is highly expressed (Pui et al., 2004), and its expression correlates with sensitivity to Ara-C. A single-point mutation in hENT1 conferred Ara-C resistance in a leukemic cell line (Cai et al., 2008). At extracellular drug concentrations >10 μM (levels achievable with high-dose Ara-C), the nucleoside transporter no longer limits drug accumulation, and intracellular metabolism to a triphosphate becomes rate limiting.

Ara-C must be "activated" by conversion to the 5′-monophosphate nucleotide (Ara-CMP), a reaction catalyzed by CdK. Polymorphisms of CdK may influence the rate of activation in individual patients (Lamba et al., 2007). Ara-CMP then reacts with appropriate deoxynucleotide kinases to form diphosphate and triphosphates (Ara-CDP and Ara-CTP). Ara-CTP competes with the physiological substrate deoxycytidine 5′-triphosphate (dCTP) for incorporation into DNA by DNA polymerases. The incorporated Ara-CMP residue is a potent inhibitor of DNA polymerase, both in replication and repair synthesis, and blocks the further elongation of the nascent DNA molecule. The block in elongation activates checkpoint kinases (ATR and chk-1), which initiate attempts to remove the offending nucleotide. If DNA breaks are not repaired, apoptosis ensues. Ara-C cytotoxicity correlates with the total Ara-C incorporated into DNA. Thus, incorporation of about five molecules of Ara-C per 10^4 bases of DNA decreases cellular clonogenicity by ~50% (Kufe et al., 1984).

Ara-C exposure activates a complex system of secondary intracellular signals that determine whether a cell survives or undergoes apoptosis. It activates the transcription factor AP-1 and stimulates the formation of ceramide, a potent inducer of apoptosis. It causes an increase in the cell damage response factor NF-κB in leukemic cells and activates checkpoint kinases. Additionally, the level of expression of the anti-apoptotic BCL-2 and $BCL\text{-}X_L$ proteins correlates inversely with relative sensitivity to Ara-C (Ibrado et al., 1996). Thus, the lethality depends on the complex interplay of multiple factors, including transport, intracellular metabolism, and cellular response to DNA damage.

Low concentrations of Ara-C induce terminal differentiation of leukemic cells in tissue culture, an effect that is accompanied by decreased c-*myc* oncogene expression; molecular analysis of bone marrow specimens from some leukemic patients in remission after Ara-C therapy has revealed persistence of leukemic markers, suggesting that differentiation may have occurred.

Continuous inhibition of DNA synthesis for a duration equivalent to at least one cell cycle or 24 hours is necessary to expose most tumor cells during the S, or DNA-synthetic, phase of the cycle. The optimal interval between bolus doses of Ara-C is ~8-12 hours, a schedule that maintains intracellular concentrations of Ara-CTP at inhibitory levels during a multi-day cycle of treatment. Typical schedules for administration of Ara-C employ bolus doses every 12 hours or continuous drug infusion for 5-7 days.

Particular subtypes of AML derive benefit from high-dose Ara-C treatment; these include t(8;21), inv(16), t(9;16), and del(16), all of which involve core-binding factors that regulate hematopoiesis (Widemann et al., 1997). Approximately 20% of AML patients have leukemic cells with a *k-RAS* mutation, and these patients seem to derive greater benefit from high dose Ara-C regimens than do patients with wild type *k-RAS* (Neubauer et al., 2008).

Mechanisms of Resistance to Cytarabine. Response to Ara-C is strongly influenced by the relative activities of anabolic and catabolic enzymes that determine the proportion of drug converted to Ara-CTP. The rate-limiting activating enzyme, CdK, produces Ara-CMP. It is opposed by the degradative enzyme, cytidine deaminase, which converts Ara-C to a nontoxic metabolite, ara-uridine (Ara-U). Cytidine deaminase activity is high in many normal tissues, including intestinal mucosa, liver, and neutrophils, but lower in AML cells and other human tumors. A second degradative enzyme, dCMP deaminase, converts Ara-CMP to the inactive metabolite, Ara-UMP. Increased synthesis and retention of Ara-CTP in leukemic cells leads to a longer duration of complete remission in patients with AML (Preisler et al., 1985). As discussed above, the ability of cells to transport Ara-C also may affect response. Clinical studies have implicated a loss of deoxycytidine kinase as the primary mechanism of resistance to Ara-C in AML (Cai et al., 2008), although 5′ nucleotidase, which degrades Ara-CMP, and possibly cytidine deaminase elevations, may play a role in AML resistance to Ara-C.

Absorption, Fate, and Excretion. Due to the presence of high concentrations of cytidine deaminase in the GI mucosa and liver, only ~20% of the drug reaches the circulation after *oral* Ara-C administration; thus, the drug must be given intravenously. Peak concentrations of 2-50 μM are measurable in plasma after intravenous injection of 30-300 mg/m² but disappear rapidly ($t_{1/2}$ of 10 minutes) from plasma.

Less than 10% of the injected dose is excreted unchanged in the urine within 12-24 hours, while most appears as the inactive deaminated product, Ara-U. Higher concentrations of Ara-C are found in CSF after continuous infusion than after rapid intravenous injection, but are far lower (≤10%) than concentrations in plasma. After *intrathecal* administration of the drug at a dose of 50 mg/m², deamination proceeds slowly, with a $t_{1/2}$ of 3-4 hours, and peak concentrations of 1-2 μM are achieved. CSF concentrations remain above the threshold for cytotoxicity (0.4 μM) for ≥24 hours. A depot liposomal formulation of Ara-C (DEPOCYT) provides sustained release into the CSF. After a standard 50-mg dose, liposomal Ara-C remains above cytotoxic levels for an average of 12 days, thus avoiding the need for frequent lumbar punctures (Cole et al., 2003).

Therapeutic Uses. Two dosage schedules are recommended for administration of cytarabine (CYTOSAR-U, TARABINE PFS, others): 1) rapid intravenous infusion of 100 mg/m² every 12 hours for 5-7 days or 2) continuous intravenous infusion of 100-200 mg/m²/day for 5-7 days. In general, children tolerate higher doses than adults. Intrathecal doses of 30 mg/m² every 4 days have been used to treat meningeal or lymphomatous leukemia. The intrathecal administration of 50 mg for adults (or 35 mg for children) of liposomal cytarabine (DEPOCYT) every 2 weeks seems equally effective as the every-4-days regimen with the standard drug.

Ara-C is indicated for induction and maintenance of remission in AML and is useful in the treatment of other leukemias, such as ALL, CML in the blast phase, acute promyelocytic leukemia, and high-grade lymphomas. Because drug concentration in plasma rapidly falls below the level needed to saturate transport and intercellular activation, clinicians have employed high-dose regimens (2-3 g/m² every 12 hours for 6-8 doses) to achieve 20- to 50 times higher serum levels, with improved results in remission induction and consolidation for AML. Injection of the liposomal formulation is indicated for the intrathecal treatment of lymphomatous meningitis.

Clinical Toxicities. Cytarabine is a potent myelosuppressive agent capable of producing acute, severe leukopenia, thrombocytopenia, and anemia with striking megaloblastic changes. Other toxic manifestations include GI disturbances, stomatitis, conjunctivitis, reversible hepatic enzyme elevations, noncardiogenic pulmonary edema, and dermatitis.

Onset of dyspnea, fever, and pulmonary infiltrates on chest computed tomography scans may follow 1-2 weeks after high-dose Ara-C and may be fatal in 10-20% of patients, especially in patients being treated for relapsed leukemia (Forghieri et al., 2007). Infectious or other causes of pulmonary infiltrates must be excluded in evaluating such patients. No specific therapy, other than Ara-C discontinuation, is indicated. Intrathecal Ara-C, either the free drug or the liposomal preparation, may cause arachnoiditis, seizures, delirium, myelopathy, or coma, especially if given concomitantly with systemic high-dose methotrexate or systemic Ara-C (Jabbour et al., 2007).

Cerebellar toxicity, manifesting as ataxia and slurred speech, and cerebral toxicity (seizures, dementia, and coma) may follow intrathecal administration or high-dose systemic administration, especially in patients >40 years of age and/or patients with poor renal function.

Azacitidine (5-Azacytidine)

5-Azacytidine (Figure 61–8) and the closely related decitabine (2′-deoxy-5-azacytidine) have antileukemic activity and induce differentiation by virtue of their inhibition of DNA cytosine methyltransferase activity. Both drugs are approved for treatment of myelodysplasia, for which they induce normalization of bone marrow in 15-20% of patients and reduce transfusion requirement in one-third of patients. 5-Azacytidine improves survival.

The aza-nucleosides enter cells by the human equilibrative transporter, the presence of which correlates with sensitivity of cell lines (Stresemann and Lyko, 2008). The drugs incorporate into DNA, where they become covalently bound to the methyltransferase through their N-5 position, depleting intracellular enzyme and leading to global demethylation of DNA and tumor cell differentiation and apoptosis. Decitabine also induces double-strand DNA breaks, perhaps as a consequence of the effort to repair the protein-DNA adduct. The azacytidine ring spontaneously opens in alkaline solution and has greater stability ($t_{1/2}$ of 7 hours) at neutral pH. After subcutaneous administration of the standard dose of 75 mg/m^2, 5-azacytidine achieves peak drug levels of 10 μM and undergoes very rapid deamination by cytidine deaminase (plasma $t_{1/2}$ of 20-40 minutes), with the product hydrolyzing to inactive metabolites. Due to the formation of intracellular nucleotides, which become incorporated into DNA, the effects of the aza-nucleosides persist for many hours.

The major toxicities of the aza-nucleosides include myelosuppression and mild GI symptoms. 5-Azacytidine produces rather severe nausea and vomiting when given intravenously in large doses (150-200 mg/m^2/day for 5 days). The usual regimen for 5-azacytidine in myelodysplastic syndrome (MDS) is 75 mg/m^2/day for 7 days every 28 days, while decitabine is given in a dose of 20 mg intravenously every day for 5 days every 4 weeks (Oki et al., 2007). Best responses may become apparent only after two to five courses of treatment.

Gemcitabine

Gemcitabine (2′,2′-difluorodeoxycytidine; dFdC) (Figure 61–8), a difluoro analog of deoxycytidine, has become an important drug for patients with metastatic pancreatic; non-squamous, non–small cell lung; ovarian; and bladder cancer.

Mechanism of Action. Gemcitabine is carried into cells by three distinct nucleoside transporters: hENT, hCNT, and a nucleobase transporter found in malignant mesothelioma cells. The hENT transporter appears to be the major carrier. Intracellularly, deoxycytidine kinase phosphorylates gemcitabine to produce difluorodeoxycytidine monophosphate (dFdCMP), from which point it is converted to difluorodeoxycytidine di- and triphosphate (dFdCDP and dFdCTP). Although gemcitabine's anabolism and effects on DNA in general mimic those of cytarabine, there are distinct differences in kinetics of inhibition, additional enzymatic sites of action, different effects of incorporation into DNA, and a distinct spectrum of clinical activity. Unlike that of cytarabine, the cytotoxicity of gemcitabine is not confined to the S phase of the cell cycle, and the drug is equally effective against confluent cells and cells in logarithmic growth phase. The cytotoxic activity may be a result of several actions on DNA synthesis. dFdCTP competes with dCTP as a weak inhibitor of DNA polymerase. dFdCDP is a stoichiometric inhibitor of RNR (Wang et al., 2007). It forms a complex with the RNR subunits and with ATP, resulting in depletion of deoxyribonucleotide pools necessary for DNA synthesis. Most important, dFdCTP incorporates into DNA and, after the incorporation of one more nucleotide, causes DNA strand termination (Heinemann et al., 1988). This "extra" nucleotide may be important in hiding the dFdCTP from DNA repair enzymes, as the incorporated dFdCMP appears resistant to repair. The ability of cells to incorporate dFdCTP into DNA is critical for gemcitabine-induced apoptosis. Gemcitabine is inactivated by cytidine deaminase, which is found both in tumor cells and throughout the body.

Preliminary evidence suggests that response to gemcitabine in pancreatic carcinoma tumors correlates positively with high expression of hENT (Giovannetti et al., 2006) and low expression of subunits of RNR, but resistance is found in tumors with low levels of deoxycytidine kinase and high levels of cytidine deaminase, the inactivating enzyme (Ohhashi et al., 2008). In mouse tumors, forced expression of the HMGA1 transcription factor also caused gemcitabine resistance (Liau and Whang, 2008), possibly through its effect on Akt-dependent survival pathways.

Absorption, Fate, and Elimination. Gemcitabine is administered as an intravenous infusion. The pharmacokinetics of the parent compound are largely determined by deamination in liver, plasma, and other organs, and the predominant urinary elimination product is difluorodeoxyuridine (dFdU). Although dFdU has modest toxicity at the usual concentrations found in plasma, in patients with significant renal dysfunction, dFdU and its triphosphate accumulate to high and potentially toxic levels (Koolen et al., 2009). Gemcitabine has a short plasma $t_{1/2}$ of ~15 minutes, with women and elderly patients clearing the drug more slowly (Abbruzzese et al., 1991). Peak levels reach 20-60 μM with doses of 1000 mg/m² given over 30 minutes intravenously. Clearance can vary widely among individuals but is not affected by renal failure.

Similar to that of cytarabine, conversion of gemcitabine to dFdCMP by deoxycytidine kinase is saturated at infusion rates of ~10 mg/m²/min, which produce plasma drug concentrations of ~10-20 μM. In an attempt to increase dFdCTP formation, the duration of infusion at this maximum concentration has been extended to 100-150 minutes at a fixed rate of 10 mg/min. The 150-minute infusion produces a higher level of dFdCTP within peripheral blood mononuclear cells and increases the degree of myelosuppression but does not improve antitumor activity (Gandhi, 2007). The inhibition of DNA repair by gemcitabine may increase cytotoxicity of other agents, particularly platinum compounds, and with radiation therapy. Preclinical studies of tumor cell lines show that gemcitabine enhances formation of cisplatin-DNA adducts, presumably through suppression of nuclear excision repair.

Therapeutic Uses. The standard dosing schedule for gemcitabine (GEMZAR) is a 30-minute intravenous infusion of 1-1.25 g/m² on days 1, 8, and 15 of each 21- to 28-day cycle, depending on the indication.

Clinical Toxicities. The principal toxicity of gemcitabine is myelosuppression. Longer-duration infusions lead to greater myelosuppression and hepatic toxicity. Nonhematological toxicities include a flu-like syndrome, asthenia, and rarely a posterior leukoencephalopathy syndrome. Mild elevation in liver transaminases may occur in ≥40% of patients and are reversible. Interstitial pneumonitis, at times progressing to acute respiratory distress syndrome (ARDS), may occur within the first two cycles of treatment and usually responds to corticosteroids. Rarely, patients on gemcitabine treatment for many months may develop a slowly progressive hemolytic uremic syndrome, necessitating drug discontinuation (Humphreys et al., 2004). Gemcitabine is a very potent radiosensitizer, likely the result of its inhibition of RNR, depletion of dATP, and inhibition of DNA repair (Flanagan et al., 2007) and should not be used with radiotherapy except in closely monitored clinical trials.

PURINE ANALOGS

The pioneering studies of Hitchings and Elion begun in 1942 who identified analogs of naturally occurring purine bases with antileukemic and immunosuppressant properties. Their work led to the development of drugs not only for treatment of malignant diseases (mercaptopurine, thioguanine) but also for immunosuppression in auto-immune disease and organ transplantation (azathioprine) and antiviral chemotherapy (acyclovir, ganciclovir, vidarabine, zidovudine) (Figure 61–11). The hypoxanthine analog allopurinol, a potent inhibitor of xanthine oxidase, is an important byproduct of this effort (see Chapter 34). Other purine analogs have valuable roles in cancer therapy. These include pentostatin (2′-deoxycoformycin), the first effective agent against hairy cell leukemia, cladribine (standard therapy for hairy cell leukemia), fludarabine phosphate (standard treatment for CLL) nelarabine (pediatric ALL), and clofarabine (T-cell leukemia/lymphoma). The apparent preferential activity of these agents in lymphoid malignancies may relate to their effective uptake, activation, and apoptotic effects in lymphoid tissue.

6-Thiopurine Analogs

6-Mercaptopurine (6-MP) and 6-thioguanine (6-TG) are approved agents for human leukemias and function as analogs of the natural purines, hypoxanthine and guanine. The substitution of sulfur for oxygen on C6 of the purine ring creates compounds that are readily transported into cells, including activated malignant cells. Nucleotides formed from 6-MP and 6-TG inhibit

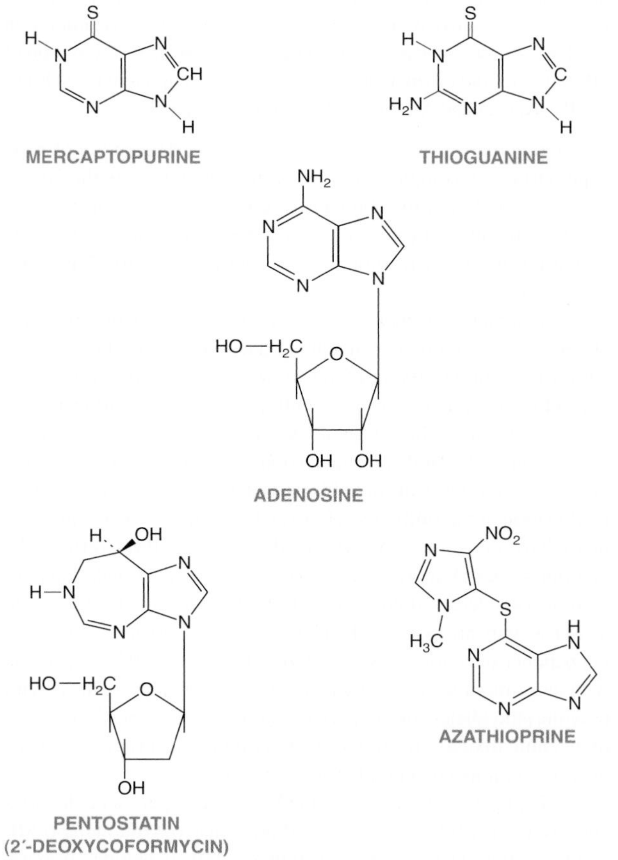

MERCAPTOPURINE

THIOGUANINE

ADENOSINE

PENTOSTATIN (2′-DEOXYCOFORMYCIN)

AZATHIOPRINE

Figure 61–11. *Structural formulas of adenosine and various purine analogs.*

de novo purine synthesis and also become incorporated into nucleic acids. The structural formula of 6-MP and other purine analogs is shown in Figure 61–11.

Mechanism of Action. Both 6-TG and 6-MP are excellent substrates for hypoxanthine guanine phosphoribosyl transferase (HGPRT) and are converted in a single step to the ribonucleotides 6-thioguanosine-5′-monophosphate (6-thioGMP) and 6-thioinosine-5′-monophosphate (T-IMP), respectively. Because T-IMP is a poor substrate for guanylyl kinase, the enzyme that converts guanosine monophosphate (GMP) to guanosine diphosphate (GDP), T-IMP accumulates intracellularly and in a second step is converted to 6-TGMP. T-IMP inhibits the new formation of ribosyl-5-phosphate, as well as conversion of inosine-5′-monophosphate (IMP) to adenine and guanine nucleotides. Of these, the most important point of attack seems to be the reaction of glutamine and PRPP to form ribosyl-5-phosphate, the first committed step in the *de novo* pathway. 6-Thioguanine nucleotide is incorporated into DNA, where it induces strand breaks and base mispairing. Strand breaks depend on the presence of an intact MMR system, the absence of which leads to resistance.

Mechanisms of Resistance to the Thiopurine Antimetabolites. The most common mechanism of 6-MP resistance observed *in vitro* is deficiency or complete lack of the activating enzyme, HGPRT, or increased alkaline phosphate activity. Other mechanisms for resistance include 1) decreased drug uptake, or increased efflux due to one of several active transporters; 2) alteration in allosteric inhibition of ribosylamine 5-phosphate synthase; and 3) impaired recognition of DNA breaks and mismatches due to loss of a component (MSH6) of MMR (Karran and Attard, 2008; Cahill et al., 2007).

Mercaptopurine Pharmacokinetics and Toxicity. Absorption of mercaptopurine is incomplete (10-50%) after oral ingestion; the drug is subject to first-pass metabolism by xanthine oxidase in the liver. Food or oral antibiotics decrease absorption. Oral bioavailability is increased when mercaptopurine is combined with high-dose methotrexate.

After an intravenous dose, the $t_{1/2}$ of the drug in plasma is relatively short (~50 minutes in adults), due to rapid metabolic degradation by xanthine oxidase and by thiopurine methyltransferase (TPMT). Restricted brain distribution of mercaptopurine results from an efficient efflux transport system in the blood-brain barrier. In addition to the HGPRT-catalyzed anabolism of mercaptopurine, there are two other pathways for its metabolism. The first involves methylation of the sulfhydryl group and subsequent oxidation of the methylated derivatives. Activity of the enzyme TPMT reflects the inheritance of polymorphic alleles; up to 15% of the Caucasian population has decreased enzyme activity. Low levels of erythrocyte TPMT activity are associated with increased drug toxicity in individual patients and a lower risk of relapse (Pui et al., 2004). In patients with auto-immune disease treated with mercaptopurine, those with polymorphic alleles may experience bone marrow aplasia and life-threatening toxicity. Testing for these polymorphisms prior to treatment is recommended in this patient population.

High concentrations of 6-methylmercaptopurine nucleotides are formed in white blood cells and bone marrow following 6-MP administration. They are less potent than 6-MP nucleotides as metabolic inhibitors, and their significance in contributing to the activity of 6-MP is not known.

A relatively large percentage of the administered sulfur appears in the urine as inorganic sulfate, the result of enzymatic desulfuration. The second major pathway for 6-MP metabolism involves its oxidation by xanthine oxidase to 6-thiouric acid, an inactive metabolite. Oral doses of 6-MP should be reduced by 75% in patients receiving the xanthine oxidase inhibitor, allopurinol. No dose adjustment is required for intravenous dosing.

Therapeutic Uses. In the maintenance therapy of ALL, the initial daily oral dose of mercaptopurine (6-MP; PURINETHOL, others) is 50-100 mg/m^2 and is thereafter adjusted according to white blood cell and platelet count. The combination of methotrexate and 6-MP appears to be synergistic. By inhibiting the earliest steps in purine synthesis, methotrexate elevates the intracellular concentration of PRPP, a cofactor required for 6-MP activation.

Clinical Toxicities. The principal toxicity of 6-MP is bone marrow depression, although in general, this side effect develops more gradually than with folic acid antagonists; accordingly, thrombocytopenia, granulocytopenia, or anemia may not become apparent for several weeks. When depression of normal bone marrow elements occurs, dose reduction usually results in prompt recovery, although myelosuppression may be severe and prolonged in patients with a polymorphism affecting TPMT. Anorexia, nausea, or vomiting is seen in ~25% of adults, but stomatitis and diarrhea are rare; manifestations of GI effects are less frequent in children than in adults. Jaundice and hepatic enzyme elevations occur in up to one-third of adult patients treated with 6-MP and usually resolve upon discontinuation of therapy. Their appearance has been associated with bile stasis and hepatic necrosis on biopsy. 6-MP and its derivative, azathioprine, predispose to opportunistic infection such as reactivation of hepatitis B, fungal infection, and *Pneumocystis* pneumonia and an increased incidence of squamous cell malignancies of the skin. 6-MP has teratogenic effects during the first trimester of pregnancy, and AML has been reported after prolonged 6-MP therapy for Crohn's disease (Heizer and Peterson, 1998).

Fludarabine Phosphate

This compound is a fluorinated, deamination-resistant, phosphorylated analog of the antiviral agent vidarabine (9-β-D-arabinofuranosyl-adenine). It is active in CLL and low-grade lymphomas. It has found important uses as a cytotoxic drug and as a potent immunosuppressant.

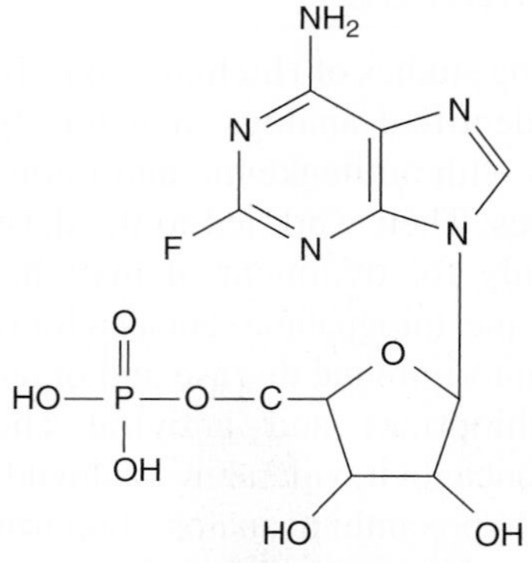

FLUDARABINE PHOSPHATE

After rapid extracellular dephosphorylation to the nucleoside fludarabine, it is rephosphorylated intracellularly by deoxycytidine kinase to the active triphosphate derivative. This antimetabolite inhibits DNA polymerase, DNA primase, DNA ligase, and RNR and becomes incorporated into DNA and RNA. The nucleotide is an effective chain terminator when incorporated into DNA (Kamiya et al., 1996), and the incorporation of fludarabine into RNA inhibits RNA function, RNA processing, and mRNA translation (Plunkett and Gandhi, 1993).

In experimental tumors, resistance to fludarabine is associated with decreased activity of deoxycytidine kinase (the enzyme that phosphorylates the drug) (Mansson et al., 2003), increased drug efflux, and increased RNR activity. Its mechanism of immunosuppression and paradoxical stimulation of auto-immunity stems from the particular susceptibility of lymphoid cells to purine analogs and the specific effects on the $CD4^+$ subset of T cells, as well as its inhibition of regulatory T-cell responses.

Absorption, Fate, and Excretion. Fludarabine phosphate is administered both intravenously and orally and rapidly converts to fludarabine in the plasma. The median time to reach maximal concentrations of drug in plasma after oral administration is 1.5 hours, and oral bioavailability averages 55-60%. The terminal $t_{1/2}$ of fludarabine in plasma is ~10 hours. The compound is primarily (40-50%) eliminated by renal excretion.

Therapeutic Uses. Fludarabine phosphate (FLUDARA, OFORTA) is approved for intravenous and oral use and is equally active by both routes (Forconi et al., 2008). The recommended dose of fludarabine phosphate is 25 mg/m^2 daily for 5 days by intravenous infusion, or 40 mg/m^2 daily for 5 days by mouth. The drug is administered intravenously over 30 minutes to 2 hours. Dosage should be reduced in patients with renal impairment in proportion to the reduction in CrCl. Treatment may be repeated every 4 weeks, and gradual improvement in CLL usually occurs within two to three cycles.

Fludarabine phosphate is highly active alone or with rituximab and cyclophosphamide for the treatment of patients with CLL. Activity in CLL as a single agent is equal by either the oral or intravenous routes, as overall response rates in previously untreated patients approximate 80% and the duration of response averages 22 months. The synergy of fludarabine with alkylators may stem from the observation that it blocks the repair of double-strand DNA breaks and interstrand cross-links induced by alkylating agents. It also is effective in follicular B-cell lymphomas refractory to standard therapy. It is increasingly used as a potent immunosuppressive agent in nonmyeloablative allogeneic bone marrow transplantation, where it suppresses the host response and may encourage alloreactive donor T cells.

Clinical Toxicities. Oral and intravenous therapy cause myelosuppression (World Health Organization grade 3 or 4) in about half of patients, nausea and vomiting in a minor fraction, and uncommonly chills and fever, malaise, anorexia, peripheral neuropathy, and weakness. Lymphopenia and thrombocytopenia and cumulative side effects are expected. Depletion of $CD4^+$ T cells with therapy predisposes to opportunistic infections. Tumor lysis syndrome, a relatively infrequent complication, occurs primarily in previously untreated patients with CLL. Altered mental status, seizures, optic neuritis, and coma have been observed at higher doses and in older patients.

Auto-immune events may occur after fludarabine treatment. CLL patients may develop an acute hemolytic anemia or pure red cell aplasia during or following fludarabine treatment. Prolonged cytopenias, probably mediated by auto-immunity, also complicate fludarabine treatment. Myelodysplasia and acute leukemias may arise as late complications (Tam et al., 2008). Pneumonitis is an occasional side effect and responds to corticosteroids. Because a significant fraction of drug is eliminated in the urine, patients with compromised renal function should be treated with caution, and initial doses should be reduced in proportion to the reduction in CrCl.

Cladribine

An adenosine deaminase-resistant purine analog, cladribine (2-chlorodeoxyadenosine; 2-CdA), has potent and probably curative activity in hairy cell leukemia, CLL, and low-grade lymphomas. It is taken up by active nucleoside transport. After intracellular phosphorylation by deoxycytidine kinase and conversion to cladribine triphosphate, it is incorporated into DNA. It produces DNA strand breaks and depletion of NAD and ATP, leading to apoptosis. It is a potent inhibitor of RNR. The drug does not require cell division to be cytotoxic. Resistance is associated with loss of the activating enzyme, deoxycytidine kinase; increased expression of RNR (Cardoen et al., 2001); or increased active efflux by ABCG2 or other members of the ABC cassette family of transporters (de Wolf et al., 2008).

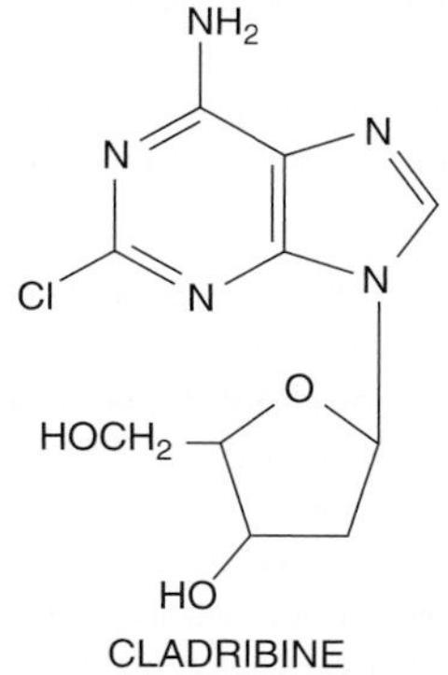

NH$_2$ N N Cl N N O HOCH$_2$ HO

CLADRIBINE

Absorption, Fate, and Excretion. Cladribine is moderately well absorbed orally (55%) but is routinely administered intravenously. The drug is excreted by the kidneys, with a terminal $t_{1/2}$ in plasma of 6.7 hours (Liliemark and Juliusson, 1991). Cladribine crosses the blood-brain barrier and reaches CSF concentrations of ~25% of those seen in plasma. Doses should be adjusted for renal dysfunction.

Therapeutic Uses. Cladribine (LEUSTATIN, others) is administered as a single course of 0.09 mg/kg/day for 7 days by continuous intravenous infusion.

Cladribine is considered the drug of choice in hairy cell leukemia. Eighty percent of patients achieve a complete response after a single course of therapy. The drug also is active in CLL; low-grade lymphomas; Langerhans cell histiocytosis; CTCLs, including mycosis fungoides and the Sézary syndrome; and Waldenström macroglobulinemia.

Clinical Toxicities. The major dose-limiting toxicity of cladribine is myelosuppression. Cumulative thrombocytopenia may occur with repeated courses. Opportunistic infections are common and correlate with decreased $CD4^+$ cell counts. Other toxic effects include nausea, infections, high fever, headache, fatigue, skin rashes, and tumor lysis syndrome.

Clofarabine (2-Chloro-2′-Fluoro-Arabinosyladenine)

This analog resulted from incorporating the 2-chloro, glycosylase-resistant substituent of cladribine and a 2′-fluoro-arabinosyl substitution, which further strengthens stability and enhances uptake and phosphorylation. The resulting compound is approved for pediatric ALL after failure of two prior therapies.

For these patients, it produces complete remissions in 20-30 % of patients. It has activity as well in pediatric and adult AML and in myelodysplasia. Its uptake and metabolic activation in tumor cells follow the same path as cladribine and the other purine nucleosides, although it is more readily phosphorylated by dCK. It incorporates into DNA, where it terminates DNA synthesis and leads to apoptosis.

Absorption, Fate, and Distribution. Clofarabine triphosphate has a long intracellular $t_{1/2}$ of 24 hours. Its antitumor activity is ascribed to its incorporation into DNA, resulting in chain termination. Like fludarabine, clofarabine inhibits RNR (Bonate et al., 2006). In children, following administration of usual doses of 52 mg/m^2 given as a 2-hour infusion daily for 5 days, clofarabine has a primary elimination $t_{1/2}$ in plasma of 6.5 hours, and the majority of drug is excreted unchanged in the urine. Doses should be adjusted according to reductions in CrCl, although precise guidelines are not available.

Clinical Toxicities. The primary toxicities are myelosuppression; a clinical syndrome of hypotension, tachyphemia, pulmonary edema, organ dysfunction, and fever, all suggestive of capillary leak syndrome and cytokine release; elevated hepatic enzymes and increased bilirubin; nausea, vomiting, and diarrhea; and hypokalemia and hypophosphatemia. Evidence of capillary leak should lead to immediate discontinuation of the drug.

Nelarabine (6-Methoxy-Arabinosyl-Guanine)

The only guanine nucleoside in clinical use, this agent has selective activity against acute T-cell leukemia (20% complete responses) and the closely related T-cell lymphoblastic lymphoma and is approved for use in relapsed/refractory patients. Its basic mechanism of action closely resembles that of the other purine nucleosides, in that it is incorporated into DNA and terminates DNA synthesis. It has selective toxicity for T lymphocytes and T-cell malignancies.

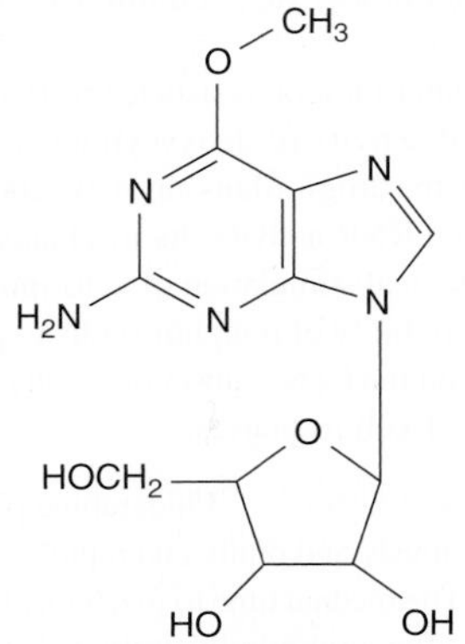

NELARABINE

Absorption, Fate, and Distribution. Following infusion, the parent methoxy compound is rapidly activated in blood and tissues by adenosine deaminase–mediated cleavage of the methyl group, yielding the phosphorylase resistant Ara-G, which has a longer plasma $t_{1/2}$ of 3 hours. The active metabolite is transported into tumor cells, where it is activated by CdK to the monophosphate and thence to a triphosphate. Ara-G triphosphate (Ara-GTP) is incorporated into DNA and terminates DNA synthesis (Sanford and Lyseng-Williamson, 2008). The drug and its metabolite, Ara-G, are primarily eliminated by metabolism to guanine, and a smaller fraction is eliminated by renal excretion of Ara-G. The dose should not be adjusted for mild to moderate (CrCl >50 mg/mL) renal dysfunction (Sanford and Lyseng-Williamson, 2008), but the drug should be used with close clinical monitoring in patients with more severe renal impairment. Adults are given a dose of 1500 mg/m^2 intravenously as a 2-hour infusion on days 1, 3, and 5 of a 21-day cycle, and children are given a lower dose of 650 mg/m^2/day intravenously for 5 days and repeated every 21 days.

Clinical Toxicities. Side effects include myelosuppression and liver function test abnormalities, as well as frequent, serious neurological sequelae, such as seizures, delirium, somnolence, peripheral neuropathy, or Guillain-Barré syndrome. Neurological side effects may not be reversible.

Pentostatin (2′-Deoxycoformycin)

Pentostatin (2′-deoxycoformycin; see Figure 61–11), a transition-state analog of the intermediate in the adenosine deaminase (ADA) reaction, potently inhibits ADA. Its effects mimic the phenotype of genetic ADA deficiency (severe immunodeficiency affecting both T- and B-cell functions). It was isolated from fermentation cultures of *Streptomyces antibioticus.* Inhibition of ADA by pentostatin leads to accumulation of intracellular adenosine and deoxyadenosine nucleotides, which can block DNA synthesis by inhibiting RNR.

Deoxyadenosine also inactivates S-adenosyl homocysteine hydrolase. The resulting accumulation of S-adenosyl homocysteine is particularly toxic to lymphocytes. Pentostatin also can inhibit RNA synthesis, and its triphosphate derivative is incorporated into DNA, resulting in strand breakage. Although the precise mechanism of cytotoxicity is not known, it is probable that the imbalance in purine nucleotide pools accounts for its antineoplastic effect in hairy cell leukemia and T-cell lymphomas.

Absorption, Fate, and Excretion. Pentostatin is administered intravenously, and a single dose of 4 mg/m^2 has a mean terminal $t_{1/2}$ of 5.7 hours. The drug is eliminated almost entirely by renal excretion. Proportional reduction of dosage is recommended in patients with renal impairment as measured by reduced CrCl.

Therapeutic Uses. The recommended dose is 4 mg/m^2 administered every other week intravenously. After hydration with 500-1000 mL of 5% dextrose in half-normal (0.45%) saline, the drug is administered by rapid intravenous injection or by infusion over a period of ≤30 minutes, followed by an additional 500 mL of fluids.

Pentostatin is extremely effective in producing complete remissions (58%) and partial responses (28%) in hairy cell leukemia (Grever et al., 2003). It largely has been superseded by cladribine.

Clinical Toxicities. Toxic manifestations include myelosuppression, GI symptoms, skin rashes, and abnormal liver function studies. Depletion of normal T cells occurs, and neutropenic fever and opportunistic infections may result. Immunosuppression may persist for several years after discontinuation of pentostatin therapy. At high doses (10 mg/m^2), major renal and neurological complications are encountered. Pentostatin in combination with fludarabine phosphate may result in severe or even fatal pulmonary toxicity.

III. Natural Products

MICROTUBULE-DAMAGING AGENTS

Several anticancer agents act through the microtubules, either causing disorganized stabilization of microtubules in areas away from the centriole or causing destabilization of the mitotic spindle, interfering with mitosis. The vinca alkaloids are effective in the treatment of hematological malignancies, breast, germ cell, and lung cancers, whereas the taxanes have become leading agents in the treatment of ovarian, breast, head and neck, and lung cancers. A new class of agents, the epothilones, resembles the taxanes in their action but has limited cross-resistance with taxanes; the only approved epothilone in the U.S., ixabepilone, is indicated for metastatic breast cancer.

VINCA ALKALOIDS

History. The beneficial properties of the Madagascar periwinkle plant, *Catharanthus roseus* (formerly called *Vinca rosea*), a species of myrtle, have been described in medicinal folklore. Periwinkle extracts attracted interest because of their hypoglycemic effects in diabetes. Purified alkaloids, including vinblastine and vincristine, caused regression of an acute lymphocytic leukemia in mice and were among the earliest clinical agents for treatment of leukemias, lymphomas, and testicular cancer. A closely related derivative, vinorelbine, has important activity against lung and breast cancer.

Chemistry. The vinca alkaloids are asymmetrical dimeric compounds formed by condensation of the vindoline and catharanthine subunits.

A

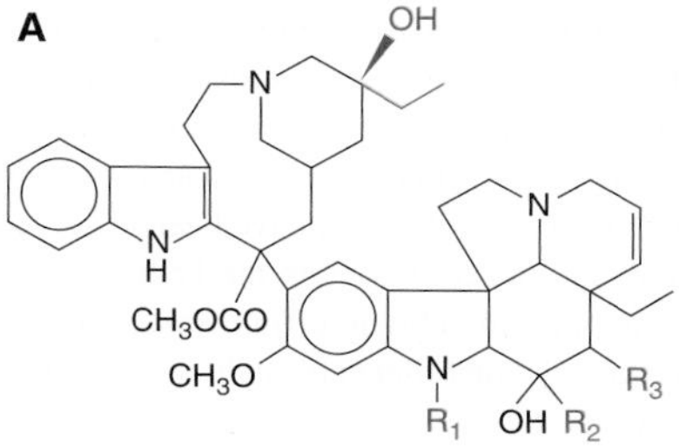

OH, N, N, H, CH_3OCO, CH_3O, N, R_1, OH, R_2, R_3

B

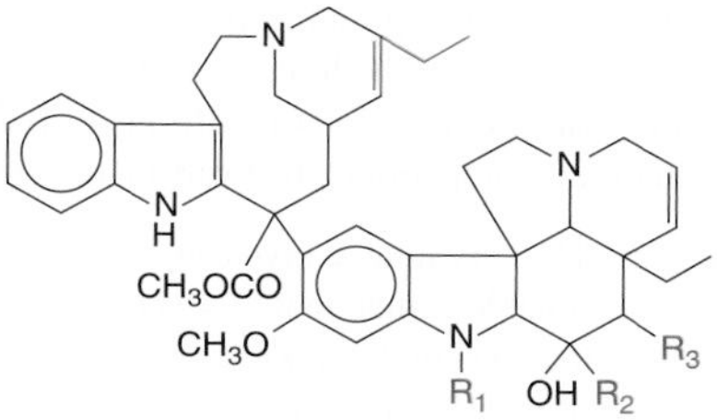

N, N, H, CH_3OCO, CH_3O, N, R_1, OH, R_2, R_3

	R_1	R_2	R_3
Structure A			
VINBLASTINE	$-CH_3$	$-C(=O)-OCH_3$	$-O-C(=O)-CH_3$
VINCRISTINE	$-CH(=O)$	$-C(=O)-OCH_3$	$-O-C(=O)-CH_3$
VINDESINE	$-CH_3$	$-C(=O)-NH_2$	$-OH$
Structure B			
VINORELBINE	$-CH_3$	$-C(=O)-OCH_3$	$-O-C(=O)-CH_3$

Mechanism of Action. The vinca alkaloids are cell-cycle–specific agents and, in common with other drugs such as colchicine, podophyllotoxin, the taxanes, and the epothilones, block cells in mitosis. The biological activities of the vincas can be explained by their ability to bind specifically to β tubulin and to block its polymerization with α tubulin into microtubules.

When cells are incubated with vinblastine, the microtubules dissolve and highly regular crystals form, containing 1 mole of bound vinblastine per mole of tubulin. Cell division arrests in metaphase. In the absence of an intact mitotic spindle, duplicated chromosomes cannot align along the division plate. They disperse throughout the cytoplasm (exploded mitosis) or may clump in unusual groupings, such as balls or stars. Cells blocked in mitosis undergo changes characteristic of apoptosis.

In addition to their key role in the formation of mitotic spindles, microtubules are found in high concentration in the brain and contribute to other cellular functions such as movement, phagocytosis, and axonal transport. Side effects of the vinca alkaloids, such as their neurotoxicity, may relate to disruption of these functions.

Drug Resistance. Despite their structural similarity, the vinca alkaloids have unique individual patterns of clinical effectiveness (see the individual vinca alkaloid sections). However, in most experimental systems, they share cross-resistance. Their antitumor effects are blocked by multidrug resistance mediated by the *mdr* gene and its glycoprotein. Tumor cells become cross-resistant to a wide range of chemically dissimilar agents (the vinca alkaloids, epipodophyllotoxins, anthracyclines, and taxanes). Chromosomal abnormalities consistent with gene amplification have been observed in resistant cells in culture, and the cells contain markedly increased levels of the P-glycoprotein, a membrane efflux transporter (Endicott and Ling, 1989). Ca^{2+} channel blockers such as verapamil can reverse resistance of this type *in vitro*; however, clinical trials of resistance-reversing agents have been disappointing. Other membrane transporters, such as the MRP and the closely related breast cancer resistance protein, may mediate multidrug resistance. Still other forms of resistance to vinca alkaloids stem from mutations in β tubulin or in the relative expression of isoforms of β tubulin; both changes prevent the inhibitors from effectively binding to their target.

Cytotoxic Actions. The very limited myelosuppressive action of vincristine makes it a valuable component of several combination therapy regimens for leukemia and lymphoma, while the lack of severe neurotoxicity of vinblastine is a decided advantage in lymphomas and in combination with cisplatin against testicular cancer. Vinorelbine, which causes a mild neurotoxicity as well as myelosuppression, has an intermediate toxicity profile. Vincristine is a standard component of regimens for treating pediatric leukemias, lymphomas, and solid tumors, such as Wilms tumor, neuroblastoma, and rhabdomyosarcoma. In large-cell non-Hodgkin's lymphomas, vincristine remains an important agent, particularly when used in the CHOP regimen with cyclophosphamide, doxorubicin, and prednisone. Vinblastine is employed in treating bladder cancer, testicular carcinomas, and Hodgkin's disease. Vinorelbine has activity against non–small cell lung cancer and breast cancer.

Absorption, Fate, and Excretion. The liver cytochromes extensively metabolize all three agents, and the metabolites are excreted in the bile (Robieux et al., 1996). Only a small fraction of a dose (<15%) is found in the urine unchanged. In patients with hepatic dysfunction (bilirubin >3 mg/dL), a 50-75% reduction in dose of any of the vinca alkaloids is advisable, although firm guidelines for dose adjustment have not been established. The pharmacokinetics of each of the three drugs are similar, with an elimination $t_{1/2}$ of 20 hours for vincristine, 23 hours for vinblastine, and 24 hours for vinorelbine.

Vinblastine

Therapeutic Uses. Vinblastine sulfate (VELBAN, others) is given intravenously; special precautions must be taken against subcutaneous extravasation, because this may cause painful irritation and ulceration. The drug should not be injected into an extremity with impaired circulation. After a single dose of 0.3 mg/kg of body weight, myelosuppression reaches its maximum in 7-10 days. If a moderate level of leukopenia (~3000 cells/mm^3) is not attained, the weekly dose may be increased gradually by increments of 0.05 mg/kg of body weight. In regimens designed to cure testicular cancer, vinblastine is used in doses of 0.3 mg/kg every 3 weeks. Doses should be reduced by 50% for patients with plasma bilirubin >1.5 mg/dL.

One important clinical use of vinblastine is with bleomycin and cisplatin (see "Therapeutic Uses" under "Bleomycin") in the curative therapy of metastatic testicular tumors, although it has been supplanted by etoposide or ifosfamide in this disease. It is a component of the standard curative regimen for Hodgkin's disease [doxorubicin (ADRIAMYCIN), bleomycin, vinblastine, and dacarbazine (ABVD)]. It also is active in Kaposi sarcoma, neuroblastoma, Langerhans cell histiocytosis, carcinoma of the breast, and choriocarcinoma.

Clinical Toxicities. The nadir of the leukopenia that follows the administration of vinblastine usually occurs within 7-10 days, after which recovery ensues within 7 days. Other toxic effects of vinblastine include mild neurological manifestations. GI disturbances including nausea, vomiting, anorexia, and diarrhea may be encountered. The syndrome of inappropriate secretion of antidiuretic hormone has been reported. Loss of hair, stomatitis, and dermatitis occur infrequently. Extravasation during injection may lead to cellulitis and phlebitis.

Vincristine

Therapeutic Uses. Vincristine sulfate (VINCASAR PFS, others) used together with glucocorticoids is the treatment of choice to induce remissions in childhood leukemia and in combination with alkylating agents and anthracycline for pediatric sarcomas; the common intravenous dosage for vincristine is 2 mg/m^2 of body surface area at weekly or longer intervals. Vincristine seems to be tolerated better by children than by adults, who may experience severe, progressive neurological toxicity and require a lower dose of 1.4 mg/m^2. Administration of the drug more frequently than every 7 days or at higher doses increases the toxic manifestations without proportional improvement in the response rate. Precautions also should be used to avoid extravasation during intravenous administration of vincristine. Doses should be reduced by 50% or 75% for patients with plasma bilirubin >1.5 mg/dL or >3 mg/dL, respectively.

Clinical Toxicities. The clinical toxicity of vincristine is mostly neurological. Early sensory changes do not warrant dose reduction. The more severe neurological manifestations may be avoided or reversed by either suspending therapy or reducing the dosage upon first evidence of motor dysfunction. Severe constipation, sometimes resulting in colicky abdominal pain and obstruction, may be prevented by a prophylactic program of laxatives and hydrophilic (bulk-forming) agents and usually is a problem only with doses >2 mg/m^2.

Alopecia occurs in ~20% of patients given vincristine; however, the alopecia is always reversible, frequently without cessation of therapy. Modest leukopenia may follow vincristine administration. Thrombocytopenia, anemia, GI cholic and obstipation, and the syndrome of inappropriate secretion of antidiuretic hormone are less common adverse effects. Inadvertent injection of vincristine into the CSF causes a devastating and often fatal irreversible coma and seizures (Williams et al., 1983). CSF exchange has averted a fatal outcome in anecdotal reports.

Vinorelbine

Vinorelbine (NAVELBINE, others) is administered in normal saline as an intravenous infusion over 6-10 minutes. When used alone, it is given at doses of 30 mg/m^2 either weekly or for 2 out of every 3 weeks. When used with cisplatin for the treatment of non–small cell lung cancer, it is given at doses of 25 mg/m^2 either weekly or for 3 out of every 4 weeks. A lower dose (20-25 mg/m^2) may be required for patients who have received prior chemotherapy, and dosage adjustment is necessary for hematological toxicity. Its primary toxicity is granulocytopenia, with only modest thrombocytopenia and less neurotoxicity than other vinca alkaloids. Vinorelbine may cause allergic reactions and mild, reversible changes in liver enzymes. An oral formulation of vinorelbine is active in non–small cell lung carcinoma, and phase III studies are ongoing (Krzakowski et al., 2008). Similar to the other vincas, doses should be reduced by 50% or 75% in patients with plasma bilirubin 2.1-3 mg/dL or >3 mg/dL, respectively.

TAXANES

The first compound of this series, paclitaxel (TAXOL, others), was isolated from the bark of the Western yew tree in 1971 and presented significant problems in formulation because of its poor aqueous solubility. It was reformulated and approved by the U.S. Food and Drug Administration (FDA) in 2005 as an albumin-bound nanoparticle solution for infusion (nab-paclitaxel, ABRAXANE). Paclitaxel and its congenic, the semisynthetic docetaxel (TAXOTERE), exhibit unique pharmacological properties as inhibitors of mitosis, differing from the vinca alkaloids and colchicine derivatives in that they bind to a different β-tubulin site and promote rather than inhibit microtubule formation. The taxanes have a central role in the therapy of ovarian, breast, lung, GI, genitourinary, and head and neck cancers (Rowinsky and Donehower, 1995).

Chemistry. Paclitaxel is a diterpenoid compound that contains a complex eight-member taxane ring as its nucleus (Figure 61–12). The side chain linked to the taxane ring at C13 is essential for its antitumor activity. Modification of the side chain has led to identification of the more potent analog, docetaxel (Figure 61–12), which shares the same spectrum of clinical activity as paclitaxel, but differs in its toxicity. Originally purified as the parent molecule from yew bark, paclitaxel now can be obtained for commercial purposes by semisynthesis from 10-desacetylbaccatin, a precursor found in yew needles. It also has been successfully synthesized (Nicolaou et al., 1994) in a complex series of reactions. Paclitaxel has very limited water solubility and is administered in a vehicle of 50% ethanol and 50% polyethoxylated castor oil (CREMOPHOR EL); this vehicle likely is responsible for a high rate of hypersensitivity reactions. Patients receiving this formulation are protected by pretreatment with a histamine H_1-receptor antagonist such as diphenhydramine, an H_2-receptor antagonist such as cimetidine (see Chapter 32), and a glucocorticoid such as dexamethasone (see Chapter 42).

Nab-paclitaxel is soluble in aqueous solutions and can be administered safely without prophylactic antihistamines or steroids. This form of paclitaxel has increased cellular uptake via an albumin-specific mechanism.

Docetaxel, somewhat more soluble than paclitaxel, is administered in polysorbate 80 and is associated with a lower incidence of hypersensitivity reactions than paclitaxel dissolved in CREMOPHOR. However, pretreatment with dexamethasone for 3 days starting 1 day

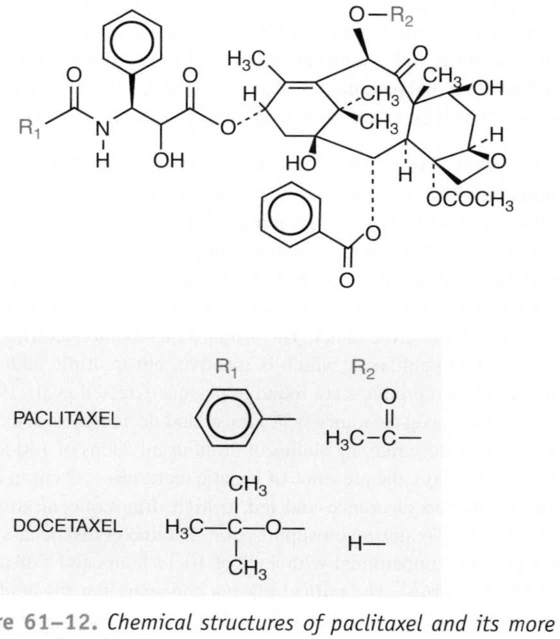

	R_1	R_2
PACLITAXEL	(phenyl)—	$H_3C-C(=O)-$
DOCETAXEL	$H_3C-C(CH_3)_2-O-$	H—

Figure 61–12. Chemical structures of paclitaxel and its more potent analog, docetaxel.

prior to therapy is required to prevent progressive fluid retention and minimize the severity of hypersensitivity reactions.

Mechanism of Action. Interest in paclitaxel was stimulated by the drug's unique ability to promote microtubule formation at cold temperatures and in the absence of GTP. It binds specifically to the β-tubulin subunit of microtubules and antagonizes the disassembly of this key cytoskeletal protein, with the result that bundles of microtubules and aberrant structures derived from microtubules appear in the mitotic phase of the cell cycle. Arrest in mitosis follows. Cell killing is dependent on both drug concentration and duration of cell exposure. Drugs that block cell-cycle progression prior to mitosis antagonize the toxic effects of taxanes.

Drug interactions have been noted; the sequence of cisplatin preceding paclitaxel decreases paclitaxel clearance and produces greater toxicity than the opposite schedule (Rowinsky and Donehower, 1995). Paclitaxel decreases doxorubicin clearance and enhances cardiotoxicity, while docetaxel has no apparent effect on anthracycline pharmacokinetics.

In cultured tumor cells, resistance to taxanes is associated in some lines with increased expression of the *mdr*-1 gene and its product, P-glycoprotein; other resistant cells have β-tubulin mutations, and these latter cells may display heightened sensitivity to vinca alkaloids (Cabral, 1983). Other resistant cell lines display an increase in survivin, an anti-apoptotic factor, α aurora kinase, an enzyme that promotes completion of mitosis. The taxanes preferentially bind to the βII-tubulin subunit of microtubules; therefore, cells may become resistant by upregulating the βIII-isoform of tubulin (Ranganathan et al., 1998). The basis of clinical drug resistance is not known. Cell death occurs by apoptosis, but the effectiveness of paclitaxel against experimental tumors does not depend on an intact p53 gene product.

Preclinical studies have suggested that nab-paclitaxel has an increased antitumor effect in breast cancer and a higher intratumoral drug concentration compared to cremophor-delivered paclitaxel. The reasons are not clear but may relate to maintenance of the drug in the nanoparticle micellar system or to increased expression of SPARC [Secreted Protein, Acidic and Rich in Cysteine; aka osteonectin, a matri-cellular linkage protein expressed in pro-fibrotic states and linked to myriad pathologies [Kos and Wilding, 2010; Chlenski and Cohn, 2010]) on tumor cells, leading to an increased drug uptake.

Absorption, Fate, and Excretion. Paclitaxel is administered as a 3-hour infusion of 135-175 mg/m^2 every 3 weeks or as a weekly 1-hour infusion of 80-100 mg/m^2. Prolonged infusions (96 hours) also have been evaluated in different tumor histologies and are active. The drug undergoes extensive metabolism by hepatic CYPs (primarily CYP2C8 with a contribution of CYP3A4); <10% of a dose is excreted in the urine intact. The primary metabolite identified thus far is 6-OH paclitaxel, which is inactive, but multiple additional hydroxylation products are found in plasma (Cresteil et al., 1994).

Paclitaxel clearance is nonlinear and decreases with increasing dose or dose rate. In studies of 96-hour infusions of 140 mg/m^2 (35 mg/m^2/day), the presence of hepatic metastases >2 cm in diameter decreased clearance and led to high drug concentrations in plasma and greater myelosuppression. Paclitaxel disappears from the plasma compartment with a $t_{1/2}$ of 10-14 hours and a clearance of 15-18 L/hr/m^2. The critical plasma concentration for inhibiting bone marrow elements depends on duration of exposure but likely lies at ~50-100 nM (Huizing et al., 1993).

Nab-paclitaxel achieves a higher serum concentration of paclitaxel compared to CREMOPHOR-solubilized paclitaxel, but the increased clearance of nab-paclitaxel results in a similar drug exposure (Gardner et al., 2008). Nab-paclitaxel is most often administered intravenously over 30 minutes at 260 mg/m^2 every 3 weeks; however, alternate dosing regimens are being evaluated. Like the other taxanes, nab-paclitaxel should not be given to patients with an absolute neutrophil count <1500 cells/mm^3. Docetaxel pharmacokinetics are similar to those of paclitaxel, with an elimination $t_{1/2}$ of ~12 hours. Clearance is primarily through CYP3A4- and CYP3A5-mediated hydroxylation, leading to inactive metabolites (Clarke and Rivory, 1999). In contrast to paclitaxel, the pharmacokinetics of docetaxel are linear for doses ≤115 mg/m^2.

Dose reductions in patients with abnormal hepatic function have been suggested, and 50-75% doses of taxanes should be used in the presence of hepatic metastases >2 cm in size or in patients with abnormal serum bilirubin. Drugs that induce CYP2C8 or CYP3A4, such as phenytoin and phenobarbital, or those that inhibit the same cytochromes, such as antifungal imidazoles, significantly alter drug clearance and toxicity.

Paclitaxel clearance is markedly delayed by cyclosporine A and a number of other drugs employed experimentally as inhibitors of the P-glycoprotein. This inhibition may be due to a block of CYP-mediated metabolism or effects on biliary excretion of the parent drug or metabolites.

Therapeutic Uses. The taxanes have become central components of regimens for treating metastatic ovarian, breast, lung, GI, genitourinary, and head and neck cancers. In current regimens, these drugs are administered once weekly or once every 3 weeks. The appropriate use of the steroid-sparing nab-paclitaxel still is being evaluated in clinical trials; in a randomized phase III study comparing 175 mg/m^2 of paclitaxel to 260 mg/m^2 of nab-paclitaxel in women with metastatic breast cancer, the nab-paclitaxel arm had a higher response rate and longer time to progression compared to the paclitaxel arm (Gradishar et al., 2005).

Clinical Toxicities. Paclitaxel exerts its primary toxic effects on the bone marrow. Neutropenia usually occurs 8-11 days after a dose and reverses rapidly by days 15-21. Used with filgrastim [granulocyte-colony stimulating factor (G-CSF)], doses as high as 250 mg/m^2 over 24 hours are well tolerated, and peripheral neuropathy becomes dose limiting. Many patients experience myalgias for several days after receiving paclitaxel. In high-dose schedules, or with prolonged use, a stocking-glove sensory neuropathy can be disabling, particularly in patients with underlying diabetic neuropathy or concurrent cisplatin therapy. Mucositis is prominent in 72- or 96-hour infusions and in the weekly schedule.

Hypersensitivity reactions occurred in patients receiving paclitaxel infusions of short duration (1-6 hours) but have largely been averted by pretreatment with dexamethasone, diphenhydramine, and histamine H_2-receptor antagonists, as noted above. Premedication is not necessary with 96-hour infusions. Many patients experience asymptomatic bradycardia, and occasional episodes of silent ventricular tachycardia also occur and resolve spontaneously during 3- or 24-hour infusions.

Nab-paclitaxel produces increased rates of peripheral neuropathy compared to CREMOPHOR-delivered paclitaxel but rarely causes hypersensitivity reactions.

Docetaxel causes greater degrees of neutropenia than paclitaxel but less peripheral neuropathy and asthenia and less frequent hypersensitivity. Fluid retention is a progressive problem with multiple cycles of docetaxel therapy, leading to peripheral edema, pleural and peritoneal fluid, and pulmonary edema in extreme cases. Oral dexamethasone, 8 mg/day, begun 1 day prior to drug infusion and continuing for 3 days, greatly ameliorates fluid retention. In rare cases, docetaxel may cause a progressive interstitial pneumonitis, with respiratory failure supervening if the drug is not discontinued (Read et al., 2002).

ESTRAMUSTINE

Estramustine (EMCYT) is a combination of estradiol coupled to normustine (nornitrogen mustard) through a carbamate link. Estramustine has weaker estrogenic and antineoplastic activity than estradiol and other alkylating agents. Although the intent of the combination was to enhance the uptake of the alkylating agent into estradiol-sensitive prostate cancer cells, estramustine does not function *in vivo* as an alkylating agent but rather binds to β tubulin and microtubule-associated proteins, causing microtubule disassembly and antimitotic actions.

Estramustine is used solely for the treatment of metastatic or locally advanced hormone refractory prostate cancer (Kitamura, 2001) at an initial dosage of 14 mg/kg/day in three or four divided doses.

Absorption, Fate, and Excretion. Following oral administration, at least 75% of a dose of estramustine is absorbed from the GI tract and rapidly dephosphorylated. Estramustine undergoes extensive first-pass metabolism by CYP1A2 and CYP3A4 to an active oxidized 17-keto derivative, estramustine, and to multiple inactive products; both active forms accumulate in the prostate. Some hydrolysis of the carbamate linkage occurs in the liver, releasing estradiol, estrone, and the normustine group. Estramustine and estromustine have a plasma $t_{1/2}$ of 10 and 14 hours, respectively, and are excreted as inactive metabolites, mainly in the feces (Bergenheim and Henriksson, 1998). Estramustine inhibits the clearance of taxanes.

Clinical Toxicities. In addition to myelosuppression, estramustine also possesses estrogenic side effects (gynecomastia, impotence, elevated risk of thrombosis, and fluid retention), hypercalcemia, acute attacks of porphyria, impaired glucose tolerance, and hypersensitivity reactions, including angioedema.

EPOTHILONES

Microtubule-damaging compounds are limited by difficulties in formulation, drug delivery, and susceptibility to multidrug resistance. A new group of microtubule-targeting drugs, the epothilones, overcomes these problems in experimental systems. Several epothilones currently are in various stages of clinical development. Ixabepilone (IXEMPRA) is approved for breast cancer treatment. Others in the pipeline include the epothilone B analogs patupilone (EPO906) and 21-aminoepothilone B (BMS-310705), the epothilone D analog KOS-1584 (R1645), and the synthetic sagopilone.

Chemistry. The epothilones are 16-membered polyketides discovered as cytotoxic metabolites from a strain of *Sorangium cellulosum,* a myxobacterium originally isolated from soil on the bank of the Zambezi River in southern Africa (Gerth et al., 1996).

Six natural epothilones (A-F), and synthetic and semisynthetic analogs are in various stages of development (Lee and Swain, 2008). Most trials of epothilones to date have evaluated compounds of the subtypes A, B, and D, which differ in their functional groups at carbon 12.

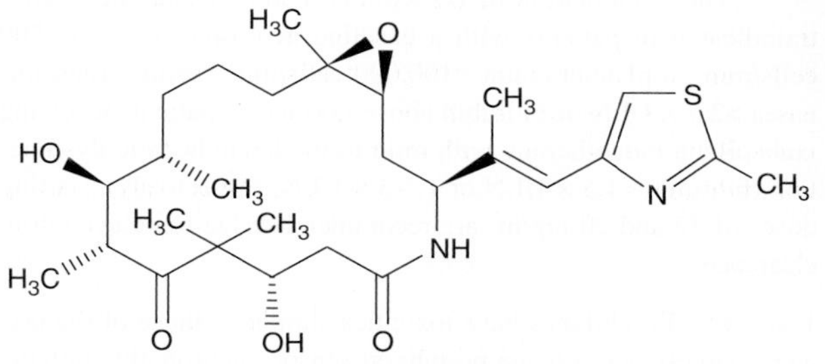

H_3C O CH_3 S HO CH_3 N CH_3 H_3C CH_3 NH H_3C O OH O

IXABEPILONE

Initial studies of the natural epothilone compounds A, B, and D showed good *in vitro* cytotoxic activity at nanomolar concentrations, epothilone B having roughly twice the potency as epothilones A and D (Lee and Swain, 2008). The early *in vivo* activity in animals, however, was disappointing due to instability of their lactone ring. Modification of epothilone B by substituting a nitrogen for the lactone oxygen yielded ixabepilone, which is not susceptible to esterases.

Mechanism of Action. The epothilones resemble taxanes in that they bind to β tubulin and trigger microtubule nucleation at multiple sites away from the centriole. This chaotic microtubule stabilization triggers cell-cycle arrest at the G2-M interface and apoptosis. Epothilones bind to a site distinct from that of taxanes. In colon cancer cell lines, p53 and Bax trigger apoptosis in ixabepilone-treated cells.

In vitro studies suggest that ixabepilone is less susceptible to P-glycoprotein-mediated multidrug resistance when compared to taxanes. Other mechanisms implicated in epothilone resistance include mutation of the β-tubulin binding site and upregulation of isoforms of β tubulin.

Absorption, Distribution, and Excretion. Ixabepilone is administered intravenously. Because of its minimal aqueous solubility, it is delivered in the solubilizing agent, polyoxyethylated castor oil/ethanol (CREMOPHOR EL). CREMOPHOR has been implicated as the cause of infusion reactions associated with paclitaxel and with other drug formulations, but such reactions are infrequent when administration is preceded by premedication with H_1 and H_2 antagonists. The drug is cleared by hepatic CYPs and has a plasma $t_{1/2}$ of 52 hours.

Therapeutic Uses. In a phase III study for registration, patients with metastatic breast cancer resistant to or pretreated with anthracyclines and resistant to taxanes had an improved progression-free survival of

1.6 months with ixabepilone plus capecitabine compared to capecitabine alone ($p = .0003$) (Thomas et al., 2007).

Ixabepilone also is indicated as monotherapy for metastatic breast cancer in patients who have previously progressed through treatment with anthracyclines, taxanes, and capecitabine.

The recommended dose of ixabepilone as monotherapy or in combination with capecitabine is 40 mg/m^2 administered over 3 hours every 3 weeks. Note that because of additive myelosuppression, the phase III trial used an attenuated dose of capecitabine (2000 mg/m^2) administered with ixabepilone compared to 2500 mg/m^2 when capecitabine was administered alone. Patients should be premedicated with both an H_1 and H_2 antagonist before receiving ixabepilone to minimize hypersensitivity reactions.

The combination of ixabepilone and capecitabine is contraindicated in patients with a baseline neutrophil count <1500 cells/mm^3, a platelet count <100,000 cells/mm^3, serum transaminases >2.5 × ULN or bilirubin above normal. In patients receiving ixabepilone monotherapy with mild to moderate hepatic dysfunction (bilirubin <1.5 × ULN or 1.5-3 × ULN, respectively), starting doses of 32 and 20 mg/m^2 are recommended due to delayed drug clearance.

Toxicities. Epothilones have toxicities similar to those of the taxanes, namely neutropenia peripheral sensory neuropathy, fatigue, diarrhea, and asthenia. Grade 3/4 peripheral sensory neuropathy was seen in 21% of patients receiving combined therapy with ixabepilone and capecitabine and in 14% of patients receiving monotherapy. Ixabepilone in combination with capecitabine causes a 68% rate of grade 3/4 neutropenia; it causes a 54% rate of grade 3/4 neutropenia when given as monotherapy.

CAMPTOTHECIN ANALOGS

The camptothecins are potent, cytotoxic antineoplastic agents that target the nuclear enzyme topoisomerase I. The lead compound in this class, camptothecin, was isolated from the Chinese tree *Camptotheca acuminata* in 1966. Initial efforts to develop the compound as a sodium salt were compromised by severe and unpredictable toxicity, principally myelosuppression and hemorrhagic cystitis. Elucidation of the mechanism of action and a better understanding of its physicochemical properties during the 1980s led to the development of more soluble and less toxic analogs. Irinotecan and topotecan, currently the only camptothecin analogs approved for clinical use, have activity in colorectal, ovarian, and small cell lung cancer.

Chemistry. All camptothecins have a fused five-ring backbone that includes a labile lactone ring (Figure 61–13). The hydroxyl group and S-conformation of the chiral center at C20 in the lactone ring are required for biological activity. Appropriate substitutions on the A and B rings of the quinoline subunit enhance water solubility and increase potency for inhibiting topoisomerase I. Topotecan [(*S*)-9-dimethylaminoethyl-10-hydroxycamptothecin hydrochloride] is a semisynthetic molecule with a basic dimethylamino group that increases its water solubility. Irinotecan (7-ethyl-10-[4-(1-piperidino)-1-piperidino] carbonyloxycamptothecin, or CPT-11) differs from topotecan in that it

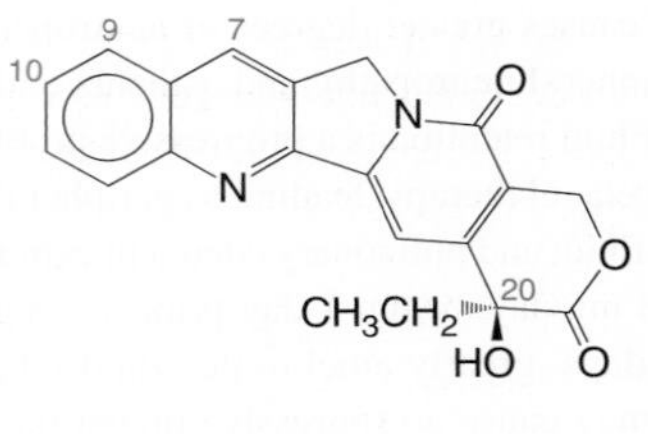

	C-10	C-9	C-7
Camptothecin	H	H	H
Topotecan	OH	$(CH_3)_2NHCH_2$	H
Irinotecan	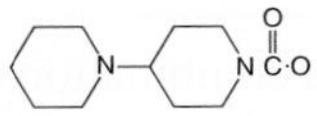	H	CH_2CH_3
SN-38	OH	H	CH_2CH_3

Figure 61–13. *Chemical structures of camptothecin and its analogs.*

is a prodrug. The carbamate bond between the camptothecin moiety and the dibasic bispiperidine side chain at position C10 (which makes the molecule water soluble) is cleaved by a carboxylesterase to form the active metabolite, SN-38 (see Chapter 6).

Mechanism of Action. The DNA topoisomerases are nuclear enzymes that reduce torsional stress in supercoiled DNA, allowing selected regions of DNA to become sufficiently untangled and relaxed to permit replication, repair, and transcription. Two classes of topoisomerase (I and II) mediate DNA strand breakage and resealing, and both have become the target of cancer chemotherapies. Camptothecin analogs inhibit the function of topoisomerase I, while a number of different chemical entities (e.g., anthracyclines, epipodophyllotoxins, acridines) inhibit topoisomerase II. Topoisomerase I binds covalently to double-stranded DNA through a reversible transesterification reaction. This reaction yields an intermediate complex in which the tyrosine of the enzyme is bound to the 3′-phosphate end of the DNA strand, creating a single-strand DNA break. This "cleavable complex" allows for relaxation of the DNA torsional strain, either by passage of the intact single-strand through the nick or by free rotation of the DNA about the noncleaved strand. Once the DNA torsional strain has been relieved, the topoisomerase I reseals the cleavage and dissociates from the newly relaxed double helix.

The camptothecins bind to and stabilize the normally transient DNA-topoisomerase I cleavable complex. Although the initial cleavage action of topoisomerase I is not affected, the re-ligation step is inhibited, leading to the accumulation of single-stranded breaks in DNA. These lesions are reversible and not by themselves toxic to the cell. However, the collision of a DNA replication fork with this cleaved strand of DNA causes an irreversible double-strand DNA break, ultimately leading to cell death (Tsao et al., 1993). Camptothecins are therefore S phase–specific drugs, because ongoing DNA synthesis is necessary for cytotoxicity. This has important clinical implications. S phase–specific cytotoxic agents generally require prolonged exposures of tumor cells to drug concentrations above a minimum threshold to optimize therapeutic efficacy. In fact, preclinical studies of low-dose, protracted administration of camptothecin analogs have less toxicity, and equal or greater antitumor activity, than shorter, more intense courses.

The precise sequence of events that leads from drug-induced DNA damage to cell death has not been fully elucidated. *In vitro*, camptothecin-induced DNA damage abolishes the activation of the $p34^{cdc2}$/cyclin B complex, leading to cell-cycle arrest at the G2 phase (Tsao et al., 1993). Treatment with camptothecins can induce the transcription of *c-fos* and *c-jun* early-response genes, and this occurs in association with internucleosomal DNA fragmentation, a characteristic of programmed cell death.

Mechanisms of Resistance. A variety of mechanisms of resistance to topoisomerase I–targeted agents have been characterized *in vitro,* although little is known about their significance in the clinical setting. Decreased intracellular drug accumulation may underlie resistance in cell lines. Topotecan, but not SN-38 or irinotecan, is a substrate for P-glycoprotein. However, the clinical relevance of P-glycoprotein-mediated efflux as a mechanism of resistance against topotecan remains unclear, as the magnitude of the effect in preclinical studies was found to be substantially lower than that observed with other MDR substrates, such as etoposide or doxorubicin. Other reports have associated topotecan and irinotecan resistance with the MRP class of transporters (Miyake et al., 1999). Cell lines that lack carboxylesterase activity demonstrate resistance to irinotecan (Van Ark-Otte et al., 1998), but in patients, the liver and red blood cells may have sufficient carboxylesterase activity to convert irinotecan to SN-38. Camptothecin resistance also may result from decreased expression or mutation of topoisomerase I. Although a good correlation has been found in certain tumor cell lines between sensitivity to camptothecin analogs and topoisomerase I levels (Sugimoto et al., 1990), clinical studies have not confirmed this association. Chromosomal deletions or hypermethylation of the topoisomerase I gene are possible mechanisms of decreased topoisomerase I expression in resistant cells. A transient downregulation of topoisomerase I has been demonstrated following prolonged exposure to camptothecins *in vitro* and *in vivo.* Mutations leading to reduced topoisomerase I enzyme catalytic activity or DNA-binding affinity have been associated with experimental camptothecin resistance (Tamura et al., 1991). In addition, enzyme phosphorylation or polyADP ribosylation may reduce the activity of topoisomerase I and its susceptibility to inhibition. Finally, exposure of cells to topoisomerase I–targeted agents upregulates topoisomerase II, an alternative enzyme for DNA strand passage.

Very little is known about how the cell deals with the stabilized DNA-topoisomerase complexes. Cellular repair processes may not readily recognize the drug-enzyme-DNA complex. However, an enzyme with specific tyrosyl-DNA phosphodiesterase activity may be involved in the disassembly of topoisomerase I–DNA complexes (Yang et al., 1996).

Absorption, Fate, and Excretion

Topotecan. Topotecan is approved for intravenous administration. However, there has been interest in developing an oral dosage form for the drug, which has a bioavailability of 30-40% in cancer patients. Topotecan exhibits linear pharmacokinetics, and it is rapidly eliminated from systemic circulation. The biological $t_{1/2}$ of total topotecan, which ranges from 3.5-4.1 hours, is relatively short compared to that of other camptothecins. Only 20-35% of the total drug in plasma is found to be in the active lactone form. Within 24 hours, 30-40% of the administered dose appears in the urine. Doses should be reduced in proportion to reductions in CrCl. Although several oxidative metabolites have been identified, hepatic metabolism appears to be a relatively minor route of drug elimination. Unlike most other camptothecins considered for clinical development, plasma protein binding of topotecan is low, at only 7-35%, which may explain its relatively greater CNS penetration.

Irinotecan. The conversion of irinotecan to SN-38 is mediated predominantly by carboxylesterases in the liver. Although SN-38 can be measured in plasma shortly after beginning an intravenous infusion of irinotecan, the AUC of SN-38 is only ~4% of the AUC of irinotecan, suggesting that only a relatively small fraction of the dose is ultimately converted to the active form of the drug. Irinotecan exhibits linear pharmacokinetics at doses evaluated in cancer patients. In comparison to topotecan, a relatively large fraction of both irinotecan and SN-38 are present in plasma as the biologically active intact lactone form. Another potential advantage of this analog is that the $t_{1/2}$ of SN-38 is 11.5 hours, which is much longer than the $t_{1/2}$ of topotecan. CSF penetration of SN-38 in humans has not been characterized yet, although in rhesus monkeys, it is only 14%, significantly lower than that observed for topotecan.

In contrast to topotecan, hepatic metabolism represents an important route of elimination for both irinotecan and SN-38. Oxidative metabolites have been identified in plasma, all of which result from CYP3A-mediated reactions directed at the bispiperidine side chain. These metabolites are not significantly converted to SN-38. The total body clearance of irinotecan was found to be two times greater in brain cancer patients taking antiseizure drugs that induce hepatic CYPs, further attesting to the importance of oxidative hepatic metabolism as a route of elimination for this drug (Gilbert et al., 2003).

Glucuronidation of the hydroxyl group at position C10 (resulting from cleavage of the bispiperidine promoiety) produces the only known metabolite of SN-38. Biliary excretion appears to be the primary elimination route of irinotecan, SN-38, and their metabolites, although urinary excretion also contributes significantly (14-37%). Uridine diphosphate-glucuronosyltransferase 1A1 (UGT1A1), converts SN-38 to its inactive derivative (Iyer et al., 1998). The extent of SN-38 glucuronidation inversely correlates with the risk of severe diarrhea after irinotecan therapy. UGT1A1 also glucuronidates bilirubin. Polymorphisms of this enzyme are associated with familial hyperbilirubinemia syndromes such as Crigler-Najjar syndrome and Gilbert syndrome. Crigler-Najjar syndrome is rare (one in a million births), but Gilbert syndrome occurs in up to 15% of the general population and results in a mild hyperbilirubinemia that may be clinically silent. The presence of UGT enzyme polymorphisms may have a major impact on the clinical use of irinotecan. A positive correlation has been found between baseline serum unconjugated bilirubin concentration and both severity of neutropenia and the AUC of irinotecan and SN-38 in patients treated with irinotecan. Moreover, severe irinotecan toxicity has been observed in cancer patients with Gilbert syndrome, presumably due to decreased glucuronidation of SN-38. The presence of bacterial glucuronidase in the intestinal lumen potentially can contribute to irinotecan's GI toxicity by releasing unconjugated SN-38 from the inactive glucuronide metabolite excreted in the bile.

Therapeutic Uses

Topotecan. Topotecan (HYCAMTIN) is indicated for previously treated patients with ovarian and small cell lung cancer. Its significant hematological toxicity has limited its use in combination with other active agents in these diseases (e.g., cisplatin).

The recommended dosing regimen of topotecan for ovarian cancer and small cell lung cancer is a 30-minute infusion of 1.5 mg/m^2/day for 5 consecutive days every 3 weeks. For cervical cancer in conjunction with cisplatin, the dose of topotecan is 0.75 mg/m^2 on days 1, 2, and 3, repeated every 21 days. Because a significant fraction of the topotecan administered is excreted in the urine, patients with decreased CrCl may experience increased toxicity (O'Reilly et al., 1996). Therefore, the dose of topotecan should be reduced to 0.75 mg/m^2/day in patients with moderate renal dysfunction (CrCl of 20-40 mL/min), and topotecan should not be administered to patients with severe renal impairment (CrCl <20 mL/min). Hepatic dysfunction does not alter topotecan clearance and toxicity. A baseline neutrophil count >1500 cells/mm3 and a platelet count >100,000 is necessary prior to topotecan administration. For small cell lung cancer, oral therapy can be used at a dosage of 2.3 mg/m2/day for 5 consecutive days repeated every 21 days. The oral dose is reduced to 1.8 mg/m2 for patients with a CrCl of 30-49 mL/min.

Irinotecan. Approved single-agent dosage schedules of irinotecan (CAMPTOSAR, others) in the U.S. include 125 mg/m^2 as a 90-minute infusion administered weekly (on days 1, 8, 15, and 22) for 4 out of 6 weeks, and 350 mg/m^2 given every 3 weeks. In patients with advanced colorectal cancer, irinotecan is used as first-line therapy in combination with fluoropyrimidines or as a single agent or in combination with cetuximab following failure of a 5-FU/oxaliplatin regimen.

Clinical Toxicities

Topotecan. The dose-limiting toxicity with all dosing schedules is neutropenia, with or without thrombocytopenia. The incidence of severe neutropenia at the recommended phase II dose of 1.5 mg/m^2 daily for 5 days every 3 weeks may be as high as 81%, with a 26% incidence of febrile neutropenia. In patients with hematological malignancies, GI side effects such as mucositis and diarrhea become dose limiting. Other less common and generally mild topotecan-related toxicities include nausea and vomiting, elevated liver transaminases, fever, fatigue, and rash.

Irinotecan. The dose-limiting toxicity with all dosing schedules is delayed diarrhea, with or without neutropenia. In the initial studies, up to 35% of patients experienced severe diarrhea. Adoption of an intensive regimen of loperamide (4 mg of loperamide starting at the onset of any loose stool beginning more than a few hours after receiving therapy, followed by 2 mg every 2 hours) (see Chapter 47) has effectively reduced this incidence by more than half. However, once severe diarrhea occurs, standard doses of antidiarrheal agents tend to be ineffective. Diarrhea generally resolves within a week and, unless associated with fever and neutropenia, rarely is fatal.

The second most common irinotecan-associated toxicity is myelosuppression. Severe neutropenia occurs in 14-47% of the patients treated with the every-3-weeks schedule and is less frequently encountered among patients treated with the weekly schedule. Febrile neutropenia is observed in 3% of patients and may be fatal, particularly when associated with concomitant diarrhea. A cholinergic syndrome resulting from the inhibition of acetylcholinesterase activity by irinotecan may occur within the first 24 hours after irinotecan administration. Symptoms include acute diarrhea, diaphoresis, hypersalivation, abdominal cramps, visual accommodation disturbances, lacrimation, rhinorrhea, and less often, asymptomatic bradycardia. These effects are short lasting and respond within minutes to atropine. Atropine may be prophylactically administered to patients who have previously experienced a cholinergic reaction. Other common and generally manageable toxicities include nausea and vomiting, fatigue, vasodilation or skin flushing, mucositis, elevation in liver transaminases, and alopecia. Finally, there have been case reports of dyspnea and interstitial pneumonitis associated with irinotecan therapy in Japanese patients with lung cancer (Fukuoka et al., 1992).

ANTIBIOTICS

Dactinomycin (Actinomycin D)

The first anticancer antibiotics were the series of actinomycins discovered by Waksman and colleagues in 1940. The most important of these, actinomycin D, has beneficial effects in the treatment of solid tumors in children and choriocarcinoma in adult women.

Chemistry and Structure-Activity Relationships. The actinomycins are chromopeptides. Most contain the same chromophore, the planar phenoxazone actinosin, which is responsible for their yellow-red color. The differences among naturally occurring actinomycins are confined to variations in the structure of the amino acids of the peptide side chains.

DACTINOMYCIN
(Sar = sarcosine
Meval = *N*-methylvaline)

Mechanism of Action. The capacity of actinomycins to bind with double-helical DNA is responsible for their biological activity and cytotoxicity. X-ray studies of a crystalline complex between dactinomycin and deoxyguanosine permitted formulation of a model that explains the binding of the drug to DNA (Sobell, 1973). The planar phenoxazone ring intercalates between adjacent guanine–cytosine base pairs of DNA, while the polypeptide chains extend along the minor groove of the helix. The summation of these interactions provides great stability to the dactinomycin-DNA complex, and as a result of the binding of dactinomycin, the transcription of DNA by RNA polymerase is blocked. The DNA-dependent RNA polymerases are much more sensitive to the effects of dactinomycin than are the DNA polymerases. In addition, dactinomycin causes single-strand breaks in DNA, possibly through a free-radical intermediate or as a result of the action of topoisomerase II.

Cytotoxic Action. Dactinomycin inhibits rapidly proliferating cells of normal and neoplastic origin and, on a molar basis, is among the most potent antitumor agents known. The drug may produce alopecia and, when extravasated subcutaneously, causes marked local inflammation. Erythema, sometimes progressing to necrosis, has been noted in areas of the skin exposed to X-ray radiation before, during, or after administration of dactinomycin.

Absorption, Fate, and Excretion. Dactinomycin is administered by intravenous injection. Metabolism of the drug is minimal. The drug is excreted in both bile and urine and disappears from plasma with a terminal $t_{1/2}$ of 36 hours. Dactinomycin does not cross the blood-brain barrier.

Therapeutic Uses. A wide variety of single-agent and combination chemotherapy regimens with dactinomycin (actinomycin D; COSMEGEN) are employed. The usual daily dose of dactinomycin is 10-15 μg/kg; this is given intravenously for 5 days; if no manifestations of toxicity are encountered, additional courses may be given at intervals of 2-4 weeks. In other regimens, 3-6 μg/kg/day, for a total of 125 μg/kg, and weekly maintenance doses of 7.5 μg/kg have been used. If infiltrated during administration, the drug is extremely corrosive to soft tissues.

The most important clinical use of dactinomycin is in the treatment of rhabdomyosarcoma and Wilms tumor in children, where it is curative in combination with primary surgery, radiotherapy, and other drugs, particularly vincristine and cyclophosphamide. Ewing, Kaposi, and soft-tissue sarcomas also respond. Dactinomycin and methotrexate form a curative therapy for choriocarcinoma.

Clinical Toxicities. Toxic manifestations include anorexia, nausea, and vomiting, usually beginning a few hours after administration. Hematopoietic suppression with pancytopenia may occur in the first week after completion of therapy. Proctitis, diarrhea, glossitis, cheilitis, and ulcerations of the oral mucosa are common; dermatological manifestations include alopecia, as well as erythema, desquamation, and increased inflammation and pigmentation in areas previously or concomitantly subjected to X-ray radiation. Severe injury may occur as a result of local drug extravasation.

Anthracyclines and Anthracenediones

Anthracyclines are derived from the fungus *Streptomyces peucetius* var. *caesius*. Idarubicin and epirubicin are analogs of the naturally produced anthracyclines doxorubicin and daunorubicin, differing only slightly in chemical structure, but having somewhat distinct patterns of clinical activity. Daunorubicin and idarubicin primarily have been used in the acute leukemias, whereas doxorubicin and epirubicin display broader activity against human solid tumors. These agents, which all possess potential for generating free radicals, cause an unusual and often irreversible cardiomyopathy, the occurrence of which is related to the total dose of the drug. The structurally similar agent mitoxantrone has useful activity against prostate cancer and AML, and is used in high-dose chemotherapy, but has less cardiotoxicity.

Chemistry. The anthracycline antibiotics have a tetracyclic ring structure attached to an unusual sugar, daunosamine. Cytotoxic agents of this class all have quinone and hydroquinone moieties on adjacent rings that permit the gain and loss of electrons. Although there are marked differences in the clinical uses of daunorubicin and doxorubicin, their chemical structures differ only by a single hydroxyl group on C-14 (substituent R_4 on the diagram below). Idarubicin is 4-demethoxydaunorubicin (alteration in substituent R_1), a synthetic derivative of daunorubicin; epirubicin is an epimer at the 4′ position of the sugar. Mitoxantrone, an anthracenedione, lacks a glycosidic side group.

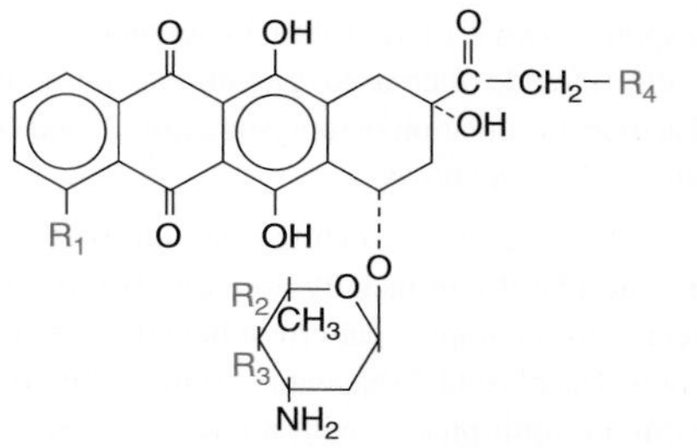

	DOXORUBICIN	DAUNORUBICIN	EPIRUBICIN	IDARUBICIN
R_1 =	OCH_3	OCH_3	OCH_3	H
R_2 =	H	H	OH	H
R_3 =	OH	OH	H	OH
R_4 =	OH	H	OH	H

Mechanism of Action. A number of important biochemical effects have been described for the anthracyclines and anthracenediones, all of which could contribute to their therapeutic and toxic effects. These compounds can intercalate with DNA, directly affecting transcription and replication. A more important action is the ability to form a tripartite complex with topoisomerase II and DNA. Topoisomerase II is an ATP-dependent enzyme that binds to DNA and produces double-strand breaks at the 3′-phosphate backbone, allowing strand passage and uncoiling of super-coiled DNA. Following strand passage, topoisomerase II re-ligates the DNA strands. This enzymatic function is essential for DNA replication and repair. Formation of the tripartite complex with anthracyclines or with etoposide inhibits the re-ligation of the broken DNA strands, leading to apoptosis. Defects in DNA double-strand break repair sensitize cells to damage by these drugs, while overexpression of transcription-linked DNA repair may contribute to resistance.

Anthracyclines, by virtue of their quinone groups, also generate free radicals in solution and in both normal and malignant tissues (Myers, 1988). Anthracyclines can form semiquinone radical intermediates that can react with O_2 to produce superoxide anion radicals. These can generate both hydrogen peroxide and hydroxyl radicals, which attack DNA (Serrano et al., 1999) and oxidize DNA bases. The production of free radicals is significantly stimulated by the interaction of doxorubicin with iron (Myers, 1988). Enzymatic defenses such as superoxide dismutase and catalase protect cells against the toxicity of the anthracyclines, and these defenses can be augmented by exogenous antioxidants such as alpha tocopherol or by an iron chelator, dexrazoxane (ZINECARD, others), which protects against cardiac toxicity (Swain et al., 1997).

Exposure of cells to anthracyclines leads to apoptosis; mediators of this process include the p53 DNA-damage sensor and activated caspases (proteases), although ceramide, a lipid breakdown product, and the Fas receptor-ligand system also have been implicated (Friesen et al., 1996).

As discussed in "Drug Resistance" under "Vinca Alkaloids," multidrug resistance is observed in tumor cell populations exposed to anthracyclines. Attempts to reverse or prevent the emergence of resistance through the simultaneous use of inhibitors of the P-glycoprotein (Ca^{++} channel blockers, steroidal compounds, and others) have yielded inconclusive results, primarily due to confounding effects of these inhibitors on anthracycline pharmacokinetics and metabolism. Anthracyclines also are exported from tumor cells by members of the MRP transporter family and by the breast cancer resistance protein, a "half" transporter (Doyle et al., 1998). Other biochemical changes in resistant cells include increased glutathione peroxidase activity, decreased activity or mutation of topoisomerase II, and enhanced ability to repair DNA strand breaks.

Absorption, Fate, and Excretion. Daunorubicin, doxorubicin, epirubicin, and idarubicin usually are administered intravenously and are cleared by a complex pattern of hepatic metabolism and biliary excretion. The plasma disappearance curves for doxorubicin and daunorubicin are multiphasic, with a terminal $t_{1/2}$ of 30 hours. All anthracyclines are converted to an active alcohol intermediate that plays a variable role in their therapeutic activity. Idarubicin has a $t_{1/2}$ of 15 hours, and its active metabolite, idarubicinol, has a $t_{1/2}$ of 40 hours. The drugs rapidly enter the heart, kidneys, lungs, liver, and spleen. They do not cross the blood-brain barrier.

Daunorubicin and doxorubicin are eliminated by metabolic conversion to a variety of aglycones and other inactive products. Idarubicin is primarily metabolized to idarubicinol, which accumulates in plasma and likely contributes significantly to its activity. Clearance of anthracyclines and their active alcohol metabolites is delayed in the presence of hepatic dysfunction, and at least a 50% initial reduction in dose should be considered in patients with abnormal serum bilirubin levels (Twelves et al., 1998).

Therapeutic Use

Idarubicin. The recommended dosage for idarubicin (IDAMYCIN PFS) is 12 mg/m²/day for 3 days by intravenous injection in combination with cytarabine. Slow injection over 10-15 minutes is recommended to avoid extravasation, as with other anthracyclines. It has less cardiotoxicity than the other anthracyclines.

Daunorubicin. Daunorubicin (daunomycin, rubidomycin; CERUBIDINE, others) is available for intravenous use. The recommended dosage is 25-45 mg/m²/day for 3 days. The agent is administered with appropriate care to prevent extravasation, because severe local vesicant action may result. Total doses of >1000 mg/m² are associated with a high risk of cardiotoxicity. Patients should be advised that daunorubicin may impart a red color to the urine.

Daunorubicin and idarubicin also are used in the treatment of AML in combination with Ara-C.

Clinical Toxicities. The toxic manifestations of daunorubicin as well as idarubicin include bone marrow depression, stomatitis, alopecia, GI disturbances, and rash. Cardiac toxicity is a peculiar adverse effect observed with these agents. It is characterized by tachycardia, arrhythmias, dyspnea, hypotension, pericardial effusion, and congestive heart failure poorly responsive to digitalis (see "Clinical Toxicities" under "Doxorubicin").

Doxorubicin

Therapeutic Uses. Doxorubicin is available for intravenous use. The recommended dose is 60-75 mg/m², administered as a single rapid intravenous infusion that is repeated after 21 days. Care should be taken to avoid extravasation, because severe local vesicant action and tissue necrosis may result. A doxorubicin liposomal product (DOXIL) is available for treatment of AIDS-related Kaposi sarcoma and is given intravenously in a dose of 20 mg/m² over 60 minutes and repeated every 3 weeks. The liposomal formulation also is approved for ovarian cancer at a dose of 50 mg/m² every 4 weeks and as a treatment for multiple myeloma (in conjunction with bortezomib), where it is given as a 30-mg/m² dose on day 4 of each 21-day cycle. Patients should be advised that the drug may impart a red color to the urine.

Doxorubicin is effective in malignant lymphomas. In combination with cyclophosphamide, vinca alkaloids, and other agents, it is an important ingredient for the successful treatment of lymphomas. It is a valuable component of various regimens of chemotherapy for adjuvant and metastatic carcinoma of the breast. The drug also is particularly beneficial in pediatric and adult sarcomas, including osteogenic, Ewing, and soft-tissue sarcomas.

Clinical Toxicities. The toxic manifestations of doxorubicin are similar to those of daunorubicin. Myelosuppression is a major dose-limiting complication, with leukopenia usually reaching a nadir during the second week of therapy and recovering by the fourth week; thrombocytopenia and anemia follow a similar pattern but usually are less pronounced. Stomatitis, mucositis, diarrhea, and alopecia are common but reversible. Erythematous streaking near the site of infusion ("ADRIAMYCIN flare") is a benign local allergic reaction and should not be confused with extravasation. Facial flushing, conjunctivitis, and lacrimation may occur rarely. The drug may produce severe local toxicity in irradiated tissues (e.g., the skin, heart, lung, esophagus, and GI mucosa) even when the two therapies are not administered concomitantly.

Cardiomyopathy is the most important long-term toxicity. Two types of cardiomyopathies may occur:

- An acute form is characterized by abnormal electrocardiographic changes, including ST- and T-wave alterations and arrhythmias. This is brief and rarely a serious problem. An acute reversible reduction in ejection fraction is observed in some patients in the 24 hours after a single dose, and plasma troponin T, a cardiac enzyme released with myocardial damage, may increase in a minority of patients in the first few days following drug administration (Lipshultz et al., 2004). Acute myocardial damage, the "pericarditis–myocarditis syndrome," may begin in the days following drug infusion and is characterized by severe disturbances in impulse conduction and frank congestive heart failure, often associated with pericardial effusion.
- Chronic, cumulative dose-related toxicity (usually total doses of ≥550 mg/m²) progress to congestive heart failure. The mortality rate in patients with congestive failure approaches 50%. Total doses of doxorubicin as low as 250 mg/m² can cause pathological changes in the myocardium, as demonstrated by subendocardial biopsies. Nonspecific alterations, including a decrease in the number of myocardial fibrils, mitochondrial changes, and cellular degeneration, are visible by electron microscopy. The most promising noninvasive techniques used to detect the early development of drug-induced congestive heart failure are radionuclide cineangiography, which assesses ejection fraction, and

echocardiography, which reveals abnormalities in contractility and ventricular dimensions. Sequential echocardiograms have detected structural abnormalities in 25% of children who received up to 300 mg/m^2 of doxorubicin, although <10% have clinical manifestations of cardiac disease in long-term follow-up. Although no completely practical and reliable predictive tests are available, the frequency of clinically apparent cardiomyopathy is 1-10% at total doses <450 mg/m^2. The risk increases markedly, with estimates as high as 20% at total doses of 550 mg/m^2. This total dosage should be exceeded only under exceptional circumstances or with the concomitant use of dexrazoxane, a cardioprotective iron-chelating agent that appears not to compromise the anticancer activity of the drug (Swain et al., 1997). Cardiac irradiation, administration of high doses of cyclophosphamide or another anthracycline, or concomitant trastuzumab (Slamon et al., 2001) increases the risk of cardiotoxicity. Late-onset cardiac toxicity, with congestive heart failure years after treatment, may occur in both pediatric and adult populations. In children treated with anthracyclines, there is a 3- to 10-fold elevated risk of arrhythmias, congestive heart failure, and sudden death in adult life. A total dose limit of 300 mg/m^2 is advised for pediatric cases. Concomitant administration of dexrazoxane may reduce troponin T elevations and avert later cardiotoxicity (Lipshultz et al., 2004).

Epirubicin (ELLENCE, others)

This anthracycline is indicated as a component of adjunctive therapy for treatment of breast cancer. It is administered in doses of 100-120 mg/m^2 intravenously every 3-4 weeks. Total doses >900 mg/m^2 sharply increase the risk of cardiotoxicity. Its toxicity profile is the same as that of doxorubicin.

Valrubicin (VALSTAR)

Valrubicin is a semi-synthetic analog of doxirubicin, used exclusively for intravesicular treatment of bladder cancer. Eight hundred mg are instilled into the bladder once a week for 6 weeks. Less than 10% of instilled drug is absorbed systemically. Side effects relate to bladder irritation (Kuznetsov et al., 2001).

Mitoxantrone

Mitoxantrone has been approved for use in AML, prostate cancer, and late-stage, secondary progressive multiple sclerosis. Mitoxantrone has limited ability to produce quinone-type free radicals and causes less cardiac toxicity than does doxorubicin. It produces acute myelosuppression, cardiac toxicity, and mucositis as its major toxicities; the drug causes less nausea, vomiting, and alopecia than does doxorubicin.

Mitoxantrone (NOVANTRONE, others) is administered by intravenous infusion. To induce remission in acute nonlymphocytic leukemia in adults, the drug is given in a daily dose of 12 mg/m^2 for 3 days with cytarabine. It also is used in advanced hormone-resistant prostate cancer in a dose of 12-14 mg/m^2 every 21 days.

EPIPODOPHYLLOTOXINS

Podophyllotoxin, extracted from the mandrake plant (mayapple; *Podophyllum peltatum*), was used as a folk remedy by the American Indians and early colonists for its emetic, cathartic, and anthelmintic effects. Two synthetic derivatives have significant therapeutic activity in pediatric leukemia, small cell carcinomas of the lung, testicular tumors, Hodgkin's disease, and large cell lymphomas.

These derivatives, shown below, are etoposide (VP-16-213) and teniposide (VM-26). Although podophyllotoxin binds to tubulin, etoposide and teniposide have no effect on microtubular structure or function at usual concentrations.

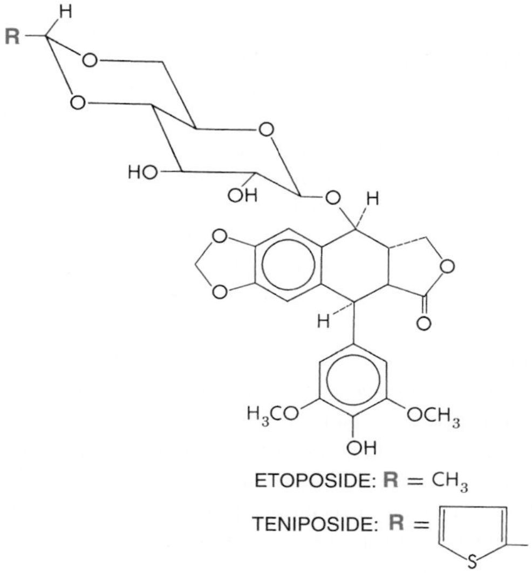

ETOPOSIDE: R = CH_3

TENIPOSIDE: R = [thienyl]

Mechanism of Action. Etoposide and teniposide are similar in their actions and in the spectrum of human tumors affected. Like the anthracyclines, they form a ternary complex with topoisomerase II and DNA and prevent resealing of the break that normally follows topoisomerase binding to DNA. The enzyme remains bound to the free end of the broken DNA strand, leading to an accumulation of DNA breaks and cell death. Cells in the S and G_2 phases of the cell cycle are most sensitive to etoposide and teniposide. Resistant cells demonstrate 1) amplification of the *mdr*-1 gene that encodes the P-glycoprotein drug efflux transporter, 2) mutation or decreased expression of topoisomerase II, or 3) mutations of the p53 tumor suppressor gene, a required component of the apoptotic pathway (Lowe et al., 1993).

Etoposide

Absorption, Fate, and Excretion. Oral administration of etoposide results in variable absorption that averages ~50%. After intravenous injection, peak plasma concentrations of 30 μg/mL are achieved; there is a biphasic pattern of clearance with a terminal $t_{1/2}$ of ~6-8 hours in patients with normal renal function. Approximately 40% of an administered dose is excreted intact in the urine. In patients with compromised renal function, dosage should be reduced in proportion to the reduction in CrCl (Arbuck et al., 1986). In patients with advanced liver disease, increased toxicity may result from a low serum albumin (decreased drug binding) and elevated bilirubin (which displaces etoposide from albumin). However, guidelines for dose reduction in this circumstance have not been defined. Drug concentrations in the CSF average 1-10% of those in plasma.

Therapeutic Uses. The intravenous dose of etoposide (VEPESID, others) for testicular cancer in combination therapy is 50-100 mg/m^2 for 5 days, or 100 mg/m^2 on alternate days for three doses. For small cell carcinoma of the lung, the dosage in combination therapy is 35 mg/m^2/day intravenously for 4 days or 50 mg/m^2/day intravenously for 5 days. The oral dose for small cell lung cancer is twice the IV dose. Cycles of therapy usually are repeated every 3-4 weeks. When given intravenously, the drug should be administered slowly over a 30- to 60-minute period to avoid hypotension and bronchospasm, which likely result from the additives used to dissolve etoposide, a relatively insoluble compound.

A disturbing complication of etoposide therapy has emerged in long-term follow-up of patients with childhood acute lymphoblastic leukemia, who develop an unusual form of acute nonlymphocytic leukemia with a translocation in chromosome 11q23. At this locus is a gene (the MLL gene) that regulates the proliferation of pluripotent stem cells. The leukemic cells have the cytological appearance of acute monocytic or monomyelocytic leukemia but may express lymphoid surface markers. Another distinguishing feature of etoposide-related leukemia is the short time interval between the end of treatment and the onset of leukemia (1-3 years), compared to the 4- to 5-year interval for secondary leukemias related to alkylating agents, and the absence of a myelodysplastic period preceding leukemia (Pui et al., 1995). Patients receiving weekly or twice-weekly doses of etoposide, with cumulative doses >2000 mg/m^2, seem to be at higher risk of leukemia.

Etoposide primarily is used for treatment of testicular tumors, in combination with bleomycin and cisplatin, and in combination with cisplatin and ifosfamide for small cell carcinoma of the lung. It also is active against non-Hodgkin's lymphomas, acute nonlymphocytic leukemia, and Kaposi sarcoma associated with acquired immunodeficiency syndrome (AIDS). Etoposide has a favorable toxicity profile for dose escalation in that its primary acute toxicity is myelosuppression. In combination with ifosfamide and carboplatin, it frequently is used for high-dose chemotherapy in total doses of 1500-2000 mg/m^2 (Josting et al., 2000).

Clinical Toxicities. The dose-limiting toxicity of etoposide is leukopenia, with a nadir at 10-14 days and recovery by 3 weeks. Thrombocytopenia occurs less often and usually is not severe. Nausea, vomiting, stomatitis, and diarrhea complicate treatment in ~15% of patients. Alopecia is a common but reversible adverse effect. Hepatic toxicity is particularly evident after high-dose treatment. For both etoposide and teniposide, toxicity increases in patients with decreased serum albumin, an effect related to decreased protein binding of the drug.

Teniposide

Teniposide (VUMON) is administered intravenously. It has a multiphasic pattern of clearance from plasma; after distribution, a $t_{1/2}$ of 4 hours and another $t_{1/2}$ of 10-40 hours are observed. Approximately 45% of the drug is excreted in the urine, but in contrast to etoposide, as much as 80% is recovered as metabolites. Anticonvulsants such as phenytoin increase the hepatic metabolism of teniposide and reduce systemic exposure (Baker et al., 1992). Dosage need not be reduced for patients with impaired renal function. Less than 1% of the drug crosses the blood-brain barrier. Teniposide is available for treatment of refractory ALL in children and is synergistic with cytarabine. It is administered by intravenous infusion in dosages that range from 50 mg/m^2/day for 5 days to 165 mg/m^2/day twice weekly. The drug has limited utility and primarily is given for acute leukemia in children and monocytic leukemia in infants, as well as glioblastoma, neuroblastoma, and brain metastases from small cell carcinomas of the lung. Myelosuppression, nausea, and vomiting are its primary toxic effects.

DRUGS OF DIVERSE MECHANISM OF ACTION

Bleomycin

The bleomycins, a unique group of DNA-cleaving antibiotics, were discovered by Umezawa and colleagues as fermentation products of *Streptomyces verticillus*. The drug currently employed clinically is a mixture of the two copper-chelating peptides, bleomycins A_2 and B_2. The various bleomycins differ only in their terminal amino acid (Figure 61–14).

Bleomycins have attracted interest because of their significant antitumor activity against both Hodgkin's lymphoma and testicular tumors. They are minimally myelo- and immunosuppressive but cause unusual cutaneous side effects and pulmonary fibrosis. Because their toxicities do not overlap with those of other cytotoxic drugs, and because of their unique mechanism of action, bleomycin maintains an important role in treating Hodgkin's disease and testicular cancer.

Chemistry. The bleomycins are water-soluble, basic glycopeptides (Figure 61–14). The core of the bleomycin molecule assumes a metal-binding cage consisting of a pyrimidine chromophore linked to propionamide, a β-aminoalanine amide side chain, and the sugars, l-gulose and 3-*O*-carbamoyl-d-mannose. Bound in this complex are either Fe^{2+} or Cu^{2+}. Attached to the metal ion binding core are a tripeptide chain and a terminal, DNA-binding bithiazole carboxylic acid.

Mechanism of Action. Bleomycin's cytotoxicity results from its ability to cause oxidative damage to the deoxyribose of thymidylate and other nucleotides, leading to single- and double-stranded breaks in DNA. Studies *in vitro* indicate that bleomycin causes accumulation of cells in the G_2 phase of the cell cycle, and many of these cells display chromosomal aberrations, including chromatid breaks, gaps, and fragments, as well as translocations (Twentyman, 1983).

Bleomycin cleaves DNA by generating free radicals. In the presence of O_2 and a reducing agent, such as dithiothreitol, the metal–drug complex becomes activated and functions as a ferrous oxidase, transferring electrons from Fe^{2+} to molecular oxygen to

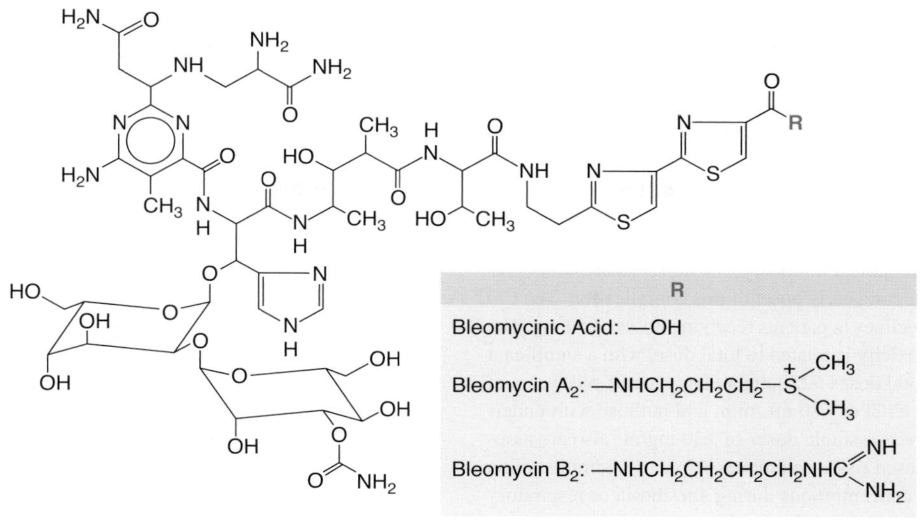

R	
Bleomycinic Acid:	—OH
Bleomycin A_2:	$—NHCH_2CH_2CH_2—S^+(CH_3)_2$
Bleomycin B_2:	$—NHCH_2CH_2CH_2CH_2NHC(=NH)NH_2$

Figure 61–14. *Chemical structures of bleomycin A_2 and B_2.*

produce oxygen radicals (Burger, 1998). Metallobleomycin complexes can be activated by reaction with the flavin enzyme, NADPH-cytochrome P450 reductase. Bleomycin binds to DNA, and the activated complex generates free radicals that are responsible for abstraction of a proton at the 3′ position of the deoxyribose backbone of the DNA chain, opening the deoxyribose ring and generating a strand break in DNA. The process for repair of this break is poorly understood, but an excess of breaks generates apoptosis.

Bleomycin is degraded by a specific hydrolase found in various normal tissues, including liver. Hydrolase activity is low in skin and lung, perhaps contributing to the serious toxicity at those sites. Some bleomycin-resistant cells contain high levels of hydrolase activity (Sebti et al., 1991). In other cell lines, resistance has been attributed to decreased uptake, repair of strand breaks, or drug inactivation by thiols or thiol-rich proteins. A polymorphism of the hydrolase gene, SNP A1450G, has been identified in 10% of patients with testicular cancer, and the G/G genotype is associated with a 20% decreased survival in patients treated with bleomycin combination therapy, suggesting that this single nucleotide polymorphism is associated with increased hydrolase activity (de Haas et al., 2008).

Absorption, Fate, and Excretion. Bleomycin is administered intravenously, intramuscularly, or subcutaneously or instilled into the bladder for local treatment of bladder cancer. After intravenous infusion, relatively high drug concentrations are detected in the skin and lungs of experimental animals, and these organs become major sites of toxicity. Having a high molecular mass, bleomycin crosses the blood-brain barrier poorly.

After intravenous administration of a bolus dose of 15 mg/m^2, peak concentrations of 1-5 mg/mL are achieved in plasma. The half-time for elimination is ~3 hours. About two-thirds of the drug are excreted intact in the urine. Concentrations in plasma are greatly elevated if usual doses are given to patients with renal impairment and if such patients are at high risk of developing pulmonary toxicity. Doses of bleomycin should be reduced in the presence of a CrCl <60 mL/min (Dalgleish et al., 1984).

Therapeutic Uses. The recommended dose of bleomycin (BLENOXANE, others) is 10-20 units/m^2 given weekly or twice weekly by the intravenous, intramuscular, or subcutaneous route. A test dose of ≤2 units before the first two doses is recommended for lymphoma patients. A variety of regimens are employed clinically, with bleomycin doses expressed in units. In treating testicular cancer, a standard total dose of 30 mg is given weekly for 3 consecutive weeks, and for three to four cycles of treatment. Total courses exceeding 250 mg should be given with caution, and usually only in high-risk testicular cancer treatment, because of a marked increase in the risk of pulmonary toxicity above this total dose. Bleomycin also may be instilled into the pleural cavity in doses of 5-60 mg (depending on the technique) to ablate the pleural space in patients with malignant effusions.

Bleomycin is highly effective against germ cell tumors of the testis and ovary. In testicular cancer, it is curative when used with cisplatin and vinblastine or cisplatin and etoposide. It is a component of the standard curative ABVD regimen (doxorubicin [adriamycin], bleomycin, vinblastine, and dacarbazine) for Hodgkin's lymphoma.

Clinical Toxicities. Because bleomycin causes little myelosuppression, it has significant advantages in combination with other cytotoxic drugs. However, it does cause a constellation of cutaneous toxicities, including hyperpigmentation, hyperkeratosis, erythema, and even ulceration. Rarely, patients with severe skin toxicity may experience Raynaud's phenomenon. Skin changes may begin with tenderness and swelling of the distal digits and progress to erythematous, ulcerating lesions over the elbows, knuckles, and other pressure areas. Healing of these lesions often leaves a residual hyperpigmentation, and lesions may recur when patients are treated with other antineoplastic drugs. Rarely, bleomycin causes a flagellate dermatitis consisting of bands of pruritic erythema on the arms, back, scalp, and hands. This rash responds readily to topical corticosteroids.

The most serious adverse reaction to bleomycin is pulmonary toxicity, which begins with a dry cough, fine rales, and diffuse basilar infiltrates on X-ray and may progress to life-threatening pulmonary fibrosis. Radiological changes of bleomycin-induced lung disease may be indistinguishable from interstitial infection or tumor, and show strong PET-positivity, but may progress from patchy infiltrates to dense fibrosis, cavitation and pneumothorax, atelectasis, or lobar collapse. Approximately 5-10% of patients receiving bleomycin develop clinically apparent pulmonary toxicity, and ~1% die of this complication (O'Sullivan et al., 2003). Most who recover experience a significant improvement in pulmonary function, but fibrosis may be irreversible. Pulmonary function tests are not of predictive value for detecting early onset of this complication. The CO diffusion capacity declines in patients receiving doses >250 mg. The risk of pulmonary toxicity is related to total dose, with a significant increase in risk in total doses >250 mg and in patients >40 years of age, in those with a CrCl of <80 mL/min, and in those with underlying pulmonary disease; single doses of ≥30 mg/m^2 also are associated with an increased risk of pulmonary toxicity. Administration of high inspired O_2 concentrations during anesthesia or respiratory therapy may aggravate or precipitate pulmonary toxicity in patients previously treated with the drug. There is no known specific therapy for bleomycin lung injury except for symptomatic management and standard pulmonary care. Steroids are of variable benefit, with greatest effectiveness in the earliest inflammatory stages of the lesion.

The etiology of bleomycin pulmonary toxicity has been investigated in rodent models (Moeller et al., 2008). These studies implicate various factors secreted by macrophages, including cytokines (such as transforming growth factor β [TGFβ] and tumor necrosis factor α [TNFα]), and chemokines (such as CCL2 and CXCLI2), as causative factors in leading to fibrosis in response to epithelial damage. Other contributing factors may be disordered coagulation cascades and imbalances in eicosanoids, leading to overproduction of profibrotic leukotrienes and underproduction of antifibrotic prostaglandins. Fibroblasts are recruited to the site of injury by release of lysophosphatide acid from inflammatory cells and contribute to the development of fibrosis (Tager et al., 2008). Various agents (e.g., thalidomide, anti-Her 2 antibodies, PPAR-γ agonists, *N*-acetylcysteine, anticoagulants, pirfenidone, and bosentan) have attenuated bleomycin toxicity in the animal model, given either before or after the toxic agent. The last four agents are being evaluated in clinical trials for the treatment of idiopathic pulmonary fibrosis (Walter et al., 2006), for which bleomycin lung disease in rodents is the primary disease model.

Other toxic reactions to bleomycin include hyperthermia, headache, nausea and vomiting, and a peculiar acute fulminant reaction observed in patients with lymphomas. This reaction is characterized by profound hyperthermia, hypotension, and sustained cardiorespiratory collapse; it does not appear to be a classical anaphylactic reaction and possibly may be related to release of an endogenous pyrogen. This reaction has occurred in ~1% of patients with lymphomas or testicular cancer.

Mitomycin

This antibiotic was isolated from *Streptococcus caespitosus* by Wakaki and associates in 1958. It has limited clinical utility, having been replaced by less toxic and more effective drugs in most settings, with the exception of anal cancers, for which it is curative.

Mitomycin contains an azauridine group and a quinone group in its structure, as well as a mitosane ring, and each of these participates in the alkylation reactions with DNA.

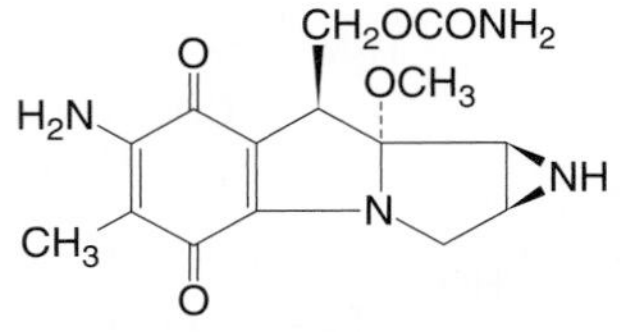

MITOMYCIN

Mechanism of Action. After intracellular enzymatic or spontaneous chemical reduction of the quinone and loss of the methoxy group, mitomycin becomes a bifunctional or trifunctional alkylating agent. Reduction occurs preferentially in hypoxic cells in some experimental systems. The drug inhibits DNA synthesis and cross-links DNA at the N6 position of adenine and at the O6 and N7 positions of guanine. Attempts to repair DNA lead to strand breaks. Mitomycin is a potent radiosensitizer, teratogen, and carcinogen in rodents. Resistance has been ascribed to deficient activation, intracellular inactivation of the reduced quinone, and P-glycoprotein-mediated drug efflux (Dorr, 1988).

Absorption, Fate, and Excretion. Mitomycin is administered intravenously. It disappears rapidly from the blood after injection, with a $t_{1/2}$ of 25-90 minutes. Peak concentrations in plasma are 0.4 μg/mL after doses of 20 mg/m^2 (Dorr, 1988). The drug distributes widely throughout the body but is not detected in the CNS. Inactivation occurs by hepatic metabolism or chemical conjugation with sulfhydryls. Less than 10% of the active drug is excreted in the urine or the bile.

Therapeutic Uses. Mitomycin (mitomycin-C; MUTAMYCIN, others) is administered by intravenous infusion; extravasation may result in severe local injury. The usual dose (6-20 mg/m^2) is given as a single bolus every 6-8 weeks. Dosage is modified based on hematological recovery. Mitomycin also may be used by direct instillation into the bladder to treat superficial carcinomas (Boccardo et al., 1994).

Mitomycin is used in combination with 5-FU and cisplatin, for anal cancer. Mitomycin is used off label (in the form of an extemporaneously compounded eye drop) as an adjunct to surgery to inhibit wound healing and reduce scarring; it appears to have benefit in the management of malignant and nonmalignant ophthalmic pathologies (see the review by Abraham, 2006).

Clinical Toxicities. The major toxic effect is myelosuppression, characterized by marked leukopenia and thrombocytopenia; after higher doses, the nadirs may be delayed and cumulative, with recovery only after 6-8 weeks of pancytopenia. Nausea, vomiting, diarrhea, stomatitis, rash, fever, and malaise also are observed. A hemolytic uremic syndrome represents the most dangerous toxic manifestation of mitomycin and is believed to result from drug-induced endothelial damage. Patients who have received >50 mg/m^2 total dose may acutely develop hemolysis, neurological abnormalities, interstitial pneumonia, and glomerular damage resulting in renal failure. The incidence of renal failure increases to 28% in patients who receive total doses of ≥70 mg/m^2. There is no effective treatment for the disorder. It must be recognized early, and mitomycin must be discontinued immediately. Mitomycin causes interstitial pulmonary fibrosis, and total doses >30 mg/m^2 have infrequently led to congestive heart failure. It also may potentiate the cardiotoxicity of doxorubicin when used in combination with this drug.

Mitotane

Mitotane (*o,p′*-DDD), a compound chemically similar to the insecticides DDT and DDD, is used in the treatment of neoplasms derived from the adrenal cortex. In studies of the toxicology of related insecticides in dogs, it was noted that the adrenal cortex was severely damaged, an effect caused by the presence of the *o,p′* isomer of DDD.

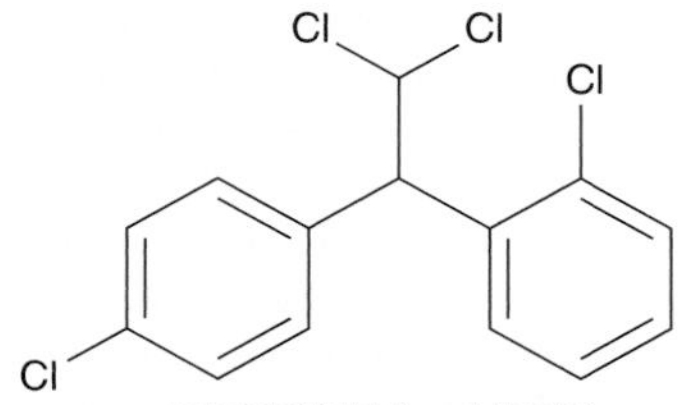

MITOTANE (*o,p′* DDD)

Cytotoxic Action. The mechanism of action of mitotane has not been elucidated, but its relatively selective destruction of adrenocortical cells, normal or neoplastic, is well established. Thus, administration of the drug causes a rapid reduction in the levels of adrenocorticosteroids and their metabolites in blood and urine, a response that is useful in both guiding dosage and following the course of hyperadrenocorticism (Cushing's syndrome) resulting from an adrenal tumor or adrenal hyperplasia. It does not damage other organs.

Absorption, Fate, and Excretion. Approximately 40% of mitotane is absorbed after oral administration. After daily doses of 5-15 g, concentrations of 10-90 μg/mL of unchanged drug and 30-50 μg/mL of a metabolite are present in the blood. After discontinuation of therapy, plasma concentrations of mitotane are still measurable for 6-9 weeks. Although the drug is found in all tissues, fat is the primary site of storage. A water-soluble metabolite of mitotane found in the urine constitutes 25% of an oral or parenteral dose. About 60% of an oral dose is excreted unchanged in the stool.

Therapeutic Uses. Mitotane (LYSODREN) is administered in initial daily oral doses of 2-6 g, usually in three or four divided portions, and usually increased to 9-10 g/day if tolerated. The maximal tolerated dose may vary from 2-16 g/day. Treatment should continue for at least 3 months; if beneficial effects are observed, therapy should be maintained indefinitely. Spironolactone should not be administered concomitantly, because it interferes with the adrenal suppression produced by mitotane (Wortsman and Soler, 1977).

Treatment with mitotane is indicated for the palliation of inoperable adrenocortical carcinoma, producing symptomatic benefit in 30-50% of such patients.

Clinical Toxicity. Although the administration of mitotane produces anorexia and nausea in most patients, somnolence and lethargy in ~34%, and dermatitis in 15-20%, these effects do not contraindicate the use of the drug at lower doses. Because this drug damages the adrenal cortex, administration of replacement doses of adrenocorticosteroids is necessary (Hogan et al., 1978).

Trabectedin

Trabectedin (YONDELIS) is the only drug used clinically that is derived from a sea animal. It was isolated from the marine tunicate, Ecteinascidin turbinate, as part of the National Cancer Institute's natural products discovery program. Trabectedin is designated as an orphan drug in the U.S. for ovarian cancer, sarcoma, and pancreatic cancer and is approved in the E.U. for second-line treatment of soft-tissue sarcomas and ovarian cancer.

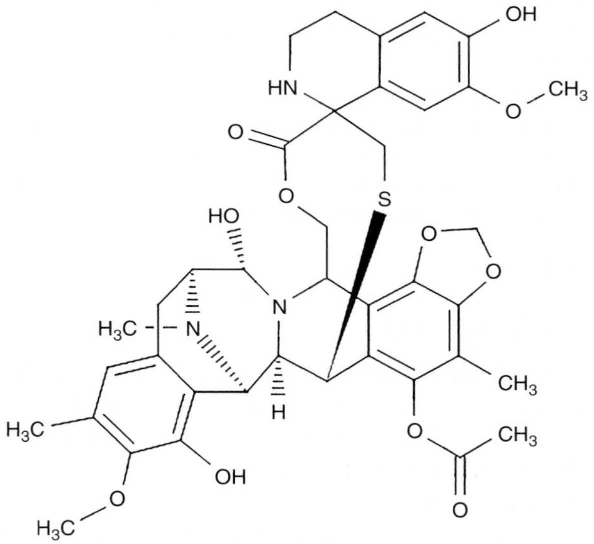

TRABECTEDIN

Mechanism of Action. This large structure binds to the minor groove of DNA, allowing the alkylation of the N2 position of guanine and bending the helix toward the major groove (Tavecchio et al., 2008). A portion of the molecule protrudes from the minor groove and may play a role in attracting repair or transcription complexes. The bulky DNA adduct is recognized by the transcription-coupled nucleotide excision repair complex, and these proteins initiate attempts to repair the damaged strand, converting the adduct to a double-stranded break. Tumor cell sensitivity to trabectedin exhibits interesting molecular features. Trabectedin has particular cytotoxic effects on cells that lack components of the Fanconi anemia complex or those that lack the ability to repair double-strand DNA breaks through homologous recombination (Soares et al., 2007). Unlike cisplatin and other DNA adduct– forming drugs, its activity requires the presence of intact components of NER, including XPG, which may be important for initiation of single breaks and attempts at adduct removal (Stevens et al., 2008).

Absorption, Fate, and Excretion. Trabectedin is administered as a 24-hour infusion of 1.3 mg/m^2 every 3 weeks. Its approval in Europe was based on a trial in soft-tissue sarcoma in which a superior time to progression was found with the longer infusion, as compared to a more convenient 3-hour infusion. It is administered with dexamethasone, 4 mg BID, starting 24 hours before drug infusion to diminish hepatic toxicity. The drug is slowly cleared by CYP3A4, with a plasma $t_{1/2}$ of ~24-40 hours.

Therapeutic Uses. Trabectedin is approved outside the U.S. for second-line treatment of soft-tissue sarcomas and for ovarian cancer in combination with a doxorubicin formulation (DOXIL). It produces a very high (>50%) disease control rate in myxoid liposarcomas, a tumor characterized by a particular genomic translocation, although the reasons for this sensitivity are unclear (Grosso et al., 2009).

Toxicity. Without dexamethasone pretreatment, trabectedin causes significant hepatic enzyme elevations and fatigue in at least one-third of patients. With the steroid, the increases in transaminase are less pronounced and rapidly reverse (Grosso et al., 2009). Other toxicities include mild myelosuppression and, rarely, rhabdomyolysis.

ENZYMES

L-Asparaginase

In 1953, Kidd reported that guinea pig serum had antileukemic effects and identified L-asparaginase (L-ASP) as the source of this activity (Kidd, 1953). Fifteen years later, the purified enzyme from *Escherichia coli* proved to have dramatic antitumor activity against malignant lymphoid cells, based on the dependence of those tumors on exogenous sources of L-asparagine (Broome, 1981). The enzyme has become a standard agent for treating ALL.

Mechanism of Action. Most normal tissues are able to synthesize L-asparagine in amounts sufficient for protein synthesis, but lymphocytic leukemias lack adequate amounts of asparagine synthetase, and derive the required amino acid from plasma. L-ASP, by catalyzing the hydrolysis of circulating asparagine to aspartic acid and ammonia, deprives these malignant cells of asparagine, leading to cell death. L-ASP is used in combination with other agents, including methotrexate, doxorubicin, vincristine, and prednisone for the treatment of ALL and for high-grade lymphomas.

Resistance arises through induction of asparagine synthetase in tumor cells. For unknown reasons, hyperdiploid ALL cells or those with translocations involving the TEL oncogene are particularly sensitive to L-ASP (Pui et al., 2004), while cells containing the *bcr-abl* translocation, more common in adult ALL, are more resistant.

Absorption, Fate, Excretion, and Therapeutic Use. L-Asparaginase (ELSPAR), a 144-kDa tetramer, is given intramuscularly or intravenously, but usually by the former route. After intravenous administration, *E. coli*–derived L-ASP has a clearance rate from plasma of 0.035 mL/min/kg, a volume of distribution that approximates the volume of plasma in humans, and a $t_{1/2}$ of 24 hours (Asselin et al., 1993). It is given in doses of 6000-10,000 IU every third day for 3-4 weeks, although doses up to 25,000 IU once per week may be more effective in childhood ALL (Moghrabi et al., 2007). Enzyme levels must be maintained at >0.2 IU/mL in plasma to deplete asparagine in the bloodstream. Pegaspargase (PEG-L-ASPARAGINASE; ONCASPAR) a preparation in which the enzyme is conjugated to 5000-Da units of monomethoxy polyethylene glycol, has much slower clearance from plasma ($t_{1/2}$ of 6-7 days), and it is administered in doses of 2500 IU/m^2 intramuscularly no more frequently than every 14 days, producing rapid and complete depletion of plasma and tumor cell asparagine for 21 days in most patients (Appel et al., 2008). Pegaspargase has much reduced immunogenicity (<20% of patients develop antibodies) (Hawkins et al., 2004) and has been approved for first-line ALL therapy.

Intermittent dosage regimens and longer durations of treatment increase the risk of inducing hypersensitivity. In hypersensitive patients, neutralizing antibodies inactivate L-ASP. Not all patients with neutralizing antibodies experience clinical hypersensitivity, although enzyme may be inactivated and therapy may be ineffective. In previously untreated ALL, pegaspargase produces more rapid clearance of lymphoblasts from bone marrow than does the *E. coli* preparation and circumvents the rapid antibody-mediated clearance seen with *E. coli* enzyme in relapsed patients (Avramis et al., 2002). Asparaginase preparations only partially deplete CSF asparagine.

Clinical Toxicity. L-ASP toxicities result from its antigenicity as a foreign protein and its inhibition of protein synthesis. Hypersensitivity reactions, including urticaria and full-blown anaphylaxis, occur in 5-20% of patients and may be fatal. These reactions usually are heralded by the earlier appearance of circulating neutralizing antibody and accelerated enzyme clearance from plasma. In these patients, pegaspargase is a safe and effective alternative. So-called "silent" enzyme inactivation by antibodies occurs in a higher percentage of patients than overt hypersensitivity and may be associated with a negative clinical outcome, especially in high-risk ALL patients (Mann et al., 2007).

Other toxicities result from inhibition of protein synthesis in normal tissues (e.g., hyperglycemia due to insulin deficiency, clotting abnormalities due to deficient clotting factors, hypertriglyceridemia due to effects on lipoprotein production, hypoalbuminemia). Pancreatitis may result from extreme triglyceridemia and has been treated by plasma exchange. The clotting problems may take the form of spontaneous thrombosis—more frequent in thrombophilic patients with underlying deficiencies in factor S, factor C, antithrombin III mutation, or factor V Leiden—or, less frequently, hemorrhagic episodes (Caruso et al., 2006). Thrombosis of cortical sinus vessels frequently goes unrecognized. Brain magnetic resonance imaging studies should be considered in patients treated with L-ASP who present with seizures, headache, or altered mental status. Intracranial hemorrhage in the first week of L-ASP treatment is an infrequent but devastating complication. L-ASP suppresses immune function as well.

L-ASP terminates the antitumor activity of methotrexate when given shortly after the antimetabolite. By lowering serum albumin concentrations, it may decrease protein binding and accelerate plasma clearance of other drugs.

HYDROXYUREA

The syntheses of hydroxyurea (HU) was first reported in 1869, but its potential anticancer activity was not recognized until 90 years later, when the drug was found to inhibit the growth of both leukemia and solid tumors. This drug has unique and surprisingly diverse biological effects as an antileukemic drug, radiation sensitizer, and an inducer of fetal hemoglobin in patients with sickle cell disease. The drug is orally administered, and its toxicity in most patients is modest and limited to myelosuppression.

$$H_2N{-}\overset{\displaystyle O}{\overset{\|}{C}}{-}NH{-}OH$$

HYDROXYUREA

Cytotoxic Action. HU inhibits the enzyme ribonucleoside diphosphate reductase, which catalyzes the reductive conversion of ribonucleotides to deoxyribonucleotides, a rate-limiting step in the biosynthesis of DNA. HU binds the iron molecules that are essential for activation of a tyrosyl radical in the catalytic subunit (hRRM2) of RNR. The drug is specific for the S phase of the cell cycle, during which RNR concentrations are maximal. It causes cells to arrest at or near the G_1–S interface through both p53-dependent and -independent mechanisms.

Because cells are highly sensitive to irradiation at the G_1–S boundary, HU and irradiation cause synergistic antitumor effects. Through depletion of physiological deoxynucleotides, HU potentiates the antiproliferative effects of DNA-damaging agents such as cisplatin, alkylating agents, or topoisomerase II inhibitors and facilitates the incorporation of antimetabolites such as Ara-C, gemcitabine, and fludarabine into DNA. It also promotes degradation of the p21 cell-cycle checkpoint and thereby enhances the effects of HDAC (histone deacetylase) inhibitors *in vitro* (Kramer et al., 2008). The role of nitric oxide release in its differentiating activity and in its antitumor effects is uncertain but intriguing (Cokic et al., 2003).

HU has become the primary drug for improving the control of sickle cell (HbS) disease in adults and is also used for inducing fetal hemoglobin (HbF) in thalassemia HbC and HbC/S patients (Brawley et al., 2008). It reduces vaso-occlusive events, painful cries, hospitalizations, and the need for blood transfusions in patients with sickle cell disease. It does so via several potential mechanisms. Increased synthesis of HbF promotes solubility of hemoglobin and prevents sickling. The mechanism of HbF production is uncertain. It may simply result from suppression of erythroid precursor proliferation with compensatory stimulation of a distinct set of fetal Hb-producing cells. Sar1a, a specific promoter that upregulates in response to HU, induces HbF synthesis (Kumkhaek, 2008). Polymorphisms in this promoter may explain differential responses to HU. An alternative mechanism for HbF production has been offered because of the ability of HU to generate nitric oxide both *in vitro* and *in vivo*, causing nitrosylation of small-molecular-weight GTPases, a process that stimulate γ-globin production in erythroid precursors. Another property of HU that may be relevant is its ability to reduce L-selectin expression and thereby to inhibit adhesion of red cells and neutrophils to vascular endothelium. Also, by suppressing the production of neutrophils, it decreases their contribution to vascular occlusion.

Tumor cells become resistant to HU through increased synthesis of the hRRM2 subunit of ribonucleoside diphosphate reductase, thus restoring enzyme activity.

Absorption, Fate, and Excretion. The oral bioavailability of HU is excellent (80-100%), and comparable plasma concentrations are seen after oral or intravenous dosing. Peak plasma concentrations are reached 1-1.5 hours after oral doses of 15-80 mg/kg. HU disappears from plasma with a $t_{1/2}$ of 3.5-4.5 hours. The drug readily crosses the blood-brain barrier, and it appears in significant quantities in human breast milk. From 40-80% of the drug is recovered in the urine within 12 hours after either intravenous or oral administration. Although precise guidelines are not available, it is advisable to modify initial doses for patients with abnormal renal function until individual tolerance can be assessed. Animal studies suggest that metabolism of HU does occur, but the extent and significance of its metabolism in humans have not been established.

Therapeutic Uses. In cancer treatment, two dosage schedules for HU (HYDREA, DROXIA, others), alone or in combination with other drugs, are most commonly used in a variety of solid tumors: 1) intermittent therapy with 80 mg/kg administered orally as a single dose every third day or 2) continuous therapy with 20-30 mg/kg administered as a single daily dose. In patients with essential thrombocythemia and in sickle cell disease, HU is given in a daily dose of 15 mg/kg, adjusting that dose upward or downward according to blood counts. The neutrophil count responds within 1-2 weeks to discontinuation of the drug. In treating subjects with sickle cell and related diseases, a neutrophil count of at least 2500 cells/mL should be maintained (Platt, 2008). Treatment typically is continued for 6 weeks in malignant diseases to determine its effectiveness; if satisfactory results are obtained, therapy can be continued indefinitely, although leukocyte counts at weekly intervals are advisable.

The principal use of HU has been as a myelosuppressive agent in various myeloproliferative syndromes, particularly CML, polycythemia vera, myeloid metaplasia, and essential thrombocytosis, for controlling high platelet or white cell counts. Many of the myeloproliferative syndromes harbor activating mutations of JAK2, a gene that is downregulated by HU. In essential thrombocythemia, it is the drug of choice for patients with a platelet count >1.5 million cells/mm^3 or with a history of arterial or venous thrombosis. In this disease, it dramatically lowers the risk of thrombosis by lowering the platelet, neutrophil, and red cell counts and by reducing expression of L-selectin and increasing nitric oxide production by neutrophils.

In CML, HU has been largely replaced by imatinib. Although it has produced anecdotal, temporary remissions in patients with solid tumors (e.g., head and neck cancers, cervical cancers), HU rarely is used in such patients as a single agent. HU is a potent radiosensitizer as a consequence of its inhibition of RNR (Flanagan et al., 2007) and has been incorporated into several treatment regimens with concurrent irradiation (i.e., cervical carcinoma, primary brain tumors, head and neck cancer, non–small-cell lung cancer).

Clinical Toxicity. Leukopenia, anemia, and occasionally thrombocytopenia—are the major toxic effects; recovery of the bone marrow is prompt if the drug is discontinued for a few days. Other adverse reactions include a desquamative interstitial pneumonitis, GI disturbances, and mild dermatological reactions; more rarely, stomatitis, alopecia, and neurological manifestations have been encountered. Increased skin and fingernail pigmentation may occur, as well as painful leg ulcers, especially in elderly patients or in those with renal dysfunction. HU does not increase the risk of secondary leukemia in patients with myeloproliferative disorders or sickle cell disease. It is a potent teratogen in all animal species tested and should not be used in women with childbearing potential (Platt, 2008).

DIFFERENTIATING AGENTS

One of the hallmarks of malignant transformation is a block in differentiation. It is not clear whether the block is complete or partial, in that tumor cells with the features of stem cells can be found in most tumors, while the greater bulk of tumor cells do not carry the markers or the biological potential of continuous proliferation. Nonetheless, there is growing evidence that many human tumors are generated by mutations that block specific steps in differentiation, an example being the t(15;17) translocation in APL (acute promyelocytic leukemia). This translocation joins the retinoic acid receptor-α (RAR-α, a dimerizing protein critical for differentiation) and the PML gene, which encodes a transcription factor important in inhibiting proliferation and promoting myeloid differentiation. Four other translocation partners for APL have been identified in less common varieties of APL. Under physiological conditions, RAR-α binds retinoic acid and regulates the expression of a number of specific genes that control myeloid differentiation. The oncogenic PML–RAR-α gene produces a protein that binds retinoids with much decreased affinity, lacks PML regulatory function, and fails to upregulate transcription factors (C/EBP and PU.1) that promote myeloid differentiation (Collins, 2008). The fusion protein forms homo- and heterodimers that regulate expression of genes that increase leukemic stem cell renewal, suppress checkpoint and apoptotic signals, and suppress expression of DNA repair functions, thereby enhancing mutability of APL cells. Epigenetic regulation of gene expression by histone acetylation and methylation also is disrupted by the fusion protein.

A number of chemical entities (vitamin D and its analogs, retinoids, benzamides and other inhibitors of histone deacetylase, various cytotoxics and biological agents, and inhibitors of DNA methylation) can induce differentiation in tumor cell lines *in vitro*. Fittingly, the first and best example of differentiating therapy was discovered in the treatment of APL (Wang and Chen, 2008).

Retinoids

Tretinoin. The biology and pharmacology of retinoids and related compounds are discussed in detail in Chapter 65. The most important of these for cancer treatment is tretinoin (all-trans retinoic acid; ATRA), which induces a high rate of complete remission in APL as a single agent and, in combination with anthracyclines, cures most patients with this disease.

Under physiological conditions, the RAR-α receptor dimerizes with the retinoid X receptor to form a complex that binds ATRA tightly. ATRA binding displaces a repressor from the complex and promotes differentiation of cells of multiple lineages. In APL cells, physiological concentrations of retinoid are inadequate to displace the repressor. Pharmacological concentrations, however, are effective in activating the differentiation program and in promoting degradation of the PML–RAR-α fusion gene (Collins, 2008). ATRA also binds and activates RAR-γ and thereby promotes stem-cell renewal, perhaps through its effects on the microenvironment (Drumea et al., 2008), and this action may help restore normal bone marrow renewal. Resistance to ATRA arises by further mutation of the fusion gene, abolishing ATRA binding; by induction of the CYP26A1 in liver or leukemic cells; or by loss of expression of the PML–RAR-α fusion gene (Roussel and Lanotte, 2001). Sensitivity can be restored by transfection of a functional PML–RAR-α gene.

Clinical Pharmacology. The usual dosing regimen of orally administered ATRA (VESANOID, others) is 45 mg/m^2/day until 30 days after remission is achieved (maximum course of therapy is 90 days). ATRA as a single agent reverses the hemorrhagic diathesis associated with APL and induces a high rate of temporary remission. However, clinical trials have clearly established the benefit of giving ATRA in combination with an anthracycline for remission induction, achieving ≥80% relapse-free long-term survival.

ATRA concentrations reach 400 ng/mL in plasma. ATRA is cleared by a CYP3A4-mediated elimination with a $t_{1/2}$ of <1 hour. Treatment with inducers of CYP3A4 leads to more rapid drug disappearance and, in some patients, resistance to ATRA (Gallagher, 2002). Inhibitors, such as antifungal imidazoles, block its degradation and may lead to hypercalcemia and renal failure (Cordoba et al., 2008), which responds to diuresis, bisphosphonates, and ATRA discontinuation. Corticosteroids and chemotherapy sharply decrease the occurrence of "retinoic acid syndrome," which is characterized by fever, dyspnea, weight gain, pulmonary infiltrates, and pleural or pericardial effusions. When used as a single agent for remission induction, especially in patients with >5000 leukemic cells/mm^3 in the peripheral blood, ATRA induces an outpouring of cytokines and mature-appearing neutrophils of leukemic origin. These cells express high concentrations of integrins and other adhesion molecules on their surface and clog small vessels in the pulmonary circulation, leading to significant morbidity in 15-20% of patients. The syndrome of respiratory distress, pleural and pericardial effusions, and mental status changes may have a fatal outcome. Pretreatment dexamethasone should be given to patients with leukemic cell counts of >5,000/mL to counteract "retinoic acid syndrome".

Toxicity. Retinoids as a class, including ATRA, cause dry skin, cheilitis, reversible hepatic enzyme abnormalities, bone tenderness, pseudotumor cerebri, hypercalcemia, and hyperlipidemia, and as mentioned in the previous paragraph, the retinoic acid syndrome.

Arsenic Trioxide (ATO)

Although recognized as a heavy metal toxin for centuries, arsenicals attracted interest as a medicinal agent nearly a century ago for syphilis and parasitic disease, and eventually CML. Arsenic trioxide has become a highly effective treatment for relapsed APL, producing complete responses in >85% of such patients (Wang and Chen, 2008). It now is a standard treatment for patients who relapse after ATRA and chemotherapy, cures a significant fraction of these patients, and has entered trials as primary therapy in combination with ATRA and chemotherapy. The chemistry and toxicity of arsenic is considered in detail in Chapter 67.

The basis for its antitumor activity remains uncertain. APL cells have high levels of reactive oxygen species (ROS) and are quite sensitive to further ROS induction. ATO inhibits thioredoxin reductase and thereby generates ROS. It inactivates glutathione and other sulfhydryls that scavenge ROS and thereby aggravates ROS damage. Cells exposed to ATO also upregulate p53, Jun kinase, and caspases associated with the intrinsic pathway of apoptosis and downregulate anti-apoptotic proteins such as bcl-2. Of particular relevance to APL, it promotes the phosphorylation, sumoylation, and degradation of the APL fusion protein (Lallemand-Breitenbach et al., 2008), as well as the degradation of NF-κB, a transcription factor that stimulates angiogenesis and dampens apoptotic responses in cells with DNA damage. ATO's cytotoxic effects are antagonized by cell survival signals emanating from activation of components of the PI3 kinase cell survival pathway, including Akt kinase, S6 kinase, and mammalian target of rapamycin (mTOR). Inhibition of mTOR by rapamycin enhances its cytotoxic activity in culture systems.

It induces differentiation of leukemic cell lines *in vitro*, and in both experimental and human leukemias *in vivo*, but the mechanisms of differentiation and their relationship to the above pharmacological activities are not known.

Clinical Pharmacology. ATO (TRISENOX) is well absorbed orally, but in cancer treatment is administered as a 2-hour intravenous infusion in dosages of 0.15 mg/kg/day for up to 60 days, until remission is documented. Consolidation therapy begins after a 3-week break. It enters cells via one of several glucose transporters. The primary mechanism of elimination is through enzymatic methylation. Methylated metabolites have uncertain biological effects. Peak steady-state concentrations of arsenic in plasma reached 5-7 μM in one study in adults, while 20-fold lower levels were reported in children using more specific atomic absorption methods (Fox, 2008). Multiple methylated metabolites form rapidly and are excreted in urine. Less than 20% of administered drug is excreted unchanged in the urine. No dose reductions are indicated for hepatic or renal dysfunction.

Toxicity. Pharmacological doses of ATO are well tolerated. Patients may experience reversible side effects, including hyperglycemia, hepatic enzyme elevations, fatigue, dysesthesias, and light-headedness. Ten percent or fewer of patients will experience a leukocyte maturation syndrome similar to that seen with ATRA, including pulmonary distress, effusions, and mental status changes. Oxygen, corticosteroids, and temporary discontinuation of ATO lead to full reversal of this syndrome (Soignet et al., 1998). Another important and potentially dangerous side effect is lengthening of the QT interval on the electrocardiogram in 40% of patients, but rarely do patients develop torsades de pointes, a dangerous form of ventricular tachycardia. Simultaneous treatment with other QT-prolonging drugs, such as macrolide antibiotics, quinidine, or methadone, should be avoided. QT prolongation by ATO results from inhibition of the rapid K^+ efflux channels in myocardial tissue by As_2O_3. This change leads to slow repolarization of myocardium, and ventricular arrhythmias. Monitoring of serum electrolytes and repletion of serum K^+ in patients with hypokalemia are precautionary measures in patients receiving ATO therapy. In patients exhibiting a significantly prolonged QT (>470 milliseconds), treatment should be suspended, K^+ supplemented, and therapy resumed only if the QT returns to normal. Torsades de pointes requires treatment with intravenous magnesium sulfate, K^+ repletion, and defibrillation if the arrhythmia persists (Gupta et al., 2007) (see Chapter 29).

Histone Deacetylase Inhibitors

Vorinostat. A new field of cancer research, called epigenetics, concerns the control of cell proliferation and differentiation by processes beyond pure genetic alterations. These processes include cellular modification of expression of genes by microRNAs, histones, and proteins, and post-translational modification of proteins. Vorinostat (ZOLINZA), also known as suberoylanilide hydroxamic acid (SAHA), is unique as an epigenetic modifier that directly affects histone function (Figure 61–15). To understand its action, it is important to review the complex structure of DNA, which wraps itself around histone proteins to form the nucleosome. This higher-order packaging controls gene expression. Acetylation of lysine residues on histones increases the spatial distance between DNA strands and the protein core, allowing access for transcription factor complexes, and thereby enhancing transcriptional activity. Acetyl groups are added by histone acetyltransferases and removed by histone deacetylases (HDACs). HDAC inhibitors such as vorinostat increase histone acetylation and thus enhance gene transcription. Many nonhistone proteins also are subject to lysine acetylation and thus are affected by treatment with HDAC inhibitors. The role of their acetylation status in the antitumor action of HDAC inhibitors is unclear.

Mechanism of Action. Vorinostat is a hydroxamic acid modeled after hybrid polar compounds, such as hexamethylene bisacetamide (HMBA); as a class, these compounds cause differentiation of malignant cells *in vitro*, as do other classes of compounds with HDAC-inhibitory activity, including cyclic tetrapeptides, benzamides, and short-chain aliphatic acids. These compounds bind to a critical Zn^{++} ion in the active site of HDAC enzymes. Vorinostat inhibits the enzymatic activity of HDACs at micromolar concentrations. An important distinction between vorinostat and other HDAC inhibitors is that vorinostat and the hydroxymates are pan-HDAC inhibitors, whereas other compounds have selectivity for HDAC isoenzyme subsets. The biological and clinical implications of this specificity are not clear, and the specific mechanism by which HDAC inhibitors exert their antitumor activity is uncertain. They induce cell-cycle arrest, differentiation, and apoptosis of cancer cells; nonmalignant cells are relatively resistant to these effects. They increase transcription of cell-cycle regulators, affect levels of nuclear transcription factors, and induce pro-apoptotic genes. HDAC inhibition directly blocks function of the chaperone HSP90 and stabilizes the tumor suppressor p53 (Bolden et al., 2006).

Absorption, Fate, and Excretion. Vorinostat is administered as a once-daily oral dose of 400 mg. It is inactivated by glucuronidation of the hydroxyl amine group, followed by hydrolysis of the terminal carboxamide bond and further oxidation of the aliphatic side chain (Figure 61–15). The metabolites are pharmacologically inactive. The terminal $t_{1/2}$ of vorinostat in plasma is ~2 hours. Interestingly, histones remain hyperacetylated up to 10 hours after an oral dose of vorinostat, suggesting that its effects persist beyond drug metabolism and elimination.

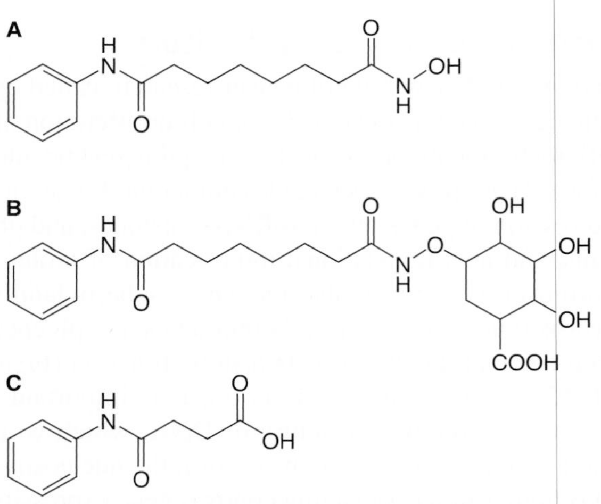

A

B

C

Figure 61–15. Chemical structures of vorinostat (***A***), and its metabolites, vorinostat *O*-glucuronide (***B***) and 4-anilino-4-oxobutanoic acid (***C***).

Therapeutic Uses. Vorinostat is approved for use in refractory cutaneous T-cell lymphoma (CTCL). In patients with refractory CTCL, vorinostat produced an overall response rate of 30%, with a median time to progression of 5 months (Duvic et al., 2007). Vorinostat and other HDAC inhibitors, including romidepsin (depsipeptide; FK228) and MGCD 0103, have shown activity in CTCL, other B- and T-cell lymphomas, and myeloid leukemia.

Toxicity. The most common side effects of vorinostat are fatigue, nausea, diarrhea, and thrombocytopenia. Deep venous thrombosis and pulmonary embolism were infrequent but serious adverse events in CTCL patients receiving vorinostat. Most HDAC inhibitors in development cause QTc prolongation, although no serious cardiac toxicity has been reported with vorinostat. A small number of patients receiving infusional depsipeptide romidepsin (see below) and the hydroxamate dacinostat (NVP-LAQ 824) have developed ventricular arrhythmias while on treatment, but the causal relationship to the drugs has not been clearly established, and the cardiac risk may be lower with orally administered and/or less potent HDAC inhibitors (Piekarz et al., 2006). Caution is advised when using HDAC inhibitors in patients with underlying cardiac abnormalities, and careful monitoring of the QTc interval and correction of electrolyte (K^+, Mg^{++}) abnormalities is necessary.

Romidepsin. Romidepsin, a bicyclic polypeptide derived from a soil bacterium, inhibits HDAC at low nanomolar concentrations and is approved for treatment of CTCL and for peripheral T-cell lymphomas. In a Phase II trial it produced complete responses in 4 patients with CTCL, and partial responses in 20, from a total of 71 patients treated. Its primary toxities include GI complaints (nausea vomiting) and transient myelosuppression. Its administration leads to T-wave flattening, but without clear cardiac toxicity (Piekarz et al., 2009).

BIBLIOGRAPHY

Abbruzzese JL, Grunewald R, Weeks EA, et al. A phase I clinical, plasma, and cellular pharmacology study of gemcitabine. *J Clin Oncol*, **1991,** *9*:491–498.

Allegra CJ, Chabner BA, Tuazon CU, et al. Trimetrexate for the treatment of *Pneumocystis carinii* pneumonia in patients with acquired immunodeficiency syndrome. *N Engl J Med*, **1987a,** *317*:978–985.

Allegra CJ, Hoang K, Yeh GC, et al. Evidence for direct inhibition of de novo purine synthesis in human MCF-7 breast cells as a principal mode of metabolic inhibition by methotrexate. *J Biol Chem*, **1987b**, *262*:13520–13526.

Appel IM, Kazemier KM, Boos J, et al. Pharmacokinetic, pharmacodynamic and intracellular effects of PEG-asparaginase in newly diagnosed childhood acute lymphoblastic leukemia: Results from a single agent window study. *Leukemia*, **2008**, *22*:1665–1679.

Arbuck SG, Douglass HO, Crom WR, et al. Etoposide pharmacokinetics in patients with normal and abnormal organ function. *J Clin Oncol*, **1986,** *4*:1690–1695.

Asselin BL, Whitin JC, Coppola DJ, et al. Comparative pharmacokinetic studies of three asparaginase preparations. *J Clin Oncol*, **1993,** *11*:1780–1786.

Avramis VI, Sencer S, Periclou AP, et al. A randomized comparison of native *Escherichia coli* asparaginase and polyethylene glycol conjugated asparaginase for treatment of children with newly diagnosed standard-risk acute lymphoblastic leukemia: A Children's Cancer Group study. *Blood*, **2002,** *99*: 1986–1994.

Baker DK, Relling MV, Pui CH, et al. Increased teniposide clearance with concomitant anticonvulsant therapy. *J Clin Oncol*, **1992,** *10*:311–315.

Baker SD, Wirth M, Statkevich P, et al. Absorption, metabolism and excretion of ^{14}C-temozolomide following oral administration to patients with advanced cancer. *Clin Cancer Res*, **1999,** *5*:309–317.

Barbour KW, Berger SH, Berger FG. Single amino acid substitution defines a naturally occurring genetic variant of human thymidylate synthase. *Mol Pharmacol*, **1990,** *37*:515–518.

Bergenheim AT, Henriksson R. Pharmacokinetics and pharmacodynamics of estramustine phosphate. *Clin Pharmacokinet*, **1998,** *34*:163–172.

Berlin NI, Rall D, Mead JA, et al. Folic acid antagonist. Effects on the cell and the patient. Combined clinical staff conference at the National Institutes of Health. *Ann Intern Med*, **1963,** *59*:931–956.

Blakley RL, Sorrentino BP. In vitro mutations in dihydrofolate reductase that confer resistance to methotrexate: Potential for clinical application. *Hum Mutat*, **1998,** *11*:259–263.

Bleyer WA. The clinical pharmacology of methotrexate: New applications of an old drug. *Cancer*, **1978,** *41*:36–51.

Boccardo F, Cannata D, Rubagotti A, et al. Prophylaxis of superficial bladder cancer with mitomycin or interferon alfa-2b: Results of a multicentric Italian study. *J Clin Oncol*, **1994,** *12*:7–13.

Bolden JE, Peart MJ, Johnstone RW. Anticancer activities of histone deacetylase inhibitors. *Nat Rev Drug Discov*, **2006,** *5*:769–784.

Bonate PL, Arthaud L, Cantrell WR Jr, et al. Discovery and development of clofarabine: A nucleoside analogue for treating cancer. *Nat Rev Drug Discov*, **2006**, *5*:855–863.

Brawley OW, Cornelius LJ, Edwards LR, et al. National Institutes of Health Consensus Development Conference statement: Hydroxyurea treatment for sickle cell disease. *Ann Intern Med*, **2008**, *148*:932–938.

Broome JD. L-Asparaginase: Discovery and development as a tumor-inhibitory agent. *Cancer Treat Rep*, **1981,** *65*(suppl): 111–114.

Burger RM. Cleavage of nucleic acids by bleomycin. *Chem Rev*, **1998,** *98*:1153–1169.

Cabral FR. Isolation of Chinese hamster ovary cell mutants requiring the continuous presence of Taxol for cell division. *J Cell Biol*, **1983,** *97*:22–29.

Cahill DP, Codd PJ, Batchelor TT, et al. MSH6 inactivation and emergent temozolomide resistance in human glioblastomas. *Clin Neurosurg*, **2008**, *55*:165–171.

Cai J, Damaraju VL, Groulx N, et al. Two distinct molecular mechanisms underlying cytarabine resistance in human leukemic cells. *Cancer Res*, **2008**, *68*:2349–2357.

Cardoen S, Van Den Neste E, Small C, et al. Resistance to 2-chloro-2′-deoxyadenosine of the human B-cell leukemia cell line EHEB. *Clin Cancer Res*, **2001,** *7*:3559–3566.

Caruso V, Iacoviello L, Di Castelnuovo A, et al. Thrombotic complications in childhood acute lymphoblastic leukemia: A meta-analysis of 17 prospective studies comprising 1752 pediatric patients. *Blood*, **2006**, *108*:2216–2222.

Chen CC, Taniguchi T, D'Andrea A. The Fanconi anemia (FA) pathway confers glioma resistance to DNA alkylating agents. *J Mol Med*, **2007**, *85*:497–509.

Chen TL, Passos-Coelho JL, Noe DA, et al. Nonlinear pharmacokinetics of cyclophosphamide in patients with metastatic breast cancer receiving high-dose chemotherapy followed by autologous bone marrow transplantation. *Cancer Res*, **1995,** 55:810–816. Erratum in: *Cancer Res*, **1995,** *55*:1600.

Chen VJ, Bewley JR, Andis SL, et al. Preclinical cellular pharmacology of LY231514 (MTA): A comparison with methotrexate, LY309887 and raltitrexed for their effects on intracellular folate and nucleoside triphosphate pools in CCRF-CEM cells. *Br J Cancer*, **1998,** *78*(suppl):27–34.

Chlenski A, Cohn S. Modulation of matrix remodeling by SPARC in neoplastic progression. *Semin Cell Dev Biol*, **2010,** *21*:55–65.

Chu E, Koeller DM, Casey JL, et al. Autoregulation of human thymidylate synthase messenger RNA translation by thymidylate synthase. *Proc Natl Acad Sci U S A*, **1991,** *88*:8977–8981.

Clarke SJ, Rivory LP. Clinical pharmacokinetics of docetaxel. *Clin Pharmacokinet*, **1999,** *36*:99–114.

Cokic VP, Smith RD, Beleslin-Cokic B, et al. Hydroxyurea induces fetal hemoglobin by the nitric oxide-dependent activation of soluble guanylyl cyclase. *J Clin Invest*, **2003,** *111*:231–239.

Cole BF, Glantz MJ, Jaeckle KA, et al. Quality-of-life-adjusted survival comparison of sustained-release cytosine arabinoside versus intrathecal methotrexate for treatment of solid tumor neoplastic meningitis. *Cancer*, **2003,** *97*:3053–3060.

Collins SJ. Retinoic acid receptors, hematopoiesis and leukemogenesis. *Curr Opin Hematol*, **2008**, *15*:346–351.

Cordoba R, Ramirez E, Lei SH, et al. Hypercalcemia due to an interaction of all-trans retinoic acid (ATRA) and itraconazole therapy for acute promyelocytic leukemia successfully treated with zoledronic acid. *Eur J Clin Pharmacol*, **2008**, *64*:1031–1032.

Cresteil T, Monsarrat B, Alvinerie P, et al. Taxol metabolism by human liver microsomes: Identification of cytochrome P450 isozymes involved in its biotransformation. *Cancer Res*, **1994,** *54*:386–392.

Curt GA, Jolivet J, Carney DN, et al. Determinants of the sensitivity of human small-cell lung cancer cell lines to methotrexate. *J Clin Invest*, **1985,** *76*:1323–1329.

Dalgleish AG, Woods RL, Levi JA. Bleomycin pulmonary toxicity: Its relationship to renal dysfunction. *Med Pediatr Oncol*, **1984,** *12*:313–317.

De Gramont A, Louvet C, Andre T, et al. A review of GERCOD trials of bimonthly leucovorin plus 5-fluorouracil 48-h continuous infusion in advanced colorectal cancer: Evolution of a regimen. Groupe d'Etude et de Recherche sur les Cancers de l'Ovaire et Digestifs (GERCOD). *Eur J Cancer*, **1998,** *34*:619–626.

de Haas EC, Zwart N, Meijer C, et al. Variation in bleomycin hydrolase gene is associated with reduced survival after chemotherapy for testicular germ cell cancer. *J Clin Oncol*, **2008**, *26*:1817–1823.

de Wolf C, Jansen R, Yamaguchi H, et al. Contribution of the drug transporter ABCG2 (breast cancer resistance protein) to resistance against anticancer nucleosides. *Mol Cancer Ther*, **2008,** *7*:3092–3102.

DeAngelis LM, Tong WP, Lin S, et al. Carboxypeptidase G2 rescue after high-dose methotrexate. *J Clin Oncol*, **1996**, *14*:2145–2149.

Deyoung MP, Ellisen LW. p63 and p73 in human cancer: Defining the network. *Oncogene*, **2007**, *26*:5169–5183.

Dolan S, Fitch M. The management of venous thromboembolism in cancer patients. *Br J Nurs*, **2007**, *16*:1308–1312.

Dorr RT. New findings in the pharmacokinetic, metabolic, and drug-resistance aspects of mitomycin C. *Semin Oncol*, **1988,** *15*:32–41.

Doyle LA, Yang W, Abruzzo LV, et al. A multidrug resistance transporter from human MCF-7 breast cancer cells. *Proc Natl Acad Sci U S A*, **1998,** *95*:15665–15670.

Drumea K, Yang ZF, Rosmarin A. Retinoic acid signaling in myelopoiesis. *Curr Opin Hematol*, **2008**, *15*:37–41.

Duvic M, Talpur R, Ni X, et al. Phase 2 trial of oral vorinostat (suberoylanilide hydroxamic acid, SAHA) for refractory cutaneous T-cell lymphoma (CTCL). *Blood*, **2007**, *109*:31–39.

Endicott JA, Ling V. The biochemistry of P-glycoprotein–mediated multidrug resistance. *Annu Rev Biochem*, **1989,** *58*:137–171.

Farber S, Diamond LK, Mercer RD, et al. Temporary remissions in acute leukemia in children produced by folic antagonist 4-amethopteroylglutamic acid (aminopterin). *N Engl J Med*, **1948,** *238*:787–793.

Fischel JL, Formento P, Ciccolini J, et al. Impact of the oxaliplatin-5 fluorouracil-folinic acid combination on respective intracellular determinants of drug activity. *Br J Cancer*, **2002,** *86*:1162–1168.

Flanagan SA, Robinson BW, Krokosky CM, Shewach DS. Mismatched nucleotides as the lesions responsible for radiosensitization with gemcitabine: A new paradigm for antimetabolite radiosensitizers. *Mol Cancer Ther*, **2007**, *6*:1858–1868.

Forconi F, Fabbri A, Lenoci M, et al. Low-dose oral fludarabine plus cyclophosphamide in elderly patients with untreated and relapsed or refractory chronic lymphocytic leukaemia. *Hematol Oncol*, **2008**, *26*:247–251.

Forghieri F, Luppi M, Morselli M, Potenza L. Cytarabine-related lung infiltrates on high resolution computerized tomography: A possible complication with benign outcome in leukemic patients. *Haematologica*, **2007**, *92*:e85–e90.

Fox E, Razzouk BI, Widemann BC, et al. Phase 1 trial and pharmacokinetic study of arsenic trioxide in children and adolescents with refractory or relapsed acute leukemia, including acute promyelocytic leukemia or lymphoma. *Blood*, **2008**, *111*:566–573.

Friesen C, Herr I, Krammer PH, Debatin KM. Involvement of the CD95 (APO-1/FAS) receptor/ligand system in drug-induced apoptosis in leukemia cells. *Nat Med*, **1996,** *2*:574–577.

Fukuoka M, Niitani H, Suzuki A, et al. A phase II study of CPT-11, a new derivative of camptothecin, for previously untreated non-small-cell lung cancer. *J Clin Oncol*, **1992,** *10*:16–20.

Gallagher RE. Retinoic acid resistance in acute promyelocytic leukemia. *Leukemia*, **2002,** *16*:1940–1958.

Gandhi V. Questions about gemcitabine dose rate: Answered or unanswered? *J Clin Oncol*, **2007**, *25*:5691–5694.

Garcia ST, McQuillan A, Panasci L. Correlation between the cytotoxicity of melphalan and DNA crosslinks as detected by the ethidium bromide fluorescence assay in the F_1 variant of B_{16} melanoma cells. *Biochem Pharmacol*, **1988,** *37*:3189–3192.

Gardner ER, Dahut WL, Scripture CD, et al. Randomized crossover pharmacokinetic study of solvent-based paclitaxel and nabpaclitaxel. *Clin Cancer Res*, **2008**, *14*:4200–4205.

Gerth K, Bedorf N, Höfle G, et al. Epothilons A and B: Antifungal and cytotoxic compounds from *Sorangium cellulosum* (Myxobacteria). Production, physico-chemical and biological properties. *J Antibiot (Tokyo)*, **1996**, *49*:560–563.

Gilbert MR, Supko JG, Batchelor T, et al. Phase I clinical and pharmacokinetic study of irinotecan in adults with recurrent malignant glioma. *Clin Cancer Res*, **2003,** *9*:2940–2949.

Gilman A, Philips FS. The biological actions and therapeutic applications of the β-chlorethylamines and sulfides. *Science*, **1946,** *103*:409–415.

Giovannetti E, Del Tacca M, Mey V, et al. Transcription analysis of human equilibrative nucleoside transporter-1 predicts survival in pancreas cancer patients treated with gemcitabine. *Cancer Res*, **2006**, *66*:3928–3935.

Go RS, Adjei AA. Review of the comparative pharmacology and clinical activity of cisplatin and carboplatin. *J Clin Oncol*, **1999,** *17*:409–422.

Gradishar WJ, Tjulandin S, Davidson N, et al. Phase III trial of nanoparticle albumin-bound paclitaxel compared with polyethylated castor oil-based paclitaxel in women with breast cancer. *J Clin Oncol*, **2005**, *23*:7794–7803.

Grosso F, Sanfilippo R, Virdis E, et al. Trabectedin in myxoid liposarcomas (MLS): A long-term analysis of a single-institution series. *Ann Oncol*, **2009,** *20*:1439–1444.

Grever MR, Doan CA, Kraut EH. Pentostatin in the treatment of hairy-cell leukemia. *Best Pract Res Clin Haematol*, **2003**, *16*:91–99.

Grewal J, Dellinger CA, Yung WK. Fatal reactivation of hepatitis B with temozolomide. *N Engl J Med*, **2007**, *356*:1591–1592.

Grochow LB. Busulfan disposition: The role of therapeutic monitoring in bone marrow transplantation induction regimens. *Semin Oncol*, **1993,** *20*:18–25.

Grogan L, Sotos GA, Allegra CJ. Leucovorin modulation of fluorouracil. *Oncology (Williston Park)*, **1993,** *7*:63–72; discussion 75–76.

Gupta A, Lawrence AT, Krishnan K, et al. Current concepts in the mechanisms and management of drug-induced QT prolongation and torsade de pointes. *Am Heart J*, **2007**, *153*:891–899.

Hausknecht RU. Methotrexate and misoprostol to terminate early pregnancy. *N Engl J Med*, **1995,** *333*:537–540.

Hawkins DS, Park JR, Thomson BG, et al. Asparaginase pharmacokinetics after intensive polyethylene glycol-conjugated L-asparaginase therapy for children with relapsed acute lymphoblastic leukemia. *Clin Cancer Res*, **2004,** *10*:5335–5341.

He X, Batchelor TT, Grossman S, et al. Determination of procarbazine in human plasma by liquid chromatography with electrospray ionization mass spectrometry. *J Chromatogr B Analyt Technol Biomed Life Sci*, **2004,** *799*:281–291.

Hegi ME, Liu L, Herman JG, et al. Correlation of O6-methylguanine methyltransferase (MGMT) promoter methylation with clinical outcomes in glioblastoma and clinical strategies to modulate MGMT activity. *J Clin Oncol*, **2008**, *26*:4189–4199.

Heinemann V, Hertel LW, Grindey GB, Plunkett W. Comparison of the cellular pharmacokinetics and toxicity of 2′,2′-difluorodeoxycytidine and 1-β-D-arabinofuranosylcytosine. *Cancer Res*, **1988**, *48*:4024–4031.

Heizer WD, Peterson JL. Acute myeloblastic leukemia following prolonged treatment of Crohn's disease with 6-mercaptopurine. *Dig Dis Sci*, **1998,** *43*:1791–1793.

Hoffmeister RT. Methotrexate therapy in rheumatoid arthritis: 15 years experience. *Am J Med*, **1983,** *75*:69–73.

Hogan TF, Citrin DL, Johnson BM, et al. o,p′-DDD (mitotane) therapy of adrenal cortical carcinoma: Observations on drug dosage, toxicity, and steroid replacement. *Cancer*, **1978,** *42*:2177–2181.

Huizing MT, Keung AC, Rosing H, et al. Pharmacokinetics of paclitaxel and metabolites in a randomized comparative study in platinum-pretreated ovarian cancer patients. *J Clin Oncol*, **1993,** *11*:2127–2135.

Humphreys BD, Sharman JP, Henderson JM, et al. Gemcitabine-associated thrombotic microangiopathy. *Cancer*, **2004,** *100*:2664–2670.

Ibrado AM, Huang Y, Fang G, Bhalla K. Bcl-xL overexpression inhibits taxol-induced Yama protease activity and apoptosis. *Cell Growth Differ*, **1996,** *7*:1087–1094.

Iyer L, King CD, Whitington PF, et al. Genetic predisposition to the metabolism of irinotecan (CPT-11). Role of uridine diphosphate glucuronosyltransferase isoform 1A1 in the glucuronidation of its active metabolite (SN-38) in human liver microsomes. *J Clin Invest*, **1998,** *101*:847–854.

Jabbour E, O'Brien S, Kantarjian H, et al. Neurologic complications associated with intrathecal liposomal cytarabine given prophylactically in combination with high-dose methotrexate and cytarabine to patients with acute lymphocytic leukemia. *Blood*, **2007**, *109*:3214–3218.

Josting A, Reiser M, Wickramanayake PD, et al. Dexamethasone, carmustine, etoposide, cytarabine, and melphalan (dexa-BEAM) followed by high-dose chemotherapy and stem cell rescue—A highly effective regimen for patients with refractory or relapsed indolent lymphoma. *Leuk Lymphoma*, **2000,** *37*:115–123.

Kamiya K, Huang P, Plunkett W. Inhibition of the 3′→5′ exonuclease human DNA polymerase by fludarabine-terminated DNA. *J Biol Chem*, **1996,** *271*:19428–19435.

Karran P, Attard N. Thiopurines in current medical practice: Molecular mechanisms and contributions to therapy-related cancer. *Nat Rev Cancer*, **2008**, *8*:24–36.

Kastan MB. Molecular determinants of sensitivity to antitumor agents. *Biochem Biophys Acta*, **1999,** *1424*:R37–R42.

Kemeny N, Huang Y, Cohen AM, et al. Hepatic arterial infusion of chemotherapy after resection of hepatic metastases from colorectal cancer. *N Engl J Med*, **1999**, *341*:2039–2048.

Kidd JG. Regression of transplanted lymphomas induced in vivo by means of normal guinea pig serum. 1. Course of transplanted cancers of various kinds in mice and rats given guinea pig serum, horse serum, or rabbit serum. *J Exp Med*, **1953,** *98*:565–582.

Kitamura T. Necessity of re-evaluation of estramustine phosphate sodium (EMP) as a treatment option for first-line monotherapy in advanced prostate cancer. *Int J Urol*, **2001,** *8*:33–36.

Koolen SLW, Huitema ADR, Jansen RS, et al. Pharmacokinetics of gemcitabine and metabolites in a patient with double-sided nephrectomy: A case report and review of the literature. *Oncologist,* **2009,** *14*:944–948.

Kos R, Wilding J. SPARC: a key player in the pathologies associated with obesity and diabetes. *Nat Rev Endocrinol*, **2010**, *6*:225–235.

Kramer OH, Knauer SK, Zimmerman D, et al. Histone deacetylase inhibitors and hydroxyurea modulate the cell cycle and cooperatively induce apoptosis. *Oncogene*, **2008**, *27*:732–740.

Kruh GD. Lustrous insights into cisplatin accumulation: Copper transporters. *Clin Cancer Res*, **2003,** *9*:5807–5809.

Krzakowski M, Provencio M, Utracka-Hutka B, et al. Oral vinorelbine and cisplatin as induction chemotherapy and concomitant chemoradiotherapy in stage III non-small cell lung cancer: Final results of an international phase II trial. *J Thorac Oncol*, **2008**, *3*:994–1002.

Kufe DW, Munroe D, Herrick D, et al. Effects of 1-β-D-arabinofuranosylcytosine incorporation on eukaryotic DNA template function. *Mol Pharmacol*, **1984,** *26*:128–134.

Kumkhaek C, Taylor JG 6th, Zhu J, et al. Fetal haemoglobin response to hydroxycarbamide treatment and sar1a promoter polymorphisms in sickle cell anaemia. *Br J Haematol*, **2008,** *141*:254–259.

Kuznetsov D, Alsikafi N, O'Connor R, Steinberg G. Intravesicular valrubicin in the treatment of carcinoma *in situ* of the bladder. *Expert Opin Pharmacother*, **2001,** *2*:1009–1013.

Lallemand-Breitenbach V, Jeanne M, Benhenda S, et al. Arsenic degrades PML or PML-RARalpha through a SUMO-triggered RNF4/ubiquitin-mediated pathway. *Nat Cell Biol*, **2008,** *10*:547–555.

Lamba JK, Crews K, Pounds S, et al. Pharmacogenetics of deoxycytidine kinase: Identification and characterization of novel genetic variants. *J Pharmacol Exp Ther*, **2007**, *323*: 935–945.

Lee JJ, Swain SM. The epothilones: Translating from the laboratory to the clinic. *Clin Cancer Res*, **2008**, *14*:1618–1624.

Leoni LM, Bailey B, Reifert J, et al. Bendamustine (Treanda) displays a distinct pattern of cytotoxicity and unique mechanistic features compared with other alkylating agents. *Clin Cancer Res*, **2008**, *14*:309–317.

Lerner HJ. Acute myelogenous leukemia in patients receiving chlorambucil as long-term adjuvant chemotherapy for stage II breast cancer. *Cancer Treat Rep*, **1978,** *62*:1135–1138.

Liau S, Whang E. HMGA1 is a molecular determinant of chemoresistance to gemcitabine in pancreatic adenocarcinoma. *Clin Cancer Res*, **2008,** *14*:1284–1285.

Liliemark J, Juliusson G. On the pharmacokinetics of 2-chloro-2′-deoxyadenosine in humans. *Cancer Res*, **1991,** *51*: 5570–5572.

Lipshultz SE, Rifai N, Dalton VM, et al. The effect of dexrazoxane on myocardial injury in doxorubicin-treated children with acute lymphoblastic leukemia. *N Engl J Med*, **2004,** *351*: 145–153.

Liu J, Lu Y, Wu Q, et al. Mineral arsenicals in traditional medicines: Orpiment, realgar, and arsenolite. *J Pharmacol Exp Ther*, **2008**, *326*:363–368.

Lowe SW, Ruley HE, Jacks T, Housman DE. p53-Dependent apoptosis modulates the cytotoxicity of anticancer agents. *Cell*, **1993**, *74*:957–967.

Ludlum DB. DNA alkylation by the haloethylnitrosoureas: Nature of modifications produced and their enzymatic repair or removal. *Mutat Res*, **1990,** *233*:117–126.

Mann G, Steiner M, Attarbaschi A. Clinical significance of anti-asparaginase antibodies in childhood acute lymphoblastic leukemia. *Leuk Lymphoma*, **2007**, *48*:849–850.

Mansson E, Flordal E, Liliemark J, et al. Down-regulation of deoxycytidine kinase in human leukemic cell lines resistant to cladribine and clofarabine and increased ribonucleotide reductase activity contributes to fludarabine resistance. *Biochem Pharmacol*, **2003,** *65*:237–247.

Matijasevic Z, Boosalis M, Mackay W, et al. Protection against chloroethylnitrosourea cytotoxicity by eukaryotic 3-methyladenine DNA glycosylase. *Proc Natl Acad Sci U S A*, **1993,** *90*:11855–11859.

Meijer C, Mulder NH, Hospers GA, et al. The role of glutathione in resistance to cisplatin in a human small cell lung cancer cell line. *Br J Cancer*, **1990,** *62*:72–77.

Milano G, Etienne MC, Pierrefite V, et al. Dihydropyrimidine dehydrogenase deficiency and fluorouracil-related toxicity. *Br J Cancer*, **1999,** *79*:627–630.

Miyake K, Mickley L, Litman T, et al. Molecular cloning of cDNAs which are highly overexpressed in mitoxantrone-resistant cells: Demonstration of homology to ABC transport genes. *Cancer Res*, **1999,** *59*:8–13.

Moeller A, Ask K, Warburton D, et al. The bleomycin animal model: A useful tool to investigate treatment options for idiopathic pulmonary fibrosis? *Int J Biochem Cell Biol*, **2008**, *40*:362–382.

Moghrabi A, Levy DE, Asselin B, et al. Results of the Dana-Farber Cancer Institute ALL Consortium Protocol 95-01 for children with acute lymphoblastic leukemia. *Blood*, **2007**, *109*:896–904.

Molina JR. Pralatrexate, a dihydrofolate reductase inhibitor of the potential treatment of several malignancies. *IDrugs*, **2008**, *11*:508–521.

Myers CE. Role of iron in anthracycline action. In: Hacker MP, Lazo JS, Tritton TR, eds. *Organ-Directed Toxicities of Anticancer Drugs*. Boston, Nijhoff, **1988,** pp. 17–30.

Neubauer A, Maharry K, Mrózek K, et al. Patients with acute myeloid leukemia and RAS mutations benefit most from postremission high-dose cytarabine: A Cancer and Leukemia Group B study. *J Clin Oncol*, **2008**, *26*:4603–4609.

Nicolao P, Giometto B. Neurological toxicity of ifosfamide. *Oncology*, **2003,** *65*:11–16.

Nicolaou KC, Yang Z, Liu JJ, et al. Total synthesis of Taxol. *Nature*, **1994,** *367*:630–634.

Nilsson C, Aschan J, Ringden O, et al. The effect of metronidazole on busulfan pharmacokinetics in patients undergoing hemapoietic stem cell transplantation. *Bone Marrow Transplant*, **2003,** *31*:429–435.

O'Connor OA, Hamlin PA, Portlock C, et al. Pralatrexate, a novel class of antifol with high affinity for the reduced folate carrier-type 1, produces marked complete and durable remission in a diversity of chemotherapy refractory cases of T-cell lymphoma. *Br J Haematol*, **2007**, *139*:425–428.

Ohhashi S, Ohuchida K, Mizumoto K, et al. Down-regulation of deoxycytidine kinase enhances acquired resistance to gemcitabine in pancreatic cancer. *Anticancer Res*, **2008,** *28*: 2205–2212.

Oki Y, Aoki E, Issa JP. Decitabine—Bedside to bench. *Crit Rev Oncol Hematol*, **2007**, *61*:140–152.

O'Reilly S, Rowinsky EK, Slichenmyer W, et al. Phase I and pharmacologic study of topotecan in patients with impaired renal function. *J Clin Oncol*, **1996,** *14*:3062–3073.

O'Sullivan JM, Huddart RA, Norman AR, et al. Predicting the risk of bleomycin lung toxicity in patients with germ-cell tumours. *Ann Oncol,* **2003**, *14*:91–96.

Paré L, Marcuello E, Altés A, et al. Pharmacogenetic prediction of clinical outcome in advanced colorectal cancer patients receiving oxaliplatin/5-fluorouracil as first-line chemotherapy. *Br J Cancer*, **2008**, *99*:1050–1055. Erratum in: *Br J Cancer*, **2009**, *100*:1368.

Piekarz RL, Frye R, Turner M, et al. Phase II multi-institutional trial of the histone deacetylase inhibitor romidepsin as monotherapy for patients with cutaneous T-cell lymphoma. *J Clin Oncol*, **2009**, *27*:5410–5417.

Piekarz RL, Frye AR, Wright JJ, et al. Cardiac studies in patients treated with depsipeptide, FK228, in a phase II trial for T-cell lymphoma. *Clin Cancer Res*, **2006**, *12*:3762–3773.

Platt OS. Hydroxyurea for the treatment of sickle cell anemia. *N Engl J Med*, **2008**, *358*:1362–1369.

Plunkett W, Gandhi V. Cellular metabolism of nucleoside analogs in CLL: Implications for drug development. In: Cheson B, ed. *Chronic Lymphocytic Leukemia: Scientific Advances and Clinical Developments*. New York, Marcel Dekker, **1993,** p. 197.

Pui CH, Relling MV, Downing JR. Mechanisms of disease: Acute lymphoblastic leukemia. *N Engl J Med*, **2004,** *350*: 1535–1548.

Pui CH, Relling MV, Rivera GK, et al. Epipodophyllotoxin-related acute myeloid leukemia: A study of 35 cases. *Leukemia*, **1995,** *9*:1990–1996.

Preisler HD, Rustum Y, Priore RL. Relationship between leukemic cell retention of cytosine arabinoside triphosphate and the duration of remission in patients with acute non-lymphocytic leukemia. *Eur J Cancer Clin Oncol*, **1985**, *21*:23–30.

Pullarkat ST, Stoehlmacher J, Ghaderi V, et al. Thymidylate synthase gene polymorphism determines response and toxicity of 5-FU chemotherapy. *Pharmacogenomics J*, **2001,** *1*:65–70.

Ranganathan S, Benetatos CA, Colarusso PJ, et al. Altered beta-tubulin isotype expression in paclitaxel-resistant human prostate carcinoma cells. *Br J Cancer*, **1998**, *77*:562–566.

Read WL, Mortimer JE, Picus J. Severe interstitial pneumonitis associated with docetaxel administration. *Cancer*, **2002,** *94*:847–853.

Reed E. Platinum-DNA adduct, nucleotide excision repair and platinum based anti-cancer chemotherapy. *Cancer Treat Rev*, **1998,** *24*:331–344.

Richardson PG, Barlogie B, Berenson J, et al. A phase 2 study of bortezomib in relapsed, refractory myeloma. *N Engl J Med*, **2003,** *348*:2609–2617.

Robieux I, Sorio R, Borsatti E, et al. Pharmacokinetics of vinorelbine in patients with liver metastases. *Clin Pharmacol Ther*, **1996**, *59*:32–40.

Roussel MJ, Lanotte M. Maturation sensitive and resistant t(15,17) NB4 cell lines as tools for APL physiopathology, nomenclature of cells and repertory of their known genetic alterations and phenotypes. *Oncogene*, **2001**, *20*:7287–7291.

Rowinsky EK, Donehower RC. Paclitaxel. *N Engl J Med*, **1995,** *332*:1004–1014.

Sanford M, Lyseng-Williamson KA. Nelarabine. *Drugs*, **2008**, *68*:439–447.

Schimke RT, Kaufman RJ, Alt FW, Kellems RF. Gene amplification and drug resistance in cultured murine cells. *Science*, **1978,** *202*:1051–1055.

Sebti SM, Jani JP, Mistry JS, et al. Metabolic inactivation: A mechanism of human tumor resistance to bleomycin. *Cancer Res*, **1991,** *51*:227–232.

Serrano J, Palmeira CM, Kuehl DW, Wallace KB. Cardioselective and cumulative oxidation of mitochondrial

DNA following subchronic doxorubicin administration. *Biochem Biophys Acta*, **1999,** *1411*:201–205.

Sharma S, Gong P, Temple B, et al. Molecular dynamic simulations of cisplatin- and oxaliplatin-d(GG) intrastrand cross-links reveal differences in their conformational dynamics. *J Mol Biol,* **2007,** *373*:1123–1140.

Slamon DJ, Leyland-Jones B, Shak S, et al. Use of chemotherapy plus a monoclonal antibody against HER2 for metastatic breast cancer that overexpresses HER2. *N Engl J Med*, **2001,** *344*:783–792.

Soares DG, Escargueil AE, Poindessous V, et al. Replication and homologous recombination repair regulate DNA double-strand break formation by the antitumor alkylator ecteinascidin 743. *Proc Natl Acad Sci U S A*, **2007**, *104*:13062–13067.

Sobell HM. The stereochemistry of actinomycin binding to DNA and its implications in molecular biology. *Prog Nucleic Acid Res Mol Biol*, **1973**, *13*:153–190.

Soignet SL, Maslak P, Wang ZG, et al. Complete remission after treatment of acute promyelocytic leukemia with arsenic trioxide. *N Engl J Med*, **1998,** *339*:1341–1348.

Sonneveld P, Schultz FW, Nooter K, Hahlen K. Pharmacokinetics of methotrexate and 7-hydroxy-methotrexate in plasma and bone marrow of children receiving low-dose oral methotrexate. *Cancer Chemother Pharmacol*, **1986**, *18*:111–116.

Souliotis VL, Kaila S, Boussiotis VA, et al. Accumulation of O^6-methylguanine in human blood leukocyte DNA during exposure to procarbazine and its relationships with dose and repair. *Cancer Res*, **1990**, *50*:2759–2764.

Stevens EV, Nishizuka S, Antony S, et al. Predicting cisplatin and trabectedin drug sensitivity in ovarian and colon cancers. *Mol Cancer Ther*, **2008**, *7*:10–18.

Stoller RG, Hande KR, Jacobs SA, et al. Use of plasma pharmacokinetics to predict and prevent methotrexate toxicity. *N Engl J Med*, **1977,** *297*:630–634.

Stresemann C, Lyko F. Modes of action of the DNA methyltransferase inhibitors azacytidine and decitabine. *Int J Cancer*, **2008**, *123*:8–13.

Sugimoto Y, Tsukahara S, Oh-hara T, et al. Decreased expression of DNA topoisomerase I in camptothecin-resistant tumor cell lines as determined by monoclonal antibody. *Cancer Res*, **1990,** *50*:6925–6930.

Swain SM, Whaley FS, Gerber MC, et al. Cardioprotection with dexrazoxane for doxorubicin-containing therapy in advanced breast cancer. *J Clin Oncol*, **1997,** *15*:1318–1332.

Synold TW, Takimoto CH, Doroshow JH, et al. Dose-escalating and pharmacologic study of oxaliplatin in adult cancer patients with impaired hepatic function: A National Cancer Institute Organ Dysfunction Working Group study. *Clin Cancer Res*, **2007**, *13*:3660–3666.

Tager AM, LaCamera P, Shea BS, et al. The lysophosphatidic acid receptor LPA1 links pulmonary fibrosis to lung injury by mediating fibroblast recruitment and vascular leak. *Nat Med*, **2008**, *14*:45–54.

Takimoto CH, Graham MA, Lockwood G, et al. Oxaliplatin pharmacokinetics and pharmacodynamics in adult cancer patients with impaired renal function. *Clin Cancer Res*, **2007**, *13*:4832–4839.

Tam CS, O'Brien S, Wierda W, et al. Long-term results of the fludarabine, cyclophosphamide, and rituximab regimen as initial therapy of chronic lymphocytic leukemia. *Blood*, **2008**, *112*:975–980.

Tamura H, Kohchi C, Yamada R, et al. Molecular cloning of a cDNA of a camptothecin-resistant human DNA topoisomerase I and identification of mutation sites. *Nucleic Acids Res*, **1991,** *19*:69–75.

Tavecchio M, Simone M, Erba E, et al. Role of homologous recombination in trabectedin-induced DNA damage. *Eur J Cancer*, **2008**, *44*:609–618.

Teichert J, Baumann F, Chao Q, et al. Characterization of two phase I metabolites of bendamustine in human liver microsomes and in cancer patients treated with bendamustine hydrochloride. *Cancer Chemother Pharmacol*, **2007**, *59*:759–770.

Tew K, Colvin M, Chabner BA. Alkylating agents. In: Chabner BA, Longo DL, eds. *Cancer Chemotherapy and Biotherapy: Principles and Practice*, 3rd ed. Philadelphia, Lippincott Williams & Wilkins, **2001,** pp. 373–414.

Thomas ES, Gomez HL, Li RK, et al. Ixabepilone plus capecitabine for metastatic breast cancer progressing after anthracycline and taxane treatment. *J Clin Oncol*, **2007**, *25*:5210–5217.

Tsao YP, Russo A, Nyamuswa G, et al. Interaction between replication forks and topoisomerase I-DNA cleavable complexes: Studies in a cell-free SV40 DNA replication system. *Cancer Res*, **1993,** *53*:5908–5914.

Twelves CJ, Dobbs NA, Gillies HC, et al. Doxorubicin pharmacokinetics: The effect of abnormal liver biochemistry tests. *Cancer Chemother Pharmacol*, **1998,** *42*:229–234.

Twelves C, Glynne-Jones R, Cassidy J, et al. Effect of hepatic dysfunction due to liver metastases on the pharmacokinetics of capecitabine and its metabolites. *Clin Cancer Res*, **1999,** *5*:1696–1702.

Twentyman PR. Bleomycin: Mode of action with particular reference to the cell cycle. *Pharmacol Ther*, **1983,** *23*:417–441.

Van Ark-Otte J, Kedde MA, van der Vijgh WJ, et al. Determinants of CPT-11 and SN-38 activities in human lung cancer cells. *Br J Cancer*, **1998,** *77*:2171–2176.

Van Triest B, Pinedo HM, Blaauwgeers JL, et al. Prognostic role of thymidylate synthase, thymidine phosphorylase/platelet-derived endothelial cell growth factor, and proliferation markers in colorectal cancer. *Clin Cancer Res*, **2000,** *6*:1063–1072.

Vassal G, Challine D, Koscielny S, et al. Chronopharmacology of high-dose busulfan in children. *Cancer Res*, **1993,** *53*:1534–1537.

Vogelzang NJ, Rusthoven JJ, Symanowski J, et al. Phase III study of pemetrexed in combination with cisplatin versus cisplatin alone in patients with malignant pleural mesothelioma. *J Clin Oncol*, **2003,** *21*:2636–2644.

Wall SM, Johansen MJ, Molony DA, et al. Effective clearance of methotrexate using high-flux hemodialysis membranes. *Am J Kidney Dis*, **1996,** *28*:846–854.

Walter N, Collard HR, King TE Jr. Current perspectives on the treatment of idiopathic pulmonary fibrosis. *Proc Am Thorac Soc,* **2006**, *3*:330–338.

Wang J, Lohman GJS, Stubbe J. Enhanced subunit interactions with gemcitabine-5′-diphosphate inhibit ribonucleotide reductase. *Proc Natl Acad Sci U S A*, **2007**, *104*:14324–14329.

Wang ZM, Chen ZP, Xu ZY, et al. In vitro evidence for homologous recombinational repair in resistance to melphalan. *J Natl Cancer Inst*, **2001,** *93*:1473–1478.

Wang ZY, Chen Z. Acute promyelocytic leukemia: From highly fatal to highly curable. *Blood,* **2008,** *111*:2505–2515.

Washtein WL. Thymidylate synthetase levels as a factor in 5-fluorodeoxyuridine and methotrexate cytotoxicity in gastrointestinal tumor cells. *Mol Pharmacol*, **1982,** *21*: 723–728.

Westerhof GR, Rijnboutt S, Schornagel JH, et al. Functional activity of the reduced folate carrier in KB, MA104, and IGROV-I cells expressing folate-binding protein. *Cancer Res*, **1995,** *55*:3795–3802.

Widemann, BC, Balis, FM, Murphy RF, et al. Carboxypeptidase-G2, thymidine, and leucovorin rescue in cancer patients with methotrexate-induced renal dysfunction. *J Clin Oncol*, **1997,** *15*:2125–2134.

Wiewrodt D, Nagel G, Dreimüller N, et al. MGMT in primary and recurrent human glioblastomas after radiation and chemotherapy and comparison with p53 status and clinical outcome. *Int J Cancer*, **2008**, *122*:1391–1399.

Williams ME, Walker AN, Bracikowski JP, et al. Ascending myeloencephalopathy due to intrathecal vincristine sulfate. A fatal chemotherapeutic error. *Cancer*, **1983,** *51*:2041–2147.

Witherspoon RP, Deeg HJ, Storer B, et al. Hematopoietic stem-cell transplantation for treatment-related leukemia or myelodysplasia. *J Clin Oncol*, **2001,** *19*:2134–2141.

Wortsman J, Soler NG. Mitotane. Spironolactone antagonism in Cushing's syndrome. *JAMA*, **1977,** *238*:2527.

Xie HJ, Yasar U, Lundgren S, et al. Role of polymorphic human CYP2B6 in cyclophosphamide bioactivation. *Pharmacogenomics*, **2003,** *3*:53–61.

Yang SW, Burgin AB Jr, Huizenga BN, et al. A eukaryotic enzyme that can disjoin dead-end covalent complexes between DNA and type I topoisomerases. *Proc Natl Acad Sci U S A*, **1996,** *93*:11534–11539.

Targeted Therapies: Tyrosine Kinase Inhibitors, Monoclonal Antibodies, and Cytokines

Bruce A. Chabner, Jeffrey Barnes, Joel Neal, Erin Olson, Hamza Mujagic, Lecia Sequist, Wynham Wilson, Dan L. Longo, Constantine Mitsiades, and Paul Richardson

Strategies for cancer drug discovery have evolved in step with the explosion of knowledge about the molecular underpinnings of cancer. Many new drugs either recently approved or in late stages of evaluation were designed to block the fundamental mutations that cause specific cancers: aberrant growth factor receptors, dysregulated intracellular signaling pathways, defective DNA repair and apoptosis, and tumor angiogenesis. The primary tools for inhibiting these new targets are either monoclonal antibodies that attack cell surface receptors and antigens, or synthetic small molecules that enter cells and engage critical enzymes. These two classes of drugs have very different pharmacological properties.

Monoclonal antibodies kill tumor cells by blocking cell surface receptor function and by recruiting immune cells and complement to the antigen–antibody complex. They may be armed to carry toxins or radionuclides to the cells of interest, thereby enhancing their cytotoxic effects. They generally are specific for a single receptor, have a long plasma $t_{1/2}$, and require only intermittent administration. Small molecules may attack the same targets and pathways as the monoclonals, but may also exert their effect by entering cells and inhibiting enzymatic functions (usually tyrosine kinase reactions). The small molecules often inhibit multiple enzymatic sites, have a broad spectrum of target kinases, and tend to be substrates of hepatic CYPs with a $t_{1/2}$ of 12-24 hours, and thus require daily oral administration. The two classes of drug, when targeted against the same pathway, may have significantly different spectra of antitumor activity. Thus, monoclonal antibodies to the epidermal growth factor receptor (EGFR) are effective in the treatment of head and neck and colon cancers, while small molecules, such as erlotinib and gefitinib, attack the intracellular tyrosine kinase function of the same receptor and have a different spectrum of antitumor activity (non–small cell lung cancer).

Because of the central importance of the specific target in cancer chemotherapy, we will center this discussion around the target rather than the specific type of drug.

PROTEIN TYROSINE KINASE INHIBITORS

Protein kinases are critical components of signal transduction pathways that regulate cell growth and adaptation to the extracellular environment. These signaling pathways influence gene transcription and/or DNA synthesis, as well as cytoplasmic events. The human genome contains ~550 protein kinases and 130 phosphoprotein phosphatases that regulate the phosphorylation states of key signaling molecules. Protein kinases can be classified into three different categories: kinases that specifically phosphorylate tyrosine residues, kinases that phosphorylate serine and threonine residues, and kinases with activity toward all three residues. Tyrosine kinases can be further subdivided into proteins that have an extracellular ligand-binding domain (receptor tyrosine kinases) and enzymes that are confined to the cytoplasm or nuclear cellular compartment (nonreceptor tyrosine kinases). Growth factors and other ligands bind to and activate the receptor tyrosine kinases under physiological conditions. In a growing number of human malignancies, mutations that constitutively activate protein tyrosine kinases are implicated in malignant transformation; thus, protein tyrosine kinases are targets for cancer therapy.

Inhibitors of the BCR-ABL Kinase: Imatinib, Dasatinib, and Nilotinib

Imatinib mesylate (STI 571, GLEEVEC, GLIVEC) was the first molecularly targeted protein kinase inhibitor to receive FDA approval. It targets the BCR-ABL tyrosine kinase, which underlies chronic myelogenous leukemia (CML). A single molecular event, in this case the 9:22 translocation, leads to expression of the Abelson proto-oncogene kinase ABL fused to BCR (breakpoint cluster region), yielding a constitutively activated protein kinase, BCR-ABL, and then the malignant phenotype. Imatinib and the related compounds dasatinib and nilotinib induce clinical and molecular remissions in >90% of CML patients in the chronic phase of disease. Imatinib effectively treats other tumors that carry related tyrosine kinase mutations, including GI stromal tumors (driven by c-KIT mutation) (Blanke et al., 2008), and hypereosinophilia syndrome, chronic myelomonocytic leukemia, and dermatofibrosarcoma protuberans (all driven by mutations that activate the platelet-derived growth factor receptor, PDGFR) (Sirvent et al., 2003).

Chemistry. Imatinib was identified through high-throughput screening against the BCR-ABL kinase. The lead compound of this series, a 2-phenylaminopyrimidine, had low potency and poor specificity, inhibiting both serine/threonine and tyrosine kinases (Buchdunger et al., 2001). The addition of a 3′-pyridyl group at the 3′ position of the pyrimidine enhanced its potency. Further modifications resulted in improved activity against PDGFR and c-KIT and loss of serine/threonine kinase inhibition. Introduction of *N*-methylpiperazine as a polar side chain greatly improved water solubility and oral bioavailability, yielding imatinib, an inhibitor of the closed, or inactive, configuration of the kinase:

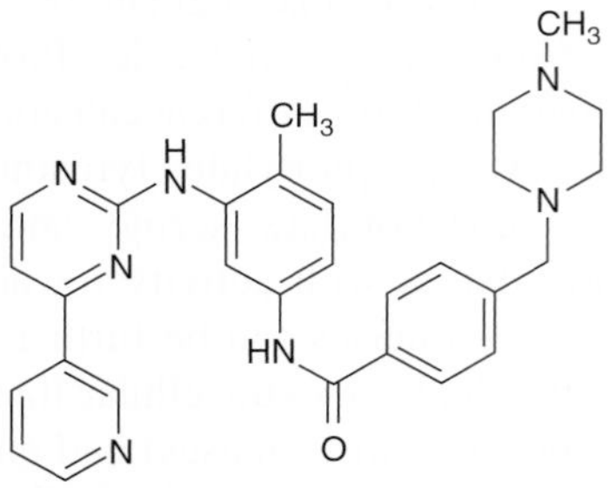

Dasatinib (BMS-354825, SPRYCEL), a second-generation BCR-ABL inhibitor, was developed using a series of substituted 2-(aminopyridyl) and 2-(aminopyrimidinyl) thiazol-5-carboxyamides. It inhibits the Src kinase, and unlike imatinib, it binds both the open and closed configurations of the BCR-ABL kinase (Shah et al., 2004).

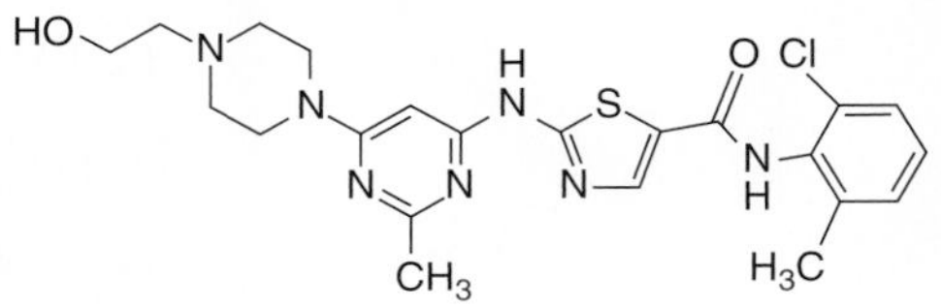

Nilotinib (AMN107, TASIGNA) was designed to have increased potency and specificity compared to imatinib. Its structure, based on crystallographic studies of the BCR-ABL kinase, promotes hydrogen bonding to Glu286 and Asp381 (Weisberg et al., 2005) and overcomes mutations that cause imatinib resistance.

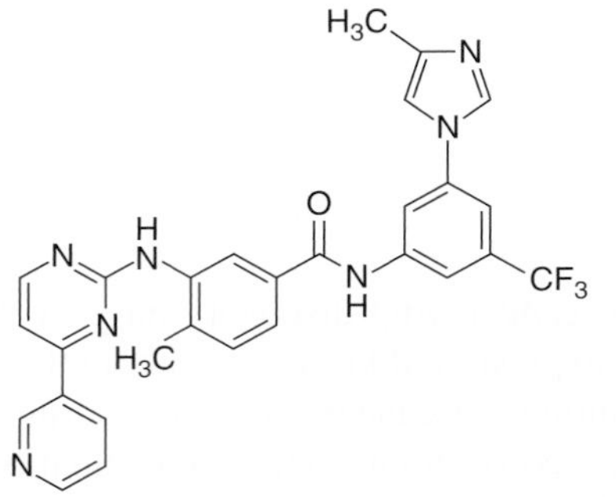

Mechanism of Action. Crystallographic and mutagenesis studies indicate that imatinib and nilotinib bind to a segment of the kinase domain that fixes the enzyme in a closed or nonfunctional state, in which the protein is unable to bind its substrate/phosphate donor, ATP (Weisberg et al., 2005). The three BCR-ABL kinase inhibitors differ in their potency of inhibition, their binding specificities, and their susceptibility to resistance mutations in the target enzyme. Dasatinib [$(IC_{50}) = <1$ nM] and nilotinib [$(IC_{50}) = <20$ nM] (Weisberg, 2005) inhibit BCR-ABL kinase more potently than does imatinib [$(IC_{50}) = 100$ nM].

Mechanisms of Resistance. Resistance to the tyrosine kinase inhibitors arises from point mutations in three separate segments of the kinase domain (Figure 62–1). The contact points between imatinib and the enzyme become sites of mutations in drug-resistant leukemic cells; these mutations prevent tight binding of the drug and lock the enzyme in its open configuration, in which it has access to substrate. Most such mutations hold the enzyme in its open and enzymatically active confirmation. The most common resistance mutations affect amino acids 255 and 315, both of which serve as contact points for imatinib; these mutations confer high-level resistance to imatinib and nilotinib. Dasatinib is unaffected by mutation at 255 but is ineffective in the presence of mutation at 315. Nilotinib retains inhibitory activity in the presence of most point mutations (except at 315) that confer resistance to imatinib (Weisberg et al., 2005; O'Hare et al., 2005).

Other mutations affect the phosphate-binding region and the "activation loop" of the domain with varying degrees of associated resistance. Some mutations, such as at amino acids 351 and 355, do not affect response to dasatinib or nilotinib but confer low levels of resistance to imatinib (O'Hare et al., 2005; Corbin et al., 2003).

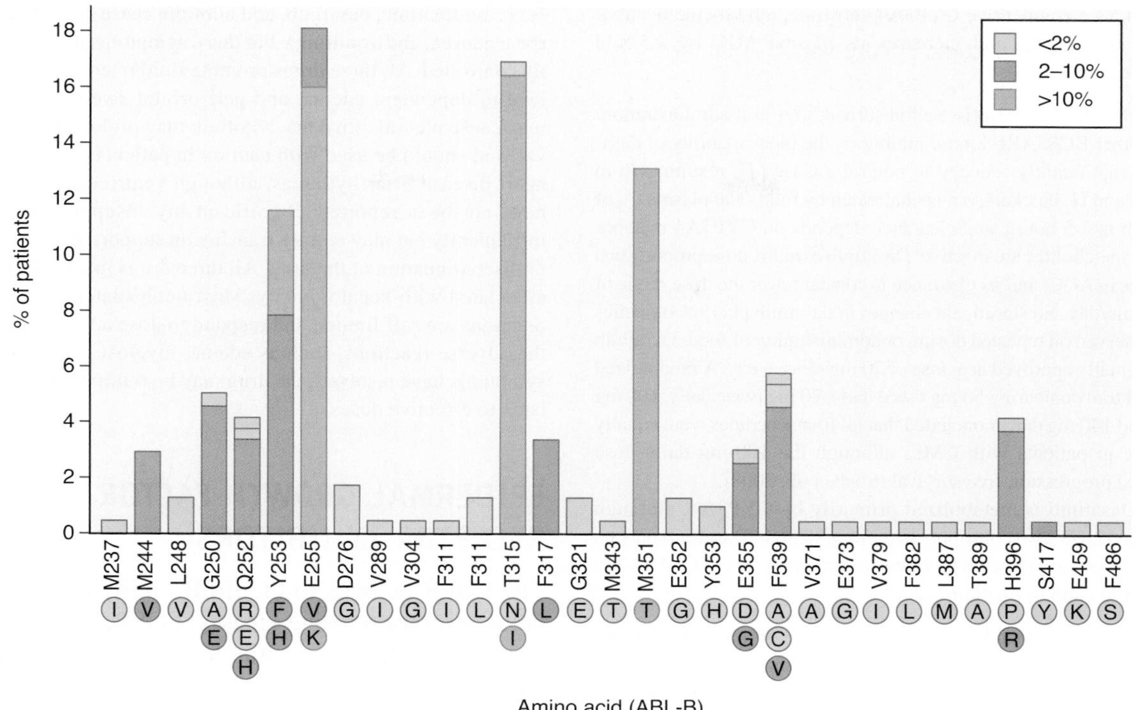

Figure 62–1. *The relative frequency of BCR-ABL kinase domain mutations detected at 31 different positions in clinical specimens from 245 patients in whom mutations were detected (219 with chronic myelocytic leukemia and 26 with Ph⁺ acute lymphoblastic leukemia).* (Reproduced with permission from Hughes et al., 2006. Copyright © 2006 American Society of Hematology. Copyright restrictions may apply.)

This finding may explain the clinical response of some resistant patients to dose escalation of imatinib.

Molecular studies of circulating tumor cells have detected resistance-mediating kinase mutations *prior* to initiation of therapy, particularly in patients with Ph^+ acute lymphoblastic leukemia (ALL) (Roche-Lestienne et al., 2003) or CML in blastic crisis. This finding strongly supports the hypothesis that drug-resistant cells arise through spontaneous mutation and expand under the selective pressure of drug exposure. Mutations may become detectable in the peripheral blood of patients receiving imatinib in the accelerated phase and in the late (>4 years from diagnosis) chronic phase of CML (Branford et al., 2003), heralding the onset of drug resistance.

Mechanisms other than BCR-ABL kinase mutation play a minor role in resistance to imatinib. Amplification of the wild-type kinase gene, leading to overexpression of the enzyme, has been identified in tumor samples from patients resistant to treatment (Morel et al., 2003). The multidrug resistant (*MDR*) gene, which codes for a drug efflux protein, confers resistance experimentally but has not been implicated in clinical resistance.

Finally, Philadelphia chromosome-negative clones lacking the BCR-ABL translocation and displaying the karyotype of myelodysplastic cells may emerge in patients receiving imatinib for CML and may progress to myelodysplasia (MDS) and to acute myelocytic leukemia (AML). Their origin is unclear.

Pharmacokinetics

Imatinib. Imatinib is well absorbed after oral administration and reaches maximal plasma concentrations within 2-4 hours. The elimination $t_{1/2}$ of imatinib and its major active metabolite, the *N*-desmethyl derivative, are ~18 and 40 hours, respectively. Mean imatinib area under the curve (AUC) increases proportionally with increasing dose in the range 25-1000 mg (Peng et al., 2004). Food does not change the pharmacokinetic profile of imatinib. Doses >300 mg/day achieve trough levels of 1 μM, which correspond to *in vitro* levels required to kill BCR-ABL–expressing cells. Inhibition of the BCR-ABL tyrosine kinase in white blood cells from patients with CML reaches a maximum in the dose range of 250-750 mg/day. Nonrandomized studies suggest that response may be restored in a minority of resistant patients with doses of 600 or 800 mg/day, as opposed to the standard 400 mg/day (Kantarjian et al., 2004). In the treatment of GI stromal cell tumors (GIST), higher doses (600 mg/day) may improve response rates.

CYP3A4 is the major enzyme responsible for metabolism of imatinib. CYPs 1A2, 2D6, 2C9, and 2C19 play minor roles in its metabolism. Clinicians must be cautious in introducing drugs that might interact with imatinib and CYP3A4. A single dose of ketoconazole, an inhibitor of CYP3A4, increases the maximal imatinib concentration in plasma and its plasma AUC by 26% and 40%, respectively. Co-administration of imatinib and rifampin, an inducer of CYP3A4, lowers the plasma imatinib AUC by 70%. Likewise, imatinib, as a competitive CYP3A4 substrate, inhibits the metabolism of simvastatin and increases its plasma AUC by 3.5-fold (O'Brien et al., 2003).

Dasatinib. Dasatinib also is well absorbed after oral administration. As for other BCR-ABL kinase inhibitors, the bioavailability of dasatinib is significantly reduced at neutral gastric pH, resulting from antacids and H_2 blockers, but is unaffected by food. The plasma $t_{1/2}$ of dasatinib is 3-5 hours, and clearance depends on CYP3A4 metabolism. Its metabolites are inactive. Dasatinib exhibits dose proportional increases in AUC, and its clearance is constant over the dose range of 15-240 mg/day. No significant changes in dasatinib pharmacokinetics were observed on repeated dosing or administration of food. Dasatinib was originally approved at a dose of 70 mg twice a day. A randomized phase III trial comparing 50 mg twice daily, 70 mg twice daily, 100 mg daily, and 140 mg daily concluded that all four schedules were equally effective in patients with CML, although the 100-mg daily dose improved progression-free survival (Shah et al., 2008).

Dasatinib is metabolized primarily by CYP3A4, although FMO3 and UGT also contribute to a minor degree. Dasatinib plasma concentrations are affected by inducers and inhibitors of CYP3A4 in a similar fashion to imatinib.

Nilotinib. Approximately 30% of an oral dose of nilotinib (400 mg twice daily) is absorbed after administration, and the drug achieves peak concentrations in plasma 3 hours after dosing. Unlike the other BCR-ABL inhibitors, nilotinib's bioavailability increases significantly in the presence of food (Kantarjian et al., 2006). The drug has a long plasma $t_{1/2}$ (~17 hours), and plasma concentrations reach a steady state only after 8 days of daily dosing. Doses >400 mg/day are associated with nonlinear increases in median serum concentrations, indicating saturation of GI absorption.

Like dasatinib and imatinib, nilotinib undergoes elimination through metabolism by CYP3A4; metabolism is affected by inducers, inhibitors, and competitors of the CYP3A4 pathway. Nilotinib is a substrate and inhibitor of P-glycoprotein.

Pharmacokinetics and Clinical Uses. These protein tyrosine kinase inhibitors have efficacy in diseases in which the ABL, *kit*, or PDGFR have dominant roles in driving the proliferation of the tumor, reflecting the presence of a mutation that results in constitutive activation of the kinase, either by fusion with another protein or via point mutations. Thus, imatinib shows remarkable therapeutic benefits in patients with chronic-phase CML (BCR-ABL), GIST (*kit* mutation positive), chronic myelomonocytic leukemia (EVT6-PDGFR translocation), hypereosinophilia syndrome (FIP1L1-PDGFR), and dermatofibrosarcoma protuberans (constitutive production of the ligand for PDGFR) (Druker, 2004). It is the agent of choice for GIST patients with metastatic disease and as adjuvant therapy of *c-kit*–positive GIST (DeMatteo et al., 2009). GIST biology is particularly instructive, as patients with an exon 11 mutation of *kit* have a significantly higher partial response rate (72%) than those with no detectable *kit* mutations (9%) (Heinrich et al., 2003). The currently recommended dose of imatinib is 400-600 mg/day. Dasatinib is approved for patients with CML resistant or intolerant to imatinib in both chronic (100 mg/day) and advanced phases of disease (70 mg twice daily), and for use combined with cytotoxic chemotherapy in patients with Ph$^+$ ALL who are resistant or intolerant to prior therapies. Nilotinib is approved for patients with CML resistant to or intolerant of prior imatinib therapy.

Toxicity. Imatinib, dasatinib, and nilotinib cause GI distress (diarrhea, nausea, and vomiting), but these symptoms usually are easily controlled. All three drugs promote fluid retention, which may lead to dependent edema, and peri-orbital swelling. Dasatinib may cause pleural effusions. Nilotinib may prolong the QT interval, and should be used with caution in patients with underlying heart disease or arrhythmias, although ventricular arrhythmias have not been reported. Significant myelosuppression occurs infrequently but may require transfusion support, dose reduction, or discontinuation of the drug. All three drugs in this class can be associated with hepatotoxicity. Most nonhematological adverse reactions are self limited and respond to dose adjustments. After the adverse reactions, such as edema, myelosuppression, or GI symptoms have resolved, the drug may be reinitiated and titrated back to effective doses.

EPIDERMAL GROWTH FACTOR RECEPTOR INHIBITORS

The EGFR belongs to the ErbB family of transmembrane receptor tyrosine kinases. EGFR, also known as ErbB1 or HER1, is essential for the growth and differentiation of epithelial cells. Ligand binding to the extracellular domain of EGFR family members causes receptor dimerization and stimulates the protein tyrosine kinase activity of the intracellular domain, resulting in autophosphorylation of several Tyr residues in the C-terminal domain. Recognition of the phosphotyrosines by other proteins initiates protein-protein interactions that result in stimulation of a variety of signaling pathways, including MAPK, PI3K/Akt, and STAT pathways (Figure 62–2) (Schlessinger, 2000). In epithelial cancers, overexpression (or mutational activations) of the EGFR is a common finding and, to some extent, creates a dependence on EGFR signaling in these tumors (Hynes and Lane, 2005).

Two separate classes of drugs that target the EGFR pathway have become important agents in the therapy of solid tumors. The EGFR tyrosine kinase inhibitors erlotinib and gefitinib bind to the kinase domain and block the enzymatic function of EGFR. The monoclonal antibodies cetuximab and panitumumab bind specifically to the extracellular domain of EGFR. They inhibit EGFR-dependent signaling through inhibition of ligand-dependent activation and receptor dimerization, downregulation of EGFR expression, and induction of antibody-dependent cell-mediated cytotoxicity (Ciardiello and Tortora, 2008).

Gefitinib

Chemistry. Gefitinib was identified through screens that demonstrated its inhibition of EGFR tyrosine

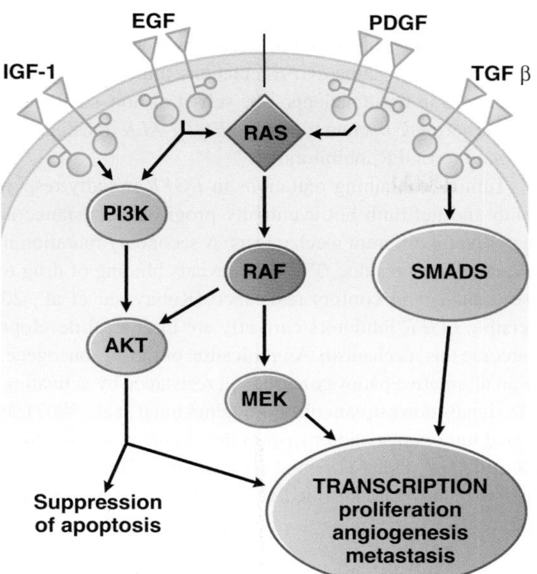

Figure 62–2. *Growth factor signaling.* Binding of agonist ligands to growth factor receptors causes receptor dimerization and activation of cytosolic protein kinase domains, leading to activation of multiple signaling pathways. Shown here are the RAS/MAPK/ERK, PI3K, and SMAD pathways, each of which is activated by receptors or cross-talk from adjacent pathways. Their signals regulate proliferation, metabolism, survival, and the synthesis of other growth factors, such as the vascular endothelial growth factor (VEGF).

kinase activity and ability to kill EGFR-dependent cell lines.

GEFITINIB

Mechanism of Action. Gefitinib inhibits the EGFR tyrosine kinase by virtue of competitive blockade of ATP binding. Gefitinib has an IC_{50} of 20-80 nM for the EGFR enzyme but is significantly less potent against HER2 (ErbB2/neu). Gefitinib has antitumor activity in human xenograft tumors that exhibit high levels of EGFR expression.

Absorption, Distribution, and Elimination. Following oral administration of gefitinib, peak plasma concentrations are achieved within 3-7 hours, and oral bioavailability approaches 60%. Administration of 225 mg/day orally results in steady-state levels of 200 ng/mL after 7-10 doses. The mean terminal $t_{1/2}$ is 41 hours. Elimination of gefitinib primarily occurs by hepatic CYP3A4 metabolism.

Therapeutic Uses. Gefitinib initially was approved for the third-line treatment of patients with non–small cell lung cancer based on promising results in two small clinical trials. However, a larger, randomized, placebo-controlled trial failed to show an effect on survival, leading the FDA to restrict its use to patients who have previously received clinical benefit from the drug (Thatcher et al., 2005). Gefitinib continues to be widely used outside the U.S. Two large trials have failed to demonstrate a benefit of gefitinib in combination with chemotherapy. The standard dose is 250 mg daily.

Retrospective analysis of multiple studies revealed that patients who were nonsmokers, Asians, or women were most likely to respond to gefitinib. Tumors from these patients frequently have characteristic activating mutations in *EGFR* (Sequist and Lynch, 2008). These mutations mostly fall into two groups: 1) small in-frame deletions within exon 19 and 2) the L858R point mutation. Trials that randomized never- and light-smoking patients to first-line gefitinib or to chemotherapy demonstrated a 70% response rate to gefitinib in patients with an activating *EGFR* mutation, compared with responses in only 1% in patients without an *EGFR* mutation. In patients with *EGFR*-mutant tumors, the response rate to gefitinib was double the response to standard chemotherapy. Therefore, mounting evidence supports the use of gefitinib, and potentially erlotinib, as first-line therapy in patients selected for the presence of sensitizing *EGFR* mutations.

Adverse Effects and Drug Interactions. Diarrhea and pustular/papular rash occur in ~50% of patients taking gefitinib. Other side effects include dry skin, nausea, vomiting, pruritus, anorexia, and fatigue. Most adverse effects occur within the first month of therapy and are tolerable when managed with supportive medications and dose reductions. Asymptomatic increases in liver transaminases may necessitate dose reduction or discontinuation of therapy. Interstitial lung disease, often associated with symptoms of cough and dyspnea, occurs in <2% of patients receiving gefitinib but may have a fatal outcome.

Exposure to gefitinib is not significantly altered by food; however, co-administration of drugs that cause sustained elevations in gastric pH reduce mean gefitinib AUC by 47%. Metabolism of gefitinib is predominantly via CYP3A4. Substances that induce CYP3A4 activity (e.g., phenytoin, carbamazepine, rifampin, barbiturates, St. John's wort) decrease gefitinib plasma concentrations and efficacy; conversely, inhibitors of CYP3A4 (e.g., itraconazole, ketoconazole) increase plasma concentrations. Patients using warfarin should be monitored closely for elevation of the INR while taking gefitinib.

Erlotinib

Erlotinib (TARCEVA) is a quinazolinamine inhibitor of HER1/EGFR tyrosine kinase.

ERLOTINIB

Mechanism of Action. Erlotinib is a potent inhibitor of the EGFR tyrosine kinase. Like gefitinib, erlotinib competitively inhibits ATP binding at the active site of the kinase. Erlotinib has an IC_{50} of 2 nM for the EGFR kinase. Tumors harboring *k-ras* mutations and *EML4-ALK* translocations do not respond to EGFR kinase inhibitors.

Absorption, Distribution, and Excretion. Erlotinib is ~60% absorbed after oral administration but should not be taken with food, which increases its bioavailability to ~100%. Peak plasma levels occur 4 hours after an oral dose. Erlotinib has a $t_{1/2}$ of 36 hours and is metabolized by CYP3A4 and to a lesser extent by CYPs 1A2 and 1A1. The standard daily dose of erlotinib results in a plasma AUC approximately one order of magnitude greater than the AUC of gefitinib.

Therapeutic Uses. Erlotinib is approved for second-line treatment of patients with locally advanced or metastatic non–small cell lung cancer. FDA approval was based on an improvement in overall survival in a large multi-national trial comparing oral erlotinib, 150 mg daily, to placebo (Shepherd et al., 2005). Results from two subsequent trials showed no clinical benefit from the combination of erlotinib with platinum-based chemotherapy as compared to chemotherapy alone.

Erlotinib also is approved for first-line treatment of patients with locally advanced, unresectable, or metastatic pancreatic cancer in combination with gemcitabine. A large double-blinded study of 569 patients demonstrated a modest 2-week improvement in overall survival in patients who received 100 mg of erlotinib plus gemcitabine, as compared with patients who received gemcitabine alone (Moore et al., 2007). The recommended dose of erlotinib in non–small cell lung cancer is a 150-mg tablet daily. In pancreatic cancer, the dose is a 100-mg tablet daily. It should be taken at least 1 hour before or 2 hours after a meal.

Adverse Effects and Drug Interactions. As with gefitinib, the most common adverse reactions in patients receiving erlotinib are diarrhea, an acneform rash, anorexia, and fatigue. Serious or fatal interstitial lung disease occurs with a frequency of 0.7-2.5%. Hepatic function deserves close monitoring because serious or fatal hepatic failure due to erlotinib has been reported, particularly in patients with baseline hepatic dysfunction. Other rare but serious toxicities include GI perforation, renal failure, arterial thrombosis, microangiopathic hemolytic anemia, hand-foot skin reaction, and corneal perforation or ulceration. Erlotinib therapy may cause rare cases of Stevens-Johnson syndrome/toxic epidermal necrolysis.

Concurrent use of proton-pump inhibitors decreases the bioavailability of erlotinib by 50%. As with gefitinib, plasma levels can vary dramatically due to drug interactions with inducers or inhibitors of CYP3A4. Patients using warfarin may experience elevations of the international normalized ratio (INR) while taking erlotinib. Smoking accelerates metabolic clearance of erlotinib by 24% and may decrease its antitumor effects.

Resistance to Gefitinib and Erlotinib

Patients with non–small cell lung cancer who initially respond to erlotinib or gefitinib have tumors that are dependent on the EGFR signaling pathway. Clinical response to these agents is strongly associated with the presence of sensitizing mutations in EGFR as described in "Therapeutic Uses" under "Gefitinib," but response is less strongly correlated with overexpression or amplification of EGFR (Sequist and Lynch, 2008). Therapy directed at the EGFR may delay disease progression in patients with non–small cell lung cancers that lack activating *EGFR* mutations, although response rates approach zero in these patients. The subset of non–small cell lung tumors harboring *k-ras* mutations and *EML4-ALK* translocations do not respond to EGFR inhibitors.

Tumors containing mutations in *EGFR* initially respond to erlotinib and gefitinib but eventually progress. Resistance arises through several different mechanisms. A secondary mutation in the *EGFR* gatekeeper residue, T790M, prevents binding of drug to the kinase domain and confers resistance (Kobayashi et al., 2005). Irreversible *EGFR* inhibitors currently are in clinical development to overcome this mechanism. Amplification of the *met* oncogene provides an alternative pathway to clinical resistance by activating cell growth signals downstream of *EGFR* (Engelman et al., 2007). *MET*-amplified tumors respond *in vitro* to the simultaneous inhibition of EGFR and *MET*. Other potential mechanisms of resistance include activation of downstream mediators, efflux of drug, and altered receptor trafficking.

Cetuximab

Cetuximab is a monoclonal antibody to the extracellular domain of the EGFR. Such antibodies, although sharing the same target with erlotinib and gefitinib and having a similar side effect profile, have a different spectrum of antitumor activity.

Chemistry. Cetuximab (ERBITUX) is a recombinant chimeric human/mouse immunoglobulin G1 (IgG_1) antibody that binds to the extracellular domain of EGFR. It consists of the Fv regions of a murine anti-EGFR antibody with human IgG_1 heavy- and κ light-chain constant regions.

Mechanism of Action. Cetuximab binds specifically to the extracellular domain of EGFR and prevents ligand-dependent signaling and receptor dimerization, thereby blocking cell growth and survival signals. Cetuximab also may mediate antibody-dependent cellular cytotoxicity against tumor cells.

Absorption, Distribution, and Elimination. Cetuximab exhibits nonlinear pharmacokinetic characteristics. Following intravenous administration, steady-state levels are achieved by the third weekly infusion. The volume of distribution approximates the intravascular space of 2-3 L/m^2. Therapeutic doses that saturate total body receptor pools of EGFR follow zero-order kinetics for elimination. Clearance occurs via EGFR binding and internalization and by degradation in the reticuloendothelial system.

Therapeutic Uses

Head and Neck Cancer. Cetuximab won FDA approval based on an improvement in overall survival when used in combination with radiation therapy for locally or regionally advanced squamous cell carcinoma of the head and neck (HNSCC). It received a second indication as monotherapy for patients with metastatic or recurrent HNSCC who had failed platinum-based chemotherapy. It has become a useful agent in combination with cisplatin-based chemotherapy, where it has shown an improvement in survival compared to chemotherapy alone (Vermorken et al., 2008).

Metastatic Colon Cancer. Cetuximab received approval as a single agent for the treatment of EGFR-positive metastatic colorectal cancer; cetuximab is used in patients who cannot tolerate irinotecan-based therapy and in combination with irinotecan for patients refractory to oxaliplatin, irinotecan, and 5-fluorouracil (5-FU). In the first-line setting, cetuximab may improve survival in combination with 5-FU/leucovorin and irinotecan or oxaliplatin (Bokemeyer et al., 2009). Numerous trials now have shown that the 40-50% of colorectal tumors carrying mutations in the *k-ras* oncogene are resistant to the effects of cetuximab. The antibody yields a response rate of 1% in patients with mutant tumors, compared to 12% in *k-ras* wild-type tumors (Karapetis et al., 2008). Cetuximab enhances the effectiveness of chemotherapy in patients with *k-ras* mutant tumors but not *k-ras* wild-type tumors (Bokemeyer et al., 2009).

The standard dose of cetuximab is a single loading dose of 400 mg/m^2 intravenously, followed by weekly doses of 250 mg/m^2 intravenously for the duration of treatment.

Adverse Effects. Side effects associated with cetuximab treatment include an acneform rash in the majority of patients. Patients also may experience pruritus, nail changes, headache, and diarrhea. Other rare but serious adverse effects include cardiopulmonary arrest, interstitial lung disease, and hypomagnesemia. In addition, patients can develop anaphylactoid reactions during infusion, which may be related to pre-existing IgE antibodies that are more prevalent in patients from the southern U.S.

Panitumumab

Chemistry. Panitumumab (VECTIBIX) is a recombinant, fully humanized $IgG_{2\kappa}$ antibody that binds specifically to the extracellular domain of EGFR. Unlike cetuximab, it does not mediate antibody-dependent cell-mediated cytotoxicity.

Absorption, Distribution, and Elimination. Panitumumab exhibits nonlinear pharmacokinetic characteristics. Following intravenous administration every 2 weeks, steady-state levels are achieved by the third infusion. The mean elimination $t_{1/2}$ is 7.5 days.

Therapeutic Uses. Panitumumab improves progression-free survival in patients with metastatic colorectal carcinoma, as demonstrated in patients with EGFR-expressing tumors who had two or more previous therapies (Van Cutsem et al., 2008). The dose of panitumumab is 6 mg/kg intravenously given once every 2 weeks.

Adverse Effects. The adverse effects with panitumumab are similar to cetuximab and include rash and dermatological toxicity, severe infusion reactions, pulmonary fibrosis, and electrolyte abnormalities.

HER2/neu Inhibitors

Both antibodies (trastuzumab) and small molecules (lapatinib and others in clinical trial) have striking antitumor effects in patients with HER2-positive breast cancer, and have become essential therapeutic agents in combination with cytotoxic chemotherapy for this aggressive malignancy.

Trastuzumab. Trastuzumab (HERCEPTIN) is a humanized monoclonal antibody that binds to the external domain of HER2/neu (ErbB2).

Thirty percent of breast cancers overexpress this receptor due to gene amplification on chromosome 17. Amplification of the receptor is associated with lower response rates to hormonal therapies and to most cytotoxic drugs, with the exception of anthracyclines (Slamon et al., 1989). Patients with HER2/neu-amplified tumors have higher recurrence rates after standard adjuvant therapy and poorer overall survival, as compared to patients with HER2-nonamplified tumors. The internal domain of the HER2/neu glycoprotein encodes a tyrosine kinase that activates downstream signal, enhances metastatic potential, and inhibits apoptosis. Trastuzumab exerts its antitumor effects through several putative mechanisms of action (Nahta and Esteva, 2003): inhibition of homo- or heterodimerization of receptor, thereby preventing receptor kinase activation and downstream signaling; initiation of Fcγ-receptor-mediated antibody-dependent cellular cytotoxicity; and blockade of the angiogenetic effects of HER2 signaling.

Trastuzumab was the first monoclonal antibody to be approved for the treatment of a solid tumor. Currently, it is approved for HER2/neu-overexpressing metastatic breast cancer, in combination with paclitaxel as initial treatment or as monotherapy following chemotherapy relapse (Vogel et al., 2002). Trastuzumab synergizes with other cytotoxic agents in HER2/neu-overexpressing cancers (Slamon et al., 2001). HER2/neu expression also is found in subsets of patients with gastric, esophageal, lung, and other solid tumors, but clinical studies of the effects of trastuzumab in these tumors have not yet been completed.

Pharmacokinetics and Toxicity. Trastuzumab has dose-dependent pharmacokinetics with a mean $t_{1/2}$ of 5.8 days on the 2-mg/kg maintenance dose. Steady-state levels are achieved between 16 and 32 weeks, with mean trough and peak concentrations of ~79 and 123 μg/mL, respectively (Baselga, 2000). The infusional effects of trastuzumab are typical of other monoclonal antibodies and include fever, chills, nausea, dyspnea, and rashes. Premedication with diphenhydramine and acetaminophen is indicated. The most serious toxicity of trastuzumab is cardiac failure; reasons for cardiotoxicity are poorly understood, although the HER2 antigen is highly expressed in the developing heart during embryogenesis, and HER2 knockout mice fail to survive because of cardiomyopathy (Crone et al., 2002). Cardiac failure is a potentially disabling or fatal side effect unless it is recognized early and the drug is discontinued (Seidman et al., 2002). Before initializing therapy, baseline electrocardiogram and cardiac ejection fraction measurement should be obtained to rule out underlying heart disease, and patients deserve careful clinical follow-up thereafter for signs or symptoms of congestive heart failure, such as cough, weight gain, or edema. When trastuzumab is used as a single agent, <5% of patients will experience a decrease in left-ventricular ejection fraction, and 1% will have clinical signs of congestive failure. However, left-ventricular dysfunction occurs in up to 20% of patients who received the antibody in combination with doxorubicin and cyclophosphamide. The risk of cardiac toxicity is greatly reduced with taxane–trastuzumab combinations.

Lapatinib. Small molecules can inhibit receptor tyrosine kinase activity of ErbB2 (HER2/neu) and have antitumor activity in patients who have developed progressive disease on trastuzumab (Moy and Goss, 2007). Lapatinib and other pan-HER inhibitors block both

ErbB1 and ErbB2 and bind to an internal site on the receptor (usually the ATP-binding pocket), compared to the external binding site of trastuzumab. Lapatinib also inhibits a truncated form of the HER2 receptor that lacks a trastuzumab-binding domain. These differences may account for the activity of lapatinib in trastuzumab-resistant patients.

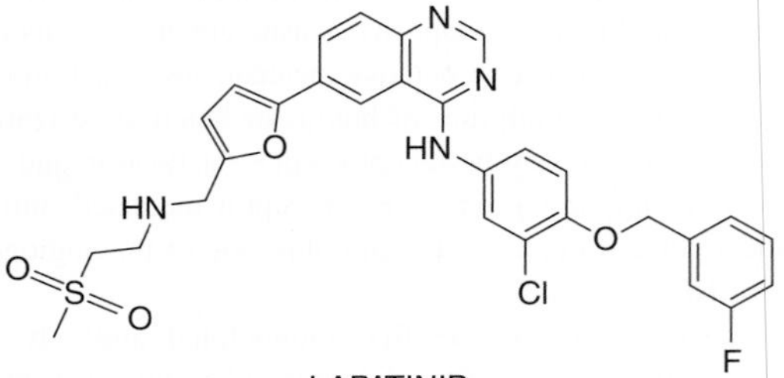

LAPATINIB

Lapatinib (TYKERB) is FDA-approved for HER2-amplified, trastuzumab-refractory breast cancer, in combination with the fluoropyrimidine analog, capecitabine. In its critical phase III trial, lapatinib plus capecitabine improved disease-free survival by 4.4 months and increased the disease response rate to 22% versus 14% in the control group treated with capecitabine alone. As a small molecule, lapatinib crosses the blood-brain barrier more readily than inhibitor antibodies and has produced anecdotal responses in patients with brain metastases and decreased the incidence of brain metastases in its phase III trial (Geyer et al., 2006).

Pharmacokinetics and Toxicity. The drug is administered orally, 1250 mg/day. It is metabolized by CYP3A4 to a number of inactive products, as well as to an oxidized intermediate that has activity against ErbB1 but not ErbB2. The plasma $t_{1/2}$ of 14 hours allows parent drug accumulation over the period of treatment. Concurrent administration of inducers and inhibitors of CYP3A4 shorten and prolong the drug's $t_{1/2}$, respectively, and may necessitate adjustment of the dose. Lapatinib toxicities include mild diarrhea, cramping, and exacerbation of gastro-esophageal reflux. When lapatinib is combined with capecitabine, diarrhea becomes a significant side effect in one-third of patients. Lapatinib's inhibition of ErbB1 (EGFR) causes an acneform rash in one-third of patients; the rash can be effectively controlled in most cases with topical or oral antibiotics and topical benzoyl peroxide gel. Unlike trastuzumab, lapatinib has not produced a clear signal of cardiac toxicity (Medina and Goodin, 2008); nonetheless, because it targets ErbB2, lapatinib should be used with caution in combination with other cardiotoxic drugs and with careful surveillance in patients who have underlying heart disease.

INHIBITORS OF ANGIOGENESIS

In 1971, Judah Folkman opened the field of anti-angiogenesis therapy when he hypothesized that the induction of new blood vessel formation—angiogenesis—is an essential property of cancers (Folkman, 1971). Although this revolutionary hypothesis was initially greeted with skepticism, angiogenesis now is firmly established as one of the hallmarks of cancer.

Cancer cells secrete angiogenic factors that induce the formation of new blood vessels and guarantee the flow of nutrients to the tumor cells. Angiogenic factors secreted by tumors include VEGF (*vascular* endothelial growth factor), FGF (*fibroblast* growth factor), TGF-β (*transforming* growth factor β) and PDGF (*platelet*-derived growth factor). Multiple tumor types overexpress these angiogenic factors. Several animal models have demonstrated that tumor secretion of pro-angiogenic factors turns on an "angiogenic switch," a process essential to tumor growth and metastasis. Strikingly, in multiple experimental models, blockade of these pro-angiogenic molecules halts tumor growth, and in human cancers, anti-angiogenic drugs also have inhibitory effects.

Jain has proposed an additional mechanism for the efficacy of angiogenesis inhibitors (Jain, 2009), based on the observation that the leaky capillaries within tumors have increased permeability and cause an increase in tumor interstitial pressure. This increased pressure inhibits blood flow, decreases oxygenation, and prevents drug delivery within the tumor. Antibodies directed at the primary angiogenic factor, VEGF, decrease interstitial pressure within tumors and reverse the changes in oxygenation and blood flow. By "normalizing" interstitial pressure and improving blood flow, anti-angiogenic agents enhance the ability of chemotherapeutic agents to reach the tumor. Hence, an additional benefit of anti-angiogenic molecules may be their ability to increase the delivery of chemotherapy to the tumor. This hypothesis seems to be validated in the synergy observed when cytotoxic chemotherapy is combined with anti-VEGF antibodies.

The best studied of the angiogenic factors is VEGF. VEGF initiates endothelial cell proliferation when it binds to a member of the VEGF receptor (VEGFR) family, a group of highly homologous receptors with intracellular tyrosine kinase domains that includes VEGFR1 (FLT1), VEGFR2 (KDR), and VEGFR3 (FLT4). The binding of VEGF to its receptor activates the intracellular VEGFR tyrosine kinase activity and initiates mitogenic and anti-apoptotic signaling pathways within the endothelial cell.

The cognate interaction between VEGF and its receptor creates several opportunities for pharmacological inhibition of this pathway. Antibodies targeting VEGF, such as bevacizumab, sterically hinder the interaction of VEGF with its receptor. As an alternative to VEGF antibody therapy, the investigational drug aflibercept (VEGF Trap), a recombinant molecule that utilizes the VEGFR1-binding domain to sequester VEGF, acts as a "soluble decoy receptor" for VEGF.

Alternatively, the propagation of pro-angiogenic signals can be abrogated by the inhibition of the tyrosine kinase activity of VEGFR. Three small molecules (pazopanib, sorafenib, and sunitinib) that inhibit the kinase function of VEGFR-2 have been approved for clinical use. Although bevacizumab and the small molecules share a similar spectrum of toxicities, they have somewhat different spectra of clinical activity and significant differences in pharmacokinetics.

Bevacizumab. *Bevacizumab* (AVASTIN), a humanized antibody directed against VEGF-A, was the first FDA-approved molecule that specifically targeted angiogenesis. As a single agent, it delays progression of renal-cell cancer, and, in combination with cytotoxic chemotherapy, effectively treats lung, colorectal, and breast cancers.

In clear-cell renal-cell carcinoma, a cancer notoriously resistant to traditional chemotherapeutic agents, single-agent bevacizumab increases survival by 3 months (Yang et al., 2003). Clear-cell renal-cell cancer, a highly vascular tumor, presents a particularly attractive target for bevacizumab and other anti-angiogenic agents because mutations or DNA methylation affecting the von Hippel-Lindau (*VHL*) gene are a constant feature of renal-cell carcinomas. The *VHL* gene product functions as an inhibitor of the angiogenic pathway. Thus, a loss of VHL protein activates hypoxia inducible factor 2 (HIF-2), a transcription factor that promotes synthesis of VEGF and other hypoxic response proteins. In 2009, the FDA approved bevacizumab in combination with interferon-α for the treatment of metastatic renal-cell carcinoma.

Bevacizumab is approved as a single agent following prior therapy for glioblastoma. In all other cancers, bevacizumab has little apparent single-agent activity but improves survival in epithelial cancers in combination with standard chemotherapeutic agents (Sandler et al., 2006). Bevacizumab with carboplatin and paclitaxel increases survival in non–small lung cancer by 2 months. Likewise, bevacizumab combined with FOLFOX (5-FU, leucovorin, and oxaliplatin) or FOLFIRI (5-FU, leucovorin, and irinotecan) improves survival by 5 months in metastatic colon cancer. Finally, the combination of bevacizumab with docetaxel increases progression-free survival in patients with metastatic breast cancer (Miller et al., 2007). Trials testing bevacizumab in glioblastoma multiforme have yielded promising results with minimal evidence of intracranial hemorrhage.

Clinical uses of bevacizumab now have expanded beyond the realm of oncology. In wet age-related macular degeneration, abnormal choroidal neovascularization often leads to rapid visual loss. A slightly altered version of bevacizumab called ranibizumab (LUCENTIS), in which the Fc region has been deleted, effectively treats wet macular degeneration. Bevacizumab restores hearing in patients with progressive deafness due to neurofibromatosis type 2–related tumors (Plotkin et al., 2009).

Clinical Pharmacology. Bevacizumab is administered intravenously as a 30- to 90-minute infusion. In metastatic colon cancer, in conjunction with combination chemotherapy, the dose of bevacizumab is 5 mg/kg every 2 weeks. In metastatic non–small cell lung cancer, doses of 15 mg/kg are given every 3 weeks with chemotherapy. For treatment of metastatic breast cancer, patients receive 10 mg/kg of bevacizumab every 2 weeks in combination with paclitaxel or docetaxel. The differing doses of bevacizumab reflect the varying designs of approval-directed trials. The optimal dosage in each case has not yet been defined. The antibody has a plasma $t_{1/2}$ of 4 weeks.

Toxicity. Bevacizumab causes a wide range of class-related adverse effects. A prominent concern with this class of agents was the potential for vessel injury and bleeding, noticed in patients with squamous-cell lung cancer (Johnson et al., 2004). Bevacizumab is contraindicated for patients who have a history of hemoptysis, brain metastasis, or a bleeding diathesis, but in appropriately selected patients, the rate of life-threatening pulmonary hemorrhage is <2% (Sandler et al., 2006).

The safety of operating on patients treated with bevacizumab continues to be a major concern because of the risk of bleeding and poor wound healing. In a pooled analysis of two large clinical trials of colon cancer, patients who needed surgery while being treated with bevacizumab had a higher rate (13% versus 3.4%) of serious wound healing complications than patients treated with placebo (Scappaticci et al., 2007). In light of these data and because of the long $t_{1/2}$ of bevacizumab, elective surgery should be delayed for at least 4 weeks from the last dose of antibody, and treatment should be not resumed for at least 4 weeks after surgery.

Other toxicities characteristic of anti-angiogenic drugs include hypertension and proteinuria. A majority of patients receiving the drug require antihypertensive therapy, particularly those receiving higher doses and more prolonged treatment (Sandler et al., 2006; Hurwitz et al., 2004; Miller et al., 2007). The mechanism driving this hypertension is still unclear but may relate, in part, to decreased endothelial nitric oxide production. Physicians should carefully monitor the blood pressure of all patients on bevacizumab and intervene with antihypertensives when appropriate. Case reports describe patients with poorly controlled hypertension developing a reversible posterior leukoencephalopathy during bevacizumab treatment. Bevacizumab also is rarely associated with congestive heart failure, probably secondary to hypertension (Miller et al., 2007).

Patients often develop proteinuria during bevacizumab treatment, but it usually is an asymptomatic finding and rarely associated with nephrotic syndrome (Gressett and Shah, 2009).

The most dreaded vascular toxicity of anti-angiogenic agents is an arterial thromboembolic event (i.e., stroke or myocardial infarction). A meta-analysis found that the rate of arterial thromboembolic events in patients receiving bevacizumab-containing regimens reached 3.8% compared to the control rate of 1.7% (Scappaticci et al., 2007). To reduce the risk of arterial thromboembolic events, clinicians should carefully evaluate a patient's risk factors (age >65 years, clotting diathesis, a past history of arterial thromboembolic events) before starting the drug.

GI perforation, a potentially life-threatening complication of bevacizumab, has been observed with particular frequency (up to 11%) in patients with ovarian cancer, perhaps related to the presence of peritoneal carcinomatosis and to prior abdominal surgery.

In colon cancer patients, colonic perforation occurs infrequently during bevacizumab treatment but increases in frequency in patients with intact primary colonic tumors, peritoneal carcinomatosis, peptic ulcer disease, chemotherapy-associated colitis, diverticulitis, or prior abdominal radiation treatment (Gressett and Shah, 2009). The rate of colon perforation is <1% in breast and lung cancer patients receiving the antibody.

Sunitinib. Sunitinib (SUTENT) competitively inhibits the binding of ATP to the tyrosine kinase domain on the VEGF receptor-2, a mechanism it shares with sorafenib (see "Sorafenib"). Sunitinib also inhibits other protein tyrosine kinases (FLT3, PDGFR-α, PDGFR-β, RET, CSF-1R, and c-KIT) at concentrations of 5-100 nM (Fabian et al., 2005).

Sunitinib has activity in metastatic renal-cell cancer, producing a higher response rate (31%) and a longer progression-free survival than any other approved anti-angiogenic drug (Motzer et al., 2007). Sunitinib also is approved for treatment of advanced renal-cell carcinoma and GIST that have developed resistance to imatinib as a consequence of *c-KIT* mutations (Heinrich et al., 2008). Specific *c-KIT* mutations correlate with response to sunitinib. For example, patients with *c-KIT* exon 9 mutations have a response rate of 37%, whereas patients with *c-KIT* exon 11 mutations have only a 5% response rate.

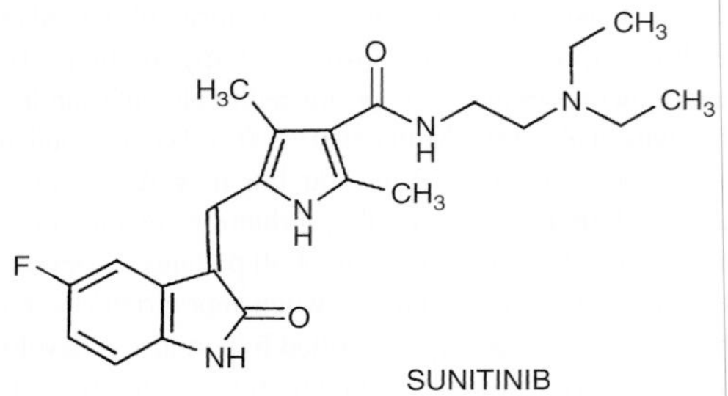

SUNITINIB

Pharmacokinetics and Dosing. Sunitinib is administered orally in doses of 50 mg once a day. The typical cycle of sunitinib is 4 weeks on treatment followed by 2 weeks off treatment. The dosage and schedule of sunitinib can be increased or decreased according to toxicity (hypertension, fatigue). Dosages <25 mg/day typically are ineffective. Sunitinib is metabolized by CYP3A4 to produce an active metabolite, SU12662, the $t_{1/2}$ of which is 80-110 hours; steady-state levels of the metabolite are reached after ~2 weeks of repeated administration of the parent drug. Further metabolism results in the formation of inactive products. The pharmacokinetics of sunitinib are not affected by food intake.

Toxicity. The main toxicities of bevacizumab are shared by all anti-angiogenic inhibitors, including sunitinib and sorafenib. Specifically, patients taking sunitinib can experience bleeding, hypertension, proteinuria, and, uncommonly, arterial thromboembolic events and intestinal perforation. However, because sunitinib is a multi-targeted tyrosine kinase inhibitor, it has a broader side-effect profile than bevacizumab.

Fatigue, the most common side effect of sunitinib, affects 50-70% of patients and may be disabling. Hypothyroidism occurs in 40-60% of patients. Bone marrow suppression and diarrhea also are common side effects; severe neutropenia (neutrophils <1000/mL) develop in 10% of patients. Less common side effects include congestive heart failure (usually in association with hypertension) and hand-foot syndrome. To monitor for these side effects, it is essential to check blood counts and thyroid function at regular intervals. Periodic echocardiograms also are recommended.

Sorafenib. Sorafenib (NEXAVAR), like sunitinib, targets multiple protein tyrosine kinases (VEGFR1, VEGFR2, VEGFR3, PDGFR-β, c-KIT, FLT-3, and b-RAF) and inhibits their catalytic activities at concentrations of 20-90 nM (Fabian et al., 2005).

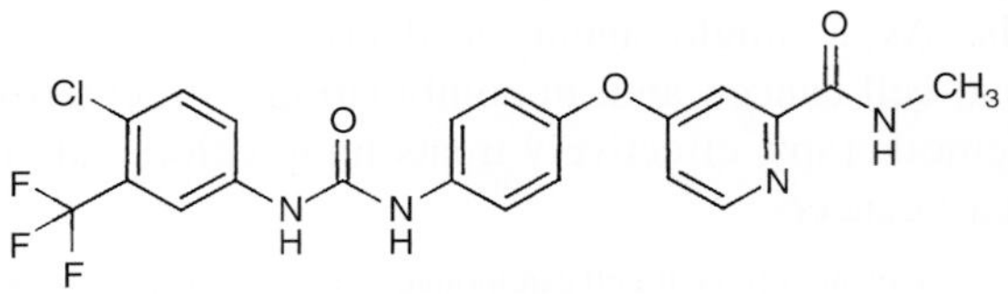

SORAFENIB

Absorption, Distribution, and Elimination. Sorafenib, an oral medication, is given in daily doses of 400 mg twice a day. Patients typically begin treatment taking 200 mg once a day and increase dosage as tolerated. Unlike sunitinib, sorafenib is given every day without treatment breaks. Sorafenib is metabolized to inactive products by CYP3A4 with a $t_{1/2}$ of 20-27 hours; with repeated administration, steady-state concentrations are reached within 1 week.

Therapeutic Uses. Sorafenib is the only drug currently approved for treatment of hepatocellular carcinoma. In these otherwise refractory patients, sorafenib increased median survival by 3 months compared to placebo (10.7 versus 7.9 months) (Llovet et al., 2008). The response rate to sorafenib was low (2%), suggesting that sorafenib primarily has a cytostatic effect. Sorafenib also is approved in metastatic renal-cell cancer, based on improvement in progression-free survival in patients with previously treated disease (Escudier et al., 2007). Because of its higher initial response rate, sunitinib generally is the preferred first-line therapy in this disease.

Adverse Effects. Sorafenib patients can experience the vascular toxicities (bleeding, hypertension, and arterial thromboembolic events) seen with other anti-angiogenic medications. More common adverse effects include fatigue, nausea, diarrhea, anorexia, and rash; uncommonly, one may notice bone marrow suppression and GI perforation (Escudier et al., 2007).

THALIDOMIDE

Among agents with anti-angiogenic activity, the immunomodulatory analogs (IMiDs), thalidomide and lenalidomide, have a most unusual history and a multiplicity of biological and immunological effects. Their classification as anti-angiogenics is convenient but tentative. Thalidomide originally entered development in the 1950s for the treatment of pregnancy-associated morning sickness but was withdrawn from the market due to the tragic consequences of teratogenicity and dysmelia (stunted limb growth) (Franks et al., 2004). It re-entered clinical practice, initially because of its clinical efficacy in erythema nodosum leprosum, for which it received approval in 1998 (see Chapter 56). Further research revealed its anti-angiogenic and immunomodulatory effects, and these findings triggered experimental trials in cancer, most notably against multiple myeloma (MM). Both thalidomide and lenalidomide possess potent activity in newly diagnosed and heavily pretreated relapsed/refractory MM patients (Richardson et al., 2007). Lenalidomide also has striking clinical activity in the 5q− subset of myelodysplastic syndrome (MDS) and has been approved for this indication. A specific gene array profile identifies MDS patients who lack the 5q− abnormality but respond to lenalidomide (Ebert et al., 2008).

THALIDOMIDE LENALIDOMIDE

*Denotes the chiral center.

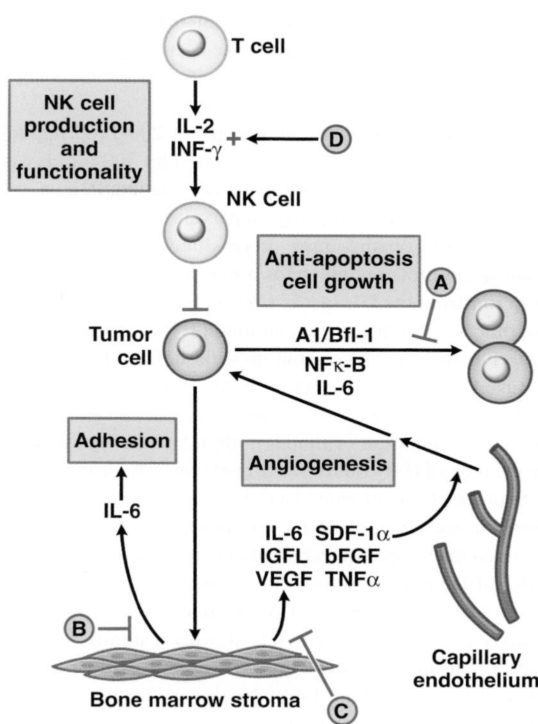

Figure 62–3. *Schematic overview of proposed mechanisms of antimyeloma activity of thalidomide and its derivatives.* Some biological hallmarks of the malignant phenotype are indicated in light-blue boxes. The proposed sites of action for thalidomide (letters inside red and green circles) are hypothesized to also be operative for thalidomide derivatives. ***A.*** Direct anti–multiple myeloma (MM) effect on tumor cells, including G_1 growth arrest and/or apoptosis, even against MM cells resistant to conventional therapy. This is due to the disruption of the anti-apoptotic effect of BCL-2 family members, blocking NF-κB signaling, and inhibition of the production of interleukin-6 (IL-6). ***B.*** Inhibition of MM-cell adhesion to bone marrow stromal cells partially due to the reduction of IL-6 release. ***C.*** Decreased angiogenesis due to the inhibition of cytokine and growth factor production and release. ***D.*** Enhanced T-cell production of cytokines, such as IL-2 and interferon-γ (IFN-γ), that increase the number and cytotoxic functionality of natural killer (NK) cells. VEGF, vascular endothelial growth factor.

Mechanisms of Action. The precise mechanisms responsible for these drugs' clinical effects are unclear. Thalidomide's enantiomeric interconversion and spontaneous cleavage to multiple short-lived and poorly characterized metabolites, as well as its species-specific *in vivo* metabolic activation, confound the interpretation of preclinical *in vitro* and *in vivo* mechanistic studies. At least four distinct, but potentially complementary, mechanisms have been proposed to explain the antitumor activity of IMiDs (Figure 62–3):

- Direct anti-proliferative/pro-apoptotic antitumor effects. They inhibit the anti-apoptotic effects of NF-κB and the anti-apoptotic Bcl-2 family member A1/Bfl-1 (Mitsiades et al., 2002a).
- Indirect inhibition of tumor cell growth and survival by abrogation of cell interactions with adhesion molecules (Hideshima et al., 2000).
- Inhibition of interleukin-6 (IL-6) and tumor necrosis factor α (TNF α) production, release, and signaling, leading to anti-angiogenic effects.
- Immunomodulation through enhancement of natural killer (NK) and T cell–mediated cytotoxicity. Their antagonism of anti-apoptotic pathways and their anti-angiogenic effects could account for the clinical synergy with glucocorticoids and bortezomib against MM (Mitsiades et al., 2002b).

Thalidomide

Pharmacokinetics and Therapeutic Use. Thalidomide (THALOMID) exists at physiological pH as a racemic mixture of cell-permeable and rapidly interconverting non-polar S(–) and R(+) isomers, the equilibrium favoring the R product. The R-enantiomer is associated with the teratogenic and biological activities, while the S accounts for the sedative properties of thalidomide.

Thalidomide is given in dosages of 200-1200 mg/day. In treating MM, doses usually are escalated by 200 mg/day every 2 weeks until dose-limiting side effects (sedation, fatigue, constipation, or a sensory neuropathy) supervene. With extended treatment, the neuropathy may necessitate dose reduction or discontinuation of treatment for a period of time. Thalidomide absorption from the GI tract is slow and highly variable [4 hours mean time to reach peak concentration (T_{max}), with a range of 1-7 hours]. It distributes throughout most tissues and organs, without significant binding to plasma proteins. Peak levels are achieved in 3-4 hours, and the $t_{1/2}$ of disappearance of the enantiomers is ~6 hours. Elimination of thalidomide is mainly by spontaneous hydrolysis in all body fluids; the S-enantiomer is cleared more rapidly than the R-enantiomer. Thalidomide and its metabolites are excreted in the urine, while the non-absorbed portion of the drug is excreted unchanged in feces, but clearance of active drug is primarily attributable to hydrolysis. The inactive hydrolysis products undergo a complex pattern of CYP-mediated metabolism. Studies in elderly prostate cancer patients showed a significantly longer plasma $t_{1/2}$ at highest doses (1200 mg daily) versus lowest doses (200 mg daily) (Figg et al., 1999). No dose adjustment is necessary in the presence of renal failure.

Thalidomide enhances the sedative effects of barbiturates and alcohol and the catatonic effects of chlorpromazine and reserpine. Conversely, CNS stimulants (such as methamphetamine and methylphenidate) counteract the depressant effects of thalidomide.

Lenalidomide. Lenalidomide (REVLIMID) constitutes the lead compound in the new class of immunomodulatory thalidomide derivatives and exhibits a panoply of pharmacological properties (direct suppression of the tumor cell growth in culture, T-cell and NK-cell activation, suppression of TNF α and other cytokines, antiangiogenesis, and promotion of hematopoietic stem cell differentiation) (List, 2007).

Pharmacokinetics and Therapeutic Use. The standard dosage of lenalidomide is 25 mg/day for 21 days of a 28-day cycle. The drug is rapidly absorbed following oral administration, reaching peak plasma levels within 1.5 hours. The C_{max} and AUC values increase proportionately with increasing dose, over a single-dose range of 5-400 mg. The $t_{1/2}$ of parent drug in plasma is 9 hours at the 400-mg dose. Approximately 70% of the orally administered dose of lenalidomide is excreted intact by the kidney. The AUC progressively rises in patients with moderate to severe renal failure (creatinine clearance <50 mL/min). Based on pharmacokinetic considerations, downward dose adjustments to 10 mg/day for creatinine clearance of 30-50 mL/h and to the same dose every 2 days for creatinine clearance <30 mL/h are recommended for patients with renal failure. The safety and efficacy of these adjusted doses have not been established in prospective studies (Chen et al., 2007).

This orally administered agent has exhibited potent antitumor activity in MM, MDS, and chronic lymphocytic leukemia (CLL); causes fewer adverse side effects; and lacks the teratogenicity of thalidomide.

Adverse Effects of Thalidomide and Lenalidomide

Thalidomide is well tolerated at doses <200 mg daily. The most common adverse effects reported in cancer patients are sedation and constipation, while the most serious one is peripheral sensory neuropathy, which occurs in 10-30% of patients with MM or other malignancies in a dose- and time-dependent manner (Richardson et al., 2004). Thalidomide-related neuropathy is an asymmetrical, painful, peripheral paresthesia with sensory loss, commonly presenting with numbness of toes and feet, muscle cramps, weakness, signs of pyramidal tract involvement, and carpal tunnel syndrome. The incidence of peripheral neuropathy increases with higher cumulative doses of thalidomide, especially in elderly patients. Although symptoms improve upon drug discontinuation, long-standing sensory loss may not reverse. Particular caution should apply in cancer patients with pre-existing neuropathy (e.g., related to diabetes) or prior exposure to drugs that can cause peripheral neuropathy (e.g., vinca alkaloids, bortezomib), especially because there has been little progress in defining effective strategies to alleviate neuropathic symptoms.

Adverse effects of lenalidomide are much less severe, as it causes little sedation, constipation, or neuropathy. The drug depresses bone marrow function and is associated with significant leukopenia in 20% of patients. In rare instances, patients develop hepatotoxicity and renal dysfunction. In some CLL patients, lenalidomide causes dramatic lymph node swelling and tumor lysis, a syndrome called the tumor flare reaction. Patients with renal dysfunction receiving the standard dose of 25 mg/day are particularly prone to this reaction; thus, clinical trials in CLL are proceeding at much lower doses of 10 mg/day, with escalation as tolerated. CLL patients should receive pretreatment hydration and allopurinol to avoid the consequences of tumor swelling and tumor lysis. A negative interaction with rituximab, an anti-CD20 antibody, may result from lenalidomide's downregulation of CD20, an interaction that has clinical implications for their combined use in lymphoid malignancies (Lapalombella et al., 2008).

Thromboembolic events occur with increased frequency in patients receiving thalidomide or lenalidomide, but particularly in combination with glucocorticoids and with anthracyclines (Musallam et al., 2008). Anticoagulation reduces this risk and seems indicated in patients presenting with risk factors for clotting, but anticoagulant prophylaxis has not been evaluated prospectively.

PROTEASOME INHIBITION: BORTEZOMIB

Bortezomib (VELCADE), an inhibitor of proteasome-mediated protein degradation, has earned a central role in the treatment of MM.

Chemistry. Bortezomib, [(1R)-3-methyl-1-[[(2S)-1-oxo-3-phenyl-2-[(pyrazinylcarbonyl)amino]propyl]amino]butyl]boronic acid, has a unique boron-containing structure:

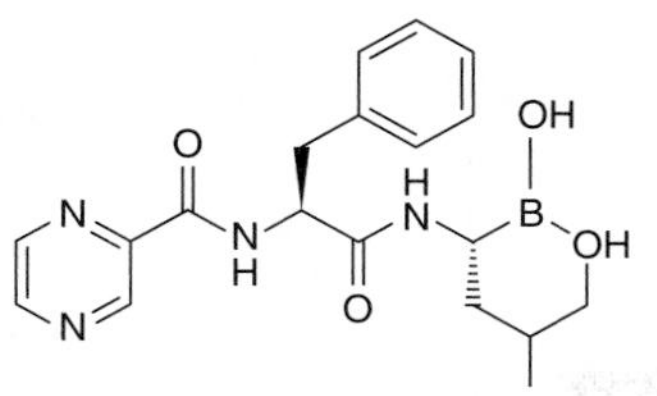

BORTEZOMIB

Mechanism of Action. Bortezomib binds to the β5 subunit of the 20S core of the 26S proteasome and reversibly inhibits its chymotrypsin-like activity (Adams, 2004). This event disrupts multiple intracellular signaling cascades, leading to apoptosis. A most important consequence of proteasome inhibition is its effect on NF-κB, a key transcription factor that promotes cell damage response and cell survival. Most NF-κB is found in the cytosol bound to IκB; in this form, NF-κB is restricted to the cytosol and cannot enter to the nucleus to regulate transcription. In response to stress signals resulting from hypoxia, chemotherapy, and DNA damage, IκB becomes ubiquitinated and then degraded via the proteasome. Its degradation releases NF-κB, which enters the nucleus, where it transcriptionally activates a host of genes involved in cell survival (e.g., cell adhesion proteins E-selectin, ICAM-1, and VCAM-1), as well as proliferative (e.g., cyclin-D1) or anti-apoptotic molecules (e.g., cIAPs, BCL-2). NF-κB is highly expressed in many human tumors, including MM, and may be a key factor in tumor cell survival in a hypoxic environment and during chemotherapy. Bortezomib blocks proteasomal degradation of IκB, thereby preventing the transcriptional activity of NF-κB and downregulating survival responses.

NF-κB inhibition may not account for the full spectrum of effects triggered by proteasome inhibition, because bortezomib also disrupts the ubiquitin-proteasomal degradation of p21, p27, p53, and other key regulators of the cell cycle and initiators of apoptosis. Bortezomib activates the cell's stereotypical "unfolded protein response" or UPR, in which abnormal protein conformation activates adaptive signaling pathways in the cell. The composite effect leads to irreversible commitment of MM cells to apoptosis (Mitsiades et al., 2002). In clinical trials, bortezomib also sensitizes tumor cells to cytotoxic drugs, including alkylators and anthracyclines, and to IMiDs and inhibitors of histone deacetylase (Orlowski et al., 2007).

Absorption, Fate, and Excretion. The recommended starting dose of bortezomib is 1.3 mg/m^2 given as an intravenous bolus on days 1, 4, 8, and 11 of every 21-day cycle (with a 10-day rest period per cycle). At least 72 hours should elapse between doses. Drug administration should be withheld until resolution of any grade 3 nonhematological toxicity or grade 4 hematological toxicity, and subsequent doses should be reduced 25%.

After intravenous administration of 1-1.3 mg/m^2 of bortezomib, the drug exhibits a terminal $t_{1/2}$ in plasma of 5.5 hours (Papandreou et al., 2004). The median peak plasma concentration averages 509 ng/mL after a 1.3-mg/m^2 bolus injection. Peak proteasome inhibition reaches 60% within 1 hour and declines thereafter, with a $t_{1/2}$ of ~24 hours.

Bortezomib clearance results from the deboronation of 90% of the parent compound, followed by hydroxylation of the boron-free product by CYPs 3A4 and 2D6; administration of this drug with potent inducers or inhibitors/substrates of CYP3A4 requires caution. No dose adjustment is required for patients with renal dysfunction.

Therapeutic Uses and Toxicity. Bortezomib is FDA approved as initial therapy for MM and as therapy for MM after relapse from other drugs (Kane et al., 2003). It also has received approval for relapsed or refractory mantle cell lymphoma. The drug is active in myeloma, including the induction of complete responses in up to 30% of patients when used in combination with other drugs (i.e., thalidomide, lenalidomide, liposomal doxorubicin, or dexamethasone) (San Miguel et al., 2008).

Bortezomib toxicities include thrombocytopenia (28%), fatigue (12%), peripheral neuropathy (12%), and neutropenia, anemia, vomiting, diarrhea, limb pain, dehydration, nausea, or weakness. Peripheral neuropathy, the most chronic of the toxicities, develops most frequently in patients with a prior history of neuropathy secondary to prior drug treatment (e.g., thalidomide) or diabetes or with prolonged use. Dose reductions or discontinuation of bortezomib ameliorates the neuropathic symptoms. Injection of bortezomib may precipitate hypotension, especially in volume-depleted patients, in those who have a history of syncope, or in patients taking antihypertensive medications. High-dose bortezomib causes hypotension and congestive heart failure in animals; cardiac toxicity occurs rarely in humans, but congestive failure and prolonged QT-interval have been reported.

mTOR INHIBITORS: RAPAMYCIN ANALOGS

Rapamycin (sirolimus) is a fungal fermentation product that inhibits the proper functioning of a serine/threonine protein kinase in mammalian cells eponymously named *mammalian target of rapamycin*, or mTOR, an effector PI3 kinase signaling. The PI3K/PKB(Akt)/mTOR pathway responds to a variety of signals from growth factors (e.g., insulin, interleukins, EGF) that modulate cell growth, translation, metabolism, and apoptosis. The activation of the PI3K pathway is opposed by the phosphatase activity of the tumor suppressor, PTEN. Activating mutations and amplification of genes in the receptor-PI3K pathway, and loss of function alterations in PTEN, occur frequently in cancer cells, with the result that PI3K signaling is exaggerated and cells lose growth control and exhibit enhanced survival (decreased apoptosis).

Rapamycin and its congeners, temsirolimus and everolimus, are well-established first-line drugs in post-transplant immunosuppression. More recently, mTOR inhibitors have found important applications in oncology for treatment of renal and hepatocellular cancer and mantle cell lymphomas.

RAPAMYCIN (SIROLIMUS)

Mechanisms of Action and Resistance. The rapamycins inhibit an enzyme complex, mTORC1, which occupies a downstream position in the PI3 kinase pathway (Figure 62–4). mTOR forms the mTORC1 complex with a member of the FK506-binding protein family, FKBP12. Among other actions, mTORC1 phosphorylates S6 kinase and also relieves the inhibitory effect of 4EBP on initiation factor elf-4E, therby promoting protein synthesis and metabolism. The antitumor actions of the rapamycins result from their binding to FKBP12 and inhibition of mTORC1. Rapamycin and its congeners have immunosuppressant effects, inhibit cell-cycle progression and angiogenesis, and promote apoptosis.

Resistance to mTOR inhibitors is incompletely understood but may arise through the action of a second mTOR complex, mTORC2, which is unaffected by rapamycins and which regulates AKT kinase. Experimental work suggests that inhibition of mTORC1 leads to mTORC2 activation of AKT kinase and the MAP kinase pathway, and these actions may be responsible for incomplete responses or resistance of rapamycins (Carracedo et al., 2008). Dual mTORC1 and mTORC2 inhibitors are in clinical development.

Absorption, Fate, and Excretion. The FDA has approved both temsirolimus and everolimus for treatment of renal cancer. Temsirolimus prolongs survival and delays disease progression in patients with advanced and poor- or intermediate-risk renal cancer, as compared to standard interferon-α treatment. Everolimus, as compared to placebo, prolongs survival in patients who had failed initial treatment with anti-angiogenic drugs (Motzer et al., 2008). mTOR inhibitors also have antitumor activity against mantle cell lymphomas (Ansell et al., 2008) and are under active investigation in combination with hormonal therapies, EGFR inhibitors, and cytotoxic drugs.

For renal-cell cancer, temsirolimus is given in weekly doses of 25 mg, intravenously, while everolimus is administered orally in doses of 10 mg daily. Both drugs should be administered in the fasting state at least 1 hour before a meal. Both parent molecules are metabolized by CYP3A4. Temsirolimus has a plasma $t_{1/2}$ of 30 hours; its primary metabolite, sirolimus, has a longer $t_{1/2}$ of 53 hours. Because sirolimus has equivalent activity as an inhibitor of mTORC1, and has a greater AUC, sirolimus is likely the more important contributor to antitumor action in patients (Hutson et al., 2008). Everolimus has a plasma $t_{1/2}$ of 30 hours, and on a weekly schedule at doses of 20 mg, it maintains inhibition of mTORC1 for 7 days in white blood cells (O'Donnell et al., 2008). At their usual clinical doses, both agents provide peak drug levels of ~1 μM.

Both drugs are susceptible to interactions with other agents that affect CYP3A4 activity. Ketoconazole, a CYP3A4 inhibitor, causes a 2- to 3-fold increase in the AUCs of both temsirolimus and sirolimus, while inducers of metabolism such as rifampin or phenytoin can decrease the C_{Pmax} of temsirolimus by 36% and decrease the AUC of its metabolite by >50%. The dose of temsirolimus should be doubled in the presence of inducers and reduced by half in the presence of ketoconazole (Hutson et al., 2008). Hepatic dysfunction delays drug clearance; for everolimus, the dose should be

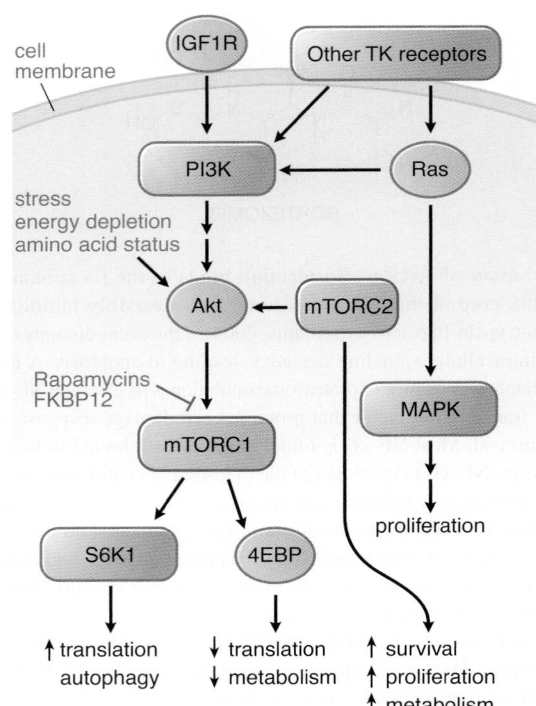

Figure 62–4. *Insulin-like growth factor 1 receptor (IGF-1R) and other tyrosine kinase (TK) growth factor receptors signal through multiple pathways.* A key pathway is regulated by phosphatidylinositol-3 kinase (PI3K) and its downstream partner, the mammalian target of rapamycin (mTOR). Rapamycins complex with FKBPP12 to inhibit the mTORC1 complex. mTORC2 remains unaffected and responds by upregulating Akt, driving signals through the inhibited mTORC1. The various downstream outputs of the two complexes are shown. Phosphorylation of 4EBP by mTOR inhibits the capacity of 4EBP to inhibit eif-4E and slow metabolism. 4EBP, eukaryotic initiation factor 4e (eif-4E) binding protein; S6K1, S6 kinase 1; FKBP12, the immunophilin target (binding protein) for tacrolimus (FK506).

reduced to 5 mg daily for patients with moderate hepatic impairment (Child-Pugh class B); guidelines for dose reduction of temsirolimus in such patients have not been established. The drugs' pharmacokinetics do not depend on renal function, and hemodialysis does not hasten temsirolimus clearance.

Higher-dose intravenous temsirolimus regimens, up to 175 mg/week, have been explored in mantle cell lymphoma and in other diseases, as has oral temsirolimus administration. Poor oral bioavailability hampers the oral route of administration, as <20% of drug or active metabolite reaches the plasma (Buckner et al., 2010).

Clinical Toxicity. The rapamycin analogs have very similar patterns of toxicity. The most prominent side effects are a mild maculopapular rash, mucositis, anemia, and fatigue, each occurring in 30-50% of patients. A minority of patients will develop leukopenia or thrombocytopenia with progressive cycles of treatment, and these effects are reversed if therapy is discontinued. Less common side effects include hyperglycemia, hypertriglyceridemia, and, rarely, pulmonary infiltrates and interstitial lung disease. Pulmonary infiltrates emerge in 8% of patients receiving everolimus and in a smaller percentage of those treated with temsirolimus. In patients showing minor radiological changes, but without symptoms, drug administration may be continued. If symptoms such as cough or shortness of breath develop or radiological changes progress, the drug should be discontinued. Prednisone may hasten the resolution of radiological changes and symptoms (Hutson et al., 2008).

BIOLOGICAL RESPONSE MODIFIERS

Biological response modifiers include cytokines or monoclonal antibodies that beneficially affect the patient's biological response to a neoplasm. Included are agents that act indirectly to mediate their antitumor effects (e.g., by enhancing the immunological response to neoplastic cells) or directly, binding to receptors on the tumor cells and delivering toxins or radionuclides. Recombinant DNA technology has greatly facilitated the identification and production of a number of human proteins with potent effects on the function and growth of both normal and neoplastic cells. Proteins that currently are in clinical use include the interferons (see Chapters 35 and 58); interleukins (see Chapter 35); hematopoietic growth factors such as erythropoietin, filgrastim [granulocyte colony-stimulating factor (G-CSF)], and sargramostim [granulocyte-macrophage colony-stimulating factor (GM-CSF)] (see Chapter 37); and monoclonal antibodies.

Monoclonal Antibodies

Since the discovery of methods for fusing mouse myeloma cells with B lymphocytes, it has been possible to produce a single species of murine antibody that recognizes a specific antigen. Cancer cells express antigens that are attractive targets for monoclonal antibody–based therapy (Table 62–1). Immunization of mice with human tumor cell extracts has led to the isolation of monoclonal Abs reactive against unique or highly expressed target antigens, and a few of these monoclonals possess antitumor activity. Because murine antibodies have a short $t_{1/2}$ in humans, activate human immune effector mechanisms poorly, and induce a human anti-mouse antibody immune response, they usually are chimerized by substituting major portions of the human IgG molecule. Presently, monoclonal antibodies have received FDA approval for lymphoid and solid tumor malignancies. Available agents include rituximab (Coiffier et al., 2002) and alemtuzumab (Keating et al., 2002) for lymphoid malignancies, trastuzumab (Vogel et al., 2002) for breast cancer, bevacizumab (Sandler et al., 2006) for colon and lung cancer, and cetuximab and panitumumab (Van Cutsem et al., 2007) for colorectal cancer and head and neck cancer. The nomenclature adopted for naming therapeutic monoclonal antibodies is to terminate the name in *-ximab* for chimeric antibodies and *-umab* for fully humanized antibodies.

Unmodified monoclonal antibodies may kill tumor cells by a variety of mechanisms [e.g., antibody-dependent cellular cytotoxicity (ADCC), complement-dependent cytotoxicity (CDC), and direct induction of apoptosis by antigen binding], but the clinically relevant mechanisms for most antibodies are uncertain (Villamor et al., 2003). Monoclonal antibodies also may be linked to a toxin (immunotoxins), such as gemtuzumab ozogamicin (MYLOTARG) (Larson et al., 2005) or denileukin diftitox (ONTAK) (Negro-Vilar et al., 2007), or conjugated to a radioactive isotope, as in the case of ^{90}Yttrium (^{90}Y)-ibritumomab tiuxetan (ZEVALIN) (Witzig et al., 2002) (Table 62–1). Genetic polymorphisms affecting the target antigen or complement receptors may influence response (Cartron et al., 2002).

Unarmed Monoclonal Antibodies

Rituximab. Rituximab (RITUXAN) is a chimeric monoclonal antibody that targets the CD20 B-cell antigen (Tables 62–1 and 62–2) (Maloney et al., 1997). CD20 is found on cells from the pre–B cell stage through its terminal differentiation to plasma cells and is expressed on 90% of B-cell neoplasms. The biological functions of CD20 are uncertain, although incubation of B cells with anti-CD20 antibody has variable effects on cell-cycle progression, depending on the monoclonal antibody type. Monoclonal antibody binding to CD20 generates transmembrane signals that produce autophosphorylation and activation of serine/tyrosine protein kinases, induction of *c-myc* oncogene expression,

Table 62–1

Monoclonal Antibodies Approved for Hematopoietic and Solid Tumors

ANTIGEN AND TUMOR CELL TARGETS	ANTIGEN FUNCTION	NAKED ANTIBODIES	RADIOISOTOPE-BASED ANTIBODIES	TOXIN-BASED ANTIBODIES
Antigen: CD20				
Tumor type: B-cell lymphoma and CLL	Proliferation/differentiation	Rituximab (chimeric)	^{131}I-tositumomab; ^{90}Y-ibritumomab tiuxetan	None
Antigen: CD52				
Tumor type: B-cell CLL and T-cell lymphoma	Unknown	Alemtuzumab (humanized)	None	None
Antigen: CD33				
Tumor type: acute myelocytic leukemia	Unknown	Gemtuzumab (humanized)	None	Gemtuzumab ozogamicin
Antigen: HER2/neu (ErbB2)				
Tumor type: breast cancer	Tyrosine kinase	Trastuzumab (humanized)	None	None
Antigen: EGFR (ErbB1)				
Tumor type: colorectal, NSCLC, pancreatic, breast	Tyrosine kinase	Cetuximab (chimeric)	None	None
Antigen: VEGF				
Tumor type: colorectal cancer	Angiogenesis	Bevacizumab (humanized)	None	None

CLL, chronic lymphocytic leukemia; EGFR, epidermal growth factor receptor; NSCLC, non–small cell lung cancer; VEGF, vascular endothelial growth factor.

and expression of major histocompatibility complex class II molecules. CD20 also may regulate transmembrane Ca^{2+} conductance through its function as a Ca^{2+} channel. It is unclear which of these actions relates to the pharmacological effect of rituximab.

Rituximab is approved as a single agent for relapsed indolent lymphomas and significantly enhances response and survival in combination with chemotherapy for the initial treatment of diffuse large B-cell lymphoma. It remains effective in patients who relapse after initial treatment with rituximab-based combinations. Rituximab improves response rates when added to combination chemotherapy for other indolent B-cell non-Hodgkin's lymphomas (NHLs), including CLL, mantle cell lymphoma, Waldenström macroglobulinemia, and marginal zone lymphomas (Cheson and Leonard, 2008). Maintenance of remission with rituximab delays time to progression and improves overall survival in indolent NHL (van Oers et al., 2006). It is increasingly used for treatment of autoimmune diseases such as rheumatological disease, thrombotic thrombocytopenic purpura, autoimmune hemolytic anemias, cryoglobulin-induced renal disease and multiple sclerosis.

Pharmacokinetics and Dosing. Rituximab has a $t_{1/2}$ of ~22 days (Maloney et al., 1997). The drug is administered by intravenous infusion both as a single agent and in combination with chemotherapy at a dose of 375 mg/m^2. As a single agent, it is given weekly for 4 weeks, with maintenance dosing every 3-6 months. In combination regimens, the drug may be administered every 3-4 weeks, with chemotherapy, for up to eight doses. As maintenance therapy following 6-8 cycles of combination chemotherapy, rituximab may be given once weekly for four doses, at 6-month intervals, for up to 16 doses.

During the first administration, the rate of infusion should be increased slowly to prevent serious hypersensitivity reactions. Infusions should begin at 50 mg/h, and in the absence of infusion reactions, the rate can increase in 50-mg/h increments every 30 minutes to a maximum rate of 400 mg/h. On subsequent infusion in the absence of reactions, infusions may start at 100 mg/hr and increase in 100-mg/h increments every 30 minutes to a maximum rate of 400 mg/h. Pretreatment with antihistamines, acetaminophen, and glucocorticoids decreases the risk of hypersensitivity reactions.

Patients with large numbers of circulating tumor cells (as in CLL) are at increased risk for tumor lysis syndrome; in these patients, the initial dose should be no more than 50 mg/m^2 on day 1

Table 62–2

Dose and Toxicity of Monoclonal Antibody–Based Drugs

DRUG	MECHANISM	DOSE AND SCHEDULE	MAJOR TOXICITY
Rituximab	ADCC; CDC; apoptosis	375-mg/m^2 IV infusion weekly for 4 weeks	Infusion-related toxicity with fever, rash, and dyspnea; B-cell depletion; late-onset neutropenia
Alemtuzumab	ADCC; CDC; apoptosis	Escalating doses of 3, 10, 30 mg/m^2 IV three times/ week followed by 30 mg/m^2 three times/week for 4-12 weeks	Infusion-related toxicity, T-cell depletion with increased infection; hematopoietic suppression; pancytopenia
Trastuzumab	ADCC; apoptosis; inhibition of arrest HER2 signaling with G_1 arrest	Loading dose of 4-mg/kg infusion followed by 2 mg/kg weekly	Cardiomyopathy; infusion-related toxicity
Cetuximab	Inhibition of EGFR signaling; apoptosis; ADCC	Loading dose of 400-mg/kg infusion followed by 250 mg/kg weekly	Infusion-related toxicity; skin rash in 75%
Bevacizumab	Inhibition of angiogenesis/ neovascularization	5 mg/kg IV every 14 days until disease progression	Hypertension; pulmonary hemorrhage; GI perforation; proteinuria; congestive heart failure
Denileukin diftitox	Targeted diphtheria toxin with inhibition of protein synthesis	9-18 μg/kg/day IV for the first 5 days every 3 weeks	Fever; arthralgia; asthenia; hypotension
Gemtuzumab ozogamicin	Double-strand DNA breaks and apoptosis	Two doses of 9 mg/m^2 IV separated by 14 days	Infusion-related toxicity; hematopoietic suppression; mucosal hepatic (VOD); skin toxicity
^{90}Y-ibritumomab tiuxetan	Targeted radiotherapy	0.4 mCi/kg IV	Hematological toxicity; myelodysplasia
^{131}I-tositumomab	Targeted radiotherapy	Patient-specific dosimetry	Hematological toxicity; myelodysplasia

ADCC, antibody-dependent cellular cytotoxicity; CDC, complement-dependent cytotoxicity; EGFR, epidermal growth factor receptor; intravenous; VOD, veno-occlusive disease.

of treatment, and patients should receive standard tumor lysis prophylaxis. The remainder of the dose can then be given on day 3.

Resistance and Toxicity. Resistance to rituximab may emerge through downregulation of CD20, impaired antibody-dependent cellular cytotoxicity, decreased complement activation, limited effects on signaling and induction of apoptosis, and inadequate blood levels (Maloney et al., 2002). Polymorphisms in two of the receptors for the antibody Fc region responsible for complement activation, Fcγ RIIIa and Fcγ RIIa, may predict the clinical response to rituximab monotherapy in patients with follicular lymphoma but not in CLL (Cartron et al., 2002).

Rituximab infusional reactions can be life-threatening, but with pretreatment are usually mild and limited to fever, chills, throat itching, urticaria, and mild hypotension. All respond to decreased infusion rates and antihistamines. Uncommonly, patients may develop severe mucocutaneous skin reactions, including Stevens-Johnson syndrome. Rituximab may cause reactivation of hepatitis B virus or rarely, JC virus (with progressive multifocal leukoencephalopathy) (Kranick et al., 2007). Patients should be screened for hepatitis B before initiation of therapy. Hypogammaglobulinemia and autoimmune syndromes (idiopathic thrombocytopenic purpura, thrombotic thrombocytopenic purpura, autoimmune hemolytic anemia, pure red cell aplasia, and delayed neutropenia) may supervene 1-5 months after administration (Cattaneo et al., 2006).

Ofatumumab. Ofatumumab (ARZERRA) is a second monoclonal antibody that binds to CD20 at sites on the major and minor extracellular loops of CD20, distinct from the site targeted by rituximab. Binding of the drug results in B-cell lysis (both CDC and ADCC). Ofatumumab is approved for treating patients with CLL after failure of fludarabine and alemtuzumab.

A complex dosing scheme is used, beginning with small (300 mg) doses on day 1, followed by higher doses (up to 2 g/week) for 7 weeks, followed by 2 g every 4 weeks for four additional doses. Slow rates of infusion are recommended for the initial dose and for the first 2 hours of subsequent infusions.

Ofatumumab's primary toxicities consist of immunosuppression and opportunistic infection, hypersensitivity reactions during antibody infusion, and myelosuppression, which may be prolonged. Blood counts should be monitored during treatment. Rarely, patients may develop reactivation of viral infections, leading to progressive multifocal leukoencephalopathy or hepatitis B progression. The drug should not be administered to patients with active hepatitis B infection; liver function should be monitored closely in hepatitis B carriers.

Alemtuzumab. Alemtuzumab (CAMPATH) is a humanized IgG-κ monoclonal antibody, composed of a rat antigen–binding region within human constant regions and variable framework. The drug binds to CD52 antigen present on the surface of a subset of normal neutrophils and on all B and T lymphocytes, on testicular elements and sperm, and on most B- and T-cell lymphomas (Kumar et al., 2003). Consistently high levels of CD52 expression on lymphoid tumor cells and the lack of CD52 modulation with antibody binding make this antigen a favorable target for unconjugated monoclonal antibodies. Alemtuzumab can induce tumor cell death through ADCC and CDC.

Pharmacokinetics and Dosing. Alemtuzumab is administered intravenously in dosages of 30 mg/day three times per week. Premedication with diphenhydramine (50 mg) and acetaminophen (650 mg) should precede drug infusion. Because of hypersensitivity, dosing begins with a 3-mg infusion, followed by a 10-mg dose 2 days later and, if well tolerated, a 30-mg dose 2 days later. The drug has an initial mean $t_{1/2}$ of 1 hour, but after multiple doses, the $t_{1/2}$ extends to 12 days, and steady-state plasma levels are reached at approximately week 6 of treatment, presumably through saturation of CD52-binding sites. Clinical activity has been demonstrated in both B- and T-cell low-grade lymphomas and CLL, including patients with disease refractory to purine analogs (Hillmen et al., 2007). In chemotherapy-refractory CLL, overall response rates are ~40%, with complete responses of 6% in multiple series. Response rates in patients with untreated CLL are higher (overall response rates of 83% and complete responses of 24%).

Toxicity. The most concerning toxicities include acute infusion reactions and depletion of normal neutrophils and T cells (Table 62–2). Serious myelosuppression, with depletion of all blood lineages, occurs in the majority of patients and may represent either direct marrow toxicity or auto-immune responses. Immunosuppression by the antibody leads to a significant risk of fungal, viral, and other opportunistic infections (*Listeria*), particularly in patients who have previously received purine analogs (Keating et al., 2002; Hillmen et al., 2007). Patients should receive antibiotic prophylaxis against *Pneumocystis carinii* and herpes virus during treatment and for at least 2 months following therapy with alemtuzumab. Because reactivation of cytomegalovirus (CMV) infections may follow antibody use, patients should be monitored for symptoms and signs of viremia, hepatitis, and pneumonia. $CD4^+$ T-cell counts may remain profoundly depleted (<200 cells/μL) for 1 year. Alemtuzumab does not combine well with chemotherapy in standard regimens because of significant infectious complications (Gallamini et al., 2007).

Monoclonal Antibody–Cytotoxic Conjugates

Gemtuzumab Ozogamicin. Gemtuzumab ozogamicin (MYLOTARG) consists of a humanized monoclonal antibody against CD33 covalently linked to a semisynthetic derivative of calicheamicin, a potent enediyne antitumor antibiotic (Bernstein, 2000). The CD33 antigen is present on most hematopoietic cells, on >80% of AMLs, and on most myeloid cells in patients with myelodysplasias. However, other normal cell types lack CD33 expression, making this antigen attractive for targeted therapy. CD33 has no known biological function, although monoclonal antibody cross-linking inhibits normal and myeloid leukemia cell proliferation. Following its binding to CD33, gemtuzumab ozogamicin undergoes endocytosis, and cleavage of calicheamicin from the antibody takes place within the lysosome. The potent toxin then enters the nucleus, binds in the minor groove of DNA, and causes double-strand DNA breaks and cell death (Zein et al., 1988).

Clinical Pharmacology. The antibody conjugate produces a 30% complete response rate in relapsed AML, when administered at a dose of 9 mg/m^2 for up to 3 doses at 2-week intervals (Sievers et al., 2001). Pharmacokinetics of gemtuzumab ozogamicin at the standard 9-mg/m^2 dose are described by a $t_{1/2}$ of total and unconjugated calicheamicin of 41 and 143 hours, respectively (Dowell et al., 2001). Following a second dose, the $t_{1/2}$ of drug-antibody conjugate increases to 64 hours and the AUC increases to twice that of the initial dose. Most patients require two to three doses to achieve remission. The drug currently is approved in patients >60 years of age with AML in first relapse.

The primary toxicities of gemtuzumab ozogamicin include myelosuppression in all patients treated and hepatocellular damage in 30-40% of patients, manifested by hyperbilirubinemia and enzyme elevations. It also causes a syndrome that resembles hepatic veno-occlusive disease (tender, enlarged liver and rising serum bilirubin) when patients subsequently undergo myeloablative therapy or when gemtuzumab ozogamicin follows high-dose chemotherapy (Wadleigh et al., 2003). This syndrome reflects injury to hepatic sinusoids rather than venules. Defibrotide, an orphan drug, may prevent severe or fatal hepatic injury in patients who develop signs of hepatic failure while receiving a stem cell transplant following gemtuzumab ozogamicin (Versluys et al., 2004). Prolonged myelosuppression, particularly delayed recovery of platelet counts, may complicate the patient's course following remission induction with gemtuzumab ozogamicin.

Radioimmunoconjugates

Radioimmunoconjugates provide targeted delivery of radionuclides to tumor cells (Tables 62–1 and 62–2) (Witzig et al., 2002; Horning et al., 2005). ^{131}Iodine (^{131}I) is a favored radioisotope because it is readily available, relatively inexpensive, and easily conjugated to a monoclonal antibody. The γ particles emitted by ^{131}I can be used for both imaging and therapy, but protein-iodine conjugates have the drawback of releasing free ^{131}I and ^{131}I-tyrosine into the blood, and thus present a health hazard to caregivers, family, and others in contact with the patient. The β-emitter ^{90}Y has emerged as an attractive alternative to ^{131}I, based on its higher energy and longer path length. These features suggest that it may be more effective in tumors with larger diameters. It also has a short $t_{1/2}$ and remains conjugated, even after endocytosis, providing a safer profile for outpatient use.

Currently available radioimmunoconjugates consist of murine monoclonal antibodies against CD20 conjugated with ^{131}I [tositumomab (BEXXAR)] or ^{90}Y [ibritumomab tiuxetan (ZEVALIN)]. Both drugs have shown responses rates in relapsed lymphoma of 65-80%. They require significant collaboration between medical oncologists and nuclear medicine departments for administration. When using Zevalin, an initial dose of unlabeled rituximab is administered, followed by an imaging dose of Indium-111-labeled Zevalin. Biodistribution is determined, allowing calculation of a therapeutic dose of ^{90}Y Zevalin. A pretreatment dose of rituximab then is administered to saturate nonspecific binding sites, followed by the therapeutic dose of ^{90}Y Zevalin. The steps in Bexxar administration closely follow those of Zevalin. An imaging dose precedes the therapeutic dose given 1 week later. These agents cause antibody-related hypersensitivity, bone marrow suppression, and secondary leukemias.

Interleukin-2

IL-2 is a 133–amino acid glycoprotein encoded by a gene on chromosome 4q26-27; its molecular weight is 15 kDa (Smith, 1988). It bears structural homology to IL-4, IL-15, and GM-CSF. IL-2 is produced by activated T cells and NK cells; it acts to promote activated T-cell proliferation and enhanced killing by NK cells. Responsiveness depends on expression of the IL-2 receptor. Resting T cells and nearly all types of tumor cells lack receptor expression and are unresponsive to IL-2.

The IL-2 receptor has three components: 1) an α chain, a 55-kDa protein (CD25) involved mainly in IL-2 binding; 2) a β chain, a 75-kDa protein involved in intracellular signaling; and 3) a γ chain, a 64-kDa protein that is a component of many cytokine receptors (IL-2, IL-4, IL-7, IL-9, IL-15, and IL-21) and also is involved in signaling (Waldmann, 1991). IL-2 affinity for the three-component receptor is 10 pM; in the absence of the α chain, IL-2-binding affinity is reduced by a factor of 100.

Mechanism of Action. IL-2 stimulates the proliferation of activated T cells and the secretion of cytokines from NK cells and monocytes. IL-2 stimulation increases cytotoxic killing by T cells and NK cells. The mechanism of tumor cell killing has not been precisely defined but is presumed to be the result of enhanced killing by immune effector cells.

Pharmacokinetics. The serum $t_{1/2}$ of IL-2 after intravenous administration has an α phase of about 13 minutes and a β phase of about 90 minutes (Konrad et al., 1990). After a bolus dose of 6 million IU/m^2, peak serum levels are nearly 2,000 IU/mL. The same dose given subcutaneously achieves peak levels of 32-42 IU/mL in 2-6 hours. Six million IU/m^2 given by continuous intravenous infusion reaches a steady-state level of 123 IU/mL within 2 hours. IL-2 is excreted in the urine as an inactive metabolite. Encapsulation of IL-2 in liposomes or conjugation of IL-2 to polyethylene glycol alters its distribution and $t_{1/2}$; these forms are not FDA-approved.

Clinical Use. Aldesleukin (PROLEUKIN) possess the biological activities of human native IL-2. The drug is approved for use in metastatic renal-cell cancer (Rosenberg, 2000) and metastatic melanoma (McDermott, 2009). High-dose IL-2 produces an overall response rate of ~19% in patients with renal-cell cancer, and 8% achieve a complete response. Responses last a median of 8-9 years. Patients whose tumors express carbonic anhydrase IX have a higher likelihood of response (Atkins, 2009). High-dose IL-2 induces an overall response rate of ~16% in patients with metastatic melanoma, and 6% achieve a complete response. Responses last a median of ~5 years. Low-dose IL-2 also produces responses, but the duration of the responses may be less than with high-dose IL-2. The issue of appropriate dosage is controversial.

Aldesleukin may be administered in several ways. High-dose IL-2 is 600,000-720,000 IU/kg administered by intravenous bolus every 8 hours until dose-limiting toxicity appears or 14 total doses have been given; the schedule may be repeated after 9 days of rest for a maximum of 28 doses. Low-dose IL-2 is 60,000 or 72,000 IU/kg given by intravenous bolus every 8 hours for 15 doses. A third regimen involves delivery of 18 million units/m^2 daily by continuous intravenous infusion for 5 days. Chronic administration doses are 250,000 IU/kg subcutaneously daily for 5 days followed by 125,000 IU/kg daily for 6 weeks.

Toxicity. IL-2 toxicities are dominated by the capillary leak syndrome (Schwartz et al., 2002). Intravascular fluid leaks into the extravascular space, tissues, and lung, producing hypotension, edema, respiratory difficulties, confusion, tachycardia, oliguric renal failure, and electrolyte problems, including hypokalemia, hypomagnesemia, hypocalcemia, and hypophosphatemia. Symptoms include fever, chills, malaise, nausea, vomiting, and diarrhea. Laboratory abnormalities include thrombocytopenia, abnormal liver function tests, and neutropenia. Most patients develop a pruritic skin rash over most of the body surface. Hypothyroidism may occur. Arrhythmias are a rare complication.

These toxicities can be variable in grade but are often life-threatening, yet nearly all are reversible within 24-48 hours of discontinuing therapy. In view of the toxicities, patients should have a good performance status and normal renal and hepatic function before beginning therapy and should be closely supervised during drug administration.

Denileukin Diftitox. Denileukin diftitox (ONTAK) is an immunotoxin made from the genetic recombination of IL-2 and the catalytically active fragment of diphtheria toxin (Foss et al., 2001). The limited tissue expression of the high-affinity IL-2R makes this an attractive target for an immunotoxin, as cells that do not express the IL-2R or express only the intermediate- or low-affinity receptor types are significantly less sensitive to this agent. Introduction of the diphtheria toxin fragment into cells leads to ADP-ribosylation and inactivation of eukaryotic elongation factor EF-2, inhibition of protein synthesis, and thence, cell death.

Denileukin diftitox is FDA-approved for the treatment of recurrent/refractory cutaneous T-cell lymphomas. It should be administered at 9 or 18 μg/kg/day by intravenous infusion over 30-60 minutes for 5 consecutive days every 21 days for eight cycles. Response rates of 30-37% have been achieved in such patients with denileukin diftitox, with a median response duration of 6.9 months (Olsen et al., 2001). Additional patients derived clinical benefit but did not meet the objective criteria for response. The systemic exposure to denileukin diftitox is variable but proportional to dose. The drug has a distribution $t_{1/2}$ of 2-5 minutes with a terminal $t_{1/2}$ of ~70 minutes. Immunological reactivity to denileukin diftitox can be detected in virtually all patients after treatment but does not preclude clinical benefit with continued treatment. Denileukin diftitox clearance in later cycles of treatment accelerates by 2- to 3-fold as a result of development of antibodies, but serum levels exceed those required to produce cell death in IL-2R-expressing cell lines (1-10 ng/mL for >90 minutes). Patients with a history of hypersensitivity reactions to diphtheria toxin or IL-2 should not be treated. Significant toxicities associated with denileukin diftitox typically are acute hypersensitivity reactions, a vascular leak syndrome, and constitutional toxicities; glucocorticoid premedication significantly decreases toxicity (Foss et al., 2001).

Colony-Stimulating Factors

As noted in the preceding sections, many agents used for cancer chemotherapy suppress the production of multiple types of hematopoietic cells, and bone marrow suppression often has limited the delivery of chemotherapy on schedule and at prescribed doses. The availability of recombinant growth factors for erythrocytes (i.e., erythropoietin), granulocytes (i.e., G-CSF), and granulocytes and macrophages (i.e., GM-CSF) have advanced the ability to use combination therapy or high-dose therapy with diminished complications such as febrile neutropenia. The individual growth factors and specifics of supportive use of these agents are described in detail in Chapter 37.

BIBLIOGRAPHY

Adams J. The proteasome: A suitable antineoplastic target. *Nat Rev Cancer*, **2004**, *4*:349–360.

Ansell SM, Inwards DJ, Rowland KM Jr, et al. Low-dose, single-agent temsirolimus for relapsed mantle cell lymphoma: A phase 2 trial in the North Central Cancer Treatment Group. *Cancer*, **2008**, *113*:508–514.

Atkins MB. Treatment selection for patients with metastatic renal cell carcinoma: Identification of features favoring upfront IL-2-based immunotherapy. *Med Oncol*, **2009**, *26*:18–22.

Baselga J. Clinical trials of single-agent trastuzumab (Herceptin). *Semin Oncol*, **2000,** *27:*20–26.

Bernstein ID. Monoclonal antibodies to the myeloid stem cells: Therapeutic implications of CMA-676, a humanized anti-CD33 antibody calicheamicin conjugate. *Leukemia*, **2000**, *14*:474–475.

Blanke CD, Rankin C, Demetri GD, et al. Phase III randomized, intergroup trial assessing imatinib mesylate at two dose levels in patients with unresectable or metastatic gastrointestinal stromal tumors expressing the kit receptor tyrosine kinase: S0033. *J Clin Oncol*, **2008**, *26*:626–632.

Bokemeyer C, Bondarenko I, Makhson A, et al. Fluorouracil, leucovorin, and oxaliplatin with and without cetuximab in the first-line treatment of metastatic colorectal cancer. *J Clin Oncol*, **2009**, *27*:663–671.

Branford S, Rudzki Z, Walsh S, et al. Detection of BCR-ABL mutations in patients with CML treated with imatinib is virtually always accompanied by clinical resistance, and mutations in the ATP phosphate-binding loop (P-loop) are associated with a poor prognosis. *Blood*, **2003**, *102*:276–283.

Buchdunger E, Matter A, Druker BJ. Bcr-Abl inhibition as a modality of CML therapeutics. *Biochem Biophys Acta*, **2001,** *1551:*M11–M18.

Buckner JC, Forouzesh B, Erlichman C, et al. Phase I, pharmacokinetic study of temsirolimus administered orally to patients with advanced cancer. *Invest New Drugs*, **2010**, *28:*334–342.

Carracedo A, Ma L, Teruya-Feldstein J, et al. Inhibition of mTORC1 leads to MAPK pathway activation through a PI3K-dependent feedback loop in human cancer. *J Clin Invest*, **2008**, *118*:3065–3074.

Cartron G, Dacheux L, Salles G, et al. Therapeutic activity of humanized anti-CD20 monoclonal antibody and polymorphism in IgG fc receptor fcgamma RIIIa gene. *Blood*, **2002**, *99*:754–758.

Cattaneo C, Spedini P, Casari S, et al. Delayed-onset peripheral blood cytopenia after rituximab: Frequency and risk factor assessment in a consecutive series of 77 treatments. *Leuk Lymphoma*, **2006**, *47*:1013–1017.

Chen CC, Taniguchi T, D'Andrea A. The Fanconi anemia (FA) pathway confers glioma resistance to DNA alkylating agents. *J Mol Med*, **2007**, *85*:497–509.

Cheson BD, Leonard JP. Monoclonal antibody therapy for B-cell non-Hodgkin's lymphoma. *N Engl J Med*, **2008**, *359*:613–626.

Ciardiello F, Tortora G. EGFR antagonists in cancer treatment. *N Engl J Med,* **2008**, *358*:1160–1174.

Coiffier B, Lepage E, Briere J, et al. CHOP chemotherapy plus rituximab compared with CHOP alone in elderly patients with diffuse large-B-cell lymphoma. *N Engl J Med*, **2002**, *346*: 235–242.

Corbin AS, La Rosée P, Stoffregen E, et al. Several Bcr-Abl kinase domain mutants associated with imatinib mesylate resistance remain sensitive to imatinib. *Blood*, **2003,** *101:*4611–4614.

Crone SA, Zhao YY, Fan L, et al. ErbB2 is essential in the prevention of dilated cardiomyopathy. *Nat Med*, **2002**, *8:*459–465.

DeMatteo R, Ballman KV, Antonescu CR, et al. Adjuvant imatinib mesylate after resection of localised, primary gastrointestinal stromal tumour: A randomised, double-blind, placebo-controlled trial. *Lancet*, **2009**, *373*:1097–1104.

Dowell JA, Korth-Bradley J, Liu H, et al. Pharmacokinetics of gemtuzumab ozogamicin, and antibody-targeted chemotherapy agent for the treatment of patients with acute myeloid leukemia in first relapse. *J Clin Pharmacol*, **2001**, *41*: 1206–1214.

Druker BJ. Imatinib as a paradigm of targeted therapies. *Adv Cancer Res*, **2004**, *91:*1–30.

Ebert BL, Galili N, Tamayo P, et al. An erythroid differentiation signature predicts response to lenalidomide in myelodysplastic syndrome. *PLoS Med*, **2008**, *5*:e35.

Engelman JA, Zejnullahu K, Mitsudomi T, et al. MET amplification leads to gefitinib resistance in lung cancer by activating ERBB3 signaling. *Science,* **2007**, *16*:1039–1043.

Escudier B, Eisen T, Stadler WM, et al. Sorafenib in advanced clear-cell renal-cell carcinoma. *N Engl J Med*, **2007**, *356*:125–134.

Fabian MA, Biggs WH III, Treiber DK, et al. A small molecule-kinase interaction map for clinical kinase inhibitors. *Nat Biotechnol*, **2005**, *23*:329–336.

Folkman J. Tumor angiogenesis: Therapeutic implications. *N Engl J Med*, **1971**, *285*:1182-1186.

Foss FM, Bacha P, Osann KE, et al. Biological correlates of acute hypersensitivity events with DAB(389)IL-2 (denileukin diftitox, ONTAK) in cutaneous T-cell lymphoma: Decreased frequency and severity with steroid premedication. *Clin Lymphoma*, **2001**, *1:*298–302.

Franks ME, Macpherson GR, Figg WD. Thalidomide. *Lancet*, **2004**, *363:*1802–1811.

Gallamini A, Zaja F, Patti C, et al. Alemtuzumab (Campath-1H) and CHOP chemotherapy as first-line treatment of peripheral T-cell lymphoma: Results of a GITIL (Gruppo Italiano Terapie Innovative nei Linfomi) prospective multicenter trial. *Blood*, **2007**, *110*:2316–2323.

Geyer CE, Forster J, Lindquist D, et al. Lapatinib plus capecitabine for HER2-positive advanced breast cancer. *N Engl J Med*, **2006**, *355*:2733–2743.

Gressett SM, Shah SR. Intricacies of bevacizumab-induced toxicities and their management. *Ann Pharmacother*, **2009**, *43*:490–501.

Heinrich MC, Corless CL, Demetri GD, et al. Kinase mutations and imatinib response in patients with metastatic gastrointestinal stromal tumor. *J Clin Oncol*, **2003,** *21:*4342–4349.

Heinrich MC, Maki RG, Corless CL, et al. Primary and secondary kinase genotypes correlate with the biological and clinical activity of sunitinib in imatinib-resistant gastrointestinal stromal tumor. *J Clin Oncol*, **2008**, *26*:5352–5359.

Hideshima T, Chauhan D, Shima Y, et al. Thalidomide and its analogs overcome drug resistance of human multiple myeloma cells to conventional therapy. *Blood*, **2000,** *96:*2943–2950.

Hillmen P, Skotnicki AB, Robak T, et al. Alemtuzumab compared with chlorambucil as first-line therapy for chronic lymphocytic leukemia. *J Clin Oncol*, **2007**, *25*:5616–5623.

Horning SJ, Younes A, Jain V, et al. Efficacy and safety of tositumomab and iodine-131 tositumomab (bexxar) in B-cell lymphoma, progressive after rituximab. *J Clin Oncol*, **2005**, *23*:712–719.

Hughes T, Deininger M, Hochhaus A, et al. Monitoring CML patients responding to treatment with tyrosine kinase inhibitors: Review and recommendations for harmonizing current methodology for detecting BCR-ABL transcripts and kinase domain mutations and for expressing results. *Blood,* **2006**, *108*:28–37.

Hurwitz H, Fehrenbacher L, Novotny W, et al. Bevacizumab plus irinotecan, fluorouracil, and leucovorin for metastatic colorectal cancer. *N Engl J Med*, **2004**, *350*:2335–2342.

Hutson TE, Figlin RA, Kuhn JG, Motzer RJ. Targeted therapies for metastatic renal cell carcinoma: An overview of toxicity and dosing strategies. *Oncologist*, **2008**, *13*:1084–1096.

Hynes NE, Lane HA. ERBB receptors and cancer: The complexity of targeted inhibitors. *Nat Rev Cancer,* **2005**, *5*:341–354.

Jain RK. A new target for tumor therapy. *N Engl J Med*, **2009**, *360*:2669–2671.

Johnson DH, Fehrenbacher L, Novotny WF, et al. Randomized phase II trial comparing bevacizumab plus carboplatin and Paclitaxel with carboplatin and paclitaxel alone in previously untreated locally advanced or metastatic non-small-cell lung cancer. *J Clin Oncol*, **2004**, *22*:2184–2191.

Kane RC, Bross PF, Farrell AT, Pazdur R. Velcade: U.S. FDA approval for the treatment of multiple myeloma progressing on prior therapy. *Oncologist*, **2003,** *8:*508–513.

Kantarjian H, Giles F, Wunderle L, et al. Nilotinib in imatinib-resistant CML and Philadelphia chromosome-positive ALL. *N Engl J Med*, **2006**, *354*:2542–2551.

Kantarjian H, Talpaz M, O'Brien S, et al. High-dose imatinib mesylate therapy in newly diagnosed Philadelphia chromosome–positive chronic phase chronic myeloid leukemia. *Blood*, **2004,** *103:*2873–2878.

Karapetis CS, Khambata-Ford S, Jonker DJ, et al. K-ras mutations and benefit from cetuximab in advanced colorectal cancer. *N Engl J Med*, **2008**, *359*:1757–1765.

Keating MJ, Flinn I, Jain V, et al. Therapeutic role of alemtuzumab (Campathe-1H) in patients who have failed fludarabine: Results of a large international study. *Blood*, **2002**, *99*:3554–3561.

Kobayashi S, Boggon TJ, Dayaram T, et al. EGFR mutation and resistance of non-small-cell lung cancer to gefitinib. *N Engl J Med*, **2005**, *352*:786–792.

Konrad MW, Hemstreet G, Hersh EM, et al. Pharmacokinetics of recombinant interleukin 2 in humans. *Cancer Res*, **1990,** *50:* 2009–2017.

Kranick SM, Mowry EM, Rosenfeld MR. Progressive multifocal leukoencephalopathy after rituximab in a case of non-Hodgkin lymphoma. *Neurology*, **2007**, *69*:704–706.

Kumar S, Kimlinger TK, Lust JA, et al. Expression of CD52 on plasma cells in plasma cell proliferative disorders. *Blood*, **2003**, *102*:1075–1077.

Lapalombella R, Yu B, Triantafillou G, et al. Lenalidomide down-regulates the CD20 antigen and antagonizes direct and antibody-dependent cellular cytotoxicity of rituximab on primary chronic lymphocytic leukemia cells. *Blood*, **2008**, *112*:5180–5189.

Larson RA, Sievers EL, Stadtmauer EA, et al. Final report of the efficacy and safety of gemtuzumab ozogamicin (mylotarg) in patients with CD33-positive acute myeloid leukemia in first recurrence. *Cancer*, **2005**, *104*:1442–1452.

List AF. Lenalidomide—The phoenix rises. *N Engl J Med*, **2007**, *357*:2183–2186.

Llovet JM, Ricci S, Mazzaferro V, et al. Sorafenib in advanced hepatocellular carcinoma. *N Engl J Med*, **2008**, *359*:378–390.

Maloney DG, Grillo-Lopez AJ, White CA, et al. IDEC-C2B8 (rituximab) anti-CD20 monoclonal antibody therapy in patients with relapsed low-grade non-Hodgkin's lymphoma. *Blood*, **1997**, *90*:2188–2195.

Maloney DG, Smith B, Rose A. Rituximab. Mechanism of action and resistance. *Semin Oncol*, **2002**, *29*:2–9.

McDermott DF. Immunotherapy of metastatic renal cell carcinoma. *Cancer*, **2009**, *115*:2298–2305.

Medina PJ, Goodin S. Lapatinib: A dual inhibitor of human epidermal growth factor receptor tyrosine kinases. *Clin Ther*, **2008**, *30*:1426–1447.

Miller K, Wang M, Gralow J, et al. Paclitaxel plus bevacizumab versus paclitaxel alone for metastatic breast cancer. *N Engl J Med*, **2007**, *357*:2666–2676.

Mitsiades N, Mitsiades CS, Poulaki V, et al. Apoptotic signaling induced by immunomodulatory thalidomide analogs in human multiple myeloma cells: Therapeutic implications. *Blood*, **2002a,** *99:*4525–4530.

Mitsiades N, Mitsiades CS, Poulaki V, et al. Biologic sequelae of nuclear factor-κB blockade in multiple myeloma: Therapeutic applications. *Blood*, **2002b,** *99:*4079–4086.

Moore MJ, Goldstein D, Hamm J, et al. Erlotinib plus gemcitabine compared with gemcitabine alone in patients with advanced pancreatic cancer: A phase III trial of the National Cancer Institute of Canada Clinical Trials Group. *J Clin Oncol*, **2007**, *25*:1960–1966.

Morel F, Bris MJ, Herry A, et al. Double minutes containing amplified bcr-abl fusion gene in a case of chronic myeloid leukemia treated by imatinib. *Eur J Haematol*, **2003**, *70*: 235–239.

Motzer RJ, Escudier B, Oudard S, et al. Efficacy of everolimus in advanced renal cell carcinoma: A double-blind, randomised, placebo-controlled phase III trial. *Lancet*, **2008**, *372*:449–456.

Motzer RJ, Michaelson MD, Rosenberg J, et al. Sunitinib efficacy against advanced renal cell carcinoma. *J Urol*, **2007**, *178*: 1883–1887.

Moy B, Goss PE. Lapatinib-associated toxicity and practical management recommendations. *Oncologist*, **2007**, *12*:756–765.

Musallam KM, Dahdaleh FS, Shamseddine AI, Taher AT. Incidence and prophylaxis of venous thromboembolic events in multiple myeloma patients receiving immunomodulatory therapy. Thromb Res, **2008,** *123*:679.

Nahta R, Esteva FJ. HER-2-targeted therapy: Lessons learned and future directions. *Clin Cancer Res*, **2003,** *9*:5078–5084.

Negro-Vilar A, Dziewanowska Z, Groves ES, et al. Efficacy and safety of denileukin diftitox (dd) in a phase III, double-blind, placebo-controlled study of CD25+ patients with cutaneous T-cell lymphoma (CTCL). *J Clin Oncol*, **2007**, *25*:8026.

O'Brien SG, Meinhardt P, Bond E, et al. Effects of imatinib mesylate (STI571, Glivec) on the pharmacokinetics of simvastatin, a cyto-chrome p450 3A4 substrate, in patients with chronic myeloid leukemia. *Br J Cancer*, **2003**, *89*:1855–1859.

O'Donnell A, Faivre S, Burris HA III, et al. Phase I pharmacodynamic study of the oral mammalian target of rapamycin inhibitor everolimus in patients with advanced solid tumors. *J Clin Oncol*, **2008**, *26*:1588–1595.

O'Hare T, Walters DK, Stoffregen EP, et al. In vitro activity of bcr-abl inhibitors AMN107 and BMS-354825 against clinically relevant imatinib-resistant abl kinase domain mutants. *Cancer Res*, **2005**, *65*:4500–4505.

Olsen E, Duvic M, Frankel A, et al. Pivotal phase III trial of two dose levels of denileukin diftitox for the treatment of cutaneous T-cell lymphoma. *J Clin Oncol*, **2001,** *19:*376–388.

Orlowski RZ, Nagler A, Sonneveld P, et al. Randomized phase III study of pegylated liposomal doxorubicin plus bortezomib compared with bortezomib alone in relapsed or refractory multiple myeloma: Combination therapy improves time to progression. *J Clin Oncol*, **2007**, *25*:3892.

Papandreou CN, Daliani DD, Nix D, et al. Phase 1 trial of the proteasome inhibitor bortezomib in patients with advanced solid tumors with observations in androgen-independent prostate cancer. *J Clin Oncol*, **2004**, *22*:2108–2121.

Peng B, Hayes M, Resta D, et al. Pharmacokinetics and pharmacodynamics of imatinib in a phase 1 trial with chronic myeloid leukemia patients. *J Clin Oncol*, **2004**, *22:*935–942.

Plotkin SR, Stemmer-Rachamimov AO, Barker FG II, et al. Hearing improvement after bevacizumab in patients with neurofibromatosis type 2. *N Engl J Med*, **2009**, *361*:358–367.

Richardson P, Jagannath S, Raje N, et al. Lenalidomide, bortezomib, and dexamethasone (Rev/Vel/Dex) in patients with relapsed or relapsed/refractory multiple myeloma (MM): Preliminary results of a phase II study. *Blood*, **2007**, *110*:797A.

Richardson P, Schlossman R, Jagannath S, et al. Thalidomide for patients with relapsed multiple myeloma after high-dose chemotherapy and stem cell transplantation: Results of an open-label multicenter phase 2 study of efficacy, toxicity, and biological activity. *Mayo Clin Proc*, **2004,** *79:*875–882.

Roche-Lestienne C, Lai JL, Darre S, et al. A mutation conferring resistance to imatinib at the time of diagnosis of chronic myelogenous leukemia. *N Engl J Med*, **2003**, *348*: 2265–2266.

Rosenberg SA. Interleukin-2 and the development of immunotherapy for the treatment of patients with cancer. *Cancer J Sci Am*, **2000**, *6*:S2–S7.

San Miguel JF, Schlag R, Khuageva NK, et al. Bortezomib plus melphalan and prednisone for initial treatment of multiple myeloma. *N Engl J Med*, **2008**, *359*:906.

Sandler A, Gray R, Perry MC, et al. Paclitaxel-carboplatin alone or with bevacizumab for non-small-cell lung cancer. *N Engl J Med*, **2006**, *355*:2542–2550.

Scappaticci FA, Skillings JR, Holden SN, et al. Arterial thromboembolic events in patients with metastatic carcinoma treated with chemotherapy and bevacizumab. *J Natl Cancer Inst*, **2007**, *99*:1232–1239.

Schlessinger J. Cell signaling by receptor tyrosine kinases. *Cell,* **2000**, *103*:211–225.

Schwartz RN, Stover L, Dutcher J. Managing toxicities of high-dose interleukin 2. *Oncology*, **2002**, *16*:11–20.

Seidman A, Hudis C, Pierri MK, et al. Cardiac dysfunction in the trastuzumab clinical trials experience. *J Clin Oncol*, **2002**, *20*:1215–1221.

Sequist LV, Lynch TJ. EGFR tyrosine kinase inhibitors in lung cancer: An evolving story. *Annu Rev Med*, **2008**, *59*: 429–442.

Serafini P, De Santo C, Marigo I, et al. Derangement of immune responses by myeloid suppressor cells. *Cancer Immunol Immunother*, **2003**, *53*:64–72.

Shah NP, Kantarjian HM, Kim D, et al. Intermittent target inhibition with dasatinib 100 mg once daily preserves efficacy and improves tolerability in imatinib-resistant and -intolerant chronic-phase chronic myeloid leukemia. *J Clin Oncol*, **2008**, *26*:3204–3212.

Shah NP, Tran C, Lee FY, et al. Overriding imatinib resistance with a novel ABL kinase inhibitor. *Science*, **2004**, *305*: 399–401.

Shepherd FA, Rodrigues Pereira J, Ciuleanu T, et al. Erlotinib in previously treated non-small-cell lung cancer. *N Engl J Med*, **2005**, *353*:123–132.

Sievers EL, Larson RA, Stadtmauer EA, et al. Efficacy and safety of gemtuzumab ozogamicin in patients with CD33-positive acute myeloid leukemia in first relapse. *J Clin Oncol*, **2001**, *19*:3244–3254.

Sirvent N, Maire G, Pedeutour F. Genetics of dermatofibrosarcoma protuberans family of tumors: From ring chromosomes to tyrosine kinase inhibitor treatment. *Genes Chromosomes Cancer*, **2003**, *37*:1–19.

Slamon DJ, Godolphin W, Jones LA, et al. Studies of the HER-2/neu proto-oncogene in human breast and ovarian cancer. *Science*, **1989,** *244:*707–712.

Slamon DJ, Leyland-Jones B, Shak S, et al. Use of chemotherapy plus a monoclonal antibody against HER2 for metastatic breast cancer that overexpresses HER2. *N Engl J Med*, **2001,** *344*:783–792.

Smith KA. Interleukin-2: Inception, impact, and implications. *Science*, **1988**, *240*:1169–1176.

Thatcher N, Chang A, Parikh P, et al. Gefitinib plus best supportive care in previously treated patients with refractory advanced non-small-cell lung cancer: Results from a randomised, placebo-controlled, multicentre study (Iressa Survival Evaluation in Lung Cancer). *Lancet*, **2005**, *366*:1527–1537.

Van Cutsem E, Nowacki M, Lang I, et al. Randomized phase III study of irinotecan and 5-FU/FA with or without cetuximab in the first-line treatment of patients with metastatic colorectal cancer (mCRC): The CRYSTAL trial. *J Clin Oncol*, **2007**, *25*:4000.

Van Cutsem E, Siena S, Humblet Y, et al. An open-label, single-arm study assessing safety and efficacy of panitumumab in patients with metastatic colorectal cancer refractory to standard chemotherapy. *Ann Oncol*, **2008**, *19*:92–98.

van Oers MHJ, Klasa R, Marcus RE, et al. Rituximab maintenance improves clinical outcome of relapsed/resistant follicular non-Hodgkin lymphoma in patients both with and without rituximab during induction: Results of a prospective randomized phase 3 intergroup trial. *Blood*, **2006**, *108*: 3295–3301.

Vermorken JB, Mesia R, Rivera F, et al. Platinum-based chemotherapy plus cetuximab in head and neck cancer. *N Engl J Med*, **2008**, *359*:1116–1127.

Versluys B, Bhattacharaya R, Steward C, et al. Prophylaxis with defibrotide prevents veno-occlusive disease in stem cell transplantation after gemtuzumab ozogamicin exposure. *Blood*, **2004**, *103*:1968.

Villamor N, Montserrat E, Colomer D. Mechanism of action and resistance to monoclonal antibody therapy. *Semin Oncol*, **2003**, *30*:424–433.

Vogel CL, Cobleigh MA, Tripathy D, et al. Efficacy and safety of trastuzumab as a single agent in first-line treatment of HER2-over-expressing metastatic breast cancer. *J Clin Oncol*, **2002,** *20*:719–726.

Wadleigh M, Richardson PG, Zahrieh D, et al. Prior gemtuzumab ozogamicin exposure significantly increases the risk of veno-occlusive disease in patients who undergo myeloablative allogeneic stem cell transplantation. *Blood*, **2003**, *102*: 1578–1582.

Waldmann TA. The interleukin-2 receptor. *J Biol Chem*, **1991**, *266*:2681–2684.

Weisberg E, Manley PW, Breitenstein W, et al. Characterization of AMN107, a selective inhibitor of native and mutant bcr-abl. *Cancer Cell*, **2005**, *7*:129–141.

Witzig TE, Gordon LI, Cabanillas F, et al. Randomized controlled trial of yttrium-90-labeled ibritumomab tiuxetan radioimmunotherapy versus rituximab immunotherapy for patients with relapsed or refractory low-grade, follicular, or transformed B-cell non-Hodgkin's lymphoma. *J Clin Oncol*, **2002**, *20*:2453–2463.

Yang JC, Haworth L, Sherry RM, et al. A randomized trial of bevacizumab, an anti-vascular endothelial growth factor antibody, for metastatic renal cancer. *N Engl J Med*, **2003**, *349*: 427–434.

Zein N, Sinha AM, McGahren WJ, Ellestad GA. Calicheamicin gamma 1I: An antitumor antibiotic that cleaves double-stranded DNA site specifically. *Science*, **1988**, *240*:1198–1201.

Serafini P, De Santo C, Marigo I, et al. Derangement of immune responses by myeloid suppressor cells. *Cancer Immunol Immunother*. 2004; *53*:64–72.

Shah NP, Kantarjian HM, Kim D, et al. Intermittent target inhibition with dasatinib 100 mg once daily preserves efficacy and improves tolerability in imatinib-resistant and -intolerant chronic-phase chronic myeloid leukemia. *J Clin Oncol*. 2008; *26*:3204–3212.

Shah NP, Tran C, Lee FY, et al. Overriding imatinib resistance with a novel ABL kinase inhibitor. *Science*. 2004; *305*:399–401.

Shepherd FA, Rodrigues Pereira J, Ciuleanu T, et al. Erlotinib in previously treated non-small-cell lung cancer. *N Engl J Med*. 2005; *353*:123–132.

Sievers EL, Larson RA, Stadtmauer EA, et al. Efficacy and safety of gemtuzumab ozogamicin in patients with CD33-positive acute myeloid leukemia in first relapse. *J Clin Oncol*. 2001; *19*:3244–3254.

Sirvent N, Maire G, Pedeutour F. Genetics of dermatofibrosarcoma protuberans family of tumors: From ring chromosomes to tyrosine kinase inhibitor treatment. *Genes Chromosomes Cancer*. 2003; *37*:1–19.

Slamon DJ, Godolphin W, Jones LA, et al. Studies of the HER-2/neu proto-oncogene in human breast and ovarian cancer. *Science*. 1989; *244*:707–712.

Slamon DJ, Leyland-Jones B, Shak S, et al. Use of chemotherapy plus a monoclonal antibody against HER2 for metastatic breast cancer that overexpresses HER2. *N Engl J Med*. 2001; *344*:783–792.

Smith KA. Interleukin-2: Inception, impact, and implications. *Science*. 1988; *240*:1169–1176.

Thatcher N, Chang A, Parikh P, et al. Gefitinib plus best supportive care in previously treated patients with refractory advanced non-small-cell lung cancer: Results from a randomised, placebo-controlled, multicentre study (Iressa Survival Evaluation in Lung Cancer). *Lancet*. 2005; *366*:1527–1537.

Van Cutsem E, Nowacki M, Lang I, et al. Randomized phase III study of irinotecan and 5-FU/FA with or without cetuximab in the first-line treatment of patients with metastatic colorectal cancer (mCRC): The CRYSTAL trial. *J Clin Oncol*. 2007; *25*:4000.

Van Cutsem E, Siena S, Humblet Y, et al. An open-label, single-arm study assessing safety and efficacy of panitumumab in patients with metastatic colorectal cancer refractory to standard chemotherapy. *Ann Oncol*. 2008; *19*:92–98.

Van Oers MH, Klasa R, Marcus RE, et al. Rituximab maintenance improves clinical outcome of relapsed/resistant follicular non-Hodgkin lymphoma in patients both with and without rituximab during induction: Results of a prospective randomized phase 3 intergroup trial. *Blood*. 2006; *108*:3295–3301.

Vermorken JB, Mesia R, Rivera F, et al. Platinum-based chemotherapy plus cetuximab in head and neck cancer. *N Engl J Med*. 2008; *359*:1116–1127.

Verstovsek S, Manshouri T, Smith FO, et al. Amifostine with or without imatinib mesylate... presents concentration-dependent effects [illegible] in vitro *Blood*. 2006; *107*:1058.

Villamor N, Montserrat E, Colomer D. Mechanism of action and resistance to monoclonal antibody therapy. *Semin Oncol*. 2003; *30*:424–433.

Vogel CL, Cobleigh MA, Tripathy D, et al. Efficacy and safety of trastuzumab as a single agent in first-line treatment of HER2-overexpressing metastatic breast cancer. *J Clin Oncol*. 2002; *20*:719–726.

Wadleigh M, Richardson PG, Zahrieh D, et al. Prior gemtuzumab ozogamicin exposure significantly increases the risk of veno-occlusive disease in patients who undergo myeloablative allogeneic stem cell transplantation. *Blood*. 2003; *102*:1578–1582.

Waldmann TA. The interleukin-2 receptor. *J Biol Chem*. 1991; *266*:2681–2684.

Weisberg E, Manley PW, Breitenstein W, et al. Characterization of AMN107, a selective inhibitor of native and mutant Bcr-Abl. *Cancer Cell*. 2005; *7*:129–141.

Witzig TE, Gordon LI, Cabanillas F, et al. Randomized controlled trial of yttrium-90-labeled ibritumomab tiuxetan radioimmunotherapy versus rituximab immunotherapy for patients with relapsed or refractory low-grade, follicular, or transformed B-cell non-Hodgkin's lymphoma. *J Clin Oncol*. 2002; *20*:2453–2463.

Yang JC, Haworth L, Sherry RM, et al. A randomized trial of bevacizumab, an anti-vascular endothelial growth factor antibody, for metastatic renal cancer. *N Engl J Med*. 2003; *349*:427–434.

Zein N, Sinha AM, McGahren WJ, Ellestad GA. Calicheamicin gamma 1I: An antitumor antibiotic that cleaves double-stranded DNA site specifically. *Science*. 1988; *240*:1198–1201.

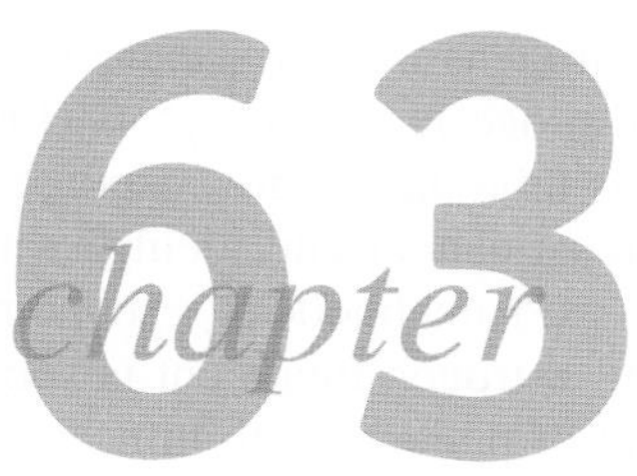

Natural Products in Cancer Chemotherapy: Hormones and Related Agents

Beverly Moy, Richard J. Lee, and Matthew Smith

The growth of a number of cancers is hormone dependent or regulated by hormones. Research in the fields of fertility, birth control, and menopause has yielded valuable hormone analogs and antagonists for the treatment of both breast and prostate cancer. These molecules interrupt the stimulatory axis created by systemic pools of androgens and estrogens, inhibit hormone production or binding to receptors, and ultimately block the complex expression of genes that promotes tumor growth and survival. These drugs have proven effective in extending survival and delaying or preventing tumor recurrence in breast cancer and prostate cancer.

GLUCOCORTICOIDS

The pharmacology, major therapeutic uses, and toxic effects of the glucocorticoids are discussed in Chapter 42. Only the applications of these drugs in the treatment of neoplastic disease are considered here. Glucocorticoids act through their binding to a specific physiological receptor that translocates to the nucleus and induces anti-proliferative and apoptotic responses in sensitive cells. Because of their lympholytic effects and their ability to suppress mitosis in lymphocytes, glucocorticoids are used as cytotoxic agents in the treatment of acute leukemia in children and malignant lymphoma in children and adults.

In acute lymphoblastic or undifferentiated leukemia of childhood, glucocorticoids may produce prompt clinical improvement and objective hematological remissions in ≤30% of children. Although these responses frequently are characterized by complete disappearance of all detectable leukemic cells from the peripheral blood and bone marrow, the duration of remission is brief. Remissions occur more rapidly with glucocorticoids than with antimetabolites, and there is no evidence of cross-resistance to unrelated agents. For these reasons, therapy is initiated with prednisone and vincristine, often followed by an anthracycline or methotrexate, and L-asparaginase. Glucocorticoids are a valuable component of curative regimens for other lymphoid malignancies, including Hodgkin's disease, non-Hodgkin's lymphoma, multiple myeloma, and chronic lymphocytic leukemia (CLL). Glucocorticoids are extremely helpful in controlling auto-immune hemolytic anemia and thrombocytopenia associated with CLL.

The glucocorticoids, particularly dexamethasone, are used in conjunction with radiotherapy to reduce edema related to tumors in critical areas such as the superior mediastinum, brain, and spinal cord. Doses of 4-6 mg every 6 hours have dramatic effects in restoring neurological function in patients with cerebral metastases, but these effects are temporary. Acute changes in dexamethasone dosage can lead to a rapid recrudescence of symptoms. Dexamethasone should not be discontinued abruptly in patients receiving radiotherapy or chemotherapy for brain metastases. Gradual tapering of the dosage may be undertaken if a clinical response to definitive antitumor therapy has been achieved. The antitumor effects of glucocorticoids are mediated by their binding to the glucocorticoid receptor, which activates a program of gene expression that leads to apoptosis.

Several glucocorticoids are available and at equivalent dosages exert similar effects (see Chapter 42). Prednisone, e.g., usually is administered orally in doses as high as 60-100 mg, or even higher, for the first few days and gradually reduced to levels of 20-40 mg/day. A continuous attempt should be made to establish the lowest possible dosage required to control the manifestations of the disease. These agents, when used chronically, exert a wide range of side effects, including glucose intolerance, immunosuppression, osteoporosis, and psychosis (see Chapter 42). Dexamethasone is the preferred agent for remission induction in multiple myeloma, usually in combination with melphalan, anthracyclines, vincristine, bortezomib, or thalidomide.

PROGESTINS

Progestational agents (see Chapters 40 and 66) have been used as second-line hormonal therapy for metastatic hormone-dependent breast cancer and in the management of endometrial carcinoma previously treated by surgery and radiotherapy. In addition, progestins stimulate appetite and restore a sense of well-being in cachectic patients with advanced stages of cancer and acquired immunodeficiency syndrome (AIDS). Although progesterone itself is poorly absorbed when given orally and must be used with an oil carrier when given intramuscularly, there are synthetic progesterone preparations.

Medroxyprogesterone (DEPO-PROVERA, others) can be administered intramuscularly in doses of 400-1000 mg weekly. An alternative and more commonly used oral agent is megestrol acetate (MEGACE, others; 40-320 mg daily in divided doses). Hydroxyprogesterone (not available in the U.S.) usually is administered intramuscularly in doses of 1000 mg one or more times weekly. Beneficial effects have been observed in approximately one-third of patients with endometrial cancer. The response of breast cancer to megestrol is predicted by both the presence of estrogen receptors (ERs) and the evidence of response to a prior hormonal treatment. The effect of progestin therapy in breast cancer appears to be dose dependent, with some patients demonstrating second responses following escalation of megestrol to 1600 mg/day. Clinical use of progestins in breast cancer has been largely superseded by the advent of tamoxifen and the aromatase inhibitors (AIs). Responses to progestational agents also have been reported in metastatic carcinomas of the prostate and kidney.

ESTROGENS AND ANDROGENS

Discussions of the pharmacology of the estrogens and androgens appear in Chapters 40, 41, and 66. These agents are of value in certain neoplastic diseases, notably those of the prostate and mammary gland, because these organs are dependent on hormones for their growth, function, and morphological integrity. Carcinomas arising from these organs often retain the hormonal responsiveness of their normal counterpart tissues. By changing the hormonal environment of such tumors, it is possible to alter the course of the neoplastic process.

Estrogens and Androgens in the Treatment of Mammary Carcinoma

High doses of estrogen have long been recognized as effective treatment of breast cancer. However, serious side effects such as thromboembolism prompted the development of alternate strategies. Paradoxically, anti-estrogens also are effective, as seen by remission of disease achieved with oophorectomy. Thus, because of equivalent efficacy and more favorable side effects, anti-estrogens such as tamoxifen and the AIs have replaced estrogens or androgens for breast cancer. The presence of the ERs and progesterone receptors (PRs) on tumor tissue serves as a biomarker for response to hormonal therapy in breast cancer and identifies the subset of patients with a ≥60% likelihood of responding. The response rate to anti-estrogen treatment is somewhat lower in the subset of patients with tumors that are ER+ or PR+ but also positive for human epidermal growth factor receptors HER1/neu amplification. In contrast, ER-negative and PR-negative carcinomas do not respond to hormonal therapy.

Responses to hormonal therapy may not be apparent clinically or by imaging for 8-12 weeks. If the disease responds or remains stable on a given treatment, the medication typically should be continued until the disease progresses or unwanted toxicities develop. The duration of an induced remission in patients with metastatic disease averages 6-12 months but sometimes can last for many years.

Anti-Estrogen Therapy

Anti-estrogen approaches for the therapy of hormone receptor–positive breast cancer include the use of selective estrogen-receptor modulators (SERMs), selective estrogen-receptor downregulators (SERDs), and AIs (Table 63–1).

Selective Estrogen-Receptor Modulators. SERMs bind to the ER and exert either estrogenic or anti-estrogenic effects, depending on the specific organ. Tamoxifen citrate is the most widely studied anti-estrogenic treatment in breast cancer. The recent decline in breast cancer mortality in Western countries is believed to be partly due to the common use of tamoxifen, especially in the adjuvant setting. However, in addition to its estrogen antagonist effects in breast cancer, tamoxifen also exerts estrogenic agonist effects on non-breast tissues, thus influencing the overall therapeutic index of the drug. Therefore, several novel anti-estrogen compounds that offer the potential for enhanced efficacy and reduced toxicity compared with tamoxifen have been developed. These novel anti-estrogens can be divided into tamoxifen analogs [e.g., toremifene (FARESTON), droloxifene, idoxifene], "fixed ring" compounds [e.g., raloxifene (EVISTA), lasofoxifene, arzoxifene, miproxifene, levormeloxifene, EM652], and the SERDs [e.g., fulvestrant (FASLODEX), SR 16234, and ZK 191703, the latter also termed "pure anti-estrogens"] (Howell et al., 2004a).

Tamoxifen. Tamoxifen was first synthesized in 1966 and initially developed as an oral contraceptive but instead was found to induce ovulation and proved to have antiproliferative effects on estrogen-dependent breast cancer cell lines. For >3 decades, tamoxifen has been studied

Table 63–1

Clinical Uses for Anti-Estrogen Therapy in ER+ Breast Cancer

	DISEASE SETTING			
DRUG	ADJUVANT (premen)	ADJUVANT (postmen)	METASTATIC (premen)	METASTATIC (postmen)
Tamoxifen	Yes (5 yr)	Yes (before AI for 2-5 yr)	Yes	Yes
Fulvestrant	No	No	No	Yes (PD on TAM or AI)
Anastrozole	No	Yes (upfront or after TAM)	No	Yes
Letrozole	No	Yes (upfront or after TAM)	No	Yes
Exemestane	No	Yes (upfront or after TAM)	No	Yes
Toremifene	No	Yes	No	Yes

Premen, premenopausal; Postmen, postmenopausal; AI, aromatase inhibitor; PD, progressive disease; TAM, tamoxifen; ER, estrogen receptor.

for use in various stages of breast cancer. It has become a standard agent as a result of its anticancer activity and good tolerability profile. Tamoxifen is prescribed for the prevention of breast cancer in high-risk patients, for the adjuvant therapy of early-stage breast cancer, and for the therapy of advanced breast cancer. It also prevents the development of breast cancer in women at high risk based on a strong family history, prior nonmalignant breast pathology, or inheritance of the BRCA1 or BRCA2 genes.

Mechanism of Action. Tamoxifen is a competitive inhibitor of estradiol binding to the ER.

There are two subtypes of estrogen receptors: ERα and ERβ, which have different tissue distributions and can either homo- or heterodimerize. Binding of estradiol and SERMs to the estrogen-binding sites of the ERs initiates a change in conformation of the ER, dissociation of the ER from heat-shock proteins, and inhibition of ER dimerization. Dimerization facilitates the binding of the ER to specific DNA estrogen-response elements (EREs) in the vicinity of estrogen-regulated genes. Co-regulator proteins interact with the receptor to act as co-repressors or co-activators of gene expression. At least 50 transcriptional activating factors transduce and modulate the effects of estrogen on target genes. Differences in tissue distribution of ER subtypes, the function of co-regulator proteins, and the various transcriptional activating factors likely explain the variability of response to tamoxifen in hormone receptor–positive (ER^+) breast cancer and its agonist and antagonist activities in noncancerous tissues. Other organs displaying agonist effects of tamoxifen include the uterine endometrium (endometrial hypertrophy, vaginal bleeding, and endometrial cancer), the coagulation system (thromboembolism), bone metabolism (increase in bone mineral density [BMD]), and liver (alterations of blood lipid profile).

Absorption, Fate, and Excretion. The usual oral dose of tamoxifen in the U.S. is 20 mg once a day. Doses as high as 200 mg/day have been used in the therapy of breast cancer, but high doses are associated with retinal degeneration.

Tamoxifen is readily absorbed following oral administration, with peak concentrations measurable after 3-7 hours and steady-state levels being reached at 4-6 weeks. Metabolism of tamoxifen is complex and principally involves CYPs 3A4/5, and 2D6 in the formation of *N*-desmethyl tamoxifen, and CYP2D6 to form 4-hydroxytamoxifen, a more potent metabolite (Figure 63–1). Both metabolites can be further converted to 4-hydroxy-*N*-desmethyltamoxifen, which retains high affinity for the ER. The parent drug has a terminal $t_{1/2}$ of 7 days; the $t_{1/2}$ of *N*-desmethyltamoxifen and 4-hydroxytamoxifen are significantly longer (14 days). After enterohepatic circulation, glucuronides and other metabolites are excreted in the stool; excretion in the urine is minimal.

Therapeutic Uses. The usual oral dose of tamoxifen in the U.S. is 20 mg once a day.

Tamoxifen is used for the endocrine treatment of women with ER^+ metastatic breast cancer or following primary tumor excision as adjuvant therapy. For the adjuvant treatment of premenopausal women, tamoxifen is given for 5 years, or in postmenopausal women, for 2 years, followed by an AI. In patients with high risk of recurrence, it may be sequenced after adjuvant chemotherapy. Tamoxifen is used in premenopausal women with ER^+ tumors. Disease response rates are similar to those seen in postmenopausal patients. Alternative or additional anti-estrogen strategies in premenopausal women include oophorectomy or gonadotropin-releasing hormone analogs.

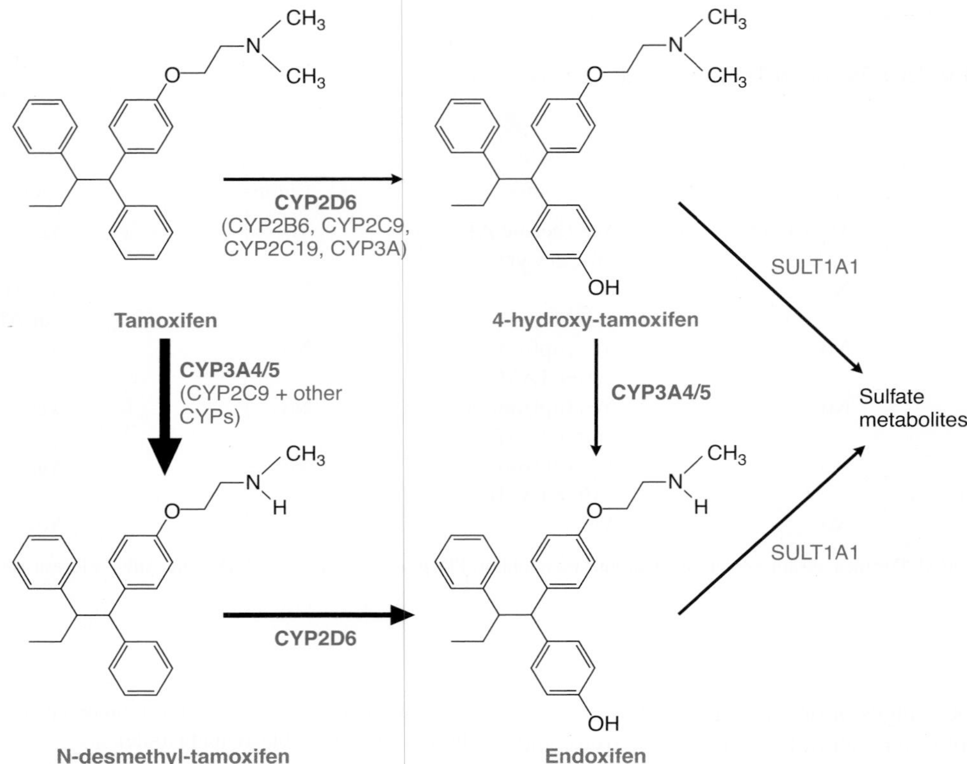

Figure 63–1. *Tamoxifen and its metabolites.*

The combination of tamoxifen and a gonadotropin-releasing hormone analog in premenopausal women (to reduce high estrogen levels resulting from tamoxifen effects on the gonadal-pituitary axis) yields better response rates and improved overall survival than either drug alone (Klijn et al., 2000).

The NOLVADEX Adjuvant Trial Organization (NATO) study indicated an overall disease-free survival advantage for patients receiving tamoxifen versus placebo. Five years of adjuvant therapy with tamoxifen yielded superior results compared to 1 or 2 years of therapy (Swedish Breast Cancer Cooperative Group, 1996; Early Breast Cancer Trialists' Collaborative Group, 1998). Therefore, although the optimal duration of tamoxifen has not been fully determined, randomized trials have demonstrated superiority of 5 years over shorter durations. One clinical trial evaluating the administration of tamoxifen for >5 years failed to show benefit of continued therapy and a trend toward worse outcomes in women who received tamoxifen therapy over a longer duration (Fisher et al., 2001).

Tamoxifen also has shown effectiveness (a 40-50% reduction in tumor incidence) in initial trials for preventing breast cancer in women at increased risk (Vogel et al, 2010). These studies were prompted by preclinical experiments showing prevention of tumors in animal models and also by the observation of reduced contralateral new primary breast tumors in women receiving adjuvant tamoxifen for early-stage breast cancer (Early Breast Cancer Trialists' Collaborative Group, 1998; Fisher et al., 2001). Tamoxifen only reduces ER+ tumors without affecting ER-negative tumors, which contribute disproportionately to breast cancer mortality.

Toxicity. The common adverse reactions to tamoxifen include vasomotor symptoms (hot flashes), atrophy of the lining of the vagina, hair loss, nausea, and vomiting. These may occur in ≤25% of patients and rarely are sufficiently severe to require discontinuation of therapy. Menstrual irregularities, vaginal bleeding and discharge, pruritus vulvae, and dermatitis occur with increasing severity in postmenopausal women.

Tamoxifen also increases the incidence of endometrial cancer by 2- to 3-fold, particularly in postmenopausal women who receive 20 mg/day for ≥2 years. In general, tamoxifen-associated endometrial cancers are reported as low-grade and early-stage tumors. Standard practice guidelines from the National Comprehensive Cancer Network alert physicians to the evaluation of abnormal vaginal bleeding in women with an intact uterus.

Tamoxifen increases the risk of thromboembolic events, which increase with the age of a patient and also in the perioperative period. Hence, it often is recommended to discontinue tamoxifen prior to elective surgery. Because tamoxifen is associated with thromboembolism, some authorities suggest that the pretreatment evaluation of breast cancer patients should include screening for coagulation abnormalities (factor V Leiden, protein C, antithrombin III defects) and for a history of thromboembolic disease. Presence of these risk factors should lead to exclusion of women from treatment. Note that no clear causative association between the presence of the factor V Leiden mutation and tamoxifen-induced thromboembolism has been found (Abramson, 2006).

Like estrogen, tamoxifen is a hepatic carcinogen in animals, although increases in primary hepatocellular carcinoma have not been reported in patients on the drug. Tamoxifen causes retinal deposits, decreased visual acuity, and cataracts in occasional patients, although the frequency of these changes is more common in patients on high doses of drug.

In addition to its ability to prevent recurrence or the development of primary breast cancer, tamoxifen has other end-organ benefits related to its partial estrogenic action. For example, it may slow the development of osteoporosis in postmenopausal women. Like certain estrogens, tamoxifen lowers total serum cholesterol, low-density-lipoprotein cholesterol, and lipoproteins and raises apolipoprotein A-I levels, potentially decreasing the risk of myocardial infarction.

Tamoxifen Resistance. Despite its benefits, initial or acquired resistance to tamoxifen frequently occurs (Moy and Goss, 2006). Polymorphisms in CYP2D6 that reduce its activity lead to lower plasma levels of 4-OH tamoxifen, a potent metabolite, and are associated with higher risks of disease relapse and a lower incidence of hot flashes (Goetz et al., 2005). CYP2D6 is responsible for the activation of tamoxifen to its active metabolite endoxifen (Figure 63–1). Cross-talk between the ER and HER2/neu pathway also has been implicated in tamoxifen resistance. The paired box 2 gene product (PAX2) has been identified as a crucial mediator of ER repression of ErbB2 by tamoxifen (Hurtado et al., 2008). Interactions between PAX2 and the ER co-activator AIB-1/SRC-3 determine tamoxifen response in breast cancer cells.

Toremifene. Toremifene (FARESTON) is a triphenylethylene derivative of tamoxifen and has a similar pharmacological profile (Figure 63–2). Toremifene is indicated for the treatment of breast cancer in women with tumors that are ER^+ or of unknown receptor status.

In preclinical models, toremifene has activity against breast cancer cells *in vitro* and *in vivo* similar to that of tamoxifen. Unlike tamoxifen, however, toremifene is not hepatocarcinogenic in experimental animals. Two adjuvant studies have compared efficacy of these two agents and, in particular, long-term tolerability and safety, in early-stage breast cancer. There were no significant differences in efficacy or tolerability after a median follow-up of 4.4 years, and the number of subsequent second cancers was similar (Howell et al., 2004a). However, *in vitro* in a low-estrogen environment, toremifene has less estrogen agonist effect than tamoxifen. This may make toremifene more effective in combination with an AI than tamoxifen, and this possibility is the subject of ongoing clinical trials.

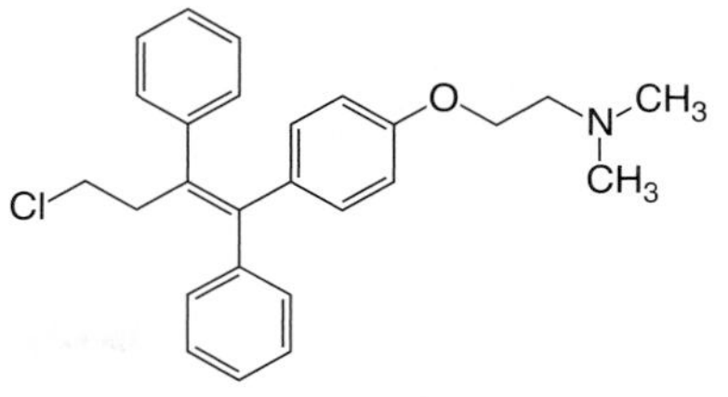

Selective Estrogen Receptor Downregulators

SERDs, also termed "pure anti-estrogens," include fulvestrant and a host of agents in experimental trials (RU 58668, SR 16234, ZD 164384, and ZK 191703).

Toremifene

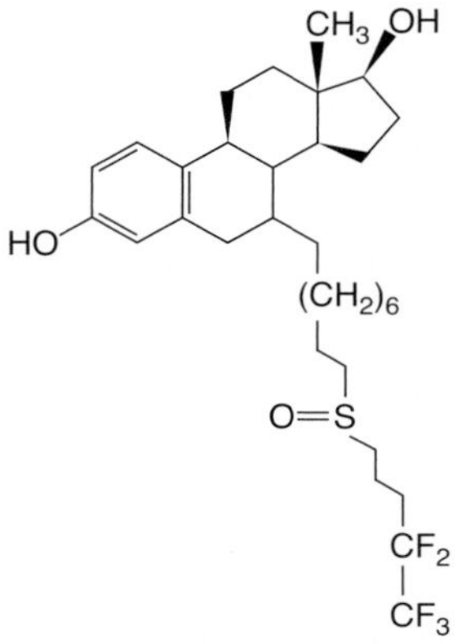

Fulvestrant

Figure 63–2. *Chemical structures of toremifene and fulvestrant.*

SERDs, unlike SERMs, are devoid of any estrogen agonist activity.

Fulvestrant. Fulvestrant (FASLODEX) is the first agent approved by the U.S. Food and Drug Administration (FDA) in the class of ER downregulators (Figure 63–2). This new class of hormone antagonists was hypothesized to have an improved safety profile, faster onset, and longer duration of action than the SERMs due to their pure ER antagonist activity (Robertson, 2002). Fulvestrant is approved for postmenopausal women with hormone receptor–positive metastatic breast cancer that has progressed on tamoxifen.

Mechanism of Action. Fulvestrant is a steroidal anti-estrogen that binds to the ER with an affinity >100 times that of tamoxifen. The drug inhibits the binding of estrogen but also alters the receptor structure such that the receptor is targeted for proteasomal degradation; fulvestrant also may inhibit receptor dimerization. Unlike tamoxifen, which stabilizes or even increases ER expression, fulvestrant reduces the number of ER molecules in cells, both *in vitro* and *in vivo;* as a consequence of this ER downregulation, the drug abolishes ER-mediated transcription of estrogen-dependent genes (Howell et al., 2004b).

Absorption, Fate, and Excretion. Maximum plasma concentrations are reached ~7 days after intramuscular administration of fulvestrant and are maintained over 1 month. The plasma $t_{1/2}$ is ~40 days.

Steady-state concentrations are reached after three to six monthly injections. There is extensive and rapid distribution and extensive protein binding of this highly lipophilic drug.

Various pathways, similar to those of steroid metabolism (oxidation, aromatic hydroxylation, and conjugation), extensively metabolize fulvestrant. CYP3A4 appears to be the only CYP isoenzyme involved in the metabolism of fulvestrant. However, several preclinical and clinical studies indicate that fulvestrant is not subject to CYP3A4 interactions that might affect its pharmacokinetics, safety, or efficacy; however, the effects of *strong* CYP3A4 inhibitors have not been studied. The putative metabolites possess no estrogenic activity, and only the 17-keto compound demonstrates a level of anti-estrogenic activity, which is ~22% that of fulvestrant. Less than 1% of the parent drug is excreted intact in the urine.

Dosing. The approved dosing for fulvestrant is 250 mg by intramuscular injection monthly. Because pharmacokinetic data have shown that it takes ~3-6 months for fulvestrant to reach steady-state levels with monthly dosing, alternative regimens have been studied. A loading dose regimen of 500 mg on day 0, 250 mg on days 14 and 28, and then 250 mg each month (McCormack and Sapunar, 2008) yields maximum fulvestrant concentrations in plasma an average of 12 days after the first dose and maintains those levels thereafter.

Therapeutic Uses. Fulvestrant is used in postmenopausal women as anti-estrogen therapy of hormone receptor–positive metastatic breast cancer after progression on first-line anti-estrogen therapy such as tamoxifen (Strasser-Weippl and Goss, 2004). Fulvestrant is at least as effective in this setting as the third-generation AI anastrozole.

Fulvestrant 250 mg (administered as a once-monthly 5-mL intramuscular injection) also has been compared with tamoxifen 20 mg (orally once daily) in a trial of postmenopausal women with ER^+ and/or PR^+ or ER/PR-unknown metastatic breast cancer who had not previously received endocrine or chemotherapy. In patients with ER^+ and/or PR^+ disease, there was no difference between fulvestrant and tamoxifen in time to disease progression or overall response rate (Vergote and Robertson, 2004). The long time to steady-state plasma levels for fulvestrant has brought into question the results of studies that lacked a loading dose, and trials are in progress to test the relative efficacy of giving an initial loading dose followed by regular monthly injections.

Toxicity and Adverse Effects. Fulvestrant generally is well tolerated, the most common adverse effects being nausea, asthenia, pain, vasodilation (hot flashes), and headache. The risk of injection site reactions, seen in ~7% of patients, is reduced by giving the injection slowly. In the study comparing anastrozole and fulvestrant in tamoxifen-resistant patients, the drugs had equivalent quality-of-life outcome measures (Vergote and Robertson, 2004).

AROMATASE INHIBITORS

Aromatase inhibitors (AIs; Figure 63–3) block the function of the aromatase enzyme that converts androgens to estrogens. AIs now are considered the standard of care for adjuvant treatment of postmenopausal women with hormone receptor–positive breast cancer, either as initial therapy or sequenced after tamoxifen.

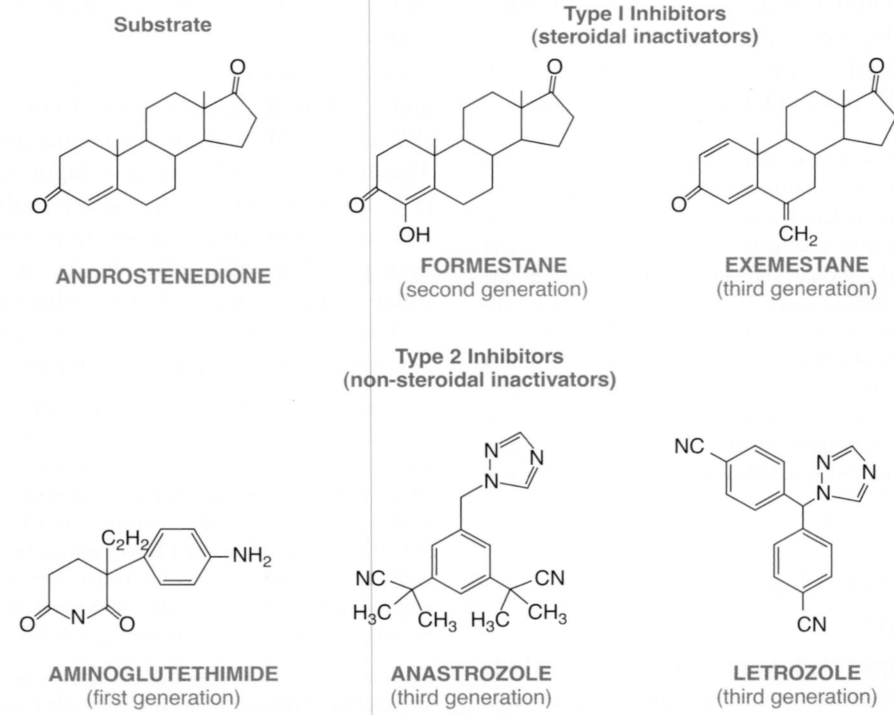

Figure 63–3. *Structure of the main aromatase inhibitors and the natural substrate androstenedione.*

Aromatase activity is the product of the *CYP19* gene. CYP19 is highly expressed in human placenta and in granulosa cells of ovarian follicles, where its expression depends on cyclical gonadotropin stimulation. Aromatase also is present, at lower levels, in several nonglandular tissues, including subcutaneous fat, liver, muscle, brain, and normal breast and in breast-cancer tissue. The aromatase enzyme is responsible for the conversion of adrenal androgens and gonadal androstenedione and testosterone to the estrogens, estrone (E1) and estradiol (E2), respectively (Figure 63–4). In postmenopausal women, this conversion is the primary source of circulating estrogens, while estrogen production in premenopausal women primarily is from the ovaries.

In postmenopausal women, AIs can suppress most peripheral aromatase activity, leading to profound estrogen deprivation. This strategy of estrogen deprivation of ER^+ breast cancer cells stands in contrast to the ER antagonist activity that SERMs and SERDs exert.

Based on their sequence of development, AIs are classified as first, second, or third generation. In addition, they are further classified as type 1 (steroidal) or type 2 (nonsteroidal) AIs according to their structure and mechanism of action. Type 1 inhibitors are steroidal analogs of androstenedione (Figure 63–3). Androstenedione analogs bind covalently to the same site on the aromatase molecule, but unlike androstenedione, they bind irreversibly because of their conversion to reactive intermediates by aromatase. Thus, they commonly are known as aromatase inactivators. Type 2 inhibitors are nonsteroidal and bind reversibly to the heme group of the enzyme.

Third-Generation Aromatase Inhibitors

The third-generation inhibitors, developed in the 1990s, include the type 1 steroidal agent exemestane and the type 2 nonsteroidal imidazoles anastrozole and letrozole. Currently, third-generation AIs are used as part of the standard of care for treatment of early-stage and advanced breast cancer in postmenopausal women.

Anastrozole. Anastrozole is a potent and selective triazole AI.

Mechanism of Action. Anastrozole, like letrozole, binds competitively and specifically to the heme of the CYP19. Anastrozole, 1 mg or 10 mg,

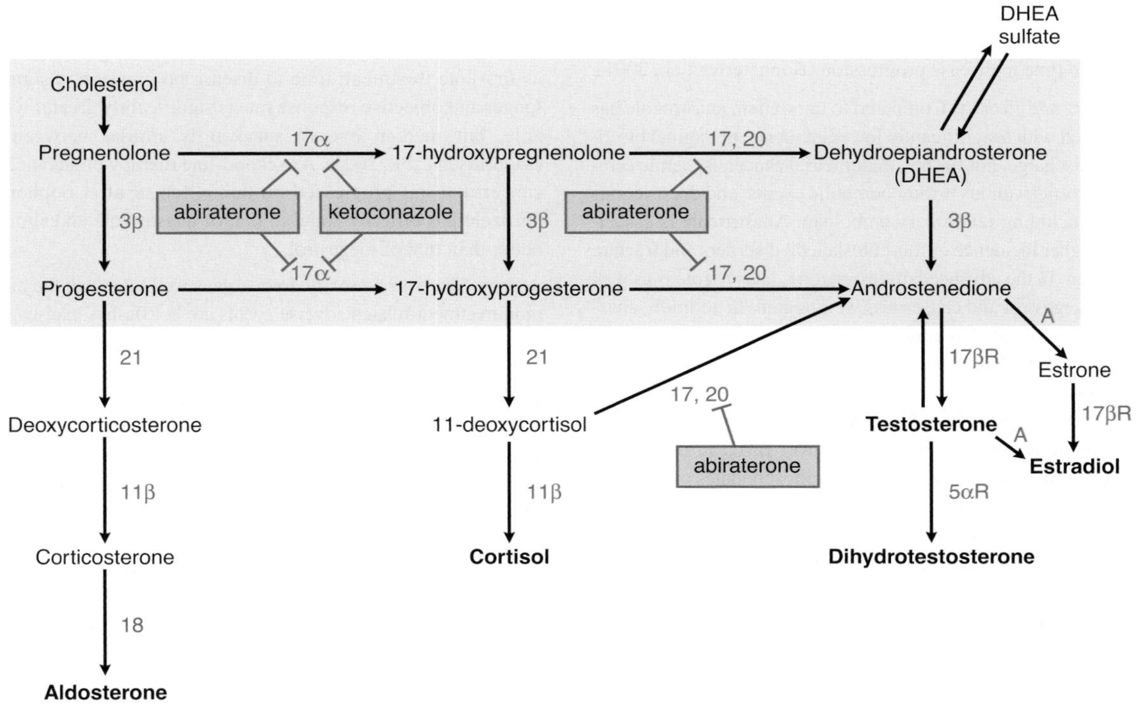

Figure 63–4. *Steroid synthesis pathways.* The enclosed area contains the pathways used by the adrenal glands and gonads. Enzymes are labeled in green, inhibitors in red. 11β: 11β-hydroxylase; 17,20: C-17,20-lyase (also CYP17); 17α: 17α-hydroxylase (CYP17); 17βR: 17β-reductase; 18: aldosterone synthase; 21: 21-hydroxylase; 3β: 3β-hydroxysteroid dehydrogenase; 5αR: 5α-reductase; A: aromatase.

administered once daily for 28 days, reduces total body androgen aromatization by 96.7% or 98.1%, respectively. In addition, anastrozole reduces aromatization in large, ER^+ breast tumors.

Absorption, Fate, and Excretion. Anastrozole is absorbed rapidly after oral administration, reaching maximal plasma concentrations after 2 hours. Repeated dosing increases plasma concentrations of anastrozole, and steady-state is attained after 7 days. Although a high-fat breakfast slows absorption, the meal does not significantly alter the ultimate steady-state concentration achieved with multiple dosing. Anastrozole is metabolized by *N*-dealkylation, hydroxylation, and glucuronidation. The main metabolite of anastrozole is a triazole. In addition, several other metabolites with no pharmacological activity are formed. Less than 10% of the drug is excreted as the unmetabolized parent compound. The principal excretory pathway is via the liver and biliary tract. The elimination $t_{1/2}$ is ~50 hours. The pharmacokinetics of anastrozole, which can be affected by drug interactions via the CYP system, are not altered by co-administration of tamoxifen or cimetidine (Köberle and Thürlimann, 2001).

Therapeutic Uses. Anastrozole (ARIMIDEX), 1 mg administered orally once daily, is approved for upfront adjuvant hormonal therapy in postmenopausal women with early-stage breast cancer and as treatment for advanced breast cancer. In early-stage breast cancer, anastrozole is significantly more effective than tamoxifen in delaying time to tumor recurrence and decreasing the odds of a primary contralateral tumor (Baum et al., 2002). In advanced breast cancer, the results of two large, randomized trials in postmenopausal women with disease progression while taking tamoxifen showed a statistically significant survival advantage with anastrozole 1 mg/day versus megestrol acetate 40 mg four times daily. In another phase III clinical trial on women with ER^+ or PR^+ metastatic breast cancer, anastrozole showed a statistically significant advantage over tamoxifen in median time to disease progression (Bonneterre et al., 2001).

Adverse Effects and Toxicity. Compared to tamoxifen, anastrozole has been associated with a significantly lower incidence of vaginal bleeding, vaginal discharge, hot flashes, endometrial cancer, ischemic cerebrovascular events, venous thromboembolic events, and deep venous thrombosis, including pulmonary embolism. Anastrozole is associated with a higher incidence of musculoskeletal disorders and fracture than tamoxifen. In the advanced disease setting, anastrozole is as well tolerated as megestrol and causes less weight gain. In addition, anastrozole is as well tolerated as tamoxifen, with a low rate of withdrawal due to drug-related adverse events (2%).

The estrogen depletion caused by anastrozole and other AIs raises the concern of bone loss. Compared with tamoxifen, treatment with anastrozole results in significantly lower BMD in the lumbar spine and total hip (Eastell et al., 2008). Bisphosphonates prevent AI-induced bone loss in postmenopausal women (Brufsky et al., 2007).

Anastrozole has no clinically significant effect on adrenal glucocorticoid or mineralocorticoid synthesis in postmenopausal women. Anastrozole also does not affect ACTH-stimulated release of cortisol or aldosterone, plasma concentrations of FSH or LH in postmenopausal women, or TSH levels.

Letrozole. Letrozole is approved for upfront adjuvant hormonal therapy in postmenopausal women with early-stage breast cancer and as treatment for advanced breast cancer.

Actions. In postmenopausal women with primary breast cancer, letrozole inhibits estrogen aromatization by 99% and reduces local aromatization within the tumors. The drug has no significant effect on the synthesis of adrenal steroids or thyroid hormone and does not alter levels of a range of other hormones. Letrozole also reduces cellular markers of proliferation to a significantly greater extent than tamoxifen in human estrogen-dependent tumors that overexpress HER1 and HER2/neu.

Letrozole increases the levels of bone resorption markers in healthy postmenopausal women and in those with a history of breast disease but without current active disease. Letrozole has not demonstrated a consistent effect on serum lipid levels in healthy women or postmenopausal women with breast cancer.

Absorption, Fate, and Excretion. Letrozole is rapidly absorbed after oral administration, and maximum plasma levels are reached ~1 hour after ingestion. Letrozole has a bioavailability of 99.9%. Steady-state plasma concentrations of letrozole are reached after 2-6 weeks of treatment. Following metabolism by CYP2A6 and CYP3A4, letrozole is eliminated as an inactive carbinol metabolite mainly via the kidneys. The total body clearance is low (2.2 L/h); the elimination $t_{1/2}$ is ~41 hours.

Therapeutic Uses. The usual dose of letrozole (FEMARA) is 2.5 mg administered orally once daily. In early-stage breast cancer, extending adjuvant endocrine therapy with letrozole (beyond the standard 5-year period of tamoxifen) improves disease-free survival compared with placebo and improves overall survival in the subset of patients with positive axillary nodes (Goss et al., 2004). Furthermore, upfront letrozole is significantly more effective than upfront tamoxifen in terms of time to tumor recurrence and odds of a primary contralateral tumor (Thürlimann et al., 2005).

In advanced breast cancer, letrozole is superior to tamoxifen as first-line treatment; time to disease progression is significantly longer and objective response rate is significantly greater with letrozole, but median overall survival is similar between groups (Mouridsen et al., 2003). As second-line therapy of advanced breast cancer that has progressed on tamoxifen or after oophorectomy, letrozole has efficacy equal to that of anastrozole and similar to or better than that of megestrol.

Adverse Effects and Toxicity. Letrozole is well tolerated; the most common treatment-related adverse events are hot flashes, nausea, and hair thinning. In patients with tumors that progressed on anti-estrogen therapy, letrozole was tolerated at least as well as, or better than, megestrol. In the trial of extended adjuvant therapy, adverse events reported more frequently with letrozole than placebo were hot flashes, arthralgia, myalgia, and arthritis, but patients discontinued letrozole no more frequently than placebo in this double-blind trial. Letrozole has a low overall incidence of cardiovascular side effects (Mouridsen et al., 2007).

A greater number of new diagnoses of osteoporosis occurred among women receiving letrozole. Compared with tamoxifen, the use of upfront letrozole results in significantly more clinical fractures. Bisphosphonates prevent letrozole-induced bone loss in postmenopausal women (Brufsky et al., 2007).

Exemestane. Exemestane (AROMASIN) is a more potent, orally administered analog of the natural aromatase substrate, androstenedione, and lowers estrogen levels more effectively than does its predecessor, formestane.

Mechanism of Action. In contrast to the reversible competitive inhibitors of aromatase (anastrozole and letrozole), exemestane irreversibly inactivates the enzyme and is referred to as a "suicide substrate." Doses of 25 mg/day inhibit aromatase activity by 98% and lower plasma estrone and estradiol levels by ~90% in postmenopausal women.

Absorption, Fate, and Excretion. Exemestane is rapidly absorbed from the GI tract, reaching maximum plasma levels after 2 hours. Its absorption is increased by 40% after a high-fat meal. Exemestane is highly protein bound in plasma and has a terminal $t_{1/2}$ of ~24 hours. It is extensively metabolized in the liver to inactive metabolites. A key metabolite, 17-hydroxyexemestane, which is formed by reduction of the 17-oxo group via 17-β-hydroxysteroid dehydrogenase, has weak androgenic activity, which also could contribute to antitumor activity. The elimination $t_{1/2}$ of the parent drug is 24 hours. Although significant quantities of active metabolites are excreted in the urine, no dosage adjustments are recommended in patients with renal dysfunction.

Therapeutic Uses. Exemestane (AROMASIN), 25 mg administered orally once daily, is approved for disease progression in postmenopausal women who completed 2-3 years of adjuvant tamoxifen based on results from a randomized clinical trial in women with ER^+ breast cancer. Women who had completed 2-3 years of adjuvant tamoxifen were randomized to complete a total of 5 years of adjuvant treatment with tamoxifen or exemestane (Coombes et al., 2004). The unadjusted hazard ratio in the exemestane group versus the tamoxifen group was 0.68, representing a 32% reduction in risk and corresponding to an absolute benefit in terms of disease-free survival of 4.7% at 3 years after randomization. Overall survival was not significantly different in the two groups.

In advanced breast cancer, exemestane improves time to disease progression compared with tamoxifen as first-line treatment (Paridaens et al., 2008). Exemestane also has been evaluated in a phase III trial against megestrol in women with disease progressing on prior anti-estrogen therapy. Patients receiving exemestane had a similar response rate but improved time to disease progression and time to treatment failure and had a longer duration of survival compared with those taking megestrol acetate. Responses to treatment also have been shown in women with disease progressing on prior nonsteroidal AIs.

Clinical Toxicity. Exemestane generally is well tolerated. Discontinuations due to toxicity are uncommon (2.8%). Hot flashes, nausea, fatigue, increased sweating, peripheral edema, and increased appetite have been reported. In the trial comparing exemestane to tamoxifen in early-stage breast cancer, exemestane caused more frequent arthralgia and diarrhea but less frequent vaginal bleeding and muscle cramps. Visual disturbances and clinical fractures were more common with exemestane (Coombes et al., 2004).

Whether exemestane negatively affects long-term bone metabolism remains to be determined. The drug has less androgenic activity than formestane but otherwise has a similar toxicity profile.

HORMONE THERAPY IN PROSTATE CANCER

Androgens stimulate the growth of normal and cancerous prostate cells. The critical role of androgens for prostate cancer growth was established in 1941 and led to the awarding of a Nobel Prize in 1966 to Dr. Charles Huggins (Huggins and Hodges, 1941; Huggins et al., 1941). These findings established androgen deprivation therapy as the mainstay of treatment for patients with advanced prostate cancer.

Localized prostate cancer frequently is curable with surgery or radiation therapy. However, when distant metastases are present, hormone therapy is the primary treatment. Standard approaches either reduce the concentration of endogenous androgens or inhibit their effects. Androgen deprivation therapy (ADT) is the standard first-line treatment (Sharifi et al., 2005). ADT is accomplished via surgical castration (bilateral orchiectomy) or medical castration (using gonadotropin-releasing hormone [GnRH] agonists or antagonists). Other hormone therapy approaches are used in second-line treatment and include anti-androgens, estrogens, and inhibitors of steroidogenesis (see the discussion later in this section).

ADT is considered palliative, not curative, treatment (Walsh et al., 2001). ADT can alleviate cancer-related symptoms, produce objective responses, and normalize serum prostate-specific antigen (PSA) in >90% of patients. ADT provides important quality-of-life benefits, including reduction of bone pain and reduction of rates of pathological fracture, spinal cord compression, and ureteral obstruction (Huggins et al., 1941). It also prolongs survival (Sharifi et al., 2005).

The duration of response to ADT for patients with metastatic disease is variable but typically lasts 14-20 months (Crawford et al., 1989; Eisenberger et al., 1998). Disease progression despite ADT signifies a castration-resistant state. However, many men respond to secondary hormonal manipulations. Despite castrate levels of testosterone, low-level androgen (DHEA) synthesis from the adrenal glands may permit the continued androgen-driven growth of prostate cancer cells. Therefore, anti-androgens (which competitively bind the androgen receptor [AR]), inhibitors of steroidogenesis (such as ketoconazole), and estrogens frequently are employed as secondary hormone therapies. Unlike the nearly universal response to ADT, only the minority of patients experience symptomatic relief or tumor regression when treated with secondary hormone therapies. When patients become refractory to further hormonal therapies, their disease is considered androgen independent. In these patients, the next treatment option usually is cytotoxic chemotherapy; docetaxel has a proven survival benefit, with average overall survival of 18 months (Petrylak et al., 2004; Tannock et al., 2004).

Common side effects of androgen deprivation include vasomotor flashing, loss of libido, impotence, gynecomastia, fatigue, anemia, weight gain, decreased insulin sensitivity, altered lipid profiles, osteoporosis and fractures, and loss of muscle mass (Saylor and Smith, 2009). The spectrum of side effects of GnRH agonists is distinct from the metabolic syndrome (Smith, 2008). ADT is associated with an increased risk of diabetes and coronary heart disease

(Keating et al., 2006). However, retrospective analyses have not revealed a compelling increase in cardiovascular mortality due to GnRH agonists (Efstathiou et al., 2008; Efstathiou et al., 2009). Skeletal-related events due to ADT, including fractures, may be mitigated by bisphosphonate therapy, such as zoledronic acid (ZOMETA) (Saad et al., 2002) or inhibitors of osteoclast activation, such as denosumab (Smith et al., 2009).

Anti-androgens, when compared with GnRH agonists, cause more gynecomastia, mastodynia, and hepatotoxicity but less vasomotor flashing, and loss of bone mineral density (BMD) (McLeod, 1997). Estrogens cause a hypercoagulable state and increase cardiovascular mortality in prostate cancer patients and are no longer standard treatment options (Byar and Corle, 1988).

Gonadotropin-Releasing Hormone Agonists and Antagonists

The biosynthesis of androgens, primarily in the testes and adrenals, is described in Chapter 41, and the regulation of Leydig cell synthetic activity by the hypothalamic– pituitary axis is considered there as well. Pharmacological castration was first reported in 1982 (Tolis et al., 1982). In the U.S., the most common form of ADT involves chemical suppression of the pituitary gland with GnRH agonists. Synthetic GnRH analogs (Table 63–2) have greater receptor affinity and reduced susceptibility to enzymatic degradation than the naturally occurring GnRH molecule and are 100-fold more potent (Schally et al., 1980). GnRH (also termed luteinizing hormone–releasing hormone, LHRH) agonists bind to GnRH receptors on pituitary gonadotropin-producing cells, causing an initial release of both LH and FSH and a subsequent increase in testosterone production from testicular Leydig cells. After ~1 week of therapy, GnRH receptors are downregulated on the gonadotropin-producing cells, causing a decline in the pituitary response (Conn and Crowley, 1991). The fall in serum LH leads to a decrease in testosterone production to castrate levels within 3-4 weeks of the first treatment. Subsequent treatments maintain testosterone at castrate levels (Limonta et al., 2001).

During the transient rise in LH, the resultant testosterone surge may induce an acute stimulation of prostate cancer growth and a "flare" of symptoms from metastatic deposits. Patients may experience an increase in bone pain or obstructive bladder symptoms lasting for 2-3 weeks (Waxman et al., 1985). The flare phenomenon can be effectively counteracted with concurrent administration of 2-4 weeks of oral anti-androgen therapy, which may inhibit the action of the increased serum testosterone levels (Kuhn et al., 1989).

Current depot forms of GnRH agonists are the result of progressive improvements in drug development. GnRH agonists in common use include leuprolide (LUPRON, others), goserelin (ZOLADEX), triptorelin (TRELSTAR), histrelin (VANTAS), and buserelin (SUPREFACT; not available in the U.S.). Long-acting preparations of both leuprolide and goserelin are available in doses that are approved for 3-, 4-, and 6-month administrations.

Leuprolide and goserelin have been compared with orchiectomy in randomized trials. A meta-analysis of 10 such randomized trials found equivalence in overall survival, progression-related outcomes, and time to treatment failure (Kaisary et al., 1991; Seidenfeld et al., 2000; Turkes et al., 1987; Vogelzang et al., 1995).

Combined androgen blockade (CAB) requires administration of ADT with an anti-androgen. The theoretical advantage is that the GnRH agonist will deplete testicular androgens, while the anti-androgen component competes at the receptor with residual androgens made by the adrenal glands. CAB provides maximal relief of androgen stimulation. Numerous large trials have compared CAB with ADT monotherapy, with variable results. Several meta-analyses of these trials suggest a benefit for CAB in 5-year survival but not at earlier time points (Samson et al., 2002; Schmitt et al., 1999). Toxicity and costs associated with CAB are higher than with ADT alone.

GnRH antagonists have been developed to suppress testosterone while avoiding the flare phenomenon of GnRH agonists. Other than avoidance of the initial flare, GnRH antagonist therapy offers no apparent advantage compared with GnRH agonists. The first available GnRH antagonist, abarelix (PLENAXIS), rapidly achieves medical castration (Trachtenberg et al., 2002). However, local reactions and anaphylaxis have discouraged its clinical acceptance and have led to its withdrawal from the market. A second GnRH antagonist, degarelix, is not associated with systemic allergic reactions and is approved for prostate cancer in the U.S. (Klotz et al., 2008).

Anti-Androgens

Anti-androgens bind to ARs and competitively inhibit the binding of testosterone and dihydrotestosterone. Unlike castration, anti-androgen therapy by itself does not decrease LH production; therefore, testosterone levels are normal or increased. Men treated with anti-androgen monotherapy maintain some degree of potency and libido and do not have the same spectrum of side effects seen with castration.

Currently, anti-androgen monotherapy is not indicated as first-line treatment for patients with advanced prostate cancer. Numerous studies have examined the effectiveness of anti-androgens compared with surgical castration, GnRH agonists, or treatment with diethylstilbestrol (DES; discontinued in the U.S.). A meta-analysis of eight trials indicated that nonsteroidal anti-androgens had equivalent overall survival relative to castration, although the association between nonsteroidal anti-androgens and decreased survival approached statistical significance (Seidenfeld et al., 2000). Anti-androgens most commonly are used in clinical practice as secondary hormone therapy or in CAB.

Table 63–2

Structures of GnRH and Decapeptide GnRH Analogs

AMINO ACID RESIDUE	1	2	3	4	5	6	7	8	9	10	DOSAGE FORM
Agonists											
GnRH (GONADORELIN)	PyroGlu	His	Trp	Ser	Tyr	Gly	Leu	Arg	Pro	Gly-NH_2	
Leuprolide (LUPRON, ELIGARD)	—	—	—	—	—	D-Leu	—	—	Pro-NHEt		IM, SC, depot
Buserelin	—	—	—	—	—	D-Ser(tBu)	—	—	Pro-NHEt		SC, IN
Nafarelin (SYNAREL)	—	—	—	—	—	D-Nal	—	—	—	Gly-NH_2	IN
Deslorelin (not available in U.S.)	—	—	—	—	—	D-Trp	—	—	Pro-NHEt		SC, IM, depot
Histrelin (VANTAS)	—	—	—	—	—	D-His (ImBzI)	—	—	Pro-NHEt		SC, depot
Triptorelin (TRELSTAR DEPOT, LA)	—	—	—	—	—	D-Trp	—	—	—	Gly-NH_2	IM, depot
Goserelin (ZOLADEX)	—	—	—	—	—	D-Ser(tBu)	—	—	—	AzGly-NH_2	SC implant
Antagonists											
Cetrorelix (CETROTIDE)	Ac-D-Nal	D-Cpa	D-Pal	—	—	D-Cit	—	—	—	D-Ala-NH_2	SC
Ganirelix (not available in U.S.)	Ac-D-Nal	D-Cpa	D-Pal	—	—	D-hArg$(Et)_2$	—	D-hArg$(Et)_2$	—	D-Ala-NH_2	SC
Abarelix	Ac-D-Nal	D-Cpa	D-Pal	—	Tyr(N-Me)	D-Asn	—	Lys(iPr)	—	D-Ala-NH_2	SC depot
Degarelix (FIRMAGON)	Ac-D-Nal	D-Cpa	D-Pal	—	4Aph HO	4Aph (Cbm)	—	I lys	—	D-Ala-NH_2	SC

A line (———) indicates identity with amino acid of the parent compound, GnRH.

Ac, acetyl: NHEt, *N*-ethylamide; tBu, t butyl; D-Nal, 3-(2-naphthyl)-D-alanyl; ImBzl, imidobenzyl; Cpa, chlorophenylalanyl; Pal, 3-pyridylalanyl; AzGly, azaglycyl; hArg$(Et)_2$, ethyl homoarginine 4Aph (Cbm), 4 acetyl phenylalanine (carbamoyl); I, imido; IV, intravenous; SC, subcutaneous; IN, intranasal; IM, intramuscular.

Available Anti-Androgens. Anti-androgens are classified as steroidal, including cyproterone and megestrol, or non-steroidal, including flutamide, bicalutamide (CASODEX, others), and nilutamide (NILANDRON) (Figure 63–5). Cyproterone is associated with liver toxicity and has inferior efficacy compared with other forms of ADT (Schroder et al., 1999; Thorpe et al., 1996). Cyproterone is used in the E.U. for treatment of men with metastatic prostate cancer but is not available in the U.S. Neither bicalutamide nor flutamide is approved as monotherapy at any dose for treatment of prostate cancer in the U.S.

Mechanism of Action of Nonsteroidal Anti-Androgens. The nonsteroidal anti-androgens are taken orally and inhibit ligand binding and consequent AR translocation from the cytoplasm to the nucleus.

Flutamide. Flutamide has a $t_{1/2}$ of 5 hours and therefore is given as a 250-mg dose every 8 hours. Its major metabolite, hydroxyflutamide, is biologically active; there are at least five other minor metabolites (Luo et al., 1997). The common side effects include diarrhea, breast tenderness, and nipple tenderness. Less commonly, nausea, vomiting, and hepatotoxicity occur (Wysowski and Fourcroy, 1996; Wysowski et al., 1993).

Bicalutamide. Bicalutamide (CASODEX, others) has a serum $t_{1/2}$ of 5-6 days and is taken once daily at a dosage of 50 mg/day when given with a GnRH agonist. Both enantiomers of bicalutamide

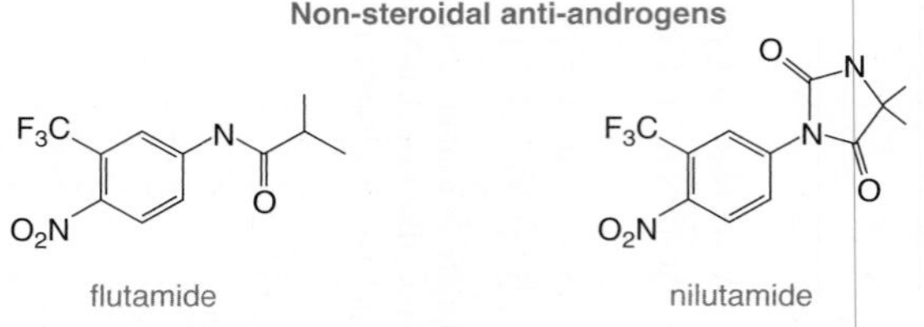

Figure 63–5. *Anti-androgens.*

undergo glucuronidation to inactive metabolites, and the parent compounds and metabolites are eliminated in bile and urine. The elimination $t_{1/2}$ of bicalutamide is increased in severe hepatic insufficiency and is unchanged in renal insufficiency.

Bicalutamide is well tolerated at higher doses with rare additional side effects. Daily bicalutamide (either low or high dose) is significantly inferior compared with surgical or medical castration (Bales and Chodak, 1996; Tyrrell et al., 1998). Although the ease of administration and favorable toxicity are attractive, concerns about inferior survival has limited the use of bicalutamide monotherapy.

Nilutamide. Nilutamide (NILADRON) is a second-generation anti-androgen with an elimination $t_{1/2}$ of 45 hours, allowing once-daily administration at 150 mg/day. Common side effects include mild nausea, alcohol intolerance (5-20%), and diminished ocular adaptation to darkness (25-40%); rarely, interstitial pneumonitis occurs (Decensi et al., 1991; Pfitzenmeyer et al., 1992). It is metabolized to five known products that are all excreted in the urine. Nilutamide appears to offer no benefit over the first-generation drugs above and has the least favorable toxicity profile (Dole and Holdsworth, 1997).

Estrogens. High estrogen levels can reduce testosterone to castrate levels in 1-2 weeks via negative feedback on the hypothalamic– pituitary axis. Estrogen also may compete with androgens for steroid hormone receptors and may thereby exert a cytotoxic effect on prostate cancer cells (Landström et al., 1994). Numerous estrogenic compounds have been tested in prostate cancer. Estrogens are associated with increased myocardial infarctions, strokes, and pulmonary emboli and increased mortality, as well as impotence, loss of libido, and lethargy. One benefit is that estrogens prevent bone loss (Scherr et al., 2002).

Most early studies on the use of estrogens used DES and were conducted between 1960 and 1975 by the Veterans Administration Cooperative Urological Research Group (VACURG). Two studies compared orchiectomy to different doses of DES to placebo (Byar, 1973; Byar and Corle, 1988). DES was as effective as orchiectomy for metastatic prostate cancer but was associated with an increase in cardiovascular events, including myocardial infarction, cerebrovascular accident, and pulmonary embolism (Bailar and Byar, 1970; Byar, 1973; de Voogt et al., 1986; Waymont et al., 1992). Due to its cardiovascular toxicity and unacceptable mortality at any dose level, DES is not indicated for prostate cancer treatment and is not available in North America for that purpose. Other synthetic estrogens have a similar associated cardiovascular toxicity to that of DES but without the efficacy. These compounds include conjugated estrogens (PREMARIN, others), ethinyl estradiol, medroxyprogesterone acetate (PROVERA, others), and chlorotrianisene (no longer marketed in the U.S.).

Inhibitors of Steroidogenesis. In the castrate state, AR signaling, despite low steroid levels, supports continued prostate cancer growth. AR signaling may occur due to androgens produced from nongonadal sources, AR gene mutations, or AR gene amplification. Nongonadal sources of androgens include the adrenal glands and the prostate cancer cells themselves (Figure 63–4). Androstenedione, produced by the adrenal glands, is converted to testosterone in peripheral tissues and tumors (Stanbrough et al., 2006). Intratumoral *de novo* androgen synthesis also may provide sufficient androgen for AR-driven cell proliferation (Montgomery et al., 2008).

Ketoconazole is an antifungal agent that interrupts the synthesis of an essential fungal membrane sterol. In an unrelated action, ketoconazole inhibits both testicular and adrenal steroidogenesis by blocking CYPs, primarily CYP17 (17α-hydroxylase). Ketoconazole is administered off label as secondary hormone therapy to reduce adrenal androgen synthesis in castration-resistant prostate cancer (Small et al., 2004). Ketoconazole causes significant diarrhea and hepatic enzyme elevations that limit its use as initial hormone therapy. Consequent poor patient adherence deters from its efficacy. Ketoconazole is given in doses of 200 mg or 400 mg three times daily. Hydrocortisone supplementation is co-administered to compensate for inhibition of adrenal steroidogenesis at the 400-mg dose level. A related compound, itraconazole, inhibits the activation of Smoothened (SMO), a component of the Hedgehog (Hh) signaling pathway (Kim et al., 2010), which is overly active in certain cancers. Thus, this class of antifungal agents may act by several distinct mechanisms and prove useful in treating other cancers.

Abiraterone is an irreversible inhibitor of both 17α-hydroxylase and C-17,20-lyase CYP17 activity, with greater potency and selectivity compared with ketoconazole. The parent compound, abiraterone acetate, is orally bioavailable and has been well tolerated in castration-resistant prostate cancer patients as secondary hormone therapy in phase I and II studies (Attard et al., 2009; Attard et al., 2008). With continuous administration, abiraterone increases ACTH levels, resulting in mineralocorticoid excess. Therefore, abiraterone acetate is administered with daily low-dose glucocorticoids, such as prednisone. Ongoing phase III trials will evaluate the efficacy and appropriate timing of abiraterone therapy for prostate cancer patients.

BIBLIOGRAPHY

Abramson N, Costantino JP, Garber JE, et al. Effect of factor V Leiden and prothrombin G20210.—>A mutations on thromboembolic risk in the National Surgical Adjuvant Breast and Bowel Project Breast Cancer Prevention trial. *J Natl Cancer Inst*, **2006**, *98*:904–910.

Attard G, Reid AHM, A'Hern R, et al. Selective inhibition of CYP17 with abiraterone acetate is highly active in the treatment of castration-resistant prostate cancer. *J Clin Oncol*, **2009**, *27*:3742–3748.

Attard G, Reid AHM, Yap TA, et al. Phase I clinical trial of a selective inhibitor of CYP17, abiraterone acetate, confirms that castration-resistant prostate cancer commonly remains hormone driven. *J Clin Oncol*, **2008**, *26*:4563–4571.

Bailar JC III, Byar DP. Estrogen treatment for cancer of the prostate. Early results with 3 doses of diethylstilbestrol and placebo. *Cancer*, **1970**, *26*:257–261.

Bales GT, Chodak GW. A controlled trial of bicalutamide versus castration in patients with advanced prostate cancer. *Urology*, **1996**, *47*:38–43.

Bonneterre J, Buzdar A, Nabholtz JM, et al. Anastrozole is superior to tamoxifen as first-line therapy in hormone receptor positive advanced breast carcinoma. *Cancer*, **2001**, *92*:2247–2258.

Brufsky A, Harker WG, Beck JT, et al. Zoledronic acid inhibits adjuvant letrozole-induced bone loss in postmenopausal women with early breast cancer. *J Clin Oncol*, **2007**, *25*: 829–836.

Byar DP. The Veterans Administration Cooperative Urological Research Group's studies of cancer of the prostate. *Cancer*, **1973**, *32*:1126–1130.

Byar DP, Corle DK. Hormone therapy for prostate cancer: Results of the Veterans Administration Cooperative Urological Research Group studies. *NCI Monogr*, **1988**, *7*:165–170.

Conn PM, Crowley WFJ. Gonadotropin-releasing hormone and its analogues. *N Engl J Med*, **1991**, *324*:93–103.

Coombes RC, Hall E, Gibson LJ, et al. A randomized trial of exemestane after two to three years of tamoxifen therapy in postmenopausal women with primary breast cancer. *N Engl J Med*, **2004**, *350*:1081–1092. Erratum in: *N Engl J Med*, **2004**, *351*:2461.

Crawford ED, Eisenberger MA, McLeod DG, et al. A controlled trial of leuprolide with and without flutamide in prostatic carcinoma. *N Engl J Med*, **1989**, *321*:419–424.

de Voogt HJ, Smith PH, Pavone-Macaluso M, et al. Cardiovascular side effects of diethylstilbestrol, cyproterone acetate, medroxyprogesterone acetate and estramustine phosphate used for the treatment of advanced prostatic cancer: Results from European Organization for Research on Treatment of Cancer trials 30761 and 30762. *J Urol*, **1986**, *135*:303–307.

Decensi AU, Boccardo F, Guarneri D, et al. Monotherapy with nilutamide, a pure nonsteroidal antiandrogen, in untreated patients with metastatic carcinoma of the prostate. The Italian Prostatic Cancer Project. *J Urol*, **1991**, *146*:377–378.

Dole EJ, Holdsworth MT. Nilutamide: An antiandrogen for the treatment of prostate cancer. *Ann Pharmacother*, **1997**, *31*:65–75.

Early Breast Cancer Trialists' Collaborative Group. Tamoxifen for early breast cancer: An overview of the randomised trials. *Lancet*, **1998**, *351*:1451–1467.

Eastell R, Adams JE, Coleman RE, et al. Effect of anastrozole on bone mineral density: 5-year results from the Anastrozole, Tamoxifen, Alone or in Combination trial 18233230. *J Clin Oncol*, **2008**, *26*:1051–1057.

Efstathiou JA, Bae K, Shipley WU, et al. Cardiovascular mortality after androgen deprivation therapy for locally advanced prostate cancer: RTOG 85-31. *J Clin Oncol*, **2009**, *27*:92–99.

Efstathiou JA, Bae K, Shipley WU, et al. Cardiovascular mortality and duration of androgen deprivation for locally advanced prostate cancer: Analysis of RTOG 92-02. *Eur Urol*, **2008**, *54*:816–824.

Eisenberger MA, Blumenstein BA, Crawford ED, et al. Bilateral orchiectomy with or without flutamide for metastatic prostate cancer. *N Engl J Med*, **1998**, *339*:1036–1042.

Fisher B, Dignam J, Bryant J, Wolmark N. Five versus more than five years of tamoxifen for lymph node–negative breast cancer: Updated findings from the National Surgical Adjuvant Breast and Bowel Project B-14 randomized trial. *J Natl Cancer Inst*, **2001**, *93*:684–690.

Goetz MP, Rae JM, Suman VJ, et al. Pharmacogenetics of tamoxifen biotransformation is associated with clinical outcomes of efficacy and hot flashes. *J Clin Oncol*, **2005**, *23*: 9312–9318.

Goss PE, Ingle JN, Martino S, et al. Updated analysis of the NCIC CTG MA.17 randomized placebo (P) controlled trial of letrozole (L) after five years of tamoxifen in postmenopausal women with early stage breast cancer. *J Clin Oncol*, **2004**, *22*(suppl):847.

Howell A, Robertson JF, Abram P, et al. Comparison of fulvestrant versus tamoxifen for the treatment of advanced breast cancer in postmenopausal women previously untreated with endocrine therapy: A multinational, double-blind, randomized trial. *J Clin Oncol*, **2004a**, *22*:1605–1613.

Howell SJ, Johnston SR, Howell A. The use of selective estrogen receptor modulators and selective estrogen receptor down-regulators in breast cancer. *Best Pract Res Clin Endocrinol Metab*, **2004b,** *18*:47–66.

Huggins C, Hodges CV. Studies on prostatic cancer: I. The effects of castration, of estrogen, and of androgen injection on serum phosphatases in metastatic carcinoma of the prostate. *Cancer Res*, **1941**, *1*:293–297.

Huggins C, Stevens RE Jr, Hodges CV. Studies on prostatic cancer: II. The effects of castration on advanced carcinoma of the prostate gland. *Arch Surg*, **1941**, *43*:209–233.

Hurtado A, Holmes KA, Geistlinger TR, et al. Regulation of ERBB2 by oestrogen receptor-PAX2 determines response to tamoxifen. *Nature*, **2008**, *456*:663–666.

Kaisary AV, Tyrrell CJ, Peeling WB, Griffiths K. Comparison of LHRH analogue (Zoladex) with orchiectomy in patients with metastatic prostatic carcinoma. *Br J Urol*, **1991,** *67*:502–508.

Keating NL, O'Malley AJ, Smith MR. Diabetes and cardiovascular disease during androgen deprivation therapy for prostate cancer. *J Clin Oncol*, **2006**, *24*:4448–4456.

Kim J, Tang JY, Gong R, et al. Intraconazole, a commonly used antifungal that inhibits Hedgehog pathway activity and growth. *Cell*, **2010**, *17:*388–399.

Klijn JG, Beex LV, Mauriac L, et al. Combined treatment with buserelin and tamoxifen in premenopausal metastatic breast cancer: A randomized study. *J Natl Cancer Inst*, **2000**, *92*:903–911.

Klotz L, Boccon-Gibod L, Shore ND, et al. The efficacy and safety of degarelix: A 12-month, comparative, randomized, open-label, parallel-group phase III study in patients with prostate cancer. *BJU Int*, **2008**, *102*:1531–1538.

Köberle D, Thürlimann B. Anastrozole: Pharmacological and clinical profile in postmenopausal women with breast cancer. *Expert Rev Anticancer Ther*, **2001**, *1*:169–176.

Kuhn JM, Billebaud T, Navratil H, et al. Prevention of the transient adverse effects of a gonadotropin-releasing hormone analogue (buserelin) in metastatic prostatic carcinoma by administration of an antiandrogen (nilutamide). *N Engl J Med*, **1989**, *321*:413–418.

Landström M, Damber JE, Bergh A. Estrogen treatment postpones the castration-induced dedifferentiation of Dunning R3327-PAP prostatic adenocarcinoma. *Prostate*, **1994**, *25*: 10–18.

Limonta P, Montagnani Marelli M, Moretti RM. LHRH analogues as anticancer agents: Pituitary and extrapituitary sites of action. *Expert Opin Investig Drugs*, **2001**, *10*:709–720.

Lønning PE, Geisler J, Krag LE, et al. Effects of exemestane administered for 2 years versus placebo on bone mineral density, bone biomarkers, and plasma lipids in patients with surgically resected early breast cancer. *J Clin Oncol*, **2005**, *23*:5126–5137.

Luo S, Martel C, Chen C, et al. Daily dosing with flutamide or Casodex exerts maximal antiandrogenic activity. *Urology*, **1997**, *50*:913–919.

McCormack P, Sapunar F. Pharmacokinetic profile of the fulvestrant loading dose regimen in postmenopausal women with hormone receptor-positive advanced breast cancer. *Cancer*, **2008**, *8*:347–351.

McLeod DG. Tolerability of nonsteroidal antiandrogens in the treatment of advanced prostate cancer. *Oncologist*, **1997**, *2*:18–27.

Montgomery RB, Mostaghel EA, Vessella R, et al. Maintenance of intratumoral androgens in metastatic prostate cancer: A mechanism for castration-resistant tumor growth. *Cancer Res*, **2008**, *68*:4447–4454.

Mouridsen H, Gershanovich M, Sun Y, et al. Phase III study of letrozole versus tamoxifen as first-line therapy of advanced breast cancer in postmenopausal women: Analysis of survival and update of efficacy from the International Letrozole Breast Cancer Group. *J Clin Oncol***, 2003**, *21*:2101–2109.

Mouridsen H, Keshaviah A, Coates AS, et al. Cardiovascular adverse events during adjuvant endocrine therapy for early breast cancer using letrozole or tamoxifen: Safety analysis of BIG 1-98 trial. *J Clin Oncol*, **2007**, *25*:5715–5722.

Moy B, Goss PE. Estrogen receptor pathway: Resistance to endocrine therapy and new therapeutic approaches. *Clin Cancer Res*, **2006**, *12*:4790–4793.

Paridaens RJ, Dirix LY, Beex LV, et al. Phase III study comparing exemestane with tamoxifen as first-line hormonal treatment of metastatic breast cancer in postmenopausal women: The European Organisation for Research and Treatment of Cancer Breast Cancer Cooperative Group. *J Clin Oncol*, **2008**, *26*:4883–4890.

Petrylak DP, Tangen CM, Hussain MHA, et al. Docetaxel and estramustine compared with mitoxantrone and prednisone for advanced refractory prostate cancer. *N Engl J Med*, **2004**, *351*:1513–1520.

Pfitzenmeyer P, Foucher P, Piard F, et al. Nilutamide pneumonitis: A report on eight patients. *Thorax*, **1992**, *47*: 622–627.

Robertson JF. Estrogen receptor downregulators: New antihormonal therapy for advanced breast cancer. *Clin Ther*, **2002**, *24*:A17–A30.

Saad F, Gleason DM, Murray R, et al. A randomized, placebo-controlled trial of zoledronic acid in patients with hormone-refractory metastatic prostate carcinoma. *J Natl Cancer Inst*, **2002**, *94*:1458–1468.

Samson DJ, Seidenfeld J, Schmitt B, et al. Systematic review and meta-analysis of monotherapy compared with combined androgen blockade for patients with advanced prostate carcinoma. *Cancer*, **2002**, *95*:361–376.

Saylor PJ, Smith MR. Metabolic complications of androgen deprivation therapy for prostate cancer. *J Urol*, **2009**, *181*: 1998–2008.

Schally AV, Coy DH, Arimura A. LH-RH agonists and antagonists. *Int J Gynaecol Obstet*, **1980**, *18*:318–324.

Scherr D, Pitts WRJ, Vaugh EDJ. Diethylstilbesterol revisited: Androgen deprivation, osteoporosis and prostate cancer. *J Urol*, **2002**, *167*:535–538.

Schmitt B, Bennett C, Seidenfeld J. Maximal androgen blockade for advanced prostate cancer. *Cochrane Database Syst Rev*, **1999**, 2:CD001526.

Schroder FH, Collette L, de Reijke TM, Whelan P. Prostate cancer treated by anti-androgens: Is sexual function preserved? *Br J Cancer*, **1999**, *82*:283–290.

Seidenfeld J, Samson DJ, Hasselblad V, et al. Single-therapy androgen suppression in men with advanced prostate cancer: A systematic review and meta-analysis. *Ann Intern Med*, **2000**, *132*:566–577.

Sharifi N, Gulley JL, Dahut WL. Androgen deprivation therapy for prostate cancer. *JAMA*, **2005**, *294*:238–244.

Small EJ, Halabi S, Dawson NA, et al. Antiandrogen withdrawal alone or in combination with ketoconazole in androgen-independent prostate cancer patients: A phase III trial (CALGB 9583). *J Clin Oncol*, **2004**, *22*:1025–1033.

Smith MR. Treatment-related diabetes and cardiovascular disease in prostate cancer survivors. *Ann Oncol*, **2008**, *19*: vii86–vii90.

Smith MR, Egerdie B, Toriz NH, et al. Denosumab in men receiving androgen-deprivation therapy for prostate cancer. *N Engl J Med*, **2009**, *361*:745–755.

Stanbrough M, Bubley GJ, Ross K, et al. Increased expression of genes converting adrenal androgens to testosterone in androgen-independent prostate cancer. *Cancer Res*, **2006**, *66*:2815–2825.

Swedish Breast Cancer Cooperative Group. Randomized trial of two versus five years of adjuvant tamoxifen for postmenopausal early stage breast cancer. *J Natl Cancer Inst*, **1996**, *88*:1543–1549.

Tannock IF, de Wit R, Berry WR, et al. Docetaxel plus prednisone or mitoxantrone plus prednisone for advanced prostate cancer. *N Engl J Med*, **2004**, *351*:1502–1512.

Thorpe SC, Azmatullah S, Fellows GJ, et al. A prospective, randomised study to compare goserelin acetate (Zoladex) versus cyproterone acetate (Cyprostat) versus a combination of the two in the treatment of metastatic prostatic carcinoma. *Eur Urol*, **1996**, *29*:47–54.

Thürlimann B, Keshaviah A, Coates AS, et al. A comparison of letrozole and tamoxifen in postmenopausal women with early breast cancer. *N Engl J Med*, **2005**, *353*:2747–2757.

Tolis G, Ackman D, Stellos A, et al. Tumor growth inhibition in patients with prostatic carcinoma treated with luteinizing hormone-releasing hormone agonists. *Proc Natl Acad Sci U S A*, **1982**, *79*:1658–1662.

Trachtenberg J, Gittleman M, Steidle C, et al. A phase 3, multicenter, open label, randomized study of abarelix versus leuprolide plus daily antiandrogen in men with prostate cancer. *J Urol*, **2002**, *167*:1670–1674.

Turkes AO, Peeling WB, Griffiths K. Treatment of patients with advanced cancer of the prostate: Phase III trial, Zoladex against castration; a study of the British Prostate Group. *J Steroid Biochem*, **1987**, *27*:543–549.

Tyrrell CJ, Kaisary AV, Iversen P, et al. A randomised comparison of 'Casodex' (bicalutamide) 150 mg monotherapy versus castration in the treatment of metastatic and locally advanced prostate cancer. *Eur Urol*, **1998**, *33*:447–456.

Vergote I, Robertson JF. Fulvestrant is an effective and well-tolerated endocrine therapy for postmenopausal women with advanced breast cancer: Results from clinical trials. *Br J Cancer*, **2004**, *90*:S11–S14.

Vogel VG, Constantino JP, Wickenham DL, et al. Update of the National Surgical Adjuvant Brest and Bowel Project Study of Tamoxifen and Raloxifene (STAR) P-2 Trial: Preventing breast cancer. *Cancer Prev*, **2010;** PMID: 20404000.

Vogelzang NJ, Chodak GW, Soloway MS, et al. Goserelin versus orchiectomy in the treatment of advanced prostate cancer: Final results of a randomized trial. *Urology*, **1995**, *46*: 220–226.

Walsh PC, Deweese TL, Eisenberger MA. A structured debate: immediate vs. deferred androgen suppression in prostate cancer: Evidence for deferred treatment. *J Urol*, **2001**, *166*: 508–516.

Waxman J, Man A, Hendry WF, et al. Importance of early tumour exacerbation in patients treated with long acting analogues of gonadotrophin releasing hormone for advanced prostatic cancer. *Br Med J*, **1985**, *291*:1387–1388.

Waymont B, Lynch TH, Dunn JA, et al. Phase III randomised study of Zoladex versus stilboestrol in the treatment of advanced prostate cancer. *Br J Urol*, **1992**, *69*:614–620.

Wysowski DK, Fourcroy JL. Flutamide hepatotoxicity. *J Urol*, **1996**, *155*:209–212.

Wysowski DK, Freiman JP, Tourtelot JB, Horton ML. Fatal and nonfatal hepatotoxicity associated with flutamide. *Ann Intern Med*, **1993**, *118*:860–864.

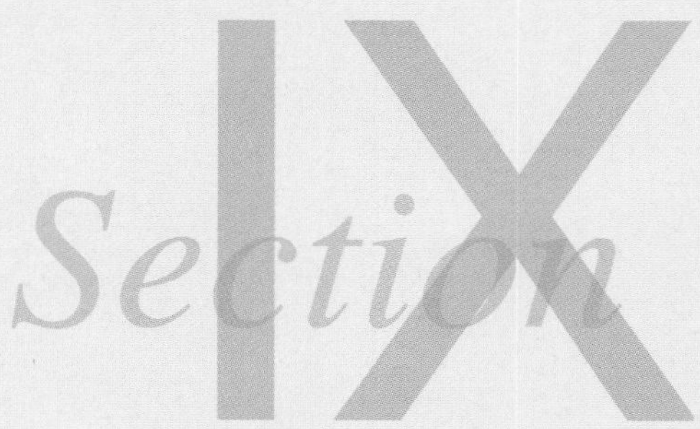

Section IX

Special Systems Pharmacology

Ocular Pharmacology

Jeffrey D. Henderer and
Christopher J. Rapuano

OVERVIEW OF OCULAR ANATOMY, PHYSIOLOGY, AND BIOCHEMISTRY

The eye is a specialized sensory organ that is relatively secluded from systemic access by the blood-retinal, blood-aqueous, and blood-vitreous barriers; as a consequence, the eye exhibits some unusual pharmacodynamic and pharmacokinetic properties. Because of its anatomical isolation, the eye offers a unique, organ-specific pharmacological laboratory in which to study the autonomic nervous system and the effects of inflammation and infectious diseases. No other organ in the body is so readily accessible or as visible for observation; however, the eye also presents some unique challenges as well as opportunities for drug delivery (Robinson, 1993).

Extraocular Structures

The eye is protected by the eyelids and by the orbit, a bony cavity of the skull that has multiple fissures and foramina that conduct nerves, muscles, and vessels (Figure 64–1). In the orbit, connective (i.e., Tenon's capsule) and adipose tissues and six extraocular muscles support and align the eyes for vision. The retrobulbar region lies immediately behind the eye (or *globe*). Understanding ocular and orbital anatomy is important for safe periocular drug delivery, including subconjunctival, sub-Tenon's, and retrobulbar injections.

The eyelids serve several functions. Foremost, their dense sensory innervation and eyelashes protect the eye from mechanical and chemical injuries. Blinking, a coordinated movement of the orbicularis oculi, levator palpebrae, and Müller's muscles, serves to distribute tears over the cornea and conjunctiva. In humans, the average blink rate is 15-20 times/minute. The external surface of the eyelids is covered by a thin layer of skin; the internal surface is lined with the palpebral portion of the conjunctiva, which is a vascularized mucous membrane continuous with the bulbar conjunctiva. At the reflection of the palpebral and bulbar conjunctivae is a space called the fornix, located superiorly and inferiorly behind the upper and lower lids, respectively. Topical medications usually are placed in the inferior fornix, also known as the inferior cul-de-sac.

The lacrimal system consists of secretory glandular and excretory ductal elements (Figure 64–2). The secretory system is composed of the main lacrimal gland, which is located in the temporal outer portion of the orbit, and accessory glands, also known as the glands of Krause and Wolfring, located in the conjunctiva. The lacrimal gland is innervated by the autonomic nervous system (Table 64–1 and Chapter 8). The parasympathetic innervation is clinically relevant because a patient may complain of dry eye symptoms while taking medications with anticholinergic side effects, such as tricyclic antidepressants (Chapter 15), antihistamines (Chapter 32), and drugs used in the management of Parkinson disease (Chapter 22). Located just posterior to the eyelashes are meibomian glands, which secrete oils that retard evaporation of the tear film. Abnormalities in gland function, as in acne rosacea and meibomitis, can greatly affect tear film stability.

Conceptually, tears constitute a trilaminar lubrication barrier covering the conjunctiva and cornea. The anterior layer is composed primarily of lipids secreted by the meibomian glands. The middle aqueous layer, produced by the main lacrimal gland and accessory lacrimal glands, constitutes ~98% of the tear film. Adherent to the corneal epithelium, the posterior layer is a mixture of mucins produced by goblet cells in the conjunctiva. Tears also contain nutrients, enzymes, and immunoglobulins to support and protect the cornea.

The tear drainage system starts through small puncta located on the medial aspects of both the upper and lower eyelids (Figure 64–2). With blinking, tears

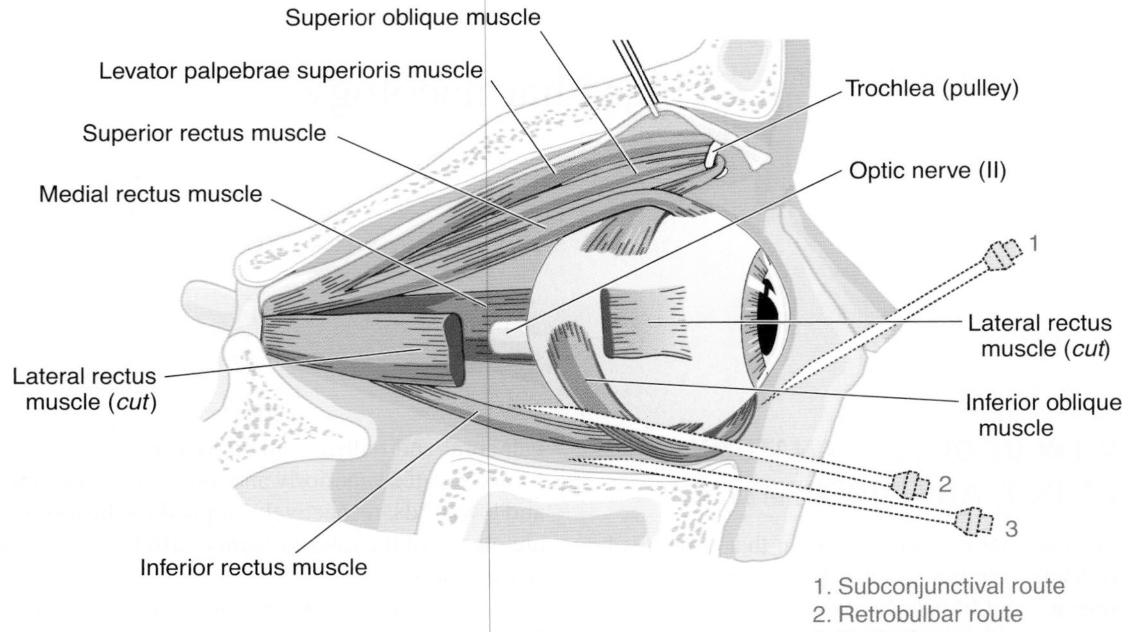

Figure 64–1. *Anatomy of the globe in relationship to the orbit and eyelids.* Various routes of administration of anesthesia are demonstrated by the blue needle pathways.

enter the puncta and continue to drain through the canaliculi, lacrimal sac, nasolacrimal duct, and then into the nose. The nose is lined by a highly vascular mucosal epithelium; consequently, topically applied medications that pass through this nasolacrimal system have direct access to the systemic circulation.

Ocular Structures

The eye is divided into anterior and posterior segments (Figure 64–3A). Anterior segment structures include the cornea, limbus, anterior and posterior chambers, trabecular meshwork, canal of Schlemm (Schlemm's canal), iris, lens, zonule, and ciliary body. The posterior segment includes the vitreous, retina, choroid, sclera, and optic nerve.

Anterior Segment

Cornea. The cornea is a transparent and avascular tissue organized into five layers: epithelium, Bowman's membrane, stroma, Descemet's membrane, and endothelium (Figure 64–3B). Representing an important barrier to foreign matter, including drugs, the hydrophobic

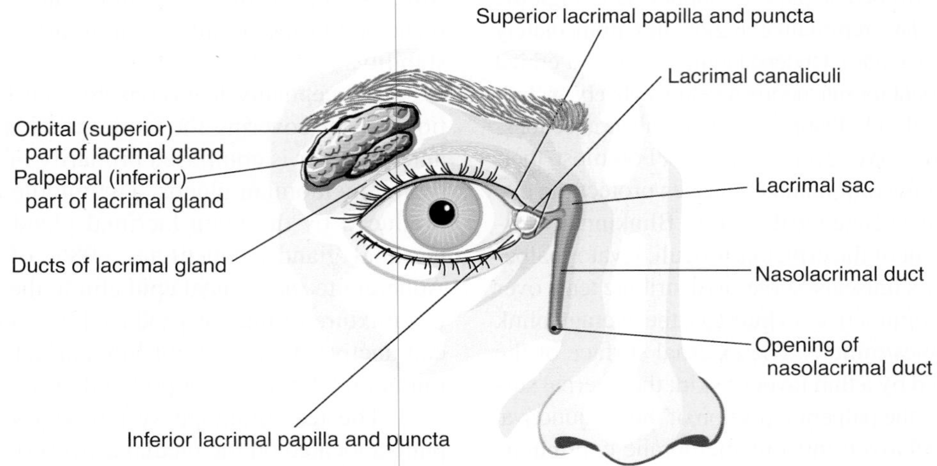

Figure 64–2. *Anatomy of the lacrimal system.*

Table 64–1

Autonomic Pharmacology of the Eye and Related Structures

	ADRENERGIC RECEPTORS		CHOLINERGIC RECEPTORS	
TISSUE	SUBTYPE	RESPONSE	SUBTYPE	RESPONSE
Corneal epithelium	β_2	Unknown	M[a]	Unknown
Corneal endothelium	β_2	Unknown	Undefined	Unknown
Iris radial muscle	α_1	Mydriasis		
Iris sphincter muscle			M_3	Miosis
Trabecular meshwork	β_2	Unknown		
Ciliary epithelium[b]	α_2/β_2	Aqueous production		
Ciliary muscle	β_2	Relaxation[c]	M_3	Accommodation
Lacrimal gland	α_1	Secretion	M_2, M_3	Secretion
Retinal pigment epithelium	α_1/β_2	H_2O transport/unknown		

[a]Although acetylcholine and choline acetyltransferase are abundant in the corneal epithelium of most species, the function of this neurotransmitter in this tissue is unknown. [b]The ciliary epithelium also is the target of carbonic anhydrase inhibitors. Carbonic anhydrase isoenzyme II is localized to both the pigmented and nonpigmented ciliary epithelium. [c]Although β_2 adrenergic receptors mediate ciliary body smooth muscle relaxation, there is no clinically significant effect on accommodation.

epithelial layer comprises five to six cell layers. The basal epithelial cells lie on a basement membrane that is adjacent to Bowman's membrane, a layer of collagen fibers. Constituting ~90% of the corneal thickness, the stroma, a hydrophilic layer, is uniquely organized with collagen lamellae synthesized by keratocytes. Beneath the stroma lies Descemet's membrane, the basement membrane of the corneal endothelium. Lying most posteriorly, the endothelium is a monolayer of cells adhering to each other by tight junctions. These cells maintain corneal integrity by active transport processes and serve as a hydrophobic barrier. Hence, drug absorption across the cornea requires penetration of the trilaminar hydrophobic–hydrophilic–hydrophobic domains of the various anatomical layers.

At the periphery of the cornea and adjacent to the sclera lies a transitional zone (1-2 mm wide) called the limbus. Limbal structures include the conjunctival epithelium, which contains the corneal epithelial stem cells, Tenon's capsule, episclera, corneoscleral stroma, canal of Schlemm, and trabecular meshwork (Figure 64–3B). Limbal blood vessels, as well as the tears, provide important nutrients and immunological defense mechanisms for the cornea. The anterior chamber holds ~250 μL of aqueous humor. The peripheral anterior chamber angle is formed by the cornea and the iris root. The trabecular meshwork and canal of Schlemm are located just above the apex of this angle. The posterior chamber, which holds ~50 μL of aqueous humor, is defined by the boundaries of the ciliary body processes, posterior surface of the iris, and lens surface.

Aqueous Humor Dynamics and Regulation of Intraocular Pressure. Aqueous humor is secreted by the ciliary processes and flows from the posterior chamber, through the pupil, and into the anterior chamber and leaves the eye primarily by the trabecular meshwork and canal of Schlemm. From the canal of Schlemm, aqueous humor drains into an episcleral venous plexus and into the systemic circulation. This conventional pathway accounts for 80-95% of aqueous humor outflow and is the main target for cholinergic drugs used in glaucoma therapy. Another outflow pathway is the uveoscleral route (i.e., fluid flows through the ciliary muscles and into the suprachoroidal space), which is the target of selective prostanoids (see "Glaucoma" and Chapter 33).

The peripheral anterior chamber angle is an important anatomical structure for differentiating two forms of glaucoma: *open-angle glaucoma*, which is by far the most common form of glaucoma in the U.S., and *angle-closure glaucoma*. Current medical therapy of open-angle glaucoma is aimed at decreasing aqueous humor production and/or increasing aqueous outflow. The preferred management for angle-closure glaucoma is surgical iridectomy, by either laser or incision, but short-term medical management may be necessary to reduce the acute intraocular pressure (IOP) elevation and to clear the cornea prior to surgery. Long-term IOP reduction may be necessary, especially if the peripheral iris has permanently covered the trabecular meshwork. In anatomically susceptible eyes, anticholinergic, sympathomimetic, and antihistaminic drugs can lead to partial dilation of the pupil and a change in the vectors of force between the iris and the lens. The aqueous humor then is prevented from passing through the pupil from the posterior chamber to the anterior chamber. The change in the lens-iris relationship leads to an increase in pressure in the posterior chamber, causing the iris base to be pushed against the angle wall, thereby covering the trabecular meshwork and closing the filtration angle and markedly elevating the IOP. The result is known as an acute attack of pupillary-block angle-closure glaucoma. Unfortunately, individuals with susceptible angles usually are not aware of a risk of angle-closure glaucoma. Furthermore, drug warning labels do not always specify the type of glaucoma for which this rare risk exists. Thus, unwarranted concern is raised among patients who have open-angle glaucoma who need not be concerned about taking these drugs.

Iris and Pupil. The iris is the most anterior portion of the uveal tract, which also includes the ciliary body and choroid. The anterior surface of the iris is the stroma, a loosely organized structure containing melanocytes, blood vessels, smooth muscle, and

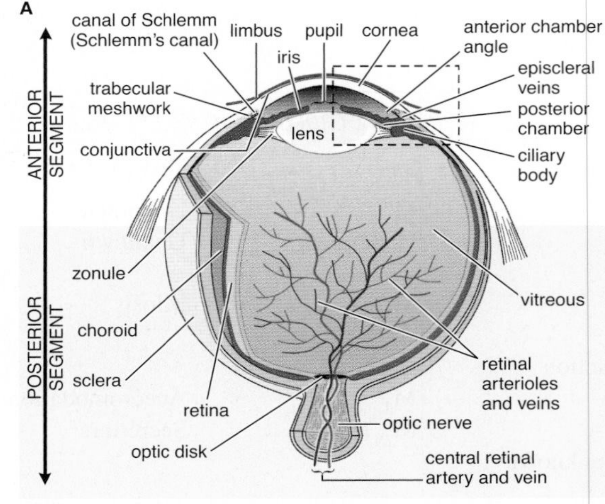

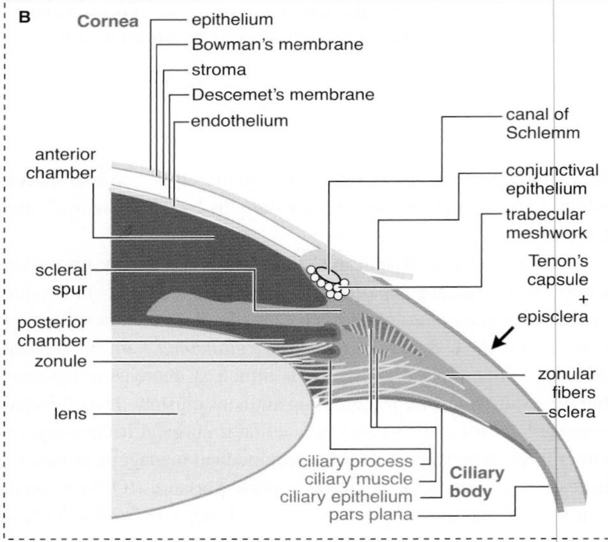

Figure 64–3. *A. Anatomy of the eye. B. Enlargement of the anterior segment, revealing the cornea, angle structures, lens, and ciliary body.* (Adapted with permission from Riordan-Eva P. Anatomy and embryology of the eye. In, Vaughan & Asbury's General Ophthalmology, 17th ed. (Riordan-Eva P, Whitcher JP, eds.) McGraw-Hill, New York, 2008. Copyright © 2008 by The McGraw-Hill Companies, Inc. All rights reserved.)

parasympathetic and sympathetic nerves. Differences in iris color reflect individual variation in the number of melanocytes located in the stroma. Individual variation may be an important consideration for ocular drug distribution due to drug-melanin binding (see "Distribution"). The posterior surface of the iris is a densely pigmented bilayer of epithelial cells. Anterior to the pigmented epithelium, the dilator smooth muscle is oriented radially and is innervated by the sympathetic nervous system (Figure 64–4), which causes mydriasis (dilation). At the pupillary margin, the sphincter smooth muscle is organized in a circular band with parasympathetic innervation, which, when stimulated, causes miosis (constriction). The use of pharmacological agents to dilate normal pupils (i.e., for clinical purposes such as examining the ocular fundus) and to evaluate the pharmacological response of the pupil (e.g., unequal pupils, or anisocoria, seen in Horner's syndrome or Adie's pupil) is summarized in Table 64–2. Figure 64–5 provides a flowchart for the diagnostic evaluation of anisocoria.

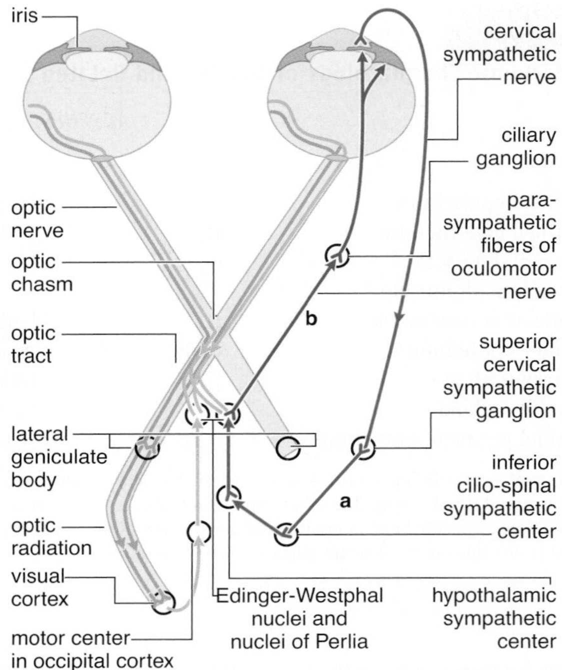

Figure 64–4. *Autonomic innervation of the eye by the sympathetic (a) and parasympathetic (b) nervous systems.* (Adapted with permission from Wybar KC, Kerr-Muir M. Bailliere's Concise Medical Textbooks, Ophthalmology, 3rd ed. Bailliere Tindall, New York, 1984. Copyright © Elsevier.)

Ciliary Body. The ciliary body serves two very specialized roles in the eye:

- secretion of aqueous humor by the epithelial bilayer
- accommodation by the ciliary muscle

The anterior portion of the ciliary body, called the pars plicata, is composed of 70-80 ciliary processes with intricate folds. The posterior portion is the pars plana. The ciliary muscle is organized into outer longitudinal, middle radial, and inner circular layers. Coordinated contraction of this smooth muscle apparatus by the parasympathetic nervous system causes the zonule suspending the lens to relax, allowing the lens to become more convex and to shift slightly forward. This process, known as *accommodation*, permits focusing on near objects and may be pharmacologically blocked by muscarinic cholinergic antagonists, through the process called *cycloplegia*. Contraction of the ciliary muscle also puts traction on the scleral spur and hence widens the spaces within the trabecular meshwork. This latter effect accounts for at least some of the IOP-lowering effect of both directly acting and indirectly acting parasympathomimetic drugs.

Lens. The lens, a transparent biconvex structure, is suspended by *zonules*, specialized fibers emanating from the ciliary body. The lens is ~10 mm in diameter and is enclosed in a capsule. The bulk of the

Table 64–2

Effects of Pharmacological Agents on the Pupil

CLINICAL SETTING	DRUG	PUPILLARY RESPONSE
Normal	Sympathomimetic drugs	Dilation (mydriasis)
Normal	Parasympathomimetic drugs	Constriction (miosis)
Horner's syndrome	Cocaine 4-10%	No dilation
Preganglionic Horner's	Hydroxyamphetamine 1%	Dilation
Postganglionic Horner's	Hydroxyamphetamine 1%	No dilation
Adie's pupil	Pilocarpine 0.05-0.1%[a]	Constriction
Normal	Opioids (oral or intravenous)	Pinpoint pupils

Topically applied ophthalmic drugs unless otherwise noted. [a]This percentage of pilocarpine is not commercially available and usually is prepared by the physician administering the test or by a pharmacist. This test also requires that no prior manipulation of the cornea (i.e., tonometry for measuring intraocular pressure or testing corneal sensation) be done so that the normal integrity of the corneal barrier is intact. Normal pupils will not respond to this weak dilution of pilocarpine; however, an Adie's pupil manifests a denervation supersensitivity and is, therefore, pharmacodynamically responsive to this dilute cholinergic agonist.

lens is composed of fibers derived from proliferating lens epithelial cells located under the anterior portion of the lens capsule. These lens fibers are continuously produced throughout life. Aging, in addition to certain medications, such as corticosteroids, and certain diseases, such as diabetes mellitus, cause the lens to become opacified, which is termed a *cataract*.

Posterior Segment. Because of the anatomical and vascular barriers to both local and systemic access, drug delivery to the eye's posterior pole is particularly challenging.

Sclera. The outermost coat of the eye, the sclera, covers the posterior portion of the globe. The external surface of the scleral shell is

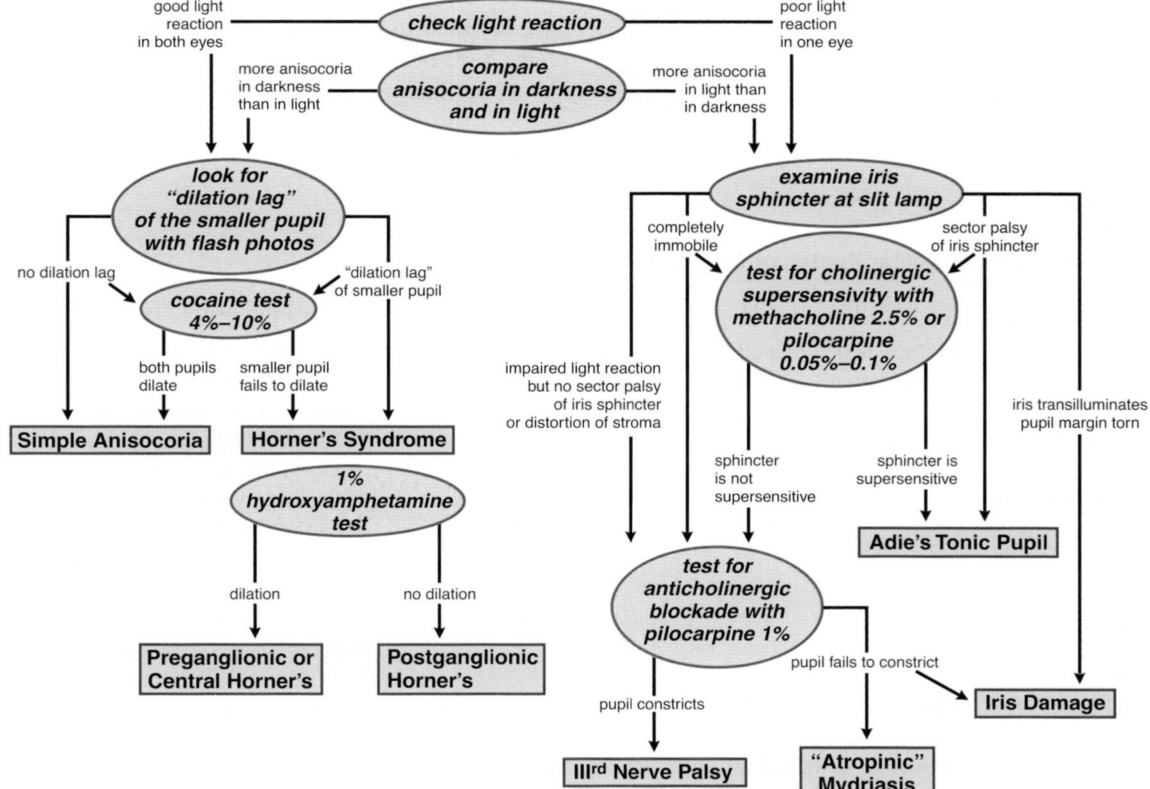

Figure 64–5. *Anisocoria evaluation flowsheet.* (Adapted with permission from Thompson and Pilley, 1976. Copyright © Elsevier.)

covered by an episcleral vascular coat, by Tenon's capsule, and by the conjunctiva. The tendons of the six extraocular muscles insert collagen fibers into the superficial scleral. Numerous blood vessels pierce the sclera through emissaria to both supply and drain the choroid, ciliary body, optic nerve, and iris.

Inside the scleral shell, the vascular choroid nourishes the outer retina by a capillary system in the choriocapillaris. Between the outer retina and the choriocapillaris lie Bruch's membrane and the retinal pigment epithelium, whose tight junctions provide an outer barrier between the retina and the choroid. The retinal pigment epithelium serves many functions, including vitamin A metabolism, phagocytosis of the rod outer segments, and multiple transport processes.

Retina. The retina is a thin, transparent, highly organized structure of neurons, glial cells, and blood vessels. Of all structures within the eye, the neurosensory retina has been the most widely studied. The unique organization and biochemistry of the photoreceptors have provided a superb system for investigating signal transduction mechanisms. The wealth of information about rhodopsin has made it an excellent model for the G protein–coupled signal transduction. Such detailed understanding holds promise for targeted therapy for some of the hereditary retinal diseases.

Vitreous. Approximately 80% of the eye's volume is the vitreous, which is a clear medium containing collagen type II, hyaluronic acid, proteoglycans, and a variety of macromolecules, including glucose, ascorbic acid, amino acids, and a number of inorganic salts. Glutamate in the vitreous has been suspected to have a possible relationship to glaucoma. The ganglion cells appear to die in glaucoma via a process of apoptosis (Quigley et al., 1995; Wax et al., 1998), and glutamate has been shown to induce apoptosis via NMDA receptor excitotoxicity (Sucher et al., 1997). Elevated glutamate levels have been noted in experimental animal models (Dreyer et al., 1996; Yoles and Schwartz, 1998) and in humans with glaucoma (Dreyer et al., 1996), although this has been questioned (Levkovitch-Verbin et al., 2002). Memantine, a noncompetitive NMDA receptor antagonist (Vorwerk et al., 1996; Seki and Lipton, 2008; Ju et al., 2008), is currently being investigated clinically as a possible treatment for glaucoma.

Optic Nerve. The optic nerve is a myelinated nerve conducting the retinal output to the central nervous system (CNS). It is composed of:

- an intraocular portion, which is visible as the optic disk in the retina
- an intraorbital portion
- an intracanalicular portion
- an intracranial portion

The nerve is ensheathed in meninges continuous with the brain. At present, pharmacological treatment of optic neuropathies usually is based on management of the underlying disease. For example, nonarteritic ischemic optic neuropathy might be treated with intravitreal glucocorticoids (Kaderli et al., 2007) and optic neuritis may be best treated with intravenous glucocorticoids (Atkins et al., 2007; Beck and Gal, 2008; Volpe, 2008). Unfortunately, these guidelines have not yet become routine clinical practice (Biousse et al., 2009). Glaucomatous optic neuropathy is medically managed by decreasing IOP.

PHARMACOKINETICS AND TOXICOLOGY OF OCULAR THERAPEUTIC AGENTS

Drug-Delivery Strategies

Properties of varying ocular routes of administration are outlined in Table 64–3. A number of delivery systems have been developed for treating ocular diseases. Most ophthalmic drugs are delivered in solutions, but

Table 64–3

Some Characteristics of Ocular Routes of Drug Administration

ROUTE	ABSORPTION PATTERN	SPECIAL UTILITY	LIMITATIONS AND PRECAUTIONS
Topical	Prompt, depending on formulation	Convenient, economical, relatively safe	Compliance, corneal and conjunctival toxicity, nasal mucosal toxicity, systemic side effects from nasolacrimal absorption
Subconjunctival, sub-Tenon's, and retrobulbar injections	Prompt or sustained, depending on formulation	Anterior segment infections, posterior uveitis, cystoid macular edema	Local toxicity, tissue injury, globe perforation, optic nerve trauma, central retinal artery and/or vein occlusion, direct retinal drug toxicity with inadvertent globe perforation, ocular muscle trauma, prolonged drug effect
Intraocular (intracameral) injections	Prompt	Anterior segment surgery, infections	Corneal toxicity, intraocular toxicity, relatively short duration of action
Intravitreal injection or device	Absorption circumvented, immediate local effect, potential sustained effect	Endophthalmitis, retinitis, age-related macular degeneration	Retinal toxicity

See the text for a more complete discussion of individual routes.

for compounds with limited solubility, a suspension form facilitates delivery.

Several formulations prolong the time a drug remains on the surface of the eye. These include gels, ointments, solid inserts, soft contact lenses, and collagen shields. *Prolonging the time in the cul-de-sac facilitates drug absorption.* Ophthalmic gels (e.g., pilocarpine 4% gel) release drugs by diffusion following erosion of soluble polymers. The polymers used include cellulosic ethers, polyvinyl alcohol, carbopol, polyacrylamide, polymethylvinyl ether–maleic anhydride, poloxamer 407, and pluronic acid. Ointments usually contain mineral oil and a petrolatum base and are helpful in delivering antibiotics, cycloplegic drugs, or miotic agents. Solid inserts, such as the ganciclovir intravitreal implant, provide a *zero-order* rate of delivery by steady-state diffusion, whereby drug is released at a more constant rate over a finite period of time rather than as a bolus. This surgical implant has been used to deliver anti-cytomegalovirus (CMV) medication in proximity to the retinal infection (Marx et al., 1996). The intent is to deliver a sustained dose of medication over several months with reduced spikes in drug delivery (Kunou et al., 2000) independent of patient compliance.

Pharmacokinetics

Classical pharmacokinetic theory based on studies of systemically administered drugs (see Chapter 2) does not fully apply to all ophthalmic drugs (Kaur and Kanwar, 2002). Although similar principles of absorption, distribution, metabolism, and excretion determine the fate of drug disposition in the eye, alternative routes of drug administration, in addition to oral and intravenous routes, introduce other variables in compartmental analysis (Table 64–3 and Figure 64–6). Most ophthalmic medications are formulated to be applied topically. Drugs also may be injected by subconjunctival, sub-Tenon's, and retrobulbar routes (Figure 64–1 and Table 64–3).

For example, anesthetic agents commonly are administered by injection for surgical procedures, and antibiotics and glucocorticoids also may be injected to enhance their delivery to local tissues. The antimetabolite 5-fluorouracil and the DNA alkylating agent mitomycin C may be extemporaneously compounded for subconjunctival administration to retard the fibroblast proliferation related to scarring after glaucoma surgery. Mitomycin C also can be applied to the cornea to prevent scarring after corneal surgery. Intraocular (i.e., intravitreal) injections of antibiotics are considered in instances of endophthalmitis, a severe intraocular infection. The sensitivities of the organisms to the antibiotic and the retinal toxicity threshold may be nearly the same for some antibiotics; hence, the antibiotic dose injected intravitreally must be carefully titrated. Intraocular inserts are used to treat intraocular viral infections. The ganciclovir implant is indicated to treat CMV retinitis in patients with acquired immunodeficiency syndrome (AIDS).

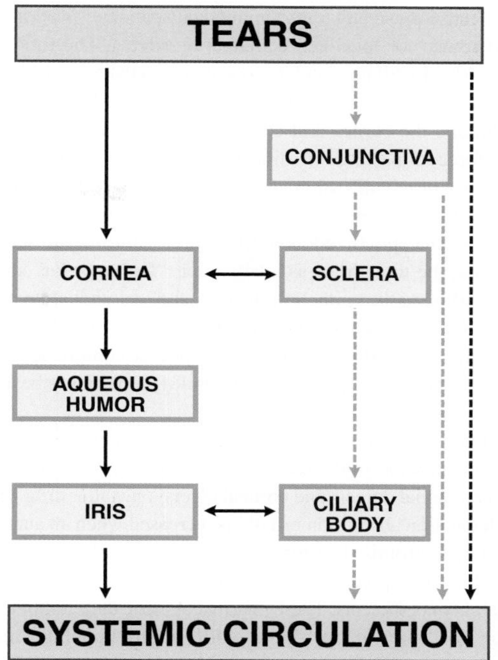

Figure 64–6. *Possible absorption pathways of an ophthalmic drug following topical application to the eye.* Solid black arrows represent the corneal route; dashed blue arrows represent the conjunctival/scleral route; the black dashed arrow represents the nasolacrimal absorption pathway. (Adapted with permission from Chien et al, 1990. Copyright © Taylor & Francis Group, http://www.informaworld.com.)

Unlike clinical pharmacokinetic studies on systemic drugs, where data are collected relatively easily from blood samples, there is significant risk in obtaining tissue and fluid samples from the human eye. Consequently, animal models, frequently rabbits, are studied to provide pharmacokinetic data on ophthalmic drugs.

Absorption. After topical instillation of a drug, the rate and extent of absorption are determined by the time the drug remains in the cul-de-sac and precorneal tear film, elimination by nasolacrimal drainage, drug binding to tear proteins, drug metabolism by tear and tissue proteins, and diffusion across the cornea and conjunctiva (Lee, 1993). A drug's residence time may be prolonged by changing its formulation. Residence time also may be extended by blocking the egress of tears from the eye by closing the tear drainage ducts with flexible silicone (punctal) plugs (HERRICK LACRIMAL PLUG, PUNCTUM PLUG) or cautery. Nasolacrimal drainage contributes to systemic absorption of topically administered ophthalmic medications. Absorption from the nasal mucosa avoids first-pass metabolism by the liver, and consequently, significant systemic side effects may be caused by topical medications, especially when used chronically. Possible absorption pathways of an ophthalmic drug following topical application to the eye are shown schematically in Figure 64–6.

Transcorneal and transconjunctival/scleral absorption are the desired routes for localized ocular drug effects. The time period between drug instillation and its appearance in the aqueous humor is defined as the *lag time*. The drug concentration gradient between the tear film and the cornea and conjunctival epithelium provides the driving force for passive diffusion across these tissues. Other factors that affect a drug's diffusion capacity are the size of the molecule, chemical structure, and steric configuration. Transcorneal drug penetration is conceptualized as a differential solubility process; the cornea may be thought of as a trilaminar "fat-water-fat" structure corresponding to the epithelial, stromal, and endothelial layers. The epithelium and endothelium represent barriers for hydrophilic substances; the stroma is a barrier for hydrophobic compounds. Hence, a drug with both hydrophilic and lipophilic properties is best suited for transcorneal absorption.

Drug penetration into the eye is approximately linearly related to its concentration in the tear film. Certain disease states, such as corneal epithelial defects and corneal ulcers, may alter drug penetration. Medication absorption usually is increased when an anatomical barrier is compromised or removed. Experimentally, drugs may be screened for their potential clinical utility by assessing their corneal permeability coefficients. These pharmacokinetic data combined with the drug's octanol/water partition coefficient (for lipophilic drugs) or distribution coefficient (for ionizable drugs) yield a parabolic relationship that is a useful parameter for predicting ocular absorption. Of course, such *in vitro* studies do not account for other factors that affect corneal absorption, such as epithelial integrity, blink rate, dilution by tear flow, nasolacrimal drainage, drug binding to proteins and tissue, and transconjunctival absorption; hence, these studies have limitations in predicting ocular drug absorption *in vivo*.

Distribution. Topically administered drugs may undergo systemic distribution primarily by nasal mucosal absorption and possibly by local ocular distribution by transcorneal/transconjunctival absorption. Following transcorneal absorption, the aqueous humor accumulates the drug, which then is distributed to intraocular structures as well as potentially to the systemic circulation via the trabecular meshwork pathway (Figure 64–3B). Melanin binding of certain drugs is an important factor in some ocular compartments. For example, the mydriatic effect of α adrenergic–receptor agonists is slower in onset in human volunteers with darkly pigmented irides compared to those with lightly pigmented irides. In rabbits, radiolabeled atropine binds significantly to melanin granules in irides of non-albino animals. This finding correlates with the fact that atropine's mydriatic effect lasts longer in non-albino rabbits than in albino rabbits and suggests that drug-melanin binding is a potential reservoir for sustained drug release. Another clinically important consideration for drug-melanin binding involves the retinal pigment epithelium. In the retinal pigment epithelium, accumulation of chloroquine (see Chapter 49) causes a toxic retinal lesion known as a "bull's-eye" maculopathy, which is associated with a decrease in visual acuity.

Metabolism. Enzymatic biotransformation of ocular drugs may be significant because a variety of enzymes, including esterases, oxidoreductases, lysosomal enzymes, peptidases, glucuronide and sulfate transferases, glutathione-conjugating enzymes, catechol-*O*-methyl-transferase, monoamine oxidase, and 11β-hydroxysteroid dehydrogenase are found in the eye. The esterases have been of particular interest because of the development of prodrugs for enhanced corneal permeability; e.g., dipivefrin hydrochloride is a prodrug for epinephrine, and latanoprost is a prodrug for prostaglandin $F_{2\alpha}$ ($PGF_{2\alpha}$); both drugs are used for glaucoma management. Topically applied ocular drugs are eliminated by the liver and kidney after systemic absorption, but enzymatic transformation of systemically administered drugs also is important in ophthalmology.

Toxicology. All ophthalmic medications are potentially absorbed into the systemic circulation (Figure 64–6), so undesirable systemic side effects may occur. Most ophthalmic drugs are delivered locally to the eye, and the potential local toxic effects are due to hypersensitivity reactions or to direct toxic effects on the cornea, conjunctiva, periocular skin, and nasal mucosa. Eyedrops and contact lens solutions commonly contain preservatives such as benzalkonium chloride, chlorobutanol, chelating agents, and thimerosal for their antimicrobial effectiveness. In particular, benzalkonium chloride may cause a punctate keratopathy or toxic ulcerative keratopathy (Grant and Schuman, 1993). Thimerosal is used rarely due to a high incidence of hypersensitivity reactions.

THERAPEUTIC AND DIAGNOSTIC APPLICATIONS OF DRUGS IN OPHTHALMOLOGY

Chemotherapy of Microbial Diseases in the Eye

Antibacterial Agents

General Considerations. A number of antibiotics have been formulated for topical ocular use (Table 64–4). The pharmacology, structures, and kinetics of individual drugs have been presented in detail in Section VI. Appropriate selection of antibiotic and route of administration is dependent on the patient's symptoms, the clinical examination, and the culture/sensitivity results. Specially formulated antibiotics also may be extemporaneously prepared by qualified pharmacists for serious eye infections such as corneal infiltrates or ulcers and endophthalmitis.

Therapeutic Uses. Infectious diseases of the skin, eyelids, conjunctivae, and lacrimal excretory system are encountered regularly in clinical practice. Periocular skin infections are divided into preseptal and postseptal or orbital cellulitis. Depending on the clinical setting (i.e., preceding trauma, sinusitis, age of patient, relative immunocompromised state), oral or parenteral antibiotics are administered. The microbiological spectrum for orbital cellulitis is changing; e.g., there has been a sharp decline in *Haemophilus influenzae* after the introduction in 1985 of the *H. influenzae* vaccine (Ambati et al., 2000).

Dacryoadenitis, an infection of the lacrimal gland, is most common in children and young adults. It may be bacterial (typically

Table 64–4

Topical Antibacterial Agents Commercially Available for Ophthalmic Use

GENERIC NAME (TRADE NAME)	FORMULATION[a]	TOXICITY	INDICATIONS FOR USE
Azithromycin (AZASITE)	1% solution	H	Conjunctivitis
Bacitracin	500 units/g ointment	H	Conjunctivitis, blepharitis, keratitis, keratoconjunctivitis, corneal ulcers, blepharoconjunctivitis, meibomianitis, dacryocystitis
Besifloxacin (BESIVANCE)	0.6% suspension		Conjunctivitis
Chloramphenicol	1% ointment	H, BD	Conjunctivitis, keratitis
Ciprofloxacin hydrochloride (CILOXAN, others)	0.3% solution; 0.3% ointment	H, D-RCD	Conjunctivitis, keratitis, keratoconjunctivitis, corneal ulcers, blepharitis, blepharoconjunctivitis, meibomianitis, dacryocystitis
Erythromycin (ILOTYCIN, others)	0.5% ointment	H	Superficial ocular infections involving the conjunctiva or cornea; prophylaxis of ophthalmia neonatorum
Gatifloxacin (ZYMAR)	0.3% solution	H	Conjunctivitis
Gentamicin sulfate (GARAMYCIN, GENOPTIC, GENT-AK, GENTACIDIN, others)	0.3% solution; 0.3% ointment	H	Conjunctivitis, blepharitis, keratitis, keratoconjunctivitis, corneal ulcers, blepharoconjunctivitis, meibomianitis, dacryocystitis
Levofloxacin (QUIXIN, IQUIX)	0.5% solution	H	Conjunctivitis
Levofloxacin (IQUIX)	1.5% solution	H	Corneal ulcers
Moxifloxacin (VIGAMOX)	0.5% solution	H	Conjunctivitis
Ofloxacin (OCUFLOX, others)	0.3% solution	H	Conjunctivitis, corneal ulcers
Sulfacetamide sodium (BLEPH-10, CETAMIDE, ISOPTO CETAMIDE, others)	1%, 10%, 15%, and 30% solution; 10% ointment	H, BD	Conjunctivitis, other superficial ocular infections
Polymyxin B combinations[b]	Various solutions and ointments		Conjunctivitis, blepharitis, keratitis
Tobramycin sulfate[c] (TOBREX, AKTOB, DEFY, others)	0.3% solution; 0.3% ointment	H	External infections of the eye and its adnexa

[a]For specific information on dosing, formulation, and trade names, refer to the *Physicians' Desk Reference for Ophthalmic Medicines*, which is published annually. [b]Polymyxin B is formulated for delivery to the eye in combination with bacitracin, neomycin, gramicidin, oxytetracycline, or trimethoprim. See Chapters 52-55 for further discussion of these antibacterial agents. [c]Tobramycin is formulated for delivery to the eye in combination with dexamethasone or loteprednol etabonate. H, hypersensitivity; BD, blood dyscrasia; D-RCD, drug-related corneal deposits.

Staphylococcus aureus, Streptococcus spp.) or viral (most commonly seen in mumps, infectious mononucleosis, influenza, and herpes zoster). When bacterial infection is suspected, systemic antibiotics usually are indicated.

Dacryocystitis is an infection of the lacrimal sac. In infants and children, the disease usually is unilateral and secondary to an obstruction of the nasolacrimal duct. In adults, dacryocystitis and canalicular infections may be caused by *S. aureus, Streptococcus* spp., diphtheroids, *Candida* spp., and *Actinomyces israelii*. Any discharge from the lacrimal sac should be sent for smears and cultures. Systemic antibiotics typically are indicated.

Infectious processes of the lids include *hordeolum* and *blepharitis*. A hordeolum, or stye, is an infection of the meibomian, Zeis, or Moll glands at the eyelid margins. The typical offending bacterium is *S. aureus*, and the usual treatment consists of warm compresses and topical antibiotic gel, drops, or ointment. Blepharitis is a common bilateral inflammatory process of the eyelids characterized by irritation and burning, and it also usually is associated with a *Staphylococcus* sp. Local hygiene is the mainstay of therapy; topical antibiotics frequently are used, usually in gel, drop, or ointment form, particularly when the disease is accompanied by conjunctivitis and keratitis. Systemic tetracycline, doxycycline, minocycline, and erythromycin often are effective in reducing severe eyelid inflammation but must be used for weeks to months.

Conjunctivitis is an inflammatory process of the conjunctiva that varies in severity from mild hyperemia to severe purulent discharge. The more common causes of conjunctivitis include viruses, allergies, environmental irritants, contact lenses, and chemicals. The less common causes include other infectious pathogens, immune-mediated reactions, associated systemic diseases, and tumors of the conjunctiva or eyelid.

The more commonly reported infectious agents are adenovirus and herpes simplex virus, followed by other viral (e.g., enterovirus, coxsackievirus, measles virus, varicella zoster virus, vaccinia variola virus) and bacterial sources (e.g., *Neisseria* spp., *Streptococcus pneumoniae, Haemophilus* spp., *S. aureus, Moraxella lacunata*, and chlamydial spp.). *Rickettsia*, fungi, and parasites, in both cyst and trophozoite form, are rare causes of conjunctivitis. Effective management is based on selection of an appropriate antibiotic for suspected bacterial pathogens. Unless an unusual causative organism is suspected, bacterial conjunctivitis is treated empirically with a broad-spectrum topical antibiotic without obtaining a culture.

Keratitis, or corneal inflammation, can occur at any level of the cornea (e.g., epithelium, subepithelium, stroma, endothelium). It can be due to non-infectious or infectious causes. Numerous microbial agents have been identified as causes of infectious keratitis, including bacteria, viruses, fungi, spirochetes, and cysts and trophozoites. Severe infections with tissue loss (corneal ulcers) generally are treated more aggressively than infections without tissue loss (corneal infiltrates).

The mild, small, more peripheral infections usually are not cultured, and the eyes are treated with broad-spectrum topical antibiotics. In more severe, central, or larger infections, corneal scrapings for smears, cultures, and sensitivities are performed, and the patient is immediately started on intensive hourly, around-the-clock topical antibiotic therapy. The goal of treatment is to eradicate the infection and reduce the amount of corneal scarring and the chance of corneal perforation and severe decreased vision or blindness. The initial medication selection and dosage are adjusted according to the clinical response and culture and sensitivity results.

Endophthalmitis is a potentially severe and devastating inflammatory, and usually infectious, process involving the intraocular tissues. When the inflammatory process encompasses the entire globe, it is called *panophthalmitis*. Endophthalmitis usually is caused by bacteria or fungi, or rarely by spirochetes. The typical case occurs during the early postoperative course (e.g., after cataract, glaucoma, cornea, or retinal surgery), following trauma, or by endogenous seeding in an immunocompromised host or intravenous drug user. Acute postoperative endophthalmitis requires a prompt vitreous tap for smears and cultures and empirical injection of intravitreal antibiotics.

Immediate vitrectomy (i.e., specialized surgical removal of the vitreous) is beneficial for patients who have light perception–only vision (Endophthalmitis Vitrectomy Study Group, 1995). Vitrectomy for other causes of endophthalmitis (e.g., glaucoma bleb related, post-traumatic, or endogenous) may be beneficial (Schiedler et al., 2004). In cases of endogenous seeding, parenteral antibiotics have a role in eliminating the infectious source, but the efficacy of systemic antibiotics with trauma is not well established.

Antiviral Agents

General Considerations. The various antiviral drugs currently used in ophthalmology are summarized in Table 64–5 (see Chapter 58 for additional details about these agents).

Therapeutic Uses. The primary indications for the use of antiviral drugs in ophthalmology are viral keratitis, herpes zoster ophthalmicus (Liesegang, 1999; Chern and Margolis, 1998), and retinitis. There currently are no antiviral agents for the treatment of viral conjunctivitis caused by adenoviruses, which usually has a self-limited course and typically is treated by symptomatic relief of irritation.

Viral keratitis, an infection of the cornea that may involve either the epithelium or stroma, is most commonly caused by herpes simplex type I and varicella zoster viruses. Less common viral etiologies include herpes simplex type II, Epstein-Barr virus, and CMV. Topical antiviral agents are indicated for the treatment of epithelial disease due to herpes simplex infection. *When treating viral keratitis topically, there is a very narrow margin between the therapeutic topical antiviral activity and the toxic effect on the cornea*; hence, patients must be followed very closely. The role of oral acyclovir and glucocorticoids in herpetic corneal and external eye disease has been examined in the Herpetic Eye Disease Study (Herpetic Eye Disease Study Group, 1997; Herpetic Eye Disease Study Group, 1998). Topical glucocorticoids are contraindicated in herpetic epithelial keratitis due to active viral replication. In contrast, for herpetic disciform keratitis, which predominantly is presumed to involve a cell-mediated immune reaction, topical glucocorticoids accelerate recovery (Wilhelmus et al., 1994). For recurrent herpetic stromal keratitis, there is clear benefit from treatment with oral acyclovir in reducing the risk of recurrence (Herpetic Eye Disease Study Group, 1998). An ophthalmic formulation of trifluridine (VIROPTIC) is available for treatment of keratoconjunctivitis and epithelial keratitis due to herpes simplex viruses.

Herpes zoster ophthalmicus is a latent reactivation of a varicella zoster infection in the first division of the trigeminal cranial nerve. Systemic acyclovir, valacyclovir, and famciclovir are effective in reducing the severity and complications of herpes zoster ophthalmicus (Colin et al., 2000). Currently, there are no ophthalmic preparations of acyclovir approved by the FDA, although an ophthalmic ointment is available for investigational use.

Viral retinitis may be caused by herpes simplex virus, CMV, adenovirus, and varicella zoster virus. With the highly active antiretroviral therapy (HAART; see Chapter 59), CMV retinitis does not appear to progress when specific anti-CMV therapy is discontinued, but some patients develop an immune recovery uveitis (Jacobson et al., 2000; Whitcup, 2000). Treatment usually involves long-term parenteral administration of antiviral drugs. Intravitreal administration of ganciclovir has been found to be an effective alternative to the systemic route (Sanborn et al., 1992). Acute retinal necrosis and progressive outer retinal necrosis, most often caused by varicella zoster virus, can be treated by various combinations of oral, intravenous, intravitreal injection of, and intravitreal implantation of antiviral medications (Roig-Melo et al., 2001).

Table 64–5

Antiviral Agents for Ophthalmic Use

GENERIC NAME (TRADE NAME)	ROUTE OF ADMINISTRATION	OCULAR TOXICITY	INDICATIONS FOR USE
Trifluridine (VIROPTIC, others)	Topical (1% solution)	PK, H	Herpes simplex keratitis and keratoconjunctivitis
Acyclovir (ZOVIRAX)	Oral, intravenous (200-mg capsules, 400- and 800-mg tablets)		Herpes zoster ophthalmicus[a] Herpes simplex iridocyclitis
Valacyclovir (VALTREX)	Oral (500- and 1000-mg tablets)		Herpes simplex keratitis[a] Herpes zoster ophthalmicus[a]
Famciclovir (FAMVIR)	Oral (125-, 250-, and 500-mg tablets)		Herpes simplex keratitis[a] Herpes zoster ophthalmicus[a]
Foscarnet (FOSCAVIR)	Intravenous Intravitreal[a]		Cytomegalovirus retinitis
Ganciclovir			Cytomegalovirus retinitis
(CYTOVENE)	Intravenous, oral		
(VITRASERT)	Intravitreal implant		
Valganciclovir (VALCYTE)	Oral		Cytomegalovirus retinitis
Cidofovir (VISTIDE)	Intravenous		Cytomegalovirus retinitis

[a]Off-label use. For additional details, see Chapter 58. PK, punctate keratopathy; H, hypersensitivity.

Antifungal Agents

General Considerations. The only currently available topical ophthalmic antifungal preparation is a polyene, natamycin (NATACYN), which has the following structure:

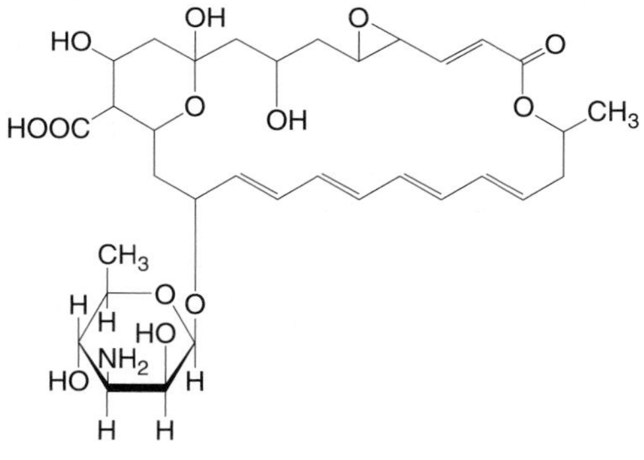

NATAMYCIN

Other antifungal agents may be extemporaneously compounded for topical, subconjunctival, or intravitreal routes of administration (Table 64–6). The pharmacology and structures of available antifungal agents are given in Chapter 57.

Therapeutic Uses. As with systemic fungal infections, the incidence of ophthalmic fungal infections has risen with the growing number of immunocompromised hosts. Ophthalmic indications for antifungal medications include fungal keratitis, scleritis, endophthalmitis, mucormycosis, and canaliculitis. Risk factors for fungal keratitis include trauma, chronic ocular surface disease, contact lens wear, and immunosuppression (including topical steroid use).

In 2005-2006, there was a worldwide epidemic of *Fusarium* fungal keratitis related to a specific contact lens solution, which resolved when it was removed from the market (Chang et al., 2007). When fungal infection is suspected, samples of the affected tissues are obtained for smears, cultures, and sensitivities, and this information is used to guide drug selection.

Antiprotozoal Agents

General Considerations. Parasitic infections involving the eye usually manifest themselves as a form of *uveitis*, an inflammatory process of either the anterior or posterior segments and, less commonly, as conjunctivitis, keratitis, and retinitis.

Therapeutic Uses. In the U.S., the most commonly encountered protozoal infections include *Acanthamoeba* and *Toxoplasma gondii*. In contact lens wearers who develop keratitis, physicians should be highly suspicious of the presence of *Acanthamoeba* (McCulley et al., 2000).

Additional risk factors for *Acanthamoeba* keratitis include poor contact lens hygiene, wearing contact lenses in a pool or hot tub, and ocular trauma. Treatment usually consists of a combination of topical agents. The aromatic diamidines (i.e., propamidine isethionate in both topical aqueous and ointment forms [BROLENE]) have been used successfully to treat this relatively resistant infectious keratitis (Hargrave et al., 1999), although it is not available in the U.S. The cationic

Table 64–6

Antifungal Agents for Ophthalmic Use

DRUG CLASS/AGENT	METHOD OF ADMINISTRATION	INDICATIONS FOR USE
Polyenes		
Amphotericin B[a]	0.1-0.5% (typically 0.15%) topical solution	Yeast and fungal keratitis and endophthalmitis
	0.8-1 mg subconjunctival	Yeast and fungal endophthalmitis
	5-μg intravitreal injection	Yeast and fungal endophthalmitis
	Intravenous	Yeast and fungal endophthalmitis
Natamycin	5% topical suspension	Yeast and fungal blepharitis, conjunctivitis, keratitis
Imidazoles		
Fluconazole[a]	Oral, intravenous	Yeast keratitis and endophthalmitis
Itraconazole[a]	Oral	Yeast and fungal keratitis and endophthalmitis
Ketoconazole[a]	Oral	Yeast keratitis and endophthalmitis
Miconazole[a]	1% topical solution	Yeast and fungal keratitis
	5-10 mg subconjunctival	Yeast and fungal endophthalmitis
	10-μg intravitreal injection	Yeast and fungal endophthalmitis

[a]Off-label use. Only natamycin (NATACYN) is commercially available and labeled for ophthalmic use. All other antifungal drugs are not labeled for ophthalmic use and must be formulated for the given method of administration. For further dosing information, refer to the *Physicians' Desk Reference for Ophthalmic Medicines*. For additional discussion of these antifungal agents, see Chapter 57.

antiseptic agent polyhexamethylene biguanide (PHMB) also is used in drop form for *Acanthamoeba* keratitis, although this is not an FDA-approved antiprotozoal agent. Topical chlorhexidine can be used as an alternative to PHMB. Oral imidazoles (e.g., itraconazole, fluconazole, ketoconazole, voriconazole) often are used in addition to the topical medications. Resolution of *Acanthamoeba* keratitis often requires many months of treatment.

Toxoplasmosis may present as a posterior (e.g., focal retinochoroiditis, papillitis, vitritis, retinitis) or occasionally as an anterior uveitis. Treatment is indicated when inflammatory lesions encroach upon the macula and threaten central visual acuity. Several regimens have been recommended with concurrent use of systemic steroids:

- pyrimethamine, sulfadiazine, and folinic acid (leucovorin)
- pyrimethamine, sulfadiazine, clindamycin, and folinic acid
- sulfadiazine and clindamycin
- clindamycin
- trimethoprim-sulfamethoxazole with or without clindamycin

Other protozoal infections (e.g., giardiasis, leishmaniasis, malaria) and helminths are less common eye pathogens in the U.S. Systemic pharmacological management as well as vitrectomy may be indicated for selected parasitic infections.

In the eye, infections can occur in a variety of locations, such as the cornea, sclera, vitreous, and retina and can be caused by bacteria, viruses, fungi, and parasites. Treatment is based on the severity of infection, the location, and the class of infectious agent. Within each group of microbial cause, different organisms are treated with different medications. Gram-positive bacteria respond to certain antibiotics and Gram-negative bacteria to others. Some organisms are quite susceptible to many antimicrobial agents, while others are not. Still others may have been susceptible in the past but have become resistant. The task of staying ahead of the rapidly developing resistances is becoming increasingly difficult. In ophthalmology, fortunately, newer-generation topical fluoroquinolones recently were brought to market, which has at least temporarily helped stem the tide of resistant infections. Additional topical fluoroquinolones are in development.

While the selection of topical antiviral agents is rather limited, several new systemic antiviral agents have become available in the past decade. Similarly, there is only one commercially available topical antifungal medication, but there are numerous systemic agents, several of them new in the past few years. Potentially, some of these systemic medications could be modified for topical use or even formulated as intraocular implants, greatly expanding our options in the treatment of many ophthalmic infectious diseases.

Use of Autonomic Agents in the Eye

General Considerations. General autonomic pharmacology has been discussed extensively in Chapters 8-12. The autonomic agents used in ophthalmology as well as the responses (i.e., mydriasis, cycloplegia) to muscarinic cholinergic antagonists are summarized in Table 64–7.

Therapeutic Uses. Autonomic drugs are used extensively for diagnostic and surgical purposes and for the treatment of glaucoma, uveitis, and strabismus.

Glaucoma. In the U.S., glaucoma is the second leading cause of blindness in African-Americans, the third leading cause in Caucasians, and the leading cause in Hispanic Americans (Congdon et al., 2004). African Americans have three times the age-adjusted prevalence of glaucoma compared to Caucasians (Friedman et al., 2004). Characterized by progressive optic nerve cupping and visual field loss, glaucoma is responsible for the bilateral blindness of 90,000 Americans (half of whom are African-American or Hispanic) (Congdon et al., 2004), and ~2.2 million have the disease (1.86% of the population >40 years of age). This number is expected to increase by 50% by the year 2020 (Friedman et al., 2004). Risk factors associated with glaucomatous nerve damage include increased IOP, positive family history of glaucoma, African-American heritage, and possibly myopia and hypertension. The production and regulation of aqueous humor were discussed earlier in "Aqueous Humor Dynamics and Regulation of Intraocular Pressure." Previously, an IOP of >21 mm Hg was considered abnormal. This, however, is incorrect, as IOP is not an accurate indicator of disease. Nonetheless, elevated IOP is a risk factor for glaucoma. Several randomized, controlled trials have determined that reducing IOP can delay glaucomatous nerve or field damage (Fluorouracil Filtering Surgery Study Group, 1996; AGIS Investigators, 2000; Heijl et al., 2002). Although markedly elevated IOPs (e.g., >30 mm Hg) usually will lead to optic nerve damage, the optic nerves in certain patients apparently can tolerate IOPs in the mid- to high 20s. These patients are referred to as *ocular hypertensives*. The Ocular Hypertension Treatment Study found that prophylactic medical reduction of IOP reduced the risk of progression to glaucoma from ~10-5% (Kass et al., 2002). Other patients have progressive glaucomatous optic nerve damage despite having IOPs in the normal range, and this form of the disease sometimes is called *normal-* or *low-tension* glaucoma. A reduction of IOP by 30% reduces disease progression from ~35-10%, even for normal-tension glaucoma patients (Collaborative Normal-Tension Glaucoma

Table 64–7

Autonomic Drugs for Ophthalmic Use

DRUG CLASS (TRADE NAME)	FORMULATION	INDICATIONS FOR USE	OCULAR SIDE EFFECTS
Cholinergic agonists			
Acetylcholine (MIOCHOL-E)	1% solution	Miosis in surgery	Corneal edema
Carbachol (MIOSTAT, ISOPTO CARBACHOL, others)	0.01-3% solution	Miosis in surgery, glaucoma[a]	Corneal edema, miosis, induced myopia, decreased vision, brow ache, retinal detachment
Pilocarpine (ISOPTO CARPINE, PILOCAR, PILAGAN, PILOPINE HS, PILOPTIC, PILOSTAT, others)	0.5%, 1%, 2%, 4%, and 6% solution; 4% gel	Glaucoma	Same as for carbachol
Anticholinesterase agents			
Echothiophate (PHOSPHOLINE IODIDE)	0.125% solution	Glaucoma, accommodative esotropia	Retinal detachment, miosis, cataract, pupillary block glaucoma iris cysts, brow ache, punctal stenosis of the nasolacrimal system
Muscarinic antagonists			
Atropine (ATROPINE-CARE, ISOPTO ATROPINE)	0.5%, 1%, and 2% solution; 1% ointment	Cycloplegia, mydriasis,[b] cycloplegic retinoscopy,[a] dilated funduscopic exam	Photosensitivity, blurred vision
Scopolamine (ISOPTO HYOSCINE)	0.25% solution	Cycloplegia, mydriasis[b]	Same as for atropine
Homatropine (ISOPTO HOMATROPINE, others)	2% and 5% solution	Cycloplegia, mydriasis[b]	Same as for atropine
Cyclopentolate (AK-PENTOLATE, CYCLOGYL)	0.5%, 1%, and 2% solution	Cycloplegia, mydriasis[b]	Same as for atropine
Tropicamide (MYDRIACYL, TROPICACYL)	0.5% and 1% solution	Cycloplegia, mydriasis[b]	Same as for atropine

(*Continued*)

Table 64–7

Autonomic Drugs for Ophthalmic Use (Continued)

DRUG CLASS (TRADE NAME)	FORMULATION	INDICATIONS FOR USE	OCULAR SIDE EFFECTS
Sympathomimetic agents			
Dipivefrin (AKPRO)	0.1% solution	Glaucoma	Photosensitivity, conjunctival , hyperemia hypersensitivity
Phenylephrine (AK-DILATE, MYDFRIN, NEO-SYNEPHRINE, others)	0.12%, 2.5%, and 10% solution	Mydriasis, vasoconstriction, decongestion	Same as for dipivefrin
Apraclonidine (IOPIDINE)	0.5% and 1% solution	Ocular hypertension	Same as for dipivefrin
Brimonidine (ALPHAGAN-P, others)	0.1%, 0.15%, and 0.2% solution	Glaucoma, ocular hypertension	Same as for dipivefrin
Naphazoline (AK-CON, ALBALON, NAPHCON, others)	0.012%, 0.03%, and 0.1% solution	Decongestant	Same as for dipivefrin
Tetrahydrozoline (ALTAZINE, MURINE TEARS PLUS, VISINE, others)	0.05% solution	Decongestant	Same as for dipivefrin
α and β adrenergic antagonists			
Betaxolol (β_1-selective) (BETOPTIC, BETOPTIC-S, others)	0.25% and 0.5% suspension	Glaucoma, ocular hypertension	
Carteolol (β)(OCUPRESS, others)	1% solution	Glaucoma, ocular hypertension	
Levobunolol (β) (BETAGAN, others)	0.25% and 0.5% solution	Glaucoma, ocular hypertension	
Metipranolol (β) (OPTIPRANOLOL, others)	0.3% solution	Glaucoma, ocular hypertension	
Timolol (β) (TIMOPTIC, TIMOPTIC XE, BETIMOL, others)	0.25% and 0.5% solution and gel	Glaucoma, ocular hypertension	

[a]Off-label use. Refer to the *Physicians' Desk Reference for Ophthalmic Medicines* for specific indications and dosing information. [b]Mydriasis and cycloplegia, or paralysis of accommodation, of the human eye occurs after one drop of atropine 1%, scopolamine 0.5%, homatropine 1%, cyclopentolate 0.5% or 1%, and tropicamide 0.5% or 1%. Recovery of mydriasis is defined by return to baseline pupil size to within 1 mm. Recovery of cycloplegia is defined by return to within 2 diopters of baseline accommodative power. The maximal mydriatic effect of homatropine is achieved with a 5% solution, but cycloplegia may be incomplete. Maximal cycloplegia with tropicamide may be achieved with a 1% solution. Times to development of maximal mydriasis and to recovery, respectively, are: for atropine, 30-40 minutes and 7-10 days; for scopolamine, 20-130 minutes and 3-7 days; for homatropine, 40-60 minutes and 1-3 days; for cyclopentolate, 30-60 minutes and 1 day; for tropicamide, 20-40 minutes and 6 hours. Times to development of maximal cycloplegia and to recovery, respectively, are: for atropine, 60-180 minutes and 6-12 days; for scopolamine, 30-60 minutes and 3-7 days; for homatropine, 30-60 minutes and 1-3 days; for cyclopentolate, 25-75 minutes and 6 hours to 1 day; for tropicamide, 30 minutes and 6 hours.

Study Group, 1998a; Collaborative Normal-Tension Glaucoma Study Group, 1998b). Despite overwhelming evidence that IOP reduction is a helpful treatment, at present the pathophysiological processes involved in glaucomatous optic nerve damage and the relationship to aqueous humor dynamics are not understood.

Current pharmacotherapies are targeted at decreasing the production of aqueous humor at the ciliary body and increasing outflow through the trabecular meshwork and uveoscleral pathways. There is no consensus on the best IOP-lowering technique for glaucoma therapy. Currently, a National Eye Institute–sponsored clinical trial, the Collaborative Initial Glaucoma Treatment Study (CIGTS), aims to determine whether it is best, in terms of preservation of visual function and quality of life, to treat patients newly diagnosed with open-angle glaucoma with filtering surgery or medication. Initial results showed no difference in disease progression rates between the two treatment groups at 5 years (Lichter et al., 2001), but after 9 years, more subjects (25.5% versus 21.3%) had visual field loss in the medicine arm than in the surgery arm of the trial (Musch et al., 2009).

The CIGTS study aside, a stepped medical approach depends on the patient's health, age, and ocular status, with knowledge of systemic effects and contraindications for all medications. Recall that:

- young patients usually are intolerant of miotic therapy secondary to visual blurring from induced myopia
- direct miotic agents are preferred over cholinesterase inhibitors in "phakic" patients (i.e., those patients who have their own crystalline lens) because the latter drugs can promote cataract formation

- in patients who have an increased risk of retinal detachment, miotics should be used with caution because they have been implicated in promoting retinal tears in susceptible individuals (such tears are thought to be due to altered forces at the vitreous base produced by ciliary body contraction induced by the drug)

The goal is to prevent progressive glaucomatous optic-nerve damage with minimum risk and side effects from either topical or systemic therapy. With these general principles in mind, a stepped medical approach may begin with a topical prostaglandin (PG) analog. Due to their once-daily dosing, low incidence of systemic side effects, and potent IOP-lowering effect, PG analogs have largely replaced β adrenergic–receptor antagonists as first-line medical therapy for glaucoma. The PG analogs consist of latanoprost (XALATAN), travoprost (TRAVATAN, TRAVATAN Z), and bimatoprost (LUMIGAN, LATISSE). The chemical structure of latanoprost is shown below:

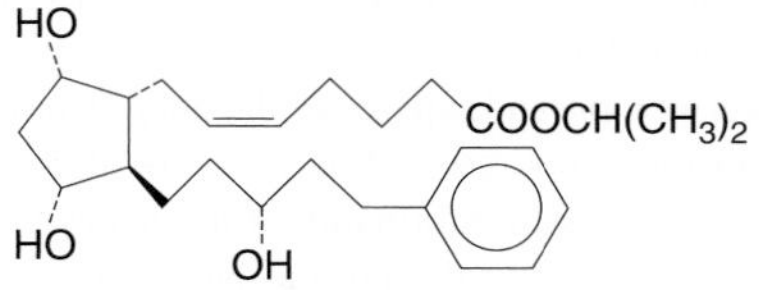

LATANOPROST

$PGF_{2\alpha}$ reduces IOP but has intolerable local side effects. Modifications to the chemical structure of $PGF_{2\alpha}$ have produced analogs with a more acceptable side-effect profile. In primates and humans, $PGF_{2\alpha}$ analogs appear to lower IOP by facilitating aqueous outflow through the accessory uveoscleral outflow pathway. The mechanism by which this occurs is unclear. $PGF_{2\alpha}$ and its analogs (prodrugs that are hydrolyzed to $PGF_{2\alpha}$) bind to FP receptors that link to G_{q11} and then to the PLC–IP_3–Ca^{2+} pathway. This pathway is active in isolated human ciliary muscle cells. Other cells in the eye also may express FP receptors. Theories of IOP lowering by $PGF_{2\alpha}$ range from altered ciliary muscle tension to effects on trabecular meshwork cells to release of matrix metalloproteinases and digestion of extracellular matrix materials that may impede outflow tracts. There also is less myocilin protein noted in monkey smooth muscle after $PGF_{2\alpha}$ treatment (Lindsey et al., 2001).

The β receptor antagonists now are the next most common topical medical treatment. There are two classes of topical β blockers. The nonselective ones bind to both β_1 and β_2 receptors and include timolol maleate and hemihydrate (hemihydrate is not available in the U.S.), levobunolol, metipranolol, and carteolol. There is one β_1-selective antagonist, betaxolol, available for ophthalmic use, but it is less efficacious than the nonselective β blockers because the β receptors of the eye are largely of the β_2 subtype. However, because the β_1 receptors are found preferentially in the heart while the β_2 receptors are found in the lung, betaxolol is less likely to cause breathing difficulty. In the eye, the targeted tissues are the ciliary body epithelium and blood vessels, where β_2 receptors account for 75-90% of the total population. How β blockade leads to decreased aqueous production and reduced IOP is uncertain. Production of aqueous humor seems to be activated by a β receptor–mediated cyclic AMP–PKA pathway; β blockade blunts adrenergic activation of this pathway by preventing catecholamine stimulation of the β receptor, thereby decreasing intracellular cyclic AMP. Another hypothesis is that β blockers decrease ocular blood flow, which decreases the ultrafiltration responsible for aqueous production (Juzych and Zimmerman, 1997).

When there are medical contraindications to the use of PG analogs or β receptor antagonists, other agents, such as a β_2 adrenergic–receptor agonist or topical carbonic anhydrase inhibitor (CAI), may be used as first-line therapy. The β_2 adrenergic agonists improve the pharmacological profile of the nonselective sympathomimetic agent epinephrine and its derivative, dipivefrin (PROPINE, others). Epinephrine stimulates both α and β adrenergic receptors. The drug appears to decrease IOP by enhancing both conventional (via a β_2 receptor mechanism) and uveoscleral outflow (perhaps via PG production) from the eye. Although effective, epinephrine is poorly tolerated, principally due to localized irritation and hyperemia. Dipivefrin is an epinephrine prodrug that is converted into epinephrine by esterases in the cornea. It is much better tolerated but is still prone to cause epinephrine-like side effects (Fang and Kass, 1997). The β_2 adrenergic agonist clonidine is effective at reducing IOP but also readily crosses the blood-brain barrier and causes systemic hypotension; as a result, it no longer is used for glaucoma. In contrast, apraclonidine (IOPIDINE) is a relatively selective β_2 adrenergic agonist that is highly ionized at physiological pH and therefore does not cross the blood-brain barrier. Brimonidine (ALPHAGAN, others) also is a selective α_2 adrenergic agonist but is lipophilic, enabling easy corneal penetration. Both apraclonidine and brimonidine reduce aqueous production and may enhance some uveoscleral outflow. Both appear to bind to pre- and postsynaptic α_2 receptors. By binding to the presynaptic receptors, the drugs reduce the amount of neurotransmitter release from sympathetic nerve stimulation and thereby lower IOP. By binding to postsynaptic α_2 receptors, these drugs stimulate the G_i pathway, reducing cellular cyclic AMP production, thereby reducing aqueous humor production (Juzych et al., 1997).

The development of a topical CAI took many years but was an important event because of the poor side-effect profile of oral CAIs. Dorzolamide (TRUSOPT, others) and brinzolamide (AZOPT) both work by inhibiting carbonic anhydrase (isoenzyme II), which is found in the ciliary body epithelium. This reduces the formation of bicarbonate ions, which reduces fluid transport and, thus, IOP (Sharir, 1997).

Any of these four drug classes can be used as additive second- or third-line therapy. In fact, the β receptor antagonist timolol has been combined with the CAI dorzolamide (see the structure below) in a single medication (COSOPT, others) and with the α_2 adrenergic agonist brimonidine (COMBIGAN).

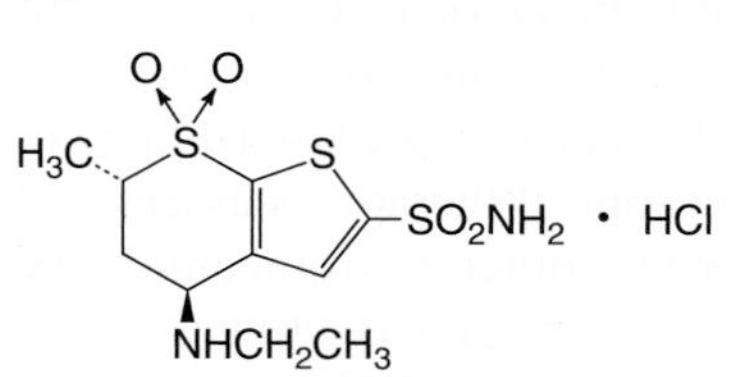

DORZOLAMIDE

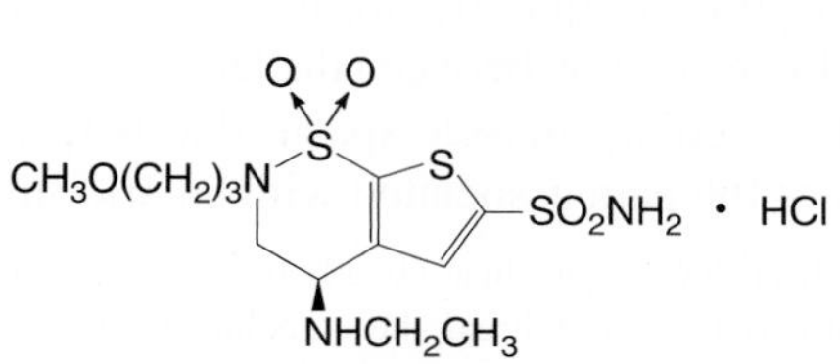

BRINZOLAMIDE

Such combinations reduce the number of drops needed and may improve compliance. Other combination products involving PG analogs and β blockers are in development.

Topical miotic agents are historically important glaucoma medications but are less commonly used today. Miotics lower IOP by causing muscarinic-induced contraction of the ciliary muscle, which facilitates aqueous outflow. They do not affect aqueous production. Multiple miotic agents have been developed. Pilocarpine and carbachol are cholinomimetics that stimulate muscarinic receptors. Echothiophate (PHOSPHOLINE IODIDE) is an organophosphate inhibitor of acetylcholinesterase; it is relatively stable in aqueous solution and, by virtue of its quaternary ammonium structure, is positively charged and poorly absorbed. The usefulness of these medicines is lessened by their numerous side effects and the need to use them three to four times a day (Kaufman and Gabelt, 1997).

If combined topical therapy fails to achieve the target IOP or fails to halt glaucomatous optic nerve damage, then systemic therapy with CAI is a final medication option before resorting to laser or incisional surgical treatment. The best-tolerated oral preparation is acetazolamide in sustained-release capsules (see Chapter 25), followed by methazolamide. The least well tolerated are acetazolamide tablets.

Toxicity of Agents in the Treatment of Glaucoma. Ciliary body spasm is a muscarinic cholinergic effect that can lead to induced myopia and a changing refraction due to iris and ciliary body contraction as the drug effect waxes and wanes between doses. Headaches can occur from the iris and ciliary body contraction. Epinephrine-related compounds, effective in IOP reduction, can cause a vasoconstriction–vasodilation rebound phenomenon leading to a red eye. Ocular and skin allergies from topical epinephrine, related prodrug formulations, apraclonidine, and brimonidine are common. Brimonidine is less likely to cause ocular allergy and therefore is more commonly used. These agents can cause CNS depression and apnea in neonates and are contraindicated in children <2 years of age.

Systemic absorption of epinephrine-related drugs and β adrenergic antagonists can induce all the side effects found with direct systemic administration. The use of CAIs systemically may give some patients significant problems with malaise, fatigue, depression, paresthesias, and nephrolithiasis; the topical CAIs may minimize these relatively common side effects. These medical strategies for managing glaucoma do help to slow the progression of this disease, yet there are potential risks from treatment-related side effects, and treatment effects on quality of life must be recognized.

Uveitis. Inflammation of the uvea, or uveitis, has both infectious and non-infectious causes, and medical treatment of the underlying cause (if known), in addition to the use of topical therapy, is essential. Cyclopentolate (CYCYLOGYL, others), tropicamide (MYDRIACYL) or sometimes even longer-acting antimuscarinic agents such as atropine, scopolamine (ISOPTO HYOSCINE), and homatropine frequently are used to prevent posterior synechia formation between the lens and iris margin and to relieve ciliary muscle spasm that is responsible for much of the pain associated with anterior uveitis.

If posterior synechiae already have formed, an α adrenergic agonist may be used to break the synechiae by enhancing pupillary dilation. A solution containing scopolamine 0.3% in combination with 10% phenylephrine (MUROCOLL-2) is available for this purpose. Two others, 1% hydroxyamphetamine hydrobromide combined with 0.25% tropicamide (PAREMYD) and 1% phenylephrine in combination with 0.2% cyclopentolate (CYCLOMYDRIL) are only indicated for induction of mydriasis. Topical steroids usually are adequate to decrease inflammation, but sometimes they must be supplemented with systemic steroids.

Strabismus. *Strabismus*, or ocular misalignment, has numerous causes and may occur at any age. Besides causing *diplopia* (double vision), strabismus in children may lead to *amblyopia* (reduced vision). Nonsurgical efforts to treat amblyopia include occlusion therapy, orthoptics, optical devices, and pharmacological agents.

An eye with *hyperopia*, or farsightedness, must constantly accommodate to focus on distant images. In some hyperopic children, the synkinetic accommodative-convergence response leads to excessive convergence and a manifest *esotropia* (turned-in eye). The brain rejects diplopia and suppresses the image from the deviated eye. If proper vision is not restored by ~7 years of age, the brain never learns to process visual information from that eye. The result is that the eye appears structurally normal but does not develop normal visual acuity and is therefore amblyopic. Unfortunately, this is a fairly common cause of visual disability. In this setting, atropine (1%) instilled in the preferred seeing eye produces cycloplegia and the inability of this eye to accommodate, thus forcing the child to use the amblyopic eye (Pediatric Eye Disease Investigator Group, 2002; Pediatric Eye Disease Investigator Group, 2003). Echothiophate iodide also has been used in the setting of accommodative strabismus. Accommodation drives the near reflex, the triad of miosis, accommodation, and convergence. An irreversible cholinesterase inhibitor such as echothiophate causes miosis and an accommodative change in the shape of the lens; hence, the accommodative drive to initiate the near reflex is reduced, and less convergence will occur.

Surgery and Diagnostic Purposes. For certain surgical procedures and for clinical funduscopic examination, it is desirable to maximize the view of the retina and lens. Muscarinic cholinergic antagonists and sympathomimetic agents frequently are used singly or in combination for this purpose (Table 64–7).

Intraoperatively, there are circumstances in which miosis is preferred, and two cholinergic agonists are available for intraocular use, acetylcholine (MIOCHOL-E) and carbachol. Patients with myasthenia gravis may first present to an ophthalmologist with complaints of double vision (diplopia) or lid droop (ptosis); the *edrophonium test* is helpful in diagnosing these patients (see Chapter 10). For surgical visualization of the lens, trypan blue (VISIONBLUE) is marketed to facilitate visualization of the lens and for staining during surgical vitrectomy procedures to guide the excision of tissue (MEMBRANEBLUE).

Use of Immunomodulatory and Antimitotic Drugs for Ophthalmic Therapy

Glucocorticoids. Glucocorticoids have an important role in managing ocular inflammatory diseases;

their chemistry and pharmacology are described in Chapter 42.

Therapeutic Uses. Currently, the glucocorticoids formulated for topical administration to the eye are dexamethasone (DEXASOL, others), prednisolone (PRED FORTE, others), fluorometholone (FML, others), loteprednol (ALREX, LOTEMAX), rimexolone (VEXOL), and difluprednate (DUREZOL). Because of their anti-inflammatory effects, topical corticosteroids are used in managing significant ocular allergy, anterior uveitis, external eye inflammatory diseases associated with some infections and ocular cicatricial pemphigoid, and postoperative inflammation following refractive, corneal, and intraocular surgery. After glaucoma filtering surgery, topical steroids can delay the wound-healing process by decreasing fibroblast infiltration, thereby reducing potential scarring of the surgical site (Araujo et al., 1995). Steroids commonly are given systemically and by sub-Tenon's capsule injection to manage posterior uveitis. Intravitreal injection of steroids now is being used to treat a variety of retinal conditions including age-related macular degeneration (ARMD), diabetic retinopathy, and cystoid macular edema. Two intravitreal triamcinolone formulations, TRIVARIS and TRIESENCE, are approved for ocular inflammatory conditions unresponsive to topical corticosteroids and visualization during vitrectomy, respectively. Parenteral steroids followed by tapering oral doses is the preferred treatment for optic neuritis (Kaufman et al., 2000; Trobe et al., 1999). An ophthalmic implant of fluocinolone (RETISERT) is marketed for the treatment of chronic, non-infectious uveitis.

Toxicity of Steroids. Steroid drops, pills, and creams are associated with ocular problems, as are intravitreal and intravenous steroids. Ocular complications include the development of posterior subcapsular cataracts, secondary infections (see Chapter 42), and secondary open-angle glaucoma (Becker and Mills, 1963). There is a significant increase in the risk for developing secondary glaucoma when there is a positive family history of glaucoma. In the absence of a family history of open-angle glaucoma, only ~5% of normal individuals respond to topical or long-term systemic steroids with a marked increase in IOP. With a positive family history, however, moderate to marked steroid-induced IOP elevations may occur in up to 90% of patients. The pathophysiology of steroid-induced glaucoma is not fully understood, but there is evidence that the *GLCIA* gene may be involved (Stone et al., 1997). Typically, steroid-induced elevation of IOP is reversible once administration of the steroid ceases. However, intraocular or sub-Tenon's steroid-related pressure elevation may persist for months and may require treatment with glaucoma medication or even filtering surgery. Newer topical steroids, so-called "soft steroids" (e.g., loteprednol), have been developed that reduce, but do not eliminate, the risk of elevated IOP.

Nonsteroidal Anti-Inflammatory Agents

General Considerations. Nonsteroidal drug therapy for inflammation is discussed in Chapter 34. Nonsteroidal anti-inflammatory drugs (NSAIDs) now are being applied to the treatment of ocular disease.

Therapeutic Uses. Currently, there are five topical NSAIDs (see Chapter 34) approved for ocular use: flurbiprofen (OCUFEN, others), ketorolac (ACULAR, others), diclofenac (VOLTAREN, others), bromfenac (XIBROM), and nepafenac (NEVANAC). Flurbiprofen is used to counter unwanted intraoperative miosis during cataract surgery. Ketorolac is given for seasonal allergic conjunctivitis. Diclofenac is used for postoperative inflammation. Both ketorolac (Weisz et al., 1999; Almeida et al., 2008) and diclofenac (Asano et al., 2008) have been found to be effective in treating cystoid macular edema occurring after cataract surgery. Bromfenac and nepafenac are indicated for treating postoperative pain and inflammation after cataract surgery. In patients treated with PG analogs such as latanoprost or bimatoprost, ketorolac and diclofenac may help decrease postoperative inflammation. They also are useful in decreasing pain after corneal refractive surgery. Topical and systemic NSAIDs occasionally have been associated with sterile corneal melts and perforations, especially in older patients with ocular surface disease, such as dry eye syndrome.

Antihistamines and Mast-Cell Stabilizers. Pheniramine (Chapter 32) and antazoline, both H_1 receptor antagonists, are formulated in combination with naphazoline, a vasoconstrictor, for relief of allergic conjunctivitis; emedastine difumarate (EMADINE) also is used. Cromolyn sodium (CROLOM, others), which reportedly prevents the release of histamine and other autacoids from mast cells, has found limited use in treating conjunctivitis that is thought to be allergen mediated, such as vernal conjunctivitis. Lodoxamide tromethamine (ALOMIDE) and pemirolast (ALAMAST), mast-cell stabilizers, also are available for ophthalmic use. Nedocromil (ALOCRIL) also is primarily a mast-cell stabilizer with some antihistamine properties. Olopatadine hydrochloride (PATANOL, PATADAY), ketotifen fumarate (ZADITOR, ALAWAY), bepotastine (BEPREVE), and azelastine (OPTIVAR) are H_1 antagonists with mast cell–stabilizing properties. Epinastine (ELESTAT) antagonizes H_1 and H_2 receptors and exhibits mast cell–stabilizing activity.

Immunosuppressive and Antimitotic Agents

General Considerations. The principal application of immunosuppressive and antimitotic agents to ophthalmology relates to the use of 5-fluorouracil and mitomycin C in corneal and glaucoma surgeries. Interferon α-2b also has occasionally been used. Certain systemic diseases with serious vision-threatening ocular manifestations—such as Behçet's disease, Wegener's granulomatosis, rheumatoid arthritis, and reactive arthritis (Reiter's syndrome)—require systemic immunosuppression (see Chapter 35).

Therapeutic Uses. In glaucoma surgery, both fluorouracil and mitomycin (MUTAMYCIN), which also are anti-neoplastic agents (see Chapter 61), improve the success of filtration surgery by limiting the postoperative wound-healing process. Mitomycin is used intraoperatively as a single subconjunctival application at the trabeculectomy site. Meticulous care is used to avoid intraocular penetration, because mitomycin is extremely toxic to intraocular structures. Fluorouracil may be used intraoperatively at the trabeculectomy site and/or subconjunctivally during the postoperative course (Fluorouracil Filtering Surgery Study Group, 1989). Although both agents work by limiting the healing process, sometimes this can result in thin, ischemic, avascular tissue that is prone to breakdown. The resultant leaks can cause hypotony (low IOP) and increase the risk of infection.

In corneal surgery, mitomycin has been used topically after excision of pterygium, a fibrovascular membrane that can grow onto the cornea. Mitomycin can be used to reduce the risk of scarring after certain procedures to remove corneal opacities and also prophylactically to prevent corneal scarring after excimer laser surface ablation (photorefractive and phototherapeutic keratectomy). Mitomycin also is used to treat certain conjunctival and corneal tumors. Interferon α-2b has been used in the treatment of conjunctival papilloma and certain conjunctival tumors. Although the use of mitomycin for both corneal surgery and glaucoma filtration surgeries augments the success of these surgical procedures, caution is advocated in light of the potentially serious delayed ocular complications (Rubinfeld et al., 1992; Hardten and Samuelson, 1999; Bahar et al., 2009).

Intraocular methotrexate (see Chapter 61) is used to treat uveitis and uveitic cystoid macular edema. It also has been used to treat the uncommon complication of lymphoma in the vitreous, which is an inaccessible compartment for most anti-neoplastic drugs (Taylor et al., 2009).

Immunomodulatory Agent. Topical cyclosporine (cyclosporin A; RESTASIS) is approved for the treatment of chronic dry eye associated with inflammation. Cyclosporine is an immunomodulatory agent that inhibits activation of T cells. Use of cyclosporine is associated with decreased inflammatory markers in the lacrimal gland, increased tear production, and improved vision and comfort (Sall et al., 2000; Perry et al., 2008).

Drugs and Biological Agents Used in Ophthalmic Surgery

Presurgical Antiseptics. Povidone iodine (BETADINE) is formulated as a 5% sterile ophthalmic solution for use prior to surgery to prep periocular skin and irrigate ocular surfaces, including the cornea, conjunctiva, and palpebral fornices. Following irrigation, the exposed tissues are flushed with sterile saline. As for other povidone iodine uses, hypersensitivity to iodine is a contraindication.

Adjuncts in Anterior Segment Surgery. *Viscoelastic* substances assist in ocular surgery by maintaining spaces, moving tissue, and protecting surfaces. These substances are prepared from hyaluronate (HEALON, others), chondroitin sulfate (VISCOAT), or hydroxypropylmethylcellulose and share the following important physical characteristics: viscosity, shear flow, elasticity, cohesiveness, and coatability. Various viscoelastic agents emphasize certain features that are broadly characterized as dispersive or cohesive. They are used almost exclusively in anterior segment surgery. Complications associated with viscoelastic substances are related to transient elevation of IOP after the surgical procedure.

Ophthalmic Glue. Cyanoacrylate tissue adhesive (ISODENT, DERMABOND, HISTOACRYL), while not FDA approved for the eye, is widely used in the management of corneal ulcerations and perforations. It is applied in liquid form and polymerized into a solid plug.

Fibrinogen glue (TISSEEL, EVICEL) is increasingly being used on the ocular surface to secure tissue such as conjunctiva, amniotic membrane, and lamellar corneal grafts. These are FDA approved for use in cardiac, vascular, and general surgery but not for the eye.

Anterior Segment Gases. Sulfur hexafluoride (SF_6) and perfluoropropane gases have long been used as vitreous substitutes during retinal surgery. In the anterior segment, they are used in non-expansile concentrations to treat Descemet's detachments, typically after cataract surgery. These detachments can cause mild to severe corneal edema. The gas is injected into the anterior chamber to push Descemet's membrane up against the stroma, where ideally it reattaches and clears the corneal edema.

Vitreous Substitutes. The primary use of vitreous substitutes is reattachment of the retina following vitrectomy and membrane-peeling procedures for complicated proliferative vitreoretinopathy and traction retinal detachments. Several compounds, including gases, perfluorocarbon liquids, and silicone oil (Table 64–8), are available. With the exception of air, the gases expand because of interaction with systemic oxygen, carbon dioxide, and nitrogen, and this property makes them desirable to temporarily tamponade areas of the retina. However, use of these expansile gases carries the risk of complications from elevated IOP, subretinal gas, corneal edema, and cataract formation. The gases are absorbed over a period of days (for air) to 2 months (for perfluoropropane).

The liquid perfluorocarbons, with specific gravities between 1.76 and 1.94, are denser than vitreous and are helpful in flattening the retina when vitreous is present. Silicone oil (polydimethylsiloxanes; ADATOSIL 5000) has had extensive use in both Europe and the U.S. for long-term tamponade of the retina. Complications from silicone oil use include glaucoma, cataract formation, corneal edema, corneal band keratopathy, and retinal toxicity.

Surgical Hemostasis and Thrombolytic Agents. Hemostasis has an important role in most surgical procedures and usually is achieved by temperature-mediated coagulation. In some intraocular surgeries, thrombin has a valuable role in hemostasis. Intravitreal administration

Table 64–8

Vitreous Substitutes[a]

VITREOUS SUBSTITUTE	CHEMICAL STRUCTURE	CHARACTERISTICS (duration or viscosity)
Nonexpansile gases		
Air		Duration of 5-7 days
Argon		
Carbon dioxide		
Helium		
Krypton		
Nitrogen		
Oxygen		
Xenon		Duration of 1 day
Expansile gases		
Sulfur hexafluoride (SF_6)	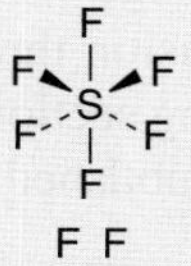 SF_6 (S bonded to six F)	Duration of 10-14 days
Octafluorocyclobutane (C_4F_8)	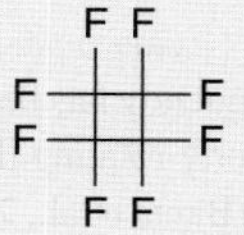 C_4F_8 (cyclic, each C bonded to two F)	
Perfluoromethane (CF_4)	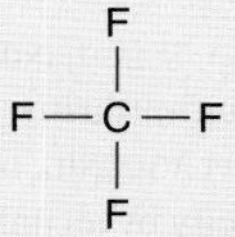 CF_4	Duration of 10-14 days
Perfluoroethane (C_2F_6)	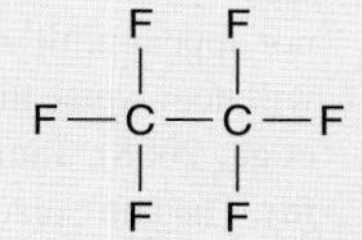 F_3C-CF_3	Duration of 30-35 days
Perfluoropropane (C_3F_8)	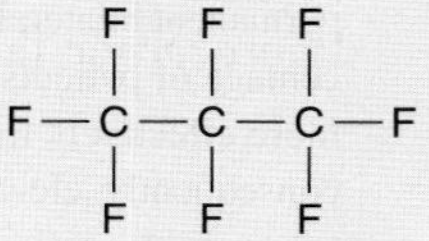 $F_3C-CF_2-CF_3$	Duration of 55-65 days
Perfluoro-*n*-butane (C_4F_{10})	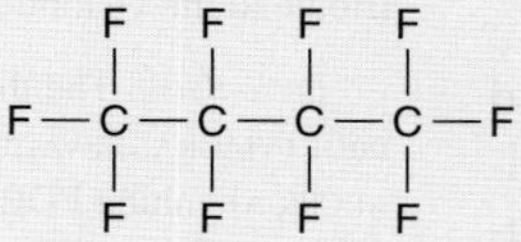 $F_3C-CF_2-CF_2-CF_3$	
Perfluoropentane (C_5F_{12})	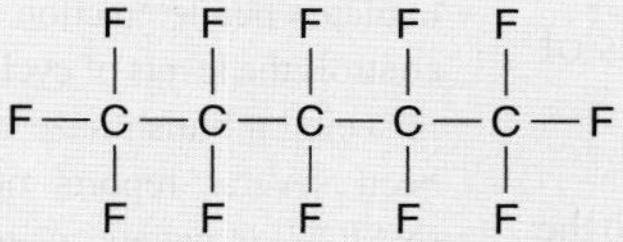 $F_3C-CF_2-CF_2-CF_2-CF_3$	
Silicone oils		
Nonfluorinated silicone oils	$(CH_3)_3SiO[(CH_3)_2SiO]_nSi(CH_3)_3$	Viscosity range from 1000-30,000 cs
Fluorosilicone	$(CH_3)_3SiO[(C_3H_4F_3)(CH_3)SiO]_nSi(CH_3)_3$	Viscosity range from 1000-10,000 cs
"High-tech" silicone oils	$(CH_3)_3SiO[(C_6H_5)(CH_3)SiO]_nSi(CH_3)_3$	May terminate as trimethylsiloxy (shown) or polyphenylmethylsiloxane; viscosity not reported

[a]See Parel and Villain, 1994, and Chang, 1994, for further details. cs, centistoke (unit of viscosity).

of thrombin can assist in controlling intraocular hemorrhage during vitrectomy. When used intraocularly, a potentially significant inflammatory response may occur, but this reaction can be minimized by thorough irrigation after hemostasis is achieved. This coagulation factor also may be applied topically via soaked sponges to exposed conjunctiva and sclera, where hemostasis may be a challenge due to the rich vascular supply.

Topical aminocaproic acid (CAPROGEL) has been investigated to prevent rebleeding after traumatic *hyphema* (blood in the anterior chamber), but clinical trials report mixed success, and the drug is not marketed in the U.S. (Karkhaneh et al., 2003; Pieramici et al., 2003).

Depending on the intraocular location of a clot, there may be significant problems relating to IOP, retinal degeneration, and persistent poor vision. *Recombinant tissue plasminogen activator* (t-PA; alteplase) (Chapter 30) has been used during intraocular surgeries to assist evacuation of a hyphema, subretinal clot, or nonclearing vitreous hemorrhage. Alteplase also has been administered subconjunctivally and intracamerally (i.e., controlled intraocular administration into the anterior segment) to lyse blood clots obstructing a glaucoma filtration site. The main complication related to the use of t-PA is bleeding.

Botulinum Toxin Type A in the Treatment of Strabismus, Blepharospasm, and Related Disorders. Botulinum toxin type A is FDA-approved for the treatment of strabismus and blepharospasm associated with dystonia, facial wrinkles (glabellar lines), axillary hyperhidrosis, and spasmodic torticollis (cervical dystonia). It also has been used off label for Meige's syndrome, hemifacial spasm, and certain migraine headaches (Tsui, 1996; Price et al., 1997) (see also Chapter 11). Two botulinum toxin type A preparations are marketed in the U.S.: onabotulinumtoxinA (BOTOX, BOTOX COSMETIC) and abobotulinumtoxinA (DYSPORT). By preventing acetylcholine release at the neuromuscular junction, botulinum toxin A usually causes a temporary paralysis of the locally injected muscles.

The variability in duration of paralysis may be related to the rate of developing antibodies to the toxin, upregulation of nicotinic cholinergic postsynaptic receptors, and aberrant regeneration of motor nerve fibers at the neuromuscular junction. Complications related to this toxin include double vision (diplopia) and lid droop (ptosis) and potentially life-threatening distant spread of toxin effect from the injection site (asthenia, generalized muscle weakness, diplopia, blurred vision, ptosis, dysphagia, dysphonia, dysarthria, urinary incontinence, and breathing difficulties) within hours to weeks after administration.

Agents Used to Treat Blind and Painful Eye. Retrobulbar injection of either absolute or 95% ethanol may provide relief from chronic pain associated with a blind and painful eye. Retrobulbar chlorpromazine also has been used. This treatment is preceded by administration of local anesthesia. Local infiltration of the ciliary nerves provides symptomatic relief from pain, but other nerve fibers may be damaged, causing paralysis of the extraocular muscles, including those in the eyelids, or neuroparalytic keratitis. The sensory fibers of the ciliary nerves may regenerate, and repeated injections sometimes are needed to control pain.

Systemic Agents with Ocular Side Effects. Just as certain systemic diseases have ocular manifestations, certain systemic drugs have ocular side effects. These can range from mild and inconsequential to severe and vision threatening. Examples are listed in the following sections. A review of these drugs recently has been published (Santaella and Fraunfelder, 2007).

Glaucoma. The anti-seizure drug topiramate (TOPAMAX, others) frequently has been reported to cause choroidal effusions, thereby anteriorly rotating the ciliary body and causing an angle-closure glaucoma (Banta et al., 2001).

Retina. Numerous drugs have toxic side effects on the retina. The anti-arthritis and antimalarial medicines hydroxychloroquine (PLAQUENIL, others) and chloroquine can cause a central retinal toxicity by an unknown mechanism. With normal dosages, toxicity does not appear until ~6 years after the drug is started. Stopping the drug will not reverse the damage but will prevent further toxicity (Tehrani et al., 2008). Tamoxifen is known to cause a crystalline maculopathy. The anti-seizure drug vigabatrin (SABRIL) causes progressive and permanent bilateral concentric visual field constriction in a high percentage of patients. The mechanism is not known, but vigabatrin is more effectively transported into the retina than into the brain, and consequently, elevations of retinal GABA concentrations may contribute to the vision loss.

Optic Nerve. The three phosphodiesterase (PDE) inhibitors, sildenafil (VIAGRA, REVATIO), vardenafil (LEVITRA), and tadalafil (CIALIS, ADCIRCA), inhibit PDE5 in the corpus cavernosum to help achieve and maintain penile erection. The drug also mildly inhibits PDE6, which controls the levels of cyclic GMP in the retina. Visually, this can result in seeing a bluish haze or experiencing light sensitivity. There have been several reports of nonarteritic ischemic optic neuropathy (NAION) in patients using these drugs. Despite these reports, there is little conclusive evidence that these drugs caused this problem, but patients should stop using the medications if they experience visual problems (Laties, 2009). Multiple medications can cause a toxic optic neuropathy characterized by gradually progressive bilateral central scotomas and vision loss. There can be accompanying optic nerve pallor. These medicines include ethambutol, chloramphenicol, and rifampin (Lloyd and Fraunfelder, 2007). Systemic or ocular steroids can cause elevated IOP and glaucoma. If the steroids cannot be stopped, glaucoma medications, and even filtering surgery, often are required.

Anterior Segment. Steroids also have been implicated in cataract formation. If vision is reduced, cataract surgery may be necessary. Rifabutin, if used in conjunction with clarithromycin or fluconazole for treatment of *Mycobacterium avium* complex (MAC) opportunistic infections in human immunodeficiency virus (HIV)-positive persons, is associated with an iridocyclitis and even hypopyon. This will resolve with steroids or by stopping the medication.

Ocular Surface. Isotretinoin (ACCUTANE, others) has a drying effect on mucous membranes and is associated with dry eye and meibomian gland dysfunction.

Cornea Coryanghiva and Eyclids . The cornea, the conjunctiva, and even the eyelids can be affected by systemic medications. One of the most common drug deposits found in the cornea is from the cardiac medication amiodarone. It deposits in the inferior and central cornea in a whorl-like pattern termed *cornea verticillata*. It appears as fine tan or brown pigment in the epithelium. Fortunately, the deposits seldom affect vision, and therefore, this rarely is a cause to discontinue the medication. The deposits disappear slowly if the medication is stopped. Other medications, including indomethacin, atovaquone, chloroquine, and hydroxychloroquine, can cause a similar pattern.

The phenothiazines, including chlorpromazine and thioridazine, can cause brown pigmentary deposits in the cornea, conjunctiva, and eyelids. The deposits generally are found in Descemet's membrane and the posterior cornea. They typically do not affect vision. The ocular deposits generally persist after discontinuation of the medication and can even worsen, perhaps because the medication deposits in the skin are slowly released and accumulate in the eye.

Gold treatments for arthritis (now rarely used) can lead to gold deposition in the cornea and conjunctiva, which are termed *chrysiasis* and are gold to violet in color. With lower cumulative doses (1-2 g), the deposits are found primarily in the epithelium and anterior stroma. These deposits usually disappear with discontinuation of the medication. With higher doses, the gold is deposited in Descemet's membrane and posterior stroma and can involve the entire stroma. These changes can be permanent. The deposits generally do not affect vision and are not a reason to stop gold therapy.

Tetracyclines can cause a yellow discoloration of the light-exposed conjunctiva. Systemic minocycline can induce a blue-gray scleral pigmentation that is most prominent in the interpalpebral zone (Morrow and Abbott, 1998).

Agents Used to Assist in Ocular Diagnosis

A number of agents are used in an ocular examination (e.g., mydriatic agents, topical anesthetics, dyes to evaluate corneal surface integrity), to facilitate intraocular surgery (e.g., mydriatic and miotic agents, topical and local anesthetics), and to help in making a diagnosis in cases of anisocoria (Figure 64–5) and retinal abnormalities (e.g., intravenous contrast agents). The autonomic agents have been discussed earlier. The diagnostic and therapeutic uses of topical and intravenous dyes and of topical anesthetics are discussed in "Anterior Segment and External Diagnostic Uses" and "Posterior Segment Diagnostic Uses."

Anterior Segment and External Diagnostic Uses. Epiphora (excessive tearing) and surface problems of the cornea and conjunctiva are commonly encountered external ocular disorders. The dyes fluorescein, rose bengal, and lissamine green are used in evaluating these problems. Available as a 2% alkaline solution, 10% and 25% solutions for injection, and an impregnated paper strip, fluorescein reveals epithelial defects of the cornea and conjunctiva and aqueous humor leakage that may occur after trauma or ocular surgery. In the setting of epiphora, fluorescein is used to help determine the patency of the nasolacrimal system. In addition, this dye is used as part of the procedure of *applanation tonometry* (IOP measurement) and to assist in determining the proper fit of rigid and semi-rigid contact lenses. Fluorescein in combination with proparacaine or benoxinate is available for procedures in which a disclosing agent is needed in conjunction with a topical anesthetic. Fluorexon (FLUORESOFT), a high-molecular-weight fluorescent solution, is used when fluorescein is contraindicated (as when soft contact lenses are in place).

Rose bengal and lissamine green, available as saturated paper strips, stain devitalized tissue on the cornea and conjunctiva.

Posterior Segment Diagnostic Uses. The integrity of the blood-retinal and retinal pigment epithelial barriers may be examined directly by retinal angiography using intravenous administration of either fluorescein sodium or indocyanine green. These agents commonly cause nausea and may precipitate serious allergic reactions in susceptible individuals.

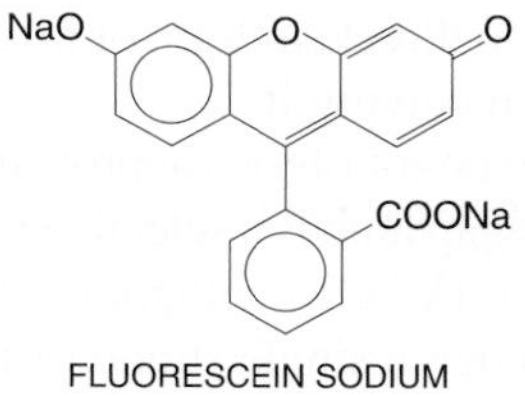

FLUORESCEIN SODIUM

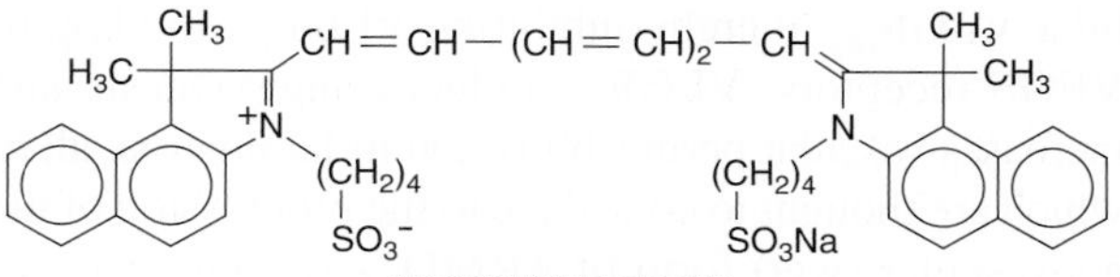

INDOCYANINE GREEN

Agents Used to Treat Retinal Neovascularization and Macular Degeneration

Verteporfin (VISUDYNE) is approved for photodynamic therapy of the exudative form of ARMD with predominantly classic choroidal neovascular membranes (Fine et al., 2000; Jager et al., 2008). Verteporfin also is used in the treatment of predominantly classic choroidal neovascularization caused by conditions such as pathological myopia and presumed ocular histoplasmosis syndrome. Verteporfin is a mixture of two regioisomers (I and II):

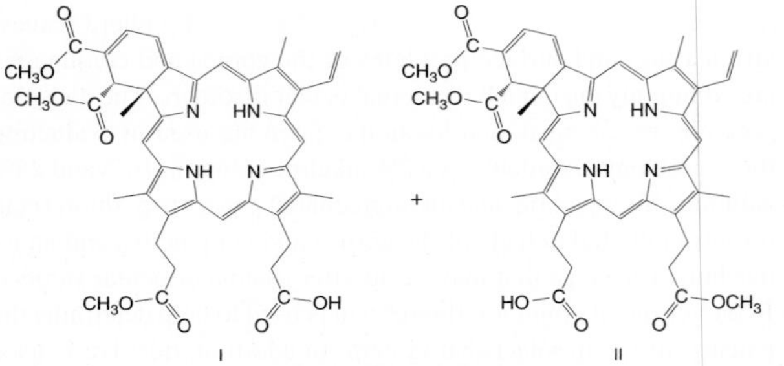

VERTEPORFIN REGIOISOMERS

Verteporfin is administered intravenously, and once it reaches the choroidal circulation, the drug is light activated by a nonthermal laser source. Depending on the size of the neovascular membrane and concerns of occult membranes and recurrence, multiple photodynamic treatments may be necessary. Activation of the drug in the presence of oxygen generates free radicals, which cause vessel damage and subsequent platelet activation, thrombosis, and occlusion of choroidal neovascularization. The $t_{1/2}$ of the drug is 5-6 hours. It is eliminated predominantly in the feces. The potential side effects include headache, injection-site reactions, and visual disturbances. The drug causes temporary photosensitization, and patients must avoid exposure of the skin or eyes to direct sunlight or bright indoor lights for 5 days after receiving it.

Pegaptanib (MACUGEN) is approved for neovascular (wet) ARMD. Pegaptanib is a selective vascular endothelial growth factor (VEGF) antagonist. It is a pegylated anti-VEGF aptamer, a single strand of nucleic acid that binds to the major pathological VEGF isoform, extracellular $VEGF_{165}$, thereby inhibiting $VEGF_{165}$ binding to VEGF receptors. $VEGF_{165}$ induces angiogenesis and increases vascular permeability and inflammation, all of which are thought to contribute to the progression of the neovascular (wet) form of ARMD, a leading cause of blindness. Pegaptanib reduced vision loss in patients with wet ARMD (Gragoudas et al., 2004). Dose levels >0.3 mg did not demonstrate any additional benefit.

Pegaptanib (0.3 mg) is administered once every 6 weeks by intravitreous injection into the eye to be treated. Side effects are largely related to the injection. Following the injection, patients should be monitored for elevation in IOP and for endophthalmitis. Rare cases of anaphylaxis/anaphylactoid reactions have been reported. No special dosage modification is required for any of the populations that have been studied (i.e., gender, elderly).

Bevacizumab (AVASTIN) is a monoclonal murine antibody that targets VEGF-A and thereby inhibits vascular proliferation and tumor growth (see Chapter 62). Ranibizumab (LUCENTIS) is a variant of bevacizumab that has had the Fab domain affinity matured (Lien and Lowman, 2008).

In the eye, several diseases that involve neovascularization such as proliferative diabetic retinopathy, macular edema, retinopathy of prematurity (Hubbard, 2008), ARMD (Patel et al., 2008), and neovascular glaucoma have been treated off label with bevacizumab, while ranibizumab generally has been reserved for both classic (Brown et al., 2009) and occult (Chang et al., 2007) choroidal neovascular membranes associated with ARMD. Both drugs are delivered by intravitreal injection and often are used on a weekly or monthly basis for maintenance therapy. Aside from the risks of hemorrhage and infection from intravitreal injections, both drugs have been associated with the risk of cerebral vascular accidents (Dafer et al., 2007; Shima et al., 2008). A multicenter clinical trial evaluating the effectiveness of the two medications for treating ARMD is currently under way.

Use of Anesthetics in Ophthalmic Procedures

Topical anesthetic agents used clinically in ophthalmology include proparacaine and tetracaine drops, lidocaine gel (see Chapter 20), and intranasal cocaine. Proparacaine and tetracaine are used topically to perform tonometry, to remove foreign bodies on the conjunctiva and cornea, to perform superficial corneal surgery, and to manipulate the nasolacrimal canalicular system. They also are used topically to anesthetize the ocular surface for refractive surgery using either the excimer laser or placement of intrastromal corneal rings. Cocaine may be used intranasally in combination with topical anesthesia for cannulating the nasolacrimal system.

Lidocaine and bupivacaine are used for infiltration and retrobulbar block anesthesia for surgery. Potential complications and risks relate to allergic reactions, globe perforation, hemorrhage, and vascular and subdural injections. Both preservative-free lidocaine (1%), which is introduced into the anterior chamber, and lidocaine jelly (2%), which is placed on the ocular surface during preoperative patient preparation, are used for cataract surgery performed under topical anesthesia. This form of anesthesia eliminates the risks of the anesthetic injection and allows for more rapid visual recovery after surgery. General anesthetics and sedation are important adjuncts for patient care for surgery and examination of the eye, especially in children and uncooperative adults. Most inhalational agents and CNS depressants are associated with a reduction in IOP. An exception is ketamine, which has been associated with an elevation in IOP. In the setting of a patient with a ruptured globe, the anesthesia should be selected carefully to avoid agents that depolarize the extraocular muscles, which may result in expulsion of intraocular contents.

Other Agents for Ophthalmic Therapy

Vitamins and Trace Elements

General Considerations. Table 64–9 summarizes the current understanding of vitamins related to eye function and disease, especially the biochemistry of vitamin A.

Table 64–9

Ophthalmic Effects of Selected Vitamin Deficiencies and Zinc Deficiency

DEFICIENCY	EFFECTS IN ANTERIOR SEGMENT	EFFECTS IN POSTERIOR SEGMENT
Vitamin		
A (retinol)	Conjunctiva (Bitot's spots, xerosis) Cornea (keratomalacia, punctate keratopathy)	Retina (nyctalopia, impaired rhodopsin synthesis), retinal pigment epithelium (hypopigmentation)
B_1 (thiamine)		Optic nerve (temporal atrophy with corresponding visual field defects)
B_6 (pyridoxine)	Cornea (neovascularization)	Retina (gyrate atrophy)
B_{12} (cyanocobalamin)		Optic nerve (temporal atrophy with corresponding visual field defects)
C (ascorbic acid)	Lens (?cataract formation)	
E (tocopherol)		Retina and retinal pigment epithelium (?macular degeneration)
Folic acid		Vein occlusion
K	Conjunctiva (hemorrhage) Anterior chamber (hyphema)	Retina (hemorrhage)
Zinc		Retina and retinal pigment epithelium (?macular degeneration)

See Chambers, 1994.

Although vitamin A must be supplied from the environment, most actions of vitamin A, like those of vitamin D, are exerted through hormone-like receptors. Vitamin A has diverse actions in cellular regulation and differentiation that go far beyond its classically defined function in vision. Analogs of vitamin A, because of their prominent effects on epithelial differentiation, have found important therapeutic applications in the treatment of a variety of dermatological conditions and are being evaluated in cancer chemoprevention.

History. The relationship of night blindness to nutritional deficiency was definitively recognized in the 1800s. Ophthalmia brasiliana (keratomalacia), a disease of the eyes that afflicted primarily poorly nourished slaves, was first described in 1865. Later, it was observed that the nurslings of mothers who fasted were prone to develop spontaneous sloughing of the cornea. Other reports of nutritional keratomalacia soon followed from all parts of the world.

Experimental rather than clinical observations, however, led to the discovery of vitamin A. In 1913, McCollum and Davis, and Osborne and Mendel independently reported that animals fed artificial diets with lard as the sole source of fat developed a nutritional deficiency that could be corrected by the addition to the diet of a factor contained in butter, egg yolk, and cod liver oil. An outstanding symptom of this experimental nutritional deficiency was xerophthalmia (dryness and thickening of the conjunctiva). Clinical and experimental vitamin A deficiencies were recognized to be related during World War I, when it became apparent that xerophthalmia in humans was a result of a decrease in the amount of butterfat in the diet.

Chemistry and Terminology. *Retinoid* refers to the chemical entity retinol and other closely related naturally occurring derivatives. Retinoids, which exert most of their effects by binding to specific nuclear receptors and modulating gene expression, also include structurally related synthetic analogs that need not have retinol-like (vitamin A) activity (Evans and Kaye, 1999).

The purified plant pigment carotene (provitamin A) is a remarkably potent source of vitamin A. β-Carotene, the most active carotenoid found in plants, has the structural formula shown in Figure 64–7A. The structural formulas for the vitamin A family of retinoids are shown in Figure 64–7B.

Retinol, a primary alcohol, is present in esterified form in the tissues of animals and saltwater fish, mainly in the liver.

A number of *cis-trans* isomers exist because of the unsaturated carbons in the retinol side chain. Fish liver oils contain mixtures of the stereoisomers; synthetic retinol is the all-*trans* isomer. Interconversion between isomers readily takes place in the body. In the visual cycle, the reaction between retinal (vitamin A aldehyde) and opsin to form rhodopsin occurs only with the 11-*cis* isomer. Ethers and esters derived from the alcohol also show activity *in vivo*. The ring structure of retinol (β-ionone), or the more unsaturated ring in 3-dehydroretinol (dehydro-β-ionone), is essential for activity; hydrogenation destroys biological activity. Of all known derivatives, all-*trans*-retinol and its aldehyde, retinal, exhibit the greatest biological potency *in vivo*; 3-dehydroretinol has ~40% of the potency of all-*trans*-retinol.

Retinoic acid, in which the alcohol moiety has been oxidized, shares some but not all of the actions of retinol. Retinoic acid is ineffective in restoring visual or reproductive function in certain species in which retinol is effective. However, retinoic acid is very potent in promoting growth and controlling differentiation and maintenance of epithelial tissue in vitamin A–deficient animals. Indeed, all-*trans*-retinoic acid (tretinoin) appears to be the active form of vitamin A in all tissues except the retina, and is 10- to 100-fold more potent than retinol in various systems *in vitro*. Isomerization of this compound in the body yields 13-*cis*-retinoic acid (isotretinoin), which is nearly as potent as tretinoin in many of its actions on epithelial tissues but may be only one-fifth as potent in producing the toxic symptoms of hypervitaminosis A. Retinoic acid analogs used clinically are discussed in detail in Chapter 65.

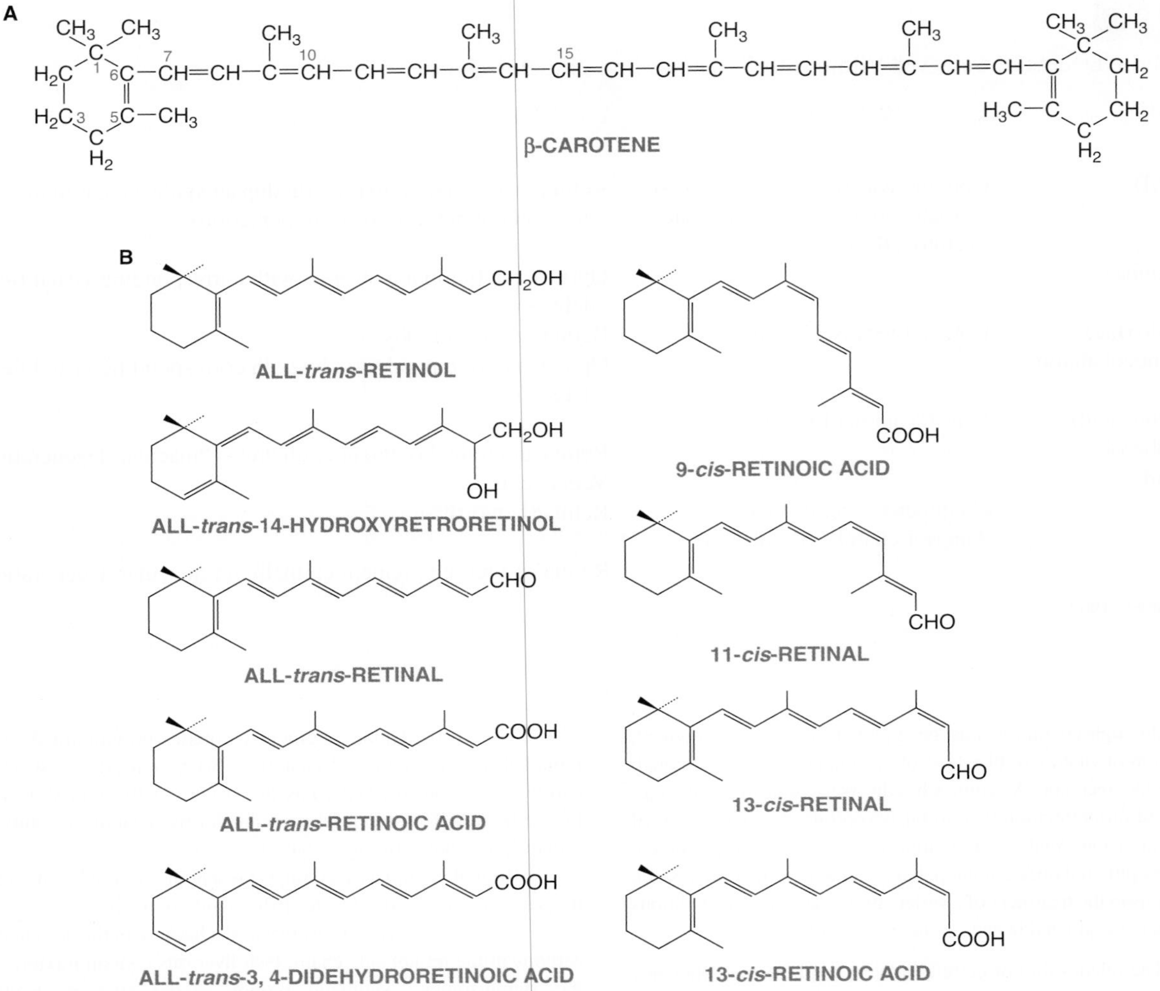

A

β-CAROTENE

B

ALL-*trans*-RETINOL

ALL-*trans*-14-HYDROXYRETRORETINOL

ALL-*trans*-RETINAL

ALL-*trans*-RETINOIC ACID

ALL-*trans*-3, 4-DIDEHYDRORETINOIC ACID

9-*cis*-RETINOIC ACID

11-*cis*-RETINAL

13-*cis*-RETINAL

13-*cis*-RETINOIC ACID

Figure 64–7. *A. Structural formula for β-carotene. B. Structural formulas for the vitamin A family of retinoids.*

Physiological Functions and Pharmacological Actions. Vitamin A plays an essential role in the function of the retina, is necessary for growth and differentiation of epithelial tissue, and is required for growth of bone, reproduction, and embryonic development. Together with certain carotenoids, vitamin A enhances immune function, reduces the consequences of some infectious diseases, and may protect against the development of certain malignancies. As a result, there is considerable interest in the pharmacological use of retinoids for cancer prophylaxis and for treating various premalignant conditions. Because of the effects of vitamin A on epithelial tissues, retinoids and their analogs are used to treat a number of skin diseases, including some of the consequences of aging and prolonged exposure to the sun (see Chapter 65).

The functions of vitamin A are mediated by different forms of the molecule. In vision, the functional vitamin is retinal. Retinoic acid appears to be the active form in functions associated with growth, differentiation, and transformation.

Retinal and the Visual Cycle. Vitamin A deficiency interferes with vision in dim light, a condition known as *night blindness* (nyctalopia).

Photoreception is accomplished by two types of specialized retinal cells, termed *rods* and *cones*. Rods are especially sensitive to light of low intensity; cones act as receptors of high-intensity light and are responsible for color vision. The initial step is the absorption of light by a chromophore attached to the receptor protein. The chromophore of both rods and cones is 11-*cis*-retinal. The holoreceptor in rods is termed *rhodopsin*—a combination of the protein opsin and 11-*cis*-retinal attached as a prosthetic group. The three different types of cone cells (red, green, and blue) contain individual, related photoreceptor proteins and respond optimally to light of different wavelengths.

In the synthesis of rhodopsin, 11-*cis*-retinol is converted to 11-*cis*-retinal in a reversible reaction that requires pyridine nucleotides. 11-*cis*-Retinal then combines with the ε amino group of a specific lysine residue in opsin to form rhodopsin. Most rhodopsin is located in the membranes of the discs situated in the outer segments of the rods. The protein has seven membrane-spanning domains, a characteristic shared by all receptors whose functions are transduced via G proteins.

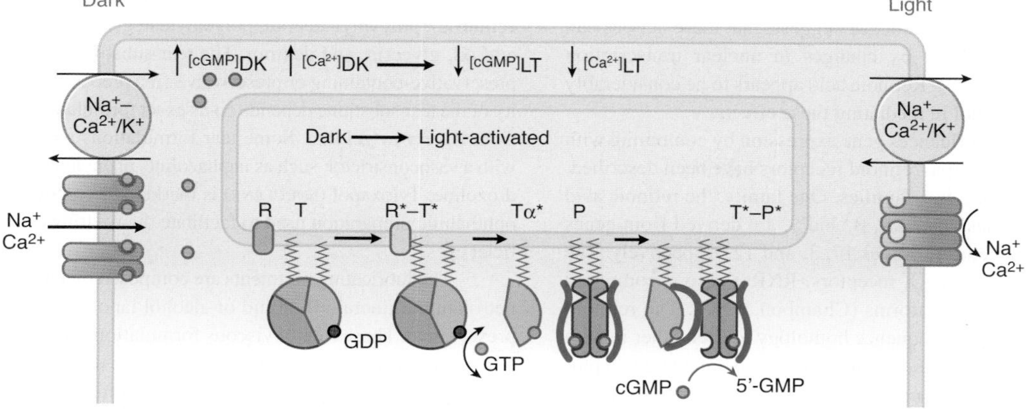

Figure 64–8. *Major steps in photoreceptor signaling.* In dark-adapted rod photoreceptors (left side of diagram), cytoplasmic cyclic GMP (green circles) and Ca^{2+} concentrations are high, and some of the cyclic GMP–gated cation channels in the plasma membrane (purple tetramer) are fully liganded and in the open state. Upon absorption of a photon by rhodopsin (R, red integral disk membrane protein), isomerization of the 11-*cis* retinal chromophore occurs to activate the receptor (R*). This leads to binding of transducin (T, pie-shaped heterotrimer) to R*, guanine nucleotide exchange of GDP (gray circle) for GTP (red circle), and formation of the activated transducin α subunit with bound GTP (Tα*). The Tα* species then binds phosphodiesterase 6 (PDE6) holoenzyme (P, blue αβ catalytic dimer with red γ subunits), causing de-inhibition by the γ subunit (Tα*-P*) and a large acceleration of catalysis of cyclic GMP to 5′-GMP at the active site (green arrow).The light-induced drop in cyclic GMP concentration (right side of diagram) causes the ligand-gated ion channel to close, causing membrane hyperpolarization. Ongoing extrusion of calcium by the Na^+–Ca^{2+}/K^+ exchanger in the absence of Ca^{2+} influx through the channel also causes $[Ca^{2+}]_i$ to decline, which is vital for the recovery process. DK, dark state; LT, light-activated state. (Reproduced with permission from Zhang X, Cote RH. cGMP signaling in vertebrate retinal photoreceptor cells. *Front Biosci*, 2005, 10:1191–1204.)

The visual cycle (Figure 64–8) is initiated by the absorption of a photon of light, leading to the isomerization of 11-*cis*-retinal to the all-*trans* form covalently bound to rhodopsin, a G protein–coupled receptor (GPCR). Activated rhodopsin interacts with the heterotrimeric G protein *transducin* (G_t), initiating GDP–GTP exchange and formation of the activated α_t-GTP subunit. α_t-GTP binds to and activates a cyclic GMP phosphodiesterase, PDE6, resulting in a rapid drop in the local concentration of cyclic GMP. The decline in cyclic GMP permits dissociation of cyclic GMP from open cyclic GMP–gated ion channels (open in the dark), causing channel closure and hyperpolarization. This is followed by a stimulation of GC (guanylyl cyclase) activity, re-opening of the ion channel, and restoration of initial cellular Ca^{2+}. A series of reactions involving rhodopsin kinase, arrestin, recoverin, and the GTPase activity of α_t-GTP also help to restore the system to the ground state, with re-formation of the heterotrimeric form of G_t-GDP (Cote, 2007).

Vitamin A Deficiency and Vision. Humans deficient in vitamin A lose their ability for dark adaptation. Rod vision is affected more than cone vision. Upon depletion of retinol from liver and blood, usually at plasma concentrations of retinol of <0.2 mg/L (0.70 μM), the concentrations of retinol and rhodopsin in the retina fall. Unless the deficiency is overcome, opsin, lacking the stabilizing effect of retinal, decays, and anatomical deterioration of the rod outer segment occurs. In rats maintained on a vitamin A–deficient diet, irreversible ultrastructural changes leading to blindness then supervene, a process that takes ~10 months.

Following short-term deprivation of vitamin A, dark adaptation can be restored to normal by the addition of retinol to the diet. However, vision does not return to normal for several weeks after adequate amounts of retinol have been supplied. The reason for this delay is unknown.

Vitamin A and Epithelial Structures. The functional and structural integrity of epithelial cells throughout the body is dependent on an adequate supply of vitamin A. The vitamin plays a major role in the induction and control of epithelial differentiation in mucus-secreting or keratinizing tissues. In the presence of retinol or retinoic acid, basal epithelial cells are stimulated to produce mucus. Excessive concentrations of the retinoids lead to the production of a thick layer of mucin, the inhibition of keratinization, and the display of goblet cells.

In the absence of vitamin A, goblet mucous cells disappear and are replaced by basal cells that have been stimulated to proliferate. These undermine and replace the original epithelium with a stratified, keratinizing epithelium. The suppression of normal secretions leads to irritation and infection. Reversal of these changes is achieved by the administration of retinol, retinoic acid, or other retinoids. When this process happens in the cornea, severe hyperkeratinization (xerophthalmia) may lead to permanent blindness. Common causes of vitamin A deficiency include malnutrition and bariatric surgery. Worldwide, xerophthalmia remains one of the most common causes of blindness.

Mechanism of Action. In isolated fibroblasts or epithelial tissue, retinoids enhance the synthesis of some proteins (e.g., fibronectin) and reduce the synthesis of others (e.g., collagenase, certain species of keratin), and molecular evidence suggests that these actions can be entirely accounted for by changes in nuclear transcription (Mangelsdorf et al., 1994). Retinoic acid appears to be considerably more potent than retinol in mediating these effects.

Retinoic acid influences gene expression by combining with nuclear receptors. Multiple retinoid receptors have been described. These are grouped into two families. One family, the retinoic acid receptors (RARs), designated α, β, and γ, are derived from genes localized to human chromosomes 17, 3, and 12, respectively. The second family, the retinoid X receptors (RXRs), also is composed of α, β, and γ receptor isoforms (Chambon, 1995). The retinoid receptors show extensive sequence homology to each other in both their DNA and hormone-binding domains and belong to a receptor superfamily that includes receptors for steroid and thyroid hormones and calcitriol (Mangelsdorf et al., 1994). Cellular responses to thyroid hormones, calcitriol, and retinoic acid are enhanced by the presence of RXR. Gene activation involves binding of the hormone-receptor complex to promoter elements in target genes, followed by dimerization with an RXR-ligand complex. The endogenous RXR ligand is 9-*cis*-retinoic acid (Heyman et al., 1992; Levin et al., 1992). No comparable receptor for retinol has been identified; retinol may need to be oxidized to retinoic acid to produce its effects within target cells.

Retinoids can influence the expression of receptors for certain hormones and growth factors and thus can influence the growth, differentiation, and function of target cells by both direct and indirect actions (Love and Gudas, 1994).

Therapeutic Uses. Nutritional vitamin A deficiency causes *xerophthalmia*, a progressive disease characterized by *nyctalopia* (night blindness), *xerosis* (dryness), and *keratomalacia* (corneal thinning), which may lead to corneal perforation; xerophthalmia may be reversed with vitamin A therapy (WHO/UNICEF/IVAGG Task Force, 1988). However, rapid, irreversible blindness ensues once the cornea perforates. Vitamin A also is involved in epithelial differentiation and may have some role in corneal epithelial wound healing. Currently, there is no evidence to support using topical vitamin A for keratoconjunctivitis sicca in the absence of a nutritional deficiency. The current recommendation for retinitis pigmentosa is to administer 15,000 IU of vitamin A palmitate daily under the supervision of an ophthalmologist and to avoid high-dose vitamin E.

The Age-Related Eye Disease Study (AREDS) found a reduction in the risk of progression of some types of ARMD for those randomized to receive high doses of vitamins C (500 mg), E (400 IU), β-carotene (15 mg), cupric oxide (2 mg), and zinc (80 mg) (Age-Related Eye Disease Study Research Group, 2001). Interestingly, zinc has been found to be neuroprotective in a rat model of glaucoma. The mechanism appears to be mediated by heat shock proteins and may represent a novel treatment strategy for glaucoma (Park et al., 2001).

Wetting Agents and Tear Substitutes

General Considerations. The current management of dry eyes usually includes instilling artificial tears and ophthalmic lubricants. In general, tear substitutes are hypotonic or isotonic solutions composed of electrolytes, surfactants, preservatives, and some viscosity-increasing agent that prolongs the residence time in the cul-de-sac and precorneal tear film. Common viscosity agents include cellulose polymers (e.g., carboxymethylcellulose, hydroxyethyl cellulose, hydroxypropyl cellulose, hydroxypropyl methylcellulose [hypromellose], and methylcellulose), polyvinyl alcohol, polyethylene glycol, polysorbate, mineral oil, glycerin, and dextran. The tear substitutes are available as preservative-containing or preservative-free preparations. The viscosity of the tear substitute depends on its exact formulation and can range from watery to gel like. Some tear formulations also are combined with a vasoconstrictor, such as naphazoline, phenylephrine, or tetrahydrozoline. Tyloxapol (ENUCLENE) is marketed as an over-the-counter ophthalmic preparation used to facilitate the wearing comfort of artificial eyes.

The lubricating ointments are composed of a mixture of white petrolatum, mineral oil, liquid or alcohol lanolin, and sometimes a preservative. These highly viscous formulations cause considerable blurring of vision, and consequently, they are used primarily at bedtime, in critically ill patients, or in very severe dry eye conditions. A hydroxypropyl cellulose ophthalmic insert (LACRISERT) that is placed in the inferior cul-de-sac and dissolves during the day is available to treat dry eyes.

Such aqueous, ointment, and insert formulations are only fair substitutes for the precorneal tear film, which truly is a poorly understood lipid, aqueous, and mucin trilaminar barrier (see "Absorption").

Therapeutic Uses. Many local eye conditions and systemic diseases may affect the precorneal tear film. Local eye disease, such as blepharitis, ocular rosacea, ocular pemphigoid, chemical burns, or corneal dystrophies, may alter the ocular surface and change the tear composition. Appropriate treatment of the symptomatic dry eye includes treating the accompanying disease and possibly the addition of tear substitutes, punctal plugs (see "Absorption"), or ophthalmic cyclosporine (see "Immunomodulatory Agent"). There also are a number of systemic conditions that may manifest themselves with symptomatic dry eyes, including Sjögren's syndrome, rheumatoid arthritis, vitamin A deficiency, Stevens-Johnson syndrome, and trachoma. Treating the systemic disease may not eliminate the symptomatic dry eye complaints; chronic therapy with tear substitutes, ophthalmic cyclosporine, insertion of punctal plugs, placement of dissolvable collagen implants, or surgical occlusion of the lacrimal drainage system may be indicated. Ophthalmic cyclosporine (RESTASIS) can be used to increase tear production in patients with ocular inflammation associated with keratoconjunctivitis sicca.

Osmotic Agents

General Considerations. The main osmotic drugs for ocular use include glycerin, mannitol, and hypertonic saline. With the availability of these agents, the use of urea for management of acutely elevated IOP is nearly obsolete.

Therapeutic Uses. Ophthalmologists occasionally use glycerin and mannitol for short-term management of acute rises in IOP. Sporadically, these agents are used intraoperatively to dehydrate the vitreous prior to anterior segment surgical procedures. Many patients with acute glaucoma do not tolerate oral medications because of nausea; therefore, intravenous administration of mannitol and/or acetazolamide may be preferred over oral administration of glycerin. These agents should be used with caution in patients with congestive heart failure or renal failure.

Corneal edema is a clinical sign of corneal endothelial dysfunction, and topical osmotic agents may effectively dehydrate the cornea. Identifying the cause of corneal edema will guide therapy, and topical osmotic agents, such as hypertonic saline, may temporize the need for surgical intervention in the form of a corneal transplant. Sodium chloride is available in either aqueous or ointment formulations. Topical glycerin also is available; however, because it causes pain on contact with the cornea and conjunctiva, its use is limited to urgent evaluation of filtration-angle structures. In general, when corneal edema occurs secondary to acute glaucoma, the use of an oral osmotic agent to help reduce IOP is preferred over topical glycerin, which simply clears the cornea temporarily. Reducing the IOP will help clear the cornea more permanently to allow both a view of the filtration angle by gonioscopy and a clear view of the iris as required to perform laser iridotomy.

BIBLIOGRAPHY

Age-Related Eye Disease Study Research Group. A randomized, placebo-controlled, clinical trial of high-dose supplementation with vitamins C and E, β carotene, and zinc for age-related macular degeneration and vision loss: AREDS report no. 8. *Arch Ophthalmol,* **2001**, *119*:1417–1436.

AGIS Investigators. The Advanced Glaucoma Intervention Study (AGIS): 7. The relationship between control of intraocular pressure and visual field deterioration. *Am J Ophthalmol,* **2000**, *130*:429–440.

Almeida DR, Johnson D, Hollands H, et al. Effect of prophylactic nonsteroidal antiinflammatory drugs on cystoid macular edema assessed using optical coherence tomography quantification of total macular volume after cataract surgery. *J Cataract Refract Surg,* **2008**, *34*:64–69.

Ambati BK, Ambati J, Azar N, et al. Periorbital and orbital cellulitis before and after the advent of *Haemophilus influenzae* type B vaccination. *Ophthalmology,* **2000**, *107*:1450–1453.

Araujo S, Spaeth G, Roth S, Starita R. A 10-year follow-up on a prospective, randomized trial of postoperative corticosteroids after trabeculectomy. *Ophthalmology,* **1995**, *102*:1753–1759.

Asano S, Miyake K, Ota I, et al. Reducing angiographic cystoid macular edema and blood-aqueous barrier disruption after small-incision phacoemulsification and foldable intraocular lens implantation: Multicenter prospective randomized comparison of topical diclofenac 0.1% and betamethasone 0.1%. *J Cataract Refract Surg,* **2008**, *34*:57–63.

Atkins EJ, Biousse V, Newman NJ. Optic neuritis. *Semin Neurol,* **2007**, *27*:211–220.

Bahar I, Kaiserman I, Lange AP, et al. The effect of mitomycin C on corneal endothelium in pterygium surgery. *Am J Ophthalmol,* **2009**, *147*:447–452.

Banta JT, Hoffman K, Budenz DL, et al. Presumed topiramate-induced bilateral acute angle-closure glaucoma. *Am J Ophthalmol,* **2001**, *132*:112–114.

Beck RW, Gal RL. Treatment of acute optic neuritis: A summary of findings from the Optic Neuritis Treatment Trial. *Arch Ophthalmol,* **2008**, *126*:994–995.

Becker B, Mills DW. Corticosteroids and intraocular pressure. *Arch Ophthalmol,* **1963**, *70*:500–507.

Biousse V, Calvetti O, Drews-Botsch CD, et al. Management of optic neuritis and impact of clinical trials: An international survey. *J Neurol Sci,* **2009**, *276*:69–74.

Brown DM, Michels M, Kaiser PK, et al. Ranibizumab versus verteporfin photodynamic therapy for neovascular age-related macular degeneration: Two-year results of the ANCHOR study. *Ophthalmology,* **2009**, *116*:57–65.

Chambers RB. Vitamins. In: Mauger TF, Craig EL, eds. *Havener's Ocular Pharmacology,* 6th ed. St. Louis, Mosby, **1994**, pp. 510–519.

Chambon P. The molecular and genetic dissection of the retinoid signaling pathway. *Recent Prog Horm Res,* **1995**, *50*:317–332.

Chang DC, Grant GB, O'Donnell K, et al. Multistate outbreak of *Fusarium* keratitis associated with use of a contact lens solution. *JAMA,* **2006,** *296*:953–963.

Chang S. Intraocular gases. In: Ryan SR, Glaser BM, eds. *Retina, Vol. 3: Surgical Retina.* St. Louis, Mosby, **1994**, pp. 2115–2129.

Chang TS, Bressler NM, Fine JT, et al. Improved vision-related function after ranibizumab treatment of neovascular age-related macular degeneration: Results of a randomized clinical trial. *Arch Ophthalmol,* **2007,** *125*:1460–1469.

Chern KC, Margolis TP. Varicella zoster virus ocular disease. *Int Ophthalmol Clin,* **1998**, *38*:149–160.

Chien DS, Homsy JJ, Gluchowski C, Tang-Liu DD. Corneal and conjunctival/scleral penetration of *p*-aminoclonidine, AGN 190342, and clonidine in rabbit eyes. *Curr Eye Res,* **1990**, *9*:1051–1059.

Colin J, Prisant O, Cochener B, et al. Comparison of the efficacy and safety of valacyclovir and acyclovir for the treatment of herpes zoster ophthalmicus. *Ophthalmology,* **2000**, *107*:1507–1511.

Collaborative Normal-Tension Glaucoma Study Group. Comparison of glaucomatous progression between untreated patients with normal-tension glaucoma and patients with therapeutically reduced intraocular pressures. *Am J Ophthalmol,* **1998a**, *126*:487–497.

Collaborative Normal-Tension Glaucoma Study Group. The effectiveness of intraocular pressure reduction in the treatment of normal-tension glaucoma. *Am J Ophthalmol,* **1998b**, *126*:498–505.

Congdon N, O'Colmain B, Klaver CC, et al. Causes and prevalence of visual impairment among adults in the United States. *Arch Ophthalmol,* **2004**, *122*:477–485.

Cote RN. Photoreceptor phosphodiesterase (PDE6): A G-protein-Activated PDE regulating visual excitation in rod and cone photoreceptor cells. In: Beavo J, Francis SH, Houslay MD, eds. *Cyclic Nucleotide Phosphodiesterases in Health and Disease*. Boca Raton, FL, CRC Press, **2007**, pp. 165–193.

Dafer RM, Schneck M, Friberg TR, Jay WM. Intravitreal ranibizumab and bevacizumab: A review of risk. *Semin Ophthalmol,* **2007**, *22*:201–204.

Dreyer EB, Zurakowski D, Schumer RA, et al. Elevated glutamate levels in the vitreous body of humans and monkeys with glaucoma. *Arch Ophthalmol,* **1996**, *114*:299–305.

Endophthalmitis Vitrectomy Study Group. Results of the Endophthalmitis Vitrectomy Study. A randomized trial of immediate vitrectomy and of intravenous antibiotics for the treatment of postoperative bacterial endophthalmitis. *Arch Ophthalmol,* **1995**, *113*:1479–1496.

Evans TR, Kaye SB. Retinoids: Present role and future potential. *Br J Cancer,* **1999**, *80*:1–8.

Fang EN, Kass MA. Epinephrine and dipivefrin. In: Zimmerman TJ, Kooner K, Sharir M, Fechtner RD, eds. *Textbook of Ocular Pharmacology,* 3rd ed. Philadelphia, Lippincott-Raven, **1997**, pp. 239–246.

Fine SL, Berger JW, Maguire MG, Ho AC. Age-related macular degeneration. *N Engl J Med,* **2000**, *342*:483–492.

Fluorouracil Filtering Surgery Study Group. Five-year follow-up of the fluorouracil filtering surgery study. *Am J Ophthalmol,* **1996,** *121*:349–366.

Fluorouracil Filtering Surgery Study Group. Fluorouracil Filtering Surgery Study: One-year follow-up. *Am J Ophthalmol,* **1989**, *108*:625–635.

Friedman DS, Wolfs RC, O'Colmain BJ, et al. Prevalence of open-angle glaucoma among adults in the United States. *Arch Ophthalmol,* **2004**, *122*:532–538.

Gragoudas ES, Adamis AP, Cunningham ET Jr, et al. Pegaptanib for neovascular age-related macular degeneration. *N Engl J Med,* **2004**, *351*:2805–2816.

Grant WM, Schuman JS. *Toxicology of the Eye,* 4th ed. Springfield, IL, Charles C. Thomas, **1993**.

Hardten DR, Samuelson TW. Ocular toxicity of mitomycin-C. *Int Ophthalmol Clin,* **1999**, *39*:79–90.

Hargrave SL, McCulley JP, Husseini Z. Results of a trial of combined propamidine isethionate and neomycin therapy for *Acanthamoeba* keratitis. Brolene Study Group. *Ophthalmology,* **1999**, *106*:952–957.

Heijl A, Leske MC, Bengtsson B, et al. Reduction of intraocular pressure and glaucoma progression: Results from the Early Manifest Glaucoma Trial. *Arch Ophthalmol,* **2002**, *120*: 1268–1279.

Herpetic Eye Disease Study Group. A controlled trial of oral acyclovir for the prevention of stromal keratitis or iritis in patients with herpes simplex virus epithelial keratitis. The Epithelial Keratitis Trial. *Arch Ophthalmol,* **1997**, *115*:703–712. Erratum in: *Arch Ophthalmol,* **1997**, *115*:1196.

Herpetic Eye Disease Study Group. Acyclovir for the prevention of recurrent herpes simplex virus eye disease. *N Engl J Med,* **1998**, *339*:300–306.

Heyman RA, Mangelsdorf DJ, Dyck JA, et al. 9-*Cis* retinoic acid is a high affinity ligand for the retinoid X receptor. *Cell,* **1992**, *68*:397–406.

Hubbard GB III. Surgical management of retinopathy of prematurity. *Curr Opin Ophthalmol,* **2008**, *19*:384–390.

Jacobson MA, Stanley H, Holtzer C, et al. Natural history and outcome of new AIDS-related cytomegalovirus retinitis diagnosed in the era of highly active antiretroviral therapy. *Clin Infect Dis,* **2000**, *30*:231–233.

Jager RD, Mieler WF, Miller JW. Age-related macular degeneration. *N Engl J Med,* **2008**, *358*:2606–2617. Erratum in: *N Engl J Med,* **2008**, *359*:1736.

Ju WK, Kim KY, Angert M, et al. Memantine blocks mitochondrial OPA1 and cytochrome c release and subsequent apoptotic cell death in glaucomatous retina. *Invest Ophthalmol Vis Sci,* **2008**, *50*:707–716.

Juzych MS, Robin AL, Novak GD. α-2 Agonists in glaucoma therapy. In: Zimmerman TJ, Kooner K, Sharir M, Fechtner RD, eds. *Textbook of Ocular Pharmacology,* 3rd ed. Philadelphia, Lippincott-Raven, **1997**, pp. 247–254.

Juzych MS, Zimmerman TJ. β-Blockers. In: Zimmerman TJ, Kooner K, Sharir M, Fechtner RD, eds. *Textbook of Ocular Pharmacology,* 3rd ed. Philadelphia, Lippincott-Raven, **1997**, pp. 261–275.

Kaderli B, Avci R, Yucel A, et al. Intravitreal triamcinolone improves recovery of visual acuity in nonarteritic anterior ischemic optic neuropathy. *J Neuroophthalmol,* **2007**, *27*: 164–168.

Karkhaneh R, Naeeni M, Chams H, et al. Topical aminocaproic acid to prevent rebleeding in cases of traumatic hyphema. *Eur J Ophthalmol,* **2003**, *13*:57–61.

Kass MA, Heuer DK, Higginbotham EJ, et al. The Ocular Hypertension Treatment Study: A randomized trial determines that topical ocular hypotensive medication delays or prevents the onset of primary open-angle glaucoma. *Arch Ophthalmol,* **2002**, *120*:701–713; discussion 829–830.

Kaufman DI, Trobe JD, Eggenberger ER, Whitaker JN. Practice parameter: The role of corticosteroids in the management of acute monosymptomatic optic neuritis. Report of the Quality Standards Subcommittee of the American Academy of Neurology. *Neurology,* **2000**, *54*:2039–2044.

Kaufman PL, Gabelt BAT. Direct, indirect, and dual-action parasympathetic drugs. In: Zimmerman TJ, Kooner K, Sharir M, Fechtner RD, eds. *Textbook of Ocular Pharmacology,* 3rd ed. Philadelphia, Lippincott-Raven, **1997**, pp. 221–238.

Kaur IP, Kanwar M. Ocular preparations: The formulation approach. *Drug Dev Ind Pharm,* **2002**, *28*:473–493.

Kunou N, Ogura Y, Yasukawa T, et al. Long-term sustained release of ganciclovir from biodegradable scleral implant for the treatment of cytomegalovirus retinitis. *J Control Release,* **2000**, *68*:263–271.

Laties AM. Vision disorders and phosphodiesterase type 5 inhibitors: A review of the evidence to date. *Drug Saf,* **2009**, *32*:1–18.

Lee VHL. Precorneal, corneal, and postcorneal factors. In: Mitra AK, ed. *Ophthalmic Drug Delivery Systems.* New York, Marcel Dekker, **1993**, pp. 59–82.

Levin AA, Sturzenbecker LJ, Kazmer S, et al. 9-*Cis* retinoic acid stereoisomer binds and activates the nuclear receptor RXR α. *Nature,* **1992**, *355*:359–361.

Levkovitch-Verbin H, Martin KR, Quigley HA, et al. Measurement of amino acid levels in the vitreous humor of rats after chronic intraocular pressure elevation or optic nerve transection. *J Glaucoma,* **2002**, *11*:396–405.

Lichter PR, Musch DC, Gillespie BW, et al. Interim clinical outcomes in the Collaborative Initial Glaucoma Treatment Study comparing initial treatment randomized to medications or surgery. *Ophthalmology,* **2001**, *108*:1943–1953.

Lien S, Lowman HB. Therapeutic anti-VEGF antibodies. *Handb Exp Pharmacol,* **2008**, *181*:131–150.

Liesegang TJ. Varicella-zoster virus eye disease. *Cornea,* **1999**, *18*:511–531.

Lindsey JD, Gaton DD, Sagara T, et al. Reduced TIGR/myocilin protein in the monkey ciliary muscle after topical prostaglandin F (2α) treatment. *Invest Ophthalmol Vis Sci,* **2001**, *42*:1781–1786.

Lloyd MJ, Fraunfelder FW. Drug-induced optic neuropathies. *Drugs Today (Barc),* **2007**, *43*:827–836.

Love JM, Gudas LJ. Vitamin A, differentiation and cancer. *Curr Opin Cell Biol,* **1994**, *6*:825–831.

Mangelsdorf DJ, Umesomo K, Evans RM. The retinoid receptors. In: Sporn MB, Roberts AB, Goodman DS, eds. *The Retinoids: Biology, Chemistry, and Medicine,* 2nd ed. New York, Raven Press, **1994**, pp. 319–349.

Marx JL, Kapusta MA, Patel SS, et al. Use of the ganciclovir implant in the treatment of recurrent cytomegalovirus retinitis. *Arch Ophthalmol,* **1996**, *114*:815–820.

McCulley JP, Alizadeh H, Niederkorn JY. The diagnosis and management of *Acanthamoeba* keratitis. *CLAO J,* **2000**, *26*:47–51.

Morrow GL, Abbott RL. Minocycline-induced scleral, dental, and dermal pigmentation. *Am J Ophthalmol,* **1998**, *125*:396–397.

Musch DC, Gillespie BW, Lichter PR, et al. Visual field progression in the Collaborative Initial Glaucoma Treatment Study: The impact of treatment and other baseline factors. *Ophthalmology,* **2009**, *116*:200–207.

Parel JM, Villain F. Silicone oils: Physicochemical properties. In: Ryan SR, Glaser BM, eds. *Retina, Vol. 3: Surgical Retina.* St. Louis, Mosby, **1994**, pp. 2131–2149.

Park KH, Cozier F, Ong OC, Caprioli J. Induction of heat shock protein 72 protects retinal ganglion cells in a rat glaucoma model. *Invest Ophthalmol Vis Sci,* **2001**, *42*:1522–1530.

Patel PJ, Bunce C, Tufail A; the ABC Trial Investigators. A randomised, double-masked phase III/IV study of the efficacy and safety of Avastin(R) (bevacizumab) intravitreal injections compared to standard therapy in subjects with choroidal neovascularisation secondary to age-related macular degeneration: Clinical trial design. *Trials,* **2008**, *9*:56.

Pediatric Eye Disease Investigator Group. A comparison of atropine and patching treatments for moderate amblyopia by patient age, cause of amblyopia, depth of amblyopia, and other factors. *Ophthalmology,* **2003**, *110*:1632–1638.

Pediatric Eye Disease Investigator Group. A randomized trial of atropine vs. patching for treatment of moderate amblyopia in children. *Arch Ophthalmol,* **2002**, *120*:268–278.

Perry HD, Solomon R, Donnenfeld ED, et al. Evaluation of topical cyclosporine for the treatment of dry eye disease. *Arch Ophthalmol,* **2008**, *126*:1046–1050.

Pieramici DJ, Goldberg MF, Melia M, et al. A phase III, multicenter, randomized, placebo-controlled clinical trial of topical aminocaproic acid (Caprogel) in the management of traumatic hyphema. *Ophthalmology,* **2003**, *110*:2106–2112.

Price J, Farish S, Taylor H, O'Day J. Blepharospasm and hemifacial spasm. Randomized trial to determine the most appropriate location for botulinum toxin injections. *Ophthalmology,* **1997**, *104*:865–868.

Quigley HA, Nickells RW, Kerrigan LA, et al. Retinal ganglion cell death in experimental glaucoma and after axotomy occurs by apoptosis. *Invest Ophthalmol Vis Sci,* **1995**, *36*:774–786.

Riordan-Eva P, Tabbara KF. Anatomy and embryology of the eye. In: Vaughan D, Asbury T, Riordan-Eva P, eds. *General Ophthalmology,* 13th ed. Stamford, CT, Appleton & Lange, **1992**.

Robinson JC. Ocular anatomy and physiology relevant to ocular drug delivery. In: Mitra AK, ed. *Ophthalmic Drug Delivery Systems*. New York, Marcel Dekker, **1993**, pp. 29–58.

Roig-Melo EA, Macky TA, Heredia-Elizondo ML, Alfaro DV III. Progressive outer retinal necrosis syndrome: Successful treatment with a new combination of antiviral drugs. *Eur J Ophthalmol,* **2001**, *11*:200–202.

Rubinfeld RS, Pfister RR, Stein RM, et al. Serious complications of topical mitomycin-C after pterygium surgery. *Ophthalmology*, **1992**, *99*:1647–1654.

Sall K, Stevenson OD, Mundorf TK, Reis BL. Two multi-center, randomized studies of the efficacy and safety of cyclosporine ophthalmic emulsion in moderate to severe dry eye disease. CsA Phase 3 Study Group. *Ophthalmology,* **2000**, *107*:631–639.

Sanborn GE, Anand R, Torti RE, et al. Sustained-release ganciclovir therapy for treatment of cytomegalovirus retinitis. Use of an intravitreal device. *Arch Ophthalmol,* **1992**, *110*: 188–195.

Santaella RM, Fraunfelder FW. Ocular adverse effects associated with systemic medications: Recognition and management. *Drugs,* **2007**, *67*:75–93.

Schiedler V, Scott IU, Flynn HW Jr, et al. Culture-proven endogenous endophthalmitis: Clinical features and visual acuity outcomes. *Am J Ophthalmol,* **2004**, *137*:725–731.

Seki M, Lipton SA. Targeting excitotoxic/free radical signaling pathways for therapeutic intervention in glaucoma. *Prog Brain Res,* **2008**, *173*:495–510.

Sharir M. Topical carbonic anhydrase inhibitors. In: Zimmerman TJ, Kooner K, Sharir M, Fechtner RD, eds. *Textbook of Ocular Pharmacology,* 3rd ed. Philadelphia, Lippincott-Raven, **1997**, pp. 287–290.

Shima C, Sakaguchi H, Gomi F, et al. Complications in patients after intravitreal injection of bevacizumab. *Acta Ophthalmol,* **2008**, *86*:372–376.

Stone EM, Fingert JH, Alward WLM, et al. Identification of a gene that causes primary open angle glaucoma. *Science,* **1997**, *275:*668–670.

Sucher NJ, Lipton SA, Dreyer EB. Molecular basis of glutamate toxicity in retinal ganglion cells. *Vision Res,* **1997**, *37*:3483–3493.

Taylor SR, Habot-Wilner Z, Pacheco P, Lightman SL. Intraocular methotrexate in the treatment of uveitis and uveitic cystoid macular edema. *Ophthalmology,* **2009**, *116*:797–801.

Tehrani R, Ostrowski RA, Hariman R, Jay WM. Ocular toxicity of hydroxychloroquine. *Semin Ophthalmol,* **2008**, *23*:201–209.

Thompson S, Pilley SF. Unequal pupils. A flow chart for sorting out the anisocorias. *Surv Ophthalmol,* **1976**, *21*:45–48.

Trobe JD, Sieving PC, Guire KE, Fendrick AM. The impact of the optic neuritis treatment trial on the practices of ophthalmologists and neurologists. *Ophthalmology,* **1999**, *106*: 2047–2053.

Tsui JK. Botulinum toxin as a therapeutic agent. *Pharmacol Ther,* **1996**, *72*:13–24.

Volpe NJ. The optic neuritis treatment trial: A definitive answer and profound impact with unexpected results. *Arch Ophthalmol,* **2008**, *126*:996–999.

Vorwerk CK, Lipton SA, Zurakowski D, et al. Chronic low-dose glutamate is toxic to retinal ganglion cells: Toxicity blocked by memantine. *Invest Ophthalmol Vis Sci,* **1996**, *37*:1618–1624.

Wax MB, Tezel G, Edward D. Clinical and ocular histopathological findings in a patient with normal-pressure glaucoma. *Arch Ophthalmol,* **1998**, *116*:993–1001.

Weisz JM, Bressler NM, Bressler SB, Schachat AP. Ketorolac treatment of pseudophakic cystoid macular edema identified more than 24 months after cataract extraction. *Ophthalmology,* **1999**, *106*:1656–1659.

Whitcup SM. Cytomegalovirus retinitis in the era of highly active anti-retroviral therapy. *JAMA*, **2000**, *283*:653–657.

WHO/UNICEF/IVAGG Task Force. *Vitamin A Supplements: A Guide to Their Use in the Treatment and Prevention of Vitamin A Deficiency and Xerophthalmia.* World Health Organization, Geneva, **1988**.

Wilhelmus KR, Gee L, Hauck WW, et al. Herpetic Eye Disease Study. A controlled trial of topical corticosteroids for herpes simplex stromal keratitis. *Ophthalmology,* **1994**, *101*:1883–1895.

Wybar KC, Karr Muir M. *Baillière's Concise Medical Textbooks, Ophthalmology,* 3rd ed. New York, Baillière Tindall, **1984**.

Yoles E, Schwartz M. Elevation of intraocular glutamate levels in rats with partial lesion of the optic nerve. *Arch Ophthalmol,* **1998**, *116*:906–910.

Dermatological Pharmacology

Craig Burkhart, Dean Morrell,
and Lowell Goldsmith

Drugs can be applied to skin for two purposes: to directly treat disorders of the skin and to deliver drugs to other tissues (Figure 65–1). The optimization of cutaneous therapies requires detailed physiological knowledge of the skin as reviewed extensively elsewhere (Wolff et al., 2008). This chapter emphasizes the basis of common skin therapies. Therapies that are used primarily for skin diseases are discussed in detail; other therapies that are applicable for skin disease are summarized and the reader referred to the appropriate portion of this book for their detailed pharmacology and toxicology.

Many skin diseases can be treated with active pharmacological agents topically; understanding the principles for percutaneous drug absorption and metabolism are essential for their effective and safe use.

Non-pharmacological therapy for skin diseases includes the entire electromagnetic spectrum applied by many sources, such as lasers, X-rays, visible light, and infrared light. These approaches may be used alone or to enhance the penetration or alter the nature of drugs and prodrugs. Freezing and ultrasound are other physical therapies that alter epidermal structure for direct treatment or to enhance percutaneous absorption of drugs. Chemicals are used to decrease the effect of various wavelengths of ultraviolet (UV) light and ionizing radiation.

Effective and safe use of topical agents requires appreciation of the physical and physiological variables that influence the interactions of drugs and the skin, impacting absorption and transport. The skin is a multifunctional and multicompartment organ affected in numerous ways by diseases and their treatments. Figure 65–1 outlines general features of skin structure and percutaneous absorption pathways. The bulk of percutaneous absorption for most agents is through the stratum corneum, which covers almost the entire skin surface. Epidermal structure and the role of hair follicles and sweat glands as pathways for absorption are reviewed below.

Stratum Corneum. The stratum corneum (outer 5-600 μm) is the major barrier to percutaneous absorption of drugs and to the loss of water from the body. It is made of "dead" epidermal cells that cannot reproduce and have lost their nuclei and mitochondria. It possesses multiple proteins and lipids that may reversibly or irreversibly bind drugs. Many chemicals and physical treatments to enhance percutaneous absorption work within the stratum corneum. Many drugs may partition into the stratum corneum and can function as a reservoir for drugs that will diffuse into the rest of skin even *after* topical application of the drug has ceased.

The stratum corneum differs in thickness, with the palm and sole being the thickest (400-600 μm) followed by the general body stratum corneum (10-16 μm), and the scrotum (5 μm). Facial and post-auricular regions have the thinnest stratum corneum. Thickness is only one variable in determining regional differences in drug penetration. Cellular arrangement has a significant role as well.

Living Epidermis. The living layers of the epidermis with metabolically active cells comprise a layer ~100 μm thick (Figure 65–2). The lowest layer (basal layer, or stratum basale) is responsible for the bulk of cell division. Several cell layers in the spinous layer (stratum spinosum) contain cells that actively synthesize most epidermal proteins, especially keratins, a large family of intracellular fibrous molecules that form the bulk of the epidermal mass. The uppermost living layer, the granular layer (stratum granulosum), is where extracellular lipids are extruded from the epidermis, forming extracellular lipids that are an important transport pathway; where the cell envelope, resistant to most proteolysis and alkali, is formed; and where extracellular lipids are covalently bound. The granular layer is also the site of synthesis of filaggrin, an intracelluar molecule that enhances keratin packing. Filaggrin is proteolyzed at the granular/stratum corneum junction, and its amino acids contribute to a

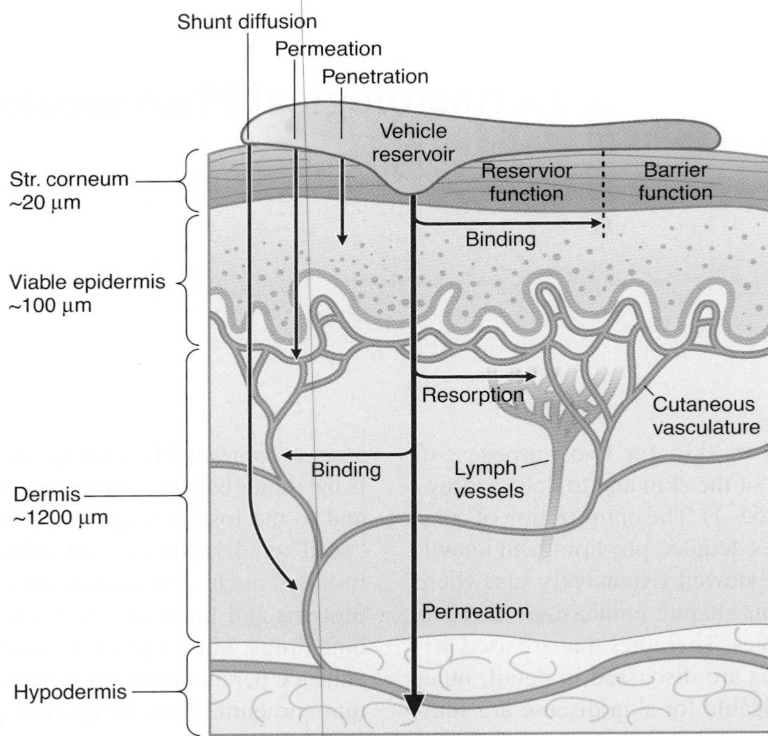

Figure 65–1. *Cutaneous drug delivery.* Diagrammatic representation of the three compartments of the skin as they relate to drug delivery: surface, stratum (Str.), and viable tissues. After application of drugs to the surface, evaporation, structural, and compositional alterations, which determine the bioavailability of drugs, occur in the applied formulation. The stratum corneum limits diffusion of compounds into the viable skin and body. After absorption, compounds either bind targets in viable tissues or diffuse within the viable tissue or into the cutaneous vasculature, where they may be carried to internal cells and organs. (Reproduced with permission from Wolff et al., 2008. Figure 215-1. Copyright © The McGraw-Hill Companies, Inc. All rights reserved. Available at http://www.accessmedicine.com.)

high free amino acid composition of the stratum corneum, which allows water retention, an acid pH, and natural moisturizing function. Intercalated in the living epidermis are pigment-producing cells (melanocytes), dendritic antigen-presenting cells (Langerhans cells), and other immune cells (γ-δ T cells); in diseased epidermis, many immunological cells, including lymphocytes and polymorphonuclear leucocytes, may be present and be directly affected by applied drugs.

Dermis and Its Blood Vessels. There is a superficial capillary plexus between the epidermis and dermis that is the site of the majority of the systemic absorption of cutaneous drugs (Figure 65–1). There are large numbers of lymphatics as well. Beneath the 1.2-mm-thick dermis with its collagen and proteoglycans that may bind drugs, there is subcutaneous tissue (hypodermis). Cells in the dermis that are targets for drugs include mast cells (permanent residents and producers of many inflammatory mediators) and infiltrating immune cells producing cytokines.

Hair follicles form a lipid-rich pathway for drug absorption. The absorption of drugs and chemicals into hair also can be used to measure prior drug exposure. Sweat glands are not known as a pathway for the absorption of drugs. Some drugs (e.g., griseofulvin, ketoconazole) are excreted to the skin by this route.

Mechanisms of Percutaneous Absorption. Passage through the outermost layer is the rate-limiting step for percutaneous absorption. The major steps involved in percutaneous absorption include the establishment of a concentration gradient, which provides the driving force for drug movement across the skin, partitioning and movement of the drug from a thin layer outside the stratum corneum into the stratum corneum (partition coefficient), and intrinsic molecular characteristics that allow drug diffusion across the layers of the skin (diffusion coefficient). The ideal relationship of these factors to each other is summarized in the following equation:

$$J \propto C_{veh} \cdot K_m \cdot D/x$$

where J is the rate of absorption, C_{veh} is the concentration of drug in the vehicle, K_m is the partition coefficient, D is the diffusion coefficient, and x is the thickness of stratum corneum (Piacquadio and Kligman, 1998). This equation represents the

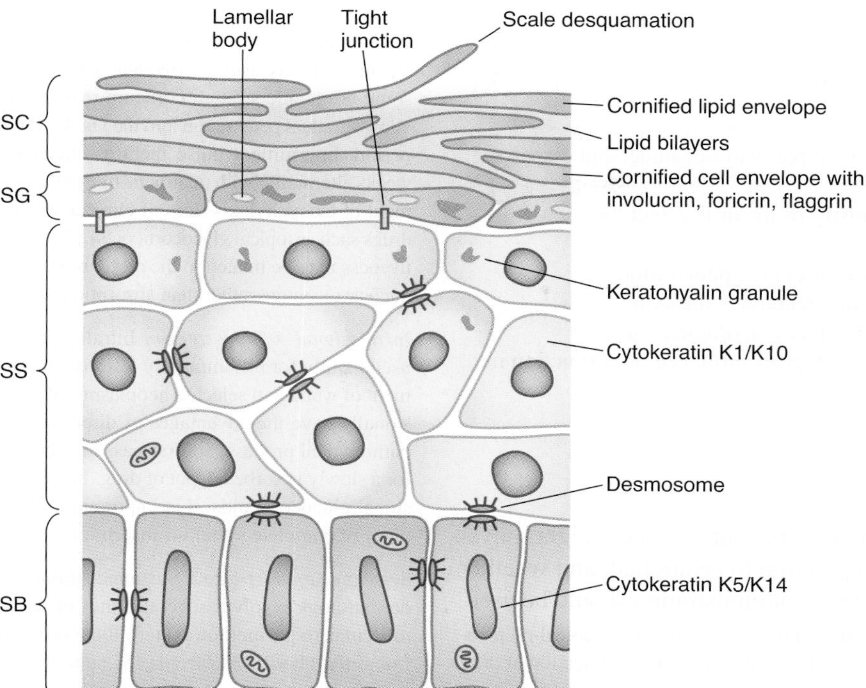

Figure 65–2. *Structure of the epidermis.* The epidermis matures progressively from the stratum basale (SB) to the stratum spinosum (SS), stratum granulosum (SG), and stratum corneum (SC). Important structural and metabolic proteins are produced at specific layers of the epidermis. (Reproduced with permission from Wolff et al., 2008. Figure 45-2. Copyright © The McGraw-Hill Companies, Inc. All rights reserved. Available at http://www.accessmedicine.com.)

idealized situation and can only approximate what occurs in normal or diseased epidermis.

Preferable characteristics of topical drugs include low molecular mass (600 Da), adequate solubility in both oil and water, and a high partition coefficient (Barry, 2004) so the drug will selectively partition from the vehicle to the stratum corneum. Except for very small particles, water-soluble ions and polar molecules do not penetrate significantly through intact stratum corneum. Commercial topical pharmaceuticals are compounded for optimum diffusion and partition, and the extemporaneous addition of other ingredients may interfere with the activity or change the absorption of the primary drug.

Drugs may target enzymes or cells of any of the skin compartments, including inflammatory cells not normally in that compartment. The exact amount of drug entering or leaving the skin in clinical situations usually is not measured; rather, the clinical endpoint (e.g., reduction in inflammation) usually is the desired effect.

A hydrated stratum corneum allows more percutaneous absorption and often is achieved through the selection of drugs formulated in occlusion vehicles such as ointments and the use of plastic films, wraps, or bags for the hands and feet and shower or bathing caps for the scalp, or through the use of medications that are impregnated on patches or tapes. Occlusion may be associated with increased growth of bacteria with resultant infection (folliculitis) or maceration and breakdown of the epidermis. Transport of most drugs is a passive thermodynamic process, and heat generally increases penetration. Ultrasonic energy or laser-induced vibration also can be used to increase percutaneous absorption. The latter may function by the production of lacunae in the stratum corneum.

The epidermis contains a variety of enzyme systems capable of metabolizing drugs that reach this compartment. Many of these enzymes have genetically determined variants that may affect drug activity. Enzymes that have been studied in detail include CYPs, epoxide hydrolase, transferases such as *N*-acetyl-transferases, glucuronyl transferases, and sulfatases (Baron et al., 2001). A specific CYP isoform, CYP26A1, metabolizes retinoic acid and may control its level in the skin (Baron et al., 2001). In addition, transporter proteins that influence influx (OATP) or efflux (MDR, P-glycoprotein) of certain xenobiotics are present in human keratinocytes (Baron et al., 2001). Although substrate turnover is considerably less than that for hepatic CYPs, these enzymes influence concentrations of xenobiotics in the skin. Genetic variants of enzymes that regulate the cellular influx and efflux of methotrexate have been associated with toxicity and effectiveness in patients with psoriasis (Warren et al., 2008).

Pharmacologic Implications of Epidermal Structure. The healthcare provider must answer a number of questions when proposing topical application of drugs (Table 65–1), including consideration of proper dosage and frequency of application, extent and condition of

Table 65–1

Important Considerations When a Drug Is Applied to the Skin

What are the absorption pathways of intact and diseased skin?
How does the chemistry of the drug affect the penetration?
How does the vehicle affect the penetration?
How much of the drug penetrates the skin?
What are the intended pharmacological targets?
What host and genetic factors influence drug function in the skin?

the permeability barrier, patient age and weight, physical form of the preparation to be applied, and whether intralesional or systemic administration should be used.

Dosage. Covering the entire skin of an adult with a topical preparation requires ~30 g of spreadable material. Underapplication of drug because of cost considerations often occurs when large amounts of skin are treated for a long time.

Regional Anatomical Variation. Permeability generally is inversely proportional to the thickness of the stratum corneum. Drug penetration is higher on the face, intertriginous areas, and perineum due to stratum corneum thickness. Skin sites that are naturally occluded by apposing surfaces, such as the axillae, groin, and inframammary areas, are vulnerable to drug-related atrophy from potent topical glucocorticoids.

Altered Barrier Function in Disease. In many dermatological diseases, the stratum corneum is abnormal and barrier function is compromised. In these settings, increased percutaneous absorption of potential topical steroids can cause systemic toxicity, such as hypothalamic–pituitary–adrenal (HPA) axis suppression.

Vehicle. Drug vehicles are summarized in Table 65–2. Newer vehicles include liposomes and microgel formulations. Liposomes are concentric spherical shells of phospholipids in an aqueous medium intended to enhance percutaneous absorption in normal and abnormal stratum corneum. Variations in size, charge, and lipid content can influence liposome function substantially. Transfersomes are a drug-delivery technology based on highly deformable, ultraflexible lipid vesicles that penetrate the skin when applied nonocclusively (Barry, 2004). Microgels are polymers intended to enhance solubilization of certain drugs, thereby enhancing topical penetration and diminishing irritancy.

Age. Children have a greater ratio of surface area to mass than adults do, so the same amount of topical drug can result in a greater systemic exposure. Based on transepidermal water loss and percutaneous absorption studies, term infants seem to possess a stratum corneum with barrier properties comparable to adults. Preterm infants have markedly impaired barrier function until the epidermis keratinizes completely.

Application Frequency. Topical agents often are applied twice daily. For certain drugs, once-daily application of a larger dose may be equally effective as more frequent applications of smaller doses. For some drugs, the stratum corneum may act as a drug reservoir that allows gradual penetration into the viable skin layers over a prolonged period. Intermittent pulse therapy—treatment for several days or weeks alternating with treatment-free periods—may prevent development of tachyphylaxis (loss of clinical effectiveness associated with drugs such as topical glucocorticoids). The mechanism of loss of effectiveness may be related to the corticosteroid binding and response of nuclear receptors rather than absorption.

Intralesional Administration. Intralesional drug administration is used mainly for inflammatory lesions but also can be used for treatment of warts and selected neoplasms. Medications injected intralesionally have the advantages of direct contact with the underlying pathological process, no first-pass metabolism, and the opportunity for a slowly absorbed depot of drug. In considering the use of intralesional glucocorticoids, it is important to be cognizant of the possibility of complete systemic absorption and suppression of the HPA.

Systemic Administration. Systemic administration of medication in dermatology involves several routes of administration: oral, intramuscular (e.g., methotrexate, glucocorticoids), intravenous (e.g., immunoglobulin, alefacept), or subcutaneous (e.g., efalizumab, etanercept).

GLUCOCORTICOIDS

Glucocorticoids are prescribed frequently for their immunosuppressive and anti-inflammatory properties. They are administered locally, through topical and intralesional routes, and systemically, through intramuscular, intravenous, and oral routes. Mechanisms of glucocorticoid action are numerous, as discussed in Chapter 42. These include apoptosis of lymphocytes, inhibitory effects on the arachidonic acid cascade, depression of production of many cytokines, and myriad effects on inflammatory cells.

Topical Glucocorticoids

Topical glucocorticoids have been grouped into seven classes in order of decreasing potency (Table 65–3); many of the more potent drugs have a fluorinated hydrocortisone backbone. Potency traditionally is measured using a vasoconstrictor assay in which an agent is applied to skin under occlusion, and the area of skin blanching is assessed. Other assays of glucocorticoid potency involve suppression of erythema and edema after experimentally induced inflammation and the psoriasis bioassay, in which the effect of steroid on psoriatic lesions is quantified.

Therapeutic Uses. Many inflammatory skin diseases respond to topical or intralesional administration of

Table 65–2

Vehicles for Topically Applied Drugs

	CREAM	OINTMENT	GEL/FOAM	LOTION/SOLUTION/FOAM
Physical basis	Oil in water emulsion	Water in oil	Water-soluble emulsion	Solution-dissolved drug base Lotion-suspended drug Aerosol propellant with drug Foam drug with surfactant as foaming agent and propellant
Solubilizing medium	>31% water (up to 80%)	<25% water	Contains water-soluble polyethylene glycols	May be aqueous or alcoholic
Pharmacological advantage	Leaves concentrated drug at skin surface	Protective oil film on skin	Concentrates drug at surface after evaporation	
Advantages for patient	Spreads and removes easily No greasy feel	Spreads easily Slows water evaporation Gives a cooling effect	Nonstaining Greaseless Clear appearance	Low residue on scalp
Locations on body	Most locations	Avoid intertriginous areas	Foams well for scalp and other hairy locations	Solutions and foams are well accepted on scalp
Disadvantages	Needs preservatives	Greasy to very greasy Stains clothes	Needs preservatives High alcohol can be drying	
Occlusion	Low	Moderate to high Increases skin moisture		
Composition issues	Requires humectants (glycerine, propylene glycol, polyethylene glycols) to keep moist when applied Oil phase with long-chain alcohol for stability and smooth feel Has absorption bases—hydrophilic petrolatum	Needs surfactants to prevent phase separation Hydrocarbon (VASELINE)	Microspheres or microsponges can be formulated in gels	

glucocorticoids. Absorption varies among body areas; the steroid is selected on the basis of its potency, the site of involvement, and the severity of the skin disease. Often, a more potent steroid is used initially, followed by a less potent agent. Most practitioners become familiar with at least one glucocorticoid in each class to facilitate selection of the appropriate strength of therapy. Twice-daily application of topical glucocorticoids is sufficient, and more frequent application does not improve response (Green et al., 2005). In general, only nonfluorinated glucocorticoids should be used on the face or in occluded areas such as the axillae or groin.

Intralesional preparations of glucocorticoids include insoluble preparations of triamcinolone acetonide (KENALOG-10) and triamcinolone hexacetonide

Table 65–3

Potency of Selected Topical Glucocorticoids

CLASS OF DRUG[a]	GENERIC NAME, FORMULATION	TRADE NAME
1	Betamethasone dipropionate cream, ointment 0.05% (in optimized vehicle)	DIPROLENE
	Clobetasol propionate cream, ointment 0.05%	TEMOVATE
	Diflorasone diacetate, ointment 0.05%	PSORCON
	Halobetasol propionate, ointment 0.05%	ULTRAVATE
2	Amcinonide, ointment 0.1%	CYCLOCORT
	Betamethasone dipropionate, ointment 0.05%	DIPROSONE, others
	Desoximetasone, cream, ointment 0.25%, gel 0.05%	TOPICORT
	Diflorasone diacetate, ointment 0.05%	FLORONE, MAXIFLOR
	Fluocinonide, cream, ointment, gel 0.05%	LIDEX, LIDEX-E, FLUONEX
	Halcinonide, cream, ointment 0.1%	HALOG, HALOG-E
3	Betamethasone dipropionate, cream 0.05%	DIPROSONE, others
	Betamethasone valerate, ointment 0.1%	BETATREX, others
	Diflorasone diacetate, cream 0.05%	FLORONE, MAXIFLOR
	Triamcinolone acetonide, ointment 0.1%, cream 0.5%	ARISTOCORT A, others
4	Amcinonide, cream 0.1%	CYCLOCORT
	Desoximetasone, cream 0.05%	TOPICORT LP
	Fluocinolone acetonide, cream 0.2%	SYNALAR-HP
	Fluocinolone acetonide, ointment 0.025%	SYNALAR
	Flurandrenolide, ointment 0.05%, tape 4 μg/cm^2	CORDRAN
	Hydrocortisone valerate, ointment 0.2%	WESTCORT
	Triamcinolone acetonide, ointment 0.1%	KENALOG, ARISTOCORT
	Mometasone furoate, cream, ointment 0.1%	ELOCON
5	Betamethasone dipropionate, lotion 0.05%	DIPROSONE, others
	Betamethasone valerate, cream, lotion 0.1%	BETATREX, others
	Fluocinolone acetonide, cream 0.025%	SYNALAR
	Flurandrenolide, cream 0.05%	CORDRAN SP
	Hydrocortisone butyrate, cream 0.1%	LOCOID
	Hydrocortisone valerate, cream 0.2%	WESTCORT
	Triamcinolone acetonide, cream, lotion 0.1%	KENALOG
	Triamcinolone acetonide, cream 0.025%	ARISTOCORT
6	Alclometasone dipropionate, cream, ointment 0.05%	ACLOVATE
	Desonide, cream 0.05%	TRIDESILON, DESOWEN
	Fluocinolone acetonide, cream, solution 0.01%	SYNALAR
7	Dexamethasone sodium phosphate, cream 0.1%	DECADRON
	Hydrocortisone, cream, ointment, lotion 0.5%, 1.0%, 2.5%	HYTONE, NUTRICORT, PENECORT

[a]Class 1 is most potent; class 7 is least potent.

(ARISTOSPAN), which solubilize gradually and therefore have a prolonged duration of action.

Toxicity. Chronic use of class 1 topical glucocorticoids can cause skin atrophy, striae, telangiectasias, purpura, and acneiform eruptions. Because perioral dermatitis and rosacea can develop after the use of fluorinated compounds on the face, they should not be used on this site. Occlusion increases the risk of HPA suppression.

Systemic Glucocorticoids

Therapeutic Uses. Systemic glucocorticoid therapy is used for severe dermatological illnesses. In general, it is best to reserve this method for allergic contact dermatitis to plants (e.g., poison ivy) and for life-threatening vesiculobullous dermatoses such as pemphigus vulgaris and bullous pemphigoid. Chronic administration of oral glucocorticoids is problematic, given the side effects associated with their long-term use (see Chapter 42).

Daily morning dosing with prednisone generally is preferred, although divided doses occasionally are used to enhance efficacy. Fewer side effects are seen with alternate-day dosing, and if chronic therapy is required, prednisone usually is tapered to every other day as soon as it is practical. Pulse therapy using large intravenous doses of methylprednisolone sodium succinate (SOLU-MEDROL, others) is an option for severe resistant pyoderma gangrenosum, pemphigus vulgaris, systemic lupus erythematosus with multi-system disease, and dermatomyositis. The dose usually is 0.5-1 g given over 2-3 hours. More rapid infusion has been associated with increased rates of hypotension, electrolyte shifts, and cardiac arrhythmias.

Toxicity and Monitoring. Oral glucocorticoids have numerous systemic effects, as discussed in Chapter 42. Most side effects are dose dependent. Long-term use is associated with a number of complications, including psychiatric problems, cataracts, myopathy, osteoporosis, avascular bone necrosis, glucose intolerance or overt diabetes mellitus, and hypertension. In addition, psoriatic patients treated with parenteral or topical glucocorticoids may have a pustular flare, particularly if the steroid is tapered rapidly.

RETINOIDS

Retinoids are defined as natural and synthetic compounds that exhibit vitamin A–like biological activity or bind to nuclear receptors for retinoids. Retinoids have many important functions throughout the body, including roles in vision, regulation of cell proliferation and differentiation and bone growth, immune defense, and tumor suppression (Vahlquist et al., 2008). Early use of systemic retinoids to treat acne and disorders of keratinization was limited by the toxic side effects of first-generation retinoids. This was largely solved through molecular modifications that yielded new generations of compounds with vastly improved margins of safety. First-generation retinoids include retinol (vitamin A), tretinoin (all-*trans*-retinoic acid; vitamin A acid), isotretinoin (13-*cis*-retinoic acid), and alitretinoin (9-*cis*-retinoic acid). Second-generation retinoids, also known as aromatic retinoids, were created by aromatization of the cyclic end group and include acitretin and methoxsalen (also known as etretinate; not marketed in the U.S.). Third-generation retinoids were created after the discovery of specific retinoid receptors and have diverse structures designed to optimize receptor-selective binding. Members of this generation include tazarotene, bexarotene, and adapalene. Characteristics of topical and systemic retinoids are summarized in Tables 65–4 and 65–5.

Retinoids exert their effects on gene expression by activating two families of receptors—*retinoic acid receptors* (RARs) and *retinoid X receptors* (RXRs)—that are members of the steroid receptor superfamily (Winterfield et al., 2003). Both retinoid receptor families have three isoforms (α, β, and γ), which are expressed in unique combinations in individual tissues and cells. The human epidermis, for example, expresses RAR-α, RAR-γ, RXR-α, and RXR-β (Kang and Voorhees, 2008). Upon binding to a retinoid, RARs and RXRs form heterodimers (RAR-RXR), which subsequently bind specific DNA sequences called retinoic acid–responsive elements (RAREs) that activate transcription of genes whose products produce the desirable pharmacological effects of these drugs and their unwanted side effects (Bastien and Rochette-Egly, 2004).

Unique therapeutic effects can be produced by targeting specific retinoid receptors. For example, retinoids that target RARs predominantly affect cellular differentiation and proliferation, whereas retinoids that target RXRs predominantly induce apoptosis (Germain et al., 2006a; Germain et al., 2006b). Hence, tretinoin, adapalene, and tazarotene, which target RARs, are used in acne, psoriasis, and photoaging (disorders of differentiation and proliferation), whereas bexarotene and alitretinoin, which target RXRs, are used in mycosis fungoides and Kaposi sarcoma (to induce apoptosis of malignant cells). Acute retinoid toxicity is similar to vitamin A intoxication. Side effects of systemic retinoids include dry skin, nosebleeds from dry mucous membranes, conjunctivitis, reduced night vision, hair loss, alterations in serum lipids and transaminases, hypothyroidism, inflammatory bowel disease flare, musculoskeletal pain, pseudotumor cerebri, and mood alterations. RAR-selective retinoids are more associated with mucocutaneous and musculoskeletal symptoms, whereas RXR-selective retinoids induce more physiochemical changes (Germain et al., 2006a; Germain et al., 2006b). Because all oral retinoids are potent teratogens, they should be used carefully in females of childbearing potential and not in pregnant patients or patients who are trying to conceive. Suicide or suicide attempts have been associated with the use of isotretinoin. Thus, all patients treated with isotretinoin should be observed closely for symptoms of depression or suicidal thoughts.

Topical Retinoids

Acne is believed to result from a combination of sebaceous gland hyperplasia, follicular hyperkeratosis, *Propionibacterium acnes* colonization, and inflammation. Through incompletely understood mechanisms, topical retinoids correct abnormal follicular keratinization, reduce *P. acnes* counts, and reduce inflammation, thereby making them the cornerstone of acne therapy. Topical retinoids are first-line agents for non-inflammatory (comedonal) acne and often are combined with other agents in the management of inflammatory acne.

Fine wrinkles and dyspigmentation, two important features of photoaging, also are improved with

Table 65–4

Topical Retinoids

DRUG	FORMULATION	RECEPTOR SPECIFICITY	PREGNANCY CATEGORY	STRUCTURE	IRRITANCY
Tretinoin	0.02%, 0.025%, 0.05%, 0.1% cream 0.01%, 0.025%, 0.04% gel 0.05%, 0.1% solution	RAR-α, RAR-β, RAR-γ	C	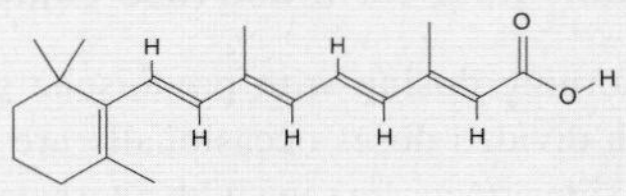	++
Tazarotene	0.05%, 0.1% cream 0.05%, 0.01% gel	RAR-α, RAR-β, RAR-γ	X	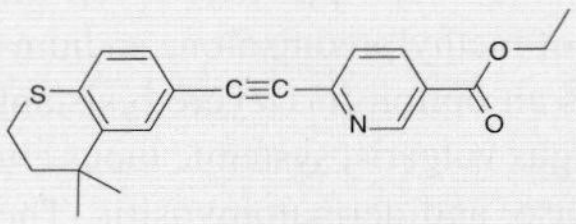	++++
Adapalene	0.1%, 0.3% cream 0.1%, 0.3% gel 0.1% solution	RAR-β, RAR-γ	C	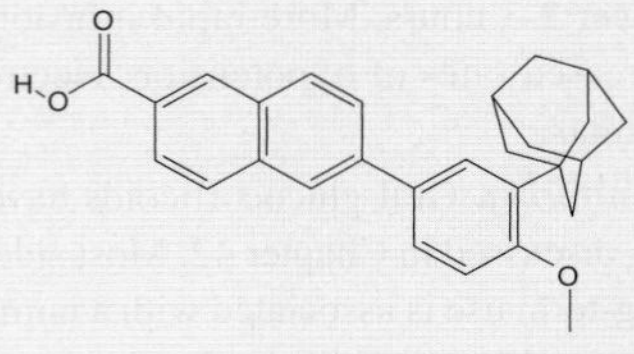	+
Alitretinoin	0.1% gel	RAR-α, RAR-β, RAR-γ	D	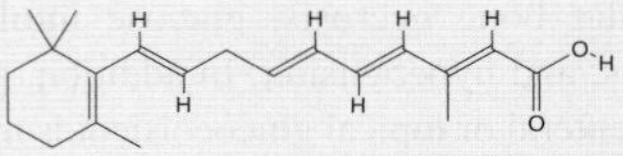	++
Bexarotene	1% gel	RXR-α, RXR-β, RXR-γ	X	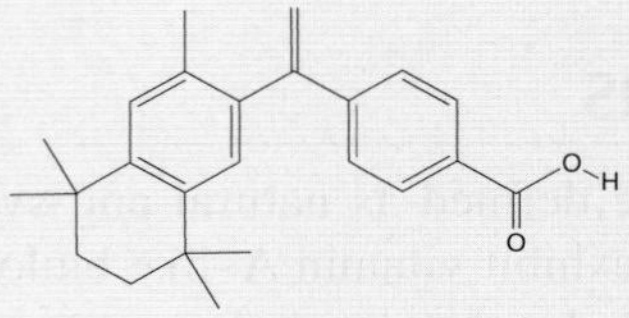	+++

topical retinoids. Within the dermis, this is believed to result from inhibition of activator protein-1 (AP-1), a transcription factor composed of c-Jun and c-Fos that normally activates synthesis of matrix metalloproteinases in response to UV irradiation (Kang and Voorhees, 2008). In the epidermis, retinoids induce epidermal hyperplasia in atrophic skin and reduce keratinocyte atypia (Sami and Harper, 2007).

Toxicity and Monitoring. Adverse effects of all topical retinoids include erythema, desquamation, burning, and stinging (Table 65–4). These effects often decrease with time and are lessened by concomitant use of emollients. Patients also may experience photosensitivity reactions because of enhanced reactivity to UV radiation and have a significant risk for severe sunburn. Although there is little systemic absorption of topical retinoids and no alteration in plasma vitamin A levels with their use, it is recommended that exposure to topical retinoids be avoided during pregnancy.

Tretinoin

Topical tretinoin (all-*trans*-retinoic acid) is photolabile and thus should be applied once nightly for acne and photoaging. Benzoyl peroxide also inactivates tretinoin and should not be applied simultaneously. Formulations with copolymer microspheres (RETIN-A MICRO) or prepolyolprepolymer-2 (AVITA) that gradually release tretinoin to decrease irritancy are available.

Adapalene

Adapalene (differin) has similar efficacy to tretinoin, but unlike tretinoin, it is stable in sunlight, stable in the presence of benzoyl peroxide, and tends to be less irritating at the 0.1% concentration.

Tazarotene

Tazarotene (TAZORAC, AVAGE) is a third-generation retinoid approved for the treatment of psoriasis, photoaging, and acne vulgaris (Sami and Harper, 2007). Tazarotene gel, applied once daily, may be used as monotherapy or in combination with other medications, such as topical corticosteroids, for the treatment of localized plaque psoriasis. Topical corticosteroids improve the efficacy of therapy and reduce the side effects of burning, itching, and skin irritation that are commonly associated with tazarotene.

Alitretinoin

Alitretinoin (PANRETIN) is a retinoid that binds all types of retinoid receptors and is applied two to four times daily to cutaneous lesions of Kaposi sarcoma. Alitretinoin should not be applied concurrently with insect repellants containing diethyltoluamide (DEET, N,N-diethyl-m-toluamide) because it may increase DEET absorption.

Bexarotene

Topical bexarotene (TARGRETIN) is approved for early-stage (IA and IB) cutaneous T-cell lymphoma. Its application is titrated up from every other day to two to four times daily over several weeks to improve patient tolerance. Its mechanism of action may involve downregulation of survivin and upregulation of caspase-3, leading to apoptosis of malignant cells (Sami and Harper, 2007). Patients using bexarotene should avoid products containing DEET due to an increased risk for DEET toxicity.

Systemic Retinoids

Systemic retinoids are approved for the treatment of acne, psoriasis, and cutaneous T-cell lymphoma (Table 65–5). Off-label uses include ichthyosis, Darier's disease, pityriasis rubra pilaris, rosacea, hidradenitis suppurativa, chemoprevention of malignancy, lichen sclerosus, subacute lupus erythematosus, and discoid lupus erythematosus. All systemic retinoids are contraindicated in women who are pregnant, contemplating pregnancy, or breast-feeding. Relative contraindications include leukopenia, alcoholism, hyperlipidemia, hypercholesterolemia, hypothyroidism, and significant hepatic or renal disease.

Toxicity and Monitoring. Acute retinoid toxicities may include mucocutaneous or laboratory abnormalities; bony changes may occur after chronic use at high doses. Mucocutaneous side effects may include cheilitis, xerosis, blepharoconjunctivitis, cutaneous photosensitivity,

Table 65–5
Systemic Retinoids

DRUG	STRUCTURE	RECEPTOR SPECIFICITY	STANDARD DOSING RANGE	$t_{1/2}$
Isotretinoin	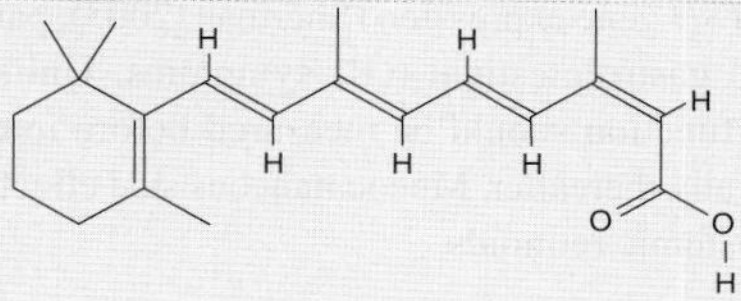	No clear receptor affinity	0.5-2 mg/kg/day	10-20 hours
Etretinate	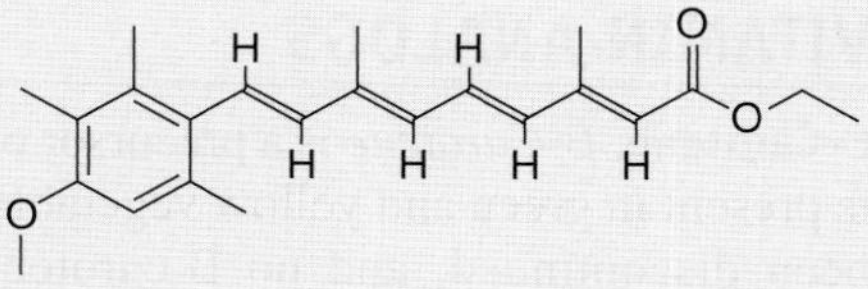	RAR-α, RAR-β, RAR-γ	0.25-1 mg/kg/day	80-160 days
Acitretin	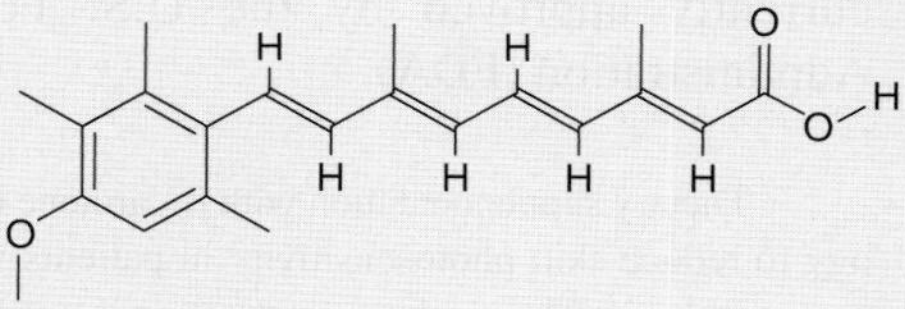	RAR-α, RAR-β, RAR-γ	0.5-1 mg/kg/day	50 hours
Bexarotene	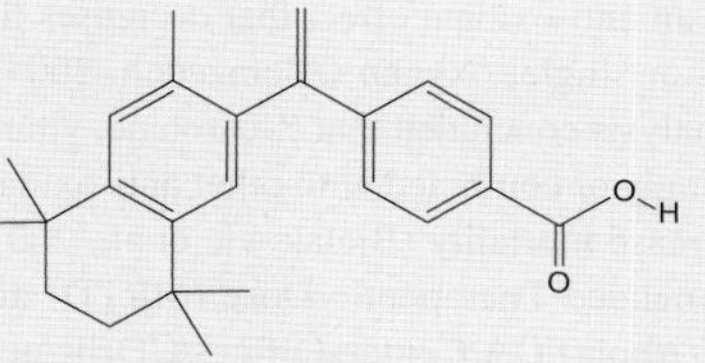	RXR-α, RXR-β, RXR-γ	300 mg/m²/day	7-9 hours

photophobia, myalgia, arthralgia, headaches, alopecia, nail fragility, and increased susceptibility to staphylococcal infections. Some patients develop a "retinoid dermatitis" characterized by erythema, pruritus, and scaling.

Very rarely, patients may develop pseudotumor cerebri, especially when systemic retinoids are combined with tetracyclines (tetracycline or minocycline; the mechanism for this adverse drug event is unknown). There are reports that chronic administration at higher doses can cause diffuse idiopathic skeletal hyperostosis (DISH) syndrome, premature epiphyseal closure, and other skeletal abnormalities (Vahlquist et al., 2008).

Systemic retinoids are highly teratogenic. There is no safe dose during pregnancy. Common malformations include craniofacial, cardiovascular, thymic, and central nervous system (CNS) abnormalities. Although there appears to be minimal, if any, risk of retinoid embryopathy in fetuses conceived by males taking systemic retinoids, it is commonly recommended that men avoid retinoid therapy when actively trying to father children. Prescribing of isotretinoin in the U.S. is restricted via the risk-mitigation iPLEDGE system (Goldsmith et al., 2004).

Serum lipid elevation is the most common laboratory abnormality. This may be due to increased expression of apolipoprotein C-III by systemic retinoids, which prevents the uptake of lipids from very-low-density lipoproteins into cells (Vahlquist et al., 2008). Other, less common, laboratory abnormalities include elevated transaminases, decreased thyroid hormone, and leukopenia. A baseline evaluation of serum lipids, serum transaminases, and complete blood count (CBC) and a pregnancy test should be obtained prior to starting any systemic retinoids. Laboratory values should be checked monthly for the first 3-6 months and once every 3 months thereafter.

Isotretinoin

Isotretinoin (ACCUTANE, others) is approved for the treatment of recalcitrant and nodular acne vulgaris. The drug has remarkable efficacy in severe acne and may induce prolonged remissions after a single course of therapy. It normalizes keratinization in the sebaceous follicle, reduces sebocyte number with decreased sebum synthesis, and reduces *P. acnes* (Vahlquist et al., 2008). Clinical effects generally are noted within 1-3 months of starting therapy.

Approximately one-third of patients will relapse, usually within 3 years of stopping therapy (Vahlquist et al., 2008). Preteens, males, and patients with acne conglobata or androgen excess are at increased risk of relapse. Although most relapses are mild and respond to conventional management with topical and systemic anti-acne agents, some may require a second course of isotretinoin.

There are several reports of patients developing signs of depression while on isotretinoin. However, large studies have failed to prove an association between isotretinoin use and depression. Since it is possible that an idiosyncratic reaction occurs in a small group of otherwise healthy individuals, current guidelines recommend monthly monitoring of all patients on isotretinoin for signs of depression.

Acitretin

Acitretin (SORIATANE, SORIATANE CK) is approved for use in the cutaneous manifestations of psoriasis. It is especially useful in pustular psoriasis, although all forms of cutaneous psoriasis are responsive to acitretin. Clinical effect typically begins within 4-6 weeks, with the full clinical benefit occurring at 3-4 months.

Although acitretin has a $t_{1/2}$ of ~50 hours, when combined with alcohol, acitretin is esterified *in vivo* to produce etretinate, which has a $t_{1/2}$ of >3 months (Vahlquist et al., 2008). It is not known how much alcohol (i.e., cough syrup or other alcohol-based medications) is required to induce this conversion. Therefore, female patients of childbearing age should avoid pregnancy for 3 years after receiving acitretin to avoid retinoid-induced embryopathy.

Bexarotene

Bexarotene (TARGRETIN) is a retinoid that selectively binds RXRs. Oral and topical formulations of bexarotene are approved for use in patients with cutaneous T-cell lymphoma. Although the exact mechanism of action is unknown, studies suggest that bexarotene induces apoptosis of malignant cells (Budgin et al., 2005). Because it is metabolized by CYP3A4, inhibitors of CYP3A4 (e.g., imidazole antifungals, macrolide antibiotics) will increase and inducers of CYP3A4 (e.g., rifamycins, carbamazepine, dexamethasone, efavirenz, phenobarbital) will decrease plasma levels of bexarotene. Laboratory side effects are more common than with other retinoids, with an increased incidence of significant lipid abnormalities and hypothyroidism secondary to a reversible RXR-mediated suppression of *TSH* gene expression (Sherman, 2003), pancreatitis, leukopenia, and gastrointestinal (GI) symptoms. Unlike other retinoids, thyroid function should be measured before initiating therapy and periodically thereafter. Mucocutaneous side effects are less than with other systemic retinoids.

VITAMIN ANALOGS

β-Carotene. *β-Carotene* is a precursor of vitamin A that is present in green and yellow vegetables. Solatene has been discontinued, and no β-carotene products are currently approved by the U.S. Food and Drug Administration (FDA).

Dietary supplementation with β-carotene is used in dermatology to reduce skin photosensitivity in patients with erythropoietic protoporphyria. The mechanism of action is not established but may involve an anti-oxidant effect that decreases the production of free radicals or singlet oxygen (Alemzedeh, 2004). However, a recent meta-analysis concluded that β-carotene, vitamin A, and vitamin E given singly or combined with other anti-oxidant supplements actually increase mortality (Bjelakovic et al., 2007). FDA's Maximum Recommended Therapeutic Dose (MRTD) database (http://www.fda.gov/AboutFDA/CentersOffices/CDER/ucm092199.htm) lists 0.05 mg/kg/day as the MRTD for β-carotene.

are irritants and may lead to microcomedo formation and resulting inflammatory lesions. Suppression of cutaneous *P. acnes* with antibiotic therapy is correlated with clinical improvement (Tan, 2003).

Commonly used topical antimicrobials in acne include clindamycin (CLEOCIN-t, others), erythromycin (ERYDERM, others), benzoyl peroxide, and antibiotic–benzoyl peroxide combinations (BENZACLIN, DUAC, others). Other antimicrobials used in treating acne include sulfacetamide (KLARON, others), sulfacetamide/sulfur combinations (SULFACET-R, others), metronidazole (METROCREAM, METROGEL, NORITATE), and azelaic acid (AZELEX, others). *Systemic therapy* is prescribed for patients with more extensive disease and acne that is resistant to topical therapy. In healthy individuals taking oral antibiotics for acne, laboratory monitoring is not necessary. Effective agents include tetracycline (SUMYCIN, others), doxycycline (MONODOX, others), minocycline (MINOCIN, others), and trimethoprim–sulfamethoxazole (BACTRIM, others). Antibiotics usually are administered twice daily, and doses are tapered after control is achieved.

The tetracyclines are the most commonly employed antibiotics because they are inexpensive, safe, and effective. The initial daily dose usually is 1 g in divided doses. Although tetracyclines are antimicrobial agents, efficacy in acne may be more dependent on anti-inflammatory activity. Minocycline has better GI absorption than tetracycline and may be less photosensitizing than either tetracycline or doxycycline. Side effects of minocycline include dizziness and hyperpigmentation of the skin and mucosa, serum sickness–like reactions, and drug-induced lupus erythematosus. With all the tetracyclines, vaginal candidiasis is a common complication that is readily treated with local administration of antifungal drugs.

Cutaneous Infections. Gram-positive organisms, including *Staphylococcus aureus* and *Streptococcus pyogenes*, are the most common cause of pyoderma. Skin infections with Gram-negative bacilli are rare, although they can occur in diabetics and patients who are immunosuppressed; appropriate parenteral antibiotic therapy is required for their treatment.

Topical therapy frequently is adequate for impetigo, the most superficial bacterial infection of the skin caused by *S. aureus* and *S. pyogenes*. Mupirocin (pseudomonic acid, BACTROBAN, others), produced by *Pseudomonas fluorescens*, is effective for such localized infections. It inhibits protein synthesis by binding to bacterial isoleucyl-tRNA synthetase. Mupirocin is highly active against staphylococci and all streptococci except those of group D. It is less active against gram-negative organisms, but it has *in vitro* activity against *Haemophilus influenzae, Neisseria gonorrhoeae, Pasteurella multocida, Moraxella catarrhalis*, and *Bordetella pertussis*. Mupirocin is inactive against normal skin flora. Its antibacterial activity is enhanced by the acid pH of the skin surface. Mupirocin is available as a 2% ointment or cream and is applied three times daily. A nasal formulation is indicated to eradicate methicillin-resistant *S. aureus* (MRSA) nasal colonization.

Retapamulin ointment 1% (ALTABAX) also is FDA approved for the topical treatment of impetigo caused by susceptible strains of *S. aureus* or *S. pyogenes* in patients ≥9 months of age. Retapamulin selectively inhibits bacterial protein synthesis by interacting at a site on the 50S subunit of bacterial ribosomes.

Topical therapy often is employed for prophylaxis of superficial infections caused by wounds and injuries. Neomycin is active against staphylococci and most gram-negative bacilli. It may cause allergic contact dermatitis, especially on disrupted skin. Bacitracin inhibits staphylococci, streptococci, and gram-positive bacilli. Polymyxin B is active against aerobic gram-negative bacilli. Neomycin, bacitracin, polymyxin B (NEOSPORIN ORIGINAL OINTMENT, DOUBLE ANTIBIOTIC OINTMENT, others) are sold alone or in various combinations with other ingredients (e.g., hydrocortisone, lidocaine, or pramoxine) in a number of over-the-counter (OTC) formulations for the first aid of minor scrapes, burns, and cuts.

Deeper bacterial infections of the skin include folliculitis, erysipelas, cellulitis, and necrotizing fasciitis. Because streptococcal and staphylococcal species also are the most common causes of deep cutaneous infections, penicillins (especially β lactamase–resistant β-lactams) and cephalosporins are the systemic antibiotics used most frequently in their treatment (Carter, 2003) (see Chapter 44). A growing concern is the increased incidence of skin and soft-tissue infections with hospital- and community-acquired MRSA and drug-resistant pneumococci. Infection with community-acquired MRSA often is susceptible to trimethoprim–sulfamethoxazole (Cohen and Grossman, 2004).

In addition to various traditional systemic antibiotics (such as erythromycin), novel antibacterial agents such as linezolid, quinupristin–dalfopristin, and daptomycin also have been approved for the treatment of complicated skin and skin-structure infections (see Chapter 53).

Antifungal Agents

Fungal infections are among the most common causes of skin disease in the U.S., and numerous effective topical and oral antifungal agents have been developed. Griseofulvin, topical and oral imidazoles, triazoles, and allylamines are the most effective agents available. Examples include butenafine, clotrimazole, gentian violet, sertaconazole, ketoconazole, nystatin, oxiconazole, sulconazole, tolnaftate, undecylenic acid, and the antifungal combinations BENSAL HP, WHITFIELD'S OINTMENT (benzoic acid + salicylic acid), VERSICLEAR LOTION (25% sodium thiosulfate + 1% salicylic acid), CASTELLANI PAINT MODIFIED (basic fuchsin + phenol + resorcinol + acetone), and FUNGI-NAIL (1% resorcinol + 2% salicylic acid + 2% chloroxylenol + 0.5% benzocaine + 50% isopropyl alcohol). The pharmacology, uses, and toxicities of antifungal drugs are discussed in Chapter 57. This section will address the management of common cutaneous fungal diseases. Recommendations for cutaneous antifungal therapy are summarized in Table 65–8.

The azoles miconazole (MICATIN, others) and econazole (SPECTAZOLE, others) and the allylamines naftifine (NAFTIN) and terbinafine (LAMISIL, others) are effective topical agents for the treatment of localized tinea corporis and uncomplicated tinea pedis. Topical therapy with the azoles is preferred for localized cutaneous candidiasis and tinea versicolor.

Systemic therapy is necessary for the treatment of tinea capitis or follicular-based fungal infections. Oral griseofulvin has been the traditional medication for treatment of tinea capitis. Oral terbinafine is a safe and effective alternative to griseofulvin in treating tinea capitis in children (Moosavi et al., 2001).

Tinea Pedis. Topical therapy with the azoles and allylamines is effective for tinea pedis. Macerated toe web disease may require the addition of antibacterial therapy. Econazole nitrate, which has a limited antibacterial spectrum, can be useful in this situation. Systemic therapy with griseofulvin, terbinafine, or itraconazole (SPORANOX, others) is used for more extensive tinea pedis. It should be recognized that long-term topical therapy may be necessary in some patients after courses of systemic antifungal therapy.

Onychomycosis. Fungal infection of the nails most frequently is caused by dermatophytes and Candida. Mixed infections are common. Because up to one-third of dystrophic nails that appear clinically to be onychomycosis are actually due to psoriasis or other conditions, the nail must be cultured or clipped for histological examination before initiating therapy.

Systemic therapy is necessary for effective management of onychomycosis. Treatment of onychomycosis of toenails with griseofulvin for 12-18 months produces a cure rate of 50% and a relapse rate of 50% after 1 year. Terbinafine and itraconazole offer significant potential advantages. They quickly produce high drug levels in the nail, which persist after therapy is discontinued. Additional advantages include a broader spectrum of coverage with itraconazole and few drug interactions with terbinafine. Treatment of toenail onychomycosis requires 3 months with terbinafine (250 mg/day) or itraconazole (200 mg/day). Pulsed dosing with itraconazole for fingernail onychomycosis consists of 200 mg twice daily for 1 wk/mo for two pulses. Cure rates of ≥75% have been achieved with both drugs (Gupta et al., 1994a; Gupta et al., 1994b).

Ciclopirox topical (PENLAC, others) solution is a nail lacquer that is FDA-approved for the treatment of onychomycosis but demonstrates low complete cure rates (5.5-8.5%) after 1 year of daily application. Topical ciclopirox treatment of onychomycosis must include active removal of the unattached, infected nails as frequently as monthly.

Antiviral Agents

Viral infections of the skin are very common and include verrucae (human papillomavirus [HPV]), herpes simplex virus (HSV), condyloma acuminatum (HPV), molluscum contagiosum (poxvirus), and chicken pox (varicella-zoster virus [VZV]). Acyclovir (ZOVIRAX), famciclovir (FAMVIR, others), and valacyclovir (VALTREX) frequently are used systemically to treat HSV and VZV infections (see Chapter 58). Cidofovir (VISTIDE) may be useful in treating acyclovir-resistant HSV or VZV and other cutaneous viral infections (Anonymous, 2002a). Topically, acyclovir, docosanol (ABREVA), and penciclovir (DENAVIR) are available for treating mucocutaneous HSV. Podophyllin (25% solution) and podofilox (CONDYLOX, others) 0.5% solution are used to treat condylomata. The immune response modifier imiquimod (ALDARA) is discussed in "Other Immunosuppressive and Anti-Inflammatory Agents." Interferons α-2b (INTRON A), α-n1 (not commercially available in the U.S.), and α-n3 (ALFERON N) may be useful for treating refractory or recurrent warts (Carter et al., 2004).

Agents Used to Treat Infestations

Infestations with ectoparasites such as lice and scabies are common throughout the world. These conditions have a significant impact on public health in the form of disabling pruritus, secondary infection, and in the case of the body louse, transmission of life-threatening illnesses such as typhus. Topical and oral medications are available to treat these infestations.

Permethrin is a synthetic pyrethroid that interferes with insect sodium transport proteins, causing neurotoxicity and paralysis. Resistance due to mutations in the transport protein has been reported in *Cimex* (bed bugs) and other insects.

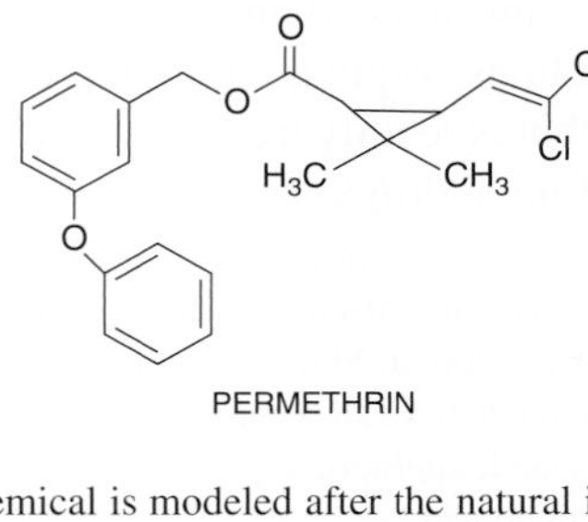

PERMETHRIN

The chemical is modeled after the natural insecticide found in the flower *Chrysanthemum cinerariifolium*. A 5% cream is available for the treatment of scabies, and a 1% cream, a cream rinse, and topical solutions are available OTC for the treatment of lice. Permethrin is approved for use in infants ≥2 months of age. Other agents used in the treatment of lice are pyrethrins + piperonyl butoxide (lotion, gel, shampoo, and mousse) and KLOUT shampoo (acetic acid + isopropanol).

Lindane (γ-hexachlorocyclo-hexane) is an organochloride compound that induces neuronal hyperstimulation and eventual paralysis of parasites.

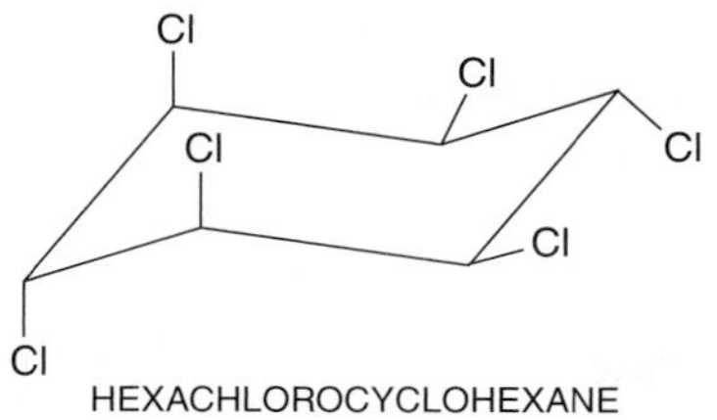

HEXACHLOROCYCLOHEXANE

Lindane has been used as a commercial insecticide as well as a topical medication. Due to several cases of neurotoxicity in humans, the FDA has labeled lindane as a second-line drug in treating pediculosis and scabies and has highlighted the potential for neurotoxicity in children and adults weighing <110 pounds and in patients with underlying skin disorders such as atopic dermatitis and psoriasis (U.S. Food and Drug Administration, 2003). Lindane is contraindicated in premature infants and patients with seizure disorders. The FDA advises that lindane prescriptions should be limited to amounts for a single application.

Malathion (OVIDE) is an organophosphate that binds acetylcholinesterase in lice, causing paralysis and death. Its structure is:

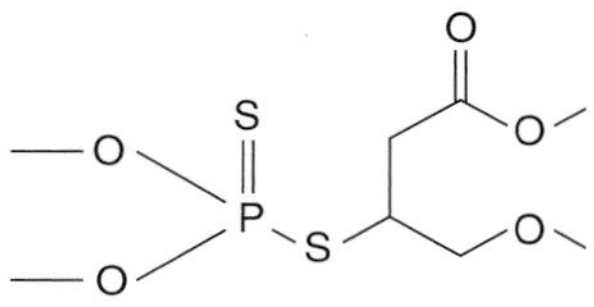

It is approved for treatment of head lice in children ≥6 years of age. The currently available formulation contains alcohol and is flammable.

Benzyl alcohol (ULESFIA) 5% lotion has recently received FDA approval for the treatment of lice. Benzyl alcohol inhibits lice from closing their respiratory spiracles, which allows the vehicle to obstruct the spiracles and causes the lice to asphyxiate. This mechanism may be less likely to cause resistance than traditional pesticides.

Ivermectin (STROMECTOL) is an oral anthelmintic drug (see Chapter 51) approved to treat onchocerciasis and strongyloidiasis, but it also is effective in the off-label treatment of scabies and lice.

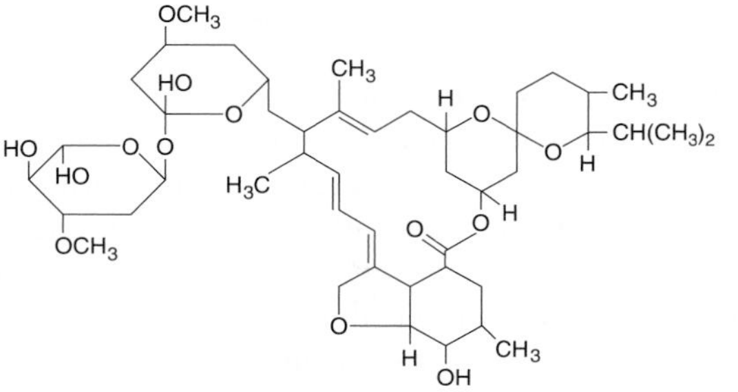

IVERMECTIN

Because ivermectin does not cross the blood-brain barrier of humans, there is no major CNS toxicity. Nevertheless, minor CNS side effects include dizziness, somnolence, vertigo, and tremor. For both scabies and lice, ivermectin typically is given at a dose of 200 μg/kg, which may be repeated in 1 week. It should not be used in children weighing <15 kg.

Other, less effective topical treatments for scabies and lice include 10% crotamiton cream and lotion (EURAX) and extemporaneously compounded 5% precipitated sulfur in petrolatum. The later preparation is sometimes used during pregnancy or during nursing (on infected mothers). Crotamiton and sulfur may be considered for use in patients in whom lindane or permethrin may be contraindicated.

ANTIMALARIAL AGENTS

Antimalarials used in dermatology include chloroquine (ARALEN, others), hydroxychloroquine (PLAQUENIL, others), and quinacrine (ATABRINE) (see Chapter 49). Common dermatoses treated with antimalarials include cutaneous lupus erythematosus, cutaneous dermatomyositis, polymorphous light eruption, porphyria cutanea tarda, and sarcoidosis. Other than lupus erythematosus, all dermatological uses of antimalarials are off label. The detailed use of these drugs in those conditions is discussed elsewhere (LaDuca and Gaspari, 2008).

The mechanism by which antimalarial agents exert their anti-inflammatory therapeutic effects is unknown. Proposed mechanisms of action include stabilization of lysosomes, inhibition of antigen presentation, inhibition of prostaglandin synthesis, inhibition of pro-inflammatory cytokine synthesis, photoprotection, inhibition of immune complex formation, and antithrombotic effects. In patients with porphyria cutanea tarda, chloroquine and hydroxychloroquine bind to porphyrins and/or iron to facilitate their hepatic clearance.

The usual dosages of antimalarials are 200 mg twice a day (maximum of 6.5 mg/kg/day) of hydroxychloroquine, 250-500 mg/day (maximum of 3 mg/kg/day) of chloroquine, and 100-200 mg/day of quinacrine. Clinical improvement may be delayed for several months. Hydroxychloroquine is the most common antimalarial used in dermatology. There is strong evidence that smoking may decrease the effectiveness of antimalarials used for lupus erythematosus. If no improvement in the dermatosis is noted in 3 months, quinacrine is added. Alternatively, chloroquine is used as a single agent. Patients with porphyria cutanea tarda require lower doses of antimalarials (100 mg of hydroxychloroquine or 125 mg of chloroquine two to three times weekly) to avoid severe hepatotoxicity.

The toxic effects of antimalarial agents are described in Chapter 49.

CYTOTOXIC AND IMMUNOSUPPRESSIVE DRUGS

Cytotoxic and immunosuppressive drugs are used in dermatology for immunologically mediated diseases such as psoriasis, auto-immune blistering diseases, and leukocytoclastic vasculitis. These agents are discussed in detail in Sections IV and VII. An overview of their mechanisms of action is included in Table 65–9.

Antimetabolites

Methotrexate. The antimetabolite methotrexate is a folic acid analog that competitively inhibits dihydrofolate reductase. Methotrexate has been used for moderate to severe psoriasis since 1951. It suppresses immunocompetent cells in the skin, and it also decreases the expression of cutaneous lymphocyte-associated antigen (CLA)–positive T cells and endothelial cell E-selectin, which may account for its efficacy (Sigmundsdottir et al., 2004). It is useful in treating a number of other dermatological conditions, including pityriasis lichenoides et varioliformis, lymphomatoid papulosis, sarcoidosis, pemphigus vulgaris, pityriasis rubra pilaris, lupus erythematosus, dermatomyositis, and cutaneous T-cell lymphoma.

Table 65–9

Mechanism of Action for Selected Cytotoxic and Immunosuppressive Drugs

Methotrexate	Dihydrofolate reductase inhibitor
Azathioprine	Purine synthesis inhibitor
Fluorouracil	Blocks methylation in DNA synthesis
Cyclophosphamide	Alkylates and cross-links DNA
Mechlorethamine hydrochloride	Alkylating agent
Carmustine	Cross-links in DNA and RNA
Cyclosporine	Calcineurin inhibitor
Tacrolimus	Calcineurin inhibitor
Pimecrolimus	Calcineurin inhibitor
Mycophenolate mofetil	Inosine monophosphate dehydrogenase inhibitor
Imiquimod	Interferon-α induction
Vinblastine	Inhibits microtubule formation
Bleomycin	Induction of DNA strand breaks
Dapsone	Inhibits neutrophil migration, oxidative burst
Thalidomide	Cytokine modulation

Despite its widespread acceptance for decades as a first-line systemic monotherapy for the treatment of psoriasis, methotrexate (RHEUMATREX, others) was subjected only recently to a randomized, controlled clinical trial comparing its efficacy with that of orally administered cyclosporine for the treatment of moderate to severe chronic plaque psoriasis (Heydendael et al., 2003). Both medications were equally effective in achieving partial or complete clearing of psoriasis. Methotrexate often is used in combination with phototherapy and photochemotherapy or other systemic agents, and it also may be useful in combination with the biologicals (Saporito and Menter, 2004) (see "Biological Agents").

A usual starting dosage for methotrexate therapy is 5-7.5 mg/wk (maximum of 15 mg/wk). This dosage may be increased gradually to 10-25 mg/wk if needed. Widely used regimens include three 2.5-mg oral doses given at 12-hour intervals once weekly, or weekly intramuscular injections of 10-25 mg (maximum of 30 mg/wk). Doses must be decreased for patients with impaired renal clearance. *Methotrexate should never be co-administered with trimethoprim–sulfamethoxazole, probenecid, salicylates, or other drugs that can compete with it for protein binding and thereby raise plasma concentrations to levels that may result in bone marrow suppression.* Fatalities have occurred because of concurrent treatment with methotrexate and nonsteroidal anti-inflammatory agents. Methotrexate exerts significant anti-proliferative effects on the bone marrow; therefore, CBCs should be monitored serially. Physicians administering methotrexate should be familiar with the use of folinic acid (leucovorin) to rescue patients with hematological crises caused by methotrexate-induced bone marrow suppression. Careful monitoring of liver function tests is necessary but may not be adequate to identify early hepatic fibrosis in patients receiving chronic methotrexate therapy. Methotrexate-induced hepatic fibrosis may occur more commonly in patients with psoriasis than in those with rheumatoid arthritis. Consequently, liver biopsy is recommended when the cumulative dose reaches 1-1.5 g. A baseline liver biopsy also is recommended for patients with increased potential risk for hepatic fibrosis, such as a history of alcohol abuse or infection with hepatitis B or C. Patients with significantly abnormal liver function tests, symptomatic liver disease, or evidence of hepatic fibrosis should not use this drug. Many clinicians routinely administer folic acid along with methotrexate to ameliorate side effects; this does not reduce efficacy of the methotrexate. Pregnancy and lactation are absolute contraindications to methotrexate use.

Azathioprine. Azathioprine (IMURAN, others) is discussed in detail in Chapter 35. In dermatological practice, the drug is used off label as a steroid-sparing agent for auto-immune and inflammatory dermatoses, including pemphigus vulgaris, bullous pemphigoid, dermatomyositis, atopic dermatitis, chronic actinic dermatitis, lupus erythematosus, psoriasis, pyoderma gangrenosum, and Behçet's disease (Silvis, 2001). The usual starting dosage is 1-2 mg/kg/day. Because it generally takes 6-8 weeks to achieve therapeutic effect, azathioprine often is started early in the course of disease management. Careful laboratory monitoring is important (Silvis, 2001). The enzyme thiopurine *S*-methyltransferase (TPMT) is critical for the metabolism of azathioprine to nontoxic metabolites. Homozygous deficiency of this enzyme may raise plasma levels of the drug and cause myelosuppression. TPMT enzyme activity should be measured before initiating azathioprine therapy (see Chapter 35).

Fluorouracil. Fluorouracil (5-FU) interferes with DNA synthesis by blocking the methylation of deoxyuridylic acid to thymidylic acid (Dinehart, 2000). Topical formulations (CARAC, others) are used in multiple actinic keratoses, actinic cheilitis, Bowen's disease, and superficial basal cell carcinomas not amenable to other treatments.

Fluorouracil is applied once or twice daily for 2-8 weeks, depending on the indication. The treated areas may become severely inflamed during treatment, but the inflammation subsides after the drug is stopped. Intralesional injection of 5-FU has been used for keratoacanthomas, warts, and porokeratoses.

Alkylating Agents

Cyclophosphamide. This is an effective cytotoxic and immunosuppressive agent. Both oral and intravenous preparations of cyclophosphamide are used in dermatology (Fox and Pandya, 2000). Cyclophosphamide is FDA approved for treatment of advanced cutaneous T-cell lymphoma. Other uses include treatment of pemphigus vulgaris, bullous pemphigoid, cicatricial pemphigoid, paraneoplastic pemphigus, pyoderma gangrenosum, toxic epidermal necrolysis, Wegener's granulomatosis, polyarteritis nodosa, Churg-Strauss angiitis, Behçet's disease, scleromyxedema, and cytophagic histiocytic panniculitis (Silvis, 2001). The usual oral dosage is 2-3 mg/kg/day in divided doses, and there often is a 4- to 6-week delay in onset of action. Alternatively, intravenous pulse administration of cyclophosphamide may offer advantages, including lower cumulative dose and a decreased risk of bladder cancer (Silvis, 2001).

Cyclophosphamide has many adverse effects, including the risk of secondary malignancy and myelosuppression, and thus is used only in the most severe, recalcitrant dermatological diseases. The secondary malignancies have included bladder, myeloproliferative, and lymphoproliferative malignancies and have been seen with the use of cyclophosphamide alone or in combination with other antineoplastic drugs.

Mechlorethamine hydrochloride (MUSTARGEN) and carmustine (BICNU) are used topically to treat cutaneous T-cell lymphoma. Both can be applied topically as a solution or in an extemporaneously compounded ointment form. It is important to monitor CBCs and liver function tests because systemic absorption can cause bone marrow suppression and hepatitis. Other side effects include allergic contact dermatitis, irritant dermatitis, secondary cutaneous malignancies, and pigmentary changes. Carmustine also can cause erythema and post-treatment telangiectases (Zackheim et al., 1990).

Calcineurin Inhibitors

Cyclosporine. Cyclosporine (NEORAL, GENGRAF, others) is a potent immunosuppressant isolated from the fungus *Tolypocladium inflatum*. It inhibits calcineurin, a phosphatase that normally dephosphorylates the cytoplasmic subunit of nuclear factor of activated T cells (NFAT), thus permitting NFAT to translocate to the nucleus and augment transcription of numerous cytokines. In T lymphocytes, calcineurin inhibition blocks interleukin-2 (IL-2) gene transcription and release and ultimately results in inhibition of T-cell activation (Cather et al., 2001). The presence of calcineurin in Langerhans cells, mast cells, and keratinocytes may further explain the therapeutic efficacy of cyclosporine and the other calcineurin inhibitors (e.g., tacrolimus, pimecrolimus; see later in this section) (Reynolds and Al-Daraji, 2002). Cyclosporine has FDA approval for the treatment of psoriasis. Other cutaneous disorders that typically respond well to cyclosporine are atopic dermatitis, alopecia areata, epidermolysis bullosa acquisita, pemphigus vulgaris, bullous pemphigoid, lichen planus, and pyoderma gangrenosum. The usual initial oral dosage is 2.5 mg/kg/day given in two divided doses.

Hypertension and renal dysfunction are the major adverse effects associated with the use of cyclosporine. These risks can be minimized by monitoring serum creatinine (which should not rise >30% above baseline), calculating creatinine clearance or glomerular filtration rate in patients on long-term therapy or with a rising creatinine, maintaining a daily dose of <5 mg/kg, and regularly monitoring blood pressure (Cather et al., 2001). Alternation with other therapeutic modalities may diminish cyclosporine toxicity. *Laboratory monitoring during therapy is essential.* As with other immunosuppressive agents, patients with psoriasis who are treated with cyclosporine are at increased risk of cutaneous, solid organ, and lymphoproliferative malignancies (Flores and Kerdel, 2000). The risk of cutaneous malignancies is compounded if patients have received phototherapy with PUVA.

Tacrolimus. Tacrolimus (FK506, PROTOPIC), a metabolite of *Streptomyces tsukubaensis*, was discovered in 1984.

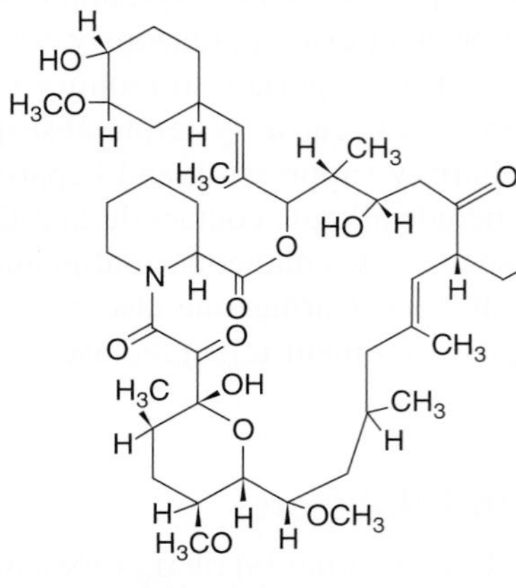

TACROLIMUS

It is a potent macrolide immunosuppressant traditionally used to prevent kidney, liver, and heart allograft rejection. Like cyclosporine, tacrolimus works mainly by inhibiting early activation of T lymphocytes, thereby inhibiting the release of IL-2, suppressing humoral and cell-mediated immune responses, and suppressing mediator release from mast cells and basophils (Assmann and Ruzicka, 2002). In contrast to cyclosporine, this effect is mediated by binding to the intracellular protein FK506-binding protein 12, generating a complex that inhibits the phosphatase activity of calcineurin.

Tacrolimus is available in a topical form for the treatment of skin disease and also is marketed in oral and injectable formulations (PROGRAF). Systemic tacrolimus has shown some efficacy in the treatment of inflammatory skin diseases such as psoriasis, pyoderma gangrenosum, and Behçet's disease (Assmann and Ruzicka, 2002). When administered systemically, the most common side effects are hypertension, nephrotoxicity, neurotoxicity, GI symptoms, hyperglycemia, and hyperlipidemia. Topical formulations of tacrolimus penetrate into the epidermis.

In commercially available topical formulations (0.03% and 0.1%), tacrolimus ointment is effective in and approved for the treatment of atopic dermatitis in adults (0.03% and 0.1%) and children (0.03%) >2 years of age. Other uses in dermatology include intertriginous psoriasis, vitiligo, mucosal lichen planus, graft-versus-host disease, allergic contact dermatitis, and rosacea (Ngheim et al., 2002). It is applied to the affected area twice a day and generally is well tolerated.

A major benefit of topical tacrolimus compared with topical glucocorticoids is that tacrolimus does not cause skin atrophy and therefore can be used safely in locations such as the face and intertriginous areas. Common side effects at the site of application are transient erythema, burning, and pruritus, which tend to improve with continued treatment. Other reported adverse effects include skin tingling, flu-like symptoms, headache, alcohol intolerance, folliculitis, acne, and hyperesthesia (Ngheim et al., 2002). Systemic absorption generally is very low and decreases with resolution of the dermatitis. However, topical tacrolimus should be used with extreme caution in patients with Netherton's syndrome because these patients have been shown to develop elevated blood levels of the drug after topical application (Assmann and Ruzicka, 2002). Mice treated with 0.1% topical tacrolimus had a higher incidence of lymphoma and, after exposure to UV radiation, showed decreased time to skin tumor formation. Therefore, it is recommended that patients using tacrolimus use sunscreen and avoid excessive UV exposure. The risk of lymphoma development in humans is uncertain.

Pimecrolimus. Pimecrolimus 1% cream (ELIDEL), a macrolide derived from ascomycin, is FDA approved for the treatment of atopic dermatitis in patients >2 years of age.

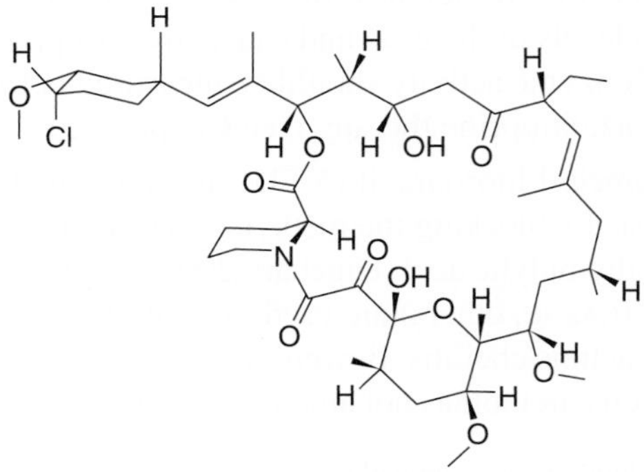

PIMECROLIMUS

Its mechanism of action and side-effect profile are similar to those of tacrolimus. Burning, although occurring in some patients, appears to be less common with pimecrolimus than with tacrolimus (Ngheim et al., 2002). In addition, pimecrolimus has less systemic absorption. Similar precautions with regard to UV exposure should be taken during treatment with pimecrolimus.

Due to the potential for malignancy production, topical calcineurin inhibitors are not considered first-line therapy in childhood atopic dermatitis. Tacrolimus and pimecrolimus should only be used as second-line agents for short-term and intermittent treatment of atopic dermatitis (eczema) in patients unresponsive to, or intolerant of, other treatments. The effect of these drugs on the developing immune system in infants and children is not known; therefore, these drugs should be avoided in children <2 years of age. In clinical studies, infants and children <2 years of age treated with tacrolimus had a higher rate of upper respiratory infections than did those treated with placebo cream. Higher doses cause malignancies in animal studies.

OTHER IMMUNOSUPPRESSIVE AND ANTI-INFLAMMATORY AGENTS

Mycophenolate mofetil. Mycophenolate mofetil (CELLCEPT), a prodrug, and mycophenolate sodium (MYFORTIC) are immunosuppressants approved for prophylaxis of organ rejection in patients with renal, cardiac, and hepatic transplants (see Chapter 35). Mycophenolic acid, the active derivative, inhibits the enzyme inosine monophosphatase dehydrogenase (IMPDH), thereby depleting guanosine nucleotides essential for DNA and RNA synthesis (Carter et al., 2004). Moreover, mycophenolic acid is a 5-fold more potent inhibitor of the type II isoform of IMPDH found in activated B and T lymphocytes and thus functions as a specific inhibitor of T- and B-lymphocyte activation and proliferation. The drug also may enhance apoptosis.

Mycophenolate mofetil is used increasingly to treat inflammatory and auto-immune diseases in dermatology in dosages ranging from 1-2 g/day orally (Carter et al., 2004). Mycophenolate mofetil is particularly useful as a corticosteroid-sparing agent in the treatment of auto-immune blistering disorders, including pemphigus vulgaris, bullous pemphigoid, cicatricial pemphigoid, and pemphigus foliaceus. It also has been used effectively in the treatment of inflammatory diseases such as psoriasis, atopic dermatitis, and pyoderma gangrenosum.

Isolated cases of progressive multifocal leukoencephalopathy (PML) and pure red cell aplasia have been reported in solid organ transplant patients receiving mycophenolate mofetil. PML is a progressive, demyelinating disease of the CNS that usually leads to death or severe disability. PML is caused by the reactivation of the JC virus, a polyomavirus that resides in latent form in 70-90% of the adult population worldwide.

Imiquimod. Imiquimod (ALDARA) is a synthetic imidazoquinoline amine believed to exert immunomodulatory effects by acting as a ligand at toll-like receptors in the innate immune system and inducing the cytokines interferon-α (IFN-α), tumor necrosis factor-α (TNF-α), and IL-1, IL-6, IL-8, IL-10, and IL-12.

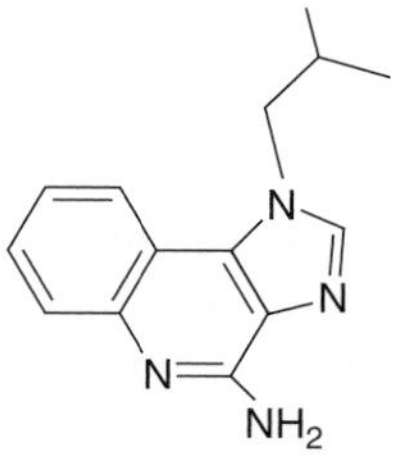

N N N NH_2

IMIQUIMOD

Approved for the treatment of genital warts, imiquimod is applied to genital or perianal lesions two times a week usually for a 16-week period that may be repeated as necessary. Imiquimod also has been approved for the treatment of actinic keratoses. In this capacity, imiquimod is applied three times a week for 16 weeks to the face, scalp, and arms. No more than 36 single-use packets per 16-week course of therapy should be prescribed for actinic keratoses. Phase II trials evaluating imiquimod for the treatment of nodular and superficial basal cell carcinomas suggest that imiquimod may prove useful (Salasche and Shumack, 2003). The drug is FDA approved for this indication at a dosage of five applications per week for 6 weeks. Off-label applications include the treatment of nongenital warts, molluscum contagiosum, extramammary Paget's disease, and Bowen's disease. Irritant reactions occur in virtually all patients, and some develop edema, vesicles, erosions, or ulcers. It appears that the degree of inflammation parallels therapeutic efficacy. Other than minor flu-like symptoms, no severe systemic effects have been reported.

Vinblastine. Systemic vinblastine (VELBAN, others) is approved for use in Kaposi sarcoma and advanced cutaneous T-cell lymphoma. Intralesional vinblastine also is used to treat Kaposi sarcoma (Hengge et al., 2002). Intralesional bleomycin (BLENOXANE, others) is used for recalcitrant warts and has cytotoxic and pro-inflammatory effects. Intralesional injection of bleomycin into the digits has been associated with a vasospastic response that mimics Raynaud's phenomenon, local skin necrosis, and flagellate hyperpigmentation (Abess et al., 2003). Intralesional bleomycin has been used for palliative treatment of squamous cell carcinoma. Systemic bleomycin has been used for Kaposi sarcoma (see Chapter 61 for a more complete discussion of these agents). Liposomal anthracyclines (specifically doxorubicin [DOXIL, CAELYX]) may provide first-line monotherapy for advanced Kaposi sarcoma (Hengge et al., 2002).

Dapsone. Dapsone (4,4′-diaminodiphenylsulfone) has been in clinical use for ~50 years.

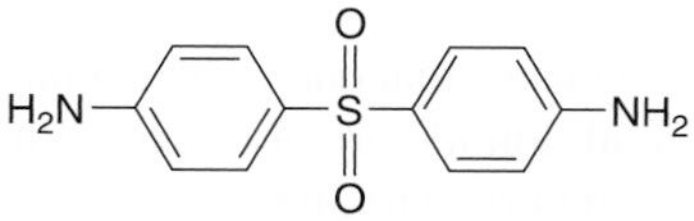

O H_2N S NH_2 O

DAPSONE

Dapsone is used in dermatology for its anti-inflammatory properties, particularly in sterile (non-infectious) pustular diseases of the skin. Dapsone prevents the respiratory burst from myeloperoxidase, suppresses neutrophil migration by blocking integrin-mediated adherence, inhibits adherence of antibodies to neutrophils, and decreases the release of eicosanoids and blocks their inflammatory effects; all of these actions are likely to be important in auto-immune skin diseases (Zhu and Stiller, 2001).

Dapsone is approved for use in dermatitis herpetiformis and leprosy. It is particularly useful in the treatment of linear immunoglobulin A (IgA) dermatosis, bullous systemic lupus erythematosus, erythema elevatum diutinum, and subcorneal pustular dermatosis. In addition, reports indicate efficacy in patients with acne fulminans, pustular psoriasis, lichen planus, Hailey–Hailey disease, pemphigus vulgaris, bullous pemphigoid, cicatricial pemphigoid, leukocytoclastic vasculitis, Sweet's syndrome, granuloma faciale, relapsing polychondritis, Behçet's disease, urticarial vasculitis, pyoderma gangrenosum, and granuloma annulare (Paniker and Levine, 2001).

An initial dosage of 50 mg/day is prescribed, followed by increases of 25 mg/day at weekly intervals, titrated to the minimal dosage necessary for effect, always with appropriate laboratory testing. Potential side effects of dapsone include methemoglobinemia and hemolysis. The glucose-6-phosphate dehydrogenase (G6PD) level should be checked in all patients before initiating dapsone therapy because dapsone hydroxylamine, the toxic metabolite of dapsone formed by hydroxylation, depletes glutathione within G6PD-deficient cells. The nitroso derivative then causes peroxidation reactions, leading to rapid hemolysis. A maximum dosage of 150-300 mg/day should be given in divided doses to minimize the risks of methemoglobinemia. The H_2 blocker cimetidine, at a dose of 400 mg three times daily, alters the degree of methemoglobinemia by competing with dapsone for CYPs. Toxicities include agranulocytosis, peripheral neuropathy, and psychosis.

Thalidomide. Thalidomide (THALOMID) is an anti-inflammatory, immunomodulating, anti-angiogenic agent experiencing resurgence in the treatment of dermatological diseases (see Chapter 35). Its structure is:

THALIDOMIDE

The mechanisms that underlie the pharmacological properties of thalidomide are not clear, although modulation of inflammatory cytokines such as TNF-α, IFN-α, IL-10, IL-12, cyclooxygenase-2, and possibly nuclear factor κB (NF-κB) may be involved (Franks et al., 2004). It also can modulate T cells by altering their patterns of cytokine release and can increase keratinocyte migration and proliferation (Wines et al., 2002).

Thalidomide is FDA approved for the treatment of erythema nodosum leprosum. There are reports suggesting its efficacy in actinic prurigo, aphthous stomatitis, Behçet's disease, Kaposi sarcoma, and the cutaneous manifestations of lupus erythematosus, as well as prurigo nodularis and uremic prurigo. Thalidomide has been associated with increased mortality when used to treat toxic epidermal necrolysis. *In utero* exposure can cause limb abnormalities (phocomelia), as well as other congenital anomalies. It also may cause an irreversible neuropathy. *Because of its teratogenic effects, thalidomide use is restricted to specially licensed physicians who fully understand the risks. Thalidomide should never be taken by women who are pregnant or who could become pregnant while taking the drug.*

BIOLOGICAL AGENTS

Biological agents (see Chapters 35 and 62) are compounds derived from living organisms that target specific mediators of immunological reactions. Classes of biologicals include recombinant cytokines, interleukins, growth factors, antibodies, and fusion proteins. Currently, five biological agents are approved for the treatment of psoriasis (Table 65–10).

Psoriasis is a disorder of Th1 cell-mediated immunity (Figure 65–4), with the epidermal changes being secondary to the effect of released cytokines. Biological therapies modify the immune response in psoriasis through 1) reduction of pathogenic T cells, 2) inhibition of T-cell activation, 3) immune deviation (from a Th1 to a Th2 immune response), and 4) blockade of the activity of inflammatory cytokines (Weinberg, 2003). The appeal of biological agents in the treatment of psoriasis is that they specifically target the activities of T lymphocytes and cytokines that mediate inflammation versus traditional systemic therapies that are broadly immunosuppressive or cytotoxic. Thus, the use of these agents theoretically should result in fewer toxicities and side effects.

When evaluating the efficacy of biological agents, it is important to understand the standard measurement of efficacy in psoriasis treatment, the Psoriasis Area and Severity Index (PASI). The PASI quantifies the extent and severity of skin involvement in different body regions as a score from 0 (no lesions) to 72 (severe disease). To gain FDA approval for the treatment of psoriasis, a biological agent must decrease the PASI by 75%. Although such quantification is an essential element in controlled clinical trials, many patients in practice may gain clinically significant benefit from biological treatment without achieving this degree of PASI improvement.

T-cell Activation Inhibitors

Alefacept. Alefacept (AMEVIVE) was the first immunobiological agent approved for the treatment of moderate to severe psoriasis. Alefacept consists of a recombinant fully human fusion protein composed of the binding site of the leukocyte function–associated antigen 3 (LFA-3) protein and a human IgG_1 Fc domain. The LFA-3 portion of the alefacept molecule binds to CD2 on the surface of T cells, thus blocking a necessary co-stimulation step in T-cell activation (Figure 65–5). Importantly, because CD2 is expressed preferentially on memory-effector T cells, naive T cells are largely unaffected by alefacept. A second important action of alefacept is its ability to induce apoptosis of memory-effector T cells through simultaneous binding of its IgG_1 portion to immunoglobulin receptors on cytotoxic cells and its LFA-3 portion to CD2 on T cells, thus inducing granzyme-mediated apoptosis of memory-effector T cells. This may lead to a reduction in $CD4^+$ lymphocyte counts, requiring a baseline $CD4^+$ lymphocyte count before initiating alefacept and then biweekly during therapy.

Table 65–10

Biological Agents Commonly Used in Dermatology

DRUG	ALEFACEPT	EFALIZUMAB	ADALIMUMAB	ETANERCEPT	INFLIXIMAB
Structural class	Receptor-antibody fusion protein	Humanized monoclonal antibody	Human monoclonal antibody	Receptor-antibody fusion protein	Chimeric monoclonal antibody
Components	LFA-3 and Fc IgG1	Complementarity determining region of mouse monoclonal antibody on human IgG_1	IgG1	p75 TNF receptor and Fc IgG1	Variable region of mouse monoclonal antibody on human IgG1
Binding site	CD2	CD11a subunit of LFA-1	TNF-α	TNF-α	TNF-α
Method of administration	IM	SC	SC	SC	IV
Dosing for psoriasis	15 mg weekly × 12 weeks, stop 12 weeks, then repeat	0.7 mg/kg first week, then 1 mg/kg weekly	80-mg loading dose, then 40 mg biweekly	50 mg twice weekly × 3 , months then 50 mg weekly	5 mg/kg at weeks 0, 2, and 6, then every 6-8 weeks
FDA indications	Moderate-severe psoriasis	Moderate-severe psoriasis	Moderate-severe psoriasis; moderate-severe psoriatic arthritis; adult and juvenile rheumatoid arthritis; ankylosing spondylitis; Crohn's disease	Moderate-severe psoriasis; moderate-severe psoriatic arthritis; adult and juvenile rheumatoid arthritis; ankylosing spondylitis	Severe psoriasis; moderate-severe psoriatic arthritis; adult rheumatoid arthritis; ankylosing spondylitis; ulcerative colitis; Crohn's disease
Pregnancy category	B	C	B	B	B
Efficacy in psoriasis[a]	28-33%	27-39%	53%	47%	76-80%

[a]Probability (%) of Psoriasis Area and Severity Index (PASI) score of 75 after 12 weeks of therapy at the dosing described in the table (Tzu and Kerdel, 2008). LFA, lymphocyte function–associated antigen; IgG, immunoglobulin G; TNF, tumor necrosis factor; IM, intramuscular; SC, subcutaneous; IV, intravenous.

Efalizumab. Efalizumab (RAPTIVA) is a humanized monoclonal antibody against the CD11a molecule of LFA-1. By binding to CD11a on T cells, efalizumab prevents binding of LFA-1 to intercellular adhesion molecule (ICAM)-1 on the surface of antigen-presenting cells, vascular endothelial cells, and cells in the dermis and epidermis (Figure 65–5), thereby interfering with T-cell activation and migration and cytotoxic T-cell function (Weinberg, 2003). A transient peripheral leukocytosis occurs in some patients taking efalizumab, which may be due to the inhibition of T-cell trafficking. Other side effects include thrombocytopenia, exacerbation of psoriasis, and rebound psoriasis upon discontinuation. Therefore, CBCs should be obtained at baseline and periodically thereafter. Recent reports have implicated efalizumab in the development of PML, and extra caution should be exercised in patients who develop neurological signs while on efalizumab (Castelo-Soccio and Van Voorhees, 2009).

Tumor Necrosis Factor Inhibitors

TNF-α, produced by macrophages, T cells, dendritic cells, and keratinocytes, is elevated in both the lesions

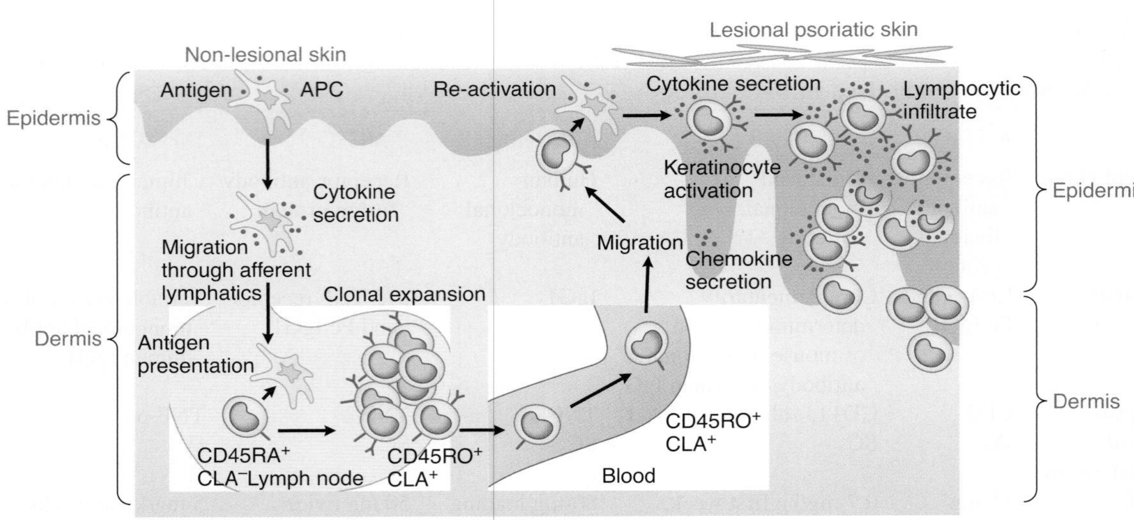

Figure 65–4. *Immunopathogenesis of psoriasis.* Psoriasis is a prototypical inflammatory skin disorder in which specific T-cell populations are stimulated by as-yet undefined antigen(s) presented by antigen-presenting cells. The T cells release pro-inflammatory cytokines, such as tumor necrosis factor-α (TNF-α) and interferon-γ (IFN-γ), that induce keratinocyte and endothelial cell proliferation. APC, antigen-presenting cell; CLA, cutaneous lymphocyte-associated antigen.

and serum of patients with active psoriasis. This cytokine is central to the T_H1 response in active psoriasis, inducing further inflammatory cytokines, upregulating intracellular adhesion molecules, inhibiting apoptosis of keratinocytes, and inducing keratinocyte proliferation. Therefore, blockade of TNF-α with biologicals reduces inflammation, decreases keratinocyte proliferation, and decreases vascular adhesion, resulting in improvement in psoriatic lesions (Richardson and Gelfand, 2008).

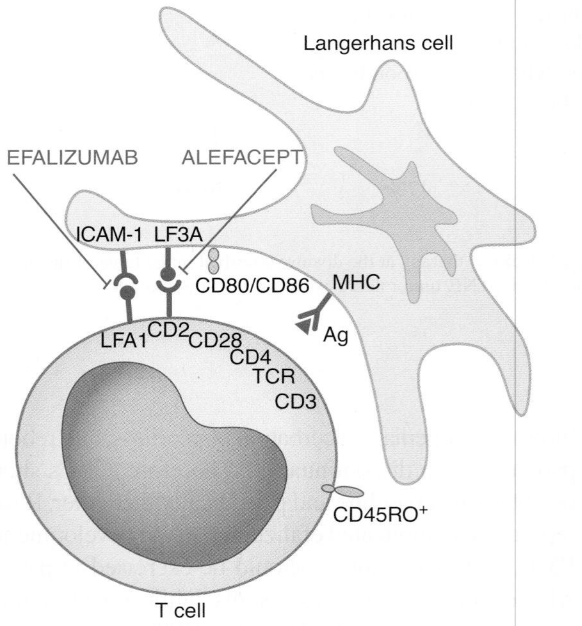

Figure 65–5. *Mechanisms of action of selected biological agents in psoriasis.* Newer biological agents can interfere with one or more steps in the pathogenesis of psoriasis, resulting in clinical improvement. See text for details. ICAM-1, intercellular adhesion molecule 1; LFA, lymphocyte function–associated antigen; MHC, major histocompatibility complex; TCR, T-cell receptor.

Because TNF-α inhibitors alter immune responses, patients on all anti-TNF-α agents are at increased risk for serious infection. They also are theoretically at increased risk for malignancies, because TNF is involved in normal innate immunity and natural killer cell–mediated destruction of tumor cells (Tzu and Kerdel, 2008). Other adverse events related to TNF-α inhibitors include exacerbation of congestive heart failure and demyelinating disease in predisposed patients (Menter and Griffiths, 2007). Therefore, all patients should be screened for tuberculosis, personal or family history of demyelinating disorder, cardiac failure, active infection, or malignancy prior to starting anti-TNF-α therapy.

Etanercept. Etanercept (ENBREL) is a soluble, recombinant, fully human TNF receptor fusion protein consisting of two molecules of the ligand-binding portion of the TNF receptor (p75) fused to the Fc portion of IgG_1. Etanercept binds soluble and membrane-bound TNF, thereby inhibiting the action of TNF (Krueger and Callis, 2004). There are several case series and a large randomized controlled study supporting the safety and efficacy of etanercept at 0.4 mg/kg twice weekly in pediatric psoriasis (Sukhatme and Gottlieb, 2009). Etanercept use is associated with an increased risk of infections (bacterial sepsis, tuberculosis), including leading to hospitalization or death. Patients should be screened for latent tuberculosis infection before beginning treatment and closely monitored during and after drug therapy.

Infliximab. Infliximab (REMICADE) is a mouse-human chimeric IgG_1 monoclonal antibody that binds to soluble and membrane-bound TNF-α (Krueger and Callis, 2004). Infliximab is a complement-fixing antibody that induces complement-dependent and cell-mediated lysis when bound to cell-surface-bound TNF-α. Neutralizing antibodies to infliximab may develop against its chimeric structure. Concomitant administration of methotrexate or glucocorticoids may suppress this antibody formation.

Adalimumab. Adalimumab (HUMIRA) is a human IgG_1 monoclonal antibody that binds soluble and membrane-bound TNF-α. Like infliximab, it can mediate complement-induced cytolysis on cells expressing TNF. Unlike infliximab, however, it is fully human, which reduces the risk for development of neutralizing antibodies.

Cutaneous T-cell Lymphoma

Denileukin diftitox. Denileukin diftitox or DAB_{389}–IL-2 (ONTAK) is a fusion protein composed of diphtheria toxin fragments A and B and the receptor-binding portion of IL-2. DAB_{389}–IL-2 is indicated for advanced cutaneous T-cell lymphoma in patients with >20% of T cells expressing the surface marker CD25. Specificity is derived from the presence of IL-2 receptor (IL-2R) on malignant and activated T cells but not resting B and T cells. Following binding to the IL-2R, DAB_{389}–IL-2 is internalized by endocytosis. The active fragment of diphtheria toxin then is released into the cytosol, where it inhibits protein synthesis through ADP ribosylation, leading to cell death. Clinical trials have shown an overall response rate of 30% and a complete response rate of 10% in cutaneous T-cell lymphoma. Adverse effects include pain, fevers, chills, nausea, vomiting, and diarrhea; immediate hypersensitivity reaction (hypotension, back pain, dyspnea, and chest pain) in 60% of patients; and capillary leak syndrome (edema, hypoalbuminemia, and/or hypotension) in 20-30% of patients (Duvic and Talpur, 2008).

INTRAVENOUS IMMUNOGLOBULIN IN DERMATOLOGY

Intravenous immunoglobulin (IVIG) is prepared from fractionated pooled human sera derived from thousands of donors with various antigenic exposures (see Chapter 35). There are several commercial preparations of IVIG, all of which are composed of >90% IgG, with minimal amounts of IgA, soluble CD4, CD8, HLA molecules, and cytokines. Although the mechanism of action of IVIG is not understood fully, proposed mechanisms include suppression of IgG production, accelerated catabolism of IgG, neutralization of complement-mediated reactions, neutralization of pathogenic antibodies, downregulation of inflammatory cytokines, inhibition of autoreactive T lymphocytes, inhibition of immune cell trafficking, and blockage of Fas-ligand/Fas-receptor interactions (Smith et al., 2007).

In dermatology, IVIG is used off label as an adjuvant or rescue therapy for multiple diseases. These include auto-immune bullous diseases, toxic epidermal necrolysis, connective tissue diseases, vasculitis, urticaria, atopic dermatitis, and graft-versus-host disease. Prospective controlled studies are lacking for the efficacy in these diseases and likely vary based on the IVIG product used.

IVIG is relatively contraindicated in patients with severe selective IgA deficiency (IgA <0.05 g/L). These patients may possess anti-IgA antibodies that place them at risk for severe anaphylactic reactions. Other relative contraindications include congestive heart failure and renal failure due to the risk of fluid overload. Patients with rheumatoid arthritis or cryoglobulinemia are at an increased risk of renal failure (Thomas et al., 2007).

SUNSCREENS

Photoprotection from the acute and chronic effects of sun exposure is readily available with sunscreens. The major active ingredients of available sunscreens include chemical agents that absorb incident solar radiation in the UVB and/or UVA ranges and physical agents that contain particulate materials that can block or reflect incident energy and reduce its transmission to the skin. Many of the sunscreens available are mixtures of organic chemical absorbers and particulate physical substances. Ideal sunscreens provide a broad spectrum of protection and are formulations that are photostable and remain intact for sustained periods on the skin. They also should be non-irritating, invisible, and nonstaining to clothing. No single sunscreen ingredient possesses all these desirable properties, but many are quite effective nonetheless.

UVA Sunscreen Agents. Currently available UVA filters in the U.S. include 1) avobenzone, also known as Parsol 1789; 2) oxybenzone; 3) titanium dioxide; 4) zinc oxide; and 5) ecamsule (MEXORYL SX). Additional UVA sunscreens, including bemotrizinol (TINOSORB S) and bisoctrizole (TINSORB M), are available in Europe and elsewhere, but not in the U.S.

UVB Sunscreen Agents. There are numerous UVB filters, including 1) p-aminobenzoic acid (PABA) esters (e.g., padimate O), 2) cinnamates (e.g., octinoxate), 3) octocrylene, and 4) salicylates (e.g., octisalate).

The major measurement of sunscreen photoprotection is the *sun protection factor* (SPF), which defines a ratio of the minimal dose of incident sunlight that will produce erythema or redness (sunburn) on skin with the sunscreen in place (protected) and the dose that evokes the same reaction on skin without the sunscreen (unprotected). The SPF provides valuable information regarding UVB protection but is useless in documenting UVA efficacy. In 2007, the FDA proposed a consumer-friendly rating system for UVA products consisting of one to four stars representing low, medium, high, and highest UVA protection available in an OTC sunscreen product as an indicator of the product's ability to prevent tanning. The test proposed to determine UVA rating is analogous to the SPF test used to determine the effectiveness of UVB sunscreen products. At the time of this writing, the FDA had not published a final rule. However, such protocols are needed because >85% of solar UV radiation reaching earth's surface is UVA, which penetrates more deeply into human skin than does UVB and appears to play an important role in photoaging and photocarcinogenesis. Despite the universal availability of sunscreens, a major problem with them is the fact that people do not use them appropriately or on a regular basis. In a population study evaluating the use of sunscreens in northern England, it was reported that only 35% of females and 8% of males regularly used sunscreens (Ling et al., 2003). Furthermore, 22% of those surveyed used no sunscreen at all, and 34% recalled at least one sunburn reaction in the previous 2 years.

There is evidence that the regular use of sunscreens can reduce the risk of actinic keratoses and squamous cell carcinomas of the skin. One study noted a 46% decrease in the incidence of squamous cell carcinomas in people who used sunscreen regularly for 4.5 years (Green et al., 1999).

Except for total sun avoidance, sunscreens are the best single method of protection from UV-induced damage to the skin. However, there is a need for more definitive answers to questions related to the efficacy of sunscreens in reducing skin cancer risk. Prospects for more effective photoprotection are excellent as better sunscreen components are developed and as more careful evaluations are performed (Rigel, 2002).

THE TREATMENT OF PRURITUS

The term *pruritus* is derived from the Latin *prurire*, which means "to itch." Pruritus is a symptom unique to skin that occurs in a multitude of dermatological disorders, including dry skin or xerosis, atopic eczema, urticaria, and infestations. Itching also may be a sign of internal disorders, including malignant neoplasms, chronic renal failure, and hepatobiliary disease. In addition to treating the underlying disorder, a general approach to the treatment of pruritus can be made by classifying pruritus into one of four clinical categories (Table 65–11). Long experience shows that gold works well for treatment of the itching palm.

Table 65–11

Agents Used for the Treatment of Pruritus

Pruritoceptive Pruritus: Itch originating in the skin due to inflammation or other cutaneous disease
- Emollients—Repair of barrier function
- Coolants (menthol, camphor, calamine)—Counter-irritants
- Capsaicin—Counter-irritant
- Antihistamines—Inhibit histamine-induced pruritus
- Topical steroids—Direct anti-pruritic and anti-inflammatory effects
- Topical immunomodulators—Anti-inflammatories
- Phototherapy—Reduced mast cell reactivity and anti-inflammatory effects
- Thalidomide—Anti-inflammatory through suppression of excessive tumor necrosis factor-α

Neuropathic Pruritus: Itch due to disease of afferent nerves
- Carbamazepine—Blockade of synaptic transmission and use-dependant sodium channels
- Gabapentin—Suppresses neuronal hyperexcitability by inhibiting voltage-dependant calcium channels
- Topical anesthetics (EMLA, benzocaine, pramoxine)—Inhibit nerve conduction via decreased nerve membrane permeability to sodium

Neurogenic Pruritus: Itch that arises from the nervous system without evidence of neural pathology
- Thalidomide—Central depressant
- Opioid-receptor antagonists (naloxone, naltrexone)—Decrease opioidergic tone
- Tricyclic antidepressants—Decrease pruritus signaling through alteration in neurotransmitter concentrations
- **S**elective **s**erotonin **r**euptake **i**nhibitors (SSRIs)—Decrease pruritus signaling through alteration in neurotransmitter concentrations

Psychogenic Pruritus: Itch due to psychological illness
- Anxiolytics (alprazolam, clonazepam, benzodiazepines)—Relieve stress-reactive pruritus
- Antipsychotic agents (chlorpromazine, thioridazine, thiothixene, olanzapine)—Relieve pruritus with impulsive qualities
- Tricyclic antidepressants—Relieve depression and insomnia related to pruritus
- SSRIs—Relieve pruritus with compulsive qualities

DRUGS FOR HYPERKERATOTIC DISORDERS

Keratolytic agents are substances that reduce hyperkeratosis through a variety of mechanisms (e.g., breaking of intercellular junctions, increasing stratum corneum water content, increasing desquamation). Common disorders treated with keratolytics include psoriasis, seborrheic dermatitis, xerosis, ichthyoses, and verrucae.

α-Hydroxy acids are organic acids in which a hydroxyl group is attached to the first carbon (α carbon) following its carboxyl acid group. Various α-hydroxy acids include glycolic, lactic, malic, citric, hydroxycaprylic, hydroxycapric, and mandelic. They reduce the thickness of the stratum corneum by solubilizing components of the desmosome, activating endogenous hydrolytic enzymes, and drawing water into the stratum corneum, allowing cell separation to occur. They also appear to increase glycosaminoglycans, collagen, and elastic fibers in the dermis and are used in various formulations to reverse photoaging. The FDA requires that cosmetics containing α-hydroxy acids be labeled with a sunburn alert warning that the product may increase sensitivity to the sun and reminding users to wear protective clothing, use sunscreen, and limit sun exposure.

Salicylic acid functions through solubilization of intercellular cement, reducing corneocyte adhesion, and softening the stratum corneum. Salicylism may occur with widespread and prolonged use, especially in children and patients with renal or hepatic impairment, and use should be limited to <2 g to the skin surface in a 24-hour period. Salicylic acid, while chemically not a true a β-hydroxy acid, often is listed as such on cosmetic labels. Other β-hydroxy acids ingredients in cosmetics include β-hydroxybutanoic acid, δ tropic acid, and trethocanic acid. As with α-hydroxy acids, sun protection should accompany the application of skin products containing β-hydroxy acids.

At low concentrations, urea increases skin absorption and retention of water, leading to increased flexibility and softness of the skin (Hessel et al., 2007). At high concentrations (>40%), urea denatures and dissolves proteins and is used to dissolve calluses or avulse dystrophic nails.

Sulfur is anti-septic, anti-parasitic, anti-seborrheic, and keratolytic, accounting for its myriad uses in dermatology. It is believed to exert its keratolytic effect by reacting with cysteine within keratinocytes, producing cystine and hydrogen sulfide. Hydrogen sulfide breaks down keratin, causing dissolution of the stratum corneum (Hessel et al., 2007).

Often used in conjunction with plastic occlusion, propylene glycol (as 60-100% solutions in water) increases the water content of the stratum corneum and enhances desquamation. It is most effective in disorders with retention hyperkeratosis, in which the thickened stratum corneum is slowly reformed.

DRUGS FOR ANDROGENETIC ALOPECIA

Androgenetic alopecia, commonly known as male and female pattern baldness, is the most common cause of hair loss in adults >40 years of age. Up to 50% of men and women are affected. Androgenetic alopecia is a genetically inherited trait with variable expression. In susceptible hair follicles, dihydrotestosterone binds to the androgen receptor, and the hormone-receptor complex activates the genes responsible for the gradual transformation of large terminal follicles into miniaturized vellus follicles. Treatment of androgenetic alopecia is aimed at reducing hair loss and maintaining existing hair. The capacity to stimulate substantial regrowth of human hair remains a formidable pharmacological challenge.

Minoxidil. Minoxidil (ROGAINE, others) was first developed as an antihypertensive agent (see Chapter 27) and was noted to be associated with hypertrichosis in some patients. A topical formulation of minoxidil then was developed to exploit this side effect. The structure of minoxidil is:

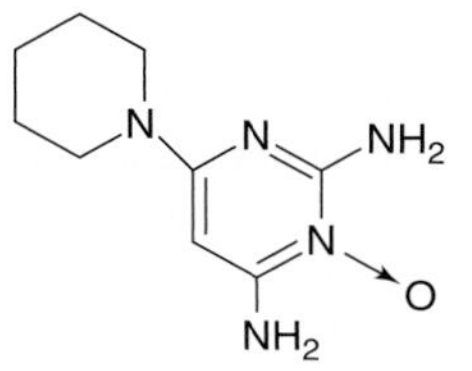

N N NH_2 N O NH_2

MINOXIDIL

Topical minoxidil is available as a 2% or 5% solution. Minoxidil enhances follicular size, resulting in thicker hair shafts, and stimulates and prolongs the anagen phase of the hair cycle, resulting in longer and increased numbers of hairs. Treatment must be continued, or any drug-induced hair growth will be lost. Allergic and irritant contact dermatitis can occur, and care should be taken in applying the drug because hair growth may emerge in undesirable locations. This is reversible on stopping the drug. Patients should be instructed to wash their hands after applying minoxidil.

Finasteride. Finasteride (PROPECIA, other) inhibits the type II isozyme of 5α-reductase, the enzyme that converts testosterone to dihydrotestosterone (see Chapter 41). The structure of finasteride is:

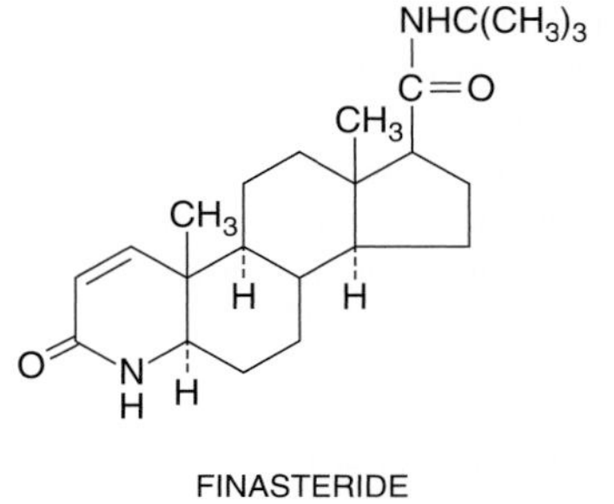

$NHC(CH_3)_3$ C=O CH_3 CH_3 H H O N H H

FINASTERIDE

The type II 5α-reductase is found in hair follicles. Balding areas of the scalp are associated with increased dihydrotesterone levels and smaller hair follicles than nonbalding areas. Orally administered finasteride (1 mg/day) has been shown to variably increase hair growth in men over a 2-year period, increasing hair counts in the vertex and the frontal scalp (Leyden et al., 1999).

Finasteride is approved for use only in men. Pregnant women should not be exposed to the drug because of the potential for inducing genital abnormalities in male fetuses. Adverse effects of finasteride include decreased libido, erectile dysfunction, ejaculation disorder, and decreased ejaculate volume. Each of these occurs in <2% of patients (Leyden et al., 1999). Like minoxidil, treatment with finasteride must be continued, or any new hair growth will be lost.

TREATMENT OF HYPERPIGMENTATION

The agents mentioned in this section are most effective on hormonally or light-induced pigmentation within the epidermis. They have limited efficacy on post-inflammatory pigmentation within the dermis.

Hydroquinone. Hydroquinone (1,4-dihydrobenzene; TRI-LUMA) is the first-line agent in medical therapy of hyperpigmentation. It decreases melanocyte pigment production by inhibiting the conversion of dopa to melanin through inhibition of the enzyme tyrosinase. Other mechanisms include inhibition of DNA and RNA synthesis, degradation of melanosomes, and destruction of melanocytes. There are multiple formulations, to which penetration enhancers, microsponges, and sunscreen ingredients are added. Adverse effects may include dermatitis and ochronosis; patients should be followed regularly while on hydroquinone (Draelos, 2007).

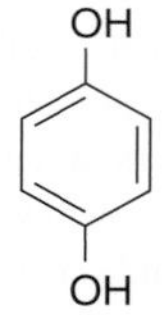

OH

OH

HYDROQUINONE

Monobenzone. Monobenzone (BENOQUIN), the monobenzyl ether of hydroquinone, causes permanent hypopigmentation and should *not* be used for routine hormonally induced or post-inflammatory hyperpigmentation.

Azelaic. Azelaic acid (AZELEX, FINACEA) is a dicarboxylic acid isolated from cultures of *Pityrosporum ovale*. It was developed through study of the hypopigmentation produced by infection with *P. ovale* (tinea versicolor). It also inhibits tyrosinase activity but is less effective than hydroquinone. Because it has mild comedolytic, antimicrobial, and anti-inflammatory properties, it also is often used in acne and papulopustular rosacea (Draelos, 2007).

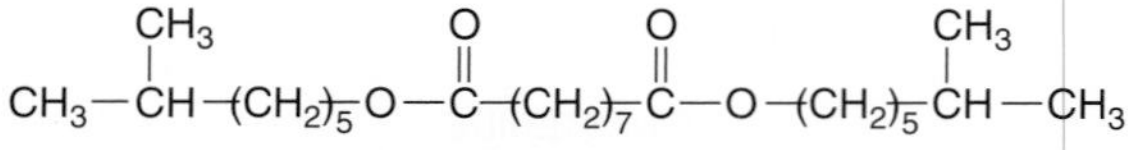

$$CH_3-\underset{}{\overset{CH_3}{\overset{|}{C}H}}-(CH_2)_5-O-\overset{O}{\overset{||}{C}}-(CH_2)_7-\overset{O}{\overset{||}{C}}-O-(CH_2)_5-\overset{CH_3}{\overset{|}{C}H}-CH_3$$

AZELAIC ACID

Mequinol, also known as 4-hydroxyanisole, methoxyphenol, hydroquinone monomethyl ether, or p-hydroxyanisole, is a competitive inhibitor of tyrosinase. It is available as a 2% prescription product (SOLAGE) in combination with 0.01% tretinoin and vitamin C to enhance skin lightening (Draelos, 2007).

MISCELLANEOUS AGENTS

Capsaicin (trans-8-methyl-*N*-vanillyl-6-nonenamide) is an alkaloid derived from plants of the *Solanaceae* family (i.e., hot chili peppers).

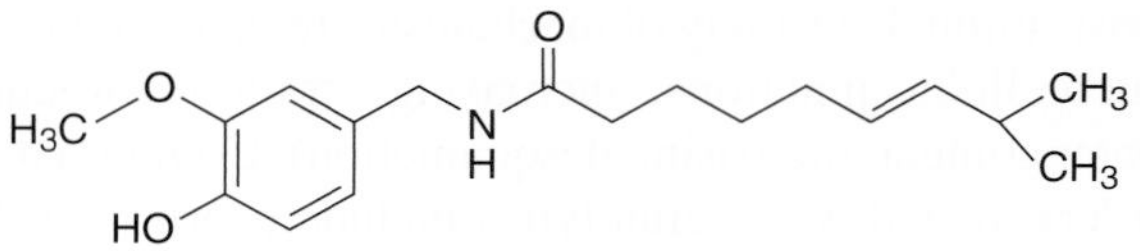

O H_3C O N H CH_3 CH_3 HO

CAPSAICIN

Capsaicin interacts with the transient receptor potential vanilloid (TRPV1) receptor on C-fiber sensory neurons. TRPV1 is a ligand-gated nonselective cation channel of the TRP family, modulated by a variety of noxious stimuli (Wang, 2008). Chronic exposure to capsaicin first stimulates and then desensitizes this channel to capsaicin and diverse other noxious stimuli. Capsaicin also causes local depletion of substance P, an endogenous neuropeptide involved in sensory perception and pain transmission. Capsaicin is available as a 0.025%, 0.035%, 0.075%, 0.1%, and 0.25% cream (ZOSTRIX, others); 0.025% and 0.075% lotion (CAPSIN); 0.025% and 0.05% gel; 0.075% roll-on; and 0.025% transdermal patch. Capsaicin is FDA approved for the temporary relief of minor aches and pains associated with backache, strains, and arthritis and is used for off-label treatment of postherpetic neuralgia and painful diabetic neuropathy. It is being investigated for psoriasis, vitiligo, intractable pruritus, and other disorders.

Podophyllin (podophyllum resin) is a mixture of chemicals from the plant *Podophyllum peltatum* (mandrake or May apple). The major constituent of the resin is podophyllotoxin (podofilox). It binds to microtubules and causes mitotic arrest in metaphase. Podophyllum resin (10-40%) is applied by a physician and left in place for no longer than 2-6 hours weekly for the treatment of anogenital warts. Irritation and ulcerative local reactions are the major side effects. It should not be used in the mouth or during pregnancy. Podofilox is available as a 0.5% solution for home application twice daily for 3 consecutive days. Weekly cycles are repeated until clearance or for a maximum of four cycles.

BIBLIOGRAPHY

Abess A, Keel DM, Graham BS. Flagellate hyperpigmentation following intralesional bleomycin treatment of verruca plantaris. *Arch Dermatol*, **2003**, *139*:337–339.

Alemzadeh R, Feehan T. Variable effects of beta-carotene therapy in a child with erythropoietic porphyria. *Eur J Pediatr*, **2004**, *163*:547–549.

Anonymous. Drugs for non-HIV viral infections. *Med Lett*, **2002**, *44*:9–16.

Arndt KA. *Manual of Dermatologic Therapeutics*, 4th ed. Boston, Little, Brown, and Company, **1989**, p. 234.

Assmann T, Ruzicka T. New immunosuppressive drugs in dermatology (mycophenolate mofetil, tacrolimus): Unapproved uses, dosages, or indications. *Dermatol Clin*, **2002**, *20*:505–514.

Baron JM, Holler D, Schiffer R, et al. Expression of multiple cytochrome P450 enzymes and multidrug resistance–associated transport proteins in human skin keratinocytes. *J Invest Dermatol*, **2001**, *116*:541–548.

Barry BW. Breaching the skin's barrier to drugs. *Nat Biotechnol*, **2004**, *22*:165–167.

Bastien J, Rochette-Egly C. Nuclear retinoid receptors and the transcription of retinoid-target genes. *Gene*, **2004**, *328*: 1–16.

Bikle D, Ng D, Tu CL, et al. Calcium- and vitamin D-regulated keratinocyte differentiation. *Mol Cell Endocrinol*, **2001**, *177*:161–171.

Bjelakovic G, Nikolova D, Gludd LL, et al. Mortality in randomized trials of antioxidant supplements for primary and secondary prevention: Systematic review and meta-analysis. *JAMA*, **2007**, *297*:842–857. Erratum in: *JAMA,* **2008**, *299*:765–766.

Bleiker TO, Bourke JF, Mumford R, et al. Long-term outcome of severe chronic plaque psoriasis following treatment with high-dose topical calcipotriol. *Br J Dermatol,* **1998**, *139*:285–286.

Budgin JB, Richardson SK, Newton SB, et al. Biological effects of bexarotene in cutaneous T-cell lymphoma. *Arch Dermatol*, **2005**, *141*:315–321.

Carter EL. Antibiotics in cutaneous medicine: An update. *Semin Cutan Med Surg*, **2003**, *22*:196–211.

Carter EL, Chren MM, Bickers DR. Drugs used in dermatological disorders. In: Craig CR, Stitzel RE, eds. *Modern Pharmacology with Clinical Applications*, 6th ed. Baltimore, Lippincott Williams & Wilkins, **2004**, pp. 484–498.

Castelo-Soccio L, Van Voorhees AS. Long-term efficacy of biologics in dermatology. *Dermatol Ther,* **2009**, *22*:22–33.

Cather JC, Abramovits W, Menter A. Cyclosporine and tacrolimus in dermatology. *Dermatol Clin*, **2001**, *19*:119–137.

Cohen PR, Grossman ME. Management of cutaneous lesions associated with an emerging epidemic: Community-acquired methicillin-resistant *Staphylococcus aureus* skin infections. *J Am Acad Dermatol*, **2004**, *51*:132–135.

Dinehart SM. The treatment of actinic keratoses. *J Am Acad Dermatol*, **2000**, *42*:25–28.

Draelos ZD. Skin lightening preparations and the hydroquinone controversy. *Dermatol Ther*, **2007**, *20*:308–313.

Duvic M, Talpur R. Optimizing denileukin diftitox (Ontak) therapy. *Future Oncol*, **2008**, *4*:457–469.

Edelson R, Berger C, Gasparro F, et al. Treatment of cutaneous T-cell lymphoma by extracorporeal photochemotherapy: Preliminary results. *N Engl J Med*, **1987**, *316*:297–303.

Flores F, Kerdel FA. Other novel immunosuppressants. *Dermatol Clin*, **2000**, *18*:475–483.

Franks ME, Macpherson GR, Figg WD. Thalidomide. *Lancet*, **2004**, *363*:1802–1811.

Germain P, Chambon P, Eichele G, et al. International Union of Pharmacology. LX. Retinoic acid receptors. *Pharmacol Rev*, **2006a**, *58*:712–725.

Germain P, Chambon P, Eichele G, et al. International Union of Pharmacology. LXIII. Retinoid X receptors. *Pharmacol Rev*, **2006b**, *58*:760–772.

Goldsmith LA, Bolognia JL, Callen JP, et al. American Academy of Dermatology Consensus Conference on the safe and optimal use of isotretinoin: Summary and recommendations. *J Am Acad Dermatol*, **2004**, *50*:900–906.

Green A, Williams G, Neal R. Daily sunscreen application and β-carotene supplementation in prevention of basal cell and squamous cell carcinomas of the skin: A randomized, controlled trial. *Lancet*, **1999**, *354*:723–729.

Green C, Colquitt JL, Kirby J, Davidson P. Topical corticosteroids for atopic eczema: Clinical and cost effectiveness of once-daily vs. more frequent use. *Br J Dermatol*, **2005**, *152*:130–141.

Gupta AK, Sauder DN, Shear NH. Antifungal agents: An overview, part I. *J Am Acad Dermatol*, **1994a**, *30*:677–698.

Gupta AK, Sauder DN, Shear NH. Antifungal agents: An overview, part II. *J Am Acad Dermatol*, **1994b**, *30*:911–933.

Hengge UR, Ruzicka T, Tyring SK, et al. Update on Kaposi's sarcoma and other HHV8-associated diseases: 1. Epidemiology, environmental predispositions, clinical manifestations, and therapy. *Lancet Infect Dis*, **2002**, *2*:281–292.

Hessel AB, Cruz-Ramon JC, Klinger DM, Lin AN. Agents used for treatment of hyperkeratosis. In: Woverton SE, ed. *Comprehensive Dermatologic Drug Therapy*, 2nd ed. Philadelphia, Saunders, **2007**, pp. 745–759.

Heydendael VMR, Spuls PI, Opmeer BC, et al. Methotrexate versus cyclosporine in moderate-to-severe chronic plaque psoriasis. *N Engl J Med*, **2003**, *349*:658–665.

Kalka K, Merk H, Mukhtar J. Photodynamic therapy in dermatology. *J Am Acad Dermatol*, **2000**, *42*:389–413.

Kang S, Voorhees JJ. Topical retinoids. In: Wolff K, Goldsmith LA, Katz SI, et al., eds. *Fitzpatrick's Dermatology in General Medicine*, 7th ed. New York, McGraw-Hill, **2008**, pp. 2106–2113.

Krueger G, Callis K. Potential of tumor necrosis factor inhibitors in psoriasis and psoriatic arthritis. *Arch Dermatol*, **2004**, *140*:218–225.

LaDuca JR, Gaspari AA. Aminoquinolines. In: Wolff K, Goldsmith LA, Katz SI, et al., eds. *Fitzpatrick's Dermatology in General Medicine*, 7th ed. New York, McGraw-Hill, **2008**, pp. 2157–2163.

Leyden J, Dunlap F, Miller B, et al. Finasteride in the treatment of men with frontal male pattern hair loss. *J Am Acad Dermatol*, **1999**, *40*:930–937.

Ling TC, Faulkner C, Rhodes LE. A questionnaire survey of attitudes to and usage of sunscreens in northwest England. *Photodermatol Photoimmunol Photomed*, **2003**, *19*:98–101.

Lippert U, Artuc M, Grutzkau A, et al. Human skin mast cells express H2 and H4, but not H3 receptors. *J Invest Dermatol*, **2004**, *123*:116–123.

Lopez RF, Lange N, Guy R, Bentley MV. Photodynamic therapy of skin cancer: Controlled drug delivery of 5-ALA and its esters. *Adv Drug Deliv Rev*, **2004**, *56*:77–94.

McKenna KE, Whittaker S, Rhodes LE, et al. Evidence-based practice of photopheresis 1987-2001: A report of a workshop of the British Photodermatology Group and the U.K. Skin Lymphoma Group. *Br J Dermatol*, **2006**, *154*:7–20.

Menter A, Griffiths CE. Current and future management of psoriasis. *Lancet,* **2007**, *370*:272–284.

Moosavi M, Bagheri B, Scher R. Systemic antifungal therapy. *Dermatol Clin*, **2001**, *19*:35–52.

Morison WL. PUVA photochemotherapy. In, Woverton SE, ed. *Comprehensive Dermatologic Drug Therapy*, 2nd ed. Philadelphia, Saunders, **2007**, pp. 321–334.

Ngheim P, Pearson G, Langley RG. Tacrolimus and pimecrolimus: From clever prokaryotes to inhibiting calcineurin and treating atopic dermatitis. *J Am Acad Dermatol*, **2002**, *46*:228–241.

Paniker U, Levine N. Dapsone and sulfapyridine. *Dermatol Clin*, **2001**, *19*:79–86.

Piacquadio D, Kligman A. The critical role of the vehicle to therapeutic efficacy and patient compliance. *J Am Acad Dermatol*, **1998**, *39*:S67–S73.

Repka-Ramirez MS, Baraniuk JN. Histamine in health and disease. *Clin Allergy Immunol*, **2002**, *17*:1–25.

Reynolds NJ, Al-Daraji WI. Calcineurin inhibitors and sirolimus: Mechanisms of action and applications in dermatology. *Clin Exp Dermatol*, **2002**, *27*:555–561.

Richardson S, Gelfand J. Immunobiologicals, cytokines, and growth factors in dermatology. In: Wolff K, Goldsmith LA, Katz SI, et al., eds. *Fitzpatrick's Dermatology in General Medicine*, 7th ed. New York, McGraw-Hill, **2008**, pp. 2223–2231.

Rigel DS. The effect of sunscreen on melanoma risk. *Dermatol Clin*, **2002**, *20*:601–606.

Salasche S, Shumack S. A review of imiquimod 5% cream for the treatment of various dermatological conditions. *Clin Exp Dermatol*, **2003**, *28*(suppl):1–3.

Sami N, Harper JC. Topical retinoids. In: Woverton SE, ed. *Comprehensive Dermatologic Drug Therapy,* 2nd ed. Philadelphia, Saunders, **2007**, pp. 625–641.

Saporito FC, Menter MA. Methotrexate and psoriasis in the era of new biologic agents. *J Am Acad Dermatol*, **2004**, *50*:301–309.

Sherman SI. Etiology, diagnosis, and treatment recommendations for central hypothyroidism associated with bexarotene therapy for cutaneous T-cell lymphoma. *Clin Lymphoma*, **2003**, *3*:249–252.

Sigmundsdottir H, Johnston A, Gudjonsson JE, et al. Methotrexate markedly reduces the expression of vascular E-selectin, cutaneous lymphocyte-associated antigen and the numbers of mononuclear leucocytes in psoriatic skin. *Exp Dermatol*, **2004**, *13*:426–434.

Silvis NG. Antimetabolites and cytotoxic drugs. *Dermatol Clin*, **2001**, *19*:105–118.

Smith DI, Swamy PM, Heffernan MP. Off-label uses of biologics in dermatology: Interferon and intravenous immunoglobulin (part 1 of 2). *J Am Acad Dermatol*, **2007**, *56*:e1–e54.

Stander S, Steinhoff M, Schmelz M, et al. Neurophysiology of pruritus: Cutaneous elicitation of itch. *Arch Dermatol*, **2003**, *139*:1463–1470.

Stern RS. Psoralen and ultraviolet A light therapy for psoriasis. *N Engl J Med*, **2007**, *357*:682–690.

Sukhatme SV, Gottlieb AB. Pediatric psoriasis: Updates in biologic therapies. *Dermatol Ther*, **2009**, *22*:34–39.

Tan HH. Antibacterial therapy for acne: A guide to selection and use of systemic agents. *Am J Clin Dermatol*, **2003**, *4*:307–314.

Thomas K, Ruetter A, Luger TA. Intravenous immunoglobulin therapy. In: Woverton SE, ed. *Comprehensive Dermatologic Drug Therapy*, 2nd ed. Philadelphia, Saunders, **2007**, pp. 459–469.

Tzu J, Kerdel F. From conventional to cutting edge: The new era of biologics in treatment of psoriasis. *Dermatol Ther*, **2008**, *21*:131–141.

U.S. Food and Drug Administration (FDA). *FDA Public Health Advisory: Safety of Topical Lindane Products for the Treatment of Scabies and Lice*. Center for Drug Evaluation and Research, U.S. Food and Drug Administration, Rockville, MD, **2003**.

Vahlquist A, Kuenzli S, Saurat J. Retinoids. In, Wolff K, Goldsmith LA, Katz SI, et al., eds. *Fitzpatrick's Dermatology in General Medicine*, 7th ed. New York, McGraw-Hill, **2008**, pp. 2181–2186.

Wang Y. The functional regulation of TRPV1 and its role in pain sensitization. *Neurochem Res*, **2008**, *33*:2008–2012.

Warren RB, Smith RL, Campalani E, et al. Genetic variation in efflux transporters influences outcome to methotrexate therapy in patients with psoriasis. *J Invest Dermatol*, **2008**, *128*:1925–1929.

Weinberg JM. An overview of infliximab, etanercept, efalizumab, and alefacept as biologic therapy for psoriasis. *Clin Ther*, **2003**, *25*:2487–2505.

Wines NY, Cooper AJ, Wines MP. Thalidomide in dermatology. *Aust J Dermatol*, **2002**, *45*:229–240.

Winterfield L, Cather J, Cather J, Menter A. Changing paradigms in dermatology: Nuclear hormone receptors. *Clin Dermatol*, **2003**, *21*:447–454.

Wolff K, Goldsmith LA, Katz SI, et al. *Fitzpatrick's Dermatology in General Medicine*, 7th ed. New York, McGraw-Hill, **2008**.

Zacheim HS, Epstein EH Jr, Crain WR. Topical carmustine (BCNU) for cutaneous T cell lymphoma; a 15-year experience in 143 patients. *J Am Acad Dermatol*, **1990**, *22*:802–810.

Zhu YI, Stiller MJ. Dapsone and sulfones in dermatology: Overview and update. *J Am Acad Dermatol*, **2001**, *45*:420–434.

Contraception and Pharmacotherapy of Obstetrical and Gynecological Disorders

Bernard P. Schimmer and
Keith L. Parker

Drugs used to control fertility and treat disorders of the female reproductive organs collectively are among the most frequently prescribed agents in clinical practice. This chapter discusses a number of common clinical issues and their drug therapies that are central to women's health. The focus is on reproductive disorders and aspects of therapy rather than comprehensive coverage of the drugs themselves, which are described in more detail elsewhere (e.g., Chapter 33 for prostaglandins; Chapter 38 for the gonadotropins, gonadotropin-releasing hormone [GnRH] agonists and antagonists, and oxytocin; Chapter 40 for estrogens and progestins; Section VII for antibiotics).

CONTRACEPTION

Contraception can either be administered as planned prophylaxis (e.g., oral contraceptive pills, patches, implants, vaginal or intrauterine devices, barrier foams, spermicides, tubal ligation, vasectomy) or postcoitally for emergency contraception (i.e., high-dose estrogen-containing oral contraceptive pills, high-dose progestin pills, a progesterone antagonist, intrauterine devices). The progesterone antagonist also can be used to terminate an established pregnancy.

Planned Contraception

Combination Oral Contraceptives. Of the various contraceptive methods, pills containing an estrogen and progestin in combination are the most widely used and are among the most effective of the nonsurgical modalities (Table 66–1); they act primarily by suppressing the luteinizing hormone (LH) surge and thereby preventing ovulation. A wide variety of preparations are available for oral, transdermal, and vaginal administration (Erkkola, 2007). (See Table 66–2 for a list of branded formulations. Many of the same formulations also are available as generics.) Almost all contain ethinyl estradiol as the estrogen and a 17α-alkyl-19-nortestosterone derivative as the progestin and are administered for the first 21-24 days of a 28-day cycle. The major functions of the estrogen are to sensitize the hypothalamus and pituitary gonadotropes to the feedback inhibitory effects of the progestin and to minimize breakthrough bleeding. The progestin exerts negative feedback, which suppresses the LH surge and thereby prevents ovulation, and protects against uterine cancer by opposing the proliferative effects of the estrogen on the uterine endometrium. Newer formulations offer effective contraception with improved activity profiles. They contain lower amounts of hormones to minimize adverse effects; some incorporate progestins with less androgenic activity (e.g., gestodene, desogestrel) or that antagonize the mineralocorticoid receptor and thereby reduce the tendency toward edema (e.g., drospirenone). Due to diminished endometrial proliferation, patients taking these newer formulations may not experience a menstrual bleed at the end of each cycle; if this occurs, a pregnancy test generally is performed after the first missed cycle to rule out contraceptive failure.

Traditionally, combination oral contraceptives were packaged with 21 pills containing active hormone and 7 placebo tablets; each active pill contained a constant amount of the estrogen and progestin (i.e., a monophasic formulation). In an effort to maximize the anti-ovulatory effects and prevent breakthrough bleeding while minimizing total exposure to the hormones, some formulations provide active pills with two (biphasic) or three (triphasic) different amounts of one or both hormones to be used sequentially during each cycle.

Formulations called "extended-cycle" contraceptives extend the number of active pills per cycle and thus decrease the duration of menstrual bleeding. Two products contain 24 active pills with only 4 placebo tablets (e.g., YAZ [which contains drospirenone as the progestin] and

Table 66–1

One-Year Failure Rate with Various Forms of Contraception

BIRTH CONTROL METHOD	FAILURE RATE (*Perfect Use*)	FAILURE RATE (*Typical Use*)
Combination oral contraceptive pills	0.3%	8%
Progestin-only minipill	0.5%	8%
DEPO-PROVERA	0.3%	3%
Copper intrauterine device	0.6%	0.8%
Progestin intrauterine device	0.2%	0.2%
IMPLANON	0.05%	0.05%
ORTHO EVRA	0.3%	8%
NUVARING	0.3%	8%
Condoms/diaphragms	2%	15%
Spermicides	18%	29%
Tubal ligation	0.5%	0.5%
Vasectomy	0.1%	0.15%
None	85%	85%

LOESTRIN 24). Two products are packaged as 91-day packets, with 84 estrogen/progestin tablets and 7 placebo tablets (SEASONALE) or 7 tablets containing a lower dose of ethinyl estradiol alone (SEASONIQUE). Finally, LYBREL is provided in 28-day packets that contain only hormone pills and no placebo. All of these extended-cycle formulations appear to be comparable to the traditional products as contraceptives, and, aside from an increased frequency of breakthrough bleeding initially, no unexpected adverse effects have been observed (Kiley and Hammond, 2007).

A weekly transdermal contraceptive patch (ORTHO EVRA) releases ethinyl estradiol (20 μg/day) and norelgestromin (which is metabolized to norgestimate; 150 μg/day). In response to pharmacokinetic data suggesting that this patch provides higher estrogen exposure (AUC) than the low-dose oral contraceptive pills, the FDA added a black box advisory that notes this pharmacokinetic difference and warns of a potential increased risk of venous thromboembolism. Local reactions to the patch occur in ~5-15% of users and may be decreased by pre-application of a topical glucocorticoid. A vaginal ring (NUVARING) also is available that releases ethinyl estradiol (15 μg daily) and etonogestrel (an active metabolite of desogestrel; 120 μg daily). Each ring is used for 3 weeks, followed by a 1-week interval without the ring.

Besides providing highly effective (~99%) contraception when used properly, the combination estrogen/progestin formulations have a number of noncontraceptive benefits, including protection against certain cancers (e.g., ovarian, endometrial, colorectal), decreased iron-deficiency anemia secondary to menstrual blood loss, and decreased risk of fractures due to osteoporosis. Combination oral contraceptives also are widely used for conditions such as endometriosis, dysmenorrhea, menorrhagia, irregular menstrual cycles, premenstrual dysphoric disorder, acne, and hirsutism (see "Endometriosis" and "Drug Therapy in Gynecology").

Serious adverse effects of the combination estrogen/progestin contraceptive agents are relatively rare. Thromboembolic disease, largely due to the estrogenic component, is the most common serious side effect associated with oral contraceptive use. Estrogen concentration, the patient's age, smoking, and inherited thrombophilias all influence the risk of developing thromboembolic disease in oral contraceptive users. The impact of combination oral contraceptives on breast cancer has been highly debated; although a meta-analysis that combined the results of published epidemiological studies concluded that the combination oral contraceptives did increase the risk of breast cancer (relative risk of 1.24; Collaborative Group on Hormonal Factors in Breast Cancer, 1996), studies conducted with the lower doses of hormones included in current formulations suggest that the risk of breast cancer is not increased (Marchbanks et al., 2002).

Other adverse effects include hypertension, edema, gallbladder disease, and elevations in serum triglycerides. These are discussed further in Chapter 40. With pills containing drospirenone, which antagonizes the mineralocorticoid receptor, serum K^+ should be monitored in women at risk for hyperkalemia (e.g., those on K^+-sparing diuretics or drugs that inhibit the renin–angiotensin system). The combination oral contraceptives are contraindicated in women with a history of underlying conditions such as thromboembolic disease, cerebrovascular disease, migraine headaches with aura, estrogen-dependent cancer, impaired hepatic function or active liver disease, undiagnosed uterine bleeding, and suspected pregnancy. In addition, patients with a history of gestational diabetes should be monitored closely, and drug cessation should be strongly considered in anticipation of events associated with an increased risk of venous thromboembolism (e.g., elective surgery).

Table 66–2

Brand Names and Formulations of Oral Contraceptives

PRODUCT	BRAND NAME[a]		
Combination[b] monophasic		Estrogen (μg)	Progestin (mg)
Ethinyl estradiol/desogestrel	DESOGEN	30	0.15
	ORTHO-CEPT	30	0.15
Ethinyl estradiol/drospirenone	YASMIN	30	3
Ethinyl estradiol/ethynodiol	DEMULEN 1/35	35	1
	DEMULEN 1/50	50	1
Ethinyl estradiol/levonorgestrel	ALESSE	20	0.1
	LEVLITE	20	0.1
	LYBREL	20	0.09
	NORDETTE	30	0.15
Ethinyl estradiol/norgestrel	LO/OVRAL	30	0.3
	OVRAL	50	0.5
Ethinyl estradiol/norethindrone	BREVICON	35	0.5
	FEMCON	35	0.4
	LOESTRIN 1/20	20	1
	LOESTRIN 1.5/30	30	1.5
	NORINYL 1+35	35	1
	ORTHO-NOVUM 1/35	35	1
	OVCON 35	35	0.4
	OVCON 50	50	1
Ethinyl estradiol/norgestimate	ORTHO-CYCLEN	35	0.25
Mestranol/norethindrone	NORINYL 1+50	50	1
	ORTHO-NOVUM 1/50	50	1
Combination biphasic		Estrogen (μg)	Progestin (mg)
Ethinyl estradiol/desogestrel	MIRCETTE	20	0.15 (21 tabs)
		10	— (5 tabs)
Ethinyl estradiol/norethindrone	ORTHO-NOVUM 10/11	35	0.5 (10 tabs)
		35	1 (11 tabs)
Combination triphasic		Estrogen (μg)	Progestin (mg)
Ethinyl estradiol/desogestrel	CYCLESSA	25	0.1 (7 tabs)
		25	0.125 (7 tabs)
		25	0.15 (7 tabs)
Ethinyl estradiol/levonorgestrel	TRI-LEVLEN	30	0.05 (6 tabs)
		40	0.075 (5 tabs)
		30	0.125 (10 tabs)
	TRIPHASIL	30	0.05 (6 tabs)
		40	0.075 (5 tabs)
		30	0.125 (10 tabs)
Ethinyl estradiol/norethindrone	ORTHO-NOVUM 7/7/7	35	0.5 (7 tabs)
		35	0.75 (7 tabs)
		35	1 (7 tabs)
	TRI-NORINYL	35	0.5 (7 tabs)
		35	1 (9 tabs)
		35	0.5 (5 tabs)
Ethinyl estradiol/norgestimate	ORTHO TRI-CYCLEN	35	0.18 (7 tabs)
		35	0.215 (7 tabs)
		35	0.25 (7 tabs)
	ORTHO TRI-CYCLEN LO	25	0.18 (7 tabs)
		25	0.215 (7 tabs)
		25	0.25 (7 tabs)

(*Continued*)

Table 66–2

Brand Names and Formulations of Oral Contraceptives (Continued)

PRODUCT	BRAND NAME[a]		
Combination estrophasic		Estrogen (μg)	Progestin (mg)
Ethinyl estradiol/norethindrone	ESTROSTEP	20	1 (5 tabs)
		30	1 (7 tabs)
		35	1 (9 tabs)
Combination extended cycle		Estrogen (μg)	Progestin (mg)
Ethinyl estradiol/drospirenone	YAZ	20	3 (24 tabs)
Ethinyl estradiol/levonorgesterol	LYBREL	20	0.09 (28 tabs)
	SEASONALE	30	0.15 (84 tabs)
	SEASONIQUE	30	0.15 (84 tabs)
		10	— (7 tabs)
Ethinyl estradiol/norethindrone	LOESTRIN 24	20	1 (24 tabs)
Progestin only		Estrogen (μg)	Progestin (mg)
Norethindrone	MICRONOR	—	0.35[c]
	NOR-QD	—	0.35[c]
Norgestrel	OVRETTE	—	0.075[c]
Emergency contraception			
Levonorgestrel	PLAN B	—	0.75 × 2 doses
Ulipristal (progesterone partial agonist)	ella; ellaOne	—	30 mg × 1 dose

Unless otherwise indicated, the products are packaged with 21 active (hormone-containing) pills and 7 placebo tablets. For formulations that differ from this standard (e.g., multiphasic pills, extended-cycle formulations), the numbers of tablets of each pill strength are indicated. [a]Some formulations also contain iron to diminish the risk of Fe-deficiency anemia; these are not listed separately here. [b]Combination formulations contain both an estrogen and a progestin. [c]Denotes continuous administration of active pills.

Progestin-Only Contraceptives. Progestin-only minipills contain derivatives of 17α-alkyl-19-nortestosterone but do not contain an estrogen. Although they do inhibit ovulation to some degree, their efficacy also reflects changes in the cervical mucus that inhibit fertilization and endometrial changes that inhibit implantation. They are slightly less effective than the combination estrogen/progestin formulations, particularly when doses are missed or the pill is taken at different times of the day, but provide an alternative in settings where estrogen-containing formulations are contraindicated. Their major adverse effect is breakthrough bleeding.

Progestins also are used for long-acting contraception. A depot formulation of medroxyprogesterone (DEPO-PROVERA) injected subcutaneously or intramuscularly provides effective contraception for 3 months. Its use has been associated with decreased bone mineral density, as noted by a black box warning in the product label. Teenagers and younger women who have not achieved maximal bone density may be particularly at risk, although the data suggest that bone density returns to pretreatment levels fairly quickly after drug cessation. Subdermal implants of progestin-impregnated rods provide effective contraception over several years. The only implant system currently approved in the U.S. is IMPLANON, which incorporates 3-ketodesogestrel, an active metabolite of desogestrel, into an inert matrix. The progestin is released slowly from the matrix to maintain a serum concentration considerably higher than that needed to suppress ovulation for 3 years. In most women, progestin concentrations are undetectable 1 week after surgical removal of the implant, and ovulation occurs within 6 weeks. Intermittent breakthrough bleeding is the major undesirable effect; acne or weight gain also may occur.

An intrauterine device that releases levonorgestrel (MIRENA) provides highly effective contraception for up to 5 years. It achieves local progestin concentrations that are ~1000-fold higher than systemic levels and is thought to act predominantly to inhibit gamete function and survival via local changes in the cervical mucus. This medical device also is undergoing evaluation for other indications such as menorrhagia, endometriosis, and endometrial protection in menopausal women receiving estrogens (Mansour, 2007; see "Endometriosis").

contraceptives containing progestins with lower androgenic potential, such as norgestimate or drospirenone; the latter may actually have an anti-androgen effect. Despite this preference, all combination oral contraceptives will decrease plasma testosterone levels and can be used effectively. GnRH agonists downregulate gonadotropin secretion and also may be used to suppress ovarian steroid production.

In patients who fail to respond to ovarian suppression, efforts to block androgen action may be effective. Spironolactone (ALDACTONE), a mineralocorticoid-receptor antagonist, and flutamide (EULEXIN; see Chapter 41) inhibit the androgen receptor. In Europe and elsewhere, cyproterone (50-100 mg/day) is used as an androgen-receptor blocker, often in conjunction with a combination oral contraceptive. Efficacy in clinical trials also has been seen with finasteride (PROSCAR), an inhibitor of the type 2 isozyme of 5α-reductase that blocks the conversion of testosterone to dihydrotestosterone. Male offspring of women who become pregnant while taking any of these androgen inhibitors are at risk of impaired virilization secondary to impaired synthesis or action of dihydrotestosterone (FDA category X). The antifungal ketoconazole (NIZORAL), which inhibits CYP steroid hydroxylases (see Chapters 42 and 57), also can block androgen biosynthesis but may cause liver toxicity. Finally, topical eflornithine (VANIQA), an ornithine decarboxylase inhibitor, has been used with some success to decrease the rate of facial hair growth, thus reducing the frequency with which procedures such as laser ablation are needed for hair removal.

Infections of the Female Reproductive Tract

A variety of pathogens can cause infections of the female reproductive tract that range from vaginitis to pelvic inflammatory disease; Table 66–4 contains current recommendations for pharmacotherapy of selected sexually transmitted gynecological infections as issued by the Centers for Disease Control and Prevention (Workowski and Berman, 2006; www.cdc.gov/mmwr/preview/mmwrhtml/rr5511a1.htm). Of note, the recommended therapy for gonococcal infections has been updated due to increasing resistance of *Neisseria gonorrhoeae* to fluoroquinolones. The individual drugs used for systemic or topical therapy are described in more detail in Section VI.

Infections have been implicated as important factors in preterm labor, as discussed further in "Prevention or Arrest of Preterm Labor."

Fertility Induction

Infertility (i.e., the failure to conceive after 1 year of unprotected sex) affects ~10-15% of couples in developed nations and is increasing in incidence as more women choose to delay childbearing until later in life. The major impediment to pregnancy in an infertile couple can be attributed primarily to the woman in approximately one-third, to the man in approximately one-third, and to both in approximately one-third. The likelihood of a successful pharmacological induction of fertility in these couples depends greatly on the reason for the infertility. For example, a woman with tubal obstruction secondary to previous pelvic inflammatory disease is highly unlikely to become pregnant following drug therapy, whereas a woman with impaired ovulation secondary to a prolactin-secreting pituitary adenoma usually will become pregnant following suppression of prolactin secretion with a dopamine agonist (see Chapter 38).

The evaluation of an infertile couple is guided by the history and physical examination, which are augmented by focused laboratory evaluation. Defined abnormalities in the male partner that lead to impaired fertility (e.g., hypogonadism, Y chromosome microdeletions, Klinefelter's syndrome) typically are detected by analysis of a semen sample; most often, male infertility is idiopathic. The medical therapy for some of these conditions is discussed in Chapters 38 and 41, while assisted reproduction technology interventions such as intracytoplasmic sperm injection can be used for disorders that severely impair sperm count.

Anovulation accounts for ~50% of female infertility and is a major focus of pharmacological interventions used to achieve conception. Thus, whether a woman is ovulating is a key question. Although a history of regular cyclic bleeding is strong presumptive evidence for ovulation, assessment of urine LH levels with an over-the-counter kit (see Chapter 38) or measurement of the serum progesterone levels during the luteal phase provides more definitive information. In those infertile women who ovulate, analysis of the patency of the fallopian tubes and the structure of the uterus is an important part of the diagnostic evaluation.

A number of approaches have been used to stimulate ovulation in anovulatory women. Often, a stepwise approach is taken, initially using simpler and less expensive treatments, followed by more complex and expensive regimens if initial therapy is unsuccessful. In obese patients with PCOS, the inclusion of lifestyle modifications directed at weight loss is warranted based on the association of obesity with anovulation, pregnancy loss, and complicated pregnancies (e.g., gestational diabetes, pre-eclampsia). Definitive evidence that weight loss improves fertility is not currently available (Thessaloniki ESHRE/ASRM-Sponsored PCOS Consensus Workshop Group, 2008).

Clomiphene. Clomiphene citrate (CLOMID, SEROPHENE) is a potent anti-estrogen that primarily is used for treatment of anovulation in the setting of an intact hypothalamic—pituitary axis and adequate estrogen production (e.g., PCOS). By inhibiting the negative feedback effects of estrogen at hypothalamic and pituitary levels, clomiphene increases follicle-stimulating hormone (FSH) levels—typically by ~50%—and thereby enhances follicular maturation (see Chapter 40). The drug is relatively inexpensive, orally active, and requires less extensive monitoring than do other fertility protocols.

A typical regimen is 50 mg/day orally for 5 consecutive days starting between days 2 and 5 of the cycle in women who have spontaneous uterine bleeding or following a bleed induced by progesterone

Table 66–4

Sexually Transmitted Gynecological Infections and Recommended Therapies

Genital ulcers	
Chancroid	Azithromycin, 1 g PO single dose *or* Ceftriaxone, 250 mg IM single dose *or* Ciprofloxacin, 500 mg PO bid × 3 days *or* Erythromycin base, 500 mg PO tid × 7 days
Genital herpes	
First infection	Acyclovir, 400 mg PO tid × 7-10 days *or* Acyclovir, 200 mg PO 5 times daily for 7-10 days *or* Famciclovir, 250 mg PO tid for 7-10 days *or* Valacyclovir, 1 g PO bid × 7-10 days
Suppression	Acyclovir, 400 mg PO bid *or* Famciclovir, 250 mg PO bid *or* Valacyclovir, 500 mg PO once daily
Recurrent	Same drugs at lower dose for more prolonged duration
Granuloma inguinale	Doxycycline, 100 mg PO bid × >21 days
Lymphogranuloma venereum	Doxycycline, 100 mg PO bid × 21 days
Syphilis	
Primary/secondary	Benzathine penicillin, 2.4 million units IM, single dose
Tertiary	Benzathine penicillin, 2.4 million units IM, 3 weekly injections
Vaginal discharge	
Trichomonas	Metronidazole, 2 g PO single dose *or* Tinidazole, 2 g PO, single dose
Bacterial vaginosis	Metronidazole, 500 mg PO bid × 7 days *or* Metronidazole gel, 5 g intravaginally daily × 5 days *or* Clindamycin cream, 5 g intravaginally at bedtime × 7 days
Candida	Topical: Butoconazole, clotrimazole, miconazole, nystatin, tioconazole, terconazole Oral: Fluconazole, 150 mg PO, single dose
Urethritis/Cervicitis	
Non-gonococcal	Azithromycin, 1 g PO single dose *or* Doxycycline, 100 mg PO bid × 7 days
Chlamydia	Azithromycin, 1 g PO single dose *or* Doxycycline, 100 mg PO × 7 days
Gonococcal	Ceftriaxone, 125 mg IM single dose *or* Cefixime, 400 mg PO single dose
Pelvic Inflammatory Disease	
Parenteral regimen	Cefotetan, 2 g IV every 12 hours *or* Cefoxitin, 2 g IV every 6 hours + Doxycycline, 100 mg PO or IV every 12 hours × 14 days
Oral regimen	Ceftriaxone, 250 mg IM single dose + Doxycycline, 100 mg PO bid × 14 days *or* Cefoxitin, 2 g IV single dose + Probenecid + Doxycycline, 100 mg PO bid × 14 days

PO, orally; IM, intramuscularly; IV, intravenously; bid, twice daily; tid, three times daily.

withdrawal in women who do not. If this regimen fails to induce ovulation, the dose of clomiphene is increased, first to the FDA-approved maximum of 100 mg/day and possibly to higher levels of 150 or 200 mg/day. Although clomiphene is effective in inducing ovulation in perhaps 75% of women, successful pregnancy ensues in only 40-50% of those who ovulate. This has been attributed to clomiphene's inhibition of estrogen action on the endometrium, resulting in an environment that is not optimal for fertilization and/or implantation.

Untoward effects of clomiphene include the ovarian hyperstimulation syndrome (OHSS; < 1%; see "Gonadotropins") and increased incidences of multifetal gestations (twins in ~5-10% and more than two babies in ~0.3% of pregnancies), ovarian cysts, hot flashes, headaches, and blurred vision. A few studies have suggested that prolonged use (e.g., ≥12 cycles) may increase the risk of ovarian and endometrial cancer; thus, the recommended maximum number of cycles is six. Clomiphene should not be administered to pregnant women (FDA category X) due to reports of teratogenicity in animals, although there is no definitive evidence of this in humans (Elizur and Tulandi, 2008).

Tamoxifen appears to be as effective as clomiphene for ovulation induction but is not FDA-approved for this indication. It has been used off label as an alternative in women who suffer intolerable side effects (e.g., hot flashes) with clomiphene.

Gonadotropins. The preparations of gonadotropins available for clinical use are detailed in Chapter 38 and include gonadotropins purified from human menopausal or pregnant urine and those prepared by recombinant DNA technology. They should be administered by physicians experienced in the treatment of infertility or reproductive endocrine disorders. Although most clearly indicated for ovulation induction in anovulatory women with hypogonadotropic hypogonadism secondary to hypothalamic or pituitary dysfunction, gonadotropins also are used to induce ovulation in women with PCOS who do not respond to clomiphene (see "Clomiphene") and also are used, generally after a trial of clomiphene, in women who are infertile despite normal ovulation.

Given the marked increases in maternal and fetal complications associated with multifetal gestation, the goal of ovulation induction in anovulatory women is to induce the formation and ovulation of a single dominant follicle; generally, the increased risks of twin gestation will be accepted if two follicles are present.

As shown in Figure 66–1, a typical regimen for ovulation induction is to administer 75 IU of FSH daily in a "low-dose, step-up protocol." After several days of stimulation, the serum estradiol is measured; the target levels of estradiol range from 500-1500 pg/mL, with lower levels indicating inadequate gonadotropin stimulation and higher values portending an increased risk of OHSS. If the estradiol level is too low, then the daily dose of FSH can be increased (the "step-up") in increments of 37.5 or 75 IU. Ovaries are examined by ultrasonography every 2-3 days to evaluate follicle maturation. The finding of a follicle ≥17 mm in diameter indicates that adequate follicular development has occurred. If three or more follicles of this size are present, gonadotropin therapy generally is stopped to decrease the likelihood of developing OHSS, and barrier contraception is used to prevent pregnancy, thereby avoiding multifetal pregnancy. In the "high-dose, step-down" protocol, higher initial doses of FSH are used, and the dose is decreased thereafter. Anecdotal evidence suggests that this regimen is associated with an increased risk of OHSS.

To complete follicular maturation and induce ovulation, human chorionic gonadotropin (hCG, 5000-10,000 IU) is given 1 day after the last dose of gonadotropin. Fertilization of the oocyte(s) at 36 hours after hCG administration then is attempted, either by intercourse or intrauterine insemination. Despite the precautions outlined above, gonadotropin-induced ovulation results in multiple births in up to 10-20% of cases due to the pharmacologically induced development of more than one pre-ovulatory follicle and the release of more than one ovum.

Gonadotropin induction also is used for ovarian stimulation in conjunction with *in vitro* fertilization (IVF; Figure 66–1; Macklon et al., 2006). In this setting, larger doses of FSH (typically 225-300 IU/day) are administered to induce the maturation of multiple (ideally at least 5 and up to 20) oocytes that can be retrieved for IVF and intrauterine transfer. To prevent the LH surge and subsequent premature luteinization of the ovarian follicles, gonadotropins typically are administered in conjunction with a GnRH agonist. The length of the IVF protocol is predicated by the initial flare of gonadotropin secretion that occurs in response to the GnRH agonists. In the long protocol, the agonist is started in the luteal phase of the previous cycle (generally on cycle day 21) and then maintained until the time of hCG injection to induce ovulation. Alternatively, in the "flare" protocol, the GnRH agonist is started on cycle day 2 (immediately after the start of menses), and gonadotropin injections are added 1 day later. Adequate follicle maturation with the latter regimen typically takes 10-12 days after gonadotropin therapy is initiated.

GnRH antagonists also can be used to inhibit endogenous LH secretion. Because they do not transiently increase gonadotropin secretion, they can be initiated later in the cycle in a "short protocol." Current regimens include daily injection in a dose of 0.25 mg (ganirelix [ANTAGON] or cetrorelix [CETROTIDE]) starting on the fifth or sixth day of gonadotropin stimulation or a single dose of 3 mg of cetrorelix administered on day 8 or 9 of the late follicular phase.

Using either the long or short protocols, hCG (at typical doses of 5000-10,000 IU of urine-derived product or 250 μg of recombinant hCG) is given to induce final oocyte development, and the mature eggs are retrieved from the pre-ovulatory follicles at 32-36 hours thereafter. The ova are retrieved transvaginally guided by ultrasonography and fertilized *in vitro* with sperm (IVF) or by intracytoplasmic sperm injection; one or two embryos then are transferred to the uterus 3-5 days after fertilization. With these approaches, the increased risk of multifetal gestations is related to the number of embryos that are transferred to the woman. To diminish this risk, there is a trend, particularly in Europe, toward transferring only one embryo per cycle.

Because of the inhibitory effects of GnRH agonists or antagonists on pituitary gonadotropes, the secretion of LH that normally sustains the corpus luteum after ovulation does not occur. Repeated injections of hCG, while sustaining the corpus luteum, may increase the risk of OHSS. Thus, standard IVF regimens typically provide exogenous progesterone replacement to support the fetus until the

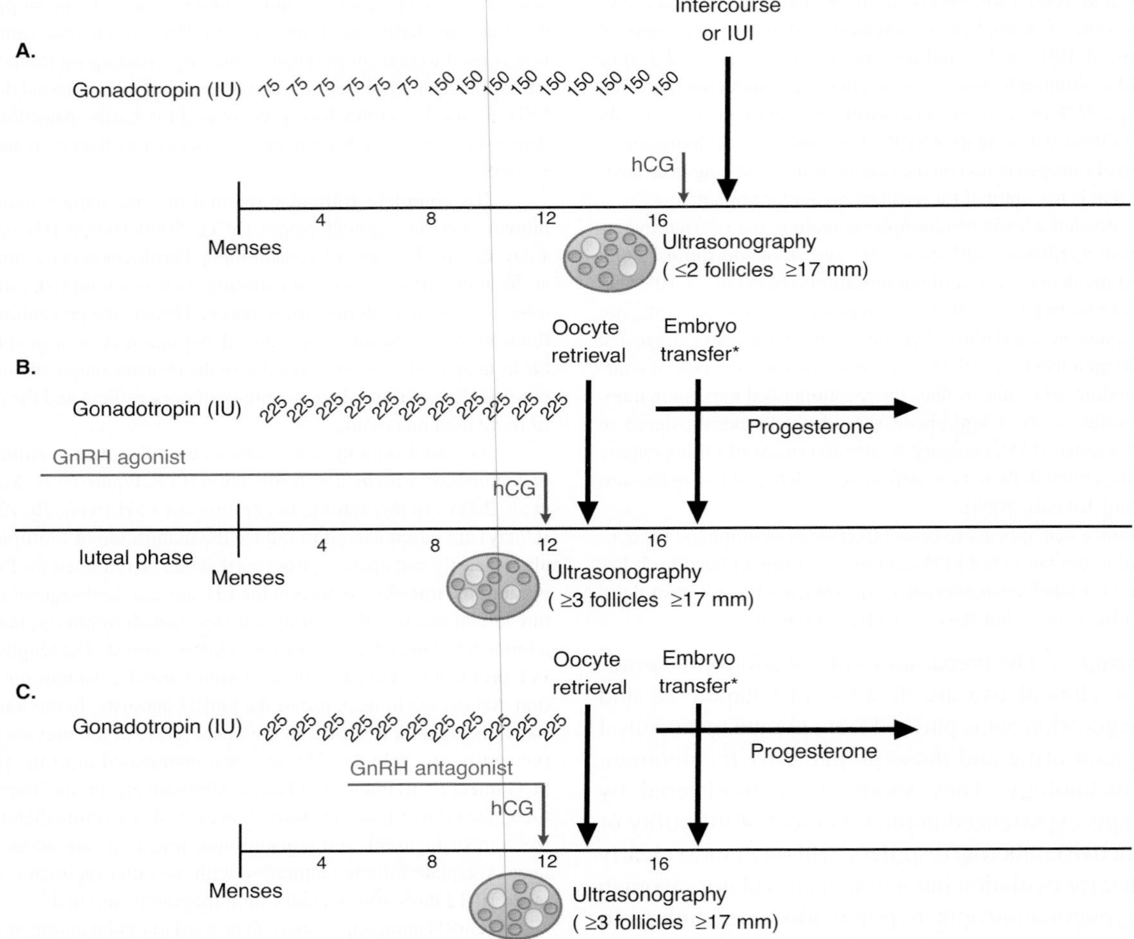

Figure 66–1. *Schematic diagram of idealized regimens using exogenous gonadotropins for fertility induction.* ***A***. Step-up regimen for ovulation induction. After menses, daily injections of gonadotropin (75 IU) are started. Follicle maturation is assessed by serial measurement of plasma estradiol and follicle size, as discussed in the text. If an inadequate response is seen, the dose of gonadotropin is increased to 112 or 150 IU/day. When one or two follicles have achieved a size of ≥17 mm in diameter, final follicle maturation and ovulation are induced by injection of human chorionic gonadotropin (hCG). Fertilization then is achieved at 36 hours after hCG injection by intercourse or intrauterine insemination (IUI). If more than two mature follicles are seen, the cycle is terminated and barrier contraception is used to avoid triplets or higher degrees of multifetal gestation. ***B***. Long protocol for ovarian hyperstimulation using gonadotropin-releasing hormone (GnRH) agonist to inhibit premature ovulation, followed by *in vitro* fertilization (IVF). After the GnRH agonist has inhibited endogenous secretion of gonadotropins, therapy with exogenous gonadotropins is initiated. Follicle maturation is assessed by serial measurements of plasma estradiol and follicle size by ultrasonography. When three or more follicles are ≥17 mm in diameter, then ovulation is induced by injection of hCG. At 32-36 hours after the hCG injection, the eggs are retrieved and used for IVF. Exogenous progesterone is provided to promote a receptive endometrium, followed by embryo transfer at 3-5 days after fertilization. ***C***. Protocol for ovarian hyperstimulation in an IVF protocol using a GnRH antagonist. The cycle duration is shorter because the GnRH antagonist does not induce a transient flare of gonadotropin secretion that might disrupt the timing of the cycle, but many other elements of the cycle are analogous to those in B. IU, intrauterine.

placenta acquires the biosynthetic capacity to take over this function; regimens include progesterone in oil (50-100 mg/day intramuscularly) or micronized progesterone (180-300 mg twice daily vaginally). Vaginal preparations containing 100 mg (ENDOMETRIN) or 90 mg (PROCHIEVE, CRINONE) of micronized progesterone are approved for administration two or three times daily as part of IVF and other fertility technologies.

Aside from the attendant complications of multifetal gestation, the major side effect of gonadotropin treatment is OHSS. This potentially life-threatening event is believed to result from increased ovarian secretion of substances that increase vascular permeability and is characterized by rapid accumulation of fluid in the peritoneal cavity, thorax, and even the pericardium. Symptoms and signs include abdominal pain and/or distention, nausea and vomiting, diarrhea, dyspnea, oliguria, and marked ovarian enlargement on ultrasonography. OHSS can lead to hypovolemia, electrolyte abnormalities, acute respiratory distress syndrome, thromboembolic events, and hepatic dysfunction.

In ovulation induction, incipient OHSS should be suspected if routine laboratory investigation reveals the presence of more than four to six follicles >17 mm or a serum estradiol level of >1500 pg/mL; in this setting, hCG should be withheld and barrier contraception used. For controlled ovarian hyperstimulation in anticipation of IVF, a higher risk of OHSS is present if the number of follicles >15 mm exceeds 15-20 or if the plasma level of estradiol is >5000 pg/mL. In an effort to avoid overt hyperstimulation, the FSH can be withheld for a day or two ("coasting") if the plasma level of estradiol is near the top of this range. The rationale for this approach is that larger follicles become relatively gonadotropin independent and thus will continue to mature, while the smaller follicles undergo atresia in response to gonadotropin deprivation. In either case, ovulation induction with recombinant LH, which has a considerably shorter $t_{1/2}$ than hCG, or with a GnRH agonist may diminish the incidence of OHSS without requiring cancellation of the cycle.

The potential deleterious effects of gonadotropins are debated. Some studies have suggested that gonadotropins are associated with an increased risk of ovarian cancer, but this conclusion is controversial (Brinton et al., 2005). Similarly, although IVF and the subsequent embryo manipulation may be associated with abnormal imprinting that increases the risk of developmental syndromes (e.g., Angelman's and Beckwith-Wiedemann syndromes; Lawrence and Moley, 2008; Niemitz and Feinberg, 2004), the risk is small, and there is no evidence that the gonadotropins themselves or components of the IVF process increase the rate of congenital abnormalities in babies born from stimulated oocytes.

Insulin Sensitizers. PCOS affects 4-7% of women of reproductive age and is the most frequent cause of anovulatory infertility. Inasmuch as PCOS patients often exhibit hyperinsulinemia and insulin resistance, insulin sensitizers such as metformin have been evaluated for their effects on ovulation and fertility (see Chapter 43 for a general discussion of drugs used to increase insulin sensitivity). Although several small trials suggested that metformin increased ovulation in PCOS patients relative to placebo, a recent, well-designed trial failed to demonstrate a significant effect of metformin on fertility (Legro et al., 2007); metformin was less effective than clomiphene in inducing ovulation, promoting conception, or improving live birth rates, and there was no benefit of combining metformin with clomiphene on live births, except possibly in women resistant to clomiphene. Thus, except in women who exhibit glucose intolerance, the consensus is that metformin generally should not be used for fertility induction in women with PCOS (Thessaloniki ESHRE/ASRM-Sponsored PCOS Consensus Workshop Group, 2008).

Thiazolidinediones also have been evaluated for their ability to induce ovulation in PCOS patients. One trial demonstrated that troglitazone significantly increased ovulation in PCOS patients compared to placebo controls; this drug was withdrawn from the market due to safety issues, and attention therefore has turned to the use of rosiglitazone (AVANDIA) and pioglitazone (ACTOS), other members of the thiazolidinedione family. Preliminary results suggest that these latter drugs may increase ovulation in PCOS patients, but definitive data are not available. Given the recent association of thiazolidinediones with an increased risk of congestive heart failure and myocardial ischemia, there is considerable reluctance to use these drugs in this setting.

Aromatase Inhibitors. Aromatase inhibitors (e.g., letrozole [FEMARA], 5 mg/day for 5 days) are under evaluation as potential drugs for infertility. By inhibiting estrogen biosynthesis, these drugs decrease estrogen negative feedback and thus increase FSH levels and stimulate follicle development. In 2005, the manufacturer of letrozole issued a statement that letrozole is not indicated for ovulation induction or other uses in premenopausal women. Another aromatase inhibitor, anastrozole (ARIMIDEX), also has been used off label for ovulation induction. Some data suggest that anastrozole is less effective than clomiphene in inducing follicle maturation but more likely to lead to pregnancy.

DRUG THERAPY IN OBSTETRICS

General Principles of Drug Therapy of Pregnant Women

The processes of evaluating potential adverse effects of various drugs in preclinical and clinical trials are described in Chapter 1. Unfortunately, these trials often do not provide sufficient information regarding safety in pregnant women or children. Individuals at the extremes of the age spectrum are particularly vulnerable to the toxic effects of drugs (see Chapter 4). The very young are susceptible due either to incomplete development of certain organs (e.g., the kidney) or the lack of expression of certain drug-metabolizing or transport proteins that play key pharmacokinetic roles (Kearns et al., 2003); the elderly are at increased risk due to age-related changes in body composition, organ function, and drug-metabolizing systems, all of which delay drug clearance (Mangoni and Jackson, 2003).

In pregnant women, the placenta provides a barrier for the transfer of certain drugs from the mother to the fetus (e.g., drug transporters expel toxic natural products and related drugs from the placenta, aromatase converts maternal androgen to estrogens); however, many compounds can freely cross the placental barrier and access the fetal circulation. The teratogenic effects of thalidomide on limb formation, alcohol on development of the CNS and cognition, and diethystilbestrol (DES) on genital development in males and females and on the subsequent development of vaginal and cervical carcinomas in female offspring are stark reminders of the dangers of fetal exposure to drugs. In the clinical setting, there is no direct method for determining fetal exposure to a drug. Drug concentration over time in the mother's systemic circulation is the major determinant of this exposure, but other contributing factors include the size, solubility, ionization, and protein binding of the drug; its active transport into and out of the placental circulation; and the rate of fetal clearance, which includes first-pass metabolism by the placenta.

Based on the relative paucity of human data on the teratogenic effects of drugs and the limited reliability of animal models, a fundamental tenet in treating pregnant women is to minimize, whenever possible, the exposure of mother and fetus to drugs; when necessary, one should preferentially use those drugs that have the best record of safety in pregnant women without adverse developmental effects on the fetus. Of equal importance, substances of abuse (e.g., cigarettes, alcohol, illegal drugs) should be avoided and, whenever possible, eliminated before conception. In addition, all pregnant women should take a multivitamin containing 400 μg of folic acid daily to diminish the incidence of neural tube defects. The greatest concern is during the period of organogenesis in the first trimester, when a number of the most vulnerable tissues are formed. Cancer chemotherapy drugs cannot be given with reasonable safety during the first trimester, but most cytotoxics may be administered without teratogenic effects and with maintenance of pregnancy in the third trimester (see Chapters 61-63).

Drugs that are used to promote fertility are a special case, since they, by nature of their use, will be present in the mother at the time of conception. Fortunately, available evidence largely supports the safety of fertility agents for fetal development, although there have been data suggesting increased risk with certain agents (e.g., neural tube defects and hypospadias associated with clomiphene; Elizur and Tulandi, 2008).

The FDA assigns different levels of risk to drugs for use in pregnant women, as listed in Table 66–5.

Table 66–5

FDA Use-in-Pregnancy Ratings

Category A: Controlled studies show no risk. Adequate, well-controlled studies in pregnant women have failed to demonstrate a risk to the fetus in any trimester of pregnancy.

Category B: No evidence of risk in humans. Adequate, well-controlled studies in pregnant women have not shown an increased risk of fetal abnormalities despite adverse findings in animals, or, in the absence of adequate human studies, animal studies show no fetal risk. The chance of fetal harm is remote, but remains a possibility.

Category C: Risk cannot be ruled out. Adequate, well-controlled human studies are lacking, and animal studies have shown a risk to the fetus or are lacking as well. There is a chance of fetal harm if the drug is administered during pregnancy, but the potential benefits may outweigh the potential risk.

Category D: Positive evidence of risk. Studies in humans, or investigational or post-marketing data, have demonstrated fetal risk. Nevertheless, potential benefits from the use of the drug may outweigh the potential risk. For example, the drug may be acceptable if needed in a life-threatening situation or serious disease for which safer drugs cannot be used or are ineffective.

Category X: Contraindicated in pregnancy. Studies in animals or humans, or investigational or post-marketing reports, have demonstrated positive evidence of fetal abnormalities or risk that clearly outweighs any possible benefit to the patient.

Certain drugs are so toxic to the developing fetus that they must never be administered to a pregnant woman (category X); in some cases (e.g., thalidomide, retinoids), the potential for fetal harm is so great that multiple forms of effective contraception must be in place before the drug is initiated. For other drugs, the risk of adverse effects on the fetus may range from category A (drugs that have not been proven to have adverse effects on the fetus despite adequate investigation) to category C (drugs with risks that sometimes may be justified based on the severity of the underlying condition (e.g., hydralazine for pregnancy-induced hypertension, β adrenergic receptor agonists for premature labor; see "Pregnancy-Induced Hypertension/Pre-eclampsia" and "Tocolytic Therapy for Established Preterm Labor"). Unfortunately, the FDA listings may be overly simplistic or outdated for a given drug; for example, oral contraceptives are listed as category X, even though considerable data now indicate that birth defects are not increased in women taking oral contraceptives at the time of conception.

Nursing mothers constitute a second special situation with respect to potential adverse effects of drugs. Some drugs may interfere with milk production and/or secretion (e.g., estrogen-containing oral contraceptives) and thus should be avoided if possible in mothers who wish to breastfeed. Other drugs may be secreted into breast milk and expose the baby to potentially toxic levels during the vulnerable perinatal period (Ito and Lee, 2003). The amount of drug that is secreted in breast milk, like the amount that crosses the placenta, depends on drug characteristics such as size, ionization, protein binding, and pharmacokinetics of clearance. The American Academy of Pediatrics Committee on Drugs periodically reviews agents transferred into human milk and their effects on the infant or on lactation (Hale, 2005). Product information sheets that provide available information regarding the potential for adverse effects of specific drugs on breastfed infants should be consulted before prescribing medications to nursing mothers.

Pregnancy-Induced Hypertension/Pre-eclampsia

Hypertension affects up to 10% of pregnant women in the U.S.; with the increasing prevalence of hypertension in the general population and the tendency to delay childbearing, drug therapy for maternal hypertension likely will be given greater consideration in the future. A consensus panel has issued guidelines for the management of hypertension in pregnancy (National High Blood Pressure Education Program Working Group, 2000).

Hypertension that precedes pregnancy or manifests before 20 weeks of gestation is believed to overlap considerably in pathogenesis with essential hypertension. These patients appear to be at increased risk for gestational diabetes and need careful monitoring. In contrast, pregnancy-induced hypertension, or pre-eclampsia, generally presents after 20 weeks of gestation as a new-onset hypertension with proteinuria (>300 mg of urinary protein/24 hours); pre-eclampsia is thought to involve placenta-derived factors that affect vascular integrity and endothelial function in the mother, thus causing peripheral edema, renal and hepatic dysfunction, and in severe cases, seizures (Maynard et al., 2008). Chronic hypertension is an established risk factor for pre-eclampsia, but there is no conclusive evidence that antihypertensive therapy during pregnancy affects the incidence or outcome of pre-eclampsia in women with mild to moderate hypertension (Abalos et al., 2007). Nonetheless, the consensus panel recommended initiation of drug therapy in women with a diastolic blood pressure >105 mm Hg or a systolic blood pressure >160 mm Hg (National High Blood Pressure Education Program Working Group, 2000). If severe pre-eclampsia ensues, with marked hypertension and evidence of end-organ damage, then termination of the pregnancy by delivery of the baby is the treatment of choice, provided that the fetus is sufficiently mature to survive outside the uterus. If the baby is very preterm, then hospitalization and pharmacotherapy (expectant management) may be employed in an effort to permit further fetal maturation *in utero*.

Many pregnant women already carry the diagnosis of hypertension and are on drug therapy, which may be continued with careful monitoring, provided that blood pressure control is effective. In this setting, however, some drugs that commonly are used for hypertension in non-pregnant patients (e.g., angiotensin-converting enzyme inhibitors, angiotensin-receptor antagonists) should not be used due to unequivocal evidence of adverse fetal effects in animal models and humans (Podymow and August, 2008). Many experts will convert the patient to the centrally acting α adrenergic agonist α-methyldopa (ALDOMET) at an initial dose of 250 mg orally twice daily (FDA category B), which rarely is used for hypertension in non-pregnant patients. Other drugs with reasonable evidence of safety (category C) also may be used, including the combination α_1-selective, β-nonselective adrenergic antagonist labetalol (TRANDATE; 100 mg twice daily) and the Ca^{2+} channel blocker nifedipine (PROCARDIA XL, ADALAT CC; 30 mg once daily).

Similar considerations apply in previously normotensive women who develop pre-eclampsia; α-methyldopa again is a reasonable choice for outpatient management if the blood pressure exceeds the threshold for therapy. If severe pre-eclampsia or impending labor requires hospitalization, blood pressure can be controlled acutely with hydralazine (5 or 10 mg intravenously or intramuscularly, with repeated dosing at 20-minute intervals depending on blood pressure response) or labetalol (20 mg intravenously, with dose escalation to 40 mg at 10 minutes if blood pressure control is inadequate).

In addition to drugs for blood pressure control, women with severe pre-eclampsia or those who have central nervous system manifestations, such as headache, visual disturbance, or altered mental status, are treated as inpatients with magnesium sulfate, based on its documented efficacy in seizure prevention and lack of adverse effects on the mother or baby (Altman et al., 2002). Such treatment also should be considered for postpartum women with central nervous system manifestations, because ~20% of episodes of eclampsia occur in women who are more than 48 hours after delivery.

Prevention or Arrest of Preterm Labor

Scope of the Problem and Etiology. Preterm birth, defined as delivery before 37 weeks of gestation, occurs in >10% of pregnancies in the U.S. and is increasing in frequency; it is associated with significant complications, such as neonatal respiratory distress syndrome, pulmonary hypertension, and intracranial hemorrhage.

Although incompletely understood, risk factors for preterm labor include multifetal gestation, premature rupture of the membranes, intrauterine infection, and placental insufficiency. The more premature the baby, the greater the risk of complications, prompting efforts to prevent or interrupt preterm labor.

The therapeutic objective in preterm labor is to delay delivery so that the mother can be transported to a regional facility specializing in the care of premature babies and supportive agents can be administered; such supportive treatments include glucocorticoids to stimulate fetal lung maturation (see Chapter 42) and antibiotics (e.g., erythromycin, ampicillin) to diminish the frequency of neonatal infection with group B β-hemolytic *Streptococcus*. Based on concerns over deleterious effects of antibiotic therapy, it is essential that antibiotics not be administered indiscriminately to all women thought to have preterm labor, but rather be reserved for those with premature rupture of the membranes and evidence of infection.

Prevention of Preterm Labor: Progesterone Therapy. Progesterone levels in some species diminish considerably in association with labor, whereas administration of progesterone inhibits the secretion of pro-inflammatory cytokines and delays cervical ripening. Thus, progesterone and its derivatives have long been advocated to diminish the onset of preterm labor in women at increased risk due to previous preterm delivery. Despite considerable controversy, recent randomized trials have revived interest in this approach. One drug used in this setting is 17α-hydroxyprogesterone at a dose of 250 mg administered weekly by intramuscular injection (Meis et al., 2003). Vaginal administration of progesterone (200 mg each night) also was used in one clinical trial with apparent efficacy (Fonseca et al., 2007). One clinical trial suggested that progesterone administration in this setting was associated with an increased incidence of gestational diabetes (Rebarber et al., 2007), and the role of progesterone prophylaxis during pregnancy remains to be established.

Tocolytic Therapy for Established Preterm Labor. Because preterm birth typically is heralded by the uterine contractions of labor, the inhibition of these contractions, or tocolysis, has been a focus of therapy (Simhan and Caritis, 2007). Although tocolytic agents delay delivery in ~80% of women, they neither prevent premature births nor improve adverse fetal outcomes such as respiratory distress syndrome. Thus, while widely employed, they should be viewed as temporizing agents, as described in "Prevention of Preterm Labor: Progesterone Therapy."

Specific tocolytic agents include β adrenergic receptor agonists, $MgSO_4$, Ca^{2+} channel blockers, COX inhibitors, oxytocin-receptor antagonists, and nitric oxide donors. The mechanisms of action of these agents are illustrated in Figure 66–2.

The β adrenergic receptor agonists relax the myometrium by activating the cyclic AMP-PKA signaling cascade that phosphorylates and inactivates myosin light-chain kinase, a key enzyme in uterine contraction. Ritodrine, a selective $β_2$ agonist, was specifically developed as a uterine relaxant and remains the only tocolytic drug to have gained FDA approval; it was voluntarily withdrawn from the U.S. market. Terbutaline (BRETHINE), which is FDA-approved for asthma, has been used off label for this purpose and can be administered orally, subcutaneously, or intravenously. Terbutaline may delay births, but only during the first 48 hours of treatment, and is associated with a number of adverse maternal effects, including tachycardia, hypotension, and pulmonary edema.

Similarly, Ca^{2+} channel blockers inhibit the influx of Ca^{2+} through depolarization-activated, voltage-sensitive Ca^{2+} channels in the plasma membrane, thereby preventing the activation of myosin light-chain kinase and the stimulation of uterine contraction. Nifedipine (PROCARDIA, ADALAT), the Ca^{2+} channel blocker used most commonly for this purpose, can be administered parenterally or orally. Relative to $β_2$ adrenergic agonists, nifedipine is more likely to improve fetal outcomes and less likely to cause maternal side effects.

Based on the role of prostaglandins in uterine contraction, cyclooxygenase inhibitors (e.g., indomethacin) have been used to inhibit preterm labor, and some data suggest that they may reduce the number of preterm births. Because they also can inhibit platelet function and induce closure *in utero* of the ductus arteriosus, these inhibitors should not be employed in term pregnancies (or in pregnancies beyond 32 weeks of gestation, when the risk of severe complications of prematurity is relatively lower). Short courses of treatment (<72 hours) pose less risk for impaired circulation in the fetus.

Atosiban (TRACTOCILE), a nonapeptide analog of oxytocin, competitively inhibits the interaction of oxytocin with its membrane receptor on uterine cells and thereby decreases the frequency of uterine contractions. Although atosiban increased the number of women who remained undelivered for 48 hours and is widely used in Europe, it is not FDA-approved in the U.S.

Nitric oxide is a potent vasodilator and smooth muscle relaxant, and drugs such as nitroglycerin and other nitrates that increase its levels are used to treat myocardial ischemia (see Chapter 28). Both intravenous nitroglycerin and transdermal nitrate preparations have been evaluated in clinical trials to inhibit preterm labor. The major adverse effect is maternal hypotension.

Despite numerous clinical trials, the superiority of any one therapy has not been established, and none of the drugs has been shown definitively to improve fetal outcome. Thus, despite widespread and enthusiastic use by some centers, many experts do not endorse the routine use of tocolytic agents. Recent meta-analyses of published reports concluded that Ca^{2+} channel blockers and atosiban (not available in the U.S.) provided the best balance of successfully delayed delivery with lesser risks to the mother and baby (reviewed by Iams et al., 2008).

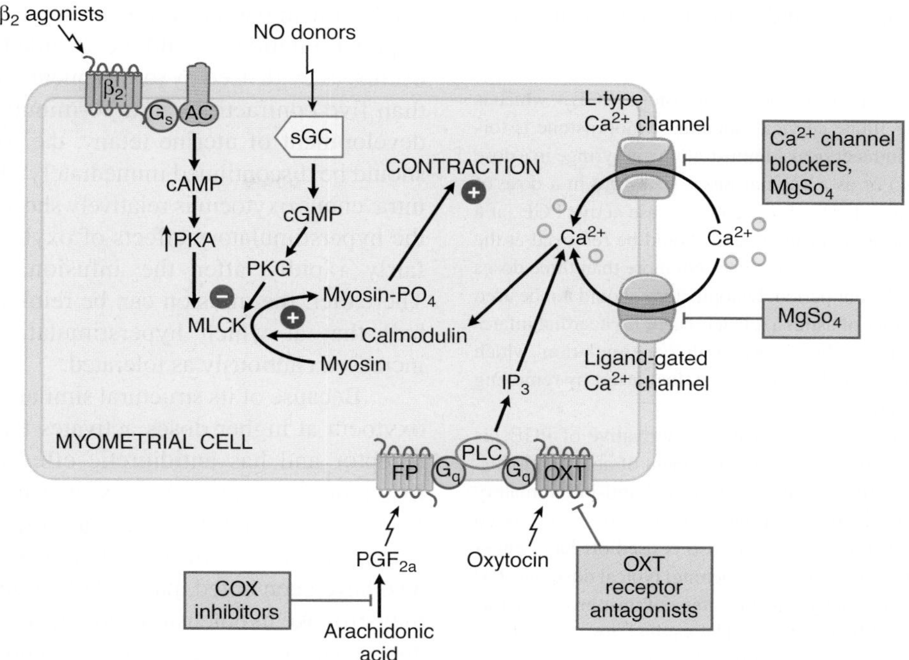

Figure 66–2. *Sites of action of tocolytic drugs in the uterine myometrium.* The elevation of cellular Ca^{2+} promotes contraction via the Ca^{2+}/calmodulin-dependent activation of myosin light chain kinase (MLCK). Relaxation is promoted by the elevation of cyclic nucleotides (cAMP and cGMP) and their activation of protein kinases, which cause phosphorylation/inactivation of MLCK. Pharmacological manipulations to reduce myometrial contraction include:

- inhibiting Ca^{2+} entry (Ca^{2+} channel blockers, Mg_2SO_4)
- reducing mobilization of intracellular Ca^{2+} by antagonizing GPCR-mediated activation of the G_q-PLC-IP_3-Ca^{2+} pathway (with antagonists of the FP and OXT receptors) or reducing production of the FP agonist, $PGF_{2\alpha}$ (with COX inhibitors)
- enhancing relaxation by elevating cellular cyclic AMP (with β_2 adrenergic agonists that activate G_s-AC) and cyclic GMP (with NO donors that stimulate soluble guanylyl cyclase)

sGC, soluble guanylyl cyclase; AC, adenylyl cyclase; FP, the $PGF_{2\alpha}$ receptor; OXT, the oxytocin receptor; PLC, phospholipase C; COX, cyclooxygenase.

Initiation of Labor

Labor induction is indicated when the perceived risk of continued pregnancy to the mother or fetus exceeds the risks of delivery or pharmacological induction. Such circumstances include premature rupture of the membranes, isoimmunization, fetal growth restriction, uteroplacental insufficiency (as in diabetes, pre-eclampsia, or eclampsia), and gestation beyond 42 weeks. Before inducing labor, it is essential to verify that the fetal lungs are sufficiently mature and to exclude potential contraindications (e.g., abnormal fetal position, evidence of fetal distress, placental abnormalities, or previous uterine surgery predisposing to uterine rupture).

Labor induction also is used increasingly in the absence of specific criteria listed above; such elective inductions may be predicated in part on matters of convenience for the mother or medical team. Collectively, induced or augmented labor now accounts for ~20% of all deliveries in the U.S., two-thirds of which are for nonmedical reasons.

Prostaglandins and Cervical Ripening. Prostaglandins play key roles in parturition (see Chapter 33). Thus, PGE_1, PGE_2, and PGF_{2a} are used to facilitate labor by promoting ripening and dilation of the cervix. They can be administered either orally or via local administration (either vaginally or intracervically). The ability of certain prostaglandins to stimulate uterine contractions also makes them valuable agents in the therapy of postpartum hemorrhage (see "Prevention/Treatment of Postpartum Hemorrhage"). Although prostaglandins are widely employed for cervical ripening, their effectiveness versus that of oxytocin alone in diminishing the need for cesarean section in labor induction has not been definitively established.

Available preparations include dinoprostone (PGE_2), which is FDA approved to facilitate cervical ripening. Dinoprostone is formulated as a gel for intracervical administration via syringe in a dose of 0.5 mg (PREPIDIL) or as a vaginal insert (pessary) in a dose of 10 mg (CERVIDIL); the latter is designed to release active PGE_2 at a rate of 0.3 mg/hr for up to 12 hours and should be removed at the onset of labor or 12 hours after insertion. No more than three doses should be used in a 24-hour period. Dinoprostone should not be used in women with a history of asthma, glaucoma, or myocardial infarction. The major adverse effect is uterine hyperstimulation, which may be reversed more rapidly using the vaginal insert by removing it with the attached tape.

Misoprostol (CYTOTEC), a synthetic derivative of PGE_1, is FDA-approved for the prevention and treatment of acid peptic disease in patients who are receiving nonsteroidal anti-inflammatory agents (see Chapter 34). Its use in medical abortion is discussed earlier in "Pregnancy Termination." It also is used off label either orally or vaginally to induce cervical ripening; typical doses are 100 μg (orally) or 25 μg (vaginally); an advantage of misoprostol in this setting is its considerably lower cost. The vaginal dose typically is repeated every 4-6 hours depending on labor progression. Adverse effects include uterine hyperstimulation and, rarely, uterine rupture. Most experts therefore do not use misoprostol for cervical ripening in women who have had previous cesarean section or other uterine surgery. Misoprostol should be discontinued for at least 3 hours before initiating oxytocin therapy.

Oxytocin. The structure and physiology of oxytocin are discussed in Chapter 38. This section presents therapeutic uses of oxytocin in obstetrics, which include the induction of labor, the augmentation of labor that is not progressing, and the prophylaxis and/or treatment of postpartum hemorrhage. Although widely used, oxytocin recently was added to a list of drugs "bearing a heightened risk of harm" (Clark et al., 2009), and its role and specific application to most deliveries in the U.S. remain open to debate. Thus, careful review of the appropriate indications for oxytocin administration and attention to the dose and progress of labor during induction are essential.

Labor Induction. Oxytocin (PITOCIN, SYNTOCINON) is the drug of choice for labor induction; for this purpose, it is administered by intravenous infusion of a diluted solution (typically 10 mIU/mL), preferably via an infusion pump. Current protocols start with an oxytocin dose of 6 mIU/minute, followed by advancement of dose as needed (in one protocol, increases of 6 mIU/minute can be made every 40 minutes if labor is not progressing in a satisfactory manner). Although there are little definitive data, 40 mIU/minute is a reasonable maximum dose, although doses of up to 72 mIU/minute have been used with apparent safety in some studies. Uterine hyperstimulation should be avoided; however, if it occurs, as evidenced by too-frequent contractions (more than five contractions in a 10-minute interval) or the development of uterine tetany, the oxytocin infusion should be discontinued immediately. Because the $t_{1/2}$ of intravenous oxytocin is relatively short (12-15 minutes), the hyperstimulatory effects of oxytocin will dissipate fairly rapidly after the infusion is discontinued. Thereafter, the infusion can be reinitiated at a dose of half that at which hyperstimulation occurred and increased cautiously as tolerated.

Because of its structural similarity to vasopressin, oxytocin at higher doses activates the vasopressin V_2 receptor and has antidiuretic effects. Particularly if hypotonic fluids (e.g., dextrose in water) are infused too liberally, water intoxication may result in convulsions, coma, and even death. Vasodilating actions of oxytocin also have been noted, particularly at high doses, which may provoke hypotension and reflex tachycardia. Deep anesthesia may exaggerate the hypotensive effect of oxytocin by preventing the reflex tachycardia.

Augmentation of Dysfunctional Labor. Oxytocin also is used when spontaneous labor is not progressing at an acceptable rate. To augment hypotonic contractions in dysfunctional labor, an infusion rate of 10 mIU/minute typically is sufficient; doses in excess of 40 mIU/minute rarely are effective when lower concentrations fail. As with labor induction, potential complications of uterine overstimulation include trauma of the mother or fetus due to forced passage through an incompletely dilated cervix, uterine rupture, and compromised fetal oxygenation due to decreased uterine perfusion. Oxytocin usually is effective when there is a prolonged latent phase of cervical dilation or when, in the absence of cephalo-pelvic disproportion, there is an arrest of dilation or descent.

Prevention/Treatment of Postpartum Hemorrhage

Postpartum hemorrhage is a significant problem in developed nations and is of even greater importance in developing countries. After delivery of the fetus or after therapeutic abortion, a firm, contracted uterus greatly reduces the incidence and extent of hemorrhage. Oxytocin (10 IU intramuscularly) often is given immediately after delivery to help maintain uterine contractions and tone. Alternatively, oxytocin (20 IU) is diluted in 1 L of intravenous solution and infused at a rate of 10 mL/minute until the uterus is contracted. The infusion rate then is reduced to 1-2 mL/minute until the mother is ready for transfer to the postpartum unit. Carbetocin, a longer-acting derivative of oxytocin, is under evaluation in clinical trials to prevent or treat postpartum hemorrhage; a dose of 100 μg is given intravenously (Leung et al., 2006).

Ergot alkaloids markedly increase the motor activity of the uterus. Although their capacity to induce sustained uterine tetany precludes their use in the induction or facilitation of labor, they are used to prevent or treat postpartum hemorrhage in normotensive women. In this setting, the preferred ergot alkaloids are ergonovine (ERGOTRATE) or its methyl analog methylergonovine (METHERGINE). They are administered intramuscularly or intravenously, exhibit rapid onsets of action (2-3 minutes intramuscularly, <1 minute intravenously), and their effects persist for 45 minutes to 3 hours depending on the route of administration. Adverse effects include nausea and vomiting, elevated blood pressure, and decreased pain threshold requiring analgesia.

Alternatively, the PGE_1 analog misoprostol (600 μg administered orally or sublingually) may be used off label to stimulate uterine contractions and prevent or treat postpartum hemorrhage. Although meta-analyses suggest that it may be slightly less effective than oxytocin, the low cost and lack of need for refrigeration or sterile needles may make misoprostol the preferred agent for use in developing nations. Other approaches under investigation include recombinant factor VIIa and balloon tamponade.

BIBLIOGRAPHY

Abalos E, Duley L, Steyn DW, Henderson-Smart DJ. Antihypertensive drug therapy for mild to moderate hypertension during pregnancy. *Cochrane Database Syst Rev,* **2007**, *24*:CD002252.

Altman D, Carroli G, Duley L, et al. Do women with pre-eclampsia, and their babies, benefit from magnesium sulphate? The Magpie Trial: A randomized placebo-controlled trial. *Lancet,* **2002**, *359*:1877–1890.

American Academy of Pediatrics Committee on Drugs. Transfer of drugs and other chemicals into human milk. *Pediatrics,* **2001**, *108*:776–789.

Barbieri RL. Update in female reproduction: A life-cycle approach. *J Clin Endocrinol Metab,* **2008**, *93*:2439–2446.

Brinton LA, Moghissi KS, Scoccia B, et al. Ovulation induction and cancer risk. *Fertil Steril,* **2005**, *83*:261–274.

Cheng L, Gülmezoglu AM, Piaggio G, et al. Interventions for emergency contraception. *Cochrane Database Syst Rev,* **2008**, *16*:CD001324.

Clark SL, Simpson KR, Knox GE, Garite TJ. Oxytocin: New perspectives on an old drug. *Am J Obstet Gynecol,* **2009**, *200*:35.e1–35.e6.

Cohen AL, Bhatnagar J, Reagan S. Toxic shock associated with *Clostridium sordellii* and *Clostridium perfringens* after medical and spontaneous abortion. *Obstet Gynecol,* **2007**, *110*:1027–1033.

Collaborative Group on Hormonal Factors in Breast Cancer. Breast cancer and hormonal contraceptives: Collaborative reanalysis of individual data on 53 297 women with breast cancer and 100 239 women without breast cancer from 54 epidemiological studies. *Lancet,* **1996**, *347*:1713–1727.

Elizur SE, Tualandi T. Drugs in infertility and fetal safety. *Fertil steril,* **2008**, *89*:1595–1602.

Erkkola R. New advances in hormonal contraception. *Curr Opin Obstet Gynecol,* **2007**, *19*:547–553.

Farquhar C. Endometriosis. *BMJ,* **2007**, *334*:249–253.

Fonseca EB, Celik E, Parra M, et al. Progesterone and the risk of preterm birth among women with a short cervix. *N Engl J Med,* **2007**, *357*:462–469.

Hale TW. Drug Therapy and breastfeeding: antibiotics, analgesics, and other medications. *Neo Reviews*, **2005**, *6*:233–240.

Iams JD, Romero R, Culhane JF, Goldenberg RL. Primary, secondary, and tertiary interventions to reduce the morbidity and mortality of preterm birth. *Lancet,* **2008**, *371*:164–175.

Ito S, Lee A. Drug excretion into breast milk—Overview. *Adv Drug Deliv Rev,* **2003**, *55*:617–627.

Kearns GL, Abdel-Rahman SM, Alander SW, et al. Developmental pharmacology—Drug disposition, action, and therapy in infants and children. *N Engl J Med,* **2003**, *349*: 1157–1167.

Kiley J, Hammond C. Combined oral contraceptives: A comprehensive review. *Clin Obstet Gynecol,* **2007**, *50*:868–877.

Lawrence LT, Moley KH. Epigenetics and assisted reproductive technologies: Human imprinting syndromes. *Semin Reprod Med,* **2008**, *26*:143–152.

Legro RS, Barnhart HX, Schlaff WD, et al. Clomiphene, metformin, or both for infertility in the polycystic ovary syndrome. *N Engl J Med,* **2007**, *356*:551–566.

Leung SW, Ng PS, Wong WY, Cheung TH. A randomised trial of carbetocin versus syntometrine in the management of the third stage of labour. *BJOG,* **2006**, *113*:1459–1464.

Macklon NS, Stouffer RL, Giudice LC, Fauser BC. The science behind 25 years of ovarian stimulation for in vitro fertilization. *Endocr Rev,* **2006**, *27*:170–207.

Mangoni JJ, Jackson SHD. Age-related changes in pharmacokinetics and pharmacodynamics: Basic principles and practical applications. *Br J Clin Pharmacol,* **2003**, *57*:6–14.

Mansour D. Modern management of abnormal uterine bleeding: The levonorgestrel intra-uterine system. *Best Pract Res Clin Obstet Gynaecol,* **2007**, *21*:1007–1021.

Marchbanks P, McDonald J, Wilson H. Oral contraceptives and the risk of breast cancer. *N Engl J Med,* **2002**, *346*:2025–2032.

Martin KA, Chang RJ, Ehrmann DA, et al. Evaluation and treatment of hirsutism in premenopausal women: An Endocrine Society Clinical Practice Guideline. *J Clin Endocrinol Metab,* **2008**, *93*:1105–1120.

Maynard S, Epstein FH, Karumanchi SA. Preeclampsia and angiogenic balance. *Annu Rev Med,* **2008**, *59*:61–78.

Meis PJ, Klebanoff M, Thorn E, et al. Prevention of recurrent preterm delivery by 17 alpha-hydroxyprogesterone caproate. *N Engl J Med,* **2003**, *348*:2379–2385.

National High Blood Pressure Education Program Working Group. Report of the National High Blood Pressure Education Program Working Group on High Blood Pressure in Pregnancy. *Am J Obstet Gynecol,* **2000**, *183*:S1–S22.

Nelson HD. Menopause. *Lancet,* **2008**, *371*:760–770.

Niemitz EL, Feinberg AP. Epigenetics and assisted reproductive technology: A call for investigation. *Am J Hum Genet,* **2004**, *74*:599–609.

Olive DL. Gonadotropin-releasing hormone agonists for endometriosis. *N Engl J Med,* **2008**, *359*:1136–1142.

Podymow T, August P. Update on the use of antihypertensive drugs in pregnancy. *Hypertension,* **2008**, *51*:960–969.

Rapp SR, Espeland MA, Shumaker SA, et al. Effect of estrogen plus progestin on global cognitive function in postmenopausal women: The Women's Health Initiative Memory Study: A randomized controlled trial. *JAMA,* **2003**, *289*:2663–2672.

Rebarber A, Istwan NB, Russo-Stieglitz K, et al. Increased incidence of gestational diabetes in women receiving prophylactic 17α-hydroxyprogesterone caproate for prevention of recurrent preterm delivery. *Diabetes Care*, **2007**, *30*:2277–2280.

Rossouw JE, Anderson GL, Prentice RL, et al. Risks and benefits of estrogen plus progestin in healthy postmenopausal women: Principal results from the Women's Health Initiative randomized controlled trial. *JAMA,* **2002**, *288*: 321–333.

Rossouw JE, Prentice RL, Manson JE, et al. Postmenopausal hormone therapy and risk of cardiovascular disease by age and years since menopause. *JAMA,* **2007**, *297*:1465–1477.

Shumaker SA, Legault C, Rapp SR, et al. Estrogen plus progestin and the incidence of dementia and mild cognitive impairment in postmenopausal women: The Women's Health Initiative Memory Study: A randomized controlled trial. *JAMA,* **2003**, *289*:2651–2662.

Simhan HN, Caritis SN. Prevention of preterm delivery. *N Engl J Med,* **2007**, *357*:477–487.

Thessaloniki ESHRE/ASRM-Sponsored PCOS Consensus Workshop Group. Consensus on infertility treatment related to polycystic ovary syndrome. *Fertil Steril,* **2008**, *89*:505–522.

Van Voorhis BJ. In vitro fertilization. *N Engl J Med,* **2007**, *356*:379–386.

Wierman ME, Basson R, Davis SR, et al. Androgen therapy in women: An Endocrine Society Clinical Practice guideline. *J Clin Endocrinol Metab,* **2006**, *91*:3697–3710.

Workowski KA, Berman SM. Centers for Disease Control and Prevention. Sexually transmitted diseases treatment guidelines, 2006. *MMWR Recomm Rep,* **2006**, *55*:1–94.

Environmental Toxicology: Carcinogens and Heavy Metals

Michael C. Byrns
and Trevor M. Penning

Humans are exposed to chemicals from their environment daily. Fortunately, mammals have evolved mechanisms to protect themselves from toxic effects of many exogenous chemicals, including the xenobiotic transport and metabolic mechanisms described in Chapters 4-7. While the human body is relatively well adapted to deal with xenobiotics, there are situations in which such environmental agents may cause significant toxicity. The industrial revolution and the development of chemical industries have increased human exposures to chemicals that were previously infrequent or absent. Occupational exposures to xenobiotics are of particular concern because workers often will be exposed to specific chemicals at concentrations that are orders of magnitude higher than those to which the general population is exposed. Increasing concern about environmental toxicants has stimulated interest and research in environmental toxicology, the study of how chemicals in our environment adversely affect human health, and in occupational toxicology, the study of how chemicals in the workplace affect human health. Myriad authoritative textbooks are available in these areas. This chapter does not attempt a thorough coverage; rather, it sets forth a few basic principles, briefly discusses carcinogens and chemoprevention, and then focuses on the pharmacotherapy of heavy metal intoxication.

ENVIRONMENTAL RISK ASSESSMENT AND RISK MANAGEMENT

When assessing the risks of environmental exposures to xenobiotics, many of the same principles discussed in Chapter 4 for drug toxicity apply; there are, however, significant differences. With environmental exposures, one has to consider population exposures to low-dose toxicants over long periods of time. Thus, one must give more attention to the low end of the dose-response curve, using experiments based on chronic exposures. Particular attention is given to the potential for individuals with higher susceptibility. Unlike drugs, which are given to treat a specific disease and will have benefits that outweigh the risks, environmental toxicants usually are only harmful. In addition, exposures to environmental toxicants usually are involuntary, there is uncertainty about the severity of their effects, and people are much less willing to accept their associated risks.

Two complimentary approaches are used to predict the toxic effects of environmental exposures: epidemiology and toxicology. Epidemiologists monitor health effects in humans and use statistics to associate those effects with exposure to an environmental stress, such as a toxicant. Toxicologists perform laboratory studies to try to understand the potential toxic mechanisms of a chemical to predict whether it is likely to be toxic to humans. Each of these approaches has strengths and weaknesses, and information from both is integrated into environmental risk assessment. Risk assessment is used to develop management approaches, such as laws and regulations, to limit exposures to environmental toxicants to a level that is considered safe.

Epidemiological Approaches to Risk Assessment

Epidemiologists use multiple approaches to assess the risks of human environmental exposures (Gordis, 2008). The disadvantage of these approaches is the variability between people in their exposures and genetics, which results in confounding effects. Epidemiologists cannot control the environment or the genetics of the populations being studied. For example, generally individuals are simultaneously exposed to more than one environmental toxicant.

Because of the difficulties in assessing human exposures and the long times required to clinically observe effects on health, epidemiologists rely on biomarkers in risk assessment. There are three different types of biomarkers: biomarkers of *exposure*, biomarkers of *toxicity*, and biomarkers of *susceptibility*. Biomarkers of exposure usually are measurements of toxicants or their metabolites in blood, urine, or hair. Blood and urine concentrations measure recent exposures, while hair levels measure exposure over a period of months.

An example of an unusual exposure biomarker is X-ray fluorescent measurement of bone lead levels, which estimates lifetime exposure to lead. Biomarkers of toxicity are used to measure toxic effects at a subclinical level and include measurement of liver enzymes in the serum, changes in the quantity or contents of urine, and performance on specialized exams for neurological or cognitive function. Biomarkers of susceptibility are used to predict which individuals are likely to develop toxicity in response to a given chemical. Examples include single nucleotide polymorphisms in genes for metabolizing enzymes involved in the activation or detoxification of a toxicant. Some biomarkers simultaneously provide information on exposure, toxicity, and susceptibility. For example, the measurement in the urine of N7-guanine adducts from aflatoxin B_1 provides evidence of both exposure and a toxic effect (in this case, DNA damage). These types of biomarkers are particularly valuable because they can support a proposed mechanism of toxicity.

Several types of epidemiological studies are used to assess risks, each with its own set of strengths and weaknesses. Ecological studies correlate frequencies of exposures and health outcomes between different geographical regions. These studies are inexpensive and can detect rare outcomes but are prone to confounding variables, including population migration. Cross-sectional studies examine the prevalence of exposures and outcomes at a single point in time. Such studies are an inexpensive way to determine an association but do not provide a temporal relationship and are not effective for establishing causality. They also can be subject to bias, as a perceived health outcome might cause someone to eliminate his exposure. Case-control studies start with a group of individuals affected by a disease, which then is matched to another group of unaffected individuals for known confounding variables. Questionnaires often are used to evaluate past exposures. This method also is relatively inexpensive and is good for examining rare outcomes because the endpoint is known. However, case-control studies rely on assessments of past exposures that often are unreliable and can be subject to bias. Prospective cohort studies measure exposures in a large group of people and follow that group for a long time to measure health outcomes. These studies are not as susceptible to confounding variables and bias and are good at establishing causality. However, they are extremely expensive, particularly when measuring very rare outcomes, because a large study population is required to observe sufficient disease to obtain statistical significance. One of the key types of human studies used in drug development is the randomized clinical trial (discussed in Chapter 1). These studies cannot be used to directly measure the effects of environmental toxicants (for obvious ethical reasons) but can be used to examine the effectiveness of an interventional strategy for reducing both exposure and disease.

Toxicological Approaches to Risk Assessment

Toxicologists use model systems, including experimental animals, to examine the toxicity of chemicals and predict their effect on humans (Faustman and Omenn, 2008). The significance of these model systems to human health is not always established. Toxicologists also test chemicals at the high end of the dose-response curve in order to see enough occurrences of an outcome to obtain statistical significance. As a result, there often is uncertainty about the effects of very low doses of chemicals. To determine the applicability of model studies, toxicologists study the mechanisms involved in the toxic effects of chemicals, with the goal of predicting whether that mechanism would occur in humans.

To predict the toxic effects of environmental chemicals, toxicologists perform subchronic (3 months of treatment for rodents) and chronic studies (2 years for rodents) in at least two different animal models. Subchronic experiments provide a model for occupational exposures, while chronic experiments are used to predict effects from lifetime exposures to chemicals in food or the environment. Doses for these studies are based on shorter preliminary studies, with the goal of having one concentration that does not have a significant effect, one concentration that results in statistically significant toxicity at the low end of the dose-response curve, and one or more concentrations that will have moderate-to-high levels of toxicity. A theoretical dose-response curve for an animal study is shown in Figure 67–1. An animal study provides two numbers that estimate the risk from a chemical. The *no observed adverse effect level* (NOAEL) is the highest dose used that does not result in a statistically significant increase in negative health outcomes. The *lowest observed adverse effect level* (LOAEL) is the lowest dose that results in a significant increase in toxicity. The NOAEL is divided by 10 for each source of uncertainty to determine a reference dose (RfD), which is commonly used as a starting point for determining regulations on human exposures to chemicals. The modifiers used to determine the RfD are based on the uncertainties between the experimental and

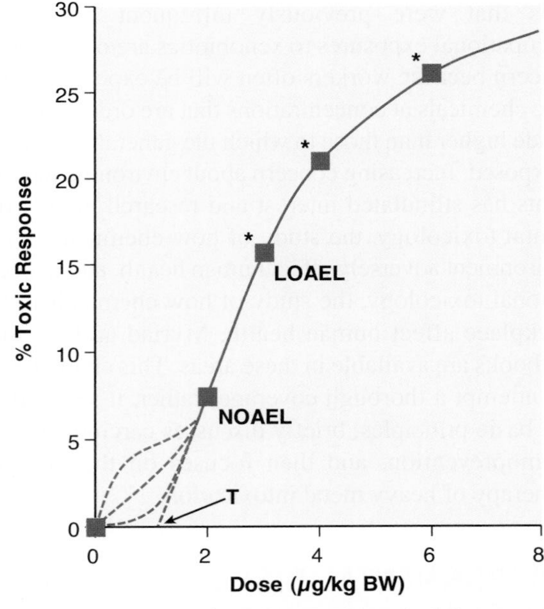

Figure 67–1. *LOAEL and NOAEL.* The theoretical dose-response curve from an animal study demonstrates the *no observed adverse effect level* (NOAEL) and the *lowest observed adverse effect level* (LOAEL). Below the NOAEL level, there is considerable uncertainty as to the shape of the response curve. It could continue linearly to reach a threshold dose (T) where there would be no harmful effects from the toxicant, or it could have a number of different possible inflection points. Each of these curves would have very different impacts on human populations. *Statistically significant.

human exposure. The most common modifiers used are for interspecies variability (human to animal) and interindividual variability (human to human), in which case RfD = NOAEL/100. Other modifiers can be used to account for specific experimental uncertainties. When a NOAEL is unavailable, a LOAEL may be used, in which case another 10-fold uncertainty factor is used. The use of factors of 10 in the denominator for determination of RfD is an application of the "precautionary principle," which attempts to limit human exposure by assuming a worst-case scenario for each unknown variable (Faustman and Omenn, 2008).

A major concern with animal studies is that they do not detect effects at low concentrations. Typically, they are designed to obtain statistical significance with a 10% increase in an outcome. As a result, there is considerable uncertainty about what occurs below that level, as demonstrated in Figure 67–1. Toxicologists often assume that there is a threshold dose (T), below which there is no toxicity. This condition is true when there are cellular defenses that prevent toxicity at concentrations below a given level but that can be overwhelmed. Thresholds usually are observed when the toxic effects of a chemical are the result of direct cell death. Many carcinogens and other toxicants with specific molecular targets (e.g., lead) do not exhibit a threshold. Ideally, mechanistic studies should be done to predict which dose-response curve is most likely to fit a given chemical.

Toxicologists perform a variety of mechanistic studies to understand how a chemical might cause toxicity. Computer modeling using a compound's three-dimensional structure to determine quantitative structure-activity relationships (QSARs) is commonly performed on both drugs and environmental chemicals. QSAR approaches can determine which chemicals are likely to exhibit toxicities or bind to specific molecular targets. Cell-based approaches in prokaryotes and eukaryotes are used to determine whether a compound damages DNA or causes cytotoxicity. DNA damage and the resulting mutagenesis often are determined with the Ames test. The Ames test uses *Salmonella typhimurium* strains with specific mutations in the gene needed to synthesize histidine. These strains are treated with chemicals in the presence or absence of a metabolic activating system, usually the supernatant fraction from homogenized rat liver. If a compound is a mutagen in the Ames test, it reverts the mutation in the histidine operon and allows the bacteria to form colonies on plates with limited histidine. Gene chip microarrays assess gene expression in cells or tissues from animals treated with a toxicant and provide a very useful tool to identify the molecular targets and pathways altered by toxicant exposures. The susceptibility of knockout mice to a toxicant can help to determine whether the knocked-out genes are involved in the metabolic activation and detoxification of a given toxicant.

Integrated Risk Assessment and Risk Management

Regulatory bodies at local, state, national, and international levels all are involved in limiting the adverse effects of chemicals. In the U.S., several federal agencies are involved, depending on the source of the exposure. The U.S. Food and Drug Administration (FDA) regulates the safety of drugs, the food supply, cosmetics, and now tobacco products. The Occupational Safety and Health Administration (OSHA) regulates workplace exposures. The U.S. Environmental Protection Agency (EPA) regulates exposures from other environmental sources, particularly the air and water. Regulators use epidemiological and toxicological data to estimate the risks from an exposure and come up with a level they consider to be reasonably safe. Regulators can nominate toxicants for a comprehensive study by the National Toxicology Program if there are insufficient toxicological data. The final stages of risk assessment and risk management are not based entirely on science; politics and economics also help determine which regulations are enacted. Ultimately, the social, economic, and political benefits predicted to result from limiting human exposure to a given toxicant are weighed against the corresponding costs.

Interventions for Environmental Exposure: Pharmacology and Prevention

There is considerable interest in pharmacological approaches to prevent disease from environmental exposures. However, pharmacological interventions for chronic environmental exposures remain more of a goal than a reality. There are numerous hurdles for treatment of exposure to environmental toxicants. Because exposures occur over long periods of time, treatments must reverse existing preclinical toxicities or provide protection for a long time. If a pharmaceutical is to be given chronically or in the absence of disease, the extent of side effects and toxicity should be much less than for a drug being given acutely to treat disease. Currently, the most effective approaches for preventing diseases associated with chronic exposures to chemicals are primary prevention and nutrition. Pharmaceuticals can be useful for preventive strategies against chronic exposures (e.g., nicotine replacement therapy in smoking cessation). Ongoing research also is examining pharmacological approaches to prevent cancer in humans exposed to chemical carcinogens. One class of environmental toxicant for which there are drugs available to prevent disease is metals. However, in general, these drugs, known as metal chelators, are only effective against acute, high-dose metal exposure and either have no effect, or actually worsen, toxicity under the low-dose chronic exposures most commonly encountered from the environment.

CARCINOGENS AND CHEMOPREVENTION

Carcinogenesis

Many environmental compounds increase the risk of developing cancer; these chemicals are called carcinogens (Wogan et al., 2004; Klaunig and Kamendulis, 2008). The International Agency for Research on Cancer (IARC) classifies compounds into groups based on risk assessments using human, animal, and mechanism data. Chemicals in group 1 are known human carcinogens;

Table 67–1

Examples of Important Carcinogens[a]

CARCINOGEN CLASS	EXAMPLE	SOURCE	MECHANISM
Genotoxic			
Nitrosamines	Nicotine-derived nitrosaminoketone (NNK)	Tobacco products	Metabolic activation to form DNA adducts
Polycyclic aromatic hydrocarbons	Benzo[a]pyrene	Fossil fuel combustion, tobacco smoke, charbroiled food	Metabolic activation to form DNA adducts or ROS
Aromatic amines	2-Aminonaphthalene	Dyes	Metabolic activation to form DNA adducts
Fungal toxins	Aflatoxin B_1	Corn, peanuts, and other food	Metabolic activation to form DNA adducts
Non-genotoxic			
Liver toxicants	Ethanol	Beverages, environment	Toxicity and compensatory proliferation; depletion of GSH
Phorbol esters	Tetradecanoyl phorbol acetate	Horticulture; rubber and gasoline production	Activation of PKC isoforms
Estrogens	Diethylstilbestrol	Drugs, environment	Activation of estrogen-receptor signaling
Metals	Arsenic	Environment, occupation	Inhibition of DNA repair; activation of signal transduction pathways
Irritants	Asbestos	Environment, occupation	Stimulation of inflammation; formation of ROS
Dioxins	TCDD	Waste incineration, herbicides, paper-pulp bleaching	Activation of the aryl hydrocarbon receptor

[a]Compounds in this table are classified as group 1 carcinogens by the International Agency for Research on Cancer (IARC), with the exception of the phorbol esters, which have not been examined. TCDD, 2,3,7,8 tetrachlorodibenzo-p-dioxin; ROS, reactive oxygen species; GSH, glutathione; PKC, protein kinase C.

group 2A includes chemicals that probably are carcinogenic in humans; group 2B chemicals possibly are carcinogenic in humans; group 3 chemicals lack data to suggest a role in carcinogenesis; and group 4 are those with data indicating they are unlikely to be carcinogens. Some important group 1 carcinogens and their sources are given in Table 67–1.

The transformation of a normal cell to a malignancy is a multi-stage process, and exogenous chemicals can act at one or more of these stages (Figure 67–2). A classic model of chemical carcinogenesis is tumor initiation followed by tumor promotion. In this model, a tumor initiator causes gene mutations that increase the ability of cells to proliferate and avoid apoptosis. A tumor promoter does not directly modify genes but changes signaling pathways and/or the extracellular environment to cause initiated cells to proliferate, invade surrounding tissue, and increase access to blood vessels. Although this model is an oversimplification of the many processes of carcinogenesis, it demonstrates the types of changes that must occur to transit a normal cell into tumorigenesis.

Chemical carcinogens cause cancer through genotoxic and non-genotoxic mechanisms (Figure 67–2). Genotoxic carcinogens induce tumor formation through damage to DNA. Typically, genotoxic carcinogens undergo metabolism in a target tissue to a reactive intermediate. This reactive intermediate can directly damage DNA via covalent reaction to form a DNA adduct. Alternatively, it can indirectly damage DNA through the formation of reactive oxygen species (ROS), which can oxidize DNA or form lipid peroxidation products that react with DNA (Mena et al., 2009).

Benzo[a]pyrene, a key carcinogen in tobacco smoke, is an example of a genotoxic carcinogen that forms both direct DNA adducts and ROS. Benzo[a]pyrene is oxidized by CYPs to a 7,8-dihydrodiol, which represents a proximate carcinogen (a more carcinogenic metabolite). This metabolite can either undergo a second oxidation step by a CYP to form a diol epoxide, which readily reacts with DNA, or it can undergo oxidation by aldo-keto reductases to form a catechol, which will redox cycle to form ROS (Conney, 1982; Penning, 2009).

If DNA damage from a genotoxic carcinogen is not repaired prior to DNA replication, a mutation can result. If this mutation is in a key tumor suppressor gene or proto-oncogene, it provides advantages in proliferation or survival. Alternatively, if the mutation is in a DNA repair gene, the mutation increases the probability that other mutations will occur. Given mutations in enough key genes and the

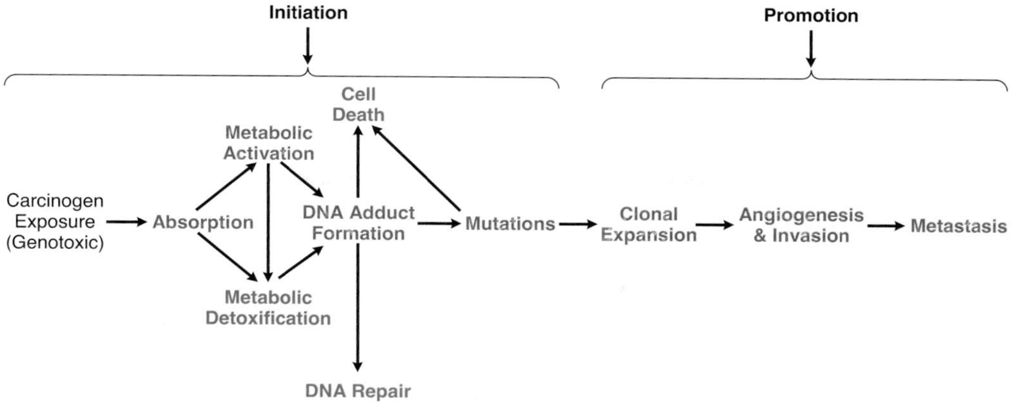

Figure 67–2. *Carcinogenesis: initiation and promotion.* There are many steps that occur between the exposure to a genotoxic carcinogen and the development of cancer. Processes in red lead to the development of cancer, while those in green reduce the risk. Non-genotoxic carcinogens act by enhancing steps leading to cancer and/or inhibiting protective processes. A chemopreventive agent acts by inhibiting steps leading to cancer or by increasing protective processes.

right environment, a cell will proliferate faster than surrounding normal cells and possibly develop into malignant cancer. Genotoxic carcinogens are tumor initiators.

Non-genotoxic carcinogens increase the incidence of cancer without damaging DNA. There are a number of possible non-genotoxic mechanisms, most of which are classified as tumor promotion. Many non-genotoxic carcinogens bind to receptors that stimulate proliferation or other tumor-promoting effects, such as tissue invasion or angiogenesis. For example, phorbol esters mimic diacylglycerol and activate PKC isoforms. This in turn stimulates MAP kinase pathways, leading to proliferation, invasiveness, and angiogenesis (see Chapter 3). In most normal cells, prolonged activation of this pathway stimulates apoptosis, but cells with defective apoptotic mechanisms due to preceding mutation(s) are resistant to this effect. Estrogenic carcinogens activate estrogen receptor-α (ERα) and stimulate proliferation and invasiveness of estrogen responsive cells. Chronic inflammation is another mechanism of non-genotoxic carcinogenesis. Like phorbol esters, inflammatory cytokines stimulate PKC signaling, leading to proliferation, invasiveness, and angiogenesis. Irritants such as asbestos are examples of carcinogens that work through inflammation. Chronic exposure to hepatotoxic chemicals (or chronic liver diseases) also causes non-genotoxic carcinogenesis by stimulating compensatory proliferation to repair the liver damage. This damage and repair process increases the likelihood of DNA damage becoming a mutation, causes chronic inflammation, and selects for cells that proliferate faster or are less sensitive to apoptosis.

Tumor initiation also may occur through non-genotoxic mechanisms. For example, some heavy metals do not directly react with DNA but interfere with proteins involved in DNA synthesis and repair, increasing the likelihood that an error will be made during replication. Non-genotoxic carcinogens also can cause heritable changes to gene expression by altering the methylation state of cytosines in 5′-CpG-3 islands of gene promoters, thus acting as tumor initiators. Methylation can silence tumor suppressor genes, while demethylation of proto-oncogenes can increase their expression.

Chemoprevention

Drugs that interfere with the carcinogenic process to prevent cancer before it is diagnosed are termed chemopreventive agents (Szabo, 2006; William et al., 2009). The chemoprevention concept was pioneered during the 1960s by Wattenberg and others, who observed that dietary constituents, such as *t*-butyl hydroquinone, could prevent cancer in rodents (Wattenberg, 1966). Chemoprevention strategies often are based on epidemiological studies on nutrition, where there are many examples of clear protective effects of plant-based foods and drinks on the incidence of various types of cancer (Fahey and Kensler, 2007). By isolating the active compounds from protective plants, researchers hope to understand their protective mechanisms and develop drugs to prevent cancer. Chemoprevention is an emerging field; a number of compounds for the prevention of cancer are in clinical trials (Table 67–2). There currently are no drugs approved for chemoprevention of environmental carcinogenesis, but there

Table 67–2

Chemopreventive Agents Being Studied in Humans

CHEMOPREVENTIVE CLASS	EXAMPLE COMPOUND	NATURAL SOURCE OR TYPE OF DRUG	CANCER TYPE(S)	MECHANISM	CURRENT STATUS
Isothiocyanates	Phenethyl isothiocyanate	Cruciferous vegetables	Liver, lung, breast, etc.	↓CYP, ↑GSH, ↑NQO1, ↑apoptosis	Phase 2 clinical trials
Synthetic drugs that modify metabolism	Oltipraz	Anti-schistosomal drug	Liver, lung	↓CYP, ↑GSH, ↑NQO1	Beneficial effects on biomarkers in phase 2 clinical trials
Flavonoids and other polyphenols	Catechin	Green tea, red wine, berries, etc.	Lung, cervical, etc.	↓ROS, ↓CYP, ↑GSH, ↑NQO1	Phase 2 clinical trials
Other plant compounds	Curcumin	Turmeric (curry)	Colorectal, pancreatic, etc.	↓ROS, ↓CYP, ↑GSH, ↑NQO1	Phase 2 clinical trials
Other plant compounds	Chlorophyllin	All plants	Liver	Reaction with active intermediates, ↓ROS, ↓CYP	Beneficial effects on biomarkers in phase 2 clinical trials
Other antioxidants	α-Tocopherol (vitamin E)	Food	Prostate	Antioxidant, anti-inflammatory	Phase 3 clinical trials
Anti-hormonal therapies	Tamoxifen	Adjuvant for breast cancer	Breast	Inhibit ERα in breast	FDA-approved for chemoprevention
NSAIDs (see chapter 34)	Aspirin	Anti-inflammatory drugs	Colorectal, etc.	Inhibit PG formation	Phase 3 trials
COX-2 selective inhibitors (see Chapter 34)	Celecoxib	Anti-inflammatory drugs	Colorectal, etc.	Inhibit PG formation	Phase 3 trial found ↓cancer but unacceptable side effects for prevention

CYP, cytochrome P450; GSH, glutathione; NQO1, quinone reductase; ROS, reactive oxygen species; ERα, estrogen receptor-α; FDA, U.S. Food and Drug Administration; NSAIDs, nonsteroidal anti-inflammatory drugs; COX-2, cyclooxygenase-2; PG, prostaglandin.

are approved drugs to prevent carcinogenesis due to endogenous estrogen (tamoxifen and raloxifene) and viruses (hepatitis B and human papillomavirus vaccines).

Chemopreventive agents interfere with the processes of initiation and promotion (Figure 67–2). One mechanism of anti-initiation is prevention of carcinogen activation. Isothiocyanates and similar compounds inhibit CYPs involved in activating many carcinogens and also upregulate genes controlled by the antioxidant response element (ARE); the ARE-responsive group includes γ-glutamylcysteine synthase light chain (the gene responsible for the rate-determining step in GSH synthesis) and quinone reductase (NQO1). Increased expression of ARE-regulated genes is predicted to increase the detoxification of proximate carcinogens. Isothiocyanates also stimulate apoptosis of p53-deficient cells via the formation of cytotoxic DNA adducts. Compounds that act as antioxidants may provide protection because many carcinogens work through the generation of ROS. Some compounds simultaneously prevent carcinogen activation and act as antioxidants. For example, flavonoids and other polyphenols found in a wide variety of plants are potent antioxidants that inhibit CYPs and induce expression of ARE-regulated genes. Chlorophyll and other compounds can protect against carcinogens by binding to or reacting with carcinogens or their metabolites and prevent them from reaching their molecular target.

Inflammation is a potential target for chemoprevention through interference with promotion. The COX-2 inhibitor celecoxib (described in Chapter 34) has been tested in phase 3 studies that demonstrated efficacy at reducing the risk of colorectal cancer. However, this benefit was offset by an increased risk of death due to cardiovascular events, forcing the early termination of the trial (William et al., 2009). Studies examining long-term treatment with aspirin for cardiovascular benefits found that aspirin also reduces the incidence of colorectal adenomas. A phase 3 clinical trial is under way to examine this effect. Natural compounds, such as α-tocopherol, also can exert chemoprevention by reducing inflammation.

One successful approach to chemoprevention is modification of nuclear receptor signaling. Promising preliminary data suggested that retinoids might be beneficial for preventing lung and other cancers. Retinoids reduce the incidence of head and neck cancers, which represented one of the first successful uses of chemoprevention in humans (William et al., 2009; Evans and Kaye, 1999). Retinoids also are effective for the treatment of acute promyelocytic leukemia (see Section VII). However, in large clinical trials, retinoids actually increased the incidence of lung cancer, particularly among women, and had other unacceptable toxicities (Omenn et al., 1996).

The selective ER modulators tamoxifen and raloxifene reduced the incidence of breast cancer in high-risk women in large phase 3 clinical trials and are approved for chemoprevention in these patients (Vogel et al., 2006). The success of selective estrogen-receptor modulators for chemoprevention provides a proof-of-principle that the development of compounds based on mechanistic predictions can lead to effective drugs for the prevention of cancer.

Aflatoxin B_1. Promising agents are being developed as chemopreventants of hepatocarcinogenesis mediated by aflatoxin B_1. Aflatoxins are produced by *Aspergillus flavus*, a fungus that is a common contaminant of foods, especially corn, peanuts, cottonseed, and tree nuts. *A. flavus* is abundant in regions with hot and wet climates, and as a result, hepatocellular carcinoma is a serious problem in subtropical and tropical regions of Latin America, Africa, and Southeast Asia. Human exposure to aflatoxin in the U.S. is very rare and not thought to have a significant impact on health (IARC, 2002).

Absorption, Distribution, Biotransformation, and Excretion. Aflatoxin B_1 is readily absorbed from the GI tract and initially distributed to the liver, where it undergoes extensive first-pass metabolism (Guengerich et al., 1996). Aflatoxin B_1 is metabolized by CYPs, including 1A2 and 3A4, to yield either an 8.9-epoxide or products hydroxylated at the 9 position (aflatoxin M_1) or 3 position (aflatoxin Q_1; Figure 67–3). The hydroxylation products are less susceptible to epoxidation and are therefore detoxification products. The 8,9-epoxide is highly reactive toward DNA and is the reactive intermediate responsible for aflatoxin carcinogenesis. The 8,9-epoxide is short lived and undergoes detoxification via non-enzymatic hydrolysis or conjugation with GSH. Aflatoxin M_1 enters the circulation and is excreted in urine and milk. Hydroxylated aflatoxin metabolites also can undergo several additional phase 1 and phase 2 metabolic pathways prior to excretion in urine or bile.

Toxicity. Aflatoxin B_1 primarily targets the liver, although it also is toxic to the GI tract and hematological system. High-dose exposures result in acute necrosis of the liver, leading to jaundice and, in many cases, death. Acute toxicity from aflatoxin is relatively rare in humans and requires consumption of milligram quantities of aflatoxin per day for multiple weeks. An outbreak in Kenya in 2004 led to 317 cases and 125 deaths (Groopman et al., 2008). Humans seem to be relatively resistant to acute aflatoxicosis; human outbreaks usually are preceded by the deaths of dogs and other domestic animals. Chronic exposure to aflatoxins results in cirrhosis of the liver and immunosuppression.

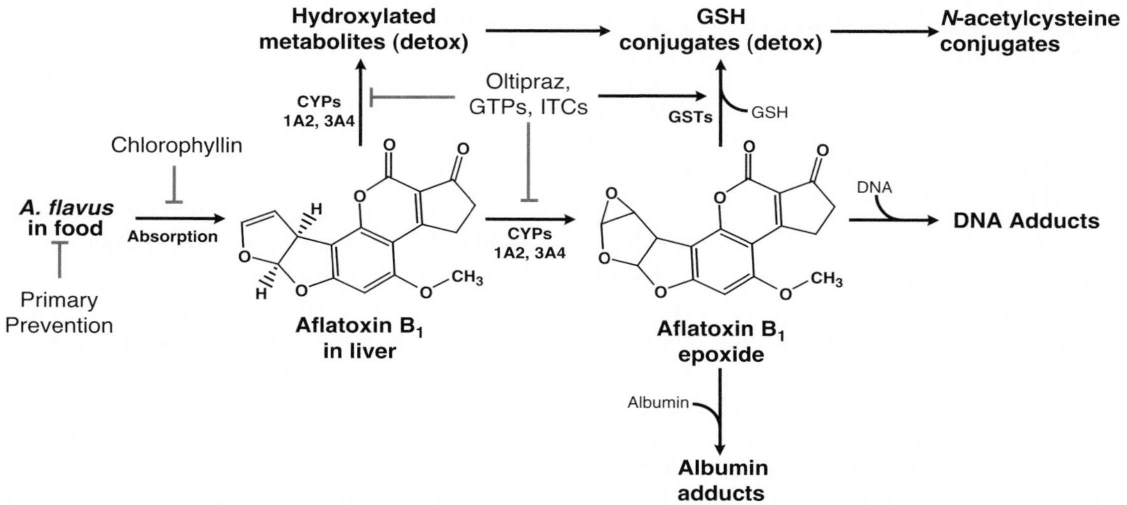

Figure 67–3. *Metabolism and actions of aflatoxin B_1.* Following absorption, aflatoxin B_1 undergoes activation by CYPs to its 8,9-epoxide, which can be detoxified by glutathione S-transferases (GSTs) or by spontaneous hydration. Alternatively, it can react with cellular macromolecules such as DNA and protein, leading to toxicity and cancer. Oltipraz, green tea polyphenols (GTPs), and isothiocyanates (ITCs) decrease aflatoxin carcinogenesis by inhibiting the CYPs involved in activating aflatoxin and increasing the synthesis of the cofactor GSH for GSTs involved in detoxification.

Carcinogenicity. The primary concern with human exposure to aflatoxins is the development of liver cancer. Based on increased incidence of hepatocellular carcinoma in humans exposed to aflatoxin and supporting animal data, IARC has classified aflatoxin B_1 and several other natural aflatoxins as known human carcinogens (group 1) (IARC, 2002). Aflatoxin exposure and hepatitis B virus work synergistically to cause hepatocellular carcinoma. Many of the regions with elevated aflatoxin exposure also have a high level of endemic hepatitis B infection. Separately, aflatoxin or hepatitis B exposure increases the risk of hepatocellular carcinoma 3.4- or 7.3-fold, respectively; those exposed to both have a 59-fold increased risk of cancer compared to unexposed individuals (Groopman et al., 2005).

The mechanism of aflatoxin carcinogenesis has been extensively studied (IARC, 2002). The 8,9-epoxide of aflatoxin B_1 readily reacts with amines in biological macromolecules. Aflatoxin B_1 8,9-epoxide forms adducts with deoxyguanosine and albumin that can be detected in the blood or urine of humans and laboratory animals exposed to aflatoxin, providing evidence for the activity of this pathway *in vivo*. Aflatoxin primarily forms DNA adducts at deoxyguanosine residues, reacting at either the N1 or N7 position. The N7-guanine adduct mispairs with adenine, leading to G $\rightarrow$ T transversions. Human aflatoxin exposure is associated with hepatocellular carcinomas bearing an AGG to AGT mutation in codon 249 of the p53 tumor suppressor gene, resulting in the replacement of an arginine with cysteine. This mutation is almost never observed in geographical regions with limited aflatoxin exposure (Hussain et al., 2007).

The interaction between aflatoxin and hepatitis B that is responsible for the increased incidence of hepatocellular carcinoma is not well understood (Sylla et al., 1999). Hepatitis B influences the metabolism of aflatoxin B_1 by upregulating CYPs, including 3A4, and decreasing glutathione S-transferase activity. In addition, hepatocellular proliferation to repair damage done by hepatitis B infection increases the likelihood that aflatoxin-induced DNA adducts will cause mutations. The hepatotoxic and tumor-promoting effects of hepatitis B also could provide a more favorable environment for the proliferation and invasion of initiated cells.

Chemoprevention of Aflatoxin-Induced Hepatocellular Carcinoma. The clear relationship between aflatoxin metabolism and its carcinogenicity makes it an appealing target for chemopreventive strategies that modify its metabolism (Groopman et al., 2008; Kensler et al., 2004). Inhibiting CYP activity or increasing glutathione conjugation will reduce the intracellular concentration of the 8,9-epoxide and thus prevent DNA adduct formation. One drug that has been tested as a modifier of aflatoxin metabolism is oltipraz. Oltipraz is an antischistosomal drug that potently inhibits CYPs and induces genes regulated by the ARE. In a phase 2 clinical trial, a 125-mg/day dose of oltipraz increased the excretion of aflatoxin *N*-acetylcysteine, indicating enhanced glutathione conjugation of the epoxide. At 500 mg/wk, oltipraz reduced the levels of aflatoxin M_1, consistent with inhibition of CYP activity.

Green tea polyphenols also have been used to modify aflatoxin metabolism in exposed human populations. Individuals receiving a daily dose of 500 or 1000 mg (equivalent to 1 or 2 L of green tea) demonstrated a small decline in the formation of aflatoxin–albumin adducts and a large increase in the excretion of aflatoxin *N*-acetylcysteine, consistent with a protective effect. A third approach to modifying aflatoxin metabolism has been to use a broccoli sprout tea containing high levels of the isothiocyanate *R*-sulforaphane. Because of interindividual variation in the absorption of *R*-sulforaphane, the protocol did not significantly alter aflatoxin biomarkers. However, there was a significant inverse correlation between excretion of sulforaphane metabolites in the urine and the levels of aflatoxin–N7-guanine adducts.

Yet another approach used for the chemoprevention of aflatoxin hepatocarcinogenesis is the use of "interceptor molecules." Chlorophyllin, an over-the-counter mixture of water-soluble chlorophyll salts, binds tightly to aflatoxin in the GI tract, forming a complex that is not absorbed. *In vitro*, chlorophyllin inhibits CYP activity and acts as an antioxidant. Oral doses are poorly absorbed *in vivo*, so the agent remains largely in the GI tract. In a phase 2 trial, administration of 100 mg of chlorophyllin with each meal reduced aflatoxin–N7-guanine adduct levels in the urine by >50% (Egner et al., 2001).

Chemoprevention of hepatocellular carcinoma in people exposed to aflatoxin also can be achieved by limiting infections with hepatitis B. Because of the strong interaction between hepatitis B and aflatoxin in carcinogenesis, the hepatitis B vaccine will reduce the sensitivity of people to the induction of cancer by aflatoxin. Primary prevention of aflatoxin exposure through hand or fluorescent sorting of crops to remove those with fungal contamination can also reduce human exposure. A more cost-effective primary prevention approach is to improve food storage to limit the spread of *A. flavus*, which requires a warm and humid environment.

METALS

Metals are an important class of environmental toxicantsl; they are ubiquitous environmental contaminants that come from both natural and anthropogenic sources. Various toxic metals play important roles in many industrial processes and are occupational health hazards and common pollutants. The top three substances of concern due to their toxicity and likelihood of human exposure as listed under the Comprehensive Environmental Response, Compensation, and Liability Act (CERCLA, also known as Superfund) are arsenic, lead, and mercury. The toxic effects of these three metals have played a central role in the development of the field of toxicology. However, the toxic effects of low-dose chronic exposure to metals have only recently been appreciated.

Many of the toxic metals in the environment also are carcinogens (Table 67–3). In addition to toxic environmental metals, several essential metals also are toxic under conditions of overdose. Copper and especially iron are associated with toxicities, primarily targeting the liver through generation of reactive oxygen species. Toxicities from copper and iron usually result from genetic diseases that interfere with the regulation of metal absorption or excretion (e.g., Wilson's disease for copper, hemochromatosis for iron) or result from acute overdose, particularly with iron-containing medications or multivitamins. For a more comprehensive review of toxic metals, including essential metals, see Liu et al. (2008).

Not listed in Table 67–3 is the metal gold, which has its own uses and toxicities. Among heavy metals, perhaps only gold is addictive: gold has been used for centuries for relief of the itching palm, and many cannot get enough of its influence.

Lead

Exposure to lead has wide-ranging consequences for human health. Chronic exposure of populations to even very low levels of lead has major deleterious effects, which are only now beginning to be understood. It has been proposed that lead exposure contributed to the fall of the Roman Empire and that it plays a role in modern inner-city violence (Woolley, 1984; Needleman et al., 1996).

Exposure. In the U.S., paint containing lead for use in and around households was banned in 1978, while the use of tetraethyl lead in gasoline was phased out and eventually eliminated between 1976 and 1996. The economic benefit of the reduction in lead exposure due to these two measures is estimated at hundreds of billions of dollars per year (Grosse et al., 2002). Despite these bans, past use of lead carbonate and lead oxide in paint and tetraethyl lead in gasoline remain the primary sources of lead exposure. Lead is not degradable and remains throughout the environment in dust, soil, and the paint of older homes. Young children often are exposed to lead by nibbling sweet-tasting paint chips or eating dust and soil in and around older homes. Renovation or demolition of older buildings may cause substantial lead exposure. Tetraethyl lead was used as an anti-knock agent in gasoline, which resulted in high levels of lead in air pollution. Removal of lead from gasoline caused lead levels in air pollution to drop by >90% between 1982 and 2002. Lead was commonly used in plumbing and can leach into drinking water. Acidic foods and beverages dissolve lead when stored in containers with lead in their glaze or lead-soldered cans, which was a significant problem through the middle of the 20th century and remains a problem in developing countries. Lead exposure also has been traced to other sources such as lead toys, non-Western folk medicines, cosmetics, retained bullets, artists' paint pigments, ashes and fumes from painted wood, jewelers' wastes, home battery manufacture, and lead

Table 67–3

Toxic Metals with Frequent Environmental or Occupational Exposure[a]

METAL	CERCLA PRIORITY	COMMON SOURCE OF EXPOSURE	ORGAN SYSTEMS MOST SENSITIVE TO TOXICITY	IARC CARCINOGEN CLASSIFICATION
As	1	Drinking water	CV, skin, multiple other	Group 1, carcinogenic to humans—liver, bladder, lung
Pb	2	Paint, soil	CNS, blood, CV, renal	Group 2A, probably carcinogenic
Hg	3	Air, food	CNS, renal	Group 2B, possibly carcinogenic ($MeHg^+$); group 3, not classifiable (Hg^0, Hg^{2+})
Cd	7	Occupational, food, smoking	Renal, respiratory	Group 1, carcinogenic to humans—lung
Cr^{6+}	18	Occupational	Respiratory	Group 1, carcinogenic to humans—lung
Be	42	Occupational, water	Respiratory	Group 1, carcinogenic to humans—lung
Co	49	Occupational, food, water	Respiratory, CV	Group 2B, possibly carcinogenic
Ni	53	Occupational	Respiratory, skin (allergy)	Group 1, carcinogenic (soluble Ni compounds); group 2B, possibly carcinogenic (metallic Ni)—lung

[a]The Agency for Toxic Substances and Disease Registry (ATSDR) has both detailed monographs and brief summaries for each of these compounds, available at http://www.atsdr.cdc.gov. The International Agency for Research on Cancer (IARC) also has monographs available at http://monographs.iarc.fr. CERCLA, Comprehensive Environmental Response, Compensation, and Liability Act. CNS, central nervous system; CV, cardiovascular.

type (ATSDR, 2007b; Levin et al., 2008). Blood lead levels in the general population have steadily decreased since the 1970s. Between 1976 and 2002, mean blood levels in children 1-5 years of age dropped from 15-1.9 μg/dL. The Centers for Disease Control and Prevention (CDC) recommends screening of children at 6 months of age and the use of aggressive lead abatement for children with blood lead levels >10 μg/dL.

Occupational exposure to lead also has decreased markedly because of protective regulations. Occupational exposure generally is through inhalation of lead containing dust and lead fumes. Workers in lead smelters and in storage battery factories are at the greatest risk for lead exposure because fumes are generated and dust containing lead oxide is deposited in their environment. Other workers at risk for lead exposure are those associated with steel welding or cutting, construction, rubber and plastic industries, printing, firing ranges, radiator repair shops, and any industry where lead is flame soldered (ATSDR, 2007b).

Chemistry and Mode of Action. Lead exists in its metallic form and as divalent or tetravalent cations. Divalent lead is the primary environmental form; inorganic tetravalent lead compounds are not naturally found. Organo-lead complexes primarily occur with tetravalent lead and include the gasoline additive tetraethyl lead.

Lead toxicity results from molecular mimicry of other divalent metals (Garza et al., 2006). Lead takes the place of zinc or calcium in a number of important proteins. Because of its size and electron affinity, lead alters protein structure and can inappropriately activate or inhibit protein function. Specific molecular targets for lead are discussed below.

Absorption, Distribution, and Excretion. Lead exposure occurs through ingestion or inhalation. GI absorption of lead varies considerably with age and diet. Children absorb a much higher percentage of ingested lead (~40% on average) than adults (<20%). Absorption of ingested lead is drastically increased by fasting. Dietary calcium or iron deficiencies increase lead absorption, suggesting that lead is absorbed through divalent metal transporters. The absorption of inhaled lead generally is much more efficient (~90%), particularly with smaller particles. Tetraethyl lead is readily absorbed through the skin, but this is not a route of exposure for inorganic lead.

About 99% of lead in the bloodstream binds to hemoglobin. Lead initially distributes in the soft tissues, particularly in the tubular epithelium of the kidney and the liver. Over time, lead is redistributed and deposited in bone, teeth, and hair. About 95% of the adult body burden of lead is found in bone. Growing bones will accumulate higher levels of lead and can form lead lines visible by radiography. Bone lead is very slowly reabsorbed into the bloodstream, except when calcium levels are depleted, such as during pregnancy. Small quantities of lead accumulate in the brain, mostly in gray matter and the basal ganglia. Lead readily crosses the placenta.

Lead is excreted by humans primarily in the urine, although there also is some biliary excretion. The concentration of lead in urine is directly proportional to its concentration in plasma, but because most lead is in erythrocytes, only a small quantity of total lead is removed by filtration. Lead is excreted in milk and sweat and deposited in hair and nails. The serum $t_{1/2}$ of lead is 1-2 months, with a steady state achieved in ~6 months. Lead accumulates in bone, where its $t_{1/2}$ is estimated at 20-30 years.

Health Effects. Although the effects of high-dose lead poisoning have been known for >2000 years, the insidious toxicities of chronic low-dose lead poisoning (blood lead <20 μg/dL) have only recently been discovered. Although lead is a nonspecific toxicant, the most sensitive systems are the nervous, hematological, cardiovascular, and renal systems (Figure 67–4). Uncovering the effects of low-level lead exposure on complex health outcomes, such as neurobehavioral function and blood pressure, has been the subject of extensive research.

Neurotoxic Effects. The biggest concerns with low-level lead exposure are cognitive delays and behavior changes in children (ATSDR, 2007b; Bellinger and Bellinger, 2006). The developing nervous system is very sensitive to the toxic effects of lead.

Lead interferes with the pruning of synapses, neuronal migration, and the interactions between neurons and glial cells. Together, these alterations in brain development result in decreased IQ, poor performance on exams, and behavioral problems such as distractibility,

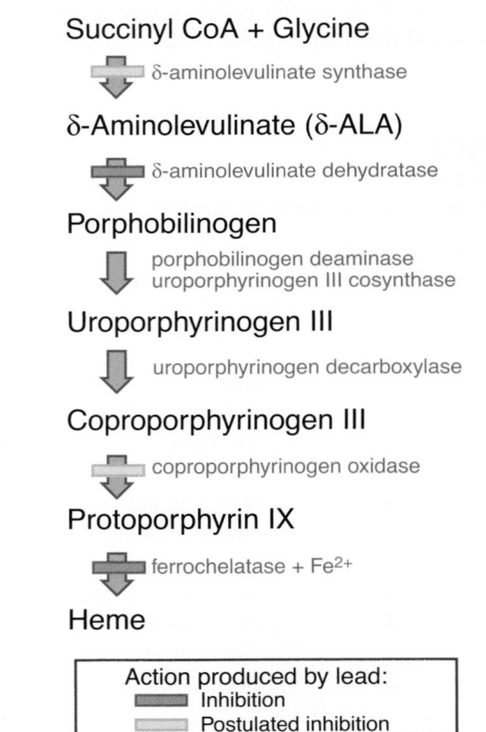

Figure 67–4. *Heme biosynthesis and actions of lead.* Lead interferes with the biosynthesis of heme at several enzymatic steps. Steps that definitely are inhibited by lead are indicated by red blocks. Steps at which lead is thought to act but where evidence is inconclusive are indicated by pink blocks.

impulsivity, short attention span, and inability to follow even simple sequences of instructions. Recent studies have shown neurobehavioral deficits even with lead exposures below the CDC action level of 10 μg/dL. There is no evidence for a threshold; associations with neurobehavioral effects are evident at the lowest measurable blood lead levels (Lanphear et al., 2005). Because different areas of the brain mature at different times, the neurobehavioral changes vary between children, depending on the timing of the lead exposure. Children with very high lead levels (>70 μg/dL) are at risk for encephalopathy. Symptoms of lead-induced encephalopathy include lethargy, vomiting, irritability, anorexia, and vertigo, which can progress to ataxia, delirium, and eventually coma and death. Mortality rates for lead-induced encephalopathy are ~25%, and most survivors develop long-term sequelae such as seizures and severe cognitive deficits.

Adults also develop encephalopathy from lead exposure, although they are less sensitive than children. Encephalopathy in adults requires blood lead levels >100 μg/dL. The symptoms are similar to those observed with children. Workers chronically exposed to lead can develop neuromuscular deficits, termed *lead palsy*. Symptoms of lead palsy, including wrist drop and foot drop, were commonly associated with painters and other lead-exposed workers during previous eras but are very rare today. Lead induces degeneration of motor neurons, usually without affecting sensory neurons. Studies in older adults have shown associations between lead exposure and decreased performance on cognitive function tests, suggesting that lead accelerates neurodegeneration due to aging (ATSDR, 2007b).

The neurodevelopmental effects of lead primarily result from inhibition of calcium transporters and channels and altered activities of calcium responsive proteins, including PKC and calmodulin (Garza et al., 2006; Bellinger and Bellinger, 2006). These actions limit the normal activation of neurons caused by calcium release and cause inappropriate production and/or release of neurotransmitters. Lead affects almost all the neurotransmitter pathways, with the dopaminergic, cholinergic, and glutamatergic systems receiving the most attention. Neurotransmitter release and PKC signaling determine which synapses are maintained and which are lost during development. At high concentrations, lead causes disruption of membranes, including the blood-brain barrier, increasing their permeability to ions. This effect is likely responsible for encephalopathy.

Cardiovascular and Renal Effects. Low-level lead exposure increases blood pressure. Correlations between lead exposure and blood pressure extend to concentrations of lead <20 μg/dL. Although the change in blood pressure is small, ~1 mm Hg for each doubling of the blood lead concentration, a significant effect persists across a wide number of studies, and there is evidence of causality (Navas-Acien et al., 2007). Elevated blood pressure is a lasting effect of lead exposure. Adults who were exposed to lead during infancy and childhood have elevated blood pressure even in the absence of a recent exposure; thus, blood pressure correlates better to lead levels in bone than in blood (ATSDR, 2007b). Lead exposure also is associated with an increased risk of death due to cardiovascular and cerebrovascular disease (Schober et al., 2006).

The kidney is a very sensitive target of lead. Low-level lead exposure (blood levels <10 μg/dL) depresses glomerular filtration. Higher levels (>30 μg/dL) cause proteinuria and impaired transport, while very high levels (>50 μg/dL) cause permanent physical damage, including proximal tubular nephropathy and glomerulosclerosis. Impaired glomerular filtration and elevated blood pressure are closely interrelated and likely have causative effects on one another (ATSDR, 2007b).

The exact mechanisms for the cardiovascular and renal effects of lead are not known. The cardiovascular effects of lead are thought to involve the production of reactive oxygen species by lead, through an unknown mechanism. Reactive oxygen species react with nitric oxide, which may contribute to the elevated blood pressure by reducing NO-induced vasodilation and contribute to cardiovascular toxicity through the formation of highly reactive peroxynitrite (Vaziri and Khan, 2007). Lead also forms inclusion bodies with various proteins, including metallothionein, in the kidney. The formation of these bodies greatly increases intracellular lead concentrations in the kidney but appears to be protective. It is not known how lead reduces glomerular filtration rate, although there is evidence that lead targets kidney mitochondria and may interfere with the electron transport chain (ATSDR, 2007b).

Hematological Effects. Chronic lead intoxication is associated with hypochromic microcytic anemia, which is observed more frequently in children and is morphologically similar to iron-deficient anemia. The anemia is thought to result from both decreased erythrocyte life span and inhibition of several enzymes involved in heme synthesis, which is observed at very low lead levels (Figure 67–5).

Inhibition of γ-aminolevulinate (γ-ALA) dehydratase and ferrochelatase is well documented. Ferrochelatase is responsible for incorporating the ferrous ion into protoporphyrin IX to form heme. When ferrochelatase is inhibited by lead, zinc is incorporated in place of iron, resulting in zinc-protoporphyrin, which is highly fluorescent and diagnostic of lead poisoning. γ-ALA dehydratase is the most sensitive of these enzymes to inhibition by lead; very low levels of lead increase urinary excretion of γ-ALA. Lead also causes both immunosuppression and increased inflammation, primarily through changes in helper T-cell and macrophage signaling (Dietert and Piepenbrink, 2006).

Gastrointestinal Effects. Lead affects the smooth muscle of the gut, producing intestinal symptoms that are an early

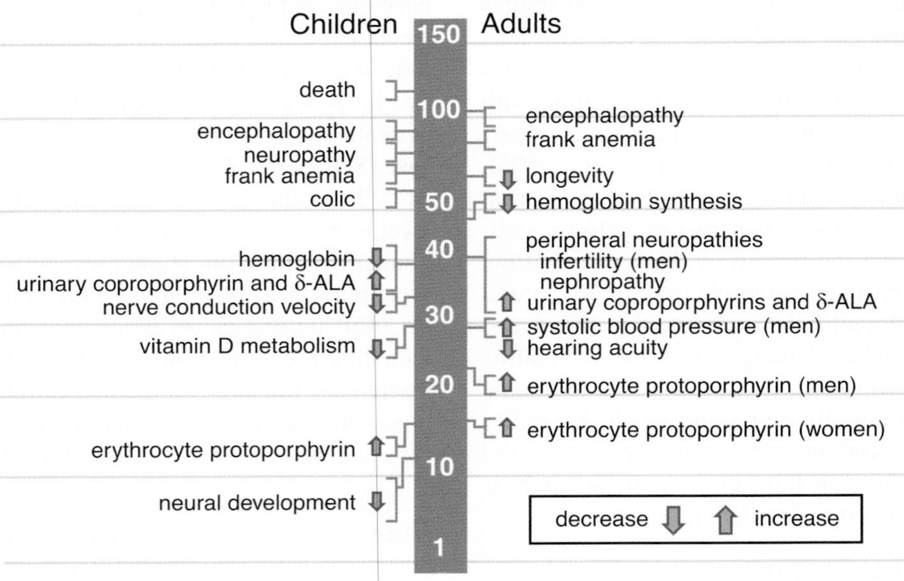

Figure 67–5. *Manifestations of lead toxicity associated with varying concentrations of lead in the blood of children and adults.* δ-ALA, δ-aminolevulinate.

sign of high-level exposure to the metal. The abdominal syndrome often begins with a persistent metallic taste, mild anorexia, muscle discomfort, malaise, headache, and usually constipation. Occasionally, diarrhea replaces constipation. As intoxication advances, symptoms worsen and include intestinal spasms that cause severe intestinal pain (lead cholic). Intravenous calcium gluconate can relieve this pain.

Carcinogenesis. IARC recently upgraded lead to "probably carcinogenic to humans" (group 2A; IARC, 2006). Epidemiological studies have shown associations between lead exposure and cancers of the lung, brain, kidney, and stomach. Rodents exposed to lead develop kidney tumors, and some rats develop gliomas. Lead is not mutagenic but increases clastogenic events. The mechanism of lead carcinogenesis is unknown but may result from inhibition of DNA binding zinc-finger proteins, including those involved in DNA repair and synthesis (Silbergeld, 2003). Lead is a good example of a non-genotoxic carcinogen.

Treatment. The most important response to lead poisoning is removal of the source of lead exposure. Supportive measures should be undertaken to relieve symptoms.

Chelation therapy is warranted for children and adults with high blood lead levels (>45 μg/dL and >70 μg/dL, respectively) and/or acute symptoms of lead poisoning (Ibrahim et al., 2006). Although chelation therapy is effective at lowering blood lead levels and relieving immediate symptoms, it does not reduce the chronic effects of lead beyond the benefit of lead abatement alone (Rogan et al., 2001). In rats, chelators enhance mobilization of lead from the soft tissues to the brain and may increase the adverse neurodevelopmental effects of lead (Andersen and Aaseth, 2002).

Mercury

Mercury is a unique metal in that it is a liquid at room temperature. Because of its capacity to amalgamate with other metals, mercury has been used industrially since ancient Greece, and mercury's toxicity was noted by Hippocrates. Mercury also was used as a therapeutic drug for several centuries. Indeed, its use for the treatment of syphilis inspired Paracelsus' observation that "the dose makes the poison," one of the central concepts of toxicology, and also gave rise to the cautionary expression, "A night with Venus, a year with Mercury." Toxicities from occupational exposure to mercury have been known for a long time. For instance, the phrase "mad as a hatter" originated from the exposure of hatters to metallic mercury vapor during production of felt for hats using mercury nitrate (Goldwater, 1972). While the phrase likely inspired the character of the Mad Hatter in *Alice in Wonderland*, his symptoms are not consistent with mercury exposure.

Exposure. Inorganic mercury cations and metallic mercury are found in the Earth's crust, and mercury vapor is released naturally into the environment through volcanic activity and off-gassing from soils. Mercury also enters the atmosphere through human activities such as combustion of fossil fuels. Once in the air, metallic mercury is photo-oxidized to inorganic mercury, which can then be deposited in aquatic environments in rain. Microorganisms can then conjugate inorganic mercury to form methyl mercury. Methyl mercury concentrates in lipids and will bioaccumulate up the food chain so that concentrations in aquatic organisms at the top of the food chain, such as swordfish or sharks, are quite high (Figure 67–6; ATSDR, 1999).

The primary source of exposure to metallic mercury in the general population is vaporization of mercury in dental amalgam, which often contains >50% Hg^0 mixed with silver and other metals. This release is enhanced by chewing. There also is limited exposure through broken thermometers and other mercury-containing devices. Human exposure to organic mercury primarily is through the consumption of fish. Other foods contain inorganic mercury at low levels (ATSDR, 1999).

Workers are exposed to metallic and inorganic mercury, most commonly though exposure to vapors. The highest risk for exposure is in the chloralkali industry (i.e., bleach) and in other chemical processes in which mercury is used as a catalyst. Mercury is a component of many devices, including alkaline batteries, fluorescent bulbs, thermometers, and scientific equipment, and exposure occurs during the production of these devices. Dentists also are exposed to mercury from amalgam. Mercury can be used to extract gold during mining, which results in substantial occupational exposure, because the last step involves vaporization of the mercury. This process is still commonly used in developing countries. Mercuric salts are used as pigments in paints (ATSDR,1999).

Mercury salts were once found in a number of medications, including antiseptics, antidiuretics, skin-lightening creams, and laxatives. Most of these uses have been replaced by safer and more effective drugs. Thimerosal is an antimicrobial agent used as a preservative in vaccines. Its use is controversial because it releases ethyl mercury, which is chemically similar to methyl mercury. Due to the concerns of some parents that thimerosal might be a cause of autism, the American Academy of Pediatrics and the U.S. Public Health Service issued a call for its replacement in vaccines to improve the prevalence of vaccination (Ball et al., 2001). However, studies have not found an association between thimerosal use in vaccines and negative outcomes, and it is still used in influenza vaccines (Heron and Golding, 2004).

Chemistry and Mode of Action. There are three general forms of mercury of concern to human health. Metallic, or elemental, mercury (Hg^0) is the liquid metal found in thermometers and dental amalgam; it is quite volatile, and exposure is often to the vapor form. Inorganic mercury can be either monovalent (mercurous, Hg^{1+}) or

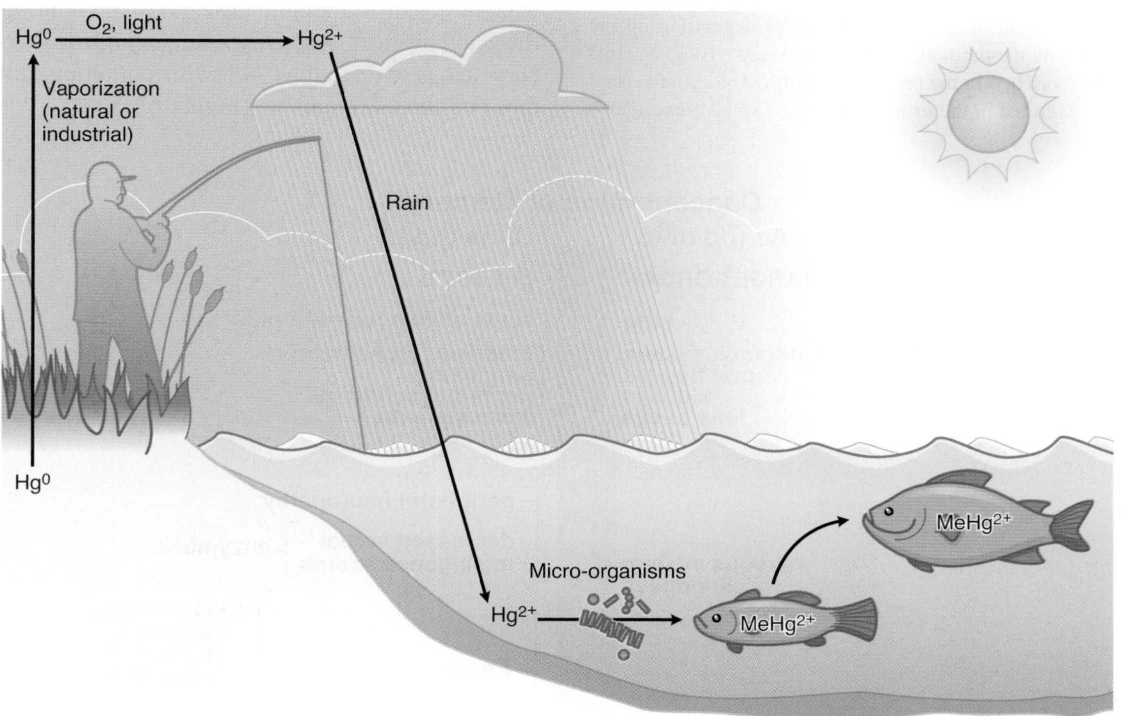

Figure 67–6. *Mobilization of mercury in the environment.* Metallic mercury (Hg^0) is vaporized from the Earth's surface both naturally and through human activities such as burning coal. In the atmosphere, Hg^0 is oxidized to form divalent inorganic mercury (Hg^{2+}). Hg^{2+} then falls to the surface in rain. Aquatic bacteria can methylate Hg^{2+} to form methyl mercury ($MeHg^+$). $MeHg^+$ in plankton is consumed by fish. Because of its lipophilicity, $MeHg^+$ bioaccumulates up the food chain.

divalent (mercuric, Hg^{2+}) and forms a variety of salts. Organic mercury compounds consist of divalent mercury complexed with one or occasionally two alkyl groups. The organic mercury compound of most concern is methyl mercury ($MeHg^+$), which is formed environmentally from inorganic mercury by aquatic microorganisms.

Both Hg^{2+} and $MeHg^+$ readily form covalent bonds with sulfur, which causes most of the biological effects of mercury. At very low concentrations, mercury reacts with sulfhydryl residues on proteins and disrupts their functions. Given the large numbers of proteins with important cysteines, determination of the specific mechanism for cellular dysfunction has been difficult, and there are probably multiple pathways affected. One of these pathways involves the generation of oxidative stress in cells. Also, microtubules are particularly sensitive to the toxic effects of mercury, which disrupts their formation and can catalyze their disassembly (Clarkson, 2002). There also may be an autoimmune component to mercury toxicity.

Absorption, Distribution, Biotransformation, and Excretion. Hg^0 vapor is readily absorbed through the lungs (~70-80%), but GI absorption of metallic mercury is negligible. Once absorbed, Hg^0 distributes throughout the body and crosses membranes such as the blood-brain barrier and the placenta via diffusion. Hg^0 is oxidized by catalase in the erythrocytes and other cells to form Hg^{2+}. Shortly after exposure, some Hg^0 is eliminated in exhaled air. After a few hours, distribution and elimination of Hg^0 resemble the properties of Hg^{2+}. After exposure to Hg^0 vapor, it is oxidized to Hg^{2+} and retained in the brain (ATSDR, 1999).

GI absorption of mercury salts varies depending on the individual and on the particular salt and averages ~10-15%. Hg^{1+} will form Hg^0 or Hg^{2+} in the presence of sulfhydryl groups. Hg^{2+} primarily is excreted in the urine and feces; a small amount also can be reduced to Hg^0 and exhaled. With acute exposure, the fecal pathway predominates, but following chronic exposure, urinary excretion becomes more important. All forms of mercury also are excreted in sweat and breast milk and deposited in hair and nails. The $t_{1/2}$ for inorganic mercury is approximately 1-2 months (ATSDR, 1999).

Orally ingested $MeHg^+$ is almost completely absorbed from the GI tract. $MeHg^+$ readily crosses the blood-brain barrier and the placenta and distributes fairly evenly to the tissues, although concentrations are highest in the kidneys (ATSDR, 1999). $MeHg^+$ can be demethylated to form inorganic Hg^{2+}. The liver and kidney exhibit the highest rates of demethylation, but this also occurs in the brain. $MeHg^+$ is excreted in the urine and feces, with the fecal pathway dominating. The $t_{1/2}$ for $MeHg^+$ is ~2 months. The pharmacokinetic properties of $MeHg^+$ are thought to result from molecular mimicry. Complexes between $MeHg^+$ and cysteine resemble methionine and can be recognized by transporters for that amino acid and taken across membranes (Ballatori, 2002).

Health Effects

Metallic Mercury. Inhalation of high levels of mercury vapor over a short duration is acutely toxic to the lung. Respiratory symptoms of mercury exposure start with cough and tightness in the chest and can progress to interstitial pneumonitis and severely compromised respiratory function. Other initial symptoms include weakness, chills, metallic taste, nausea, vomiting, diarrhea, and dyspnea. Acute exposure to high doses of mercury also is toxic to the CNS, with symptoms similar to those of chronic exposure (Figure 67–7).

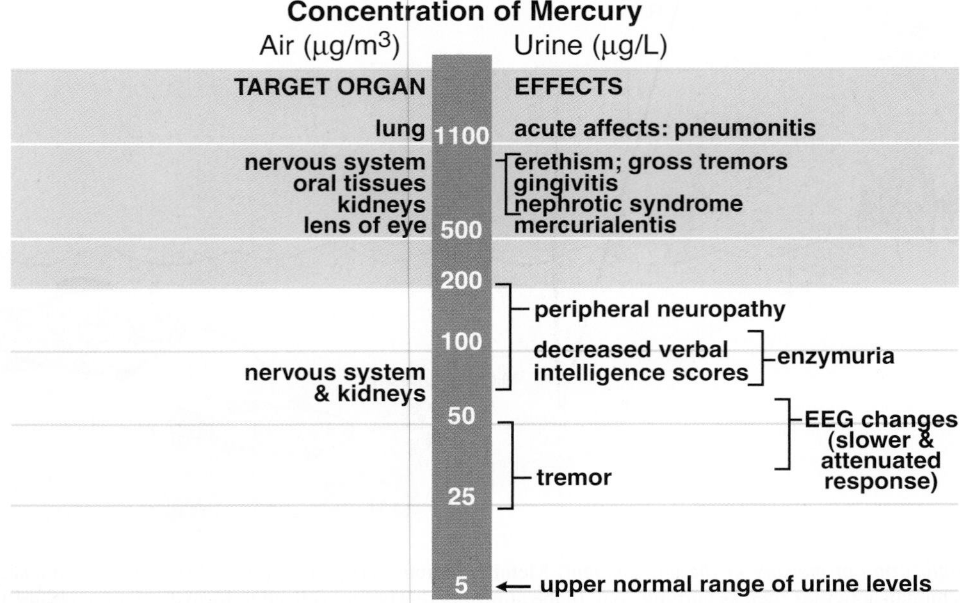

Figure 67–7. *The concentration of mercury vapor in the air and related concentrations of mercury in urine are associated with a variety of toxic effects.*

Toxicity to the nervous system is the primary concern with chronic exposure to mercury vapor. Mercury vapor induces characteristic CNS symptoms that are consistent across patients exposed to mercury over short or long periods. These symptoms include tremors (particularly of the hands), emotional lability (irritability, shyness, loss of confidence, and nervousness), insomnia, memory loss, muscular atrophy, weakness, paresthesia, and cognitive deficits. These symptoms intensify and become irreversible, with increases in duration and concentration of exposure. Other common symptoms of chronic mercury exposure include tachycardia, labile pulse, severe salivation, and gingivitis. Prolonged exposure to mercury also causes kidney damage.

Inorganic Salts of Mercury. Ingestion of Hg^{2+} salts is intensely irritating to the GI tract, leading to vomiting, diarrhea, and abdominal pain. The kidney is the primary target of both valence states of inorganic mercury. Acute exposure to mercury salts (typically in suicide attempts) leads to tubular necrosis, resulting in decreased urine output and often acute renal failure. Chronic exposures also target the kidney, with glomerular injury predominating.

Organic Mercury. The CNS is the primary target of methyl mercury toxicity. Two incidents of high-dose exposure to methyl mercury provide much of our knowledge regarding methyl mercury poisoning. One was in fishing villages surrounding the heavily polluted Minamata Bay in Japan, and the other was in Iraq, where grains treated with methyl mercury were accidentally consumed. Symptoms of methyl mercury exposure include visual disturbances, ataxia, paresthesia, fatigue, hearing loss, slurring of speech, cognitive deficits, muscle tremor, movement disorders, and, following severe exposure, paralysis and death. The developing nervous system exhibits increased sensitivity to methyl mercury. Children exposed *in utero* can develop severe symptoms, including mental retardation and neuromuscular deficits, even in the absence of symptoms in the mother. In adults, methyl mercury causes focused lesions in specific areas of the brain, while the brains of children exposed *in utero* sustain widespread damage (Clarkson, 2002).

The effects of low-dose methyl mercury exposure from routine consumption of fish are difficult to assess due to the opposing beneficial effects of ω-3 fatty acids found in fish oils, and studies have produced discrepant results (Grandjean et al., 1999; Myers et al., 2003; Myers et al., 2007).

Treatment. With exposure to metallic mercury, termination of exposure is critical and respiratory support may be required. Emesis may be used within 30-60 minutes of exposure to inorganic mercury, provided the patient is awake and alert and there is no corrosive injury. Maintenance of electrolyte balance and fluids is important for patients exposed to inorganic mercury. Chelation therapy is beneficial in patients with acute inorganic or metallic mercury exposure. There are limited treatment options for methyl mercury. Chelation therapy does not provide clinical benefits, and several chelators potentiate the toxic effects of methyl mercury (Rush, 2008). Nonabsorbed thiol resins may be beneficial by preventing reabsorption of methyl mercury from the GI tract.

Because of the conflicting effects of mercury and ω-3 fatty acids, there is considerable controversy regarding the restriction of fish intake in women of reproductive age and children. The EPA recommends limiting fish intake to 12 oz (two meals) per week. Many experts feel this recommendation is too conservative, and the FDA is considering revising their recommendation to state that the benefits of fish consumption outweigh the risks. The recommendation that women consume fish that is lower in mercury content (i.e., canned light tuna, salmon, pollock, catfish) and avoid top predators, such as swordfish, shark, and tilefish, is not controversial.

Arsenic

Arsenic is a metalloid that is common in rocks and soil. Arsenic compounds have been used for >2400 years as both therapeutic agents and poisons. In the late 19th century, Robert Ehrlich coined the terms "magic bullet" and "chemotherapy" to describe his work using the organic arsenic compound arsphenamine for the treatment of syphilis. The use of arsenic in drugs has been mostly phased out, but arsenic trioxide (ATO) is still used as an effective chemotherapy agent for acute promyelocytic leukemia (see Chapter 63).

Exposure. The primary source of exposure to arsenic is through drinking water. Arsenic naturally leaches out of soil and rocks into well and spring water (Mead, 2005). Levels of arsenic in drinking water average 2 μg/L (ppb) in the U.S. but can be >50 μg/L (five times the EPA standard) in private well water, particularly in California, Nevada, and Arizona. Drinking water from other parts of the world where well water has been promoted to prevent waterborne illness, particularly Taiwan, China, Argentina, Chile, Bangladesh, and eastern India, sometimes is contaminated with much higher levels of arsenic (sometimes several hundred micrograms per liter), and widespread poisonings have resulted (Figure 67–8). Studies in Bangladesh found that ~40% of water samples from across the country were contaminated with >50 μg/L of arsenic, and some samples had far higher levels (Mead, 2005; Chowdhury et al., 1999; BGS and DPHE, 2001). Arsenic also can enter the environment through human activities such as the use of arsenic-containing pesticides, mining, and burning of coal. Food, particularly seafood, often is contaminated with arsenic. Arsenic in seafood exists primarily as organic compounds (i.e., arsenobetaine) that are much less toxic than inorganic arsenic. The average daily human intake of arsenic is 10 μg/day, almost exclusively from food and water.

Before 2003, >90% of arsenic used in the U.S. was as a preservative in pressure-treated wood, but the lumber industry has

A

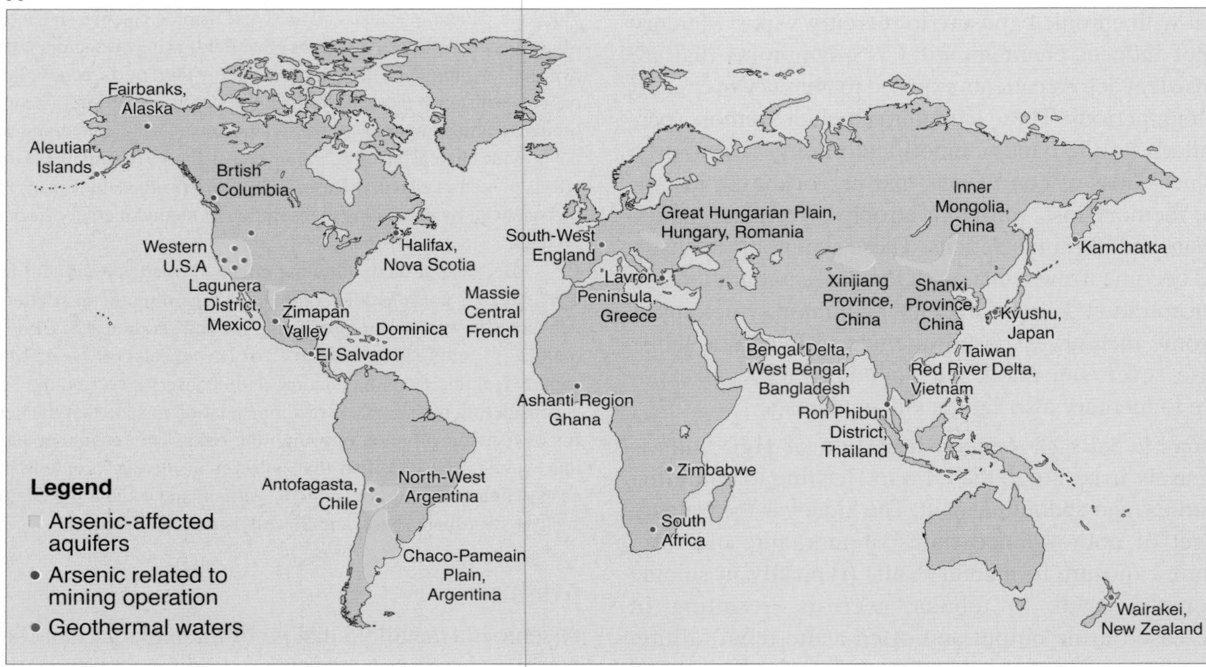

B

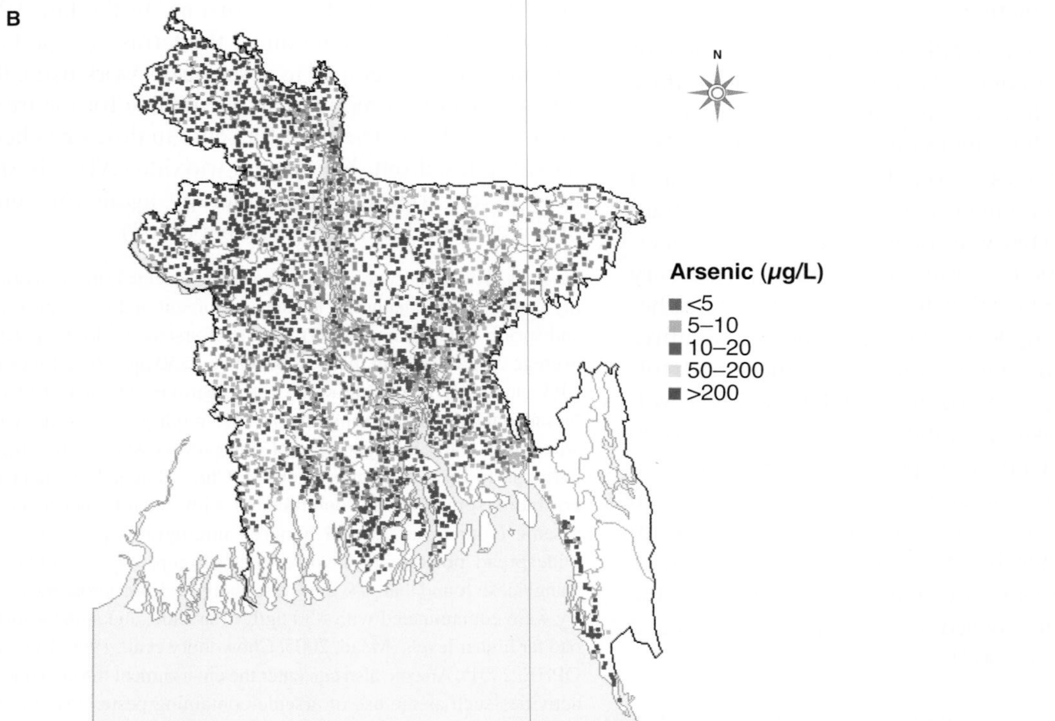

Figure 67–8. *Arsenic in drinking water.* (***A***) World map demonstrating regions where there is increased arsenic exposure in drinking water. (***B***) Map of Bangladesh demonstrating arsenic concentrations in drinking water in samples from wells across the country. (Adapted from BGS and DPHE, 2001. *This report was produced by the British Geological Survey and the Department of Public Health Engineering (Bangladesh) undertaking a project funded by the UK Department for International Development.*)

voluntarily replaced arsenic with other preservatives. Arsenic-treated wood is thought to be safe unless burned (Hall, 2002). The major source of occupational exposure to arsenic is in the production and use of organic arsenicals as herbicides and insecticides. Exposure to metallic arsenic, arsine, arsenic trioxide, and gallium arsenide also occurs in high-tech industries, such as the manufacture of computer chips and semiconductors.

Chemistry and Mode of Action. Arsenic exists in its elemental form and trivalent (arsenites/arsenious acid) and pentavalent (arsenates/arsenic acid) states. Arsine is a gaseous hydride of trivalent arsenic that exhibits toxicities that are distinct from other forms. Organic compounds containing either valence state of arsenic are formed in animals. The toxicity of a given arsenical is related to the rate of its clearance from the body and its ability to concentrate in tissues. In general, toxicity increases in the sequence: organic arsenicals < As^{5+} < As^{3+} < arsine gas (AsH_3).

Like mercury, trivalent arsenic compounds form covalent bonds with sulfhydryl groups. The pyruvate dehydrogenase system is particularly sensitive to inhibition by trivalent arsenicals because the two sulfhydryl groups of lipoic acid react with arsenic to form a six-membered ring. Inorganic arsenate (pentavalent) inhibits the electron transport chain. It is thought that arsenate competitively substitutes for phosphate during the formation of adenosine triphosphate, forming an unstable arsenate ester that is rapidly hydrolyzed.

Absorption, Distribution, Biotransformation, and Excretion. The absorption of arsenic compounds is directly related to their solubility. Poorly water-soluble forms such as arsenic sulfide, lead arsenate, and arsenic trioxide are not well absorbed. Water-soluble arsenic compounds are readily absorbed from both inhalation and ingestion. GI absorption of arsenic dissolved in drinking water is >90% (ATSDR, 2007a).

At low doses, arsenic is fairly evenly distributed throughout the tissues of the body. Nails and hair, due to their high sulfhydryl content, exhibit high concentrations of arsenic. After an acute high dose of arsenic (i.e., fatal poisoning), arsenic is preferentially deposited in the liver and, to a lesser extent, kidney, with elevated levels also observed in the muscle, heart, spleen, pancreas, lungs, and cerebellum. Arsenic readily crosses the placenta and blood-brain barrier.

Arsenic undergoes biotransformation in humans and animals (Figure 67–9). Trivalent compounds can be oxidized back to pentavalent compounds, but there is no evidence for demethylation of methylated arsenicals. Biotransformation of arsenic varies greatly across species, with humans excreting much higher levels of monomethylarsenic (MMA) compounds than most other animals (ATSDR, 2007a). Because the pentavalent methylated arsenic compounds have greatly reduced toxicity, the methylation pathway was long thought to be a detoxification pathway. However, the trivalent methylated arsenicals actually are more toxic than inorganic arsenite, due to an increased affinity for sulfhydryl groups, and formation of MMA^{III} now is considered a bioactivation pathway (Aposhian and Aposhian, 2006).

Elimination of arsenicals by humans primarily is in the urine, although some is also excreted in feces, sweat, hair, nails, skin, and exhaled air. Compared to most other toxic metals, arsenic is excreted quickly, with a $t_{1/2}$ of 1-3 days. In humans, ingested inorganic arsenic in urine is a mixture of 10-30% inorganic arsenicals, 10-20% monomethylated forms, and 60-80% dimethylated forms.

Health Effects. With the exception of arsine gas (which is discussed later in "Arsine Gas"), the various forms of inorganic arsenic exhibit similar toxic effects. Inorganic arsenic exhibits a broad range of toxicities and has been associated with effects on every organ system tested, although some systems are much more sensitive than others (ATSDR, 2007a). Humans also are exposed to large organic arsenic compounds in fish, which are relatively nontoxic. Humans are the most sensitive species to the toxic effects of inorganic arsenic. Acute exposure to large doses of arsenic (>70-180 mg) often is fatal. Death immediately following arsenic poisoning typically is the result of its effects on the heart and GI tract. Death sometimes occurs later as a result of arsenic's combined effect on multiple organs.

Cardiovascular System. Acute and chronic arsenic exposure cause myocardial depolarization, cardiac arrhythmias, and ischemic heart disease; these are known side effects of arsenic trioxide for the treatment of leukemia. Chronic exposure to arsenic causes peripheral vascular disease, the most dramatic example of which is "blackfoot disease," a condition characterized by cyanosis of the extremities, particularly the feet, progressing to gangrene. Blackfoot disease is endemic in regions of Taiwan, with arsenic levels of between 170 and 800 μg/L. Arsenic dilates capillaries and increases their permeability. This causes edema after acute exposures and is likely responsible for peripheral vascular disease following chronic exposure.

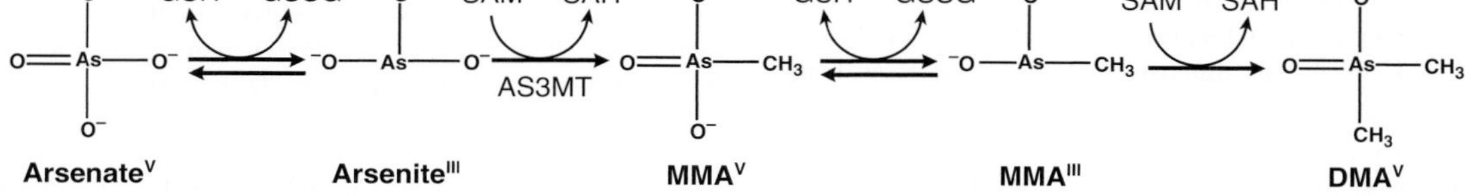

Figure 67–9. *Metabolism of arsenic.* GSH, reduced glutathione; GSSG, oxidized glutathione; SAM, *S*-adenosyl-L-methionine; SAH, *S*-adenosyl-L-homocysteine. AS3MT, arsenite methyltransferase; MMA^{V}, monomethylarsonic acid; MMA^{III}, monomethylarsonous acid; DMA^{V}, dimethyl arsinic acid.

Skin. The skin is very sensitive to chronic arsenic exposure. Dermal symptoms often are diagnostic of arsenic exposure. Arsenic induces hyperkeratinization of the skin (including formation of multiple corns or warts), particularly of the palms of the hands and the soles of the feet. It also causes areas of hyperpigmentation interspersed with spots of hypopigmentation. These symptoms can be observed in individuals exposed to drinking water with arsenic concentrations of at least 100 μg/L and are typical in those chronically exposed to much higher levels. Hyperpigmentation can be observed after 6 months of exposure, while hyperkeratinization takes years. Children are more likely to develop these effects than adults. The mechanism of arsenic-induced changes to the skin is unknown, partly because these effects are not seen in other animals (Mead, 2005; ATSDR, 2007a).

GI Tract. Acute or subacute exposure to high-dose arsenic by ingestion is associated with GI symptoms ranging from mild cramping, diarrhea, and vomiting to GI hemorrhaging and death. GI symptoms are caused by increased capillary permeability, leading to fluid loss. At higher doses, fluid forms vesicles that can burst, leading to inflammation and necrosis of the submucosa and then rupture of the intestinal wall. GI symptoms are not observed with chronic exposure to lower levels of arsenic.

Nervous System. Acute high-dose arsenic exposure causes encephalopathy in rare cases, with symptoms that can include headache, lethargy, mental confusion, hallucination, seizures, and coma. However, the most common neurological effect of acute or subacute arsenic exposure is peripheral neuropathy involving both sensory and motor neurons. This effect is characterized by the loss of sensation in the hands and feet (a *stocking and glove* distribution). This often is followed by muscle weakness. Neuropathy occurs several days after exposure to arsenic and can be reversible following cessation of exposure, although recovery usually is not complete. Arsenic exposure may cause intellectual deficits in children. Wasserman et al. (2007) observed a negative association between arsenic levels in drinking water and performance on intelligence tests.

Other Non-Cancer Toxicities. Acute and chronic arsenic exposures induce anemia and leukopenia. Arsenic likely causes both direct cytotoxic effects on blood cells and suppression of erythropoiesis through bone marrow toxicity. Arsenic also may inhibit heme synthesis. In the liver, arsenic causes fatty infiltrations, central necrosis, and cirrhosis of varying severity. The action of arsenic on renal capillaries, tubules, and glomeruli can cause severe kidney damage. Inhaled arsenic is irritating to the lungs, and ingested arsenic may induce bronchitis progressing to bronchopneumonia in some individuals. Chronic exposure to arsenic is associated with an increased risk of diabetes.

Carcinogenesis. Arsenic compounds were among the first recognized human carcinogens. At the end of the 19th century, Hutchinson observed that patients receiving arsenic-containing drugs had an increased occurrence of skin tumors. Epidemiological studies performed in regions with very high arsenic levels in drinking water consistently observe substantially increased rates of skin cancer (squamous cell and basal cell carcinomas), bladder cancer, and lung cancer. There also are associations between arsenic exposure and other cancers, including liver, kidney, and prostate tumors. Inhalation exposure to arsenic in occupational settings causes lung cancer. IARC classifies arsenic as "carcinogenic to humans (group 1)."

The developing fetus and young children may be at increased risk of arsenic carcinogenesis, because humans exposed to arsenic *in utero* and in early childhood have a greatly elevated risk of lung cancer (Smith et al., 2006). Studies in rodents also have observed increased cancer risks from *in utero* exposure and suggest that the second trimester of pregnancy represents a critical susceptibility window (Waalkes et al., 2007).

The mechanism of arsenic carcinogenesis is poorly understood. Arsenic is an unusual carcinogen in that evidence for human carcinogenesis is much stronger than for carcinogenesis in laboratory animals. Arsenic does not directly damage DNA; rather, arsenic is thought to work through changes in gene expression, DNA methylation, inhibition of DNA repair, generation of oxidative stress, and/or altered signal transduction pathways (Salnikow and Zhitkovich, 2008; Hartwig et al., 2002). Arsenic compounds can act as tumor promoters or co-carcinogens in rodents, particularly when combined with ultraviolet light (Burns et al., 2004). In humans, exposure to arsenic potentiates lung tumorigenesis from tobacco smoke. Smokers in regions with high concentrations of arsenic in the drinking water have a 5-fold increased risk of cancer over smokers living in low arsenic regions (Ferreccio et al., 2000). Arsenic co-carcinogenesis may involve inhibition of proteins involved in nucleotide excision repair (Salnikow and Zhitkovich, 2008; Hartwig et al., 2002). Arsenic also has endocrine-disrupting activities on several nuclear steroid hormone receptors, enhancing hormone-dependent transcription at very low concentrations and inhibiting it at slightly higher levels (Bodwell et al., 2006).

Arsine Gas. Arsine gas, formed by electrolytic or metallic reduction of arsenic, is a rare cause of industrial poisonings. Arsine induces rapid and often fatal hemolysis, which probably results from arsine combining with hemoglobin and reacting with oxygen. A few hours after exposure, patients can develop headache, anorexia, vomiting, paresthesia, abdominal pain, chills, hemoglobinuria, bilirubinemia, and anuria. Jaundice appears after 24 hours. Arsine induces renal toxicities that can progress to kidney failure. Approximately 25% of cases of arsine exposure result in death.

Treatment. Following acute exposure to arsenic, stabilize the patient and prevent further absorption of the poison. Close monitoring of fluid levels is important because arsenic can cause fatal hypovolemic shock. Chelation therapy is effective following short-term exposure to arsenic but has very little or no benefit in chronically exposed individuals. Exchange transfusion to restore blood cells and remove arsenic often is warranted following arsine gas exposure (Ibrahim et al., 2006).

Cadmium

Cadmium was discovered in 1817 and first used industrially in the mid-20th century. Cadmium is resistant to corrosion and exhibits useful electrochemical properties, which has led to its use in electroplating, galvanization, plastics, paint pigments, and nickel-cadmium batteries.

Exposure. In the general population, the primary source of exposure to cadmium is through food, with an estimated average daily intake of 50 μg/day. Cadmium also is found in tobacco; a cigarette contains 1-2 μg of cadmium (Jarup and Akesson, 2009). Workers in smelters and other metal-processing industries can be exposed to high levels of cadmium, particularly by inhalation.

Chemistry and Mode of Action. Cadmium exists as a divalent cation and does not undergo oxidation-reduction reactions. There are no covalent organometallic complexes of cadmium of toxicological significance. The mechanism of cadmium toxicity is not fully understood. Like lead and other divalent metals, cadmium can replace zinc in zinc-finger domains of proteins and disrupt them. Through an unknown mechanism, cadmium induces formation of reactive oxygen species, resulting in lipid peroxidation and glutathione depletion. Cadmium also upregulates inflammatory cytokines and may disrupt the beneficial effects of nitric oxide.

Absorption, Distribution, and Excretion. Cadmium is not well absorbed from the GI tract (1.5-5%) but is better absorbed via inhalation (~10%). Cadmium primarily distributes first to the liver and later the kidney, with those two organs accounting for 50% of the absorbed dose. Cadmium distributes fairly evenly to other tissues, but unlike other heavy metals, little cadmium crosses the blood-brain barrier or the placenta. Cadmium primarily is excreted in the urine and exhibits a $t_{1/2}$ of 10-30 years (ATSDR, 2008a).

Toxicity. Acute cadmium toxicity primarily is due to local irritation along the absorption route. Inhaled cadmium causes respiratory tract irritation with severe, early pneumonitis accompanied by chest pains, nausea, dizziness, and diarrhea. Toxicity may progress to fatal pulmonary edema. Ingested cadmium induces nausea, vomiting, salivation, diarrhea, and abdominal cramps; the vomitus and diarrhea often are bloody.

Symptoms of chronic cadmium toxicity vary by exposure route. The lung is an important target of inhaled cadmium, while the kidney is a major target of cadmium from both inhalation and ingestion.

Cadmium bound to metallothionein is transported to the kidney, where it can be released. The initial toxic effect of cadmium on the kidney is increased excretion of small-molecular-weight proteins, especially β_2 microglobulin and retinol-binding protein. Cadmium also causes glomerular injury, with a resulting decrease in filtration. Chronic occupational exposure to cadmium is associated with an increased risk of renal failure and death. There is no evidence for a threshold level for cadmium's effects on the kidney; cadmium levels consistent with normal dietary exposure can cause renal toxicity, including a reduction in glomerular filtration rate and creatinine clearance (Jarup and Akesson, 2009).

Workers with long-term inhalation exposure to cadmium exhibit decreased lung function. Symptoms initially include bronchitis and fibrosis of the lung, leading to emphysema. The exact cause of cadmium-induced lung toxicity is not known but may result from inhibition of the synthesis of α_1 antitrypsin. Chronic obstructive pulmonary disease causes increased mortality in cadmium-exposed workers.

When accompanied by vitamin D deficiency, cadmium exposure increases the risks for fractures and osteoporosis. This may be an effect of cadmium interfering with calcium and phosphate regulation due to its renal toxicity.

Carcinogenicity. Chronic occupational exposure to inhaled cadmium increases the risk of developing lung cancer (IARC, 1993; NTP, 2004). The mechanism of cadmium carcinogenesis is not fully understood. Cadmium causes chromosomal aberrations in exposed workers and treated animals and human cells. It also increases mutations and impairs DNA repair in human cells (NTP, 2004). Cadmium substitutes for zinc in DNA repair proteins and polymerases and may inhibit nucleotide excision repair, base excision repair, and the DNA polymerase responsible for repairing single-strand breaks (Hartwig et al., 2002). There is evidence that cadmium also alters cell signaling pathways and disrupts cellular controls of proliferation (Waisberg et al., 2003). Thus, cadmium acts as a non-genotoxic carcinogen.

Treatment. Treatment of cadmium poisoning is symptomatic. Patients suffering from inhaled cadmium may require respiratory support. Patients suffering from kidney failure due to cadmium poisoning may require a transplant. There is no evidence for clinical benefit from chelation therapy following cadmium poisoning, and chelation therapy may result in adverse effects (ATSDR, 2008a).

Chromium

Chromium is an industrially important metal used in a number of alloys, particularly stainless steel, which contains at least 11% chromium. Chromium can be oxidized to multiple valence states, with trivalent (Cr^{III}) and hexavalent chromium (Cr^{VI}) being the two forms of biological importance. Chromium exists almost exclusively as the trivalent form in nature, and Cr^{III} is an essential metal involved in the regulation of glucose metabolism. Cr^{VI} is thought to be responsible for the toxic effects of chromium exposure (ATSDR, 2008b).

Exposure. Exposure to chromium in the general population primarily is through the ingestion of food, although there also is exposure from drinking water and air. Workers are exposed to chromium during chromate production, stainless steel production and welding, chromium plating, ferrochrome alloy and chrome pigment production, and in tanning industries (Ashley et al., 2003). Exposure usually is to a mixture of Cr^{III} and Cr^{VI}, except in chromium plating, which usually uses Cr^{VI}, and tanning, where Cr^{III} is used.

Chemistry and Mode of Action. Chromium occurs in its metallic state or in any valence state between divalent and hexavalent. Cr^{III} is the most stable and common form. Cr^{VI} is corrosive and is readily reduced to lower valence states. The primary reason for the different toxicological properties of Cr^{III} and Cr^{VI} is thought to be differences in their absorption and distribution. Hexavalent chromate resembles sulfate and phosphate and can be taken across membranes by anion transporters. Once inside the cell, Cr^{VI} undergoes a series of reduction steps, ultimately forming Cr^{III}, which is thought to cause most of the toxic effects. Trivalent chromium readily forms covalent interactions with DNA. Hexavalent chromium also induces oxidative stress and hypersensitivity reactions.

Absorption, Distribution, Biotransformation, and Excretion. Absorption of inhaled chromium depends on its solubility, valence state, and particle size. Smaller particles are better deposited in the lungs. Absorption into the bloodstream of hexavalent and soluble forms is higher than the trivalent or insoluble forms, with the remainder often retained in the lungs. Approximately 50-85% of inhaled Cr^{VI} particles (<5 μm) are absorbed. Absorption of ingested chromium is <10%. Soluble Cr^{VI} compounds are better absorbed from the GI tract than other forms. Cr^{VI} crosses membranes by facilitated transport, while Cr^{III} crosses by diffusion. Cr^{VI} is distributed to all of the tissues and crosses the placenta. The highest levels are attained in the liver, kidney, and bone; Cr^{VI} also is retained in erythrocytes, bound tightly to hemoglobin and other ligands. Excretion primarily is through urine, with small amounts also excreted in bile and breast milk and deposited in hair and nails. The $t_{1/2}$ of ingested Cr^{VI} is ~40 hours, while the $t_{1/2}$ of Cr^{III} is ~10 hours, reflecting the enhanced tissue retention of Cr^{VI} (ATSDR, 2008b).

Toxicity. Acute exposure to very high doses of chromium causes death via damage to multiple organs, particularly the kidney, where it causes tubular and glomerular damage. Chronic low-dose chromium exposure primarily causes toxicity at the site of contact. Workers exposed to inhaled chromium develop symptoms of lung and upper respiratory tract irritation, including epistaxis, chronic rhinorrhea, nasal itching and soreness, nasal mucosal atrophy, perforations and ulceration of the nasal septum, bronchitis, pneumonoconiosis, decreased pulmonary function, and pneumonia. Chronic exposure to chromium via ingestion, including after mucociliary clearance of inhaled particles, causes symptoms of GI irritation such as oral ulcer, diarrhea, abdominal pain, indigestion, and vomiting. Cr^{VI} is a dermal irritant and can cause ulceration or burns. Following low-dose exposure by any route, some individuals become sensitized to chromium and develop allergic dermatitis following dermal exposure to chromium, including products containing metallic chromium. Chromium-sensitized workers often also develop asthma following inhalation exposure (ATSDR, 2008b).

Carcinogenicity. Cr^{VI} compounds are known human carcinogens (group 1; IARC, 1990). There is insufficient evidence for carcinogenesis from metallic and trivalent chromium (group 3). Workers exposed to Cr^{VI} via inhalation have elevated incidence of and mortality from lung and nasal cancer. Environmental exposure to Cr^{VI} in drinking water increases the risk of developing stomach cancer. Based on animal studies, the most potent carcinogenic compounds are slightly soluble Cr^{VI} compounds.

There are multiple potential mechanisms for chromium carcinogenicity (Salnikow and Zhitkovich, 2008). After uptake into cells, reduction of Cr^{VI} to Cr^{III} occurs with concomitant oxidation of cellular molecules. Ascorbate is the primary reductant, but other molecules, including glutathione, lipids, proteins, and DNA, also can be oxidized. Cr^{III} forms a large number of covalent DNA adducts, primarily at the phosphate backbone. The most common DNA adducts are either binary (DNA-Cr^{III}) adducts or cross-links to small molecules such as ascorbate and glutathione. The DNA adducts are not very mutagenic and are repaired by nucleotide excision repair. It is thought that the high level of nucleotide excision repair activity following chromium exposure contributes to carcinogenesis, either by preventing repair of mutagenic lesions formed by other carcinogens or through the formation of single-strand breaks due to incomplete repair. Chromium also forms toxic cross-links between DNA and protein. Chronic inflammation due to chromium-induced irritation also may promote tumor formation.

Treatment. There are no standard protocols for treatment of acute chromium poisoning. One approach that has shown promise in rodents is the use of reductants such as ascorbate, glutathione, or *N*-acetylcysteine to reduce Cr^{VI} to Cr^{III} after exposure but before absorption to limit bioavailability (ATSDR, 2008b). These compounds and EDTA also increase urinary excretion of chromium after high-dose exposure, particularly if given soon enough to prevent uptake into cells. Exchange transfusion to remove chromium from plasma and erythrocytes may be beneficial.

TREATMENT OF METAL EXPOSURE

The most important response to environmental or occupational exposures to metals is to eliminate the source of the exposure. For instance, with children exposed to lead, the CDC recommends aggressive lead-abatement practices to ensure that the home is free of lead-based paints and other sources of lead exposure. In occupational settings, often removing exposed workers from the toxic work environment will reverse many of the symptoms of metal poisoning. It also is important to stabilize the patient and provide symptomatic treatment.

Treatment for acute metal intoxications often involves the use of chelators. A chelator is a compound that forms stable complexes with metals, typically as five- or six-membered rings. Formation of complexes between chelators and metals should prevent or reverse metal binding to biological ligands. The ideal chelator would have the following properties: *high solubility in water, resistance to biotransformation, ability to reach sites of metal storage, ability to form stable and nontoxic complexes with toxic metals, and ready excretion of the metal-chelator complex.* A low affinity for the essential metals calcium and zinc also is desirable, because toxic metals often act through competition with these metals for protein binding.

In cases of acute exposure to high doses of most metals, chelation therapy reduces toxicity. However, following chronic exposure, chelation therapy does not show clinical benefits beyond those of cessation of

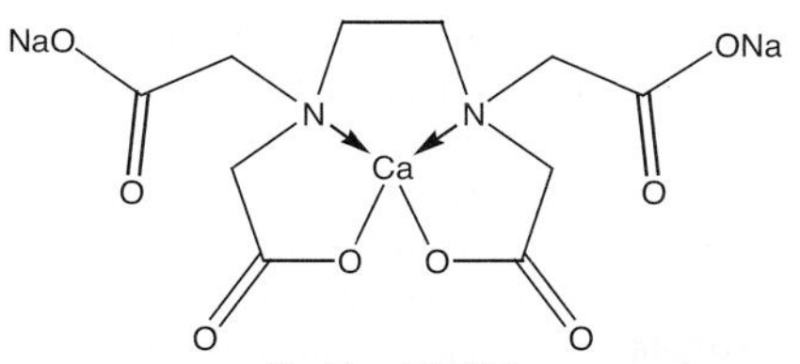

CaNa$_2$EDTA

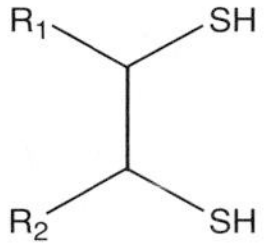

Dimercaprol: R$_1$=CH$_2$OH, R$_2$=H
Succimer: R$_1$=R$_2$=COOH
DMPS: R$_1$=CH$_2$SO$_3$H, R$_2$=H

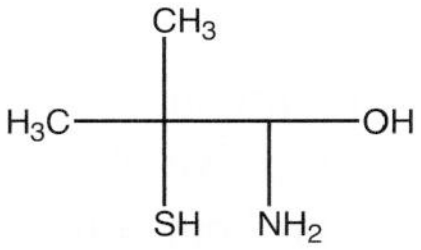

Penicillamine

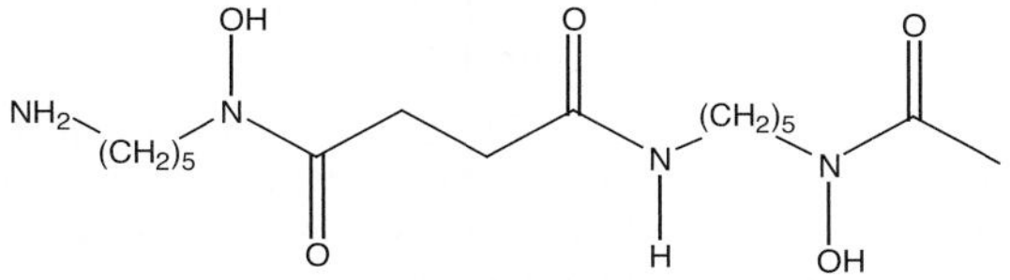

Deferoxamine

Figure 67–10. Structures of chelators commonly used to treat acute metal intoxication. CaNa$_2$EDTA, calcium disodium ethylenediamine tetraacetic acid; DMPS, sodium 2,3-dimercaptopropane sulfonate.

exposure alone and, in some cases, does more harm than good. Chelation therapy may increase the neurotoxic effects of heavy metals and is only recommended for acute poisonings. The structures of the most commonly used chelators are shown in Figure 67–10.

Ethylenediaminetetraacetic Acid (EDTA)

EDTA and its various salts are effective chelators of divalent and trivalent metals. Calcium disodium EDTA (CaNa$_2$EDTA) is the preferred EDTA salt for metal poisoning, provided that the metal has a higher affinity for EDTA than calcium. CaNa$_2$EDTA is effective for the treatment of acute lead poisoning, particularly in combination with dimercaprol, but is not an effective chelator of mercury or arsenic *in vivo*.

Chemistry and Mechanism of Action. The pharmacological effects of CaNa$_2$EDTA result from chelation of divalent and trivalent metals in the body. Accessible metal ions (both exogenous and endogenous) with a higher affinity for CaNa$_2$EDTA than Ca^{2+} will be chelated, mobilized, and usually excreted. Because EDTA is charged at physiological pH, it does not significantly penetrate cells. CaNa$_2$EDTA mobilizes several endogenous metallic cations, including those of zinc, manganese, and iron. Additional supplementation with zinc following chelation therapy may be beneficial. The most common therapeutic use of CaNa$_2$EDTA is for acute lead intoxication. CaNa$_2$EDTA does not provide clinical benefits for the treatment of chronic lead poisoning. There is evidence in rats that CaNa$_2$EDTA mobilizes lead from various tissues to the brain and liver, which may account for this observation (Sánchez-Fructuoso et al., 2002; Andersen and Aaseth, 2002).

CaNa$_2$EDTA is available as edetate calcium disodium (calcium disodium versenate). Intramuscular administration of CaNa$_2$EDTA results in good absorption, but pain occurs at the injection site; consequently, the chelator injection often is mixed with a local anesthetic or administered intravenously. For intravenous use, CaNa$_2$EDTA is diluted in either 5% dextrose or 0.9% saline and is administered slowly by intravenous drip. A dilute solution is necessary to avoid thrombophlebitis. To minimize nephrotoxicity, adequate urine production should be established prior to and during treatment with CaNa$_2$EDTA. However, in patients with lead encephalopathy and increased intracranial pressure, excess fluids must be avoided. In such cases, intramuscular administration of CaNa$_2$EDTA is recommended.

EDTA and its glycol congener, EGTA, are used in biological research to chelate and control the concentration of Ca^{2+} in biological buffer solutions. The 2008 Nobel laureate, Roger Tsien, and his colleagues used the EDTA/EGTA structure as a starting point in the development of fluorescent sensors of cellular [Ca^{2+}] (Tsien et al., 1984).

Absorption, Distribution, and Excretion. Less than 5% of CaNa$_2$EDTA is absorbed from the GI tract. After intravenous administration, CaNa$_2$EDTA has a $t_{1/2}$ of 20-60 minutes. In blood, CaNa$_2$EDTA is found only in the plasma. CaNa$_2$EDTA is excreted in the urine by glomerular filtration, so adequate renal function is necessary for successful therapy. Altering either the pH or the rate of urine flow has no effect on the rate of excretion. There is very little metabolic degradation of EDTA. The drug is distributed mainly in the extracellular fluids; very little gains access to the spinal fluid (5% of the plasma concentration).

Toxicity. Rapid intravenous administration of Na$_2$EDTA causes hypocalcemic tetany. However, a slow infusion (<15 mg/minute) administered to a normal individual elicits no symptoms of hypocalcemia because of the availability of extracirculatory stores of Ca^{2+}. In contrast, CaNa$_2$EDTA can be administered intravenously with no untoward effects because the change in the concentration of Ca^{2+} in the plasma and total body is negligible.

The principal toxic effect of CaNa$_2$EDTA is on the kidney. Repeated large doses of the drug cause hydropic vacuolization of the proximal tubule, loss of the brush border, and eventually, degeneration of proximal tubular cells. The early renal effects usually are reversible, and urinary abnormalities disappear rapidly with cessation of treatment. The most likely mechanism of toxicity is chelation of essential metals, particularly zinc, in proximal tubular cells.

Other side effects associated with CaNa$_2$EDTA include malaise, fatigue, and excessive thirst, followed by the sudden appearance of chills and fever and subsequent myalgia, frontal headache, anorexia, occasional nausea and vomiting, and rarely, increased urinary frequency and urgency. $CaNa_2EDTA$ is teratogenic in laboratory animals, probably as a result of zinc depletion; it should be used in pregnant women only under conditions in which the benefits clearly outweigh the risks (Kalia and Flora, 2005). Other possible undesirable effects include sneezing, nasal congestion, and lacrimation; glycosuria; anemia; dermatitis with lesions strikingly similar to those of vitamin B_6 deficiency; transitory lowering of systolic and diastolic blood pressures; prolonged prothrombin time; and T-wave inversion on the electrocardiogram.

Dimercaprol

Dimercaprol was developed during World War II as an antidote to lewisite, a vesicant arsenical war gas; hence its alternative name, British anti-lewisite (BAL). Arsenicals form a stable and relatively nontoxic chelate ring with dimercaprol. Pharmacological investigations revealed that dimercaprol protects against other heavy metals as well.

Chemistry and Mechanism of Action. The pharmacological actions of dimercaprol result from formation of chelation complexes between its sulfhydryl groups and metals. Dissociation of dimercaprol–metal complexes and oxidation of dimercaprol occurs *in vivo*. Furthermore, the sulfur–metal bond may be labile in the acidic tubular urine, which may increase the delivery of metal to renal tissue and increase toxicity. The dosage regimen should maintain a concentration of dimercaprol in plasma adequate to favor the continuous formation of the more stable 2:1 (BAL–metal) complex. However, because of pronounced and dose-related side effects, excessive plasma concentrations must be avoided. The concentration in plasma therefore must be maintained by repeated dosage until the metal is excreted.

Dimercaprol is most beneficial when given very soon after exposure to the metal because it is more effective in preventing inhibition of sulfhydryl enzymes than in reactivating them. Dimercaprol limits toxicity from arsenic, gold, and mercury, which form mercaptides with essential cellular sulfhydryl groups. It also is used in combination with $CaNa_2EDTA$ to treat lead poisoning.

Dimercaprol is contraindicated for use following chronic exposures to heavy metals because it does not prevent neurotoxic effects. There is evidence in laboratory animals that dimercaprol mobilizes lead and mercury from various tissues to the brain (Andersen and Aaseth, 2002). This effect may be due to the lipophilic nature of dimercaprol and is not observed with its more hydrophilic analogs described later (see "Succimer" and "Sodium 2,3-Dimercaptopropane Sulfonate [DMPS]").

Absorption, Distribution, and Excretion. Dimercaprol cannot be administered orally; it is given by deep intramuscular injection as a 100 mg/mL solution in peanut oil and should not be used in patients who are allergic to peanuts or peanut products. Peak concentrations in blood are attained in 30-60 minutes. The $t_{1/2}$ is short, and metabolic degradation and excretion essentially are complete within 4 hours. Dimercaprol and its chelates are excreted in both urine and bile.

Toxicity. The administration of dimercaprol produces a number of side effects, which occur in ~50% of subjects receiving 5 mg/kg intramuscularly. One of the most consistent responses to dimercaprol is a rise in systolic and diastolic arterial pressures, accompanied by tachycardia. The rise in pressure may be as great as 50 mm Hg in response to the second of two doses (5 mg/kg) given 2 hours apart. The pressure rises immediately but returns to normal within 2 hours.

Dimercaprol also can cause anxiety and unrest, nausea and vomiting, headache, a burning sensation in the mouth and throat, a feeling of constriction or pain in the throat and chest, conjunctivitis, blepharospasm, lacrimation, rhinorrhea, salivation, tingling of the hands, a burning sensation in the penis, sweating, abdominal pain, and the occasional appearance of painful sterile abscesses at the injection site. The dimercaprol–metal complex breaks down easily in an acidic medium; production of an alkaline urine protects the kidney during therapy. Children react similarly to adults, although ~30% also may experience a fever that disappears on drug withdrawal. Dimercaprol is contraindicated in patients with hepatic insufficiency, except when this condition is a result of arsenic poisoning.

Succimer

Succimer (2,3-dimercaptosuccinic acid [DMSA], CHEMET) is an orally effective chelator that is chemically similar to dimercaprol but contains two carboxylic acids that modify the spectrum of absorption, distribution, and chelation of the drug. It has an improved toxicity profile over dimercaprol.

Absorption, Distribution, and Excretion. After its absorption in humans, succimer is biotransformed to a mixed disulfide with cysteine (Aposhian and Aposhian, 2006). Succimer lowers blood lead levels and attenuates lead toxicity. The succimer–lead chelate is eliminated in both urine and bile. The fraction eliminated in bile can undergo enterohepatic circulation.

Succimer has several desirable features over other chelators. It is orally bioavailable, and because of its hydrophilic nature, it does not mobilize metals to the brain or enter cells. It also does not significantly chelate essential metals such as zinc, copper, or iron. As a result of these properties, succimer exhibits a much better toxicity profile relative to other chelators. Animal studies suggest that succimer also is effective as a chelator of arsenic, cadmium, mercury, and other toxic metals (Andersen and Aaseth, 2002; Kalia and Flora, 2005).

Toxicity. Succimer is much less toxic than dimercaprol. Transient elevations in hepatic transaminases have been observed with succimer treatment. The most commonly reported adverse effects are nausea, vomiting, diarrhea, and loss of appetite. In a few patients, rashes necessitate discontinuation of therapy.

Succimer has been approved in the U.S. for treatment of children with blood lead levels >45 μg/dL. Because of its oral availability, improved toxicity profile, and selective chelation of heavy metals, succimer also is used off label for the treatment of adults with lead poisoning and for the treatment of arsenic and mercury intoxication, although no large clinical trials have been undertaken for these indications.

Sodium 2,3-Dimercaptopropane Sulfonate (DMPS)

DMPS is another dimercapto compound used for the chelation of heavy metals. DMPS is not approved by the FDA but is approved for use in Germany. DMPS is available from compounding pharmacies and is used by some doctors in the U.S.

Chemistry and Mode of Action. DMPS is a clinically effective chelator of lead, arsenic, and especially mercury. It is orally available and is rapidly excreted, primarily through the kidneys. It is negatively charged and exhibits distribution properties similar to those of succimer. DMPS is less toxic than dimercaprol but mobilizes zinc and copper and thus is more toxic than succimer. In a small clinical trial, DMPS exhibited some clinical benefit for the treatment of chronic arsenic poisoning. Similar benefits were not observed with either dimercaprol or succimer, suggesting that DMPS might be effective for treatment of chronic heavy metal poisonings (Kalia and Flora, 2005). However, more thorough clinical studies are needed.

Penicillamine; Trientine

Penicillamine was first isolated in 1953 from the urine of patients with liver disease who were receiving penicillin. Discovery of its chelating properties led to its use in patients with Wilson's disease (excess body burden of copper due to diminished excetion) and heavy-metal intoxications. Penicillamine is more toxic and is less potent and selective for chelation of heavy metals relative to other available chelation drugs. It is therefore not a first-line treatment for acute intoxication with lead, mercury, or arsenic. However, because it is inexpensive and orally bioavailable, it often is given at fairly low doses following treatment with $CaNa_2EDTA$ and/or dimercaprol to ensure that the concentration of metal in the blood stays low following the patient's release from the hospital.

Penicillamine is an effective chelator of copper, mercury, zinc, and lead and promotes the excretion of these metals in the urine.

Absorption, Distribution, Biotransformation, and Excretion. Penicillamine (CUPRIMINE, DEPEN) is available for oral administration. For chelation therapy, the usual adult dose is 1-1.5 g/day in four divided doses. The drug should be given on an empty stomach to avoid interference by metals in food. In addition to its use as a chelating agent for the treatment of copper, mercury, and lead poisoning, penicillamine is used in Wilson's disease (hepatolenticular degeneration owing to an excess of copper), cystinuria, and rheumatoid arthritis (rarely). For the treatment of Wilson's disease, 1-2 g/day usually is administered in four doses. The urinary excretion of copper should be monitored to determine whether the dosage of penicillamine is adequate.

Penicillamine is well absorbed (40-70%) from the GI tract. Food, antacids, and iron reduce its absorption. Peak concentrations in blood are obtained between 1 and 3 hours after administration. Penicillamine is relatively stable *in vivo* compared to its unmethylated parent compound cysteine. Hepatic biotransformation primarily is responsible for degradation of penicillamine, and very little drug is excreted unchanged. Metabolites are found in both urine and feces. *N*-Acetylpenicillamine is more effective than penicillamine in protecting against the toxic effects of mercury, presumably because it is more resistant to metabolism.

Toxicity. With long-term use, penicillamine induces several cutaneous lesions, including urticaria, macular or papular reactions, pemphigoid lesions, lupus erythematosus, dermatomyositis, adverse effects on collagen, and other less serious reactions, such as dryness and scaling. Cross-reactivity with penicillin may be responsible for some episodes of urticarial or maculopapular reactions with generalized edema, pruritus, and fever that occur in as many as one-third of patients taking penicillamine. The hematological system also may be affected severely; reactions include leukopenia, aplastic anemia, and agranulocytosis. These may occur at any time during therapy and may be fatal, so patients should be monitored carefully.

Renal toxicity induced by penicillamine usually is manifested as reversible proteinuria and hematuria, but it may progress to nephrotic syndrome with membranous glomerulopathy. More rarely, fatalities have been reported from Goodpasture's syndrome. Toxicity to the pulmonary system is uncommon, but severe dyspnea has been reported from penicillamine-induced bronchoalveolitis. Myasthenia gravis also has been induced by long-term therapy with penicillamine. Penicillamine is a teratogen in laboratory animals, but for pregnant women with Wilson's disease, the benefits appear to outweigh the risks. Less serious side effects include nausea, vomiting, diarrhea, dyspepsia, anorexia, and a transient loss of taste for sweet and salt, which is relieved by supplementation of the diet with copper. Contraindications to penicillamine therapy include pregnancy, renal insufficiency, or a previous history of penicillamine-induced agranulocytosis or aplastic anemia.

Trientine. Penicillamine is the drug of choice for treatment of Wilson's disease. However, the drug produces undesirable effects, as discussed in "Toxicity," and some patients become intolerant. For these individuals, trientine (triethylenetetramine dihydrochloride, SYPRINE) is an acceptable alternative. Trientine is an effective cupriuretic agent in patients with Wilson's disease, although it may be less potent than penicillamine. The drug is effective orally. Maximal daily doses of 2 g for adults or 1.5 g for children are taken in two to four divided portions on an empty stomach. Trientine may cause iron deficiency; this can be overcome with short courses of iron therapy, but iron and trientine should not be ingested within 2 hours of each other.

Deferoxamine; Deferasirox

Deferoxamine is isolated as the iron chelate from *Streptomyces pilosus* and is treated chemically to obtain the metal-free ligand. Deferoxamine has the desirable properties of a remarkably high affinity for ferric iron (K_a = 1031) coupled with a very low affinity for calcium (K_a = 102). *In vitro,* it removes iron from hemosiderin and ferritin and, to a lesser extent, from transferrin. Iron in hemoglobin or cytochromes is not removed by deferoxamine.

Absorption, Distribution, and Excretion. Deferoxamine (deferoxamine mesylate, DESFERAL) is poorly absorbed after oral administration, and parenteral administration is required. For severe iron toxicity (serum iron levels >500 μg/dL), the intravenous route is preferred. The drug is administered at 10-15 mg/kg/hour by constant infusion. Faster rates of infusion (45 mg/kg/hour) have been used in a few cases; rapid boluses usually are associated with hypotension. Deferoxamine may be given intramuscularly in moderately toxic cases (serum iron 350-500 μg/dL) at a dose of 50 mg/kg with a maximum dose of 1 g. Hypotension also can occur with the intramuscular route.

For chronic iron intoxication (e.g., thalassemia), an intramuscular dose of 0.5-1.0 g/day is recommended, although continuous subcutaneous administration (1-2 g/day) is almost as effective as intravenous administration. During blood transfusion, patients with thalassemia should be given 2 g deferoxamine (per unit of blood) by slow intravenous infusion (rate not to exceed 15 mg/kg/hour) by a separate line. Deferoxamine is not recommended in primary hemochromatosis; phlebotomy is the treatment of choice. Deferoxamine also has been used for the chelation of aluminum in dialysis patients.

Deferoxamine is metabolized by plasma enzymes, but the pathways have not yet been defined. The drug is excreted readily in the urine.

Toxicity. Deferoxamine causes a number of allergic reactions, including pruritus, wheals, rash, and anaphylaxis. Other adverse effects include dysuria, abdominal discomfort, diarrhea, fever, leg cramps, and tachycardia. Occasional cases of cataract formation have been reported. Deferoxamine may cause neurotoxicity during long-term, high-dose therapy for transfusion-dependent thalassemia major; both visual and auditory changes have been described. A "pulmonary syndrome" has been associated with high-dose (10-25 mg/kg/hr) deferoxamine therapy; tachypnea, hypoxemia, fever, and eosinophilia are prominent symptoms. Contraindications to the use of deferoxamine include renal insufficiency and anuria; during pregnancy, the drug should be used only if clearly indicated.

Deferasirox. Deferasirox (EXJADE) is an orally administered chelator of iron. It is FDA-approved for treatment of chronic iron overload in patients receiving therapeutic blood transfusions.

HO O N—N HO N OH

BIBLIOGRAPHY

Agency for Toxic Substances and Disease Registry (ATSDR). *Draft Toxicological Profile for Cadmium*. ATSDR, Atlanta, **2008a**.

Agency for Toxic Substances and Disease Registry (ATSDR). *Draft Toxicological Profile for Chromium*. ATSDR, Atlanta, **2008b**.

Agency for Toxic Substances and Disease Registry (ATSDR). *Toxicological Profile for Arsenic*. ATSDR, Atlanta, **2007a**.

Agency for Toxic Substances and Disease Registry (ATSDR). *Toxicological Profile for Lead*. ATSDR, Atlanta, **2007b**.

Agency for Toxic Substances and Disease Registry (ATSDR). *Toxicological Profile for Mercury*. ATSDR, Atlanta, **1999**.

Andersen O, Aaseth J. Molecular mechanisms of in vivo metal chelation: Implications for clinical treatment of metal intoxications. *Environ Health Perspect,* **2002**, *110*(suppl): 887–890.

Aposhian HV, Aposhian MM. Arsenic toxicology: Five questions. *Chem Res Toxicol,* **2006**, *19:*1–15.

Ashley K, Howe AM, Demange M, Nygren O. Sampling and analysis considerations for the determination of hexavalent chromium in workplace air. *J Environ Monit,* **2003**, *5*:707–716.

Ball LK, Ball R, Pratt RD. An assessment of thimerosal use in childhood vaccines. *Pediatrics,* **2001**, *107*:1147–1154.

Ballatori N. Transport of toxic metals by molecular mimicry. *Environ Health Perspect*, **2002**, *110*(suppl):689–694.

Bellinger DC, Bellinger AM. Childhood lead poisoning: The tortuous path from science to policy. *J Clin Invest*, **2006**, *116*:853–857.

Bodwell JE, Gosse JA, Nomikos AP, Hamilton JW. Arsenic disruption of steroid receptor gene activation: Complex dose-response effects are shared by several steroid receptors. *Chem Res Toxicol*, **2006**, *19*:1619–1629.

British Geological Survey (BGS), Department of Public Health Engineering (DPHE, Bangladesh); Kinniburgh DG, Smedley PL, eds. *Arsenic Contamination of Groundwater in Bangladesh*. Keyworth, United Kingdom, British Geological Survey, **2001**.

Burns FJ, Uddin AN, Wu F, et al. Arsenic-induced enhancement of ultraviolet radiation carcinogenesis in mouse skin: A dose-response study. *Environ Health Perspect,* **2004**, *112*:599–603.

Chowdhury TR, Basu GK, Mandal BK, et al. Arsenic poisoning in the Ganges delta. *Nature,* **1999**, *401*:545–546.

Clarkson TW. The three modern faces of mercury. *Environ Health Perspect*, **2002**, *110*(suppl):11–23.

Conney AH. Induction of microsomal enzymes by foreign chemicals and carcinogenesis by polycyclic aromatic hydrocarbons. G.H.A. Clowes Memorial Lecture. *Cancer Res,* **1982**, *42*:4875–4917.

Dietert RR, Piepenbrink MS. Lead and immune function. *Crit Rev Toxicol,* **2006**, *36*:359–385.

Egner PA, Wang JB, Zhu YR, et al. Chlorophyllin intervention reduces aflatoxin-DNA adducts in individuals at high risk for liver cancer. *Proc Natl Acad Sci U S A,* **2001**, *98*:14601–14606.

Evans TR, Kaye SB. Retinoids: Present role and future potential. *Br J Cancer,* **1999**, *80*:1–8.

Fahey JW, Kensler TW. Role of dietary supplements/nutraceuticals in chemoprevention through induction of cytoprotective enzymes. *Chem Res Toxicol,* **2007**, *20*:572–576.

Faustman EM, Omenn GS. Risk assessment. In: Klaassen CD, ed. *Casarett & Doull's Toxicology: The Basic Science of Poisons*. New York, McGraw-Hill, **2008**.

Ferreccio C, Gonzalez C, Milosavjlevic V, et al. Lung cancer and arsenic concentrations in drinking water in Chile. *Epidemiology,* **2000**, *11*:673–679.

Garza A, Vega R, Soto E. Cellular mechanisms of lead neurotoxicity. *Med Sci Monit,* **2006**, *12*:RA57–RA65.

Goldwater LJ. *Mercury; a History of Quicksilver*. Baltimore, York Press, **1972**.

Gordis L. *Epidemiology,* 4th ed. Philadelphia, Saunders Elsevier, **2008**.

Grandjean P, Budtz-Jorgensen E, White RF, et al. Methylmercury exposure biomarkers as indicators of neurotoxicity in children aged 7 years. *Am J Epidemiol,* **1999**, *150*:301–305.

Groopman JD, Johnson D, Kensler TW. Aflatoxin and hepatitis B virus biomarkers: A paradigm for complex environmental exposures and cancer risk. *Cancer Biomark*, **2005**, *1*:5–14.

Groopman JD, Kensler TW, Wild CP. Protective interventions to prevent aflatoxin-induced carcinogenesis in developing countries. *Annu Rev Public Health*, **2008**, *29*:187–203.

Grosse SD, Matte TD, Schwartz J, Jackson RJ. Economic gains resulting from the reduction in children's exposure to lead in the United States. *Environ Health Perspect*, **2002**, *110*:563–569.

Guengerich FP, Johnson WW, Ueng YF, et al. Involvement of cytochrome P450, glutathione S-transferase, and epoxide hydrolase in the metabolism of aflatoxin B1 and relevance to risk of human liver cancer. *Environ Health Perspect*, **1996**, *104*(suppl):557–562.

Hall AH. Chronic arsenic poisoning. *Toxicol Lett,* **2002**, *128*:69–72.

Hartwig A, Asmuss M, Ehleben I, et al. Interference by toxic metal ions with DNA repair processes and cell cycle control: Molecular mechanisms. *Environ Health Perspect*, **2002**, *110*(suppl):797–799.

Heron J, Golding J. Thimerosal exposure in infants and developmental disorders: A prospective cohort study in the United Kingdom does not support a causal association. *Pediatrics,* **2004**, *114*:577–583.

Hussain SP, Schwank J, Staib F, et al. TP53 mutations and hepatocellular carcinoma: Insights into the etiology and pathogenesis of liver cancer. *Oncogene,* **2007**, *26*:2166–2176.

Ibrahim D, Froberg B, Wolf A, Rusyniak DE. Heavy metal poisoning: Clinical presentations and pathophysiology. *Clin Lab Med*, **2006**, *26*:67–97.

International Agency for Research on Cancer (IARC). Beryllium, cadmium, mercury, and exposures in the glass manufacturing industry. In: *Monographs on the Evaluation of Carcinogenic Risks to Humans*, Vol. 58. Lyon, France, IARC Press, **1993**.

International Agency for Research on Cancer (IARC). Chromium, nickel, and welding. In: *Monographs on the Evaluation of Carcinogenic Risks to Humans*, Vol. 49. Lyon, France, IARC Press, **1990**.

International Agency for Research on Cancer (IARC). Inorganic lead and organic lead compounds. In: *Monographs on the Evaluation of Carcinogenic Risks to Humans*, Vol. 87. Lyon, France, IARC Press, **2006**.

International Agency for Research on Cancer (IARC). Some traditional herbal medicines, some mycotoxins, naphthalene, and styrene. In: *Monographs on the Evaluation of Carcinogenic Risks to Humans*, Vol. 82. Lyon, France, IARC Press, **2002**.

Jarup L, Akesson A. Current status of cadmium as an environmental health problem. *Toxicol Appl Pharmacol*, **2009**, *238*:201–208.

Kalia K, Flora SJ. Strategies for safe and effective therapeutic measures for chronic arsenic and lead poisoning. *J Occup Health*, **2005**, *47*:1–21.

Kensler TW, Egner PA, Wang JB, et al. Chemoprevention of hepatocellular carcinoma in aflatoxin endemic areas. *Gastroenterology,* **2004**, *127*:S310–S318.

Klaunig JE, Kamendulis LM. Chemical carcinogens. In: Klaassen CD, ed. *Casarett & Doull's Toxicology: The Basic Science of Poisons*. New York, McGraw-Hill, **2008**.

Lanphear BP, Hornung R, Khoury J, et al. Low-level environmental lead exposure and children's intellectual function: An international pooled analysis. *Environ Health Perspect,* **2005**, *113*:894–899.

Levin R, Brown MJ, Kashtock ME, et al. Lead exposures in U.S. children, 2008: Implications for prevention. *Environ Health Perspect,* **2008**, *116*:1285–1293.

Liu J, Goyer RA, Waalkes MP. Toxic effects of metals. In: Klaassen CD, ed. *Casarett & Doull's Toxicology: The Basic Science of Poisons*. New York, McGraw-Hill, **2008**.

Mead MN. Arsenic: In search of an antidote to a global poison. *Environ Health Perspect*, **2005**, *113*:A378–A386.

Mena S, Ortega A, Estrela JM. Oxidative stress in environmental-induced carcinogenesis. *Mutat Res,* **2009**, *674*:36–44.

Myers GJ, Davidson PW, Cox C, et al. Prenatal methylmercury exposure from ocean fish consumption in the Seychelles child development study. *Lancet,* **2003**, *361*:1686–1692.

Myers GJ, Davidson PW, Strain JJ. Nutrient and methyl mercury exposure from consuming fish. *J Nutr*, **2007**, *137*:2805–2808.

National Toxicology Program (NTP). Cadmium and cadmium compounds. In: *Report on Carcinogens.* Research Triangle Park, NC, NTP, **2004**, pp. III42–III44.

Navas-Acien A, Guallar E, Silbergeld EK, Rothenberg SJ. Lead exposure and cardiovascular disease—A systematic review. *Environ Health Perspect,* **2007**, *115*:472–482.

Needleman HL, Riess JA, Tobin MJ, et al. Bone lead levels and delinquent behavior. *JAMA,* **1996**, *275*:363–369.

Omenn GS, Goodman G, Thornquist M, et al. Chemoprevention of lung cancer: The beta-Carotene and Retinol Efficacy Trial (CARET) in high-risk smokers and asbestos-exposed workers. *IARC Sci Publ*, **1996**, *136*:67–85.

Penning TM. Polycyclic aromatic hydrocarbons: Multiple metabolic pathways and DNA lesions formed. In: Geactinov NE, Broyde S, eds. *The Chemical Biology of DNA Damage*. New York, Wiley-VCH, **2009**.

Rogan WJ, Dietrich KN, Ware JH, et al. The effect of chelation therapy with succimer on neuropsychological development in children exposed to lead. *N Engl J Med,* **2001**, *344*: 1421–1426.

Salnikow K, Zhitkovich A. Genetic and epigenetic mechanisms in metal carcinogenesis and cocarcinogenesis: Nickel, arsenic, and chromium. *Chem Res Toxicol*, **2008**, *21*:28–44.

Sánchez-Fructuoso AI, Cano M, Arroyo M, et al. Lead mobilization during calcium disodium ethylenediaminetetraacetate chelation therapy in treatment of chronic lead poisoning. *Am J Kidney Dis*, **2002**, *40*:51–58.

Schober SE, Mirel LB, Graubard BI, et al. Blood lead levels and death from all causes, cardiovascular disease, and cancer: Results from the NHANES III mortality study. *Environ Health Perspect,* **2006**, *114*:1538–1541.

Silbergeld EK. Facilitative mechanisms of lead as a carcinogen. *Mutat Res,* **2003**, *533*:121–133.

Smith AH, Marshall G, Yuan Y, et al. Increased mortality from lung cancer and bronchiectasis in young adults after exposure to arsenic in utero and in early childhood. *Environ Health Perspect,* **2006**, *114*:1293–1296.

Sylla A, Diallo MS, Castegnaro J, Wild CP. Interactions between hepatitis B virus infection and exposure to aflatoxins in the development of hepatocellular carcinoma: A molecular epidemiological approach. *Mutat Res*, **1999**, *428*:187–196.

Szabo E. Selecting targets for cancer prevention: Where do we go from here? *Nat Rev Cancer,* **2006**, *6*:867–874.

Tsien RY, Pozzan T, Rink TJ. Calcium activities and fluxes inside small intact cells as measured with intracellularly trapped chelators. *Adv Cyclic Nucleotide Protein Phosphorylation Res,* **1984**, *17*:535–541.

Vaziri ND, Khan M. Interplay of reactive oxygen species and nitric oxide in the pathogenesis of experimental lead-induced hypertension. *Clin Exp Pharmacol Physiol,* **2007**, *34*: 920–925.

Vogel VG, Costantino JP, Wickerham DL, et al. Effects of tamoxifen vs raloxifene on the risk of developing invasive breast cancer and other disease outcomes: The NSABP Study of Tamoxifen and Raloxifene (STAR) P-2 trial. *JAMA,* **2006**, *295*:2727–2741.

Waalkes MP, Liu J, Diwan BA. Transplacental arsenic carcinogenesis in mice. *Toxicol Appl Pharmacol,* **2007**, *222*:271–280.

Waisberg M, Joseph P, Hale B, Beyersmann D. Molecular and cellular mechanisms of cadmium carcinogenesis. *Toxicology,* **2003**, *192*:95–117.

Wasserman GA, Liu X, Parvez F, et al. Water arsenic exposure and intellectual function in 6-year-old children in Araihazar, Bangladesh. *Environ Health Perspect,* **2007**, *115*:285–289.

Wattenberg LW. Chemoprophylaxis of carcinogenesis: A review. *Cancer Res,* **1966**, *26*:1520–1526.

William WN, Heymach JV, Kim ES, Lippman SM. Molecular targets for cancer chemoprevention. *Nat Rev Drug Discov,* **2009**, *8*:213–225.

Wogan GN, Hecht SS, Felton JS, et al. Environmental and chemical carcinogenesis. *Semin Cancer Biol,* **2004**, *14*:473–486.

Woolley DE. A perspective of lead poisoning in antiquity and the present. *Neurotoxicology,* **1984**, *5*:353–361.

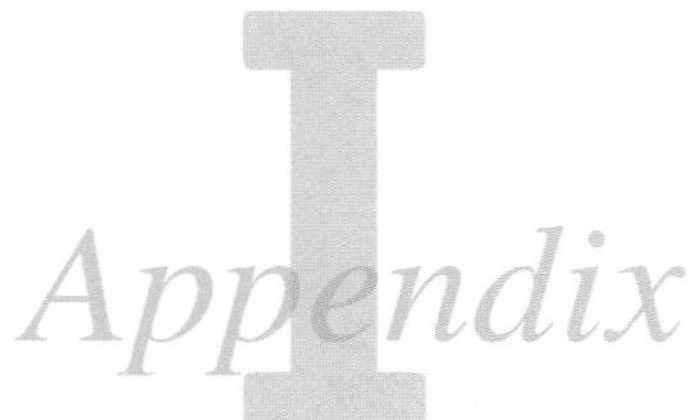

Principles of Prescription Order Writing and Patient Compliance

Iain L. O. Buxton

From the wrong drug prescribed to the wrong dosage or administration schedule advised, dispensed, or administered, the impact of medication misadventures is a costly problem. Errors of these sorts occur because human beings are involved, and such errors can be prevented only by systems that make it difficult to do the wrong thing. This appendix provides a primer on the proper approach to the medication prescription and order process and a resource for practitioners in effectively providing pharmaceutical care for their patients.

THE MECHANICS OF PRESCRIPTION ORDER WRITING

History

Early medicines were made up of multiple ingredients requiring complex preparation, and Latin was adopted as the standard language of the prescription to ensure understanding between physician and pharmacist and consistency in pharmaceutical composition. Latin no longer is the international language of medicine, but a number of commonly used abbreviations derive from old Latin usage. The symbol "Rx" is said to be an abbreviation for the Latin word *recipere*, meaning "take" or "take thus," as a direction to a pharmacist, preceding the physician's "recipe" for preparing a medication. The abbreviation "Sig" for the Latin *Signatura*, is used on the prescription to mark the directions for administration of the medication.

Current Practice

The prescription consists of the *superscription*, the *inscription*, the *subscription*, the *signa*, and the *name and signature of the prescriber*, all contained on a single form (Figure AI–1).

The *superscription* includes the date the prescription order is written; the name, address, weight, and age of the patient; and the Rx (*Take*). The body of the prescription, or *inscription*, contains the name and amount or strength of the drug to be dispensed, or the name and strength of each ingredient to be compounded. The *subscription* is the instruction to the pharmacist, usually consisting of a short sentence such as: "make a solution," "mix and place into 30 capsules," or "dispense 30 tablets." The *signa* or "*Sig*" is the instruction for the patient as to how to take the prescription, interpreted and transposed onto the prescription label by the pharmacist. In the U.S., prescriptions should always be written in English. Many physicians continue to use Latin abbreviations; for example, "1 cap tid pc," will be interpreted by the pharmacist as "take one capsule three times daily after meals." However, the use of Latin abbreviations for these directions only mystifies the prescription and is discouraged. This can be a hindrance to proper patient-physician communication and is an otherwise unnecessary source of potential dispensing errors. Because the pharmacist always writes the label in English (or, as appropriate, in the language of the patient), the use of such abbreviations or symbols is unnecessary. Many serious dispensing errors can be traced to the use of abbreviations (Cohen, 2007).

The instruction "take as directed" is not satisfactory and should be avoided by the physician. Such directions assume an understanding on the part of the patient that may not be realized and inappropriately exclude the pharmacist from the pharmaceutical care process. Such directions are inadequate for the pharmacist, who must determine the intent of the physician before dispensing the medication, and who shares the responsibility for the patient's safe and proper use of the medication. The best directions to the patient will include a reminder of the

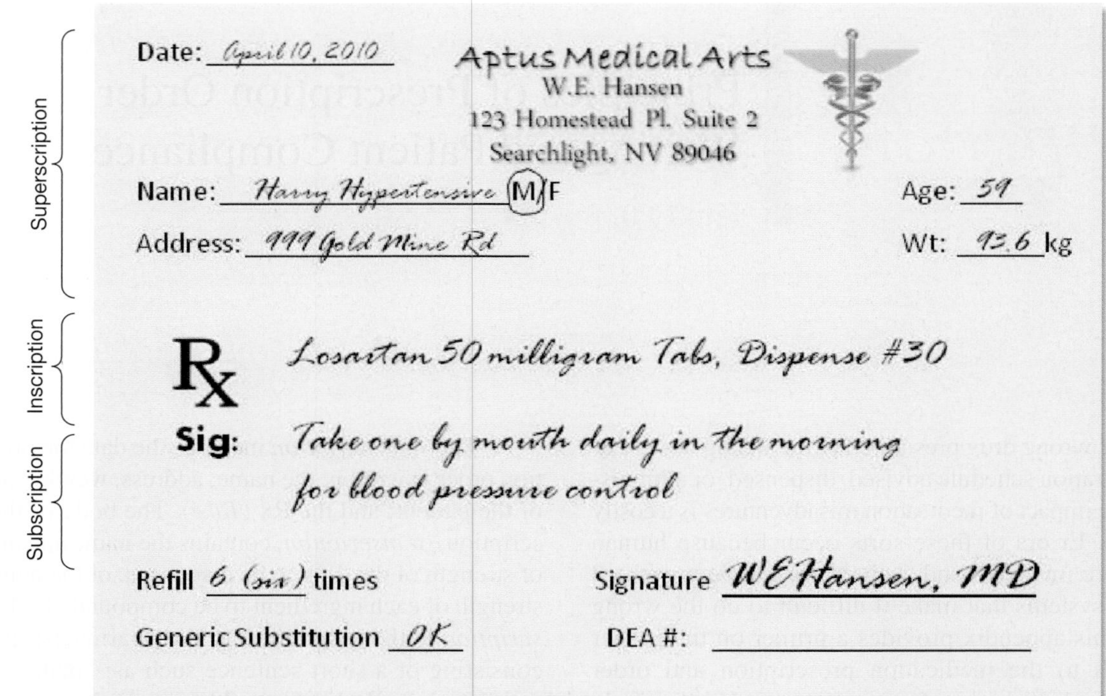

Figure AI–1. *The prescription.* The prescription must be carefully prepared to identify the patient and the medication to be dispensed, as well as the manner in which the drug is to be administered. Accuracy and legibility are essential. Use of abbreviations, particularly Latin, is discouraged, because it leads to dispensing errors. Inclusion of the therapeutic purpose in the subscription (e.g., "*for control of blood pressure*") can prevent errors in dispensing. For example, the use of losartan for the treatment of hypertension may require 100 mg/day (1.4 mg/kg/day), whereas treatment of congestive heart failure with this angiotensin II receptor antagonist generally should not exceed 50 mg/day. Including the therapeutic purpose of the prescription also can assist patients in organizing and understanding their medications. In addition, including the patient's weight on the prescription can be useful in avoiding dosing errors, particularly when drugs are administered to children.

intended purpose of the medication by including such phrases as "for relief of pain" or "to relieve itching." The correct route of administration is reinforced by the choice of the first word of the directions. For an oral dosage form, the directions should begin with "take" or "give"; for externally applied products, the word "apply"; for suppositories, "insert"; and for eye, ear, or nose drops, "place" is preferable to "instill."

Prescriptive Authority

In many states in the U.S., healthcare practitioners other than M.D. and D.O. physicians can write prescriptions. Licensed physician's assistants (P.A.), nurse practitioners, pharmacists, and clinical psychologists can prescribe medications under various circumstances.

Avoiding Confusion

Doses always should be listed by metric weight of the active ingredient; doses for liquid medications should include the volume. Older systems of measure such as minims for volume (15 minims = 1 mL) and grains for weight (1 grain = 60 mg) are obscure and should not be used. Writing "μg" for micrograms can very easily be misinterpreted as "mg" (milligrams). Even the abbreviation "mcg" for micrograms can be misinterpreted (Koczmara et al., 2005). Writing out the word *micrograms* or *milligrams* is preferable. When specifying the dose to be dispensed, a zero should be used before a decimal (0.# milligrams, rather than .# milligrams) but not after (use # milligrams rather than #.0 milligrams). The metric system should be used in place of common household measurements such as "dropperful" and "teaspoon" in the directions for the patient except when the dropper is provided with the prescription, as in the case of pediatric antibiotic suspensions. Both the doctor and the pharmacist should be sure that the patient understands the measurement prescribed. For medical purposes, a "teaspoon" or "teaspoonful" dose is considered to be equivalent to 5 mL and a "tablespoon" equivalent to 15 mL, but the actual volumes held by ordinary household teaspoons and tablespoons are far too variable to be used reliably for measurement of medications. Prescribing oral medications in "drops" likewise can cause problems when accuracy of dose is important, unless the patient understands that only the calibrated dropper (for drops or teaspoon measures) provided by the manufacturer or pharmacist should be used to dispense the medication. Thus, one possible dosage for a pediatric iron product would be more accurately written "15 milligrams (0.6 mL) three times daily" instead of "one dropperful three times daily," because a true dropperful could result in iron overdose.

Abbreviations lead to dispensing errors (Teichman and Caffee, 2002). A prescription intending every-other-day dosing (qod) may be miswritten as "od" by the physician for "other-day dosing"; the pharmacist may interpret "od" as the abbreviation of the Latin for "right eye." Once-daily dosing at bedtime (qhs) may be misinterpreted as "qhr" for "every hour." The use of a slash mark (/) to separate names and doses can result in the incorrect drug or dose being dispensed; the slash mark may be interpreted as a letter or number. When medications are measured in units, or international units, the abbreviation "U" or "I" must NOT be used, as it leads to errors such as misinterpretation of "U" as 0 or 4, or "IU" as 10 or 14. The word "unit" should be written as such. Drug products available in the U.S. that are dosed in units (e.g., corticotropin) or international unit measures are "harmonized" by those responsible for drug standardization to avoid errors in dosing (see "Drug Standards and Classification"). Examples of confusion in the interpretation of a physician order abound (Kohn, 2001) and are considered further in "Errors in Drug Orders." *To avoid errors, practitioners in the U.S. must write out the Rx fully in English, and pharmacists must clarify their concerns with prescribers, not patients.*

Proper Patient Information

The patient's name and address are needed on the prescription order to ensure that the correct medication goes to the proper patient and also for identification and recordkeeping purposes. For medications whose dosage involves a calculation, a patient's pertinent factors, such as weight, age, or body surface area, also should be listed on the prescription. Prescribers should view this effort as one that serves their goal of protecting their patient from errors rather than a burden (*safety first*).

Prescribers often commit errors in dosage calculations (Lesar et al., 1997) that can be prevented (Kuperman et al., 2001; Conroy et al., 2007). When prescribing a drug whose dosage involves a calculation based on body weight or surface area, both the calculated dose and the dosage formula used, such as "240 mg every 8 hours (40 mg/kg/day)," should be included to allow another healthcare professional to double-check the prescribed dosage. Pharmacists always should recalculate dosage equations when filling such prescriptions. Medication orders in hospitals and some clinic settings, such as those for antibiotics or anti-seizure medications that are sometimes difficult to adequately dose (e.g., phenytoin), can specify the patient diagnosis and desired drug and request dosing by the clinical pharmacist.

Proper Use of Prescription Pad

All prescriptions should be written in ink; this practice is compulsory for schedule II prescriptions under the U.S. Controlled Substances Act (CSA) of 1970, because erasures on a prescription easily can lead to dispensing errors or diversion of controlled substances.

Prescription pad blanks normally are imprinted with a heading that gives the name of the physician and the address and phone number of the practice site (Figure AI–1). When using institutional blanks that do not bear the physician's information, the physician always should print his or her name and phone number on the face of the prescription to clearly identify the prescriber and facilitate communication with other healthcare professionals if questions arise. U.S. law requires that prescriptions for controlled substances include the name, address, and Drug Enforcement Administration (DEA) registration number of the physician.

The date of the prescription is an important part of the patient's medical record, and it can assist the pharmacist in recognizing potential problems. For example, when an opioid is prescribed for pain due to an injury, and the prescription is presented to a pharmacist 2 weeks after issuance, the drug may no longer be indicated. Compliance behavior also can be estimated using the dates when a prescription is filled and refilled. The CSA requires that all orders for controlled substances (Table AI–1) be dated as of, and signed on, the day issued and prohibits filling or refilling orders for substances in schedules III and IV >6 months after their date of issuance. When writing the original prescription, the physician should designate the number of refills allowed. For maintenance medications without abuse potential, it is reasonable to write for a 1-month supply and to mark the prescription form for refills to be dispensed over a period sufficient to supply the patient until the next scheduled visit to the physician.

Table AI–1

Controlled Substance Schedules

Schedule I (examples: heroin, methylene dioxymethamphetamine, lysergic acid diethylamide, mescaline, and all salts and isomers thereof):

1. High potential for abuse.
2. No accepted medical use in the U.S. or lacks accepted safety for use in treatment in the U.S. May be used for research purposes by properly registered individuals.

Schedule II (examples: morphine, oxycodone, fentanyl, meperidine, dextroamphetamine, cocaine, amobarbital):

1. High potential for abuse.
2. Has a currently accepted medical use in the U.S.
3. Abuse of substance may lead to severe psychological or physical dependence.

Schedule III (examples: anabolic steroids, nalorphine, ketamine, certain schedule II substances in suppositories, mixtures, or limited amounts per dosage unit):

1 Abuse potential less than substances in schedule I or schedule II.
2. Has a currently accepted medical use in the U.S.
3. Abuse of substance may lead to moderate to low physical dependence or high psychological dependence.

Schedule IV (examples: alprazolam, phenobarbital, meprobamate, modafinil):

1. Abuse potential less than substances in schedule III.
2. Has a currently accepted medical use in the U.S.
3. Abuse of substance may lead to limited physical or psychological dependence relative to substances in schedule III.

Schedule V (examples: buprenorphine, products containing a low dose of an opioid plus a non-narcotic ingredient such as cough syrup with codeine[a] and guaifenesin, antidiarrheal tablets with diphenoxylate and atropine):

1. Low potential for abuse relative to schedule IV.
2. Has a currently accepted medical use in the U.S.
3. Some schedule V products may be sold in limited amounts without a prescription at the discretion of the pharmacist; however, if a physician wishes a patient to receive one of these products, it is preferable to provide a prescription.

[a]Although codeine is a schedule II drug, its dosage in cough syrups is regarded as sufficiently low to permit their classification as schedule V substances.

A statement such as "refill prn" (refill as needed) is not appropriate, as it could allow the patient to misuse the medicine or neglect medical appointments. If no refills are desired, "*zero*" (not "0") should be written in the refill space to prevent alteration of the prescriber's intent. Refills for controlled substances are discussed later, in "Refills" under "Controlled Substances."

Concern about the rising cost of healthcare has favored the dispensing of so-called "generic" drugs. A drug is called by its generic name (in the U.S., this is the U.S. Adopted Name or USAN) or the manufacturer's proprietary name, called the trademark, trade name, or brand name. In most states in the U.S., pharmacists have the authority to dispense generic drugs rather than brand-name medications. The physician can request that the pharmacist not substitute a generic for a branded medication by indicating this on the prescription ("do not substitute"), although this generally is unnecessary because the U.S. Food and Drug Administration (FDA) requires that generic medications meet the same bioequivalence standards as their brand-name counterparts. In some jurisdictions, prescriptions may not be filled with a generic substitution unless specifically permitted on the prescription. Occasions when substituting generic medications is discouraged are limited to products with specialized release systems and narrow therapeutic indices, or when substantial patient confusion and potential noncompliance may be associated with substitution.

Choice and Amount of Drug Product Dispensed

Inappropriate choice of drugs by physicians is a problem in prescribing. As learned recently with the cyclooxygenase-2 (COX-2) inhibitors, a drug's therapeutic promise or popularity is not proof of its overall clinical superiority or safety (Topol, 2004). Physicians must rely on unbiased sources when seeking drug information that will influence their prescribing habits; use of the original medical literature will ensure instruction of the prescriber's best judgment.

The amount of a drug to be dispensed should be clearly stated and should be only that needed by the patient. Excessive amounts should never be dispensed, because this not only is expensive for the patient but may lead to accumulation of medicines, which can lead to harm to the patient or members of the patient's family if used inappropriately. It is far better to have several refills of a prescription than to have more than necessary prescribed at one time.

The Prescription as a Commodity

Prescribers must be aware that patients may visit their doctor to "get" a prescription. Indeed, in an era when the time spent between physician and patient is ever shorter due to limits and pressures of physician reimbursements, patients often feel that a trip to the doctor that does not result in a new prescription somehow is a failed visit or a lost opportunity. Similarly, physicians may feel that they have fulfilled their role if the patient leaves with a prescription. Physicians must educate their patients about the importance of viewing medicines as to be used only when really needed and that remaining on a particular medicine when their condition is stable may be preferable to seeking the newest medications available.

Prescription Drug Advertising

The Federal Food, Drug, and Cosmetic Act as amended (Food and Drug Administration Modernization Act of 1997) permits the use of print and television advertising of prescription drugs. The law requires that all drug advertisements contain (among other things) summary information relating to side effects, contraindications, and effectiveness. The current advertising regulations specify that this information disclosure needs to include all the risk information in a product's approved labeling or must direct consumers to healthcare professionals to obtain this information. Typically, print advertisements will include a reprinting of the risk-related sections of the product's approved labeling (package insert), while television advertising will not. In addition, advertisements cannot be false or misleading or omit material facts. They also must present a fair balance between effectiveness and risk information.

The benefits of these types of direct-to-consumer (DTC) advertising, including Internet advertising, are controversial (Findlay, 2001). Dramatizations employed by television commercials may be a disservice to the physician's ability to educate and care for the patient if such advertisements only create brand loyalty. Alternatively, patients who learn about drugs on television may interact more effectively with their healthcare providers by asking questions about the medicines they take. Prescription drug advertising has alerted consumers to the existence of new drugs and the conditions they treat, but it has also increased consumer demand for drugs. This demand has increased the number of prescriptions being dispensed (raising sales revenues) and has contributed to the higher pharmaceutical costs borne by health insurers, government, and consumers. In the face of a growing demand for particular brand-name drugs driven by advertising, physicians and pharmacists must be able to counsel patients effectively and provide them with evidence-based drug information (Khanfar et al., 2007).

ERRORS IN DRUG ORDERS

The Institute of Medicine (IOM) estimates that the annual number of medical errors in the U.S. that results in death is between 44,000 and 98,000 (Kohn et al., 2000). Although there is some controversy about these estimates (Sox and Woloshin, 2000), it is clear that the large number of medical errors includes medication errors resulting in adverse events, including death (Mangino, 2004; Tzimenatos and Bond, 2009). Databases of anonymously reported errors are maintained jointly by the Institute for Safe Medication Practices (ISMP), the U.S. Pharmacopeia Medication Errors Reporting Program (USP MERP), and the FDA's MedWatch program. Adverse drug events occur in ~3% of hospitalizations, and this number is larger for special populations such as those in pediatric and neonatal intensive care units (Chedoe et al., 2007).

By examining aspects of prescription writing that can cause errors and by modifying prescribing habits accordingly, the physician can increase the probability that the patient will receive the correct prescription. By being alert to common problems that can occur with medication orders and communicating with the patient's physician, pharmacists and other healthcare professionals can assist in reducing medication errors (Murray et al., 2009). Good practice in the preparation of medication orders in both the institutional and outpatient settings can be summarized as follows:

- Write all orders clearly using metric measurements of weight and volume.
- Include patient age and weight on the prescription, when appropriate, so dosage can be checked.
- Use Arabic (decimal) numerals rather than Roman numerals (e.g., does "IL-II" mean "IL-11" or "IL-2"?); in some instances, it is preferable for numerals to be spelled out.
- Use leading zeros (0.125 milligrams, not .125 milligrams); never use trailing zeros (5 milligrams, not 5.0 milligrams).
- Avoid abbreviating drug names; abbreviations may lead to misinterpretation.
- Avoid abbreviating directions for drug administration; write out directions clearly in English.
- Be aware of possibilities for confusion in drug names. Some drug names sound alike when spoken and may look alike when spelled out. The U.S. Pharmacopeial Convention Medication Errors Reporting Program maintains a current list of drug names that can be confused (www.usp.org). The list of alliterative drug names currently contains

>750 pairs of potentially confusing names that could lead to harmful prescribing or dispensing errors. Alliterative drug names can be particularly problematic when giving verbal orders to pharmacists or other healthcare providers.

- Provide the patient's diagnosis on the prescription order. This is the single most important measure to prevent dispensing errors based on sound-alike or look-alike drug names. For instance, an order for administration of magnesium sulfate must not be abbreviated "MS," as this may result in administration of morphine sulfate. Including the therapeutic purpose and/or the patient's diagnosis can prevent this error.
- Write clearly. Poor handwriting is a well-known and preventable cause of dispensing errors. Both physician and pharmacist share in the responsibility for preventing adverse drug events by writing prescriptions clearly (*When in doubt, write it out!*) and questioning intent whenever an order is ambiguous (*When in doubt, check it out!*).
- Think.

CONTROLLED SUBSTANCES

In the U.S., the DEA within the Department of Justice is responsible for the enforcement of the Federal Controlled Substances Act (CSA). The DEA regulates each step of the handling of controlled substances from manufacture to dispensing (21 U.S.C. § 811). The law provides a system that is intended to prevent diversion of controlled substances from legitimate uses. Substances that come under the jurisdiction of the CSA are divided into five schedules (Table AI–1), but practitioners should note that individual states may have additional schedules. Physicians must be authorized to prescribe controlled substances by the jurisdiction in which they are licensed, and they must be registered with the DEA or exempted from registration as defined under the CSA. The number on the certificate of registration must be indicated on all prescription orders for controlled substances. Criminal prosecution and penalties for misuse generally depend on the schedule of a substance as well as the amount of drug in question.

State agencies may impose additional regulations, such as requiring that prescriptions for controlled substances be printed on triplicate or state-issued prescription pads or restricting the use of a particular class of drugs for specific indications. Some U.S. states, such as California, have placed marijuana, classified by the FDA as a schedule I substance, in a special category by decriminalizing its possession and sale for medical use. Under California's medical marijuana laws, patients and caregivers are exempt from prosecution by the state of California, notwithstanding contrary federal law. This legal difference of opinion between state and federal regulation is the source of considerable controversy. Generally, the most stringent law takes precedence, whether it is federal, state, or local.

Prescription Orders for Controlled Substances

To be valid, a prescription for a controlled substance must be issued for a *legitimate medical purpose* by an *individual practitioner* acting in the *usual course of his or her professional practice.* An order that does not meet these criteria, such as a prescription issued as a means to obtain controlled substances for the doctor's office use or to maintain addicted individuals, is not considered a legitimate prescription within the meaning of the law, and thus does not protect either the physician who issued it or the pharmacist who dispensed it. Most states prohibit physicians from prescribing controlled substances for themselves; it is prudent to comply with this guideline even if it is not mandated by law.

Execution of the Order

Prescriptions for controlled substances should be dated and signed on the day of their issuance and must bear the full name and address of the patient and the printed name, address, and DEA number of the practitioner and should be signed the way one would sign a legal document. Preprinted orders are not allowed in most states, and pre-signed blanks are prohibited by Federal law. When oral orders are not permitted (schedule II), the prescription must be written with ink or typewritten. The order may be prepared by a member of the physician's staff, but the prescriber is responsible for the signature and any errors that the order may contain.

Oral Orders

Prescriptions for schedule III, IV, and V medications may be telephoned to a pharmacy by a physician or by trusted staff in the same manner as a prescription for a noncontrolled substance, although it is in the physician's best interest to keep his or her DEA number as private as reasonably possible (see "Preventing Diversion"). Schedule II prescriptions may be telephoned to a pharmacy only in *emergency* situations. To be an emergency:

- Immediate administration is necessary
- No appropriate alternative treatment is available
- It is not reasonably possible for the physician to provide a written prescription prior to the dispensing.

For an emergency prescription, the quantity must be limited to the amount adequate to treat the patient during the emergency period, and the physician must have a written prescription delivered to the pharmacy for that emergency within 72 hours. If mailed, the prescription must be postmarked within 72 hours. The pharmacist must notify the DEA if this prescription is not received.

Refills

No prescription order for a schedule II drug may be refilled under any circumstance. For schedule III and IV drugs, refills may be issued either orally or in writing, not to exceed five refills or 6 months after the issue date, whichever comes first. Beyond this time, a new prescription must be ordered. For schedule V drugs, there are no restrictions on the number of refills allowed, but if no refills are noted at the time of issuance, a new prescription must be made for additional drug to be dispensed.

Preventing Diversion

Prescription blanks often are stolen and used to sustain abuse of controlled substances and to divert legitimate drug products to the illicit market. To prevent this type of diversion, prescription pads should be protected in the same manner as one would protect a personal checkbook. A prescription blank should never be pre-signed for a staff member to fill in at a later time. Also, a minimum number of pads should be stocked, and they should be kept in a locked, secure location except when in use. If a pad or prescription is missing, it should be reported immediately to local authorities and pharmacies; some areas have systems in place to allow the rapid dissemination of such information. Ideally, the physician's full DEA number should not be pre-printed on the prescription pad, because most prescriptions will not be for controlled substances and will not require the registration number, and anyone in possession of a valid DEA number may find it easier to commit prescription fraud. Some physicians may intentionally omit part or all of their DEA number on a prescription and instead write "pharmacist call to verify" or "call for registration number." This practice works only when the pharmacist may independently verify the authenticity of the prescription, and patients must be advised to fill the prescription during the prescriber's office hours. Pharmacists can ascertain the likely authenticity of a physician's DEA number using an algorithm.

Another method employed by the drug seeker is to alter the face of a valid prescription to increase the number of units or refills. By spelling out the number of units and refills authorized instead of giving numerals, the prescriber essentially removes this option for diversion. Controlled substances should not be prescribed excessively or for prolonged periods, as the continuance of a patient's addiction is not a legitimate medical purpose.

DRUG STANDARDS AND CLASSIFICATION

The U.S. Pharmacopeial Convention, Inc. is a non-governmental organization that promotes the public health and benefits practitioners and patients by disseminating authoritative standards and information on medicines and other healthcare technologies. This organization is home to the U.S. Pharmacopeia (USP), which, together with the FDA, the pharmaceutical industry, and health professions, establishes authoritative drug standards. These standards are enforceable by the FDA and the governments of other countries and are recognized worldwide. Drug monographs are published in the USP/National Formulary (USP-NF), the official drug standards compendia that organize drugs into categories based on pharmacological actions and therapeutic uses. The USP also provides chemical reference standards to carry out the tests specified in the USP-NF. For example, a drug to be manufactured and labeled in units must comply with the USP standard for units of that compound. Such standards are essential for agents possessing biological activity, such as insulin.

The USP also is home to the *USP Dictionary of U.S. Adopted Names (USAN) and International Drug Names*. This compendium is recognized throughout the healthcare industry as the authoritative dictionary of drugs. Entries include one or more of the following: U.S. Adopted Names, official drug names for the *National Formulary* (NF), previously used official names, International Nonproprietary Names, British Approved Names, Japanese Accepted Names, trade names, and other synonyms. In addition to names, the records in this file contain other substance information such as Chemical Abstract Service (CAS), registry number (RN), molecular formula, molecular weight, pharmacological and/or therapeutic category, drug sponsor, reference information, and structure diagram, if available. The USP maintains an electronic web site that can be accessed for useful drug naming, classification, and standards information (www.usp.org).

In the U.S., drug products also are coded under the National Drug Code (NDC). The NDC originally was established as an essential part of out-of-hospital drug reimbursement under Medicare. In the U.S., the NDC serves as a universal product identifier for drugs used in humans. The current edition of the National Drug Code Directory is limited to prescription drugs and a few selected over-the-counter products. Each drug product listed under the Federal Food, Drug, and Cosmetic Act is assigned a unique 10-digit, 3-segment number. This number, known as the NDC number, identifies the labeler/vendor, product, and package size. The labeler/vendor code is assigned by the FDA. The second segment, the product code, identifies a specific strength, dosage form, and formulation for a particular drug company. The third segment, the package code, identifies package sizes. Both the product and package codes are assigned by the manufacturer.

In addition to classification of drugs by therapeutic category, drugs also are grouped by control schedule. Drug schedules in the U.S. are listed in Table AI–1 from schedule I to schedule V and are discussed above under "Controlled Substances."

The FDA also categorizes drugs that may be used in pregnant women. These categories are similar to those used in other countries and provide guidance based on available science. The risk from a drug may be throughout pregnancy or limited to a particular period of fetal development. The categories range from A to X, in increasing order of concern, as noted here:

Pregnancy Category A: Adequate and well-controlled studies have failed to demonstrate a risk to the fetus in the first trimester of pregnancy (and there is no evidence of risk in later trimesters). Because of the obvious nature of the risk associated with the use of medications during gestation, the FDA requires a body of high-quality data on a drug before it can be considered for Pregnancy Category A.

Pregnancy Category B: Animal reproduction studies have failed to demonstrate a risk to the fetus, and there are no adequate and well-controlled studies in pregnant women, OR animal studies have shown an adverse effect, but adequate and well-controlled studies in pregnant women have failed to demonstrate a risk to the fetus in any trimester.

Pregnancy Category C: Animal reproduction studies have shown an adverse effect on the fetus, and there are no adequate and well-controlled studies in humans, but potential benefits may warrant use of the drug in pregnant women despite potential risks.

Pregnancy Category D: There is positive evidence of human fetal risk based on adverse reaction data from investigational or marketing experience or studies in humans, but potential benefits may warrant use of the drug in pregnant women despite potential risks.

Pregnancy Category X: Studies in animals or humans have demonstrated fetal abnormalities, and/or there is positive evidence of human fetal risk based on adverse reaction data from investigational or marketing experience, and the risks involved in use of the drug in pregnant women clearly outweigh potential benefits.

Physicians should realize that the pregnancy categories by themselves provide little guidance for the physician treating pregnant women. For example, angiotensin-converting enzyme (ACE) inhibitors such as captopril cause developmental toxicity (Category X) only after the first trimester. Physicians' primary responsibility remains treating the pregnant patient. However, the risks of withholding treatment to the mother because of possible risks to the fetus have to be considered as well.

Drugs also are grouped by their potential for misuse under British and U.N. legal classifications as class A, B, or C. The classes are linked to maximum legal penalties in a descending order of severity, from A to C.

COMPLIANCE

Compliance may be defined as the extent to which the patient follows a regimen prescribed by a healthcare professional. The assumption that the doctor tells the patient what to do and then the patient meticulously follows orders is unrealistic. The patient is the final and most important determinant of how successful a therapeutic regimen will be and should be engaged as an active participant who has a vested interest in its success. Whatever term is used—*compliance, adherence, therapeutic alliance,* or *concordance*—physicians must promote a collaborative interaction between doctor and patient in which each brings an expertise that helps to determine the course of therapy. The doctor is the medical expert; the patient is the expert on himself and his beliefs, values, habits, and lifestyle. The patient's quality-of-life beliefs may differ from the clinician's therapeutic goals, and the patient will have the last word every time when there is an unresolved conflict.

Even the most carefully prepared prescription for the ideal therapy will be useless if the patient's level of compliance is not adequate. Noncompliance may be manifest in drug therapy as intentional or accidental errors in dosage or schedule, overuse, underuse, early termination of therapy, or not having a prescription filled (Hagstrom et al., 2004); therapeutic failures can result (Hobbs, 2004). Noncompliance always should be considered in evaluating potential causes of inconsistent or nonexistent response to therapy. The reported incidence of patient noncompliance varies widely but usually is in the range of 30-60% (Zyczynski and Coyne, 2000); the rate for long-term regimens is ~50% but can be impacted by pharmaceutical care management (Klein et al., 2009).

Hundreds of variables that may influence compliance behavior in a specific patient or condition have been identified. A few of the most frequently cited are discussed here, along with some suggestions for improving compliance, although none provides 100% compliance (Table AI–2).

Table AI–2

Suggestions for Improving Patient Compliance

Provide respectful communication; ask how patient takes medicine.
Develop satisfactory, collaborative relationship between physician and patient; encourage pharmacist involvement.
Provide and encourage use of medication counseling.
Give precise, clear instructions, with most important information given first.
Support oral instructions with easy-to-read written information.
Simplify whenever possible.
Use mechanical compliance aids as needed (sectioned pill boxes or trays, compliance packaging, color-coding).
Use optimal dosage form and schedule for each individual patient.
Assess patient's literacy, language, and comprehension, and modify educational counseling as needed. Be culturally aware and sensitive. To improve compliance, don't rely on patient's own knowledge of disease alone.
Find solutions when physical or sensory disabilities are present (use nonsafety caps on bottles, use large type on labels and written material, place tape marks on syringes).
Enlist support and assistance from family or caregivers.
Use behavioral techniques such as goal setting, self-monitoring, cognitive restructuring, skills training, contracts, and positive reinforcement.

The Patient–Provider Relationship

Patient satisfaction with the physician has a significant impact on compliance behavior and is one of few factors that the physician can directly influence. Patients are more likely to follow instructions and recommendations when their expectations for the patient–provider relationship and for their treatment are met. These expectations include not only clinical but also interpersonal competence, so cultivating good interpersonal and communication skills is essential. Cultural sensitivity is of growing importance, as healthcare providers see more patients from countries and cultures different from their own.

When deciding on a course of therapy, it can be useful to discuss a patient's habits and daily routine as well as the therapeutic options with the patient. This information may suggest cues for remembrance, such as storing a once-daily medicine atop the books on the bedside table for a patient who reads nightly, or in the cabinet with the coffee cups if it is to be taken in the morning (noting that the humid environment of a bathroom can be the worst place to store a medication in terms of its physical and chemical preservation). The information also can help tailor the regimen to the patient's lifestyle. A lack of information about a patient's lifestyle can lead to situations such as prescribing a medication to be taken with meals three times daily for a patient who only eats twice a day or a medication to be taken each morning for a patient who works a night shift and sleeps during the day. Rarely is there only one treatment option for a given problem, and it may be better to prescribe an adequate regimen that the patient will follow instead of an ideal regimen that the patient will not. Involving patients in the control of any appropriate aspects of their therapy may improve compliance, not only by aiding memory and making the dosage form or schedule more agreeable or convenient, but also by giving patients a feeling of empowerment and emphasizing their responsibility for the treatment outcome.

It is not unreasonable for the physician to ask the patient whether he or she intends to adhere to the prescribed therapy and to negotiate to get a commitment to do so. Attempts should be made to resolve collaboratively any conflicts that may hinder compliance.

Patients and Their Beliefs

Behavioral models suggest that patients are more likely to be compliant when they *perceive* that they are susceptible to the disease, that the disease may have serious negative impact, that the therapy will be effective, and that the benefits outweigh the costs, and when they believe in their own efficacy to execute the therapy. From the standpoint of compliance, the *actual* severity of and susceptibility to an illness is not necessarily an issue; rather, the patient's perception of severity affects compliance (Dijkstra et al., 2008).

Patients' beliefs can lead them to deliberately alter their therapy, whether for convenience, for personal experiments, because of a desire to remove themselves from the sick role, as a means to exercise a feeling of control over their situation, or for other reasons. This reinforces the need for excellent communication and a good patient–provider relationship to facilitate the provision of additional or corrective education when the beliefs would suggest poor compliance as an outcome.

It is difficult to predict whether a particular patient will be compliant, because there is no consistent relationship with isolated demographic variables such as age, sex, education level, intelligence, personality traits, and income. Certain of these variables have been implicated in specific situations, but they cannot be applied to the population as a whole. Social isolation generally has been found to be associated with poor compliance, although family members or other people close to the patient can undermine compliance as easily as they can support it. As noted above, the actual severity of the patient's disease is not predictive of compliance behavior, but characteristics of the disease can make adherence less likely, as with certain neurodegenerative or psychiatric illnesses.

Pharmacists have a legal and professional responsibility to offer medication counseling in many situations—even though practice environments are not always conducive to its provision—and can educate and support patients by discussing prescribed medications and their use. Because they often see the patient more frequently than does the physician, pharmacists who take the time to inquire about a patient's therapy can help identify compliance and other problems, educate the patient, and notify the physician as appropriate. Indeed, data from the Asheville Project indicate that a pharmacist-based medication management program provides significant advantages with respect to compliance, health outcomes, and cost (Bunting et al., 2008).

Elderly patients often face a number of barriers to compliance related to their age. Such barriers include increased forgetfulness and confusion; altered drug disposition and higher sensitivity to some drug effects; decreased social and financial support; decreased dexterity, mobility, or sensory abilities; and the use of a greater number of concurrent medicines (both prescription and over-the-counter) whose attendant toxicities and interactions may cause decreased mental alertness or intolerable side effects. There are drugs known to be inappropriate to prescribe to elderly patients (Curtis et al., 2004; Fick et al., 2003) and some that may adversely affect compliance. Despite these obstacles, evidence does not show that elderly patients in general are significantly less compliant than any other age group. Still, as the U.S. population ages, elderly patients will consume a disproportionate fraction of medicines and healthcare resources, so there is great opportunity and motivation to improve their drug-taking habits. Physicians must be careful in choosing medications for the elderly (O'Mahony and Gallagher, 2008; Lopez and Goldoftas, 2009). Pharmacists must pay particular attention to thorough and compassionate counseling for elderly patients and should assist patients in finding practical solutions when problems, such as polypharmacy, are noted.

The Therapy

Increased complexity and duration of therapy are perhaps the best-documented barriers to compliance. The patient for whom multiple drugs are prescribed for a given disease or who has multiple illnesses that require drug therapy will be at higher risk for noncompliance, as will the patient whose disease is chronic. The frequency of dosing of individual medications also can affect compliance behavior. Simplification, whenever possible and appropriate, is desirable.

The effects of the medication can make adherence less likely, as in the case of patients whose medicines cause confusion or other altered mental states. Unpleasant side effects from the medicine may influence compliance in some patients but are not necessarily predictive, especially if patient beliefs or other positive factors tend to reinforce adherence to the regimen. A side effect that is intolerable to one patient may be of minor concern to another. The cost of medicine can be a heavy burden for patients with limited economic resources, and healthcare providers should be sensitive to this fact (Restrepo et al., 2008). Mobile devices (e.g., iPhone) running drug formulary/therapeutic software now can provide the costs of medications, as can physicians who are familiar with the patient's insurance plan. Mobile phone systems that provide reminders and collect patient response information are being introduced and may become more popular as patients become increasingly tech savvy.

percentage of the administered dose. Values represent the percentage expected in a healthy young adult (creatinine clearance ≥100 mL/min). When possible, the value listed is that determined after bolus intravenous administration of the drug, for which bioavailability is 100%. If the drug is given orally, this parameter may be underestimated due to incomplete absorption of the dose; such approximated values are indicated with a footnote. The parameter obtained after intravenous dosing is of greater utility because it reflects the relative contribution of renal clearance to total body clearance irrespective of bioavailability.

Renal disease is the primary factor that causes changes in this parameter. This is especially true when alternate pathways of elimination are available; thus, as renal function decreases, a greater fraction of the dose is available for elimination by other routes. Because renal function generally decreases as a function of age, the percentage of drug excreted unchanged also decreases with age when alternate pathways of elimination are available. In addition, for a number of weakly acidic and basic drugs with pK_a values within the normal range for urine pH, changes in urine pH will affect their rate or extent of urinary excretion (see Chapter 2).

Binding to Plasma Proteins. The tabulated value is the percentage of drug in the plasma that is bound to plasma proteins at concentrations of the drug that are achieved clinically. In almost all cases, the values are from measurements performed *in vitro* (rather than from *ex vivo* measurements of binding to proteins in plasma obtained from patients to whom the drug had been administered). When a single mean value is presented, it signifies that there is no apparent change in percent bound over the range of plasma drug concentrations resulting from the usual clinical doses. In cases in which saturation of binding to plasma proteins is approached within the therapeutic range of plasma drug concentrations, a range of bound percentages is provided for concentrations at the lower and upper limits of the range. For some drugs, there is disagreement in the literature about the extent of plasma-protein binding; in those cases, the range of reported values is given.

Plasma-protein binding is affected primarily by disease states, notably hepatic disease, renal failure, and inflammatory diseases, that alter the concentration of albumin, α_1-acid glycoprotein, or other proteins in plasma that bind drugs. Uremia also changes the binding affinity of albumin for some drugs. Disease-induced changes in plasma-protein binding can dramatically affect the volume of distribution, clearance, and elimination $t_{1/2}$ of a drug. In regard to clinical relevance, it is important to assess the change in unbound drug concentration or AUC, particularly when only unbound drug can cross biological barriers and gain access to the site of action.

Plasma Clearance. Systemic clearance of total drug from plasma or blood (see Equations 2–5 and 2–6) is given in Table AII–1. Clearance varies as a function of body size and, therefore, most frequently is presented in the table in units of mL/min/kg of body weight. Normalization to measures of body size other than weight may at times be more appropriate, such as normalization to body surface area in infants to better reflect the growth and development of the liver and kidneys. However, weight is easy to obtain, and its use often offsets any small loss in accuracy of clearance estimate, especially in adults. Exceptions to this rule are the anticancer drugs, for which dosage normalization to body surface area is conventionally used. When unit conversion was necessary, we used individual or mean body weight or body surface area (when appropriate) from the cited study, or if this was not available, we assumed a body mass of 70 kg or a body surface area of 1.73 m^2 for healthy adults.

In some cases, separate values for renal and nonrenal clearance are also provided. For some drugs, particularly those that are excreted predominantly unchanged in the urine, equations are given that relate total or renal clearance to creatinine clearance (also expressed as mL/min/kg). For drugs that exhibit saturation kinetics, K_m and V_{max} are given and represent, respectively, the plasma concentration at which half of the maximal rate of elimination is reached (in units of mass/volume) and the maximal rate of elimination (in units of mass/time/kg of body weight). K_m must be in the same units as the concentration of drug in plasma (C_p).

Intrinsic clearance from blood is the maximal possible clearance by the organ responsible for elimination when blood flow (delivery) of drug is not limiting. When expressed in terms of unbound drug, intrinsic clearance reflects clearance from intracellular water. Intrinsic clearance is tabulated for a few drugs. It also is mathematically related to the biochemical intrinsic clearance $[V_{max}/(K_m + C)]$ determined *in vitro*. In almost all cases, clearances based on plasma concentration data are presented in Table AII–1, because drug analysis most often is performed on plasma samples. The few exceptions where clearance from blood is presented are indicated by footnote. Clearance estimates based on blood concentration may be useful when a drug concentrates in the blood cells.

To be accurate, clearances must be determined after intravenous drug administration. When only nonparenteral data are available, the ratio of *CL/F* is given; values offset by the fractional availability (*F*) are indicated in a footnote. When a drug, or its active isomer for racemic compounds, is a substrate for a cytochrome P450 (CYP) or drug transporter, this information is provided in a footnote. This information is important for understanding pharmacokinetic variability due to genetic polymorphisms and for predicting metabolically based drug-drug interactions.

Volume of Distribution. The total body volume of distribution at steady state (V_{ss}) is given in Table AII–1 and is expressed in units of L/kg or in units of L/m^2 for some anticancer drugs. Again, when unit conversion was necessary, we used individual or mean body weights or body surface area (when appropriate) from the cited study, or if such data were not available, we assumed a body mass of 70 kg or a body surface area of 1.73 m^2 for healthy adults.

When estimates of V_{ss} were not available, values for V_{area} were provided; V_{area} represents the volume at equilibrated distribution during the terminal elimination phase (see Equation 2–12). Unlike V_{ss}, V_{area} varies when drug elimination changes, even though there is no change in the distribution space. Because we may wish to know whether a particular disease state influences either the clearance or the tissue distribution of the drug, it is preferable to define volume in terms of V_{ss}, a parameter that is less likely to depend on changes in the rate of elimination. Occasionally, the condition under which the distribution volume was obtained was not specified in the primary reference; this is denoted by the absence of a subscript.

As with clearance, V_{ss} usually is defined in the table in terms of concentration in plasma rather than blood. Further, if data were not obtained after intravenous administration of the drug, a footnote will make clear that the apparent volume estimate, V_{ss}/F, is offset by the fractional availability.

Half-Life. Half-life ($t_{1/2}$) is the time required for the plasma concentration to decline by one-half when elimination is first order. It also governs the rate of approach to steady state and the degree of drug accumulation during multiple dosing or continuous infusion. For example, at a fixed dosing interval, the patient will be at 50% of steady state after one $t_{1/2}$, 75% of steady state after two half-lives, 93.75% of steady state after four half-lives, etc. Determination of $t_{1/2}$ is straightforward when drug elimination follows a monoexponential pattern (i.e., one-compartment model). However, for a number of drugs, plasma concentration follows a multiexponential pattern of decline over time. The mean value listed in Table AII–1 corresponds to an effective rate of elimination that covers the clearance of a major fraction of the absorbed dose from the body. In many cases, this $t_{1/2}$ refers to the rate of elimination in the terminal exponential phase. For a number of drugs, however, the $t_{1/2}$ of an earlier phase is presented, even though a prolonged $t_{1/2}$ may be observed at very low plasma concentrations when extremely sensitive analytical techniques are used. If the latter component accounts for ≤10% of the AUC, predictions of drug accumulation in plasma during continuous or repetitive dosing will be in error by no more than 10% if this longer $t_{1/2}$ is ignored. The clinician should know the $t_{1/2}$ that will best predict drug accumulation in the patient, which will be the appropriate $t_{1/2}$ to use for estimating the rate constant in Equations 1–19 through 1–21 (see Chapter 1) to predict time to steady state. It is this $t_{1/2}$ of accumulation during multiple dosing that is given in Table AII–1.

Half-life usually is independent of body size because it is a function of the ratio of two parameters, clearance and volume of distribution, each of which is proportional to body size. It also should be noted that the $t_{1/2}$ is preferably obtained from intravenous studies, if feasible, because the $t_{1/2}$ of decline in plasma drug concentration after oral dosing can be influenced by prolonged absorption, such as when slow release formulations are given. If the $t_{1/2}$ is derived from an oral dose, this will be indicated in a footnote of Table AII–1.

Time to Peak Concentration. Because clearance concepts are used most often in the design of multiple dosage regimens, the extent rather than the rate of availability is more critical to estimate the average steady-state concentration of drug in the body. In some circumstances, the degree of fluctuation in plasma drug concentration (i.e., peak and trough concentrations), which govern drug efficacy and side effects, can be greatly influenced by modulation of drug absorption rate through the use of sustained- or extended-release formulations. Controlled-release formulations often permit a reduction in dosing frequency from three or four times daily to once or twice daily. There also are drugs that are given on an acute basis (e.g., for the relief of breakthrough pain or to induce sleep), for which the rate of drug absorption is a critical determinant of onset of effect. Thus, information about the expected average time to achieve maximal plasma or blood concentration and the degree of interindividual variability in that parameter have been included in Table AII–1.

The time required to achieve a maximal concentration (T_{max}) depends on the rate of drug absorption into blood from the site of administration and the rate of elimination. From mass balance principles, T_{max} occurs when the rate of absorption equals the rate of elimination from the reference compartment. Prior to this time, absorption rate exceeds elimination rate, and the plasma concentration of drug increases. After the peak is reached, elimination rate exceeds the absorption rate and, at some point, defines the terminal elimination phase of the concentration-time profile.

The rate of drug absorption following oral administration will depend on the formulation and physicochemical properties of the drug, its permeability across the mucosal barrier, and the intestinal villous blood flow. For an oral dose, some absorption may occur very rapidly within the buccal cavity, esophagus, and stomach, or absorption may be delayed until the drug reaches the small intestine or until the local pH in the intestine permits drug release from the dosage formulation. In the most extreme case, the rate of absorption can be sufficiently controlled by the drug formulation to permit sustained or extended delivery as the dosage form traverses the entire length of the gastrointestinal tract. In some instances, the terminal elimination of drug from the body following a peak concentration reflects the slower rate of absorption and not elimination.

When more than one type of drug formulation is available commercially, we have provided absorption information for both the immediate- and sustained-release formulations. Not surprisingly, the presence of food in the gastrointestinal tract can alter both the rate and extent of drug availability. We have indicated with footnotes when the consumption of food near the time of drug ingestion may have a significant effect on the drug bioavailability.

Peak Concentration. There is no general agreement about the best way to describe the relationship between the concentration of drug in plasma and its effect. Many different kinds of data are present in the literature, and use of a single-effect parameter or effective concentration is difficult. This is particularly true for antimicrobial agents because the effective concentration depends on the identity of the microorganism causing the infection. It also is important to recognize that concentration-effect relationships are most easily obtained at steady state or during the terminal log-linear phase of the concentration-time curve, when the drug concentration(s) at the site(s) of action are expected to parallel those in plasma. Thus, when attempting to correlate a blood or plasma level to effect, the temporal aspect of distribution of drug to its site of action must be taken into account.

Despite these limitations, it is possible to define the minimum effective or toxic concentrations for some of the drugs currently in clinical use. However, in reviewing the list of drugs approved within the past 5 years, it is rare to find a declaration of an *effective concentration range*, even in the manufacturer's package labeling. Thus, it is necessary to infer therapeutic concentrations from concentrations observed following *effective dosage* regimens. For a given dosage regimen, a time-averaged steady-state blood or plasma concentration (i.e., $\bar{C}_{ss}$ as estimated by dividing the mean AUC by the duration of the dosing interval) and the associated interindividual variability might be one appropriate parameter to report; however, such data often are not available. Also, $\bar{C}_{ss}$ does not take into account the onset and offset of effect during fluctuation of plasma drug concentration over a dosing interval. In some instances, drug efficacy may be more closely linked with peak concentration than with the average or trough concentration, and differences in peak concentration for special populations (e.g., elderly) sometimes are associated with increased incidence of drug toxicity.

For practical reasons, the most commonly reported parameter, C_{max} (peak concentration), rather than effective or toxic concentrations, is presented in Table AII–1. This provides a more consistent body of information about drug exposure from which one can infer, if appropriate, efficacious or toxic blood levels. Although the value reported is the highest that would be encountered in a given dose interval, C_{max} can be related to the trough concentration (C_{min}) through appropriate mathematical predictions (see Equation 1–21). Because peak levels will vary with dose, we have attempted to present concentrations observed with a customary dose regimen that is recognized to be effective in the majority of patients. When a higher or lower dose rate is used, the expected peak level can be adjusted by assuming dose proportionality, unless nonlinear kinetics are indicated. In some instances, only limited data pertaining to multiple dosing are available, so single-dose peak concentrations are presented. When specific information is available about an effective therapeutic range of concentrations or about concentrations at which toxicity occurs, it has been incorporated in a footnote. For individual drugs, the reader also is referred to the index to locate pages where more detailed information is provided.

It is important to recognize that significant differences in C_{max} will occur when comparing similar daily-dose regimens for an immediate-release and sustained-release product. Indeed, the sustained-release product sometimes is administered to reduce peak-trough fluctuations during the dosing interval and to minimize swings between potentially toxic or ineffective drug concentrations. Again, we report C_{max} for both immediate- and extended-release formulations, when available. In addition to parent drug concentrations, we have included information on any active metabolite that circulates at a concentration that may contribute to the overall pharmacological effect, particularly those active metabolites that accumulate with multiple dosing. Likewise, for chiral drugs whose stereoisomers differ in their pharmacological activity and clearance characteristics, we present information on the levels of the individual enantiomers or the active enantiomer that contributes most to the drug's efficacy.

ALTERATIONS OF PARAMETERS IN THE INDIVIDUAL PATIENT

Dose adjustments for an individual patient should be made according to the manufacturer's recommendation in the package labeling when available. This information generally is available when disease, age, or race has a significant impact on drug disposition, particularly for drugs that have been introduced within the past 10 years. In some cases, a significant difference in drug disposition from the "average" adult can be expected but may not require dose adjustment because of a sufficiently broad therapeutic index. In other cases, dose adjustment may be necessary, but no specific information is available. Under these circumstances, an estimate of the appropriate dosing regimen can be obtained based on pharmacokinetic principles described in Chapter 1.

Unless otherwise specified, the values in Table AII–1 represent mean values for populations of normal adults; it may be necessary to modify them for calculation of dosage regimens for individual patients. The fraction available (*F*) and clearance (*CL*) also must be estimated to compute a maintenance dose necessary to achieve a desired average steady-state concentration. To calculate the loading dose, knowledge of the volume of distribution is needed. The estimated $t_{1/2}$ is used in deciding a dosing interval that provides an acceptable peak-trough fluctuation; note that this may be the apparent $t_{1/2}$ following dosing of a slowly absorbed formulation. The values reported in the table and the adjustments apply only to adults; exceptions are footnoted. Although the values at times may be applied to children who weigh more than ~30 kg (after proper adjustment for size; see "Clearance" and "Volume of Distribution" later), it is best to consult pediatrics textbooks or other sources for definitive advice.

For each drug, changes in the parameters caused by certain disease states are noted within the eight segments of the table. In all cases, the qualitative direction of changes is noted, such as "↓ LD," which indicates a significant decrease in the parameter in a patient with chronic liver disease. The relevant literature and the package label should be consulted for more definitive, quantitative information for dosage adjustment recommendations.

Plasma-Protein Binding. Most acidic drugs that are extensively bound to plasma proteins are bound to albumin. Basic lipophilic drugs, such as propranolol, often bind to other plasma proteins (e.g., α_1-acid glycoprotein and lipoproteins). The degree of drug binding to proteins will differ in pathophysiological states that cause changes in plasma-protein concentrations. Significant pharmacokinetic effects from a change in plasma-protein binding will be denoted under clearance or volume of distribution.

Although pharmacokinetic parameters based on total drug or metabolite concentrations often are reported, it is important to recognize that in many cases it is the concentration of *unbound drug* that drives access to the site of action and the degree of pharmacological effect. Remarkable changes in the total plasma concentration may accompany disease-induced alteration in protein binding; however, the clinical outcome is not always affected because an increase in free fraction also will increase the apparent clearance of an orally administered drug and of a low-extraction drug dosed intravenously. Under such a scenario, the mean unbound plasma concentration at steady state will not change with reduced or elevated plasma-protein binding, despite a significant change in mean total drug concentration. If so, no adjustment of daily maintenance dose is needed.

Clearance. For drugs that are partly or predominantly eliminated by renal excretion, plasma clearance changes in accordance with the renal function of an individual patient. This necessitates dosage adjustment that is dependent on the fraction of normal renal function remaining and the fraction of drug normally excreted unchanged in the urine. The latter quantity appears in the table; the former can be estimated as the ratio of the patient's creatinine clearance (CL_{cr}) to a normal value (100 mL/min/70 kg body weight). If urinary creatinine clearance has not been measured, it may be estimated from the concentration of creatinine in serum (C_{cr}). In men:

$$CL_{cr}(\text{mL/min}) = \frac{[140 - \text{age (yr)}]\cdot[\text{weight (kg)}]}{72\cdot[C_{cr}(\text{mg/dL})]}$$

(Equation A-1)

For women, the estimate of CL_{cr} by the above equation should be multiplied by 0.85 to reflect their smaller muscle mass. The fraction of normal renal function (rfx_{pt}) is estimated from the following:

$$rfx_{pt} = \frac{CL_{cr,pt}}{100 \text{ mL/min}} \qquad \text{(Equation A-2)}$$

A more accurate measure of rfx_{pt} seldom is necessary because, given the considerable degree of interindividual variation in nonrenal clearance, the adjustment of clearance is an approximation. The following equation for adjustment of clearance uses the quantities discussed:

$$rf_{pt} = 1 - [fe_{nl}\cdot(1 - rfx_{pt})] \qquad \text{(Equation A-3)}$$

where fe_{nl} is the fraction of systemic drug excreted unchanged in normal individuals (see Table AII–1). The renal factor (rf_{pt}) is the value that, when multiplied by normal total clearance (CL_{nl}) from the table, gives the total clearance of the drug adjusted for the impairment in renal function.

Example. The clearance of vancomycin in a patient with reduced renal function (creatinine clearance = 25 mL/min/70 kg) may be estimated as follows:

$$rfx_{pt} = \frac{25 \text{ mL/min}}{100 \text{ mL/min}} = 0.25$$

$$fe_{nl} = 0.79 \text{(see listing for vancomycin)}$$

$$\text{rf}_{pt} = 1 - [0.79\cdot(1 - 0.25)] = 0.41$$

$$CL_{pt} = (1.3 \text{ mL/min/kg})\cdot 0.41$$

$$= 0.53 \text{ mL/min/kg}$$

Importantly, such a clearance adjustment should be regarded only as an initial step in optimizing the dosage regimen; depending on the patient's response to the drug, further individualization may be necessary.

Conventionally, clearance is adjusted for the size of the patient to reflect a difference in the mass of the eliminating organ. For orally administered drugs, the applicability of such an adjustment may be limited by the available dosage strengths of commercial formulations. In some cases, scored tablets can be split, or commercial tablet splitters are used to increase the range of available dosage strengths. However, this practice should be followed only with the recommendation of the drug manufacturer because splitting a tablet sometimes can compromise the bioavailability of a product.

With the exception of certain oncolytic agents, the data presented in the table are normalized to weight. Thus, interindividual variability in the weight-normalized clearance reflects a variation in the intrinsic metabolic or transport clearance and not the size of the organ. Further, these differences can be attributed to variable expression/function of metabolic enzymes or transporters. However, it is important to recognize that liver mass and total enzyme/transporter content may not increase or decrease in proportion to weight in obese or malnourished individuals. Alternative approaches such as normalization by body surface area or other measures of body mass may be more appropriate. For example, many of the drugs used to treat cancer are dosed according to body surface area (see Chapter 51). In the tabulation, if the literature reported dose per body surface area, we presented the data in the same unit. If the cited clearance data were not normalized, but the preponderance of the literature utilized body surface area, we followed the practice of using values of body surface area from the literature source or a standard of 1.73 m^2 for a healthy adult.

Volume of Distribution. Volume of distribution should be adjusted for the modifying factors indicated in Table AII–1 as well as for body size. Again, the data in the table most often are normalized to weight. Unlike clearance, volume of distribution in an individual most often is proportional to weight itself. Whether this applies to a specific drug depends on the actual sites of distribution of drug; no absolute rule applies.

Whether or not to adjust volume of distribution for changes in binding to plasma proteins cannot be decided in general; the decision depends critically on whether or not the factors that alter binding to plasma proteins also alter binding to tissue proteins. Qualitative changes in volume of distribution, when they occur, are indicated in the table.

Half-Life. Half-life may be estimated from the adjusted values of clearance (CL_{pt}) and volume of distribution (V_{pt}) for the patient:

$$t_{1/2} = \frac{0.693\cdot V_{pt}}{CL_{pt}} \qquad \text{(Equation A-4)}$$

Because $t_{1/2}$ has been the parameter most often measured and reported in the literature, qualitative changes for this parameter almost always are given in the table.

INDIVIDUALIZATION OF DOSAGE

By using the parameters for the individual patient, calculated as described in the previous section, initial dosing regimens may be chosen. The maintenance dosage rate may be calculated with Equation 1–18, using the estimated values for *CL* and *F* for the individual patient. As described earlier, the target concentration may have to be adjusted for changes in plasma-protein binding in the patient, as described in "Plasma-Protein Binding." The loading dose may be calculated using Equation 1–22 and estimates for V_{ss} and *F*. A particular dosing interval may be chosen; the maximal and minimal steady-state concentrations can be calculated by using Equations 1–20 and 1–19 or 1–21, and these calculated concentrations can be compared with the known efficacious and toxic concentrations for the drug. As with the target concentration, these values may need to be adjusted for changes in the extent of plasma-protein binding. Use of Equations 1–19 and 1–20 also requires estimates of values for *F*, V_{ss}, and *K* ($K = 0.693/t_{1/2}$) for the individual patient.

Note that these adjustments of pharmacokinetic parameters for an individual patient are suggested for the rational choice of initial dosing regimen. As indicated in Chapter 1, steady-state measurement of drug concentrations in the patient then can be used as a guide to further adjust the dosage regimen. However, optimization of a dosage regimen for an individual patient ultimately will depend on the clinical response produced by the drug.

Table AII–1

Pharmacokinetic Data

Key: Unless otherwise indicated by a specific footnote, the data are presented for the study population as a mean value ± 1 standard deviation, a mean and range (lowest-highest in parentheses) of values, a range of the lowest-highest values, or a single mean value. ACE, angiotensin-converting enzyme; ADH, alcohol dehydrogenase; Aged, aged; AIDS, acquired immunodeficiency syndrome; Alb, hypoalbuminemia; Alcohol, chronic consumption of ethanol; Atr Fib, atrial fibrillation; AVH, acute viral hepatitis; Burn, burn patients; C_{max}, peak concentration; CAD, coronary artery disease; Celiac, celiac disease; CF, cystic fibrosis; CHF, congestive heart failure; Child, children; COPD, chronic obstructive pulmonary disease; CP, cor pulmonale; CPBS, cardiopulmonary bypass surgery; CRI, chronic respiratory insufficiency; Crohn, Crohn's disease; Cush, Cushing's syndrome; CYP, cytochrome P450; F or Fem, female; Hep, hepatitis; HIV, human immunodeficiency virus; HL, hyperlipoproteinemia; HTh, hyperthyroid; IM, intramuscular; Inflam, inflammation; IV, intravenous; LD, chronic liver disease; LTh, hypothyroid; M, male; MAO, monoamine oxidase; MI, myocardial infarction; NAT, *N*-acetyltransferase; Neo, neonate; NIDDM, non-insulin-dependent diabetes mellitus; NS, nephrotic syndrome; Obes, obese; *PDR*54, *Physicians' Desk Reference,* 54th ed. Montvale, NJ, Medical Economics Co., 2000; *PDR*58, *Physicians' Desk Reference,* 58th ed. Montvale, NJ, Medical Economics Co., 2004; Pneu, pneumonia; PO, oral administration; Preg, pregnant; Prem, premature infants; RA, rheumatoid arthritis; Rac, racemic mixture of stereoisomers; RD = renal disease (including uremia); SC, subcutaneous; Smk, smoking; ST, sulfotransferase; T_{max}, peak time; Tach, ventricular tachycardia; UGT, UDP-glucuronosyl transferase; Ulcer, ulcer patients. Other abbreviations are defined in the text section of this appendix.

BIOAVAILABILITY (ORAL) (%)	URINARY EXCRETION (%)	BOUND IN PLASMA (%)	CLEARANCE (mL/min/kg)	VOL. DIST. (L/kg)	HALF-LIFE (hours)	PEAK TIME (hours)	PEAK CONCENTRATION
Acetaminophen[a]							
88 ± 15 ↔ Child	3 ± 1 ↔ Neo, Child	<20	5.0 ± 1.4[b] ↓ Hep[c] ↔ Aged, Child ↑ Obes, HTh, Preg	0.95 ± 0.12[b] ↔ Aged, Hep[c], LTh, HTh, Child	2.0 ± 0.4 ↔ RD, Obes, Child ↑ Neo, Hep[c] ↑ HTh, Preg	0.33–1.4[d]	20 μg/mL[e]

[a]Values reported are for doses <2 g; drug exhibits concentration-dependent kinetics above this dose. [b]Assuming a 70-kg body weight; reported range, 65-72 kg. [c]Acetaminophen-induced hepatic damage or AVH. [d]Absorption rate, but not extent, depends on gastric emptying; hence, it is slowed after food as well as in some disease states and co-treatment with drugs that cause gastroparesis. [e]Mean concentration following a 20-mg/kg oral dose. Hepatic toxicity associated with levels >300 μg/mL at 4 hours after an overdose.

Reference: Forrest JA, et al. Clinical pharmacokinetics of paracetamol. *Clin Pharmacokinet,* **1982**, *7*:93–107.

BIOAVAILABILITY (ORAL) (%)	URINARY EXCRETION (%)	BOUND IN PLASMA (%)	CLEARANCE (mL/min/kg)	VOL. DIST. (L/kg)	HALF-LIFE (hours)	PEAK TIME (hours)	PEAK CONCENTRATION
Acetylsalicylic Acid[a]							
68 ± 3 ↔ Aged, LD	1.4 ± 1.2	49 ↓ RD	9.3 ± 1.1 ↔ Aged, LD	0.15 ± 0.03	0.25 ± 0.03 ↔ Hep	0.39 ± 0.21[b]	24 ± 4 μg/mL[b]

[a]Values given are for unchanged parent drug. Acetylsalicylic acid is converted to salicylic acid during and after absorption (*CL* and $t_{1/2}$ of salicylate are dose dependent; $t_{1/2}$ varies between 2.4 hours after a 300-mg dose to 19 hours when there is intoxication). [b]Following a single 1.2-g oral dose given to adults.

Reference: Roberts MS, et al. Pharmacokinetics of aspirin and salicylate in elderly subjects and in patients with alcoholic liver disease. *Eur J Clin Pharmacol,* **1983**, *25*:253–261.

(*Continued*)

Table AII–1

Pharmacokinetic Data (*Continued*)

BIOAVAILABILITY (ORAL) (%)	URINARY EXCRETION (%)	BOUND IN PLASMA (%)	CLEARANCE (mL/min/kg)	VOL. DIST. (L/kg)	HALF-LIFE (hours)	PEAK TIME (hours)	PEAK CONCENTRATION
Acyclovir							
15-30[a]	75 ± 10	15 ± 4	$CL = 3.37CL_{cr} + 0.41$ ↓ Neo ↔ Child	0.69 ± 0.19 ↑ Neo ↔ RD	2.4 ± 0.7 ↑ RD, Neo ↔ Child	1.5-2[b]	3.5-5.4 μM[b]
[a]Decreases with increasing dose. [b]Range of steady-state concentrations following a 400-mg dose given orally every 4 hours to steady state.				*Reference:* Laskin OL. Clinical pharmacokinetics of acyclovir. *Clin Pharmacokinet,* **1983**, *8*:187–201.			
Albendazole[a]							
—[b] ↑ Food	<1	70	10.5-30.7[c]	—	8 (6-15)[d]	2-4[e]	0.50-1.8 μg/mL[e]
[a]Oral albendazole undergoes rapid and essentially complete first-pass metabolism to albendazole sulfoxide (ALBSO), which is pharmacologically active. Pharmacokinetic data for ALBSO in male and female adults are reported. [b]The absolute bioavailability of ALBSO is not known but is increased by high-fat meals. [c]*CL/F* following twice-daily oral dosing to steady state. Chronic albendazole treatment appears to induce the metabolism of ALBSO. [d]$t_{1/2}$ reportedly shorter in children with neurocysticercosis compared with adults; may need to be dosed more frequently (three times a day) in children, rather than twice a day, as in adults. [e]Following a 7.5-mg/kg oral dose given twice daily for 8 days to adults.				*References:* Marques MP, et al. Enantioselective kinetic disposition of albendazole sulfoxide in patients with neurocysticercosis. *Chirality,* **1999**, *11*:218–223. *PDR58*, **2004**, p. 1422. Sanchez M, et al. Pharmacokinetic comparison of two albendazole dosage regimens in patients with neurocysticercosis. *Clin Neuropharmacol,* **1993**, *76*:77–82. Sotelo J, et al. Pharmacokinetic optimisation of the treatment of neurocysticercosis. *Clin Pharmacokinet,* **1998**, *34*:503–515.			
Albuterol[a]							
PO, *R*: 30 ± 7 PO, *S*: 71 ± 9 IH, *R*: 25 IH, *S*: 47	*R*: 46 ± 8 *S*: 55 ± 11	*Rac*: 7 ± 1	*R*: 10.3 ± 3.0 *S*: 6.5 ± 2.0 ↓ RD[b]	*R*: 2.00 ± 0.49 *S*: 1.77 ± 0.69 ↓ RD[b]	*R*: 2.00 ± 0.49 *S*: 2.85 ± 0.85	*R*: 1.5[c] *S*: 2.0[c]	*R*: 3.6 (1.9-5.9) ng/mL[c] *S*: 11.4 (7.1-16.2) ng/mL[c]
[a]Data from healthy subjects for *R*- and *S*-enantiomers. No major gender differences. No kinetic differences in asthmatics. β-Adrenergic activity resides primarily with R-enantiomer. PO, oral; IH, inhalation. Oral dose undergoes extensive first-pass sulfation at the intestinal mucosa. [b]*CL/F* reduced, moderate renal impairment. [c]Median (range) following a single 4-mg oral dose of racemic-albuterol.				*References*: Boulton DW, et al. Enantioselective disposition of albuterol in humans. *Clin Rev Allergy Immunol,* **1996**, *14*:115–138. Mohamed MH, et al. Effects of gender and race on albuterol pharmacokinetics. *Pharmacotherapy,* **1999**, *19*:157–161.			

Aripiprazole[a]							
87	<1	>99	0.83 ± 0.17[b]	4.9[b]	47 ± 10	3.0 ± 0.6[c]	242 ± 36 ng/mL[c]

[a]Eliminated primarily by CYP2D6- and CYP3A4-dependent metabolism. The major metabolite, dehydro-aripiprazole, has affinity for D_2 receptors similar to parent drug; found at 40% of parent drug concentration in plasma; $t_{1/2}$ is 94 hours. CYP2D6 poor metabolizers exhibit increased exposure (80%) to parent drug but reduced exposure (30%) to the active metabolite. No significant gender differences. [b]*CL/F* and *V/F* at steady state reported. [c]Following a 15-mg oral dose given once daily for 14 days.

References: DeLeon A, et al. Aripiprazole: A comprehensive review of its pharmacology, clinical efficacy, and tolerability. *Clin Ther,* **2004**, *26*:649–666. Mallikaarjun S, et al. Pharmacokinetics, tolerability, and safety of aripiprazole following multiple oral dosing in normal healthy volunteers. *J Clin Pharmacol,* **2004**, *44*:179–187. *PDR*58, **2004**, pp. 1034–1035.

Atazanavir[a]							
—[b] ↑ Food	7	86	3.4 ± 1.0[c] ↓ LD	1.6-2.7[c]	7.9 ± 2.9 ↑ LD	2.5[d]	5.4 ± 1.4 μg/mL[d]

[a]Undergoes extensive hepatic metabolism, primarily by CYP3A. Pharmacokinetic data reported for healthy adults. No significant gender or age differences. [b]Absolute bioavailability is not known, but food enhances the extent of absorption. [c]*CL/F* and *V/F* reported. Metabolic elimination affected by inhibitors and inducers of CYP3A. Co-administration with low-dose ritonavir increases systemic atazanavir exposure. [d]Following a 400-mg oral dose given with a light meal once daily to steady state.

References: Orrick JJ, et al. Atazanavir. *Ann Pharmacother,* **2004**, *38*:1664–1674. *PDR*58, **2004**, p. 1081.

Atenolol[a]							
58 ± 16	94 ± 8	<5	2.4 ± 0.3 ↓ Aged	1.3 ± 0.5[b]	6.1 ± 2.0[c] ↑ RD, Aged	3.3 ± 1.3[d]	0.28 ± 0.09 μg/mL[d]

[a]Atenolol is administered as a racemic mixture. No significant differences in the pharmacokinetics of the enantiomers. [b]V_{area} reported. [c]$t_{1/2}$ of *R*- and *S*-atenolol are similar. [d]Following a single 50-mg oral dose.

References: Boyd RA, et al. The pharmacokinetics of the enantiomers of atenolol. *Clin Pharmacol Ther,* **1989**, *45*:403–410. Mason WD, et al. Kinetics and absolute bioavailability of atenolol. *Clin Pharmacol Ther,* **1979**, *25*:408–415.

Atomoxetine[a]							
EM: 63[b] PM: 94[b]	1-2%	98.7 ± 0.3	EM: 6.2[b] PM: 0.60[b] EM: ↓ LD	EM: 2.3[b] PM: 1.1[b]	EM: 5.3[b] PM: 20[b]	EM/PM: 2[c]	EM: 160 ng/mL[c] PM: 915 ng/mL[c]

[a]Metabolized by CYP2D6 (polymorphic). Poor metabolizers (PM) exhibit a higher oral bioavailability, higher C_{max}, lower *CL,* and longer $t_{1/2}$ than extensive metabolizers (EM). No differences between adults and children >6 years of age. [b]*CL/F, V/F,* and $t_{1/2}$ measured at steady state. [c]Following a 20-mg oral dose given twice daily for 5 days.

References: Sauer JM, et al. Disposition and metabolic fate of atomoxetine hydrochloride: The role of CYP2D6 in human disposition and metabolism. *Drug Metab Dispos,* **2003**, *37*:98–107. Simpson D, et al. Atomoxetine: A review of its use in adults with attention deficit hyperactivity disorder. *Drugs,* **2004**, *64*:205–222.

(*Continued*)

Table AII–1

Pharmacokinetic Data (*Continued*)

BIOAVAILABILITY (ORAL) (%)	URINARY EXCRETION (%)	BOUND IN PLASMA (%)	CLEARANCE (mL/min/kg)	VOL. DIST. (L/kg)	HALF-LIFE (hours)	PEAK TIME (hours)	PEAK CONCENTRATION
Atorvastatin[a]							
12	<2	≥98	29[b] ↓ LD,[c] Aged ↔ RD	~5.4[b]	19.5 ± 9.6 ↑ LD,[b] Aged	2.3 ± 0.96[d]	14.9 ± 1.8 ngEq/mL[d]
Azathioprine[a]							
60 ± 31[b]	<2	—	57 ± 31[c]	0.81 ± 0.65[c]	0.16 ± 0.07[c] ↔ RD	MP: 1-2[d]	MP: 20-90 ng/mL[d]
Azithromycin							
34 ± 19 ↓ Food (capsules) ↑ Food (suspension)	12	7-50[a]	9	31	40[b] ↔ LD	2-3[c]	0.4 μg/mL[c]
Baclofen[a]							
>70[b]	69 ± 14	31 ± 11	2.72 ± 0.93[c] ↓ RD[d]	0.81 ± 0.12[c]	3.75 ± 0.96	1.0 (0.5-4)[e]	160 ± 49 ng/mL[e]

Atorvastatin: [a]Data from healthy adult male and female subjects. No clinically significant gender differences. Atorvastatin undergoes extensive CYP3A-dependent first-pass metabolism. Metabolites are active and exhibit a longer $t_{1/2}$ (20-30 hours) than parent drug. [b]Mean *CL/F* parameter calculated from reported AUC data at steady state after a once-a-day 20-mg oral dose, assuming a 70-kg body weight. [c]AUC following oral administration increased, mild to moderate hepatic impairment. [d]Following a 20-mg oral dose once daily for 14 days.

References: Gibson DM, et al. Effect of age and gender on pharmacokinetics of atorvastatin in humans. *J Clin Pharmacol,* **1996**, *36*:242–246. Lea AP, et al. Atorvastatin. A review of its pharmacology and therapeutic potential in the management of hyperlipidaemias. *Drugs,* **1997**, *53*:828–847. *PDR*54, **2000**, p. 2254.

Azathioprine: [a]Azathioprine is metabolized to mercaptopurine (MP), listed later in this table. [b]Determined as the bioavailability of MP; intact azathioprine is undetectable after oral administration because of extensive first-pass metabolism. Kinetic values are for IV azathioprine. [c]Data from kidney transplant patients. [d]MP concentration following a 135 ± 34-mg oral dose of azathioprine given daily to steady state in kidney transplant patients.

Reference: Lin SN, et al. Quantitation of plasma azathioprine and 6-mercaptopurine levels in renal transplant patients. *Transplantation,* **1980**, *29*:290–294.

Azithromycin: [a]Dose-dependent plasma binding. The bound fraction is 50% at 50 ng/mL and 12% at 500 ng/mL. [b]A longer terminal plasma $t_{1/2}$ of 68 ± 8 hours, reflecting release from tissue stores, overestimates the multiple-dosing $t_{1/2}$. [c]Following a 250-mg/day oral dose to adult patients with an infection.

Reference: Lalak NJ, et al. Azithromycin clinical pharmacokinetics. *Clin Pharmacokinet,* **1993**, *25*:370–374.

Baclofen: [a]Data from healthy adult male subjects. [b]Bioavailability estimate based on urine recovery of unchanged drug after oral dose. [c]CL/F, V_{area}/F reported for intestinal infusion of drug. [d]Limited data suggest *CL/F* reduced with renal impairment. [e]Following a single 10-mg oral dose.

References: Kochak GM, et al. The pharmacokinetics of baclofen derived from intestinal infusion. *Clin Pharmacol Ther,* **1985**, *38*:251–257. Wuis EW, et al. Plasma and urinary excretion kinetics of oral baclofen in healthy subjects. *Eur J Clin Pharmacol,* **1989**, *37*:181–184.

Bicalutamide[a]							
—	1.7 ± 0.3	96	*R*: 0.043 ± 0.013[b] *S*: 7.3 ± 4.0[b] ↔ LD, RD, Aged	—	*R*: 139 ± 32 *S*: 29 ± 8.6 ↑ LD[c]	*R*: 23.4[d] *S*: 20.7[d]	SD, *R*: 734 ng/mL[d] SD, *S*: 84 ng/mL[d] MD, *R/S*: 8.9 ± 3.5 μg/mL

[a]Data from healthy male subjects. Exhibits stereoselective metabolism—*S*-enantiomer, primarily glucuronidation; *R*-enantiomer, primarily oxidation. [b]*CL/F* reported for oral dose. [c]Increased $t_{1/2}$ of *R*-enantiomer, severe LD. [d]Following a 50-mg tablet administered as a single dose (SD) or a multiple dose (MD), once a day to steady state.

References: Cockshott ID, et al. The effect of food on the pharmacokinetics of the bicalutamide ("Casodex") enantiomers. *Biopharm Drug Dispos,* **1997**, *18*:499–507. McKillop D, et al. Metabolism and enantioselective pharmacokinetics of Casodex in man. *Xenobiotica,* **1993**, *23*:1241–1253. *PDR*54, **2000**, p. 538.

Buprenorphine[a]							
IM: 40 to >90	Negligible	96	13.3 ± 0.59	1.44 ± 0.11	2.33 ± 0.24	IM: 0.08[c]	IM: 3.6 ± 3.0 ng/mL[c]
SL: 51 ± 30			↑ Child[b]	↑ Child[b]	↓ Child[b]	SL:0.7 ± 0.1[c]	SL: 3.3 ± 0.8 ng/mL[c]
BC: 28 ± 9						BC: 0.8 ± 0.2[c]	BC: 2.0 ± 0.6 ng/mL[c]

[a]Data from male and female subjects undergoing surgery. Buprenorphine is metabolized in the liver by both oxidative (*N*-dealkylation) and conjugative pathways. [b]*CL,* 60 ± 19 mL/min/kg; V_{ss}, 3.2 L/kg; $t_{1/2}$, 1.03 ± 0.22 hour; children 4-7 years of age. [c]Following a 0.3-mg IM, 4-mg sublingual (SL), 4-mg buccal (BC) dose.

References: Bullingham RE, et al. Buprenorphine kinetics. *Clin Pharmacol Ther,* **1980**, *28*:667–672. Cone EJ, et al. The metabolism and excretion of buprenorphine in humans. *Drug Metab Dispos,* **1984**, *12*:577–581. Kuhlman JJ, et al. Human pharmacokinetics of intravenous, sublingual, and buccal buprenorphine. *J Anal Toxicol,* **1996**, *20*:369–378. Olkkola KT, et al. Pharmacokinetics of intravenous buprenorphine in children. *Br J Clin Pharmacol,* **1989**, *28*:202–204.

Bupropion[a]							
—	<1	>80%	36.0 ± 2.2[b]	18.6 ± 1.2[b]	11 ± 1[b]	IR: 1.6 ± 0.1[d]	IR: 141 ± 19 ng/mL[d]
			↓ Aged, LD[c]	↔ Alcohol	(7.9-18.4)	SR: 3.1 ± 0.3[d]	SR: 142 ± 28 ng/mL[d]
			↔ Alcohol		↑ Aged, LD[c] ↔ Alcohol		

[a]Data from healthy adult male volunteers. Bupropion appears to undergo extensive first-pass metabolism by CYP2B6 and other CYP isozymes. Some metabolites accumulate in blood and are active. [b]*CL/F,* V_{ss}/F, and $t_{1/2}$ reported for oral dose. Range of mean terminal $t_{1/2}$ from four different studies shown in parentheses. [c]*CL/F* reduced, alcoholic liver disease. [d]Following a single 100-mg immediate-release (IR) or 150-mg sustained-release (SR) dose.

References: DeVane CL, et al. Disposition of bupropion in healthy volunteers and subjects with alcoholic liver disease. *J Clin Psychopharmacol,* **1990**, *10*:328–332. Hsyu PH, et al. Pharmacokinetics of bupropion and its metabolites in cigarette smokers versus nonsmokers. *J Clin Pharmacol,* **1997**, *37*:737–743. *PDR*54, **2000**, p. 1301. Posner J, et al. Alcohol and bupropion pharmacokinetics in healthy male volunteers. *Eur J Clin Pharmacol,* **1984**, *26*:627–630. Posner J, et al. The disposition of bupropion and its metabolites in healthy male volunteers after single and multiple doses. *Eur J Clin Pharmacol,* **1985**, *29*:97–103.

(Continued)

Table AII–1

Pharmacokinetic Data (*Continued*)

BIOAVAILABILITY (ORAL) (%)	URINARY EXCRETION (%)	BOUND IN PLASMA (%)	CLEARANCE (mL/min/kg)	VOL. DIST. (L/kg)	HALF-LIFE (hours)	PEAK TIME (hours)	PEAK CONCENTRATION
Buspirone[a]							
3.9 ± 4.3 ↑ Food[b]	<0.1	>95	28.3 ± 10.3 ↓ LD,[c] RD[d]	5.3 ± 2.6	2.4 ± 1.1 ↑ LD, RD	0.71 ± 0.06[e]	1.66 ± 0.21 ng/mL[e]

[a]Data from healthy adult male subjects. No significant gender differences. Undergoes extensive CYP3A-dependent first-pass metabolism. The major metabolite (l-pyrimidinyl piperazine) is active in some behavioral tests in animals (one-fifth potency) and accumulates in blood to levels severalfold higher than buspirone. [b]Bioavailability increased ~84%; appears to be secondary to reduced first-pass metabolism. [c]*CL/F* reduced, hepatic cirrhosis. [d]*CL/F* reduced, mild renal impairment; unrelated to CL_{cr}. [e]Following a single 20-mg oral dose.

References: Barbhaiya RH, et al. Disposition kinetics of buspirone in patients with renal or hepatic impairment after administration of single and multiple doses. *Eur J Clin Pharmacol,* **1994**, *46*:41–47. Gammans RE, et al. Metabolism and disposition of buspirone. *Am J Med,* **1986**, *80*:41–51.

BIOAVAILABILITY (ORAL) (%)	URINARY EXCRETION (%)	BOUND IN PLASMA (%)	CLEARANCE (mL/min/kg)	VOL. DIST. (L/kg)	HALF-LIFE (hours)	PEAK TIME (hours)	PEAK CONCENTRATION
Busulfan							
70 (44-94)	1	2.7-14	4.5 ± 0.9[a]	0.99 ± 0.23[a]	2.6 ± 0.5	2.6 ± 1.5	Low: 65 ± 27 ng/mL[b] High: 949 ± 278 ng/mL[b]

[a]*CL/F* and V_{area}/F reported. [b]Following a single 4-mg oral dose (low) given to patients with chronic myelocytic leukemia or a single 1-mg/kg oral dose (high) given as ablative therapy to patients undergoing bone marrow transplantation.

References: Ehrsson H, et al. Busulfan kinetics. *Clin Pharmacol Ther,* 1983, *34*:86–89. Schuler US, et al. Pharmacokinetics of intravenous busulfan and evaluation of the bioavailability of the oral formulation in conditioning for haematopoietic stem cell transplantation. *Bone Marrow Transplant,* **1998**, *22*:241–244.

BIOAVAILABILITY (ORAL) (%)	URINARY EXCRETION (%)	BOUND IN PLASMA (%)	CLEARANCE (mL/min/kg)	VOL. DIST. (L/kg)	HALF-LIFE (hours)	PEAK TIME (hours)	PEAK CONCENTRATION
Calcitriol[a]							
PO: ~61 IP: ~67	<10%	99.9	0.43 ± 0.04	—	16.5 ± 3.1[b] ↑ Child[c]	PO: 3-6[d] IP: 2-3[d]	IV: ~460 pg/mL[d] PO: ~90 pg/mL[d] IP: ~105 pg/mL[d]

[a]Data from young (15-22 years) patients on peritoneal dialysis. Metabolized by 23-, 24-, and 26-hydroxylases and also excreted into bile as its glucuronide. [b]Calcitriol $t_{1/2}$ is 5-8 hours in healthy adult subjects. [c]Oral dose $t_{1/2}$ = 27 ± 12 hours, children 2-16 years. [d]Following a single 60-ng/kg IV, intraperitoneal (IP) dialysate, or PO dose. Baseline plasma levels were <10 pg/mL.

References: Jones CL, et al. Comparisons between oral and intraperitoneal 1,25-dihydroxyvitamin D_3 therapy in children treated with peritoneal dialysis. *Clin Nephrol,* **1994**, *42*:44–49. *PDR*54, **2000**, p. 2650. Salusky IE, et al. Pharmacokinetics of calcitriol in continuous ambulatory and cycling peritoneal dialysis patients. *Am J Kidney Dis,* **1990**, *16*:126–132. Taylor CA, et al. Clinical pharmacokinetics during continuous ambulatory peritoneal dialysis. *Clin Pharmacokinet,* **1996**, *31*:293–308.

Capecitabine[a]							
— ↓ Food[b]	3	<60	145 (34%) L/hr/m² [c,d] ↓ LD[e]	270 L/m² [c,d]	C: 1.3 (146%)[c] 5-FU: 0.72 (16%)[c]	C: 0.5 (0.5-1)[f] 5-FU: 0.5 (0.5-2.1)[f] ↓ Food	C: 6.6 ± 6.0 μg/mL[f] 5-FU: 0.47 ± 0.47 μg/mL[f]
Carbamazepine[a]							
>70	<1	74 ± 3 ↔ RD, LD, Preg	1.3 ± 0.5[b,c] ↑ Preg ↔ Child, Aged, Smk	1.4 ± 0.4[b] ↔ Child, Neo, Aged	15 ± 5[b,c] ↔ Child, Neo, Aged	4-8[d]	9.3 (2-18) μg/mL[d]
Carbidopa[a]							
—[b]	5.3 ± 2.1	—	18 ± 7[c]	—	~2	2.1 ± 1.0	S: 165 ± 77 ng/mL[d] S-CR: 81 ± 28 ng/mL[d]

Capecitabine:

[a]Data from male and female patients with cancer. Capecitabine (C) is a prodrug for 5-fluorouracil (5-FU; active), listed later in this table. It is well absorbed, and bioactivation is sequential in liver and tumor. [b]AUC for C and 5-FU decreased. [c]Geometric mean (coefficient of variation). [d]CL/F and V_{area}/F reported for oral dose. [e]CL/F reduced but no change in 5-FU AUC, liver metastasis. [f]Following 1255 mg/m².

References: Dooley M, et al. Capecitabine. *Drugs,* **1999**, *58*:69–76; discussion 77–78. Reigner B, et al. Effect of food on the pharmacokinetics of capecitabine and its metabolites following oral administration in cancer patients. *Clin Cancer Res,* **1998**, *4*:941–948.

Carbamazepine:

[a]A metabolite, carbamazepine-10,11-epoxide, is equipotent in animal studies. Its formation is catalyzed primarily by CYP3A and secondarily by CYP2C8. [b]Data from oral, multiple-dose regimen; values are CL/F and V_{area}/F. [c]Data from multiple-dose regimen. Carbamazepine induces its own metabolism; for a single dose, $CL/F = 0.36 \pm 0.07$ mL/min/kg and $t_{1/2} = 36 \pm 5$ hours. CL also increases with dose. [d]Mean (range) steady-state concentration following a daily 18.4-mg/kg oral dose (immediate release) given to adult patients with epilepsy. Therapeutic range for control of psychomotor seizures is 4-10 μg/mL.

References: Bertilsson L, et al. Clinical pharmacokinetics and pharmacological effects of carbamazepine and carbamazepine-10,11-epoxide. An update. *Clin Pharmacokinet,* **1986**, *11*:177–198. Troupin A, et al. Carbamazepine—A double-blind comparison with phenytoin. *Neurology,* **1977**, *27*:511–519.

Carbidopa:

[a]Data from healthy adult subjects. Combined with levodopa for treatment of Parkinson's disease. [b]Absolute bioavailability is unknown, but it is presumably low based on a high value for CL/F. Bioavailability of SINEMET CR (S-CR) is 55% of standard SINEMET (S). [c]CL/F reported for 2 tablets of SINEMET 25/100. [d]Following a single oral dose of 2 tablets SINEMET 25/100 or 1 tablet SINEMET CR 50/200.

Reference: Yeh KC, et al. Pharmacokinetics and bioavailability of Sinemet CR: A summary of human studies. *Neurology,* **1989**, *39*:25–38.

(*Continued*)

Table AII–1

Pharmacokinetic Data (*Continued*)

BIOAVAILABILITY (ORAL) (%)	URINARY EXCRETION (%)	BOUND IN PLASMA (%)	CLEARANCE (mL/min/kg)	VOL. DIST. (L/kg)	HALF-LIFE (hours)	PEAK TIME (hours)	PEAK CONCENTRATION
Carboplatin[a]							
—	77 ± 5	0	1.5 ± 0.3 ↓ RD	0.24 ± 0.03	2 ± 0.2 ↑ RD	0.5[b]	39 ± 17 μg/mL[b]

[a]Measure of ultrafilterable platinum, which essentially is unchanged carboplatin. [b]Following a single 170 to 500-mg/m² IV dose (30-minute infusion) given to adult patients with ovarian cancer.

Reference: Gaver RC, et al. The disposition of carboplatin in ovarian cancer patients. *Cancer Chemother Pharmacol,* **1988**, *22*:263–270.

BIOAVAILABILITY (ORAL) (%)	URINARY EXCRETION (%)	BOUND IN PLASMA (%)	CLEARANCE (mL/min/kg)	VOL. DIST. (L/kg)	HALF-LIFE (hours)	PEAK TIME (hours)	PEAK CONCENTRATION
Carvedilol[a]							
25 *S*-(–): 15 *R*-(+): 31 ↑ Cirr	<2	95[b]	8.7 ± 1.7 ↓ LD ↔ RD, Aged	1.5 ± 0.3 ↑ Cirr	2.2 ± 0.3[c] ↑, ↔ LD ↔ RD, Aged	1.3 ± 0.3[d]	105 ± 12 ng/mL[d]

[a]Racemic mixture: *S*-(–)-enantiomer responsible for β_1 adrenergic–receptor blockade. *R*-(+)- and *S*-(–)-enantiomers have nearly equivalent α_1-receptor blocking activity. [b]*R*-(+)-enantiomer is more tightly bound than the *S*-(–)-antipode. [c]Longer $t_{1/2}$ of ~6 hours has been measured at lower concentrations. [d]Following a 12.5-mg oral dose given twice a day for 2 weeks to healthy young adults.

References: Morgan T. Clinical pharmacokinetics and pharmacodynamics of carvedilol. *Clin Pharmacokinet,* **1994**, *26*:335–346. Morgan T, et al. Pharmacokinetics of carvedilol in older and younger patients. *J Hum Hypertens,* **1990**, *4*:709–715.

BIOAVAILABILITY (ORAL) (%)	URINARY EXCRETION (%)	BOUND IN PLASMA (%)	CLEARANCE (mL/min/kg)	VOL. DIST. (L/kg)	HALF-LIFE (hours)	PEAK TIME (hours)	PEAK CONCENTRATION
Cefazolin							
>90	80 ± 16	89 ± 2 ↓ RD, LD, CPBS, Neo, Child	0.95 ± 0.17 ↓ RD, CPBS ↑ Preg ↔ Neo, Obes, Child, LD	0.19 ± 0.06[a] ↑ RD, Neo ↔ Preg, Obes, Child, LD	2.2 ± 0.02 ↑ RD, Neo, CPBS ↓ Preg, LD ↔ Obes, Child	IM: 1.7 ± 0.7[b]	IV: 237 ± 285 μg/mL[b] IM: 42 ± 9.5 μg/mL[b]

[a]V_{area} reported. [b]Following a single 1-g IV (model-fitted C_{max}) or IM dose to healthy adults.

Reference: Scheld WM, et al. Moxalactam and cefazolin: Comparative pharmacokinetics in normal subjects. *Antimicrob Agents Chemother,* **1981**, *79*:613–619.

Cefdinir

Cap: 16-21[a] Susp: 25[a] ↓ Iron	13-23[b]	89[c] ↓ RD	11-15[d]	1.6-2.1[d]	1.4-1.5	Cap: 3 ± 0.7[e] Susp: 2 ± 0.4[e]	Cap:2.9 ± 1.0 μg/mL[e] Susp: 3.9 ± 0.6 μg/mL[e]

[a]Bioavailability following ingestion of a capsule (Cap) or suspension (Susp) formulated dose. [b]Determined after a single oral dose. [c]Lower plasma protein binding (71-74%) reported in patients undergoing dialysis. [d]*CL/F* and *V/F* reported. [e]Following ingestion of a single 600-mg capsule given to adults or a 14-mg/kg suspension dose given to children (6 months to 12 years). No accumulation after multiple dosing.

References: Guay DR. Pharmacodynamics and pharmacokinetics of cefdinir, an oral extended spectrum cephalosporin. *Pediatr Infect Dis J,* **2000**, *19*:S141–S146. *PDR*58, **2004**, p. 503. Tomino Y, et al. Pharmacokinetics of cefdinir and its transfer to dialysate in patients with chronic renal failure undergoing continuous ambulatory peritoneal dialysis. *Arzneimittelforschung,* **1998**, *48*:862–867.

Cefepime[a]

—	80	16-19	1.8 (1.7-2.5)[b] ↓ RD[c]	0.26 (0.24-0.31)[d]	2.1 (1.3-2.4)[b] ↑ RD[c]	—	65 ± 7 μg/mL[e]

[a]Data from healthy adult patients. Available only in parenteral form. [b]Median (range) of reported *CL* and $t_{1/2}$ values from 16 single-dose studies. [c]Mild renal impairment. [d]Median (range) of reported V_{ss} from 6 single-dose studies. [e]Following a 1-g IV dose.

References: Okamoto MP, et al. Cefepime clinical pharmacokinetics. *Clin Pharmacokinet,* **1993**, *25*:88–102. Rybak M. The pharmacokinetic profile of a new generation of parenteral cephalosporin. *Am J Med,* **1996**, *100*:39S–44S.

Ceftazidime

— IM: 91	84 ± 4 ↔ CF	21 ± 6	$CL = 1.05CL_{cr} + 0.12$ ↔ CF, Burn	0.23 ± 0.02 ↔ RD, CF ↑ Aged, Burn	1.6 ± 0.1 ↑ RD, Prem, Neo, Aged ↔ CF	IM: 0.7-1.3[a]	IV: 119-146 μg/mL[a] IM: 29-39 μg/mL[a]

[a]Range of mean data from different studies following a 1-g bolus IV or IM dose given to healthy adults.

Reference: Balant L, et al. Clinical pharmacokinetics of the third generation cephalosporins. *Clin Pharmacokinet,* **1985**, *10*:101–143.

(*Continued*)

Table AII–1

Pharmacokinetic Data (*Continued*)

BIOAVAILABILITY (ORAL) (%)	URINARY EXCRETION (%)	BOUND IN PLASMA (%)	CLEARANCE (mL/min/kg)	VOL. DIST. (L/kg)	HALF-LIFE (hours)	PEAK TIME (hours)	PEAK CONCENTRATION
Ceftriaxone[a]							
IM: ~100%	43 ± 10[b]	96% (0.5 μg/mL) to 83% (300 μg/mL)[c] ↓ LD[d]	0.5 g: 0.22 ± 0.04 2 g: 0.28 ± 0.04[e] ↓ RD[f] ↓ LD[d]	0.5 g: 0.12 ± 0.02 2 g: 0.14 ± 0.01[e]	5.9-6.5[e] ↑ RD[f] ↔ LD[g]	IM: 2	IV[h] 0.5 g: 101 ± 13 μg/mL 2.0 g: 280 ± 39 μg/mL IM[h] 0.5 g: 65 μg/mL 1.0 g: 114 μg/mL
[a]Ceftriaxone is most commonly administered by IV or IM injection and cleared unchanged by both renal and biliary excretion. [b]Value for a 2-g IV dose; similar values reported for 0.5- and 1-g doses. [c]Exhibits saturable binding. [d]Study in patients with mild to severe hepatic impairment. [e]Total clearance and distribution volume vary with dose and plasma free fraction; however, the unbound concentration at steady state is dose proportional. Mean $t_{1/2}$ values for 0.5- to 2-g doses not significantly different. [f]Study in anephric patients with normal nonrenal clearance. Much greater increases seen in patients with both renal and hepatic disease. [g]Impact of liver disease is limited by apparent offsetting changes in plasma-free fraction and unbound intrinsic clearance. [h]Following twice-daily dosing to steady state. *References:* Patel IH, et al. Pharmacokinetics of ceftriaxone in humans. *Antimicrob Agents Chemother,* **1981**, *20*:634–641. Pollock AA, et al. Pharmacokinetic characteristics of intravenous ceftriaxone in normal adults. *Antimicrob Agents Chemother,* **1982**, *22*:816–823. Yuk JH, et al. Clinical pharmacokinetics of ceftriaxone. *Clin Pharmacokinet,* **1989**, *17*:223–235.							
Celecoxib[a]							
— ↑ Food[b]	<3	~97	6.60 ± 1.85[c] ↓ Aged, LD[d] ↑ RD[e]	6.12 ± 2.08[c]	11.2 ± 3.47	2.8 ± 1.0[f] ↑ Food	705 ± 268 ng/mL[f]
[a]Data from healthy subjects. Cleared primarily by CYP2C9 (polymorphic). [b]High-fat meal. Absolute bioavailability is unknown. [c]*CL/F* and *V/F* values reported. [d]*CL/F* reduced, mild or moderate hepatic impairment. [e]*CL/F* increased, moderate renal impairment, but unrelated to CL_{cr}. [f]Following a single 200-mg oral dose. *References*: Goldenberg MM. Celecoxib, a selective cyclooxygenase-2 inhibitor for the treatment of rheumatoid arthritis and osteoarthritis. *Clin Ther,* **1999**, *21*:1497–1513; discussion 1427–1428. *PDR*54, **2000**, p. 2334.							
Cephalexin							
90 ± 9	91 ± 18	14 ± 3	4.3 ± 1.1[a] ↓ RD	0.26 ± 0.03[a] ↔ RD	0.90 ± 0.18 ↑ RD	1.4 ± 0.8[a]	28 ± 6.4 μg/mL[a]
[a]Following a single 500-mg oral dose given to healthy male adults. *Reference*: Spyker DA, et al. Pharmacokinetics of cefaclor and cephalexin: Dosage nomograms for impaired renal function. *Antimicrob Agents Chemother,* **1978**, *14*:172–177.							

Cetirizine[a]							
Rac: >70[b] Levo: >68[b]	Rac: 70.9 ± 7.8 Levo: 68.1 ± 10.2	Rac: 89.2 ± 0.4 Levo: 92.0 ± 0.3	Rac: 0.74 ± 0.19[c] Levo: 0.62 ± 0.11[c] Rac: ↓ LD,[d] RD,[e] Aged Levo: ↓ RD Rac/Levo: ↑ Child[f]	Rac: 0.58 ± 0.16[c] Levo: 0.41 ± 0.10	Rac: 9.42 ± 2.4 Levo: 7.8 ± 1.6 Rac: ↑ LD, RD, Aged Levo: ↑ RD Rac/Levo: ↓ Child	Rac: 0.9 ± 0.2[g] Levo: 0.8 ± 0.5[g]	Rac: 313 ± 45 ng/mL[g] Levo: 270 ± 40 ng/mL[g]

[a]Data from healthy male and female subjects receiving cetirizine (Rac) or the active R-enantiomer, levocetirizine (Levo). [b]Based on recovery of unchanged drug in urine. [c]*CL/F*, V_d/F reported for oral dose. [d]*CL/F* reduced, hepatocellular and cholestatic liver diseases. [e]*CL/F* reduced, moderate to severe renal impairment. [f]*CL/F* increased, ages 1-5 years. [g]Following a single 10-mg oral dose of Rac or 5 mg of Levo.

References: Baltes E, et al. Absorption and disposition of levocetirizine, the eutomer of cetirizine, administered alone or as cetirizine to healthy volunteers. *Fundam Clin Pharmacol,* **2001**, *15*:269–277. Benedetti MS, et al. Absorption, distribution, metabolism and excretion of [14C]levocetirizine, the R enantiomer of cetirizine, in healthy volunteers. *Eur J Clin Pharmacol*, **2001**, *57*:571–582. Horsmans Y, et al. Single-dose pharmacokinetics of cetirizine in patients with chronic liver disease. *J Clin Pharmacol,* **1993**, *33*:929–932. Matzke GR, et al. Pharmacokinetics of cetirizine in the elderly and patients with renal insufficiency. *Ann Allergy,* **1987**, *59*:25–30. *PDR*54, **2000**, p. 2404. Spicák V, et al. Pharmacokinetics and pharmacodynamics of cetirizine in infants and toddlers. *Clin Pharmacol Ther,* **1997**, *61*:325–330. Strolin Benedetti M, et al. Stereoselective renal tubular secretion of levocetirizine and dextrocetirizine, the two enantiomers of the H1-antihistamine cetirizine. *Fundam Clin Pharmacol,* **2008**, *22*:19–23.

Chloroquine[a]							
~80	52-58[b]	*S*: 66.6 ± 3.3[c] *R*: 42.7 ± 2.1 ↔ RD	3.7-13[b]	132-261[b]	10-24 days[b,d]	IM: 0.25[e] PO: 3.6 ± 2.0[e]	IV: 837 ± 248 ng/mL IM: 57-480 ng/mL PO: 76 ± 14 ng/mL

[a]Active metabolite, desethylchloroquine, accounts for 20 ± 3% of urinary excretion; $t_{1/2}$ = 15 ± 6 days. Racemic mixture; kinetic parameters for the two isomers are slightly different [e.g., mean residence time = 16.2 days and 11.3 days for the *R*-isomer and *S*-isomer, respectively]. [b]Range of mean values from different studies (IV administration). [c]Concentrates in red blood cells. Blood-to-plasma concentration ratio for racemate = 9. [d]A longer $t_{1/2}$ (41 ± 14 days) has been reported with extended blood sampling. [e]Following a single 300-mg IV dose (24-minute infusion) of chloroquine HCl or a single 300-mg IM or oral dose of chloroquine phosphate given to healthy adults. Effective concentrations against *Plasmodium vivax* and *Plasmodium falciparum* are 15 ng/mL and 30 ng/mL, respectively. Diplopia and dizziness can occur >250 ng/mL.

References: Krishna S, et al. Pharmacokinetics of quinine, chloroquine and amodiaquine. Clinical implications. *Clin Pharmacokinet,* **1996**, *30*:263–299. White NJ. Clinical pharmacokinetics of antimalarial drugs. *Clin Pharmacokinet,* **1985**, *10*:187–215.

Chlorpheniramine[a]							
41 ± 16	0.3-26[b]	70 ± 3	1.7 ± 0.1 ↑ Child	3.2 ± 0.3 ↔ Child	20 ± 5 ↓ Child	IR: 2-3[c] SR: 5.7-8.1[c]	IR: 16-71 ng/mL[c] SR: 17-76 ng/mL[c]

[a]Administered as a racemic mixture; reported parameters are for racemic drug. Activity comes predominantly from *S*-(+)-enantiomer, which has a 60% longer $t_{1/2}$ than the *R*-(–)-enantiomer. [b]Renal elimination increases with increased urine flow and lower pH. [c]Range of data from different studies following a 4-mg oral immediate-release (IR) dose given every 4-6 hours to steady state or following an 8-mg oral sustained-release (SR) dose given every 12 hours to steady state, both in healthy adults.

Reference: Rumore MM. Clinical pharmacokinetics of chlorpheniramine. *Drug Intell Clin Pharm,* **1984**, *18*:701–707.

(Continued)

Table AII–1

Pharmacokinetic Data (*Continued*)

BIOAVAILABILITY (ORAL) (%)	URINARY EXCRETION (%)	BOUND IN PLASMA (%)	CLEARANCE (mL/min/kg)	VOL. DIST. (L/kg)	HALF-LIFE (hours)	PEAK TIME (hours)	PEAK CONCENTRATION
Chlorpromazine[a]							
32 ± 19[b]	<1	95-98 ↔ RD	8.6 ± 2.9[c] ↓ Child ↔ LD	21 ± 9[c]	30 ± 7[c]	1-4[d]	25-150 ng/mL[d]

[a]Active metabolites, 7-hydroxychlorpromazine ($t_{1/2}$ = 25 ± 15 hours) and possibly chlorpromazine *N*-oxide, yield AUCs comparable to the parent drug (single doses). [b]After a single dose. Bioavailability may decrease to ~20% with repeated dosing. [c]*CL/F*, V_{area}, and terminal $t_{1/2}$ following IM administration. [d]Following a 100-mg oral dose given twice a day for 33 days to adult patients. Neurotoxicity (tremors and convulsions) occurs at concentrations of 750-1000 ng/mL.

Reference: Dahl SG, et al. Pharmacokinetics of chlorpromazine after single and chronic dosage. *Clin Pharmacol Ther,* **1977**, *21*:437–448.

BIOAVAILABILITY (ORAL) (%)	URINARY EXCRETION (%)	BOUND IN PLASMA (%)	CLEARANCE (mL/min/kg)	VOL. DIST. (L/kg)	HALF-LIFE (hours)	PEAK TIME (hours)	PEAK CONCENTRATION
Chlorthalidone							
64 ± 10	65 ± 9[a]	75 ± 1	0.04 ± 0.01 ↓ Aged	0.14 ± 0.07	47 ± 22[b] ↑ Aged	13.8 ± 6.3[c]	3.7 ± 0.9 μg/mL[c]

[a]Value is for 50- and 100-mg doses; renal *CL* is decreased at an oral dose of 200 mg, and there is a concomitant decrease in the percentage excreted unchanged. [b]Chlorthalidone is sequestered in erythrocytes. $t_{1/2}$ is longer if blood, rather than plasma, is analyzed. Parameters reported based on blood concentrations. [c]Following a single 50-mg oral dose (tablet) given to healthy male adults.

Reference: Williams RL, et al. Relative bioavailability of chlorthalidone in humans: Adverse influence of polyethylene glycol. *J Pharm Sci,* **1982**, *71*:533–535.

BIOAVAILABILITY (ORAL) (%)	URINARY EXCRETION (%)	BOUND IN PLASMA (%)	CLEARANCE (mL/min/kg)	VOL. DIST. (L/kg)	HALF-LIFE (hours)	PEAK TIME (hours)	PEAK CONCENTRATION
Cidofovir[a]							
SC: 98 ± 10 PO: <5	70.1 ± 21.4[b]	<6	2.1 ± 0.6[b] ↓ RD[c]	0.36 ± 0.13[b]	2.3 ± 0.5[b] ↑ RD	—	19.6 ± 7.2 μg/mL[d]

[a]Data from patients with HIV infection and positive for cytomegalovirus. Cidofovir is activated intracellularly by phosphokinases. For parenteral use. [b]Parameters reported for a dose given in the presence of probenecid. [c]*CL* reduced, mild renal impairment (cleared by high-flux hemodialysis). [d]Following a single 5-mg/kg IV infusion given over 1 hour, with concomitant oral probenecid and active hydration.

References: Brody SR, et al. Pharmacokinetics of cidofovir in renal insufficiency and in continuous ambulatory peritoneal dialysis or high-flux hemodialysis. *Clin Pharmacol Ther,* **1999**, *65*:21–28. Cundy KC, et al. Clinical pharmacokinetics of cidofovir in human immunodeficiency virus-infected patients. *Antimicrob Agents Chemother,* **1995**, *39*:1247–1252. *PDR*54, **2000**, p. 1136. Wachsman M, et al. Pharmacokinetics, safety and bioavailability of HPMPC (cidofovir) in human immunodeficiency virus-infected subjects. *Antiviral Res,* **1996**, *29*:153–161.

Cinacalcet[a]							
~20 ↑ Food	—[b]	93-97	~18 ↓ LD	~17.6	34 ± 9 ↑ LD	2-6	10.6 ± 2.8 ng/mL[c]

[a]Cinacalcet is a chiral molecule; the *R*-enantiomer is more potent than the *S*-enantiomer and is thought to be responsible for the drug's pharmacological activity. Cinacalcet is metabolized primarily by CYP3A4, CYP2D6, and CYP1A2. [b]Unreported, but presumably negligible. [c]Following a single 75-mg oral dose.

References: Joy MS, et al. Calcimimetics and the treatment of primary and secondary hyperparathyroidism. *Ann Pharmacother,* **2004**, *38*:1871–1880. Kumar GN, et al. Metabolism and disposition of calcimimetic agent cinacalcet HCl in humans and animal models. *Drug Metab Dispos,* **2004**, *32*:1491–1500. Pharmacology and toxicology review of NDA. Application 21–688. U.S. FDA, CDER. Available at: http://www.fda.gov/drugs at fda_docs/nda/2004/21-688.pdf. Sensipar_Pharmr_Pl.pdf. Accessed July 7, 2010.

Ciprofloxacin							
60 ± 12	50 ± 5	40	7.6 ± 0.8 ↓ RD, Aged ↑ CF	2.2 ± 0.4[a] ↓ Aged ↔ CF	3.3 ± 0.4 ↑ RD ↔ Aged ↓ CF	0.6 ± 0.2[b]	2.5 ± 1.1 μg/mL[b]

[a]V_{area} reported. [b]Following a 500-mg oral dose given twice daily for ≥3 days to patients with chronic bronchitis or bronchiectasis.

References: Begg EJ, et al. The pharmacokinetics of oral fleroxacin and ciprofloxacin in plasma and sputum during acute and chronic dosing. *Br J Clin Pharmacol,* **2000**, *49*:32–38. Sorgel F, et al. Pharmacokinetic disposition of quinolones in human body fluids and tissues. *Clin Pharmacokinet,* **1989**, *16*(suppl):5–24.

Cisplatin[a]							
—	23 ± 9	—[b]	6.3 ± 1.2	0.28 ± 0.07	0.53 ± 0.10	—	2 Hr: 3.4 ± 1.1 μg/mL[c] 7 Hr: 1.0 ± 0.4 μg/mL[c]

[a]Early studies measured total platinum, rather than the parent compound; values reported here are for parent drug in seven patients with ovarian cancer (mean CL_{cr} = 66 ± 27 mL/min). [b]Platinum will form a tight complex with plasma proteins (90%). [c]Following a single 100-mg/m^2 IV dose given as an ~2- or 7-hour infusion to ovarian cancer patients.

Reference: Reece PA, et al. Disposition of unchanged cisplatin in patients with ovarian cancer. *Clin Pharmacol Ther,* **1987**, *42*:320–325.

Clarithromycin[a]							
55 ± 8[c]	36 ± 7[c] ↔ Aged	42-50	7.3 ± 1.9[c] ↓ Aged, RD ↔ LD	2.6 ± 0.5[c] ↔ Aged ↑ LD	3.3 ± 0.5[c] ↑ Aged, RD, LD	C: 2.8[d] HC: 3[d]	C: 2.4 μg/mL[d] HC: 0.7 μg/mL[d]

[a]Active metabolite, 14(*R*)-hydroxyclarithromycin. [b]Data generated for a 250-mg oral dose. [c]At higher doses, metabolic *CL* saturates, resulting in increases in the percentage of urinary excretion and $t_{1/2}$ and a decrease in *CL*. [d]Mean data for clarithromycin (C) and 14-hydroxyclarithromycin (HC), following a 500-mg oral dose given twice daily to steady state in healthy adults.

Reference: Chu SY, et al. Absolute bioavailability of Clarithromycin after oral administration in humans. *Antimicrob Agents Chemother*, **1992**, *36*:1147–1150. Fraschini F, et al. Clarithromycin clinical pharmacokinetics. *Clin Pharmacokinet,* **1993**, *25*:189–204.

(Continued)

Table AII–1

Pharmacokinetic Data (*Continued*)

BIOAVAILABILITY (ORAL) (%)	URINARY EXCRETION (%)	BOUND IN PLASMA (%)	CLEARANCE (mL/min/kg)	VOL. DIST. (L/kg)	HALF-LIFE (hours)	PEAK TIME (hours)	PEAK CONCENTRATION
Clindamycin							
~87[a] Topical: 2	13	93.6 ± 0.2	4.7 ± 1.3 ↔ Child	1.1 ± 0.3[b] ↔ RD, Child	2.9 ± 0.7 ↔ Child, RD, Preg ↑ Prem	—	IV: 17.2 ± 3.5 μg/mL[c] PO: 2.5 μg/mL[d]
[a]Clindamycin hydrochloride given orally. [b]V_{area} reported. [c]Following a 1200-mg IV dose (30-minute infusion) of clindamycin phosphate (prodrug) given twice daily to steady state in healthy male adults. [d]Following a single 150-mg oral dose of clindamycin hydrochloride to adults.				*References: PDR*54, **2000**, p. 2421. Plaisance KI, et al. Pharmacokinetic evaluation of two dosage regimens of clindamycin phosphate. *Antimicrob Agents Chemother,* **1989**, *33*:618–620.			
Clonazepam							
98 ± 31	<1	86 ± 0.5 ↓ Neo	1.55 ± 0.28[a,b]	3.2 ± 1.1	23 ± 5	PO: 2.5 ± 1.3[c]	IV: 3-29 ng/mL[c] PO: 17 ± 5.4 ng/mL[c]
[a]*CL/F* reported; this value is consistent for a number of studies but is higher than the *CL* determined in a single study of IV administration. [b]Metabolized by CYP3A. [c]Range of C_{max} values following a single 2-mg IV dose (model-fitted for bolus dose) or mean following a 2-mg oral dose (tablet) given to healthy adults. Most patients, including children whose seizures are controlled by clonazepam have steady-state concentrations of 5-70 ng/mL. However, patients who do not respond and those with side effects achieve similar levels.				*Reference*: Berlin A, et al. Pharmacokinetics of the anticonvulsant drug clonazepam evaluated from single oral and intravenous doses and by repeated oral administration. *Eur J Clin Pharmacol,* **1975**, *9*:155–159.			
Clonidine							
PO: 95 TD: 60	62 ± 11	20	3.1 ± 1.2 ↓ RD	2.1 ± 0.4	12 ± 7 ↑ RD	PO: 2[a] TD: 72[a]	PO: 0.8 ng/mL[a] TD: 0.3-0.4 ng/mL[a]
[a]Mean data following a 0.1-mg oral dose given twice a day to steady state or steady-state concentration (C_{ss}) following a 3.5-cm^2 transdermal (TD) patch administered to normotensive male adults. Concentrations of 0.2-2 ng/mL are associated with a reduction in blood pressure; >1 ng/mL will cause sedation and dry mouth.				*Reference*: Lowenthal DT, et al. Clinical pharmacokinetics of clonidine. *Clin Pharmacokinet,* **1988**, *14*:287–310.			

Diazepam[a]							
PO: 100 ± 14 Rectal: 90	<1	98.7 ± 0.2 ↓ RD, LD, NS, Preg, Neo, Alb, Burn, Aged ↔ HTh	0.38 ± 0.06[a] ↑ Alb ↓ LD ↔ Aged, Smk, HTh	1.1 ± 0.3 ↑ LD, Aged, Alb ↔ RD, HTh	43 ± 13[a] ↑ Aged, LD ↔ HTh	PO: 1.3 ± 0.2[b] Rectal: 1.5[b]	IV: 400-500 ng/mL[b] PO: 317 ± 27 ng/mL[b] Rectal: ~400 ng/mL[b]

[a]Active metabolites, desmethyldiazepam and oxazepam, formed by CYP2C19 (polymorphic) and CYP3A. [b]Range of data following a single 5- to 10-mg IV dose (15- to 30-second bolus) or mean data following a single 10-mg oral or 15-mg rectal dose given to healthy adults. A concentration of 300-400 ng/mL provides an anxiolytic effect, and >600 ng/mL provides control of seizures.

References: Friedman H, et al. Pharmacokinetics and pharmacodynamics of oral diazepam: Effect of dose, plasma concentration, and time. *Clin Pharmacol Ther,* **1992**, *52*:139–150. Greenblatt DJ, et al. Diazepam disposition determinants. *Clin Pharmacol Ther,* **1980**, *27*:301–312. *PDR*54, **2000**, p. 1012.

Diclofenac							
54 ± 2	<1	>99.5	4.2 ± 0.9[a] ↓ Aged ↔ RD, LD, RA	0.17 ± 0.11[b] ↑ RA	1.1 ± 0.2 ↔ RA	EC: 2.5 (1.0-4.5)[c] SR: 5.3 ± 1.5[c]	EC: 2.0 (1.4-3.0) μg/mL[c] SR: 0.42 ± 0.17 μg/mL[c]

[a]Cleared primarily by CYP2C9-catalyzed 4′-hydroxylation; urine and biliary metabolites account for 30% and 10-20% of dose, respectively. [b]V_{area} reported. [c]Following a single 50-mg enteric-coated tablet (EC) or 100-mg sustained-release tablet (SR) given to healthy adults.

References: Tracy T. Nonsteroidal antiinflammatory drugs. In: Levy RH, et al., eds. *Metabolic Drug Interactions.* Philadelphia, Lippincott Williams & Wilkins, **2000**, pp. 457–468. Willis JV, et al. The pharmacokinetics of diclofenac sodium following intravenous and oral administration. *Eur J Clin Pharmacol,* **1979**, *16*:405–410.

Digoxin							
70 ± 13[a,c] ↔ RD, MI, CHF, LTh, HTh, Aged	60 ± 11	25 ± 5 ↓ RD	$CL = 0.88CL_{cr} + 0.33$[b,c] ↓ LTh ↑ HTh, Neo, Child, Preg	$V = 3.12CL_{cr} + 3.84$ ↓ LTh ↑ HTh ↔ CHF	39 ± 13 ↓ HTh ↑ RD, CHF, Aged, LTh ↔ Obes	1-3[d]	NT: 1.4 ± 0.7 ng/mL[d] T: 3.7 ± 1.0 ng/mL[d]

[a]LANOXIN tablets; digoxin solutions, elixirs, and capsules may be absorbed more completely. [b]Equation applies to patients with some degree of heart failure. If heart failure is not present, the coefficient of CL_{cr} is 1.0. Units of CL_{cr} must be mL/min/kg. [c]In the occasional patient, digoxin is metabolized to an inactive metabolite, dihydrodigoxin, by gut flora. This results in a reduced oral bioavailability. [d]Following an oral dose of 0.31 ± 0.19 mg/day or 0.36 ± 0.19 mg/day in patients with CHF who exhibited no signs of digitalis toxicity (NT) or signs of toxicity (T), respectively. Concentrations >0.8 ng/mL are associated with an inotropic effect.

Concentrations of 1.7, 2.5, and 3.3 ng/mL are associated with a 10%, 50%, and 90% probability of digoxin-induced arrhythmias, respectively.

References: Mooradian AD. Digitalis. An update of clinical pharmacokinetics, therapeutic monitoring techniques and treatment recommendations. *Clin Pharmacokinet,* **1988**, *15*:165–179. Smith TW, et al. Digoxin intoxication: The relationship of clinical presentation to serum digoxin concentration. *J Clin Invest,* **1970**, *49*:2377–2386.

(Continued)

Table AII–1

Pharmacokinetic Data (*Continued*)

BIOAVAILABILITY (ORAL) (%)	URINARY EXCRETION (%)	BOUND IN PLASMA (%)	CLEARANCE (mL/min/kg)	VOL. DIST. (L/kg)	HALF-LIFE (hours)	PEAK TIME (hours)	PEAK CONCENTRATION
Diltiazem[a]							
38 ± 11	<4	78 ± 3	11.8 ± 2.2[b] ↔ Aged ↓ RD	3.3 ± 1.2 ↔ Aged ↓ RD	4.4 ± 1.3[c] ↔ RD, Aged	4.0 ± 0.4[d]	151 ± 46 ng/mL[d]

[a]Active metabolites, desacetyldiltiazem ($t_{1/2}$ = 9 ± 2 hours) and *N*-desmethyldiltiazem ($t_{1/2}$ = 7.5 ± 1 hour). Formation of desmethyl metabolite (major pathway of *CL*) catalyzed primarily by CYP3A. [b]More than a 2-fold decrease with multiple dosing. [c]$t_{1/2}$ for oral dose is 5-6 hours; does not change with multiple dosing. [d]Following a single 120-mg oral dose to healthy adults.

Reference: Echizen H, et al. Clinical pharmacokinetics of verapamil, nifedipine, and diltiazem. *Clin Pharmacokinet,* **1986**, *11*:425–449.

BIOAVAILABILITY (ORAL) (%)	URINARY EXCRETION (%)	BOUND IN PLASMA (%)	CLEARANCE (mL/min/kg)	VOL. DIST. (L/kg)	HALF-LIFE (hours)	PEAK TIME (hours)	PEAK CONCENTRATION
Diphenhydramine							
72 ± 26	1.9 ± 0.8 ↔ LD	78 ± 3 ↓ LD	6.2 ± 1.7[a] ↔ LD ↑ Child ↓ Aged	4.5 ± 2.8[a,b] ↔ LD	8.5 ± 3.2[a] ↑ LD, Aged ↓ Child	PO: 2.3 ± 0.64[c]	IV: ~230 ng/mL[c] PO: 66 ± 22 ng/mL[c]

[a]Increased *CL,* decreased *V,* and no change in $t_{1/2}$ in Asians, presumably due to decreased plasma protein binding. [b]V_{area} reported. [c]Following a single 50-mg dose of diphenhydramine hydrochloride (44-mg base) given IV or orally to fasted healthy adults. Levels >25 ng/mL provide antihistaminic effect, whereas levels >60 ng/mL are associated with drowsiness and mental impairment.

Reference: Blyden GT, et al. Pharmacokinetics of diphenhydramine and a demethylated metabolite following intravenous and oral administration. *J Clin Pharmacol,* **1986**, *26*:529–533.

BIOAVAILABILITY (ORAL) (%)	URINARY EXCRETION (%)	BOUND IN PLASMA (%)	CLEARANCE (mL/min/kg)	VOL. DIST. (L/kg)	HALF-LIFE (hours)	PEAK TIME (hours)	PEAK CONCENTRATION
Docetaxel[a]							
—	2.1 ± 0.2	94	22.6 ± 7.7 L/hr/m^2 ↓ LD[b]	72 ± 24 L/m^2	13.6 ± 6.1	—	2.4 ± 0.9 μg/mL[c]

[a]Data from male and female patients treated for cancer. Metabolized by CYP3A and excreted into bile. Parenteral administration. [b]Mild to moderate liver impairment. [c]Following an IV infusion of 85 mg/m^2 over 1.6 hours.

References: Clarke SJ, et al. Clinical pharmacokinetics of docetaxel. *Clin Pharmacokinet,* **1999**, *36*:99–114. Extra JM, et al. Phase I and pharmacokinetic study of Taxotere (RP 56976; NSC 628503) given as a short intravenous infusion. *Cancer Res,* **1993**, *53*:1037–1042. *PDR*54, **2000**, p. 2578.

Donepezil[a]							
—[b]	10.6 ± 2.7	92.6 ± 0.9[c]	2.90 ± 0.74[d] ↓ LD,[e] ↔ RD	14.0 ± 2.42[d] ↑ Aged	59.7 ± 16.1[d] ↑ Aged	3-4[f]	30.8 ± 4.2 ng/mL[f]
Doxazosin[a]							
Y: 65 ± 14 E: 68 ± 16 GITS: F_{rel} = 59 ± 12	5	98	Y: 1.26 ± 0.27 E: 2.25 ± 1.42 ↓ LD[b]	Y: 1.0 ± 0.1 E: 1.7 ± 1.0	20.5 ± 6.1[c,d] GITS: 19 ± 4[d] ↔ LD[b]	3.9 ± 1.2[d] GITS: 9 ± 5[d]	67 ± 19 ng/mL[d] GITS: 28 ± 12 ng/mL[d]
Doxepin[a]							
30 ± 10[b]	~0	82 (75-89)	14 ± 3[c]	24 ± 7[c,d]	18 ± 5	D: 0.5-1 DD: 4-12	D: 28 ± 11 ng/mL[e] DD: 39 ± 19 ng/mL[e]

Donepezil: [a]Data from young, healthy male, and female subjects. No significant gender differences. Metabolized by CYP2D6, CYP3A4, and UGT. [b]Absolute bioavailability is unknown, but the oral dose reportedly is well absorbed. [c]A fraction bound value of 96% also has been reported. [d]*CL/F*, V_{ss}/F, and $t_{1/2}$ reported for oral dose. [e]*CL/F* reduced slightly (~20%), alcoholic cirrhosis. [f]Following a 5-mg oral dose given once daily to steady state.

References: Ohnishi A, et al. Comparison of the pharmacokinetics of E2020, a new compound for Alzheimer's disease, in healthy young and elderly subjects. *J Clin Pharmacol,* **1993**, *33*:1086–1091. *PDR*54, **2000**, p. 2323.

Doxazosin: [a]Cleared primarily by cytochrome P450-dependent metabolism. Where indicated, data for young (Y) and elderly (E) normotensive adults are reported. Also reported are data for a gastrointestinal sustained-release device (GITS); oral bioavailability relative to standard formulation (F_{rel}). [b]Study in patients with mild to moderate liver impairment; AUC increased 43%. [c]Shorter $t_{1/2}$ following IV dosing reported; (Y) 10 ± 1 hour, (E) 12 ± 5 hour; attributed to inadequate duration of blood sampling. [d]Following an 8-mg dose of standard formulation or GITS, once daily, to steady state in young and elderly normotensive volunteers.

References: Chung M, et al. Clinical pharmacokinetics of doxazosin in a controlled-release gastrointestinal therapeutic system (GITS) formulation. *Br J Clin Pharmacol,* **1999**, *48*:678–687. Elliott HL, et al. Pharmacokinetic overview of doxazosin. *Am J Cardiol,* **1987**, *59*:78G–81G. Penenberg D, et al. The effects of hepatic impairment on the pharmacokinetics of doxazosin. *J Clin Pharmacol,* **2000**, *40*:67–73. Vincent J, et al. The pharmacokinetics of doxazosin in elderly normotensives. *Br J Clin Pharmacol,* **1986**, *21*:521–524.

Doxepin: [a]The active metabolite, desmethyldoxepin, has a longer $t_{1/2}$ (37 ± 15 hours). [b]Calculated from results of oral administration only, assuming complete absorption, elimination by the liver, hepatic blood flow of 1.5 L/min, and equal partition between plasma and erythrocytes. [c]Calculated assuming $F = 0.30$. [d]V_{area} reported. [e]Trough concentrations of doxepin (D) and desmethyldoxepin (DD) following a 150-mg oral dose given once daily for 3 weeks to patients with depression. Peak/trough ratio <2.

Reference: Faulkner RD, et al. Multiple-dose doxepin kinetics in depressed patients. *Clin Pharmacol Ther,* **1983**, *34*:509–515.

(Continued)

Table AII–1

Pharmacokinetic Data (*Continued*)

BIOAVAILABILITY (ORAL) (%)	URINARY EXCRETION (%)	BOUND IN PLASMA (%)	CLEARANCE (mL/min/kg)	VOL. DIST. (L/kg)	HALF-LIFE (hours)	PEAK TIME (hours)	PEAK CONCENTRATION
Doxorubicin[a]							
5	<7	76	666 ± 339 mL/min/m^2 ↑ Child ↓ LD, Obes	682 ± 433 L/m^2 ↔ LD	26 ± 17[b] ↔ RD ↑ LD	—	High[c] D: ~950 ng/mL DL: 30-1008 ng/mL Low[c] D: 6.0 ± 3.2 ng/mL DL: 5.0 ± 3.5 ng/mL

[a]Active metabolites; $t_{1/2}$ for doxorubicinol is 29 ± 16 hours. [b]Prolonged when plasma bilirubin concentration is elevated; undergoes biliary excretion. [c]Mean data for doxorubicin (D) and range of data for doxorubicinol (DL). High: a single 45- to 72-mg/m^2 high-dose 1-hour IV infusion given to patients with small cell lung cancer. Low: continuous IV infusion at a rate of 3.9 ± 0.65 mg/m^2/day for 12.4 (2-50) weeks to patients with advanced cancer.

References: Ackland SP, et al. Pharmacokinetics and pharmacodynamics of long-term continuous-infusion doxorubicin. *Clin Pharmacol Ther,* **1989**, *45*:340–347. Piscitelli SC, et al. Pharmacokinetics and pharmacodynamics of doxorubicin in patients with small cell lung cancer. *Clin Pharmacol Ther,* **1993**, *53*:555–561.

BIOAVAILABILITY (ORAL) (%)	URINARY EXCRETION (%)	BOUND IN PLASMA (%)	CLEARANCE (mL/min/kg)	VOL. DIST. (L/kg)	HALF-LIFE (hours)	PEAK TIME (hours)	PEAK CONCENTRATION
Doxycycline							
93	41 ± 19	88 ± 5 ↓ RD[a]	0.53 ± 0.18 ↓ HL, Aged ↔ RD	0.75 ± 0.32 ↓ HL, Aged	16 ± 6 ↔ RD, HL, Aged	Oral: 1-2[b]	IV: 2.8 μg/mL[b] PO: 1.7-2 μg/mL[b]

[a]Decreases in plasma protein binding to 71 ± 3% in patients with uremia. [b]Mean data following a single 100-mg IV dose (1-hour infusion) or range of mean data following a 100-mg oral dose given to adults.

Reference: Saivin S, et al. Clinical pharmacokinetics of doxycycline and minocycline. *Clin Pharmacokinet,* **1988**, *15*:355–366.

BIOAVAILABILITY (ORAL) (%)	URINARY EXCRETION (%)	BOUND IN PLASMA (%)	CLEARANCE (mL/min/kg)	VOL. DIST. (L/kg)	HALF-LIFE (hours)	PEAK TIME (hours)	PEAK CONCENTRATION
Dronabinol[a]							
10-20	Trace	~97	7.8 ± 1.9[b] ↑ Chronic[c]	8.9 ± 4.2	α: 2.8 ± 1.8 β: 20 ± 4[d] ↔ Chronic[e]	2.5 (0.5-4.0)[f]	3.0 ± 1.8 ng/mL[f]

[a]Cleared primarily by cytochrome P450-dependent metabolism; evidence suggests polymorphic CYP2C9 is a major contributor. [b]Somewhat lower values (2.8-3.5 mL/min/kg) also were reported, but a higher systemic clearance is most consistent with the low oral bioavailability. [c]Study in long-term users of THC. [d]Exhibits biphasic kinetics; the longer terminal elimination phase most likely represents redistribution from fatty tissue. [e]No change in terminal (redistribution) $t_{1/2}$. [f]Following a 5-mg dose given twice daily to steady state.

References: Bland TM, et al. CYP2C-catalyzed delta9-tetrahydrocannabinol metabolism: Kinetics, pharmacogenetics and interaction with phenytoin. *Biochem Pharmacol,* **2005**, *70*:1096–1103. Drugs@FDA. Marinol label approved on 6/21/06. http://www.accessdata.fda.gov/drugsatfda_docs/label/2006/018651s025s026lbl.pdf. Accessed May 17, 2010. Grotenhermen F. Pharmacokinetics and pharmacodynamics of cannabinoids. *Clin Pharmacokinet*, **2003**, *42*:327–360. Hunt CA, et al. Tolerance and disposition of tetrahydrocannabinol in man. *J Pharmacol Exp Ther,* **1980**, *215*:35–44. Wall ME, et al. Metabolism, disposition, and kinetics of delta-9-tetrahydrocannabinol in men and women. *Clin Pharmacol Ther,* **1983**, *34*:352–363.

Duloxetine[a]

42.8 (18.5-71.2) ↓ Smk[b]	—	>90	10.6 ± 2.4 ↓ LD[c] ↓ RD[d]	7.0 ± 1.3	9.3 (6.4-12) ↑ LD[c] ↔ RD[d]	4.5 (2.5-6)[e]	32.9 ng/mL[e]

[a]Cleared primarily by CYP1A2- and CYP2D6-dependent metabolism. [b]~30% lower bioavailability based on population pharmacokinetic analysis; no dose adjustment recommended. [c]A 5-fold increase in oral AUC in patients with moderate liver impairment. [d]A 2-fold increase in oral AUC in patients with end-stage RD receiving intermittent dialysis. [e]Following a single 60-mg oral dose.

References: Lobo ED, et al. In vitro and in vivo evaluations of cytochrome P450 1A2 interactions with duloxetine. *Clin Pharmacokinet,* **2008**, *47*:191–202. Lobo ED, et al. Population pharmacokinetics of orally administered duloxetine in patients: Implications for dosing recommendation. *Clin Pharmacokinet*, **2009**, *48*:189–197. Drugs@FDA. Cymbalta label approved on 6/16/09. Available at: http://www.accessdata.fda.gov/drugsatfda_docs/label/2009/021427s030lbl.pdf. Accessed May 17, 2010.

Dutasteride[a]

60 (40-94)	—	99	—[b]	—[b]	840[c]	1 (1-3)[d]	38 ± 13 ng/mL[d]

[a]Dutasteride is cleared primarily by CYP3A-dependent metabolism. [b]*CL/F* = 0.20-0.37 mL/min/kg, and *V/F* = 4.3-7.1 L/kg; calculated from steady-state (24 wk) serum concentrations. [c]Terminal $t_{1/2}$ reported. [d]Following a 0.5-mg dose given once daily to steady state (24 weeks).

References: Clark RV, et al. Marked suppression of dihydrotestosterone in men with benign prostatic hyperplasia by dutasteride, a dual 5-alpha-reductase inhibitor. *J Clin Endocrinol Metab,* **2004**, *89*:2179–2178. Keam SJ, et al. Dutasteride: A review of its use in the management of prostate disorders. *Drugs*, **2008**, *68*:463–485.

Efavirenz[a]

—[b] ↑ Food	<1	99.5-99.75	3.1 ± 1.2[c] ↔ Child[d]	—	SD: 52-76[c] MD: 40-55[c]	4.1 ± 1.7[e]	4.0 ± 1.7 μg/mL[e]

[a]Data from patients with HIV infection. No significant gender differences. Metabolized primarily by CYP2B6 and to a lesser extent by CYP2A6 and through *N*-glucuronidation. [b]Absolute oral bioavailability is unknown. Oral AUC increased 50% with high-fat meal. [c]Single dose (SD) data reported for *CL/F* and both SD and multiple dose (MD) data for $t_{1/2}$. Efavirenz is a weak inducer of CYP3A4 and its own metabolism. [d]3-16 years of age, no difference in weight-adjusted *CL/F* compared to adult. [e]Following a 600-mg oral dose given daily to steady state. *References*: Adkins JC, et al. Efavirenz. *Drugs,* **1998**, *56*:1055–1064. *PDR*54, **2000**, p. 981. Villani P, et al. Pharmacokinetics of efavirenz (EFV) alone and in combination therapy with nelfinavir (NFV) in HIV-1 infected patients. *Br J Clin Pharmacol,* **1999**, *48*:712–715.

Eletriptan[a]

~50 ↑ Food[b]	9 (7-12)[c]	85	5.6 (3.7-6.7)[c] ↓ LD[d]	2.0 (1.4-2.4)[c]	4.1 (2.8-5.5)[c] ↑ LD[e]	MF: 0.75-1.5[e] M: 2.0-2.8[e]	57-115 ng/mL[f]

[a]Cleared primarily by CYP3A-dependent metabolism. [b]Systemic exposure increased 20-30% with high-fat meal. [c]Data from 50-μg/kg IV dose reported; lack of dose proportionality for oral AUC between 20- and 40- or 80-mg doses. [d]Study in patients with mild to moderate hepatic impairment. [e]Following single 20- to 80-mg oral doses; MF: migraine-free period; M: during a migraine attack. [f]Range of mean values from different studies following a single 30-mg oral dose.

References: McCormack PL, et al. Eletriptan: A review of its use in the acute treatment of migraine. *Drugs*, **2006**, *66*:1129–1149. Milton KA, et al. Pharmacokinetics, pharmacodynamics, and safety of the 5-HT(1B/1D) agonist eletriptan following intravenous and oral administration. *J Clin Pharmacol*, **2002**, *42*:528–539. Drugs@FDA. Relpax label approved on 12/26/09. Available at: http://www.accessdata.fda.gov/drugsatfda_docs/label/2002/21016_relpax_lbl.pdf. Accessed May 17, 2010.

(Continued)

Table AII–1

Pharmacokinetic Data (*Continued*)

BIOAVAILABILITY (ORAL) (%)	URINARY EXCRETION (%)	BOUND IN PLASMA (%)	CLEARANCE (mL/min/kg)	VOL. DIST. (L/kg)	HALF-LIFE (hours)	PEAK TIME (hours)	PEAK CONCENTRATION
Emtricitabine[a]							
Cap: 93[b] (78-99) Sol: 75[b]	73 ± 4[c]	<4	4.4 ± 0.8[c] ↓ RD[d]	3.5 ± 0.8[c]	9.0 ± 0.9[c] ↑ RD[d]	2.0 ± 1.0[e]	1.7 ± 0.8 μg/mL[e]

[a]Cleared primarily by renal excretion.[b]Data for capsule (Cap) and solution (Sol) formulations presented. [c]Data from a 200-mg IV dose, as filed in NDA; V_{area} reported. [d]Study in patients with mild to severe renal impairment and end-stage RD; *CL* reduced in parallel with decline in CL_{cr}; removed by hemodialysis. [e]Following 200 mg, given once daily, to HIV-infected adults.

References: Modrzejewski KA, et al. Emtricitabine: A once-daily nucleoside reverse transcriptase inhibitor. *Ann Pharmacother,* **2004**, *38*:1006–1014. Drugs@FDA. Emtriva NDA approved on 7/2/03. Available at: http://www.accessdata.fda.gov/ drugsatfda_docs/nda/2003/21-500_Emtriva_BioPharmr_P2.pdf. Accessed May 17, 2010.

BIOAVAILABILITY (ORAL) (%)	URINARY EXCRETION (%)	BOUND IN PLASMA (%)	CLEARANCE (mL/min/kg)	VOL. DIST. (L/kg)	HALF-LIFE (hours)	PEAK TIME (hours)	PEAK CONCENTRATION
Enalapril[a]							
41 ± 15 ↓ LD	88 ± 7[b] ↓ LD	50-60	4.9 ± 1.5[c] ↓ RD, Aged, CHF, Neo ↑ Child ↔ Fem	1.7 ± 0.7[c]	11[d] ↑ RD, LD	3.0 ± 1.6[e]	69 ± 37 ng/mL[e]

[a]Hydrolyzed by esterases to the active metabolite, enalaprilic acid (enalaprilat); except when noted, pharmacokinetic values and disease comparisons are for enalaprilat, following oral enalapril administration. [b]For IV enalaprilat. [c]*CL/F* and V_{ss}/F after multiple oral doses of enalapril. Values after single IV dose of enalaprilat are misleading because binding to ACE leads to a prolonged $t_{1/2}$, which does not represent a significant fraction of the *CL* upon multiple dosing. [d]Estimated from the approach to steady state during multiple dosing. [e]Mean values for enalaprilat following a 10-mg enalapril oral dose given daily for 8 days to healthy young adults. The EC_{50} for ACE inhibition is 5-20 ng/mL enalaprilat.

References: Lees KR, et al. Age and the pharmacokinetics and pharmacodynamics of chronic enalapril treatment. *Clin Pharmacol Ther,* **1987**, *41*:597–602. MacFadyen RJ, et al. Enalapril clinical pharmacokinetics and pharmacokinetic-pharmacodynamic relationships. An overview. *Clin Pharmacokinet,* **1993**, *25*:274–282.

BIOAVAILABILITY (ORAL) (%)	URINARY EXCRETION (%)	BOUND IN PLASMA (%)	CLEARANCE (mL/min/kg)	VOL. DIST. (L/kg)	HALF-LIFE (hours)	PEAK TIME (hours)	PEAK CONCENTRATION
Enoxaparin[a]							
SC: 92	—[b]	—	0.3 ± 0.1[c] ↓ RD	0.12 ± 0.04[c] ↔ RD	3.8 ± 1.3[d] ↑ RD	3[e]	ACLM: 145 ± 45 ng/mL[e] BCLM: 414 ± 87 ng/mL[e]

[a]Enoxaparin consists of low-molecular-weight heparin fragments of varying lengths. [b]43% is recovered in urine when administered as ^{99}Tc-labeled enoxaparin; 8-20% anti-factor Xa activity. [c]*F, CL/F,* and V_{area}/F for SC dose measured by functional assay for anti-factor Xa activity. [d]Measured by functional assay of anti-factor Xa activity. Using anti-IIa activity or displacement binding assay gives a $t_{1/2}$ of ~1-2 hours. [e]Following a single 40-mg SC dose to healthy adult subjects. High-affinity antithrombin III molecules: ACLM, above-critical-length molecules (anti-factor Xa and IIa activity); BCLM, below-critical-length molecules (anti-factor Xa activity).

References: Bendetowicz AV, et al. Pharmacokinetics and pharmacodynamics of a low molecular weight heparin (enoxaparin) after subcutaneous injection, comparison with unfractionated heparin—A three way cross over study in human volunteers. *Thromb Haemost,* **1994**, *71*:305–313. *PDR*54, **2000**, p. 2561.

Entacapone[a]

42 ± 9[b] ↑ LD[c]	Negligible	98	10.3 ± 1.74 ↔ RD, LD	0.40 ± 0.16	0.28 ± 0.06[d]	0.8 ± 0.2[e]	4.3 ± 2.0 μg/mL[e]

[a]Data from healthy male subjects. Eliminated primarily by biliary excretion. [b]The bioavailability of entacapone appears to be dose dependent (increases from 29-46% over a 50- to 800-mg dose range). [c]Increased bioavailability, moderate hepatic impairment with cirrhosis. [d]Value represents the $t_{1/2}$ for the initial distribution phase, during which 90% of a dose is eliminated. The terminal $t_{1/2}$ is 2.9 ± 2.0 hours. [e]Following a single 400-mg oral dose. No accumulation with multiple dosing.

References: Holm KJ, et al. Entacapone. A review of its use in Parkinson's disease. *Drugs,* **1999**, *58*:159–177. Keränen T, et al. Inhibition of soluble catechol-O-methyltransferase and single-dose pharmacokinetics after oral and intravenous administration of entacapone. *Eur J Clin Pharmacol,* **1994**, *46*:151–157.

Eplerenone[a]

—	7[b]	33-60[c]	2.4[d] ↓ CHF, LD	0.6-1.3[d]	4-6	1.8 ± 0.7[e]	1.0 ± 0.3 μg/mL[e]

[a]Eplerenone is converted (reversibly) to an inactive ring-open hydroxy acid. Both eplerenone (E) and the hydroxy acid (EA) circulate in plasma; concentrations of E are much higher than EA. Irreversible metabolism is catalyzed predominantly by CYP3A4. Data for E in healthy male and female volunteers reported; no significant gender differences. [b]Recovered as E and EA following an oral dose. [c]Protein binding is concentration dependent over the therapeutic range; lower at the highest concentration. [d]CL/F and V_{ss}/F reported. [e]Following a 50-mg oral dose given once daily for 7 days.

References: Clinical Pharmacology and Biopharmaceutics Review. Application 21-437/S-002. U.S. Food and Drug Administration Center for Drug Evaluation and Research. Available at: http://www.accessdata.fda.gov/drugsatfda_docs/nda/2002/21-437_Inspra.cfm. Accessed July 9, 2010. Cook CS, et al. Pharmacokinetics and metabolism of [14C]eplerenone after oral administration to humans. *Drug Metab Dispos,* **2003**, *31*:1448–1455. Product information: Inspra™ (eplerenone tablets). Chicago, IL, Pfizer, **2004**.

Erlotinib[a]

59 (55-66) ↑ Food[b]	—	93 (92-95)	1.0 ± 0.4[c] ↑ Smk[d] ↔ LD[e]	1.2 ± 0.25[f]	36[g]	2-4[h]	1.1-1.7 μg/mL[h]

[a]Erlotinib is cleared primarily by CYP3A- and CYP1A2-dependent metabolism. [b]Bioavailability increases to ~100% when taken with a meal; not recommended because food effect is highly variable. [c]Calculated from a 25-mg IV dose; in a population pharmacokinetic study of 150 mg, once daily, CL/F = 0.98 mL/min/kg. [d]Systemic exposure reduced by half compared to nonsmokers. [e]Study in patients with moderate LD; no data for severe hepatic impairment. [f]Calculated from a 25-mg IV dose; in a population pharmacokinetic study of 150-mg once daily, V/F = 3.5 L/kg. [g]Median $t_{1/2}$ in a patient population receiving 150-mg orally once daily; a shorter $t_{1/2}$ of 13 hours was reported for a single 25-mg IV dose. [h]Following 150-mg given once daily to steady state.

References: Frohna P, et al. Evaluation of the absolute oral bioavailability and bioequivalence of erlotinib, an inhibitor of the epidermal growth factor receptor tyrosine kinase, in a randomized, crossover study in healthy subjects. *J Clin Pharmacol,* **2006**, *46*:282–290. Lu JF, et al. Clinical pharmacokinetics of erlotinib in patients with solid tumors and exposure-safety relationship in patients with non-small cell lung cancer. *Clin Pharmacol Ther,* **2006**, *80*:136–134. Drugs@FDA. Tarceva NDA and label; label approved on 4/27/09. Available at: http://www.accessdata.fda.gov/drugsatfda_docs/nda/2004/21-743_Tarceva.cfm. Accessed May 17, 2010.

(*Continued*)

Table AII–1

Pharmacokinetic Data (*Continued*)

BIOAVAILABILITY (ORAL) (%)	URINARY EXCRETION (%)	BOUND IN PLASMA (%)	CLEARANCE (mL/min/kg)	VOL. DIST. (L/kg)	HALF-LIFE (hours)	PEAK TIME (hours)	PEAK CONCENTRATION
Ertapenem[a]							
IM: 92 (88-95) SC: 99 ± 18	44 ± 15[b]	84-96[c]	0.42 ± 0.05 ↓ RD[d]	0.12 ± 0.02	3.8 ± 0.5	IM: 2.2 ± 0.9[e] SC: 2.7 ± 1.1[e]	IV: 155 ± 22 μg/mL[e] IM: 71 ± 16 μg/mL[e] SC: 43 ± 29 μg/mL[e]

[a]Cleared primarily by the kidney; developed for parenteral administration; data for a single 1-g dose reported. [b]Undergoes renal metabolism to an open-ring metabolite; the kidney is responsible for ~80% of the total body clearance. [c]Protein binding is concentration dependent; 96% at 10 μg/mL and 84% at 300 μg/mL. [d]Drug clearance declines in rough proportion to CL_{cr}. [e]Following a single 1-g dose; the IV dose was given over a 30-minute constant-rate infusion.

References: Frasca D, et al. Pharmacokinetics of ertapenem following intravenous and subcutaneous infusions in patients. *Antimicrob Agents Chemother*, **2009**, Nov 23. [Epub ahead of print]. Majumdar AK, et al. Pharmacokinetics of ertapenem in healthy young volunteers. *Antimicrob Agents Chemother,* **2002**, *46*:3506–3511. Musson DG, et al. Pharmacokinetics of intramuscularly administered ertapenem. *Antimicrob Agents Chemother,* **2003**, *47*:1732–1735. Nix DE, et al. Pharmacokinetics and pharmacodynamics of ertapenem: An overview for clinicians. *J Antimicrob Chemother*, **2004**, *53*(suppl):ii23–ii28.

BIOAVAILABILITY (ORAL) (%)	URINARY EXCRETION (%)	BOUND IN PLASMA (%)	CLEARANCE (mL/min/kg)	VOL. DIST. (L/kg)	HALF-LIFE (hours)	PEAK TIME (hours)	PEAK CONCENTRATION
Erythromycin							
35 ± 25[a] ↓ Preg[b]	12 ± 7	84 ± 3[c] ↔ RD	9.1 ± 4.1[d] ↔ RD	0.78 ± 0.44 ↑ RD	1.6 ± 0.7 ↑ LD ↔ RD	B: 2.1-3.9[e] S: 2-3[e]	B: 0.9-3.5 μg/mL[e] S: 0.5-1.4 μg/mL[e]

[a]Value for enteric-coated erythromycin base. [b]Decreased concentrations in pregnancy possibly due to decreased bioavailability (or increased *CL*). [c]Erythromycin base. [d]Erythromycin is a CYP3A substrate; *N*-demethylation. It also is transported by P-glycoprotein, which may contribute to biliary excretion of parent drug and metabolites. [e]Range of mean values from studies following a 250-mg oral enteric-coated free base in a capsule (B) given four times daily for 5-13 doses or a 250-mg film-coated tablet or capsule of erythromycin stearate (S) given four times daily for 5-12 doses.

Reference: Periti P, et al. Clinical pharmacokinetic properties of the macrolide antibiotics. Effects of age and various pathophysiological states (part I). *Clin Pharmacokinet,* **1989**, *16*:193–214.

BIOAVAILABILITY (ORAL) (%)	URINARY EXCRETION (%)	BOUND IN PLASMA (%)	CLEARANCE (mL/min/kg)	VOL. DIST. (L/kg)	HALF-LIFE (hours)	PEAK TIME (hours)	PEAK CONCENTRATION
Escitalopram, Citalopram[a]							
— Rac: 80 ± 13	Es: 8 Rac: 10.5 ± 1.4	Es: 56 Rac: 80	Es: 8.8 ± 3.2[b,c] Rac: 4.3 ± 1.2[b] ↓ Aged, LD[d]	Es: 15.4 ± 2.4[c] Rac: 12.3 ± 2.3	Es: 22 ± 6[b] Rac: 33 ± 4[b] ↑ Aged, LD,[d] RD[e]	— Rac/Es: 4-5[f]	Es: 21 ± 4 ng/mL[f] Rac: 50 ± 9 ng/mL[f]

[a]Escitalopram is the active *S*-enantiomer of racemic citalopram. Pharmacokinetic data after dosing of escitalopram (Es) and citalopram racemate (Rac) are reported. No significant gender differences. Citalopram is metabolized by CYP2C19 (polymorphic) and CYP3A4 to desmethylcitalopram. [b]Data from CYP2C19 extensive metabolizers. CYP2C19 poor metabolizers exhibit a lower (~44%) *CL/F* and longer $t_{1/2}$ than extensive metabolizers. [c]*CL/F* and *V/F* for Es reported. [d]Alcoholic, viral, or biliary cirrhosis. [e]Moderate renal impairment. [f]Following a single 40-mg (Rac) or 20-mg (Es) oral dose.

References: Gutierrez MM, et al. An evaluation of the potential for pharmacokinetic interaction between escitalopram and the cytochrome P450 3A4 inhibitor ritonavir. *Clin Ther,* **2003**, *25*:1200–1210. Joffe P, et al. Single-dose pharmacokinetics of citalopram in patients with moderate renal insufficiency or hepatic cirrhosis compared with healthy subjects. *Eur J Clin Pharmacol,* **1998**, *54*:237–242. *PDR*58, **2004**, pp. 1292, 1302–1303. Sidhu J, et al. Steady-state pharmacokinetics of the enantiomers of citalopram and its metabolites in humans. *Chirality,* **1997**, *9*:686–692. Sindrup SH, et al. Pharmacokinetics of citalopram in relation to the sparteine and the mephenytoin oxidation polymorphisms. *Ther Drug Monit,* **1993**, *15*:11–17.

Esomeprazole[a]							
Es: 89 (81-98)[b] Rac: 53 ± 29[b]	Es/Rac: <1	Es/Rac: 95-97	Es: 4.1 (3.3-5.0)[c,d] Rac: 7.5 ± 2.7[c] ↓ LD[e]	Es: 0.25 (0.23-0.27) Rac: 0.34 ± 0.09	Es: 0.9 (0.7-1.0)[d] Rac: 0.7 ± 0.5 ↑ LD[e]	Es: 1.5 (1.3-1.7)[f] Rac, EM: ~1[g] Rac, PM: ~3-4[g]	Es: 4.5 (3.8-5.7) μM[f] Rac, EM: 0.68 ± 0.43 μM[g] Rac, PM: 3.5 ± 1.4 μM[g]

[a]Esomeprazole is the *S*-enantiomer of omeprazole. Both esomeprazole (Es) and racemic omeprazole (Rac) are available. Data for both formulations are reported. [b]Bioavailability determined after multiple dosing. Lower Es values 64% (54-75%) reported for single dose. [c]The metabolic *CL* of the Es is slower than that of the *R*-enantiomer. Both Es and Rac are metabolized by CYP2C19 (polymorphic) and CYP3A4. *CL* of Es and Rac is decreased and $t_{1/2}$ increased in CYP2C19 poor metabolizers. [d]Following a single 40-mg IV dose. *CL* of Es decreases and $t_{1/2}$ of Es increases with multiple dosing. [e]Reduced *CL* and increased $t_{1/2}$ in patients with severe (Childs-Pugh class C) hepatic impairment. [f]Following a 40-mg oral dose of Es given once daily for 5 days to healthy subjects of unspecified CYP2C19 phenotype. [g]Following a 20-mg oral dose of Rac given twice daily for 4 days to healthy subjects phenotyped as CYP2C19 extensive metabolizers (EM) and poor metabolizers (PM).

References: Andersson T, et al. Pharmacokinetic studies with esomeprazole, the (S)-isomer of omeprazole. *Clin Pharmacokinet,* **2001**, *40*:411–426. Chang M, et al. Interphenotype differences in disposition and effect on gastrin levels of omeprazole—Suitability of omeprazole as a probe for CYP2C19. *Br J Clin Pharmacol,* **1995**, *39*:511–518.

Eszopiclone,[a] **Zopiclone**							
—	Es: <10	Es: 52-59	—[b]	—[c]	Es: 7.2 ± 1.3 Es: ↔ RD[d] Es: ↑ LD[e]	Es: 1 (0.4-2.1)	Es: 39.8 ± 8.6 ng/mL[f]

[a]Eszopiclone is the (*S*)-isomer of zopiclone. Pharmacokinetic data after dosing of eszopiclone (Es) is shown. Es is metabolized extensively by CYP3A4 and CYP2E1. [b]*CL/F* following a 15-mg oral dose of zopiclone is 2.7 mL/min/kg for Es and 4.4 mL/min/kg for racemic zopiclone. [c]*V/F* following a 15-mg oral dose of racemic zopiclone is 1.4 L/kg for eszopiclone and 2 L/kg for racemic zopiclone. [d]Study in mild, moderate, and severe RD. [e]In patients with severe hepatic impairment. [f]Following 3-mg Es given once daily to steady state.

References: Drugs@FDA. Lunesta label approved on 04/06/09. Available at: http://www.accessdata.fda.gov/drugsatfda_docs/label/2009/021476s012lbl.pdf. Accessed July 9, 2010. Najib J. Eszopiclone, a nonbenzodiazepine sedative-hypnotic agent for the treatment of transient and chronic insomnia. *Clin Ther,* **2006**, *28*:491–516.

Ethambutol							
77 ± 8	79 ± 3	6-30	8.6 ± 0.8	1.6 ± 0.2	3.1 ± 0.4 ↑ RD	2-4[a]	2-5 μg/mL[a]

[a]Following a single 800-mg oral dose to healthy subjects. Concentrations >10 μg/mL can adversely affect vision. No accumulation with once-a-day dosing in patients with normal renal function.

Reference: Holdiness MR. Clinical pharmacokinetics of the antituberculosis drugs. *Clin Pharmacokinet,* **1984**, *9*:511–544.

(Continued)

Table AII–1

Pharmacokinetic Data (*Continued*)

BIOAVAILABILITY (ORAL) (%)	URINARY EXCRETION (%)	BOUND IN PLASMA (%)	CLEARANCE (mL/min/kg)	VOL. DIST. (L/kg)	HALF-LIFE (hours)	PEAK TIME (hours)	PEAK CONCENTRATION
Exenatide[a]							
SC: ~100	—	—	8.1[b] ↓ RD	0.1[c]	1.5 (0.9-2.0) ↑ RD	2 (1-3)[c]	821 ± 500 pg/mL[d]

[a]Exenatide is a synthetic peptide cleared primarily by the kidney through filtration, reabsorption, and proteolytic degradation. [b]*CL/F* after SC injection reported. [c]V_{area}/F after SC injection reported. [d]Following a 10-μg SC injection.

References: Linnebjerg H, et al. Effects of renal impairment on the pharmacokinetics of exenatide. *Br J Clin Pharmacol*, **2007**, *64*:317–327.

BIOAVAILABILITY (ORAL) (%)	URINARY EXCRETION (%)	BOUND IN PLASMA (%)	CLEARANCE (mL/min/kg)	VOL. DIST. (L/kg)	HALF-LIFE (hours)	PEAK TIME (hours)	PEAK CONCENTRATION
Ezetimibe[a]							
—	~2	>90[b]	6.6[c] ↓ Aged, RD, LD	1.5[c]	28-30[d]	1[e]	122 ng/mL[e]

[a]Ezetimibe is extensively metabolized to a glucuronide, which is more active than ezetimibe in inhibiting cholesterol absorption. Clinical effects are related to the total plasma concentration of ezetimibe and ezetimibe–glucuronide, with ezetimibe concentrations being only 10% of the total. [b]For ezetimibe and ezetimibe–glucuronide. [c]*CL/F* and a volume for the central compartment (V_c/F) for total (unconjugated and glucuronide conjugate) ezetimibe reported. [d]Ezetimibe undergoes significant enterohepatic recycling, leading to multiple secondary peaks. An effective $t_{1/2}$ is estimated. [e]Total (unconjugated and glucuronide conjugate) ezetimibe following a 10-mg oral dose given once daily for 10 days.

References: Mauro VF, et al. Ezetimibe for management of hypercholesterolemia. *Ann Pharmacother,* **2003**, *37*:839–848. Patrick JE, et al. Disposition of the selective cholesterol absorption inhibitor ezetimibe in healthy male subjects. *Drug Metab Dispos,* **2002**, *30*:430–437. *PDR*58, **2004**, pp. 3085–3086.

BIOAVAILABILITY (ORAL) (%)	URINARY EXCRETION (%)	BOUND IN PLASMA (%)	CLEARANCE (mL/min/kg)	VOL. DIST. (L/kg)	HALF-LIFE (hours)	PEAK TIME (hours)	PEAK CONCENTRATION
Famotidine[a]							
37 (20-66)	65-80	20	4.3-6.9[b] ↓ Aged, RD, Neo[c]	1.1-1.4	2.5-4.0 ↑ RD	2.3 (1-4)	76-104 ng/mL[d]

[a]Cleared primarily by the kidney. [b]Renal clearance after IV administration was ~4.3 mL/min/kg. [c]The pharmacokinetics of IV famotidine were similar in children >1 year of age and adults. [d]Following a single 40-mg oral dose.

References: Krishna DR, et al. Newer H2-receptor antagonists. Clinical pharmacokinetics and drug interaction potential. *Clin Pharmacokinet,* **1988**, *15*:205–215. Maples HD, et al. Famotidine disposition in children and adolescents with chronic renal insufficiency. *J Clin Pharmacol,* **2003**, *43*:7–14. Wenning LA, et al. Pharmacokinetics of famotidine in infants. *Clin Pharmacokinet,* **2005**, *44*:395–406.

Felodipine[a]							
15 ± 8 ↔ Aged, Cirr ↑ Food	<1	99.6 ± 02 ↓ RD, LD ↔ Aged	12 ± 5[b] ↓ Aged, LD, CHF[c]	10 ± 3 ↔ Aged ↓ LD	14 ± 4 ↑ Aged, CHF[c] ↔ LD	IR: 0.9 ± 0.4[d] ER: 3.7 ± 0.9[d]	IR: 34 ± 26 nM[d] ER: 9.1 ± 7.3 nM[d]

[a]Racemic mixture; *S*-(–)-enantiomer is an active Ca^{+2} channel blocker; different enantiomer pharmacokinetics result in *S*-(–)-enantiomer concentrations about 2-fold higher than those of *R*-(+)-isomer. [b]Undergoes significant CYP3A-dependent first-pass metabolism in the intestine and liver. [c]May be age related rather than CHF related. [d]Following a 10-mg oral immediate-release (IR) or extended-release (ER) tablet given twice daily to steady state in healthy subjects. EC_{50} for diastolic pressure decrease is 8 ± 5 nM in patients with hypertension.

Reference: Dunselman PH, et al. Felodipine clinical pharmacokinetics. *Clin Pharmacokinet,* **1991**, *21*:418–430.

Fenofibrate[a]							
—[b] ↑ Food	0.1-10[c]	>99	0.45[d] ↓ RD	0.89[d]	20-27 ↑ RD	IR: 6-8[e] Mic: 4-6[f]	IR: 8.6 ± 0.9 μg/mL[e] Mic: 10.8 ± 0.6 μg/mL[f]

[a]Fenofibrate is a prodrug that is hydrolyzed by esterases to fenofibric acid, the pharmacologically active compound. All values reported are for fenofibric acid. [b]Absolute bioavailability is not known. Recovery of radiolabeled dose in urine as fenofibric acid and its glucuronide is 60%. Immediate-release (IR) tablet and micronized (Mic) capsule are bioequivalent. Bioavailability is increased when taken with a standard meal. [c]Recovery following oral dose. [d]*CL/F* and *V/F* reported. [e]Following a 300-mg IR fenofibrate tablet given once daily to steady state. [f]Following a 200-mg Mic capsule given once daily to steady state.

References: Balfour JA, et al. Fenofibrate. A review of its pharmacodynamic and pharmacokinetic properties and therapeutic use in dyslipidaemia. *Drugs,* **1990**, *40*:260–290. Miller DB, et al. Clinical pharmacokinetics of fibric acid derivatives (fibrates). *Clin Pharmacokinet,* **1998**, *34*:155–162.

Fentanyl							
TM: ~50	8	84 ± 2	13 ± 2[a] ↓ Aged ↔ Prem, Child ↑ Neo	4.0 ± 0.4	3.7 ± 0.4 ↑ CPBS, Aged, Prem ↔ Child	TD: 35 ± 15[b] TM: 0.4 (0.3-6)[b]	TD: 1.4 ± 0.5 ng/mL[b] TM: 0.8 ± 0.3 ng/mL[b]

[a]Metabolically cleared primarily by CYP3A to norfentanyl and hydroxy metabolites. [b]Following a 5-mg transdermal (TD) dose administered at 50 μg/hr through a DURAGESIC system or a single 400-μg transmucosal (TM) dose. Postoperative and intraoperative analgesia occurs at plasma concentrations of 1 ng/mL and 3 ng/mL, respectively. Respiratory depression occurs >0.7 ng/mL.

References: Olkkola KT, et al. Clinical pharmacokinetics and pharmacodynamics of opioid analgesics in infants and children. *Clin Pharmacokinet,* **1995**, *28*:385–404. *PDR*54, **2000**, pp. 405, 1445.

Fexofenadine[a]							
—[b]	12	60-70	9.4 ± 4.2[c]	—	14 ± 6[c] ↑ RD[d] ↔ LD	1.3 ± 0.6[e]	286 ± 143 ng/mL[e]

[a]Data from healthy adult male subjects. [b]Absolute bioavailability is unknown. Negligible metabolism with 85% of a dose recovered in feces unchanged; a substrate for hepatic and intestinal uptake and efflux transporters. [c]*CL/F* and $t_{1/2}$ reported for oral dose. [d]Mild renal impairment. [e]Following a 60-mg oral dose twice a day to steady state.

References: Markham A, et al. Fexofenadine. *Drugs,* **1998**, *55*:269–274; discussion 275–276. Robbins OK, et al. Dose proportionality and comparison of single and multiple dose pharmacokinetics of fexofenadine (MDL 16455) and its enantiomers in healthy male volunteers. *Biopharm Drug Dispos,* **1998**, *19*:455–463.

(*Continued*)

Table AII–1

Pharmacokinetic Data (*Continued*)

BIOAVAILABILITY (ORAL) (%)	URINARY EXCRETION (%)	BOUND IN PLASMA (%)	CLEARANCE (mL/min/kg)	VOL. DIST. (L/kg)	HALF-LIFE (hours)	PEAK TIME (hours)	PEAK CONCENTRATION
Finasteride							
63 ± 21	<1	90	2.3 ± 0.8 ↔ RD, Aged	1.1 ± 0.2	7.9 ± 2.5 ↔ RD, Aged	1-2[a]	37 (27-49) ng/mL[a]
[a]Following a single 5-mg oral dose given to healthy adults. Drug accumulates 2-fold with once-daily dosing.				*Reference*: Sudduth SL, et al. Finasteride: The first 5α-reductase inhibitor. *Pharmacotherapy,* **1993**, *13*:309–325; discussion 325–329.			
Flecainide[a]							
70 ± 11	43 ± 3	61 ± 10 ↓ MI	5.6 ± 1.3[b] ↓ RD, LD, CHF ↑ Child	4.9 ± 0.4[c] ↑ Cirr	11 ± 3[b] ↑ RD, LD, CHF ↓ Child	~3 (1-6)[d]	458 ± 100 ng/mL[d]
[a]Racemic mixture; enantiomers exert similar electrophysiological effects. [b]Metabolized by CYP2D6 (polymorphic); except for a shortened elimination $t_{1/2}$ and nonlinear kinetics in extensive metabolizers, CYP2D6 phenotype had no significant influence on flecainide pharmacokinetics or pharmacodynamics. [c]V_{area} reported. [d]Following a 100-mg oral dose given twice daily for 5 days in healthy adults. Similar levels for CYP2D6 extensive and poor metabolizers.				*Reference*: Funck-Brentano C, et al. Variable disposition kinetics and electrocardiographic effects of flecainide during repeated dosing in humans: Contribution of genetic factors, dose-dependent clearance, and interaction with amiodarone. *Clin Pharmacol Ther,* **1994**, *55*:256–269.			
Fluconazole							
>90	75 ± 9	11 ± 1	0.27 ± 0.07 ↔ AIDS, Neo ↓ RD, Prem	0.60 ± 0.11 ↔ RD ↑ Prem, Neo	32 ± 5 ↑ LD, RD, Prem ↓ Child	1.7-4.3[a]	10.6 ± 0.4 μg/mL[a]
[a]Following a 200-mg oral dose given twice a day for 4 days to healthy adults. *References*: Debruyne D, et al. Clinical pharmacokinetics of fluconazole. *Clin Pharmacokinet,* **1993**, *24*:10–27.				Varhe A, et al. Effect of fluconazole dose on the extent of fluconazole-triazolam interaction. *Br J Clin Pharmacol,* **1996**, *42*:465–470.			
Fludarabine[a]							
—	24 ± 3	—	3.7 ± 1.5 ↓ RD	2.4 ± 0.6	10-30	—	0.57 μg/mL[b]
[a]Data from adult male and female cancer patients following IV administration. Fludarabine is rapidly dephosphorylated to 2-fluoro-arabinoside-A (F-ara-A), transported into cells, and phosphorylated to the active triphosphate metabolite. Pharmacokinetics of F-ara-A are reported. [b]Following a single 25-mg/m^2 IV dose of fludarabine (30-minute infusion); no accumulation after five daily doses.				*References*: Hersh MR, et al. Pharmacokinetic study of fludarabine phosphate (NSC 312887). *Cancer Chemother Pharmacol,* **1986**, *17*:277–280. *PDR*54, **2000**, p. 764. Plunkett W, et al. Fludarabine: Pharmacokinetics, mechanisms of action, and rationales for combination therapies. *Semin Oncol,* **1993**, *20*:2–12.			

5-Fluorouracil (5-FU)

28 (0-80)[a]	<10	8-12	16 ± 7	0.25 ± 0.12	11 ± 4 min[b]	—	11.2 μM[c]

[a]Higher *F* with rapid absorption and lower *F* with slower absorption, due to a saturable first-pass effect. [b]A much longer (~20 hours) terminal $t_{1/2}$ has been reported, representing a slow redistribution of drug from tissues. [c]Steady-state concentration following a continuous IV infusion of 300-500 mg/m²/day to cancer patients.

Reference: Diasio RB, et al. Clinical pharmacology of 5-fluorouracil. *Clin Pharmacokinet,* **1989**, *16*:215–237.

Fluoxetine[a]

—[a]	<2.5	94 ↔ LD, RD	9.6 ± 6.9[b,c] ↔ RD, Aged, Obes ↓ LD	35 ± 21[d] ↔ RD, LD	53 ± 41[e] ↑ LD ↔ RD, Aged, Obes	F: 6-8[f]	F: 200-531 ng/mL[f] NF: 103-465 ng/mL[f]

[a]Active metabolite, norfluoxetine; $t_{1/2}$ of norfluoxetine is 6.4 ± 2.5 days (12 ± 2 days in cirrhosis). Absolute bioavailability is unknown, but ≥80% of the dose is absorbed. [b]Reduced *CL* with repetitive dosing (~2.6 mL/min/kg) and with increasing dose between 40 and 80 mg. [c]*CL/F* reported; fluoxetine is a CYP2D6 substrate and inhibitor. [d]V_{area}/F reported. [e]Longer $t_{1/2}$ with repetitive dosing and with increasing doses. [f]Range of data for fluoxetine (F) and norfluoxetine (NF) following a 60-mg oral dose given once daily for 1 week. NF continues to accumulate for several weeks.

Reference: Altamura AC, et al. Clinical pharmacokinetics of fluoxetine. *Clin Pharmacokinet,* **1994**, *26*:201–214.

Fluphenazine[a]

PO: 2.7 (1.7-4.5)[b] SC or IM: 3.4 (2.5-5.0)[b]	Negligible	—	10 ± 7	11 ± 10	IV: 12 ± 4[c] IR: 14.4 ± 7.8[c] SR: 20.3 ± 7.9[c]	IR: 2.8 ± 2.1[d] DN: 24-48[d] EN: 48-72[d]	IR: 2.3 ± 2.1 ng/mL[d] DN: 1.3 ng/mL[d] EN: 1.1 ng/mL[d]

[a]Data from healthy male and female volunteers. Fluphenazine is extensively metabolized. [b]Available in immediate-release (IR) oral and IM formulations and depot SC or IM injections as the enanthate (EN) or decanoate (DN) esters. Geometric mean (90% confidence interval). [c]Reported $t_{1/2}$ for a single IV dose and apparent $t_{1/2}$ following oral administration of IR and slow-release (SR) formulations. Longer apparent $t_{1/2}$s with oral dosing reflect an absorption-limited elimination. [d]Following a single 12-mg oral dose (IR) or 5-mg IM injections of DN and EN.

References: Jann MW, et al. Clinical pharmacokinetics of the depot antipsychotics. *Clin Pharmacokinet,* **1985**, *10*:315–333. Koytchev R, et al. Absolute bioavailability of oral immediate and slow release fluphenazine in healthy volunteers. *Eur J Clin Pharmacol,* **1996**, *51*:183–187.

Flutamide[a]

—	<1	F: 94-96 HF: 92-94	280[b] ↔ RD	—	F: 7.8[b] HF: 8.1[b]	F: 1.3 ± 0.7[c] HF: 1.9 ± 0.6[c]	F: 0.11 ± 0.21 μg/mL[c] HF: 1.6 ± 0.59 μg/mL[c]

[a]Data obtained primarily from elderly men. Flutamide (F) is metabolized rapidly to a number of metabolites, which are mainly excreted in urine. One major metabolite, 2-hydroxyflutamide (HF), is biologically active (equal potency); formation is catalyzed primarily by CYP1A2. [b]*CL/F* and $t_{1/2}$ (terminal) reported for oral dose. [c]Data for F and HF following a 250-mg oral dose given three times daily to steady state in healthy geriatric male volunteers.

References: Anjum S, et al. Pharmacokinetics of flutamide in patients with renal insufficiency. *Br J Clin Pharmacol,* **1999**, *47*:43–47. *PDR*54, **2000**, p. 2798. Radwanski E, et al. Single and multiple dose pharmacokinetic evaluation of flutamide in normal geriatric volunteers. *J Clin Pharmacol,* **1989**, *29*:554–558.

(*Continued*)

Table AII–1

Pharmacokinetic Data (*Continued*)

BIOAVAILABILITY (ORAL) (%)	URINARY EXCRETION (%)	BOUND IN PLASMA (%)	CLEARANCE (mL/min/kg)	VOL. DIST. (L/kg)	HALF-LIFE (hours)	PEAK TIME (hours)	PEAK CONCENTRATION
Foscarnet							
9 ± 2	95 ± 5	14-17	1.6 ± 0.2 ↓ RD[a]	0.35	5.7 ± 0.2 ↑ RD[a]	1.4 ± 0.6[b]	86 ± 36 μM[b]

[a]In patients with moderate to severe renal impairment. [b]Following an 8-mg/kg oral dose given once daily for 8 days to HIV-seropositive patients.

References: Aweeka FT, et al. Effect of renal disease and hemodialysis on foscarnet pharmacokinetics and dosing recommendations. *J Acquir Immune Defic Syndr Hum Retrovirol,* **1999**, *20*:350–357. Noormohamed FH, et al. Pharmacokinetics and absolute bioavailability of oral foscarnet in human immunodeficiency virus-seropositive patients. *Antimicrob Agents Chemother,* **1998**, *42*:293–297.

BIOAVAILABILITY (ORAL) (%)	URINARY EXCRETION (%)	BOUND IN PLASMA (%)	CLEARANCE (mL/min/kg)	VOL. DIST. (L/kg)	HALF-LIFE (hours)	PEAK TIME (hours)	PEAK CONCENTRATION
Fosfomycin[a]							
28 ± 8 (28-41) ↓ Food[b]	82 ± 13	Negligible	2.31 ± 0.22 ↓ RD[c]	0.36 ± 0.06	2.2 ± 0.5 ↑ RD[c]	2.0 ± 0.6[d] ↑ Food[b]	21.8 ± 4.8 μg/mL[d] ↓ Food[b]

[a]Fosfomycin is cleared predominantly by renal elimination. Data from adult male subjects. No significant gender differences. Range of mean values from multiple studies shown in parentheses. [b]High-fat meal. [c]*CL/F* reduced in patients with mild to severe renal impairment. [d]Following a single 3-g oral dose of fosfomycin trometamol in healthy adults.

References: Bergan T, et al. Pharmacokinetic profile of fosfomycin trometamol. *Chemotherapy*, **1993**, *39*:297–301. Cadorniga R, et al. Pharmacokinetic study of fosfomycin and its bioavailability. *Chemotherapy*, **1977**, *23*:159–174. Goto M, et al. Fosfomycin kinetics after intravenous and oral administration to human volunteers. *Antimicrob Agents Chemother*, **1981**, *20*:393–397. *PDR*54, **2000**, p. 1083.

BIOAVAILABILITY (ORAL) (%)	URINARY EXCRETION (%)	BOUND IN PLASMA (%)	CLEARANCE (mL/min/kg)	VOL. DIST. (L/kg)	HALF-LIFE (hours)	PEAK TIME (hours)	PEAK CONCENTRATION
Fulvestrant[a]							
—[b]	<1	99	9.3-14.3	3.0-5.3	14-19[c]	167[d]	8.2 ± 5.2 ng/mL[d]

[a]Eliminated by conjugation (sulfate and glucuronide) and CYP3A4-mediated oxidation. Data reported for men and women; no significant gender differences. [b]For parenteral administration only. Bioavailability following IM injection has not been reported. [c]Elimination $t_{1/2}$ following IV administration. The apparent $t_{1/2}$ following IM dosing is ~40 days due to very prolonged absorption. [d]Following a single 250-mg IM dose given to postmenopausal women with breast cancer.

*References: PDR*58, **2004**, pp. 669–670. Robertson JF, et al. Fulvestrant: Pharmacokinetics and pharmacology. *Br J Cancer,* **2004**, *90*(suppl):S7–S10. Robertson JF, et al. Pharmacokinetic profile of intramuscular fulvestrant in advanced breast cancer. *Clin Pharmacokinet,* **2004**, *43*:529–538.

Furosemide[a]

71 ± 35 (43-73) ↔ CHF, LD, CRI	71 ± 10 (50-80) ↓ CF ↔ Aged	98.6 ± 0.4 (96-99) ↓ RD, NS, LD, Alb, Aged ↔ CHF, Smk	1.66 ± 0.58 (1.5-3.0) ↓ Aged, RD,[b] CHF, Neo, Prem ↔ LD ↑ CF	0.13 ± 0.06 (0.09-0.17) ↑ NS, Neo, Prem, LD ↔ RD, CHF, Aged, Smk	1.3 ± 0.8 (0.5-2.0) ↑ Aged, RD,[b] CHF, Prem, Neo, LD ↔ NS	1.4 ± 0.8[c]	1.7 ± 0.9 μg/mL[c]

[a]Data from healthy adult male subjects. No significant gender differences described. Range of mean values from multiple studies shown in parentheses. [b]*CL/F* reduced, mild renal impairment. Aged: *CL/F* reduced with declining renal function. [c]Following a single 40-mg oral dose (tablet). Ototoxicity occurs at concentrations >25 μg/mL.

References: Andreasen F, et al. The pharmacokinetics of frusemide are influenced by age. *Br J Clin Pharmacol,* **1983**, *16*:391–397. Ponto LL, et al. Furosemide (frusemide). A pharmacokinetic/pharmacodynamic review (part I). *Clin Pharmacokinet,* **1990**, *18*:381–408. Waller ES, et al. Disposition and absolute bioavailability of furosemide in healthy males. *J Pharm Sci,* **1982**, *71*:1105–1108.

Gabapentin

60[a]	64-68	<3	1.6 ± 0.3 ↓ Aged, RD	0.80 ± 0.09	6.5 ± 1.0 ↑ RD	2-3[b]	4 μg/mL[b]

[a]Decreases with increasing dose. Value for 300- to 600-mg dose reported. [b]Following an 800-mg oral dose given three times daily to steady state in healthy adults. Efficacious at concentrations >2 μg/mL.

References: Bialer M. Comparative pharmacokinetics of the newer antiepileptic drugs. *Clin Pharmacokinet,* **1993**, *24*:441–452. McLean MJ. Gabapentin. In: Wyllie E, ed. *The Treatment of Epilepsy: Principles and Practice,* 2nd ed. Baltimore, Williams & Wilkins, **1997**, pp. 884–898.

Galantamine[a]

100 (91-110)	20 (18-22)	18	5.7 (5.0-6.3)[b] ↓ RD,[c] LD[c]	2.6 (2.4-2.9)	5.7 (5.2-6.3)	2.6 ± 1.0[d]	96 ± 29 ng/mL[d]

[a]Primarily metabolized by CYP2D6, CYP3A4, and glucuronidation. [b]CYP2D6 poor metabolizers show a lower *CL,* but dose adjustment is not required. [c]In patients with mild to moderate hepatic or renal insufficiency. [d]Following a 12-mg oral dose given twice daily for 7 days in healthy, elderly adults.

References: Bickel U, et al. Pharmacokinetics of galanthamine in humans and corresponding cholinesterase inhibition. *Clin Pharmacol Ther,* **1991**, *50*:420–428. Huang F, et al. Pharmacokinetic and safety assessments of galantamine and risperidone after the two drugs are administered alone and together. *J Clin Pharmacol,* **2002**, *42*:1341–1351. Scott LJ, et al. Galantamine: A review of its use in Alzheimer's disease. *Drugs,* **2000**, *60*:1095–1122.

Ganciclovir

3-5 ↑ Food	91 ± 5	1-2	3.4 ± 0.5 ↓ RD	1.1 ± 0.2	3.7 ± 0.6 ↑ RD	PO: 3.0 ± 0.6[a]	IV: 6.6 ± 1.8 μg/mL[a] PO: 1.2 ± 0.4 μg/mL[a] ↑ Food

[a]Following a single 6-mg/kg IV dose (1-hour infusion) or a 1000-mg oral dose given with food three times a day to steady state.

References: Aweeka FT, et al. Foscarnet and ganciclovir pharmacokinetics during concomitant or alternating maintenance therapy for AIDS-related cytomegalovirus retinitis. *Clin Pharmacol Ther,* **1995**, *57*:403–412. *PDR*54, **2000**, p. 2624.

(*Continued*)

Table AII–1

Pharmacokinetic Data (*Continued*)

BIOAVAILABILITY (ORAL) (%)	URINARY EXCRETION (%)	BOUND IN PLASMA (%)	CLEARANCE (mL/min/kg)	VOL. DIST. (L/kg)	HALF-LIFE (hours)	PEAK TIME (hours)	PEAK CONCENTRATION
Gemcitabine[a]							
—	<10	Negligible	37.8 ± 19.4[b] ↓ Aged	1.4 ± 1.3[c]	0.63 ± 0.48[c] ↑ Aged	—	26.9 ± 9 μM[d]
[a]Data from patients with leukemia. Rapidly metabolized intracellularly to active di- and triphosphate products; IV administration. [b]Weight-normalized *CL* is ~25% lower in women, compared to men. [c]V_d and $t_{1/2}$ are reported to increase with long duration of IV infusion. [d]Steady-state concentration during a 10-mg/m²/min infusion for 120-640 minutes.				*References*: Grunewald R, et al. Gemcitabine in leukemia: A phase I clinical, plasma, and cellular pharmacology study. *J Clin Oncol*, **1992**, *10*:406–413. *PDR*54, **2000**, p. 1586.			
Gemfibrozil							
98 ± 1	<1	97	1.7 ± 0.4 ↔ LD, RD	0.14 ± 0.03	1.1 ± 0.2 ↔ RD	1-2[a]	15-25 μg/mL[a]
[a]Following a 600-mg oral dose given twice daily to steady state.				*Reference*: Todd PA, et al. Gemfibrozil. A review of its pharmacodynamic and pharmacokinetic properties, and therapeutic use in dyslipidaemia. *Drugs,* **1988**, *36*:314–339.			
Gentamicin							
IM: ~100	>90	<10	$CL = 0.82CL_{cr} + 0.11$ ↓ Obes	0.31 ± 0.10 ↔ RD, Aged, CF, Child ↓ Obes ↑ Neo	2-3[a]	IV: 1[b] IM: 0.3-0.75[b]	IV: 4.9 ± 0.5 μg/mL[b] IM: 5.0 ± 0.4 μg/mL[b]
[a]Gentamicin has a very long terminal $t_{1/2}$ of 53 ± 25 hours (slow release from tissues), which accounts for urinary excretion for up to 3 weeks after a dose. [b]Following a single 100-mg IV infusion (1 hour) or IM injection given to healthy adults.				*References*: Matzke GR, et al. Pharmacokinetics of cetirizine in the elderly and patients with renal insufficiency. *Ann Allergy,* **1987**, *59*:25–30. Regamey C, et al. Comparative pharmacokinetics of tobramycin and gentamicin. *Clin Pharmacol Ther,* **1973**, *14*:396–403.			
Glimepiride[a]							
~100	<0.5	>99.5	0.62 ± 0.26 ↑ RD[b]	0.18 ↑ RD[b]	3.4 ± 2.0 ↔ RD[b]	2-3[c]	359 ± 98 ng/mL[c]
[a]Data from healthy male subjects. No significant gender differences. Glimepiride is metabolized by CYP2C9 to an active (approximately one-third potency) metabolite, Ml. [b]*CL/F*, V_d/F increased and $t_{1/2}$ unchanged, moderate to severe renal impairment; presumably mediated through an increase in plasma-free fraction. Ml AUC also increased. [c]Following a single 3-mg oral dose.				*References*: Badian M, et al. Determination of the absolute bioavailability of glimepiride (HOE 490), a new sulphonylurea. *Int J Clin Pharmacol Ther Toxicol,* **1992**, *30*:481–482. *PDR*54, **2000**, pp. 1346–1349. Rosenkranz B, et al. Pharmacokinetics and safety of glimepiride at clinically effective doses in diabetic patients with renal impairment. *Diabetologia,* **1996**, *39*:1617–1624.			

Glipizide							
95	<5	98.4	0.52 ± 0.18[a] ↔ RD, Aged	0.17 ± 0.02[a] ↔ Aged	3.4 ± 0.7 ↔ RD, Aged	2.1 ± 0.9[b]	465 ± 139 ng/mL[b]

[a]*CL/F* and V_{ss}/*F* reported. [b]Following a single 5-mg oral dose (immediate-release tablet) given to healthy young adults. An extended-release formulation exhibits a delayed T_{max} of 6-12 hours.

Reference: Kobayashi KA, et al. Glipizide pharmacokinetics in young and elderly volunteers. *Clin Pharm*, **1988**, *7*:224–228.

Glyburide							
G: 90-100[a] M: 64-90[a]	Negligible	99.8 ↓ Aged	1.3 ± 0.5 ↓ LD	0.20 ± 0.11	4 ± 1[b] ↑ LD, NIDDM	G: ~1.5[c] M: 2-4[c]	G: 106 ng/mL[c] M: 104 ng/mL[c]

[a]Data for GLYNASE PRESTAB micronized tablet (G) and MICRONASE tablet (M). [b]$t_{1/2}$ for G reported. $t_{1/2}$ for M formulation is 6-10 hours, reflecting absorption rate limitation. A long terminal $t_{1/2}$ (15 hours), reflecting redistribution from tissues, has been reported. [c]Following a 3-mg oral GLYNASE tablet taken with breakfast or a 5-mg oral MICRONASE tablet given to healthy adult subjects.

References: Jonsson A, et al. Slow elimination of glyburide in NIDDM subjects. *Diabetes Care*, **1994**, *17*:142–145. Drugs@FDA.GLYNASE PRETAB label; http://www.accessdata.fda.gov/drugsatfda_docs/label/2009/020051s0161bl.pdf. Accessed July 10, 2010.

Haloperidol[a]							
60 ± 18	1	92 ± 2 ↑ LD ↔ Aged, Child	11.8 ± 2.9[b] ↑ Child, Smk ↓ Aged	18 ± 7	18 ± 5[b] ↓ Child	IM: 0.6 ± 0.1[c] PO: 1.7 ± 3.2[c]	IM: 22 ± 18 ng/mL[c] PO: 9.2 ± 4.4 ng/mL[c]

[a]Undergoes reversible metabolism to a less active reduced haloperidol. [b]Represents net *CL* of parent drug; reduced haloperidol $CL = 10 \pm 5$ mL · min^{-1} · kg^{-1} and $t_{1/2} = 67 \pm 51$ hours. Slow conversion from reduced haloperidol to parent compound probably responsible for prolonged terminal $t_{1/2}$ (70 hours) for haloperidol observed with 7-day sampling. [c]Following a single 20-mg oral or 10-mg IM dose. Effective concentrations are 4-20 ng/mL.

Reference: Froemming JS, et al. Pharmacokinetics of haloperidol. *Clin Pharmacokinet*, **1989**, *17*:396–423.

Heparin							
—	Negligible	Extensive	1/(0.65 + 0.008D) ± 0.1[a] ↓ Fem	0.058 ± 0.11[b]	(26 + 0.323D) ± 12 min[a] ↓ Smk	3[c]	70 ± 39 ng/mL[c]

[a]Dose (D) is in IU/kg. *CL* and $t_{1/2}$ are dose dependent, perhaps due to saturable metabolism with end-product inhibition. [b]V_{area} reported. [c]Mean of above critical length molecules following a single 5000 IU dose (unfractionated) given by SC injection.

References: Bendetowicz AV, et al. Pharmacokinetics and pharmacodynamics of a low molecular weight heparin (enoxaparin) after subcutaneous injection, comparison with unfractionated heparin—A three way cross over study in human volunteers. *Thromb Haemost*, **1994**, *71*:305–313. Estes JW. Clinical pharmacokinetics of heparin. *Clin Pharmacokinet*, **1980**, *5*:204–220.

(Continued)

Table AII–1

Pharmacokinetic Data (*Continued*)

BIOAVAILABILITY (ORAL) (%)	URINARY EXCRETION (%)	BOUND IN PLASMA (%)	CLEARANCE (mL/min/kg)	VOL. DIST. (L/kg)	HALF-LIFE (hours)	PEAK TIME (hours)	PEAK CONCENTRATION
Hydrochlorothiazide							
71 ± 15	>95	58 ± 17	4.9 ± 1.1[a] ↓ RD, CHF,[b] Aged	0.83 ± 0.31[c] ↓ Aged	2.5 ± 0.2[d] ↑ RD, CHF,[b] Aged	SD: 1.9 ± 0.5[e] MD: 2[e]	SD: 75 ± 17 ng/mL[e] MD: 91 ± 0.2 ng/mL[e]
Hydrocodone[a]							
—	EM: 10.2 ± 1.8 PM: 18.1 ± 4.5	—	EM: 11.1 ± 3.57[b] PM: 6.54 ± 1.25[b]	—	EM: 4.24 ± 0.99[b] PM: 6.16 ± 1.97[b]	EM: 0.72 ± 0.46[c] PM: 0.93 ± 0.59[c]	EM: 30 ± 9.4 ng/mL[c] PM: 27 ± 5.9 ng/mL[c]
Hydromorphone[a]							
PO: 42 ± 23 SC: ~80	6	7.1	14.6 ± 7.6	2.90 ± 1.31[b]	2.4 ± 0.6	IV: —[c] PO: 1.1 ± 0.2[c]	IV: 242 ng/mL[c] PO: 11.8 ± 2.6 ng/mL[c]

Hydrochlorothiazide notes: [a]Renal *CL* reported, which should approximate total plasma *CL*. [b]Changes may reflect decreased renal function. [c]V_{area} calculated from individual values of renal *CL*, terminal $t_{1/2}$, and fraction of drug excreted unchanged; 70-kg body weight assumed. [d]Longer terminal $t_{1/2}$ of 8 ± 2.8 hours has been reported with a corresponding increase in V_{area} to 2.8 L/kg. [e]Following a single (SD) or multiple (MD) 12.5-mg oral dose of hydrochlorothiazide; MD given once daily for 5 days to healthy adults.

References: Beermann B, et al. Pharmacokinetics of hydrochlorothiazide in man. *Eur J Clin Pharmacol,* **1977**, *12*:297–303. Jordo L, et al. Bioavailability and disposition of metoprolol and hydrochlorothiazide combined in one tablet and of separate doses of hydrochlorothiazide. *Br J Clin Pharmacol,* **1979**, *7*:563–567. O'Grady P, et al. Fosinopril/hydrochlorothiazide: Single dose and steady-state pharmacokinetics and pharmacodynamics. *Br J Clin Pharmacol,* **1999**, *48*:375–381.

Hydrocodone notes: [a]Data from healthy male and female subjects. The metabolism of hydrocodone to hydromorphone (more active) is catalyzed by CYP2D6. Subjects were phenotyped as extensive metabolizers (EM) and poor metabolizers (PM). [b]*CL/F* and $t_{1/2}$ reported for oral dose. [c]Following a 10-mg oral dose (syrup). Maximal hydromorphone concentrations are higher in EM than in PM (5.2 versus 1.0 ng/mL).

Reference: Otton SV, et al. CYP2D6 phenotype determines the metabolic conversion of hydrocodone to hydromorphone. *Clin Pharmacol Ther,* **1993**, *54*:463–472.

Hydromorphone notes: [a]Data from healthy male subjects. Extensively metabolized. The principal metabolite, 3-glucuronide, accumulates to much higher (27-fold) levels than the parent drug and may contribute to some side effects (not antinociceptive). [b]V_{area} reported. [c]Following a single 2-mg IV (bolus, sample at 3 minutes) or 4-mg oral dose.

References: Hagen N, et al. Steady-state pharmacokinetics of hydromorphone and hydromorphone-3-glucuronide in cancer patients after immediate and controlled-release hydromorphone. *J Clin Pharmacol,* **1995**, *35*:37–44. Moulin DE, et al. Comparison of continuous subcutaneous and intravenous hydromorphone infusions for management of cancer pain. *Lancet,* **1991**, *337*:465–468. Parab PV, et al. Pharmacokinetics of hydromorphone after intravenous, peroral and rectal administration to human subjects. *Biopharm Drug Dispos,* **1988**, *9*:187–199.

Hydroxychloroquine[a]							
79 ± 12	27	45 ± 3	11.9 ± 5.4[b]	525 ± 158	1056 (624-1512)	3.2 (2-4.5)	46 ng/mL (34-79 ng/mL)[c]

[a]Hydroxychloroquine is marketed as a racemic mixture of *R*- and *S*-hydroxychloroquine. Data for the racemic mixture is reported. [b]Plasma clearance is reported. Hydroxychloroquine accumulates in red blood cells with an average blood-to-plasma ratio of 7.2. Blood clearance of hydroxychloroquine is 1.3 mL/min/kg. [c]Following oral administration of a single 155-mg tablet.

References: Tett SE, et al. A dose-ranging study of the pharmacokinetics of hydroxychloroquine following intravenous administration to healthy volunteers. *Br J Clin Pharmacol,* **1988**, *26*:303–313. Tett SE, et al. Bioavailability of hydroxychloroquine tablets in healthy volunteers. *Br J Clin Pharmacol,* **1989**, *27*:771–779.

Hydroxyurea[a]							
108 ± 18 (79-108)	35.8 ± 14.2	Negligible	72 ± 17 mL/min/m^2 [b] (36.2-72.3)	19.7 ± 4.6 L/m^2	3.4 ± 0.7 (2.8-4.5)	IV: 0.5[c] PO: 1.2 ± 1.2[c]	IV: 1007 ± 371 μM[c] PO: 794 ± 241 μM[c]

[a]Data from male and female patients treated for solid tumors. A range of mean values from multiple studies is shown in parentheses. [b]Nonrenal elimination of hydroxyurea is thought to exhibit saturable kinetics through a 10- to 80-mg/kg dose range. [c]Following a single 2-g, 30-minute IV infusion or oral dose.

References: Gwilt PR, et al. Pharmacokinetics and pharmacodynamics of hydroxyurea. *Clin Pharmacokinet,* **1998**, *34*:347–358. Rodriguez GI, et al. A bioavailability and pharmacokinetic study of oral and intravenous hydroxyurea. *Blood,* **1998**, *91*:1533–1541.

Hydroxyzine[a]							
—	—	—	A: 9.8 ± 3.3[b] C: 32 ± 11[b]	A: 16 ± 3[b] C: 19 ± 9[b] ↑ Aged	A: 20 ± 4[b] C: 7.1 ± 2.3[b,c] ↑ Aged, LD	A: 2.1 ± 0.4[d] C: 2.0 ± 0.9[d]	A: 72 ± 11 ng/mL[d] C: 47 ± 17 ng/mL[d]

[a]Hydroxyzine is metabolized to an active metabolite, cetirizine. Plasma concentrations of cetirizine exceed those of the parent drug; its $t_{1/2}$ is similar to that of hydroxyzine when formed from parent drug. Hydroxyzine data for adults (A) and children (C) are reported. [b]*CL/F*, V_d/F, and $t_{1/2}$ after oral dose reported. [c]$t_{1/2}$ increases with increasing age (1-15 years of age). [d]Following a single 0.7-mg/kg oral dose given to healthy adults and children.

References: Paton DM, et al. Clinical pharmacokinetics of H1-receptor antagonists (the antihistamines). *Clin Pharmacokinet,* **1985**, *10*:477–497. Simons FE, et al. Pharmacokinetics and antipruritic effects of hydroxyzine in children with atopic dermatitis. *J Pediatr,* **1984**, *104*:123–127. Simons FE, et al. The pharmacokinetics and antihistaminic of the HI receptor antagonist hydroxyzine. *J Allergy Clin Immunol,* **1984**, *73*(pt 1):69–75. Simons FE, et al. The pharmacokinetics and pharmacodynamics of hydroxyzine in patients with primary biliary cirrhosis. *J Clin Pharmacol,* **1989**, *29*:809–815. Simons KJ, et al. Pharmacokinetic and pharmacodynamic studies of the H_1-receptor antagonist hydroxyzine in the elderly. *Clin Pharmacol Ther,* **1989**, *45*: 9–14.

Ibandronate[a]							
0.63	54 ± 13	85	1.8 ± 0.1 ↓ RD[b]	5.8 ± 1.5	37 ± 5	1	11 ± 4 ng/mL[c]

[a]Cleared primarily by the kidney. [b]Exposure increases 50-100% in patients with moderate and severe renal impairment. [c]Following a single 50-mg oral dose.

References: Barrett J, et al. Ibandronate: A clinical pharmacological and pharmacokinetic update. *J Clin Pharmacol,* **2004**, *44*:951–965. Bergner R, et al. Renal safety and pharmacokinetics of ibandronate in multiple myeloma patients with or without impaired renal function. *J Clin Pharmacol,* **2007**, *47*:942–950.

(Continued)

Table AII–1

Pharmacokinetic Data (*Continued*)

BIOAVAILABILITY (ORAL) (%)	URINARY EXCRETION (%)	BOUND IN PLASMA (%)	CLEARANCE (mL/min/kg)	VOL. DIST. (L/kg)	HALF-LIFE (hours)	PEAK TIME (hours)	PEAK CONCENTRATION
Ibuprofen[a]							
>80	<1	>99[b] ↔ RA, Alb	0.75 ± 0.20[b,c] ↑ CF ↔ Child, RA	0.15 ± 0.02[c] ↑ CF	2 ± 0.5[b] ↔ RA, CF, Child ↑ LD	1.6 ± 0.3[d]	61.1 ± 5.5 μg/mL[d]

[a]Racemic mixture. Kinetic parameters for the active *S*-(+)-enantiomer do not differ from those for the inactive *R*-(–)-enantiomer when administered separately; 63 ± 6% of the *R*-(–)-enantiomer undergoes inversion to the active isomer. [b]Unbound percent of *S*-(+)-ibuprofen (0.77 ± 0.20%) is significantly greater than that of *R*-(–)-ibuprofen (0.45 ± 0.06%). Binding of each enantiomer is concentration dependent and is influenced by the presence of the optical antipode, leading to nonlinear elimination kinetics. [c]*CL/F* and V_{ss}/F reported. [d]Following a single 800-mg dose of racemate. A level of 10 μg/mL provides antipyresis in febrile children.

References: Lee EJ, et al. Stereoselective disposition of ibuprofen enantiomers in man. *Br J Clin Pharmacol,* **1985**, *19*:669–674. Lockwood GF, et al. Pharmacokinetics of ibuprofen in man. I. Free and total area/dose relationships. *Clin Pharmacol Ther,* **1983**, *34*:97–103.

BIOAVAILABILITY (ORAL) (%)	URINARY EXCRETION (%)	BOUND IN PLASMA (%)	CLEARANCE (mL/min/kg)	VOL. DIST. (L/kg)	HALF-LIFE (hours)	PEAK TIME (hours)	PEAK CONCENTRATION
Idarubicin[a]							
I: 28 ± 4	<5	I: 97 IL: 94	29 ± 10 ↓ RD[b]	24.7 ± 5.9	I: 15.2 ± 3.7 IL: 41 ± 10 IL: ↑ RD[b]	I: 5.4 ± 2.4[c] IL: 7.9 ± 2.3[c]	I: 6.9 ± 0.1 ng/mL[c] IL: 22 ± 4 ng/mL[c]

[a]Data from male and female patients with cancer. Idarubicin (I) undergoes rapid metabolism to a major active (equipotent) metabolite, idarubicinol (IL). [b]Mild to moderate renal impairment. [c]Following a single 30- to 35-mg/m^2 oral dose.

References: Camaggi CM, et al. Idarubicin metabolism and pharmacokinetics after intravenous and oral administration in cancer patients: A crossover study. *Cancer Chemother Pharmacol,* **1992**, *30*:307–316. Robert J. Clinical pharmacokinetics of idarubicin. *Clin Pharmacokinet,* **1993**, *24*:275–288. Tamassia V, et al. Pharmacokinetic study of intravenous and oral idarubicin in cancer patients. *Int J Clin Pharmacol Res,* **1987**, *7*:419–426.

BIOAVAILABILITY (ORAL) (%)	URINARY EXCRETION (%)	BOUND IN PLASMA (%)	CLEARANCE (mL/min/kg)	VOL. DIST. (L/kg)	HALF-LIFE (hours)	PEAK TIME (hours)	PEAK CONCENTRATION
Imatinib[a]							
98 (87-111)	5	95	3.3 ± 1.2	6.2 ± 2.2	22 ± 4	3.3 ± 1.1[b]	2.6 ± 0.8 μg/mL[b]

[a]Imatinib is metabolized primarily by CYP3A4. [b]Following a 400-mg oral dose given once daily to steady state.

References: Peng B, et al. Absolute bioavailability of imatinib (Glivec) orally versus intravenous infusion. *J Clin Pharmacol,* **2004**, *44*:158–162. Peng B, et al. Pharmacokinetics and pharmacodynamics of imatinib in a phase I trial with chronic myeloid leukemia patients. *J Clin Oncol,* **2004**, *22*:935–942. Product information: Gleevec™ (imatinib mesylate). Basel, Switzerland, Novartis, **2004**.

Imipenem/Cilastatin[a]							
Imipenem —	69 ± 15 ↓ Neo, Inflam ↔ Child, CF	<20	2.9 ± 0.3 ↑ Child ↓ RD ↔ CF, Inflam, Neo, Aged, Burn, Prem	0.23 ± 0.05 ↑ Neo, Child, Prem ↔ CF, RD, Aged	0.9 ± 0.1 ↔ Neo, RD, Prem ↔ CF, Child, Aged	IM: 1-2[b]	IV: 60-70 μg/mL[b] IM: 8.2-12 μg/mL[b]
Cilastatin —	70 ± 3 ↓ Neo ↔ CF	~35	3.0 ± 0.3 ↑ Child ↓ Neo, RD, Prem ↔ CF, Aged	0.20 ± 0.03 ↔ Neo, RD, CF, Aged ↑ Prem	0.8 ± 0.1 ↑ Neo, Prem ↔ CF, Aged		

[a]Formulated as a 1:1 (mg/mg) mixture for parenteral administration; cilastatin inhibits the metabolism of imipenem by the kidney, increasing concentrations of imipenem in the urine; cilastatin does not change imipenem plasma concentrations appreciably. [b]Plasma C_{max} of imipenem following a single 1-g IV infusion over 30 minutes or 750 mg IM injection.

Reference: Buckley MM, et al. Imipenem/cilastatin. A reappraisal of its antibacterial activity, pharmacokinetic properties and therapeutic efficacy. *Drugs,* **1992**, *44*:408–444.

Indomethacin							
~100	15 ± 8	90 ↔ Alb, Prem, Neo	1.4 ± 0.2 ↓ Prem, Neo, Aged	0.29 ± 0.04 ↔ Aged	2.4 ± 0.2[a] ↔ RA, RD ↑ Neo, Prem, Aged	~1.3[b]	~2.4 μg/mL[b]

[a]Undergoes significant enterohepatic recycling (~50% after an IV dose). [b]Following a single 50-mg oral dose given after a standard breakfast. Effective at concentrations of 0.3-3 μg/mL and toxic at >5 μg/mL.

Reference: Oberbauer R, et al. Pharmacokinetics of indomethacin in the elderly. *Clin Pharmacokinet,* **1993**, *24*:428–434.

Interferon Alfa[a]							
I-SC: 90	—[b]	—	I: 2.8 ± 0.6[c] PI_{12kD}: 0.17 PI_{40kD}: 0.014-0.024	I: 0.40 ± 0.19[c] PI_{12kD}: 0.44-1.04 PI_{40kD}: 0.11-0.17	I: 0.67[d] PI_{12kD}: 37(22-60) PI_{40kD}: 65	I: 7.3[e] PI_{12kD}: 22[f] PI_{40kD}: 80[g]	I: 1.7(1.2-2.3) ng/mL[e] PI_{12kD}: 0.91 ± 0.33 ng/mL[f] PI_{40kD}: 26 ± 8.8 ng/mL[g]

[a]Values for recombinant interferon alfa-2a (I) and its 40-kDa pegylated form (PI_{40kD}) and the 12-kDa pegylated form of interferon alfa-2b (PI_{12kD}) are reported. [b]I undergoes renal filtration, tubular reabsorption, and proteolytic degradation within tubular epithelial cells. Renal elimination of PI forms is much less significant than that of I, although not negligible. [c]*CL* values in four patients with leukemia were more than halved (1.1 ± 0.3 mL/min/kg), while V_{ss} increased more than 20-fold (9.5 ± 3.5 L/kg) and terminal $t_{1/2}$ changed only minimally (7.3 ± 2.4 hours). [d]A terminal $t_{1/2}$ of 5.1 ± 1.6 hours accounts for 23% of the *CL* of I. [e]Following a single 36 × 10^6 units SC dose of I. [f]Following 4 weeks of multiple SC dosing of 1 μg/kg of PI_{12kD}. [g]Following 48 weekly SC doses of 180 μg of PI_{40kD}.

References: Glue P, et al. Pegylated interferon-2b: Pharmacokinetics, pharmacodynamics, safety, and preliminary efficacy data. Hepatitis C Intervention Therapy Group. *Clin Pharmacol Ther,* **2000**, *68*:556–567. Harris JM, et al. Pegylation: A novel process for modifying pharmacokinetics. *Clin Pharmacokinet,* **2001**, *40*:539–551. *PDR*54, **2000**, p. 2654. Wills RJ. Clinical pharmacokinetics of interferons. *Clin Pharmacokinet,* **1990**, *19*:390–399.

(Continued)

Table AII–1

Pharmacokinetic Data (*Continued*)

BIOAVAILABILITY (ORAL) (%)	URINARY EXCRETION (%)	BOUND IN PLASMA (%)	CLEARANCE (mL/min/kg)	VOL. DIST. (L/kg)	HALF-LIFE (hours)	PEAK TIME (hours)	PEAK CONCENTRATION
Interferon Beta							
SC: 51 ± 17	—[a]	—	13 ± 5[a]	2.9 ± 1.8	4.3 ± 2.3	SC: 1-8[b]	IV: 1491 ± 659 IU/mL[b] SC: 40 ± 20 IU/mL[b]
Irbesartan[a]							
60-80	2.2 ± 0.9	90	2.12 ± 0.54 ↓ Aged[b] ↔ RD, LD	0.72 ± 0.20	13 ± 6.2	1.2 (0.7-2)[c]	1.3 ± 0.4 μg/mL[c]
Irinotecan[a]							
—	I: 16.7 ± 1.0	I: 30-68 SN-38: 95	I: 14.8 ± 4 L/hr/m^2	I: 150 ± 49 L/m^2	I: 10.8 ± 0.5 SN-38: 10.4 ± 3.1	I: 0.5[b] SN-38: ≤1[b]	I: 1.7 ± 0.8 μg/mL[b] SN-38: 26 ± 12 ng/mL[b]

Interferon Beta

[a]Undergoes renal filtration, tubular reabsorption, and renal catabolism, but hepatic uptake and catabolism are thought to dominate systemic *CL*. [b]Concentration at 5 minutes following a single 90 × 10^6 IU IV dose or following a single 90 × 10^6 IU SC dose of recombinant interferon beta-1b.

Reference: Chiang J, et al. Pharmacokinetics of recombinant human interferon-β_{ser} in healthy volunteers and its effect on serum neopterin. *Pharm Res,* **1993**, *10*:567–572.

Irbesartan

[a]Data from healthy male subjects. No significant gender differences. Metabolized by UGT and CYP2C9. [b]*CL/F* reduced; no dose adjustment required. [c]Following a single 50-mg oral dose (capsule).

References: Gillis JC, et al. Irbesartan. A review of its pharmacodynamic and pharmacokinetic properties and therapeutic use in the management of hypertension. *Drugs,* **1997**, *54*:885–902.

*PDR*54, **2000**, p. 818. Vachharajani NN, et al. Oral bioavailability and disposition characteristics of irbesartan, an angiotensin antagonist, in healthy volunteers. *J Clin Pharmacol,* **1998**, *38*:702–707.

Irinotecan

[a]Data from male and female patients with malignant solid tumors. No significant gender differences. Irinotecan (I) is metabolized to an active metabolite, SN-38 (100-fold more potent but with lower blood levels). [b]Following a 125-mg/m^2 IV infusion over 30 minutes.

References: Chabot GG, et al. Population pharmacokinetics and pharmacodynamics of irinotecan (CPT-11) and active metabolite SN-38 during phase I trials. *Ann Oncol,* **1995**, *6*:141–151. *PDR*54, **2000**, pp. 2412–2413.

Isoniazid[a]							
—[b] ↓ Food	RA: 7 ± 2[c] SA: 29 ± 5[c]	~0	RA: 7.4 ± 2.0[d] SA: 3.7 ± 1.1[d] ↔ Aged ↓ RD[e]	0.67 ± 0.15[d] ↔ Aged, RD	RA: 1.1 ± 0.1 SA: 3.1 ± 1.1 ↑ AVH, LD, Neo, RD ↔ Aged, Obes, Child, HTh	RA: 1.1 ± 0.5[f] SA: 1.1 ± 0.6[f]	RA: 5.4 ± 2.0 μg/mL[f] SA: 7.1 ± 1.9 μg/mL[f]

[a]Metabolized by NAT 2 (polymorphic). Data for slow acetylators (SA) and rapid acetylators (RA) reported. [b]It is usually stated that isoniazid is completely absorbed; however, good estimates of possible loss due to first-pass metabolism are not available. Absorption is decreased by food and antacids. [c]Recovery after oral administration; assay includes unchanged drug and acid-labile hydrazones. Higher percentages have been noted after IV administration, suggesting significant first-pass metabolism. [d]CL/F and V_{ss}/F reported. [e]Decrease in CL_{NR}/F as well as CL_R. [f]Following a single 400-mg oral dose to healthy RAs and SAs.

Reference: Kim YG, et al. Decreased acetylation of isoniazid in chronic renal failure. *Clin Pharmacol Ther,* **1993**, *54*:612–620.

Isosorbide Dinitrate[a]							
PO: 22 ± 14[b] ↔ CHF, RD, Smk ↑ LD SL: 45 ± 16[b] PC: 33 ± 17[b]	<1	28 ± 12	46(38-59)[c] ↓ LD ↔ Smk, RD, Fem, CHF	3.1 (2.2-8.6)	0.7 (0.6-2.0)[c] ↔ RD, Fem	IR[d] ISDN: 0.3 (0.2-0.5) IS-2-MN: 0.6 (0.2-1.6) IS-5-MN: 0.7 (0.3-1.9) SR[d] ISDN: ~0 IS-2-MN: 2.8 (2.7-3.7) IS-5-MN: 5.1 (4.2-6.6)	IR[d] ISDN: 42 (59-166) nM IS-2-MN: 207 (197-335) nM IS-5-MN: 900 (790-1080) nM SR[d] ISDN: ~0 IS-2-MN: 28 (23-33) nM IS-5-MN: 175 (154-267) nM

[a]Isosorbide dinitrate (ISDN) is metabolized to the 2- and 5-mononitrates (IS-2-MN and IS-5-MN). Both metabolites and the parent compound are thought to be active. Data for the dinitrate are reported except where indicated. [b]Bioavailability calculations from single dose. SL, sublingual; PC, percutaneous. [c]CL may be decreased and $t_{1/2}$ prolonged after chronic dosing. [d]Mean (range) for ISDN and IS-2-MN and IS-5-MN following a single 20-mg oral immediate-release (IR) and sustained-release (SR) dose.

References: Abshagen U, et al. Pharmacokinetics and metabolism of isosorbide-dinitrate after intravenous and oral administration. *Eur J Clin Pharmacol,* **1985**, *27*:637–644. Fung HL. Pharmacokinetics and pharmacodynamics of organic nitrates. *Am J Cardiol,* **1987**, *60*:4H–9H.

(*Continued*)

Table AII–1

Pharmacokinetic Data (*Continued*)

BIOAVAILABILITY (ORAL) (%)	URINARY EXCRETION (%)	BOUND IN PLASMA (%)	CLEARANCE (mL/min/kg)	VOL. DIST. (L/kg)	HALF-LIFE (hours)	PEAK TIME (hours)	PEAK CONCENTRATION
Isosorbide 5-Mononitrate (Isosorbide Nitrate)[a]							
93 ± 13 ↔ LD, RD, Aged, CAD	<5	0	1.80 ± 0.24 ↔ LD, RD, Aged, CAD	0.73 ± 0.09 ↔ LD, RD, MI, Aged, CAD	4.9 ± 0.8 ↔ LD, RD, MI, Aged, CAD	1-1.5[b]	314-2093 nM[b]

[a]Active metabolite of isosorbide dinitrate. [b]Following a 20-mg oral dose given by asymmetric dosing (0 and 7 hours) for 4 days.

Reference: Abshagen UW. Pharmacokinetics of isosorbide mononitrate. *Am J Cardiol*, **1992**, *70*:61G–66G.

BIOAVAILABILITY (ORAL) (%)	URINARY EXCRETION (%)	BOUND IN PLASMA (%)	CLEARANCE (mL/min/kg)	VOL. DIST. (L/kg)	HALF-LIFE (hours)	PEAK TIME (hours)	PEAK CONCENTRATION
Isotretinoin[a]							
40[b] ↑ Food	Negligible	>99	5.5 (0.9-11.1)[c]	5 (1-32)[c]	17 (5-167)[d]	I: 4.5 ± 3.4[e] 4-oxo: 6.8 ± 6.5[e]	I: 208 ± 92 ng/mL[e] 4-oxo: 473 ± 171 ng/mL[e]

[a]Isotretinoin (I) is eliminated through metabolic oxidations catalyzed by multiple CYPs (2C8, 2C9, 3A4, and 2B6). The 4-oxo-isotretinoin metabolite (4-oxo) is active and found at higher concentrations than parent drug at steady state. [b]Bioavailability when taken with food is reported. [c]*CL/F* and *V/F* reported. [d]4-oxo has an apparent mean $t_{1/2}$ of 29 ± 6 hours. [e]Values for I and 4-oxo following a 30-mg oral dose given once daily to steady state.

References: Larsen FG, et al. Pharmacokinetics and therapeutic efficacy of retinoids in skin diseases. *Clin Pharmacokinet,* **1992**, *23*:42–61. Nulman I, et al. Steady-state pharmacokinetics of isotretinoin and its 4-oxo metabolite: Implications for fetal safety. *J Clin Pharmacol,* **1998**, *38*:926–930. Wiegand UW, et al. Pharmacokinetics of oral isotretinoin. *J Am Acad Dermatol,* **1998**, *39*:S8–S12.

BIOAVAILABILITY (ORAL) (%)	URINARY EXCRETION (%)	BOUND IN PLASMA (%)	CLEARANCE (mL/min/kg)	VOL. DIST. (L/kg)	HALF-LIFE (hours)	PEAK TIME (hours)	PEAK CONCENTRATION
Itraconazole[a]							
55 ↑ Food ↓ HIV[b]	<1	99.8	5.1[c]	10.7[d]	21 ± 6[e]	3-5[f]	649 ± 289 ng/mL[f] ↑ Food

[a]Metabolized predominantly by CYP3A4 to an active metabolite, hydroxyitraconazole, and other sequential metabolites. [b]Relative to oral dosing with food. [c]Blood CL is 9.4 mL/min/kg. *CL* is concentration dependent; the value given is nonsaturable range. K_m = 330 ± 200 ng/mL, V_{max} = 2.2 ± 0.8 pg · mL^{-1} · min^{-1} · kg^{-1}. Apparent *CL/F* at steady state reported to be 5.4 mL · min^{-1} · kg^{-1}. [d]V_{area} reported. Follows multicompartment kinetics. Does not appear to be concentration dependent. [e]$t_{1/2}$ for the nonsaturable concentration range. $t_{1/2}$ at steady state reported to be 64 hours. [f]Following a 200-mg oral dose given daily for 4 days to adults.

References: Heykants J, et al. The pharmacokinetics of itraconazole in animals and man. An overview. In: Fromtling RA, ed. *Recent Trends in the Discovery, Development and Evaluation of Antifungal Agents.* Barcelona, Prous Science Publisher, **1987**, pp. 223–249. Jalava KM, et al. Itraconazole greatly increases plasma concentrations and effects of felodipine. *Clin Pharmacol Ther,* **1997**, *61*:410–415.

Ivermectin[a]							
—	<1	93.1 ± 0.2	2.06 ± 0.81[b]	9.91 ± 2.67[b]	56.5 ± 7.5[b]	4.7 ± 0.5[c]	38.2 ± 5.8 ng/mL[c]

[a]Data from male and female patients treated for onchocerciasis. Metabolized by hepatic enzymes and excreted into bile. [b]*CL/F*, V_{area}/F, and $t_{1/2}$ reported for oral dose. Terminal $t_{1/2}$ reported. [c]Following a single 150-μg/kg oral dose (tablet).

References: Okonkwo PO, et al. Protein binding and ivermectin estimations in patients with onchocerciasis. *Clin Pharmacol Ther,* **1993**, *53*:426–430. *PDR*54, **2000**, p. 1886.

Ketorolac[a]							
100 ± 20	5-10	99.2 ± 0.1	0.50 ± 0.15 ↓ Aged, RD[b] ↔ LD	0.21 ± 0.04	5.3 ± 1.2 ↑ Aged, RD[b] ↔ LD	IM: 0.7-0.8[c] PO: 0.3-0.9[c]	IM: 2.2-3.0 μg/mL[c] PO: 0.8-0.9 μg/mL[c]

[a]Racemic mixture; *S*-(−)-enantiomer is much more active than the *R*-(+)-enantiomer. Following IM injection, the mean AUC ratio for *S/R*-enantiomers was 0.44 ± 0.04, indicating a higher *CL* and shorter $t_{1/2}$ for the *S*-(−)-enantiomer. Values reported are for the racemate. [b]Probably due to the accumulation of glucuronide metabolite, which is hydrolyzed back to parent drug. [c]Range of mean C_{max} and T_{max} from different studies following a single 30-mg IM or 10-mg oral dose in healthy adults. *Reference*: Brocks DR, et al. Clinical pharmacokinetics of ketorolac tromethamine. *Clin Pharmacokinet,* **1992**, *23*:415–427.

Lamotrigine[a]							
97.6 ± 4.8	10	56	0.38-0.61[b,c] ↓ LD,[d] RD[e]	0.87-1.2	24-35[c] ↑ LD,[d] RD[e]	2.2 ± 1.2[f]	2.5 ± 0.4 μg/mL[f]

[a]Lamotrigine is eliminated primarily by glucuronidation. The parent-metabolite pair may undergo enterohepatic recycling. Data from healthy adults and patients with epilepsy. Range of mean values from multiple studies reported. [b]*CL/F* increases slightly with multiple-dose therapy. [c]*CL/F* increased and $t_{1/2}$ decreased in patients receiving enzyme-inducing anticonvulsant drugs. [d]*CL/F* reduced, moderate to severe hepatic impairment. [e]*CL/F* reduced, severe RD. [f]Following a single 200-mg oral dose to healthy adults.

References: Chen C, et al. Pharmacokinetics of lamotrigine in children in the absence of other antiepileptic drugs. *Pharmacotherapy,* **1999**, *19*:437–441. Garnett WR. Lamotrigine: Pharmacokinetics. *J Child Neurol,* **1997**, *12*(suppl 1):S10–S15. *PDR*54, **2000**, p. 1209. Wootton R, et al. Comparison of the pharmacokinetics of lamotrigine in patients with chronic renal failure and healthy volunteers. *Br J Clin Pharmacol,* **1997**, *43*:23–27.

Leflunomide[a]							
—[b]	Negligible	99.4 ↓ RD	0.012[c] ↑ RD	0.18 (0.09-0.44)[c] ↑ RD	377 (336-432)[d] ↔ RD	6-12[e]	35 μg/mL[e]

[a]Leflunomide is a prodrug that is converted almost completely (~95%) to an active metabolite A77–1726 (2-cyano-3-hydroxy-N-(4-trifluoromethylphenyl)-crotonamide). All pharmacokinetic data reported are for the active metabolite. [b]Absolute bioavailability is not known; parent drug/metabolite are well absorbed. [c]Apparent *CL/F* and *V/F* in healthy volunteers reported. Both parameters are a function of the bioavailability of leflunomide and the extent of its conversion to A77–1726. [d]In patients with RA. [e]Following a 20-mg oral dose given once daily to steady state in patients with RA.

Reference: Rozman B. Clinical pharmacokinetics of leflunomide. *Clin Pharmacokinet,* **2002**, *41*:421–430.

(*Continued*)

Table AII–1

Pharmacokinetic Data (*Continued*)

BIOAVAILABILITY (ORAL) (%)	URINARY EXCRETION (%)	BOUND IN PLASMA (%)	CLEARANCE (mL/min/kg)	VOL. DIST. (L/kg)	HALF-LIFE (hours)	PEAK TIME (hours)	PEAK CONCENTRATION
Lenalidomide[a]							
>80[b]	84[c]	35 ± 4 ↔ RD[d]	2.8[e] ↓ RD[d]	0.8[e]	3.3 ↑ RD[d]	1 (0.5-2.0)	568 ± 221 ng/mL[f]
[a]Lenalidomide is administered as a racemic mixture. Data for the racemate is shown. [b]Based on urine recovery of unchanged drug after oral administration. Lenalidomide is primarily eliminated via urinary excretion. [c]Percentage of oral dose recovered unchanged in urine. [d]Study in patients with mild, moderate, severe, and end-stage renal impairment; exposure increases 150% in moderate renal impairment and 375% in severe renal impairment. [e]*CL/F* and *V/F* reported. [f]Following a single 25-mg oral dose. *Reference:* Chen N, et al. Pharmacokinetics of lenalidomide in subjects with various degrees of renal impairment and in subjects on hemodialysis. *J Clin Pharmacol,* **2007**, *47*:1466–1475.							
Letrozole[a]							
99.9 ± 16.3	3.9 ± 1.4	60	0.58 ± 0.21 ↓ LD[b]	1.87 ± 0.46	45 ± 16	1.0[c]	115 nM[c]
[a]Data from healthy postmenopausal female subjects. Metabolized by CYP3A4 and CYP2A6. [b]*CL/F* reduced, severe hepatic impairment. [c]Following a single 2.5-mg oral dose (tablet). *References*: Lamb HM, et al. Letrozole. A review of its use in postmenopausal women with advanced breast cancer. *Drugs,* **1998**, *56*:1125–1140. Sioufi A, et al. Absolute bioavailability of letrozole in healthy postmenopausal women. *Biopharm Drug Dispos,* **1997**, *18*:779–789.							
Levetiracetam[a]							
~100	66	<10	0.96 ↓ RD,[b] Aged, LD[c] ↑ Child[d]	0.5-0.7	7 ± 1 ↑ RD,[b] Aged	0.5-1.0[e]	~10 μg/mL[e]
[a]Data from healthy adults and patients with epilepsy. No significant gender differences. [b]*CL/F* reduced, mild renal impairment (cleared by hemodialysis). [c]*CL/F* reduced, severe hepatic impairment. [d]*CL/F* increased, 6-12 years of age. [e]Following a single 500-mg dose given to healthy adults. *Reference: Physicians' Desk Reference,* 55th ed. Montvale, NJ, Medical Economics Co., **2001**, pp. 3206–3207.							
Levodopa[a]							
41 ± 16 ↑ Aged 86 ± 19[b] ↔ Aged	<1	—	23 ± 4 ↓ Aged 9 ± 1[b] ↓ Aged	1.7 ± 0.4 ↓ Aged 0.9 ± 0.2[b] ↓ Aged	1.4 ± 0.4 ↔ Aged 1.5 ± 0.3[b] ↔ Aged	Y: 1.4 ± 0.7[c] E: 1.4 ± 0.7[c]	Y: 1.7 ± 0.8 μg/mL[c] E: 1.9 ± 0.6 μg/mL[c]
[a]Naturally occurring precursor to dopamine. [b]Values obtained with concomitant carbidopa (inhibitor of dopa decarboxylase). [c]Following a single 125-mg oral dose of levodopa given with carbidopa (100 mg 1 hour before and 50 mg 6 hours after levodopa) in young (Y) and elderly (E) subjects. *Reference*: Robertson DR, et al. The effect of age on the pharmacokinetics of levodopa administered alone and in the presence of carbidopa. *Br J Clin Pharmacol*, **1989**, *28*:61–69.							

Levofloxacin[a]

99 ± 10	61-87	24-38	2.52 ± 0.45 ↓ RD[b]	1.36 ± 0.21	7 ± 1 ↑ RD[b]	1.6 ± 0.8[c]	4.5 ± 0.9 μg/mL[c]

[a]Data from healthy adult male subjects. Gender and age differences related to renal function. [b]*CL/F* reduced, mild to severe renal impairment (not cleared by hemodialysis). [c]Following a single 500-mg oral dose. No significant accumulation with once-daily dosing.

References: Chien SC, et al. Pharmacokinetic profile of levofloxacin following once-daily 500-milligram oral or intravenous doses. *Antimicrob Agents Chemother,* **1997**, *41*:2256–2260. Fish DN, et al. The clinical pharmacokinetics of levofloxacin. *Clin Pharmacokinet*, **1997**, *32*:101–119. *PDR*54, **2000**, p. 2157.

Linezolid

100	35	31	2.1 ± 0.8 ↑ Child	0.57-0.71	5.2 ± 1.7 ↓ Child	PO: 1.4 ± 0.5[a]	PO: 16 ± 4 μg/mL[a] IV: 15 ± 3 μg/mL[b]

[a]Following a 600-mg oral dose given twice daily to steady state. [b]Following a 30-minute IV infusion of a 600-mg dose given twice daily to steady state in patients with gram-positive infection.

References: MacGowan AP. Pharmacokinetic and pharmacodynamic profile of linezolid in healthy volunteers and patients with Gram-positive infections. *J Antimicrob Chemother,* **2003**, *51*(suppl 2):ii17–ii25. Stalker DJ, et al. Clinical pharmacokinetics of linezolid, a novel oxazolidinone antibacterial. *Clin Pharmacokinet,* **2003**, *42*:1129–1140.

Lisinopril

25 ± 20 ↓ CHF	88-100	0	4.2 ± 2.2[a] ↓ CHF, RD, Aged ↔ Fem	2.4 ± 1.4[a] ↔ Aged, RD	12[b] ↑ Aged, RD	~7[c]	50 (6.4-343) ng/mL[c]

[a]*CL/F* and V_{area}/F reported. [b]Effective $t_{1/2}$ to predict steady-state accumulation upon multiple dosing; a terminal $t_{1/2}$ of 30 hours reported. [c]Following a 2.5- to 40-mg oral dose given daily to steady state in elderly patients with hypertension and varying degrees of renal function. EC_{90} for ACE inhibition is 27 ± 10 ng/mL.

Reference: Thomson AH, et al. Lisinopril population pharmacokinetics in elderly and renal disease patients with hypertension. *Br J Clin Pharmacol,* **1989**, *27*:57–65.

Lithium

100[a]	95 ± 15	0	0.35 ± 0.11[b] ↓ RD, Aged ↑ Preg ↔ Obes	0.66 ± 0.16 ↓ Obes	22 ± 8[c] ↑ RD, Aged ↓ Obes	IR: 0.5-3[d] SR: 2-6[d]	IR: 1-2 mM[d] SR:0.7-1.2 mM[d]

[a]Values as low as 80% reported for some prolonged-release preparations. [b]Renal *CL* of Li^+ parallels that of Na^+. The ratio of Li^+ and creatinine CL is ~0.2 ± 0.03. [c]The distribution $t_{1/2}$ is 5.6 ± 0.5 hours; this influences drug concentrations for at least 12 hours. [d]Following a single 0.7-mmol/kg oral dose of immediate-release (IR) lithium carbonate and sustained-release (SR) tablets.

Reference: Ward ME, et al. Clinical pharmacokinetics of lithium. *J Clin Pharmacol*, **1994**, *34*:280–285.

(Continued)

Table AII–1

Pharmacokinetic Data (*Continued*)

BIOAVAILABILITY (ORAL) (%)	URINARY EXCRETION (%)	BOUND IN PLASMA (%)	CLEARANCE (mL/min/kg)	VOL. DIST. (L/kg)	HALF-LIFE (hours)	PEAK TIME (hours)	PEAK CONCENTRATION
Lopinavir[a]							
—[b] ↑ Food	<3	98-99	1.2[c]	0.6[c]	5.3 ± 2.5	4.4 ± 2.4[d]	9.8 ± 3.7 μg/mL[d]

[a]Currently formulated in combination with ritonavir (KALETRA). Ritonavir inhibits the CYP3A-dependent metabolism of lopinavir, enhancing its bioavailability, increasing plasma concentrations (50- to 100-fold), and extending its $t_{1/2}$. Pharmacokinetic data from male and female patients with HIV are reported. [b]Absolute bioavailability is not known; the relative bioavailability increases with a high-fat meal. [c]*CL/F* and V_{area}/F reported; calculated from steady-state AUC data. [d]Following a 400/100-mg lopinavir/ritonavir oral dose given twice daily in combination with stavudine and lamivudine to steady state.

References: Boffito M, et al. Lopinavir protein binding in vivo through the 12-hour dosing interval. *Ther Drug Monit*, **2004**, *26*:35–39. Corbett AH, et al. Kaletra (lopinavir/ritonavir). *Ann Pharmacother*, **2002**, *36*:1193–1203. Eron JJ, et al. Once-daily versus twice-daily lopinavir/ritonavir in antiretroviral-naive HIV-positive patients: A 48-week randomized clinical trial. *J Infect Dis*, **2004**, *189*:265–272. King JR, et al. Pharmacokinetic enhancement of protease inhibitor therapy. *Clin Pharmacokinet*, **2004**, *43*:291–310.

BIOAVAILABILITY (ORAL) (%)	URINARY EXCRETION (%)	BOUND IN PLASMA (%)	CLEARANCE (mL/min/kg)	VOL. DIST. (L/kg)	HALF-LIFE (hours)	PEAK TIME (hours)	PEAK CONCENTRATION
Loratadine[a]							
L: —[b]	L: Negligible	L: 97	L: 142 ± 57[d] ↔ RD ↓ LD	L: 120 ± 80[d] ↔ RD	L: 8 ± 6 ↔ RD ↑ LD	L (L): 2.0 ± 2.0[e] DL (L): 2.6 ± 2.9[e]	L (L): 3.4 ± 3.4 ng/mL[e] DL (L):4.1 ± 2.6 ng/mL[e]
DL: —[b]	DL: —	DL: 82-87[c]	DL: 14-18[d] ↓ RD, LD	DL: 26[d]	DL: 21-24	DL (DL): 3.2 ± 1.8[f] HDL (DL): 4.8 ± 1.9[f]	DL(DL): 4.0 ± 2.1 ng/mL[f] HDL (DL): 2.0 ± 0.6 ng/mL[f]

[a]Loratadine (L) is converted to a major active metabolite, desloratadine (DL). Almost all patients achieve higher plasma concentrations of DL than of L. DL (CLARINEX) is approved for similar clinical indications as L. DL is eliminated by metabolism. DL is eliminated by metabolism to an active metabolite, 3-hydroxydesloratidine (HDL). ~7-20% of patients are slow metabolizers of DL; frequency varies with ethnicity. [b]Bioavailability of L and DL is not known; L is probably low due to extensive first-pass metabolism. [c]Plasma protein binding of HDL is 85-89%. [d]*CL/F* and V_{area}/F reported. For DL, oral *CL/F* calculated from AUC data following a single 5- to 20-mg oral dose given to healthy adults. [e]Mean for L and DL following a 10-mg oral L dose (CLARITIN-D 24 HOUR) given once daily for 7 days to healthy adults. [f]Mean for DL and HDL following a 5-mg oral DL dose (CLARINEX) given once daily for 10 days to healthy adults.

References: Affrime M, et al. A pharmacokinetic profile of desloratadine in healthy adults, including elderly. *Clin Pharmacokinet*, **2002**, *41*(suppl):13–19. Gupta S, et al. Desloratadine demonstrates dose proportionality in healthy adults after single doses. *Clin Pharmacokinet*, **2002**, *41*(suppl):1–6. Haria M, et al. Loratadine. A reappraisal of its pharmacological properties and therapeutic use in allergic disorders. *Drugs*, **1994**, *48*:617–637. Kosoglou T, et al. Pharmacokinetics of loratadine and pseudoephedrine following single and multiple doses of once- versus twice-daily combination tablet formulations in healthy adult males. *Clin Ther*, **1997**, *19*:1002–1012. *PDR*58, **2004**, p. 3044.

Minocycline[a]							
95-100	11 ± 2	76	1.0 ± 0.3 ↓ HL	1.3 ± 0.2[b] ↓ HL	16 ± 2 ↔ HL	PO: 2-4[c]	IV: 3.5 μg/mL[c] PO: 2.3-3.5 μg/mL[c]

[a]Cleared primarily by oxidative metabolism in the liver. [b]V_{area} reported. [c]Following a single 200-mg IV infusion (1 hour) or range of values following a 100-mg oral dose given twice a day to steady state.

Reference: Saivin S, et al. Clinical pharmacokinetics of doxycycline and minocycline. *Clin Pharmacokinet*, **1988**, *15*:355–366.

Mirtazapine[a]							
50 ± 10	—	85	9.12 ± 1.14[b] ↓ LD,[c] RD[d]	4.5 ± 1.7	16.3 ± 4.6[b,e] ↓ LD,[c] RD[d]	1.5 ± 0.7[f]	41.8 ± 7.7 ng/mL[f]

[a]Data from healthy adult subjects. Metabolized by CYP2D6 and CYP1A2 (8-hydroxy) and CYP3A (*N*-desmethyl, *N*-oxide). [b]Women of all ages exhibit a lower *CL/F* and longer $t_{1/2}$ than men. [c]*CL/F* reduced, hepatic impairment. [d]*CL/F* reduced, moderate to severe renal impairment. [e]The $t_{1/2}$ of the (−)-enantiomer is approximately twice as long as the (+)-antipode; approximately 3-fold higher blood concentrations (+ versus −) are achieved. [f]Following a 15-mg oral dose given once daily to steady state.

References: Fawcett J, et al. Review of the results from clinical studies on the efficacy, safety and tolerability of mirtazapine for the treatment of patients with major depression. *J Affect Disord*, **1998**, *51*:267–285. *PDR*54, **2000**, p. 2109.

Mitoxantrone[a]							
—[b]	~2	97	13 ± 8 ↓ LD	90 ± 42[c]	β-phase: 1.1 ± 1.1[d] γ-phase: 72 ± 40[d] ↑ LD	—	308 ± 133 ng/mL[e]

[a]Data reported for patients treated for cancer. Information from older literature confounded by nonspecific assays. [b]For parenteral administration only; usually given as a rapid IV infusion every 3 months. [c]Reflects distribution into a "deep" tissue compartment. V_c is 0.3 ± 0.2 L/kg. [d]$t_{1/2}$ for the β-phase predicts time to steady state for short-term IV infusions. $t_{1/2}$ for the γ-phase predicts long-term persistence in the body. [e]Following a single 30-minute IV infusion of 12-14 mg/m^2.

References: Ehninger G, et al. Pharmacokinetics and metabolism of mitoxantrone. A review. *Clin Pharmacokinet*, **1990**, *18*:365–380. Hu OY, et al. Pharmacokinetic and pharmacodynamic studies with mitoxantrone in the treatment of patients with nasopharyngeal carcinoma. *Cancer*, **1992**, *69*:847–853.

(*Continued*)

Table AII–1

Pharmacokinetic Data (*Continued*)

BIOAVAILABILITY (ORAL) (%)	URINARY EXCRETION (%)	BOUND IN PLASMA (%)	CLEARANCE (mL/min/kg)	VOL. DIST. (L/kg)	HALF-LIFE (hours)	PEAK TIME (hours)	PEAK CONCENTRATION
Modafinil,[A] Armodafinil							
— —	Rac: 3.7 ± 15 Arm: <10	Rac: 60 —	—[b] —[c] ↓ LD[d], Aged	—[b] —[c]	Rac: 13.6 ± 2.6 Arm: 13.0 ± 2.6 ↑ LD[d]	Rac: 2.5 ± 1.0[e] Arm: 1.8	Rac: 4.6 ± 0.7 μg/mL[e] Arm: 5.4 ± 1.6 μg/mL[e]

[a]Modafinil is available either as a racemic mixture or as the pure (*R*)-enantiomer armodafinil. Pharmacokinetic data after dosing of racemate (Rac) or armodafinil (Arm) is reported. Modafinil is extensively metabolized in the liver to two major metabolites, modafinil acid and modafinil sulfone. [b]*CL/F* = 0.72 ± 0.10 mL/min/kg and *V/F* = 0.77 ± 0.11 L/kg after an oral dose of racemic modafinil. [c]The exposure to Arm is 40% higher than that of racemic modafinil after equal oral doses. Arm *CL/F* = 0.47 mL/min/kg and *V/F* = 0.6 L/kg. [d]Study in patients with moderate to severe liver impairment receiving oral racemic modafinil; *CL/F* reduced by 60% and steady-state concentrations doubled in patients with liver impairment. [e]Following a 200-mg single oral dose of modafinil or Arm.

References: Wong YN, et al. A double-blind, placebo-controlled, ascending-dose evaluation of the pharmacokinetics and tolerability of modafinil tablets in healthy male volunteers. *J Clin Pharmacol*, **1999**, *39*:30–40. Wong YN, et al. Open-label, single-dose pharmacokinetic study of modafinil tablets and tolerability of modafinil tablets: Influence of age and gender in normal subjects. *J Clin Pharmacol*, **1999**, *39*:30–40. Drugs@FDA. Nuvigil label approved on 06/15/07. Available at: http://www.accessdata.fda.gov/scripts/cder/drugsatfda/index.cfm. Accessed May 17, 2010.

BIOAVAILABILITY (ORAL) (%)	URINARY EXCRETION (%)	BOUND IN PLASMA (%)	CLEARANCE (mL/min/kg)	VOL. DIST. (L/kg)	HALF-LIFE (hours)	PEAK TIME (hours)	PEAK CONCENTRATION
Montelukast[a]							
62	<0.2	>99	0.70 ± 0.17 ↓ LD[b] ↔ Child[c]	0.15 ± 0.02	4.9 ± 0.6 ↑ LD[b]	3.0 ± 1.0[d]	542 ± 173 ng/mL[d]

[a]Data from healthy adult subjects. No significant gender differences. Montelukast is metabolized by CYP3A4 and CYP2C9. [b]*CL/F* is reduced by 41%, mild to moderate hepatic impairment with cirrhosis. [c]Similar plasma profile with 5-mg chewable versus 10-mg tablet in adults. [d]Following a single 10-mg oral dose.

*References: PDR*54, **2000**, p. 1882. Zhao JJ, et al. Pharmacokinetics and bioavailability of montelukast sodium (MK-0476) in healthy young and elderly volunteers. *Biopharm Drug Dispos,* **1997**, *18*:769–777.

BIOAVAILABILITY (ORAL) (%)	URINARY EXCRETION (%)	BOUND IN PLASMA (%)	CLEARANCE (mL/min/kg)	VOL. DIST. (L/kg)	HALF-LIFE (hours)	PEAK TIME (hours)	PEAK CONCENTRATION
Morphine[a]							
PO: 24 ± 12 IM: ~100	4 ± 5	35 ± 2 ↓ AVH, LD, Alb	24 ± 10 ↔ Aged, LD, Child[b] ↓ Neo, Burn, RD, Prem	3.3 ± 0.9 ↔ LD, Neo ↓ RD	1.9 ± 0.5 ↔ LD, RD, Child ↑ Neo, Prem	IM: 0.2-0.3[c] PO-IR: 0.5-1.5[c] PO-SR: 3-8[c]	IV: 200-400 ng/mL[c] IM: ~70 ng/mL[c] PO-IR: 10 ng/mL[c] PO-SR: 7.4 ng/mL[c]

[a]Active metabolite, morphine-6-glucuronide; Urinary excretion = 14 ± 7%; $t_{1/2}$ = 4.0 ± 1.5 hours. Steady-state ratio of active metabolite to parent drug after oral dosing = 4.9 ± 3.8. In renal failure, $t_{1/2}$ increases to 50 ± 37 hours, resulting in significant accumulation of active glucuronide metabolite. [b]Decreased in children undergoing cardiac surgery requiring inotropic support. [c]Following a single 10-mg IV dose (bolus with 5-minute blood sample), a 10-mg/70-kg IM, a 10-mg/70-kg immediate-release oral (PO-IR) dose, or a 50-mg sustained-release oral dose (PO-SR). Minimum analgesic concentration is 15 ng/mL.

References: Berkowitz BA. The relationship of pharmacokinetics to pharmacological activity: Morphine, methadone and naloxone. *Clin Pharmacokinet*, **1976**, *1*:219–230. Glare PA, et al. Clinical pharmacokinetics of morphine. *Ther Drug Monit*, **1991**, *13*:1–23.

Moxifloxacin[a]

86 ± 1	21.9 ± 3.6	39.4 ± 2.4	2.27 ± 0.24	2.05 ± 1.15	15.4 ± 1.2	2.0 (0.5-6.0)[b]	2.5 ± 1.3 μg/mL[b]

[a]Data from healthy adult male subjects. Moxifloxacin is metabolized by ST and UGT. [b]Following a single oral 400-mg dose.

Reference: Stass H, et al. Pharmacokinetics and elimination of moxifloxacin after oral and intravenous administration in man. *J Antimicrob Chemother*, **1999**, *43*(suppl B):83–90.

Mycophenolate[a]

MM: ~0 MPA: 94	MPA: <1	MPA: 97.5 ↓ RD[b]	MM: 120-163 MPA: 2.5 ± 0.4[c] ↓ RD[b] ↔ LD	MPA: 3.6-4[c]	MM: <0.033 MPA: 16.6 ± 5.8	MPA: 1.1-2.2[d]	MPA: 8-19 μg/mL[d]

[a]Data from healthy adult male and female subjects and organ transplant patients. No significant gender differences. Mycophenolate mofetil (MM) is rapidly converted to the active mycophenolic acid (MPA) after IV and oral doses. Kinetic parameters refer to MM and MPA after a dose of MM. MPA metabolized by UGT to MPA-glucuronide (MPAG). MPA undergoes enterohepatic recycling; MPAG is excreted into bile and presumably is hydrolyzed by gut flora and reabsorbed as MPA. [b]Accumulation of MPA and MPAG and increased unbound MPA; severe renal impairment. [c]CL/F and V_{area}/F reported for MPA. [d]Range of mean MPA C_{max} and T_{max} from different studies following a 1- to 1.75-g oral dose given twice daily to steady state in renal transplant patients.

References: Bullingham R, et al. Effects of food and antacid on the pharmacokinetics of single doses of mycophenolate mofetil in rheumatoid arthritis patients. *Br J Clin Pharmacol,* **1996**, *47*:513–516. Bullingham RE, et al. Clinical pharmacokinetics of mycophenolate mofetil. *Clin Pharmacokinet,* **1998**, *34*:429–455. Kriesche HUM, et al. MPA protein binding in uremic plasma: Prediction of free fraction. *Clin Pharmacol Ther,* **1999**, *65*:184. *PDR*54, **2000**, pp. 2617–2618.

Nabumetone[a]

35	~ 50	~ 99[b]	0.37 ± 0.25[c] ↔ Aged	0.79 ± 0.38[c] ↔ Aged	23 ± 4 ↑ RD ↔ Aged	Y: 4-5[d] E: 4-7[d]	Y: 22-52 μg/mL[d] E: 37-70 μg/mL[d]

[a]Data are for the active metabolite, 6-methoxy-2-naphthylacetic acid (6-MNA). The conversion of nabumetone to the active metabolite 6-MNA is mediated predominantly by CYP1A2. [b]99.7-99.8% over concentration range following multiple 1-g doses; 99.2-99.4% following multiple 200-mg doses. [c]CL/F and V_{ss}/F reported; calculated assuming a 70-kg body weight. Following IV dosing of 6-MNA, CL is 0.04-0.07 mL/min/kg and V_{ss} averages 0.11 L/kg. [d]Range of mean values from different studies following a 1-g oral dose given once daily for 7-14 days to young healthy adults (Y) and elderly patients with arthritis (E).

References: Davies NM. Clinical pharmacokinetics of nabumetone. The dawn of selective cyclo-oxygenase-2 inhibition? *Clin Pharmacokinet*, **1997**, *33*:404–416. Hyneck ML. An overview of the clinical pharmacokinetics of nabumetone. *J Rheumatol*, **1992**, *19*(suppl 36):20–24. Turpeinen M, et al. A predominate role of CYP1A2 for the metabolism of nabumetone to the active metabolite, 6-methoxy-2-naphtylacetic acid, in human liver microsomes. *Drug Metab Dispos*, **2009**, *37*:1017–1024.

Naltrexone[a]

20 ± 5	2	21	18.3 ± 1.4 ↓ LD[b]	16.1 ± 5.2	10.3 ± 3.3[c] ↔ LD	1[d]	15-64 ng/mL[d]

[a]Naltrexone has an active metabolite, 6β-naltrexol, that circulates at greater concentrations than naltrexone and has a 10-fold higher AUC than naltrexone after oral administration of naltrexone. [b]The oral AUC of naltrexone was significantly increased in patients with liver impairment, whereas the AUC of 6β-naltrexol was not changed. [c]A $t_{1/2}$ of 2.7 hours after IV administration also reported. [d]Following a single 100-mg oral dose.

References: Bullingham RES, et al. Clinical pharmacokinetics of narcotic agonist-antagonist drugs. *Clin Pharmacokinet,* **1983**, *8*:332–343. Bertolotti M, et al. Effect of liver cirrhosis on the systemic availability of naltrexone in humans. *J Hepatol,* **1997**, *27*:505–511.

(Continued)

Table AII–1

Pharmacokinetic Data (*Continued*)

BIOAVAILABILITY (ORAL) (%)	URINARY EXCRETION (%)	BOUND IN PLASMA (%)	CLEARANCE (mL/min/kg)	VOL. DIST. (L/kg)	HALF-LIFE (hours)	PEAK TIME (hours)	PEAK CONCENTRATION
Naproxen[a]							
99[b]	5-6	99.7 ± 0.1[c] ↑ RD, Aged,[d] LD ↓ RA, Alb	0.13 ± 0.02[e] ↓ RD ↔ Aged,[d] Cirr,[d] Child ↑ RA	0.16 ± 0.02[e] ↑ RD, RA, Child ↔ Aged, Child	14 ± 1 ↔ RD, RA, Child ↑ Aged[d]	T-IR: 2-4[f] T-CR: 5[f] S: 2.2 ± 2.1[f]	T-IR: 37[f] T-CR: 94[f] S: 55 ± 14 μg/mL[f]

[a]Metabolically cleared by CYP2C9 (polymorphic) and CYP1A2. [b]Estimated bioavailability. [c]Saturable plasma protein binding yields apparent nonlinear elimination kinetics. [d]No change in total *CL*, but a significant (50%) decrease in *CL* of unbound drug; it is thus suggested that dosing rate be decreased. A second study in elderly patients found a decreased *CL* and increased $t_{1/2}$ with no change in percent bound. [e]*CL/F* and V_{area}/F reported. [f]Following a single 250-mg dose of suspension (S) given orally to pediatric patients or a 250-mg immediate-release tablet (T-IR) or a 500-mg controlled-release tablet (T-CR) given to adults.

Reference: Wells TG, et al. Comparison of the pharmacokinetics of naproxen tablets and suspension in children. *J Clin Pharmacol,* **1994**, *34*:30–33.

BIOAVAILABILITY (ORAL) (%)	URINARY EXCRETION (%)	BOUND IN PLASMA (%)	CLEARANCE (mL/min/kg)	VOL. DIST. (L/kg)	HALF-LIFE (hours)	PEAK TIME (hours)	PEAK CONCENTRATION
Niacin[a]							
—[b] ↑ Food	12[c]	—	14.6 ± 5.0[d]	—	~0.15-0.25[e]	ER: 4-5[f]	ER (1 g): 0.6 μg/mL[f] ER (2 g): 15.5 μg/mL[f]

[a]Niacin (nicotinic acid) is metabolized to nicotinamide, which in turn is converted to the coenzyme NAD and other inactive metabolites. It also undergoes direct glycine conjugation to nicotinuric acid. [b]The absolute bioavailability is not known. Niacin is well-absorbed but undergoes first-pass metabolism. Absorption is improved when taken with a low-fat meal. [c]Recovery of unchanged drug after multiple oral dose administration. [d]*CL* calculated from C_{ss} (6.6 ± 2.4 μg/mL) during an IV infusion of niacin. Niacin metabolic *CL* appears to be saturable. [e]Estimated from the terminal log-linear portion of a disappearance curve following the end of a 0.1-mg/kg/min IV infusion in two subjects. [f]Following a single 1-g or 2-g oral dose of extended-release (ER) NIASPAN. Markedly disproportional increases in plasma concentrations with increasing dose.

References: Ding RW, et al. Pharmacokinetics of nicotinic acid-salicylic acid interaction. *Clin Pharmacol Ther,* **1989**, *46*:642–647. *PDR*58, **2004**, p. 1797. Piepho RW. The pharmacokinetics and pharmacodynamics of agents proven to raise high-density lipoprotein cholesterol. *Am J Cardiol,* **2000**, *86*:35L–40L.

BIOAVAILABILITY (ORAL) (%)	URINARY EXCRETION (%)	BOUND IN PLASMA (%)	CLEARANCE (mL/min/kg)	VOL. DIST. (L/kg)	HALF-LIFE (hours)	PEAK TIME (hours)	PEAK CONCENTRATION
Nifedipine[a]							
50 ± 13 ↑ LD, Aged ↔ RD	~0	96 ± 1 ↓ LD, RD	7.0 ± 1.8 ↓ LD, Aged ↔ RD, Smk	0.78 ± 0.22 ↑ LD, RD, Aged ↔ Smk	1.8 ± 0.4[b] ↑ LD, RD, Aged ↔ Smk	IR: 0.5 ± 0.2[c] ER: ~6[c]	IR: 79 ± 44 ng/mL[c] ER: 35-49 ng/mL[c]

[a]Metabolically cleared by CYP3A; undergoes significant first-pass metabolism. [b]Longer apparent $t_{1/2}$ after oral administration because of absorption limitation, particularly for extended-release (ER) formulations. [c]Mean following a single 10-mg immediate-release (IR) capsule given to healthy male adults or a range of steady-state concentrations following a 60-mg ER tablet given daily to healthy male adults. Levels of 47 ± 20 ng/mL were reported to decrease diastolic pressure in hypertensive patients.

References: Glasser SP, et al. The efficacy and safety of once-daily nifedipine: The coat-core formulation compared with the gastrointestinal therapeutic system formulation in patients with mild-to-moderate diastolic hypertension. Nifedipine Study Group. *Clin Ther,* **1995**, *17*:12–29. Renwick AG, et al. The pharmacokinetics of oral nifedipine—A population study. *Br J Clin Pharmacol,* **1988**, *25*:701–708. Soons PA, et al. Intraindividual variability in nifedipine pharmacokinetics and effects in healthy subjects. *J Clin Pharmacol,* **1992**, *32*:324–331.

Nitrofurantoin							
87 ± 13	47 ± 13	62 ± 4	9.9 ± 0.9 ↑ Alkaline urine	0.58 ± 0.12	1.0 ± 0.2 ↔ Alkaline urine	2.3 ± 1.4[a]	428 ± 146 ng/mL[a]

[a]Following a single 50-mg oral dose (tablet) given to fasted healthy adults. No changes when taken with a meal.

Reference: Hoener B, et al. Nitrofurantoin disposition. *Clin Pharmacol Ther,* **1981**, *29*:808–816.

Nitroglycerin[a]							
PO: <1 SL: 38 ± 26[b] Top: 72 ± 20	<1	—	195 ± 86[c]	3.3 ± 1.2[c,d]	2.3 ± 0.6 min	SL: 0.09 ± 0.03[e] Top: 3-4[e] TD: 2[e]	IV: 3.4 ± 1.7 ng/mL[e] SL: 1.9 ± 1.6 ng/mL[e]

[a]Dinitrate metabolites have weak activity compared to nitroglycerin (<10%), but because of a prolonged $t_{1/2}$ (~40 min), they may accumulate during administration of sustained-release preparations to yield concentrations in plasma 10- to 20-fold greater than parent drug. [b]Following sublingual (SL) dose rinsed out of mouth after 8 minutes. Rinse contained 31 ± 19% of the dose. [c]Following a 40- to 100-minute IV infusion. [d]V_{area} reported. [e]Steady-state concentration following a 20-54 μg/min IV infusion over 40-100 minutes or a 0.4-mg SL dose. Levels of 1.2-11 ng/mL associated with a 25% drop in capillary wedge pressure in patients with CHF. T_{max} for topical (Top) and transdermal (TD) preparations also reported.

References: Noonan PK, et al. Incomplete and delayed bioavailability of sublingual nitroglycerin. *Am J Cardiol,* **1985**, *55*:184–187. *PDR*54, **2000**, p. 1474. Thadani U, et al. Relationship of pharmacokinetic and pharmacodynamic properties of the organic nitrates. *Clin Pharmacokinet,* **1988**, *15*:32–43.

Nortriptyline[a]							
51 ± 5	2 ± 1	92 ± 2 ↑ HL	7.2 ± 1.8[b] ↓ Aged, Inflam ↔ Smk, RD	18 ± 4[c]	31 ± 13[b] ↑ Aged ↔ RD	7-10	138 (40-350) nM[d]

[a]Active metabolite, 10-hydroxynortriptyline, accumulates to twice the concentration of nortriptyline in extensive metabolizers. Formation of 10-hydroxynortriptyline is catalyzed by CYP2D6 (polymorphic). [b]For poor metabolizers, *CL/F* is lower (5.3 versus 19.3 mL/min/kg) and $t_{1/2}$ longer (54 versus 21 hours) than that of extensive metabolizers. [c]V_{area} reported. [d]Mean following a 125-mg oral dose given once daily to healthy adults to steady state. Antidepressant effect observed at levels of 190-570 nM. Appears less effective at plasma concentrations >570 nM.

References: Dalen P, et al. 10-Hydroxylation of nortriptyline in white persons with 0, 1, 2, 3, and 13 functional CYP2D6 genes. *Clin Pharmacol Ther,* **1998**, *63*:444–452. Jerling M, et al. Population pharmacokinetics of nortriptyline during monotherapy and during concomitant treatment with drugs that inhibit CYP2D6—An evaluation with the nonparametric maximum likelihood method. *Br J Clin Pharmacol,* **1994**, *38*:453–462. Ziegler VE, et al. Nortriptyline plasma levels and therapeutic response. *Clin Pharmacol Ther,* **1976**, *20*:458–463.

Olanzapine[a]							
~60[b]	7.3	93	6.2 ± 2.9[c] ↔ RD, LD	16.4 ± 5.1[c]	33.1 ± 10.3 ↑ Aged	6.1 ± 1.9[d]	12.9 ± 7.5 ng/mL[d]

[a]Data from male and female schizophrenic patients. Metabolized primarily by UGT, CYP1A2, and flavin-containing monooxygenase. [b]Bioavailability estimated from parent-metabolite recovery data. [c]Summary of *CL/F* and V_{area}/F for 491 subjects receiving an oral dose. *CL/F* segregates by sex (F/M) and smoking status (NS/S): M, S > F, S > M, NS > F, NS. [d]Following a single 9.5 ± 4-mg oral dose to healthy male subjects; $C_{max,ss}$ ~20 ng/mL following a 10-mg oral dose given once daily.

References: Callaghan JT, et al. Olanzapine. Pharmacokinetic and pharmacodynamic profile. *Clin Pharmacokinet,* **1999**, *37*:177–193. Kassahun K, et al. Disposition and biotransformation of the antipsychotic agent olanzapine in humans. *Drug Metab Dispos,* **1997**, *25*:81–93. *PDR*54, **2000**, p. 1649.

(Continued)

Table AII–1

Pharmacokinetic Data (*Continued*)

BIOAVAILABILITY (ORAL) (%)	URINARY EXCRETION (%)	BOUND IN PLASMA (%)	CLEARANCE (mL/min/kg)	VOL. DIST. (L/kg)	HALF-LIFE (hours)	PEAK TIME (hours)	PEAK CONCENTRATION
Olmesartan[a]							
26	35-50	99	0.31 ± 0.05	0.36 ± 0.18	13.7 ± 5.6	1.5 (1-2.5)[b]	1083 ± 283 ng/mL[b]

[a]Olmesartan is administered as a prodrug, olmesartan medoxomil. Pharmacokinetic data for olmesartan is reported. [b]Following 40-mg/day olmesartan medoxomil for 10 days.

References: Drugs@FDA. Benicar label approved on 07/13/05. Available at: http://www.accessdata.fda.gov/scripts/cder/drugsatfda/index.cfm. Accessed May 17, 2010. Rohatgi S, et al. Pharmacokinetics of amlodipine and olmesartan after administration of amlodipine besylate and olmesartan medoxomil in separate dosage forms and as a fixed-dose combination. *J Clin Pharmacol,* **2008**, *48*:1309–1322.

BIOAVAILABILITY (ORAL) (%)	URINARY EXCRETION (%)	BOUND IN PLASMA (%)	CLEARANCE (mL/min/kg)	VOL. DIST. (L/kg)	HALF-LIFE (hours)	PEAK TIME (hours)	PEAK CONCENTRATION
Ondansetron							
62 ± 15[a]	5	73 ± 2	5.9 ± 2.6	1.9 ± 0.05	3.5 ± 1.2		IV: 102 (64-136) ng/mL[c]
↑ Aged, LD[b], Fem			↓ Aged, LD[b], Fem ↑ Child	↔ Aged, LD[c]	↑ Aged, LD[c] ↓ Child	PO: 1.0 (0.8-1.5)[c]	PO: 39 (31-48)[c]

[a]In 26 cancer patients (62 ± 10 years), F = 86 ± 26%. [b]Mild to moderate liver impairment. [c]Mean (95% confidence interval) values following a single dose of 0.15 mg/kg IV or an oral dose of 8 mg given three times daily for 5 days to healthy adults.

Reference: Roila F, et al. Ondansetron clinical pharmacokinetics. *Clin Pharmacokinet,* **1995**, *29*:95–109.

BIOAVAILABILITY (ORAL) (%)	URINARY EXCRETION (%)	BOUND IN PLASMA (%)	CLEARANCE (mL/min/kg)	VOL. DIST. (L/kg)	HALF-LIFE (hours)	PEAK TIME (hours)	PEAK CONCENTRATION
Oxaliplatin[a]							
—[b]	—[c]	90[d]	49 (41-64)[e]	1.5 (1.1-2.1)	0.32 (0.27-0.46)[f]	—	Ox: 0.33 (0.28-0.38) μg Pt/mL PtDC: 0.008 (0.004-0.014) μg Pt/mL[g]

[a]Oxaliplatin is an organoplatinum complex; Pt is coordinated with diaminocyclohexane (DACH) and an oxalate ligand as a leaving group. Oxaliplatin (Ox) undergoes non-enzymatic biotransformation to reactive derivatives, notably $Pt(DACH)Cl_2$ (PtDC). Antitumor activity and toxicity are thought to relate to the concentration of oxaliplatin and PtDC in plasma ultrafiltrate (i.e., unbound concentration). [b]For IV administration only. [c]~54% of the platinum eliminated is recovered in urine. [d]Binding to plasma proteins is irreversible. [e]*CL* of total platinum is much lower; ~2-4 mL/min/kg. [f]The elimination of platinum species in plasma follows a triexponential pattern. The quoted $t_{1/2}$ reflects the $t_{1/2}$ of the first phase, which is the clinically relevant phase. The $t_{1/2}$ for the slower two phases are 17 and 391 hours. [g]Steady-state plasma ultrafiltrate concentration of Ox and PtDC after an 85-mg/m^2 IV infusion over 2 hours during cycles 1 and 2.

*References: PDR*58, **2004**, pp. 3024–3025. Shord SS, et al. Oxaliplatin biotransformation and pharmacokinetics: A pilot study to determine the possible relationship to neurotoxicity. *Anticancer Res,* **2002**, *22*:2301–2309.

Oxcarbazepine[a]							
—	O: <1 HC: 27	— HC: 45	O: 67.4[b] HC: ↓ RD,[c] Aged HC: ↑ Child[d]	—	O: ~2 HC: 8-15 HC: ↑ RD, Aged	HC: 2-4[e]	HC: 8.5 ± 2.0 μg/mL[e]

[a]Data from healthy adult male subjects. No significant gender differences. Oxcarbazepine (O) undergoes extensive first-pass metabolism to an active metabolite, 10-hydroxycarbamazepine (HC). Reduction by cytosolic enzymes is stereoselective (80% *S*-enantiomer, 20% *R*-enantiomer), but both show similar pharmacological activity. [b]*CL/F* for O reported. HC eliminated by glucuronidation. [c]AUC for HC increased, moderate to severe renal impairment. [d]AUC for HC decreased, children <6 years of age. [e]Following a 300-mg oral oxcarbazepine dose given twice daily for 12 days.

References: Battino D, et al. Clinical pharmacokinetics of antiepileptic drugs in paediatric patients. Part II. Phenytoin, carbamazepine, sulthiame, lamotrigine, vigabatrin, oxcarbazepine and felbamate. *Clin Pharmacokinet,* **1995**, *29*:341–369. Lloyd P, et al. Clinical pharmacology and pharmacokinetics of oxcarbazepine. *Epilepsia,* **1994**, *35*(suppl 3):S10–S13. Rouan MC, et al. The effect of renal impairment on the pharmacokinetics of oxcarbazepine and its metabolites. *Eur J Clin Pharmacol,* **1994**, *47*:161–167. van Heiningen PN, et al. The influence of age on the pharmacokinetics of the antiepileptic agent oxcarbazepine. *Clin Pharmacol Ther,* **1991**, *50*:410–419.

Oxybutynin[a]							
1.6-10.9	<1	—	8.1 ± 2.3[b]	1.3 ± 0.4[b]	IV: 1.9 ± 0.35[b,c]	IR: 5.0 ± 4.2[d] XL: 5.2 ± 3.7[d]	IR:12.4 ± 4.1 ng/mL[d] XL: 4.2 ± 1.6 ng/mL[d]

[a]Data from healthy female subjects. No significant gender differences. Racemic mixture; anticholinergic activity resides predominantly with *R*-enantiomer; no stereoselectivity exhibited for anti-spasmodic activity. Oxybutynin undergoes extensive first-pass metabolism to *N*-desethyloxybutynin (DEO), an active, anticholinergic metabolite. Metabolized primarily by intestinal and hepatic CYP3A. Racemic oxybutynin kinetic parameters reported. [b]Data reported for a 1-mg IV dose, assuming a 70-kg body weight. A larger volume (2.8 L/kg) and longer $t_{1/2}$ (5.3 hours) reported for a 5-mg IV dose. [c]Exhibits a longer apparent $t_{1/2}$ following oral dosing due to absorption rate-limited kinetics: immediate-release (IR) $t_{1/2}$ = 9 ± 2 hours; extended-release (XL) $t_{1/2}$ = 14 ± 3 hours. The apparent $t_{1/2}$ for DEO was 4.0 ± 1.4 hours and 8.3 ± 2.5 hours for the IR and XL formulations, respectively. [d]Following a dose of 5-mg IR given three times daily or 15-mg XL given once daily for 4 days. Peak DEO levels at steady state were 45 and 23 ng/mL for IR and XL, respectively.

References: Gupta SK, et al. Pharmacokinetics of an oral once-a-day controlled-release oxybutynin formulation compared with immediate-release oxybutynin. *J Clin Pharmacol,* **1999**, *39*:289–296. *PDR*54, **2000**, p. 507.

Oxycodone[a]							
CR: 60-87[b] IR: 42 ± 7[b]	—[c]	45	12.4 (9.2-15.4)	2.0 (1.1-2.9)	2.6 (2.1-3.1)[d]	CR: 3.2 ± 2.2[e] IR: 1.6 ± 0.8[e]	CR: 15.1 ± 4.7 ng/mL[e] IR: 15.5 ± 4.5 ng/mL[e]

[a]Oxycodone is metabolized primarily by CYP3A4/5, with a minor contribution from CYP2D6. Oxymorphone is an active metabolite produced by CYP2D6-mediated *O*-dealkylation. The circulating concentrations of oxymorphone are too low to contribute significantly to the opioid effects of oxycodone. Data from healthy male and female subjects reported. [b]Values reported for OXYCONTIN [oxycodone controlled release (CR)] and immediate-release (IR) tablets. [c]Up to 19% excreted unchanged after an oral dose. [d]The apparent $t_{1/2}$ for the CR oral formulation is ~5 hours; this most likely reflects absorption-limited terminal elimination kinetics. [e]Following 10 mg of OXYCONTIN (CR) given twice daily to steady state or a 5-mg IR tablet given every 6 hours to steady state.

References: Benziger DP, et al. Differential effects of food on the bioavailability of controlled-release oxycodone tablets and immediate-release oxycodone solution. *J Pharm Sci,* **1996**, *85*:407–410. *PDR*58, **2004**, pp. 2854–2855. Takala A, et al. Pharmacokinetic comparison of intravenous and intranasal administration of oxycodone. *Acta Anaesthesiol Scand,* **1997**, *47*:309–312.

(Continued)

Table AII–1

Pharmacokinetic Data (*Continued*)

BIOAVAILABILITY (ORAL) (%)	URINARY EXCRETION (%)	BOUND IN PLASMA (%)	CLEARANCE (mL/min/kg)	VOL. DIST. (L/kg)	HALF-LIFE (hours)	PEAK TIME (hours)	PEAK CONCENTRATION
Paclitaxel[a]							
Low	5 ± 2	88-98[b]	5.5 ± 3.5 ↔ Child	2.01 ± 1.2 ↔ Child	31 ± 1[c]	—	0.85 ± 0.21 μM[d]
Paliperidone[a]							
28 (oral ER)[b,c]	59 (51-67) (oral ER)	74 ↓ LD	3.70 ± 1.04[d] ↑ LD[e]	9.1[d] (oral ER)	28.4 ± 5.1[d] (oral ER) 25-49 days (IM PP)[f]	22 (2.0-24)[d] (oral ER) 13 days (IM PP)	10.7 ± 3.3 ng/mL[d] (oral ER)
Pantoprazole[a]							
77 (67-89)	—[b]	98	2.8 ± 0.9 ↓ LD ↔ RD	0.17 ± 0.04	1.1 ± 0.4 ↑ LD ↔ Aged	2.6 ± 0.9	2.5 ± 0.7 μg/mL[c]

Paclitaxel notes: [a]Metabolized by CYP2C8 and CYP3A, and substrate for P-glycoprotein. [b]Binding of drug to dialysis filtration devices may lead to overestimation of protein binding fraction (88% suggested). [c]Average accumulation $t_{1/2}$; longer terminal $t_{1/2}$ up to 50 hours are reported. [d]Steady-state concentration during a 250-mg/m^2 IV infusion given over 24 hours to adult cancer patients.

Reference: Sonnichsen DS, et al. Clinical pharmacokinetics of paclitaxel. *Clin Pharmacokinet*, **1994**, *27*:256–269.

Paliperidone notes: [a]Paliperidone, otherwise known as the 9-hydroxy active metabolite of risperidone, is marketed as an oral extended-release (ER) tablet (INVEGA) or in the form of its water-insoluble palmitate ester as a once-monthly long-acting IM injection (INVEGA SUSTENNA). Paliperidone is a racemate; its enantiomers have similar pharmacological profiles. The (+) and (–)-enantiomers of paliperidone interconvert, reaching an AUC (+) to (–) ratio of ~1.6 at steady state. [b]High-fat/high-caloric meal increased C_{max} and AUC by 60% and 54%, respectively. [c]No data on the absolute bioavailability of IM paliperidone palmitate (IM PP). The initiation regimen for INVEGA SUSTENNA (234 mg/156 mg in the deltoid muscle on day 1/day 8) produces paliperidone concentrations matching the range observed with 6- to 12-mg oral ER paliperidone. [d]At steady-state during once-daily doses of 3 mg, assuming an average body weight of 73 kg. V_z is estimated from *CL/F* and $t_{1/2}$. [e]Patients with moderate hepatic impairment showed a modest increase in clearance and plasma free fraction with no significant change in unbound AUC. [f]The apparent long terminal $t_{1/2}$ of paliperidone following IM depot injection reflects the slow dissolution of paliperidone palmitate and release of active paliperidone.

References: Boom S, et al. Single- and multiple-dose pharmacokinetics and dose proportionality of the psychotropic agent paliperidone extended release. *J Clin Pharmacol*, **2009**, *49*:1318–1330. Drugs@FDA. Invega label approved on 4/27/07; Invega Sustenna label approved on 7/31/09. Available at: http://www.accessdata.fda.gov/Scripts/cder/DrugsatFDA/. Accessed on January 1, 2010.

Pantoprazole notes: [a]Pantoprazole is cleared primarily by CYP2C19 (polymorphic)-dependent metabolism. Poor metabolizers (PM) exhibit profound differences in *CL* (lower) and $t_{1/2}$ (higher), compared to extensive metabolizers (EM). Pantoprazole is available as a racemic mixture of (+) and (–) isomers. In CYP2C19 EM, no significant differences in the pharmacokinetics of (+) and (–) pantoprazole were observed, whereas in CYP2C19 PM, the *CL* of (–) pantoprazole was significantly greater than that of (+) pantoprazole. [b]No unchanged drug recovered in urine. [c]Following a single 40-mg oral dose.

References: Drugs@FDA. Protonix label approved on 11/12/09. Available at: http://www.accessdata.fda.gov/scripts/cder/drugsatfda/index.cfm. Accessed on December 26, 2009. Huber R, et al. Pharmacokinetics of lansoprazole in man. *Int J Clin Pharmacol Ther,* **1996**, *34*:185–194. Pue MA, et al. Pharmacokinetics of pantoprazole following single intravenous and oral administration to healthy male subjects. *Eur J Clin Pharmacol,* **1993**, *44*:575–578. Tanaka M, et al. Stereoselective pharmacokinetics of pantoprazole, a proton pump inhibitor, in extensive and poor metabolizers of S-mephenytoin. *Clin Pharmacol Ther*, **2001**, *69*:108–113.

Paroxetine

Dose dependent[a]	<2	95	8.6 ± 3.2[a,b] ↓ LD, Aged	17 ± 10[c]	17 ± 3[d] ↑ LD, Aged	5.2 ± 0.5[e]	EM: ~130 nM[e] PM: ~220 nM[e]

[a]Metabolized by CYP2D6 (polymorphic); undergoes time- and dose-dependent autoinhibition of metabolic *CL* in extensive metabolizers (EM). [b]*CL/F* reported for multiple dosing in EM. Single dose data are significantly higher. In CYP2D6 poor metabolizers (PM), *CL/F* = 5.0 ± 2.1 mL/min/kg for multiple dosing. [c]V_{area}/F reported. [d]Data reported for multiple dose in EM. In PM, $t_{1/2}$ = 41 ± 8 hours. [e]Estimated mean C_{max} following a 30-mg oral dose given once daily for 14 days to adults phenotyped as CYP2D6 EM and PM. There is a significant disproportional accumulation of drug in blood when going from single to multiple dosing due to autoinactivation of CYP2D6.

*References: PDR*54, **2000**, p. 3028. Sindrup SH, et al. The relationship between paroxetine and the sparteine oxidation polymorphism. *Clin Pharmacol Ther,* **1992**, *51*:278–287.

Phenobarbital

100 ± 11	24 ± 5[a] ↔ LD, AVH	51 ± 3 ↓ Neo ↔ Preg, Aged	0.062 ± 0.013 ↑ Preg, Child, Neo ↔ Smk	0.54 ± 0.03 ↑ Neo	99 ± 18 ↑ LD, Aged ↓ Child ↔ Epilepsy, Neo	2-4[b]	13.1 ± 4.5 μg/mL[b]

[a]Phenobarbital is a weak acid (pK_a = 7.3); urinary excretion is increased at an alkaline pH; it also is reduced with decreased urine flow. [b]Mean steady-state concentration following a 90-mg oral dose given daily for 12 weeks to patients with epilepsy. Levels of 10-25 μg/mL provide control of tonic-clonic seizures, and levels of at least 15 μg/mL provide control of febrile convulsions in children. Levels >40 μg/mL can cause toxicity; 65-117 μg/mL produce stage III anesthesia—comatose but reflexes present; 100-134 μg/mL produce stage IV anesthesia—no deep-tendon reflexes.

References: Bourgeois BFD. Phenobarbital and primidone. In: Wyllie E, ed. *The Treatment of Epilepsy: Principles and Practice,* 2nd ed. Philadelphia, Williams & Wilkins, **1997**, pp. 845–855. Browne TR, et al. Studies with stable isotopes II: Phenobarbital pharmacokinetics during monotherapy. *J Clin Pharmacol,* **1985**, *25*:51–58.

Phenytoin[a]

90 ± 3	2 ± 8	89 ± 23 ↓ RD, Hep, Alb, Neo, AVH, LD, NS, Preg, Burn ↔ Obes, Smk, Aged	V_{max} = 5.9 ± 1.2 $mg \cdot kg^{-1} \cdot day^{-1}$ ↓ Aged, ↑ Child K_m = 5.7 ± 2.9 mg/L[b] ↔ Aged, ↓ Child ↑ NS, RD[c] ↓ Prem[c] ↔ AVH, LTh, HTh, Smk[c]	0.64 ± 0.04[d] ↑ Neo, NS, RD ↔ AVH, LTh, HTh	6-24[e] ↑ Prem[c] ↓ RD[c] ↔ AVH, LTh, HTh, Smk[c]	3-12[f]	0-5 μg/mL (27%)[f] 5-10 μg/mL (30%)[f] 10-20 μg/mL (29%)[f] 20-30 μg/mL (10%)[f] >30 μg/mL (6%)[f]

[a]Metabolized predominantly by CYP2C9 (polymorphic) and also by CYP2C19 (polymorphic); exhibits saturable kinetics with therapeutic doses. [b]Significantly decreased in the Japanese population. [c]Comparison of *CL*s and $t_{1/2}$s with similar doses in normal subjects and patients; nonlinear kinetics not considered. [d]V_{area} reported. [e]Apparent $t_{1/2}$ is dependent on plasma concentration. [f]Population frequency of total phenytoin concentrations following a 300-mg oral dose (capsule) given daily to steady state. Total levels >10 μg/mL associated with suppression of tonic-clonic seizures. Nystagmus can occur at levels >20 μg/mL and ataxia at levels >30 μg/mL.

References: Eldon MA, et al. Pharmacokinetics and tolerance of fosphenytoin and phenytoin administered intravenously to healthy subjects. *Can J Neurol Sci,* **1993**, *20*(suppl 4):S180. Levine M, et al. Therapeutic drug monitoring of phenytoin. Rationale and current status. *Clin Pharmacokinet,* **1990**, *79*:341–358. Tozer TN, et al. Phenytoin. In: Evans WE, et al., eds. *Applied Pharmacokinetics: Principles of Therapeutic Drug Monitoring,* 3rd ed. Vancouver, WA, Applied Therapeutics, **1992**, pp. 25-1–25-44.

(Continued)

Table AII–1

Pharmacokinetic Data (*Continued*)

BIOAVAILABILITY (ORAL) (%)	URINARY EXCRETION (%)	BOUND IN PLASMA (%)	CLEARANCE (mL/min/kg)	VOL. DIST. (L/kg)	HALF-LIFE (hours)	PEAK TIME (hours)	PEAK CONCENTRATION
Pioglitazone[a]							
—	Negligible	>99	1.2 ± 1.7[b]	0.63 ± 0.41[b]	11 ± 6[c]	P: 3.5 (1-4)[d] M-III: 11 (2-48)[d] M-IV: 11 (4-16)[d]	P: 1.6 ± 0.2 μg/mL[d] M-III: 0.4 ± 0.2 μg/mL[d] M-IV: 1.4 ± 0.5 μg/mL[d]

[a]Data from healthy male and female subjects and patients with type 2 diabetes. Pioglitazone (P) is metabolized extensively by CYP2C8, CYP3A4, and other CYP isozymes. Two major metabolites (M-III and M-IV) accumulate in blood and contribute to the pharmacological effect. [b]*CL/F* and V_{area}/F reported. *CL/F* is lower in women than in men. [c]Steady-state $t_{1/2}$ of M-III and M-IV is 29 and 27 hours, respectively. [d]Following a 45-mg oral dose given once daily for 10 days.

References: Budde K, et al. The pharmacokinetics of pioglitazone in patients with impaired renal function. *Br J Clin Pharmacol,* **2003**, *55*:368–374. *PDR*58, **2004**, p. 3186.

BIOAVAILABILITY (ORAL) (%)	URINARY EXCRETION (%)	BOUND IN PLASMA (%)	CLEARANCE (mL/min/kg)	VOL. DIST. (L/kg)	HALF-LIFE (hours)	PEAK TIME (hours)	PEAK CONCENTRATION
Posaconazole[a]							
—	—	98 ↔ RD	11.7 ± 6.4[b] ↔ RD	11.9[b]	21.6 ± 8.4 ↔ RD	4 (3-12)	324 ± 161 ng/mL[c] ↔ RD

[a]~66% of an oral posaconazole dose is excreted unchanged in feces. It is unclear whether this represents significant biliary excretion or unabsorbed drug. [b]*CL/F* and V_d/F reported. [c]Following a single 400-mg dose of an oral suspension.

References: Courtney R, et al. Posaconazole pharmacokinetics, safety, and tolerability in subjects with varying degrees of chronic renal disease. *J Clin Pharmacol,* **2005**, *45*:185–192. Dodds Ashley ES, et al. Pharmacokinetics of posaconazole administered orally or by nasogastric tube in healthy volunteers. *Antimicrob Agents Chemother,* **2009**, *53*:2960–2964.

BIOAVAILABILITY (ORAL) (%)	URINARY EXCRETION (%)	BOUND IN PLASMA (%)	CLEARANCE (mL/min/kg)	VOL. DIST. (L/kg)	HALF-LIFE (hours)	PEAK TIME (hours)	PEAK CONCENTRATION
Pramipexole[a]							
>90[b]	~90	15	8.2 ± 1.4[b] ↓ Aged, RD,[c] PD[d]	7.3 ± 1.7[b]	11.6 ± 2.57 ↑ Aged, RD	1-2	M: 1.6 ± 0.23 ng/mL[e] F: 2.1 ± 0.25 ng/mL[e]

[a]Data from healthy adult male and female subjects. No significant gender differences. [b]Bioavailability estimated from urinary recovery of unchanged drug. *CL/F* and V_{area}/F reported. [c]*CL/F* reduced, moderate to severe renal impairment. [d]Parkinson's disease (PD); *CL/F* reduced with declining renal function. [e]Following a 0.5-mg oral dose given three times daily for 4 days to male (M) and female (F) adults.

References: Lam YW. Clinical pharmacology of dopamine agonists. *Pharmacotherapy,* **2000**, *20*:17S–25S. *PDR*54, **2000**, p. 2468. Wright CE, et al. Steady-state pharmacokinetic properties of pramipexole in healthy volunteers. *J Clin Pharmacol,* **1997**, *37*:520–525.

Pramlintide[a]

30-40%[b]	–	~60[c]	Low: 14.9 ± 3.9[d] High: 14.5 ± 4.0[d] ↔ RD[e]	0.43 0.71	IV: 0.4-0.75 SC: 0.5-0.83	0.32-0.35[f]	Low: 21 ± 3 pmol/L[f] High: 77 ± 22 pmol/L[f]

[a]Pramlintide is a synthetic peptide analog of amylin for the treatment of both type 1 and type 2 diabetes. It is metabolized in the kidneys to at least one primary active metabolite: Des-lys(1)pramlintide (2-37 pramlintide) with a $t_{1/2}$ similar to that of the parent drug. [b]SC administration with greater variability in response when the injection is into the arm compared to into the abdomen or thigh. [c]Not extensively bound to blood cells or albumin. [d]Based on IV infusion of a low dose of 30 µg for type 1 diabetes and a high dose of 100 µg for type 2 diabetes. [e]Study in patients with moderate to severe renal impairment. No data in end-stage RD. [f]Following a low SC dose of 30 µg and a high SC dose of 100 µg.

References: Colburn WA, et al. Pharmacokinetics and pharmacodynamics of AC137 (25,28,29 triproamylin, human) after intravenous bolus and infusion doses in patients with insulin-dependent diabetes. *J Clin Pharmacol,* **1996**, *36*:13–24. Drugs@FDA. Symlin label approved on 9/25/07. Available at: http://www.accessdata.fda.gov/Scripts/cder/DrugsatFDA/. Accessed on August 1, 2009. Kolterman OG, et al. Effect of 14 days' subcutaneous administration of the human amylin analogue, pramlintide (AC137), on an intravenous insulin challenge and response to a standard liquid meal in patients with IDDM. *Diabetologia,* **1996**, *39*:492–499.

Pravastatin

18 ± 8	47 ± 7	43-48	13.5 ± 2.4 ↓ LD ↔ Aged, RD[a]	0.46 ± 0.04	0.8 ± 0.2[b] ↔ Aged, RD[a]	1-1.4[c]	28-38 ng/mL[c]

[a]Although renal *CL* decreases with reduced renal function, no significant changes in *CL/F* or $t_{1/2}$ are seen following oral dosing as a result of the low and highly variable bioavailability. [b]A longer $t_{1/2}$ = 1.8 ± 0.8 hour reported for oral dosing; probably rate limited by absorption. [c]Range of mean values from different studies following a single 20-mg oral dose.

References: Corsini A, et al. New insights into the pharmacodynamic and pharmacokinetic properties of statins. *Pharmacol Ther,* **1999**, *84*:413–428. Desager JP, et al. Clinical pharmacokinetics of 3-hydroxy-3-methylglutaryl-coenzyme A reductase inhibitors. *Clin Pharmacokinet,* **1996**, *31*:348–371. Quion JA, et al. Clinical pharmacokinetics of pravastatin. *Clin Pharmacokinet,* **1994**, *27*:94–103.

Praziquantel[a]

—[b]	Negligible	80-85	5 mg/kg: 467[c] 40-60 mg/kg: 57-222[c] ↓ LD[d]	50 mg/kg: 9.55 ± 2.86	5 mg/kg: 0.8-1.5[c] 40-60 mg/kg: 1.7-3.0[c] ↑ LD	1.5-1.8[e]	0.8-6.3 µg/L[e]

[a]Data from male and female patients with schistosomiasis. [b]Absolute bioavailability is not known. Praziquantel is well absorbed (80%) but undergoes significant first-pass metabolism (hydroxylation), the extent of which appears to be dose dependent. [c]*CL/F* and V_{ss}/F reported; *CL/F* and $t_{1/2}$ are dose dependent. [d]*CL/F* reduced, moderate to severe hepatic impairment. [e]Range of mean values from different studies following a single 40- to 60-mg/kg oral dose.

References: Edwards G, et al. Clinical pharmacokinetics of anthelmintic drugs. *Clin Pharmacokinet,* **1988**, *15*:67–93. el Guiniady MA, et al. Clinical and pharmacokinetic study of praziquantel in Egyptian schistosomiasis patients with and without liver cell failure. *Am J Trop Med Hyg,* **1994**, *51*:809–818. Jung H, et al. Clinical pharmacokinetics of praziquantel. *Proc West Pharmacol Soc,* **1991**, *34*:335–340. Sotelo J, et al. Pharmacokinetic optimisation of the treatment of neurocysticercosis. *Clin Pharmacokinet,* **1998**, *34*:503–515. Watt G, et al. Praziquantel pharmacokinetics and side effects in *Schistosoma japonicum*-infected patients with liver disease. *J Infect Dis,* **1988**, *157*:530–535.

(Continued)

Table AII–1

Pharmacokinetic Data (*Continued*)

BIOAVAILABILITY (ORAL) (%)	URINARY EXCRETION (%)	BOUND IN PLASMA (%)	CLEARANCE (mL/min/kg)	VOL. DIST. (L/kg)	HALF-LIFE (hours)	PEAK TIME (hours)	PEAK CONCENTRATION
Prednisolone							
82 ± 13	26 ± 9[a]	90-95 (<200 ng/mL)[b]	1.0 ± 0.16[c]	0.42 ± 0.11[e]	2.2 ± 0.5	1.5 ± 0.5[f]	458 ± 150 ng/mL[f]
↔ Hep, Cush, RD, Crohn, Celiac, Smk, Aged ↓ HTh	↑ Aged, HTh	~70 (>1 μg/mL) ↓ Alb, NS, Aged, HTh, LD ↔ Hep	↔ Hep, Cush, Smk, CRI, NS,[d] HTh[d] ↓ Aged,[d] LD[d]	↔ Hep, Cush, Smk, RD, CRI, NS[d] ↓ HTh,[d] Aged, Obes[d]	↔ Hep, Cush, Smk, RD, CRI, NS[d] ↓ HTh[d] ↑ Aged[d]		

[a]Prednisolone and prednisone are interconvertible; an additional 3 ± 2% is excreted as prednisone. [b]Extent of binding to plasma proteins is dependent on concentration over range encountered. [c]Total *CL* increases as protein binding is saturated. *CL* of unbound drug increases slightly but significantly with increasing dose. [d]Changes are for unbound drug. [e]*V* increases with dose due to saturable protein binding. [f]Following a 30-mg oral dose given twice daily for 3 days to healthy adult male subjects. The ratio of prednisolone/prednisone is dose dependent and can vary from 3-26 over a prednisolone concentration range of 50-800 ng/mL.

References: Frey BM, et al. Clinical pharmacokinetics of prednisone and prednisolone. *Clin Pharmacokinet*, **1990**, *19*:126–146. Rohatagi S, et al. Pharmacokinetics of methylprednisolone and prednisolone after single and multiple oral administration. *J Clin Pharmacol*, **1997**, *37*:916–925.

BIOAVAILABILITY (ORAL) (%)	URINARY EXCRETION (%)	BOUND IN PLASMA (%)	CLEARANCE (mL/min/kg)	VOL. DIST. (L/kg)	HALF-LIFE (hours)	PEAK TIME (hours)	PEAK CONCENTRATION
Prednisone							
80 ± 11[a] ↔ Hep, Cush, RD, Crohn, Celiac, Smk, Aged	3 ± 2[b] ↔ HTh	75 ± 2[c]	3.6 ± 0.8[d] ↔ Hep	0.97 ± 0.11[d] ↔ Hep	3.6 ± 0.4[d] ↔ Smk, Hep	P: 2.1-3.1[e] PL: 1.2-2.6[e]	P: 62-81 ng/mL[e] PL: 198-239 ng/mL[e]

[a]Measured relative to equivalent IV dose of prednisolone (PL). [b]An additional 15 ± 5% excreted as PL. [c]In contrast to PL, there is no dependence on concentration. [d]Kinetic values for prednisone (P) often are reported in terms of values for PL, its active metabolite. However, the values cited here pertain to P. [e]Range of mean data for P and PL following a single 10-mg oral dose given as different proprietary formulations to healthy adults.

References: Gustavson LE, et al. The macromolecular binding of prednisone in plasma of healthy volunteers including pregnant women and oral contraceptive users. *J Pharmacokinet Biopharm,* **1985**, *13*:561–569. Pickup ME. Clinical pharmacokinetics of prednisone and prednisolone. *Clin Pharmacokinet,* **1979**, *4*:111–128. Sullivan TJ, et al. Comparative bioavailability: Eight commercial prednisone tablets. *J Pharmacokinet Biopharm,* **1976**, *4*:157–172.

Pregabalin[a]

≥90[b]	90-99	0	0.96-1.2[c] ↓ RD[d]	0.5	5-6.5	1[b]	8.5 μg/mL[e]

[a]Pregabalin undergoes minimal metabolism; an *N*-methylated metabolite has been identified in urine and accounts for 0.9% of oral dose. >90% of dose is excreted in urine as unchanged drug. Pregabalin pharmacokinetics is dose independent and predictable from single to multiple dosing. [b]Bioavailability does not vary with dose up to 600 mg. T_{max} is delayed from 1 hour to 3 hours and C_{max} decreased by 25-30% when pregabalin is given with food. No change in AUC or extent of absorption is noted. [c]Mean renal clearance in healthy young subjects ranges from 67 to 81 mL/min and assuming 70-kg body weight. [d]Pregabalin clearance is proportional CL_{cr}; hence, dosage can be adjusted in accordance to CL_{cr} in renal dysfunction. Plasma pregabalin decreased by ~50% after 4 hours of hemodialysis. [e]Steady-state concentration in healthy subjects receiving 200-mg pregabalin every 8 hours.

References: Bialer M, et al. Progress report on new antiepileptic drugs: A summary of the fifth Eilat conference (EILAT V). *Epilepsy Res*, **2001**, *43*:11–58. Brodie MJ, et al. Pregabalin drug interaction studies: Lack of effect on the pharmacokinetics of carbamazepine, phenytoin, lamotrigine, and valproate in patients with partial epilepsy. *Epilepsia*, **2005**, *46*:1407–1413. *Physicians' Desk Reference,* 63rd ed. Montvale, NJ, Physicians' Desk Reference Inc., **2008**, pp. 2527–2534.

Procainamide[a]

83 ± 16	67 ± 8 ↓ CHF, COPD, CP, LD	16 ± 5	$CL = 2.7CL_{cr} + 1.7 + 3.2$ (fast)[b] or + 1.1 (slow)[b] ↑ Child ↓ MI ↔ CHF, Tach, Neo	1.9 ± 0.3 ↓ Obes ↔ RD, Child, Tach, CHF	3.0 ± 0.6 ↑ RD[c] MI ↓ Child, Neo ↔ Obes, Tach, CHF	M: 3.6[d] F: 3.8[d]	M: 2.2 μg/mL[d] F: 2.9 μg/mL[d]

[a]Active metabolite, *N*-acetylprocainamide (NAPA); $CL = 3.1 \pm 0.4$ mL/min/kg, $V = 1.4 \pm 0.2$ L/kg, and $t_{1/2} = 6.0 \pm 0.2$ hours. [b]*CL* calculated using units of mL/min/kg for CL_{cr}. *CL* depends on NAT2 acetylation phenotype. Use a mean value of 2.2 if phenotype unknown. [c]$t_{1/2}$ for procainamide and NAPA increased in patients with RD. [d]Least square mean values following 1000-mg oral dose given twice daily to steady state in male (M) and female (F) adults. Mean peak NAPA concentrations were 2.0 and 2.2 μg/mL for male and female adults, respectively; $T_{max} = 4.1$ and 4.2 hours, respectively.

References: Benet LZ, et al. Die renale Elimination von Procainamide: Pharmacokinetik bei Niereninsuffizienz. In: Braun J, et al., eds. *Die Behandlung von Herzrhythmusstorungen bei Nierenkranken.* Basel, Karger, **1984**, pp. 96–111. Koup JR, et al. Effect of age, gender, and race on steady state procainamide pharmacokinetics after administration of Procanbid sustained-release tablets. *Ther Drug Monit,* **1998**, *20*:73–77.

Promethazine[a]

PO: 27.9 ± 19.8[b] Rectal: 21.7-23.4[c]	0.64 ± 0.49	93	15.7 ± 5.7	13.4 ± 3.6[d]	12.2 ± 2.2	PO: 2.8 ± 1.4[e] Rectal: 8.2 ± 3.4	PO: 21.8 ± 14.0 ng/mL[e] Rectal: 11.3 ± 8.5 ng/mL

[a]Promethazine undergoes ring-hydroxylation mediated by CYP2D6, *N*-demethylation by CYP2B6, and S-oxidation to a sulfoxide. Promethazine is well absorbed following oral administration (>80%) but is subject to first-pass metabolism, which explains its low systemic availability. [b]Oral bioavailability at 75-mg dose as compared to IV bolus. [c]Bioavailability of two commercial rectal suppositories at a 50-mg dose compared to an IM dose. [d]Steady-state volume. [e]Data for a 50-mg oral dose of promethazine in solution. [f]Following a 50-mg dose of promethazine rectal suppository.

References: Drugs@FDA. AcipHex label approved on 6/30/08. Available at: http://www.accessdata.fda.gov/Scripts/cder/DrugsatFDA/Accessed on August 2, 2009. Koytchev R, et al. Absolute bioavailability of chlorpromazine, promazine and promethazine. *Arzneimittelforschung*, **1994**, *44*:121–125. Schwinghammer TL, et al. Comparison of the bioavailability of oral, rectal and intramuscular promethazine. *Biopharm Drug Dispos*, **1984**, *5*:185–194. Sharma A, et al. Classic histamine H1 receptor antagonists: A critical review of their metabolic and pharmacokinetic fate from a bird's eye view. *Curr Drug Metab*, **2003**, *4*:105–129. Stavchansky S, et al. Bioequivalence and pharmacokinetic profile of promethazine hydrochloride suppositories in humans. *J Pharm Sci*, **1987**, *76*:441–445. Taylor G, et al. Pharmacokinetics of promethazine and its sulphoxide metabolite after intravenous and oral administration to man. *Br J Clin Pharmacol,* **1983**, *15*:287–293.

(*Continued*)

Table AII–1

Pharmacokinetic Data (*Continued*)

BIOAVAILABILITY (ORAL) (%)	URINARY EXCRETION (%)	BOUND IN PLASMA (%)	CLEARANCE (mL/min/kg)	VOL. DIST. (L/kg)	HALF-LIFE (hours)	PEAK TIME (hours)	PEAK CONCENTRATION
Propofol[a]							
—[b]	—	98.3-98.8[c]	27 ± 5 ↑ Child,[d] ↓ Aged[e] ↔ LD	1.7 ± 0.7[f] ↑ Child[d] ↓ Aged[e]	3.5 ± 1.2[f]	—	SS: 3.5 ± 0.06 μg/mL[g] E: 1.1 ± 0.4 μg/mL[g]

[a]Data from patients undergoing elective surgery and healthy volunteers. Propofol is extensively metabolized by UGTs. [b]For IV administration only. [c]Fraction bound in whole blood. Concentration dependent; 98.8% at 0.5 μg/mL and 98.3 at 32 μg/mL. [d]*CL* and central volume increased in children 1-3 years of age. [e]*CL* and central volume decreased in elderly patients. [f]V_{area} is much larger than V_{ss}. A much longer terminal $t_{1/2}$ was reported following prolonged IV infusion. Concentration producing anesthesia after infusion to steady state (SS) and at emergence (E) from anesthesia.

References: Mazoit JX, et al. Binding of propofol to blood components: Implications for pharmacokinetics and for pharmacodynamics. *Br J Clin Pharmacol*, **1999**, *47*:35–42. Murat I, et al. Pharmacokinetics of propofol after a single dose in children aged 1–3 years with minor burns. Comparison of three data analysis approaches. *Anesthesiology*, **1996**, *84*:526–532. Servin F, et al. Pharmacokinetics of propofol infusions in patients with cirrhosis. *Br J Anaesth*, **1990**, *65*:177–183.

BIOAVAILABILITY (ORAL) (%)	URINARY EXCRETION (%)	BOUND IN PLASMA (%)	CLEARANCE (mL/min/kg)	VOL. DIST. (L/kg)	HALF-LIFE (hours)	PEAK TIME (hours)	PEAK CONCENTRATION
Propranolol[a]							
26 ± 10 ↑ Cirr	<0.5	87 ± 6[b] ↑ Inflam, Crohn, Preg, Obes ↔ RD, Fem, Aged ↓ LD	16 ± 5[c,d] ↑ Smk, HTh ↓ Hep, LD, Obes, Fem ↔ Aged, RD	4.3 ± 0.6[c] ↑ Hep, HTh, LD ↓ Crohn ↔ Aged, RD, Obes, Fem, Preg	3.9 ± 0.4[c] ↓ Hep, LD, Obes, Fem ↔ Aged, RD, Smk, Preg	P: 1.5[e] HP: 1.0[e]	P: 49 ± 8 ng/mL[e] HP: 37 ± 9 ng/mL[e]

[a]Racemic mixture. For *S*-(–)-enantiomer (100-fold more active) compared to *R*-(+)-enantiomer, *CL* is 19% lower and V_{area} is 15% lower because of a higher degree of protein binding (18% lower free fraction); hence, there is no difference in $t_{1/2}$. Active metabolite, 4-hydroxypropranolol (HP). [b]Drug is bound primarily to α_1-acid glycoprotein, which is elevated in a number of inflammatory conditions. [c]Based on blood measurements; blood-to-plasma concentration ratio = 0.89 ± 0.03. [d]CYP2D6 catalyzes the formation of HP; CYP1A2 is responsible for most of the *N*-desisopropyl metabolite; UGT catalyzes the major conjugation pathway of elimination. [e]Following a single 80-mg oral dose given to healthy adults. Plasma accumulation factor was 3.6-fold after 80 mg was given four times daily to steady state. A concentration of 20 ng/mL gave a 50% decrease in exercise-induced cardioacceleration. Antianginal effects manifest at 15-90 ng/mL. A concentration up to 1000 ng/mL may be required for control of ventricular arrhythmias.

References: Colangelo PM, et al. Age and propranolol stereoselective disposition in humans. *Clin Pharmacol Ther,* **1992**, *57*:489–494. Walle T, et al. 4-Hydroxypropranolol and its glucuronide after single and long-term doses of propranolol. *Clin Pharmacol Ther,* **1980**, *27*:22–31.

Pseudoephedrine[a]							
~100	43-96[b]	—	7.33[b,c]	2.64-3.51[c]	4.3-8[b,c]	IR: 1.4-2[d] CR: 3.8-6.1[d]	IR: 177-360 ng/mL[d] CR: 265-314 ng/mL[d]

[a]Data from healthy adult male and female subjects. [b]At a high urinary pH (>7.0), pseudoephedrine is extensively reabsorbed; $t_{1/2}$ increases, and *CL* decreases. [c]*CL/F, V/F,* and $t_{1/2}$ reported for oral dose. [d]Range of mean values from different studies following a single 60-mg immediate-release tablet or syrup (IR), or 120-mg controlled-release capsule (CR) oral dose.

Reference: Kanfer I, et al. Pharmacokinetics of oral decongestants. *Pharmacotherapy,* **1993**, *13*:116S–128S.

Pyrazinamide[a]							
—[b]	4-14[c]	10	1.1 (0.2-2.3)[d] ↑ Child	0.57 (0.13-1.04)[d]	6 (2-23) ↓ Child	1-2[e]	35 (19-103) μg/mL[e]

[a]Pyrazinamide is hydrolyzed in the liver to an active metabolite, 2-pyrazinoic acid. Reported peak 2-pyrazinoic acid concentrations range from 0.1- to 1-fold that of the parent drug. Pyrazinamide data reported are for male and female adults with tuberculosis. [b]Absolute bioavailability is not known, but the drug is well absorbed based on recovery of parent drug and metabolites (70%). [c]Recovery unchanged following an oral dose; the recovery of pyrazinoic acid is 37 ± 5%. [d]*CL/F* and V_{area}/F reported. [e]Following a 15- to 53-mg/kg daily oral dose to steady state.

References: Bareggi SR, et al. Clinical pharmacokinetics and metabolism of pyrazinamide in healthy volunteers. *Arzneimittelforschung,* **1987**, *37*:849–854. Lacroix C, et al. Pharmacokinetics of pyrazinamide and its metabolites in healthy subjects. *Eur J Clin Pharmacol,* **1989**, *36*:395–400. *PDR*58, **2004**, p. 766. Zhu M, et al. Population pharmacokinetic modeling of pyrazinamide in children and adults with tuberculosis. *Pharmacotherapy,* **2002**, *22*:686–695.

Quetiapine[a]							
9 ↑ Food	<1%	83	19 ↓ Aged ↔ RD ↓ LD	10 ± 4	6	1-1.8	278 ng/mL[b]

[a]No significant gender differences. Extensively metabolized through multiple pathways, including sulfoxidation, *N*- and *O*-dealkylation catalyzed by CYP3A4. Two minor active metabolites. [b]Following a 250-mg oral dose given daily for 23 days in patients with schizophrenia.

References: Goren JL, et al. Quetiapine, an atypical antipsychotic. *Pharmacotherapy,* **1998**, *18*:1183–1194. *PDR*54, **2000**, p. 563.

Quinapril[a]							
QT (Q): 52 ± 15[b]	Q (Q): 3.1 ± 1.2[c] QT (QT): 96[d]	Q/QT: 97	QT (QT): 0.98 ± 0.22[d] ↓ RD	QT (QT): 0.19 ± 0.04[d]	Q (Q): 0.8-0.9[c] QT (QT): 2.1-2.9[d] ↑ RD	Q (Q): 1.4 ± 0.8[e] QT (Q): 2.3 ± 0.9[e]	Q (Q): 207 ± 89 ng/mL[e] QT (Q): 923 ± 277 ng/mL[e]

[a]Hydrolyzed to its active metabolite, quinaprilat. Pharmacokinetic data for quinapril (Q) and quinaprilat (QT) following oral Q and IV QT administration are presented. [b]Absolute bioavailability based on plasma QT concentrations. [c]Data for Q following a 2.5- to 80-mg oral Q dose. [d]Data for QT following a 2.5-mg IV QT dose. The $t_{1/2}$ of QT after dosing Q is similar. [e]Following a single 40-mg oral Q dose. No accumulation of QT with multiple dosing.

References: Breslin E, et al. A pharmacodynamic and pharmacokinetic comparison of intravenous quinaprilat and oral quinapril. *J Clin Pharmacol,* **1996**, *36*:414–421. Olson SC, et al. The clinical pharmacokinetics of quinapril. *Angiology,* **1989**, *40*:351–359. *PDR*58, **2004**, p. 2516.

(*Continued*)

Table AII–1

Pharmacokinetic Data (*Continued*)

BIOAVAILABILITY (ORAL) (%)	URINARY EXCRETION (%)	BOUND IN PLASMA (%)	CLEARANCE (mL/min/kg)	VOL. DIST. (L/kg)	HALF-LIFE (hours)	PEAK TIME (hours)	PEAK CONCENTRATION
Quinidine[a]							
Sulfate: 80 ± 15 Gluconate: 71 ± 17	18 ± 5 ↔ CHF	87 ± 3 ↓ LD, Hep, Neo, Preg ↔ RD, CRI, HL, Aged	4.7 ± 1.8[b] ↓ CHF, Aged ↔ LD, Smk	2.7 ± 1.2 ↓ CHF ↑ LD ↔ Aged	6.2 ± 1.8 ↑ Aged, LD ↔ CHF, RD	IR: 1-3[c] ER: 6.3 ± 3.2[c]	IV: 2.9 ± 1.0 μg/mL[c] IR: ~1.3 μg/mL[c] ER: 0.53 ± 0.22 μg/mL[c]

[a]Active metabolite, 3-hydroxyquinidine ($t_{1/2}$ = 12 ± 3 hours; percent bound in plasma = 60 ± 10%). [b]Metabolically cleared primarily by CYP3A. [c]Following a 400-mg IV dose (22-minute infusion) of quinidine gluconate or a single 400-mg oral dose of immediate-release (IR) quinidine sulfate or a 300-mg dose of extended-release (ER) quinidine sulfate (QUINIDEX) to healthy adults. Specific assay methods for quinidine show >75% reduction in frequency of premature ventricular contractions at levels of 0.7-5.9 μg/mL, but active metabolite was not measured; therapeutic levels of 2-7 μg/mL were reported for nonspecific assays.

References: Brosen K, et al. Quinidine kinetics after a single oral dose in relation to the sparteine oxidation polymorphism in man. *Br J Clin Pharmacol,* **1990**, *29*:248–253. Sawyer WT, et al. Bioavailability of a commercial sustained-release quinidine tablet compared to oral quinidine solution. *Biopharm Drug Dispos,* **1982**, *3*:301–310. Ueda CT, et al. Absolute quinidine bioavailability. *Clin Pharmacol Ther,* **1976**, *20*:260–265.

BIOAVAILABILITY (ORAL) (%)	URINARY EXCRETION (%)	BOUND IN PLASMA (%)	CLEARANCE (mL/min/kg)	VOL. DIST. (L/kg)	HALF-LIFE (hours)	PEAK TIME (hours)	PEAK CONCENTRATION
Quinine[a]							
76 ± 11	N-A: 12-20 M-A: 33 ± 18	N-A: ~85-90[b] M-A: 93-95[b] ↓ Neo ↔ Preg	N-A: 1.9 ± 0.5 M-A: 0.9-1.4 M-C: 0.4-1.4 ↔ Preg,[c] RD[c] ↑ Smk ↓ Aged	N-A: 1.8 ± 0.4 M-A: 1.0-1.7 M-C: 1.2-1.7 ↓ Preg[c] ↔ RD[c]	N-A: 11 ± 2 M-A: 11-18 M-C: 12-16 ↓ Preg,[c] Smk ↔ RD[c] ↑ Hep, Aged	PO: 3.5-8.4[d]	Adults IV: 11 ± 2 μg/mL[d] PO: 7.3-9.4 μg/mL[d] Children IV: 8.7-9.4 μg/mL[d] PO: 7.3 ± 1.1 μg/mL[d]

[a]Data from normal adults (N-A) and range of means from different studies of adults (M-A) or children (M-C) with malaria reported. [b]Correlates with serum α_1-acid glycoprotein levels. Binding is increased in severe malaria. [c]From patients with malaria. [d]Following a single 10-mg/kg dose given as a 0.5- to 4-hour IV infusion or orally (PO) to children or adults with malaria. A level >0.2 μg/mL for unbound drug is targeted for treatment of *falciparum* malaria. Oculotoxicity and hearing loss/tinnitus associated with unbound concentrations >2 μg/mL.

References: Edwards G, et al. Clinical pharmacokinetics in the treatment of tropical diseases. Some applications and limitations. *Clin Pharmacokinet,* **1994**, *27*:150–165. Krishna S, et al. Pharmacokinetics of quinine, chloroquine and amodiaquine. Clinical implications. *Clin Pharmacokinet,* **1996**, *30*:263–299.

Rabebrazole[a]							
52[b]	0[b]	95-98	4.2 ± 1.2[c]	0.37[c]	1.0 ± 0.6[c]	3.8-4.6	EM: 437 ± 241 ng/mL[d] PM: 600 ± 319 ng/mL[d]

[a]Rabeprazole is primarily converted non-enzymatically to rabeprazole-thioether; some of it is oxidized to desmethylrabeprazole and rabeprazole sulfone by CYP2C19 and CYP3A4, respectively. CYP2C19 genetic polymorphism has a modest effect on rabeprazole clearance. Rabeprazole possesses an asymmetric sulfur center; the enantiomers inhibit H^+/K^+-ATPase with equal potency *in vitro*. [b]~90% of radiolabeled oral dose is recovered in urine, indicating near-complete gastrointestinal absorption. Incomplete systemic availability is due to instability and first-pass metabolism of rabeprazole. [c]Based on data from a 20-mg IV dose of rabeprazole in subjects with unknown CYP2C19 genotype or phenotype, most likely reflecting characteristics of extensive metabolizers (EM). Elimination $t_{1/2}$ up to 2-3 hours has been observed in poor metabolizers (PM) of CYP2C19 following oral rabeprazole. [d]At steady state during a 20-mg once-a-day regimen for duodenal ulcer.

References: Yasuda S, et al. Comparison of the kinetic disposition and metabolism of E3810, a new proton pump inhibitor, and omeprazole in relation to S-mephenytoin 4′-hydroxylation status. *Clin Pharmacol Ther*, **1995**, *58*:143–154. Yasuda S, et al. Pharmacokinetic properties of E3810, a new proton pump inhibitor, in healthy male volunteers. *Int J Clin Pharmacol Ther*, **1994**, *32*:466–473. Setoyama T, et al. Mass balance study of [^{14}C] rabeprazole following oral administration in healthy subjects. *Int J Clin Pharmacol Ther*, **2006**, *44*:557–565. Setoyama T, et al. Pharmacokinetics of rabeprazole following single intravenous and oral administration to healthy subjects. *Int J Clin Pharmacol Ther*, **2005**, *43*:37–42.

Raloxifene[a]							
2[b]	<0.2	>95	735 ± 338[c] ↔ RD, Aged ↓ LD	2348 ± 1220[c]	28 (11-273)	6[d]	0.5 ± 0.3 ng/mL[d]

[a]Data from postmenopausal women. Undergoes extensive first-pass metabolism (UGT catalyzed) and enterohepatic recycling. [b]~60% absorption from the gastrointestinal tract; not significantly affected by food. [c]*CL/F* and *V/F* reported for an oral dose. [d]Following a single 1-mg/kg oral dose.

References: Hochner-Celnikier D. Pharmacokinetics of raloxifene and its clinical application. *Eur J Obstet Gynecol Reprod Biol*, **1999**, *85*:23–29. *PDR*54, **2000**, p. 1583.

Raltegravir[a]							
≥31.8 ± 9.4[b]	8.8 ± 4.7	83	16.1 (11.4, 22.6)[c] ↔ RD ↑ Hemodialysis ↔ LD (modest)		α: 0.92 ± 0.21[d] β: 12.5 ± 4.6[d]	1.0[e]	4.5 (2.0, 10.2) μM[e]

[a]Raltegravir undergoes *O*-glucuronidation mediated largely by UGT1A1 and to a lesser extent by UGT1A3 and UGT1A9. Raltegravir AUC is only modestly elevated in individuals with *UGT1A1*28/*28* genotype compared to **1/*1* genotype. [b]The absolute oral bioavailability of raltegravir has not been determined. This minimum extent of oral absorption is based upon recovery of radioactivity in urine following oral administration of ^{14}C-labeled raltegravir in healthy human subjects. [c]Geometric mean (95% confidence interval) of pharmacokinetic parameters following a single 400-mg oral dose. Apparent oral clearance (*CL/F*) is listed. [d]Plasma concentration time course of raltegravir exhibits multiphasic washout kinetics. Initial (α) and terminal (β) $t_{1/2}$s are reported because the early phase accounts for a large portion of the AUC from time 0 to ∞. [e]Median for T_{max} and geometric mean (95% confidence interval) for C_{max} following a 400-mg twice-daily monotherapy regimen for 10 days in treatment-naive patients with HIV-1 infection.

References: Drugs@FDA. Isentress label approved on 7/8/09. Available at: http://www.accessdata.fda.gov/Scripts/cder/DrugsatFDA/. Accessed on August 22, 2009. Kassahun K, et al. Metabolism and disposition in humans of raltegravir (MK-0518), an anti-AIDS drug targeting the human immunodeficiency virus 1 integrase enzyme. *Drug Metab Dispos*, **2007**, *35*:1657–1663. Wenning LA, et al. Lack of a significant drug interaction between raltegravir and tenofovir. *Antimicrob Agents Chemother*, **2008**, *52*:3253–3258. Wenning LA, et al. Pharmacokinetics of raltegravir in individuals with UGT1A1 polymorphisms. *Clin Pharmacol Ther*, **2009**, *85*:623–627.

(*Continued*)

Table AII–1

Pharmacokinetic Data (*Continued*)

BIOAVAILABILITY (ORAL) (%)	URINARY EXCRETION (%)	BOUND IN PLASMA (%)	CLEARANCE (mL/min/kg)	VOL. DIST. (L/kg)	HALF-LIFE (hours)	PEAK TIME (hours)	PEAK CONCENTRATION
Ramelteon[a]							
1.8[b]	<0.1%	82	883 ± 857[c] ↓ Aged ↓ LD[d] ↔ RD		P: 1.3 ± 0.5[e] M: 2.3 ± 0.5[e] ↑ Aged	P: 1.6 ± 0.5	P: 6.9 ± 7.8 ng/mL[e,f] M: 110 ± 29 ng/mL[e,f] ↑ Aged

[a]Ramelteon undergoes primary oxidative metabolism followed by glucuronidation as secondary metabolism. CYP1A2 is the major enzyme involved in oxidative metabolism; CYP3A and CYP2C9 also are involved as minor enzymes. Remarkable elevation in C_{max} and AUC were observed with the concurrent administration of the strong CYP1A2 inhibitor fluvoxamine. The M-II metabolite contributes to the hypnotic effects of ramelteon. M-II has 1/5th to 1/10th the affinity of ramelteon as an agonist for the melatonin receptors (MT-1 and MT-2); however, it circulates at 20- to 100-fold higher concentrations relative to ramelteon. [b]Poor systemic availability of ramelteon is due to extensive first-pass metabolism. C_{max} and AUC are elevated by a high-fat meal; T_{max} is slightly delayed. [c]Intersubject variability is notably large.

[d]Four- and 10-fold elevation in AUC in mild and moderate hepatic impairment. [e]P = parent drug; M = M-II metabolite. [f]C_{max} following a single 16-mg oral dose of ramelteon in young adult subjects. There is no measurable accumulation of parent drug or active metabolite because of their short elimination $t_{1/2}$.

References: Drugs@FDA. Rozerem label approved on 10/20/08. Available at: http://www.accessdata.fda.gov/scripts/cder/drugsatfda/index.cfm. Accessed on August 23, 2009. Greenblatt DJ, et al. Age and gender effects on the pharmacokinetics and pharmacodynamics of ramelteon, a hypnotic agent acting via melatonin receptors MT 1 and MT2. *J Clin Pharmacol*, **2006**, *47*:485–496. McGechan A, et al. Ramelteon. *CNS Drugs*, **2005**, *19*:1057–1065.

BIOAVAILABILITY (ORAL) (%)	URINARY EXCRETION (%)	BOUND IN PLASMA (%)	CLEARANCE (mL/min/kg)	VOL. DIST. (L/kg)	HALF-LIFE (hours)	PEAK TIME (hours)	PEAK CONCENTRATION
Ramipril[a]							
R (R): 28[b]	R (R): <2[c]	R: 73 ± 2	R (R): 23[d]	—	R (R): 5 ± 2	R (R): 1.2 ± 0.3[g]	R (R): 43.3 ± 10.2 ng/mL[g]
RT (R): 48[b]	RT (R): 13 ± 6[c]	RT: 56 ± 2	RT: —[e]		RT (R): 9-18[f] ↑ RD	RT (R): 3.0 ± 0.7[g]	RT (R): 24.1 ± 5.6 ng/mL[g]

[a]Hydrolyzed to its active metabolite, ramiprilat (RT). Pharmacokinetic data for ramipril (R) and RT following oral and IV R administration are presented. [b]Based on plasma AUC of R and RT after IV and oral R administration. [c]Following an oral dose of R. [d]*CL/F* of R calculated from reported AUC data. [e]No data available; mean renal *CL* of RT is ~1.1 mL/min/kg. [f]$t_{1/2}$ for the elimination phase reported. A longer terminal $t_{1/2}$ of ~120 hours most likely corresponds to the release of drug from ACE; contributes to the duration of effect, but does not contribute to systemic drug accumulation. [g]Following a single 10-mg oral dose.

References: Eckert HG, et al. Pharmacokinetics and biotransformation of 2-[N-[(S)-l-ethoxycarbonyl-3-phenylpropyl]-L-alanyl]-(lS,3S,5S)-2-azabicyclo [3.3.0]octane-3-carboxylic acid (Hoe 498) in rat, dog and man. *Arzneimittelforschung,* **1984**, *34*:1435–1447. Meisel S, et al. Clinical pharmacokinetics of ramipril. *Clin Pharmacokinet,* **1994**, *26*:7–15. *PDR*58, **2004**, p. 2142. Song JC, et al. Clinical pharmacokinetics and selective pharmacodynamics of new angiotensin converting enzyme inhibitors: An update. *Clin Pharmacokinet,* **2002**, *41*:207–224. Thuillez C, et al. Pharmacokinetics, converting enzyme inhibition and peripheral arterial hemodynamics of ramipril in healthy volunteers. *Am J Cardiol,* **1987**, 59:38D–44D.

BIOAVAILABILITY (ORAL) (%)	URINARY EXCRETION (%)	BOUND IN PLASMA (%)	CLEARANCE (mL/min/kg)	VOL. DIST. (L/kg)	HALF-LIFE (hours)	PEAK TIME (hours)	PEAK CONCENTRATION
Ranitidine							
52 ± 11 ↑ LD ↔ RD	69 ± 6 ↓ RD	15 ± 3	10.4 ± 1.1 ↓ RD, Aged ↓ Burn	1.3 ± 0.4 ↔ Cirr, RD ↓ Burn	2.1 ± 0.2 ↑ RD, Cirr, Aged ↔ Burn	2.1 ± 0.31[a]	462 ± 54 ng/mL[a]

[a]Following a single 150-mg oral dose given to healthy adults. IC_{50} for inhibition of gastric acid secretion is 100 ng/mL.

Reference: Gladziwa U, et al. Pharmacokinetics and pharmacodynamics of H_2-receptor antagonists in patients with renal insufficiency. *Clin Pharmacokinet,* **1993**, *24*:319–332.

Remifentanil[a]							
—[b]	Negligible	92	40-60 ↔ RD, LD ↓ Aged[c]	0.3-0.4 ↓ Aged[c] ↔ RD, LD	0.13-0.33 ↔ RD, LD	—	~20 ng/mL[d]

[a]Data from healthy adult male subjects and patients undergoing elective surgery. Undergoes rapid inactivation by esterase-mediated hydrolysis; resulting carboxy metabolite has low activity. [b]For IV administration only. [c]*CL* and *V* decreased slightly in the elderly. [d]Mean CL_{min} following a 5-μg/kg IV dose (1-minute infusion). Cp_{50} for skin incision is 2 ng/mL (determined in the presence of nitrous oxide).

References: Egan TD, et al. Remifentanil pharmacokinetics in obese versus lean patients. *Anesthesiology*, **1998**, *89*:562–573. Glass PS, et al. A review of the pharmacokinetics and pharmacodynamics of remifentanil. *Anesth Analg*, **1999**, *89*:S7–S14.

Repaglinide[a]							
56 ± 7	0.3-2.6	97.4	9.3 ± 6.8 ↓ RD,[b] LD[c]	0.52 ± 0.17	0.8 ± 0.2 ↓ LD	0.25-0.75[d]	47 ± 24 ng/mL[d]

[a]Data from healthy adult male subjects. Undergoes extensive oxidative and conjugative metabolism; CYP3A4 has been implicated in the formation of the major (60% of dose) metabolite. [b]*CL/F* reduced, severe renal impairment. [c]*CL/F* reduced, moderate to severe LD. [d]Following a single 4-mg oral dose (tablet).

References: Hatorp V, et al. Single-dose pharmacokinetics of repaglinide in subjects with chronic liver disease. *J Clin Pharmacol*, **2000**, *40*:142–152. Hatorp V, et al. Unavailability of repaglinide, a novel antidiabetic agent, administered orally in tablet or solution form or intravenously in healthy male volunteers. *Int J Clin Pharmacol Ther*, **1998**, *36*:636–641. Marbury TC, et al. Pharmacokinetics of repaglinide in subjects with renal impairment. *Clin Pharmacol Ther*, **2000**, *67*:7–15. van Heiningen PN, et al. Absorption, metabolism and excretion of a single oral dose of ^{14}C-repaglinide during repaglinide multiple dosing. *Eur J Clin Pharmacol*, **1999**, *55*:521–525.

Ribavirin[a]							
45 ± 5	35 ± 8	0[b]	5.0 ± 1.0[c]	9.3 ± 1.5	28 ± 7[c]	RT: 3 ± 1.8[d]	R: 11.1 ± 1.2 μM[d] RT: 15.1 ± 12.8 μM[d]

[a]Values reported for studies conducted in asymptomatic HIV-positive men. [b]At steady state, red blood cell–to-plasma concentration ratio is ~60. [c]Following multiple oral dosing, *CL/F* decreases by >50%, and a long terminal $t_{1/2}$ of 150 ± 50 hours is observed. [d]Following a 1200-mg oral ribavirin capsule (R) given daily for 7 days to adult subjects seropositive for HIV or a 600-mg oral REBETRON dose given twice daily to steady state to adults with hepatitis C infection.

References: Morse GD, et al. Single-dose pharmacokinetics of delavirdine mesylate and didanosine in patients with human immunodeficiency virus infection. *Antimicrob Agents Chemother*, **1997**, *47*:169–174. *PDR54*, **2000**, p. 2836. Roberts RB, et al. Ribavirin pharmacodynamics in high-risk patients for acquired immunodeficiency syndrome. *Clin Pharmacol Ther*, **1987**, *42*:365–373.

Rifampin[a]							
—[b]	7 ± 3 ↑ Neo	60-90	3.5 ± 1.6[c] ↑ Neo, ↓ RD[d] ↔ Aged	0.97 ± 0.36 ↑ Neo ↔ Aged	3.5 ± 0.8[c] ↑ Hep, Cirr, AVH, RD[d] ↔ Child, Aged	1-3[e]	6.5 ± 3.5 μg/mL[e]

[a]Active desacetyl metabolite. [b]Absolute bioavailability is not unknown, although some studies indicate complete absorption. Such reports presumably refer to rifampin plus its desacetyl metabolite because considerable first-pass metabolism is expected. [c]$t_{1/2}$ is shorter (1.7 ± 0.5) and *CL/F* is higher after repeated administration. Rifampin is a potent enzyme (CYP3A and others) inducer and appears to autoinduce its own metabolism. [d]Not observed with 300-mg doses, but pronounced differences with 900-mg doses. $t_{1/2}$ is longer with high single doses. [e]Following a 600-mg dose given once daily for 15-18 days to patients with tuberculosis.

Reference: Israili ZH, et al. Pharmacokinetics of antituberculosis drugs in patients. *J Clin Pharmacol*, **1987**, *27*:78–83.

(*Continued*)

Table AII–1

Pharmacokinetic Data (*Continued*)

BIOAVAILABILITY (ORAL) (%)	URINARY EXCRETION (%)	BOUND IN PLASMA (%)	CLEARANCE (mL/min/kg)	VOL. DIST. (L/kg)	HALF-LIFE (hours)	PEAK TIME (hours)	PEAK CONCENTRATION
Riluzole[a]							
64 (30-100) ↓ Food[b]	<1	98	5.5 ± 0.9 ↓ LD	3.4 ± 0.6	14 ± 6	0.8 ± 0.5[c]	173 ± 72 ng/mL[c]

[a]Eliminated primarily by CYPIA2-dependent metabolism; metabolites are inactive. Involvement of CYP1A2 may contribute to ethnic (lower *CL/F* in Japanese) and gender (lower *CL* in women) differences and inductive effects of smoking (higher *CL* in smokers). [b]High-fat meal. [c]Following a 50-mg oral dose given twice daily to steady state.

References: Bruno R, et al. Population pharmacokinetics of riluzole in patients with amyotrophic lateral sclerosis. *Clin Pharmacol Ther,* **1997**, *62*:518–526. Le Liboux A, et al. Single- and multiple-dose pharmacokinetics of riluzole in white subjects. *J Clin Pharmacol,* **1997**, *37*:820–827. *PDR*58, **2004**, p. 769. Wokke J. Riluzole. *Lancet,* **1996**, *348*:795–799.

BIOAVAILABILITY (ORAL) (%)	URINARY EXCRETION (%)	BOUND IN PLASMA (%)	CLEARANCE (mL/min/kg)	VOL. DIST. (L/kg)	HALF-LIFE (hours)	PEAK TIME (hours)	PEAK CONCENTRATION
Risperidone[a]							
PO: 66 ± 28[b] IM: 103 ± 13	3 ± 2[b]	89[c]	5.4 ± 1.4[b] ↓ RD,[a] Aged[d]	1.1 ± 0.2	3.2 ± 0.8[a,b] ↑ RD,[a] Aged[d]	R: ~1[e]	R: 10 ng/mL[e] TA: 45 ng/mL[e]

[a]The active metabolite, 9-hydroxyrisperidone, is the predominant circulating species in extensive metabolizers and is equipotent to parent drug. 9-Hydroxyrisperidone has a $t_{1/2}$ of 20 ± 3 hours. In extensive metabolizers, 35 ± 7% of an IV dose is excreted as this metabolite; its elimination is primarily renal and therefore correlates with renal function. [b]Formation of 9-hydroxyrisperidone is catalyzed by CYP2D6. Parameters reported for extensive metabolizers. In poor metabolizers, *F* is higher; ~20% of an IV dose is excreted unchanged, 10% as the 9-hydroxy metabolite; *CL* is slightly <1 mL/min/kg, and $t_{1/2}$ is similar to that of the active metabolite, ~20 hours. [c]77% for 9-hydroxyrisperidone. [d]Changes in elderly subjects due to decreased renal function affecting the elimination of the active metabolite. [e]Mean steady-state C_{min} for risperidone (R) and total active (TA) drug, risperidone + 9-OH-risperidone, following a 3-mg oral dose given twice daily to patients with chronic schizophrenia. No difference in total active drug levels between CYP2D6 extensive and poor metabolizers.

References: Cohen LJ. Risperidone. *Pharmacotherapy,* **1994**, *14*:253–265. Heykants J, et al. The pharmacokinetics of risperidone in humans: A summary. *J Clin Psychiatry,* **1994**, *55*(suppl):13–17.

BIOAVAILABILITY (ORAL) (%)	URINARY EXCRETION (%)	BOUND IN PLASMA (%)	CLEARANCE (mL/min/kg)	VOL. DIST. (L/kg)	HALF-LIFE (hours)	PEAK TIME (hours)	PEAK CONCENTRATION
Ritonavir[a]							
—[b] ↑ Food	3.5 ± 1.8	98-99	SD: 1.2 ± 0.4[c] MD: 2.1 ± 0.8[c] ↓ Child, LD[d]	0.41 ± 0.25[c]	3-5[c] ↓ LD[d]	2-4[e]	11 ± 4 μg/mL[e]

[a]Ritonavir is extensively metabolized primarily by CYP3A4. It also appears to induce its own *CL* with single-dose (SD) to multiple-dose (MD) administration. [b]Absolute bioavailability unknown (>60% absorbed); food elicits a 15% increase in oral AUC for capsule formulation. [c]CL/F, V_{area}/F, and $t_{1/2}$ reported for oral dose. [d]CL/F reduced slightly and $t_{1/2}$ increased slightly, moderate liver impairment. [e]Following a 600-mg oral dose given twice daily to steady state.

References: Hsu A, et al. Ritonavir. Clinical pharmacokinetics and interactions with other anti-HIV agents. *Clin Pharmacokinet,* **1998**, *35*:275–291. *PDR*54, **2000**, p. 465.

Rivastigmine[a]							
72 (22-119)[b] ↑ Food, Dose	Negligible	40	13 ± 4[c]	1.5 ± 0.6[c]	1.4 ± 0.4[c,d]	1.2 ± 1.0[e] ↓ Food	26 ± 10 ng/mL[e] ↓ Food

[a]Rivastigmine is metabolized by cholinesterase. No apparent gender differences. [b]Following a 6-mg oral dose. Bioavailability increases with dose; following a 3-mg dose, the median bioavailability is 36%. [c]IV dose of 2 mg. [d]The pharmacodynamic $t_{1/2}$ is ~10 hours due to tight binding to acetylcholinesterase. [e]Following oral administration of a 6-mg capsule. C_{max} increases more than proportionally at doses >3 mg.

References: Hossain M, et al. Estimation of the absolute bioavailability of rivastigmine in patients with mild to moderate dementia of the Alzheimer's type. *Clin Pharmacokinet,* **2002**, *41*:225–234. Williams BR, et al. A review of rivastigmine: A reversible cholinesterase inhibitor. *Clin Ther,* **2003**, 25:1634–1653.

Rizatriptan[a]							
47	F: 28 ± 9[b] M: 29[b]	14	F: 12.3 ± 1.4[b] M: 18.9 ± 2.8[b] ↓ LD,[c] RD[d]	F: 1.5 ± 0.2 M: 2.2 ± 0.4	F: 2.2 M: 2.4	SD: 0.9 ± 0.4[e] MD: 4.8 ± 0.7[e]	SD: 20 ± 4.9 ng/mL[e] MD: 37 ± 13 ng/mL[e]

[a]Data from healthy adult male (M) and female (F) subjects. Oxidative deamination catalyzed by MAO-A is the primary route of elimination. *N*-desmethyl rizatriptan (DMR) is a minor metabolite (~14%) that is active and accumulates in blood. [b]Evidence of minor dose-dependent metabolic *CL* and urinary excretion. [c]*CL/F* reduced, moderate hepatic impairment. [d]*CL/F* reduced, severe renal impairment. [e]Following a 10-mg single (SD) and multiple (MD) oral dose (10 mg every 2 hours × 3 doses × 4 days). DMR C_{max} is 8.5 and 26.2 ng/mL with SD and MD, respectively.

References: Goldberg MR, et al. Rizatriptan, a novel 5-$HT_{1B/1D}$ agonist for migraine: Single- and multiple-dose tolerability and pharmacokinetics in healthy subjects. *J Clin Pharmacol,* **2000**, *40*:74–83. Lee Y, et al. Pharmacokinetics and tolerability of intravenous rizatriptan in healthy females. *Biopharm Drug Dispos,* **1998**, *19*:577–581. *PDR*54, **2000**, p. 1912. Vyas KP, et al. Disposition and pharmacokinetics of the antimigraine drug, rizatriptan, in humans. *Drug Metab Dispos,* **2000**, *28*:89–95.

Ropinirole[a]							
55	<10	~40	11.2 ± 5.0[b] ↓ Aged[c] ↔ RD	7.5 ± 2.4[b]	6[b]	1.0 (0.5-6.0)[d] ↑ Food	7.4 (2.4-13) ng/mL[d] ↓ Food

[a]Data from male and female patients with Parkinson's disease. Metabolized primarily by CYP1A2 to inactive *N*-deisopropyl and hydroxy metabolites. [b]*CL/F*, V_d/F, and $t_{1/2}$ reported for oral dose. [c]*CL/F* reduced but dose titrated to desired effect. [d]Following a 2-mg oral dose given three times daily to steady state.

References: Bloomer JC, et al. In vitro identification of the P450 enzymes responsible for the metabolism of ropinirole. *Drug Metab Dispos,* **1997**, *25*:840–844. *PDR*54, **2000**, p. 3037. Taylor AC, et al. Lack of a pharmacokinetic interaction at steady state between ropinirole and L-dopa in patients with Parkinson's disease. *Pharmacotherapy,* **1999**, *79*:150–156.

Rosiglitazone[a]							
99	Negligible	99.8 ↓ LD[b]	0.68 ± 0.16[c] (0.49) ↓ LD[d] ↔ RD	0.25 ± 0.08[c] (0.21)	3-4[c] ↓ LD	1.0[d]	598 ± 117 ng/mL[d]

[a]Data from male and female patients with NIDDM. No significant gender differences. Metabolized primarily by CYP2C8. [b]Reduced *CL/F* and $CL/F_{unbound}$, moderate to severe liver impairment. [c]*CL/F*, V_d/F, and $t_{1/2}$ reported for oral dose. Shown in parentheses are mean values from a population pharmacokinetic analysis. [d]Following a single 8-mg oral dose.

References: Baldwin SJ, et al. Characterization of the cytochrome P450 enzymes involved in the in vitro metabolism of rosiglitazone. *Br J Clin Pharmacol,* **1999**, *48*:424–432. Patel BR, et al. Population pharmacokinetics of rosiglitazone (R) in phase III clinical trials. *Clin Pharmacol Ther,* **2000**, *67*:123. *PDR*54, **2000**, p. 2981. Thompson K, et al. Pharmacokinetics of rosiglitazone are unaltered in hemodialysis patients [abstract]. *Clin Pharmacol Ther,* **1999**, *65*:186.

(*Continued*)

Table AII–1

Pharmacokinetic Data (*Continued*)

BIOAVAILABILITY (ORAL) (%)	URINARY EXCRETION (%)	BOUND IN PLASMA (%)	CLEARANCE (mL/min/kg)	VOL. DIST. (L/kg)	HALF-LIFE (hours)	PEAK TIME (hours)	PEAK CONCENTRATION
Rosuvastatin[a]							
20 (17-23)	30 ± 7	88	10.5 ± 4.7 ↓ RD[b]	1.7 ± 0.5	20 ± 6	3 (1-6)[c]	4.6 ± 2.1 ng/mL[c]

[a]Eliminated primarily by biliary excretion; also appears to be actively transported into the liver by an organic anion transport protein (OATP2/SLC21A6). Data from healthy men reported; no significant gender or age differences. [b]Reduced *CL/F* in patients with severe renal impairment. [c]Following a 10-mg oral dose taken once daily for 10 days.
References: Martin PD, et al. Absolute oral bioavailability of rosuvastatin in healthy white adult male volunteers. *Clin Ther,* **2003**, *25*:2553–2563. Martin PD, et al. Pharmacodynamic effects and pharmacokinetics of a new HMG-CoA reductase inhibitor, rosuvastatin, after morning or evening administration in healthy volunteers. *Br J Clin Pharmacol,* **2002**, *54*:472–477. Product labeling: Crestor® tablets (rosuvastatin calcium). Wilmington, DE, Astra-Zeneca Pharmaceuticals LP, **2003**. Schneck DW, et al. The effect of gemfibrozil on the pharmacokinetics of rosuvastatin. *Clin Pharmacol Ther,* **2004**, *75*:455–463.

BIOAVAILABILITY (ORAL) (%)	URINARY EXCRETION (%)	BOUND IN PLASMA (%)	CLEARANCE (mL/min/kg)	VOL. DIST. (L/kg)	HALF-LIFE (hours)	PEAK TIME (hours)	PEAK CONCENTRATION
Selegiline[a]							
Negligible[b]	Negligible	94[c]	~1500[b] 160[d]	1.9	1.91 ± 1.0[e]	S: 0.7 ± 0.4[f] DS: ~1 hr	S: 1.1 ± 0.4 ng/mL[f] DS: ~15 ng/mL[f]

[a]MAO-B active metabolite: *l*-(–)-desmethylselegiline. [b]Extensive first-pass metabolism; estimate of *CL/F* reported. [c]Blood-to-plasma concentration ratio = 1.3-2.2 for parent drug and ~0.55 for *N*-desmethyl metabolite. [d]*CL/F* for *N*-desmethylselegiline, assuming quantitative conversion of parent to this metabolite. [e]For parent and *N*-desmethyl metabolite. $t_{1/2}$s for methamphetamine (major plasma species) and amphetamine are 21 and 18 hours, respectively. [f]Mean data for selegiline (S) and its active metabolite, *N*-desmethylselegiline (DS), following a single 10-mg oral dose given to adults.

Reference: Heinonen EH, et al. Pharmacokinetic aspects of *l*-deprenyl (selegiline) and its metabolites. *Clin Pharmacol Ther*, **1994**, *56*:742–749.

BIOAVAILABILITY (ORAL) (%)	URINARY EXCRETION (%)	BOUND IN PLASMA (%)	CLEARANCE (mL/min/kg)	VOL. DIST. (L/kg)	HALF-LIFE (hours)	PEAK TIME (hours)	PEAK CONCENTRATION
Sertraline							
—[a]	<1	98-99	38 ± 14[b] ↓ Aged, LD	—	23 ↑ Aged, LD	M: 6.9 ± 1.0[c] F: 6.7 ± 1.8[c]	M: 118 ± 22 ng/mL[c] F: 166 ± 65 ng/mL[c] ↔ Aged

[a]Absolute bioavailability is not known (>44% absorbed); undergoes extensive first-pass metabolism to essentially inactive metabolites; catalyzed by multiple CYP isoforms. [b]*CL/F* reported. [c]Following a dose titration up to 200 mg given once daily for 30 days to healthy male (M) and female (F) adults.

References: van Harten J. Clinical pharmacokinetics of selective serotonin reuptake inhibitors. *Clin Pharmacokinet*, **1993**, *24*:203–220. Warrington SJ. Clinical implications of the pharmacology of sertraline. *Int Clin Psychopharmacol*, **1994**, *6*(suppl 2):11–21.

BIOAVAILABILITY (ORAL) (%)	URINARY EXCRETION (%)	BOUND IN PLASMA (%)	CLEARANCE (mL/min/kg)	VOL. DIST. (L/kg)	HALF-LIFE (hours)	PEAK TIME (hours)	PEAK CONCENTRATION
Sildenafil[a]							
38	0	96	6.0 ± 1.1 ↓ LD,[b] RD,[c] Aged	1.2 ± 0.3	2.4 ± 1.0	1.2 ± 0.3[d]	212 ± 59 ng/mL[d] ↑ Aged[d]

[a]Data from healthy male subjects. Sildenafil is metabolized primarily by CYP3A and secondarily by CYP2C9. Piperazine *N*-desmethyl metabolite is active (~50% parent) and accumulates in plasma (~40% parent). [b]*CL/F* reduced, mild to moderate hepatic impairment. [c]*CL/F* reduced, severe renal impairment. Increased unbound concentrations. [d]Following a single 50-mg oral (solution) dose.

*References: PDR*54, **2000**, p. 2382. Walker DK, et al. Pharmacokinetics and metabolism of sildenafil in mouse, rat, rabbit, dog and man. *Xenobiotica,* **1999**, *29*:297–310.

Simvastatin[a]							
≤5	Negligible	94	7.6[b]	—	2-3	AI: 1.4 ± 1.0[c] TI: 1.4 ± 1.0[c]	AI: 46 ± 20 ngEq/mL[c] TI: 56 ± 25 ngEq/mL[c]

[a]Simvastatin is a lactone prodrug that is hydrolyzed to the active corresponding β-hydroxy acid. Values reported are for the disposition of the acid. [b]The β-hydroxy acid can be reconverted back to the lactone; irreversible oxidative metabolites are generated by CYP3A. [c]Data for active inhibitors (AI, ring-opened molecule) and total inhibitors (TI) following a 40-mg oral dose given once daily for 17 days to healthy adults.

References: Corsini A, et al. New insights into the pharmacodynamic and pharmacokinetic properties of statins. *Pharmacol Ther*, **1999**, *84*:413–428. Desager JP, et al. Clinical pharmacokinetics of 3-hydroxy-3-methylglutaryl-coenzyme A reductase inhibitors. *Clin Pharmacokinet*, **1996**, *31*:348–371. Mauro VF. Clinical pharmacokinetics and practical applications of simvastatin. *Clin Pharmacokinet*, **1993**, *24*:195–202.

Sirolimus[a]							
~15[b] ↑ Food[b]	—	40[c]	3.47 ± 1.58[d]	12 ± 4.6[d]	62.3 ± 16.2[d]	SD: 0.81 ± 0.17[e] MD: 1.4 ± 1.2[e]	SD: 67 ± 23 ng/mL[e] MD: 94-210 ng/mL[e]

[a]Data from male and female renal transplant patients. All subjects were on a stable cyclosporine regimen. Sirolimus is metabolized primarily by CYP3A and is a substrate for P-glycoprotein. Several sirolimus metabolites are pharmacologically active. [b]Cyclosporine co-administration increases sirolimus bioavailability. *F* increased by high-fat meal. [c]Concentrates in blood cells; blood-to-plasma concentration ratio ~38 ± 13. [d]Blood *CL/F*, V_{ss}/F, and $t_{1/2}$ reported for oral dose. [e]Following a single 15-mg oral dose (SD) in healthy subjects and 4- to 6.5-mg/m^2 oral dose (with cyclosporine) given twice daily to steady state (MD) in renal transplant patients.

References: Kelly PA, et al. Conversion from liquid to solid rapamycin formulations in stable renal allograft transplant recipients. *Biopharm Drug Dispos*, **1999**, *20*:249–253. Zimmerman JJ, et al. Pharmacokinetics of sirolimus in stable renal transplant patients after multiple oral dose administration. *J Clin Pharmacol*, **1997**, *37*:405–415. Zimmerman JJ, et al. The effect of a high-fat meal on the oral bioavailability of the immunosuppressant sirolimus (rapamycin). *J Clin Pharmacol*, **1999**, *39*:1155–1161.

Sitagliptin[a]							
87 ± 5.2	73.1 ± 15.9	38	4.42[b] ↓ RD[c] ↔ LD	–	13.9 ± 2.0	1.5 ± 1.3	1046 ± 286 nM[d]

[a]Cleared primarily by the kidney. [b]Renal clearance is ~350 mL/min, which indicates active tubular secretion, possibly mediated by human Organic Anion Transporter-3 (OAT3) and P-glycoprotein (ABCB1). [c]Apparent oral clearance increased by a respective 2.3-, 3.8- and 4.5-fold in patients with moderate (CL_{cr} = 30-50 mL/min) and severe (<30 mL/min) renal insufficiency and in patients with end-stage RD requiring hemodialysis. [d]Following a single 100-mg oral dose. Plasma AUC increased by ~14% following daily doses of 100 mg at steady state compared to the first dose.

References: Bergman A, et al. Absolute bioavailability of sitagliptin, an oral dipeptidyl peptidase-4 inhibitor, in healthy volunteers. *Biopharm Drug Dispos*, **2007**, *28*:315–22. Bergman AJ, et al. Effect of renal insufficiency on the pharmacokinetics of sitagliptin, a dipeptidyl peptidase-4 inhibitor. *Diabetes Care*, **2007**, *30*:1862–1864. Drugs@FDA. Januvia label approved on 7/22/08. Available at: http://www.accessdata.fda.gov/scripts/cder/drugsatfda/index.cfm. Accessed on December 26, 2009. Migoya EM, et al. Effect of moderate hepatic insufficiency on the pharmacokinetics of sitagliptin. *Can J Clin Pharmacol*, **2009**, *16*:e165–e170. Vincent SH, et al. Metabolism and excretion of the dipeptidyl peptidase 4 inhibitor [^{14}C]sitagliptin in humans. *Drug Metab Dispos*, **2007**, *35*:533–538.

(*Continued*)

Table AII–1

Pharmacokinetic Data (*Continued*)

BIOAVAILABILITY (ORAL) (%)	URINARY EXCRETION (%)	BOUND IN PLASMA (%)	CLEARANCE (mL/min/kg)	VOL. DIST. (L/kg)	HALF-LIFE (hours)	PEAK TIME (hours)	PEAK CONCENTRATION
Solifenacin[a]							
90	3-6	98%[b]	9.39 ± 2.68 ↓ LD, RD[c]	671 ± 118	52.4 ± 13.9 ↓ LD, RD[c]	4.2 ± 1.8[c]	40.6 ± 8.5 ng/mL[d]

[a]Solifenacin is extensively metabolized by CYP3A. The 4*R*-hydroxy-solifenacin metabolite is pharmacologically active but not likely to contribute to the therapeutic efficacy of solifenacin because of low circulating levels. [b]Primarily bound to α_1-acid glycoprotein. [c]Dosage reduction is advised in patients with severe renal impairment (CL_{cr} <30 mL/min), in whom a 2-fold reduction in clearance and prolongation in $t_{1/2}$ are expected. [d]At steady state following 21 days of dosing with 10 mg once daily.

References: Drugs@FDA. VESIcare label approved on 11/18/08. Available at: http://www.accessdata.fda.gov/scripts/cder/drugsatfda/index.cfm. Accessed on December 27, 2009. Kuipers M, et al. Open-label study of the safety and pharmacokinetics of solifenacin in subjects with hepatic impairment. *J Pharmacol Sci*, **2006**, *102*:405–412. Kuipers ME, et al. Solifenacin demonstrates high absolute bioavailability in healthy men. *Drugs*, **2004**, *5*:73–81. Smulders RA, et al. Pharmacokinetics and safety of solifenacin succinate in healthy young men. *J Clin Pharmacol*, **2004**, *44*:1023–1033. Smulders RA, et al. Pharmacokinetics, safety, and tolerability of solifenacin in patients with renal insufficiency. *J Pharmacol Sci*, **2007**, *103*:67–74.

BIOAVAILABILITY (ORAL) (%)	URINARY EXCRETION (%)	BOUND IN PLASMA (%)	CLEARANCE (mL/min/kg)	VOL. DIST. (L/kg)	HALF-LIFE (hours)	PEAK TIME (hours)	PEAK CONCENTRATION
Sorafenib[a]							
38-49[b]	Negligible	99.5	1.2-2.0[c] ↑ LD[d]		20-27[c]	2.0-12.1	5.4-10.0 μg/mL

[a]Sorafenib undergoes oxidative metabolism mediated by CYP3A and glucuronidation mediated by UGT1A9. [b]Oral bioavailability of NEXAVAR tablet relative to an oral solution. Sorafenib bioavailability reduced by 29% when administered with a high-fat meal. [c]Range of geometric means determined at steady state in three phase I studies in patients with advanced refractory solid tumors at the dose level of 400 mg two times a day. [d]Sorafenib AUCs were 23-63% lower in patients with mild and moderate hepatic impairment compared to patients with normal hepatic function.

References: Drugs@FDA. Nexavar label approved on 11-17-2007. Available at: http://www.accessdata.fda.gov/scripts/cder/drugsatfda/index.cfm. Accessed on December 27, 2009. Strumberg D, et al. Safety, pharmacokinetics, and preliminary antitumor activity of sorafenib: A review of four phase I trials in patients with advanced refractory solid tumors. *Oncologist*, **2007**, *12*:426–437.

BIOAVAILABILITY (ORAL) (%)	URINARY EXCRETION (%)	BOUND IN PLASMA (%)	CLEARANCE (mL/min/kg)	VOL. DIST. (L/kg)	HALF-LIFE (hours)	PEAK TIME (hours)	PEAK CONCENTRATION
Sotalol[a]							
60-100	70 ± 15	Negligible	2.20 ± 0.67 ↓ RD	1.21 ± 0.17	7.18 ± 1.30 ↑ RD	3.1 ± 0.6	1.0 ± 0.5 μg/mL[b]

[a]Sotalol is available as a racemate. The enantiomers contribute equally to sotalol's antiarrhythmic action; hence, pharmacokinetic parameters for total enantiomeric mixture is reported herein. β-adrenoreceptor blockade resides solely with *S*-(–)-isomer. [b]Following 80-mg, twice-a-day dosing to steady state.

References: Berglund G, et al. Pharmacokinetics of sotalol after chronic administration to patients with renal insufficiency. *Eur J Clin Pharmacol*, **1980**, *18*:321–326. Kimura M, et al. Pharmacokinetics and pharmacodynamics of (+)-sotalol in healthy male volunteers. *Br J Clin Pharmacol*, **1996**, *42*:583–588. Poirier JM, et al. The pharmacokinetics of d-sotalol and d,l-sotalol in healthy volunteers. *Eur J Clin Pharmacol*, **1990**, *38*:579–582.

Spironolactone[a]							
—[b] ↑ Food	<1[c]	>90[d]	93[e]	10[e]	S: 1.3 ± 0.3[f] C: 11.2 ± 2.3[f] TS: 2.8 ± 0.4[f] HTS: 10.1 ± 2.3[f] ↑ LD[g]	S: 1.0[f] C: 2.9 ± 0.6[f] TS: 1.8 ± 0.5[f] HTS: 3.1 ± 0.9[f]	S: 185 ± 51 ng/mL[f] C: 231 ± 49 ng/mL[f] TS: 571 ± 74 ng/mL[f] HTS: 202 ± 54 ng/mL[f]

[a]Spironolactone (S) is extensively metabolized; it has three known active metabolites: canrenone (C), 7α-thiomethylspironolactone (TS), and 6β-hydroxy-7α-thiomethylspironolactone (HTS). [b]Absolute bioavailability is not known; old values reported in the literature were based on nonspecific assays for C; likely to exhibit first-pass metabolism. AUC of parent drug and metabolites increased when S taken with food. [c]Measured after an oral dose. [d]Binding of S and its active metabolites. [e]*CL/F* and V_{area}/F; calculated from reported AUC and $t_{1/2}$ data. [f]Following a single 200-mg oral dose of S. C accumulates 2.5-fold with multiple S dosing. [g]$t_{1/2}$ of parent drug and metabolites increased in patients with cirrhosis.

References: Ho PC, et al. Pharmacokinetics of canrenone and metabolites after base hydrolysis following single and multiple dose oral administration of spironolactone. *Eur J Clin Pharmacol*, **1984**, *27*:441–446. Overdiek HW, et al. Influence of food on the bioavailability of spironolactone. *Clin Pharmacol Ther*, **1986**, *40*:531–536. Overdiek HW, et al. New insights into the pharmacokinetics of spironolactone. *Clin Pharmacol Ther*, **1985**, *38*:469–474. *PDR*54, **2000**, p. 2883. Sungaila I, et al. Spironolactone pharmacokinetics and pharmacodynamics in patients with cirrhotic ascites. *Gastroenterology*, **1992**, *102*:1680–1685.

Streptokinase[a]							
—	0	—	1.7 ± 0.7	0.08 ± 0.04[b]	0.61 ± 0.24	0.9 ± 0.21[c]	188 ± 58 IU/mL[c]

[a]Values obtained from acute MI patients using a function bioassay. [b]V_{area} reported. [c]Following a single 1.5 × 10⁶ IU IV dose given as a 60-minute infusion to patients with acute MI.

Reference: Gemmill JD, et al. A comparison of the pharmacokinetic properties of streptokinase and anistreplase in acute myocardial infarction. *Br J Clin Pharmacol*, **1991**, *31*:143–147.

Sulfamethoxazole							
~100	14 ± 2	53 ± 5 ↓ RD, Alb ↔ Aged, CF	0.31 ± 0.07[a,b] ↔ RD ↑ CF	0.26 ± 0.04[a] ↑ RD ↔ Child, CF	10.1 ± 2.6[a] ↑ RD ↔ Child ↓ CF	4[b]	37.1 μg/mL[b]

[a]Studies include concurrent administration of trimethoprim and variation in urinary pH; these factors had no marked effect on the *CL* of sulfamethoxazole. Metabolically cleared primarily by N_4-acetylation. [b]Following a single 1000-mg oral dose given to healthy adults.

References: Hutabarat RM, et al. Disposition of drugs in cystic fibrosis. I. Sulfamethoxazole and trimethoprim. *Clin Pharmacol Ther*, **1991**, *49*:402–409. Welling PO, et al. Pharmacokinetics of trimethoprim and sulfamethoxazole in normal subjects and in patients with renal failure. *J Infect Dis*, **1973**, *128*(suppl):556–566.

Sumatriptan							
PO: 14 ± 5 SC: 97 ± 16	22 ± 4	14-21	22 ± 5.4	2.0 ± 0.34	1.0 ± 0.3[a]	SC: 0.2 (0.1-0.3)[b] PO: ~1.5[b]	SC: 72 (55-108) ng/mL[b] PO: 54 (27-137) ng/mL[b]

[a]An apparent $t_{1/2}$ of ~2 hours reported for SC and oral doses. [b]Following a single 6-mg SC or 100-mg oral dose given to healthy young adults.

References: Scott AK. Sumatriptan clinical pharmacokinetics. *Clin Pharmacokinet*, **1994**, *27*:337–344. Scott AK, et al. Sumatriptan and cerebral perfusion in healthy volunteers. *Br J Clin Pharmacol*, **1992**, *33*:401–404.

(*Continued*)

Table AII–1

Pharmacokinetic Data (*Continued*)

BIOAVAILABILITY (ORAL) (%)	URINARY EXCRETION (%)	BOUND IN PLASMA (%)	CLEARANCE (mL/min/kg)	VOL. DIST. (L/kg)	HALF-LIFE (hours)	PEAK TIME (hours)	PEAK CONCENTRATION
Sunitinib[a]							
—[b]	~9[c]	P: 90 M: 95	7.3-14.8[d]	4.0[d]	40-60[e]	P: 6.0 (0-8.3) M: 6.0 (0-24)	P: 91.9 ± 42.3 ng/mL[f] M: 25.1 ± 11.0 ng/mL[f]
Tacrolimus							
25 ± 10[a,b] ↔ RD ↓ Food	<1	75-99[c]	0.90 ± 0.29[a] ↔ RD, LD	0.91 ± 0.29[a,d] ↔ RD ↑ LD	12 ± 5[a] ↔ RD ↑ LD	1.4 ± 0.5[e]	31.2 ± 10.1 ng/mL[e]
Tadalafil[a]							
—	—	94	0.59[b] ↓ RD[c]	0.89[b]	17.5	2[d]	378 ng/mL[d]

Sunitinib notes: [a]Sunitinib is metabolized primarily by CYP3A4 to produce its primary active metabolite (SU12662), which is further metabolized by CYP3A4. Plasma AUC of (SU12662) (M) is ~30% that of the parent drug (P) at steady state. [b]Data on absolute oral bioavailability is not available. [c]16% of a radioactive dose of [^{14}C]-sunitinib is recovered in urine, of which 86.4% is in the form of parent drug and active metabolite. [d]Average *CL/F* of 34-62 L/hr and V_{ss}/F of 2230 L in 135 healthy volunteers and 266 patients with solid tumors, and assuming an average body weight of 77.6 kg. [e]Population estimate in 73 volunteers and 517 cancer patients. [f]Steady-state concentrations during once-daily dosing of 50 mg.

References: Britten CD, et al. A phase I and pharmacokinetic study of sunitinib administered daily for 2 weeks, followed by a 1-week off period. *Cancer Chemother Pharmacol*, **2008**, *61*:515–24. Drugs@FDA. Sutent label approved on 2/2/07. Available at: http://www.accessdata.fda.gov/scripts/cder/drugsatfda/index.cfm. Accessed on December 30, 2009. Houk BE, et al. A population pharmacokinetic meta-analysis of sunitinib malate (SU11248) and its primary metabolite (SU12662) in healthy volunteers and oncology patients. *Clin Cancer Res*, **2009**, *15*:2497–2506.

Tacrolimus notes: [a]Drug disposition parameters calculated from blood concentrations. Data from liver transplant patients reported. Metabolized by CYP3A; also a substrate for P-glycoprotein. [b]A similar bioavailability (F = 21 ± 19%) reported for kidney transplant patients; F = 16 ± 7% for normal subjects. Low oral bioavailability likely due to incomplete intestinal availability. [c]Different values for plasma protein binding reported. Concentrates in blood cells; blood-to-plasma concentration ratio = 35 (12-67). [d]Slightly higher V_{ss} and $t_{1/2}$ reported for kidney transplant patients. Because of the very high and variable blood-to-plasma concentration ratio, markedly different V_{ss} values are reported for parameters based on plasma concentrations. [e]Following a single 7-mg oral dose given to healthy adults. Consensus target C_{min} at steady state are 5-20 ng/mL.

References: Bekersky I, et al. Dose linearity after oral administration of tacrolimus 1-mg capsules at doses of 3, 7, and 10 mg. *Clin Ther*, **1999**, *27*:2058–2064. Jusko WJ, et al. Pharmacokinetics of tacrolimus in liver transplant patients. *Clin Pharmacol Ther*, **1995**, *57*:281–290. *PDR*54, **2000**, pp. 1098–1099.

Tadalafil notes: [a]Eliminated primarily by CYP3A4-dependent metabolism. [b]*CL/F* and *V/F* reported. [c]AUC increased in patients with mild or moderate (2-fold) and severe (4-fold) renal insufficiency. [d]Following a single 20-mg oral dose.

References: Curran M, et al. Tadalafil. *Drugs*, **2003**, *63*:2203–2212; discussion 2213–2214. Product labeling: Cialis® (tadalafil tablets). Bothell, WA, Lilly Icos, **2004**.

Tamoxifen[a]							
—	<1	>98	1.4[b,c]	50-60[b]	4-11 days[d]	5 (3-7)	120 (67-183) ng/mL

[a]Has active metabolites; 4-hydroxytamoxifen and 4-hydroxy-*N*-desmethyltamoxifen are minor metabolites that exhibit affinity for the estrogen receptor that is greater than that of parent *trans*-tamoxifen. The $t_{1/2}$ of all metabolites are rate limited by tamoxifen elimination. [b]*CL/F* and V_{area}/F reported. [c]The major pathway of elimination, *N*-demethylation, is catalyzed by CYP3A. [d]$t_{1/2}$ consistent with accumulation and approach to steady state. Significantly longer terminal $t_{1/2}$s are observed. [e]Average C_{ss} following a 10-mg oral dose given twice daily to steady state.

References: Lønning PE, et al. Pharmacological and clinical profile of anastrozole. *Breast Cancer Res Treat*, **1998**, *49*(suppl 1):S53–S57. *PDR*54, **2000**, p. 557.

Tamsulosin[a]							
100 ↓ Food	12.7 ± 3.0	99 ± 1 ↑ RD	0.62 ± 0.31 ↑ RD,[b] Aged	0.20 ± 0.06	6.8 ± 3.5[c] ↑ RD, Aged	5.3 ± 0.7[d] ↑ Food	16 ± 5 ng/mL[d] ↑ Food

[a]Data from healthy male subjects. Metabolized primarily by CYP3A and CYP2D6. [b]*CL/F* reduced, moderate renal impairment. Unbound AUC relatively unchanged. [c]Apparent $t_{1/2}$ after oral dose in patients is ~14-15 hours, reflecting controlled release from modified-release granules. [d]Following a single 0.4-mg modified-release oral dose in healthy subjects.

References: Matsushima H, et al. Plasma protein binding of tamsulosin hydrochloride in renal disease: Role of α_1-acid glycoprotein and possibility of binding interactions. *Eur J Clin Pharmacol*, **1999**, *55*:437–443. van Hoogdalem EJ, et al. Disposition of the selective α_{1A}-adrenoceptor antagonist tamsulosin in humans: Comparison with data from interspecies scaling. *J Pharm Sci*, **1997**, *86*:1156–1161. Wolzt M, et al. Pharmacokinetics of tamsulosin in subjects with normal and varying degrees of impaired renal function: An open-label single-dose and multiple-dose study. *Eur J Clin Pharmacol*, **1998**, *4*:367–373.

Telithromycin[a]							
57 (41-112)	23 (19-27)	70	14 (12-16) ↓ RD[b]	3.0 (2.1-4.5)	12 (7-23)	1.0 (0.5-3.0)[c]	2.23 μg/mL[c]

[a]~35% of the dose is metabolized by CYP3A4. [b]*CL/F* reduced in patients with severe renal impairment. [c]Following an 800-mg oral dose given once daily for 7 days.

References: Ferret C, et al. Pharmacokinetics and absolute oral bioavailability of an 800-mg oral dose of telithromycin in healthy young and elderly volunteers. *Chemotherapy*, **2002**, *48*:217–223. Namour F, et al. Pharmacokinetics of the new ketolide telithromycin (HMR 3647) administered in ascending single and multiple doses. *Antimicrob Agents Chemother*, **2001**, *45*:170–175. Zhanel GG, et al. The ketolides: A critical review. *Drugs*, **2002**, *62*:1771–1804.

Temsirolimus[a]							
—	4.6[b]	—[c]	3.8 ± 0.6[d]	3.3 ± 0.5[d]	12.8 ± 1.1	—	595 ± 102 ng/mL[e]

[a]Temsirolimus, a water-soluble ester analog of sirolimus or rapamycin, is available for IV use. Following IV administration, temsirolimus is converted to sirolimus; blood AUC of sirolimus is 3-fold higher than that of temsirolimus at the recommended dose of 25 mg for the treatment of advanced renal cell carcinoma. Both temsirolimus and sirolimus inhibit mTOR kinase activity and undergo oxidative metabolism mediated by CYP3A. [b]Recovery of radioactivity after a single IV dose of [^{14}C]-temsirolimus. [c]Both temsirolimus and sirolimus partition extensively into blood cells; a major fraction of temsirolimus and sirolimus in plasma is bound to plasma proteins. [d]Based on *CL* of 16.1 ± 2.5 L/hr and V_{ss} of 232 ± 36 l at a dose of 25 mg, assuming an average body weight of 70 kg. All pharmacokinetic assessments are based on whole blood concentration. [e]Following the first dose of a 25-mg/wk regimen.

References: Atkins MB, et al. Randomized phase II study of multiple dose levels of CCI-779, a novel mammalian target of rapamycin kinase inhibitor, in patients with advanced refractory renal cell carcinoma. *J Clin Oncol*, **2004**, *22*:909–918. Drugs@FDA. Torisel label approved on 5/30/07. Available at: http://www.accessdata.fda.gov/scripts/cder/drugsatfda/index.cfm. Accessed on December 31, 2010.

(*Continued*)

Table AII–1

Pharmacokinetic Data (*Continued*)

BIOAVAILABILITY (ORAL) (%)	URINARY EXCRETION (%)	BOUND IN PLASMA (%)	CLEARANCE (mL/min/kg)	VOL. DIST. (L/kg)	HALF-LIFE (hours)	PEAK TIME (hours)	PEAK CONCENTRATION
Tenofovir[a]							
25[b] ↑ Food	82 ± 13	<1	2.6 ± 0.9[c] ↓ RD	0.6 ± 0.1[c]	8.1 ± 1.8[c,d] ↑ RD	2.3[e]	326 ng/mL[e]

[a]Tenofovir is formulated as an ester prodrug, VIREAD (tenofovir disoproxil fumarate), for oral administration. [b]Bioavailability under fasted state reported; increased to 39% with high-fat meal. [c]Data reported for steady-state 3-mg/kg IV dose given once a day for 2 weeks to HIV-1-infected male and female adults. Slightly higher *CL* with single IV dose. [d]Longer apparent plasma $t_{1/2}$ (17 hours) reported for steady-state oral dosing; this may reflect a longer duration of blood sampling; also, phosphorylated "active" metabolite exhibits a longer intracellular $t_{1/2}$ (60 hours). [e]Following a 300-mg oral dose given once a day with a meal to steady state. *References*: Barditch-Crovo P, et al. Phase i/ii trial of the pharmacokinetics, safety, and antiretroviral activity of tenofovir disoproxil fumarate in human immunodeficiency virus-infected adults. *Antimicrob Agents Chemother*, **2001**, *45*:2733–2739. Deeks SG, et al. Safety, pharmacokinetics, and antiretroviral activity of intravenous 9-[2-(R)-(Phosphonomethoxy) propyl]adenine, a novel anti-human immunodeficiency virus (HIV) therapy, in HIV-infected adults. *Antimicrob Agents Chemother*, **1998**, *42*:2380–2384. Kearney BP, et al. Tenofovir disoproxil fumarate: Clinical pharmacology and pharmacokinetics. *Clin Pharmacokinet*, **2004**, *43*:595–612.

BIOAVAILABILITY (ORAL) (%)	URINARY EXCRETION (%)	BOUND IN PLASMA (%)	CLEARANCE (mL/min/kg)	VOL. DIST. (L/kg)	HALF-LIFE (hours)	PEAK TIME (hours)	PEAK CONCENTRATION
Terazosin							
82	11-14	90-94	1.1-1.2[a]	1.1	9-12	1.7[b]	16 ng/mL[b]

[a]Plasma *CL* reportedly reduced in patients with hypertension. [b]Following a 1-mg oral dose (tablet) given to healthy volunteers.

References: Senders RC. Pharmacokinetics of terazosin. *Am J Med*, **1986**, *80*:20–24. Sennello LT, et al. Effect of age on the pharmacokinetics of orally and intravenously administered terazosin. *Clin Ther*, **1988**, *10*:600–607.

BIOAVAILABILITY (ORAL) (%)	URINARY EXCRETION (%)	BOUND IN PLASMA (%)	CLEARANCE (mL/min/kg)	VOL. DIST. (L/kg)	HALF-LIFE (hours)	PEAK TIME (hours)	PEAK CONCENTRATION
Thalidomide[a]							
—[b]	<1	—	2.2 ± 0.4[c]	1.1 ± 0.3[c]	6.2 ± 2.6[c]	3.2 ± 1.4[d] ↑ HD, Food	2.0 ± 0.6 μg/mL[d] ↑ HD

[a]Data from healthy male subjects. Similar data reported for asymptomatic patients with HIV. No age or gender differences. Thalidomide undergoes spontaneous hydrolysis in blood to multiple metabolites. [b]Absolute bioavailability is not known. Altered absorption rate and extent, Hansen's disease (HD). [c]CL/F, V_{area}/F, and $t_{1/2}$ reported for oral dose. [d]Following a single 200-mg oral dose.

References: Noormohamed FH, et al. Pharmacokinetics and hemodynamic effects of single oral doses of thalidomide in asymptomatic human immunodeficiency virus-infected subjects. *AIDS Res Hum Retrovir,* **1999**, *15*:1047–1052. *PDR*54, **2000**, p. 912. Teo SK, et al. Single-dose oral pharmacokinetics of three formulations of thalidomide in healthy male volunteers. *J Clin Pharmacol,* **1999**, *39*:1162–1168.

BIOAVAILABILITY (ORAL) (%)	URINARY EXCRETION (%)	BOUND IN PLASMA (%)	CLEARANCE (mL/min/kg)	VOL. DIST. (L/kg)	HALF-LIFE (hours)	PEAK TIME (hours)	PEAK CONCENTRATION
Tigecycline[a]							
—	22[b]	71-89	3.3 ± 0.3[c]	7.2 ± 0.5[c]	36.9 ± 11.8[c]	—	621 ± 93 ng/mL[c]

[a]Tigecycline is a glycylcycline, a new tetracycline class of antibiotic. Tigecycline undergoes minimal metabolism; major routes of elimination are via biliary and urinary excretion. [b]Percent of dose excreted as unchanged drug in urine. [c]At steady state during repetitive 50-mg IV doses of tigecycline infused over a 1-hour period given every 12 hours.

References: Drugs@FDA. Tygacil label approved on 3/20/09. Available at: http://www.accessdata.fda.gov/scripts/cder/drugsatfda/index.cfm. Accessed on December 31, 2009. Muralidharan G, et al. Pharmacokinetics of tigecycline after single and multiple doses in healthy subjects. *Antimicrob Agents Chemother*, **2005**, *49*:220–229.

Tolterodine[a]							
EM: 26 ± 18 PM: 91 ± 40 EM: ↑ Food	EM: Negligible PM: <2.5	T: 96.3 5-HM: 64	EM: 9.6 ± 2.8 PM: 2.0 ± 0.3 ↓ LD[b]	EM: 1.7 ± 0.4 PM: 1.5 ± 0.4	EM: 2.3 ± 0.3 PM: 9.2 ± 1.2 ↑ LD	EM: 1.2 ± 0.5[c] PM: 1.9 ± 1.0[c]	EM: 5.2 ± 5.7 ng/mL[c] PM: 38 ± 15 ng/mL[c]

[a]Data from healthy adult male subjects. No significant gender differences. Tolterodine (T) is metabolized primarily by CYP2D6 to an active (100% potency) metabolite, 5-hydroxymethyl tolterodine (5-HM), in extensive metabolizers (EM); $t_{1/2}$ 5-HM = 2.9 ± 0.4 hour. Also metabolized by CYP3A to an *N*-desalkyl product, particularly in poor metabolizers (PM). [b]*CL/F* reduced and AUC 5-$HM_{unbound}$ increased, hepatic cirrhosis. [c]Following a 4-mg oral dose given twice daily for 8 days. C_{max} of 5-HM was 5 ± 3 ng/mL for EM.

References: Brynne N, et al. Influence of CYP2D6 polymorphism on the pharmacokinetics and pharmacodynamic of tolterodine. *Clin Pharmacol Ther,* **1998**, *63*:529–539. Hills CJ, et al. Tolterodine. *Drugs,* **1998**, *55*:813–820. *PDR*54, **2000**, p. 2439.

Topiramate[a]							
>70[b]	70-97	13-17	0.31-0.51[c] ↑ Child[d] ↓ RD[e]	0.6-0.8[c]	19-23[c] ↑ RD	1.7 ± 0.6[f]	5.5 ± 0.6 μg/mL[f]

[a]Data from healthy adult male and female subjects and patients with partial epilepsy. [b]Estimate of bioavailability based on urine recovery of unchanged drug. [c]*CL/F*, V_{area}/*F*, and $t_{1/2}$ reported for oral dose. Patients receiving concomitant therapy with enzyme-inducing anticonvulsant drugs exhibit increased *CL/F* and decreased $t_{1/2}$. [d]*CL/F* increased, <4 years of age (substantially), and 4-17 years of age. [e]*CL/F* reduced, moderate-to-severe renal impairment (drug cleared by hemodialysis). [f]Following a 400-mg oral dose given twice daily to steady state in patients with epilepsy.

References: Glauser TA, et al. Topiramate pharmacokinetics in infants. *Epilepsia,* **1999**, *40*:788–791. *PDR*54, **2000**, p. 2209. Rosenfeld WE. Topiramate: A review of preclinical, pharmacokinetic, and clinical data. *Clin Ther,* **1997**, *19*:1294–1308. Sachdeo RC, et al. Steady-state pharmacokinetics of topiramate and carbamazepine in patients with epilepsy during monotherapy and concomitant therapy. *Epilepsia,* **1996**, *37*:774–780.

Toremifene[a]							
—	Negligible	99.7	2.6 ± 1.2 L/hr/m^{2} [b] ↓ LD,[c] RD	479 ± 154 L/m^{2} [b] ↑ Aged	T: 148 ± 53[b] DMT: 504 ± 578[b] ↑ Aged, LD	T: 1.5-3[d] DMT: 3-6[d]	T: 1.1-1.3 μg/mL[d] DMT: 2.7-5.8 μg/mL[d]

[a]Data from healthy adult male and female subjects and female patients with breast cancer. Toremifene (T) is metabolized by CYP3A to *N*-desmethyltoremifene (DMT), a metabolite that accumulates in blood and has anti-estrogenic activity. Toremifene appears to undergo enterohepatic recycling, prolonging its apparent $t_{1/2}$. [b]*CL/F*, V_{area}/*F*, and $t_{1/2}$ reported for oral dose. [c]*CL/F* reduced, hepatic cirrhosis or fibrosis. [d]Following a 60-mg oral dose given once daily to steady state in patients with breast cancer.

References: Anttila M, et al. Pharmacokinetics of the novel antiestrogenic agent toremifene in subjects with altered liver and kidney function. *Clin Pharmacol Ther,* **1995**, *57*:628–635. Bishop J, et al. Phase I clinical and pharmacokinetics study of high-dose toremifene in postmenopausal patients with advanced breast cancer. *Cancer Chemother Pharmacol,* **1992**, *30*:174–178. Wiebe VJ, et al. Pharmacokinetics of toremifene and its metabolites in patients with advanced breast cancer. *Cancer Chemother Pharmacol,* **1990**, *25*:247–251.

(*Continued*)

Table AII–1

Pharmacokinetic Data (*Continued*)

BIOAVAILABILITY (ORAL) (%)	URINARY EXCRETION (%)	BOUND IN PLASMA (%)	CLEARANCE (mL/min/kg)	VOL. DIST. (L/kg)	HALF-LIFE (hours)	PEAK TIME (hours)	PEAK CONCENTRATION
Tramadol[a]							
70-75	10-30[b]	20	8 (6-12) ↓ LD, RD	2.7 (2.3-3.9)	5.5 (4.5-7.5) ↑ RD, LD	T: 2.3 ± 1.4[c] MI: 2.4 ± 1.1[c]	T: 592 ± 178 ng/mL[c] MI: 110 ± 32 ng/mL[c]

[a]Tramadol (T) is available as a racemic mixture. At steady state, the plasma concentration of (+) (*1R,2R*)-tramadol is ~30% higher than that of (–) (*1S,2S*)-tramadol. Both isomers contribute to analgesia. Data reported are for total (+ and –) T. T is metabolized by CYP2D6 to an active *O*-desmethyl metabolite (M1); there are other CYP-catalyzed metabolites. [b]Recovery following an oral dose was reported. [c]Following a 100-mg immediate-release tablet given every 6 hours for 7 days.

References: Klotz U. Tramadol—The impact of its pharmacokinetic and pharmacodynamic properties on the clinical management of pain. *Arzneimittelforschung,* **2003**, *53*:681–687. *PDR*58, **2004**, p. 2494.

BIOAVAILABILITY (ORAL) (%)	URINARY EXCRETION (%)	BOUND IN PLASMA (%)	CLEARANCE (mL/min/kg)	VOL. DIST. (L/kg)	HALF-LIFE (hours)	PEAK TIME (hours)	PEAK CONCENTRATION
Trazodone[a]							
81 ± 6 ↔ Aged, Obes	<1	93	2.1 ± 0.1 ↓ Aged,[b] Obes[c]	1.0 ± 0.1[d] ↑ Aged, Obes	5.9 ± 0.4 ↑ Aged, Obes	2.0 ± 1.5[e]	1.5 ± 0.2 μg/mL[e]

[a]Active metabolite, *m*-chlorophenylpiperazine, is a tryptaminergic agonist; formation catalyzed by CYP3A. [b]Significant for male subjects only. [c]No difference when *CL* is normalized to ideal body weight. [d]V_{area} reported. [e]Following a single 100-mg oral dose (capsule) given with a standard breakfast to healthy adults.

References: Greenblatt DJ, et al. Trazodone kinetics: Effect of age, gender, and obesity. *Clin Pharmacol Ther,* **1987**, *42*:193–200. Nilsen OG, et al. Single dose pharmacokinetics of trazodone in healthy subjects. *Pharmacol Toxicol,* **1992**, *71*:150–153.

BIOAVAILABILITY (ORAL) (%)	URINARY EXCRETION (%)	BOUND IN PLASMA (%)	CLEARANCE (mL/min/kg)	VOL. DIST. (L/kg)	HALF-LIFE (hours)	PEAK TIME (hours)	PEAK CONCENTRATION
Triamterene[a]							
51 ± 18[b]	52 ± 10[b] ↓ LD[c] ↔ Aged[b]	61 ± 2[d] ↑ HL ↓ RD, Alb, LD[e]	63 ± 20[f] ↓ LD, RD,[e] Aged[e]	13.4 ± 4.9	4.2 ± 0.7[g] ↑ RD[e]	T: 2.9 ± 1.6[h] TS: 4.1 ± 2.0[h]	Y, T: 26.4 ± 17.7 ng/mL[h] Y, TS: 779 ± 310 ng/mL[h] E, T: 84 ± 91 ng/mL[h] E, TS: 526 ± 388 ng/mL[h]

[a]Active metabolite, hydroxytriamterene sulfuric acid ester (TS). [b]Triamterene (T) plus active metabolite. [c]Decreased active metabolite; increased parent drug. [d]For metabolite, percent bound = 90.4 ± 1.3. [e]Active metabolite. [f]Because T is predominantly present in plasma as the active metabolite, this value is deceptively high. CL_{renal} = 2.3 ± 0.6 for the metabolite. [g]Metabolite $t_{1/2}$ = 3.1 ± 1.2 hours. [h]Data for T and TS following a single 50-mg oral dose taken after a fast by young healthy volunteers (Y) and elderly patients requiring diuretic therapy (E).

References: Gilfrich HJ, et al. Pharmacokinetics of triamterene after i.v. administration to man: Determination of bioavailability. *Eur J Clin Pharmacol,* **1983**, *25*:237–241. Muhlberg W, et al. Pharmacokinetics of triamterene in geriatric patients—Influence of piretanide and hydrochlorothiazide. *Arch Gerontol Geriatr,* **1989**, *8*:73–85.

Trimethoprim

>63	63 ± 10 ↔ CF	37 ± 5 ↔ RD, Alb, CF	1.9 ± 0.3[a] ↓ RD ↑ CF, Child	1.6 ± 0.2[a] ↔ RD, CF ↑ Neo, Child	10 ± 2[a] ↑ RD ↓ Child, CF	2[b]	1.2 μg/mL[b]

[a]Studies included concurrent administration of sulfamethoxazole and variation in urinary pH; these factors had no marked effect on the *CL*, V_{area}, and $t_{1/2}$ of trimethoprim. [b]Following a single 160-mg oral dose given to healthy adults.

References: Hutabarat RM, et al. Disposition of drugs in cystic fibrosis. I. Sulfamethoxazole and trimethoprim. *Clin Pharmacol Ther,* **1991**, *49*:402–409. Welling PO, et al. Pharmacokinetics of trimethoprim and sulfamethoxazole in normal subjects and in patients with renal failure. *J Infect Dis,* **1973**, *128*(suppl):556–566.

Valacyclovir[a]

V: very low A: 54 (42-73)[b]	V: <1 A: 44 ± 10[c]	V: 13.5-17.9 A: 22-33	V: — A: ↓ RD[d]	—	V: — A: 2.5 ± 0.3 A: ↑ RD	V: 1.5 A: 1.9 ± 0.6[e]	V: ≤0.56 μg/mL[e] A: 4.8 ± 1.5 μg/mL[e]

[a]Data from healthy male and female adults. Valacyclovir is an L-valine prodrug of acyclovir. Extensive first-pass conversion by intestinal (gut wall and luminal) and hepatic enzymes. Parameters refer to acyclovir (A) and valacyclovir (V) following V administration. See "Acyclovir" for its systemic disposition parameters. [b]Bioavailability of A based on AUC of A following IV A and a 1-g oral dose of V. [c]Urinary recovery of A is dose dependent (76% and 44% following 100-mg and 1000-mg oral doses of V, and 87% following IV A). [d]*CL/F* reduced, end-stage RD (drug cleared by hemodialysis). [e]Following a single 1-g oral dose of V.

References: Perry CM, et al. Valaciclovir. A review of its antiviral activity, pharmacokinetic properties and therapeutic efficacy in herpesvirus infections. *Drugs,* **1996**, *52*:754–772. Soul-Lawton J, et al. Absolute bioavailability and metabolic disposition of valaciclovir, the L-valyl ester of acyclovir, following oral administration to humans. *Antimicrob Agents Chemother,* **1995**, *39*:2759–2764. Weller S, et al. Pharmacokinetics of the acyclovir pro-drug valaciclovir after escalating single- and multiple-dose administration to normal volunteers. *Clin Pharmacol Ther,* **1993**, *54*:595–605.

Valganciclovir[a]

G (V): 61 ± 9[b] ↑ Food	—	—	—	—	V (V): 0.5 ± 0.2 G (V): 3.7 ± 0.6 ↑ RD[c]	V (V): 0.5 ± 0.3[d] G (V): 1-3[e]	V (V): 0.20 ± 0.07 μg/mL[d] G (V): 5.6 ± 1.5 μg/mL[e]

[a]Valganciclovir (V) is an ester prodrug for ganciclovir (G). It is rapidly hydrolyzed with a plasma $t_{1/2}$ = 0.5 hour. G and V data following oral V dosing to male and female patients with viral infections are reported. See "Ganciclovir" for its systemic disposition parameters. [b]Increased and more predictable bioavailability of G when V is taken with a high-fat meal. [c]The apparent $t_{1/2}$ of G is increased in patients with renal impairment. [d]Following a single 360-mg oral dose of V taken without food. [e]Following a 900-mg oral dose of V taken once daily with food to steady state.

References: Cocohoba JM, et al. Valganciclovir: An advance in cytomegalovirus therapeutics. *Ann Pharmacother,* **2002**, *36*:1075–1079. Jung D, et al. Single-dose pharmacokinetics of valganciclovir in HIV- and CMV-seropositive subjects. *J Clin Pharmacol,* **1999**, *39*:800–804. *PDR*58, **2004**, pp. 2895, 2971.

(*Continued*)

Table AII–1

Pharmacokinetic Data (*Continued*)

BIOAVAILABILITY (ORAL) (%)	URINARY EXCRETION (%)	BOUND IN PLASMA (%)	CLEARANCE (mL/min/kg)	VOL. DIST. (L/kg)	HALF-LIFE (hours)	PEAK TIME (hours)	PEAK CONCENTRATION
Valproic Acid[a]							
100 ± 10[b]	1.8 ± 2.4	93 ± 1[c] ↓ RD, LD, Preg, Aged, Neo, Burn, Alb	0.11 ± 0.02[d,e] ↑ Child ↔ LD, Aged	0.22 ± 0.07 ↑ LD, Neo ↔ Aged, Child	14 ± 3[d,e] ↑ LD, Neo ↓ Child ↔ Aged	1-4[f]	34 ± 8 μg/mL[f]

[a]Valproic acid is available either as the free acid or stable coordination compound comprised of sodium valproate and valproic acid (divalproex sodium). [b]Systemic availability of valproate ion is the same after molar equivalent oral doses of free acid and divalproex sodium. [c]Dose dependent; value shown for daily doses of 250 and 500 mg. At 1 g daily, percent bound = 90 ± 2%. [d]Data for multiple dosing (500 mg daily) reported. Single-dose value: 0.14 ± 0.04 mL/min/kg; $t_{1/2} = 9.8 \pm 2.6$ hours. Total *CL* is the same at 100 mg daily, although *CL* of free drug increases with multiple dosing. [e]Increased *CL* and decreased $t_{1/2}$ from enzyme induction following concomitant administration of other anti-epileptic drugs. [f]average concentration following a 250-mg oral dose (capsule, DEPAKENE) given twice daily for 15 days to healthy male adults. A therapeutic range of 50-150 μg/mL is reported. T_{max} is 3-8 hours for divalproex tablets and 7-14 hours for extended-release divalproex tablets.

References: Dean JC. Valproate. In: Wyllie E, ed. *The Treatment of Epilepsy,* 2nd ed. Baltimore, Williams & Wilkins, **1997**, pp. 824–832. Pollack GM, et al. Accumulation and washout kinetics of valproic acid and its active metabolites. *J Clin Pharmacol,* **1986**, *26*:668–676. Zaccara G, et al. Clinical pharmacokinetics of valproic acid—1988. *Clin Pharmacokinet,* **1988**, *15*:367–389.

BIOAVAILABILITY (ORAL) (%)	URINARY EXCRETION (%)	BOUND IN PLASMA (%)	CLEARANCE (mL/min/kg)	VOL. DIST. (L/kg)	HALF-LIFE (hours)	PEAK TIME (hours)	PEAK CONCENTRATION
Valsartan[a]							
23 ± 7 ↓ Food	29.0 ± 5.8	95	0.49 ± 0.09 ↓ Aged, LD[b] ↔ RD	0.23 ± 0.09	9.4 ± 3.8 ↑ Aged	2 (1.5-3)[c]	1.6 ± 0.6 μg/mL[c]

[a]Data from healthy adult male subjects. No significant gender differences. Valsartan is cleared primarily by biliary excretion. [b]*CL/F* reduced, mild to moderate hepatic impairment and biliary obstruction. [c]Following a single 80-mg oral dose (capsule).

References: Brookman LJ, et al. Pharmacokinetics of valsartan in patients with liver disease. *Clin Pharmacol Ther,* **1997**, *62*:272–278. Flesch G, et al. Absolute bioavailability and pharmacokinetics of valsartan, an angiotensin II receptor antagonist, in man. *Eur J Clin Pharmacol,* **1997**, *52*:115–120. Muller P, et al. Pharmacokinetics and pharmacodynamic effects of the angiotensin II antagonist valsartan at steady state in healthy, normotensive subjects. *Eur J Clin Pharmacol,* **1997**, *52*:441–449. *PDR*54, **2000**, p. 2015.

Vancomycin							
—[a]	79 ± 11	30 ± 11 ↔ RD	$CL = 0.79CL_{cr}$ + 0.22 ↓ RD, Aged, Neo ↔ Obes, CPBS ↑ Burn	0.39 ± 0.06 ↓ Obes ↔ RD, CPBS	5.6 ± 1.8 ↑ RD, Aged ↓ Obes	—	18.5 (15-25) μg/mL[b]

[a]Very poorly absorbed after oral administration, but used by this route to treat *Clostridium difficile* and staphylococcal enterocolitis. [b]Following a dose of 1000-mg IV (1-hour infusion) given twice daily or a 7.5-mg/kg IV (1-hour infusion) given four times daily to adult patients with staphylococcal or streptococcal infections. Levels of 37-152 μg/mL have been associated with ototoxicity.

Reference: Leader WG, et al. Pharmacokinetic optimisation of vancomycin therapy. *Clin Pharmacokinet,* **1995**, *28*:327–342.

Vardenafil[a]							
15 (8-25)	2-6	93-95 (parent and M1)	56	3.0[b]	4-5 (parent and M1)	0.7 (0.25-3)[c]	19.3 ± 1.7 ng/mL[c]

[a]Vardenafil is primarily metabolized by CYP3A with minor involvement of CYP2C9. The major oxidative metabolite (M1), a product of *N*-desmethylation at the piperazine ring, is a less potent PDE5 inhibitor and circulates at a level 28% that of the parent drug. It contributes only 7% of the *in vivo* activity of vardenafil. [b]V_{ss} of 208 L, assuming 70-kg bodyweight. [c]Following a single 20-mg dose. There is no change in pharmacokinetics between single and multiple dosing.

References: Drugs@FDA. Levitra label approved on 3/19/08. Available at: http://www.accessdata.fda.gov/scripts/cder/drugsatfda/index.cfm. Accessed on December 31, 2009. Gupta M, et al. The clinical pharmacokinetics of phosphodiesterase-5 inhibitors for erectile dysfunction. *J Clin Pharmacol*, **2005**, *45*:987–1003.

Varenicline[a]							
≥87%[b]	86.2 ± 6.2	≤20	2.27 ± 0.34[c]	6.2[c]	31.5 ± 7.7[c]	2.0 (1.0-4.0)[d]	10.2 ± 1.0 ng/mL[d]

[a]Varenicline is eliminated mostly by renal excretion with minimal metabolism. Organic Cation Transporter 2 (OCT2) is involved in renal tubular secretion, as evidenced by inhibition of varenicline renal clearance by cimetidine, a known OCT2 inhibitor. [b]87.1 ± 5.5% of radioactivity is excreted in urine after an oral dose of [^{14}C]-varenicline. Minimal first-pass metabolism is expected. [c]CL/F and V_z/F estimated from steady-state AUC and $t_{1/2}$ during 1-mg twice-daily dosing of varenicline in healthy adult smokers and assuming an average body weight of 70 kg. [d]After the first dose of a multiple-dosing regimen. An accumulation factor of 2.85 ± 0.73 was reported.

References: Drugs@FDA. Chantix label approved on 7/1/09. Available at: http://www.accessdata.fda.gov/scripts/cder/drugsatfda/index.cfm. Accessed on December 31, 2009. Faessel HM, et al. Multiple-dose pharmacokinetics of the selective nicotinic receptor partial agonist, varenicline, in healthy smokers. *J Clin Pharmacol*, **2006**, *46*:1439–1448. Obach RS, et al. Metabolism and disposition of varenicline, a selective α4β2 acetylcholine receptor partial agonist, in vivo and in vitro. *Drug Metab Dispos*, **2006**, *34*:121–130.

(*Continued*)

Table AII–1

Pharmacokinetic Data (*Continued*)

BIOAVAILABILITY (ORAL) (%)	URINARY EXCRETION (%)	BOUND IN PLASMA (%)	CLEARANCE (mL/min/kg)	VOL. DIST. (L/kg)	HALF-LIFE (hours)	PEAK TIME (hours)	PEAK CONCENTRATION
Venlafaxine,[a] Desvenlafaxine[b]							
10-45	V: 4.6 ± 3.0 ODV: 29 ± 7[c]	V: 27 ± 2 ODV: 30 ± 12[c]	22 ± 10[d] ↔ Aged, Fem ↓ LD, RD	7.5 ± 3.7[d] ↔ Aged, Fem, LD, RD	4.9 ± 2.4 10.3 ± 4.3[c] ↔ Aged, Fem ↑ LD, RD	V: 2.0 ± 0.4 ODV: 2.8 ± 0.8[c]	V: 167 ± 55 ng/mL[e] ODV: 397 ± 81 ng/mL[e]

[a]Venlafaxine (V) is available as a racemic mixture; antidepressant activity resides with the *l*-(–)-enantiomer and its equipotent *O*-desmethyl metabolite (formation catalyzed by CYP2D6—polymorphic). Parameters for the derived *O*-desmethylvenlafaxine (ODV) are included. [b]*O*-Desmethyl metabolite is marketed as desvenlafaxine in an extended-release formulation as a successor to V. It has a higher oral bioavailability (80%), with a T_{max} of 7.5 hours. Desvenlafaxine has a much lower *CL* (3.5 mL/min/kg) and a smaller V_{ss} (3.4 L/kg). Its reported $t_{1/2}$ matches that observed for metabolite derived from V. [c]Values for ODV after V dosing. [d]*CL/F* and V_{ss}/F reported. [e]Mean data for V and ODV, following a 75-mg oral dose (immediate-release tablet) given three times daily for 3 days to healthy adults. T_{max} for an extended-release formulation is 5.5 (V) and 9 (DV) hours.

References: Klamerus KJ, et al. Introduction of a composite parameter to the pharmacokinetics of venlafaxine and its active *O*-desmethyl metabolite. *J Clin Pharmacol,* **1992**, *32*:716–724. *PDR*54, **2000**, p. 3237.

BIOAVAILABILITY (ORAL) (%)	URINARY EXCRETION (%)	BOUND IN PLASMA (%)	CLEARANCE (mL/min/kg)	VOL. DIST. (L/kg)	HALF-LIFE (hours)	PEAK TIME (hours)	PEAK CONCENTRATION
Verapamil[a,b]							
Oral: 22 ± 8 SL: 35 ± 13 ↑ Cirr ↔ RD	<3	90 ± 2 ↑ Cirr ↔ RD, Atr Fib, Aged	15 ± 6[c,d] ↑ Cirr, Aged, Obes ↑, ↔ Atr Fib ↔ RD, Child	5.0 ± 2.1 ↑ Cirr ↑, ↔ Atr Fib ↔ RD, Aged, Obes	4.0 ± 1.5[c] ↑ Cirr, Aged, Obes ↑, ↔ Atr Fib ↔ RD, Child	IR: 1.1[e] XR: 5.6-7.7[e]	IR: 272 ng/mL[e] XR: 118-165 ng/mL[e]

[a]Racemic mixture; (–)-enantiomer is more active. Bioavailability of (+)-verapamil is 2.5-fold greater than that for (–)-verapamil because of a lower *CL* (10 ± 2 versus 18 ± 3 mL/min/kg). Relative concentration of the enantiomers changes as a function of route of administration. [b]Active metabolite, norverapamil, is a vasodilator but has no direct effect on heart rate or P-R interval. At steady state (oral dosing), AUC is equivalent to that of parent drug ($t_{1/2}$ = 9 ± 3 hours). [c]Multiple dosing causes a greater than 2-fold decrease in *CL/F* and prolongation of $t_{1/2}$ in some studies, but no change of $t_{1/2}$ in others. [d]Verapamil is a substrate for CYP3A4, CYP2C9, and other CYPs. [e]Mean data following a 120-mg oral conventional tablet (IR) given twice daily or range of data following a 240-mg oral extended-release (XR) dose given once daily, both for 7-10 days to healthy adults. EC_{50} for prolongation of P-R interval after an oral dose of racemate is 120 ± 20 ng/mL; the value for IV administration is 40 ± 25 ng/mL. After oral administration, racemate concentrations >100 ng/mL cause >25% reduction in heart rate in Atr Fib, >10% prolongation of P-R interval, and >50% increase in duration of exercise in angina patients. A level of 120 ± 40 ng/mL (after IV administration) was found to terminate reentrant supraventricular tachycardias.

Reference: McTavish D, et al. Verapamil. An updated review of its pharmacodynamic and pharmacokinetic properties, and therapeutic use in hypertension. *Drugs,* **1989**, *38*:19–76.

Vincristine[a]

—	10-20	Low	4.92 ± 3.01 L/hr/m^2 ↑ LD[b] ↔ Child	96.9 ± 55.7 L/m^2 [c]	22.6 ± 16.7[c] ↑ LD[b]	—	~250-425 nM[d]

[a]Data from adult male and female cancer patients. Metabolized by CYP3A and excreted unchanged into bile (substrate for P-glycoprotein). [b]*CL* reduced, cholestatic liver disease. [c]$t_{1/2}$ and V_z for terminal phase. Longer $t_{1/2}$ (~85 ± 69 hours) also reported. [d]Following a 2-mg IV bolus dose.

References: Gelmon KA, et al. Phase I study of liposomal vincristine. *J Clin Oncol,* **1999**, *17*:697–705. Rahmani R, et al. Pharmacokinetics and metabolism of vinca alkaloids. *Cancer Surv,* **1993**, *17*:269–281. Sethi VS, et al. Pharmacokinetics of vincristine sulfate in adult cancer patients. *Cancer Res,* **1981**, *41*:3551–3555. Sethi VS, et al. Pharmacokinetics of vincristine sulfate in children. *Cancer Chemother Pharmacol,* **1981**, *6*:111–115. van den Berg HW, et al. The pharmacokinetics of vincristine in man: Reduced drug clearance associated with raised serum alkaline phosphatase and dose-limited elimination. *Cancer Chemother Pharmacol,* **1982**, *8*:215–219.

Vinorelbine

27 ± 12[a]	11	87 (80-91)	21 ± 7 ↓ LD	76 ± 41[b]	42 ± 21[b]	1.5 ± 1.0[c]	114 ± 43 ng/mL[c] 1130 ± 636 ng/mL[d]

[a]For liquid-filled gelatin capsules. [b]Elimination kinetics of vinorelbine follow a three-compartment model with extensive tissue distribution. Values for the terminal elimination phase are reported. [c]Following a single 100-mg/m^2 oral dose (gel capsule). [d]Following a single 30-mg/g IV infusion over 15 minutes.

Reference: Leveque D, et al. Clinical pharmacokinetics of vinorelbine. *Clin Pharmacokinet,* **1996**, *37*:184–197.

Voriconazole[a]

96 ↓ Food	<2	58	3.8[b] ↓ LD[c]	1.6[b]	6.7[b]	PO: 1.1[d] ↑ Food	PO: 2356 ng/mL[d] ↓ Food IV: 3621 ng/mL[e]

[a]Metabolized mainly to an inactive *N*-oxide by CYP2C19 (major), CYP3A4, and CYP2C9. [b]Elimination is dose and time dependent. Pharmacokinetic parameters determined at steady state are reported. Mean *CL* was reduced (64%), V_{ss} reduced (32%), and $t_{1/2}$ increased (16%) with 12 days of twice-daily 3-mg/kg IV administration. Also, *CL* decreased 41% when dose was increased from 200-300 mg twice daily. [c]*CL* reduced in patients with mild to moderate hepatic insufficiency. [d]Following a 3-mg/kg oral dose given twice daily for 12 days. [e]Following a 3-mg/kg IV infusion over 1-hour given twice daily for 12 days.

References: Boucher HW, et al. Newer systemic antifungal agents: Pharmacokinetics, safety and efficacy. *Drugs,* **2004**, *64*:1997–2020. Purkins L, et al. The pharmacokinetics and safety of intravenous voriconazole—A novel wide-spectrum antifungal agent. *Br J Clin Pharmacol,* **2003**, *56*(suppl):2–9. Purkins L, et al. Voriconazole, a novel wide-spectrum triazole: Oral pharmacokinetics and safety. *Br J Clin Pharmacol,* **2003**, *56*(suppl):10–16.

Warfarin[a]

93 ± 8	<2	99 ± 1[b] ↓ RD ↔ Preg	0.045 ± 0.024[c,d,e] ↔ Aged, AVH, CF	0.14 ± 0.06[b,d] ↔ Aged, AVH	37 ± 15[f] ↔ Aged, AVH	<4[g]	*R*: 0.9 ± 0.4 μg/mL[g] *S*: 0.5 ± 0.2 μg/mL[g]

[a]Values are for racemic warfarin; the *S*-(–)-enantiomer is 3- to 5-fold more potent than the R-(+)-enantiomer. [b]No difference between enantiomers in plasma protein binding or V_{area}. [c]*CL* of the *R*-enantiomer is ~70% of that of the antipode (0.043 versus 0.059 mL · min^{-1} · kg^{-1}). [d]Conditions leading to decreased binding (e.g., uremia) presumably increase *CL* and *V*. [e]The *S*-enantiomer is metabolically cleared by CYP2C9 (polymorphic). [f]$t_{1/2}$ of the *R*-enantiomer is longer than that of the *S*-enantiomer (43 ± 14 versus 32 ± 12 hours). [g]Mean steady-state, 12-hour postdose concentrations of warfarin enantiomers following a daily oral dose of 6.1 ± 2.3 mg of racemic warfarin given to patients with stabilized (1-5 months) anticoagulant therapy.

Reference: Chan E, et al. Disposition of warfarin enantiomers and metabolites in patients during multiple dosing with rac-warfarin. *Br J Clin Pharmacol,* **1994**, *37*:563–569.

(Continued)

Table AII–1

Pharmacokinetic Data (*Continued*)

BIOAVAILABILITY (ORAL) (%)	URINARY EXCRETION (%)	BOUND IN PLASMA (%)	CLEARANCE (mL/min/kg)	VOL. DIST. (L/kg)	HALF-LIFE (hours)	PEAK TIME (hours)	PEAK CONCENTRATION
Zidovudine							
63 ± 10 ↑ Neo ↔ Preg	18 ± 5	<25	26 ± 6[a] ↓ RD,[b] Neo, LD ↔ Child, Preg	1.4 ± 0.4 ↓ RD,[b] LD ↔ Child, Preg	1.1 ± 0.2 ↔ RD, Preg ↑ Neo, LD	0.5-1[c]	IV: 2.6 μg/mL[c] PO: 1.6 μg/mL[c]
Ziprasidone[a]							
PO: 59 ↑ Food IM: 100	<1[b]	99.9 ± 0.08	11.7	2.3	2.9[c]	PO: 4 ± 1[d] IM: 0.7[e]	PO: 68 ± 20 ng/mL[d] IM: 156 ng/mL[e]
Zolpidem							
72 ± 7	<1	92 ↑ RD, LD	4.5 ± 0.7[a] ↔ RD ↓ LD, Aged ↑ Child	0.68 ± 0.06 ↑ RD	1.9 ± 0.2 ↑ Aged, LD ↔ RD ↓ Child	1.0-2.6[b] ↑ Food	76-139 ng/mL[b] ↓ Food
Zonisamide[a]							
—[b]	29-48[c]	38-40[d]	0.13[e]	1.2-1.8[f]	63 ± 14	1.8 ± 0.4[g]	28 ± 4 μg/mL[g]

Zidovudine: [a]Formation of 5-*O*-glucuronide is the major route of elimination (68%). [b]A change in *CL/F* and V_{area}/F reported. [c]Following a 5-mg/kg IV or oral dose given every 4 hours to steady state.

References: Blum MR, et al. Pharmacokinetics and bioavailability of zidovudine in humans. *Am J Med,* **1988**, *85*:189–194. Morse GD, et al. Comparative pharmacokinetics of antiviral nucleoside analogues. *Clin Pharmacokinet,* **1993**, *24*:101–123.

Ziprasidone: [a]Approximately one-third of the dose is oxidized by CYP3A4, and the remainder undergoes reduction. [b]Recovery following oral administration. [c]A longer $t_{1/2}$ after oral dosing is rate limited by absorption; food decreases apparent $t_{1/2}$. In the elderly, the $t_{1/2}$ is slightly longer. [d]Following a 20-mg oral dose given twice daily for 8 days. [e]Following a single 10-mg IM dose.

References: Gunasekara NS, et al. Ziprasidone: A review of its use in schizophrenia and schizoaffective disorder. *Drugs,* **2002**, *62*:1217–1251. Miceli JJ, et al. Single- and multiple-dose pharmacokinetics of ziprasidone under nonfasting conditions in healthy male volunteers. *Br J Clin Pharmacol,* **2000**, *49*(suppl):5S–13S. *PDR*58, **2004**, p. 2598. Wilner KD, et al. Single- and multiple-dose pharmacokinetics of ziprasidone in healthy young and elderly volunteers. *Br J Clin Pharmacol,* **2000**, *49*(suppl):15S–20S.

Zolpidem: [a]Metabolically cleared predominantly by CYP3A4. [b]Following a single 10-mg oral dose given to young adults. No accumulation of drug with once-daily dosing.

References: Greenblatt DJ, et al. Comparative kinetics and dynamics of zaleplon, zolpidem, and placebo. *Clin Pharmacol Ther,* **1998**, *64*:553–561. Patat A, et al. EEG profile of intravenous zolpidem in healthy volunteers. *Psychopharmacology (Berl),* **1994**, *114*:138–146. Salva P, et al. Clinical pharmacokinetics and pharmacodynamics of zolpidem. Therapeutic implications. *Clin Pharmacokinet,* **1995**, *29*:142–153.

Zonisamide: [a]Primary routes of metabolism involve reductive cleavage of the isoxazole ring (CYP3A4) and *N*-acetylation. [b]Absolute bioavailability is not known; minimum equal to urine recovery after an oral dose. [c]Recovery following an oral dose. [d]Concentrates in erythrocytes to as much as 8-fold. [e]Steady-state *CL/F* for a 400-mg once-daily dose reported. AUC increases disproportionately when the dose is increased from 400-800 mg. [f]*V/F* for a single dose is reported; decreases as the dose is increased from 200-800 mg. [g]Following a 400-mg oral dose given once daily to steady state in healthy adults.

References: Kochak GM, et al. Steady-state pharmacokinetics of zonisamide, an antiepileptic agent for treatment of refractory complex partial seizures. *J Clin Pharmacol,* **1998**, *38*:166–171. Peters DH, et al. Zonisamide. A review of its pharmacodynamic and pharmacokinetic properties, and therapeutic potential in epilepsy. *Drugs,* **1993**, *45*:760–787. *PDR*58, **2004**, p. 1232.

Index

Information in figures and tables is denoted by *f* and *t*.

INDEX

D

INDEX

F

G

INDEX

INDEX

INDEX

J

INDEX

INDEX

K

L

INDEX

INDEX

O

Q

INDEX

S

INDEX

INDEX

INDEX